HISTOLOGY for PATHOLOGISTS

FIFTH EDITION

Stacey E. Mills, MD

W.S. Royster Professor of Pathology
Chief of Anatomic Pathology
Director of Surgical Pathology and Cytopathology
University of Virginia Health System
Charlottesville, Virginia

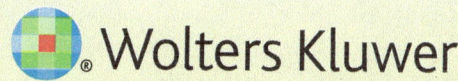

Philadelphia • Baltimore • New York • London
Buenos Aires • Hong Kong • Sydney • Tokyo

Acquisitions Editor: Ryan Shaw
Development Editor: Sean McGuire
Editorial Coordinators: Kayla Smull
Marketing Manager: Julie Sikora
Production Project Manager: Bridgett Dougherty
Design Coordinator: Joan Wendt
Manufacturing Coordinator: Beth Welsh
Prepress Vendor: Aptara, Inc.

Copyright © 2020 Wolters Kluwer.

All rights reserved. This book is protected by copyright. No part of this book may be reproduced or transmitted in any form or by any means, including as photocopies or scanned-in or other electronic copies, or utilized by any information storage and retrieval system without written permission from the copyright owner, except for brief quotations embodied in critical articles and reviews. Materials appearing in this book prepared by individuals as part of their official duties as U.S. government employees are not covered by the above-mentioned copyright. To request permission, please contact Wolters Kluwer at Two Commerce Square, 2001 Market Street, Philadelphia, PA 19103, via email at permissions@lww.com, or via our website at shop.lww.com (products and services).

Printed in the United States of America

Library of Congress Cataloging-in-Publication Data

Names: Mills, Stacey E., editor.
Title: Histology for pathologists / [edited by] Stacey E. Mills.
Description: 5e. | Philadelphia : Wolters Kluwer, [2020] | Includes
    bibliographical references and index.
Identifiers: LCCN 2018044561 | ISBN 9781496398949 (hardback)
Subjects: | MESH: Histology | Pathology
Classification: LCC QM551 | NLM QS 504 | DDC 611/.018–dc23
LC record available at https://lccn.loc.gov/2018044561

This work is provided "as is," and the publisher disclaims any and all warranties, express or implied, including any warranties as to accuracy, comprehensiveness, or currency of the content of this work.

This work is no substitute for individual patient assessment based upon healthcare professionals' examination of each patient and consideration of, among other things, age, weight, gender, current or prior medical conditions, medication history, laboratory data and other factors unique to the patient. The publisher does not provide medical advice or guidance and this work is merely a reference tool. Healthcare professionals, and not the publisher, are solely responsible for the use of this work including all medical judgments and for any resulting diagnosis and treatments.

Given continuous, rapid advances in medical science and health information, independent professional verification of medical diagnoses, indications, appropriate pharmaceutical selections and dosages, and treatment options should be made and healthcare professionals should consult a variety of sources. When prescribing medication, healthcare professionals are advised to consult the product information sheet (the manufacturer's package insert) accompanying each drug to verify, among other things, conditions of use, warnings and side effects and identify any changes in dosage schedule or contraindications, particularly if the medication to be administered is new, infrequently used or has a narrow therapeutic range. To the maximum extent permitted under applicable law, no responsibility is assumed by the publisher for any injury and/or damage to persons or property, as a matter of products liability, negligence law or otherwise, or from any reference to or use by any person of this work.

shop.lww.com

Contributors

Sylvia L. Asa, MD, PhD
Professor
Department of laboratory Medicine and Pathobiology
University of Toronto
Toronto, Ontario

Kristen A. Atkins, MD
Professor
Department of Pathology
University of Virginia School of Medicine
Charlottesville, Virginia

Hikmat Al-Ahmadie, MD
Assistant Attending
Department of Pathology
Memorial Sloan Kettering Cancer Center
New York, New York

Leomar Y. Ballester, MD, PhD
Assistant Professor
Department of Pathology and Laboratory Medicine
University of Texas Health Science Center at Houston
Houston, Texas

Karoly Balogh, MD
Associate Professor of Pathology
Harvard Medical School
Beth Israel Deaconess Medical Center
Boston, Massachusetts

José E. Barreto, MD
Attending Pathologist
Instituto de Patología e Investigación
Asunción, Paraguay

Kurt Benirschke, MD[†]
Emeritus Professor
Department of Pathology
UC San Diego School of Medicine
San Diego, California

Gerald J. Berry, MD
Professor of Pathology
Director of Cardiac and Pulmonary Pathology
Director of Anatomic Pathology
Stanford University
Stanford, California

John S.J. Brooks, MD
Chair
Department of Pathology
Pennsylvania Hospital of University of Pennsylvania
    Health System
Philadelphia, Pennsylvania

Sofía Cañete-Portillo, MD
Research collaborator
Instituto de Patología e Investigación
Asunción, Paraguay

Maria Luisa Carcangiu, MD
Director UO 1 Anatomic Pathology
Department of Pathology
Fondazione IRCCS Istituto Nazionale dei Tumori
Milan, Italy

J. Aidan Carney, MD, PhD
Emeritus
Department of Laboratory Medicine and Pathology
Mayo Clinic College of Medicine and Science
Rochester, Minnesota

Darryl Carter, MD
Professor Emeritus
Department of Pathology
Yale School of Medicine
New Haven, Connecticut

William L. Clapp, MD
Director, Renal Pathology
Professor, Department of Pathology, Immunolgy
    and Laboratory Medicine
University of Florida School of Medicine
Gainesville, Florida

Laura C. Collins, MBBS
Vice Chair of Anatomic Pathology
Director of Breast Pathology
Beth Israel Deaconess Medical Center
Professor
Department of Pathology
Harvard Medical School
Boston, Massachusetts

Julian Conejo-Mir, MD, PhD
Head Professor and Chairman
Medical & Surgical Dermatology Department
Hospital Universitario Virgen del Rocio
University of Sevilla
Spain

[†]Deceased

Contributors

James R. Conner, MD, PhD
Assistant Prof Laboratory Medicine and Pathobiology
University of Toronto Pathologist
Mt Sinai Hospital Toronto
Ontario, Canada

Antonio L. Cubilla, MD
Emeritus Professor Of Pathology
Universidad Nacional de Asuncion
Director
Instituto de Patología e Investigación
Asunción, Paraguay

Thomas J. Cummings, MD
Professor
Department of Pathology
Duke University School of Medicine
Durham, North Carolina

Gerald R. Cunha, PhD
Professor of Anatomy, Professor of Obstetrics
 & Gynecology, Professor of Urology
Department of Urology
University of California San Francisco School of Medicine
San Francisco, California

Ronald A. DeLellis, MD
Consultant Pathologist
Department of Pathology
Lifespan Academic Medical Center
Providence, Rhode Island

Javier Dominguez-Cruz, MD
Dermatologist, Investigation Unit
Dermatology Department
Hospital Universitario Virgen del Rocio
Sevilla, Spain

Samson W. Fine, MD
Associate Attending Pathologist
Department of Pathology
Memorial Sloan Kettering Cancer Center
New York, New York

Gregory N. Fuller, MD, PhD
Professor
Department of Pathology
University of Texas MD Anderson Cancer Center
Houston, Texas

Patrick J. Gallagher, MD, PhD, FRCPath
Senior Clinical Lecturer
Centre for Medical Education
Bristol University Medical School
Bristol, United Kingdom

C. Blake Gilks, MD
Professor
Department of Pathology and Laboratory Medicine
University of British Columbia Faculty of Medicine
Vancouver, British Columbia

Joel K. Greenson, MD
Professor of Pathology
Department of Pathology
University of Michigan Medical School
Ann Arbor, Michigan

Krisztina Z. Hanley, MD
Associate Professor
Department of Pathology
Emory University School of Medicine
Atlanta, Georgia

Ralph H. Hruban, MD
Baxley Professor and Director
Department of Pathology
The Johns Hopkins University School of Medicine
Baltimore, Maryland

Seung-Mo Hong, MD, PhD
Professor
Department of Pathology
Asan Medical Center
University of Ulsan College of Medicine
Seoul, Republic of Korea

Muhammad T. Idrees, MD
Associate Professor
Director immunohistochemistry
Department of Pathology
Indiana University
Indianapolis, IndianaBest

Andrew Kanik, MD
Medical Director of Histopathology and Director
 of Dermatopathology
Department of Dermatopathology
CBLPath, Inc.
Rye Brook, New York

Darcy A. Kerr, MD
Assistant Professor
Department of Pathology
University of Miami Miller School of Medicine
Miami, Florida

David S. Klimstra, MD
Chairman
Department of Pathology
Memorial Sloan Kettering Cancer Center
New York, New York

Contributors

Günter Klöppel, MD
Professor Emeritus
Department of Pathology
Consultation Center for Pancreatic and Endocrine Tumors
Technical University Munich
Munich, Germany

S.H. Kroft, MD
Professor and Interim Chair
Department of Pathology
Medical College of Wisconsin
Milwaukee, Wisconsin

Takeshi Kurita, PhD
Associate Professor of Cancer Biology and Genetics
Department of Cancer Biology and Genetics
Ohio State University College of Medicine
Columbus, Ohio

Steven H. Lewis, MD, FCAP, FACOG
Clinical Professor of Pathology and Faculty Associate
 Bioethics and Humanities
Department of Pathology
University of Colorado Anschutz Medical Campus
Aurora, Colorado

Megan G. Lockyer, DO
Staff Pathologist
Department of Pathology
AmeriPath Cleveland
Oakwood Village, Ohio

M. Beatriz S. Lopes, MD, PhD
Professor of Neuropathology and Neurological Surgery
Department of Pathology
University of Virginia School of Medicine
Charlottesville, Virginia

Fiona Maclean, MBBS
Clinical Associate Professor
Department of Clinical Medicine
Macquarie University, Sydney
Deputy Director
Department of Anatomical Pathology
Douglass Hanly Moir Pathology
Macquarie Park, Sydney

Shamlal Mangray, MBBS
Director, Pediatric Pathology
Department of Pathology
Lifespan Academic Medical Center
Providence, Rhode Island

Fernando Martínez-Madrigal, MD
Pathologist
Department of Pathology
Instituto Mexicano del Seguro Social
Morelia, Mexico

Jesse K. McKenney, MD
Pathologist
Department of Pathology
Cleveland Clinic
Cleveland, Ohio

Ozgur Mete, MD, FRCPC
Associate Professor
Department of Pathology
University Health Network
University of Toronto
Toronto, Ontario, Canada

Stacey E. Mills, MD
W.S. Royster Professor of Pathology
Chief of Anatomic Pathology
Director of Surgical Pathology and Cytopathology
University of Virginia Health System
Charlottesville, Virginia

Attilio Orazi, MD, FRCPath
Professor and Chairman Department of Pathology
Texas Tech University Health Care Sciences
P.L. Foster School of Medicine
El Paso, Texas

Carlos Ortiz-Hidalgo, MD
Professor of Histology
Department of Tissue and Cell Biology
Universidad Panamericana Escuela de Ciencias de la Salud
Mexico City
Histopathologist
Department of Anatomical Pathology
Hospital y Fundación Medica Sur
Mexico City, Mexico

Christopher N. Otis, MD
Professor of Pathology
Department of Pathology
University of Massachusetts Medical School—Baystate
Springfield, Massachusetts

David A. Owen, MB, BCh, FRCPC
Professor Emeritus
Pathology and Laboratory Medicine
University of British Columbia Faculty of Medicine
Vancouver, British Columbia

Liron Pantanowitz, MD
Professor of Pathology
Department of Pathology
University of Pittsburgh Medical Center
Pittsburgh, Pennsylvania

Robert E. Petras, MD
Managing Director
AmeriPath Institute of Gastrointestinal Pathology and
 Digestive Disease
AmeriPath Cleveland
Oakwood Village, Ohio

Meredith E. Pittman, MD
Assistant Professor
Department of Pathology and Laboratory Medicine
NewYork-Presbyterian Hospital/Weill Cornell Medicine
New York, New York

Miriam D. Post, MD
Associate Professor
Department of Pathology
University of Colorado Anschutz Medical Campus
Aurora, Colorado

Alan D. Proia, MD, PhD
Professor
Department of Pathology
Duke University School of Medicine
Durham, North Carolina

Victor E. Reuter, MD
Vice Chairman
Department of Pathology
Memorial Sloan Kettering Cancer Center
New York, New York

Robert H. Riddell, MD, FRCPC, FRCPath
Prof Laboratory Medicine and Pathobiology
University of Toronto Pathologist
Mt Sinai Hospital Toronto
Ontario, Canada

Stanley J. Robboy, MD
Professor of Pathology and Professor of Obstetrics
 and Gynecology
Department of Pathology
Duke University School of Medicine
Durham, North Carolina

Andrew E. Rosenberg, MD
Professor, Vice Chair
Director of Bone and Soft Tissue Pathology
Department of Pathology
Miller School of Medicine
University of Miami
Miami, Florida

Stuart J. Schnitt
Chief of Breast Oncologic Pathology
Dana-Farber/Brigham and Women's Cancer Center
Senior Pathologist
Brigham and Women's Hospital
Professor of Pathology
Harvard Medical School
Boston, Massachusetts

Mercedes Sendín-Martín, MD
Dermatologist
Department of Dermatology
Hospital Universitario Virgen del Rocio
Sevilla, Spain

Carlie S. Sigel, MD
Assistant Attending Pathologist
Department of Pathology
Memorial Sloan Kettering Cancer Center
New York, New York

Edward B. Stelow, MD
Professor of Pathology
Department of Pathology
University of Virginia School of Medicine
Charlottesville, Virginia

Kyle C. Strickland, MD, PhD
Assistant Professor of Pathology
Department of Pathology
Duke University School of Medicine
Durham, North Carolina

Arief A. Suriawinata, MD
Section Chief of Anatomic Pathology
Department of Pathology and Laboratory Medicine
Dartmouth-Hitchcock Medical Center
Lebanon, New Hampshire

David Suster, MD
Pathologist
Department of Pathology
Massachusetts General Hospital
Harvard Medical School
Boston, Massachusetts

Saul Suster, MD
Professor and Chairman
Department of Pathology & Laboratory Medicine
Froedtert and the Medical College of Wisconsin
Froedtert Hospital
Milwaukee, Wisconsin

Swan N. Thung, MD
Director of Liver Pathology
Department of Pathology
Mount Sinai Hospital
New York, New York

Arthur S. Tischler, MD
Professor
Department of Pathology
Tufts University School of Medicine
 & Tufts Medical Center
Boston, Massachusetts

Satish K. Tickoo, MD
Attending Pathologist
Department of Pathology
Memorial Sloan Kettering Cancer Center
New York, New York

Humberto E. Trejo Bittar, MD
Assistant Professor of Pathology
Department of Pathology/Thoracic and Autopsy Pathology
University of Pittsburgh Medical Center
Pittsburgh, Pennsylvania

Lawrence True, MD
Professor
Department of Pathology
University of Washington School of Medicine
Seattle, Washington

Thomas M. Ulbright, MD
Lawrence M. Roth Emeritus Professor of Pathology & Laboratory Medicine
Indiana University School of Medicine
Indianapolis, Indiana

Paul van der Valk, MD, PhD
Professor
Department of Pathology
University of Amsterdam Medical Centers
VU University Medical Center
Amsterdam, The Netherlands

Allard C. van der Wal, MD, PhD
Professor
Faculty of Medicine
University of Amsterdam
Clinical Pathologist
Academic Medical Center
Amsterdam, The Netherlands

J. Han J.M. van Krieken, PhD
Professor
Department of Pathology
Radboudumc
Nijmegen, The Netherlands

Elsa F. Velazquez, MD
Vice President and Director
Department of Dermatopathology
Inform Diagnostics
Needham, Massachusetts
Clinical Assistant Professor of Dermatology
Tufts University School of Medicine
Boston, Massachusetts

Hannes Vogel, MD
Professor
Department of Pathology
Stanford Medicine
Stanford, California

Roy O. Weller, MD, PhD, FRCPath
Emeritus Professor of Neuropathology
Clinical Neurosciences
University of Southampton School of Medicine
Emeritus Consultant Neuropathologist
Cellular Pathology (Neuropathology)
Southampton University Hospitals Trust
Southampton, United Kingdom

Bruce M. Wenig, MD
Senior Member
Department of Anatomic Pathology
H. Lee Moffitt Cancer Center and Research Institute
Tampa, Florida

Maria Westerhoff, MD
Associate Professor
Department of Pathology
University of Michigan Medical School
Ann Arbor, Michigan

Rhonda K. Yantiss, MD
Professor of Pathology and Laboratory Medicine
Chief, Gastrointestinal Pathology Service
New York-Presbyterian Hospital/Weill Cornell Medical Center
New York, New York

Samuel A. Yousem, MD
E. Leon Barnes Professor of Anatomic Pathology
Department of Pathology
University of Pittsburgh Medical Center
Pittsburgh, Pennsylvania

Hala El-Zimaity, MD
Pathologist
Dynacare Laboratories
University of Brampton
Toronto Ontario, Canada

Preface

The fourth edition of Histology for Pathologists was published in 2012 and, as before, it is again reasonable to ask if "normal" has changed enough in the ensuing 6 years to justify a new edition. The answer, of course, is that normal has not changed at all (evolution is indeed a slow process!) but our perception of normal continues to expand and improve. In particular, we have developed many new immunohistochemical markers, and the ever-growing spectrum of their expression in normal tissues provides insights into pathologic processes arising from or differentiating toward these tissues. We also continue to recognize new variations of normal that cause diagnostic confusion and touch on the interface between normal and disease. Accordingly, the fifth edition brings incremental but valuable improvements in our perceptions of human histology.

This new edition also brings quite a few new authors and their fresh perspectives. The chapters on Joints, Anus, Vulva, Parathyroid, and Paraganglia, in particular, have been greatly revised in this new edition because of new senior authorship. Many more chapters include new junior authors who bring a fresh approach of their own.

As with prior editions of this text, its goal remains to bridge the gap between the histology of normality and pathologic alterations. Although the text emphasizes normal histology and normal features that may be confused with pathologic conditions, prepathologic conditions and pathologic processes confused with normal are briefly discussed in most chapters. It is this pathologic perspective that continues to set Histology for Pathologists apart from standard histology texts written by anatomists. Considerable effort has been expended to improve and update the illustrations, adding new ones whenever appropriate.

We believe that the fifth edition of this text is the best yet and that it will continue to provide valuable aid to both the neophyte pathology trainee and the experienced anatomic pathologist.

Stacey E. Mills, MD

Preface to the First Edition

Histology textbooks exist in abundance. Some are classics of their kind and have gone through innumerable editions over many years. They have served pathologists well, for the most part, especially in terms of strict tissue and cell histology. There is, however, a borderline between histology and pathology in which information for the pathologist is often lacking.

With this textbook we made an attempt to fill the gap. The significance and function of many histologic structures in terms of pathologic interpretation is often absent or obscure. In particular, variations of the norm related to such variables as age, sex, and race are often not clarified in conventional textbooks. For example, the chapter on Paraganglia notes that the connective tissue between the lobules in the carotid body increases with age. Another example related to age is in the pediatric kidney chapter, where it is noted that the glomeruli of fetuses are disproportionately large and are rarely seen in a state of histologic "immaturity." While the chapter on the myofibroblast details the location, staining, ultrastructure, and cytoskeletal protein composition of this unusual cell, we also learn of its importance in the desmoplastic reaction in cancerous tissue and, most importantly, that it is not found in carcinomas which are still in situ.

Some gross observations occasionally will be found as lagniappe, such as the notation that in patients with congenital absence of a kidney, the ipsilateral adrenal will be round rather than angulated. Another example would be that there is a crease in the earlobe associated with coronary artery disease.

Variations in staining reactions are considered, such as the failure of factor VIII to stain renal glomerular vessels. One finds that intestinal endocrine cells can be detected with hematoxylin and eosin (sic) stains by the infranuclear location of the granules. Uncommonly known fixation artifacts are uncovered; for example, the prickle-cell layer (with the so-called intercellular bridges) is actually a retraction artifact of the plasma membranes with the desmosomes remaining relatively fixed.

In most chapters, "prepathologic" considerations are emphasized, while in others the developed pathologic alterations related to the norm represent the major thrust of the chapter.

Some comments will be perceived as gratuitous, such as the remark in the Penis chapter to the effect that "the prepuce could be a mistake of nature." Furthermore, we learn that the "collagen fibers are wavy in the flaccid state and become straight during erection."

The pathology neophyte as well as the many esteemed and experienced pathologists will find helpful information in this book.

Stephen S. Sternberg, MD

Acknowledgments

The chapter authors are the heart and soul of this text and their efforts over multiple editions have made this book the asset to pathologists that it has become. My own contributions would not have been possible without the support of my friends and family, especially my wife, Linda. Our daughters, Elizabeth and Anne, now with families of their own, continue to be sources of pride, inspiration and insight about all things beyond pathology. I remain indebted to my early mentors, Ben Sturgill, Shannon Allen, Bob Fechner, and Phil Cooper who got me started on the right path; to Dick Kempson my "adopted" west coast mentor and good friend; and to all my colleagues at the University of Virginia and our trainees from whom I continue to learn.

Stacey E. Mills, MD

Contents

Contributors iii
Preface ix
Preface to the First Edition xi
Acknowledgments xiii

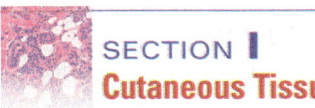
SECTION I
Cutaneous Tissue

1 Skin 3
   Andrew Kanik

2 Nail 31
   Julian Conejo-Mir, Javier Dominguez-Cruz, and Mercedes Sendín-Martín

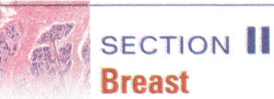
SECTION II
Breast

3 Breast 69
   Laura C. Collins and Stuart J. Schnitt

SECTION III
Musculoskeletal System

4 Bone 87
   Darcy A. Kerr and Andrew E. Rosenberg

5 Joints 113
   Fiona Maclean

6 Adipose Tissue 133
   John S.J. Brooks

7 Skeletal Muscle 166
   Hannes Vogel

8 Blood Vessels 190
   Patrick J. Gallagher and Allard C. van der Wal

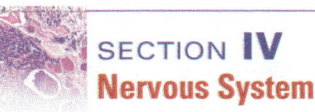
SECTION IV
Nervous System

9 Central Nervous System 219
   Gregory N. Fuller and Leomar Y. Ballester

10 Pituitary and Sellar Region 270
    M. Beatriz S. Lopes

11 Peripheral Nervous System 300
    Carlos Ortiz-Hidalgo and Roy O. Weller

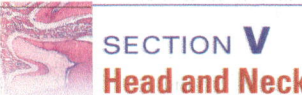
SECTION V
Head and Neck

12 Eye and Ocular Adnexa 335
    Alan D. Proia and Thomas J. Cummings

13 The Ear and Temporal Bone 362
    Bruce M. Wenig

14 Mouth, Nose, and Paranasal Sinuses 396
    Liron Pantanowitz and Karoly Balogh

15 Larynx and Pharynx 424
    Stacey E. Mills

16 Major Salivary Glands 440
    Fernando Martínez-Madrigal

SECTION VI
Thorax and Serous Membranes

17 Lungs 469
    Humberto E. Trejo Bittar and Samuel A. Yousem

18 Thymus 506
    David Suster and Saul Suster

19 Heart 529
    Gerald J. Berry

20 Serous Membranes 551
    Darryl Carter, Lawrence True, and Christopher N. Otis

xv

SECTION VII
Alimentary Tract

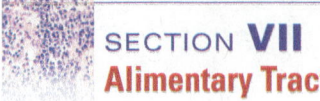

21 **Esophagus** 573
    James R. Conner, Hala El-Zimaity, and Robert H. Riddell

22 **Stomach** 601
    David A. Owen

23 **Small Intestine** 615
    Megan G. Lockyer and Robert E. Petras

24 **Colon** 640
    Maria Westerhoff and Joel K. Greenson

25 **Appendix** 664
    Megan G. Lockyer and Robert E. Petras

26 **Anal Canal** 677
    Meredith E. Pittman and Rhonda K. Yantiss

27 **Liver** 692
    Arief A. Suriawinata and Swan N. Thung

28 **Gallbladder and Extrahepatic Biliary System** 719
    Edward B. Stelow and Seung-Mo Hong

29 **Pancreas** 738
    Carlie S. Sigel, Ralph H. Hruban, Günter Klöppel, and David S. Klimstra

SECTION VIII
Hematopoietic System

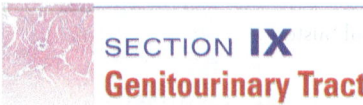

30 **Lymph Nodes** 783
    Paul van der Valk

31 **Spleen** 799
    J. Han J.M. van Krieken and Attilio Orazi

32 **Bone Marrow** 813
    S.H. Kroft

SECTION IX
Genitourinary Tract

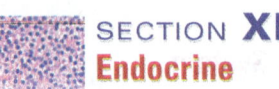

33 **Kidney** 855
    William L. Clapp

34 **Urinary Bladder, Ureter, and Renal Pelvis** 949
    Victor E. Reuter, Hikmat Al-Ahmadie, and Satish K. Tickoo

35 **Prostate** 964
    Samson W. Fine and Jesse K. McKenney

36 **Testis and Excretory Duct System** 981
    Muhammad T. Idrees and Thomas M. Ulbright

37 **Penis and Distal Urethra** 1009
    Elsa F. Velazquez, José E. Barreto, Sofía Cañete-Portillo, and Antonio L. Cubilla

SECTION X
Female Genital System

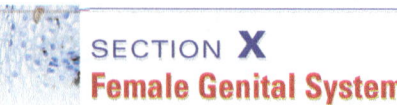

38 **Vulva** 1031
    Krisztina Z. Hanley

39 **Vagina** 1047
    Stanley J. Robboy, Gerald R. Cunha, Takeshi Kurita, and Kyle C. Strickland

40 **Normal Histology of the Uterus and Fallopian Tubes** 1059
    Kristen A. Atkins

41 **Ovary** 1107
    C. Blake Gilks

42 **Placenta** 1137
    Steven H. Lewis, Miriam D. Post, and Kurt Benirschke

SECTION XI
Endocrine

43 **Thyroid** 1175
    Maria Luisa Carcangiu

44 **Parathyroids** 1201
    Sylvia L. Asa and Ozgur Mete

45 **Adrenal** 1225
    J. Aidan Carney

46 **Neuroendocrine** 1249
    Ronald A. DeLellis and Shamlal Mangray

47 **Paraganglia** 1274
    Arthur S. Tischler and Sylvia L. Asa

Index 1297

SECTION I

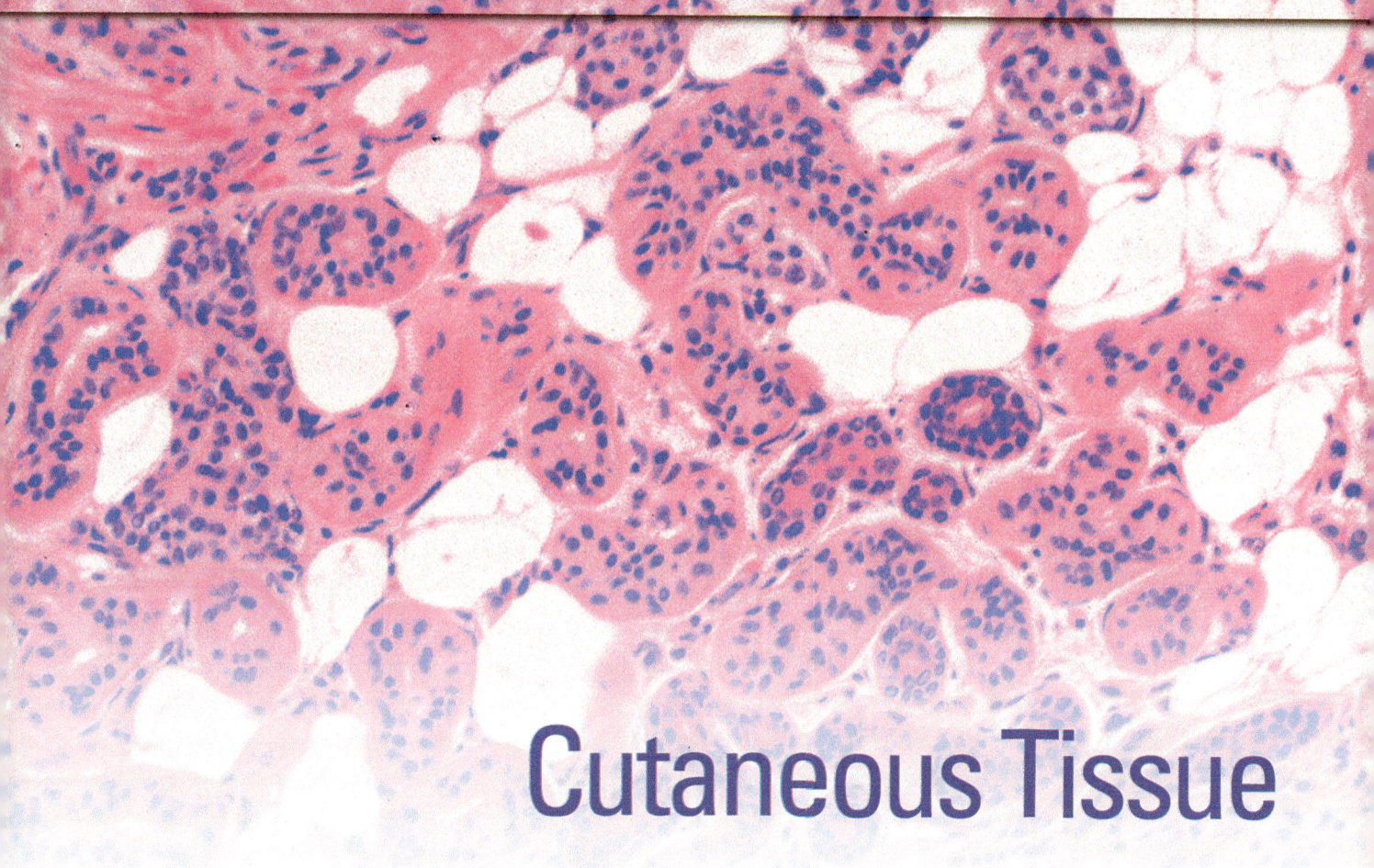

Cutaneous Tissue

Skin

Andrew Kanik

- EMBRYOLOGY 3
  - Epidermis 3
  - Dermis 4
  - Epithelial Skin Appendages 4
- HISTOMORPHOLOGY 5
  - Epidermis 5
  - Dermis 15
  - Subcutaneous Tissue 16
  - Blood Vessels, Lymphatics, Nerves, and Muscle 16
- HISTOLOGIC DIFFERENCES OF SKIN WITH AGE 18
  - Newborns and Children 18
  - Elderly 18
- HISTOLOGIC VARIATIONS ACCORDING TO ANATOMIC SITES 18
- PATHOLOGIC CHANGES FOUND IN BIOPSIES AND INTERPRETED AS "NORMAL SKIN" 20
- SPECIMEN HANDLING 21
- ARTIFACTS 21
- STAINING METHODS 22
  - Histochemical Stains 22
  - Immunofluorescence 23
  - Immunohistochemical Stains/Molecular Studies 23
- REFERENCES 27

The skin accounts for about 15% of the total body weight and is the largest organ of the body. It is composed of three layers: (a) epidermis, (b) dermis, and (c) the subcutaneous adipose tissue. Each component has its unique and complex structure and function (1–3), with variations according to age, gender, race, and anatomic location. Functions of the skin are extremely diverse. It serves as a mechanical barrier against external physical, chemical, and biologic noxious substances and as an immunologic organ. It participates in body temperature and electrolyte regulation. It is an important organ of sensuality and psychological well-being. In addition, it is a vehicle that expresses not only primary diseases of the skin, but also diseases of the internal organs. An understanding of the skin's normal histology is essential to the understanding of pathologic conditions.

EMBRYOLOGY

Epidermis

Basic knowledge of the embryology of the skin is important because it helps to understand some postnatal pathology.

The ectoderm gives rise to epidermis and its appendages. The mesoderm provides the mesenchymal elements of the dermis and subcutaneous fat (4). Developmental abnormalities in the ectoderm produce among others a variety of syndromes grouped under the umbrella term of ectodermal dysplasias (5).

Initially, the embryo is covered by a single layer of ectodermal cells which by the 6th to 8th week of development differentiates into two layers, the basal layer and an overlying second layer called periderm. Because of mitotic activity, the basal layer becomes the germinative layer and additional rows of cells develop from this proliferating layer, forming a multilayer of cells between the ectoderm and periderm (4). By the 23rd week, keratinization has taken place in the upper stratum, and the cells of the periderm have already been shed (4,6,7). Of interest is that the CD30 antigen, considered to be restricted to tumor cells of Hodgkin disease and anaplastic large cell lymphoma, participates in the terminal differentiation of many fetal tissues including the skin (8).

Cell junction proteins are expressed in the early two-layered embryonic epidermis and as early as the 8th week of estimated gestational age (9). By the end of the first trimester, the dermoepidermal junction with its components is ultrastructurally similar to that of mature skin (10). Thus, the characteristic neonatal epidermis is well developed by the 4th month.

Keratinocytes constitute 90% to 95% of the cells in the epidermis. The rest of the epidermal cells are nonkeratinocytes, and they include melanocytes, Langerhans cells, and Merkel cells. The nonkeratinocytes are seen in the epidermis of 8- to 10-week-old embryos. The precursor cells of melanocytes migrate from the neural crest to the dermis and then to the epidermis, where they differentiate into melanocytes during the first 3 months of development. During this migration, melanocytes can reside in other organs and tissues. Ultrastructurally, recognizable melanosomes in melanocytes may be seen in the fetal epidermis at 8 to 10 weeks of gestational age (11).

Langerhans cells are derived from the CD34+ hematopoietic precursor cell of the bone marrow. The characteristic cytoplasmic marker, the Birbeck granule, is seen ultrastructurally in 10-week-old embryos (12). The expression of a more characteristic immunohistochemical marker, CD1a, is completed by 12 to 13 weeks of estimated gestational age (12,13).

Merkel cells can also be seen in the epidermis of 8- to 10-week-old embryos. The origin of Merkel cells is debatable. Some have suggested a neural crest derivation (14), whereas others suggest epidermal origin through a process of differentiation from neighboring keratinocytes (15,16,17). Merkel cells in the epidermis are initially numerous and later diminish with increasing gestational age (18).

Dermis

The dermis is derived from the primitive mesenchyme underlying the surface ectoderm. The papillary and reticular dermis are recognized by 15 weeks of intrauterine life (19,20).

As described by Breathnach (19), three types of cells are recognized in 6- to 14-week-old embryos. Type I cells are stellate-dendritic cells with long, slender processes. These are the most numerous primitive mesenchymal cells and probably give rise to the endothelial cells and the pericytes. Type II cells have less extensive cell processes; the nucleus is round and the cytoplasm contains large vacuoles. They are classified as phagocytic macrophages of yolk-sac origin. Type III cells are round with little or no membrane extension, but they contain numerous vesicles, some with an internal content suggestive of granule secretory type of cells. These cells could be melanoblasts on their way to the epidermis, or they could be precursors of mast cells; Schwann cells associated with neuroaxons, but lacking basal lamina, are also identified during this period.

The type II mesenchymal cells are rarely seen after week 14 of development. However, another cell type with ultrastructure of histiocyte or macrophage is frequently seen during this time. Well-formed mast cells are also seen in the dermis.

In 14 to 21 weeks of development, fibroblasts are numerous and active. Fibroblasts are recognized as elongated spindle cells with abundant rough endoplasmic reticulum. They are the fundamental cells of the dermis and synthesize all types of fibers and ground substance (1). Type III collagen fibers are abundantly present in the matrix of fetus, whereas type I collagen fibers are more prominent in adult skin (20). Elastic fibers appear in the dermis after the collagen fiber during the 22nd week of gestational age; and, by week 32, a well-developed network of elastic fibers is formed in the dermis.

Initially, the dermis is organized into somites, but soon this segmental organization ends and the dermis of the head and neck and extremities organizes into dermatomes along the segmental nerves that are being formed (21). From the 24th week to term, fat cells develop in the subcutaneous tissue from the primitive mesenchymal cells.

Epithelial Skin Appendages

Most epithelial cells of skin appendages derive from follicular epithelial stem cells localized in the basal layer of epidermis at the prominent bulge region of the developing human fetal hair follicles. Furthermore, such multipotent stem cells may represent the ultimate epidermal stem cell (22). In 10-week-old embryos, mesenchymal cells of the developing dermis interact with epidermal basal cells. These epidermal cells grow both downward to the dermis and upward through the epidermis to form the opening of the hair canal. As the growing epithelial cells reach the subcutaneous fat, the lower portion becomes bulbous and partially encloses the mesenchymal cells descending with them to form the dermal papillae of the hair follicle, this structure plays an important role in the future processes of hair follicle regeneration (23). The descending epidermal cells around the dermal papillae constitute the matrix cells from which the hair layers and inner root sheath will develop. The outer root sheath derives from downward growth of the epidermis. The first hairs appear by the end of the 3rd gestational month as lanugo hair around the eyebrow and the upper lip. The lanugo hair is shed around the time of birth. The developing hair follicle gives rise to the sebaceous and apocrine glands.

The sebaceous glands originate as epithelial buds from the outer root sheath of the hair follicles and are developed at approximately the 13th to 15th gestational weeks (24). Differentiated sebaceous glands with a hair protruding through the skin surface are present at the 18th week of gestational age (25). They respond to maternal hormones and are well developed at the time of birth.

The apocrine glands also develop as epithelial buds from the outer sheath of the hair follicles in 5- to 6-month-old fetuses (21) and continue into late embryonic life as long as new hair follicles develop.

The eccrine glands develop from the fetal epidermis independent of the hair follicles (21). Initially, they are seen as regularly spaced undulations of the basal layer. At 14 to 15 weeks, the tips of the primordial eccrine glands have reached the deep dermis, forming the eccrine coils (26). At the same time, the eccrine epithelium grows upward into the epidermis. The primordial eccrine epithelium acquires a lumen by the 7th to 8th fetal month, and thus the first eccrine unit is formed. Both ducts and secretory portions are lined by two layers of cells. The two layers in the secretory segment undergo further differentiation; the luminal cells into tall columnar secretory cells, and the basal layer into secretory cells or myoepithelial cells. The first glands are formed on the palms and soles by the 4th month, then in the axillae in the 5th month, and finally on the rest of the hairy skin (27).

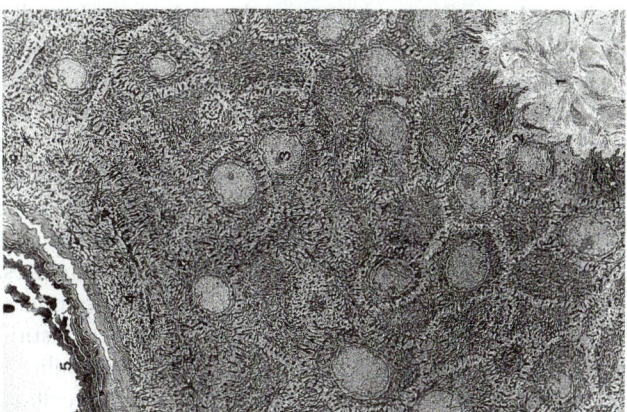

FIGURE 1.1 Electron micrograph of normal epidermis and portion of papillary dermis (×2,100) (*1*, papillary dermis; *2*, basal cells; *3*, squamous layer; *4*, granular layer; *5*, cornified layer).

HISTOMORPHOLOGY

Epidermis

The epidermis is a stratified and keratinizing squamous epithelium that dynamically renews itself maintaining its normal thickness by the process of desquamation. The cells in the epidermis include (a) keratinocytes, (b) melanocytes, (c) Langerhans cells, (d) Toker cells (in certain anatomic locations), and (e) Merkel cells. In addition, the epidermis contains the openings for the eccrine ducts (acrosyringium) and hair follicles. Recent immunohistochemical studies have demonstrated that the epidermis contains free nerve axons in association with Langerhans cells (28).

Keratinocytes

The keratinocytes of the epidermis are stratified into four orderly layers from bottom to top: (a) the basal layer (stratum basale, germinativum), (b) the squamous layer (prickle cell layer or stratum spinosum), (c) the granular layer (stratum granulosum), and (d) the cornified or horny layer (stratum corneum) (Fig. 1.1). In histologic sections, the dermoepidermal junction has an irregular contour because of the upward extension of the papillary dermis to form the dermal papillae. The portion on the epidermis separating the dermal papillae are the rete ridges (Fig. 1.2).

The transcription factor p63 plays an important role in this orderly arrangement and continuous development of the pre- and postnatal skin (29).

> **THE BASAL LAYER** Basal cells are the mitotically active cells that give rise to the other keratinocytes. Histologically, basal cells are seen as a single layer of cells above the basement membrane that show minor variations in size, shape, and melanin content. Basal cells are columnar or cuboidal, with a basophilic cytoplasm. The nucleus is round or oval, with coarse chromatin and indistinct nucleolus. Basal cells contain melanin in their cytoplasm as a result of pigment transfer from neighboring melanocytes. Basal cells are connected to each other and to keratinocytes by specialized regions (known as desmosomes) located in the plasma cell membranes. They are aligned perpendicular to the subepidermal basement membrane and attached to it by modified desmosomes, hemidesmosomes.

Certain dermatitides involving the basal layer produce vacuolar alteration of the basal cells, which may progress to the formation of subsequent subepidermal vesicles as seen in diseases such as graft-versus-host disease, lupus erythematosus, and erythema multiforme.

> **THE SQUAMOUS LAYER** The squamous layers are composed of approximately 5 to 10 layers of cells with keratinocytes larger than the basal cells. The suprabasal keratinocytes are polyhedral, have a somewhat basophilic cytoplasm, and a round nucleus. Again, melanin is seen scattered in many of these keratinocytes, where it provides protection from the damaging effect of ultraviolet light. The more superficial

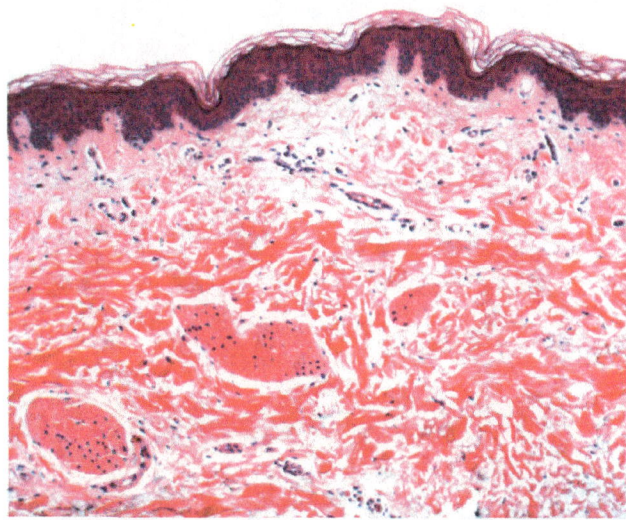

FIGURE 1.2 Normal skin showing stratified epidermis with rete ridges, papillary dermis, and reticular dermis (H&E).

cells are larger, flattened, eosinophilic, and oriented parallel to the surface. The keratinocytes contain one or two conspicuous nucleoli and tonofilaments within the cytoplasm.

The squamous layer is also called the spinous or prickle cell layer because of the characteristic appearance by light microscopy of short projections extending from cell to cell. These projections are the result of retraction of the plasma membrane during tissue processing, whereas the desmosomes remain relatively fixed and correlate with intercellular bridges.

Desmosomes are composed of a variety of polypeptides, desmogleins and desmocollins as transmembrane constituents and the desmoplakin, plakoglobin, and plakophilin as cytoplasmic components. In addition, other intercellular junctions (such as gap junctions and adherens junctions) are distinct from desmosomes in composition and distribution and provide alternative cell-to-cell adhesion mechanisms (30). An intercellular space of constant dimension is present between each cell; acid and neutral mucopolysaccharides are present in the intercellular spaces as indicated by special stains. The pemphigus antigens are localized in the cell membranes (31) or in the desmosomes of these cells (32).

Occasionally, Toker cells with clear or pale cytoplasm are seen in the squamous layer. It is important to distinguish these cells from the neoplastic cells of Paget disease. Benign clear cells have a pyknotic nucleus surrounded by a clear halo and a narrow rim of clear cytoplasm (Fig. 1.3). They lack the pleomorphism, nuclear morphology, and intensity of the chromatin staining seen in Paget cells (Fig. 1.4). Regardless of gender (33), these benign

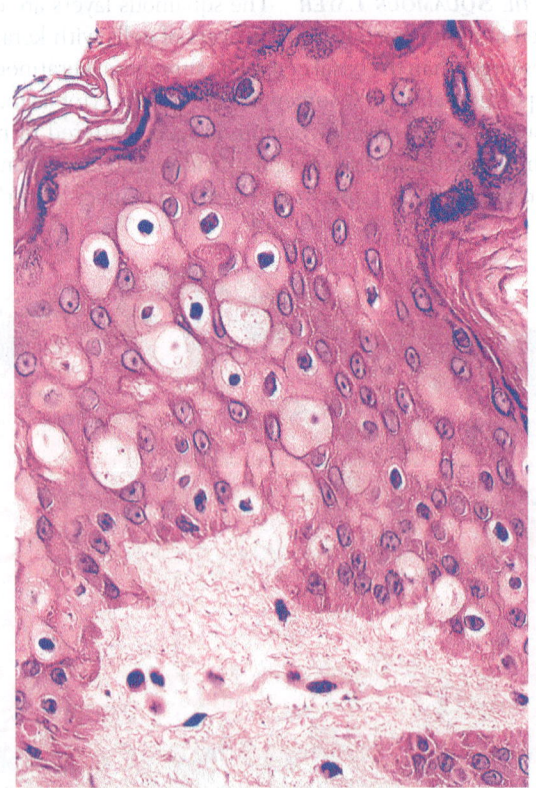

FIGURE 1.3 Clear cells of the nipple epidermis.

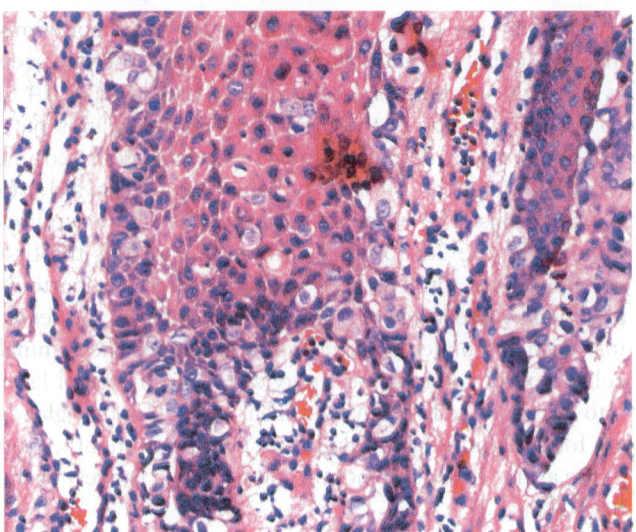

FIGURE 1.4 Paget cells in extramammary Paget disease.

clear cells are often seen in the epidermis of the nipple, the accessory nipple (34,35), and the pubic regions or in the milk-line distribution (36). In the nipple, these clear cells, also called Toker cells, have been considered to be non-neoplastic ductal epithelial cells, although some authors hypothesized that these cells might be the precursors of mammary or extramammary Paget diseases (35,37). Those outside of the nipple are considered to be the result of either abnormal keratinization or aberrant derivatives of eccrine or apocrine sweat gland epithelial cells (38–40). They may present as hypopigmented macules or papules in a rare disorder called clear cell papulosis. The immunohistochemical staining pattern of benign clear cells may resemble that of Paget cells in that they react with the cytokeratin 7 (CK7) but differ from Paget cells in that they are usually negative for GCDFP-15. However, emphasis should be made that morphologic distinction is the most important manner to differentiate both cells.

Common inflammatory changes seen in the squamous layer are (a) spongiosis—intercellular edema (e.g., allergic contact dermatitis), (b) acanthosis—thickening of the epidermis (e.g., psoriasis), (c) atrophy—thinning of the epidermis (e.g., discoid lupus erythematosus), (d) acantholysis—detachment of keratinocytes because of changes involving intercellular junctions (e.g., pemphigus), and (e) dyskeratosis—abnormal keratinization (e.g., squamous carcinoma).

> **THE GRANULAR LAYER** The granular layer is composed of one to three layers of flattened cells lying parallel to the skin surface. The cytoplasm contains intensely basophilic-stained granules known as the keratohyalin granules. In contrast, trichohyalin granules (produced by the inner root sheath of hair follicles) are stained red on routine hematoxylin and eosin (H&E)-stained sections. The keratohyalin granules are histidine rich and are the precursors to the protein filaggrin, which promotes aggregation of keratin filaments in the cornified layer.

Histologic observation of this layer can provide key findings in certain entities such as increase (e.g., lichen planus) and decrease (e.g., psoriasis) in the thickness of the granular layer.

Keratinocytes, located between the squamous layer and the granular layer, contain small membrane-coating granules known as lamellar granules (also called Odland bodies or keratinosomes). They are composed of the acid hydrolase and neutral sugars conjugated with proteins and lipids. These granules, present both intra- and extracellularly, are approximately 300 nm in diameter and are not visible by light microscopy. Their functions are to provide epidermal lipids, increase the barrier property of the cornified layer against water loss, and aid in the desquamation process. This interface between the squamous and the granular layer is also the site of synthesis and storage of cholesterol (41).

> **The Cornified Layer** The cornified layer is composed of multiple layers of polyhedral eosinophilic keratinocytes that lack a nucleus and cytoplasmic organelles. These cells are the most differentiated cells of the keratinization system. They are composed entirely of high–molecular-weight keratin filaments. In formalin-fixed section, the cornified layers are arranged in a basket-weave pattern (Fig. 1.5). These cells eventually shed from the surface of the skin. The process of keratinization takes 20 to 45 days.

In histologic sections taken from the skin of the palms and soles, a homogenous eosinophilic zone, known as the stratum lucidum is present in the lowest portion of the cornified layer (above the granular layer). This additional layer is rich in extracellular elements such as energetic enzymes and SH groups adding to the normal functional barrier of the skin (42).

Common abnormalities of the cornified layer are (a) hyperkeratosis—increased thickness in the cornified layer (e.g., ichthyosis), (b) parakeratosis—presence of nuclei in the cornified layer (as usually seen in actinic keratosis), and (c) presence of fungal organisms (superficial dermatophytosis).

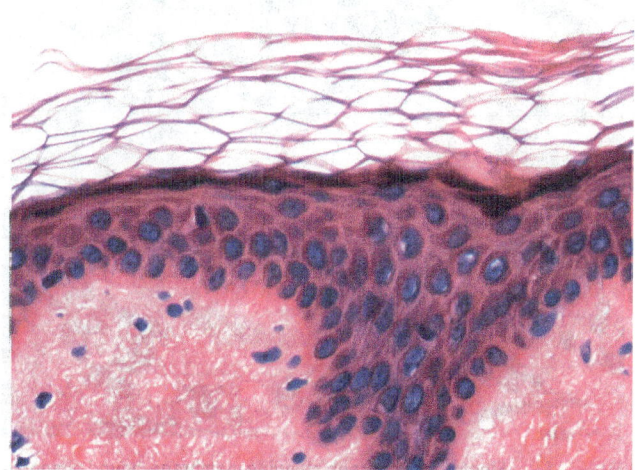

FIGURE 1.5 Basket-weave pattern of the cornified layer (also in Fig. 1.2).

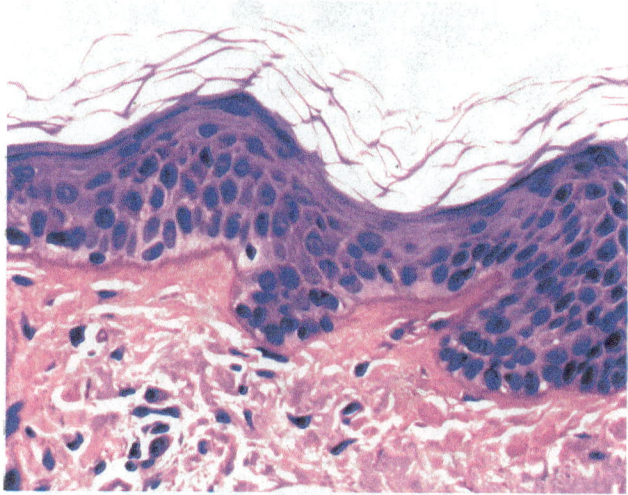

FIGURE 1.6 PAS-positive basement membrane.

Basement Membrane Zone

The basement membrane zone separates the epidermal basal layer from the dermis. It is seen by light microscopy as a continuous, undulating, and thin periodic acid–Schiff (PAS)-stained layer (Fig. 1.6). By electron microscopy, the basal cells are attached to the basal lamina by hemidesmosomes. Ultrastructurally, the basement membrane zone is composed of four distinct structures, from top to bottom (Fig. 1.7) (43):

1. The plasma membrane of the basal cells containing the hemidesmosomes. Bullous pemphigoid antigen 1 is localized in the intracellular component of hemidesmosomes.

2. The lamina lucida, an electron-lucent area with anchoring filaments containing various laminin isoforms (44). Bullous pemphigoid antigen 2 (type XVII collagen) is associated with the transmembrane component of hemidesmosome-anchoring filament complexes in the lamina lucida. It is also the site of the blister in dermatitis herpetiformis (45).

3. The lamina densa, an electron-dense area composed of mainly type IV collagen.

4. The sublamina densa zone, or pars fibroreticularis, contains mainly the anchoring fibrils (46) (type VII collagen) that attach the basal lamina to the connective tissue of the dermis. Antibodies against epidermolysis bullosa acquisita react with the carboxy terminus of type VII collagen (47,48).

Inflammatory conditions of the basement membrane can be seen by light microscopy as thickening (e.g., discoid lupus erythematosus) or by the formation of subepidermal vesicles (e.g., bullous pemphigoid).

Melanocytes

Melanocytes are dendritic cells that derive from the neural crest. During migration from the neural crest, melanocytes may localize in other epithelia. In the epidermis,

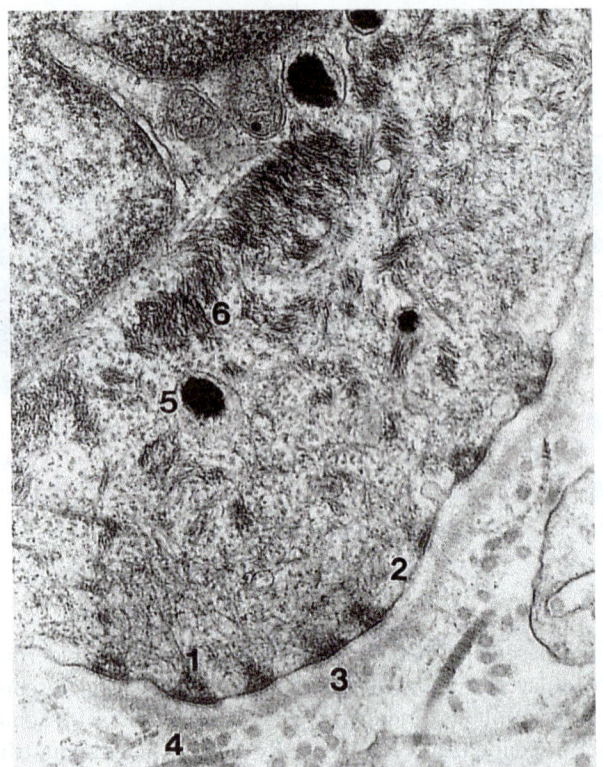

FIGURE 1.7 Ultrastructure of basement membrane (×37,800) (*1*, hemidesmosome; *2*, lamina lucida; *3*, lamina densa; *4*, lamina reticularis; *5*, melanin; *6*, tonofilaments).

the melanocytes are localized in the basal layer, and their dendritic processes extend in all directions. The dendritic nature of normal melanocytes is usually not seen in routine H&E-stained sections. In H&E preparations, melanocytes are composed of elongated or ovoid nuclei surrounded by a clear space (Fig. 1.8). They are usually smaller than the neighboring basal keratinocytes. Melanocytes do not contain tonofilaments and do not attach to basal cells with desmosomes. However, anchoring filaments extend from the plasma membrane of these melanocytes to the basal lamina. Laminin-5, a component of anchoring filaments, may be a ligand for melanocyte attachment to the basement membrane in vivo (49). In addition, melanocytes that are close to the basal lamina have structures resembling hemidesmosomes of basal keratinocytes (50).

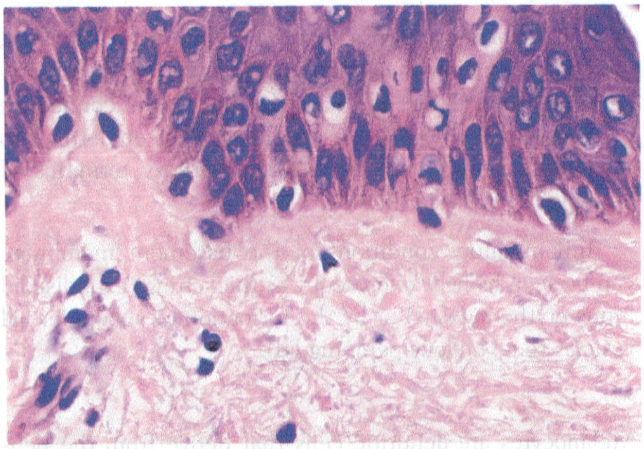

Melanocytes produce and secrete melanin. Melanin can be red (pheomelanin) or yellow-black (eumelanin). The most important function of melanin is to protect against the injurious effects of nonionizing ultraviolet irradiation.

Melanin is formed through a complex metabolic process in which tyrosinase is the main catabolic enzyme, using tyrosine as substrate. The synthesis of melanin takes place in melanosomes, lysosome-related organelles. In the early stages of development, melanosomes are membrane-limited vesicles, located in the Golgi-associated endoplasmic reticulum. The maturation of melanosomes undergoes four stages. Stage I melanosomes are round without melanin. These are seen in balloon cell melanoma. Stage II through stage IV melanosomes are ellipsoidal with numerous longitudinal filaments. Melanin deposits start at stage II. In stage III, melanin deposits are prominent. Stage IV melanosomes are fully packed, with melanin obscuring the internal structures.

The developing melanosomes, with their content of melanin, are transferred to the neighboring basal keratinocytes and hair follicular cells. The mechanism of melanin transfer is a complex process (51,52), with the end result being phagocytosis of the tip of melanocytic dendrites by the keratinocytes (Fig. 1.9) in a process called pigment donation (53).

The number of melanocytes in normal skin is constant in all races, the ratio being 1 melanocyte for every 4 to 10 basal keratinocytes. Alteration of this ratio is important in the diagnosis of certain pigmented lesions such as malignant melanoma of the lentigo maligna type and etiologies of clinical hypopigmentation such as vitiligo.

FIGURE 1.8 Melanocytes in the basal layer, composed of ovoid nuclei within a clear space.

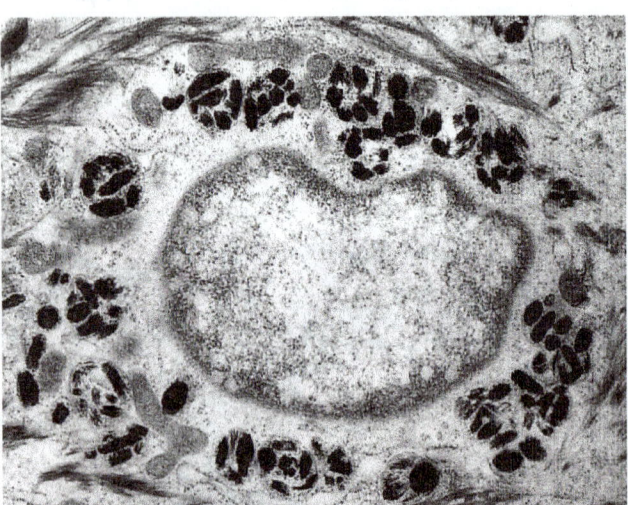

FIGURE 1.9 Electron micrograph showing membrane-bound phagocytized melanin in keratinocyte (×19,200).

The color of the skin is determined by the number and size of melanosomes present both in keratinocytes and melanocytes—and not by the number of melanocytes. The number of melanocytes decreases with age. As a result, the availability of melanin to keratinocytes diminishes, so the skin becomes lighter in color and the incidence of skin cancer increases because of the lack of protection that melanin provides.

Melanin is both argentaffin and argyrophilic. It can be recognized by Fontana–Masson silver stains. In addition, melanocytes and their dendritic processes are identified by the dopa reaction in histologic slides prepared from frozen sections and in paraffin-embedded sections with immunohistochemical stains with S100 protein. The latter is highly sensitive but not specific for cells of melanocytic lineage. The S100 protein can be detected in various types of cells, such as Langerhans cells, Schwann cells, eccrine, and apocrine gland cells. Melanocytes can also be identified with monoclonal antibodies Melan-A/MART-1 (Melanoma Antigens Recognized by T cells-1), a melanocytic differentiation marker. The Melan-A/MART-1 antigen is expressed in normal melanocytes, common nevi, Spitz nevi, and malignant melanoma. Under normal conditions, the melanoma-associated antigen HMB-45 does not react with adult melanocytes (54). It is expressed in embryonic melanocytes, hair bulb melanocytes and activated melanocytes (55). It is usually seen reacting with most melanoma cells, Spitz nevi, the junctional component of common nevi, and dysplastic nevi.

An absence or significant decrease in the number of melanocytes is seen in vitiligo. In albinism, there is a defect in the synthesis of melanin, but the number of melanocytes is normal in a skin biopsy. Melanocytic hyperplasia is seen in lentigo, benign, and malignant melanocytic neoplasms, and as a reaction pattern in a variety of neoplastic and non-neoplastic conditions (e.g., dermatofibroma). In a freckle, there is an increase in pigment donation to adjacent keratinocytes rather than melanocytic hyperplasia.

Langerhans Cells

Langerhans cells (LCs), discovered by Paul Langerhans in 1868, are mobile, dendritic, antigen-presenting cells present in all stratified epithelium and predominantly in the mid to upper parts of the squamous layer. In H&E-stained sections, LCs can be suggested as they appear to lie within lacunae having darkly stained nuclei with indented, reniform shape at high magnification (Fig. 1.10). As with melanocytes, their dendritic nature cannot be seen in routine sections. Langerhans cells can be recognized by histoenzymatic stains for adenosine triphosphatase (ATPase); they can also be detected in formalin-fixed, paraffin-embedded tissue using immunoreactivity for S100 protein and, more specifically, the antibody to the CD1a antigen (Fig. 1.11). With histoenzymatic and immunohistochemical stains, the extensive dendritic nature of LCs becomes evident.

By electron microscopy, LCs show no desmosomes, tonofilaments, or melanosomes. They contain small vesicles,

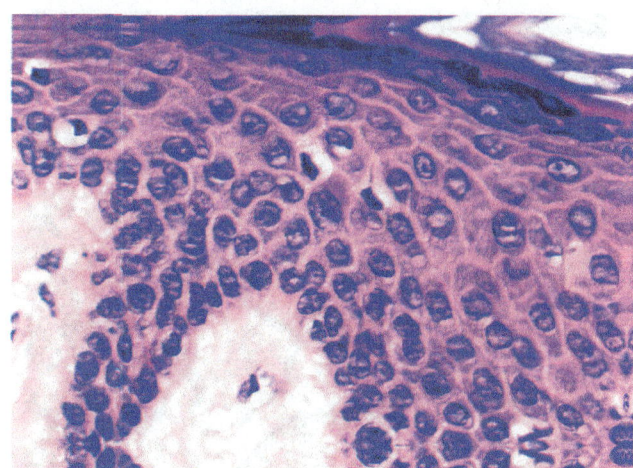

FIGURE 1.10 H&E section of possible Langerhans cells composed of elongated nuclei surrounded by a clear space in the mid epidermis.

multivesicular bodies, lysosomes, and the characteristic Birbeck granule (Fig. 1.12) (56), a rod-shaped organelle varying in size from 100 nm to 1 μm (57). It has a centrally striated density and an occasional bulb at one end with a unique tennis-racket appearance. Langerhans cells are also present in epithelia, lymphoid organs, and dermis and are increased in the skin in a variety of inflammatory conditions, such as contact dermatitis, where they can be seen as minute nodular aggregates in the epidermis. Langerhans cell granulomatosis is a reactive lesion most commonly seen in bones but also appearing at other sites.

Merkel Cells

Merkel cells (MCs), first described by F.S. Merkel in 1875, are scattered and irregularly distributed in the basal cell layer in the epidermis. They may group together in clusters coupled with enlarged terminal sensory nerve fibers to form slowly adapting mechanoreceptors; within the epidermis, they mediate tactile sensation (58–60). They are located in higher concentration in the glabrous skin of the digits, lips, and oral cavity, in the outer root sheath of hair follicles (61), and in the tactile hair disks (62).

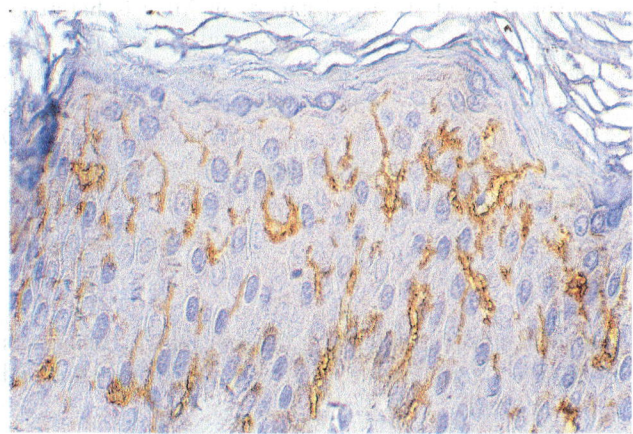

FIGURE 1.11 CD1a-specific reaction of Langerhans cells. Note the dendritic processes.

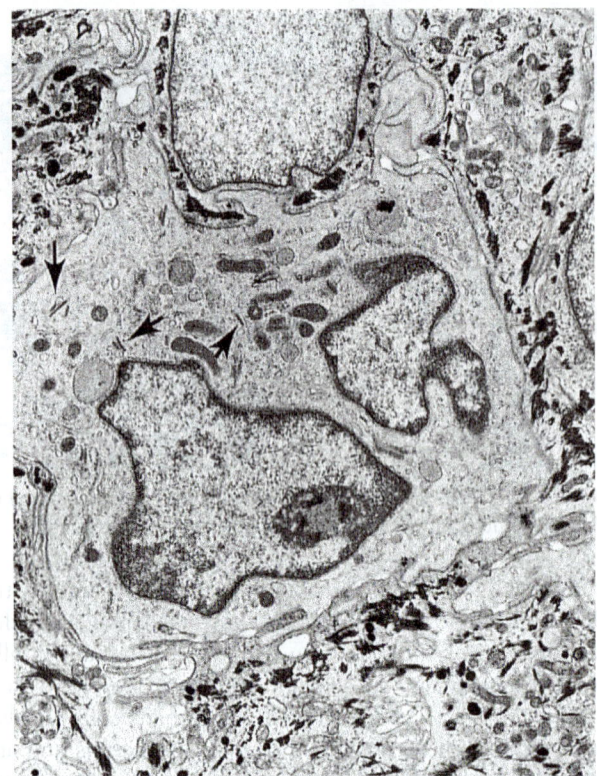

FIGURE 1.12 Electron micrograph of a Langerhans cell containing Birbeck granules (*arrows*) and multisegmented nucleus (×8,000).

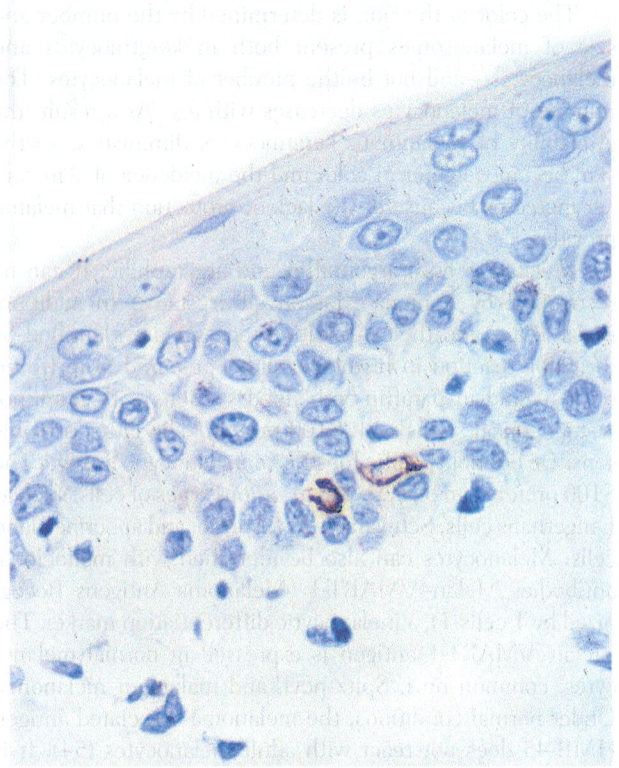

FIGURE 1.13 Cytokeratin 20 staining a Merkel cell in the basal layer of the epidermis.

Merkel cells are not recognized in routine histologic preparations. Electron microscopy and immunostaining are required for their identification. By electron microscopy, MCs are attached to adjacent keratinocytes by desmosomes. They have scant cytoplasm, invaginated nuclei, a parallel array of cytokeratin filaments in the paranuclear zone, and the characteristic membrane-bound dense core granules that are often, but not always, related to unmyelinated neurites.

By immunostaining techniques, normal and neoplastic MCs may express neuron-specific enolase, chromogranin, synaptophysin, neural cell adhesion molecule, and various neuropeptides and other substances (63–65). However, the expression of these substances in MCs is heterogeneous and variable. The constant pattern seen in MCs is the presence of paranuclear aggregates of cytokeratins (15,65,66), which include low–molecular-weight keratins 8, 18, 19, and 20. The most specific cytokeratin is CK20 because, in addition to MCs, they are expressed in simple epithelial cells and not in adjacent keratinocytes (67,68) (Fig. 1.13).

Pilar Unit

The pilar unit is composed of the hair follicle, sebaceous gland, arrector pili muscle, and (when present) eccrine and apocrine glands.

> **HAIR FOLLICLE** The hair follicle is divided into three segments from top to bottom: (a) the infundibulum, which extends from the opening of the hair follicle in the epidermis to the opening of the sebaceous duct; (b) the isthmus, which extends from the opening of the sebaceous duct to the insertion of the arrector pili muscle; and (c) the inferior segment, which extends to the base of the follicle. The inferior segment is bulbous and encloses a vascularized component of the dermis referred to as follicular (dermal) papilla of the hair follicle (Fig. 1.14).

The microanatomy and function of the hair follicle are very complex. The cells of the hair matrix differentiate along six cell linings. Beginning from the innermost layer, they are (a) the hair medulla; (b) the hair cortex; (c) the hair cuticle; and (d) three concentric layers of the inner root sheath, which are the cuticle of the inner root sheath, Huxley layer, and Henle layer.

The inner root sheath of the hair follicle is surrounded by the outer root sheath (Fig. 1.15), which is composed of clear cells. These glycogen-rich cells are seen in some of the neoplasm with hair follicular differentiation (e.g., trichilemmoma). A PAS-positive basement membrane separates the outer root sheath from the surrounding connective tissue. Thus, the hair shaft is formed from the bulb region that occupies the hair follicular canal.

Dendritic melanocytes are present only in the upper half of the bulb, whereas inactive (amelanotic) melanocytes are present in the outer root sheath. These melanocytes can become active after injury, migrating into the upper portion of the outer root sheath and to the regenerating epidermis.

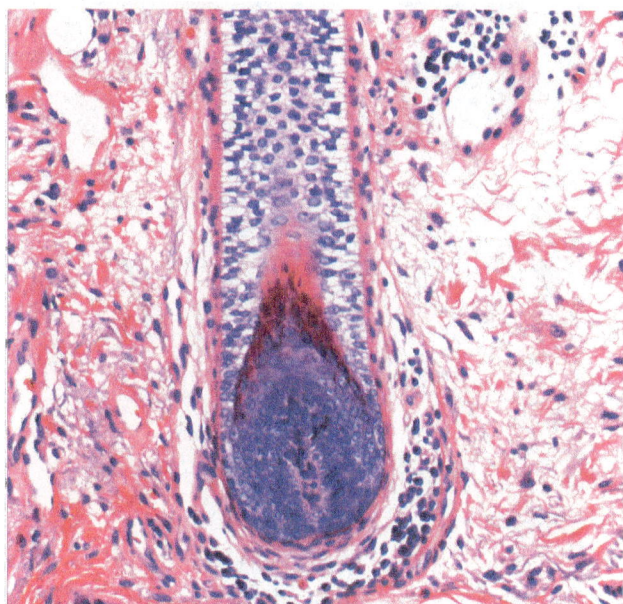

FIGURE 1.14 Inferior segment of the hair follicle, showing the hair papilla.

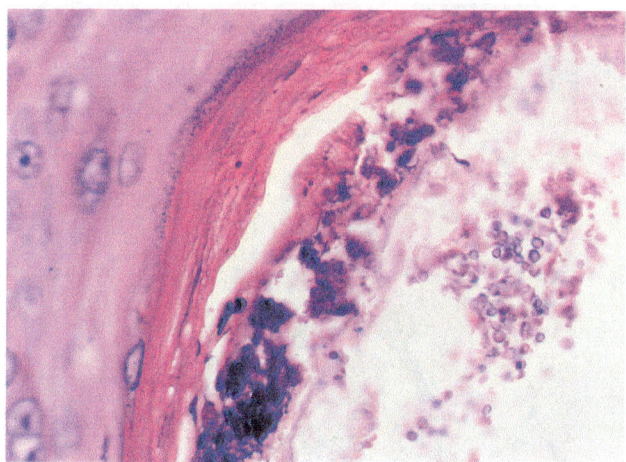

FIGURE 1.16 Yeasts of *Pityrosporum* in the follicular infundibulum.

At the level of the isthmus, the cells of the inner root sheath disintegrate and disappear, whereas the cells of the outer root sheath begin an abrupt sequence of keratinization. This process is called trichilemmal keratinization (69). Trichohyalin granules are red in routine H&E-stained sections, as opposed to the blue granules of the keratohyalin of epidermal keratinization and of the epithelium of the follicular infundibulum of the hair follicle. The staining features of these granules permit neoplasms and cysts to be distinguished from either pilar or epidermal origin.

Under normal circumstances, microorganisms like *Staphylococcus epidermis*, *Pityrosporum* yeast (Fig. 1.16), and the *Demodex folliculorum* mites (Fig. 1.17) are encountered in the follicular infundibulum.

The mantle hair of Pinkus (70) is a hair follicle in which proliferation of basaloid epithelioid cells emanating from the infundibulum is seen. Sebaceous proliferation is present in those cords (Fig. 1.18). The significance of this hair follicle is not known.

The hair growth is in lifelong cyclic transformation. Hormones and their receptors play prominent roles in hair cycle regulation (71). Three phases are recognized: (a) anagen—active growth phase; (b) catagen—involuting phase (apoptosis-driven regression); and (c) telogen—relative resting phase. The histologic features previously described correspond to the anagen hair.

During the catagen phase, mitosis and melanin synthesis cease at the level of the hair bulb. The hair bulb is then replaced by a cornified sac formed by retraction of the outer root sheath around the hair bulb, and a club hair is formed. A thick glassy basement membrane surrounds the hair

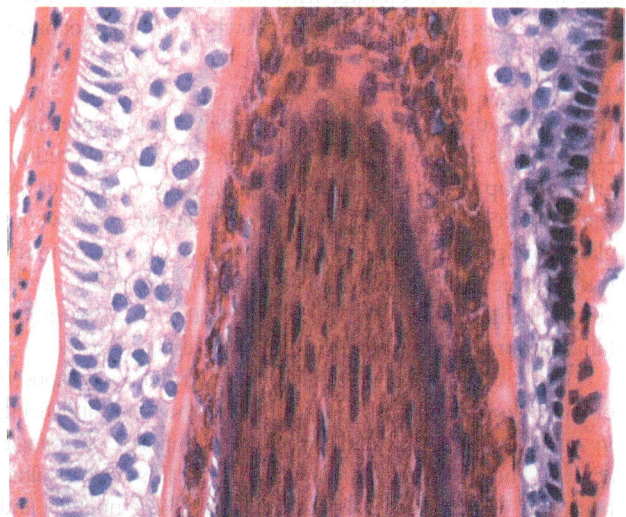

FIGURE 1.15 Hair follicle showing the hair shaft (**center**) surrounded by the inner root sheath, which contains trichohyalin granules. The outer root sheath is composed of clear cells.

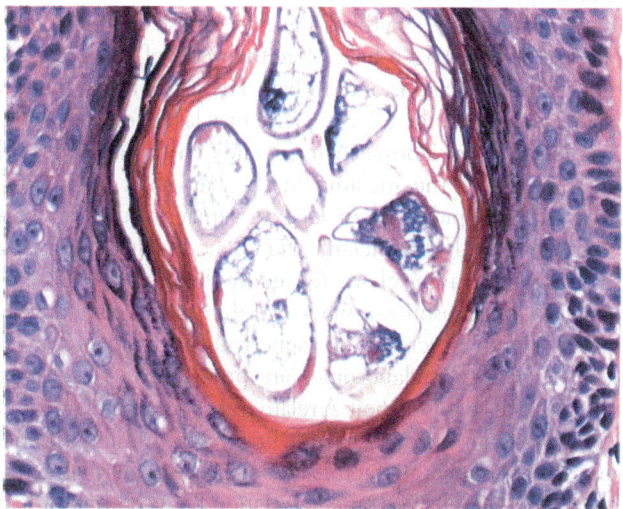

FIGURE 1.17 *Demodex folliculorum* mites in the follicular infundibulum.

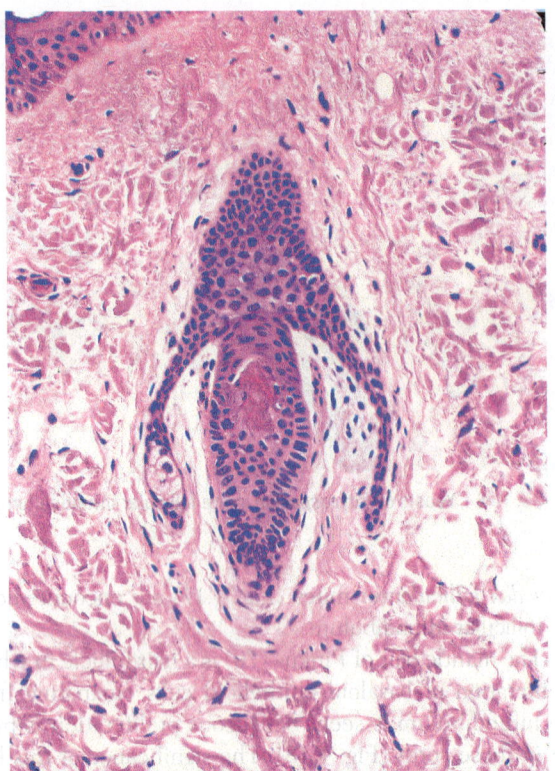

FIGURE 1.18 Mantle hair of Pinkus with lateral extensions containing sebaceous cells.

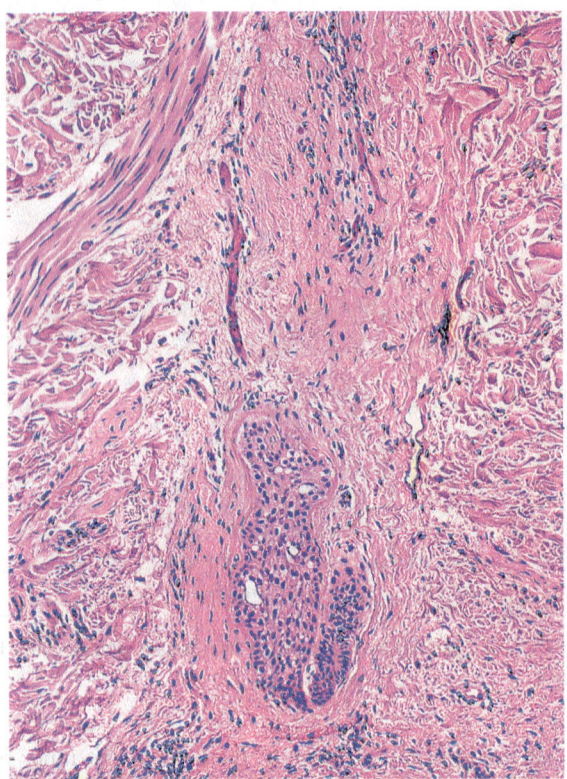

FIGURE 1.19 Catagen–telogen hair follicle located entirely within the dermis.

follicle. Apoptosis of single cells in the outer root sheath is a characteristic finding during the catagen phase.

During the telogen phase, the club hair and its cornified sac retract even further to the insertion of the arrector pili muscle, leaving behind the dermal papilla, which is connected to the retracted hair follicle by a fibrous tract (Fig. 1.19) (21). When the cycle is complete, a new anagen phase begins with the formation of new hair matrix.

The duration of the normal hair cycle varies. The anagen phase is measured in years for the scalp, but it is measured in shorter periods of time for the anagen cycle in other regions of the body. The length of the hair is also related to the amount of the anagen hair. More than 80% of the hair present in normal scalp is anagen hair. The catagen phase takes 2 to 3 weeks and the telogen phase may last a few months.

The color of normal hair depends on the amount and distribution of the melanin in the hair shaft (21). Normal human epidermal melanocytes may synthesize both eumelanin and pheomelanin (72). The melanins in black hair are eumelanin (characterized by the presence of ellipsoidal eumelanosomes), while those in red hair are mainly pheomelanin (ascribed to spherical pheomelanosomes) (72,73). Fewer melanosomes are produced in the bulbar melanocytes of blond hair. A relative absence of melanin and fewer melanosomes are seen in gray hair. Multiple internal or external regulatory factors are involved in hair pigmentation. There might be some correlation between tryptophan content and tyrosinase expression with hair color (74,75).

Another structure related to the pilar unit is the hair or pilar disk (the Haarscheibe). The Haarscheibe is a specialized spot in close vicinity to hairs. This structure is usually not recognized on routine histologic section. It may present as an acanthotic elevation of the epidermis, limited by two elongated rete ridges laterally (1). The epidermis in this area has more Merkel cells in the basal layer, and the dermal component is well vascularized, containing myelinized nerve fibers in contact with Merkel cells (21,63). It is considered as a highly sensitive, slowly adapting mechanoreceptor (1,76).

› **SEBACEOUS GLANDS** The sebaceous glands are holocrine glands associated with hair follicles. Their secretions are made up of disintegrated cells. The palms and soles are the only regions devoid of sebaceous glands. Sebaceous glands are prominent in facial skin. They are also seen in the buccal mucosa, vermilion of the lip (Fordyce spot), areola surrounding the nipple (Montgomery tubercles), prepuce, labia minora, and, at times, in the parotid gland.

The sebaceous glands are lobulated structures composed of multiple acini in some locations like the head and neck; in other sites, such as chest, they are composed of a single acinus. The periphery of the lobules contains the germinative cells, which are cuboidal and flat with large nucleoli and basophilic cytoplasms without lipid droplets. As differentiation occurs, several inner layers show lipid droplet accumulation in the cytoplasm until they fill the cell.

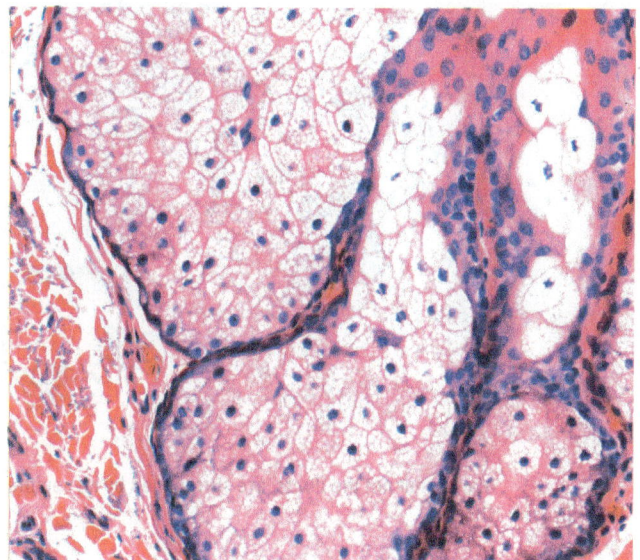

FIGURE 1.20 Sebaceous glands with peripheral germinative cells and, toward the center, the differentiated vacuolated cells.

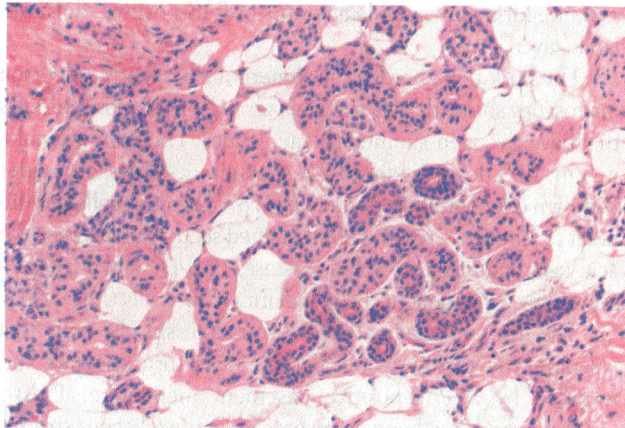

FIGURE 1.21 Eccrine lobule containing fat, glands, and ducts.

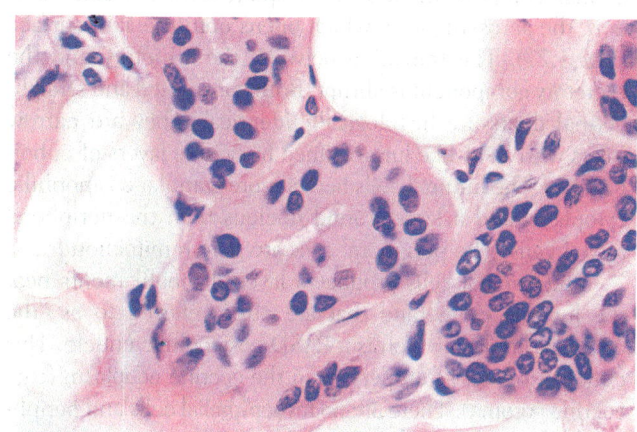

FIGURE 1.22 Clear cells of the eccrine glands.

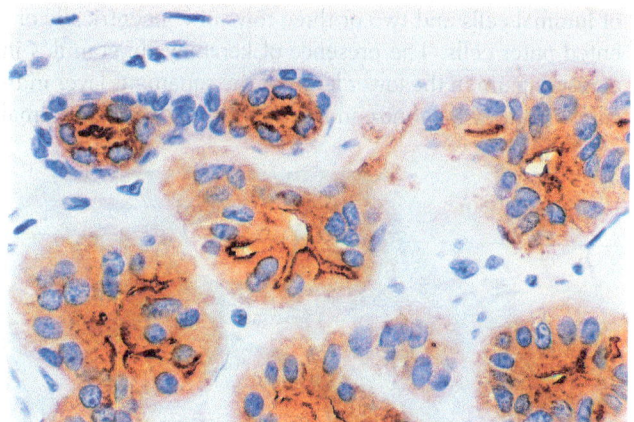

FIGURE 1.23 Intercellular canaliculi (anti-CEA).

The more differentiated cells (sebocytes) have a characteristic multivacuolated cytoplasm (Fig. 1.20). The nucleus is centrally located and scalloped due to the lipid imprints. The more differentiated cells disintegrate and discharge the cellular debris (sebum) into the excretory duct, which opens into the hair follicle in the lower portion of the infundibulum. The excretory duct is short, shared by several lobules, and lined by keratinized squamous epithelium.

Within sebaceous glands, the germinative cells express appreciable quantities of keratins. Mature sebocytes demonstrate cytoplasmic reactivity for high–molecular-weight keratins and epithelial membrane antigen with adipophilin showing membranous and vesicular reactivity of lipids.

› Eccrine Glands The eccrine glands are the true sweat glands responsible for thermoregulation. They are found in higher concentration in palms, soles, forehead, and axillae and have dual secretory and excretory functions.

The secretory portion of an eccrine gland is a convoluted tube located in the dermis, in the interface with the subcutaneous tissue, and rarely, within the subcutaneous tissue. In cross sections, it appears that several glandular structures with a central lumen form the secretory coils. These are seen as lobular structures often surrounded by fat even when located within the dermis (Fig. 1.21).

Three types of cells are identified in the eccrine coil: clear cells, dark cells, and myoepithelial cells. The clear cells are easily seen in H&E-stained sections (Fig. 1.22). They rest directly on the basement membrane and on the myoepithelial cells. Clear cells are composed of pale or finely granular cytoplasms with a round nucleus usually seen in the center of the cell. Deep invaginations of the luminal membranes of adjacent clear cells form intercellular canaliculi lined with microvilli (Fig. 1.23) (77). The intercellular canaliculi often persist in neoplasms derived from eccrine glands. The clear cells contain abundant mitochondria and variable amounts of PAS-positive, diastase-labile glycogen.

The dark cells border the lumen of the glands. Electron microscopy shows that they contain abundant secretory granules that have glycogen-staining characteristics. They contain sialomucin, PAS positive, diastase resistant mucopolysaccharides and high concentration of proteins (78). The dark cells are difficult to identify in routine H&E-stained sections. However, the acid-fast, Periodic acid-Schiff-diastase (PAS-D), and S100 protein stains will highlight the granularity of the cells (Fig. 1.24).

The myoepithelial cells are contractile spindle cells that surround the secretory coil (Fig. 1.25). In turn, they are surrounded by a PAS-positive basement membrane. Elastic fibers, fat, and small nerves are present in the adjacent stroma.

The excretory component of the eccrine gland is composed of three segments: (a) a convoluted duct in close association with the secretory unit (Fig. 1.26), (b) a straight dermal component, and (c) a spiral intraepidermal portion, the acrosyringium, which opens onto the skin surface (Fig. 1.27). The transition between the secretory and the excretory component is abrupt. Both convoluted and straight dermal ducts are histologically identical. They are narrow tubes with a slit-like lumina lined by double layers of cuboidal cells. The luminal cells have a more granular eosinophilic cytoplasm and a larger round nucleus than the peripheral row of cells. The peripheral cells are rich in mitochondria.

The luminal cells produce a layer of tonofilaments near the luminal membrane that are often referred to as "the cuticular border," which is a PASD eosinophilic cuticle. This cuticular border often persists in the eccrine neoplasm (e.g., eccrine poroma). There are no myoepithelial cells and peripheral hyalin basement membrane zone in the eccrine ducts.

The intraepidermal segment of the eccrine duct, known as acrosyringium, has a unique symmetrical and helicoidal course in the epidermis with its length correlated to the thickness of the epidermis (40). It consists of a single layer of luminal cells and two or three rows of concentrically oriented outer cells. The presence of keratohyalin granules in acrosyringium in the lower levels of the squamous layer indicates that they keratinize independently. The intraepidermal

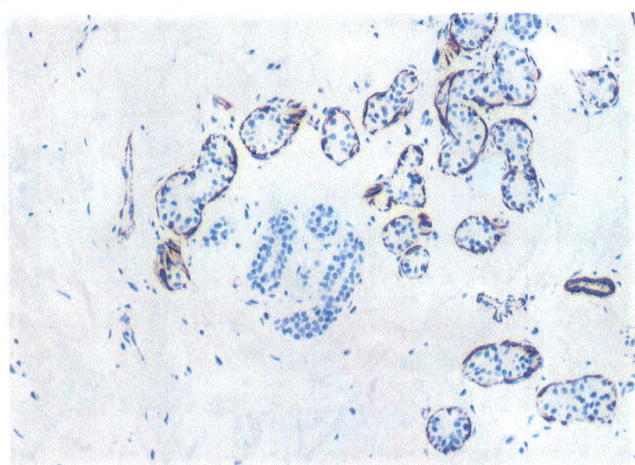

FIGURE 1.25 Glands, but not the ducts, are surrounded by myoepithelial cells (anti-HHF35).

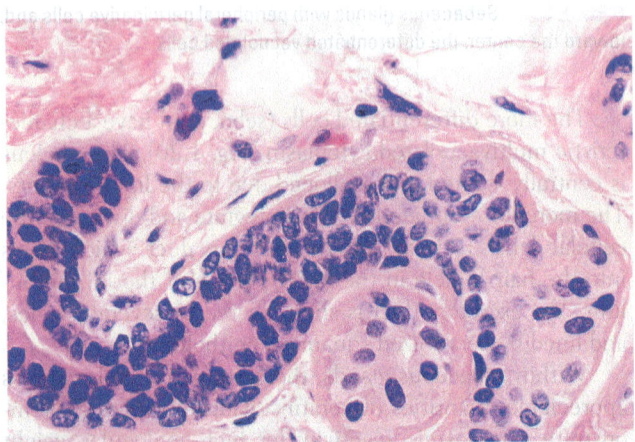

FIGURE 1.26 Eccrine duct. Note the abrupt transition from the secretory portion.

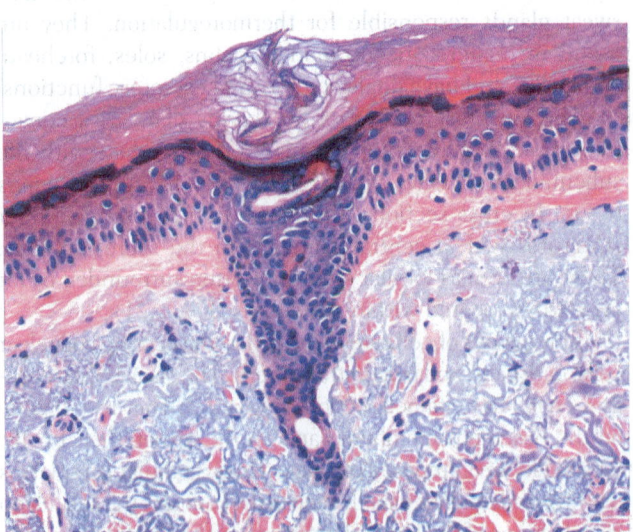

FIGURE 1.27 Acrosyringium.

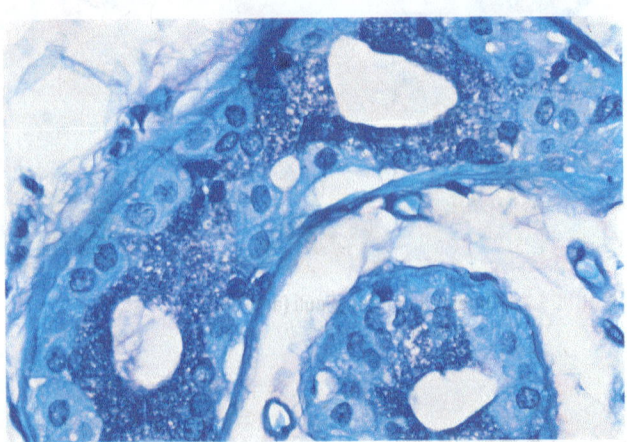

FIGURE 1.24 Dark cells with granular cytoplasm (acid-fast stain).

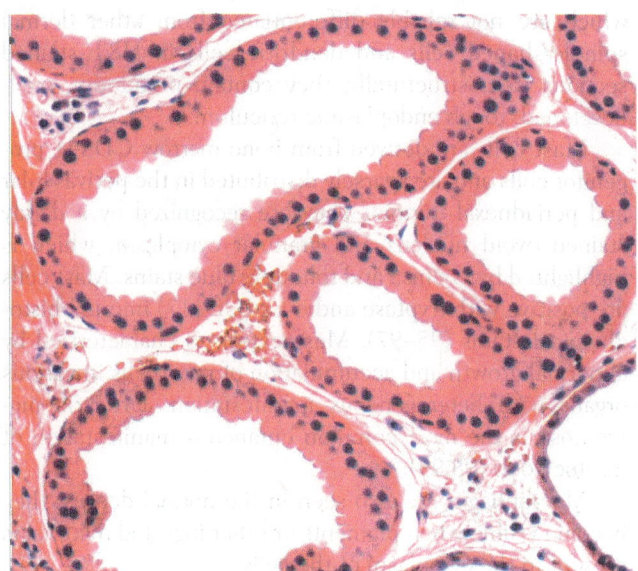

FIGURE 1.28 Secretory apocrine glands.

A third type of sweat gland, the so-called "apoeccrine glands" of the human axillae (80), is composed of a dilated secretory portion that, by electron microscopy, is indistinguishable from the apocrine glands; however, they retain the intercellular canaliculi, as well as the dark cells of the eccrine glands. The duct does not open in the hair follicle but in the epidermis. These glands, which develop from eccrine glands during puberty, account for as much as 45% of all axillary sweat glands in a young person. Recently, it was reported that the obstruction of intraepidermal apoeccrine sweat ducts by apoeccrine secretory cells might be the possible cause of Fox–Fordyce disease (81).

Dermis

The dermis is a dynamic, supportive connective tissue harboring cells, fibrous tissue, and ground substances with adnexal structures and vascular and nerve plexuses running through it (1). The dermis (Fig. 1.29) consists of two zones, the papillary and the reticular dermis. The adventitial dermis (82) combines the papillary and the periadnexal dermis.

The papillary and periadnexal dermis can be recognized by a loose meshwork of thin, poorly organized collagen composed of predominantly type III collagen (83–85) mixed with some type I collagen and a delicate branching network of fine elastic fibers. The papillary dermis also contains abundant ground substance, fibroblasts, and the capillaries of the superficial arterial and venous plexuses.

The reticular dermis is thicker than the papillary dermis and is composed of multiple layers of well-organized thick bundles of collagens, predominantly type I collagen, mostly arranged parallel to the surface. These layers are built from overlapping of individual fibers of uniform size. The plates are oriented randomly in different directions (86). There are also thick elastic fibers with fragmented appearance

lumen is lined by acellular eosinophilic cuticle before keratinization (3,21). Melanin granules are absent.

> **APOCRINE GLANDS** The apocrine gland (Fig. 1.28) has a coiled secretory portion and an excretory (ductal) component. The secretory portion is much longer than its eccrine counterpart; and it may reach 200 μm in diameter, compared with 20 μm for the eccrine glands. The secretory glands are located in the subcutaneous fat or in the deep dermis. They are lined by one layer of cuboidal, columnar, or flat cells (luminal cells), and an outer layer of myoepithelial cells, which is surrounded by a PAS-positive basement membrane. The luminal cells are composed of eosinophilic cytoplasm, which may contain lipid, iron, lipofuscin, PASD granules, and a large nucleus located near the base of the cell. Detached fragments of apical cytoplasm are found in the lumen of the glands. The secretion from apocrine glands releases secretory materials accompanied with loss of a part of cytoplasm (79), although other forms of secretion have been observed, including merocrine (granular contents within numerous vesicles are released without loss of cytoplasm) and holocrine type (the entire cell is secreted into the glandular lumen) (79).

Similar to the eccrine duct, the excretory (ductal) component of the apocrine gland has a double layer of cuboidal cells. Microvilli are identified on the surface of the luminal cells and keratin filaments are present in their cytoplasms, the latter giving the eosinophilic hyalin appearance to the inner lining of the duct. No myoepithelial cells and peripheral basement membrane are identified in the excretory duct. Apocrine glands are always connected to a pilosebaceous follicle. The intrafollicular or intraepidermal portion of the apocrine duct is straight other than the spiral as seen in acrosyringium.

Apocrine glands are mostly located in the axillary, anogenital areas, mammary region, eyelids (Moll glands), and external ear canal (ceruminous glands), and their presence is characteristic in nevus sebaceus of Jadassohn.

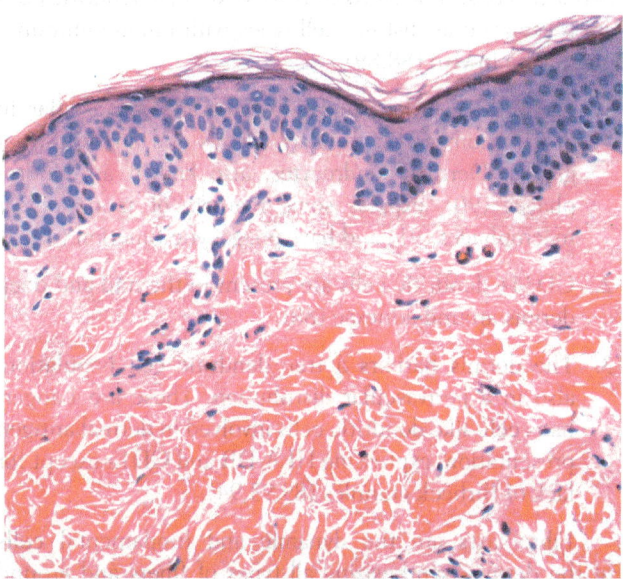

FIGURE 1.29 Papillary and reticular dermis.

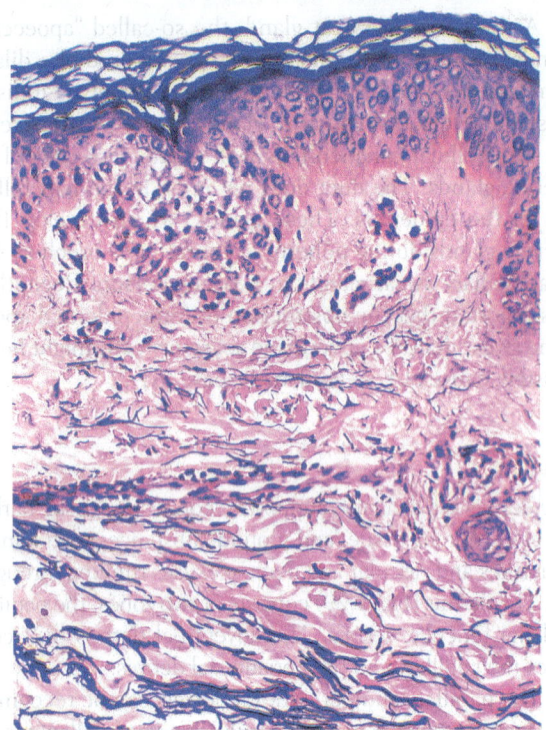

FIGURE 1.30 Distribution of elastic fibers. Elastic fibers are thin and branching in the papillary dermis and thick and fragmented in the reticular dermis.

detected by special elastic tissue stains (Fig. 1.30). Some ground substance and the vessels of the deep plexuses are also present in the reticular dermis.

The resident cells in the dermis mainly include dermal dendritic cells, fibroblasts, and mast cells. Dermal dendritic cells are a group of cells with immunophenotypic and functional heterogeneity located in the dermis and possessing a dendritic morphology (87). There are multiple subsets of dendritic cells. At least three types of dermal dendritic cells are recognized as distinct cell types with unique immunophenotype in vivo (88,89).

1. Factor XIIIa+ dermal dendrocytes are perivascular in distribution in the papillary dermis and around sweat glands. Dermal dendrocytes, also known as dendrophages (90), express some markers of mononuclear macrophages (91) and have phagocytic function (92).

2. CD34+ dendritic cells are present in the mid and deep dermis around adnexae (88).

3. The dermis harbors a true dendritic cell population, also in a perivascular distribution. These are Langerhans cell–like dendritic cells involved in dermal antigen presentation, expressing HLA-DR and CD1a except for lack of Birbeck granules (89,93,94).

Fibroblasts are the dynamic and fundamental cells of the dermis, synthesizing all types of fibers and ground substances. They appear as spindle-shaped or stellate cells, which are not reliably differentiated from other dermal spindle-shaped cells and dendritic cells in H&E-stained sections. Ultrastructurally, they contain prominent, well-developed, rough endoplasmic reticulum.

Mast cells are derived from bone marrow CD34+ progenitor cells and are sparsely distributed in the perivascular and periadnexal dermis. They are recognized by a darkly stained ovoid nucleus and granular cytoplasm, which is highlighted by Giemsa and toluidine blue stains. Mast cells are positive with tryptase and c-kit (CD117) immunohistochemical stains (95–97). Mastocytosis is characterized by abnormal growth and accumulation of mast cells in various organs with heterogeneous manifestation. Urticaria pigmentosa is the most common cutaneous manifestation of mastocytosis (98,99).

Macrophages are also seen in the normal dermis; they become visible when pigments or other ingested material is present in the cytoplasm of the cells.

Besides fibrous tissue and cellular components, the dermis also contains amorphous ground substance filling the spaces between fibers and dermal cells. It mainly consists of glycosaminoglycans or acid mucopolysaccharides (the nonsulfated acid mucopolysaccharides [predominantly hyaluronic acid] and, to a lesser degree, sulfated acid mucopolysaccharide [largely chondroitin sulfate]). The ground substance is present in small amounts and is seen as empty spaces between collagen bundles in routine H&E-stained sections; it is also easily identified with Alcian blue and toluidine blue special stains. In pathologic conditions, such as lupus erythematosus, granuloma annulare, and dermal mucinosis, the excessive quantity of ground substance produced can be seen without the aid of special stains as strings of bluish material.

Subcutaneous Tissue

Subcutaneous tissue, also called subcutis or hypodermis, is crucial in thermal regulation, insulation, provision of energy, and protection from mechanical injuries. It is composed of mature adipose tissue arranged into lobules. The mature adipocytes within the lobules are round cells rich in cytoplasmic lipids, which compress the nucleus to the side of the cell membrane. The adipocytes express S100 protein and vimentin in immunohistochemical stains. These lobules of mature adipocytes are separated by the thin bands of dermal connective tissue that constitute the interlobular septa (Fig. 1.31). Thus, inflammatory changes involving the subcutaneous tissue can be divided into septal panniculitis (e.g., erythema nodosum) and lobular panniculitis (e.g., panniculitis associated with pancreatitis).

Blood Vessels, Lymphatics, Nerves, and Muscle

The large arteries that supply the skin are located in the subcutaneous tissue, usually within the interlobular septa and are accompanied by large veins. Smaller arteries, venules,

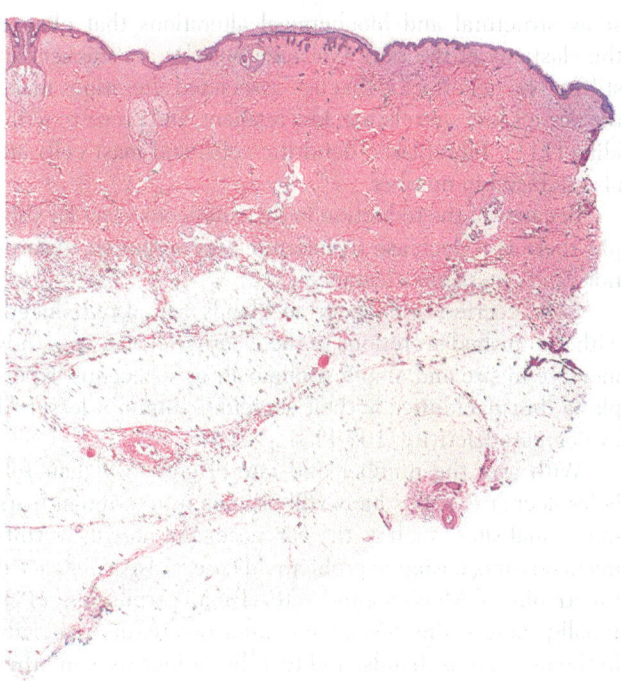

FIGURE 1.31 Septa and lobules of subcutaneous fat.

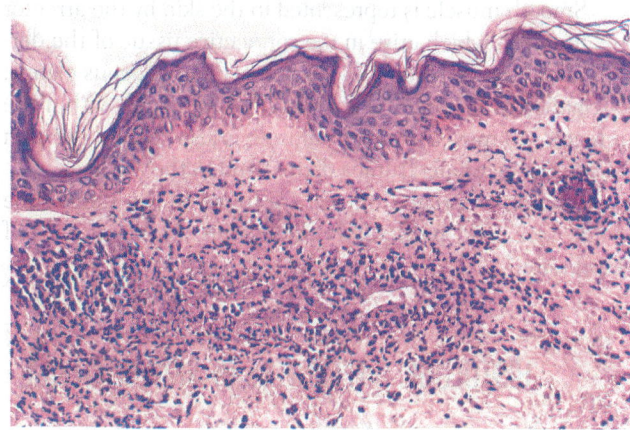

FIGURE 1.32 Vasculitis. Case of leukocytoclastic vasculitis showing damage to the capillary wall.

and capillaries constitute the main vasculature seen in the dermis and within the lobules of the subcutaneous fat.

A network of these smaller vessels is located in the papillary dermis (superficial plexus) and in the deep reticular dermis (deep plexus). Superficial vascular plexuses separate the papillary dermis from the reticular dermis, whereas the deep vascular plexuses define the boundary between the reticular dermis and subcutaneous tissue. The division of superficial and deep plexuses is important in the classification and recognition of many inflammatory diseases of the skin in which characteristic infiltrates are located around the superficial, deep, or superficial and deep plexuses.

Vasculitis is the inflammatory process that involves the blood vessels. It is important to remember that strict criteria are applied for the diagnosis of cutaneous vasculitis. They include (a) the presence of an inflammatory cell infiltrate within the vessel wall, and (b) the presence of vascular injury. Features of vascular injury range from edema, extravasation of erythrocytes, leukocytoclasis and thrombi in the lumina of the vessel to fibrinoid necrosis and/or destruction of the blood vessel wall (Fig. 1.32). However, it is important to note that fibrinoid necrosis of the vessel wall is essential for the diagnosis of true vasculitis. Perivascular inflammation alone is not a sign of vasculitis.

Mainly in the acral skin, special arteriovenous anastomosing structures known as glomera are present in the reticular dermis. Each glomus is composed of an arterial segment (the Sucquet–Hoyer canals) connected directly with venous segments. Each Sucquet–Hoyer canal is surrounded by four to six layers of glomus cells, which are considered as vascular smooth muscle cells serving as a sphincter. The glomera appear to be involved in thermal regulation.

The lymphatics of the skin (100) accompany the venules and are also located in the deep and superficial plexuses. Unless valves are seen within these vessels, their recognition in routine sections is impossible. Under normal conditions, they are surrounded by a cuff of elastic fibers.

Large nerve bundles are seen in the subcutaneous fat and in the deep reticular dermis; however, small nerve fibers are present throughout the skin, reaching the papillary dermis.

In sections of the palm and sole, some sensory nerves form nerve ending organs. Meissner corpuscles are seen in the papillary dermis, which is composed of several parallel layers of Schwann cells containing an axon; they function as rapid mechanical receptors for the sense of touch. In weight-bearing areas, the Vater–Pacini corpuscles consist of concentrically arranged Schwann cells with an axon and are located in the deep dermis and subcutaneous fat. They serve as receptors for sense of deep pressure and vibration (Fig. 1.33).

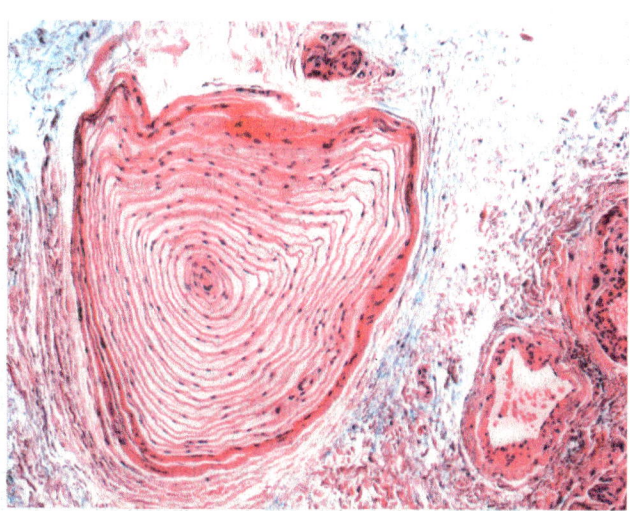

FIGURE 1.33 Vater–Pacini corpuscle.

Smooth muscle is represented in the skin by the arrector pili muscles, which arise in the connective tissue of the dermis and insert into hair follicles below the sebaceous glands. Melanocytes of congenital nevus are often seen within the arrector pili muscle. Smooth muscle is also seen in the skin of external genitalia (tunica dartos) and in the areolae.

Strands of striated muscle are found in the skin of the neck, face, and particularly the eyelids as the muscle of expression.

HISTOLOGIC DIFFERENCES OF SKIN WITH AGE

Newborns and Children

The epidermis of newborns and children is usually of the same thickness as in adults, with the exception of the acral skin. There is a greater density of melanocytes and Langerhans cells.

The dermis is more cellular than in the adult with a higher concentration of ground substance. The number of eccrine glands is higher at birth, while apocrine glands are not well developed until after puberty (101). The sebaceous glands are developed in children, but sebaceous secretion begins at puberty under the influence of androgen stimulation (102).

The adipocytes of the subcutaneous tissue in newborns and children are thin walled and larger than the adult adipocytes. In addition to white fat as seen in adults, infants possess brown fat, which initially comprises up to 5% of body weight, then diminishes with age and virtually disappears by adulthood. Brown adipocytes are rich in mitochondria and contain multiple lipid droplets of varying size in the cytoplasm with centrally located nuclei. Brown fat contains an abundance of blood-filled capillaries and is of particular importance in neonates because it has the ability to produce heat (thermogenesis) by degrading fat molecules into fatty acids (103,104).

Elderly

In the elderly, the histologic differences are mainly due to atrophy and reduction of most cutaneous elements (105,106). The cells of the epidermis are arranged haphazardly because of aberrant proliferation of the basal cell layer, which may predispose to the development of neoplasms (107). There is a marked decrease in the number of melanocytes and in the number of melanosomes, leading to reduced pigmentation (108,109) and, consequently, more exposure to the damaging effects of ultraviolet light. The Langerhans cells also decrease in number and function with advanced age, which increases the damaging effects of contactants and partially contributes to age-associated deterioration of immune function (110).

In the elderly, the dermis is thinned, relatively acellular, and avascular. The dermal collagen, elastin, and ground substance are altered and reduced (105,109). Elastic fibers show structural and biochemical alterations that change the elasticity of the skin. Collagen bundles are thicker but stiffer. The net effect is that age-associated alterations make the dermis less stretchable, less resilient, and prone to wrinkling (111). Fibroblasts, dendritic cells, and mast cells are also reduced in number.

Because of the reduction in the cutaneous vascular supply, there is a decrease in inflammatory response, absorption, and cutaneous clearance (112).

Both eccrine and apocrine glands are also reduced, with diminished secretions in the elderly. Sebaceous glands increase in size and manifest clinically as sebaceous hyperplasia, but paradoxically their secretory output is lessened by decreased activity (105,113).

With age, the number and rate of growth of hair follicles decrease, vellus hairs will develop into terminal hairs in unusual sites, such as the ear, nose, and nostrils, resulting in possible cosmetic problems. There is also a decreased functioning of Meissner and Vater–Pacini corpuscles (114). Finally, there is diminished subcutaneous tissue especially in the face, shins, hands, and feet, but it increases in other areas, particularly the abdomen in men and the thighs in women (105).

The pathologic hallmark of extrinsic aging is solar elastosis (Fig. 1.34), whereas wrinkling is due to the intrinsic factors mentioned previously (115).

HISTOLOGIC VARIATIONS ACCORDING TO ANATOMIC SITES

Regional variations of the normal histomorphology are important to recognize so as to avoid the misinterpretation of variation as abnormality.

The normal scalp and other dense hair–containing regions show hair follicles extending through the dermis

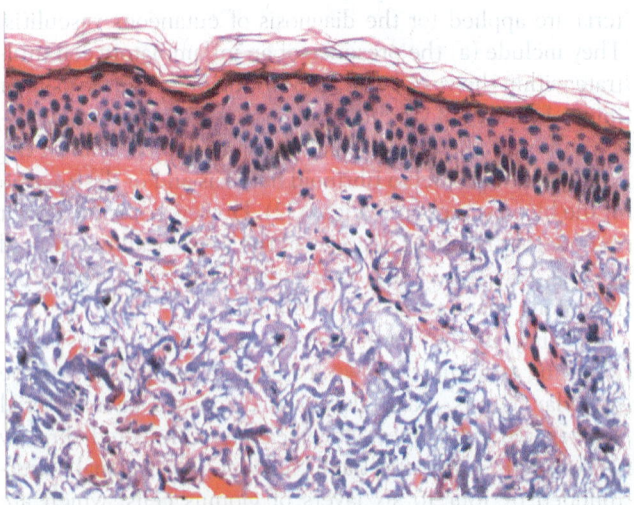

FIGURE 1.34 Solar elastosis in the dermis.

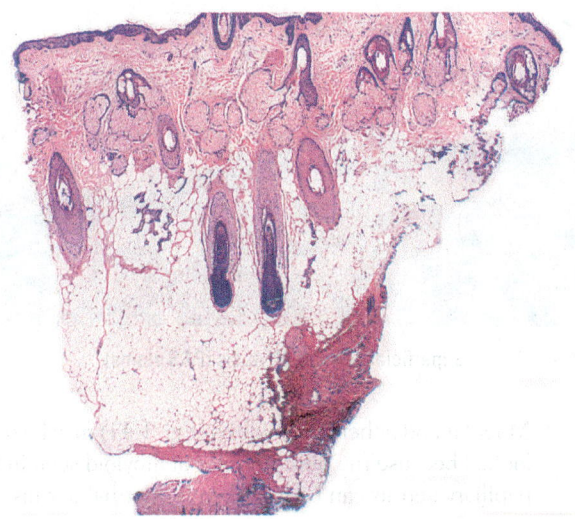

FIGURE 1.35 Section of scalp showing hair follicles extending into the subcutaneous tissue.

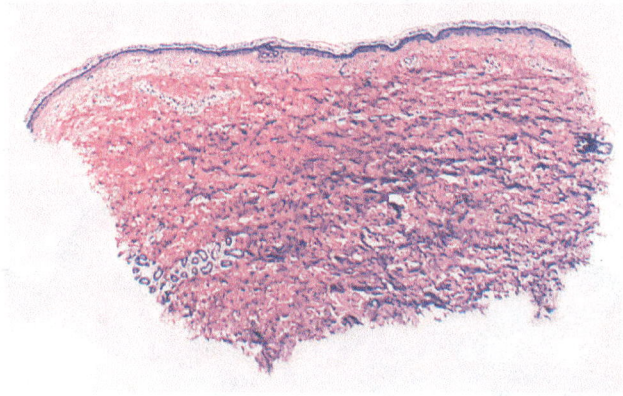

FIGURE 1.37 Section of skin of the back showing the normal reticular dermis.

into the subcutaneous fat (Fig. 1.35). This is usually not seen in areas with less concentration of hair. Abundant vellus hair is seen in sections taken from the skin of the ear. The skin of the face shows characteristically many pilosebaceous units (Fig. 1.36), and large sebaceous glands are seen on the nose.

The squamous layer of the eyelid epidermis is thin and composed of two to three layers of cells and basaloid epithelial buds. Modified apocrine glands (Moll glands) and vellus hairs are seen in the dermis.

Sections taken from the skin of the trunk, especially the back, show a normally thickened reticular dermis when compared with other sites (Fig. 1.37). Unawareness of this normal variation may lead to the erroneous diagnosis of processes producing thick collagen, such as scleroderma. The skin around the umbilicus also shows thick and fibrotic dermis (Fig. 1.38).

The palms and soles contain stratum lucidum and show a thick, compact cornified layer with loss of the characteristic basket-weave pattern (Fig. 1.39). In addition, there are numerous eccrine units, nerve end organs, and glomus structures seen in the dermis. There are no pilosebaceous units. Sections of the skin of the lower leg may show thicker blood vessels in the papillary dermis as a result of gravity and stasis (Fig. 1.40). Smooth muscle fibers are seen in the dermis of the skin of external genitalia and areola of the nipple. Cutaneous–mucosal junctions may lack granular and cornified layers, and cells of the squamous layers are larger, with higher glycogen content.

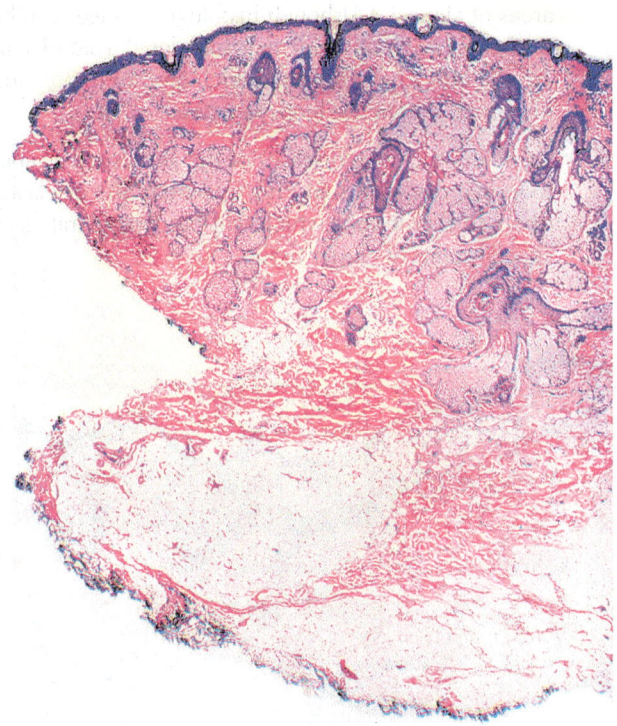

FIGURE 1.36 Skin of face with pilosebaceous units.

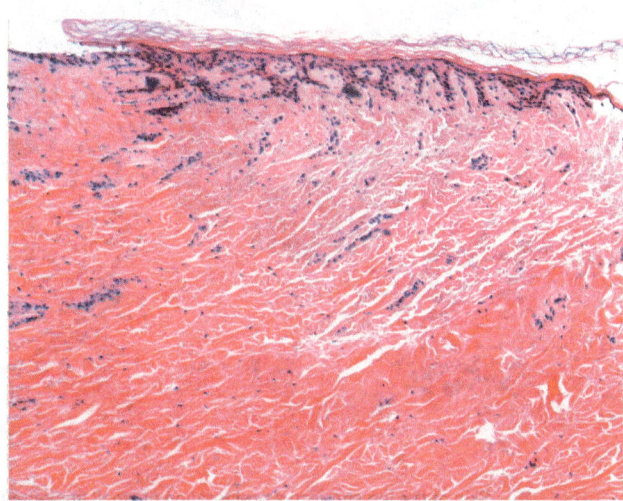

FIGURE 1.38 Umbilicus with dermal fibrosis.

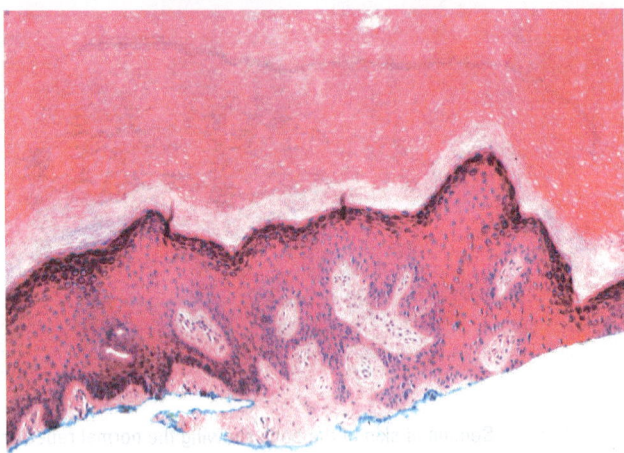

FIGURE 1.39 Histologic section of the palm with compact cornified layers and stratum lucidum.

PATHOLOGIC CHANGES FOUND IN BIOPSIES AND INTERPRETED AS "NORMAL SKIN"

Biopsies taken from clinically abnormal skin lesions may be interpreted histologically as normal because of the presence of subtle changes. The following are some examples.

- Dermatophytosis is seen in the cornified layer (Fig. 1.41) of an otherwise normal skin.
- A thick or absent granular layer may indicate an abnormal process of keratinization like psoriasis or an ichthyosiform dermatosis.
- Vitiligo (Figs. 1.42 and 1.43) may give the histologic impression of normal skin unless one searches for melanocytes and melanin.

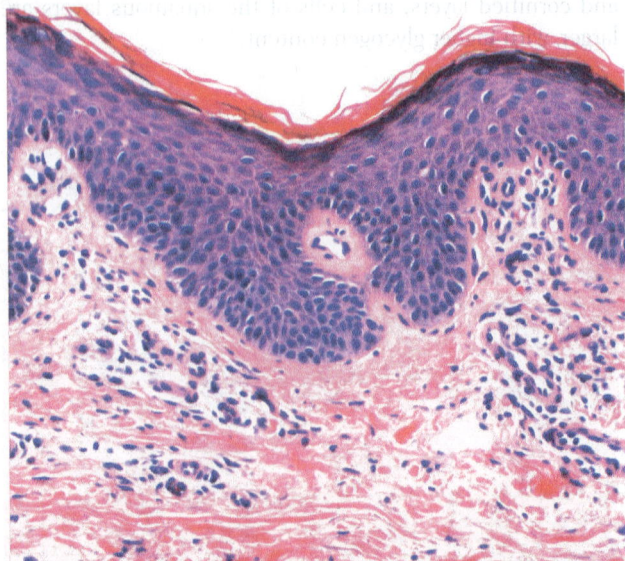

FIGURE 1.40 Skin of the leg showing a proliferation of small thickened blood vessels secondary to stasis.

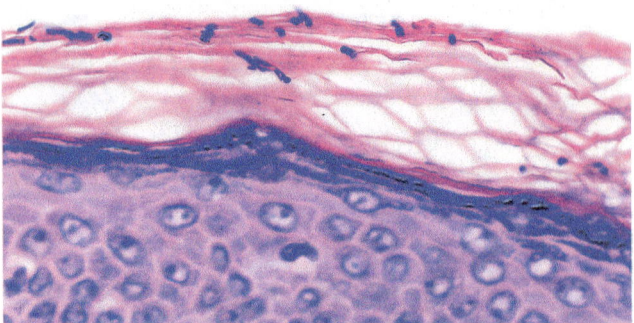

FIGURE 1.41 Superficial dermatophytosis (PAS stains).

- Macular and lichen amyloidosis (Fig. 1.44) may be overlooked because the pink globules of amyloid seen in the papillary dermis can be mistaken for normal dermis.
- Urticaria (Fig. 1.45) may produce only edema, which in routine sections is seen as separation of the collagen bundles in the dermis. Similar dermal changes are noted in the case of dermal mucinosis, in which deposition of mucinous material may be inconspicuous in routine sections. Special stains for mucin such as Alcian blue pH 2.5 or colloidal iron will be helpful.
- In telangiectasia macularis eruptive perstans, a subtype of cutaneous mastocytosis, the changes may be quite subtle and are composed of dilated blood vessels in the upper dermis with a scant infiltrate of mast cells. The infiltrate must be confirmed with appropriate stains for mast cells such as CD117.
- Trichotillomania is a hair-pulling habit resulting in areas of alopecia. Although histologic changes can be numerous (21), at times hair follicles devoid of hair are the only changes seen, which give an impression of normal skin in the biopsy material.
- Some degenerative diseases of the skin, such as anetoderma, can represent only as partial loss of elastic fibers in the dermis, which will be demonstrated by special stains of elastic tissue.

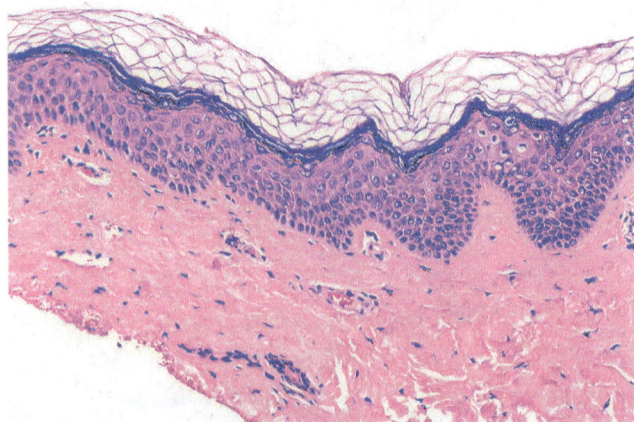

FIGURE 1.42 Vitiligo. Note the absence of basal melanocytes.

CHAPTER 1: Skin

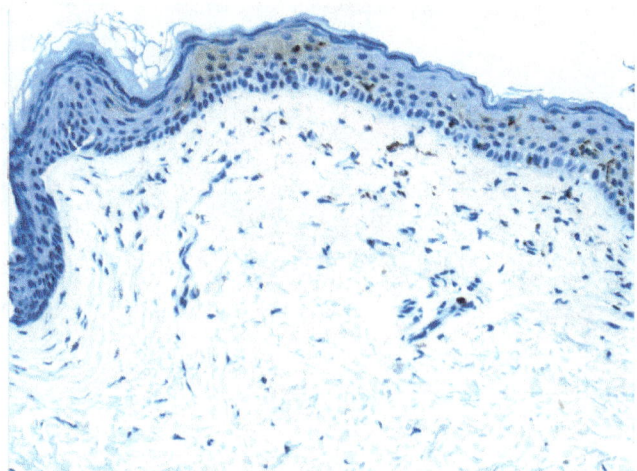

FIGURE 1.43 Vitiligo. S100 protein stains show the absence of basal melanocytes.

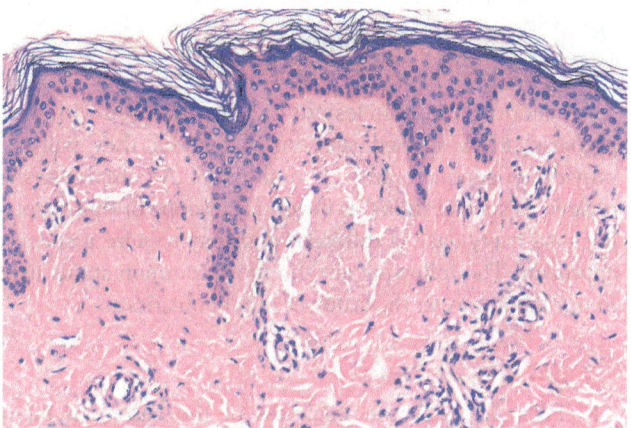

FIGURE 1.44 Lichen amyloidosis composed of pink globules in the papillary dermis.

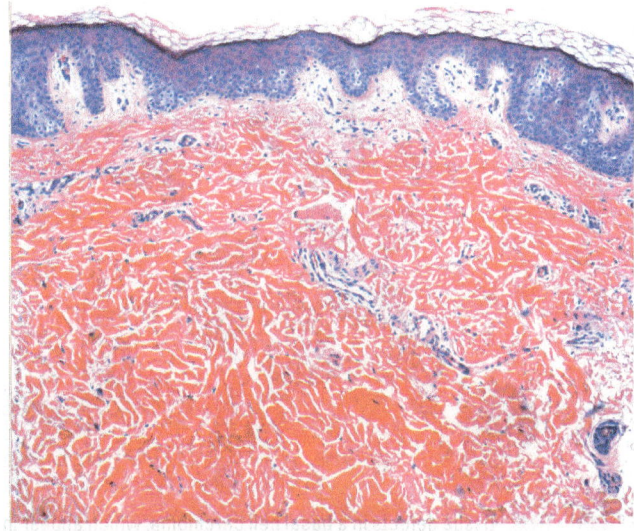

FIGURE 1.45 Urticaria shows only dermal edema.

- The so-called "connective tissue nevus" representing a hamartoma with an overproduction of collagen bundles and increased, normal, or decreased elastic tissue in the dermis is another condition that can be erroneously interpreted as normal skin.

Other conditions that might be missed as "normal skin" include café au lait spots, cutis laxa (elastolysis), myxoedema, scleromyxedema, and more. Therefore, the clinical information combined with careful histologic examination, sometimes special stains, or immunohistochemical studies of the biopsy material is crucial to avoid misinterpretation of skin disorders as normal tissue.

SPECIMEN HANDLING

Once the biopsy is done, the specimen should be placed in formalin fixative immediately for the purpose of routine histologic examination. Specimens needed for direct immunofluorescent study ideally should be placed in Michel medium or, alternatively, put in saline-moistened gauze if it is going to be processed within 24 hours. Specimens required for flow cytometry, molecular studies, and electron microscopy are sent fresh in saline-soaked gauze or in the appropriate transport media; they should be processed as soon as possible. If the specimens are excisional biopsies or larger surgical material, proper sharing of the specimen is done, always with consideration that histology has priority if no prior diagnosis exists for that particular patient.

Punch and shave biopsies are described grossly and either embedded intact or sectioned, depending on the size of the biopsy. Then the specimen is embedded on "edge" (vertical). Five levels are usually obtained for histologic examination.

Excisional biopsies and surgical specimens obtained for neoplasm are described grossly, and the entire deep and lateral margins of the specimen are inked before sectioning. The margins are evaluated by cutting along all margins or, most commonly, by entirely "bread loafing" the specimen (Fig. 1.46). The entire neoplasm is also evaluated using the bread-loafing technique.

ARTIFACTS

Poor histologic preparation as a result of artifacts will hamper the evaluation of slides by the pathologists. These artifacts can be the result of various factors.

1. Fixation problems such as poor or no fixation of the specimen before cutting, old solutions being used, insufficient fixation time, or inadequate volume of fixative (ideally, the specimen must be properly fixed in a solution 15 to 20 times the volume of the specimen) (116)

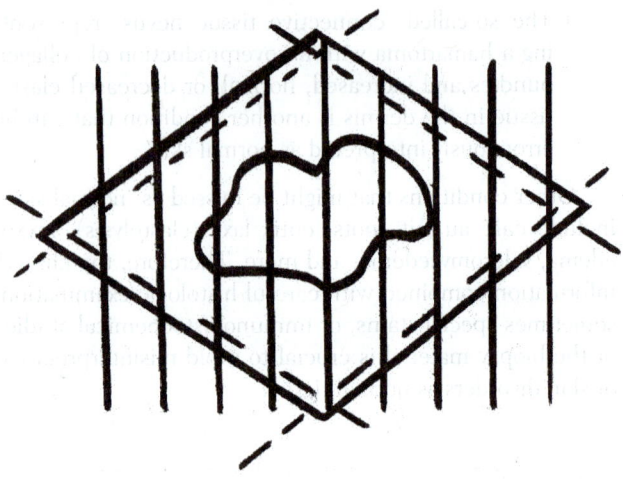

FIGURE 1.46 The entire neoplasm in the center of the lesion is examined by "bread loafing" the specimen; the deep margin is also evaluated. The lateral margins are included in each section submitted for histologic evaluation, or they can be submitted separately by cutting them along the depicted interrupted lines.

2. Improper monitoring of the multiple steps involved in the preparation of a slide, such as cutting, temperature of the water bath, freshness of the staining solutions employed, and other factors
3. Artifacts produced at the time of excision, such as cautery (Fig. 1.47) and excessive squeezing of the specimen
4. Specimens stored at low temperatures, giving freezing artifacts (Fig. 1.48)
5. Artifacts characteristically seen in certain pathologic processes, such as tissue holes in basal cell carcinoma (Fig. 1.49) and the lack of epidermis in sections from toxic epidermal necrolysis

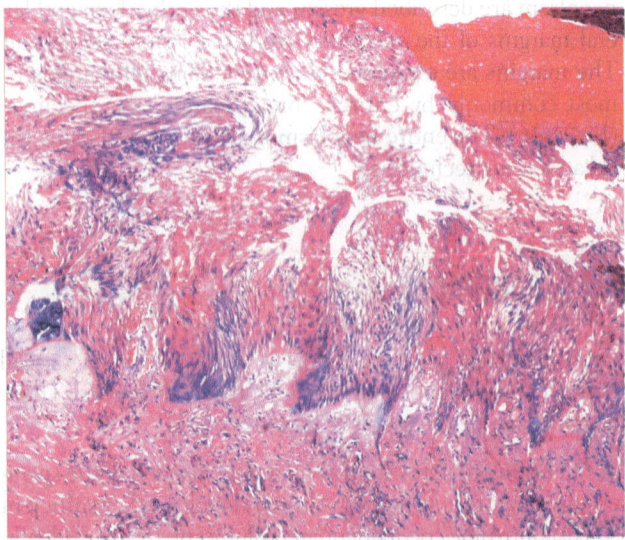

FIGURE 1.47 Cautery effect with vertical elongation of keratinocytes; such a sample is difficult to evaluate.

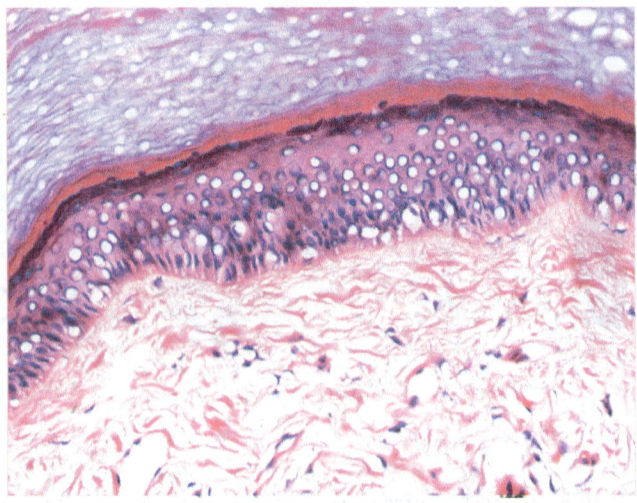

FIGURE 1.48 Freezing artifacts of a specimen with vacuolar changes in the epidermis.

STAINING METHODS

The majority of the skin lesions can be diagnosed with well-prepared H&E-stained sections. However, they will not provide an adequate answer in all cases. A comprehensive review of "special stains" is beyond the scope of this chapter because every case is different and may require a specific approach. The following are the most common stains used in our laboratory in the study of cutaneous tissue.

Histochemical Stains

1. PAS: To study the thickness of the basement membrane, for glycogen (diastase liable) and fungal organisms (diastase resistant)

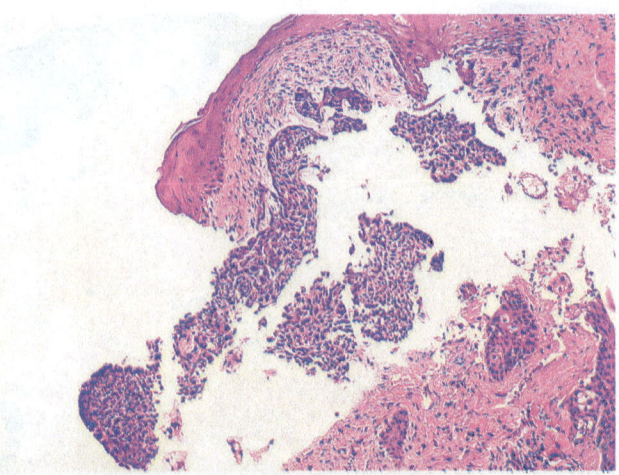

FIGURE 1.49 Tissue defects in a basal cell carcinoma, which appear in the spaces after multiple sections were performed.

2. Gomori methenamine silver (GMS): For fungal organisms and cutaneous *Pneumocystis carinii*
3. Ziehl–Neelsen and Fite stains: For acid-fast organisms
4. Gram stains: For bacteria
5. Steiner and Warthin–Starry stains: In cases of bacillary angiomatosis and for spirochetes, although the latter immunohistochemical method is preferred
6. Giemsa: For mast cells and protozoan organisms, such as *Leishmania*
7. Mucicarmine: For epithelial complex acid mucin as well as capsule of *Cryptococcus* fungus
8. Alcian blue: For acid mucopolysaccharides (pH 2.5), sulfated mucopolysaccharides (pH 1.0), and acid complex connective tissue mucin (pH 0.5)
9. Congo red: For amyloid
10. Elastic van Gieson (EVG): For elastic fibers
11. Fontana–Masson: For melanin
12. von Kossa: For calcium

Immunofluorescence

Immunofluorescence plays an important role in the diagnosis and evaluation of skin disorders such as lupus erythematosus, vasculitis, and autoimmune blistering diseases. Specimens are provided to the laboratory either immediately following biopsy on saline-soaked gauze or preferable in Michel transport medium. Michel transport medium is not a fixative, but a solution which stabilizes proteins for immunofluorescence. It is made up of citric acid, ammonium sulfate, N-ethylmaleimide, and magnesium sulfate and maintains at room temperature the isotonicity and pH of the tissue (7.0 to 7.2). Specimens that have been fixed in formalin are not able to be processed for immunofluorescent studies. Specimens that have been placed in Michel transport medium and then processed for routine H&E staining show a recognizable artifact in which there is a loss of nuclear detail. Immunofluorescent studies are either direct, using the patient's tissue, or indirect, using the serum of patients and a control tissue containing the relevant target molecules (human skin, monkey esophagus). Direct immunofluorescent studies are performed on cryostat sections of skin using fluorescein isothiocyanate (FITC)–conjugated antisera to immunoglobulins A, G, and M, as well as fibrinogen and complement (C3). Normal nonspecific staining includes autofluorescence of dermal components such as elastic fibers, internal elastic laminae surrounding small- to medium-sized arteries, and necrotic keratinocytes (colloid bodies). Basement membrane material may show weak autofluorescence with IgG and needs to be distinguished from true positive staining noted in disorders such as pemphigoid and lupus. Also many nonimmunobullous and nonautoimmune disorders such as actinic keratosis, rosacea, and polymorphous light eruption along with marked solar elastosis can show weak often discontinuous linear or granular staining that must be distinguished from true positive basement membrane deposition. In addition, nonspecific staining can be seen in serum crust, spongiotic epidermis, and linear zones surrounding blood vessels that have increased vascular permeability. These nonspecific staining patterns tend to involve all FITC-labeled immunoglobulins rather than specific disease-associated ones.

Immunohistochemical Stains/Molecular Studies

Immunohistochemistry is the process of detecting cellular and fibrillar antigens (e.g., proteins) in tissue section. The antigens may be cytoplasmic, membranous, or nuclear and show cellular events such as apoptosis or altered proliferation. Most commercially available antibodies can be used on formalin-fixed tissue. Most immunohistochemical studies utilize either a DAB detection kit ("brown stain") or an alkaline phosphatase detection kit ("red stain") (Fig. 1.50), the latter which is especially helpful in the diagnosis of pigmented melanocytic lesions (Figs. 1.51 and 1.52). Positive or negative reactivity of the antibodies tested often depends on variables such as quality and duration of fixation as well as the use of additional steps such as protease digestion and antigen retrieval.

Although a separate positive control slide is standard for each immunohistochemistry stain, this does not guarantee that the stain has worked properly for the patient's tissue. Interpretation of immunohistochemical studies relies on knowledge of normal skin components that can serve as internal positive controls (Table 1.1).

Immunohistochemistry is now widely used as an aid in the diagnosis of difficult cases where there is a defined differential. Examples include pigmented actinic keratosis and melanoma in situ (lentigo maligna), reactive and neoplastic T-cell infiltrates, benign cutaneous lymphoid hyperplasia

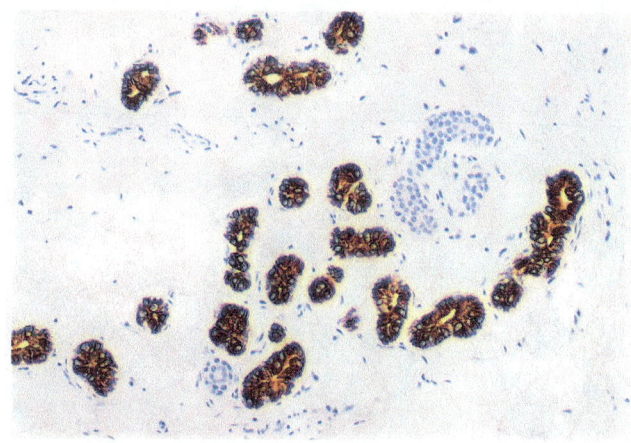

FIGURE 1.50 CAM5.2 immunostaining. The secretory glands but not the ducts are stained.

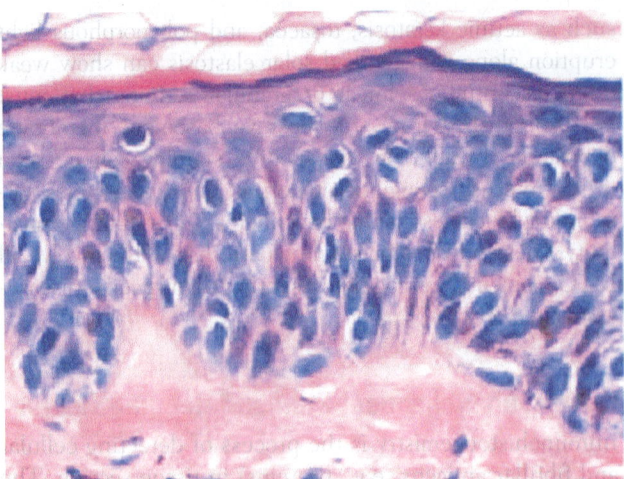

FIGURE 1.51 Normal melanocytes with brown melanin pigment. This coloration is identical to that of the diaminobenzidine chromogen often used with immunohistochemistry, making distinction of a positive immunostain versus background melanin difficult.

(pseudolymphoma) and B-cell lymphoid neoplasms, atypical melanocytic proliferations and melanoma, basal cell carcinoma and squamous cell carcinoma, intraepidermal pagetoid proliferations, and poorly differentiated epithelioid and spindle cell tumors. Some commonly used panels in our laboratory are shown in Tables 1.2 and 1.3.

There are numerous cytokeratins available ranging from cocktails of high–molecular-weight or low–molecular-weight cytokeratins to individual cytokeratins. High–molecular-weight cytokeratins 34βe12 and 5/6 are reactive with epidermal and follicular keratinocytes along with eccrine and apocrine sweat glands. As cytokeratin 5/6 is found primarily in mesothelium and other lining type epithelia such as epidermis and squamous mucosa, it is a particularly useful antibody in differentiating metastases from primary cutaneous tumors, either epidermal or adnexal (117). We have also found these cytokeratins to be helpful in the diagnosis/detection of poorly differentiated squamous cell and infiltrating/morpheaform basal cell carcinomas in fibrotic and inflamed dermis. Cytokeratin 20 is a heavy-weight cytokeratin which shows a specific perinuclear (Golgi) dot-like staining pattern in cutaneous neuroendocrine (Merkel cells) carcinomas. Cytokeratin 7 shows similar dot-like perinuclear reactivity with extracutaneous (metastatic) neuroendocrine carcinomas. Low–molecular-weight cytokeratins such as CAM5.2 and cytokeratin 7 are reactive with secretory glandular cells found in sebaceous apocrine and eccrine glands and are valuable in the diagnosis of Paget disease along with adnexal carcinomas (Fig. 1.50).

Other antibodies useful in the diagnosis of epithelial tumors include BerEp4, p63, p40, adipophilin, and FXIIIa (AC-1A1). BerEp4 is an epithelial antibody used in differentiating basal cell from squamous cell carcinomas, as well as aiding in differentiating microcystic adnexal carcinoma from basal cell carcinoma (118,119). p63 and p40 are proliferation antibodies, which show nuclear staining of many cutaneous malignancies. While both are particularly helpful in the diagnosis of spindle cell/sarcomatoid squamous cell carcinomas (120), p40 has been shown to be as sensitive as and more specific than p63 (121). Adipophilin is an antibody to a surface protein of intracellular lipid material. Membranous and cytoplasmic vesicular pattern staining of adipophilin has been reported as useful in differentiating sebaceous tumors, particularly intraepithelial sebaceous carcinomas from other pagetoid neoplasms. Of note, granular adipophilin staining is nonspecific and can be noted in pagetoid squamous cell carcinoma (122). FXIIIa (AC-1A1), a nuclear marker for sebaceous differentiation, has recently been reported as an even more sensitive and specific antibody for the differentiation of sebaceous neoplasms from squamous and other clear cell neoplasms (123).

Melanocytic antibodies include the highly sensitive S100 protein and SOX10 immunostain along with antibodies specific to melanocytes such as Melan-A/MART-1, HMB-45, and tyrosinase. Melan-A/MART-1 and tyrosinase are antibodies associated with pre-melanosomes and are present in both benign and malignant neoplasms. HMB-45 reactivity is limited to activated melanocytes and melanocytes with abundant melanin (blue nevus cells, type A nevus cells). This latter fact is utilized in differentiating atypical nonneoplastic dermal nevomelanocytic proliferations from melanoma. With the exception of a blue nevus, most nonneoplastic nevomelanocytic proliferations show an absence or loss of HMB-45 reactivity upon descent into the dermis. Conversely most melanomas show no loss of HMB-45 reactivity (124,125). Other antibodies useful in the diagnosis of malignant melanocytic lesions are the nuclear proliferation antibody Ki-67 (126) and p16 (127). Similar to HMB-45, benign nevomelanocytic lesions show a low to absent Ki-67 positivity while many melanocytic malignancies show an increased Ki-67 staining pattern (127). p16 is the opposite,

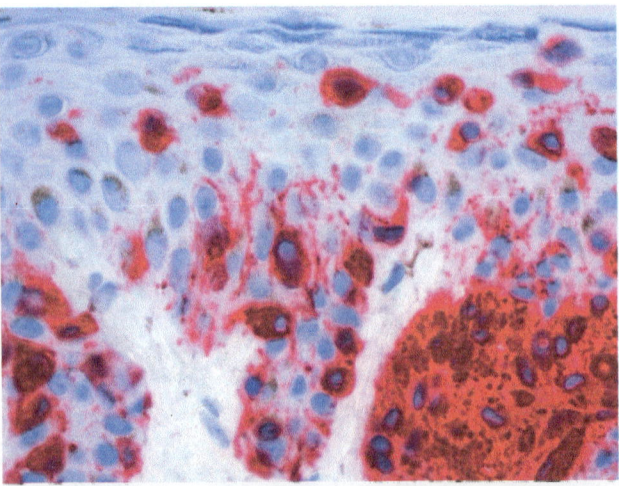

FIGURE 1.52 Proliferating melanocytes decorated with MART-1 and alkaline phosphate detection.

TABLE 1.1
Epithelial, Melanocytic, and Mesenchymal Antibodies

Epithelial Antibodies

Cytokeratins	AE1:AE3	Appendage and epidermal keratinocytes
	34βe12	Epidermal and follicular keratinocytes
	CAM5.2	Apocrine, eccrine, and sebaceous glands
	Cytokeratin 5/6	Lining epithelium of skin and squamous mucosa
	Cytokeratin 7	Apocrine, eccrine, and sebaceous glands
	Cytokeratin 19	Apocrine and eccrine glands
	Cytokeratin 20	Normal epidermal basal layer Merkel cells
p63		Basal and suprabasal epidermal keratinocytes, matrix and outer root sheath of hair follicles, sebaceous gland basal cells and myoepithelial cells of sweat glands
p40		Basal and suprabasal epidermal keratinocytes, matrix and outer root sheath of hair follicles, sebaceous gland basal cells and myoepithelial cells of sweat glands
EMA		Perineural cells, sometimes epidermis, sebocytes, luminal surfaces, and lateral borders of sweat glands
BerEp4		Matrical and outer root sheath follicular keratinocytes and apocrine/eccrine glands
CEA		Eccrine and apocrine gland luminal surfaces
Androgen receptor		Sebaceous glands
Adipophilin		Sebaceous glands, adipose tissue
FXIIIa (AC-1A1)		Nuclei of sebocytes

Melanocyte Antibodies

S100	Nevomelanocytes, nerves, adipose tissue, Langerhans cells, some dermal histiocytes/dendrocytes, and myoepithelial cells
SOX10	Schwann cells, melanocytes along with myoepithelial cells in breast and salivary gland tissue; normal mast cells also can be positive
Melan-A/MART-1	Nevomelanocytes
HMB-45	Activated melanocytes and pigmented melanocytes (blue nevus, type A nevus cells)
Tyrosinase	Nevomelanocytes
MITF	Nevomelanocytes, lymphocytes, smooth muscle cells, mast cells, fibroblasts, and Schwann cells

Mesenchymal Antibodies

Vascular endothelium	CD31	Vascular endothelium
	CD34	Vascular endothelium
	FVIII	Vascular endothelium and serum
	FLI-1	Vascular endothelium and small lymphocytes
	D2-40	Lymphatic endothelium
Muscle	SMA (alpha smooth muscle)	Myofibroblasts, smooth muscle
	HHF-35 (muscle common actin)	Myofibroblasts, smooth muscle
	Desmin	Smooth muscle
Neural/neuroendocrine	CD56	Small dermal nerves
	S100	Nevomelanocytes, nerves, adipose tissue, Langerhans cells, some dermal histiocytes/dendrocytes, and myoepithelial cells
	Cytokeratin 20	Merkel cells
	Chromogranin	Merkel cells and nerves and some cells in eccrine/apocrine glands
	Synaptophysin	Merkel cells, nerves, and some cells in eccrine/apocrine glands
Fibroblast	CD10	Fibroblast proliferation and follicular center lymphocytes
	CD34	Mesenchymal and dendritic interstitial cells in dermis and around nerves, vascular endothelium, hematopoietic stem cells
	FXIIIa	Dermal dendrocytes
CD117		Mast cells, immature Langerhans cells, basal layer keratinocytes, and melanocytes

EMA, epithelial membrane antigen; CEA, carcinoembryonic antigen; MITF, microphthalmia-associated transcription factor.

showing loss of staining in most malignant melanocytic lesions (128). However, of note is that not all melanomas show increased Ki-67 reactivity and/or loss of p16 reactivity and by themselves these findings are not diagnostic of malignancy (129,130).

Melanocytic antibodies are also useful in the diagnosis of atypical dermal spindle cell malignancies and atypical epidermal proliferations. Desmoplastic/spindle cell melanomas show variable reactivity with MART-1/Melan-A and are always negative for HMB-45. S100 and SOX10 are

TABLE 1.2 BCC versus SCC

	34βe12	EMA	BerEp4
Basal cell carcinoma	+	−	+
Squamous cell carcinoma	+	+	−

often the only melanocytic antibodies which are positive, with SOX10 showing greater sensitivity for spindle melanocytic proliferation than S100 (131). Of note, like S100, SOX10 is not specific for neural/melanocytic lesions, with positivity noted in both breast carcinomas and salivary gland lesions as well as mast cells (132). MART-1/Melan-A and other melanocytic immunostains are useful in differentiating pigmented atypical keratinocytic epidermal proliferation (pigmented actinic keratosis) from atypical junctional melanocytic proliferations (melanoma in situ/ lentigo maligna) (133).

Antibodies which are reactive with varied normal mesenchymal elements within the dermis and subcutis are useful when identifying their neoplastic counterparts. Vascular neoplasms, both benign and malignant, may be reactive with endothelial antibodies CD31, CD34, FVIII, FLI-1, and D2-40. Of these, CD31 is the most specific with FLI-1 showing more specificity for epithelioid angiosarcoma. FVIII often shows nonspecific staining of perivascular tissue, as it is associated with von Willebrand factor and is present not only in lining endothelial cells but in the surrounding extravascular plasma. CD34 is the least specific as it is also reactive with mesenchymal and dendritic interstitial cells in the dermis and around nerves. D2-40 is specifically reactive with lymphatic endothelium and can be used to confirm metastatic tumor within lymphatic vasculature. Although not reactive with any normal skin component, herpes virus type 8 (HHV8) antibody is useful in the diagnosis of Kaposi sarcoma (134). However, in some populations where this virus is endemic, it can be seen in non-Kaposi sarcoma vascular and fibroblastic proliferations (135). Smooth muscle antibodies, alpha smooth muscle actin (SMA), and HHF-35 (muscle common actin) are reactive with both vascular myoepithelium and arrector pili muscles with desmin limited to only smooth muscles. Fibrous tumors such as dermatofibroma and dermatofibrosarcoma protuberans may be differentiated with a combination of FXIIIa (dermatofibromas) and CD34 (dermatofibrosarcoma protuberans) (136). CD10 is a nonspecific antibody which in addition to reactivity with hematopoietic cells is also reactive with mesenchymal and dendritic interstitial cells in the dermis. Neural tumors show reactivity with S100 along with NKI/C3. In addition, S100 is positive with both cartilaginous and adipose tumors.

Hematologic antibodies are used to define both the cell type in an inflammatory infiltrate as well as whether the infiltrate is reactive or malignant. Lymphoid markers include all available CD antibodies for the characterization of T-cell and B-cell reactive and neoplastic proliferations. Histiocytic antibodies include CD68 and CD163 for non–Langerhans cell histiocytes and CD1a and S100 for Langerhans cells and tumors. CD117 is positive for mast cells as well as immature Langerhans cells, basal layer keratinocytes and melanocytes. Neuroendocrine cells are limited in normal skin to Merkel cells and eccrine sweat glands and can be demonstrated with chromogranin and synaptophysin. As mentioned above, Merkel cells are positive with cytokeratin 20. An immunohistochemical panel for the diagnosis of neuroendocrine tumors includes cytokeratin 7, cytokeratin 20, TTF-1, napsin, synaptophysin, and chromogranin.

Antibodies that demonstrate cell proliferation and apoptosis such as Ki-67 and p53 are valuable in differentiating actively proliferating malignancies and dysplasias from the histologic atypical appearing benign counterparts. Ki-67 is useful in the diagnosis of melanomas and follicular center lymphomas from atypical nevi and pseudolymphomas, respectively (137,138,139). Ki-67 in combination with p53 is also helpful in the diagnosis of keratinocytes dysplasia in sun-damaged skin (actinic keratosis and in situ squamous cell carcinoma) (140).

Immunostains and in situ hybridization have become valuable in diagnosing or confirming infectious agents within the skin. There are immunostain antibodies specific for herpes simplex virus (I and II), varicella-zoster virus, herpes virus type 8, Cytomegalovirus, spirochete, and *Mycobacterium*. Of note, the immunostain for spirochete while specific for *Treponema pallidum* does show cross reactivity with other spirochete organisms such as borreliosis (141). In situ hybridization is currently used for the diagnosis of high- and low-risk human papillomavirus (HPV) condyloma accuminata lesions (Fig. 1.53).

Recent molecular studies utilizing polymerase chain reaction (PCR) and fluorescent in situ hybridization (FISH) have been utilized to assist in differentiating true neoplastic lesion from reactive or non-neoplastic mimickers. PCR molecular biologic clonality studies in combination with immunohistochemical phenotyping have become useful in aiding the differentiation of reactive and neoplastic T-cell and B-cell proliferations. However, there are reports

TABLE 1.3 Intraepidermal Atypical Pagetoid Cells

	MART-1	34βe12	CK7	p63	CAM5.2
Pagetoid Bowen disease	−	+	−	+	−
Melanoma	+	−	−	+/−	−
Paget/extramammary Paget	−	+/−	+	−	+
Sebaceous carcinoma	−	+/−	+	+	+

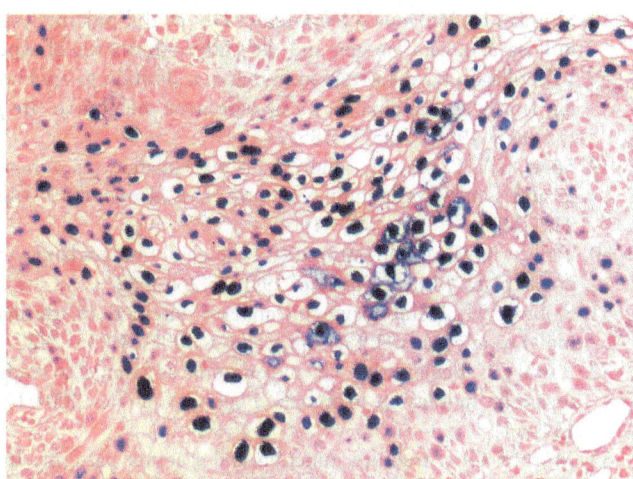

FIGURE 1.53 In situ hybridization with low-risk HPV 6 in a warty lesion.

of false-negative gene rearrangements (pseudoclonality). T-cell pseudoclonality can be seen in inflammatory dermatoses, such as lichen planus, pityriasis lichenoides, and lichen sclerosus along with histologic neoplastic mimickers such as lymphomatoid drug eruption and nickel contact dermatitis (142). B-cell pseudoclonality has been reported in some insect bite reactions and drug reactions (143).

FISH testing for DNA copy number abnormalities in chromosome regions associated with melanoma are utilized as an ancillary diagnostic test for differentiating benign melanocytic lesions from melanomas. The loci-tested RREB1 at 6p25 (gained in melanoma), MYB at 6q23 (gain or loss in melanoma), CEP6 (centromere 6), and CCND1 at 11q13 (gained in melanoma) have shown high sensitivity and specificity in this regard. Of note, 10% of metastatic melanomas are reported to show negative FISH results (144). Conversely, positive results have been reported in benign melanocytic lesions such as Spitz nevi and other borderline lesions due to some benign lesions showing polyploidy/tetraploidy (145,146).

REFERENCES

1. Kanitakis J. Anatomy, histology and immunohistochemistry of normal human skin. *Eur J Dermatol* 2002;12:390–399.
2. Montagna W, Parakkal PF. *The Structure and Function of the Skin*. 3rd ed. New York: Academic Press; 1974.
3. Montagna W, Freedberg IM, eds. Cutaneous biology 1950–1975. *J Invest Dermatol* 1976;67:1–230.
4. Murphy GF. Histology of the skin. In: Elder DE, Elenitsas R, Johnson BL Jr, Murphy GF, eds. *Lever's Histopathology of the Skin*. 9th ed. Philadelphia, PA: Lippincott Williams & Wilkins; 2005.
5. Visinoni AF, Lisboa-Costa T, Pagnan NA, et al. Ectodermal dysplasias: Clinical and molecular review. *Am J Med Genet A* 2009;149A(9):1980–2002.
6. Breathnach AS. Embryology of human skin. A review of ultrastructural studies. *J Invest Dermatol* 1971;57:133–143.
7. Holbrook KA, Odland GF. The fine structure of developing human epidermis: Light, scanning and transmission electron microscopy of the periderm. *J Invest Dermatol* 1975;65: 16–38.
8. Tamiolakis D, Papadopoulos N, Lambropoulou M, et al. Ber-H2 (CD30) Immunohistochemical staining of human fetal tissue. *Int J Biol Sci* 2005;1:135–140.
9. Hentula M, Peltonen J, Peltonen S. Expression profiles of cell-cell and cell-matrix junction proteins in developing human epidermis. *Arch Dermatol Res* 2001;293:259–267.
10. Smith LT, Sakai LY, Burgeson RE, et al. Ontogeny of structural component at the dermal–epidermal junction in human embryonic and fetal skin: The appearance of anchoring fibrils and type VII collagen. *J Invest Dermatol* 1988;90: 480–485.
11. Sagebiel RW, Rorsman H. Ultrastructural identification of melanocytes in early human embryos [abstract]. *J Invest Dermatol* 1970;54:96.
12. Foster CA, Holbrook KA, Farr AG. Ontogeny of Langerhans cells in human embryonic and fetal skin: Expression of HLA-DR and OKT-6 determinants. *J Invest Dermatol* 1986;86: 240–243.
13. Foster CA, Holbrook KA. Ontogeny of Langerhans cells in human embryonic and fetal skin: Cell densities and phenotypic expression relative to epidermal growth. *Am J Anat* 1989;184: 157–164.
14. Winkelmann RK, Breathnach AS. The Merkel cell. *J Invest Dermatol* 1973;60:2–15.
15. Moll R, Moll I, Franke WW. Identification of Merkel cells in human skin by specific cytokeratin antibodies: Changes of cell density and distribution in fetal and adult plantar epidermis. *Differentiation* 1984;28:136–154.
16. Moll I, Lane AT, Franke WW, et al. Intraepidermal formation of Merkel cells in xenografts of human fetal skin. *J Invest Dermatol* 1990;94:359–364.
17. Polakovicoca S, Seidenberg H, Mikusova R, et al. Merkel cell—review on developmental, functional and clinical aspects. *Bratisl Lek Listy (Abstract)* 2011;112:80–87.
18. Boot PM, Rowden G, Walsh N. The distribution of Merkel cells in human fetal and adult skin. *Am J Dermatopathol* 1992;14:391–396.
19. Breathnach AS. Development and differentiation of dermal cells in man. *J Invest Dermatol* 1978;71:2–8.
20. Smith LT, Holbrook KA, Madri JA. Collagen types I, III, and V in human embryonic and fetal skin. *Am J Anat* 1986;175: 507–521.
21. Mehregan AH, Hashimoto K, Mehregan DA, et al. Normal structure of the skin. In: Mehregan AH, Hashimoto K, Mehregan DA, Mehregan DR, eds. *Pinkus' Guide to Dermatohistopathology*. 6th ed. Norwalk, CT: Appleton & Lange; 1995.
22. Lavker RM, Sun TT, Oshima H, et al. Hair follicle stem cells. *J Investig Dermatol Symp Proc* 2003;8:28–38.
23. Matsuzaki T, Yoshizato K. Role of hair papilla on induction and regeneration processes of hair follicles. *Wound Repair Regen* 1998;6:524–530.
24. Downig DT, Stewart ME, Strauss JJ. Biology of sebaceous glands. In: Fitzpatrick TB, Eisen AZ, Wolff K, Freedberg IM, Austen KF, eds. *Dermatology in General Medicine. Vol 1*. 3rd ed. New York: McGraw-Hill; 1987:185–190.
25. Muller M, Jasmin JR, Monteil RA, et al. Embryology of the hair follicle. *Early Hum Dev* 1991;26:159–166.

26. Hashimoto K, Gross BG, Lever WF. The ultrastructure of the skin of human embryos. I. The intraepidermal eccrine sweat duct. *J Invest Dermatol* 1965;45:139–151.
27. Montagna W. Embryology and anatomy of the cutaneous adnexa. *J Cutan Pathol* 1984;11:350–351.
28. Hosoi J, Murphy GF, Egan CL, et al. Regulation of Langerhans cell function by nerves containing calcitonin gene-related peptide. *Nature* 1993;363:159–163.
29. Koster M. p63 in skin development and ectodermal dysplasias. *J Invest Dermatol* 2010;130:2352–2358.
30. Ishiko A, Matsunaga Y, Masunaga T, et al. Immunomolecular mapping of adherens junction and desmosomal components in normal human epidermis. *Exp Dermatol* 2003;12:747–754.
31. Wolff K, Schreiner E. Ultrastructural localization of pemphigus autoantibodies within the epidermis. *Nature* 1971;229:59–61.
32. Stanley JR, Klaus-Kovtun V, Sampaio SA. Antigenic specificity of fogo selvagem autoantibodies is similar to North American pemphigus foliaceus and distinct from pemphigus vulgaris autoantibodies. *J Invest Dermatol* 1986;87:197–201.
33. Val-Bernal JF, Diego C, Rodriquez-Villar D, et al. The nipple-areola complex epidermis: A prospective systematic study in adult autopsies. *Am J Dermatopathol* 2010;32:787–793.
34. Toker C. Clear cells of the nipple epidermis. *Cancer* 1970;25:601–610.
35. Willman JH, Golitz LE, Fitzpatrick JE. Clear cells of Toker in accessory nipples. *J Cutan Pathol* 2003;30:256–260.
36. Kumarasinghe SP, Chin GY, Kumarasinghe MP. Clear cell papulosis of the skin: A case report from Singapore. *Arch Pathol Lab Med* 2004;128:e149–e152.
37. Marucci G, Betts CM, Golouh R, et al. Toker cells are probably precursors of Paget cell carcinoma: A morphological and ultrastructural description. *Virchows Arch* 2002;441(2):117–123.
38. Kuo TT, Chan HL, Hsueh S. Clear cell papulosis of the skin. A new entity with histogenetic implications for cutaneous Paget's disease. *Am J Surg Pathol* 1987;11:827–834.
39. Tschen JA, McGavran MH, Kettler AH. Pagetoid dyskeratosis: A selective keratinocytic response. *J Am Acad Dermatol* 1988;19:891–894.
40. Kim YC, Mehregan DA, Bang D. Clear cell papulosis: An immunohistochemical study to determine histogenesis. *J Cutan Pathol* 2002;29:11–14.
41. Elias PM. Epidermal lipids, barrier function, and desquamation. *J Invest Dermatol* 1983;80(suppl):44s–49s.
42. Zirra AM. The functional significance of the skin's stratum lucidum. *Morphol Embryol (Bucur)* 1976;22:9–12.
43. Katz SI. The epidermal basement membrane zone—structure, ontogeny, and role in disease. *J Am Acad Dermatol* 1984;11:1025–1037.
44. Foidart JM, Bere EW Jr, Yaar M, et al. Distribution and immunoelectron microscopic localization of laminin, a noncollagenous basement membrane glycoprotein. *Lab Invest* 1980;42:336–342.
45. Smith JB, Taylor TB, Zone JJ. The site of blister formation in dermatitis herpetiformis is within the lamina lucida. *J Am Acad Dermatol* 1992;27:209–213.
46. Leblond CP, Inoue S. Structure, composition, and assembly of basement membrane. *Am J Anat* 1989;185:367–390.
47. Woodley DT, Burgeson RE, Lunstrum G, et al. Epidermolysis bullosa acquisita antigen is the globular carboxyl terminus of type VII procollagen. *J Clin Invest* 1988;81:683–687.
48. Shimizu H, McDonald JN, Gunner DB, et al. Epidermolysis bullosa acquisita antigen and the carboxy terminus of type VII collagen have a common immunolocalization to anchoring fibrils and lamina densa of basement membrane. *Br J Dermatol* 1990;122:577–585.
49. Scott GA, Cassidy L, Tran H, et al. Melanocytes adhere to and synthesize laminin-5 in vitro. *Exp Dermatol* 1999;8:212–221.
50. Tarnowski WM. Ultrastructure of the epidermal melanocyte dense plate. *J Invest Dermatol* 1970;55:265–268.
51. Seiberg M. Keratinocyte–melanocyte interactions during melanosome transfer. *Pigment Cell Res* 2001;14:236–242.
52. Barral DC, Seabra MC. The melanosome as a model to study organelle motility in mammals. *Pigment Cell Res* 2004;17:111–118.
53. Murphy GF. Structure, function and reaction patterns. In: Murphy GF, ed. *Dermatopathology*. Philadelphia, PA: WB Saunders; 1995.
54. Gown AM, Vogel AM, Hoak D, et al. Monoclonal antibodies specific for melanocytic tumors distinguish subpopulations of melanocytes. *Am J Pathol* 1986;123:195–203.
55. Kanitakis J. Immunohistochemistry of normal skin. In: Kanitakis J, Vassileva S, Woodley D, eds. *Diagnostic Immunohistochemistry of the Skin. An Illustrated Text*. London, UK: Chapman & Hall Medical; 1998:38–51.
56. Birbeck NS, Breathnach AS, Everall JD. An electron microscope study of basal melanocytes and high-level clear cells (Langerhans cells) in vitiligo. *J Invest Dermatol* 1961;37:51–64.
57. Niebauer G, Krawczyk W, Wilgram GF. The Langerhans cell organelle in Letterer Siwe's disease. *Arch Klin Exp Dermatol* 1970;239:125–137.
58. Halata Z, Grim M, Baumann KI. The Merkel cell: Morphology, developmental origin, function. *Cas Lek Cesk* 2003;142:4–9.
59. Halata Z, Grim M, Bauman KI. Friedrich Sigmund Merkel and his "Merkel cell," morphology, development, and physiology: Review and new results. *Anat Rec A Discov Mol Cell Evol Biol* 2003;271:225–239.
60. Tachibana T, Nawa T. Recent progress in studies on Merkel cell biology. *Anat Sci Int* 2002;77:26–33.
61. Santa Cruz DJ, Bauer EA. Merkel cells in the outer follicular sheath. *Ultrastruct Pathol* 1982;3:59–63.
62. Camisa C, Weissmann A. Friedrich Sigmund Merkel Part II. The cell. *Am J Dermatopathol* 1982;4:527–535.
63. Gu J, Polak JM, Van Noorden S, et al. Immunostaining of neuron-specific enolase as a diagnostic tool for Merkel cell tumors. *Cancer* 1983;52:1039–1043.
64. Leff EL, Brooks JS, Trojanowski JQ. Expression of neurofilament and neuron-specific enolase in small cell tumors of skin using immunohistochemistry. *Cancer* 1985;56:625–631.
65. Rosen ST, Gould VE, Salwen HR, et al. Establishment and characterization of a neuroendocrine skin carcinoma cell line. *Lab Invest* 1987;56:302–312.
66. van Muijen GN, Ruiter DJ, Warnaar SO. Intermediate filaments in Merkel cell tumors. *Hum Pathol* 1985;16:590–595.
67. Wang NP, Zee S, Zarbo RJ, et al. Coordinate expression of cytokeratins 7 and 20 defines unique subsets of carcinomas. *Appl Immunohistochem* 1995;3:99–107.
68. Moll I, Kuhn C, Moll R. Cytokeratin 20 is a general marker of cutaneous Merkel cells while certain neuronal proteins are absent. *J Invest Dermatol* 1995;104:910–915.

69. Headington JT. Transverse microscopic anatomy of the human scalp. A basis for a morphometric approach to disorders of the hair follicle. *Arch Dermatol* 1984;120:449–456.
70. de Viragh PA. The 'mantle hair of Pinkus.' A review on the occasion of its centennial. *Dermatology* 1995;191:82–87.
71. Alonso LC, Rosenfield RL. Molecular genetic and endocrine mechanisms of hair growth. *Horm Res* 2003;60:1–13.
72. Nakagawa H, Imokawa G. Characterization of melanogenesis in normal human epidermal melanocytes by chemical and ultrastructural analysis. *Pigment Cell Res* 1996;9:175–178.
73. Jimbow K, Ishida O, Ito S, et al. Combined chemical and electron microscopic studies of pheomelanosomes in human red hair. *J Invest Dermatol* 1983;81:506–511.
74. Biasiolo M, Bertazzo A, Costa CV, et al. Correlation between tryptophan and hair pigmentation in human hair. *Adv Exp Med Biol* 1999;467:653–657.
75. Burchill SA, Ito S, Thody AJ. Effects of melanocyte-stimulating hormone on tyrosinase expression and melanin synthesis in hair follicular melanocytes of the mouse. *J Endocrinol* 1993;137:189–195.
76. Smith KR Jr. The Haarscheibe. *J Invest Dermatol* 1977;69:68–74.
77. Baron DA, Briggman JV, Spicer SS. Tubulocisternal endoplasmic reticulum in human eccrine sweat glands. *Lab Invest* 1984;51:233–243.
78. Sbarbati A, Osculati A, Morroni M, et al. Electron spectroscopic imaging of secretory granules in human eccrine sweat glands. *Eur J Histochem* 1994;38:327–330.
79. Schaumburg-Lever G, Lever WF. Secretion from human apocrine glands: An electron microscopic study. *J Invest Dermatol* 1975;64:38–41.
80. Sato K, Leidal R, Sato F. Morphology and development of an apoeccrine sweat gland in human axillae. *Am J Physiol* 1987;252:R166–R180.
81. Kamada A, Saga K, Jimbow K. Apoeccrine sweat duct obstruction as a cause for Fox-Fordyce disease. *J Am Acad Dermatol* 2003;48:453–455.
82. Reed RJ, Ackerman AB. Pathology of the adventitial dermis. Anatomic observations and biologic speculations. *Hum Pathol* 1973;4:207–217.
83. Meigel WN, Gay S, Weber L. Dermal architecture and collagen type distribution. *Arch Dermatol Res* 1977;259:1–10.
84. Junqueira LC, Montes GS, Martins JE, et al. Dermal collagen distribution. A histochemical and ultrastructural study. *Histochemistry* 1983;79:397–403.
85. Sorrell JM, Caplan AI. Fibroblast heterogeneity: More than skin deep. *J Cell Sci* 2004;117(pt 5):667–675.
86. McNeal JE. Scleroderma and the structural basis of skin compliance. *Arch Dermatol* 1973;107:699–705.
87. Nestle FO, Nickoloff BJ. A fresh morphological and functional look at dermal dendritic cells. *J Cutan Pathol* 1995;22:385–393.
88. Narvaez D, Kanitakis J, Faure M, et al. Immunohistochemical study of CD34-positive dendritic cells of human dermis. *Am J Dermatopathol* 1996;18:283–288.
89. Kanitakis J. Immunohistochemistry of normal human skin. *Eur J Dermatol* 1998;8:539–547.
90. Nickoloff BJ, Griffiths CE. Not all spindled-shaped cells embedded in a collagenous stroma are fibroblasts: Recognition of the "collagen-associated dendrophage." *J Cutan Pathol* 1990;17:252–254.
91. Headington JT. The dermal dendrocyte. *Adv Dermatol* 1986;1:159–171.
92. Headington JT, Cerio R. Dendritic cells and the dermis: 1990. *Am J Dermatopathol* 1990;12:217–220.
93. Sepulveda-Merrill C, Mayall S, Hamblin AS, et al. Antigen-presenting capacity in normal human dermis is mainly subserved by CD1a+ cells. *Br J Dermatol* 1994;131:15–22.
94. Meunier L, Gonzalez-Ramos A, Cooper KD. Heterogeneous populations of class II MHC+ cells in human dermal cell suspensions. Identification of a small subset responsible for potent dermal antigen-presenting cell activity with features analogous to Langerhans cells. *J Immunol* 1993;151:4067–4080.
95. Walls AF, Jones DB, Williams JH, et al. Immunohistochemical identification of mast cells in formaldehyde-fixed tissue using monoclonal antibodies specific for tryptase. *J Pathol* 1990;162:119–126.
96. Arber DA, Tamayo R, Weiss LM. Paraffin section detection of the c-kit gene product (CD117) in human tissues: Value in the diagnosis of mast cell disorders. *Hum Pathol* 1998;29:498–504.
97. Longley BJ, Reguera MJ, Ma Y. Classes of c-KIT activating mutations: Proposed mechanisms of action and implications for disease classification and therapy. *Leuk Res* 2001;25:571–576.
98. Metcalfe DD, Akin C. Mastocytosis: Molecular mechanisms and clinical disease heterogeneity. *Leuk Res* 2001;25:577–582.
99. Valent P, Horny HP, Escribano L, et al. Diagnostic criteria and classification of mastocytosis: A consensus proposal. *Leuk Res* 2001;25:603–625.
100. Ryan TJ, Mortimer PS, Jones RL. Lymphatics of the skin. Neglected but important. *Int J Dermatol* 1986;25:411–419.
101. Johnson BL, Honig PJ, Jaworsky C, eds. *Pediatric Dermatopathology*. Newton, MA: Butterworth-Heinemann; 1994.
102. Pochi PE, Strauss JS, Downing DT. Age-related changes in sebaceous gland activity. *J Invest Dermatol* 1979;73:108–111.
103. Klaus S. Functional differentiation of white and brown adipocytes. *Bioessays* 1997;19:215–223.
104. Klaus S. Adipose tissue as a regulator of energy balance. *Curr Drug Targets* 2004;5:241–250.
105. Fenske NA, Lober CW. Structural and functional changes of normal aging skin. *J Am Acad Dermatol* 1986;15(pt 1):571–585.
106. Smith L. Histopathologic characteristics and ultrastructure of aging skin. *Cutis* 1989;43:414–424.
107. Patterson JAK. Structural and physiologic changes in the skin with age. In: Patterson JAK, ed. *Aging and Clinical Practice: Skin Disorders, Diagnosis and Treatment*. New York: Igaku-Shoin; 1989.
108. Kurban RS, Bhawan J. Histologic changes in skin associated with aging. *J Dermatol Surg Oncol* 1990;16:908–914.
109. Montagna W, Carlisle K. Structural changes in ageing skin. *Br J Dermatol* 1990;122(suppl 35):61–70.
110. Sauder DN. Effect of age on epidermal immune function. *Dermatol Clin* 1986;4:447–454.
111. Lavker RM, Zheng PS, Dong G. Morphology of aged skin. *Clin Geriatr Med* 1989;5:53–67.
112. Balin AK, Pratt LA. Physiological consequences of human skin aging. *Cutis* 1989;43:431–436.
113. Bolognia JL. Aging skin. *Am J Med* 1995;98:99S–103S.
114. Cerimele D, Celleno L, Serri F. Physiological changes in ageing skin. *Br J Dermatol* 1990;122(suppl 35):13–20.

115. Rongioletti F, Rebora A. Fibroelastolytic patterns of intrinsic skin aging: Pseudoxanthoma-elasticum-like papillary dermal elastolysis and white fibrous papulosis of the neck. *Dermatology* 1995;191:19–24.
116. Mondragon G, Nygaard F. Routine and special procedures for processing biopsy specimens of lesions suspected to be malignant melanomas. *Am J Dermatopathol* 1981;3:265–272.
117. Plumb SJ, Argenyi ZB, Stone MS, et al. Cytokeratin 5/6 immunostaining in cutaneous adnexal neoplasms and metastatic adenocarcinoma. *Am J Dermatopathol* 2004;26(6):447–451.
118. Tellechea O, Reis JP, Domingues JC, et al. Monoclonal antibody Ber EP4 distinguishes basal-cell carcinoma from squamous-cell carcinoma of the skin. *Am J Dermatopathol* 1993;15(5):452–455.
119. Krahl D, Sellheyer K. Monoclonal antibody Ber-EP4 reliably discriminates between microcystic adnexal carcinoma and basal cell carcinoma. *J Cutan Pathol* 2007;34(10):782–787.
120. Dotto JE, Glusac EJ. p63 is a useful marker for cutaneous spindle cell squamous cell carcinoma. *J Cutan Pathol* 2006;33(6):413–417.
121. Alomari AK, Glusac EJ, McNiff JM. P40 is a more specific marker than p63 for cutaneous poorly differentiated squamous cell carcinoma. *J Cutan Pathol* 2014;41(11):839–845.
122. Ostler DA, Prieto VG, Reed JA, et al. Adipophilin expression in sebaceous tumors and other cutaneous lesions with clear cell histology: an immunohistochemical study of 117 cases. *Mod Pathol* 2010;23(4):567–573.
123. Tjarks BJ, Pownell BR, Evans C, et al. Evaluation and comparison of staining patterns of factor XIIIa (AC-1A1), adipophilin and GATA3 in sebaceous neoplasia. *J Cutan Pathol* 2018;45:1–7.
124. Schaumburg-Lever G, Metzler G, Kaiserling E. Ultrastructural localization of HMB-45 binding site. *J Cutan Pathol* 1991;18(6):432–435.
125. Magro CM, Crowson AN, Mihm MC Jr. Unusual variants of malignant melanoma. *Mod Pathol* 2006;19:S41–S70.
126. Soyer HP. Ki 67 immunostaining in melanocytic skin tumors. Correlation with histologic parameters. *J Cutan Pathol* 1991;18(4):264–272.
127. Nasr MR, El-Zammar O. Comparison of pHH3, Ki-67, and survivin immunoreactivity in benign and malignant melanocytic lesions. *Am J Dermatopathol* 2008;39(2):117–122.
128. Al Dhaybi R, Agoumi M, Gagné I, et al. A marker of differentiation between childhood malignant melanomas and Spitz nevi. *J Am Acad Dermatol* 2011;64(2):357–363.
129. Blokhin E, Pulitzer M, Busam KJ. Immunohistochemical expression of P16 in desmoplastic melanoma. *J Cutan Pathol* 2013;40(9):796–800.
130. Mason A, Wititsuwannakul J, Klump VR, et al. Expression of p16 along does not differentiate between Spitz nevi and Spitzoid melanomas. *J Cutan Pathol* 2012;39(12):1062–1074.
131. Karamchandani JR, Nielsen TO, van de Rijn M, et al. Sox10 and S100 in the diagnosis of soft-tissue neoplasms. *Appl Immunohistochem Mol Morphol* 2012;20(5):445–450.
132. Miettinen M, McCue PA, Sarlomo-Rikala M, et al. Sox10 – A marker for not only Schwannian and melanocytic neoplasms but also myoepithelial cell tumors of soft tissue. A systematic analysis of 5134 tumors. *Am J of Surg Pathol* 2015;39(6):826–835.
133. Helm K, Findeis-Hosey J. Immunohistochemistry of pigmented actinic keratoses, actinic keratoses, melanomas in situ and solar lentigines with Melan-A. *J Cutan Pathol* 2008;35:931–934.
134. Pantanowitz L, Pinkus GS, Dezube BJ, et al. HHV8 is not limited to Kaposi's sarcoma. *Mod Pathol* 2005;18:1148–1150.
135. Patel RM, Goldblum JR, Hsi ED. Immunohistochemical detection of human herpes virus-8 latent nuclear antigen-1 is useful in the diagnosis of Kaposi sarcoma. *Mod Pathol* 2004;17:456–460.
136. Altman DA, Nickoloff BJ, Fivenson DP. Differential expression of factor XIIIa and CD34 in cutaneous mesenchymal tumors. *J Cutan Pathol* 1993;20:154–158.
137. Scholzen T, Gerdes J. The Ki-67 protein: From the known and the unknown. *J Cell Physiol* 2000;182:311–322.
138. Li LX, Crotty KA, McCarthy SW, et al. A zonal comparison of MIB1-Ki67 immunoreactivity in benign and malignant melanocytic lesions. *Am J Dermatopathol* 2000;22:489–495.
139. Abdelsayed RA, Guijarro-Rojas M, Ibrahim NA, et al. Immunohistochemical evaluation of basal cell carcinoma and trichoepithelioma using Bcl-2, Ki67, PCNA and P53. *J Cutan Pathol* 2000;27:169–175.
140. Talghini S, Halimi M, Baybordi H. Expression of P27, Ki67 and P53 in squamous cell carcinoma, actinic keratosis and Bowen disease. *Pak J Biol Sci* 2009;12(12):929–933.
141. Pavlidskey P, Seminario-Vidal L, McKay KM. Spirochete immunostaining is not just for syphilis: diagnostic utility in borreliosis. *J Cutan Pathol* 2015;42:370–372.
142. Alessi E, Coggi A, Venegoni L, et al. The usefulness of clonality for the detection of cases clinically and/or histopathologically not recognized as cutaneous T-cell lymphoma. *Br J Dermatol* 2005;153:368–371.
143. Boer A, Tirumalae R, Bresch M, et al. Pseudoclonality in cutaneous pseudolymphomas: a pitfall in interpretation of rearrangement studies. *Br J Dermatol* 2008;159:394–402.
144. Hindi Z, Sidiropouos M, Al Habeeb A, et al. Fluorescence in situ hybridization (FISH) copy number abnormalities at 6p (REBI), 6q (MYB) and 11q (CCND1) reliably distinguish metastatic versus benign melanocytic lesions. *J Dermatol Res Ther* 2016;2:017.
145. Gerami P, Li G, Pouryazdanparast P, et al. A highly specific and discriminatory FISH assay for distinguishing between benign and malignant melanocytic neoplasms. *Am J Surg Pathol* 2012;36:808–817.
146. North JP, Garrido MC, Kolaitis NA, et al. Fluorescence in situ hybridization as an ancillary tool in the diagnosis of ambiguous melanocytic neoplasms: a review of 804 cases. *Am J Surg Pathol* 2014;38:824–831.

Nail

Julian Conejo-Mir ■ Javier Dominguez-Cruz ■ Mercedes Sendín-Martín

HISTORY 31	Merkel Cells 51
EMBRYOLOGY 32	Melanocytes 51
GENETIC AND NAIL KERATINS 34	Immunology and Inflammatory Cells 53
GROSS ANATOMY 37	ULTRASTRUCTURAL ANATOMY 53
MICROSCOPIC ANATOMY 39	CONFOCAL MICROSCOPY OF NAIL 55
The Nail Plate 39	OTHER TISSUES OF THE NAIL UNIT 56
Proximal Nail Fold 40	Dermis 56
Matrix 41	Bone 58
Nail Bed 43	Blood Supply 58
Hyponychium 45	NAIL GROWTH 59
Lateral Nail Folds 45	HANDLING AND PROCESSING OF THE NAIL 61
IMMUNOHISTOCHEMISTRY OF THE NAIL UNIT 46	REFERENCES 61
Nail Plate 46	
Keratinocytes 46	

Fingernails are an important epithelial miniorgan system of the hand, with a complex anatomical structure well described in the last decades. They are important in certain animals for the prehension and capture of prey. In primates and humans, the nail has two different functions: as a protective plate and enhances sensation of the fingertip. The protection function of the fingernail is commonly known, but the sensation function is equally important. The fingertip has many nerve endings in it allowing us to receive volumes of information about objects we touch. The nail acts as a counterforce to the fingertip providing even more sensory input when an object is touched.

Although most pathologic specimens from the nail show well-known changes such as psoriasis, lichen planus, and the characteristic malignant tumors, a broad spectrum of other changes may be found. For the pathologist, knowledge of the normal histology and its more common variations is important in establishing a correct diagnosis. Unfortunately, much of the literature on the nail can be troublesome and confusing because a great profusion of names and concepts exists and has changed over the years; also, many newer concepts of the embryology, physiology, genetic, immunohistochemistry, and nail growth mechanism find their way slowly into textbooks. In particular, this chapter can provide a great service to the general pathologist and dermatopathologist by being aware of the anatomy and unique histology, even when performing micrographic Mohs surgery on the nail area.

This chapter emphasizes those observations and theories related to clinical pathology.

HISTORY

Historical interest can be traced to the works of Galen in the second-century BC when he noticed the nail's resemblance to hair structure. However, the real study of the nail begins at the end of the 19th century, mostly by Germans like Zander (1), Kolliker (2), and Unna (3). The first studies dealt with embryology and anatomy and their comparison to birds and primates (1,4,5). After the initial spark of interest, the nail literature was enriched by many authors, both on the embryology and the anatomy of the human nail (6,7). Due to the technical shortcomings of their time, the authors interpreted the nail plate as formed entirely by the matrix cells and concluded that other adjacent structures did not contribute in the formation of the plate.

During the 1950s, Lewis (8) challenged this view and published his idea of the "nail unit," consisting of a dorsal, intermediate, and ventral nail, with differentiation based on the use of a silver-proteinate stain. In 1963, Zaias (9) extended the concept of the "nail unit," including the proximal nail fold (PNF), the matrix, the nail bed, and the hyponychium, all of which contribute to the formation of the nail. During the last 25 years, most studies on the nail have fundamentally tried to explain its biochemistry and physiology, with emphasis on analyzing nail growth; also considered were ultrastructure and, most recently, the immunohistochemistry of the nail.

Difficult biopsy access, as well as the complicated orientation and specimen handling, with the resulting difficulties of interpretation, are the main reasons why there are few histologic and histopathologic studies on the nail (10).

EMBRYOLOGY

Whereas the embryonic development of the fetal skin has been divided into eight stages, using scanning electron microscopy (11), the embryonic development of the nail shows only five stages (12,13): (a) plate phase; (b) fibrillar phase; (c) granular phase; (d) squamous phase; and (e) definitive nail phase or end phase (Table 2.1).

TABLE 2.1

Comparison of the Different Stages of Nail Development With the Epidermis of the Embryo Using Scanning Electron Microscopy

Nail Unit[a]	Embryonic/Fetal Skin[b]	Development
Plaque phase	Indifferent epithelium phase Flattened surface phase Elevated surface phase	7–10 weeks
Fibrilar phase	Incipient bleb formation phase	2.5–3 months
Granular phase	Single bleb formation phase	3–4 months
Squamous phase	Complex bleb formation phase	4–5 months
Definitive nail phase	Cornification phase	Up to 5 months

[a]Suchard R. Des modifications des cellules de la matrice et du lit de l'ongle dans quelques cas pathologiques. *Arch Physiol (Paris)* 1882;2:44–45.
[b]Holbrook KA, Odland GF. The fine structure of the developing human epidermis: light, scanning, and transmission electron microscopy of the periderm. *J Invest Dermatol* 1975;65:16–38.

The earliest recognizable fingers are seen in 42- to 45-day-old embryos (16-mm crown rump), while the toes lag somewhat and are seen at 52 to 54 days of age (18.5 mm) (14).

Studies using optical microscopy showed that the ungual morphogenesis begins at the embryonic age of 10 weeks, with a smooth, shiny quadrangular surface delineated by continuous shallow grooves. This surface of the phalanx is the "primary nail base" of Zander (1) or "primary nail field" of Zaias (9), delimited proximally by a transversal groove: the proximal nail groove. Studies performed using scanning electron microscopy showed that the formation of the nail begins very early, at the embryonic age of 7 weeks, with an accumulation of strongly active cells, abundant mitosis, and cellular damage, followed by necrosis, with the presence of T lymphocytes in the primary nail base (Fig. 2.1). This phenomenon, named apoptosis, occurs in all the epidermal accumulated cells following a transversal band in the dorsal area of the distal third of the fingers. Apoptosis of these epidermal cells is the most important step in the nail's development because it permits an immediate epidermal invagination identical to the one in the hair follicle except for one difference; in the hair follicle, the process starts at the age of 2.5 to 3 months. We observed apoptosis in nail development in this first phase only. Yet, the two processes are so identical that, sometimes, the layers of the nail have been compared with those of the hair follicle. The result is the formation of a transversal groove, which subsequently becomes the PNF.

An interesting feature of the first stage is the excessive size of the primitive nail plate (2.5 to 3 months), nearly occupying the total distal third part of the finger. This plate stays attached to its surroundings through some periungual-fixing filaments (Fig. 2.2). At the age of 11 weeks, all the folds are already formed, both the proximal and lateral nail folds. The transversal distal fold, corresponding to the hyponychium, is completely keratinized at the age of 3.5 months (Fig. 2.3). Afterward, the epidermal cells of the nail field suffer a process of keratin formation, different from the rest of the embryo. The result is a keratinized structure, covering the whole nail bed from the age of 14 weeks on, sometimes confused by some authors with a false nail (Fig. 2.4) (8,9). The production of the true nail plate starts from the matrix cells, located in the proximal nail groove and the most proximal portion of the nail bed. Its presence in the proximal fold is visible from the fifth month of intrauterine life on, the histochemical confirmation of its formation being the presence of sulfhydryl radicals (15).

The nail unit at this stage shows grooves form by invaginations of primitive ectoderm in regions that will become nail folds. These grooves delimit rectangular areas at distal aspects of the dorsa of fingers and toes where nail plates will be situated subsequently. These areas are covered by primitive epithelium, that approximately at the 14th week of intrauterine life (Fig. 2.5) appears composed of a basal layer of primitive germinative cells, three or four layers of primitive keratinocytes with clear or pale cytoplasm,

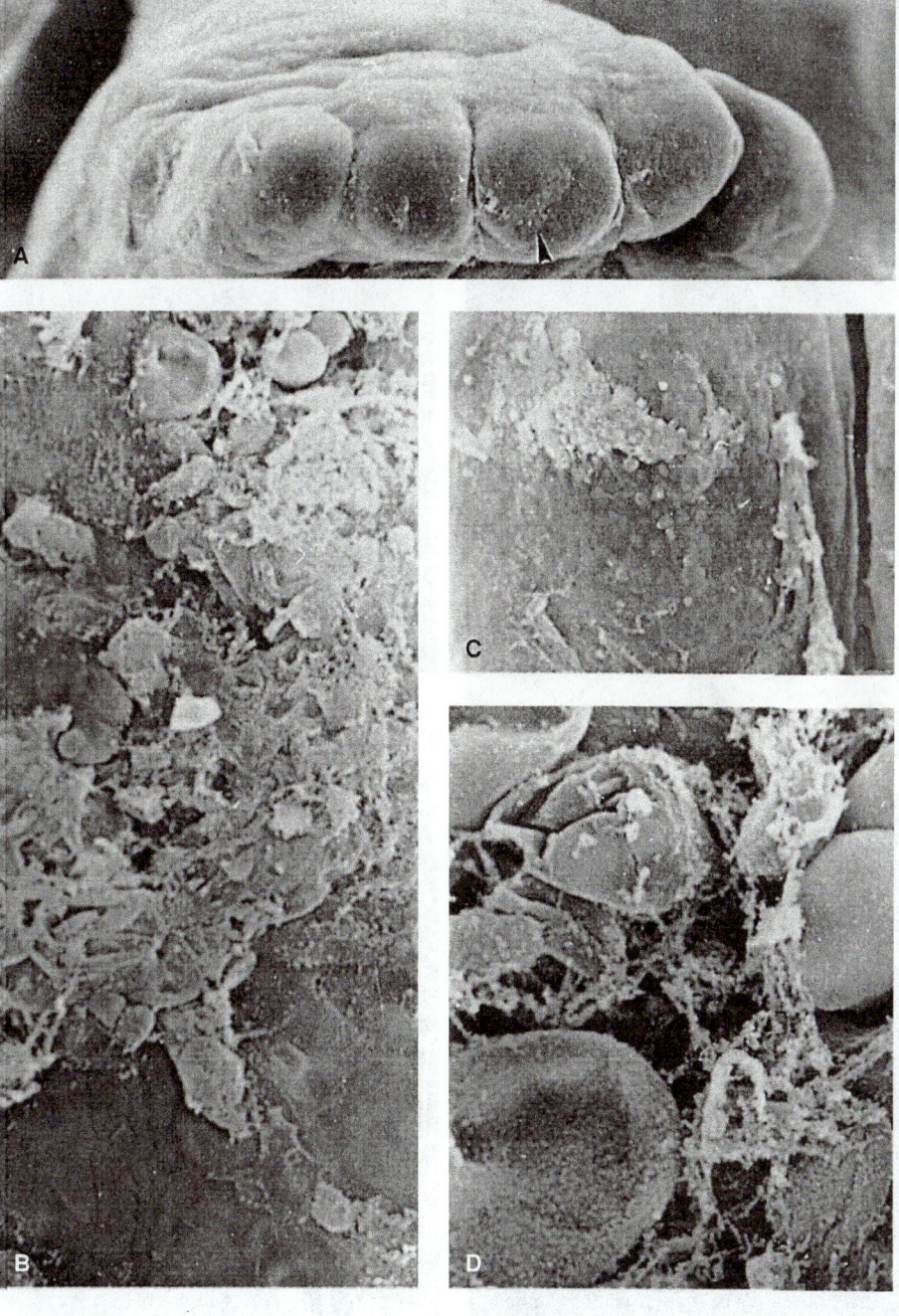

FIGURE 2.1 Development of the human nail exhibited through scanning electron microscopy (13). Plaque phase: Foot of a 7-week-old human embryo. The fingers are already defined but have no interphalangeal folds (**A**, ×50). On the third toe, you can see distally poorly structured material accumulated (*arrow* in **A**, ×50) that corresponds to apoptotic cells, which limits the future proximal nail fold (**B**, ×500; **C**, ×100). Close-up view of the apoptotic cells: Amorphous extracellular material appears with numerous vesicles of keratohyalin which are different phases of their evolution (**D**, ×1,500).

and a thin and eosinophilic acellular layer at the surface. This primitive epithelium covering the dorsum of a distal phalanx develops two clusters of epithelial cells at their proximal and distal ends. The proximal bud of primitive epithelial basaloid cells proliferates backward and downward, descending at an angle into the subjacent primitive mesenchymal tissue. The superficial part of this wedge of epithelial cells will become the PNF and the deeper part will eventuate in the dorsal and intermediate nail matrices. At the junction between the superficial and deeper parts, there is a crease of cornified cells that will be the cuticle of the fully developed nail. At this stage of development, the primitive mesenchymal tissue underlying the future nail is a highly cellular tissue with abundant ground substance. At this time, the future distal phalanx is represented by primitive cartilaginous tissue with the earliest evidences of focal calcification. Distally, the primitive epithelium forms another cluster of cells with a distal ridge that will become the hyponychium.

From the fifth month on, the definitive nail plate starts to grow in a distal sense until it reaches the hyponychium at the time of birth. The growth mechanism of the definitive nail is discussed later in the section entitled "Nail Growth."

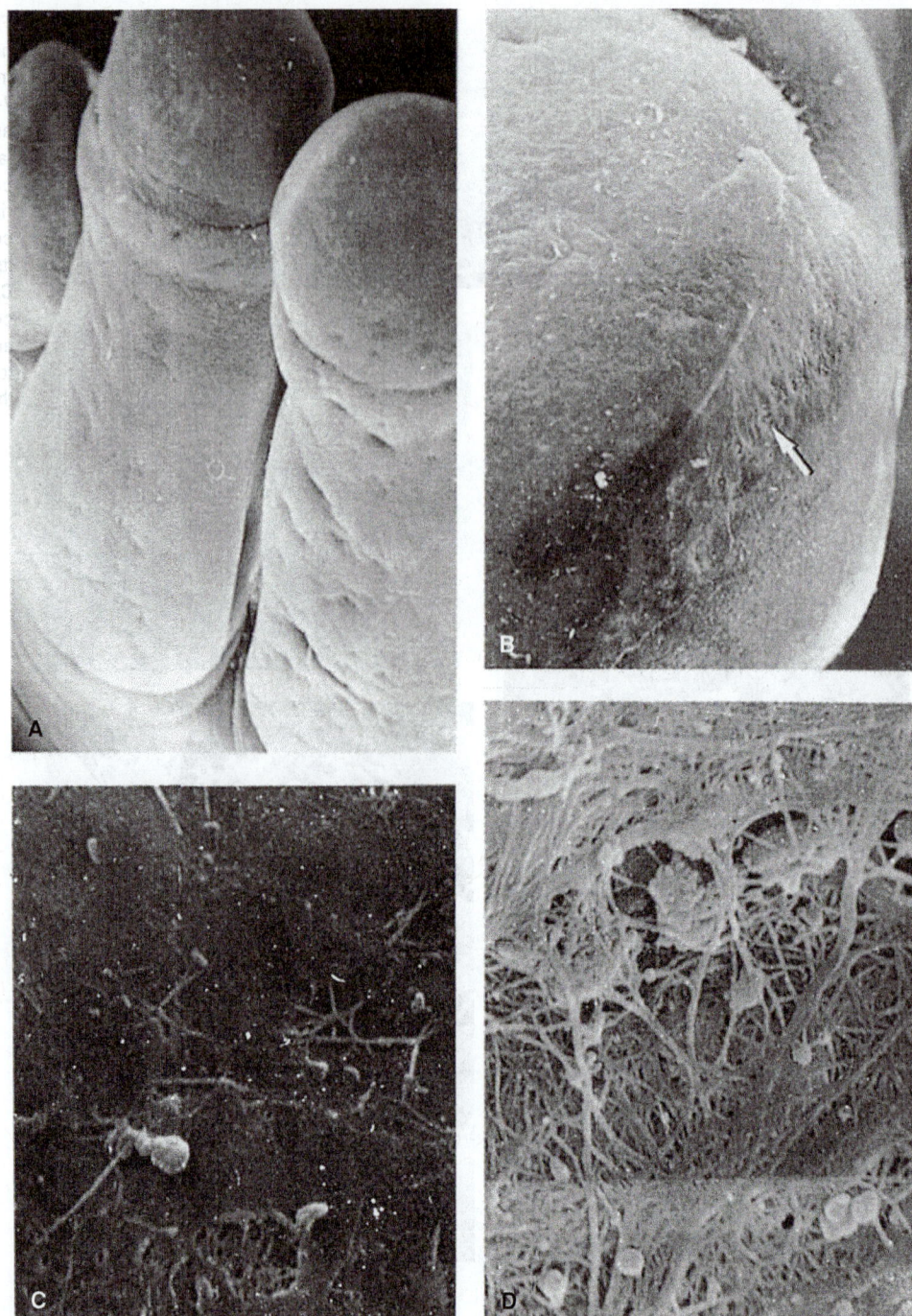

FIGURE 2.2 Fibrillar phase: Fingers of the hand of a 3-month-old embryo. The ungual region is perfectly delimited by the proximal nail fold (**A**, ×40). The ungual region is delimited by multiple fibrillar formations (*arrow* in **B**, ×150). Different morphology is seen in the nail bed surface (**C**, ×2,400). Detail of the fibrillar attachment of the nail region to the neighboring tissue (**D**, ×2,400).

GENETIC AND NAIL KERATINS

Keratin epithelial cells possess three cytoskeletal systems: actin microfilaments, microtubules, and keratin intermediate filaments. The protective structural role of keratins was clearly revealed in the early 1990s, when mutations in human keratin genes were discovered in a variety of human genetic diseases characterized by fragility and/or overgrowth (hyperkeratosis) of specific epithelial tissues (16). It is not precisely known how mutations in these keratins lead to hyperkeratosis of the nail, but fragility of the underlying nail bed keratinocytes presumably leads to release of cytokines and other inflammatory factors that act upon the proliferative cells of the nail matrix and produce overgrowth of the nail (17). Shotgun proteomic analysis of the human nail plate identified 144 proteins in the samples from Caucasian volunteers, with identifying more than 300 constituents of the isopeptide cross-linked proteome and even certain posttranslational modifications. The 30 identified proteins

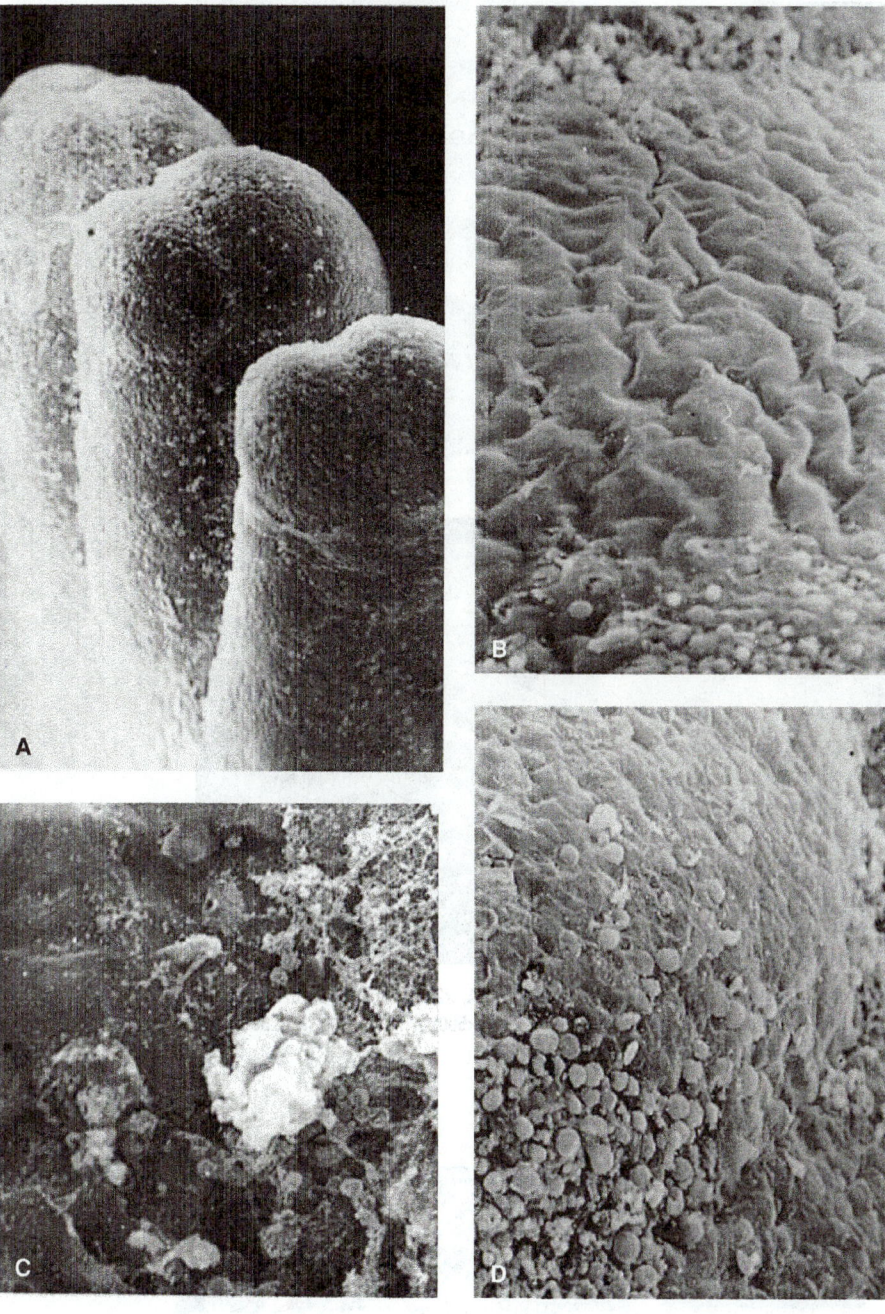

FIGURE 2.3 Granular phase: Fingers of the hand of 4.5-month-old embryo. All fingers show a granular aspect (**A**, ×40). The nail bed has an undulating surface covered by keratin scales (**B**, ×400). The hyponychium zone is occupied by numerous keratohyalin vesicles (**C**, ×400; **D**, ×150).

solubilized by detergent and reducing agents, 90% of the total nail plate mass, were primarily keratins and keratin-associated proteins. Keratins comprise a majority of the detergent-insoluble fraction as well, but numerous cytoplasmic membranes, and junctional proteins and histones were also identified, indicating broad use by transglutaminases of available proteins as substrates for cross-linking (18,19). Keratins are a large family of intermediate filament proteins encoded by more than 50 distinct genes in humans (20). About half of these are the epithelial keratins that are found in soft epithelial tissues of the human body. The rest are the trichocyte or high sulfur hard keratins of which hair and nail are composed. Both epithelial keratins and hard keratins can be further subdivided into type I and type II proteins, on the basis of their size, charge, and amino acid sequence characteristics (21). Recent work has shown that the human hair keratin family consists of nine type I and six type II members, whose genes are organized as distinct clusters within the type I and type II epithelial keratin gene domains on chromosomes 17q21.2 and 12q13.3, respectively (17–21). The functional type I (K9–K23; Ha1–Ha8) and type II keratin genes (K1–K8; Hb1–Hb6) are each clustered on distinct chromosomes in the human and mouse genomes. The pair-wise and differentiation-related regulation of most type I and type II keratin genes provides a unique handle to track differentiation within epithelial tissue (22,23). A family-wide,

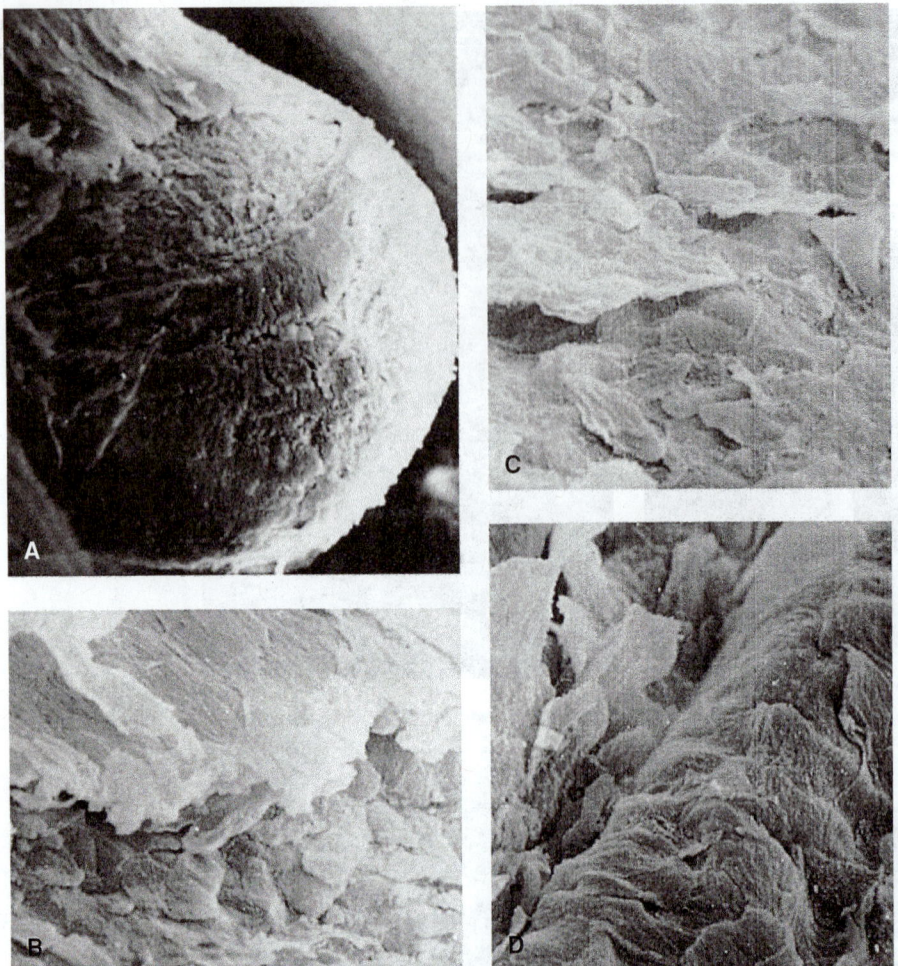

FIGURE 2.4 Squamous phase: Index finger of 5.5-month-old fetus (**A**, ×200). The keratinization process is complete in the nail bed surface, simulating a false nail (**C**, ×500). The cuticle (**B**, ×500) and hyponychium are also completely developed (**D**, ×500).

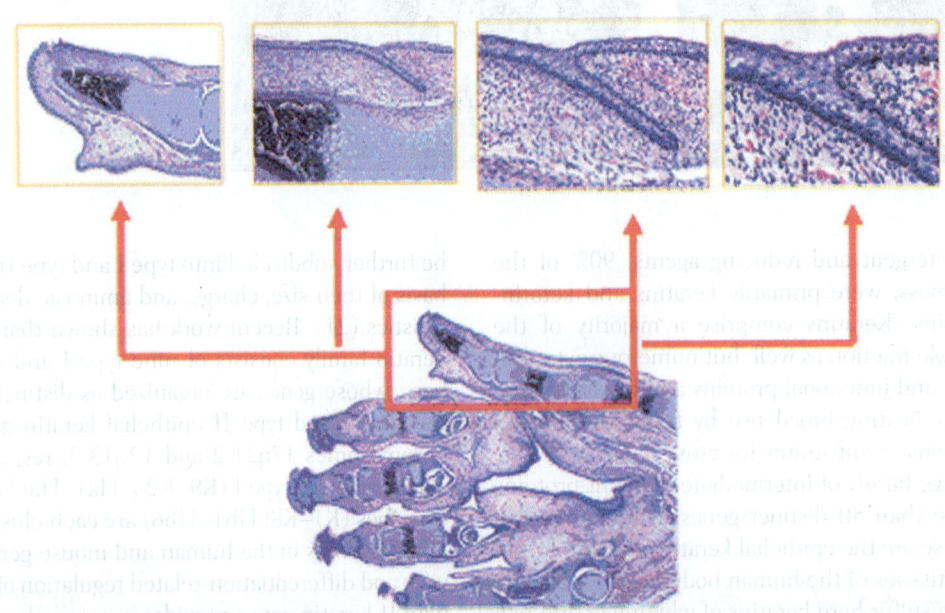

FIGURE 2.5 Sagittal section of a fetal hand of 16 weeks, with special close-up views of the nail matrix area.

crucial function of keratin filaments is to endow epithelial cells with the ability to withstand mechanical and other forms of stress.

The pattern of the keratins in the nail unit differs from that of the follicle in two points: the lack of an IRS-like compartment and of the companion layer (24). The expression of K6hf was observed almost exclusively in the nail bed. K6 and K16 were expressed in the eponychium, the apical matrix, and the nail bed, but not in the ventral matrix. Distribution of K6 and K16 was essentially suprabasal. On the basis of morphologic and biochemical considerations, the distal nail unit can be divided into three segments. The nail bed, which represents the main segment of distal nail unit, does not differentiate into a thin, orthokeratinizing surface. The nail isthmus is typified by a peculiar mode of keratinization (i.e., a compartment of pale, nucleated corneocytes), which is closely adherent to the inferior border of the nail plate, including its distal free edge. The nail isthmus presents a profile of keratin expression in transition between the nail bed and the hyponychium. The keratin pattern of the nail bed, including K6hf and Ki-67, is maintained. However, the nail isthmus differs from the nail bed in that K10 is only present in the nail isthmus (23). The morphologic aspect and the pattern of expression of K5, K17, K6, K16, and K75 suggested a differentiation toward the nail bed and the nail isthmus (24).

Accordingly, mutations in keratin genes are responsible for a number of genetically based fragility disorders involving specific cell types(s) in skin and other epithelia (24–26). Among type I keratin genes, *K17* stands out in multiple ways. In mouse embryonic skin, it is first expressed in ectodermal cells committing to a nonepidermal cell fate (i.e., all appendages and periderm) in response to mesenchymal induction (27). Concomitant with skin maturation, *mK17* expression becomes restricted to specific cell layers and compartments within all major types of epithelial appendages. Both *hK17* and *mK17* can be coregulated with distinct type II keratin genes (e.g., *K5, K6a, K6b, K6hf*) in mature epithelial settings (23). In addition to its constitutive expression in epithelial appendages, *K17* expression is induced in mature interfollicular epidermis subjected to various types of acute challenges (e.g., injury, UV exposure, inflammation) (27) or during diseases (e.g., psoriasis, basal cell carcinoma). Mutations affecting a particular segment of *hK17*'s coding sequence can cause distinct disorders of the skin, related to ectodermal dysplasias (16,17).

GROSS ANATOMY

It was first noted early in the 20th century that the nail unit was comparable in several respects to a hair follicle sectioned longitudinally and laid on its side (28–30). Various types of differently keratinizing epidermis make up the nail. What is commonly termed "the nail plate" is the horny

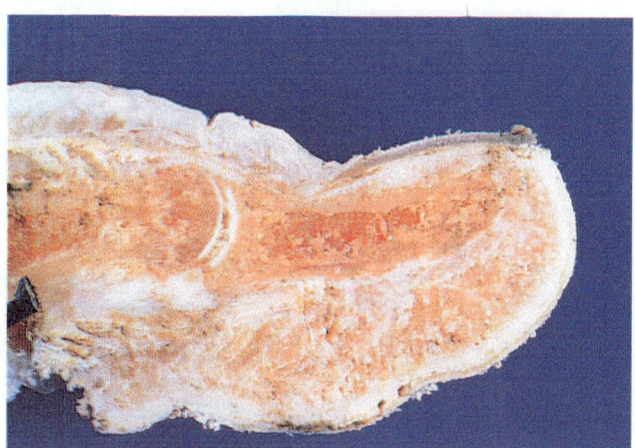

FIGURE 2.6 Sagittal section of an adult thumb, in which it is possible to observe the relations of the nail unit with the adjacent tissues.

end product of the most important epithelial component, the matrix. Usually, this nail plate is slightly convex or flat, rectangular, and of varying sizes between approximately 1 × 1 and 2 × 3 cm, depending on the finger (Figs. 2.6 to 2.8). In the hand, this is usually 25% to 50% of the dorsal surface of the fingertips, whereas in the big toe it occupies about 75%. The nail is translucent and becomes rosy from the underlying vascular network. However, change of colors (erythronychia, melanonychia) can be observed in the nail plate and may indicate inflammatory diseases (lichen planus, lupus erythematosus); benign or malignant neoplasm, mainly subungual melanoma; and scarring of the dermis. The white appearance of nails in leukonychia seems to be due to an abnormal keratinization of cells originating from the proximal nail matrix (PNM), leading to the presence of abundant intracellular vacuoles and to a lesser compactness of keratins. Gene mapping within

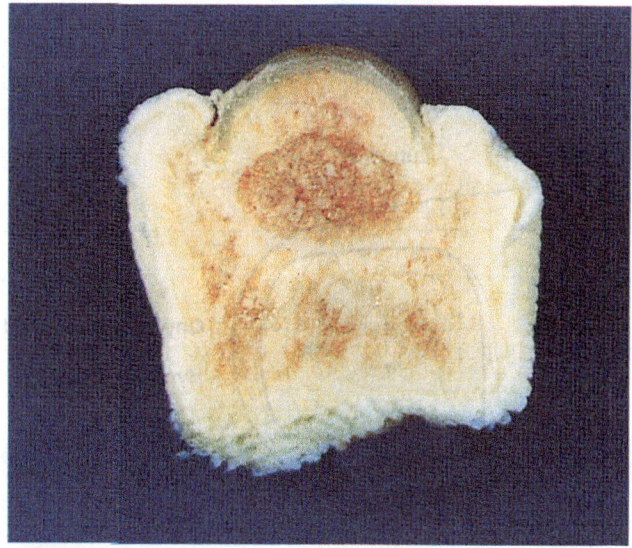

FIGURE 2.7 Cross section of an adult finger. The nail plate lies on nail bed, and the lateral border is overlapped by lateral nail fold.

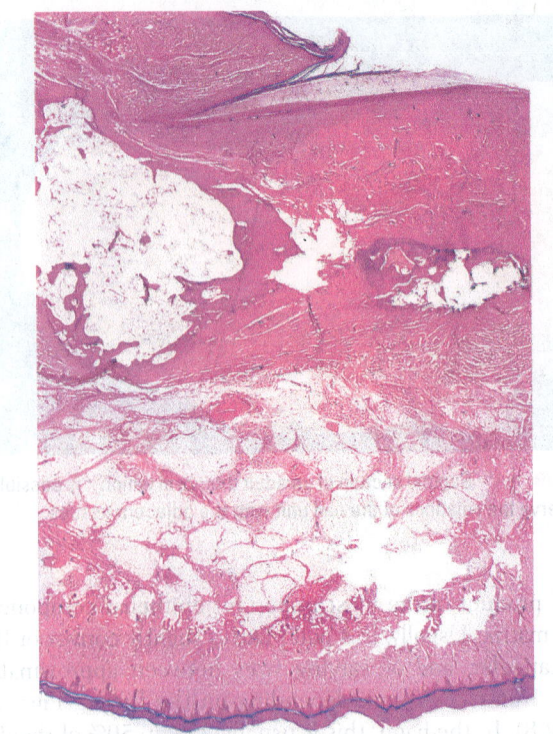

FIGURE 2.8 Histologic sagittal section of a finger.

this chromosomal region includes gene coding for type II (basic) cytokeratins and hard keratins, and the gene defect resides on chromosome 12q13 (31).

In the proximal portion, there is an arch called lunula. The thickness of the nail plate is 0.5 mm in women and 0.6 mm in men (32). The nail plate is delimited by three folds: two lateral and one proximal (Fig. 2.9). If the nail plate is avulsed, the grooves become visible where the nail plate rested. These potential spaces are only real spaces in abnormal conditions of the nail, as in paronychia. In the lateral nail grooves the epidermal lining does not contribute to the formation of the nail plate, except in the most proximal portions where it becomes continuous with the epidermis of the proximal groove or matrix.

The PNF is the most important one, since, as we shall note later, its contribution to the formation of the nail plate is fundamental (33). This fold shows two portions: a dorsal portion, lodging the matrix, and a ventral portion. Twenty-five percent of the total surface of the nail plate is located under the ventral portion of the PNF. Terminal tendon of the digital extensor is closely related with this area and the thin nature and proximity with the nail matrix must be kept in mind during surgery (34). A white crescent-shaped lunula can project from under the PNF. It is usual on the thumbs and common on other fingers and on large toenails. The lunula is the most distal portion of the matrix and determines the shape of the free edge of the nail plate. The color of the lunula is partly due to the effect of light scattered by the nucleated cells of the keratogenous zone of the matrix and partly due to the thick layer of epithelial cells making up the matrix (33,35). At the point of separation of the nail plate and the nail bed, the subungual epidermis may be modified as the sole horn (36). In humans, this structure may only be vestigial: its original significance only being evident from comparative anatomical studies. However, in certain diseases, it could be the seat of distal subungual hyperkeratosis or parakeratosis, for example, in pachyonychia congenita and pityriasis rubra pilaris (37). The distal limit of the ungual layer is the hyponychium, determining the formation of the distal fold, a keratinized structure that continues until the fingertips. A subungual extension of the hyponychium and obliteration of the distal groove is named pterygium inversum unguis (38). This term was coined because of the similarity between the behavior of the hyponychium and the eponychium in classic cases of pterygium unguis. On close examination, two further distal zones can often be identified: the distal yellow-white margin and, immediately proximal to this, the onychodermal band (39). This band is a barely perceptible narrow transverse band, 0.5- to 1.5-mm wide, that is more prominent in acrocyanosis. The exact anatomical basis for the onychodermal band is not known, but it appears to have a different blood supply from the main body of the nail bed (40). It is possible to explore it through a strong compression of the distal zone of the finger, leaving behind a white band. The band's color can occasionally be modified by diseases (37,41). Several studies have been published about the exploration of the nail apparatus. Although ultrasound transmission can be useful for studying the nail plate thickness (42), magnetic resonance imaging (MRI) permits the detection of subungual lesions smaller than 1 mm in diameter (43). Specific causes of injury including homicide, abuse, neglect, assault, self-inflicted injury, suicide, torture, poisoning, and bioterrorism have been studied in nails (27).

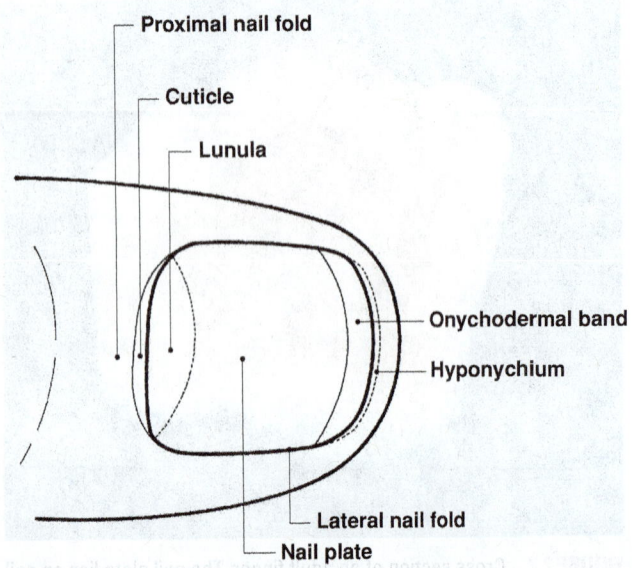

FIGURE 2.9 Schematic diagram of the nail, including nomenclature.

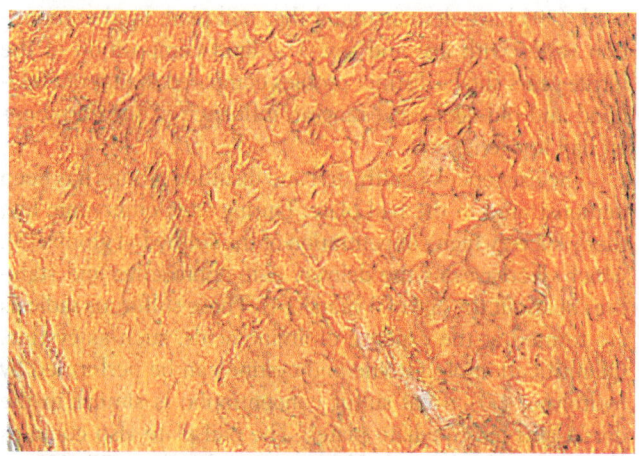

FIGURE 2.10 Horizontal section of the dorsal nail plate. Corneocytes show a polyhedral disposition, with rounded corners; the cells do not contain nuclei or elements (VVG stain).

MICROSCOPIC ANATOMY

The Nail Plate

Microscopically, the nail plate consists of closely packed, adherent, interdigitating corneocytes lacking nuclei or organelles (Figs. 2.10 and 2.11). Many intercellular links including tight, intermediate, and desmosomal junctions are present (44). The nail plate is made up of three layers: a thin dorsal layer, a thick intermediate layer, and the ventral layer from the nail bed. The cells of the surface of the nail plate overlap, slanting from "proximal-dorsal to distal-volar." For this reason, the dorsal surface of the nail plate is smooth, whereas the palmar surface is irregular, showing longitudinal striations. This can also be observed with optical microscopy, as well as with scanning electron microscopy (45) and x-ray microdiffraction (46). With this latter technique, Garson et al. (46) demonstrated three different layers in the nail plate characterized by different orientations of the keratin molecules from the outer to the inner side of human nail. These layers were associated with the histologic dorsal, intermediate, and ventral plates. The hair-like type alpha-keratin filaments (81 Å in diameter) are only present in the intermediate layer (accounting for approximately two-thirds of the nail width) and are perfectly oriented perpendicular to the growth axis, in the nail plane. Keratin filaments of stratum corneum (epidermis) type, found in the dorsal and ventral cells, are oriented in two privileged directions; parallel and perpendicular to the growth axis. This "sandwich" structure in the corneocytes and the strong intercellular junctions gives the nail high mechanical rigidity and hardness, both in the curvature direction and in the growth direction. Lipid bilayers (49-Å thick) parallel to the nail surface fill certain ampullar dilations of the dorsal plate and intercellular spaces in the ventral plate. Using x-ray microdiffraction, they also showed that onychomycosis disrupts the keratin structure, probably during the synthesis phase. No keratohyalin granules were seen, but acidophilic masses, called pertinax bodies of Lewis and Montgomery, are occasionally seen in older age groups.

Hamilton et al. (47) believed that the progressive increase in the thickness of the nail plate with age is attributable to

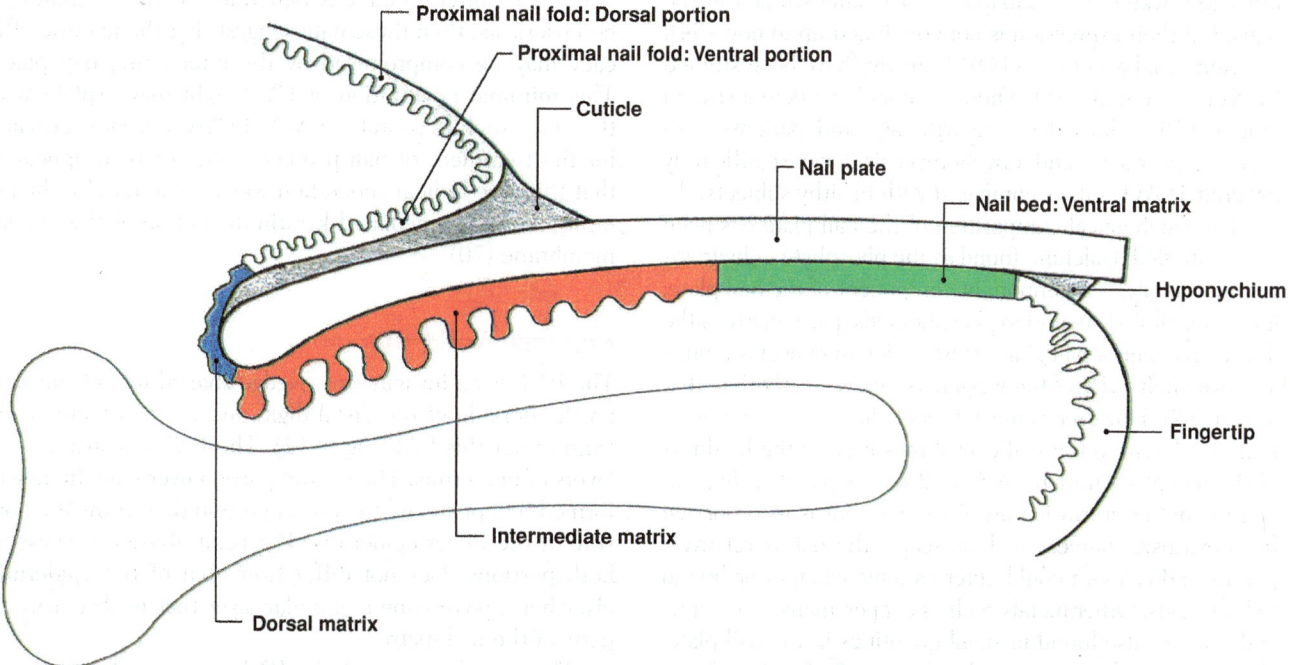

FIGURE 2.11 Schematic diagram of a sagittal section through the nail unit.

the increasing size of the cells in the plate, consecutive to the frictional loss of nail; however, Johnson and Shuster (48) studied in 20 normal great toenails the determinant of final nail thickness and length at its point of detachment at the onychodermal band. They confirmed that the increase of nail thickness with age is independent of the frictional traumatisms on the plate. Cutting tests showed that fracture of the nail plate occurred because the energy to cut nails transversely, at approximately 3 kJ m^{-2}, was about half that needed (~6 kJ m^{-2}) to cut them longitudinally (49).

Corneocytes of the human nail plate have been studied by German et al. (50). Corneocytes of the dorsal nail plates of normal nails are irregular and polyhedral, non-nucleated, and show distinctly irregular networks. These horny cells from nail plates increase in size with age: Babies have small cells, adults have significantly larger cells, and aged subjects have significantly larger cells than the adults. These authors also commented that the faster-than-normal-growing nail plates yield smaller cells; for example, corneocytes from psoriatic patients are smaller than normal, whereas corneocytes from slow-growing nails, such as from persons having lichen planus or dyskeratosis congenita, are larger than normal.

Frequent gap junctions were observed near the area where lamellar granules were discharging their contents, and it was suggested that a certain substance might be able to pass through the nail plate through such intercellular channels. Perhaps such channels explain the greater permeability of the nail plate to polar molecules compared with the permeability of the skin (51). The water content of human nail plates have been determined using a portable near-infrared spectrometer with an InGaAs photodiode array detector and PLS regression by Egawa et al. (52).

Chemical composition shows that a normal nail contains 18% water (53). Aquaporins are being studied in the nails, but their expression is not concluded up to now (54). Transonychial water loss (TOWL) in vivo have been studied by Nuutinen et al. (55). These authors have demonstrated that TOWL values decrease with age and patients with eczema, psoriasis, and onychomycosis have significantly lowered TOWL values compared with healthy subjects.

The biochemical composition of the nail plate has been widely studied. Calcium, found as the phosphate in hydroxyapatite crystals, is an important component of the nail plate; it is intracellularly bound to phospholipids, particularly in the dorsal and ventral nail plates (56). Calcium concentration is approximately 0.1% of the weight, 10 times greater than that in hair (57). However, some authors believe that the proportion of calcium in the nail contributes little to the hardness of the nail plate in men (39,58). Also, it is possible that calcium is not an intrinsic part of the nail but is incorporated from extrinsic sources, such as soaps; the nail is relatively porous and calcium could enter as ionic calcium or bound to fatty acids. Other metals such as copper, manganese, zinc, and iron are also found in small quantities in the nail plate, although their function is still unknown (58,59). Lipids are also an important component of the nail plate. Helmdach et al. (59) have demonstrated that nail plate lipid composition varies with age and sex: The lipid composition of the fertile years shows distinct profiles compared to that of childhood and old age, suggesting an influence of sex hormones on nail lipogenesis.

The existence of sulfhydryl and disulfide groups has been demonstrated in the nail plate. During early embryonic life, there is a very high concentration of the sulfhydryl groups (9), which decreases as the delivery date approaches and stabilizes at about the age of 3 years (14). These sulfurous radicals are formed at the expense of amino acids, such as cystine. Quantification of cysteine and cystine can be performed by hydrolysis (60). Total sulfur concentration is similar in the dorsal and intermediate plates. The nail plate also contains glutamic acid, serine, and less tyrosine than hair (57–60).

In certain diseases, the quantity of various organic and metallic components of the nail plate can be increased. A brief listing is presented for reference: total nonprotein nitrogen, urea nitrogen, ammonia nitrogen, and uric acid in gout (61); creatinine in chronic renal failure (62); sodium in cystic fibrosis (63,64); calcium in older subjects (48,57); copper in Wilson disease (65); arsenic as a biomarker to arsenic exposure in the endemic areas (66); and morphine, 6-acetylmorphine, and cocaine in drug abusers (67).

An analysis of the keratin of the nail plate revealed the following (68): (a) alpha-fibrillar, low sulfur protein; (b) globular, high sulfur matrix protein; and (c) high glycine–tyrosine-rich matrix protein. All these fractions are also present in hair. The hardness of nail is due to the high sulfur matrix protein, contrasting with the relatively soft keratin of the epidermis.

The nail plate completely blocked the UV-B light and only a minimal amount of UV-A light penetrated the nails. If UV is required to directly penetrate the nail to treat nail bed psoriasis, then these data suggest that therapeutic efficacy may be compromised by the intervening nail plate. This minimal penetration of UV-A light may explain why therapies such as psoralen-UV-A (PUVA) have low efficacy for the treatment of nail psoriasis (69). Thus, it appeared that this free radical generation was fundamental in facilitating the redox-mediated keratin disruption of the ungual membrane (70).

Proximal Nail Fold

The PNF is an invaginating, wedge-shaped fold of the skin on the dorsum of the distal digit, and the nail plate arises from under this fold (Fig. 2.12). The PNF consists of two layers of epidermis: The ventral portion overlying the newly formed nail plate and the dorsal portion that forms the dorsum of the finger epidermis. The keratinization process in both portions does not differ from that of the epidermis elsewhere, possessing a granular layer that is absent in all parts of the nail matrix.

The dorsal portion of the PNF consists of a continuation of the epidermis and dermis of the dorsal digit with

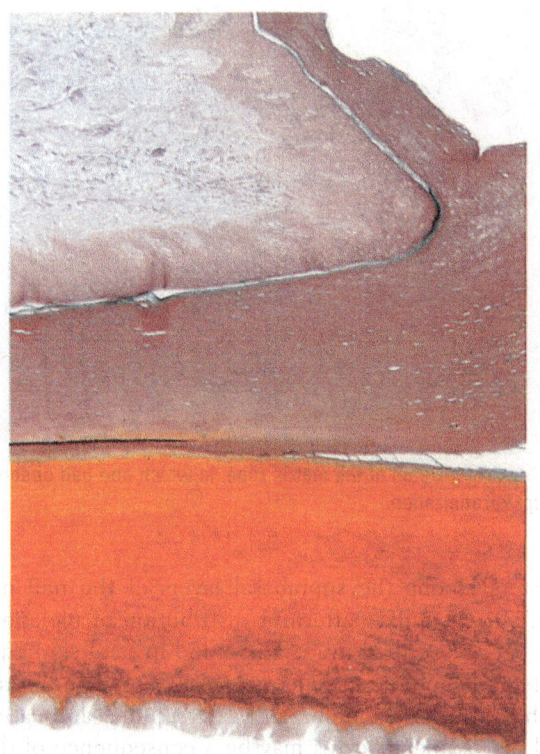

FIGURE 2.12 Proximal nail fold with its two portions: Dorsal portion, with identical histologic pattern to the skin of the dorsum of the distal digit; ventral portion, overlying the nail plate. Note the great thickness of the stratum corneum of this epithelium (MF stain).

sweat glands, but no follicles or sebaceous glands. At the distal tip, a thick corneal layer called the cuticle shows on the dorsal surface of the nail plate (Fig. 2.13). Its function is the protection of the nail base, particularly the germinative matrix. Loss of the cuticle often allows acute and chronic inflammatory and infective processes to involve the nail matrix, leading to secondary nail plate dystrophies.

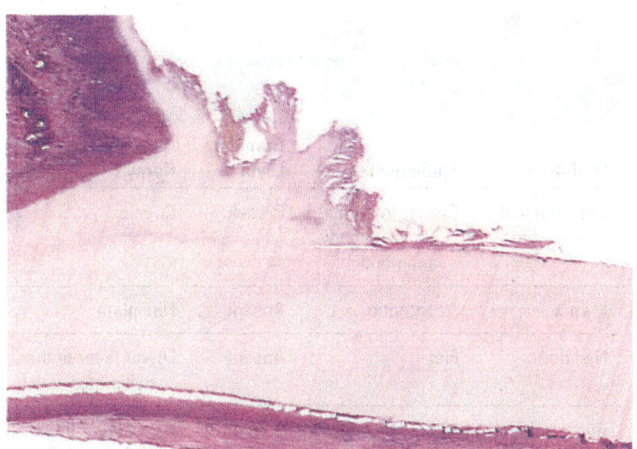

FIGURE 2.13 Detail of the cuticle. At the distal tip, the proximal nail fold shows a thick corneal layer (cuticle) on the dorsal surface of the nail plate.

The ventral portion is thick skinned, has no appendages, and is closely attached on the dorsal surface of the nail plate. The epithelium of the ventral surface of the PNF has been called eponychium (9,35,37). Diseases that affect the ventral portion of the PNF can affect the newly formed nail plate. For this reason, some authors think that the PNF contributes to form the superficial layer of the nail plate. In particular, the apparition of pits and grooves (Beau line) on the nail is due to parakeratotic and growth detention phenomena, respectively, in the ventral portion of the PNF.

Matrix

The ventral surface of the PNF forms the roof of the proximal nail groove; the nail matrix forms its floor, and the nail plate lies between the two. The matrix is divided into three parts (8,9,37): dorsal, intermediate, and ventral. Of these, the dorsal and, above all, the intermediate portions play an important role in nail plate formation. In particular, the true matrix is the intermediate portion. For this reason, when we discuss the histology of the matrix, we are fundamentally referring to the intermediate portion. The ventral portion corresponds to the nail bed; the controversy about its participation in the formation of the definitive nail plate is discussed in "Nail Growth."

The main body of the matrix is composed of epithelial cells, with melanocytes, Merkel cells (MCs), and Langerhans cells scattered among the epithelial cells.

Epithelial Cells

The matrix is an easily identified thick squamous epithelium, situated immediately below the ventral portion of the PNF (Fig. 2.14). Its main feature is its thickness, with between 8 and 15 mamelons (protuberances) (Fig. 2.15). Its undulation can only be seen for a few millimeters, flattening itself in the area corresponding to the nail bed. As in the epidermis of the skin, the matrix possesses a very active germinative basal layer of immature basaloid cells, producing keratinocytes which differentiate, harden, die, and contribute to the nail plate (Fig. 2.16). The nail plate is formed by a process that involves flattening of the basal cells of the matrix, fragmentation of nuclei, and condensation of the cell cytoplasm to form horny flat cells. An important histologic feature is the lack of granular layer. Acanthosis and papillomatosis are only seen in the nail unit in the matrix and, distally, in the hyponychium (Table 2.2).

Melanocytes

In order to have a better knowledge of nail histology, it is important to understand not only the normal nail anatomy but also the melanocytic density of nail unit epithelium. The nail matrix possesses melanocytes, just as the hair matrix does. The matrix of Caucasian patients contains sparse, poorly developed melanocytes (Figs. 2.17 and 2.18) (71,72). It is difficult to observe melanocytes in the proximal matrix zone using light microscopy, but their numbers

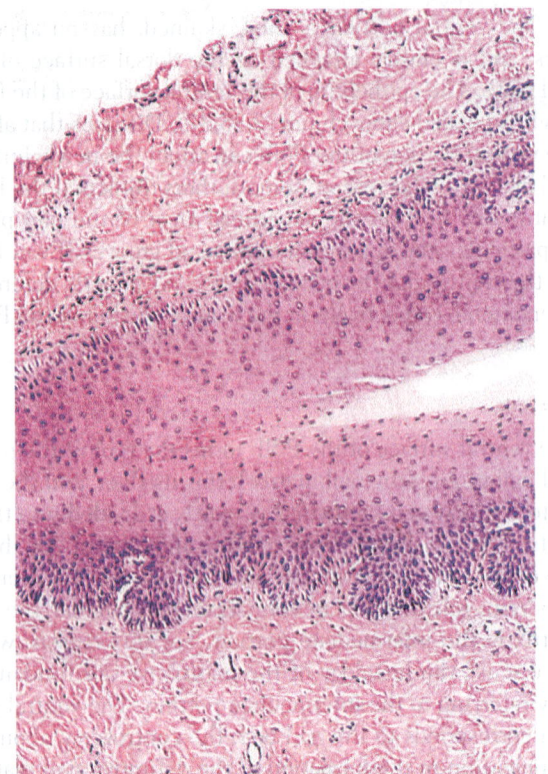

FIGURE 2.14 Histologic appearance of the matrix angle, formed by the ventral portion of the nail fold and the dorsal and the intermediate matrix.

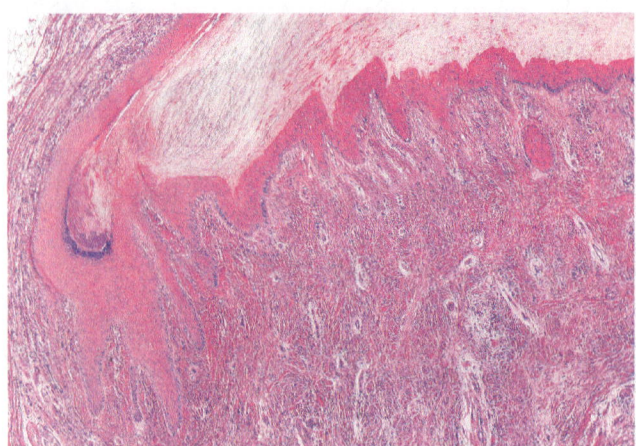

FIGURE 2.16 Detail of the matrix zone, in which one can observe the abrupt keratinization.

are progressively increased distally. Nevertheless, the number of melanocytes is always lower in the matrix than in normal skin (72–76).

There are distinct differences in the distribution of melanocytes in adult skin and nail matrix. Immunostaining of nail matrix melanocytes revealed that they are not singly interspersed between the keratinocytes of the basal layer, but that they are frequently arranged in small clusters among the suprabasal layers of the nail matrix (76,77). A similar pattern of distribution of melanocytes has been described in fetal skin and in fetal skin equivalents, in which the melanocytes are grouped and localized both basally and suprabasally. The suprabasal location of nail matrix melanocytes may be a consequence of differences in the distribution of adhesion molecules in the nail epithelium (76,77).

Higashi and Saito (78) demonstrated that the number of melanocytes and the intensity of the dopa reaction in them were much greater in the distal than the proximal matrix. The melanocyte count in normal epidermis was reported to be 400 per 2.784 mm^2 (77,78), while the range was 208 to 576 in the distal areas of the intermediate nail matrix (78).

Ultraviolet rays and trauma are factors that could influence a more extensive distribution in the distal zone (79,80). In some races such as Japanese, the matrix contains several hundred well-developed melanocytes per millimeter (81). Also, it seems that melanocytes of the nail matrix in Oriental

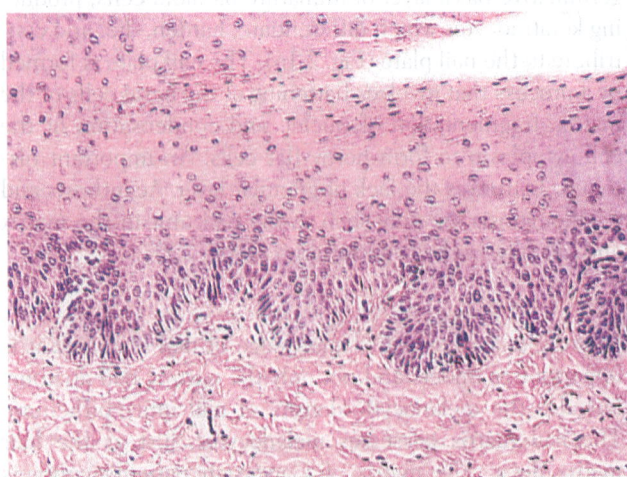

FIGURE 2.15 Detail of matrix epithelium. This zone shows an acanthotic epithelium, with germinative basal cells keratinocytes and scarce melanocytes.

TABLE 2.2

Histologic Characteristic Features of Each Zone of the Nail Unit

Nail Area	Epithelium	Granular Layer	Horny End Product
Proximal nail fold	Similar to normal skin or slightly acanthotic	Present	Cuticle
Matrix	Acanthotic	Absent	Nail plate
Nail bed	Flat	Absent	Lower layer of the nail plate
Hyponychium	Acanthotic	Present	Horny layer in the under surface of the distal nail, similar to cuticle

Langerhans and Merkel Cells

Langerhans and MCs have also been identified in the matrix (73) although their signification is unknown. Studies of the Langerhans cells in the nail matrix are almost absent. Nevertheless, interesting studies about the MCs have been recently published. Moll and Moll (82) studied the MCs in ontogenesis of human nails, using immunohistochemical stains with cytokeratins 18 and 20 in human fetuses of 9 to 22 weeks of life. These authors have concluded that the number of MCs are detected very early (9 weeks) in the matrix primordium. However, MCs were found to decrease in number with aging of the fetuses: at 12 to 15 weeks, MCs were only seen in the PNF, and were essentially absent from the epithelium of the ventral matrix and nail bed in the adult

Lunula

The intermediate matrix continues forward with a visible, white half-moon–shaped area called lunula. The lunula is shown to be linked to a well-defined area in the underlying dermis with a specific histology and microvascularization. Although always present, it cannot be seen in some fingers but is most visible in the thumbs. The typical white color is related to some histologic features of this area. Lewin (32) confirmed that the opacity of the proximal nail plate, the relative avascularity of the subepidermal layer, and the loose texture of the dermal collagen are responsible for its color. Samman (83,84) thought that it was a combination of incomplete keratinization in the nail plate and loose connective tissue in the underlying tissue. Zaias (85) believed that the nail plate would be thinner in the lunula because it coincides with the keratogenous zone, the zone of cytoplasmic condensation in the matrix just before cells form the nail plate. The length of the subnail matrix area distal to the free edge of the PNF is highly correlated with the length of the lunula (86).

Other special histologic features of this zone of the matrix, including a different chemical composition of the nail plate and a different distribution of the dermal fibers, have been related to the typical white color of the lunula (87,88), although not one of these factors has been confirmed. We do not even know the exact function of the lunula.

Nail Bed

The nail bed begins where the intermediate matrix ends, and some authors prefer to designate the ventral matrix as the site (37,87). A histologic appreciation of the end of the intermediate matrix and the beginning of the nail bed is very easy. The nail bed epidermal layer is usually a flat epithelium no more than three- or four-cell thick, without melanocytes (Figs. 2.19 and 2.20). The transition zone from living keratinocytes to dead ventral nail plate cells is abrupt, occurring in the space of one horizontal cell layer, very similar to what occurs in the Henle layer of the internal root sheath of the hair follicle (89).

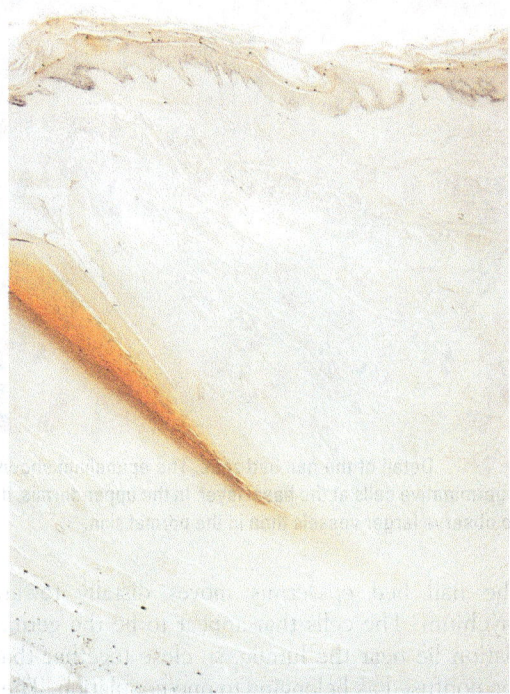

FIGURE 2.17 Observe the notable hyperpigmentation of the basal layer in the pulp of the finger in contrast with the absence of pigmentation in the nail matrix (Fontana stain).

races have larger dendritic processes than Caucasians. Pigment, therefore, arrives in the nail plate as in the keratinized cells of the stratum corneum and hair cortex (79). Nail pigmentation is most evident in African Americans in whom it is commonly seen as longitudinal linear streaks, although this anomalous distribution of pigmentation can also be seen in pathologic states, such as subungual pigmented nevi and melanomas in the matrix zone (80). Abundant melanosomes of these subjects have a protective UV effect, since variations in racial pigmentation are due to the number and size of melanosomes produced (81).

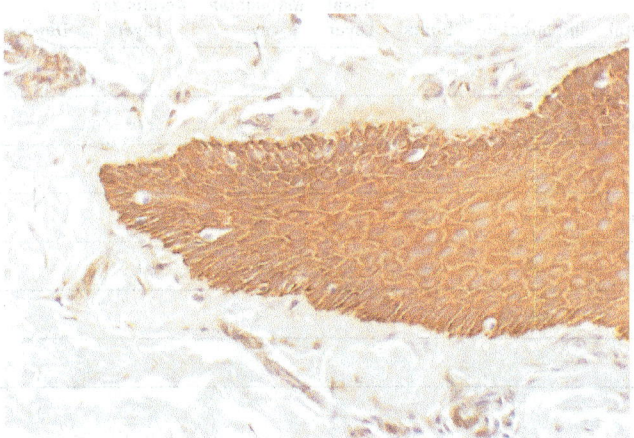

FIGURE 2.18 Melanocytes in the nail matrix, not staining with cytokeratin antibody, are scarce in number (cytokeratin antibody).

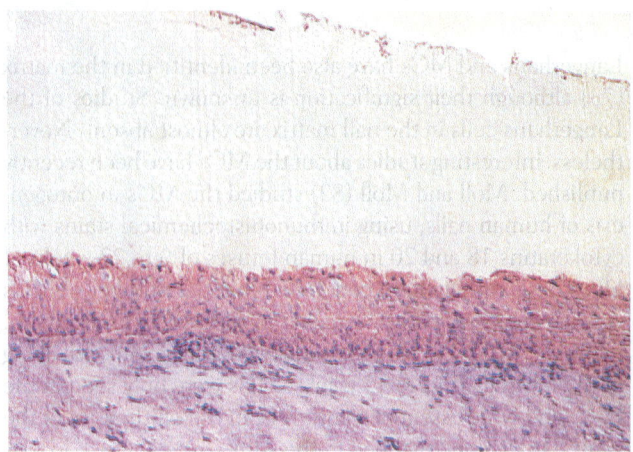

FIGURE 2.19 Nail bed. Note the flat epithelium with an interdigitated upper zone.

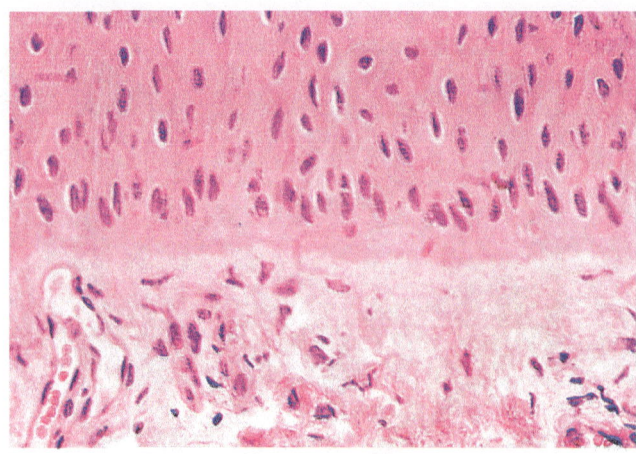

FIGURE 2.20 Detail of the nail bed zone. The epithelium shows a few active germinative cells at the basal layer. In the upper dermis, it is possible to observe larger vessels than in the normal skin.

During its early development, the nail bed exhibits a keratinization process differing from the adult's, with a prominent granular layer at 17 to 20 weeks of development. However, after birth, the nail bed, like the matrix, keratinizes without a granular layer. It is less active than the matrix, with a longer turnover time than the matrix and skin (89). A thin parakeratotic keratin is produced, apparently dragged forward by the nail plate growing over it, rather than becoming incorporated into the nail.

In the nail bed, the dermis fits into the longitudinal and parallel nail bed ridges in tongue-and-groove fashion. The fine capillaries of the nail bed run in these parallel dermal ridges, and disruption of these accounts for the splinter hemorrhages commonly seen in normal and disease states (40). There is no fat tissue in the nail bed, although scattered dermal fat cells may be visible microscopically.

The nail bed epidermis moves distally toward the hyponychium. The cells that appear to be the germinative population lie near the lunula, so close together that they may be confused as belonging to one population. The distal movement from this position may also help explain why during development, the nail bed epidermis seems to lose keratohyaline granule layers from a proximal-to-distal direction concomitantly with the formation of the primitive nail plate (90). The nail bed shows a granular layer in some pathologic states, in which the activity in the nail bed is greatly increased, such as occurs in onychogryphosis, pachyonychia congenita, and psoriasis (91); in these cases, the horny cells produced push the nail plate upward and give it a claw-like appearance. Histochemical studies of the nail bed prove the presence of bound phospholipids in the nail bed epidermis (Table 2.3). Bound cysteine can be detected in the transition

TABLE 2.3
Histochemistry of the Nail[a]

	Matrix		Nail Bed		Nail Plate			Nail Folds—Hyponychium			
	Dorsal	Intermediate	Basal Layer	Malpighian Layer	Ventral	Intermediate	Dorsal	Basal Layer	Malpighian Layer	Keratinized Layer	Dermis
Glycogen	−	−	−	+/−	−	−	−	−	+/−	−	
Mucopoly saccharide	+	+	+/−	+	++	−	+	+/−	+	+/−	+
Ribonucleic acid	+	+	+	+	−	−	−	+	+	−	
Sulfhydryl groups					++	++	+		+	+	
Acid phosphatase	+		+/−	+/−	+	++	−	+	+	+	
Alkaline phosphatase	−				−	−	−			+	+
Amylophosphorylase	+	+	+	−	−	−					
Cholinesterase											+

[a]Baran R, Dawber RPR, eds. *Diseases of the Nail and Their Management*. Oxford: Blackwell Scientific;1984:1–21; Jarrett A, Spearman RI. The histochemistry of the human nail. *Arch Dermatol* 1966;94:652–657.

zones: Acid phosphatase and nonspecific esterase are absent in the dorsal and intermediate zones (37,56).

Immunohistochemical studies have demonstrated that nail bed expressed all the target antigens found in the normal nonappendageal basement membrane (92). In particular, there was normal expression of the epidermal-associated antigens, the 220- and 180-kDa bullous pemphigoid antigens and the α-6 β-4 integrin. There was also normal expression of the lamina lucida antigens LH39, GB3, and laminin. Sinclair et al. (93) pointed out that the dermal-associated components, namely the 285-kDa linear immunoglobulin A (IgA) antigen, the extracellular matrix glycoproteins, chondroitin sulfate, type VII collagen and its closely associated proteins, and the poorly characterized antigen for LH24 and LH39 were all normally expressed. All the former data were also found in the PNF, nail matrix, and hyponychium. The presence of antimicrobial peptides in nails, mainly cathelicidin LL-37, demonstrated by immunostaining, with activity against relevant nail pathogens may account for the ability of the nail unit to resist infection in the absence of direct access to the cellular immune system (94).

Hyponychium

The most distal portion of the nail bed is the hyponychium, representing the union between the nail bed and the fingertips; its histologic characteristics are rather peculiar. This transition zone presents a notable change of appearance after a few millimeters because the epithelium undergoes keratinization similar to that of the epidermis (Fig. 2.21). The result is marked acanthosis and papillomatosis with the crests oriented almost horizontally; this is associated with normal appendages (Fig. 2.22). An area of abundant keratohyaline granules is present, and the horny layer produced tends to accumulate under the free edge of the nail plate, producing a keratin horn similar to the cuticle. The hyponychium is the first site of keratinization in the nail unit (8,9,11–13) and of all epidermis in the embryo (95). The

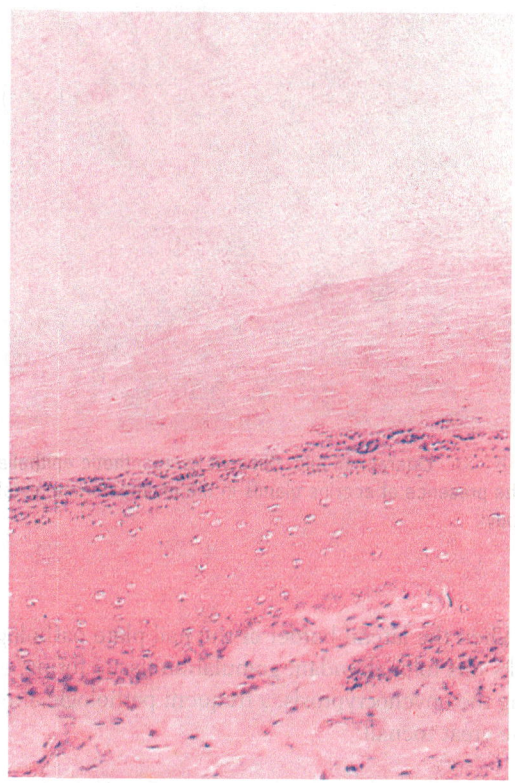

FIGURE 2.22 Detail of the hyponychium zone. Note the great keratin layer under the nail plate and the visible granular layer. The epithelium shows an acanthotic aspect, with transversal papillae.

function of this anatomical formation is to render the nail bed impermeable to protect it from external agents (96). If this structure fails, dermatophyte invasions will be frequent, producing onychomycosis (97).

Terry (39) describes an intermediate zone between the nail bed and the hyponychium, which he called onychodermal band. Terry speculated that this area, normally from 0.5- to 1.5-mm wide, had a blood supply different from the remainder of the nail bed, a fact later confirmed by other authors (40). For this reason, the color is paler than the pink nail bed and has a slightly amber tinge with a translucent quality. The onychodermal band occasionally changes its color, especially in cirrhosis and other chronic diseases (37,41).

Lateral Nail Folds

The lateral nail folds have a structure similar to the adjacent skin but are normally devoid of dermatoglyphic markings and pilosebaceous glands. Acanthosis and papillomatosis of the epithelium are present, similar to that of the hyponychium. Keratinization within the nail folds proceeds by keratohyalin formation in the granular layer (Fig. 2.23). The epidermis lining of these grooves does not contribute to the formation of the nail plate, except in the most proximal portions of the grooves, where it becomes continuous with the epidermis of the PNF or matrix.

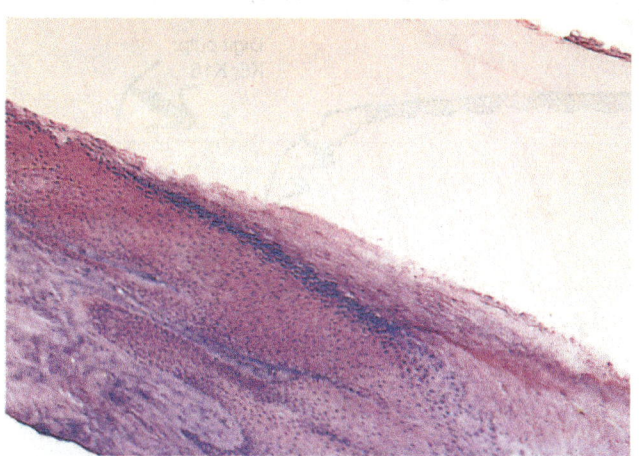

FIGURE 2.21 Hyponychium zone. The most important feature of this zone is the great accumulation of keratin under the distal nail plate.

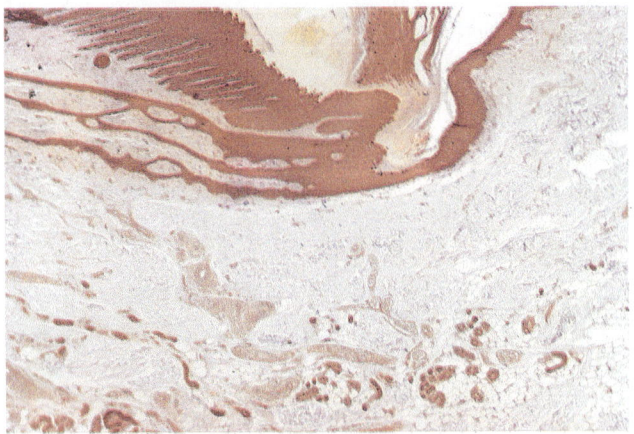

FIGURE 2.23 Lateral nail fold. Observe its acanthotic epithelial layer and the presence of eccrine glands in the middle dermis (cytokeratin antibody).

When the lateral border of the nail plate pathologically breaks this fold, abundant granulation tissue forms, constituting the onychocryptosis, a frequent pathologic alteration of the great toenail.

IMMUNOHISTOCHEMISTRY OF THE NAIL UNIT

Nail Plate

The cornified envelope of the epidermis is formed by several precursor proteins, including involucrin, keratolinin, loricrin, pancornulin, sciellin, 195-kDa protein, keratin, and filaggrin. Baden and Kvedar (98) have demonstrated that in the nail, monoclonal antibodies show the presence of pancornulin in the nail fold and proximal matrix, while sciellin was detected in the nail fold, matrix, and bed. Similarly, in studies of the human nails (which contain hard keratins), the use of immunofluorescence, immunoblotting, and PCR have shown that trichohyalin, a 200-kDa protein of the inner root sheath and medulla, was present in the ventral matrix, but not in the nail bed; a few scattered cells stained for trichohyalin were observed within the nail plate (99).

Heid et al. (100) studied the keratin expression patterns observed in the human fetal nail matrix and revealed that the nail develops from both skin- and hair-type differentiating cells. Kitahara and Ogawa (101) demonstrated that AE1/AE3 antibody reacted with the dorsal nail matrix. As AE1/AE3 antibody recognized hard keratins which are characteristics of differentiation in hair, these results show that adult nail develops in such a way that hair-type differentiation is confined to the ventral nail matrix, supporting Heid et al. results (102,103).

Keratinocytes

Expression of keratins in the different compartments within the nail unit has been demonstrated in some recent articles (17,104–112). The characteristics of the different keratins found at different sites could be relevant to our understanding of the biology of the normal nail and changes seen in several diseases.

Analysis of human nail plate by gel electrophoresis demonstrates a range of keratins of two characteristic types,

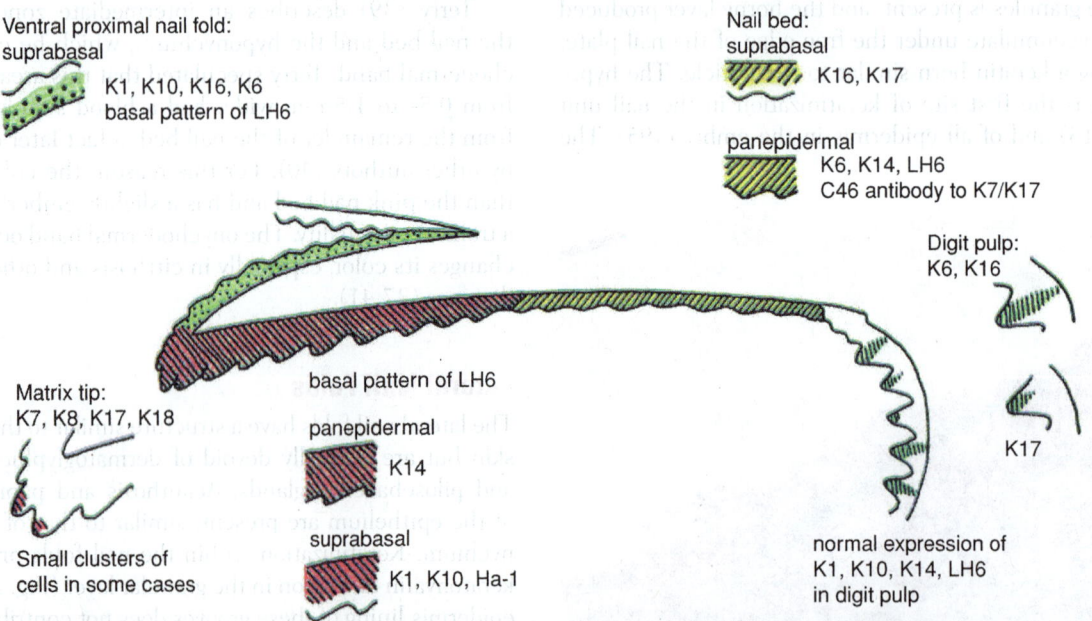

FIGURE 2.24 Keratin expression in the normal nail unit: Markers of regional differentiation. From De Berker D, Wojnarowska F, Sviland L, et al. Keratin expression in the normal nail unit: markers of regional differentiation. *Br J Dermatol* 2000;142:89–96.

as we commented formerly (see before "Genetic and Nail Keratins"). "Soft" or epithelial keratins represent the major structural intermediate filament isolated from human skin, but constitute only 10% to 20% of the keratin found in nails (101). "Hard" keratins, characteristic of hair and nail differentiation, which exist in the same acid–base heterodimer configuration as soft epithelial keratins, but have additional resilience.

Molecular classification of hard keratin proteins on gel electrophoresis describes eight major (Ha1–4 and Hb1–4) and two minor (Hax and Hbx) proteins, all of which are probably present in the human nail (100). This family has been extended by genome analysis into at least seven type I Ha keratins and six type II Hb keratins. Further keratins and their isoforms are likely to be discovered. In addition to the hard keratins, epithelial keratins isolated from the nail plate include K1, K10, K5, K14, K6, K16, K17, and K19 from fetal nail (17,100) (Fig. 2.24). Ha1 is one of the major hard keratins found in nail, where hard keratin represents 80% to 90% of nail keratin.

Pancytokeratin antibodies can be used to demonstrate keratins in the nail. AE-1/AE-3 is a keratin cocktail that detects CK1–8, 10, 14–16, and 19 (Fig. 2.25). The most evident positive for cytokeratin in nail region is to CK5–8 (Fig. 2.26) and CK-14 stains (Fig. 2.27). Cytokeratin 15, 19, and 20 are poorly expressed in the nail matrix (Fig. 2.28). It is very interesting that CK-KL1 stain is very positive to the dorsal nail matrix epithelium but negative in the ventral nail matrix (Fig. 2.29). Epithelial membrane antigen (EMA) stains, can demonstrate some isolated positive areas in the nail bed (Fig. 2.30). In the same way, claudin-1 (CLDN1) is a major component of the tight junction structure and plays an important role in cell–cell adhesion. This former stain is very positive, expressed in the upper layers of the nail matrix epithelium (Fig. 2.31).

Berker et al. (17) found a low expression of the differentiation-specific keratins K1 and K10 in the keratogenous zone of the ventral matrix, and no expression in the nail bed. However, Perrin et al. have reported the absence of keratin 10 from both the nail matrix and nail bed (104). Keratins K6, K16, and K17 are normally found in hyperproliferative epidermis, such as in psoriasis or in wound healing (105). Studies of proliferative compartments in the nail unit suggest that the nail bed is not a major contributor to the nail plate. It may be that the ventral aspect of the PNF and not the nail bed is the source of nail plate K6 and K16, and the matrix and not the nail bed provides K17. K14 is synthesized in the basal layer and K14 protein was detected throughout the epithelium, as has been noted in other tissues. However, the marker of basal keratin conformation, LH6, was also seen throughout the nail bed. This is unusual and may reflect the absence of the expression of the suprabasal keratins K1 and K10, which are thought to obscure the epitopes detected by LH6 in normal stratified epithelium. This persistence of LH6 antigen is also seen in the outer root sheath of the hair follicle, which is also the site of expression of K16, K6, and K17 (106), supporting the analogy drawn between the nail bed and outer root sheath (107). However, expression of K1 and K10 is found to a degree in the upper outer root sheath superficial to the level of the sebaceous gland.

The absence of K1 and K10 from the nail bed correlates with a reduction in terminal differentiation. Lack of cornification is also seen in mucosal epithelium in combination with the presence of K16 and K17. However, mucosal differentiation is defined by the presence of K4 and K13, which was absent in the nail bed (108).

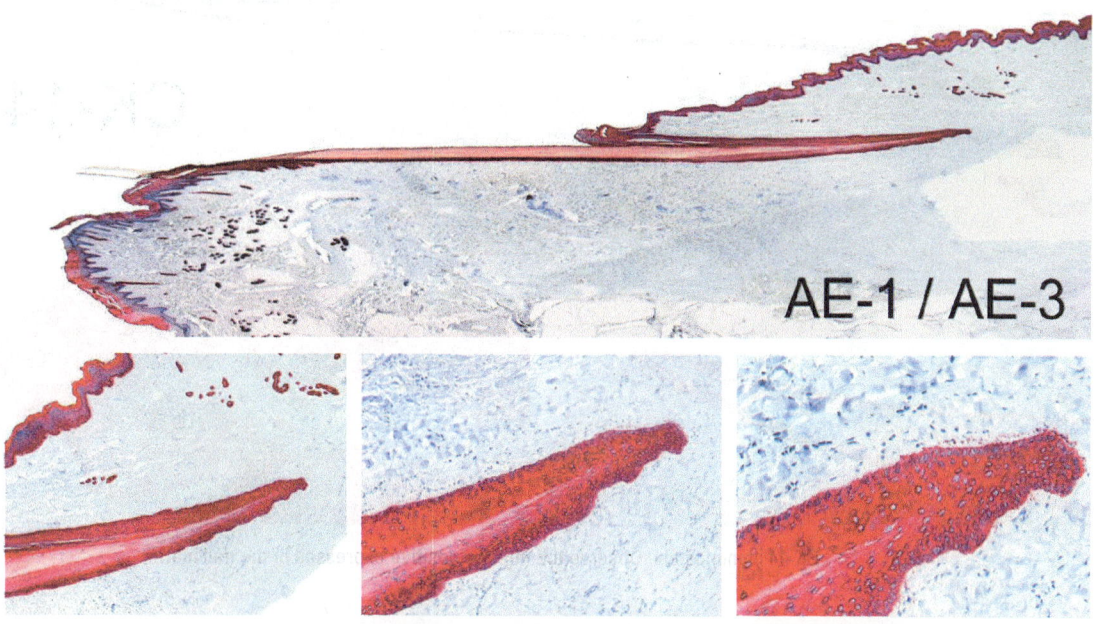

FIGURE 2.25 Pan-keratin AE-1/AE-3 in normal nail matrix.

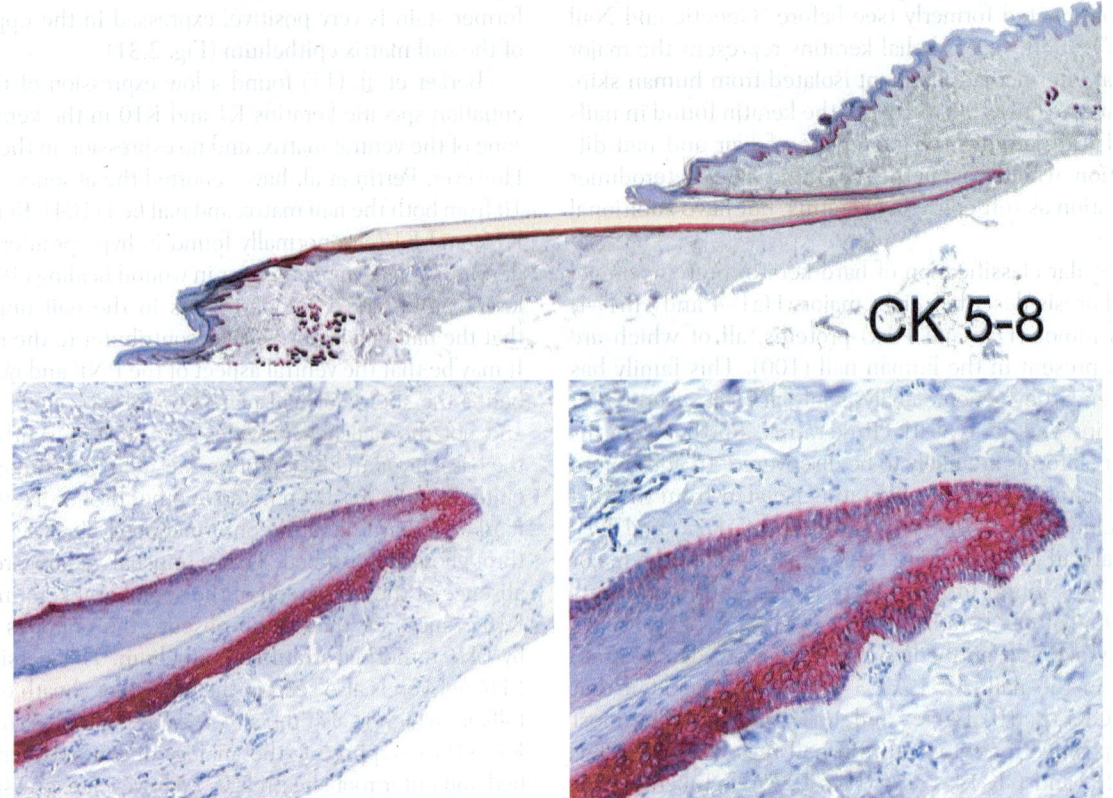

FIGURE 2.26 CK-5–8 immunostain.

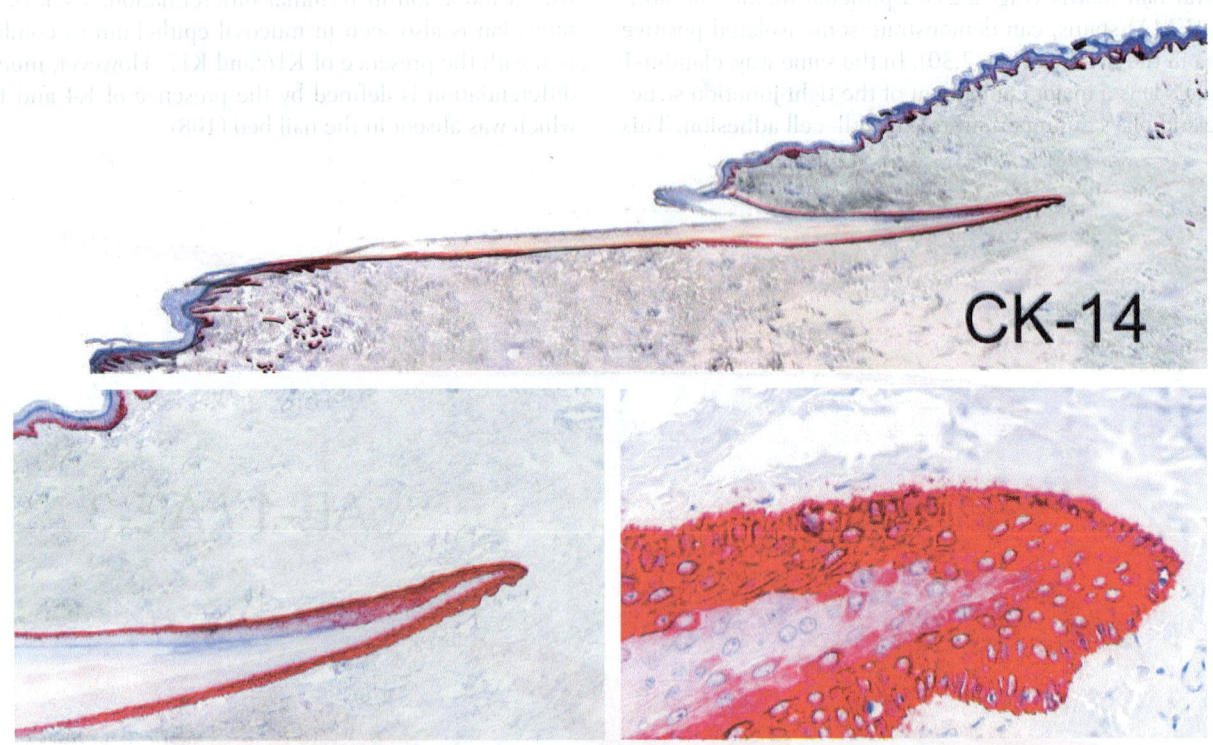

FIGURE 2.27 CK-14 immunostain. Observe the intense positive expressed in the nail matrix.

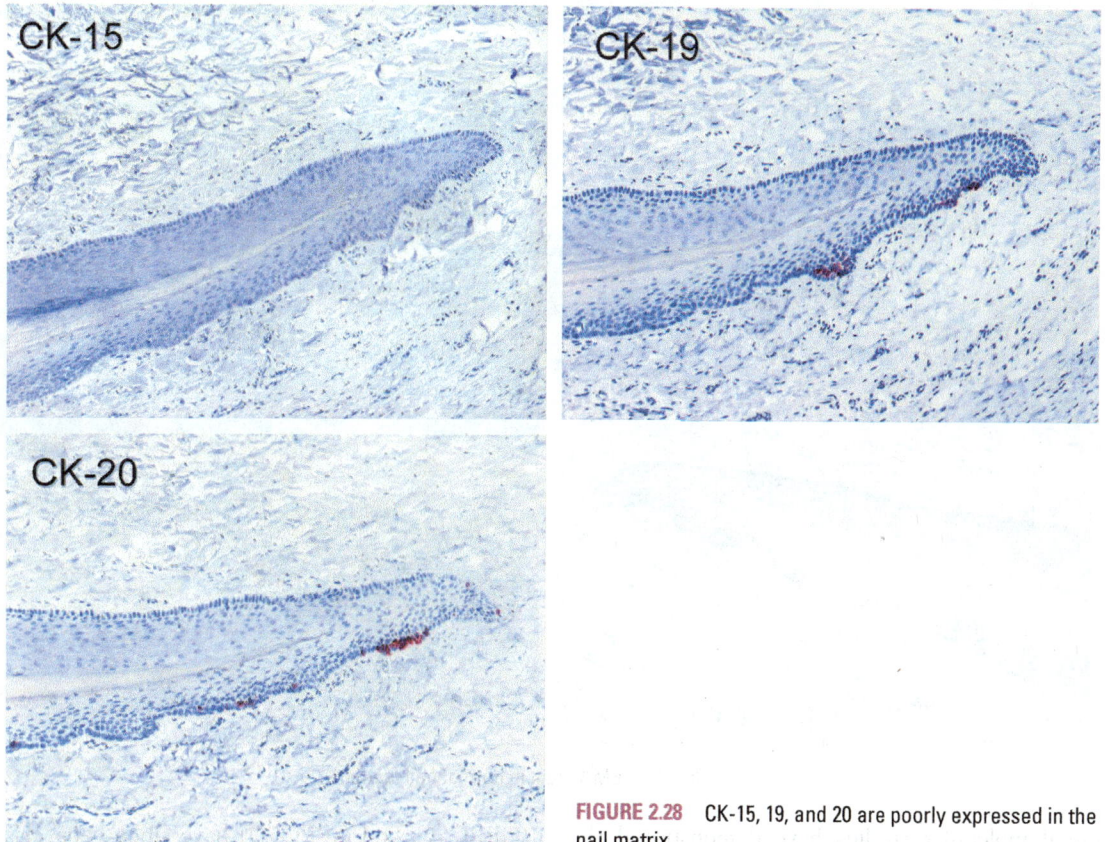

FIGURE 2.28 CK-15, 19, and 20 are poorly expressed in the nail matrix.

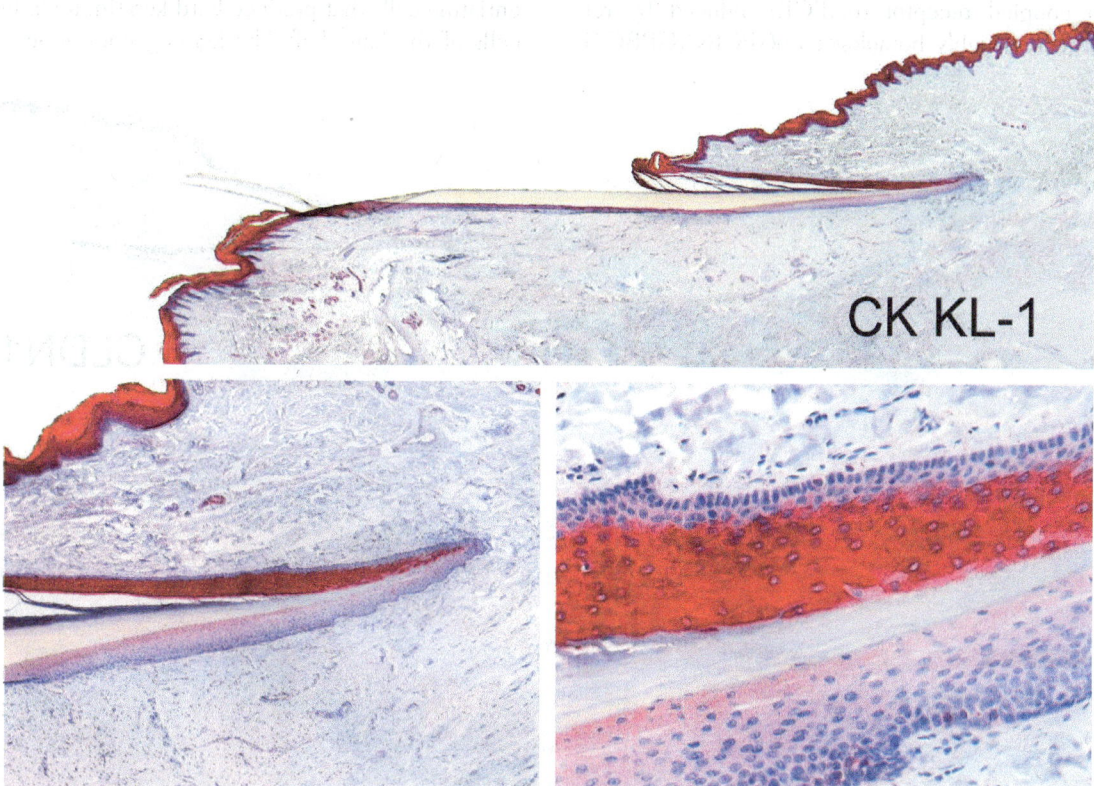

FIGURE 2.29 CK-KL1 immunostain demonstrated an intense positive to the dorsal nail matrix, but negative in the ventral nail matrix epithelium.

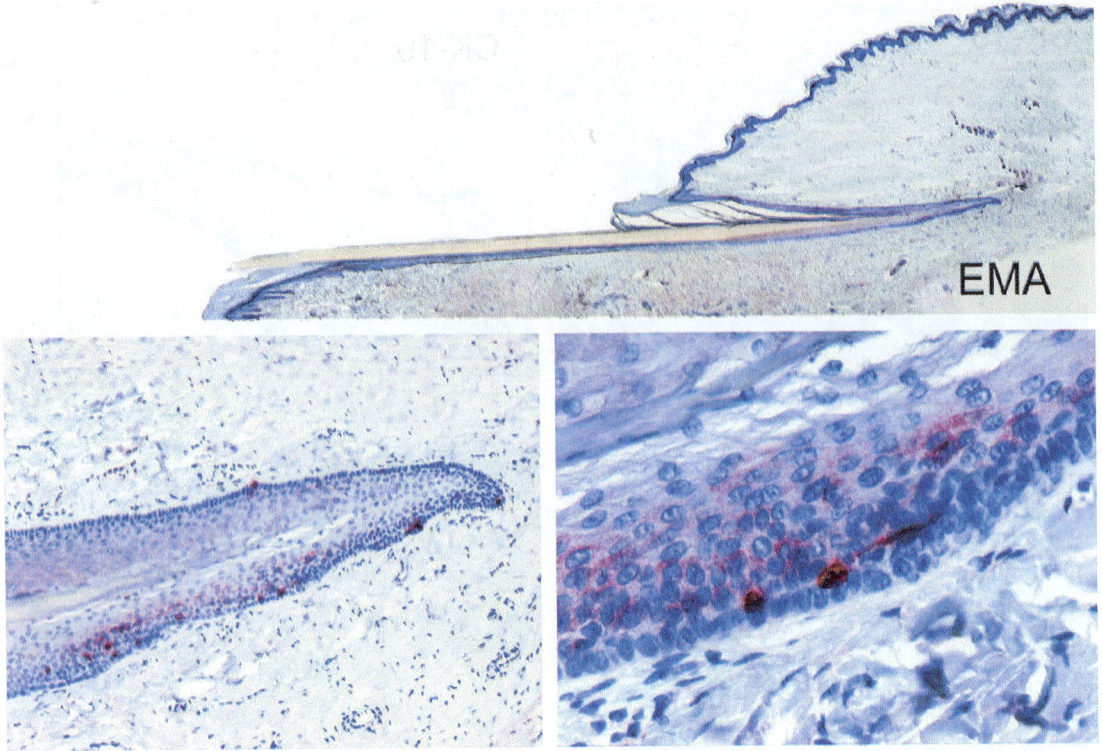

FIGURE 2.30 EMA stain in normal nail matrix.

Additional molecular studies have demonstrated the homology between hair and nail keratins (109). Retinoic acid-inducible gene-1 was originally identified as an orphan G-protein coupled receptor (oGPCR) induced by retinoic acid. Three highly homologous oGPCRs (GPRC5B, GPRC5C, and GPRC5D) have since been classified into the RAIG1 family. Inoue et al. (109) studied the distribution of GPRC5D, and found that it is expressed in differentiating cells that produce hard keratin, including cortical cells of the hair shaft, the keratogenous zone of the nail,

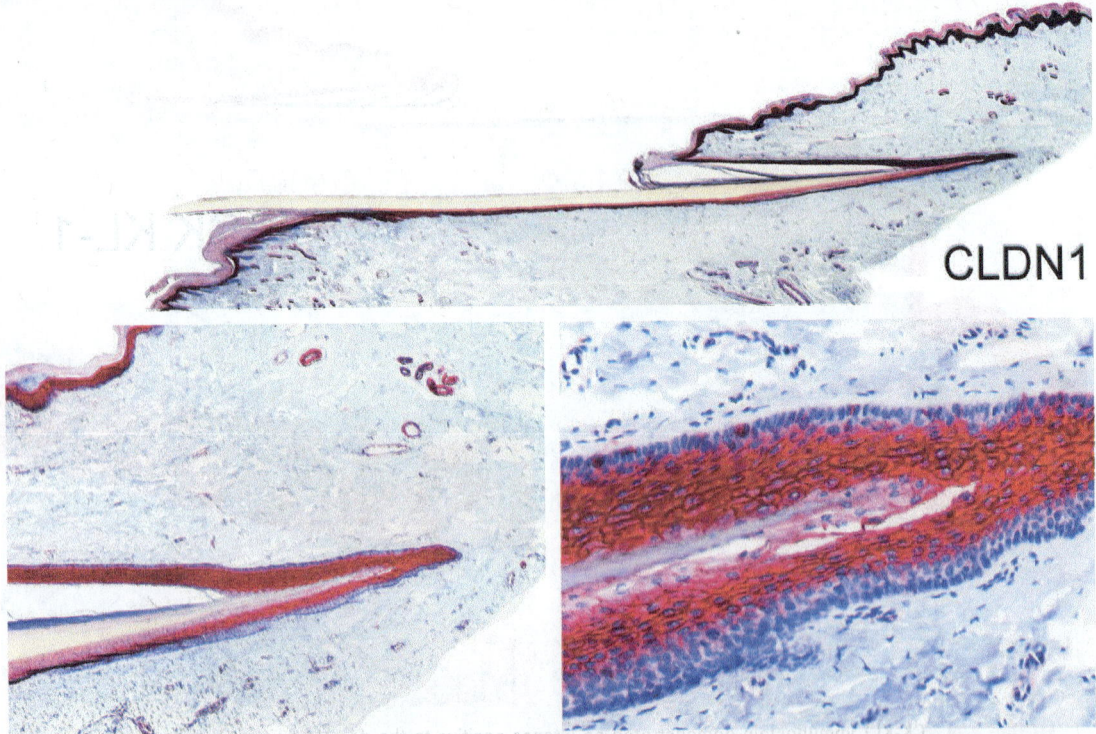

FIGURE 2.31 Claudin-1 (CLDN-1) is very positive in the upper layers of the nail matrix epithelium.

and in a central region of the filiform papillae of the tongue. The differentiation inducer, all-trans retinoic acid, induces GPRC5D expression in cultured hair bulb cells. Since the tissue distribution of GPRC5D indicates a relationship with hard keratins that constitute the major structural proteins of hard epithelial tissues, they investigated the effect of GPRC5D on acid hard keratins. Analyses of cultured cells showed that transient overexpression resulted in suppression of Ha3 and stimulation of Ha4 hair keratin gene expression. The expression was maintained in the hair follicles of winged helix nude-deficient (nude) mice, suggesting that this gene is regulated by a signal pathway different from that of hair keratin synthesis. These data provide a framework for understanding the molecular mechanisms of GPRC5D function in hard keratinization.

Matrical fibroblasts are essential in the expression of hard keratin by matrical keratinocytes. Okazaki et al. (110) demonstrated that even in non–nail-matrical keratinocyte expression of hard keratin could be induced by nail-matrical fibroblasts. These investigators constructed three different skin equivalents: (a) ventral keratinocytes (from the ventral side of the digit) were cocultured with ventral fibroblasts (group A); (b) ventral keratinocytes were cocultured with nail-matrical fibroblasts (group B); and (c) nail-matrical keratinocytes were cocultured with ventral fibroblasts (group C). Immunohistochemical examinations with anti–hard keratin antibody (HKN-7) revealed hard keratin expression in groups B and C. This study indicated extrinsic hard keratin induction in non–nail-matrical keratinocytes by nail-matrical fibroblasts and suggests that non–nail-matrical epidermal grafts may be effective in the treatment of deepithelized nail injuries.

Human carcinoembryonic antigen (CEA) and CEA-related molecules play an important role in adhesion of the nail plate to the nail bed. Egawa et al. (111) demonstrated that a CEA family antigen with NCA (CD66c)-like immunoreactivity was strongly expressed in the keratinocytes distributed in the upper epithelial cell layers of the major central portions of the nail bed, to which the nail plate is firmly bonded. This expression was stronger at the more distal portion of the nail bed, and was absent in the nail matrix, the hyponychium, and the lateral folds. The results are interesting because the nail plate is firmly bonded to the nail bed, less so proximal to the matrix margin, and it has been shown that the bed epithelium travels at the same speed as the nail plate, indicating that the bed epithelium has a proximal site of origin and a distal end.

Plasminogen activator inhibitor type 2 (PAI-2) was detected in the differentiating cells of the matrix and nail bed (112). These authors have suggested that this inhibitor may confer protection against programmed cell death. This consistent, selective distribution of PAI-2 in the postmitotic, maturing cells prior to terminal keratinization and death suggests that: (a) PAI-2 may be considered as a differentiation marker for many epithelial cell types; and (b) PAI-2 is appropriately positioned to protect epithelial cells from premature demise (112).

Recently, a special mesenchyme containing onychofibroblast has been described in the nail matrix and nail bed by Lee Y et al. (113). This mesenchyme is immunohistochemically and histologically different from the rest of the nail dermis, and it has been given the name of onychodermis. The presence of CD10 (cell surface metalloprotease) has only been detected in this matrix and bed nail dermis and not in the dermis of the rest of the nail. The exact function of CD10 in the matrix and the nail bed is not clearly defined (114). CD13 is another protein that is frequently expressed together with CD10 in other tissues, and also appears in this specialized mesenchyme, both in bed and in nail matrix, although it is expressed with greater intensity in the latter. It is thought that this onychodermis containing onychofibroblasts plays an important role in the genesis of the nail and interact with the stem cells of the nail matrix (115).

The presence of β-catenin in the nail matrix has also recently been described. This protein, which is part of the Wingless/Integrated (Wnt)/β-catenin signaling pathway, had been described in the hair matrix cells, so it was known to play an important role in the morphogenesis of hair. Kim et al. (116) have reported for the first time the presence of β-catenin in the nucleus and cytoplasm of the cells of the nail matrix, which means that both structures (the hair matrix and the nail matrix) have similar properties.

Merkel Cells

Lacour et al. (117), in a double indirect immunofluorescence and immunoelectron microscopy with the monoclonal antibody Troma-1, have only found MCs in the PNF of the adults, with a concentration greater than 50 MCs/mm^2.

Immunohistochemically, keratins K8 and K18 have been used as markers of MCs (82). MCs have neuroendocrine characteristics and are of uncertain function, although their prominence in the nail unit in the early stages of fetal development has been noted, and a role in ontogenesis has been proposed. The number and location of cells demonstrating K8 and K18, which included the rete ridges of the digit pulp, suggested that these cells were MCs rather than contributing directly to nail plate formation.

Melanocytes

Melanocyte immunostains find a scarce number of melanocytes in the normal nail matrix. In this way, S-100, HMB-45, and Melan-A may demonstrate isolated cells in this area (Fig. 2.32). Tosti et al. (118), have studied the melanocyte characterization of the normal nail matrix, using immunohistochemistry techniques. These authors found nail matrix melanocytes reacted with the antibodies anti-PEP1, anti-Pep8, and anti-TMP1, which recognize the tyrosinase-related protein-1, the tyrosinase-related protein-2 (DOPA-chrome tautomerase), and the tyrosinase-related protein encoded by pMT4 (Table 2.4). This confirms that, even if

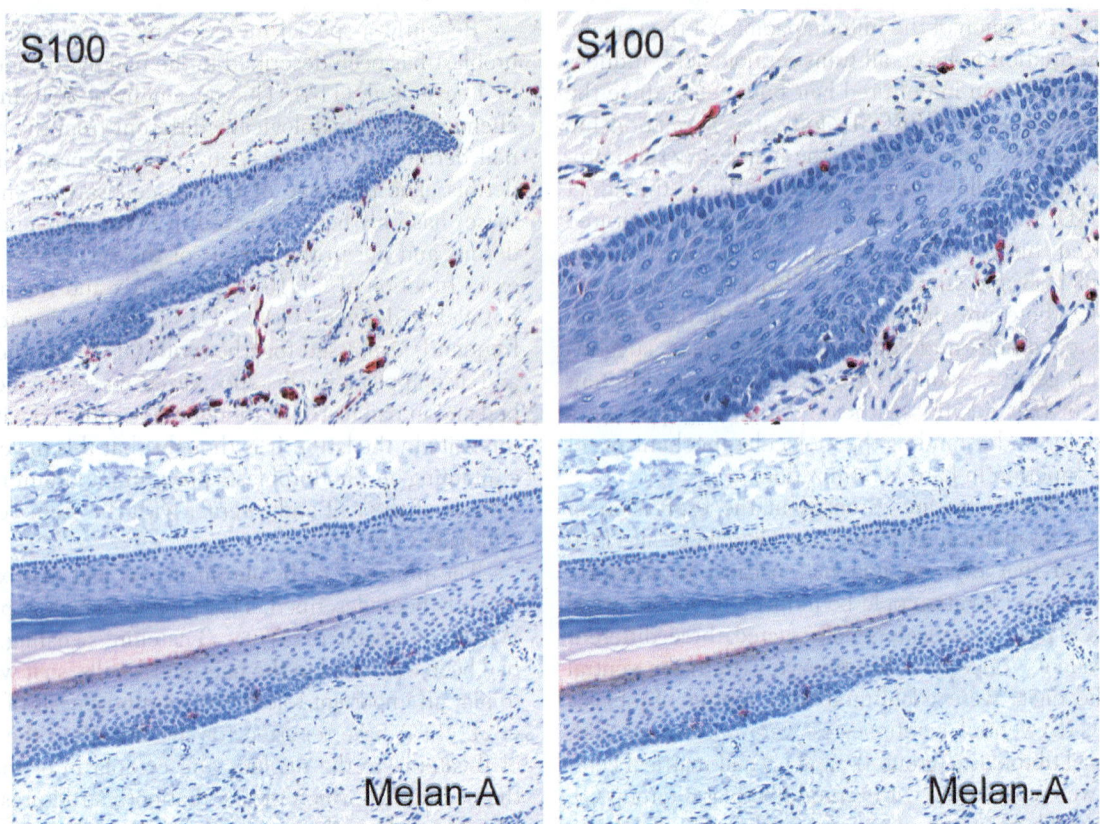

FIGURE 2.32 S-100 and Melan-A immunostains in the nail matrix.

normally quiescent, nail matrix melanocytes possess the key enzymes responsible for the formation of melanin pigment (119).

Expression of integrins in the nail matrix has been studied by Cameli et al. (120). These authors found that α-2-β-1 and α-3-β-1 expression differ in nail matrix epithelium. In the nail matrix, these integrins are not only expressed on the basal layer, but also on the fourth to fifth suprabasal layers, with suprabasal expression gradually decreasing from the distal to the proximal matrix (Table 2.5). As in the normal human epidermis, α-1, α-4, and α-5 integrin subunits are not expressed in the nail matrix; in the same way, ICAM-1, the ligand of LFA1, was negative in the matrix cells. The expression of β-1 subunits in the suprabasal layers of the nail matrix indicates a very strong cohesion between nail matrix cells, this probably revealing them to be an essential prerequisite for the development of a compact nail plate. Cultures of nail matrix cells may represent a useful model to study the biologic properties of nail structure (121).

As melanocytes of the human pigmentary unit show deficient classical MHC class I expression (122), we investigated the human leukocyte antigen (HLA)-A/B/C expression on melanocytes in nail matrix. Melanocytes in the PNF and nail bed were strongly HLA-A/B/C+. In contrast, PNM melanocytes displayed no HLA-A/B/C immunoreactivity. This reflects the situation in the (MHC class I-negative) human hair follicle matrix (123) and further supports the notion that the human nail matrix is a site of relative immune privilege.

Comparable with the hair follicle (124,125), lack of MHC class I expression on nail melanocytes may prevent attacks by autoreactive CD8+ T cells on melanocyte-associated antigens in PNM. Collapse of nail immune privilege and a concomitant ectopic upregulation of MHC class I expression on nail melanocytes, for example, in patients with alopecia areata may expose melanocytes to immune recognition and cytotoxic autoimmune attack (124).

TABLE 2.4 Immunostaining of Human Nail Melanocytes[a]

Antibody	Reactive to	Species	Nail Matrix Melanocytes
Anti-PEP1	Tyrosine-related protein-1	Rabbit	++
Anti-PEP8	Tyrosine-related protein-2 (DOPA-chrome tautomerase)	Rabbit	+
HMB-45	Glycoconjugate present in immature melanosomes	Mouse	++
TMH-1	Tyrosinase-related protein encoded by pMT4	Mouse	+

[a]Tosti A, Cameli N, Piraccini BM, et al. Characterization of nail matrix melanocytes with anti-PEP1, anti-PEP8, TMH-1 and HMB-45 antibodies. *J Am Acad Dermatol* 1994;31:193–196.

TABLE 2.5
Integrin Expression in Human Nail Matrix[a]

	α-1	α-2	α-3	α-4	α-5	α-6	α-v	β-1	β-4	ICAM-1
Basal membrane zone	−	−	−	−	−	+++	−	−	+++	−
Basal layer	−	++	++	−	−	++	++	++	++	−
Suprabasal layer (ventral matrix)	−	++	++	−	−	−	+	++	−	−
Suprabasal layers (dorsal matrix)	−	+	+	−	−	−	+	+	−	−
Keratogenous zone	−	−	−	−	−	−	−	−	−	−

[a]Cameli N, Picardo M, Tosti A, et al. Expression of integrins in human nail matrix. *Br J Dermatol* 1994;130:583–588.

Immunology and Inflammatory Cells

The nail apparatus is constantly exposed to environmental damage. It requires effective immune responses to combat infection, while avoiding the loss of nail production and regeneration by autoaggressive immunity. Ito et al. (125) have well described the immunology of the human nail apparatus.

Compared with other regions of nail epithelium, HLA-A/B/C expression is prominently downregulated on both keratinocytes and melanocytes of the PNM, whereas HLA-G(+) is upregulated here. Together with the expression of macrophage migration inhibitory factor in PNM, this may serve to inhibit a natural killer (NK) cell attack on major histocompatibility complex class Ia-negative PNM, and also displays strong immunoreactivity for potent, locally generated immunosuppressants such as transforming growth factor-β1, α-melanocyte stimulating hormone, insulin-like growth factor-1, and adrenocorticotropic hormone, exhibits unusually few CD1a(+), CD4(+), or CD8(+), NK, and mast cells.

In the same way, Ito et al. (122,125) found important immunologic differences between the nail apparatus and the pilosebaceous unit in man:

- $β_2$ microglobulin is not detected in the proximal epithelium of human hair follicle, but was positive in the PNF.

- In contrast to the strongly MHC class I+ and $β_2$ microglobulin + mesenchyme of the human hair follicle, the nail immune privilege appears to extend to the periungual mesenchyme, especially around the PNF, as the latter is also MHC class I-negative and shows a greatly reduced number of T, Langerhans, and NK cells.

- HLA-G is strongly expressed in the nail matrix, but has not been reported in human hair matrix and was also not found by us in sections of normal human scalp skin.

MHC class II and CD 209 expression on CD1a(+) cells in and around the proximal matrix is reduced, indicating diminished antigen-presenting capacity. Thus, the nail immune system strikingly differs from the skin immune system, but shows intriguing similarities to the hair follicle immune system, including the establishment of an area of relative immune privilege in the PNF. This nail immune privilege may offer a relative safeguard against autoimmunity. But, the localized intraepithelial defect of innate and adaptive immunity in the PNM revealed here also may impede effective anti-infection defense.

Bcl-2 immunostain is very positive in the ventral nail matrix epithelium; however, p53 and Ki-67 stains were poorly expressed in this area (Fig. 2.33).

On the other hand, chronic and acute inflammatory nail disorders because of infection or irritation (maceration, chemical damage) affect primarily the PNF not the PNM. Therefore, it is conceivable that the relative immune privilege of the PNM may serve to suppress inflammatory/autoimmune damage to the most critical component of the actual "nail factory" to promote the survival chances of a species by protecting it from a loss of claws, hooves, or nails because of proinflammatory environmental insults (maceration, trauma, chemical irritation, bacterial and fungal infection), and to quickly restore the vital use of these skin appendages by limiting swelling and pain after nail trauma or infection.

ULTRASTRUCTURAL ANATOMY

Very few studies of the normal ultrastructural morphology of the nail exist (10–13,44,45,72–75,79,90), because of varied difficulties (73): (a) achieving proper fixation and adequate penetration of epoxy resin into the nail plate; (b) obtaining ultrathin sections; and (c) securing the high-voltage electron beam necessary to penetrate through extraordinarily hard tissue and availability of 100- to 200-kV machines.

The proximal end of the human toenail is composed of several layers of epithelial cells. Hashimoto et al. (72–75) make the distinction between a proximal dorsal, apical, and ventral matrix, although noting that there are few differences between them. They found that the cells composing the proximal matrix were: (a) relatively small, elongated basal cells attached to the basal lamina; (b) relatively large,

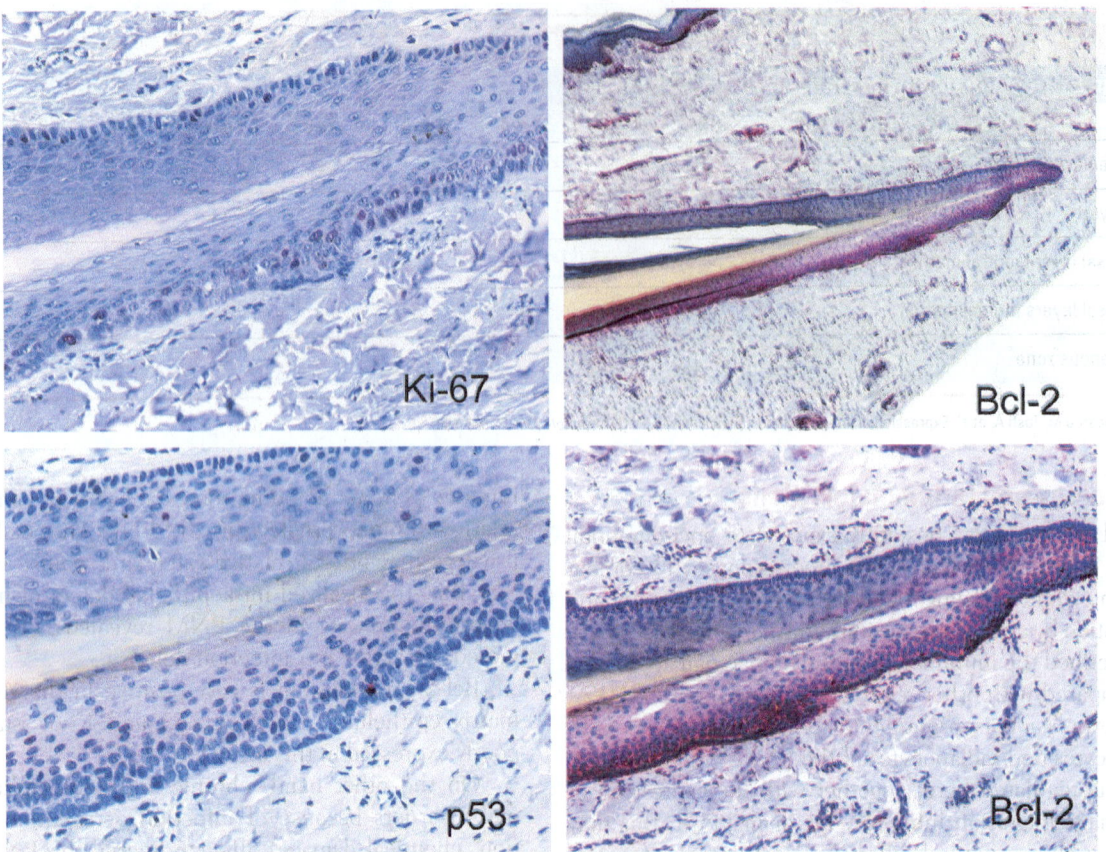

FIGURE 2.33 Ki-67, Bcl-2, and p53 immunostains.

round, or polygonal squamous cells filling the more central portion of the matrix; (c) melanocytes; (d) Langerhans cells; and (e) MCs.

Moreover, there exists a system of attachment to the dermis, showing the surface of the basal cell with frequent finger-like elongations that interdigitate with the papillary dermis (Fig. 2.34). This results in the formation of numerous micropapillae, with bundles of very fine fibrils (11 to 12 mm). The subjacent dermis of the matrix zone shows poor vascularity and scarce collagen fibers, with abundant basic matrix.

The basal cells are very active, with frequent mitotic figures. They showed an elongated nucleus and cytoplasm with numerous, slender projections (or villi) intricately interdigitated with neighboring cells. Tonofibrils were also seen as a perinuclear ring with an interposition of the nuclear clear zone in which the majority of mitochondria, transferred melanosomes, and occasional centrioles are located. The suprabasal matrix cells are also round, with frequent mitotic figures. In general, the long axes of these cells were oriented axiodistally, suggesting the direction of their migration. Large intercellular spaces were often seen between these suprabasal cells. The extensive interdigitation of the peripheral villi as seen in the basal cells disappeared and

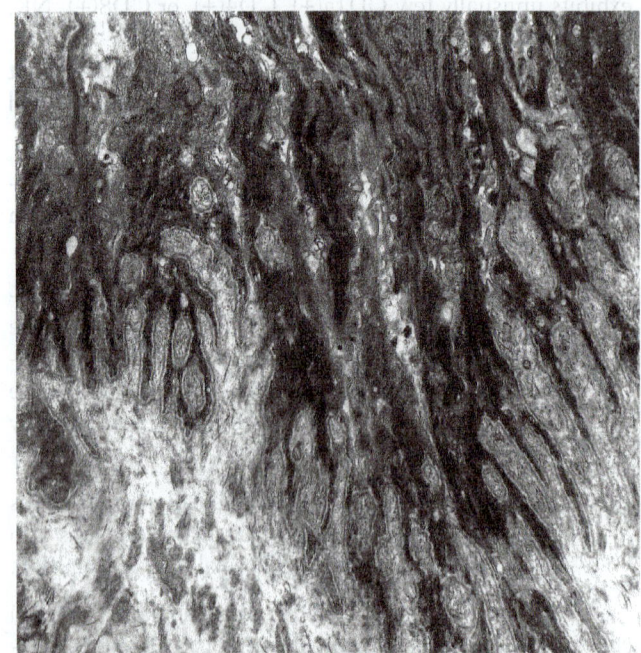

FIGURE 2.34 Ultrastructural appearance of the dermoepidermal junction of the intermediate matrix. The basal layer shows an accentuated digitiform distribution, with multiple intermediate filaments (×7,000).

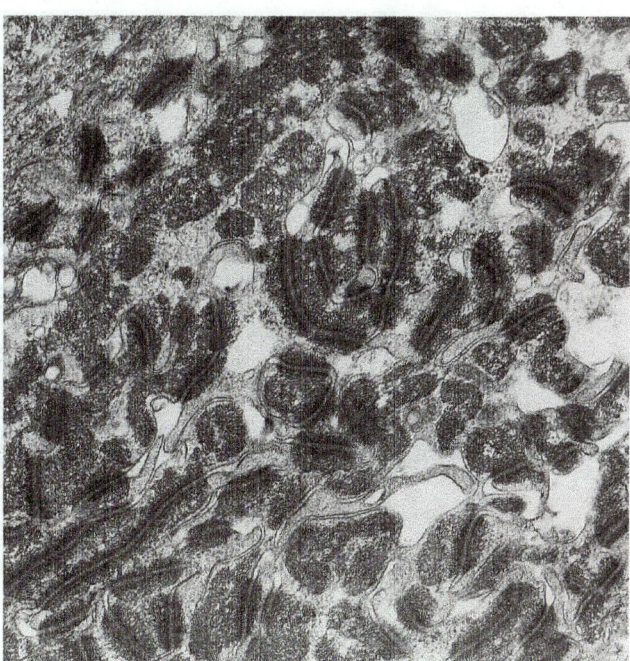

FIGURE 2.35 Detail of the desmosomal junctions of the suprabasal layer. They are bigger and more abundant than in a normal epidermis (×12,000).

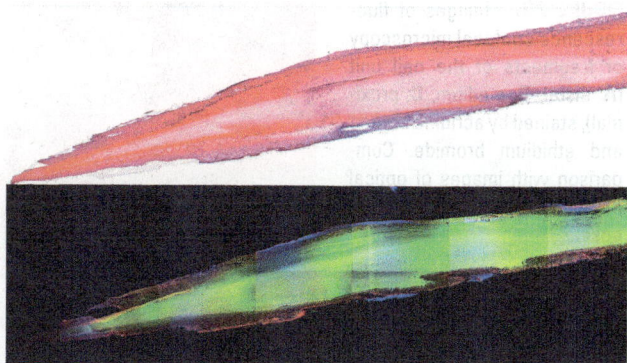

FIGURES 2.36 Image of fluorescence confocal microscopy of the nail unit, stained by acridine orange and ethidium bromide. Comparison with images of optical microscopy with hematoxylin-eosin.

multiple desmosomal junctions alone connected these cells (Fig. 2.35).

Abundant desmosomes can be seen in the intermediate layers with high condensations of intermediate fibrils. The aspect of the intermediate layer of the nail matrix is similar to the upper layers of the normal epidermis. The cells have lost their organelles, and their cytoplasm is nearly filled with tonofibrils. For this reason, the keratinization process is very abrupt, passing from three to four cellular lines to completely keratinized corneocytes.

CONFOCAL MICROSCOPY OF NAIL

Confocal microscopy (CM) is a high-resolution emerging imaging technique that can be used to explore the entire body surface, including skin, mucosa, hair and nails. This technique can be performed on the nail in vivo, or on nail fragments extirpated (ex vivo). Stains can also be applied to improve the differentiation of structures by fluorescence. This process is known as fluorescence CM (Figs. 2.36 and 2.37).

The nail plate transparency allows a deep penetration of CM that can image up to the nail bed in case of thin nails. The cost of CM is a limit for a wide use of this technology. Then, there is the limited penetration depth of about 400 to 500 lm, that does not allow to clearly image in vivo the nail bed and reach the nail matrix. The convex surface of the nail and the concavity of the transition between the nail plate and the surrounding skin make difficult to place and hold the device during in vivo imaging. The nail plate can be scanned from the surface to the lower part adjacent to the underlying nail bed. Three different layers can be differentiated by CM according to the intensity of the reflection. The superficial layer shows a brighter reflection, followed by a zone with slightly poorer signal, followed again by a brighter zone in the deepest part. The transition to the underlying nail bed is visible only in thin nails (<500 μm) and displayed in wave-like structures, which are directed toward the fingertip (126). The transition between the skin and the proximal part of the nail plate is characterized by a stripe corresponding to the cuticle, and by stellate figures corresponding to the membranes of keratinocytes sectioned obliquely on the skin side.

CM could play a role in the diagnosis of onychomycosis and melanonychia (127). Dermatophytes can be easily observed in nail plate as network of lengthy structures with high reflection and the typical shape of hyphae. CM has been shown to be useful in discriminating benign versus malignant melanocytic lesions of the skin, and can image melanocytes of the Hutchinson sign, but cannot penetrate in the nail matrix in vivo, to allow a diagnosis of subungueal melanoma in case of melanonychia. It is unable to directly explore the nail matrix located deep under the eponychium. However, it also helps in case of melanonychia to distinguish subungueal melanoma from lentigo and nevi because the matrix can be observed by reclining the eponychium (128).

CM has showed to be useful to confirm the diagnosis of periungueal and subungueal pyogenic granuloma, by showing a lobulated proliferation of capillary-sized vessels with possible secondary ulceration, hemorrhage, and inflammatory infiltrate. CM could be used in the future as a noninvasive procedure for the investigation of different inflammatory nail diseases, such as psoriasis and lichen planus (129). As a consequence, CM could reduce the number of nail biopsies in the diagnosis of nail disorder (130).

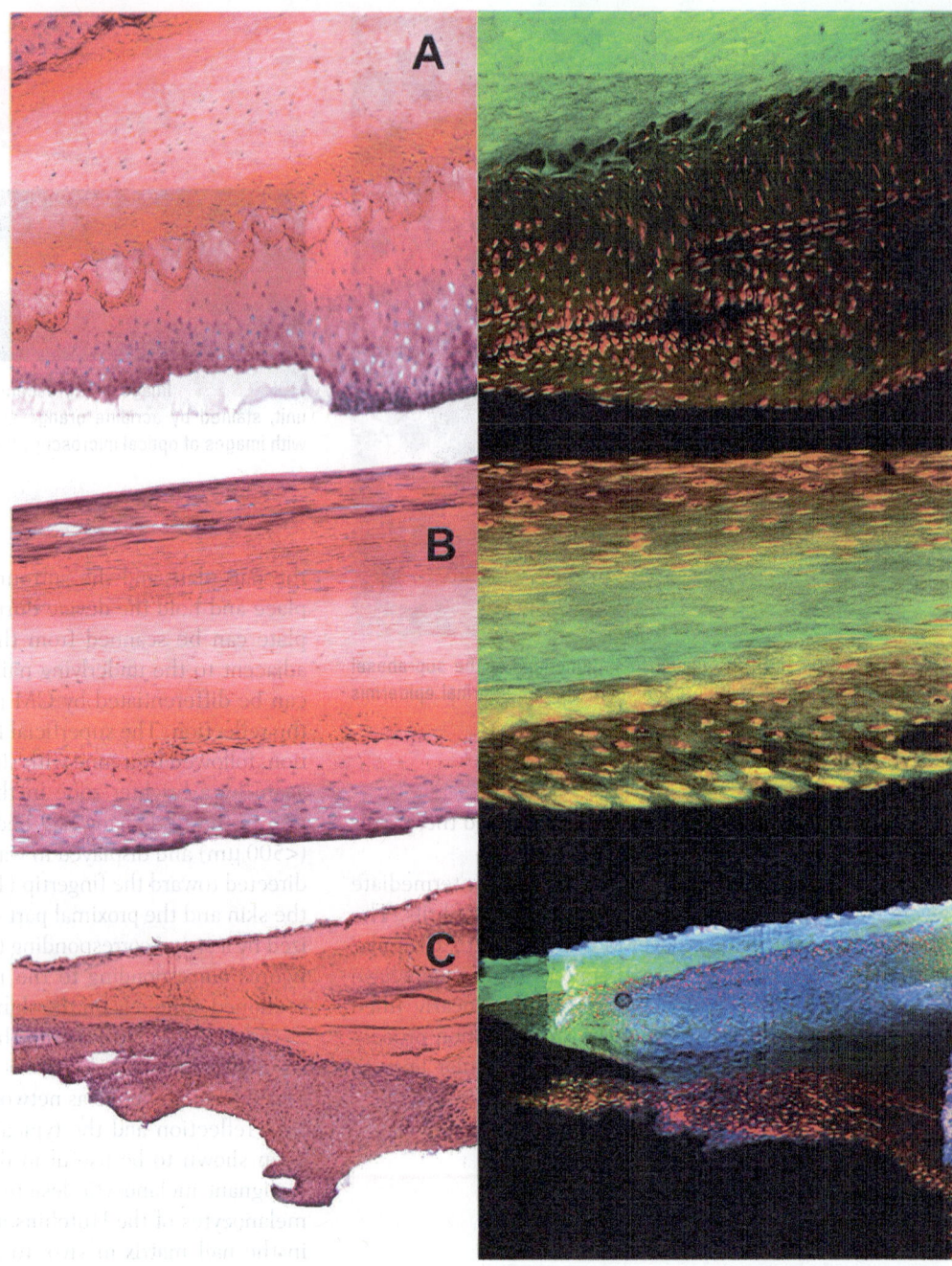

FIGURE 2.37 Images of fluorescence confocal microscopy of fragments of the nail unit (**A**: distal, **B**: medium, **C**: proximal), stained by acridine orange and ethidium bromide. Comparison with images of optical microscopy with hematoxylin-eosin.

OTHER TISSUES OF THE NAIL UNIT

Dermis

The dermal component of the nail structures is a very specialized tissue, unique in that it is limited by the underlying phalanx and closely associated with its vasculature and nerve supply. There is no subcutaneous tissue, as previously noted.

Dermis, epithelium, and nail plate in the nail bed present special histologic features due to the great traction that is supported. The dermis is very thick with a dense collagen layer. These fibers are vertically situated in the proximal zone of the nail bed (Fig. 2.38) and inclined at 45 degrees in the zone adjacent to the hyponychium (Fig. 2.39). Collagen-IV immunostains demonstrate an intense positive in this area (Fig. 2.40). Their mission is to attach the nail plate directly with the phalangeal periosteum. Conversely, the nail plate and the nail bed are quite firmly attached to each other, more so than the nail plate to the matrix, and this seems to be accomplished by the striking, deep longitudinal ridges and furrows of the nail surface of the nail plate. The nail bed has a unique, longitudinal, tongue-and-groove spatial arrangement of papillary dermal papillae and epidermal rete ridges. This feature is easily observed in

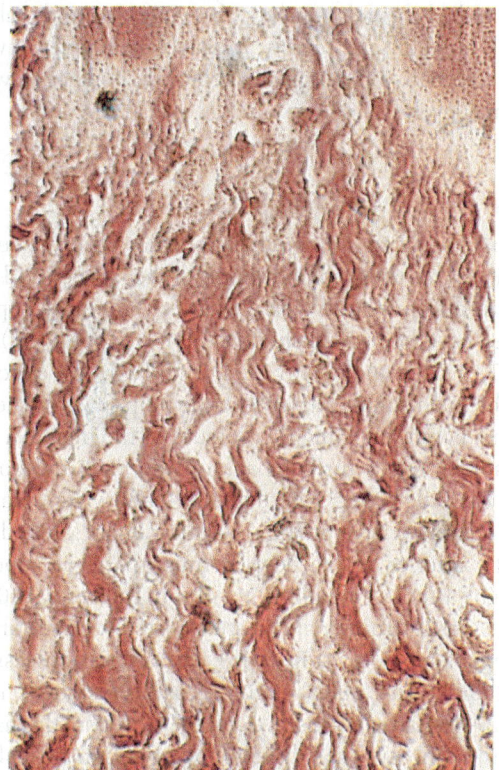

FIGURE 2.38 Collagen fibers of the proximal nail bed. Observe the peculiar vertical disposition (reticulin stain, ×**400**).

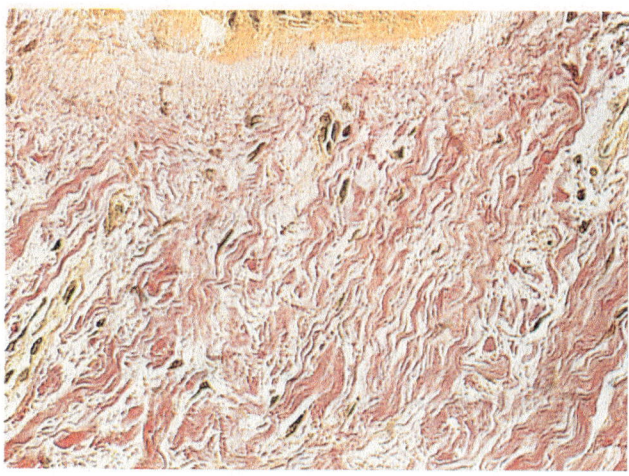

FIGURE 2.39 Collagen fibers of the distal nail bed. Observe the peculiar inclined disposition (VVG stain).

transverse sections, in which this arrangement is appreciated as a serrated interdigitation of the ventral surface of the nail, papillae, and rete. These furrows can be seen very well macroscopically just after avulsion of the nail plate, but they are also beautifully shown microscopically by optical microscope (Figs. 2.41 and 2.42) (90).

It has been recently introduced that the nail dermis has a specialized mesenchyme expressing CD10, called onychodermis (containing onychofibroblasts), which contains onychofibroblasts that may play an important role in the genesis of the nail, through interaction with the stem cells of the nail matrix (116,131).

There are few studies about the nerve supply of the nail. The matrix and nail bed present sparse nerve endings and few Vater–Pacini (132) and Meissner corpuscles

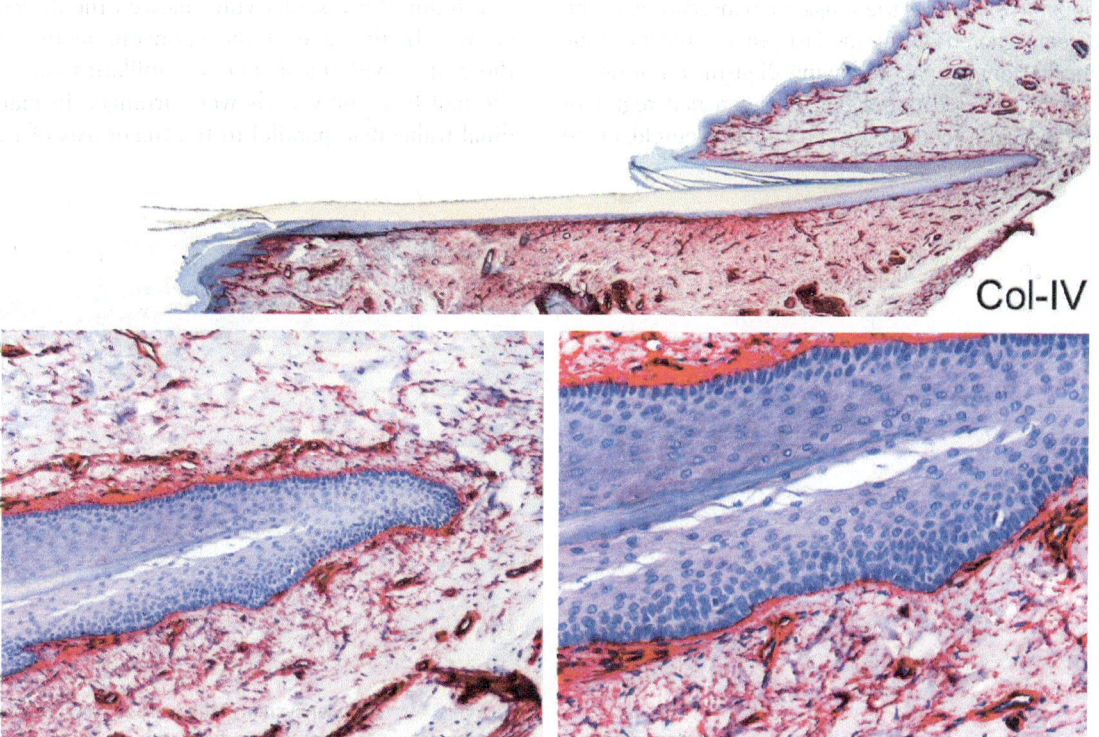

FIGURE 2.40 Collagen-IV (Col-IV) immunostains of the nail matrix.

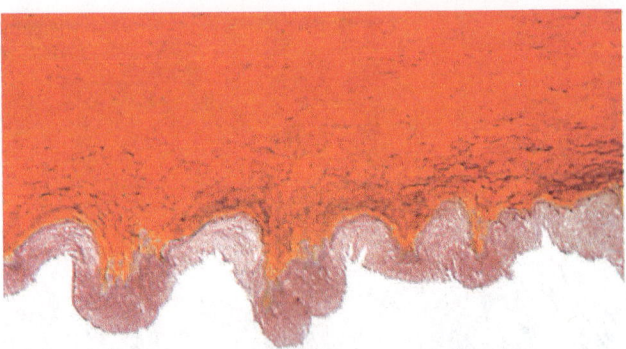

FIGURE 2.41 Transverse section of the nail plate. Note the serrated lower surface of the nail plate (MF stain).

(133). Intraepithelial nerve fibers were described at the beginning of this century (132), but other authors (134) were unable to confirm the description. Experimental studies have established that for digit-tip regrowth, the major nerve supply is not needed but the nail organ is needed. Nail organ of regrowing fetal digit-tips has been shown to produce Msx, a transcription factor associated with limb bud outgrowth (135).

The hyponychium is the area with greater abundance of nerve endings of the nail, and with abundant Meissner and Merkel–Ranvier corpuscles, as in the lateral nail folds (134). This histologic feature gives the hyponychium an important role in the fine sensibility of the finger.

Bone

The nail apparatus includes the subjacent bone. Although the bone has been ignored during the last years, a recent study of postamputational repair following digit-tip amputation revealed an unexpected correlation between nail regrowth and bone regrowth. In this way, Zhao and Neufeld (136) have studied this relationship, observing that in the absence of nail, bone did not regrow at distal levels, and conversely, when the nail was surgically retained, bone regrew from proximal levels.

Blood Supply

The nail has a rich vascularization that deserves separate mention. The arterial blood supply of the nail bed and matrix is derived from paired digital arteries. The most important studies have been published by Flint in 1955 (137), Ryan in 1973 (138), and Smith et al. in 1991 (139) concluding that the main supply passes into the pulp space of the distal phalanx before reaching the dorsum of the digit. An accessory supply arises further back on the digit and does not enter the pulp space. The digital arterial system manifests three characteristic anatomic features: (a) arched anastomotic arteries in the deep dermis; (b) more superficial terminal arteries branching to supply the rete (140); and (c) the great tortuosity of the arterial architecture subjacent to the nail apparatus (Fig. 2.43). The arteries possess inner longitudinal and outer circular coats of smooth muscle (Fig. 2.44). Oxygen-sensitive microelectrodes (tip diameter ~5 μm) to measure the distribution of pO_2 in dermal papillae of the finger nail folds of healthy human subjects have been developed by Wang et al. (141).

The vasculature in the nail bed is unique in that it must supply a vascular structure between two hard surfaces, the nail plate and the bone. Studies with scanning electron microscopy revealed special vascular patterns of nail microcirculation (142). In the eponychium and perionychium, the vascular villi followed the direction of nail growth. In the face of the eponychium in contact with the nail, a wide-mesh net of capillaries was evident. In the nail bed, the vessels were arranged in many longitudinal trabeculae parallel to the major axis of the digit. In

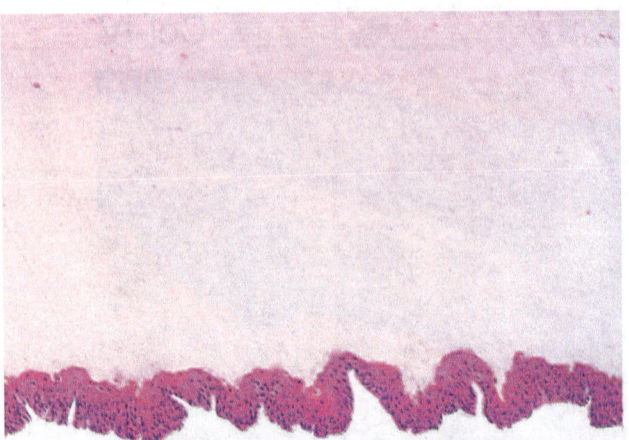

FIGURE 2.42 Avulsed nail plate. Observe the sinusoidal form of the nail bed epithelium attached to the lower surface of the nail plate.

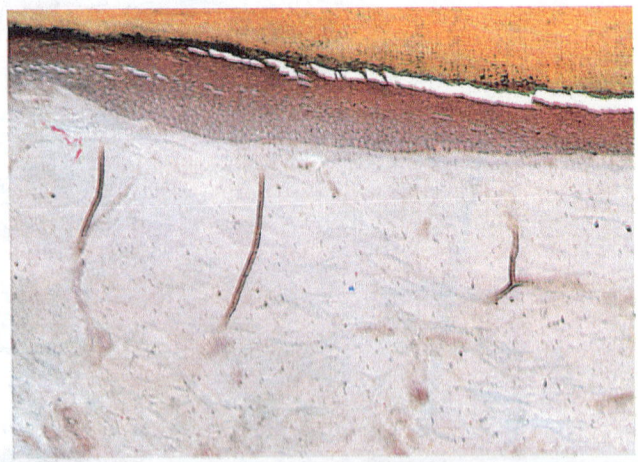

FIGURE 2.43 Vascular system of the nail bed. This zone has a rich vascular supply, with numerous vertical arteries; branches of the arched arteries of the deep dermis (MF stain).

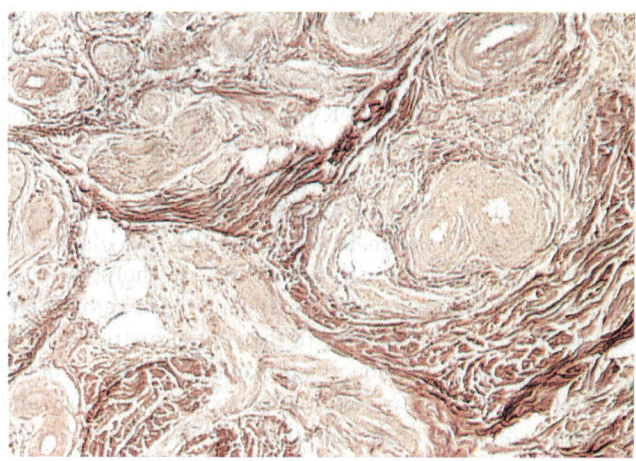

FIGURE 2.44 Detail of the rich vascular supply of the nail bed (reticulin stain).

the root of the nail, many columnar vessels characterized by multiple angiogenic buttons on their surface may be observed.

The venous drainage is achieved by two veins, one on each side of the nail plate, in the PNFs (140). The capillary network is easily seen in the PNF with a magnifying lens, and is seen in more detail with an ophthalmoscopic or capillary microscope. It is essentially the same as the network of the skin but the capillary loops are more horizontal and visible throughout their length. Certain diseases can modify its normal structure and a simple clinical examination or by widefield nail fold microscopy can be very useful as an aid in diagnosis (142–147).

Nailfold capillaroscopy (NFC) is an in vivo, noninvasive, and inexpensive imaging technique that allows direct observation of the capillary network in living tissues throughout the intact skin (148). It represents the best method to analyze micro/cardiovascular abnormalities in rheumatic diseases such as scleroderma, lupus, dermatomyositis, and others, helping with the diagnoses and prognoses of these diseases (149).

NAIL GROWTH

The rate of growth of the nail plate has been studied extensively. Normal nail growth varies between 0.1 and 1.12 mm per day, or 1.9 to 4.4 mm per month (150,151). This growth, however, is not the same in all fingers or toes. For example, fingernails grow faster than toenails. Whereas a normal fingernail grows out completely in approximately 6 months, a normal toenail takes 12 to 18 months to do the same (84), although nails grow faster when regenerating after avulsion (37).

Several physiologic circumstances can cause variations in the nail growth (Table 2.6). Nail growth is quicker in males (37), during the day than during the night, during pregnancy (152), in persons who bite their nails (41), and in summer or warm climates (153). Conversely, nails grow more slowly in females, during the night, in toes, in winter, after age 20 (154), and during lactation (152).

Nail growth is also altered in several diseases (Table 2.6) (155–160). Nails grow quicker with psoriasis (155), pityriasis

TABLE 2.6 Physiologic and Pathologic Variations That Influence Nail Growth

Physiologic		Pathologic	
Increased	Decreased	Increased	Decreased
Men	Women	Psoriasis	Fever
Daytime	Night	Pityriasis rubra pilaris	Poor nutrition
Summer	Winter	Hyperthyroidism	Hypothyroidism
Pregnancy	First day of life	A-V shunts	Decreased blood supply
Third digit	First and fifth digits	Idiopathic onycholysis in women	Kwashiorkor
Right hand[a]	Left hand[a]	Epidermolytic hyperkeratosis	Beau lines
Youth	Old age	Hyperpituitarism	Denervation/immobilization
Nail biting		Morgagni–Stewart–Morel sd	Acute infection
Avulsion		Brittle nail sd. *Medications:* calcium, vitamin D, benoxaprofen, biotin, cysteine, oral contraceptives, L-dopa, fluconazole, itraconazole, terbinafine, etretinate	Chronic disease, smoking, onychomycosis, yellow nail sd, lichen planus, relapsing polychondritis *Medications:* methotrexate, azathioprine, cyclosporine, lithium, retinoids, sulfonamides, heparin

[a]In a person's dominant right hand.
sd, syndrome.

rubra pilaris (96), etretinate treatment (156), and hyperthyroidism (37); nails grow slower in cases of immobilization or paralysis (157), local ischemic conditions (150), cytostatic therapy (37), denutrition (158), hypothyroidism (154), and yellow nail syndrome (159). In the case of a sudden decrease in nail growth, for example, in acute infections (151), a transverse band will appear afterward, depressed in the proximal line called Beau line. However, patients with unilateral toenail onychomycosis did not support the hypothesis that slow nail growth rate is a predisposing factor for this onychomycosis (160). The absence of K1 and K10 from healthy nail bed may also be related to the adherence of the overlying nail. In simple terms, the nail plate might be interpreted as the suprabasal layer of the nail bed, containing keratins not produced by the nail bed, but affording barrier function, or some other properties associated with K1, K10, and Ha1. The presence of these overlying keratins might be responsible for the lack of a granular layer and associated absence of K1 and K10. In diseases such as onychomycosis and psoriasis, where nail plate adherence is lost, a granular layer forms alongside expression of K1 and K10 (101–103,160). The rate of growth of the nail plate is determined by the turnover rate of the matrix cells. Shortly after death, matrix cells do not incorporate tritiated thymidine in their nuclei; the cells appear to be incapable of DNA synthesis and cell division, and, therefore, the nail does not grow (89). Previous reports of nail growth after death are, in fact, erroneous. Apparent growth, caused by severe postmortem drying and shrinking of the soft tissues around the nail plate, is what was observed (161). The question of where the nail plate is formed is still controversial (162). The first theories at the beginning of the century pointed toward a complete formation by the matrix (3). Years later, Lewis (8), however, concluded that the nail plate was the product of three different matrices on the basis of staining of the nail plate with a silver-protein stain and the morphology of keratinizing cells. Lewis's hypothesis was supported by differential staining of the nail plate (8), by differential interference contrast microscopy (69–72), and by ultrastructural observation of keratohyalin granules in embryonic nail (72). Lewis's hypothesis, however, has been extensively reviewed. Zaias and Alvarez (89) used radioautography to show that the nail plate was formed exclusively by the matrix in normal conditions; Samman (163) and Norton (162) confirmed it by following the incorporation of H-labeled glycine and thymidine in human toenails; and Caputo and Dadati (44) reported that, ultrastructurally, the nail plate was a homogeneous structure with no evidence of formation from three different matrices. To add one final bit to the confusion, Samman (163) suggests that although under normal conditions the nail plate is made exclusively by the matrix, in certain pathologic conditions, the nail bed adds a ventral nail to the undersurface of the nail plate. Nevertheless, a study using antibodies to the antigen Ki-67 and to proliferating cell nuclear antigen suggested a low degree of proliferation in the normal nail bed, indicating its minimal or nonexistent contribution to the nail plate (164). Kato published a case with an ectopic nail at the palmar tip, with a vertical growth. In this case, the PNF promotes upward growth of the nail plate, in the absence of a proper nail bed (165). Recently, Sellheyer K proposed that at least during embryogenesis the proximal ventral nail fold represents the niche for the nail stem cells (166).

Perrin et al. (104) have clearly demonstrated that the ventral matrix is the main source of the nail plate. The coexpression of hHb5 with K5 and K17 in the uppermost cell layers of the basal compartment and the lowermost layers of the keratogenous zone of the ventral matrix prompts us to designate this region, the prekeratogenous zone of the ventral matrix. The two alternating types of histology and keratin expression in the dorsal matrix identify this region as a transitional zone between the eponychium and the apical matrix. In addition, the mixed scenario of hair and epithelial keratins, including demonstrable amounts of K10, in superficial cells of the apical matrix, lends support to the notion that the dorsal portion of the nail is generated by the apical matrix (104). However, some authors believe that the nail bed epithelium produces a significant 20% portion of the nail plate and thus, include the nail bed in the generative portion of the nail (167). Interestingly, indirect immunofluorescence studies in the fetal nail by means of pan-anti-type I and pan-anti-type II hair keratin antibodies revealed a positive staining in a broad band of suprabasal cells of the nail bed epithelium. However, exclusion of hair keratins hHa1, hHb5, hHb1, hHb6, and hHa4 from the adult nail bed epithelium clearly identifies the matrix as the sole origin of the nail plate (104,168). It has previously been speculated that a few so-called "horn cells" may be added by the nail bed epithelium to the underside of the nail plate. This study confirmed the occurrence of clearly visible K5/17-positive nail bed cells in the lower nail plate, we believe that these cells represent sectioning artifacts. Transverse nail sections, stained for either K5/17 or hHb5, showed that the boundary between the nail bed epithelium and the nail plate is extremely undulated and that the resulting narrow-spaced folds and ridges exhibit a distinctly varying height. Therefore, it is evident that already slight deviations from a vertical angle of section through the nail bed region may reveal K5-positive cells in the nail plate, which in reality stem from the tip of an adjacent epithelial fold of the bed epithelium. Collectively, these data emphasize that the nail bed epithelium does not actively contribute to the formation of the nail plate (Fig. 2.45) (17,100,104–112). Otherwise, Leung Y et al. examined the regenerative potential of the perinail region and discovered a previously unidentified population of K15-positive LRCs within the PNF with self-renewal capabilities. Physiologically, these cells display bifunctional SC qualities and contribute to both the nail structure and perinail epidermis long term; however, upon injury, the homeostatic balance is tilted toward nail regeneration (169).

An important controversy is why nails grow out instead of up. Kligman postulated that the cul-de-sac of the proximal

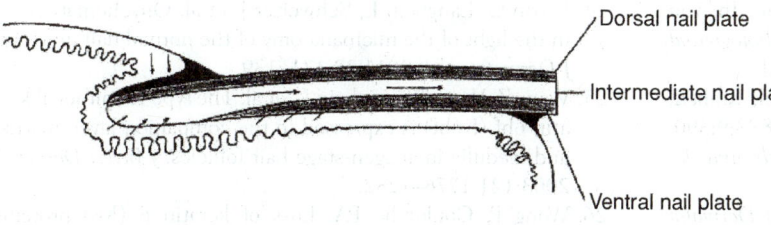

FIGURE 2.45 Schematic diagram of nail growth.

nail groove forced the cells of the matrix to grow out (170,171). To confirm his theory he transplanted nail matrix to the forearm, producing a vertical cylinder of hard keratin that had histologic characteristics of the nail. Hashimoto et al. (72) stated later that the long axis of matrix cells in embryonic nail was directed upward and distally.

Another important question is why the nail bed accompanies the nail plate in its growth. A well-known fact is that a hemorrhage, which occurs between the plate and bed, grows forward with the plate. If the plate merely moved over the bed, the blood would not move; therefore, the upper part of the bed must move out with the plate. Some authors, such as Krantz (172), Kligman (170,171), and Zaias (85), tried to study this phenomenon in an experimental way. Of all theories, the one by Zaias is most acceptable at present: He believes that the proximal nail bed moves out, either by pressure by advancing plate or because of trauma, but that the distal nail bed and hyponychium do not move.

Technical advances in molecular and cellular biology have been updating our understanding of the field of epithelial stem cells and on the nail unit too. The location of the stem cells in the nail is still under study and is controversial (173,174). Recently, in tamoxifen-inducible lineage tracing of transgenic mice under the control of the keratin 14 (K14) promoter, the K14-positive basal epidermal cells (both the nail matrix cells and the nail bed cells) were labeled with LacZ (175). The LacZ positive cells that emanate linearly and distally from the PNM persisted much longer than those from the distal nail matrix and the nail bed. This finding indicates that the PNM included nail stem cells. On the other hand, a recent study examined embryonic and fetal nail samples through the use of stem cell markers (including cytokeratin 15), and proposed that the PNF represents the fundamental niche where nail stem cells are located, at least during nail embryogenesis (166).

HANDLING AND PROCESSING OF THE NAIL

The major problem of the nail unit is the difficulty of tissue selection and the need for proper orientation of the specimen. These problems are the reason for the small number of histologic studies. The first important point is how to take a biopsy of the nail unit (170–172,176–184). The best way of studying a biopsy of the nail is to ascertain that it includes the complete thickness of the nail unit (which means nail plate, bed, and subjacent dermis); these can be sectioned transversely. Nail can be biopsied with a punch or with an elliptical excision, and sometimes in this process the lesion might be completely eliminated (181–183,185). Nail matrix biopsy is useful to confirm or exclude malignant melanoma. The nail plate can be avulsed or a punch biopsy can be taken through the nail plate (185). If one wishes to eliminate the nail plate before taking the biopsy, special care has to be taken about nail avulsion because if it has been avulsed without care, the epithelium of the bed or matrix may become separated and the undersurface may remain attached to the plate and distort the true histopathologic picture. The ideal biopsy technique for the nail is a longitudinal biopsy (160,185), which includes the hyponychium, the nail bed, and matrix with overlying plate, and the PNF and cuticle. The second point is the orientation of the specimen for cutting. In all cases, the surgeon should alert the pathologist on the submission form as to the way the specimen was obtained, whether a particular orientation is needed, and whether a piece of the nail plate is included.

The third point is how to treat the specimen in the laboratory. If the nail plate is present in the specimen, it will be too hard for ready cutting with a microtome unless some method of softening is used. Several techniques have been reported for this issue (186) including 10% formalin followed by routine processing (8), potassium bichromate, sodium sulfate, or sodium bisulfate and water followed by decalcification with nitric acid and embedding in collodion (187). Other methods include placing fragments of the nail in a solution of thioglycolate at 37° C for 5 days, or using 10% to 20% hydrogen peroxide for 5 to 6 days. Afterwards nail is fixed by boiling in formalin 1 minute, before cutting 10 to 15 μm sections (188). For specimens with nail plate, the most commonly used softening methods, were Mollifex Gurr (VWR Int. Ltd.), potassium hydroxide solution 10% applied to the surface of the paraffin-embedded specimen, and potassium thioglycolate 10% (186).

REFERENCES

1. Zander R. Untersuchungen uber den Verhornungsprogress 1. Die Histogenese des Nagels beim menschlichen Fetus. *Arch Anat Entwick* 1886;1:273.
2. Kolliker A. Die entwicklung des menschlichen Nagels. *Z Wiss Zool* 1988;1:1–12.

3. Unna PG. Entwicklungsgeschichte und Anatomie. In: von Ziemssen HW, ed. *Handbook der Speciellen Pathologieund Therapie*. Leipzig: F.C.W. Vogel; 1882: vol. 14, pt.1.
4. Boas JEV. Ein Beitrag zur Morphologie der Nagel, Kralien, Hufe and Klauen der Saugetiere. *Morphol Jahrb* 1883;9:390.
5. Henle J. *Das Wachstrum des menschlichen Nagels und des Pferdehufs*. Gottingen: Dieterich; 1884.
6. Branca A. Notes sur la structure de l'ongle. *Ann Dermatol Syphiligr (Paris)* 1910;1:353–371.
7. Clark WE, Buxton LH. Studies in nail growth. *Br J Dermatol* 1938;50:221–235.
8. Lewis BL. Microscopic studies of fetal and mature nail and surrounding soft tissue. *AMA Arch Derm Syphilol* 1954;70(6): 732–747.
9. Zaias N. Embryology of the human nail. *Arch Dermatol* 1963; 87:37–53.
10. Horner KL, Gasbarre CC. Special considerations for Mohs micrographic surgery on the eyelids, lips, genitalia, and nail unit. *Dermatol Clin* 2011;29:311–317.
11. Holbrook KA, Odland GF. The fine structure of the developing human epidermis: light, scanning, and transmission electron microscopy of the periderm. *J Invest Dermatol* 1975;65:16–38.
12. Conejo-Mir JS, Ambrosiani J, Dorado M. *Analisis De La Morfogénesis Ungueal. Estudio Con Microscopio Electronica De Barrido En El Embrion Humano*. Barcelona: Isdin; 1985:1–8.
13. Conejo-Mir JS, Ambrosiani J, Dorado M, et al. *Human Nail Development. A Scanning Electron Microscopy Study*. Abstract book of the Meeting of the American Society of Dermatopathology, Washington DC; 1988.
14. Suchard R. Des modifications des celluies de la matrice et du lit de l'ongle dans quelques cas pathologiques. *Arch Physiol (Paris)* 1882;2:445.
15. Ogura R, Knox JM, Griffin AC, et al. The concentration of sulfhydryl and disulfide in human epidermis, hair and nail. *J Invest Dermatol* 1962;38:69–75.
16. Irvine AD, McLean WH. Human keratin diseases: the increasing spectrum of disease and subtlety of phenotype-genotype correlation. *Br J Dermatol* 1999;140:815–828.
17. De Berker D, Wojnarowska F, Sviland L, et al. Keratin expression in the normal nail unit: markers of regional differentiation. *Br J Dermatol* 2000;142:89–96.
18. Rice RH, Xia Y, Alvarado RJ, et al. Proteomic analysis of human nail plate. *J Proteome Res* 2010;3:6752–6758.
19. Rice RH. Proteomic analysis of hair shaft and nail plate. *J Cosmet Sci* 2011;62:229–236.
20. Hesse M, Magin TM, Weber K. Genes for intermediate filament proteins and the draft sequence of the human genome: Novel keratin genes and a surprisingly high number of pseudogenes related to keratin genes 8 and 18. *J Cell Sci* 2001; 114:2569–2575.
21. Smith TA, Strelov SV, Burkhard P, et al. Sequence comparisons of intermediate filament chains: evidence of a unique functional/structural role for coiled-coil segment 1A and linker L1. *J Struct Biol* 2002;137:128–145.
22. Fuchs E. Keratins and the skin. *Annu Rev Cell Dev Biol* 1995;11:123–153.
23. Perrin C. Expression of follicular sheath keratins in the normal nail with special reference to the morphological analysis of the distal nail unit. *Am J Dermatopathol* 2007;29: 543–550.
24. Perrin C, Langbein L, Schweizer J, et al. Onychomatricoma in the light of the microanatomy of the normal nail unit. *Am J Dermatopathol* 2011;33:131–139.
25. Wang Z, Wong P, Langbein L, et al. The type II epithelial keratin 6hf (K6hf) is expressed in the companion layer, matrix, and medulla in anagen-stage hair follicles. *J Invest Dermatol* 2003;121:1276–1282.
26. Wong P, Coulombe PA. Loss of keratin 6 (K6) proteins reveals a function for intermediate filaments during wound repair. *J Cell Biol* 2003;163:327–337.
27. Reddy K, Lowenstein EJ. Forensics in dermatology: part II. *J Am Acad Dermatol* 2011;64:811–824; quiz 825–826.
28. Baran R, Dawber RP, Haneke E. Hair and nail relationship. *Skinmed* 2005;4:18–23.
29. Sehgal VN, Aggarwal AK, Srivastava G, et al. Nail biology, morphologic changes, and clinical ramifications: part I. *Skinmed* 2011;9:39–46.
30. de Berker DA, Perrin C, Baran R. Localized longitudinal erythronychia: diagnostic significance and physical explanation. *Arch Dermatol* 2004;140:1253–1257.
31. Norgett EE, Wolf F, Balme B, et al. Hereditary 'white nails': a genetic and structural study. *Br J Dermatol* 2004;151:65–72.
32. Lewin K. The normal fingernail. *Br J Dermatol* 1965;77: 421–430.
33. Pinkus F. The development of the integument. In: Kleibel F, Mali F, eds. *Manual of Human Embryology. Chapter 10*. Philadelphia, PA: Lippincott; 1910.
34. Schweitzer TP, Rayan GM. The terminal tendon of the digital extensor mechanism: part I, anatomic study. *J Hand Surg Am* 2004;29:898–902.
35. Le Groos Clark WB. The problems of the claw in primates. *Proc Zool Soc* 1936;106:1–24.
36. Pinkus F. Der Nagel. In: Jadassohns J, ed. *Handbuch, der Haut und Geschlechtskrankeilen*. Berlin: Springer-Verlag; 1927.
37. Baran R, Dawber RPR. *Diseases of the Nail and their Management*. Oxford: Blackwell Scientific; 1984:1–21.
38. Caputo R, Cappio F, Rigoni C, et al. Pterygium inversum unguis. Report of 19 cases and review of the literature. *Arch Dermatol* 1993;129:1307–1309.
39. Terry RB. The onychodermal hand in health and disease. *Lancet* 1955;1:179–181.
40. Martin BF, Platts MM. A histological study of the nail region in normal human subjects and in those showing splinter hemorrhages of the nail. *J Anat* 1959;93:323–330.
41. Raffle EJ. Terry's nails. *Lancet* 1984;1:1131.
42. Finlay AY, Moseley H, Duggan TC. Ultrasound transmission time: an in vivo guide to nail thickness. *Br J Dermatol* 1987; 117:765–770.
43. Goettmann S, Drape JL, Lidy-Peretti I, et al. Magnetic resonance imaging: a new tool in the diagnosis of tumors of the nail apparatus. *Br J Dermatol* 1994;130:701–710.
44. Caputo R, Dadati E. Preliminary observations about the ultrastructure of the human nail plate treated with thioglycolic acid. *Arch Klin Exp Dermatol* 1968;231:344–354.
45. Forslind B, Thyresson N. On the structure of the normal nail. A scanning electron microscope study. *Arch Dermatol Forsch* 1975;251:199–204.
46. Garson JC, Baltenneck F, Leroy F, et al. Histological structure of human nail as studied by synchrotron X-ray microdiffraction. *Cell Mol Biol* 2000;46:1025–1034.

47. Hamilton JB, Tereda H, Mestler GE. Studies of growth throughout the lifespan in Japanese: growth and size of nails and their relationship to age, sex, heredity, and other factors. *J Gerontol* 1955;10:401–415.
48. Johnson M, Shuster S. Determinants of nail thickness and length. *Br J Dermatol* 1994;130:195–198.
49. Farren L, Shayler S, Ennos AR. The fracture properties and mechanical design of human fingernails. *J Exp Biol* 2004; 207(Pt 5):735–741.
50. Germann H, Barran W, Plewig G. Morphology of corneocytes from human nail plates. *J Invest Dermatol* 1980;74:115–118.
51. Walters KA, Flynn GL, Marvel JR. Physicochemical characterization of the human nail. I. Pressure sealed apparatus for measuring nail plate permeabilities. *J Invest Dermatol* 1981; 76:76–79.
52. Egawa M, Fukuhara T, Takahashi M, et al. Determining water content in human nails with a portable near-infrared spectrometer. *Appl Spectrosc* 2003;57:473–478.
53. Duarte AF, Correia O, Baran R. Nail plate cohesion seems to be water independent. *Int J Dermatol* 2009;48:193–195.
54. Osorio G, Bernabéu J, Echevarría M, et al. Acuaporinas: moléculas revelación en cosmética y oncología cutánea. *Piel* 2009;24:192–199.
55. Nuutinen J, Harvima I, Lahtinen M-R, et al. Water loss through the lip, nail, eyelid skin, scalp skin and axillary skin measured with a closed-chamber evaporation principle. *Br J Dermatol* 2003;148(4):839–841.
56. Jarrett A, Spearman RI. The histochemistry of the human nail. *Arch Dermatol* 1966;94:652–657.
57. Pautard FG. Mineralization of keratin and its comparison with enamel matrix. *Nature* 1963;199:531–535.
58. Forslind B, Wroblewski R, Afzelius BA. Calcium and sulphur location in human nail. *J Invest Dermatol* 1976;67: 273–275.
59. Helmdach M, Thielitz A, Ropke EM, et al. Age and sex variation in lipid composition of human fingernail plates. *Skin Pharmacol Appl Skin Physiol* 2000;13:111–119.
60. Sass JO, Skladal D, Zelger B, et al. Trichothiodystrophy: quantification of cysteine in human hair and nails by application of sodium azide-dependent oxidation to cysteic acid. *Arch Dermatol Res* 2004;296:188–191.
61. Bolliger A, Gross R. Non-keratin of human toenails. *Aust J Exp Biol Med Sci* 1953;31:127–130.
62. Levitt JI. Creatinine concentration of human fingernail and toenail clippings. Application in determining the duration of renal failure. *Ann Intern Med* 1966;64:312–327.
63. Goldblum RW, Derby S, Lerner AB. The metal content of skin, nails and hair. *J Invest Dermatol* 1953;20:13–18.
64. Kopito L, Mahmoodian A, Townley RR, et al. Studies in cystic fibrosis: analysis of nail clippings for sodium and potassium. *N Engl J Med* 1965;272:504–509.
65. Martin SM. Copper content of hair and nails of normal individuals and of patients with hepatolenticular degeneration. *Nature* 1964;202:903–904.
66. Mandal BK, Ogra Y, Anzai K, et al. Speciation of arsenic in biological samples. *Toxicol Appl Pharmacol* 2004;198: 307–318.
67. Cingolani M, Scavella S, Mencarelli R, et al. Simultaneous detection and quantitation of morphine, 6-acetylmorphine, and cocaine in toenails: comparison with hair analysis. *J Anal Toxicol* 2004;28:128–131.
68. Gillespie JM, Frenkel MJ. The diversity of keratins. *Comp Biochem Physiol* 1974;47B:339–349.
69. Stern DK, Creasey AA, Quijije J, et al. UV-A and UV-B penetration of normal human cadaveric fingernail plate. *Arch Dermatol* 2011;147:439–441.
70. Khengar RH, Brown MB, Turner RB, et al. Free radical facilitated damage of ungual keratin. *Free Radic Biol Med* 2010;49:865–871.
71. Ruben BS. Pigmented lesions of the nail unit: clinical and histopathologic features. *Semin Cutan Med Surg* 2010;29: 148–158.
72. Hashimoto K, Gross BG, Nelson R, et al. The ultrastructure of the skin of human embryos. 3. The formation of the nail in 16–18 week old embryos. *J Invest Dermatol* 1966;47:205–217.
73. Hashimoto K. Ultrastructure of the human toenails. 1. Proximal nail matrix. *J Invest Dermatol* 1971;56:235–246.
74. Hashimoto K. Ultrastructure of the human toenail. II. Keratinization and formation of the marginal band. *J Ultrastruct Res* 1971;36:391–410.
75. Hashimoto K. Ultrastructure of the human toenail. Cell migration, keratinization and formation of the intercellular cement. *Arch Dermatol Forsch* 1971;240:1–22.
76. Higashi N. Melanocytes of nail matrix and nail pigmentation. *Arch Dermatol* 1968;97:570–574.
77. Scott GA, Haake AR. Keratinocytes regulate melanocyte number in human fetal and neonatal skin equivalents. *J Invest Dermatol* 1991;97:776–781.
78. Higashi N, Saito T. Horizontal distribution of dopa-positive melanocytes in the nail matrix. *J Invest Dermatol* 1969;53: 163–165.
79. Jimbow K, Takahashi M, Sato S, et al. Ultrastructural and cytochemical studies on melanogenesis in melanocytes of normal human hair matrix. *J Electron Microsc (Tokyo)* 1971;20: 87–92.
80. Feibleman CE, Stoll H, Maize JC. Melanomas of the palm, sole and nail bed: a clinicopathologic study. *Cancer* 1980;46: 2492–2504.
81. Baran R, Juhlin L. Photoonycholysis. *Photodermatol Photoimmunol Photomed* 2002;18:202–207.
82. Moll I, Moll R. Merkel cells in ontogenesis of human nails. *Arch Dermatol Res* 1993;285:366–371.
83. Samman PD. The ventral nail. *Arch Dermatol* 1961;84: 192–195.
84. Samman PD. *The Nail in Disease*. 3rd ed. London: Heinemann Medical Books; 1978.
85. Zaias N. The movement of the nail bed. *J Invest Dermatol* 1967;48:402–403.
86. Drapé JL, Wolfram-Gabel W, Idy-Peretti I, et al. The lunula: a magnetic resonance imaging approach to the subnail matrix area. *J Invest Dermatol* 1996;106:1081–1085.
87. Dawber RPR, Baran R. The nails. In: Rook A, Wilkinson DS, Ebling FJG, Champion RH, Burton JL, eds. *Textbook of Dermatology*. Oxford: Blackwell Scientific; 1986:2039–2044.
88. Burrows MT. The significance of the lunula of the nail. *Johns Hopkins Hosp Res* 1919;18:357–361.
89. Zaias N, Alvarez J. The formation of the primate nail plate. An autoradiographic study in squirrel monkeys. *J Invest Dermatol* 1968;51:120–126.
90. Meyer JC, Grundmand HP. Scanning electron microscopic investigation of the healthy nail and its surrounding tissue. *J Cutan Pathol* 1984;11:74–79.

91. Omura EF. Histopathology of the nail. *Dermatol Clin* 1985; 3:531–541.
92. Sehgal VN, Aggarwal AK, Srivastava G, et al. Nail biology, morphologic changes, and clinical ramifications: part II. *Skinmed* 2011;9:103–107.
93. Sinclair RD, Wojnarowska F, Leigh IM, et al. The basement zone of the nail. *Br J Dermatol* 1994;131:499–505.
94. Dorschner RA, Lopez-Garcia B, Massie J, et al. Innate immune defense of the nail unit by antimicrobial peptides. *J Am Acad Dermatol* 2004;50:343–348.
95. Holbrook KA. Human epidermal embryogenesis. *Int J Dermatol* 1979;18:329–356.
96. Runne U, Orfanos CE. The human nail: structure, growth and pathological changes. *Curr Probl Dermatol* 1981;9: 102–149.
97. Zaias N. Onychomycosis. *Arch Dermatol* 1972;105:263–274.
98. Baden H, Kvedar JC. Epithelial cornified envelope precursors are in the hair follicle and nail. *J Invest Dermatol* 1993;101: 72S–74S.
99. O'Keefe EJ, Hamilton EH, Lee SC, et al. Trichohyalin: a structural protein of hair, tongue, nail and epidermis. *J Invest Dermatol* 1993;101:65S–71S.
100. Heid HW, Moll I, Franke WW. Pattern of expression of trichocytic and epithelial cytokeratins in mammalian tissues. II. Concomitant and mutually exclusive synthesis of trichocytic and epithelial cytokeratins in diverse human and bovine tissues (hair follicle, nail bed and matrix, lingual papilla, thymic reticulum). *Differentiation* 1988;37:215–230.
101. Kitahara T, Ogawa H. The expression and characterization of human nail keratin. *J Dermatol Sci* 1991;2:402–406.
102. Kitahara T, Ogawa H. Cultured nail keratinocytes express hard keratins characteristic of nail and hair in vivo. *Arch Dermatol Res* 1992;284:253–256.
103. Kitahara T, Ogawa H. Coexpression of keratins characteristics of skin and hair differentiation in nail cells. *J Invest Dermatol* 1993;100:171–175.
104. Perrin C, Langbein L, Schweizer J. Expression of hair keratins in the adult nail unit: an immunohistochemical analysis of the onychogenesis in the proximal nail fold, matrix and nail bed. *Br J Dermatol* 2004;151(2):362–371.
105. Kitahara T, Ogawa H. Cellular features of differentiation in the nail. *Microsc Res Tech* 1997;38:436–442.
106. Lane EB, Wilson CA, Hughes BR, et al. Stem cells in hair follicles. Cytoskeletal studies. *Ann N Y Acad Sci* 1991;642: 197–213.
107. Stark HJ, Breitkreutz D, Limat A, et al. Keratins of the human hair follicle: "hyperproliferative" keratins consistently expressed in outer root sheath cells in vivo and in vitro. *Differentiation* 1987;35:236–248.
108. McLean WHI, Epithelial Genetics Group. Genetic disorders of palm skin and nail. *J Anat* 2003;202:133–141.
109. Inoue S, Nambu T, Shimomura T. The RAIG family member, GPRC5D, is associated with hard-keratinized structures. *J Invest Dermatol* 2004;122:565–573.
110. Okazaki M, Yoshimura K, Fujiwara H, et al. Induction of hard keratin expression in non-nail-matrical keratinocytes by nail-matrical fibroblasts through epithelial-mesenchymal interactions. *Plast Reconstr Surg* 2003;111:286–290.
111. Egawa K, Kuroki M, Inoue Y, et al. Nail bed keratinocytes express an antigen of the carcinoembryonic antigen family. *Br J Dermatol* 2000;143:79–83.
112. Lavker RM, Risse B, Brown H, et al. Localization of plasminogen activator inhibitor type 2 (PAI-2) in hair and nail: Implications for terminal differentiation. *J Invest Dermatol* 1998;110:917–924.
113. Lee DY, Park JH, Shin HT, et al. Onychodermis (specialized nail mesenchyme) containing onychofibroblasts in horizontal sections of the nail unit. *Br J Dermatol* 2012;166(5): 1127–1129.
114. Lee KJ, Kim WS, Lee JH, et al. CD10, a marker for specialized mesenchymal cells (onychofibroblasts) in the nail unit. *J Dermatol Sci* 2006;42(1):65–67.
115. Park JH, Lee DY, Jang KT, et al. CD13 is a marker for onychofibroblasts within nail matrix onychodermis: comparison of its expression patterns in the nail unit and in the hair follicle. *J Cutan Pathol* 2017;44(11):909–914.
116. Kim CR, Shin HT, Park JH, et al. Nuclear and cytoplasmic localization of β-catenin in the nail-matrix cells and in an onychomatricoma. *Clin Exp Dermatol* 2013;38(8): 917–920.
117. Lacour JP, Dubois D, Pisani A, et al. Anatomical mapping of Merkel cells in normal human adult epidermis. *Br J Dermatol* 1991;125:535–542.
118. Tosti A, Cameli N, Piraccini BM, et al. Characterization of nail matrix melanocytes with anti-PEP1, anti-PEP8, TMH-1 and HMB-45 antibodies. *J Am Acad Dermatol* 1994;31: 193–196.
119. Guerrero-Fernandez J, Garcia-Ascaso MT, Guerrero Vazquez J. Pigmentation band on toenail. *An Pediatr (Barc)* 2004;61: 455–456.
120. Cameli N, Picardo M, Tosti A, et al. Expression of integrins in human nail matrix. *Br J Dermatol* 1994;130:583–588.
121. Picardo M, Tosti A, Marchese C, et al. Characterization of cultured nail matrix cells. *J Am Acad Dermatol* 1994;30: 434–440.
122. Ito T, Ito N, Bettermann A, et al. Collapse and restoration of MHC class I-dependent immune privilege: exploiting the human hair follicle as a model. *Am J Pathol* 2004;164: 623–634.
123. Paus R, Nickoloff BJ, Ito T. A "hairy" privilege. *Trends Immunol* 2005;26:32–40.
124. Chuong CM, Noveen A. Phenotypic determination of epithelial appendages: genes, developmental pathways, and evolution. *J Investig Dermatol Symp Proc* 1999;4:307–311.
125. Ito T, Meyer KC, Ito N, et al. Immune privilege and the skin. *Curr Dir Autoimmun* 2008;10:27–52.
126. Sattler E, Kaestle R, Rothmund G, et al. Confocal laser scanning microscopy, optical coherence tomography and transonychial water loss for in vivo investigation of nails. *Br J Dermatol* 2012;166:740–746.
127. Hongcharu W, Dwyer P, Gonzalez S, et al. Confirmation of onychomycosis by in vivo confocal microscopy. *J Am Acad Dermatol* 2000;42:214–216.
128. Moscarella E, Longo C, Zalaudek I, et al. Dermoscopy and confocal microscopy clues in the diagnosis of psoriasis and porokeratosis. *J Am Acad Dermatol* 2013;69:e231–e233.
129. Cinotti E, Fouilloux B, Perrot JL, et al. Confocal microscopy for healthy and pathological nail. *J Eur Acad Dermatol Venereol* 2014;28:853–858.
130. Kaufman SC, Beuerman RW, Greer DL. Confocal microscopy: a new tool for the study of the nail unit. *J Am Acad Dermatol* 1995;32:668–670.

131. Sellheyer K, Nelson P. The concept of the onychodermis (specialized nail mesenchyme): an embryological assessment and a comparative analysis with the hair follicle. *J Cutan Pathol* 2013;40:463–471.
132. Doigel AS. Die nerbenendigungen im nagelbett des Menschen. *Arch Mikr Anat* 1904;64:173–188.
133. Martino L. Sulia innervazione dell'apparato ungueale. *Boll Soc Ital Biol Sper* 1942;1(7):488–489.
134. Winkelmann RK. *Nerve Endings in Normal and Pathologic Skin*. Springfield, IL: Charles C Thomas; 1960:100.
135. Reginelli AD, Wang YQ, Sassoon D, et al. Digit tip regeneration correlates with regions of Msx1 (Hox 7) expression in fetal and newborn mice. *Development* 1995;121:1065–1076.
136. Zhao W, Neufeld DA. Bone regrowth in young mice stimulated by nail organ. *J Exp Zool* 1995;271:155–159.
137. Flint MH. Some observations on the vascular supply of the nail bed and terminal segments of the finger. *Br J Plast Surg* 1955;8:186–189.
138. Ryan TJ. In: Jarret A, ed. *The Physiology and Pathophysiology of the Skin*. Vol II. London: Academic Press; 1973;612: 658–659.
139. Smith DO, Oura C, Kimura C, et al. Artery anatomy and tortuosity in the distal finger. *J Hand Surg Am* 1991;16:297–302.
140. Hale AR, Burch GE. The arteriovenous anastomoses and blood vessels of the human finger. *Medicine* 1960;39: 191–240.
141. Wang W, Winlove CP, Michel CC. Oxygen partial pressure in outer layers of skin of human finger nail folds. *J Physiol* 2003;549:855–863.
142. Sangiorgi S, Manelli A, Congiu T, et al. Microvascularization of the human digit as studied by corrosion casting. *J Anat* 2004;2:123–131.
143. Ross JB. Nail fold capillaroscopy—a useful aid in the diagnosis of collagen vascular diseases. *J Invest Dermatol* 1966;47: 282–285.
144. Gilje O, Kierland R, Baldes EJ. Capillary microscopy in the diagnosis of dermatologic diseases. *J Invest Dermatol* 1954;22: 199–206.
145. Ohtsuka T, Yamakage A, Miyachi Y. Statistical definition of nailfold capillary pattern in patients with psoriasis. *Int J Dermatol* 1994;33:779–782.
146. Vaz JL, Dancour MA, Bottino DA, et al. Nailfold videocapillaroscopy in primary antiphospholipid syndrome (PAPS). *Rheumatology* 2004;43:1025–1027.
147. Mugii N, Hasegawa M, Matsushita T, et al. Association between nail-fold capillary findings and disease activity in dermatomyositis. *Rheumatology (Oxford)* 2011;50:1091–1098.
148. Bertolazzi C, Cutolo M, Smith V, et al. State of the art on nailfold capillaroscopy in dermatomyositis and polymyositis. *Semin Arthritis Rheum*. 2017;47(3):432–444.
149. Cutolo M, Sulli A, Secchi ME, et al. Nailfold capillaroscopy is useful for the diagnosis and follow-up of autoimmune rheumatic diseases. A future tool for the analysis of microvascular heart involvement? *Rheumatology* 2006;45(Suppl 4): 43–46.
150. Bean WB. Nail growth: 30 years of observation. *Arch Intern Med* 1974;134:497–502.
151. Sibinga MS. Observations on growth of fingernails in health and disease. *Pediatrics* 1959;24:225–233.
152. Halban J, Spitzer MZ. On the increased growth of nails in pregnancy. *Monatsschr Gerburtshilfe Gynaekol* 1929;82:25.
153. Geoghegan B, Roberts DF, Sampford MR. A possible climatic effect on nail growth. *J Appl Physiol* 1958;13:135–138.
154. Orentreich N, Markofsky J, Vogelman JH. The effect of aging on the rate of linear nail growth. *J Invest Dermatol* 1979;73:126–130.
155. Landherr G, Braun-Falco O, Hofmann C, et al. Fingernagelwachstum bei Psoriatikern unter puvatherapie. *Hautarzt* 1982;33:210–213.
156. Baran R. Action therapeutique et complications due retinoique aromatique sur l'appareil ungueal. *Ann Dermatol Venereol* 1982; 109:367–371.
157. Fleckman P. Anatomy and physiology of the nail. *Dermatol Clin* 1985;3:373–381.
158. Geyer AS, Onumah N, Uyttendaele H, et al. Modulation of linear nail growth to treat disease of the nail. *J Am Acad Dermatol* 2004;50:229–234.
159. Pavlidakey GP, Hashimoto K, Blurn D. Yellow nail syndrome. *J Am Acad Dermatol* 1984;11:509–512.
160. Yu HJ, Kwon HM, Oh DH, et al. Is slow nail growth a risk factor for onychomycosis? *Clin Exp Dermatol* 2004;29: 415–418.
161. Zaias N. Nails. Components, growth and composition of the nail. In: Demis J, Dobson RL, McGuire J, eds. *Clinical Dermatology*. Vol. 1. New York: Harper & Row; 1980;3l: 1–6.
162. Norton LA. Incorporation of thymidine-methyl-H3 and glycine-2-H3 in the nail matrix and bed of humans. *J Invest Dermatol* 1971;56:61–68.
163. Samman PD. The human toe nail. Its genesis and blood supply. *Br J Dermatol* 1959;71:296–302.
164. Berker D, Angus B. Proliferative compartments in the normal nail unit. *Br J Dermatol* 1996;135:555–9.
165. Kato N. Vertically growing ectopic nail. *J Cutan Pathol* 1992;19:445–447.
166. Sellheyer K, Nelson P. The ventral proximal nail fold: stem cell niche of the nail and equivalent to the follicular bulge—a study on developing human skin. *J Cutan Pathol*. 2012;39(9):835–843.
167. Johnson M, Comaish JS, Shuster S. Nail is produced by the normal nail bed: a controversy resolved. *Br J Dermatol* 1991;125:27–29.
168. De Berker D, Mawhinney B, Sviland L. Quantification of regional matrix nail production. *Br J Dermatol* 1996;134: 1083–1086.
169. Leung Y, Kandyba E, Chen YB, et al. Bifunctional ectodermal stem cells around the nail display dual fate homeostasis and adaptive wounding response toward nail regeneration. *Proc Natl Acad Sci U S A*. 2014;111(42):15114–15119.
170. Kligman AM. Nails. In: Pillsbury DM, Shelley WB, Kligman AM, eds. *Dermatology*. Philadelphia, PA: WB Saunders; 1956:80–86.
171. Kligman AM. Why do nails grow out instead of up? *Arch Dermatol* 1961;84:313–315.
172. Krantz W. Beitrag zur anatomie des nagels. *Dermatol Z* 1932; 64:239–242.
173. Cotsarelis G, Sun TT, Lavker RM. Label-retaining cells reside in the bulge area of pilosebaceous unit: implications for follicular stem cells, hair cycle, and skin carcinogenesis. *Cell* 1990;61:1329–1337.
174. Ohyama M. Hair follicle bulge: a fascinating reservoir of epithelial stem cells. *J Dermatol Sci* 2007;46:81–89.

175. Takeo M, Chou WC, Sun Q, et al. Wnt activation in nail epithelium couples nail growth to digit regeneration. *Nature* 2013;499:228–232.
176. Parent D, Achten G, Stouffs-Vanhoof F. Ultrastructure of the normal human nail. *Am J Dermatopathol* 1985;7:529–535.
177. Baran R, Sayag J. Nail biopsy–why, when, where, how? *J Dermatol Surg Oncol* 1976;2:322–324.
178. Bennet RG. Technique of biopsy of nails. *J Dermatol Surg Oncol* 1976;2:325–326.
179. Stone OJ, Barr RJ, Herten RJ. Biopsy of the nail area. *Cutis* 1978;21:257–260.
180. Scher RK. Biopsy of the matrix of a nail. *J Dermatol Surg Oncol* 1980;6:19–21.
181. Scher RK. Longitudinal resection of nails for purposes of biopsy and treatment. *J Dermatol Surg Oncol* 1980;6:805–807.
182. Rich P. Nail biopsy: indications and methods. *J Dermatol Surg Oncol* 1992;18(8):673–682.
183. Hwa C, Kovich OI, Stein JA. Achieving hemostasis after nail biopsy using absorbable gelatin sponge saturated in aluminum chloride. *Dermatol Surg* 2011;37:368–369.
184. Luna LG. Preparation of tissues. In: Luna LG, ed. *Manual of Histologic Staining Methods of the Armed Forces Institute of Pathology*. 3rd ed. New York: McGraw-Hill; 1968:1–11.
185. Rich P. Nail biopsy: indications and methods. *Dermatol Surg*. 2001;27(3):229–34.
186. Wlodek C, Lecerf P, Andre J, et al. An international survey about nail histology processing techniques. *J Cutan Pathol* 2017;44:749–756.
187. Baran R, de Berker DAR, Holzberg M, Thomas L. *Diseases of the Nails and their Management*. 4th ed. Chichester, UK: Wiley-Blackwell; 2012.
188. Alkiewicz J, Pfister R. *Atlas der Nagelkrankheiten*. Stuttgart, Germany: Schattauer-Verlag; 1976.

SECTION II

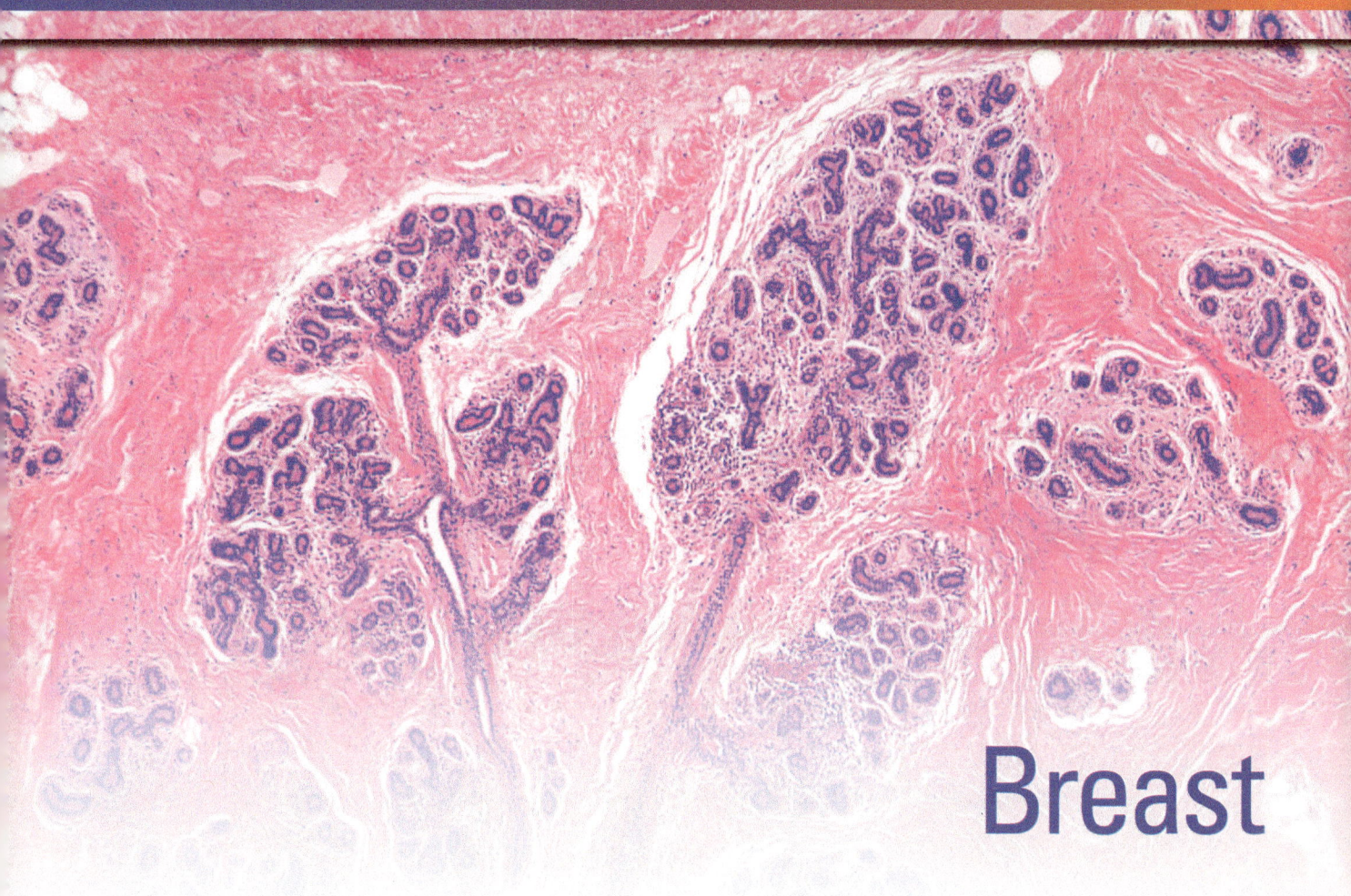

Breast

Breast

Laura C. Collins ■ Stuart J. Schnitt

EMBRYOLOGY 69	THE ADULT MALE BREAST 80
ADOLESCENCE 70	BIOLOGIC MARKERS, IMMUNOPHENOTYPE, AND MOLECULAR BIOLOGY 80
THE ADULT FEMALE BREAST 71	Estrogen Receptor and Progesterone Receptor 80
PREGNANCY AND LACTATION 78	Other Biomarkers and Immunophenotypic Features 81
	Molecular Markers 81
MENOPAUSE 79	CONCLUSION 81
BLOOD SUPPLY 79	REFERENCES 81
LYMPHATIC DRAINAGE 80	

Advances in breast imaging have provided a variety of noninvasive means to assist in the evaluation of patients with breast disorders (1–4). Nevertheless, at the present time, histologic examination of tissue specimens remains the cornerstone for the diagnosis of breast diseases, and an understanding of normal breast histology is essential for accurate evaluation of such specimens. It should be noted, however, that what constitutes "normal" histology in the breast varies according to gender, age, menopausal status, phase of the menstrual cycle, pregnancy, and lactation, among other factors. Therefore, determination of whether a given breast specimen is normal or shows pathologic alterations must take these variables into consideration.

EMBRYOLOGY

Development of the human mammary gland begins during the 5th week of gestation, at which time thickenings of the ectoderm appear on the ventral surface of the fetus. These mammary ridges, also known as milk lines, extend from the axilla to the groin. Except for a small area in the pectoral region, the bulk of these ridges normally regress as the fetus continues to develop. Failure of regression of other portions of the milk lines can result in the appearance in postnatal life of ectopic mammary tissue or accessory nipples anywhere along the milk lines; this phenomenon is most commonly encountered in the axilla, inframammary fold, and vulva (5–7).

The earliest stages of breast development are largely independent of sex steroid hormones (8). After the 15th week of gestation, the developing breast exhibits transient sensitivity to testosterone, which acts primarily on the mesenchyme. Under the influence of testosterone, the mesenchyme condenses around an epithelial stalk on the chest wall to form the breast bud, the site of mammary gland development. Solid epithelial columns then develop within the mesenchyme, and these ultimately give rise to the lobes or segments of the mammary gland. Portions of the fetal papillary dermis encase the developing epithelial cords and eventually give rise to the vascularized fibrous connective tissue that surrounds and invests the mammary ducts and lobules. The more collagen-rich reticular dermis extends into the breast to form the suspensory ligaments of Cooper, which attach the breast parenchyma to the skin. Portions of the mesenchyme differentiate into fat within the collagenous stroma between the 20th and 32nd weeks of gestation.

This chapter is an update of a previous version authored by Laura C. Collins and Stuart J. Schnitt.

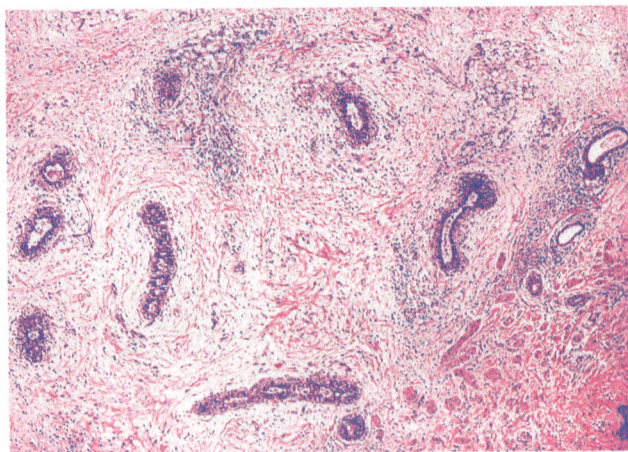

FIGURE 3.1 Breast tissue from an infant showing ducts embedded in a loose connective tissue stroma. The stromal mononuclear cells are hematopoietic elements, indicative of persistent extramedullary hematopoiesis. (Courtesy of Theonia Boyd, MD, Children's Hospital, Boston, MA)

During the last 8 weeks of gestation, the epithelial cords canalize and branch, forming lobuloalveolar structures as a result of mesenchymal paracrine effects. A depression in the epidermis, the mammary pit, forms at the convergence of the lactiferous ducts. The nipple forms by evagination of the mammary pit near the time of birth.

During the last few weeks of gestation the fetal mammary gland is responsive to maternal and placental steroid hormones, and, as a result, the epithelial cells in the acinar units exhibit secretory activity. At the time of birth, withdrawal of the maternal and placental sex steroids stimulates prolactin secretion, which in turn stimulates colostrum secretion. Both male and female neonates exhibit palpable enlargement of the breast bud. As the serum levels of maternal and placental sex steroid hormones and prolactin decline during the first month of life, secretory activity ends, and the gland regresses and becomes inactive. At this stage, and until puberty, the breast consists primarily of lactiferous ducts that exhibit some branching without evidence of progressive alveolar differentiation, although some rudimentary lobular structures may persist.

Another feature that may be seen in the fetal breast is extramedullary hematopoiesis, and this may persist in the periductal stroma until 4 months of age (Fig. 3.1) (9).

ADOLESCENCE

Adolescent breast development in the female begins with the onset of puberty and the cyclic secretion of estrogen and progesterone. However, a variety of other steroid and peptide hormones are also required for proper mammary gland development (Table 3.1) (8). The ducts elongate, branch, and develop a thickened epithelium primarily due to the influence of estrogen (Fig. 3.2) (10). The process

TABLE 3.1 Major Steroid and Peptide Hormonal Influences on the Breast

Hormone	Effects
Estrogen	Required for ductal growth and branching during adolescence Required for lobuloalveolar growth during pregnancy Required for induction of progesterone receptor Not necessary for maintenance of secretion or lactation
Progesterone	Required for lobuloalveolar differentiation and growth Probable mitogen in normal estrogen-primed breast Not necessary for ductal growth and branching
Testosterone	Stimulates breast mesenchyme during fetal development Causes mesenchymal destruction of mammary epithelium during critical period of testosterone sensitivity
Glucocorticoids	Required for maximal ductal growth Enhances lobuloalveolar growth during pregnancy
Insulin	Enhanced ductal-alveolar growth Enhances protein synthesis in mammary epithelium Required for secretory activity (with glucocorticoids and prolactin)
Prolactin	Stimulates epithelial growth after parturition Required for initiation and maintenance of lactation
Human placental lactogen	Able to substitute for prolactin in epithelial growth and differentiation Stimulates alveolar growth and lactogenesis in second half of pregnancy
Growth hormone	Required for ductal growth and branching during adolescence May contribute to lobuloacinar growth during pregnancy
Thyroid hormone	Increases epithelial response to prolactin May enhance lobuloacinar growth

Adapted from McCarty KS, Nath M. Breast. In: Sternberg SS, ed. *Histology for Pathologists*. Philadelphia, PA: Lippincott-Raven; 1997: 71–82.

of ductal growth and branching is largely independent of progesterone. There is an increase in the density of periductal connective tissue, also as a result of relative estrogen dominance. Deposition of stromal adipose tissue occurs, and it is this adipose tissue that is largely responsible for the enlargement and protrusion of the breast disk at this time. Cyclical exposure to progesterone following exposure to estrogen during ovulatory cycles promotes lobuloacinar growth, as well as connective tissue growth. Although the majority of breast development occurs during puberty, this process continues into the third decade, and terminal differentiation of the breast is only induced by pregnancy.

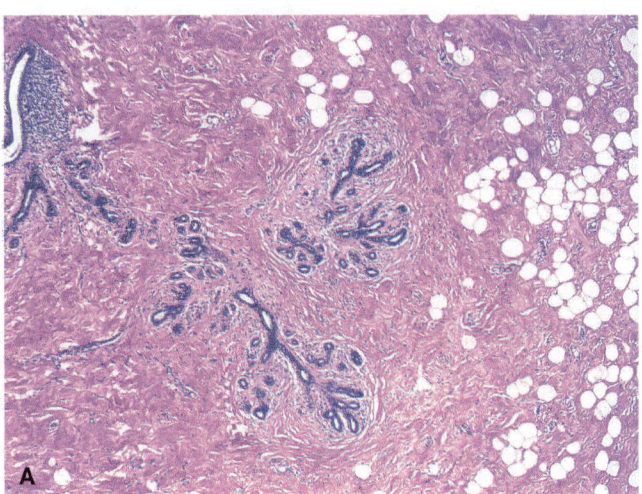 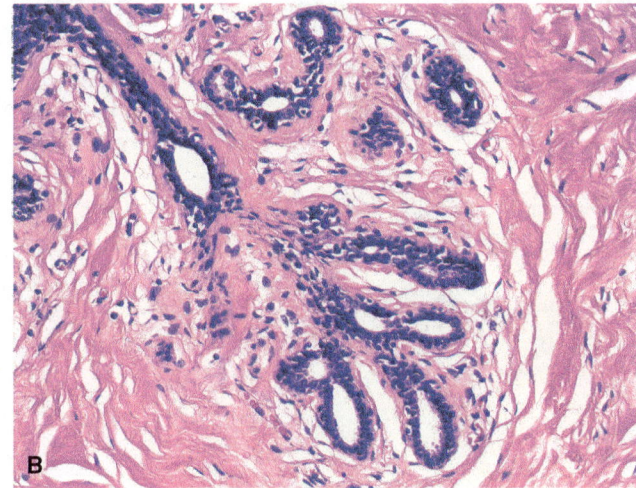

FIGURE 3.2 Adolescent breast tissue composed of branching ducts with rudimentary lobule development (type 1 lobules). The stroma consists of a mixture of fibrous connective tissue and adipose tissue. **A:** Scanning magnification. **B:** High power.

The adolescent male breast is composed of fibroadipose tissue and ducts lined by low cuboidal cells.

THE ADULT FEMALE BREAST

The size of the breast is greatly influenced by the individual's body habitus since the breast is a major repository for fat; it can range in size from 30 g to more than 1,000 g. The breast lies on the anterior chest wall over the pectoralis major muscle and typically extends from the 2nd to the 6th rib in the vertical axis and from the sternal edge to the mid-axillary line in the horizontal axis. Breast tissue also projects into the axilla as the tail of Spence. The breast extends laterally over the serratus anterior muscle and inferiorly over the external oblique muscle and the superior rectus sheath. The breast lies within a space in the superficial fascia, which is continuous with the cervical fascia superiorly and the superficial abdominal fascia of Cooper inferiorly. The only boundary of the breast that is anatomically well defined is the deep surface where it abuts the pectoralis fascia. However, despite this macroscopic demarcation, microscopic foci of glandular tissue may extend into and even through the pectoral fascia and may traverse the other anatomic boundaries described above. The clinical significance of this observation is that even total mastectomy does not result in removal of all glandular breast tissue. Bundles of dense fibrous connective tissue, the suspensory ligaments of Cooper, extend from the skin to the pectoral fascia and provide support to the breast.

The adult female breast consists of a series of ducts, ductules, and lobular acinar units embedded within a stroma that is composed of varying amounts of fibrous and adipose tissue. The stroma comprises the major portion of the nonlactating adult breast, and the relative proportions of fibrous tissue and adipose tissue vary with age and among individuals (Fig. 3.3).

The ductal-lobular system of the breast is arranged in the form of segments, or lobes. While these segments can be readily appreciated by injecting the ductal system with dyes or radiologic contrast agents (Fig. 3.4), they are anatomically poorly defined, and no obvious boundaries can be appreciated between these segments during surgery, upon gross inspection of mastectomy specimens, or on histologic examination. In addition, these segments show considerable individual variation with regard to their extent and distribution (11), and the ramifications of individual segments may overlap. The segmental nature of some neoplastic processes in the breast, particularly ductal carcinoma in situ, is now widely appreciated. This recognition, in conjunction with observations in developmental anatomy and morphology, has led to the development of the "sick lobe" hypothesis of breast cancer (12,13). This theory postulates that early breast carcinoma (ductal carcinoma in situ) is a lobar disease, often isolated to a single ductal system (or lobe). Thus, surgical resection of the involved lobe or segment is an important therapeutic goal. Unfortunately, since it is not possible for the surgeon to define intraoperatively the boundaries of the involved segment, performing a "segmentectomy" to remove the entirety of a diseased segment is at this time more of a theoretical concept than a practically attainable goal.

Each segment consists of a branching structure that has been likened to a flowering tree (Fig. 3.5) (14). The lobules represent the flowers, draining into ductules and ducts (twigs and branches), which, in turn, drain into the collecting ducts (trunk) that open onto the surface of the nipple. Just below the nipple, the ducts expand to form lactiferous sinuses. The sinuses terminate in cone-shaped ampullae just below the surface of the nipple.

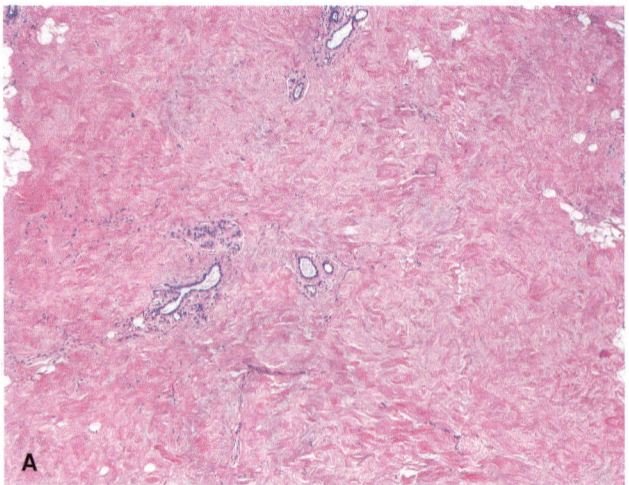 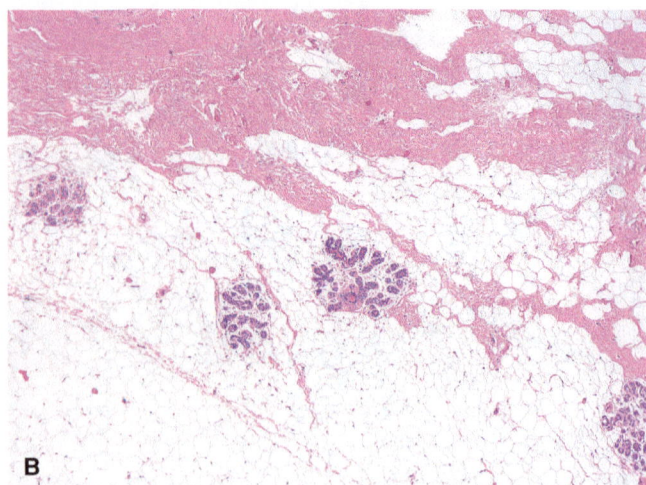

FIGURE 3.3 The stroma is the predominant component of the nonlactating breast and consists of varying amounts of collagen and adipose tissue. **A:** Low-power view of breast with dense, fibrotic stroma. **B:** Low-power view of breast with predominantly fatty stroma.

The actual number of segments in the breast and their relationship to each other has long been a matter of debate. Most textbooks indicate that there are 15 to 20 ductal orifices on the nipple surface and suggest that this corresponds to the number of ductal systems, segments, or lobes in the breast (5,6,15,16). In contrast, a number of mammary duct injection studies have suggested that there are only between 5 and 15 discrete breast ductal systems or segments in each breast. The discrepancy between the number of ductal orifices on the nipple and the actual number of breast segments or ductal systems may be explained by the fact that some of the orifices on the nipple represent openings of sebaceous glands or other nonductal tubular structures that do not contribute to the ductal-lobular anatomy of the breast. Another possibility is that some lactiferous ducts bifurcate immediately prior to entering the nipple or end blindly (16,17). The issue of anastomoses between ductal systems is also unresolved. One study indicated that, while ductal systems may lie in close proximity to one another and even intertwine within a particular quadrant, they do not interconnect (16). However, anastomoses between ductal systems have been reported by others (18).

FIGURE 3.4 Ductogram (galactogram). Performed by injecting contrast material into an orifice of a lactiferous duct at the nipple, a ductogram demonstrates the complex ramifications of a single mammary ductal system (also known as a segment or lobe).

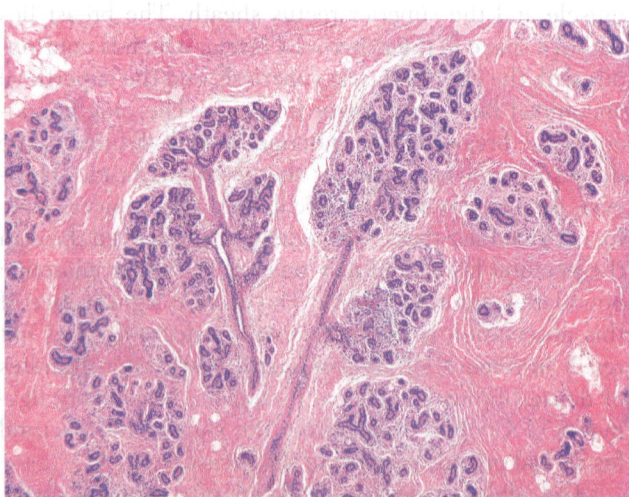

FIGURE 3.5 Microanatomy of normal adult female breast tissue showing extralobular ducts, terminal ducts, and lobules, the latter composed of groups of small glandular structures, the acini.

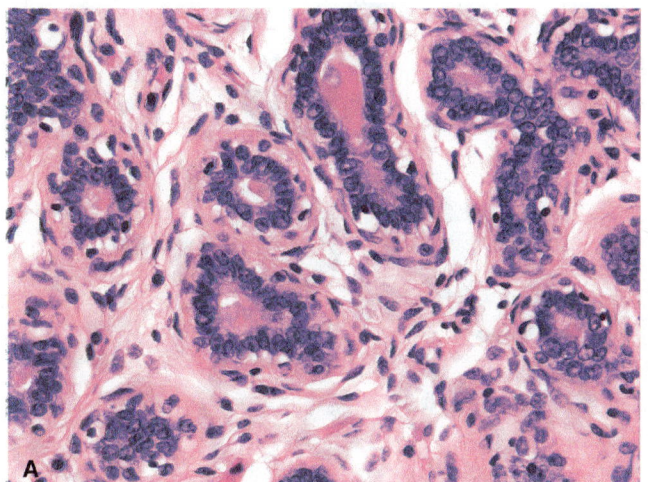
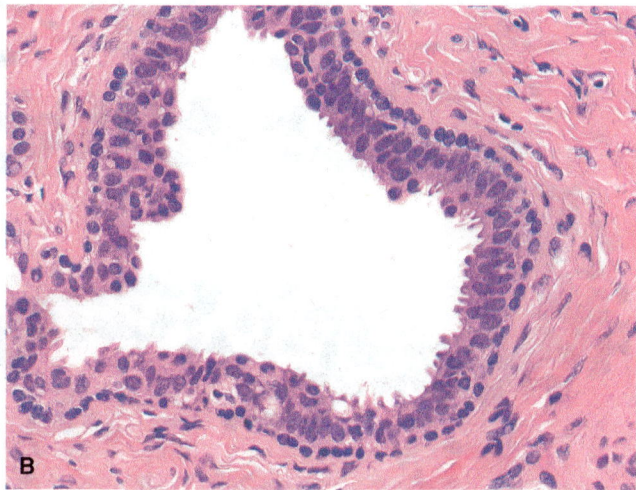

FIGURE 3.6 The mammary ductal-lobular system is lined by a dual cell population, an inner epithelial cell layer and an outer layer of myoepithelial cells. **A:** High-power view of a lobule. The myoepithelial cells surrounding the acinar epithelial cells are variably conspicuous. **B:** High-power view of an extralobular duct, showing distinct epithelial and myoepithelial cell layers.

The epithelium throughout the ductal-lobular system is bilayered, consisting of an inner (luminal) epithelial cell layer and an outer (basal) myoepithelial cell layer. The importance of this double cell layer cannot be overemphasized because it is one of the main guides used to distinguish benign from malignant lesions (19). The luminal epithelial cells of the resting breast ducts and lobules are cuboidal to columnar in shape and typically have pale eosinophilic cytoplasm and relatively uniform oval nuclei. These epithelial cells express a variety of low–molecular-weight cytokeratins, including cytokeratins 7, 8, 18, and 19 (20–24).

The outer (or myoepithelial) cell layer, although always present, is variably distinctive (Fig. 3.6). Myoepithelial cells range in appearance from barely discernible, flattened cells with compressed nuclei to prominent epithelioid cells with abundant clear cytoplasm. In some cases, the myoepithelial cells have a myoid appearance featuring a spindle cell shape and dense, eosinophilic cytoplasm, reminiscent of smooth muscle cells (Fig. 3.7). Even when inconspicuous on hematoxylin- and eosin-stained sections, myoepithelial cells can readily be demonstrated using immunohistochemical stains for a variety of markers, including actins, calponin, smooth muscle myosin heavy chain, p63, CD10, and p75 among others (Fig. 3.8) (25–30). However, these markers vary in both sensitivity and specificity for myoepithelium as well as in their expression by location within the terminal duct lobular unit (TDLU). Myoepithelial cells express high–molecular-weight cytokeratins 5/6, 14, and 17 (20–24,31), but the expression of cytokeratin 14 is restricted to the myoepithelial cells of the large ducts and terminal ducts;

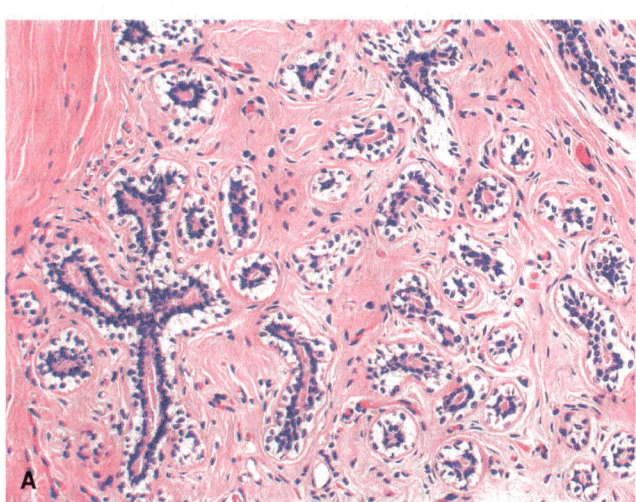
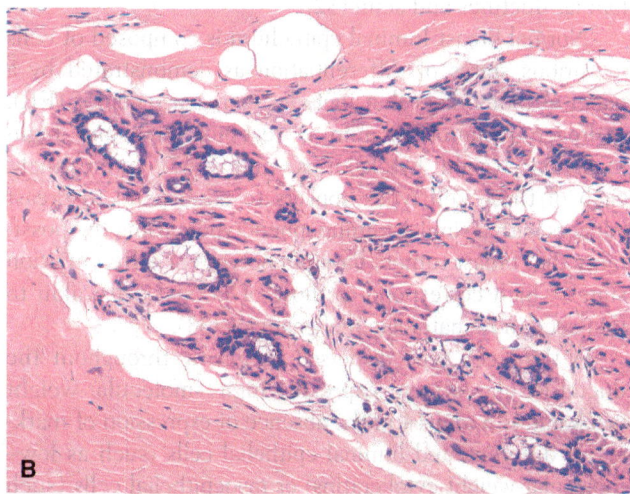

FIGURE 3.7 Myoepithelial cells can vary in their histologic appearance. **A:** Myoepithelial cells in this lobule show prominent cytoplasmic clearing. **B:** In this lobule, the myoepithelial cells show myoid features.

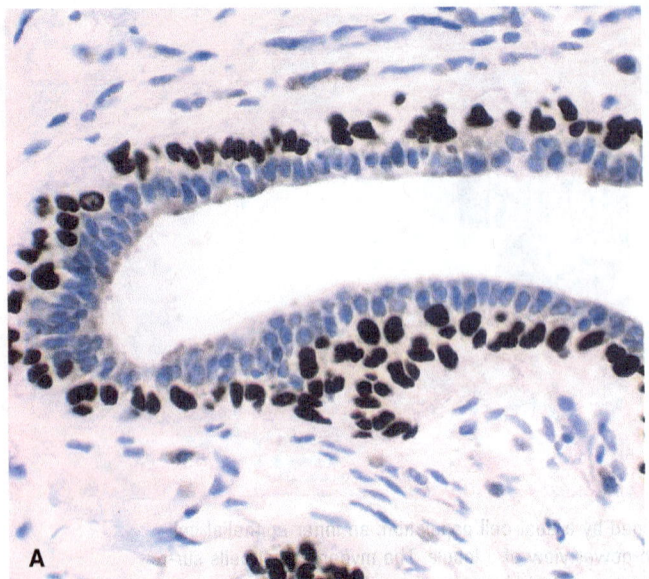
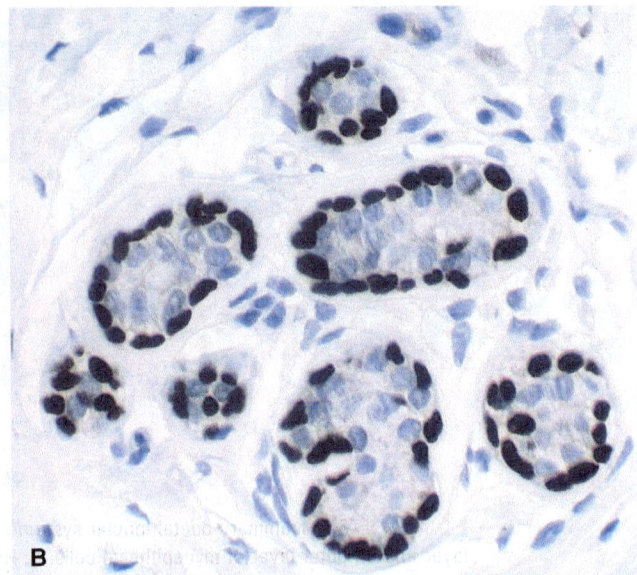
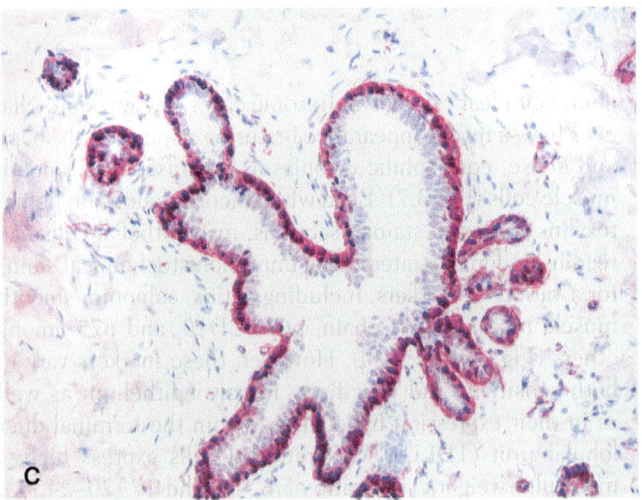

FIGURE 3.8 Extralobular duct (**A**) and lobule (**B**) immunostained for p63. The myoepithelial cells show strong nuclear reactivity, whereas the epithelial cell nuclei are negative. **C:** Double immunostain for smooth muscle actin (red cytoplasmic staining) and p63 (brown nuclear staining) highlight the myoepithelial cells around this mammary duct. Note the lack of staining of the epithelial cells for both p63 and smooth muscle actin.

expression is not seen in myoepithelial cells of the intralobular ductules and acini (32).

Normal breast luminal epithelium is composed of cells in various states of differentiation as demonstrated by a panel of biomarkers that includes estrogen receptor (ER), androgen receptor, vitamin D receptor, low- and high-molecular–weight cytokeratins, and Ki67. Interestingly, each of these cell types appears to correspond to breast cancers with a similar immunophenotype, raising the possibility that breast tumors have phenotypes or differentiation states which correspond to those of normal cells, akin to that seen in hematologic malignancies (33).

A third cell type dispersed irregularly throughout the ductal-lobular system expresses high—molecular-weight cytokeratins 5 and 14 in the absence of expression of markers of differentiated luminal epithelial cells (such as low–molecular-weight cytokeratins) or myoepithelial cells (such as smooth muscle actin). These cells have been postulated to represent progenitor cells capable of differentiating into both luminal epithelial cells and myoepithelial cells (34). The relationship of these putative "progenitor" cells to mammary stem cells is an unresolved issue (34,35). However, it is clear that the cells with the characteristic features of stem cells (i.e., self-renewal and the ability to differentiate down different cell lineages to form all of the cell types found in the mature tissue) do exist in the breast. Mammary stem cells appear to be important in both breast development (36) and mammary carcinogenesis (35,37,38). Phenotypic features that have been associated with the mammary stem cell population include lack of expression of ER and progesterone receptor (PR), high expression of CD44, low or absent expression of CD24 and expression of aldehyde dehydrogenase 1 (ALDH1) (38,39), although the most accurate combination of markers to reliably identify mammary stem cells is unresolved at this time.

A basal lamina consisting of type IV collagen and laminin surrounds the mammary ducts, ductules, and acini (21,40). This basal lamina is present outside of the myoepithelial

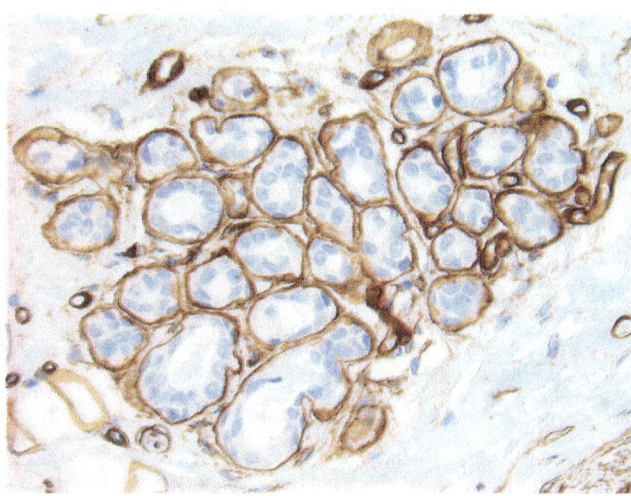

FIGURE 3.9 Immunostain for type IV collagen highlights the basal lamina around the acini of a lobule.

cell layer and serves to demarcate the breast ductal-lobular system from the surrounding stroma (Fig. 3.9). Beyond the basal lamina, the extralobular ducts exhibit a zone of fibroblasts and capillaries. Elastic tissue is normally present in variable amounts around ducts and is generally more prominent in older than in younger women. Elastic fibers are not typically seen around the terminal ducts or lobular acini.

The lobule, together with its terminal duct, has been called the TDLU. This represents the structural and functional unit of the breast. During lactation, epithelial cells in both the terminal duct and lobule undergo secretory changes. Thus, the terminal ducts are responsible for both secretion and transport of the secretions to the extra-lobular portion of the ductal system (15). Subgross anatomic studies have shown that most lesions originally termed "ductal" (e.g., cysts, ductal epithelial hyperplasià, and ductal carcinoma in situ) actually arise from the TDLU, which "unfolds" with coalescence of the acini to produce larger structures resembling ducts. The majority of pathologic changes in the breast, including in situ and invasive carcinomas, are generally considered to arise from the TDLU (14,41). Indeed, the only common lesion thought to arise from large- or medium-sized ducts rather than from the TDLU is solitary intraductal papilloma (Fig. 3.10).

The normal lobule consists of a variable number of blind-ending terminal ductules, also called acini, each with its typical double cell layer. The lobular acini are invested by a loose, fibrovascular intralobular stroma with varying numbers of lymphocytes, plasma cells, macrophages, and mast cells. This specialized intralobular stroma is sharply demarcated from the surrounding denser, more highly collagenized, paucicellular interlobular stroma, and stromal adipose tissue (Fig. 3.11). One feature of note that is sometimes encountered in the extralobular stroma is the presence of multinucleated giant cells (42). Their significance is unknown; and, while they may present a disturbing appearance, they should not be mistaken for the malignant cells of an invasive carcinoma (Fig. 3.12).

The size of mammary lobules and number of acini per lobule are extremely variable. Russo et al. have described four lobule types (43–45). Type 1 lobules are the most rudimentary and are most prevalent in prepubertal and nulliparous women, comprising 65% to 80% of the lobules in this group (Fig. 3.2). These lobules are comprised primarily of ducts with sprouting alveolar buds. However in practice, it is not possible to reliably distinguish type 1 lobules (i.e., those that have not fully developed) from those in which the number of acini is reduced due to involution. Type 1 lobules gradually evolve to more mature structures (type 2 and type 3 lobules) through the development of additional alveolar buds. The number of alveolar buds per lobule increases from approximately 11 in type 1 lobules to 47 and 80 in type 2 and 3 lobules, respectively. Recent data suggest that the histologic appearance of normal lobules may influence the risk of subsequent breast cancer. In particular, women whose breast tissue exhibits predominantly type 1 lobules or lobules that have undergone involution have a reduced risk of subsequent breast cancer compared to women with predominantly type 3 lobules or those that have not undergone involution (46–48). While there is

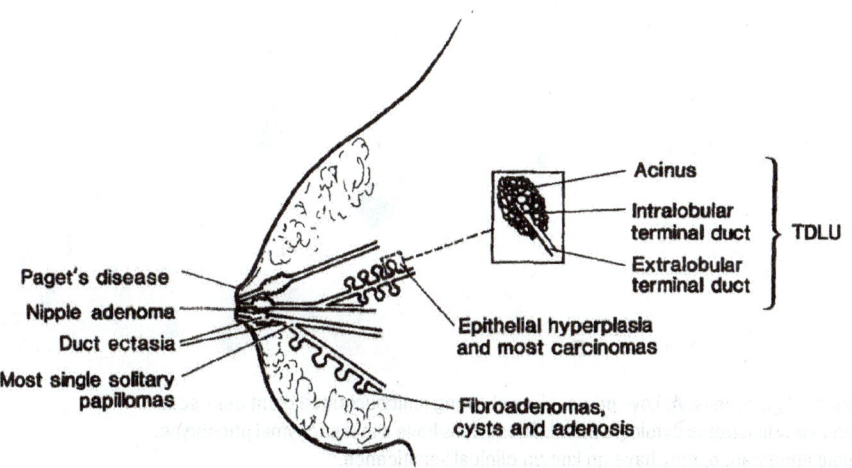

FIGURE 3.10 A schematic representation of the breast, indicating the sites of origin of pathologic lesions. (Reprinted from Schnitt SJ, Millis RR, Hanby AM, et al. The breast. In: Mills SE, Carter D, Greeson JK, Oberman HA, Reuter VE, Stoler MH, eds. *Sternberg's Diagnostic Surgical Pathology*. 4th ed. Philadelphia, PA: Lippincott Williams & Wilkins; 2004:323–398.)

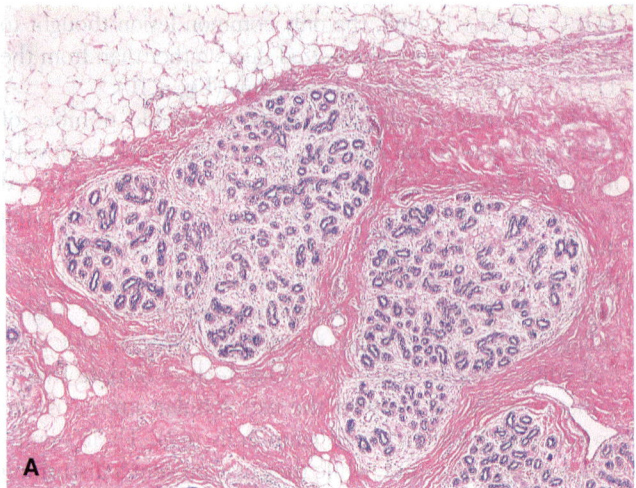
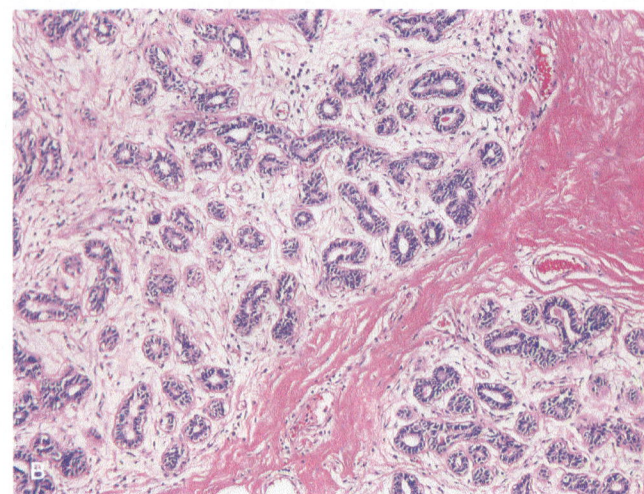

FIGURE 3.11 Intralobular and extralobular stroma. **A:** Low-power view of several lobules that are invested by loose, intralobular stroma. The interlobular stroma is composed primarily of dense collagen with admixed adipose tissue. **B:** Higher-power view contrasts loose intralobular stroma with more collagenized interlobular stroma.

some evidence to suggest the stage of involution is consistent across the breast and may provide an additional assessment of risk, the value of reporting the predominant lobular type in clinical practice remains to be determined (49).

The lobules exhibit morphologic changes during the menstrual cycle, and these are seen in both the epithelial and stromal components (50–53). These changes are summarized in Table 3.2. While the changes that occur during the menstrual cycle are variable among lobules in the same breast, even among immediately adjacent lobules, a dominant morphologic pattern is typically present in each phase. However, these menstrual cycle–related changes are subtle when compared with the dramatic alterations seen during pregnancy and lactation and when compared with the menstrual cycle–related changes seen in the endometrium.

Occasionally, the TDLU epithelial cells show prominent clear cell change in the cytoplasm. This may be seen in both premenopausal and postmenopausal women and appears to be unrelated to pregnancy or exogenous hormone use (54).

The nipple–areola complex is a circular area of skin that exhibits increased pigmentation and contains numerous sensory nerve endings. The nipple is placed centrally and is elevated above the surrounding areola. The tip of the nipple contains 15 to 20 orifices. However, as discussed earlier, the number of such openings may not correlate directly with the number of breast segments. In the nonlactating breast, these duct openings typically possess keratin plugs. The areola surface exhibits numerous small, rounded elevations, the tubercles of Montgomery.

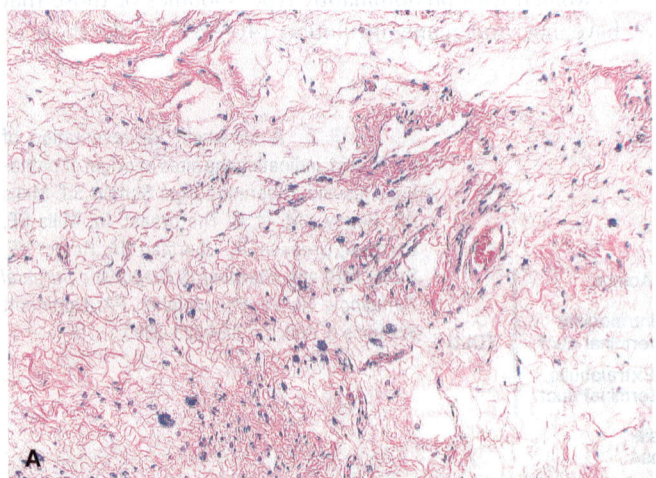
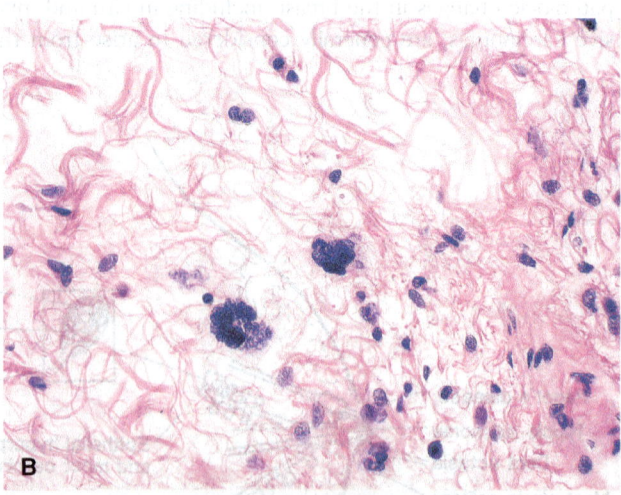

FIGURE 3.12 Multinucleated stromal giant cells. **A:** Low-power view showing multinucleated giant cells scattered in the stroma. **B:** High-power view illustrates cytologic detail. These cells have a mesenchymal phenotype. Despite their worrisome histologic appearance, they have no known clinical significance.

TABLE 3.2
Histologic Changes in Lobules During the Menstrual Cycle

Menstrual Cycle Phase	Epithelium	Acinar Lumina	Intralobular Stroma
Early follicular	*Cells:* single cell type (small, polygonal cells with pale eosinophilic cells); myoepithelial cells inconspicuous *Orientation:* poor *Secretion:* none *Mitoses/apoptosis:* rare	Largely closed and inapparent	Dense, cellular, with plump fibroblasts
Late follicular	*Cells:* three cell types, including luminal basophilic cells, intermediate pale cells (as seen in early follicular phase), and myoepithelial cells with clear cytoplasm *Orientation:* radial around lumen *Secretion:* none *Mitoses/apoptosis:* rare	Well-defined	Less cellular and more collagenized than in early luteal phase
Early luteal	*Cells:* three cell types, including luminal basophilic cells with minimal apical snouting, intermediate pale cells, and myoepithelial cells with prominent cytoplasmic vacuolization and ballooning *Orientation:* radial around lumen *Secretion:* slight *Mitoses/apoptosis:* rare	Open, enlarged compared to follicular phase, with slight secretion	Loose
Late luteal	*Cells:* three cell types, including luminal basophilic cells with prominent apical snouting, intermediate pale cells and myoepithelial cells with prominent cytoplasmic vacuolization *Orientation:* radial around lumen *Secretion:* active apocrine secretion from luminal cells *Mitoses/apoptosis:* frequent (peak of mitotic activity)	Open, with secretion	Loose, edematous, congested blood vessels
Menstrual	*Cells:* two cell types, including luminal basophilic cells with scant cytoplasm and less apical snouting than in late luteal phase, and myoepithelial cells with extensive cytoplasmic vacuolization *Orientation:* radial around lumen *Secretion:* resorbing *Mitoses/apoptosis:* rare	Distended with secretion	Dense, cellular

Adapted from McCarty KS, Nath M. Breast. In: Sternberg SS, ed. *Histology for Pathologists*. Philadelphia, PA: Lippincott-Raven; 1997: 71–82.

Both the nipple and areola are covered by keratinizing, stratified squamous epithelium, and this extends for a short distance into the terminal portions of the lactiferous ducts. The epidermis of the nipple–areola complex may contain occasional clear cells that are cytologically benign and that must not be confused with Paget cells (Fig. 3.13) (55,56). Some of these cells represent clear keratinocytes, whereas others are thought to be derived from epidermally located mammary ductal epithelium (Toker cells) (56).

The proximal ramifications of the mammary ductal system that are present in the dermis of the nipple typically have a pleated or serrated contour (Fig. 3.14). These ducts are surrounded by a stroma rich in circular and longitudinal smooth muscle bundles, collagen, and elastic fibers (Fig. 3.15). Occasionally, lobules may be seen in the nipple (57). Simple mammary ducts are also present throughout the dermis of the areola, even at its periphery, and these

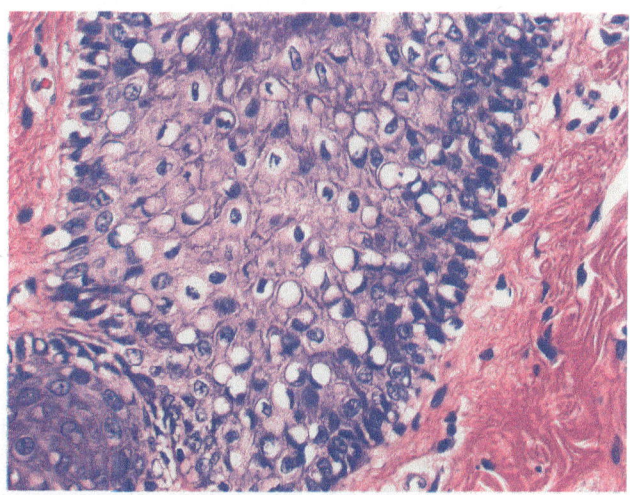

FIGURE 3.13 Clear cells in nipple epidermis. In some cells, the clearing is extreme, with formation of large intracytoplasmic vacuoles. These cells should not be mistaken for the cells of Paget disease.

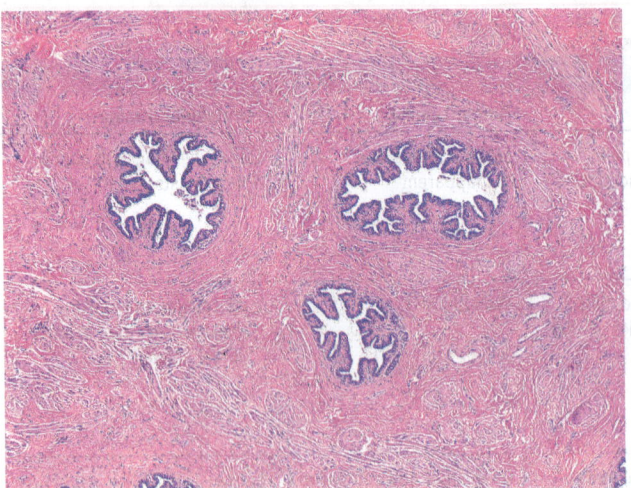

FIGURE 3.14 Cross section through the nipple. The irregular, pleated, or serrated contour of the nipple ducts is evident.

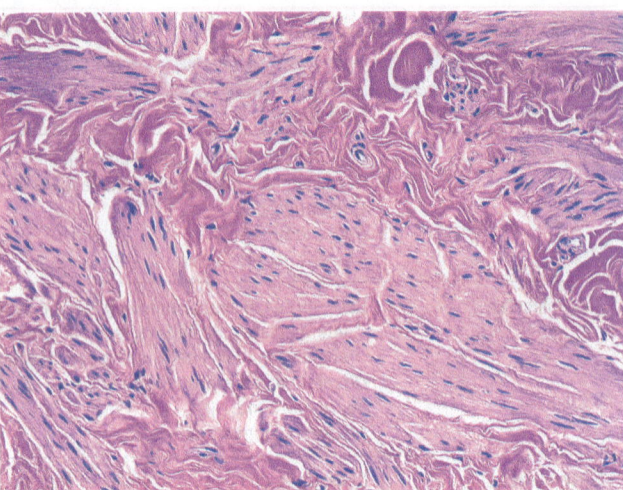

FIGURE 3.15 High-power view of nipple dermis/stroma, demonstrating prominent bundles of smooth muscle fibers.

may extend to within less than 1 mm of the basal layer of the epidermis (58).

While the nipple–areola complex lacks pilosebaceous units and hairs except at the periphery of the areola, the dermis contains numerous sebaceous glands. Some of these glands open directly onto the surface of the nipple and areola, whereas others drain into a lactiferous duct or share a common ostium with a lactiferous duct. The tubercles of Montgomery represent a unit consisting of a sebaceous apparatus and an associated lactiferous duct (Fig. 3.16) (59). During pregnancy, these tubercles become increasingly prominent. Apocrine sweat glands may also be seen in the dermis of the nipple and areola.

Another finding that may occasionally be encountered within the breast parenchyma is the presence of intramammary lymph nodes (60,61). These lymph nodes may be identified as an incidental finding in breast tissue removed because of another abnormality, or they may be seen as densities on mammograms (62).

PREGNANCY AND LACTATION

It is not until pregnancy that full development of the breast occurs in humans. During pregnancy, epithelial cell proliferation resumes. There is a dramatic increase in the number of lobules, as well as in the number of acinar units within each lobule secondary to epithelial cell proliferation and lobuloalveolar differentiation under the influence of estrogen, progesterone, prolactin, and growth hormone; growth is further enhanced by adrenal glucocorticoids and insulin. This lobular development and expansion occurs at the expense of both the intralobular and extralobular stroma. By

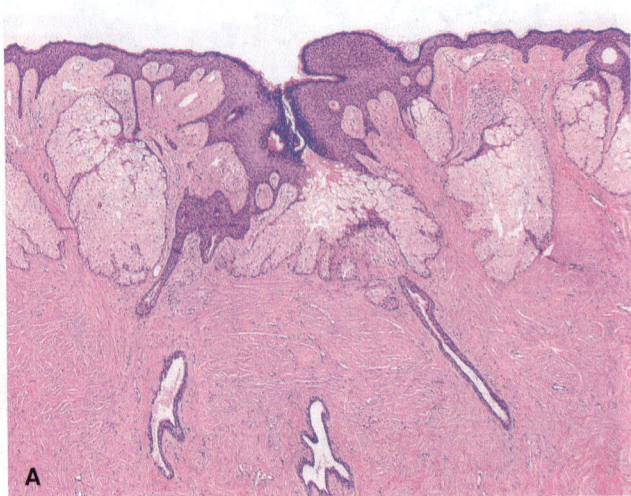
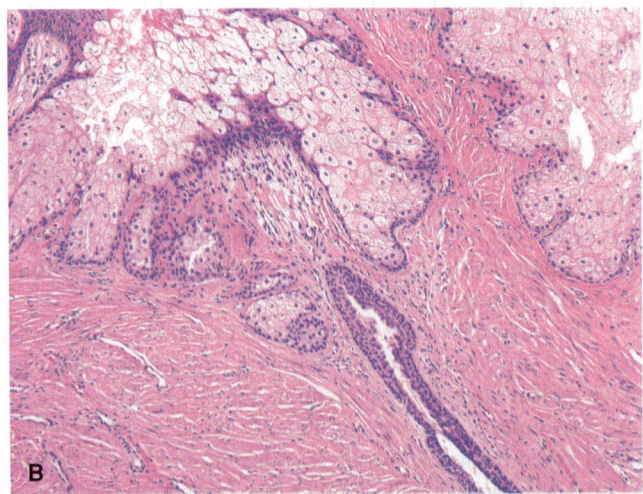

FIGURE 3.16 Montgomery areolar tubercle. **A:** Low-power view. **B:** Higher-power view. These tubercles are units composed of a lactiferous duct and associated sebaceous gland.

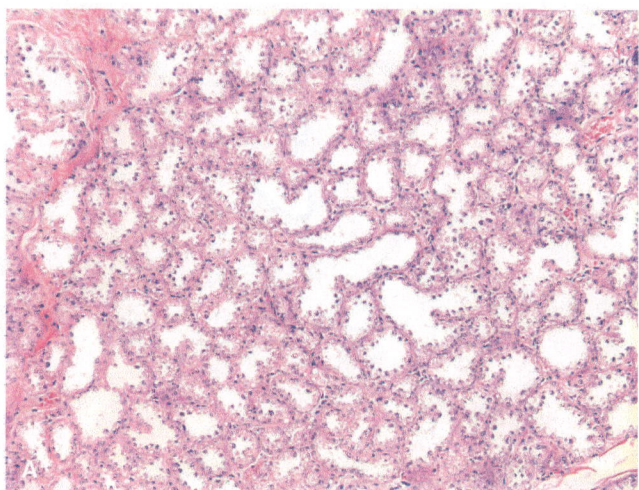
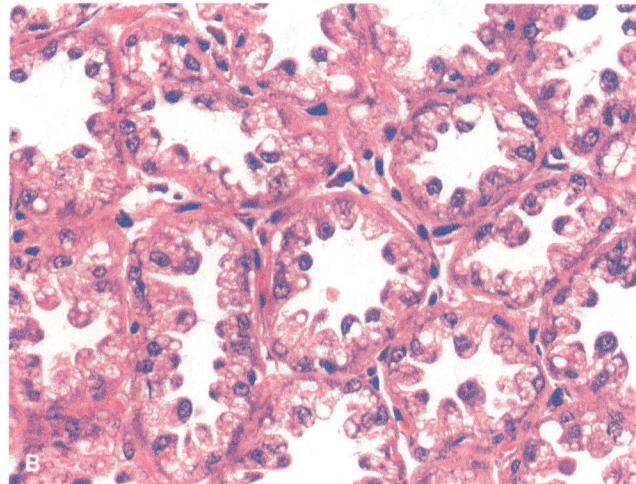

FIGURE 3.17 Lactating breast tissue. **A:** There are numerous acini in this lobule, and these are enlarged and dilated. There is minimal intervening stroma. **B:** Higher-power view illustrates prominent epithelial cell enlargement, cytoplasmic vacuolization, and protrusion of cells into the acinar lumen. Some of the cells have a hobnail appearance. Myoepithelial cells are inconspicuous.

the end of the first trimester, there is grossly evident breast enlargement, superficial venous dilatation, and increased pigmentation of the areola.

During the second and third trimesters, lobular growth continues, and the acinar units begin to appear monolayered. The myoepithelial cells in the acini are difficult to discern at this time due to the increase in size and volume of the epithelial cells, but they remain clearly evident in the extralobular ducts. The cytoplasm of the epithelial cells becomes vacuolated, and secretion accumulates in the greatly expanded lobules. After parturition, the lactating breast is characterized by distension of the lobular acini as a result of abundant accumulated secretory material and prominent epithelial cell cytoplasmic vacuolization. Many of the epithelial cells have a bulbous or hobnail appearance and protrude into the acinar lumina (Fig. 3.17). Myoepithelial cells remain attenuated and inconspicuous. The florid changes seen in pregnancy and lactation can be alarming to the inexperienced observer; areas of infarction, which occasionally occur in the pregnant breast, may compound the problem (63).

When lactation ceases, the lobules involute and return to their normal resting appearance. Involution usually proceeds unevenly and takes several months. Involuting lobules are irregular in contour and are frequently infiltrated by lymphocytes and plasma cells (64,65). Occasionally, an isolated lobule showing secretory changes may be seen in the breasts of women who are not pregnant; this phenomenon may occur in the nulliparous woman as well.

MENOPAUSE

During the postmenopausal period, with the reduction of estrogen and progesterone levels, there is involution and atrophy of the mammary TDLUs, with reduction in the size and complexity of the acini, and there is loss of the specialized intralobular stroma (66,67). Ducts may become variably ectatic. The postmenopausal breast is characterized by a marked reduction in glandular tissue and collagenous stroma, often with a concomitant increase in stromal adipose tissue. The end stage of menopausal involution is typified by remnants of the TDLUs, typically composed of ducts with atrophic acini, surrounded by hyalinized connective tissue or embedded within adipose tissue with little or no surrounding stroma (Fig. 3.18).

BLOOD SUPPLY

The principal arterial supply to the breast is provided by the internal mammary and lateral thoracic arteries. Perforating branches of the internal mammary artery provide the blood supply to approximately 60% of the breast, mainly the medial and central portions. Approximately 30% of the breast, mainly the upper and outer portions, receives blood from the lateral thoracic artery. Branches of the thoracoacromial, intercostal, subscapular, and thoracodorsal arteries make minor contributions to the mammary blood supply (7).

Venous drainage of the breast, as in other locations, shows considerable individual variation but largely follows the arterial system. There is a superficial venous complex that runs transversely from lateral to medial in the subcutaneous tissue. These vessels then drain into the internal thoracic vein. Deep venous drainage of the breast is via three routes: the perforating branches of the internal thoracic vein, branches of the axillary vein, and tributaries of the

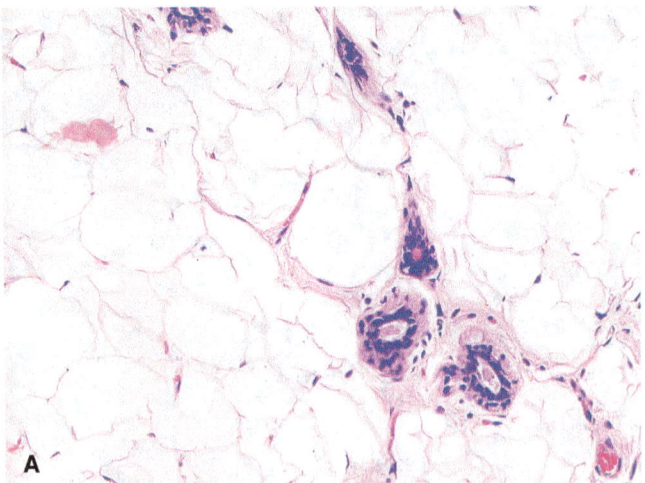
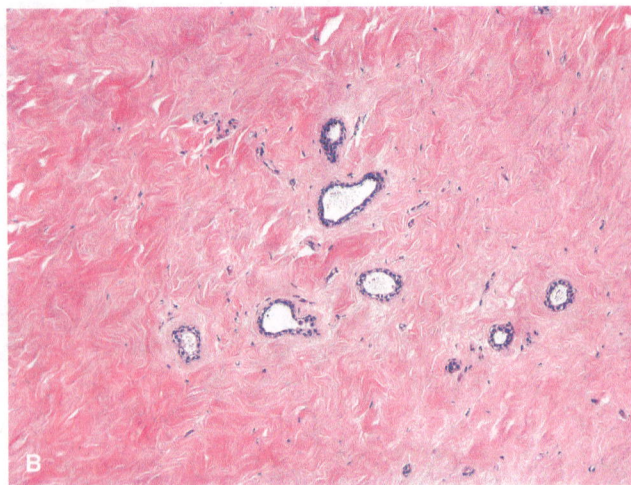

FIGURE 3.18 Postmenopausal breast tissue. **A:** This sample consists primarily of fatty stroma with a few atrophic ductules. **B:** In this specimen, a few residual, atrophic lobular acini are evident in a fibrotic stroma, which has replaced the normal, loose intralobular stroma.

intercostal veins, which drain posteriorly into the vertebral veins and the vertebral plexus (8,68).

LYMPHATIC DRAINAGE

Lymphatic drainage of the breast occurs through four routes: cutaneous, axillary, internal thoracic, and posterior intercostal lymphatics. The cutaneous lymphatic drainage system consists of both a superficial plexus of channels that lie within the dermis overlying the breast and a deeper network of lymphatic channels that runs with the mammary ducts in the subareolar area. Most of these cutaneous channels drain to the ipsilateral axilla. Cutaneous lymphatics from the inferior aspect of the breast may drain to the epigastric plexus and ultimately to the lymphatic channels of the liver and intra-abdominal lymph nodes.

There are three lymphatic drainage pathways in the mammary parenchyma. The most important drainage basin for lymphatic flow from the breast is the axilla, and the axillary lymph nodes receive the vast majority of the lymph drained. The internal thoracic lymphatic route carries less than 10% of the lymphatic flow from the breast and ultimately terminates in the internal mammary lymph nodes (7). Drainage eventually empties into the great veins via the thoracic duct, the lower cervical nodes, or the jugular–subclavian confluence. The third and least important route of mammary lymphatic drainage is the posterior intercostal lymphatics, which drain into the posterior intercostal lymph nodes. An understanding of the lymphatic drainage of the breast is of particular importance in the current era of sentinel lymph node biopsy since this explains the occasional finding of sentinel lymph nodes outside of the axilla (5,7,8).

THE ADULT MALE BREAST

The adult male breast, like the female breast, is composed of glandular epithelial elements embedded in a stroma that is composed of varying amounts of collagen and adipose tissue. However, in contrast to the adult female breast, the epithelial elements of the male breast normally consist of branching ducts without lobule formation.

BIOLOGIC MARKERS, IMMUNOPHENOTYPE, AND MOLECULAR BIOLOGY

Estrogen Receptor and Progesterone Receptor

It is now known that there are at least two different ERs, ERα and ERβ; ERα has been far more extensively studied. Using immunohistochemistry, ERα expression can be demonstrated in the nuclei of both ductal and lobular epithelial cells, with a higher proportion in lobules than in ducts. However, even in the lobules, only a small proportion of the cells show ERα immunoreactivity. Most often, ERα-positive cells in the lobules are distributed singly, admixed with and surrounded by ERα-negative cells (Fig. 3.19) (69). Furthermore, there is considerable heterogeneity in staining for ERα among lobules in the same breast. Of interest, in breast tissue from premenopausal women, there is generally an inverse relationship between expression of ERα and markers of cell proliferation. In particular, most ERα-positive cells do not show expression of the proliferation-related antigen Ki-67, and Ki-67–positive cells are typically ERα-negative. The proportion of ERα-positive cells gradually increases with age but remains relatively stable after the menopause. The incidence of lobules showing contiguous

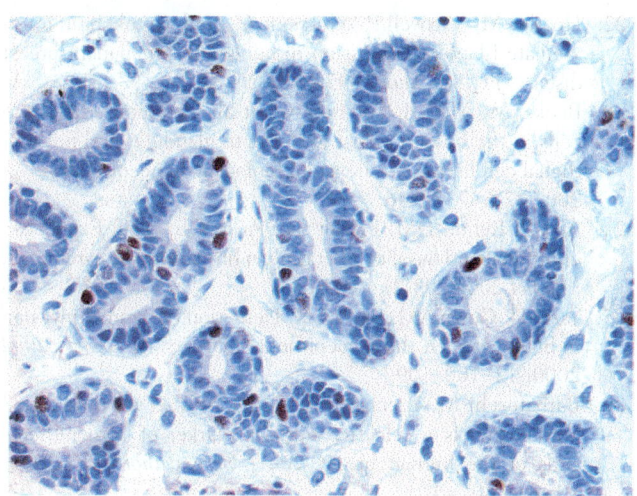

FIGURE 3.19 Immunostain for estrogen receptor-α (ERα) in a normal lobule. A minority of epithelial cells show nuclear staining.

patches of ERα-positive cells also increases with age and with involutional changes (69). In addition, the proportion of ERα-positive proliferating cells increases with age (69). In premenopausal women, ERα expression varies with the phase of the menstrual cycle, being higher in the follicular than in the luteal phase (70). Myoepithelial cells do not show ERα immunoreactivity (33).

A second form of ER, ERβ, is also expressed in normal breast tissue. Expression of ERβ has been observed not only in epithelial cells of ducts and lobules, but also in myoepithelial cells, endothelial cells, and stromal cells (70–73). The expression of this form of ER does not seem to vary with the phase of the menstrual cycle. It has been speculated that the relative levels of ERβ and ERα may be important in determining the risk of breast cancer development, and that higher levels of ERβ relative to ERα are protective against neoplastic progression in the breast (71). However, additional studies are needed to more clearly elucidate the role of ERβ in normal breast physiology and in breast cancer pathogenesis and to determine which ERβ isoform provides the greatest specificity in this regard (74).

Expression of PR has not been as extensively studied in normal breast tissue as has ER. Like ERα, PR is expressed in the nuclei of ductal and lobular epithelium. However, in contrast to ERα expression, PR expression does not seem to vary with the menstrual cycle phase (70).

Other Biomarkers and Immunophenotypic Features

Expression of a wide variety of biomarkers has been studied in benign breast tissue (75) and a comprehensive review of these is beyond the scope of this chapter. However, a couple of these merits brief mention, though the clinical significance of the findings is as yet uncertain. Rarely, normal breast epithelium may show HER2 protein overexpression, p53 protein accumulation, or *p53* mutations. Of note p53 alterations have been identified more frequently in normal epithelium adjacent to breast carcinomas that are ER, PR and HER2 negative ("triple negative"), and/or in *BRCA1* mutation carriers raising the possibility that this "p53 signature" may confer a predisposition to p53-associated— high-grade carcinomas (76,77).

The antiapoptotic protein bcl-2 is consistently expressed by normal breast epithelial cells (78). S-100 protein is strongly expressed by normal myoepithelial cells and variably expressed by mammary epithelial cells (79). Epithelial cells also show variable expression for casein (80), α-lactalbumin (81), gross cystic disease fluid protein-15 (82), mammaglobin (83), GATA-3 and c-Kit (CD117) (84), among other proteins. As noted earlier, cytokeratins 7, 8, 18, and 19 (20–24) are typically expressed by epithelial cells, whereas myoepithelial cells express cytokeratins 5/6, 14, and 17 (20–24,31).

Molecular Markers

The ability to evaluate DNA, RNA, and protein using the modern tools of molecular biology, particularly when guided by such techniques as laser capture microdissection (85), are enhancing our understanding of breast tumorigenesis and may even serve to redefine what constitutes "normal." For example, a number of studies have shown that histologically normal TDLUs can exhibit an abnormal genotype, characterized by loss of heterozygosity (86,87), allelic imbalance (88,89) at various chromosomal loci, or altered gene expression profiles (90). At this time, however, the significance of these genetic and molecular alterations in histologically normal breast tissue remains to be determined. Studies of normal breast tissue using these techniques will also help to further define the presence and nature of progenitor cells or stem cells and their role in breast development and carcinogenesis (23,91–93), as well as patterns of gene and protein expressions that distinguish normal from abnormal breast tissue and cells (94–97).

CONCLUSION

The histologic features of the normal breast are dynamic and vary with age and hormonal milieu, among other factors. An understanding of normal breast histology is essential to permit the reliable distinction between physiologic changes and pathologic alterations.

REFERENCES

1. Jochelson M. Breast cancer imaging: the future. *Semin Oncol* 2001;28(3):221–228.

2. Leung JW. New modalities in breast imaging: digital mammography, positron emission tomography, and sestamibi scintimammography. *Radiol Clin North Am* 2002;40(3):467–482.
3. Koomen M, Pisano ED, Kuzmiak C, et al. Future directions in breast imaging. *J Clin Oncol* 2005;23(8):1674–1677.
4. Hylton N. Magnetic resonance imaging of the breast: opportunities to improve breast cancer management. *J Clin Oncol* 2005;23(8):1678–1684.
5. Rosen PP. *Rosen's Breast Pathology*. 3rd ed. Philadelphia, PA: Lippincott Williams & Wilkins; 2009.
6. Tavassoli FA. Normal development and anomalies. In: Tavassoli FA, ed. *Pathlogy of the Breast*. 2nd ed. Stamford, CT: Appelton and Lange; 1999:1–25.
7. Osborne MP. Breast anatomy and development. In: Harris JR, Lippman ME, Morrow M, Osborne CK, eds. *Diseases of the Breast*. 4th ed. Philadelphia, PA: Lippincott Williams and Wilkins; 2010:3–11.
8. McCarty KS, Nath M. Breast. In: Sternberg SS, ed. *Histology for Pathologists*. Philadelphia, PA: Lippincott-Raven; 1997:71–82.
9. Anbazhagan R, Bartek J, Monaghan P, et al. Growth and development of the human infant breast. *Am J Anat* 1991;192(4):407–417.
10. Monaghan P, Perusinghe NP, Cowen P, et al. Peripubertal human breast development. *Anat Rec* 1990;226(4):501–508.
11. Going JJ, Moffat DF. Escaping from Flatland: clinical and biological aspects of human mammary duct anatomy in three dimensions. *J Pathol* 2004;203(1):538–544.
12. Going JJ, Mohun TJ. Human breast duct anatomy, the 'sick lobe' hypothesis and intraductal approaches to breast cancer. *Breast Cancer Res Treat* 2006;97(3):285–291.
13. Tot T. The theory of the sick breast lobe and the possible consequences. *Int J Surg Pathol* 2007;15(4):369–375.
14. Jensen HM. Breast pathology, emphasizing precancerous and cancer-associated lesions. In: Bulbrook RO, Taylor DJ, eds. *Commentaries on Research in Breast Disease*. Vol. 2. New York: Alan R. Liss; 1981:41–86.
15. Page OL, Anderson TJ. *Diagnostic Histopathology of the Breast*. Edinburgh: Churchill Livingstone; 1987.
16. Love SM, Barsky SH. Anatomy of the nipple and breast ducts revisited. *Cancer* 2004;101(9):1947–1957.
17. Rusby JE, Brachtel EF, Michaelson JS, et al. Breast duct anatomy in the human nipple: three-dimensional patterns and clinical implications. *Breast Cancer Res Treat* 2007;106(2):171–179.
18. Ohtake T, Kimijima I, Fukushima T, et al. Computer-assisted complete three-dimensional reconstruction of the mammary ductal/lobular systems: implications of ductal anastomoses for breast-conserving surgery. *Cancer* 2001;91(12):2263–2272.
19. Schnitt SJ, Millis RR, Hanby AM, et al. The Breast. In: Mills SE, ed. *Diagnostic Surgical Pathology*. 4th ed. Philadelphia, PA: Lippincott, Williams & Wilkins; 2004:323–395.
20. Jarasch ED, Nagle RB, Kaufmann M, et al. Differential diagnosis of benign epithelial proliferations and carcinomas of the breast using antibodies to cytokeratins. *Hum Pathol* 1988;19(3):276–289.
21. Bocker W, Bier B, Freytag G, et al. An immunohistochemical study of the breast using antibodies to basal and luminal keratins, alpha-smooth muscle actin, vimentin, collagen IV and laminin. Part I: Normal breast and benign proliferative lesions. *Virchows Arch A Pathol Anat Histopathol* 1992;421(4):315–322.
22. Heatley M, Maxwell P, Whiteside C, et al. Cytokeratin intermediate filament expression in benign and malignant breast disease. *J Clin Pathol* 1995;48(1):26–32.
23. Bocker W, Moll R, Poremba C, et al. Common adult stem cells in the human breast give rise to glandular and myoepithelial cell lineages: a new cell biological concept. *Lab Invest* 2002;82(6):737–746.
24. Abd El-Rehim DM, Pinder SE, Paish CE, et al. Expression of luminal and basal cytokeratins in human breast carcinoma. *J Pathol* 2004;203(2):661–671.
25. Yaziji H, Gown AM, Sneige N. Detection of stromal invasion in breast cancer: the myoepithelial markers. *Adv Anat Pathol* 2000;7(2):100–109.
26. Barbareschi M, Pecciarini L, Cangi MG, et al. p63, a p53 homologue, is a selective nuclear marker of myoepithelial cells of the human breast. *Am J Surg Pathol* 2001;25(8):1054–1060.
27. Moritani S, Kushima R, Sugihara H, et al. Availability of CD10 immunohistochemistry as a marker of breast myoepithelial cells on paraffin sections. *Mod Pathol* 2002;15(4):397–405.
28. Yeh IT, Mies C. Application of immunohistochemistry to breast lesions. *Arch Pathol Lab Med* 2008;132(3):349–358.
29. Bhargava R, Dabbs DJ. Use of immunohistochemistry in diagnosis of breast epithelial lesions. *Adv Anat Pathol* 2007;14(2):93–107.
30. Popnikolov NK, Cavone SM, Schultz PM, et al. Diagnostic utility of p75 neurotrophin receptor (p75NTR) as a marker of breast myoepithelial cells. *Mod Pathol* 2005;18(12):1535–1541.
31. Nielsen TO, Hsu FD, Jensen K, et al. Immunohistochemical and clinical characterization of the basal-like subtype of invasive breast carcinoma. *Clin Cancer Res* 2004;10(16):5367–5674.
32. Going JJ. *Normal Breast*. In: O'Malley FP, Pinder SE, Goldblum JR, eds. Philadelphia, PA: Churchill, Livingstone, Elsevier; 2006:55–65.
33. Santagata S, Thakkar A, Ergonul A, et al. Taxonomy of breast cancer based on normal cell phenotype predicts outcome. *J Clin Invest* 2014;124(2):859–870.
34. Boecker W, Weigel S, Handel W, et al. The normal breast. In: Boecker W, ed. *Preneoplasia of the Breast: A New Conceptual Approach to Proliferative Breast Disease*. Munich: Elsevier; 2006:2–27.
35. Cariati M, Purushotham AD. Stem cells and breast cancer. *Histopathology* 2008;52(1):99–107.
36. Shackleton M, Vaillant F, Simpson KJ, et al. Generation of a functional mammary gland from a single stem cell. *Nature* 2006;439(7072):84–88.
37. Morimoto K, Kim SJ, Tanei T, et al. Stem cell marker aldehyde dehydrogenase 1-positive breast cancers are characterized by negative estrogen receptor, positive human epidermal growth factor receptor type 2, and high Ki67 expression. *Cancer Sci* 2009;100(6):1062–1068.
38. Zhou L, Jiang Y, Yan T, et al. The prognostic role of cancer stem cells in breast cancer: A meta-analysis of published literatures. *Breast Cancer Res Treat* 2010;122(3):795–801.
39. Al-Hajj M, Wicha MS, Benito-Hernandez A, et al. Prospective identification of tumorigenic breast cancer cells. *Proc Natl Acad Sci U S A* 2003;100(7):3983–3988.
40. Barsky SH, Siegal GP, Jannotta F, et al. Loss of basement membrane components by invasive tumors but not by their benign counterparts. *Lab Invest* 1983;49(2):140–147.

41. Wellings SR, Jensen HM, Marcum RG. An atlas of subgross pathology of the human breast with special reference to possible precancerous lesions. *J Natl Cancer Inst* 1975;55(2):231–273.
42. Rosen PP. Multinucleated mammary stromal giant cells: a benign lesion that simulates invasive carcinoma. *Cancer* 1979;44(4):1305–1308.
43. Russo J, Russo IH. Development of the human mammary gland. In: Neville MC, Daniel CW, eds. *The Mammary Gland Development, Regulation and Function*. New York: Plenum Press; 1987:67–93.
44. Russo J, Rivera R, Russo IH. Influence of age and parity on the development of the human breast. *Breast Cancer Res Treat* 1992;23(3):211–218.
45. Russo J, Romero AL, Russo IH. Architectural pattern of the normal and cancerous breast under the influence of parity. *Cancer Epidemiol Biomarkers Prev* 1994;3(3):219–224.
46. Baer HJ, Collins LC, Connolly JL, et al. Lobule type and subsequent breast cancer risk: Results from the Nurses' Health Studies. *Cancer* 2009;115(7):1404–1411.
47. Milanese TR, Hartmann LC, Sellers TA, et al. Age-related lobular involution and risk of breast cancer. *J Natl Cancer Inst* 2006;98(22):1600–1607.
48. Radisky DC, Visscher DW, Frank RD, et al. Natural history of age-related lobular involution and impact on breast cancer risk. *Breast Cancer Res Treat* 2016;155(3):423–430.
49. Vierkant RA, Hartmann LC, Pankratz VS, et al. Lobular involution: Localized phenomenon or field effect? *Breast Cancer Res Treat* 2009;117(1):193–196.
50. Vogel PM, Georgiade NG, Fetter BF, et al. The correlation of histologic changes in the human breast with the menstrual cycle. *Am J Pathol* 1981;104(1):23–34.
51. Longacre TA, Bartow SA. A correlative morphologic study of human breast and endometrium in the menstrual cycle. *Am J Surg Pathol* 1986;10(6):382–393.
52. Ramakrishnan R, Khan SA, Badve S. Morphological changes in breast tissue with menstrual cycle. *Mod Pathol* 2002;15(12):1348–1356.
53. Anderson TJ. Normal breast: myths, realities, and prospects. *Mod Pathol* 1998;11(2):115–119.
54. Tavassoli FA, Yeh IT. Lactational and clear cell changes of the breast in nonlactating, nonpregnant women. *Am J Clin Pathol* 1987;87(1):23–29.
55. Toker C. Clear cells of the nipple epidermis. *Cancer* 1970;25(3):601–610.
56. Kohler S, Rouse RV, Smoller BR. The differential diagnosis of pagetoid cells in the epidermis. *Mod Pathol* 1998;11(1):79–92.
57. Rosen PP, Tench W. Lobules in the nipple. Frequency and significance for breast cancer treatment. *Pathol Annu* 1985;20(Pt 2):317–322.
58. Schnitt SJ, Goldwyn RM, Slavin SA. Mammary ducts in the areola: implications for patients undergoing reconstructive surgery of the breast. *Plast Reconstr Surg* 1993;92(7):1290–1293.
59. Smith DM, Jr., Peters TG, Donegan WL. Montgomery's areolar tubercle. A light microscopic study. *Arch Pathol Lab Med* 1982;106(2):60–63.
60. Egan RL, McSweeney MB. Intramammary lymph nodes. *Cancer* 1983;51(10):1838–1842.
61. Jadusingh IH. Intramammary lymph nodes. *J Clin Pathol* 1992;45(11):1023–1026.
62. Svane G, Franzen S. Radiologic appearance of nonpalpable intramammary lymph nodes. *Acta Radiol* 1993;34(6):577–580.
63. Oberman HA. Breast lesions confused with carcinoma. In: McDivitt R, Oberman H, Ozello L, ed. *The Breast*. Baltimore, MD: Williams and Wilkins; 1984:1–3.
64. Battersby S, Anderson TJ. Proliferative and secretory activity in the pregnant and lactating human breast. *Virchows Arch A Pathol Anat Histopathol* 1988;413(3):189–196.
65. Battersby S, Anderson TJ. Histological changes in breast tissue that characterize recent pregnancy. *Histopathology* 1989;15(4):415–419.
66. Hutson SW, Cowen PN, Bird CC. Morphometric studies of age related changes in normal human breast and their significance for evolution of mammary cancer. *J Clin Pathol* 1985;38(3):281–287.
67. Cowan DF, Herbert TA. Involution of the breast in women aged 50–104 years: A histopathological study of 102 cases. *Surg Pathol* 1989;2(4):323–333.
68. Rosen PP. *Rosen's Breast Pathology*. 2nd ed. Philadelphia, PA: Lippincott Williams & Wilkins; 2001:381–404.
69. Shoker BS, Jarvis C, Sibson DR, et al. Oestrogen receptor expression in the normal and pre-cancerous breast. *J Pathol* 1999;188(3):237–244.
70. Shaw JA, Udokang K, Mosquera JM, et al. Oestrogen receptors alpha and beta differ in normal human breast and breast carcinomas. *J Pathol* 2002;198(4):450–457.
71. Shaaban AM, O'Neill PA, Davies MP, et al. Declining estrogen receptor-beta expression defines malignant progression of human breast neoplasia. *Am J Surg Pathol* 2003;27(12):1502–1512.
72. Speirs V, Walker RA. New perspectives into the biological and clinical relevance of oestrogen receptors in the human breast. *J Pathol* 2007;211(5):499–506.
73. Younes M, Honma N. Estrogen receptor β. *Arch Pathol Lab Med* 2011;135(1):63–66.
74. Haldosen LA, Zhao C, Dahlman-Wright K. Estrogen receptor beta in breast cancer. *Mol Cell Endocrinol* 2014;382(1):665–672.
75. Krishnamurthy S, Sneige N. Molecular and biologic markers of premalignant lesions of human breast. *Adv Anat Pathol* 2002;9(3):185–197.
76. Wang X, Stolla M, Ring BZ, et al. p53 alteration in morphologically normal/benign breast tissue in patients with triple-negative high-grade breast carcinomas: breast p53 signature? *Hum Pathol* 2016;55:196–201.
77. Wang X, El-Halaby AA, Zhang H, et al. P53 alteration in morphologically normal/benign breast luminal cells in BRCA carriers with or without history of breast cancer. *Hum Pathol* 2017;68:22–25.
78. Siziopikou KP, Prioleau JE, Harris JR, et al. bcl-2 expression in the spectrum of preinvasive breast lesions. *Cancer* 1996;77(3):499–506.
79. Egan MJ, Newman J, Crocker J, et al. Immunohistochemical localization of S100 protein in benign and malignant conditions of the breast. *Arch Pathol Lab Med* 1987;111(1):28–31.
80. Earl HM, McIlhinney RA, Wilson P, et al. Immunohistochemical study of beta- and kappa-casein in the human breast and breast carcinomas, using monoclonal antibodies. *Cancer Res* 1989;49(21):6070–6076.

81. Bailey AJ, Sloane JP, Trickey BS, et al. An immunocytochemical study of alpha-lactalbumin in human breast tissue. *J Pathol* 1982;137(1):13–23.
82. Mazoujian G, Pinkus GS, Davis S, et al. Immunohistochemistry of a gross cystic disease fluid protein (GCDFP-15) of the breast. A marker of apocrine epithelium and breast carcinomas with apocrine features. *Am J Pathol* 1983;110(2):105–112.
83. Sasaki E, Tsunoda N, Hatanaka Y, et al. Breast-specific expression of MGB1/mammaglobin: an examination of 480 tumors from various organs and clinicopathological analysis of MGB1-positive breast cancers. *Mod Pathol* 2007;20(2): 208–214.
84. Chui X, Egami H, Yamashita J, et al. Immunohistochemical expression of the c-kit proto-oncogene product in human malignant and non-malignant breast tissues. *Br J Cancer* 1996; 73(10):1233–1236.
85. Simone NL, Paweletz CP, Charboneau L, et al. Laser capture microdissection: Beyond functional genomics to proteomics. *Mol Diagn* 2000;5(4):301–307.
86. Deng G, Lu Y, Zlotnikov G, et al. Loss of heterozygosity in normal tissue adjacent to breast carcinomas. *Science* 1996;274(5295):2057–2059.
87. Lakhani SR, Chaggar R, Davies S, et al. Genetic alterations in 'normal' luminal and myoepithelial cells of the breast. *J Pathol* 1999;189(4):496–503.
88. Larson PS, de las Morenas A, Cupples LA, et al. Genetically abnormal clones in histologically normal breast tissue. *Am J Pathol* 1998;152(6):1591–1598.
89. Larson PS, de las Morenas A, Bennett SR, et al. Loss of heterozygosity or allele imbalance in histologically normal breast epithelium is distinct from loss of heterozygosity or allele imbalance in co-existing carcinomas. *Am J Pathol* 2002; 161(1):283–290.
90. Graham K, Ge X, de Las Morenas A, et al. Gene expression profiles of estrogen receptor-positive and estrogen receptor-negative breast cancers are detectable in histologically normal breast epithelium. *Clin Cancer Res* 2011;17(2):236–246.
91. Dontu G, Al-Hajj M, Abdallah WM, et al. Stem cells in normal breast development and breast cancer. *Cell Prolif* 2003; 36(Suppl 1):59–72.
92. Sarrio D, Franklin CK, Mackay A, et al. Epithelial and mesenchymal subpopulations within normal basal breast cell lines exhibit distinct stem cell/progenitor properties. *Stem Cells* 2012; 30(2):292–303.
93. Keller PJ, Arendt LM, Skibinski A, et al. Defining the cellular precursors to human breast cancer. *Proc Natl Acad Sci U S A* 2012;109(8):2772–2777.
94. Sgroi DC, Teng S, Robinson G, et al. In vivo gene expression profile analysis of human breast cancer progression. *Cancer Res* 1999;59(22):5656–5661.
95. Perou CM, Jeffrey SS, van de Rijn M, et al. Distinctive gene expression patterns in human mammary epithelial cells and breast cancers. *Proc Natl Acad Sci U S A* 1999;96(16): 9212–9217.
96. Emmert-Buck MR, Strausberg RL, Krizman DB, et al. Molecular profiling of clinical tissue specimens: feasibility and applications. *Am J Pathol* 2000;156(4):1109–1115.
97. Espina V, Geho D, Mehta AI, et al. Pathology of the future: Molecular profiling for targeted therapy. *Cancer Invest* 2005; 23(1):36–46.

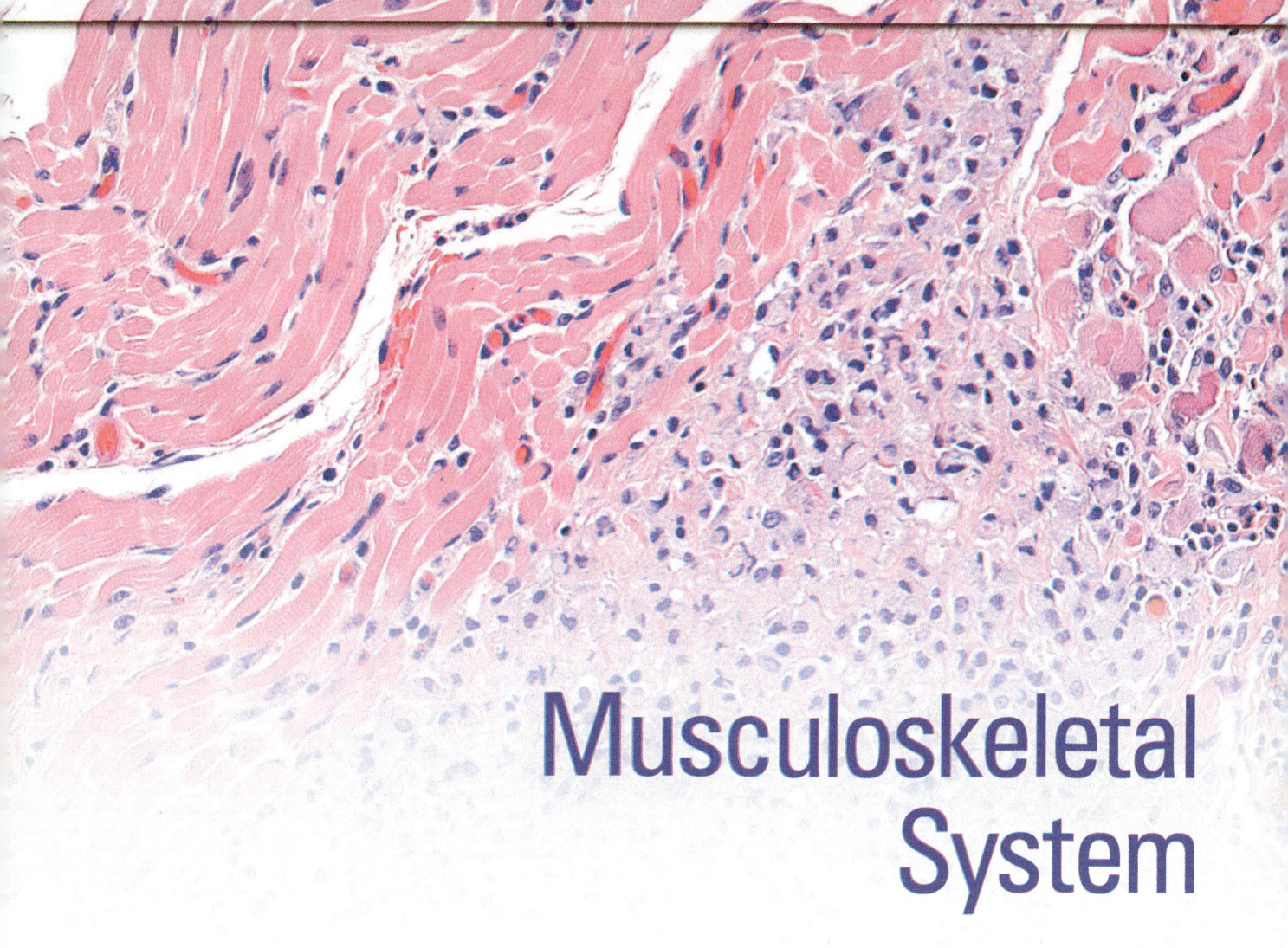

SECTION III

Musculoskeletal System

Bone

Darcy A. Kerr ■ Andrew E. Rosenberg

BONE—THE ORGAN: GROSS AND MICROSCOPIC ANATOMY 89	**BONE FORMATION, GROWTH, AND REMODELING** 101
Woven and Lamellar Bone 90	Endochondral Ossification 101
Cortical (Compact) Bone 91	Intramembranous Ossification 108
Cancellous (Trabecular or Spongy) Bone 94	Modeling and Remodeling 108
Periosteum 94	**BONE—HISTOLOGIC ARTIFACTS** 109
Vascular Supply and Innervation 95	**REFERENCES** 110
Bone Marrow 96	
BONE—THE TISSUE: ORGANIC AND INORGANIC COMPONENTS 96	
Organic Components 96	
Inorganic Components 100	

The skeletal system is vital to life. It plays an essential role in mineral metabolism, movement, protection of viscera, endocrine regulation of critical biologic processes (ion homeostasis, energy metabolism, male phenotype, and fertility), and the storage and nourishment of the hematopoietic marrow. The skeletal system is composed of 206 parts (213 if the 9 fused vertebrae of the sacrum and coccyx are counted individually), namely, the individual bones of the body. Bones are living structures that undergo constant remodeling throughout life. The unique biology of the skeletal system is related to its growth and development, ability to change its structure, function, and metabolism in response to biomechanical and systemic demands, and successfully repair itself in the setting of skeletal injury.

The term "bone" refers to a specialized type of mesenchymal connective tissue or structures composed of bone tissue. The bone tissue along with the cartilage, fibrous tissue, fat, blood vessels, nerves, and hematopoietic elements form the individual bones. In humans, the separate bones together with their articulations form the skeleton. Anatomically, the skeleton can be divided into the *axial* skeleton, which includes the skull, vertebral column, ribs, sternum, and hyoid, and the *appendicular* (or *peripheral*) skeleton, which consists of the upper and lower limbs and the pelvis. The *acral* skeleton refers to the bones of the hands and feet (Table 4.1).

- The bone, whether referring to an organ or a type of connective tissue, is a unique biphasic blend of organic (cells and proteins) and inorganic elements (calcium hydroxyapatite). Developing and adult bones have a distinct gross appearance due to their hierarchical structure (Fig. 4.1) composed of mineralized organic matrix (collagen and noncollagenous proteins), deposited in a woven or lamellar pattern, and cells that in combination are arranged into compact or trabecular bone. The ultimate quality, quantity, and architecture of these components confer important biologic properties which are influenced by the mechanical function and the applied forces to the bone. The ability of the bone tissue to alter its mass and structure in response to its biomechanical environment is known as the Wolff law. The contributions of bone to mineral homeostasis, primarily calcium and phosphorous homeostasis, are crucial to life, and the structural characteristics of bone are fundamental to locomotion, acting as levers for muscle action and organ protection. In addition, bones form the framework of our bodies, thereby giving it size and shape and provide a storehouse and

---

This chapter is an update of a previous version authored by Andrew E. Rosenberg and Sanford I. Roth.

TABLE 4.1 Location, Type, and Method of Formation of Bones of the Skeleton

Skeletal Region	Bone	Type (Based on Shape and Size)	Method of Formation[a]
Axial	Skull[b]	Flat and irregular	Intramembranous
	Mandible	Irregular	Endochondral
	Maxilla	Irregular	Endochondral
	Clavicle	Flat	Endochondral
	Sternum	Flat	Endochondral
	Vertebral column	Irregular	Endochondral
	Ribs	Flat	Endochondral
	Hyoid	Irregular	Endochondral
Appendicular	Limbs	Tubular—long	Endochondral
	Pelvis	Flat	Endochondral
Acral	Metacarpals	Cuboid	Endochondral
	Carpals	Tubular—short	Endochondral
	Metatarsals	Cuboid	Endochondral
	Tarsals	Tubular—short	Endochondral

[a]Cortices of all bones are formed by intramembranous ossification.
[b]Frontal, parietal, and parts of the occipital bones.

nurturing environment for the hematopoietic elements. Lastly, the cells of the bone have been shown to play an important role in energy metabolism, the renal excretion of phosphate, and development and maturation of the male phenotype. Accordingly, the four basic functions of bones are (1) storage and metabolism of elements, minerals, and ions, (2) mechanical structures for movement and protection of viscera, (3) a home for hematopoietic tissue, and (4) an endocrine organ that helps regulate important biologic processes.

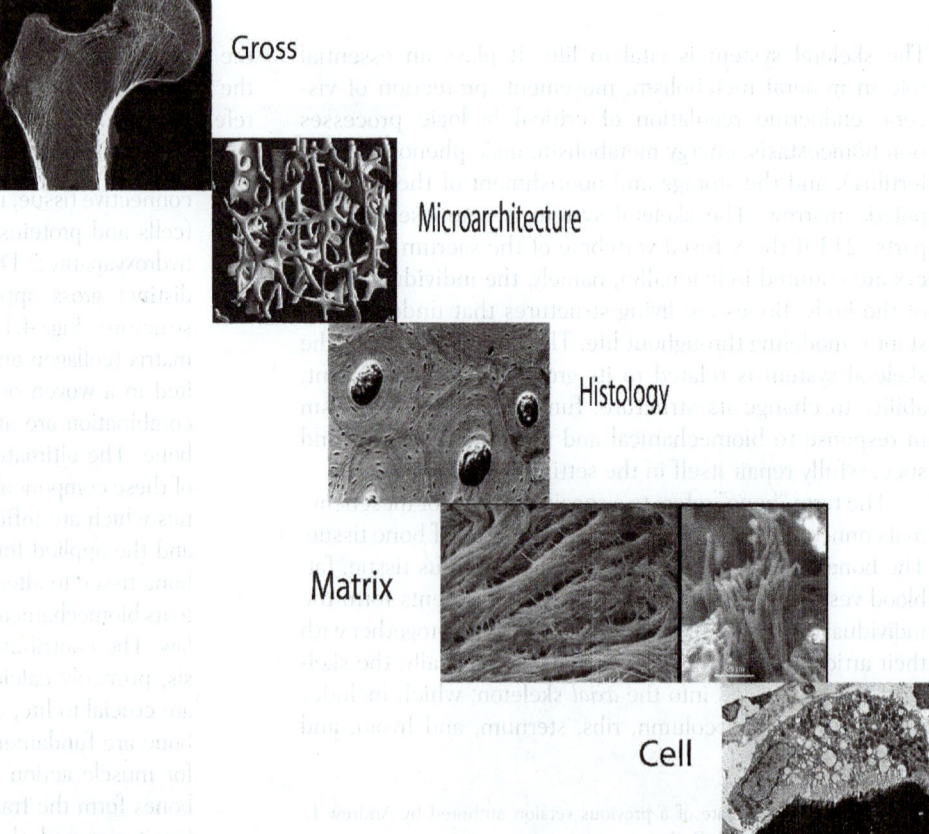

FIGURE 4.1 The hierarchical structure of bone. Gross. A cross-section of the head and upper diaphysis of a macerated femur with the soft tissue removed. The cortex of the metaphysis and diaphysis is of varying thickness depending upon the stress placed upon the bone. The trabeculae of the head follow the lines of stress. Microarchitecture. The cross-linking of the trabeculae demonstrated by micro CT. Histology. A microscopic section of the compact bone of the cortex showing haversian systems and circumferential and interstitial lamellae. Matrix. Bundles of collagen fibers by scanning electron microscopy of two macerated areas of bone in which the mineral has been removed. Cell. An electron micrograph of an osteoclast on the surface of a trabecula. (Courtesy of Bauxstein ML, PhD. Department of Orthopaedics, Beth Israel Deaconess Medical Center, Boston MA.)

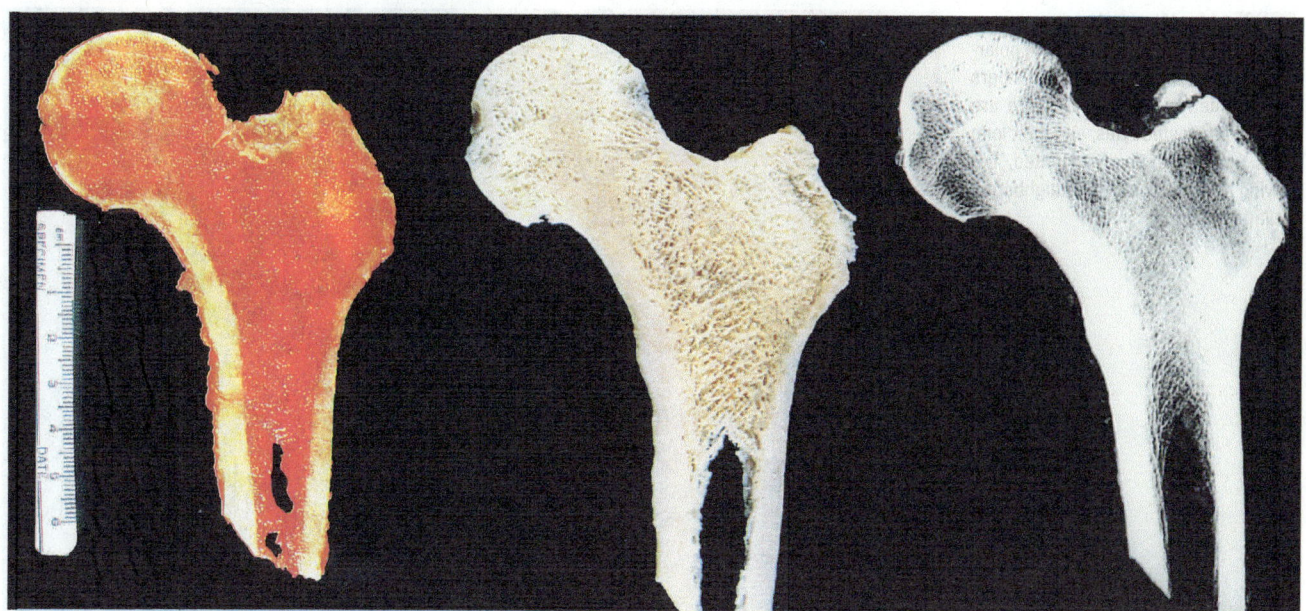

FIGURE 4.2 Gross (*left*) and macerated (*center*) longitudinally cut specimen and the accompanying x-ray (*right*) of a proximal femur, including the head, neck, and upper diaphysis sectioned in the frontal plane. The cortex defines the outer limits of the bone and is thickest along the medial surface (*left*) of the neck and diaphysis, where load bearing is greatest. The medullary cavity is filled with bony trabeculae and red hematopoietic and yellow fatty marrow. The trabeculae are aligned along the lines of stress; this is especially prominent in the medial portion. The horizontal line at the base of the head on the x-ray represents the accrual of bone that occurred during closure of the epiphyseal growth plate.

BONE—THE ORGAN: GROSS AND MICROSCOPIC ANATOMY

Bones are rigid (but not brittle), lightweight, usually cylindrical structures that have a relatively high tensile strength. Tan-white and smooth surfaced, they are the hardest and strongest structures of the body, being as strong as cast iron but one-third of the weight as a result of their unique structure. Bones are reinforced, asymmetric, hollow structures (Fig. 4.2) designed to provide a maximum strength-to-weight ratio.

Bones vary greatly in size and shape and these characteristics form the classification of individual bones. There are bones that are flat (bilaminar plates), cuboid, irregular, and the most common group are those that are tubular, both long and short (Table 4.1). Tubular bones are further subdivided anatomically along their long axis into the epiphysis, the metaphysis, and the diaphysis (1). The epiphysis extends from the base of the articular surface to the point where significant narrowing of the bone diameter begins. During development a secondary center of ossification is often formed in the epiphysis. The metaphysis is the portion of the bone in which there is a significant decrease in the bone diameter. The diaphysis or shaft extends from the base of one metaphysis (the point where the decrease in the bone diameter ceases) to the base of the opposing metaphysis (Fig. 4.3). In an immature or growing bone, the metaphysis contains the cartilaginous growth plate (the physis). Apophyses are anatomic sites that have secondary centers of ossification and growth plates to produce a protuberance to which tendons and muscles attach, such as the greater and lesser trochanters of the femur. The medical and forensic determination of the

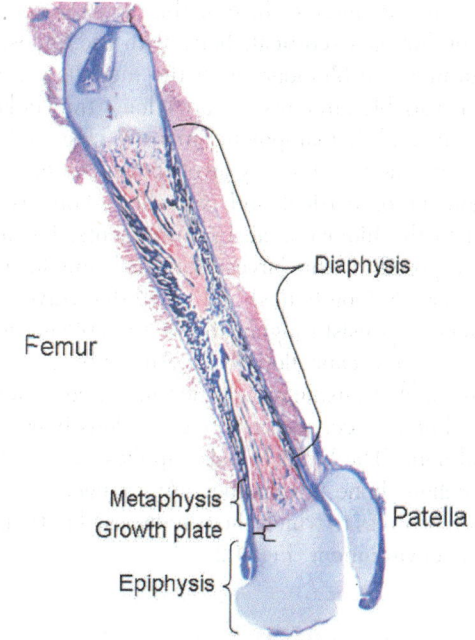

FIGURE 4.3 Longitudinal whole mount of an immature femur and patella prior to the formation of the secondary centers of ossification. The long bone is composed of the proximal and distal epiphyses, metaphyses, and growth plates (physes), and the intervening diaphysis.

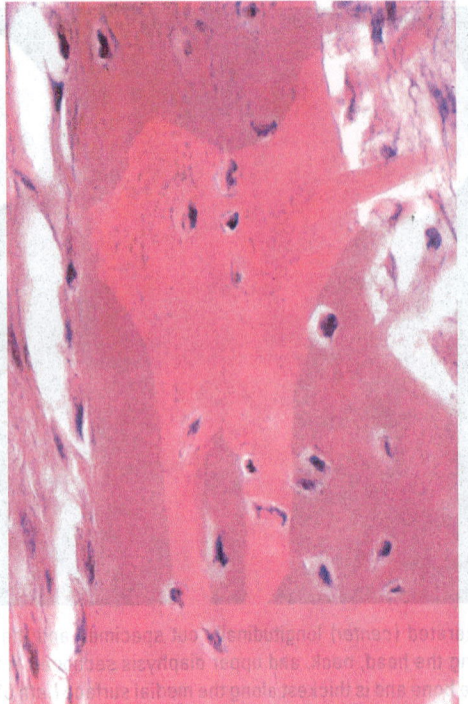
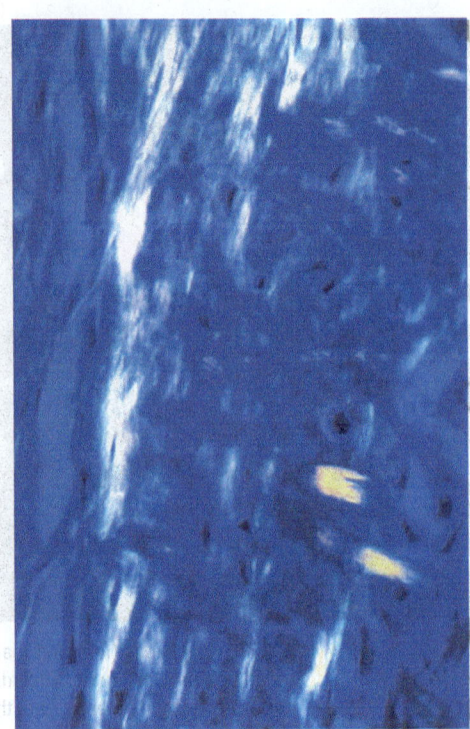

FIGURE 4.4 Woven bone seen on H&E-stained slide (*left*) and with polarized light (*right*). The collagen fibers are oriented in all planes. There are many plump osteocytes, and their long axes appear randomly oriented, following the direction of the neighboring collagen fibers.

skeletal age and the prediction of ultimate growth utilize the amount and localization of bone ossification, the degree of maturation of the growth plates, the formulation and size of the secondary ossification centers, and the degree and amount of remodeling (see later).

Despite their differences in size and shape, all bones are of similar composition and generally have a periosteum attached to the outer surface of the cortex, a cortex composed of compact (cortical) bone with the endosteal surface forming the boundary with the medullary canal that contains variable amounts of cancellous (trabecular) bone with fatty and hematopoietic marrow (Fig. 4.2), blood vessels, and nerves. For any given bone, the quantity and arrangement of cortical and cancellous bone is directly related to the biomechanical requirements. For instance, bones exposed to the largest torsional and load-bearing forces (usually long bones) and those that serve a protective function consist roughly of 80% to 100% cortical bone and 0% to 20% cancellous bone. In contrast, bones that predominately transmit weight-bearing forces, such as the vertebral bodies, consist of 80% cancellous bone and 20% cortical bone. The Wolff law also applies to the trabeculae of cancellous bone in that they are arranged according to the lines of stress to which they are exposed in their biomechanical environment (Fig. 4.2).

Woven and Lamellar Bone

Histologically, bone tissue, regardless of whether it is cortical or cancellous, normal or part of a pathologic process, is categorized into woven and lamellar types on the basis of the organization of its type I collagen fibers which are the major structural proteins of bone tissue. In woven bone, the collagen fibers are arranged in a seemingly haphazard feltwork (Fig. 4.4), while in lamellar bone they are deposited in parallel arrays (Fig. 4.5) either longitudinally or circumferentially around haversian canals forming osteons or haversian systems.

The woven bone is fabricated during periods of rapid bone formation. It composes parts of both the cortex and the trabeculae of the developing bony skeleton during embryogenesis and portions of bones in the growing infant

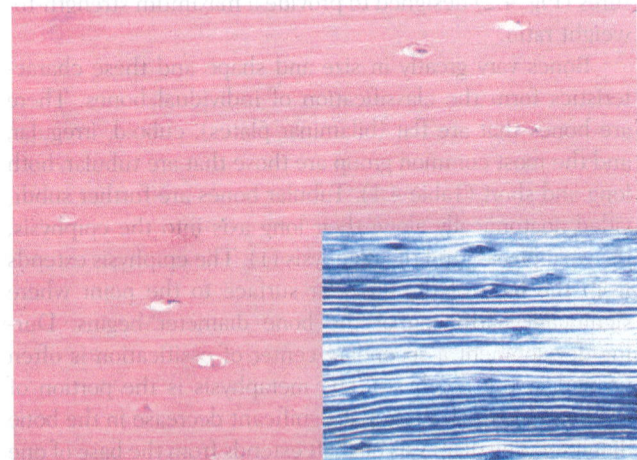

FIGURE 4.5 Lamellar bone as seen on H&E-stained slide and with polarization (*inset*). The collagen fibers are arranged in parallel arrays. There are comparatively fewer osteocytes, and they are oriented in the same direction as the collagen fibers.

and the adolescent. It may also be the predominant type of bone that is formed in various reactive (fracture-callus, infection-involucrum) and neoplastic (Codman triangle, matrix of bone-forming neoplasms) conditions. The woven bone is hypercellular, and the osteocytes and their lacunae are large and appear to be oriented in a haphazard fashion as the long axes of the cells parallel the seemingly random arrangement of the neighboring collagen fibers (Fig. 4.4). The mineral content of woven bone is higher than that of the lamellar bone. Overall, this structural organization enables woven bone to resist forces equally in all directions and facilitates rapid formation, mineralization, and resorption. These factors explain why woven bone is weaker, less rigid, and more flexible than the lamellar bone.

Normally, the entire mature skeleton is composed solely of lamellar bone. The lamellar bone, in contrast to the woven bone, is synthesized more slowly, is less cellular, and the osteocytes and their lacunae are smaller and distributed in a more organized fashion as their long axes are parallel to the more regular collagen lamellae (Fig. 4.5). In addition, the process of mineralization of the lamellar bone differs from that of the woven bone in that it occurs more slowly and continues long after the organic matrix is initially deposited. Subsequently, the mineral content increases as a result of enlargement and increase in the number of the apatite crystals. Microradiographs of undemineralized sections reveal varying densities, with the oldest bone being the most heavily mineralized (Fig. 4.6). Since the mineral and collagen fibers are well organized and intimately bound to one another, lamellar bone has greater rigidity and tensile strength and less elasticity than the woven bone.

Both lamellar and woven bone are made by osteoblasts in discrete quantities or units and are deposited only in an appositional fashion. Osteoblasts first synthesize and secrete a layer of unmineralized type I collagen (osteoid) and noncollagenous proteins on a surface of mineralized cartilage, previously formed bone, or collagen, and then regulate its mineralization. Discrete units of lamellar bone deposited by cohorts of osteoblasts are separated from one another by cement lines also known as reversal lines. Cement lines are deposited by osteoblasts on the surface of the bone subsequent to osteoclast bone resorption. They manifest as thin (1 to 5 μm) and intensely basophilic linear structures on conventional hematoxylin and eosin (H&E) histologic slides (Fig. 4.7). Evidence suggests that they are composed of areas of mineral-rich collagen and noncollagenous proteins (2). Some investigators have suggested that cement lines represent a residuum of mineralized "ground substance" that is secreted during the initial reversal phase in the formation of a new bone (3).

Cortical (Compact) Bone

The cortical bone, also known as dense compact bone, is hard and tan-white (Figs. 4.2 and 4.8). Its thickness depends on its location and mechanical requirements, being thickest in areas exposed to large torsional and weight-bearing forces, such as the medial region of the middiaphysis of the femur, and thinnest where the transmission of weight-bearing and torsional forces is smallest, as seen adjacent to articular surfaces and within vertebral bodies (Fig. 4.2).

During the early stages of growth and development, the cortical bone is constructed entirely of the woven bone. Over time, it is gradually remodeled until in the mature skeleton it is composed of pure lamellar bone. The adult cortical bone is composed of three different architectural patterns of the lamellar bone: circumferential, concentric, and interstitial (Fig. 4.7). The circumferential lamellae form outer and inner envelopes to the cortex and consist of several subperiosteal and endosteal layers that are oriented parallel to the long axis of the bone. They are the first cortical lamellae to be deposited, and in young individuals comprise almost the entire cortex. As mechanical stress on the bone increases with age, many of the circumferential lamellae (except for several lamellae just beneath the periosteum and along the endosteum) are replaced by the concentric lamellae of the haversian systems (Figs. 4.7 and 4.9 to 4.12).

Haversian systems, or osteons, are created by osteoclastic resorption of the circumferential lamellae that usually begins on the endosteal surface of the cortex, and less frequently on the periosteal surface. The bone resorption proceeds perpendicular or at an angle to the long axis of the bone forming a canal (the Volkmann canal) (Figs. 4.10 and 4.11). The numerous osteoclasts situated in the leading edge of the canal are known as the "cutting cone," and the canal they generate becomes filled with vessels, nerves, and mesenchymal cells (including stem cells) enmeshed in a loose connective tissue stroma. Within a short distance, the osteoclastic activity becomes concentrated on one side of the canal; and, as a consequence, the direction of the newly formed canal (haversian) becomes aligned with the long axis of the bone. The burrowing osteoclasts elongate the canal,

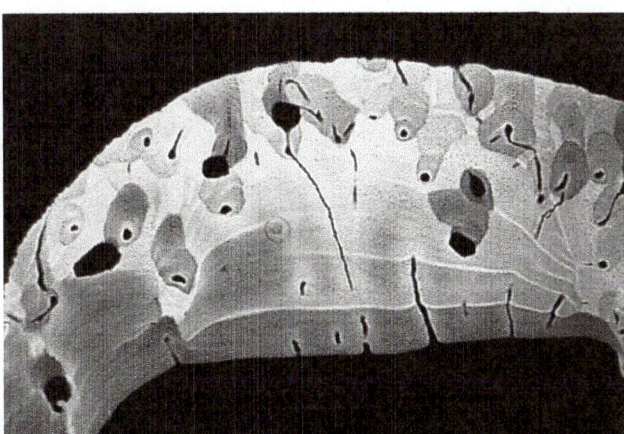

FIGURE 4.6 Microradiograph of the cortex of a 2-month-old female. There are various degrees of mineralization, with the radiolucent areas (*dark*) being the most recently deposited and least mineralized. The radiodense portions (*light*) represent the oldest areas of formation and the most mineralized.

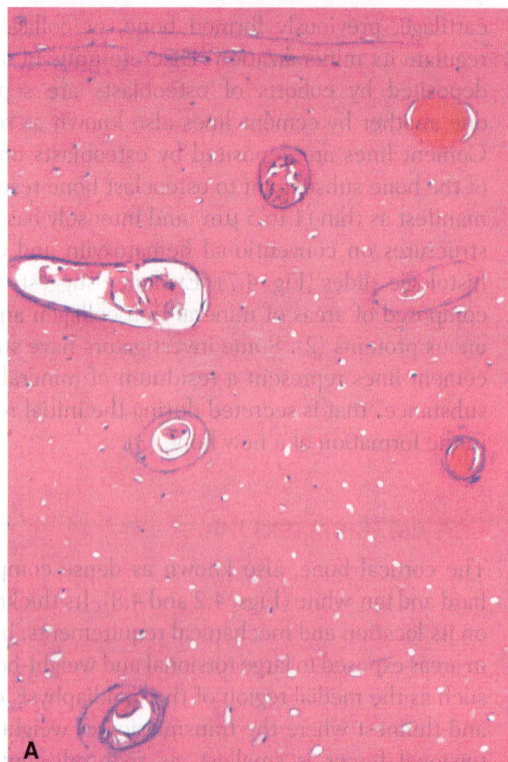
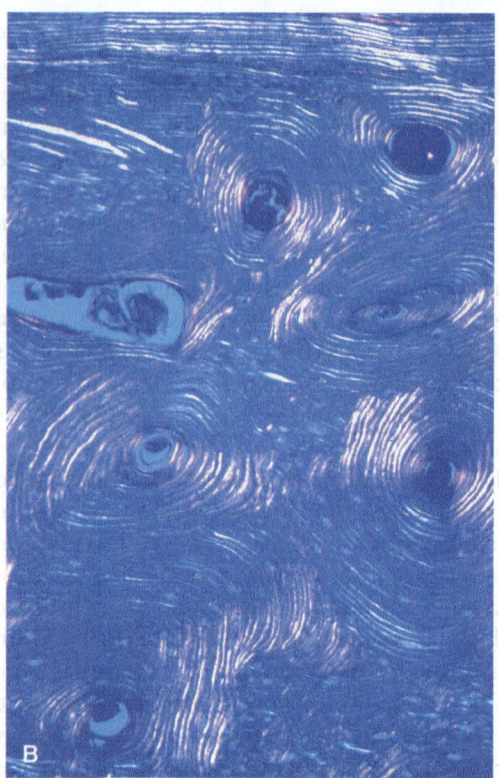

FIGURE 4.7 Cross-sections of cortex with circumferential, concentric, and interstitial lamellae. The circumferential lamellae are beneath the periosteum, the concentric lamellae surround the haversian canals containing blood vessels, and the interstitial lamellae fill the intervening spaces. Scattered intensely basophilic cement lines are present, tethering the units of lamellar bone. **A:** H&E stain. **B:** Polarized light.

and in their wake newly formed osteoblasts deposit lamellae of the bone in a target-like, or concentric fashion. The collagen fibers in any one lamella are oriented parallel to each other; however, their pitch is slightly different from those in adjacent lamellae, and this enhances the biomechanical strength of the cortex. The accrual of concentric lamellae over time reduces the diameter of the haversian canal so that in the end it is small and contains nutritional blood vessels and nerve twigs (Fig. 4.9). Together, these elements define a haversian or osteonal system.

Mature haversian canals are long and cylindrical, range from 25 to 125 μm in diameter (average 50 μm), and are widest nearest the medullary cavity. They form an intricate, branching, spiraling, and interconnecting network that courses throughout the cortex. The number of haversian systems in a particular bone is variable and is determined by age, the amount of mechanical stress and weight that

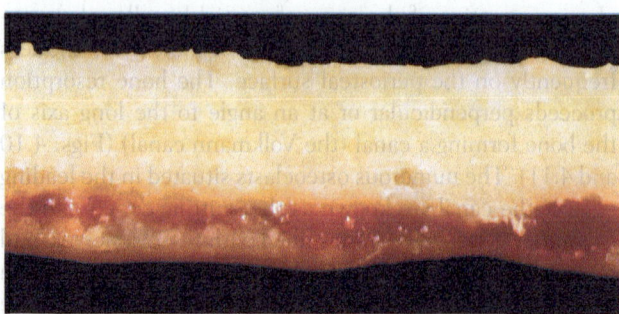

FIGURE 4.8 Photograph of a longitudinal section through a flat bone. The inner cortex is tan-white and solid. The round hole within it represents the pathway of the nutrient artery. The red area is the central bone marrow.

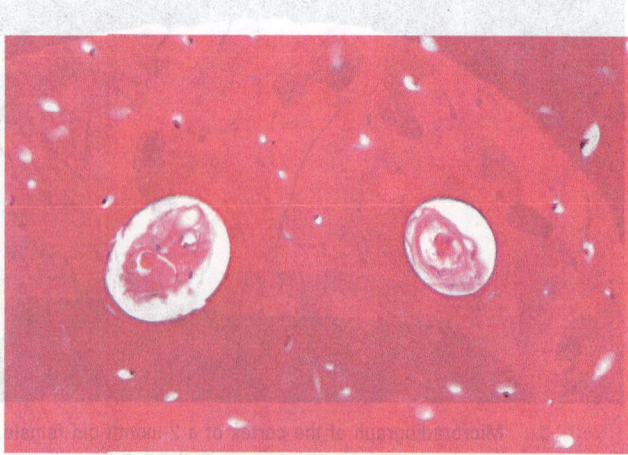

FIGURE 4.9 Two adjacent mature haversian systems containing the central canal, blood vessels, and surrounding concentric lamellae. Empty lacunae are seen in areas of the interstitial lamellae.

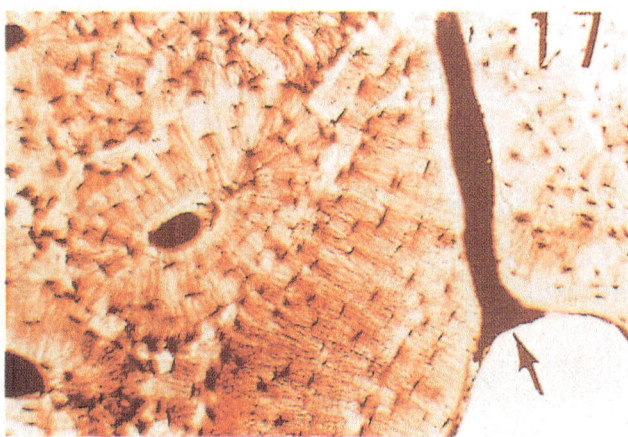

FIGURE 4.10 Ground, unstained section of mineralized, compact, cortical bone. The arrow points to a Volkmann canal arising from the endosteum. Canaliculi connect the lacunae in adjacent circumferential lamellae. (Courtesy of Glimcher MJ, Roth SI, Schiller AL, as part of a course in Pathophysiology of Bone for the Harvard Medical School, Boston, MA.)

the bone is subjected to over time, and other biologic and genetic factors (3,4).

Individual haversian systems are relatively self-contained metabolic units because nutritional support of their cells, especially the bone cells, depends upon the process of diffusion from their central vessels. Consequently, osteocyte viability is not sustainable beyond a certain distance from the vessels, which imposes a biologic limit on the maximal number of lamellae contained within any haversian system. Also, the integrated network of osteocytes is generally limited to the osteon within which it develops, as osteocytic cytoplasmic processes usually contact only those that dwell in the same system (Fig. 4.12).

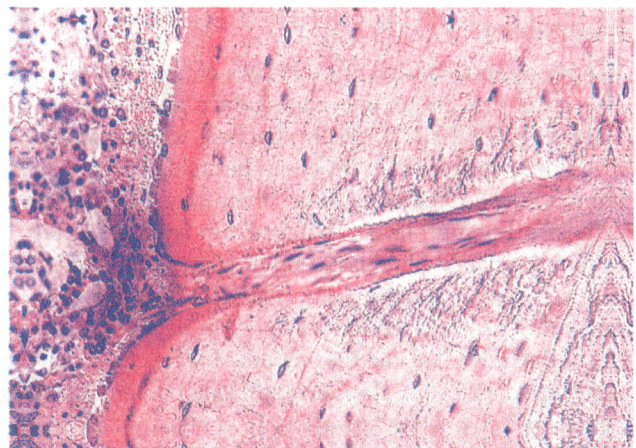

FIGURE 4.11 A forming Volkmann canal coursing through the cortex of the bone. The canal is angled with respect to the bone lamellae and is filled with connective tissue. Osteoid and osteoblasts, indicating new bone formation, are present around the endosteal opening of the canal, but none are seen in the canal. The cortex shows circumferential lamellar bone with regularly placed osteocytes (Undemineralized bone section).

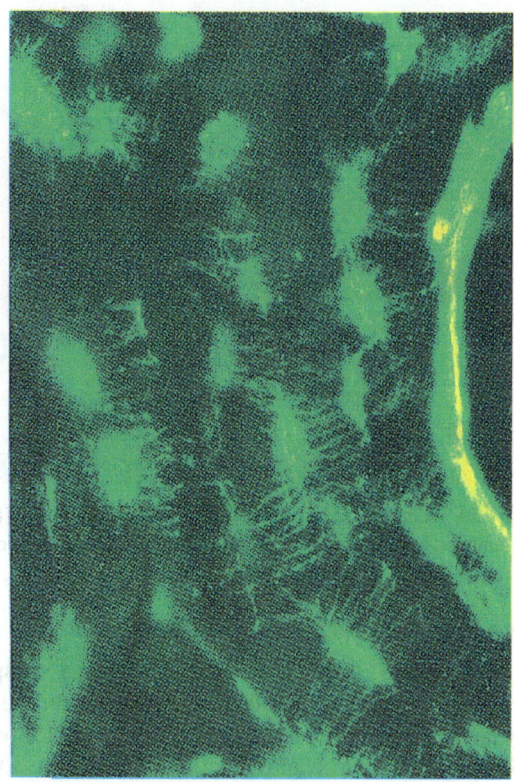

FIGURE 4.12 An undemineralized section of the cortical bone, stained in vivo, with tetracycline. A layer of tetracycline appears at the mineralization front of the haversian system where a new bone is being formed. The osteocyte lacunae and the canaliculi of their connecting dendritic processes are visible as bright green areas. The lacunae of the adjacent interstitial regions (left upper and lower corners) do not connect with the haversian cells surrounding the haversian canal (dark area right center) (unstained, fluorescent light).

The bone filling the spaces between the haversian systems is known as the interstitial bone. The interstitial lamellae represent the remnants of circumferential lamellae of previously formed haversian systems that have become partially destroyed by osteoclastic activity. They are irregular, geometric-shaped units of lamellar bone (Figs. 4.7 and 4.9) that help "glue," or anneal haversian systems to one another—this arrangement is important in maintaining cortical integrity. The osteocytes confined to the interstitial lamellae may lose their access to nutritional sources and consequently undergo necrosis, leaving behind empty lacunae.

Cement lines denote the physical boundaries of every haversian system and unit of interstitial bone. As the bone ages and is subject to varying forces and remodeling, more haversian systems develop which replace pre-existing interstitial lamellae and older haversian systems which subsequently become newly created interstitial lamellae.

The endosteum is the loose areolar connective tissue that immediately abuts the osteoblasts along the inner surface of the cortex and along the medullary surfaces of the trabeculae.

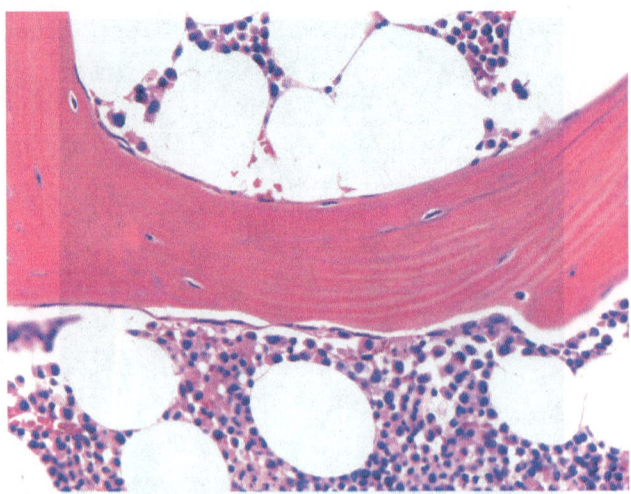

FIGURE 4.13 A mature trabecula composed of lamellar bone. The collagen lamellae are oriented parallel to the long axis of the trabecula.

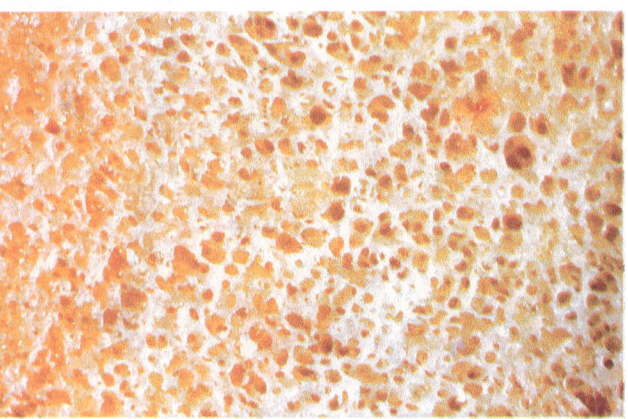

FIGURE 4.15 Gross photograph of a macerated portion of the cancellous bone. The trabeculae (*white areas*) are forming interconnecting plates.

Cancellous (Trabecular or Spongy) Bone

Cancellous bone, also known as the trabecular or spongy bone, is tan-white, fenestrated, and located within the medullary cavity (Figs. 4.1 and 4.2). It is composed of interconnecting plates and struts of trabecular bone. In the adult, it is the fourth type of lamellar bone with the lamellae oriented parallel to the long axis of a trabecula (Figs. 4.13 and 4.14). In developing bone, the cancellous bone is composed of significant amounts of woven bone; it has a central core of calcified cartilage (primary spongiosa) when initially formed in infants and children and in reparative bone containing cartilage. Enlargement of trabeculae occurs via the process of appositional growth which indicates that the newly formed bone is deposited on pre-existing trabecular surfaces. Adult cancellous bone is lamellar and it is oriented in relation to lines of mechanical stress to provide support and distribute large weight-bearing forces along a variety of different pathways (Fig. 4.2). Accordingly, cancellous bone is most abundant in the weight-bearing ends of bones, such as the epiphyses and vertebral bodies, and is present in only small amounts in the middiaphysis of tubular bones. Small trabeculae are avascular, while larger ones may contain small haversian-like systems, including concentric lamellae. The surfaces of mature trabeculae are typically lined by quiescent osteoblasts or surface-lining cells and adjacent endosteal connective tissue (Fig. 4.14).

In three dimensions, the trabeculae are usually interconnecting plates (Fig. 4.15) and their global surface area is very large, approaching the square footage of three football fields, which facilitates remodeling and the ability of the skeleton to rapidly respond to the metabolic demands of the body. The mature trabeculae are heavily mineralized with a thin (1 to 3 μm) layer of osteoid beneath the relatively inactive flattened osteoblasts.

Periosteum

The periosteum consists of a thin layer of tan-white connective tissue that covers the outer surface of all cortices. In children it is relatively loosely attached, whereas in adults it is firmly anchored to the bone. In children, the periosteum is constructed of an outer fibrous layer and an inner cellular (cambium) layer. The cambium layer is composed of spindle-shaped fibroblasts and osteoprogenitor cells and mature polyhedral osteoblasts (Fig. 4.16). In general, the number of osteoprogenitor cells present depending on the age of the individual and the amount of bone cell activity in any particular region; they are especially numerous during periods of active bone formation. In contrast, in adults the periosteum appears largely as a fibrous layer. The fibrous layer contains fibroblasts and broad type I collagen fibers that are continuous with those of the joint capsule, tendons, and muscle fascia. At tendoligamentous insertion sites (Fig. 4.17), the collagen fibers of the tendoligamentous structure pierce the periosteum and become anchored in the bone where they are known as Sharpey fibers.

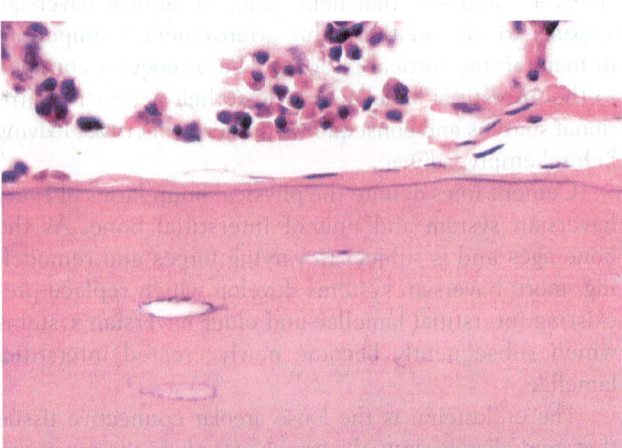

FIGURE 4.14 Quiescent osteoblasts lining a trabecular surface of the lamellar bone.

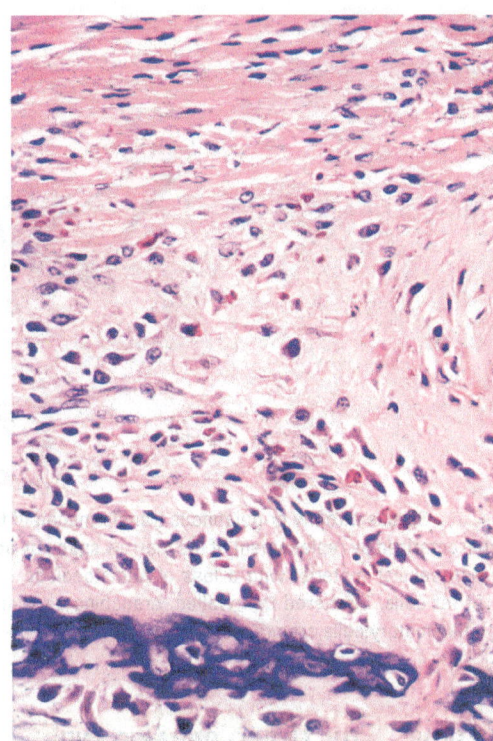

FIGURE 4.16 The outer fibrous layer of a fetal periosteum consists of thick bundles of horizontally oriented collagen fibers. The inner cellular cambium layer contains spindle-shaped osteoprogenitor cells. The maturing osteoblasts steadily become more polyhedral and acquire increasing amounts of amphophilic cytoplasm. A portion of intramembranous woven bone is seen forming the new cortex. The hematoxylin-positive area staining blue is mineralized, while the pink area above is the unmineralized osteoid.

Vascular Supply and Innervation

Bones are vascular organs and receive their blood supply from three main sources (a) large nutrient arteries (one to two per bone), (b) metaphyseal and epiphyseal vessels, and (c) periosteal vessels. Nutrient arteries enter long bones in the diaphysis, traverse the cortex through the foramina, and divide into ascending and descending branches within the medullary cavity. Smaller branch arteries, arterioles, capillaries, venules, and veins (Fig. 4.18) course throughout the medullary cavity, nourish the fatty and hematopoietic marrow, and extend into haversian canals, where they supply the inner two-thirds of the cortex. At the ends of growing bones, they terminate as small arteries that give rise to capillary loops at the bases of epiphyseal growth plates. The epiphyseal and metaphyseal vessels access the bone through small apertures and provide blood flow to regions of the epiphysis and metaphysis in the mature skeleton and to the secondary centers of ossification during active endochondral ossification. The periosteal vessels are small and are believed to nourish the outer third of the cortex. The venous drainage system of the bone is composed of medullary sinusoids that empty into a central venous sinus, which merges with nutrient veins.

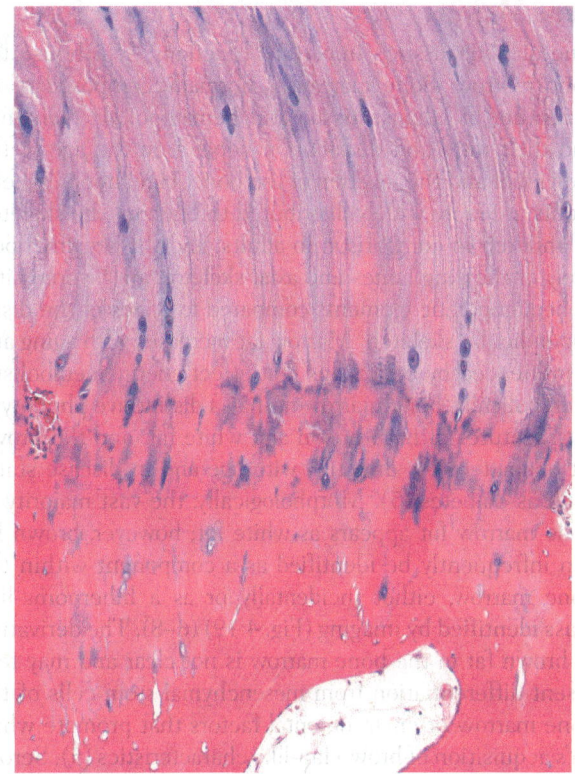

FIGURE 4.17 Dense regular connective tissue inserts into the bone at the tendoligamentous insertion site or enthesis.

Bones are innervated largely by nonmyelinated nerves derived from the autonomic nervous system that function to control blood flow. Larger nerve branches are usually associated with arterial vessels (Fig. 4.18), whereas small groups of fibers can be found adjacent to vessels in haversian systems. Nerves supplying the periosteum contain sensory elements and are the source of the sensation of bone pain.

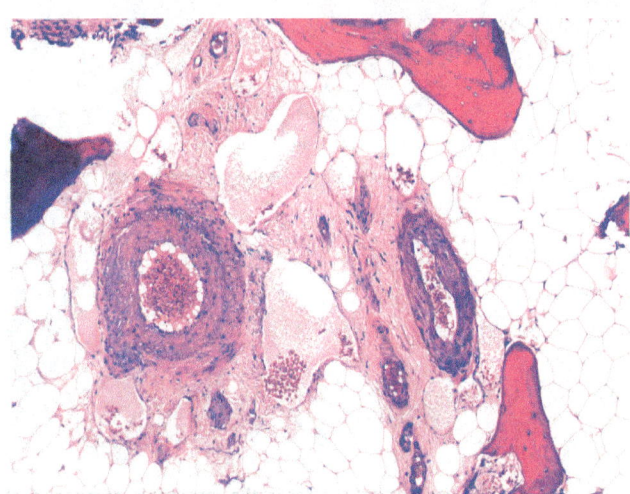

FIGURE 4.18 Small arteries, surrounded by dilated capillaries and nerves, in an area of fatty marrow.

Bone Marrow

One of bone tissue's important functions is to house the bone marrow. Bone marrow is normally composed of an admixture of adipose tissue and hematopoietic elements, and their ratio and distribution depend on the age of the individual and the location of the bone. Hematopoietic elements are more widely distributed throughout the skeleton in children in comparison to adults, and the proximal portions of the long bones and axial skeleton are favored sites of hematopoietic elements compared to bones of the distal appendicular skeleton. Marrow fat increases with aging and is influenced by conditions that affect energy metabolism. Metabolically, bone marrow fat has a distinctive phenotype with features of both brown and white fat, and the brown fat characteristics diminish with age and in disease states such as diabetes (5). Morphologically, the vast majority of bone marrow fat appears as white fat; however, brown fat can infrequently be identified as a component within the bone marrow, either incidentally or as a hibernoma-like mass identified by imaging (Fig. 4.19) (6–8). The derivation of brown fat in the bone marrow is not clear and may represent differentiation from mesenchymal stem cells of the bone marrow or environmental factors that promote white fat's acquisition of brown fat–like characteristics (5). Serous atrophy of the bone marrow, also known as gelatinous transformation of the bone marrow, occurs in a wide variety of conditions including malnutrition (cachexia or anorexia nervosa), immunosuppression, chronic heart or kidney failure, malignancy, and cytotoxic therapy. Grossly, the marrow has a gelatinous consistency, and histologically, it manifests as an increase in extracellular gelatinous material (hyaluronic acid–rich mucopolysaccharides) not normally present in the bone marrow and a decrease in the amount of hematopoietic elements and the number and size of adipocytes (Fig. 4.20) (9–12).

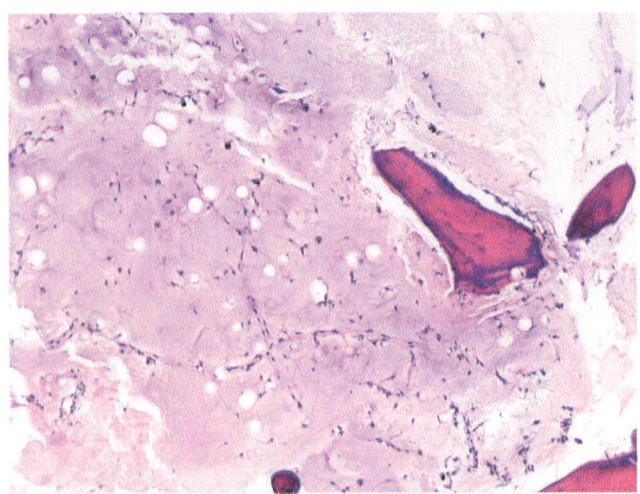

FIGURE 4.20 Serous atrophy or gelatinous transformation of the marrow is characterized by replacement of the marrow space by abundant myxoid extracellular material with a loss of hematopoietic cells and atrophy of fat cells. Scattered thin-walled, branching capillaries and chronic inflammatory cells are present.

BONE—THE TISSUE: ORGANIC AND INORGANIC COMPONENTS

The special biphasic amalgamation of organic and inorganic materials found in bone distinguishes it from all other tissues in the body. The organic component consists of proteins and bone cells, and the inorganic element is a specialized, calcium-poor form of apatite, resembling hydroxyapatite $[Ca_{10}(PO_4)_6(OH)_2]$ in which the hydroxyl residues are replaced by phosphate and carbonate ions. The integration of the mineral phase with the organic matrix (primarily collagen) provides the bone with hardness, strength, and limited elasticity (13).

Organic Components

Proteins

The organic component accounts for approximately 35% of the wet weight of the bone; and of this, collagen is responsible for 90%. Collagen is the primary structural protein of the bone, is produced by osteoblasts, and the overwhelming majority (90%) is type I (14); type III, V, and fibril-associated collagens with interrupted triple helices (FACIT) collagens are present in trace amounts. FACIT collagens are nonfibrillar collagens that organize and stabilize the extracellular matrix and include collagens IX, XII, XIV, XIX, XX, and XXI (15). Type III collagen may be increased in pathologic conditions (16). In addition to their contribution to structural support, the numerous, large type I collagen molecules anchor many of the other constituents (17).

The noncollagenous proteins are grouped according to their function as adhesion proteins, calcium-binding proteins, mineralization proteins, enzymes, cytokines, growth factors,

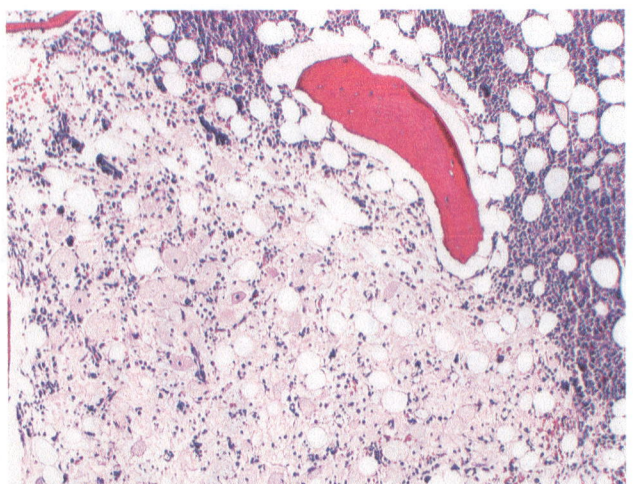

FIGURE 4.19 The majority of the fat in the marrow is composed of white fat; however, foci of brown fat may occasionally be seen, present here in association with a region of decreased hematopoiesis.

and receptors (18,19). These proteins mediate all aspects of bone cell activity and are extremely important to the biologic success of the bone as a tissue. Many of these substances are synthesized and secreted by osteoblasts, and others are derived and concentrated from the serum (18). Approximately 25% of these noncollagenous proteins are exogenously derived (15). An important osteoblast-produced noncollagenous protein is osteocalcin, which functions as a hormone that is involved in the regulation of glucose and insulin metabolism as well as male development and fertility (20). Osteocalcin is made by both osteoblasts and osteoclasts, and its quantification in serum has made it an important clinical marker of bone turnover (17,21).

Osteoprogenitor Cells

Osteoprogenitor cells are derived from tissue-bound mesenchymal stem cells. These mesenchymal stem cells also have the capability to form adipocytes, chondrocytes, myocytes, and fibroblasts. The mesenchymal stem cells are located in the perianlage tissue of fetuses, periosteum, haversian systems, and Volkmann and medullary canals. Osteoprogenitor cells are primitive committed mesenchymal cells that have the capacity to produce only osteoblasts. The process of osteoblast differentiation and maturation is complex and involves a variety of different elements including transcription factors such as the Runt domain–containing transcription factor 2 (RUNX2), Osterix (OSX), and activating transcription factor 4 (ATF4), as well as signaling pathways such as Wnt and Notch (Table 4.2) (22–27). By light microscopy, osteoprogenitor cells appear as generic spindle cells and do not have any distinguishing morphologic features; therefore, they cannot be identified with certainty in routine histologic sections (Figs. 4.16, 4.21, and 4.22), except by immunohistochemistry. Since the bone can be formed in the skin, soft tissue, muscle, and viscera in both experimental and pathologic conditions, osteoprogenitor cells or inducible stem cells are likely to be present in these sites as well.

Osteoblasts

Osteoblasts are vital to the bone tissue and are the cells responsible for the production, transport, and arrangement of most of the components of the organic matrix (osteoid). In addition, they initiate and regulate matrix mineralization and use autocrine and paracrine mechanisms to control the activity of neighboring osteoblasts, osteocytes, and osteoclasts (14,17–19,22,28). Immunohistochemical and biochemical studies reveal the presence of alkaline phosphatase, osteopontin, and osteocalcin within their cytoplasm, receptor activator for nuclear factor κβ (RANK) ligand (RANKL) (see section Osteoclasts) in their cytoplasm and cell membranes, and receptors for parathyroid hormone (PTH), prostaglandins, vitamin D_3, estrogens, and cytokines on their cell membranes (14,17–19,22,28).

Osteoblasts cover all bone surfaces and their lifespan may range from months to many years. Their metabolic state is closely related to their morphology; they are spindle-shaped

TABLE 4.2 Important Regulators of Osteoblast Differentiation and Function

Transcription Factor	Actions and Regulation
RUNX2	Promotes osteoblast differentiation. Regulation: actions promoted by MAF, TAZ, SATB2, MSX2, BAPX1, RB, GLI2, DLX5 and inhibited by Twist, HAND2, STAT1, Schnurri-3, ZPF521, HOXA2, HES, HEY, and GLI3
OSX	Promotes osteoblast differentiation, required downstream of RUNX2. Regulation: actions promoted NFATC1 and inhibited by p53
ATF4	Promotes mature osteoblast functions. Regulation: actions promoted SATB2 and inhibited by FIAT

Signaling Pathway	Actions and Regulation
Wnt	Promotes osteoblast differentiation
Notch	Inhibits osteoblast differentiation
BMP signaling	Stimulates osteoblast differentiation and function
FGF signaling	Promotes preosteoblast proliferation, stimulates osteoblast differentiation and function

RUNX2, runt-related transcription factor 2; MAF, macrophage activating factor; TAZ, transcriptional coactivator with PDZ-binding motif; SATB2, special AT-rich sequence-binding 2; MSX2, Msh homeobox 2; BAPX1, bagpipe homeobox protein homologue 1; RB, retinoblastoma; GLI2, Gli transcription factor 2; DLX5, distal-less homeobox 5; Twist, twist-related protein; HAND2, heart and neural crest derivatives expressed 2; STAT1, signal transducer and activator of transcription 1; Schnurri-3, Schnurri-3 zinc finger protein; ZPF521, zinc-finger protein 521; HOXA2, homeobox A2; HES, hairy and enhancer of split; HEY, HES-related with YRPW motif; GLI3, Gli transcription factor 3; OSX, osterix; NFATC1, nuclear factor of activated T cells cytoplasmic 1; p53, tumor protein p53; ATF4, activating transcription factor 4; SATB2, special AT-rich sequence-binding protein 2; FIAT, factor-inhibiting ATF4-mediated transcription; Wnt, Wingless-related integration site; Notch, Notch type-1 transmembrane protein; BMP, bone morphogenic protein; FGF, fibroblast growth factor.

when quiescent and large and polyhedral when rapidly producing the bone. Metabolically active osteoblasts vary in size from 10 to 80 μm (average 20 to 30 μm) and have abundant amphophilic to basophilic cytoplasm that is in intimate contact with the bone (Figs. 4.21 and 4.22). Multiple cytoplasmic processes extend from the cells into and through

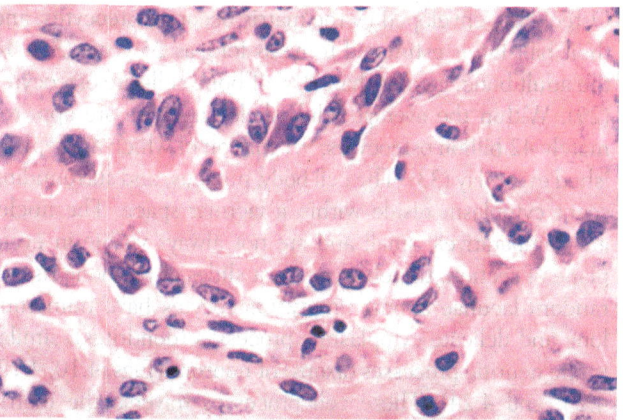

FIGURE 4.21 Metabolically active osteoblasts lining a trabecula of woven bone. Some osteoblasts are in various stages of being surrounded by matrix and becoming osteocytes. Spindle cells in the connective tissue adjacent to the trabecula may represent osteoprogenitor cells.

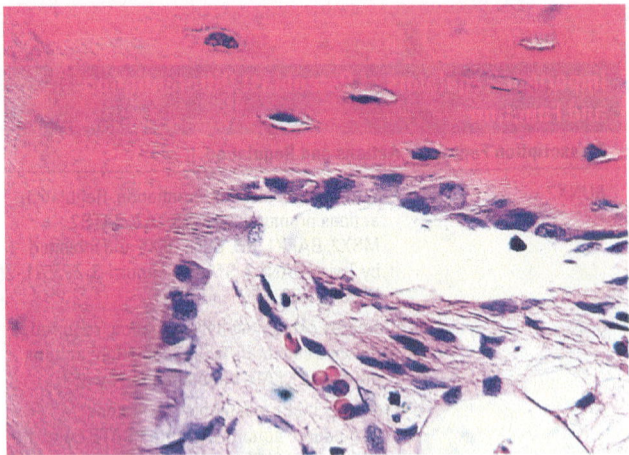

FIGURE 4.22 Metabolically active osteoblasts forming the lamellar bone. A thin layer of osteoid cannot be identified in these demineralized sections. At the right of the micrograph, the osteoblasts are becoming inactive, flattened, and being incorporated into the bone as osteocytes. The osteocytes of the lamellar bone are spindle shaped. The dendrites are identifiable extending from the osteoblast bodies into the bone.

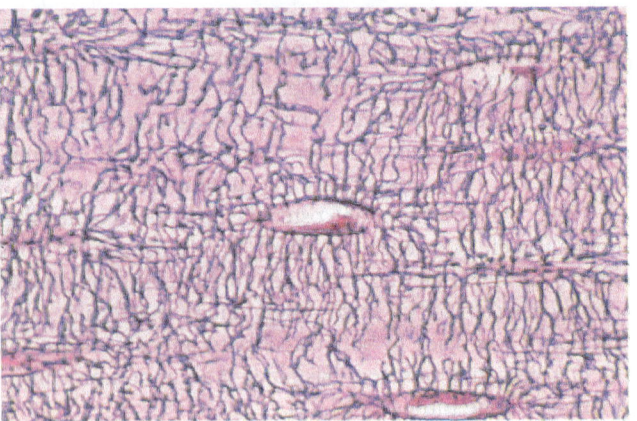

FIGURE 4.23 Osteocytes within lacunar spaces. Numerous cell processes course through the matrix and contact those of neighboring osteocytes.

the bone (Fig. 4.22), contacting adjacent osteoblasts and osteocytes via nexus (gap) junctions. The nuclei of active osteoblasts are polarized away from the matrix surface and often have a conspicuous nucleolus and a prominent perinuclear halo that represents a well-developed Golgi apparatus (Fig. 4.21). Approximately 60% to 80% of osteoblasts undergo apoptosis; the remaining osteoblasts either become osteocytes surrounded by the matrix or flatten and elongate as their synthetic activity diminishes and ultimately, they remain as a cellular lining of the bone surfaces (29) (Figs. 4.14 and 4.22).

Ultrastructurally, the cytoplasm of productive osteoblasts contains extensive, granular endoplasmic reticulum, a large, prominent Golgi apparatus, and numerous mitochondria, and lysosomes (30). In contrast, the cytoplasm of inactive osteoblasts resembles that of quiescent fibroblasts (31).

Osteocytes

Osteoblasts enveloped by the matrix become osteocytes, and their half-life is estimated to be as long as 25 years (32). In the adult bone, greater than 90% of bone cells are osteocytes (29). Within the average adult skeleton, there are approximately 42 billion osteocytes, 9.1 million of which are replenished every day (33). The cell body, nucleus, and surrounding scant cytoplasm reside within a lacunar space. The nuclei are comparatively small and are not always visible in every plane of section; therefore, in most slides of the bone tissue, random lacunae appear empty. Osteocytes have numerous long and delicate cytoplasmic processes (dendrites), similar to the neuritic processes (axons) of neurons (Figs. 4.10, 4.12, 4.23, and 4.24). These cell processes traverse the matrix through small tunnels termed *canaliculi* and provide a very large surface area of contact between the osteocyte and the matrix and extracellular fluid that bathes each cell. It is estimated that the adult skeleton contains 3.7 trillion osteocyte dendritic projections with a total length of 175,000 km, forming 23 trillion cellular connections (33). Osteocyte cell processes connect to those of neighboring osteocytes and to surface osteoblasts via gap junctions. Gap junctions facilitate the transfer of small molecules and biologically generated electrical potentials from cell to cell. In this manner, osteocytes communicate with one another and form a complex and integrated network throughout the bone tissue (Fig. 4.24). Osteocytes are thought to function as sensor cells in the bone that can mediate the effects of mechanical loading through their extensive communication network.

The number, size, shape, and position of osteocytes vary according to the type of bone they inhabit. In woven bone, they are numerous, large, and plump (Fig. 4.4). Their arrangement appears disorganized because their long axes parallel the direction of the neighboring collagen fibers, which in sections of the woven bone appears random. In lamellar bone, osteocytes are comparatively fewer in number, smaller, more spindle shaped, and appear in sections to be more regularly organized because the cells are oriented in the same direction as the surrounding lamellae (Fig. 4.5). Age is another factor that affects osteocyte quantity as osteocyte apoptosis increases with aging, leading to decreased osteocyte density (29).

The repertoire of biologic activity possessed by osteocytes helps them maintain the bone tissue and allows the bone to be responsive to the mechanical and metabolic demands of the body. As mechanosensory cells, they translate mechanical forces into biologic activity (32,34). The detection of physical forces stimulates osteocytes to produce and release intercellular messengers that target precursor cells, osteoblasts, and osteoclasts (32,35). These cells, in turn, respond by remodeling the bone regionally and allowing it to change its mass and structure according to demands of the external physical environment (Wolff law). The widespread distribution of osteocytes and their cell processes is fundamental to another important role of theirs, namely, mineral homeostasis (29). Osteocytes generate and

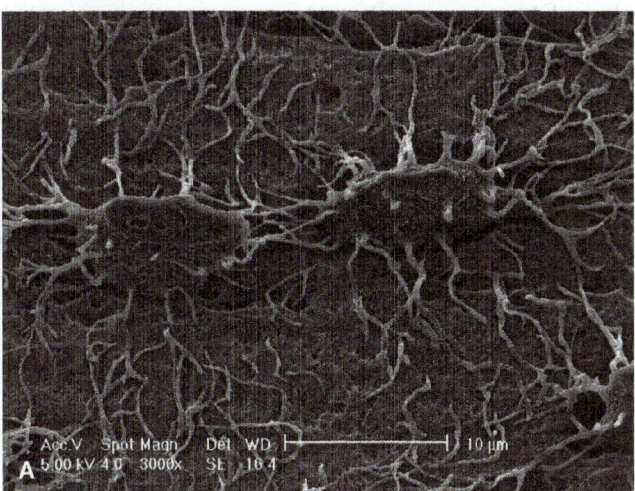 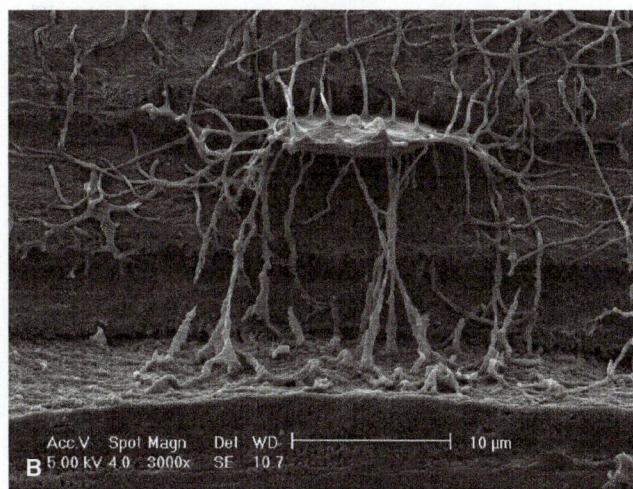

FIGURE 4.24 The osteocyte lacuno-canalicular network demonstrating the contact of cytoplasmic processes of two adjacent osteocytes in the bone (**A**) and an intraosseous osteocyte connecting with an osteoblast on the bone surface (**B**). Osteocyte cell processes (dendrites) pass through the canalicular network. The images are scanning electron micrographs of resin-embedded acid-etched mouse bone samples. (With permission from Bonewald LF. Generation and function of osteocyte dendritic processes. *J Musculoskelet Neuronal Interact* 2005;5(4):321–324.)

respond to microfluxes in ion concentrations and mediate the exchange of calcium and other ions between the bone matrix and extracellular fluid. In certain conditions, they may even be able to rapidly release calcium and phosphorus from the mineralized matrix by a process termed *osteocytic osteolysis*, which manifests histologically as enlarged lacunar spaces (36). In addition, osteocytes produce fibroblast growth factor-23 (FGF-23), which negatively regulates PTH and is a hormone essential in the regulation of serum phosphorus by modulating the reabsorption of phosphorus in the renal tubule (29,37). They also control osteoblastic activity through the secretion of sclerostin, which inhibits osteoblastic bone formation through Wnt/β-catenin pathway, and osteoclast activity through secretion of RANKL and osteoprotegerin (OPG) (29).

Osteoclasts

Osteoclasts are terminally differentiated, multinucleated cells responsible for bone resorption. They are mobile effector cells that have a lifespan of only several weeks. By the time they are recognizable by light microscopy, they are mature, biologically active, and can be found residing within resorption pits (Howship lacunae) produced by their digestion of mineralized bone matrix (Fig. 4.25).

Osteoclasts are 40 to 100 μm in diameter and are polarized with one portion of the cell membrane intimately attached to the bone and the remainder exposed to the extracellular fluid in its microenvironment. The segment of cell membrane that actually adheres or seals to the bone is laden with $\alpha_V\beta_3$ integrins. The integrins bind to specific extracellular bone matrix proteins (vitronectin, osteopontin, and bone sialoprotein) previously deposited by osteoblasts, and in this manner the osteoclast can anchor to the bone surface. In the cytoplasm, there is a network of interconnecting actin filaments that extends from the site where the osteoclast cell membrane attaches to the bone (clear zone) directly to the nuclei (31). On average, osteoclasts have 4 to 20 nuclei, though the number may range from 2 to as many as 100. In normal circumstances,

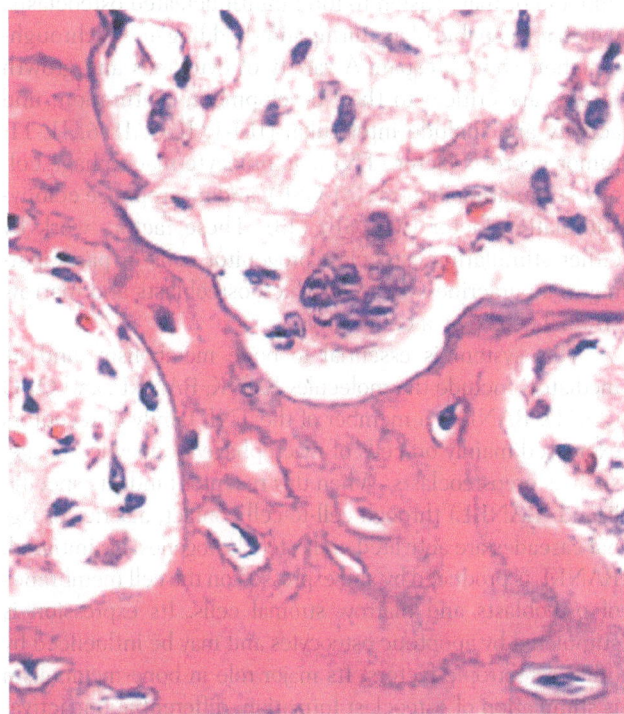

FIGURE 4.25 Osteoclast located within a resorption pit (Howship lacuna) on a trabecula.

however, the amount is usually not greater than 12. The nuclei and adjacent prominent Golgi apparatus tend to congregate away from the bone-resorbing surface, and are surrounded by abundant amphophilic cytoplasm.

The cytoplasm in the vicinity of the resorbing surface is rich in tartrate-resistant acid phosphatase, carbonic anhydrase, and membrane-bound lysosomes (38). The adjacent cell membrane, which also directly apposes the bone-resorbing surface, has numerous finger-like extensions that effectively increase its surface area and form the so-called brush border.

The lysosomes fuse with the brush border and release their contents into the resorption pit, which begins the actual process of bone digestion. Metabolic activation of osteoclasts is initiated by anchorage, and this process generates a stimulatory signal that is transmitted to the nuclei by the actin network. The nuclei, now activated, orchestrate the complex and transitory cytoplasmic and cell-membrane modifications required for bone digestion. Importantly, mineralized bone or cartilage is more efficiently resorbed by osteoclasts than nonmineralized bone or cartilage. Focal, or partial, demineralization of collagen fibers appears to be one of the first steps in matrix resorption and is followed by catabolism of noncollagenous proteins and, lastly, the degradation of collagen fibers themselves. Once osteoclast activity ceases and the cell moves to another targeted site, macrophages move into the base of the resorption pit and phagocytize the organic remnants.

Osteoclasts are derived from mononuclear, hematopoietic progenitor cells of the granulocytic-macrophage colony-forming units (GM-CFU) and macrophage colony-forming units (M-CFU) (39,40). The mononuclear preosteoclasts undergo primary fusion to form multinucleated osteoclasts, which are capable of acquiring and shedding nuclei throughout their short lifespan. A variety of cytokines and growth factors are critical to their development, maturation, and activity and include interleukin (IL)-1, IL-3, IL-6, IL-11, tumor necrosis factor (TNF), granulocyte-macrophage colony-stimulating factor (GM-CSF), and macrophage colony-stimulating factor (M-CSF) (40). These factors work by either stimulating osteoclast progenitor cells or participating in a paracrine system in which osteoblasts and marrow stromal cells play a central role.

This system is essential to bone metabolism, and its mediators include the molecules RANK, RANKL, and OPG (29,41). RANK is a member of the TNF family of receptors expressed mainly on cells of macrophage/monocytic lineage, such as preosteoclasts. When this receptor binds its specific ligand (RANKL) through cell-to-cell contact, a series of signal cascades are activated and osteoclastogenesis is initiated. RANKL is produced by and expressed on the cell membranes of osteoblasts and marrow stromal cells. Its expression is stimulated by apoptotic osteocytes and may be influenced by other osteotropic factors. Its major role in bone metabolism is stimulation of osteoclast formation, differentiation, activation, and survival. The actions of RANKL can be blocked by another member of the TNF family of receptors, OPG, which is a soluble protein produced by a number of tissues, including bone, hematopoietic marrow cells, and immune cells. OPG inhibits osteoclastogenesis by acting as a decoy receptor that binds to RANKL, thus preventing the interaction of RANK with RANKL (29). The interplay between bone cells and these molecules permits osteoblasts and stromal cells to control osteoclast development. This ensures the tight coupling of bone formation and resorption vital to the success of the skeletal system and provides a mechanism for a wide variety of biologic mediators (hormones, cytokines, and growth factors) to influence the homeostasis of bone tissue.

Inorganic Components

Mineral

The bone is composed of approximately 65% mineral. The primary mature inorganic mineral of the bone is a calcium-deficient variant of hydroxyapatite $[Ca_{10}(PO_4)_6(OH)_2]$, in which the hydroxyl groups have been largely replaced by phosphate and carbonate groups (13,15). It is the body's major reservoir for calcium and phosphate and contains more than 99% of the body's calcium and 85% of the body's phosphorus. Also harbored within the bone crystals are 95% of the body's sodium, 50% of the body's magnesium, and trace amounts of other essential minerals (42,43).

The bone is hypothesized to contain two distinct types of mineral, one manifesting as granular, electron-dense bands within the collagen fibrils and the other as needle or filament-like crystals that reside in the interfibrillar spaces. The deposition mechanism and chemical interactions between the collagen matrix and calcium phosphate apatite nanocrystals remain to be clarified (44,45). Two main theories seek to explain the mineralization of collagen: the hole zone theory, where initial mineralization begins in holes within the collagen fibrils, and the superhelix theory, where mineralization takes place along collagen fibrils arranged in a parallel array (46). However, the use of newer, less invasive tissue sectioning methods reveals that most mineral is extrafibrillar rather than deposited on collagen, forming mineral lamellae of polycrystalline plates arranged circumferentially around collagen fibrils (47).

Bone mineralization is divided into two stages: primary and secondary mineralization. Primary mineralization is a fast process (occurring over several days) that is biologically fine-tuned and is controlled by osteoblasts secreting abundant collagen fibrils, noncollagenous proteins, and matrix vesicles. Ca^{2+} and PO_4^{3-} are transported into matrix vesicles, the small extracellular, plasma membrane–bound vesicles where mineral is first observed through membrane transporters and enzymes. This influx initiates calcium phosphate nucleation followed by crystal growth. Initially amorphous, crystals are then converted into mature crystalline structures of calcium phosphate, principally hydroxyapatite. The mature calcium phosphate crystals elongate radially until they penetrate the membranes of the matrix vesicles and continue to grow outward to form calcifying nodules, needle-shaped minerals crystals in globular arrangements that still retain some transporters and enzymes. Surrounding organic compounds such as osteopontin, osteocalcin, and matrix gla protein regulate subsequent growth of the calcifying nodules, and collagen becomes mineralized, beginning at the site of contact with the calcifying nodule. It is estimated that 60% to 70% of the minerals are deposited by primary mineralization. Secondary mineralization is a slower process (occurring over several months) that ultimately achieves the full mineral load of the bone. This stepwise process leads to the mosaic-like pattern of bone mineralization seen on microradiographs (Fig. 4.6). The biologic and ultrastructural mechanisms behind secondary mineralization are not known with certainty, but it is hypothesized that osteocytes regulate the transportation of Ca^{2+} and PO_4^{3-}, leading to their physical and chemical deposition (44,46).

Once the crystals are deposited in the bone, they remain there for days to years, only to be dissolved at a future time during bone resorption, when the calcium and phosphorous are released into the extracellular fluid and become available for other biologic activities. Initial mineralization of osseous organic matrix takes approximately 2 weeks; therefore, the surfaces of the bone are covered by a layer of unmineralized organic matrix, called the osteoid (Figs. 4.11, 4.21, and 4.22). The width of this layer is dependent on the relative rate of bone formation. In inactive regions, the bone is nearly fully mineralized and is covered by a thin osteoid seam (1 to 5 μm in thickness), whereas in foci of rapid bone deposition, the osteoid layer may be more than several times thicker. The actual zone of mineralization can be detected by the systemic administration of the antibiotic tetracycline, which binds to the bone at the mineralization front and can be visualized with fluorescent microscopy (Fig. 4.12).

BONE FORMATION, GROWTH, AND REMODELING

From the time that skeleton formation begins in the embryo until the stage that adult stature is attained, the bones of the body undergo a marked increase in size, refinement of their shape, and enhancement of their contour. The bone is a rigid structure that cannot grow interstitially and only enlarges by the apposition of a new bone on its surface. Appositional growth alone is adequate for portions of the skeleton that enlarge slowly during maturation, such as the skull, and the diameter of long bones; however, it is insufficient for bones that must increase in size at a more rapid rate, such as the length of long and short tubular bones of the extremities, the vertebrae, and the ribs. The cartilage, in contrast, exhibits both appositional and interstitial growth; that is, it increases its volume and enlarges in all dimensions by adding new cells and elaborating the freshly synthesized extracellular matrix. Consequently, the growth in length of tubular bones in embryos and prepubertal children occurs as the growing cartilage is replaced by bone, with the majority of the increase in bone length derived from the cartilage primordium represented in the anlage and growth plate (physis).

The genetic code for skeletal morphogenesis is encrypted in the homeobox genes. Homeobox genes contain the DNA library of a repository of transcriptional regulators essential for growth and differentiation. The expression of homeobox genes occurs in a specific order and temporal sequence; and, regarding the skeletal system, homeobox gene activation results in the generation of localized cellular condensations of primitive mesenchyme at the sites of future bones. The mesenchymal condensations are the earliest precursors of individual bones and are critical to the formation of the skeleton. They begin to develop just prior to day 40 of gestation and, depending upon their anatomic location, are derived from cells that migrate from the cranial neural crest (craniofacial skeleton), paraxial mesoderm (axial skeleton), or the lateral plate mesoderm (appendicular skeleton) (48–50). Shortly after being formed, usually by the 7th week of gestation, the mesenchymal cells in the condensation begin to alter their genetic expression and assume the morphology of matrix-forming cells. Those cells that mature into chondrocytes form a cartilage model or anlage of the future bone, which is fundamental to the process of endochondral ossification, whereas those that develop directly into osteoblasts produce bone via the mechanism of intramembranous ossification. The mature bone tissue formed from either endochondral or intramembranous ossification is grossly and histologically indistinguishable.

Endochondral Ossification

Initially, the newly formed cartilage anlage is avascular and has the crude shape of the adult bone (Fig. 4.26 and 4.27). The mesenchyme surrounding the anlage forms the perichondrium (Fig. 4.26), which is the precursor to the

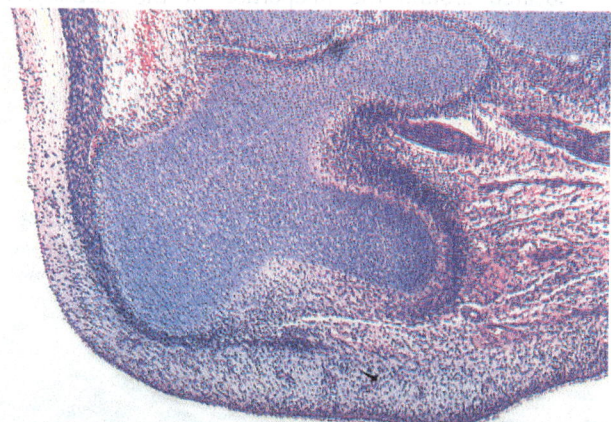

FIGURE 4.26 Photomicrograph of cartilage anlage of the os calcis (calcaneus). The cartilage model is the approximate shape of the adult bone. The attachment site of the Achilles tendon and the tibial–calcaneal joint are present.

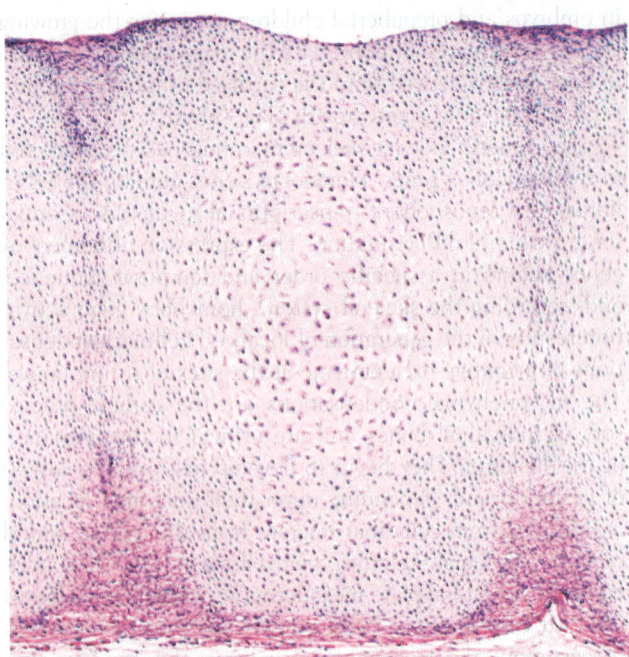

FIGURE 4.27 Sagittal section through vertebral body composed of cartilage anlage. The chondrocytes in the center are undergoing hypertrophy.

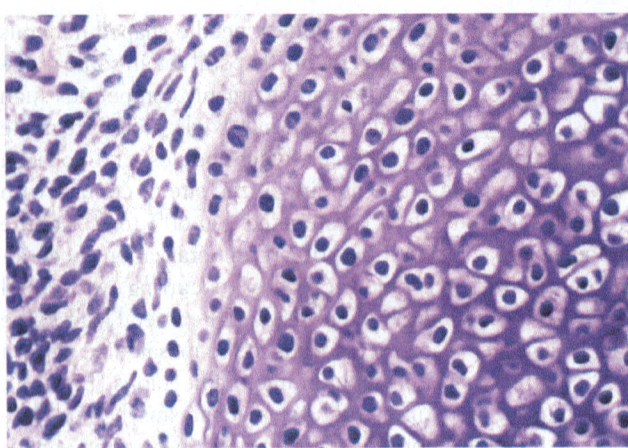

FIGURE 4.29 Cells of mesenchymal condensation surrounding an area in which they have differentiated into hyaline cartilage anlage. The chondrocytes show early hypertrophy.

periosteum that develops once ossification begins (see later). This process is initiated in each bone at a specific time, and this temporal sequence is the same in all humans.

Growth of the anlage occurs both interstitially and appositionally as a result of the proliferation of chondrocytes and the accumulation of secreted extracellular matrix (Figs. 4.28 and 4.29). The matrix is composed of proteoglycans and type II collagen with smaller amounts of collagen types IX, X, XI, and XIII (13). As this process continues, three events occur at very nearly the same stage of development in every bone (51):

1. The mesenchymal stems cells of the perichondrium, located around the midportion of the cartilaginous shaft, produce a layer of osteoblasts that deposit a collar of woven mineralized bone on the surface of the anlage. This heralds the transformation of the perichondrium into the periosteum. The periosteum, osteoblasts, and the thin surface layer of bone delineate the middle region of the diaphysis and form the primary center of ossification (Figs. 4.30 to 4.34).

2. The chondrocytes in the center of the anlage shaft, encased by the periosteal shell of the bone, begin to

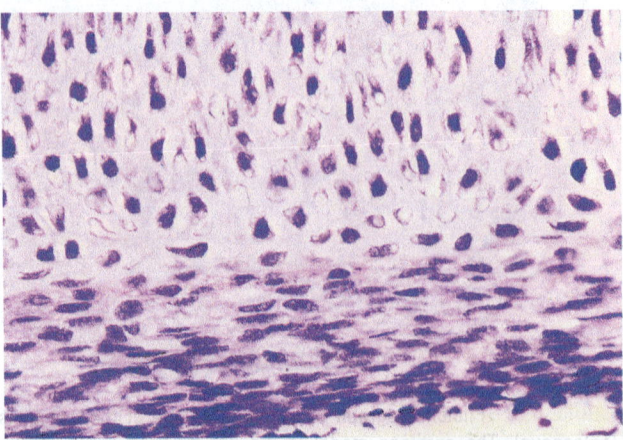

FIGURE 4.28 Cartilage anlage of the femur in an embryo. The perichondrium is in intimate contact with the cartilage.

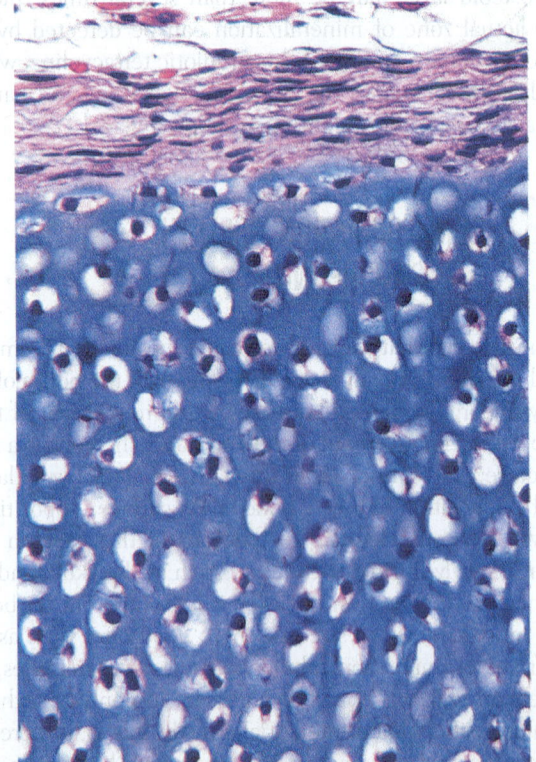

FIGURE 4.30 The perichondrium about the diaphysis of a cartilage anlage containing hypertrophied chondrocytes.

CHAPTER 4: Bone

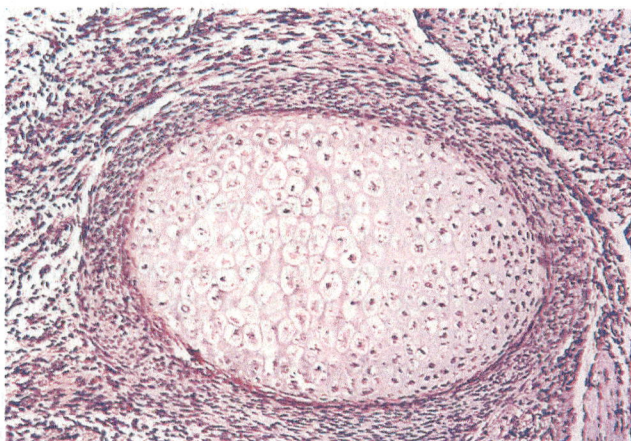

FIGURE 4.31 Cross-section of the diaphysis of an embryonic femur. The thin, collar-like primary center of ossification is between the hypertrophying chondrocytes and the periosteal cells.

undergo biologic changes and hypertrophy and swell (Figs. 4.29 to 4.33). The chondrocyte enlargement is accompanied by an increase in intracellular glycogen and in the deposition of type X collagen in the vicinity of the chondrocyte. Soon thereafter the chondrocytes undergo apoptotic necrosis. Concurrently, the surrounding matrix mineralizes, largely via matrix vesicles derived from the chondrocytes. Some matrix crystallization mineralization may occur within the "holes" of the collagen fibers.

3. A capillary network originating from periosteal vessels forms and, with the aid of osteoclastic (chondroclastic) resorption, penetrates the woven bone of the primary center of ossification (Fig. 4.34) into the mineralized cartilage. The capillaries are the precursor to the future nutrient vessels and are accompanied by pericytes and other primitive mesenchymal cells, including immature osteoprogenitor and osteoclast progenitor cells.

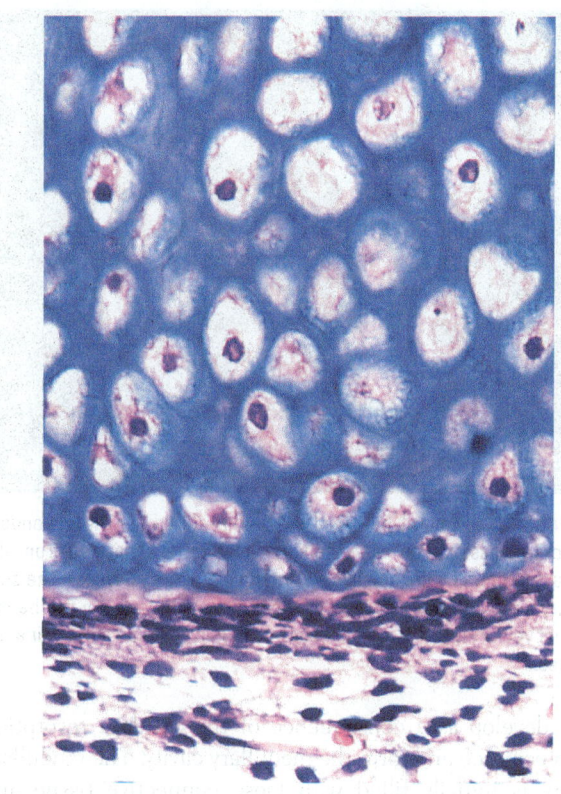

FIGURE 4.33 Primary center of ossification. A thin pink layer of osteoid, containing flattened osteocytes, separates the hypertrophied chondrocytes from the periosteal osteoblasts.

As the cartilaginous core of the bone undergoes continued resorption, osteoblasts derived from perivascular stem cells deposit layers of osteoid on the residual longitudinally oriented struts of mineralized cartilage. These trabeculae, composed of a central cartilaginous core covered by a rim of woven bone, are the first (or primary) trabeculae formed, and together they form the primary spongiosa. The spaces

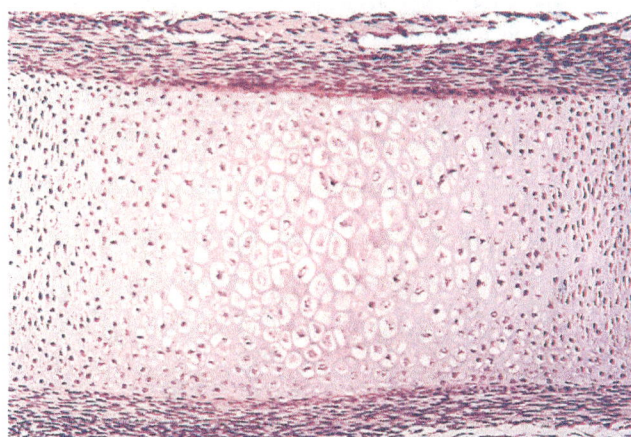

FIGURE 4.32 Longitudinal section of the primary center of ossification in an embryonic femur. The cellular layer of the periosteum is producing osteoblasts, which have formed a layer of pink osteoid. The outer spindle cells of the periosteum are oriented longitudinally along the femoral shaft. The underlying chondrocytes show hypertrophy.

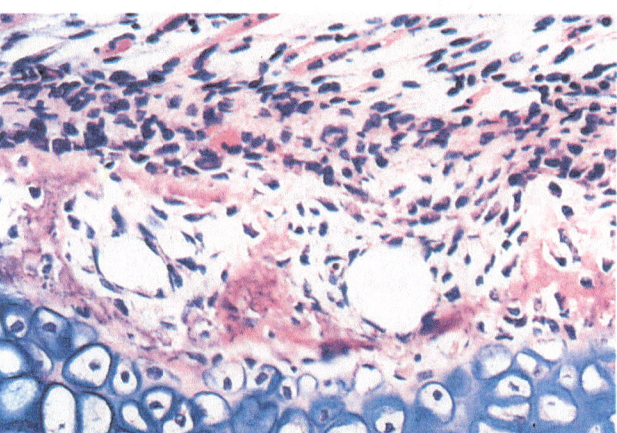

FIGURE 4.34 Primary center of ossification with capillary proliferation indicating the early formation of the nutrient artery. Between these capillaries, new trabecular membranous woven bone is being formed in the cambium layer of the periosteum. The outer fibrous layer of the periosteum is more cellular than in the adult.

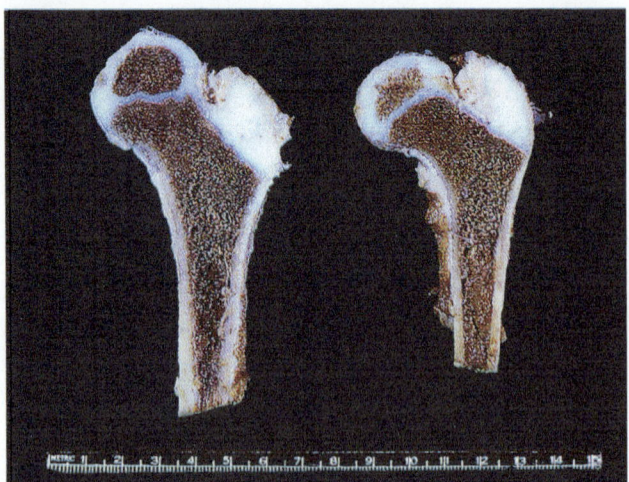

FIGURE 4.35 Femoral heads of a 3.5-year-old male. The secondary centers of ossification in the femoral heads are separated from the primary centers by the epiphyseal growth plates (the physes). The secondary center of ossification of the apophysis of the greater trochanter has not yet formed. The metaphyses and diaphyses resemble their adult shapes.

tissue and hematopoietic elements. This complex process begins within the center of the shaft and progresses toward both ends of the bone as the bone lengthens (see later). When complete with primary trabeculae and an adjacent secondary center of ossification (see later), the entrapped cartilage is recognized as the growth plate (the physis) (Figs. 4.35 to 4.38). Longitudinal growth of bones occurs at the physis so that markers placed in both the diaphysis or metaphysis and the epiphysis will separate with bone growth while markers placed only in the diaphysis will remain the same distance apart.

The fully developed growth plate (physis) is structured and has been divided into five merging regions that correspond to different stages of chondrocyte maturation (Figs. 4.36 to 4.39). As the chondrocytes pass through the different stages, they do not literally move within the matrix but mature in the position they occupy when first formed. Important regulators of this sequence of chondrocyte growth and maturation include the *Indian hedgehog* gene (Ihh), PTH, parathyroid hormone–related protein (PTHrP), fibroblast growth factor (FGF), RUNX2 and RUNX3, and bone morphogenic proteins (BMPs) (Table 4.3) (52–57). The zones include (a) a region of resting or reserve chondrocytes located nearest to the ends of the bone; (b) a region of proliferating chondrocytes that become arranged in spiral columns; (c) a region of chondrocyte hypertrophy; (d) a region

that develop as a consequence of the cartilage resorption then coalesce and form the medullary cavity. The medullary cavity is initially filled with loose connective tissue and eventually becomes occupied by varying amounts of adipose

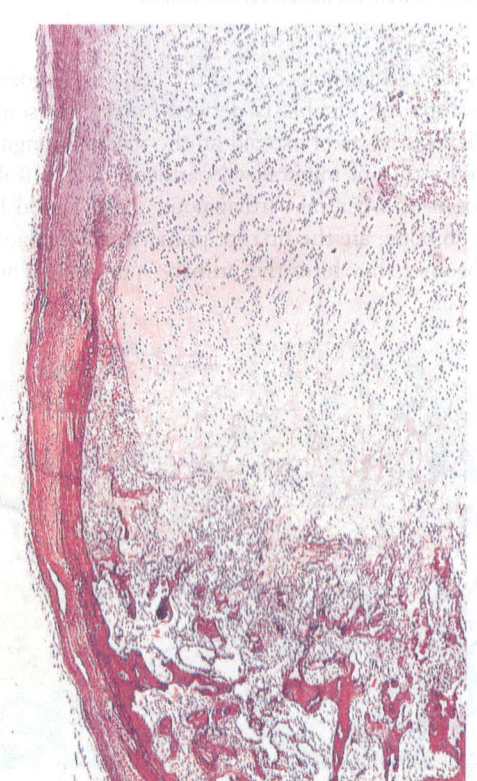

FIGURE 4.36 The epiphyseal growth plate of the costochondral junction from a 2-month-old male. The growth plate is surrounded by the ring of Ranvier. No secondary center is present. Primary trabeculae with central cartilaginous cores are seen in the metaphysis and upper diaphysis.

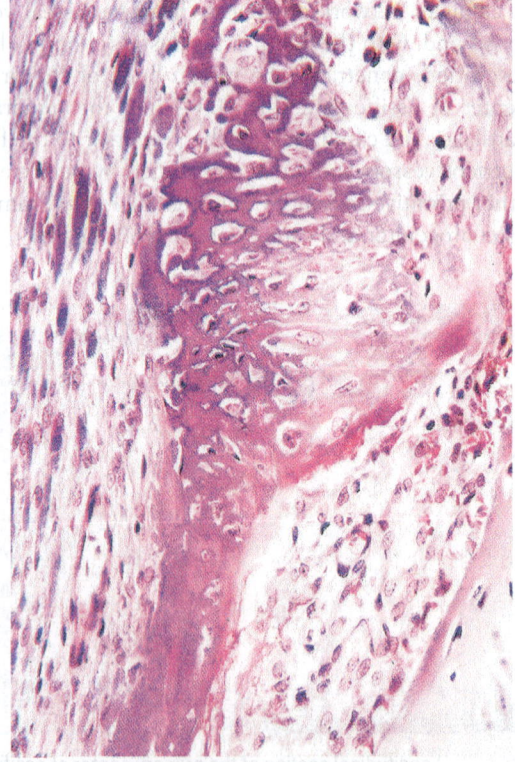

FIGURE 4.37 The ring of Ranvier, composed of a bone that forms by the process of intramembranous ossification beneath the periosteum on the left and delineates the peripheral portion of the epiphyseal growth plate near the metaphysis.

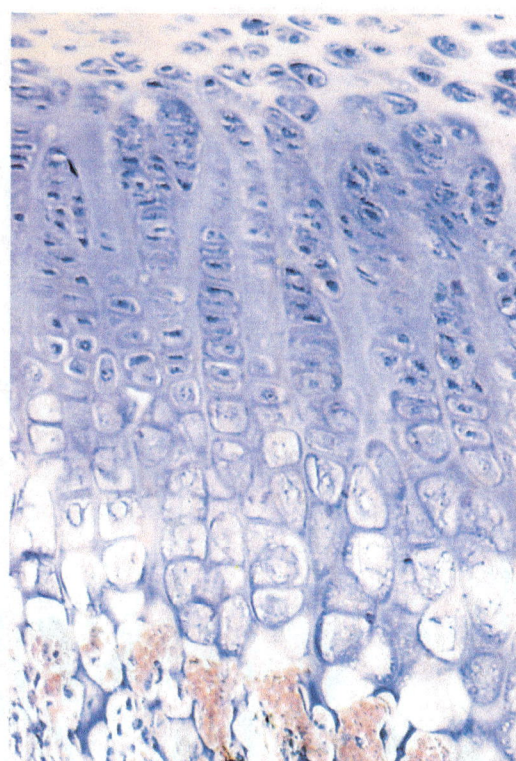

FIGURE 4.38 The maturing epiphyseal growth plate showing the reserve zone (*top*), the proliferating zone, the hypertrophied zone, and zone of mineralization of the cartilage. The primary trabeculae are oriented vertically and are supporting the base of the growth plate.

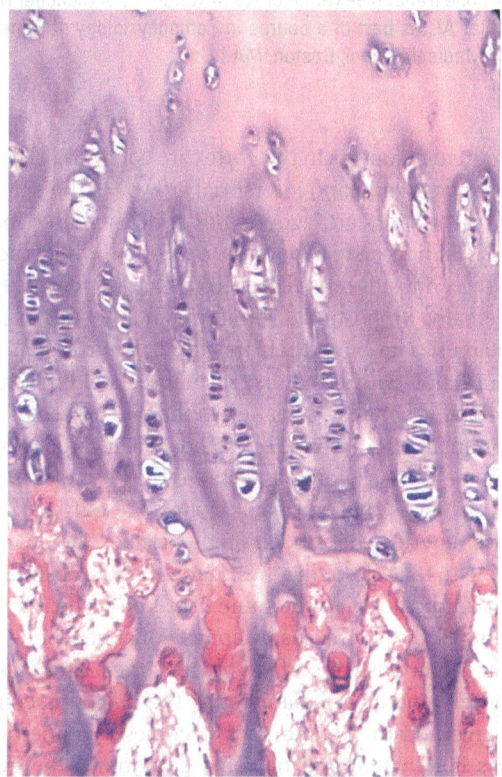

FIGURE 4.39 The junction between the mineralized cartilage columns and the primary trabeculae with the mineralized cartilage cores covered by a layer of woven bone.

TABLE 4.3

Important Local and Systemic Regulators of the Growth Plate

Factor	Actions and Regulation
Local Effects	
Ihh	Master regulator of chondrocyte differentiation. Stimulates PTHrP, regulates resting zone to proliferative zone chondrocytes, stimulates proliferation, determines transition from proliferating to hypertrophic chondrocytes. Regulation: CSPG-binding influences its distribution throughout growth plate; positively regulated by BMPs, negatively regulated by dEF1.
PTHrP	Maintains proliferative chondrocytes in the proliferative pool. Regulation: positively regulated by ADAMTS12 and ADAMTS17.
Cyclin D1	Transitions cells from G1 to S phase.
RUNX2 and RUNX3	Promote chondrocyte differentiation.
TGF-β	Promotes differentiation and matrix synthesis
C/EBP(β)	Promotes differentiation of chondrocytes from proliferative to hypertrophic.
Pannexin3	Promotes differentiation of chondrocytes from proliferative to hypertrophic.
Capn4	Modulates terminal cell differentiation.
SDF-1	Enhances chondrocyte hypertrophy.
SOX9	Proliferation and differentiation of the fetal growth plate; negatively regulates vascularization, cartilage resorption, and trabecular bone formation.
FGFs	Inhibit proliferation.
Vitamin D3	Organization of growth plate, mineralization, and longitudinal bone growth.
CNP	Promotes chondrogenesis by stimulating expression of cell adhesion molecules and glycosaminoglycans.
Systemic Effects	
Growth hormone (GH)	Longitudinal bone growth. Stimulates production of IGF-1.
Glucocorticoids	Suppress bone growth. Thought to be mediated through disturbance of the GH/IGF-1 axis.
Thyroid hormone	Promotes chondrocyte hypertrophy and terminal differentiation through Wnt/β-catenin signaling, stimulates the IGF-1 pathway.
Estrogens and Androgens	Increase skeletal growth in early puberty, fuse growth plate in late puberty.

Ihh, Indian hedgehog; PTHrP, parathyroid hormone–related protein; CSPG, chondroitin sulfate proteoglycan; BMPs, bone morphogenic proteins; dEF1, d-crystallin enhancer factor 1; ADAMTS12, a disintegrin and metalloproteinase with thrombospondin motifs 12; ADAMTS17, a disintegrin and metalloproteinase with thrombospondin motifs 17; RUNX, runt-related transcription factor; TGF-β, transforming growth factor beta; C/EBP(β), CCAAT/enhancing binding protein-β; Capn4, Calpain-4; SDF-1, stromal cell–derived factor 1; SOX9, sex-determining region Y-box 9; FGFs, fibroblast growth factors; CNP, C-type natriuretic peptide; IGF-1, insulin-like growth factor-1; Wnt/β-catenin, canonical Wingless-related integration site/beta-catenin signaling pathway.

of chondrocyte apoptotic necrosis and matrix mineralization; and (e) a region of cartilage resorption by osteoclasts (chondroblasts) that tunnel into the mineralized matrix.

The chondrocytes in the reserve zone are relatively small, round or oval, surrounded by abundant matrix and those at its base give rise to those that form the zone of proliferation. The chondrocytes in the zone of proliferation are flattened, undergo cell division, become arranged in spiral columns, and elaborate the extracellular matrix. In the zone of hypertrophy, the chondrocytes enlarge with the cytoplasmic volume increasing 10 times resulting in a transverse diameter of up to 30 µm, and the cells model the surrounding matrix as they increase in size (51). In the zone of mineralization or calcifying cartilage, the chondrocytes secrete matrix vesicles that are derived from the cell membrane which controls mineralization of the surrounding extracellular matrix. The number of longitudinally oriented chondrocytes that is associated with calcified matrix is 3 to 5 cells, and measures approximately 90 to 150 µm in length (58). As the matrix mineralizes, the chondrocytes undergo rapid necrosis in the last row of lacunae before the ossification front. This process is associated with the release of cytokines that attracts the ingrowth of endothelial cells and osteoclasts that tunnel into the mineralized matrix digesting the transverse septae of matrix that separates the chondrocytes from one another and leave behind residual longitudinal struts of mineralized cartilage that parallel the long axis of the bone. The orientation of the struts is determined by the pre-existing columnar arrangement of the chondrocytes in the proliferative and hypertrophied zones (Figs. 4.36 and 4.38). This columnar arrangement is thought to be controlled by a combination of physical or mechanical properties of the extracellular matrix and signaling molecules in the resting zone, specifically those involved in the noncanonical frizzled pathway. Primary cilia may also help create polarization gradients and transduce Ihh signaling (52). The mineralized cartilaginous struts act as scaffolding for newly deposited woven bone and form the primary trabeculae (Figs. 4.38 to 4.40).

In a growing long bone, the rate of resorption of mineralized cartilage at the chondro-osseous junction is balanced by the rate of chondrocyte proliferation in the zone of proliferation. It is estimated that chondrocytes spend an average of several days in the proliferating zone and in the zone of hypertrophy (59). Evidence suggests that in an individual column of chondrocytes four to seven cells die per day. Studies have found that in the costochondral junction of newborn infants there are 12.6 ± 1.0 chondrocytes per column, and of these 39.6% ± 6.9% are proliferating chondrocytes, and that the number of chondrocytes per column decrease with age (60). The rate of growth differs for each physeal plate and is greatest in the growth plate of the distal femur, followed by that of the proximal tibia. In diseases in which mineralization of the cartilage is impaired (rickets), removal of the cartilage is delayed, and the zone of hypertrophy becomes massively and irregularly thickened. While most tubular long bones have two epiphyseal growth plates, other bones (such as the ribs and some of the phalanges, carpals, tarsals, metacarpals, and metatarsals) have only a single physis. The growth plates, located at the diaphyseal–epiphyseal junctions of the bones, are delineated peripherally by a circumferential, thin collar of membrane bone that is a continuation of the primary center of ossification and is called the ring of Ranvier (Figs. 4.36 and 4.37) (61).

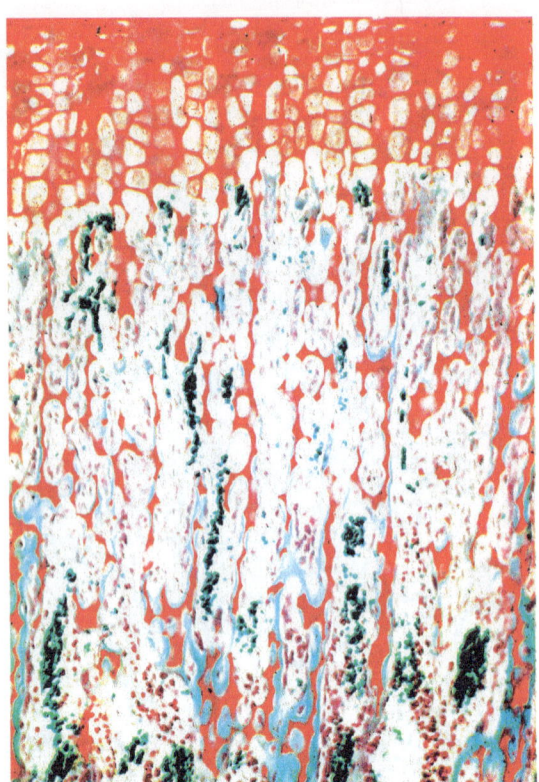

FIGURE 4.40 Longitudinal section of the epiphyseal growth plate, showing the zone of mineralization of the cartilage (*orange*) and the cartilage struts are being covered by a thin layer of osteoid (*blue-green*). Capillaries with numerous erythrocytes (*green*) are present between the primary bone trabeculae (Goldner stain). (Courtesy of Glimcher MJ, Roth SI, Schiller AL, as part of a course in Pathophysiology of Bone for the Harvard Medical School, Boston, MA.)

Dramatic changes in the cortex are concurrent with continued appositional and interstitial growth of the epiphyseal and growth plate cartilage. As the bone increases in diameter, the subperiosteal bone is deposited while the bone along the endosteum is resorbed so that the cortical thickness remains proportionally uniform and the medullary cavity enlarges. The bone that first forms the cortex is woven in nature; but, within the first several years of life, the fabricated bone is lamellar. Variation in the rate of formation and resorption alters the shape of the bone. This process is most pronounced in a region just distal to the base of the growth plate, known as the "cut back" zone. The cut back zone is rich in subperiosteal osteoclasts that reduce the diameter of the bone to that of the diaphysis, and this results in "funnelization" of the bone. At the same time, the cortical thickness is maintained or increases by appositional new bone formation on the endosteal surface of the cortex. During growth and development, the diameter of the diaphysis continues to enlarge and in specific sites becomes asymmetric. This process is dynamic and not only determines the eventual diameter of the bone but controls the thickness and contour of the cortex and the arrangement of the trabeculae (Wolff law). Conditions altering the balance of bone formation and

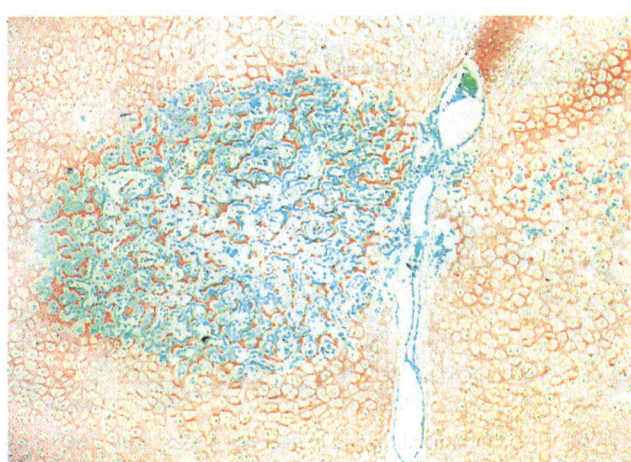

FIGURE 4.41 Photomicrograph of the secondary center of ossification of the femoral head. The nutrient vessels from the ligamentum teres are seen. Osteoid (*green*) is seen on the cartilage trabeculae (*orange*) in the spherical center (Goldner stain).

resorption may cause abnormally thickened or significantly thinned (osteoporotic) cortices.

In most long bones, a similar process subsequently develops in the epiphysis, and this region is the secondary center of ossification (Figs. 4.35 and 4.41). A few long bones have a similar growth center in the apophyses. The maturation and replacement of the cartilage anlage in a secondary center is identical to that which occurs in the diaphysis except that the maturation proceeds from the center centrifugally, toward the periphery. This means that the growing area of the secondary center is, at first, a sphere. Eventually, the enlarging primary and secondary centers of ossification approach one another, entrapping a cylindrical segment of residual cartilage anlage and delineating the final form of the physeal plate.

Continual growth of the primary and secondary centers of ossification results in the mergence of their reserve zones. At this time, a plate of bone demarcating the secondary center from the forming growth plate is deposited. From then on, the centrifugal growth of the epiphysis is hemispheric. The cartilage located at the base of the true articular cartilage is responsible for progressive epiphyseal enlargement, and it has the architectural organization of a physis. Variation in the subarticular growth results in concordance of the shapes of the ends of articulating bones. The epiphysis receives its nutrition primarily from blood vessels within the bone and its adjacent periosteum, whereas, the true articular cartilage is nourished by the synovial fluid.

In the apophyseal cartilage, located on the surface of the bone, a secondary-like center of ossification appears and is responsible for the development of the apophyseal bone of the iliac crests, the greater and lesser trochanters of the femur (Fig. 4.35), and the tibial tuberosities, to name a few.

Once endochondral ossification is well underway at the growth plate, modeling of the newly formed bone begins. The primary spongiosa undergoes complete osteoclastic resorption, and the secondary trabeculae composed solely of lamellar bone are deposited. The expanding medullary cavity becomes largely free of spicules of cancellous bone in much of the diaphysis and fills with adipose tissue and the hematopoietic marrow. Subperiosteal bone deposition and endosteal resorption of the cortex maintains a proper, tubular shape, and mechanical forces exerted by weight-bearing and muscle attachments alter the rate of these processes in specific regions, which help sculpt the contour of the bone.

Several hormones, including PTH, growth hormone, somatomedins, thyroid hormone, androgens, estrogens, and adrenal cortical hormones, are essential regulators of bone growth (54) (Table 4.3). At puberty, low doses of androgens and estrogens cause an increase in cell division in the proliferative zone of the growth plate and the secondary center of ossification. This is accompanied by an increase in the rate of cartilage maturation, mineralization, osteoclastic removal, and formation of primary trabeculae. In toto, these effects produce the so-called growth spurt seen at puberty. As estrogen and androgen levels increase and growth hormone and somatomedin levels fall off, chondrocyte proliferation decreases while maturation and bone formation proceed. This leads to a diminution or thinning of the growth plate, and eventually all of the cartilage of the growth plate undergoes complete endochondral ossification (Fig. 4.42), leaving little or no evidence of its previous existence. The fusion of the growth plate occurs as the hypertrophic chondrocytes furthest from the physis undergo cell death, a process that historically has been attributed to apoptosis but morphologically resembles hypoxia and necrosis and may not involve classical apoptotic pathways molecularly (52,62). At this time, the growth plate is considered closed, and all additional bone growth is appositional. An imprinted gene network is thought to be responsible for

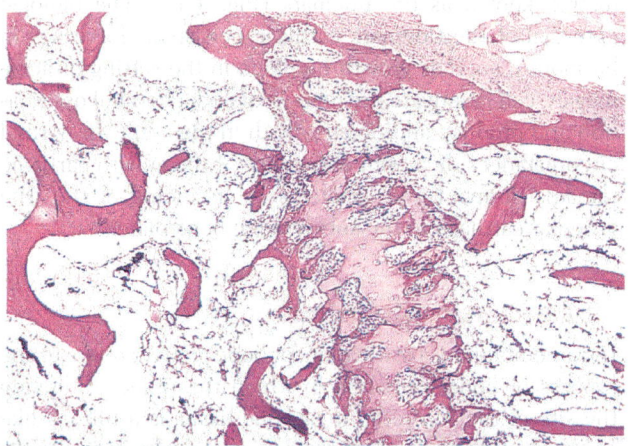

FIGURE 4.42 The closing epiphyseal growth plate in a 16-year-old boy. The periphery of the plate has been bridged by bone connecting the metaphysis and the secondary center of ossification. Cellular proliferation in the physis has ceased while the maturation process continues. The secondary center of ossification is at the left of the micrograph above the remnant of the physis.

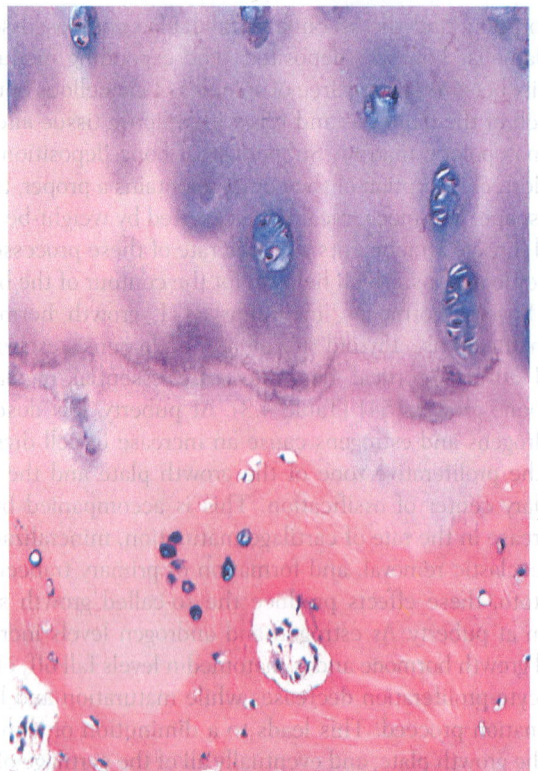

FIGURE 4.43 Section of the base of articular cartilage in the region of the tidemark. The tidemark separates the articular nonmineralized cartilage (*above*) from the mineralized cartilage remnant of the physis and the lamellar bone of the subchondral plate (*below*).

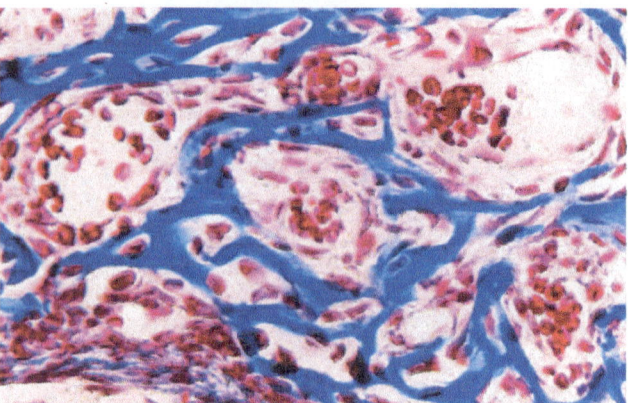

FIGURE 4.44 Intramembranous bone from a fetal skull. The osteoblasts are large along the randomly formed trabeculae. The osteocytes and their lacunae are large, round, and irregularly spaced in the trabeculae (trichrome stain).

growth deceleration (52). Cessation of growth of the secondary centers of ossification occurs in a similar fashion. However, a remnant of mineralized growth cartilage, which is the tidemark cartilage, persists at the base of the articular surface. It is demarcated from the true articular cartilage by a thin undulating layer of more densely mineralized matrix, known as the tidemark (Fig. 4.43). The biologic potential of the tidemark cartilage persists as increases in hormones, such as growth hormone in the setting of acromegaly, can reactivate the process of endochondral ossification and produce additional growth in the adult. In normal circumstances, however, the vestige of the growth cartilage remains dormant and functions as an anchor of the true articular cartilage to the subchondral bone plate.

Intramembranous Ossification

Intramembranous ossification, or bone growth, refers to the process of bone formation in which the tissue occupying the site of the future bone or bone tissue is a fibrous-like membrane. The membrane is rich in osteoprogenitor cells and in normal situations develops from the mesenchymal condensations in the developing embryo, the periosteum in the fetus, child, and adult, and the thin layer of fibrous tissue adjacent to all active bone-forming sites. The osteoprogenitor cells within the membrane produce offspring that differentiate into mature osteoblasts that directly deposit the bone matrix (Figs. 4.21 and 4.44). Large portions of the flat bones of the skull, including the frontal, parietal, occipital, and temporal bones, form by this process. Also, since the cortices of all bones are largely created by osteoblasts derived from the cambium layer of the periosteum, all bones, in at least some part, are formed by intramembranous ossification. Growth of the membranous bone occurs only by the apposition of the new bone, and the medullary cavities of membranous bones are created and maintained by endosteal osteoclastic activity. Initially, the marrow spaces of these bones are composed of highly vascularized loose connective tissue, which is eventually replaced by adipose and hematopoietic tissues.

Modeling and Remodeling

The processes of bone formation and resorption are tightly coupled, and their balance determines the skeletal mass at any point in time (50). As the skeleton grows and enlarges (undergoes modeling) during childhood and young adulthood, bone formation predominates, whereas after the third or fourth decades bone resorption prevails. The breakdown and renewal of the bone fundamental to the formation and maintenance of the skeleton is called remodeling. Remodeling is a dynamic process involving the removal and replenishment of both cortical and trabecular bones; it continues throughout life to maintain bone mass, skeletal integrity, and skeletal function (63). This process is complex and at least partially controlled by the central nervous system through hormones (such as leptin and serotonin) and by mechanically induced microdamage. It depends on the integrated actions of osteoblasts, osteocytes, and osteoclasts (64). Together these cells form the functional or basic multicellular unit of bone (BMU, or bone remodeling unit of Frost) and, in adults, are responsible for remodeling approximately 10% of the skeleton on an annual basis (Figs. 4.45 and 4.46) (65).

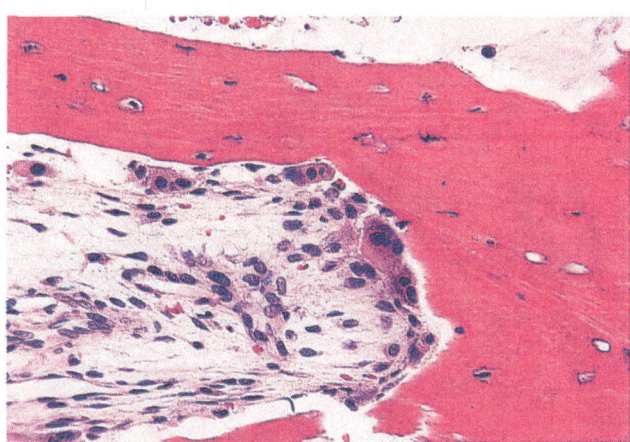

FIGURE 4.45 Basic multicellular unit of a bone (bone remodeling unit of Frost). Osteoclasts form the leading edge of the bone resorption ("the cutting cone"), and just behind them are mononuclear macrophages and osteoblasts. The newly created space is filled with a vascular loose connective tissue.

the diminished bone mass in postmenopausal osteoporosis, hyperparathyroidism, and hyperthyroidism results from increased osteoclastic bone resorption, which is not adequately compensated for by an appropriate amount of new bone formation. The lytic lesions in early Paget disease or those caused by metastases and myeloma result from localized increased osteoclastic bone resorption, which is significantly greater in amount than any new bone that is deposited. The goal of therapy for this broad spectrum of diseases is to restore the bone mass, balance bone formation and resorption, and protect and maintain structural integrity.

Approximately 1 million BMUs are active at any one time to execute this substantial remodeling, and they likely first target sites that are experiencing fatigue and microdamage (63). The process may begin on any bony surface and incorporates three phases of cell activity: activation, bone resorption, and bone formation.

Many pathologic conditions of the bone result from abnormalities in bone remodeling. These disorders may be generalized, in the form of a metabolic bone disease, or localized to small regions of the skeleton or individual bones. For instance,

BONE—HISTOLOGIC ARTIFACTS

Several common artifacts may be seen in histologic sections of the bone, and awareness of them can facilitate accurate interpretations. The high mineral content of the bone requires that it be decalcified during routine histologic processing. Multiple decalcifying agents are available, and they can be categorized as strong acids (such as hydrochloric acid), weak acids (such as formic acid), chelating agents (such as ethylenediaminetetraacetic acid [EDTA]), or combinations thereof (66). If preservation of DNA and RNA is necessary, decalcification in EDTA is recommended. Specimens must be well fixed in formalin before the decalcification procedure, or the histology will be suboptimal. Exposure of tissue to decalcification agents prior to appropriate fixation can lead to poor cellular preservation, such as artifactual cytoplasmic vacuolization (Fig. 4.47). Overdecalcification can lead to very pale stained sections, making it difficult to appreciate the nuclear detail (Fig. 4.48). Underdecalcification leads to problems cutting bone tissue on the microtome, resulting in thick sections that fold,

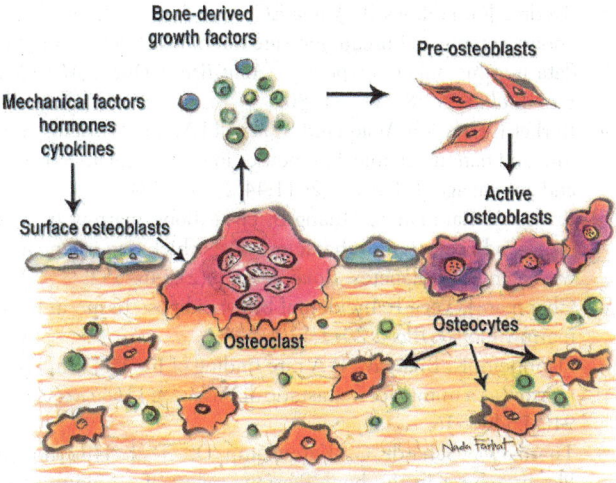

FIGURE 4.46 Illustration of the basic multicellular unit of bone, or bone remodeling unit of Frost. Osteocytes sense mechanical forces through their intricately connected network of dendrites. Mechanical factors, hormones, or cytokines stimulate resting surface osteoblasts to secrete cytokines that activate osteoclasts. Osteoclastic bone resorption through tartrate-resistant acid phosphatase within resorption lacunae releases bone-derived growth factors that stimulate precursor cells to differentiate into active osteoblasts. New osteoblastic bone fills the resorbed lacunae, ultimately coupling bone resorption with bone formation. (Courtesy of Nada Farhat.)

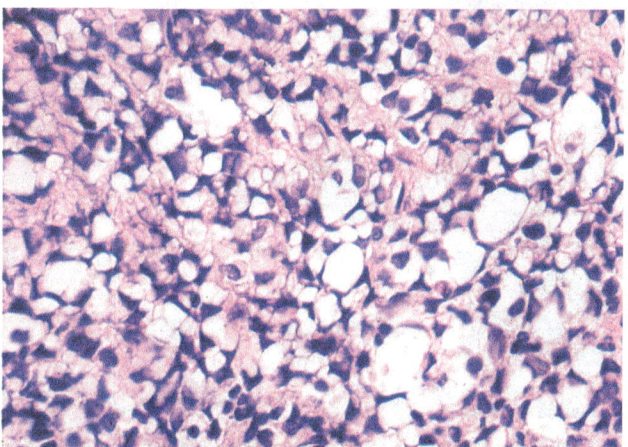

FIGURE 4.47 Bone biopsy specimen that was exposed to a decalcification agent prior to being well fixed in formalin (in this case, simultaneous exposure). While the cells represent large lymphoid cells of a large cell lymphoma, artifactual vacuolization of the cytoplasm mimics an adenocarcinoma with signet ring cells.

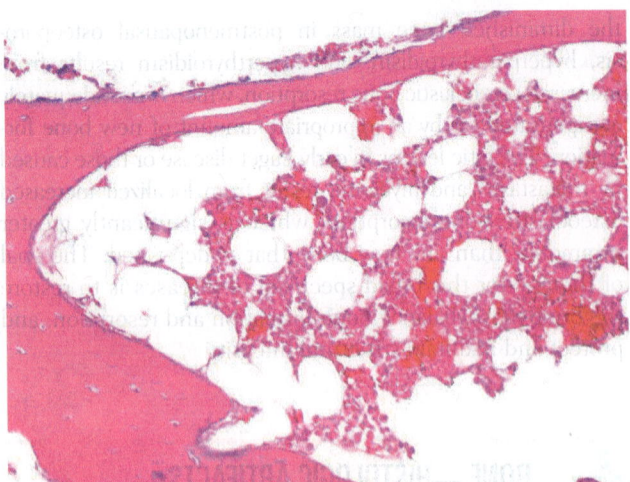

FIGURE 4.48 Trabecular bone and marrow with overdecalcification artifact. The marrow elements have limited hematoxylin staining, leading to pale nuclei and poor contrast between the nucleus and cytoplasm. The specific hematopoietic cell subtypes are more difficult to distinguish from one another.

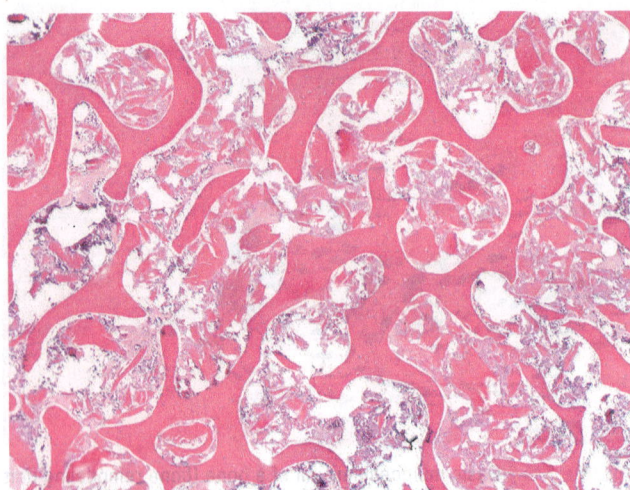

FIGURE 4.50 Bone dust manifests as irregular fragments of cortical bone or amorphous pink-purple tissue and can be mistaken for osteonecrosis or necrotic tumor.

frequently leading to physical separation of the bone and the surrounding soft tissue causing the tissue to mimic a vascular neoplasm (Fig. 4.49). Bone dust is another common artifact, present as a consequence of the force required to cut through (typically cortical) bone either as a part of a medical procedure, from core biopsies to orthopedic saws or reamers, or as a part of sectioning the specimen in the pathology laboratory. Bone dust appears as irregular fragments of cortical bone or amorphous pink-purple tissue and can mimic bone necrosis (Fig. 4.50).

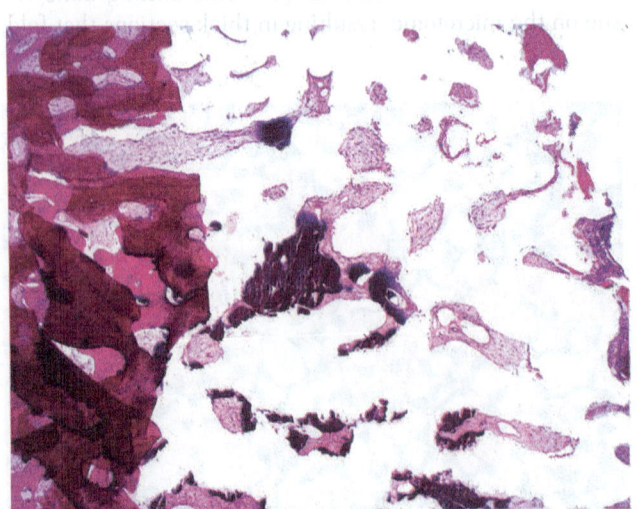

FIGURE 4.49 A section of cancellous bone without decalcification. The bone does not cut well on the microtome, leading to folding and thickening of the tissue section and retraction or separation of the bone from the adjacent tissue. In this case, the separation of the folded bone on the left from the vascular tissue within the marrow space may mimic a vascular neoplasm.

REFERENCES

1. Burdan F, Szumilo J, Korobowicz A, et al. Morphology and physiology of the epiphyseal growth plate. *Folia Histochem Cytobiol* 2009;47(1):5–16.
2. Milovanovic P, Vom Scheidt A, Mletzko K, et al. Bone tissue aging affects mineralization of cement lines. *Bone* 2018;110:187–93.
3. Skedros JG, Holmes JL, Vajda EG, et al. Cement lines of secondary osteons in human bone are not mineral-deficient: new data in a historical perspective. *Anat Rec A Discov Mol Cell Evol Biol* 2005;286(1):781–803.
4. Burket J, Gourion-Arsiquaud S, Havill LM, et al. Microstructure and nanomechanical properties in osteons relate to tissue and animal age. *J Biomech* 2011;44(2):277–284.
5. Krings A, Rahman S, Huang S, et al. Bone marrow fat has brown adipose tissue characteristics, which are attenuated with aging and diabetes. *Bone* 2012;50(2):546–552.
6. Chapman J, Vega F. Incidental brown adipose tissue in bone marrow biopsy. *Blood* 2017;130(7):952.
7. Dannheim K, Bhargava P. A rare finding of brown fat in bone marrow as a mimic for metastatic disease. *Am J Hematol* 2016;91(5):545–546.
8. Thorns C, Schardt C, Katenkamp D, et al. Hibernoma-like brown fat in the bone marrow: report of a unique case. *Virchows Arch* 2008;452(3):343–345.
9. Boutin RD, White LM, Laor T, et al. MRI findings of serous atrophy of bone marrow and associated complications. *Eur Radiol* 2015;25(9):2771–2778.
10. Chan N, Ho C, Yip SF. Cardiac cachexia causing extensive serous degeneration of bone marrow. *Br J Haematol* 2017;178(5):660.
11. Bohm J. Gelatinous transformation of the bone marrow: the spectrum of underlying diseases. *Am J Surg Pathol* 2000;24(1):56–65.

12. Sung CW, Hsieh KL, Lin YH, et al. Serous degeneration of bone marrow mimics spinal tumor. *Eur Spine J* 2017; 26(Suppl 1):80–84.
13. Gorski JP. Biomineralization of bone: a fresh view of the roles of non-collagenous proteins. *Front Biosci (Landmark Ed)* 2011; 16:2598–2621.
14. Neve A, Corrado A, Cantatore FP. Osteoblast physiology in normal and pathological conditions. *Cell Tissue Res* 2011; 343(2):289–302.
15. Clarke B. Normal bone anatomy and physiology. *Clin J Am Soc Nephrol* 2008;3(Suppl 3):S131–S139.
16. Veis A, Sabsay B. The collagen of mineralized matrices. In: Peck WA, ed. *Bone and Mineral Research*. Amsterdam: Elsevier; 1988:1–63.
17. Camozzi V, Vescini F, Luisetto G, et al. Bone organic matrix components: their roles in skeletal physiology. *J Endocrinol Invest* 2010;33(7 Suppl):13–15.
18. Allori AC, Sailon AM, Warren SM. Biological basis of bone formation, remodeling, and repair-part II: extracellular matrix. *Tissue Eng Part B Rev* 2008;14(3):275–283.
19. Allori AC, Sailon AM, Warren SM. Biological basis of bone formation, remodeling, and repair-part I: biochemical signaling molecules. *Tissue Eng Part B Rev* 2008;14(3):259–273.
20. Oury F, Sumara G, Sumara O, et al. Endocrine regulation of male fertility by the skeleton. *Cell* 2011;144(5):796–809.
21. DiGirolamo DJ, Clemens TL, Kousteni S. The skeleton as an endocrine organ. *Nat Rev Rheumatol* 2012;8(11):674–683.
22. Chau JF, Leong WF, Li B. Signaling pathways governing osteoblast proliferation, differentiation and function. *Histol Histopathol* 2009;24(12):1593–1606.
23. Zhou H, Mak W, Zheng Y, et al. Osteoblasts directly control lineage commitment of mesenchymal progenitor cells through Wnt signaling. *J Biol Chem* 2008;283(4):1936–1945.
24. Komori T. Regulation of bone development and maintenance by Runx2. *Front Biosci* 2008;13:898–903.
25. Soltanoff CS, Yang S, Chen W, et al. Signaling networks that control the lineage commitment and differentiation of bone cells. *Crit Rev Eukaryot Gene Expr* 2009;19(1):1–46.
26. Deng ZL, Sharff KA, Tang N, et al. Regulation of osteogenic differentiation during skeletal development. *Front Biosci* 2008; 13:2001–2021.
27. Long F. Building strong bones: molecular regulation of the osteoblast lineage. *Nat Rev Mol Cell Biol* 2011;13(1): 27–38.
28. Burger C, Zhou HW, Wang H, et al. Lateral packing of mineral crystals in bone collagen fibrils. *Biophys J* 2008;95(4): 1985–1992.
29. Chen H, Senda T, Kubo KY. The osteocyte plays multiple roles in bone remodeling and mineral homeostasis. *Med Mol Morphol* 2015;48(2):61–68.
30. Baron R. Anatomy and ultrastructure of bone. In: Favus MJ, ed. *Primer on the Metabolic Bone Diseases and Disorders of Mineral Metabolism*. Philadelphia, PA: Lippincott Williams & Wilkins; 1999:3–10.
31. Marks SC Jr, Popoff SN. Bone cell biology: the regulation of development, structure, and function in the skeleton. *Am J Anat* 1988;183(1):1–44.
32. Bonewald LF. The amazing osteocyte. *J Bone Miner Res* 2011; 26(2):229–238.
33. Buenzli PR, Sims NA. Quantifying the osteocyte network in the human skeleton. *Bone* 2015;75:144–150.
34. Rochefort GY, Pallu S, Benhamou CL. Osteocyte: the unrecognized side of bone tissue. *Osteoporos Int* 2010;21(9):1457–1469.
35. Nakashima T, Hayashi M, Fukunaga T, et al. Evidence for osteocyte regulation of bone homeostasis through RANKL expression. *Nat Med* 2011;17(10):1231–1234.
36. Belanger LF. Osteocytic osteolysis. *Calcif Tissue Res* 1969; 4(1):1–12.
37. Juppner H. Phosphate and FGF-23. *Kidney Int* 2011;79(S121): S24–S7.
38. Teitelbaum SL. Bone resorption by osteoclasts. *Science* 2000; 289(5484):1504–1508.
39. Takahashi N, Maeda K, Ishihara A, et al. Regulatory mechanism of osteoclastogenesis by RANKL and Wnt signals. *Front Biosci (Landmark Ed)* 2011;16:21–30.
40. Edwards JR, Mundy GR. Advances in osteoclast biology: old findings and new insights from mouse models. *Nat Rev Rheumatol* 2011;7(4):235–243.
41. Boyce BF, Yao Z, Xing L. Functions of nuclear factor kappaB in bone. *Ann N Y Acad Sci* 2010;1192:367–375.
42. Glimcher MJ. The nature of the mineral phase of bone: biological and clinical implications. In: Avioli LV, Kranem SM, eds. *Metabolic Bone Disease and Clinically Related Disorders*. San Diego, CA: Academic Press; 1998:23–50.
43. Robey PG, Bianco P, Termine JD. The cellular biology and molecular biochemistry of bone formation. In: Coe FL, Favus MJ, eds. *Disorders of Bone and Mineral Metabolism*. New York, NY: Raven Press; 1992:241–263.
44. Rey C, Combes C. What bridges mineral platelets of bone? *Bonekey Rep* 2014;3:586.
45. Bonucci E. Bone mineralization. *Front Biosci (Landmark Ed)* 2012;17:100–128.
46. Hasegawa T. Ultrastructure and biological function of matrix vesicles in bone mineralization. *Histochem Cell Biol* 2018;149(4):289–304.
47. Schwarcz HP. The ultrastructure of bone as revealed in electron microscopy of ion-milled sections. *Semin Cell Dev Biol* 2015;46:44–50.
48. Lefebvre V, Bhattaram P. Vertebrate skeletogenesis. *Curr Top Dev Biol* 2010;90:291–317.
49. Yang Y. Skeletal morphogenesis during embryonic development. *Crit Rev Eukaryot Gene Expr* 2009;19(3):197–218.
50. Olsen BR, Reginato AM, Wang W. Bone development. *Annu Rev Cell Dev Biol* 2000;16:191–220.
51. Mackie EJ, Ahmed YA, Tatarczuch L, et al. Endochondral ossification: how cartilage is converted into bone in the developing skeleton. *Int J Biochem Cell Biol* 2008;40(1):46–62.
52. Lui JC, Nilsson O, Baron J. Recent research on the growth plate: Recent insights into the regulation of the growth plate. *J Mol Endocrinol* 2014;53(1):T1–T9.
53. Chen H, Ghori-Javed FY, Rashid H, et al. Runx2 regulates endochondral ossification through control of chondrocyte proliferation and differentiation. *J Bone Miner Res* 2014;29(12): 2653–2665.
54. Karimian E, Chagin AS, Savendahl L. Genetic regulation of the growth plate. *Front Endocrinol (Lausanne)* 2011;2:113.
55. Hirai T, Chagin AS, Kobayashi T, et al. Parathyroid hormone/parathyroid hormone-related protein receptor signaling is required for maintenance of the growth plate in postnatal life. *Proc Natl Acad Sci U S A* 2011;108(1):191–196.
56. Wuelling M, Vortkamp A. Chondrocyte proliferation and differentiation. *Endocr Dev* 2011;21:1–11.

57. Marino R. Growth plate biology: new insights. *Curr Opin Endocrinol Diabetes Obes* 2011;18(1):9–13.
58. Jerome C, Hoch B. Skeletal system. In: Treuting PM, Dintzis SM, Montine KS, eds. *Comparative Anatomy and Histology*. Waltham, MA: Academic Press; 2012:53–70.
59. Farnum CE, Wilsman NJ. Determination of proliferative characteristics of growth plate chondrocytes by labeling with bromodeoxyuridine. *Calcif Tissue Int* 1993;52(2):110–119.
60. Gruber HE, Rimoin DL. Quantitative histology of cartilage cell columns in the human costochondral junction: findings in newborn and pediatric subjects. *Pediatr Res* 1989;25(2):202–204.
61. Langenskiold A. Role of the ossification groove of Ranvier in normal and pathologic bone growth: a review. *J Pediatr Orthop* 1998;18(2):173–177.
62. Emons J, Chagin AS, Hultenby K, et al. Epiphyseal fusion in the human growth plate does not involve classical apoptosis. *Pediatr Res* 2009;66(6):654–659.
63. Eriksen EF. Cellular mechanisms of bone remodeling. *Rev Endocr Metab Disord* 2010;11(4):219–227.
64. Karsenty G, Oury F. The central regulation of bone mass, the first link between bone remodeling and energy metabolism. *J Clin Endocrinol Metab* 2010;95(11):4795–4801.
65. Pogoda P, Priemel M, Rueger JM, et al. Bone remodeling: new aspects of a key process that controls skeletal maintenance and repair. *Osteoporos Int* 2005;16(Suppl 2):S18–S24.
66. Dimenstein IB. Bone grossing techniques: helpful hints and procedures. *Ann Diagn Pathol* 2008;12(3):191–198.

Joints

Fiona Maclean

THE NORMAL JOINT 113	**TISSUE RESPONSE TO INJURY** 124
Diarthrodial Joint 113	Cartilage 124
Amphiarthrodial Joint 115	Bone 126
THE NORMAL JOINT TISSUES 116	Ligaments and Tendons 129
Articular Cartilage 116	Synovial Membrane 129
Synovial Membrane 121	Synovial Fluid 130
Ligaments and Tendons 122	**REFERENCES** 130
THE ARTHRITIC JOINT 122	
Alteration in Shape 124	

Bone, cartilage, ligaments, and tendons have a mechanical function, providing movement, stability, and protection. Unlike organs such as the liver or kidneys, which are composed mainly of cellular elements with a metabolic function, the connective tissues are largely formed from extracellular material. This material (or matrix) is made up of substances that resist the tensile and compressive forces to which they are subjected. The cellular component of the connective tissues provides for their growth and maintenance.

THE NORMAL JOINT

"Norms are recognized as such only through infractions. Functions are revealed only by their breakdown"
—GEORGES CANGUILHEM
LE NORMAL ET LE PATHOLOGIQUE (PARIS, 1966)

The joint is a functioning unit comprising the ends of contiguous bones together with their soft tissue components, including cartilage, ligaments, and synovium. There are three types of joints. The most common is the diarthrodial joint, which is a mobile unit between two bones. Hyaline cartilage covers the articulating surfaces of the diarthrodial joints, with the exception of the sternoclavicular and temporomandibular joints, which are covered by fibrocartilage. The second type is the amphiarthrodial joint, typified by the intervertebral disc and characterized by limited mobility. The third type is the fibrous synarthroses, such as the skull sutures, which are nonmovable joints and will not be discussed further.

Diarthrodial Joint
In the normal diarthrodial joint, the opposed articular surfaces move painlessly over each other within the required range of motion, with the load distributed across joint tissues. Conversely, clinical joint dysfunction is characterized by instability, loss of motion, maldistribution of load, and pain.

Normal joint function depends on the shape (geometry) of the joint, the mechanical properties of the various tissues that compose the joint, and the integrity of the joint, including its neuromuscular control.

The Shape
Perhaps the most obvious feature of any joint is the shape of its articulating surfaces. In general, one surface is convex and the other concave. The convex side usually has the

---

This chapter is an update of a previous version authored by Peter G. Bullough.

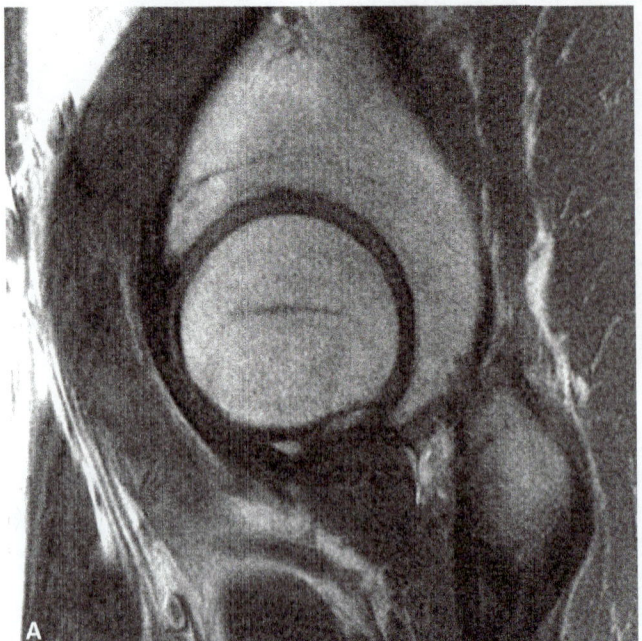 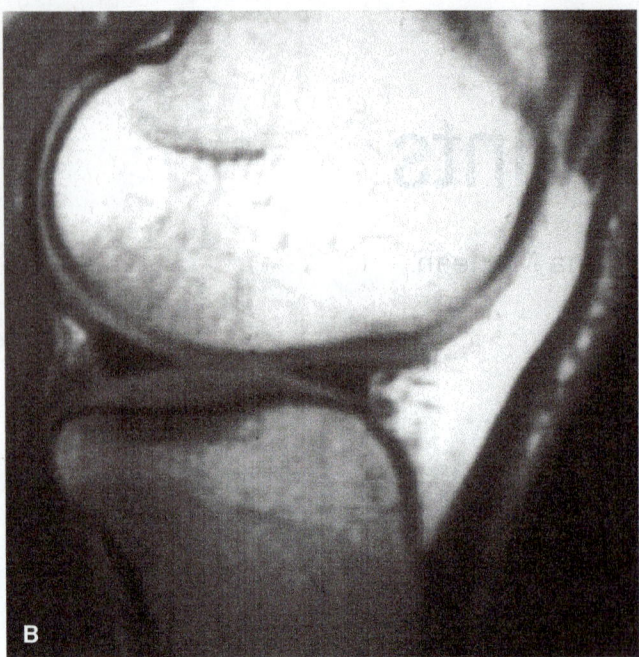

FIGURE 5.1 A: Sagittal section through the hip joint seen by magnetic resonance imaging (MRI) shows a close fit between the acetabulum and femoral head. B: Lateral MRI of a normal knee shows the gross incongruity of the articular surfaces. This is partially corrected by the interposed menisci, which act as load-bearing structures.

greater surface area. These complementary shapes permit the normal range of motion and provide stability and equal loading. Some joints fit together almost exactly (e.g., the hip and ankle) (1), whereas other joints (e.g., the knee and finger joints) show greater incongruence (Fig. 5.1). The position of greatest congruence of any joint is referred to as its close-packed position (2).

In some joints, such as the knee, the incongruences of the surfaces are partially compensated by the intra-articular fibrocartilaginous menisci (3). Removal or damage to the menisci results in significant consequences. The same is true of the labrum of the hip joint, which may be regarded as an extension of the articular surface of the acetabulum.

In most joints, the initial contact between the articular surfaces is at the joint periphery. The tissues that make up the articulating surfaces undergo elastic deformation when loaded. As the load increases, the surfaces come into increasing contact with more even distribution of the load (Fig. 5.2).

These mechanical factors together with the movement of the joint, mix and circulate the synovial fluid, which is essential to the metabolism of the chondrocytes, as the articular cartilage is avascular.

The Mechanical Properties of the Extracellular Matrices

In 1743, William Hunter (4) noted that: The articulating cartilages are most happily contrived to all purposes of motion in those parts. By their uniform surface, they move upon one another with ease; by their soft, smooth, and slippery surface, mutual abrasion is prevented; by their

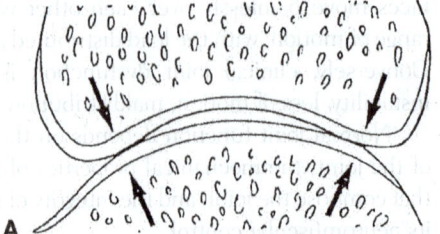 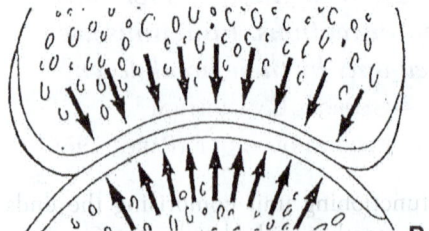

FIGURE 5.2 A: Light load. At rest and under light load, limited contact at the joint periphery assures access for synovial fluid to the joint space. B: Increased load. With increasing load, deformation of the bone and cartilage allows increased contact of the cartilage surfaces and an equitable distribution of the load. Cyclical loading permits circulation of the synovial fluid in the joint and between the articular surfaces to provide for the metabolic needs of the cartilage.

flexibility, the contiguous surfaces are constantly adapted to each other and the friction diffused equally over the whole; by their elasticity, the violence of any shock, which may happen in running, jumping, etc., is broken and gradually spent, which must have been extremely pernicious, if the hard surfaces of bones had been immediately contiguous.

These biomechanical properties of articular cartilage are determined by the extracellular matrices. Connective tissues such as bone, cartilage, and ligaments have a unique composition and structural organization that enable specific mechanical function. Following trauma, disturbances in the structure and/or composition of the extracellular matrix of articular cartilage may result in joint dysfunction.

The connective tissue matrices are remodeled by their intrinsic cells (i.e., fibroblasts, osteoblasts, osteoclasts, and chondrocytes). In maintaining their physicochemical and mechanical properties, the metabolism of these cells are subject to highly sensitive local and systemic feedback systems.

Collagen fibers, the principal extracellular component of connective tissues, are made up of bundles of fibrils, which are composed of stacked molecules formed from polypeptide chains arranged in a helical pattern. The fibrillar collagens provide tensile strength. There are also non–fiber-forming collagens that have varying functions, such as acting as binding sites for other matrix components (type IX collagen) or facilitating calcification (type X collagen) (5). Type I collagen is the most common form of collagen in tendon, ligaments, and bone. Type II collagen gives articular cartilage its tensile strength and, together with the proteoglycans (PGs), is essential for maintaining the tissue's volume and shape (6).

Connective tissues are also subjected to compression. In bone, the compressive load is resisted by hydroxyapatite. A mucoid filler between the collagen fibers of cartilage provides compressive strength as well as its viscoelastic properties. This filler is composed of large negatively charged macromolecular PG aggregates.

PGs are a group of heterogeneous molecules, consisting of protein chains and attached carbohydrates, which have a sticky gel-like quality. The major PG in cartilage is aggrecan (7), containing a protein core to which carbohydrate side chains (keratan and chondroitin sulfate) are attached. The highly charged PG molecules attract water and swell considerably. However, within the cartilage, the expansion of the PGs is restricted by the collagen network. When cartilage is loaded, some water is extruded and PGs are further compressed. Removal of the load permits the absorption of water and nutrients into the tissue.

Aggrecan shows age-related changes including decreased size and changes in chemical structure altering the stiffness and water content of the cartilage (8). In addition to aggrecan, the extracellular matrix of cartilage contains many noncollagenous proteins and PGs, whose precise functions are only just beginning to be understood. These molecules may serve a structural and/or regulatory role. The recognition of genetic disorders in which synthesis of the matrix molecules is affected has given insights into their functional role (9).

Prolonged physical activity can cause the total cartilage thickness to decrease by about 5%, although the changes are not uniform throughout the tissue. For example, the superficial zone can experience significant fluid exudation and consolidation in the range of 60%, while the radial zone experiences relatively little fluid flow and consolidation. These changes alter the synthesis and degradation of matrix proteins. Long-term, even minor differences in these cellular processes may affect the micro- and macromorphology of articular cartilage.

Capsular, Pericapsular Tissues and Muscular Control

Through the perception of touch, temperature, pain, and position, there is continuous sensory feedback regarding our movements. Correct joint function is thus dependent on intact ligaments, muscles, and nerves. As recognized by Charcot, a breakdown of neuromuscular coordination can lead to profound arthritis (10).

Amphiarthrodial Joint

The intervertebral disc is a fibrocartilaginous complex that forms the articulation between the vertebral bodies. It can be divided into two components: the outermost fibrous ring (annulus fibrosus) and the innermost gelatinous core (nucleus pulposus). It contributes spinal mobility and stability, as well as allowing for the transmission of load.

The annulus, when viewed from above, contains fibrous tissue layers arranged in concentric circles. Each layer extends obliquely from vertebral body to vertebral body, with the fibers of each layer running in opposing directions. This arrangement of alternating oblique layers allows for controlled motion that is universal in direction (rotation, flexion, and extension) but restricted in degree (Fig. 5.3).

The fibers of the annulus are attached by Sharpey fibers to the bony endplates of the adjacent vertebral bodies. The fibers are stronger and more numerous in the anterior and lateral aspects of the disc than in the posterior aspect. As a result, the anterior annulus is almost twice the thickness of the posterior annulus. Due to this variation in thickness, the nucleus pulposus typically occupies an eccentric position within the disc space, closer to the posterior margin. The tissue of the nucleus is separated from that of the bone above and below by a clearly defined layer of hyaline cartilage (Fig. 5.4).

On microscopic examination, the nucleus pulposus shows chondrocytes and stellate and fusiform cells suspended in a loose fibromyxoid matrix rich in PGs. Because no blood vessels are present in most of the adult disc tissue, nutrients must travel by diffusion from the disc margins. A restricted flow of nutrients to the nucleus and inner annulus contributes to disc degeneration. Disc height is not the same in all segments of the spine, with the cervical and thoracic discs being flatter than those of the lumbar region.

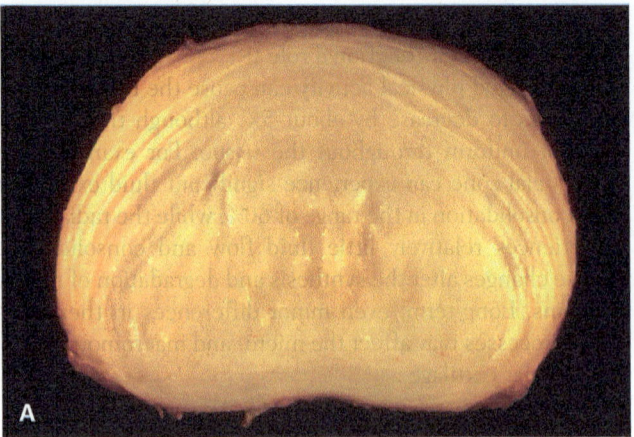
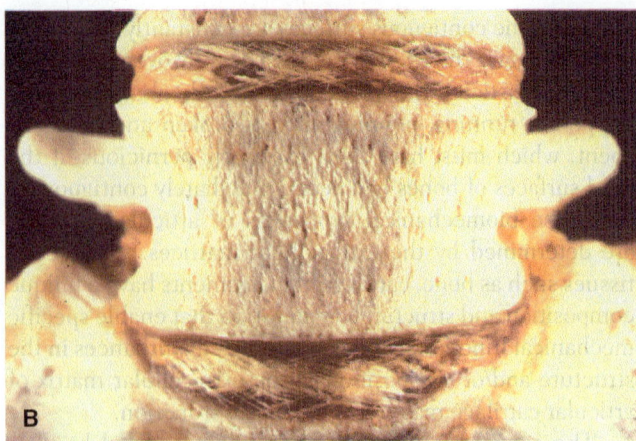

FIGURE 5.3 **A:** Photograph of an intervertebral disc seen in cross section. Note the layers of circumferential fibers that make up the annulus fibrosus and the well-demarcated bulging central mass of the nucleus pulposus. Note also the decreasing width of the annulus from anterior (*top*) to posterior (*bottom*). **B:** In this desiccated specimen of the lower lumbar spine, the alternating oblique orientation of the collagen fibers in the annulus can be appreciated.

There is also a variation in disc height from front to back, relative to the curvature of the spine. Age-related dehydration results in disc thinning.

THE NORMAL JOINT TISSUES

Articular Cartilage

Morphology

The articular ends of the bones are covered by hyaline cartilage, which is nerveless, bloodless, firm, and yet pliable. When pressure is applied to hyaline cartilage, it temporarily deforms (11). During development, cartilage is a precursor of the bony skeleton, and it is the means by which the bones increase in length via endochondral ossification at the cartilaginous growth plate (physis).

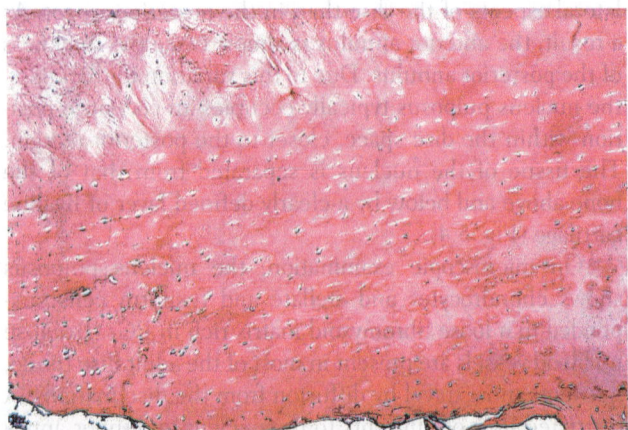

FIGURE 5.4 The nucleus pulposus of the disc (*top*) is separated from the bone (*bottom*) by a dense layer of hyaline cartilage, as demonstrated in this photomicrograph (H&E stain, ×4 objective).

In young people, hyaline cartilage is translucent and bluish-white; in older individuals, it is opaque and slightly yellow (Fig. 5.5) (12). This change in the appearance of the articular cartilage is also seen in other connective tissues and is related to a number of factors, including dehydration, increased numbers of collagen cross-linkages, and the possible accumulation of lipofuscin pigment.

On microscopic examination, articular cartilage is characterized by its abundant glassy (hyaline) extracellular matrix with isolated cells located in lacunar spaces (Fig. 5.6). It has four zones: superficial (I), intermediate (II), deep (III), and calcified (IV). In the superficial layer, the cells are flat. In the intermediate zone, the cells form radial groups that follow the pattern of collagen deposition. In the deep zone, the cells are hypertrophied; and in the calcified zone adjacent to the bone, the cells are nonviable (Figs. 5.7 and 5.8).

Within the mineralized bone matrix, the osteocytes are connected to one another by means of cytoplasmic processes. This arrangement is not present within the cartilage. The chondrocytes depend on the diffusion of solutes through the extracellular matrix for their metabolism. The matrix of the deep calcified zone of the articular cartilage forms a barrier to the passage of solutes from the subchondral bone. The articular cartilage is dependent on the diffusion of nutrients and metabolites between the synovial fluid and the articular surface (13).

The principal orientation of collagen fibers in articular cartilage is vertical through most of its thickness and horizontal at the surface (Fig. 5.9) (14). Electron microscopic studies have shown closely packed collagen fibers at the joint surface, which are arranged parallel to the surface. The collagen content of cartilage progressively diminishes from superficial to deep. In deep layers, collagen fibers are vertically aligned, more widely separated, and thicker, forming a web of arch-shaped structures (15). The collagen

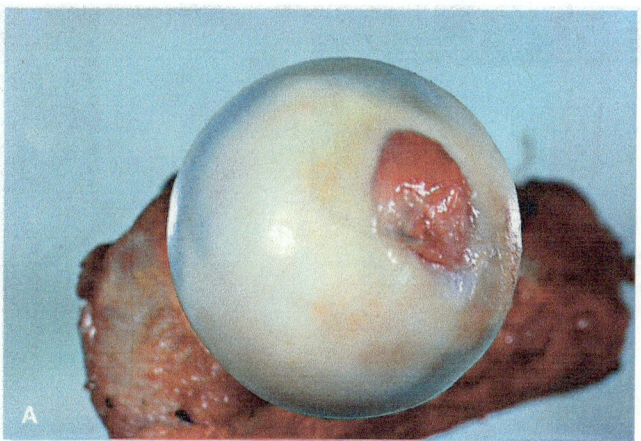
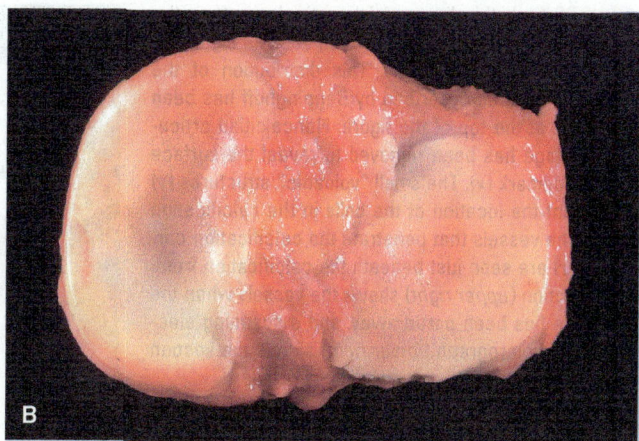

FIGURE 5.5 **A:** A femoral head, resected from a 16 year old, demonstrates the blue–white translucency of young healthy cartilage. **B:** For comparison, the tibial plateau of a 50 year old. The cartilage is smooth and healthy in appearance but is more yellowish in color and opaque in quality than that of the 16 year old.

fibers are continuous with those in the calcified layer. There is discontinuity, however, with the underlying subchondral bone. This network reflects the local stresses and strains in the articular cartilage (16). The principal orientation of the collagen fibers in the menisci of the knee is circumferential, reflecting the tension that occurs during normal loading. Occasional radially disposed fibers are present, acting to resist longitudinal splitting of the menisci resulting from undue compression (Fig. 5.10) (17).

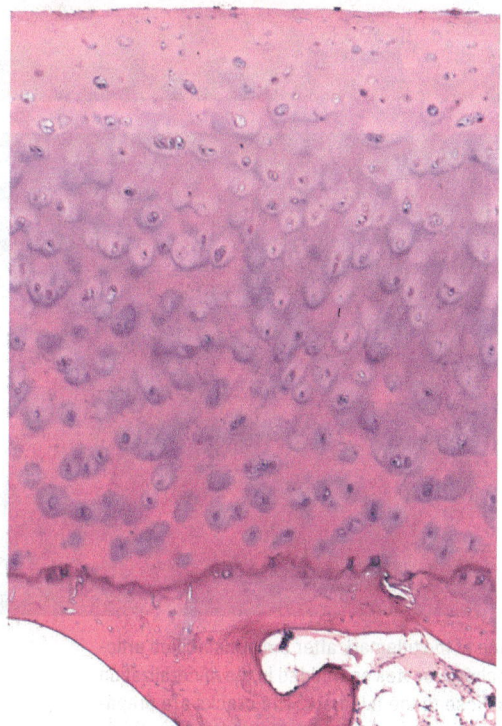

FIGURE 5.6 Photomicrograph of normal articular cartilage obtained from the femoral condyle of a middle-aged individual (H&E stain, ×4 objective).

The distribution of PGs in the cartilage matrix is related to the local mechanical requirements and varies from joint to joint. In general, PG distribution is more even in children than in adults. The surface layers contain much less PG than the deeper layers. In the deeper layers, the concentration is higher around the chondrocytes (the pericellular matrix) than between them (the intercellular matrix) (Fig. 5.11) (18).

In histologic sections, the junction between the calcified cartilage and the noncalcified cartilage is marked by a basophilic line known as the tidemark (Fig. 5.12). This basophilic line is not seen in the developing skeleton. In older individuals (over 60 years of age), replication of the tidemark is usually evident and in osteoarthritic joints, replication may be marked (Fig. 5.13). Mechanical failure in the deep cartilage rarely gives rise to separation at the bone–cartilage interface. When failure occurs, it is often seen as a horizontal cleft at the tidemark, reflecting the change in the rigidity of the cartilage at this junction. Adult articular cartilage is bordered by the subchondral bone plate, with an irregular interface, somewhat like a jigsaw puzzle. Calcification of this region contributes to its rigid structure (Fig. 5.14).

The insertions of ligaments and tendons into the bone are also calcified, and their adhesion is affected by this arrangement. These structures are dynamic, reflecting growth in skeletally immature individuals and continuous bone turnover in mature individuals.

The chondrocytes embedded in the cartilage matrix are responsible for synthesis and maintenance of the extracellular tissue. They vary in size, shape, and number, both from the superficial to the deep layers and in different anatomic locations (19). In general, cells at the cartilage surface are more numerous, flatter, smaller, and oriented parallel to the cartilage surface (20). In the middle zones, chondrocytes are more spherical and arranged in columns. This vertical arrangement reflects the orientation of collagen fibers present. The pericellular matrix

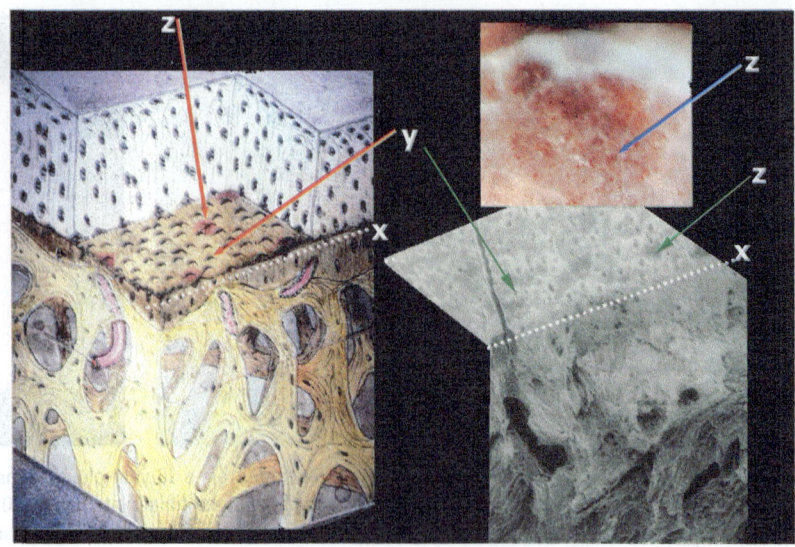

FIGURE 5.7 In this diagram of the articular surface, the organization of the articular surface seen on Figure 5.6 is shown diagrammatically. This distribution of the collagen arcades described by Benninghoff has been drawn in at the top of the figure. Noncalcified articular cartilage has been removed to reveal the surface of the tidemark (*x*). The small "volcanic" structures (*y*) represent the location of the cells in the calcification front. The vessels that penetrate the calcification cartilage (*z*) are seen just beneath the calcification front. A dissection (*upper right*) shows the vessels when the cartilage has been pared away, and a scanning electron photomicrograph (*lower right*) shows the section from which the diagram was reconstructed.

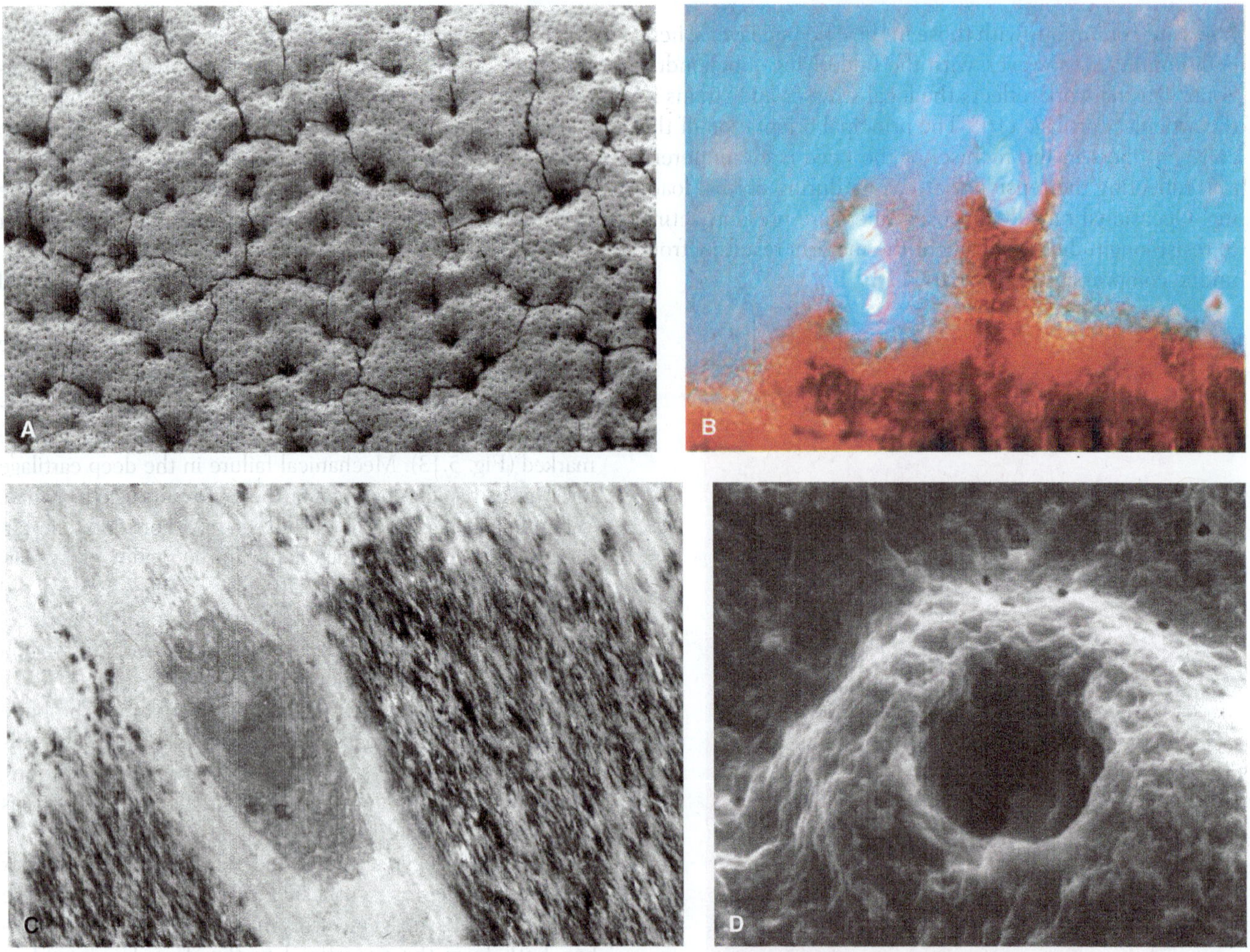

FIGURE 5.8 **A:** Scanning electron photomicrograph of the surface of the tidemark after the noncalcified articular cartilage had been digested away. The small dots represent chondrocytes embedded in the mineralization front (tidemark). The larger voids result from underlying vessels close to the tidemark. The cracks are preparation artifact. **B:** The appearance of chondrocytes embedded in this surface is shown in a cross-sectional image of an H&E section, photomicrographed using polarized light. The same sample (as in **B**) is shown in **C** as in a transmission electron and in **D** as a higher-power scanning image. It is hypothesized that this layer of embedded chondrocytes regulates the rate of active calcification at the tidemark.

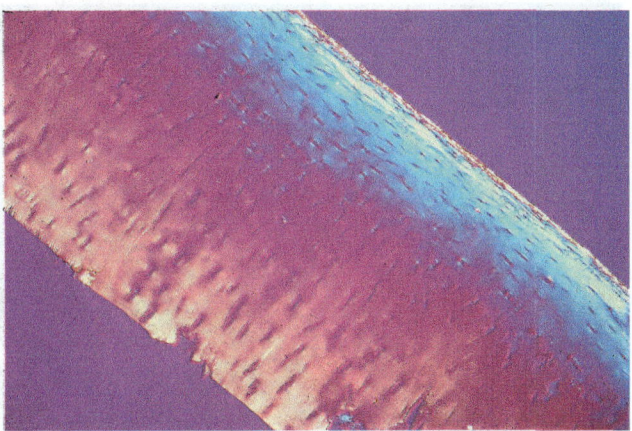

FIGURE 5.9 In this polarized-light photomicrograph, the surface collagen fibers can be visualized as blue, the deeper collagen fibers (which are perpendicular) as yellow. Collagen cannot be seen in the intermediate area because the fibers in this zone are decussating as in the model of Benninghoff arcade shown in Figure 5.7 (×4 objective).

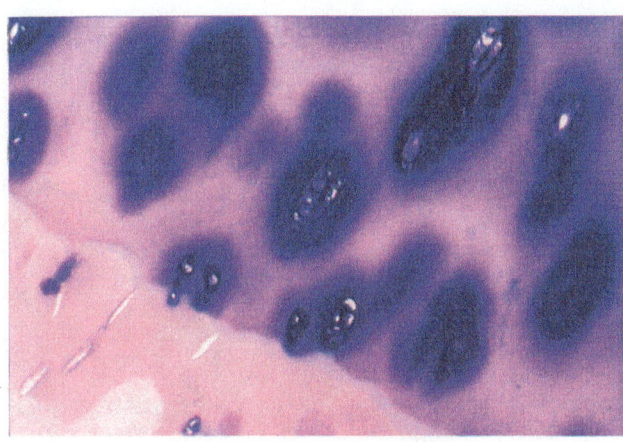

FIGURE 5.11 Portion of cartilage showing intense metachromasia around the chondrocytes in the deep part of the noncalcified cartilage. This represents staining of the proteoglycan. There is much less staining in the interterritorial matrix than around the cell. Even less staining is seen in the calcified cartilage (methylene blue stain, ×25 objective).

layer is rich in PGs and contains hyaluronic acid, with relatively little collagen. Around this layer is a basket-like structure composed of cross-linked type VI collagen which provides a protective framework and helps maintain equal hydrostatic pressure. In chondrocytes, mitochondria are sparse—reflecting their comparatively low rates of oxygen consumption. Cells in the deeper noncalcified zone have the most prominent endoplasmic reticulum and Golgi apparatus, indicating active protein synthesis. The cell membrane makes no connection with the processes of other chondrocytes. Small membrane-bound vesicles are visible in the extracellular matrix adjacent to the chondrocytes. These have been thought to play a role in the calcification of cartilage matrix (21).

Apart from hyaline cartilage, two other forms of cartilage are recognized, fibrocartilage and elastic cartilage. The matrix of fibrocartilage contains and a high proportion of type I collagen. Fibrocartilage is present in the menisci of the knee, in the annulus fibrosus, at the insertions of ligaments and tendons, and on the inner side of tendons as they angle around pulleys (e.g., at the malleoli). In all of these locations, the structures are subjected to compressive and tensile forces.

Elastic cartilage, on the other hand, contains a high proportion of elastin in the matrix and is present in the

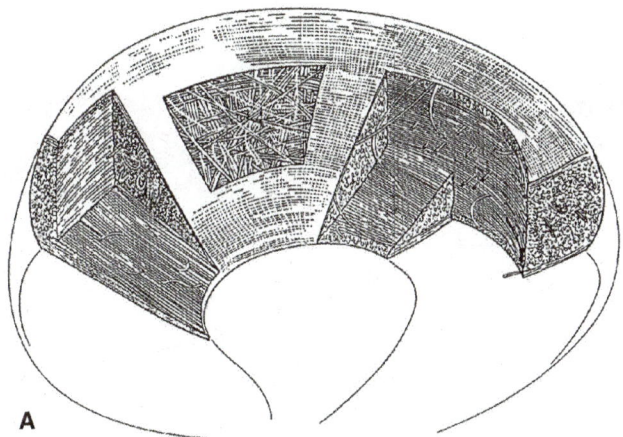
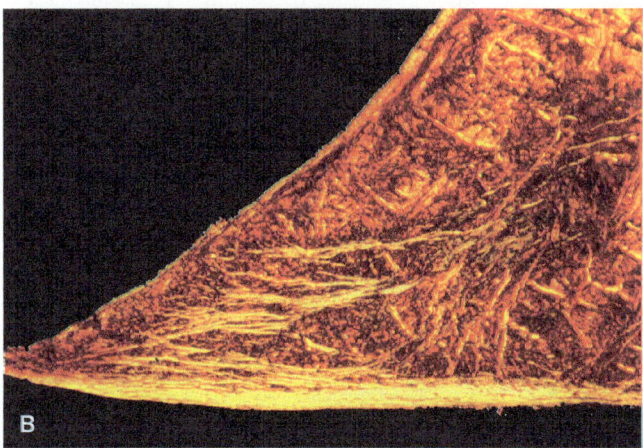

FIGURE 5.10 **A:** A drawing to illustrate the distribution of collagen fibers in the meniscus. The majority of the fibers are circumferentially distributed to resist the tension generated in the meniscus when the knee is under compressive load. The radially distributed fibers are most obvious on the tibial surface of the meniscus. **B:** Photomicrograph of a cross section of meniscus seen with polarized light. The tibial surface is the bottom edge where most of the fibers are radially arranged (×1 objective). (Modified from Bullough PG, Munuera L, Murphy J, et al. The strength of the menisci of the knee as it relates to their fine structure. *J Bone Joint Surg Br* 1970;52:564–567, with permission.)

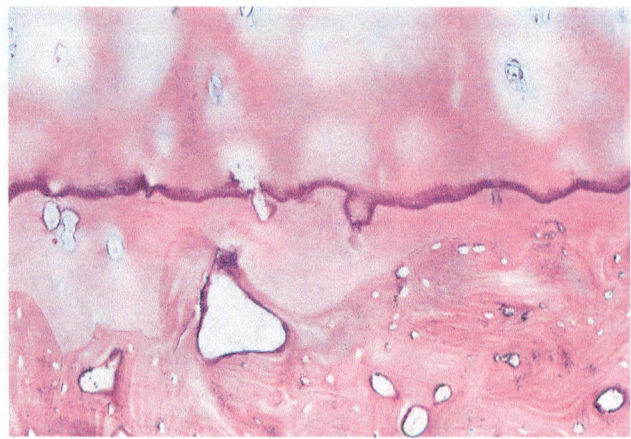

FIGURE 5.12 Photomicrograph of the deep and calcified layers of the articular cartilage. The deep layer is separated from the calcified layer by a basophilic line referred to as the "tidemark," which represents the mineralizing front (H&E stain, ×4 objective).

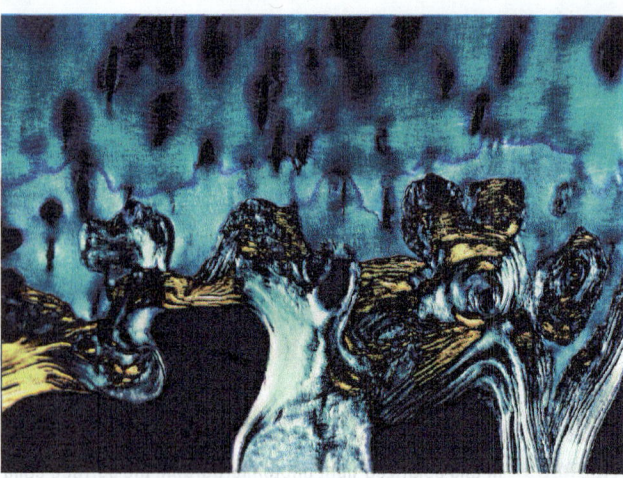

FIGURE 5.14 In this photomicrograph, taken with polarized light, the irregularity of the interface between the subchondral bone and the overlying calcified cartilage is obvious. The functional keying of the bone and cartilage depends on the two tissues having equal rigidity (×4 objective).

ligamentum flavum, external ear, and epiglottis (Fig. 5.15). Compared to collagen, elastin has much greater elasticity; this is particularly important in the ligaments of the spinal canal, which makes flexion of the vertebral column possible.

The mechanical functions of fibrocartilage and elastic cartilage are very different from those of hyaline cartilage. Hyaline cartilage mainly resists compressive forces, whereas the others function principally to resist tension, with some element of compression.

Cartilage Turnover and Articular Remodeling

Wolff law states that both bone density and bone architecture correlate with the magnitude and direction of applied load. At the articular end of a bone, the subchondral bone trabeculae are remodeled to accommodate optimal load distribution.

Endochondral ossification is an important mechanism for both bone growth and remodeling. In the epiphyseal growth plate, calcified cartilage is invaded by blood vessels from the metaphyseal bone and is subsequently replaced by bone synthesized by osteoblasts. This process also occurs in adult articular joints. Thus, throughout life, the calcified cartilage is slowly replaced by new subarticular bone (Fig. 5.16).

The tidemark advances into the noncalcified cartilage at a rate in equilibrium with the rate of absorption of the calcified cartilage from the subarticular bone (22). The articular

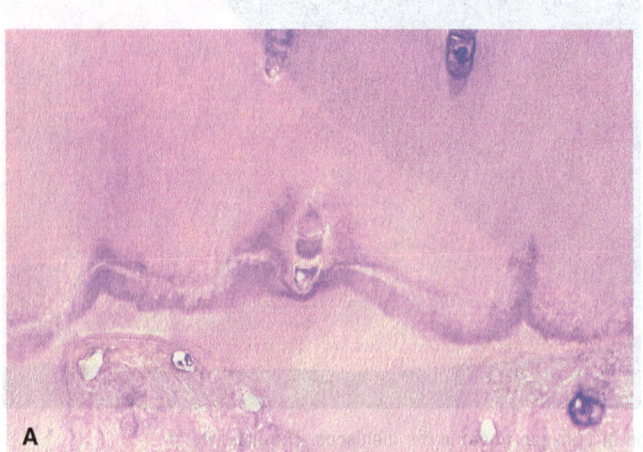
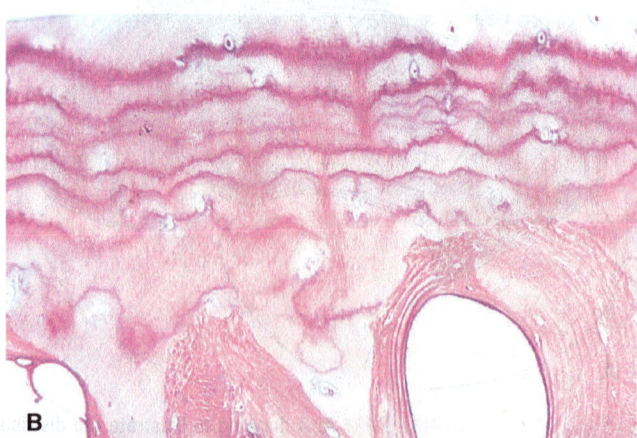

FIGURE 5.13 A: Photomicrograph demonstrating accelerated mineralization with a replicated tidemark. The mineralization front is almost certainly under cellular control; here, a chondrocyte is seen caught up in the tidemark (H&E stain, ×25 objective). **B:** In most areas of normal cartilage, only one tidemark is observed. However, in an early stage of osteoarthritis, seen here, multiple tidemarks indicating rapid advance of the mineralization front can often be seen (H&E stain, ×10 objective).

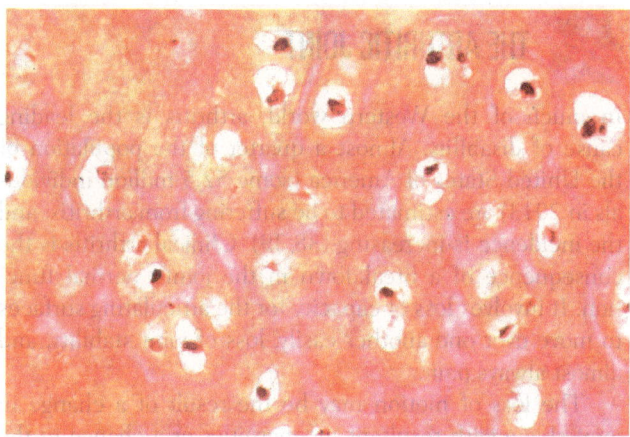

FIGURE 5.15 Photomicrograph of ear cartilage. Although the cells resemble those seen in hyaline cartilage, the matrix contains many elastic fibers that appear red in this section (phloxine and tartrazine stain, ×25 objective).

cartilage is not a static tissue and the joint undergoes continuous remodeling, with the extracellular matrix and the chondrocytes replaced throughout life. Apoptosis plays an important role in this process, similar to that of joint development during fetal life (23,24).

There are regional variations in morphologic, biochemical, and biomechanical components of weight-bearing joints. Variation in cartilage thickness is present in most joints. Stiffness in different areas of the femoral head is related to PG and water content (25). Stiffness and cartilage thickness affect the mechanical properties of the calcified cartilage and the underlying cancellous bone (26).

Within the knee joint, the morphology varies depending on whether there is a meniscal covering or not (27). In sites where the meniscus is present, the cartilage is firm and smooth. Where the meniscus is deficient, the cartilage has a rough surface and soft matrix. Even in young adults, cartilage that is not covered by meniscus shows matrix softening and superficial fibrillation (28). These naturally occurring variations are likely related to joint loading. Normally in the knee, load is transmitted through the meniscus and onto the tibial cartilage. The exposed cartilage remains relatively unloaded. Similar areas of disuse atrophy have been described around the rim of the radial head, in the roof of the acetabulum, and on the perifoveal and inferomedial aspects of the femoral head (29). Changes in the immediate environment of the joint lead to alterations of the cartilage matrix (30). Thus, immobilization or unloading of a joint results in decreased synthesis of glycosaminoglycans. Conversely, exercise appears to increase synthesis (31). Low levels of mechanical stress are associated with enhanced catabolic activity, whereas normal stress is associated with anabolic activity. Under high stress, the chondrocytes are unable to adapt. There is a window of physiologic stress above or below which the chondrocytes cannot maintain an adequate functional matrix.

Histomorphogenesis of Articular Cartilage

A key feature in joint development is the formation of the superficial, transitional, and radial zones through the cartilage thickness. The characteristics of these zones have been correlated with the changing pressure, shape, and fluid flow (32). However, unlike muscle and bone, the thickness of articular cartilage may not entirely depend upon mechanical stimulation (33).

Synovial Membrane

The synovial membrane lines the inner surface of the joint capsule and all other noncartilaginous intra-articular structures. In addition, synovial membranes line the bursae, which permit freedom of movement for adjacent structures and tendon sheaths.

Synovial membrane consists of two components. The first of these is the cellular lining surrounding the joint space. This surface is smooth, moist, and glistening, with a few small villi and fringelike folds. The second component is a supportive backing layer (34). The surface lining the joint space is normally relatively inconspicuous and consists of a single layer of synoviocytes (Fig. 5.17). The subsynovium comprises fibrovascular tissue with scattered histiocytes and mast cells.

Electron microscopic studies have shown two main types of synoviocytes. Type A cells have macrophage-like features, with phagocytic functions. Type B cells secrete synovial fluid hyaluronate. Normal synovium contains 25% type A and 75% type B cells (35).

The synovial membrane has three principal functions: secretion, phagocytosis, and regulation of the movement of metabolites into the synovial fluid. These metabolites provide for the metabolic requirements of the joint chondrocytes.

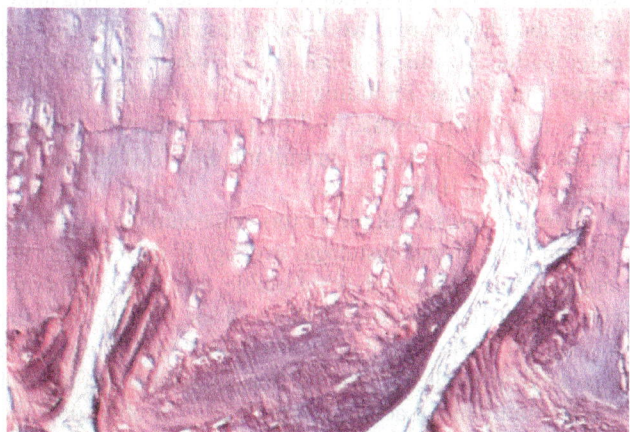

FIGURE 5.16 In this photomicrograph, two vessels can be seen that have extended into the calcified layer of cartilage. Around the circumference of each of these vessels, a thin layer of lamellar bone can be appreciated. By means of continuing endochondral ossification, the articular bone end is continuously modeled (H&E stain, ×10 objective).

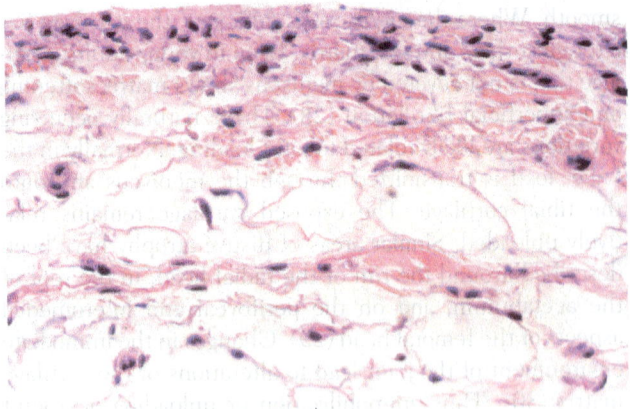

FIGURE 5.17 Photomicrograph of normal synovium. The ratio of fat to fibrous tissue varies depending on the joint and the location within the joint (H&E, ×10 objective).

Ligaments and Tendons

Ligaments, which are structures that join together two adjacent bones, are formed mainly of collagen. The arrangement of the collagen bundles within a particular ligament may be complex, reflecting the motion required at that joint. The collagen fibers calcify where they enter the bone, interdigitating with the underlying bone.

Tendons are specialized connective tissues that enable muscles to concentrate or extend their action. The Achilles tendon is an example of a tendon that concentrates the power of several bulky muscles to one area of insertion. Conversely, the long tendons of the hands and feet extend the effect of distant muscles. Adjacent to the insertion point, there is chondroid metaplasia, with the cells in lacunae-like spaces (36). This is due to the tendons entering the bone at an acute angle with resultant shear and compressive forces inducing metaplastic changes (Fig. 5.18). Some muscles have short, fan-shaped insertions without an obvious tendon—for example, the paravertebral and the gluteal muscles.

Normal tendons contain relatively sparse tenocytes scattered in a longitudinal pattern between the collagen bundles (Fig. 5.19). There is a slight gradient in the cell population, with the muscular portion of the tendon being more cellular than the distal insertion. Wherever a tendon turns a corner, it is restrained under a pulley and has a surrounding synovial sheath.

The surfaces of the flexor tendons of the hand are covered by a single layer of synovial cells (the endotenon) and a similar layer covers the parietal surface (the epitenon). In the palm of the hand, the tendons are covered by a fine vascular adventitia (paratenon) nourished by vessels from the deep palmar arch (37).

The feeding arteries to the tendons of the hands and feet are long, coiled vessels that can stretch as the tendons move. The sensory nerve supply to tendons is relatively abundant, with free ramifications. The nerve endings provide feedback regarding tendon tension, allowing for proprioceptive impulses.

THE ARTHRITIC JOINT

In much of the Western world, arthritis is the leading cause of disability. Almost a quarter of the population of the United States of America (some 52.5 million individuals in 2013) are estimated to be suffering from arthritis, and the incidence is increasing (38,39). Clinical arthritis is the consequence of a breakdown in the joint's normal function. It involves loss of capacity for the articulating surfaces to move over one another easily, loss of joint stability, and almost always pain.

The loss of motion may be the result of a change in joint shape with resultant incongruities or a change in the tissue matrices affecting their mechanical properties. Instability may be due to alterations in ligamentous support and neuromuscular control. Pain may originate in the bone as a result of maldistribution of load; in the synovium as a result of reactive synovitis; or in the muscle as a consequence of reflex spasm.

Malfunction of a joint results from acute or chronic morbid conditions that produce any of the following (Fig. 5.20):

- Anatomic alterations in the shape of the articulating surfaces (e.g., fracture, increased remodeling, Paget disease, or endocrine disturbances including acromegaly and hyperparathyroidism) (40)
- Loss of structural integrity of the joint (e.g., by enzymatic destruction in inflammatory arthritis or, more commonly, traumatic injury which may be acute in nature or low grade and repetitive)
- Alterations in the mechanical properties of the tissue matrices (e.g., brittle collagen as occurs in ochronosis)

Arthritis can be considered as either noninflammatory, as typified by osteoarthritis (OA), or inflammatory which encompasses seropositive arthritis (rheumatoid arthritis), seronegative arthritis (spondyloarthropathies including ankylosing spondylosis, reactive arthritis, psoriatic arthritis, and enteropathic arthritis; systemic lupus erythematosus; crystal deposition disease including gout and calcium pyrophosphate deposition disease [CPPD]), or infective arthritis (septic [usually bacterial], granulomatous [mycobacterial], or vector borne [Lyme disease]).

In many cases, multiple factors come into play and there is often clinical and histologic overlap. If the changes are long-standing enough, it is inevitable that OA is superimposed upon the pre-existing morphologic changes, making assessment of the initial etiology difficult (41). Pre-existing structural anomalies including developmental dysplasia of the hip and femoral acetabular impingement often underlie development of OA, especially in young individuals (42). OA can be seen secondary to subchondral insufficiency fracture which usually occurs in older individuals subsequent to loading of regions of low bone density. Subchondral insufficiency fracture as a cause of OA was long overlooked, possibly due

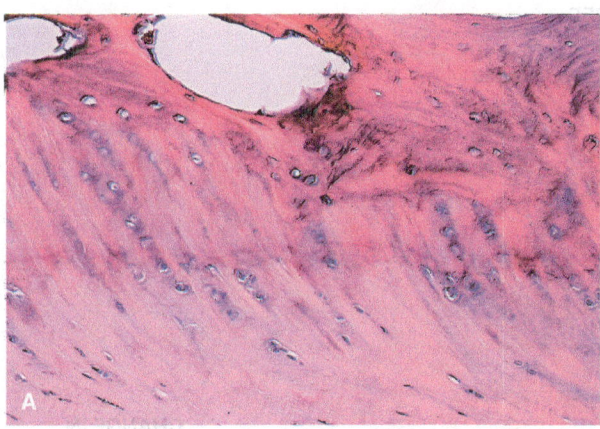
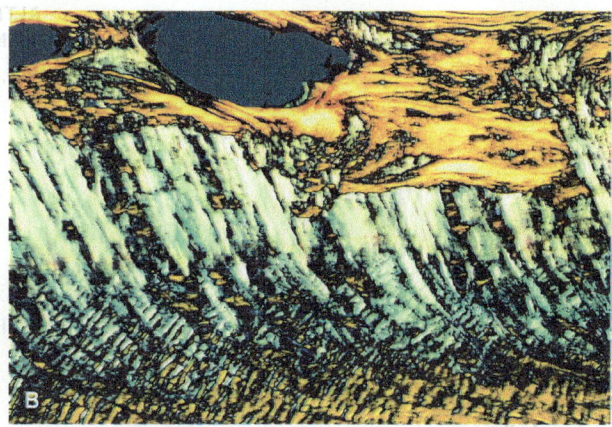
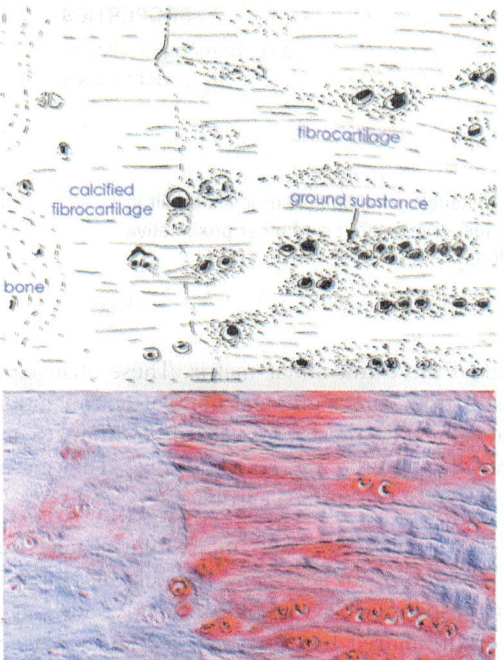

FIGURE 5.18 **A:** Photomicrograph of a ligamentous insertion using transmitted white light (H&E stain, ×10 objective). **B:** Polarized light. The portion of the ligament that interfaces with the bone is calcified, and the edge of the calcified portion of the ligament is marked by a basophilic line (tidemark) that represents the mineralization front. Note the similarity with the bone–cartilage interface illustrated in Figure 5.14. **C:** A higher-powered view to demonstrate the rounded cells lying in lacunae, which are seen at the insertion site of both ligaments and tendons (fibrocartilaginous metaplasia). The red staining in the matrix indicates the presence of proteoglycans (safranin O stain, ×25 objective).

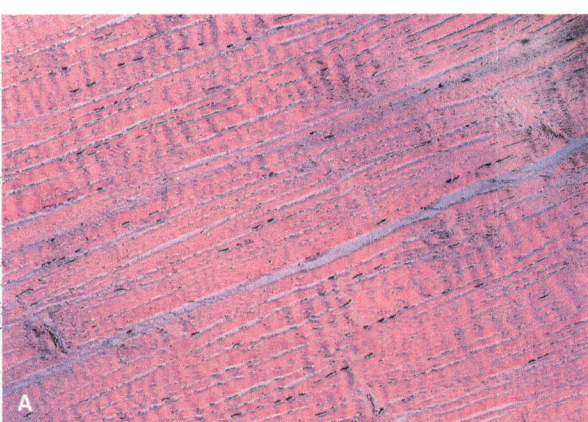
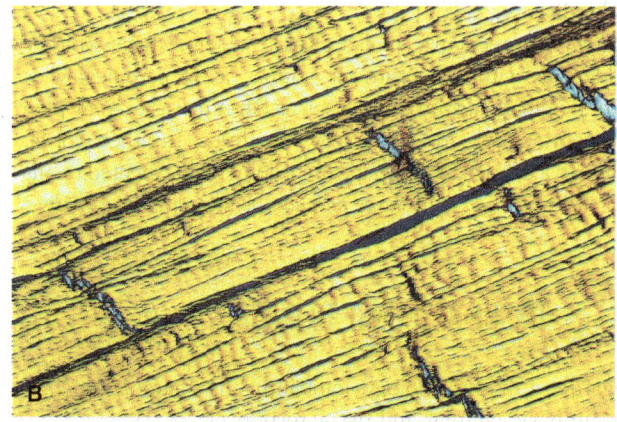

FIGURE 5.19 Photomicrograph of the same field of a tendon that has been photographed in transmitted light (**A**) and in polarized light (**B**). Both images demonstrate the scant and elongated fibroblasts lying between the dense parallel collagen bundles characteristic of tendon (H&E stain, ×4 objective).

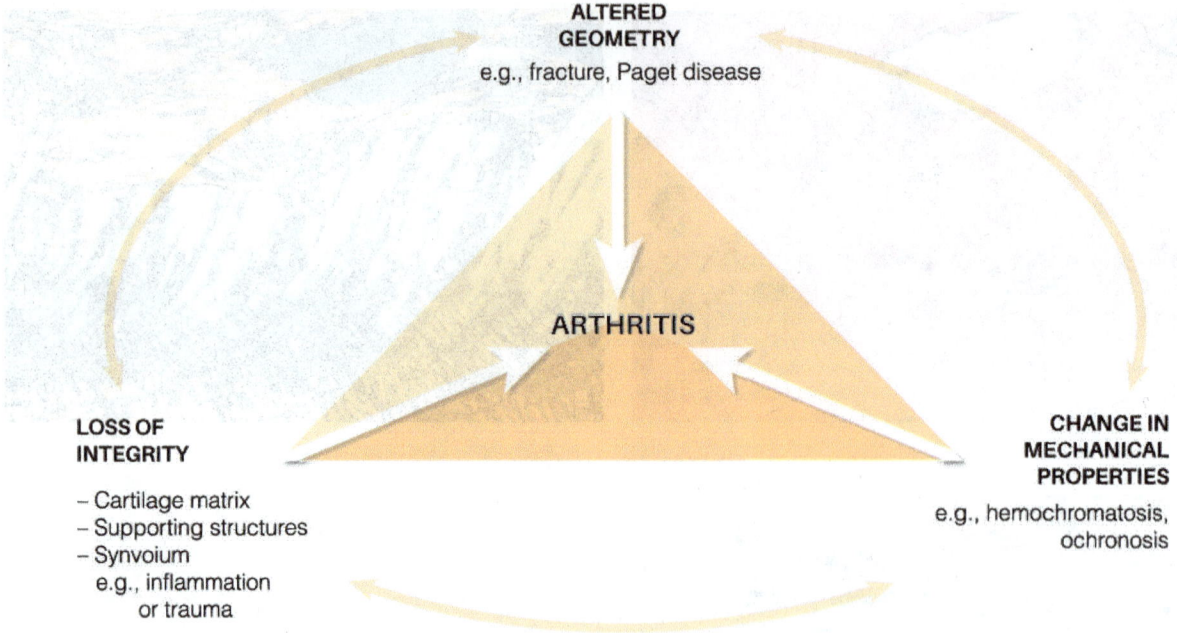

FIGURE 5.20 Causes of arthritis. Changes to shape, constituent materials, and support of joints result in arthritis. Multiple factors are usually present. (Reprinted from Maclean FM. Arthritis and other proliferative joint diseases. *Diagn Histopathol* 2016;22(10):369–377, with permission.)

to the fact that it often clinically and radiologically mimics avascular necrosis. It is frequently the cause underlying rapidly destructive OA (43). While OA has long been considered to be a noninflammatory process, recent studies have shown that there is an inflammatory component (44).

Alteration in Shape

A change in joint shape is characteristic of most forms of arthritis. In the inflammatory arthritides, tissue loss results from destruction. On the other hand, although bone and cartilage loss play an important part in the osteoarthritic process, it is the addition of new bone and cartilage in the form of osteophytes that is one of the characteristic features of the disease.

We now recognize that a change in joint shape—either sudden, as with a fracture, or gradual, as in acromegaly or other metabolic disturbances such as Paget disease—may play an important role in the etiology of arthritis. In other words, although a change in the shape of the joint is an expected result of arthritis, *a change in shape may also be the cause of arthritis.*

TISSUE RESPONSE TO INJURY

Regardless of the etiology, joint injury is characterized by certain basic cellular and tissue responses.

- There is usually macroscopic and microscopic evidence of both degeneration and repair in the cells and in the extracellular matrix. These changes may result from direct physical injury, from alteration in the cellular synthesis of the matrix, or from enzymatic breakdown of the matrix constituents. They are most apparent in the surface cartilage (45).

- In the vascularized tissues, injury from whatever cause is followed by an acute and then chronic inflammatory response of a variable degree. As a result, the necrotic injured tissue is removed and replaced by granulation tissue, resulting in fibrous scar. In nonvascularized tissue, such as cartilage, an inflammatory response and subsequent scarring cannot occur.

Cartilage

Macroscopic evidence of injury to cartilage is evident only in the extracellular matrix, and one of the earliest findings is a disruption of the collagen fibers at the articular surface, which becomes deficient (46). Three patterns of macroscopic alteration can be identified: fibrillation (generally age related), erosion, and cracking (both of which are probably trauma related) (47). The term *fibrillation* is used to describe replacement of the normally smooth, shiny surface by a surface similar to cut velvet. The "pile" of the fibrillated area may be short or shaggy. The junction between the fibrillated area and the adjacent normal-appearing cartilage is distinct (Fig. 5.21).

Fibrillation is not only seen in the context of prior mechanical abrasion in cases of OA, but is also possibly related to underloading of the cartilage, being identified in well-defined

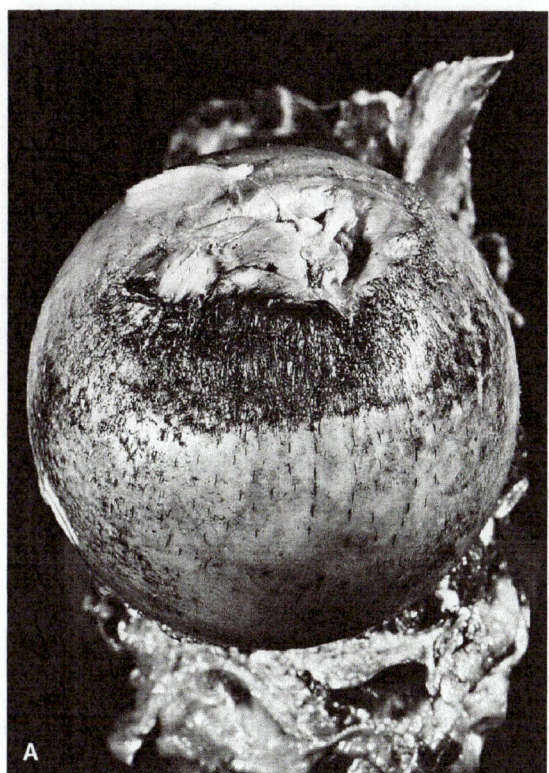
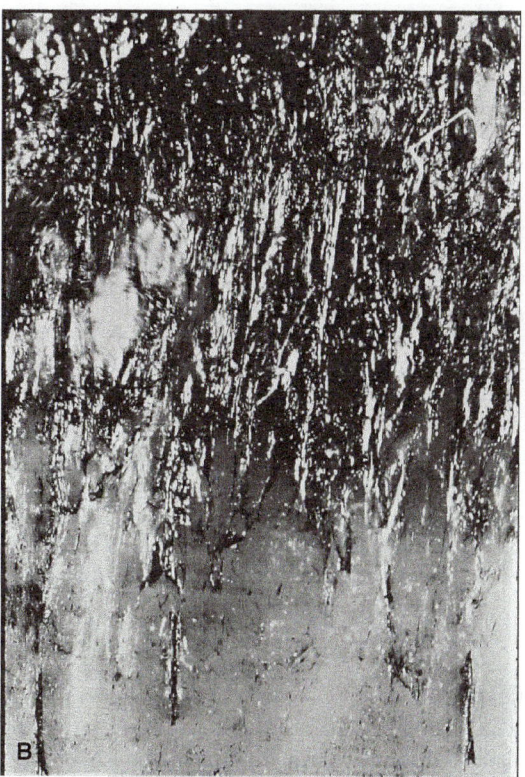

FIGURE 5.21 **A:** Photograph to demonstrate superficial fibrillation of the cartilage on the femoral head in the perifoveal region. The fibrillated cartilage has been highlighted by India ink. **B:** In a close-up photograph, pin splits in the cartilage seem to follow the orientation of the collagen fibers in the fibrillated area.

areas affecting particular locations in certain joints, present in everyone from an early age (35). In established cases of OA, the changes are however more marked being characterized by deeper clefts and areas of chondrocyte cloning.

Cartilage *erosion* is characteristic of progressive degenerative changes in the joint. The base of the erosion is initially contoured or smooth, but as further damage occurs, it may eventually be so extensive as to completely denude the joint surface of its covering cartilage layer (eburnation). The last and least common form of cartilage injury is deep *cracking* of the cartilage which results from severe impact loading. These cracks extend vertically into the cartilage and microscopically often have a horizontal component (Fig. 5.22).

In considering the pathogenesis of these three histologic types of cartilage matrix damage in the early stages of OA, it is important to recognize that they may affect the opposed articular surfaces in different areas and to different degrees. This is in marked contrast to eburnation, in which both of the opposed surfaces are affected. Thus, in many cases fibrillation and other cartilage alteration cannot be ascribed solely to abrasion.

Articular cartilage is largely composed of type II collagen and aggrecan; however, multiple minor collagens additionally contribute to the extracellular matrix. Apart from their structural roles, they also contribute biologic function, participating in the turnover of articular cartilage (48). The protease degradation products identified from these minor collagens have the potential to perform as biomarkers of disease (48). Chondrocyte necrosis can be identified when focal ghost outlines of the chondrocytes are present. Less often, all of the chondrocytes are seen to be necrotic (Fig. 5.23).

Cartilage regeneration is reflected by the histologic response of both matrix and cells. Chondrocyte cloning may be prominent and when the tissue is stained with toluidine blue, there is often intense metachromasia of the surrounding

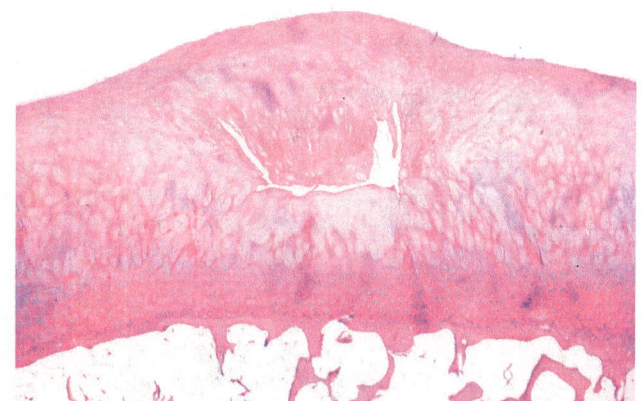

FIGURE 5.22 Photomicrograph demonstrating deep cracking of the cartilage matrix. The lesion shown is characteristic of a blister-like lesion, which is seen in many cases of chondromalacia patellae (H&E stain, ×4 objective).

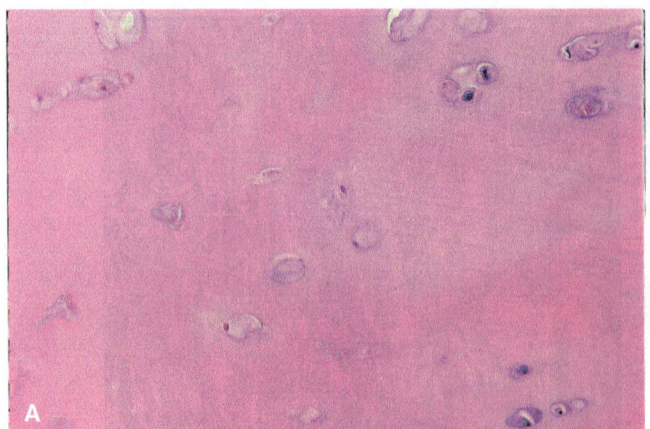
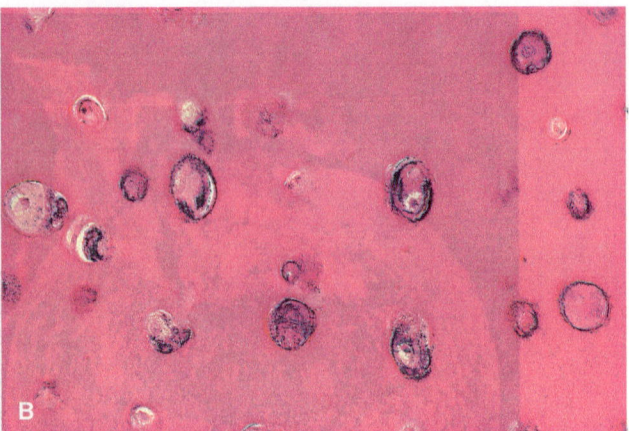

FIGURE 5.23 **A:** A photomicrograph to demonstrate focal chondrocyte necrosis. In cases of degenerative arthritis, focal areas of necrosis (such as seen here) are common. Rarely, the necrosis is extensive. In inflammatory arthritis, chondrocyte necrosis is also common and often associated with an irregular lysis of the matrix around the necrotic cells, the so-called Weichselbaum lacunae (H&E stain, ×10 objective). **B:** Photomicrograph to demonstrate focal calcification around necrotic chondrocytes in the deep zone of the cartilage (H&E stain, ×25 objective).

matrix reflecting increased PG synthesis. This process can be thought of as "intrinsic" repair (Fig. 5.24) (49).

In a damaged joint, cartilage repair may also be initiated from the joint margin or the subchondral bone. Repair initiated at the joint margin consists of a cellular layer of cartilage extending over the joint surface. This cartilage is usually much more cellular and the chondrocytes are evenly distributed (Fig. 5.25). On microscopic examination, this may be easily overlooked. Examination under polarized light will clearly demonstrate the discontinuity between the collagen network of the repair cartilage and that of the preexisting cartilage (Fig. 5.26).

In osteoarthritic joints, there are frequently pits in the bone surface from which protrude small nodules of fibrocartilage which arise in the marrow spaces of the subchondral bone. The fibrocartilage may extend over the previously denuded surface to form a continuous layer of repair tissue. Most specimens of OA reveal both intrinsic and extrinsic repair (50).

Bone

Arthritis affects not only the articular cartilage, but also the underlying bone and the structures around the joint. As the articular cartilage is eroded from the surface, the underlying bone is subjected to increasingly localized overloading. In subarticular bone that has been denuded, there is proliferation of osteoblasts and formation of new bone, which occurs both on the surfaces of existing intact trabeculae and around microfractures (Fig. 5.27) (51). In x-rays of arthritic joints, this new bone appears as sclerosis. Areas of focal pressure necrosis may be identified (Fig. 5.28). This should be differentiated from avascular necrosis which itself leads

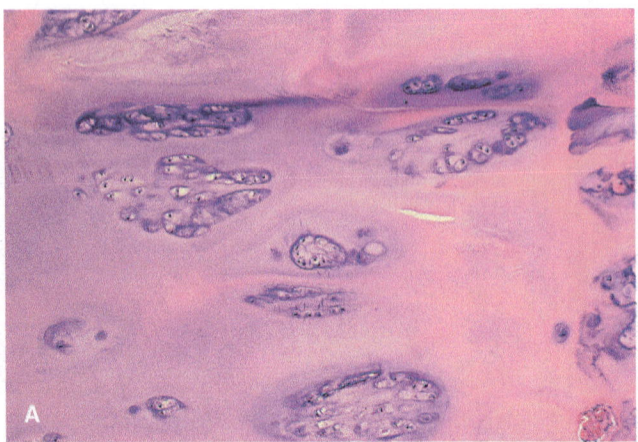
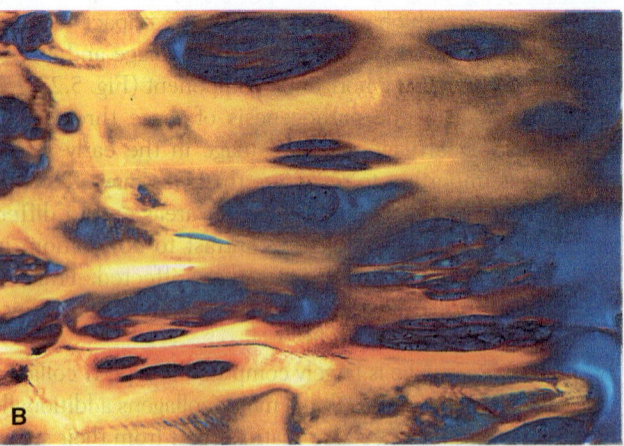

FIGURE 5.24 **A:** Photomicrograph to demonstrate clones of regenerating chondrocytes. Note the basophilia around the clones, which correspond to increased proteoglycan synthesis by the cells (H&E stain, ×10 objective). **B:** When examined by polarized light, the proliferating clones are visibly displacing the existing collagen matrix.

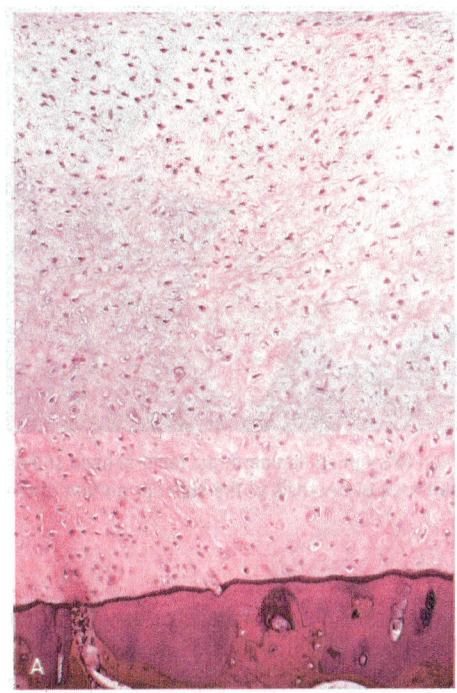 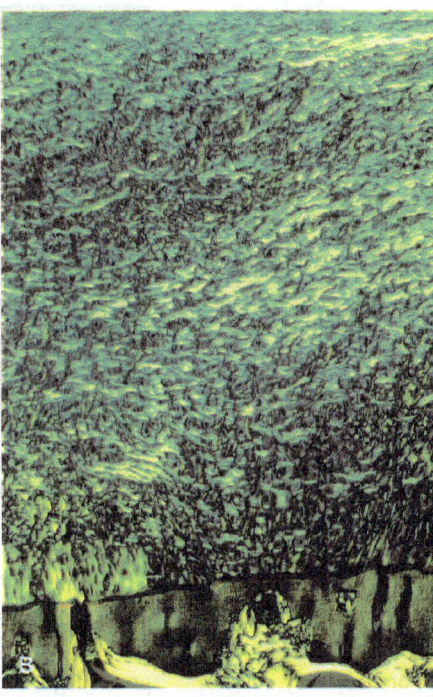

FIGURE 5.25 A: A section through the articular surface of an arthritic joint demonstrates extrinsic reparative fibrocartilage, which extends to the tidemark of the original articular hyaline cartilage (H&E stain, ×10 objective). **B:** The same field photographed with polarized light shows the discontinuity of the collagen between the calcified zone and the reparative cartilage.

to secondary OA. In clinical practice, differentiation may be difficult (52). A clue is whether the involved osteonecrotic bony trabeculae are sclerotic or not, with the former usually seen in the context of OA with secondary osteonecrosis.

Subarticular cysts are usually seen only where the overlying cartilage is absent. Such cysts are common in cases of OA and are believed to result from transmission of intra-articular pressure through defects in the articular surface into the marrow space of the subchondral bone (53). The cysts increase in size until the pressure within them equals the intra-articular pressure. Cysts may also occur because of focal tissue necrosis (54). In cases of rheumatoid arthritis, periarticular radiologic "cysts" may be associated with erosion of the marginal subchondral bone by the diseased synovium, and in gout by tophaceous deposits of monosodium urate crystals.

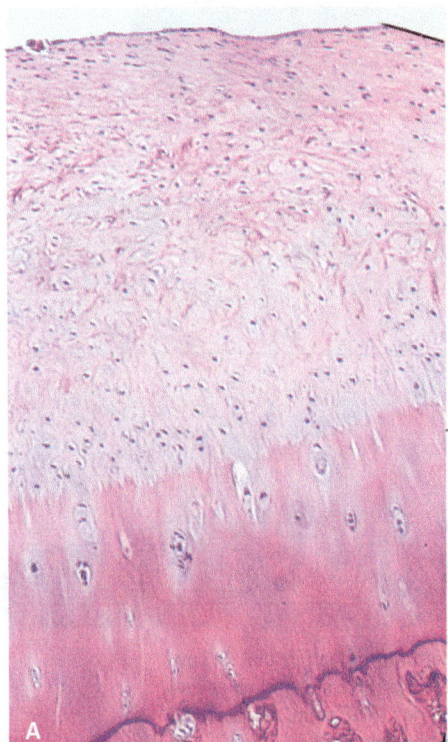 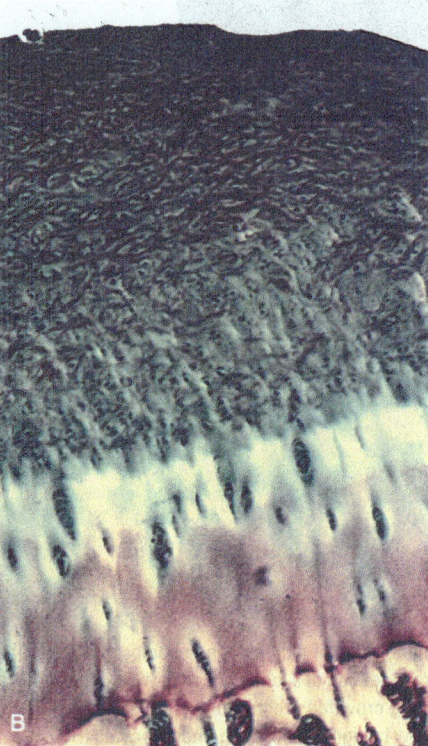

FIGURE 5.26 A: Photomicrograph showing reparative cartilage extending over pre-existing damaged cartilage (H&E stain, ×4 objective). **B:** Same field photographed with polarized light.

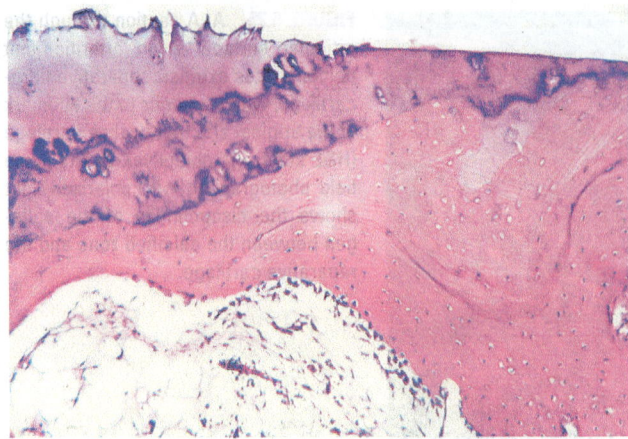

FIGURE 5.27 Photomicrograph of the edge of an eburnated area of bone in a case of osteoarthritis. There is a very prominent layer of osteoblasts covering the sclerotic bone that underlies the area denuded of cartilage (H&E stain, ×4 objective).

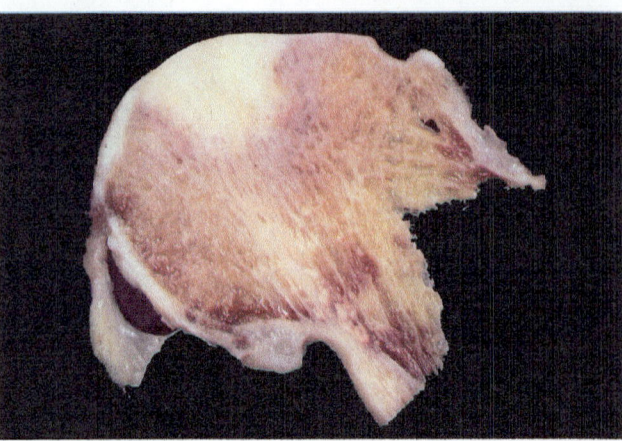

FIGURE 5.28 A section through an osteoarthritic femoral head shows a large wedge-shaped area of necrosis of the superior portion of the head.

Separated fragments of bone and cartilage from a damaged joint surface may become incorporated into the synovial membrane and digested, or they may remain free as loose bodies in the joint cavity. Under certain circumstances, proliferation of cartilage cells occurs at the surface of these loose bodies and consequently they grow larger (Fig. 5.29). In histologic sections, it is possible to visualize periodic extension of this central calcification

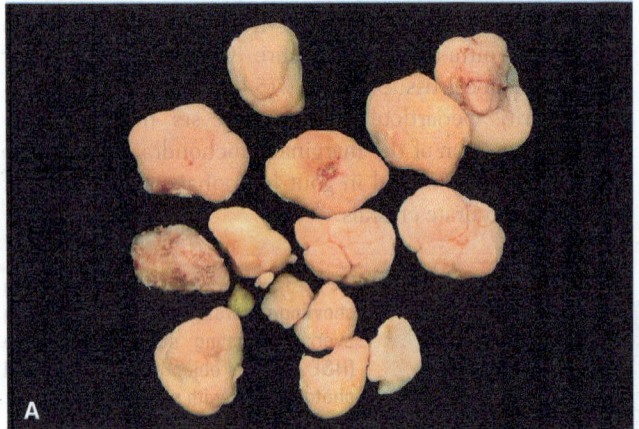
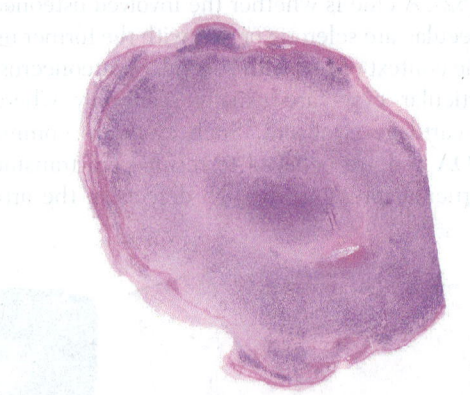
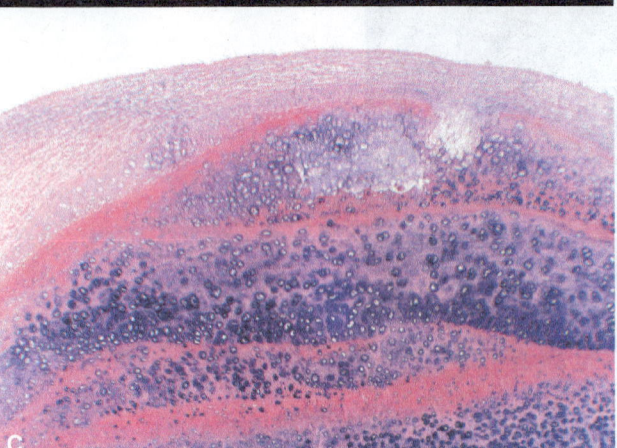
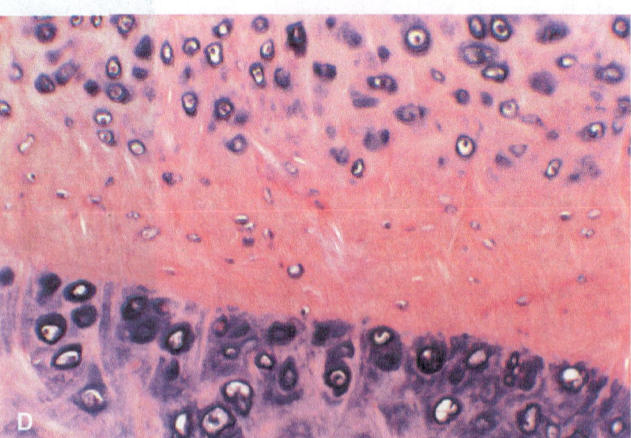

FIGURE 5.29 **A:** Gross photograph of multiple loose bodies in a case of osteoarthritis of the hip joint. **B:** Low-power photograph of a cross section of a loose body showing concentric growth rings (H&E stain, ×1 objective). **C:** Photomicrograph showing crowded proliferating chondrocytes and a growth ring (H&E stain, ×4 objective). **D:** Photomicrograph to show benign proliferating chondrocytes (H&E stain, ×25 objective).

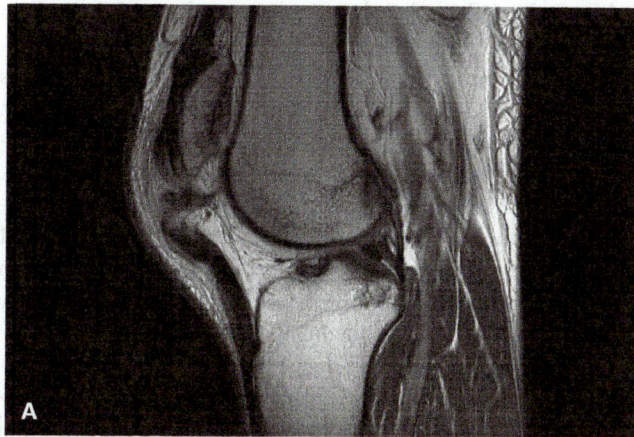
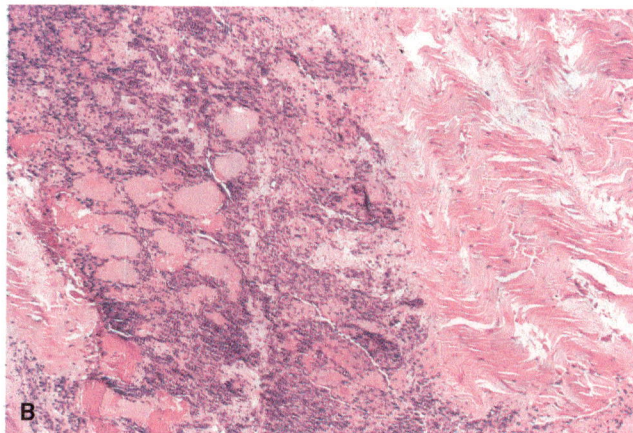
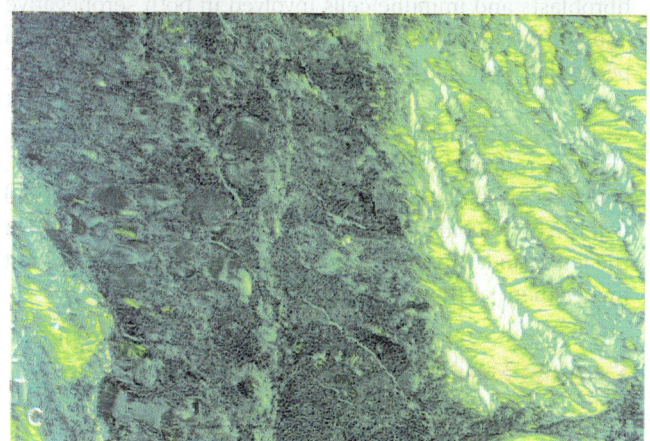

FIGURE 5.30 **A:** A magnetic resonance image of a knee shows rupture of the patellar ligament. **B:** Photomicrograph to demonstrate an area in a ligament where a laceration has occurred. The well-oriented collagen of the lacerated ligament is clearly demarcated from the resultant defect, which can be seen to have been filled with a vascularized cellular fibrous scar tissue (H&E stain, ×10 objective). **C:** Same field photographed with polarized light.

in the form of concentric rings, which increase in number as the loose body grows, appearing somewhat akin to the rings of a tree trunk. Sometimes the loose bodies reattach to the synovial membrane, in which case they are invaded by blood vessels.

Although loose bodies can be identified in many forms of arthritis, they are especially prominent in neuropathic (Charcot) joints and in other types of rapidly destructive OA. Occasionally, in cases of OA, the loose bodies are so numerous that they must be distinguished from those that occur in primary synovial chondromatosis (55) and are often termed "secondary" synovial chondromatosis.

Ligaments and Tendons

Microscopic evidence of both lacerations and repair by scar tissue is common in the ligamentous and capsular tissue around an arthritic joint. These changes are readily recognized by the use of polarized microscopy, which highlights alterations in collagen organization (Fig. 5.30). Low-grade repetitive trauma results in changes to both ligaments and tendons, including increases in cellularity and myxoid ground substance. When tenocytes proliferate they may form runs of cells (Fig. 5.31). Zones of chondroid metaplasia may be apparent.

Synovial Membrane

Injury and breakdown of cartilage and bone result in particulate debris within the joint cavity. This is removed from the synovial fluid by type A cells of the synovial membrane. The membrane becomes hypertrophic and hyperplastic, with a

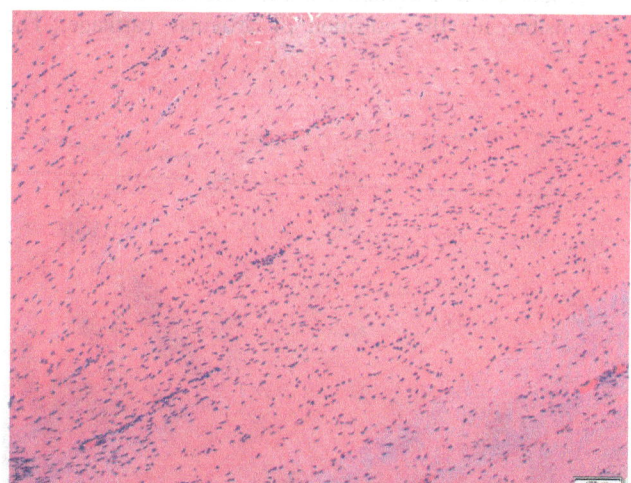

FIGURE 5.31 Photomicrograph demonstrating the linear arrangement of proliferating tenocytes between collagen bundles on a background of increased myxoid ground substance (H&E stain, ×40 objective).

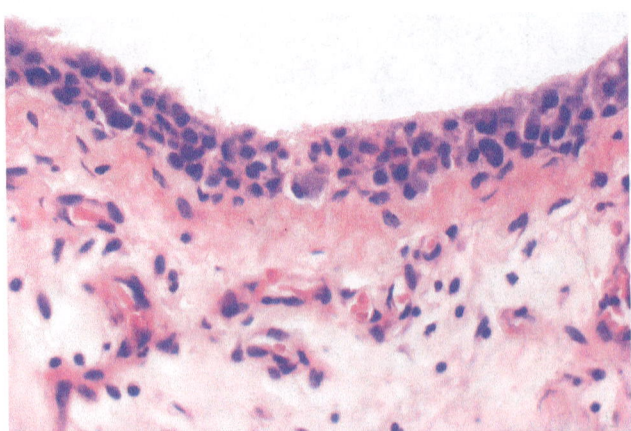

FIGURE 5.32 Photomicrograph of the synovium removed from the joint of a patient with a moderate degree of osteoarthritis reveals not only hypertrophy of the synovial lining cells but also hyperplasia that has resulted in a piling up of the synoviocytes. In the subsynovial tissue, there is increased vascularity and a mild chronic inflammatory infiltrate (H&E stain, ×25 objective).

villiform architecture. The breakdown products of the cartilage and bone matrix evoke an inflammatory response (Fig. 5.32). Thus, chronic inflammation can be expected in the synovial membrane of arthritic joints, even when the injury has been purely mechanical. Inflammation is especially prominent where there has been rapid tissue breakdown.

There may be a similarity between the degree of inflammatory response in some cases of severe OA and rheumatoid arthritis (56). In OA the synovial inflammation is the result of cartilage breakdown, whereas in rheumatoid arthritis the synovial inflammation is the cause of cartilage breakdown. Extension of hyperplastic synovium onto the articular surface of the joint (i.e., a pannus) is a common finding even in OA (Fig. 5.33). However, the extent and aggressiveness of the pannus with associated cartilage damage is generally much less marked in OA than in rheumatoid arthritis.

Under normal conditions, the synovial membrane is responsible for the nutrition of articular cartilage. The chronically inflamed and scarred synovial membrane of an arthritic joint functions less effectively than that of a normal joint. The hypertrophied and hyperplastic synovium is also likely to be traumatized as it extends into the joint cavity. Thickening of the joint capsule is a marker of disease in general, rather than being specific for a particular etiology (57). Evidence of bleeding into the joint, with subsequent hemosiderotic synovitis may be present. The orange-brown color of the villous synovium should not be confused with the swollen papillary synovium of tenosynovial giant cell tumor (formerly known as pigmented villonodular synovitis).

In recent years, there has been an increasing appreciation for the function of stromal cells in disease pathogenesis. There are complex interactions between synovial fibroblasts and immune cells involved in both seronegative and seropositive arthropathies. In rheumatoid arthritis, in particular, synovial fibroblasts participate in joint destruction (58). They function as innate immune cells and interact with other inflammatory cells (T cells, B cells, monocytes, and macrophages), as well as cartilage, endothelial cells, and osteoclasts. It is likely that further research in this field will further elucidate the etiology of the diseases that affect the joints and offer some explanation for the pattern of joint involvement of those conditions (58).

Synovial Fluid

Examination of synovial fluid is extremely helpful in the diagnosis of arthritis, both for determining the cause and chronicity of the disease. Whatever the cause of arthritis, the synovial fluid is altered. Normal synovial fluid is viscous, pale yellow, and clear. Even in large joints the volume is small. In cases of inflammatory arthritis, there is an increased volume of synovial fluid with a high count of inflammatory cells. The amount of hyaluronic acid is markedly diminished, leading to decreased viscosity. In degenerative arthritis, the amount of hyaluronic acid is increased, resulting in an extremely viscous fluid.

Interestingly, in the post-arthroplasty setting, there is formation of a pseudocapsule with regeneration of the synovial lining, resulting in production of synovial fluid facilitating function of the implanted joint. Although this fluid is less viscous than in a native joint, the protein and phospholipid concentrations are maintained (59).

Polarized microscopic examination of synovial fluid is additionally the gold standard for detection of a crystal deposition disease (gout or CPPD).

REFERENCES

1. Hammond BT, Charnley J. The sphericity of the femoral head. *Med Biol Eng* 1967;5:445–453.
2. Bullough P, Goodfellow J, O'Conner J. The relationship between degenerative changes and load-bearing in the human hip. *J Bone Joint Surg Br* 1973;55:746–758.

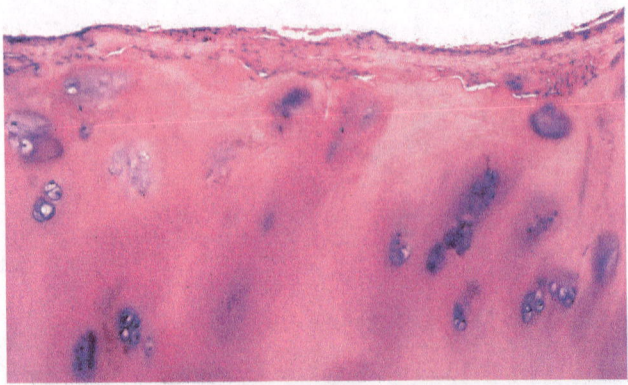

FIGURE 5.33 Photomicrograph of a portion of the articular surface of a femoral head in a case of osteoarthritis. A fibrous pannus extends over the articular surface (H&E stain, ×10 objective).

3. Bullough PG, Walker PS. The distribution of load through the knee joint and its possible significance to the observed patterns of articular cartilage breakdown. *Bull Hosp Joint Dis* 1976;37:110–123.
4. Hunter W. On the structure and disease of articulating cartilages. *Phil Trans* 1743;42:514–521.
5. Mayne R, Irwin MH. Collagen types in cartilage. In: Kuettner KE, Schleyerbach R, Hascall VC, eds. *Articular Cartilage Biochemistry*. New York: Raven Press; 1986:23.
6. Hulmus DJ. Collagen, diversity and synthesis. In: Fratzl P, ed. *Collagen: Structure and Mechanics*. New York: Springer; 2010:15–48..
7. Watanabe H, Yamada Y, Kimata K. Roles of aggrecan, a large chondroitin sulfate proteoglycan, in cartilage structure and function. *J Biochem* 1998;124:687–693.
8. Kiani C, Chen L, Wu YJ, et al. Structure and function of aggrecan. *Cell Res* 2002;12:19–32.
9. Roughley PJ. Articular cartilage and changes in arthritis: Non-collagenous proteins and proteoglycans in the extracellular matrix of cartilage. *Arthritis Res* 2001;3:342–347.
10. Smith MM, Gosh P. Experimental models of osteoarthritis. In: Moskowitz RW, Howell DS, Goldberg VM, et al., eds. *Osteoarthritis: Diagnosis and Medical/Surgical Management*. 3rd ed. Philadelphia, PA: WB Saunders; 2001:171–200.
11. Kempson GE. Mechanical properties of articular cartilage. In: Freeman MAR, ed. *Adult Articular Cartilage*. 2nd ed. London: Pitman Medical; 1973.
12. Van der Korst JK, Skoloff L, Miller EJ. Senescent pigmentation of cartilage and degenerative joint disease. *Arch Pathol* 1968; 86:40–47.
13. Maroudas A, Bullough P, Swanson SA, et al. The permeability of articular cartilage. *J Bone Joint Surg Br* 1968;50: 166–177.
14. Benninghoff A. Form und Bau der Gelenkknorpel in ihren Beziehungen zur Funktion. II. Der Aufbau des Gelenkknorpels in seinen Beziehungen zur Funktion. *Z Zellforsch Mikrosk Anat* 1925;2:783–862.
15. Muir H, Bullough P, Maroudas A. The distribution of collagen in human articular cartilage with some of its physiological implications. *J Bone Joint Surg Br* 1970;52:554–563.
16. Wilson W, van Donkelaar CC, van Rietbergen B, et al. Stresses in the local collagen network of articular cartilage: a poroviscoelastic fibril-reinforced finite element study. *J Biomech* 2004;37:357–366.
17. Bullough PG, Munuera L, Murphy J, et al. The strength of the menisci of the knee as it relates to their fine structure. *J Bone Joint Surg Br* 1970;52:564–567.
18. Maroudas A, Evans H, Almeida L. Cartilage of the hip joint. Topographical variation of glycosaminoglycan content in normal and fibrillated tissue. *Ann Rheum Dis* 1973;32:1–9.
19. Stockwell RA, Meachim G. The chondrocytes. In: Freeman MAR, ed. *Adult Articular Cartilage*. London: Pitman Medical; 1973.
20. Stockwell RA. The interrelationship of cell density and cartilage thickness in mammalian articular cartilage. *J Anat* 1971;109: 411–421.
21. Anderson HC. Calcification processes. *Pathol Annu* 1980; 15(Pt 2):45–75.
22. Boskey AL, Bullough PG, Dmitrovsky E. The biochemistry of the mineralization front. *Metab Bone Dis Relat Res* 1980;2S: 61–67.
23. Mitrovic D. Regression of normally constituted articular cavities in paralyzed chick embryos [in French]. *C R Acad Sci Hebd Seances Acad Sci D* 1972;274:288–291.
24. Mori C, Nakamura N, Kimura S, et al. Programmed cell death in the interdigital tissue of the fetal mouse limb is apoptosis with DNA fragmentation. *Anat Rec* 1995;242:103–110.
25. Kempson GE. *Mechanical Properties of Human Articular Cartilage* [doctoral thesis]. London: University of London; 1970.
26. Dar FH, Aspden RM. A finite element model of an idealized diarthrodial joint to investigate the effects of variation in the mechanical properties of the tissues. *Proc Inst Mech Eng H* 2003;217:341–348.
27. Bullough PG, Yawitz PS, Tafra L, et al. Topographical variations in the morphology and biochemistry of adult canine tibial plateau articular cartilage. *J Orthop Res* 1985;3:1–16.
28. Bennet GA, Waine H, Bauer W. *Changes in the Knee Joint at Various Ages: With Particular Reference to the Nature and Development of Degenerative Joint Disease*. New York: Commonwealth Fund; 1942.
29. Goodfellow JW, Bullough PG. The pattern of ageing of the articular cartilage of the elbow joint. *J Bone Joint Surg Br* 1967;49:175–181.
30. Palmoski MJ, Brandt KD. Effects of static and cyclic compressive loading on articular cartilage plugs in vitro. *Arthritis Rheum* 1984;27:675–681.
31. Palmoski M, Perricone E, Brandt KD. Development and reversal of a proteoglycan aggregation defect in normal canine knee cartilage after immobilization. *Arthritis Rheum* 1979;22: 508–517.
32. Wong M, Carter DR. Articular cartilage functional histomorphology and mechanobiology: A research perspective. *Bone* 2003;33:1–13.
33. Eckstein F, Faber S, Muhlbauer R, et al. Functional adaptation of human joints to mechanical stimuli. *Osteoarthritis Cartilage* 2002;10:44–50.
34. Henderson B, Pettipher ER. The synovial lining cell: Biology and pathobiology. *Semin Arthritis Rheum* 1985;15:1–32.
35. Barland P, Novikoff AB, Hamerman D. Electron microscopy of the human synovial membrane. *J Cell Biol* 1962;14:207–220.
36. Cooper RR, Misol S. Tendon and ligament insertion. A light and electron microscopic study. *J Bone Joint Surg Am* 1970; 52:1–20.
37. Lundborg G, Myrhage R. The vascularization and structure of the human digital tendon sheath as related to flexor tendon function. An angiographic and histological study. *Scand J Plast Reconstr Surg* 1977;11:195–203.
38. Barbour KE, Helmick CG, Theis KA, et al. Prevalence of doctor-diagnosed arthritis and arthritis-attributable activity limitation–United States, 2010–2012. *MMWR Morb Mortal Weekly Rep* 2013;62:869–873.
39. Hootman JM, Helmick CG, Barbour KE, et al. Updated projected prevalence of self-reported doctor-diagnosed arthritis and arthritis-attributable activity limitation among US adults, 2015–2040. *Arthritis Rheumatol* 2016;68:1582–1587.
40. Johanson NA. Endocrine arthropathies. *Clin Rheum Dis* 1985; 11:297–323.
41. Maclean FM. Arthritis and other proliferative joint diseases. *Diagn Histopathol* 2016;22(10):369–377.
42. Ganz R, Leunig M, Leunig-Ganz K, et al. The etiology of osteoarthritis of the hip: An integrated mechanical concept. *Clin Orthop Relat Res* 2008;466:264–272.

43. Yamamoto T, Schneider R, Bullough PG. Insufficiency subchondral fracture of the femoral head. *Am J Surg Pathol* 2000; 24:464–468.
44. Rahmati M, Mobasheri A, Mozafari M. Inflammatory mediators in osteoarthritis: A critical review of the state-of-the-art, current prospects, and future challenges. *Bone* 2016; 85:81–90.
45. Rieppo J, Toyras J, Nieminen MT, et al. Structure-function relationships in enzymatically modified articular cartilage. *Cells Tissues Organs* 2003;175:121–132.
46. Collins DH. *The Pathology of Articular and Spinal Diseases*. London: Edward Arnold; 1949.
47. Heine J. Über die Arthritis deformans. *Virchows Arch Path Anat* 1926;260:521–663.
48. Luo Y, Sinkeviciute D, He Y, et al. The minor collagens in articular cartilage. *Protein Cell* 2017;8:560–572.
49. Nakata K, Bullough PG. The injury and repair of human articular cartilage: A morphological study of 192 cases of coxarthrosis. *Nihon Seikeigeka Gakkai Zasshi* 1986;60: 763–775.
50. Macys JR, Bullough PG, Wilson PD Jr. Coxarthrosis: A study of the natural history based on a correlation of clinical, radiographic, and pathologic findings. *Semin Arthritis Rheum* 1980; 10:66–80.
51. Christensen SB. Osteoarthrosis. Changes of bone, cartilage and synovial membrane in relation to bone scintigraphy. *Acta Orthop Scand Suppl* 1985;214:1–43.
52. Franchi A, Bullough PG. Secondary avascular necrosis in coxarthrosis: A morphologic study. *J Rheumatol* 1992;19:1263–1268.
53. Landells JW. The bone cysts of osteoarthritis. *J Bone Joint Surg Br* 1953;35-B:643–649.
54. Rhaney K, Lamb DW. The cysts of osteoarthritis of the hip: A radiological and pathological study. *J Bone Joint Surg Br* 1955; 37-B:663–675.
55. Villacin AB, Brigham LN, Bullough PG. Primary and secondary synovial chondrometaplasia: Histopathologic and clinicoradiologic differences. *Hum Pathol* 1979;10:439–451.
56. Ito S, Bullough PG. Synovial and osseous inflammation in degenerative joint disease and rheumatoid arthritis of the hip. A histometric study. *Transactions of the American Orthopedic Research Society*. Proceedings of the 25th Annual ORS; 1979;199.
57. Rakhra KS, Bonura AA, Nairn R, et al. Is the hip capsule thicker in diseased hips? *Bone Joint Res* 2016;5:586–593.
58. Ospelt C. Synovial fibroblasts in 2017. *RMD Open* 2017;3: e000471.
59. Kung MS, Markantonis J, Nelson SD, et al. The synovial lining and synovial fluid properties after joint arthroplasty. *Lubricants* 2015;3:394–412.

Adipose Tissue

John S.J. Brooks

TYPES OF FAT CELLS 134	Cellulite 144
WHITE FAT 134	Ischemia 145
Prenatal Development 134	Metaplasia 146
Molecular Biology 136	**LIPODYSTROPHY** 146
Postnatal Development 136	**ADIPOCYTES IN ORGANS** 147
Gender Differences 136	Fatty Infiltration 147
Functions 136	**FAT BIOPSY FOR AMYLOID** 147
Regulation 137	**INFLAMMATIONS** 147
Gross Aspects 138	Fat Necrosis 147
Histology 138	Calciphylaxis 149
Ultrastructure 138	Panniculitis 149
BROWN FAT 139	Mesenteritis 149
Prenatal Development 139	Lipogranuloma 150
Postnatal Development 140	**TUMORS AND TUMOR-LIKE LESIONS** 150
Function 140	Brown Fat Lesions 150
Regulation 140	White Fat Lesions 150
Histology 141	Special Lipoma Types 155
Beige Fat 141	Lipoblastoma 155
Stem Cells 141	**CYTOGENETICS OF LIPOMAS** 155
HISTOCHEMISTRY 141	**SYNDROMES ASSOCIATED WITH FATTY LESIONS (INCLUDING LIPOMATOSIS)** 156
Enzyme Histochemistry 141	**MIMICS OF FAT CELLS** 156
Lipid Histochemistry 142	Mature Fat Cells 156
IMMUNOHISTOCHEMISTRY 143	Lipoblasts 157
Obesity 143	**REFERENCES** 158
ADIPOCYTE LESIONS 144	
Terminology 144	
Degeneration 144	
Atrophy 144	

In compiling this chapter, our intention was to provide practicing surgical pathologists with both a description of normal and abnormal adipose tissue and a reference source. We were inclusive in our approach and considered all bodily lesions containing mature fat appropriate for discussion regardless of site. The section on development should provide a deeper understanding for the diagnostician and a starting point for the researcher. Collected and detailed as a group are the fatty infiltrations of organs, the inflammations affecting fat, the hamartomas and mesenchymomas, and the lipomas and variants thereof. Up-to-date definitions are provided where necessary. Importantly, we have also summarized clinical

---

This chapter is an update of a previous version authored by Patricia M. Perosio.

and genetic syndromes in which fat cells may participate. Unusual but distinctive histologies are enumerated, such as may occur in starvation, pancreatic fat necrosis, and true lipodystrophy. All topics are well referenced, hopefully providing the reader with a valuable resource. In short, we have attempted to describe not only as many lesions as possible, not just primary fatty entities, but also anything extraneous within adipose tissue or confused with it.

TYPES OF FAT CELLS

Until recently, it was commonly believed there were only two types of fat cells, namely white adipocytes (white adipose tissue [WAT]) and brown adipocytes (brown adipose tissue [BAT]). However, efforts to uncover the functions of fat cells in obesity have discovered a third type of fat cell, or at least a third functional state or class which has been termed "beige" or "brite." These beige adipocytes result from stimuli to white adipocytes and appear in anatomical sites corresponding to WAT (see Beige Fat below).

WHITE FAT

Prenatal Development

The morphology of developing adipose tissue has been studied in detail. By examining serial sections obtained from 805 human fetuses of various ages, Poissonnet et al. (1) have determined that prior to the second trimester of pregnancy, adipose tissue primordia cannot be identified by light microscopy. After 14 weeks' gestation, aggregates of mesenchymal cells are seen condensed around proliferating primitive blood vessels. They refer to these findings as stage II in the development of adipose tissue (Fig. 6.1). Prior to this time, future adipose tissue is characterized by loose spindle cells and ground substance (stage I). Later on, capillaries continue to proliferate into a rich network, around which preadipocytes become stellate and organized into a mesenchymal lobule (stage III). These preadipocytes do not contain lipid. With further development, fine lipid vacuoles characteristic of stage IV accumulate within cytoplasm (Fig. 6.2). Continued proliferation of the components of the lobule results in the formation of densely packed aggregates of vacuolated fat cells with a rich capillary vascular network. Finally, condensation of perilobular mesenchyme at the periphery of the lobule results in formation of fibrous interlobular septa in stage V. This process occurs over the 10-week period between the 14- and 24-week gestation periods. From approximately 24 to 29 weeks, the number of fat lobules is relatively constant. Continued growth occurs mainly because of proliferation of capillaries and adipocytes, causing an increase in the size of the fat lobules (Fig. 6.2).

The same sequence of development of adipose tissue occurs at all sites throughout the body (2). The earliest white fat lobules appear first in the face, neck, breast, and abdominal wall at 14 weeks' gestation. By 15 weeks, they

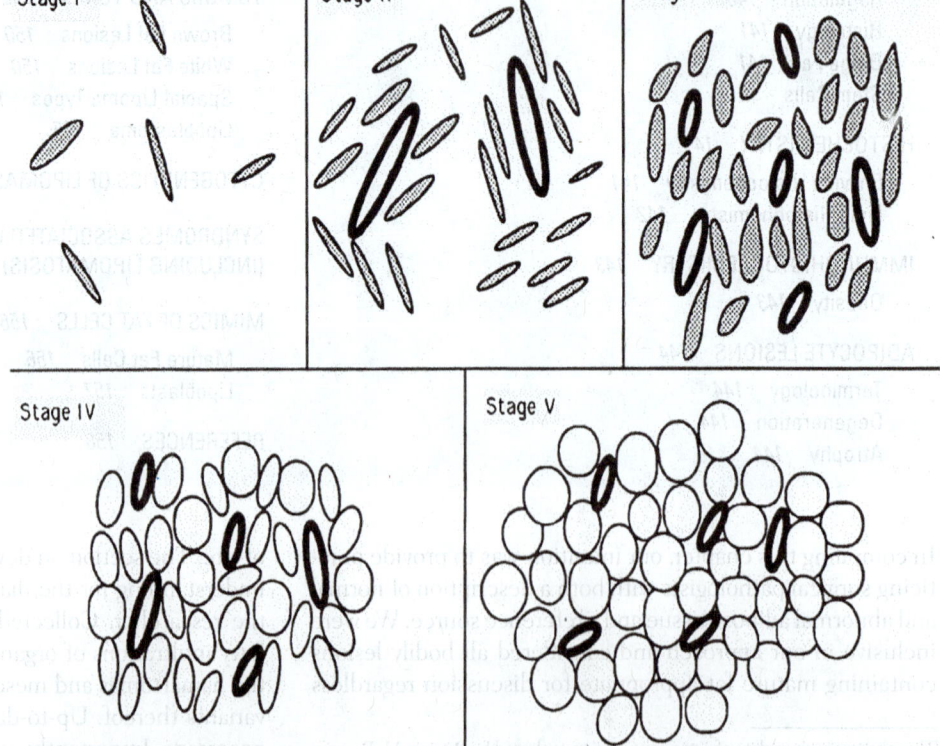

FIGURE 6.1 Developmental stages of adipose tissue. Stage I: Stellate cells (*stippled*) embedded in amorphous ground substance. Stage II: As angiogenesis begins, mesenchymal cells (*stippled*) condense around the blood vessels (*bold ovals*). Stage III: A rich capillary network develops from each vessel, forming a glomerulus-like network around which each lobule forms. The preadipocytes become more stellate. Stage IV: With accumulation of lipid, these adipocytes, with multiple small lipid droplets, become closely packed around the capillaries. Stage V: Further accumulation of lipid with many unilocular cells (*clear circles*) is evident. The perilobular mesenchyme condenses into interlobular septa at this stage.

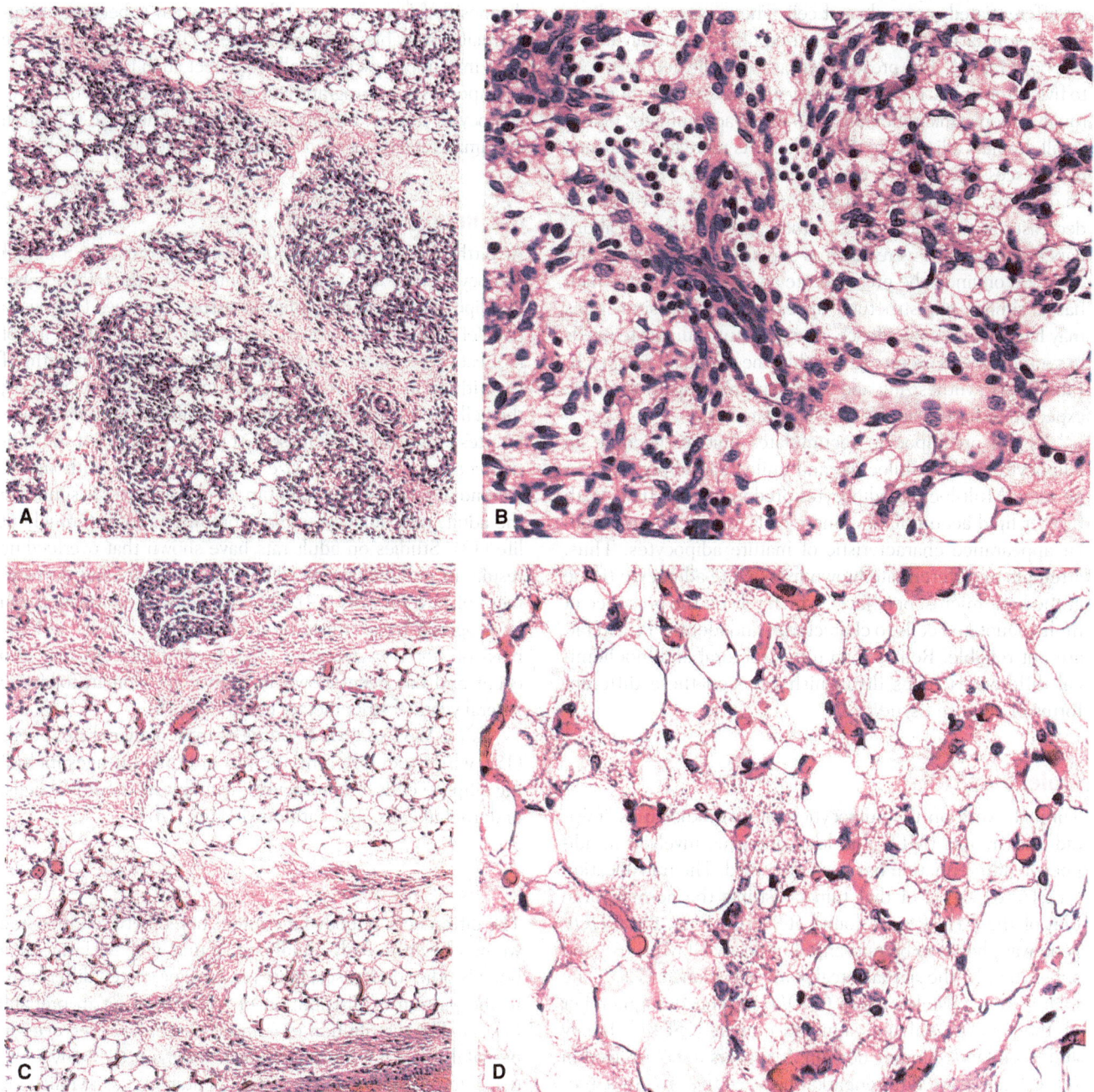

FIGURE 6.2 Fetal fat. **A:** Fat lobules from a 25-week fetus with a myxoid quality and prominent vasculature. **B:** At high power, both univacuolated and multivacuolated cells are noted together with small capillaries. By 37 weeks, the lobules are more developed (**C**) and many of the cells are univacuolated (**D**).

are also evident over the back and shoulders. Development in the upper and lower extremities and anterior chest begins around the 16th week. By the end of the 23rd week, a layer of subcutaneous fat completely covers the extremities.

There is a very close association of adipocyte development and angiogenesis. Fat appears first in well-vascularized regions, such as the shoulder joint, before differentiation can be identified in the less well-supplied adjacent subcutaneous tissue. There is also an important physiologic significance to this close anatomic relationship. Lipoprotein lipase (LPL),

the hormone responsible for transfer of triglyceride from circulating lipoproteins to adipose tissue, is synthesized by adipocytes and transferred to the luminal surface of the capillary endothelium (3). Thus, this close spatial relationship provides efficient transfer of enzyme and lipid.

Because of this close developmental association of capillaries and adipocytes, some have proposed that the adipocyte precursor, or preadipocyte, actually is derived from endothelial cells (4). Others have felt that the preadipocyte may be a perivascular reticulum cell, perivascular fibroblast-like cell, or undifferentiated mesenchymal cell. The presumptive adipocyte precursor has been characterized ultrastructurally in the newborn rat (5). The preadipocyte is a spindle cell with four to five cytoplasmic extensions along its long axis and abundant rough endoplasmic reticulum (ER). Lipid accumulates first as small droplets adjacent to the nucleus. As more lipid appears, it coalesces into a single large vacuole, and the cell takes on an oval then, finally, a round shape. The amount of rough ER decreases as the cell matures. Although cell shape and abundance of rough ER were taken as supportive evidence for the common origin of the preadipocyte and the fibroblast, which has a similar ultrastructural appearance, these similarities may have been a coincidence. The immature adipocyte needs to synthesize and excrete LPL—thus the abundant rough ER. Fibroblasts synthesizing and secreting procollagen would be expected to have a similar array of organelles.

As the preadipocyte accumulates lipid to become an adipocyte, both multilocular and unilocular adipocytes can be seen. Multilocular adipocytes predominate at first. With further lipid accumulation, more cells assume the unilocular appearance characteristic of mature adipocytes. Thus, attempts to differentiate brown from white adipocyte tissue at the light microscopic level, which rely on the presence of multivacuolated cells to characterize and identify brown fat, are not reliable. Reliance on ultrastructural and biochemical differences helps distinguish between these different forms of adipose tissue.

Molecular Biology

Through work on the adipocytic neoplasm known as "myxoid liposarcoma (MLS)," at least one gene involved in adipocytic differentiation has been identified. The translocation t(12;16)(q13;p11) of that tumor disrupts the normal function of the *CHOP* gene found at 12q13. First, the *CHOP* gene was shown to be rearranged in nearly all MLS (6), and subsequently, the actual breakpoint was cloned (7,8). The *CHOP* gene, also known as *GADD153*, encodes a member of the CCAAT/enhancer-binding protein (C/EBP) family and has a DNA-binding domain. It appears to be involved in normal adipocyte differentiation because the protein it produces may be a dominant inhibitor of other C/EBP transcription factors known to be important in cell proliferation (9). Members of this C/EBP group are highly expressed in fat and are involved in the differentiation of fibroblasts into adipocytes and in the growth arrest of terminally differentiated adipocytes (6). *CHOP* itself is induced in the differentiation of 3T3-L1 cells to adipocytes. In the neoplasm, the translocation results in a fusion gene involving *CHOP* and *TLS* (translocated in liposarcoma), an RNA-binding gene with much similarity structurally and functionally to the *EWS* gene of Ewing sarcoma. Presumably, the lack of the normal inhibitory function of an intact *CHOP* gene allows the fatty tumor to proliferate unchecked. The use of both Southern blots and fluorescent in situ hybridization (FISH) techniques in detecting the rearranged gene will have usefulness in the diagnosis of fatty tumors. Likewise, when it becomes commercially available, antibody to the CHOP protein might be used immunohistochemically to detect such tumors.

Apoptosis, or programmed cell death, probably occurs in adipocytic tissues, but studies localizing the BCL-2 protein in human fetal tissues fail to mention its detection in fat (10).

Postnatal Development

At birth, the average-size infant has approximately 5 billion adipocytes (11). This represents only 16% of the total number of adipocytes in adults. Adipose tissue continues to grow in parallel with general growth throughout the first 10 years of life. Fat cells enlarge significantly during the first 6 months of life without much increase in cell number (12). Until puberty, the cell size remains fairly constant while the number of adipocytes progressively increases. At puberty, there is a substantial increase in adipocyte size and number (12). Although at the end of puberty the total number of adipocytes is similar to the adult, new adipocytes may continue to form throughout life (13). Studies on adult rats have shown that overfeeding results in proliferation of adipocyte precursors and development of new fat cells (14). De novo adipocyte formation can be triggered by overdistention of existing fat cells and the mass of stored triglycerides (15). Loss of fat cells may also occur and has been shown in overweight women following several years of strict dietary restriction (16).

Adult WAT may be a source of mesenchymal stem cells (17), which can differentiate into multiple lineages including adipose cells, chondrocytes, osteoblasts, neuronal cells, endothelial cells, and cardiomyocytes (18).

Gender Differences

The differences in body fat content noted between men and women begin in early childhood. Young girls are fatter than boys. Studies on fetuses, however, have not noted differences in the pattern of distribution or quantity of fat in prenatal life (1). The distribution of adipose tissue, however, even in prenatal life is not homogeneous throughout the body. Gender differences in the distribution of adipose tissue following puberty are well known and thought to be related to steroid hormone secretion (12). In humans, estrogens and progesterone induce an increase in trochanteric fat. The localization of more fat in the lower body in women results in the so-called gynecoid habitus. These same deposits are reduced by androgens in men, resulting in an android distribution of fat. The percentage of body fat also differs in men and women. Males reach a peak in body fat content during early adolescence, whereas women continue to accumulate fat relative to body weight throughout the teen years.

Functions

WAT is the body's largest energy store and it possesses the enzymes necessary for the uptake and release of triglycerides.

Briefly, triglycerides circulate in the blood in the form of chylomicrons from the intestine and very low-density lipoproteins from the liver (19). LPL present on the luminal surface of endothelial cells hydrolyzes the triglyceride to release free fatty acids. This enzyme is synthesized by adipocytes and transferred to the endothelial cells. Most of the free fatty acids are taken up by the fat cells and re-esterified to glycerol phosphate within the adipocyte to form triacylglycerol, which is then stored within the cell's lipid droplet. The fat is mobilized through the action of hormone-sensitive lipase, which hydrolyzes stored triglycerides. The released free fatty acids may be reesterified or released to the circulation and bound to albumin for transfer to other cells.

Until recently, the main endocrine function of adipose tissue was thought to be the conversion of androstenedione to estrone, the major source of estrogen in men and postmenopausal women. The aromatase action, however, has been localized to the stromal cell fraction of adipose tissue and not the adipocyte (20). More recently, a dynamic role of adipose tissue has emerged with expression of several hormones, growth factors, and cytokines identified in adipocytes, stromal cells, and macrophages that are localized to adipose tissue. These include leptin, a regulator of energy expenditure and appetite; interleukin-6 (IL-6), which may play a role in the metabolic syndrome; and several important regulators of glucose and lipid metabolism, the complement cascade, and the fibrinolytic system.

Leptin, the protein product of the *ob* gene, is synthesized exclusively by adipocytes and acts on the hypothalamus to increase energy expenditure and decrease appetite (21). This pathway is well established in rats. In humans, fasting lowers serum leptin levels and increases appetite (22). Unfortunately, elevated or rising levels of leptin do not show the reverse effect, and leptin has not been shown to have an antiobesity action in humans. The majority of obese individuals have elevated serum leptin levels, proportional to the amount of adipose tissue, and it is postulated that humans are leptin resistant (23). Leptin receptors are present on most tissues, and leptin may play a role outside the adipose tissue to accelerate wound healing, increase vascular tone, and inhibit bone formation (24).

Cytokines are secreted by adipocytes, stromal cells, and resident macrophages. IL-6 is made by adipocytes and macrophages, and adipose tissue accounts for approximately 30% of circulating IL-6 in humans (25). Like leptin, serum IL-6 levels are highly correlated with percent body fat. The IL-6 released from intra-abdominal stores enters the portal circulation. Hepatic triglyceride secretion is stimulated by IL-6, and this may contribute to the hypertriglyceridemia seen with visceral obesity (24). IL-6 also stimulates hepatic secretion of acute phase reactants, increases platelet number and activity, and increases expression of endothelial adhesion molecules. There are ongoing investigations of the role this cytokine (which is derived in large part from adipose tissue) plays in the metabolic syndrome and the risk of cardiovascular disease in obesity.

Adipocytes also secrete C3 and adipsin, the proteins of the alternate complement pathway (26). Plasminogen activator inhibitor 1 (PAI-1) is a potent inhibitor of the fibrinolytic system and favors the development of thromboemboli. Insulin induces expression of PAI-1 by adipocytes, and elevated levels are seen with obesity (27).

Mitochondrial dysfunction in adipocytes may be related to the development of obesity and the diabetes epidemic and appears to be involved in HIV treatment–associated lipodystrophy (28).

Regulation

WAT contains numerous receptors for hormones, cytokines, catecholamines, and lipoproteins. Catecholamines acting through α-2 receptors inhibit lipolysis, and a predominance of α-2 receptors in gluteal fat of women is thought to impact maintenance of these fat stores despite weight loss (19). Regional differences in LPL levels also occur in women. Gluteal fat in premenopausal women tends to have high LPL levels, and these regions contain larger fat cells. Such regional differences disappear after menopause and are not present in obese men (29,30). This suggests that the sex steroids also play a role in adipose tissue distribution and activity. Both androgens and estrogen modulate *ob* gene expression and control adipose tissue development (31,32). Androgens are antiadipogenic and estrogens proadipogenic. These may play a role in the regional differences in fat distribution and the development of the android and gynecoid patterns of obesity.

Insulin stimulates lipogenesis and glucose uptake while inhibiting fat breakdown. Insulin and glucocorticoids stimulate DNA synthesis in cultured human adipocytes and conversion of preadipocytes to mature adipocytes. These effects are enhanced on cells obtained from obese, as compared with lean, people. Estradiol-17β has also been shown to stimulate division of cultured preadipocytes obtained from both men and women. Progesterone acts in vitro to stimulate both preadipocyte division and LPL activity (33). This dual role facilitates triglyceride accumulation in women. Fibroblast growth factor 1, secreted by adipose-derived microvascular endothelial cells, stimulates preadipocyte differentiation and accumulation of triglycerides (34).

Tumor necrosis factor alpha (TNF-α) and IL-6 have the opposite effect and are implicated along with leptin in the weight loss and anorexia of chronic wasting illnesses and cancer (35,36). TNF-α is expressed in preadipocytes and acts to block differentiation to mature adipocytes through CCAAT/enhancer-binding protein alpha (C/EBP-α) (37). It also suppresses LPL and stimulates the mobilization of fatty acids. The TNF-α induces the release of IL-6 and leptin from adipose tissue, and the action of these cytokines is closely interrelated.

In addition to adipocyte function, fat cell size and number are also regulated. Numerous studies using tritiated

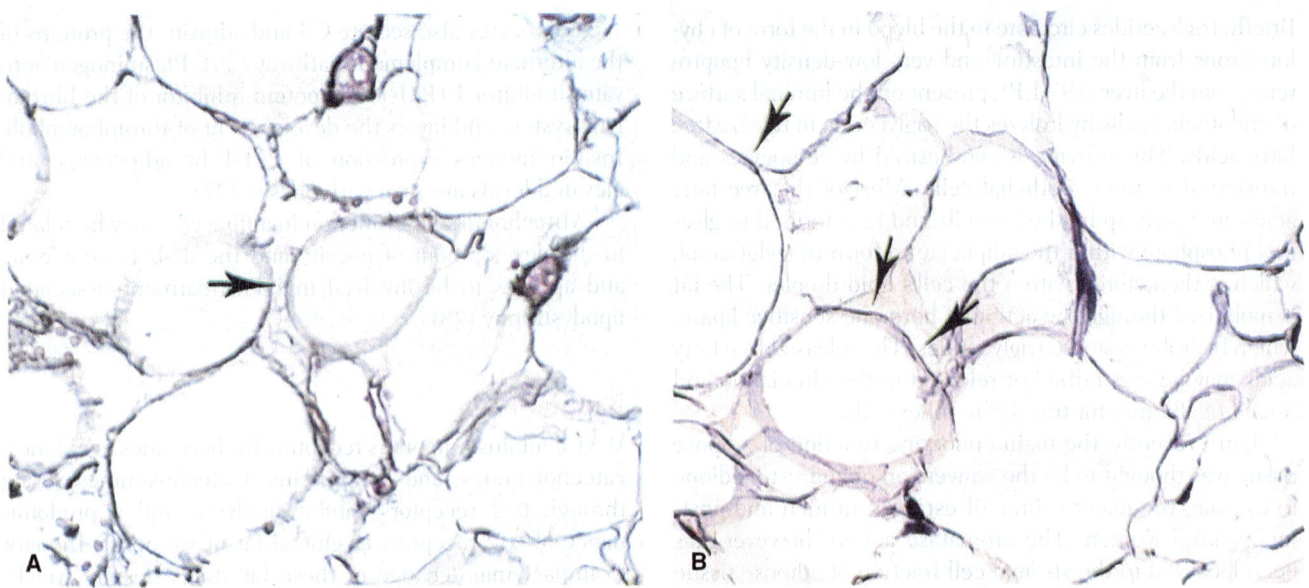

FIGURE 6.3 Normal adult adipocyte. **A:** On a reticulin stain, each adipocyte is outlined by reticulin (*arrow*), which is present outside the cytoplasm. **B:** The same is true on PAS stain, where the basement membrane is highlighted (*arrows*) and encompasses the pale residue of cytoplasm remaining after fixation and embedding.

thymidine incorporation as a marker for cell division in adipose tissue have been done in rats to identify mitotically active cells within fat. Mature lipid-laden adipocytes are generally considered to be incapable of cell differentiation because of the absence of mitotic figures seen histologically in normal adipose tissue. Sampling fat from rats injected with tritiated thymidine at 1 day and 3 days of age, which are then sacrificed at various times up to 5 months of age, has shown that the number of labeled cells in subcutaneous fat initially rises because of cell proliferation. The concentration of radioactivity then falls, probably as a result of a dilutional effect resulting from continued cell division (38). This study, however, failed to distinguish adipocyte from stromal labeling. Similar studies had been performed on rats in which the subcutaneous tissue is separated into stromal and adipose components. In one study, the specific radioactivity of the adipocyte fraction did not increase until 2 to 5 days after injection (39). Thus, they concluded that DNA synthesis occurs in non–lipid-laden cells or preadipocytes. As these cells accumulate lipid, labeled cells are detected within the adipocyte fraction.

Gross Aspects

Fatty tissue is typically homogeneous, bright cadmium-like yellow, with a glistening and greasy surface texture, and finely divided by faint septa. Any variation in color indicates a pathologic process: white to white/yellow in fat necrosis, paler yellows in many lipomas, reddish tinge to orange/yellow in angiolipoma, definite gray/white to whitish streaks in spindle cell lipoma, and white/yellow to white nodules in liposarcoma.

Histology

Microscopically, a mature white fat cell is spherical and measures up to 120 μm in diameter (40). The cytoplasm is compressed at the perimeter of the cell, and only a thin rim of cell membrane is evident on hematoxylin–eosin (H&E)-stained sections. Reticulin and periodic acid–Schiff (PAS) stains highlight the adipocyte basement membrane (Fig. 6.3). The cytoplasm is displaced by a single lipid vacuole, and the cells are fairly uniform in size (Fig. 6.4). The nucleus, although oval, is thin and small with finely distributed chromatin; when seen in profile, a central minute clear vacuole may be seen within the nucleus (Fig. 6.4). Normal subcutaneous fat is finely divided into ill-defined lobules by thin bands of collagen (Fig. 6.5).

Ultrastructure

The ultrastructure of developing adipocytes has previously been discussed. In brief, a spindle shape with abundant ER and small spherical mitochondria characterizes preadipocytes (40). Lipid accumulates as small perinuclear inclusions that coalesce to form larger lipid droplets. The mitochondria become filamentous and the ER less prominent. In a mature adipocyte, the nucleus is flattened against the cytoplasmic membrane by a large lipid droplet. There is only a thin, tenuous rim of cytoplasm that surrounds it. Pinocytotic vesicles are seen in variable numbers but are very numerous following periods of starvation. Adjacent to the cell membrane are deposits of basement membrane. Capillaries are closely opposed to the adipocyte basement membrane. Only rarely have nerves been identified adjacent

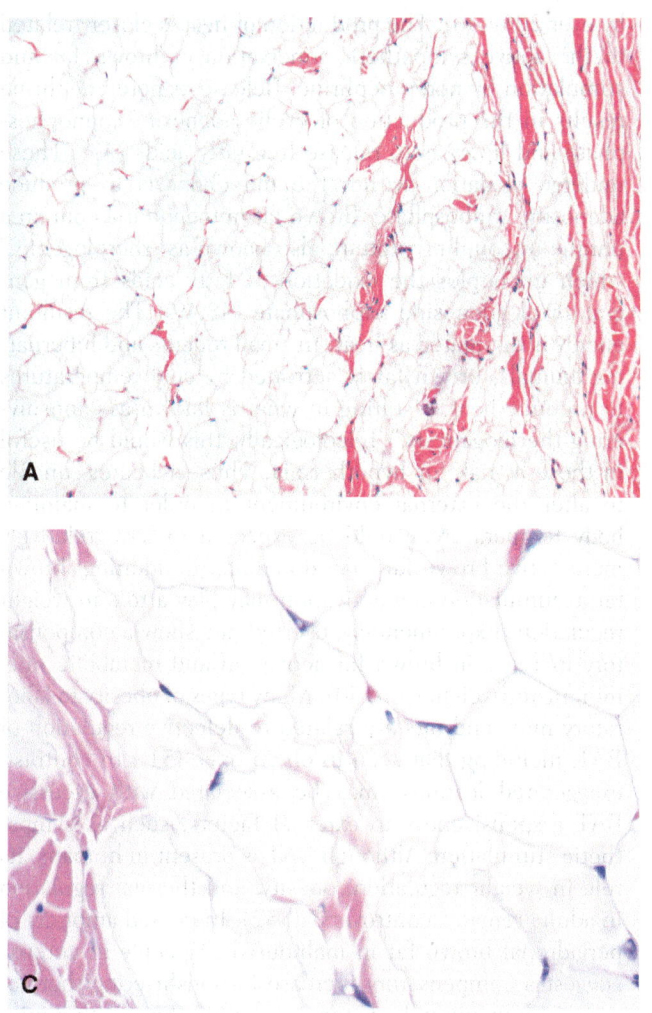
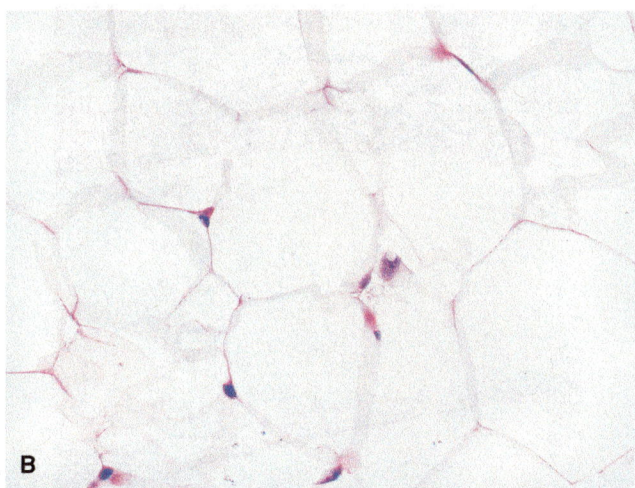

FIGURE 6.4 **A:** At medium power, the size of subcutaneous adipocytes appears relatively uniform. **B:** At high power, pale areas represent portions of basement membrane and cytoplasm cut on the bias. Nuclei of capillary endothelial cells are present at intersections between multiple cells. **C:** In contrast to other nuclei, an ideal section of an adipocyte nucleus shows a pale character due to its thin nature and the common central vacuole, or "Locherne." The wrinkled cell outlines are an artifact occasionally seen, the result of improper fixation.

to white fat cells, although they may be seen in intercellular collagenous septa.

BROWN FAT

Prenatal Development

The development of brown adipose tissue (BAT) has been studied in animal models. The brown adipocyte precursors are spindle cells closely related to a network of capillaries (41). As the cells and vessels proliferate, they are organized into lobules by connective tissue septa. As the cells accumulate lipid, they initially are unilocular. However, with further lipid accumulation, multiple cytoplasmic lipid vacuoles appear. As in white fat, the close association of developing adipocytes and blood vessels has led some to speculate that adipocytes actually develop from endothelial cells. Although similar ultrastructural features are cited as supportive evidence of theory, more recent investigations have attributed these similarities to a common origin from undifferentiated mesenchyme. In fact, ultrastructural and biochemical studies that have examined developing BAT have shown that unique features such as large mitochondria and a unique mitochondrial protein are found early in development and distinguish brown from white fat. Recent studies suggest that brown fat precursors may also be recruited directly from WAT and skeletal muscle (42).

Fetal necropsy studies have identified lobules of developing brown fat in the human fetus (43). The largest of these are from the posterior cervical, axillary, suprailiac, and perirenal regions. Those in the neck and axillae are closely associated with the major blood vessels of these regions in such a way that they extend along the course of the cervical blood vessels into the root of the neck. The suprailiac collections lie deep to the abdominal muscles, yet superficial to the peritoneum, and invest the anterior abdominal wall to the diaphragm. Intermediate-sized brown fat pads are seen in the interscapular paralateral trapezius and deltoid regions. Small collections are evident in the intercostal area. In this study, no difference was noted in distribution between the sexes or among the races. The amount of brown fat increases in proportion to growth throughout life. Deposits are well established by the 5th month of gestation.

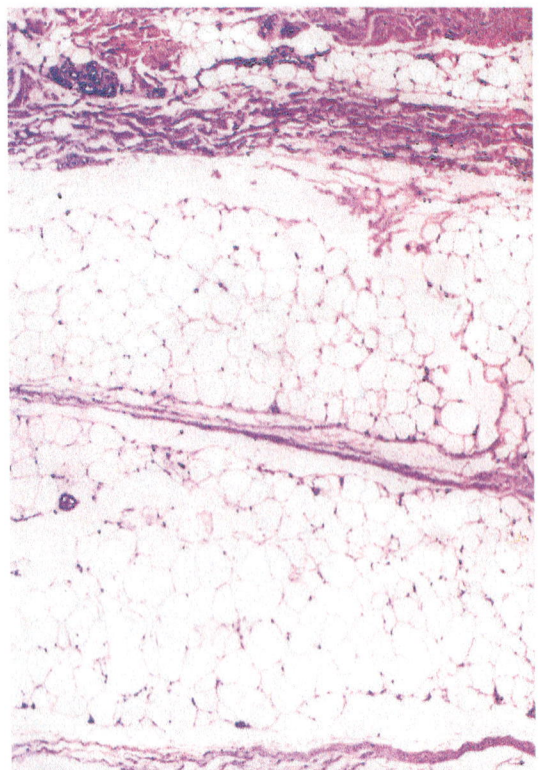

FIGURE 6.5 Adult subcutaneous fat lobule with associated microvasculature; note the thin and delicate fibrous tissue septa.

Postnatal Development

The presence of brown fat beyond the neonatal period in humans has been debated. An autopsy study by Heaton (44), however, has identified lobules of brown fat throughout life to the eighth decade. Brown fat is most widely distributed in young children and, over the next several decades, gradually disappears from most sites. In children younger than 10 years, identifiable deposits of brown fat were identified in the interscapular region, around the neck vessels and muscles, around the structures of the mediastinum, and adjacent to the lung hila. Intra-abdominal and retroperitoneal deposits were noted around the kidneys, pancreas, spleen, mesocolon, and omentum, as well as in the anterior abdominal wall. The extremities were not sampled. Although brown fat disappeared from most areas, it was found to persist around the kidneys, adrenals, and aorta and within the mediastinum and neck throughout adult life. As in fetal life, no difference in distribution based on gender was noted.

Function

The main function of BAT is heat production. It has been estimated that the maximal aerobic capacity per gram of tissue is almost 10 times that of skeletal muscle (45). It has been estimated that even in humans the small quantities of brown fat present are capable of raising heat production by over 20% (46). The production of heat is closely related to the active sympathetic innervation of brown fat and stimulation by norepinephrine. Release of norepinephrine results in the production of cyclic adenosine monophosphate and lipolysis to release free fatty acids (47). These undergo oxidation within the mitochondria to produce adenosine triphosphate. Brown fat mitochondria contain a unique uncoupling protein, also known as "thermogenin," which uncouples the oxidation of fatty acids from generation of adenosine triphosphate (48,49). The resultant energy is dissipated as heat. In small rodents and hibernating animals, brown fat is activated by cold temperatures to produce heat, resulting in what is known as "nonshivering thermogenesis." Teleologically, this would be useful in those at risk for hypothermia. Thus, neonates, unable to alter the external environment in order to maintain body temperature, would be expected to have relatively more active brown fat than do adults. In addition, brown fat accumulation and activation may play a role in weight regulation. Experimentally, overfed rats show a compensatory increase in brown fat activation and metabolic rate, minimizing weight gain (50). Many types of obesity in laboratory mice and rats are related to defective regulation of BAT, including that seen in ob/ob mice (51). In contrast, exaggerated leanness may be associated with excessive BAT responsiveness to external factors, such as sympathetic stimulation. Although BAT is present in humans, its role in weight regulation, obesity, and thermal regulation in adults remains controversial (52). Increased amounts of periadrenal brown fat in malnourished people at autopsy suggest a compensatory increase in nonshivering thermogenesis to maintain body temperature in those with diminished subcutaneous fat and cachexia (53).

Regulation

Unlike white fat, brown fat is highly innervated and regulated by sympathetic stimulation. Nerves enter each lobe and branch within the interlobular septa, running along the vessels to terminate on the fat cells (54). Brown fat cells have numerous β-1 and β-2 adrenoreceptors that regulate lipolysis and thermogenesis (47). The α-adrenoreceptors, although present, probably do not act directly in heat production. Norepinephrine may also act to increase the number and character of brown fat cells. Using continuous infusions of norepinephrine, Mory et al. (55) have shown that such chronic sympathetic stimulation results in increased cellularity, increased protein content, and increased mitochondrial density in brown fat. Because of this close association of sympathetic activity and brown fat activity, several investigators have used pheochromocytoma as a model to study brown fat activities in humans. These studies have provided evidence supportive of early autopsy studies. Functional BAT was identified in adults with pheochromocytomas that had similar biochemical features to the better-characterized BAT of rodents (56).

Hormones also play a role in brown fat regulation, but it is minor in comparison to the sympathetic system. Thyroid hormone, although active in regulating metabolic rate, has little importance in diet-induced or nonshivering thermogenesis (47). Insulin stimulates glucose intake into BAT. Both cortisol and gonadal steroid hormones inhibit thermogenesis, thus promoting energy conservation.

Histology

The term *brown fat* was applied to this tissue because of its characteristic gross appearance. It is incorrect to refer to it as "fetal" fat because it is present throughout life. The abundant vascularity and numerous mitochondria within the cells impart a characteristic reddish-brown color to the tissue. Brown fat has a glandular lobulated appearance. This is in contrast to the more diffuse growth pattern of white fat. Histologically, brown fat is organized into lobules of cells that are made up of adipocytes, capillaries, nerves, and connective tissue. These are surrounded by a thin, fibrous capsule containing blood vessels, nerves, and scattered white adipose cells (57). The cells are polygonal in shape, with a mixture of multivacuolated and univacuolated cells (Fig. 6.6). The occurrence of both cell types is emphasized, and their presence in developing white fat initially confused studies on its origin. The multivacuolated cell, characteristic of brown fat, has a highly granular cytoplasm with numerous lipid inclusions. Its granular appearance is due to the numerous mitochondria necessary for thermogenesis. The nucleus is spherical and often centrally located, although a large lipid inclusion may displace it toward the periphery of the cell or, rarely, to the extreme perimeter (as in white fat). Small nucleoli are common. The unilobular cells are indistinguishable histologically from the mature signet-ring cell–type white adipocytes but are different ultrastructurally. On average, the size of the brown fat cells is smaller than that of white adipocytes, approximately 25 to 40 μm. In animals that hibernate, marked seasonal variation in cell size has been noted. Both exposures to cold and starvation result in lipid depletion, causing reduction in cell size and wrinkling of the cell membrane.

Brown adipose cells are surrounded by a network of collagen fibers that contain numerous minute nerve axons and blood vessels. Nonmyelinated axons terminate on the fat cells, providing an avenue for direct sympathetic regulation. The vascularity is quite prominent with numerous capillaries coursing between the adipocytes. It is estimated in rats that the vascularity of brown fat is four to six times greater than that of white fat (57).

Beige Fat

Cells that resemble brown adipocytes may appear after thermogenic stimuli at anatomical sites corresponding to WAT, in a process called "browning" of WAT. This third class of fat cells appearing in WAT derive from precursor cells different from those in classical BAT and are closer to the white adipocyte cell lineage and are often called "inducible, beige, or brite" (58–60). In combating the obesity epidemic, efforts to increase the expenditure of thermogenic energy by brown fat has become a new strategy. It became clear that brown adipocytes originate from a precursor shared with skeletal muscle that expresses Myf5-Cre, while all white adipocytes originate from Myf5-negative precursors (60). However, the situation is more complicated because subsets of white adipocytes may also arise from Myf5-Cre–expressing precursors. Hypothetical models of the lineage of adipocytes have been developed to include these beige fat cells (60). These beige cells appear in WAT in response to cold or beta-adrenergic agonists, especially in certain locations like inguinal (ingWAT) and retroperitoneal (rWAT), possibly by transdifferentiation. Suffice it to say that these discoveries may lead to better understanding of obesity and perhaps a therapy based on biologic pathways.

Stem Cells

Adipose tissue contains not only mature adult cells, but also stem cells. These adipose-derived stem cells are a common source of research and have been shown to generate pericytes, chondrocytes, endothelial cells, and Schwann cells, and have been used for repair of ischemic muscle (61–63).

HISTOCHEMISTRY

Enzyme Histochemistry

In development, enzyme histochemistry within developing adipocytes is related to the stage of adipocyte differentiation. In fact, in some systems, such as the rat, it is

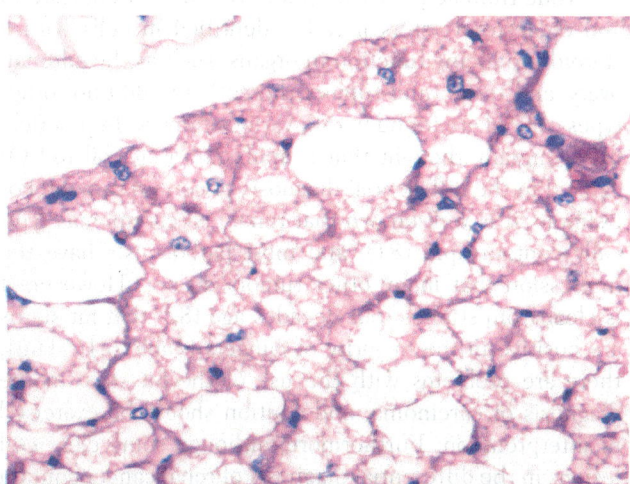

FIGURE 6.6 Normal adult brown fat. Nearly all cells have centrally placed nuclei and multivacuolated cytoplasm. Rare cells (*top left*) are nonvacuolated. An arborizing thin capillary network is noted.

clear that enzymatic differentiation of adipocytes precedes morphologic differentiation (64,65). In regions destined to become adipose tissue, undifferentiated morphology is initially present without a capillary bed and without any enzymatic capacity. Subsequently, immature cells or what can be termed "preadipocytes" exist in the form of spindle cells within an area containing a capillary bed. These cells lack any lipid or a basal lamina and have a large complement of enzymatic activity, but they lack the capability to release fat as a result of the absence of esterase (lipase). In mature lobules, adipocytes in the form of rounded cells now contain lipid, a basal lamina, and a well-developed capillary bed; the entire complement of enzymatic activity is present, including NADH-tetrazolium reductase, ADPH-tetrazolium reductase, and glucose-6-phosphate dehydrogenase (G6PDH). Malate dehydrogenase (NADP) activity is acquired only by late-stage adipocytes (64). Hausman demonstrated the presence of such enzymatic differentiation before the assumption of an obviously rounded cell shape consistent with an adipocyte.

LPL is an enzyme found at high concentration in fatty tissues. It is involved in the transport of serum triglycerides into adipocytes in the form of fatty acids. However, it can be found in other tissues such as skeletal muscles (66,67) and cardiac muscle (68), where it may be localized to endothelial cells. Concentration in fat is directly related to the serum insulin concentration.

Lipid Histochemistry

Lipids in adipose tissue are generally identified using various stains, such as oil red O and Sudan IV (64,69–73). It should be noted that lipids are lost in formaldehyde after prolonged fixation, and thus, cases to be tested using frozen cryostat sections of fixed material should be obtained as soon as possible. Of the two time-honored lipid stains mentioned, oil red O gives the more intense stain and is more rapid to perform. Sudan black B may stain nonlipid substances (such as coagulated proteins) nonspecifically. As a rule, neutral fats are detected using these fat stains. However, a differential staining pattern between neutral fats and fatty acid components and phospholipids can be obtained with the Nile blue sulfate stain (74); with this stain, neutral fat stains pink to red, and fatty acids and phospholipids stain bluish. The lipid composition of fatty tissues may also be investigated using new techniques such as the hot-stage polarizing-light microscopic method (75).

The normal composition of lipid in WAT consists of 99% triglycerides in the form of neutral fat and less than 1% in the form of phospholipid, cholesterol, and fatty acids (63). In less-differentiated adipocytes, such as those found in liposarcomas, there is a shift away from neutral fat to phospholipids and cholesterol (74). Unfortunately, lipid stains appear to have little use in the everyday examination of adipocyte lesions. The droplets seen on the stains may represent nonspecific staining, and various other mesenchymal lesions may contain lipid (72). An exception is the distinction between lesions with artificial vacuoles, such as epithelioid smooth muscle lesions, which are negative with fat stains.

Intracellular Lipid in Nonadipocytes

Lipid may accumulate in various other cell types and in nonadipocytic tumors.

Steatosis

According to *Stedman's Medical Dictionary* (76), steatosis has two main meanings: adiposis and fatty degeneration (e.g., steatosis cordis = fatty degeneration of heart). These terms (and the terms used in various pathology texts) are unclear, and the distinction between intracellular lipid accumulation and adipocyte infiltration of organs is not made. When nonadipocytes store lipid intracellularly, the phrase *lipid accumulation* is accurate; in the liver, the term *steatosis* is used; and, in major pathology texts (77,78), the term appears to be applied solely to the hepatocyte. However, intracytoplasmic lipid can be found within other solid organs, such as the heart (in the myocardial fibers in hypoxia (77)) and the kidney (in the renal tubule in diabetes, poisonings, Reye syndrome (79)). Theoretically, there is no reason why these processes cannot be referred to as myocardial or renal tubular steatosis. Regardless, in referring to intracellular lipid accumulation, terms such as *lipid accumulation* or *steatosis* are preferable to unclear and archaic designations, such as *adiposis* or *fatty degeneration*. Discussion of adipocyte infiltration of organs is found later (see the section entitled Syndromes Associated With Fatty Lesions [including Lipomatosis]).

Lipid accumulation may occur in the placenta after prolonged parenteral nutrition; there, it takes the form of foamy vacuoles within the syncytial and Hofbauer cells of the chorionic villi (80).

Aside from adipocytes, lipid in the form of cholesterol and cholesterol esters may be identified in cells with a steroid-producing function in organs, such as the adrenal, ovary, and testis (and tumors thereof). In addition, other types of lipid are found within various tumors. In practice, it is generally thought that a lipid stain (e.g., oil red O) can aid in the differential diagnosis of certain tumors. For example, it is well known that renal cell carcinomas typically contain lipid (81), and most pathologists have the impression that many other tumors do not. However, it is clear from studies four decades ago (82) that fat stains are positive in the majority of cancers (Table 6.1). Thus, there are problems with the use of the fat stain in the diagnosis of carcinoma, and caution should be exercised in interpretation. Furthermore, although some clear cell lesions in the differential diagnosis of renal cancer contain glycogen (benign sugar tumor of lung) (83), others such as xanthoma of bone (84) contain lipid—and thus a fat stain is of no assistance.

TABLE 6.1	
Oil Red O—Positive Carcinomas[a]	
Squamous cell carcinoma	Ovarian carcinoma
Gastric carcinoma	Breast carcinoma
Lung carcinomas	Prostatic carcinoma
Renal cell carcinoma	Thyroid carcinoma
Lymphoma, large cell	Myeloma

[a]For the majority of cancer types, a high percentage of the tumors listed showed a positive reaction.
Elizalde N, Korman S. Cytochemical studies of glycogen, neutral mucopolysaccharides, and fat in malignant tissues. *Cancer* 1968;21:1061–1068.

IMMUNOHISTOCHEMISTRY

Currently, there is no commercially available specific immunohistochemical marker for adipose tissue. However, an adipocyte lipid-binding protein, p422 or aP2, is a protein expressed exclusively in preadipocytes late in adipogenesis. Preliminary studies with an antibody to aP2 demonstrate that it stains only lipoblasts and brown fat cells and is capable of identifying liposarcomas selectively (85). This may be quite useful diagnostically in the future.

Adipocytes and tumors thereof stain positively for vimentin, and in our experience, adipocytic tumors have been negative for cytokeratin, desmin, and muscle-specific actin. In 1983, Michetti et al. (86) were the first to describe S100 immunoreactivity in adipocytes, specifically of rat origin. The S100 protein was extracted and shown to be identical to that found in the rat brain. Ultrastructurally, S100 reactivity was widely dispersed within adipocyte cytoplasm but was not found within mitochondria, lipid droplets, or most of the ER. In a similar ultrastructural study, Haimoto et al. (87) identified S100 protein in the plasma membranes, in membranes of microvesicles, and within polysomes. The Golgi apparatus was negative for this marker, although some reactivity was found within the rough ER. During the process of lipolysis in fat cells, Haimoto et al. (87) noted a change in the distribution of S100 antigen and suggested that S100 protein molecules interact with free fatty acids, indicating that this protein may act as a carrier protein for free fatty acids.

The S100 protein is a highly acidic calcium-binding protein of molecular weight 21,000. It consists of two polypeptide chains (α and β) and may occur as dimers in three ways: S100a (α, β), S100b (β, β), or S100ao (α, α) (88). When fat cells have been analyzed, they have been shown to contain only S100b (β form), like Schwann cells (88,89). In the routine practice of immunohistochemistry, adipose tissue reacts in a variable fashion (Fig. 6.7), accounting for some negative reactions observed by Kahn et al. (90). Although lipomas and liposarcomas are reported to be

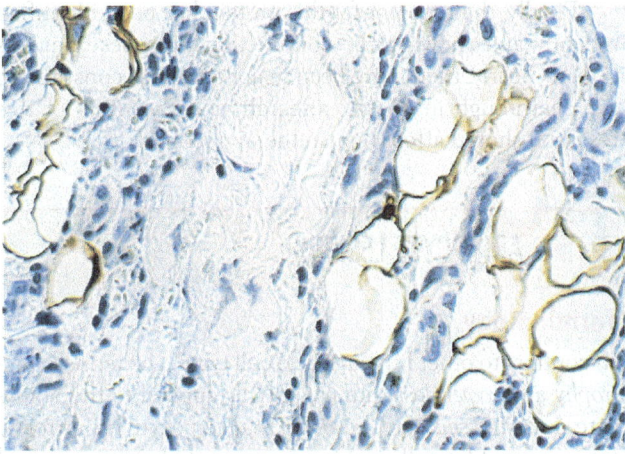

FIGURE 6.7 S100 immunohistochemistry. Reactivity is seen both in the nuclei and in the cytoplasm surrounding the lipid droplets. Such S100-positive results appear to vary considerably from case to case, probably reflecting fixation differences.

frequently positive with S100 (91–94), in our experience, this has not been true. Regardless of fixation with formalin or Bouin solution, very few liposarcomas have exhibited S100 immunoreactivity.

Adipocytic lesions do not stain with antibodies to neuron-specific enolase (95).

Brown fat also exhibits S100 protein reactivity but curiously may also express the endothelial marker CD31, a potential pitfall (96).

Obesity

Human obesity is thought to be approximately 60% genetic in origin, with multiple genetic and environmental factors involved (97). The role of BAT was briefly alluded to earlier, and new research continues to underscore its importance. For example, in transgenic mice engineered to lack BAT, obesity develops routinely (98). In mice, the genetics of obesity are clearer than in humans. A team at the Rockefeller University led by Dr. Friedman first reported the identification of the *ob* mouse gene and showed that mutations of it are associated with the development of obesity (99). These same researchers have located the human counterpart (*OB* gene) (99) and mapped its location to chromosome 7 (100). The human protein produced by this gene has 84% homology with the mouse protein, appears to be a hormone secreted by adipose tissue, and likely functions as part of a pathway to regulate body fat. If, indeed, a defective hormone is responsible for some forms of obesity, then there is an immediate therapy available in the form of fully intact native hormone. In 1995, several research groups (101–103) have shown that injection of the ob protein into mice causes the animals to lose weight and maintain their weight loss. Even obesity due to a nongenetic defect like excess diet fat is corrected by the ob protein, now called "leptin."

Finally, the receptor for this protein has been identified recently and shown to be nonfunctional in obese animals (104). Clearly, there have been major advances constituting a breakthrough in obesity research, and the fruits of this research should affect human therapy soon.

ADIPOCYTE LESIONS

Terminology

In contrast to other human tissue cell types, the terms *hypertrophy* and *hyperplasia* are not usually applied to the adipocyte. It is stressed here, however, that adipocyte hypertrophy (or increased fat cell size) is a recognized phenomenon and is found, for example, in obesity. Enlarged, or hypertrophic, fat cells (>120 μm or so) can also be identified in neoplasia (lipoma and liposarcoma) where cells appear to have three or four times the normal diameter (e.g., >300 μm). Hyperplasia (or an increased number of adipocytes), in contrast to widespread belief, is a definite occurrence. Again, it is common in obese patients, but it may also be seen in organ-based infiltrations; these are a type of site-specific adipocyte hyperplastic processes. Mature adipocytes are incapable of regeneration, and new fat cells are added through in situ mesenchymal cell differentiation recruited from primitive perivascular cells. No disease or change involving adipocytes can appropriately be termed a "degeneration (as mentioned earlier)," other than liquefaction with necrosis. Atrophy of adipocytes may be seen in malnutrition, starvation, or as the effect of chemotherapy (see the section entitled Atrophy). The appearance of mature fat cells as small foci in unusual places is termed *metaplasia* and is discussed in a later section. Localized new growths of either pure adipocytes or mixtures of adipocytes in other tissue constitute neoplasia and are presumably clonal entities.

Degeneration

In the condition sclerema adiposum neonatorum, the subcutaneous fat is grossly and microscopically abnormal. Rubbery plaques are due to fat necrosis and degenerative individual fat cells with intracellular needle-shaped crystals (105). This fat crystallization is brown and can be highlighted by polarization. Such crystals apparently may also be identified in up to 30% of stillbirths as a general degeneration following intrauterine demise (105). In another disease, Neu–Laxova syndrome, a defect in lipid metabolism, causes a lard-like appearance to the adipose tissue and is lethal.

Atrophy

The changes in fat lobules during starvation or malnutrition are particularly noticeable in the subcutaneous region or the omentum. Individual fat cells are reduced in size and fat content, and those without much lipid take on a rounded or epithelioid appearance (106). In the extreme, lobules of these epithelioid cells can simulate tumor nodules histologically (Fig. 6.8). The cytoplasm is variable in amount and is eosinophilic or granular with or without small lipid vacuoles of differing size, depending on the severity of the malnutrition. Some cells have a multivacuolated appearance. The intervening region between cells is constituted by homogeneous eosinophilic or amphophilic myxoid ground substance (Fig. 6.8) that is probably an extract of serum, although stimulation of proteoglycan matrix by the process of starvation (107) is possible. As part of this involution process, lipofuscin is deposited within the shrinking cells (Fig. 6.8). Importantly, each lobule retains its overall oval shape, although markedly reduced in size and considerably separated from other lobules (Fig. 6.8). In extreme cachexia, only streaks of tissue remain.

Nearly identical changes can also be seen in the WAT of fasted animals. As the cells gradually lose their lipid, the single lipid droplet breaks up into multiple vacuoles. Gradually, all lipid disappears. These cells become small and ovoid in shape, sometimes measuring only 15 μm in diameter (108). There is an apparent expansion of pericellular collagen in such a way that these cells appear as clusters of mesenchymal cells in fibrous stroma. Similarly, in cachexia, the fat cells are reduced in volume but not in number (109). Ultrastructurally, multiple pinocytotic vesicles are seen clustered along the entire cell membrane (57). Lipid is not seen within these vesicles, and their significance is unknown.

In the bone marrow, chemotherapy causes changes referred to as serous atrophy or gelatinous transformation (110,111). The majority of the fat cells have been destroyed, leaving scattered adipocytes of varying size remaining. No lobular appearance is present in the marrow, but the interstitial compartment is composed of the same eosinophilic myxoid substance described previously, again probably consisting of serum fluid and proteins. Droplets of lipid scattered about are also found and, upon regeneration, may appear as foci of lipogranulomas.

Although the microscopic features of the starvation effect on human brown fat have not been described, animals maintained on a dextrose–thiamine diet are known to show distinct morphologic changes in brown fat (40). The mitochondria are disrupted and large, irregular electron-dense inclusions are seen within the mitochondrial matrix. The cristae may assume a mosaic pattern with compartmentalization of the material. These cells revert to normal after 24 hours of a normal diet. Similar changes in white fat mitochondria have not been seen with starvation, suggesting that the active mitochondria of brown fat are particularly labile and sensitive to dietary changes.

Cellulite

The term "cellulite" is applied to the external skin when it exhibits linear depressed streaks (mattress phenomenon) or frank dimpling. Cellulite is typically found on the thigh

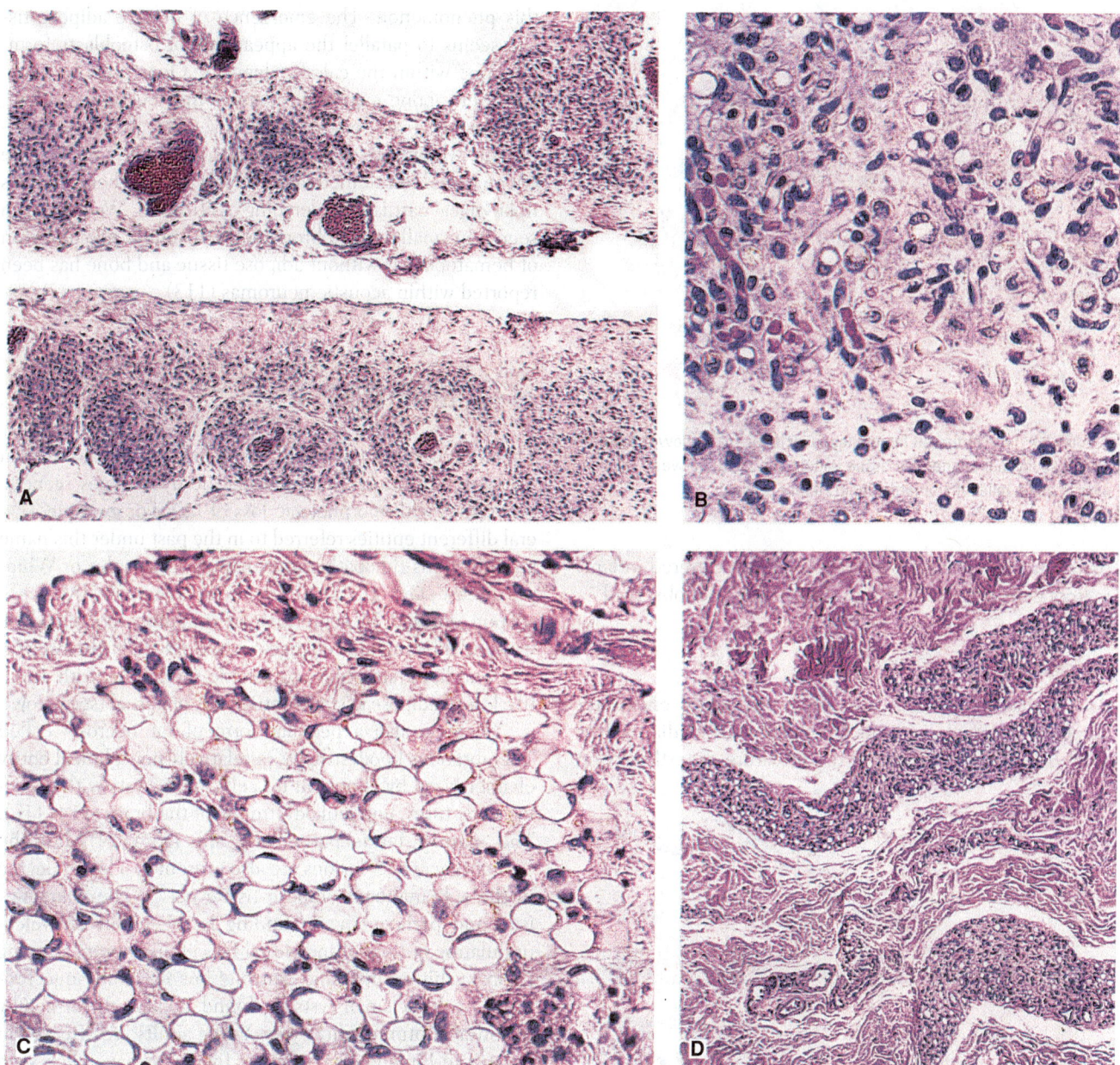

FIGURE 6.8 **A:** The extreme atrophy seen here in the omentum of a patient with anorexia nervosa may mimic tumor deposits. **B:** At high power, shrunken eosinophilic cells are seen with occasional vacuoles and lipofuscin pigment. **C:** In less severe starvation, these omental adipocytes are well recognized, although much smaller than normal size; again, note the presence of pigment. **D:** In the skin, severe cachexia secondary to a cancer resulted in marked involution of the cutaneous fat lobules, which appear only as elongated streaks.

and buttocks and is more common in females; it can be divided into incipient cellulite and full-blown cellulite. The former results from an uneven undersurface of the dermal–hypodermal interface, with fibrous tissue surrounding the protruding papillae adiposa; vertical fibrous strands of uneven thickness divide the hypodermal fat (112). In contrast, full-blown cellulite consists of a delicate meshwork of collagen fibers produced by increased hypodermal pressure of fat accumulation and increasing fat volume. Scattered CD34+ fibroblasts are seen in both forms of cellulite.

Unlike women, men have a smoother, strand-free dermal interface in the thigh and buttock areas (112).

Ischemia

Little is written about the effect of ischemia on the adipocyte. We have observed changes in the subcutaneous fat of legs removed for atherosclerotic vascular disease. They consist of accentuation of the lobular architecture by thickening of the fibrous septa; wider and more myxoid in quality,

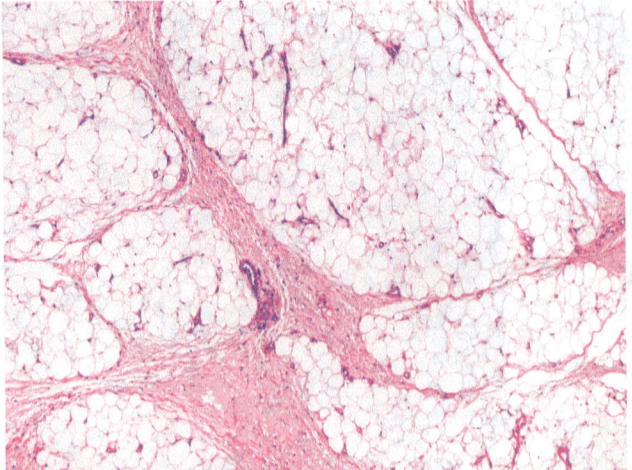

FIGURE 6.9 Accentuated fat lobules in ischemia of the lower extremity. Loose myxoid connective tissue widens the septa between lobules; edema and a mild inflammatory infiltrate are present.

the septa are edematous and also contain scattered inflammatory cells (Fig. 6.9). Actual necrosis was not observed.

Metaplasia

As surgical pathologists, we most frequently encounter adipocytic metaplasia, usually calcified, in cardiac valves (Fig. 6.10). There is little in the literature or textbooks on this phenomenon. The emergence of mature adipose tissue seems to parallel the appearance of osteoblasts forming bone within the calcific deposits. Once adipose tissue is present, bone marrow precursors may become resident, presumably from circulating cells, and cause hematopoiesis. Metaplasia is not limited to this site and may be encountered in calcified large vessels or elsewhere, such as in laryngeal cartilage undergoing ossification. We have even seen it in small ossified bronchioles. A similar phenomenon of hematopoiesis without adipose tissue and bone has been reported within acoustic neuromas (113).

LIPODYSTROPHY

This term is subject to much misunderstanding and is often misused for entities that are not true dystrophies (genetic syndromes with morphologic loss of fat). For example, several different entities referred to in the past under this name are infectious (idiopathic intestinal lipodystrophy, or Whipple disease) and others (mesenteric lipodystrophy [ML]; see section entitled Mesenteritis) are inflammatory disorders without fundamental changes in the fat cells themselves. The real lipodystrophies are genetic syndromes with selective loss of adipose tissue—entire body or partial (see below).

There is also a peculiar form of fat necrosis called "membranous lipodystrophy," a relatively new clinical entity characterized by abnormal fat cells, bone cysts with pathologic fractures, and leukodystrophy of the brain (114–116). The marrow fat is particularly affected (114), but the "membranocystic" lesions are also present to a lesser degree in the subcutaneous adipose tissue (117). The characteristic and pathognomonic finding is the highly shriveled, undulating outline of individual fat cell membranes, giving them hyalin eosinophilic convolutions or "arabesque profiles." Multiple small cysts are found, apparently formed by fusion of ruptured adipocytes. Young adults are affected in Japan and Finland primarily, but five cases have been seen in the United States (116). Its etiology and pathogenesis are unknown; it is probably related to an enzyme deficiency (114). A secondary form of membranous lipodystrophy has been described in association with lupus erythematosus and morphea profunda (117). Interestingly, the membranous changes in fat characteristic of lipodystrophy can also be seen in normal fat affected by radiation therapy (118). Another secondary disease is HIV treatment–associated lipodystrophy (28).

The genetics of lipodystrophy syndromes is now well known, and such disorders are divided into several types of congenital generalized lipodystrophy (caused by recessive mutations in genes AGPAT2, BSCL2, CAV1, and PTRF) and several forms of familial partial lipodystrophies (caused by autosomal dominant mutations in genes LMNA, PPARg, PLIN1, and AKT2; and recessive mutations can occur in genes CIDEC and LIPE) (119).

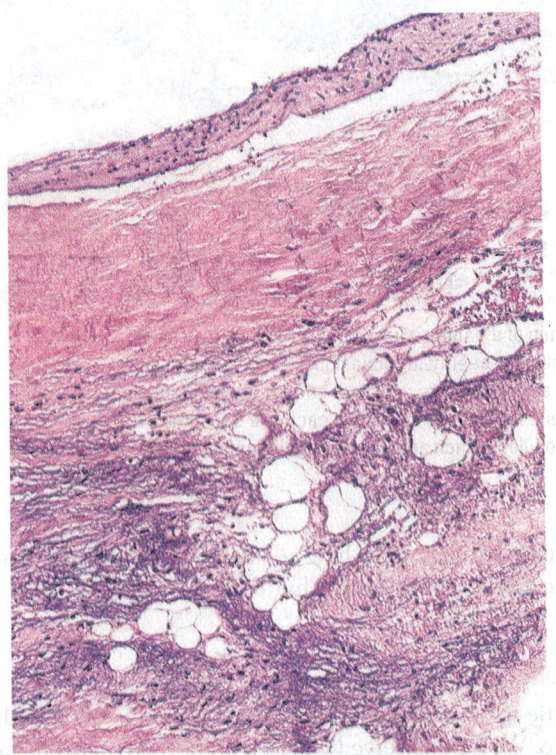

FIGURE 6.10 Fatty metaplasia of cardiac valve. Mature adipocytes are found in a myxoid background but are more commonly seen in association with calcification or ossification.

ADIPOCYTES IN ORGANS

Fatty Infiltration

As distinct from lipid accumulation or steatosis (see section entitled Steatosis), fatty infiltration is defined as the presence of mature adipose tissue in sites not normally containing fat. This is a disorder or condition relating to adipocyte cell growth and, therefore, the term *fatty degeneration* is a misnomer and incorrect. In some situations, such as within extremity muscle groups, the process of fatty infiltration is often related to atrophy of the involved site (120). This association between fatty infiltration and atrophy or involution is also noted in other organs (thymus (121), bone marrow (122), and kidney (123)) and apparently signifies the propensity for adipocytes to fill a vacuum, in a sense, left by atrophic processes (107). Whatever the stimulus may be, the adipocytes probably arise from pluripotent mesenchymal cells adjacent to blood vessels (107). The reversal of this relationship is found in the parathyroid gland, where there is an inverse relationship between parenchymal cells and adipocytes, to the point where no adipocytes are present in complete parathyroid hyperplasia.

Nonatrophic organs can also accumulate fat cells (lipomatosis), and the classic examples are the heart and the pancreas (77). In these locations, no parenchymal damage is discerned, and the process is a type of accidental lipogenesis (106). In the case of the pancreas, normal parenchymal histology and function are present even though the pancreas may be nearly invisible grossly (77,124). This type of pancreatic lipomatosis is correlated with age and obesity and also occurs in diabetics (124). The amount of pancreatic tissue is thought to be either completely normal (77) or partially depleted (124). However, true pancreatic atrophy with resultant lipomatosis also exists as a rare condition known as Shwachman syndrome (124) (see Table 6.2 in section entitled Syndromes Associated with Fatty Lesions [Including Lipomatosis]). Fatty infiltration of the heart is most often an innocuous condition with no effect on the myocardial fiber or cardiac function (77). However, there are rare exceptions in which severe adiposity has resulted in cardiac rupture (106). Another clinically important lesion is termed *lipomatous hypertrophy of the interatrial septum* (125,126), a focal enlargement that may cause sudden death, arrhythmias, or congestive failure (127,128). Be mindful that the occasional appearance of fat in endocardial biopsies in no way indicates cardiac perforation (129).

Isolated fat cells can be found within lymph nodes in childhood, but enlarged nodes with prominent fatty infiltration mainly occur in adults, particularly in obesity (123). Common in the abdomen and retroperitoneum, such "lipolymph nodes" can be mistaken for lipomas (157) or be interpreted as positive in a lymphangiogram for lymphoma or Hodgkin disease (personal observation), mimicking lymphoma relapse (158). Rarely, a lipoma or angiomyolipoma occurs in the liver (159), but those lesions should not be confused with the hepatic pseudolipoma (160). This pseudolipoma is often found as a bulge on the surface of the liver and probably represents capture of previously detached appendices epiploicae. In the mouth, fat is one of the components contributing to macroglossia in certain conditions (161).

The Ito cells of the liver are fat-containing cells along the sinuses and are a variation on normal histology (162); they may become prominent in the condition known as "lipopeliosis" (163) and may be involved in the benign neoplasm called "spongiotic pericytoma" (164).

FAT BIOPSY FOR AMYLOID

It is becoming increasingly popular to perform a subcutaneous fat biopsy for the diagnosis of amyloidosis. In such instances, the Congo red stain may reveal amyloid around blood vessels and, occasionally, between adipocytes (165–167). This procedure is at least as sensitive as the rectal biopsy (167), can identify up to 84% of cases (166), can be combined with other studies to determine amyloid type (165), and is a safe and innocuous way to make the diagnosis (166).

Biopsy analysis of adipose tissue may become important in the future to assess a given individual's storage content of toxic chemicals. Various industrial and environmental hydrocarbons are stored predominantly in fat, and subcutaneous adipose tissue deposits may be analyzed and results correlated with the development of diseases such as neoplasia.

INFLAMMATIONS

Fat Necrosis

Three histologically distinct types of fat necrosis exist: the ordinary variety secondary to trauma and other inflammation, which associated with pancreatitis and infarction of fat. Histologically, ordinary fat necrosis is typified by the presence of epithelioid histiocytes, foamy macrophages, and giant cells in adipose tissue, often surrounding and isolating individual adipocytes (Fig. 6.11). Lymphocytes and plasma cells are also found in small numbers. Occasionally, unusual crystalloids may be seen (168). Fat cells become destroyed, and the released lipid may fuse to result in a single droplet larger than the average cell or in minute droplets. This process may resolve with mild fibrosis or, if extensive, may cause cyst formation with eventual dense fibrosis and even calcification at the periphery. Such cysts with central liquefaction may be located on the buttocks and be the final result of trauma, secondary to an injection. Just beneath the cyst wall, necrotic outlines of adipocytes are usually present, signifying the origin of the end-stage cyst in fat necrosis.

TABLE 6.2
Syndromes Associated with Fatty Processes

Syndrome	Description
Diffuse mammary steatonecrosis	Fat necrosis with infarction and lipogranulomatous reaction; found in patients with large pendulous breasts (106)
Acute pancreatitis	Disseminated focal areas of fat necrosis in the subcutis; may also occur with pancreatic carcinoma (106)
Retractile mesenteritis	Fibrosis and retraction of mesentery with distortion of intestinal loops; the outcome of mesenteric panniculitis/isolated mesenteric lipodystrophy (106,130)
Weber–Christian disease (avoid term)	Historic term for a clinical syndrome with chronic inflammation, fat necrosis, and scattered acute inflammatory cells in the subcutis—"nonsuppurative panniculitis" with recurrent lesions and febrile illness; this is now known to be due to a variety of separate diseases and is a term to be avoided (131,132)
Berardinelli lipodystrophy	A minor part of a complex disorder including gigantism, hyperlipidemia, fatty cirrhosis of liver, muscular hypertrophy, and hyperpigmentation; familial (106)
Dercum disease	Multiple lipomas with pain and tenderness (106,133,134)
Fröhlich syndrome	Sexual infantilism with obesity and symmetrical or asymmetrical lipomas (a form of hypopituitarism)
Madelung disease	Symmetrical lipomatosis; associated with alcohol intake (134–136)
Gardner syndrome	Familial intestinal polyposis; subcutaneous lipomas may occur (137,138)
Multiple endocrine adenomatosis 1 (MEA-1)	Subcutaneous lipomas occur (139); a case of liposarcoma reported (140)
Shwachman syndrome	Lipomatous atrophy of the pancreas with prominent lipomatosis, maldigestion, neutropenia, and growth retardation (124)
Trite syndrome	A combination of thymolipoma, thyrolipoma, and pharyngeal lipoma (141)
Carney syndrome	Pulmonary hamartomas (which often contain fat), gastric smooth muscle tumors, and paraganglioma (142,143)
Tuberous sclerosis	Angiomyolipomas of kidney, other tumors, and hamartomas; occasionally diffuse lipomatosis (144)
Beckwith hemihypertrophy	Congenital asymmetry, some with associated Wilms tumor, occasional benign mesenchymoma with adipose tissue (145)
Familial multiple lipomas	Multiple subcutaneous lipomas (146)
Bannayan syndrome	Autosomal dominant disorder with macrocephaly, lipomas, hemangiomas, and intracranial tumors (147)
Laurence–Moon–Biedl syndrome	Congenital optic nerve atrophy, polydactyly, mental defect, and occasional adrenal lipomas (148)
Carpal tunnel syndrome	Occasionally caused by tendon sheath lipoma (149)
Fishman syndrome	Encephalocraniocutaneous lipomatosis (150,151)
Goldenhar–Gorlin syndrome	Oculoauriculovertebral dysplasia with CNS lipomas (152)
Cowden disease	GI polyposis with orocutaneous hamartomas; angiolipomas have been observed (153)
Spinal epidural lipomatosis	Fatty infiltration of epidural space (154,155); occasionally secondary to steroids (156)
Membranous lipodystrophy	Abnormal subcutaneous and bony fat with bone cysts, pathologic fractures, and leukodystrophy of brain (114–117)

An unusual type of fat necrosis forming cystic spaces has been designated *membranous fat necrosis* by Poppiti et al. (169). In this example, actual cysts are formed that contain pseudopapillary structures and central debris. Although the fat cell outlines are normal in appearance, the formation of these cysts resembles that seen in membranous lipodystrophy. Membranous fat necrosis can also occur secondary to radiation therapy (118).

Fat necrosis secondary to acute pancreatitis is histologically distinctive (Fig. 6.12). Rather than consisting of a histiocytic infiltrate, the pancreatic fat necrosis is accompanied by an infiltrate of neutrophils predominantly, and liquefaction of fat is apparent (170,171). In the center of the lesion, the infarct-like outlines of fat cells can be seen, and fat cell membranes are ruptured, releasing their contents into a central eosinophilic or basophilic material. The entire region is

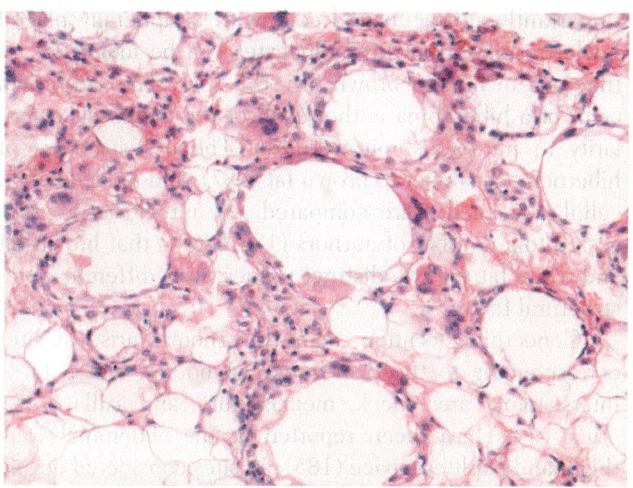

FIGURE 6.11 Fat necrosis, ordinary type. Multinucleated histiocytic giant cells surround a large lipid vacuole formed by fusion of destroyed adipocytes. Scattered lymphocytes and monocytes occupy expanded spaces between cells at top.

bordered by an acute inflammatory infiltrate. The process is thought to be secondary to the action of pancreatic lipolytic enzymes in the serum acting on susceptible foci.

The infarction type of fat necrosis, in which eosinophilic outlines of fat cells without nuclei or inflammation

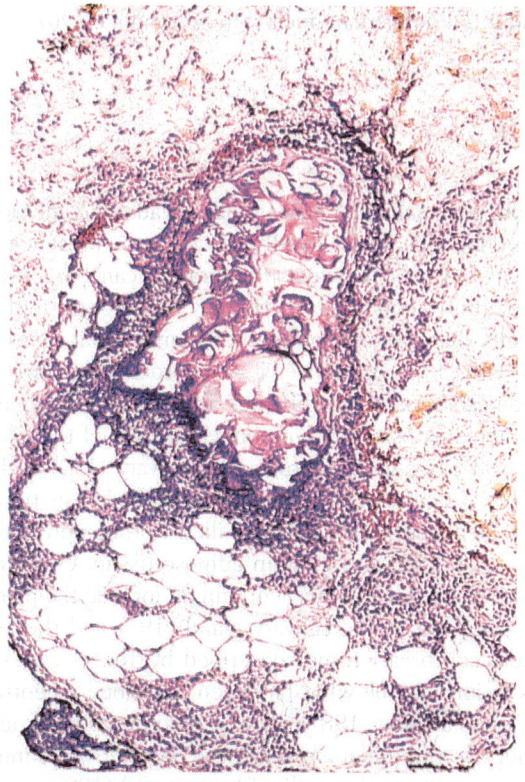

FIGURE 6.12 Fat necrosis, pancreatic type. In contrast to regular fat necrosis, numerous neutrophils are found, together with central liquefaction. The central material may give either an eosinophilic or basophilic appearance, and disrupted cell membranes can be appreciated.

are present histologically, may be seen in lipomas and in detached peritoneal tissue originating from appendices epiploicae. The lipomas containing infarction may be pedunculated with twisting, causing compromise of blood flow.

Calciphylaxis

Another disorder that often manifests itself as skin and subcutaneous fat necrosis is called "calciphylaxis"; here, the characteristic vascular necrosis with calcium precipitation will aid in the diagnosis (172). It is a painful and often lethal complication of dialysis and renal failure (173). Small vessels (including arterioles in the fat) show mural calcification and necrosis, along with thrombosis and necrosis of surrounding tissues. In some cases, an association with primary hyperparathyroidism has been reported (174).

Panniculitis

Numerous diseases and conditions may cause an inflammatory infiltrate of the subcutaneous adipose tissue, namely, a panniculitis; readers are referred to various textbooks on skin pathology for an in-depth enumeration of these. Only a few relevant points are made here. First, the condition called Weber–Christian disease, or febrile nodular nonsuppurative panniculitis of the subcutaneous fat, was described early in this century and is consistently referred to in discussions of this topic. However, it became clear in the 1960s and 1970s that this disease was not a clinically distinct entity but rather had many separate etiologies, including steroid withdrawal, diabetes mellitus, tuberculosis, pancreatic disease, and systemic lupus erythematosus (131). Thus, it is generally agreed today that Weber–Christian "disease" was a clinical description of a presentation for numerous diseases and is a term to be avoided (132).

Panniculitis, as a rule, can be divided into those that are septal and those that involve the lobules of adipose tissue (132). The character of the infiltrate is important, and note should be made of the presence of eosinophils (175), neutrophils and granulomas (176), histiocytes with lymphophagocytosis (177), or other specific changes (178). Autoimmune diseases such as scleroderma (179) and lupus (180) may be causative, indicating the importance of historical detail. Unusual causes, such as α-1–antitrypsin deficiency (132), have a characteristic histology, as does pancreatic fat necrosis (described in other texts). Even withdrawal from steroids may cause panniculitis (181).

Mesenteritis

Inflammation of the mesenteric fat is a recognizable clinical entity that has more recently been termed *mesenteric panniculitis* to signify the active inflammatory stage and *retractile mesenteritis* to signify the fibrotic stage (130). Other terms complicate the literature, but it is generally held that they all refer to the same disease process and spectrum: liposclerotic mesenteritis, sclerosing mesenteritis, ML, and Weber–Christian disease of the mesentery (see recent review by Kelly and Hwang (182)).

The process consists of a chronic inflammatory infiltrate of lymphocytes, plasma cells, foamy histiocytes, and giant cells, along with recognizable fat necrosis, edema, and a variable amount of fibrosis and calcification. Myofibroblasts proliferate and are directly involved in the pathogenesis of the retractile disease (182). While it most often thickens the mesentery (type 1 ML), it can appear as a single tumefaction at the mesenteric base (type 2 ML) or as multiple discrete nodules (type 3 ML) (183). Other space-occupying lesions, such as inflammatory pseudotumors, xanthogranulomatosis (see later), and fibromatosis, are in the differential diagnosis (158). Affected patients are usually middle-aged and predominantly male, and they complain of vague abdominal discomfort and weight loss, with more than one-half presenting with fever. Nearly one-half of them are, oddly enough, asymptomatic (182). Rare cases have been fatal, but the prognosis is generally excellent. Mass lesions regress within 2 years in about two-thirds of the patients, and any pain disappears in three-quarters of them (130). Steroids are commonly given to treat the disease, but it is unclear whether the course of the disease or the progression to fibrosis is changed (182).

Retroperitoneal xanthogranulomatosis can be due to a primary inflammatory process of the kidney, or it can represent involvement of the retroperitoneum by the mesenteritis. Many foamy histiocytes and lymphocytes are seen. Rarely, it can be associated with Erdheim–Chester disease (multisystem fibroxanthomas with bone pain and sclerotic bone lesions) (184).

Lipogranuloma

Small collections of epithelioid histiocytes with lipid droplets are commonly encountered in lymph nodes, draining the gastrointestinal tract (mesenteric, porta hepatis, retroperitoneal), and in the liver, spleen, and bone marrow. They do not imply a pancreatitis (in which necrosis should be present) or other pathologic process and are completely incidental.

TUMORS AND TUMOR-LIKE LESIONS

Brown Fat Lesions

Hibernoma

The only pathologic lesion of brown fat known to date is the hibernoma, the neoplastic counterpart given its name by Gery (185). Although many of the cells in the hibernoma are multivacuolated, some cells lack vacuoles completely and are eosinophilic and granular in appearance. Both of these cell types have a centrally placed nucleus. Importantly, univacuolated cells with peripherally placed nuclei resembling white adipocytes can be identified, as they can in normal brown fat (185,186). The red-brown color of a hibernoma is the result of the increased vascularity in numerous mitochondria. The ultrastructure of hibernoma is similar to brown fat (187), and indeed, when cellular organelles are compared, the ultrastructure suggested to a number of authors (185,186) is that brown fat and white fat are two distinct tissues, with different ultrastructural features.

Concerning location, many hibernomas arise in sites corresponding to the distribution of normal brown fat—interscapular area, neck, mediastinum, and axilla (185); other cases have been reported in the abdominal wall, thigh, and popliteal space (185), all sites considered devoid of brown fat (133). Generally, medium-sized tumors (5 to 10 cm), hibernomas may obtain a huge dimension (23 cm (188)) and are often present for years prior to excision. The tumors typically occur in young adults with a median age of 26 years, much younger than patients with ordinary lipoma (185). Interestingly, endocrine activity has been noted within these tumors, with steroid hormones (including cortisol and testosterone) detected (189). Hibernomas do not recur, but whether malignant hibernomas exist has been a controversial topic. A case having atypical mitoses and bizarre nuclei was reported by Enterline et al. (190), and a similar case with ultrastructural features was documented by Teplitz et al. (191). Recently, CD31 has been found immunohistochemically in hibernomas (96).

White Fat Lesions

Adipose Tissue Within Nonfatty Lesions

Almost any malignant tumor may invade and incorporate mature fat cells. Occasionally, however, the presence of fat cells within mesenchymal proliferation can be confusing. For example, nodular fasciitis may incorporate individual fat cells that can appear smaller than normal, mimicking lipoblasts (133). Likewise, a very prominent component of adipose tissue accompanies intramuscular hemangiomas, angiomatosis, and lymphangiomatosis of the extremities (133). Benign teratomas of the ovary (192) and lung (193,194) occasionally contain mature adipose tissue as an incidental finding. The so-called fibrous polyps of the esophagus (195) also contain adipose tissue. Other nonlipomatous tumors that may contain fat include the pleomorphic adenoma of the salivary gland (196) and the benign spindle cell breast tumor described by Toker et al. (197). This lesion may be what has been described recently as a myofibroblastoma (198) with the incorporation of adipose tissue. Even fibromatosis may have an extensive admixture of benign adipose tissue (lipofibromatosis) (199).

Perhaps by a process of cellular metaplasia, fat may also be found occasionally in the endometrium (200) or in epithelial tumors of various types (see later).

Ectopic Adipose Tissue

Ectopic fat either in cardiac valves or within organs was discussed earlier in the Metaplasia and Fatty Infiltration sections. Oddly enough, ectopic fat may occur in the dermis, where it causes a pedunculated appearance; this has been termed *nevus lipomatosis superficialis* or, more recently, *pedunculated lipofibroma* (201).

Hamartomas Containing Fat Cells

Many of us are aware that the benign pulmonary "chondroma," or "hamartoma," may contain fat (193). In fact, approximately 75% of these lesions do (202), and the presence of such a tissue foreign to the lung parenchyma supports the concept that these lesions are benign mesenchymomas (193,202). Occasionally, the lipomatous component may be so dominant as to suggest a lipoma (202,203).

Amazingly, adipose tissue can be a component of many other unusual lesions. It may be coupled with vascular, fibrous, and myofibroblastic components in multiple congenital mesenchymal hamartomas (multiple sites (204)); with undifferentiated spindle cells and fibroblasts in the fibrous hamartoma of infancy (mainly in shoulder and axillary regions (205–207)); with fibrous tissue and mature nerve in the sometimes congenital fibrolipomatous hamartoma of nerve with or without macrodactyly (palm, wrist, or fingers (208,209)); or with smooth muscle and vessels in the angiomyolipoma (210,211). These hamartomatous lesions of tuberous sclerosis will be discussed further. In another oddity, adipose tissue is one component of human tails and pseudotails (212), along with skin and other tissues.

Massive Localized Lymphedema

In morbidly obese patients, huge subcutaneous masses as large as 50 cm may form, clinically mimicking liposarcoma (213,214). Pedunculated masses of adipose tissue show dilated lymphatics and edema and thus this condition is known as massive localized lymphedema. Grossly, the fat is marbled in appearance secondary to coarse bands of fibrous tissue intersecting fat lobules. Microscopically, the adipose tissue is dissected by fibrosis simulating sclerosing liposarcoma; however, the lesion is superficial, and neither there are atypical stromal cells nor lipoblasts. In the edematous septa, scattered myofibroblasts are noted. Aside from the often postsurgical abdominal sites reported initially, massive localized lymphedema may also occur in the thigh, scrotum, and inguinal regions and be associated with hypothyroidism (214).

Mesenchymomas

Adipose tissue is a nearly constant component of what had been called "benign mesenchymomas," a term that has fallen out of favor. These growths should now be designated according to the primary component. In the past, LeBer and Stout (215) required the presence of at least two different mesenchymal elements to make a diagnosis of mesenchymoma. However, we believe that the trend has evolved in favor of diagnosing lesions with only two elements as chondrolipoma, fibrolipoma, and so on (133,134). This seems appropriate since the secondary element, usually in a lipoma, is frequently a very focal finding (as it may be in a liposarcoma). Lesions with three or more elements have been designated true mesenchymomas. For instance, a description of a trigeminal neurilemmoma (216) was really a mesenchymoma with cartilage, bone, hemangioma, schwannoma, and adipose tissue. Also, a thoracic tumor with smooth muscle, angiomatoid spaces, fibrous tissue, and adipose tissue is another mesenchymoma, reported in association with hemihypertrophy (145). Angiomyolipoma could be considered an example of a "mesenchymoma" and is frequently found in the kidney, where approximately 40% are associated with tuberous sclerosis (211). Although the fat seen here is practically always mature, rarely lipoblast-like cells may be seen in these tumors (133,217). Angiomyolipomas have also been reported in other sites, such as lymph nodes (218). In general, however, the term "mesenchymoma" should be avoided and an attempt made to classify according to the predominant cell type.

Lipomas

The distinction between adipose tissue lobules and true lipoma occasionally arises in the practice of surgical pathology, necessitating a strict definition of lipoma. Although lipoma is well described in two major texts (133,134), definitions are concise without detail. Lipoma is herein defined as a superficial or deep-circumscribed and expansile benign neoplasm composed of mature adipose tissue, which is commonly (but need not be) encapsulated. Such a definition emphasizes its well-differentiated and clonal nature (see following) and serves to distinguish most lipomas from normal fat and prominent posttraumatic skin folds, or "fat fractures" (219). As Allen (134) emphasizes, the capsule may be quite thin and poorly defined. Nonetheless, it is a crucial requirement for superficial tumors; deep lesions, on the contrary, are often nonencapsulated. When a subcutaneous lipoma is excised in a piecemeal fashion, the lesion may be diagnosed by noting the presence of portions of capsular fibrous tissue in the form of a circular arc of collagen of varying width at the edge of tissue fragments. In the absence of a clear-cut capsule or fragments thereof, a diagnosis of a superficial lipoma cannot be made.

Clinically, the majority of lipomas seen in surgical pathology are subcutaneous tumors typically in the middle-aged to elderly patient. Males and females are probably equally affected, and there are no racial differences. Most tumors are located on the trunk or upper extremities; if other sites are encountered, consideration should be given to one of the lipoma subtypes (e.g., forearm for angiolipoma, neck for spindle and pleomorphic types). Lipomas probably outnumber all other soft tissue tumors combined (133). Interesting facts about lipomas include, (a) a nearly static size after the initial growth period (133); (b) the relative rarity of lesions on the hands, feet, face, and lower leg despite the presence of fat (133); (c) hardness after the application of ice, a diagnostic sign (133); (d) the lack of size reduction in starvation (133,134); (e) a definite, but low, recurrence rate (1% to 4% (133,134)); (f) an unknown etiology; (g) a possible relation to potassium intake (220); and (h) a possible association with an increased incidence of cancer (46% (221)).

Many lesions of the subcutaneous region come to surgical pathology labeled as lipomas, and not uncommonly, a portion of these actually turn out to be something else that is frequently more interesting.

When one views normal fat histologically, the size of fat cells appears to vary somewhat due to the sectioning plane; however, the variation is relatively small (80 to 120 μm) (personal observation) (Fig. 6.4). In lipomas, including atypical lipoma (222), there is a tendency for cell size to vary more widely, with larger cells (e.g., >300 μm) being apparent. Practically, this means that a medium-power view will often disclose a two- to fivefold size range (Fig. 6.13). Normal fat has a netlike structure of fibrous tissue, wherein such dispersed fibrous bands or septa dissect the adipose tissue randomly. The fibrous tissue is thicker in quality in bodily regions exposed to pressure, such as the hands, feet, and buttocks (106). This netlike fibrous tissue arrangement is recapitulated within lipomas (Fig. 6.14), particularly at the periphery where small lobules are often found. A high degree of vascularity is a feature associated with lipogenic malignancy, but we should be aware that this refers to a visible network of capillaries, often in strings and branching arrays. However, normal adipose tissue and lipomas are likewise highly vascular, except the capillary vascular bed is more difficult to visualize. A PAS stain of a lipoma, for example, can highlight the minute but diffuse capillaries, particularly at the junctions between cells, where they are

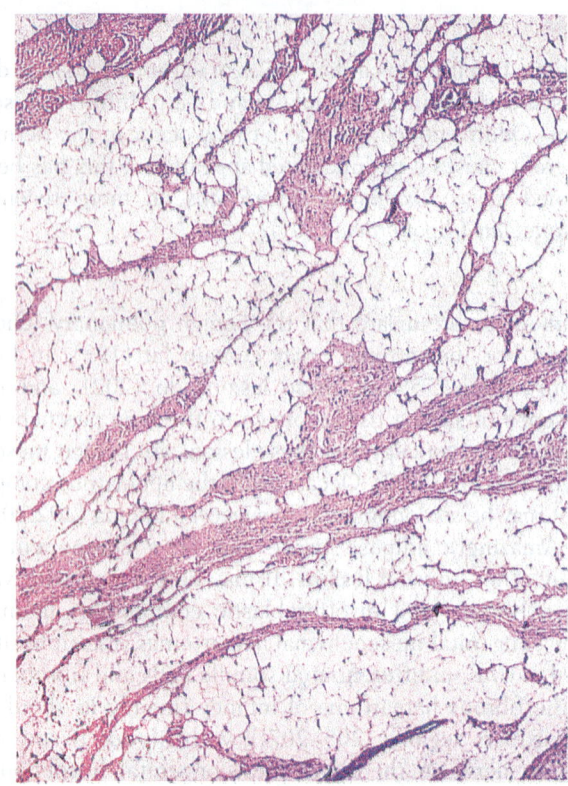

FIGURE 6.14 Lipoma with accentuated lobulation. In certain sites such as the buttock, foot, and hand (*depicted here*), thick fibrous septa are noted throughout; these correspond to the thicker septa within the normal adipose tissue in these regions.

made more difficult to see due to compression. A delicate reticulin network is also present in lipomas, contributed to by the basement membranes of both lipocytes and capillaries; each lipocyte is completely encircled by reticulin in a manner similar to normal fat cells (Fig. 6.3). Normally, lipomas have a low degree of cellularity and no nuclear atypia; the presence of either is cause for concern. Sometimes increased cellularity is due to a diffuse low-grade form of fat necrosis (Fig. 6.15). The ultrastructure of lipoma recapitulates that of its normal counterpart (223).

Myxoid Change

In rare lipomas, the mature fat cells are separated by varying amounts of a loose basophilic ground substance, probably proteoglycan (Fig. 6.16). When prominent, the lesion may be designated a *myxolipoma* or *myxoid lipoma* (133,134). The myxoid quality often raises the possibility of an MLS. However, these areas contain only widely scattered bland cells and are never hypercellular. Furthermore, the plexiform capillary network so typical of the malignant tumor is absent, as are lipoblasts. As Enzinger and Weiss (133) observed, rare cells may be vacuolated but contain bluish mucoid material.

Intramuscular Lipoma

Deep lipomas may be either intermuscular or intramuscular, with the latter unencapsulated tumors being the more

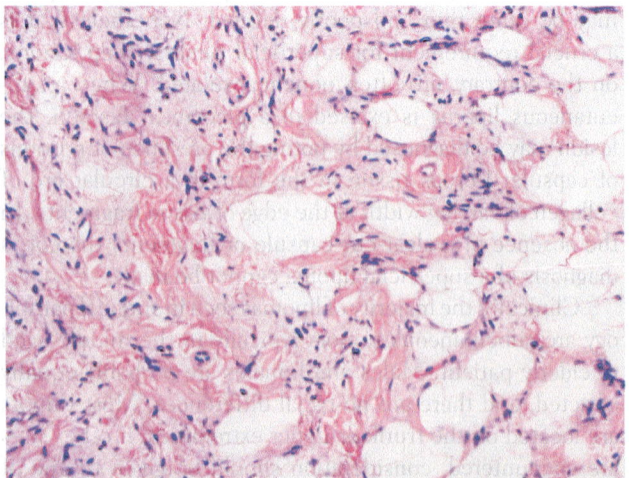

FIGURE 6.13 Variation in fat cell size in spindle cell lipoma. Some adipocytes are three to five times the size of a normal adipocyte; compare with Figure 6.4. Increased numbers of spindle cells together with collagen bands characterize this lipoma subtype, although the size variation seems to be present in all unusual types of lipoma.

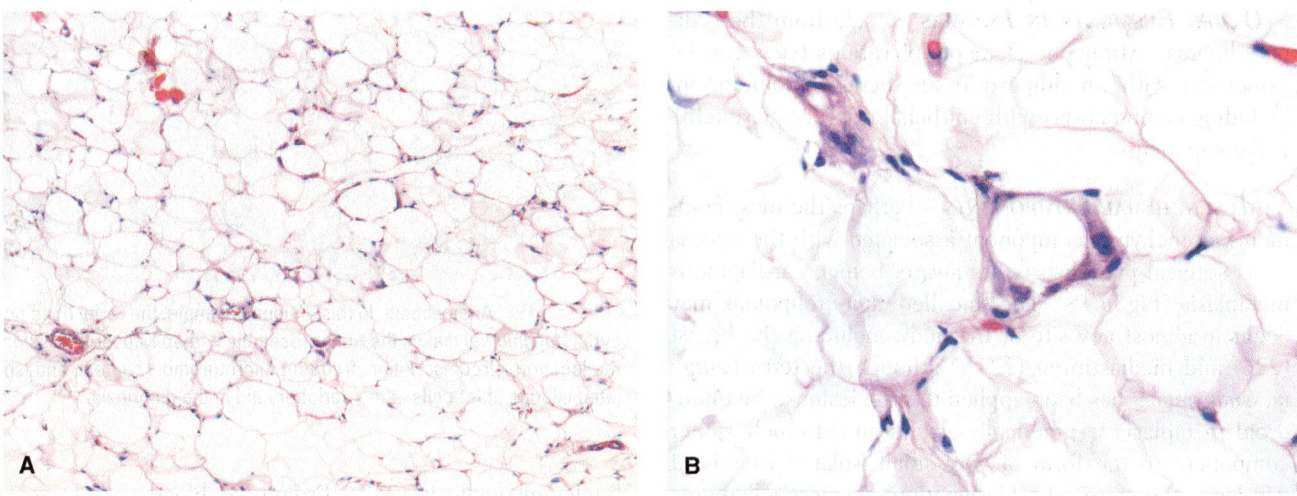

FIGURE 6.15 Lipoma. **A:** In some tumors, an increased cellularity at medium power may cause concern, but it is frequently due to a mild but diffuse fat necrosis. **B:** The lipocytes are falsely enlarged by the histiocytes without much other inflammation.

common. Intramuscular lipomas (224), also known as "infiltrating lipomas," involve the large muscles of the extremities (particularly the thigh, shoulder, and upper arm) or the paraspinal muscles. For extremity lesions, an inapparent mass may become visible upon voluntary contraction. Microscopically, the lipocytes are typically mature, and mitoses or atypical nuclei are not found. Muscle fibers are widely dispersed throughout the lesion (Fig. 6.17). Any unusual features should raise the suspicion of a well-differentiated liposarcoma (225). Often, intramuscular lipomas extend beyond the muscle fascia to involve the intervening connective tissue space. Therefore, it is often difficult to completely excise such lesions, and the recurrence rate is higher than that for ordinary subcutaneous lipoma. This has been particularly true for paraspinal intramuscular lipomas.

Intramuscular angiolipomas are lesions considered to be intramuscular hemangiomas with a variable fat content (133).

Lipoma arborescens is a special type of lipoma occurring in a joint: it has a characteristic villiform gross appearance, and the patients typically have a highly painful knee (134). The mere presence of adipose tissue on a synovial biopsy is not synonymous with this entity.

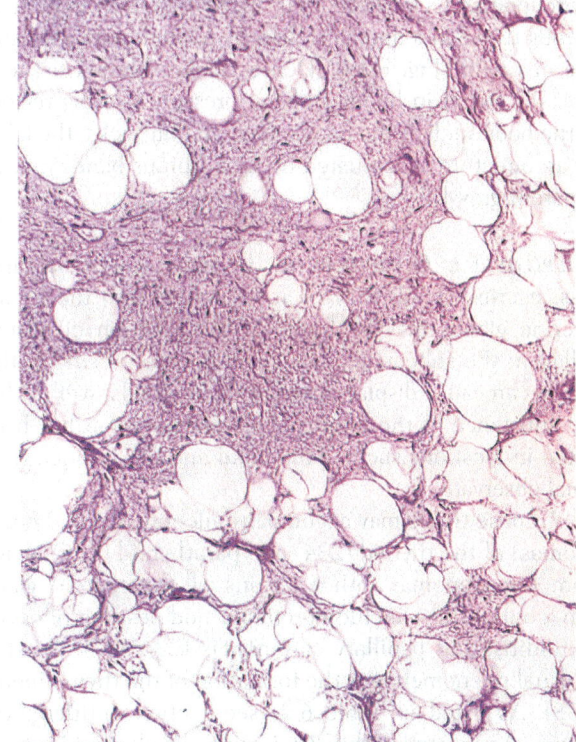

FIGURE 6.16 Lipoma with myxoid change. Features that differentiate this from myxoid liposarcoma are the lack of branching capillary vessels and significant cellularity in the myxoid component.

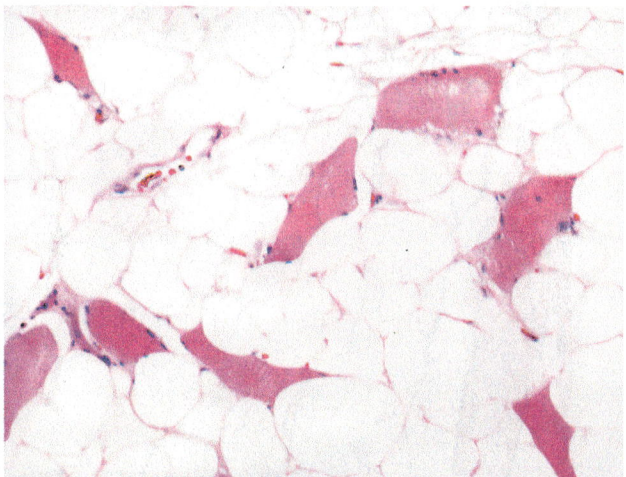

FIGURE 6.17 Lipoma, intramuscular type. The light fat cells proliferate between dark individual skeletal muscle fibers in this commonly unencapsulated tumor (trichrome stain).

› **OTHER ELEMENTS IN LIPOMAS** Aside from the ordinary lipoma, extraneous elements of various types can be associated with an adipose tissue benign proliferation, including combinations with epithelial or other mesenchymal components.

› **MESENCHYMAL COMPONENTS** Perhaps the most common mesenchymal component associated with the lipoma is, as surgical pathologists are aware, benign cartilaginous metaplasia (Fig. 6.18). The so-called chondrolipomas may occur in almost any site of the body, including the breast (226) and mediastinum (227). Although the term *benign mesenchymoma* has been applied to such lesions, the chondroid metaplasia is practically always an extremely minor component in the form of very small isolated islands of cartilage; therefore, the designation of mesenchymoma appears to be an exaggeration (as it is when cartilaginous metaplasia occurs in liposarcoma). Allen (228) also prefers to avoid the term *mesenchymoma*.

Lipochondromatosis is a recently reported entity that involves the tendons and synovium of the ankle region as a mass lesion (229). Rarely benign osteoid is also found in lipomas, either solely or coupled with cartilage (230). Some of these osteolipomas are in contact with periosteum and may be termed *periosteal lipoma* (230). Smooth muscle lesions, particularly of the uterus, may be combined with adipose tissue to produce lipoleiomyomas (231) and

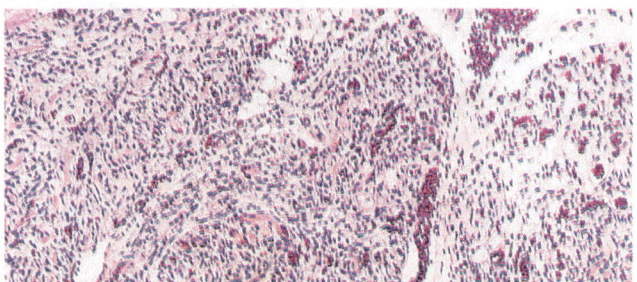

FIGURE 6.19 Angiolipoma. In this unusual example, the rarity of adipocytes (*top middle*) makes the tumor resemble a deep Kaposi-like lesion; the location, circumscription, frequent microthrombi (*center*), and isolated islands of fat cells at the periphery aid in the diagnosis.

lipoleiomyomatosis (232). Prominent blood vessels are a frequent component of superficial small subcutaneous tumors called "angiolipomas" (133). These lesions are interesting, as they may be multiple, cause pain due to frequent microthrombi, increase in size with anabolic steroids due to androgen receptors (141), and give rise to the differential diagnosis of Kaposi sarcoma when the angiomatoid component completely overcomes the lipocytic component (Fig. 6.19). These fat-poor variants are designated cellular angiolipomas (233). In such instances, the diagnosis is made by finding rare-to-scattered mature fat cells, usually at the periphery of the lesion.

Some lipomas contain an increased content of fibrous tissue. These usually superficial tumors have been called "fibrolipomas." However, it is likely that the amount of fibrous tissue in a lipoma is directly related to its anatomic site of origin (Fig. 6.14). Dense thicker fibrous tissue is typically found in lipomas of the pressure-bearing regions of the body such as the hands, feet, and buttocks; the lobular architecture accentuated by such fibrous bands may be apparent grossly.

› **EPITHELIAL COMPONENTS** In some superficial lipomas, eccrine glands may be incorporated into the lesion. Eccrine glands may be found at the junction of dermal collagen; the subcutaneous fat and lipomas arising in this region can cause displacement of these glands, well within the substance of the lipoma. This phenomenon has been noted in locations such as the hand and the buttock (personal observation).

Adipose tissue may accompany adenomas (i.e., lipoadenomas) of the thyroid (234) and parathyroid (235). Aside from lipoadenomas, other lesions of the thyroid gland may contain fat—including colloid nodules, lymphocytic thyroiditis, and papillary carcinomas (236,237). Another unusual phenomenon is the formation of the thymolipoma (238). As listed in Table 6.2 (see section entitled Syndromes Associated with Fatty Lesions [Including Lipomatosis]), an unusual lipomatous syndrome is described that consists of thyrolipoma, thymolipoma, and pharyngeal lipoma (239).

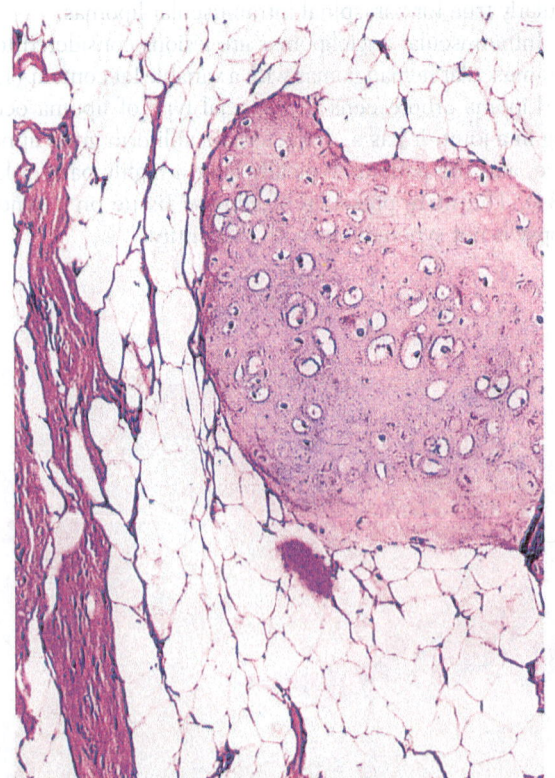

FIGURE 6.18 Chondrolipoma. Small nodules of mature cartilage are present, often very focally; this combination alone should not be labeled a mesenchymoma.

▸ LYMPHOCYTES IN LIPOMAS Occasionally, one may observe a dense perivascular lymphocytic infiltrate in scattered vessels within and outside ordinary lipomas. Although not generally described, the authors have observed this phenomenon several times and investigated the patients; they have not exhibited evidence of chronic lymphocytic leukemia or autoimmune disease. Perhaps this may represent a localized host reaction to the proliferation.

Special Lipoma Types

In the spindle cell (240–242) and pleomorphic (243,244) lipomas, the fat cells appear variable in size at low power. In spindle cell lipoma (Fig. 6.13), the spindle cell content may vary from scanty to abundant, and the nuclei of the spindle cells are wavy, resembling nerve sheath lesions. Dense fibrous tissue is also found sometimes with a keloidal quality. Similar cells may be seen in pleomorphic lipoma, which has, in addition, characteristic floret tumor giant cells (Fig. 6.20). Both of these lesions are encapsulated and have characteristic locations commonly limited to the head and the neck of elderly males. They appear to be related entities (245). Interestingly, immunoreactivity for androgen receptor has been demonstrated in the fibroblast-like spindle cells of spindle cell lipoma (246).

A tumor-like fatty mass in the periorbital region may also contain floret cells similar to pleomorphic lipoma; this entity is termed either "prolapsed orbital fat" or "subconjunctival herniated orbital fat" (247,248).

The chondroid lipoma is a well-circumscribed lesion with two elements: mature adipose tissue and focal or prominent areas containing strands and nests of eosinophilic vacuolated cells resembling chondroblasts or lipoblasts. A hyalinized myxoid matrix is also seen. This tumor is S100 protein, vimentin, and CD68 positive and may be cytokeratin positive. It occurs mainly in women in the superficial soft tissues or skeletal muscle of extremities, head, and neck. While worrisome in appearance, the lesion does not recur or metastasize (249,250).

Finally, an unusual fatty tumor of the mediastinum with elastic tissue has been described as elastofibrolipoma (251).

Lipoblastoma

Frequently, a congenital lesion, the lipoblastoma (252–258) is a benign solitary proliferation of fat, retaining the lobular architecture of developing fetal white adipose tissue. Nearly 90% of these superficial lesions occur before the age of 3 (133). Interestingly, lesions tend to mature with the age of the patient. Tumors may be predominantly myxoid with spindle cells, predominantly lipocytic, or mixed; all types have a prominent capillary bed and are often encapsulated. When mature fat cells are present, they are typically in the central portion of the lobules, in turn surrounded by collagen. In contrast, the presence of maturing adipocytes in MLS is frequently found at the periphery of the lobule (257). Thus, while these tumors bear a resemblance to MLS, there are clear differences, and the lobular accentuation with collagen is quite typical (Fig. 6.21), as is the age at presentation. Rare cells resembling brown fat or hibernoma cells have been identified in lipoblastoma (256). If these lesions are single, they should be termed *lipoblastoma* (253) and not *lipoblastomatosis* (255,258); that was the original designation given appropriately by Vellios et al. in 1958 for a diffuse form (252).

Lipoblastomatosis

Lipoblastomatosis is the proper designation for the less common diffuse form of lipoblastoma. About one-third of the patients have diffuse tumors, which (in contrast to the solitary form) are usually deeply situated, more poorly circumscribed, infiltrating muscle, and with a higher tendency to recur (253).

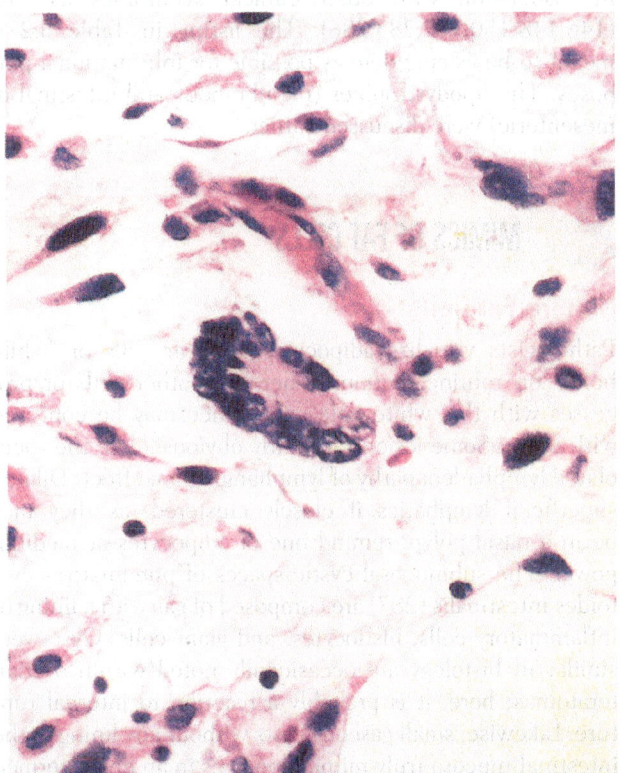

FIGURE 6.20 Floret cell. The wreath of nuclei at the periphery characterizes this cell, which is classically present in pleomorphic lipoma but may occur in some liposarcomas.

CYTOGENETICS OF LIPOMAS

Chromosomal karyotypes of lipomas have been studied (259–266) and reveal nonrandom changes involving chromosomes 3 and 12, indicative of clonality. The balanced translocation t(3;12) is a common finding (261,262), with breakpoints described at probably identical locations—q27;q13 (253) and q28;q14 (259). The breakpoint on

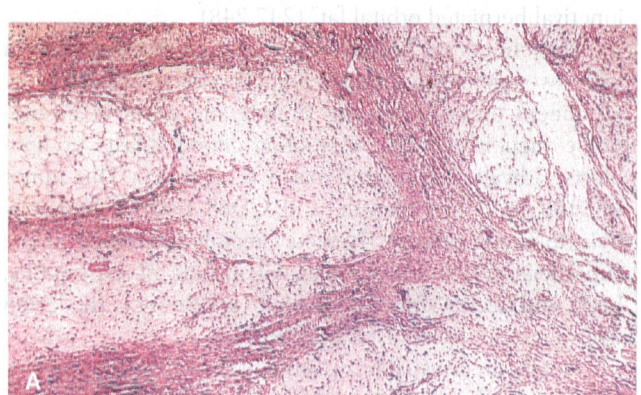
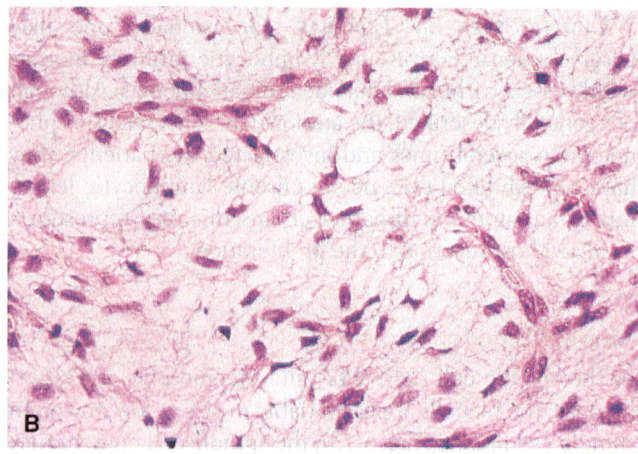

FIGURE 6.21 Lipoblastoma. **A:** At low power, a distinctly lobulated appearance can be observed. In some lobules, differentiation has started in the center. **B:** Within the myxoid lobules, small lipoblasts and spindle cells are found. The spindle cells are similar to those in developing fat (see Fig. 6.2B).

chromosome 12 is very close to the one described in the t(12;16) translocation in MLSs (261). This balanced translocation involving chromosome 12 is seen in roughly 50% of lipomas (262) and may involve other chromosomes such as 21 and 7 (262). Another one-third of lipomas show a ring chromosome (262) originally described by Heim et al. (263) as a possible rearrangement of chromosome 3; this may be a marker for lipogenic tumors. Rarely, chromosome 6 has shown an abnormality (266). Interestingly, subgroups of lipomas may show different cytogenetic changes (264).

Likewise, clonal chromosomal changes are noted in lipoblastoma with the abnormality at 8q11–q13 (267).

SYNDROMES ASSOCIATED WITH FATTY LESIONS (INCLUDING LIPOMATOSIS)

The word *lipomatosis* may appropriately refer to two separate conditions: the presence of multiple subcutaneous lipomas and the infiltration of organs or sites such as the pelvis (268,269) by adipose tissue. The bilateral multiple symmetrical lipomatosis (MSL) syndrome (Madelung disease (135,136,270–272)) is said to be frequently accompanied by a high intake of alcohol (134). However, there is increasing evidence that there is no association of MSL with alcohol abuse (154), that there may be a constitutional mitochondrial dysfunction (155), that mitochondrial DNA may be abnormal (273), that patients have plasma lipid anomalies (274), and that the cells involved may be distorted brown fat cells supportive of a neoplastic nature to MSL (275).

Lipomatosis may involve a single portion of the body, such as the face (276), the spinal epidural area (156,277–279), the mesentery (280), the mediastinum and abdomen (281), the mediastinum alone (282), the brain (150,151), and the kidney (283), as well as subcutaneous tissue (284). Syndromes relating to many of these are delineated in Table 6.2.

Lipomas, either as single or multiple tumors, may be part of various syndromes (Table 6.2), some of which are autosomal dominant (Gardner syndrome (137,138), MEA type 1 (139,140), Bannayan syndrome (147), or tuberous sclerosis (144)). Pathologists may find it interesting to note that lipomatous lesions may also occur in Cowden disease (153), Beckwith hemihypertrophy (134), and as fat within a pulmonary "hamartoma" in Carney syndrome (142,143).

Furthermore, adipose tissue lesions may be found in association with other clinical syndromes as well (146,148,150,152,285,286). The listing in Table 6.2 is meant to be as complete as possible for informational purposes. The lipodystrophies (membranous and intestinal or mesenteric) were discussed earlier.

MIMICS OF FAT CELLS

Mature Fat Cells

Pathologists visualize adipocytes as clear cells or "white holes" on routine sections. Therefore, other cells or processes with this white hole appearance may be confused with them. Some lesions are fairly obvious—like the vacuolated lymphadenopathy of lymphangiogram effect. Dilated superficial lymphatics if closely clustered, as they may be in a nasal polyp, remind one of adipocytes at medium power. The submucosal cystic spaces of pneumatosis cystoides intestinalis (287) are composed of gas with a lining of inflammatory cells, histiocytes, and giant cells. Cysts very similar in histology are occasionally noted within ovarian teratomas; here, it is probably a reaction to internal rupture. Likewise, small gaseous cysts without any lining in the intestinal mucosa truly mimic lipocytes in an entity termed *pseudolipomatosis* (287). Similar clear but artifactual vacuoles in the skin have been called "pseudolipomatosis cutis" (288). Termed *villous edema* in placental texts, this artifact

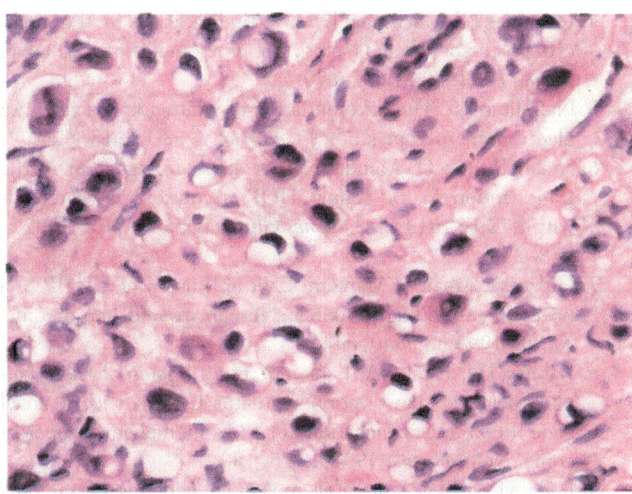

FIGURE 6.22 Adipocyte mimic. Subcutaneous metastases from either signet-ring carcinoma or melanoma (*seen here*) may rarely imitate a lipocytic tumor.

of chorionic villi gives them a pseudolipomatous appearance. Lipid-filled sinusoidal Ito cells in the liver simulate small adipocytes in vitamin A toxicity (289).

Lipoblasts

The response to the lipid-like substance silicone after the rupture of a breast implant can cause concern: when the response to the silicone is marked with sheets of histiocytes containing a single dominant vacuole, the cells resemble lipoblasts and the lesion may be mistaken for liposarcoma.

Tumors with vacuoles also cause the pathologist to consider a lipocytic origin. Metastases to the skin or subcutaneous region of signet-ring carcinoma or signet-ring melanoma (Fig. 6.22) (290) may resemble lipoblasts, and other helpful features such as nesting or spindling are not always present. Lymphomas of both B- and T-cell origin exhibiting a vacuolated or signet-ring appearance have recently been described (291–295), may mimic liposarcoma (295), and should be in the differential diagnosis of cutaneous, nodal, or retroperitoneal tumors.

Mesenchymal tumors such as epithelioid smooth muscle lesions and fibrohistiocytic neoplasms (Fig. 6.23) can be vacuolated as well, due to an artifact and proteoglycan material, respectively. These two tumor groups, particularly in the form of gastrointestinal stromal tumors and myxofibrosarcoma, probably account for the largest number of lesions mistaken for liposarcoma. In the gastrointestinal stromal tumor, the perinuclear vacuole coupled with a cellular epithelioid morphology can closely mimic the round cell or cellular MLS. In myxofibrosarcoma, vacuolated cells superficially simulate the lipoblast, but closer inspection reveals a delicate basophilic substance in the cytoplasm, apparently due to matrix production by the tumor cells (Fig. 6.23). Unusual paragangliomas with vacuoles (296,297) may also be puzzling. Other lesions most often

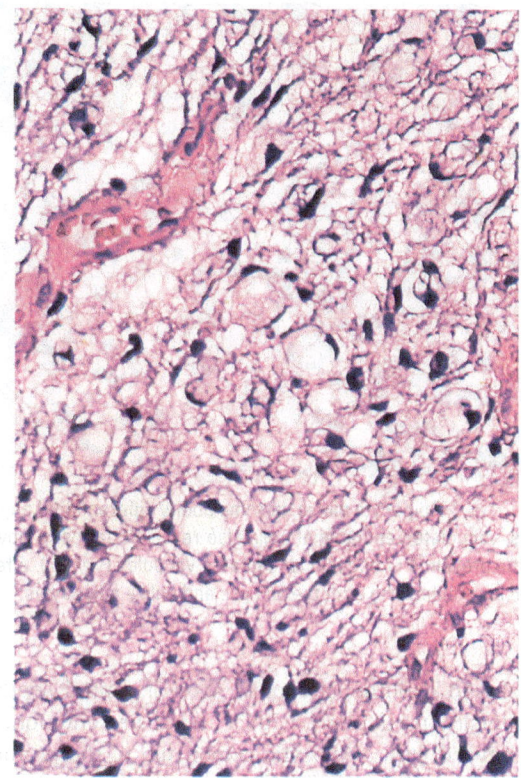

FIGURE 6.23 Lipoblast mimic. In fibrohistiocytic tumors like myxoid dermatofibrosarcoma and myxoid malignant fibrous histiocytoma, cells with a vacuolated appearance may be confused with lipoblasts; however, the vacuole contains a wispy bluish coloration due to the presence of proteoglycan matrix.

simulating lipocytes are those of endothelial origin because a true and often large vacuole is produced. Such cells may be identified in the histiocytoid hemangioma (298), in other epithelioid angiomas (299,300), in the spindle cell hemangioma (Fig. 6.24) (301), in epithelioid hemangioendothelioma (302), and in some poorly differentiated angiosarcomas (Fig. 6.25). In contrast to most large lipoblasts, the large

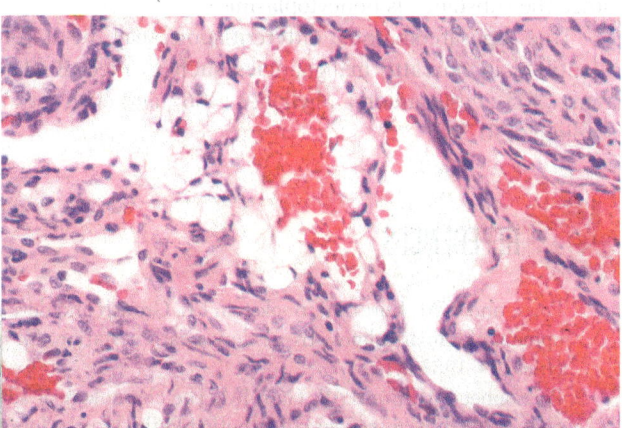

FIGURE 6.24 Adipocyte mimic. Large vacuolated cells can be found in the spindle cell hemangioma, but they are endothelial in nature and often line vascular spaces as seen here.

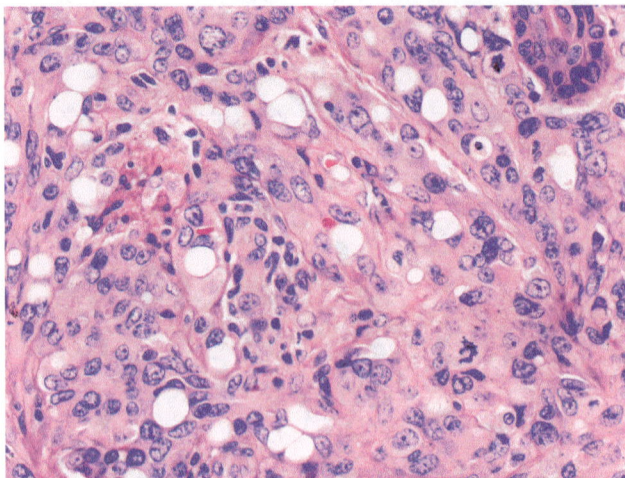

FIGURE 6.25 Adipocyte mimic. In some poorly differentiated angiosarcomas, vacuolated endothelial cells also resemble fat cells; however, note the presence of occasional septated vacuoles (*center*), a feature typical for proliferating endothelial cells and unlike adipocytes.

vacuoles in endothelial tumors show a central septation. Chordomas, particularly with a sacral presentation, may be confused with a lipocytic tumor due to the prominent vacuolization of the physaliphorous cells. The benign notochordal cell tumor has large clear vacuoles devoid of mucin and this may be mistaken for a peculiar change in vertebral body adipose tissue (303). Mesotheliomas may also be vacuolated mimicking liposarcoma (304).

The best defense against a misdiagnosis of another tumor as a lipocytic one is strict adherence to the definition of a lipoblast: a cell, occasionally large but usually small, with a vacuole or vacuoles indenting the nucleus. The requirement for nuclear indentation assures an intracellular/cytoplasmic location for the vacuole and also excludes the semicircular nuclei around small vascular channels. Extracellular vacuoles are a common phenomenon, particularly in lesions with areas of mucoid matrix, and are often mistaken for a true intracellular finding; however, the nucleus is never affected since the substance is noncytoplasmic.

True liposarcomatous differentiation may be rarely identified in nonfatty malignancies such as medulloblastoma (305), cystosarcoma phyllodes (306), and even mesothelioma (307).

REFERENCES

1. Poissonnet CM, Burdi AR, Bookstein FL. Growth and development of human adipose tissue during early gestation. *Early Hum Dev* 1983;8:1–11.
2. Poissonnet CM, Burdi AR, Garn JM. The chronology of adipose tissue appearance and distribution in the human fetus. *Early Hum Dev* 1984;10:1–11.
3. Robinson DS. In: Florkin M, Stotz EH, eds. *Comparative Biochemistry*. Vol. 18. Amsterdam: Elsevier; 1970:51–116.
4. Hausman GJ, Champion DR, Martin RJ. Search for the adipocyte precursor cell and factors that promote its differentiation. *J Lipid Res* 1980;21:657–670.
5. Napolitano L. The differentiation of white adipose cells. An electron microscope study. *J Cell Biol* 1963;18:663–679.
6. Aman P, Ron D, Mandahl N, et al. Rearrangement of the transcription factor gene CHOP in myxoid liposarcomas with t(12;16)(q13;p11). *Genes Chromosomes Cancer* 1992;5:278–285.
7. Crozat A, Aman P, Mandahl F, et al. Fusion of CHOP to a novel RNA-binding protein in human myxoid liposarcoma. *Nature* 1993;363:640–644.
8. Rabitts TH, Forster A, Larson R, et al. Fusion of the dominant negative transcription regulator CHOP with a novel gene FUS by translocation t(12;16) in malignant liposarcoma. *Nature Genet* 1993;4:175–180.
9. Ladanyi M. The emerging molecular genetics of sarcoma translocations. *Diagn Mol Pathol* 1995;4:162–173.
10. LeBrun DP, Warnke RA, Cleary ML. Expression of bcl-2 in fetal tissues suggests a role in morphogenesis. *Am J Pathol* 1993;142:743–753.
11. Martin RJ, Ramsay T, Hausman GJ. Adipocyte development. *Pediatr Ann* 1984;13:448–453.
12. Poissonnet CM, LaVelle M, Burdi AR. Growth and development of adipose tissue. *J Pediatr* 1988;113(1 Pt 1):1–9.
13. Hirsch J, Batchelor B. Adipose tissue cellularity in human obesity. *Clin Endocrinol Metab* 1976;5:299–311.
14. Faust IM. Factors which affect adipocyte formation in the rat. In: Bjorntorp P, Cairella M, Howard AN, eds. *Recent Advances in Obesity Research III. Proceedings of the 3rd International Congress on Obesity*. London: John Libbey; 1981:52–57.
15. Bjorntorp P. Adipocyte precursor cells. In: Bjorntorp P, Cairella M, Howard AN, eds. *Recent Advances in Obesity Research III. Proceedings of the 3rd International Congress on Obesity*. London: John Libbey;1981:58–69.
16. Sjostrom L, William-Olsson T. Prospective studies on adipose tissue development in man. *Int J Obes* 1981;5:597–604.
17. Nakao N, Nakayama T, Yahata T, et al. Adipose tissue derived mesenchymal stem cells facilitate hematopoiesis in vitro and in vivo. *Am J Pathol* 2010;117:547–554.
18. Witkowska-Zimny M, Walenko K. Stem cells from adipose tissue. *Cell Mol Biol Lett* 2011;16:236–257.
19. Kolata G. Why do people get fat? *Science* 1985;227:1327–1328.
20. Hirsch J, Fried SK, Edens NK, et al. The fat cell. *Med Clin North Am* 1989;73:83–96.
21. Cinti S, Frederich RC, Zingaretti C, et al. Immunohistochemical localization of leptin and uncoupling protein in white and brown adipose tissue. *Endocrinology* 1997;138:797–804.
22. Hukshorn CJ, Saris WH. Leptin and energy expenditure. *Curr Opin Clin Nutr Metab Care* 2004;7:629–633.
23. Jequier E. Leptin signaling, adiposity, and energy balance. *Ann N Y Acad Sci* 2002;967:379–388.
24. Fruhbeck G, Gomez-Ambrosi J, Muruzabal FJ, et al. The adipocyte: A model for integration of endocrine and metabolic signaling in energy metabolism regulation. *Am J Physiol Endocrinol Metab* 2001;280:E827–E847.
25. Wisse BE. The inflammatory syndrome: The role of adipose tissue cytokines in metabolic disorders linked to obesity. *J Am Soc Nephrol* 2004;15:2792–2800.

26. Choy LN, Rosen BS, Spiegelman BM. Adipsin and an endogenous pathway of complement from adipose cells. *J Biol Chem* 1992;267:12736–12741.
27. Birgel M, Gottschling-Zeller H, Rohrig K, et al. Role of cytokines in the regulation of plasminogen activator inhibitor-1 expression and secretion in newly differentiated subcutaneous human adipocytes. *Arterioscler Thromb Vasc Biol* 2000; 20:1682–1687.
28. De Pauw A, Tejerina S, Keijer J, et al. Mitochondrial (dys) function in adipocyte (de)differentiation and systemic metabolic alterations. *Am J Pathol* 2009;175:927–939.
29. Rebuffe-Scrive M, Enk L, Crona N, et al. Fat cell metabolism in different regions in women. Effect of menstrual cycle, pregnancy, and lactation. *J Clin Invest* 1985;75: 1973–1976.
30. Fried SK, Kral JB. Sex differences in regional distribution of fat cell size and lipoprotein lipase activity in morbidly obese patients. *Int J Obes* 1987;11:129–140.
31. Bjorntorp P. The regulation of adipose tissue distribution in humans. *Int J Obes Relat Metab Disord* 1996;20:291–302.
32. Kopelman PG. Effects of obesity on fat topography: Metabolic and endocrine determinants. In: Kopelman PG, Stock MJ, eds. *Clinical Obesity*. Oxford: Blackwell Science; 1998: 158–175.
33. Bjorntorp P. Fat cell distribution and metabolism. *Ann NY Acad Sci* 1987;499:66–72.
34. Hutley L, Shurety W, Newell F, et al. Fibroblast growth factor 1: A key regulator of human adipogenesis. *Diabetes* 2004;53:3097–3106.
35. Hube F, Hauner H. The role of TNF-a in human adipose tissue: Prevention of weight gain at the expense of insulin resistance? *Horm Metab Res* 1999;31:626–631.
36. Strassmann G, Fong M, Kenney JS, et al. Evidence for the involvement of interleukin 6 in experimental cancer cachexia. *J Clin Invest* 1992;89:1681–1684.
37. Stephens JM, Pekala PH. Transcriptional repression of GLUT4 and C/EBP genes in 3T3-L1 adipocytes by tumor necrosis factor-alpha. *J Biol Chem* 1991;266:21839–21845.
38. Hellman B, Hellerstrom C. Cell renewal in the white and brown fat of the rat. *Acta Pathol Microbiol Scand* 1961;51: 347–353.
39. Hollenberg CH, Vost A. Regulation of DNA synthesis in fat cells and stromal elements from rat adipose tissue. *J Clin Invest* 1969;47:2485–2498.
40. Napolitano L. The fine structure of adipose tissues. In: Reynold AE, Cahill GF, eds. *Handbook of Physiology. Section 5: Adipose Tissue*. Washington, DC: American Physical Society; 1965:109–123.
41. Nnodim JO. Development of adipose tissue. *Anat Rec* 1987; 219:331–337.
42. Schulz TJ, Huang TL, Tran TT, et al. Identification of inducible brown adipocyte progenitors residing in skeletal muscle and white fat. *Proc Natl Acad Sci U S A* 2011;108(1): 143–148.
43. Merklin RJ. Growth and distribution of human fetal brown fat. *Anat Rec* 1974;178:637–646.
44. Heaton JM. The distribution of brown adipose tissue in the human. *J Anat* 1972;112(Pt 1):35–39.
45. Girardier L. Brown fat: An energy dissipating tissue. In: Girardier L, Stock MJ, eds. *Mammalian Thermogenesis*. London: Chapman and Hall; 1983;50–98.
46. Rothwell NJ, Stock MJ. Brown adipose tissue. In: Baker PF, ed. *Recent Advances in Physiology*. Vol. 10. Edinburgh: Churchill Livingstone; 1984:349–384.
47. Rothwell NJ, Stock MJ. Whither brown fat? *Biosci Rep* 1986;6:3–18.
48. Bouillaud F, Combes-George M, Ricquier D. Mitochondria of adult human brown adipose tissue contain a 32000-Mr uncoupling protein. *Biosci Rep* 1983;3:775–780.
49. Cunningham S, Leslie P, Hopwood D, et al. The characterization and energetic potential of brown adipose tissue in man. *Clin Sci (Lond)* 1985;69:343–348.
50. Rothwell NJ, Stock MJ. A role for brown adipose tissue in diet-induced thermogenesis. *Nature* 1979;281:31–35.
51. Himms-Hagen J. Brown adipose tissue thermogenesis: Interdisciplinary studies. *FASEB J* 1990;4:2890–2898.
52. Blaza S. Brown adipose tissue in man: A review. *J R Soc Med* 1983;76:213–216.
53. Santos GC, Araujo MR, Silveira TC, et al. Accumulation of brown adipose tissue and nutritional status: A prospective study of 366 consecutive autopsies. *Arch Pathol Lab Med* 1992;116:1152–1154.
54. Cottle WH. The innervation of brown adipose tissue. In: Lindberg O, ed. *Brown Adipose Tissue*. New York: Elsevier; 1970:155–178.
55. Mory G, Bouillaud F, Combes-George M, et al. Noradrenaline controls the concentration of the uncoupling protein in brown adipose tissue. *FEBS Lett* 1984;166:393–396.
56. Ricquier D, Nechad M, Mory G. Ultrastructural and biochemical characterization of human brown adipose tissue in pheochromocytoma. *J Clin Endocrinol Metab* 1982;54: 803–807.
57. Afzelius BA. Brown adipose tissue: Its gross anatomy, histology, and cytology. In: Lindberg O, ed. *Brown Adipose Tissue*. New York: Elsevier; 1970:1–31.
58. Giralt M, Villarroya F. White, brown, beige/brite: Different adipose cells for different functions? *Endocrinology* 2013; 154(9):2992–3000.
59. Lee YH, Mottillo EP, Granneman JG. Adipose tissue plasticity from WAT to BAT and in between. *Biochim Biophys Acta* 2014;1842(3):358–369.
60. Sanchez-Gurmaches J, Guertin DA. Adipocyte lineages: Tracing back the origins of fat. *Biochim Biophys Acta* 2014; 1842(3):340–351.
61. Zhang JX, Du CY, Guo WM, et al. Adipose tissue-derived pericytes for cartilage tissue engineering. *Curr Stem Cell Res Ther* 2017;12(6):513–521.
62. Xie S, Lu F, Han J et al. Efficient generation of functional Schwann cells from adipose-derived stem cells in defined conditions. *Cell Cycle* 2017;16(9):841–851.
63. Almalki SG, Llamas Valle Y, Agrawal DK. MMP-2 and MMP-14 silencing inhibits VEGFR2 cleavage and induces the differentiation of porcine adipose-derived mesenchymal stem cells to endothelial cells. *Stem Cells Transl Med* 2017; 6(5):1385–1398.
64. Pearse AG. *Histochemistry: Theoretical and Applied*. Vol 2. 3rd ed. Baltimore, MD: Williams & Wilkins; 1972.
65. Hausman GJ. Anatomical and enzyme histochemical differentiation of adipose tissue. *Int J Obes* 1985;9(Suppl 1):1–6.
66. Lithell J, Boberg J, Hellsing K, et al. Lipoprotein-lipase activity in human skeletal muscle and adipose tissue in the fasting and the fed states. *Atherosclerosis* 1978;30:89–94.

67. Lithell H, Hellsing K, Lundqvist G, et al. Lipoprotein-lipase activity of human skeletal-muscle and adipose tissue after intensive physical exercise. *Acta Physiol Scand* 1979;105: 312–315.
68. Fielding CJ, Havel RJ. Lipoprotein lipase. *Arch Pathol Lab Med* 1977;101:225–229.
69. Zugibe FT. *Diagnostic Histochemistry*. St. Louis, MO: CV Mosby; 1970.
70. Sheehan DC, Hrapchak BB. *Theory and Practice of Histotechnology*. St. Louis, MO: CV Mosby; 1973.
71. Filipe MI, Lake BD, eds. *Histochemistry in Pathology*. Edinburgh: Churchill Livingstone; 1983.
72. Spicer SS, ed. *Histochemistry in Pathologic Diagnosis*. New York: Marcel Dekker; 1987.
73. Hausman GJ. Techniques for studying adipocytes. *Stain Technol* 1981;56:149–154.
74. Popper H, Knipping G. A histochemical and biochemical study of a liposarcoma with several aspects on the development of fat synthesis. *Pathol Res Pract* 1981;171:373–380.
75. Waugh DA, Small DM. Methods in laboratory investigation: Identification and detection of in situ cellular and regional differences of lipid composition and class in lipid-rich tissue using hot stage polarizing light microscopy. *Lab Invest* 1984; 51:702–714.
76. Stedman TL. *Stedman's Medical Dictionary*. 21st ed. Baltimore, MD: Williams & Wilkins; 1966.
77. Robbins SL, Cotran RS, Kumar V. *The Pathologic Basis of Disease*. 3rd ed. Philadelphia, PA: WB Saunders; 1984.
78. Rubin E, Farber JL, eds. *Pathology*. Philadelphia, PA: Lippincott; 1988.
79. Heptinstall RH. *Pathology of the Kidney*. 2nd ed. Boston, MA: Little, Brown & Co; 1974.
80. Jasnosz KM, Pickeral JJ, Graner S. Fat deposits in the placenta following maternal total parenteral nutrition with intravenous lipid emulsion. *Arch Pathol Lab Med* 1995;119:555–557.
81. Bennington JL. Proceedings: Cancer of the kidney: Etiology, epidemiology, and pathology. *Cancer* 1973;32:1017–1029.
82. Elizalde N, Korman S. Cytochemical studies of glycogen, neutral mucopolysaccharides and fat in malignant tissues. *Cancer* 1968;21:1061–1068.
83. Andrion A, Mazzucco G, Gugliotta P, et al. Benign clear cell (sugar) tumor of the lung: A light microscopic, histochemical, and ultrastructural study with a review of the literature. *Cancer* 1985;56:2657–2663.
84. Bertoni F, Unni KK, McLeod RA, et al. Xanthoma of bone. *Am J Clin Pathol* 1988;90:377–384.
85. Bennett JH, Shousha S, Puddle B, et al. Immunohistochemical identification of tumours of adipocytic differentiation using an antibody to aP2 protein. *J Clin Pathol* 1995;48: 950–954.
86. Michetti F, Dell'Anna E, Tiberio G, et al. Immunochemical and immunocytochemical study of S-100 protein in rat adipocytes. *Brain Res* 1983;262:352–356.
87. Haimoto H, Kato K, Suzuki F, et al. The ultrastructural changes of S-100 protein localization during lipolysis in adipocytes. An immunoelectron-microscopic study. *Am J Pathol* 1985;121:185–191.
88. Takahashi K, Isobe T, Ohtsuki Y, et al. Immunochemical study of the distribution of alpha and beta subunits of S-100 protein in human neoplasms and normal tissues. *Virchows Arch Cell Pathol* 1984;45:385–396.
89. Nakazato Y, Ishida Y, Takahashi K, et al. Immunohistochemical distribution of S-100 protein and glial fibrillary acidic protein in normal and neoplastic salivary glands. *Virchows Arch A Pathol Anat Histopathol* 1985;405:299–310.
90. Kahn HJ, Marks A, Thom H, et al. Role of antibody to S100 protein in diagnostic pathology. *Am J Clin Pathol* 1983;79: 341–347.
91. Nakajima T, Watanabe S, Sato Y, et al. An immunoperoxidase study of S-100 protein distribution in normal and neoplastic tissues. *Am J Surg Pathol* 1982;6:715–727.
92. Cocchia D, Lauriola L, Stolfi V, et al. S-100 antigen labels neoplastic cells in liposarcoma and cartilaginous tumours. *Virchows Arch A Pathol Anat Histopathol* 1983;402: 139–145.
93. Weiss SW, Langloss JM, Enzinger FM. Value of S-100 protein in the diagnosis of soft tissue tumors with particular reference to benign and malignant Schwann cell tumors. *Lab Invest* 1983;49:299–308.
94. Hashimoto H, Daimaru Y, Enjoji M. S-100 protein distribution in liposarcoma. An immunoperoxidase study with special reference to the distinction of liposarcoma from myxoid malignant fibrous histiocytoma. *Virchows Arch A Pathol Anat Histopathol* 1984;405:1–10.
95. Haimoto H, Takahashi Y, Koshikawa T, et al. Immunohistochemical localization of gamma-enolase in normal human tissues other than nervous and neuroendocrine tissues. *Lab Invest* 1985;52:257–263.
96. Rosso R, Lucioni M. Normal and neoplastic cells of brown adipose tissue express the adhesion molecule CD31. *Arch Pathol Lab Med* 2006;130:480–482.
97. Stunkard AJ, Wadden TA, eds. *Obesity: Theory and Therapy*. 2nd ed. New York: Raven Press; 1993.
98. Lowell BB, Susulic VS, Hamann A, et al. Development of obesity in transgenic mice after genetic ablation of brown adipose tissue. *Nature* 1993;366:740–742.
99. Zhang Y, Proenca R, Maffei M, et al. Positional cloning of the mouse obese gene and its human homologue. *Nature* 1994;372:425–432.
100. Green ED, Maffei M, Braden VV, et al. The human obese (OB) gene: RNA expression pattern and mapping on the physical, cytogenetic, and genetic maps of chromosome 7. *Genome Res* 1995;5:5–12.
101. Pelleymounter MA, Cullen MJ, Baker MB, et al. Effects of the obese gene product on body weight regulation in ob/ob mice. *Science* 1995;269:540–543.
102. Halaas JL, Gajiwala KS, Maffei M, et al. Weight-reducing effects of the plasma protein encoded by the obese gene. *Science* 1995;269:543–546.
103. Campfield LA, Smith FJ, Guisez Y, et al. Recombinant mouse OB protein: Evidence for a peripheral signal linking adiposity and central neural networks. *Science* 1995;269: 546–549.
104. Chua SC Jr, Chung WK, Wu-Peng XS, et al. Phenotypes of mouse diabetes and rat fatty due to mutations in the OB (leptin) receptor. *Science* 1996;271:994–996.
105. Raife T, Landas SK. Intracellular crystalline material in visceral adipose tissue: A common autopsy finding [abstract]. *Am J Clin Pathol* 1990;94:511.
106. Tedeschi CG. Pathologic anatomy of adipose tissue. In: Renold AE, Cahill GF, eds. *Handbook of Physiology. Section 5: Adipose Tissue*. Baltimore, MD: Waverly Press; 1965.

107. Manthorpe R, Helin G, Kofod B, et al. Effect of glucocorticoid on connective tissue of aorta and skin in rabbits. Biochemical studies on collagen, glycosaminoglycans, DNA and RNA. *Acta Endocrinol (Copenh)* 1974;77:310–324.
108. Napolitano LM. Observations on the fine structure of adipose cells. *Ann NY Acad Sci* 1965;131:34–42.
109. Dahlman I, Mejhert N, Linder K, et al. Adipose tissue pathways involved in weight loss of cancer cachexia. *Br J Cancer* 2010;102:1541–1548.
110. Seaman JP, Kjeldsberg CR, Linker A. Gelatinous transformation of the bone marrow. *Hum Pathol* 1978;9:685–692.
111. Wittels B. Bone marrow biopsy changes following chemotherapy for acute leukemia. *Am J Surg Pathol* 1980;4:135–142.
112. Pierard GE, Nizet JL, Pierard-Franchimont C. Cellulite: From standing fat herniation to hypodermal stretch marks. *Am J Dermatopath* 2000;22:34–37.
113. Gruskin P, Canberry JN. Pathology of acoustic neuromas. In: House WF, Leutje CM, eds. *Acoustic Tumors*. Baltimore, MD: University Park Press; 1979:85–148.
114. Wood C. Membranous lipodystrophy of bone. *Arch Pathol Lab Med* 1978;102:22–27.
115. Bird TD, Koerker RM, Leaird BJ, et al. Lipomembranous polycystic osteodysplasia (brain, bone and fat disease): A genetic cause of presenile dementia. *Neurology* 1983;33:81–86.
116. Kitajima I, Suganuma T, Murata F, et al. Ultrastructural demonstration of Maclura pomifera agglutinin binding sites in the membranocystic lesions of membranous lipodystrophy (Nasu–Hakola disease). *Virchows Arch A Pathol Anat Histopathol* 1988;413:475–483.
117. Chun SI, Chung KY. Membranous lipodystrophy: Secondary type. *J Am Acad Dermatol* 1994;31:601–605.
118. Coyne JD, Parkinson D, Baildam AD. Membranous fat necrosis of the breast. *Histopathology* 1996;28:61–64.
119. Lightbourne M, Brown RJ. Genetics of Lipodystrophy. *Endocrinol Metab Clin N Am* 2017;46:539–554.
120. Adams RD. *Diseases of Muscle: A Study in Pathology*. 3rd ed. New York: Harper & Row; 1975.
121. Rosai J, Levine GD. Tumors of the thymus. In: Firminger HI, ed. *Atlas of Tumor Pathology, 2nd Series, Fascicle 13*. Washington, DC: Armed Forces Institute of Pathology; 1976.
122. Rywlin AM. *Histopathology of the Bone Marrow*. Boston, MA: Little, Brown & Co; 1976:19.
123. Ackerman LV, Rosai J. *Surgical Pathology*. 5th ed. St Louis, MO: CV Mosby; 1974:649.
124. Seifert G. Lipomatous atrophy and other forms. In: Kloppel G, Heitz PU, eds. *Pancreatic Pathology*. New York: Churchill Livingstone; 1984.
125. Heggtveit HA, Fenoglio JJ, McAllister HA. Lipomatous hypertrophy of the interatrial septum: An assessment of 41 cases. *Lab Invest* 1976;34:318.
126. O'Connor S, Recavarren R, Nichols LC, et al. Lipomatous hypertrophy of interatrial septum: An overview. *Arch Pathol Lab Med* 2006;130:397–399.
127. McAllister HA, Fenoglio JJ. *Tumors of the Cardiovascular System*. Washington, DC: Armed Forces Institute of Pathology;1978:44–46.
128. Rokey R, Mulvagh SL, Cheirif J, et al. Lipomatous encasement and compression of the heart: Antemortem diagnosis by cardiac nuclear magnetic resonance imaging and catheterization. *Am Heart J* 1989;117:952–953.
129. Waller BF, ed. *Pathology of the Heart and Great Vessels*. New York: Churchill Livingstone; 1988.
130. Sleisenger MH, Fordtran JS, eds. *Gastrointestinal Disease: Pathophysiology, Diagnosis, Management*. 3rd ed. Philadelphia, PA: WB Saunders; 1983.
131. Macdonald A, Feiwel M. A review of the concept of Weber–Christian panniculitis with a report of five cases. *Br J Dermatol* 1968;80:355–361.
132. Sweatt HL, Hardman WJ, Solomon AR. Non-neoplastic diseases of the skin. In: Mills SE, ed. *Sternberg's Diagnostic Surgical Pathology*. 4th ed. New York: Lippincott Williams Wilkins; 2004:40–43.
133. Enzinger FM, Weiss SW. *Soft Tissue Tumors*. 2nd ed. St. Louis, MO: CV Mosby; 1988.
134. Allen P. *Tumors and Proliferations of Adipose Tissue*. New York: Masson; 1981.
135. Shugar MA, Gavron JP. Benign symmetrical lipomatosis (Madelung's disease). *Otolaryngol Head Neck Surg* 1985;93:109–112.
136. Keller SM, Waxman JS, Kim US. Benign symmetrical lipomatosis. *South Med J* 1986;79:1428–1429.
137. Scully RE, Galdabini JJ, McNeely BU. Case records of the Massachusetts General Hospital. Weekly clinicopathological exercise. Case 53–1976 (Gardner's syndrome). *N Engl J Med* 1976;295:1526–1532.
138. Scully RE, Galdabini JJ, McNeely BU. Case records of the Massachusetts General Hospital. Weekly clinicopathological exercises. Case 47–1978 (Gardner's syndrome). *N Engl J Med* 1978;299:1237–1244.
139. Snyder N III, Scurry MT, Diess WP. Five families with multiple endocrine adenomatosis. *Ann Intern Med* 1972;76:53–58.
140. Johnson GJ, Summerskill WH, Anderson VE, et al. Clinical and genetic investigation of a large kindred with multiple endocrine adenomatosis. *N Engl J Med* 1967;277:1379–1385.
141. Syed S, Brooks D, Haupt HM, et al. Anabolic steroids causing growth of benign tumors: Androgen receptor in angiolipomas. *J Am Acad Dermatol* 2007;57:899–900.
142. Carney JA. The triad of gastric epithelioid leiomyosarcoma, functioning extra-adrenal paraganglioma, and pulmonary chondroma. *Cancer* 1979;43:374–382.
143. Carney JA. The triad of gastric epithelioid leiomyosarcoma, pulmonary chondroma, and functioning extra-adrenal paraganglioma: A five-year review. *Medicine (Baltimore)* 1983;62:159–169.
144. Klein JA, Barr RJ. Diffuse lipomatosis and tuberous sclerosis. *Arch Dermatol* 1986;122:1298–1302.
145. Majeski JA, Paxton ES, Wirman JA, et al. A thoracic benign mesenchymoma in association with hemihypertrophy. *Am J Clin Pathol* 1981;76:827–832.
146. Humphrey AA, Kinsley PC. Familial multiple lipomas: Report of a family. *Arch Derm Syph* 1938;37:30–34.
147. Higginbottom MC, Schultz P. The Bannayan syndrome: An autosomal dominant disorder consisting of macrocephaly, lipomas, hemangiomas, and a risk for intracranial tumors. *Pediatrics* 1982;69:632–634.
148. Oochi N, Rikitake O, Maeda T, et al. [A case of Laurence-Moon-Biedl syndrome associated with bilateral adrenal lipomas and renal abnormalities]. *Nihon Naika Gakkai Zasshi* 1984;73:89–93.

149. Kremchek TE, Kremchek EJ. Carpal tunnel syndrome caused by flexor tendon sheath lipoma. *Orthop Rev* 1988;17:1083–1085.
150. Al-Mefty O, Fox JL, Sakati N, et al. The multiple manifestations of the encephalocraniocutaneous lipomatosis syndrome. *Childs Nerv Syst* 1987;3:132–134.
151. Brumback RA, Leech RW. Fishman's syndrome (encephalocraniocutaneous lipomatosis): A field defect of ectomesoderm. *J Child Neurol* 1987;2:168–169.
152. Aleksic S, Budzilovich G, Greco MA, et al. Intracranial lipomas, hydrocephalus and other CNS anomalies in oculoauriculovertebral dysplasia (Goldenhar–Gorlin syndrome). *Childs Brain* 1984;11:285–297.
153. Weinstock JV, Kawanishi H. Gastrointestinal polyposis with orocutaneous hamartomas (Cowden's disease). *Gastroenterology* 1978;74(5 Pt 1):890–895.
154. Boozan JA, Maves MD, Schuller DE. Surgical management of massive benign symmetric lipomatosis. *Laryngoscope* 1992;102:94–99.
155. Berkovic SF, Andermann F, Shoubridge EA, et al. Mitochondrial dysfunction in multiple symmetrical lipomatosis. *Ann Neurol* 1991;29:566–569.
156. Kaplan JG, Barasch E, Hirschfeld A, et al. Spinal epidural lipomatosis: A serious complication of iatrogenic Cushing's syndrome. *Neurology* 1989;39:1031–1034.
157. Symmers WSC. The lymphoreticular system. In: Symmers WSC, ed. *Systemic Pathology*. Vol 2. Edinburgh: Churchill Livingstone; 1978:647–651.
158. Smith T. Fatty replacement of lymph nodes mimicking lymphoma relapse. *Cancer* 1986;58:2686–2688.
159. Takayasu K, Shima Y, Muramatsu Y, et al. Imaging characteristics of large lipoma and angiomyolipoma of the liver. Case reports. *Cancer* 1987;59:916–921.
160. Pounder DJ. Hepatic pseudolipoma. *Pathology* 1983;15:83–84.
161. Shafer WG, Hine MK, Levy BM. *Development Disturbances of Oral and Paraoral Structures. A Textbook of Oral Pathology*. 4th ed. Philadelphia, PA: WB Saunders; 1983:24–25.
162. Ramadori G. The stellate cell (Ito-cell, fat-storing cell, lipocyte, perisinusoidal cell) of the liver. New insights into pathophysiology of an intriguing cell. *Virchows Arch B Cell Pathol Incl Mol Pathol* 1991;61:147–158.
163. Cha I, Bass N, Ferrell LD. Lipopeliosis: An immunohistochemical and clinicopathologic study of five cases. *Am J Surg Pathol* 1994;18:789–795.
164. Stroebel P, Mayer F, Zerban H, et al. Spongiotic pericytoma: A benign neoplasm deriving from the perisinusoidal (Ito) cells in rat liver. *Am J Pathol* 1995;146:903–913.
165. Orfila C, Giraud P, Modesto A, et al. Abdominal fat tissue aspirate in human amyloidosis: Light, electron, and immunofluorescence microscopic studies. *Hum Pathol* 1986;17:366–369.
166. Duston MA, Skinner M, Shirahama T, et al. Diagnosis of amyloidosis by abdominal fat aspiration: Analysis of four years' experience. *Am J Med* 1987;82:412–414.
167. Gertz MA, Li CY, Shirahama T, et al. Utility of subcutaneous fat aspiration for the diagnosis of systemic amyloidosis (immunoglobulin light chain). *Arch Intern Med* 1988;48:929–933.
168. Keen CE, Buk SJ, Brady K, et al. Fat necrosis presenting as obscure abdominal mass: Birefringent saponified fatty acid crystalloids as a clue to diagnosis. *J Clin Pathol* 1994;47:1028–1031.
169. Poppiti RJ Jr, Margulies M, Cabello B, et al. Membranous fat necrosis. *Am J Surg Pathol* 1986;10:62–69.
170. Bennett RG, Petrozzi JW. Nodular subcutaneous fat necrosis: A manifestation of silent pancreatitis. *Arch Dermatol* 1975;111:896–898.
171. Hughes PS, Apisarnthanarax P, Mullins F. Subcutaneous fat necrosis associated with pancreatic disease. *Arch Dermatol* 1975;111:506–510.
172. Fischer AH, Morris DJ. Pathogenesis of calciphylaxis: Study of three cases and literature review. *Hum Pathol* 1995;26:1055–1064.
173. Wilmer WA, Magro CM. Calciphylaxis: Emerging concepts in prevention, diagnosis, and treatment. *Semin Dial* 2002;15:172–186.
174. Mirza I, Chaubay D, Gunderia H, et al. An unusual presentation of calciphylaxis due to primary hyperparathyroidism. *Arch Pathol Lab Med* 2001;125:1351–1353.
175. Winkelmann RK, Frigas E. Eosinophilic panniculitis: A clinicopathologic study. *J Cutan Pathol* 1986;13:1–12.
176. Blaustein A, Moreno A, Noguera J, et al. Septal granulomatous panniculitis in Sweet's syndrome: Report of two cases. *Arch Dermatol* 1985;121:785–788.
177. Suster S, Cartagena N, Cabello-Inchausti B, et al. Histiocytic lymphophagocytic panniculitis: An unusual extranodal presentation of sinus histiocytosis with massive lymphadenopathy (Rosai–Dorfman disease). *Arch Dermatol* 1988;124:1246–1249.
178. Alegre VA, Winkelmann RK, Aliaga A. Lipomembranous changes in chronic panniculitis. *J Am Acad Dermatol* 1988;19(1 Pt 1):39–46.
179. Vincent F, Prokopetz R, Miller RA. Plasma cell panniculitis: A unique clinical and pathologic presentation of linear scleroderma. *J Am Acad Dermatol* 1989;21(2 Pt 2):357–360.
180. Izumi AK, Takiguchi P. Lupus erythematosus panniculitis. *Arch Dermatol* 1983;119:61–64.
181. Silverman RA, Newman AJ, LeVine MJ, et al. Poststeroid panniculitis: A case report. *Pediatr Dermatol* 1988;5:92–93.
182. Kelly JK, Hwang WS. Idiopathic retractile (sclerosing) mesenteritis and its differential diagnosis. *Am J Surg Pathol* 1989;13:513–521.
183. Scully RE, Galdabini JJ, McNeely BU. Lipodystrophy of mesentery (Case 30–1976). *N Engl J Med* 1976;295:214–218.
184. Eble JN, Rosenberg AE, Young RH. Retroperitoneal xanthogranulomatosis in a patient with Erdheim–Chester disease. *Am J Surg Pathol* 1994;18:843–848.
185. Seemayer TA, Knaack J, Wang NS, et al. On the ultrastructure of hibernoma. *Cancer* 1975;36:1785–1793.
186. Dardick I. Hibernoma: A possible model of brown fat histogenesis. *Hum Pathol* 1978;9:321–329.
187. Gaffney EF, Hargreaves HK, Semple E, et al. Hibernoma: Distinctive light and electron microscopic features and relationship to brown adipose tissue. *Hum Pathol* 1983;14:677–687.
188. Rigor VU, Goldstone SE, Jones J, et al. Hibernoma. A case report and discussion of a rare tumor. *Cancer* 1986;57:2207–2211.
189. Allegra SR, Gmuer C, O'Leary GP Jr. Endocrine activity in a large hibernoma. *Hum Pathol* 1983;14:1044–1052.
190. Enterline HT, Lowry LD, Richman AV. Does malignant hibernoma exist? *Am J Surg Pathol* 1979;3:265–271.

191. Teplitz C, Farrugia R, Glicksman AS. Malignant hibernoma does exist. *Lab Invest* 1980;42:58–59.
192. Talerman A. Germ cell tumors of the ovary. In: Kurman R, ed. *Blaustein's Pathology of the Female Genital Tract*. 3rd ed. New York: Springer-Verlag; 1987:689.
193. Dail DH. Uncommon tumors. In: Dale DH, Hammar SP, eds. *Pulmonary Pathology*. New York: Springer-Verlag; 1988: 847–972.
194. Ali MY, Wong PK. Intrapulmonary teratoma. *Thorax* 1964;19: 228–235.
195. Lee RG. Esophagus. In: Sternberg SS, ed. *Diagnostic Surgical Pathology*. New York: Raven Press; 1989:928.
196. Haskell HD, Butt KM, Woo SB. Pleomorphic adenoma with extensive lipometaplasia: Report of three cases. *Am J Surg Pathol* 2005;29:1389–1393.
197. Toker C, Tang CK, Whitely JF, et al. Benign spindle cell breast tumor. *Cancer* 1981;48:1615–1622.
198. Wargotz ES, Weiss SW, Norris HJ. Myofibroblastoma of the breast: Sixteen cases of a distinctive benign mesenchymal tumor. *Am J Surg Pathol* 1987;11:493–502.
199. Fetsch JF, Miettinen M, Laskin WB, et al. A clinicopathologic study of 45 pediatric soft tissue tumors with an admixture of adipose tissue and fibroblastic elements, and a proposal for classification as lipofibromatosis. *Am J Surg Pathol* 2000;24:1491–1500.
200. Nogales FF, Pavcovich M, Medina MT, et al. Fatty change in the endometrium. *Histopathology* 1992;20:362–363.
201. Nogita T, Wong TY, Hidano A, et al. Pedunculated lipofibroma: A clinicopathologic study of thirty-two cases supporting a simplified nomenclature. *J Am Acad Dermatol* 1994; 31(2 Pt 1):235–240.
202. Tomashefski JF Jr. Benign endobronchial mesenchymal tumors: Their relationship to parenchymal pulmonary hamartomas. *Am J Surg Pathol* 1982;6:531–540.
203. Palvio D, Egeblad K, Paulsen SM. Atypical lipomatous hamartoma of the lung. *Virchows Arch A Pathol Anat Histopathol* 1985;405:253–261.
204. Benjamin SP, Mercer RD, Hawk WA. Myofibroblastic contraction in spontaneous regression of multiple congenital mesenchymal hamartomas. *Cancer* 1977;40:2343–2352.
205. Enzinger FM. Fibrous hamartoma of infancy. *Cancer* 1965; 18:241–248.
206. Reye RD. A consideration of certain subdermal fibromatous tumours of infancy. *J Pathol Bacteriol* 1956;72:149–154.
207. Fletcher CD, Powell G, van Noorden S, et al. Fibrous hamartoma of infancy: A histochemical and immunohistochemical study. *Histopathology* 1988;12:65–74.
208. Silverman TA, Enzinger FM. Fibrolipomatous hamartoma of nerve: A clinocopatholigic analysis of 26 cases. *Am J Surg Pathol* 1985;9:7–14.
209. Aymard B, Bowman-Ferrand F, Vernhes L, et al. Hamartome lipofibromateux des nerfs périphériques. Etude anatomoclinique de 5 cas dont 2 avec étude ultrastructurale. *Ann Pathol* 1987;7:320–324.
210. Price EB Jr, Mostofi FK. Symptomatic angiomyolipoma of the kidney. *Cancer* 1965;18:761–774.
211. McCullough DL, Scott R, Seybold HM. Renal angiomyolipoma (hamartoma): Review of the literature and report on 7 cases. *J Urol* 1971;105:32–44.
212. Dao AH, Netsky NG. Human tails and pseudotails. *Hum Pathol* 1984;15:449–453.
213. Farshid G, Weiss SW. Massive localized lymphedema in the morbidly obese: A histologically distinct reactive lesion simulating liposarcoma. *Am J Surg Pathol* 1998;22:1277–1283.
214. Wu D, Gibbs J, Corral D, et al. Massive localized lymphedema: Additional locations and association with hypothyroidism. *Hum Pathol* 2000;31:1162–1168.
215. LeBer MS, Stout AP. Benign mesenchymomas in children. *Cancer* 1962;15:595–605.
216. Kasantikul V, Brown WJ, Netsky MG. Mesenchymal differentiation in trigeminal neurilemmoma. *Cancer* 1982;50: 1568–1571.
217. Rosai J. Case presentation at the European Society of Pathology meeting in Porto, Portugal; September 1989.
218. Brecher ME, Gill WB, Straus FH. Angiomyolipoma with regional lymph node involvement and long-term follow-up study. *Hum Pathol* 1986;17:962–963.
219. Meggitt BF, Wilson JN. The battered buttock syndrome—fat fractures. A report on a group of traumatic lipomata. *Br J Surg* 1972;59:165–169.
220. Wilson JE. Lipomas and potassium intake. *Ann Intern Med* 1989;110:750–751.
221. Solvonuk PF, Taylor GP, Hancock R, et al. Correlation of morphologic and biochemical observations in human lipomas. *Lab Invest* 1984;51:469–474.
222. Azumi N, Curtis J, Kempson R, et al. Atypical and malignant neoplasms showing lipomatous differentiation: A study of 111 cases. *Am J Surg Pathol* 1987;11:161–183.
223. Fu YS, Parker FG, Kaye GI, et al. Ultrastructure of benign and malignant adipose tissue tumors. *Pathol Annu* 1980;15(Pt 1): 67–69.
224. Kindblom L, Angervall L, Stener B, et al. Intermuscular and intramuscular lipomas and hibernomas. A clinical, roentgenologic, histologic and prognostic study of 46 cases. *Cancer* 1974;33:754–762.
225. Evans HL, Soule EH, Winkelmann RK. Atypical lipoma, atypical intramuscular lipoma, and well differentiated retroperitoneal liposarcoma: A reappraisal of 30 cases. *Cancer* 1979;43:574–584.
226. Marsh WL Jr, Lucas JG, Olsen J. Chondrolipoma of the breast. *Arch Pathol Lab Med* 1989;113:369–371.
227. Lim YC. Mediastinal chondrolipoma. *Am J Surg Pathol* 1980; 4:407–409.
228. Allen P. Letter to the case. *Pathol Res Pract* 1989;184: 444–445.
229. Hayden JW, Abellera RM. Tenosynovial lipochondromatosis of the flexor hallucis, common toe flexor, and posterior tibial tendons. *Clin Orthop Relat Res* 1989;245:220–222.
230. Katzer B. Histopathology of rare chondroosteoblastic metaplasia in benign lipomas. *Pathol Res Pract* 1989;184: 437–445.
231. Honore LH. Uterine fibrolipoleiomyoma: Report of a case with discussion of histogenesis. *Am J Obstet Gynecol* 1978; 132:635–636.
232. Brescia RJ, Tazelaar HD, Hobbs J, et al. Intravascular lipoleiomyomatosis: A report of two cases. *Hum Pathol* 1989;20:252–256.
233. Hunt SJ, Santa Cruz DJ, Barr RJ. Cellular angiolipoma. *Am J Surg Pathol* 1990;14:75–81.
234. DeRienzo D, Truong L. Thyroid neoplasms containing mature fat: A report of two cases and review of the literature. *Mod Pathol* 1989;2:506–510.

235. Perosio P, Brooks JJ, LiVolsi VA. Orbital brown tumor as the initial manifestation of a parathyroid lipoadenoma. *Surg Pathol* 1988;1:77–82.
236. Gnepp DR, Ogorzalek JM, Heffess CA. Fat-containing lesions of the thyroid gland. *Am J Surg Pathol* 1989;13:605–612.
237. Bruno J, Ciancia EM, Pingitore R. Thyroid papillary adenocarcinoma; lipomatous-type. *Virchows Arch A Pathol Anat Histopathol* 1989;414:371–373.
238. Otto HF, Loning T, Lachenmayer L, et al. Thymolipoma in association with myasthenia gravis. *Cancer* 1982;50:1623–1628.
239. Trites AE. Thyrolipoma, thymolipoma and pharyngeal lipoma: A syndrome. *Can Med Assoc J* 1966;95:1254–1259.
240. Enzinger FM, Harvey DA. Spindle cell lipoma. *Cancer* 1975;36:1852–1859.
241. Angervall L, Dahl I, Kindblom LG, et al. Spindle cell lipoma. *Acta Pathol Microbiol Scand A* 1976;84:477–487.
242. Fletcher CD, Martin-Bates E. Spindle cell lipoma: A clinicopathological study with some original observations. *Histopathology* 1987;11:803–817.
243. Shmookler BM, Enzinger FM. Pleomorphic lipoma: A benign tumor simulating liposarcoma: A clinicopathologic analysis of 48 cases. *Cancer* 1981;47:126–133.
244. Azzopardi J, Iocco J, Salm R. Pleomorphic lipoma: A tumour simulating liposarcoma. *Histopathology* 1983;7:511–523.
245. Beham A, Schmid C, Hödl S, et al. Spindle cell and pleomorphic lipoma: An immunohistochemical study and histogenetic analysis. *J Pathol* 1989;158:219–222.
246. Syed S, Martin AM, Haupt HM, et al. Frequent detection of androgen receptor in spindle cell lipoma: An explanation for this lesion's male predominance? *Arch Path Lab Med* 2008;132:81–83.
247. Ebrahimi KB, Ren S, Green WR. Floretlike cells in in situ and prolapsed orbital fat. *Ophthalmology* 2007;114:2345–2349.
248. Schmack I, Patel RM, Folpe AL, et al. Subconjunctival herniated orbital fat: A benign adipocytic lesion that may mimic pleomorphic lipoma and atypical lipomatous tumor. *Am J Surg Pathol* 2007;31:193–198.
249. Meis JM, Enzinger FM. Chondroid lipoma. A unique tumor simulating liposarcoma and myxoid chondrosarcoma. *Am J Surg Pathol* 1993;17:1103–1112.
250. Kindblom LG, Meis-Kindblom JM. Chondroid lipoma: An ultrastructural and immunohistochemical analysis with further observations regarding its differentiation. *Hum Pathol* 1995;26:706–715.
251. De Nictolis M, Goteri G, Campanati G, et al. Elastofibrolipoma of the mediastinum. A previously undescribed benign tumor containing abnormal elastic fibers. *Am J Surg Pathol* 1995;19:364–367.
252. Vellios F, Baez J, Schumacker HB. Lipoblastomatosis: A tumor of fetal fat different from hibernoma; report of a case, with observations on the embryogenesis of human adipose tissue. *Am J Pathol* 1958;34:1149–1159.
253. Chung EB, Enzinger FM. Benign lipoblastomatosis: An analysis of 35 cases. *Cancer* 1973;32:482–492.
254. Bolen JW, Thorning D. Benign lipoblastoma and myxoid liposarcoma: A comparative light- and electron-microscopic study. *Am J Surg Pathol* 1980;4:163–174.
255. Alba Greco M, Garcia RL, Vuletin JC. Benign lipoblastomatosis: Ultrastructure and histogenesis. *Cancer* 1980;45:511–515.
256. Chaudhuri B, Ronan SG, Ghosh L. Benign lipoblastoma: Report of a case. *Cancer* 1980;46:611–614.
257. Hanada M, Tokuda R, Ohnishi Y, et al. Benign lipoblastoma and liposarcoma in children. *Acta Pathol Jpn* 1986;36:605–612.
258. Dudgeon DL, Haller JA Jr. Pediatric lipoblastomatosis: Two unusual cases. *Surgery* 1984;95:371–373.
259. Turc-Carel C, Dal Cin P, Rao U, et al. Cytogenetic studies of adipose tissue tumors: I. A benign lipoma with reciprocal translocation t(3;12)(q28;q14). *Cancer Genet Cytogenet* 1986;23:283–289.
260. Heim S, Mandahl N, Kristoffersson U, et al. Reciprocal translocation t(3;12)(q27;q13) in lipoma. *Cancer Genet Cytogenet* 1986;23:301–304.
261. Sandberg AA, Turc-Carel C. The cytogenetics of solid tumors. Relation to diagnosis, classification and pathology. *Cancer* 1987;59:387–395.
262. Heim S, Mitelman F. *Cancer Cytogenetics*. New York: Alan R. Liss; 1987:240–241.
263. Heim S, Mandahl N, Kristoffersson U, et al. Marker ring chromosome—a new cytogenetic abnormality characterizing lipogenic tumors? *Cancer Genet Cytogenet* 1987;24:319–326.
264. Heim S, Mandahl N, Rydholm A, et al. Different karyotypic features characterize different clinicopathologic subgroups of benign lipogenic tumors. *Int J Cancer* 1988;42:863–867.
265. Turc-Carel C, Dal Cin P, Boghosian L, et al. Breakpoints in benign lipoma may be at 12q13 or 12q14. *Cancer Genet Cytogenet* 1988;36:131–135.
266. Sait SN, Dal Cin P, Sandberg AA, et al. Involvement of 6p in benign lipomas. A new cytogenetic entity? *Cancer Genet Cytogenet* 1989;37:281–283.
267. Dal Cin P, Sciot R, De Wever I, et al. New discriminative chromosomal marker in adipose tissue tumors. The chromosome 8q11–q13 region in lipoblastoma. *Cancer Genet Cytogenet* 1994;78:232–235.
268. Bechtold R, Shaff MI. Pelvic lipomatosis with ureteral encasement and recurrent thrombophlebitis. *South Med J* 1983;76:1030–1032.
269. Henriksson L, Liljeholm H, Lonnerholm T. Pelvic lipomatosis causing constriction of the lower urinary tract and the rectum. Case report. *Scand J Urol Nephrol* 1984;18:249–252.
270. Cinti S, Enzi G, Cigolini M, et al. Ultrastructural features of cultured mature adipocyte precursors from adipose tissue in multiple symmetric lipomatosis. *Ultrastruct Pathol* 1983;5:145–152.
271. Enzi G. Multiple symmetric lipomatosis: an updated clinical report. *Medicine (Baltimore)* 1984;63:56–64.
272. Pollock M, Nicholson GI, Nukada H, et al. Neuropathy in multiple symmetric lipomatosis. Madelung's disease. *Brain* 1988;111(Pt 5):1157–1171.
273. Klopstock T, Naumann M, Schalke B, et al. Multiple symmetric lipomatosis: Abnormalities in complex IV and multiple deletions in mitochondrial DNA. *Neurology* 1994;44:862–866.
274. Deiana L, Pes GM, Carru C, et al. Extremely high HDL levels in a patient with multiple symmetric lipomatosis. *Clin Chim Acta* 1993;223:143–147.
275. Zancanaro C, Sbarbati A, Morroni M, et al. Multiple symmetric lipomatosis. Ultrastructural investigation of the tissue and preadipocytes in primary culture. *Lab Invest* 1990;63:253–258.

276. DeRosa G, Cozzolino A, Guarino M, et al. Congenital infiltrating lipomatosis of the face: Report of cases and review of the literature. *J Oral Maxillofac Surg* 1987;45:879–883.
277. Quint DJ, Boulos RS, Sanders WP, et al. Epidural lipomatosis. *Radiology* 1988;169:485–490.
278. Vazquez L, Ellis A, Saint-Genez D, et al. Epidural lipomatosis after renal transplantation–complete recovery without surgery. *Transplantation* 1988;46:773–774.
279. Doppman JL. Epidural lipomatosis. *Radiology* 1989;171:581–582.
280. Siskind BN, Weiner FR, Frank M, et al. Steroid-induced mesenteric lipomatosis. *Comput Radiol* 1984;8:175–177.
281. Enzi G, Digito M, Marin R, et al. Mediastino-abdominal lipomatosis: Deep accumulation of fat mimicking a respiratory disease and ascites. Clinical aspects and metabolic studies in vitro. *Q J Med* 1984;53:453–463.
282. Shukla LW, Katz JA, Wagner ML. Mediastinal lipomatosis: A complication of high dose steroid therapy in children. *Pediatr Radiol* 1988;19:57–58.
283. Arora PK. Re: Non-operative diagnosis of renal sinus lipomatosis simulating tumour of the renal pelvis [letter]. *Br J Urol* 1989;63:445.
284. Rubinstein A, Goor Y, Gazit E, et al. Non-symmetric subcutaneous lipomatosis associated with familial combined hyperlipidaemia. *Br J Dermatol* 1989;120:689–694.
285. Juhlin L, Strand A, Johnsen B. A syndrome with painful lipomas, familial dysarthria, abnormal eye-movements and clumsiness. *Acta Med Scand* 1987;221:215–218.
286. Temtamy SA, Rogers JG. Macrodactyly, hemihypertrophy, and connective tissue nevi: Report of a new syndrome and review of the literature. *J Pediatr* 1976;89:924–927.
287. Petras RE. Nonneoplastic intestinal diseases. In: Mills SE, ed. *Sternberg's Diagnostic Surgical Pathology*. 4th ed. New York: Lippincott Wilkins; 2004:1519–1520.
288. Trotter MJ, Crawford RI. Pseudolipomatosis cutis: Superficial dermal vacuoles resembling fatty infiltration of the skin. *Am J Dermatopathol* 1998;20;443–447.
289. Russell RM, Boyer JL, Bagheri SA, et al. Hepatic injury from chronic hypervitaminosis a resulting in portal hypertension and ascites. *N Engl J Med* 1974;291:435–440.
290. Sheibani K, Battifora H. Signet-ring cell melanoma. A rare morphologic variant of malignant melanoma. *Am J Surg Pathol* 1988;12:28–34.
291. Iossifides I, Mackay B, Butler JJ. Signet-ring cell lymphoma. *Ultrastruct Pathol* 1980;1:511–517.
292. Hanna W, Kahn HJ, From L. Signet ring lymphoma of the skin: Ultrastructural and immunohistochemical features. *J Am Acad Dermatol* 1986;14(2 Pt 2):344–350.
293. Cross PA, Eyden BP, Harris M. Signet ring cell lymphoma of T cell type. *J Clin Pathol* 1989;42:239–245.
294. Uccini S, Pescarmona E, Ruco LP, et al. Immunohistochemical characterization of a B-cell signet ring cell lymphoma. Report of a case. *Pathol Res Pract* 1988;183:497–504.
295. Mathur DR, Ramdeo IN, Sharma SP, et al. Signet ring cell lymphoma simulating liposarcoma–a case report with brief review of literature. *Indian J Cancer* 1988;25:52–55.
296. Jacobs DM, Waisman J. Cervical paraganglioma with intranuclear vacuoles in a fine needle aspirate. *Acta Cytol* 1987;31:29–32.
297. Spagnolo DV, Paradinas FJ. Laryngeal neuroendocrine tumour with features of a paraganglioma, intracytoplasmic lumina and acinar formation. *Histopathology* 1985;9:117–131.
298. Rosai J, Gold J, Landy R. The histiocytoid hemangiomas. A unifying concept embracing several previously described entities of skin, soft tissue, large vessels, bone, and heart. *Hum Pathol* 1979;10:707–730.
299. Barnes L, Koss W, Nieland M. Angiolymphoid hyperplasia with eosinophilia: A disease that may be confused with malignancy. *Head Neck Surg* 1980;2:425–434.
300. Kung IT, Gibson JB, Bannatyne PM. Kimura's disease: A clinico-pathological study of 21 cases and its distinction from angiolymphoid hyperplasia with eosinophilia. *Pathology* 1984;16:39–44.
301. Weiss SW, Enzinger FM. Spindle cell hemangioendothelioma. A low-grade angiosarcoma resembling a cavernous hemangioma and Kaposi's sarcoma. *Am J Surg Pathol* 1986;10:521–530.
302. Weiss SW, Enzinger FM. Epithelioid hemangioendothelioma: A vascular tumor often mistaken for a carcinoma. *Cancer* 1982;50:970–981.
303. Yamaguchi T, Suzuki S, Ishiiwa H, et al. Benign notochordal cell tumors: A comparative histological study of benign notochordal cell tumors, classic chordomas, and notochordal vestiges of fetal intervertebral discs. *Am J Surg Pathol* 2004;28:756–761.
304. Shimazaki H, Aida S, Iizuka Y, et al. Vacuolated cell mesothelioma of the pericardium resembling liposarcoma: A case report. *Hum Pathol* 2000;31:767–770.
305. Chimelli L, Hahn MD, Budka H. Lipomatous differentiation in a medulloblastoma. *Acta Neuropathol (Berl)* 1991;81:471–473.
306. Powell CM, Rosen PP. Adipose differentiation in cystosarcoma phyllodes. A study of 14 cases. *Am J Surg Pathol* 1994;18:720–727.
307. Krishna J, Haqqani MT. Liposarcomatous differentiation in diffuse pleural mesothelioma. *Thorax* 1993;48:409–410.

7

Skeletal Muscle

Hannes Vogel

EMBRYOLOGY 166	GENDER, TRAINING, AND AGING 181
POSTNATAL AND DEVELOPMENTAL CHANGES 168	ARTIFACTS 183
ANATOMY 170	DIFFERENTIAL DIAGNOSIS 185
LIGHT MICROSCOPY 171	SPECIMEN HANDLING 188
ULTRASTRUCTURE 177	REFERENCES 189
SPECIAL TECHNIQUES 178	

All the individual skeletal muscles in the body taken as a whole comprise the largest organ in the body by weight and volume. Although all muscles share many common attributes, many of the more than 600 muscles differ in size, shape, and function that encompass swallowing, respiration, posture, and ocular movement. Not only is the variation in the gross anatomy of these muscles considerable, but the histologic characteristics such as fiber size and fiber type proportion vary with different sites. Since many anatomic pathologists are called upon to interpret microscopic findings in muscle as they relate to disease, a familiarity with the histology of normal muscle is the basis of any accurate assessment of this kind. Today, an understanding of muscle histology as a discipline of modern pathology is dependent on some knowledge of developmental and molecular biology.

EMBRYOLOGY

The prenatal development of skeletal muscle is orchestrated by a host of genes, transcription factors, and microRNAs, too complex to discuss in detail, although the role of several important ones will be mentioned below. Skeletal muscle develops embryologically from somitic mesodermal tissue. The paraxial mesoderm is first apparent on day 17 and is the origin of the somites that are completely formed by day 30. At this time, a series of 42 to 44 pairs of rounded somites can be found adjacent to the notochord in the midline. By the 4th week, the mesodermal somites separate into the dermatomes and segmental myotomes. The latter give rise to the muscles of the body wall. One of the important influences in the early stages of segmentation when the segmental identity of the somites is established is the expression of *Hox* genes, a family of homeobox genes that act as transcription factors involved in craniocaudal segmentation of the body.

The dorsal division of myotomes, the epimeres, represents the origin of the back muscles, whereas the ventral division, hypomeres, differentiates into the lateral and ventral muscles of the body wall, including the intercostals, abdominal obliques, and strap muscles of the neck. The muscles of the extremities arise from the limb buds that form from the lateral plate mesoderm that is also the origin of the bone, tendon, ligaments, and blood vessels. In the human embryo, the mesenchyme of the limb buds appears at about the 4th week of gestation and is subject to induction by the somites. The muscle tissue derived from somitic mesoderm invades the limb buds in week 5. At the end of the 8th week, the primordia of individual muscles can be appreciated.

Whereas limb and trunk muscles are derived from somitic mesoderm, cervical and craniobulbar muscles develop from

---

This chapter is an update of a previous version authored by Reid R. Heffner Jr. and Lucia L. Balos.

the branchial arches. Differentiation of the limb musculature follows a cephalocaudad and proximal-to-distal progression. In each limb, the somitic mesenchyme subdivides into a dorsal and ventral mass with respect to the skeletal elements. The extensor, abductor, and supinator muscles are derived from the dorsal mass, whereas the flexor, adductor, and pronator muscles originate from the ventral mass.

The so-called myogenic regulatory factors (MRFs) form a select family of transcription factors whose function and activity determine the fate of the muscle cell lineage. These genes have the function of regulating the transformation of mesenchyme into muscle tissue. The MRFs are a group of four muscle-specific proteins including myogenic determining factor (MyoD), myogenic factor-5 (Myf5), myogenin and myogenic regulatory factor 4 (MRF4) that act at multiple points in the muscle lineage to establish the skeletal muscle phenotype through the regulation of proliferation, the irreversible cell cycle arrest of precursor cells, followed by the regulated activation of sarcomeric and muscle-specific genes to facilitate differentiation and sarcomere assembly. One of the regulatory factors is *Pax-3* whose expression is highest in embryonic muscle. *Pax-3* is induced by regulatory factors such as sonic hedgehog and bone morphogenetic protein (bmp4). *Pax-3* and other factors activate MyoD, which leads to the formation of mononuclear myoblasts.

Of the mesenchymal cells that become devoted to a lineage of myogenic cells, the earliest form is the myoblast, the most immature of muscle cells. These are small, round, mononucleated cells with prominent nucleoli and evidence of mitotic activity. Myoblast cytoplasm contains no microscopically detectable filaments, but ribosomes can be identified. MyoD along with *Myf5* is required for the proliferation of myoblasts. Later in development, noggin encoded by the *Nog* gene inactivates bmp4, thereby promoting differentiation. *Pax-7* activates nuclear factor 1 X (*Nfix*), which acts like a switch, turning on fetal genes and repressing embryonic genes (1). *Nfix* activates MCK, a promoter gene in myogenesis. The B isoform of creatine kinase (BCK), which is expressed at a high level in embryonic neural tissues, is also expressed abundantly in developing striated muscle and is an early marker for skeletal myogenesis. In late myogenesis, myogenin (*Myf4*) expression is controlled by *Myf5*. Along with myoblast recognition and adherence mechanisms that rely on adhesion molecules such as M-cadherin, myogenin expression promotes myotube fusion and is ultimately important in increasing muscle mass. In turn, MRF4 is responsible for differentiation into actual myofibers. Further details of basic muscle embryology may be found elsewhere (2,3).

Masses of proliferating myoblasts represent the source of myotubes, the next step in myogenesis. They are initially indistinguishable from other differentiating mesodermal cells and are recognizable by their spindle shapes, with numerous ribosomes, Golgi apparatus, and specialized cytoskeletal proteins including slow (type 1, Myh7) and

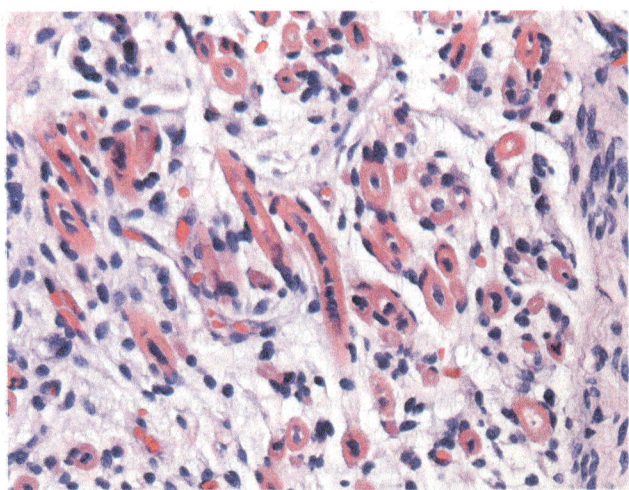

FIGURE 7.1 Myotube stage of muscle development at 14 weeks of gestational age. Myotubes typically have large central nuclei, and longitudinal sections display rows of numerous nuclei.

embryonic (Myh3) myosin heavy chains (MyHC), α-actins (cardiac [Actc1] and skeletal [Acta1]), and desmin, as well as metabolic enzymes such as β-enolase and carbonic anhydrase III (CAIII). They undergo intense proliferation and by 9 weeks of gestation are prepared to fuse with one another to form multinucleated cells called primary myotubes. They range from 8 to 50 μm in diameter, with a large central nucleus in cross section, which are in chains in longitudinal section (Fig. 7.1). The diminutive cytoplasm contains a few myofibrils, glycogen, and perinuclear mitochondria.

Cell–cell fusion encompasses several pathways including recognition, migration, adhesion, signaling, actin cytoskeletal dynamics, and membrane merger. Although many of the initial steps of myoblast fusion are similar to those of other fusogenic cell types, the elements and molecular basis of myoblast fusion have not been fully defined. Time-lapse photography and electron microscopy of myoblast fusion have provided important clues about these events. Following adhesion, electron microscopy has demonstrated that alignment occurs through the parallel apposition of the membranes of elongated myoblasts with myotubes or other myoblasts. Unilamellar vesicles are also observed in close apposition to the fusing membranes of muscle cells during development or muscle regeneration. Ultrastructurally, myoblasts are seen to have contact with each other through filopodia. Adjacent myoblasts are often joined by gap junctions. Fusing myoblasts become longitudinally oriented, a process that requires fibronectin. Interestingly, the alignment of myotubes observed in vivo does not occur in the absence of tension or deposition of aligned extracellular matrices in tissue culture. At this stage of myogenesis, groups of primitive muscle cells, including myoblasts and myotubes, are enclosed by a common basement membrane. Primary myotubes cluster in groups of 4 to 12, with spaces between clusters containing fibroblasts and probably angioblasts. In each cluster, there is usually one larger primary myotube.

There is also extensive cytoskeletal reorganization before and after fusion. Myotubes differ from myoblasts by the presence of multiple nuclei and cytoplasmic filaments. Filaments first form at the peripheral portions of the sarcoplasm and consist of 10-nm fibroblast-like fibrils that disappear during maturation. The myofibrils have a rudimentary form of sarcomeres with A and I bands and Z discs. Immunohistochemical techniques also demonstrate the presence of desmin and vimentin within myotubes. Secondary myotubes continue to arise through the successive waves of fusion of postmitotic primary myotubes. More mature secondary myotubes have a larger diameter, increased numbers of several hundred nuclei, and more prominent myofilaments. Secondary myotubes are initially encased by the same basal lamina of the parent primary myotubes, but they later separate and develop their own individual basal lamina. These cells also begin to show evidence of contractile activity. Secondary myotubes eventually give rise to muscle fibers. As they approach this stage of development, secondary myotubes cease fusing and develop acetylcholine receptor (AChR) protein on the cell surface. At first, receptor protein is diffusely distributed on the cell surface, but it later becomes focused into so-called hot spots where motor endplates will develop. Myoblast fusion occurs not only during development but throughout adulthood, as skeletal muscle growth and regeneration require the accumulation of additional nuclei within myofibers. Alterations in myoblast fusion may also contribute to muscle diseases involving loss of muscle mass.

Morphologic changes in myoblast differentiation include those of apoptosis, a regulatory process in the normal development of muscle and selected pathologic conditions including aging, disuse, and exercise (4). During embryogenesis, a necessary remodeling of muscles occurs through apoptosis, which removes "unwanted" cells or structures to make room for further maturation, just as with selected neurons. The large-diameter primary myotubes are preferentially affected. The morphologic features include misshapen nuclei and irregular chromatin condensations along the nuclear envelope, contraction of the cytoskeleton, blebbing of the cell membrane, and packaging of cytoplasmic organelles into an apoptotic body, which are common between myogenesis and apoptosis. In human fetal muscle, the programmed cell death of both primary and mature myotubes occurs between 10 and 16 weeks of gestation. The pathway to apoptosis involves the TRAIL death ligand signaling pathway (5). TRAIL binds to its upregulated receptor, DR5, initiating the caspase 8 route to apoptosis. At the same time, FLIP, a caspase 8 inhibitor, is known to be reduced. A second pathway involves mitochondrial permeability brought about by the proapoptotic members of the Bcl-2 family. This route is mediated by caspase 9. The Bcl-2/caspase 9 pathway is also important in the sarcopenia of aging during which there is a loss of myocytes. Because it is a multinucleated cell, the muscle fiber does not always undergo apoptosis in the same fashion as other cell types. Damage limited to individual myonuclei seems to be more common than death of the entire cell. Finally, the elevated expression of endogenous caspase inhibitors in muscle seems to confer relatively greater resistance to apoptosis in muscle tissue.

Mature muscle fibers differ from myotubes in that their nuclei are peripheral and their filaments are organized into sarcomeres. Muscle fibers also develop a sarcotubular system, and in time they become innervated. Immature muscle fibers often acquire multiple innervation sites, all but one of which eventually disappears. The number of myotubes declines after the 21st week of gestation so that by the time of birth, myotubes are histologically no longer conspicuous. As myotubes become fewer in number, the muscle fibers undergo histochemical differentiation, which begins in the 5th month of development. Between 15 and 20 weeks of gestation, a primitive progenitor of the checkerboard pattern emerges in which all myotubes and myofibers have high ATPase and oxidative enzyme activity. By 20 weeks of gestation, approximately 10% of fibers are larger in diameter, with both high oxidative enzyme activity and reduced ATPase activity. These fibers, which are basophilic in hematoxylin and eosin (H&E) stains, are the so-called Wohlfart type B fibers and are the earliest example of type 1 fibers to be detected in developing muscle. The remaining 90% of fibers (Wohlfart type A) correspond to type 2 fibers with enhanced ATPase activity. Although type 2A and 2B fibers are not yet visible, a few type 2C fibers that stain dark in both acid and alkaline ATPase reactions are apparent. These fibers typically immunostain with antibodies to both fast and slow myosin. The more mature checkerboard histochemical pattern, which is stimulated by the innervation of fibers, is almost completed between 26 and 30 weeks of gestation. At birth, the histochemical mosaic begins to resemble that of mature adult muscle. Approximately 80% of fibers are clearly identified as type 1 or type 2. The remaining 20% are undifferentiated fibers that have both abundant oxidative enzyme activity and stain darkly in routine ATPase reactions. A few Wohlfart type B fibers remain at birth. Type 2C fibers are not encountered.

POSTNATAL AND DEVELOPMENTAL CHANGES

During the prenatal period and childhood, muscle fibers continue to increase in length until full growth is attained. Muscle fibers lengthen in response to growth of the skeleton by virtue of two fundamental changes in the sarcomeres. Existing sarcomeres lengthen, producing longitudinal fiber growth. This mechanism may account for up to a 25% increase in fiber length and indicates that there is a relative "excess" of sarcomeres that may elongate during periods of rapid growth of the skeleton. Muscle fibers also undergo real longitudinal growth with the addition of new sarcomeres, which involves the synthesis of contractile proteins.

sets of parallel muscle fibers radiate (e.g., peroneus longus). Other muscles are simple pennate, in which only one set of parallel muscle fibers attaches obliquely on a shaft-like tendon (e.g., extensor digitorum longus). Muscles are designated as complex pennate when the muscle consists of multiple parallelograms attaching to several tendons in the muscle mass. Not all skeletal muscles follow precisely the model of parallel or pennate design. They may be triangular like the pectoralis minor, or spiral in structure like the forearm supinators. Although most muscles are attached to and are involved in moving bony skeletal structures, some voluntary muscles (such as those of the larynx and esophagus) do not have attachments to bone.

The blood supply to skeletal muscles is of paramount importance to their proper function. Accounting for 40% of body weight, skeletal muscle may require 20% of cardiac output for basal metabolic needs, which may increase drastically with vigorous exercise such as running and swimming and the use of large muscle groups. Not only is an intact supply of oxygen and substrates of importance, but also the efficient removal of metabolites such as lactic acid and carbon dioxide. It is known that the arterial supply to muscles varies somewhat with the individual. In general, the skeletal muscles are subserved by several rather than a single artery, which renders them rather resistant to ischemia from an embolus or from the disease of a single vessel. The vascular supply to skeletal muscle falls into one of the following five categories:

1. The blood supply is derived from a single nutrient artery that divides in a longitudinal fashion within the muscle itself. The medial and lateral head of the gastrocnemius is an example of such a system and represents a risk for greater damage as the consequence of arterial occlusion.

2. The muscle is supplied by several separate arteries entering the muscle along its length. Anastomoses are formed within the muscle between the territories of each artery. This pattern is typical of the soleus.

3. The blood supply arises from a single main artery that enters the belly of the muscle and subsequently forms a radiating pattern of collaterals, as in the biceps brachii.

4. In muscles such as the tibialis anterior, a pattern of anastomosing arcades is derived from a series of penetrating arteries. This vascular pattern is considered to be the most efficient form of vascularization.

5. A less efficient form of the anastomosing arcade pattern is the rectangular pattern of anastomoses formed by a series of penetrating arteries. This so-called quadrilateral pattern is seen in the extensor hallucis longus muscle.

Once a main artery enters the muscle substance, it branches into a number of primary intramuscular arteries that ramify in the epimysium and perimysium. The primary arteries, with a diameter that ranges from 80 to 360 μm, give rise to numerous secondary arterioles that run parallel to the direction of the muscle fibers. The secondary arterioles often connect to primary arteries, forming artery-to-artery anastomoses. The secondary arterioles, which range in diameter from 50 to 100 μm, typically have a thin adventitia composed of fibroblasts and collagen. The smooth muscle coat is much thinner than that of the primary arteries, usually having only two to three layers of cells. The internal elastica is prominent and continuous. The secondary arterioles branch to form terminal arterioles, which measure 15 to 50 μm in diameter. Their smooth muscle coat is usually only one layer of cells. The internal elastica becomes discontinuous and is lost in smaller vessels. The distal portions of the terminal arterioles have precapillary sphincters, which are formed from the smooth muscle cells of the media. These sphincters are found in blood vessels with an inner diameter of less than 15 μm. Footlike processes between the smooth muscle cells and the endothelium may be seen in the region of the sphincters.

As in other tissues, the arterioles end in an elaborate system of capillaries. In contrast to most other organs, a relatively small number of capillaries are open at rest in muscle. During muscle activity, there is a considerable increase in the number of open capillaries. A marked difference in capillary density is observed in different muscles, as well as in trained versus untrained subjects. Studies of capillary density reveal that the average single muscle fiber is surrounded by 1.7 capillaries. Capillary density may also be expressed as the number of capillaries per fiber, which on average in cross sections is 0.7.

The density of capillaries also reflects oxygen consumption within muscle. Therefore, increased numbers of capillaries are evident where larger numbers of type 1 fibers are present. This phenomenon is less evident in humans than in animals such as the cat, in which muscles are composed chiefly or totally of one fiber type. Thus, in the cat soleus muscle, which is composed almost entirely of type 1 fibers, the density of capillaries is 1,600/mm^2. In the gastrocnemius, a muscle with far fewer type 1 fibers, the capillary density is 600/mm^2. The capillaries within skeletal muscle travel primarily in a longitudinal direction, although they are frequently linked by short transverse branches.

Ultrastructurally, capillaries are composed of endothelial cells surrounded by a basement lamina. Occasional pericytes are encountered outside the basement membrane. Endothelial cells typically contain numerous pinocytotic vesicles. Where endothelial cells are joined, they lack tight junctions. Hence, the capillary endothelium is freely permeable to tracers such as horseradish peroxidase. The capillary pericytes are essentially smooth muscle cells that contain large numbers of filaments. The pericytes are innervated by small-diameter unmyelinated nerve fibers. The basement membrane (which lies between the endothelium and pericytes) measures 20 to 30 nm, although some thickening and reduplication of the basal lamina occur in older patients.

The nerve supply to individual skeletal muscles often enters the surface of the muscle at the belly and is accompanied by one or more major penetrating arteries. Within

New sarcomeres are known to be added at the end of fibers, usually at the myotendinous junctions. There is also evidence to suggest that new sarcomeres are not only added at the end of fibers but within internal segments as well. Studies suggest a gradual rise in the number of fibers between birth and the end of the fifth decade. In some muscles, the total increase in fibers may reach 80% to 100% of the neonatal level. The mechanism accounting for an increase in the fiber population probably involves a population of dividing stem cells that subsequently undergo fusion to produce new mature fibers.

A major aspect of growth of muscle fibers after birth relates to an increase in transverse dimension. In general, between birth and adulthood, there is an almost fivefold increase in muscle fiber diameters. For example, the average diameter of mature fibers is between 50 and 60 μm as compared to 7 μm at 20 weeks of gestational age. By birth, fiber diameters have roughly doubled to about 15 μm. The enlargement in fiber diameters does not proceed at an even rate from birth to early adulthood, when fibers obtain a maximum diameter. Instead, fiber diameters increase at a relatively slow rate until puberty, adding 2 μm each year up to age 5 years, then 3 μm per year between 5 and 9 years. By age 10 years, type 1 and 2 fibers measure between 38 and 42 μm with little variability between the average diameters. Around puberty, a burst of growth occurs whereby fibers gain their adult sizes. Type 1 fibers are typically larger than type 2 fibers in females, with the reverse noted in males.

A major revision in the histochemical profile of muscle occurs after birth. In the term infant, a checkerboard staining pattern is clearly evident in alkaline ATPase reactions. However, fiber typing is often not distinct in oxidative enzyme reactions. The emergence of type 1, 2A, and 2B fibers in oxidative preparations occurs during infancy. Undifferentiated fibers having both abundant oxidative enzyme and ATPase activity represent approximately 20% of fibers at birth. These gradually differentiate into type 1 and type 2 fibers during the first year of life. The fate of Wohlfart type B fibers, comprising about 1% of myofibers at birth, is unknown. They are not seen in biopsies of children past the age of 12 months.

The connective tissue elements of muscle are much more prominent at birth, particularly the perimysial components. Immediately after birth, the perimysium may account for up to 20% of the cross-sectional area of muscle tissue (Fig. 7.2). During early childhood, the perimysium and other connective tissue components rapidly shrink to less than 5% of the cross-sectional area, in part because of the enlargement of the muscle fibers. In the immediate postnatal period, blood vessels (especially arteries) appear excessively thickened as a result of the presence of abundant smooth muscle elements. Expansion of the luminal diameter of blood vessels in the first year of life gives the vascular elements an adult appearance. The noncontractile, supporting connective tissue contains abundant collagen and scattered fibroblasts. Foci of hematopoiesis remain

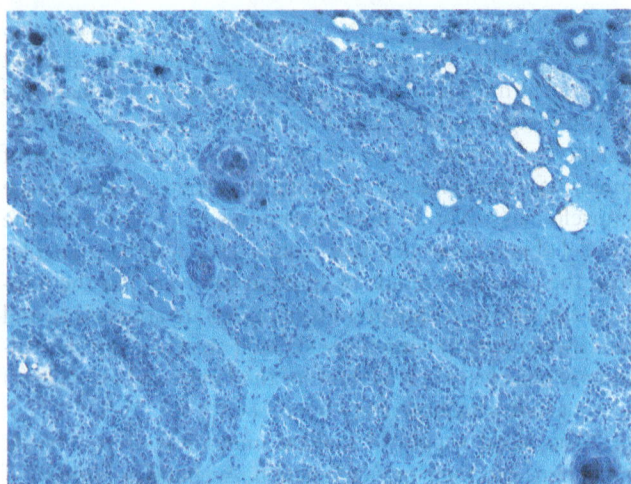

FIGURE 7.2 Infant muscle. A relative increase in perimysial connective tissue is normal (Gomori trichrome).

after birth, containing stem cells, erythroblasts, and myelocytes. These foci are more likely to be seen in the distal muscles of the extremities. They disappear within 1 month after birth.

ANATOMY

There are over 600 voluntary muscles in the human body, most of which are paired. They comprise 25% of the total body weight at birth and 40% to 50% of the total weight in adults. A greater muscle mass is encountered in males than in females. Individual muscles vary greatly in size. For example, the smallest muscle in the body, the stapedius, measures only 2 mm in length. On the contrary, the sartorius and other large muscles of the extremities measure up to 2 ft in length (61 cm). Skeletal muscles are composed of varying numbers of muscle fibers (e.g., 10,000 in lumbricals and 1,000,000 in gastrocnemius). These are connected at both ends to tendons or the epimysium.

Because the fibers work in conjunction with each other, they are aligned in the same direction. A few skeletal muscles are modeled after the lumbricals, small intrinsic muscles of the hands and feet, where all the fibers are arranged in a fusiform structure that tapers at either end at the site of tendinous insertion. The more familiar unit is a parallelogram composed of muscle fibers that insert at both ends on a flat tendon composed of dense collagen. In a parallel muscle, the fascicles are parallel to the longitudinal axis of the muscle, as in the thyrohyoid. In oblique muscles, a tendon typically runs within the muscle or on its surface, and the muscle fibers insert obliquely on the tendon. Oblique muscles are most often pennate or featherlike. Some are bipennate, much like a feather in which there is a central shaft from which a series of barbs radiate on either side. Such muscles have a central tendinous structure from which two the main nerve trunk are myelinated and unmyelinated axons. Contributions to the nerve are made from myelinated efferent motor fibers that innervate the muscle fibers; somatic afferent sensory fibers from muscle spindles, Golgi tendon organs, and pacinian corpuscles; and unmyelinated autonomic efferent fibers. At least 50% of the fibers are sensory in function. The motor fibers that innervate the myofibers demonstrate a bimodal size distribution. The large-diameter α-fibers innervate fast motor units, whereas the β-fibers are distributed to slow motor units and some intrafusal fibers of the muscle spindle. The γ-fibers, with very small diameters, supply the remainder of the muscle spindle fibers. The large motor fibers are relatively uniform in diameter, measuring between 10 and 15 µm. The small motor fibers vary from 2 to 7 µm in diameter.

As the distal motor axon approaches the muscle fiber, it is transformed into the terminal axon, which represents the proximal portion of the neuromuscular junction, or motor endplate. The neuromuscular junction, measuring about 50 µm in diameter, is composed of the presynaptic portion or terminal axon and the postsynaptic portion, which is formed by a unique region in the muscle fiber. The presynaptic and postsynaptic domains are separated by a specialized, 50-nm wide intercellular space, the synaptic cleft. The myelinated motor nerve terminates at the presynaptic region as an unmyelinated axonal segment that is enveloped by the teloglia, the distal projections of Schwann cells. The terminal axon and teloglia are covered by a layer of endoneurium, the sheath of Henle, which becomes continuous with the endomysium of the muscle fiber in the area of the motor endplate. Numerous synaptic vesicles, each 45 to 50 nm in diameter, are found in the terminal axon. The vesicles are most plentiful around thickened zones of increased electron density at the presynaptic membrane. Studies utilizing freeze–fracture electron microscopy have demonstrated that parallel pairs of double rows of intramembranous particles, measuring 10 nm in diameter, are located at these electron-dense zones. The particles are considered to represent voltage-sensitive calcium channels known as active zones.

At the postsynaptic region of the muscle fiber, the cell surface is elevated to form the hillock of Doyère, or sole plate. Within the sole plate, the sarcoplasm is granular, and a cluster of sarcolemmal nuclei is often seen. Nuclei in this location are plump and vesicular. The terminal axon ramifies in the sole plate as a series of branches called telodendria, which indent the surface of the fiber, producing gutters or troughs. The surface of the fiber at the motor endplate is undulating and redundant, creating the complex of postjunctional folds that can be demonstrated by supravital staining as the subneural apparatus of Couteaux (Fig. 7.3). The spaces between the folds denote the secondary synaptic clefts. As a result of the formation of these clefts, the surface area of the postsynaptic membrane is increased to approximately 10 times the surface area of the presynaptic portion. The postsynaptic membrane of the folds is thicker and more densely stained at the crests than

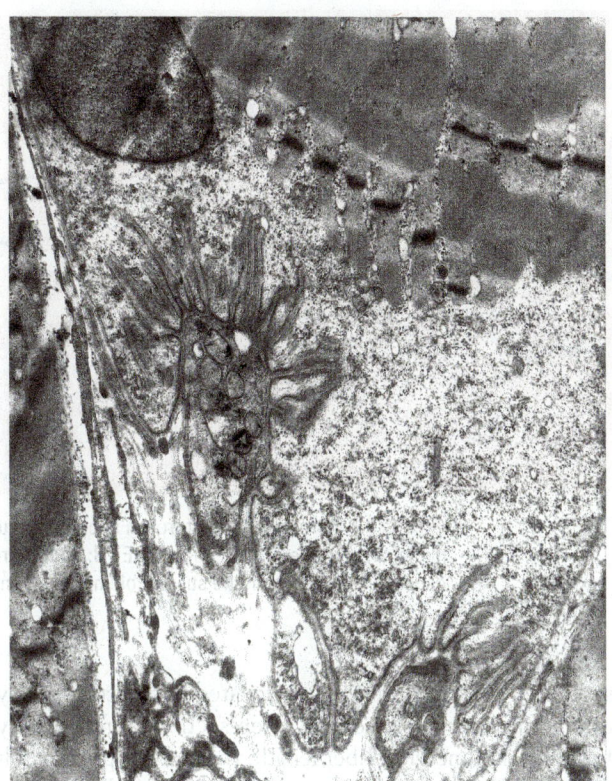

FIGURE 7.3 Electron micrograph of motor endplate. Ultrastructurally, the motor endplate consists of a terminal axon and a postsynaptic region formed by a specialized portion of the muscle fiber. The surface of the fiber is undulating, representing the postjunctional folds.

in the depths of the clefts. By electron microscopy, the juxtaneural membrane at the crests of the folds contains irregularly spaced densities measuring 11 to 14 nm in diameter. In freeze–fracture preparations, on the P face of the membrane, the crests are studded with rows of particles that are similar in size to these densities (about 10 nm). These large intramembranous particles are considered to represent the AChR, a pentameric 275-kDa glycoprotein.

LIGHT MICROSCOPY

Familiarity with the normal structure of skeletal muscle provides a useful background for the pathologist in the evaluation of muscle biopsies. Other sources offering a more comprehensive discussion of the light microscopy, histochemistry, and electron microscopy of normal muscle than is possible here are found in the literature (6–9). The muscle fiber is a multinucleated, syncytial-like unit, shaped like a long, narrow cylinder. Depending on the muscle, a single cell may be as small as 1 mm in length such as in the stapedius or several centimeters as in the sartorius. The average length of skeletal muscle cells in humans is about 3 cm. The normal adult myocyte is not perfectly round but is polygonal, producing a multifaceted profile in cross

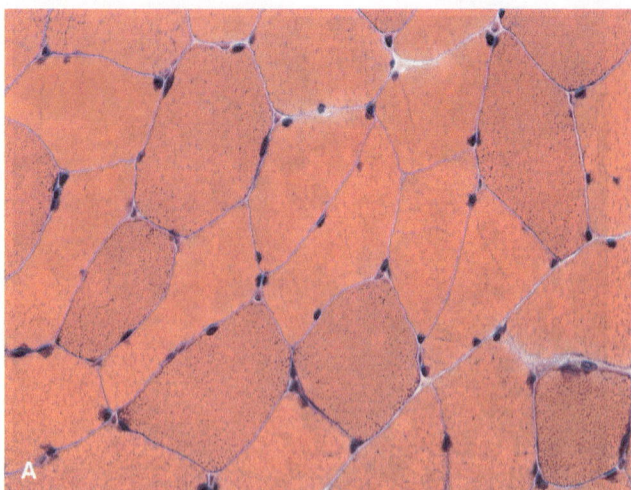
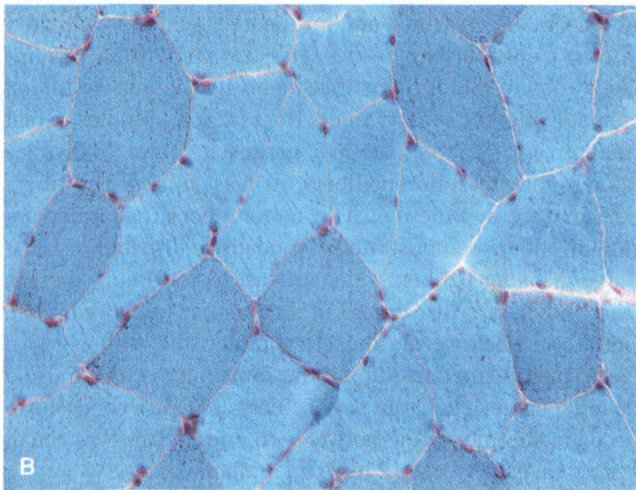

FIGURE 7.4 Cross section of frozen section of muscle. **A:** The sarcoplasm is textured and the sarcolemmal nuclei are peripheral in location (H&E). **B:** Gomori trichrome stain. Mitochondria appear as red granular areas, especially prominent in the subsarcolemmal regions of the fiber.

section. The nuclei are usually located subsarcolemmally, numbering four to six per cell when sectioned transversely. For each millimeter of fiber length, there are approximately 30 nuclei. In routine sections, the sarcolemmal nuclei are slender and flat, with an orientation that is parallel to the long axis of the fiber. These nuclei measure 5 to 12 µm in length and 1 to 3 µm in width. The nucleoli are small and not visible in many fibers. Random fibers may have internally placed nuclei but should not number greater than 3%. Increases are nonspecific but should suggest a condition involving increased turnover of myofibers. In paraffin sections stained with H&E, the sarcoplasm is light pink and textured in cross sections (Fig. 7.4A). In frozen sections that are often routine in biopsies submitted for diagnosis, muscle tissue is stained with Gomori trichrome in addition to H&E. Here, the fibers and connective tissue stain green whereas nuclei are blue-black. In most cases, the mitochondria can be identified, especially in type 1 fibers, as tiny red granules within the sarcoplasm, normally more numerous closer to subsarcolemmal regions than in the center of the fiber (Fig. 7.4B). Notable accumulations of mitochondria may be seen in subsarcolemmal regions in normal muscle, and while a reliable marker of mitochondrial proliferation, the clinical significance is unknown or doubtful. The cross-striations are best appreciated in longitudinal sections and may be accentuated by increasing the refractile index by lowering the microscope condenser (Fig. 7.5). The inability to detect cross-striations by H&E in formalin-fixed paraffin-embedded tissue or sarcotubular details in cryosections should raise the possibility of myofiber necrosis. Cross-striations are best demonstrated in periodic acid–Schiff (PAS) and PTAH stains or in resin-embedded material where alternating dark and light bands are evident (Fig. 7.6).

Red muscle, having a larger mitochondrial and lipid content and higher capillary density, depends on aerobic respiration and is designed for the fatigue resistance required for postural function or sustained activity. The color of red muscles is actually due to relatively greater myoglobin content than white muscles, which contain fewer mitochondria but abundant glycogen, rendering them better suited to anaerobic glycolytic respiration and to sudden and intermittent contraction. In vertebrates, particularly in birds, "red" muscle (e.g., soleus) can easily be distinguished from "white" (e.g., pectoralis) muscles upon external inspection, since an entire muscle in such species may be composed of either red or white fibers. Human muscles, on the

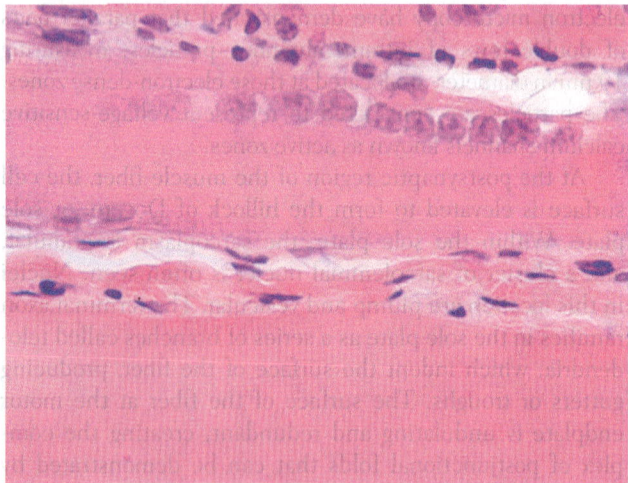

FIGURE 7.5 Longitudinal section of formalin-fixed paraffin-embedded muscle demonstrated cross striation, a valuable finding to all pathologists in recognizing skeletal muscle in diverse situations. Note the more basophilic fiber above with large vesicular nuclei within the sarcoplasm and not in the usual subsarcolemmal position, representing features of muscle fiber regeneration, usually associated with myopathic, not neuropathic, conditions (H&E).

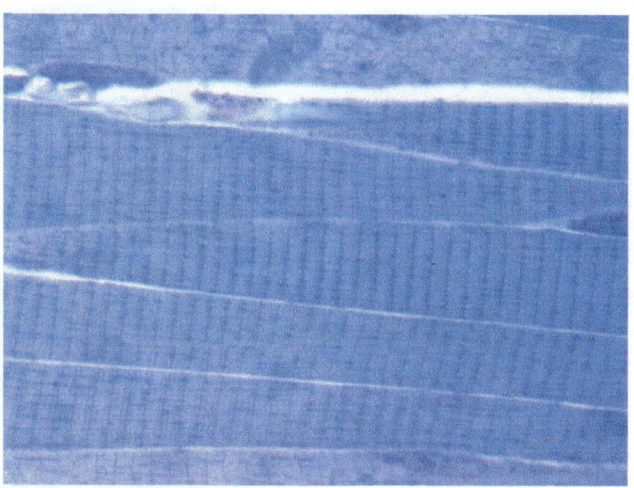

FIGURE 7.6 Resin section. Sarcomere pattern is shown in longitudinal section (toluidine blue).

contrary, contain both fiber types, which typically assume a mixed mosaic arrangement reminiscent of a checkerboard. Depending on anatomic location and function, the proportion of type 1 and type 2 fibers varies, but a typical muscle contains approximately twice as many type 2 fibers (60% to 65%) as type 1 fibers (35% to 40%). This may be conceptualized in the "average" muscle as roughly one-third portions of type 1, 2A, and 2B fibers resulting in the two-thirds majority of type 2 fibers overall.

The demonstration of the histochemical properties of the muscle fibers comprising a biopsy, which is known as fiber typing, is accomplished by applying histochemical techniques (Table 7.1). Fiber typing is best appreciated using enzyme histochemical reactions performed on frozen sections, although an H&E or trichrome stain of high quality in well-preserved muscle will allow for the discernment of darker type 1 fibers versus paler type 2 fibers (Fig. 7.4).

A number of histochemical procedures may be employed for the detection of fiber types, but the most traditional method for this purpose is the myosin ATPase reaction. By changing the pH during the procedure, a spectrum of staining reactions can be produced. In the standard or alkaline ATPase reaction, which is conducted at a pH of 9.4, two fiber types are seen. Type 2 fibers are dark in staining intensity, whereas type 1 fibers are pale (Fig. 7.7A). Fibers of intermediate staining intensity are not observed in the alkaline incubation. If the pH of the incubating solution is brought into the acidic range at pH 4.3, in what is sometimes known as the reverse ATPase reaction, the reverse staining pattern develops, whereby type 1 and 2 fibers are dark and light, respectively (Fig. 7.7B). At pH 4.6, two populations of type 2 fibers emerge: type 2A fibers are virtually unstained and type 2B fibers are intermediately stained, whereas type 1 fibers are much darker (Fig. 7.7C). These staining patterns reflect the excellent fatigue resistance of type 1 fibers versus the greater fatigability of type 2B fibers and the intermediate properties of type 2A fibers. Immunohistochemistry for fast and slow myosin is an established adjunct or replacement for ATPase enzyme histochemistry (Fig. 7.7D). It is also possible to subdivide type 2 fibers into types 2A and 2B using myosin antibodies (10). Immunohistochemistry for fiber typing may be also applicable to fixed tissues, unlike the requirement for cryosections with the ATPase technique.

All the oxidative enzyme reactions, such as the nicotinamide adenine dinucleotide tetrazolium reductase (NADH-TR), show a bimodal pattern of staining intensity, with the darker fibers containing more mitochondria corresponding to type 1 specificity. Oxidative enzyme reactions may further subdivide type 2 fibers into two categories, although the difference is subtle and not as reliable as the result of myosin ATPase enzyme histochemistry at pH 4.6. Although all muscle fibers contain glycogen and the companion enzyme phosphorylase, they are more abundant in type 2 (glycolytic) fibers. The PAS stain, a method of detecting glycogen, and the histochemical reaction for phosphorylase can be used as a means of fiber typing, although it is primarily used to investigate possible cases of enzyme deficiency (type 5 glycogen storage disease, McArdle disease). In fact, almost all stains and enzyme histochemical preparations in frozen muscle pathology may show differences between type 1 and 2 fiber staining intensities. However, staining with these techniques is not totally reliable for fiber typing. Type 1 fibers are rich in neutral lipid, which can be visualized in fat stains such as the oil red O (Fig. 7.8).

Striated muscles are partitioned into fascicles, each of which is invested by a connective tissue sheath known as the perimysium. Within this sheath, the intramuscular nerves, primary arteries, secondary and terminal arterioles, and veins travel throughout the muscle. At the innervation zone in the belly of the muscle, intramuscular nerve bundles or twigs are especially numerous (Fig. 7.9). Up to 10 myelinated nerve fibers may be present in an individual twig, which is surrounded by a thin mantle of perineurial connective tissue. The myelinated nerve fibers are perhaps best demonstrated in Gomori trichrome–stained sections, in which the bright red–colored myelin sheaths surround the unstained axons. Tangential sections of twigs may be mistaken for areas of focal fibrosis or abnormal vascular structures. Additionally, the examination of intramuscular

TABLE 7.1 Fiber Typing

Stain/Reaction	Type 1 Fibers	Type 2 Fibers
ATPase, pH 9.4	Light	Dark
NADH-TR	Dark	Light
PAS/phosphorylase	Light	Dark
Oil red O	Dark	Light

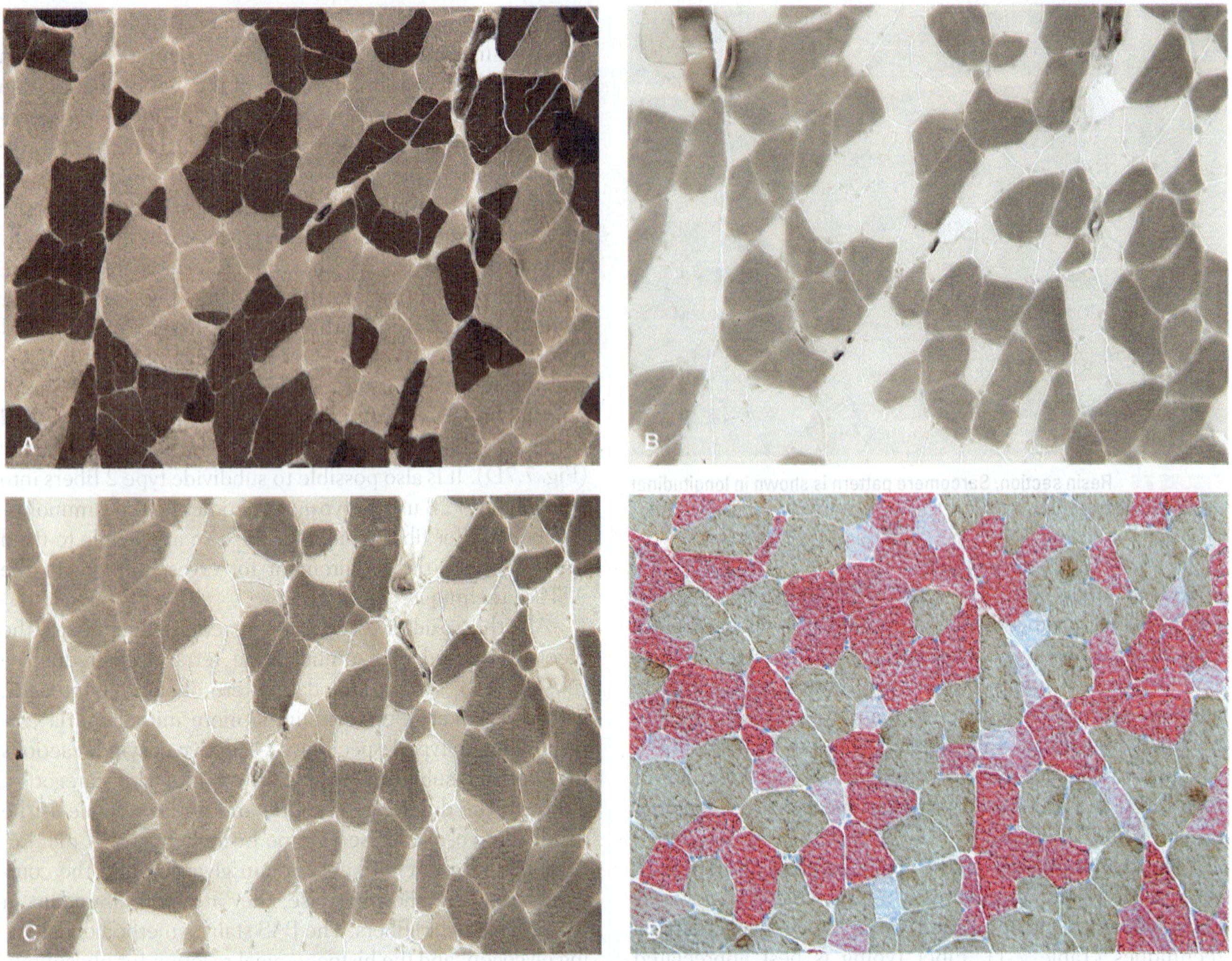

FIGURE 7.7 Skeletal muscle, fiber type determination. **A:** In the myosin ATPase reaction at pH 9.4, type 1 fibers are light and type 2 fibers are dark. **B:** At pH 4.3, the reverse staining pattern is evident. **C:** At pH 4.6, 2A and 2B fibers are distinguishable, with intermediate staining of 2B fibers, which are selectively atrophic in this case of steroid myopathy. **D:** Use of dual antimyosin antibody immunohistochemistry may also be used, showing brown staining of type 1 fibers expressing slow myosin, red-stained type 2A expressing fast myosin, and pale-staining type 2B fibers.

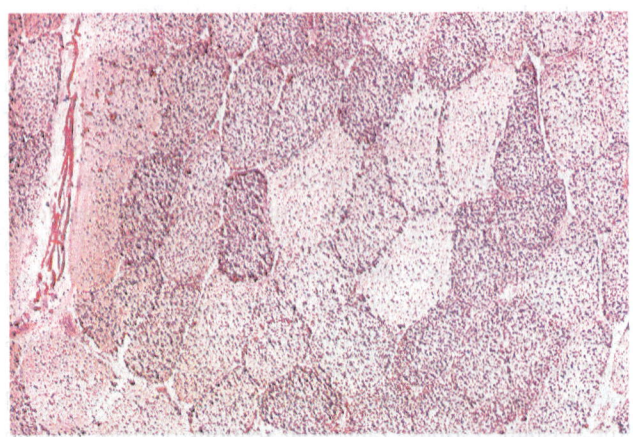

FIGURE 7.8 Lipid content of fibers as demonstrated with the oil red O stain. Type 1 oxidative fibers have a denser lipid concentration.

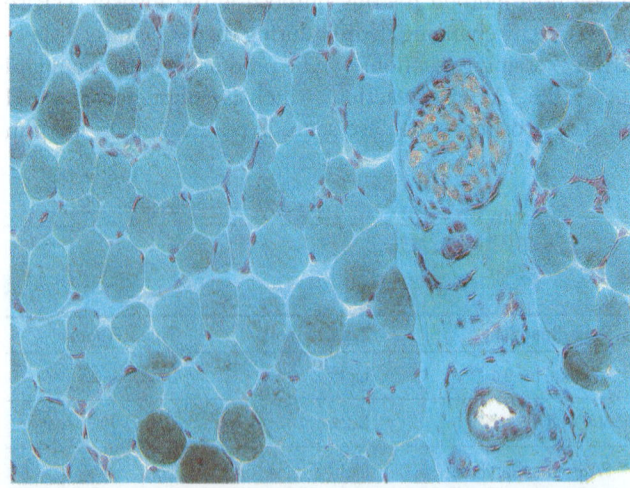

FIGURE 7.9 Intramuscular nerves. Nerve twigs contain axons surrounded by red-staining myelin sheaths (Gomori trichrome).

nerves should not be considered a reliable means to diagnose diseases of peripheral nerves, which is more appropriately accomplished through a dedicated nerve biopsy. The perimysium is a framework that lends stability to the fascicles, in part by its attachment to the epimysium. The epimysium forms septa that sequester groups of fascicles, as well as the fascia that encircles the entire muscle and merges with the dense collagenous connective tissue of the tendons.

Within each fascicle, the perimysium gives way to a normally unobtrusive network, the endomysium. Each muscle fiber may appear to be partly or completely invested by endomysium, a mesenchymal matrix composed of collagen, elastic, and reticulin fibers that support the preterminal arterioles and capillary blood supply to the fascicles. Where the muscle–tendon junction has interdigitations of the cell membrane, the interface is enlarged, transferring tension into shear stress. Two transmembrane proteins, the dystrophin–glycoprotein complex and α7β1 integrin, are especially abundant at the myotendinous junction. It is believed that the dystrophin–glycoprotein complex maintains the integrity of the sarcolemma, whereas α7β1 integrin, a receptor for laminin-2, plays a role in the organization of the basement membrane at the myotendinous junction. At the interface between muscle and either fascia or tendon, the muscle fibers become variable, often small in size, and internal nuclei are more abundant. As they attach to the tendon or fascia, the fibers are separated by dense collagenous trabeculae (Fig. 7.10). Internally placed nuclei are a usual feature of subfascial myofibers or those near myotendinous insertions, along with increased endomysial connective tissue and fiber size variability. Thus, these regions should not be interpreted to signify pathologic alterations. Therefore, the muscle biopsy should be obtained from the belly of the muscle, avoiding the tendinous insertions or subfascial muscle. However, sampling of fascia may be especially important when an inflammatory condition is suspected clinically.

Several specialized structures are found within the connective tissue–supporting framework. Muscle spindles, first described in the 19th century, were once considered to be a pathologic finding. Spindles are now known to be mechanoreceptors that sense the length and tension of skeletal muscle, governing integrated muscle activity. Although they are encountered in virtually all muscles, they are more frequently detected in smaller muscles devoted to finely coordinated activities, such as those of the hand. They are more numerous in distal than in girdle muscles. Quantitative studies have shown that 70 to 100 muscle spindles may be located in an individual muscle. Muscle spindles tend to lie in the deeper portions of the muscle, particularly in the muscle belly. They are often found where type 1 fibers are more plentiful. As the name implies, muscle spindles are fusiform in shape with a swollen center and tapering ends. They measure 3 to 4 mm in length and 200 μm in diameter. A thin fibrous capsule represents the outer boundaries of the muscle spindle. The capsule is an extension of the perimysium, where spindles are usually located. In certain muscles, such as those of the eye, face, and mouth, the capsule merges with the perimysium and is somewhat indistinct. The capsule is composed of 10 to 15 layers of flattened pavement cells that are specialized fibroblasts. The pavement cells are tightly adherent and separated only by thin layers of delicate collagen fibrils. The pavement cells are epithelial-like, in that each is surrounded by a basement membrane. As one proceeds from the equatorial region of the spindle toward the poles, the number of layers of pavement cells progressively diminishes.

Within the capsule are 3 to 15 intrafusal fibers in the typical muscle spindle (Fig. 7.11). Generally, the number of intrafusal fibers is less in small muscles than in larger axial muscles. Two distinct populations of intrafusal fibers

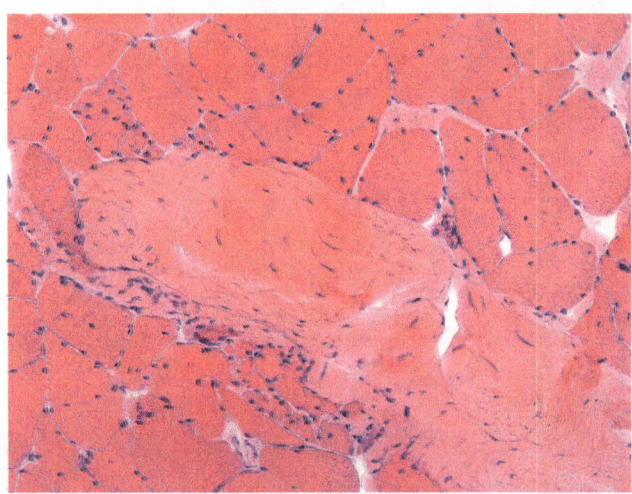

FIGURE 7.10 Subfascial muscle. At the interface, the muscle fibers normally vary in size, have internally placed nuclei, and increased endomysial connective tissue around muscle fibers (H&E).

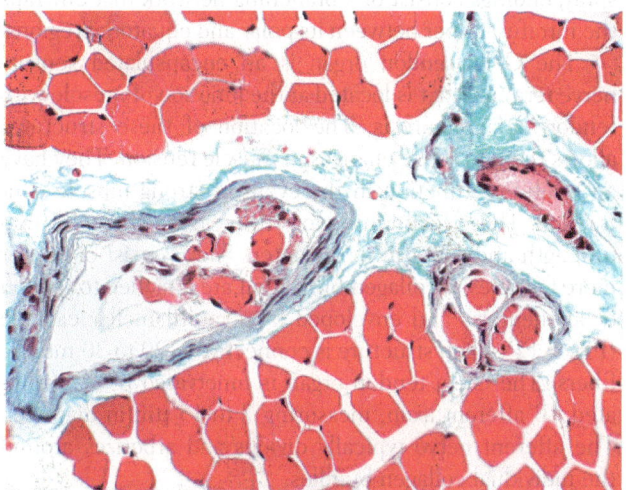

FIGURE 7.11 Muscle spindle. A fibrous capsule encloses a nerve twig and several intrafusal fibers, which are normally smaller than the extrafusal fibers (Gomori trichrome).

are found, both of which are smaller in diameter than the extrafusal fibers. The larger bag fibers, usually one to three per spindle, measure about 20 μm in diameter. The chain fibers number two to seven per spindle, with a diameter of 10 μm or less. The bag fibers are longer, sometimes extending beyond the polar ends of the capsule. They measure 4 to 8 mm in length. The chain fibers are shorter, measuring 2 to 4 mm. The bag fibers are recognized in the equatorial region of the spindle by the presence of large aggregations of nuclei. Away from the equatorial region, the nuclei remain internal or central in the bag fibers but are far less numerous. The smaller chain fibers are distinguished by a row of central nuclei, which extends along the length of the fiber. In histochemical stains, there are two types of bag fibers. Bag 1 fibers reveal considerable oxidative enzyme activity and are pale in ATPase reactions. On the contrary, bag 2 fibers, which also have high oxidative enzyme activity, reveal intermediate staining in ATPase reactions. Chain fibers, although they possess high oxidative enzyme activity, stain darkly in ATPase reactions and are considered by many to be type 2 fibers.

The innervation of muscle spindles, which is both motor and sensory, is complex and will only be summarized here. The intrafusal efferent fibers are derived from branches of β- and γ-efferent axons. The β-axons appear to terminate primarily on nuclear bag fibers. The γ-fibers supply both nuclear bag and chain intrafusal fibers. It is not uncommon for intrafusal fibers to have polyhedral innervation. Two types of sensory innervation are seen in the muscle spindle. The larger-diameter group 1A afferent fibers emanate from the equator. They originate as the annulospiral endings, a series of neural coils and spirals that attach to the nuclear bag and chain fibers. Smaller-diameter group 2 afferent fibers come from the paraequatorial regions of the spindle and are associated mainly with the so-called flower-spray endings of Ruffini. The majority of these endings project from the nuclear chain fibers. The secondary, or flower-spray, endings consist of a branching network that enwraps the intrafusal fiber between its polar and equatorial regions.

The Golgi tendon organ is an encapsulated sensory nerve terminal that is located at the junction of muscle with tendon or aponeurosis. The location of these structures allows them to sense changes in muscle tension. They have an inhibitory function in the event of strong muscle contraction. These fusiform structures measure about 1.5 mm in length and 120 μm in diameter. They consist of one or more fascicles of collagen fibrils that are attached to tendon or aponeurosis and enveloped by a multilamellar capsule (Fig. 7.12). Each structure is connected to 20 to 30 muscle fibers. The Golgi tendon organ is innervated by a myelinated 1B afferent axon, measuring 7 to 15 μm in diameter. The afferent nerve typically divides and arborizes around the individual collagen bundles.

Pacinian corpuscles are distributed widely in the subcutaneous tissues of the body, although they may also be encountered within the muscular fascial planes and

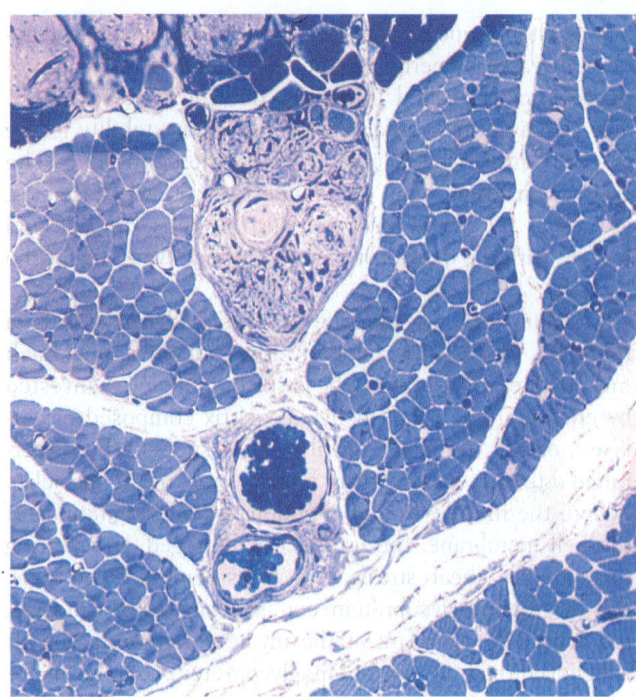

FIGURE 7.12 Golgi tendon organ. Fascicles of collagen surrounded by several nerve bundles (resin section, toluidine blue).

adjacent to tendons or aponeuroses. They are seldom seen within muscle tissue itself. In the center of the pacinian corpuscle is a central rodlike nerve terminal innervated by fast-conducting group 1 or 2 afferent axons. The central axon is surrounded by a capsule composed of concentric layers of cells (Fig. 7.13). The elongated cells forming the capsule are surrounded by basal lamina and separated by fine collagen fibrils. Pacinian corpuscles are receptor organs that are sensitive to vibration.

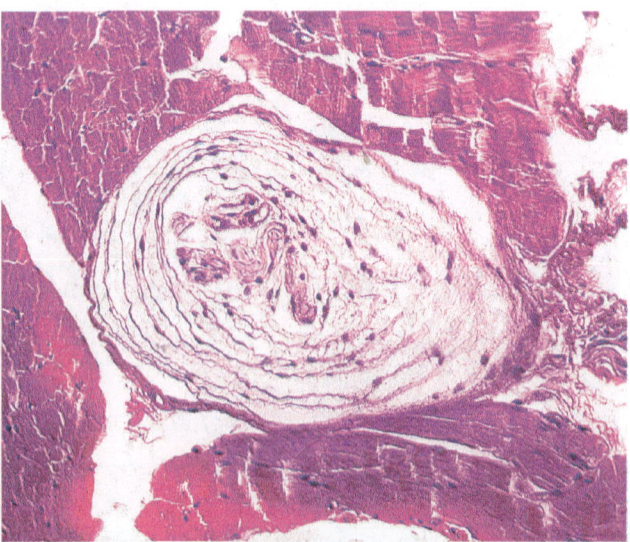

FIGURE 7.13 Pacinian corpuscle. A central nerve terminal is surrounded by a capsule composed of concentric layers of cells (H&E).

ULTRASTRUCTURE

The ultrastructural examination of skeletal muscle is conventionally performed on sections oriented longitudinally, wherein deviations from the orderly striated architecture are more easily detected than in cross sections. The sarcoplasm of each muscle fiber is divided into multiple parallel subunits, the myofibrils, which are minute, cylindroid contractile structures measuring approximately 1 μm in diameter. Myofibrils are segmented into a series of identical sarcomeres that are equal in length, whether the muscle is contracted or at rest, and are aligned in register with the sarcomeres of surrounding myofibrils. The unique periodicity of the fine structure of the muscle fiber is a function of the regimentation of this contractile system. The rectangular banding pattern within each sarcomere is produced by the arrangement of the filaments (Fig. 7.14). The Z band, which forms the lateral boundaries of the sarcomere, is an electron-dense bar-shaped structure oriented perpendicular to the long axis of the myofibril. The distance between consecutive Z bands represents the sarcomere length, an average of 2.5 to 3.0 μm. The I bands are the most electron-lucent portions of the sarcomere and stand in dramatic contrast to the dark Z bands that bisect them. The I bands are shorter in length than the moderately dense A bands located at the center of the sarcomeres. Within each sarcomere are stacks of parallel filaments that, under the electron microscope, appear to be of two types. The thicker filaments measure 15 nm in diameter and are principally composed of myosin. The thinner filaments, containing chiefly actin, are 8 nm in diameter. The thin filaments are attached to the Z band and extend across the I band, where only thin filaments are found. They penetrate the A band in which alternating thick and thin filaments are visualized. Thick filaments, on the contrary, are restricted to the A band region of the sarcomere and determine its length.

The sarcoplasmic organelles are more concentrated around the sarcolemmal nuclei and between the myofibrils.

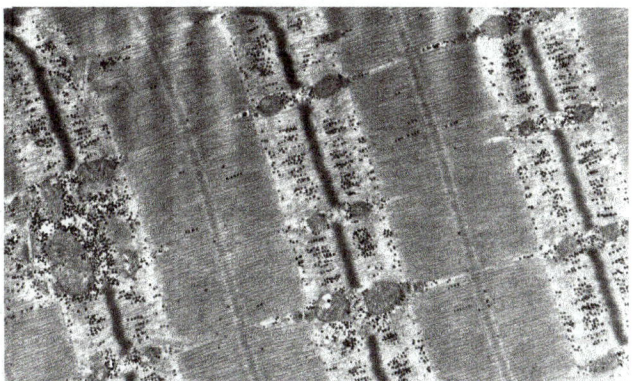

FIGURE 7.14 Ultrastructurally, the several myofibrils can be seen in register in a longitudinal section of the contractile apparatus. Each is composed of a series of sarcomeres that contain A, I, and Z band regions.

The mitochondria are somewhat variable in shape and size, although the majority of them are oval or elliptical in configuration in cross section, which belies their more elongated or tubular shapes. They are most easily recognized adjacent to the Z bands where their long axes are parallel to those of the myofibrils. Both mitochondria and lipid vacuoles are more conspicuous in oxidative fibers. Mitochondria are not normally longer than a sarcomere in length, although the exact significance of mitochondrial enlargement is nonspecific and should not equate with bona fide mitochondrial disease. Recent studies employing high-resolution, three-dimensional scanning electron microscopy have demonstrated connectivity between muscle cell mitochondria forming a reticulum connecting complex IV/COX-active subsarcolemmal paravascular mitochondria and complex V/ATP synthase–rich intramyofibrillar mitochondria.

Glycogen, composed of granules with a diameter of 15 to 30 nm, is more abundant in glycolytic fibers, particularly in the I band region of the sarcomere, but differences cannot be used to determine the fiber type at the EM level. Intermyofibrillar glycogen is more abundant in newborn skeletal muscle but is normally relatively sparse in more mature muscle. Glycogen content varies with diet and is also dependent on the amount of exertion sustained by the muscle. The sarcoplasmic reticulum (SR) and the transverse (T) tubules together comprise the sarcotubular complex, are usually more abundant in type 2 fibers, and function in the excitation–contraction coupling process. The SR, which is analogous to the endoplasmic reticulum of other cells, is an elaborate system of tubules that, by branching in all directions, surrounds the myofibrils. In contrast to the SR, which has no communication with the extracellular space, the T tubules arise as invaginations from the cell membrane. They are observed at regular intervals along the length of the fiber, particularly at the junction of the A and I bands. The T tubules encircle the myofibrils and are disposed in a predominantly transverse direction. Branches of the sarcotubular complex join together as triads at the A–I band junctions. Here, pairs of terminal cisterns derived from the SR are positioned on either side of a central T tubule. In this location, the SR tubules appear as hollow, membrane-bound profiles, whereas the T tubules are somewhat more electron dense.

In a normal muscle fiber, the nuclei (myonuclei) occur beneath the sarcolemma, although they may occasionally occur internally. Satellite cells are a separate population of myoblastic stem cells that are a source of nuclei during muscle growth, particularly hypertrophy. Satellite cells also have the capacity to synthesize new muscle after myocyte injury. Satellite cells represent approximately 10% of the myonuclei seen in cross sections of muscle. There is a decline in the number of satellite cells as a result of the aging process so that they constitute only 2% to 3% of myofiber nuclei in older individuals. Satellite cells are small, mononuclear, fusiform cells that are situated beneath the basement membrane of neighboring muscle fibers. They cannot be reliably distinguished from the muscle fiber nuclei under the light microscope, but may easily be identified as immunopositive for NCAM. Satellite cells are not randomly distributed along the length of the muscle fiber and are more numerous in certain locations such as the sole plates of the neuromuscular junction and the polar regions of the muscle spindles. Ultrastructurally, the nuclei of satellite cells differ somewhat from the above-mentioned myonuclei of muscle fibers. Satellite cells lie beneath the external lamina of the muscle fiber and are separated from the fiber by their own plasma membrane and a slender gap of 50 nm or less. They are more elongated, their nuclear chromatin is peripherally dense, and nucleoli are lacking. The satellite cell nuclei are usually asymmetrical within the cytoplasm, which contains only a few filaments without evidence of sarcomere formation. The sarcoplasm also contains free ribosomes, microtubules, and centrioles, which may be associated with cilia. Where the cell membranes of the satellite cell and muscle fiber are opposed, numerous pinocytotic vesicles are seen.

SPECIAL TECHNIQUES

Perhaps more than any other tissue, skeletal muscle in humans has been studied using a wide variety of specialized techniques, in part because human muscle biopsies are frequently collected in such a way as to make both fresh, unfixed tissue and material for special studies available. In addition to routine histochemical methods that are focused primarily on the identification of fiber types, a number of other histochemical procedures have been developed on the basis of several aspects of muscle metabolism. Among these are histochemical techniques to identify various enzymes involved in glycogen metabolism and glycolysis. Familiar examples are histochemical stains for phosphorylase and phosphofructokinase.

Enzyme histochemical procedures have been developed to study mitochondrial function. Cytochrome oxidase (COX)-deficient fibers are a reliable indicator of mitochondrial dysfunction and increase in number as a function of age. COX-deficient fibers are most reliably detected through the use of combined enzyme histochemistry for COX and Succinate dehydrogenase (SDH), whereby normal fibers show dual staining and COX-deficient fibers appear in varying shades of blue (Fig. 7.15). COX-deficient fibers are increased in a variety of diseases, not only primary mitochondrial myopathies, but also in some inflammatory myopathies such as inclusion body myositis and dermatomyositis. In determining the possible pathologic significance of the number of COX-deficient fibers, the following quantification can be considered within normal limits for the listed age ranges within a 100× magnified microscopic field: 0.3 (30 to 39 years), 0.8 (40 to 49 years), 2.0 (50 to 59 years), 2.5 (60 to 69 years), 4.2 (70 to 79 years), and 6.5 (80 to 89 years). When a primary mitochondriopathy is suspected on this basis, respiratory chain complex enzyme activities may be assayed using the frozen muscle, or the mitochondrial and nuclear DNA relevant to mitochondrial function may be analyzed for pathologic point mutations and deletions.

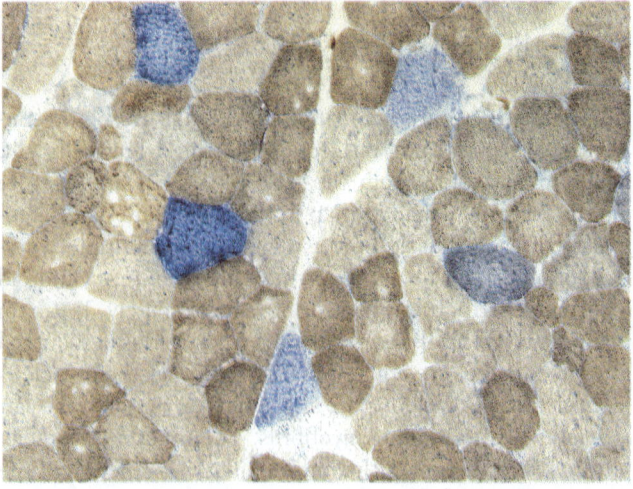

FIGURE 7.15 COX-deficient fibers are detected in a highly sensitive method by performing both the COX and SDH enzyme histochemical reactions on the same section. Fibers lacking the brown stain signifying COX activity will stain preferentially blue, marking SDH activity.

Other enzyme histochemical techniques offer particular applications in diagnosing certain myopathies or neurogenic diseases of muscle. The NADH-TR preparation highlights the cytoarchitecture of myofibers by staining the sarcotubular system, and is therefore well-suited to reveal a host of abnormalities such as target fibers in reinnervated muscle, central or multicores in those respective diseases, and a variety of nonspecific but abnormal morphologies represented by moth-eaten, lobulated, and trabecular fibers (Fig. 7.16). The nonspecific esterase preparation identifies denervated fibers in a highly sensitive manner as appearing overly dark, angular, and atrophic. The neuromuscular junction which is normally identified by esterase enzyme histochemistry may show subtle abnormalities in diseases affecting the structure such as myasthenia gravis, however is not in common usage in deference to serologic and pharmacologic means of diagnosis. The esterase preparation also carries the ancillary advantage of highlighting infiltrative inflammatory cells by virtue of the esterase present in their cytoplasm. The alkaline phosphatase reaction identifies endomysial capillaries as well as regenerating fibers. The acid phosphatase reaction is characteristic of fibers with increased lysosomal activity; its utility in recognizing acid maltase deficiency/type 2 glycogen storage disease is a classic example. The acid phosphatase reaction in perimysial connective tissue has been advocated as a means of recognizing immune myopathies with perimysial pathology (IMPP). Finally, in the workup of human disease, enzyme histochemical analysis of muscle tissue can be supplemented by biochemical analysis, specifically when histochemical techniques are unavailable.

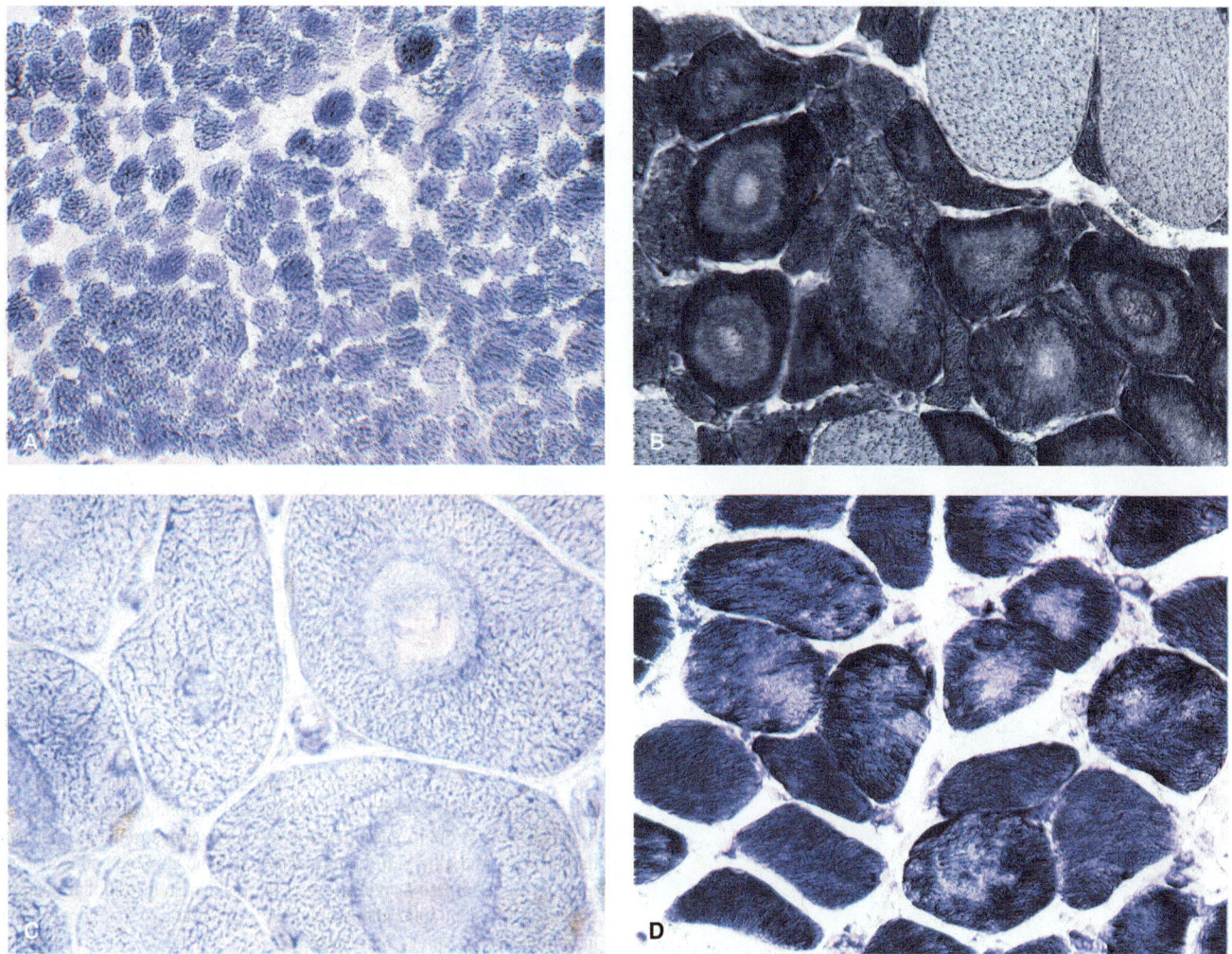

FIGURE 7.16 Aspects of NADH-TR enzyme histochemistry. **A:** Newborn muscle. Indistinct fiber typing is evident in oxidative enzyme reactions. **B:** Target fibers, with an inner unstained zone surrounded by a rim of increased enzyme activity. **C:** Central core myopathy. **D:** Moth-eaten fibers are a nonspecific finding in both myopathic and neuropathic conditions.

Immunohistochemistry is an indispensable technique in pathology that has found a niche in the study of muscle. As already described, it may serve as an adjunct or replacement to traditional myosin ATPase preparations for fiber type analysis or in cases with vague fiber type differentiation by the ATPase technique. Fibers undergoing regeneration can be detected by immunohistochemical methods: regenerating fibers contain fetal myosins and react strongly with antibodies to vimentin and desmin. Denervated fibers may show nestin immunopositivity.

Among the dystrophic myopathies, visualization of the pathogenic proteins or their loss has become a mainstream tool in myopathology. Antibodies to the C- and N-termini and rod domain of dystrophin may permit the diagnosis of Duchenne and Becker dystrophies in the approximately 30% of cases in which blood-derived DNA is not diagnostic. Several congenital and limb girdle muscular dystrophies are also diagnosable by immunohistochemistry, usually revealing partial or complete losses of the relevant protein (Fig. 7.17) (Table 7.2).

The nerve supply to muscle, including the intramuscular nerve twigs and motor endplates, cannot be adequately studied in routine samples. The anatomic location of nerve endings and endplates is variable depending on the muscle selected. They may be restricted to a narrow band across the muscle, or they may be more widely distributed throughout the muscle tissue. Some investigators prefer to biopsy shorter muscles, maximizing the chance of finding the intramuscular nerves. The external intercostal muscle has been used for this reason. Many limb muscles have a single band of terminal motor innervation that corresponds to the so-called motor point. The motor point can be identified with the use of an electrical stimulator. After the administration of local anesthesia and incision of the skin, the muscle is stimulated using a metallic electrode before any tissue is removed. The nerve endings can be located at

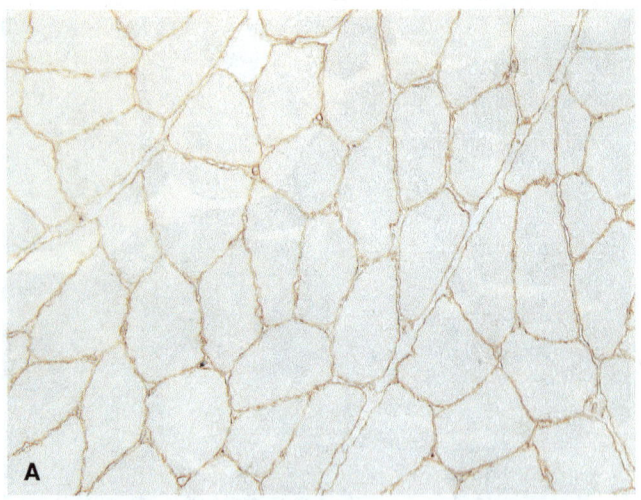
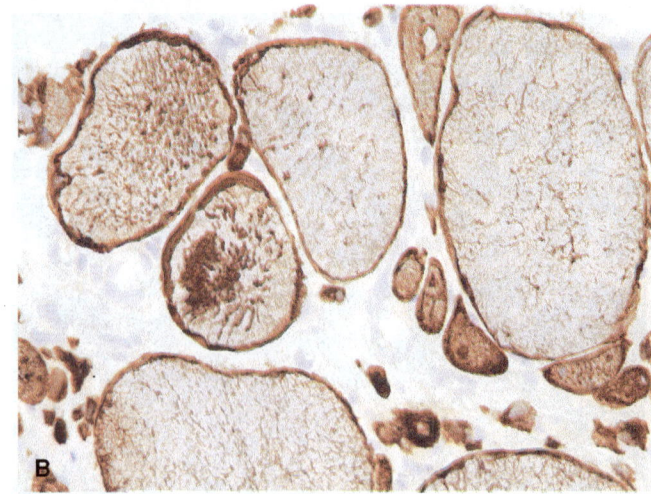
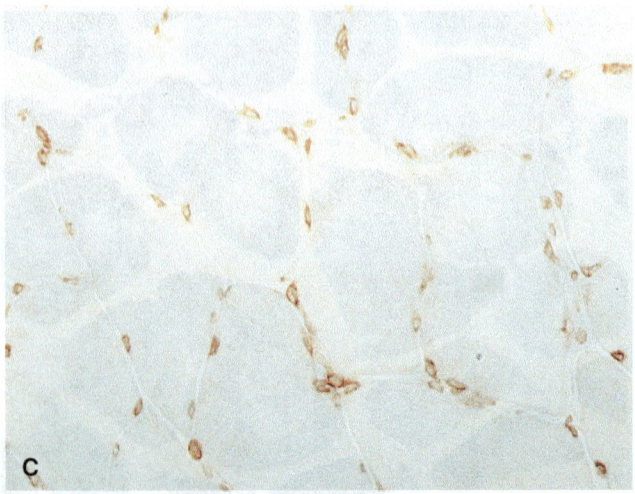

FIGURE 7.17 Immunohistochemical patterns for muscular dystrophy–related proteins. **A:** Sarcolemmal regions are normally labeled by immunostains for dystrophin, sarcoglycans, dysferlin, α-dystroglycan, merosin (laminin α2), and others. **B:** Abnormal cytoplasmic accumulations of desmin, or related proteins myotilin and αB-crystallin in myofibrillar myopathies. **C:** Normal nuclear immunopositivity for emerin, the absent protein in Emery–Dreifuss muscular dystrophy.

TABLE 7.2 Immunohistochemical Identification of Proteins in Selected Skeletal Muscle Diseases

Proteins	Muscle Disease
α-Actinin, actin, tropomyosin	Nemaline myopathies
α-Dystroglycan	Congenital muscular dystrophies of the muscle–eye–brain disorders
Caveolin	LGMD 1C; hyperCKemia; rippling muscle disease
Desmin; myotilin; α-actin; αB-crystallin	Myofibrillar AKA desmin myopathies
Dysferlin	LGMD 2B
Dystrophin, utrophin	Duchenne and Becker muscular dystrophy; Internalized in some dystrophies, i.e., myofibrillar myopathies
Emerin	Emery–Dreifuss MD
MHC-1; membrane attack complex of C5b-9 (MAC)	Inflammatory myopathies
Merosin	Congenital muscular dystrophy
Sarcoglycans	LGMD 2C–2F
SMI-31; TDP-43; LC3; αB-crystallin	Inclusion body myositis

LGMD, limb girdle muscular dystrophy.

sites where a single fascicle rather than the whole muscle contracts after stimulation with a very weak current. Once the innervation zone is established electrically, the biopsy is removed. Using a variety of techniques, different portions of the muscle innervation can be subsequently evaluated.

Vital staining with methylene blue has been used to demonstrate the intramuscular nerve twigs as well as the endplates. This technique requires that the muscle be injected with a methylene blue solution before the muscle sample is actually taken. An undesirable complication of this technique is muscle pain, which many patients experience during the injection of the dye. In order to preserve the staining of the nerve endings, the biopsy must be oxygenated for 1 hour. This technique is obviously complicated and not recommended for most laboratories. A simpler but less elegant technique for the demonstration of nerve twigs is the staining of muscle with silver methods such as Bodian stain. The postjunctional portion of the endplate can be stained enzyme histochemically for acetylcholinesterase activity. The reaction product is not restricted to the postjunctional membrane, and consequently, this is a relatively crude method of studying endplates.

More precise methods of studying endplates involve the use of α-bungarotoxin and freeze–fracture electron microscopy. α-Bungarotoxin is derived from cobra venom and binds specifically with the AChR. Immunoperoxidase techniques using α-bungarotoxin allow direct ultrastructural visualization of the postjunctional region of the motor endplate. With the use of freeze–fracture preparations, both the active zones of the presynaptic membrane and the AChRs of the postsynaptic membrane can be studied in greater detail. In certain rare disorders of the neuromuscular junction, freeze–fracture microscopy may be a useful ancillary diagnostic tool.

Finally, morphometric analysis of muscle tissue is indicated in the event that normal or abnormal findings, such as variations in fiber diameters, are minimal and subtle. In the past, morphometry has been performed manually, but more recently it has been possible to conduct morphometric analysis using a computer-based image analysis (11).

GENDER, TRAINING, AND AGING

Some of the earliest studies addressing differences between males and females with regard to muscle fiber size and composition were conducted by Brooke et al. (12). In a seminal study of the biceps muscle in six patients, they established certain principles that remain generally true concerning gender differences in skeletal muscle. Individual muscle fibers are, on average, larger in males than in females. Androgens are also thought to play a role in the size of muscle fibers in males, since it is known that testosterone supplements produce muscle fiber hypertrophy. In males, type 2 fibers are usually larger than type 1 fibers, in contrast to females where type 1 fibers tend to be of equal or greater diameter. Some of the differences between males and females are dependent on the muscles sampled. For example, studies of the biceps muscle essentially verify the findings of Brooke et al. However, examination of the vastus lateralis indicates no significant difference in diameter between type 1 and type 2 fibers in males. Another interesting conclusion from these studies addresses the question of fiber type predominance in the two sexes. With regard to the biceps muscle, males have a much higher percentage of type 2 fibers, whereas females have almost equal numbers of each. On the contrary, in the vastus lateralis, both males and females have similar proportions of type 1 and type 2 fibers.

The effect of exercise and training on skeletal muscle has been examined over the years. The results of many of these studies are conflicting, but certain general principles have emerged. It is clear that exercise and training of any type causes an increase in muscle fiber diameters. Most authorities agree that power training such as weight lifting results in remarkable hypertrophy of type 2 fibers and less, if any, enlargement of type 1 fibers. Activities that are basically anaerobic in nature promote hypertrophy of type 2 fibers, a reported finding in sprinters, and slowing of the normal age-related atrophy of type 2 fibers. In long-distance runners, for whom aerobic, fatigue-resistant metabolism is more important, type 1 fibers tend to be larger and are accompanied by greater capillary density. Elite long-distance runners may have a greater proportion of type 1 fibers, whereby runners have genetically determined fiber type compositions and little, if any, conversion of fiber types takes place during training. Furthermore, improvement in muscle function through training may be more a reflection of changes in metabolism, including mitochondrial function that is not manifested in fiber sizes and type distribution. Animal studies have shed minimal light on these questions, in part because animal muscle responds differently to exercise and training than does human muscle. In fact, animal experiments have more often clouded the issues of exercise and fiber composition instead of resolving the controversy.

During the process of aging, there is a functional and structural decline in skeletal muscle beginning in the sixth decade and accelerating after the age of 70 years. By the age of 75 years, there is a 30% to 50% decline in muscle strength, the cause of which is complex. Part of the answer lies in the reduction of fiber diameters from approximately 65 microns in the 30- to 50-year age group to around 43 microns in an 81- to 89-year age group for type 1 fibers and from 70 microns to 40 microns for type 1 fibers. The reduction in fiber diameter may be due, in part, to an alteration in growth factors, including myostatin, also known as growth differentiation factor 8 (GDF8), a member of the transforming growth factor family. Myostatin is a negative regulator of muscle, a mediator of catabolic pathways in muscle cells.

Because of the alterations in the composition of their connective tissues, associated with decreased elasticity and flexibility, and because many older patients have joint disease of varying severity, the elderly become less active with a corresponding reduction in muscle volume and contractile strength. Some experts view this condition as a form of disuse. Their conclusions are supported by the fact that aging individuals, like young patients who do not use their muscles (e.g., as a result of immobilization in a cast), have selective atrophy of type 2 fibers. The effect of poor nutrition in the elderly is probably a factor, as it is known that cachexia is accompanied by atrophy of type 2 fibers.

A second problem in the elderly population is an insidious degeneration of motor units, specifically to the anterior horn cells in the spinal cord. Due to degenerative spine disease, there is also injury to nerve roots, with subsequent radiculopathy. The integrity of the muscle fiber is closely related to the maintenance of its nerve supply. Any sustained interruption of trophic influences from the motor neuron or nerve will culminate in atrophy of the denervated muscle fiber. In acutely denervated muscle, randomly distributed small fibers are seen, although with a preference for type 2 fiber involvement. When sectioned transversely, atrophic fibers are characteristically angular or ensate (sword-like) in morphology. They appear flattened and bipolar, with tapering ends and may lie in tandem. In acute denervation, selective atrophy of type 2 fibers is commonly the only pathologic abnormality, so that the proper diagnosis of denervation requires corroborative clinical information to exclude other causes of selective type 2 myofiber atrophy such as disuse, advanced age in females, polymyalgia rheumatica, and many others. With progressive denervation, the proportion of atrophic type 1 and type 2 fibers tends to equalize.

The esterase enzyme histochemical preparation is very useful under these circumstances because denervated fibers are overly dark whereas atrophic fibers in other conditions are not (Fig. 7.18A). Atrophic fibers are also excessively dark in oxidative enzyme reactions, but such staining applies to fiber atrophy of almost any cause. Small dark fibers in oxidative preparations are probably explained by the fact that mitochondria are relatively spared or may even proliferate in the atrophic process and occupy a proportionately greater volume of sarcoplasm.

Prima facie evidence of advanced denervation is a progression from random fiber atrophy to grouped atrophy in which multiple collections of small, angular atrophic fibers are present in the biopsy sample (Fig. 7.18B). As a consequence of

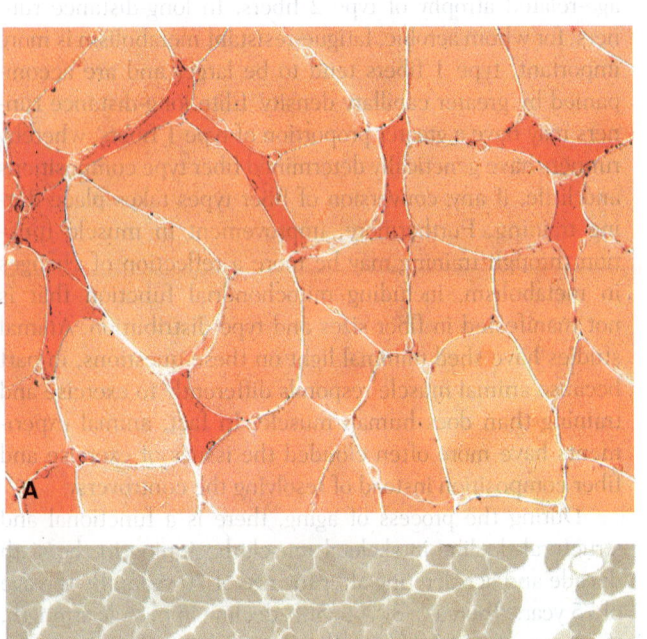

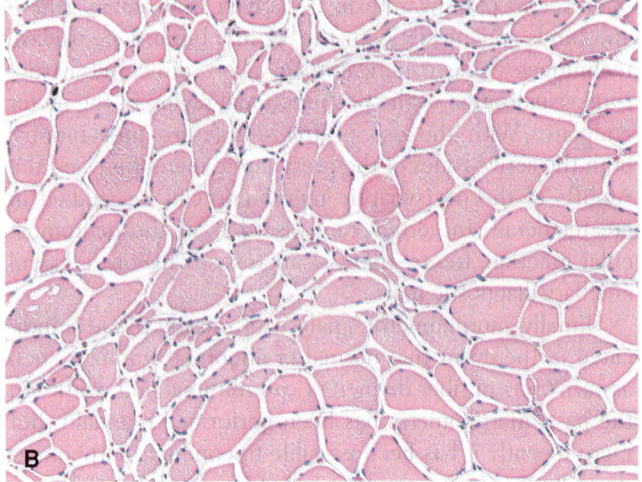

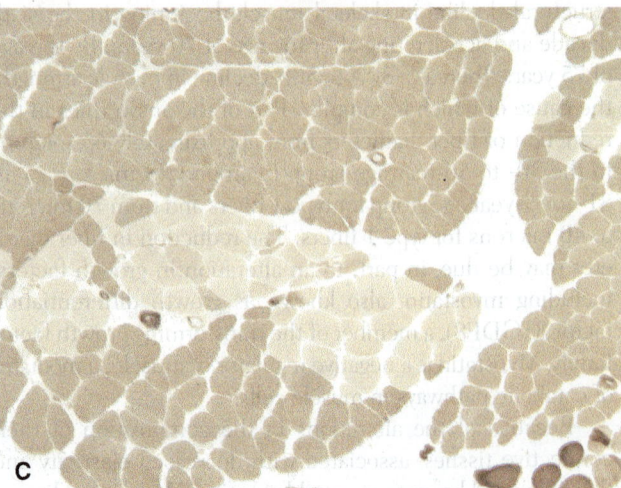

FIGURE 7.18 Neuropathic abnormalities. **A:** Neurogenic atrophy. Angular atrophic fibers, overly dark in the esterase enzyme histochemical preparation. **B:** Grouped atrophy in a confirmed case of amyotrophic lateral sclerosis. Note the compensatory hypertrophy of some fibers and the notable degree of myofiber shrinkage with formalin fixation (H&E, formalin fixed paraffin embedded). **C:** Chronic denervation with reinnervation producing fiber type grouping and alteration of the normal checkerboard staining profile, with groups, defined as a fiber completely surrounded by its own fiber type, of both types (ATPase @ pH 9.4).

chronic denervation and of reinnervation, the normal checkerboard staining profile observed in histoenzymatic reactions is lost. In an effort to reestablish the nerve supply to denervated muscle fibers, intact intramuscular nerves undergo collateral sprouting, and new synapses are formed with atrophic fibers. As motor units enlarge, reinnervated fibers occupying a large area are converted to one histochemical type. The phenomenon of type grouping (Fig. 7.18C) is explained by the fact that all muscle fibers within a single motor unit are of the same type—either type 1 or type 2—and the motor neuron, through the trophic influences of its axon and collaterals, governs the histochemical properties of its fibers. The plasticity of muscle fibers allows conversion from one histochemical type to the other when there is reinnervation by a motor neuron of the opposite type.

Along with type grouping, target fibers are pathognomonic of reinnervation. Despite their unique specificity, bona fide target fibers are present in less than 25% of cases of neuropathic disease. Although targets and central cores are similar morphologically, they differ in three ways. Although both tend to occur singly within a fiber, the target is larger in diameter. The target is limited in length, only extending across a few sarcomeres, in contrast to the central core, which may run the entire length of the fiber. Most important is the three-zone architecture of the target fiber (Fig. 7.16B). The central zone, indistinguishable at the ultrastructural level from the unstructured core, is surrounded by an intermediate zone that forms an intensely stained rim in oxidative enzyme reactions. By definition, the intermediate zone, difficult to identify in most other stains, is absent from a core. It is a zone of transition between the central zone of severe sarcoplasmic disruption and the third zone, which represents the normal portion of the muscle fiber. Targetoid fibers, which lack the intermediate zone of increased oxidative enzyme activity, are morphologically identical to core fibers. The term *core* is conventionally used in cases of congenital central core disease (Fig. 7.16C), and the term *targetoid* is applied to cores that are found in any other condition. Targetoid fibers are more commonly encountered in neurogenic atrophy than any other condition and are more frequently seen than target fibers.

ARTIFACTS

The most common artifacts are related to unsuspected or inadvertent injury to the muscle specimen in vivo (precollection phase), to collection and processing errors such as incautious handling at the time of removal, or to improper tissue holding, freezing, and sectioning. When they are linear in configuration, needle tracts, such as those produced during electromyography (EMG) studies, may easily be recognized. More often, needle tracts are cut tangentially so that the pathologist may be misled by a histologic picture of myopathy exemplified by fiber necrosis, regeneration, inflammation, and interstitial fibrosis (Fig. 7.19A). This kind of precollection artifact is generally traceable to poor communication between the physician requesting the biopsy and the individual performing the procedure, who is unaware of the previous intramuscular injections. Since routine immunizations are usually administered in the thighs of infants, it is not unusual for a diagnostic muscle biopsy in this age group to include a prior injection site. Aggregates of macrophages containing adjuvant material will be observed microscopically in such instances (Fig. 7.19B).

In an uncommon but very misleading collection error, large numbers of neutrophils are occasionally observed within the intramuscular blood vessels. These cells may be marginated and may have begun to penetrate the vascular walls to enter the perimysium or endomysium, simulating an acute vasculitis. In the absence of other pathologic changes within the specimen, the presence of neutrophils,

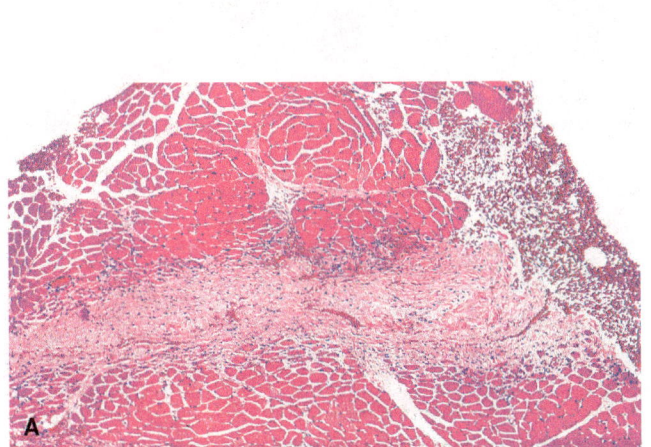
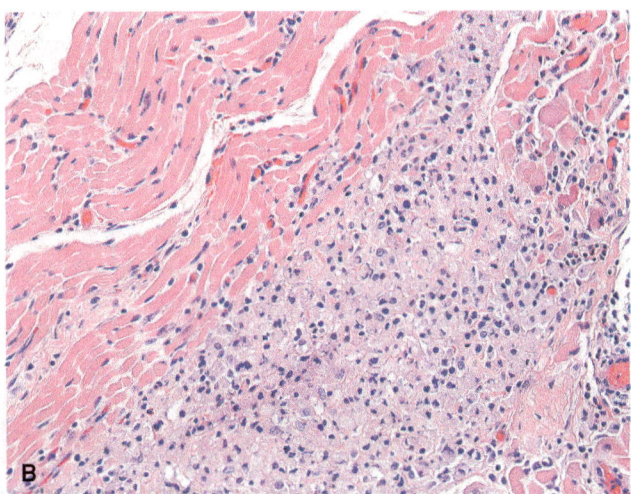

FIGURE 7.19 **A:** Needle tract. Area of injury contains necrotic fibers and a small focus of lymphocytic inflammation (H&E). **B:** Thigh immunization injection site, showing aggregates of macrophages containing adjuvant material.

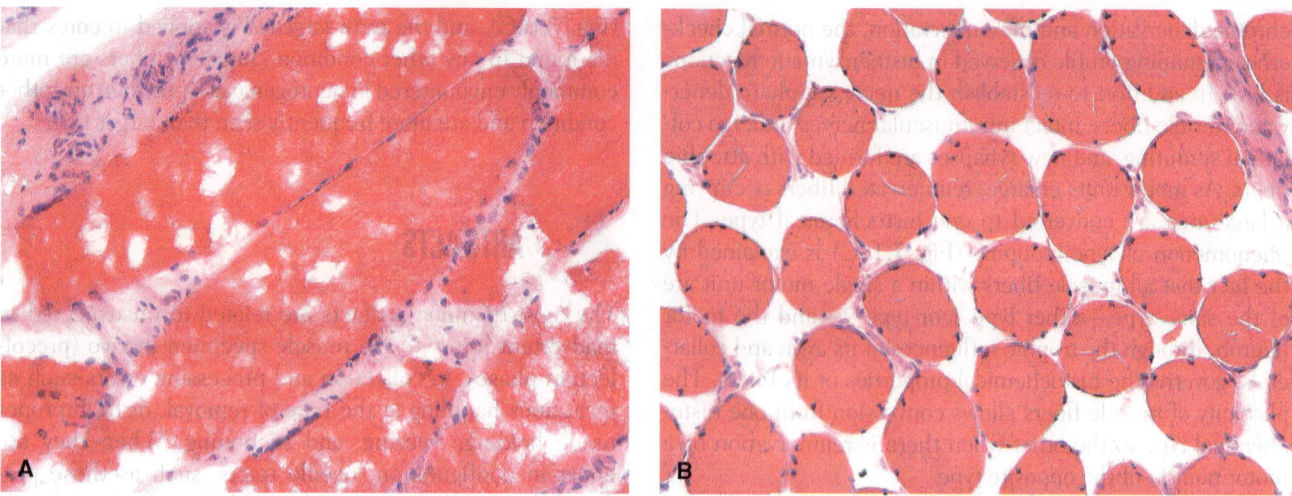

FIGURE 7.20 **A:** Vacuolar artifact. Improper freezing has caused numerous clear holes to form within the fibers (H&E). **B:** Thawing and refreezing of improperly frozen specimens may result in diminished freeze artifact but renders the fibers rounded with empty spaces between fibers, and slit-like spaces representing collapsed vacuoles.

which is abnormal in a muscle biopsy, usually means that the muscle has been tortured by crushing or squeezing by an inexperienced hand during the biopsy procedure.

Vacuolar artifact due to improper freezing technique can be minimized by using proper techniques that permit rapid freezing and by proper specimen storage to prevent thawing. Mild vacuolar artifacts may be tolerable, but large vacuoles that disrupt the sarcoplasm are especially troublesome (Fig. 7.20A). Larger vacuoles may interfere with accurate biopsy interpretation by distorting the pathologic changes in the sample or by simulating the picture of vacuolar myopathy, such as glycogen or lipid storage disease. Spaces representing freeze artifact may be considerably lessened by thawing and properly snap freezing the specimen using the method described below (Fig. 7.20B). Also, for those who use powdered gloves in specimen handling, tiny talc granules may be seen on the microscopic section, which may be confirmed by viewing the section under polarized illumination.

The so-called hyaline fibers are evident in specimens damaged by contraction artifact. These fibers are abnormally increased in diameter and rounded in configuration. Contraction artifact phenomenon is best observed in longitudinal sections where dark hypercontracted regions are separated by pale, ghostlike zones of myofibrillar disruption (Fig. 7.21A). Their sarcoplasm in both paraffin and frozen sections is smudged or glassy and more deeply stained than in normal fibers. Contraction artifact is particularly undesirable when either immunohistochemical or electron microscopic studies are needed, even if the artifact is subtle and cannot be appreciated at the light microscopic level.

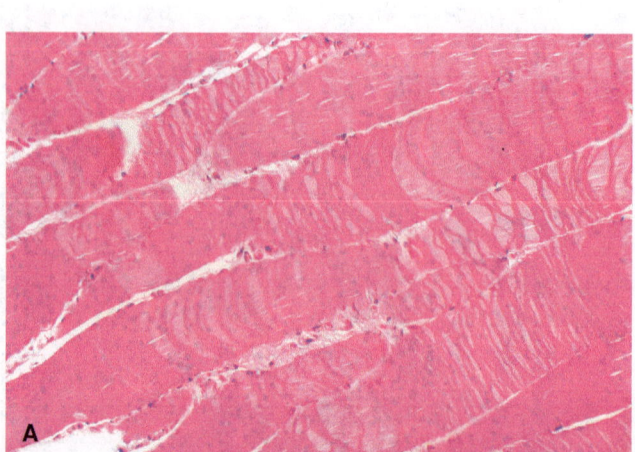
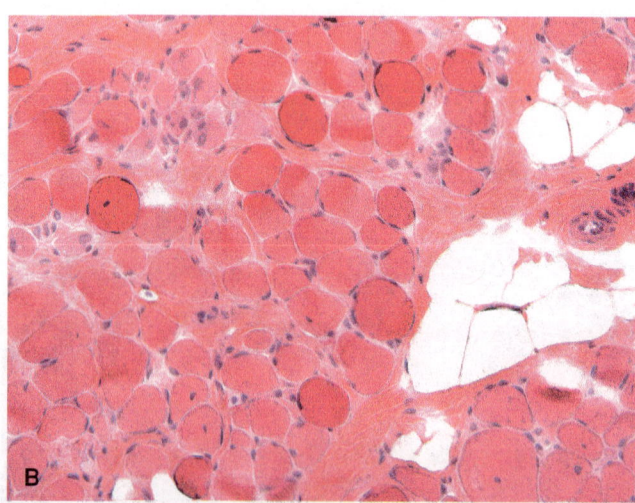

FIGURE 7.21 **A:** Contraction artifact. Dark contraction bands and lucent zones of fiber disruption are seen in longitudinally oriented fibers (H&E). **B:** Hyaline, contracted fibers. Several fibers are enlarged, rounded, with darkly stained sarcoplasm, seen in this example of Duchenne muscular dystrophy (H&E).

The detection of ultrastructural abnormalities, which is dependent on the normal alignment of the myofibrils and myofilaments, is compromised by the distortion of sarcomeric structures. An undue number of these fibers may be seen in muscle biopsies taken from infants in which the smallness of the biopsy, extracted from a correspondingly small incision, may result in excessive mechanical irritation and resulting contraction artifact. True hypercontracted, hyaline fibers in a carefully removed muscle biopsy are a common feature of Duchenne muscular dystrophy or any condition with diminished sarcolemmal integrity (Fig. 7.21B). Hyaline fiber formation may also be seen as a harbinger of in vivo necrosis of a myofiber, aside from the aforementioned iatrogenic effects described above.

Electrocautery as a means of hemostasis is a notorious cause of contraction artifact and should be strictly avoided until the biopsy is completely excised. Isometric clamping during collection is advocated by some as a means to avoid contraction artifact; however, many surgeons are unfamiliar with their use and consequently they may produce more artifact than was meant to avoid.

Excessively pale histochemical reactions can result from the degradation of enzyme systems in the sarcoplasm. Artifacts are distinguished from legitimate abnormal staining if all histochemical reactions in the biopsy are pale. Laboratories that accept transported consultation specimens should instruct the originating institution to keep the specimen cool in a sealed specimen container, on a very slightly moistened gauze or nonstick specimen pad, and ensure transport as quickly as possible. If a specimen is inadvertently exposed to melting ice or excessive amounts of saline, the excess fluid infiltrates the endomysium and perimysium simulating edema and promotes ice crystal artifact. Moreover, this hypotonic fluid produces a rat bite effect in some fibers, the result of which is a peripheral irregular defect in the fiber, looking like a bite has been taken out of the sarcoplasm.

Other artifacts are due to sectioning and staining errors. Of unknown origin is nuclear vacuolization, which seems to occur in frozen sections rather than paraffin sections (Fig. 7.22). Scattered nuclei have peripherally marginated chromatin. The center of the nuclei is clear or light pink in H&E stains. The color, greater frequency, and size distinguish this artifact from most pathologic intranuclear inclusions. A disfiguring and distracting artifact occurs in frozen sections stained with Gomori trichrome. The normal green staining of the tissue is distorted by irregular red-stained areas that interfere with interpretation of a biopsy (Fig. 7.23). This seems to be more common in specimens shipped in ice when the ice melts, leaving the exposed fresh tissue floating in water. Dark staining of the sarcoplasm in random fibers is often due to variations in section thickness. Fibers adjacent to the connective tissue of the perimysium are especially susceptible to this artifact. Inconsistencies of section thickness may be recognized when linear, band-like regions of intense staining are visible within muscle fibers. Another sectioning artifact involves wrinkling or folding of

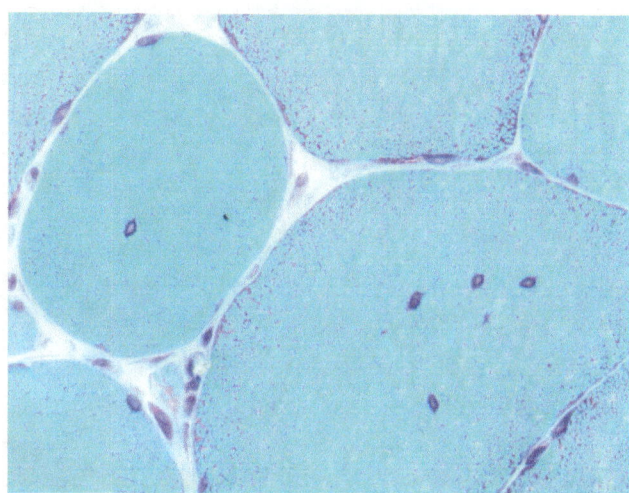

FIGURE 7.22 Nuclear vacuoles in frozen section. The vacuoles are small and round with a thick collar of chromatin as opposed to true intranuclear inclusions (H&E).

the fiber, especially evident in ATPase reactions (Fig. 7.24). The exact cause of this phenomenon sometimes called the piecrust artifact is unclear, but it has been attributed to coverslip lifting or to improper transfer of cryostat.

DIFFERENTIAL DIAGNOSIS

Several findings in skeletal muscle biopsies are normal minor variations that may be mistaken for pathologic change, or entirely nonspecific. These include internal nuclei, ring fibers, increased endomysial connective tissue, inflammation, variations in fiber diameters, lipofuscin, cytoplasmic bodies, tubular aggregates, and ragged red fibers.

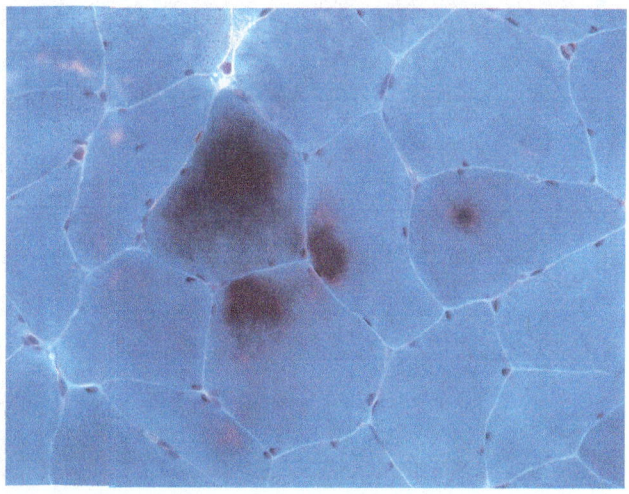

FIGURE 7.23 Of uncertain origin is an abnormal artifact in frozen section stained with Gomori trichrome. The internal detail of the sarcoplasm is distorted by a red discoloration of the normal green-staining properties of the fibers.

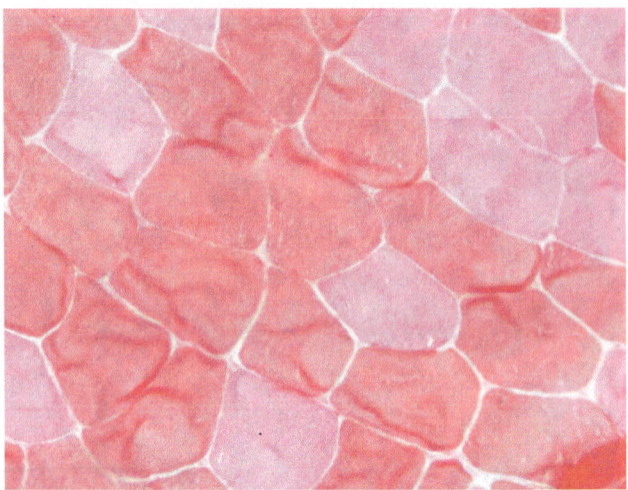

FIGURE 7.24 Piecrust artifact. Linear dark-staining creases caused by wrinkling or folding of the sarcoplasm (ATPase @ pH 9.4).

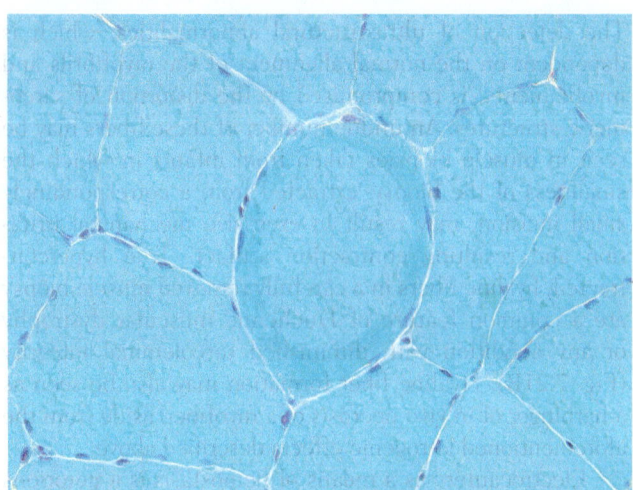

FIGURE 7.26 Ring fibers ("ringbinden"). Bundles of myofibrils are circumferentially oriented, forming rings that encircle transversely sectioned fibers (H&E).

One of the most common pathologic abnormalities in muscle biopsies is nuclear internalization (Fig. 7.25). Quantitative analyses have demonstrated that the nuclei are peripherally located in 97% to 99% of normal muscle fibers, which means that up to 3% of fibers with internal nuclei is a normal finding. In many different conditions, an increase in internal nuclei is found, typically affecting 5% to 10% of fibers and particularly those that are mildly atrophic. Nuclear internalization has no specific diagnostic significance and appears to be a reaction to virtually any type of injury, and may even be seen in neuropathic conditions. The diagnosis of myotonic dystrophy should be strongly considered if the vast majority of fibers contain internal nuclei.

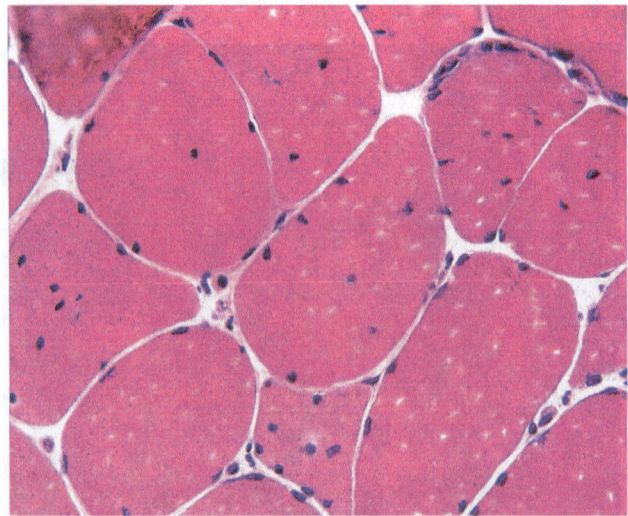

FIGURE 7.25 Nuclear internalization. Several fibers contain internal pyknotic nuclei, a common nonspecific finding if seen in less than 3% of fibers. Greater numbers may be seen in a wide variety of neuropathic and myopathic conditions (H&E).

One must exercise caution in interpreting the significance of ring fibers ("ringbinden"). The ring is formed by a bundle of peripheral myofibrils that are circumferentially oriented such that they encircle the internal portion of the sarcoplasm, which is normal in structure and orientation (Fig. 7.26). In cross sections of muscle, the ring is especially well visualized in stains where the striations of the transversely oriented peripheral myofibrils are seen in contrast to the inner sarcoplasmic contents. Rings are also seen to advantage in PTAH stains, resin sections, or under phase-contrast microscopy. Under the electron microscope, the pathologically oriented myofibrils are generally normal in structure except for hypercontraction of the sarcomeres. In properly processed, uncontracted muscle biopsies, ring fibers may be a pathologic criterion of all types of muscular dystrophy, particularly myotonic disorders, but may also signify muscle undergoing regeneration whereby reorganization of the fiber architecture involves failure to align myofibrils correctly.

Excessive quantities of endomysial connective tissue usually represent reactive fibrosis accompanying neuromuscular disease. However, as pointed out above, at the interface between muscle and tendons or fascia, abundant connective tissue is normally present and should not be regarded as reactive fibrosis. Although endomysial connective tissue is not prominent in the biopsies of infants, as indicated previously, the perimysial connective tissue far exceeds the amount present in older children and adults.

Interstitial and perivascular inflammatory cells almost always reflect clinical disease, most frequently immunologically mediated myopathies such as polymyositis or dermatomyositis. Moreover, some dystrophic myopathies are well known to display prominent inflammatory infiltrates, including facioscapulohumeral (FSH) dystrophy, merosin deficiency, and the dysferlinopathies. However, in the biopsies of infants, it is better to remember that small foci of hematopoiesis are rarely present and do not represent pathologic inflammatory infiltrates. Muscles subjected to trauma such as EMG needles may harbor foci of inflammation for months following the diagnostic study and are not clinically significant.

One of the most demanding challenges to the diagnostic pathologist is the muscle biopsy characterized by a variation in fiber diameters or by what appears to be atrophy or hypertrophy. Unconventionally biopsied muscles such as paraspinal or abdominal wall muscles may be proposed as an alternative biopsy site when spinal surgery or gastrostomy placement is planned, in order to spare the patient a separate incision. However, these muscles may display conspicuous variation in fiber diameters as a normal feature which would be abnormal in conventionally biopsied proximal muscles of the extremities. Smaller muscles, and especially those devoted to finely coordinated activities, have smaller-fiber diameters than large, bulky muscles. In evaluating fiber size, it may be necessary to measure fiber diameters. Morphometric analysis of the muscle biopsy is imperative when the changes in fiber diameters are minimal and subtle. Average fiber diameters should not vary more than 12% between type 1 and 2 fibers. While the diameter of fibers is determined by several factors, it is important to realize that there is up to 30% diminution of fiber diameters in formalin-fixed paraffin-embedded tissue as compared with cryosections.

In order to obtain statically significant morphometric data, the lesser diameter of each muscle fiber should be determined, based on a minimum number of 200 fibers in the sample. The atrophic or hypertrophic process may be selective, affecting only one fiber type, or it may be nonselective. True selective atrophy of type 1 fibers is most commonly encountered in myotonic dystrophy, but conspicuous type 1 fiber hypotrophy along with type 2 hypertrophy is a definitional feature of congenital fiber type disproportion. Type 2 fiber atrophy is a common finding in acute denervation, disuse, upper motor neuron deficit, protein malnutrition, chronic and usually high-dose corticosteroid administration, Cushing disease, myasthenia gravis, primary hyperparathyroidism, some rheumatologic disorders, aging females, and paraneoplasia (Fig. 7.27). True and characteristically extreme hypertrophy of type 1 fibers is relatively specific for infantile spinal muscular atrophy. The pattern of atrophy is important in distinguishing between normal and abnormal. Randomly distributed small or large fibers may be normal, depending on other factors discussed above. Grouped atrophy, where five or more small angular fibers cluster together is essentially diagnostic of chronic neurogenic disease (Fig. 7.18B). Perifascicular atrophy is typical of dermatomyositis and other immune myopathies with perimysial pathology.

Lipofuscin is a common finding in paranuclear and subsarcolemmal locations in muscle fibers, and are thought to originate in the intracellular degradation of waste products. It is a nonspecific finding associated with aging, but also seen in vitamin E deficiency and a wide variety of other

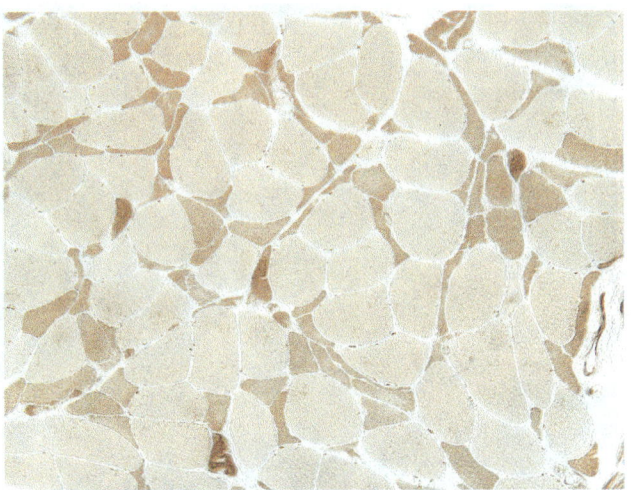

FIGURE 7.27 Type 2 fiber atrophy of an extreme degree in a case of polymyalgia rheumatica (ATPase @ pH 9.4).

myopathic conditions. Cytoplasmic bodies are easily recognizable sarcoplasmic masses composed of a central core and a pale halo, and are best visualized with the Gomori trichrome stain (Fig. 7.28). They are well documented to be associated and contiguous with varying degrees of Z-band streaming. They may be seen in a wide variety of unrelated disorders, including denervation atrophy, inflammatory myopathies, myotonic and other dystrophies, periodic paralysis, mitochondrial myopathies, and others. When seen as the predominant finding in some myopathies, the term cytoplasmic body myopathy has been used.

Ragged red fibers can be observed in the aging process. These fibers are recognized in Gomori trichrome stains performed on frozen sections, where they exhibit an irregular surface and collections of red-staining subsarcolemmal material (Fig. 7.29A). The ragged red areas represent foci of increased, often abnormal mitochondria. An SDH enzyme

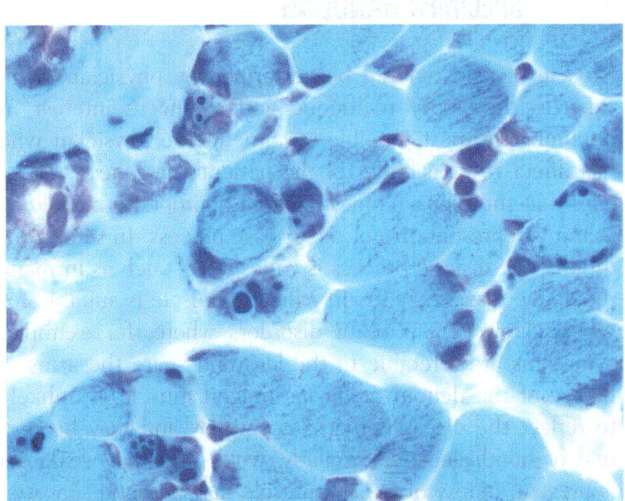

FIGURE 7.28 Cytoplasmic bodies are a highly recognizable but nonspecific find, showing red color in the Gomori trichrome stain with the characteristic haloes.

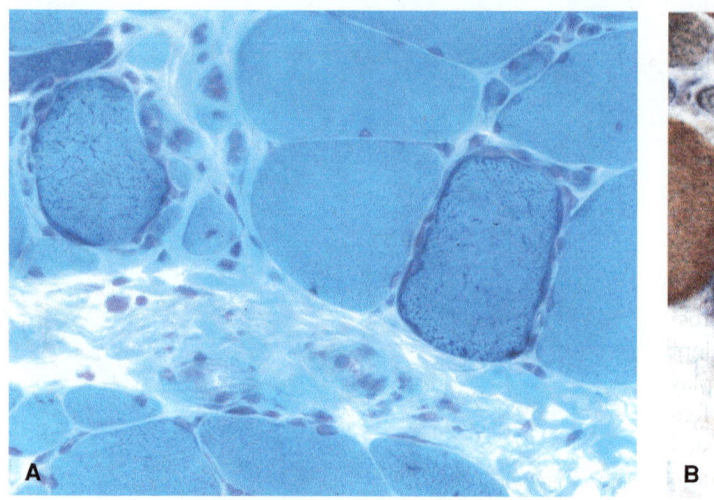
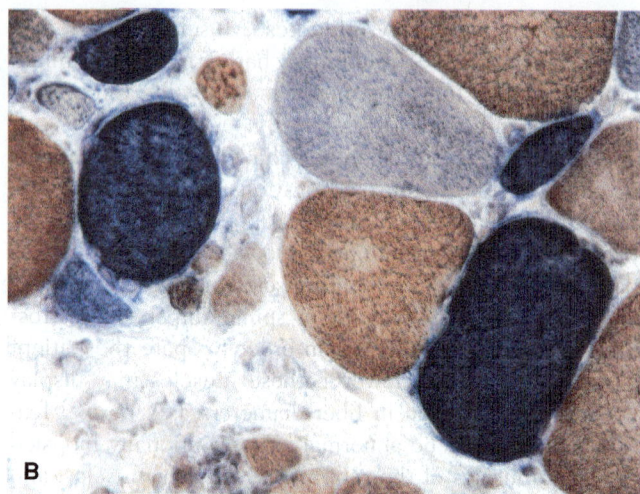

FIGURE 7.29 **A:** Ragged red fibers. Ragged red fibers are recognized in Gomori trichrome stain as having an irregular sarcolemmal surface with collections of red-staining material. **B:** The adjacent section shows the same fiber as a ragged blue fiber by the COX-SDH enzyme histochemical preparation.

histochemical preparation of a ragged red fiber yields the same evidence for subsarcolemmal mitochondrial proliferation, known as a "ragged blue fiber" (Fig. 7.29B). Ragged red or blue fibers in younger individuals are generally the hallmark of the mitochondrial myopathies, which are characterized by mitochondrial dysfunction and often mutations of mitochondrial genes. It is now known that mitochondrial damage occurs in the aging cell, including skeletal muscle, in part attributable to increased sporadic mitochondrial DNA deletions. Ragged red fibers are considered to be a reflection of this phenomenon, which may be associated with late-onset mitochondrial disease but frequently is not.

SPECIMEN HANDLING

Muscle biopsies should be performed by physicians with expertise in biopsy technique and a sincere interest in obtaining the best possible specimen. The physician who has direct responsibility for the patient's care needs to be sure that the biopsy comes from an appropriate muscle so that it is representative of the disease process. In some conditions, the disease process is widespread, such as in many metabolic diseases, and virtually any muscle is suitable for biopsy. However, in other disorders where, for example, symptoms are referable to the legs and spare the arms, a biopsy of the deltoid or biceps brachii muscle is unlikely to reflect the disease process accurately and may be normal or nondiagnostic. Similarly, when proximal weakness is present, biopsy of a distal muscle may be nondiagnostic. Moreover, whenever possible, the tissue sample should be obtained from a region in which the disease process remains active rather than quiescent. Ultrasound or MRI guidance can be useful in choosing a biopsy site, especially in inflammatory myopathies in which disease may be focal, or in dystrophic myopathies in which there may be drastic differences between involved muscles. In severely involved muscle, particularly if there is marked weakness or wasting, the pathologic findings are likely to be those of end-stage disease that may defy conclusive pathologic interpretation. Muscles subjected to previous traumatic injury, such as needle tracts incurred during EMG or intramuscular injections of medications, and muscles altered by an unrelated disease process should not be biopsied.

The special handling of the muscle biopsy is of paramount importance. Ideally, muscle biopsies are performed on weekdays when histotechnical support is available for immediate processing. Submission of the specimen "after hours" may be clinically unavoidable. When a vasculitis is suspected and rapid treatment is contemplated, such specimens can be processed for formalin fixation and paraffin embedding on an urgent basis whenever the biopsy is performed.

Ideally, two separate specimens from the same site are desirable. The major drawback to needle biopsy, which has certain advantages over open biopsy by avoiding an invasive procedure and in some cases, general anesthesia, is the limited size of the sample, although basic histologic determinations may be made in the hands of skilled histotechnologists with such small biopsies. Genetic testing may be done when an adequate amount is obtained (approximately 30 to 50 mg); however, enzyme activity assays predictably require amounts of muscle tissue (at least 150 mg), only achievable with open biopsies.

For paraffin embedding, the primary fixative for muscle biopsies is 10% formalin, buffered to a pH of 7.4 in a 0.1 M phosphate buffer. Strips of muscle 1 mm in width are dissected from the edges of the sample and postfixed in phosphate-buffered 2% glutaraldehyde for electron microscopic study. A second unfixed specimen measuring 1 × 0.5 × 0.5 cm is obtained for the preparation of frozen sections. The portion designated for cryotomy should be carefully assessed for orientation to yield cross sections. A dissecting microscope is sometimes useful toward this goal. The ideal method of rapid freezing is to cool isopentane in liquid nitrogen to below minus 100°C, into which the muscle tissue is immersed. Many laboratories place the cylinder of muscle into gum tragacanth on a cork bed, a semisolid substance that solidifies as an embedding base upon freezing. Whatever technique is employed, the condition on which the freezing technique is based is that it proceeds with extreme rapidity, within a few seconds. Freezing the tissue in a cryostat in a fashion similar to most specimens submitted for frozen section diagnosis from the operating room is contraindicated because of the propensity to cause freeze artifact. When a muscle biopsy has been suboptimally frozen and is likely to demonstrate unacceptable freeze artifact, the specimen may be thawed to room temperature and refrozen by the method outlined above, with significant resolution of freeze artifact. The unavoidable result is that the muscle fibers will assume an abnormal rounded profile with an artificial separation of the fibers by spaces not found in nature. The frozen sample should be oriented so that cross sections of muscle are cut. It is highly desirable that the histotechnologists obtain sequential and consecutive facing cryosections so that individual fibers can be tracked through the diverse stains performed. Serial frozen sections are stained with H&E, Gomori trichrome, and by the enzyme histochemical reactions ATPase (at pH 9.4, 4.3, and 4.6), NADH-TR, nonspecific esterase, and combined COX-SDH. Other stains such as PAS for glycogen, myophosphorylase, alkaline and acid phosphatase, and lipid stains are performed when indicated. Frozen tissue may also be used for biochemical analysis, for immunohistochemical preparations, and for immunofluorescence microscopy. Inasmuch as frozen tissue may be needed for future additional studies, muscle biopsies can be sealed in airtight plastic capsules or bags to prevent desiccation and freezing artifact while stored in an ultralow freezer at −70°C.

REFERENCES

1. Messina G, Biressi S, Monteverde S, et al. Nfix regulates fetal-specific transcription in developing skeletal muscle. *Cell* 2010;4:554–566.
2. Gilbert SF, Barresi MJF. *Development Biology*. 11th ed. Sunderland: Sinauer Associates; 2016.
3. Sadler TW. *Langman's Medical Embryology*. 13th ed. Philadelphia, PA: Lippincott Williams & Wilkins; 2016.
4. Adhihetty PJ, Hood DA. Mechanisms of apoptosis in skeletal muscle. *Basic Appl Myol* 2003;13:171–179.
5. O'Flaherty J, Mei Y, Freer M, et al. Signaling through the TRAIL receptor DR5/FADD pathway plays a role in the apoptosis associated with skeletal muscle myoblast differentiation. *Apoptosis* 2006;11:2103–2113.
6. Heffner RR Jr, Moore SA, Balos LL. Muscle biopsy in neuromuscular diseases. In: Mills SE, ed. *Sternberg's Diagnostic Surgical Pathology*. Vol. 1. 6th ed. Philadelphia, PA: Lippincott Williams & Wilkins; 2015:113–147.
7. Dubowitz V, Sewry CA, Oldfors A. *Muscle Biopsy. A Practical Approach*. Philadelphia, PA: Saunders Elsevier; 2013.
8. Banker BQ, Engel AG. Basic reactions of muscle. In: Engel AG, Franzini-Armstrong C, eds. *Myology: Basic and Clinical*. 3rd ed. New York: McGraw-Hill; 2004:691–747.
9. Curtis E, Sewry, C. Electron microscopy in skeletal muscle pathology. In: Stirling JW, Curry A, Eyden B, eds. *Diagnostic Electron Microscopy: A Practical Guide to Interpretation and Technique*. 1st ed. UK: John Wiley & Sons, Ltd; 2013.
10. Raheem O, Huovinen S, Suominen T, et al. Novel myosin heavy chain immunohistochemical double staining developed for the routine diagnostic separation of I, IIA and IIX fibers. *Acta Neuropathol* 2010;119:495–500.
11. Pertl C, Eblenkamp M, Pertl A, et al. A new web-based method for automated analysis of muscle histology. *BMC Musculoskelet Disord* 2013;14:26.
12. Brooke MH, Kaiser KK. Muscle fiber types: how many and what kind? *Arch Neurol* 1970;23:369–379.

8

Blood Vessels

Patrick J. Gallagher ■ Allard C. van der Wal

GROSS AND LIGHT MICROSCOPIC FEATURES 190	**Media** 208
Aorta 190	Adventitia and Supporting Cells 208
Arteries 195	Lymphatics and Veins 208
Arterioles 197	**ANTIGEN EXPRESSION OF NORMAL AND NEOPLASTIC VASCULAR TISSUE** 208
Capillaries, Sinusoids, Venules, and Lymphatics 198	Endothelium 208
Veins 199	Smooth Muscle 210
Pulmonary Arteries and Veins 199	Other Useful Antibodies for Diagnostic Vascular Pathology 213
Anastomoses, Angiodysplasias, and Vascular Malformations 202	**REFERENCES** 213
Vascular Surgery 204	
ELECTRON MICROSCOPY 206	
Endothelial Cells 206	
Inclusions of Endothelial Cells 207	

GROSS AND LIGHT MICROSCOPIC FEATURES

The normal structure of vessels, particularly the aorta, elastic and muscular arteries, and the larger veins, change progressively throughout life (Table 8.1) (1,2). These aging changes lead to increased arterial stiffness, detected clinically by alterations in pulse wave velocity (3,4). It is now clear that aging arteries are especially affected by common disorders such as atherosclerosis, hypertension, and diabetes (Table 8.2). Surgical pathologists must be fully aware not only of the nature and extent of these alterations, but also of their variation from site to site.

Aorta

The length and the breadth of the aorta increase progressively throughout life. Although there are some variations in the rate of these changes, both between men and women and from decade to decade, the process continues well into a person's 70s and 80s. This enlargement produces the characteristic unfolding of the aorta so often seen in chest radiographs; and, if the aortic valve annulus is also involved, aortic incompetence can result. Some atherosclerosis is almost inevitable in the abdominal aorta in the middle-aged and elderly, but aging changes are independent of this.

The principal components of all arteries are elastic and collagen fibers, smooth muscle cells, and a mucopolysaccharide-rich ground substance (5). In the media of the aorta and the carotid, the innominate and proximal axillary arteries elastic fibers predominate. Parallel lamellar units of elastin enclose smooth muscle cells, ground substance, and collagen (Fig. 8.1). There are about 40 lamellar units at birth and at least 50 in adult life, each measuring about 11 μm in thickness. Interconnecting bands of collagen and elastin fibers provide strength, whereas the lamellar arrangement distributes stress evenly across the wall, smoothing the cyclical pressure waves of cardiac contraction (4). The changes associated with vascular aging include progressive thickening of the aortic wall due to accumulation of smooth muscle cells and ground substance and thinning and fragmentation of elastic fibers with associated foci of fibrous tissue (collagen) and proteoglycan deposition. These changes in the structure of the extracellular matrix are thought to be the result of upregulation of genes in SMC that mediate matrix metalloproteinase production (4,6). Apoptosis can be demonstrated in a number of cell types within atheromatous plaques (7). While it is unlikely to be a key factor

TABLE 8.1 Aging Changes in Blood Vessels	
	Major Macroscopic and Histologic Features
Aorta	Progressive and linear increase in diameter with age. Eccentric or diffuse fibrous intimal thickening. Fragmentation of elastic lamellae with widening of interlamellar spaces. Focal amyloid deposits. Thickening of walls of vasa vasorum
Muscular arteries	Progressive dilatation and tortuosity. Caliber of vessels usually less in females, especially coronary arteries. Intimal fibrosis, sometimes suggesting reduplication of the internal elastic lamina. Focal fragmentation and calcification of internal elastic lamina. Increased fibrosis and hyalinization of media. No significant inflammation in atheroma-free segments
Arterioles	Intimal thickening, usually as concentric layers of fibroelastic tissue. Hyalinization of media
Capillaries	Basement membrane thickening, approximately twofold increase in thickness from puberty to old age
Venules and veins	Few detailed studies of small veins. Larger veins show intimal fibrosis and hypertrophy of both circular and longitudinal bundles

TABLE 8.2 Histologic Changes in Arteries and Arterioles	
Condition	**Major Histologic Features**
Normal adults	Minimal intimal thickening may be eccentric or diffuse. Intact internal elastic lamella, occasional small breaks only. No significant inflammation
Atherosclerosis	Eccentric fibrous intimal thickening, intimal and medial foam cell and lipid deposition. Neovascularization with intimal and medial hemorrhage. Dystrophic calcification. Adventitial aggregates of plasma cells, lymphocytes, and histiocytes. Intimal and medial aggregates of T lymphocytes, especially at shoulders of lesion. The most important complication is rupture or erosion of fibrous cap of the lesion with associated thrombus formation
Systematic hypertension	Concentric fibrous intimal thickening and medial hypertrophy, especially in arterioles. Changes pronounced in accelerated or malignant phase, with fibrinoid necrosis. Aneurysmal dilatation of intracerebral arterioles and capillaries. Increased atherosclerosis
Diabetes mellitus	Hyalin change in arterioles. Capillary microaneurysms with basement membrane thickening. Loss of pericytes; retinal neovascularization. Increased atherosclerosis in arteries
Active arteritis	Acute or chronic inflammatory cell inflammation of adventitia and media. Mural edema, reactive intimal thickening, and endothelial necrosis. Fibrinoid necrosis of wall, occasionally aneurysmal dilatation
Healed arteritis	Bizarre patterns of disordered fibrous intimal thickening. Medial scarring with patchy aggregates of chronic inflammatory cells. Abnormally prominent medial blood vessels

in the aging of the arterial wall (8) there is experimental evidence that chronic apoptosis of vascular smooth muscle cells accelerates atherosclerosis and promotes calcification and medial degeneration (9). Aging changes are the result of decades of "wear and tear." In the long term they account for the weakening that leads to aortic dilatation, especially in patients with systemic hypertension. In this respect, the effects of hypertension on the wall of arteries can be seen as accelerated aging. Vascular calcification is a common complication and, although it is most frequent in atheromatous segments, it may occur in areas where the intima is virtually devoid of plaques (10). Aortic and coronary arterial calcifications are especially common in chronic kidney disease and may, in part, be related to hyperphosphatemia (11). In its most pronounced form layers of calcifications replace large parts of the media of arteries, a condition termed Monckeberg' sclerosis (Fig. 8.2). Small amounts of amyloid can be detected in aortic atheromatous lesions of middle-aged and elderly subjects and may be derived from serum amyloid A or other apolipoproteins (12,13).

Cystic medial degeneration (CMD), originally called *medionecrosis aortae* by Erdheim, is a difficult concept, and many pathologists are unsure about the exact meaning of the term. Histologically, the condition is characterized by degeneration and fragmentation of the elastic layers of the media and formation of mucoid pools. However, it is important for surgical pathologists to recognize that there is wide variation in the extent of degeneration in biopsies of the ascending aorta (Fig. 8.1) throughout the aorta. Multiple blocks should therefore be examined. Some areas have few, if any, stainable nuclei, and this is the result of smooth muscle cell death. More recently, areas of smooth muscle cell apoptosis and disorganized proliferation, fibrosis, and angiogenesis have been described, suggesting that CMD is a process of degenerative injury and repair (9). In 1977, Schlatmann and Becker (14) showed that the histologic alterations of CMD showed a striking correlation with age and may therefore represent the normal aging process of elastic arteries. The same features are seen in hypertensive patients, who have an altered hemodynamic profile, and in genetic disorders of connective tissue, such as Marfan or some types of the Ehlers–Danlos syndrome. They have also been reported in patients with a history of cocaine abuse (15). In connective tissue disorders, CMD is more pronounced and leads to complications such as intramural hematoma formation or aortic dissection at an earlier age.

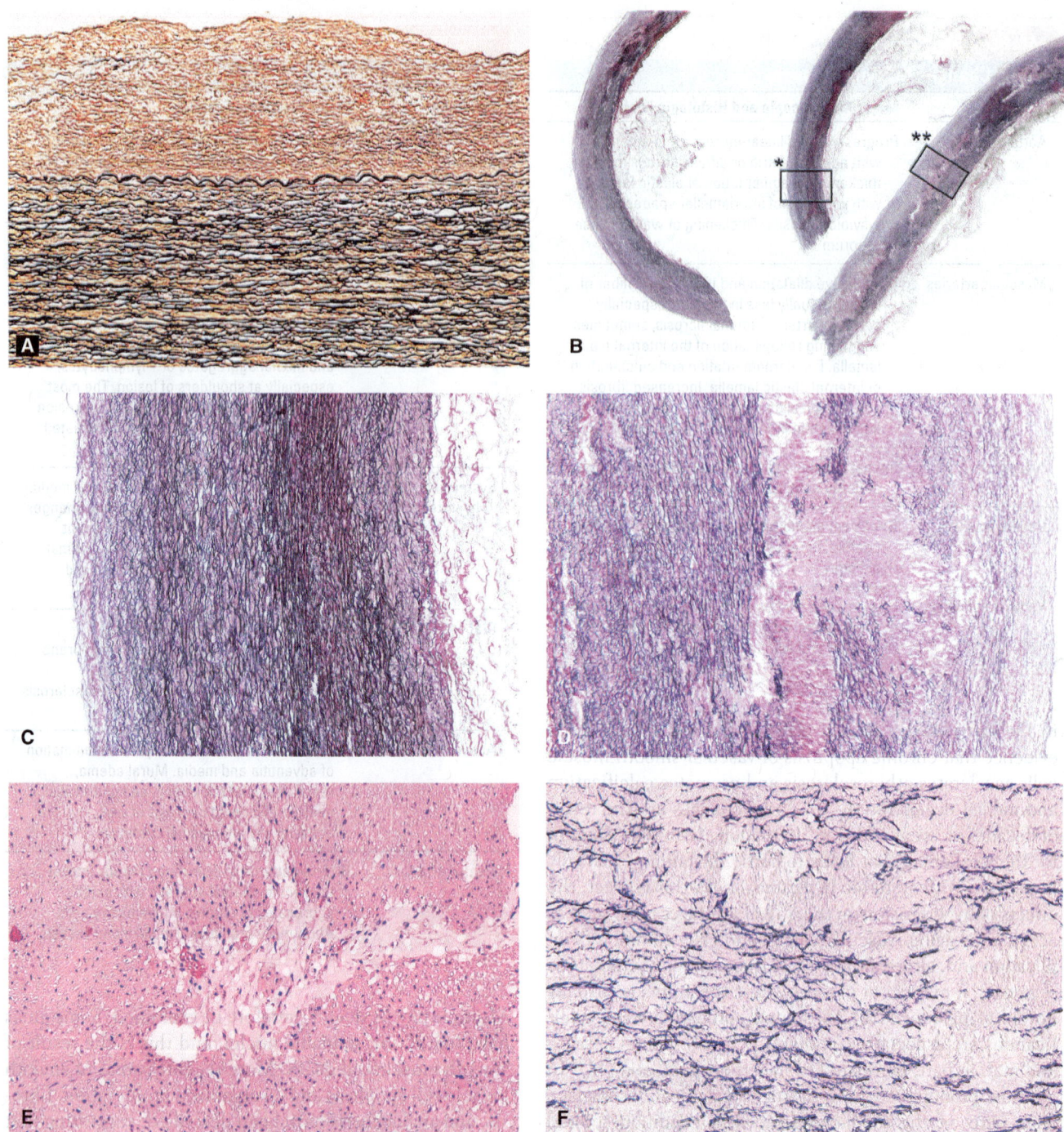

FIGURE 8.1 A: Inner half of the aortic wall of a 62-year-old man. There is a moderate degree of fibrous intimal thickening, which has no immediate clinical relevance but may predispose to atherosclerosis. There was only slight fragmentation of the elastic lamellae; the overall appearance is well within normal limits for a patient of this age (elastic van Gieson). **B:** Overview of three full-thickness cross sections through the dilated thoracic aorta of a 74-year-old man. There is marked variation in the degree of degenerative change of the media. The boxed area in the central section (enlarged in **C**) has an almost normal appearance. In contrast the boxed area on the right (enlarged in **D**) shows marked elastic degeneration. **E:** The typical appearance of cystic medial degeneration in an H&E-stained section. Note the prominent pool of mucoid material. **F:** This shows a corresponding section to **E** but is stained for elastic tissue. There is extensive loss of the normal elastic framework.

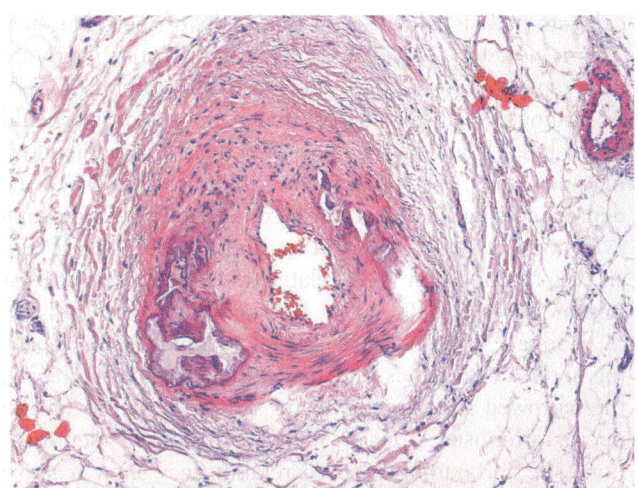

FIGURE 8.2 Arterial calcification. This muscular artery was dissected from a lower limb amputation specimen from a patient with diabetes. Note the prominent shell-like calcification of the media. This is termed Monckeberg sclerosis (hematoxylin and eosin).

Although the exact cause of CMD is unknown, it appears to be related to an imbalance between the mechanical forces imposed on the aortic wall during systole and the capacity of the aortic wall to resist these forces. The resulting shear forces may cause alterations in the secretion pattern of smooth muscle cells or their death by apoptosis. p53 accumulation, *bax* upregulation, and both vascular smooth muscle cell apoptosis and regeneration have been demonstrated in areas of cystic medial necrosis (16). In Marfan syndrome, the histologic changes suggest exaggerated aging, but there are no features that allow a specific diagnosis to be made (Fig. 8.3). The underlying genetic abnormality involves a glycoprotein, fibrillin, that is closely associated with elastin fibers. The exact functions of fibrillin and other associated glycoproteins are uncertain, but they may act as a "scaffold" on which elastin fibers are laid down. There is also growing evidence for abnormal TGFβ signaling in Marfan disease and other inherited aortopathies (17,18). There is a wide spectrum of clinical abnormalities in Marfan syndrome, and certain clinical features, such as arachnodactyly or aortic dissection, are especially common in some families (19).

Elastic fragmentation and associated medial necrosis are the most common histologic findings in both ascending and thoracic aortic aneurysms. At least 17 predominantly genetic disorders have been associated with these aneurysms in younger patients (20). Traditionally, abdominal aortic aneurysms have been considered atheromatous in origin, but this is an oversimplification. Genetic studies have provided compelling evidence for an inherited basis of this disease. Although susceptibility genes have

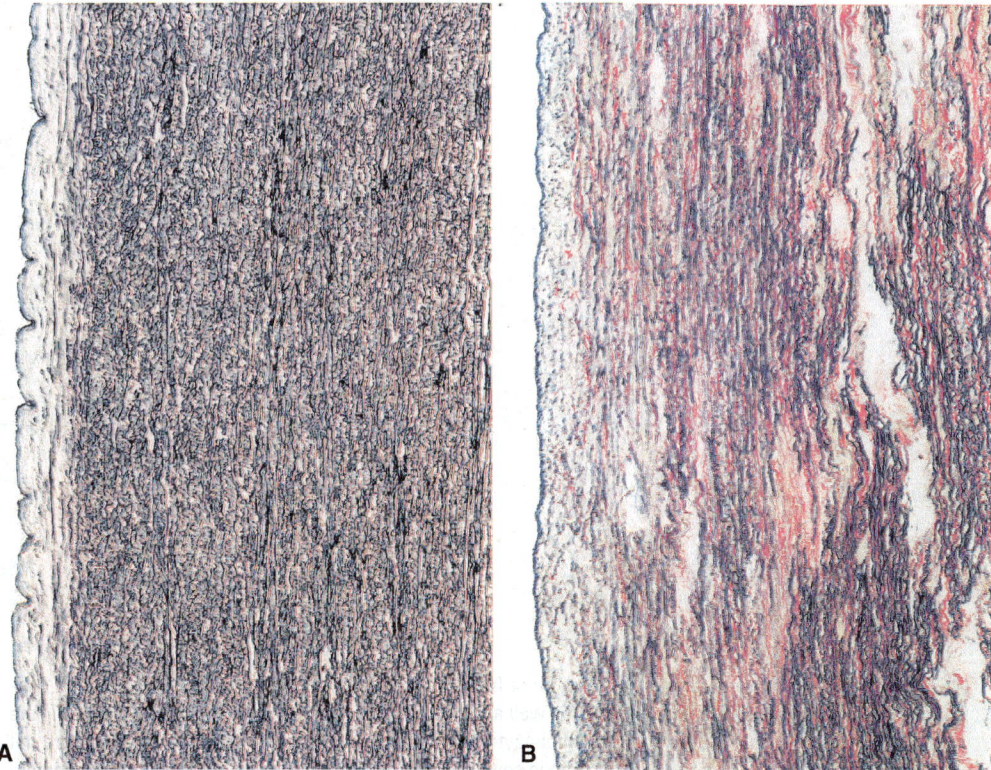

FIGURE 8.3 **A:** The normal appearance of the aortic media of a 48-year-old man. There are many parallel lamellae of elastic tissue. There is no significant intimal thickening. **B:** The aortic wall of a 31-year-old man with Marfan syndrome. The medial elastic tissue is extensively fragmented, and there is fibrosis and loose mucopolysaccharide-rich areas. Such extensive changes would be unusual even in an elderly patient (elastic van Gieson).

been described, causative gene mutations have not (21). Inheritance is usually autosomal dominant but about 25% of cases are recessive. Both males and females are affected (22). Whether the atherosclerosis is the primary cause or a secondary complication, the inflammation and medial scarring that accompany all but the earliest stages of atheroma further damage a wall already weakened by normal aging or by specific genetically determined alterations in the matrix of the aortic wall. Patchy chronic inflammatory aggregates, including lymphocytes and plasma cells, are often present in the adventitia of atheromatous segments of the aorta and coronary arteries (Fig. 8.4). In biopsies of the ascending aorta during repair of dissecting aneurysms or aortic reconstructions for root dilatation, these chronic adventitial infiltrates must not be mistaken as evidence of aortitis. Small collections of lymphocytes, macrophages, and giant cells are occasionally seen in the media of these biopsies. This is now termed isolated idiopathic aortitis. There are case reports of aortic dissection in this condition (23,24). Accordingly we always suggest that giant cell aortitis should be excluded clinically in these patients. In some abdominal aneurysms, the inflammatory infiltrates are especially dense, and surgical repair may be difficult. There is growing evidence that aortitis, periaortitis, and retroperitoneal fibrosis may be part of an IgG4-related systemic disease at least in some cases (25,26).

Cardiac surgeons have several techniques for repairing aortic coarctations and may submit samples of aorta, the narrowed aortic segment, the subclavian artery, or the ductus arteriosus (arterial duct) for histologic identification. The aorta around the coarctation may show reactive intimal thickening, even in neonates, but the underlying

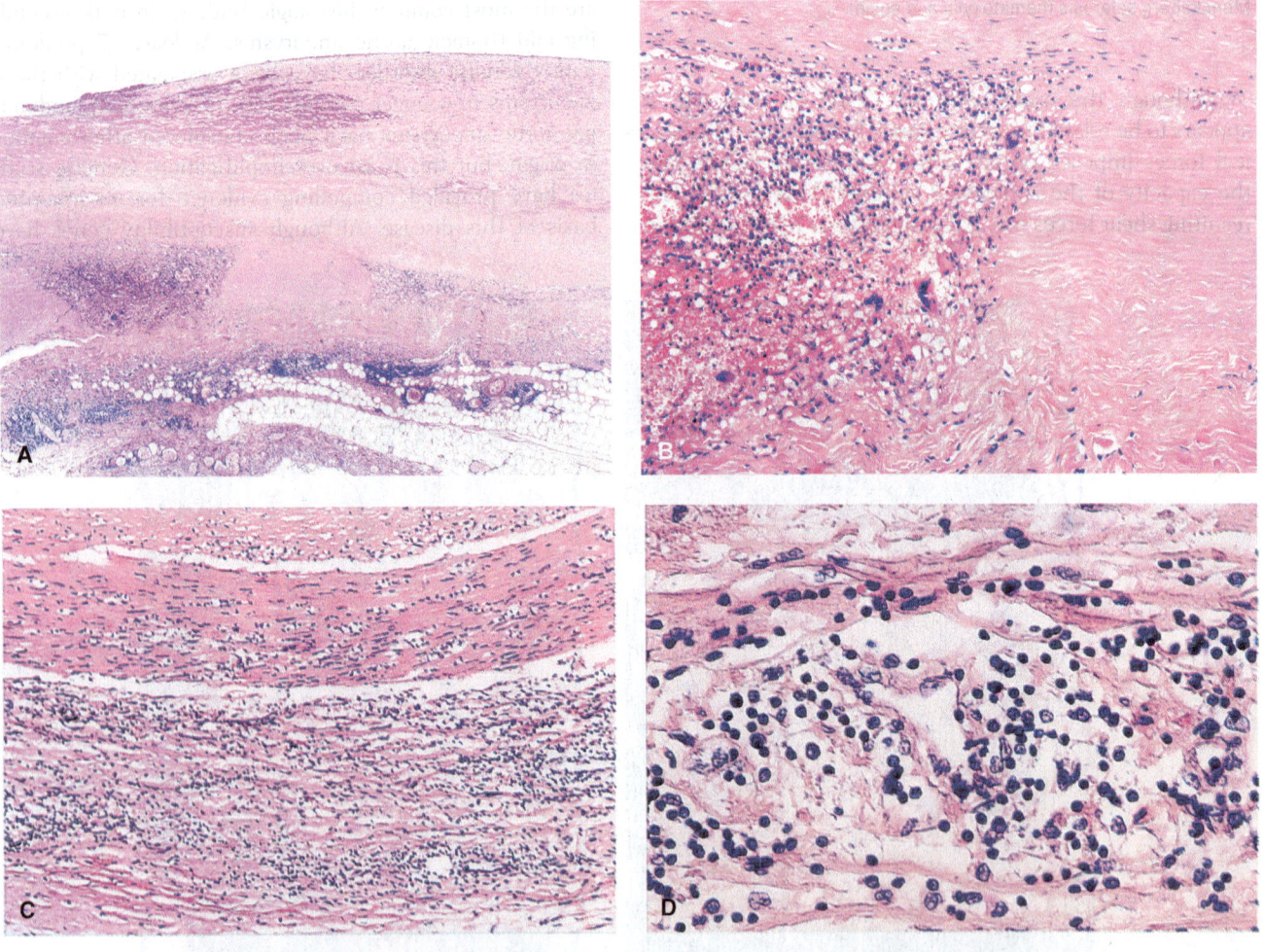

FIGURE 8.4 **A:** Low-power view of ascending aorta from a 58-year-old female with chronic aortitis and periaortitis. There is marked thickening of the aortic wall and multifocal presence of inflammatory infiltrates in the media of the artery. Also note the nodular lymphocytic infiltrates in the periadventitial tissues. They are not unique for chronic aortitis, but can also be seen in severely atherosclerotic arteries. **B:** Detail of inflammatory infiltrate showing presence of multiple giant cells (giant cell aortitis). **C** and **D:** Adventitial chronic inflammatory infiltrates in the wall of an atheromatous coronary artery. A few inflammatory cells have infiltrated into the media. The magnified view on the right confirms that most of the inflammatory cells are lymphocytes or plasma cells (hematoxylin and eosin).

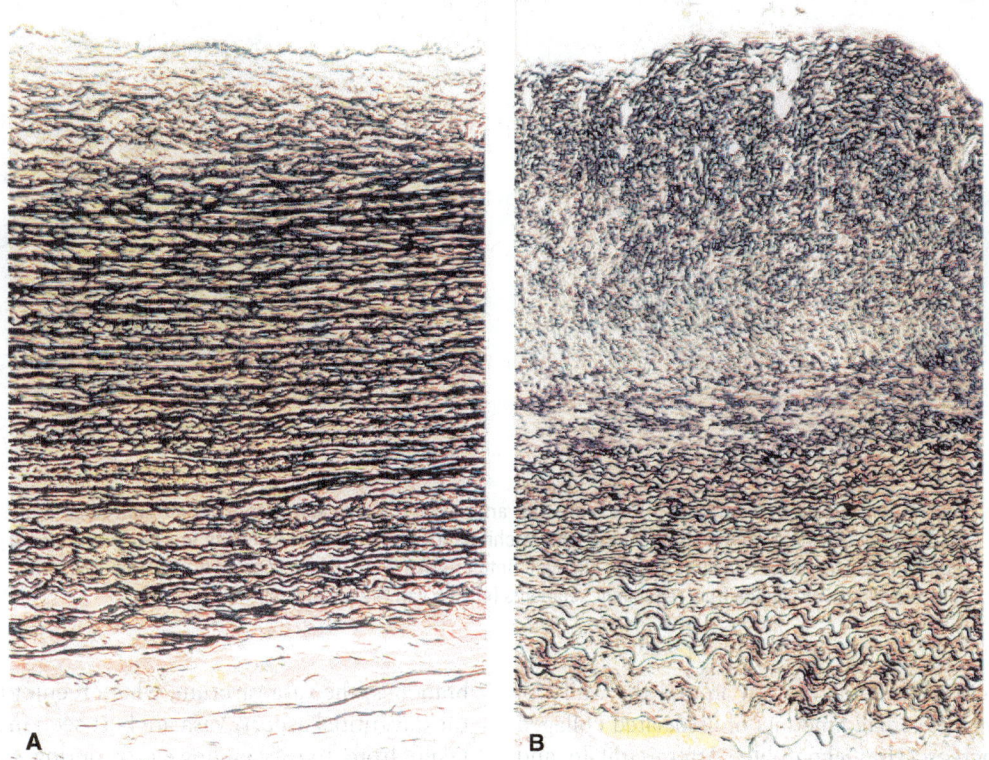

FIGURE 8.5 Coarctation of the aorta. **A:** The aortic wall distal to a coarctation in a 3-month-old child. There is slight intimal edema only. **B:** The coarctation itself; note the irregular arrangement of the intimal fibroelastic tissue (elastic van Gieson).

elastic structure is usually well preserved. The coarctation itself can have a variety of appearances. In long-standing cases, there may be dense intimal and medial fibrosis. In neonates, the intima may have a distinctly irregular pattern of fibroelastic intimal thickening, resembling some forms of arterial dysplasia (Fig. 8.5). The structure of the arterial duct changes progressively during intrauterine growth and in the postnatal period (27) and can be influenced by prostaglandin treatment. Unlike the aorta and the proximal subclavian artery, which are elastic vessels, the arterial duct has a muscular media and a defined internal elastic lamella. From 35 weeks of gestation there is progressive fragmentation of the internal elastic lamina. Small intimal cushions form which contribute to functional closure of the duct at birth. In the so-called postnatal persistent ductus arteriosus the internal elastic lamella is preserved (28).

Arteries

It is only in children and young adults that muscular arteries conform to the classical descriptions of textbooks. The intima of arteries is defined as the region from and including the endothelium to the luminal margin of the media (29). At birth, the intima is a virtual space with the endothelium closely opposed to the internal elastic lamella. This layer thickens slowly with age, either: (a) eccentrically at branching points or bifurcations; or (b) diffusely. Both types occur preferentially at sites of altered blood flow or mechanical stress, suggesting that they are adaptive changes (a response to injury). Vascular smooth muscle cells derived from the underlying media and extracellular matrix proteins accumulate in the thickened intima and may serve as a "soil" for the development of atherosclerotic plaques. For example, in the aorta and coronary arteries, the so-called atherosclerosis prone areas are those that show early diffuse or eccentric thickening.

Progressive intimal fibrosis affects nearly all arteries (Fig. 8.6), but in surgical pathology material it is especially noticeable in the spleen, myometrium, and thyroid (Fig. 8.7). As in the aorta, fragmentation of the elastic tissue, usually the internal elastic lamella, is common and is of no specific significance (Fig. 8.7). In some aging arteries, the internal lamella appears to repeatedly reduplicate, producing a pattern of concentric intimal thickening (Fig. 8.6). Small foci of calcification can be identified in otherwise normal vessels, usually just to the medial aspect of the internal elastic lamella. These aging changes, often loosely termed arteriosclerosis, have been studied most extensively in the coronary arteries, where women generally show substantially less elastic fragmentation and intimal fibrosis than do men of the same age. About 75% of the mass of the media is smooth muscle cells. These run

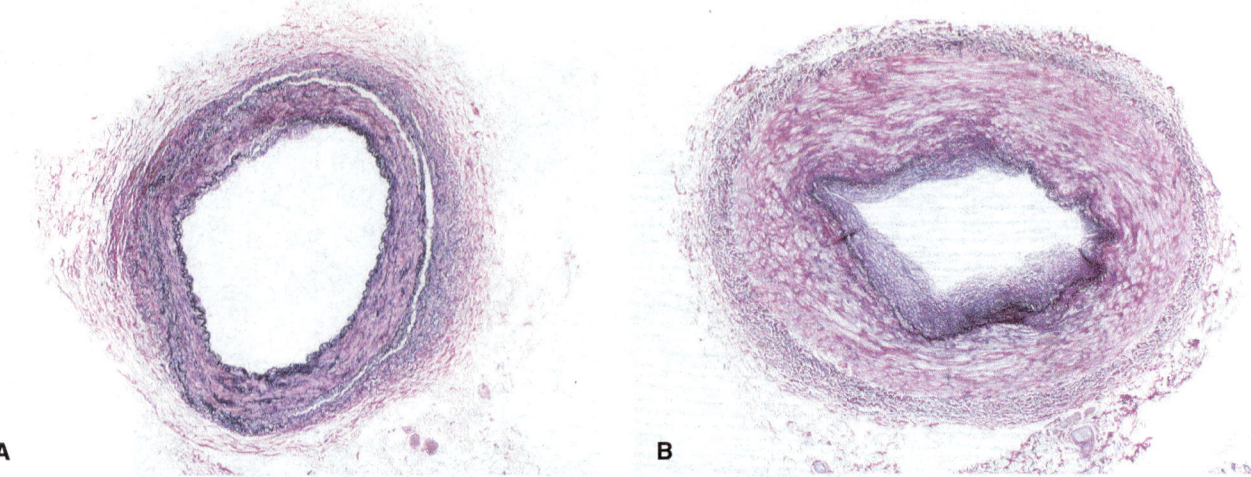

FIGURE 8.6 Transverse sections of medium-sized arteries, the mammary artery (**A**) and the radial artery (**B**). They illustrate the marked differences in the architecture of the arteries from site to site. Arteries were retrieved from the same patient, a 58-year-old man. Both arteries were used as coronary artery bypass grafts. These sections were made from redundant segments (elastic van Gieson stains).

in a spiral or circumferential pattern around the wall (5). As in the intima the small amounts of associated collagen and elastin increase throughout life. Arteries dilate and become more tortuous with increasing age, and this has a fortuitous antiocclusive effect. The caliber of the coronary arteries in middle-aged and elderly women is less than that of men. This could contribute to the poorer results recorded in women after both coronary artery surgery and coronary interventions (30). If arterial dilatation is pronounced and irregular, as in the so-called coronary artery ectasia, spontaneous thrombosis may result (31).

Nutrients reach the media of elastic or muscular arteries by direct diffusion through the intima or via small branches, the vasa vasorum, which reenter the media from the adventitial aspect. Vasa are best seen in biopsy samples taken from the ascending aorta during root repairs and sometimes have remarkably thick muscular walls (Fig. 8.8). In atheromatous arteries, there is often marked neovascular proliferation. Hemorrhage from these vessels contributes to the growth of lesions and their lipid content (32).

A modified form of the American Heart Association classification of atheromatous lesions is now widely used in studies of both coronary and carotid arteries (Table 8.3) (33). There is much interest in the concept of the so-called vulnerable plaque: Plaques at high risk for development of superimposed thrombosis or plaque hemorrhage. Several

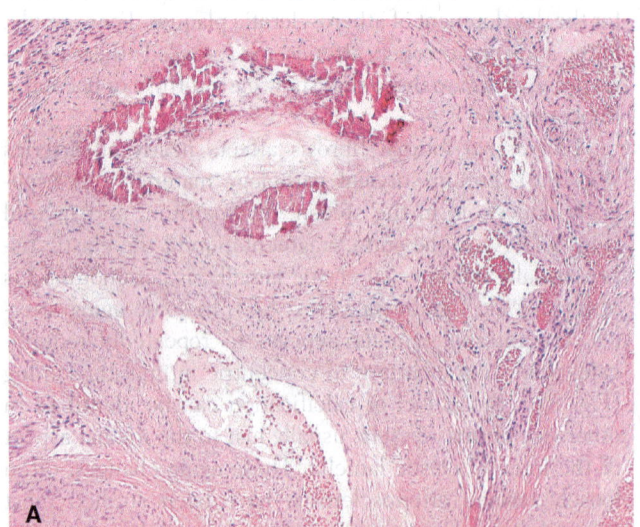 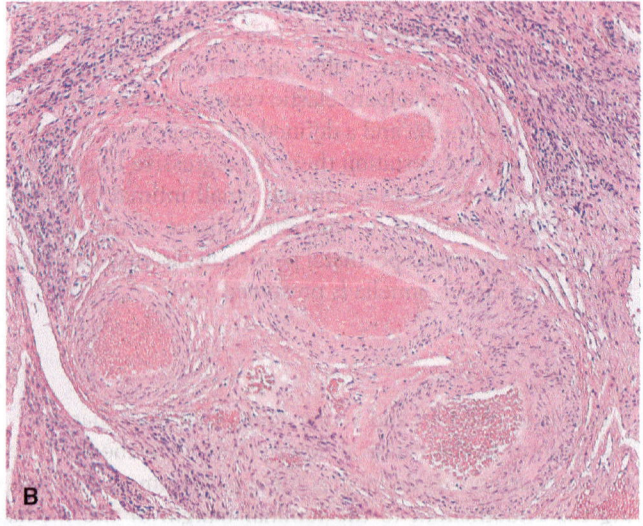

FIGURE 8.7 **A** and **B**. Aging changes in arteries. These thick-walled vessels were close to the serosa of the myometrium in a 52-year-old woman. Note the prominent calcification in **A** and the increased tortuosity in **B**. These changes have no importance. They can be seen in other sites, especially in thyroidectomy specimens.

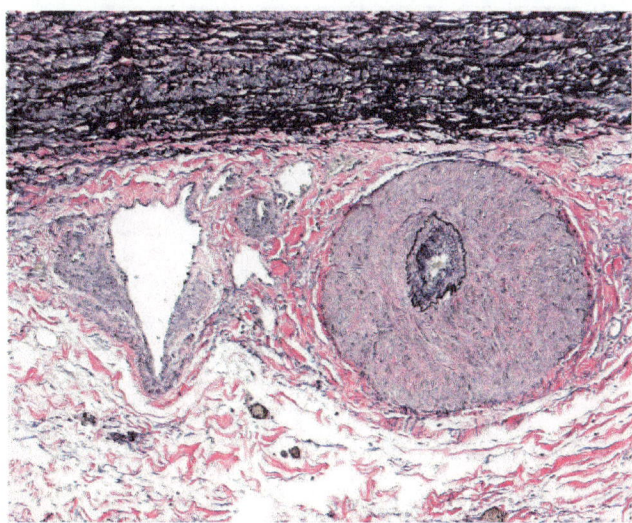

FIGURE 8.8 The aortic adventitia. The thick-walled vessel is a vasa vasorum. The thin-walled vessel (*left*) is a small vein.

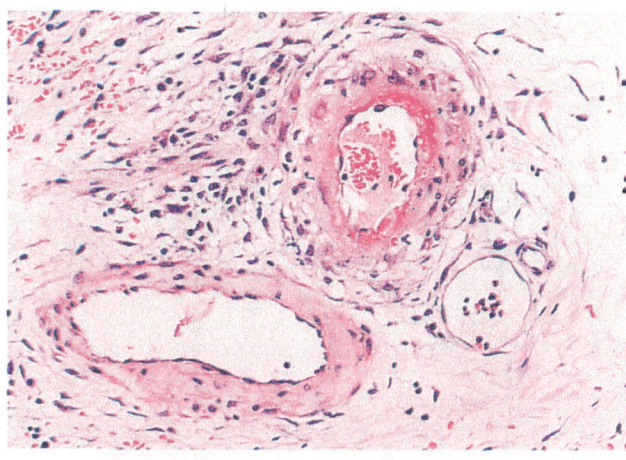

FIGURE 8.9 Florid fibrinoid necrosis in a small intestinal vessel of a girl with systemic lupus erythematosus. Fibrinoid necrosis is not a feature of normal aging or uncomplicated hypertension. It always should be regarded as pathologic. In this case, the involved vessel is probably an arteriole. Note the small vein (*lower left*) and capillary (*lower right*).

postmortem studies of coronary arteries from patients with myocardial infarction or sudden cardiac death have shown that vulnerable lesions have specific features such as a large lipid core, a thin fibrous cap, and marked inflammatory activity in the plaque tissue (34). Radiofrequency intravascular ultrasonography can identify and measure many structural features during coronary angiography. A prospective study of nearly 700 patients has shown that the lesions responsible for a second coronary event were usually thin fibrous cap atheromas (35). The pathology of recently symptomatic carotid plaques is similar to that of culprit coronary plaques, with strong correlations between macrophage instability and plaque instability (36).

Arteries in chronically inflamed tissues and within tumors often show pronounced fibrous intimal thickening, sometimes termed endarteritis obliterans (Table 8.2). In the early stages of this process, the fibrous tissue has a loose histologic appearance, and the ground substance may be basophilic. Although inflammatory or tumor cells often closely surround the adventitia, they do not usually penetrate far into the muscular wall. These changes must be carefully distinguished from those of systemic vasculitis. In general terms, vasculitis tends to affect vessels of a specific size, cause necrosis of vessel walls (Fig. 8.9) with associated hemorrhage, and leads to tissue infarction. In healed vasculitis, there is irregular fibrosis of the muscular wall (Fig. 8.10).

Arterioles

There are no specific histologic features that accurately distinguish small arteries from larger arterioles. In the coronary circulation small arteries are said to have a diameter of greater than 500 μm, prearterioles a diameter of 500 to 100 μm and true arterioles a diameter of less than 100 μm. Prearterioles are largely responsible for autoregulation of coronary blood flow while arterioles react to metabolic changes in the circulation (37). These are important physiologic differences but in biopsy material, there is so much variation in the contours of these small vessels that accurate distinction is often impossible and probably unnecessary. Larger arterioles ("prearterioles") have an obvious media and an adventitial layer of connective tissue. In the smallest arterioles, an internal elastic lamella may not be identified. The smooth muscle cells are arranged circumferentially, each cell winding around the wall several times. This is the

TABLE 8.3 Modified American Heart Association Classification of Atheromatous Lesions

Lesion	Histologic Features
Pathologic intimal thickening	Smooth muscle cell proliferation, intimal fibrosis, extracellular lipid but no lipid core or necrosis
Fibrous cap atheroma	Well-formed lipid core with thick fibrous cap, free of inflammatory cells (>80 μm coronary artery >200 μm carotid artery)
Thin fibrous cap atheroma	Thin cap of inflamed fibrous tissue with underlying lipid core
Ruptured plaque	Luminal thrombus communicating with lipid core via a ruptured fibrous cap
Eroded plaque	Luminal thrombus with endothelial ulceration; lipid core may be absent or small and does not communicate with lumen
Calcified lesions	Heavily calcified plaques with or without thrombus or lipid core

This is a simplified version of the classification of Virmani R, Kolodgie FD, Burke AP, et al. Lessons from sudden cardiac death: A comprehensive morphological classification for atherosclerotic lesions. *Arterioscler Thromb Vasc Biol* 2000;20:1262–1275.

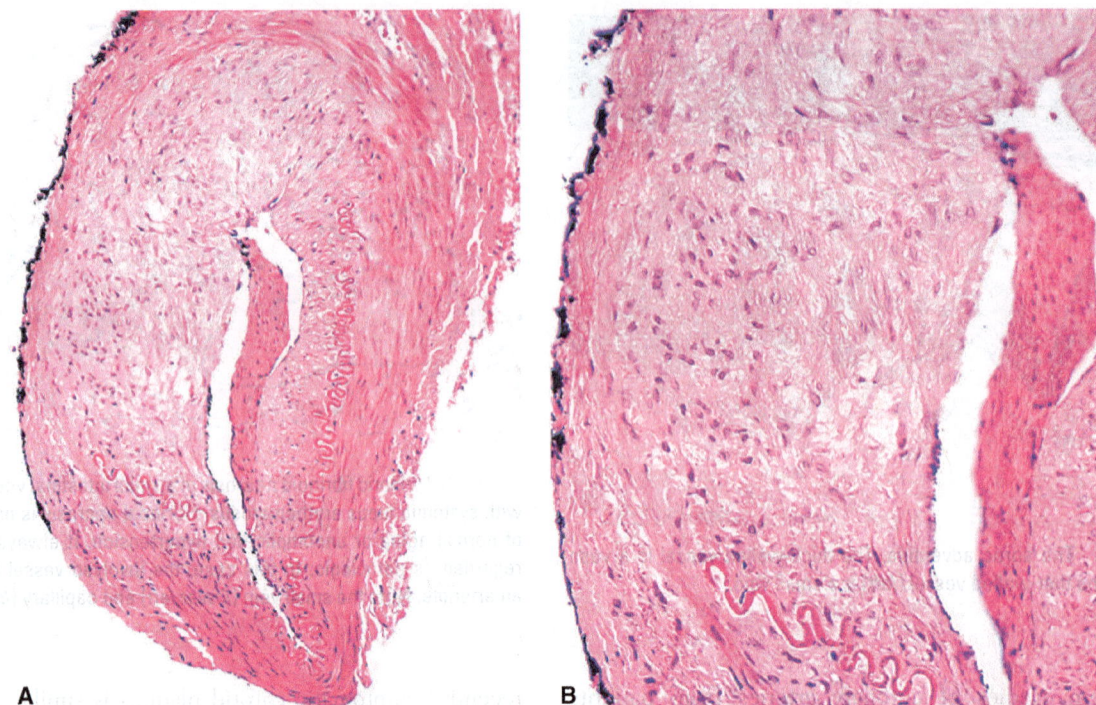

FIGURE 8.10 Healed temporal arteritis. This patient had been receiving steroid therapy for 2 weeks when this biopsy was performed. **A:** The low-power view shows irregular thickening of the wall and a loss of about 50% of the internal elastic lamella. **B:** This higher-power view shows fresh fibrous scarring of the media. Changes such as these are not part of the normal aging process.

structural basis of the precapillary sphincter. Small arterioles have a very thin adventitia but are richly supplied by sympathetic nerve fibers (5).

Hyalinization is a common lesion of arterioles and small arteries and increases with age and in conditions such as hypertension and diabetes. The glassy uniform appearance is the result of accumulation of a variety of plasma proteins and small amounts of lipids. As in arteries, reduplication of elastic tissue and intimal fibrosis are common changes in the aged. In severe long-standing benign hypertension and in the malignant phase, the arteriolar lumen can be substantially narrowed by concentric layers of fibrous tissue and smooth muscle cells, changes that are outside the normal range of aging (Table 8.1). Fibrinoid necrosis of the arteriolar media is the hallmark of malignant hypertension and some forms of acute vasculitis (Fig. 8.9). It must always be regarded as pathologic. In the earliest changes of diabetic microangiopathy, arterioles and capillaries often show prominent basement membrane thickening (38). This thickening can be readily identified in renal and peripheral nerve biopsies. Although there is physiologic evidence of small vessel disease in the heart and the peripheral vasculature, characteristic histologic changes of diabetic microangiopathy are seldom seen in these sites (39). In diabetes the amounts of type IV collagen and laminin are increased, but the proteoglycan component of the basement membrane is reduced. Albumin and immunoglobulins accumulate in these abnormal basement membranes, binding to glycosylated protein residues and contributing to the overall eosinophilic appearance.

Capillaries, Sinusoids, Venules, and Lymphatics

Capillaries, sinusoids, and small (postcapillary) venules are collectively termed exchange vessels and with arterioles form the microvascular bed, the structural basis of the microcirculation. In contrast to arterioles, capillaries have neither a muscular media nor an elastic lamella. A single but complete layer of endothelial cells lies on a basement membrane whose thickness varies from site to site. Basement membrane thickness increases with age, almost doubling in muscle capillaries from 10 to 70 years of age. There is no adventitial fibrous tissue support peripheral to this, but pericytes are present in and among the basement membrane. It is difficult to identify pericytes in routine sections, but they are easily seen by electron microscopy and, of course, stain with certain actin antibodies, especially the α_1 isoform (vascular smooth muscle actin). They provide structural support; and, because they contain several forms of myosin, they may be able to regulate blood flow. It is likely that they are involved in the synthesis of vascular basement membrane and are capable of phagocytosis. It is generally accepted that the turnover of pericytes is increased in the capillaries of diabetics, and this may contribute to the development of small vessel disease. Pericytes may also have a role in the control of peripheral insulin activity (40).

The endothelium of capillaries may have circular fenestrations that act as pores through the full thickness of the endothelial cell. Fenestrations are especially prominent in renal glomerular endothelial cells and are found in the intestinal mucosa, skin, and endocrine glands. In contrast, fenestrations are poorly developed or absent in brain, muscle, lung, and connective tissue (5).

In certain sites, such as the liver, spleen, pituitary, adrenals, and bone marrow, the vessels that connect arterioles and venules are known as sinusoids rather than capillaries. With diameters of up to 30 to 40 µm, they are generally more distended than capillaries. They have prominent fenestrations, but there are also significant gaps between endothelial cells. In the liver, there is no significant associated basement membrane.

The transition from venous capillary to muscular venule and small collecting vein is characterized by the gradual acquisition of a muscular media. The paracortical or high endothelial venules of lymph nodes have an important role in T-lymphocyte recirculation (41). The endothelial cells of postcapillary venules have a prominent cuboidal or columnar appearance, usually with an ovoid nucleus and a single central nucleolus. They stain specifically with the HECA-452 antibody (see later).

At the light microscopic level, small lymphatics closely resemble capillaries. In general terms, lymphatics have a larger diameter and a less regular cross-sectional profile (5). They begin as dilated channels with closed ends and anastomose freely. Small lymphatics have an incomplete basal lamina and lack pericytes or tight junctions. They are permeable to large proteins, cell debris, and microorganisms. Lymphatic channels have numerous valves and are often slightly distended at these sites, producing a slightly beaded appearance. Large lymphatics, such as the thoracic duct have a thin muscular media, with no clear division into circular or longitudinal coats, and a fibrous adventitia. A longitudinal muscular layer is present in the right lymphatic and thoracic ducts. Although lymphatics are present in most tissues, they are rarely found in the epidermis, nails, cornea, articular cartilage, central nervous system, or bone marrow. As detailed and illustrated later, lymphatic vessels stain specifically with the antibodies, D2-40 and LYVE-1 and VEGFR-3.

Veins

The primary function of veins is to return blood to the heart via the vena cavae. They also act as a capacitance reservoir for the vascular system, especially in the splanchnic system. In comparison to arteries of a similar diameter they have much thinner walls with a circular layer of muscle. In the saphenous, iliac, brachiocephalic, portal and renal veins and the vena cavae there is also a longitudinal muscular layer but these can be difficult to distinguish in surgical histology sections (Fig. 8.11). Placental, dural, and retinal veins and the veins of erectile tissue have very little muscle. In general, the veins of the lower limb have thicker walls than those of the arm and abdomen. Most veins have valves to prevent the reflux of blood (Fig. 8.11). In larger veins there is a well-developed fibrous adventitia. Some veins are tethered to surrounding connective tissue fascia.

The increasing use of the saphenous vein as an arterial conduit has led to a greater understanding of the normal structure of larger veins and the changes that occur in them as a result of aging (42). The connective tissue adventitia is often well developed. Saphenous veins in middle-aged and elderly patients show intimal fibrosis and longitudinal and circular muscle hypertrophy with a substantial increase in medial connective tissue (Fig. 8.11) (43). These changes must be distinguished from the form of atherosclerosis that develops in vein bypass grafts.

Pulmonary Arteries and Veins

Although the basic histologic structure of pulmonary vessels resembles that of their systemic counterparts, there are differences that reflect the much lower pressure of the pulmonary circuit. The lumina of major pulmonary arteries are widely dilated in comparison with wall thickness. The intima is hardly discernible. In an adult, the pulmonary arterial media is composed of only 10 to 15 parallel elastic lamellae, whereas, even in a young child, 40 aortic lamellae can be identified. The thickness of the pulmonary trunk is about 40% to 80% that of the aorta (Fig. 8.12).

In the systemic circulation, the transition from elastic to muscular arteries is abrupt and is usually at the point of a major arterial orifice. In contrast, even pulmonary arteries as small as 1 mm in diameter are elastic vessels. Smaller pulmonary arteries and arterioles have a thin layer of muscle enclosed by both an internal and an external layer of elastic tissue (44).

Arterioles give rise to a rich network of alveolar capillaries. Pericytes are not easily identified, and in places the endothelium and alveolar epithelium appear to share a common basement membrane. The walls of pulmonary veins are less structured than their systemic counterparts. The media is composed of a rather haphazardly arranged but roughly circular layer of connective tissue and muscle. No distinct and continuous elastic lamellae are present, and valves are said to be absent (Fig. 8.13). It can be very difficult to distinguish small pulmonary arteries and veins. We agree with others who feel that a certain distinction can only be made if the vessel can be clearly seen to be draining in a larger artery or vein (44) (Fig. 8.13A).

It can also be difficult to distinguish the early vascular changes of pulmonary hypertension from those of normal aging (Table 8.4). The initial changes in both conditions include intimal fibrosis and medial muscular hypertrophy, and each of these features is most prominent in muscular arteries and larger arterioles (45). The absence of significant changes in the larger arteries may be misleading. In long-standing pulmonary hypertension, the complex changes in muscular arteries include florid intimal thickening, marked medial hypertrophy, and prominent dilatation of small

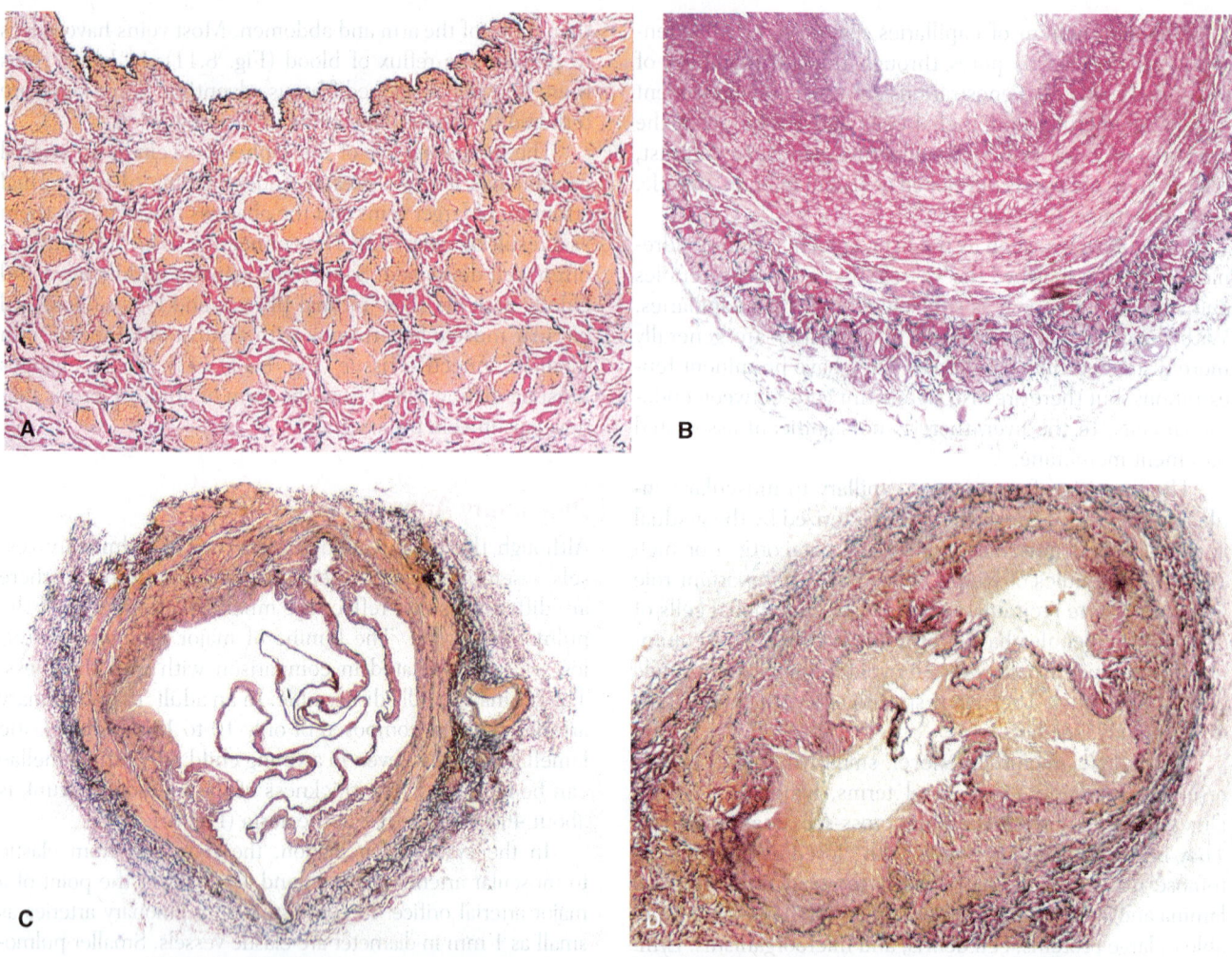

FIGURE 8.11 **A:** Renal vein from a 58-year-old woman, close to the junction with the inferior vena cava. There is no significant intimal thickening, and a thin internal elastic lamella can be identified. Note the thin layer of subendothelial collagen. The muscular wall is composed of coarse fascicles, which are not clearly arranged into circular and longitudinal layers. **B:** Detail of the wall of the proximal saphenous vein. In contrast to the renal vein the media is composed of distinct layers of circular and longitudinal smooth muscles. **C:** Cross section of normal saphenous vein. This vein is commonly used by cardiovascular surgeons for arterial bypass grafting procedures. There is a regular pattern of alternating muscle layers with some fibrous tissue and scant elastin. Note the valvular structures in the lumen of the vein. **D:** Vein affected by phlebosclerosis, showing cushions of intimal thickening fibrosis of the media and marked fibrotic thickening of the valves (elastic van Gieson).

branches of parent vessels (Fig. 8.14). In the most extreme examples, angiomatoid malformations may develop, and occasionally there is fibrinoid necrosis of the vessel wall. Mooi and Grünberg have summarized and extensively illustrated the current WHO classification of pulmonary hypertensive diseases (44). Lung biopsy is no longer used for the assessment of pulmonary hypertension in children with congenital heart disease nor in adults with primary pulmonary hypertension. However surgical pathologists must make a careful assessment of the pulmonary arteries and veins in lung biopsy specimens and be able to describe and grade these alterations accurately (45).

Aging changes in pulmonary vessels are seldom described in detail (46). In severe, long-standing cardiac failure, intimal fibrosis, medial hypertrophy, and hyalinization are prominent pulmonary venous abnormalities. Marked medial hypertrophy may confer an arterialized appearance to pulmonary veins, and they may appear to have an internal and an external elastic lamina. Multiple levels should be taken and stained for elastin and by a trichrome method. The elastic lamellae are seldom complete in these abnormal veins, and there is often more medial fibrosis than in corresponding pulmonary arteries. Even so, accurate distinction of abnormal pulmonary arteries and veins can be difficult. Extensions of atrial myocardium (myocardial sleeves) are a common finding in pulmonary veins and the vena cavae close to their junction with the heart (Fig. 8.15). Abnormal electrical activity associated with these sleeves cause ectopic beats and atrial arrhythmias, especially when the sleeves are fibrosed or infiltrated with amyloid in the elderly (47).

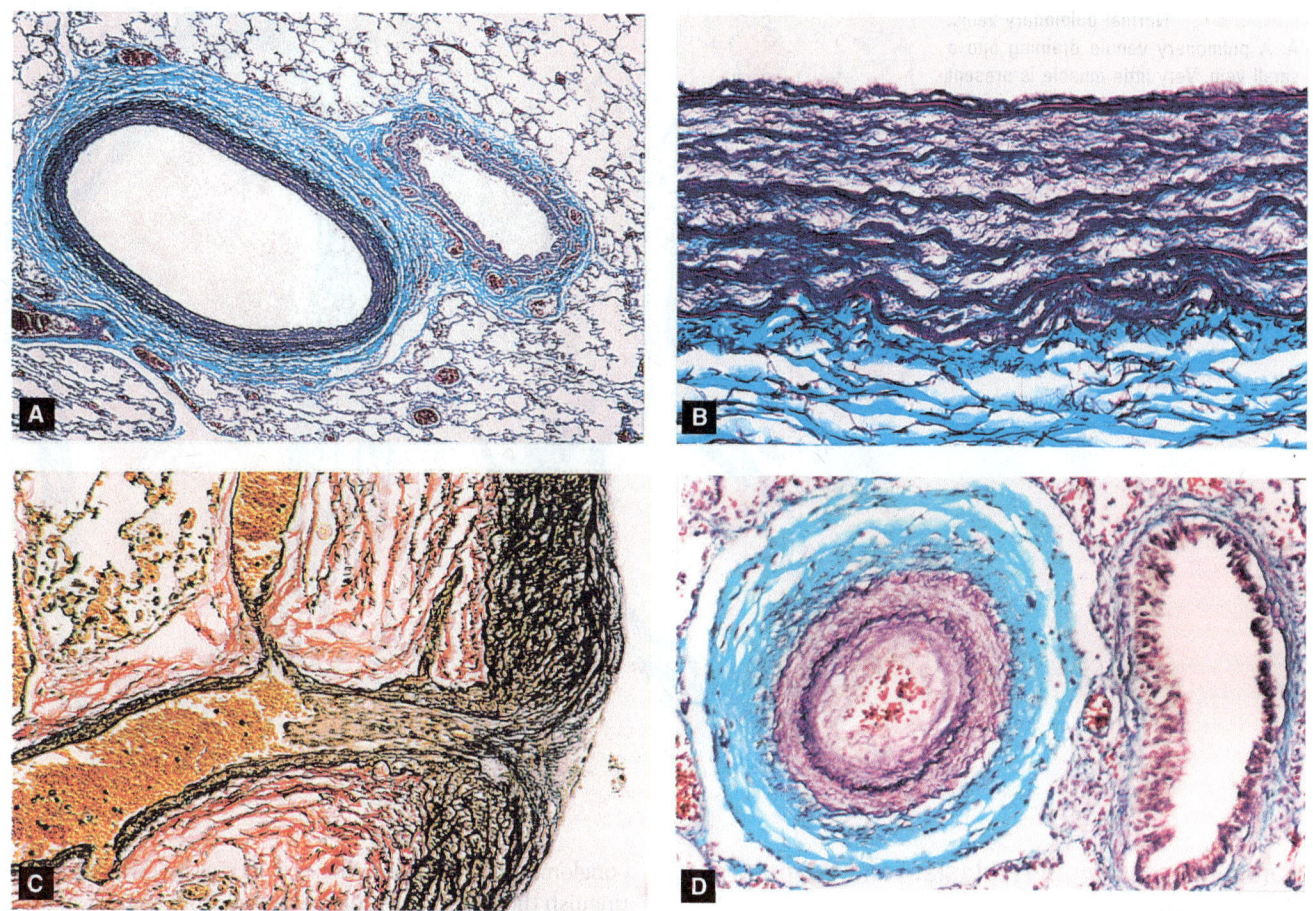

FIGURE 8.12 **A:** Elastic pulmonary artery from a 1-year-old child. The lung was inflated via the main pulmonary artery, which therefore appears much larger than the corresponding bronchus. **B:** A magnified view of the elastic wall (Gomori's trichrome). **C:** The transition from elastic to muscular pulmonary arteries in a 73-year-old man. Note the larger number of elastic lamellae. There is slight fibrous intimal thickening only (elastic van Gieson). **D:** A small pulmonary artery from a patient with long-standing pulmonary hypertension and chronic obstructive airways disease. There is hypertrophy of the muscular wall and pronounced fibrous intimal thickening (Gomori's trichrome).

TABLE 8.4
Histologic Features of Pulmonary Vessels

Vessel	Normal	Age-Related Changes	Pulmonary Hypertension
Elastic arteries (>500 μm)	Widely patent lumen, media of 10 to 15 parallel lamellae of elastic tissue	Slight intimal fibrosis; increased medial thickness due to occasional atheromatous plaques	Atherosclerosis and dilation of main pulmonary arteries; medial thickening due to hypertrophy of admixed muscular elements
Muscular arteries or arterioles	Thin muscular wall often with distinct internal and external elastic laminae	Increased muscular media, eccentric intimal fibrosis, especially in vessels less than 300 μm in diameter	Complex changes include florid intimal thickening, medial hypertrophy, dilation of small branches, angiomatoid (plexiform) lesions, and fibrinoid necrosis
Veins	Thin media of irregularly arranged fibrous tissue and muscle. No distinct elastic lamella. No valves	Few detailed studies. The media may appear hyalinized	Intimal fibrosis, medial muscular hypertrophy—occasionally sufficient to mimic appearance of arteries

FIGURE 8.13 Normal pulmonary veins. **A:** A pulmonary venule draining into a small vein. Very little muscle is present in the wall. **B:** A large pulmonary vein close to the hilum of the lung (Gomori's trichrome).

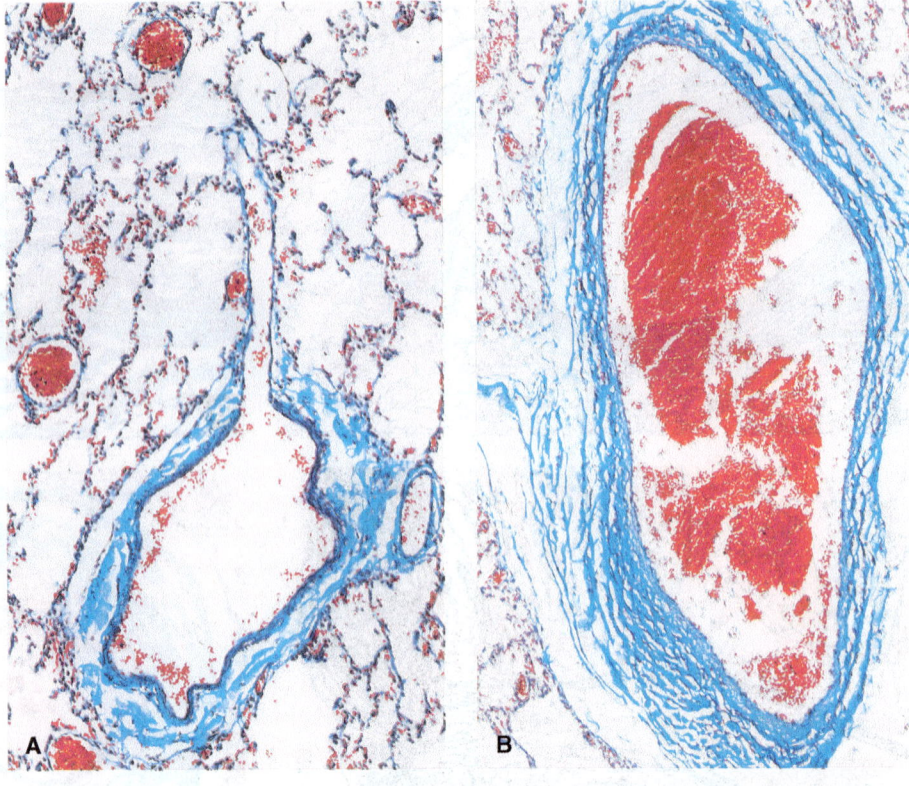

Anastomoses, Angiodysplasias, and Vascular Malformations

There is potential for anastomoses between many arteries and veins. They vary in size from about 200 to 800 μm and in some sites, such as the nail bed, have a complex structure. Occasionally, small arteriovenous anastomosis is seen in resection specimens. In the anal canal they form the so-called "anal glomeruli." In the anal canal, uterus and bladder venous plexuses may be composed of prominent conglomerates of venous channels. It may be difficult to distinguish these highly vascularized areas from angiodysplasias or hamartomatous vascular lesions (malformations). This is often the case in intestinal resections for ischemia or hemorrhage, especially when there is prominent vasocongestion (see later). Biopsies of the nasal mucosa, clitoris, and deep parts of the glans penis may include erectile vascular tissue. Highly vascular areas of interconnected vessels with aberrant smooth muscle bundles may be mistaken for angiomas or malformation, especially if there is inadequate

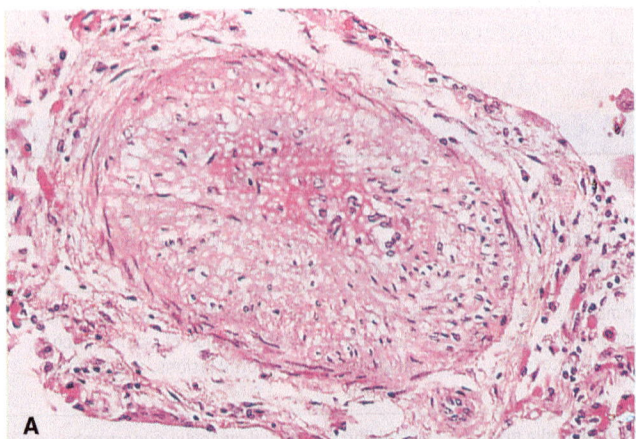
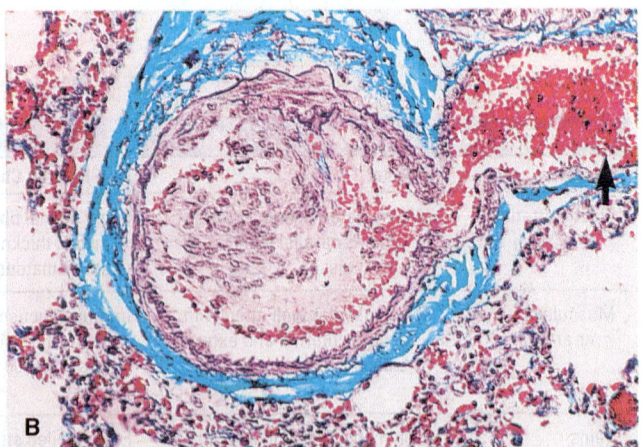

FIGURE 8.14 Advanced pulmonary hypertensive changes. **A:** There is marked hypertrophy of the medial muscle in a small pulmonary artery. **B:** An early plexiform lesion with nearby dilated thin-walled branches (*arrow*) (Gomori's trichrome).

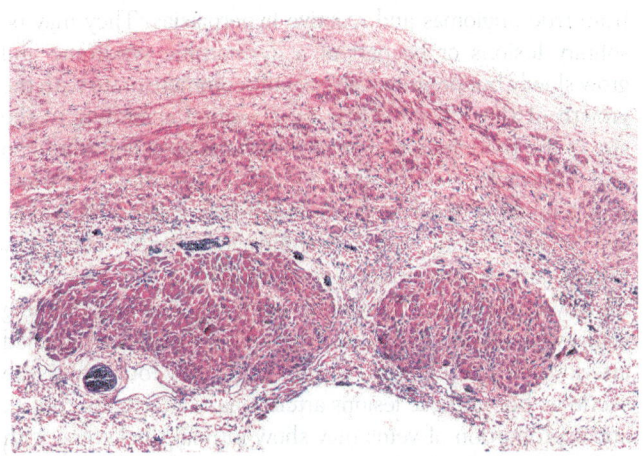

FIGURE 8.15 Myocardial sleeves in pulmonary vein. Section through a pulmonary vein close to the left atrial wall. Note the extensions of myocardial tissue along the outer aspect of vein (*arrows*). These myocardial sleeves are important sites for generation of atrial arrhythmias, especially in the elderly when the sleeves develop fibrosis or amyloid deposits.

clinical information (Fig. 8.16). There are also anastomoses between pulmonary and bronchial veins and between the portal and systemic circulations. The potential connections between the portal and systemic circulations, either in the submucosa of the esophagus or rectum or in the periumbilical or diaphragmatic region, may be massively dilated in advanced hepatic disease. Biopsies are seldom performed surgically. Peripheral glomus tumors almost certainly arise from supporting cells that surround the normal but rather complex anastomosing channels between digital arterioles and venules. Glomus cells do not express endothelial markers but, because they stain with smooth muscle actin and vimentin, may be related to vascular smooth muscle (48).

Surgical pathologists must be familiar with the normal vascular patterns of the cerebral meninges and the colonic submucosa if cerebral arteriovenous malformations and large intestinal angiodysplasia are to be accurately assessed. Each of these areas has a rich vascular supply with numerous, sometimes thick-walled, venous channels. Malformations or angiodysplasias must only be diagnosed if there

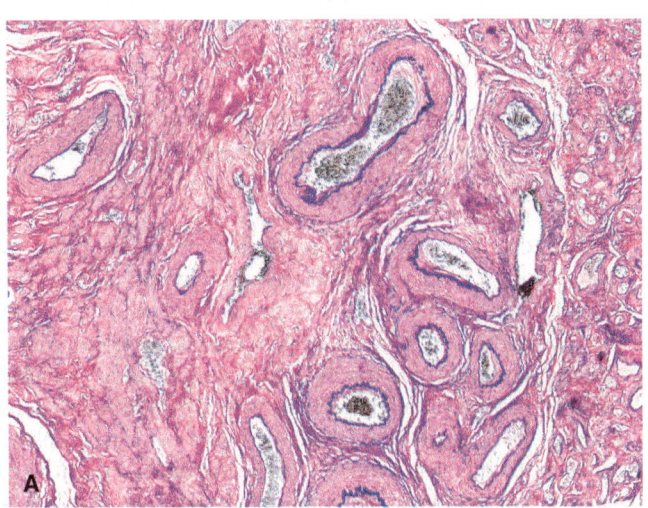
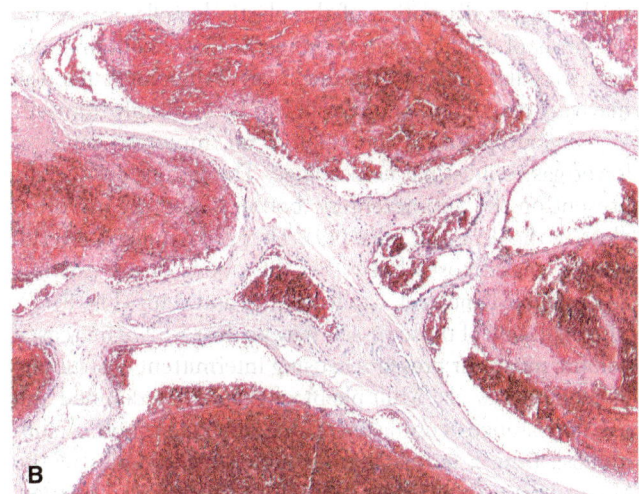
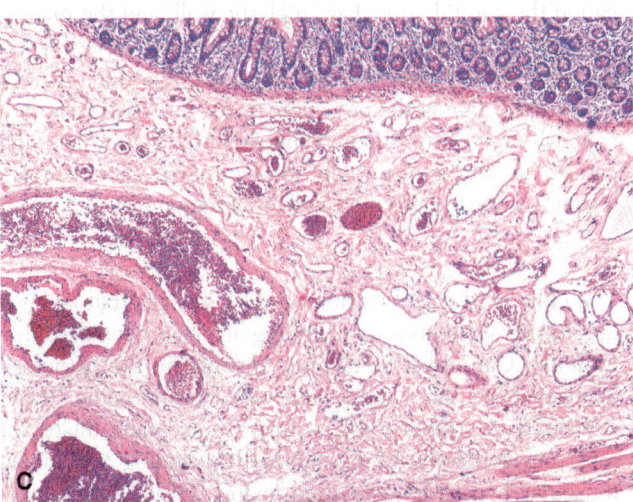

FIGURE 8.16 Highly vascularized areas in biopsy tissue that may be confused with angiomas or vascular malformations. **A:** Atrophic ovary. **B:** Hemorrhoidal tissue in the anorectal region. **C:** Dilated vessels in the submucosa of colonic resection from a patient with ischemic bowel disease.

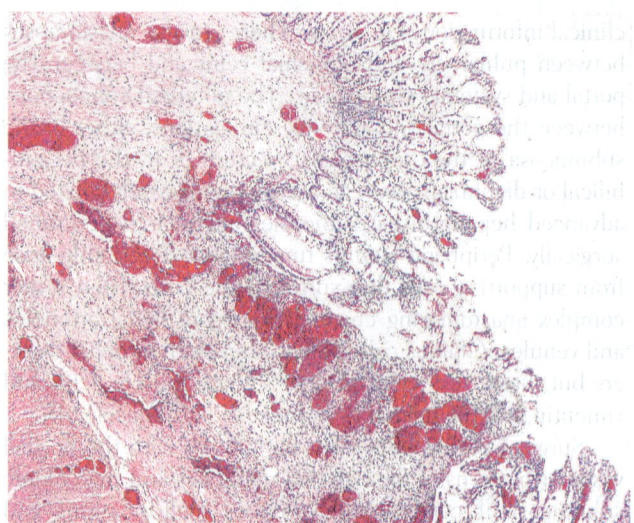

FIGURE 8.17 Angiodysplasia of the colon. Note the many dilated thin-walled blood vessels in the submucosa. Although these vessels are distended, their basic structure is unaltered.

is undoubted evidence of an abnormal vessel wall. Aging changes and atherosclerosis seldom involve the smaller leptomeningeal arteries. In arteries, eccentric fibrous intimal thickening or disruption of the elastic lamellae support a diagnosis of a malformation. Veins in these malformations have irregular contours, the thickness of their muscular wall may vary markedly, and the wall can be uniformly fibrosed.

Angiodysplasia of the colon is an important cause of lower gastrointestinal hemorrhage. The lesions are usually present on the antimesenteric border of the cecum, often close to the ileocecal valve (49). They are not direct arteriovenous anastomoses but rather dilatations of pre-existing, and previously normal, capillary rings and veins (Fig. 8.17). The dilatation of these vessels may be the result of increased colonic muscular pressure causing intermittent obstruction of draining vessels. Multiple blocks must be examined and the appearances contrasted with a control section of submucosa from a normal colon. Submucosal arteries of the large intestine may show pronounced age-related tortuosity, and this must not be interpreted as an abnormality. A proportion of cases with good clinical or radiologic evidence of angiodysplasia will not be confirmed histologically. Some cases of massive gastrointestinal hemorrhage result from abnormally large submucosal arteries. This is most common in the stomach but also has been reported in the large and small intestines. Arteries in the submucosa of the proximal portion of the stomach can arise directly from omental vessels and may have a larger caliber than superficial arteries arising from a submucosal plexus, the so-called caliber-persistent artery or Dieulafoy lesion (50).

Vascular malformations are congenital lesions composed of mature but often malformed (dysplastic) blood vessels. They result from dysregulation in the signaling pathways of vasculogenesis in early embryonic life (51), especially members of the TGFβ family (52). They must be distinguished from true angiomas and reactive hyperplasias. They may be solitary lesions or be part of a dysmorphic syndrome and grow slowly but progressively, usually commensurate with the growth of the patient. They are classified according to the size of the predominate type of vessel, the so-called Mulliken and Glowacki classification (53,54). Clinically, a distinction is made between slow- and high-flow lesions. Slow-flow lesions are usually venous malformations (55). High-flow lesions are usually arteriovenous malformations characterized by connections between feeding arteries and draining veins, without an interconnecting capillary bed, the so-called arteriovenous fistula (56). Fistulae are rarely found in tissue sections; but in these lesions arteries have a tortuous course, and a proportion of veins may show intimal thickening with collagen and elastin deposition in their walls. Pure venous malformations are composed of dilated vascular channels with walls of variable size, showing irregular degrees of attenuation and fibrosis. Complications include thrombosis with organization, papillary endothelial hyperplasia (Masson pseudotumor), and nodular calcification. In lymphatic malformations, the vascular channels vary considerably in size and may have an incomplete muscular wall. As in other vessels their endothelium stains with CD31 and CD34 antibodies and with factor VIII-related antigen.

Vascular Surgery

The changes commonly seen in vessels after surgical procedures and interventions are summarized in Table 8.5.

Endarterectomy

Patency can be restored to a partially occluded artery by drawing out a proportion of the atherosclerotic intima. The procedure is usually applied to the carotid bifurcation but occasionally to iliac, femoral, or even coronary arteries. Meta-analysis has confirmed that carotid endarterectomy is highly beneficial in symptomatic patients with 70% + atheromatous stenosis (57). Ideally, the surgeon should establish a plane between the innermost media and the intima, and the atheromatous material should be removed in its entirety. At its bifurcation the carotid artery has an elastic wall, and the material removed will include layers of elastic tissue, atheromatous debris, and thrombus. Stroke is the most important immediate complication of the procedure and is usually the result of acute thrombosis or thromboembolism. Longer-term complications are recurrent thrombosis, aneurysmal dilatation, and restenosis due to fibrous intimal proliferation (58).

Bypass Grafts

The clinical (42) and pathologic (59) changes that occur in autologous saphenous vein bypass grafts have been described in detail. Care must be taken to distinguish the pathologic changes from those associated with normal aging. When subjected to arterial pressure, many vein grafts dilate and most develop some fibrous intimal thickening and medial muscular hypertrophy. In time, many develop pronounced

TABLE 8.5 Pathologic Changes After Vascular Surgery	
Procedure	Spectrum of Histologic Change
Endarterectomy	*Acutely:* Surface platelet and fibrin deposits on inner face of surgical dissection, occasionally progressing to occlusive thrombosis. *Chronically:* Variable degrees of fibrous intimal hyperplasia, occasionally progressing to restenosis. "False" aneurysm formation
Vein bypass grafting	*Acutely:* Thrombosis, dissection at anastomosis site *Chronically:* Dilatation with fibrous intimal thickening and medial muscular hypertrophy (to be contrasted with preimplant state. Occasionally, marked intimal fibrosis with lipid deposition and hemorrhage, leading to occlusion ("vein atherosclerosis")
Internal mammary and radial artery grafting	*Acutely:* Thrombosis at anastomoses sites *Chronically:* Occasional grafts become fibrosed. Graft atherosclerosis uncommon
Angioplasty and stenting	*Acutely:* Acute inflammation, dissection, and thrombosis *Chronically:* Restenosis due to reactive fibrous intimal thickening, now reduced by drug eluting stents
Prosthetic vessels	*Acutely:* Thrombotic occlusion *Chronically:* Extensive macrophage and giant cell infiltration of fabric wall. Formation of fibrin-rich pseudointima, occasionally progressing to partial or complete occlusion. Graft failure and thrombosis

fibrous intimal thickening with areas of lipid deposition, intramural hemorrhage, and thrombosis. These appearances closely mimic atherosclerosis and are an important cause of graft failure. In one postmortem study in which saphenous vein conduits were sampled throughout their length, more than 75% narrowing was demonstrated in 11% to 26% of the segments examined (60). Intensive lipid lowering therapy can attenuate graft atherosclerosis. External synthetic sheaths are sometimes placed around vein grafts and may prevent vein wall thickening. Careful surgical harvesting of vein grafts may minimize damage to the endothelial layer (61,62). Grafts can sometimes be dilated by angioplasty, but redo coronary bypass procedures are now a significant part of the work of all cardiac surgery departments.

In cardiac surgery, coronary artery stenoses are routinely bypassed with the left or the right internal mammary artery. The origin of the artery from the subclavian artery is preserved, and it is then dissected away from the chest wall. There is usually a surrounding cuff of soft tissue, but some surgeons dissect this away, producing a so-called "skeletalized" graft (63). Long-term patency rates are superior to saphenous vein grafts. The caliber of the normal internal mammary artery is similar to that of distal coronary arteries. Pre-existing occlusive disease is present in fewer than 5% of patients, and only occasional grafts develop atheromatous obstructions. In its proximal portion, the internal mammary is an elastic artery, but the media is muscular from about the level of the 4th rib.

Segments of the radial artery are also used as free grafts. Like saphenous vein grafts, they are anastomosed proximally to the aortic root and distally to the coronary arteries. The radial artery is muscular and is invariably free of significant atheroma (Fig. 8.6).

Angioplasty

Percutaneous coronary angioplasty (PTCA) with stent emplacement is now the treatment of choice for many proximal coronary stenoses and is increasingly used as a primary intervention to open thrombosed coronary arteries after myocardial infarction (64). The mortality rate in most centers is now less than 1%, and over 90% of procedures are initially successful. The design of stents and the antiproliferative agents that they release undergo continual modification and development (65).

In order to dilate the vessel, the heavily fibrous and focally calcified atheromatous plaque must be cracked open. Only when this has occurred can the deeper intima and underlying media be distended by the inflated balloon and held open by the expandable metallic stent. Early histologic studies of patients dying soon after angioplasty demonstrated a characteristic pattern of radial tears or splits, sometimes with dissections extending into the underlying media. Stents minimize the complications of these changes. Stent thrombosis occurs in about 1% of patients within a year of stent implantation. Antiproliferative agents released from drug eluting stents may inhibit endothelialization of the stent struts (65). Restenosis is the result of fibrous intimal proliferation, thrombus formation, and an overall reduction in the size of the vessel lumen. These changes can now be visualized by either intravascular ultrasound or optical coherence tomography. These provide a virtual histology image of the arterial wall (66). If death occurs soon after the procedure, the stent can be carefully extracted from the opened artery which is then processed in the usual way. After late closure, stents can be cut with an electric diamond saw and then embedded in hard plastic (Fig. 8.18). A technique for dissolving metallic stents has also been developed (67).

Prosthetic Vessels

Vascular surgeons use various techniques to anastomose grafts to native vessels.

Grafts made of Dacron are successful in large caliber bypass procedures such as aortoiliac grafting. Expanded polytetrafluorethylene (ePTFE) is preferred for below knee grafts and in the construction of arteriovenous fistulae for chronic hemodialysis. However long-term patency rates are poor. At present prosthetic grafts are not used to bypass coronary stenosis. Acute thrombotic occlusion of prosthetic vessels is usually the result of surgical

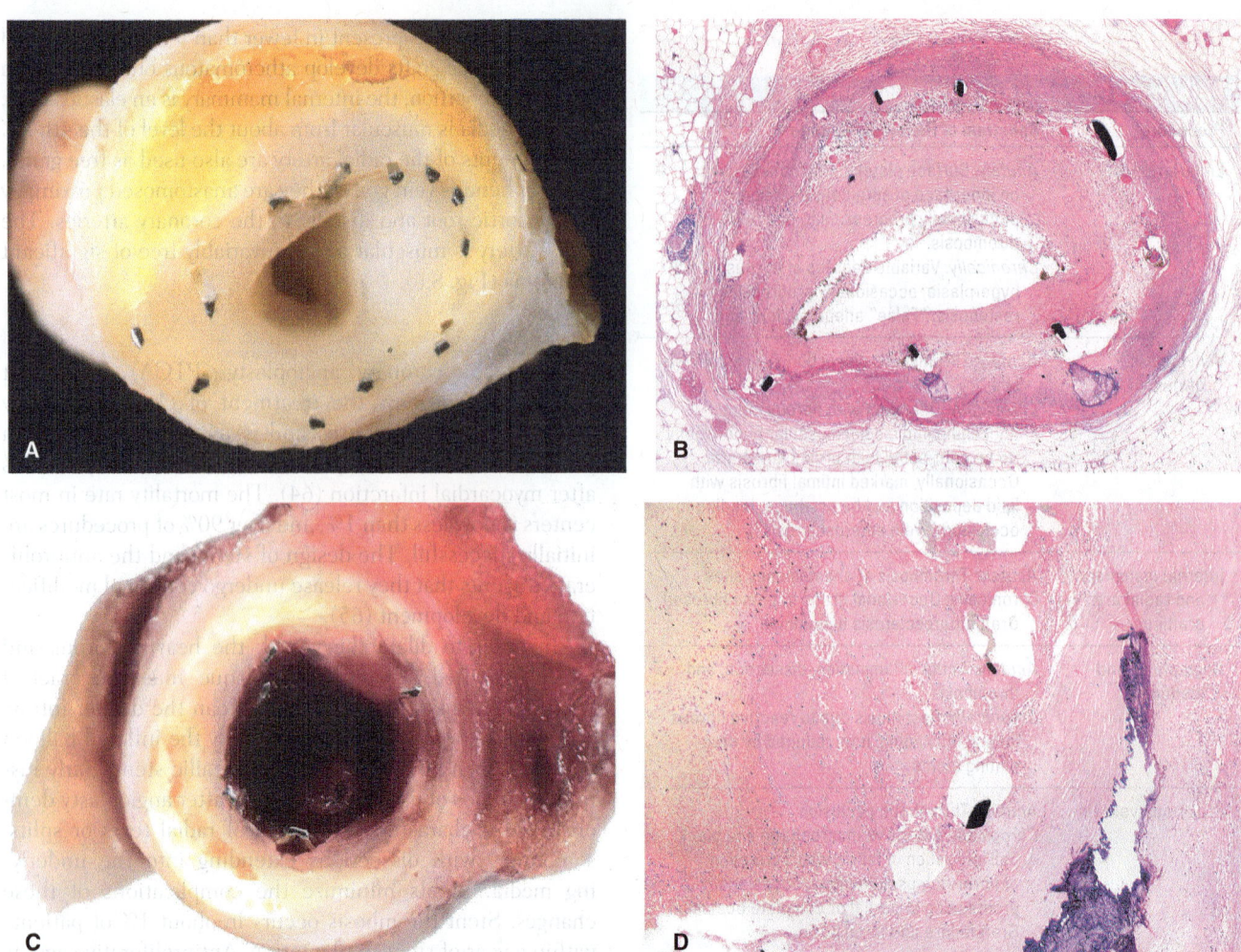

FIGURE 8.18 **A:** Macroscopic cross section of a stented coronary artery. Note the thick layer of concentric neointimal tissue that caused restenosis. The stent was cut with a diamond saw. This leaves the metal struts more or less in place, although some distortion is inevitable. **B:** Histology of the same artery after plastic embedding (BMA/MMA) shows the stent struts at the interface of fibrocellular intimal tissue and pre-existent calcified atherosclerotic plaque. **C:** Macroscopic view of cross section through coronary artery with stent affected by thrombotic occlusion. **D:** Detail of the histology of the same segment after plastic embedding, showing black stent strut and empty spaces (where the struts had been in situ) adjacent to fresh thrombus.

technique or poor flow rates. The many factors that contribute to chronic failure include inherent thrombogenicity secondary to lack of an endothelial lining and compliance mismatch between the graft and the native vessel (68). In time, prosthetic grafts develop a pseudointima. This has a jelly-like consistency and is composed of fibrin and enmeshed leukocytes. It may develop a partial endothelial lining. The most striking feature of these prosthetic vessels is the intense mononuclear and giant cell reaction that develops around the woven fibers of the graft. There is usually a moderate degree of adventitial fibrosis that binds the prosthesis to the surrounding tissues and reduces its elasticity. Long-term complications include thrombosis, particularly at flexures or surgical anastomoses, infection, and deterioration of the fibers of the graft. Modifications under study in industry include coating grafts with anticoagulants such as heparin, thrombomodulin, or hirudin, seeding grafts with endothelial cells or incorporating nitric oxide into grafts (68).

ELECTRON MICROSCOPY

Ultrastructural studies have made enormous contributions to our understanding of vascular biology. However, even surgical pathologists with a specific interest in vascular pathology have only limited experience and expertise in electron microscopy. Some of the most important ultrastructural features of vessels are summarized in Table 8.6.

Endothelial Cells

The entire vascular system is lined internally by a single layer of rather spindle-shaped endothelial cells. Small

TABLE 8.6
Ultrastructural Features of Vascular Tissues
Endothelial cells are joined by tight, adherans, or gap junctions
Transendothelial channels characterize fenestrated endothelium, as in hepatic sinusoids, glomeruli, and endocrine organs
Cytoplasmic inclusions of endothelium include lysosomes, plasmalemmal vesicles, and Weibel–Palade bodies (see Fig. 8.19).
Capillary endothelium is surrounded by basement membrane in which pericytes are embedded. There is very little basement membrane around lymphatic vessels. There are direct appositions between processes of pericytes and endothelium through gaps in the basement membrane
Smooth muscle cells are invested in basement membrane and are linked by communicating (gap) junctions. Elastin and collagen fibers may be closely opposed to the surfaces of smooth muscle cells
No significant media in small arterioles, capillaries, or lymphatics
The adventitia is composed of collagen and some elastin fibers. It has a well-developed structure in large veins but is very thin in some arteries

finger-like microvilli, 200 to 400 nm long, may be seen on the surface of endothelial cells. A thin network of membrane-bound proteoglycans and glycoproteins, the glycocalyx, coats the luminal surface of the endothelium. It varies in thickness from 0.5 μm in small capillaries to 4.5 μm in the carotid artery. The glycocalyx has important roles in vascular permeability, blood cell vessel wall interactions, and shear stress sensing. For example, the glycocalyx modulates inflammatory reactions by binding cytokine molecules and superoxide dismutase and can influence coagulation by binding proteins such as antithrombin III, thrombomodulin, and inhibitors of tissue factor. Glycocalyx proteins are responsible for transmission of shear stress signals into specific processes such as nitric oxide production (mechanotransduction). There is growing evidence that the glycocalyx is attenuated or absent in pathologic conditions such as atherosclerosis, diabetes, ischemia–reperfusion injury and smoking (69). Although endothelial cells have relatively sparse endoplasmic reticulum, a small number of free ribosomes, and an inconspicuous Golgi apparatus they produce a variety of molecules that are important in blood coagulation and the regulation of vascular tone.

Junctional complexes between endothelial cells are tight, adherens, or gap junctions (70). Tight junctions have a barrier function and help to maintain cell polarity. A variety of molecules, notably those of the claudin family create the barrier and regulate electrical resistance between cells (71). Loss of this barrier function may be important in disorders such as diabetic retinopathy (72) and in a variety of skin diseases (73). Adherens junctions regulate permeability to white cells and soluble molecules and have a role in contact inhibition (74). Gap junctions are assembled from proteins known as connexins and form channels between adjacent cells (75). Alterations in gap junction proteins have been documented in human heart disease, including arrhythmias and cardiomyopathies (76).

Inclusions of Endothelial Cells

Lysosomes are readily identified in most endothelial cells and are involved in intracytoplasmic digestion of foreign debris and products of metabolism. In many areas of the vascular system, membrane-bound vesicles measuring up to 80 to 90 nm can be identified (Fig. 8.19). They are most prominent on the abluminal surface of the endothelial cell. They were originally known as plasmalemmal vesicles but are now termed caveolae. Their functions include the sequestration and concentration of small molecules, and they contribute to the endothelial barrier function, regulation of nitric oxide synthesis, and cholesterol metabolism (77). Weibel–Palade bodies are elongated secretory organelles specific to endothelial cells (Fig. 8.19). Von Willebrand factor is stored inside Weibel–Palade bodies as tubules, but on its release forms long strings that recruit platelets to sites of endothelial injury (78).

The permeability of capillaries varies considerably from organ to organ. In some sites, such as the renal glomerulus, the hepatic sinusoids, the small intestine, and some endocrine glands, there is a rapid interchange between blood and the surrounding tissue. Some of these permeability differences are related to the exact nature of the junctions between endothelial cells, but endothelial fenestrae also have an important role in this respect. These fenestrations are in fact

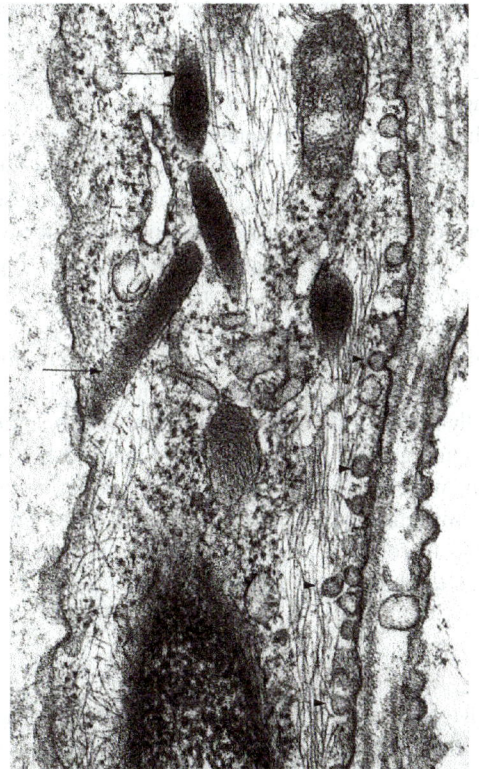

FIGURE 8.19 Transmission electron micrograph of an endothelial cell from a small subcutaneous capillary. Plasmalemmal vesicles (caveolae) are present on the abluminal surface (*arrowheads*). There are conspicuous Weibel–Palade bodies (*arrows*). Only part of the endothelial cell nucleus is included (*bottom*) (original magnification ×15,000).

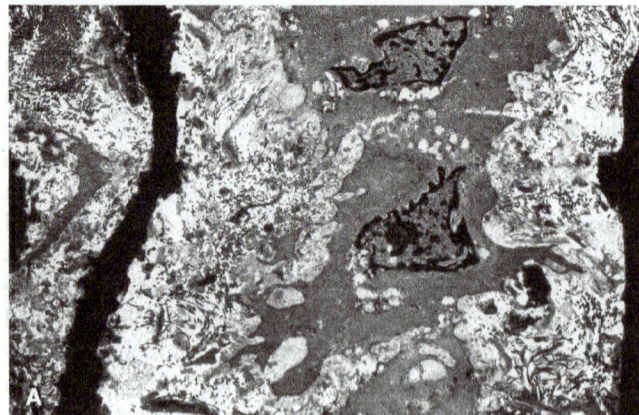 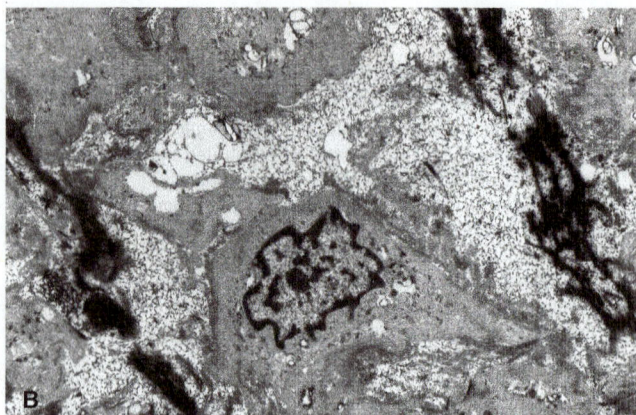

FIGURE 8.20 Transmission electron microcopy of aortic media. **A:** Normal aorta. There are musculoelastic lamellar units with regular thick elastic lamellae with numerous small extensions. Smooth muscle is present in the interlamellar space. **B:** Marfan syndrome. There is distinct thinning and fragmentation of both elastic lamellae. There is an increase in fibrillary collagen and mucoid deposits in the matrix of the interlamellar space.

the openings of irregular, and sometimes incomplete, transendothelial channels that allow the rapid interchange of fluid between the blood vessel lumen and the interstitium (79).

Media

In the human aorta, homogeneous parallel elastic lamellae alternate with layers containing smooth muscle cells and a variety of extracellular components. Smooth muscle predominates in muscular arteries. The power of contraction of smooth muscle is as great as skeletal muscle and can be maintained for longer periods with greater shortening. The structure of smooth muscle cells is maintained by the intermediate filaments vimentin and desmin, and the contractile forces are generated by actin and myosin filaments. Smooth muscle cells are arranged in parallel longitudinal bundles with the wide part of one cell opposed to the tapering part of another (Fig. 8.20). Each smooth muscle cell is covered by a basal lamina which merges with fine collagen and elastin fibers (5).

Individual smooth muscle cells are often linked by communicating (gap) junctions, but tight junctions are not generally seen. In the microcirculation and in some larger arteries and arterioles, there are gap junctions between the smooth muscle cells and the overlying endothelium (80). These myoendothelial junctions could have an important role in relaying physiologic or pharmacologic stimuli between the blood vessel lumen and the media.

Adventitia and Supporting Cells

The adventitial layer consists almost entirely of collagen and elastic fibers. The thickness of this layer varies with the size of the vessel, and it may be continuous with the surrounding connective tissue. In some medium-sized veins, it is particularly well developed but in cerebral arteries it may be as thin as 80 μm. A layer of elastic tissue, the external elastic lamella, is present at the junction of the media and adventitia.

In human material, it is seldom as pronounced as the internal elastic lamella but is prominent in many other mammalian arteries. The pericytes that are present in and among the basement membrane of capillaries and small venules superficially resemble fibroblasts. The ultrastructural appearance of their cytoplasmic filaments suggests that they are contractile, and this is further evidence that they are of mesenchymal origin.

Lymphatics and Veins

The smallest lymphatic vessels have wider lumina than blood capillaries and a discontinuous basement membrane. A variety of anchoring filaments bind the lymphatic endothelium to the surrounding collagenous tissues, perhaps providing the sort of support normally produced by basement membrane and enmeshed pericytes in capillaries. The ultrastructural appearances of venous capillaries, venules, and small veins mirror those seen at the light microscopic level.

ANTIGEN EXPRESSION OF NORMAL AND NEOPLASTIC VASCULAR TISSUE

Endothelium

Endothelial cells cover the inner surface of the entire vascular tree, arterial, venous, capillary, and lymphatic. Ongoing research on endothelial cells has revealed marked heterogeneity among the endothelium (79). There are differences in the size, shape, orientation, and antigen expression between arterial and venous endothelium. Within the heart there are differences between endothelia in the epicardial arteries, the endocardium, and myocardial capillaries. Several genes have been identified that are preferentially expressed in either arterial or venous endothelium. An increasing panel of monoclonal antibodies is available to investigate aspects of this heterogeneity, some of which may have a role in pathology.

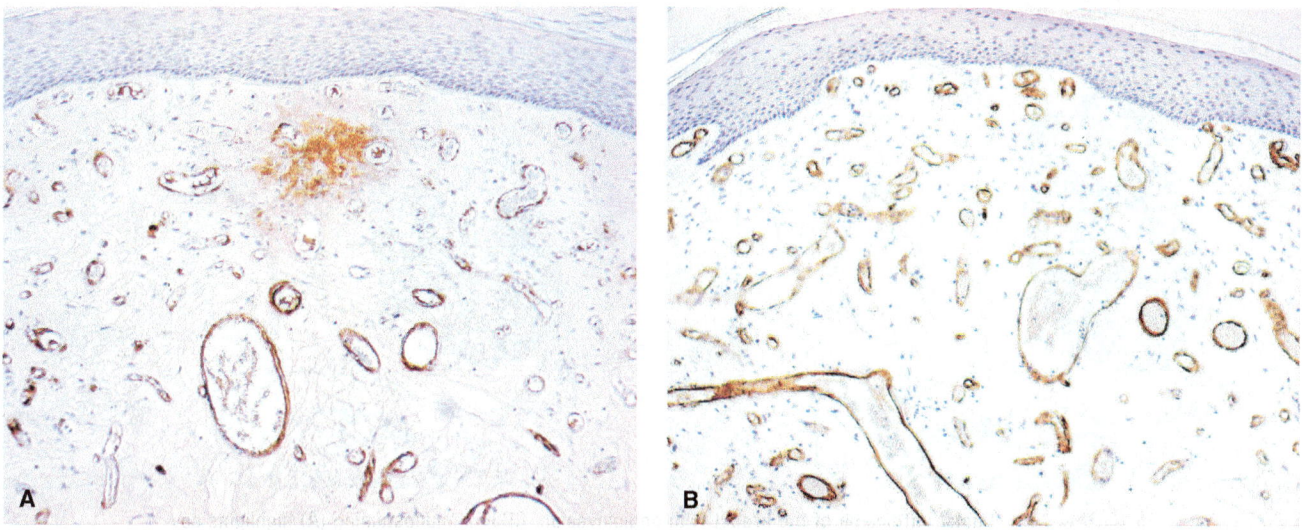

FIGURE 8.21 Staining of small vessels in a hemangioma with antibodies to factor VIII (**A**) and CD34 (**B**). As in these illustrations, the staining with CD34 is usually sharper than with factor VIII. Some nonspecific extravascular staining is often seen with factor VIII but has no significance.

At present the most widely used antibodies are directed against factor VIII, CD31, and CD34 (Fig. 8.21). Since these antigens are present in all types of endothelial cells, they are considered to be pan endothelial markers. The lectin Ulex europaeus agglutinin 1 binds to some α–L-fructose containing glycocompounds and therefore to virtually all human endothelia. The staining pattern is sometimes more intense than with factor VIII antibodies, especially in immature vessels. However, all endothelial markers cross-react to some extent with other cell components. For example, in areas of hemorrhage or thrombosis, CD31 reacts strongly with platelets, macrophages, and lymphocytes. In diseased tissues such as thin-walled microvessels in atherosclerotic plaque and at sites of vasculitis, factor VIII antibodies can produce distinct diffuse extracellular staining patterns, due to leakiness of the endothelium (Fig. 8.22). In everyday practice these antibodies are indispensable for the identification of vascular tumors such as angiomas, hemangioendotheliomas, and angiosarcomas and can be helpful in confirming that tumor deposits are in vascular or lymphatic channels, rather than in artifactual tissue spaces (Fig. 8.23).

Antibodies that recognize proteins involved in the early steps in angiogenesis include anti-endoglin (CD105) and anti-VEGF (81). CD105 is an interesting epitope, since it expresses on activated endothelial cells, especially under conditions of hypoxia. Increased expression is noted on the microvessels of tumors such as glioma and breast carcinoma and also nonneoplastic situations such as the microvessels that develop in the hypoxic environment deep in long-standing atherosclerotic plaques. In carcinomas of the breast

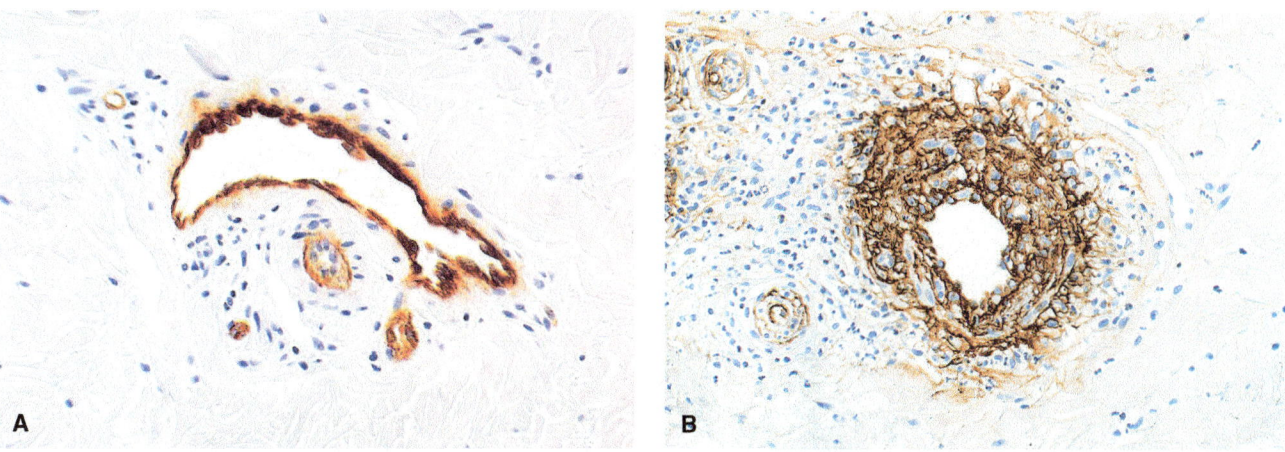

FIGURE 8.22 Staining patterns with factor VIII antibodies. **A:** Microvessel of the superior dermal vascular plexus showing sharp endothelial immunostaining. **B:** Microvessel of the superior dermal vascular plexus in case of cutaneous small vessel vasculitis. There is prominent perivascular staining due to leakage of factor VIII from damaged vessels.

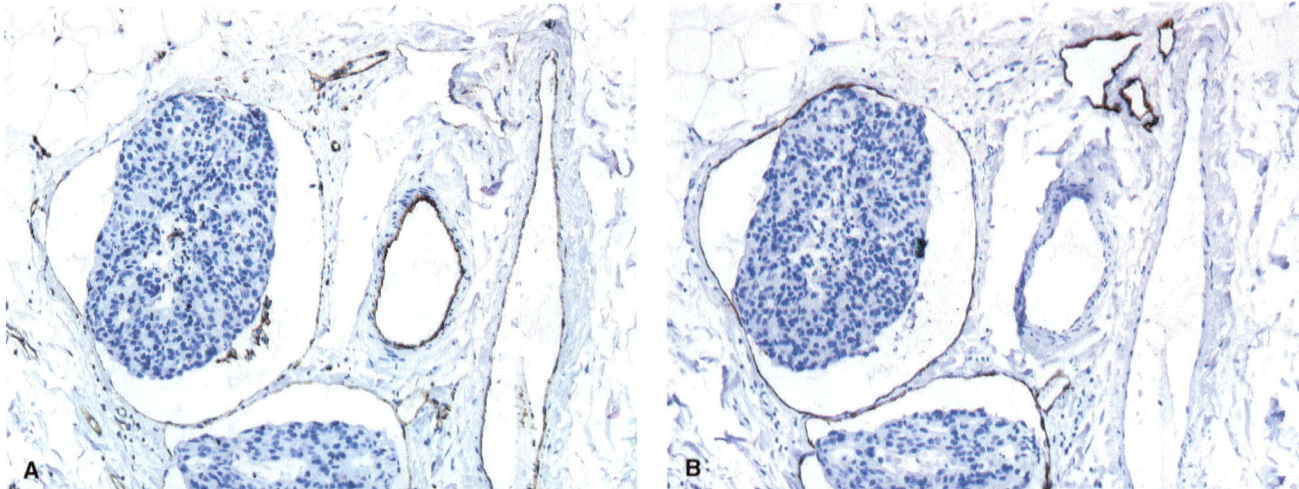

FIGURE 8.23 Ductal carcinoma of the breast with angioinvasion. CD31 immunostaining (A) highlights several empty vascular channels. Note that the spaces containing the tumor deposits do stain positively with CD31. However D2-40 immunostaining (B), which is specific for lymphatic endothelium, confirms that the tumor deposits are within lymphatics rather than tissue spaces.

a relationship between microvascular CD105 expression and invasive potential of the tumor has been observed, which appears to correlate with poor outcomes (82) (Fig. 8.24). In different sites in the vascular system, the endothelium may show marked heterogeneity in morphology, gene expression patterns, and related differences in functional status. Antibodies to glucose transporter protein 1 (GLUT-1 antibodies) react with the endothelium of cerebral capillaries, the placental vasculature, and one specific type of angioma—the juvenile capillary angioma (Fig. 8.25) (83). Another site-specific antibody is anti-HECA 452, which reacts specifically with the plump endothelial cells of high endothelial venules in lymphoid tissue and postcapillary venules in chronically inflamed tissue (Fig. 8.26) (84). In inflamed tissues and in atheromatous lesions, endothelial cells undergo profound functional alterations (endothelial activation) associated with upregulation of cell surface adhesion molecules such as ICAM-1, VCAM-1, and PECAM (CD31) or with de novo expression of leukocyte adhesion molecules such as E-selectin. D2-40, LYVE-1 and VEGFR3 stain lymphatic endothelium specifically (Fig. 8.26) (72), and D2-40 staining has confirmed the lymphatic origin of Kaposi sarcoma (Fig. 8.27) (85).

Smooth Muscle

Biochemical and immunohistologic studies have demonstrated that vascular smooth muscle has a distinctive component of contractile and intermediate filament proteins (86). In most smooth muscles, γ-smooth muscle actin and desmin predominate. In contrast, in vascular tissue there is abundant α-smooth muscle actin, and vimentin exceeds desmin. Antibodies directed against smooth muscle actin (SMA-1)

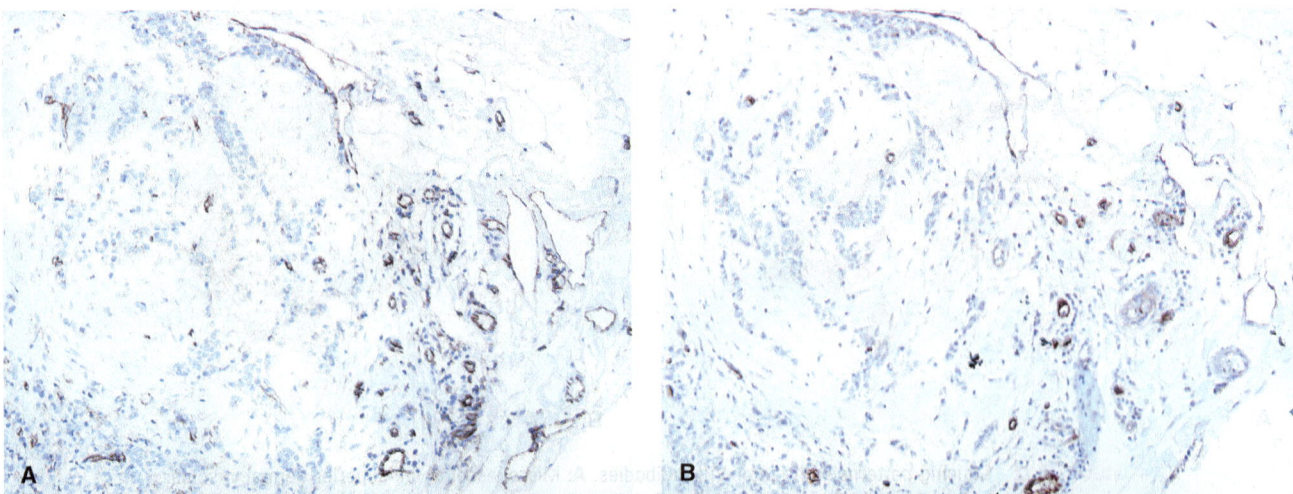

FIGURE 8.24 Microvasculature in breast carcinoma. CD31 staining (A) demonstrates a large number of microvessels. There is expression of endoglin (anti-CD105) (B) in only a subfraction of the microvessels.

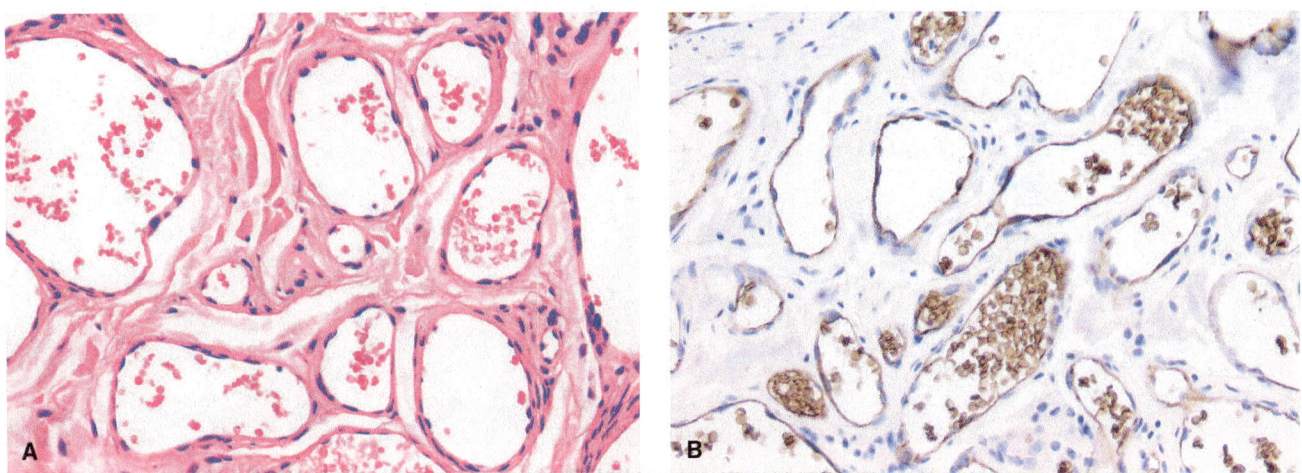

FIGURE 8.25 Site-specific staining of vascular endothelium. The vascular endothelium in this juvenile capillary hemangioma from a 3-year-old male (**A**) is specifically stained with the GLUT-1 antibody (**B**). This antibody also stains the endothelium of cerebral capillaries and the placenta. In contrast, the more commonly used endothelial antibodies such as factor VIII, CD31, and CD34 stain most types of normal and neoplastic endothelia.

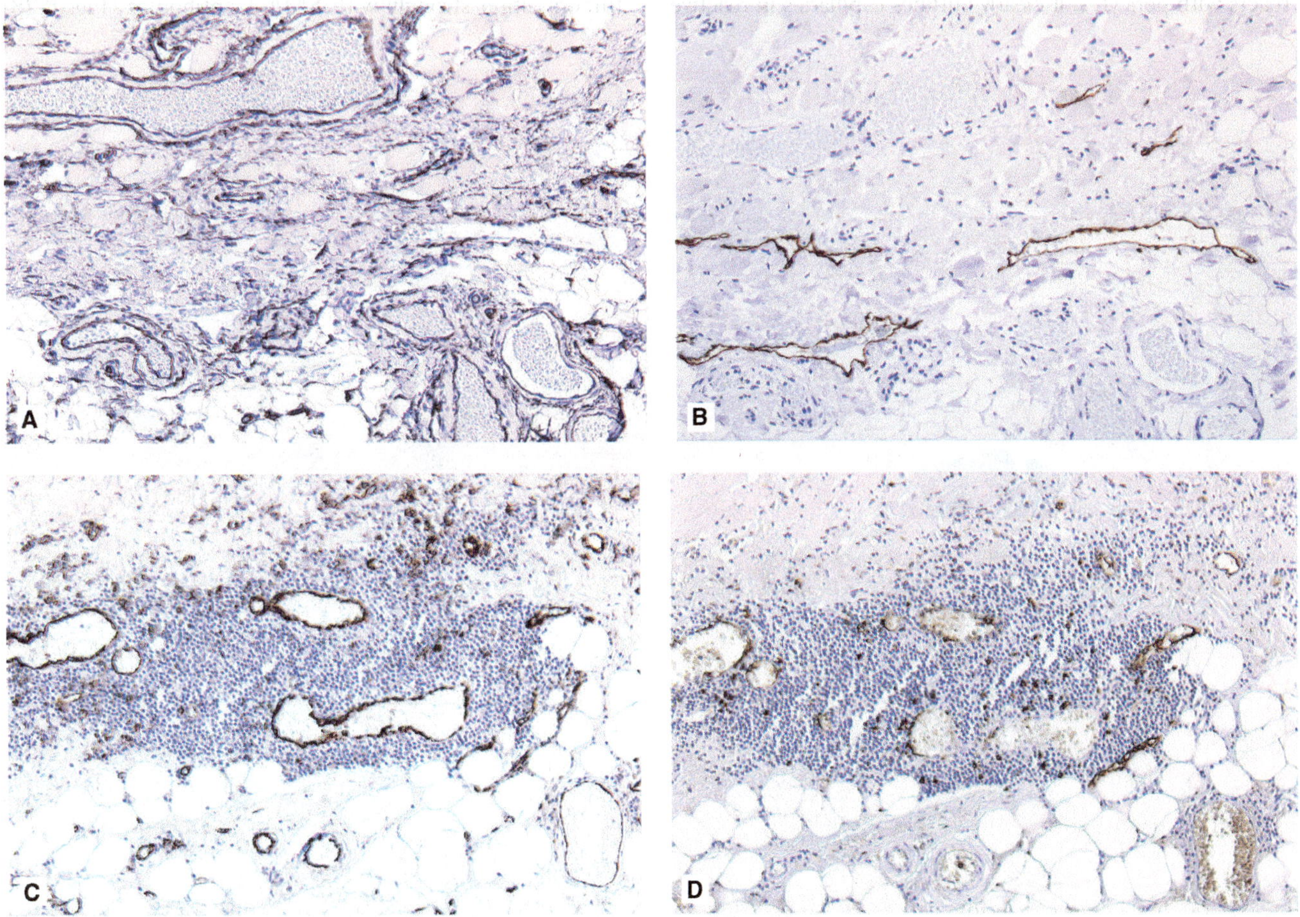

FIGURE 8.26 Immunohistochemical staining of vessels. **A** and **B** show a mixture of vessels from the subcutaneous tissues of a 68-year-old female from close to a leg ulcer: CD31 antibody staining identifies many vascular spaces (**A**), and a similar section is stained with the antibody D2-40, which recognizes lymphatic endothelium only (**B**). **C** and **D** are from a nodular inflammatory infiltrate in the aortic adventitia adjacent to a large atheromatous plaque: **C** has been stained with CD31, which recognizes most vessels, and **D** was stained with HECA-452, which recognizes high endothelial venules.

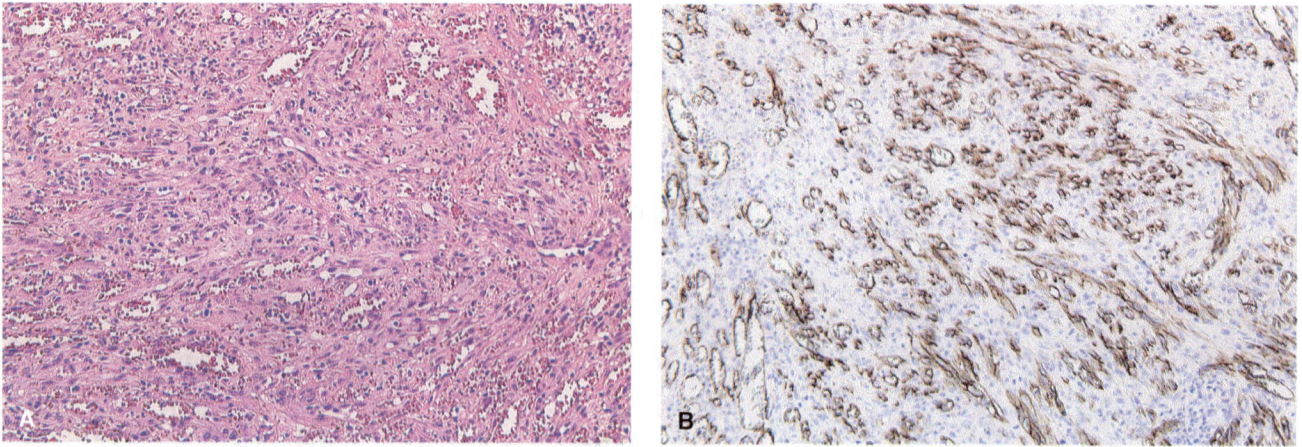

FIGURE 8.27 Kaposi sarcoma. **A** has been stained with H&E. **B** was immunostained with the D2-40 antibody, a specific marker of the lymphatic endothelium. Note the strong positive staining; LYVE-1 is another antibody that specifically stains lymphatic endothelium.

are excellent markers of medial muscle; SMA-1 recognizes the full spectrum of proliferating (or synthetic) and mature (or contractile) smooth muscle phenotypes. As SMA-1 reacts with pericytes, it clearly outlines capillaries in reactive microvascular proliferations and in pyogenic granulomas and juvenile angiomas during their growth phase. In general all benign vascular proliferations, including glomus tumors, stain strongly with SMA-1 antibodies (Fig. 8.28).

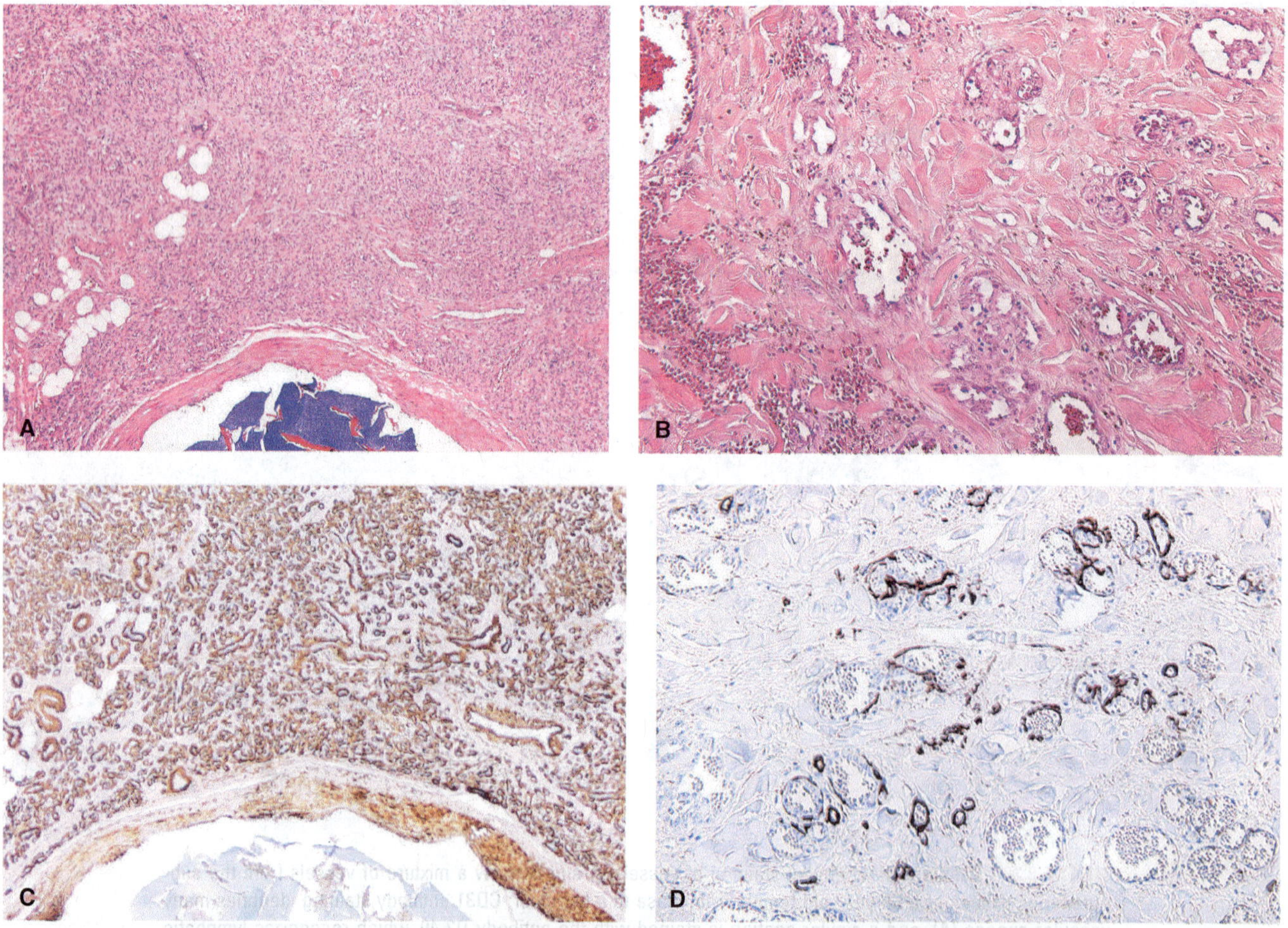

FIGURE 8.28 Patterns of staining with smooth muscle actin antibody. **A** and **C** are from a benign vascular proliferation. Note the intense staining of the walls of these small vessels. **B** and **D** are from an angiosarcoma. Only small amounts of actin are present in the walls of the malignant blood vessels (**D**).

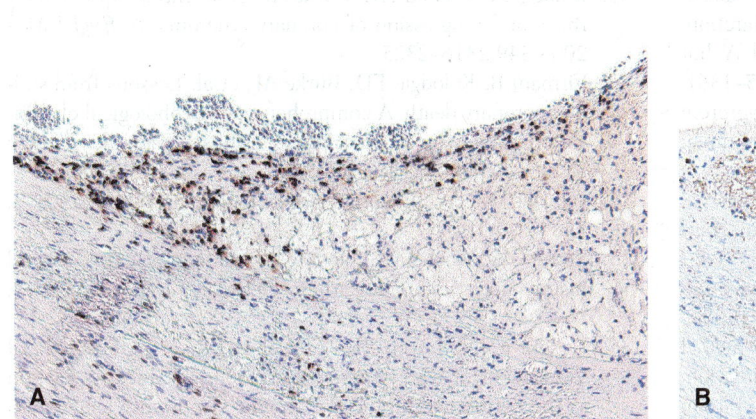
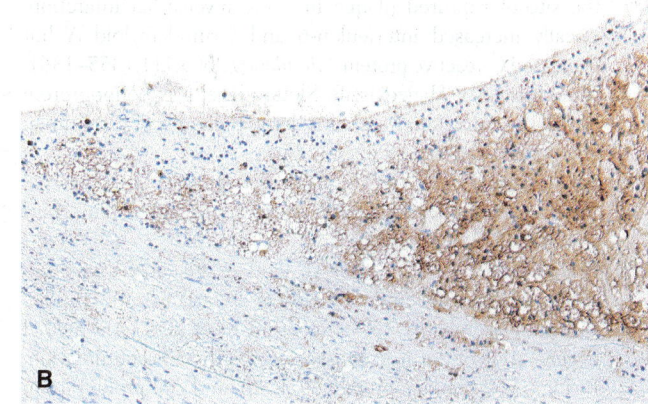

FIGURE 8.29 Immunohistochemical staining in atherosclerosis. **A:** CD3 positive lymphocytes are present at the edge of a lesion. **B:** Macrophages react for CD68.

In contrast, this staining is often incomplete or even absent in angiosarcoma, hemangiopericytoma, or Kaposi sarcoma. SMA-1 immunostaining can be helpful in the detection of early organization of thromboembolic material, especially in situations where age determination of the thrombus is required, for example investigations on sudden (coronary) cardiac death, pulmonary embolism, and in medicolegal autopsies.

Other Useful Antibodies for Diagnostic Vascular Pathology

Immunohistochemical studies of the inflammatory infiltrates in atheromatous lesions (Fig. 8.29) have contributed greatly to our understanding of the pathogenesis of atherosclerosis (87) but, as yet, have no value in everyday surgical pathology. T-lymphocyte markers, such as CD3 and CD4, may be of use in the diagnosis of vasculitis, especially temporal arteritis with minimal inflammatory activity (88). In transplant arteriosclerosis, there is a high relative proportion of CD8+ T lymphocytes, which also express granzyme B. In addition to anti-factor VIII antibodies, antifibrinogen antibodies are excellent for the demonstration of vascular leakiness and tissue damage (32,89); CD61 stains platelet aggregates in microvessels (e.g., in small vessel vasculitis (89)), angiolipomas, and coagulopathies (such as in the antiphospholipid syndrome). Glycophorin A is a specific marker of erythrocytes and their precursors in the bone marrow. The epitopes are preserved in tissues for long periods, and the antibody is valuable in the detection of old hemorrhage; for example, in completely organized pulmonary thromboemboli (90) and in atherosclerotic plaques (91).

Anti-amyloid antibodies (anti-amyloid A, anti-immunoglobulin antibodies) are used to differentiate the nature of amyloid depositions, which have a preferential distribution in vessel walls. Cerebral vascular amyloid deposits usually do not stain with these antibodies. In pathologic conditions, such as cerebral amyloid angiopathy or amyloid found occasionally in cerebral vascular malformations, the depositions show positive staining with anti-β-amyloid antibody.

REFERENCES

1. Ferrari AU, Radaelli A, Centola M. Invited review: Aging and the cardiovascular system. *J Appl Physiol (1985)* 2003;95: 2591–2597.
2. Plante GE. Impact of aging on the body's vascular system. *Metabolism* 2003;52(10 Suppl 2):31–35.
3. Lakatta EG, Levy D. Arterial and cardiac aging: Major shareholders in cardiovascular disease enterprises: Part I: Aging arteries: A 'set up' for vascular disease. *Circulation* 2003;107: 139–146.
4. Laurent S, Boutouyrie P, Lacolley P. Structural and genetic basis of arterial stiffness. *Hypertension* 2005;45: 1050–1055.
5. Kentish JC. Smooth muscle and the cardiovascular and lymphatic systems. In: Stranding S, ed. *Gray's Anatomy: The Anatomical Basis of Clinical Practice*. 40th ed. Philadelphia, PA: Churchill Livingstone Elsevier; 2008:127–144.
6. Jacob MP. Extracellular matrix remodeling and matrix metalloproteinases in the vascular wall during aging and in pathological conditions. *Biomed Pharmacother* 2003;57:195–202.
7. Kavurma MM, Bhindi R, Lowe HC, et al. Vessel wall apoptosis and atherosclerotic plaque instability. *J Thromb Haemostasis* 2005;3:465–472.
8. Boddaert J, Mallat Z, Fornes P, et al. Age and gender effects on apoptosis in the human coronary arterial wall. *Mech Ageing Dev* 2005;126:678–684.
9. Clarke MC, Littlewood TD, Figg N, et al. Chronic apoptosis of vascular smooth muscle cells accelerates atherosclerosis and promotes calcification and medial degeneration. *Circ Res* 2008;192:1529–1538.
10. Roijers RB, Debernardi N, Cleutjens JP, et al. Microcalcifications in early intimal lesions of atherosclerotic human coronary arteries. *Am J Pathol* 2011;178:2879–2887.
11. Jono S, Shioi A, Ikari Y, et al. Vascular calcification in chronic kidney disease. *J Bone Miner Metab* 2006;24:176–181.

12. Maier W, Altwegg LA, Corti R, et al. Inflammatory markers at the site of ruptured plaque in acute myocardial infarction: Locally increased interleukin-6 and serum amyloid A but decreased C-reactive protein. *Circulation* 2005;111:1355–1361.
13. Mucchiano GI, Haggqvist B, Sletten K, et al. Apolipoprotein A-1-derived amyloid in atherosclerotic plaques of the human aorta. *J Pathol* 2001;193:270–275.
14. Schlatmann TJ, Becker AE. Histologic changes in the normal aging aorta: implications for dissecting aortic aneurysm. *Am J Cardiol* 1977;39:13–20.
15. Hsue PY, Salinas CL, Bolger AF, et al. Acute aortic dissection related to crack cocaine. *Circulation* 2002;105:1592–1595.
16. Ihling C, Szombathy T, Nampoothiri K, et al. Cystic medial degeneration of the aorta is associated with p53 accumulation, Bax upregulation, apoptotic cell death, and cell proliferation. *Heart* 1999;82:286–293.
17. Gelb BD. Marfan's syndrome and related disorders—more tightly connected than we thought. *N Engl J Med* 2006;355:841–842.
18. Loeys BL, Schwarze U, Holm T, et al. Aneurysm syndromes caused by mutations in the TGF-β receptor. *N Engl J Med* 2006;355:788–798.
19. Judge DP, Dietz HC. Marfan's syndrome. *Lancet* 2005;366:1965–1976.
20. Jain D, Dietz HC, Oswald GL, et al. Causes and histopathology of ascending aortic disease in children and young adults. *Cardiovasc Pathol* 2011;20:15–25.
21. Hinterseher I, Tromp G, Kuivaniemi H. Genes and abdominal aortic aneurysm. *Ann Vasc Surg* 2011;25:388–412.
22. Kuivaniemi H, Shibamura H, Arthur C, et al. Familial aortic aneurysms: collection of 233 multiplex families. *J Vasc Surg* 2003;37:340–345.
23. Walker M, Gallagher PJ. The surgical pathology of large vessel disease. *Diagn Histopathol* 2010;16:10–16.
24. Ryder HF, Tafe LJ, Burns CM. Fatal aortic dissection due to fulminant variety of isolated aortitis. *J Clin Rheumatol* 2009;15:295–299.
25. Stone JR. Aortitis, periaortitis and retroperitoneal fibrosis, as manifestations of IgG4-related systemic disease. *Curr Opin Rheumatol* 2011;23:88–94.
26. Nirula A, Glaser SM, Kalled Sl, et al. What is IgG4? A review of the biology of a unique immunoglobulin subtype. *Curr Opin Rheumatol* 2011;23:119–124.
27. Szyszka-Mroz J, Wozniak W. A histological study of human ductus arteriosus during the last embryonic week. *Folia Morphol (Warsz)* 2003;62:365–367.
28. Anderson RH, Becker AE, Robertson WB. The arterial duct. In: Symmers WS, ed. *The Cardiovascular System Part A*. New York: Churchill Livingstone; 1993:1193, 197–202.
29. Stary HC, Blankenhorn DH, Chandler AB, et al. A definition of the intima of human arteries and of its atherosclerosis-prone regions. A report from the Committee on Vascular Lesions of the Council on Arteriosclerosis, American Heart Association. *Circulation* 1992;85:391–405.
30. Kim C, Redberg RF, Pavlic T, et al. A systematic review of gender differences in mortality after coronary artery bypass graft surgery and percutaneous interventions. *Clin Cardiol* 2007;30:491–495.
31. Antoniadis AP, Chatzizisis YS, Giannoglou GD. Pathogenetic mechanisms of coronary ectasia. *Int J Cardiol* 2008;130:335–343.
32. Kolodgie FD, Gold HK, Burke AP, et al. Intraplaque hemorrhage and progression of coronary atheroma. *N Engl J Med* 2003;349:2316–2325.
33. Virmani R, Kolodgie FD, Burke AP, et al. Lessons from sudden coronary death: A comprehensive morphological classification scheme for atherosclerotic lesions. *Arterioscler Thromb Vasc Biol* 2000;20:1262–1275.
34. van der Wal AC. Coronary artery pathology. *Heart* 2007;93:1484–1489.
35. Stone GW, Maehara A, Lansky AJ, et al. A prospective natural history study of coronary atherosclerosis. *N Engl J Med* 2011;364:226–235.
36. Redgrave JN, Lovett JK, Gallagher PJ, et al. Histological assessment of 526 symptomatic carotid plaques in relation to the nature and timing of ischemic symptoms: The Oxford plaque study. *Circulation* 2006;113:2320–2328.
37. Camici PG, Crea F. Coronary microvascular dysfunction. *N Engl J Med* 2007;356:830–840.
38. Hammes HP. Pericytes and the pathogenesis of diabetic retinopathy. *Horm Metab Res* 2005;37(Suppl 1):39–43.
39. Ashgar O, Al-Sunni A, Khavandi K, et al. Diabetic cardiomyopathy. *Clin Sci(Lond)* 2009;116:741–760.
40. Richards OC, Raines SM, Attie AD. The role of blood vessels, endothelial cells and vascular pericytes in insulin secretion and peripheral insulin action. *Endocrine Rev* 2010;31:343–363.
41. Hayasaka H, Taniguchi K, Fukai S, et al. Neogenesis and development of the high endothelial venules that mediate lymphocyte trafficking. *Cancer Sci* 2010;101:2302–2308.
42. Owens CD. Adaptive changes in autologous vein grafts for arterial reconstruction: Clinical implications. *J Vasc Surg* 2010;51:736–746.
43. Langes K, Hort W. Intimal fibrosis (phlebosclerosis) in the saphenous vein of the lower limb: A quantitative analysis. *Virchows Arch A Pathol Anat Histopathol* 1992;421:127–131.
44. Mooi WJ, Grünberg K. Histopathology of pulmonary hypertensive diseases. *Curr Diagn Pathol* 2006;12:429–440.
45. Patchefsky AS. Nonneoplastic pulmonary disease. In: Mills SE, ed. *Sternberg's Diagnostic Surgical Pathology*. 5th ed. Vol 1. Philadelphia, PA: Lippincott Williams & Wilkins; 2009:1035–1039.
46. Warnock ML, Kunzmann A. Changes with age in muscular pulmonary arteries. *Arch Pathol Lab Med* 1977;101:175–179.
47. Steiner I, Hajkova P, Kvasnicka J, et al. Myocardial sleeves of pulmonary vein and atrial fibrillation: A postmortem histopathological study on 100 subjects. *Virchows Arch* 2006;449:88–95.
48. Gombos Z, Zhang PJ. Glomus tumor. *Arch Pathol Lab Med* 2008;132:1448–1452.
49. Warkentin TE, Moore JC, Anand SS, et al. Gastrointestinal bleeding, angiodysplasia, cardiovascular disease, and acquired von Willebrand syndrome. *Transfus Med Rev* 2003;17:272–286.
50. Baxter M, Aly EH. Dieulafoy's lesion: Current trends in diagnosis and management. *Ann R Coll Surg Engl* 2010;92:548–554.
51. Boon LM, Ballieux F, Vikkula M. Pathogenesis of vascular anomalies. *Clin Plastic Surg* 2011;38:7–19.
52. Pardali E, Goumans MJ, ten Dijke P. Signaling by members of the TGF-beta family in vascular morphogenesis and disease. *Trends Cell Biol* 2010;20:556–567.
53. Mulliken JB, Glowacki J. Hemangiomas and vascular malformations in infants and children: A classification based on endothelial characteristics. *Plast Reconstr Surg* 1982;69:412–422.

54. Cahill AM, Nijs EL. Pediatric vascular malformations: Pathophysiology, diagnosis, and the role of interventional radiology. *Cardiovasc Intervent Radiol* 2011;34:691–704.
55. Dompmartin A, Vikkula M, Boon LM. Venous malformation: Update on aetiopathogenesis, diagnosis and management. *Phlebology* 2010;25:224–235.
56. Calonje E. Haemangiomas. In: Fletcher CDM, Unni KK, Mertens F, eds. *World Health Organisation Classification of Tumours: Pathology and Genetics of Tumours of Soft Tissue and Bone*. Lyon, France: IARC Press; 2002:156–158.
57. Rerkasam K, Rothwell PM. Systematic review of the operative risks of carotid endarterectomy for recently symptomatic stenosis in relation to the timing of surgery. *Stroke* 2009;40: e564–e572.
58. Riles TS, Rockman CB. Cerebrovascular disease. In: Townsend CM, Beauchamp RD, Evers BM, et al eds. *Sabiston Textbook of Surgery*. 18th ed. Philadelphia, PA: WB Saunders; 2008:1895–1899.
59. Garratt KN, Edwards WD, Kaufmann UP, et al. Differential histopathology of primary atherosclerotic and restenotic lesions in coronary arteries and saphenous vein bypass grafts: Analysis of tissue obtained from 73 patients by directional atherectomy. *J Am Coll Cardiol* 1991;17:442–448.
60. Kalan JM, Roberts WC. Morphologic findings in saphenous veins used as coronary arterial bypass conduits for longer than 1 year: Necropsy analysis of 53 patients, 123 saphenous veins, and 1865 five-millimetre segments of veins. *Am Heart J* 1990;119:1164–1184.
61. Jeremy JY, Gadsdon P, Shukla N, et al. On the biology of saphenous vein grafts fitted with external synthetic sheaths and stents. *Biomaterials* 2007;28:895–908.
62. Parang P, Arora R. Coronary vein graft disease: Pathogenesis and prevention. *Can J Cardiol* 2009;25:e57–e62.
63. Ali E, Saso S, Ahmed K, et al. When harvested for coronary artery bypass surgery, does a skeletonised or pedicled radial artery improve conduit patency? *Interact Cardiovasc Thorac Surg* 2010;10:289–292.
64. D'Souza SP, Mamas MA, Fraser DG, et al. Routine early coronary angioplasty versus ischaemia-guided angioplasty after thrombolysis in acute ST elevation myocardial infarction: A meta analysis. *Eur Heart J* 2011;32:972–982.
65. Popma JJ, Bhatt DL. Percutaneous coronary and valvular intervention. In: Bonow R, Mann DL, Zipes DP, et al., eds. *Braunwald's Heart Disease*. 9th ed. Philadelphia, PA: Elsevier Saunders; 2011:1270–1300.
66. Garcia-Garcia HM, Gonzalo N, Regar E, et al. Virtual histology and optical coherence tomography: From research to a broad clinical application. *Heart* 2009;95:1362–1374.
67. Bradshaw SH, Kennedy L, Dexter DF, et al. A practical method to rapidly dissolve metallic stents. *Cardiovasc Pathol* 2009;18:127–133.
68. Kapadia MR, Popowich DA, Kibbe MR. Modified prosthetic vascular conduits. *Circulation* 2008;117:1873–1882.
69. Reitsma S, Slaaf DW, Vink H, et al. The endothelial glycocalyx: Composition, functions, and visualization. *Pflugers Arch* 2007;454:345–359.
70. Bazzoni G, Dejana E. Endothelial cell-to-cell junctions: Molecular organization and role in vascular homeostasis. *Physiol Rev* 2004;84:869–901.
71. Van Itallie CM, Anderson JM. The molecular physiology of tight junction pores. *Physiology (Bethesda)* 2004;19:331–338.
72. Hsueh WA, Quinones MJ. Role of endothelial dysfunction in insulin resistance. *Am J Cardiol* 2003;92:10J–17J.
73. Kirschner N, Bohner C, Rachow S, et al. Tight junctions: Is there a role in dermatology. *Arch Dermatol Res* 2010;302:483–493.
74. Baum B, Georgiou M. Dynamics of adherens junctions in epithelial establishment, maintenance and remodeling. *J Cell Biol* 2011;192:907–917.
75. Maeda S, Tsukihara T. Structure of the gap junction channel and its implications for its biological functions. *Cell Mol Life Sci* 2011;68:1115–1129.
76. Hesketh GG, Van Eyk JE, Tomaselli GF. Mechanisms of gap junction traffic in health and disease. *J Cardiovasc Pharm* 2009;54:263–272.
77. Chidlow JH, Sessa WC. Caveolae, caveolins and cavins: Complex control of cellular signaling and inflammation. *Cardiovasc Res* 2010;86:219–225.
78. Valentijn KM, Sadler JE, Valentijn JA, et al. Functional architecture of Weibel–Palade bodies. *Blood* 2011;117:5033–5043.
79. Aird WC. Phenotypic heterogeneity of the endothelium. II. Representative vascular beds. *Circ Res* 2007;100:174–190.
80. Giepmans BN. Gap junctions and connexin-interacting proteins. *Cardiovasc Res* 2004;62:233–245.
81. Dales JP, Garcia S, Carpentier S, et al. Prediction of metastasis risk (11 year follow-up) using VEGF-R1, VEGF-R2, Tie-2/Tek and CD105 expression in breast cancer (n = 905). *Br J Cancer* 2004;90:1216–1221.
82. Kumar S, Ghellal A, Li C, et al. Breast carcinoma: Vascular density determined using CD105 antibody correlates with tumor prognosis. *Cancer Res* 1999;59:856–861.
83. North PE, Waner M, Mizeracki A, et al. GLUT1: A newly discovered immunohistochemical marker for juvenile hemangiomas. *Hum Pathol* 2000;31:11–22.
84. Jackson DG. Biology of the lymphatic marker LYVE-1 and applications in research into lymphatic trafficking and lymphangiogenesis. *APMIS* 2004;112:526–538.
85. Kahn HJ, Bailey D, Marks A. Monoclonal antibody D2-40, a new marker of lymphatic endothelium, reacts with Kaposi's sarcoma and a subset of angiosarcomas. *Mod Pathol* 2002;15: 434–440.
86. Desmouliere A, Chaponnier C, Gabbiani G. Tissue repair, contraction, and the myofibroblast. *Wound Repair Regen* 2005; 13:7–12.
87. Hansson GK. Inflammation, atherosclerosis and coronary artery disease. *N Engl J Med* 2005;352:1685–1695.
88. Weyand CM, Goronzy JJ. Medium- and large-vessel vasculitis. *N Engl J Med* 2003;349:160–169.
89. Meijer-Jorna LB, Mekkes JR, van der Wal AC. Platelet involvement in cutaneous small vessel vasculitis. *J Cutan Pathol* 2002;29:176–180.
90. Arbustini E, Morbini P, D'Armini AM, et al. Plaque composition in plexogenic and thromboembolic pulmonary hypertension: The critical role of thrombotic material in pultaceous core formation. *Heart* 2002;88:177–182.
91. Virmani R, Kolodgie FD, Burke AP, et al. Atherosclerotic plaque progression and vulnerability to rupture. Angiogenesis as a source of intraplaque hemorrhage. *Arterioscler Thromb Vasc Biol* 2005;25:2054–2061.

SECTION IV

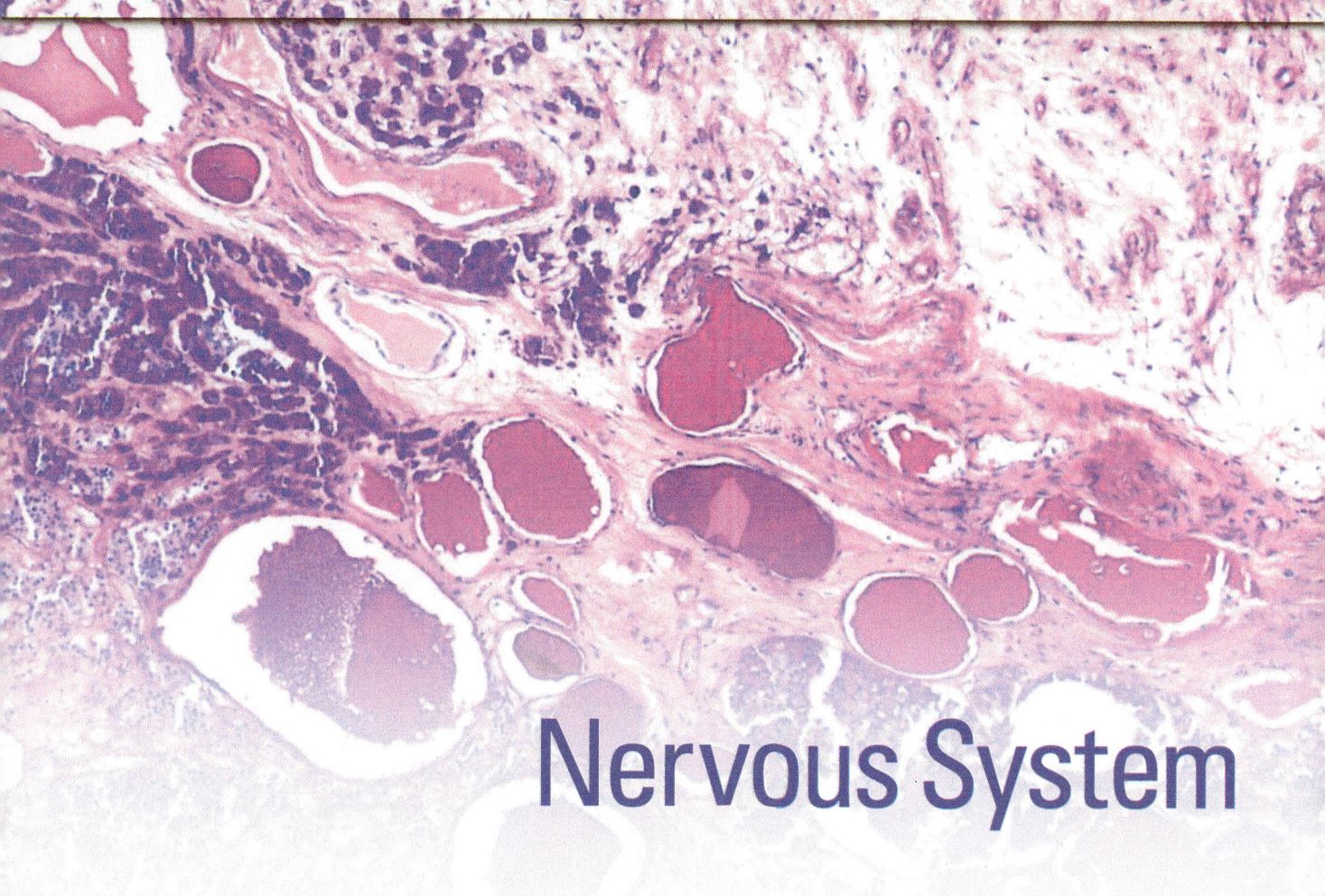

Nervous System

Central Nervous System

Gregory N. Fuller ■ Leomar Y. Ballester

INTRODUCTION 219	Olfactory Bulbs and Tracts 252
REGIONAL NEUROANATOMY 219	Choroid Plexus 253
Organization of the Spinal Cord and Brain Stem 220	Circumventricular Organs 254
CELLULAR CONSTITUENTS OF THE CENTRAL NERVOUS SYSTEM 228	INTRADURAL ELEMENTS OF THE PERIPHERAL NERVOUS SYSTEM 256
Gray Matter and White Matter 228	MENINGES 257
Neurons 230	Dura Mater (Pachymenix) 257
Astrocytes 239	Pia-arachnoid (Leptomeninges) 259
Oligodendroglia 243	Leptomeningeal Melanocytes 261
Ependyma 245	Optic Nerve 262
Microglia and the Monocyte—Macrophage System 246	FETAL BRAIN 263
Response to Injury 248	ARTIFACTS 264
SPECIALIZED ORGANS OF THE CENTRAL NERVOUS SYSTEM 249	SUGGESTED READINGS 269
Pineal Gland 249	
Median Eminence and Infundibulum 249	

INTRODUCTION

The central nervous system (CNS) is unparalleled among natural systems in terms of structural and functional complexity. As a consequence of its intricate regional architecture, heterogeneous cellular constituents, and an associated extensive and somewhat arcane lexicon, the nervous system is often viewed as a formidably Byzantine realm by many non-neuropathologists; and yet, a working familiarity with the normal morphology of this complex organ must precede competent evaluation of the many disease states that afflict it. To this end, this chapter will present the salient features of regional neuroanatomy followed by a description of the essentials of microscopic anatomy of the CNS, with special emphasis on those aspects that constitute potential diagnostic pitfalls, including normal anatomic variations, alterations associated with advancing age, reactive changes, and common artifacts. Although the focus of the book is on histology, we have included gross images of the brain to highlight key points of surface and gross anatomy that provide context to the microscopic descriptions.

REGIONAL NEUROANATOMY

We have limited this discussion of regional neuroanatomy to those principles of structural organization that are of practical value to the diagnostician, emphasizing the rudiments of neuroembryology by which the basic organization of the nervous system is best understood. Further details about topographical neuroanatomy can be found in the list of suggested readings provided at the end of the chapter.

This chapter is an update of a previous version authored by Peter C. Burger.

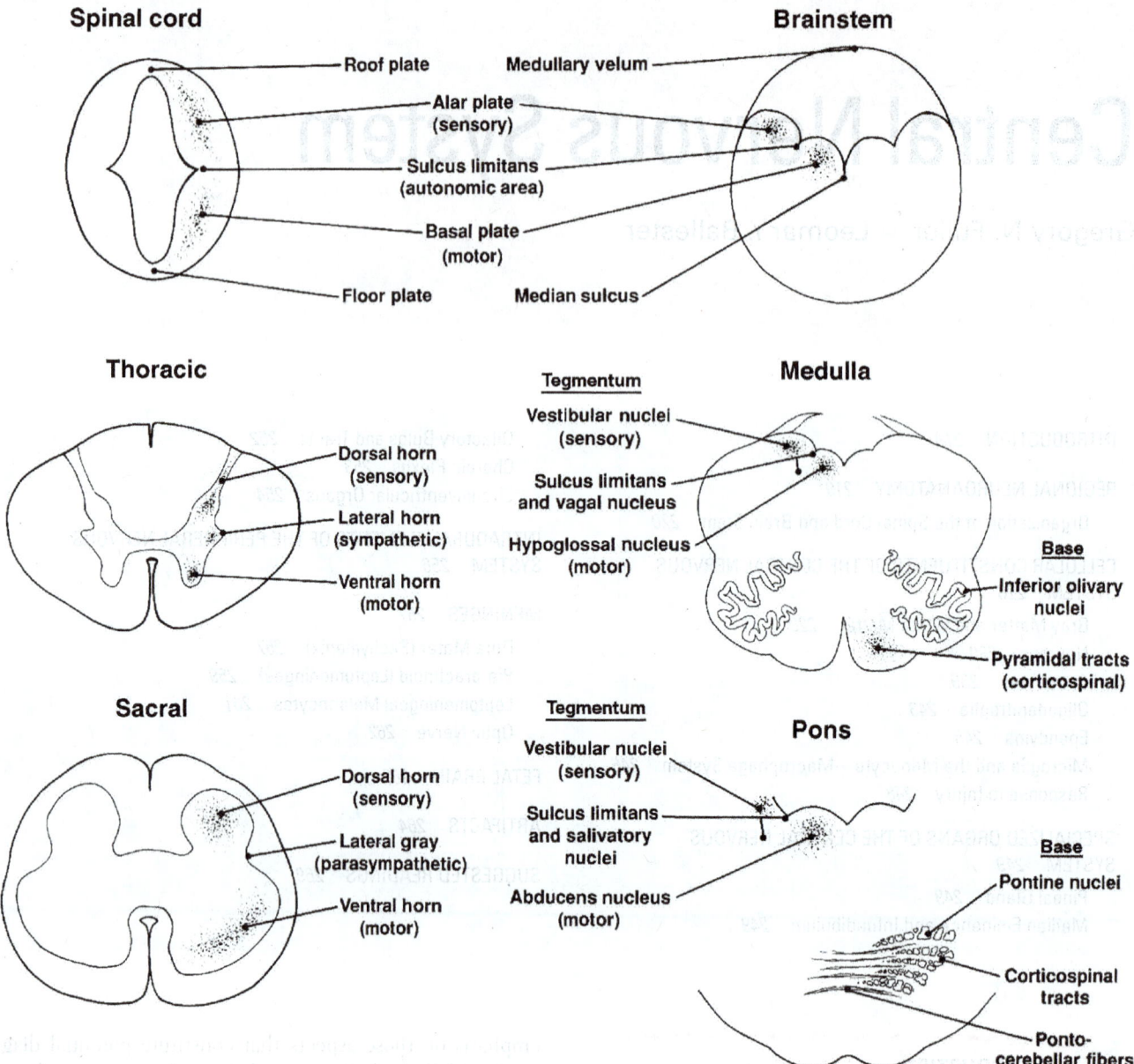

FIGURE 9.1 Structural organization of the spinal cord and brain stem. (See text for discussion.)

Organization of the Spinal Cord and Brain Stem

Embryologically, the nascent CNS begins as a hollow tube formed by the invagination of the neural plate ectoderm. This primitive cylinder is subdivided functionally into a dorsal sensory ("alar") plate and a ventral motor ("basal") plate. The two are separated by a lateral groove, termed the "sulcus limitans," along which develops the efferent autonomic system (Fig. 9.1). This primitive organizational pattern is retained, essentially unaltered, in the mature spinal cord. The central gray matter consists of: (a) dorsal horns that receive sensory input from the dorsal roots, (b) ventral horns that contain motor neurons whose axons are conducted to the somatic periphery by the ventral roots, and (c) the lateral autonomic gray matter. Spinal autonomic neurons are confined to thoracic (sympathetic) and sacral (parasympathetic) levels, forming the intermediolateral cell columns. The axons of these "preganglionic" neurons exit the spinal cord through the ventral roots, ultimately to synapse on "postganglionic" neurons in the peripheral autonomic ganglia. The sympathetic intermediolateral cell column produces a third horn of gray matter in the thoracic cord, termed "the lateral horn" (Figs. 9.1 and 9.2). The parasympathetic intermediolateral cell column occupies a similar lateral position in the sacral cord (at the S-2, S-3, and S-4 levels), but does not form a distinct horn.

Spinal Cord

The anatomy of the spinal cord varies according to the level (Fig. 9.2). Two enlargements of the ventral horns, one in the cervical region (Fig. 9.2A) and another in the lumbosacral

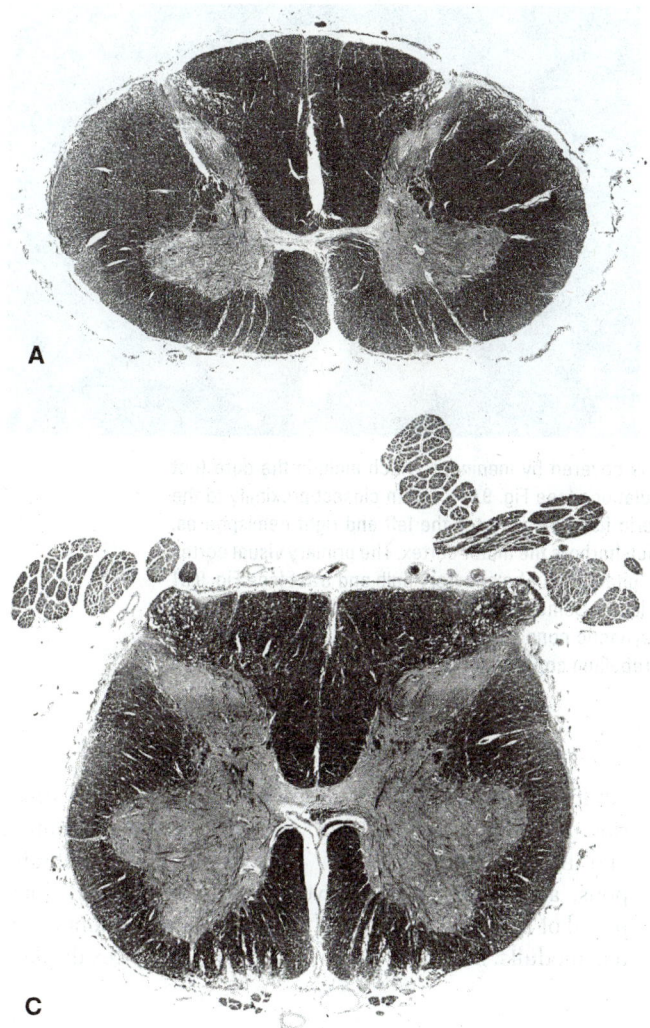
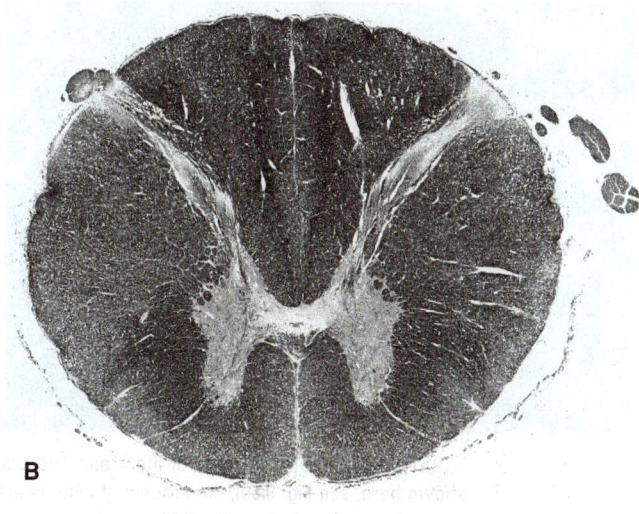

FIGURE 9.2 Spinal cord: Regional variation of spinal cord morphology is illustrated in these cross sections taken from the cervical enlargement (**A**), midthoracic cord (**B**), and lumbosacral enlargement (**C**). The cervical enlargement (**A**) is typified by an oval shape with large white matter funiculi and prominent, broad anterior gray horns which contain the motor neurons that innervate the upper extremities. In contrast, sections from thoracic cord (**B**) have a more rounded profile and exhibit small, slender, peg-like anterior gray horns. In addition, lateral horns, which house the intermediolateral cell column neurons of the sympathetic nervous system, are unique to thoracic segments (see also Fig. 9.1). The lumbosacral cord (**C**) has very large anterior gray horns (motor supply to the lower extremities) like those of the cervical enlargement, but only a very small surrounding mantle of white matter (see also Fig. 9.1).

region (Fig. 9.2C), provide motor innervation for the upper and lower extremities, respectively. In contrast, the ventral horns of the thoracic cord provide innervation for the more limited axial musculature of the trunk and are, accordingly, much smaller (Fig. 9.2B). As mentioned earlier, the lateral horns of the gray matter (sympathetic neurons) are a unique feature of the thoracic cord. The thickness of the surrounding white matter fiber bundles (termed "funiculi") also varies with the cord level, being greatest in the cervical cord, where the thickness reflects the summated accrual of ascending fiber tracts that have successively entered at lower levels, as well as the maximum content of descending tracts that are en route to lower levels, and thinnest in the lumbosacral cord. The terminus of the spinal cord, the filum terminale, is composed primarily of meningeal connective tissue in the human and is discussed separately with the pia-arachnoid (see Fig. 9.64).

Brain Stem

The brain stem (Fig. 9.3) is innately more complex than the spinal cord, but its basic organization is readily understood when viewed as a slightly modified version of the basic plan. Thus, the stem is also a neural tube, but one that has been stretched dorsally and splayed out laterally so that the ventrally located embryonic motor plate is now medial and the dorsal sensory plate is lateral (Fig. 9.1). Therefore, within the brain stem, the cranial nerve motor nuclei are located medially, the sensory nuclei laterally, and the autonomic nuclei are intermediate in position.

The brain stem can be further subcategorized in cross section into tectum, tegmentum, and base (Figs. 9.4 to 9.6). The tectum is the roof of the ventricular system, as exemplified by the superior and inferior colliculi (corpora quadrigemina) of the midbrain and the superior medullary vela of the pons and the medulla. The tegmentum forms the floor of the cerebral aqueduct and fourth ventricle, and is divisible into the medial motor and lateral sensory areas discussed previously (Fig. 9.1). The "base" is located subjacent to the tegmentum and is the most ventral portion of the stem. It is composed principally of the so-called "long tracts," that is, the descending motor pathways and ascending sensory pathways that link the spinal cord with higher neural centers. The combination of long tract signs with dysfunction

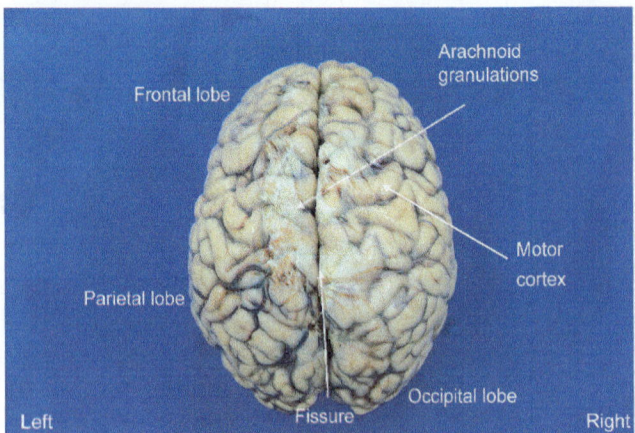
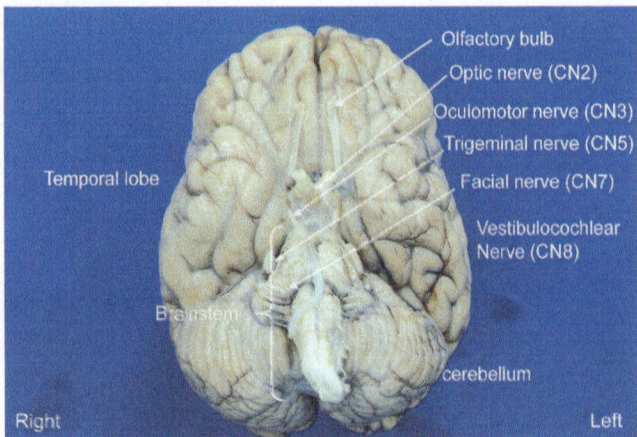

FIGURE 9.3 Surface anatomy of the brain: The brain is covered by meninges which include the dura (not shown here, see Fig. 9.60), the arachnoid with its granulations (see Fig. 9.61), and in closest proximity to the parenchyma, the pia (see Fig. 9.61). The interhemispheric fissure separates the left and right hemispheres. Anterior to the central sulcus is the prefrontal gyrus which harbors the motor cortex. The primary visual cortex (see Fig. 9.12) is located in the medial aspect of the occipital lobes. The olfactory bulb and tract (see Fig. 9.51 and 9.52) course along the inferior aspect of the frontal lobes. Some fibers from the left and right optic nerves (see Fig. 9.65) decussate in the chiasm before making synaptic connections with the lipofuscin-rich neurons of the lateral geniculate nucleus (see Fig. 9.10). The cerebellum consists of multiple folia (see Fig. 9.7), which leads to its undulated surface appearance.

of specific cranial nerves allows for the precise anatomic localization of brain stem lesions by clinical examination.

Cerebellum
Embryologically, the cerebellum arises as a dorsal outgrowth of the fetal brain stem and remains connected to it in the adult by the three pairs of cerebellar peduncles: The superior (brachium conjunctivum), middle (brachium pontis), and inferior (restiform body). They join with the midbrain, pons, and medulla, respectively. The cerebellum is composed of three structural and functional compartments: cortex, medulla, and deep nuclei (Fig. 9.7). The cortex displays

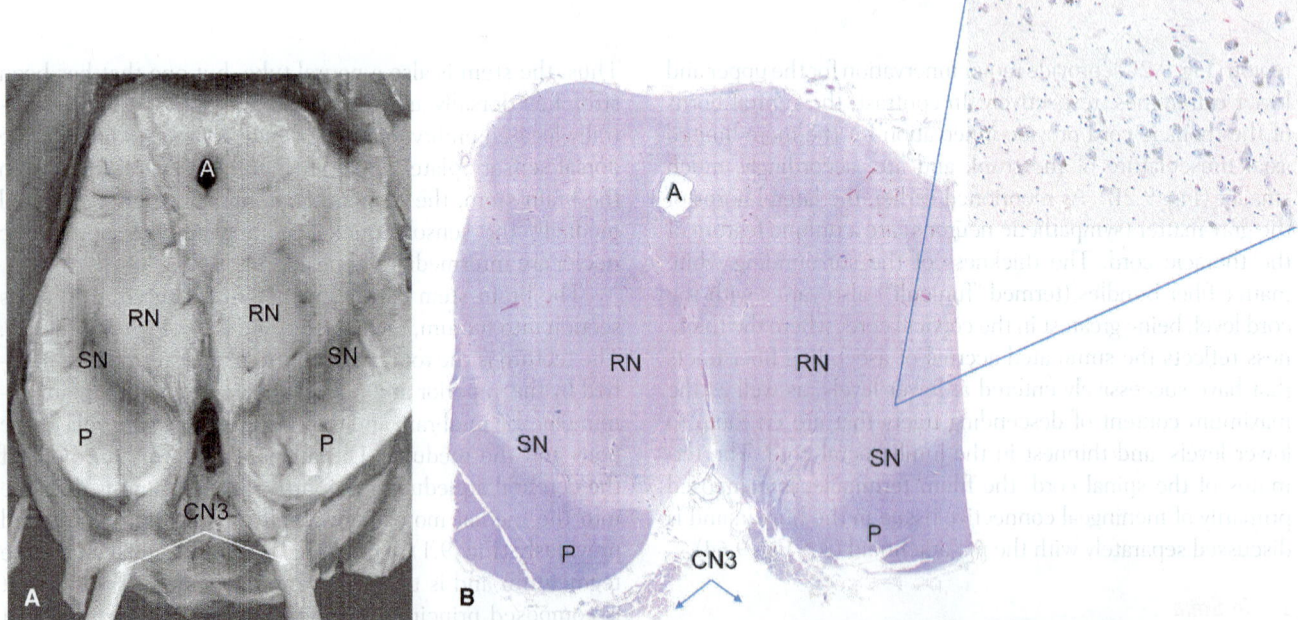

FIGURE 9.4 Midbrain: In cross section of the midbrain (**A**), the aqueduct (*A*), red nucleus (*RN*), substantia nigra (*SN*) and peduncles (*P*) are easily identified. The substantia nigra contains pigmented catecholaminergic neurons (**B**) (see Fig. 9.23).

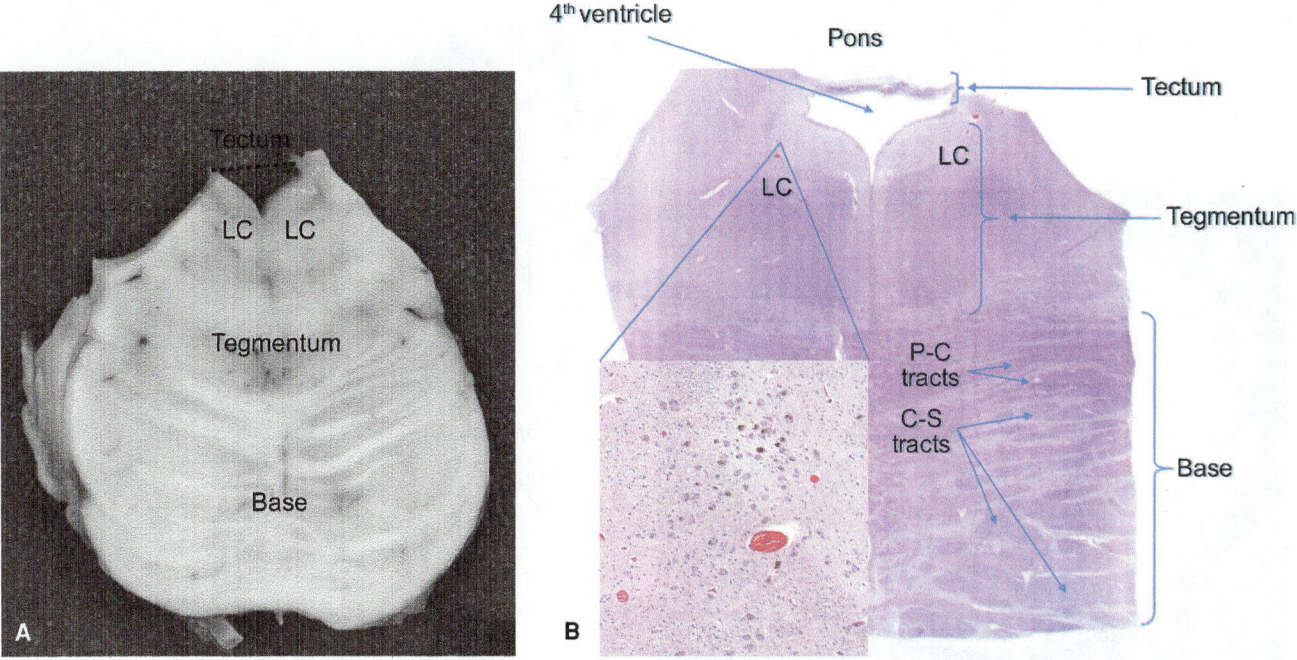

FIGURE 9.5 Pons: In cross section of the pons (**A**), the aqueduct has given rise to the fourth ventricle with its roof (tectum) and floor (tegmentum). (**B**) Two nuclei (locus ceruleus, *LC*) with pigmented catecholaminergic neurons (see Fig. 9.23) are evident on cross section of the pons. The base of the pons is formed by ponto-cerebellar tracts (*P-C*) and cortico-spinal tracts (*C-S*).

three distinct laminae: An outer hypocellular molecular layer, an intermediate single-cell thick Purkinje cell layer (described below), and a deep hypercellular granular cell layer (Fig. 9.8). Before 1 year of age, the cerebellar cortex is conspicuous for remnants of a fourth layer of small neurons, the fetal external granular cell layer, which is located immediately subjacent to pia (Fig. 9.8). The external granular cells are gradually depleted during the first year of life as they

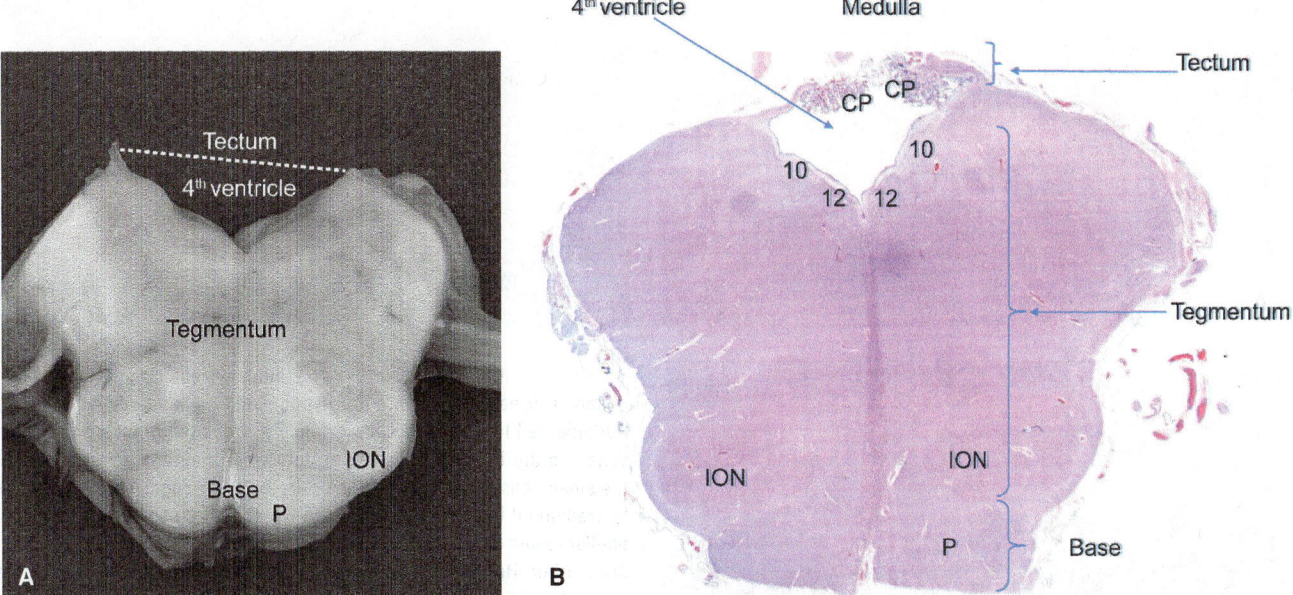

FIGURE 9.6 Medulla: In cross section of the medulla, the fourth ventricle continues, with its roof (tectum) and floor (tegmentum). Tufts of choroid plexus (see Fig. 9.53 and 9.54) can be appreciated here. The nuclei for two cranial nerves (Vagus #10 and Hypoglossal #12) can be identified microscopically in the periventricular region. Although not pigmented on gross examination, the dorsal nucleus of the vagus nerve contains pigmented neurons that can be appreciated microscopically. The convoluted inferior olivary nucleus (*ION*) is located above the peduncles (*P*).

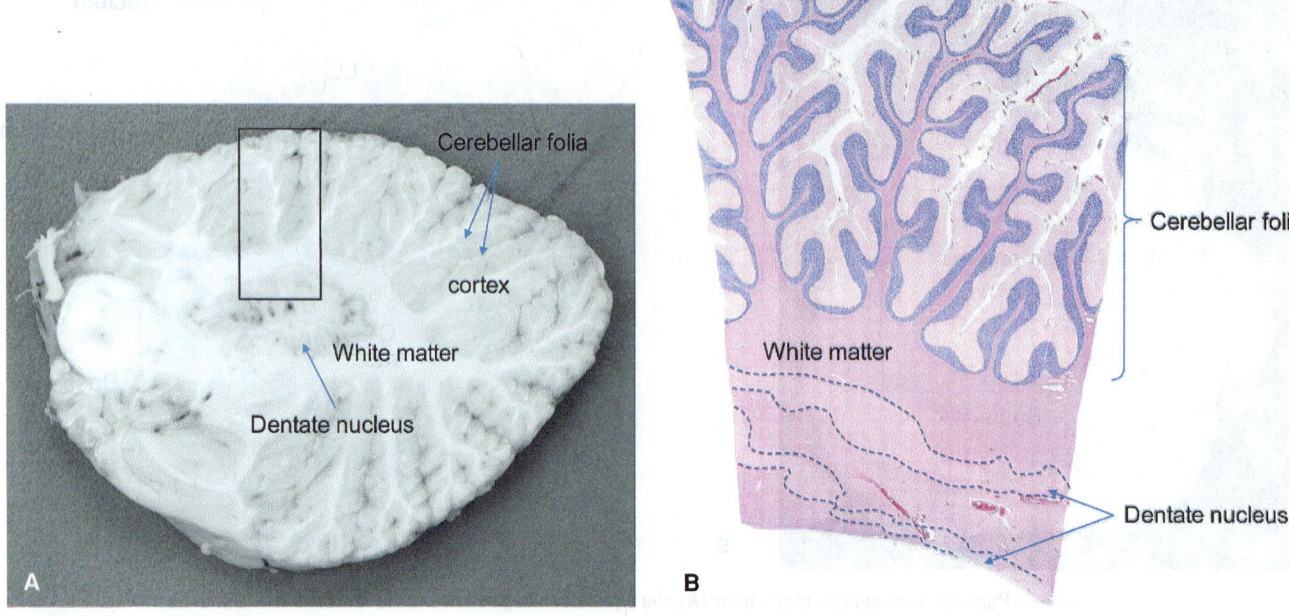

FIGURE 9.7 Cerebellum: In cross section of the cerebellum, the dentate nucleus is easily identified with the naked eye (**A**). The complex architecture of the cerebellar folia is apparent in this low magnification view of a hematoxylin and eosin-stained slide (**B**). The cell bodies of the neurons that form the dentate nucleus have a convoluted arrangement that mimics that of the ION (see Fig. 9.6).

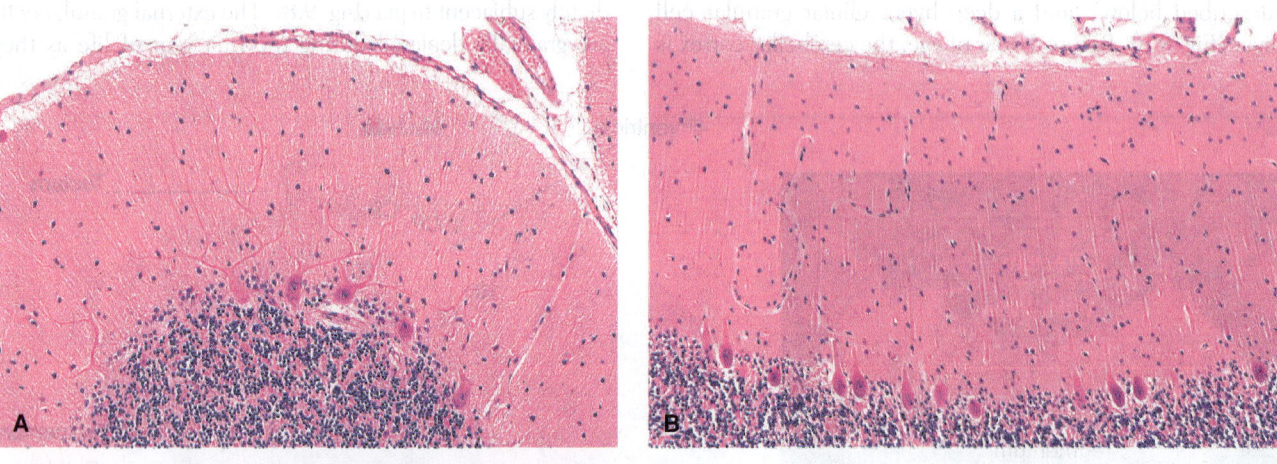

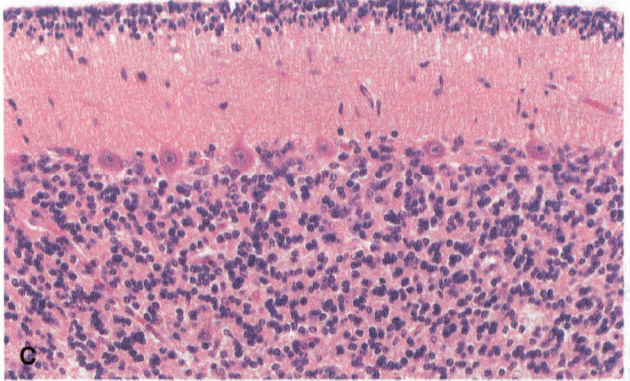

FIGURE 9.8 Cerebellar cortex: The adult cerebellar cortex is composed of three layers—an outer hypocellular molecular layer, a middle Purkinje cell layer, and an inner densely populated granular cell layer. Whereas the Purkinje cells are prototypically neuronal in appearance, the small cells of the granular layer are hardly recognizable as neurons by traditional histologic criteria (see Fig. 9.7). A cross section of a cerebellar folium (**A**) shows the typical broadly branching Purkinje cell dendritic arbor. However, sections taken parallel to the folia (**B**) reveal the streamlined "on edge" appearance of the arbor, which should not be interpreted as pathologic pruning. The fetal cerebellum (**C**) has an additional cortical lamina, the external granular layer, applied to the surface of the cortex. This pool of cells populates the internal granular cell layer during development and is, thereby, depleted by the end of the first year of postnatal life.

descend the processes of Bergmann glia to reach their final position in the internal granular cell layer. Embedded within the white matter of the cerebellar medulla are four pairs of nuclei, from medial to lateral: Fastigial, globose, emboliform, and dentate. The dentate is by far the largest, and is usually the only deep nucleus seen on routine sections (Fig. 9.7). Its serpiginous profile is strikingly similar to that of the inferior olivary nucleus of the medulla oblongata (Fig. 9.1), which is a major source of afferent fibers to the cerebellum.

The Purkinje cell dendritic arbor extends into the molecular layer like a hand with outstretched fingers. Its broad, flat palm and radiating fingers are oriented perpendicular to the long axis of the cerebellar convolutions (folia). Thus, routine folia cross sections show the typical, elaborate dendritic branching pattern, whereas longitudinal sections present a dramatically different "on edge" view of the arbor (Fig. 9.8). This should not be mistaken for pathologic dendritic tree "pruning" seen in some disease states.

Diencephalon

The diencephalon is interposed between the brain stem (midbrain, pons, and medulla) and the cerebrum. Four major divisions are recognized: Epithalamus (pineal gland and habenula), thalamus, subthalamus, and hypothalamus. The medial and lateral geniculate nuclei of the thalamus are sometimes considered together as the metathalamus. The strategic location of the thalamus is related to its major role in processing and relaying information passing between the cerebral cortex and brain stem and spinal cord. All sensory data (with the exception of olfaction) are processed by specific thalamic nuclei before distribution to the primary sensory cortices.

Of clinical significance to the pathologist, certain portions of the diencephalon immediately subjacent to the third ventricle, in particular, the large dorsomedial nuclei of the thalamus and the mammillary bodies of the hypothalamus, are often prominently involved in Wernicke encephalopathy. The lesions at these sites are postulated to account for the memory disturbance that accompanies this disorder.

Cerebrum

Supratentorially, the CNS becomes so much more complicated that it is difficult to describe in terms of any general pattern of orientation. It remains a hollow structure, but one that is no longer easy to consider as a tube of foldings and regional overgrowths. In light of this complexity, it is appropriate to review only those areas that are of particular diagnostic relevance.

Basal Ganglia

The term *basal ganglia* refers to the deep gray matter masses of the telencephalon and encompasses the caudate nucleus, putamen, globus pallidus, and amygdala (Fig. 9.9). The term *ganglion* was formerly used interchangeably with *nucleus*, and *ganglion cell* was synonymous with *neuron* to earlier neuroanatomists. With the exception of the basal ganglia, the current definition of a ganglion is now generally restricted to mean a collection of neuronal cell bodies located outside the CNS, namely, the sensory and autonomic ganglia of the peripheral nervous system. Reference to CNS neurons as *ganglion cells* is still occasionally encountered, and this historical sense of the term is reflected in the names of such neoplastic entities as *ganglioglioma, ganglioneuroma*, and *ganglion cell tumor*.

The amygdala (archistriatum) (Fig. 9.9) is located in the mesial temporal lobe immediately rostral to the hippocampus, and is functionally related to the limbic system. The remaining nuclei of the basal ganglia play an integral role in the modulation of motor function, and probably participate in other higher neural systems as well. The caudate nucleus, as the name implies, has a long tapering tail that intimately follows the curvature of the lateral ventricle (Fig. 9.9). The caudate is morphologically and functionally closely related to the putamen. These two nuclei are appropriately referred to collectively as the neostriatum, or simply striatum. For descriptive purposes, the putamen and the medially situated globus pallidus (paleostriatum or pallidum) are collectively referred to as the lentiform (lenticular) nucleus. The putamen and pallidum are separated from one another by the external medullary lamina of the pallidum, whereas the pallidum is itself divided into medial and lateral segments by the internal medullary lamina (Fig. 9.9). The globus pallidus ("pale globe") is so named because of its pale appearance in the fresh state compared to the putamen. This contrast is attributable histologically to the dense meshwork of myelinated fibers in the pallidum. In contrast, myelinated axons in the putamen are grouped into slender fascicles ("pencil bundles of Wilson") that project medially to the pallidum and to the substantia nigra (Fig. 9.9C). The histologic appearance of the lentiform nucleus is distinctive and permits unambiguous identification of even very limited amounts of tissue from this site.

The basal ganglia are prominently involved in a variety of pathologic processes, including kernicterus (literally, "nuclear jaundice") in the neonate and lacunar infarction in adults. Carbon monoxide poisoning classically produces selective necrosis of the inner segment of the pallidum. A frequent incidental finding of no diagnostic significance on routine sections of the lentiform nucleus is micronodular mineralization of small blood vessels, which is typically most prominent in the globus pallidus. Histologically, similar micronodular mineralization is also commonly seen in the hippocampus (Fig. 9.10).

Hippocampal Formation

The hippocampal formation comprises the subiculum, Ammon horn (hippocampus proper), and dentate gyrus (Fig. 9.10). In coronal sections of the medial temporal lobe, the subiculum forms the inferior base of the hippocampal formation, joining the parahippocampal gyrus with Ammon horn. Ammon horn, routinely abbreviated as CA (for cornu

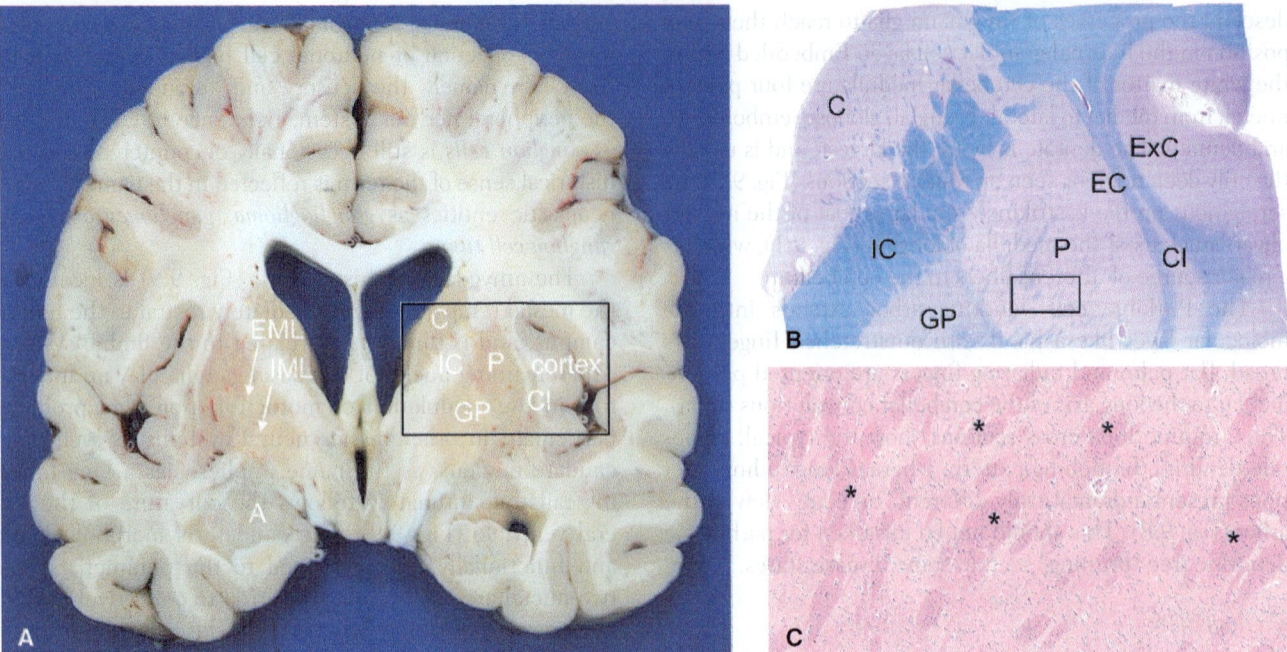

FIGURE 9.9 Basal ganglia: The gray matter of the telencephalon is broadly divisible into two components—the superficial cortical gray matter mantle and the deep gray nuclei. The latter are known as the basal ganglia, and consist of the caudate nucleus (*C*), putamen (*P*), globus pallidus (*GP*), and amygdala (**A**). The lenticular nucleus is composed of the medially situated, diffusely myelinated globus pallidus and the laterally placed putamen (**B**), whose myelinated fibers are grouped into slender fascicles known as the pencil bundles of Wilson (*asterisks*) (**C**). The internal and external medullary laminae (*IML* and *EML*, respectively) divide the globous pallidus into lateral and medial segments. The internal capsule (*IC*) separates the lenticular nucleus from the caudate and the thalamus. Lateral to the putamen there are the external capsule (*EC*), the claustrum (*Cl*), and the extreme capsule (*ExC*). Gray matter bridges occasionally span the capsule to connect the caudate and putamen, a reflection of the close functional relationship between these two nuclei. The lenticular nucleus receives its blood supply from several lenticulostriate arteries, which are direct branches of the middle cerebral artery, and is the most common site of intracerebral hypertensive hemorrhage and lacunar infarction. The large lenticulostriate artery coursing through the lateral putamen was known in former times as Charcot artery, or, more colorfully, as the artery of internal hemorrhage. The lenticulostriate vessels are often surrounded by dilated perivascular spaces that should not be mistaken for lacunar infarcts.

Ammonis), is divided into four regions, CA1 through 4, on the basis of cytologic architecture and synaptic connectivity (this nomenclature was introduced by Lorente de No in 1934). CA1 arches superiorly, forming, along with CA2, the medial floor of the temporal horn of the lateral ventricle. The dorsally situated CA2 is usually recognizable by the greater compactness of the pyramidal cell layer, as compared to CA1. CA3 forms a descending medial arch that terminates in the hilus of the dentate gyrus. The final segment of Ammon horn, CA4, lies within the hilus of the dentate gyrus and is often referred to as the end-plate. CA1, essentially equivalent to Sommer's sector, is the zone that is most sensitive to various insults, including seizures, ischemia, and Alzheimer disease changes. In contrast, the adjacent CA2 segment is known as the dorsal resistant zone, in recognition of its relative sparing compared to the other three sectors. The exquisite sensitivity of CA1 to injury, with sparing of the adjacent CA2, is routinely observed as mesial sclerosis of the hippocampus, which is seen in many temporal lobes resected for intractable epilepsy. The classic histologic description of the pattern of neuronal loss in Ammon horn was based on observations made on the brains of such epileptic patients by Wilhelm Sommer in 1880; E. Brotz coined the term *Sommer sector* in 1920.

There are several notable features that are frequently encountered incidentally in the examination of routine hippocampal sections and can be mistakenly interpreted as evidence of disease. One is an asymptomatic micronodular mineralization comparable to that seen in the pallidum. In the hippocampal formation, it is most commonly seen just outside the apex of the dentate gyrus (Fig. 9.11). A second common finding is a residual hippocampal fissure, which produces a rarefied lamina or cystic cleft that can be mistaken for a healed infarct. In addition, pyramidal neurons of Ammon horn are often dark and shrunken in autopsy material and care must be taken not to overinterpret such changes as evidence of antemortem ischemia (see Fig. 9.24).

CHAPTER 9: Central Nervous System

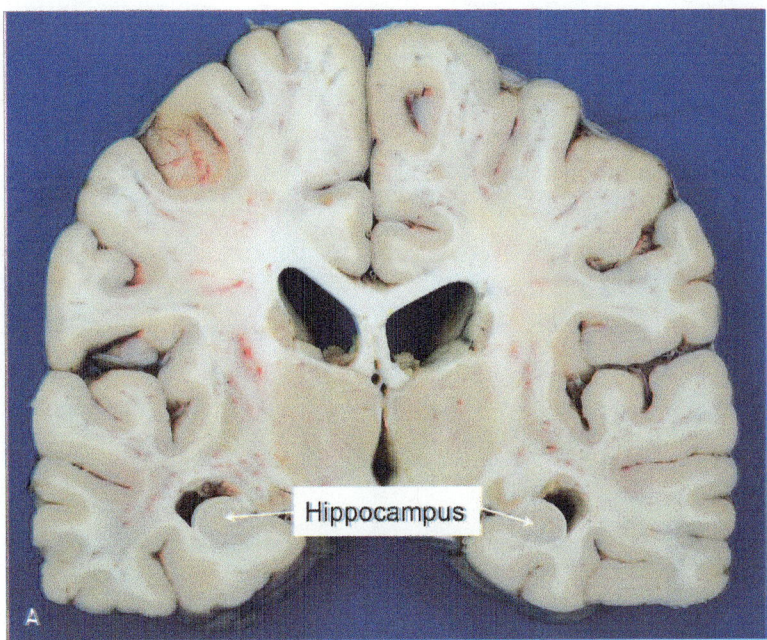
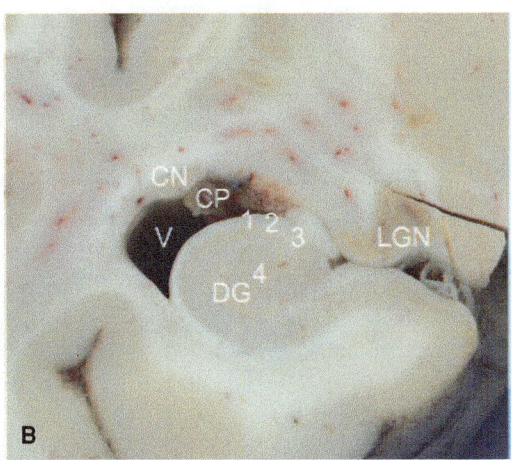
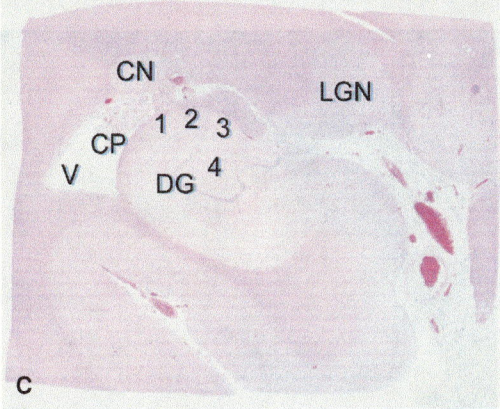

FIGURE 9.10 Hippocampal formation: The hippocampal formation (**A**) is composed of the subiculum, Ammon horn (cornu Ammonis, abbreviated as CA; divided into regions CA1-4), and the dentate gyrus (*DG*) (**B,C**). CA1 is equivalent to Sommer's sector and is the region of the hippocampus that is most sensitive to a variety of insults. In contrast, the adjacent CA2 region is known as the dorsal resistant zone. *CN*, tail of the caudate nucleus; *LGN*, lateral geniculate nucleus (note the "Napoleon's hat" profile and distinctive lamination). The tail of the lateral ventricle (*V*) is lateral to the hippocampal formation and choroid plexus (*CP*) is a common finding at this site.

Cerebral Cortex

From antiquity, neuroscientists have sought to divide the cortical mantle into discrete, functionally significant units. Early efforts yielded fanciful maps akin to those of phrenology and physiognomy. More recently, the application of light microscopy and special staining techniques for cell bodies (Nissl stains), dendritic arbors and unmyelinated axons (Golgi stains), and the myelin sheaths of myelinated axons (myelin stains such as the Weil, Weigert, and Luxol fast blue methods) have permitted a more scientific approach, although the details are beyond the scope of this chapter. In brief, the parcellation of the cortex is based on regional variation in the relative number, composition, and distribution of cortical neurons and their processes (cytoarchitectonics and myeloarchitechtonics). Many neuroanatomists have divided the cortex into a number of regions varying from 20 to more than 200, depending on the particular morphologic criteria and degree of subtlety employed. Currently, the most popular cortical map is that devised by Korbinian Brodmann in 1909. Brodmann map and the classical nomenclature for the gross anatomy of the cerebral sulci and gyri are the two systems most commonly used at present for reference purposes in the neuroanatomical and clinical literature.

Within the context of even the simplest cortical map, it is generally not possible to assign a given histologic section of cortex to a precise anatomical locus without prior knowledge of the section's provenance. However, two cortical areas do exhibit distinctive features: Primary motor cortex and primary visual cortex (Fig. 9.12). The motor cortex, located on the precentral gyrus of the frontal lobe, is distinguished by the presence of the giant pyramidal cells of Betz. Pyramidal cells generally range from 10 to 50 μm in soma height from base to origin of the apical dendrite. By comparison, Betz cells may

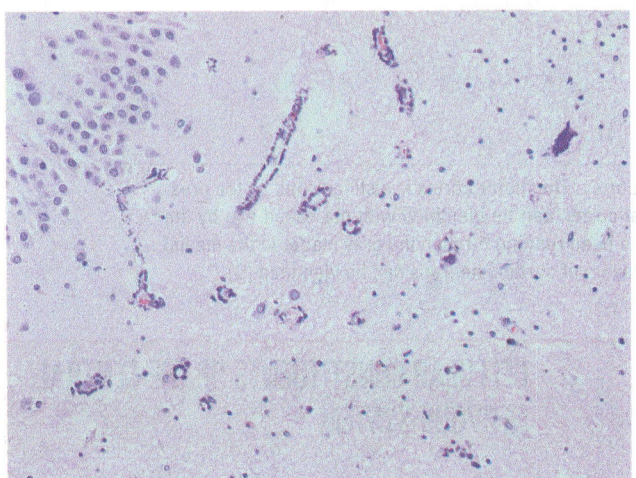

FIGURE 9.11 Micronodular mineralization: Micronodular mineralization is a common incidental finding, which is also seen in the globus pallidus.

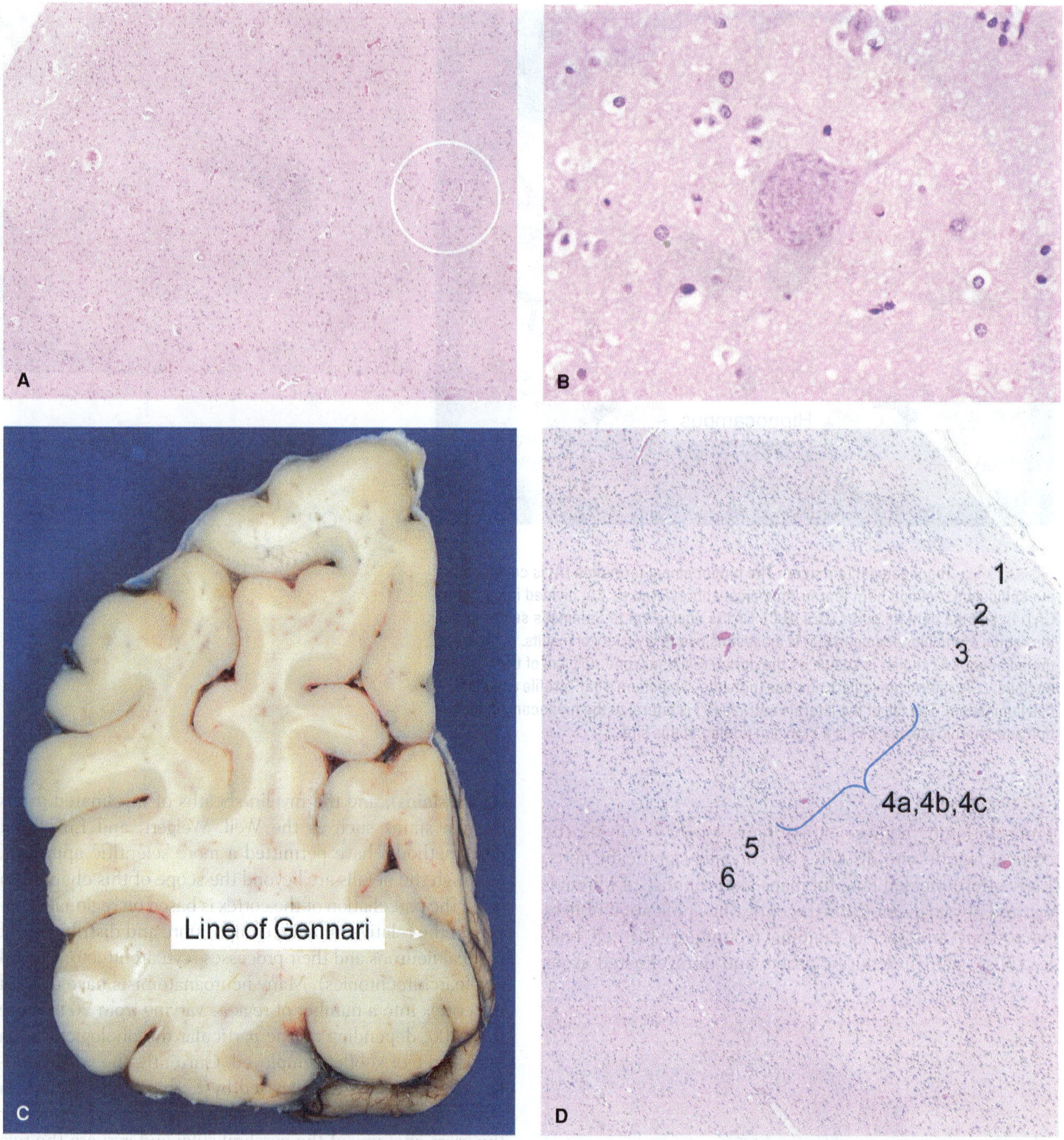

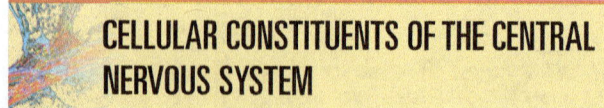

FIGURE 9.12 Primary motor cortex and primary visual cortex: The motor cortex is distinguished by the presence of the giant pyramidal cells of Betz. Primary visual cortex can be identified with the naked eye by the presence of the "external band of Baillarger" a thin white band running through the gray matter in the medial aspect of the occipital lobe (C). Microscopically the six layers of cortical neurons can be identified (D).

exceed 100 μm in soma height. The primary visual cortex, located on the banks of the calcarine fissure of the medial occipital lobe, is remarkable for the presence of a prominent "external band of Baillarger," termed the "line (or stria) of Gennari." This myelinated stratum located in lamina IV is usually visible to the naked eye and permits exact delineation of the primary visual cortex (Brodmann area 17) from the adjacent visual association cortex (Brodmann area 18).

CELLULAR CONSTITUENTS OF THE CENTRAL NERVOUS SYSTEM

Gray Matter and White Matter

By volume, most of the CNS is composed of gray matter and white matter (Fig. 9.13). Specialized types of CNS tissues

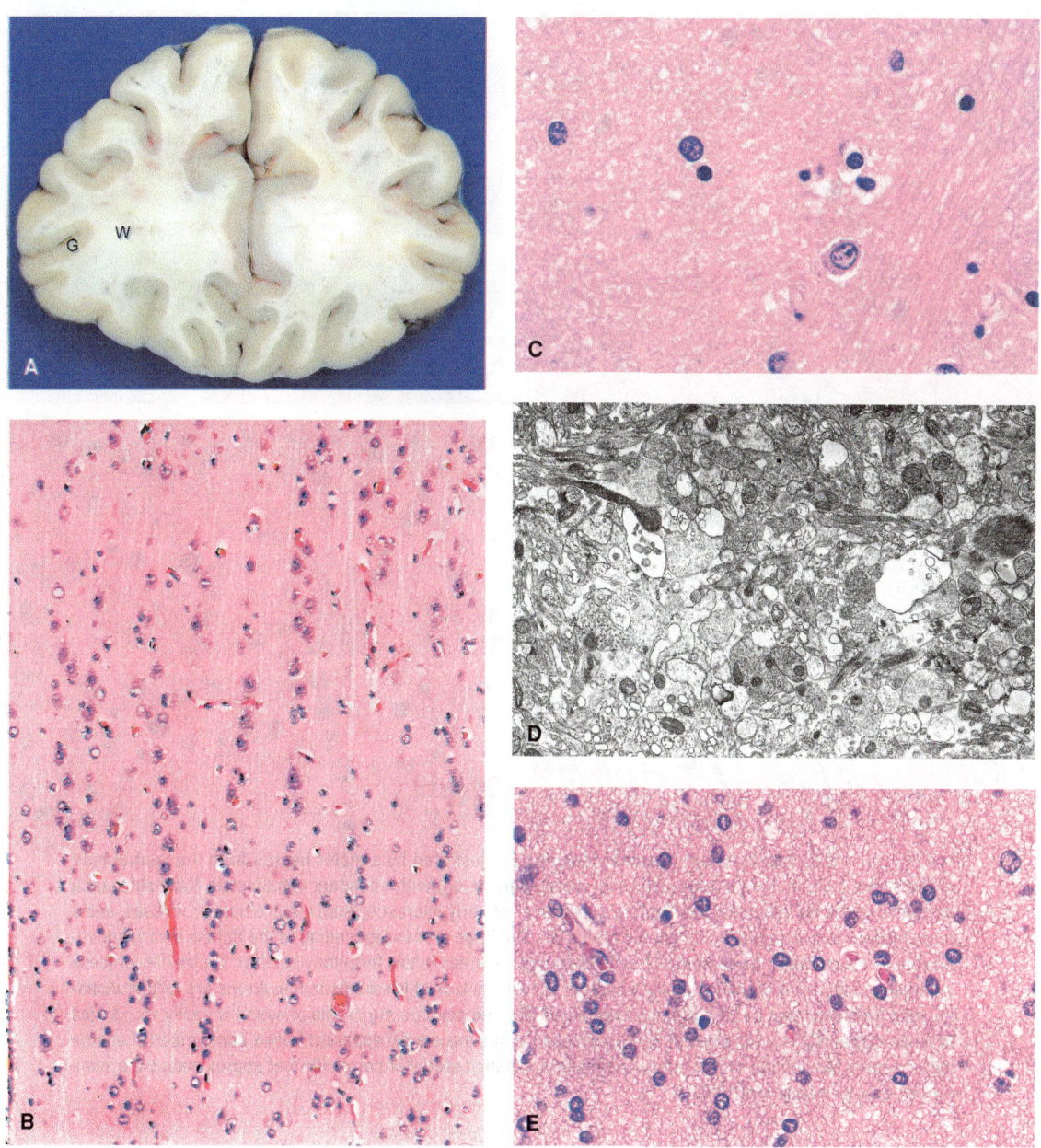

FIGURE 9.13 Gray matter and white matter: Gray (*G*) and white (*W*) matter can be distinguished with the naked eye on cross section of the brain (**A**). Gray matter contains abundant neuropil surrounding large neurons and smaller astrocytes and oligodendroglia (**B**). Neuropil is the term used for the fine amorphous eosinophilic background matrix of the CNS that fills the space between the cell bodies of the various cellular constituents as seen on H&E stains (**C**). Ultrastructural examination shows the neuropil to be composed of myriad intimately intermingling processes of the cellular constituents (**D**). White matter, in contrast, is composed primarily of oligodendroglia and the axons that they myelinate, and displays a much more uniform, homogeneous appearance (**E**).

include the choroid plexus, the pineal gland, the circumventricular organs (CVOs), and the infundibulum and neurohypophysis (discussed later). The hallmark of gray matter (Fig. 9.13B) is the presence of neuronal cell bodies embedded within a finely textured eosinophilic background termed neuropil (Fig. 9.13C,D). Neuropil (literally "nerve felt") is an interwoven meshwork of neuronal and glial cell processes. The individual neurites that compose the neuropil are not generally distinguishable in routine hematoxylin and eosin (H&E)-stained sections (Fig. 9.13C), but are resolvable at the ultrastructural level (Fig. 9.13D). White matter, in contrast, is composed primarily of myelinated axons and the supporting cells, oligodendroglia, that produce and maintain the myelin sheaths (Fig. 9.13E).

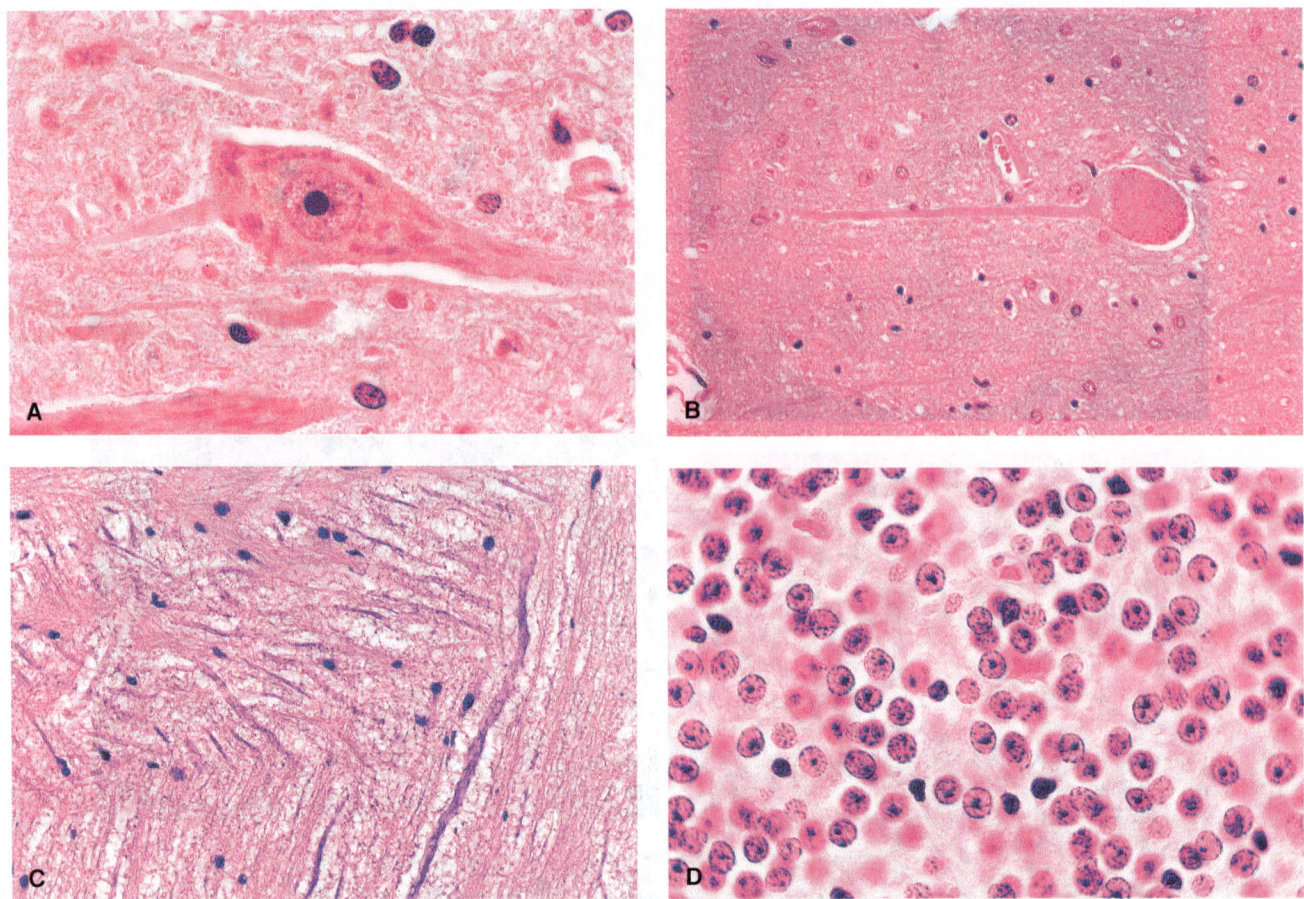

FIGURE 9.14 Neurons: Classical neuronal features, as illustrated by a motor neuron from the ventral horn of the spinal cord, include a large cell body (soma, perikaryon) with abundant cytoplasmic Nissl substance (rough endoplasmic reticulum, the "tigroid substance" of early microscopists), cytoplasmic processes, and a large nucleus with a single prominent nucleolus (**A**). The large process extending to the right is clearly recognizable as a dendrite by its content of Nissl substance, whereas in this fortuitous section, the smaller process extending to the left is identified as the neuron's axon by its lack of Nissl substance. Axons are further distinguished from dendrites by their nontapering profile (**B**). The nontapering profile of axons is easily recognized in white matter (**C**). The extremes of neuron size and shape are readily apparent from a comparison of a large motor neuron (**A**) with the small granular cell neurons of the cerebellar cortex (**D**) that approximately the same size as a motor neuron's nucleolus!

Neurons

Normal Microscopic Anatomy

The prototypical neuron is exemplified by the large multipolar Betz cells of the motor cortex, the alpha motor neurons of the ventral horn of the spinal cord, and the Purkinje cells of the cerebellum. These neurons are characterized by large perikarya (cell bodies or somas) with abundant Nissl substance (rough endoplasmic reticulum), robust dendritic arborizations, and large nuclei with prominent single nucleoli (Fig. 9.14). Such large multipolar forms, however, represent only one type of neuron; the diapason of neuronal morphologies is exceedingly broad. This is readily apparent by comparison of alpha motor neurons with granular cell neurons (Fig. 9.14A,D). These two neuronal populations typify the classical dichotomous subdivision of CNS neurons into large extroverted projection neurons with long axons (Golgi type I neurons) and small introverts that function regionally with restricted connections (Golgi type II neurons). Between these two poles is a full spectrum of neuronal sizes and shapes, with an equally impressive variety of dendritic arbor configurations. The details of the latter are generally appreciable only with special stains for neuronal processes. The cell processes of neurons are separated into two categories: Axons (Fig. 9.14C), of which each neuron only has one, and dendrites (Fig. 9.14A), which are often multiple.

With respect to morphologic variants, one unique population of CNS neurons merits brief mention. The mesencephalic nucleus of the trigeminal nerve, which is concerned chiefly with the mediation of jaw proprioception, is composed of true primary (first order) sensory neurons that possess only a single process emanating from the cell body (Fig. 9.15A). This nucleus constitutes the only intraparenchymal example

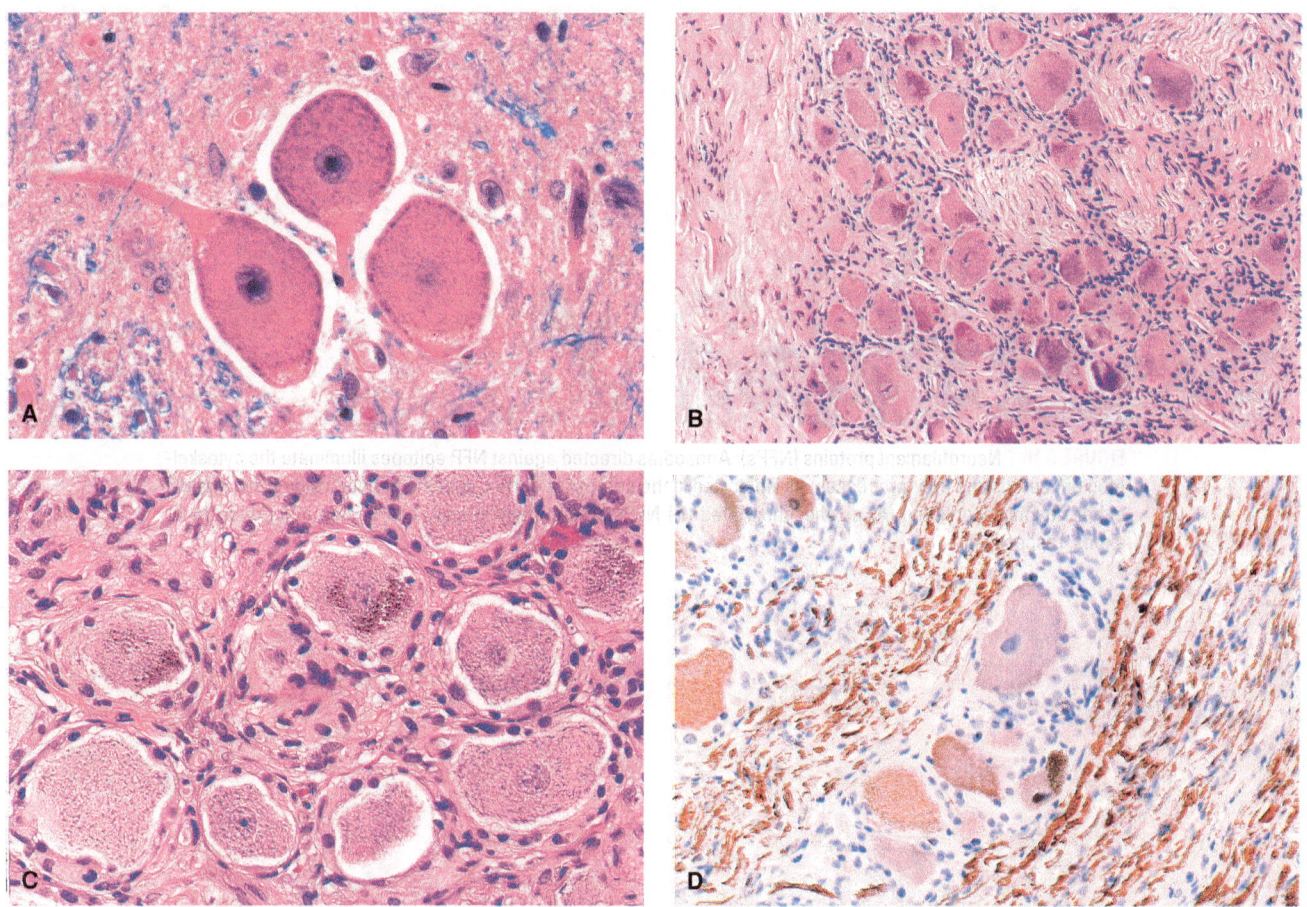

FIGURE 9.15 Unipolar neurons: Another neuronal morphologic variant is the unipolar (pseudounipolar) neuron. These large neurons possess only a single cell process, an axon, with an absence of dendrites. Unipolar neurons are primary sensory neurons and the only example of this class of neuron within the CNS is the mesencephalic nucleus of the trigeminal nerve in the upper pons and midbrain lateral to the periaqueductal gray matter (**A**). All other unipolar neurons are located in the peripheral nervous system ganglia (**B**). The dorsal root ganglia of the spinal cord provide a good example, with large unipolar neurons surrounded by satellite cells (**B**). Ganglionic neurons typically display cytoplasmic pigment (**C**) and their cell bodies and axons are strongly positive for phosphorylated neurofilament proteins (**D**).

of this class of neurons; all other primary sensory neuronal perikarya are gathered outside the CNS in the spinal and cranial nerve ganglia (Fig. 9.15B to D).

Immunohistochemistry

Antibodies have been raised against a wide variety of the many unique neuronal proteins that are being isolated and characterized at an ever-increasing rate. Most of these markers are confined to use for research purposes but several have found utility in the diagnostic laboratory. One of the earliest such markers, neuron-specific enolase (NSE), has proven notoriously unreliable as a marker of neuronal differentiation. Its use for this purpose in evaluating neoplasms of the CNS is not recommended. Antibodies directed against epitopes on the constituent proteins of neurofilaments, which are major cytoskeletal elements of the neuronal perikaryon and cytoplasmic processes, have been used extensively in both, experimental and clinical studies (Fig. 9.16). One of the most useful and widely employed neuronal markers is synaptophysin. Synaptophysin is an integral membrane protein of synaptic vesicles. In the normal nervous system, antisynaptophysin antibodies yield a diffuse, finely granular pattern throughout the gray matter neuropil (Fig. 9.17A). In addition, punctate granular decoration is seen along the cell bodies and proximal dendrites of several types of large, projection class neurons, including the Purkinje cells of the cerebellum, alpha motor neurons of the spinal cord, extraocular motor neurons of the brain stem, and Betz cells of the precentral gyrus (Fig. 9.17B). Another marker that is useful in the identification of most neurons is the antibody neuronal nuclei (NeuN) (Fig. 9.18).

Age-Related Neuronal Inclusions

A variety of inclusions, largely intracytoplasmic, appear with increasing frequency as we age. By far, the most common is lipofuscin (lipochrome or aging pigment), whose

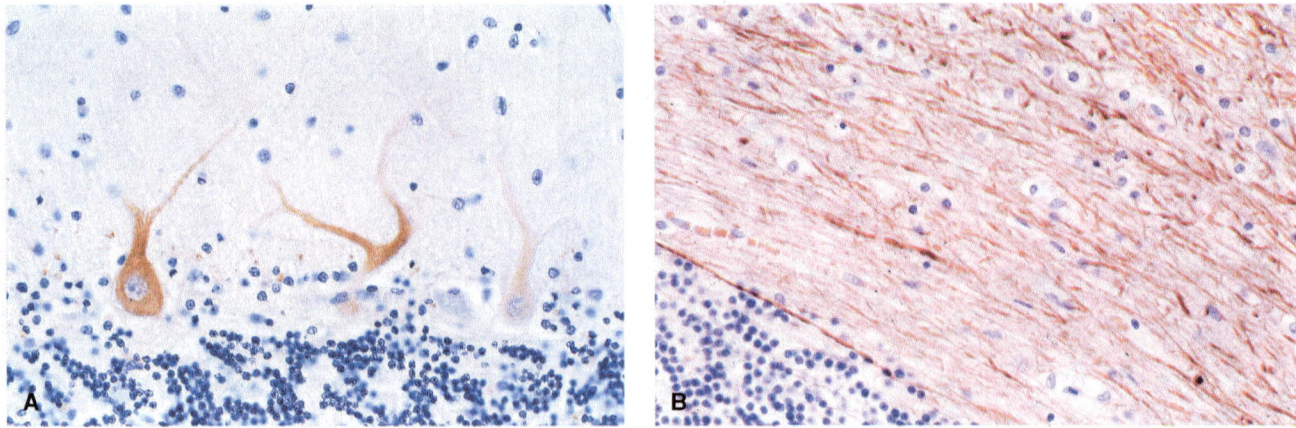

FIGURE 9.16 Neurofilament proteins (NFPs): Antibodies directed against NFP epitopes illuminate the cytoskeleton of neurons and their processes. As illustrated in the cerebellar cortex, specific antibodies directed against either nonphosphorylated (**A**) or phosphorylated (**B**) NFPs differentially identify cell bodies and dendrites or axons, respectively.

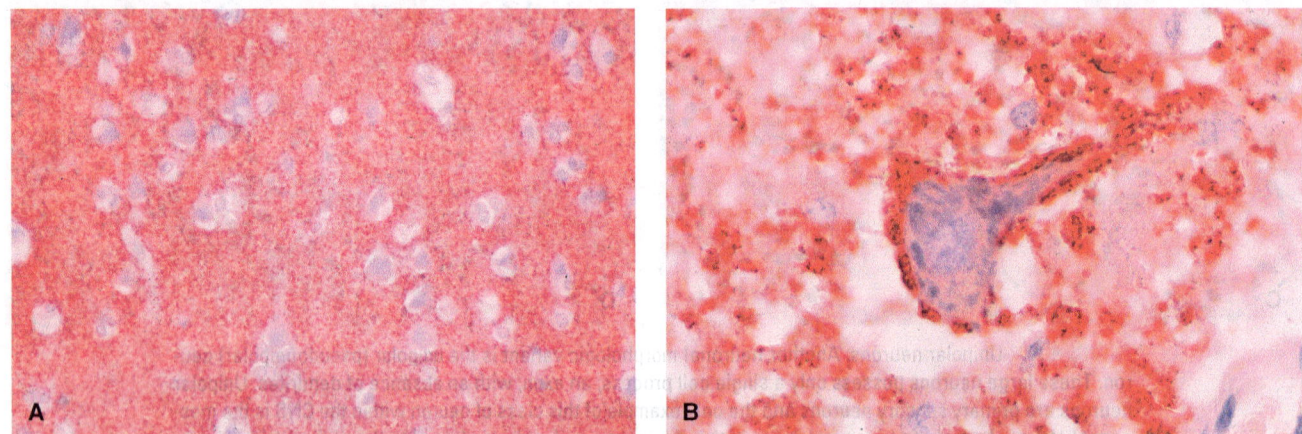

FIGURE 9.17 Synaptophysin is one of the most useful and widely employed markers of neuronal differentiation. The neuropil of gray matter, which is rich in synaptic contacts, shows a diffuse, finely granular pattern (**A**). Several specific types of large projection class neurons show prominent punctate decoration of the cell body and proximal dendrites, as illustrated here by a motor neuron in the hypoglossal nucleus of the medulla (**B**). Other groups of large neurons exhibiting this pattern of synaptophysin immunopositivity include Purkinje cells of the cerebellum, motor neurons of the ventral horn of the spinal cord, and Betz cells of the precentral gyrus in the cerebral cortex.

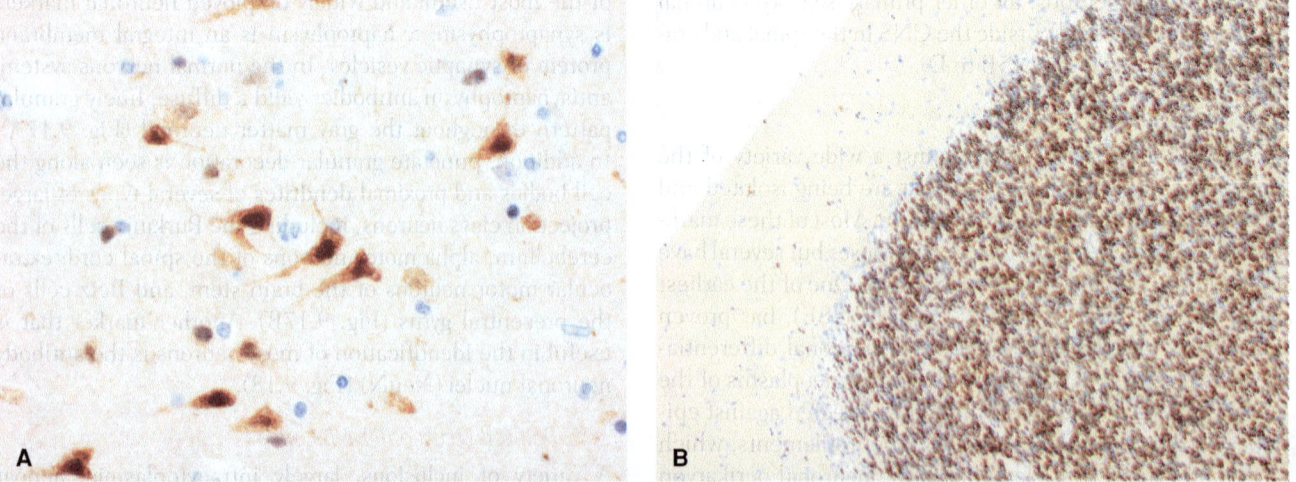

FIGURE 9.18 Neuronal nuclei: NeuN is a very useful marker for identifying neurons. The nuclear pattern of expression of this protein makes it easy to interpret (**A**). Although the neurons in the internal granular cell layer of the cerebellum are strongly positive, Purkinje cell neurons do not express this marker (**B**).

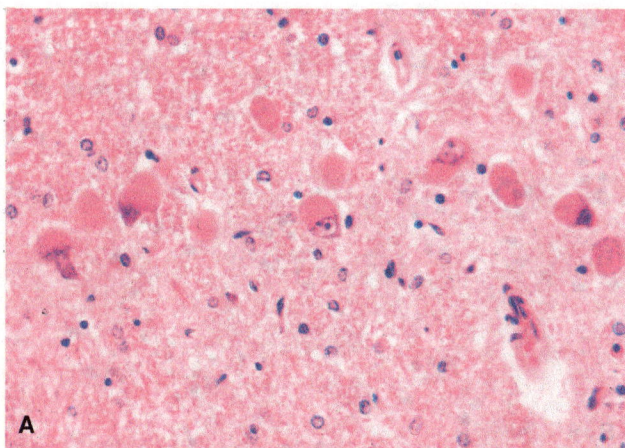 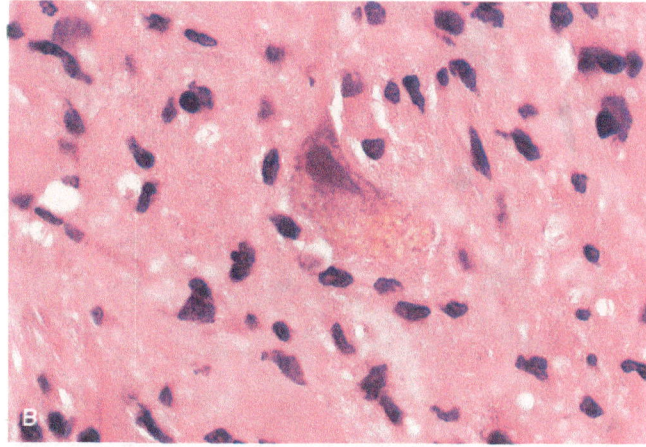

FIGURE 9.19 Lipofuscin: Prominent accumulation of lipofuscin pigment in large neurons with increasing age, as seen for example in the lateral geniculate nucleus (**A**), can result in peripheral displacement of the nucleus and Nissl substance, mimicking central chromatolysis. As a practical application of normal neurohistology, the presence of lipofuscin can sometimes aid in the identification of neurons in intraoperative frozen sections (**B**). As illustrated here, a neuron, identified by its lipofuscin content, is surrounded by tumor cells, thereby supporting a diagnosis of infiltrating glioma.

yellow-to-pale brown color is unaltered by most histologic procedures, including the H&E method (Fig. 9.19). Its autofluorescence and partial avidity for the acid-fast stain can be used to visualize differentially this "wear and tear" pigment, although little functional significance is generally assigned to lipochrome accumulation in normal aging. In larger neurons, lipofuscin may accumulate to such an extent that it displaces organelles, and creates an appearance similar to the cell swelling of central chromatolysis, described below (see Fig. 9.26). The lateral geniculate body provides an example of a densely populated nucleus whose constituent neuron's prominent accumulation of lipofuscin is often discernible macroscopically as a distinctly mahogany hue compared to adjacent cortex (see Fig. 9.10B). Interestingly, lipofuscin accumulation is not simply a function of cell size because some classes of large neurons appear comparatively immune to significant accrual, for example, the cerebellar Purkinje cells.

Functionally, more significant neuronal inclusions that may be seen in asymptomatic individuals are those associated with Alzheimer disease. They are neurofibrillary tangles, neuritic plaques, granulovacuolar degeneration (GVD), and Hirano bodies. These illustrate the often ill-defined distinction between health and disease, because these changes can be seen in the elderly, albeit in limited numbers, in the absence of antemortem disturbances of mentation. In some cases, neurofibrillary tangles may be found in asymptomatic individuals in occasional neurons of the subiculum or Ammon horn. Although silver stains greatly aid visualization and quantitation, these structures may be identified on routinely stained H&E sections if the observer is familiar with their appearance. In pyramidal cells, they appear as a slightly basophilic wisp of faintly fibrillar material that extends out into cell processes, most notably the apical dendrite, and they are often more prominent on one side of the nucleus (flame-shaped tangle; Fig. 9.20A). This morphology reflects the fact that tangles generally conform to the shape of the cell body. For example, in the pigmented neurons of the locus ceruleus, which are multipolar and lack the dominant apical dendrite of pyramidal neurons, tangles that are globular in shape are occasionally encountered as an incidental finding.

The senile plaque is also a manifestation of cell injury, but one that, like slight atherosclerosis, is not an unexpected finding in the brains of asymptomatic adults. In such individuals, the plaque is usually seen in its primitive form as a somewhat ill-defined, roughly circular region of abnormal argyrophilic neurites that is not visualized in the H&E-stained section. As the plaques mature they become visible in the latter preparation, particularly when a central core of eosinophilic amyloid appears (Fig. 9.20B). The latter can be more readily seen by Congo red, periodic acid–Schiff (PAS) staining or staining for β-amyloid. As noted earlier, both neurofibrillary tangles and neuritic plaques are more easily identified and quantitated with special techniques such as immunofluorescence or silver stains (Fig. 9.20C). Immunostains for Tau protein and β-amyloid (Fig. 9.20D) are also helpful in the identification of tangles and plaques, respectively. A finding that can also be encountered in the brain of patients with amyloid plaques is the accumulation of amyloid in the wall of meningeal and cortical blood vessels (Fig. 9.20E).

Two additional intraneuronal inclusions that are seen in Alzheimer disease, but only rarely in nondemented individuals, are GVD and Hirano bodies (Fig. 9.21). As the name implies, the inclusion of GVD consists of a dark, basophilic granule inside a small, clear vacuole. Clusters of these cytoplasmic inclusions may be present within a single neuron (Fig. 9.21A). Depending on the plane of section, Hirano

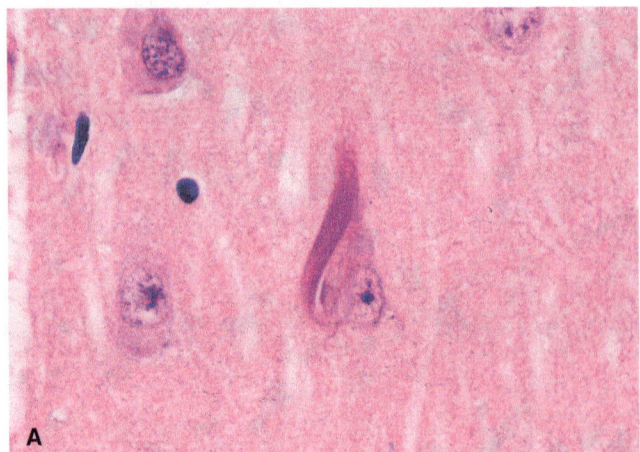
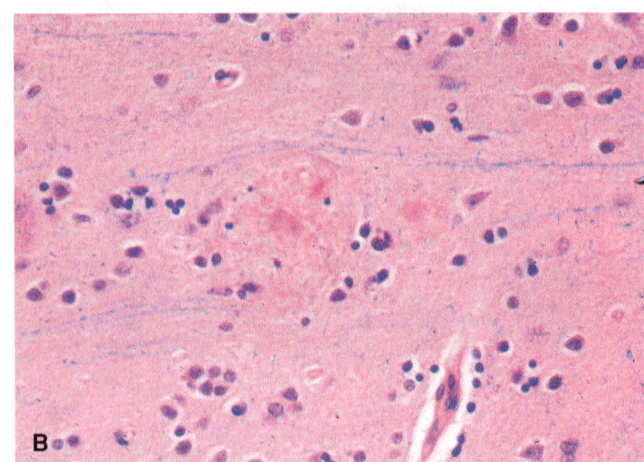
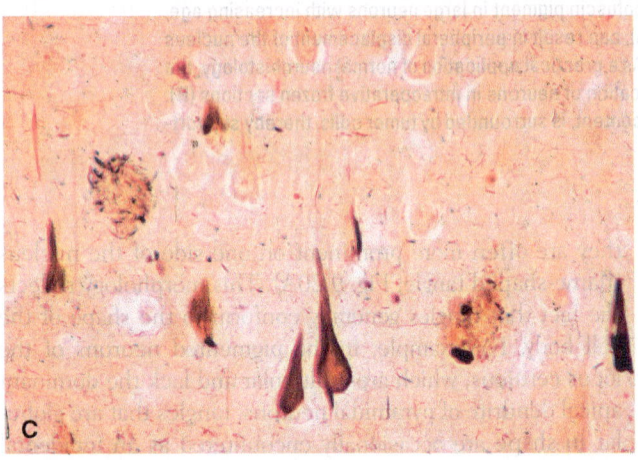

FIGURE 9.20 Neurofibrillary tangles and neuritic plaques: Neurofibrillary tangles (**A**) may be seen sporadically in the hippocampal formation of aging brains and have a fibrillary texture in H&E-stained sections. Mature senile (neuritic) plaques (**B**) deform the smooth texture of the neuropil and appear in H&E-stained sections as spherical, somewhat granular foci with a central eosinophilic core that is composed of amyloid. Note that adjacent myelinated axons are focally displaced as they pass by the plaque. In earlier stages, the plaques are less well defined and are not identifiable in H&E-stained sections. Although both neurofibrillary tangles and large mature neuritic plaques can be seen in H&E-stained sections, use of special techniques, such as silver stains (**C**), greatly facilitates visualization and quantitation.

bodies appear in H&E-stained sections as brightly eosinophilic oval, elliptical, or elongated rod-like refractile inclusions that are located either in very close apposition to a neuronal perikaryon (Fig. 9.21B), or within the neuropil. Ultrastructural examination supports localization in neuronal cell bodies and processes, and immunohistochemical studies reveal the presence of actin and actin-associated proteins. Unlike neurofibrillary tangles and neuritic plaques, both GVD and Hirano bodies exhibit a very limited neuroanatomic distribution and are, in fact, virtually confined to the hippocampal formation.

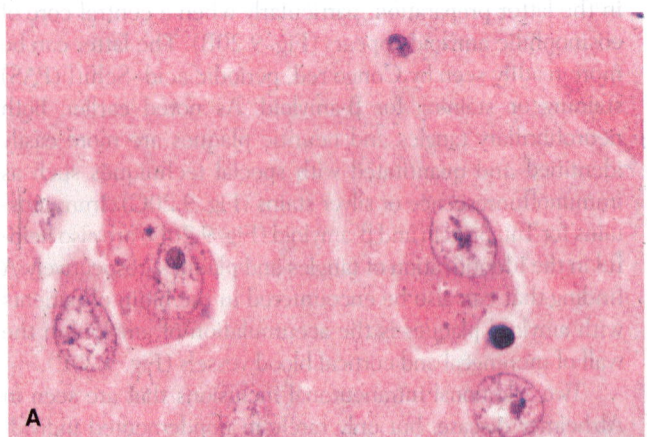
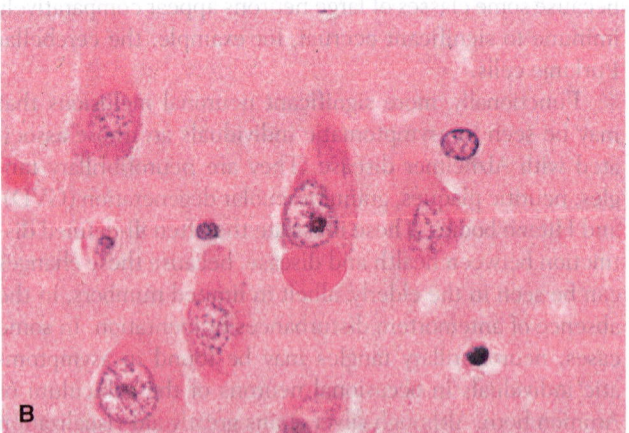

FIGURE 9.21 Granulovacuolar degeneration (of Simchowitz) (**A**) and Hirano bodies (**B**): Like neurofibrillary tangles, both of these intracytoplasmic inclusions can occasionally be seen in the hippocampal formation of normal older individuals. However, although these alterations are not pathognomonic for dementing illness, an appreciable number of affected cells should prompt a search for the evidence of Alzheimer disease in the form of a thorough examination for senile (neuritic) plaques and neurofibrillary tangles.

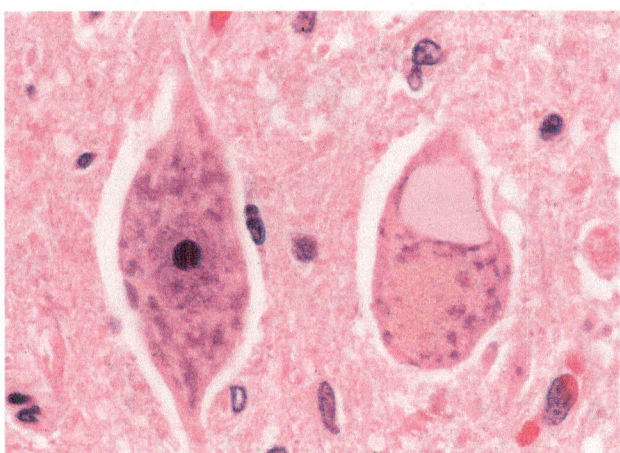

FIGURE 9.22 Hyaline (colloid) inclusion: These eye-catching inclusions, as seen in the neuron on the right, may be observed sporadically throughout the neuraxis but are most commonly encountered in the large motor neurons of the hypoglossal nuclei in the medulla (as in this micrograph). Less frequently, they may be seen in the motor neurons of the ventral horn of the spinal cord. Electron microscopic examination reveals ectatic cisternae of endoplasmic reticulum.

Encountering more than one or two cells with these alterations should raise the issue of Alzheimer disease and prompt a search for other attendant histologic features.

A particularly striking cytoplasmic inclusion occasionally encountered in routine sections of the hypoglossal nuclei of the medulla (less often in the ventral horn motor nuclei of the spinal cord) is the hyaline (colloid) inclusion (Fig. 9.22). These inclusions, which consist of ectatic cisternae of endoplasmic reticulum, are rarely seen in the first few decades of life, but appear with increasing frequency thereafter. They are occasionally mistaken by the uninformed for viral inclusions.

Catecholaminergic neurons throughout the brain stem gradually accumulate neuromelanin as a by-product of neurotransmitter synthesis. The largest and most densely populated of these nuclei is the substantia nigra ("black substance"), which contains dopaminergic neurons. The locus ceruleus ("blue spot"), which is also seen by the unaided eye, is a collection of noradrenergic neurons in the rostral pontine tegmentum. It is of practical importance that the Lewy bodies of Parkinson disease can be found in both of these neuroanatomic locales. Of the smaller and more diffusely distributed pigmented neurons, those in the vicinity of the dorsal motor nucleus of the vagus nerve in the medulla oblongata are most commonly encountered during routine histologic examination. Microscopically, neuromelanin appears as coarse, dark brown granules (Fig. 9.23A), and should not be confused with melanocytic melanin. The latter is also present in the CNS, but is confined to leptomeningeal melanocytes as discussed below (see Fig. 9.64).

Several eosinophilic inclusions may be seen in pigmented brain stem neurons. The most striking of these are the commonly encountered Marinesco bodies (Fig. 9.23B).

These bright red, hyaline-appearing structures are located within the nucleus, often adjacent to and about the same size as a nucleolus (an alternative designation is "paranucleolar body"). Multiple Marinesco bodies may occur within a single nucleus and, in some cases, a large percentage of pigmented neurons exhibit these eye-catching inclusions. In such cases, they may raise concern about a viral infection to the unaccustomed observer, but are not pathologic and have yet to be correlated with any significant process except advancing age. Two types of eosinophilic inclusions may be encountered in the cytoplasm of pigmented neurons. Clusters of diminutive acidophilic granules are occasionally noted (Fig. 9.23C) but have no pathologic significance. Lewy bodies, in contrast, are much larger, notably displace the cytoplasmic neuromelanin from which they are separated by a small clear halo, and are associated with Parkinson disease (Fig. 9.23D).

Autolysis and Basic Neuronal Reactions to Injury

As captured in their normal state by perfusion fixation or rapid immersion fixation, neurons are generally rotund with lightly eosinophilic cytoplasm that is stippled with basophilic Nissl substance in the case of the larger neurons. The surrounding glia are inconspicuous and few clear vacuoles are seen. This perfection in fixation is rarely achieved in human material, however, and virtually in all autopsy and surgical specimens, autolysis alters this ideal appearance to a greater or lesser extent. Neurons are, thereby, rendered somewhat contracted and basophilic. Nuclei are also somewhat condensed. Simultaneously, the processes of glia that surround neurons and blood vessels imbibe water to produce clear vacuoles (see Fig. 9.37). The neuronal response to injury overlaps in some cases with these autolytic changes, and it may not be possible to distinguish agonal hypotensive injury from autolysis in autopsy specimens. In the former setting, the neuronal contraction is pronounced and the perineuronal and perivascular spaces are exceptionally prominent.

There are, however, three neuronal changes that provide unequivocal evidence of antemortem injury. One is the "red" neuron, which is the sine qua non of ischemic damage. The second is central chromatolysis, and the third is ferruginization. The "red" neuron is characterized by a shrunken cell body and intense cytoplasmic eosinophilia with complete loss of Nissl basophilia (Fig. 9.24). The nucleus is dark and usually lacks a distinguishable nucleolus, but may be pale and demonstrate early karyolysis. At times, it has a somewhat fragmented look suggesting karyorrhexis, although clearly defined karyorrhexis is rare. In surgical specimens, tissue-handling artifact ("crush" artifact) also results in dark, shrunken neuronal perikarya; however, as with autolytic autopsy specimens, these cells lack the distinctive cytoplasmic eosinophilia of ischemia (Fig. 9.25).

Central chromatolysis, the second unequivocally abnormal finding, consists of a loss of central basophilic staining

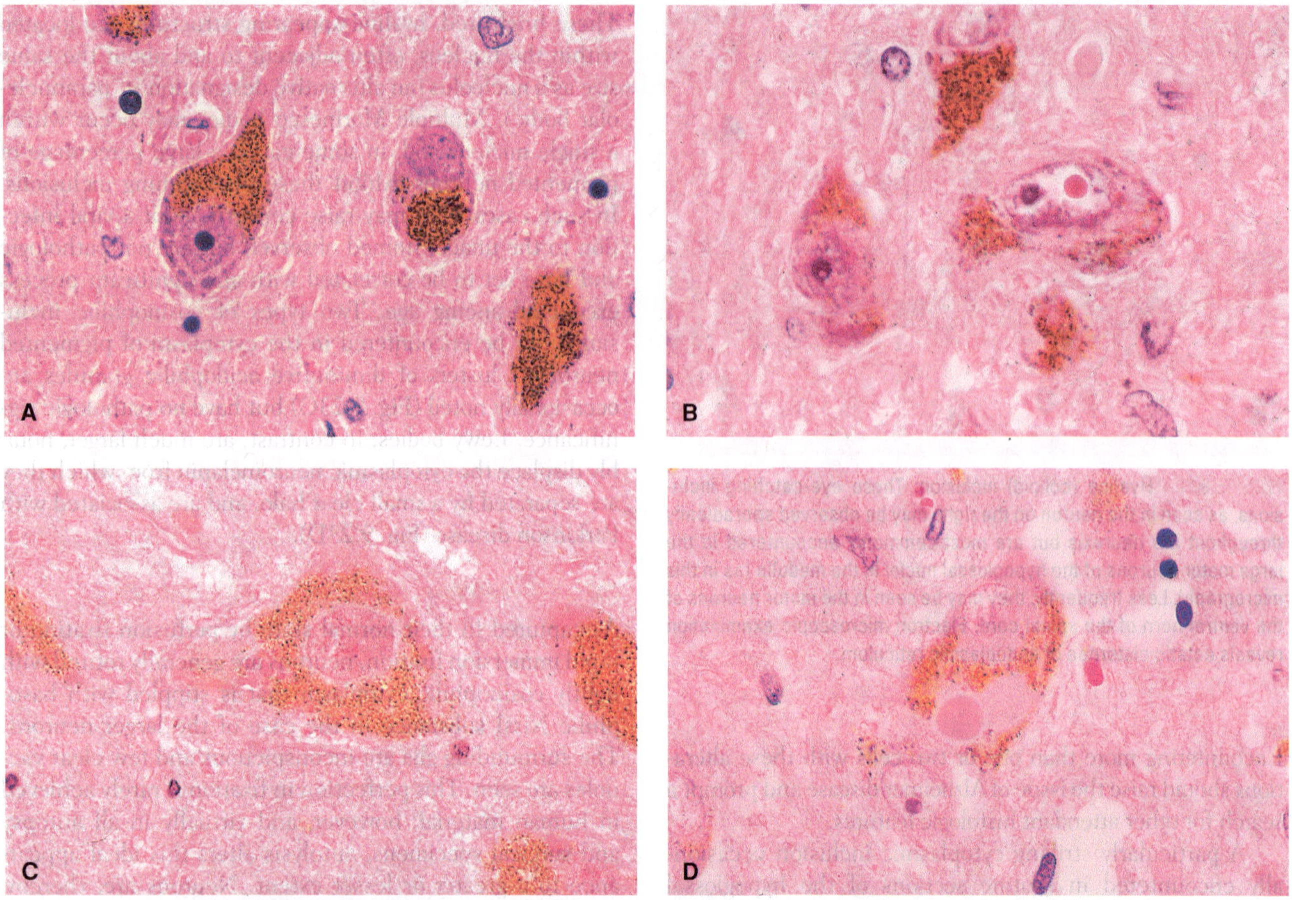

FIGURE 9.23 Pigmented neurons of the brain stem: Neuromelanin is a coarse, dark brown cytoplasmic pigment (**A**) that is formed as a by-product of catecholamine synthesis and is frequently encountered microscopically in scattered catecholaminergic neurons distributed widely throughout the brain stem. Two large populations are visible grossly: The substantia nigra ("black substance") of the midbrain and the locus ceruleus ("blue spot") of the pons. Marinesco bodies (**B**) are eosinophilic, spheroidal, paranucleolar bodies that are often observed in the nuclei of pigmented neurons, especially those of the substantia nigra. The number of Marinesco bodies increases with advancing age and can be quite striking in some individuals. They should not be mistaken for intranuclear viral inclusions. Clusters of minute intracytoplasmic eosinophilic granules (**C**), seen in this micrograph to the left of the nucleus, may occasionally catch the eye of an obsessive observer. They have no known pathologic significance and are much smaller than Lewy bodies (**D**), which are the characteristic intracytoplasmic inclusions of Parkinson disease.

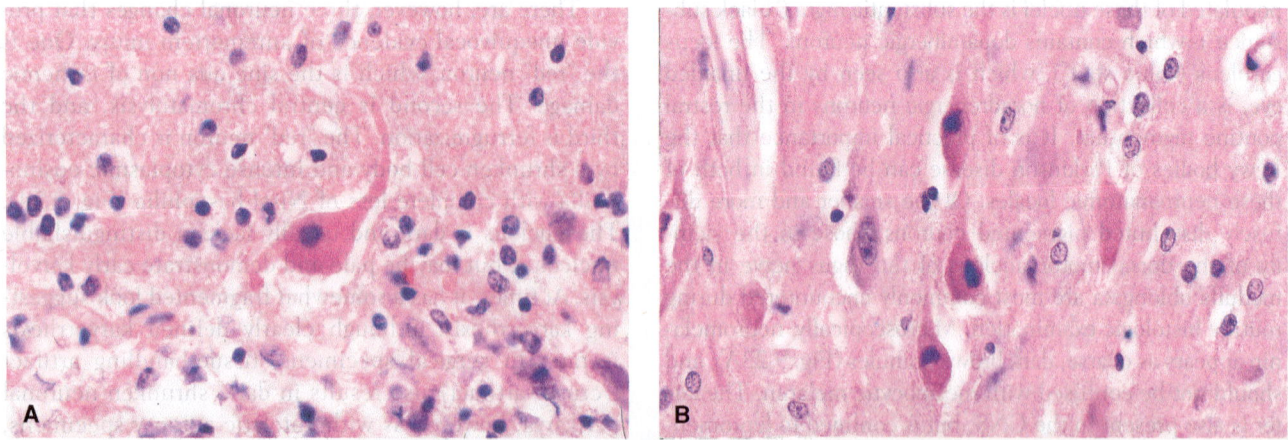

FIGURE 9.24 Ischemic injury: The sine qua non of ischemic damage to the nervous system is the so-called red neuron. As illustrated here by a Purkinje cell of the cerebellum (**A**) and pyramidal neurons of the hippocampal CA1 region (**B**), the soma (cell body) is shrunken, the cytoplasm is intensely eosinophilic, and the nucleus is pyknotic with no discernible nucleolus. It is largely the pronounced eosinophilia that distinguishes this cellular alteration from autolytic neuronal condensation, in which the cytoplasm is dark and basophilic (see Fig. 9.25).

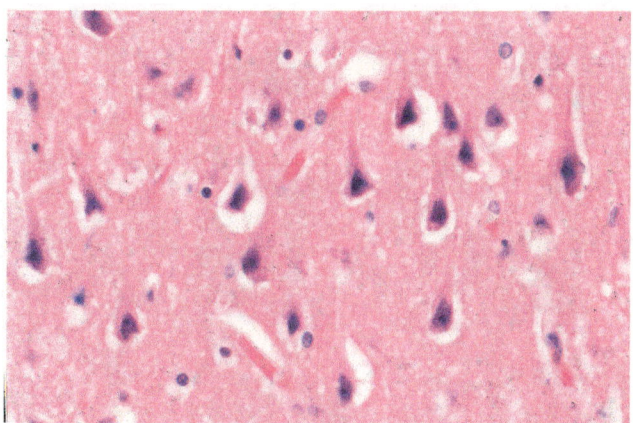

FIGURE 9.25 Neuronal contraction as a tissue-handling artifact: In contrast to ischemic insult (Fig. 9.24), in "crush artifact" the cytoplasm is dark and basophilic rather than brightly eosinophilic.

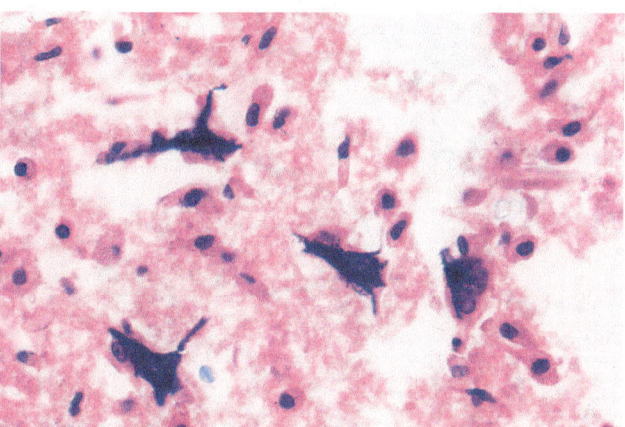

FIGURE 9.27 Mineralized (ferruginized) neurons: These encrusted relics resembling petrified tree trunks are most commonly encountered around the margins of old infarcts.

of the cell body with peripheral margination of the Nissl substance (Fig. 9.26). It is seen in a number of pathologic states (the ballooned anterior horn cells of poliomyelitis being the classical example). There are numerous mimickers that lie in wait for the unwary. For example, some normal neuronal populations, such as the supraoptic and paraventricular nuclei of the hypothalamus and the dorsal nucleus of Clarke of the thoracic spinal cord, display Nissl substance that is preferentially distributed peripherally in the soma. Other neurons, such as those of the mesencephalic nucleus of the trigeminal nerve discussed previously (see Fig. 9.15), have large, exquisitely rounded somas and, hence, mimic that aspect of chromatolysis. The giant pyramidal cells of Betz in the motor cortex are so large in comparison to surrounding neurons, that at low magnification they may give an initial impression of chromatolytic swelling. Finally, as discussed earlier, one must be careful not to mistake the accumulation of various substances that displace the Nissl substance peripherally, such as lipofuscin, for central chromatolysis (see Fig. 9.19).

A striking finding sometimes encountered near old infarcts is the presence of ferruginized or fossilized neurons, in which both perikarya and axons are encrusted by blue-staining minerals (Fig. 9.27). This arresting phenomenon is not limited to the vicinal tissue of old infarcts, although this is the most common context, nor is it confined to the adult nervous system, because prenatal insults may result in similar findings. Clusters of axons thus affected can be mistaken for fungal hyphae (Fig. 9.28).

A common reaction of axons to injury seen in a wide variety of pathologic states is the formation of localized dilatations known as axonal spheroids or axon "retraction balls" (Fig. 9.29A). These structures can be highlighted with immunohistochemical stains against the amyloid precursor protein (APP)

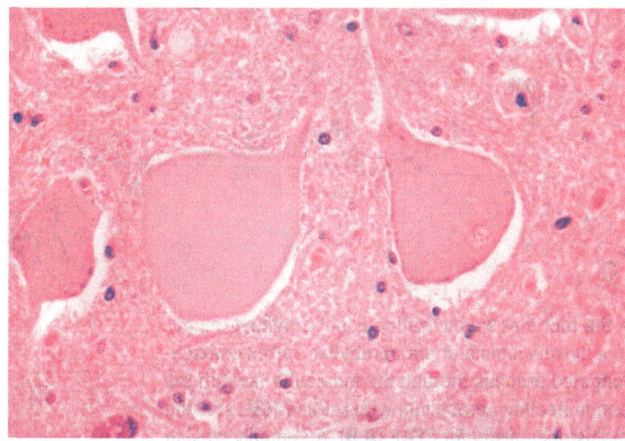

FIGURE 9.26 Central chromatolysis: Cytoplasmic hyalinization and swelling with peripheral displacement of the nucleus and lipofuscin can be a response to either intrinsic neuronal disease (such as in poliomyelitis or other viral infections) or to interruption of the axon in close proximity to the cell body. In the latter setting, the term axonal reaction is applied.

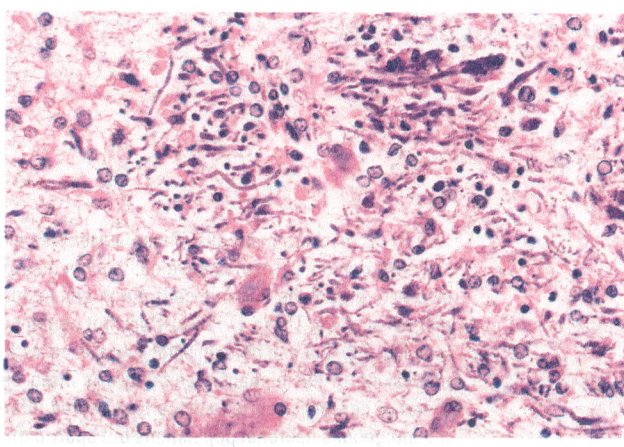

FIGURE 9.28 Mineralized axons: Clusters of mineralized axons have a superficial resemblance to fungal hyphae.

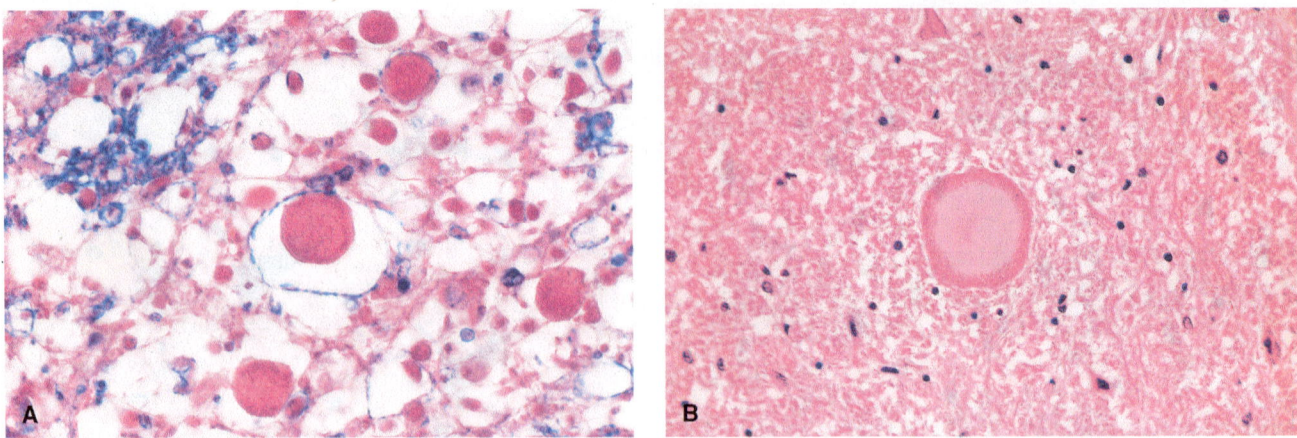

FIGURE 9.29 Axonal spheroids: Focal dilatations known as spheroids (**A**) are a common axonal reaction to injury that is seen in a wide array of pathologic conditions including radiation damage and post-traumatic diffuse axonal injury. Axonal spheroids are also frequently encountered incidentally in older individuals in the dorsal medulla oblongata (rostral fasciculus gracilis near nucleus gracilis) where, as in this example, they are often mineralized (**B**).

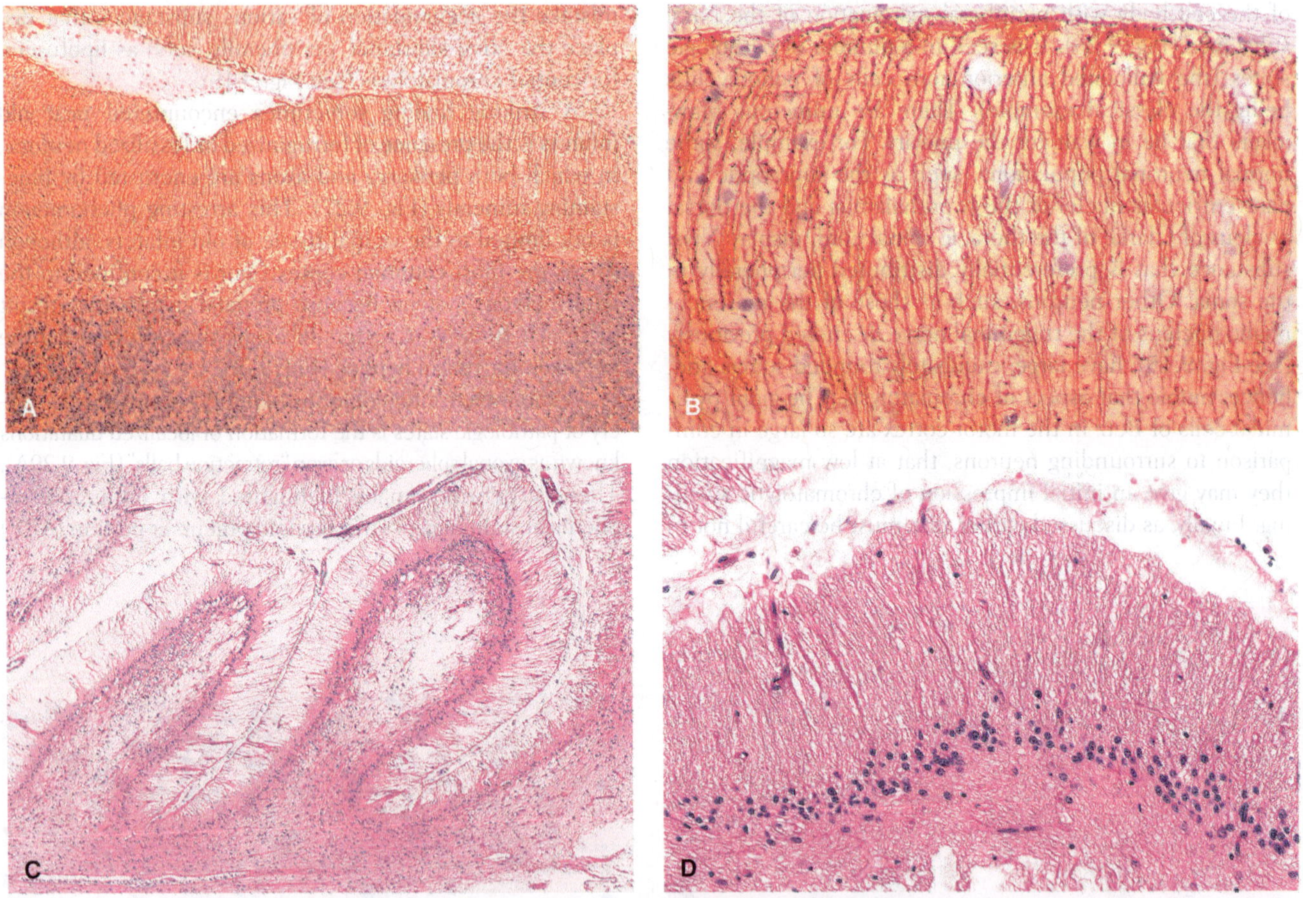

FIGURE 9.30 Bergmann glia: These astrocytes illustrate the fact that specialization is not confined to neurons. Bergmann astrocytes have cell bodies distributed in a narrow lamina of the cerebellar cortex coextensive with that of the Purkinje cells. Each cell sends an elongated process through the molecular layer to the subpial surface. These processes are not usually well seen in healthy cerebellum with routine H&E staining (see Fig. 9.8), but can be exquisitely visualized with immunohistochemistry for GFAP (**A,B**). An equally striking unmasking of this elegant architecture is often seen without the use of specialized staining techniques in areas of cerebellar cortex adjacent to healed infarcts, in which the degree of ischemia was sufficient to kill the indigenous neuronal populations but spared the more resistant Bergmann glia (**C,D**). Like other astrocytes throughout the CNS, Bergmann glia respond to ischemic insult by proliferating, resulting in an increased thickness of the cell body lamina referred to as "Bergmann gliosis" (**D**).

and ubiquitin. Ultrastructural examination shows greatly distended axis cylinders filled with bundles of neurofilaments and cellular organelles. A regional variant of this process may be observed in the granular cell layer of the cerebellum where focal dilatations of Purkinje cell axons are termed *torpedoes*. These structures are seen in a number of cerebellar degenerative diseases, as well as in normal aging. The most common site in the CNS where scattered axonal spheroids are routinely encountered as an incidental finding in aged individuals is in the rostral fasciculus gracilis of the medulla (Fig. 9.29B). Spheroids in this location are often mineralized.

Astrocytes

Normal Microscopic Anatomy

Like neurons, astrocytes are also heterogeneous. The cells of one class conform to the classic star shape, and occur as either the fibrillary or protoplasmic form. Fibrillary astrocytes populate the white matter, whereas the latter inhabit the gray matter. Other important subtypes of astrocytes include the "pilocytic" astrocytes of the periventricular region, cerebellum, spinal cord, and the Bergmann astrocytes, which are distributed in a narrow lamina between the cell bodies of Purkinje neurons in the cerebellar cortex (Fig. 9.30). In gray matter, nuclei of protoplasmic astrocytes cannot generally be distinguished from those of small neurons because the cytoplasm of both, blends imperceptibly into the surrounding neuropil and is not normally discernible as a discrete entity. In white matter, it is usually difficult in H&E-stained sections to distinguish fibrillary astrocytes from the much more numerous oligodendroglia. The nuclei of oligodendrocytes are smaller and more hyperchromatic, but usually these two cell types do not fall into two clearly defined groups. In sections stained for myelin, a very small amount of eosinophilic cytoplasm may occasionally, but not invariably, be seen surrounding normal astrocytic nuclei. This helps distinguish this cell from the oligodendrocyte whose cytoplasm, other than the myelin sheath, is not usually apparent by conventional light microscopy (see Fig. 9.38). Astrocytic cytoplasm becomes much more prominent when astrocytes respond to CNS injury, culminating in the abundant glassy cytoplasm of the gemistocyte (Fig. 9.31). To appreciate the distinctive morphology of the star cell, one must visualize its radiating processes. These thread-like extensions reach out to define a sphere of influence that is many times greater in extent than one would have suspected by looking at an H&E-stained section alone. Historically, this tinctorial feat was achieved through the technically capricious metallic impregnations, but now is accomplished with considerably greater ease and predictability by the immunohistochemical localization of glial fibrillary acidic protein (GFAP) (Fig. 9.31). In the case of the fibrillary astrocyte, processes branch infrequently, whereas those of the protoplasmic astrocyte are more numerous and divide more frequently. They are often less well stained with GFAP than the fibrillary types. Neither type of resting astrocyte is as apparent immunohistochemically as are reactive astrocytes.

The polar forms of astrocytes include the pilocytic and Bergmann types. The pilocytic astrocyte is not conspicuous in its native state, but becomes so when responding as gliosis and forming Rosenthal fibers. The latter are hyaline, often corkscrew-shaped, eosinophilic structures that are wedged within one of the cell's bipolar processes (Fig. 9.32). These structures are occasionally seen in normal brains in the hypothalamus or pineal gland, but become much more prominent in gliosis about such lesions as craniopharyngiomas, pineal cysts, cerebellar hemangioblastomas, and chronic lesions of the spinal cord.

The Bergmann astrocytes are confined to a one-to-two-cell thick lamina. Their polar processes extend to the pial surface of the cerebellum and are only faintly seen with difficulty in standard sections. Yet, they are well visualized with

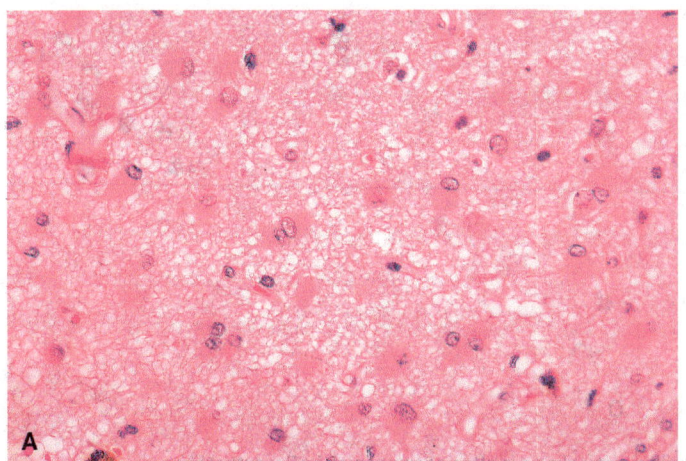
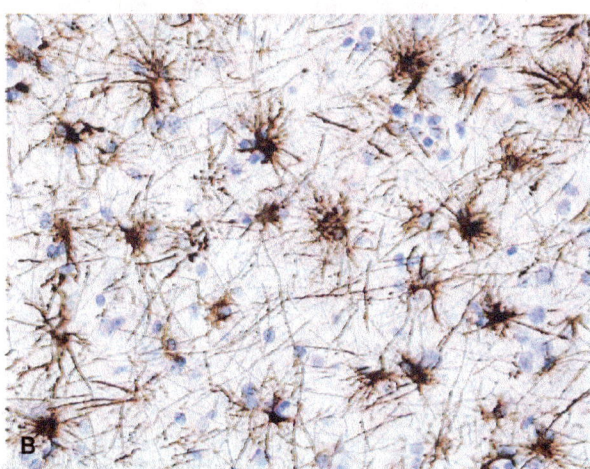

FIGURE 9.31 Reactive astrocytosis: The plainly visible cytoplasm and processes of the astrocytes seen in panel (**A**) is proof of an insult to the nervous system. Under normal conditions, only bare nuclei are usually seen. The extensive, radiating cytoplasmic processes for which the astrocyte received its name are most readily appreciated when reactive astrocytes are immunostained for GFAP (**B**). (*continued*)

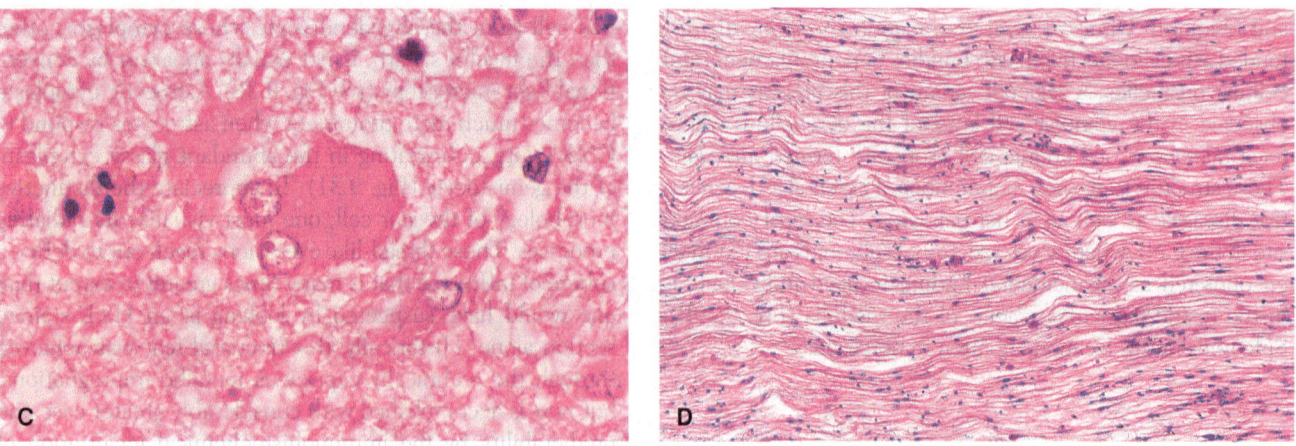

FIGURE 9.31 (*Continued*) Reactive astrocytes have been descriptively classified according to the amount and configuration of visible cytoplasm, and include the aptly named gemistocytic "laden" or "stuffed" cell (**C**), and pilocytic "hair cell" (**D**) types. Reactive gemistocytes are typical of the acute astrocytic reaction to CNS damage whereas dense fibrillary gliosis is commonly seen in longstanding lesions such as healed infarcts.

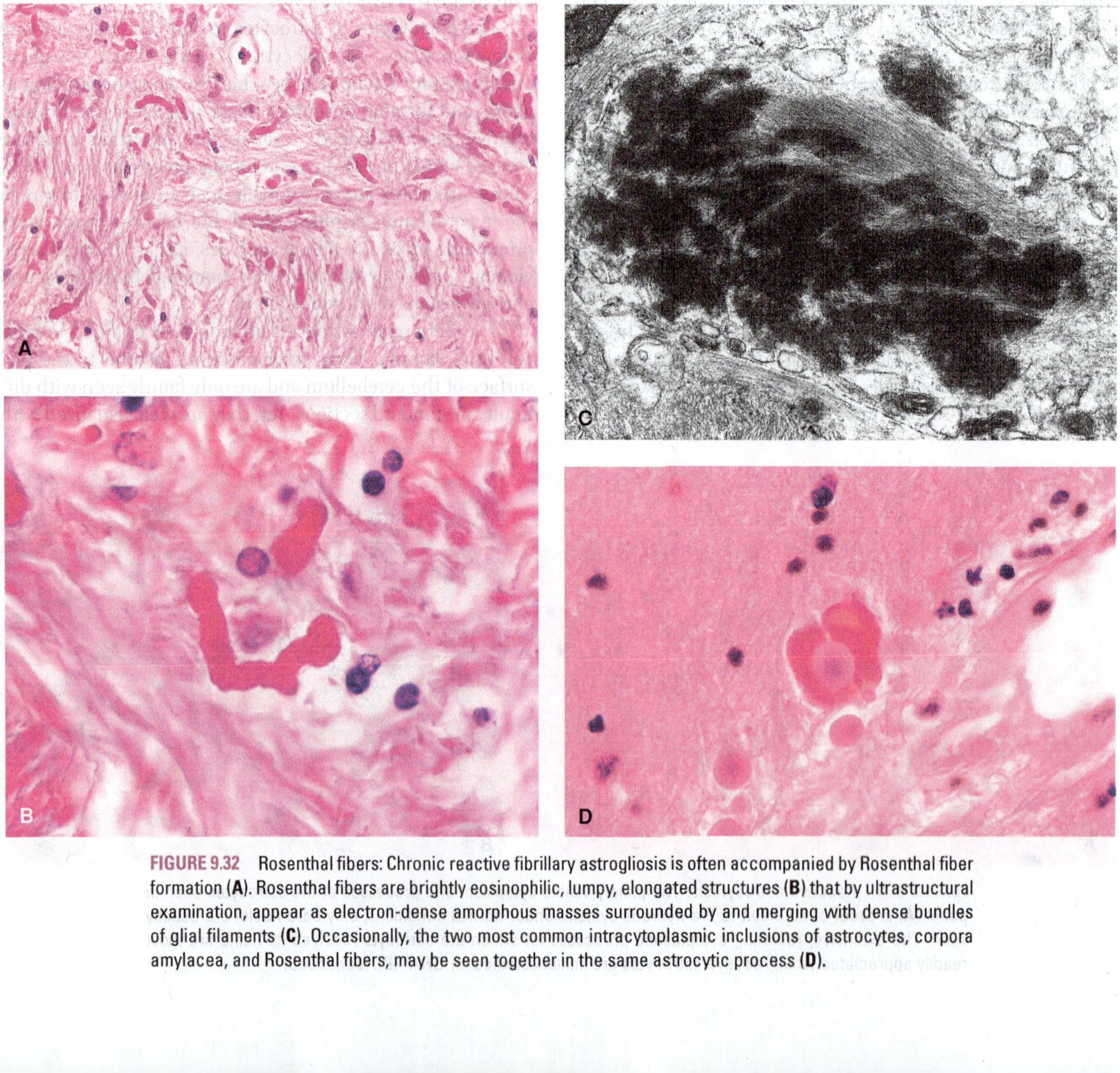

FIGURE 9.32 Rosenthal fibers: Chronic reactive fibrillary astrogliosis is often accompanied by Rosenthal fiber formation (**A**). Rosenthal fibers are brightly eosinophilic, lumpy, elongated structures (**B**) that by ultrastructural examination, appear as electron-dense amorphous masses surrounded by and merging with dense bundles of glial filaments (**C**). Occasionally, the two most common intracytoplasmic inclusions of astrocytes, corpora amylacea, and Rosenthal fibers, may be seen together in the same astrocytic process (**D**).

immunohistochemistry for GFAP and at the margins of old cerebellar infarcts (Fig. 9.30). The Bergmann glia provide an excellent illustration of astrocytic specialization. Their processes are a form of scaffold and serve as a reminder of the cooperative interplay between astrocytes and neurons during embryologic development. At that time, the small neurons of the external granular cell layer spiral down the Bergmann processes to reach their final destination in the internal granular cell layer.

Age-Related Inclusions in Astrocytes: Corpora Amylacea

The ubiquitous corpora amylacea are, by far, the most salient astrocytic inclusions encountered in routine sections. These faintly laminated, slightly basophilic polyglucosan bodies accumulate with age and are observed in greatest numbers where astrocytic foot processes are most numerous, particularly around blood vessels and beneath the pia (Fig. 9.33). The olfactory tracts of adults are also typically rich in corpora amylacea (see Fig. 9.52). The similarity between corpora amylacea and fungal yeast forms such as cryptococcus is a source of potential diagnostic error since both are strongly positive for methenamine silver, alcian blue, and PAS (Fig. 9.33). In some individuals, corpora amylacea are strikingly numerous although no pathologic significance has yet been attributed to this abundance.

Astrocytic Reactions to Injury

Although normally among the most morphologically demure of nervous system constituents (only naked nuclei are typically visible on routine H&E histology), astrocytes respond rapidly and dramatically to CNS injury. This response typically consists of two components: hypertrophy and hyperplasia. The initial hypertrophic response, an increase in cell size and cytoplasmic prominence, occurs rapidly following CNS insult. Conspicuous cytoplasm is generally indicative of reactive gliosis and constitutes prima facie evidence of CNS injury. Reactive astrocytes display a broad range of cytoplasmic quantity, from just barely perceptible to robustly embonpoint (Fig. 9.31). The latter cells are known as *gemistocytes* (literally "stuffed cells"). Gliosis may, of course, also present as an increase in the number and density of astrocytic nuclei without attendant cytoplasmic prominence. This chronic type of gliosis is frequently subtle and often requires special stains for confirmation and quantitation.

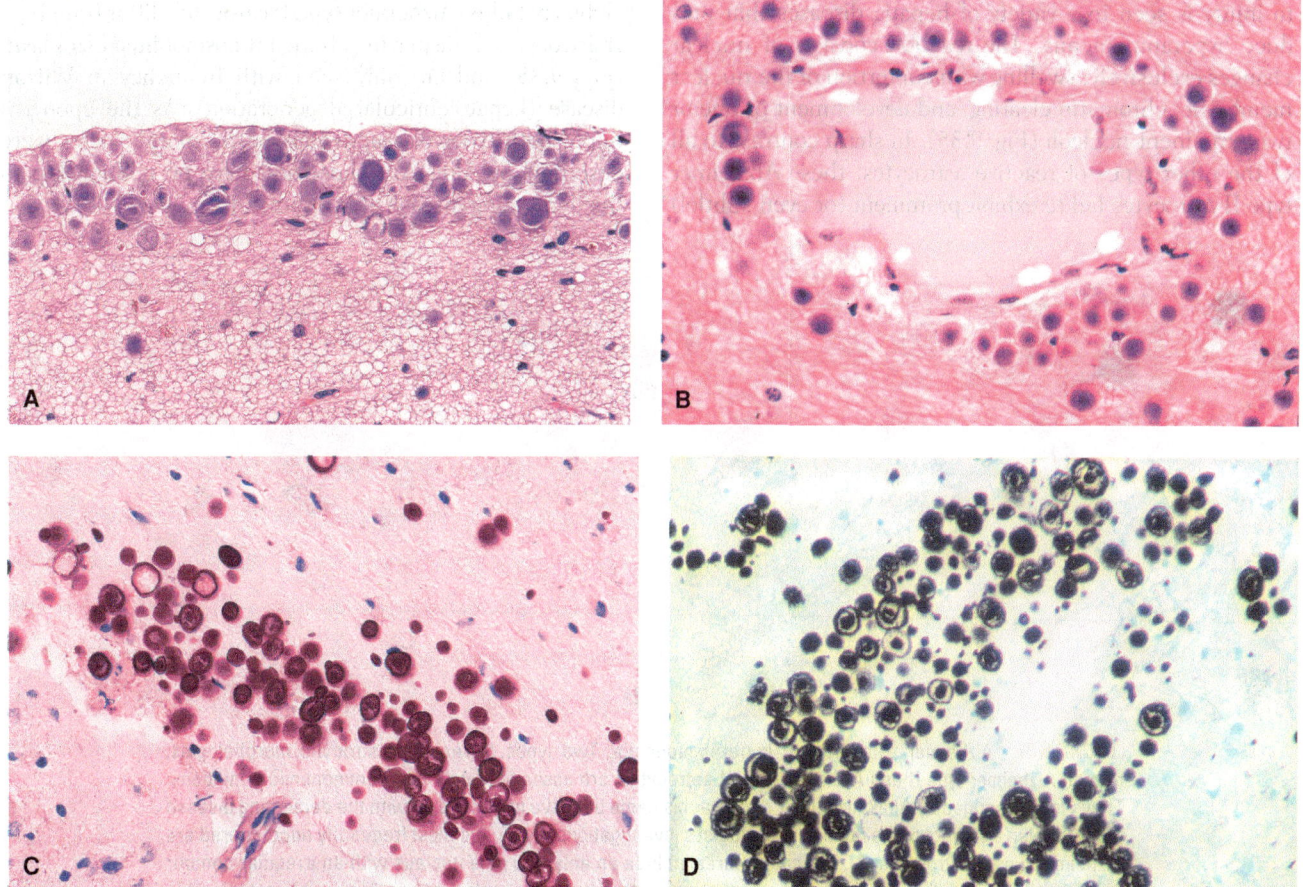

FIGURE 9.33 Corpora amylacea: These basophilic, lamellated polyglucosan bodies accumulate in astrocytic processes with age, most prominently in subpial (**A**) and perivascular (**B**) locations. Corpora amylacea can resemble fungal yeast forms and show strong positivity for fungal stains such as PAS-fungus (**C**) and Gomori methenamine silver (GMS) (**D**).

The end result of acute reactive astrogliosis, such as that accompanying cerebral infarction, is frequently a dense fibrillary gliosis (Fig. 9.31). The often-invoked analogy of the astrocyte as the "fibroblast of the CNS," that is, a ubiquitously distributed cell with mitotic capability that responds with alacrity to a wide range of deleterious stimuli, is quite apt. A distinctive cytoplasmic inclusion seen in fibrillary astrogliosis is the Rosenthal fiber (Fig. 9.32). These strikingly eosinophilic, elongated, anfractuous structures are observed in a wide variety of reactive states that share in common significant chronicity. Rosenthal fibers are also characteristic of several specific nosologic entities, including Alexander disease and, perhaps most widely known, juvenile pilocytic astrocytoma. It should be stressed, however, that Rosenthal fibers may be strikingly abundant in the chronically compressed glial stroma surrounding a large number of non-neoplastic conditions (such as syringomyelia), cysts (such as pineal cysts), and slowly expanding nonglial tumors (such as craniopharyngioma).

There are several specialized forms of reactive astrogliosis that deserve brief description. Reactive astrocytes with multiple small nuclei ("micronuclei"), termed "Creutzfeldt astrocytes," may be seen in a number of reactive or neoplastic states, but are especially typical of demyelinating processes (Fig. 9.34). A specific type of astrocytic reaction to injury is seen in a variety of hepatic diseases that produce hyperammonemia. The reaction consists of nuclear changes exclusively: swelling with contortion of the nuclear membrane, chromatin clearing, and development of one or two prominent nucleoli (Fig. 9.35). In sharp contrast to all of the other types of reactive astrocytes, these Alzheimer type II astrocytes fail to exhibit prominent (or even subtle!)

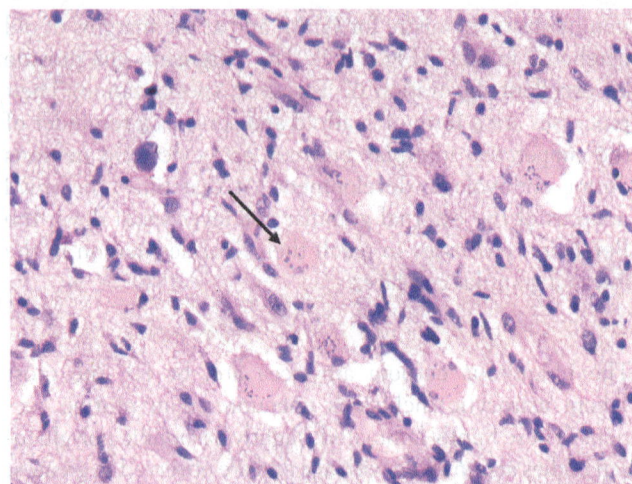

FIGURE 9.34 Granular mitoses (*white arrow*) and Creutzfeldt astrocytes (*black arrow*). These distinctive reactive astrocytes can be seen in a variety of pathologic conditions including tumors (as shown in this figure) but are particularly characteristic of demyelinating diseases.

cytoplasm by routine H&E microscopy. Alzheimer type II astrocytes may be seen throughout the neuraxis but are particularly prominent in certain locations, most notably the globus pallidus. Alzheimer type I astrocytes differ from type II astrocytes in displaying abundant eosinophilic cytoplasm (Fig. 9.35) and are only seen with frequency in Wilson disease (hepatolenticular degeneration). As the eponyms imply, both types of reactive astrocytic morphologies were described by Alois Alzheimer and have no relationship to the dementing disease of the same ilk.

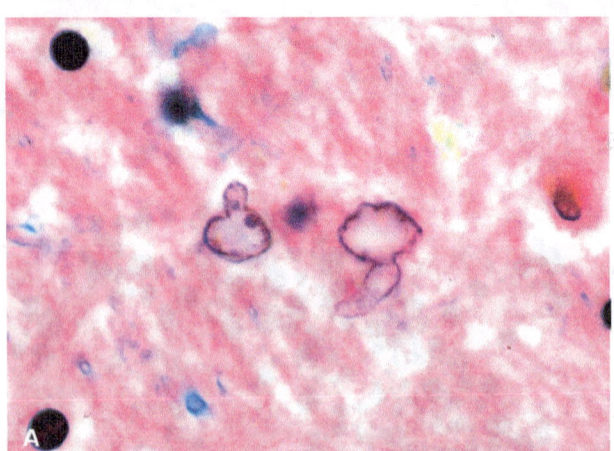
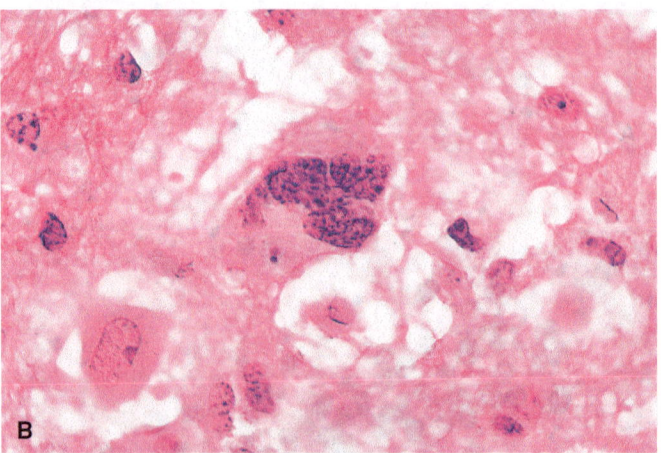

FIGURE 9.35 Alzheimer astrocytes in hyperammonemia: Two types of reactive astrocytic morphologies, termed Alzheimer type II and Alzheimer type I astrocytes, are associated with hyperammonemic conditions. They were described by Alois Alzheimer and bear his name but have nothing to do with the dementing disease that was also a subject of the famous neurologist's investigations. By far, the most frequently encountered are Alzheimer type II astrocytes (**A**). Typical features include an enlarged pale nucleus with an irregular contour and one or more small nucleoli. In marked contrast to other types of reactive astrocytes, visible cytoplasm is lacking. Alzheimer type II astrocytes are commonly seen in a wide variety of diseases that result in increased blood ammonia. In contrast, Alzheimer type I astrocytes (**B**) have large, irregularly lobulated or multiple nuclei and clearly discernible eosinophilic cytoplasm. These cells are not seen in most hyperammonemic diseases, with the exception of hepatolenticular degeneration (Wilson disease).

CHAPTER 9: Central Nervous System

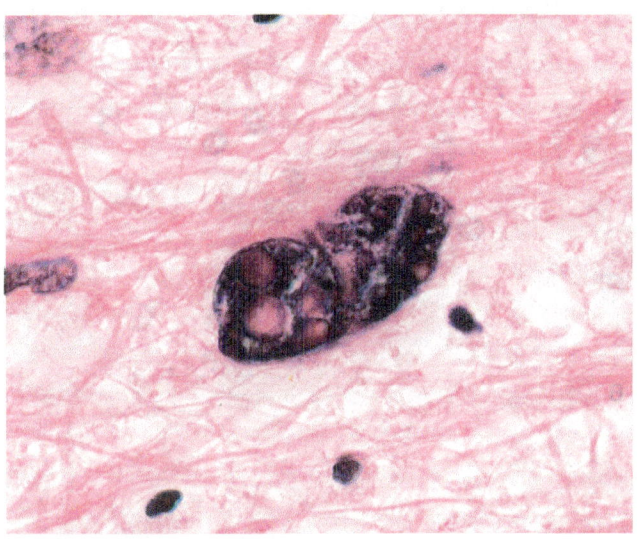

FIGURE 9.36 Bizarre reactive astrocytes of PML: Atypical-appearing reactive astrocytes are sometimes the most striking finding in a PML biopsy and can be mistaken for neoplasia by the unprepared.

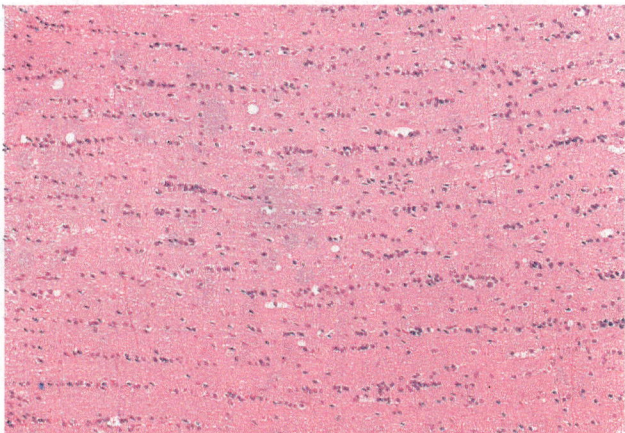

FIGURE 9.38 Oligodendroglia: As seen here in a white matter tract (the corpus callosum) cut in longitudinal section, these glia may be identified, even at low power, as rows of nuclei queuing up between fascicles of myelinated axons.

Among astrocytic reactions to injury, none is more striking than that observed in some cases of progressive multifocal leukoencephalopathy (PML). Not infrequently, the most eye-catching aspect of a PML biopsy is an alarming nuclear hyperchromatism and pleomorphism exhibited by scattered astrocytes—a vignette that has on more than one occasion elicited a mental frisson from even the most experienced observer (Fig. 9.36). Perivascular clearing is a routinely observed artifact of autolysis (Fig. 9.37). By electron microscopy, these clear spaces are revealed to be greatly dilated astrocytic perivascular foot processes. This phenomenon of water imbibition by astrocytes is seen both as an autolytic change in virtually all autopsy specimens and, when extreme, as a marker of antemortem hypoxic/ischemic injury.

Oligodendroglia

The oligodendroglia ("few branch" glia) are small cells that are active in the formation and maintenance of myelin and in the, as yet, poorly understood capacity of attending to neuronal cell bodies (satellitosis). In white matter, the oligodendrocytes' obligatory orientation to fiber pathways is occasionally made apparent by a fortuitous plane of section wherein the fascicular distribution of these cells is seen (Fig. 9.38). In gray matter, oligodendrocytes are encountered as two-to-three small, dark nuclei that are pressed against the cell membrane of larger neurons (Fig. 9.39). In surgical specimens obtained from infiltrating gliomas, these normal satellite oligodendroglia must be distinguished from infiltrating neoplastic cells that,

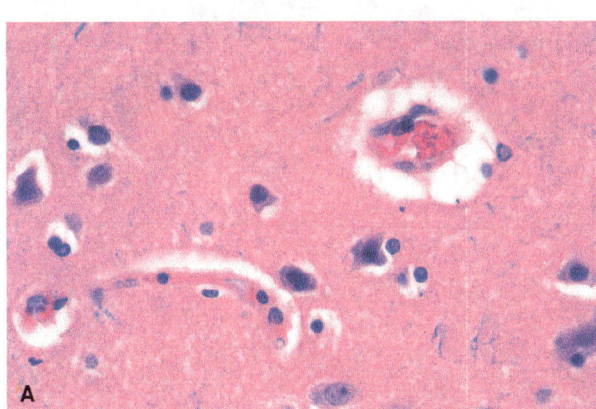

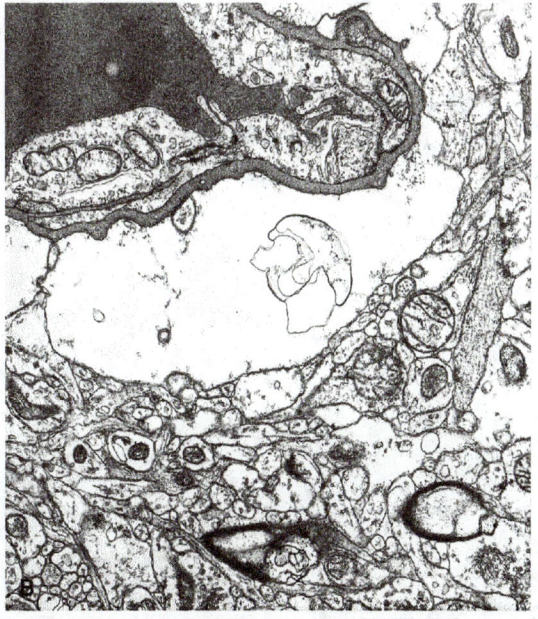

FIGURE 9.37 Perivascular astrocytic foot process swelling in autolysis: This common artifact of routine tissue processing is observed by light microscopy as apparent perivascular clearing of the neuropil (**A**). As seen by electron microscopy, the clearing is due to dilated astrocyte foot processes (**B**).

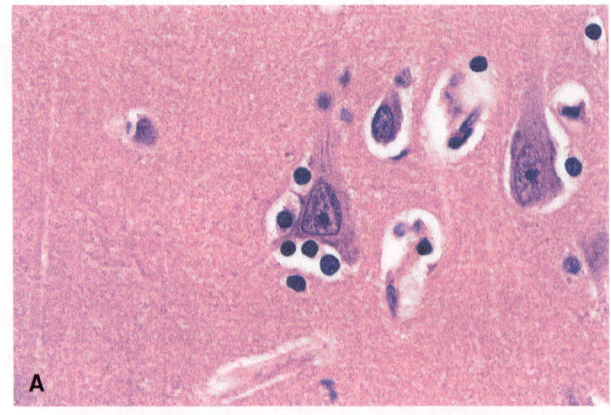
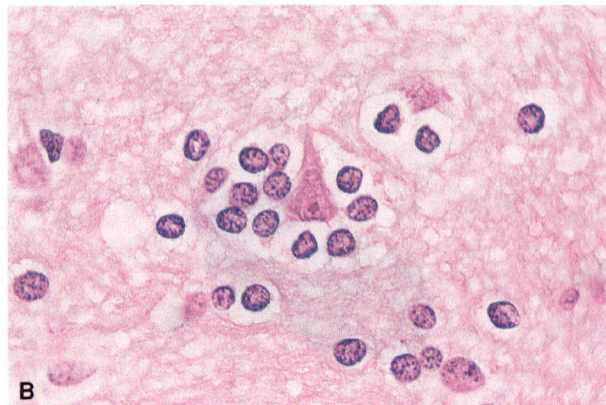
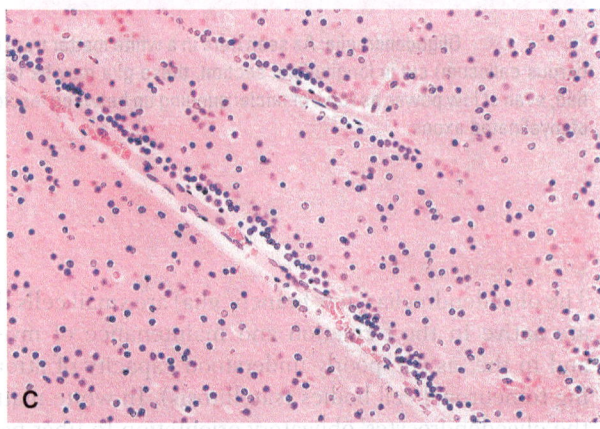

FIGURE 9.39 Perineuronal satellitosis: Normal perineuronal glia (**A**) consist primarily of oligodendroglial satellite cells, together with occasional astrocytes and microglia. This affinity of normal oligodendroglia for neuronal perikarya is often retained by their neoplastic counterparts, oligodendrogliomas, in the form of "neoplastic satellitosis" (**B**). Non-neoplastic oligodendroglial hyperplasia (**C**) can also be seen, as for example in some cases of longstanding epilepsy.

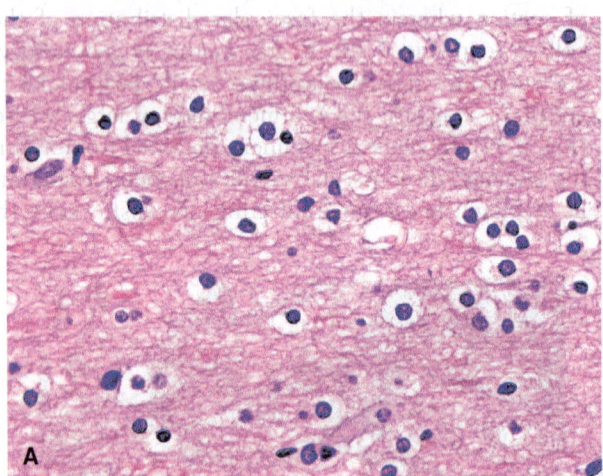
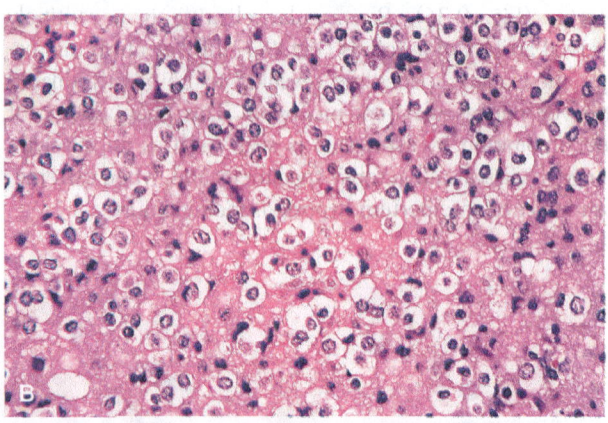
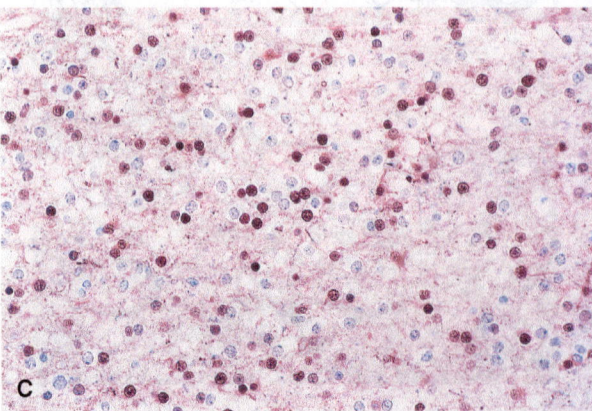

FIGURE 9.40 Oligodendroglia: In many specimens, oligodendroglia exhibit characteristic perinuclear halos (**A**). This "fried egg" appearance is an artifact of hypoxia/ischemia and delayed fixation, and is a useful diagnostic feature that is also exhibited by oligodendrogliomas (**B**). Oligodendroglia, both normal and neoplastic, typically show strong nuclear immunopositivity for S100 protein (**C**).

like their nontransformed counterparts, are attracted to the immediate perineuronal region. Both astrocytomas and oligodendrogliomas may exhibit such satellitosis, but it is most prominent in the latter neoplasm. In general, the nuclei of the neoplastic satellites are larger, more pleomorphic, and more coarsely constructed than the normal orbiting cortical oligodendrocytes.

Identification of normal oligodendroglia in both gray and white matters is greatly facilitated by these cells' perinuclear halo (the so-called fried egg appearance), which results from swelling and vacuolation of the cytoplasm (Fig. 9.40A). This is analogous to the perivascular swelling and vacuolation of astrocytic foot processes. In oligodendroglial neoplasms (oligodendrogliomas), the perinuclear halo is a well-known, distinctive, and diagnostically useful feature (Fig. 9.40B). Oligodendroglia and their neoplastic counterparts exhibit strong immunopositivity for S100 protein (Fig. 9.32C) and the transcription factor Olig2.

Ependyma

This cuboidal-to-columnar epithelium provides a lining for the CNS ventricular system (Fig. 9.41) and specializes focally as a covering for the choroid plexus (see Fig. 9.53).

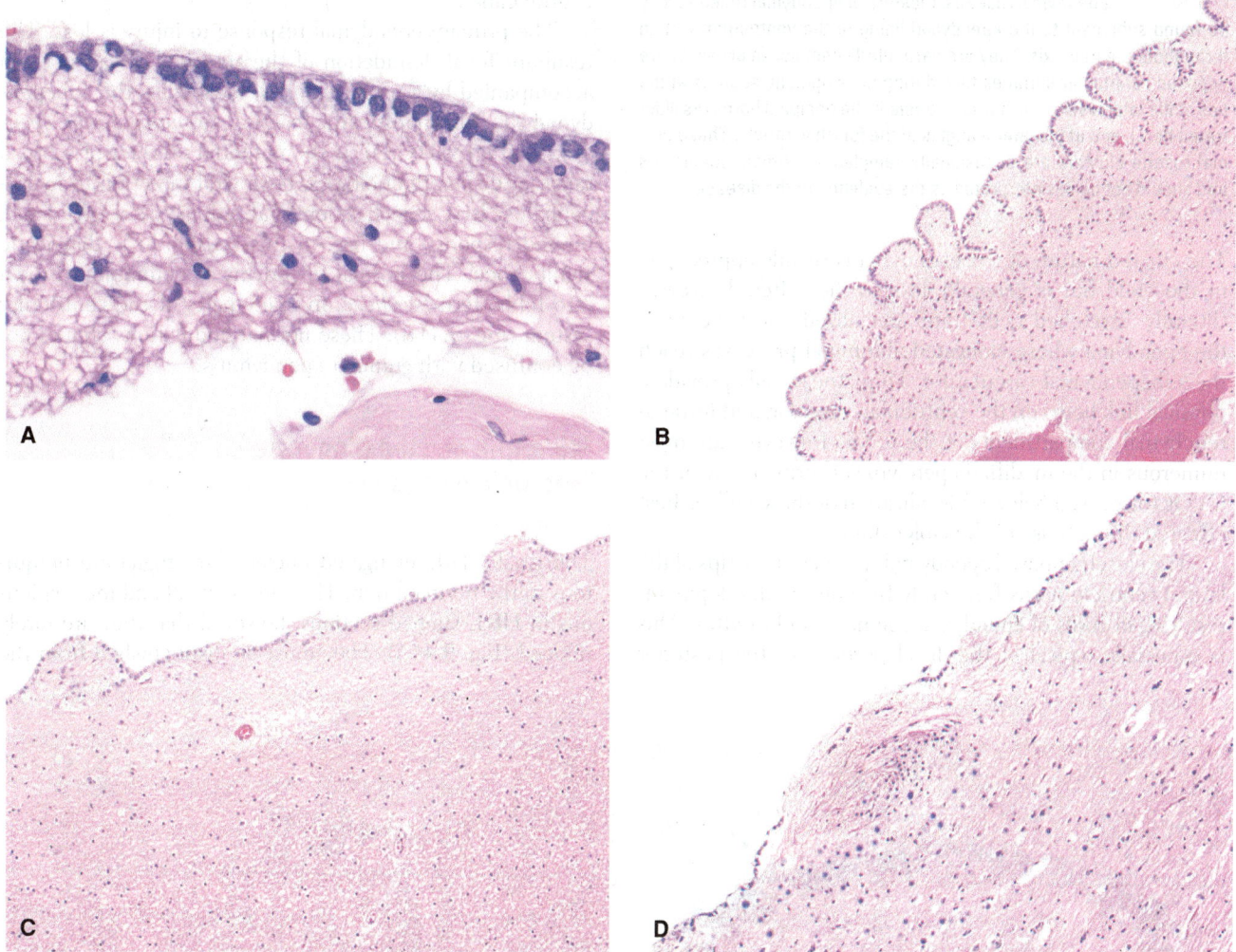

FIGURE 9.41 Ependyma and the subependymal plate: The lining of the ventricular system varies from a robust ciliated-columnar epithelium (**A**) to nearly squamous flattened cuboidal. The relative abundance of cilia and the height of the ependyma vary with anatomic location and both decrease with age. The hypocellular fibrillary zone located immediately subjacent to the ependyma is known as the subependymal plate and contains scattered glia as single cells and in small clusters. Glia of the subependymal plate respond to ependymal injury with a proliferative response termed granular ependymitis (**C,D**). Granular ependymitis, the combination of focal denudation of the ependyma, coupled with an exophytic fusiform proliferation of the subependymal glia constitutes granular ependymitis (**C,D**). Despite the implication of an inflammatory etiology inherent in the name, this common alteration can result from many diverse insults, ranging from hydrocephalus to viral infections. Normal undulations of the ependyma (**B**), termed *plicae*, should not be confused with granular ependymitis. Subependymomas originate from the glia of the ependyma and subependymal plate.

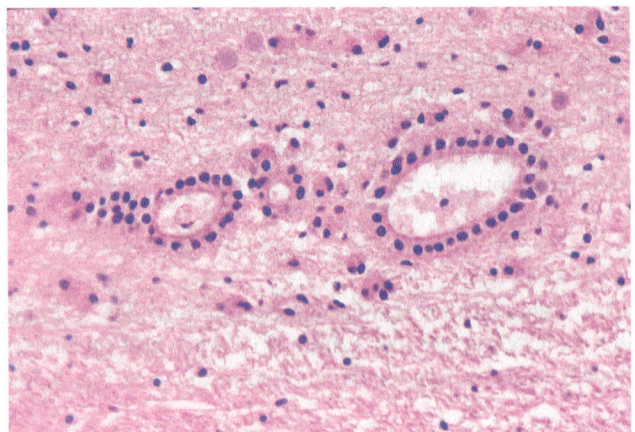

FIGURE 9.42 Ependymal rosettes: Clusters of ependymal rosettes may be found subjacent to the ependymal lining of the ventricular system throughout the neuraxis. They are particularly common in areas where opposed ventricular surfaces fuse during development, such as at the tips of the lateral ventricle horns, especially the occipital horns (as illustrated here), and at the lateral angles of the fourth ventricle. These normal rosette clusters are occasionally sampled in surgical specimens and should not be misinterpreted as the evidence of the disease.

The ciliated nature of the ependyma is readily appreciable in the child but is generally less so thereafter. Tanycytes (literally "stretched cells") are specialized constituents of the ependyma whose elongated abluminal processes reach the subependymal vasculature. Thus, these cells provide a physical link between the ventricular, vascular, and intraparenchymal compartments of the CNS. Tanycytes are most numerous in the modified ependyma covering many of the CVOs (discussed below). Visualization of these cells is best effected through use of the Golgi stain.

The closely apposed ependymal surfaces of the tips of the lateral ventricle horns frequently fuse during development, resulting in cords of ependymal cell nests and rosettes. This is especially typical of the distal portions of the posterior horns in the occipital lobes (Fig. 9.42). The white matter in such areas appears pale and can simulate the rarefaction seen after ischemic insult. Detached ependymal rosettes may be encountered subjacent to the ventricular lining at any location throughout the neuraxis.

The ependyma-lined central canal of the spinal cord is patent in the child (Fig. 9.43) but generally becomes obliterated about the time of puberty, unless obstructive hydrocephalus is present. In the latter case, the canal may remain patent and even become dilated (hydromyelia). In the normal adult, however, the spinal ependymal cells have completed their role as a generative epithelium and remain as scattered clumps and rosettes (Fig. 9.43B). Occasional sections of adult spinal cord may exhibit a focally patent central canal.

The primary ependymal response to injury is loss. The resultant focal denudation of the ventricular wall is often accompanied by a proliferation of local cells, the subependymal glia. This nonspecific reaction, termed *granular ependymitis* (Fig. 9.41C,D), is the potential product of a broad range of disparate etiologies, from viral infection to hydrocephalus. It is seen frequently at autopsy as a very focal, limited response and has, in this setting, little diagnostic significance. The normal ependyma is commonly thrown into folds, termed *plicae*, in many parts of the ventricular system (Fig. 9.41B). These normal undulations should not be confused with granular ependymitis.

Microglia and the Monocyte—Macrophage System

Normal Microscopic Anatomy

The small, dark, elongated nuclei of microglia are ubiquitous in the normal brain. They are so small and inconspicuous in H&E-stained sections, however, that they are rarely noticed (Fig. 9.44A). They must be distinguished from the

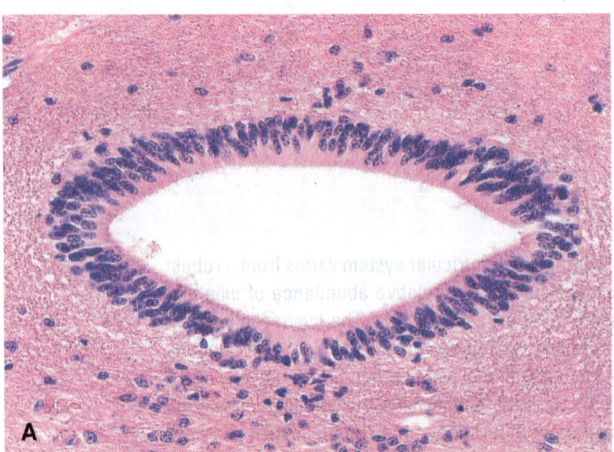
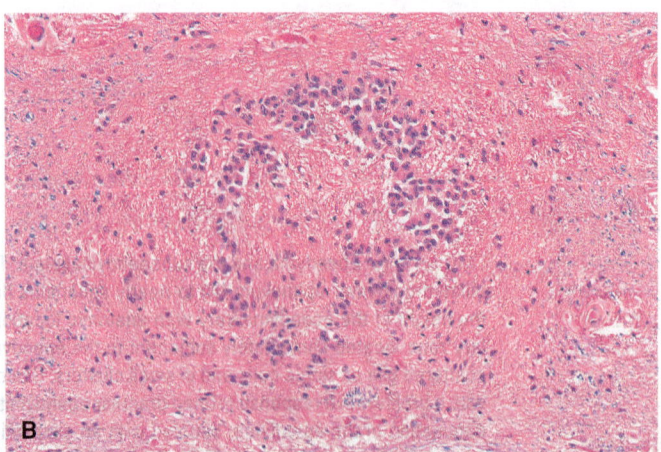

FIGURE 9.43 Central canal of the spinal cord: In the child (**A**), the central canal is widely patent and exhibits the ciliated columnar ependymal lining expected in a young individual. In contrast, the central canal of adults is typically obliterated over much of its length, with only residual small nests and occasional rosettes of ependymal cells (**B**).

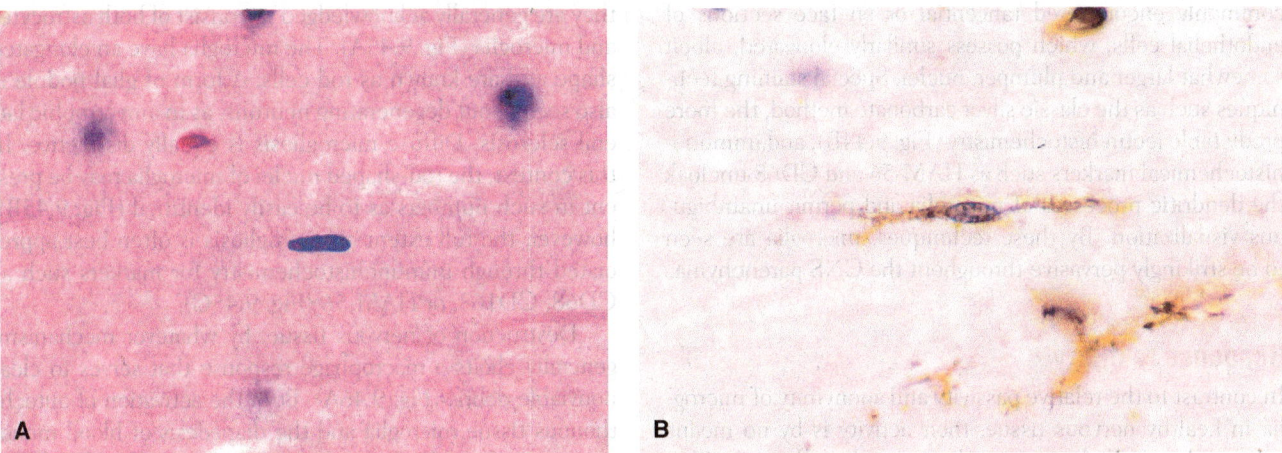

FIGURE 9.44 Microglia: These normally inconspicuous residents of the CNS parenchyma are identifiable by their classical rod-shaped nuclei on routine H&E staining (**A**). Dendritic processes, often bipolar, are vividly demonstrated by lectin staining (**B**).

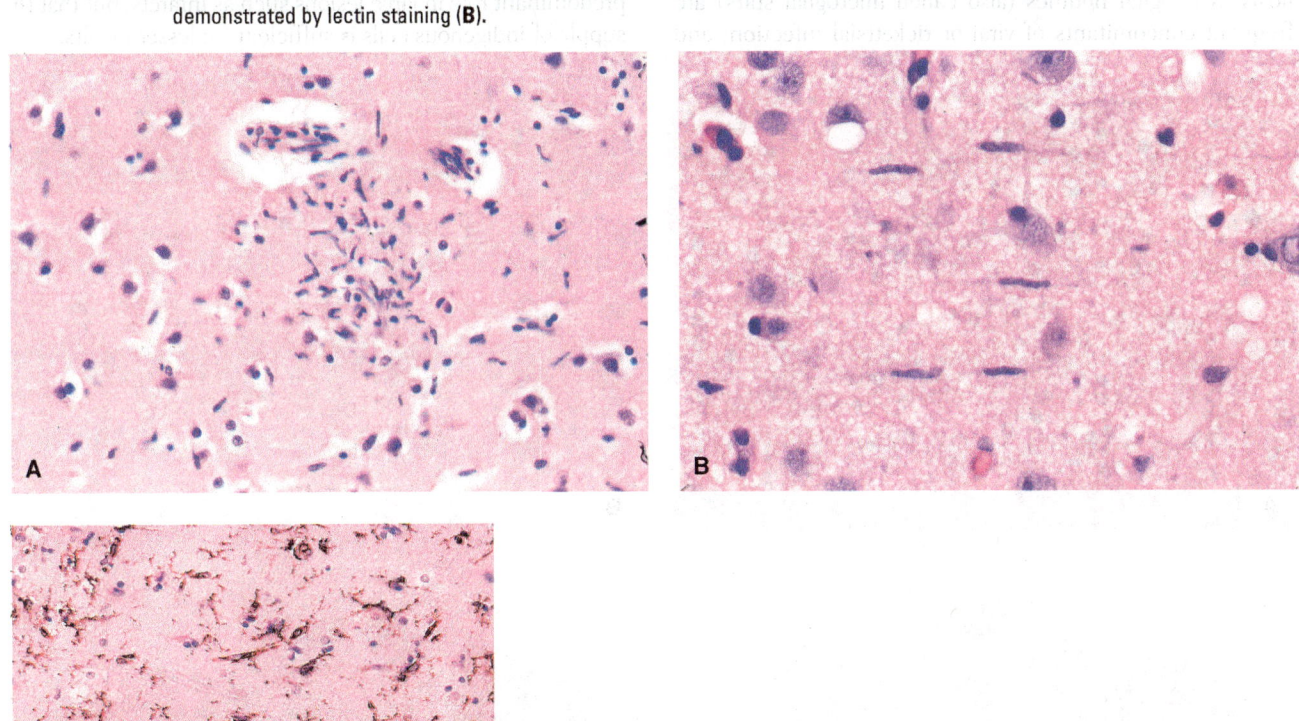

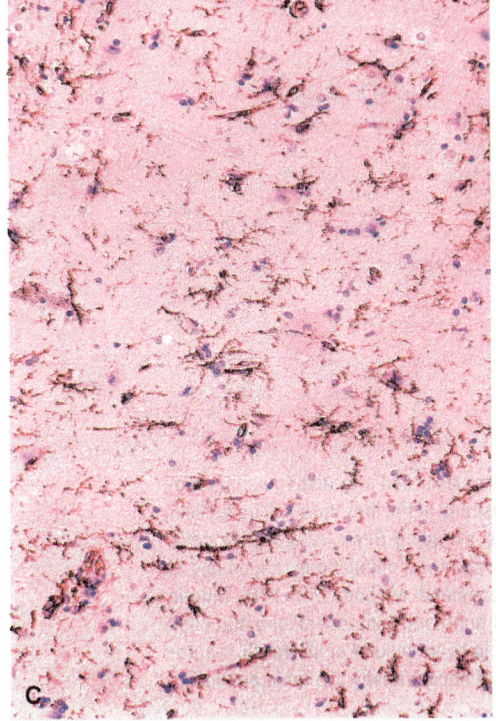

FIGURE 9.45 Microglia: Reactive microglia may assume several forms. Microglial nodules (**A**) are focal hypercellular collections of microglia together with reactive astrocytes that commonly form as a response to viral and rickettsial infections. In diffuse microgliosis (**B**), seen in a variety of conditions, including ischemia, the characteristic elongated rod-shaped nuclei can be identified on H&E-stained sections, but the true extent of their presence is more accurately visualized through immunohistochemistry, as seen here with HAM-56 (**C**).

commonly encountered tangential or en face sections of endothelial cells, which possess similarly elongated, albeit somewhat larger and plumper, nuclei. Special staining techniques such as the classic silver carbonate method, the more predictable lectin histochemistry (Fig. 9.44B), and immunohistochemical markers such as HAM-56 and CD68 uncloak the dendritic processes of microglia and permit unambiguous visualization. By these techniques, microglia are seen to be strikingly pervasive throughout the CNS parenchyma.

Response to Injury

In contrast to the relative passivity and anonymity of microglia in healthy nervous tissue, their activity is by no means subtle when called to action by parenchymal injury. Two variants are seen: microglial nodules and diffuse microgliosis. Microglial nodules (also called microglial stars) are frequent concomitants of viral or rickettsial infection; and they are generally acknowledged to consist of both astrocytes and microglia (Fig. 9.45A). The microglia have an elongated shape and are known as rod cells. A form of glial nodule is also seen about degenerating neurons, as in amyotrophic lateral sclerosis. Diffuse microgliosis is equally distinctive. In this context, the rod-shaped nuclei of microglia may be present in such numbers as to be easily identified (Fig. 9.45B); however, the full extent of microgliosis is often best appreciated through immunohistochemistry for markers such as CD68, CD163, or HAM-56 (Fig. 9.45C).

Destruction of nervous tissue, by whatever mechanism, generally elicits a macrophage response that serves to clear nonviable debris (Fig. 9.46A). Both the activation of autochthonous tissue microglia and the diapedesis of blood monocytes are sources for these scavengers. The weight of evidence suggests that the recruitment of blood monocytes plays a predominant role in large lesions such as infarcts, but that the supply of indigenous cells is sufficient for lesser insults.

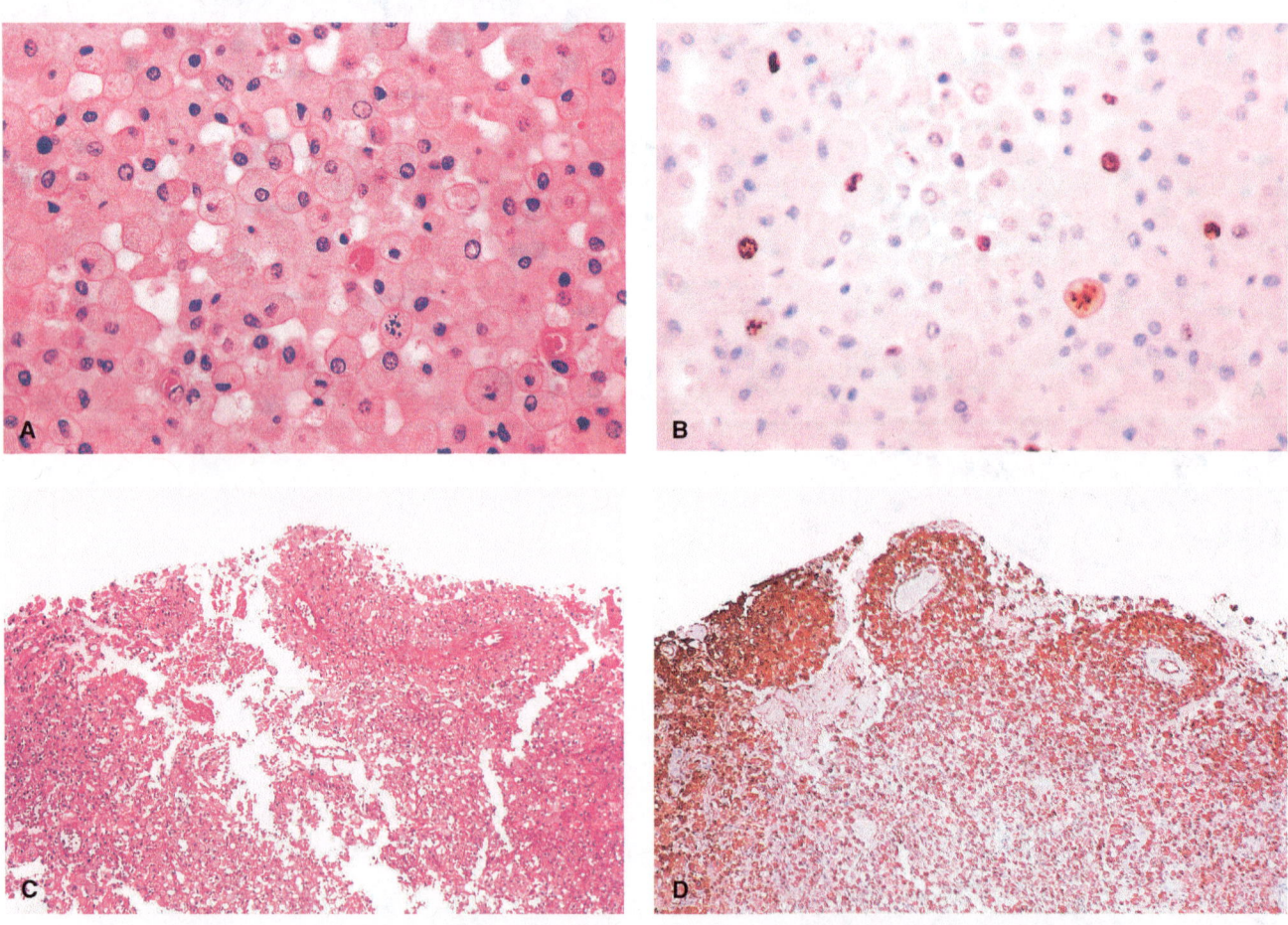

FIGURE 9.46 Macrophages: Discrete cell boundaries and vesicular cytoplasm serve to distinguish macrophages from other cellular constituents of the nervous system (**A**). Cognoscenti of the literature will be familiar with a number of colorful appellations given these cells in former times, including *Gitter cells (lattice cells)* and *compound granular corpuscles*. Macrophages are mitotically active cells and populations responding to CNS injury are readily labeled with proliferation markers such as the monoclonal antibody MIB-1 (**B**). Mitotic figures are, thus, to be expected in tissue samples from a wide range of non-neoplastic conditions that elicit a macrophage response, including infarcts and demyelinative diseases. In hypercellular biopsies (**C**), macrophages can be separated from other cellular constituents by a number of commercially available antibodies such as HAM-56, CD68, and CD163 (**D**).

Macrophages are proliferative cells (Fig. 9.46A, B). Mitotic figures will, therefore, usually be present in disease processes that elicit a macrophage response, such as infarction and demyelination. They should not be interpreted as suggestive of a neoplastic process. Macrophages often contribute substantially to the cellularity of tissue samples and, depending on preservation and fixation conditions, their identity may not always be obvious. For example, in some specimens, clearing of the macrophage cytoplasm lends an appearance similar to that of oligodendroglial cells, to the extent that, together with the attendant hypercellularity, an infiltrating glioma might be suspected. In such instances a number of antibodies, such as KP-1, Ham-56 or CD163, can be used to identify the macrophage component (Fig. 9.46C, D).

SPECIALIZED ORGANS OF THE CENTRAL NERVOUS SYSTEM

Pineal Gland

The pineal body (epiphysis or conarium) presents a singular histologic appearance among CNS tissues with a prominently lobulated architecture (Figs. 9.47 and 9.48). This glandular appearance might be mistaken for carcinoma by the unwary, and it can be difficult to distinguish the normal pineal gland from a well-differentiated pineocytoma in small surgical specimens.

Generally present in the pineal gland after puberty are corpora arenacea (acervuli cerebri or "brain sand"). These mineralized concretions accrue with age and confer the radiologic hyperdensity that, before the era of computerized tomography and magnetic resonance imaging (MRI), made the normal midline position of the pineal gland a useful radiologic landmark (Fig. 9.47). The increase in corpora arenacea with senescence is accompanied by gradual gliosis and cystic change, with attendant effacement of the lush glandular appearance of the pineal gland seen in the earlier decades of life. The ubiquitous incidental pineal cysts typically have densely gliotic walls with scattered Rosenthal fiber formation (Fig. 9.48C). The investing leptomeninges of the pineal gland contain arachnoid cell nests that occasionally give rise to meningiomas of the pineal region (Fig. 9.47). Pineocytes express strong immunopositivity for the neuronal marker synaptophysin (Fig. 9.49A). This useful phenotypic marker is retained by most pineal parenchymal neoplasms. In addition to pineocytes, the pineal gland also contains an indigenous population of astrocytes whose distribution is revealed by immunostaining for GFAP (Fig. 9.49B).

Median Eminence and Infundibulum

The median eminence, infundibulum, and neurohypophysis display a unique constellation of morphologic features that reflect their specialized neuroendocrine functions.

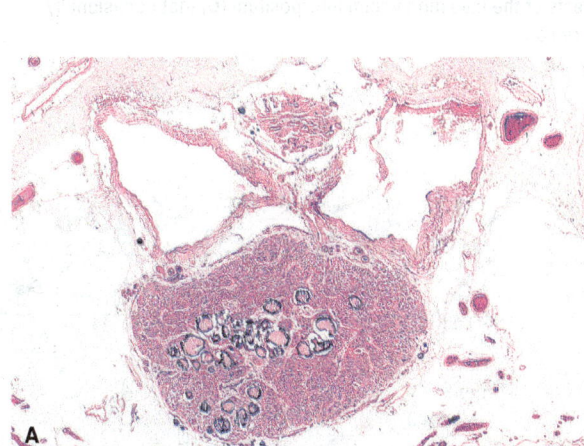
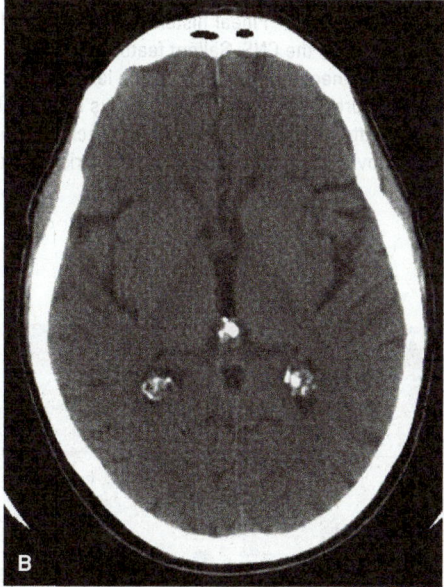

FIGURE 9.47 Pineal gland (epiphysis): Whole mount of a cross section of the pineal gland and its environs in situ (**A**) reveals the typical mineralized concretions variously referred to as corpora arenacea ("sand bodies"), acervuli cerebri ("little heaps"), or simply brain sand. Superior to the pineal gland are the paired internal cerebral veins, and between them is the suprapineal recess of the third ventricle which is lined with ependyma and often contains a tuft of choroid plexus. The loose connective tissue (redundant leptomeninges), in which all of these structures are located, is called velum interpositum. The calcification of the pineal gland increases with age and was, thereby, quite useful as a radiographic midline marker prior to the advent of contemporary high-resolution neuroimaging modalities (**B**). Also seen in this radiograph of a normal adult brain are prominently calcified tufts of choroid plexus (glomera choroidea; see Fig. 9.53) in the atria of both lateral ventricles.

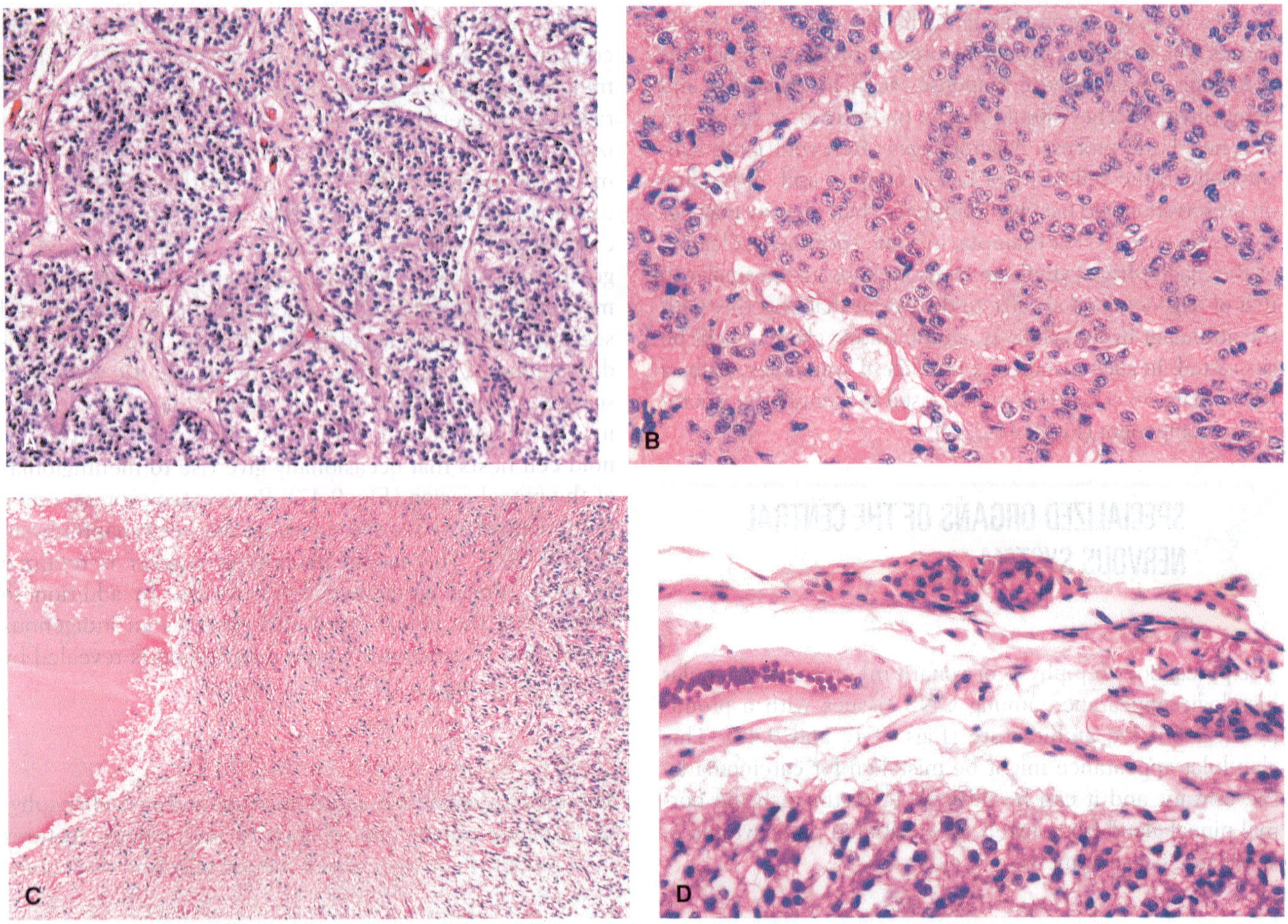

FIGURE 9.48 Pineal histology: The pineal gland has a richly glandular architecture that is unlike any other region of the CNS. Salient features include a prominent lobular organization with connective tissue septa (**A**) and pineocytic rosettes (**B**). The latter impart a distinctly neuroendocrine character. Two additional histologic features of note are the ubiquitous incidental pineal cysts, whose walls (**C**) typically exhibit astrogliosis with scattered Rosenthal fibers, and arachnoid cell nests of the investing velum interpositum (**D**) that occasionally provide a source for meningiomas arising in this region.

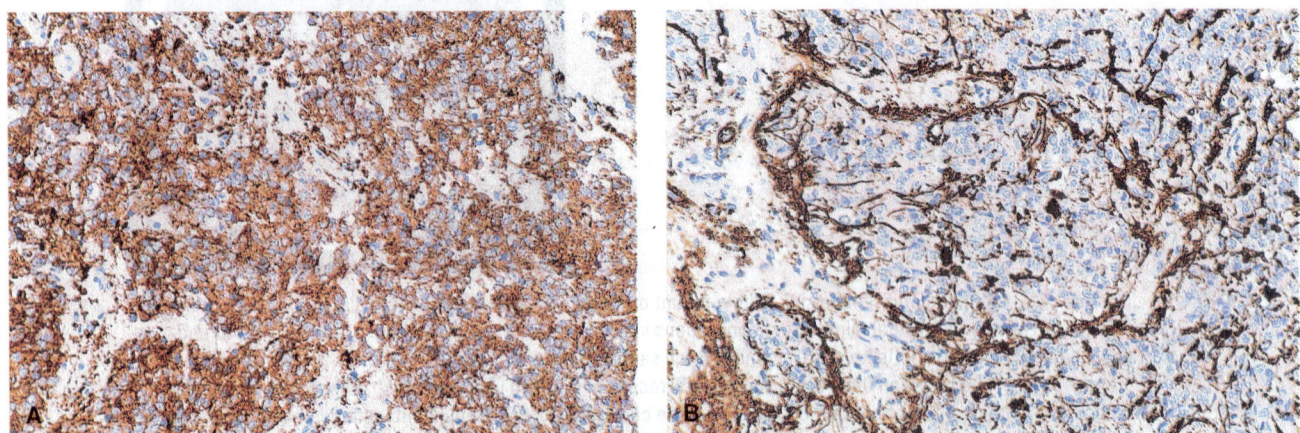

FIGURE 9.49 Pineal immunohistochemistry: Pineocytes (and their neoplastic progeny, the pineal parenchymal tumors) are strongly immunopositive for the neuronal marker synaptophysin (**A**). As expected, the indigenous populations of pineal astrocytes are well visualized with antibodies directed against GFAP (**B**).

The background stroma is highly spindled (Fig. 9.50A) and contains nodular microvascular tangles termed gomitoli (Fig. 9.50B), spherical granular bodies called Herring bodies (Fig. 9.50C, Table 9.1), which are storage sites for oxytocin and vasopressin, and scattered cells bearing lipofuscin-like brown pigment (Fig. 9.50D). The constellation of features comprising a highly spindled background, vascular tangles, and granular bodies gives this region of the CNS more than a passing resemblance to pilocytic astrocytoma. An additional incidental finding, particularly in tissue sections of the infundibulum, is the presence of small clusters of granular cells, termed granular cell tumorlets (Fig. 9.50E). The cells from the neurohypophysis express the thyroid transcription factor 1 (TTF-1) (Fig. 9.50F). This protein is not expressed by cells of the adenohypophysis, therefore, this is a useful tool for identifying tumors that

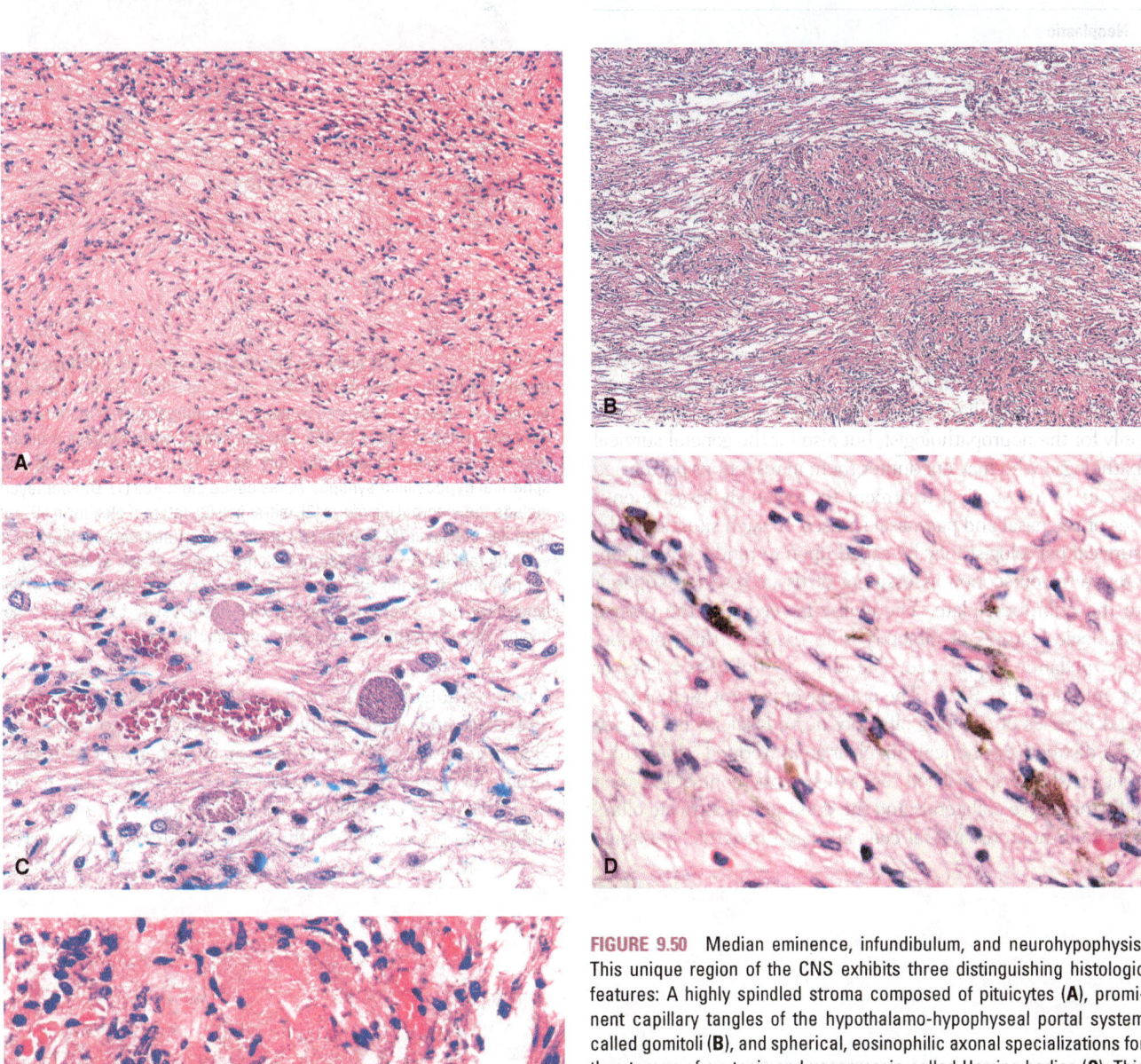

FIGURE 9.50 Median eminence, infundibulum, and neurohypophysis: This unique region of the CNS exhibits three distinguishing histologic features: A highly spindled stroma composed of pituicytes (**A**), prominent capillary tangles of the hypothalamo-hypophyseal portal system called gomitoli (**B**), and spherical, eosinophilic axonal specializations for the storage of oxytocin and vasopressin called Herring bodies (**C**). This constellation of highly spindled stroma, vascular tangles, and granular bodies bears a resemblance to pilocytic astrocytoma. The presence of lipofuscin-like pigment is also very characteristic (**D**). Small clusters of granular cells ("granular cell tumorlet") may be seen, particularly in the infundibulum (**E**), as an incidental finding, but occasionally reach a sufficient size to produce compression of the infundibulum and subsequent clinical presentation with mildly elevated serum prolactin ("stalk effect"). Cells from the neurohypophysis express thyroid transcription factor 1 (TTF-1), a useful marker for the identification of neoplasms that originate from this site (**F**). In contrast, cells from the adenohypophysis do not express TTF-1.

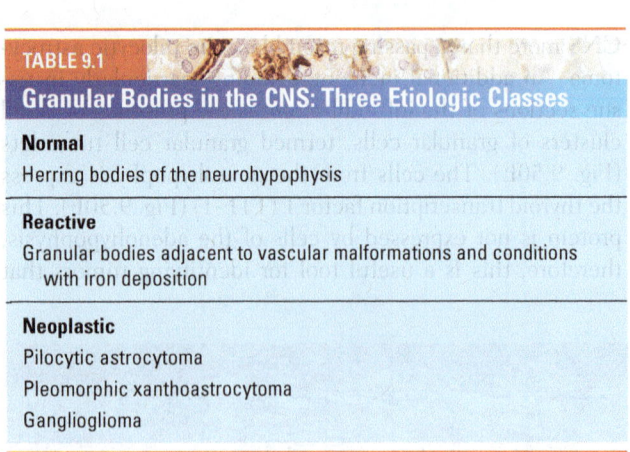

TABLE 9.1 Granular Bodies in the CNS: Three Etiologic Classes

Normal
Herring bodies of the neurohypophysis

Reactive
Granular bodies adjacent to vascular malformations and conditions with iron deposition

Neoplastic
Pilocytic astrocytoma
Pleomorphic xanthoastrocytoma
Ganglioglioma

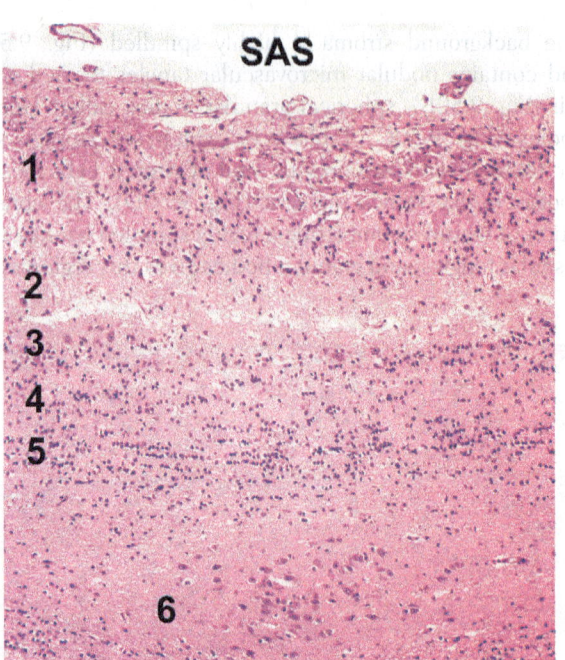

originate from the neurohypohysis; such as pituicytoma, spindle cell oncocytoma, and granular cell tumor.

Olfactory Bulbs and Tracts

The intracranial components of the olfactory apparatus (the olfactory bulbs and tracts) have a very distinctive histologic appearance. Familiarity with these structures is useful, not only for the neuropathologist, but also for the general surgical pathologist who may encounter them in resections performed as part of the surgical treatment for regionally invasive entities of the nasal and paranasal sinuses. In such situations, the surgical pathologist may be called upon to render an intraoperative frozen-section assessment of tissue resected superior to the cribriform plate. The ability to recognize the normal histologic features of olfactory bulb tissue is, thus, of more than pedantic importance. The olfactory bulb has a laminar organization (Fig. 9.51). The outer layer is composed of spindled bundles of entering olfactory nerve fascicles intermixed with distinctive spherical, anuclear areas (termed "glomeruli") that constitute specialized zones of synaptic contact between olfactory nerve collaterals and the dendrites of intrinsic olfactory bulb neurons. Mitral cells are large neurons, so-named

FIGURE 9.51 Olfactory bulb: The olfactory bulbs (see Fig. 9.3) have a very distinctive laminar organization. The most superficial layer, termed the glomerular layer (1) is covered by the leptomeninges (pia-arachnoid) and the subarachnoid space (*SAS*). The glomerular layer displays a unique architecture, with spindled olfactory nerve fascicles intermixing with spherical hypocellular synaptic zones called glomeruli (1). Deeper layers include the external plexiform (2), mitral cell (3), internal plexiform (4), and granular cell layer (5). Deeper still is the anterior olfactory nucleus (6). A working familiarity with olfactory bulb histology is essential for the surgical pathologist as this structure is frequently seen in the frozen-section laboratory during resection of superior nasal cavity tumors that may invade the cribriform plate and overlying olfactory bulbs.

for a resemblance of the perikaryon shape to a bishop's mitre. Their cell bodies are located in a lamina deep to that of the glomeruli (Fig. 9.51). The deepest layer consists of a thick lamina of granular cell neurons that are comparable in size to those of the cerebellum and dentate gyrus. The olfactory tracts (sometimes incorrectly referred to as olfactory nerves)

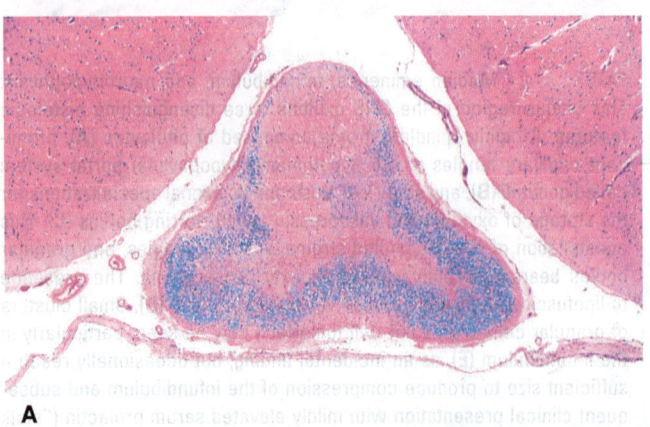
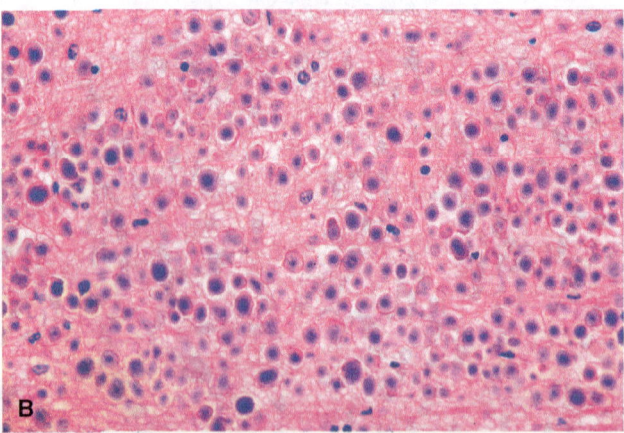

FIGURE 9.52 Olfactory tracts: The olfactory tracts contain myelinated fiber bundles and are roughly triangular in cross section (**A**). A distinctive feature of the tracts frequently observed in adults is their remarkable content of corpora amylacea (**B**).

extend posteriorly from the olfactory bulbs. They are triangular in cross section and, in adults, are notable for their profuse numbers of corpora amylacea (Fig. 9.52).

Choroid Plexus

The choroid plexus is a specialized organ of the CNS that is responsible for the production of cerebrospinal fluid. It is found in the body, atrium, and temporal horns of the lateral ventricles, in the interventricular foramina of Monro, in the roof of the third ventricle, and in the roof and lateral recesses of the fourth ventricle. The frontal and occipital horns of the lateral ventricles and the aqueduct of Sylvius are devoid of choroid plexus. The plexus is most obvious in the atria of the lateral ventricles (Fig. 9.53), where prominent bilateral tufts (glomera choroidea) are formed. Cystic xanthomatous change is a common incidental finding in these botryoid structures. The plexus is also a normal resident in the subarachnoid space of the cerebellopontine angle (CPA) cisterns, which it reaches from the lateral recesses of the fourth ventricle by protruding through the foramina of Luschka (Fig. 9.53). The paired foramina of Luschka (lateral), which open laterally into the ventral basilar CPA cisterns, are to be distinguished from the single foramen of Magendie (median), which opens in the dorsal midline into the cisterna magna.

Microscopically, choroid plexus consists of invaginated fronds of vascular leptomeninges covered by an ependyma that is modified to become a highly secretory epithelium (Fig. 9.54). The cells are larger and more cobblestoned than those of the adjacent ependyma (Fig. 9.41). In addition to collagen and blood vessels, small nests of meningothelial (arachnoid)

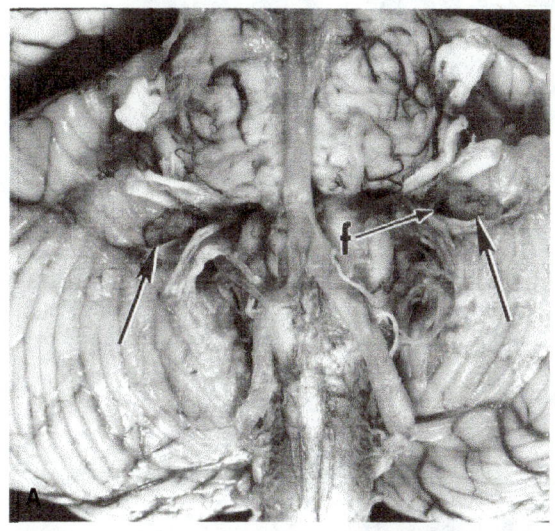

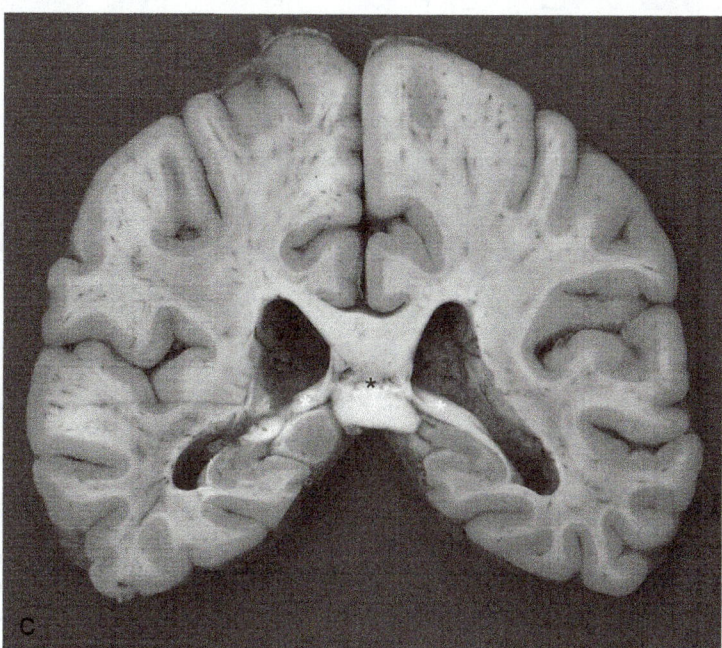

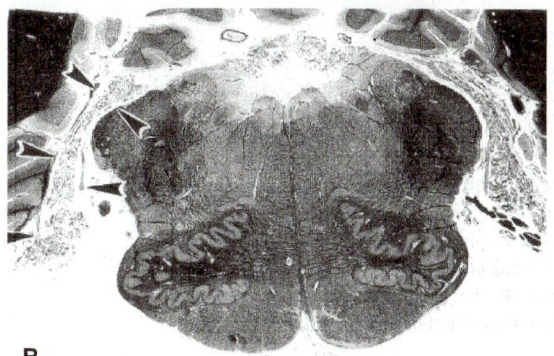

FIGURE 9.53 Choroid plexus: Choroid plexus produces the cerebrospinal fluid and is found in the lateral ventricles, foramen of Monro, roof of the third ventricle, and fourth ventricle. **A:** Small tufts of choroid plexus are normally visible on the basal surface of the brain stem in the cerebellopontine angle (*arrows*), and indicate the location of the lateral foramina of Luschka (*f*) from which they protrude. The dusty discoloration of the inferior medulla is due to the presence of leptomeningeal melanocytes (see Fig. 9.64). **B:** The ependyma-lined sleeve of the lateral recess of the fourth ventricle (*arrowheads*), together with the protruding tuft of choroid plexus, is referred to in the older literature as the "flower basket of Bochdalek" or "cornucopia." Pieces of the ependymal cuff are often seen adherent to the lateral aspect of the medulla in autopsy brain stem sections and should be recognized as a normal finding. The largest tufts of choroid plexus are called the glomera choroidea and are located in the atria of the lateral ventricles (**C**).

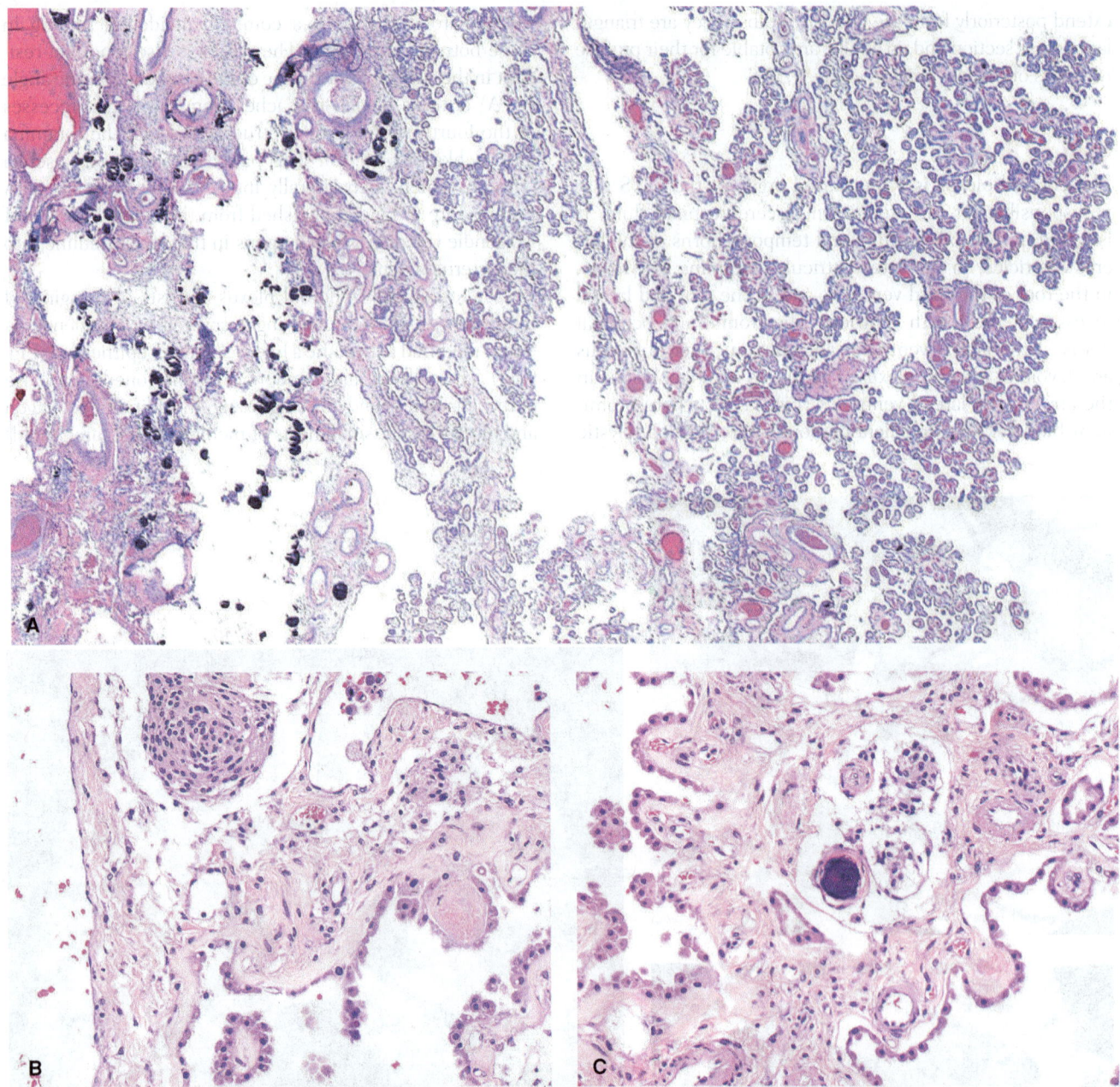

FIGURE 9.54 Choroid plexus: Histologically, choroid plexus is seen to be covered by simple cuboidal epithelium (modified ependyma) (**A**). In adults, each choroid epithelial cell bears a single prominent paranuclear cytoplasmic vacuole. An additional aging change seen in normal choroid plexus is calcification, which occurs in two forms: Nonspecific deposition of calcium salts in the collagenous stroma (A, left side of image) and as psammoma bodies (**C**). The latter arise from meningothelial cell nests (**B**) that are normally present in the choroid plexus as a result of the stroma's embryologic derivation from the pia-arachnoid meninges.

cells are common normal habitués of the choroid plexus; whorls of these cells frequently give rise to psammoma bodies (Fig. 9.54). These cells also explain the occurrence of intraventricular meningiomas. Nonspecific deposition of mineral salts also occurs commonly throughout the connective tissue core with increasing age and accounts for most of the plexuses' radiodensity. An additional aging change of no specific pathologic significance is cytoplasmic vacuolization of the ependyma-derived lining cells.

Circumventricular Organs

The CVOs comprise a diverse group of specialized CNS centers that share two anatomical features: A periventricular location and vasculature that lacks the characteristic blood–brain barrier properties found throughout the rest of the brain and the spinal cord. There are six CVOs: the pineal gland, subfornical organ, organum vasculosum of the lamina terminalis, area postrema, subcommissural organ, and the median eminence–infundibulum–neurohypophysis (Figs. 9.55 and 9.56). Of these,

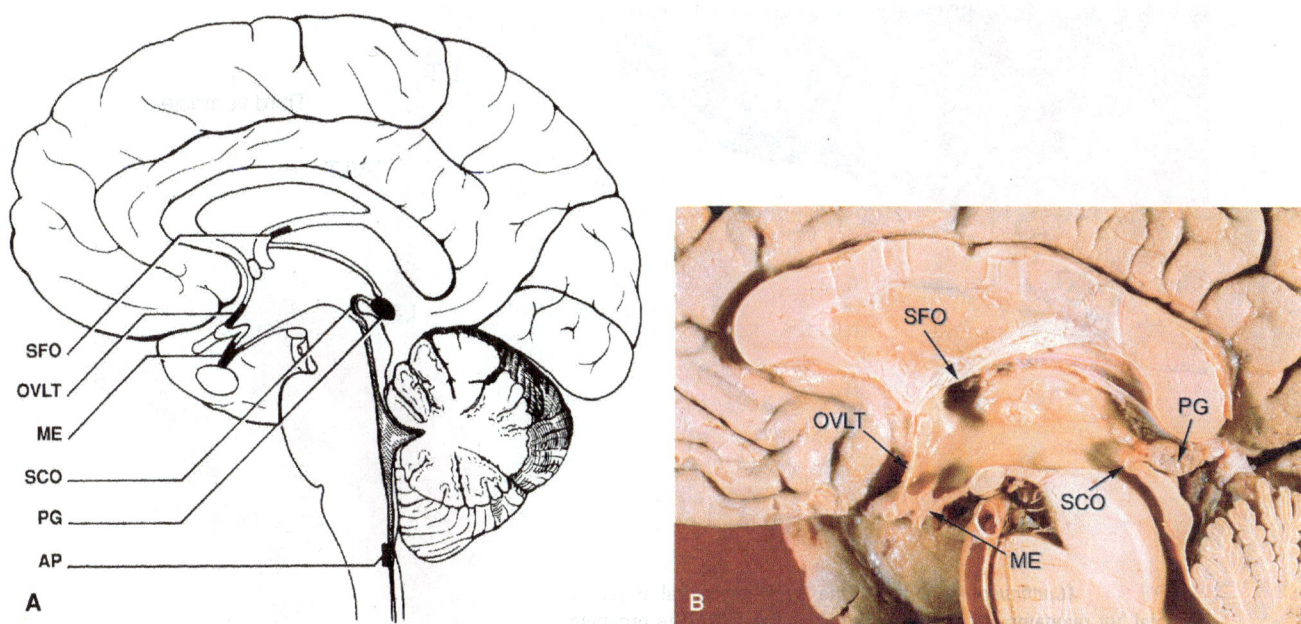

FIGURE 9.55 CVOs: As illustrated in the diagram (**A**) and mid-sagittally sectioned autopsy brain (**B**), the CVOs share a midline or paramidline position, proximity to the ventricular system, and lack of the usual blood–brain barrier. The subcommissural organ is present in the developing fetus but is vestigial in the adult. *SFO*, subfornical organ; *OVLT*, organum vasculosum of the lamina terminalis; *ME*, median eminence and infundibulum; *SCO*, subcommissural organ; *PG*, pineal gland; *AP*, area postrema.

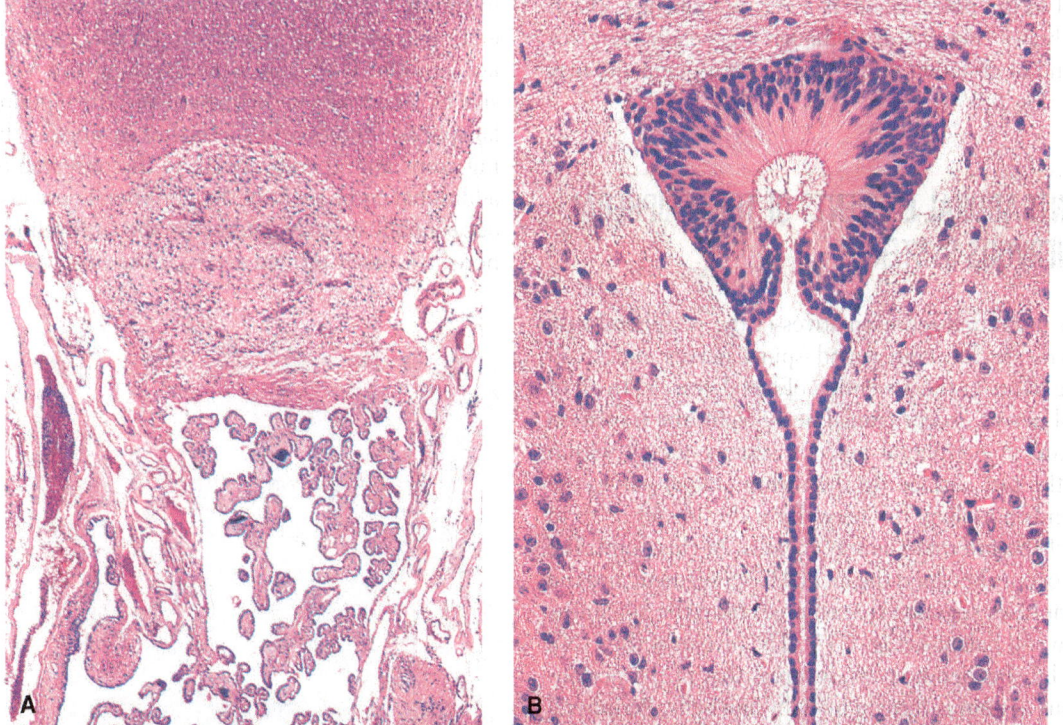

FIGURE 9.56 CVOs: Histologically, all of the CVOs except for the subcommissural organ are very similar, with a loose neuropil that is highly vascular and lacks a blood–brain barrier as illustrated by the subfornical organ (**A**). The subcommissural organ is located in the region of the pineal gland just beneath the posterior commissure in the posterior dorsal third ventricle and is highly developed in most mammalian species, as illustrated by the mouse (**B**). (*continued*)

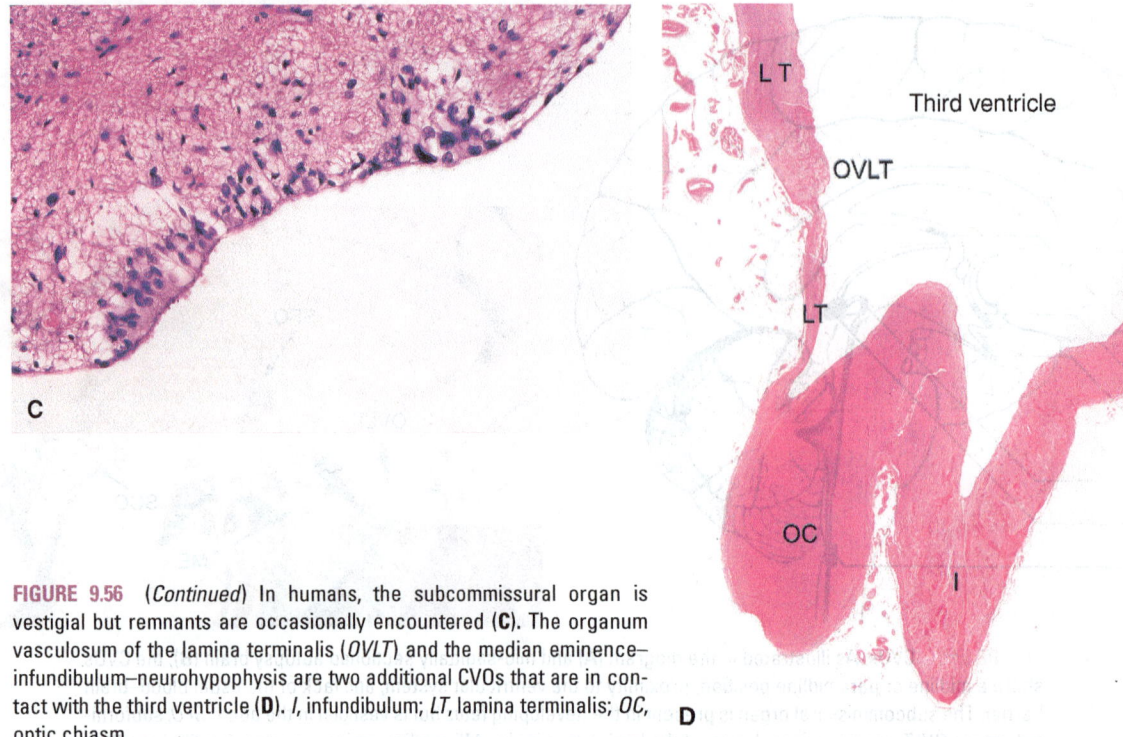

FIGURE 9.56 (*Continued*) In humans, the subcommissural organ is vestigial but remnants are occasionally encountered (**C**). The organum vasculosum of the lamina terminalis (*OVLT*) and the median eminence–infundibulum–neurohypophysis are two additional CVOs that are in contact with the third ventricle (**D**). *I*, infundibulum; *LT*, lamina terminalis; *OC*, optic chiasm.

all except the subcommissural organ are fully developed in the adult human (Fig. 9.56). The subcommissural organ, which is located on the ventral surface of the posterior commissure just caudal to the pineal gland, is a very prominent CVO in most vertebrates (Fig. 9.56B); although it generally regresses near the end of gestation in humans, vestigial remnants may be present (Fig. 9.56C).

INTRADURAL ELEMENTS OF THE PERIPHERAL NERVOUS SYSTEM

The major intradural representatives of the peripheral nervous system are the cranial and spinal nerves and small autonomic fibers in the adventitia of blood vessels. In all of the cranial nerves except cranial nerve eight, the transition from central to peripheral nervous system occurs within 2 mm of the pial surface. In the eighth cranial nerve, the CNS extends out along the nerve for a centimeter or so to the level of the internal auditory meatus. At this point, the transition occurs between the medial CNS segment and the lateral peripheral segment that emerges from the apparatus for hearing and balance (Fig. 9.57). The myelin of the CNS is formed by oligodendrocytes, whereas that of the peripheral nervous system is formed by Schwann cells. Peripheral nerve is noted for its content of interstitial collagen and the elongated nuclei of Schwann cells. Two additional intrathecal components of the peripheral nervous system may pique interest on fortuitous encounter. The first is the so-called microneuroma, which is usually found in the parenchyma of the spinal cord or, more rarely, the medulla (Fig. 9.58). These structures consist of a Gordian knot of unmyelinated axons that have been hypothesized to arise secondary to traumatic injury of peripheral nerve roots whose regenerating axons follow penetrating spinal or medullary arteries into the CNS parenchyma along the Virchow–Robin spaces. According to the hypothesis, the tapering perivascular spaces ultimately block further advance of the regenerating axons and, thereby, result in the observed neuroma. An additional component of the peripheral nervous system that occasionally arouses interest is the unmyelinated terminal nerve (variously termed *nervus terminalis, cranial nerve zero,*

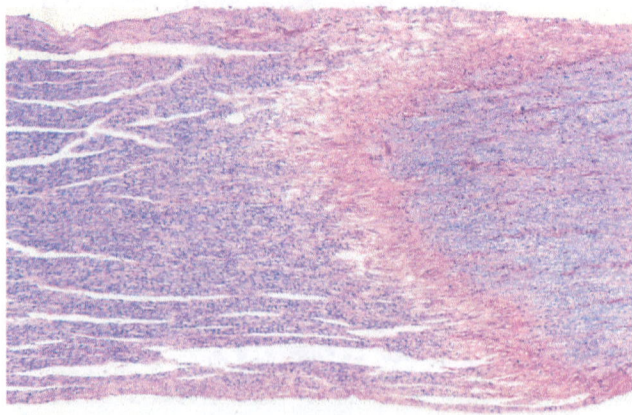

FIGURE 9.57 Transition zone from central to peripheral nervous system myelin: For cranial nerve eight (vestibulocochlear) this transition occurs in the vicinity of the internal acoustic meatus. This transition zone is also known as the "Obersteiner-Redlich zone (ORZ)."

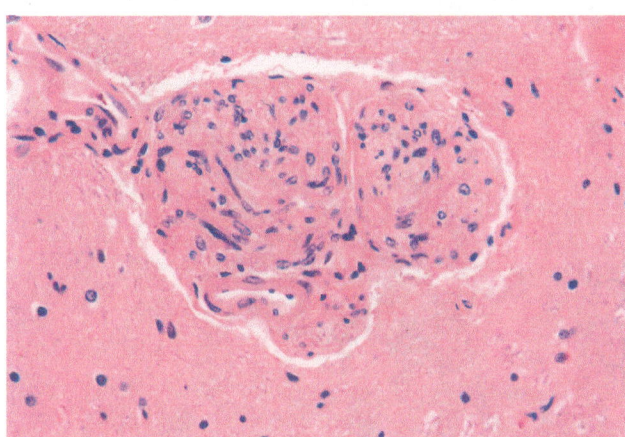

FIGURE 9.58 Microneuroma: These tangled balls of unmyelinated axons are most often encountered in the spinal cord, less often in the medulla, as an incidental finding in an otherwise unremarkable specimen.

and *cranial nerve T*), which courses in the subarachnoid space covering the gyri recti of the orbital surface of the frontal lobes (Fig. 9.59). Although usually composed of multiple small anastomosing fascicles, it occurs as a single trunk in some specimens and can be quite striking. Rarely, intrafascicular ganglion cells may be observed.

MENINGES

Dura Mater (Pachymenix)

The dura is composed of two tightly annealed layers of fibrous connective tissues (Fig. 9.60). The outer layer functions as the periosteum of the cranium, whereas the inner meningeal layer is joined to the arachnoid membrane by weak intercellular junctions and focally forms the four dural reduplications that compartmentalize the cranial cavity: The falx cerebri, falx cerebelli, tentorium cerebelli, and diaphragma sellae. The two layers of the dura separate to accommodate the dural venous sinuses (Fig. 9.60B); the inner meningeal layer is pierced by draining veins and by arachnoid villi. The latter conduct CSF back into the venous circulation and are obvious over the superior parasagittal convexities of the cerebral hemispheres where they project into the superior sagittal sinus (Fig. 9.60). They are present in all other major venous sinuses, as well. They are often observed along the posterior margin of the cerebellar hemispheres in relation to the sinus confluens and the transverse venous sinuses. Small villi are also present intraspinally. The epithelial properties of arachnoid granulations are reflected ultrastructurally in elongated, interdigitating

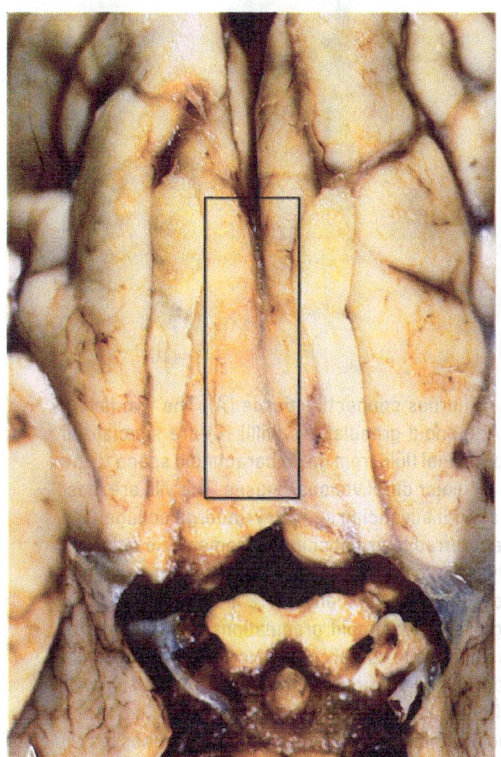

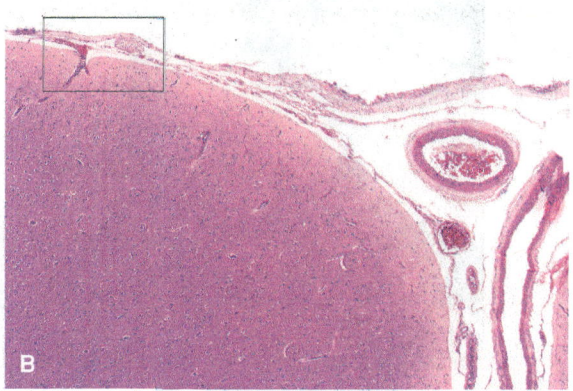

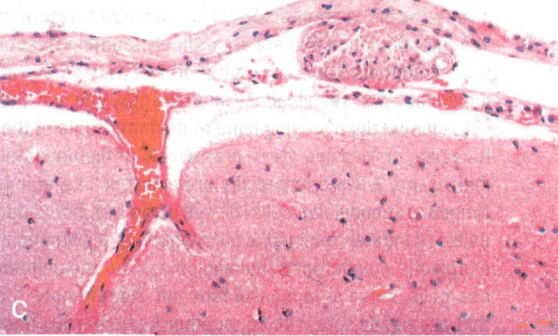

FIGURE 9.59 Cranial nerve zero: Cranial nerve zero (CN0), also known as the terminal nerve or nervus terminalis, is present in humans as a plexus of small peripheral nerve fascicles found in the subarachnoid space that covers the gyri recti that lie between the olfactory bulbs and tracts (**A**). Tissue sections taken through the gyri recti that include the overlying leptomeninges (**B**) will often include a terminal nerve fascicle cut in cross section (**C**). The small peripheral nerve fascicles of cranial nerve zero are one potential source of subfrontal schwannomas.

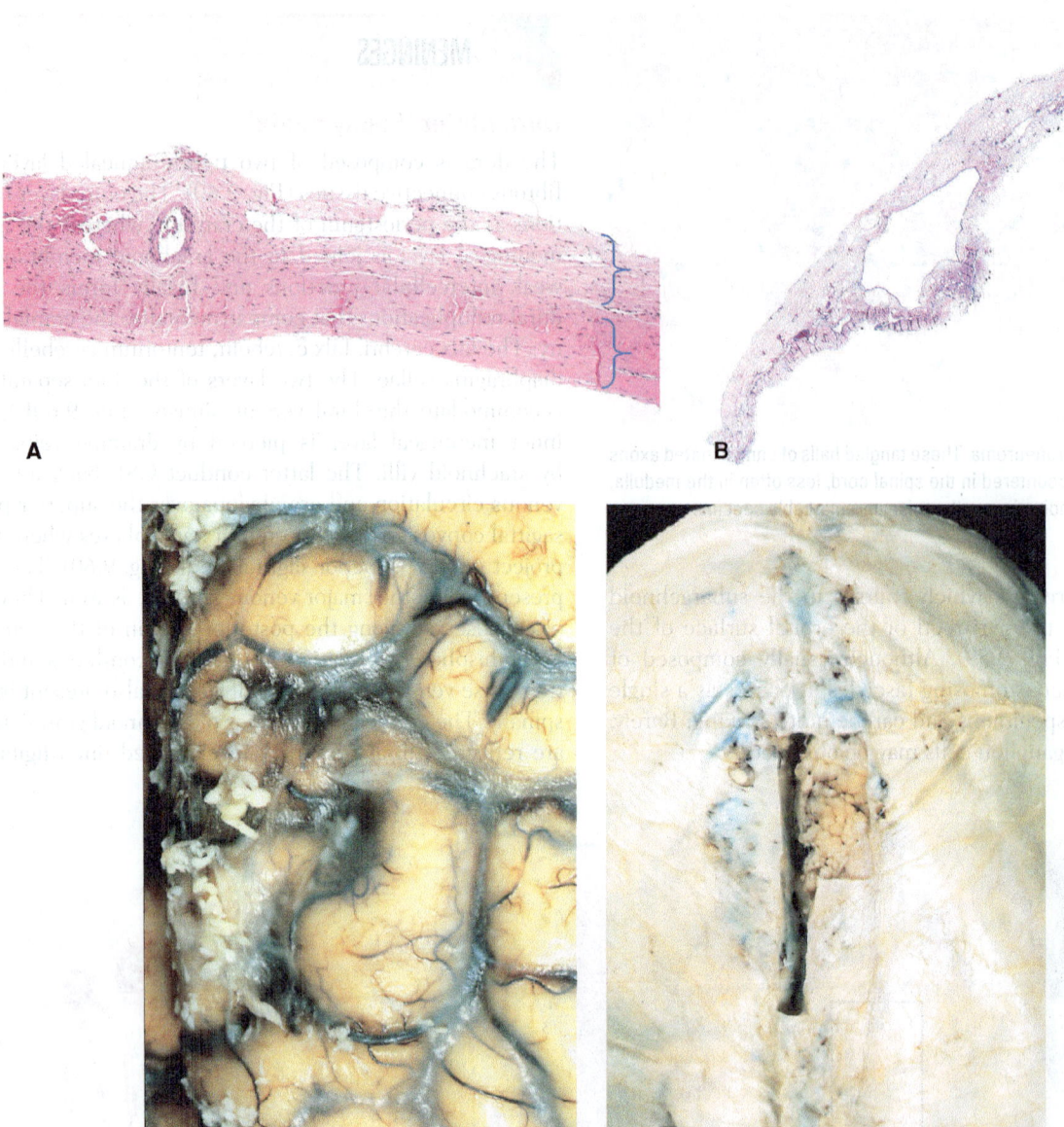

FIGURE 9.60 The dura is formed by two annealed layers of fibrous connective tissue (**A**). The two layers separate to accommodate the dural venous sinuses (**B**). Arachnoid granulations (villi) (**C**) are specialized structures of the arachnoid membrane serve to return cerebrospinal fluid from the subarachnoid space to the venous circulation and are accordingly found in relation to all major dural venous sinuses. The villi are most prominent in the superior sagittal (**D**) and transverse sinuses. With advancing age, they undergo collagenous hypertrophy, as seen in these micrographs, and may then be referred to as pacchionian bodies. The enlarged villi remodel the overlying bone of the inner table of the calvarium to produce small pits termed pacchionian foveolae, or foveolae granulares. Nests of meningothelial cells may be seen anywhere along the arachnoid membrane, but are especially prominent in the apical regions of arachnoid granulations where they are termed arachnoid cap cells (**E**), and in the arachnoid covering the orbitofrontal cortex. Normal meningothelial cells are innately inclined to form whorls and psammoma bodies, two features that are often retained by their neoplastic counterparts, meningiomas. The meningothelial cells of the arachnoid membrane, including the cap cells, serve an epithelial function. Accordingly, they possess elongated, intertwined cell processes (**F**) that are tightly spot welded together by numerous desmosomes (**G**) and exhibit strong immunopositivity for epithelial membrane antigen (EMA) (**H**). Like the tendency to form whorls and psammoma bodies, these epithelial phenotypic traits are retained by neoplastically transformed meningothelial cells and serve as useful diagnostic features of the vast majority of meningiomas which otherwise exhibit a very broad range of light microscopic morphologies. (*continued*)

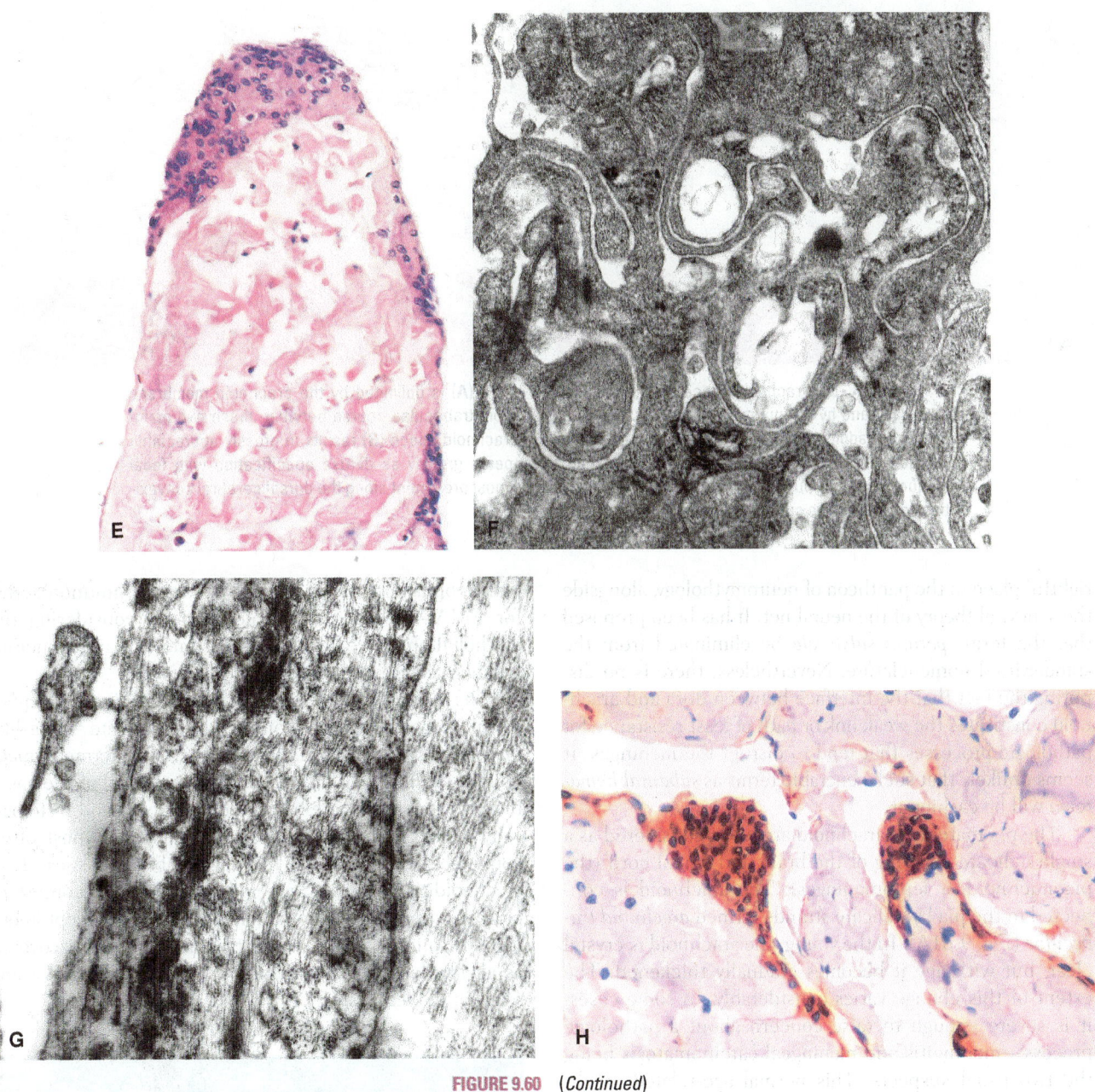

FIGURE 9.60 *(Continued)*

cell processes bonded together with desmosomes and immunohistochemically, by positivity for epithelial membrane antigen (EMA) (Fig. 9.60). These features are also characteristic of meningiomas. With age, the deposition of collagen enlarges the arachnoid villi that are then referred to as pacchionian bodies (Fig. 9.60). Such large granulations frequently press through the overlying roof of the superior sagittal sinus and its lateral lacunae to produce small pits or depressions in the inner table of the calvarium. These are known as the *foveolae granulares* or *pacchionian foveolae*. Portions of the dura, particularly the falx cerebri and parasagittal dura associated with the superior sagittal sinus, often calcify nonspecifically with age. Calcification may also be seen in association with chronic renal failure. Focal ossification is sometimes encountered as an incidental finding.

Pia-arachnoid (Leptomeninges)

The arachnoid forms a continuous sheet immediately subjacent to the dura. On the basis of descriptive and experimental ultrastructural observations, it is now generally accepted that the dura and arachnoid exist in vivo as a physically continuous tissue, with sparse but unequivocal intercellular junctions linking these two historically discrete membranes. The storied subdural space has, thus, taken its

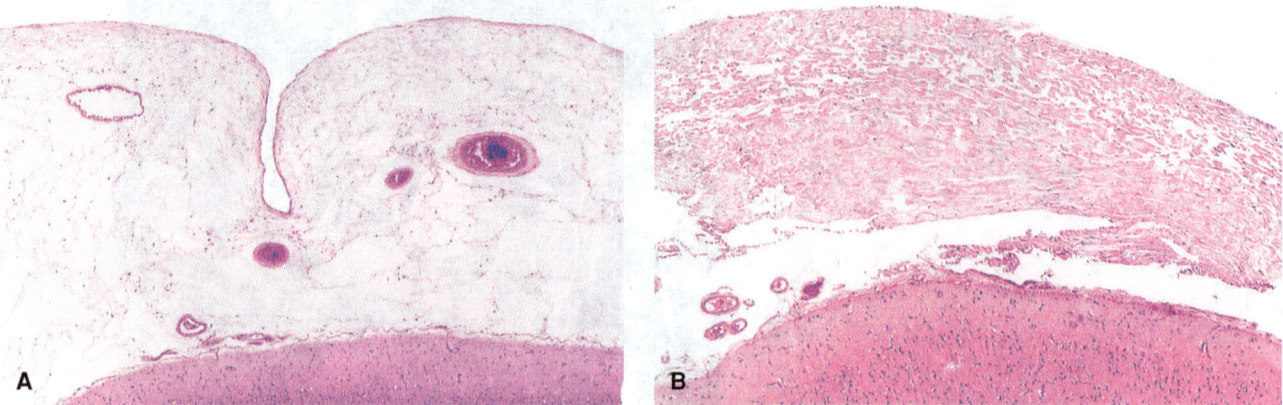

FIGURE 9.61 Subarachnoid space: The subarachnoid space (A) is delimited by the arachnoid membrane externally and by the pia mater internally. Delicate arachnoid trabeculae course between these two membranes. In adults, gradual collagen deposition in the subarachnoid space (B) results in grossly appreciable "clouding" of the leptomeninges. This aging fibrosis appears grossly as diffuse opacification with focal plaques and small punctate nodules. It is characteristically most prominent along the dorsal cerebral convexities adjacent to the superior sagittal sinus.

rightful place in the pantheon of neuromythology, alongside the syncytial theory of the neural net. It has been proposed that the term *spatium subdurale* be eliminated from the standardized nomenclature. Nevertheless, there is no disputing the fact that the interface between dura and arachnoid constitutes the weak link or path of least resistance for pathologic processes that tend to disrupt the meninges. It seems unlikely that such venerable terms as *subdural hematoma* will be cashiered.

The pia mater and arachnoid are often considered as a single delicate covering of the brain and spinal cord (the pia-arachnoid or leptomeninges). The arachnoid is connected to the pia by delicate strands termed *arachnoid trabeculae* (Fig. 9.61A). In the young, the arachnoid is crystal clear, but with age it becomes gradually thickened. The extent of this change varies considerably. In some cases, it is severe enough to raise concern about a pathologic process—meningitis and meningeal carcinomatosis being the two usual suspects. This normal age-related arachnoid thickening is typically most pronounced over the dorsal parasagittal cerebral convexities. Microscopically, it results from the deposition of dense bundles of collagen (Fig. 9.61B), analogous to the collagenous hypertrophy of arachnoid villi that occurs prominently in the same vicinity. Focal nests of arachnoid cells (also called meningothelial cells) may be seen throughout the arachnoid membrane (Fig. 9.62), but are concentrated over the arachnoid villi (arachnoid cap cells). These distinctive elements become more obvious and more clustered with advancing age and, in the adult, often form whorls with centrally placed psammoma bodies. At this point, the resemblance of these nests to those of the meningioma is inescapable. As mentioned previously, small nests of arachnoid cells are also present intraventricularly in the vascular connective tissue core of the choroid plexus (see Fig. 9.54). Both normal and neoplastic meningothelial cells are immunoreactive for EMA—an understandable property considering the epithelial phenotype of the desmosome-containing meningothelial cell (Fig. 9.60).

The dorsal leptomeninges of the thoracic and lumbosacral spinal cord occasionally contain white wafer-like plaques (Fig. 9.62), a finding that is often termed *arachnoiditis ossificans*. In fact, in most (but not all) of the cases these brittle lesions are roentgenographically and histologically devoid of bone or mineral. Rather, they most often consist of laminated and hyalinized fibrous tissues. True arachnoiditis ossificans generally occur in the context of prior symptomatic inflammation or trauma to the leptomeninges. Hyaline plaques, in contrast, are typically discovered as an incidental finding at autopsy in the absence of any relevant clinical history.

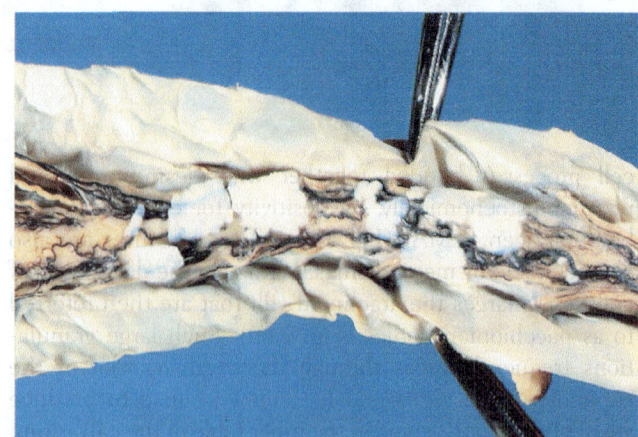

FIGURE 9.62 Hyaline plaques of the spinal leptomeninges: These plaques are common incidental findings at autopsy and occur most frequently in the dorsal spinal arachnoid, although they may occasionally be seen in the cerebral leptomeninges as well.

Like the dura, the pia is traditionally divided into two layers: The epipia, which covers the surface of the CNS parenchyma and surrounds the vasculature, and the intima pia, which extends into the CNS parenchyma as the posterior median and intermediate septa of the spinal cord. Classically, three specialized structures of the epipia are recognized: The denticulate ligaments on either side of the spinal cord, the linea splendens adjacent to the anterior spinal artery, and the filum terminale. All three structures are composed primarily of dense bundles of collagen.

The filum terminale, which forms the terminus of the spinal cord, warrants additional brief description. As noted earlier, it is composed largely of leptomeningeal collagen but also contains small blood vessels, occasional small nerve fascicles, and may harbor focal collections of adiposites in a minority of normal individuals. Most importantly, however, it is an ependymal remnant of the central canal (Fig. 9.63). This structure is the source of origin for a unique neoplasm of the conus medullaris and filum terminale: the myxopapillary ependymoma.

Leptomeningeal Melanocytes

True melanocytes like those found in the skin are normal cellular constituents of the meninges. They are typically most concentrated in the leptomeninges of the ventral aspect of the

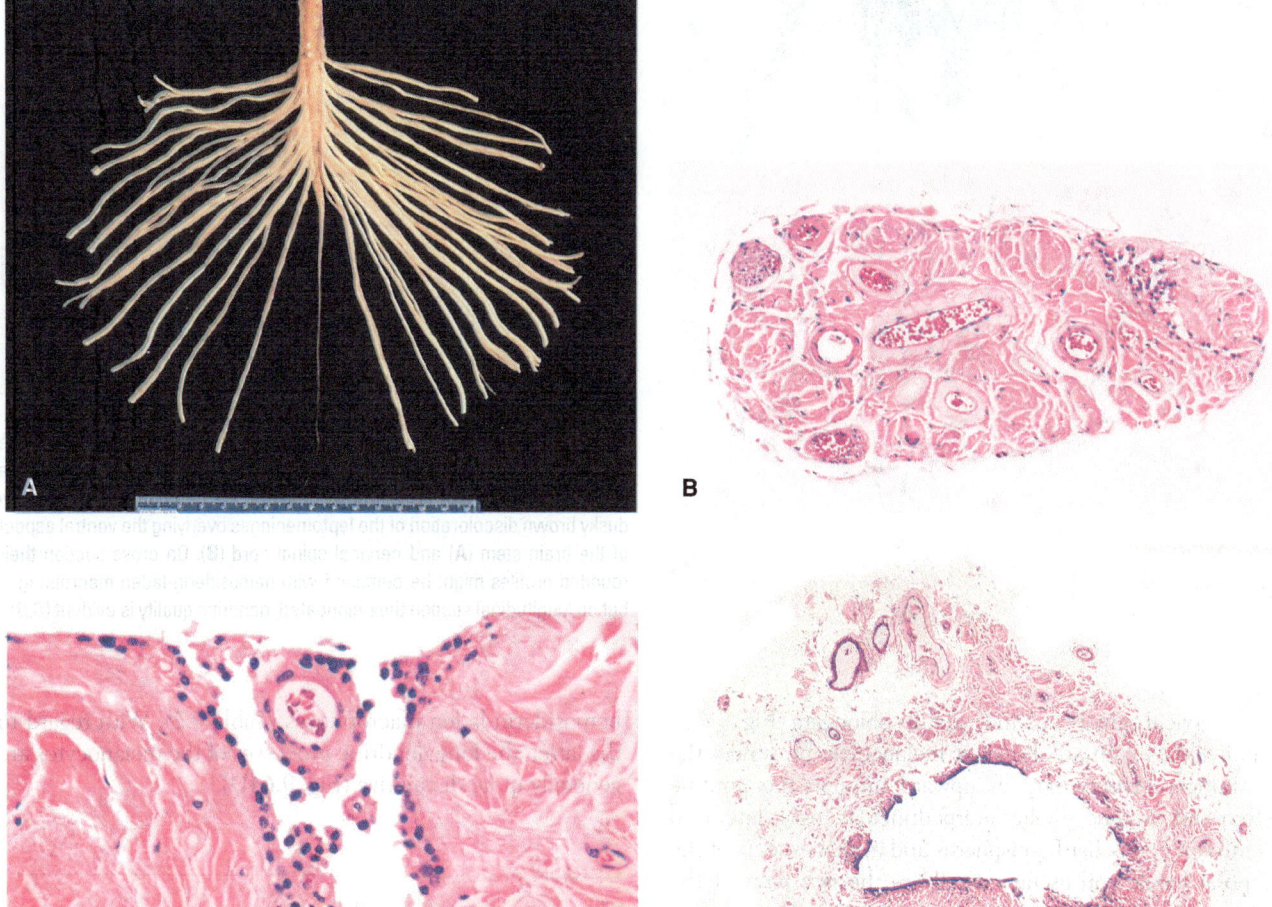

FIGURE 9.63 Filum terminale: The filum terminale is the terminus of the spinal cord and extends downward from the conus medullaris surrounded by the nerve roots of the cauda equina (**A**). As seen in cross section (**B**), the filum is composed primarily of dense collagenous tissue and contains blood vessels, small peripheral nerve fascicles, and, of significant clinical importance, a small, often eccentrically located, ependymal remnant of the central canal (*upper right*). The latter structure, shown at higher magnification in (**C**), is the origin of myxopapillary ependymoma. A remnant of the embryonic terminal ventricle of Krause (ventriculus terminalis), which consists of a focal dilatation of the central canal located in the region of the junction of the conus medullaris with the filum, may be encountered in sections from this vicinity (**D**).

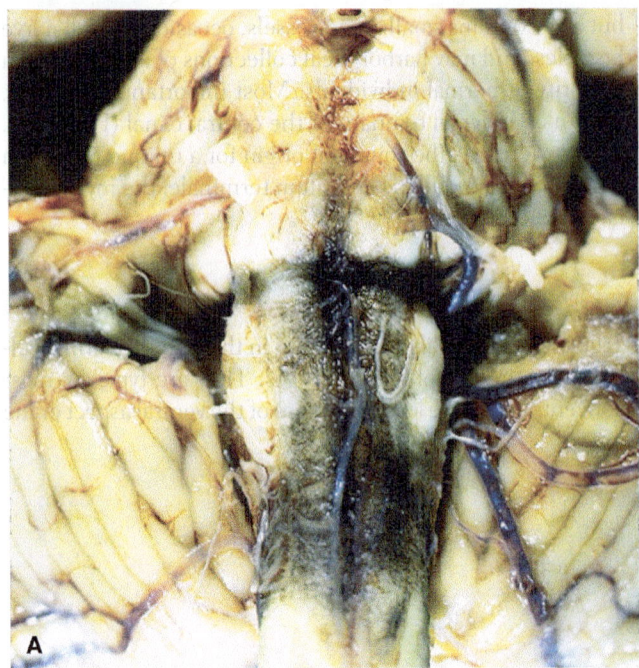
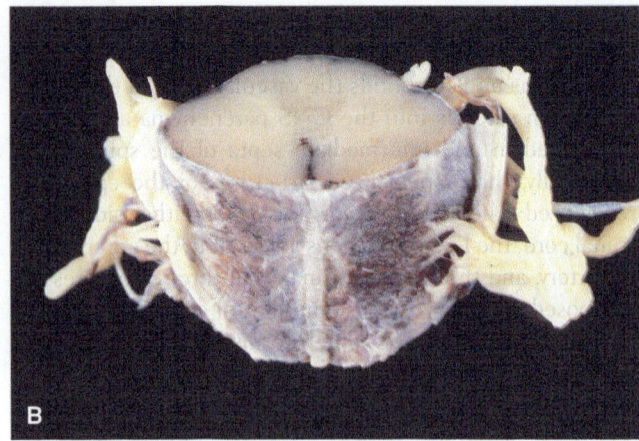
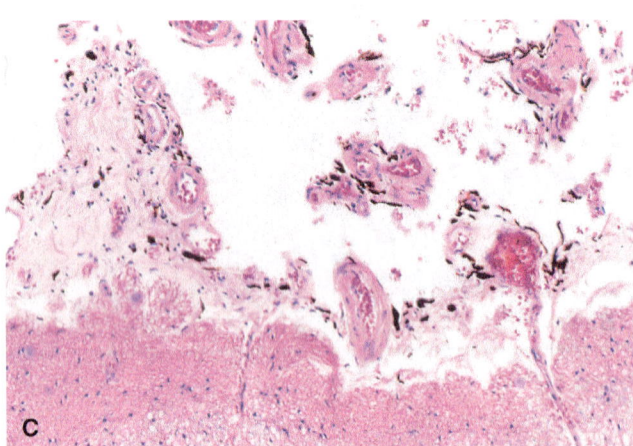
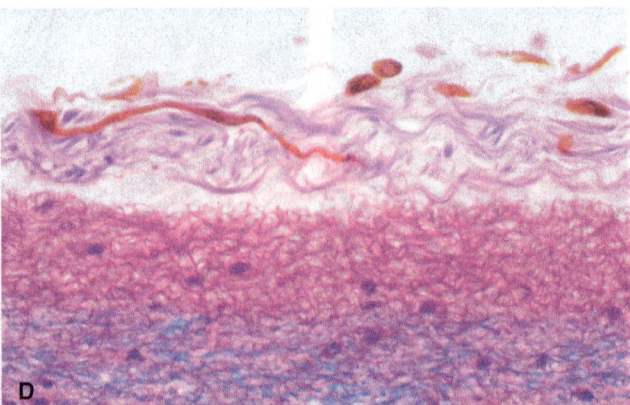

FIGURE 9.64 Leptomeningeal melanocytes: True melanocytes (not to be confused with neuromelanin-containing catecholaminergic neurons) are normal constituents of the pia-arachnoid and are often grossly visible as a dusky brown discoloration of the leptomeninges overlying the ventral aspect of the brain stem (**A**) and cervical spinal cord (**B**). On cross section their rounded profiles might be confused with hemosiderin-laden macrophages but on longitudinal section their elongated, dendritic quality is evident (**C,D**).

upper cervical spinal cord and medulla oblongata (Fig. 9.64). In individuals with an abundant melanocytic presence, the distribution territory extends upward through the pontine cistern and mesencephalic interpeduncular fossa, lateral to the inferior cerebellar hemispheres and mesial aspects of the temporal lobes, and as far rostrally as the gyri recti of the orbitofrontal cortex. It is not unusual for melanocytes to follow the investing leptomeninges of the perivascular Virchow–Robin spaces around large penetrating arteries for short distances into the CNS parenchyma. Intrinsic melanocytes of the leptomeninges may be involved in a spectrum of proliferative conditions ranging from benign melanocytoma to primary CNS melanoma, with all of these entities being exceptionally rare. In contrast, the normal presence of melanocytes in the leptomeninges must always be borne in mind when examining surgical biopsies from CNS sites known to harbor these distinctive elements; one must avoid misinterpreting them as evidence of a melanocytic neoplasm or as hemosiderin-laden macrophages (Table 9.2). With regard to the latter, the long dendritic processes of the melanocytes are generally quite distinctive (Fig. 9.64D).

Optic Nerve

The optic nerves (as well as the optic tracts and optic chiasm) are direct extensions of the CNS and not peripheral nerves. The significance of this fact is that the myelin of the optic nerves is of the central type and is produced by oligodendroglia, not Schwann cells. Thus, the optic nerves are susceptible to diseases of CNS white matter, such as multiple sclerosis. Being extensions of the CNS, the optic nerves are surrounded by the three meninges, pia mater, arachnoid, and dura mater, with the enclosed subarachnoid space (Fig. 9.65). The presence of an arachnoid layer surrounding the optic nerve explains the occurrence of optic sheath meningiomas.

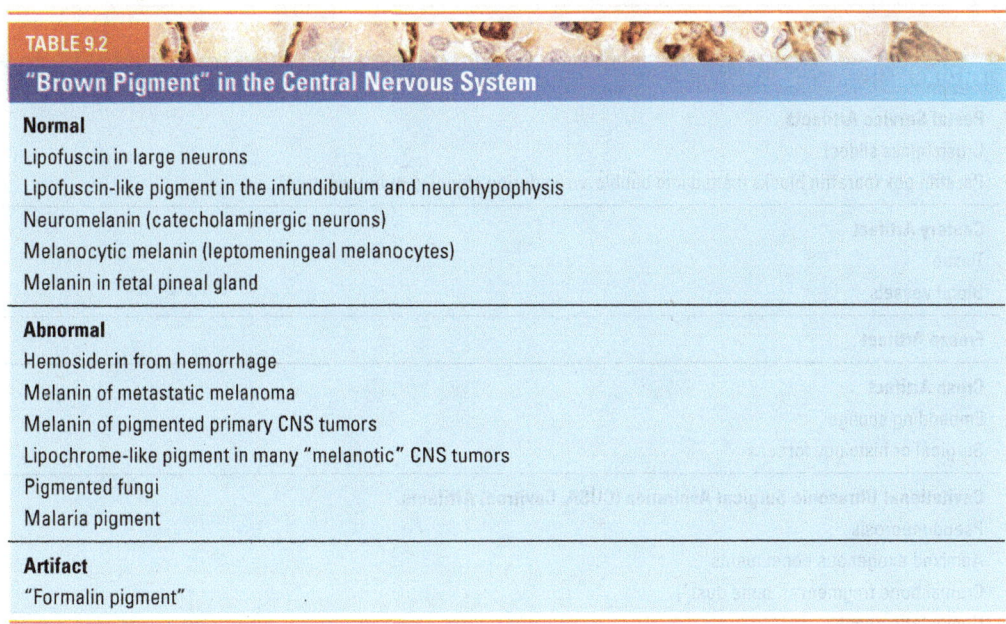

TABLE 9.2 "Brown Pigment" in the Central Nervous System

Normal
Lipofuscin in large neurons
Lipofuscin-like pigment in the infundibulum and neurohypophysis
Neuromelanin (catecholaminergic neurons)
Melanocytic melanin (leptomeningeal melanocytes)
Melanin in fetal pineal gland

Abnormal
Hemosiderin from hemorrhage
Melanin of metastatic melanoma
Melanin of pigmented primary CNS tumors
Lipochrome-like pigment in many "melanotic" CNS tumors
Pigmented fungi
Malaria pigment

Artifact
"Formalin pigment"

FETAL BRAIN

The two most distinctive histologic features of fetal brain compared to adult brain are active neurogenesis and paucity of myelin. The former is observed as a prominent, dense aggregation of neuroblasts and immature neurons in the periventricular and subpial zones. A similarly transient layer of migrating neurons in the fetal and infant cerebellum (the external granular layer) has been discussed. These generative laminae begin involuting during the latter part of gestation; remnants are present during the first year of postnatal life (see Fig. 9.3C).

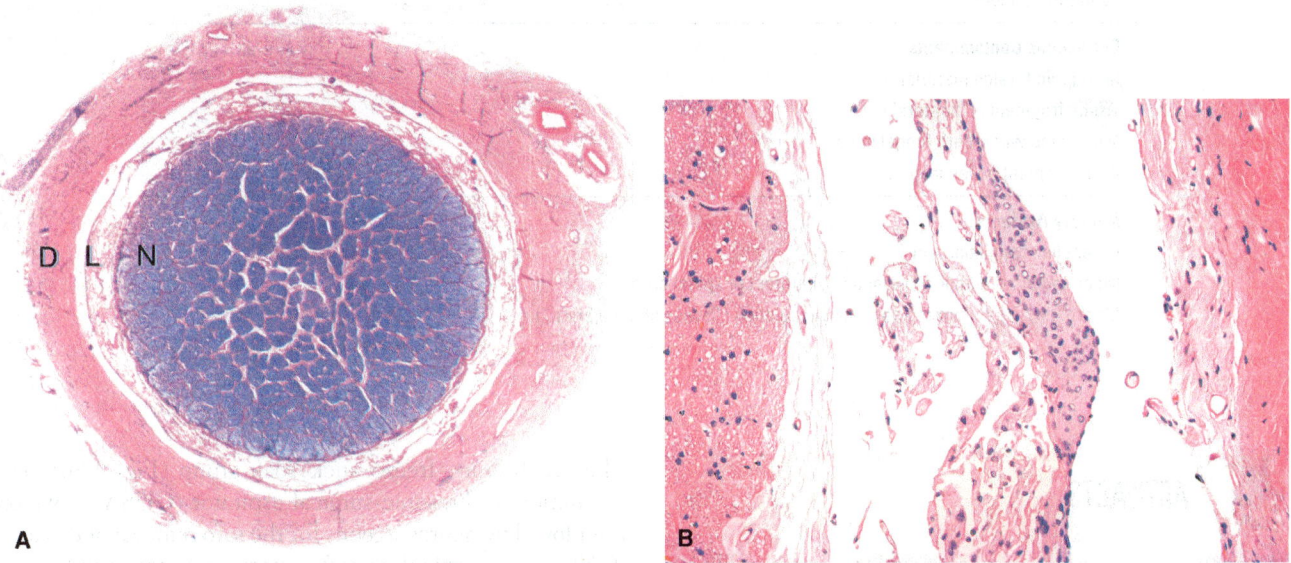

FIGURE 9.65 Optic nerve: A whole-mount cross section (**A**) reveals that the optic nerve (*N*) is surrounded by leptomeninges (*L*), which includes the pia mater and arachnoid together with the enclosed cerebrospinal fluid-containing subarachnoid space. The leptomeninges and subarachnoid space are in turn covered by the densely fibrous dura mater (*D*), which in this location, is often referred to as the optic nerve sheath. At higher magnification (**B**), leptomeningeal arachnoid cell clusters are clearly seen. The presence of arachnoid cell nests around the optic nerve must be borne in mind when examining intraoperative frozen tissue sections from this neuroanatomic vicinity.

TABLE 9.3
Artifacts

Postal Service Artifacts
Crush (glass slides)
Paraffin pox (paraffin blocks melted into bubble-wrap during shipping in hot weather)

Cautery Artifact
Tissue
Blood vessels

Freeze Artifact

Crush Artifact
Embedding sponge
Surgical or histology forceps

Cavitational Ultrasonic Surgical Aspiration (CUSA, Cavitron) Artifacts
Pseudonecrosis
Admixed exogenous constituents
Cranial bone fragments ("bone dust")
Hemostatic agents

Pseudomineralization
Bone dust
Laminar pseudomineralization

Delayed Fixation Artifact
Perinuclear halos—oligodendroglial (useful)
Perinuclear halos—neurons (mimics oligodendroglioma)
Pseudohypercellularity on smear preparations (uneven thickness mimics glioma)

Air-drying Artifact on Touch/Smear/Drag Preps

Collapsed Leptomeningeal Vessels (Mimics Vascular Malformation)

Formalin Pigment

Extraneous Contaminants
Iatrogenic foreign material
Tissue fragments ("floaters")
Microtome water bath fungal mold
Airborne plant pollen spores

Autopsy Artifacts
Cerebellar conglutination
Mechanical herniation ("toothpaste") artifact of spinal cord
Macroscopic gas-forming bacteria vacuolation ("Swiss cheese brain")

ARTIFACTS

A variety of gross and macroscopic artifacts may complicate evaluation of tissue specimens from CNS. Many of these are seen frequently in surgical neuropathology practice, while a few are limited primarily to autopsy neuropathology (Table 9.3). Artifacts can be broadly separated into those that hinder diagnostic evaluation versus those that mimic histopathologic lesions. Among the former are artifacts of the crush–burn–freeze–suck–soak group (Fig. 9.66). The cavitational ultrasonic surgical aspirator (CUSA) is widely employed by neurosurgeons for the safe removal of diseased CNS tissue, particularly soft tumors, and a trap can be used to collect the aspirated tissue and saline irrigation solution for the submission for histologic evaluation. Although microscopic examination of CUSA material can be very informative, the pathologist must be aware of the artifacts that frequently accompany such specimens, including artificial distortion and smearing, and the introduction of

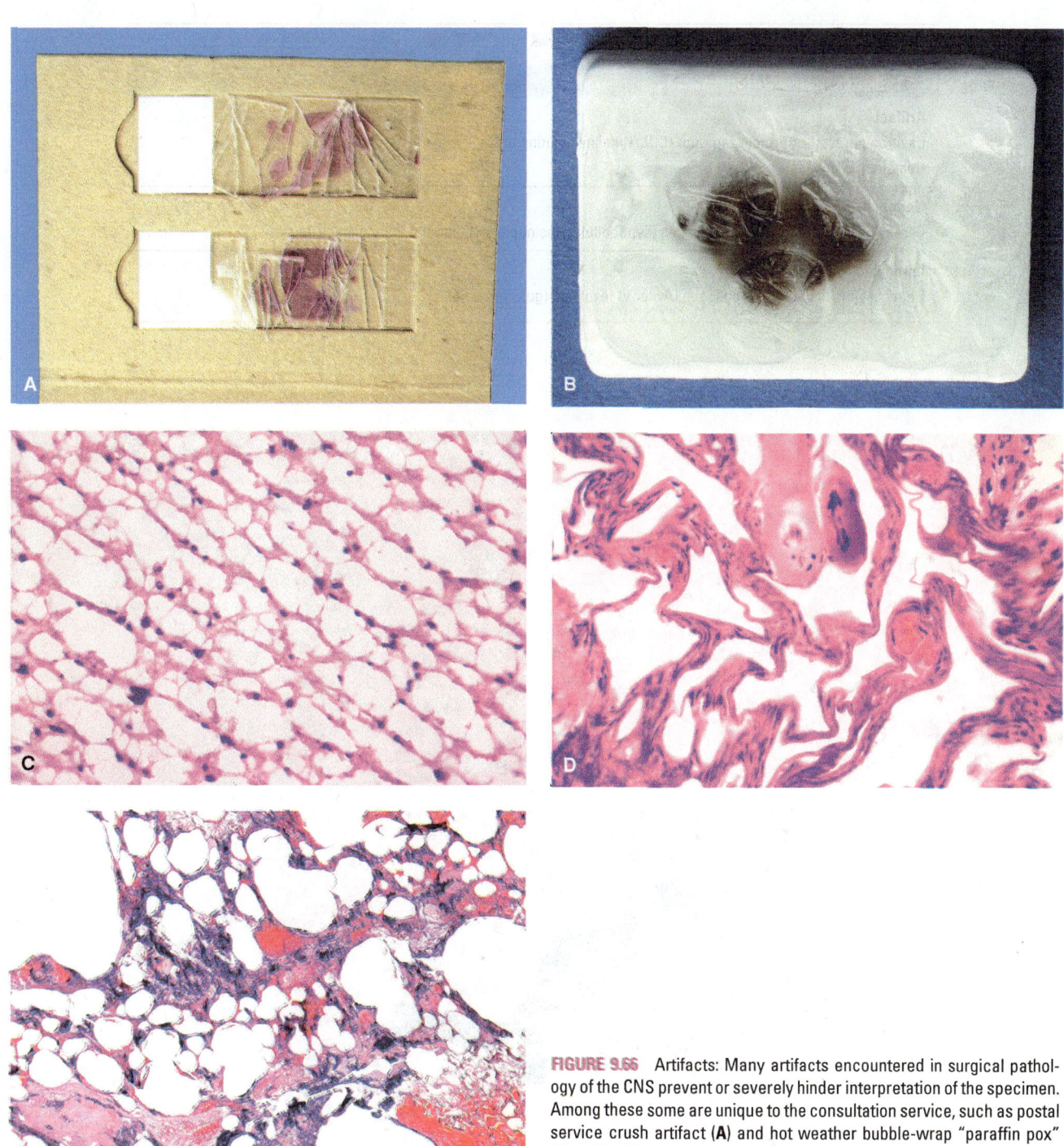

FIGURE 9.66 Artifacts: Many artifacts encountered in surgical pathology of the CNS prevent or severely hinder interpretation of the specimen. Among these some are unique to the consultation service, such as postal service crush artifact (**A**) and hot weather bubble-wrap "paraffin pox" (**B**), while others are secondary to surgical and laboratory tissue insults, such as severe freeze artifact (**C**), cautery artifact (**D**), and ultrasonic aspiration of brain tissue (**E**).

extraneous material (bone dust, hemostatic agent). CUSA artifact is one cause of pseudonecrosis in CNS tissue samples (Table 9.4). Among artifacts that mimic lesions, the most common are perinuclear halo artifact, collapsed leptomeningeal vessels, and "bone dust" (Fig. 9.67).

Iatrogenically introduced foreign material is also encountered with regularity by pathologists who examine CNS specimens and warrants brief mention (Table 9.5, Fig. 9.68). A variety of foreign agents are used to control bleeding during surgery and may be introduced preoperatively by the interventional radiologist for embolization of vascular lesions or intraoperatively by the surgeon to control hemorrhage during and after surgery. All of these agents periodically appear in tissue sections. Since they are

TABLE 9.4 Pseudonecrosis Etiologies

Artifact
Cavitron ultrasonic surgical aspirator (CUSA)/saline solution artifact
Hematoxylin absence artifact

Normal Regional Histology
Cerebellar cortex on smear preparation (hypocellular eosinophilic molecular layer mimics necrosis)

Iatrogenic
Degenerating microfibrillar collagen (Avitene) textiloma (gossypiboma)

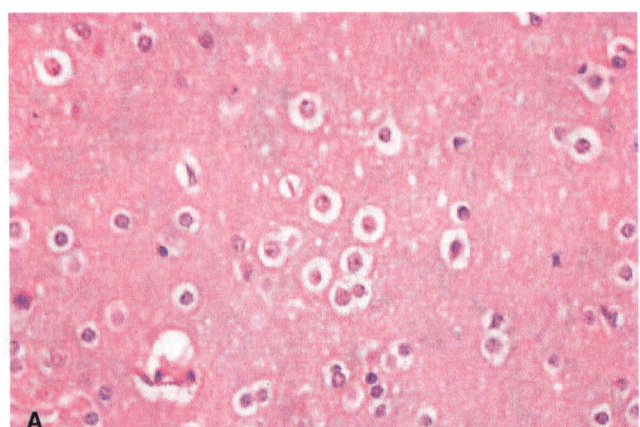
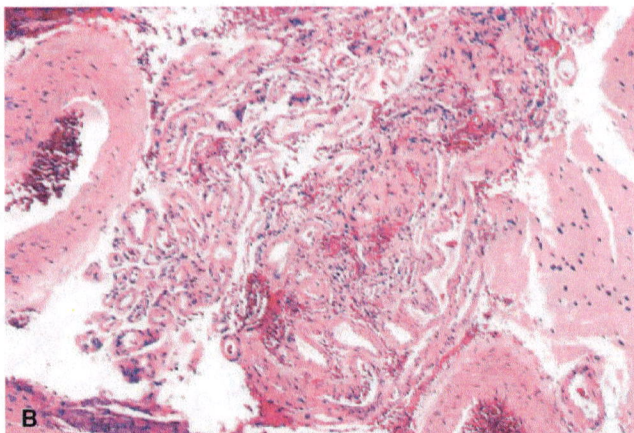
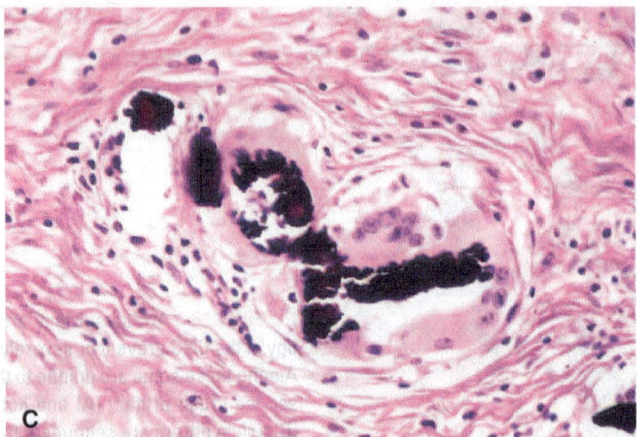

FIGURE 9.67 Artifacts: Several types of artifacts may not be recognized as artifactual in nature to the unaware and so may be particularly misleading. For example, one of the most characteristic morphologic features of normal oligodendrocytes and their derivative tumors, oligodendrogliomas, in formalin-fixed paraffin-embedded tissue sections is the presence of perinuclear halos. However, depending on fixation conditions and other factors, prominent halos may sometimes be seen around other cell types, including neurons (**A**); care must be exercised in such situations to avoid misdiagnosis. Another example of misleading artifact is the tangle of normal blood vessels that results from collapsed vascular leptomeninges (**B**). The result can mimic vascular malformation. Before rendering a diagnosis of vascular abnormality in such circumstances, the adjacent brain or spinal cord tissue should be examined for the evidence of associated features, such as gliosis, hemosiderin deposition, and granular bodies. Finally, also under the category of misleading artifact is "bone dust," which consists of microscopic fragments of cranial bone derived from the surgeon's drill that become intermixed with the tissue sample and can mimic calcification or ossification. In repeat operations, such bone dust fragments left in situ at the previous operation can be seen accompanied by a foreign body-type giant cell reaction (**C**).

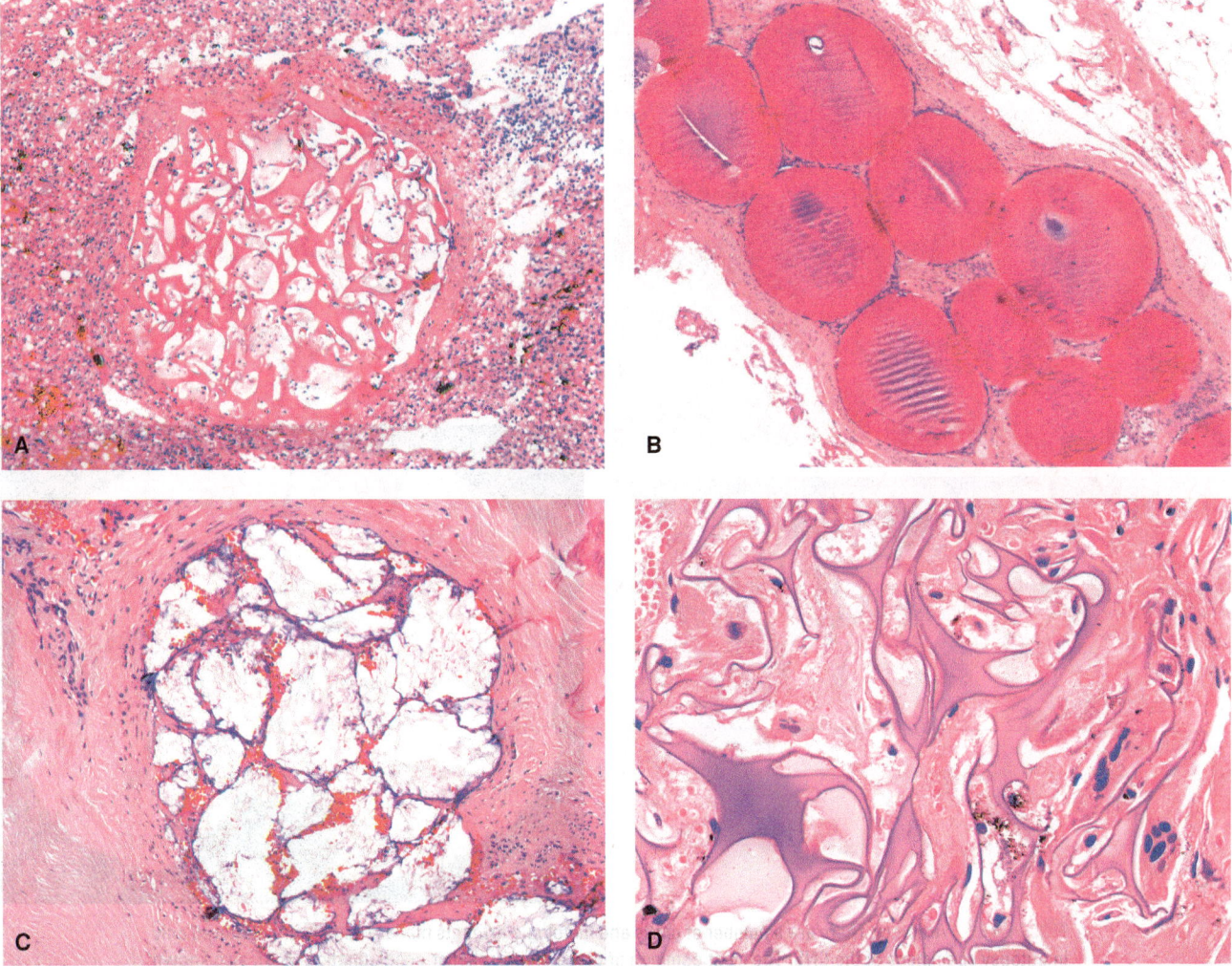

TABLE 9.5
Iatrogenically Introduced Foreign Material

Preoperative Embolic Agents
Gelatin foam (Gelfoam)
Polyvinyl alcohol particles
Acrylic microspheres (Embospheres)

Intraoperative Hemostatic Agents

Resorbable Hemostatic Agents
Gelatin foam (Gelfoam)
Oxidized cellulose (Surgicel, Oxycel)
Microfibrillar bovine collagen (Avitene)

Nonresorbable Hemostatic Agents
"Retained" cotton ball/pledgets

Surgically Introduced Therapeutic Materials
Gliadel wafers (chemotherapy)
Muslin (cotton) fabric (aneurysm wrapping)

FIGURE 9.68 Artifacts: An additional category of artifacts seen in surgical neuropathology consists of foreign material placed by the interventional radiologist or neurosurgeon and subsequently encountered by the pathologist upon tissue resection. The most common examples of this are embolic and hemostatic agents. Embolic materials are introduced by catheter prior to surgery for highly vascular lesions to reduce intraoperative bleeding; the most common are gelatin foam (**A**), acrylic resin spheres (**B**), and polyvinyl alcohol particles (**C**). Hemostatic agents, in contrast, are placed in the surgical site to stop bleeding during the operation and often left in place after closing to prevent postoperative bleeding. The most commonly employed agents are gelatin foam (**D**), oxidized cellulose (**E**), and microfibrillar bovine collagen (**F**). (*continued*)

268 SECTION IV: Nervous System

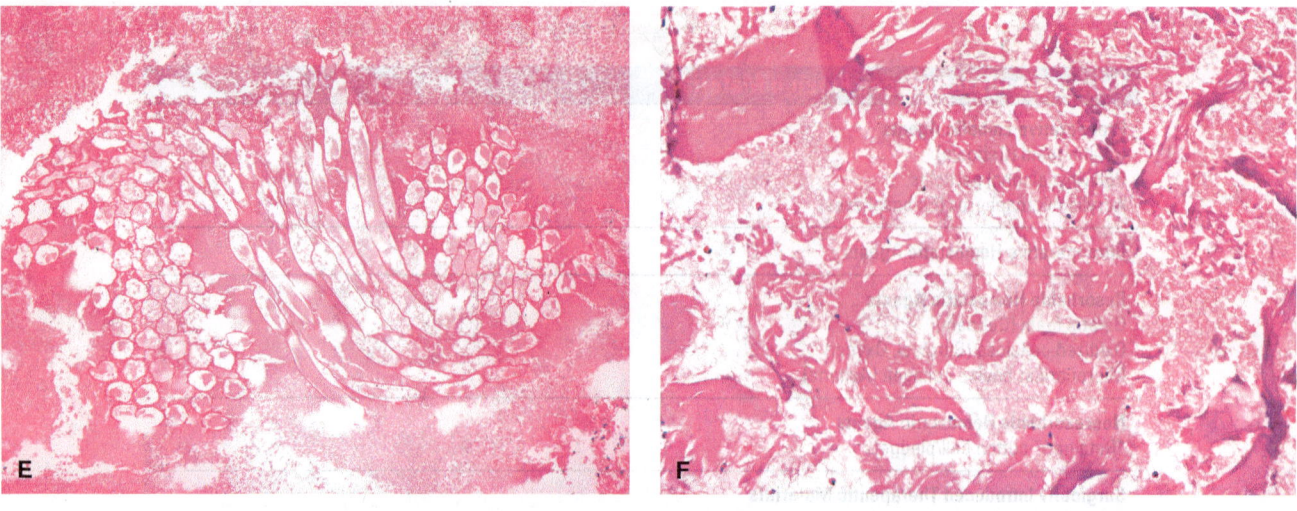

FIGURE 9.68 (*Continued*)

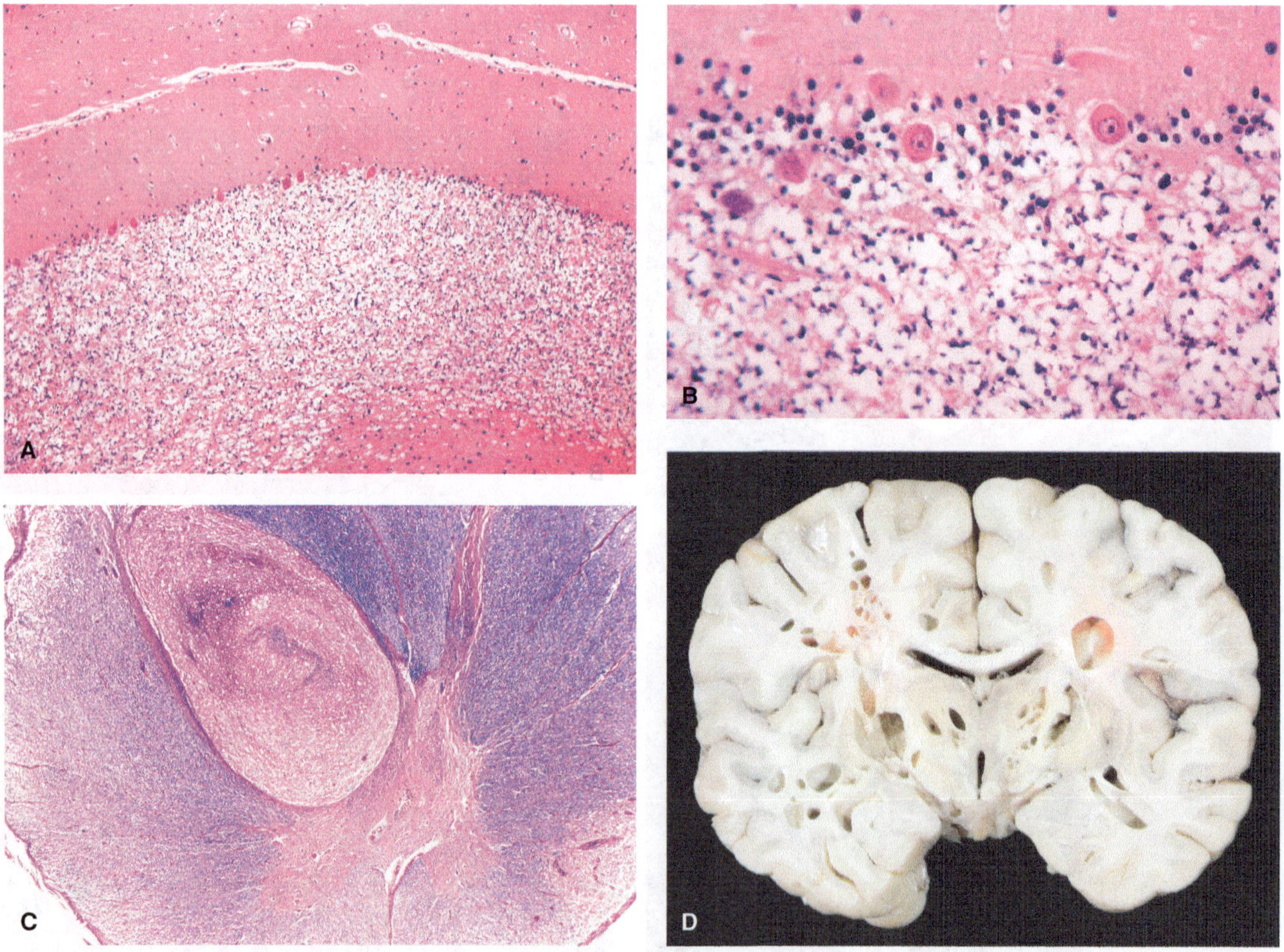

FIGURE 9.69 Artifacts: There are a number of gross and histologic artifacts that are usually encountered only in autopsy specimens of the CNS. The most common of these are cerebellar conglutination (**A,B**), also known as "etat glace," which consists of autolytic dissolution of the granular cell layer of the cerebellum; "toothpaste" or "squeeze" artifact of the spinal cord (**C**), which results from focal crushing of the cord by forceps during removal at autopsy and resultant internal herniation of the central gray matter, mimicking malformation or heterotopia; and "Swiss cheese brain" (**D**), which is a striking macroscopic vacuolization of the brain resulting from postmortem proliferation of gas-forming bacteria.

designed to be resorbable and can therefore be left in place, the morphologic appearance will vary depending on the time interval from placement at the initial surgery and subsequent resection during a second surgery (as, e.g., resection of recurrent tumor). Resorbable hemostatic agents elicit a chronic inflammatory reaction of variable intensity, which occasionally may be severe enough to create mass effect and clinical symptoms (textiloma, gossypiboma).

There are a few artifacts with which the pathologist who examines postmortem CNS specimens should be familiar (Fig. 9.69), the most common being autolysis of the cerebellar granular cell layer (cerebellar conglutination), mechanical distortion of the spinal cord produced by forceps pressure during removal ("toothpaste" artifact), and the production of cystic cavities of varying size in the brain by the postmortem proliferation of gas-forming bacteria ("Swiss cheese brain").

SUGGESTED READINGS

Neuropathology Textbooks

Burger PC. *Smears and Frozen Sections in Surgical Neuropathology*. Baltimore, MD: PB Medical Publishing; 2009.

Burger PC, Scheithauer BW. *Tumors of the Central Nervous System. AFIP Atlas of Tumor Pathology*. Washington, DC: American Registry of Pathology; 2007.

Burger PC, Scheithauer BW, Vogel FS. *Surgical Pathology of the Nervous System and its Coverings*. 4th ed. New York: Churchill Livingstone; 2002.

Ironside JW, Moss TH, Louis DN, et al. *Diagnostic Pathology of Nervous System Tumours*. New York: Churchill Livingstone; 2002.

Love S, Budka H, Ironside JW, et al. *Greenfield's Neuropathology*. 9th ed. Boca Raton, FL: Taylor and Francis Group; 2015.

McLendon RE, Bigner DD, Rosenblum M, et al. *Russell & Rubinstein's Pathology of Tumors of the Nervous System*. 7th ed. London: Arnold; 2006.

Perry A, Brat DB, eds. *Practical Surgical Neuropathology: A Diagnostic Approach*. 2nd ed. Philadelphia, PA: Elsevier; 2018.

Prayson RA. *Neuropathology*. Philadelphia, PA: Elsevier; 2005.

Neuropathology Review Books

Citow JS, Wollmann RL, MacDonald RL. *Neuropathology and Neuroradiology: A Review*. New York: Thieme; 2001.

Fuller GN, Goodman JC. *Practical Review of Neuropathology*. Philadelphia, PA: Lippincott Williams & Wilkins; 2001.

Gray F, De Girolami U, Poirer J. *Escourolle and Poirer's Manual of Basic Neuropathology*. 4th ed. Boston, MA: Butterwoth-Heinemann; 2004.

Nelson JS, Mena H, Parisi JE, et al. *Principles and Practice of Neuropathology*. 2nd ed. New York: Oxford; 2003.

Prayson RA. *Neuropathology Review*. Totowa, NJ: Humana Press; 2001.

Neuropathology Atlases

Ellison D, Love S, Chimelli L, et al. *Neuropathology*. 3rd ed. London: Mosby; 2013.

Hirano A. *Color Atlas of Pathology of the Nervous System*. 2nd ed. New York: Igaku-Shoin; 1988.

Okazaki H, Scheithauer BW. *Atlas of Neuropathology*. New York: Gower Medical; 1988.

Schochet SS, Nelson J. *Atlas of Clinical Neuropathology*. East Norwalk, CT: Appleton & Lange; 1989.

Weller RO. *Color Atlas of Neuropathology*. London: Oxford University Press; 1984.

Veterinary Neuropathology

Summers BA, Cummings JF, de Lahunta A, eds. *Veterinary Neuropathology*. St. Louis, MO: Mosby; 1995.

10
Pituitary and Sellar Region

M. Beatriz S. Lopes

EMBRYOLOGY 270	Variation in Normal Morphology of the Adenohypophysis 292
GROSS ANATOMY 271	Age-Related Changes of the Adenohypophysis 294
Bony Sella 271	Neurohypophysis 295
Meninges 272	Variation in Normal Morphology of the Neurohypophysis 296
Vasculature 273	
PHYSIOLOGY AND HISTOLOGY 277	DIFFERENTIAL DIAGNOSIS 296
Hypothalamus 277	REFERENCES 298
Adenohypophysis 283	

EMBRYOLOGY

To fully appreciate the anatomy of the pituitary (hypophysis), an understanding of its embryogenesis is essential. The gland consists of an anterior lobe (adenohypophysis), a posterior lobe (neurohypophysis), and an intermediate zone (Fig. 10.1). The development of each differs significantly.

The adenohypophysis has its origin in a thickening of oral ectoderm (1,2). During the 3rd week of gestation, this thickened plate invaginates in a cephalad direction to form the Rathke pouch, which retains its connection to the stomodeum via a narrow stalk. In the 6th week, the stalk becomes so attenuated that the pouch loses its stomodeal attachment as it comes into contact with the infundibulum. Cellular proliferation in the anterior wall of Rathke pouch gives rise to the pars distalis, the principal and largest portion of the anterior lobe. In addition, a "tonguelike" extension of the pars distalis, the pars tuberalis, grows upward to partially surround the anterior surface of the infundibulum. The posterior portion of Rathke pouch gives rise to what in humans is a thin segment of pituitary, the pars intermedia or intermediate lobe. In this zone, microcystic remnants of Rathke pouch containing colloid-like material are commonly seen (Fig. 10.1). Gross cystic dilatation of such remnants is common but infrequently produces clinically significant intermediate lobe or Rathke cleft cysts.

A remnant of the pharyngohypophysial stalk, demonstrable in fetuses and occasionally encountered in adults, comprises the pharyngeal pituitary (3). Located in the midline, beneath the mucoperiosteum of the nasopharynx, it extends from the posterior border of the vomer along the sphenoid bone. Although the full spectrum of anterior pituitary hormone–producing cells may be demonstrated in pharyngeal pituitaries, they are rarely the seat of medical or surgical disease (3).

The neurohypophysis develops from a neuroectodermal bud first noticeable in the floor of the diencephalon at 4 weeks of gestation (4). Two weeks later, the outgrowth grows ventrally to abut the posterior portion of Rathke pouch. This specialized portion of the nervous system comprises the magnocellular nuclei, their axons within the median eminence and infundibular stalk, and their terminations in the pars nervosa (posterior lobe). Oxytocin and vasopressin, as well as their carrier proteins the neurophysins, are detectable in the supraoptic (SON) and paraventricular nuclei (PVN) at 19 weeks and in the posterior lobe at 23 weeks (5).

As early as 7 to 8 weeks of gestation, the portal system begins to develop. Although by 12 weeks both the median eminence and the anterior lobe are vascularized, the circulation of the hypothalamic–pituitary portal system is not completed until 18 to 20 weeks (5).

The hypothalamus develops from a swelling in the diencephalon. Although the hypothalamic nuclei as well as the

---

This chapter is an update of a previous version authored by Bernd W. Scheithauer, Eva Horvath, Kalman Kovacs, and Peter J. Pernicone.

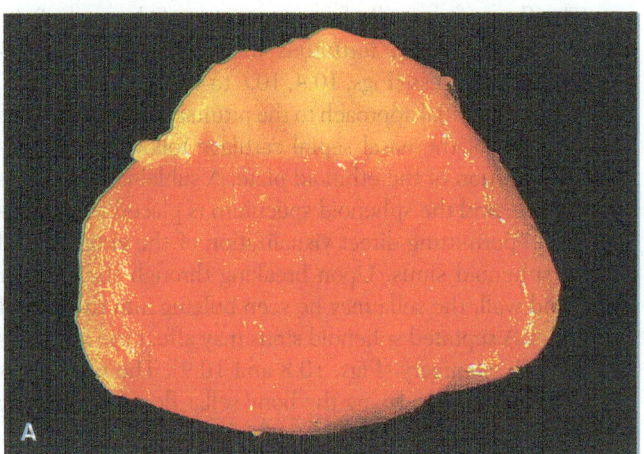 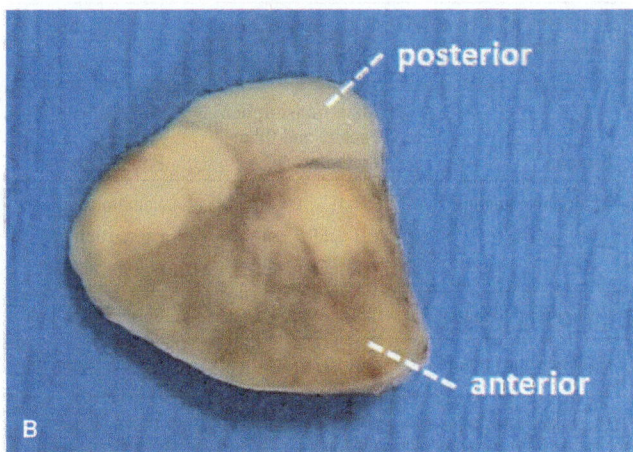

FIGURE 10.1 **A:** Normal unfixed adult pituitary gland cut in the horizontal plane. The posterior lobe is located at the top of the field. A few intermediate lobe cysts are present. The deep red color of the anterior lobe is a reflection of its extensive vascularity. **B:** Normal formalin-fixed adult pituitary gland highlighting the posterior and anterior lobes.

supraopticohypophysial tract are demonstrable at 8 weeks of gestation, unmyelinated axons growing ventrally from the magnocellular (supraoptic and paraventricular) nuclei do not reach the posterior lobe until 6 months.

By 12 weeks, a number of cartilaginous plates have fused to form the cartilaginous neurocranium (1). The body of the sphenoid bone and the sella turcica results from fusion of hypophysial cartilaginous plates located on either side of the developing pituitary. The sella is well formed by 7 weeks and matures through a process of enchondral ossification.

Rare developmental malformations of the pituitary gland, including ectopic pituitary gland in the suprasellar region and pituitary dystopia, have been reported (6,7).

The understanding of pituitary development has recently expanded as a result of the identification of molecular mechanisms that may specify cell determination and differentiation. Recent advances in pituitary development in mammals have suggested that pituitary organogenesis is controlled by a combination of sequential exogenous and endogenous signals (8–11). These signals induce the expression of interacting transcriptional regulators in temporal and spatial patterns. Pituitary cell types appear to emerge from a common pluripotent stem cell under the response of lineage-specific transcription factors and locally produced growth factors critical for determination and differentiation of specific cell type. Briefly, the early pituitary organogenesis requires three functionally oriented transcription factors, the Rathke pouch homeobox (*Rpx*) protein PAX6, the pituitary homeobox factor 1 (*Ptx1*), and the structurally related pituitary homeobox factor 2 (*Ptx2*) (11). *Pit-1* is a transcription factor that regulates the functional differentiation of the somatotrophs, lactotrophs, and thyrotrophs. For proper *Pit-1* function, there is requirement of another early determinant of pituitary differentiation, the Prophet of Pit-1 (*PROP1*).

High levels of estrogen receptors in cells that contain *Pit-1* favor prolactin (PRL) expression, whereas thyrotroph embryonic factor (TEF) induces thyroid-stimulating hormone (TSH) expression. Familial and sporadic *PROP1* mutations result in combined growth hormone (GH), PRL, TSH, and gonadotropin deficiency (12). A family of basic helix–loop–helix transcription factors, *neuroD1/b2*, and T-box family member TBX19, *Tpit*, appear to synergistically play a role in the functional differentiation for pituitary proopiomelanocortin (POMC) cell lineage and corticotroph cells. The transcription factor *PROP1* induces the pituitary development of *Pit-1*–specific lineages as well as gonadotrophs. The nuclear receptor steroidogenic factor 1 (*SF-1*), and *GATA2* are key factors for further differentiation of gonadotroph cells (13). These transcription factors have been localized in human embryonic and adult pituitary gland, and have served as diagnostic tools for characterization of pituitary adenomas in surgical pathology practice (Table 10.1). The time period of recognition of the various human pituitary hormone–producing cells during embryonal development have been well determined by immunohistochemical stains. Corticotrophs are the first cells to differentiate in the human fetal pituitary (at around 5 weeks gestational age). Somatotrophs appear around 8 to 9 weeks, followed by thyrotrophs and gonadotrophs at 12 to 15 weeks. Lactotrophs, although seen in small numbers as early as 12 weeks, are only fully recognizable at 23 weeks (5,14,15).

GROSS ANATOMY

Bony Sella

The pituitary gland is centrally situated at the base of the brain, where it lies safely nestled in the sella turcica, a saddle-shaped

TABLE 10.1
Adenohypophyseal Cell Lineage Transcription Factors

Lineage	Main Transcription Factors and Other Co-factors	Pituitary Cell
Acidophilic lineage	PIT-1	Somatotroph cell
	PIT-1, ERα	Lactotroph cell
	PIT-1, GATA-2	Thyrotroph cell
Corticotroph lineage	T-PIT	Corticotroph cell
Gonadotroph lineage	SF-1, ERα, GATA-1	Gonadotroph cell

PIT-1, pituitary-specific POU-class homeodomain transcription factor 1; ERα, estrogen receptor α; GATA-2, member of the GATA family of zinc-finger transcriptional regulatory proteins; T-PIT, T-box family member TBX19; SF-1, steroidogenic factor 1

concavity within the sphenoid bone (Figs. 10.2 to 10.4). It is attached to the hypothalamus by both the pituitary stalk and a tenuous vascular network (Figs. 10.5 to 10.7). By virtue of its location, the pituitary gland has many important anatomic relations. Anterior to the sella, the sphenoid bone forms a midline slope, the tuberculum sella, as well as a transverse indentation, the chiasmal sulcus, so named for the overlying optic chiasm (see Figs. 10.3 and 10.4). The optic canals, which transmit the optic nerves, lie anterolateral to the sulcus, whereas the optic tracts are posterolateral. In view of the pituitary's proximity to the optic apparatus, pituitary lesions that extend superiorly may cause significant visual field deficits (Figs. 10.2, 10.5 to 10.11). Specifically, compression of decussating fibers in the chiasm produces bitemporal hemianopsia, whereas compromise of an optic tract leads to homonymous hemianopsia. Suprasellar extension may cause hypothalamic dysfunction and hydrocephalus.

The floor of the sella forms a portion of the roof of the sphenoid air sinus, a fortuitous relationship that permits ready surgical access (Figs. 10.4, 10.6 to 10.12) (16). Indeed, the transsphenoidal approach to the pituitary initially involves mobilization of the nasal septal cartilage followed by resection of a portion of the ethmoid plate. A sublabial incision is then made, and the sphenoid speculum is placed in the septal space, permitting direct visualization of the anterior wall of the sphenoid sinus. Upon breaking through the anterior sphenoid wall, the sella may be seen bulging into the roof of the sinus. A septated sphenoid sinus may affect the surgeon's orientation at surgery (Figs. 10.8 and 10.9). The pituitary is then exposed by traversing the bony sellar floor and incising the dural investment around the gland.

The sloping anterior sellar wall terminates in posterolateral projections, the anterior clinoid processes (Figs. 10.3 and 10.4). Posterior to the sella, the sphenoid bone continues as the dorsum sellae, anterolateral portions of which form the posterior clinoid processes (see Figs. 10.3 and 10.4). Posterior to the dorsum sellae is situated the downward-sloping clivus, notorious as the site of predilection of chordomas (Figs. 10.3, 10.4, 10.6, and 10.7). A number of neurovascular foramina are situated in the sellar region; by name and contents from anterior to posterior, they include the foramen rotundum (maxillary nerves), ovale (mandibular nerves), spinosum (middle meningeal arteries), and lacerum (internal carotid arteries) (Fig. 10.3).

Meninges

The physical relationship of the meninges to the pituitary and sella is unusual in that the pituitary lacks a leptomeningeal investment. Periosteal dura lines the sella turcica, whereas the dura proper covers the lateral aspects of the

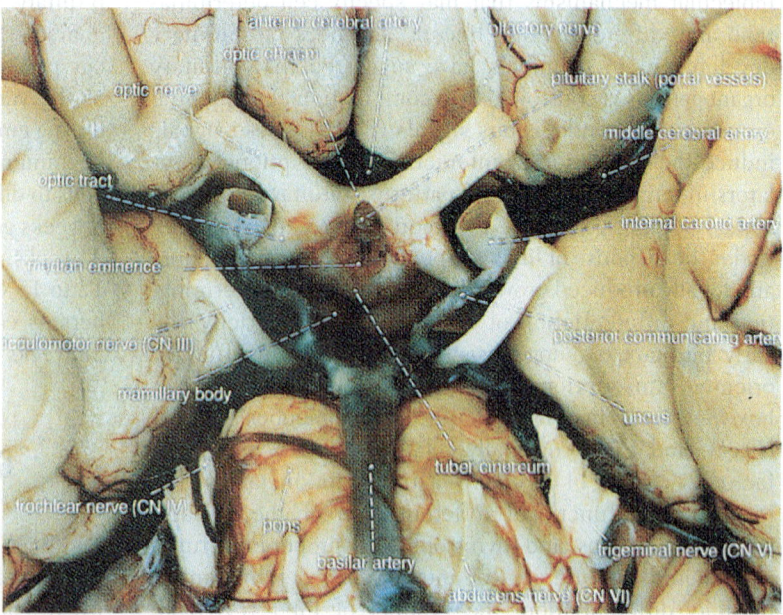

FIGURE 10.2 Ventral surface of normal brain showing the pituitary stalk and surrounding structures. The pituitary gland has been removed. The proximity of the optic chiasm to the pituitary is the basis for the visual field deficits accompanying suprasellar extension of pituitary adenomas. Visible along the posterior aspect of the stalk are tributaries of the portal system.

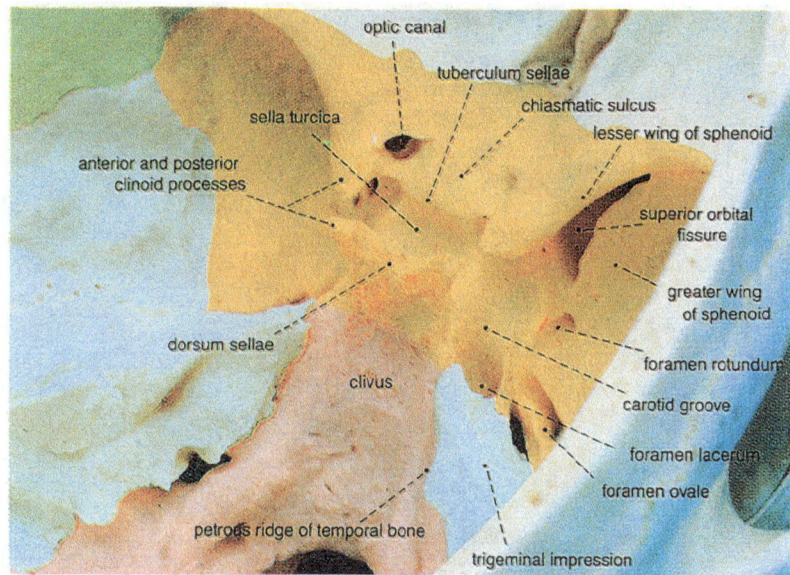

FIGURE 10.3 Oblique view of the normal skull base; the various skull bones are indicated in color. The sella turcica is centrally located with several foramina nearby. The foramen spinosum is not visible in this view. Yellow, sphenoid; pink, occipital; light blue, temporal; green, parietal; white, frontal.

cavernous sinuses and forms the sellar diaphragm. The diaphragm is usually thin at the center and thick at its periphery and possesses a variably sized central aperture through which the pituitary stalk passes (15). Leptomeninges do encircle the stalk; however, below the level of the sellar diaphragm, they reflect back upon themselves to form a circumferential channel, the infradiaphragmatic hypophysial cistern. This arrangement explains the higher incidence of development of meningiomas in the suprasellar surface of the diaphragm rather than in the intrasellar compartment.

In some individuals, the leptomeninges exhibit an important anatomic variation. It consists of extension or herniation of the arachnoid through an exceedingly large diaphragmatic opening. A deficiency of the diaphragma sellae is assumed to be a prerequisite for the formation of an empty sella. In one study, the incidence of an intrasellar arachnoidocele was found to exceed 20% (17). In such cases, transsphenoidal surgery may result in persistent cerebrospinal fluid (CSF) rhinorrhea because of inadvertent violation of the subarachnoid space. With prolonged exertion of even normal CSF pressure, enlargement of such arachnoidoceles may produce sellar enlargement and pituitary compression, the gland being reduced to a thin crescent on the posterior sellar floor (Fig. 10.13). The so-called empty sella may be present in as many as 5.5% of autopsies (18,19) and shows a distinct predilection for obese, multiparous females (Fig. 10.14). Compression of the gland and traction deformation of the pituitary stalk may cause mild to moderate hypopituitarism and hyperprolactinemia, respectively.

Vasculature

Vascular structures of major surgical significance abound in the sellar region.

The Cavernous Sinuses

The paired cavernous sinuses are situated on either side of the sella and, in part, lie lateral and superior to the sphenoid sinuses (Figs. 10.8 to 10.11). Each cavernous sinus is partially invested by dura of the middle fossa, as well as by thin bony walls of the sphenoid sinus. Venous drainage to the sinuses comes from a number of sources, including the eye (superior ophthalmic vein), brain (inferior and middle cerebral veins), and sphenoparietal sinus. Communication between right and left cavernous sinuses takes place through intercavernous sinuses bordering the anterior and posterior aspects of the sella (15). The complex thus forms a venous ring around the sella and its contents. Additional intercavernous sinuses are located along the ventral surface of the pituitary. The

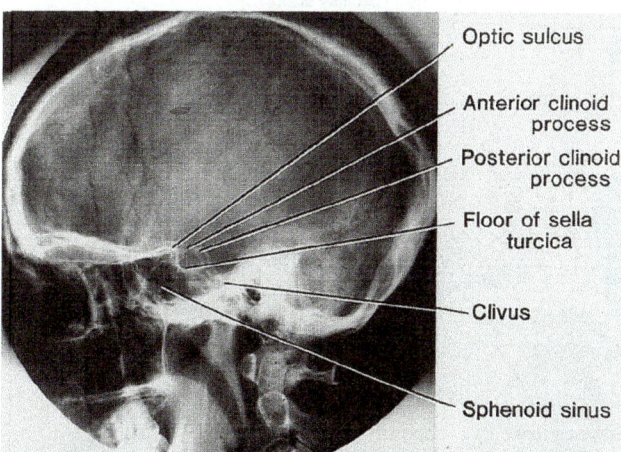

FIGURE 10.4 This normal lateral skull radiograph shows the central location of the sella turcica and surrounding bony anatomy.

FIGURE 10.5 Midline sagittal section through the brain at the level of the pituitary stalk and pituitary gland, showing the pituitary gland with surrounding structures including hypothalamus, third ventricle, optic chiasm, and sphenoid sinus.

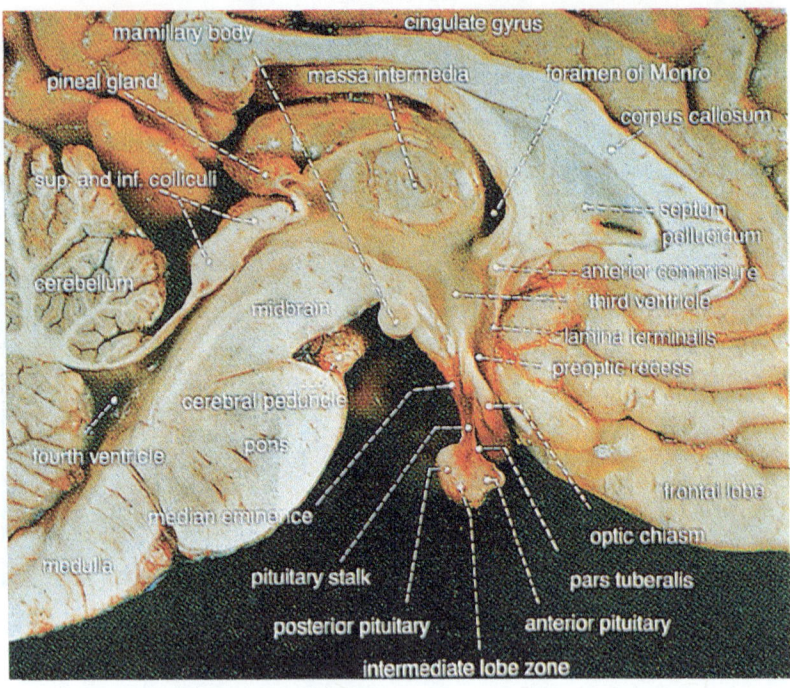

cavernous sinuses proper contain, in addition to their content of venous sinuses, a number of vital neurovascular structures (15). These include the cavernous segments of the internal carotid arteries and segments of cranial nerves III (oculomotor), IV (trochlear), V (trigeminal), and VI (abducens) (Figs. 10.8 and 10.9). Delicate areolar tissue fills the interstices between venous channels, arteries, and nerves. The location of the horizontal portions of the internal carotid arteries within the cavernous sinuses varies, not only from person to person but also from left to right. As a result, the carotids may lie immediately adjacent to the sella, in which case they may create a surgical risk (Figs. 10.8 and 10.9). Several branches of the internal carotid artery arise within the cavernous sinus, including the meningohypophysial trunk (the largest intracavernous branch), the artery of the inferior cavernous sinus, and McConnell capsular arteries (15).

Given their location, the cavernous sinuses may be directly involved by pituitary tumors. For example, extension of an invasive adenoma into the cavernous sinuses

FIGURE 10.6 Sagittal whole-mount section of normal pituitary gland and surrounding structures. The anterior (*at right*) and posterior (*at left*) lobes are clearly delineated. The pars tuberalis is the thin tongue-shaped portion of anterior lobe that extends for a short distance up the stalk. This diagram illustrates the proximity of the optic chiasm to the pituitary. Superior extension of a pituitary tumor may compress the optic chiasm with resultant visual field deficits, whereas downward extension may fill the sphenoid sinus (Luxol-Fast Blue–PAS).

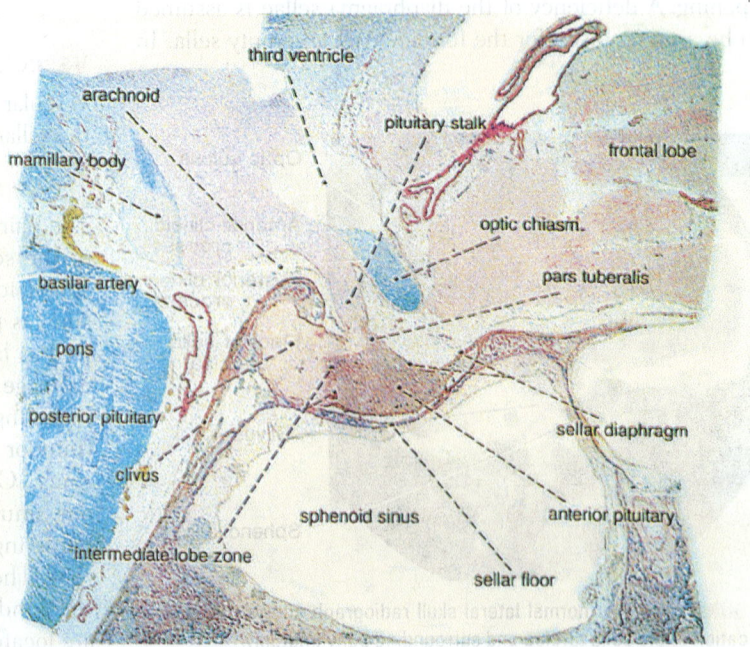

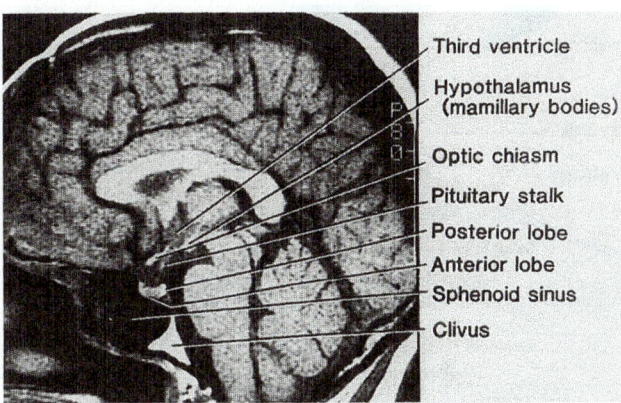

FIGURE 10.7 Magnetic resonance imaging (MRI): Sagittal view of the brain at the level of the pituitary stalk and gland. The clarity of the pituitary gland, stalk, hypothalamus, and optic chiasm is remarkable, making MRI an excellent imaging modality for the assessment of pituitary lesions. One advantage of MRI over computed tomography (CT) is the absence of bony artifact with MRI.

may produce neuropathies of cranial nerves III through VI (Fig. 10.9), including ptosis, facial pain, or diplopia.

The Arterial Supply

The principal arterial supply of the pituitary originates in two branches of the internal carotids: the superior and inferior hypophysial arteries (Fig. 10.15) (20,21). A single superior hypophysial artery springs from each carotid shortly after its entry into the cranial cavity and promptly divides into posterior and anterior branches, each of which anastomoses with the corresponding branch from the opposite side to form an arterial ring around the upper pituitary stalk. The anterior branches give rise to trabecular or loral arteries, which descend on the upper surface of the anterior lobe, course toward the pituitary stalk, and terminate in long-stalk arteries along the pars tuberalis. In their brief course along the anterior lobe, trabecular arteries each give rise to a small artery of the fibrous core (20). The posterior and anterior branches of the superior hypophysial arteries are also the source of short-stalk arteries, which penetrate the superior aspect of the pituitary stalk to run upward or downward within it.

In contrast to the superior hypophysial arteries, the inferior branches originate from the meningohypophysial trunk within the cavernous sinuses. The meningohypophysial trunk gives rise to several vessels, one of which is the inferior hypophysial artery. They contact the inferolateral portions of the gland and bifurcate into medial and lateral branches that anastomose with their opposite counterparts to form an arterial circle about the posterior lobe. Thus, branches of the inferior hypophysial arteries supply primarily the posterior lobe and lower portion of the stalk, contributing only small capsular branches to the periphery of the anterior lobe (22). Although many of the arterial branches in the pituitary stalk and infundibulum form arterioles and capillaries, some give rise to unique vascular complexes termed gomitoli (Figs. 10.15 and 10.16). These "balls of thread" consist of a central artery surrounded by a glomeruloid tangle of capillaries. The transition from central arteries to the

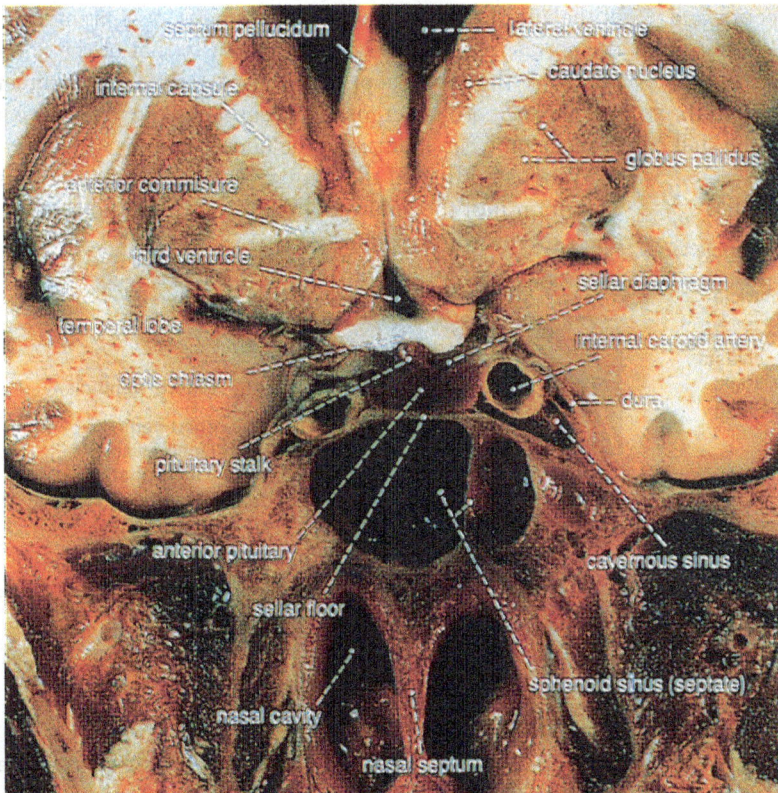

FIGURE 10.8 Coronal section of the head at the level of the pituitary stalk and gland. This photograph clearly illustrates the intimate relationships between the cavernous sinuses, the sphenoid sinus, and the pituitary gland. Invasive adenomas may extend laterally into one or both cavernous sinuses or inferiorly into the sphenoid sinus. Note the proximity of the optic chiasm to the pituitary.

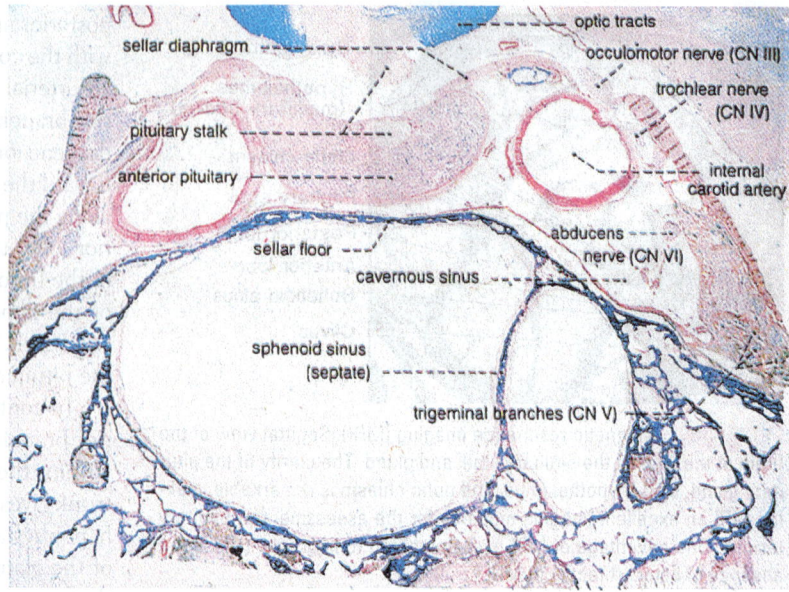

FIGURE 10.9 Coronal whole-mount view of the normal pituitary gland and surrounding structures. Note the location of cranial nerves III, IV, VI, and branches of cranial nerve V within the cavernous sinuses, a relationship explaining the occurrence of cranial nerve palsy in association with invasive pituitary adenomas. This section also illustrates the proximity of the internal carotid arteries to the pituitary gland (Luxol-Fast Blue–PAS).

capillaries is via short specialized arterioles endowed with thick smooth muscle sphincters that serve to regulate blood flow. The mixture of periarteriolar capillaries drains into an extensive pampiniform network, the portal system, which envelopes the stalk (Figs 10.2 and 10.15).

The Hypophysial Portal System

The hypophysial portal system, the critical link between hypothalamus and pituitary, takes its origin from the capillary plexus of the median eminence and stalk, which itself is derived from terminal ramifications of the superior and inferior hypophysial arteries (15). The capillary plexus in the median eminence and superior stalk, the site of uptake of hypophysiotropic (hypothalamic) factors, drains into the long portal vessels that course along the surface of the stalk to supply the majority (90%) of the anterior lobe, whereas the smaller capillary plexus in the lower stalk gives rise to the short portal vessels that descend into its central portion, including that bordering the posterior lobe (22). Distally, the portal system communicates with a delicate capillary network in the anterior lobe, which carries hypophysiotropic factors into the pituitary and conveys anterior lobe hormones to the general circulation (Fig. 10.17). Therefore, aside from a minor direct arterial supply via capsular branches of the inferior hypophysial arteries, the majority of the anterior lobe's circulation is venous, originating from the portal vessels (20–22). In contrast to that of the anterior lobe, the blood supply of the posterior lobe is direct and arterial, a characteristic that explains the predilection of metastatic carcinomas for the neural lobe.

Venous outflow of the pituitary is via collecting vessels that drain into the subhypophysial sinus, cavernous sinus, and superior circular sinus (21).

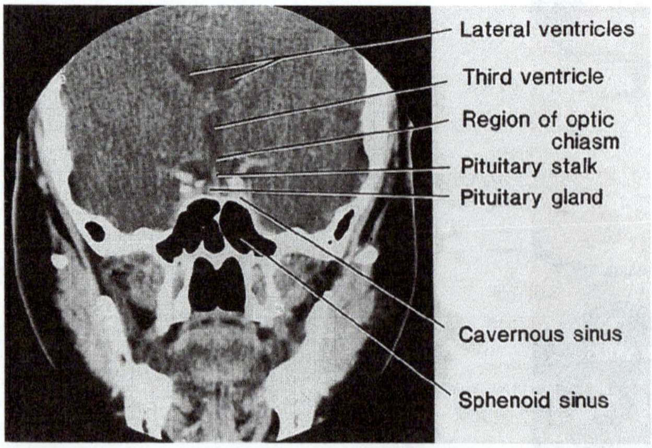

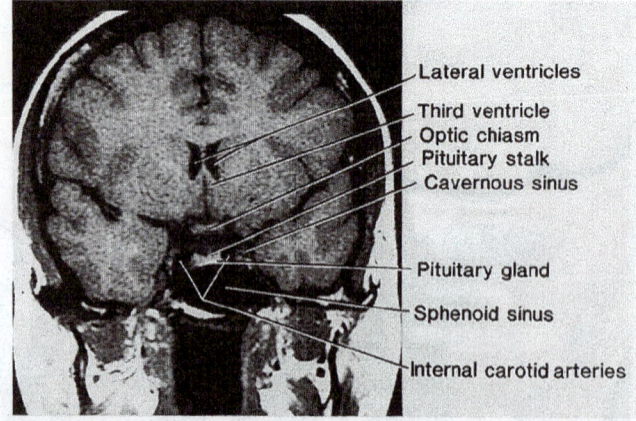

FIGURE 10.10 A computed tomographic (CT) coronal view of the normal skull and brain at the level of the pituitary stalk and gland. The CT scan is a good imaging modality for assessing the pituitary gland; however, radiologists often encounter problems with bony artifact. For this reason, MRI is superior.

FIGURE 10.11 Coronal MRI of the skull and brain at the level of the pituitary stalk and gland.

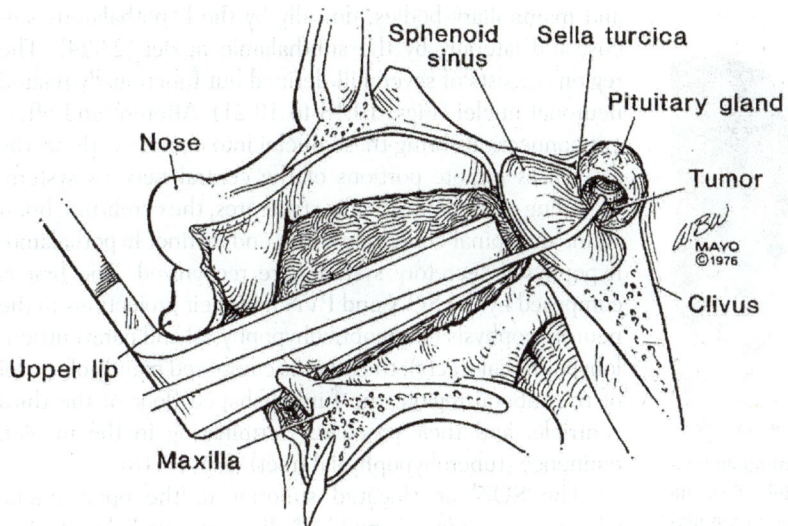

FIGURE 10.12 Transsphenoidal approach to the pituitary gland. After mobilizing the nasal septal cartilage and resecting a portion of ethmoid plate, a sublabial incision is made, and a sphenoid speculum is placed. Next, the floor of the sphenoid sinus and the floor of the sella turcica are traversed. Finally, the dural investment of the pituitary gland is incised, and the gland is exposed. This diagram illustrates a curette in place for removal of a pituitary adenoma.

PHYSIOLOGY AND HISTOLOGY

Hypothalamus

The pituitary is known to be under significant hypothalamic control. In fact, the pituitary and the hypothalamus form a complex neurohormonal circuit, a vital element for maintenance of a normal endocrine status. Weighing approximately 5 g and forming the lower walls and floor of the third ventricle, the hypothalamus lies above the pituitary to which it is connected by the pituitary stalk (Figs. 10.5 to 10.7, 10.18, and 10.19). As the name suggests, the hypothalamus lies inferior to the thalamus. Although at first glance it appears poorly demarcated, the hypothalamus is bordered anteriorly by the anterior commissure, optic chiasm, and lamina terminalis; posteriorly and superiorly by the midbrain tegmentum

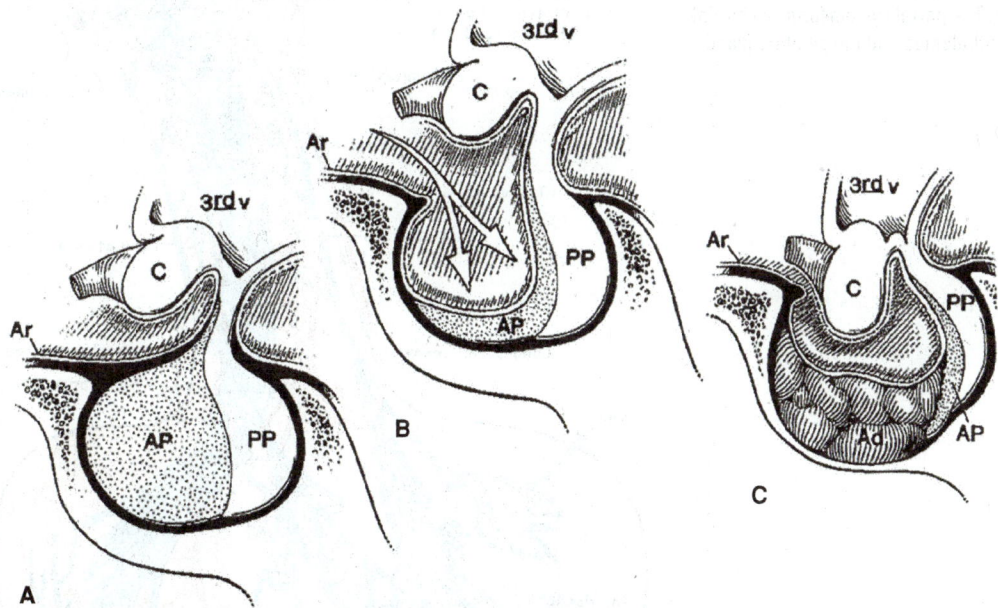

FIGURE 10.13 Illustration of normal as well as variants of the empty sella. **A (left):** The normal pituitary–sellar relationships. The leptomeninges cover the stalk and sellar diaphragm but do not extend into the sella. **B (middle):** In primary empty sella syndrome, an excessively large diaphragmatic orifice permits herniation of leptomeninges into the sella. Prolonged CSF pressure compresses the gland against the sellar floor. **C (right):** Secondary empty sella may result from infarction of a pituitary adenoma, infarction of the pituitary gland, and surgical or radioablation of the gland. (Ar, arachnoid; AP, anterior pituitary; PP, posterior pituitary; C, optic chiasm; 3rd v, third ventricle.)

SECTION IV: Nervous System

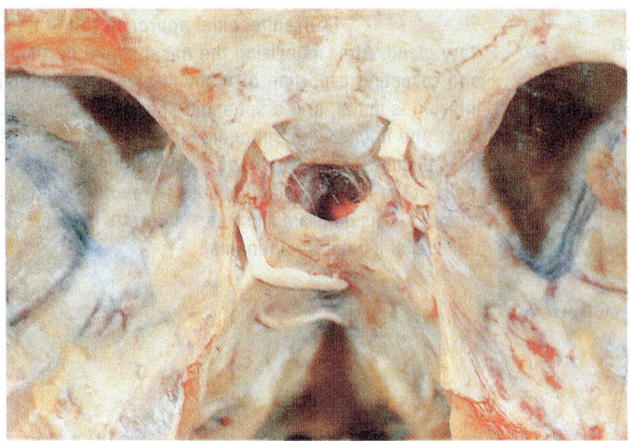

FIGURE 10.14 Superior view of the skull base, demonstrating an incidentally encountered primary empty sella. Normally in this view the upper surface of the pituitary gland would be visible through the diaphragmatic aperture, but here the sella appears empty. Only rarely is primary empty sella syndrome symptomatic. This specimen is from a 57-year-old obese diabetic woman.

FIGURE 10.15 Diagrammatic representation of the vasculature of the pituitary gland. The superior and inferior hypophysial arteries and branches of the internal carotid arteries comprise the major blood supply of the gland. Small terminal branches of the superior and inferior hypophysial arteries give rise to tangled capillary loops termed gomitoli, which drain into portal vessels. The latter traverse the length of the stalk and terminate as a capillary bed in the anterior lobe. The anterior pituitary thus receives the majority of its blood supply not from arteries but from the portal system. The portal system forms a vital link between the hypothalamus and the pituitary gland.

and mammillary bodies; dorsally by the hypothalamus sulcus; and laterally by the subthalamic nuclei (23,24). The region consists of several ill-defined but functionally related neuronal nuclei (Figs. 10.18 to 10.21). Afferent and efferent connections bring these nuclei into contact with nearby as well as remote portions of the central nervous system, including other diencephalic structures, the cerebrum, brain stem, and spinal cord. Two major and distinct hypothalamo-hypophysial secretory systems are recognized. The first is composed by the SON and PVN and their projections to the neurohypophysis (supraopticohypophysial and paraventriculohypophysial tracts); the other is composed mainly of nuclei of the tuberal region, the funnel-shaped floor of the third ventricle, and their processes terminating in the median eminence (tuberohypophysial tract) (Fig. 10.18).

The SON are located superior to the optic tracts, whereas the wedge-shaped PVN lie ventromedial to the fornix and abut the walls of the third ventricle (Fig. 10.19). Due to their predominant composition of large neurons

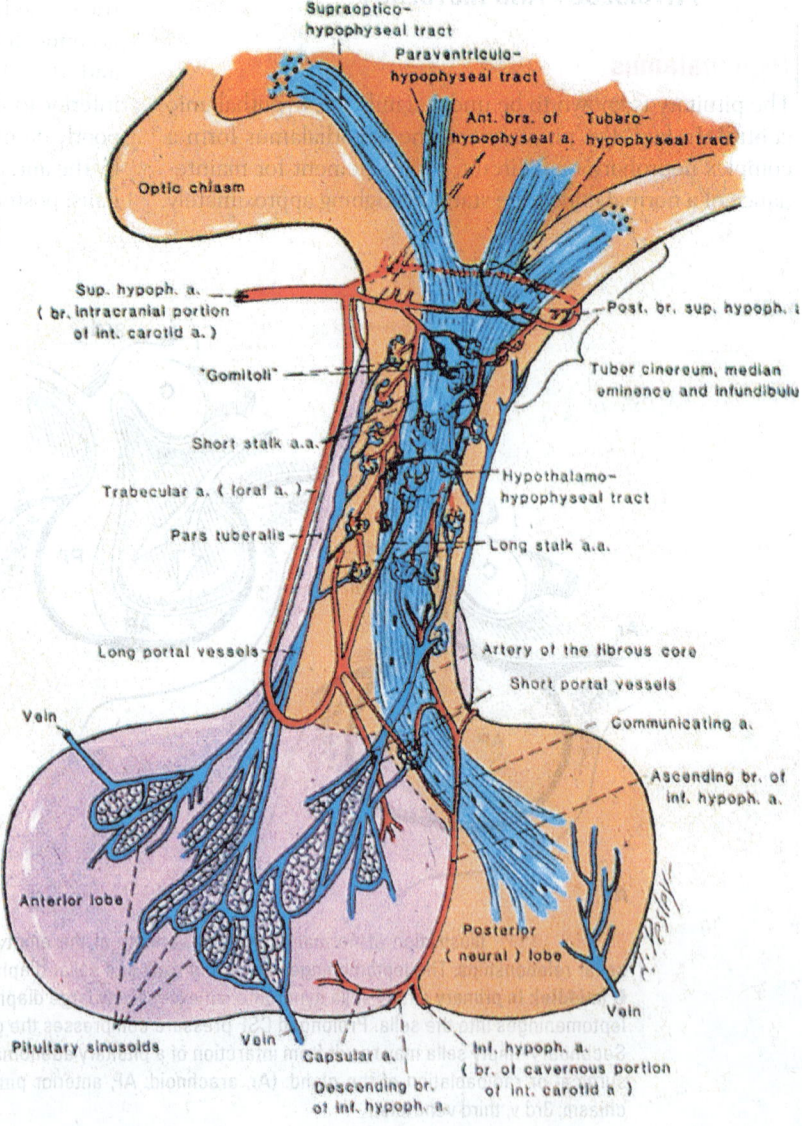

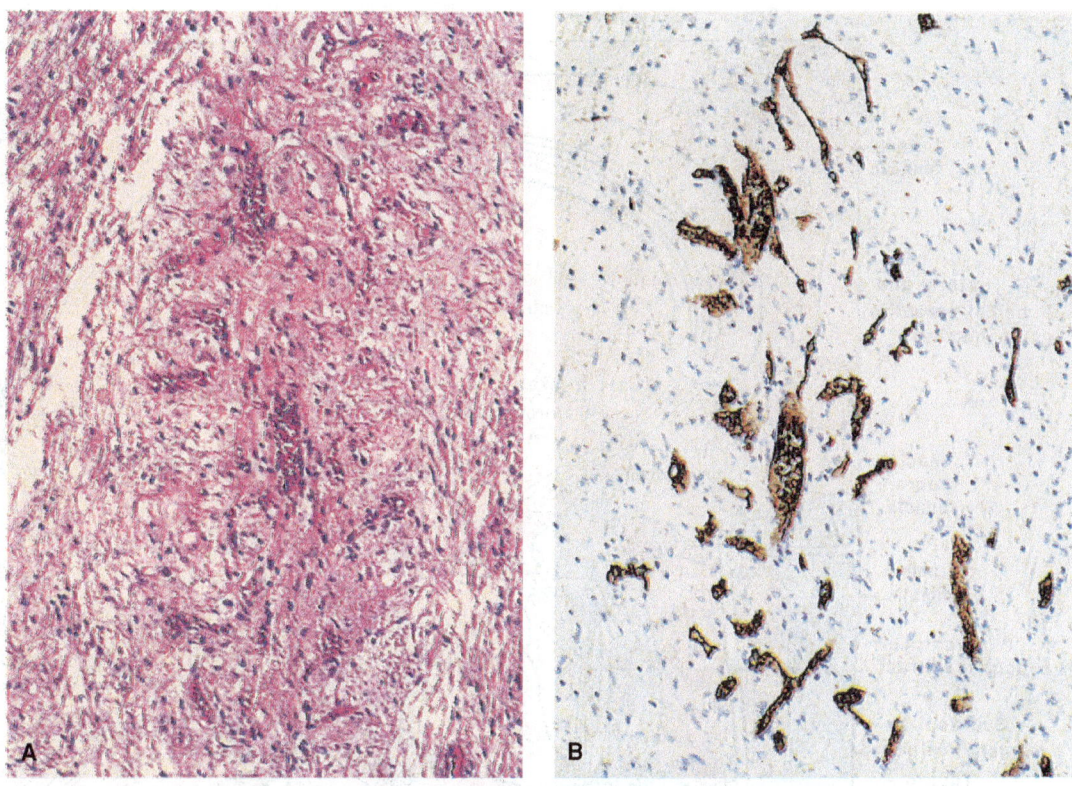

FIGURE 10.16 Gomitoli, tortuous capillary loops surrounding a central arteriole in the upper portion of the pituitary stalk. **A:** (H&E, original magnification ×100). The complex vascularity of the gomitoli is highlighted by staining with *Ulex europaeus* lectin. **B:** (immunostain, original magnification ×100).

measuring up to 25 μm, these are termed magnocellular nuclei (Fig. 10.20). Each contains vasopressin- and oxytocin-producing neurons, but only one hormone is produced by a given neuron. Their long axons form the supraopticohypophysial and paraventriculohypophysial tracts, which carry vasopressin and oxytocin (the so-called neurohypophysial hormones), as well as their respective carrier proteins, the neurophysins, to the posterior lobe of the pituitary gland.

Oxytocin and vasopressin, both nonapeptides, are synthesized mainly in the perikarya of magnocellular neurons

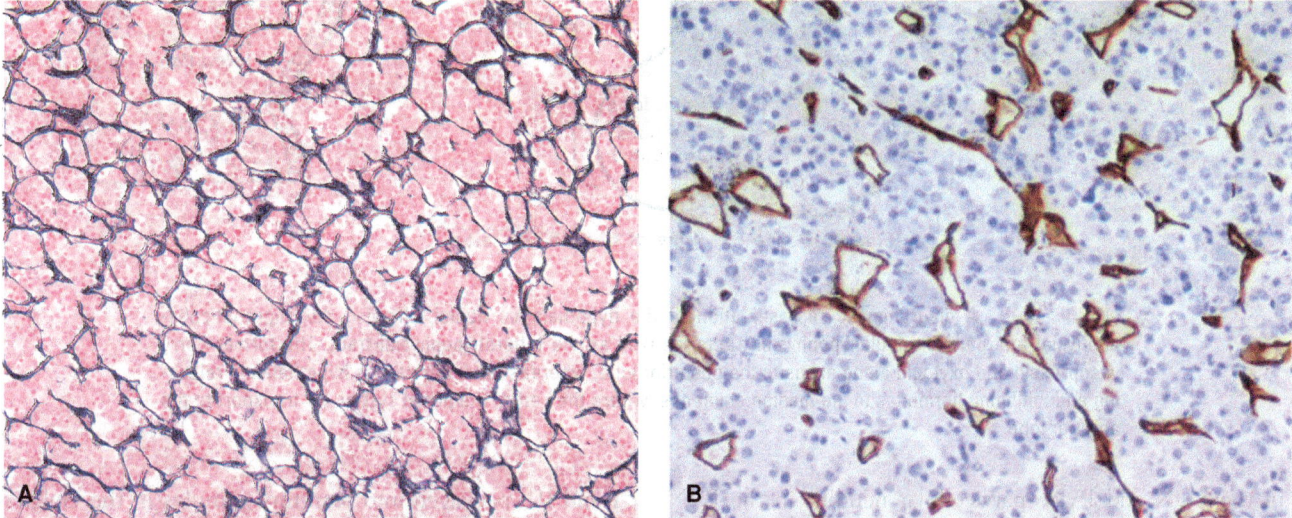

FIGURE 10.17 Adenohypophysis. **A:** The intricate capillary and connective tissue network outlined in reticulin stain. The reticulin stain is invaluable in the evaluation of pituitary adenomas, which are largely devoid of reticulin, whereas the surrounding normal gland retains it (Wilder reticulin, original magnification ×40). **B:** The capillary endothelium of the anterior lobe capillary network stains strongly for CD31 (immunostain ×100).

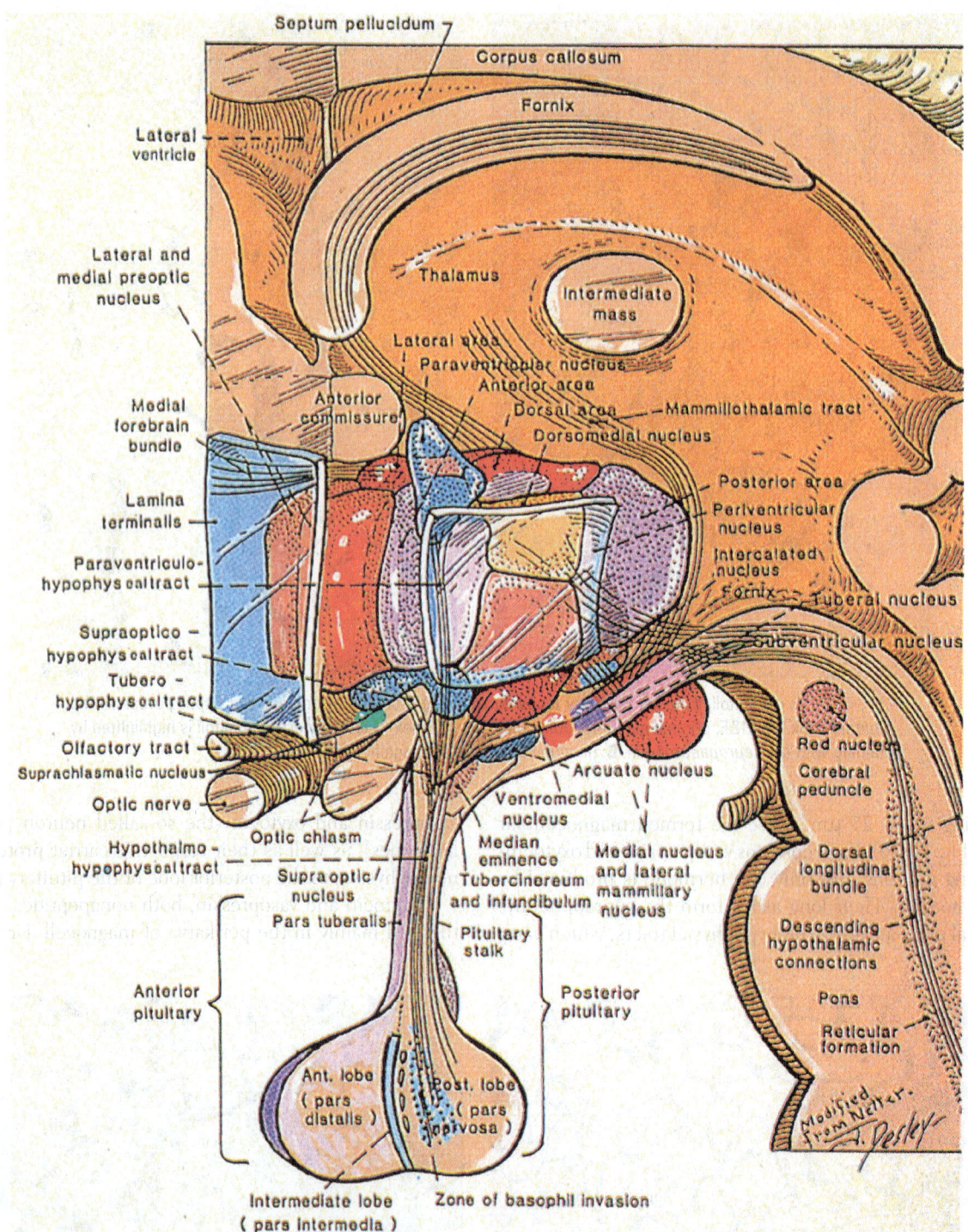

FIGURE 10.18 A diagrammatic representation of the hypothalamic nuclei, showing the supraopticohypophysial and paraventriculohypophysial tracts, as well as the tuberohypophysial tract. The former carry vasopressin and oxytocin along axons to the posterior lobe, whereas the latter carries hypothalamic releasing and inhibiting hormones to the median eminence, where they enter the portal system for transport to the anterior lobe.

in the SON and PVN; parvicellular neurons in the PVN also synthesize vasopressin. The two hormones differ by only two amino acids. Both are synthesized as a 20-kDa precursor peptide that is rapidly cleaved into the active hormone and its neurophysin carrier protein (neurophysin I and II), packaged into secretory granules in the Golgi as a hormone–neurophysin complex and secreted from nerve endings that terminate primarily in the neurohypophysis (25). Large intra-axonal accumulations of these hormones, named Herring bodies, are often visible by light microscopy

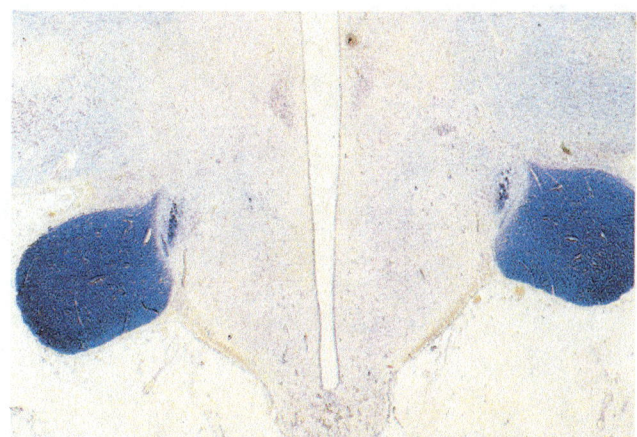

FIGURE 10.19 Coronal whole-mount section through the hypothalamus and third ventricle. The PVN are visible as darkly staining areas beneath the ependyma of the third ventricle (*upper field*), whereas the SON lie above the heavily myelinated optic tracts. The arcuate nucleus lies inferior to the base of the third ventricle (*cresyl violet*).

hormones differ by only two amino acids, oxytocin exhibits virtually no antidiuretic activity, and vasopressin has negligible oxytocic effect. Oxytocin mediates the "milk let-down reflex" by stimulating contraction of myoepithelial cells surrounding terminal mammary lobules. In addition, it serves a role in parturition, binding, and facilitating contraction in the final stages of parturition. The major physiologic role of vasopressin, also called antidiuretic hormone (ADH), is the formation of hypertonic urine. Acting via cyclic adenosine monophosphate, vasopressin increases the water permeability of renal collecting ducts, allowing the hypotonic intraductal fluid to equilibrate with the hypertonic fluid in the medullary interstitium. The results are concentrated urine and conservation of body water. Genetic mutations in either the signal peptide or VP-neurophysin give rise to central diabetes insipidus. Likewise, damage to the neurohypophysis from head trauma, surgery, inflammatory processes, or neoplasms may destroy vasopressin-producing neurons and cause diabetes insipidus.

The second component of the hypothalamohypophysial system is the tuberoinfundibular tract. Its fibers originate in a number of hypothalamic nuclei lying within the walls of the inferior third ventricle and tuberal region (Figs. 10.18, 10.19, and 10.21) (23). Products of these nuclei, targeted for the anterior pituitary, consist of releasing and inhibiting hormones. Unlike the magnocellular neurons

as round, granular structures that appear eosinophilic on hematoxylin and eosin (H&E) sections (Fig. 10.22). In transit from the hypothalamus to the posterior lobe, prohormones undergo extensive processing and cleavage to form the final products, vasopressin and oxytocin. Although these

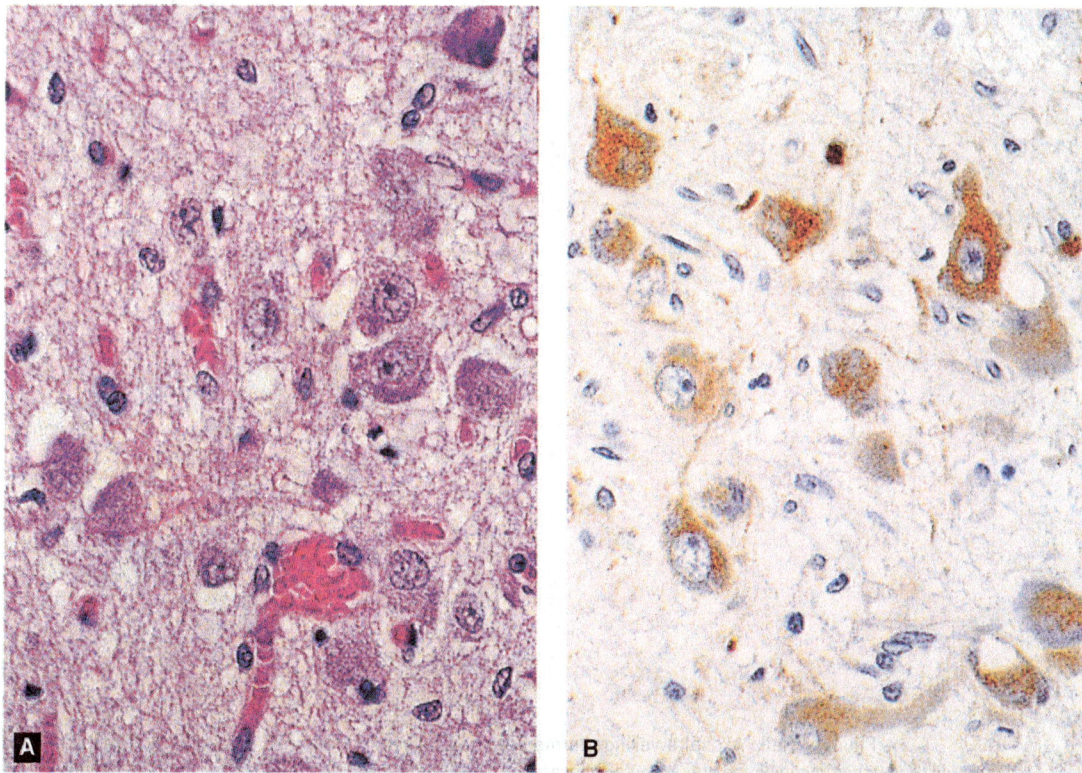

FIGURE 10.20 Paraventricular nucleus of the hypothalamus. **A:** Its high degree of vascularity is a characteristic of magnocellular nuclei (H&E, original magnification ×100). **B:** The nerve cell bodies stain positively for vasopressin (immunostain, original magnification ×100).

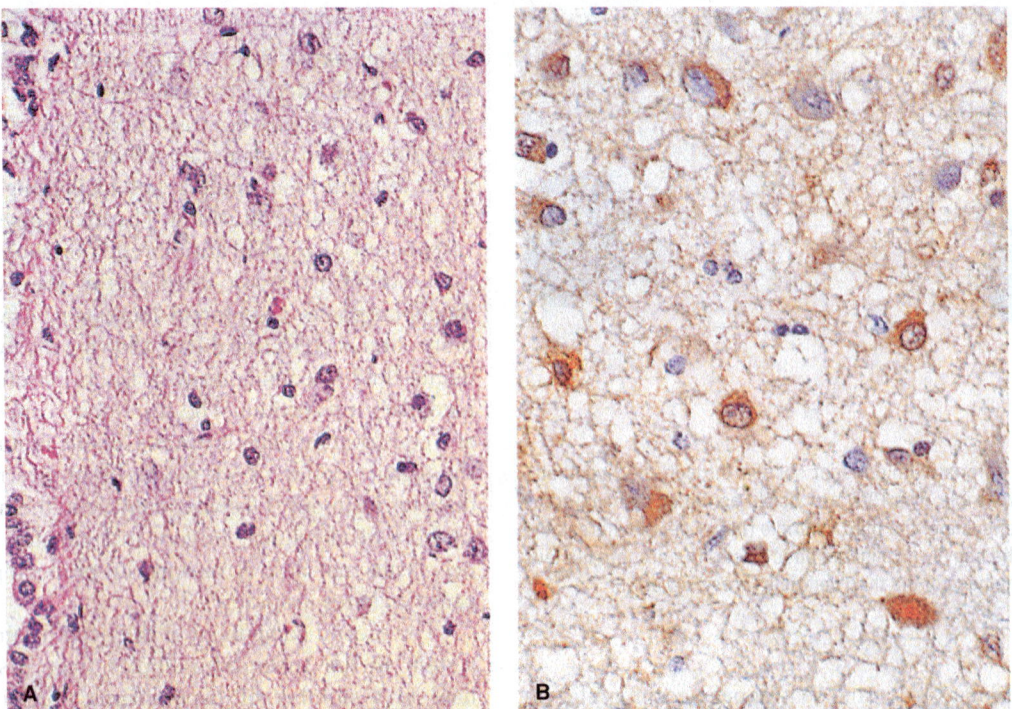

FIGURE 10.21 Periventricular nucleus. **A:** Lying beneath the ependyma of the third ventricle (**bottom left**), this ill-defined nucleus is composed of small nerve cell bodies (H&E, original magnification ×63). **B:** Its constituent neurons stain for CRH, a tropic hormone that exerts its effect on corticotrophs in the anterior lobe (immunostain, original magnification ×100).

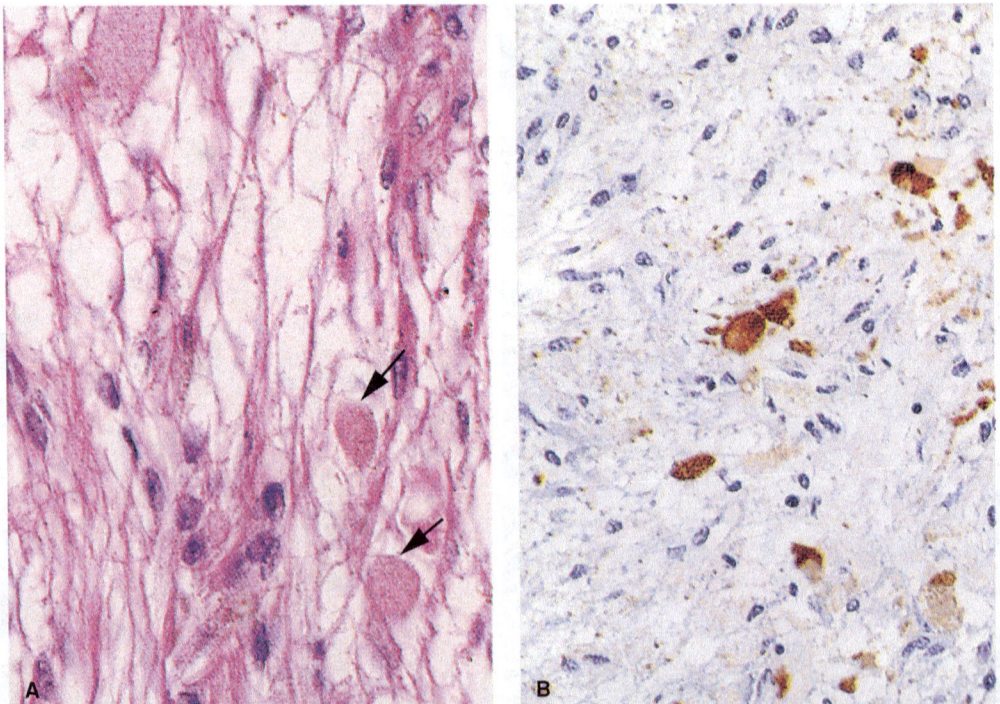

FIGURE 10.22 Pituitary stalk. Axonal swellings termed Herring bodies characterize its axons. **A:** They are distinguished by their ovoid shape and granular character on H&E (*upper left* and *lower right; arrows*). Herring bodies represent intra-axonal accumulations of oxytocin- and vasopressin-containing granules en route to the posterior lobe (H&E, original magnification ×100). **B:** Herring bodies staining for vasopressin (immunostain, original magnification ×100).

of the SON and PVN, these are small neurons and for this reason are termed parvicellular neurons (Fig. 10.21). Their processes project to the median eminence, a highly vascular zone, located in the posterior proximal portion of the pituitary stalk. Here, the hypothalamic hormones are released into the first portion of the portal system for transport to the anterior lobe. Ultrastructurally, the median eminence consists of closely packed nerve terminals containing membrane-bound neurosecretory granules. Because the terminals lie in close proximity to the fenestrated capillaries that form the origin of the portal system, the overall anatomic arrangement permits ready entry of *hypothalamic releasing* and *inhibiting hormones* and perhaps other modulators into the portal system and consequently the anterior lobe.

The hypothalamic hormones include five peptide hormones: corticotropin-releasing hormone (CRH), growth hormone–releasing hormone (GHRH), gonadotropin-releasing hormone (GnRH or LHRH), thyrotropin-releasing hormone (TRH), and somatostatin (somatotropin release–inhibiting factor) (SRIF or SST). The sites of synthesis of the various hypothalamic hormones, their characteristics, and target cells are summarized in Tables 10.2 and 10.3. In addition to these hormones, several bioactive substances produced in the hypothalamus participate in the regulation of anterior pituitary hormone secretion. The most significant one is dopamine which inhibits the secretion of PRL by pituitary lactotrophs (25).

Adenohypophysis

The pituitary is a tan to brown, bean-shaped structure varying in weight from 500 to 700 mg (Fig. 10.1). An average-sized gland of 600 mg measures about 13 × 10 × 6 mm. In general, the weight of the female pituitary is greater than that of the male (26). Among females, the gland is smaller in nulliparas than in multiparas. In pregnancy the gland enlarges significantly (up to 30%) primarily as a result of lactotroph cell hyperplasia (26). The anterior lobe comprises 80% of the pituitary and includes the pars distalis, intermedia, and tuberalis. The body and stalk of the gland are surrounded by a delicate capsule derived from the meninges (15). Staining characteristics roughly divide the pars distalis into a central mucoid wedge and two lateral wings, zones best visualized in coronal and horizontal sections.

TABLE 10.2 Pituitary Hormones and Hypothalamic Stimulatory and Inhibitory Hormones

Pituitary Hormone	Hypothalamic Hormone Stimulatory	Hypothalamic Hormone Inhibitory
GH	GHRH	Somatostatin (SRIF or SST)
PRL	TRH, VIP	Dopamine
ACTH	CRH, AVP	?
FSH/LH	GnRH	?
TSH	TRH	Somatostatin

GH, growth hormone; GHRH, growth hormone–releasing hormone; SRIF or SST, somatotropin release–inhibiting factor; PRL, prolactin; TRH, thyrotropin-releasing hormone; VIP, vasoactive intestinal peptide; ACTH, adrenocorticotropic hormone; CRH, corticotropin-releasing hormone; AVP, arginine vasopressin; FSH, follicle-stimulating hormone; GnRH, gonadotropin-releasing hormone; LH, luteinizing hormone; TSH, thyroid-stimulating hormone.

TABLE 10.3 Major Hypothalamic–Pituitary Axis Hormones

Hormone	Hypothalamic Sites	Pituitary Hormone	Target Hormone
GHRH	Arcuate nucleus	GH	IFG-1
TRH	Widely distributed in CNS with concentration in ventromedial, dorsal, and paraventricular nuclei, particularly on left	TSH	T4, T3
GnRH	Widespread distribution with concentration in the arcuate, ventromedial, dorsal, and paraventricular nuclei	FSH, Luteinizing hormone (LH)	Estrogen, Progesterone/Estrogen (Female), Testosterone (Male)
CRH	Periventricular, medial paraventricular nuclei; co-localized with arginine vasopressin	ACTH	Cortisol, DHEA
Somatostatin (SRIF or SST)	Periventricular nucleus, paraventricular (parvicellular neurons), arcuate nuclei	GH	N/A
DA	Arcuate nucleus	PRL	N/A

GHRH, growth hormone–releasing hormone; GH, growth hormone; IFG-1, insulin-like growth factor 1; TRH, thyrotropin-releasing hormone; TSH, thyroid-stimulating hormone, T4, thyroxine; T3, triiodothyronine; GnRH, gonadotropin-releasing hormone; FSH, follicle-stimulating hormone; CRH, corticotropin-releasing hormone; ACTH, adrenocorticotropic hormone; DHEA, dehydroepiandrosterone; SRIF or SST, somatotropin release–inhibiting factor; GH, growth hormone; DA, dopamine; PRL, prolactin.

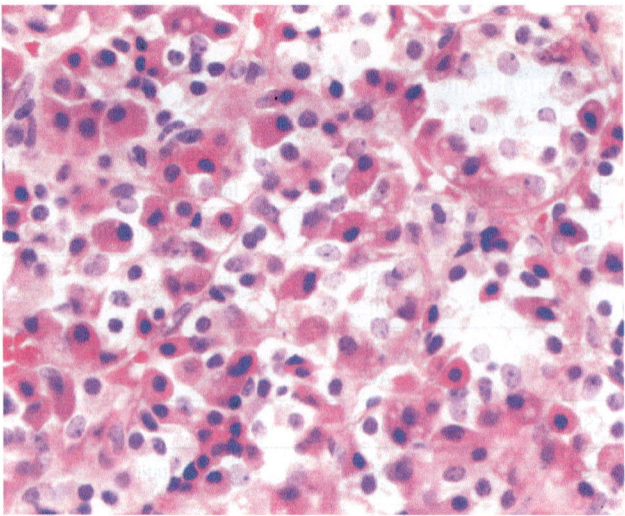

FIGURE 10.23 Anterior lobe. An H&E-stained section shows chromophobic, acidophilic, and basophilic cells. Acidophils are most numerous in the lateral wings, whereas basophils are found in greatest number in the central or mucoid wedge. The different cell types are arranged in acinar formations that can be highlighted by reticulin stain (see Fig. 10.17) (original magnification ×200).

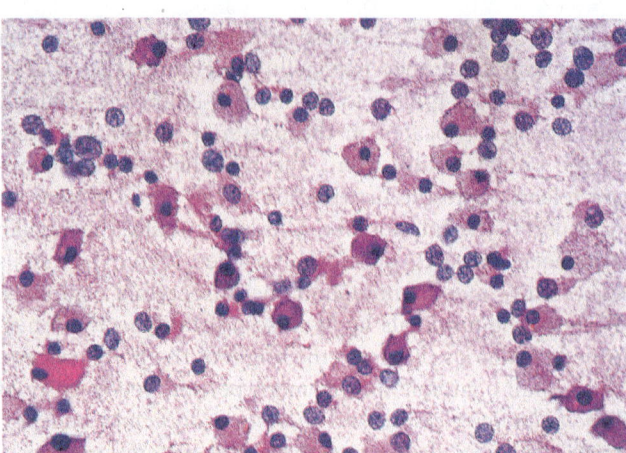

FIGURE 10.24 H&E-stained cytologic smear of the normal anterior lobe, demonstrating acidophils, chromophobes, and basophils. Delicate nuclei, inconspicuous nucleoli, and variable cytoplasmic staining characterize normal cells and permit their distinction from adenoma cells (original magnification ×100).

By light microscopy, the cells of the anterior lobe show variation, not only in size and shape, but also in their histochemical staining characteristics (Fig. 10.23 and 10.24). They are arranged in nests, cords, and small acini bounded by an interlacing capillary network that is best seen on reticulin stain (see Fig. 10.17). This architectural pattern, altered in hyperplasia and conspicuously absent in adenomas, is of considerable diagnostic significance (see Fig. 10.51).

The pars intermedia, poorly developed in humans, consists in large part of epithelium-lined spaces containing periodic acid–Schiff (PAS)-positive colloid; the constituent cells are ciliated, goblet, and a few neuroendocrine cells that may show variable immunoreactivity for pituitary hormones including adrenocorticotropic hormone (ACTH), luteinizing hormone (LH), and follicle-stimulating hormone (FSH) (Fig. 10.25) (27). These Rathke cleft remnants, the vast majority of which are microscopic in size, are present

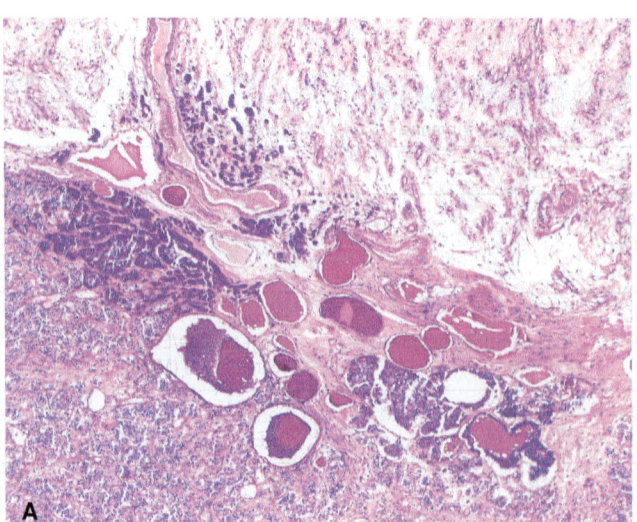
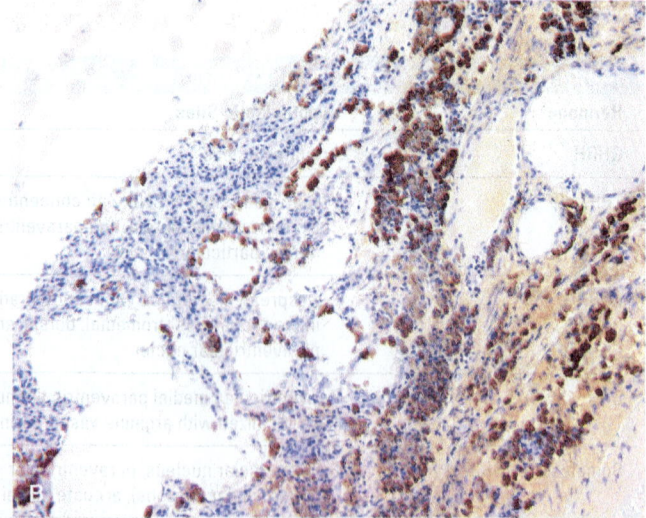

FIGURE 10.25 Intermediate lobe remnant. **A:** Intermediate lobe cysts are lined by a single layer of cuboidal to columnar epithelium that may be nonciliated, ciliated, mucin-producing cells, or neuroendocrine cells. The cyst contains an eosinophilic colloid (PAS, original magnification ×40). **B:** Many of the cells lining the cysts are neuroendocrine cells showing variable reactivity for pituitary hormones, in particular ACTH (ACTH immunostain, original magnification ×100).

in about 25% of pituitaries of autopsies (28). Cysts of the Rathke cleft are usually incidental postmortem findings; symptomatic cysts are uncommon, representing about 5% to 9% of surgical lesions of the sellar region (29).

In H&E-stained sections, three principal cell types are identified in the normal anterior lobe: acidophils (40%), basophils (10%), and chromophobes (50%) (Figs. 10.23 and 10.24). The designations reflect their staining affinities for acidic and basic dyes, with the chromophobic cells lacking affinity for either. These reactivities form the basis of an outdated classification of pituitary adenomas that offers little in specifying their hormone content or endocrine function. On the other hand, advances in immunohistochemistry permit morphologic and functional correlation (Fig. 10.26). Numerous cells in the central or mucoid wedge are basophilic and stain strongly via the PAS method. Such cells produce ACTH and TSH. In contrast, most cells in the lateral wings are acidophilic and are engaged either in GH or, less frequently, in PRL production. The essential morphologic features of the five principal cell types and the biochemical characteristics of the six hormones of the anterior pituitary are summarized in Table 10.4. Their ultrastructural features are presented in Table 10.5.

Somatotroph Cells

Somatotrophs, or GH cells, occur in greatest density in the lateral wings and comprise approximately 50% of all adenohypophysial cells. A minority of somatotroph cells are scattered throughout the median portion of the gland. They are medium-sized, ovoid cells with round, centrally located nuclei, relatively prominent nucleoli, and with abundant acidophilic granules (Fig. 10.27). Immunohistochemical stains for GH show strong and diffuse cytoplasm staining, consistent with the numerous secretory granules present at the ultrastructural level (Figs. 10.27 and 10.28). Somatotroph cells are rather stable during life, and their number, morphology, and immunoreactivity are unchanged by age.

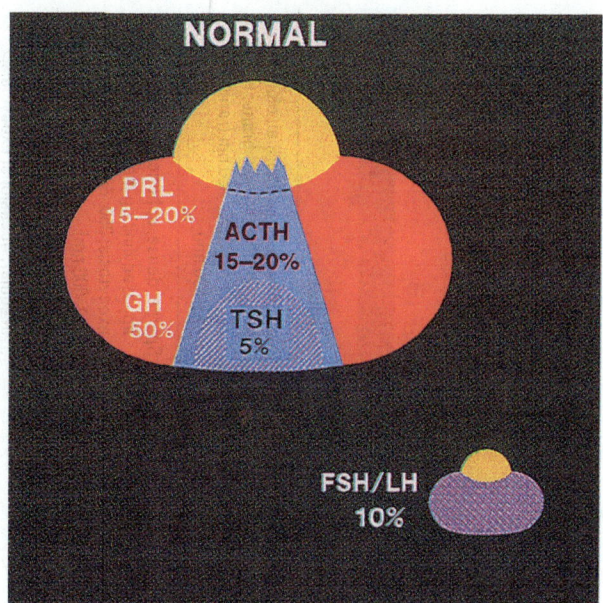

FIGURE 10.26 Preferential localization and relative frequency of functional anterior lobe cell types in the normal pituitary gland. Note that gonadotrophs (LH/FSH cells), represented in the small gland (*lower right*), are distributed diffusely and show no preferential localization.

TABLE 10.4
The Normal Anterior Pituitary: Morphologic and Functional Features of Secretory Cells

Cell Type	Product	Location	Percentage of Cells (%)	Histochemical Staining[a]	Immunoperoxidase Staining
Somatotroph[b]	GH; 21,000 dalton polypeptide	Lateral wings	50	Acidophilic; PAS (−)	GH
Lactotroph[b]	PRL; 23,500 dalton polypeptide	Resting cells: generalized; Secreting cells: posterolateral wings	15–20	Acidophilic; PAS (−)	PRL
Corticotroph	ACTH; 4,507 dalton polypeptide	Mucoid wedge	15–20	Basophilic; PAS and lead hematoxylin (+)	ACTH, β-LPH, MSH, endorphin, enkephalin
Gonadotroph	FSH and LH; 35,100 and 28,260 dalton glycoprotein	Generalized	10	Basophilic; PAS, lead hematoxylin, aldehyde fuchsin, and aldehyde thionine (+)	β-FSH, β-LH[c], α-subunit
Thyrotroph	TSH; 28,000 dalton glycoprotein	Anterior mucoid wedge	<5	Same as for gonadotroph	TSH, α-subunit

[a]The tinctorial characteristics of normal pituitary cells depend on adequate cytoplasmic granulae storage. If sparsely granulated, cells that are otherwise functional may appear nonreactive or "chromophobic."
[b]Rare acidophillic stem cells (presumed somatotroph and lactotroph precursor cells producing both GH and PRL) are present in the normal pituitary.
[c]Many gonadotrophs are capable of producing both FSH and LH, although immunohistochemical and ultrastructural evidence suggests that some gonadotrophs may produce only one hormone.
GH, growth hormone; PRL, prolactin; ACTH, adrenocorticotropic hormone; FSH and LH, follicle-stimulating hormone and luteinizing hormone; TSH, thyroid-stimulating hormone.

TABLE 10.5 The Normal Pituitary: Ultrastructural Features

Cell Type	Granularity	Cell Size and Shape	Nucleus	Cytoplasm	Golgi Complex	Rough Endoplasmic Reticulum	Granules
Somatotroph—Densely granulated (resting phase)	+++, +++++	Medium, spherical oval	Spherical and central, with prominent nucleoli	Lucent	+	+	Abundant; dense, spherical; closely apposed limiting membrane; no exocytosis; 350–600 nm (range 250–600 nm)
Somatotroph—Sparsely granulated (secretory phase)	+, ++	Medium, spherical oval	Irregular	Lucent	+++	+++ Peripherally disposed	Sparse; dense, spherical; closely apposed limiting membrane; no exocytosis; 350–600 nm (range 250–600 nm)
Lactotroph—Densely granulated (resting phase)	+++, +++++	Large, polyhedral-elongate	Oval-elongate	Lucent	+	++	Abundant; dense, spherical-oval, irregular; occasional exocytosis; 500–800 nm
Lactotroph—Sparsely granulated (secretory phase)	+, ++	Medium, polyhedral-elongate	Oval	Lucent	+++, +++++ Juxtanuclear	++++ "Nebenkern" formation	Sparse; dense, irregular; frequent normal and misplaced exocytosis 200–350 nm
Corticotroph	++, +++	Medium, oval-polygonal	Spherical, eccentric	Electron-dense; cytoplasmic cytokeratin (type I) filaments; large lysosomes	++	++, +++ Dispersed, slightly dilated	Variable density, spherical-irregular; frequently peripheral; no exocytosis; 300–350 nm (range 250–700 nm, rarely 1,000 nm)
Gonadotroph	++	Medium, oval	Spherical, eccentric	Lucent	++, +++ Prominent, globular	++, +++ Stacked or dispersed and slightly dilated	Dense, spherical; no exocytosis; 250–400 nm
Thyrotroph	+, ++	Medium, polygonal	Spherical, eccentric	Lucent; scattered lysosomes	++, +++ Globular, with numerous vesicles	+++ Short dispersed profiles	Dense, spherical; frequently peripheral; no exocytosis; 150 nm

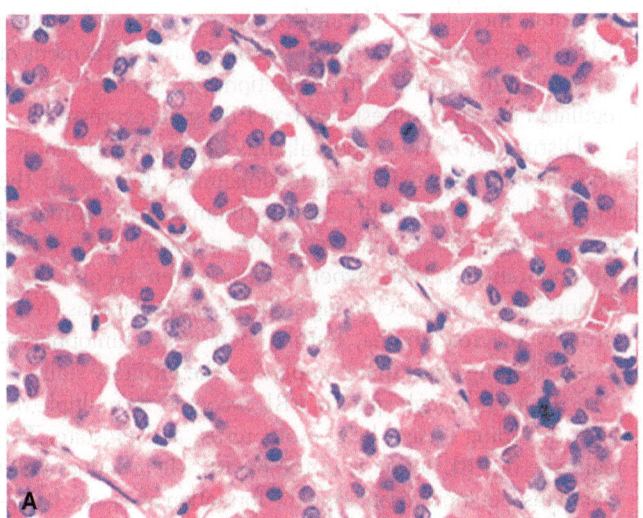 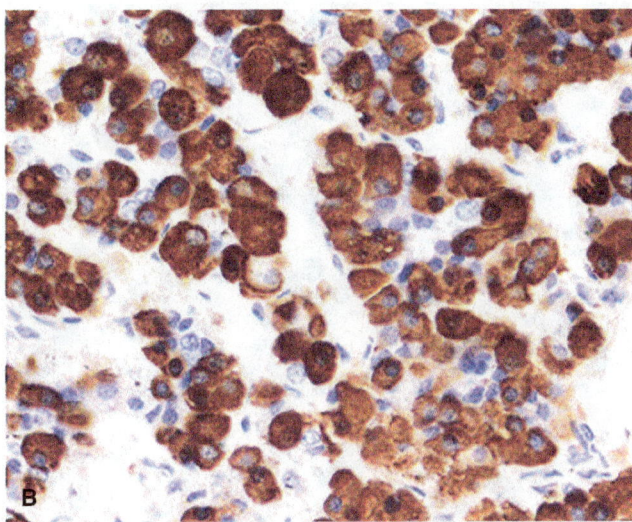

FIGURE 10.27 Somatotrophs. **A:** By H&E stain, somatotrophs are medium-sized cells with abundant, eosinophilic and granular cytoplasm. Somatotrophs comprise 50% of anterior lobe cells (original magnification ×200). **B:** The strong GH-staining reaction is a reflection of the numerous secretory granules present at the ultrastructural level (see Fig. 10.28) (GH immunostain, original magnification ×200).

The development of somatotrophs and GH transcription is determined by the expression of the nuclear transcription factor *Pit-1* (see above). Five distinct genes on chromosome 17q22 encode GH and related proteins. Two alternatively spliced peptides are produced by the pituitary GH gene (*hGH-N*), a 22-kDa GH (191 amino acids) and a less abundant 20-kDa GH molecule, both with similar biologic activity (30). During pregnancy, placental syncytiotrophoblast cells express a GH variant gene (*hGH-V*), which plays a significant role in human fetal growth and development (31).

The product of GH cells has extensive effects by direct action of GH and actions through mediators of hepatic origin called insulin-like growth factor 1 (IGF-1) (30). GH functions as the major promoter of growth but also in several other metabolic pathways, including glucose, insulin, and fatty acid. The pulsatile secretion of GH from the anterior lobe is under the control of the two hypothalamic regulatory hormones: GHRH and somatostatin (SRIF or SST). The GHRH controls GH synthesis by regulating transcription of GH mRNA via control of intracellular cyclic AMP pathway. Somatostatin appears to determine the timing and amplitude of GH pulses but has no effect on GH synthesis. IGF-1 causes negative feedback inhibition of GH release by acting at the hypothalamus and the pituitary.

Hypersecretion of GH in children causes gigantism, whereas its overproduction in adults leads to acromegaly.

Lactotroph Cells

Lactotrophs, or PRL cells, comprise approximately 20% of anterior pituitary cells and are concentrated in the posterior portions of the lateral wings. Histologically, they appear either acidophilic (densely granulated) or chromophobic (sparsely granulated). Chromophobic cells are more numerous, possess elongate processes, and, despite an abundance of endoplasmic reticulum and well-developed Golgi complexes, contain relatively few cytoplasmic granules (Figs. 10.29 and 10.30, and Table 10.5). Densely granulated lactotrophs are thought to represent a storage phase, whereas sparsely granulated cells are engaged in active secretion. A characteristic pattern of PRL staining of lactotrophs by immunohistochemistry, the so-called "Golgi pattern," is the presence of paranuclear staining corresponding to PRL in the Golgi apparatus (Fig. 10.29).

With the exception of pregnancy and lactation, there is no significant difference in PRL cell number between males and females. The doubling in volume of the pituitary during pregnancy is because of striking hyperplasia as well as hypertrophy of chromophobic lactotrophs, termed pregnancy cells. They persist until shortly after delivery or the termination

FIGURE 10.28 Densely granulated somatotrophs (GH cells) showing prominent Golgi and numerous 200- to 500-nm secretory granules (original magnification ×11,700).

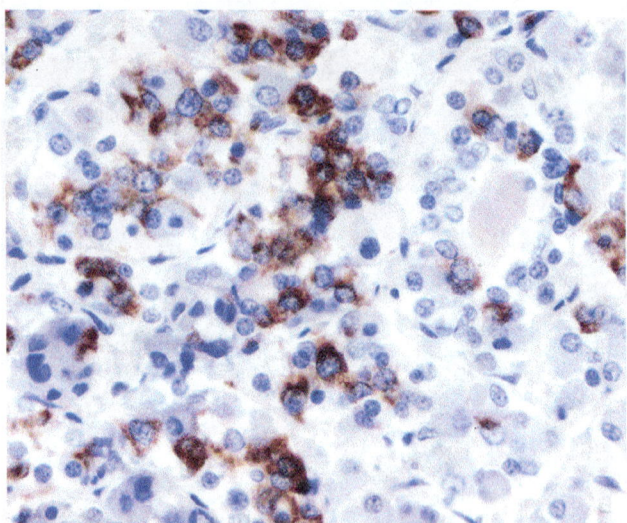

FIGURE 10.29 Lactotrophs. Lactotrophs comprise 15% to 20% of anterior lobe cells. The majority are sparsely granulated, angular cells with processes that may wrap around adjacent cells. Many lactotrophs in this field show paranuclear staining, a pattern corresponding to PRL in the Golgi apparatus (PRL immunostain, original magnification ×100).

of lactation (26). PRL cell hyperplasia also may accompany estrogen administration and hypothyroidism (30). The existence of mammosomatotrophs, cells engaged in PRL and GH production and possessing unique ultrastructural features, attests to the existence of a histogenetic relationship between PRL and GH cells (32).

PRL secretion is unique among the anterior pituitary hormones in that it is under tonic hypothalamic inhibition by dopamine (hypothalamic PRL inhibitory factor, or PIF) produced by tuberoinfundibular dopamine neurons. Dopamine type 2 (D2) receptors in lactotrophs mediate PRL inhibition. Several PRL-releasing factors participate in PRL secretion, including TRH and vasoactive intestinal peptide (VIP). Glucocorticoids, thyroid hormone and a fragment of GnRH weakly suppress PRL secretion. PRL synthesis is also regulated by effects of estrogen on PRL gene expression.

Disruption of the hypothalamus or the hypothalamic–hypophysial stalk may impede dopamine delivery to the anterior lobe, causing hyperprolactinemia, a phenomenon termed "stalk effect." This regulatory pathway accounts for the spontaneous PRL hypersecretion often secondary to compressive space-occupying sellar or parasellar mass (e.g., pituitary macroadenoma, Rathke cleft cyst, craniopharyngioma, meningioma) that compresses the pituitary stalk.

PRL acts through specific PRL receptors in multiple tissues, including breast, liver, ovary, testis, and prostate. The main site of PRL action is in the breast, where induces and maintains lactation stimulating the formation of casein, lactalbumin, lipids, and carbohydrates, all essential components of breast milk. During pregnancy, high levels of estrogen, progesterone, placental lactogen, and PRL induce acinar development and promote milk formation. As previously noted, milk secretion is under the control of oxytocin, a potent stimulator of myoepithelial cell contraction in breast tissue. PRL also decreases reproductive function and suppress sexual drive by suppressing hypothalamic GnRH and pituitary gonadotropins secretion and impairing gonadal steroidogenesis (30).

In patients with hyperprolactinemia, besides galactorrhea, decreased libido and reduced fertility are common clinical symptoms.

Corticotroph Cells

Corticotrophs, or ACTH cells, comprise 15% to 20% of adenohypophysial cells and are most numerous in the mid and posterior portions of the mucoid wedge (Fig. 10.26). Histologically, corticotroph cells are polygonal, medium- to large-sized, and basophilic (Fig. 10.31). A paranuclear vacuole that corresponds to one or several lysosomal structures at the ultrastructural level is typically seen in the cytoplasm (Fig. 10.32) (27,33). Corticotroph cells are strong PAS positive because of a carbohydrate moiety contained in POMC, the precursor molecule of ACTH. In immunostained preparations, corticotrophs show strong and diffuse cytoplasm ACTH staining (Fig. 10.31) consistent with the numerous secretory granules present at the ultrastructural level. Corticotrophs may also contain other POMC derivatives, including β-lipotropin (β-LPH), melanocyte-stimulating hormone (MSH), endorphin, and encephalin (see later) which are not of significance in the daily practice of surgical pathology. Perinuclear bundles of cytokeratin filaments are also a characteristic feature of ACTH cells (Table 10.5). Under conditions of glucocorticoid excess, either exogenous or endogenous, corticotrophs accumulate cytokeratin as a manifestation of Crooke hyaline change (Figs. 10.33 and 10.34).

ACTH, the principal product of corticotrophs, is part of a larger precursor molecule, the POMC, which is enzymatically cleaved in the anterior pituitary into β-LPH and ACTH. In the intermediate lobe, ACTH is cleaved into MSH and

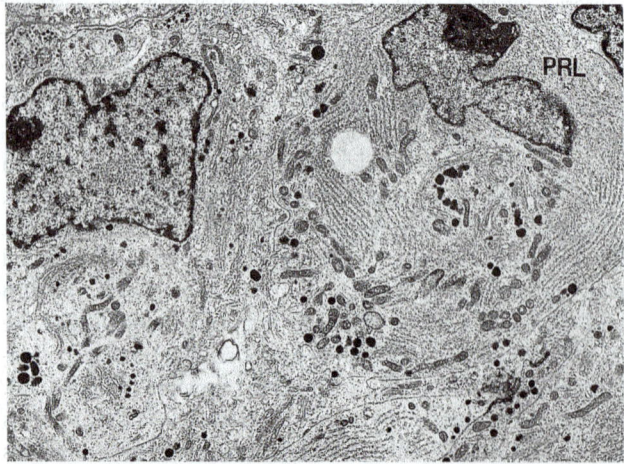

FIGURE 10.30 Sparsely granulated PRL cell. Note the abundant cisternae of rough endoplasmic reticulum and the prominent Golgi complex containing pleomorphic developing granules. Mature PRL granules range in size from 200 to 350 nm (original magnification ×8,700).

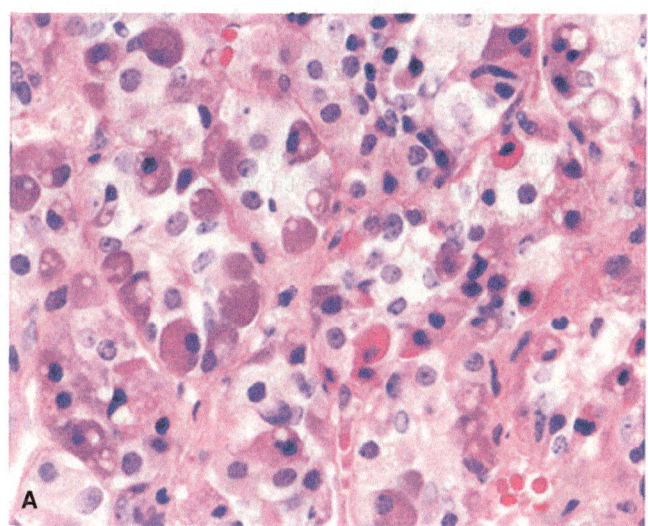
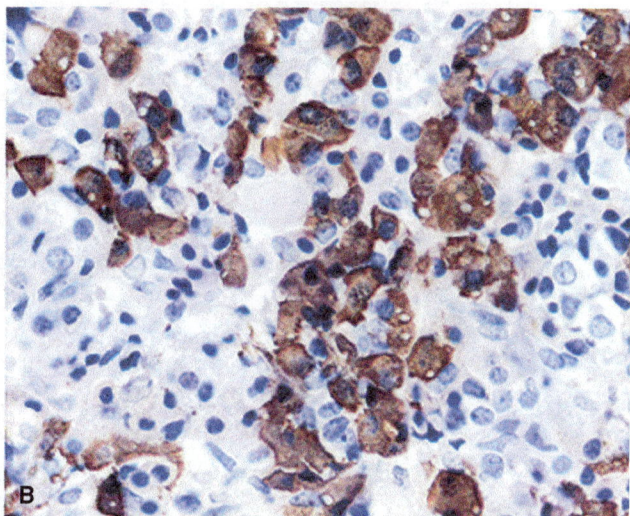

FIGURE 10.31 Corticotrophs (ACTH cells). **A:** Corticotrophs comprise about 15% to 20% of anterior lobe cells and are mainly located in the mucoid wedge. By H&E stain, corticotrophs are basophilic cells with ovoid to polyhedral shape and central nucleus. Many have a small vacuole near the nucleus, representing a massive lysosome (original magnification ×200). **B:** Note the clustering of cells, a characteristic feature of corticotrophs (ACTH immunostain, original magnification ×200).

corticotropin-like intermediate lobe protein (CLIP) (30). ACTH stimulates the adrenal cortex to secrete glucocorticoids, mineralocorticoids, and androgens. It plays a critical role in both the transport of amino acids and glucose into muscle, as well as the stimulation of insulin release from the pancreas. Pituitary ACTH secretion is regulated by hypothalamic CRH and arginine vasopressin (AVP), and proinflammatory cytokines, including interleukin-6 (IL-6), as well as leukemia inhibitory factor.

Excess secretion of ACTH, such as occurs in Cushing disease, leads to stereotypic abnormalities such as truncal obesity, hypertension, diabetes mellitus, amenorrhea, hirsutism, muscle atrophy, striae, impaired wound healing, and mental status changes. Hyperpigmentation also may occur in this setting and is because of the effects of MSH.

Thyrotroph Cells

Thyrotrophs, or TSH cells, are located primarily in the anterior part of the mucoid wedge and comprise only 5% of adenohypophysial cells (34). They are medium-sized and angular or elongate (Figs. 10.35 and 10.36). Like corticotrophs, normal TSH cells are basophilic and are PAS positive (see Table 10.5 for ultrastructural features).

TSH, like the other two glycoprotein hormones of the pituitary (LH and FSH), consists of two noncovalently bound subunits, alpha (α) and beta (β); the α-subunit is common to all three glycoprotein hormones; the β-subunit is specific for each hormone and confers biologic specificity. TSH binds to thyroid cells, inducing RNA and protein synthesis and thereby the production of thyroglobulin and thyroid hormones. Secretion of TSH is regulated by both hypothalamic hormones and circulating thyroid hormones. TRH stimulates TSH release, while thyroid hormones, dopamine, somatostatin, and glucocorticoids inhibit TSH secretion.

In the setting of primary hypothyroidism, thyrotrophs undergo hypertrophy and hyperplasia. When excessive, the response may produce sufficient hypertrophy of the pituitary gland to mimic adenoma. Pituitary adenomas that elaborate TSH are rare; most occur in the setting of hypothyroidism, although a minority results in hyperthyroidism (27,30).

Gonadotroph Cells

Gonadotrophs, or FSH and LH cells, comprise 10% of the adenohypophysis, show a strong affinity for both basic and

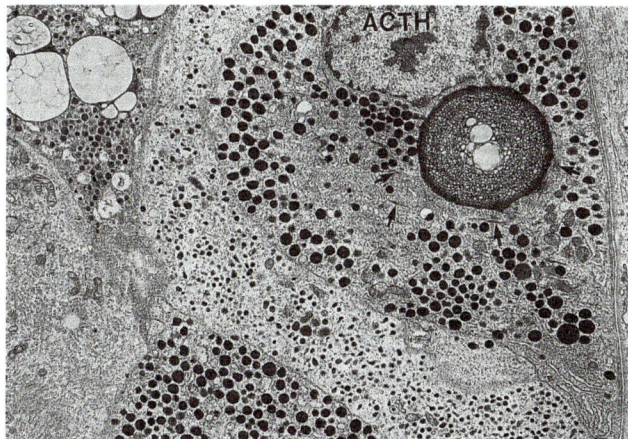

FIGURE 10.32 Corticotroph (ACTH cell). The cell contains the typical large lysosome and spherical to slightly pleomorphic and variably electron-dense secretory granules measuring 150 to 450 nm. Bundles of intermediate filaments (*arrows*) are a regular feature of corticotrophs. The adjacent cells with small granules are likely TSH cells (original magnification ×8,250).

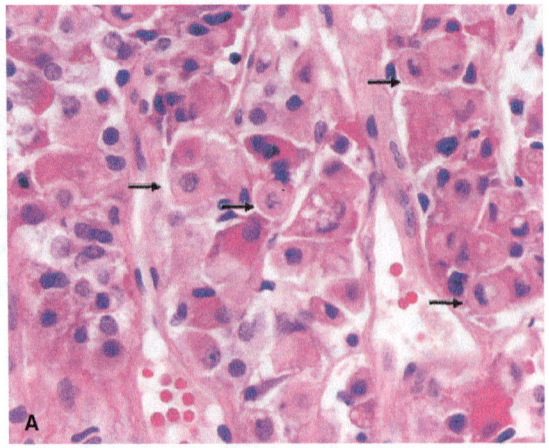
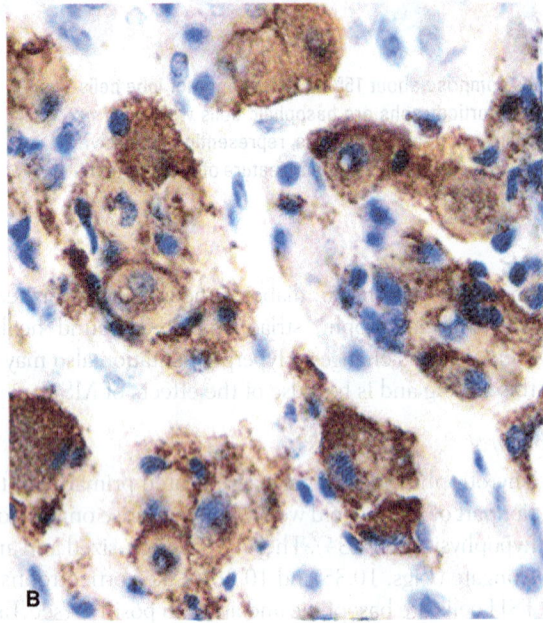
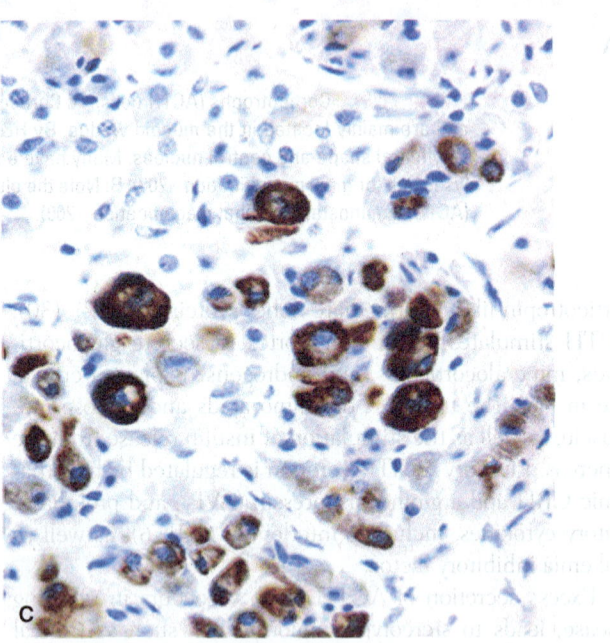

FIGURE 10.33 Crooke hyaline change. **A:** Crooke cells (*arrows*) are characterized by a conspicuous eosinophilic perinuclear ring consisting of cytokeratin (H&E, original magnification ×100). **B:** ACTH stains show central displacement of the nucleus and organelles by filament accumulation (ACTH immunostain, original magnification ×100). **C:** Staining for cytokeratin shows strong reactivity of the Crooke cells (CC immunostain, original magnification ×100).

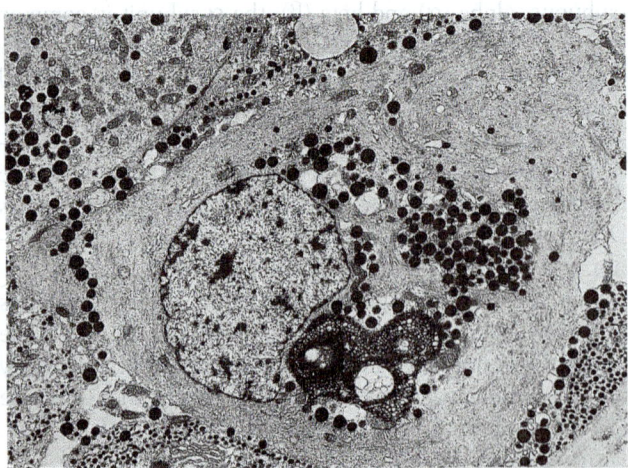

FIGURE 10.34 Crooke cell. This electron micrograph of the pituitary adjacent to a corticotroph cell adenoma displays massive accumulation of cytokeratin filament. Secretory granules are displaced to the perinuclear zone or to the periphery of the cytoplasm. Note the large lysosome in the lower portion of the field (original magnification ×6,720).

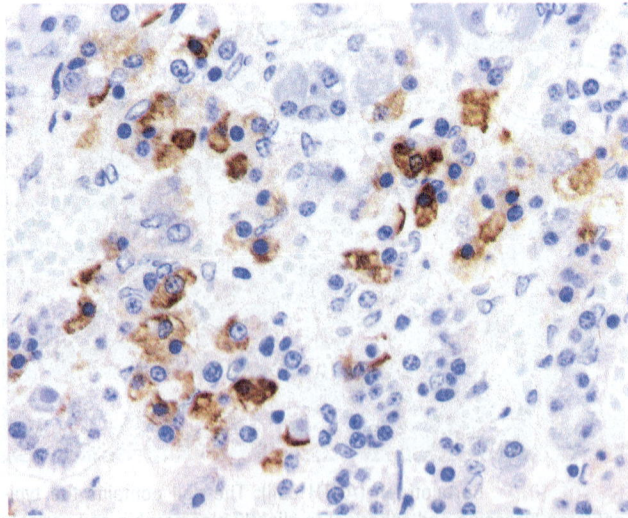

FIGURE 10.35 Thyrotroph (TSH cell). Thyrotrophs are medium-sized angulated cells with some demonstrating elongate processes. They comprise only about 5% of anterior lobe secretory cells and show strong TSH immunoreactivity (TSH immunostain, original magnification ×100).

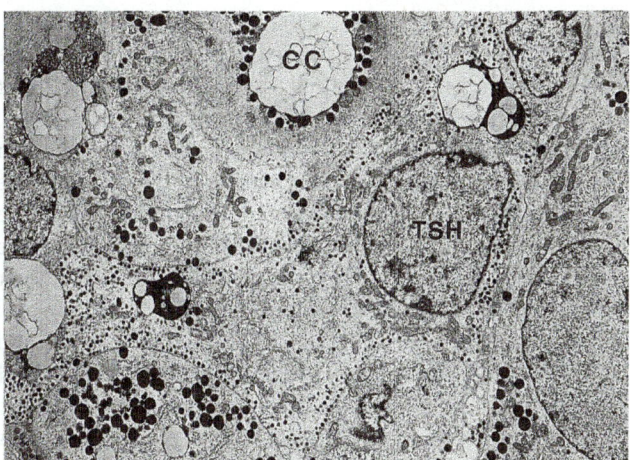

FIGURE 10.36 Thyrotroph (TSH cell). This micrograph of the normal anterior pituitary shows the characteristic elongate thyrotrophs, the large lysosomes frequently observed in cells of this type, and small (150-nm) peripherally located secretory granules. Part of a Crooke cell (*CC*) is also shown (original magnification ×5,300).

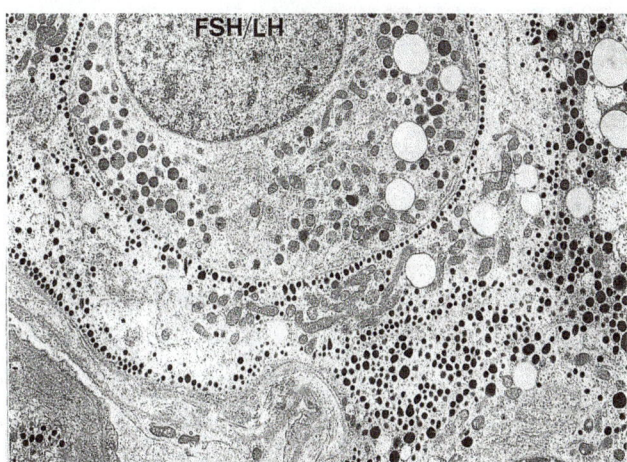

FIGURE 10.38 Gonadotroph (FSH/LH cell). The dull, low-contrast appearance of the cell is typical of gonadotrophs. Their spherical and slightly irregular secretory granules are characteristic; they have variable electron density and measure 250 to 400 nm. The cell process surrounding the gonadotroph likely belongs to a thyrotroph (original magnification ×8,250).

PAS stains, and generally are evenly distributed throughout the anterior lobe. Immunohistochemical and ultrastructural studies have shown that FSH and LH may be produced in isolation or by the same cell (Figs. 10.37 and 10.38) (see Table 10.5 for ultrastructural features) (35). Like TSH, LH and FSH are glycoprotein hormones consisting of α- and β-subunits. In the daily practice of surgical pathology, monoclonal antibodies against the specific β-subunits of LH and FSH are universally applied. In addition, antibodies against the α-subunit are useful for determination of abnormal production and/or secretion of this subunit hormone.

Both LH and FSH play distinct but essential roles in the reproductive physiology of males and females. In the female, LH is required for ovulation and follicular luteinization. In males, it stimulates interstitial Leydig cells to produce testosterone. FSH promotes follicular development in the female, whereas in the male it induces Sertoli cells to produce an androgen-binding protein.

Secretion of these hormones from the gonadotroph cells is regulated by integration of the GnRH signal and feedback effects of gonadal steroids and the peptides inhibin, follistatin, and activin (30). Hypothalamic GnRH interacts with a membrane receptor to regulate both LH and FSH release and synthesis necessary for gonadotroph cells' function. FSH synthesis is also under separate control by the gonadal peptides inhibin and activin, members of the transforming growth factor β (TGF-β) family. Inhibin selectively suppresses FSH, whereas activin stimulates FSH synthesis. In addition, estrogens act at both hypothalamic and pituitary levels to control gonadotropins secretion.

Pars Tuberalis

The pars tuberalis, an upward extension of the anterior lobe along the pituitary stalk, is composed of normal acini of pituitary cells scattered among surface portal vessels. These cells consist of mainly gonadotrophs intermixed with a few corticotrophs and thyrotrophs, histologically resembling those of pars distalis (anterior lobe) (36). They often show immunoreactivity for ACTH, FSH, LH, and α-subunit. Although in functional terms they may or may not differ from similar cells in the pars distalis (anterior lobe), these cells do show a distinct tendency to undergo squamous metaplasia (see later) (Fig. 10.39).

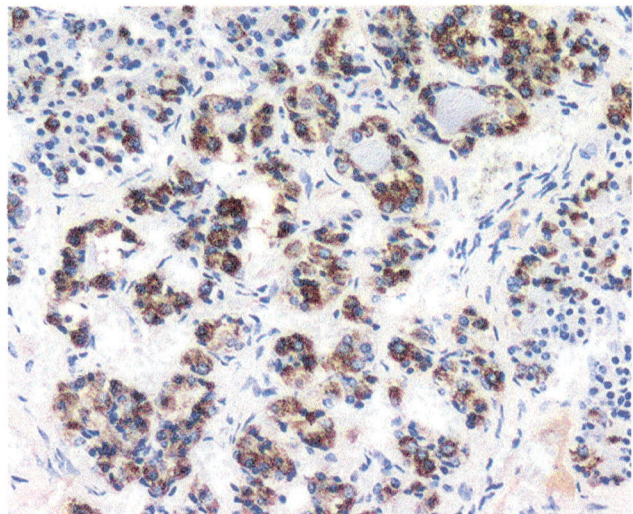

FIGURE 10.37 Gonadotroph (FSH/LH cell). Gonadotroph cells manufacture both LH and FSH. The paucity of strongly staining cells in this field reflects the fact that only 10% of anterior lobe secretory cells are gonadotrophs (FSH immunostain, original magnification ×100).

Follicles are not an uncommon feature of the normal anterior pituitary. Their functional constituent cells, termed follicular cells, appear to be derived in large part from various

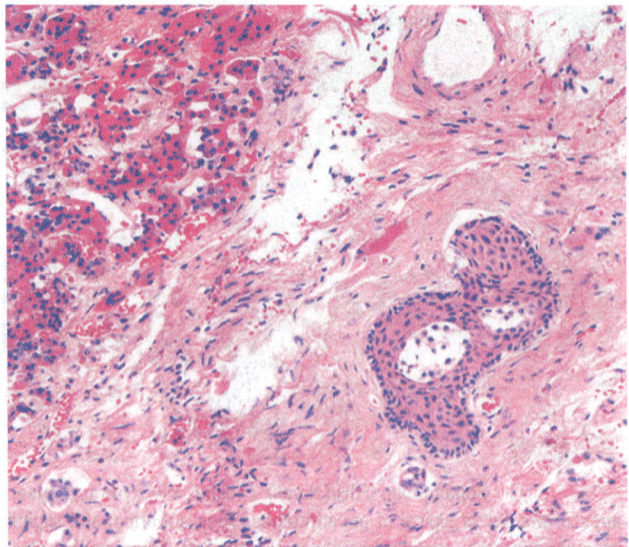

FIGURE 10.39 Anterior pituitary, pars tuberalis. Squamous metaplasia of secretory cells is a common feature of this portion of the gland.

Folliculostellate Cells

The folliculostellate cell is the sixth cellular element of the adenohypophysis, a specialized sustentacular-like cell that appears to have multiple functions related to phagocytosis, secretion of growth factors, and intercellular communication (38,39). They comprise of less than 5% of the anterior lobe cells, are scattered about the anterior lobe, and contribute to the formation of anterior lobe follicles and cysts of the intermediate lobe (39). They are readily identified by their immunoreactivity for S100 protein (Fig. 10.42), and can also be identified by glial fibrillary acidic protein (GFAP) and vimentin. They participate in regulating several activities of anterior pituitary including scavenger activity by engulfing degenerated cells and paracrine regulation of endocrine cells through the production of cytokines (such as IL-6, and leukemia inhibitory factor) and various growth factors (including basic fibroblast growth factor and vascular endothelial growth factor) (39). Additionally, ultrastructural and immunohistochemical studies on human adenomatous and non-neoplastic pituitary folliculostellate cells suggest that they may represent adult organ-specific stem cells (39,40).

secretory cells (Fig. 10.40). Ultrastructurally, they are often poorly granulated or agranular and linked by apical junctional complexes. Within follicular lumina, one often finds cellular debris (Fig. 10.41). The stimulus for follicle formation is, therefore, thought to be damage or rupture of anterior lobe secretory cells (37).

Variation in Normal Morphology of the Adenohypophysis

A number of normal histologic variations in the pituitary gland may mimic clinically significant lesions. Examples include

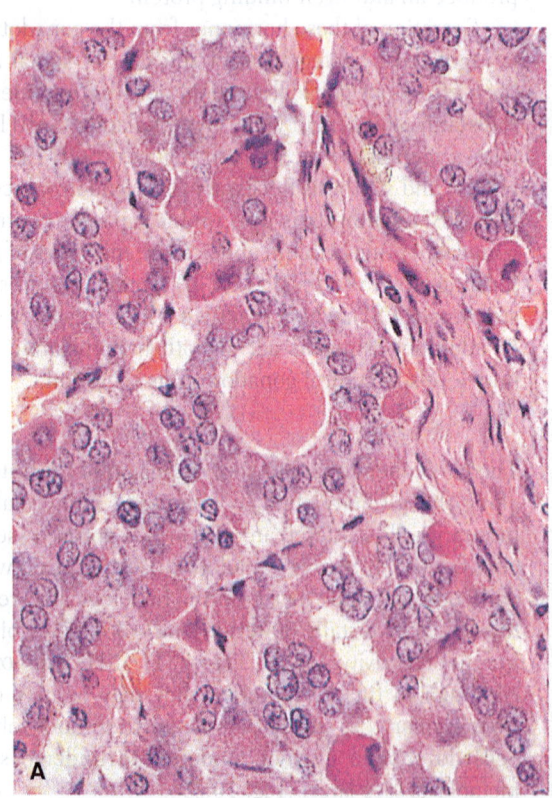
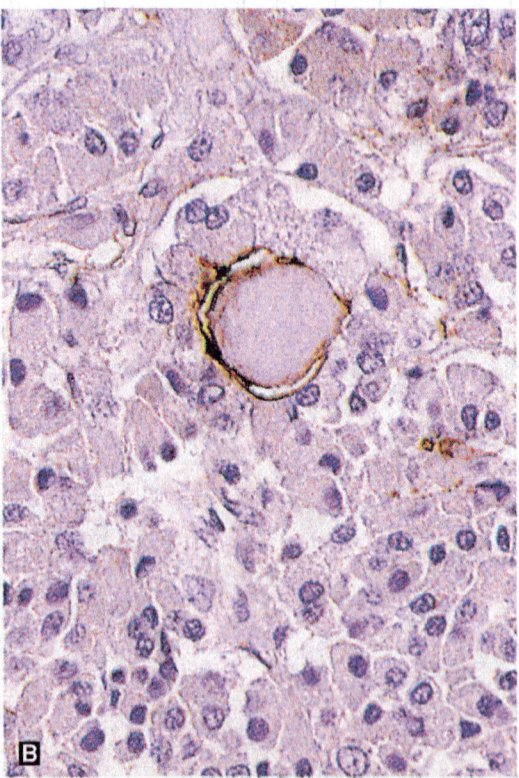

FIGURE 10.40 Anterior pituitary, follicle formation. **A:** Follicles, some containing a small quantity of colloid-like material, are commonly found in the anterior lobe (H&E, original magnification ×100). **B:** Follicles show prominent apical staining for epithelial membrane antigen (EMA) (EMA immunostain, original magnification ×100).

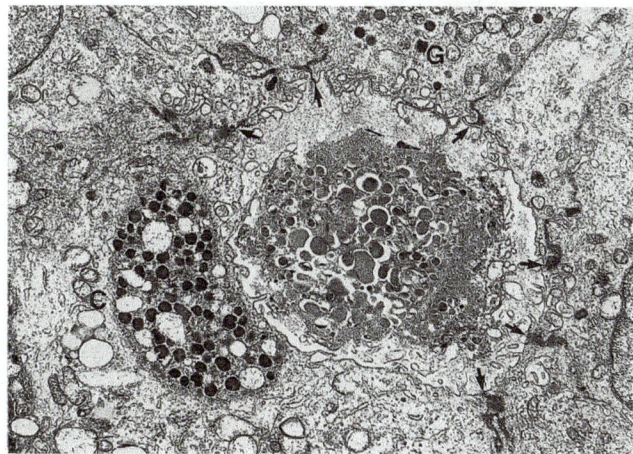

FIGURE 10.41 Electron micrograph of a pituitary follicle. This young follicle contains cell debris within its lumen. The gonadotroph (*G*), but not the corticotroph (*C*), is part of this follicle. Follicles are composed of granulated adenohypophysial cells that, through the formation of junctional complexes *(arrows)*, surround damaged adenohypophysial cells (original magnification ×12,600).

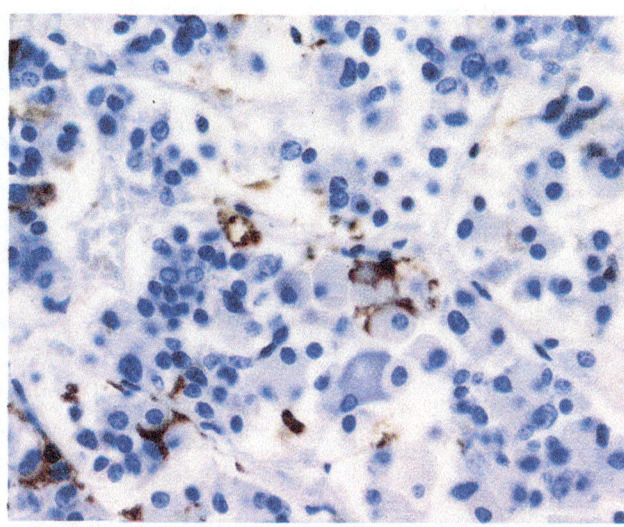

FIGURE 10.42 Anterior lobe, folliculostellate cells. Folliculostellate cells comprise less than 5% of anterior lobe cells and are scattered throughout the pituitary, including the intermediate lobe zone. Folliculostellate cells staining for S100 protein, GFAP, and vimentin (S100 immunostain, original magnification ×100).

squamous cell nests in the pars tuberalis, basophil invasion of the posterior lobe, granular cell clusters and tumorlets of the stalk and neurohypophysis, and salivary gland rests.

Squamous cell nests show a definite predilection for the pars tuberalis (Fig. 10.39); they have been found in up to 24% of autopsy cases, occur more commonly in elderly patients, and show no sex predilection (36,41). They arise through a process of metaplastic transformation from adenohypophysial cells, as evidenced by simultaneous expression of keratin and pituitary hormones, most often FSH, LH, or ACTH (36). Because squamous metaplasia also may accompany foci of ischemic infarction in the anterior lobe, it appears to be an inherent property of pituitary secretory cells.

Basophil invasion consists of corticotropic basophils extending from the pars intermedia into the neurohypophysis (Figs. 10.43 and 10.44). Basophilic invasion is more common in males and the elderly, and may at first glance mimic an adenoma. Similar to ordinary corticotrophs, these basophilic cells are immunoreactive for ACTH, and other POMC derivatives; however, they contain few cytokeratin filaments and are less susceptible to Crooke hyalinization in response to hypercortisolism (27).

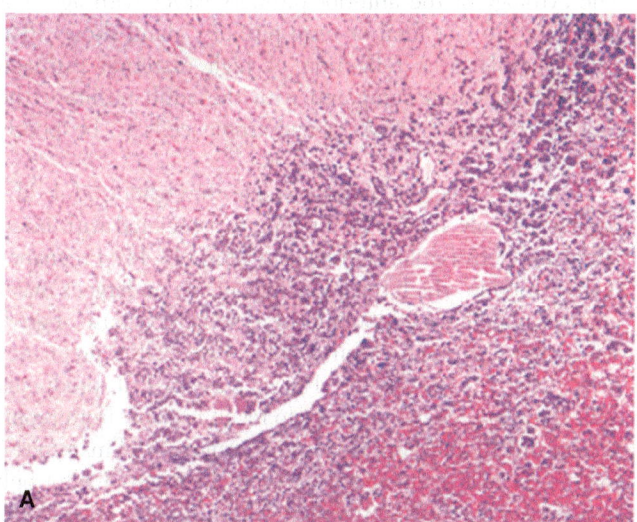
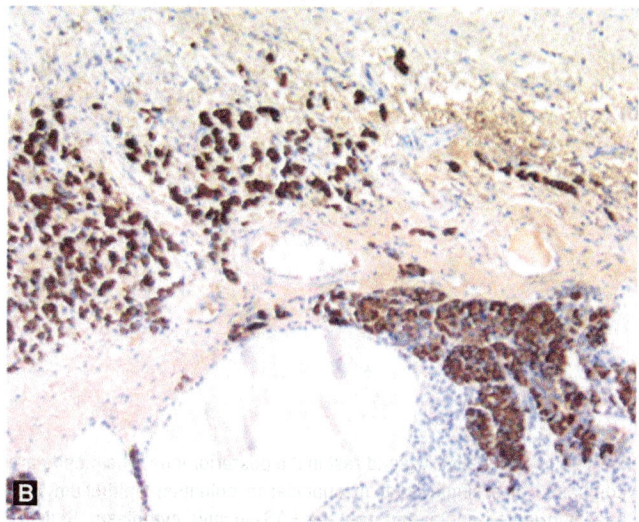

FIGURE 10.43 Basophil invasion. **A:** This subpopulation of corticotroph cells appears to infiltrate the substance of the posterior lobe (H&E, original magnification ×4). **B:** The invading cells are strongly immunoreactive for ACTH and other POMC derivative hormones (ACTH immunostain, original magnification ×40).

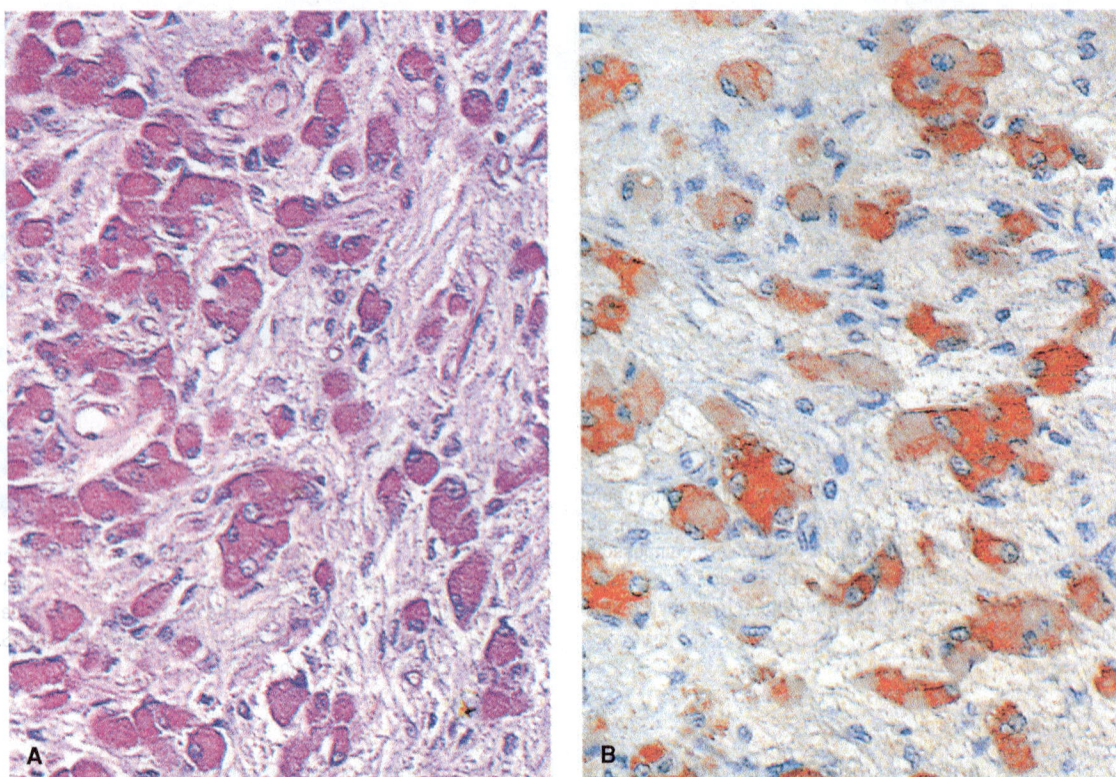

FIGURE 10.44 Basophil invasion. **A:** PAS staining (original magnification ×63). **B:** ACTH immunostain (original magnification ×63).

Salivary gland rests appear as tubular glands upon the surface or in the substance of the neurohypophysis, often just posterior to the pars intermedia (Fig. 10.45). They are composed of a single layer of cuboidal to columnar epithelium with basally oriented nuclei and finely granular, strongly PAS-positive cytoplasm. Salivary gland rests are often oncocytic. Their ultrastructural features include well-developed rough endoplasmic reticulum, secretory droplets, microvilli, and desmosomes, all of which support the contention that they are indeed salivary glands (42).

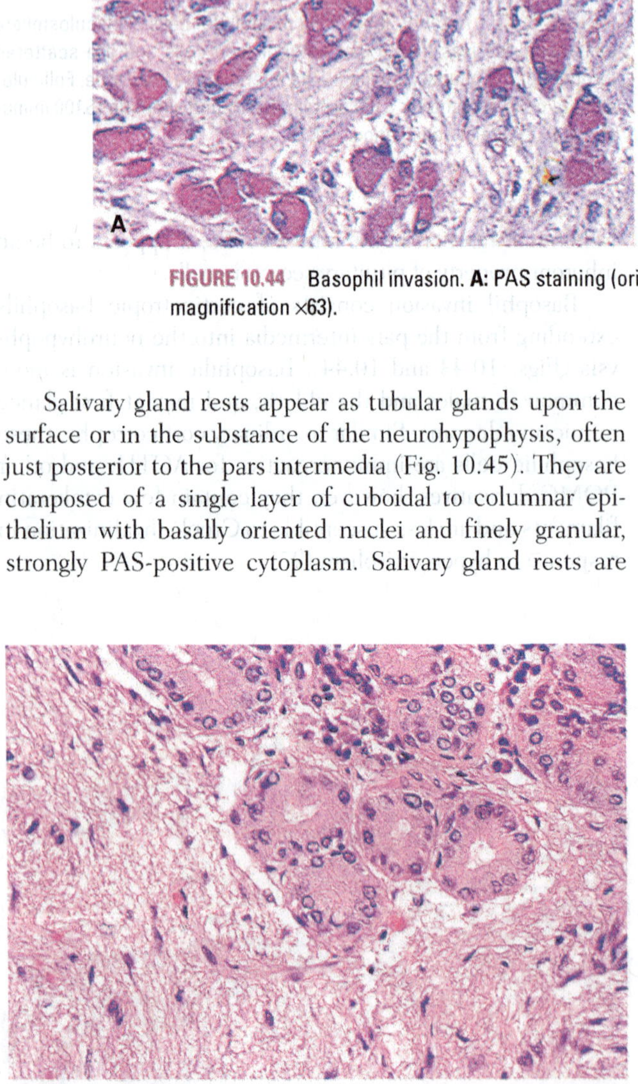

Age-Related Changes of the Adenohypophysis

The cytology of the anterior pituitary varies with age. For instance, the late fetal or term pituitary gland shows PRL cell hyperplasia, a reflection of high maternal estrogen levels. Also, when compared with the adult pituitary, the prepubertal gland shows gonadotropic cells to be poorly developed.

The gland weight remains stable throughout adult life, decreasing only slightly in the elderly associated with interstitial and perivascular fibrosis (see later) (43,44). Pregnancy is the period in which the adenohypophysis undergoes major changes resulting in a doubling of its weight because of gradual increase in large chromophobic PRL cells ("pregnancy cells") (Fig. 10.46) (26,45). The increase in PRL-producing cells during pregnancy appears to result not only from proliferation of PRL cells but also from recruitment of mammosomatotroph cells to enhance PRL production (46). Lactotroph hyperplasia gradually disappears within months after delivery or abortion. The process is often incomplete; hence, the pituitaries of multiparas are larger than those of women who were never pregnant. Pregnancy also results in a significant

FIGURE 10.45 Salivary gland rest in the posterior lobe. The glands are composed of a single layer of cuboidal to columnar epithelium with basally oriented nuclei and granular PAS-positive cytoplasm. Salivary gland rests are encountered both on the surface of or within the posterior lobe, where it abuts the intermediate lobe zone (H&E, original magnification ×63).

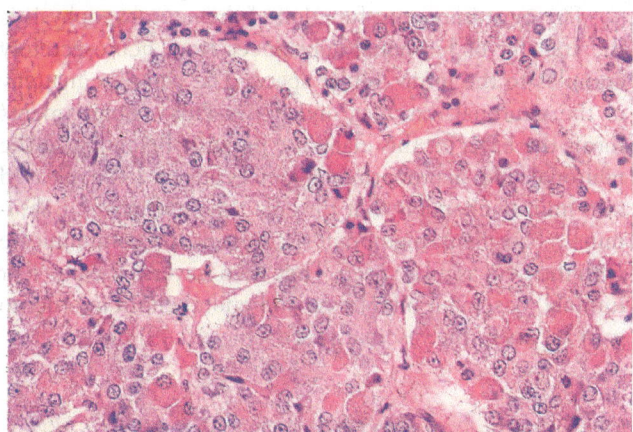

FIGURE 10.46 The pituitary in pregnancy features abundant pale chromophobic PRL cells (pregnancy cells) (H&E, original magnification ×100).

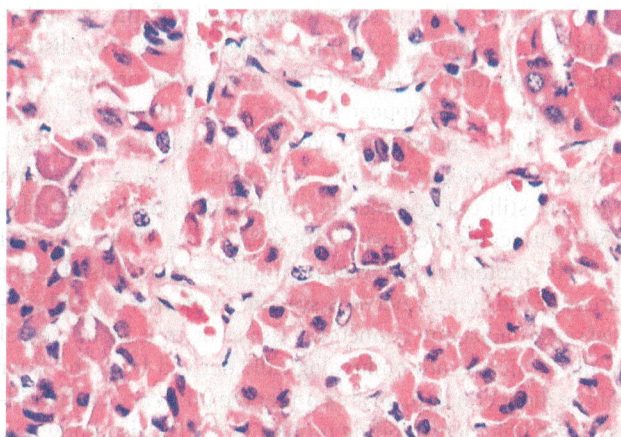

FIGURE 10.47 Perivascular fibrosis is a common feature of the aging pituitary (H&E, original magnification ×100).

decrease of gonadotropin immunoreactivity, a reflection of the production of gonadotropic hormones by the placenta.

The effects of aging on the cellular contents of several pituitary hormones have been studied. Specifically, GH and PRL cells have been shown to undergo no significant decrease in number, granularity, distribution, or immunoreactivity with increasing age (47,48). Both ACTH and TSH cells also appear to be unaffected by age, but no data are available regarding the effects of senescence on FSH and LH cells.

Fibrosis is the most frequent age-related change (43,44). It is generally perivascular in distribution (Fig. 10.47) but is on occasion patchy, suggesting a remote microinfarct. Interstitial and intracellular deposits of amyloid have been demonstrated in the majority of autopsy-derived anterior pituitaries (49). Immunohistochemically, these reacted for antiamyloid lambda (λ) light chain and amyloid P component. The mean volume percentage of such deposits is approximately 0.5% of the anterior lobe. The occurrence of amyloid and its degree of deposition were related not only to patient age but also to the prevalence of chronic obstructive pulmonary disease and to non–insulin-dependent diabetes mellitus.

Neurohypophysis

As a functional unit, the neurohypophysis consists of the infundibulum, pituitary stalk, and posterior lobe. The posterior lobe, a ventral extension of the central nervous system, is the site of release of the hypothalamic hormones oxytocin and vasopressin. Its cellular elements consist of: (1) unmyelinated axons originating from the SON and PVN and, to a lesser extent, from cholinergic neurons of the hypothalamus; (2) an extensive vascular network; and (3) specialized glial cells termed pituicytes (Fig. 10.48).

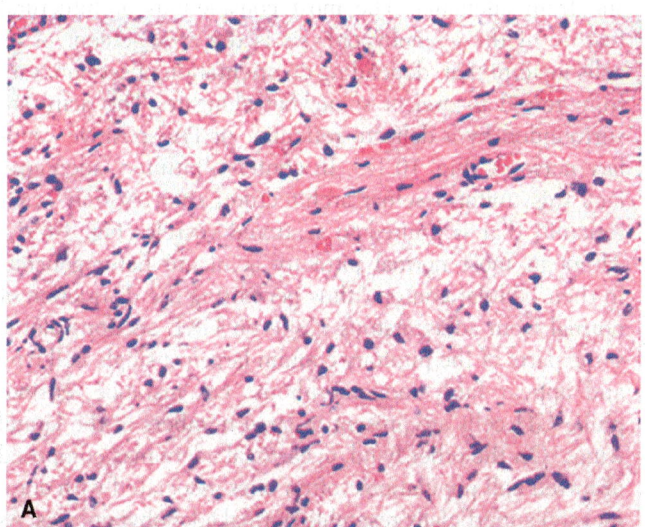
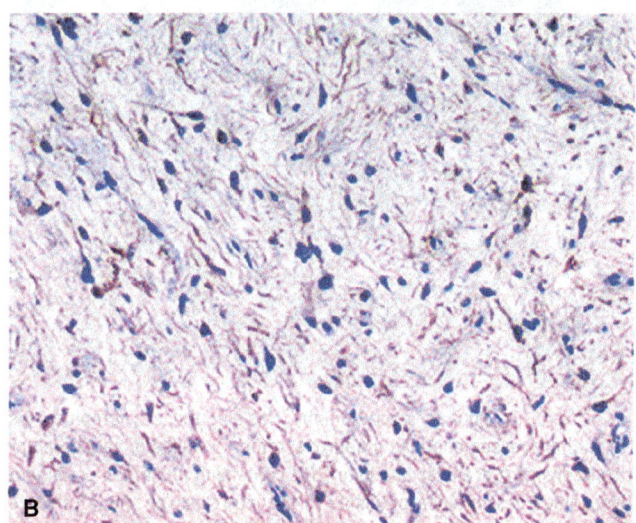

FIGURE 10.48 Posterior lobe. **A:** Pituicytes have elongated nuclei dispersed within the neuropil of the neurohypophysis (H&E, original magnification ×100). **B:** These cells stain positively for glial fibrillary acid protein (GFAP) (GFAP immunostain, original magnification ×100).

Pituicytes, the most numerous cells of the neurohypophysis, are elongated, uni- or bipolar cells that display the prolongation of the cytoplasm into one or more processes. Pituicytes appear to exist in five principal forms: major, dark, ependymal, oncocytic, and granular (50). Their morphologic diversity is thought to be a reflection of their, still not completely understood, physiologic roles (50). Pituicytes are positive for GFAP (Fig. 10.48), as well as S100 protein and vimentin. Similar to glial cells of other areas of the central nervous system, pituicytes expand processes to adjacent connective tissue or to a blood vessel wall. Pituicytes are embryologically derived from the floor of the diencephalon, an area under the influence of thyroid-specific enhancer-binding protein (T/EBP), also known as NKX2-1 or TTF-1 expression during normal development (51). Expression of TTF-1 in normal fetal and adult, and neoplastic pituicytes has been recently recognized (52).

The axons of the posterior lobe are histologically identified using silver stains and/or immunostains for neuronal markers. Focal axonal dilatations, known as Herring bodies, represent intra-axonal accumulations of posterior lobe hormones (Fig. 10.22). At the ultrastructural level, the unmyelinated axons appear as delicate fibers, measuring 0.05 to 1.0 μm in diameter, which contain longitudinal arrays of microtubules and neurofilaments. Two types of neurosecretory axons, A and B, have been described based on the morphology of their neurosecretory granules. Type A fibers, far more numerous than type B, contain 100- to 300-nm oxytocin and vasopressin granules, whereas type B fibers, likely aminergic in nature, contain granules ranging from 50 to 100 nm (53). Neurosecretory fibers are closely associated with pituicytes, their axons often being ensheathed by them (Fig. 10.49).

The most important function of the neurohypophysis is the transfer of hormonal substances from neurosecretory granules to the intravascular space. The complex anatomy of the neuronal, vascular, and perivascular compartments forms the basis for this elaborate process. Beginning at the neuronal side, neurohormonal factors appear to be released into minute channels that traverse the outermost, or abluminal, basement membrane of vessels to communicate with the perivascular space. They then traverse the inner, or luminal, basement membrane and endothelium in order to gain access to the vascular space (Fig. 10.49) (54).

Variation in Normal Morphology of the Neurohypophysis

Granular cell nests or tumorlets, most located in the stalk or posterior lobe, are found in about 6% of autopsy pituitaries and are more common among the elderly (55). Varying from scattered cells to compact tumor-like nodules, they are composed of plump cells with granular acidophilic and strongly PAS-positive cytoplasm and relatively small nuclei (Fig. 10.50). Only rarely do granular cells form clinically significant tumors (56). The origin of granular cell tumorlets and tumors of the neurohypophysis is still not completely understood, but the occasional GFAP immunoreactivity and the recently described TTF-1 expression by these lesions, have provided some evidence that these granular cell nests and tumors may originate from pituicytes (57).

DIFFERENTIAL DIAGNOSIS

The principal consideration in differential diagnosis of pituitary lesions is the distinction of normal pituitary tissue from adenoma. The most conspicuous architectural feature of the adenohypophysis is the arrangement of its cells in acini that, depending on orientation of section, vary from round to oval or somewhat elongate. The acini are surrounded by a delicate reticulin- or PAS-positive capillary network (Fig. 10.17). In contrast, pituitary adenomas lack this uniform acinar architecture, showing only scant reticulin that is limited to scattered vessels (Fig. 10.51). Although most normal pituitary acini are heterogeneous in their cellular content, thus permitting the distinction of normal from adenomatous tissue on H&E sections alone, some parts of the pituitary contain largely a single cell type and appear fairly monomorphous. For instance, eosinophilic GH cells are present in large numbers in the lateral wings. On the other hand, occasional adenomas composed of mixed cell populations (often ones associated with acromegaly) superficially resemble normal adenohypophysis. As a result, the distinction of normal from adenomatous tissue may be more easily achieved by reticulin staining than by immunohistochemistry alone.

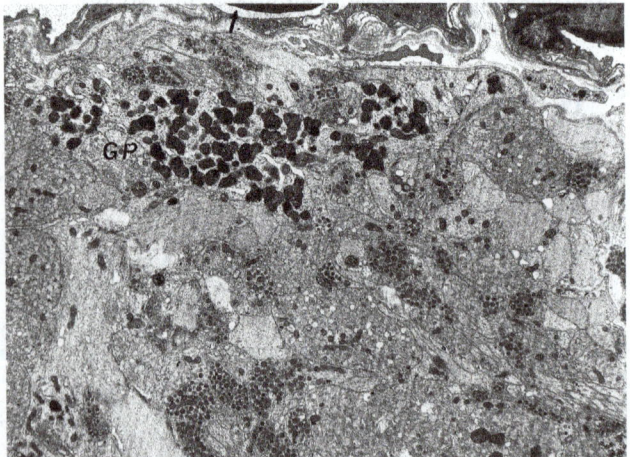

FIGURE 10.49 Pituitary, posterior lobe. This electron micrograph shows axonal processes containing neurosecretory granules of varying electron density. A granular pituicyte (*GP*) containing numerous prominent lysosomes lies in close proximity to the intravascular space (*arrow*). The intravascular space is bounded by fenestrated endothelial cells as seen here. Outside the endothelium lies the perivascular space, a region containing a variety of cell types (not shown here), including pericytes, histiocytes, fibroblasts, and mast cells (original magnification ×6,200).

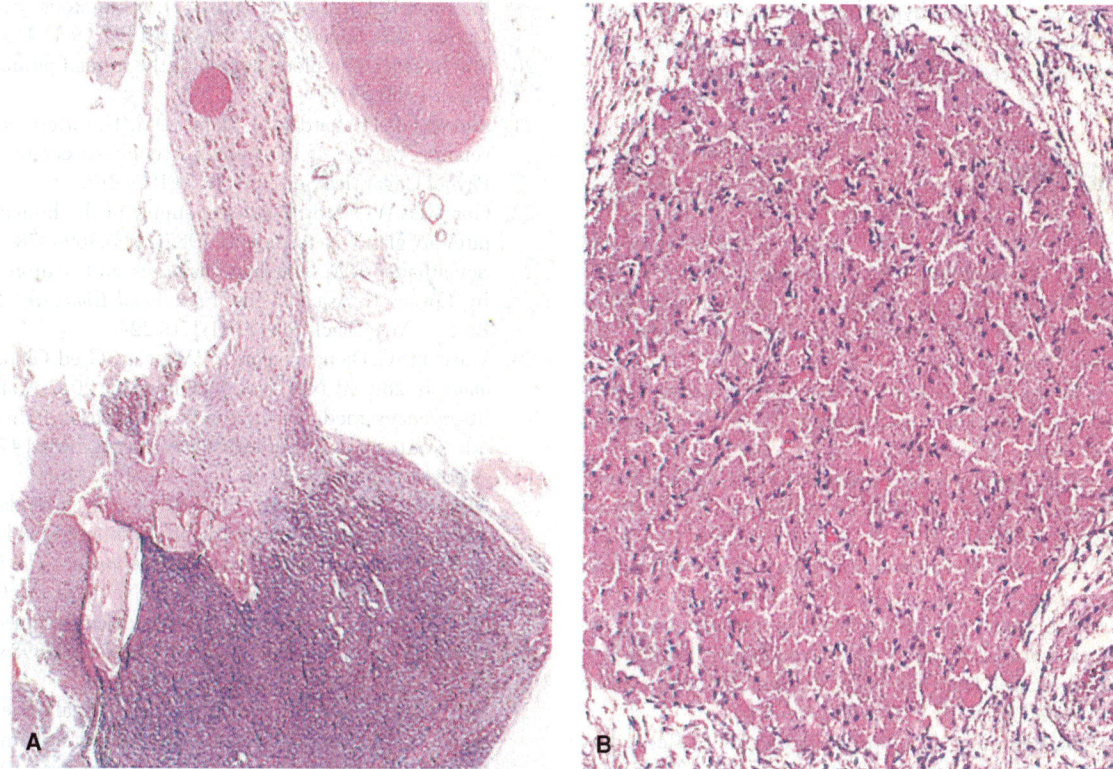

FIGURE 10.50 Pituitary stalk, granular cell tumorlets. **A:** Low-power view of the stalk shows two tumorlets. The optic chiasm is at the upper portion of the field; the anterior lobe is at the lower portion of the field (H&E, original magnification ×20). **B:** High-power view of a granular cell tumorlet. Such nodules are composed of pituicytes, modified glial cells, with abundant lysosome-rich eosinophilic cytoplasm. Tumorlets, as well as individual granular cells, are of no clinical significance (H&E, original magnification ×100).

Small biopsies of the intermediate lobe may include the so-called basophilic invasion normally seen in the posterior pituitary (Figs. 10.43 and 10.44). Since these basophilic cells are arranged diffusely or in clusters, and lack the typical acinar formation seen in the anterior pituitary, they may be mistaken for corticotroph microadenomas.

A limited biopsy of the pituitary may occasionally include intermediate zone cysts, which are normal derivatives of Rathke cleft. Correlation with radiologic and operative data usually obviates confusion with Rathke cleft cyst. Clinically significant cysts are readily evident on neuroimaging and are identified as sizable cysts by the experienced surgeon.

As previously noted above, adenohypophysial cells may undergo squamous metaplasia, particularly in the pars tuberalis. This location is only occasionally sampled in surgical specimens. Scant in extent, intimately associated with adenohypophysial cells, and cytologically benign, they are unlikely to be confused with either cysts (epidermoid or dermoid cysts) or with neoplasms (craniopharyngiomas).

In very small numbers, cytologic benign lymphocytes are seen in the intermediate zone of the normal pituitary in 10% of autopsied subjects (58). Unassociated with endocrine disease, such cells are readily distinguished from the far more widespread and dense infiltrates of lymphocytic hypophysitis or abscess.

A limited biopsy of the neurohypophysis can readily be mistaken for glioma in that the vast majority of its nucleated cells are specialized astrocytes (pituicytes). Unlike pituicytomas, the tumor most closely mimicked by posterior

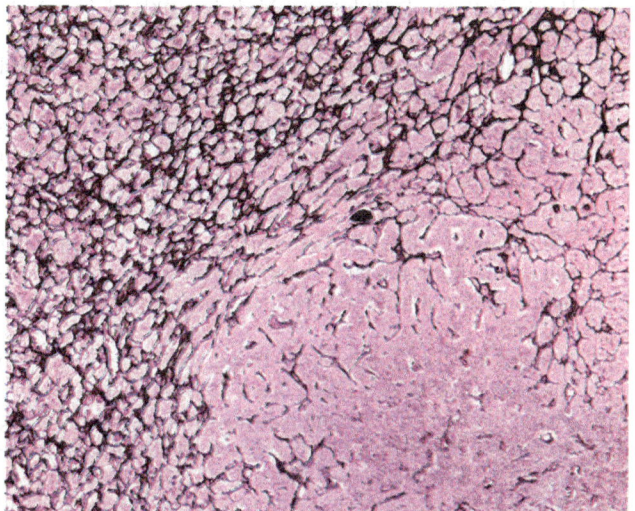

FIGURE 10.51 Disruption of the reticulin network in a pituitary adenoma. Compare the acinar pattern of the normal adenohypophysis (*upper left*) with the adenoma (*bottom right*) (Wilder reticulin, original magnification ×100).

pituitary tissue, the neurohypophysis contains large numbers of axons terminating on vessels. Of these axons, some possess PAS-positive swellings (Herring bodies).

REFERENCES

1. Moore KL. *The Developing Human: Clinically Oriented Embryology*. Philadelphia, PA: WB Saunders; 1988:170–205.
2. Falin LI. The development of human hypophysis and differentiation of cells of its anterior lobe during embryonic life. *Acta Anat (Basel)* 1961;44:188–205.
3. Hori A, Schmidt D, Rickels E. Pharyngeal pituitary: Development, malformation, and tumorigenesis. *Acta Neuropathol* 1999;98(3):262–272.
4. Solov'ev GS, Bogdanov AV, Panteleev SM, et al. Embryonic morphogenesis of the human pituitary. *Neurosci Behav Physiol* 2008;38(8):829–833.
5. Asa SL, Kovacs K. Functional morphology of the human fetal pituitary. *Pathol Annu* 1984;19 (Pt 1):275–315.
6. Hori A. Suprasellar peri-infundibular ectopic adenohypophysis in fetal and adult brains. *J Neurosurg* 1985;63(1):113–115.
7. Lennox B, Russell DS. Dystopia of the neurohypophysis: Two cases. *J Pathol Bacteriol* 1951;63(3):485–490.
8. Scully KM, Rosenfeld MG. Pituitary development: Regulatory codes in mammalian organogenesis. *Science* 2002;295(5563):2231–2235.
9. Zhu X, Rosenfeld MG. Transcriptional control of precursor proliferation in the early phases of pituitary development. *Curr Opin Genet Dev* 2004;14(5):567–574.
10. Asa SL, Ezzat S. Molecular determinants of pituitary cytodifferentiation. *Pituitary* 1999;1(3–4):159–168.
11. Lamolet B, Pulichino AM, Lamonerie T, et al. A pituitary cell-restricted T box factor, Tpit, activates POMC transcription in cooperation with Pitx homeoproteins. *Cell* 2001;104(6):849–859.
12. Mody S, Brown MR, Parks JS. The spectrum of hypopituitarism caused by PROP1 mutations. *Best Pract Res Clin Endocrinol Metab* 2002;16(3):421–431.
13. Dasen JS, O'Connell SM, Flynn SE, et al. Reciprocal interactions of Pit1 and GATA2 mediate signaling gradient-induced determination of pituitary cell types. *Cell* 1999;97(5):587–598.
14. Dubois PM, Begeot M, Dubois MP, et al. Immunocytological localization of LH, FSH, TSH and their subunits in the pituitary of normal and anencephalic human fetuses. *Cell Tissue Res* 1978;191(2):249–265.
15. Begeot M, Dubois MP, Dubois PM. Growth hormone and ACTH in the pituitary of normal and anencephalic human fetuses: Immunocytochemical evidence for hypothalamic influences during development. *Neuroendocrinology* 1977;24(3–4):208–220.
16. Dunn IF, Laws ER. Microsurgical approaches for transsphenoidal surgery. In: Laws ER, Lanzino G, eds. *Transsphenoidal Surgery*. 1st ed. Philadelphia, PA: Elsevier; 2010:120–127.
17. Bergland RM, Ray BS, Torack RM. Anatomical variations in the pituitary gland and adjacent structures in 225 human autopsy cases. *J Neurosurg* 1968;28(2):93–99.
18. Berke JP, Buxton LF, Kokmen E. The 'empty' sella. *Neurology* 1975;25(12):1137–1143.
19. Kaufman B, Chamberlin WB Jr. The ubiquitous "empty" sella turcica. *Acta Radiol Diagn (Stockh)* 1972;13(1):413–425.
20. Stanfield JP. The blood supply of the human pituitary gland. *J Anat* 1960;94:257–273.
21. Xuereb GP, Prichard MM, Daniel PM. The arterial supply and venous drainage of the human hypophysis cerebri. *Q J Exp Physiol Cogn Med Sci* 1954;39(3):199–217.
22. Gorczyca W, Hardy J. Arterial supply of the human anterior pituitary gland. *Neurosurgery* 1987;20(3):369–378.
23. Scheithauer BW. The hypothalamus and neurohypophysis. In: Kovacs K, Asa SL, eds. *Functional Endocrine Pathology*. Boston, MA: Blackwell; 1991:170–224.
24. Waxman SG. Diencephalon. In: Waxman SG, ed. *Clinical Neuroanatomy*. 28th ed. New York: McGraw-Hill; 2017. Available from http://accessmedicine.mhmedical.com.proxy01.its.virginia.edu/content.aspx?bookid=1969&sectionid=147036773. Accessed March 25, 2018.
25. Molitch ME, Schimmer BP. Introduction to endocrinology: The hypothalamic-pituitary axis. In: Brunton LL, Hilal-Dandan R, Knollmann BC, eds. *Goodman & Gilman's: The Pharmacological Basis of Therapeutics*. 13th ed. New York: McGraw-Hill; 2017. Available from http://accessmedicine.mhmedical.com.proxy01.its.virginia.edu/content.aspx?bookid=2189&sectionid=172481654. Accessed March 25, 2018.
26. Scheithauer BW, Sano T, Kovacs KT, et al. The pituitary gland in pregnancy: A clinicopathologic and immunohistochemical study of 69 cases. *Mayo Clin Proc* 1990;65(4):461–474.
27. Kovacs K, Horvath E. *Tumors of the Pituitary Gland*. Washington, DC: Armed Forces Institute of Pathology; 1986.
28. Teramoto A, Hirakawa K, Sanno N, et al. Incidental pituitary lesions in 1,000 unselected autopsy specimens. *Radiology* 1994;193(1):161–164.
29. Zada G, Lin N, Ojerholm E, et al. Craniopharyngioma and other cystic epithelial lesions of the sellar region: A review of clinical, imaging, and histopathological relationships. *Neurosurg Focus* 2010;28(4):E4.
30. Melmed S, Jameson LJ. Anterior pituitary: Physiology of pituitary hormones. In: Kasper D, Fauci A, Hauser S, et al. eds. *Harrison's Principles of Internal Medicine*. 19th ed. New York: McGraw-Hill; 2014. Available from http://accessmedicine.mhmedical.com.proxy01.its.virginia.edu/content.aspx?bookid=1130&sectionid=79751425. Accessed March 25, 2018.
31. Handwerger S, Freemark M. The roles of placental growth hormone and placental lactogen in the regulation of human fetal growth and development. *J Pediatr Endocrinol Metab* 2000;13(4):343–356.
32. Mulchahey JJ, Jaffe RB. Detection of a potential progenitor cell in the human fetal pituitary that secretes both growth hormone and prolactin. *J Clin Endocrinol Metab* 1988;66(1):24–32.
33. Horvath E, Ilse G, Kovacs K. Enigmatic bodies in human corticotroph cells. *Acta Anat (Basel)* 1977;98(4):427–433.
34. Phifer RF, Spicer SS. Immunohistochemical and histologic demonstration of thyrotropic cells of the human adenohypophysis. *J Clin Endocrinol Metab* 1973;36(6):1210–1221.
35. Phifer RF, Midgley AR, Spicer SS. Immunohistologic and histologic evidence that follicle-stimulating hormone and luteinizing hormone are present in the same cell type in the human pars distalis. *J Clin Endocrinol Metab* 1973;36(1):125–141.

36. Asa SL, Kovacs K, Bilbao JM. The pars tuberalis of the human pituitary. A histologic, immunohistochemical, ultrastructural and immunoelectron microscopic analysis. *Virchows Arch A Pathol Anat Histopathol* 1983;399(1):49–59.
37. Horvath E, Kovacs K, Penz G, et al. Origin, possible function and fate of "follicular cells" in the anterior lobe of the human pituitary. *Am J Pathol* 1974;77(2):199–212.
38. Marin F, Stefaneanu L, Kovacs K. Folliculo-stellate cells of the pituitary. *Endocr Pathol* 1991;2(4):180–192.
39. Devnath S, Inoue K. An insight to pituitary folliculo-stellate cells. *J Neuroendocrinol* 2008;20(6):687–691.
40. Horvath E, Kovacs K. Folliculo-stellate cells of the human pituitary: A type of adult stem cell? *Ultrastruct Pathol* 2002;26(4):219–228.
41. Luse SA, Kernohan JW. Squamous-cell nests of the pituitary gland. *Cancer* 1955;8(3):623–628.
42. Schochet SS Jr, McCormick WF, Halmi NS. Salivary gland rests in the human pituitary. Light and electron microscopical study. *Arch Pathol* 1974;98(3):193–200.
43. Shanklin WM. Age changes in the histology of the human pituitary. *Acta Anat (Basel)* 1953;19(3):290–304.
44. Sano T, Kovacs KT, Scheithauer BW, et al. Aging and the human pituitary gland. *Mayo Clin Proc* 1993;68(10):971–977.
45. Stefaneanu L, Kovacs K, Lloyd RV, et al. Pituitary lactotrophs and somatotrophs in pregnancy: A correlative in situ hybridization and immunocytochemical study. *Virchows Arch B Cell Pathol Incl Mol Pathol* 1992;62(5):291–296.
46. Frawley LS, Boockfor FR. Mammosomatotropes: Presence and functions in normal and neoplastic pituitary tissue. *Endocr Rev* 1991;12(4):337–355.
47. Calderon L, Ryan N, Kovacs K. Human pituitary growth hormone cells in old age. *Gerontology* 1978;24(6):441–447.
48. Kovacs K, Ryan N, Horvath E, et al. Prolactin cells of the human pituitary gland in old age. *J Gerontol* 1977;32(5):534–540.
49. Röcken C, Saeger W, Fleege JC, et al. Interstitial amyloid deposits in the pituitary gland. Morphometry, immunohistology, and correlation to diseases. *Arch Pathol Lab Med* 1995;119(11):1055–1060.
50. Takei Y, Seyama S, Pearl GS, et al. Ultrastructural study of the human neurohypophysis. II. Cellular elements of neural parenchyma, the pituicytes. *Cell Tissue Res* 1980;205(2):273–287.
51. Kimura S, Hara Y, Pineau T, et al. The T/ebp null mouse: Thyroid-specific enhancer-binding protein is essential for the organogenesis of the thyroid, lung, ventral forebrain, and pituitary. *Genes Dev* 1996;10(1):60–69.
52. Lee EB, Tihan T, Scheithauer BW, et al. Thyroid transcription factor 1 expression in sellar tumors: A histogenetic marker? *J Neuropathol Exp Neurol* 2009;68(5):482–488.
53. Seyama S, Pearl GS, Takei Y. Ultrastructural study of the human neurohypophysis. I. Neurosecretory axons and their dilatations in the pars nervosa. *Cell Tissue Res* 1980;205(2):253–271.
54. Seyama S, Pearl GS, Takei Y. Ultrastructural study of the human neurohypophysis. III. Vascular and perivascular structures. *Cell Tissue Res* 1980;206(2):291–302.
55. Luse SA, Kernohan JW. Granular-cell tumors of the stalk and posterior lobe of the pituitary gland. *Cancer* 1955;8(3):616–622.
56. Lopes MBS, Scheithauer BW, Saeger W. Granular cell tumour. In: DeLellis RA, Lloyd RV, Heitz PU, et al., eds. *World Health Organization Classification of Tumours, Pathology and Genetics of Tumours of Endocrine Organs*. Lyon: IARC Press; 2004:44–45.
57. Mete O, Lopes MB, Asa SL. Spindle cell oncocytomas and granular cell tumors of the pituitary are variants of pituicytoma. *Am J Surg Pathol* 2013;37(11):1694–1699.
58. Shanklin WM. Lymphocytes and lymphoid tissue in the human pituitary. *Anat Rec* 1951;111(2):177–191.

11

Peripheral Nervous System

Carlos Ortiz-Hidalgo ■ Roy O. Weller

DEVELOPMENT OF THE PERIPHERAL NERVOUS SYSTEM 300	CORRELATION OF NORMAL HISTOLOGY WITH THE PATHOLOGY OF PERIPHERAL NERVES 317
GROWTH OF AXONS 301	Handling and Preparation of Peripheral Nerve Biopsy and Autopsy Specimens 317
SCHWANN CELLS AND MYELINATION 301	ACKNOWLEDGMENTS 328
ANATOMY OF PERIPHERAL NERVES 302	REFERENCES 328
HISTOLOGY, IMMUNOCYTOCHEMISTRY, AND ULTRASTRUCTURE OF PERIPHERAL NERVES 303	
Components of the Nerve Sheath 303	

From a practical point of view, the pathology of peripheral nerves falls into two main categories: (a) peripheral neuropathies, which are diagnosed and treated by physicians and for which an elective nerve or muscle biopsy may be performed as a diagnostic procedure rather than as a therapeutic exercise, and (b) tumors and traumatic lesions, which are removed surgically mainly as a therapeutic measure to alleviate symptoms.

For the diagnosis of peripheral neuropathies, a detailed knowledge of the structure, immunohistochemistry and ultrastructure of peripheral nerves and clinicopathologic correlations are essential. The diagnosis of tumors and traumatic lesions, conversely, relies more on identifying the cellular components within the lesion and their interrelationships.

This chapter, therefore, concentrates first on how to identify different cellular components in normal peripheral nerves, and second, on how knowledge of the normal structure of peripheral nerves can be used to identify and assess pathologic lesions.

DEVELOPMENT OF THE PERIPHERAL NERVOUS SYSTEM

The first anatomical evidence of nervous system differentiation is the neural plate, which develops as a thickened specialized area in the middorsal ectoderm of the late gastrula stage of the developing embryo. This zone later becomes depressed along the axial midline to form a neural groove that folds inward to form the neural tube (1). Before fusion is completed, groups of cells become detached from the lateral folds of the neural plate to form the neural crests. Anteriorly, neural crests are located at the level of the presumptive diencephalon and extend backward along the whole neural tube (2).

In the peripheral nervous system, the neural crest is the source of neurons and satellite cells in the autonomic and sensory ganglia and Schwann cells; ectodermal placodes may also give rise to ganglion cells in the cranial region (1). Migrating multipotent neural crest cells and their subsequent development is determined and progressively limited, perhaps by the inductive effect of neuregulins and their ErbB receptors tyrosine kinase, by environmental factors and by relations with other cell types (1,3,4). The transcription factors Oct-6, Krox20 and SOX10, that are initially expressed in the earliest migrating neural crest cells, appear to be intimately involved in the development of Schwann cells from the neural crest (3–5). Interestingly melanoblasts also express SOX10 and it has been suggested that Schwann cell precursors associated with nerve endings could be the source of melanocytes (6). This could explain on the one hand, the association between alterations in skin pigmentation and neurologic disorders as observed in patients with neurofibromatosis type 1 (NF1), and on the other hand the presence of melanin in some schwannomas (*vide infra*) (6).

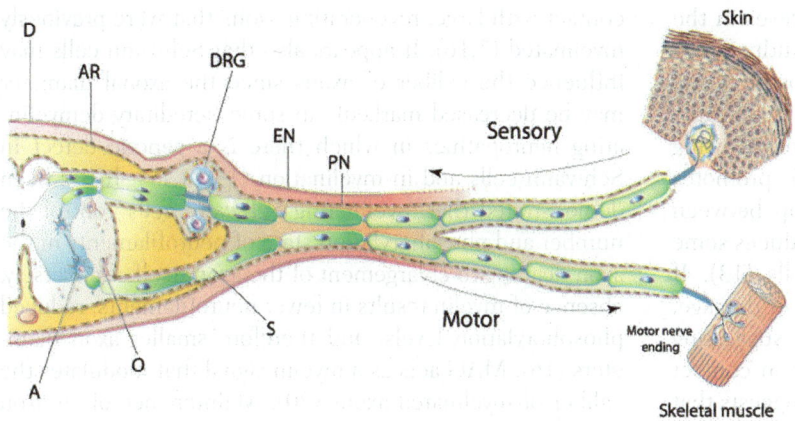

FIGURE 11.1 Anatomy of spinal nerve roots. Motor axons arising from the anterior horn cell (*A*) are initially myelinated by oligodendrocytes (*O*) and then pass into the anterior root to be myelinated by Schwann cells (*S*). Sensory nerve axons pass into the dorsal root ganglion (*DRG*) and the central extension of the sensory neuron passes via the dorsal root into the spinal cord. Arachnoid (*AR*) appears to be continuous with the perineurium of the peripheral nerve (*PN*). Dura (*D*) extends from the spinal cord to coat the roots within the intervertebral foramen, and is continuous with the epineurium (*EN*).

Many of the events that occur during the later stages of development of peripheral nerves are recapitulated during the regeneration that follows nerve damage in postnatal life. Developing neuroblasts of the dorsal root ganglia (posterior sensory root ganglia) extend neurites both centrally into the neural tube and toward the periphery. Developing motor neurons in the anterior lateral parts of the neural tube extend their neurites toward the periphery. Schwann cells become associated with the developing peripheral nerves and eventually form myelin around many of the axons (3,7). The proximal portions of the anterior horn cell axons and the central axons of the sensory ganglion cells are myelinated within the neural tube by oligodendrocytes (Fig. 11.1).

GROWTH OF AXONS

One of the major questions that has been raised is how do neuronal processes grow over long distances and arrive at specific terminal regions. Genetic determinants, growth factors, and the extracellular matrix appear to play an important role in the appropriate guidance of neuronal processes (3,7). In 1909, Ramón y Cajal proposed the concept of neurotrophic substances to explain the directionality and specificity of axonal growth in the developing nervous system. But it was not until the 1960s that nerve growth factor (NGF) was discovered by Levi-Montalcini, Cohen, and Hamburger as a target-derived neurotrophic factor that supports the survival and differentiation of sensory and autonomic ganglia in the peripheral nervous system (8). NGF is a protein composed of three subunits—alpha (α), beta (β), and gamma (γ). The γ-subunit of this complex acts as a serine protease, and cleaves the N-terminal of the β-subunit, thereby activating the protein into functional NGF (8,9). Other substances that participate in axon growth are members of the NGF family (such as brain-derived neurotrophic factor [BDNF]); neurotrophins 3 (NT-3), 4/5 (NT-4/5) and 6 (NT-6); semaphorin-3A, neuropilin-1, and ephrin (8–10). The tips of growing axons possess multiple surface receptors for soluble and bound molecules that provide information for an axon's growth course (4,10). NGF interacts with the NGF receptor on the surface of the axon and promotes motility of the growing tip of the axon by interaction with the cytoskeleton of the cell (10,11). Mitochondria, neurotubules, neurofilaments, actin filaments, and some cisternae of smooth endoplasmic reticulum are incorporated into the axonal growth cone by axoplasmic flow. In addition to its growth-promoting properties, NGF also promotes the early synthesis of neurotransmitters and stimulates myelination (8,9).

Schwann cells in the developing nerve produce NGF and possess NGF receptors on their surface membranes, but expression of these receptors diminishes markedly as the peripheral nerve matures. As NGF binds to Schwann cell receptors and becomes concentrated on the surface of the primitive Schwann cell, it provides a chemotactic stimulus for growing axons (7,10). Failure of trophic interactions between the target organ and its innervation may result in nerve dysfunction (11). Indeed, cases of human neuropathies have been attributed to deficiency of neurotrophic factors; important data that provide a rational basis for the clinical use of neurotrophic agents in peripheral neuropathies (9,11).

The extracellular matrix also plays an important role in axonal growth and guidance. The tip of the growing axon has receptors for adhesion to extracellular substances such as collagen, fibronectin, laminin, and entactin; binding of extracellular components to these receptors promotes elongation of axons and stimulates cytoskeletal protein synthesis, and therefore cell movement and axon growth (11,12). Some of these extracellular components are found within or near basement membranes surrounding Schwann cells (12).

SCHWANN CELLS AND MYELINATION

Schwann cells move freely between and around developing peripheral nerve axons, forming primitive sheaths around the neurites and growing in parallel with them. Contact with axons stimulates Schwann cell division in vitro (13).

In vivo Schwann cell multiplication virtually ceases in the normal adult animal, but mitotic activity is induced by peripheral nerve damage. It is thought that exposure of the axon to the Schwann cell following loss of myelin sheaths (demyelination) or during axonal regeneration following axonal degeneration (wallerian degeneration) promotes Schwann cell division and that the relationship between Schwann cells and axons in the normal nerve induces some sort of contact inhibition in the Schwann cells (13). If axon regeneration does not occur following axon damage, Schwann cells gradually decrease in number, suggesting that Schwann cell growth and survival depend on contact with axons (7,13). Experimental evidence also suggests that continued axon regeneration depends on the presence of Schwann cells (7,14).

By the 9th week of gestation, fascicles of the human sural nerve are identifiable and contain large axon bundles surrounded by Schwann cell processes (15,16). Between weeks 10 and 15, Schwann cells extend several long flattened processes that wrap around large clusters of fine axons. At this stage, two to four Schwann cells are located within a common basement membrane and form Schwann "families" (16).

Myelination of peripheral nerves in humans commences between the 12th and 18th weeks of gestation (16,17). Initiation of myelination depends on the diameter of the axon and its association with Schwann cells. The choice to myelinate or not is dictated to Schwann cells by the axon itself, based on the amount of type III Neuregulin 1 exposed on its membrane (17).

By the time that axons have increased in diameter to between 1.0 and 3.2 μm, they are in a 1:1 relationship with Schwann cells and have either formed mesaxons or membrane spirals with compact myelin sheaths of 3 to 15 layers (3,16,17). The reason why some nerves become myelinated and others do not is not clear. Both Schwann cells around myelinated fibers and around unmyelinated fibers are able to produce myelin but the factors that determine whether myelination occurs are unknown. Certain transcription factors, such as SOX10, Krox20 and Oct-6/Scip, are known to be involved in the myelination program (3,4,7). In Oct-6 null mice, for instance, myelination is severely delayed while in Krox20 null mice myelination fails completely (3). Schwann cells in developing and regenerating peripheral nerves also express high levels of the neurotrophin receptor p75NTR (18). Neurotrophins are a family of proteins that play a variety of functions in the development and maintenance of the peripheral nervous system (9,18). Certain glycoproteins, such as myelin-associated glycoproteins (MAGs), are believed to participate in establishing specific Schwann cell–axon interactions in the developing peripheral nervous system (19). Experimental studies have shown that axons may induce the formation of myelin if the unmyelinated sympathetic chain is grafted on to a myelinated nerve such as the saphenous nerve. Schwann cells that had not previously formed myelin will do so if they come into contact with large, regenerating axons that were previously myelinated (3,16). It appears also that Schwann cells may influence the caliber of axons since the axonal diameter may be decreased markedly in some hereditary demyelinating neuropathies in which there is a genetic defect in Schwann cells and in myelination (13,14,17). It has been demonstrated that myelinating Schwann cells control the number and phosphorylation state of neurofilaments in the axon, leading to enlargement of the axon itself. Conversely, absence of myelin results in fewer neurofilaments, reduced phosphorylation levels, and therefore smaller axon diameters (16). MAG acts as a myelin signal that modulates the caliber of myelinated axons (20). Maintenance of an axon therefore appears to depend not only on influences from the neuron cell body but also on interactions of the axon with the accompanying Schwann cells (11,13,20).

Some 70% of axons within a mixed sensory nerve such as the sural nerve are very small and will become segregated into groups of 8 to 15 axons lying in longitudinal grooves within one Schwann cell; these will form the unmyelinated (Remak) fibers within the peripheral nerve. Thus, all axons in the peripheral nervous system are invaginated into the surfaces of Schwann cells, but myelin sheaths only form around the larger axons, which represent only a small proportion of peripheral nerve fibers (16).

ANATOMY OF PERIPHERAL NERVES

An understanding of the anatomy of peripheral nerves is essential for the interpretation of clinical signs and symptoms and for planning an autopsy to investigate a patient with a peripheral neuropathy (16,21).

Major nerves, such as the sciatic and median nerves, contain motor, sensory, and autonomic nerve fibers; they are thus compound nerve trunks. It was Sir Charles Bell, who first demonstrated that motor function lay in the anterior roots; François Magendie, showed that the sensory function lay in the posterior roots. This (anterior-motor, posterior-sensory) is known as the Bell–Magendie law (16,21). Motor nerves are derived from anterior horn cells in the spinal cord or from defined nuclei in the brain stem. The initial segment of the axon lies within the central nervous system and is ensheathed by myelin formed by oligodendrocytes (Fig. 11.1). As the axons pass out of the brain stem or spinal cord, they become myelinated by Schwann cells. Anterior spinal roots join the posterior roots as they pass through the intervertebral foramina to form peripheral nerve trunks. Cranial nerves leave the skull through a number of different foramina. The junction point between oligodendrocytes and the Schwann sheath of the cranial nerves, known as Obersteiner–Redlich zone (O–Rz) or glial/Schwann junction, has some clinical significance (22). For example, the pulsatile compression of the O–Rz by a vessel in some exit foramina may be responsible for the clinical symptoms of trigeminal and glossopharyngeal neuralgia, hemifacial spasm, torticollis spasmodicus or even symptoms of essential hypertension when a vascular cross compression of the left vagus nerve occurs (22).

Motor nerves end peripherally at muscle endplates and many of the sensory nerves are associated with peripheral sensory endings. The cell bodies of sensory nerves lie outside the central nervous system in the dorsal root ganglia or in the cranial nerve ganglia (16). Each ganglion contains numerous, almost spherical neurons (ganglion cells) with their surrounding satellite cells. Such satellite cells are derived from the neural crest and have an origin similar to that of Schwann cells (23). Satellite cells have been referred to in the past by a large variety of names such as amphicyte, capsular cells, perisomatic gliocyte, or perineuronal satellite Schwann cells (16,23).

Dorsal root ganglion cells were first described by von Kölliker in 1844. They are examples of pseudounipolar cells, which means that a single, highly coiled axon, or stem process, arises from each perikaryon but, at varying distances from the neuron, there is a T- or Y-shaped bifurcation, always at a node of Ranvier, with the formation of central and peripheral axons. Thus, the initial segment of axon gives the impression that the cell is a unipolar neuron but it actually has two axons (Fig. 11.1). The central axon passes into the spinal cord either to synapse in the posterior sensory horn of gray matter or to pass directly into the dorsal columns. Peripheral axons pass into the peripheral nerves (16,21).

Autonomic nerves are either parasympathetic or sympathetic. Preganglionic parasympathetic fibers pass out of the brain stem in the III, VII, IX, and X cranial nerves and from the sacral cord in the second and third sacral nerves. Postganglionic neurons are situated near or within the structures being innervated. Sympathetic preganglionic fibers arise from neurons in the intermediolateral cell columns of gray matter in the thoracic spinal cord and pass out in thoracic anterior roots (16). These preganglionic fibers are myelinated and reach the sympathetic trunk through the corresponding anterior spinal roots and synapse with the sympathetic ganglion cells in paravertebral or prevertebral locations. The autonomic nervous system innervates viscera, blood vessels, and smooth muscle of the eye and skin (16,21).

HISTOLOGY, IMMUNOCYTOCHEMISTRY, AND ULTRASTRUCTURE OF PERIPHERAL NERVES

Components of the Nerve Sheath

Macroscopic inspection of a normal peripheral nerve reveals glistening white bundles of fascicles bound together by connective tissue. The intraneural arrangement of fascicles is variable and changes continuously throughout the length of each nerve. Damaged peripheral nerves are often gray and shrunken due to the loss of myelin. Microscopically, transverse sections of a peripheral nerve (Fig. 11.2) show how endoneurial compartments containing axons and Schwann cells are surrounded by perineurium to form individual fascicles embedded in epineurial fibrous tissue (16,21).

Epineurium

The epineurium consists of moderately dense connective tissue binding nerve fascicles together. It merges with the adipose tissue that surrounds peripheral nerves (Fig. 11.2A), particularly in the subcutaneous tissue. In addition to fibroblasts, the epineurium contains mast cells. Although mostly

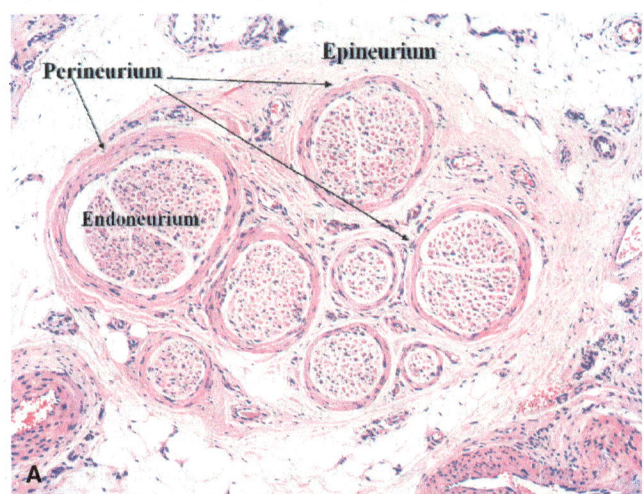 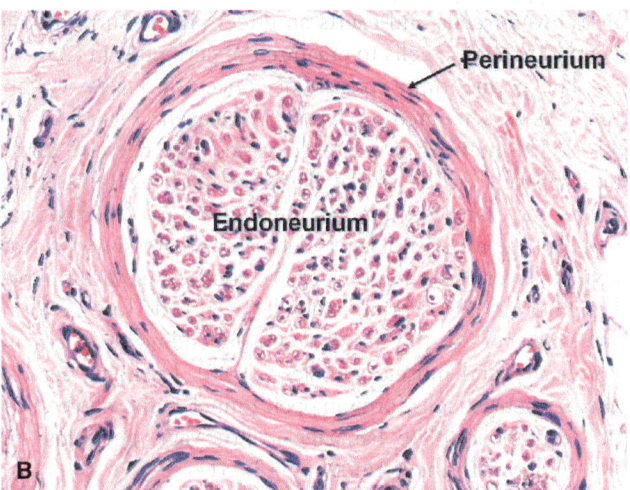

FIGURE 11.2 Peripheral nerve sheaths and compartments. **A:** A low-power view of a transverse section of a normal sural nerve. The nerve fascicles with roughly circular outlines are surrounded by perineurium and embedded in the connective tissue of the epineurium. Epineurial blood vessels (**A**) are also cut in cross section and there is adherent adipose tissue. The 1-μm sections are stained with hematoxylin and eosin (×16). **B:** The endoneurial compartment containing myelinated and nonmyelinated nerve fibers and their accompanying Schwann cells is surrounded by perineurium. Paraffin section stained with hematoxylin and eosin (×45).

composed of collagen, there are true elastic fibers composed of elaunin and oxytalan fibers in the epineurium so that when a specimen of unfixed nerve is removed from the body there is some elastic recoil of the epineurium (21,24). The amount of epineurial tissue varies and is more abundant in nerves adjacent to joints. As nerve branches become smaller to consist of only one fascicle, epineurium is no longer present. In nerves that consist of several fascicles, one or more arteries, veins, and lymphatics run longitudinally in the epineurium parallel to the nerve fascicles (the *vasa nervorum*) (16,21,25). Inflammation and occlusion of such arteries is an important cause of nerve damage in vasculitic diseases (25). The overgrowth of epineurial adipose tissue produces the so-called lipofibromatous hamartoma, which classically affects the hands and is associated with enlargement of the affected digit (26). In some nerves, such as in the sciatic nerve, there is an outermost common layer of connective tissue known as the "paraneurial component." This is a layer of connective tissue that ensheathes the entire muscle and protects muscles from friction against other muscles and bones and facilitates the gliding of the nerves during movement (27).

Perineurium

Originally described by Henle in the 19th century, the perineurium has, in the past, been known by a variety of different terms such as laminated sheath of Ranvier, mesothelium, perilemma, neurothelium, perineurothelium, and perineurial epithelium (21,28).

On the basis of the pioneer work of the 1995 Nobel Prize winners C. Nüsslein-Volhard and Wieschaus, an intercellular signaling molecule secreted by Schwann cells known as Desert Hedgehog (Dhh), was described; it functions as an important molecule in the formation of the perineurium (29). Apparently this molecule is a direct target for SOX10 in Schwann cells and exerts an effect on the surrounding connective tissue cells to organize the perineurium (29).

The perineurium consists of concentric layers of flattened cells separated by layers of collagen (Figs. 11.2 to 11.4). The number of cell layers varies from nerve to nerve and depends on the size of the nerve fascicle. In the sural nerve, for example, there are 8 to 12 layers of perineurial cells but the number of layers decreases progressively so that a single layer of perineurial cells surrounds fine distal nerve branches (21,28). Perineurial cells eventually fuse to form the outer core of the terminal sensory endings in pacinian corpuscles and muscle spindles (21,30). In motor nerves, the perineurial cells form an open funnel as the nerve ends at the motor endplate. Paraganglia of the vagus nerve may lie just underneath the perineurium (28,31).

By electron microscopy, perineurial cells are seen as thin sheets of cytoplasm containing small amounts of endoplasmic reticulum, prominent vimentin filaments, and numerous pinocytotic vesicles that open on to the external and internal surfaces of the cell. Adjacent to the plasma membrane are fibrillary patches of actin bundles

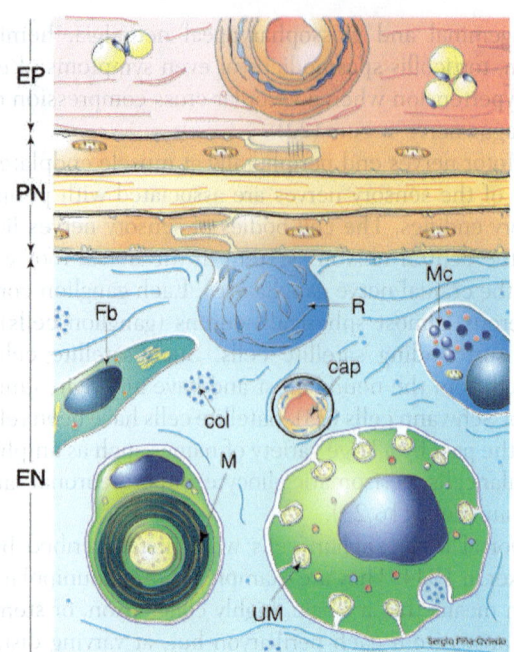

FIGURE 11.3 Diagram to show the major elements of peripheral nerve compartments. The epineurium (*EP*) contains collagen, blood vessels, and some adherent adipose tissues. The flattened cells of the perineurium (*PN*) are joined by tight junctions and form flattened layers separated by collagen fibers. Renaut bodies (*R*) project into the endoneurium (*EN*). Schwann cells forming lamellated myelin (*M*) (drawn uncompacted in this diagram) surround the larger axons. Multiple unmyelinated axons (*UM*) are invaginated into the surface of Schwann cells. Other elements include fibroblasts (*Fb*), mast cells (*Mc*), capillaries (*cap*), and collagen (*col*).

and it has been suggested that perineurium has contractile properties (21). Basement membrane is usually seen on both sides of each perineurial lamina (27,28). Numerous cell junctions, including well-formed tight junctions (*zonulae occludentes*), are present between adjacent perineurial cells and appear to be critical for the formation of the blood–nerve barrier (27,28). Claudins are integral membrane proteins that play a major role in tight junctions and are present in normal and neoplastic perineurium. In peripheral nerves, claudin-1 expression is largely limited to perineurial cells but is also present in paranodal regions and in the outer mesaxon along internodes (28,32). When tracer substances such as ferritin and horseradish peroxidase are injected into the blood, they do not enter peripheral nerves. Their entry is prevented by tight junctions in endoneurial capillaries and by the tight junctions in the inner layers of the perineurium. Thus, there is a blood–nerve barrier analogous to the blood–brain barrier. The blood–nerve barrier is present soon after birth and may prevent the entry of drugs and other substances into nerves that may otherwise interfere with or block nerve conduction (27,28). No such blood–nerve barrier exists in the dorsal root ganglia or in autonomic ganglia; these sites in the peripheral nervous system are vulnerable to certain toxins such as mercury (33).

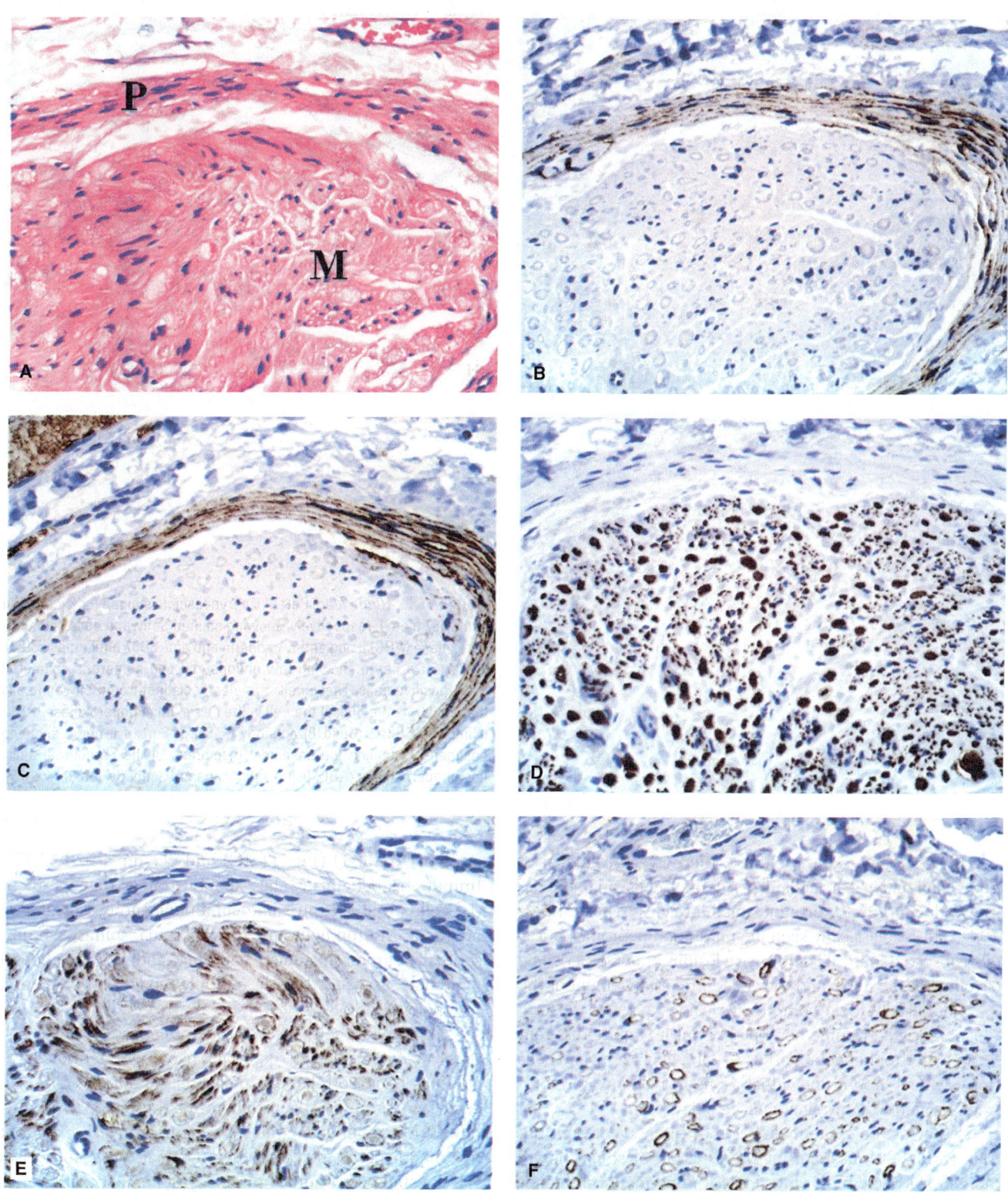

FIGURE 11.4 Immunocytochemistry of a normal peripheral nerve. **A:** Part of single nerve fascicle, cut in transverse section. Perineurium (*P*) surrounds the endoneurium containing myelinated nerve fibers (*M*). The nuclei are mainly those of Schwann cells. Paraffin section stained with hematoxylin and eosin (×160). **B** and **C:** Similar field to (**A**) stained for EMA and Glut-1, respectively. The perineurium is densely stained. Immunoperoxidase technique (ABC) with anti-EMA antibody and anti-Glut-1 antibody (×160). **D:** Part of a nerve fascicle stained for neurofilament protein. Large myelinated axons are well stained but unmyelinated axons are much smaller and more difficult to detect. Immunoperoxidase technique (ABC) using an antibody against the 80-kDa neurofilament protein (×160). **E.** Part of a nerve fascicle stained for S100 protein showing densely stained Schwann cells. Immunoperoxidase (ABC) using anti-S100 protein antibody (×160). **F** and **G:** (*continued*)

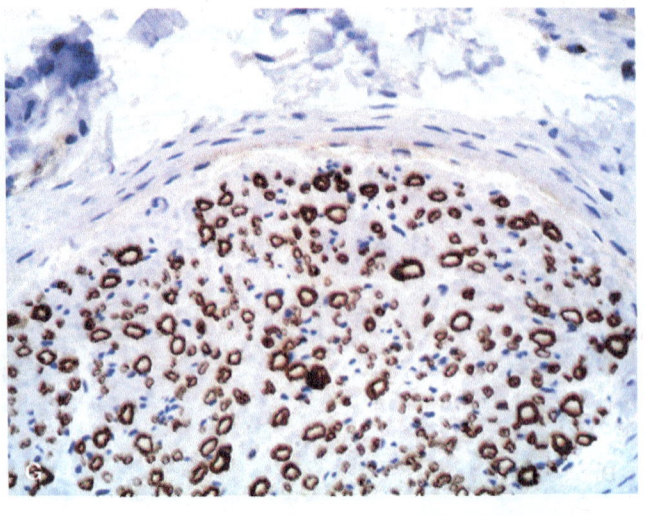
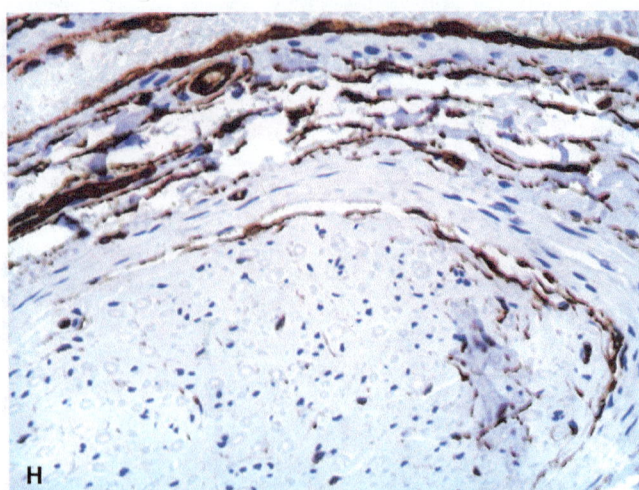
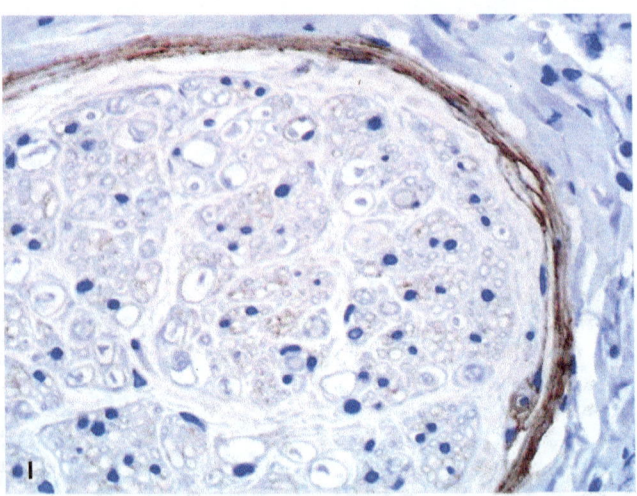

FIGURE 11.4 (*Continued*) Part of a nerve fascicle stained for E-cadherin and CD57 (Leu7), respectively, showing stained Schwann cells. Immunoperoxidase (ABC) using anti-E-cadherin and anti-CD57 antibodies (×160). **H:** Part of a nerve showing few endoneurial and numerous epineurial CD34-positive cells. These cells are clearly distinct from Schwann cells that comprise the bulk of the cell in the nerve. Immunoperoxidase (ABC) using anti-CD34 (QBend10) antibody (×160). **I:** Part of a nerve showing collagen IV staining the basement membrane of the perineurial cells. Immunoperoxidase (ABC) using anticollagen IV antibody (×160).

If the perineurium is injured, there is a breakdown of the blood–nerve barrier and perineurial cells migrate into the endoneurium to surround small fascicles of nerve fibers (34). This is classically seen in amputation neuromas but is also observed in focal compressive lesions of nerve (35). The swelling of the nerve and the concentric arrangement of the perineurial cells in the compressive lesions spawned the term "localized hypertrophic neuropathy" but it is quite different from hypertrophic neuropathy (35), in which Schwann cells form whorls around individual axons in response to recurrent segmental demyelination (see below).

Whereas the epineurial sheath of the nerve is continuous with the dura mater at the junction of spinal nerves and spinal nerve roots (Fig. 11.1), the perineurium blends with the pia-arachnoid (28). There are some morphologic similarities between the perineurium and arachnoid cells, although arachnoid cells are not usually coated by basement membrane. Immunocytochemically, perineurial cells and pia-arachnoid cells are positive for epithelial membrane antigen (EMA) (Fig. 11.4B) and vimentin but are negative for S100 protein, SOX10, and CD57 (28,36). Perineurial cells also express insulin-dependent glucose transporter protein I (Glut-1) (Fig. 11.4C) and claudin-1 (28,32,37). Immunohistochemistry has demonstrated that perineurial cells proliferate in some conditions such as traumatic neuroma, Morton neuroma, neurofibroma, solitary circumscribed neuroma, pacinian neuroma, and in the mucosal neuromas associated with multiple endocrine neoplasia (see below) (28,38).

Some tumor cells break through the perineurial sheath to grow along the perineurial space; perineurial invasion has been correlated with decreased survival times in some cancers (39). The problem for the histopathologist, however, is that sometimes perineurial invasion cannot be unequivocally determined on hematoxylin and eosin (H&E)-stained sections. Immunocytochemistry for Glut-1, EMA and claudin-1 may be used to rapidly and accurately assess the presence of perineurial invasion (28,40). Care must be taken however when examining cases of *vasitis nodosa*, in which benign proliferating ductules may be found within the perineurium and endoneurium (41). Nerve involvement has also been reported in fibrocystic disease of the breast, normal and hyperplastic prostate, and normal pancreas (41).

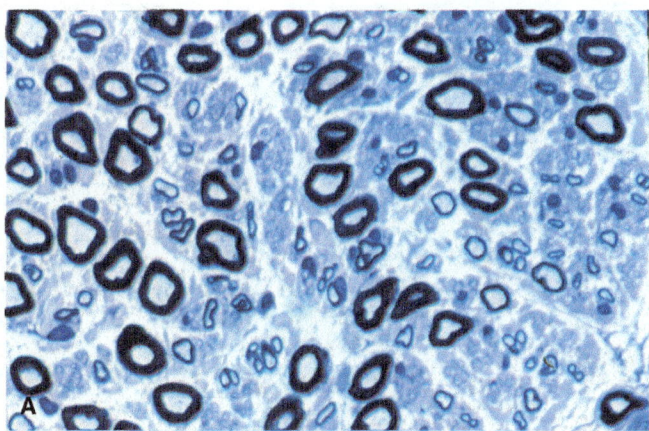 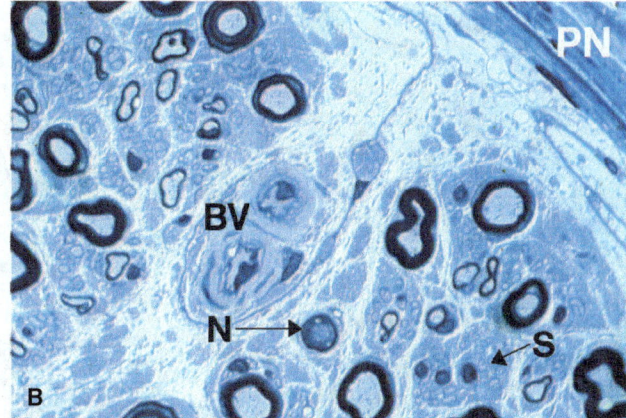

FIGURE 11.5 High-power histology of human sural nerve in transverse section. **A:** Large and small diameter myelinated fibers are seen. In a normal nerve, myelinated fibers are separated from each other but in this nerve there are also small numbers of regenerating clusters (see also Fig. 11.12B). The 1-μm resin section is stained with toluidine blue (×160). **B:** Part of a sural nerve fascicle cut in transverse section. Perineurium is at the top right (*PN*). Both large and small myelinated fibers vary in cross-sectional outline. Splits within the sheath are Schmidt–Lanterman incisures. Endoneurial blood vessel (*BV*). Section through a fiber near the node of Ranvier (*N*). Unmyelinated axons are seen as unstained circles within Schwann cells (*S*). The 1-μm resin section (×310).

Endoneurium

The endoneurium is the compartment that contains axons and their surrounding Schwann cells, collagen fibers, fibroblasts, capillaries, and a few mast cells (Figs. 11.3 to 11.5).

In cross sections of peripheral nerves, some 90% of the nuclei belong to Schwann cells, 5% to fibroblasts, and 5% to other cells (such as mast cells and capillary endothelial cells). Within the endoneurium CD34-positive bipolar cells with delicate dendritic processes (endoneurial fibroblast-like cells) have been identified and are distinct from Schwann cells (Fig. 11.4H) (42). Similar cells have been identified in peripheral nerve sheath tumors in various proportions (43). These endoneurial fibroblast-like cells are frequently located near blood vessels and under the perineurium where they are usually arranged parallel to perineurial cells and may function as phagocytes under certain conditions (42,43). In this regard, an intrinsic population of immunocompetent and potentially phagocytic cells (endoneurial macrophages) has been described within the human endoneurium that shares several lineage-related and functional markers with macrophages and may represent the peripheral counterpart of del Rio-Hortega cells (microglia) of the CNS (44).

Nerve fibers may be myelinated or unmyelinated but not all nerves have the same nerve fiber composition. Most biopsies of peripheral nerves in humans are taken from the sural nerve at the ankle and it is the composition of this nerve that has been most closely studied (45). Fibroblasts are ultrastructurally identical to fibroblasts elsewhere in the body. Mast cells are a normal constituent of the endoneurium and are also seen in sensory ganglia and in the epineurial sheath of peripheral nerves. There is an increase in the number of mast cells in some pathological conditions such as axonal (wallerian) degeneration and in some neoplastic entities such as neurofibromatosis (46). A characteristically high number of mast cells are seen in neurofibromas but they are only present in the Antoni B areas of schwannomas (47). Mast cells are thought to influence growth of neurofibromas, because some of their mediators may also act as growth factors. Apparently the inciting factor for mast cell migration into nerve sheath tumors is Kit ligand that is hypersecreted by $NF^{-/-}$ Schwann cell populations (47). Mast cell stabilizers are claimed to reduce proliferation and itching of neurofibromas (47). Following nerve injury, there is breakdown of the blood–nerve barrier as endoneurial vessels become permeable to fluid and protein; this increase in permeability may be related to the release of biogenic amines from mast cells within the endoneurium. Proteases released from mast cells have a high myelinolytic activity and may play a role in the breakdown of myelin in certain demyelinating diseases (47,48).

Collagen within the endoneurial compartment is highly organized and forms two distinct sheaths around myelinated and unmyelinated nerve fibers and their Schwann cells (Figs. 11.8 and 11.10). The outer endoneurial sheath (of Key and Retzius) is composed of longitudinally oriented large diameter collagen fibers; the inner endoneurial sheath (of Plenk and Laidlaw) is composed of fine collagen fibers oriented obliquely or circumferentially to the nerve fibers. The term neurilemma has been applied to the combined sheath formed by the basement membrane of the Schwann cell and the adjacent inner endoneurial sheath of collagen fibers (16,21). Thus the term neurilemmoma is inappropriate when used to describe tumors of Schwann cell origin (schwannomas). The longitudinal orientation of collagen fibers in the outer endoneurial sheath, together with the Schwann cell basement membrane tubes, may play an important role in guiding axons as they regenerate following peripheral nerve damage (49).

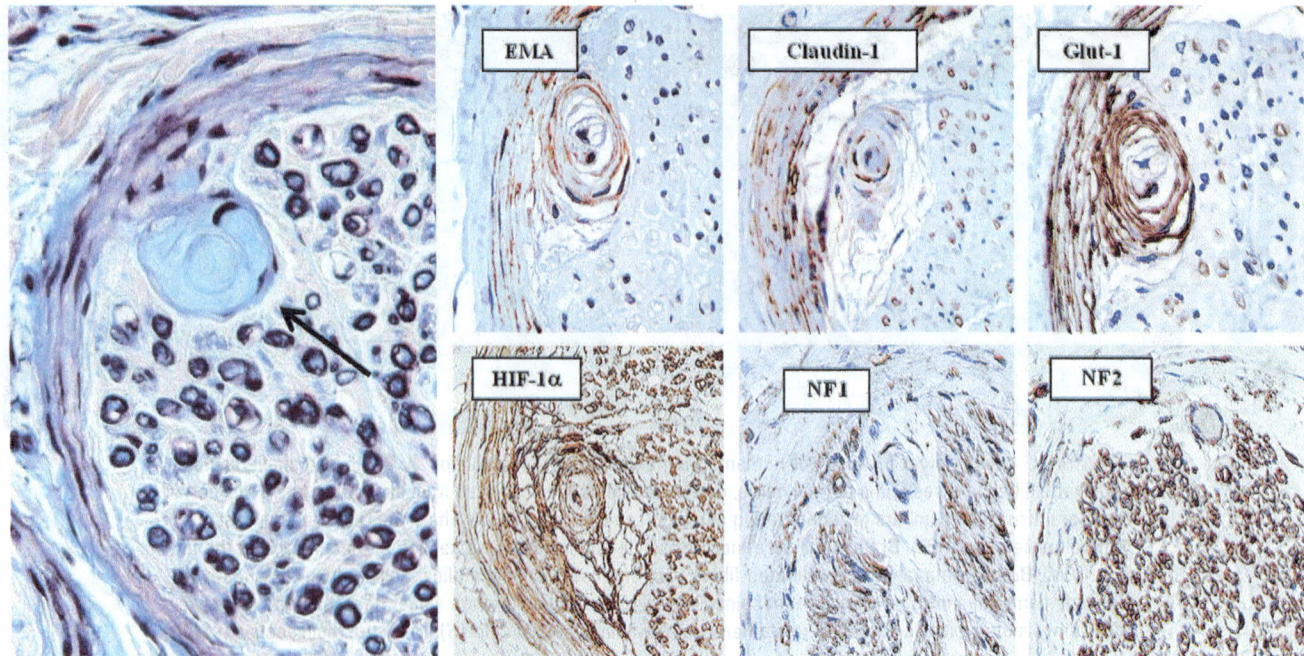

FIGURE 11.6 Nerve fascicles showing Renaut bodies (RB) (*Arrow*). **Left panel:** Russell–Movat pentachrome, showing the Renaut corpuscles in blue. Classical perineurial markers such as EMA, claudin-1 and Glut-1 are expressed in Renaut bodies. In addition HIF-1α, a transcription factor that regulates Glut-1 is also expressed in Renaut bodies and the perineurium. Expression of NF2 is also detected in Renaut bodies and scattered perineurial cells. In contrast, NF1 is negative in RB (see Ref. 51).

Renaut bodies (Figs. 11.3 and 11.6) are seen not infrequently in the endoneurium of human peripheral nerves. Described in the 19th century by the French physician J. L. Renaut, they are cylindrical (circular in cross section), hyaline structures attached to the inner aspect of the perineurium (28,50). Composed of randomly oriented collagen fibers, spidery fibroblasts and perineurial cells, Renaut bodies stain positively with Alcian blue due to the presence of acid glycosaminoglycans. The rest of the endoneurium also contains Alcian blue–positive mucoproteins (28). Renaut bodies produce extracellular matrix highly enriched in elastic fiber components and express vimentin, collagen IV, EMA, Glut-1 and claudin-1; interestingly the adjacent perineurium shows identical pattern of immunoreactivity (51). In longitudinal section, they may extend for some distance along the nerve and end in a blunt and abrupt fashion (51). These bodies are more prominent in horses and donkeys than in humans (16,21). Their precise function is not known, but Renaut himself thought that they may act as protective cushions within the nerve. They increase in number in compressive neuropathies and in a number of other neuropathies including hypothyroid neuropathy and may be a reaction to trauma (50).

Blood Supply of Peripheral Nerves

Vasa nervorum supplying peripheral nerves are derived from a series of branches from associated regional arteries. Branches from those arteries enter the epineurium (Figs. 11.2 and 11.3) to form an intercommunicating or anastomosing plexus. From that plexus, vessels penetrate the perineurium obliquely and enter the endoneurium as capillaries often surrounded by pericytes (Fig. 11.5). Tight junctions between the endothelial cells of the endoneurial capillaries constitute the blood–nerve barrier (21,34).

Complete infarction of peripheral nerves is very uncommon, probably due to the rich anastomotic connections of epineurial arteries. However, inflammation and thrombotic occlusion of epineurial arteries is seen in vasculitides (52) and occlusion by emboli occurs in patients with atherosclerotic peripheral vascular disease; both these disorders result in ischemic damage to peripheral nerves with axonal degeneration and consequent peripheral neuropathy (45).

Nerve Fibers

Most peripheral nerves contain a mixture of myelinated and unmyelinated nerve fibers. As the axons are oriented longitudinally along the nerve, quantitative estimates of the number of fibers in the nerve and their diameters are only adequately assessed in exact transverse sections. Staining techniques that can be used to identify nerve fibers and other components within peripheral nerves are summarized in Table 11.1. Longitudinal sections of peripheral nerve are less valuable than transverse sections but teased nerve fibers (see Fig. 11.15D) are very valuable for detecting segmental demyelination and remyelination and for assessing past axonal degeneration and regeneration (45).

In a transverse section of a human sural nerve there are approximately 8,000 myelinated fibers per mm^2, whereas

TABLE 11.1
Histologic Techniques for Peripheral Nerves

Technique	Application
A. General	
1. Hematoxylin and eosin (H&E)	Detection of inflammation, myelin and axons (Figs. 11.2B and 11.4A)
2. Hematoxylin–van Gieson	Collagen stains red; myelin black
3. Reticulin stains	Basement membrane around each Schwann cell in normal (e.g., Gordon–Sweet) nerve and schwannomas
4. Masson trichrome	
5. Alcian blue	Fibrinoid necrosis in vasculitis
6. Toluidine blue	Glycosaminoglycans stain blue
	(a) Mast cells in paraffin section, (b) general stain for 1-μm resin section, (c) metachromatic stain for sulfatide lipid.
B. Stains for myelin	
1. Luxol fast blue	Myelin stains blue; can be combined with silver stains for axons
2. Loyez	Myelin stains black
3. Osmium	Myelin stains black
4. Periodic acid–Schiff (PAS)	Myelin stains bright pink (good for detecting small number of nerve fibers in muscle biopsies)
5. Polarized light (frozen section)	Normal myelin, birefringent; degenerating myelin isotropic (nonbirefringent)
6. Marchi method	Degenerating myelin stains black (due to the presence of cholesterol esters); normal myelin is unstained
7. Oil red O	Degenerating myelin stains bright red; normal myelin pink
C. Stains for axons	
1. Palmgren's of Bodian's (silver stains)	Axons stains black
D. 0.5-to 1-μm sections	
1. Toluidine blue	Myelin stains black; axons unstained; Schwann cells and other cells, blue; collagen, blue (Figs. 11.5, 11.12, and 11.14A,B)
2. Toluidine blue and carbol fuschin	
3. Immunohistochemistry can be performed on these sections	Myelin stains black; axons unstained; cell and collagen, pink/blue (Fig. 11.14C)
E. Electron microscopy	(Figs. 11.8, 11.10, and 11.16)
F. Teased fibers	
1. Osmium tetraoxide stained	Myelin; nodes of Ranvier; demyelination and remyelination (Fig. 11.14D)
2. Enzyme histochemistry	
a. Mitochondrial enzymes	Schwann cytoplasm; axoplasm.
b. Acid phosphatase	Lysosomal activity with degenerating myelin
c. Polarized light	Myelin
3. Lipid histochemistry	
a. Sudan black B	Myelin
b. Oil red O	Normal and degenerating myelin
4. Immunohistochemistry	
a. S100 protein	Schwann cells (Fig. 11.4E); schwannomas, neurofibromas
b. CD57	Schwann cells (Fig. 11.4G); schwannomas, neurofibromas
c. CD56	Neurons, axons, Schwann cells; schwannomas
d. Calretinin	Schwann cells and some schwannomas
e. CD146 (Mel-CAM)	Schwann cells and some schwannomas
f. SOX10	Schwann cells, melanocytes, schwannomas, neurofibromas, and melanomas
g. GFAP (glial fibrillary acid protein)	Some schwannoma cells; possibly unmyelinated
h. PGP 9.5	Neurons, axons, Schwann and some schwannomas
i. Myelin basic protein	Myelin
j. Neurofilaments	Axons (Fig. 11.10C)
k. Epithelial membrane antigen/ Glut-1/claudin-1	Perineurium (Fig. 11.4B,C); perineuriomas
l. CD34	CD34-positive endoneurial fibroblasts (Fig. 11.4H)
m. CD68/CD163	Endoneurial macrophages
n. GAP 43	Regenerating axons

the unmyelinated axons are more numerous at 30,000 per mm² (16,53). Peripheral nerve fibers are classified as class A, class B, and class C fibers according to their size, function, and the speed at which they conduct nerve impulses. Class A fibers are myelinated and are further subdivided into six groups covering three size ranges. The largest are 10- to 20-μm diameter myelinated fibers that conduct at 50 to 100 m/sec; myelinated fibers 5 to 15 μm in diameter conduct at 20 to 90 m/sec, and 1- to 7-μm diameter myelinated fibers conduct at 12 to 30 m/sec. Class B fibers are myelinated preganglionic autonomic fibers about 3 μm in diameter and conduct at 3 to 15 m/sec. Unmyelinated fibers are small (0.2 to 1.5 μm in diameter), conduct impulses at 0.3 to 1.6 m/sec, and include postganglionic autonomic and afferent sensory fibers, including pain fibers (16,21).

Myelinated Axons

› **ULTRASTRUCTURE** Although myelinated nerve fibers can be demonstrated in paraffin sections (Fig. 11.4), they are best visualized by light microscopy in 0.5- to 1-μm thick toluidine blue–stained resin sections (Fig. 11.5). They exhibit a bimodal distribution of fiber diameter in the normal nerve with peaks at 5 and 13 μm and a range of 2 to 20 μm (16). Most axons above 3 μm in diameter are myelinated. Although along much of its length a myelinated nerve fiber has a circular outline in cross section, there is considerable variation in shape within the normal nerve, especially in the perinuclear regions and in the regions around the node of Ranvier (paranodal regions) (Fig. 11.7).

The axon itself is limited by a smooth plasma membrane (axolemma), that is separated from the encompassing Schwann cell by a 10- to 20-nm gap (periaxonal space of Klebs) (Fig. 11.8). The axonal cytoplasm (axoplasm) contains mitochondria, cisternae of smooth endoplasmic reticulum, occasional ribosomes and glycogen granules, peroxisomes, and vesicles containing neurotransmitters. The most prominent components of the axoplasm, however, are the filamentous and tubular structures. Microfilaments, 5 to 7 μm in diameter, are

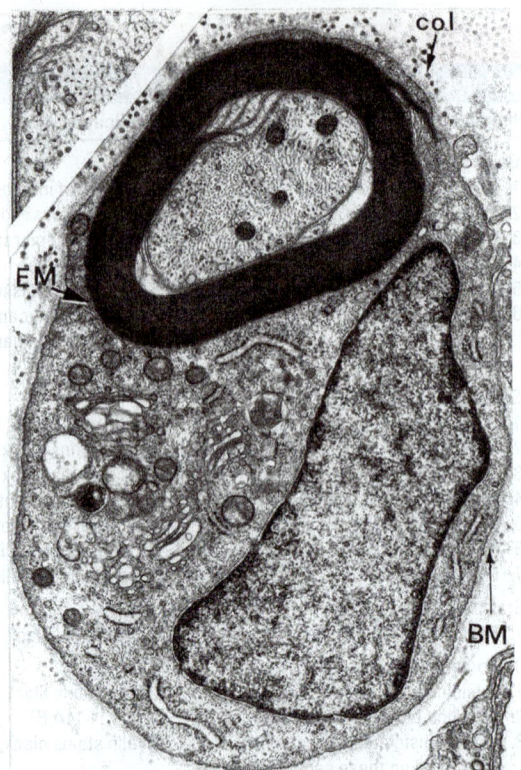

FIGURE 11.8 Transverse section of a myelinated nerve fiber in the perinuclear region. The axon contains mitochondria, small vesicles, and numerous neurofilaments and neurotubules cut in cross section (inset, *top left*). A distinct periaxonal space separates the axon from its encompassing Schwann cell. Myelin is compacted except at the external mesaxon (*EM*) and internally around the internal mesaxon near the axon itself. Part of a Schmidt–Lanterman incisure is seen on the inside of the myelin sheath. Abundant rough- and smooth-surfaced endoplasmic reticulum is seen in the perinuclear cytoplasm of the Schwann cell. A basement membrane (*BM*) surrounds the Schwann cell plasma membrane and endoneurial collagen fibers are seen cut in cross section (*col*). Electron micrograph (×18,400); inset (×40,000).

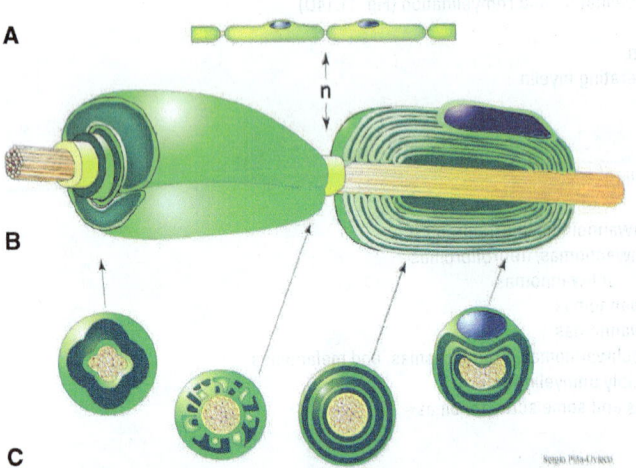

FIGURE 11.7 Diagram to show the relationships between (**A**) teased fibers, (**B**) nerve fibers in longitudinal section, and (**C**) nerve fibers in transverse section. **A:** In teased fibers, nodes of Ranvier (*n*) are separated by internodal portions of the Schwann cell and myelin sheath. The Schwann cell nucleus is roughly in the center of the internode. **B:** Longitudinal section through the node of Ranvier shows how the myelin sheath terminates as a series of end loops. The axon narrows as it passes through the node of Ranvier. **C:** Transverse sections of peripheral nerve as seen in electron micrographs and 1-μm resin sections are here related to the different portions of the internode and the node of Ranvier. From left to right, the paranodal region shows crenation of both axon and myelin sheath in larger fibers. At the node of Ranvier the axon is small and coated by radially arranged Schwann cell processes and myelin end loops. Throughout most of the internode the myelinated fiber is circular. In the region of the nucleus, the axon and the myelin sheath may be ovoid rather than circular in outline.

composed of chains of actin and comprise approximately 10% of the total axonal protein. They are virtually confined to the cortical zone of the axoplasm immediately beneath the axolemma (16).

Neurofilaments (Figs. 11.4C and 11.8) are 8- to 10-μm intermediate filaments of indeterminate length and they constitute a major filamentous component in larger axons (54). They were described originally by Ramón y Cajal and Bielschowsky as argentophilic *neurofibrillae*. In the neuronal perikaryon, neurofilaments tend to appear in multiple whorled bundles with no clear orientation to elements of the cell. In the axons, however, they appear in longitudinal, mostly parallel orientation (54). Small arm-like filaments are seen by electron microscopy. They project from the surface of the neurofilaments to form an irregular polygonal lattice. Neurofilaments are composed of protein triplets that are chemically and immunochemically distinct (54). Three major subunits are recognized and are classified according to their molecular weights of 68,000 (NF-L), 150,000 (NF-M), and 200,000 (NF-H) Daltons. Within axons, neurofilaments are phosphorylated and are immunocytochemically distinct from the nonphosphorylated filaments within neuron cell bodies. Immunocytochemistry for neurofilament protein (Fig. 11.4D) is often valuable for detecting large- or medium-sized axons in normal nerves, in traumatic lesions, in tumors involving peripheral nerves, and occasionally for detecting axonal processes in neuronal tumors (35,54). The third "filamentous" component in the axoplasm is the microtubule (neurotubule) (55). Microtubules are cylindrical (Fig. 11.8), unbranched, longitudinally oriented, hollow tubules 25 nm in diameter and composed of globular subunits of tubulin 4 to 5 nm in diameter. Periodic radial projections of high–molecular-weight proteins, that are part of the microtubule-associated proteins (MAPs), arise from the surface of the neurotubules. These arm-like projections bind neurofilaments and actin laments, and together form neurotubule–neurofilament–actin filament lattices. The three-dimensional lattices form an ordered structure in the axoplasm that appears to play an important role in axonal transport and contributes directly to the axon's shape (55). Microtubules also direct the transport of vesicular organelles between the cell body and the axon and thereby determine, in part, the composition of the axon (55).

Axoplasmic Flow

In 1906, Scott proposed that neuron cell bodies secreted "growing substances" in order to maintain the function of the axon. He suggested that such substances pass down the axon cytoplasm to the axon terminals. This suggestion was endorsed by Ramón y Cajal when he observed how regeneration occurs from the proximal stump of a damaged axon as long as continuity with the cell body is maintained (16,56). More definitive evidence of axonal transport was provided later by experimental studies using autoradiography and other techniques. Not only can labeled substances such as tritiated leucine be traced by autoradiography as they are transported along axons from the cell body, but the transport of organelles within the axon can also be directly observed by the use of dark-field microscopy or Nomarsky optics. Axoplasmic flow, the movement of different materials along the axoplasm, occurs in two directions, away from the cell body (anterograde) and toward the cell body (retrograde) (56).

Anterograde axoplasmic transport occurs at two velocities—fast and slow. Most organelles and large molecular weight substances within the axon are conveyed by fast axoplasmic transport, up to 400 mm/day. If a ligature is placed around a nerve, transported material accumulates proximal to the ligature and to some degree distal to it, due to interference with anterograde and retrograde transport, that both occur at the same rate and by the same mechanisms. The filamentous lattice component of neurotubules, neurofilaments, and actin filaments is responsible for fast axoplasmic flow, and these three elements probably act as rails along which the various transported organelles and substances move. Fast axoplasmic transport is dependent on oxidative energy mechanisms and adenosine triphosphate (ATP); it also depends on calcium and magnesium ions, and is blocked by calcium channel blocking agents. Some substances, such as trifluoperazine, that block calmodulin (calcium-activating protein) also block axoplasmic flow. Neurotubules, as an integral part of the axoplasmic transport mechanism, are depolymerized by cold and by colchicine; vincristine and vinblastine are known to bind tubulin and prevent the normal assembly of neurotubules. Such substances block fast axoplasmic flow (55,56).

Retrograde axoplasmic transport may convey information and organelles back to the cell body. In immature nerves, NGF is taken up by nerve terminals and retrogradely transported to the cell body, where it may play a role in the maturation of neurons (56). It has been suggested that the transport of such growth factors may also influence the metabolism of mature neurons and the absence of such signals from the distal part of the neuron when the axon is severed may trigger chromatolysis (56). Retrograde transport is also a pathway by which certain toxins (tetanus neurotoxin) and some metals (lead, cadmium, and mercury) may bypass the blood–brain barrier and accumulate in neurons (57). Neurotropic viruses such as herpes, rabies, and poliomyelitis may be transported to the central nervous system by retrograde transport (57). In addition to toxic neuropathies, axonal transport is defective in diabetes and peroneal muscular atrophy and probably in amyotrophic lateral sclerosis. Axoplasmic transport is reduced with age (58).

Slow axoplasmic transport at 1 to 3 mm/day concerns the distal movement of cytoskeletal elements such as neurofilaments, microtubules, and actin. It is a one-way process and neurofilaments are broken down by calcium-activated proteases at the distal end of the axon. Similarly, microtubules are depolymerized distally (59). Various toxins such as hexocarbons and their derivatives may interfere with slow axoplasmic transport so that neurofilaments accumulate and form large swellings within the axon (33,60). It is thought that neurofilaments within an axon may act primarily to maintain the bulk and the shape of large axons; neurofilaments are less numerous in small axons.

The Periaxonal Space of Klebs

As the Schwann cell enwraps the axon, it leaves a space, 12 to 14 nm wide, between the Schwann cell membrane and the axolemma (Fig. 11.8); this is the periaxonal space of Klebs (3,61). This space is in continuity with the extracellular space at the node of Ranvier through a narrow helical channel at the site where the terminal cytoplasmic processes of the Schwann cell approach the axolemma (Fig. 11.7) (16). The maintenance of the periaxonal space of Klebs appears to be mediated by an intrinsic 100-kDa MAG in the periaxonal membrane of the Schwann cell (20,61,62). This protein has a heavily glycosylated domain, with sialic acid and sulfate residues on the external surface of the plasma membrane extending into the periaxonal space; in fact, about half of the peptide of MAG is in the periaxonal space (20). Mutant mice that do not express MAG do not form a periaxonal space and the Schwann cell membrane fuses with the axolemma. Experimental studies with giant squid axons and mammalian nerve axons show that there is an increase in potassium concentration in the periaxonal space during repetitive conduction of nerve impulses. The full significance of the periaxonal space, however, is not clearly understood.

Schwann Cells

In his book on the microscopic structure of animals and plants published in Berlin in 1839, Theodore Schwann identified a vague sheath of cells within nerve fibers; these cells have subsequently borne his name as Schwann cells (peripheral nerve glia). As described previously in the section on development of peripheral nerves, Schwann cells are derived from the neural crest and migrate with growing axons into the developing peripheral nerves (3,63). Schwann cells produce NGF both in development and during regeneration and as the nerves grow, Schwann cells divide axons into groups and eventually establish 1:1 relationships with the larger fibers, that they will ultimately myelinate (16,63). Immature proliferating Schwann cells have a relatively large volume of cytoplasm compared with mature Schwann cells. The Schwann cytoplasm is rich in mitochondria, polyribosomes, Golgi cisterns, and rough endoplasmic reticulum (Fig. 11.8). The cytoskeleton within the cells includes vimentin intermediate filaments and is particularly obvious during the active proliferative and migrating phases of development and regeneration (64).

Schwann cells in a normal adult peripheral nerve are associated with both myelinated fibers and unmyelinated (Remak) fibers. There are also those Schwann cells associated with the perisynaptic region, and the so-called amphicytes that are the perineuronal satellite cells of the dorsal root ganglia and the autonomic ganglia (63). In myelinated fibers the Schwann cytoplasm is divided into two compartments: (a) around the nucleus and on the outside of the myelin sheath, and (b) that thin rim of cytoplasm on the inside of the myelin sheath and around the internal mesaxon (Fig. 11.8). Using electron microscopy, Schwann cells within a nerve can be identified by their relationship with myelinated or unmyelinated fibers. In damaged peripheral nerves, however, Schwann cells can be identified most easily by the presence of an investing basement membrane (Fig. 11.8). Other cells within the endoneurium, such as fibroblasts, do not have a basement membrane; and, although macrophages may invade the basement membrane tubes, they have a distinct ruffled border that distinguishes them from Schwann cells. Perineurial cells may be found in the endoneurial compartment, particularly in damaged nerves; they possess a basement membrane but they can be distinguished from Schwann cells by the presence of tight junctions that are not a feature of Schwann cells (3,63). With increasing age, normal Schwann cells accumulate lipofuscin and lamellated structures in the paranuclear cytoplasm in the form of Pi (π) granules of Reich. Such granules are composed of wide spaced lamellated structures and amorphous osmiophilic material; they are rich in acid phosphatase and stain metachromatically with toluidine blue in frozen sections (65). Other inclusions such as the corpuscles of Elzholz are seen in Schwann cytoplasm; these bodies are spherical, 0.5 to 2.0 μm in diameter, and stain intensely with the Marchi method. Few π granules remain in Schwann cells following nerve damage in which there has been extensive Schwann cell mitosis and proliferation (65).

In addition to an investing basal lamina, composed of laminins 1, 8, 10, fibronectin, and entactin/nidogen, Schwann cells also synthesize and secrete heparan sulfate, N-syndecan, glypican, perlecan, collagen types I, III, IV, V and XVIII, β-1 and β-4 integrin, and the protein BM-40 (3,16,63). Schwann cells can be identified in paraffin sections by immunocytochemistry and by the presence of close investment by reticulin staining. There is a rich reticulin network investing each cell, not only in the normal peripheral nerve but also in Schwann cell tumors. S100 protein in the cytoplasm and nuclei of Schwann cells can be identified by immunocytochemistry (Fig. 11.4E); this acidic protein, that is 100% soluble in ammonium sulfate at neutral pH, is a calcium-binding EF-hand type molecule, has no known function but is present in Schwann cells and not in fibroblasts or perineurial cells (66). Schwann cells are also immunolabeled using SOX10, E-cadherin (Fig. 11.4F), CD56 and CD57 (Fig. 11.4G) but perineurial cells are again negative. Calretinin, the 29-kD, calcium-binding protein that also belongs to the family of EF-hand proteins, is expressed in Schwann cells and in up to 94% of schwannomas (67). Normal and some neoplastic Schwann cells also express vimentin, PGP 9.5 and CD271 (low-affinity NGF receptor or p75 NTR—neurotrophin receptor) (68).

Occasionally, Schwann cells are labeled by anti-GFAP antibodies (36). GFAP immunoreactivity in the peripheral nervous system has been demonstrated in enteric ganglia, olfactory nerve cells and in Schwann cells in the sciatic, splenic, and vagus nerves (36,69). Schwann cells also participate in the formation, function and maintenance of neuromuscular junctions (NMJs) and Meissner corpuscles (3,30,63). These "terminal Schwann cells" may be identified by their expression of Herp-protein, which is not present in nonterminal myelinating Schwann cells (70). An interesting and peculiar intermediate glial cell type known as the olfactory ensheathing cell (OEC) is associated with neuronal processes of the olfactory bulb; OECs share astrocytic and Schwann cell phenotypes; they promote axonal regeneration and are potentially useful cells for xenotransplantation procedures (71).

Myelin

Myelin sheaths appear as slightly basophilic rings in H&E-stained transverse paraffin sections of nerve (Fig. 11.4).

They can be more prominently stained by Luxol fast blue or by hematoxylin stains such as Loyez (Table 11.1). In frozen sections, myelin is well depicted by Sudan black staining and in unstained frozen sections myelin can be identified due to its birefringence in polarized light, a technique that is particularly suitable for identifying myelin in enzyme histochemical preparations. Myelin is formed by the fusion of Schwann cell membranes and, by electron microscopy, it is seen as a regularly repeating lamellated structure with a 12- to 18-nm periodicity (72,73). On the outer and inner aspects of the sheath, external and internal mesaxons can be traced from the cell surface (Fig. 11.8). The myelin membrane is divided into two structurally and biochemically distinct domains: the compact and the noncompact myelin, each of which is characterized by a unique set of proteins. Compact myelin, for instance, contains P0, PMP-22, P2 protein and MBP, whereas noncompact myelin contains MAG, Cx32, $\alpha6\beta4$ integrin, and E-cadherin (3,17). As the external aspects of the Schwann cell membranes fuse to produce compact myelin, an interrupted interperiod (intermediate) line forms in the myelin. The more densely stained period line (major dense line) is formed by fusion of the cytoplasmic aspects of the cell membrane. A narrow cleft can be resolved between the components of the interperiod line. In myelinating Schwann cells noncompact myelin is present in paranodal loops, Schmidt–Lanterman incisures, in the nodal microvilli and in the inner and outer edges of the myelin (3,17). In these regions of noncompact myelin the cytoplasm that connects the Schwann cell perikaryon to remote parts of the myelin internode is retained (3). Several types of cell junctions, including tight, gap and adherens junctions are seen between the myelin lamellae, known as autotypic or reflexive junctions, denoting complexes between membranes of the same cell (3,17,74).

Biochemically, myelin is 75% lipid and 25% protein. The major lipids are cholesterol, sphingomyelin, and galactolipids, which are present in a rather higher proportion than they are in other cell membranes. It is the arrangement of the lipids that accounts for the liquid crystalline anisotropic nature of normal myelin sheaths that are birefringent in polarized light. Esterification of the cholesterol in degenerating myelin produces the isotropic, nonbirefringent lipid droplets that can be detected by Sudan dyes, by oil red O, and by the Marchi technique (Table 11.1). As myelin degenerates and the cholesterol becomes esterified, the ultrastructural lamellated pattern of myelin is lost and replaced by the amorphous osmiophilic globules seen in electron micrographs. More than half the protein in myelin is a transmembrane 28- to 30-kDa glycoprotein P0 (72,75); other proteins are P1 and P2. P0 mediates hemophilic adhesive interactions between Schwann cell plasma membranes; it is a key structural constituent of both the major dense line and interperiod line of compact myelin, and it is involved in myelin compaction (72,75). Numerous mutations in P0 have been described in a variety of demyelinating diseases (see below) (75).

Although the lipid composition of myelin in the peripheral nervous system is very similar to that of the central nervous system, the protein components are markedly different (76). CNS myelin has no P0 protein but has a proteolipid that is soluble in organic solvents; it also has an 18-kDa basic protein that is probably homologous with the P1 protein of peripheral nerve myelin. These biochemical differences may account for differences in the structure between peripheral and central nervous system myelin; for example, the space between the dense lines is less for CNS myelin (76,77). Biochemical differences in the proteins definitely account for the distinct antigenicities of peripheral and central nervous system myelin. Thus, injection of CNS myelin with Freund adjuvant will produce autoimmune encephalomyelitis in experimental animals with destruction of myelin in the spinal cord and brain, whereas injection of peripheral nervous system myelin with Freund adjuvant will produce autoimmune neuritis with demyelination in the peripheral nervous system.

Myelin sheaths are essential for the normal functioning of the peripheral nervous system and in those hereditary neuropathies in which myelination is defective, severe disability and retardation of development are seen (78,79). Acting as a biologic electrical insulator, myelin allows discontinuous (saltatory) and very rapid conduction of a wave of depolarization along the nerve fiber. It appears that myelination is an evolutionary adaptation that allows increased conduction velocities without excessive increases in axon diameter (17,80).

Myelination in the peripheral nervous system in humans occurs well in advance of that of the central nervous system. Although there is little myelin in human cerebral hemispheres at birth, myelin sheaths have already started to form around peripheral nerves at this time. Myelination is initiated by contact between Schwann cells and future myelinated axons (3,16,19). The Schwann cell rotates around the axon and may form 50 or more spirals, resulting in formation of the myelin sheath.

As the Schwann cell differentiates and produces a basement membrane, it acquires polarity via interaction of its cytoskeleton and some basement membrane components (mainly laminin and fibronectin) (3,21). The Schwann cell then begins to extend processes around individual axons. Once the lips of the Schwann cell start to wrap around the axon, they generate traction to pull the whole cell round and a spiral wrapping composed of many lamellae is formed (21). The importance of basement membrane formation as a prerequisite for the formation of myelin is emphasized by the lack of myelination when the basement membrane is deficient (81). MAG also plays an important role in myelination (75,82); it is present in the membranes of Schwann cells around myelinated fibers but not in those cells associated with unmyelinated fibers. MAG probably functions through its interaction with the Schwann cell cytoskeleton and this facilitates process lengthening and rotation during myelination (82). Periaxin is a 47-kDa protein constituent of the dystroglycan–dystrophin-related protein 2 complex that links the Schwann cell cytoskeleton to the extracellular matrix; it is located in the periaxonal region of Schwann cell plasma membranes and possibly interacts with MAG during myelination (83). Mutations in the periaxin gene result in the autosomal recessive demyelinating Charcot–Marie–Tooth (CMT4F) and Déjerine–Sottas diseases (79,84) (see later). As myelination proceeds, cytoplasm is expressed from the spiral of Schwann cell processes and membranes compact to form the 12- to 18-nm lamellated structure of myelin.

The length of an embryonic Schwann cell is 30 to 60 μm and it becomes associated with the length of axon in the developing nerve. As the nerve lengthens with growth of the body and limbs, so does the Schwann cell such that the length of the Schwann cell or internodal distance (Fig. 11.7) in myelinated fibers reaches some 190 μm at 18 weeks of gestation and 475 μm at birth. In the adult nerve, normal Schwann cells may extend for up to 1 mm in length along the myelinated fibers. Schwann cells associated with unmyelinated fibers lengthen to reach approximately 250 μm in the adult sural nerve. Following damage to a peripheral nerve, Schwann cell lengths revert to their embryonic length and thus give short internodes in regenerating and remyelinating nerve fibers (see Figs. 11.12 and 11.14) (16).

Schmidt–Lanterman Clefts or Incisures (S–L I)

Once viewed as artifacts, the clefts or incisures described by H. D. Schmidt and A. J. Lanterman (Fig. 11.9) are now known to be fixed components of the myelin sheath (16,21). Each Schmidt–Lanterman incisure (S–L I) consists of a continuous spiral of Schwann cytoplasm that runs from the outer (nuclear) to the inner (paraxonal) Schwann cell compartment in an oblique fashion at about 9 degrees to the long axis of the sheath. The funnel-shaped cleft splits the cytoplasmic membranes at the major dense line and forms a route for the passage of substances from the outer cytoplasmic layer through the myelin sheath to the inner cytoplasm. Near the external surface of the cleft, stacks of desmosome-like structures and gap junctions rich in Cx32, are sometimes seen, possibly maintaining the integrity of the spiral (16). The cell junction proteins, claudin-5, MUPP1, E-cadherin as well as a 155-kDa isoform of neurofascin, have been selectively detected at the S–L I (16,21). Cytoplasm in the clefts contains membrane-bound dense bodies, lysosomes, an occasional mitochondrion, intermediate filaments, and a single microtubule (Fig. 11.9) that runs circumferentially around the fiber; this microtubule may be associated with transport and with stabilization of the cytoplasmic spiral (16). The number of S–L I correlates with the diameter of the axon; the larger the fiber, the more clefts in the myelin sheath per Schwann cell. The presence of these clefts throughout myelinogenesis suggests that they are an important functional part of the sheath. It also seems obvious that they are pathways of communication between the inner and outer Schwann cell cytoplasm but their full significance remains to be elucidated.

Ramón y Cajal described longitudinal cytoplasmic channels (longitudinal bands of Cajal), similar to S–L I, that

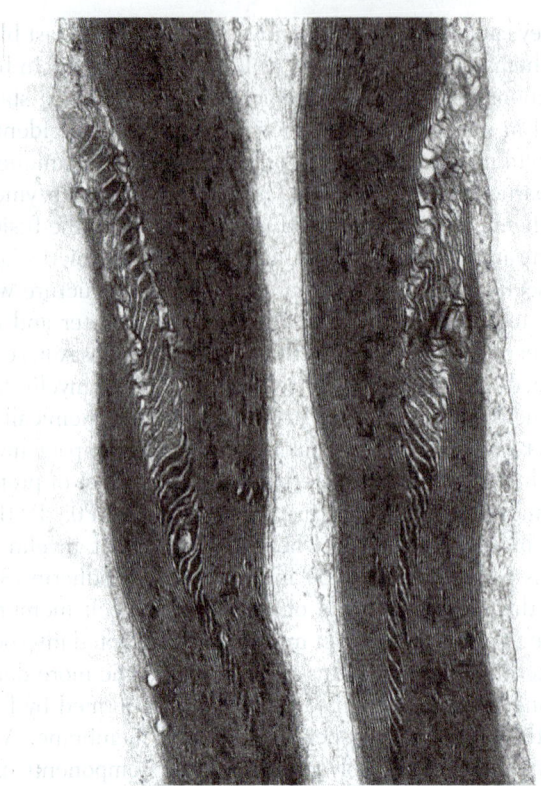

FIGURE 11.9 Longitudinal section of peripheral nerve: a Schmidt–Lanterman incisure. Blebs of cytoplasm are seen running through the myelin sheath. Densities in the cytoplasm (*top left*) suggest some form of junction between the spiral turns of the incisure. The axon is cut tangentially. (Electron micrograph (×30,000). (Reprinted from Weller RO, Cervos Navarro J. *Pathology of peripheral nerves: A practical Approach*. London:Butterworth; 1977 with permission.)

lie beneath the surface of the Schwann cell plasma membrane that are known to be separated from each other by the appositions formed by the periaxin–dystrophin-related protein 2 (Drp2) dystroglycan complex (17,85). Microtubule-based transport in these bands permits the Schwann cells to lengthen in response to axonal growth. Interestingly Schwann cells lacking longitudinal bands of Cajal are unable to keep pace with axon growth, suggesting a role in regulating the ability of Schwann cells to increase in length (17,85).

Nodes of Ranvier

With the introduction of techniques whereby individually separated or teased myelinated nerve fibers could be stained black with osmium tetroxide, a new view of nerve fibers was obtained. In his publication of 1876, Louis A. Ranvier, described and illustrated the constrictions or "*étranglements annulaires*," that are now known as the nodes of Ranvier (21,86). The functions of the node at that time were not known but Ranvier did suggest that the constrictions may prevent displacement or flow of the semiliquid myelin along the nerve fibers. He also suggested that the gap in the myelin sheath at the node of Ranvier might allow diffusion of nutrients into the axon (16).

In teased fibers stained with osmium tetroxide or viewed in polarized light, the nodal gap is readily visible, as is the bulbous swelling of the fiber on either side of the node of Ranvier (Fig. 11.15). The distance between each node along a myelinated fiber (Fig. 11.7) is approximately proportional to the thickness of the myelin sheath. In a normal adult mammalian nerve, internodal segments between the nodes of Ranvier vary from 200 to 1500 μm in length; the Schwann cell nucleus is usually sited around the middle of the internode.

Histologic study of 1-μm transverse resin sections of nerve and electron microscopic observations reveal a complex structure at the node of Ranvier and in the paranodal regions. As the axon approaches a node of Ranvier, it may become cruciform in cross section, especially in large fibers (Fig. 11.7). Deep furrows develop in the surrounding myelin sheath, and those furrows are filled with cytoplasm rich in mitochondria. As the axon passes through the node it is reduced to one-third or one-sixth of its internodal diameter although there may be a slight swelling at the midpoint of the node. Amorphous, osmiophilic material rich in ankyrin-G, NrCAM, neurofascins, and βIV-spectrin may be deposited under the axolemma (86,87). Ankyrin-binding proteins are also localized in the initial segment of the axon, the voltage-dependent sodium channel, the sodium/potassium ATPase and the sodium/calcium exchanger (88). These specialized areas of axon membrane may reflect the site of high ionic current density during transmission of a nerve impulse. Numerous ion channels are present in the nodal region of the axolemma and they are responsible for the changes in ionic milieu that occur during the conduction of nerve impulses (87). There is considerable specialization of the Schwann cell and the myelin sheath at the node of Ranvier. The myelin sheath terminates by forming dilated loop-like structures (paranodal loops) that are closely apposed to the axon surface (Fig. 11.7). Occasionally, desmosome-like structures are formed between Schwann cell terminal loops. The tight junction protein claudin-2, and the ERZ (ezrin, radizin, moesin) proteins have been identified as a ring that surrounds Na$^+$ channels at the node of Ranvier, possibly participating in the junctions formed at the outer collars of two adjacent Schwann cells at the nodal zone (89,90). The abundance of mitochondria in the paranodal cytoplasm is an indication of the high energy requirements of the node. Right in the center of the node, the myelin endloops are replaced by multiple finger-like Schwann cell processes (nodal villi) that contain F-actin and are 70 to 100 nm in diameter. The villi extend from the Schwann cells into the nodal gaps and interdigitate with processes of adjacent Schwann cells (87). This interlacing pattern of cell processes around the axon at the node of Ranvier is more prominent and complex in larger fibers.

Basement membrane from two adjacent Schwann cells is continuous over the nodal gap. Around the villous Schwann cell processes there is an electron-dense polyanionic-rich material that constitutes the extracellular matrix of the node. This gap substance creates a ring-like structure (ring of Nemiloff) and may provide an ion pool necessary for nodal function. It has been demonstrated that the gap substance contains glycosaminoglycans with cation-binding substances (16,85).

The myelin sheath acts as a biologic insulator for the internodal portion of the axons (91). Conduction of impulses along myelinated fibers proceeds in a discontinuous manner from node to node (rapid salutatory nerve conduction). Numerous sodium channels with a suggested density of approximately 100,000 per μm^2 are present on the axolemma at the node of Ranvier in contrast to the very low density of sodium channels (less than 25 per μm^2) in the internodal axon membrane; the internodal membrane may be regarded as inexcitable (16,87). Potassium channels show a complementary distribution to that of the sodium channels; they are less common than in the nodal membrane but are present in the paranodal and internodal axon membrane. Potassium channels contribute to the stabilization of the axon by preventing repetitive ring responses to a single stimulus and also help to maintain the resting potential of the myelinated fiber (87,91).

In demyelinating diseases, when the myelin sheath is stripped from the axon, there is gross slowing or cessation of nerve conduction along the affected fibers. Spread of a continuous wave of depolarization along the axon membrane is prevented due to the absence of an adequate density of sodium channels in the internodal axon membrane. Furthermore, the exposure of the internodal axon cell membrane, rich in potassium channels, will also interfere with conduction of the impulse (16,87).

Unmyelinated Axons

Unmyelinated fibers (that make up approximately 80% of the axons in most peripheral nerves) can be detected as unstained structures by light microscopy in toluidine blue–stained 0.5-μm transverse resin sections of peripheral nerve (Fig. 11.5) (16,21,63). However, at 1 to 3 μm diameter, they are almost at the limit of resolution and are only seen in good quality sections. Such fibers can be stained by silver techniques such as Palmgren or Bodian but are poorly visualized in immunocytochemical preparations using anti-neurofilament antibodies (Fig. 11.4D), probably because unmyelinated fibers contain few neurofilaments and a high proportion of microtubules.

The structure of unmyelinated fibers and their quantitation are most adequately studied by transmission electron microscopy (Fig. 11.10). They are more numerous than myelinated fibers in mixed peripheral nerves by a factor of 3 or 4:1 (25,92) and were first recognized in 1838 by the Polish physician Robert Remak as *fibriae organicae*; the Schwann cells associated with unmyelinated axons are referred to as Remak cells (7). Schwann cells have the potential to differentiate into either a myelinating or nonmyelinating ensheathing cell, depending upon the signals received from the axons that they contact, but the reason why some axons are myelinated and others are not is still unknown (7,17). A minimum caliber of 1 μm is required before an axon can be myelinated (17).

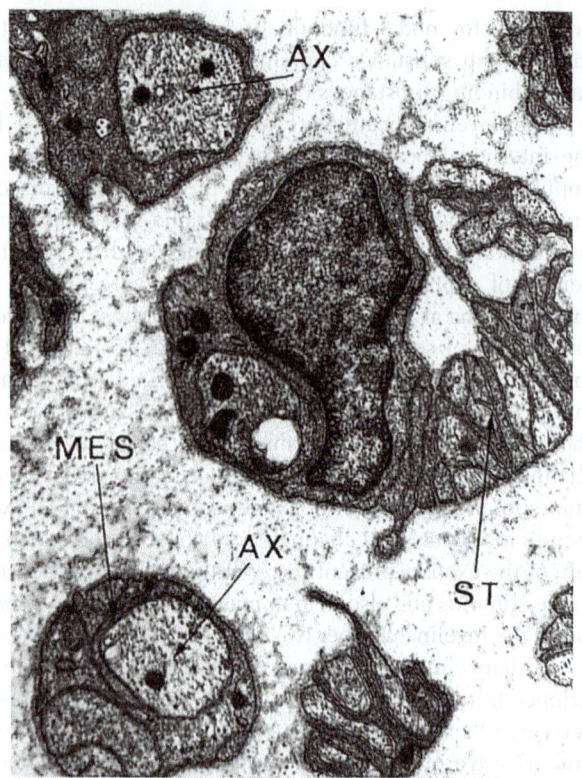

FIGURE 11.10 Unmyelinated axons (1.3 µm in diameter) cut in transverse section. The axons (*AX*) are surrounded by Schwann cells. Mesaxons (*MES*). Stacks of Schwann cell processes (*ST*) are commonly seen in adult nerves. Electron micrograph (×13,000).

Certain molecules such as L1, NCAM, integrins, and neurofascin are known to be expressed on unmyelinated axons and are downregulated during axonal myelination (7). Schwann cells around myelinated and unmyelinated axons may thus be regarded as originating from the same cell type but developing morphologic, biochemical, and physiologic differences. The main populations of axons surrounded by nonmyelinating (Remak) Schwann cells are the small nociceptive (C-type) axons, and the postganglionic sympathetic axons, and some of the preganglionic sympathetic and parasympathetic fibers (3). Axons are unmyelinated for some of their length, specifically at regions proximal to NMJs, at the most distal segments of sensory and autonomic neurons, and specialized sensory endings of the pacinian and Meissner corpuscles (3).

The cytoplasm of nonmyelinating (Remak) Schwann cells contains a Golgi apparatus, rough endoplasmic reticulum, mitochondria, microtubules, and microfilaments and may exhibit centrioles near the nucleus. Pi (π) granules, however, are not present although there are lysosomes containing acid phosphatase present in the cytoplasm. The nuclei of these cells are ellipsoid with one or more prominent nucleoli. A continuous basement membrane surrounds each cell (3). Schwann cells associated with unmyelinated fibers express different phenotypic characteristics from Schwann cells around myelinated axons. Although both types of Schwann cell contain immunocytochemically detectable vimentin intermediate filaments and S100 proteins, and almost the same basement membrane components, Schwann cells associated with unmyelinated axons are more likely to express GFAP (93). Such cells also lack MAG that is apparently necessary for segregation and myelination of axons. *Mycobacterium leprae* (Hansen bacilli) colonize nonmyelinating Schwann cells by attaching to laminin-2 and its receptor α-dystroglycan. Myelin-forming Schwann cells seem to be relatively free from infection by *M. leprae*. There is often a strong cell-mediated immune response in leprosy with extensive inflammation and peripheral nerve damage that causes paralysis and loss of sensation and frequently leads to unintentional mutilation of hands and feet (94). An important function of nonmyelinating (Remak) Schwann cells is as a reservoir of potentially mitotic cells (3). They retain the capacity to undergo mitosis in mature nerves and are prompted to divide by local myelin damage. Therefore Remak cells may be the source of new cells during nerve repair (3). Unmyelinated Schwann cells of the nerve terminal at the NMJ actively modulate synapse formation, respond to nerve conduction and neurotransmitter signaling, and play a role in the repair of the NMJ (63).

Electron microscopy of transverse sections of normal peripheral nerve shows how numerous unmyelinated axons 0.2 to 3.5 µm in diameter are associated with a single Schwann cell. Short mesaxons extend from the surface of the cell (Fig. 11.10) and the Schwann cell is separated from the axon plasma membrane by a space 10 to 15 nm wide that is analogous to the periaxonal space of Klebs seen around myelinated fibers. Although many axons may be gathered close to the cell body in the perinuclear region of the Schwann cell away from the nuclear region, single axons become more widely separated and are enclosed by thin Schwann cell processes (92) (Figs. 11.3 and 11.10). Each Schwann cell associated with unmyelinated axons in the sural nerve is between 200 and 500 µm in length. As axons pass from one Schwann cell to another, they are surrounded by flattened irregular, finger-like processes that interlock and become telescoped into the adjacent Schwann cell. The surface of the axon is therefore always in contact with the Schwann cell. In young children, only a single thin layer of Schwann cytoplasm surrounds each axon away from the nuclear region; but in adult nerves, the picture is more complex with several Schwann cell processes stacked together and associated with each unmyelinated axon (16).

Pockets of collagen bundles are frequently invaginated into the surface of Schwann cells associated with unmyelinated fibers (Fig. 11.3), particularly in aging nerves and when there is loss of unmyelinated fibers. The pockets of collagen fibers are separated from the surface of the Schwann cell by a layer of basement membrane. The significance of this phenomenon is not fully known.

Endocrine cells have been identified within the perineurium in close contact with unmyelinated nerves in the lamina propria of the appendix (95). These cells were demonstrated in 1924 by Masson and later Auböck coined the term "endocrine cell–nonmyelinated fiber complex," emphasizing the association between endocrine cells and unmyelinated fibers (95,96). These complexes are separated from the interstitial connective tissue by a common continuous basement membrane, leaving the cells in intimate contact with each other. It has been suggested that such endocrine cells could participate in the pathogenesis of the so-called neuromas of the appendix and appendiceal carcinoids (97). It is not known whether such endocrine cells exist in nerves other than those located in the wall of the appendix but there are reports of extraepithelial carcinoid tumors in stomach, small intestine, and bronchus, which suggest that there may also be endocrine cells related to nerves in these regions (96).

Interesting immunologic properties have been ascribed to Schwann cells. Numerous studies have shown that Schwann cells display a large repertoire of properties, ranging from the participation in antigen presentation, to secretion of pro- and anti-inflammatory cytokines, chemokines, and neurotrophic factors (98,99). Schwann cells express Ia determinants on their membranes and are able to present foreign antigens to specific synergic T cells (99). When Schwann cells are exposed to inflammatory cytokines they have the capacity to induce selective damage to T cells and have the potential to regulate the immune response in the peripheral nervous system (99). A role for Schwann cells has been suggested in myasthenia gravis (100).

Schwann cells also express complement receptor CR1 (CD35) and CD59, a 19- to 25-kDa glycoprotein, that binds to complement proteins C8 and C9 in the assembling cytolytic membrane attack complex (101). This may indicate that regulation of complement activation by these proteins is important in neural host defense mechanisms and may be implicated in the complement-mediated damage occurring in inflammatory demyelinating disease such as Guillian–Barré syndrome (102).

Interestingly unmyelinated (Remak) Schwann cells ensheathing sympathetic fibers within the bone marrow play an important role in hemopoietic stem cell (HSC) regulation. It has been shown that Schwann cells express bone marrow niche factor genes and the TGFβ activator molecule that converts the inactive form of TGFβ, present in the stem cells, into the active form. This in turn may downregulate lipid raft clustering, essential for HSC activation (63). It appears that the Schwann cells maintain the hibernation state of the stem cells (63).

CORRELATION OF NORMAL HISTOLOGY WITH THE PATHOLOGY OF PERIPHERAL NERVES

Handling and Preparation of Peripheral Nerve Biopsy and Autopsy Specimens

The sural nerve is the nerve that is most commonly biopsied in the investigation of peripheral neuropathies (45,103). It is

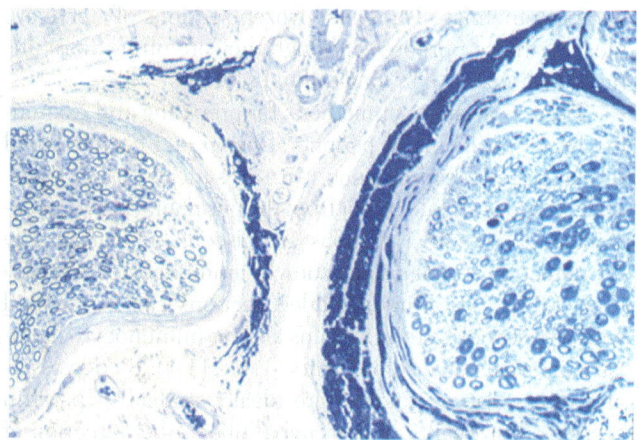

FIGURE 11.11 Histologic artifact in a peripheral nerve. In this transverse resin section, the fascicle to the left of the picture is well preserved. However, there is extensive recent hemorrhage (*center*) that occurred during the biopsy procedure; the myelinated axons in the nerve fascicle are squeezed and distorted (*right*). The 1-μm resin section is stained with toluidine blue (×40).

a sensory nerve so that in some motor neuropathies it may be totally normal, in which case examination of small branches of motor nerves within a muscle biopsy may be more fruitful (45,103). At autopsy, a wider range of motor and sensory nerves may be sampled, depending on the clinical picture. Whether taken at biopsy or autopsy, peripheral nerves are very easily damaged. The myelin sheaths are semiliquid and may be crushed by indelicate handling (Fig. 11.11). The specimen should only be gripped at one end and then gently dissected free before laying it, very gently stretched, on a piece of dry card and placing it in fixative or in liquid nitrogen for snap freezing. Fresh, frozen nerve should be used for enzyme and lipid histochemical studies whereas formalin-fixed nerve can be embedded in paraffin for the application of routine stains and immunocytochemistry (Table 11.1). Although formalin-fixed material can be used for the preparation of 0.5- to 1-μm resin-embedded sections and for electron microscopy, ideally the tissue should be fixed in glutaraldehyde and post fixed in osmium for ultrastructural studies. Teased fibers can be prepared from either glutaraldehyde- or formalin-fixed material (45,103).

The method of preparation really depends on the information sought. Frozen sections are ideal for detecting abnormal lipids, such as sulfatide in metachromatic leukodystrophy, and for detecting the cholesterol ester droplets of degenerating myelin by staining for Sudan red or oil red O. Increased lysosomal enzyme activity as in Krabbe leukodystrophy or in human and experimental neuropathies in which axonal degeneration or segmental demyelination is suspected can be detected in frozen sections stained histochemically for acid phosphatase (103). Brief formalin or glutaraldehyde fixation can be used in some cases for electron microscopic enzyme histochemistry. Frozen sections can also be used for immunofluorescence for the detection of immunoglobulin binding to myelin sheaths in paraproteinemias. Transverse frozen sections of nerve are ideal for these purposes although they are often more difficult to prepare than longitudinal sections.

There is a variety of methods for preparing and examining fixed specimens of peripheral nerve and each method reveals different information (45,103). Ideally, exact transverse sections should be cut from the peripheral nerve; occasionally, longitudinal sections are also useful particularly for detecting regenerating axons by immunocytochemistry (Fig. 11.4F). Paraffin-embedded sections can be stained with a variety of histologic stains and for immunocytochemistry to reveal nerve components (Table 11.1). Blood vessels and inflammatory exudates are ideally studied in paraffin sections, but quantitation of nerve fibers, the detection of axon degeneration and regeneration, and the assessment of segmental demyelination and remyelination are more satisfactory in 0.5- to 1-μm toluidine blue–stained resin sections or by electron microscopy. The presence of amyloid in the endoneurium or giant axons in some hereditary neuropathies and in some toxic neuropathies can be detected both in paraffin and in resin-embedded sections. Teased preparations are most useful for detecting segmental demyelination and remyelination and for assessing whether axonal degeneration and regeneration have occurred within the nerve in the past through the detection of short internodes.

Peripheral Neuropathies

The pathologic diagnosis of a peripheral neuropathy usually requires close clinicopathologic correlation and knowledge of the electrophysiologic data such as nerve conduction velocities and electromyography (84,104). Moderate slowing of nerve conduction velocities usually indicates loss of large myelinated fibers, whereas excessive slowing of conduction velocity suggests that segmental demyelination has occurred. Although there are a number of specific histopathologic features that aid in the diagnosis of peripheral neuropathy (e.g., amyloid, the presence of lepra bacilli, abnormal lipids such as sulfatide within the nerve, giant axons and vasculitis) (16,52), for the most part, assessment of peripheral nerve pathology depends on detection and quantitation of general pathologic features and good clinicopathologic correlation (45,84,103).

General Pathology of Peripheral Nerves

The general pathologic reactions of peripheral nerves are, for most practical purposes, limited to (a) axonal degeneration and regeneration and (b) segmental demyelination and remyelination. Hypertrophic changes with onion-bulb formation occur most commonly as a result of recurrent segmental demyelination and are most often seen in hereditary neuropathies.

Axonal Degeneration and Regeneration

If a neuron in the anterior horn of the gray matter of the spinal cord or in a dorsal root ganglion dies, its axon degenerates and no regeneration occurs (105). Such neuronal destruction is seen in poliomyelitis, motor neuron disease (amyotrophic lateral sclerosis), spinal muscular atrophy, and infarction of the spinal cord. Dorsal root ganglion cells may be lost in viral infections such as *Varicella zoster* or in a variety of hereditary sensory neuropathies. If an axon in a peripheral nerve is injured, for example, by trauma, entrapment, or ischemia, the distal end of the axon degenerates and subsequently regeneration occurs from the proximal stump of the damaged axon (Fig. 11.12). The success of the

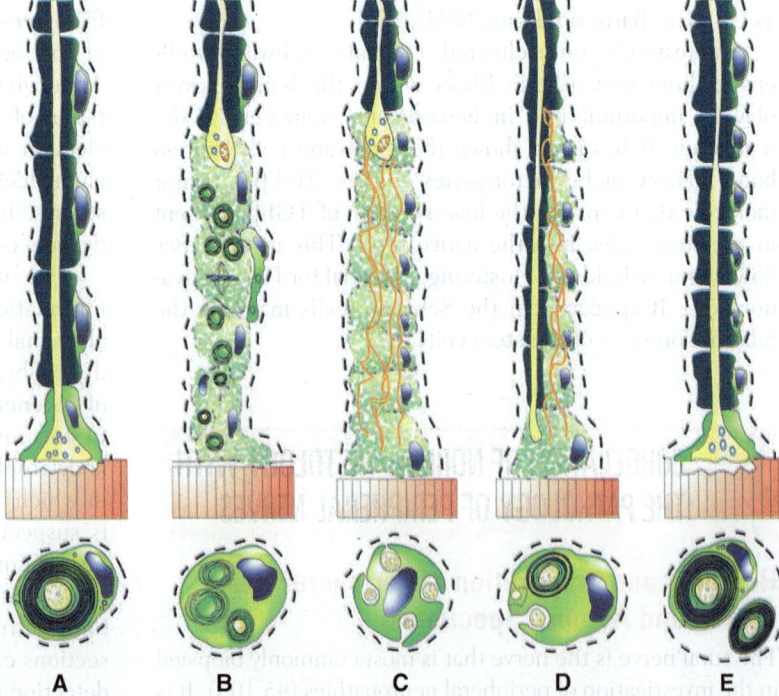

FIGURE 11.12 Diagram summarizing the events occurring during axonal degeneration and regeneration. **A:** Normal nerve. **B:** By 7 days after axonal damage, Schwann cells containing axon and myelin debris have divided to form bands of Büngner. **C:** Axon sprouts grow from the swollen end-bulb of the proximal axon. **D:** An axon becomes myelinated. **E:** Connection with the end organ is reestablished; regenerated internodes are short. (Reprinted from Weller RO, Cervos Navarro J. *Pathology of peripheral nerves: A practical Approach.* London:Butterworth; 1977 with permission.)

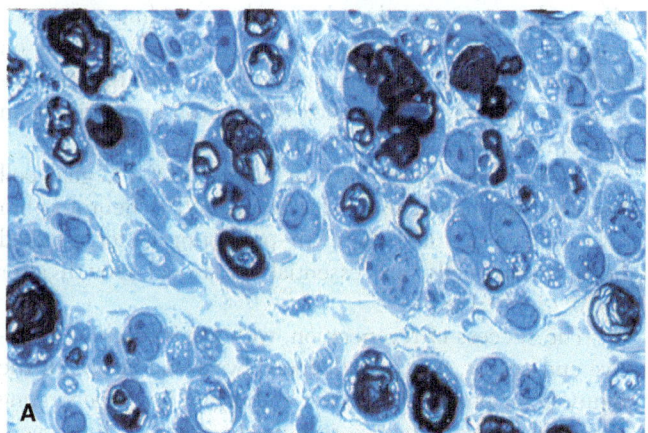 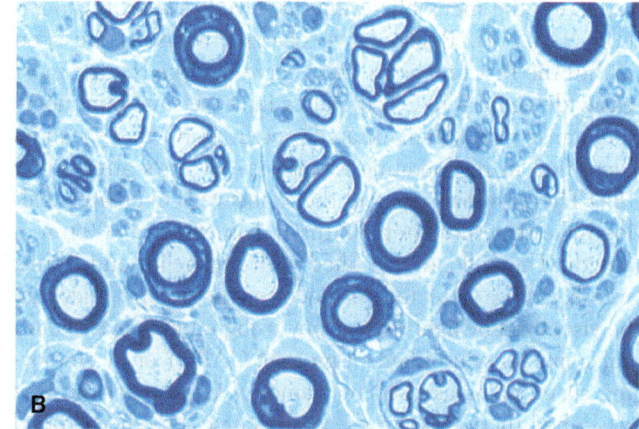

FIGURE 11.13 Axonal degeneration and regeneration in transverse sections of peripheral nerve. **A:** Axonal degeneration 4 days after nerve section. Few axons are visible and myelin is forming globules in Schwann cells and macrophages. The 1-μm section is stained with toluidine blue (×310). **B:** Axonal regeneration in a human nerve biopsy. Normal myelinated fibers are interspersed with clusters of closely associated thinly myelinated regenerating fibers (*top and bottom right*). The 1-μm section is stained with toluidine blue (×310).

regeneration depends on the distance of the site of damage from the nerve end organ (either motor endplate or sensory nerve ending) and the amount of scarring or other obstruction laid in the path of the regenerating axons.

Axonal degeneration was described by A. V. Waller in 1850 in London and the eponym wallerian degeneration is still used. Much of the fundamental work on nerve degeneration and regeneration, however, was performed by Ramón y Cajal in the early part of the 20th century (106). Twenty-four hours after nerve injury, most myelinated and nonmyelinated axons start to show degenerative changes. There is retraction of myelin from the nodes of Ranvier and dilatation of S–L I in the proximal, as well as in the distal stump. By 48 hours, myelin and axon changes become more obvious as the axon disintegrates and myelin sheaths become disrupted and form globules (Fig. 11.13) in which axon fragments are enclosed. Disintegration of the myelin appears to start with dilatation of the S–L I during the first day or two after injury (107). Myelin debris is initially birefringent and has a lamellated ultrastructure, as does normal myelin. But, as proteins break down and lysosomal enzymes become active around the myelin debris, cholesterol within the myelin is esterified to cholesterol esters and lipid debris loses its birefringence in polarized light and its lamellated ultrastructure to become amorphous globular lipid, that now stains strongly with Sudan dyes and oil red O (107,108). The Marchi technique also differentiates between normal myelin (unstained) and degenerating myelin (stained black).

During the 2nd week after nerve injury, much of the myelin debris is removed from the distal part of the nerve and regenerative features become more prominent. Axon fragments and myelin debris are broken down by both Schwann cells and macrophages (108,109). Schwann cells directly attract macrophages by secretion of different proteins, probably regulated by autocrine circuits involving the neuropoietic cytokines IL-6 and leukemia inhibitory factor (109,110). Macrophages, in addition to their phagocytic function may help to promote nerve repair through the elaboration of Schwann cell mitogens and may also affect neurons and axonal growth directly through the release of neurotrophins (109,111).

Although Schwann cell mitoses are seen as early as 24 hours after nerve injury, the peak of proliferation is between 3 and 15 days after nerve damage (112). As Schwann cells proliferate, they form columns (bands of Büngner) surrounded by basement membrane (Fig. 11.12); often redundant, old Schwann cell basement membrane is associated with these bands. Regenerating axons grow along the bands of Büngner and if regeneration fails, the bands shrink and Schwann cells may disappear and become replaced by fibrous tissue (113).

Diverse signaling molecules have been proposed to physically translocate from synapse to the nucleus known as injury signal; such transport is through a complex of proteins acting in association with neurotubules and into the cell nucleus, where gene transcription subsequently occurs (114).

Several easily detectable histologic changes occur during axonal regeneration. The neuron cell bodies in the anterior horns of the spinal cord or in the dorsal root ganglia show changes of chromatolysis during the first 3 weeks after axonal injury. The nerve cell perikaryon swells by some 20%, and the nucleus becomes eccentric as does the nucleolus. Nissl substance (a mixture of rough endoplasmic reticulum and polyribosomes) is dispersed so that the cytoplasm becomes pale when stained by H&E or by the Nissl stain. During this stage of chromatolysis, there is a marked increase in polyribosomal ribonucleic acid (RNA) with an upregulation of a number of regeneration-associated genes, including those encoding growth-associated protein 43 (GAP 43), cytoskeleton protein 23, β-tubulin and an increase in peptides such as galanin and vasointestinal polypeptide (VIP), reflecting the metabolic events involved in axon regeneration (114,115). Regenerative changes in axons are seen within the first few hours after nerve damage but are most easily detected 5 to 20 days after injury. Using immunocytochemistry, growth-associated protein 43 (GAP 43) can be identified in regenerating axons 4 to 21 days after injury (84) The proximal stump of the axon swells to create a balloon-like structure often 50 μm in diameter and 100 μm in length. The balloons are filled with organelles and fibrils, which can be detected by electron microscopy; they can be visualized by light microscopy using immunocytochemical stains for neurofilament protein, GAP 43 or by employing silver stains as used by Ramón y Cajal when he first described them. Myelin sheaths become stretched around the swollen axon balloons (109,111).

Nerve injury triggers the change of Schwann cells (myelin and nonmyelin -Remak cells) to a cell phenotype specialized to promote repair. The conversion to repair-mode Schwann cells involves dedifferentiation and reprogramming that consist of downregulation of myelin genes combined with upregulation of trophic factors and an increase of diverse cytokines as part of the innate immune response. Schwann cells collaborate with macrophages to clear myelin debris, and form regeneration columns of cells (bands of Büngner), for directing axons to their targets. This repair program is controlled by mechanisms involving the transcription factor c-Jun, which is rapidly upregulated in Schwann cells after injury. Interestingly in the absence of c-Jun, damage results in the formation of a dysfunctional repair cell, neuronal death and failure of functional recovery (116).

Starting around the 4th day after injury, multiple nerve sprouts, or neurites, extend from the axon balloon (growth cone) and grow distally at 1 to 2.5 mm/day. As the neurites enter the bands of Büngner, they become invaginated into the surface of the Schwann cell and, if growth continues, they become myelinated. Unmyelinated (Remak) fibers regenerate in a similar way, but they are smaller and no myelin sheaths form around them. Regenerating neurites can be detected in the classical way by silver staining; but, in cross sections of peripheral nerve, they are best demonstrated in 0.5- to 1-μm resin sections or by electron microscopy. Characteristically, regenerating axons form clusters encircled by a single basement membrane. In the light microscope, these clusters (Fig. 11.13) are recognized by the close association of small, thinly myelinated axons within the nerve; myelinated nerve fibers in a normal nerve are well separated from each other by endoneurial collagen (Fig. 11.5).

Axon growth and regeneration are stimulated by NGF synthesized by Schwann cells, fibroblasts and macrophages and transported back along the axon by retrograde axoplasmic transport to stimulate nerve cell protein synthesis (3,8,9,55). In addition to growth factors, there appears to be topographical affinity between regenerating axons and certain pathways; for example, it appears that regenerating tibial nerve axons grow toward the distal tibial nerve rather than toward the distal peroneal nerves. Connective tissue elements may also play a role in guiding regenerating axons (117). Neurite outgrowth–promoting factors on cell surfaces (cell adhesion molecules) or in the extracellular matrix promote extension of the axon by providing an appropriate "adhesiveness" in the substrate (3,117).

NGF, brain-derived growth factor (BDGF), glial cell line–derived neurotrophic factor (GDNF), neurotrophin (NT-3), and neurite outgrowth–promoting factor released by Schwann cells, are essential for axonal growth after injury (3,115,118).

The success of regeneration, with axons reaching effective end organs, may be influenced by several factors. If the injury is far proximal from the end organ, few regenerating axons may make effective reconnections (116). But regeneration over short distances may be very effective in the peripheral nervous system. The presence of scar tissue or discontinuity of anatomical pathways may also inhibit regeneration. A number of grafting techniques are employed to overcome this problem. If regeneration to the distal stump of a nerve is blocked by scar tissue, axons may grow outside the original course of the nerve and even back alongside the proximal stump (terminals of Perroncito) (35,119). Thus, small bundles of regenerating neurites, often surrounded by perineurial cells, form amputation neuromas in which interlacing bundles containing axons surrounded by myelin sheaths and with fine perineurial coverings can be detected microscopically. Immunocytochemistry for neurofilament proteins (axons), EMA, Glut-1 and claudin-1 (perineurial cells), and S100 and SOX10 (Schwann cells) may be very useful in establishing the structure and identity of the nerve bundles in an amputation neuroma (35,119). Immunohistochemical and radioimmunoassay data have shown focal accumulation of sodium channels within the tips of injured axons that may be responsible, in part, for the ectopic axonal excitability and the resulting abnormal sensory phenomena (pain and paresthesiae) which frequently complicate peripheral nerve injury (119). Macrophages migrate into the neuroma within the first 2 weeks after the injury and later they are seen with numerous large cytoplasmic vacuoles filled with myelin fragments. This suggests that macrophages may also participate in the genesis of chronic pain after the neuroma has formed possibly by: (a) creating demyelinating axonal regions susceptible to external stimuli, (b) by releasing substances that influence regeneration of axons, or (c) by direct action on the denuded remodeling membranes (35,119).

Axon degeneration, often with regeneration, is a feature of numerous peripheral neuropathies including those associated with diabetes, amyloidosis, infections (such as leprosy), sarcoidosis, paraneoplastic syndromes, vascular disease, and metabolic diseases (103,118). Most toxic neuropathies (33,120) result in chronic axonal degeneration at the extreme distal ends of sensory and motor nerves (distal axonopathies). The distal ends of long tracts in the spinal cord (dorsal columns and corticospinal tracts) are often affected, as well as the peripheral nerves. Timely withdrawal of the toxin may allow effective regeneration to occur, but only in the peripheral nerves, not in the spinal cord. Many peripheral neuropathies induced by the diseases itemized above are slowly progressive, so that nerve biopsies in these conditions do not usually reveal the early stages of axonal degeneration and regeneration. More frequently, the histologic picture is characterized by loss of large myelinated axons and, to a lesser extent, loss of small myelinated and unmyelinated axons. Nerve root or peripheral nerve compression, and trauma to peripheral nerve trunks result in axonal degeneration. Regeneration may be recognized in transverse sections of peripheral nerve by the presence of clusters (Fig. 11.13). In teased fiber preparations, short internodes in the distal part of the nerve indicate that axonal degeneration and regeneration have occurred in the past (16,113).

Segmental Demyelination and Remyelination

When demyelination occurs in peripheral nerves, it has a segmental distribution with each segment representing the internodal portion of an axon myelinated by one Schwann cell (Figs. 11.7 and 11.14). Such segments can be contiguous and thus demyelination may occur over long lengths of the nerve or in short sporadic segments (16). The axon remains intact except in severe demyelinating neuropathies in which secondary axonal degeneration occurs. Remyelination is often rapid and effective with restoration of nerve function. Demyelination may occur as a result of direct interference with Schwann cell metabolism as in diphtheria; myelin sheaths are broken down through the lysosomal action of Schwann cells although macrophages are later involved in the destruction of myelin debris (109,112).

Another mechanism is seen in the commonest acute demyelinating neuropathy, Guillain–Barré syndrome in which there is an immunologic attack on peripheral nerve myelin by lymphocytes and macrophages; segmental demyelination occurs and is followed by remyelination (102) (Figs. 11.14 and 11.15). Functional recovery occurs following both types of demyelination except in the most severe cases when there may be significant axonal degeneration.

The first stages of segmental demyelination are seen at the node of Ranvier, where the nodal gap becomes widened; subsequently, the whole internode of myelin may be broken down (84). This results in severe slowing of conduction of nerve impulses across the demyelinated segment and the onset of symptoms for the patient. Preserved axons remain invaginated within Schwann cells as the myelin sheaths are broken down (Figs. 11.15 and 11.16). Schwann cells proliferate and within a few days start to remyelinate the demyelinated axons by a similar mechanism to that seen during myelination in the fetus. Remyelination may be well advanced by 2 weeks after demyelination as the thickness of myelin sheaths increases and conduction velocities return to normal.

Classically, segmental demyelination can be detected in teased nerve fibers, first by the presence of widening of the gap of the node of Ranvier and then by the presence of axons devoid of myelin sheaths. Intercalated thin myelin sheaths along the axon are seen as remyelination proceeds (Fig. 11.15). In electron micrographs or in resin-embedded light microscope sections, naked axons can be recognized in transverse section and remyelinating fibers detected by the

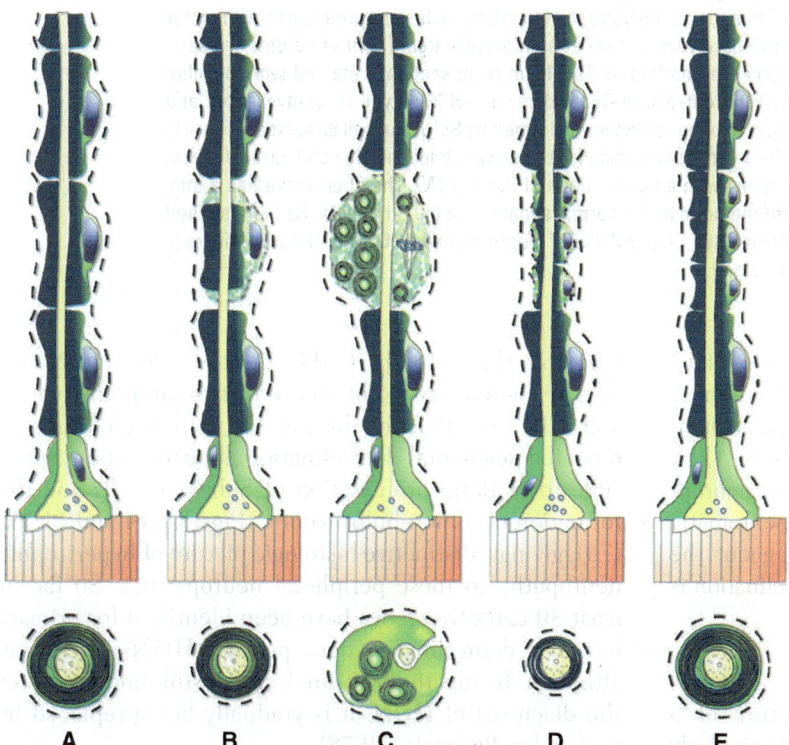

FIGURE 11.14 Summary of events occurring in primary segmental demyelination and remyelination. **A:** Normal nerve. **B:** Early segmental demyelination; retraction of paranodal myelin with widening of the nodal gap. **C:** Destruction of myelin sheath and Schwann cell mitosis. **D** and **E:** Remyelination; intercalated short segments. (Reprinted from Weller RO, Cervos Navarro J. *Pathology of peripheral nerves: A practical Approach.* London: Butterworth; 1977, with permission.)

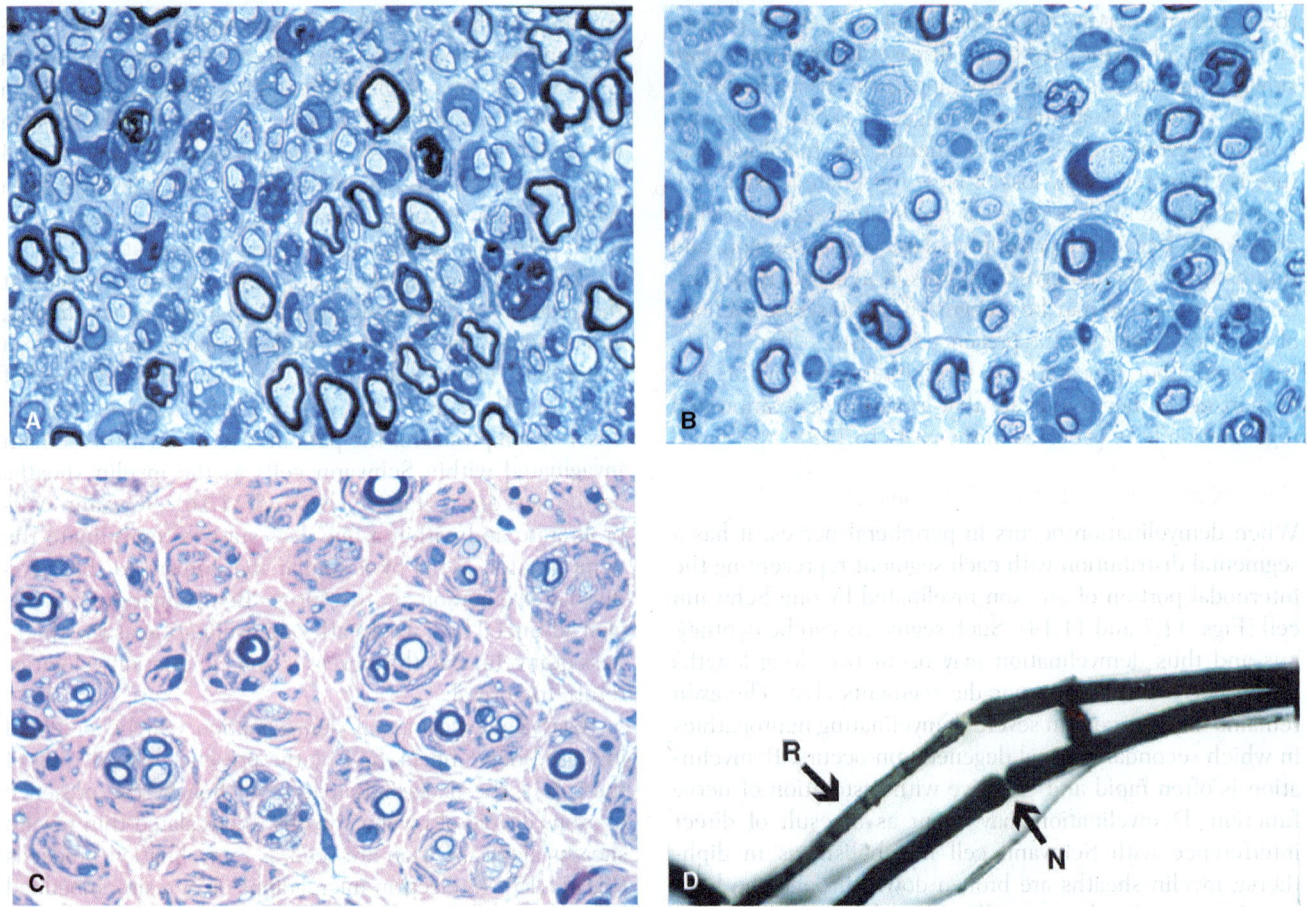

FIGURE 11.15 Segmental demyelination and remyelination. **A:** Transverse section of peripheral nerve showing early remyelination in an experimental animal. There are normal, large myelinated fibers with axons 8 to 10 μm in diameter and axons 3 to 5 μm in diameter, which have thin myelin sheaths and are remyelinating. Myelin debris is seen in Schwann cells and macrophages. The 1-μm resin section is stained with toluidine blue (×310). **B:** Nerve biopsy from a child with metachromatic leukodystrophy (sulfatide lipidosis). Large axons with either thin myelin sheaths (remyelination) or with no myelin sheath at all (demyelinated) (*right of center*) are seen in the biopsy. Unmyelinated fibers (*center*) are unaffected. The 1-μm resin section is stained with toluidine blue (×310). **C:** Hypertrophic neuropathy (Charcot–Marie–Tooth disease—HSMN type I). Demyelinated and remyelinated axons are seen at the centers of onion-bulb whorls formed by Schwann cell processes. There is abundant endoneurial collagen (*pink*). The 1-μm resin section is stained with toluidine blue and carbol fuchsin (×240). **D:** Teased fibers. Normal fiber (*lower*) with a normal node of Ranvier (*N*). The fiber above has a thin, remyelinating segment (*R*) on one side of the node and a normal segment on the other side. Osmium-stained teased fibers (×200). (Reprinted from Weller RO. *Colour Atlas of Neuropathology*. Oxford: Oxford University Press and Harvey Miller; 1984 with permission.)

presence of inappropriately thin myelin sheaths (Figs. 11.12 to 11.14). Segmental demyelination is a feature of a number of peripheral neuropathies, particularly mild vascular damage to peripheral nerves as in rheumatoid arthritis (84,121), diabetes, Guillain–Barré syndrome, occasional toxic neuropathies, and metabolic neuropathies such as metachromatic leukodystrophy (Fig. 11.15) (16,84,120). Throughout the range of neuropathies, however, segmental demyelination is less common than axonal degeneration.

Hypertrophic Neuropathy

Recurrent segmental demyelination is a feature of a number of chronic hereditary neuropathies, particularly Charcot–Marie–Tooth (CMT) disease, Déjerine–Sottas disease (hereditary motor and sensory neuropathy types I and III), and Refsum disease (79). In such diseases, repeated segmental demyelination appears to be responsible for a florid proliferation of Schwann cells and the formation of "onion-bulb" whorls (Figs. 11.14 and 11.15) (78), giving a distinctive histologic picture of hypertrophic neuropathy to these peripheral neuropathies. So far, at least 30 causative genes have been identified for primary heritable demyelinating neuropathies (HDNs) therefore, although histopathologic analysis is still important for the diagnosis of HDN, it is gradually being replaced by molecular diagnosis (79,78).

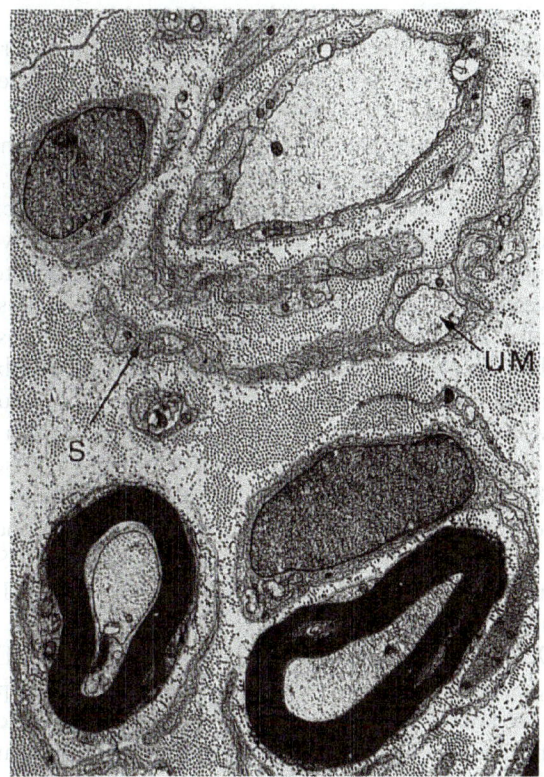

FIGURE 11.16 Demyelination. A large diameter axon (*top*) is demyelinated and devoid of a myelin sheath. A small onion-bulb whorl has formed around this axon with the encirclement by Schwann cell processes (*S*), one of which contains an unmyelinated fiber (*UM*). Thickly myelinated fibers are seen at the bottom of the picture. Electron micrograph (×6,600).

Traumatic Lesions of Peripheral Nerve

An understanding of the structure and staining reactions of normal peripheral nerve is essential for unraveling the complexities of traumatic lesions of nerve. Identification of cell types, recognition of patterns of organization, and the detection of normal elements within a traumatic lesion allow a more confident diagnosis and description to be formulated.

Amputation neuromas may develop as painful swellings at the distal ends of amputated limbs or at sites of nerve damage without amputation (35,119). They consist of disoriented bundles of axons surrounded by Schwann cells and divided into compartments by perineurial cells. In H&E-stained paraffin sections, the tubular formation of the perineurial compartments can be recognized. By immunocytochemistry, axons can be stained with antibodies to neurofilament protein and GAP 43; the Schwann cells associated with them contain S100 protein and SOX10, the perineurial cells are EMA, Glut-1, and claudin-1 positive but do not contain S100 protein or SOX10 (119). Silver stains can also be used to identify the twisted and disoriented axons. The histologic picture reflects the processes seen in the normal regeneration of peripheral nerve, but in amputation neuromas, appropriate regeneration along the distal part of the nerve is prevented.

In 1835 F Civinini from Pisa, and later in 1876 T. G. Morton, from Pennsylvania, described a neuroma that involves the plantar interdigital nerves, almost always between the third and fourth toes (Civinini–Morton metatarsalgia), and consists of small painful swellings on the nerves (35,122). Histologically, there are fibrosis and edema of the endoneurium and perineurium and the accumulation of mucosubstances similar to endoneurial glycosaminoglycans. The detection of axons and Schwann cells by immunohistochemistry is often a useful adjunct to the diagnosis of this lesion (35,119).

A pseudocyst or nerve sheath ganglion, containing mucinous material that stains with Alcian blue, may form on a peripheral nerve, generally at a site of repeated trauma. Although the fibrous capsule of the cyst and its mucinous contents may dominate the picture, damaged nerve components can usually be detected adjacent to the cyst (119).

Compressive lesions of peripheral nerves have resulted in some debate regarding their origin. Because of the resemblance of whorls within these lesions to those seen in hypertrophic neuropathies, they have been labeled "localized hypertrophic neuropathy" (35). Such lesions usually occur at sites of compression over the fibula or on the posterior interosseous nerve, although some lesions present with no obvious nerve compression. Although there are well-marked onion-bulb formations they are formed not by Schwann cells as in hypertrophic neuropathies but by perineurial cells (28,38). Such compressive lesions should not be confused with perineuromas in which immunocytochemistry has confirmed that the cell whorls are formed by EMA, Glut-1, and claudin-1–positive perineurial cells and there are abnormalities of chromosome 22 (28,38).

T.W. Beer described in 2009 a series of cutaneous reexcision specimens containing concentric proliferation of perineurial cells around nerves in the dermis in intimate association with fibrosis and/or chronic inflammation. The term reparative perineurial hyperplasia was proposed for this phenomenon that may occur in certain fibrosis associated or some traumatic conditions (123).

Palisaded encapsulated neuroma (PEN), also known as "solitary circumscribed neuroma," described by Reed in 1972, has rather distinct clinical features. Typically, it presents as a small (1 to 15 mm) solitary nodule in the area of the face with no clinical features of neurofibromatosis or type II multiple endocrine neoplasia (124). This lesion is currently viewed as a form of true neuroma. Histologically, PEN appears as one or more circumscribed nodules in the dermis, sometimes partially encapsulated by a delicate compact EMA-positive perineurial layer, and sometimes showing a plexiform or multinodular architecture (124). The process consists of a solid proliferation of tightly interwoven fascicles of Schwann cells sometimes separated by narrow gaps that create a characteristic appearance of the lesion at low magnification. The Schwann cells are often arranged as palisades and there may be numerous axons scattered throughout the lesion, best demonstrated with

Bodian silver stain or by immunohistochemistry for neurofilament proteins.

Tumors of the Peripheral Nervous System

A variety of cells and structures may be identified in tumors of the peripheral nervous system; they include perineurial cells, Schwann cells, axons, and neurons (125–127). The diagnosis frequently depends on the histologic analysis of the tumor and thus the detection of cellular components forming the tumor and their relationship with normal nerve structures (128,129).

Perineurioma is a rare true perineurial neoplasm (28,38). Perineuriomas can arise in a wide variety of sites and may exhibit different histologic patterns with extra and intraneural forms (28). Histologically, intraneural perineuriomas affect individual fascicles with concentric proliferation of spindle cells around nerve fibers in the endoneurium; extraneural (soft tissue) perineuriomas show paucicellular to cellular forms (with some cases showing dense collagenization—sclerosing perineurioma) with proliferation of spindle cells with an extremely thin and elongated profile resembling normal perineurial cells (129–131). Perineurioma cells may show granular cell change (132). Malignant perineuriomas have also been rarely reported (133). The key diagnostic finding is that the proliferating cells are labeled with EMA, Glut-1, and claudin-1, but fail to stain for S100 protein, SOX10, neurofilaments, and CD34 (28,48,128,129). Perineuriomas may be closely related to cutaneous meningioma since shared histologic features, and positive staining for vimentin and EMA in both conditions, suggest close similarities between these lesions (28).

Schwannomas are tumors of peripheral nerves composed almost entirely of Schwann cells (128,129); interestingly however, axons may be focally found, challenging the dogma concerning the absence of intratumoral axons in schwannomas (134). Neoplastic Schwann cells may produce and respond to trophic factors, particularly to the growth factor-like polypeptides known as neuregulins in an autocrine and/or paracrine fashion to promote proliferation. In fact, the presence of neuregulins in certain schwannomas has been demonstrated by immunohistochemistry (135).

Histologically, schwannomas form two basic patterns of cellular organization: (a) compact areas with elongated cells and (b) a less cellular loosely arranged area often with vacuolation and occasionally lipidization, described in 1920 by the Swedish neurologist N. R. E. Antoni and known as Antoni type A and Antoni type B patterns, respectively (136).

Neoplastic Schwann cells may exhibit different morphologies (Fig. 11.17) (128,129). Occasionally, the Schwann cells have an epithelioid appearance (epithelioid schwannomas) (137), are surrounded by an abundant myxoid stroma (nerve sheath myxoma), (138), have a high nuclear-cytoplasmic ratio (cellular schwannoma), exhibit a plexiform pattern (plexiform schwannoma), contain copious melanin (melanotic schwannomas), or exhibit xanthomatous change with many foamy cells containing oil red O positive neutral lipid (128,129). Microcystic and neuroblastoma-like variants have also been described (139). Schwannomas usually grow on the sides of nerves and do not infiltrate nerve bundles (128,129). Thus, normal nerves may be seen within the fibrous capsule that is usually present around schwannomas. Histologically, the tumor cells have elongated nuclei and long eosinophilic processes often forming palisades first described by the Uruguayan-born pathologist José Verocay and known today as Verocay bodies (140) (Fig. 11.17A). The palisades are parallel arrays of tumor nuclei separated by the eosinophilic PAS positive, processes of Schwann cells. The basement membrane investing each Schwann cell in the tumor is well demonstrated by electron microscopy but can also be demonstrated in reticulin stains by light microscopy (128,129). Collagen bundles within schwannomas may have a distinctive long-spaced appearance (Luse bodies) (141). Immunocytochemistry shows the presence of S100 protein, CD271 (low-affinity NGF receptor or p75NTR—neurotrophin receptor), CD57, CD56, calretinin, and SOX10 in schwannoma cells but they are negative for EMA (37,68,128). Schwannomas may also express transcription factors known to regulate normal Schwann cell development, such as FoxD3, and SOX9 (125). Some schwannomas associated with the spinal cord and those deep in the body or close to major joints stain by immunocytochemistry for GFAP while the superficial, subcutaneous schwannomas are negative (142). Schwann cells associated with unmyelinated fibers are more likely to express GFAP and it has been proposed that the GFAP-positive schwannomas may arise from unmyelinated nerves (3,142).

Melanin may be seen in schwannomas and by electron microscopy premelanosomes and melanosomes may be identified (128,143). Such structures emphasize the common origin of Schwann cells and melanocytes from the neural crest (6). There are two types of melanotic schwannomas. The conventional type is composed of plump spindle and epithelioid cells arranged in whorls and streaming fascicles containing melanin pigment, and the psammomatous melanotic schwannomas are mainly in autonomic/visceral locations with the same cell arrangement as melanotic schwannomas but with the additional feature of PAS-positive, von Kossa-positive, mineralized laminated calcospherites (129,144). Approximately 50% of patients with psammomatous melanotic schwannomas may have evidence of Carney complex that includes, primary pigmented nodular adrenocortical disease, pituitary-independent, primary adrenal form of hypercortisolism, lentigines, ephelides and blue nevi of the skin and mucosae, and a variety of nonendocrine and endocrine tumors such as myxomas, pituitary adenomas, testicular Sertoli cell tumor, and other benign and malignant neoplasms including tumors of thyroid and ductal adenomas of the breast (126).

Granular cell tumor (GCT) (Abrikossoff tumor) is a benign tumor of somewhat controversial histogenesis. A schwannian origin has been found to be the most accepted

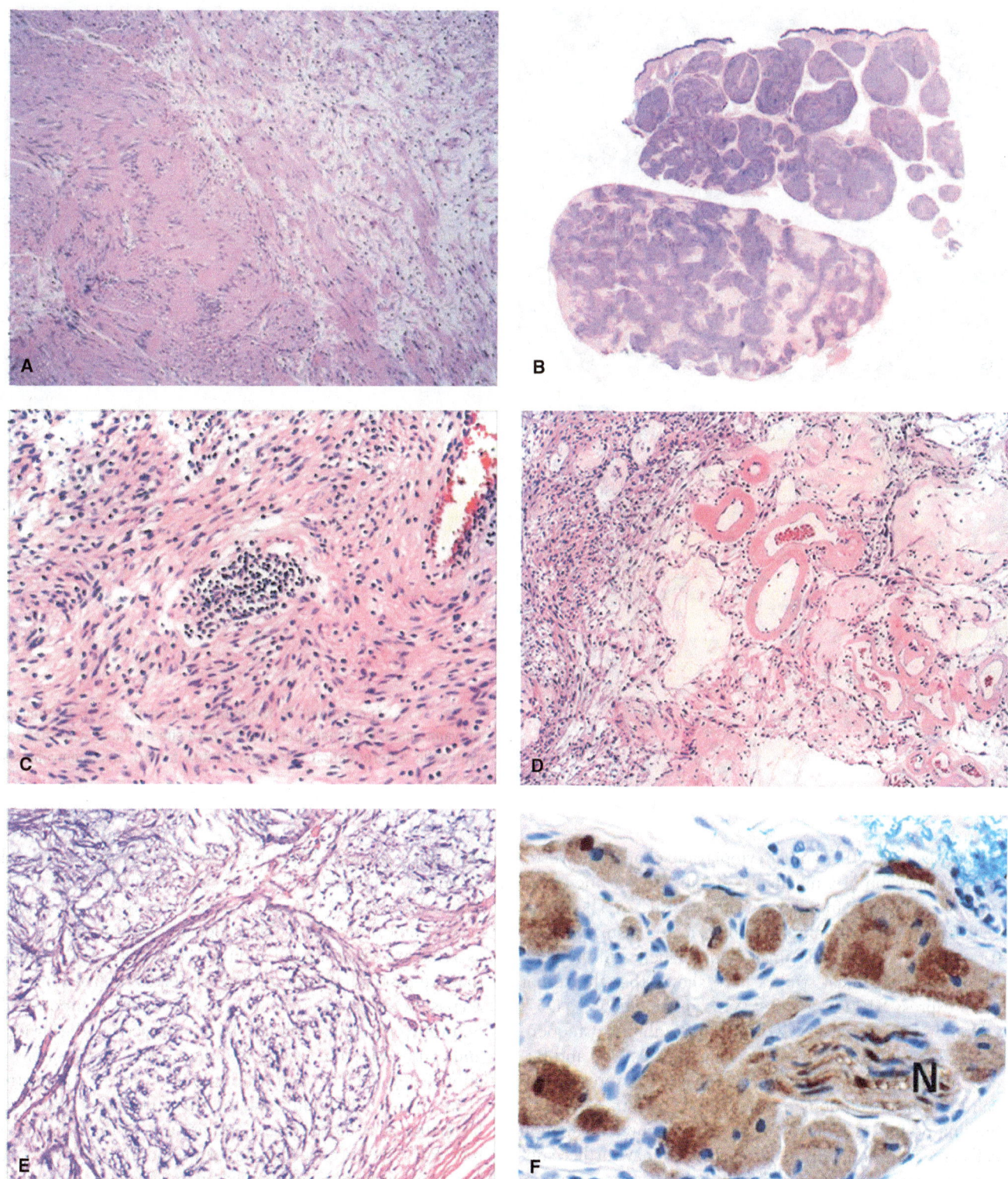

FIGURE 11.17 Panel showing the different morphology that the cell of Schwann may present in schwannomas. **A:** Benign schwannoma, showing the typical biphasic appearance with Verocay bodies. **B:** Plexiform schwannoma. **C:** Cellular schwannoma with uniform fascicular growth pattern. **D:** Ancient schwannoma. **E:** Myxoid schwannoma (nerve sheath myxoma). **F:** Granular cell schwannoma. Note the granular cells are originating from a nerve fascicle (*N*): Anti-S100 protein. (*continued*)

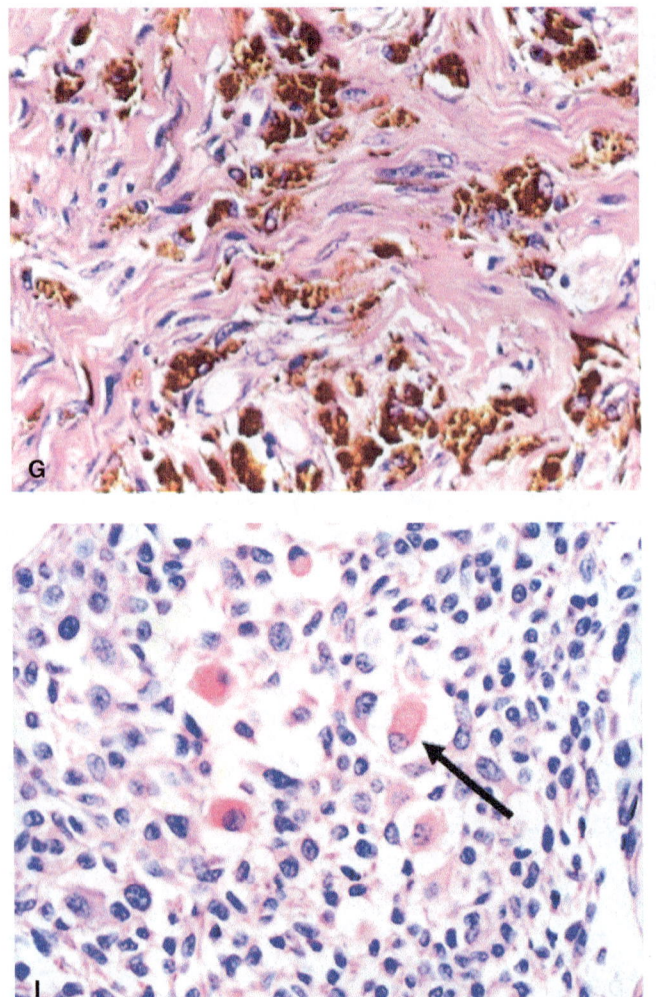
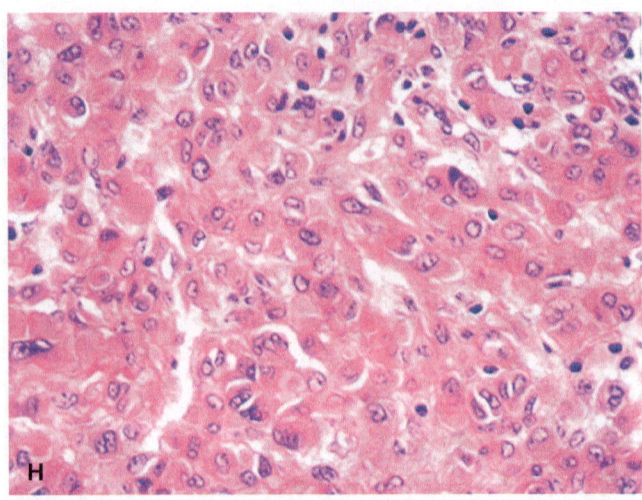

FIGURE 11.17 (*Continued*) **G:** Melanotic schwannoma. **H:** Epithelioid schwannoma. **I:** Malignant peripheral nerve sheath tumor with rhabdomyoblastic differentiation (Malignant triton tumor). Rhabdomyoblasts (*arrow*).

histogenesis (127). Granular cytoplasmic change, however, is the expression of a metabolic alteration occurring often, but not exclusively, in Schwann cells (128,127). The tumor cells have abundant granular cytoplasm and a small eccentric nucleus; they invade small nerve branches in the skin. Immunocytochemical studies have shown that the tumor cells, express S100 protein, SOX10, nestin, CD56, CD57, CD68, Actin-HHF35, NSE, PGP 9.5, α-inhibin, osteopontin, TFE3 and also occasionally express myelin (P0 and P2) and myelin-associated proteins (145,146). Expression of calretinin has been demonstrated in GCT. As this calcium-binding protein is typically expressed in neurons, ganglion cells and Schwann cells, GTC expression may further support a neuronal origin or differentiation of these tumors (147). Interestingly, calretinin positivity may be increased in the pseudoepitheliomatous hyperplasia of the squamous epithelium overlying the tumor cells seen in some cases of GCT that may indicate a role of calretinin in the interaction between GCT cells and hyperplastic epithelium (147).

Neurofibromas are complex benign lesions frequently associated with neurofibromatosis (128,129). As distinct from schwannomas, neurofibromas are diffuse lesions in the skin or around peripheral nerves that invade the peripheral nerve endoneurium and enlarge nerve branches (128,129). They also diffusely invade surrounding tissues and may cause bone destruction. Histologically, neurofibromas are as a rule not encapsulated and they contain a variety of cells that are associated with peripheral nerves; unlike schwannomas, neurofibromas are not predominantly composed of Schwann cells. Mast cells are frequently seen in the stroma and can be identified using toluidine blue or Giemsa or by antitryptase, CD117, and calretinin immunohistochemistry (128). Mast cells induce factor XIIIa–positive extracellular matrix in neurofibromas, and are one of the inflammatory cell types involved in tumor promotion (148,149). It has been hypothesized that when mast cells are lost, as seen in cases of malignant peripheral nerve sheath tumors (MPNSTs), there may be a diminution of the anticancer effect of mast cells in maintaining the benign nature of some of these proliferations (148). By immunocytochemistry, S100, SOX10, PGP 9.5, and CD57-positive Schwann cells can be detected within neurofibromas, in addition to EMA, Glut-1, and claudin-1–positive perineurial cells and CD34 endoneurial fibroblasts (36). Entrapped axons can be seen coursing through neurofibromas in immunocytochemical preparations for neurofilament protein, PGP 9.5 or in silver-stained sections. All of these cell components are set in a variable fibromyxoid stroma that in some cases may be so prominent (the myxoid part) that it may be mistaken for a myxoma or myxoid liposarcoma. Distorted structures resembling Wagner–Meissner or pacinian corpuscles are sometimes seen (pacinian neurofibromas), as well as melanin (pigmented neurofibromas) (128,129).

Neurofibromatosis is an autosomal dominant disease that is part of the group of neurocutaneous disorders, collectively known as phakomatoses (149,150). It presents as two major diseases, peripheral (type I or von Recklinghausen disease; NF1) and central (type II; NF2) (149,150). Both type I and type II are inherited as autosomal dominant traits but many cases are new mutations. Over 90% of cases of neurofibromatosis are type I; a gene defect has been located on the long arm of chromosome 17 (17q11.2) (NF1 gene) and has been linked to the locus encoding NGF (149). There is an increase in NGF in the serum of patients with this disorder (149,150). The NF1 suppressor gene which spans over 350 kb of genomic DNA and contains 60 exons, encodes a ubiquitous protein known as neurofibromin (neurofibromatosis-related protein NF1). This 2818 amino acid protein has been shown to be associated with cytoplasmic microtubules and function as a GTPase, activating Ras proteins (149,150).

A wide variety of disorders occur in patients with NF1, including elephantiasis neuromatosa, in which there are redundant folds of skin associated with plexiform neurofibromas (149,151) and, more commonly, multiple cutaneous neurofibromata. Other tumors such as gliomas, carcinoid tumors, pheochromocytomas, neuroblastomas, gastrointestinal stromal tumors, Wilms tumors, and pigmented hamartomas of the iris (Lisch nodules), are also seen in patients with this disorder (149,152).

Central or type II neurofibromatosis (NF2) is much less common than NF1 and is characterized by bilateral vestibular schwannomas; skin lesions are uncommon (152). Approximately 40% of the vestibular schwannomas in NF2 tend to have a lobular "grape-like" pattern, while this arrangement is extremely uncommon in sporadic schwannomas (149,153). A proportion of these patients have multiple tumors, including meningiomas, intramedullary spinal ependymomas and glial microhamartomas of the cerebral cortex (152). A gene deletion on chromosome 22q12 (NF2 gene) was identified in 1993 in patients with this disorder, and it is associated with abnormalities of glial growth factor and NGF activity (149,153). The NF2 gene spans 110 kb and encodes a membrane–cytoskeleton linking protein, member of the protein 4.1 family, known as merlin (for moesin–ezrin–radixin-like protein). Merlin, also known as schwannomin or neurofibromin 2, may be detected by immunohistochemistry in the cytoplasm of many cells including Schwann cells. Merlin is a tumor suppressor that exerts its function via inhibiting mitogenic receptors at the plasma membrane. The loss of function of this gene is a fundamental event in the genesis of schwannomas (154,155). Normal Schwann cells express merlin that is known to play a crucial role in cytoskeleton-associated events. It has been proposed that the mutation of NF2 may cause tumor formation through disruption of cell shape, cell matrix and cell–cell communication or signaling functions, attributed to actin cytoskeleton–plasma membrane interaction (155,156). Although multiple mutations in merlin have been identified in NF2, its molecular mechanism is not fully understood. It has been shown that merlin interacts with LRP6 and inhibits LRP6 phosphorylation, a critical step for the initiation of Wnt signaling (155). Sporadic schwannomas from non-NF2 individuals also have NF2 mutations (128,129).

Interesting nerve sheath tumors showing features of both schwannoma and neurofibromas, schwannoma and perineurioma, and neurofibroma and perineurioma (hybrid peripheral nerve tumors) have been described (157,158).

Neuronal tumors such as ganglioneuromas occur in association with autonomic ganglia in the peripheral nervous system (159). Histologically, neurons can be identified within these tumors; axons and Schwann cells may be identified by immunocytochemistry. Electron microscopy reveals the presence of 100-nm dense-core vesicles resembling catecholamine granules in the neurons. In addition to well-differentiated ganglioneuromas, primitive neuroectodermal tumors such as neuroblastoma and ganglioneuroblastomas arise within the abdomen and thorax (159). Cell types within the more primitive tumors may be difficult to identify by immunocytochemistry but electron microscopy usually reveals the presence of 100-nm dense-core catecholamine vesicles within the tumor cell cytoplasm (159).

Schwannomatosis (sometimes called neurofibromatosis type III) is a recently recognized distinct form of NF characterized by multiple (usually painful) nonvestibular schwannomas with no known constitutional NF2 mutations. Some investigators have reported that both familial and sporadic schwannomatosis may harbor mutations in the SAMRCB1 gene that regulates cell cycle, growth, and differentiation (149,160).

MPNSTs (128,161) (malignant schwannomas) are derived from specialized cells of the endoneurium and perineurium and show great histologic variation and many similarities to other soft tissue tumors (162). The term MPNST incorporates previously used terms such as neurofibrosarcoma and malignant schwannoma. Mutation in the NF1 tumor suppressor gene is the most important molecular genetic event in the development of MPNST (163,164). Malignant change in a benign schwannoma is an extremely rare event, however two forms of neurofibroma: plexiform and localized intraneural neurofibroma, are significant precursors of MPNST (161,163). Immunocytochemistry has demonstrated S100, SOX10, EMA, Glut-1, PGP 9.5 and CD56-positive cells in MPNST and occasional tumors that are EMA/Glut-1 positive and S100 protein negative have been described as MPNST with perineurial cell differentiation (161). This suggests that cells of MPNST may produce proteins characteristic of perineurial cells or of both perineurium and Schwann cells. Heterogeneity is common and so histologic sampling should include wide areas of tumor (161). Unusual elements may be encountered occasionally such as cartilages, bones, squamous elements, and muscles. MPNST may also present with malignant glands (glandular malignant schwannoma) or rhabdomyosarcoma, features that may be highlighted by immunocytochemistry for cytokeratins and desmin, respectively. In an attempt to explain the occurrence of malignant muscle differentiation (rhabdomyosarcoma) in malignant Schwannomas, Pierre Masson suggested that endoneurial cells might differentiate into muscle cells under the inductive influence of nerve cells, a situation that was thought to be operative in regenerating limbs in triton salamanders, hence the name "triton tumor" (Malignant schwannoma with rhabdomyoblastic differentiation) (161,162).

ACKNOWLEDGMENTS

We thank the staff of the Neuropathology and Cell Pathology laboratories and the Imaging Unit for Southampton University Hospitals NHS Trust, Southampton, England for their generous and expert cooperation. Special thanks are due to Margaret Harris who typed the original manuscript, to Dr. Sergio Piña-Oviedo who drew the diagrams, and to Dr. Javier Baquera-Heredia who supplied Figure 11.17F.

REFERENCES

1. Dupin E, Le Douarin NM. The neural crest, a multifaceted structure of the vertebrates. *Birth Defects Res C Embryo Today* 2014;102(3):187–209.
2. Petersen J, Adameyko I. Nerve-associated neural crest: Peripheral glial cells generate multiple fates in the body. *Curr Opin Genet Dev* 2017;45:10–14.
3. Kidd GJ, Ohno N, Trapp BD. Biology of Schwann cells. *Handb Clin Neurol* 2013;115:55–79.
4. Castelnovo LF, Bonalume V, Melfi S, et al. Schwann cell development, maturation and regeneration: A focus on classic and emerging intracellular signaling pathways. *Neural Regen Res* 2017;12(7):1013–1023.
5. Karamchandani JR, Nielsen TO, van de Rijn M, et al. Sox10 and S100 in the diagnosis of soft-tissue neoplasms. *Appl Immunohistochem Mol Morphol* 2012;20(5):445–450.
6. Graham A. Melanocyte production: Dark side of the Schwann cell. *Curr Biol* 2009;19(24):R116–R117.
7. Monk KR, Feltri ML, Taveggia C. New insights on Schwann cell development. *Glia* 2015;63(8):1376–1393.
8. Skaper SD. Nerve growth factor: A neuroimmune crosstalk mediator for all seasons. *Immunology* 2017;151(1):1–15.
9. Önger ME, Delibaş B, Türkmen AP, et al. The role of growth factors in nerve regeneration. *Drug Discov Ther* 2017;10(6):285–291.
10. Giger RJ, Hollis ER 2nd, Tuszynski MH. Guidance molecules in axon regeneration. *Cold Spring Harb Perspect Biol* 2010;2(7):a001867.
11. Madduri S, Gander B. Schwann cell delivery of neurotrophic factors for peripheral nerve regeneration. *J Peripher Nerv Syst* 2010;15(2):93–103.
12. Masu M. Proteoglycans and axon guidance: A new relationship between old partners. *J Neurochem* 2016;139(Suppl 2):58–75.
13. Taveggia C. Schwann cells-axon interaction in myelination. *Curr Opin Neurobiol* 2016;39:24–29.
14. Quintes S, Goebbels S, Saher G, et al. Neuron-glia signaling and the protection of axon function by Schwann cells. *J Peripher Nerv Syst* 2010;15(1):10–16.
15. Eid EM, Hegazy AM. Anatomical variations of the human sural nerve and its role in clinical and surgical procedures. *Clin Anat* 2011;24(2):237–245.
16. Thomas PK, Ochoa J. Microscopic anatomy of peripheral nerve fibers. In: Dyck PJ, Thomas PK, Lambert EH, et al, eds. *Peripheral Neuropathy. Vol I*. 2nd ed. Philadelphia, PA: Saunders; 1984:34–96.
17. Herbert AL, Monk KR. Advances in myelinating glial cell development. *Curr Opin Neurobiol* 2017;42:53–60.
18. Xiao J, Kilpatrick TJ, Murray SS. The role of neurotrophins in the regulation of myelin development. *Neurosignals* 2009;17(4):265–276.
19. Nave KA. Myelination and the trophic support of long axons. *Nat Rev Neurosci* 2010;11(4):275–283.
20. Han H, Myllykoski M, Ruskamo S, et al. Myelin-specific proteins: A structurally diverse group of membrane-interacting molecules. *Biofactors* 2013;39(3):233–241.
21. King R. Microscopic anatomy: Normal structure. *Handb Clin Neurol* 2013;115:7–27.
22. Alfieri A, Fleischhammer J, Strauss C, et al. The central myelin-peripheral myelin transitional zone of the nervus intermedius and its implications for microsurgery in the cerebellopontine angle. *Clin Anat* 2012;25(7):882–888.
23. Streit A. *The Cranial Sensory Nervous System: Specification of Sensory Progenitors and Placodes. In: Stem Book [Internet].* Cambridge, MA:Harvard Stem Cell Institute; 2008:1–20.
24. Tassler PL, Dellon AL, Canoun C. Identification of elastic fibers in the peripheral nerve. *J Hand Surg Br* 1994;19(1):48–54.
25. Cavanagh JG. Pathology of peripheral nerve diseases. In: Weller RO, ed. *Systemic Pathology: Nervous System Muscle and Eyes. Vol 4*. 3rd ed. Edinburgh:Churchill Livingstone; 1990:544–578.
26. Shekhani HN, Hanna T, Johnson JO. Lipofibromatous hamartoma of the median nerve: A case report. *J Radiol Case Rep* 2016;10(11):1–7.
27. Estebe JP, Atchabahian A. The nerve: A fragile balance between physiology and pathophysiology. *Eur J Anaesthesiol* 2017;34(3):118–126.
28. Piña-Oviedo S, Ortiz-Hidalgo C. The normal and neoplastic perineurium: A review. *Adv Anat Pathol* 2008;15(3):147–164.
29. Küspert M, Weider M, Müller J, et al. Desert hedgehog links transcription factor Sox10 to perineurial development. *J Neurosci* 2012;32(16):5472–5480.

30. Zimmerman A, Bai1 L, Ginty DD. The gentle touch receptors of mammalian skin. *Science* 2014;346(6212):950–954.
31. Goehler LE, Relton JK, Dripps D, et al. Vagal paraganglia bind biotinylated interleukin-1 receptor antagonist: A possible mechanism for immune-to-brain communication. *Brain Res Bull* 1997;43(3):357–364.
32. Folpe AL, Billings SD, McKenney JK, et al. Expression of claudin-1, a recently described tight junction-associated protein, distinguishes soft tissue perineurioma from potential mimics. *Am J Surg Pathol* 2002;26(12):1620–1626.
33. Katona I, Weis J. Diseases of the peripheral nerves. *Handb Clin Neurol* 2017;145:453–474.
34. Ahmed AM, Weller RO. The blood–nerve barrier and reconstitution of the perineurium following nerve grafting. *Neuropathol Appl Neurobiol* 1979;5(6):469–483.
35. Ortiz Hidalgo C, Weller RO. Traumatic and compressive lesions of peripheral nerves. In: Vallat J-M, Weis J, eds. *Peripheral Nerve Disorders. Pathology and Genetics.* UK: ISNP Wiley Blackwell; 2014:244–308.
36. MacKeever PE. Immunohistochemistry of the nervous system. In: Dabbs DJ, ed. *Diagnostic Immunohistochemistry.* 4th ed. Elsevier; 2014:762–828.
37. Piña AR, Martínez MM, de Almeida OP. Glut-1, best immunohistochemical marker for perineurial cells. *Head Neck Pathol* 2015;9(1):104–106.
38. Macarenco RS, Ellinger F, Oliveira AM. Perineurioma: A distinctive and under recognized peripheral nerve sheath neoplasm. *Arch Pathol Lab Med* 2007;131(4):625–636.
39. Tsai CY, Yeh CJ, Chao YK, et al. Perineural invasion through the sheath in posttherapy esophagectomy specimens predicts poor survival in patients with esophageal squamous cell carcinoma. *Eur J Surg Oncol* 2017;43(10):1970–1976.
40. Fogt F, Capodieci P, Loda M. Assessment of perineural invasion by Glut-1 immunohistochemistry. *Appl Immunohistochem* 1995;3:194–197.
41. Ronaghy A, Yaar R, Goldberg LJ, et al. Perineurial involvement: What does it mean? *Am J Dermatopathol* 2010;32(5):469–476.
42. Richard L, Topilko P, Magy L, et al. Endoneurial fibroblast-like cells. *J Neuropathol Exp Neurol* 2012;71(11):938–947.
43. Hirose T, Tani T, Shimada T, et al. Immunohistochemical demonstration of EMA/Glut1-positive perineurial cells and CD34-positive fibroblastic cells in peripheral nerve sheath tumors. *Mod Pathol* 2003;16(4):293–298.
44. Müller M, Leonhard C, Krauthausen M, et al. On the longevity of resident endoneurial macrophages in the peripheral nervous system: A study of physiological macrophage turnover in bone marrow chimeric mice. *J Peripher Nerv Syst* 2010;15(4):357–365.
45. King R, Ginsberg L. The nerve biopsy: Indications, technical aspects, and contribution. *Handb Clin Neurol* 2013;115:155–170.
46. Chen S, Burgin S, McDaniel A, et al. Nf1-/- Schwann cell-conditioned medium modulates mast cell degranulation by c-Kit-mediated hyperactivation of phosphatidylinositol 3-kinase. *Am J Pathol* 2010;177(6):3125–3132.
47. Staser K, Yang FC, Clapp DW. Mast cells and the neurofibroma microenvironment. *Blood* 2010;116(2):157–164.
48. Esposito B, De Santis A, Monteforte R, et al. Mast cells in Wallerian degeneration: Morphologic and ultrastructural changes. *J Comp Neurol* 2002;445(3):199–210.
49. Harris GM, Madigan NN, Lancaster KZ, et al. Nerve guidance by a decellularized fibroblast extracellular matrix. *Matrix Biol* 2017;60-61:176–189.
50. Kazamel M, Boes CJ. Renaut corpuscles or peripheral nerve infarcts? A historical overview. *Can J Neurol Sci.* 2017;44(2):184–189.
51. Piña-Oviedo S, Del Valle L, Baquera-Heredia J, et al. Imunohistochemical characterization of Renaut bodies in superficial digital nerves: Further evidence supporting their perineurial cell origin. *J Peripher Nerv Syst* 2009;14(1):22–26.
52. Collins MP, Dyck JB. Vasculitides. In: Vallat J-M, Weis J, eds. *Peripheral Nerve Disorders. Pathology and Genetics.* UK: ISNP Wiley Blackwell; 2014:175–209.
53. Lindemuth R, Ernzerhof C, Schimrigk K. Comparative morphometry of myelinated nerve fibers in the normal and pathologically altered human sural and tibial nerve. *Clin Neuropathol* 2002;21(1):29–34.
54. Yuan A, Rao MV, Veeranna et al. Neurofilaments and neurofilament proteins in health and disease. *Cold Spring Harb Perspect Biol* 2017;9(4). pii:a018309.
55. Fainikar A, Bass PW. Critical roles for microtubules in axonal development and disease. *Results Probl Cell Differ* 2009;48:47–64.
56. Tasdemir-Yilmaz OE, Segal RA. There and back again: Coordinated transcription, translation and transport in axonal survival and regeneration. *Curr Opin Neurobiol.* 2016;39:62–68.
57. Salinas S, Schlavo G, Kremer EJ. A hitchhiker's guide to the nervous system: The complex journey of viruses and toxins. *Nat Rev Microbiol* 2010;8(9):645–655.
58. Peters A. The effects of normal aging on myelin and nerve fibers: A review. *J Neurocytol* 2002;31(8–9):581–593.
59. Terada S. Where does slow axonal transport go? *Neurosci Res* 2003;47(4):367–372.
60. Cavanagh JB. Toxic and deficiency disorders. In Weller RO Ed. *Systemic Pathology: Nervous System, Muscle and Eye.* Vol. 3 3rd ed. Edinburgh:Churchill Livingstone; 1990:244–308.
61. Katalymov LL, Glukhova NV. Some characteristics of periaxonal space in myelinated nerve fibers. *Dokl Biol Sci* 2003;388:9–11.
62. Nave KA, Trapp BD. Axon-glial signaling and the glial support of axon function. *Annu Rev Neurosci* 2008;31:535–561.
63. Armati PJ, Mathey EK. An update on Schwann cell biology—immunomodulation, neural regulation and other surprises. *J Neurol Sci* 2013;333(1–2):68–72.
64. Woodhoo A, Sommers L. Development of the Schwann cell lineage: From the neural crest to the myelinated nerve. *Glia* 2008;56(14):1481–1490.
65. Weller RO, Herzog I. Schwann cell lysosomes in hypertrophic neuropathy and in normal human nerves. *Brain* 1970;93(2):347–356.
66. González-Martínez T, Pérez-Piñera P, Díaz-Esnal B, et al. S-100 proteins in the human peripheral nervous system. *Microsc Res Tech* 2003;60(6):633–638.
67. Fine SW, McCline SA, Li M. Immunohistochemical staining for calretinin is useful for differentiating schwannomas from neurofibromas. *Am J Clin Pathol* 2004;122(4):552–559.
68. Schwannomas. Avaialable from https://app.immunoquery.com/view/panel/dx?dxgroups=770&sensitivity=1&minrefs=gt1&paneltype=comprehensive. Accessed December 2017.

69. Koirala S, Reddy LV, Ko CP. Roles of glia cell in the formation, function and maintenance of the neuromuscular junction. *J Neurocytol* 2002;32(5–8):987–1002.
70. Oda R, Yaoi T, Okajima S, et al. A novel marker for terminal Schwann cells, homocysteine-responsive ER-resident protein, as isolated by a single cell PCR-differential display. *Biochem Biophys Res Commun* 2003;308(4):872–877.
71. Wewetzer K, Verdú E, Agelov DN, et al. Olfactory ensheathing glia and Schwann cells: Two of a kind? *Cell Tissue Res* 2002; 309(3):337–345.
72. Snaidero N, Simons M. Myelination at a glance. *J Cell Sci* 2014;127(Pt 14):2999–3004.
73. Salzer JL. Schwann cell myelination. *Cold Spring Harb Perspect Biol* 2015;7(8):a020529.
74. Pereira JA, Lebrun-Julien F, Suter U. Molecular mechanisms regulating myelination in the peripheral nervous system. *Trends Neurosci* 2012;35(2):123–134.
75. Nave KA, Werner HB. Myelination of the nervous system: Mechanisms and functions. *Annu Rev Cell Dev Biol* 2014;30: 503–533.
76. Garbay B, Heape AM, Sargueil F, et al. Myelin synthesis in the peripheral nervous system. *Prog Neurobiol* 2000;61(3): 267–304.
77. Simons M, Trotter J. Wrapping it up: The cell biology of myelination. *Curr Opin Neurobiol* 2007;17(5):533–540.
78. Stojkovic T. Hereditary neuropathies: An update. *Rev Neurol (Paris)* 2016;172(12):775–778.
79. Weis J, Senderek J. Introduction to the hereditary neuropathies. In: Vallat J-M, Weis J, eds. *Peripheral Nerve Disorders. Pathology and Genetics*. UK: ISNP Wiley Blackwell; 2014:59–61.
80. Werner HB. On the evolution of myelin. *Brain Res* 2016; 1641(Pt A):1–3.
81. Podratz JL, Rodriguez E, Windebank AJ. Role of the extracellular matrix in myelination of peripheral nerve. *Glia* 2001; 35(1):35–40.
82. Quarles RH. Myelin-associated glycoprotein (MAG): Past, present and beyond. *J Neurochem* 2007;100(6):1431–1448.
83. Yang Y, Shi Y. L-periaxin interacts with S-periaxin through its PDZ domain. *Neurosci Lett* 2015;609:23–29.
84. Schroeder JM, Weis J. Basic pathology of the peripheral nervous system. In: Vallat J-M, Weis J, eds. *Peripheral Nerve Disorders. Pathology and Genetics*. ISNP Wiley Blackwell; 2014:38–58.
85. Sherman DL, Wu LM, Grove M, et al. Drp2 and periaxin form Cajal bands with dystroglycan but have distinct roles in Schwann cell growth. *J Neurosci* 2012;32(27):9419–9428.
86. Rasband MN, Peles E. The nodes of Ranvier: Molecular assembly and maintenance. *Cold Spring Harb Perspect Biol* 2015;8(3):a020495.
87. Carroll SL. The molecular and morphologic structures that make saltatory conduction possible in peripheral nerve. *J Neuropathol Exp Neurol* 2017;76(4):255–257.
88. Thaxton C, Bhat M. Myelination and regional domain differentiation of the axon. *Results Probl Cell Differ* 2009;48: 1–28.
89. Alanne MH, Pummi K, Heape AM, et al. Tight junction proteins in human Schwann cell autotypic junctions. *J Histochem Cytochem* 2009;57(6):523–529.
90. Nelson AD, Jenkins PM. Axonal membranes and their domains: Assembly and function of the axon initial segment and node of Ranvier. *Front Cell Neurosci* 2017;11:136.
91. Friede RL. The significance of internode length for saltatory conduction: Looking back at the age of 90. *J Neuropathol Exp Neurol* 2017;76(4):258–259.
92. Weller RO, Cervos Navarro J. *Pathology of Peripheral Nerves: A Practical Approach*. London:Butterworth; 1977.
93. Yang Z, Wang KK. Glial fibrillary acidic protein: From intermediate filament assembly and gliosis to neurobiomarker. *Trends Neurosci* 2015;38(6):364–374.
94. Scollard DM, Truman RW, Ebenezer GJ. Mechanisms of nerve injury in leprosy. *Clin Dermatol* 2015;33(1):46–54.
95. Auböck L, Ratzenhofer M. "Extraepithelial enterochromaffin cell–nerve-fibre complexes" in the normal human appendix, and in neurogenic appendicopathy. *J Pathol* 1982;136(3): 217–226.
96. Schmidt HG, Schmid A, Domschke W. Nerve-neuroendocrine complexes in stomach mucosa in Zollinger–Ellison syndrome. *Pathologe* 1995;16(6):404–407.
97. Ruiz J, Ríos A, Oviedo MI, et al. Neurogenic appendicopathy. A report of 8 cases. *Rev Esp Enferm Dig* 2017;109(3):180–184.
98. Kieseier BC, Hu W, Hurtung H-P. Schwann cells as immunomodulatory cells. In: Armati PK, ed. *The Biolelgy of Schwan cells: Development, Differentiation and Immunomodulation*. New York: Cambridge University Press; 2007:118–125.
99. Bonetti B, Valdo P, Ossi G, et al. T-cell cytotoxicity of human Schwann cells: TNFalpha promotes fasL-mediated apoptosis and IFN gamma perforin-mediated lysis. *Glia* 2003;43(2): 141–418.
100. Petrov KA, Girard E, Nikitashina AD, et al. Schwann cells sense and control acetylcholine spillover at the neuromuscular junction by α7 nicotinic receptors and butyrylcholinesterase. *J Neurosci* 2014;34(36):11870–11183.
101. Vedeler C, Ulvestad E, Borge L, et al. Expression of CD-59 in normal human nervous tissue. *Immunology* 1994;82(4): 542–547.
102. Wijdicks EF, Klein CJ. Guillain–Barré Syndrome. *Mayo Clin Proc* 2017;92(3):467–479.
103. Brandner S. The pathological diagnosis of nerve biopsies. A practical approach. *Diagn Histopathol* 2016;22(9):333–344.
104. Bouche P. Clinical assessment and classification of peripheral nerve diseases. In: Vallat J-M, Weis J, eds. *Peripheral Nerve Disorders. Pathology and Genetics*. UK: ISNP Wiley Blackwell; 2014:1–11.
105. Geuna S, Raimondo S, Ronchi G, et al. Chapter 3: Histology of the peripheral nerve and changes occurring during nerve regeneration. *Int Rev Neurobiol* 2009;87:27–46.
106. García Segura LM. Ramón y Cajal y la neurociencia del siglo XXI. *Jano Extra* 2005;1:16–22.
107. Conforti L, Gilley J, Coleman MP. Wallerian degeneration: An emerging axon death pathway linking injury and disease. *Nat Rev Neurosci* 2014;15(6):394–409.
108. Gámez-Sánchez JA, Carty L, Iruarrizaga-Lejarreta M, et al. Schwann cell autophagy, myelinophagy, initiates myelin clearance from injured nerves. *J Cell Biol* 2015;210(1):153–168.
109. Thumm M, Simons M. Myelinophagy: Schwann cells dine in. *J Cell Biol* 2015;210(1):9–10.
110. Burnett MG, Zager EL. Pathophysiology of peripheral nerve injury: A brief review. *Neurosurg Focus* 2004;16(5):E1.
111. Carr MJ, Johnston AP. Schwann cells as drivers of tissue repair and regeneration. *Curr Opin Neurobiol* 2017;47:52–57.
112. Blesch A, Tuszynski MH. Nucleus hears axon's pain. *Nat Med* 2004;10(3):236–237.

113. Wong KM, Babetto E, Beirowski B. Axon degeneration: Make the Schwann cell great again. *Neural Regen Res* 2017; 12(4):518–524.
114. Panayotis N, Karpova A, Kreutz MR, et al. Macromolecular transport in synapse to nucleus communication. *Trends Neurosci* 2015;38(2):108–116.
115. Holahan MR. A shift from a pivotal to supporting role for the growth-associated protein (GAP-43) in the coordination of axonal structural and functional plasticity. *Front Cell Neurosci.* 2017;11:266.
116. Jessen KR, Mirsky R. The repair Schwann cell and its function in regenerating nerves. *J Physiol* 2016;594(13):3521–3531.
117. Chernousov MA, Yu WM, Chen ZL, et al. Regulation of Schwann cell function by the extracellular matrix. *Glia* 2008; 56(14):1498–1507.
118. Dyck PJ, Dyck PJB, Giannini C, et al. Peripheral nerves. In: Graham DI, Lantos PL, eds. *Greenfield's Neuropathology*. London: Arnold; 2002:551–675.
119. Antonescu CR, Scheithauer BW, Woodruff JM. Reactive lesions. Atlas of Tumor Pathology Series 4. In: *Tumors of Peripheral Nervous System*. American Registry of Pathology (AFIP); 2013:53–57.
120. Brandner S. Toxic Neuropathies. In: Vallat J-M, Weis J, eds. *Peripheral Nerve Disorders. Pathology and Genetics*. UK: ISNP Wiley Blackwell; 2014:238–246.
121. Weller RO, Bruckner FE, Chamberlain MA. Rheumatoid neuropathy: A histological and electrophysiological study. *J Neurol Neurosurg Psychiatry* 1970;33(5):592–604.
122. Stecco C, Fantoni I, Macchi V, et al. The role of fasciae in Civinini–Morton's syndrome. *J Anat* 2015;227(5):654–664.
123. Beer TW. Reparative perineurial hyperplasia: A series of 10 cases. *Am J Dermatopathol* 2009;31(1):50–52.
124. Jokinen CH, Ragsadele BD, Argenyi ZB. Expanding the clinicopathologic spectrum of palisaded encapsulated neuroma. *J Cutan Pathol* 2010;37(1):43–48.
125. Pytel P, Karrison T, Gong C, et al. Neoplasms with Schwannian differentiation express transcriptional factors known to regulate normal Schwann cell development. *Int J Surg Pathol* 2010;18(6):449–457.
126. Stratakis CA. Carney complex: A familial lentiginosis predisposing to a variety of tumors. *Rev Endocr Metab Disord* 2016;17(3):367–371.
127. Rekhi B, Jambhekar NA. Morphologic spectrum, immunohistochemical analysis, and clinical features of a series of granular cell tumors of soft tissues: A study from a tertiary referral cancer center. *Ann Diagn Pathol* 2010;14(3):162–167.
128. De Luca-Johnson J. Peripheral nerve sheath tumors: An update and review of diagnostic challenges. *Diagn Histopathol* 2016;22(11):447–457.
129. Rodriguez FJ, Folpe AL, Giannini C, et al. Pathology of peripheral nerve sheath tumors: Diagnostic overview and update on selected diagnostic problems. *Acta Neuropathol* 2012;123(3):295–319.
130. Canales-Ibarra C, Magariños G, Olsoff-Pagovich P, et al. Cutaneous sclerosing perineurioma of the digits: An uncommon soft tissue neoplasm. Report of a case with immunohistochemical analysis. *J Cutan Pathol* 2003;30(9):577–581.
131. Toussaint-Caire S, Aguilar-Donis A, Torres-Guerrero E, et al. Sclerosing acral skin perineurioma: Clinicopathologic study of ten cases (eight classical and two with xanthomatous changes). *Gac Med Mex* 2015;151(3):299–305.
132. Al-Daraji WI. Granular perineurioma: The first report of a rare distinct subtype of perineurioma. *Am J Dermatopathol* 2008;30(2):163–168.
133. Mitchell A, Scheithauer BW, Doyon J, et al. Malignant perineurioma (malignant peripheral nerve sheath tumor with perineural differentiation). *Clin Neuropathol* 2012;31(6): 424–429.
134. Nascimento AF, Fletcher CD. The controversial nosology of benign nerve sheath tumors: Neurofilament protein staining demonstrates intratumoral axons in many sporadic schwannomas. *Am J Surg Pathol* 2007;31(9):1363–1370.
135. Thaxton C, Lopera J, Bott M, et al. Neuregulin and laminin stimulate phosphorylation of the NF2 tumor suppressor in Schwann cells by distinct protein kinase A and p21-activated kinase-dependent pathways. *Oncogene* 2008;27(19):2705–2715.
136. Wippold FJ 2nd, Lubner M, Perrin RJ, et al. Neuropathology for the neuroradiologist: Antoni A and Antoni B tissue patterns. *AJNR Am J Neuroradiol* 2007;28(9):1633–1638.
137. Laskin WB, Fetsch JF, Lasota J, et al. Benign epithelioid peripheral nerve sheath tumors of the soft tissues. Clinicopathologic spectrum of 33 cases. *Am J Surg Pathol* 2005; 29(1):39–51.
138. Fetsch JF, Laskin WB, Hallman JR, et al. Neurothekeoma: An analysis of 178 tumors with detailed immunohistochemical data and long-term patient follow-up information. *Am J Surg Pathol* 2007;31(7):1103–1114.
139. Kaur K, Kakkar A, Binyaram, et al. Neuroblastoma-like schwannoma of the skull base: An enigmatic peripheral nerve sheath tumor variant. *Neuropathology* 2016;36(6):573–578.
140. Ortiz-Hidalgo C. José Verocay. Verocay neurinomas and bodies and other contributions to medicine. *Rev Neurol* 2004; 39(5):487–491.
141. Dingemans KP, Teeling P. Long-spacing collagen and proteoglycans in pathologic tissue. *Ultrastruct Pathol* 1994;18(6): 539–547.
142. Yen SH, Fields KL. A protein related to glial filaments in Schwann cells. *Ann N Y Acad Sci* 1985;455:538–551.
143. Mahmood UB, Khan FW, Fatima B, et al. Primary melanotic schwannoma with typical histology. *J Coll Physicians Surg Pak* 2016;26(8):707–709.
144. Merat R, Szalay-Quinodoz I, Laffitte E, et al. Psammomatous melanotic schwannoma: A challenging histological diagnosis. *Dermatopathology (Basel)* 2015;2(3):67–70.
145. Hoshi N, Sugino T, Suzuki T. Regular expression of osteopontin in granular cell tumor; distinct feature among Schwannian cell tumors. *Pathol Int* 2005;55(8):484–490.
146. Schoolmeester JK, Lastra RR. Granular cell tumors overexpress TFE3 without corollary gene rearrangement. *Hum Pathol* 2015;46(8):1242–1243.
147. Fine SW, Li M. Expression of calretinin and the alpha-subunit of inhibin in granular cell tumors. *Am J Clin Pathol* 2003;119(2):259–264.
148. Friedrich RE, Naber U, Glatzel M, et al. Vessel and mast cell densities in sporadic and syndrome-associated peripheral nerve sheath tumors. *Anticancer Res* 2015;35(9):4713–4722.
149. Kresak JL, Walsh M. Neurofibromatosis: A Review of NF1, NF2, and Schwannomatosis. *J Pediatr Genet* 2016;5(2): 98–104.
150. Gutmann DH, Ferner RE, Listernick RH, et al. Neurofibromatosis type 1. *Nat Rev Dis Primers* 2017;3:17004.

151. Ruggieri M, Praticò AD, Serra A, et al. Childhood neurofibromatosis type 2 (NF2) and related disorders: From bench to bedside and biologically targeted therapies. *Acta Otorhinolaryngol Ital* 2016;36(5):345–367.
152. Karajannis MA, Ferner RE. Neurofibromatosis-related tumors: Emerging biology and therapies. *Curr Opin Pediatr* 2015;27(1):26–33.
153. Neff B, Welling DB, Akhmametyeva E. The molecular biology of vestibular Schwannomas: Dissecting the pathogenic process at molecular level. *Otol Neurotol* 2006;27(2):197–208.
154. Hilton DA, Hanemann CO. Schwannomas and their pathogenesis. *Brain Pathol* 2014;24(3):205–220.
155. Kim S, Jho EH. Merlin, a regulator of Hippo signaling, regulates Wnt/β-catenin signaling. *BMB Rep* 2016;49(7):357–358.
156. Ahmad Z, Brown CM, Patel AK, et al. Merlin knockdown in human Schwann cells: Clues to vestibular Schwannoma tumorigenesis. *Otol Neurotol* 2010;31(3):460–466.
157. Michal M, Kazakov DV, Michal M. Hybrid peripheral nerve sheath tumors: A review. *Cesk Patol* 2017;53(2):81–88.
158. Ud Din N, Ahmad Z, Abdul-Ghafar J, et al. Hybrid peripheral nerve sheath tumors: Report of five cases and detailed review of literature. *BMC Cancer* 2017;17(1):349.
159. Antonescu CR, Scheithauer BW, Woodruff JM. Ganglioneuroma. Atlas of Tumor Pathology Series 4. In: *Tumors of Peripheral Nervous System*. American Registry of Pathology (AFIP); 2013:319–340.
160. Kehrer-Sawatzki H, Farschtschi S, Mautner VF, et al. The molecular pathogenesis of schwannomatosis, a paradigm for the co-involvement of multiple tumour suppressor genes in tumorigenesis. *Hum Genet* 2017;136(2):129–148.
161. Le Guellec S, Decouvelaere AV, Filleron T, et al. Malignant peripheral nerve sheath tumor is a challenging diagnosis: A systematic pathology review, immunohistochemistry, and molecular analysis in 160 patients from the French sarcoma group database. *Am J Surg Pathol* 2016;40(7):896–908.
162. Thway K, Hamarneh W, Miah AB, et al. Malignant peripheral nerve sheath tumor with rhabdomyosarcomatous and glandular elements: Rare epithelial differentiation in a triton tumor. *Int J Surg Pathol* 2015;23(5):377–383.
163. Kerezoudis P, Bydon M, Spinner RJ. Peripheral nerve sheath tumors: The "Orphan Disease" of national databases. *World Neurosurg* 2017;103:948–949.
164. Katz D, Lazar A, Lev D. Malignant peripheral nerve sheath tumor (MPNST): The clinical implications of cellular signaling pathways. *Expert Rev Mol Med* 2009;11:e30.

SECTION V

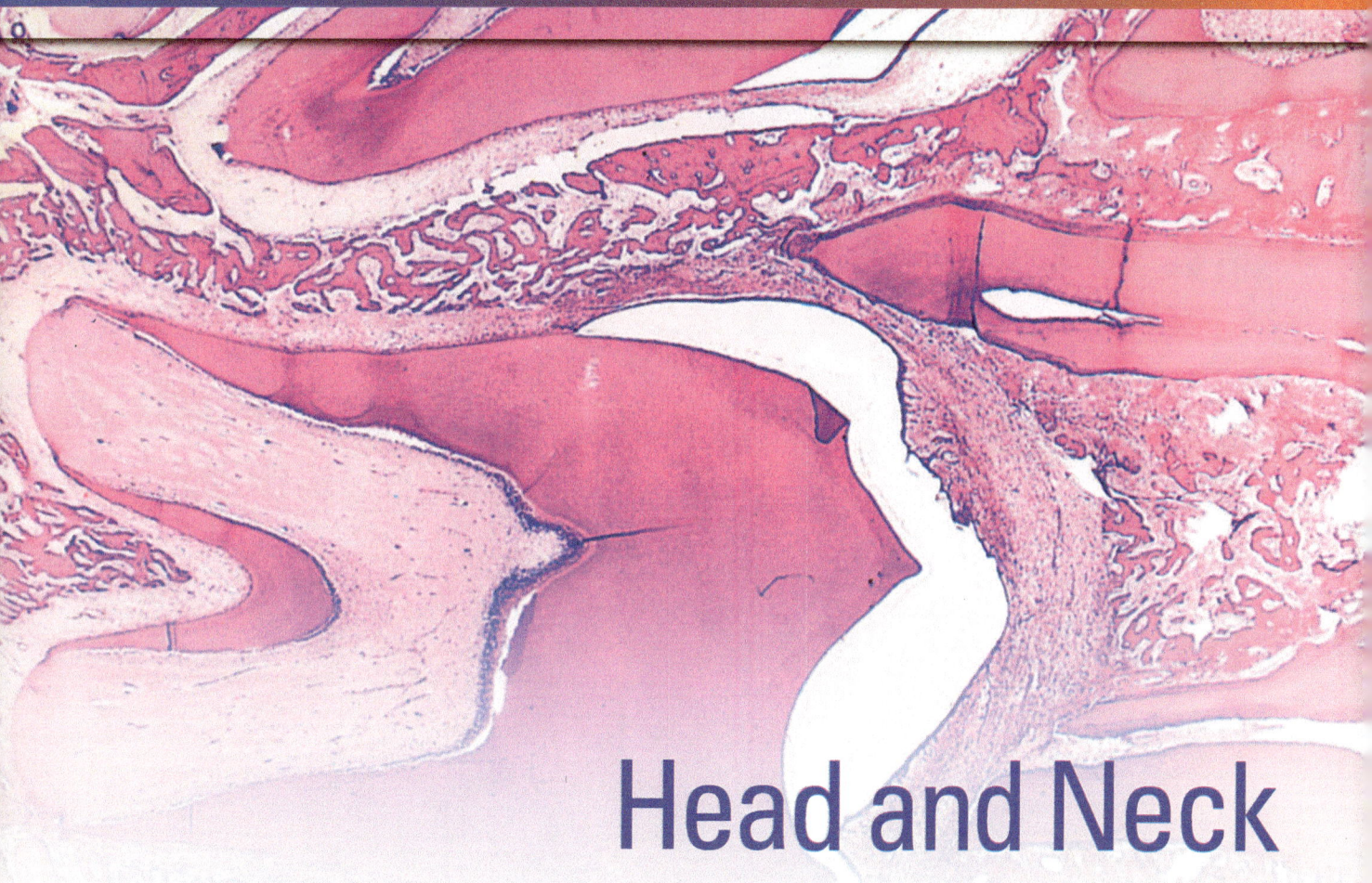

Head and Neck

Eye and Ocular Adnexa

Alan D. Proia ■ Thomas J. Cummings

CORNEA 336	THE OPTIC NERVE 352
SCLERA 339	THE CRYSTALLINE LENS 353
CORNEOSCLERAL LIMBUS 340	INTRAOCULAR COMPARTMENTS 355
CONJUNCTIVA, CARUNCLE, AND PLICA SEMILUNARIS 342	THE EYELIDS 355
THE UVEAL TRACT 343	THE ORBIT 357
The Iris 343	LACRIMAL DRAINAGE APPARATUS 357
The Ciliary Body 345	ACKNOWLEDGMENTS 360
Choroid 346	REFERENCES 360
RETINA 348	
Artifacts of the Retina 351	

The eye and surrounding tissues are subject to a wide variety of primary ocular and systemic diseases. An understanding of ocular anatomy will enable the general surgical pathologist to appreciate morphologic abnormalities and will facilitate the diagnosis of many of the pathologic conditions affecting those structures. Similar to other specimens received by the surgical pathologist, in some cases a discussion with the ophthalmologist who is submitting the tissue is important for proper handling, sectioning, and processing of the tissue. Proper handling of the tissue is required to prevent artifactually masking the diagnostic histologic features, such as the common age-related arcus lipoides.

This chapter presents an overview of the normal histology of the eye and ocular adnexa. Several excellent texts are available for more detailed information on ocular anatomy, development, and age-related changes (1–8).

The eye is roughly spherical in shape, and external measurements are routinely obtained in three dimensions. In utero, the anterior–posterior (axial) length of the eye is approximately 7 mm at 15 weeks' gestation, 10 mm at 20 weeks', and 15 mm at 30 weeks' (9,10). At birth, the anterior–posterior diameter of the eye is approximately 17 to 18 mm (11), while by the age of 3 the axial length is about 22 mm (9). In the adult, the anterior–posterior plane of the eye measures approximately 24 mm, whereas the vertical and horizontal dimensions are both about 23 to 23.5 mm, though the eyes of men tend to be slightly larger than those of women (1). The equator of the globe is located midway between the anterior and posterior poles of the eye.

Several external landmarks allow the pathologist to orient the globe and to determine whether an eye is from the right or the left side (Fig. 12.1). By establishing the nasal (medial) and temporal (lateral) sides of the globe and the superior surface of the eye, the side of the eye can easily be deduced. The six extraocular muscles (four rectus and two oblique muscles) that arise in the posterior orbit and run forward to insert upon the sclera are important in this regard. The rectus muscles arise from a fibrous ring at the apex of the orbit, the annulus of Zinn, and are enveloped by a fascial membrane that creates a cone-shaped structure posterior to the globe. The levator palpebrae superioris also arises at the orbital apex and extends anteriorly to the eyelids. Of the extraocular muscles, only the inferior oblique has a muscular insertion upon the sclera; the other muscles

---

This chapter is an update of a previous version authored by Gordon K. Klintworth and Thomas J. Cummings.

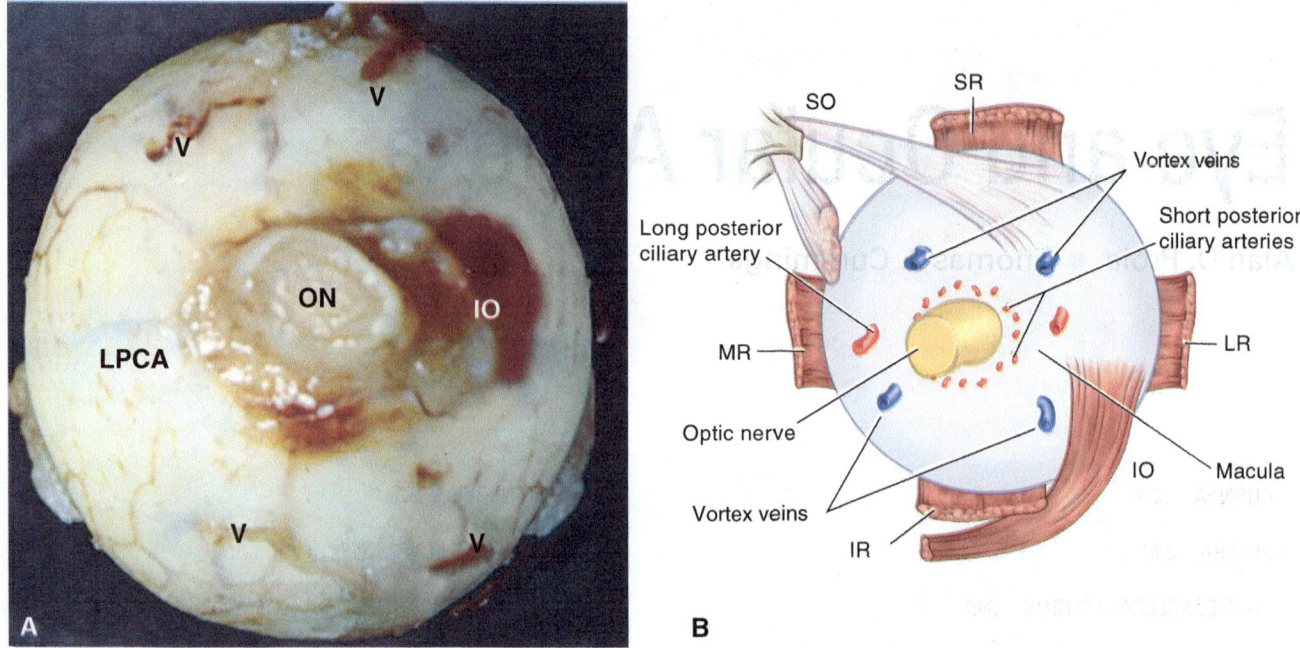

FIGURE 12.1 **A:** This posterior view of a right eye shows the transected optic nerve (*ON*) with its dura mater, the medial long posterior ciliary artery (*LPCA*), four vortex veins (*V*), and the insertion of the inferior oblique muscle (*IO*). **B:** This drawing depicts the right eye as seen from behind. Several external landmarks are useful in determining orientation of the globe. The optic nerve is located approximately 1 mm inferior to and 3 mm nasal to the posterior pole of the eye. The long posterior ciliary arteries are located in the horizontal plane and four vortex veins exit the sclera posteriorly. The superior oblique muscle (*SO*) inserts on the top of the globe, whereas the inferior oblique muscle (*IO*) inserts temporally and its fibers run posteriorly and nasally. The rectus muscles insert medially (*MR*), laterally (*LR*), inferiorly (*IR*), and superiorly (*SR*). Short posterior ciliary arteries form a ring surrounding the optic nerve. (Reproduced with permission from Freddo TF, Chaum E. *Anatomy of the Eye and Orbit. The Clinical Essentials*. Philadelphia, PA: Wolters Kluwer; 2018.)

have tendinous insertions. The extraocular muscle insertions are usually removed by the surgeon when the globe is excised (enucleated), though a short stump of the inferior oblique muscle is often present. The extraocular muscles are frequently present on eyes obtained postmortem. The superior and inferior oblique muscles are most useful in orientating the globe. The tendinous insertion of the superior oblique muscle behind the superior rectus muscle insertion indicates the top of the eye. The inferior oblique muscle inserts on the sclera temporally in the horizontal meridian, and its fibers run inferiorly toward the back of the orbit. The optic nerve is also useful in assessing orientation because it exits the globe slightly nasal to the posterior pole of the eye. Adjacent to the optic nerve, the prominent long posterior ciliary arteries course through the superficial sclera in opposite directions in a horizontal plane. Anteriorly, the dimensions of the cornea may be helpful in topographic orientation. In the adult, the cornea is usually elliptical in shape with its horizontal diameter being slightly greater than its vertical breadth. In young children this difference is less apparent.

The eye is traditionally described as having three tissue layers that surround the vitreous, the lens, and the spaces of the anterior and posterior chambers (Fig. 12.2). The outermost part of the eye is composed of the transparent cornea and the opaque sclera. The ocular middle layer, termed the "uvea" or "uveal tract," is made up of the iris, the ciliary body, and the choroid. The innermost retina is in direct contact with the vitreous body.

CORNEA

The transparent cornea occupies one-sixth of the anterior surface of the globe and refracts the entering light. Although individual variation is common, the cornea measures approximately 11.7 mm in the horizontal plane and 10.6 mm in the vertical plane (1). Centrally, the cornea is about 0.5 mm thick, but peripherally it thickens to about 0.67 mm (1). Histologically, the cornea consists of six distinct layers: (a) the epithelium, (b) the basal lamina of the epithelium, (c) the Bowman layer, (d) the stroma, (e) the Descemet membrane, and (f) the endothelium (Fig. 12.3).

The corneal epithelium, composed of stratified nonkeratinized squamous cells, is about five to seven cell layers thick. The basilar epithelial cells are polygonal in shape, and they acquire a more flattened appearance as they become displaced to the corneal surface during differentiation. In the normal cornea, even the most superficial

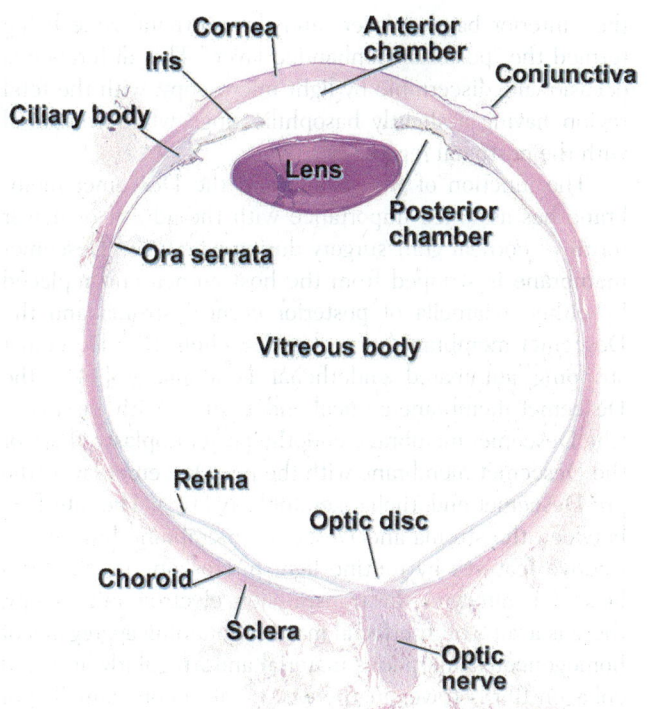

FIGURE 12.2 This photomicrograph of a histologic section of a human eye illustrates the major tissue layers of the eye, the lens, the vitreous body, and the spaces of the anterior and posterior chambers. The posterior retina exhibits artifactual detachment due to formalin fixation.

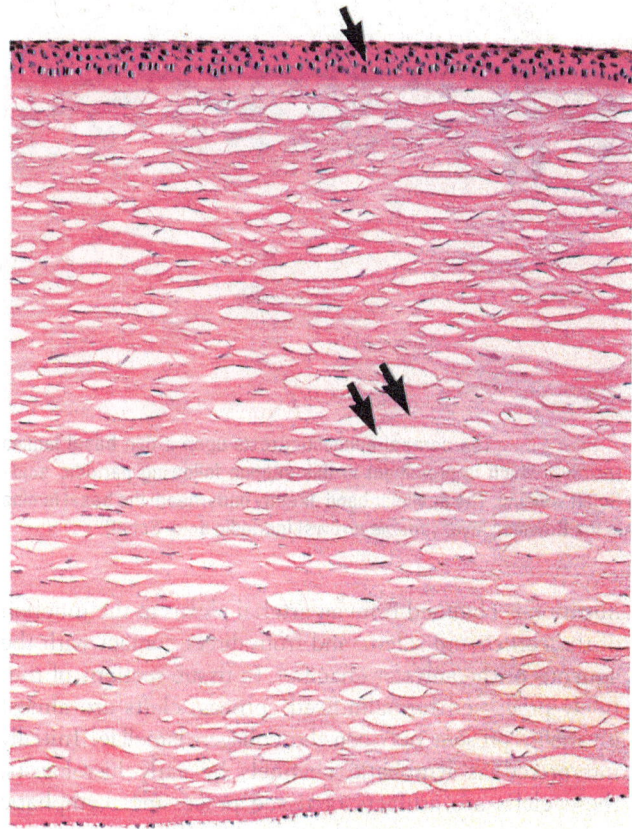

FIGURE 12.3 The stratified squamous epithelium of the cornea (*arrow*) overlies the basal lamina and the Bowman layer. The clefts within the collagenous stroma (*double arrows*) represent artifacts of tissue processing. No blood vessels or lymphatics are normally present within the cornea. The Descemet membrane and the corneal endothelium are located just posterior to the stroma (H&E).

epithelial cells retain their nuclei (Fig. 12.4). Mitotic figures are uncommon in the epithelium, but are observed in the basal cells occasionally. Some Langerhans cells are present within the corneal epithelium, and they are more abundant peripherally (12,13). Langerhans cells are most readily identified by special histochemical and immunohistochemical methods, and are not normally recognizable in routinely stained tissue sections. Apoptosis is uncommonly seen in the epithelium of the normal cornea, but it may be apparent in corneas with bullous keratopathy (corneal edema).

The corneal epithelium rests upon a basal lamina, which is difficult to see in hematoxylin and eosin (H&E)-stained tissue sections. Staining with the periodic acid–Schiff (PAS) reaction makes this layer apparent (Fig. 12.4). In certain pathologic conditions, the epithelial basal lamina assumes an intraepithelial location.

The Bowman layer is an acellular structure located just posterior to the epithelial basal lamina (Fig. 12.4). It is approximately 8 to 14 μm thick. As shown by transmission electron microscopy, the Bowman layer is not a true basement membrane but is composed of randomly oriented delicate collagen fibers. The anterior face of the Bowman layer ends distinctly at its junction with the epithelial basal lamina. Posteriorly, the Bowman layer merges inconspicuously with the underlying corneal stroma. Unmyelinated sensory nerves reach the epithelium from the stroma after crossing the Bowman layer. However, nerve processes are difficult to detect in the cornea in standard tissue sections, even with the use of special histologic techniques.

The stroma accounts for approximately 90% of the cornea's thickness. It is composed of numerous layers (lamellae) of collagen fibers embedded in a proteoglycan-rich extracellular matrix. The stroma contains keratan sulfate proteoglycans (lumican, keratocan, mimecan), as well as a galactosaminoglycan-rich proteoglycan (decorin). Transmission electron microscopy has disclosed that the corneal collagen fibers are regularly spaced and of a uniform diameter; this arrangement contributes to the transparency of the cornea. Surrounded by the stromal collagen lamellae are the corneal fibroblasts (keratocytes). The lamellae of the superficial one-third of the stroma are arranged in a less orderly fashion than those in the deeper two-thirds, and the anterior stroma is sometimes less eosinophilic than the posterior stroma (6). Other cell types are seldom identified in tissue sections of the normal corneal stroma, but rarely an occasional mononuclear leukocyte or granulocyte may be present. The normal cornea lacks blood vessels and its

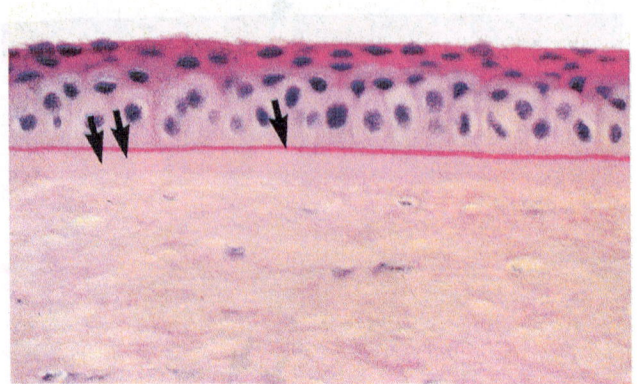

FIGURE 12.4 The corneal epithelium rests upon a thin basal lamina (*arrow*), which is prominent in this section following periodic acid–Schiff staining. The acellular band directly underneath the basal lamina is the Bowman layer (*double arrows*) (periodic acid–Schiff).

nutrition is obtained from an arterial plexus at the junction of the cornea and sclera, and from direct contact with the aqueous of the anterior chamber. In tissue sections of routinely processed formalin-fixed corneas, clefts are almost invariably present between the collagen lamellae. Initially interpreted as lymphatic channels by early histologists, these clefts are artifacts of tissue processing. Lymphatic vessels are not present in the normal cornea.

The Descemet membrane, a true basal lamina elaborated by the underlying corneal endothelial cells, begins to form during fetal life. At birth, it is approximately 3 to 4 μm thick (Fig. 12.5). Basal laminar material is continuously added to the posterior part of the Descemet membrane throughout life so that by adulthood this structure attains a thickness of approximately 10 to 12 μm. The fetal and postnatal regions of the Descemet membrane differ ultrastructurally, leading to the fetal zone also being known as

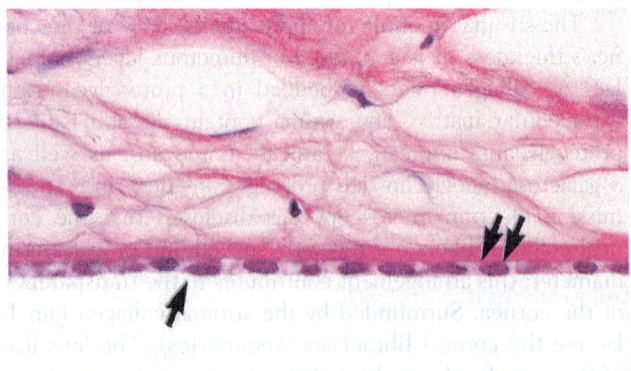

FIGURE 12.5 A thin monolayer of corneal endothelial cells (*arrow*) covers the posterior surface of the Descemet membrane (*double arrows*). These cells are in direct contact with the aqueous of the anterior chamber (H&E).

the "anterior banded layer" and the postnatal zone being termed the "posterior nonbanded layer." This difference is occasionally discernible by light microscopy, with the fetal region having a slightly basophilic tinge when compared with the postnatal region.

The junction of the stroma and the Descemet membrane has assumed importance with the advent of newer forms of corneal graft surgery during which the Descemet membrane is stripped from the host cornea and replaced by either a lamella of posterior corneal stroma and the Descemet membrane/corneal endothelium (the Descemet stripping automated endothelial keratoplasty [14]), the Descemet membrane/corneal endothelium without stroma (the Descemet membrane endothelial keratoplasty [15]), or the Descemet membrane with the pre-Descemet layer (the pre-Descemet endothelial keratoplasty [16]). The interface between the stroma and Descemet membrane has no distinctive features by routine light microscopy except for a lack of keratocytes; by transmission electron microscopy, there is a zone of interfacial matrix containing aggregates of homogeneous amorphous material and irregularly arranged collagen fibrils traversing between collagenous lamellae of the stroma and the fetal zone of the Descemet membrane (17,18). This interfacial matrix represents a cleavage zone during stripping of the Descemet membrane (18), though Dua et al. found that cleavage occurred most commonly between the last row of stromal keratocytes and an acellular layer of 5 to 8 lamellae of longitudinally, horizontally, and obliquely oriented collagen bundles that was termed "the Dua layer" (19).

The corneal endothelium (Fig. 12.5) is directly exposed to the aqueous in the anterior chamber. Although this cell layer does not line blood vessels or lymphatic spaces, the term "endothelium" is firmly entrenched in the literature. These cells function as an osmotic pump to regulate a necessary state of stromal dehydration which preserves corneal clarity. Endothelial decompensation results in corneal edema and diminished optical transparency. The corneal endothelium has been shown by immunohistochemistry to be S100 protein positive, a finding supportive of other evidence suggesting a neural crest origin (20). They react with the monoclonal antibody 2B4.14.1, which recognizes the renal Tamm–Horsfall glycoprotein (THGP) antigen, raising the possibility that the cornea expresses a molecule with homeostatic properties similar to that ascribed to THGP (21). The endothelial cells of the cornea normally form a single flattened layer and virtually never regenerate by mitosis in human eyes. The number of corneal endothelial cells decreases with advancing age (22), and it is essential to consider the patient's age when assessing whether or not the number of endothelial cells is normal. Under pathologic conditions (epithelial ingrowth and posterior polymorphous corneal dystrophy), cytokeratin-containing squamous cells replace the endothelium and form a layer that is more than one cell thick.

After the second decade of life, age-related focal excrescences (Hassall–Henle warts) commonly form on the

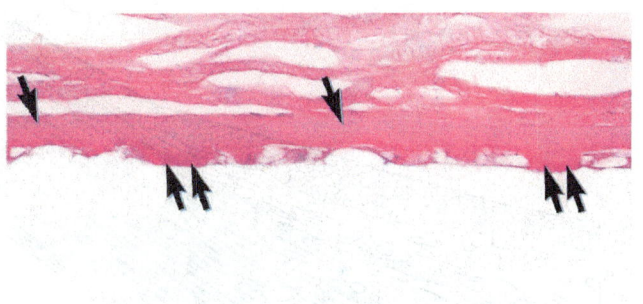

FIGURE 12.6 The Descemet membrane (*single arrows*) is located immediately posterior to the corneal stroma. Excrescences on the peripheral portion of the Descemet membrane (Hassall–Henle warts) (*double arrows*) represent an aging change. The Descemet membrane also thickens with age (H&E).

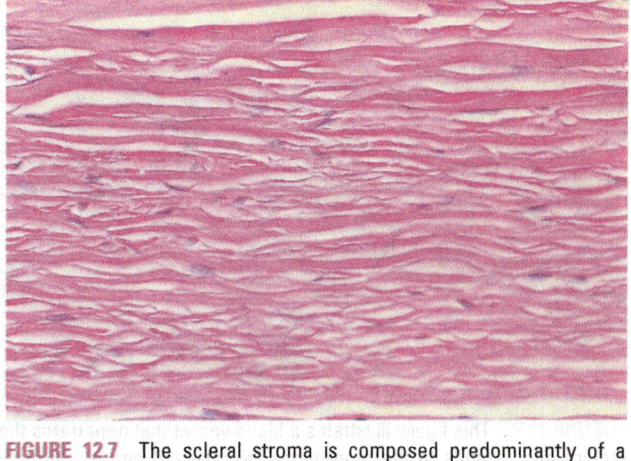

FIGURE 12.7 The scleral stroma is composed predominantly of a haphazard array of collagen bundles that vary in diameter. Scattered fibroblasts occur between the collagen bundles (H&E).

peripheral part of the Descemet membrane (Fig. 12.6). Virtually identical focal thickenings occur on the central part of the Descemet membrane (corneal guttae) under pathologic circumstances, most notably in Fuchs corneal (or Fuchs endothelial) dystrophy. The presence of excrescences on the Descemet membrane in tissue sections of corneal buttons removed at penetrating keratoplasty (full-thickness corneal transplant) is always abnormal. Hassall–Henle warts are too peripheral in location to be present in a surgically excised corneal button.

Corneal epithelium and endothelium are prone to being artifactitiously "rubbed-off" during prosection of the tissue, and it is important to distinguish this artifact from the true loss of corneal epithelium and endothelium.

SCLERA

The sclera, which accounts for approximately five-sixths of the surface area of the eye, begins at the periphery of the cornea and extends posteriorly to the optic nerve. The sclera's relatively rigid nature protects the eye from trauma and helps maintain intraocular pressure. Anteriorly, the sclera is visible underneath the transparent conjunctiva and is normally white in adults. The sclera varies in thickness, being about 0.8 mm thick near its junction with the cornea. At the insertions of the four rectus muscles (approximately 5 to 8 mm posterior to the corneoscleral junction), the sclera is at its thinnest, measuring approximately 0.3 mm. From this point posteriorly, the sclera gradually thickens and attains its maximal width of about 1.0 mm adjacent to the optic nerve.

The sclera has three components: the episclera, the stroma, and the lamina fusca. The episclera, its most superficial part, is located between the fibrous structure that envelops the globe (the Tenon capsule) and the underlying scleral stroma with which it merges. The Tenon capsule (fascia bulbi), though very well-defined anatomically (23,24), is usually difficult to recognize histologically due its thinness and the way it merges with conjunctival connective tissue anteriorly and the orbital fibroadipose tissue posteriorly (25). The episclera is composed of loosely arranged collagen fibers and fibroblasts embedded in an extracellular matrix. Occasional melanocytes and mononuclear leukocytes are also present. Anteriorly, the episclera is richly vascularized.

The largest component of the sclera is its stroma, which consists of fibrous bands of collagen, occasional elastic fibers, and scattered fibroblasts (Fig. 12.7). The corneal and scleral stroma appear similar at the light microscopic level, but when viewed by transmission electron microscopy, the individual collagen fibers within the sclera vary in diameter and are randomly arranged, in contrast to the orderly packed corneal collagen fibers of uniform diameter. This largely accounts for the opaque nature of the sclera.

Although the scleral stroma is relatively avascular, blood vessels, as well as accompanying nerves and scattered melanocytes, are present in perforating emissarial canals (Fig. 12.8). The anterior ciliary arteries perforate the sclera near the insertion of the rectus muscles. Venous channels draining the iris, ciliary body, and choroid (vortex veins) exit the sclera several millimeters posterior to the equator of the eye. The posterior ciliary arteries pass through the sclera near the optic nerve. In some individuals, a nerve in an emissarial canal near the corneoscleral junction may be prominent and attain a diameter of 1 to 2 mm. The nodular appearance of this so-called "nerve loop of Axenfeld" may mimic a neoplasm or conjunctival cyst clinically (26). To the unwary surgical pathologist, this totally normal nerve bundle may be mistaken for a neurofibroma (27).

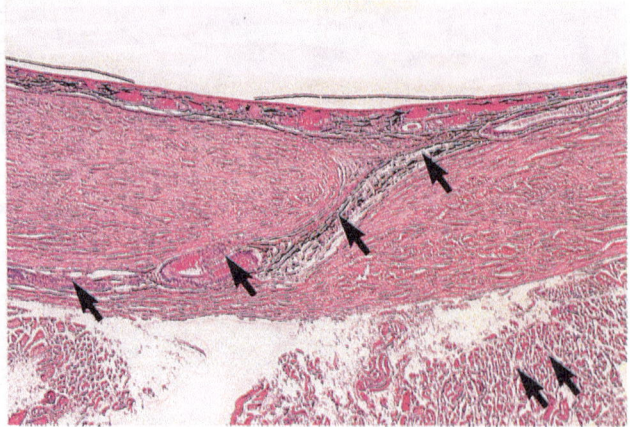

FIGURE 12.8 This figure illustrates a blood vessel that penetrates the sclera and extends to the prominently vascularized choroid through an emissarial canal (*single arrows*). Pigmented melanocytes are also present. The fibers of the inferior oblique muscle are present at the site of insertion upon the outer sclera (*double arrows*) (H&E).

The innermost layer of the sclera, the lamina fusca, contains loose collagen fibers, fibroblasts, and scattered melanocytes. It represents a region of transition between the sclera and the underlying choroid. The sclera is weakly attached to the choroid by thin fibers of collagen.

With increasing age, several histologic changes occur in the sclera. Calcium may deposit diffusely between the individual collagen fibers throughout the entire scleral stroma. Localized abnormalities, known as senile scleral plaques, may occur just anterior to the insertion of the horizontal rectus muscles. These lesions are characterized by decreased stromal cellularity, abnormal collagen, and, in advanced cases, calcification (28).

CORNEOSCLERAL LIMBUS

The corneoscleral junction, or limbus, is not a distinct anatomic site, but is a significant landmark clinically. Many surgical procedures on the anterior part of the eye are accomplished after access via an incision in the limbal area. For purposes of discussion, the trabecular meshwork and the Schlemm canal will be considered as part of the corneoscleral limbus.

The limbus is approximately 1.5 to 2.0 mm wide and separate layers of the cornea merge with components of the sclera or conjunctiva in this area (Fig. 12.9). The squamous epithelium of the cornea extends centrifugally beyond the limbus until it meets the epithelium of the bulbar conjunctiva. At the limbus, the Bowman layer of the cornea blends into the subepithelial tissues of the conjunctiva and the corneal and scleral stroma become continuous with each other. The Descemet membrane abruptly terminates in the limbal region and gives rise to the clinically significant landmark known as the Schwalbe

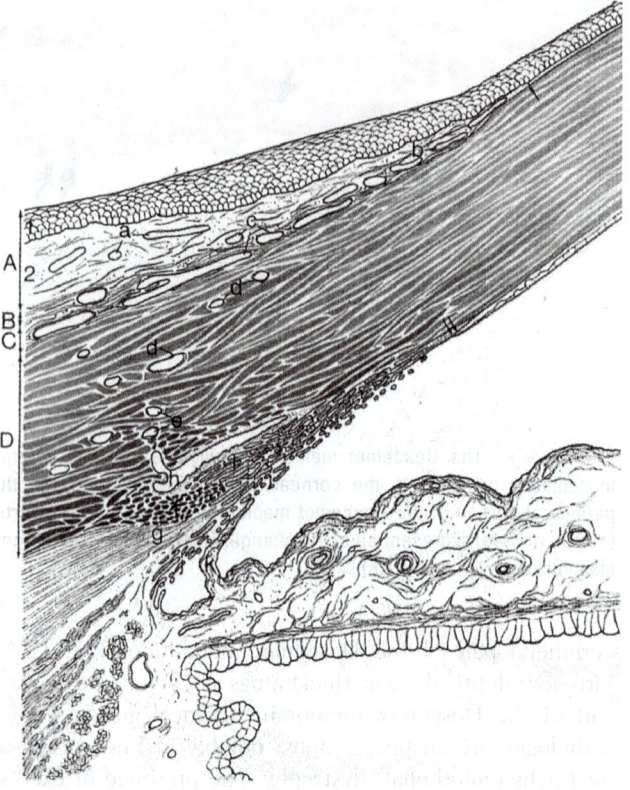

FIGURE 12.9 The corneoscleral limbus represents the junction of the peripheral cornea with the anterior sclera, and is not a distinct anatomic site. Clinically the limbus is an important landmark. The conjunctiva of the limbus (*A*) is composed of the epithelium (*1*) and stroma (*2*). The thin connective tissue layer of the Tenon capsule (*B*) overlies the episclera (*C*). The corneal and scleral stroma merge gradually in the area marked "*D*." Vessels of the conjunctival stroma (*a, b*), episclera (*c*), and limbal plexus (*d, e*) are illustrated. The projection of collagen fibers known as the scleral spur (*f*) merges with the smooth muscle fibers of the ciliary body (*g*). The Schlemm canal (*h*) and the trabecular meshwork (*i, j*) are responsible for removal of the aqueous from the eye. Occasionally, processes from the iris (*k*) insert upon the trabecular meshwork. The Bowman layer (*arrow*) and Descemet membrane (*double arrows*) both terminate in the area of the limbus. (Reproduced with permission from Hogan MJ, Alvarado JA, Weddell JE. *Histology of the Human Eye*. Philadelphia, PA: WB Saunders; 1971.)

ring. In about 15% of eyes, a prominent area of thickening is identified histologically at this site (Fig. 12.10) (6). Immediately adjacent to the Schwalbe ring is the most anterior aspect of the trabecular meshwork. Both the trabecular meshwork and the Schlemm canal constitute the apparatus responsible for the removal of the aqueous from the eye (Fig. 12.11). Aqueous drainage occurs in the angle between the anterior surface of the iris and the sclera. Histologically, the meshwork appears as a collection of finely branching and delicately pigmented connective tissue bands. The cells, which line the trabecular meshwork, are continuous with the corneal endothelium. Posteriorly, the trabecular meshwork extends to a roughly triangular projection of scleral connective tissue, known as the scleral spur.

Located slightly anterior and superficial to the trabecular meshwork is the Schlemm canal, an endothelial-lined venous channel that completely encircles the limbus. Since the Schlemm canal sometimes gives off smaller branches, two lumens are occasionally seen on histologic sections of the anterior chamber angle. Although the trabecular meshwork and the Schlemm canal appear to be in intimate contact in tissue sections, they are separated from each other by a thin layer of connective tissue and separate endothelial linings. The aqueous percolates among the delicate beams of the trabecular meshwork before becoming transported to the Schlemm canal. Ultrastructural examination of this region discloses giant cytoplasmic vacuoles in the endothelial lining of the Schlemm canal, adjacent to the trabecular meshwork. These vacuoles are thought by some to contain fluid in the process of being transported from the trabecular meshwork into the lumen of the Schlemm canal (29). Once

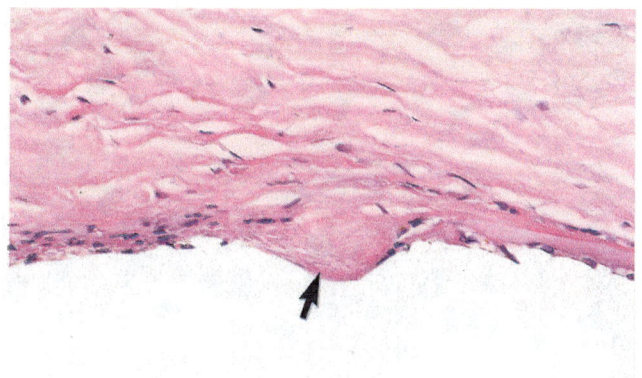

FIGURE 12.10 The Schwalbe ring is a significant clinical landmark in the limbal area and represents the peripheral termination of the Descemet membrane. Prominent Schwalbe rings (*arrow*) are identified histologically in about 15% of eyes (H&E).

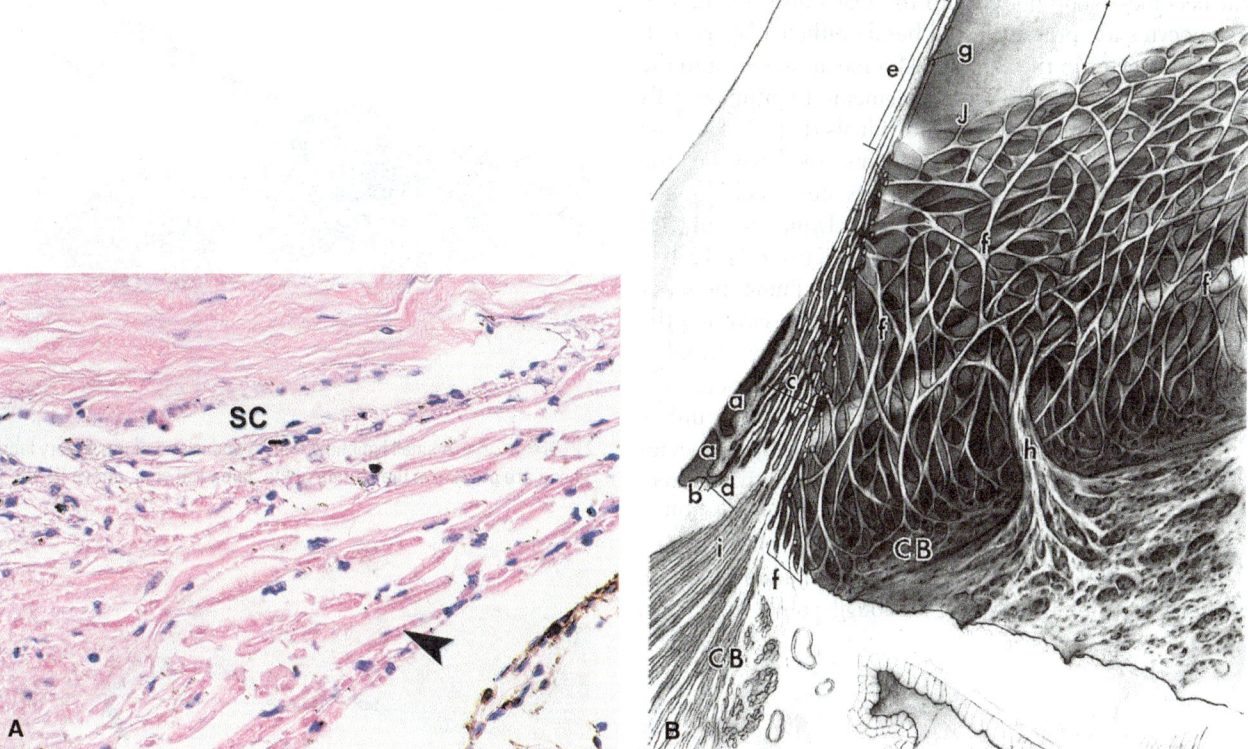

FIGURE 12.11 **A:** Located in the angle of the anterior chamber is the Schlemm canal (*SC*) and the trabecular meshwork (*arrowhead*). The Schlemm canal is an endothelial channel which enables the aqueous to drain from the eye. The aqueous reaches the Schlemm canal after percolating through the connective tissue strands of the trabecular meshwork (H&E). **B:** Structures within and near the angle of the anterior chamber are depicted in this drawing. In this illustration, the Schlemm canal (*a*) has two channels, one of which is in communication with a small collecting channel (*b*). The collecting channel is intimately associated with the limbal part of the trabecular meshwork (*c*). The scleral spur (*d*) is closely associated with the trabecular meshwork. The Descemet membrane terminates peripherally in the area denoted "*e*" and "*g*." Some components (*f*) of the trabecular meshwork arise at the ciliary body (*CB*). Isolated strands of meshwork merge with a nearby process (*h*) from the anterior surface of the iris. A muscle of the ciliary body (*i*) attaches to the trabecular meshwork as indicated by the *arrows*. The corneal endothelium merges with endothelial cells of the meshwork (*j*). (Reproduced with permission from Hogan MJ, Alvarado JA, Weddell JE. *Histology of the Human Eye*. Philadelphia, PA: WB Saunders; 1971.)

in the Schlemm canal, the aqueous drains into the episcleral venous plexus by way of numerous small collector channels. Prolonged obstruction to the outflow of the aqueous results in increased intraocular pressure and glaucoma.

CONJUNCTIVA, CARUNCLE, AND PLICA SEMILUNARIS

The conjunctiva is a thin continuous mucous membrane lining the inner surface of the eyelids and much of the anterior surface of the eye. In addition to its protective function, the conjunctiva allows the eyelids to move smoothly over the globe. The conjunctival epithelium is composed of two to five layers of cells and rests upon a basal lamina. The epithelial cells of the eyelid conjunctiva are considered stratified columnar, while those of the conjunctiva covering the eye are typically cuboidal. Within the conjunctival epithelium are goblet cells that secrete mucoid material that becomes incorporated into the tear film (Fig. 12.12). Melanocytes are present in the basal epithelial layers and, like melanocytes in the skin, transfer melanosomes into the adjacent epithelial cells. These pigmented epithelial cells are numerous in dark-skinned individuals (Fig. 12.13). The loose, fibrovascular subepithelial connective tissue of the conjunctival stroma normally contains nerve cells, melanocytes, and accessory lacrimal glands. Lymphoid follicles with germinal centers reside in the conjunctiva (Fig. 12.14), particularly in areas where the conjunctiva lining the inner surface of the eyelid merges with the portion covering the eyeball (superior and inferior fornices); scattered lymphocytes are not unusual within the conjunctiva. Hence, their presence is not indicative of chronic conjunctivitis unless both plasma cells and significant numbers of lymphocytes are present. Three distinct areas of the conjunctiva are recognized (Fig. 12.15): the palpebral conjunctiva, the bulbar conjunctiva, and the conjunctiva lining the fornices.

The morphologic attributes of the conjunctiva vary in different parts of this tissue. Although goblet cells exist

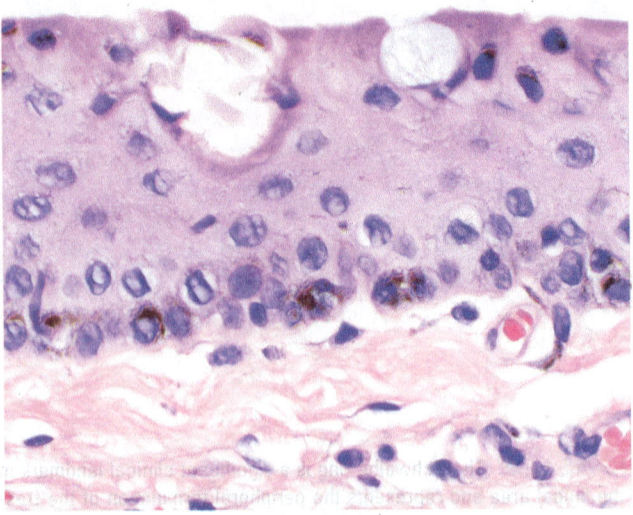

FIGURE 12.13 In dark-skinned individuals, the basal layers of the conjunctival epithelium contain intracellular melanin granules (H&E).

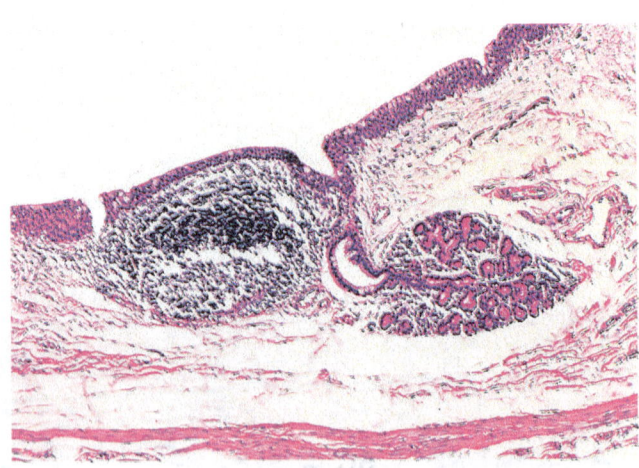

FIGURE 12.14 A small lymphoid follicle and island of accessory lacrimal tissue are present in the stroma of the palpebral conjunctiva (H&E).

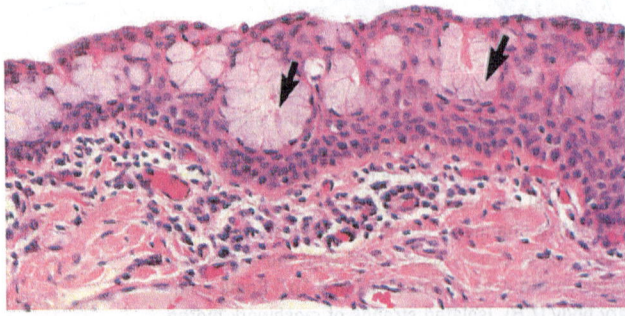

FIGURE 12.12 Goblet cells (*arrows*) are prominent in this section of conjunctival epithelium. Scattered mononuclear cells are often present in apparently healthy individuals in the underlying conjunctival stroma (H&E).

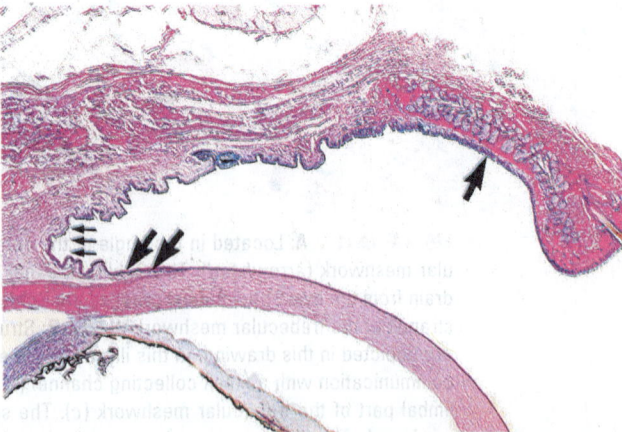

FIGURE 12.15 The conjunctiva can be divided into three parts. The palpebral conjunctiva (*arrow*) lines the posterior surface of the eyelid. The bulbar conjunctiva (*double arrows*) extends from the limbus over the anterior sclera. The bulbar and palpebral conjunctivae converge upon the conjunctiva of the superior and inferior fornices (*triple arrows*) (H&E).

throughout the conjunctival epithelium, the number varies widely and the location must be considered when trying to decide if the number of goblet cells is normal or abnormal. The goblet cell count is highest in the lower eyelid and lowest at the limbus (30). The conjunctival stroma is thickest in the fornices and bulbar areas and thinnest in the palpebral conjunctiva and at the corneoscleral limbus, where small conjunctival papillae, known as the palisades of Vogt, are evident. The palpebral conjunctiva is firmly attached to the inner surface of the eyelids, but the bulbar conjunctiva is loosely adherent to the underlying sclera by thin connective tissue strands.

The palpebral conjunctiva, which lines the posterior surface of the eyelids, extends from the fornices to the mucocutaneous junction at the eyelid margins, where the epithelium of the conjunctiva merges abruptly with the epidermis of the anterior surface of the eyelids. The palpebral conjunctiva contains several infoldings of epithelium (crypts of Henle). Islands of accessory lacrimal glands that are morphologically identical to the main tear-producing gland within the orbit occur within the palpebral conjunctiva. The subconjunctival tissue of the upper fornix may contain over 40 such glands, but fewer than 10 accessory lacrimal glands are present in the lower fornix (glands of Krause). The upper eyelids have approximately 2 to 5 accessory lacrimal glands (glands of Wolfring) located at the superior aspect of the tarsus. The bulbar conjunctiva begins at the limbus, at which point the corneal epithelium gradually becomes replaced by conjunctival epithelium and continues over the sclera to the superior and inferior fornices. There, the conjunctiva is thrown into small folds before becoming the palpebral conjunctiva.

Both the caruncle and the plica semilunaris (semilunar fold) represent specialized segments of the conjunctiva (Fig. 12.16). The caruncle is the nodular mass of fleshy tissue located in the medial interpalpebral angle of the eye. Its surface is covered by a stratified nonkeratinized squamous epithelium. The subepithelial stroma of the caruncle contains hair follicles, smooth muscle, sebaceous glands, adipose connective tissue, and occasionally, accessory lacrimal glands, as well as sweat glands. The plica semilunaris, an arc-shaped fold of conjunctiva located immediately lateral to the caruncle, is thought to be a vestigial remnant of the nictitating membrane of lower species. The histologic features of the plica semilunaris are similar to those in other areas of the conjunctiva, except that the epithelium contains abundant goblet cells and, rarely, cartilage within the stroma.

THE UVEAL TRACT

Located between the outer scleral covering and the inner retina is the uveal tract, which begins anteriorly as the iris, extends to the ciliary body, and then to the choroid posteriorly. The designated term *uvea* is derived from the Latin word *uva* (grape) because this portion of the eye was

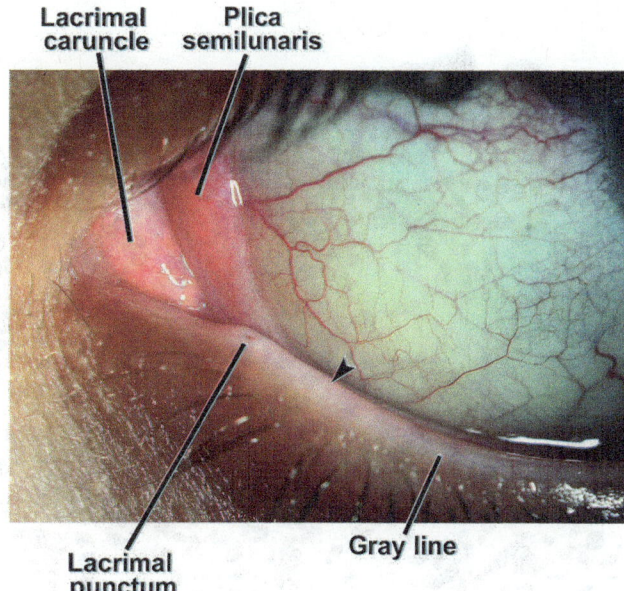

FIGURE 12.16 The caruncle and the plica semilunaris (semilunar fold) are specialized portions of the conjunctiva and are located in the medial interpalpebral angle of the eye. Before tears enter the lacrimal drainage apparatus through the lacrimal punctum, they accumulate at the medial canthus (lacrimal lake). The demarcation between the conjunctival and cutaneous portions of the eyelid is discernible clinically at the so-called "gray line." The secretions of the meibomian glands (tarsal glands) reach the surface of the eyelids at small orifices, one of which is marked with an *arrowhead*." (Courtesy of Paola Torres, COT.)

thought to somewhat resemble the dark color of a grape after the sclera and cornea are stripped from the globe.

The Iris

The iris is a thin diaphragm of tissue with a central opening, the pupil, which functions to regulate the amount of light reaching the retina (Fig. 12.17). Muscles within the iris dilate or constrict the pupil in response to sympathetic or parasympathetic nerve impulses. The diameter of the iris

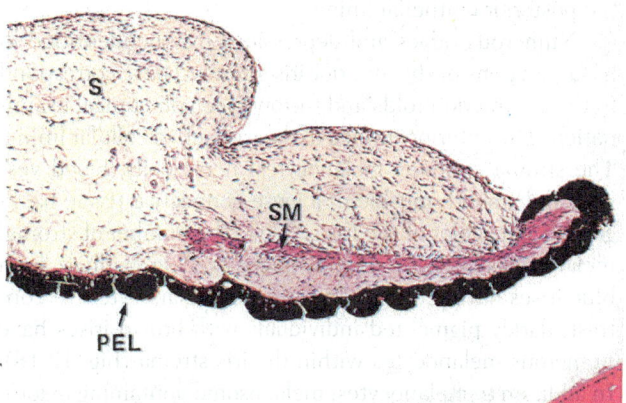

FIGURE 12.17 The iris is composed of stroma (*S*) and a posterior epithelial lining (*PEL*). The sphincter muscle (*SM*) of the iris is evident within the stroma. The pigmented posterior epithelial lining normally extends around the lip of the pupil anteriorly for a short distance (H&E).

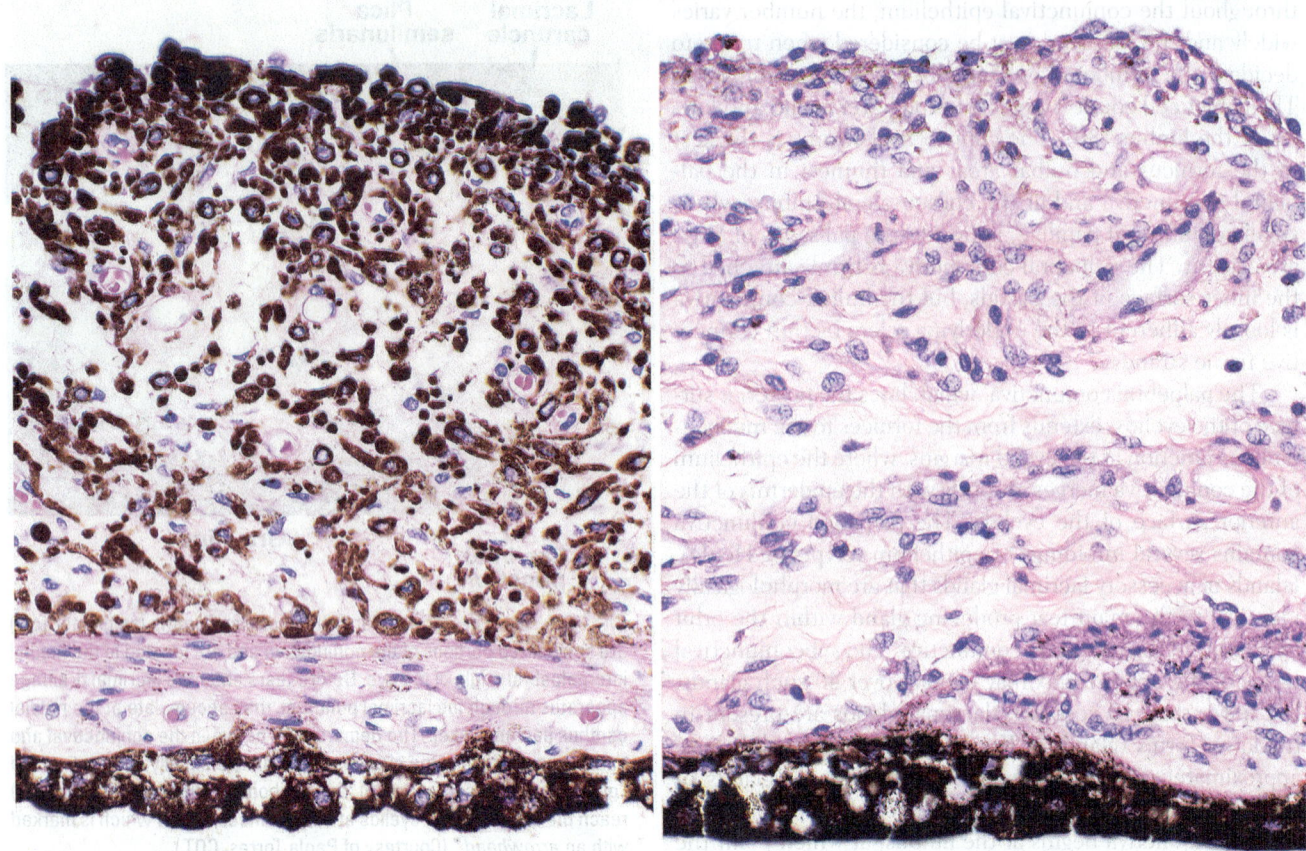

FIGURE 12.18 The color of the iris is due to the number of stromal melanocytes which are more abundant in the stroma of an individual with a brown iris (*left*) than with a blue iris (*right*). The amount of pigment in the posterior epithelial lining is similar in irises of different colors. In contrast to the posterior surface of the iris, the anterior iris lacks a cellular lining (H&E).

is approximately 21 mm, whereas the diameter of the pupil ranges from 1 to 8 mm. The iris is thinnest at its point of attachment with the ciliary body peripherally, the iris root. Normally, the iris rests gently upon the crystalline lens and, therefore, bulges slightly forward. Structurally and developmentally, the iris consists of two main parts: the stroma and the posterior epithelial lining.

Numerous ridges and depressions may be identified in tissue sections of the anterior iris stroma. These correspond to the contraction folds and furrows seen on clinical examination. The anterior surface of the iris lacks a cellular lining. The stroma contains melanocytes, nerve cells, blood vessels, and smooth muscle in a loose connective tissue background. The color of the iris is due to the number of stromal melanocytes present. Lightly pigmented individuals with blue irises have relatively few stromal melanocytes. In contrast, darkly pigmented individuals with brown irises have numerous melanocytes within the iris stroma (Fig. 12.18). In addition to melanocytes, melanosome-containing macrophages are also scattered within the iris stroma, particularly at the iris root. A thick collar of collagen fibers normally surrounds the blood vessels within the iris stroma and is especially prominent in adults. To the inexperienced observer, these normal vessels may appear to have arteriolosclerosis. In the pathologic process of iris neovascularization, thin-walled blood vessels, which lack such a collagenous coat, cover the anterior surface of the iris.

The sphincter muscle (sphincter pupillae), a bundle of circularly arranged smooth muscle innervated by parasympathetic nerves, acts to constrict the pupil. Located within the posterior stroma of the pupillary zone, the sphincter pupillae is nearly 1 mm wide. Radially oriented smooth muscle fibers with scattered cytoplasmic melanosomes are also located within the stroma of the iris (dilator pupillae). Innervated by sympathetic nerves, this muscle is active in pupil dilatation.

Posteriorly, the iris is lined by two separate, but closely apposed, epithelial layers derived from the neuroectoderm. The cells of the anterior epithelial layer, which are in direct contact with the posterior aspect of the stroma, are continuous with smooth muscle fibers of the dilator pupillae; the sphincter pupillae are of similar developmental origin. The posterior iris pigment epithelial layer is in direct contact with the aqueous of the posterior chamber. The cytoplasm of both epithelial layers contains numerous melanosomes (approximately 1 μm in diameter), which are larger than those of the iris stroma (diameter of about 0.5 μm). The number of melanosomes in the iris epithelial layers does not vary significantly between lightly and darkly pigmented individuals. In persons with ocular and oculocutaneous albinism, the pigmented epithelia, as well as the stromal melanocytes, contain fewer melanin granules than in normal individuals. The pigmented epithelia of the iris normally extend around the lip of the pupil, anteriorly, for a short distance. In certain pathologic conditions, fibrovascular tissue on the anterior surface of the iris everts the pupillary margin and pulls the pigmented epithelia onto the anterior surface of the iris. This displaced pigmented epithelium may be apparent clinically and is known as ectropion uveae.

The Ciliary Body

The middle segment of the uveal tract, the ciliary body, is located between the iris and the choroid. Situated interior to the anterior sclera, it is made up of two ring-shaped components: the pars plicata and the pars plana (Fig. 12.19). The anteriormost aspect of the ciliary body, the pars plicata begins at the scleral spur and contains approximately 70 sagittally oriented folds (approximately 2 mm long and 0.8 mm high). Continuous with these folds is the flat pars plana, which is approximately 4 mm wide, and merges posteriorly with the serrated anterior border of the retina (ora serrata). Both portions of the ciliary body consist of epithelium, stroma, and smooth muscle.

The ciliary epithelium embraces two distinct layers, both of which share a similar development derivation from neural ectoderm (Fig. 12.20). The inner epithelial layer is virtually nonpigmented and is contiguous with the aqueous of the posterior chamber. At the ora serrata, the neurosensory retina converges into the nonpigmented ciliary epithelial monolayer, which extends anteriorly until it becomes the

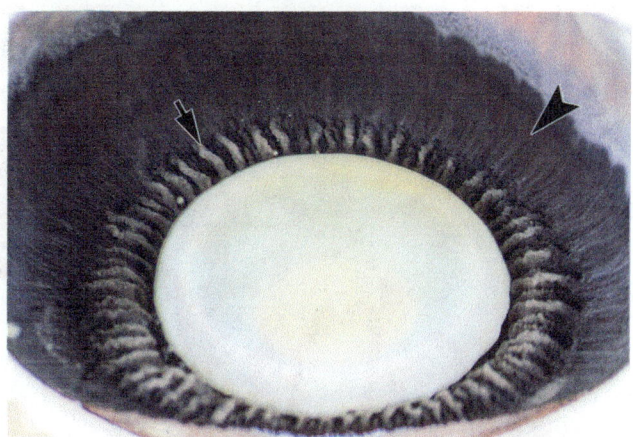

FIGURE 12.19 The lens and the ciliary body are viewed from behind in this photograph. The ciliary body has two components: the pars plicata and the pars plana. The pars plicata contains about 70 sagittally oriented folds or ciliary processes (*arrow*). The pars plicata gradually merges with the flat pars plana (*arrowhead*).

posterior epithelial layer of the iris. In contrast, the outer ciliary epithelial layer is pigmented and unites with the retinal pigment epithelium at the ora serrata. The pigmented epithelium of the ciliary body overlies a PAS-positive basal lamina that is closely adherent to the adjacent stroma. The basal lamina of the pigmented epithelium can become conspicuously thickened in diabetes mellitus. Acellular fibers, known as zonules (Fig. 12.20), attach the crests of the nonpigmented ciliary epithelium in the pars plicata to the capsule of the crystalline lens.

The stroma of the ciliary body, composed of fibroblasts, blood vessels, nerve cells, and melanocytes, is most abundant in the ciliary processes of the pars plicata, and is least plentiful in the valleys between these processes and in the pars plana. During infancy, the stroma of the ciliary body is

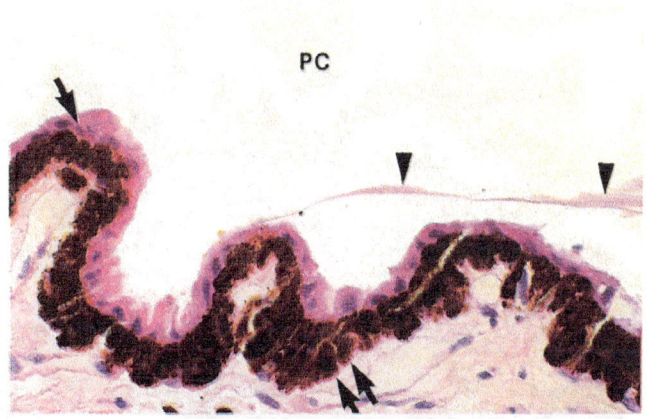 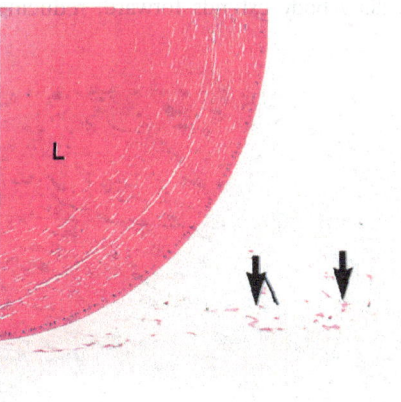 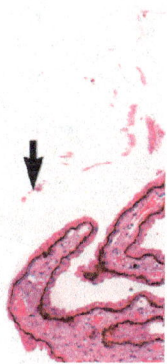

FIGURE 12.20 **Left:** The epithelium of the ciliary body has two distinct layers. The inner nonpigmented layer (*arrow*) is in direct contact with the aqueous of the posterior chamber (*PC*). The outer pigmented epithelial layer (*double arrows*) is adjacent to the underlying stroma. Acellular eosinophilic fibers (zonules) attach to the crests of the nonpigmented epithelium of the pars plicata (*arrowheads*). Zonules do not originate in the valleys between the ciliary processes (H&E). **Right:** Zonular fibers (*arrows*) span between the pars plicata of the ciliary body (on the *right*) and the lens (*L*) and hold the lens in place (H&E).

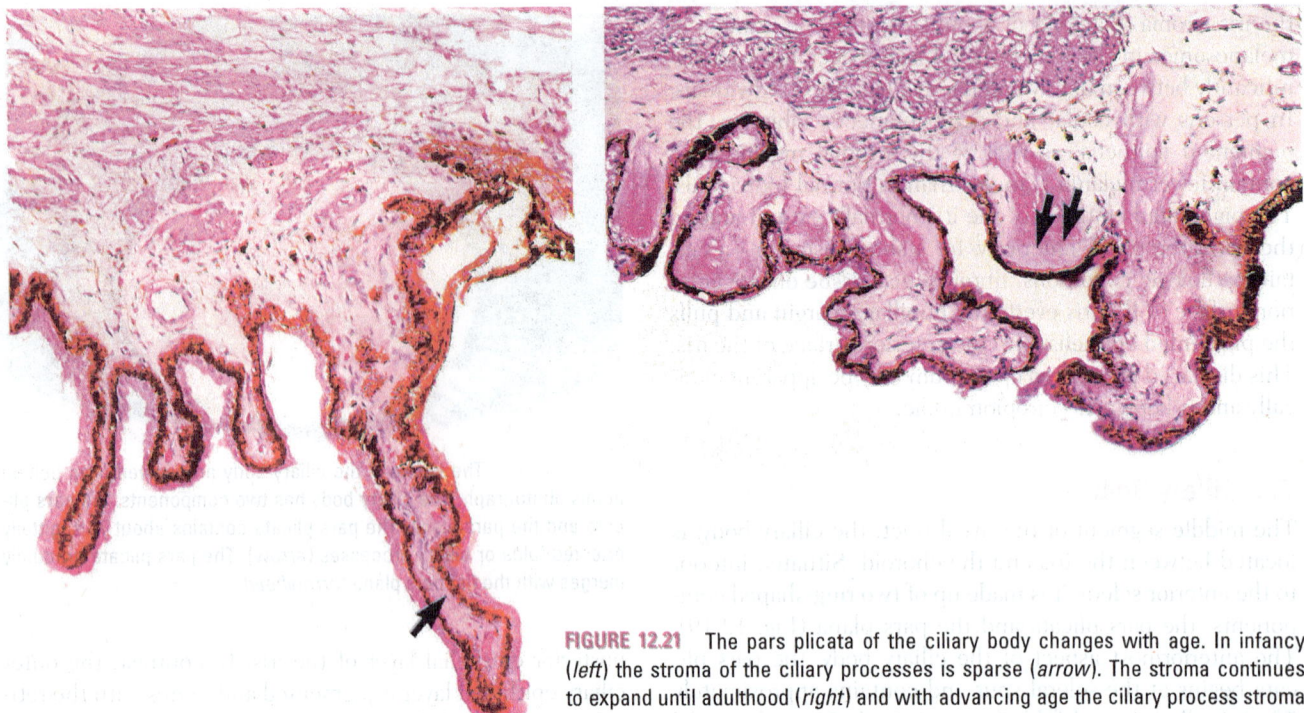

FIGURE 12.21 The pars plicata of the ciliary body changes with age. In infancy (*left*) the stroma of the ciliary processes is sparse (*arrow*). The stroma continues to expand until adulthood (*right*) and with advancing age the ciliary process stroma becomes hyalinized (*double arrows*) (*left* and *right*, H&E).

sparse (Fig. 12.21, *left*) but expands until adulthood. With advanced age, the ciliary body stroma becomes hyalinized (Fig. 12.21, *right*) and frequently calcifies.

The smooth muscle of the ciliary body (Fig. 12.22) forms three distinct bundles. The outermost muscle runs in a longitudinal or meridional direction, whereas the middle layer contains radially oriented fibers, and the innermost muscle cells are aligned in a circular fashion. In routinely processed globes, histologic differentiation of these three muscular layers is difficult. Muscles of the ciliary body attach in large part to the scleral spur. The ciliary muscle assists in accommodation. As it contracts, the ciliary body extends forward, reducing pressure on the zonules and enabling the lens to become less concave and thereby increasing its refractive power.

Choroid

The richly vascularized choroid (Fig. 12.23) extends from the ciliary body to the optic nerve. Its inner aspect is firmly adherent to the retinal pigment epithelium. The outer surface of the choroid is loosely attached to the overlying sclera. The Bruch membrane delineates the choroid from the overlying retinal pigment epithelium and is approximately 2 to 4 μm thick. Although the Bruch membrane appears as a thin eosinophilic

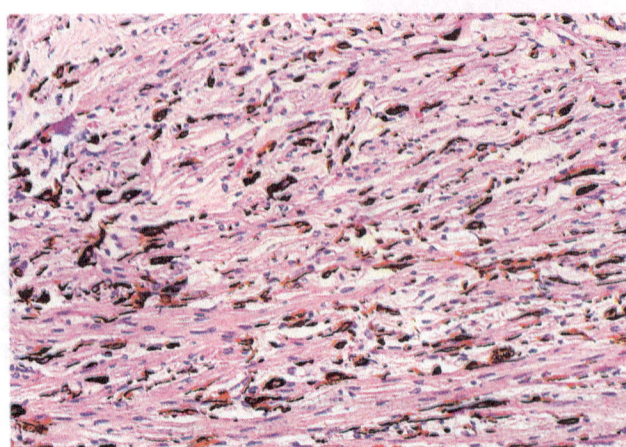

FIGURE 12.22 Smooth muscle constitutes a large portion of the ciliary body. Pigmented melanocytes are often present in between the smooth muscle bundles (H&E).

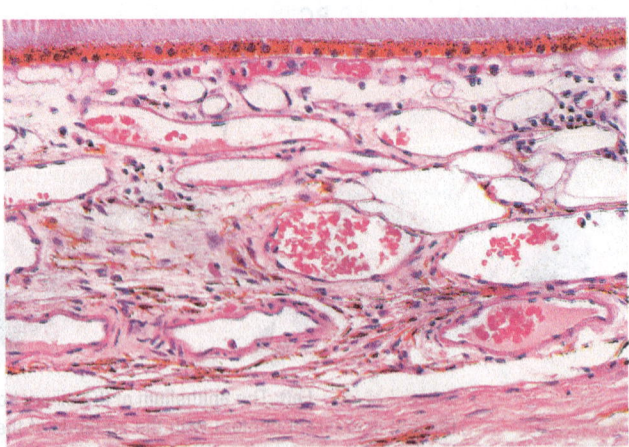

FIGURE 12.23 This photomicrograph illustrates the well-vascularized choroid. At the bottom of the figure, the choroid abuts the sclera. The single layer of retinal pigment epithelium is present at the top of the figure (H&E).

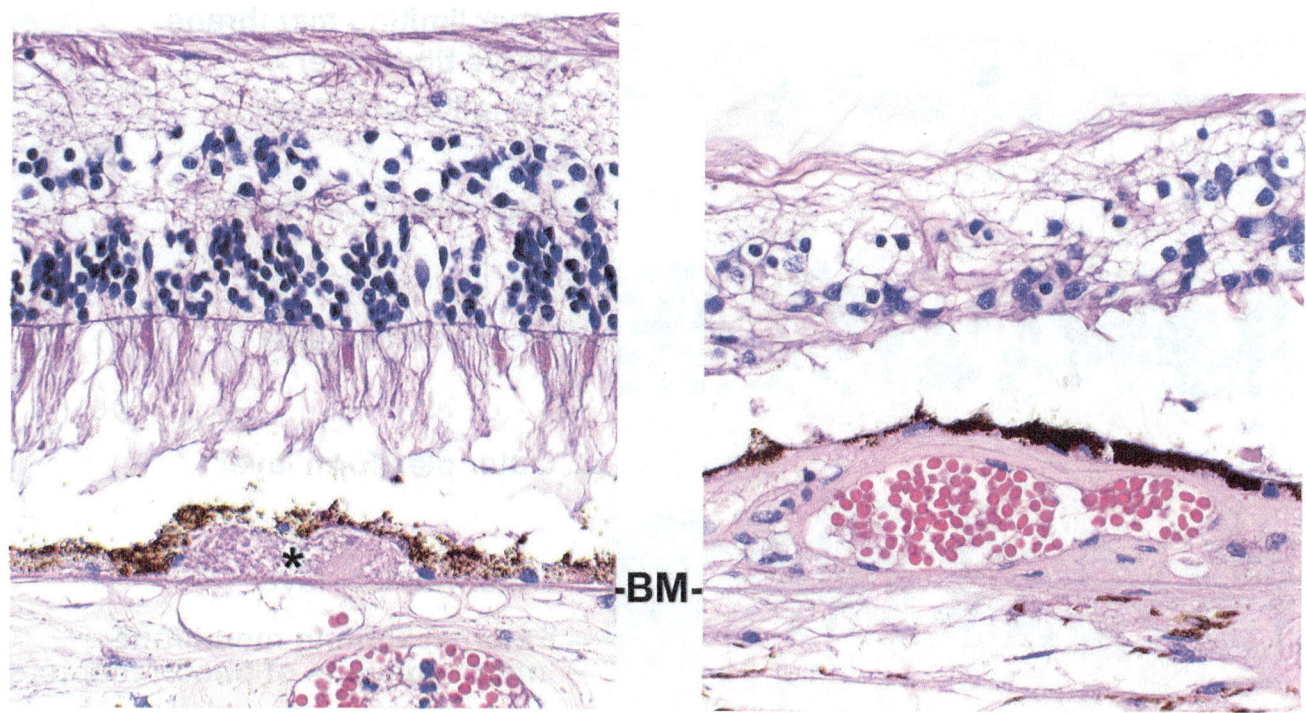

FIGURE 12.24 Left: An excrescence (*asterisk*) on the Bruch membrane (*BM*) appears to protrude into the overlying retina. Such so-called "drusen" are common as one ages and occasionally calcify (H&E). **Right:** Another very common age-related change in the eye is the development of a layer of blood vessels between the Bruch membrane and the retinal pigment epithelium (termed "choroidal neovascularization") in the peripheral choroid just posterior to the ora serrata (H&E).

layer in tissue sections, ultrastructural analysis has disclosed it to be composed of five distinct layers: the basal lamina of the overlying retinal pigment epithelium, a collagenous layer, an elastic fiber-rich component, another collagenous portion, and the basal lamina of the endothelial cells of the underlying capillary network (choriocapillaris). Located in the innermost choroidal stroma adjacent to the Bruch membrane, the choriocapillaris connects with arterial and venous channels from vessels in the outer choroidal stroma. Its function is to nourish the outer retinal layers. With age, the Bruch membrane thickens and commonly acquires focal excrescences known as drusen (Fig. 12.24, *left*). Both the drusen and the Bruch membrane may calcify. Another common, if not universal, aging change is the development of a layer of blood vessels between the Bruch membrane and the retinal pigment epithelium in the peripheral choroid just posterior to the ora serrata (Fig. 12.24, *right*) (31,32). This layer of neovascularization is usually more prominent temporally than nasally in horizontal sections through the eye (33).

The choroidal stroma is thinnest anteriorly, near the ciliary body, where it is approximately 0.1 mm thick. Posteriorly, at the optic nerve, the choroidal stroma thickens to nearly 0.22 mm. The tenuous connection between the choroidal stroma and the sclera is responsible for both the pathologic and artifactual separations often seen between these two layers in histologic sections. The stroma contains abundant pigmented melanocytes (Fig. 12.25), which are more

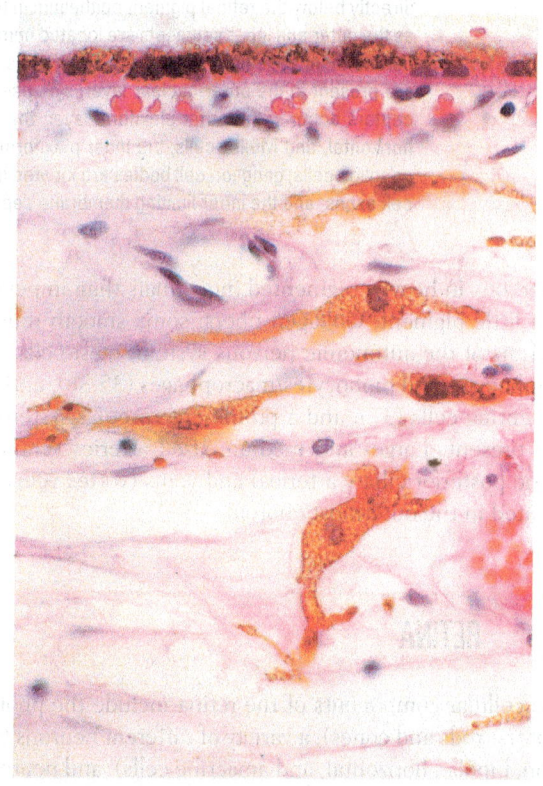

FIGURE 12.25 Numerous pigmented melanocytes are located within the choroidal stroma (H&E).

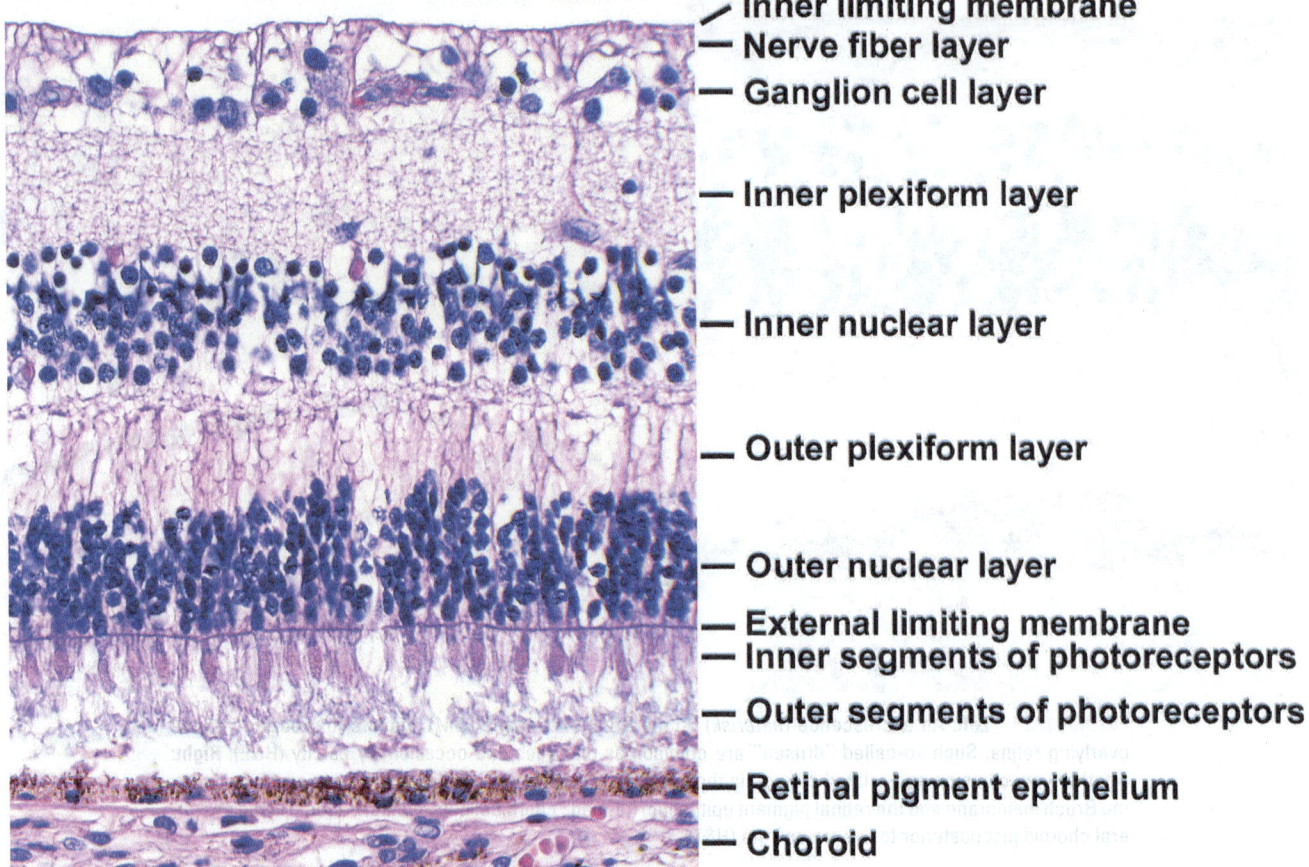

FIGURE 12.26 The cellular components of the retina are organized in well-defined layers. The choroid is directly below the retinal pigment epithelium in this figure. Specialized extensions of the photoreceptors known as the outer and inner segments are located immediately adjacent to the retinal pigment epithelium; many of the outer and inner segments are artifactually separated in this postmortem eye. Cell bodies of the photoreceptors are present in the outer nuclear layer; synapses between the bipolar cells, horizontal cells, and the photoreceptors occur in the outer plexiform layer; the inner nuclear layer embraces nuclei of the amacrine, bipolar, horizontal, and Müller cells; the inner plexiform layer contains axons and dendrites of amacrine, bipolar, and ganglion cells; ganglion cell bodies are located in the ganglion cell layer; the nerve fiber layer contains ganglion cell axons; and the inner limiting membrane separates the neurosensory retina from the vitreous.

numerous in heavily pigmented individuals than in persons with little pigment. Collagen fibers, some smooth muscle, neurons of the autonomic nervous system, mast cells (34), lymphocytes and monocytes/macrophages (35,36), antigen-presenting cells (37), and a prominent vascular system are also present. Large- and medium-sized arteries (branches of the posterior ciliary arteries) and veins (vortex veins) are situated in the outermost choroid.

RETINA

The cellular components of the retina include the photoreceptors (rods and cones), a variety of different neurons (ganglion, bipolar, horizontal, and amacrine cells), and neuroglial cells (Müller cells and astrocytes). Many of these special types of cells can only be detected with the aid of specific staining techniques. These constituents of the retina are stratified into several distinct layers (Fig. 12.26). The rods and cones comprise the outermost part of the neurosensory retina and are closely apposed to the retinal pigment epithelium. The retina's anterior boundary has a serrated edge (ora serrata), at which point it is approximately 0.1 mm thick. Cysts develop in the peripheral retina (peripheral cystoid degeneration) in virtually everyone over age 20 (Figs. 12.27 and 12.28) (38). Here, the retina converges into a single layer of nonpigmented epithelium which continues anteriorly to where it merges with the nonpigmented epithelium of the ciliary body (Fig. 12.28). Posteriorly, the retina extends to the optic nerve, where it is approximately 0.5 to 0.6 mm thick. The neurosensory retina is in direct contact with the vitreous and lies interior to the retinal pigment epithelium, which defines the outermost border of the retina.

The retinal pigment epithelium is a monolayer of cells. These epithelial cells contain numerous intracytoplasmic

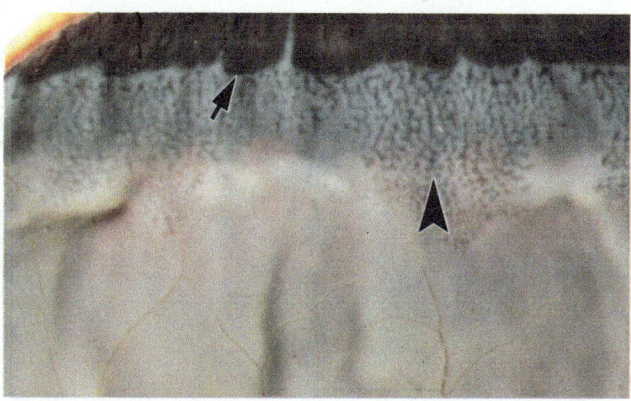

FIGURE 12.27 The ora serrata marks the anterior boundary of the retina. An almost invariable finding in the retina of all human eyes after the age of 20 is peripheral cystoid degeneration. Macroscopically, the peripheral retina immediately behind the ora serrata (*arrow*) has a vacuolated appearance (*arrowhead*).

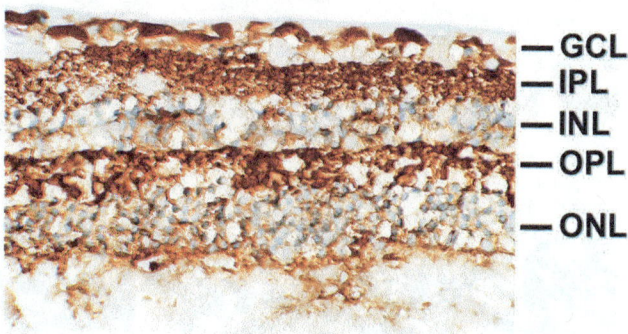

FIGURE 12.29 Synaptophysin immunopositivity is present within the ganglion cell layer (*GCL*), inner (*INL*) and outer (*ONL*) nuclear layers, and inner (*IPL*) and outer (*OPL*) plexiform layers.

melanosomes; cellular processes envelop part of the overlying rods and cones as shown by transmission electron microscopy. The phagocytic function of the retinal pigment epithelium assists in the turnover of the photoreceptor elements. Undigested products of phagolysosomes culminate in the progressively increasing number of lipofuscin granules that accumulate within the retinal pigment epithelium, with time.

Some photoreceptors are cylindrical in appearance (rods), whereas others are conical and somewhat longer and thicker (cones). Internal to the photoreceptors is the outer plexiform layer, formed from cell processes of the horizontal and bipolar cells and axonal extensions of the rods and cones. The inner nuclear layer embraces the nuclei of several cell types (the bipolar, Müller, horizontal, and amacrine cells). Constituents of the inner plexiform layer include bipolar and amacrine cell axons and dendrites of the ganglion cells. Near the vitreal aspect of the retina is the ganglion cell layer, composed predominantly of ganglion cell bodies. The axons of these large neurons make up the nerve fiber layer; these processes are usually unmyelinated, but as an incidental developmental anomaly, bundles of some nerve fibers are occasionally myelinated. In older individuals, basophilic PAS-positive intracellular rounded bodies (corpora amylacea), indistinguishable from similar structures in the brain, often accumulate in the nerve fiber layer of the retina near the optic disc. By light microscopy, two acellular zones can be distinguished within the retina: the external and internal limiting membranes. The so-called "external limiting membrane" is located between the photoreceptors and the outer nuclear layer. The membrane represents firm junctions between Müller cells and adjacent photoreceptors (zonula adherens). The basal lamina of the Müller cells accounts for the hyalin structure seen on light microscopy, and is known as the "internal limiting membrane." Similar to the neuroglial tissue of the brain, by immunohistochemistry, the neuronal cells of the retina show strong immunopositivity to synaptophysin (Fig. 12.29) and NeuN (*Neu*ronal *N*uclei) (Fig. 12.30) (39). The intensity of ganglion cell staining for synaptophysin is markedly influenced by the antibody and methods employed, and the ganglion cell staining is often much less than that of the inner and outer plexiform layers. Neurofilament protein highlights

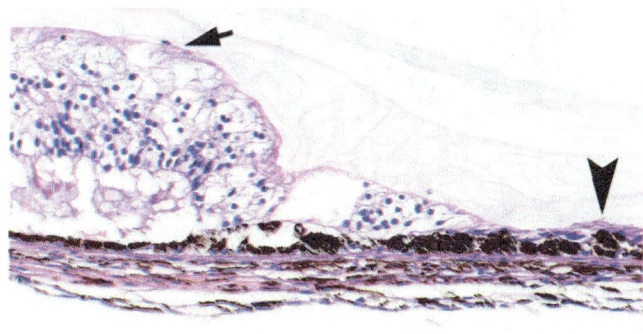 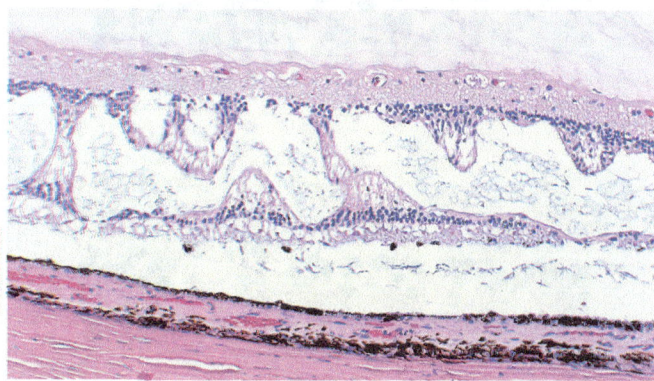

FIGURE 12.28 **Left:** At the ora serrata, the multilayered retina (*arrow*) converges with the single layer of non-pigmented epithelium of the ciliary body (*arrowhead*). The retina exhibits ischemic atrophy, a common age-related change in the peripheral retina (H&E ×50). **Right:** Microscopically, peripheral cystoid degeneration is characterized by the presence of numerous cyst-like spaces within the retina.

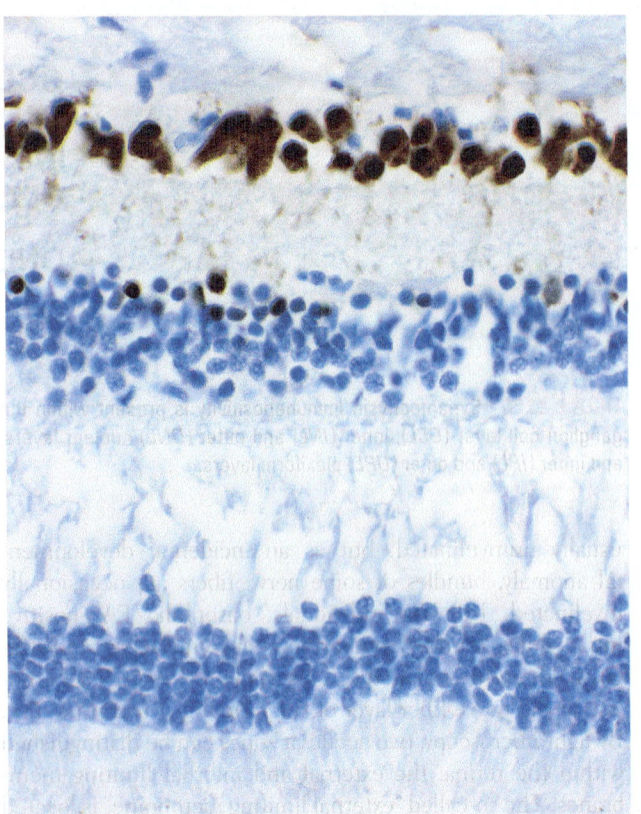

FIGURE 12.30 Reactivity with the immunohistochemical marker NeuN is restricted to neurons of the ganglion cell layer and a few cells in the inner nuclear layer.

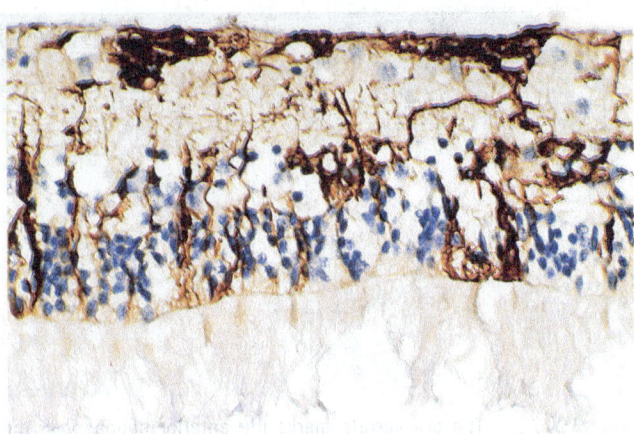

FIGURE 12.31 Antibodies to glial fibrillary acidic protein (GFAP) highlight the retinal glia and their processes.

the axons of the nerve fiber layer as they continue posteriorly to enter the optic nerve. Glial cells and their processes react with glial fibrillary acidic protein (GFAP) (Fig. 12.31).

Light passes through the entire neurosensory retina before it is converted by the photoreceptor cells into electric impulses. The impulses are eventually transmitted to the visual cortex in the occipital lobe of the brain through a complex series of intercellular connections.

The retina varies in structure in different sites (Fig. 12.32). A yellow specialized portion of the retina is

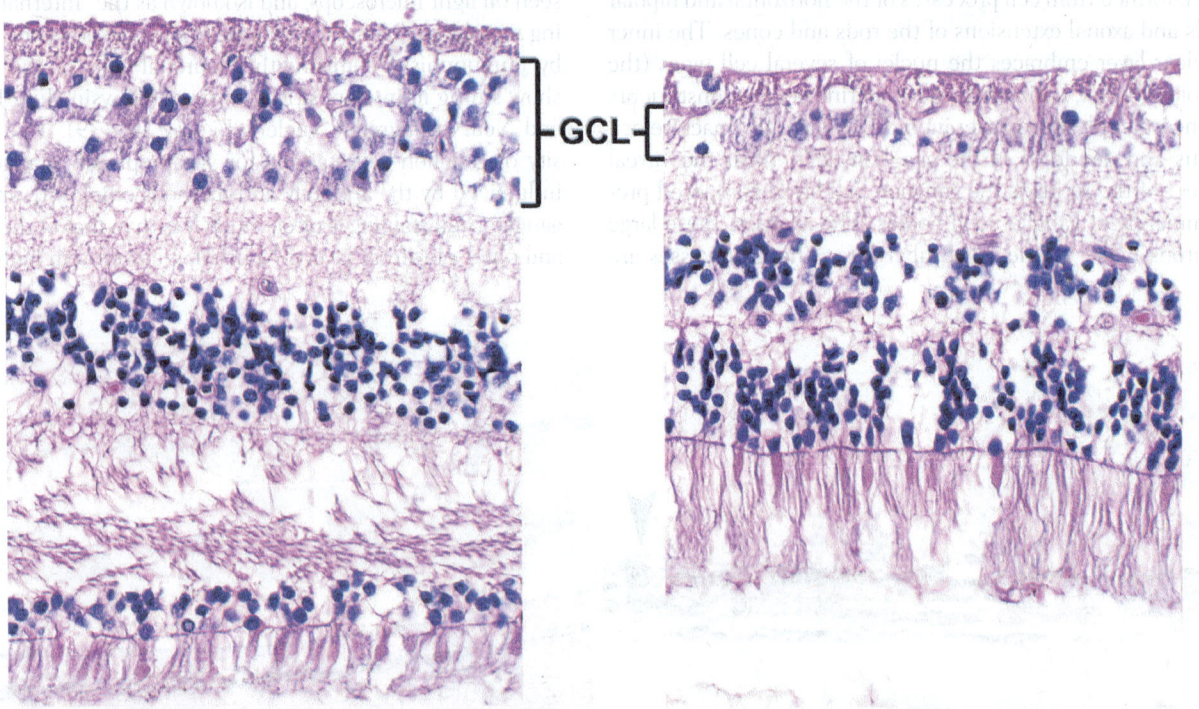

FIGURE 12.32 The retina has regional histologic variations. In the macular region (*left*), the neurosensory retina is thick and ganglion cells (*GCL*) are multilayered. In areas outside of the macula (*right*), the neurosensory retina thins and ganglion cells (*GCL*) form a single layer and then become sparse as one approaches the ora serrata (*left* and *right*, H&E).

located in the posterior pole of the eye (in an area slightly temporal to the optic disc). This is the macula lutea (yellow spot), where the bipolar and ganglion cells contain the pigment xanthophyll. In the macular region of the retina, the ganglion cells are several layers thick. The center of the macula contains a slightly depressed area (the fovea centralis) measuring almost 1.5 mm in diameter; it is responsible for most visual acuity. The walls of the fovea centralis are known as the clivus, and the precise center is designated the foveola. Blood vessels are absent in the foveola, which measures approximately 0.4 mm in diameter. The inner layers of the retina are displaced peripherally in the foveola so that only the photoreceptors, the outer nuclear layer, and the outer plexiform layer are present. Cones are located within the foveola, but rods are absent.

The microvasculature of the normal retina is composed of branches of the central retinal artery and tributaries of the central retinal vein. It contains arterioles, venules, and intervening capillaries (Fig. 12.33). In capillaries from normal individuals, endothelial cells and pericytes are present in a ratio of approximately 1:1. The retinal microvasculature is affected in hypertension, diabetes mellitus, and other conditions. Capillary microaneurysms and the loss of capillary pericytes are characteristics of diabetic retinopathy. These are best visualized in flat preparations of the retina after trypsin digestion of the retinal cells.

Artifacts of the Retina

It is necessary to distinguish a true detachment of the neurosensory retina from the retinal pigment epithelium from an artifactitious retinal detachment in the same location. True detachments of the neurosensory retina are characterized by the presence of blood or eosinophilic proteinaceous fluid in the space between the two retinal layers (Fig. 12.34), rounded edges at the site of the retinal break (if present in the section), photoreceptor elements of one

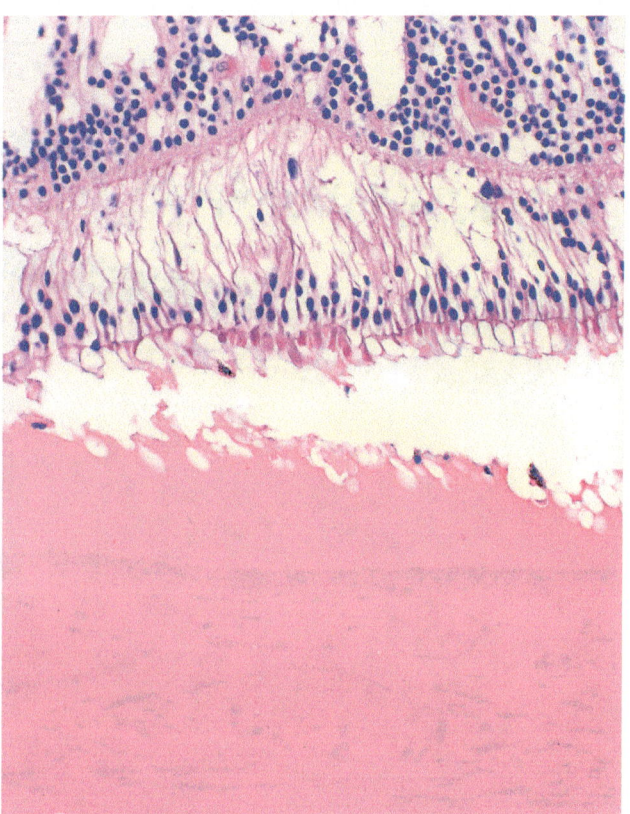

FIGURE 12.34 A feature of a true retinal detachment is the presence of eosinophilic proteinaceous fluid within the subretinal space (H&E ×20).

fold of retina adjacent to the internal limiting membrane of another fold (the Zimmerman sign), absence of photoreceptor outer segments (except in a very acute detachment), and the presence of cyst-like spaces within the detached retina. In contrast, artifactitious retinal detachments typically lack subretinal fluid that is rich in eosinophilic protein or blood, have squared-off edges at the site of the break with intact photoreceptor outer segments, and fragments of pigment epithelium cell debris are adherent to the photoreceptor outer segments (Fig. 12.35) (40).

At the ora serrata, the neurosensory retina of neonates and children folds inwardly upon itself (the Lange fold) in eyes that have been subjected to a fixative such as formalin (Fig. 12.36). This artifact of fixation is not observed in the living eye or in unfixed enucleated eyes that have been sectioned to observe the peripheral retina. The Lange fold is thought to result from traction on the peripheral retina by a shortening of the vitreous base and posterior lens zonules caused by tissue fixation. After the age of 20, the Lange fold is not observed, presumably because the peripheral retina has become firmly bound to the subjacent retinal pigment epithelium. The convexity of this artifact of fixation is directed anteriorly and axially in neonates, but in older infants and children the fold is initiated some distance from the ora serrata, apparently because of a propensity for peripheral retinal adhesions to

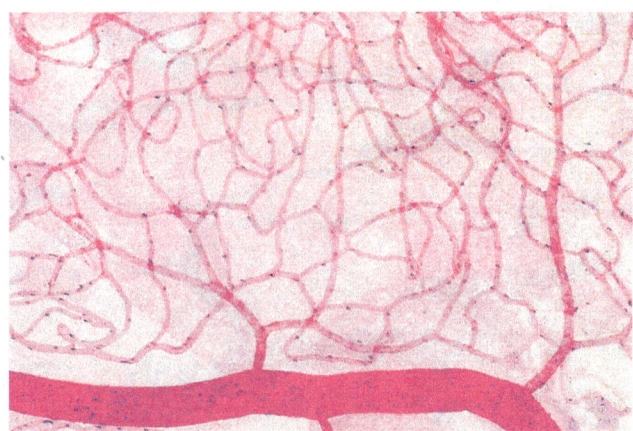

FIGURE 12.33 This flat preparation of a normal retina following trypsin digestion discloses retinal capillaries adjacent to a retinal arteriole (H&E).

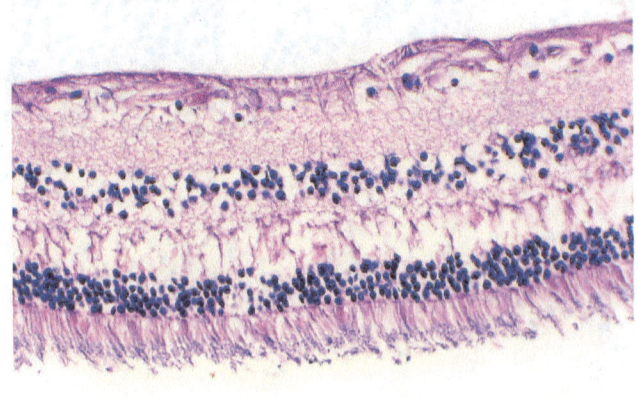

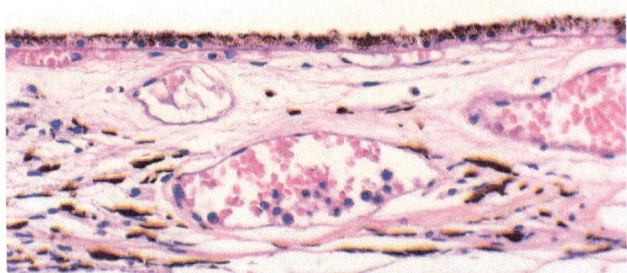

FIGURE 12.35 Artifactual retinal detachments are characterized by retinal pigment epithelium granules within the tips of the photoreceptors and the absence of subretinal eosinophilic fluid (H&E).

the subjacent retinal pigment epithelium with increasing age. In contrast to a true retinal detachment, subretinal fluid is not present between the layers of the neurosensory retina in Lange folds (41).

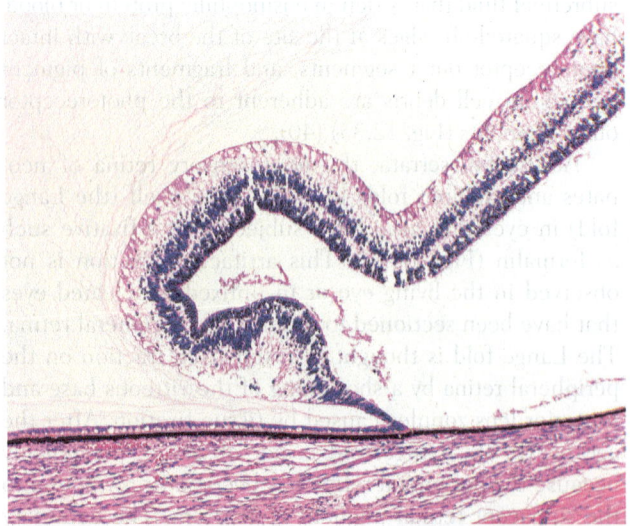

FIGURE 12.36 The Lange fold is a postmortem artifact usually seen in infant eyes. At the ora serrata the peripheral retina typically takes on a bowed or concave appearance anteriorly. The absence of subretinal fluid distinguishes this from a true retinal detachment (H&E).

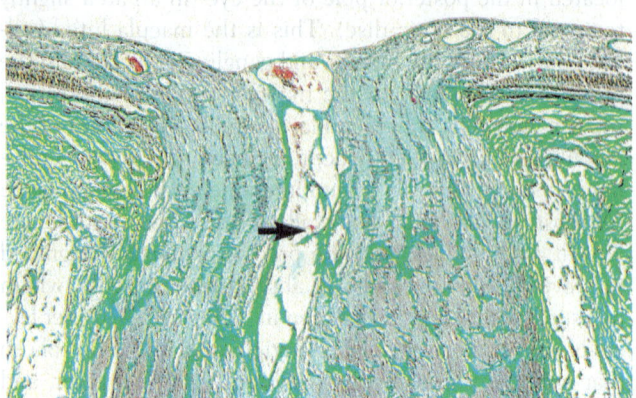

FIGURE 12.37 The optic nerve penetrates the sclera near the posterior pole of the eye. This histologic section contains the central retinal artery (*arrow*) in the central part of the optic nerve. Both the central retinal artery and the central retinal vein traverse the optic nerve until they exit the nerve about 8 to 15 mm posterior to the eyeball (Masson trichrome).

THE OPTIC NERVE

More than one million axons from the retinal nerve fiber layer converge at the optic nerve head, which accounts for the physiologic blind spot in the normal visual field and represents the beginning of the optic nerve. The central retinal artery and vein traverse the optic nerve and within a slight depression at the origin of the nerve, they are surrounded by glial tissue (Fig. 12.37). From the optic nerve head, the axons extend for approximately 1 mm to a sieve-like partition of connective tissue in the sclera (the lamina cribrosa) through which the nerve fibers pass on their way to the brain. Over one thousand nerve fiber bundles surrounded by astrocytes, oligodendroglia, and collagenous septa (Fig. 12.38) can be identified in cross sections of the optic nerve, which is a tract of the central nervous system. Like the brain, the optic nerve is surrounded by pia mater, arachnoid, and dura. Small

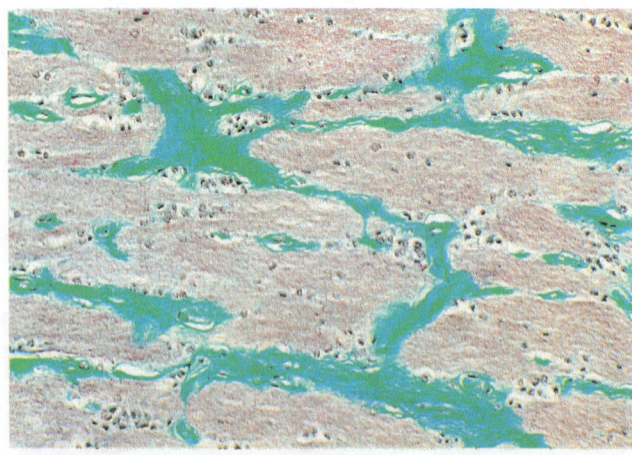

FIGURE 12.38 Nerve fiber bundles within the optic nerve are surrounded by thin collagenous septa (Masson trichrome).

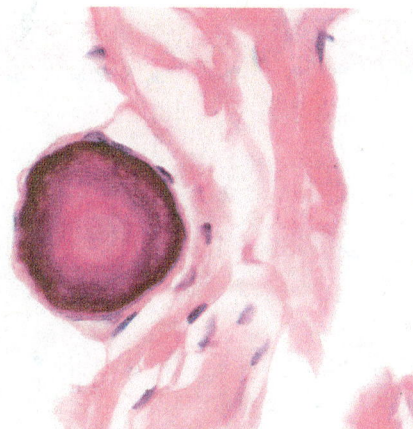

FIGURE 12.39 Laminated psammoma bodies, such as this one, are often closely associated with the meningothelial cells of the optic nerve (H&E).

focal meningothelial proliferations occasionally form within the leptomeninges surrounding the optic nerve. Some orbital meningiomas presumably arise from them. Laminated products of the meningothelial cells (psammoma bodies) sometimes occur in the arachnoid mater (Fig. 12.39). Pigmented melanocytes are sometimes encountered within the leptomeninges and the optic nerve head.

After leaving the globe, each optic nerve continues posteriorly through the orbit to its respective optic foramen, and then to the optic chiasm, before terminating in the lateral geniculate bodies.

At the level of the lamina cribrosa, the axons within the optic nerve become myelinated by concentric membranous processes of the oligodendroglia. The rather abrupt transition between myelinated and nonmyelinated nerve fibers is eminently appreciated in tissue sections stained with Luxol fast blue or other dyes with an affinity for myelin (Fig. 12.40). As the axons acquire myelin coats, the diameter of the optic nerve doubles to nearly 3 mm. Located within the central core of the optic nerve, adjacent to the globe, is the central retinal artery and vein. Both of these vascular channels exit the nerve some 8 to 15 mm posterior to the lamina cribrosa; the channels are not evident within tissue sections of the optic nerve closer to the brain. The orbital portion of the optic nerve extends some 25 mm from the lamina cribrosa to the optic foramen at the apex of the orbit. If the optic nerve becomes compressed during enucleation of the globe, some optic nerve tissue may extrude into the eye and become dislodged into the lumen of blood vessels near the optic discs, between the neurosensory retina and the retinal pigment epithelium, and even into the vitreous. Neural tissue within the optic nerve may become displaced, in a manner comparable to the "toothpaste" artifact of the spinal cord that follows a traumatic insinuation of white matter into the gray matter. This artifact should not be mistaken for ectopic intraocular nervous tissue, tumors, giant drusen, vitreous worms, or subretinal exudates (42).

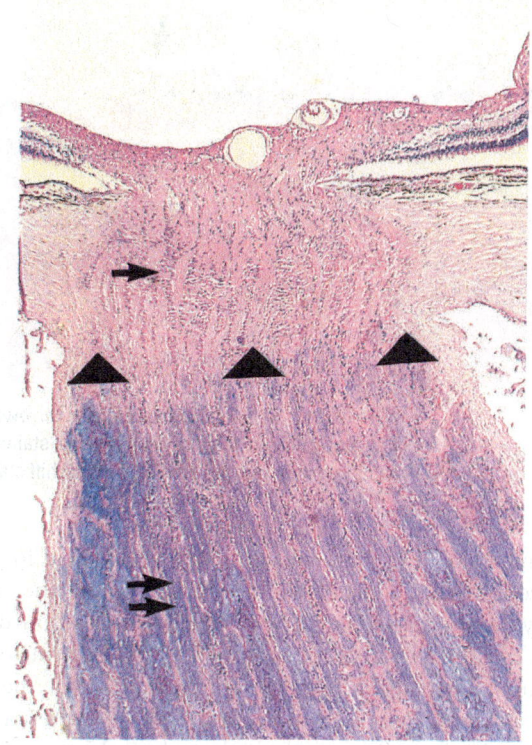

FIGURE 12.40 The abrupt transition between nonmyelinated (*arrow*) and myelinated (*double arrows*) nerve fibers of the normal optic nerve at the level of the lamina cribrosa (*arrowheads*) is dramatically illustrated in this tissue section stained with a dye that has an affinity for myelin (Luxol fast blue).

With age, corpora amylacea, similar to those in the retina and brain, may become evident in the optic nerve.

THE CRYSTALLINE LENS

The biconvex ocular lens (Fig. 12.41) is located directly behind the pupil and in front of the anterior face of the vitreous. In the adult, it measures approximately 10 mm in

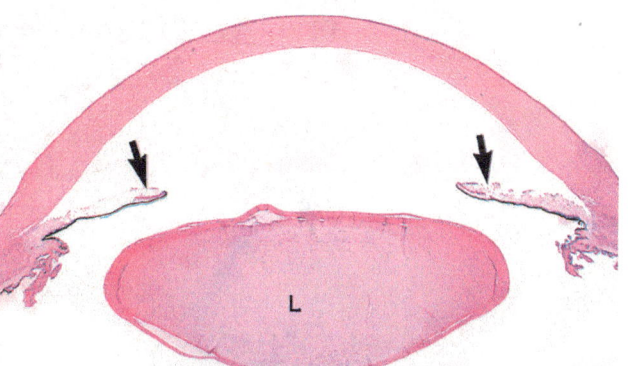

FIGURE 12.41 The crystalline lens (*L*) is situated just posterior to the pupil and iris (*arrows*) (H&E).

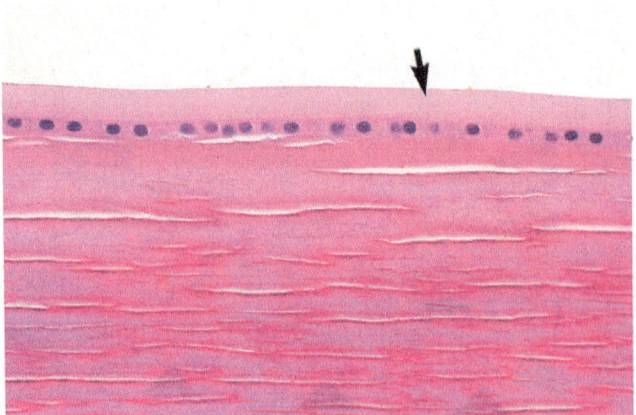 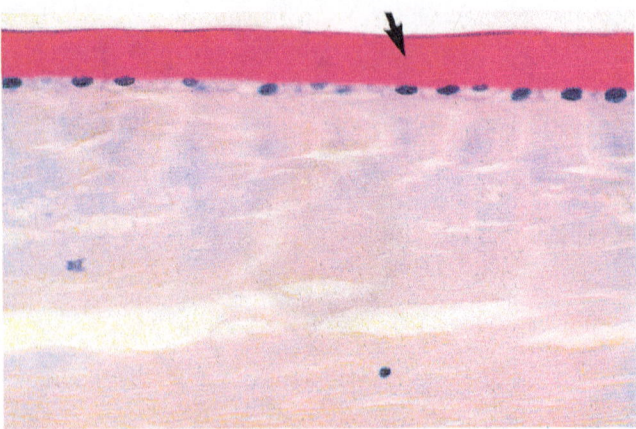

FIGURE 12.42 The anterior lens capsule (*arrow*) appears as an eosinophilic acellular band overlying a single layer of epithelial cells in hematoxylin and eosin–stained preparations (*left*). The lens capsule is rich in carbohydrate and reacts intensely with the periodic acid–Schiff stain (*arrow*) (*right*) (*left*, H&E; *right*, periodic acid–Schiff).

diameter and 4 to 5 mm in width. The lens is held in place by zonules that connect it to the pars plicata of the ciliary body. The lens is encircled by a collagen- and carbohydrate-rich capsule which serves as the site of attachment for the zonules. The capsule over the anterior surface of the lens thickens with time. At 2 to 5 years of age, the anterior capsule varies from 8 μm wide at the pole to 15 μm wide at its maximum and by 35 years of age the capsular thickness increases to 14 μm at the pole and 21 μm at its maximum (Fig. 12.42). The posterior lens capsule at 2 to 5 years of age is 2 μm at the pole and 18 μm maximally near the posterior periphery; reaches its maximum thickness at about 35 years of age (4 to 23 μm); and then diminishes to 2 to 9 μm at the age of 71 (Fig. 12.43) (3,6). Directly interior to the anterior lens capsule is a single layer of cuboidal epithelium. These cells extend to about the level of the lens equator; they do not normally exist posterior to this point. Proliferating epithelial cells elongate at the lens equator and become displaced toward the center of the lens, known as the lens nucleus, where they are retained for life. This process continues throughout life and the long slender cells are designated lens fibers. In the peripheral part of the lens near the equator, the fibers retain their nuclei, but as the fibers become displaced toward the center of the lens their nuclei disintegrate so that the center of the lens lacks nuclei. In some cataractous lenses, such as the cataract of rubella, the fibers within the center of the lens retain their nuclei.

The normally transparent lens commonly opacifies with age. Discrete globules of degenerate lens fibers may form. They are frequently accompanied by the presence of an extension of epithelial cells, posterior to the equator. The high density of the lens fibers makes it difficult to obtain histologic sections of the lens that are free from artifact.

Infant eyes can demonstrate an artifact of fixation resulting in an umbilicated, dimpled, or concave configuration of the posterior surface of the lens (Fig. 12.44) (43,44).

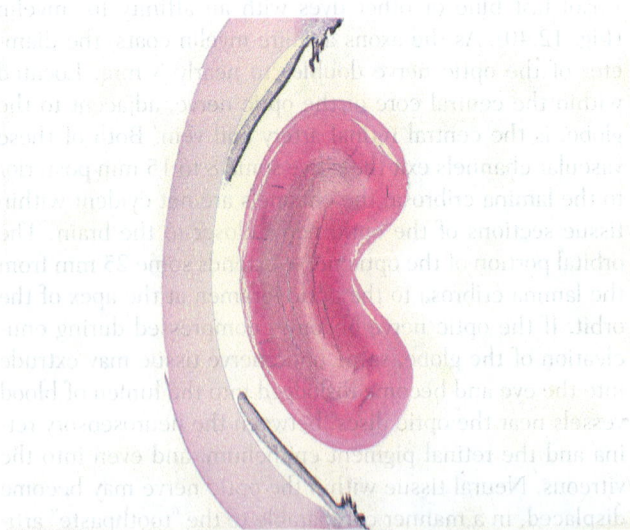

FIGURE 12.43 Posteriorly, the lens capsule (*arrow*) is thinner than anteriorly, and epithelial cells are absent (H&E).

FIGURE 12.44 Infant eye demonstrating an artifact of fixation resulting in a posterior concave or umbilicated appearance to the crystalline lens. This figure also illustrates an artifactual absence of most of the corneal epithelium, a very common finding in postmortem eyes (H&E).

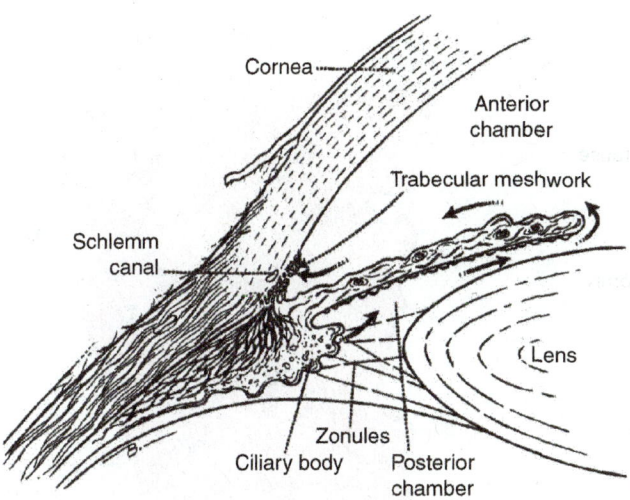

FIGURE 12.45 The anterior chamber is defined by the cornea, the anterior surface of the iris, and the pupil. The boundaries of the much smaller posterior chamber include the posterior surface of the iris, the ciliary body, and the anterior face of the vitreous. The aqueous is produced by the ciliary body and circulates from the posterior chamber through the pupil into the anterior chamber. The aqueous drains from the eye by way of the trabecular meshwork and the Schlemm canal. (Reproduced with permission from Klintworth GK, Landers MB 3rd. *The Eye. Structure and Function in Disease Monograph Series.* Baltimore, MD: Williams & Wilkins; 1976.)

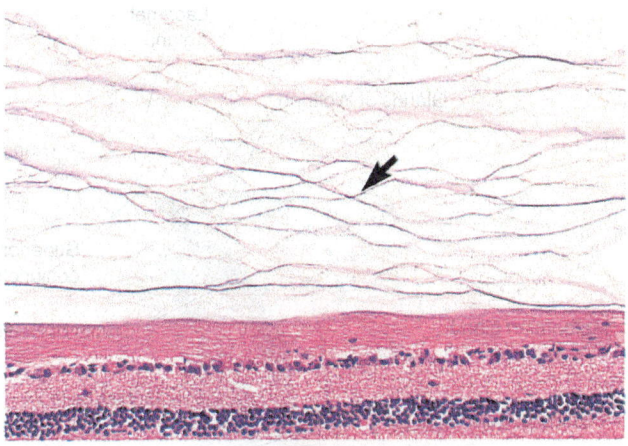

FIGURE 12.46 The vitreous (*arrow*) appears as an amorphous material, usually strands, in standard tissue sections (H&E).

INTRAOCULAR COMPARTMENTS

The eye accommodates two major fluid-containing intraocular compartments. One is filled with aqueous humor, the other with vitreous humor. The aqueous compartment is divided into an anterior and a posterior chamber (Fig. 12.45). The anterior chamber is delineated in front by the cornea, peripherally by the drainage angle of the eye, and posteriorly by the pupil and the iris. The small posterior chamber is situated between the pigmented epithelia of the iris, the ciliary body, the anterior face of the vitreous, and the lens. The aqueous humor, a watery solution that does not normally stain with routine histologic techniques, is produced by the ciliary body and flows forward through the aperture of the pupil to the anterior chamber, where it leaves the eye through the trabecular meshwork and the Schlemm canal. The anterior chamber contains approximately 0.25 mL of aqueous humor; the posterior chamber has a volume of only approximately 0.06 mL. Normal human aqueous humor has a density slightly greater than water, and like plasma, it contains protein, ascorbic acid, electrolytes, and glucose. The major differences between aqueous humor and plasma are the relatively low-protein and high-ascorbic acid concentration of aqueous, relative to plasma.

The vitreous extends from the neurosensory retina to the lens and contains a gel-like material composed of water, protein, hyaluronic acid, and a small population of cells, designated hyalocytes, that are rarely noted in standard tissue sections. These tissue macrophages are thought to synthesize collagen and hyaluronic acid. The gelatinous consistency of the vitreous is due to a framework of numerous, randomly oriented collagen fibrils. The concentration of glucose and ascorbic acid is much lower than in the aqueous, whereas the concentration of soluble protein is similar to that of the aqueous (45,46). The vitreous is attached securely to the retina at the ora serrata and near the optic disc. Occasionally, vitreous may be identified as an amorphous acellular material on H&E-stained sections (Fig. 12.46).

THE EYELIDS

The eyelids (Fig. 12.47) can be divided into cutaneous and conjunctival portions. The cutaneous segment of the eyelid is composed of a stratified squamous epidermis overlying a loosely arranged dermis, beneath which is the muscular tissue. The eyelids contain several types of skin appendages. Sebaceous glands deposit their secretions together with decomposed whole cells via ducts, into hair follicles of the eyelashes (glands of Zeis), or into ducts that open into the lid margins (meibomian glands) (Fig. 12.48). Apocrine glands, whose secretions represent the pinched-off luminal aspect of the lining acinar cells, also open into the follicles of the eyelashes (glands of Moll) (Fig. 12.49). In addition, the dermis of the eyelid contains eccrine sweat glands, which discharge secretions directly onto the skin via a convoluted duct. The subcutaneous portion of the upper and lower eyelids contains concentrically arranged skeletal muscle fibers (orbicularis oculi), but very little adipose connective tissue. The striated muscle of the palpebral portion of the levator palpebrae superioris is also present in the upper eyelid; it terminates in a dense fibrocollagenous aponeurosis. Small bundles of smooth muscle fibers (the Müller muscle) are located within the upper and lower eyelids and aid in raising the upper eyelids, lowering the lower lids, and keeping the eyelids open.

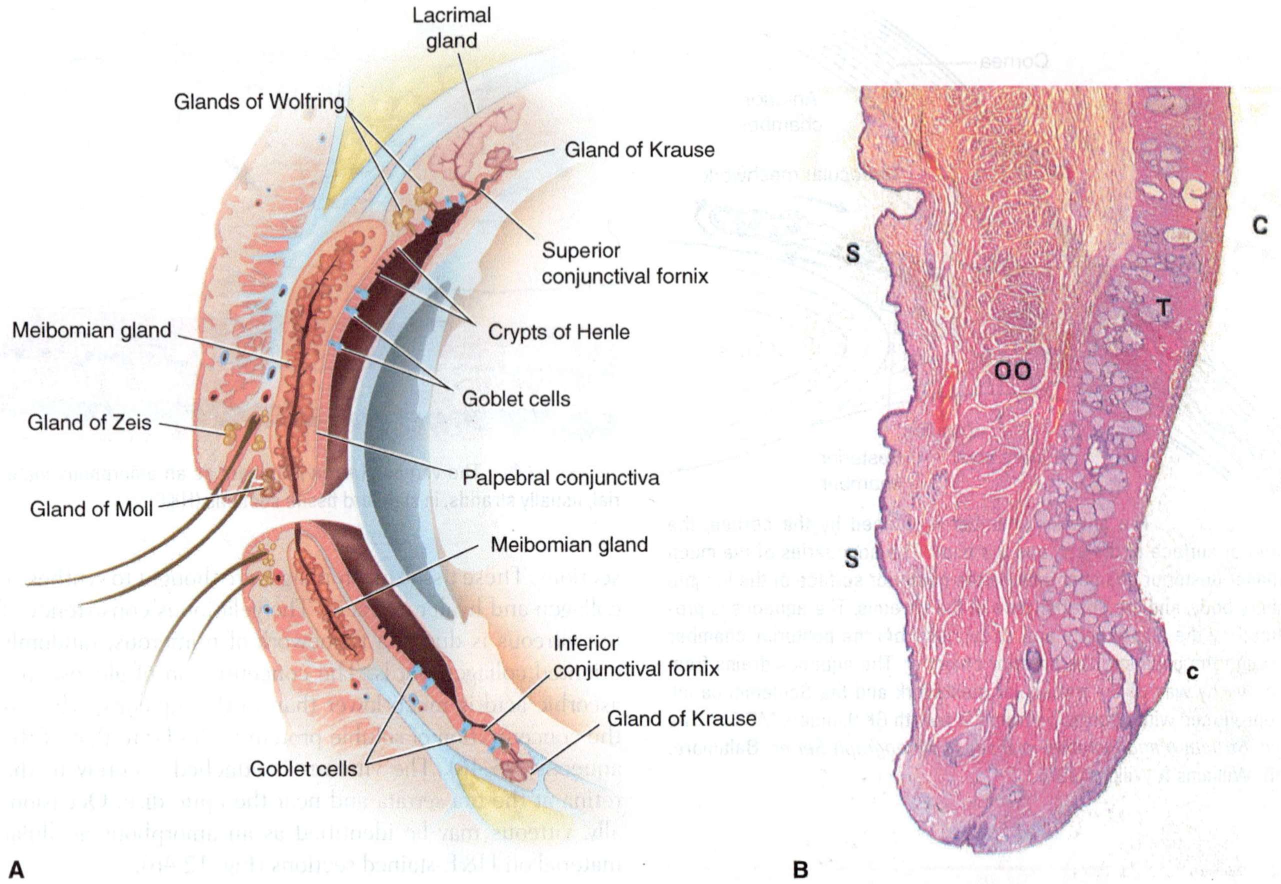

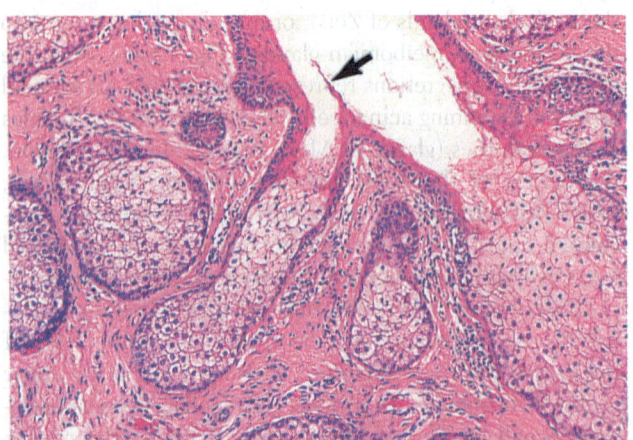

FIGURE 12.47 **A:** Components of the eyelid as illustrated in this drawing include skin, cutaneous appendages (glands of Zeiss and Moll), muscle, connective tissue, meibomian glands, conjunctiva, and accessory lacrimal gland tissue (glands of Krause and Wolfring). **B:** The skin surface (*S*), the orbicularis oculi muscle (*OO*), the tarsus (*T*), and the conjunctiva (*c*) are evident in this histologic section of an eyelid (H&E). (Figure 12.47A: Reproduced with permission from Freddo TF, Chaum E. *Anatomy of the Eye and Orbit. The Clinical Essentials*. Philadelphia, PA: Wolters Kluwer; 2018.)

The junction between the cutaneous and conjunctival parts of the eyelid is demarcated clinically by a sulcus (the gray line), located between the orifices of the meibomian glands and the eyelashes. The conjunctival portion of the eyelid is made up of dense connective tissue containing the meibomian glands (the tarsus) and the palpebral conjunctiva (Fig. 12.50). The tarsus, located immediately posterior to the muscles of the eyelid, accounts for most

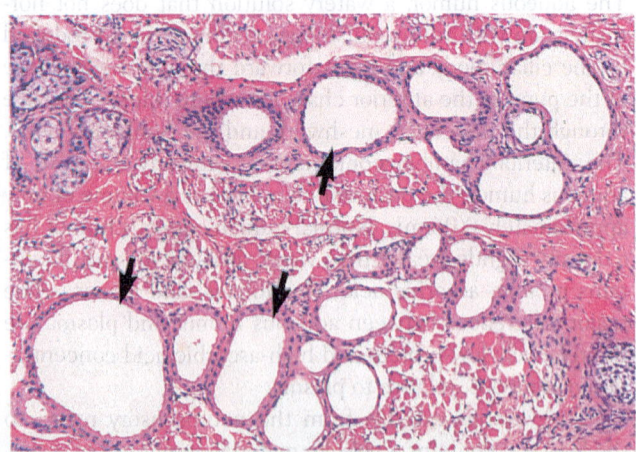

FIGURE 12.48 Modified sebaceous glands, the meibomian glands, deposit secretions into ducts opening onto the eyelids. A valve is evident (*arrow*) in this duct of a meibomian gland (H&E).

FIGURE 12.49 Apocrine glands (glands of Moll) (*arrows*) occur in the eyelid and open into the follicles of the eyelashes (H&E).

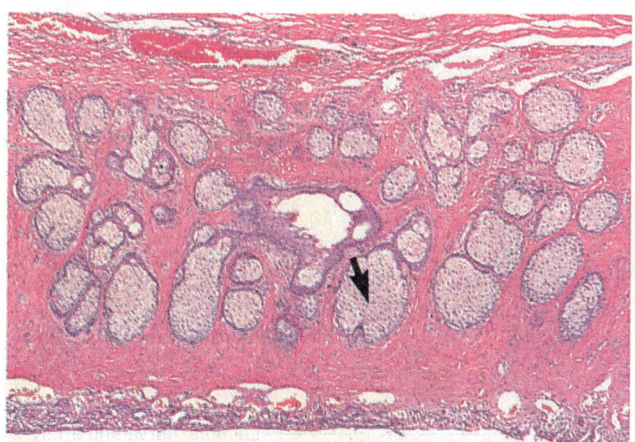

FIGURE 12.50 The tarsus, composed of dense fibrous tissue, contains the meibomian glands (*arrow*). The palpebral conjunctiva is immediately beneath the tarsus at the bottom of this figure (H&E).

of the rigidity of the eyelids and is covered posteriorly by conjunctival epithelium and a thin subepithelial stroma. As described earlier, accessory lacrimal glands are present in the palpebral conjunctiva.

The presence of more prominent subcutaneous, suborbicularis, and pretarsal fat tissue in the upper eyelid (the pretarsal fat pad) distinguishes an Asian eyelid from a Caucasian eyelid (47).

THE ORBIT

The posterior and peripheral borders of the orbit are defined by bones of the skull, face, and nose. At the anterior orbital margin, the periosteum of the orbital bones gives rise to a dense connective tissue sheet (the orbital septum) that extends forward to insert into the eyelids (Fig. 12.47). Tissue posterior to this septum is considered to be within the orbit. The human adult orbit is pyramidal and has a volume of approximately 25 cm^3, with the globe contributing about 7.2 to 8.2 cm^3 of the volume (4). The dimensions of the orbit are quite variable, but the anterior entrance is on average 3.5 cm in height and 4.0 cm in width (3). Orbital depth averages about 4.9 cm with a range from 4.1 to 5.7 cm (48). Several bony canals allow for transmission of blood vessels and nerves into and out of the orbit, posteriorly. The contents of the orbit are organized in a complex three-dimensional arrangement (Fig. 12.51). Aside from the eye, the optic nerve and its meningeal coverings, the Tenon capsule, the extraocular muscles, the lacrimal gland, blood vessels, and a delicate framework of fibroadipose connective tissue constitute the major components of the orbit.

The only epithelial structure normally present in the orbit is the lacrimal gland (Fig. 12.52). Closely apposed to the globe and situated in the superolateral aspect of the orbit, this gland is traditionally divided into two parts: a larger orbital lobe and a smaller palpebral lobe. About a dozen ducts from the lacrimal gland open into the superior conjunctival fornices and transmit their secretions into the tear film. The lacrimal gland is not encapsulated, and thin fibrovascular connective tissue septa divide the tissue into lobules composed of acini lined by columnar epithelial cells. Occasionally, some lobules extend posteriorly behind the globe. Most cells are serous in type and contain scattered intracytoplasmic fat droplets and many PAS-positive secretory granules. Myoepithelial cells, inconspicuous in routine H&E-stained sections, surround the acini and intercalated ducts (49). Mucinous cells similar to those of salivary glands are not usually present in the acini but may be identified in the ducts. Occasional lymphocytes and plasma cells are commonly present between the acini of the lacrimal gland. With increasing age, the orbital lobes of lacrimal glands in women exhibit increasing diffuse fibrosis, diffuse atrophy, and periductal fibrosis, while men have increasing periductal fibrosis of their palpebral lobes (49).

The orbit contains the cranial nerves, which innervate the extrinsic muscles of the eye (oculomotor, trochlear, and abducens nerves) and branches of the ophthalmic division of the trigeminal nerve, as well as the parasympathetic and sympathetic nerves that innervate the cornea, conjunctiva, and the muscles of the ciliary body and iris. Neurons of the ciliary ganglion, which is located near the optic nerve close to the orbital apex and which measures approximately 2 mm in diameter, receive parasympathetic and sympathetic nerve fibers.

Other constituents of the orbit include smooth muscle (Fig. 12.53) (4,50) and the arc-shaped structure (trochlea), through which the tendon of the superior oblique muscle passes before insertion upon the eyeball (Fig. 12.54). The trochlea is the only cartilaginous structure normally present in the orbit. It arises from the superior nasal aspect of the frontal bone. Smooth muscle forms the orbital muscle of Müller (4) and is present within some of the fibrous septa that are crucial for normal support and motion of the globe (4,50). The Tenon capsule contains smooth muscle within its elastic and fibrovascular tissue anteriorly but not posteriorly (25).

Lymphatic channels do not exist in the orbit according to traditional teaching, but they have now been identified using immunohistochemical staining in the extraocular muscles, lacrimal gland, and optic nerve sheath (51,52) and may possibly arise within the orbital adipose tissue as a result of inflammation (51). The orbit normally lacks lymphoid tissue but contains scattered lymphocytes. These cells presumably give rise to the monoclonal and polyclonal lymphoid proliferations that frequently develop within the orbit, creating diagnostic and prognostic difficulty for the pathologist (53,54).

LACRIMAL DRAINAGE APPARATUS

The lacrimal drainage apparatus (Fig. 12.55), composed of the puncta, canaliculi, lacrimal sac, and the nasolacrimal duct, collects the tears and drains them to the nose. Tear fluid drains toward the medial canthus and then passes

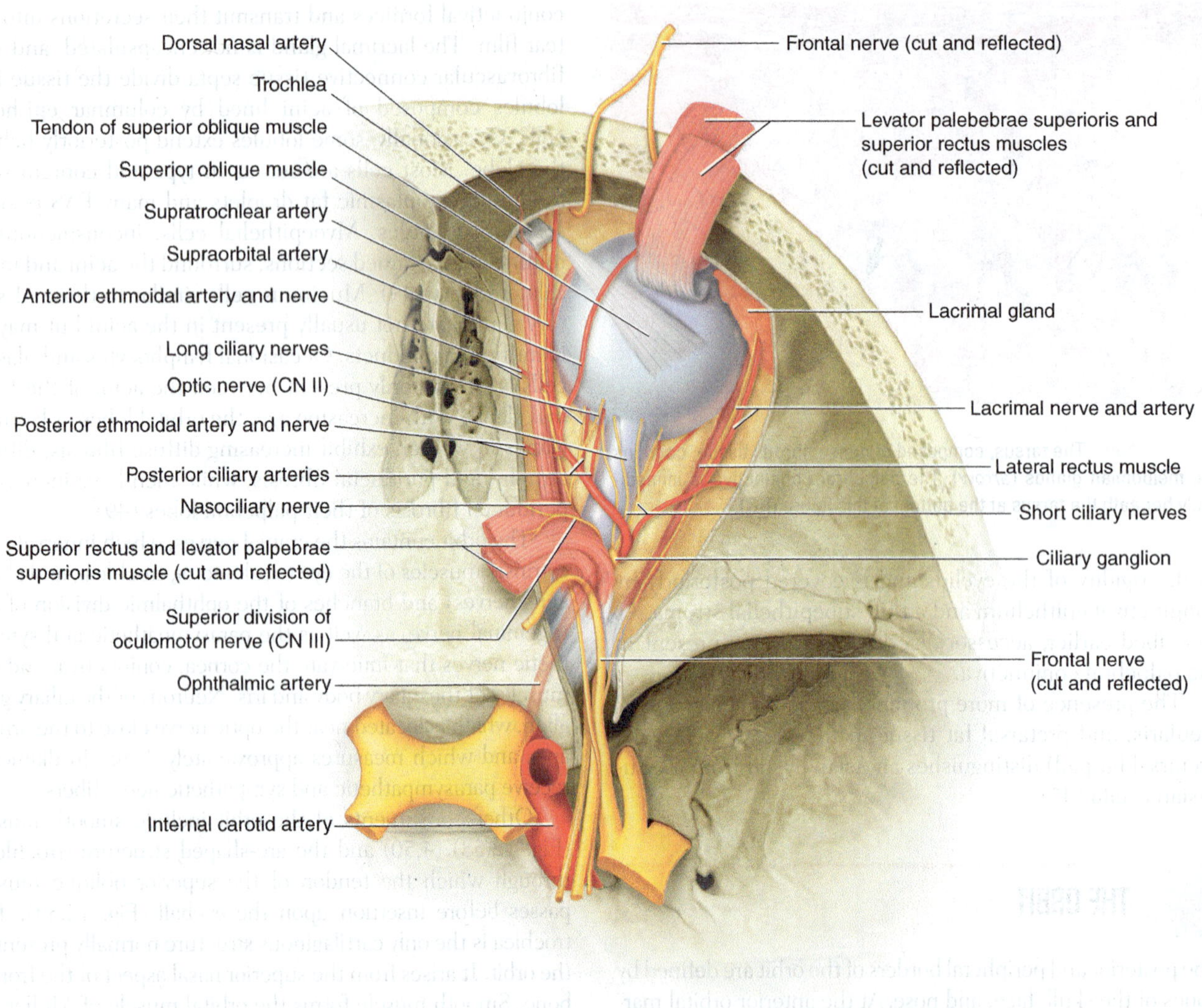

FIGURE 12.51 The bony cavity of the orbit contains the eyeball and its fibrous covering (the Tenon capsule), the cartilaginous trochlea, the lacrimal gland, the extraocular muscles, blood vessels, nerves, and fibrovascular connective tissue. The trochlea and the lacrimal gland are located within the superonasal and superotemporal aspects of the orbit, respectively. Some of the extraocular muscles originate from a ring of fibrous tissue in the posterior orbit known as the annulus of Zinn. (Reproduced with permission from Freddo TF, Chaum E. *Anatomy of the Eye and Orbit. The Clinical Essentials*. Philadelphia, PA: Wolters Kluwer; 2018.)

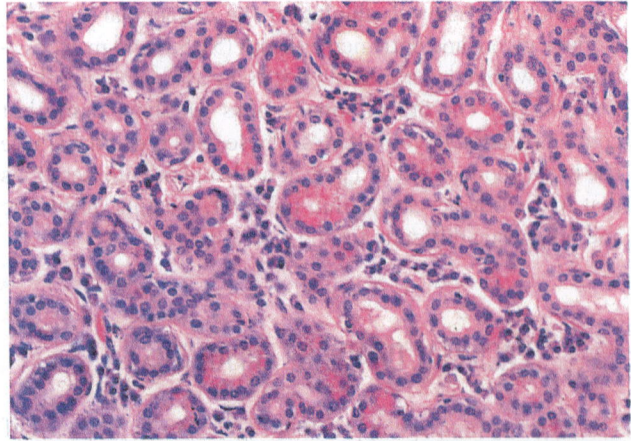

FIGURE 12.52 Acini of the lacrimal gland are lined by columnar epithelial cells. Scattered lymphocytes and plasma cells are normally present in the gland. Flattened myoepithelial cells are evident around some of the acini, such as the one near the center of the photomicrograph (H&E).

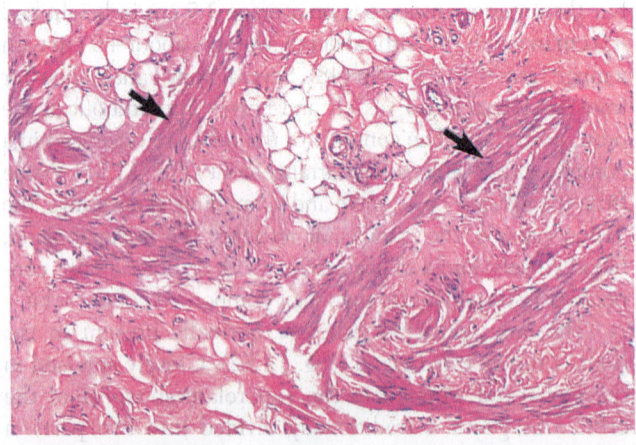

FIGURE 12.53 Fibrous septa of the orbit, critical for normal support and motion of the globe, may contain smooth muscle bundles (*arrows*) (H&E).

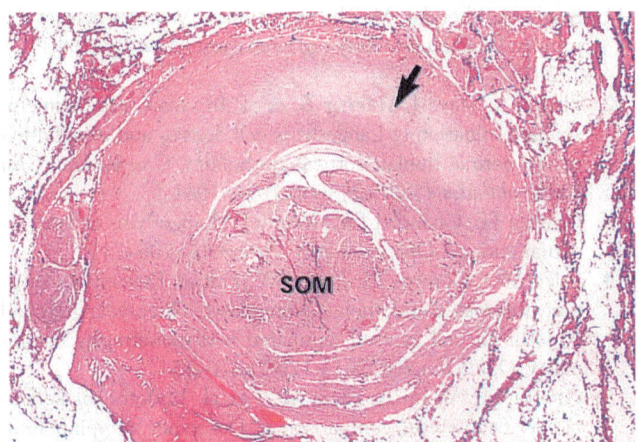

FIGURE 12.54 The arc-shaped trochlea (*arrow*), the only cartilaginous structure of the normal orbit, envelops the skeletal muscle fibers of the superior oblique muscle (*SOM*) (H&E).

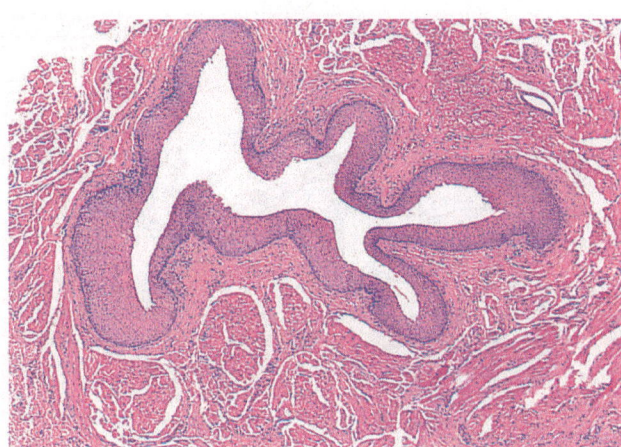

FIGURE 12.56 The lacrimal canaliculi are lined by nonkeratinizing stratified squamous epithelium and are surrounded by fibrous tissue (H&E).

through an opening in the medial aspect of each eyelid, known as the lacrimal punctum. The puncta drain into the lacrimal canaliculi, tubular structures approximately 0.5 mm in diameter. Initially, the canaliculi are oriented vertically, but within 2 mm of their origin, bend at right angles to become almost horizontal within the eyelids. The distal portions of the canaliculi exit the upper and lower eyelids.

They merge to form the lacrimal sac, which is encased by bones located in the inferomedial wall of the orbit. A duct (the nasolacrimal duct) that is nearly 1 cm long drains the lacrimal sac into the inferior nasal meatus of the nose. The epithelium lining the lacrimal drainage apparatus varies in different regions (55). In the canaliculi, it is a nonkeratinizing stratified squamous epithelium (Fig. 12.56), but in the

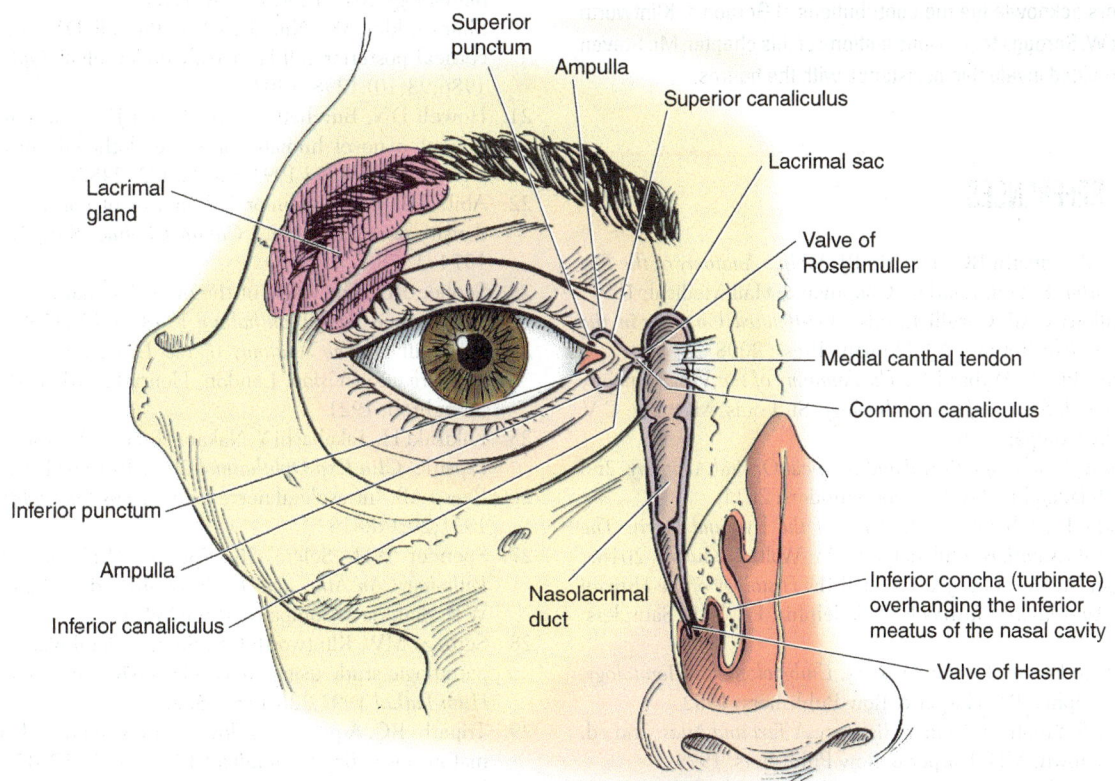

FIGURE 12.55 The lacrimal gland and drainage apparatus are illustrated here. The lacrimal gland is located in the superotemporal aspect of the orbit and contributes secretions to the tear film. Tears enter the canaliculi through the puncta and drain through the nasolacrimal sac and duct, to eventually reach the inferior meatus within the nose. (Reproduced with permission from Freddo TF, Chaum E. *Anatomy of the Eye and Orbit. The Clinical Essentials*. Philadelphia, PA: Wolters Kluwer; 2018.)

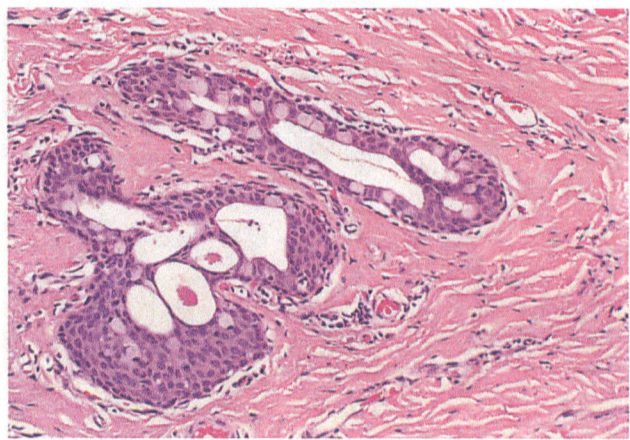

FIGURE 12.57 The epithelium of the lacrimal sacs and ducts is stratified columnar and contains goblet cells (H&E).

lacrimal sac and duct, the epithelium is stratified columnar in type, and contains mucus-secreting goblet cells surrounded by connective tissue (Fig. 12.57).

ACKNOWLEDGMENTS

The authors acknowledge the contributions of Gordon K. Klintworth and Mark W. Scroggs to previous editions of this chapter. Mr. Steven Conlon provided invaluable assistance with the figures.

REFERENCES

1. Bron AJ, Tripathi RC, Tripathi BJ. *Wolff's Anatomy of the Eye and Orbit*. 8th ed. London: Chapman & Hall Medical; 1997.
2. Cavallotti CAP, Cerulli L, eds. *Age-Related Changes in the Human Eye*. Totowa, NJ: Humana Press; 2008.
3. Duke-Elder S, Wybar KC. *The Anatomy of the Visual System, Volume II, System of Ophthalmology*. St. Louis, MO: The C.V. Mosby Company; 1961.
4. Dutton JJ. *Atlas of Clinical and Surgical Orbital Anatomy*. 2nd ed. Philadelphia, PA: Elsevier Saunders; 2011.
5. Freddo TF, Chaum E. *Anatomy of the Eye and Orbit. The Clinical Essentials*. Philadelphia, PA: Wolters Kluwer; 2018.
6. Hogan MJ, Alvarado JA, Weddell JE. *Histology of the Human Eye. An Atlas and Textbook*. Philadelphia, PA: W.B. Saunders; 1971.
7. Jakobiec FA, ed. *Ocular Anatomy, Embryology, and Teratology*. Philadelphia, PA: Harper & Row Publishers; 1982.
8. Fine BS, Yanoff M. *Ocular Histology. A Text and Atlas*. 2nd ed. Hagerstown, MD: Harper & Row Publishers; 1979.
9. Fledelius HC, Christensen AC. Reappraisal of the human ocular growth curve in fetal life, infancy, and early childhood. *Br J Ophthalmol* 1996;80(10):918–921.
10. Harayama K, Amemiya T, Nishimura H. Development of the eyeball during fetal life. *J Pediatr Ophthalmol and Strabismus* 1981;18(4):37–40.
11. Sorsby A, Sheridan M. The eye at birth: Measurement of the principal diameters in forty-eight cadavers. *J Anat* 1960;94(Pt 2):192–197.
12. Zhivov A, Stave J, Vollmar B, et al. In vivo confocal microscopic evaluation of Langerhans cell density and distribution in the normal human corneal epithelium. *Graefes Arch Clin Exp Ophthalmol* 2005;243(10):1056–1061.
13. Gillette TE, Chandler JW, Greiner JV. Langerhans cells of the ocular surface. *Ophthalmology* 1982;89(6):700–711.
14. Price MO, Gorovoy M, Price FW Jr, et al. Descemet's stripping automated endothelial keratoplasty: Three-year graft and endothelial cell survival compared with penetrating keratoplasty. *Ophthalmology* 2013;120(2):246–251.
15. Guerra FP, Anshu A, Price MO, et al. Endothelial keratoplasty: Fellow eyes comparison of Descemet stripping automated endothelial keratoplasty and Descemet membrane endothelial keratoplasty. *Cornea* 2011;30(12):1382–1386.
16. Dua HS, Said DG. Pre-Descemets endothelial keratoplasty: The PDEK clamp for successful PDEK. *Eye (Lond)* 2017;31(7):1106–1110.
17. McTigue JW. The human cornea: A light and electron microscopic study of the normal cornea and its alterations in various dystrophies. *Trans Am Ophthalmol Soc* 1967;65:591–660.
18. Schlötzer-Schrehardt U, Bachmann BO, Laaser K, et al. Characterization of the cleavage plane in Descemet's membrane endothelial keratoplasty. *Ophthalmology* 2011;118(10):1950–1957.
19. Dua HS, Faraj LA, Said DG, et al. Human corneal anatomy redefined: A novel pre-Descemet's layer (Dua's layer). *Ophthalmology* 2013;120(9):1778–1785.
20. Shamsuddin AK, Nirankari VS, Purnell DM, et al. Is the corneal posterior cell layer truly endothelial? *Ophthalmology* 1986;93(10):1298–1303.
21. Howell DN, Burchette JL Jr, Paolini JF, et al. Characterization of a novel human corneal endothelial antigen. *Invest Ophthalmol Vis Sci* 1991;32(9):2473–2482.
22. Abib FC, Barreto Junior J. Behavior of corneal endothelial density over a lifetime. *J Cataract Refract Surg* 2001;27(10):1574–1578.
23. Scobee RG. The fascia of the orbit: Its anatomy and clinical significance. *Am J Ophthalmol* 1948;31(12):1539–1553.
24. Whitnall E. *The Anatomy of the Human Orbit and Accessory Organs of Vision*. London: Henry Frowde and Hodder & Stoughton; 1921.
25. Kakizaki H, Takahashi Y, Nakano T, et al. Anatomy of Tenons capsule. *Clin Exp Ophthalmol* 2012;40(6):611–616.
26. Reese AB. Intrascleral nerve loops. *Trans Am Ophthalmol Soc* 1931;29:148–153.
27. Spencer WH. Sclera. In: Spencer WH, ed. *Ophthalmic Pathology: An Atlas and Textbook*. 4th ed. Philadelphia, PA: W.B. Saunders Company; 1996:334–371.
28. Scroggs MW, Klintworth GK. Senile scleral plaques: A histopathologic study using energy-dispersive x-ray microanalysis. *Hum Pathol* 1991;22(6):557–562.
29. Tripathi RC. Aqueous outflow pathway in normal and glaucomatous eyes. *Br J Ophthalmol* 1972;56(3):157–174.
30. Kessing SV. Mucus gland system of the conjunctiva. A quantitative normal anatomical study. *Acta Ophthalmol (Copenh)* 1968;Suppl 95:1–133.
31. Ring HG, Fujino T. Observations on the anatomy and pathology of the choroidal vasculature. *Arch Ophthalmol* 1967;78(4):431–444.

32. Friedman E, Smith TR, Kuwabara T. Senile choroidal vascular patterns and drusen. *Arch Ophthalmol* 1963;69(2):220–230.
33. Sarks SH. New vessel formation beneath the retinal pigment epithelium in senile eyes. *Br J Ophthalmol* 1973;57(12):951–965.
34. May CA. Mast cell heterogeneity in the human uvea. *Histochem Cell Biol* 1999;112(5):381–386.
35. Ezzat M, Hann C, Vuk-Pavlovic S, et al. Immune cells in the human choroid. *Br J Ophthalmol* 2008;92(7):976–980.
36. Chinnery HR, McMenamin PG, Dando SJ. Macrophage physiology in the eye. *Pflugers Arch* 2017;469(3–4):501–515.
37. Chang JH, McCluskey P, Wakefield D. Expression of toll-like receptor 4 and its associated lipopolysaccharide receptor complex by resident antigen-presenting cells in the human uvea. *Invest Ophthalmol Vis Sci* 2004;45(6):1871–1878.
38. Straatsma BR, Foss RY. Typical and reticular degenerative retinoschisis. *Am J Ophthalmol* 1973;75(4):551–575.
39. Mullen RJ, Buck CR, Smith AM. NeuN, a neuronal specific nuclear protein in vertebrates. *Development* 1992;116(1):201–211.
40. Folberg R. The eye. In: Spencer WH, ed. *Ophthalmic Pathology: An Atlas and Textbook.* 4th ed. Philadelphia, PA: W.B. Saunders Company; 1996:1–37.
41. Gartner S, Henkind P. Lange's folds: A meaningful ocular artifact. *Ophthalmology* 1981;88(12):1307–1310.
42. Zimmerman LE, Fine BS. Myelin artifacts in the optic disc and retina. *Arch Ophthalmol* 1965;74:394–398.
43. Eagle RCJ. *Eye Pathology: An Atlas and Text.* 3rd ed. Philadelphia, PA: Wolters Kluwer Health/Lippincott Williams & Wilkins; 2017.
44. Herwig MC, Müller AM, Klarmann-Schulz U, et al. Lens artifacts in human fetal eyes—the challenge of interpreting the histomorphology of human fetal lenses. *Graefes Arch Clin Exp Ophthalmol* 2014;252(1):155–162.
45. Bito LZ. The physiology and pathophysiology of intraocular fluids. *Exp Eye Res* 1977;25:273–289.
46. Reddy DV, Kinsey VE. Composition of the vitreous humor in relation to that of plasma and aqueous humors. *Arch Ophthalmol* 1960;63(4):715–720.
47. Jeong S, Lemke BN, Dortzbach RK, et al. The Asian upper eyelid: An anatomical study with comparison to the Caucasian eyelid. *Arch Ophthalmol* 1999;117(7):907–912.
48. Nitek S, Wysocki J, Reymond J, et al. Correlations between selected parameters of the human skull and orbit. *Med Sci Monit* 2009;15(12):BR370–BR377.
49. Obata H. Anatomy and histopathology of the human lacrimal gland. *Cornea* 2006;25(10 Suppl 1):S82–S89.
50. Koornneef L. New insights in the human orbital connective tissue. Result of a new anatomical approach. *Arch Ophthalmol* 1977;95(7):1269–1273.
51. Dickinson AJ, Gausas RE. Orbital lymphatics: do they exist? *Eye (Lond)* 2006;20(10):1145–1148.
52. Nakao S, Hafezi-Moghadam A, Ishibashi T. Lymphatics and lymphangiogenesis in the eye. *J Ophthalmol* 2012;2012:783163.
53. Andrew NH, Coupland SE, Pirbhai A, et al. Lymphoid hyperplasia of the orbit and ocular adnexa: A clinical pathologic review. *Surv Ophthalmol* 2016;61(6):778–790.
54. Mulay K, Honavar SG. An update on ocular adnexal lymphoma. *Semin Diagn Pathol* 2016;33(3):164–172.
55. Paulsen F. *The Human Nasolacrimal Ducts.* Berlin: Springer-Verlag; 2003.

13

The Ear and Temporal Bone

Bruce M. Wenig

EMBRYOLOGY 363

EXTERNAL EAR 363
    Embryology 363

ANATOMY 364

HISTOLOGY 365

AUDITORY EPITHELIAL MIGRATION 365

MIDDLE EAR 366
    Embryology 366

ANATOMY 367

MIDDLE EAR OSSICLES AND MUSCLES 369

EUSTACHIAN (AUDITORY) TUBE 370

HISTOLOGY 370
    Tympanic Cavity Proper 370
    Eustachian Tube 370
    Mastoid Air Cells 371
    Pneumatization of the Temporal Bone 371
    Middle Ear Ossicles 371
    Middle Ear Joints 372
    Middle Ear Muscles 373

INNER EAR 373
    Embryology 373

ANATOMY 374
    Osseous Labyrinth (Otic Capsule) 374
    Membranous Labyrinth 375
    Cochlear Duct 375
    Utricle 377
    Saccule 377
    Semicircular Canals 377
    Endolymphatic Duct and Sac 378

INNER EAR INNERVATION 378

HISTOLOGY 379
    Osseous Labyrinth 379
    Membranous Labyrinth 379
    Cochlea 379
    Semicircular Canals, Utricle, and Saccule 380
    Nerves and Paraganglia 381
    Endolymphatic Sac and Duct 382

COMPOSITION AND CIRCULATION OF THE PERILYMPH AND ENDOLYMPH 383

CONDUCTION OF SOUND 383

SELECTED ABNORMALITIES AND PATHOLOGY 384
    External Ear 384

MIDDLE EAR 385
    Otitis Media 385
    Cholesteatoma (Keratoma) 387
    Pathology 388
    Otosclerosis 389

INNER EAR 390
    Presbycusis and Other Hearing Loss 390
    Ménière Disease 391

TEMPORAL BONE DISSECTION 393

REFERENCES 394

The ear can be considered as three distinct regions or compartments to include the external ear, the middle ear and temporal bone, and the inner ear (Fig. 13.1).

The external ear consists of the auricle (pinna), external auditory canal (or meatus), and the tympanic membrane at the medial end of the auditory canal.

The middle ear cavity includes the ossicles, the eustachian tube connecting the middle ear space to the nasopharynx, and the expansion of the middle ear cavity in the form of air cells in the temporal bone.

The inner ear is embedded in the petrous portion of the temporal bone. It consists of a membranous (otic) labyrinth that lies within a dense bone referred to as the otic capsule that is excavated to form the osseous (periotic) labyrinth (1).

The inner ear is the sense organ for hearing and for balance. The external and middle ears are the sound-conducting apparatus for the auditory part of the inner ear.

EMBRYOLOGY

The external ear develops from the first branchial groove. The external auricle (pinna) forms from the fusion of the auricular hillocks or tubercles, a group of mesenchymal tissue swellings from the first and second branchial arches, that lie around the external portion of the first branchial groove (2). The external auditory canal is considered a normal remnant of the first branchial groove. The tympanic membrane forms from the first and second branchial pouches and the first branchial groove (2). The ectoderm of the first branchial groove gives rise to the epithelium on the external side, the endoderm from the first branchial pouch gives rise to the epithelium on the internal side and the mesoderm of the first and second branchial pouches gives rise to the connective tissue lying between the external and internal epithelia (Fig. 13.2) (2).

The middle ear space develops from invagination of the first branchial pouch (pharyngotympanic tube) from the primitive pharynx. The eustachian tube and the tympanic cavity develop from the endoderm of the first branchial pouch; the malleus and the stapes develop from the mesoderm of the first branchial arch (Meckel cartilage) while the incus develops from the mesoderm of the second branchial arch (Reichert cartilage) (Fig. 13.2) (2).

The first division of the ear to develop is the inner ear which appears toward the end of the first month of gestation (2,3). The membranous labyrinth, including the utricle, saccule, semicircular ducts, and cochlear duct arises from the otic vesicle (otocyst). The otic vesicle forms from the invagination of the surface ectoderm, located on either side of the neural plate, into the mesenchyme (Fig. 13.2). This invagination eventually loses its connection with the surface ectoderm. The bony labyrinth, including the vestibule, semicircular canals, and cochlea arises from the mesenchyme around the otic vesicle (2–4).

EXTERNAL EAR

Embryology

The external ear develops from the first branchial groove. The external auricle (pinna) forms from the fusion of the auricular hillocks or tubercles, a group of mesenchymal tissue swellings from the first and second branchial arches, that lie around the external portion of the first branchial groove (2). The external auditory canal is considered a

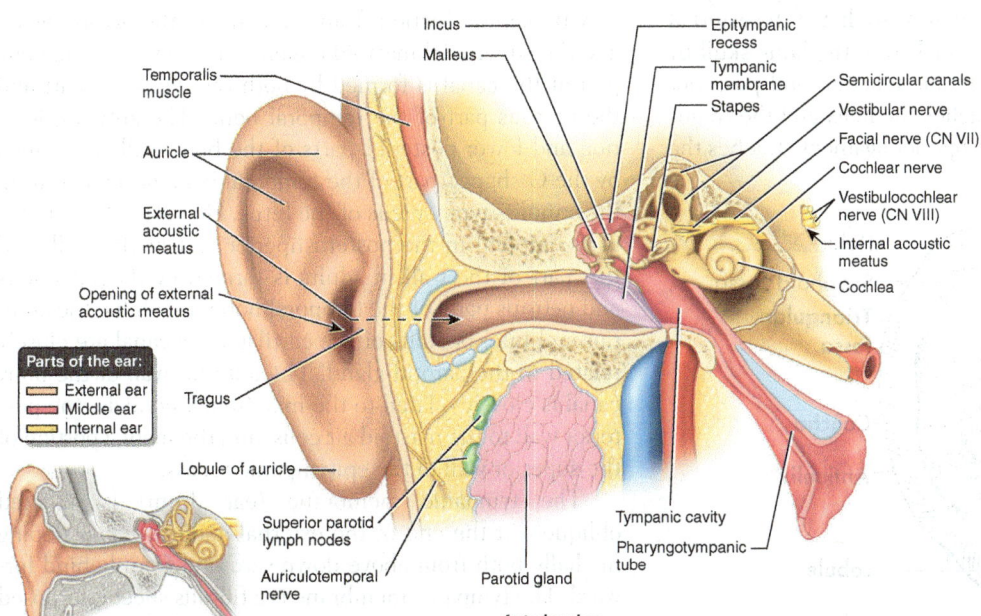

FIGURE 13.1 Parts of ear. A coronal section of the ear, with accompanying orientation figure, demonstrates that the ear has three parts: external, middle, and internal. The external ear consists of the auricle and external acoustic meatus. The middle ear is an air space in which the auditory ossicles are located. The internal ear contains the membranous labyrinth; its chief divisions are the cochlear labyrinth and the vestibular labyrinth. (Reprinted with permission from Moore KL, Dalley AF, Agur AMR. *Clinically Oriented Anatomy*. Philadelphia, PA: Wolters Kluwer Heath; 2017.)

FIGURE 13.2 Diagrammatic representation of the embryology of the epithelia of the inner, middle, and external ears.

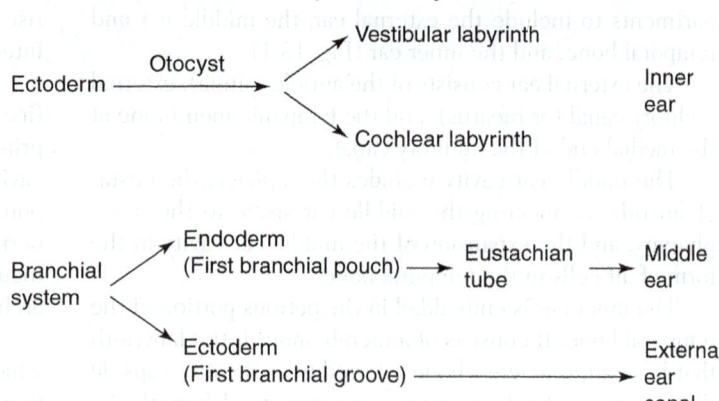

normal remnant of the first branchial groove. The tympanic membrane forms from the first and second branchial pouches and the first branchial groove (2). The ectoderm of the first branchial groove gives rise to the epithelium on the external side, the endoderm from the first branchial pouch gives rise to the epithelium on the internal side, and the mesoderm of the first and second branchial pouches gives rise to the connective tissue lying between the external and internal epithelia (Fig. 13.2) (2).

ANATOMY

The anatomy of the external ear is seen in Figure 13.3. The outer portion of the external ear includes the auricle or pinna leading into the external auditory canal. The skeleton of the auricle consists of a single plate of elastic cartilage conforming to the shape of the ear. The lobule is the only part of the auricle that is devoid of skeletal support. The cartilage of the auricle is continuous with that of the external auditory canal. The auricle is attached to the bony skull by three ligaments, including anterior, superior, and posterior (1). The anterior ligament attaches the helix and the tragus to the zygomatic process. The superior ligament attaches the spine of the helix to the superior margin of the bony external meatus. The posterior ligament attaches the medial surface (eminence) of the concha to the mastoid process. The auricle is anchored through its continuity with the cartilage of the meatus and through the skin and extrinsic muscles. The extrinsic muscles of the ear include the anterior, superior, and posterior auricular muscles. These muscles are usually functionless but may be subject to voluntary control as in ear "wiggling." There are also small intrinsic muscles in connection with the cartilage of the external ear, but they are of no apparent importance. The extrinsic and intrinsic muscles of the ear are innervated by the facial nerve.

The external auditory canal or meatus extends from the concha to its medial limit which is the external aspect of the tympanic membrane. The lateral portion of its wall consists of cartilage and connective tissue (1). The medial portion of its wall consists of bone. The cartilaginous part of the external auditory canal constitutes slightly less than half its total length. Inconstant fissures referred to as the fissures of Santorini occur in the cartilage; these fissures may transmit infection from the canal to the parotid gland and the superficial mastoid regions, or vice versa. The bony part of the canal is formed by both the tympanic part and the petrous part of the temporal bone. The anterior, inferior, and lower posterior parts of the bony wall are formed by the C-shaped part of the temporal bone developed from the annulus tympanicus of the fetus. However, the annulus is incomplete in the posterosuperior part of the wall, and this part of the wall in adults is formed by the squamous and petrous parts of the temporal bone. In adults, the anterior and inferior walls of the cartilaginous canal are closely related to the parotid gland. The anterior wall of the bony canal is closely related to the mandibular condyle, the posterior wall to the mastoid air cells, and the medial portion of the superior wall to the epitympanic recess.

The tympanic membrane (ear drum) is situated obliquely at the end of the external auditory canal sloping medially both from above downward and from behind forward. The tympanic membrane is a fibrous sheet interposed between the external auditory canal and the middle ear

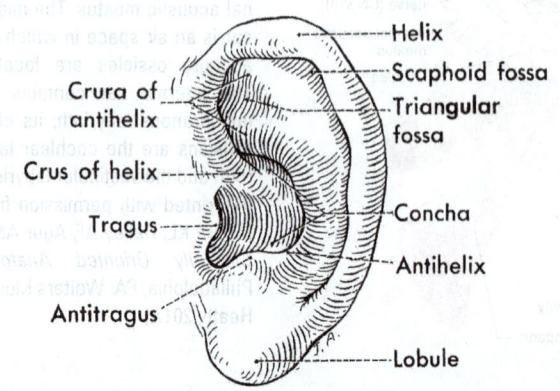

FIGURE 13.3 Anatomy of the external ear.

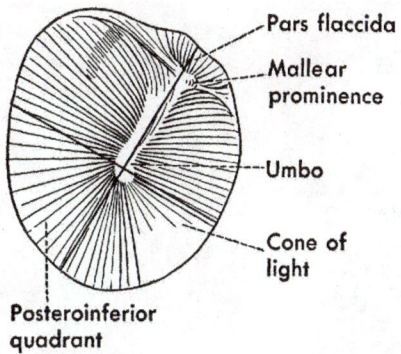

FIGURE 13.4 External (lateral) view of the tympanic membrane.

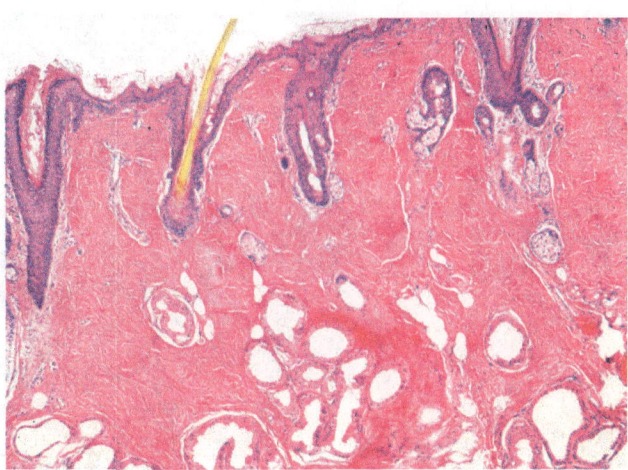

FIGURE 13.5 The auricle is a cutaneous structure histologically composed of keratinizing stratified squamous epithelium with associated cutaneous adnexal structures that include hair follicles, sebaceous glands, and eccrine sweat glands.

cavity (Fig. 13.4). The connective tissue interposed between these two layers consists of radiating fibers attached to the manubrium of the malleus that are reinforced peripherally by circular fibers. The latter are thickened at the margin of the tympanic membrane to form a fibrocartilaginous ring (annulus fibrocartilaginous) attaching the tympanic membrane to the tympanic sulcus of the temporal bone. In the upper portion of the tympanic membrane, there is a limited area where the connective tissue fibers are lacking; this area is referred to as the pars flaccida or the Shrapnell membrane. In this area, the tympanic portion of the temporal bone is deficient; this gap is referred to as the tympanic incisure or the notch of Rivinus. The remainder of the tympanic membrane in which there are intact connective tissue fibers is referred to as the pars tensa.

The outer aspect of the tympanic membrane is concave. The center of the concavity is referred to as the umbo, which is the strong point of attachment of the manubrium of the malleus to the tympanic membrane. In the anterosuperior portion of the tympanic membrane, the lateral process of the malleus is attached; from this point of attachment, the anterior and posterior mallear folds pass to the cartilaginous annulus and separate the pars flaccida from the pars tensa. In otoscopic examinations of the tympanic membrane, the bright area of light reflection present downward and forward from the umbo is referred to as the "cone of light."

HISTOLOGY

Histologically, the auricle is essentially a cutaneous structure composed of keratinizing, stratified squamous epithelium with associated cutaneous adnexal structures that include hair follicles, sebaceous glands, and eccrine sweat glands (Fig. 13.5). In addition to the hair follicles and sebaceous glands, the outer third of the external auditory canal is noteworthy due to the presence of modified apocrine glands called ceruminal glands that replace the eccrine glands seen in the auricular dermis (Fig. 13.6). Ceruminal glands produce cerumen and are arranged in clusters composed of cuboidal cells with eosinophilic cytoplasm often containing a granular, golden-yellow pigment. These cells have secretory droplets along their luminal border. Peripheral to the secretory cells are flattened myoepithelial cells. The ducts of the ceruminal glands terminate in the hair follicle or on the skin. The ducts of the ceruminal glands lack apocrine or myoepithelial cells. In the inner portion of the external auditory canal, ceruminal glands, as well as the other adnexal structures are absent.

The subcutaneous tissue is composed of fibroconnective tissue, fat, and elastic-type fibrocartilage, which gives the auricle its structural support (Fig. 13.7). The earlobe is devoid of cartilage and is replaced by a pad of adipose tissue. The perichondrium is composed of loose vascular connective tissue.

Similar to the auricle, the external auditory canal is lined by keratinizing squamous epithelium that extends to include the entire canal and covers the external aspect of the tympanic membrane. The tympanic membrane has a central bilaminated zone including lateral radially arranged and medial circularly arranged collagenous fibers (Fig. 13.8). The inner two-thirds of the external auditory canal contain bone rather than cartilage. Due to the absence of adnexal structures, there is relatively close apposition of the epithelium to the subjacent bone.

AUDITORY EPITHELIAL MIGRATION

Auditory epithelial migration represents the mechanism by which keratin is removed from the tympanic membrane. Without such a self-cleaning process, the keratin squames normally produced by the stratified squamous epithelium of the tympanic membrane would continuously build up and interfere with the conduction of sound via the tympanic

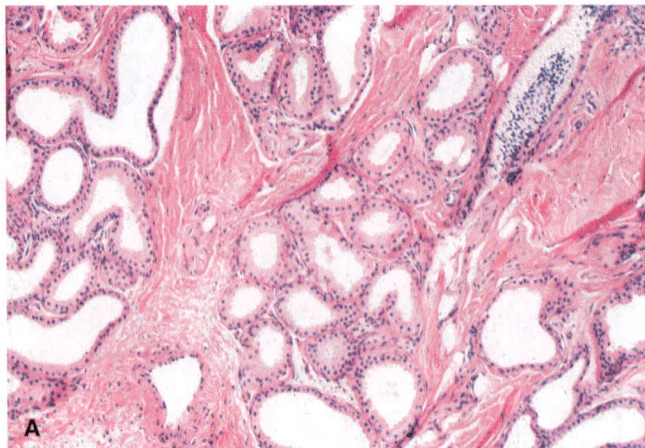
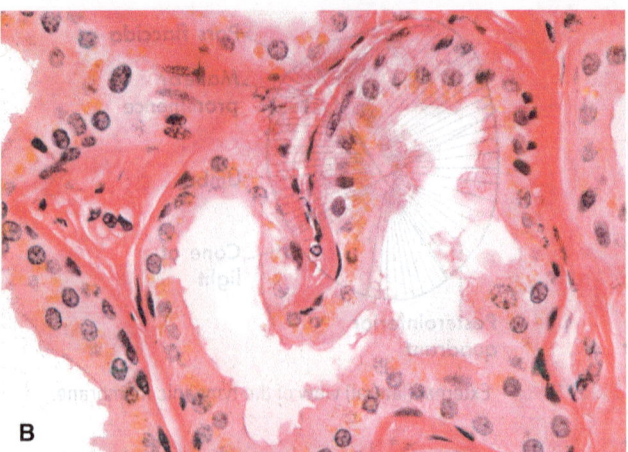

FIGURE 13.6 In addition to the hair follicles and sebaceous glands, the outer third of the external auditory canal is noteworthy due to the presence of modified apocrine glands called ceruminal glands that replace the eccrine glands seen in the auricular dermis. **A:** Ceruminal glands are submucosal in location and are arranged in clusters or lobules. **B:** Ceruminal glands are composed of a two-cell layer, including the inner or secretory cells containing intracytoplasmic cerumen appearing as granular, golden-yellow pigmentation, and flattened-appearing myoepithelial cells located peripheral to the secretory cells. Focally, the secretory cells show holocrine (decapitation) type secretion.

membrane. The entire epithelium including keratin moves from the tympanic membrane onto the deep external auditory canal. From the deep external auditory canal, the epithelium moves laterally to the junction of the deep (osseous) canal and the cartilaginous canal where it is desquamated (5–7). Auditory epithelial migration occurs in two separate and discrete pathways (Fig. 13.9) (8). In one pathway, the epithelium moves upward over the handle of the malleus then moves posterosuperiorly across the pars flaccida moving laterally over the deep canal (Fig. 13.10). The other pathway is radially moving centrifugally away from the handle of the malleus and the pars flaccida to the periphery of the tympanic membrane and then to the deep canal (Fig. 13.11). Michaels and Soucek have extensively evaluated the process of auditory epithelial migration (5–7) and correlated the

pathways to the development of the epithelia of the tympanic membrane and deep external canal in the embryo and fetus (8). The process of auditory epithelial migration has been felt to represent a possible pathogenesis for the development of cholesteatoma (see below). However, there is no definitive evidence linking auditory epithelial migration to the development of cholesteatoma (see later).

MIDDLE EAR

Embryology

The middle ear space develops from invagination of the first branchial pouch (pharyngotympanic tube) from the primitive

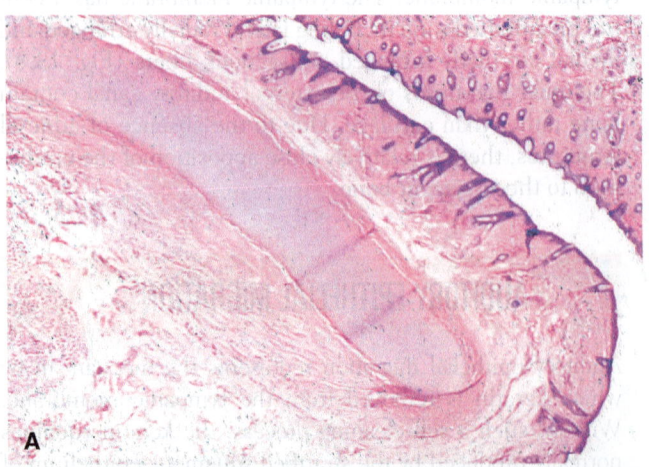
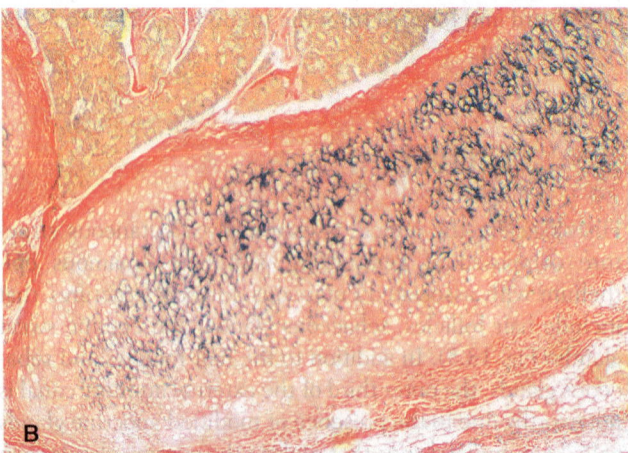

FIGURE 13.7 **A:** The cartilage of the external ear is elastic. **B:** Elastic stains show the abundant amount of elastic fibers (black staining) in the auricular cartilage.

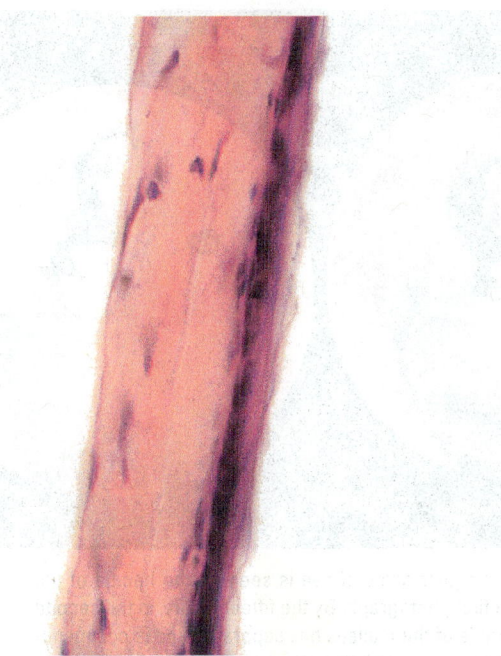
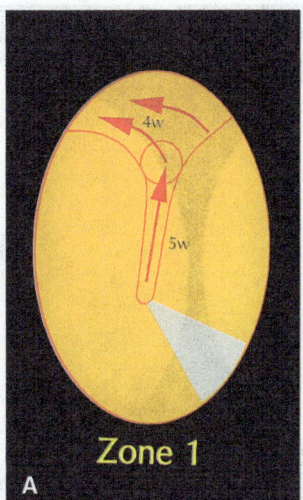
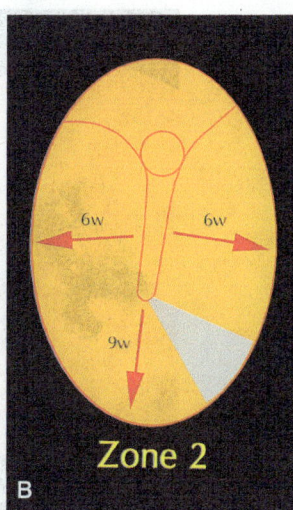

FIGURE 13.8 Section of pars tensa of tympanic membrane. The following layers may be distinguished from right to left: Stratified squamous epithelium, lamina propria, radial arrangement of collagenous fibers, circular arrangement of collagenous fibers (i.e., at right angles to former layer), lamina propria, and middle ear epithelium.

FIGURE 13.9 Summary of pathways of migration on tympanic membrane as determined by serial photography of dye markings. The tympanic membrane and adjacent deep external canal epithelium are depicted as being viewed on face. Two discrete pathways are present: (**A**) passing upward along a tongue of epithelium over the handle of the malleus to join the epithelium moving in a posterosuperior direction over the pars flaccida region (*zone 1*). **B:** A radial pathway moving centrifugally from the pars flaccida and handle of malleus regions to the periphery (*zone 2*). The times given for each region are the weeks required for the dye to be completely cleared from that region.

pharynx. The eustachian tube and the tympanic cavity develop from the endoderm of the first branchial pouch; the malleus and the incus develop from the mesoderm of the first branchial arch (Meckel cartilage) while the stapes develops from the mesoderm of the second branchial arch (Reichert cartilage) (Fig. 13.2) (2).

ANATOMY

The middle ear or the tympanic cavity lies within the temporal bone between the tympanic membrane and the squamous portions of the temporal bone laterally and the petrous portion

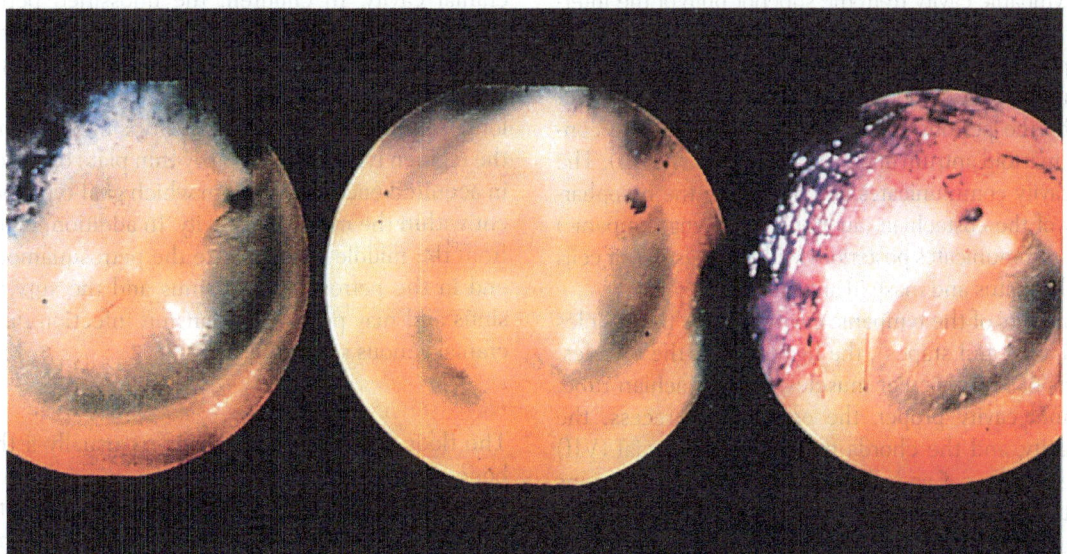

FIGURE 13.10 Pathway of auditory epithelial migration as shown by movement of blue dye daubed on the tympanic membrane. Dye is seen in the first photograph on the day at which it was daubed, just anterior and inferior to the lateral process of the malleus. In the next photograph, taken 9 days later, it has moved posteriorly and superiorly to lie over that structure. Thirteen days later, in the third photograph, it has crossed the pars flaccida region, moving in the same direction toward the external canal.

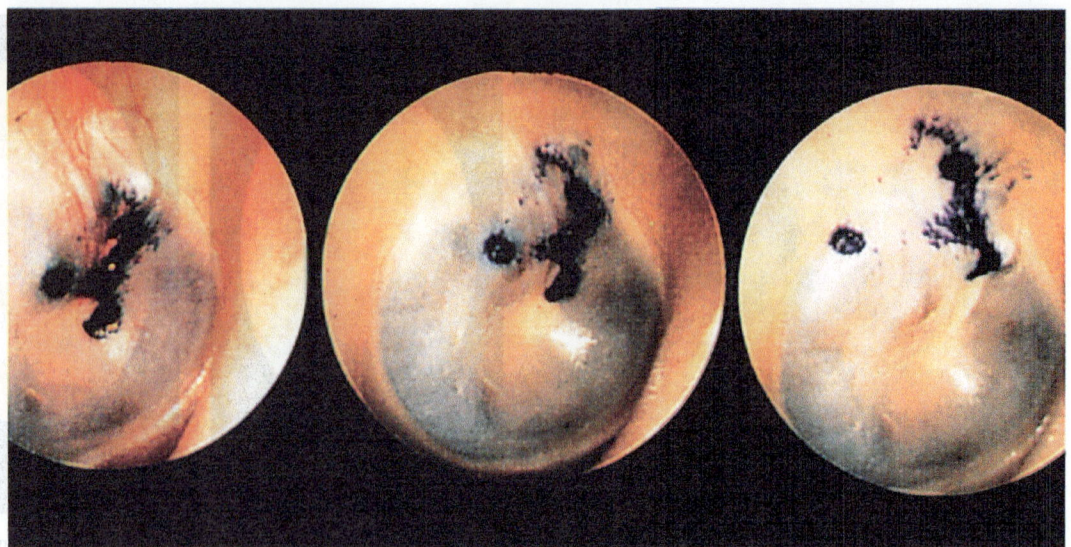

FIGURE 13.11 In this daubed tympanic membrane, an irregular array of dye is seen on the handle of the malleus region on the sixth day after its deposition, in the first photograph. By the fifteenth day, in the second photograph, a round dot that was just posterior to the handle of the malleus has separated and is commencing to travel backward, the main mass of dye moving discretely upward along the handle of the malleus. This process has advanced on the twenty-seventh day in the third photograph, the posterior dye having reached the back edge of the tympanic membrane and the large mass now being situated across the pars flaccida at an angle that has now changed to a posterosuperior one.

of the temporal bone surrounding the inner ear medially. The anatomic limits of the tympanic cavity include: (a) lateral or internal aspect made up by the tympanic membrane and squamous portion of the temporal bone, (b) medial aspect bordered by the petrous portion of the temporal bone, (c) superior (roof) delimited by the tegmen tympani, a thin plate of bone which separates the middle ear space from the cranial cavity, (d) inferior (floor) aspect bordered by a thin plate of bone separating the tympanic cavity from the superior bulb of the internal jugular vein, (e) anterior aspect delimited by a thin plate of bone separating the tympanic cavity from the carotid canal housing the internal carotid artery, and (f) posterior aspect delimited by the petrous portion of the temporal bone containing the mastoid antrum and mastoid air cells (1,9,10). The tympanic cavity communicates anteriorly with the nasopharynx by way of the eustachian (auditory or pharyngotympanic) tube and it communicates posteriorly with the mastoid air cells by way of the aditus and mastoid antrum.

The contents of the tympanic cavity include the ossicles (malleus, incus, and stapes), the ligaments of the ossicles, the tendons of the ossicular muscles, the eustachian tube, the tympanic cavity proper, the epitympanic recess, the mastoid cavity, and the chorda tympani of the facial (VII) nerve. The middle ear as well as the external ear functions as conduits for sound conduction for the auditory part of the internal ear.

Lateral Wall

The tympanic cavity extends above the level of the tympanic membrane as the epitympanic recess (attic). The head of the malleus and the body of the short process of the incus lie in this area. The epitympanic recess projects laterally above the external acoustic meatus; it is this portion of the tympanic cavity that has a part of the squamous portion of the temporal bone as its lateral wall.

Roof

The roof of the tympanic cavity is the tegmen tympani, a thin plate of bone separating the middle ear cavity from the cranial cavity. In children, the unossified petrosquamous suture of the tegmen tympani may allow the direct passage of infection from the middle ear to the meninges of the middle cranial fossa (1). In adults, especially in the setting of a long-standing history of chronic otitis media, compromise of the tegmen tympani, an already thin plate of bone may result in acquired encephalocele, in which glial-type tissue is present within the middle ear cavity. In addition, in adults, veins from the middle ear perforate the petrosquamous suture to end in the petrosquamous sinus and the superior petrosal sinus and may potentially transmit infection directly to the cranial venous sinuses (1).

Floor

The floor of the tympanic cavity is usually a thin plate of bone separating the cavity from the internal jugular vein. In the presence of a large superior bulb of the internal jugular vein, it may bulge into the middle ear and may present dehiscences (11).

Posterior Wall

The posterior wall of the tympanic cavity opens through the narrow aditus ad antrum in the wider mastoid (tympanic) antrum. Below the aditus is a relatively thin bone separating the tympanic cavity from the antrum and it is from this posterior wall that the pyramidal eminence projects with an aperture at its apex from which the tendon of the stapedius muscle is transmitted. Above and behind the pyramidal eminence, the facial nerve curves downward to change its course from horizontal to vertical. The chorda tympani, arising from the facial nerve, then enters the tympanic cavity through the canaliculus of the chorda in the posterior wall.

Anterior Wall

The lower part of the anterior wall is part of the petrous apex. This area consists of a thin plate of bone, which may be incomplete or may contain air cells, separating the cavity from the carotid canal in which the internal carotid artery is located. The upper part of the anterior wall is deficient since the canal containing the tensor tympani muscle opens in this location and immediately below this area is the tympanic orifice of the auditory tube.

Medial Wall

The medial wall of the tympanic cavity is the petrous portion of the temporal bone surrounding the internal ear and separating the middle ear cavity and the inner ear cavity.

Several markings of importance are found on its surface including the broad prominence produced by the anterior end of the lateral semicircular canal, the prominence of the facial (fallopian) canal produced by the horizontal portion of the facial nerve in its course between the inner and middle ears. The cochleariform process transmits the tendon of the tensor tympani muscle. Its apex is the landmark for the position of the turn (geniculum or external genu) between the anterolaterally and posteriorly directed horizontal portions of the facial nerve. Immediately below the facial canal is the *fossula fenestrae vestibuli* also referred to as the stapes niche, which contains the oval window, closed by the base of the stapes. Below the oval window is the promontory formed by the basal turn of the cochlea. The tympanic nerve plexus lies on the promontory. Below the back part of the promontory, the *cochlear fossula* or round window niche leads to the round window or fenestrae cochlea. Behind the promontory is a depression referred to as the sinus tympani, a site that may harbor infections and may transmit infections to the ampullary end of the posterior canal and posterior end of the lateral canal if the infection is deeply situated (1).

MIDDLE EAR OSSICLES AND MUSCLES

The middle ear bones or ossicles include the malleus, the incus, and the stapes (Fig. 13.12). The parts of the malleus include a head, upper and lower manubria (handle), lateral process, and anterior process. The malleus is closely attached to the tympanic membrane by its manubrium (handle) and its lateral process, while its head projects above the epitympanic recess to articulate with the body of the incus. The anterior (long) process (processus gracilis) of the malleus extends obliquely downward from the neck toward the tympanosquamous fissure. In infants, the anterior process may reach the tympanosquamous fissure, but in adults, the distal part is transformed to the connective tissue forming the anterior ligament of the malleus (1). The malleus is also attached to the tympanic wall by superior and lateral mallear ligaments. The lateral ligament attaches the neck of the malleus to the margin of the tympanic notch.

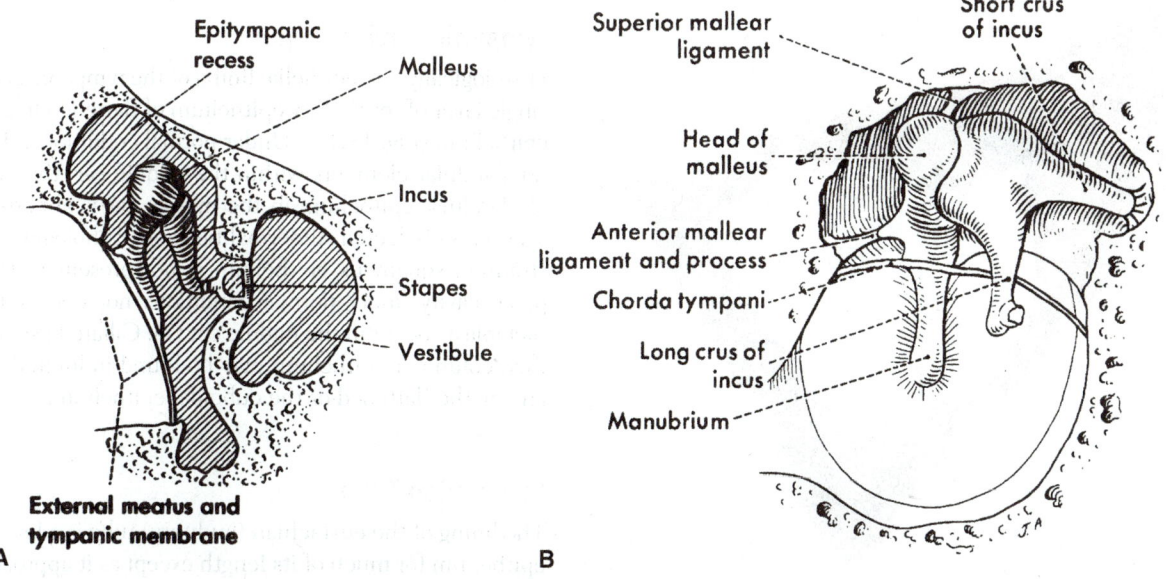

FIGURE 13.12 Diagrammatic depiction of the anatomy of the middle ear ossicles: **(A)** Frontal aspect (rotated through approximately 90 degrees) and **(B)** medial aspect.

The parts of the incus include its body, long and short processes. The body of the incus is fitted against the head of the malleus, and lies in the epitympanic recess. The short process (crus) rests in a depression referred to as the fossa of the incus that is situated in the posterior wall of the tympanic cavity below the aditus ad antrum. The long process (crus) of the incus descends parallel and slightly posteromedial to the manubrium, of the malleus, but at its lower end turns medial to articulate with the stapes (1). The incus is held in place by a posterior ligament that attaches to its short process, and by a superior ligament to attach to the body. The knob-like expansion of the long crus of the incus (at the incudomalleal joint) is referred to as the lenticular process.

The stapes is formed by its two crura, a head that lies at the junction of the crura and a footplate that lies on the oval window (Fig. 13.13). The head of the stapes articulates with the incus. From its articulation with the incus, the stapes passes almost horizontally to the oval (vestibular) window. The footplate of the stapes is attached to the oval window by the annular ligament. The latter, a ring of elastic fibers, allows movement of the stapes but seals any potential space between its footplate and the edges of the oval window.

The incudomalleolar and incudostapedial joints are synovial (diarthrodial) (see below). In addition to their ligaments, the stapes and the manubrium of the malleus have muscles attached to them. The stapedius muscle diminishes the excursion of the base of the stapes by its reflex contraction. Important functions ascribed to the stapedius muscle are to protect the inner ear from excessive sound and to improve discrimination for higher frequencies in speech. The stapedius muscle is innervated by a branch of the facial nerve.

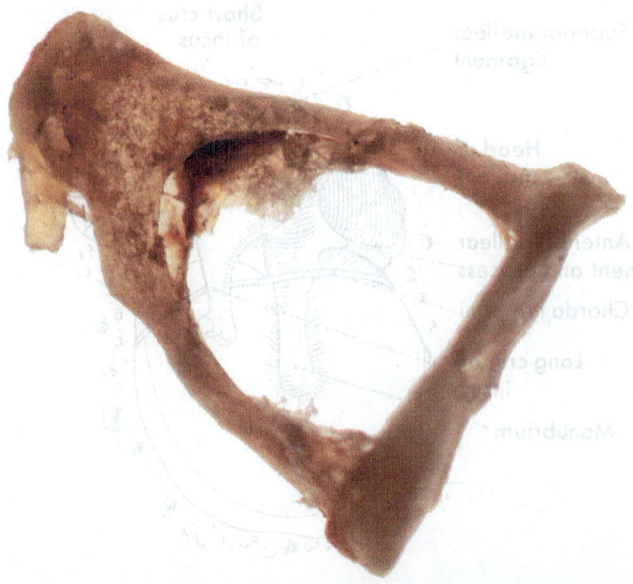

FIGURE 13.13 Intact resected stapes showing from left to right its head, two crura, and footplate.

The tensor tympani muscle draws the manubrium medially thereby tightening the tympanic membrane. The tensor tympani muscle is not only felt to primarily protect against excessive noise but also functions in conjunction with the tensor veli palatini muscle, to respond to swallowing and electric stimulation from the tongue. The action of these two muscles pump air from the tympanic cavity into the eustachian tube forcing air into the nasopharynx and helping to open the isthmus (12). The tensor tympani muscle is innervated by a branch of the mandibular nerve.

EUSTACHIAN (AUDITORY) TUBE

The eustachian tube extends from its tympanic ostium high on the anterior wall of the tympanic cavity to a nasopharyngeal ostium situated posterior to the inferior nasal concha (1). The tube is not straight but slightly S-shaped. In adults, the tympanic ostium is approximately 2 to 2.5 cm higher than the nasopharyngeal end; the tube runs downward, medially, and anteriorly to the nasopharynx. The length of the tube in adults varies from 31 to 38 mm (13). In infants, the tube is shorter, relatively wider, and more horizontal in its course and, therefore, an easier pathway for infections ascending from the nasopharynx to the tympanic cavity.

The tube can be divided into an osseous portion and a cartilaginous portion. The osseous portion or the canal has a bony wall and is the lateral or tympanic third of the tube. The anteromedial two-thirds have a cartilaginous and connective tissue wall and are referred to as the cartilaginous portion of the tube. The cartilaginous and osseous tubes meet at an obtuse angle.

HISTOLOGY

Tympanic Cavity Proper

Histologically, the epithelial lining of the tympanic cavity is a single layer of respiratory epithelium of flattened to cuboidal epithelium (Fig. 13.14). Under normal conditions, there are no glandular elements within the middle ear; the presence of glandular epithelium in the middle ear is abnormal (see section on Selected Abnormalities and Pathology). Further, stratified squamous epithelium is not present in the tympanic cavity under normal conditions nor does squamous metaplasia occur in the middle ear (7). Ciliated pseudostratified columnar epithelium may be found in limited patches among the flattened or the cuboidal epithelium.

Eustachian Tube

The lining of the eustachian (auditory) tube is a low ciliated epithelium for much of its length except as it approaches its nasopharyngeal end where it becomes ciliated pseudostratified columnar epithelium containing goblet cells. In its

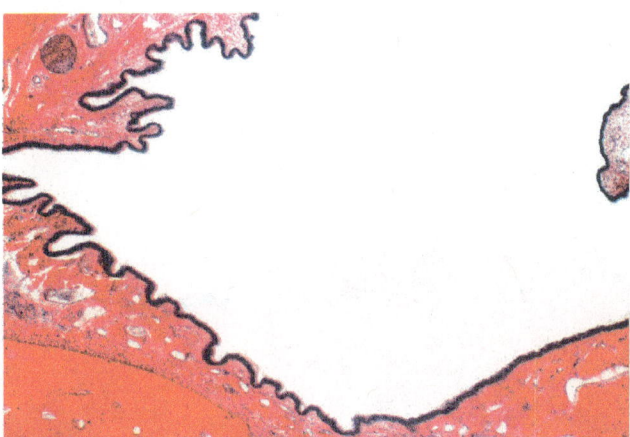

FIGURE 13.14 The epithelial lining of the tympanic cavity is a single layer of epithelium (cuboidal to respiratory). Under normal conditions glands are not identified within the tympanic cavity.

cartilaginous portion, it also contains seromucinous glands (Fig. 13.15). The eustachian tubes contain a lymphoid component, particularly in children, that is referred to as the Gerlach tubal tonsil (Fig. 13.16). Reactive hyperplasia of this lymphoid component particularly in children may close off the eustachian tube providing a desirable milieu for otitis media. The mucosa of the osseous portion of the eustachian tube is separated from the carotid canal by a thin plate of bone measuring 1 mm in thickness (7). Dehiscence of the carotid canal is fairly frequent (14). Squamous carcinoma of the middle ear or eustachian tube, a rare occurrence, may easily penetrate this area and gain access to the carotid artery with the potential for widespread dissemination (15). The cartilage of the nasopharyngeal portion of the eustachian tube is of hyaline type.

Mastoid Air Cells

The mastoid air cells represent a network of intercommunicating spaces that emanate from the tympanic cavity (7).

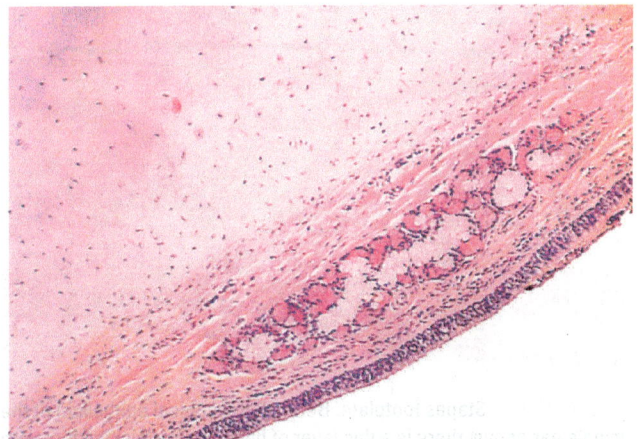

FIGURE 13.15 Cartilaginous portion of the eustachian tube with seromucinous glands.

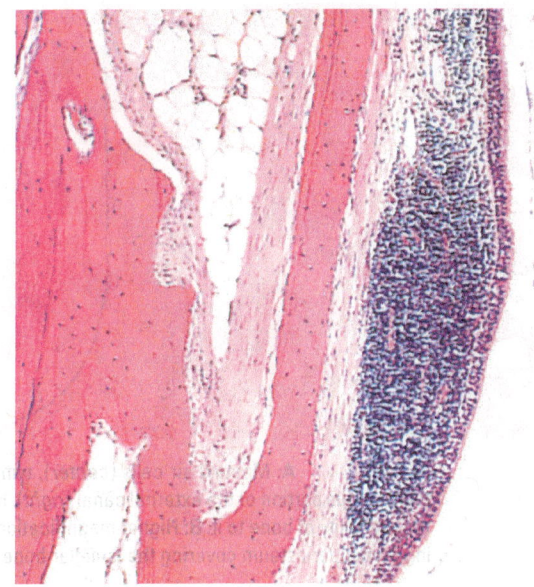

FIGURE 13.16 Mucosa of the eustachian tube. The lining is of ciliated columnar epithelium. In the lamina propria beneath, there are numerous lymphocytes, which are probably the result of inflammation.

Each air cell is lined by flattened to cuboidal epithelium which rests on periosteum that covers a thin frame of lamellar bone (Fig. 13.17).

Pneumatization of the Temporal Bone

In the newborn, the rudimentary mastoid bone contains a single air space, the antrum, surrounded by the diploic bone containing hematopoietic elements (16). As the mastoid process develops, the marrow spaces hollow out. The mesenchymal component occupying the space is resorbed and the developing air-containing cells become lined by the advancing endodermal epithelium. The mastoid process is constantly pneumatized in adults, although not in infants. The cells grow out from the antrum, as well as from each other forming complex interlocking chains of thin-walled cavities opening into each other. The antrum apparently always has air cells; the mastoid process is usually one of several types including pneumatized (containing air cells), diploic (containing marrow), mixed, (containing air cells and marrow) or sclerotic. Approximately 80% of mastoid is well-pneumatized by the age of 3 or 4 but in approximately 20% of the people, normal pneumatization fails to occur (1,17).

Middle Ear Ossicles

The middle ear ossicles develop from cartilage with a single center of ossification for bone; there is no epiphyseal ossification. The persistence of cartilage in each of the ossicles (Fig. 13.18) and the bifurcation of the stapes to form the crura with the obturator foramen between them distinguish the middle ear ossicles from other long bones (7).

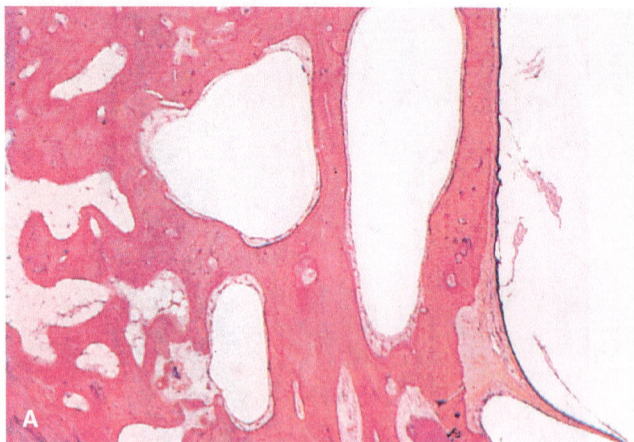
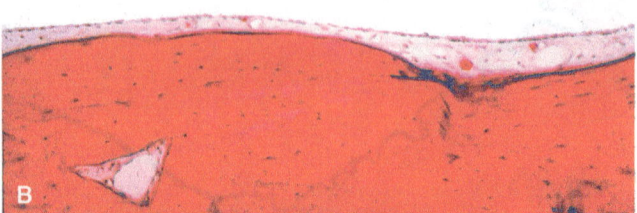

FIGURE 13.17 **A:** Mastoid air cells (*center*), tympanic membrane (*lower right*), and squamous epithelium of the osseous portion of the external canal (*right*). Note the thin covering of skin over the external ear canal and the proximity of bone to it. **B:** Higher magnification shows the very thin epithelium of the mastoid air cells resting on the periosteum covering the lamellar bone.

The head of the stapes is formed of the endochondral bone with a cartilaginous cap at the incudostapedial joint. The crura of the stapes are formed of the periosteal bone only. From the middle ear aspect of the stapes footplate to its vestibular surface, the histologic findings include the flattened-to-cuboidal epithelium of the tympanic cavity, a thin layer of bone, cartilage, and a single flattened (perilymphatic) epithelial cell layer (Fig. 13.19).

The malleus and the incus, similar to long bones, have an outer covering of the periosteal bone layer and an inner core of the endochondral bone with well-formed haversian systems. The manubrium (handle) of the malleus is predominantly covered by retained cartilage rather than the periosteal bone. The entire inner core of the manubrium, as well as the rest of the malleus is composed of the endochondral bone. The anterior process is formed in the membrane early in fetal life and merges with the malleus after its formation (7). At its superior aspect, the manubrium is separated from the tympanic membrane by a ligament covered by the middle ear epithelium. The short process of the incus shows a tip of the unossified cartilage.

Middle Ear Joints

Both the incudomalleal and incudostapedial joints are diarthrodial. Middle ear epithelium is present on the outer surface of the joint capsule and synovial membrane is present on its inner surface. The joint capsule is composed of fibrous tissue with high elastic fiber content (7). The articular disc representing the space in between the articular ends is comprised predominantly of fibrocartilage (Fig. 13.20). The articular processes of both the malleus and the incus are covered by cartilage.

The annular ligament binds the cartilaginous edge of the stapes footplate to the cartilaginous rim of the vestibular window (stapediovestibular joint) (Fig. 13.21) and is composed of fibrous tissue with elastic fibers being prominent near the ligament surfaces (18). Cartilage

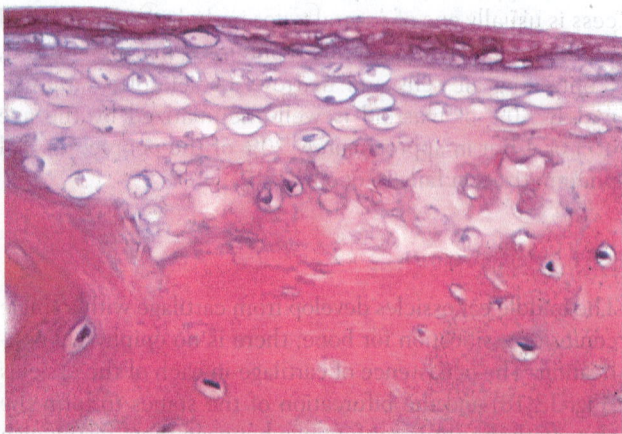

FIGURE 13.18 Stapes footplate showing persistence of cartilage.

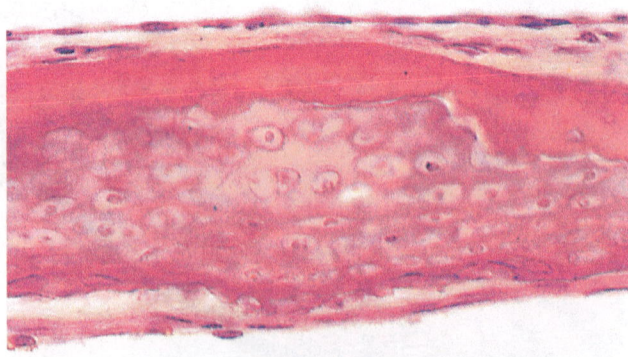

FIGURE 13.19 Stapes footplate. Beneath the cubical epithelium of the middle ear above, there is a thin layer of bone. Below this, the footplate consists of cartilage and there is a basal flattened layer of cells comprising the lining of the vestibule.

CHAPTER 13: The Ear and Temporal Bone

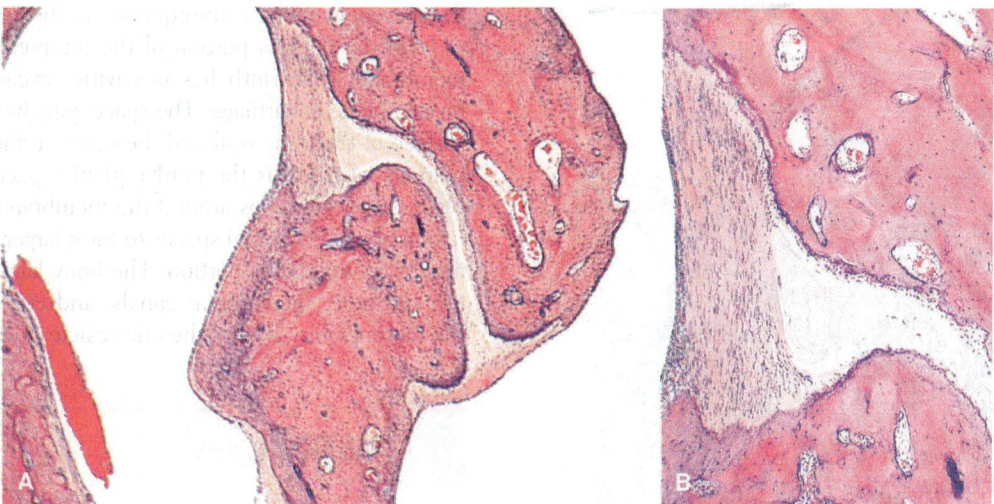

FIGURE 13.20 **A:** Incudomalleal joint. Note the joint capsule at each end of the joint. The joint space is occupied by the fibrocartilage of the articular disc. **B:** Higher power showing one end of the joint capsule and articular disc.

also covers the articular surfaces of the stapediovestibular joints.

The fissula ante fenestram is the canal linking the middle ear with the vestibule, lies in the bone just anterior to the stapediovestibular joint and develops as a slit filled with fibrous tissue often with associated cartilage (Fig. 13.22).

Middle Ear Muscles

The muscles of the middle ear including the tensor tympani and stapedius muscles are composed of a central tendon formed by elastic tissue with muscle fibers radiating from it (Fig. 13.23). This configuration has been described as feather-shaped. The tensor tympani muscle has a prominent mature adipose tissue component (Fig. 13.24) which is believed to function as insulation for the cochlea against electric effects from its contraction (7).

INNER EAR

Embryology

The first division of the ear to develop is the inner ear, which appears toward the end of the first month of gestation (2,3).

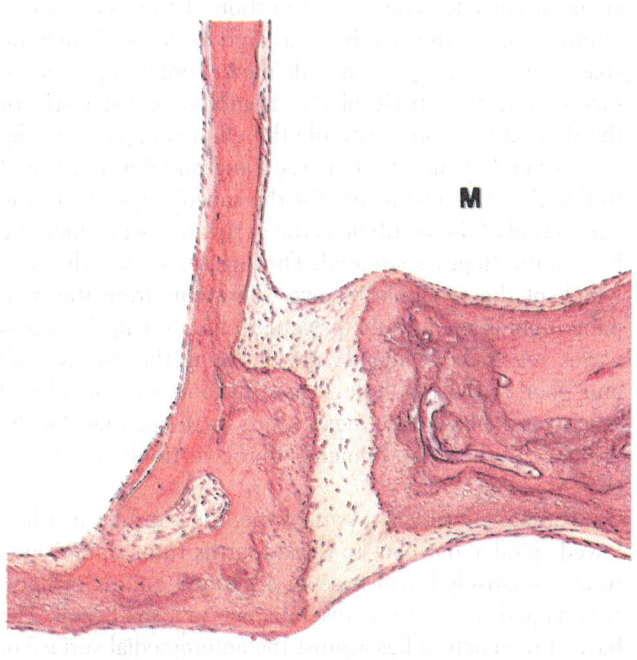

FIGURE 13.21 Stapediovestibular joint, part of footplate of stapes, adjacent bony labyrinthine wall, and crus of stapes. The footplate shows a lamina of cartilage on its vestibular surface, which is continuous with the cartilage of the stapediovestibular joint. *M*, middle ear cavity; *V*, cavity of vestibule.

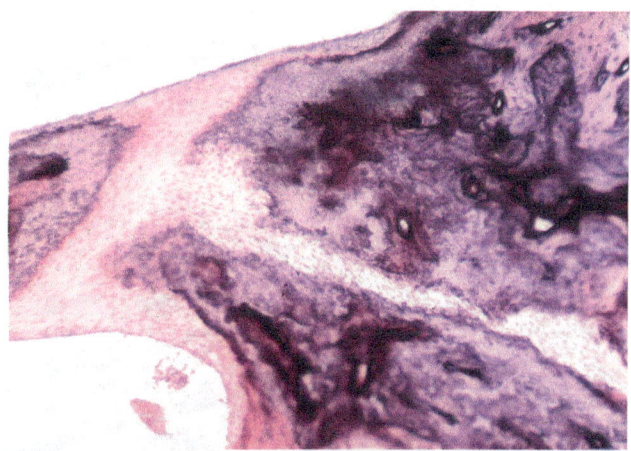

FIGURE 13.22 Fissula ante fenestram is the canal within the bone linking the middle ear with the vestibule and develops as a slit filled with fibrous tissue.

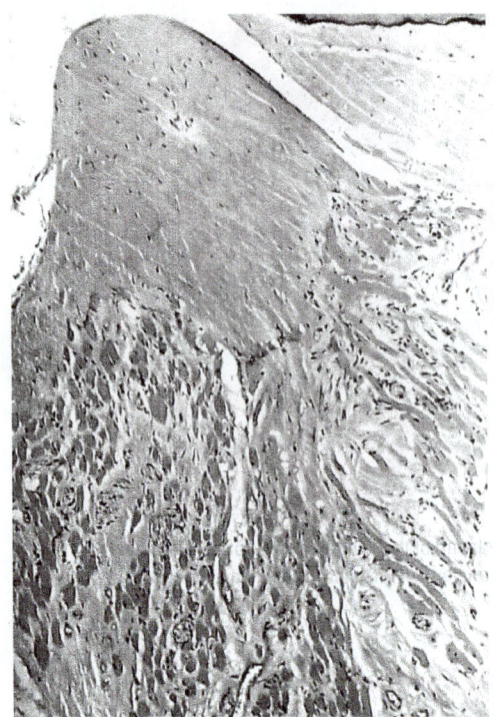

FIGURE 13.23 Stapedius muscle and tendon. The skeletal muscle fibers and fibrous bands between them radiate to a tendon.

The membranous labyrinth, including the utricle, saccule, three semicircular ducts, cochlear duct, and endolymphatic sac arises from the placodal thickening of the ectoderm to become a closed otic vesicle (otocyst). The otic vesicle forms from the invagination of the surface ectoderm, located on either side of the neural plate, into the mesenchyme (Fig. 13.2). This invagination eventually loses its connection with the surface ectoderm. The membranous labyrinth, which is essentially tubular and saccular in turn, is filled with fluid, the endolymph, or the endolymphatic fluid. The early development of the membranous labyrinth takes place in the mesenchyme and subsequently in the cartilage destined to form the petrous portion of the temporal bone (1). The membranous labyrinth lies in cavities excavated from this mesenchyme or cartilage. The space lying between the inner surface of the bony wall and the outer surface of the membranous labyrinth is the perilymphatic space. The perilymphatic space develops around the membranous labyrinth by fusion of mesenchymal spaces to form larger ones surrounding the membranous portion. The bony labyrinth, including the vestibule, semicircular canals, and cochlea arises from the mesenchyme around the otic vesicle (2–4).

ANATOMY

The internal (inner) ear, or labyrinth, is embedded within the petrous portion of the temporal bone and comprises the medial portion of the temporal bone adjacent to the cranial cavity. The inner ear contains the membranous labyrinth, which is surrounded by an osseous layer or bony shell termed the osseous (bony) labyrinth (Fig. 13.25). The membranous labyrinth contains the cochlea, which is the organ of hearing and the vestibular system, which is the system of balance (equilibrium).

Osseous Labyrinth (Otic Capsule)

The osseous labyrinth consists of the vestibular and cochlear capsule. The central portion of the osseous labyrinth cavity is the vestibule, a large ovoid perilymphatic space approximately 4 mm in diameter containing both the saccule and the utricle of the membranous labyrinth. In the floor of the bony vestibule the elliptical recess for the anterior end of the utricle is seen and anterior and lateral to this the spherical recess for the saccule is seen. In the lateral wall of the vestibule is the oval window in which the base of the stapes is situated. Through the stapes, the perilymph of the vestibule receives vibrations from the tympanic membrane and the ossicular chain set up by sound waves reach the tympanic cavity. Along the medial wall and floor of the vestibule, where it abuts the lateral end of the internal acoustic meatus, are small openings for the entrance of the nerve branches to the vestibular portion of the ear (1).

The bony cochlea, a part of the otic capsule, is a hollowed spiral about two- to three-fourths turns diminishing from a relatively broad base to a pointed cupula or apex. It is named so due to its resemblance to a snail shell. The base of the cochlea lies against the anteromedial surface of the vestibule and next to the anterior surface of the lateral (blind) end of the internal auditory canal. A central core of bone called the modiolus runs forward from the cochlea but does not reach the cupula. It is around this central core that the spiral channels of the cochlea (perilymphatic and endolymphatic) are arranged. A layer of bone arranged in a spiral

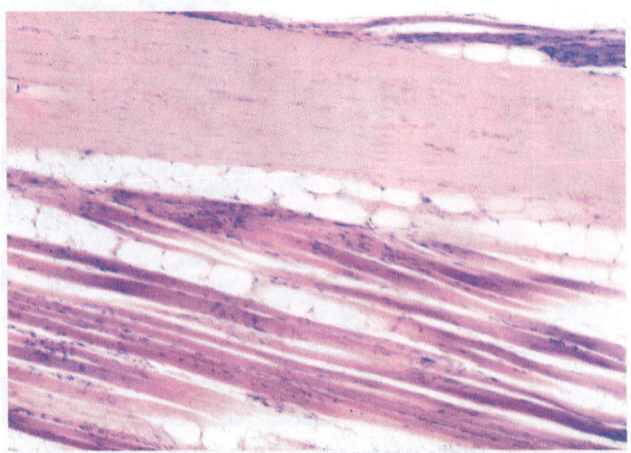

FIGURE 13.24 Tensor tympani muscle showing the presence of a mature adipose tissue component.

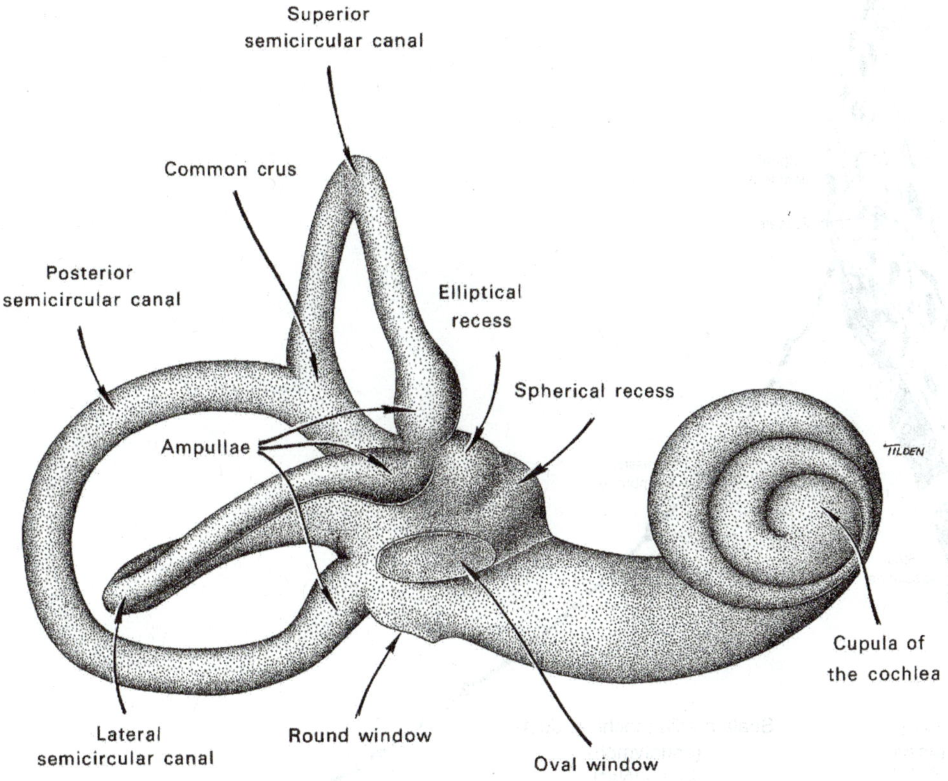

FIGURE 13.25 Schematic depicting the osseous labyrinth.

fashion unites the modiolus to the peripheral wall of the bony cochlea and separates successive spiral cavities from each other (1). The modiolus is hollow to accommodate the cochlear nerve. The base of the modiolus lies against the lateral end of the internal auditory canal to where the cochlear nerve runs.

The vestibular aqueduct extends through the otic capsule from the vestibule to the posterior cranial fossa transmitting the endolymphatic duct. The terminal end of the vestibular aqueduct is the endolymphatic sac, a dilated area that ends blindly outside the dura (1). The cochlear duct opens at one end into the lower end of the scala tympani and at the other end into the subarachnoid cavity (1). The issue as to whether the cochlear duct represents an open channel between the subarachnoid space and the perilymphatic space at the lower end of the scala tympani remains controversial (1). A possible role ascribed to the cochlear duct is to serve as part of the pressure-adjusting mechanism of the perilymph in conjunction with the round window (19–21).

Membranous Labyrinth

The membranous (otic) labyrinth is the spiral-appearing structure that resembles the shell of a snail. The principle components of the membranous labyrinth are the cochlear duct, the utricle, the saccule, the ductus reuniens, the semicircular canals with their ampullae, and the endolymphatic sac and duct.

Cochlear Duct

The membranous cochlea or cochlear duct is a cone-shaped spirally oriented membranous tube between the osseous spiral lamina and the outer osseous wall of the cochlea to which it is attached (9). The cochlear duct also referred to as the scala media lies between the scala vestibuli and the scala tympani (Fig. 13.26). These three compartments are fluid-filled. The cochlear duct, as well as the entire membranous labyrinth contains endolymph. The scala vestibuli and the scala tympani contain perilymph. The cerebrospinal fluid (CSF) communicates directly with the perilymphatic space through the cochlear aqueduct (perilymphatic duct) (Fig. 13.27). The cochlear duct contains the sensory (end) organ of hearing known as the spiral organ of Corti. The organ of Corti rests on the basilar membrane, which separates the cochlear duct from the scala tympani (Fig. 13.26). Together, the organ of Corti and the basilar membrane form the spiral membrane, which is the floor or tympanic wall of the cochlear duct. The spiral ligament is a thickened modified portion of periosteum of the bony cochlea forming the outer curved wall of the cochlea duct and adjacent parts of the scalae. The scala tympani lies below the basilar membrane while the scala vestibuli lies above the cochlear duct and is separated from it by the Reissner membrane. The Reissner membrane forms the roof of the cochlear duct. The scala tympani and scala vestibuli communicate with each other only at the apex known as the helicotrema. The scala vestibuli winds toward the apex of the cochlea at the helicotrema becoming the scala tympani, which, in turn,

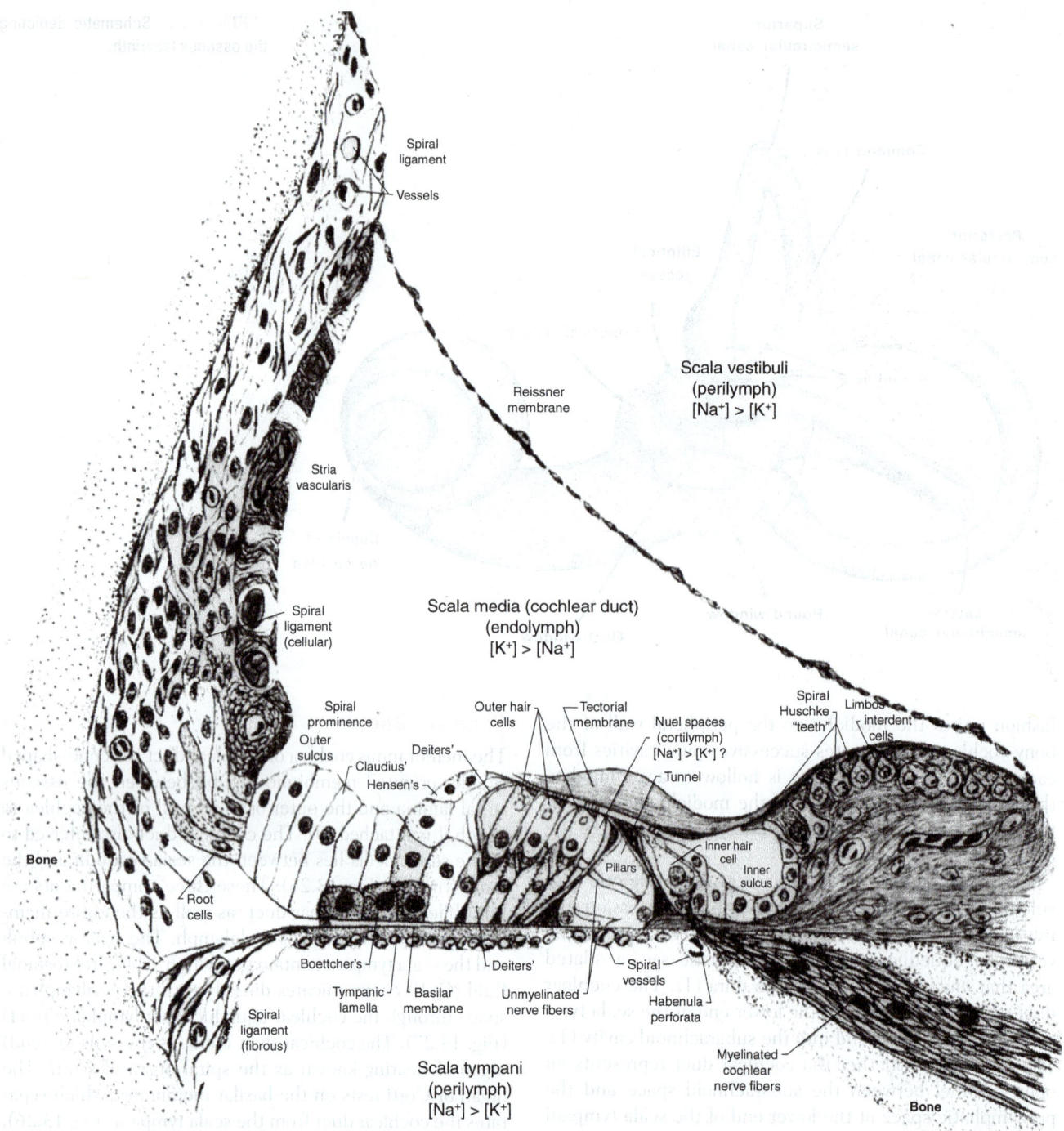

FIGURE 13.26 Schematic illustration of the membranous labyrinth, the latter containing the cochlea (organ of hearing) and the vestibular (system of balance) systems, showing the relationship between the endolymph-containing scala media (cochlear duct) and the perilymph-containing scala vestibuli and scala tympani. (From Nager GT. Anatomy of the membranous cochlea and vestibular labyrinth. In: Nager GT, ed. *Pathology of the Ear and Temporal Bone*. Baltimore, MD: Williams and Wilkins; 1993:3–48, with permission.)

coils back toward the round window (Fig. 13.28). The scala vestibuli and the scala tympani communicate with the middle ear via the oval window and round window, respectively. The scala tympani ends blindly at the round window membrane but the scala vestibuli opens up at that level into the perilymphatic space of the vestibulum. The cochlear duct connects with the vestibular system via ductus reuniens located at the saccule. In this way, the three semicircular canals that comprise the vestibular system are filled with endolymph.

CHAPTER 13: The Ear and Temporal Bone

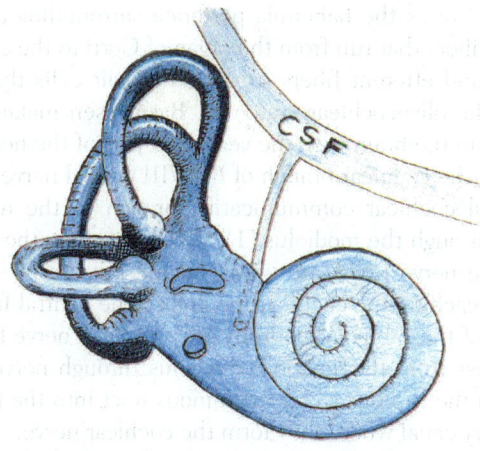

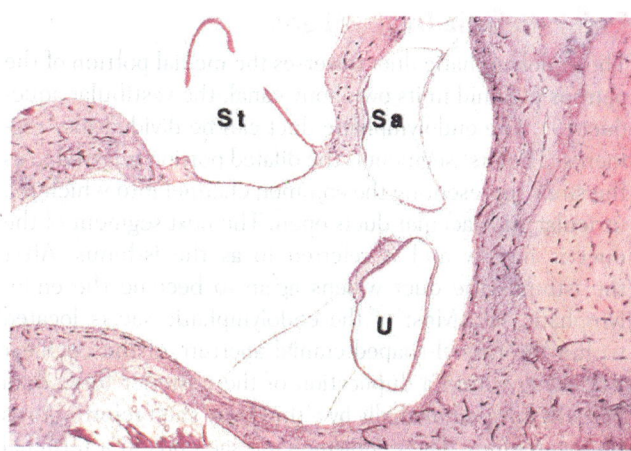

FIGURE 13.27 Schematic depicting the direct communication between the perilymphatic space and cerebrospinal fluid (*CSF*) through the cochlear aqueduct (perilymphatic duct).

FIGURE 13.29 Ventricle of a cat showing utricle (*U*) and saccule (*Sa*). *St*, stapes.

Utricle

The utricle is an elongated to oval-shaped portion of the membranous labyrinth lying superior to the saccule in the medial wall of the vestibule (Fig. 13.29). It is larger in diameter than the semicircular ducts and receives both ends of each semicircular duct (total of five) since the anterior and posterior ducts share a common opening. The macule of the utricle, located on the inferior surface of the utricle (utricular recess) is a sensory end organ. The utriculosaccular duct usually arises from the utricle and communicates with the endolymphatic duct and also connects the utricle to the saccule. As previously indicated, the three semicircular canals communicate with the utricle via openings formed by the union of the nondilated or nonampullary ends of the superior and posterior canals termed the common crus.

Saccule

The saccule is located anteromedial to the upper (anterior) end of the utricle (Fig. 13.29), and tends to be more round than the utricle. The saccule and the utricle are continuous via the utriculosaccular duct and with the cochlear duct by the ductus reuniens (also referred to as the canalis reuniens of Hansen) (1). The macule of the saccule contains the sensory nerve endings of this portion of the inner ear and is an oval thickening on the lateral wall.

Semicircular Canals

The semicircular ducts include the anterior or superior duct, the posterior duct and the lateral ducts. The end of each semicircular duct is expanded to form the ampulla. The anterior duct is directed anterolaterally, the posterior duct is directed posterolaterally, and the lateral ducts form a laterally directed angle of approximately 90 degrees between themselves. The bony or osseous canals follow a similar direction. The three semicircular canals communicate with the utricle via openings formed by the union of the nondilated or nonampullary ends of the superior and posterior canals termed the common crus. From the common crus, the anterior duct curves upward while the posterior duct curves backward and then downward. The other or (membranous) ampullary ends of the semicircular canals contain the sensory endings of the ducts. At the ampullary ends, the anterior and posterior ducts empty into the utricle. The lateral semicircular duct lies in an approximate horizontal plane; both of its ends also connect to the utricle, with the anterior end being the ampulla.

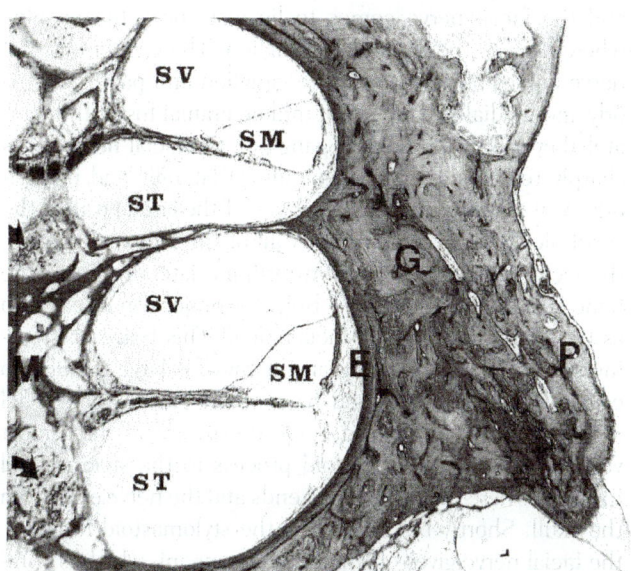

FIGURE 13.28 Cochlea, bony cochlea, and modiolus. *Arrows*, spiral ganglion cells of basal and middle coils in modiolus; *E*, endosteal layer of bone; *G*, endochondral layer containing globuli interossei; *P*, periosteal layer; *SM*, scala media; *ST*, scala tympani; *SV*, scala vestibuli.

Endolymphatic Duct and Sac

The endolymphatic duct traverses the medial portion of the petrous pyramid in its own bony canal, the vestibular aqueduct (9). The endolymphatic duct can be divided into segments. The first segment is the dilated portion referred to as the sinus representing the common channel into which the utricular and saccular ducts open. The next segment of the duct is narrow and is referred to as the isthmus. After the isthmus the duct widens again to become the endolymphatic sac. Most of the endolymphatic sac is located within the funnel-shaped cranial aperture of the cochlear duct lying within a duplication of the posterior fossa dura partially covered medially by a thin bony shelf referred to as the operculum. The endolymphatic sac ends in a terminal dilatation or fovea of the sac. Two portions of the endolymphatic sac are recognized: a proximal rugose portion with an irregular lumen caused by numerous folds of the epithelial lining and a distal portion with a smooth epithelial lining. Both the endolymphatic sac and the duct show irregularly placed thin papillary outgrowths from their epithelial base into the lumen. These may sometimes be identified on radiologic imaging in the living patient.

The membranous vestibular system contains the receptor organs for sense of motion and position. The neural structures of the inner ear, including the VIII cranial nerve (vestibulocochlear) and the VII cranial nerve (facial) enter the inner ear through the internal auditory canal.

INNER EAR INNERVATION

The nerve to the inner ear is the VIII cranial nerve variably referred to as the acoustic, auditory, or vestibulocochlear nerve. This nerve functionally consists of vestibular and cochlear divisions. In the internal auditory canal, these two parts are closely associated but at the lateral end of the canal the nerve trunk divides into three parts including two vestibular and one cochlear.

The vestibular nerve arises from the bipolar cells of the superior and inferior divisions of the (afferent) vestibular or Scarpa ganglion located at the lateral end of the internal auditory canal. Peripherally, the vestibular nerve divides into two main divisions, the superior and inferior divisions. The superior part of the ganglion gives nerves to the ampullae of the lateral and anterior (superior) canals and to the saccular and utricle maculae. The inferior part of the ganglion gives rise to a posterior ampullary nerve and a nerve to the saccule. The inferior part also gives rise to a branch to the cochlear division.

The cells of origin for the cochlear nerve form the spiral ganglion, which represents the first of the four neurons between the auditory end organ and the auditory cortex. The spiral ganglion is located in coils of the modiolus at the base of attachment of the osseous spiral lamina (Fig. 13.28). The osseous spiral lamina is a thin trabeculae of bone referred to as the habenula perforata surrounding afferent nerve fibers that run from the organ of Corti to the acoustic nerve and efferent fibers to the outer hair cells that arise from the olivocochlear system of Rasmussen making their exit from the brain with the vestibular part of the nerve and joining the cochlear branch of the VIII cranial nerve via the vestibulocochlear communicating branch or the nerve of Oort through the modiolus (1). Before reaching the modiolus, the nerve fibers are unmyelinated but are myelinated upon reaching the cochlear modiolus. The central fibers or axons of these bipolar neurons unite to form nerve bundles and pass from the cochlear modiolus through nerve channels in the osseous spiral foraminous tract into the internal auditory canal where they form the cochlear nerve.

Within the internal auditory canal, the vestibulocochlear nerve is usually connected to the facial nerve. Together the three nerves enter the posterior cranial fossa, transverse the cerebellopontine angle, and enter the brain stem at the posterior lower lateral aspect of the pons. The central auditory pathways consist of three additional neurons that form numerous connections with nuclei throughout the central nervous system as part of a complex auditory reflex system reaching the auditory cortex in the anterior transverse gyrus of the superior temporal lobe (9,10).

The facial nerve enters the temporal bone through the internal auditory meatus within the petrous portion of the temporal bone in company with (lying above) the VIII cranial nerve and the internal auditory artery. The facial nerve then passes the Bill bar, which represents a pointed bony projection separating the facial nerve from the superior division of the vestibular nerve. At the outer end of the canal, the facial nerve pierces the arachnoid and dura to enter its own bony canal, the facial canal (fallopian canal or the aqueduct of Fallopius). This canal continues for a short distance and the facial nerve comes to lie just above the cochlea where it bears the geniculate ganglion. The greater petrosal nerve comes off the geniculate ganglion and passes anteriorly and medially to enter the middle cranial fossa. Immediately beyond the geniculate ganglion, the facial nerve turns sharply (external genu or geniculum) laterally and posteriorly. As it runs backward in the bone of the lateral wall of the vestibule (which is the medial wall of the tympanic cavity), the facial nerve inclines downward and laterally where the bone surrounding it forms a bulge or projection referred to as the prominence of the facial canal. This bulge or prominence is a normal finding and it may be large enough to cover the oval window and base of the stapes. The facial nerve then makes a broad curve downward to run almost vertically through the mastoid process to the stylomastoid foramen where the facial canal ends and the nerve exits from the skull. Shortly before leaving the stylomastoid foramen, the facial nerve gives off the chorda tympani, which is composed of sensory and preganglionic motor fibers. Slightly above the stylomastoid foramen, the chorda tympani leaves the facial trunk, takes a recurrent course upward and forward in its canaliculus ("iter chordae posterius") to enter the tympanic cavity through its posterior wall. Within the tympanic cavity, it passes between the malleus and incus and leaves the tympanic membrane through a canal ("iter chordae anterius") in the pterygotympanic fissure where it joins the lingual nerve to be distributed to the anterior two-thirds of the tongue (taste buds) and to the submandibular ganglion through which postganglionic fibers reach the submandibular and sublingual salivary glands.

HISTOLOGY

Osseous Labyrinth

The cavity of osseous labyrinth (otic capsule) surrounds and replicates the outline of the membranous labyrinth lying within it. The osseous labyrinth is extremely dense and includes three layers: an outer periosteal layer, an inner layer abutting the membranous labyrinth lined by a thin layer of internal periosteum (also referred to as endosteum), a middle layer in which there is persistence of much of the calcified cartilaginous matrix referred to as globuli interossei or globuli ossei (Fig. 13.30) (7). The density of the osseous labyrinth is necessary to insulate and safeguard the delicate vibrations of the fluids contained within it and is necessary in maintaining the integrity and functions of hearing and balance (7). As noted by Michaels (7), the bone of the adult osseous labyrinth is neither lamellar nor woven bone but "somewhere in between"; in contrast to other adult bone, the osseous labyrinth lacks the normal developmental process of removal and replacement of calcified cartilaginous matrix, lacks removal and replacement of primitive bone (7).

Membranous Labyrinth

The membranous labyrinth consists of epithelium-lined channels surrounded by connective tissue. The three basic divisions of the membranous labyrinth, including the semicircular canals, the utricle and saccule, and the cochlear duct have similar structure, consisting of a specialized thickened epithelium surrounded by and attached to a fibrogelatinous membrane. The specialized epithelium consists of supporting cells and neuroepithelium or hair cells. The neuroepithelia have processes ("hairs") that project from the free edge of the cells.

Cochlea

The organ of Corti consists of neurotransmitting hair cells that rest on the basilar membrane and is arranged in a spiral like the duct itself (Fig. 13.31). The organ of Corti consists of supporting cells and hair cells. The supporting or pillar cells are of several different types. Among the more important supporting cells are the phalangeal cells which are arranged in two groups: an inner or single row of cells and an outer row of cells (cells of Deiters) formed from three to five rows of cells depending on the level of the cochlea with more rows of cells toward the apex and less rows of cells toward the base. The inner row of phalangeal cells is associated with a single layer of hair cells; the outer row of phalangeal cells alternate with rows of hair cells. The phalangeal cells get their name from the shape of the stiff processes that project from the cells contributing to the reticular membrane that covers the free surface of the organ (1). The hair cells have numerous (40 to 100 per cell) "hairs" projecting from the reticular (cuticular) surface. The outer hair cells are more sensitive, are short and wedge-shaped between the apices of the phalangeal cells in order to reach

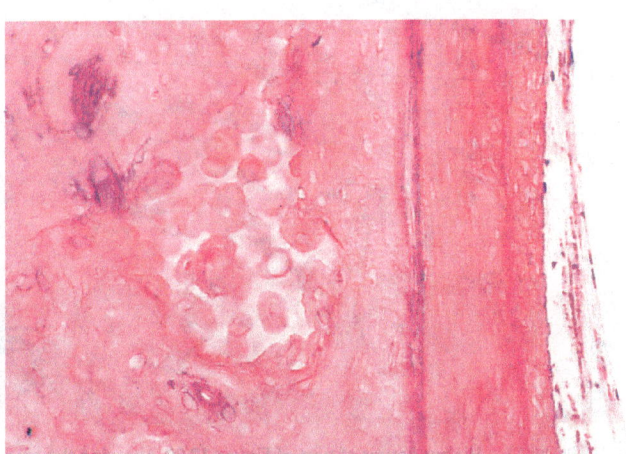

FIGURE 13.30 Globuli ossei (*left*) and endosteum (*right*) of cochlea.

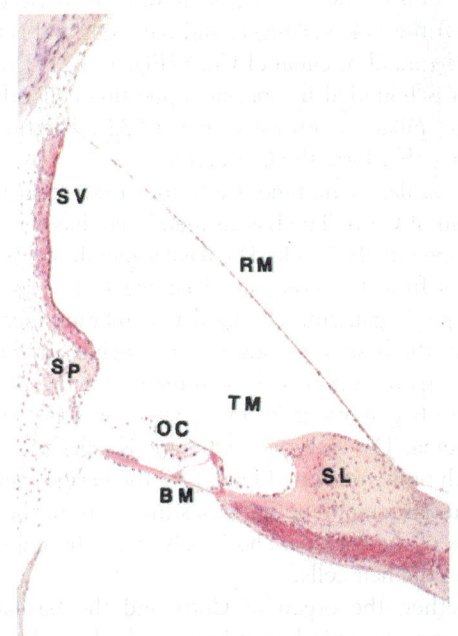

FIGURE 13.31 Scala media of a cat. *BM*, basilar membrane; *OC*, organ of Corti; *RM*, Reissner membrane; *SL*, spiral limbus; *SP*, spiral prominence; *SV*, stria vascularis; *TM*, tectorial membrane.

cochlear duct and adjacent parts of the scalae. The vestibular, or the Reissner membrane is thin and consists of two layers of cells: an inner cell layer of ectodermal origin consisting of epithelial-like clusters; an outer layer of mesodermal origin consisting of large, flat, and elongated cells (7). This membrane forms the roof of the cochlear duct. In Ménière disease (see later), the vestibular membrane bulges toward the scala vestibuli. In the outer (vertical) wall of the cochlear duct is the stria vascularis, which is supplied by 30 to 35 small arteries originating from the modiolar region of the scala vestibuli and pass outward to the lateral wall of the osseous labyrinth (Fig. 13.31) (22). It is believed to be the source of the endolymph (23). The tissue spaces of the spiral ligament serve as a site of absorption (24). The stria vascularis is altered in ototoxic conditions as it may occur secondary to the use of cisplatin, diuretic agents, and other drugs (see section on Presbycusis and Other Hearing Loss) (7).

Semicircular Canals, Utricle, and Saccule

The end of each semicircular duct is expanded to form the ampulla. The sensory endings in the ampullae of the ducts are the cristae. Each crista consists of thickened epithelium; above each crista rests a gelatinous formation of viscous protein polysaccharide called the cupola. The hairs of the neuroepithelial hair cells project into the base of the cupola. As a result of the gelatinous nature of the cupola, it may be bent by the pressure of the endolymph, which apparently stimulates the hair cells and, therefore, the nerve endings of the cristae.

The utricle and the saccule, representing the two main membranous structures of the vestibule, are lined by a sensory epithelium known as the macula (Fig. 13.33).

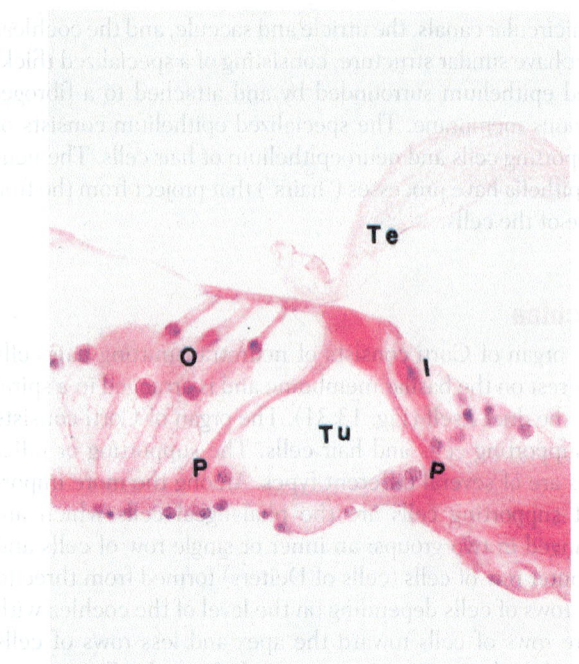

FIGURE 13.32 Higher power of the organ of Corti from Figure 13.31. *I*, inner hair cells; *O*, outer hair cells; *P*, pillar cells (walls of tunnel); *Te*, tectorial membrane; *Tu*, tunnel of Corti.

the basilar membrane and are believed to be responsible for the cochlear microphonics (1). The inner hair cells are long, less susceptible to damage than the outer hair cells and are believed to be less sensitive to sound. Intercellular spaces among the cells of the organ of Corti are apparently filled with intercellular substance. The largest of these spaces runs the entire length of the organ of Corti between inner and outer rows of phalangeal and hair cells and is referred to as the tunnel or canal of Corti (Fig. 13.32). The tunnel of Corti is bounded by special supporting cells, the inner and outer pillars (Corti rods) (Fig. 13.32). The tunnel and pillars together form the Corti arch.

The basilar membrane is a fibrous tissue that supports the organ of Corti. The basilar membrane has the tectorial membrane attached to it. The basilar membrane has fibers that pass from the bony spiral lamina to the spiral crest of the spiral ligament. The basilar membrane increases in size from the base to the apex of the cochlea, and is felt to have resonator action with deformation of the membrane by sound beginning at its lower end traveling toward the helicotrema. The tectorial membrane is a gelatinous structure with numerous fine fibers. Like the basilar membrane, the tectorial membrane increases in size from the base to the apex of the cochlea, and is believed to have a vibratory effect on the hair cells.

Together, the organ of Corti and the basilar membrane form the spiral membrane, which is the floor or tympanic wall of the cochlear duct. The spiral ligament is a thickened modified portion of periosteum of the osseous cochlea, which forms the outer or curved wall of the

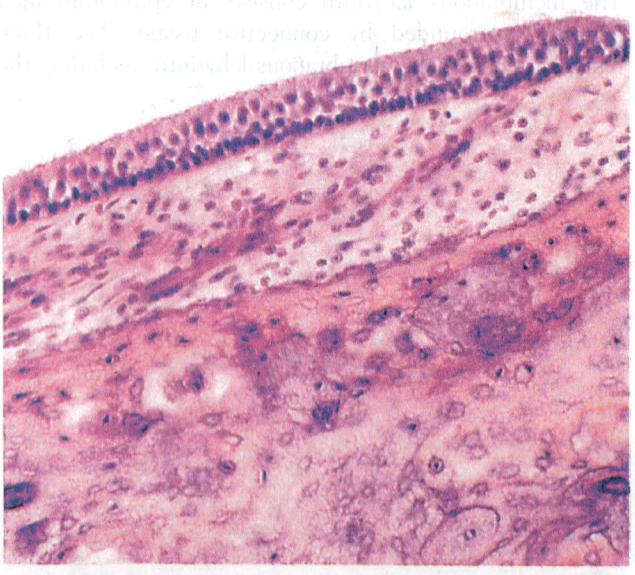

FIGURE 13.33 Higher power of part of Figure 13.29, showing the macule of the saccule.

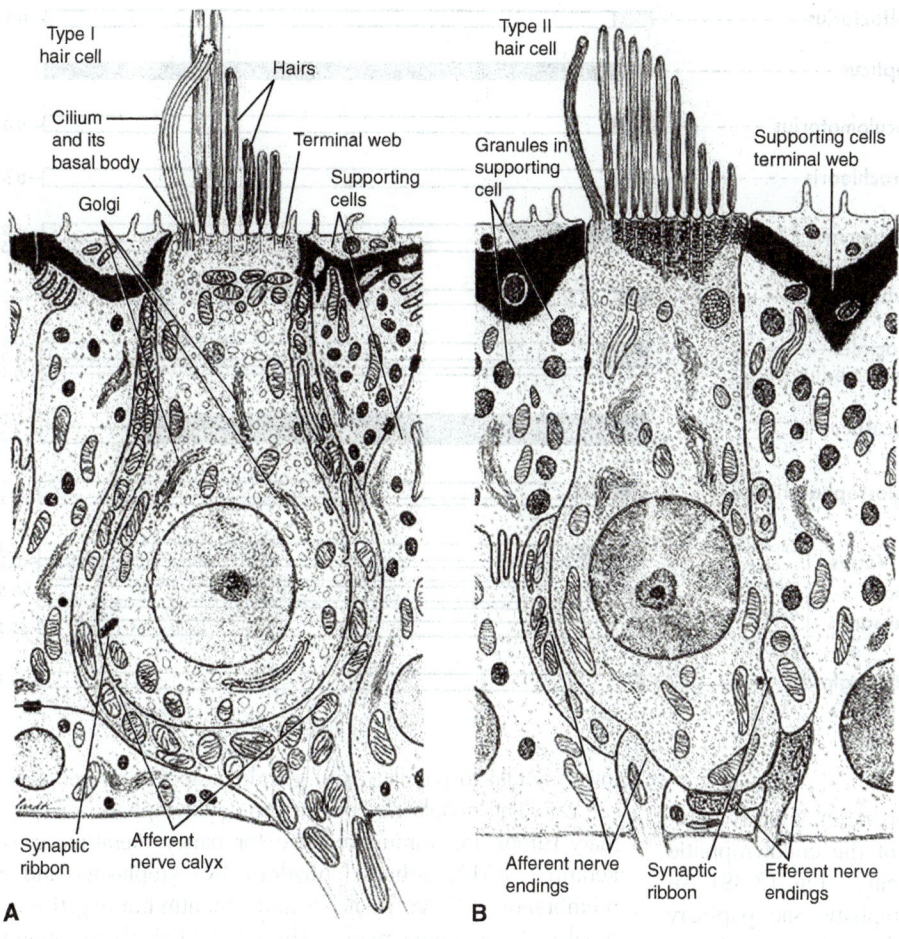

FIGURE 13.34 Schematic representation of the ultrastructure of vestibular hair cells showing the principal features of type 1 (**A**) and type 2 (**B**) hair cells and their supporting cells. (From Nager GT. Anatomy of the membranous cochlea and vestibular labyrinth. In: Nager GT, ed. *Pathology of the Ear and Temporal Bone*. Baltimore, MD: Williams and Wilkins; 1993:3–48, with permission.)

The maculae are identical to one another in structure and are similar to the cristae of the semicircular canals. By transmission electron microscopy, these sensory cells are of two types: type 1 cell is flask-shaped with a swollen basal portion; type 2 cell is cylindrical. Type 1 cells are attached to fibers of the sensory nerves by a wide chalice-like terminal and the terminal of type 2 cells is connected by button-like attachments of the nerve (Fig. 13.34) (7). The sensory epithelium consists of hair cells which, in turn, have stiff, immotile projections embedded in the gelatinous otolithic membrane. In the otolithic membrane, crystalline bodies referred to as otoliths are also embedded that contain calcium carbonate and a protein suspended in a jelly-like polysaccharide. It is only in the presence of otoliths that the maculae differ from the other sensory areas of the ear.

Nerves and Paraganglia

Most cranial and spinal nerves have glia extending only a fraction of a millimeter beyond their external origins (25,26). The optic nerve contains neuroglia throughout its length and, thereby, really is a tract of brain rather than a true nerve. The exception to the other cranial nerves is the VIII (vestibulocochlear) nerve, which typically has glia extending from 6 to 8 mm along its course (Fig. 13.35). This distribution of glia along the VIII nerve helps in explaining the greater occurrence of glial tumors on this nerve as compared to the other cranial nerves (25). The vestibular and cochlear divisions are fused near the entrance to the internal auditory meatus; at this location, the nerve changes in appearance from pale staining proximally to dark staining distally. This change in appearance is the result of the abrupt transition of the coverings of the nerve fibers from the pale staining oligodendroglia to the darker staining Schwann cells (Fig. 13.36). This glial–Schwann sheath junction of the VIII nerve is referred to as the Obersteiner–Redlich line. Acoustic neuromas (also referred to as vestibular neuromas) may arise anywhere between this junction and the cribrosa area at the fundus of the canal (27).

Paraganglia similar in structure to the carotid body are identified in the ear and may give rise to jugulotympanic paragangliomas. Most of the paraganglia are found in relation to the jugular bulb, and a minority are found under the mucosa of the medial side of the middle ear promontory (Fig. 13.37).

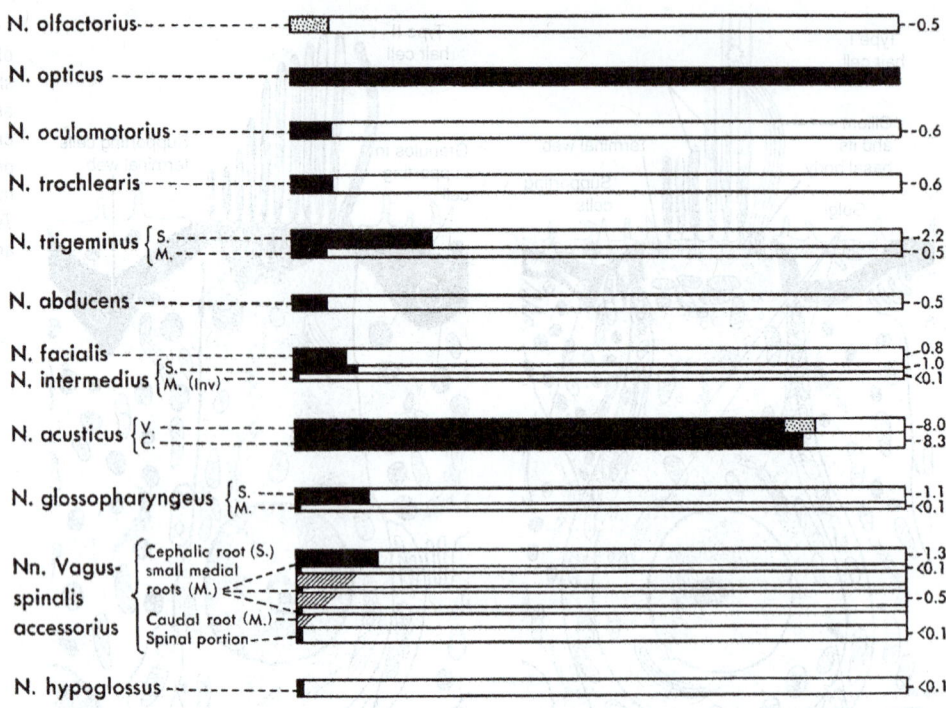

FIGURE 13.35 Schematic illustration of the cranial and spinal nerves showing that most of the nerves have glia extending for only a fraction of a millimeter beyond their external origins with the exception of the optic nerve which is really a tract of brain given the presence of neuroglia throughout its length and the VIII (vestibulocochlear) nerve. The VIII cranial nerve typically has glia extending from 6 to 8 mm along its course. (From Hollinshead WH. The cranium. In: Hollinshead WH, ed. *Anatomy for Surgeons*. 3rd ed. Philadelphia, PA: Harper and Row; 1982:26–27, with permission.)

Endolymphatic Sac and Duct

The lining epithelium of the endolymphatic duct is low cubical (Fig. 13.38) and the epithelium of the endolymphatic sac is taller and has a papillary appearance (Fig. 13.39). An aggressive neoplasm, termed endolymphatic sac papillary tumor, is presumed to originate from the endolymphatic sac epithelium (28). This tumor, initially considered to represent a low-grade malignancy (i.e., adenocarcinoma), is potentially a locally destructive but not metastatic tumor characterized by a variably appearing epithelium, including nondescript low-cuboidal to papillary and glandular-appearing neoplasm (28,29). The neoplastic cells in the endolymphatic sac papillary tumor are immunoreactive for pancytokeratins, cytokeratin 7, EMA, carbonic anhydrase IX (cytoplasmic and/or membranous), PAX8 (nuclear), and vimentin but negative for renal cell carcinoma marker (RCC), CD10, thyroglobulin, and thyroid transcription factor 1 (TTF1) (30). Patients with this tumor often describe symptoms similar to those occurring in the Ménière disease including vertigo and spinning of the room. This tumor has been found to be associated with von Hippel–Lindau disease (VHL), including the identification of the VHL gene (31–33) but may occur sporadically unassociated with VHL or any other hereditary diseases (34,35).

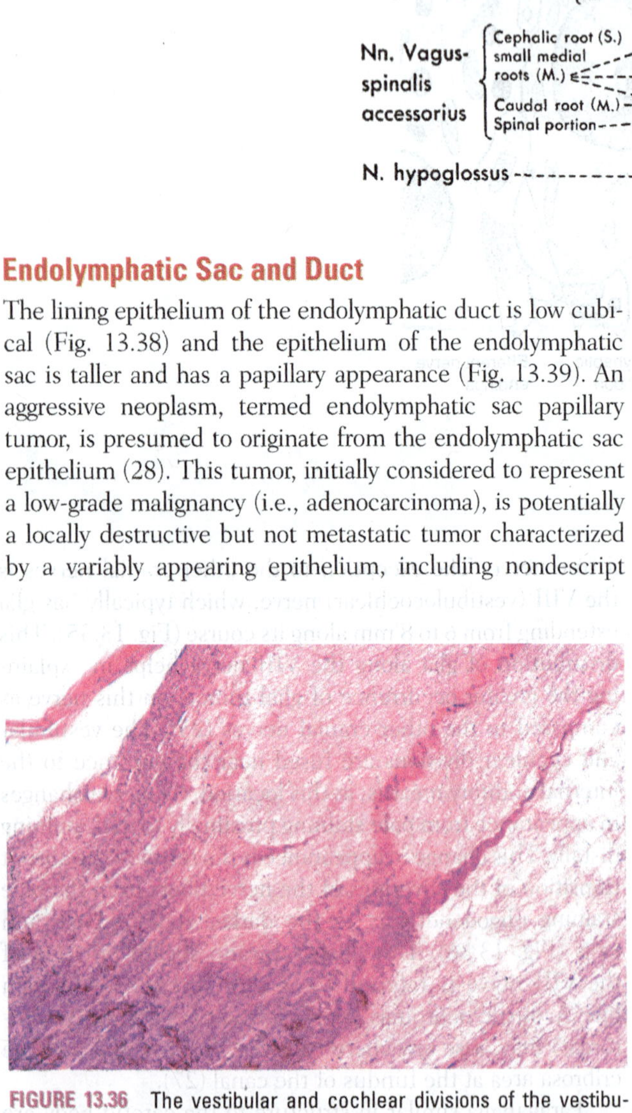

FIGURE 13.36 The vestibular and cochlear divisions of the vestibulocochlear nerve are fused near the entrance to the internal auditory meatus. At this location is the glial–Schwann sheath junction also referred to as the Obersteiner–Redlich line where the nerve changes in appearance from pale staining proximally to dark staining distally owing to the abrupt transition of the coverings of the nerve fibers from the pale staining oligodendroglia to the darker staining Schwann cells.

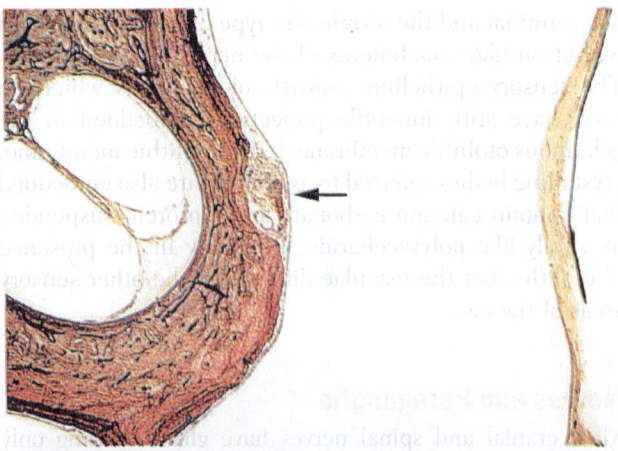

FIGURE 13.37 Normal tympanic paraganglion under mucosa of medial side of middle ear over promontory. The tympanic membrane is on the right. The Gomori reticulin stain.

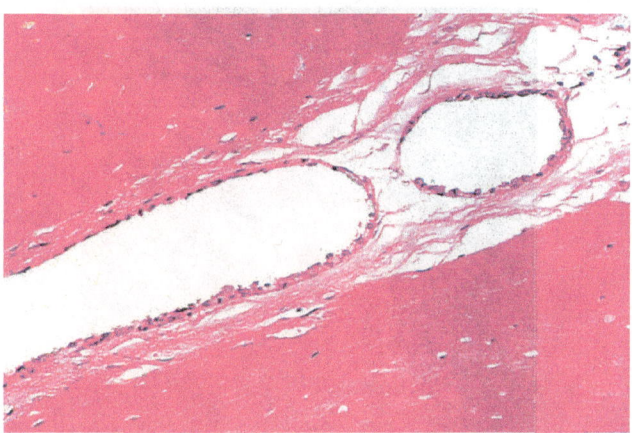

FIGURE 13.38 Endolymphatic duct within the vestibular aqueduct. The duct is lined by low cubical epithelium.

COMPOSITION AND CIRCULATION OF THE PERILYMPH AND ENDOLYMPH

Perilymph, which is partly a filtration of CSF and partly a filtration from blood vessels of the ear, has a similar chemical composition as CSF, resembling extracellular fluid with low potassium and high sodium concentrations. The similarities of perilymph and CSF support the concept that perilymph is derived from CSF. The anatomical basis for this concept is based on the consideration that because of the opening of the cochlear aqueduct (perilymphatic duct) into both the subarachnoid and perilymphatic spaces (1), an increase in CSF pressure results in flow into the labyrinth.

The perilymphatic spaces of each osseous semicircular canal are continuous on both ends with the perilymphatic space of the vestibule and this space is continuous with the scala vestibuli, which is continuous with the scala tympani at the helicotrema. All perilymphatic spaces open wide into each other. Due to areas of discontinuity or deficiency in the compact bone of the petrous portion of the temporal bone, foci of communication may exist between the perilymphatic space and other cavities. Such areas of potential communication include the middle and inner ear via the round and oval windows. In addition, the vestibular and cochlear aqueducts and the foramina for the nerves and blood vessels of the inner ear serve as potential channels between the inner ear and the cranial cavity.

Endolymph is an intracellular-like fluid containing high potassium and low sodium concentrations. Endolymph contains more than 30 times as much potassium as does perilymph or CSF but about one-tenth as much sodium (36). Endolymph has a low protein content; its protein is entirely globulin instead of an admixture of globulin and albumin (1). It has a viscosity similar to the vitreous of the eye due to its high mucopolysaccharide content. The electrolyte concentration of the endolymph is critical for normal functioning of the sensory organs. It is generally believed that the main source of endolymph is the stria vascularis, as well as the epithelium of the ampullae of the semicircular ducts as well as the epithelium of the maculae of the utricle and saccule. Recent evidence suggests that the human endolymphatic sac may have endocrine/paracrine capacity through expression of peptides with potent natriuretic activity (37). Such peptides include uroguanylin and brain natriuretic peptide, but also peptides regulating vascular tone, including adrenomedullin 2. Further, both neurophysin and oxytocin (OXT) were reported to be significantly expressed (36). The endolymphatic sac may influence the hypothalamic–pituitary–adrenal axis and may regulate vasopressin receptors and aquaporin-2 channels in the inner ear via OXT expression. In addition to its regulatory effects on inner ear endolymphatic homeostasis, the endolymphatic sac via secretion of several peptides, may also influence systemic and/or intracranial blood pressure through direct and indirect action on the vascular system and the kidney (37).

Endolymph circulates through the cochlear duct (scala media) downward to the base of the cochlea, then through the ductus reuniens into the saccule and then into the endolymphatic sac and duct where it is reabsorbed. The cochlear duct communicates with the vestibular endolymph–containing sacs through two canals so that the endolymphatic system is, like the perilymphatic system, a continuous one.

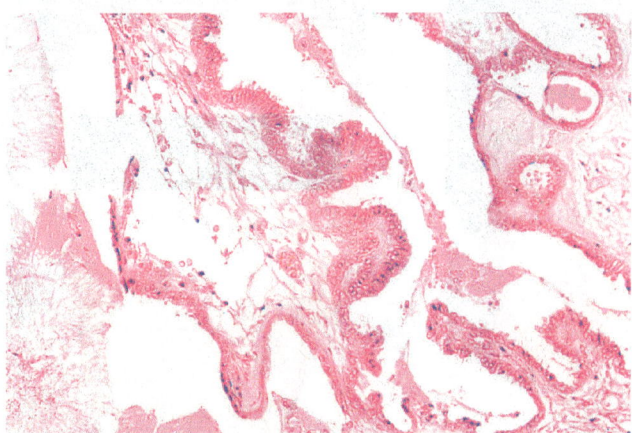

FIGURE 13.39 Endolymphatic sac, which is lined by tall columnar epithelium arranged on papillae.

CONDUCTION OF SOUND

Conduction of sound occurs via air and bone. The pinna and external auditory canal conduct sound waves in air to the tympanic membrane. Conduction of sound by air is less efficient when compared with the ossicular route. The ossicular chain, including the malleus, the incus, and the stapes, enhances the sound energy transmission by conveying vibrations from the tympanic membrane to the footplate of the stapes lying on the oval window of the vestibule which in turn is in contact with the perilymph. From the vestibular perilymph, vibrations derived from sound waves pass directly to the perilymphatic spaces of the cochlea, first via the scala vestibuli (upper compartment) ascending from the oval window and then to the scala tympani (lower compartment) descending to the round window. The walls of the endolymph-containing scala media or cochlear duct, lying in between the perilymph-containing scala vestibuli and scala tympani, receives waves of vibrations from the perilymph. Through the endolymph, the waves of vibrations affect the sensory cells of the organ of Corti, the sensory organ of sound reception located in the scala media or cochlear duct, from where it passes to the cochlear nerve with transmission via central pathways to the cerebral cortex.

SELECTED ABNORMALITIES AND PATHOLOGY

External Ear

Abnormalities of the external ear include those associated with first and second branchial arch syndromes. The first and second branchial arch syndromes include otologic and nonotologic abnormalities. The otologic manifestations or abnormalities include malformed or absent external ears, atretic external auditory canal, and impaired hearing. The nonotologic abnormalities include asymmetric facies, abnormalities of the temporomandibular joint, neuromuscular abnormalities, and associated abnormalities of the cardiovascular, renal, and central nervous systems. The

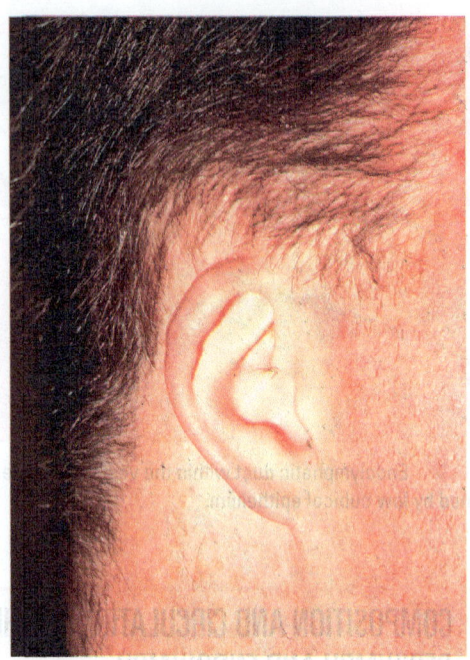

FIGURE 13.40 Individual with Down syndrome. In comparison to normal, patients with Down syndrome have external ears that are smaller, low-set, and have an incompletely developed superior helix.

Goldenhar syndrome, also known as oculoauriculovertebral dysplasia, is first and second branchial arch syndromes characterized by ear tags, preauricular pits and fissures, epidermoids, lipodermoids, and vertebral column abnormalities (38). Ear abnormalities can also be seen in association with other abnormalities, including the Down syndrome (Fig. 13.40). Cryptotia is a rare anomaly in which the superior portion of the auricle is buried in the scalp (Fig. 13.41).

FIGURE 13.41 **A, B:** Individual with cryptotia, a rare anomaly in which the superior portion of the auricle is buried in the scalp.

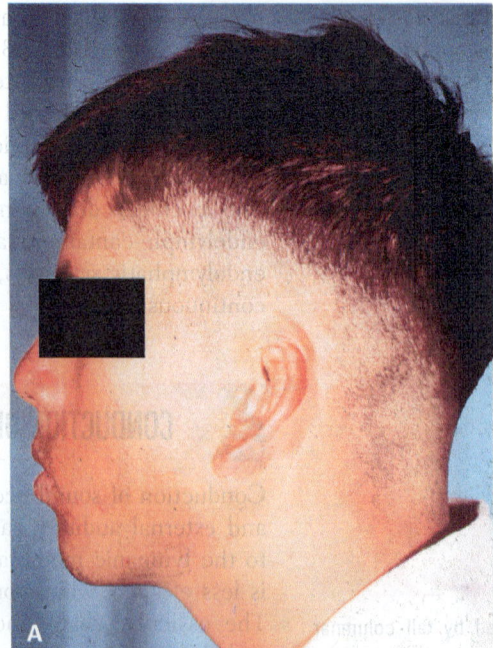
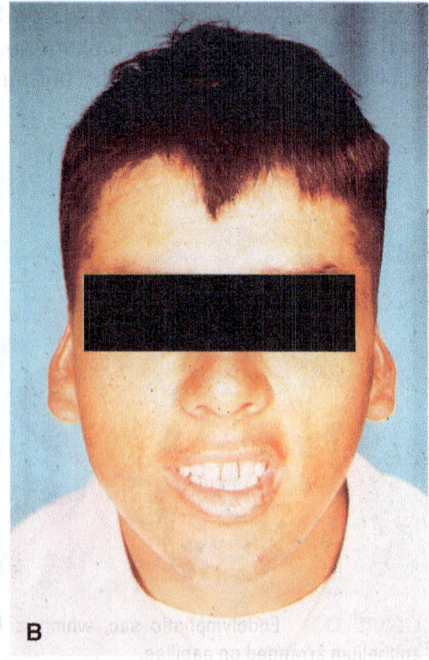

Microtia represents gross hypoplasia of the pinna with a blind or absent external auditory canal. Microtia is typically bilateral although the degree of hypoplasia may differ on the two sides. Accessory tragi, also referred to as accessory or supernumerary ears, accessory auricle, or polyotia, appear at birth, may be solitary or multiple, unilateral or bilateral, sessile or pedunculated, soft or cartilaginous, skin-covered nodules, or papules. They are located on the skin surface often anterior to the auricle and may clinically be mistaken for a papilloma. Histologically, accessory tragi recapitulate the normal external auricle and include the skin, cutaneous adnexal structures, and a central core of cartilage. Accessory tragi are thought to be related to second branchial arch anomalies. Accessory tragi may occur independent of other congenital anomalies but may occur in association with cleft palate or lip, mandibular hypoplasia, or in association with other anomalies such as the Goldenhar syndrome (oculoauriculovertebral dysplasia) (38).

In adults, diagonal earlobe crease has been associated with coronary artery disease and has been referred to as the Frank sign (39). The crease runs diagonally backward and downward across the lateral surface of the earlobe from the external meatus (Fig. 13.42). Depending on the extent and depth of the crease, three grades have been assigned with grade 1 being the least obvious appearing crease, grade 2 including a superficial crease across 100% of the earlobe or a deep crease across 50% of the earlobe, and grade 3 represented by a deep crease along 100% of the earlobe. Bilateral grades 2 and 3 creases are associated with a significantly higher risk of death from atherosclerosis and myocardial infarction (40).

MIDDLE EAR

Otitis Media

Otitis media is either an acute or a chronic infectious disease of the middle ear space. Otitis media is predominantly, but not exclusively, a childhood disease. The most common microorganisms implicated in causing disease of the middle ear are *Streptococcus pneumoniae* and *Haemophilus influenzae* (41). Otoscopic examination reveals a hyperemic, opaque, bulging tympanic membrane with limited mobility; purulent otorrhea may be present. Bilateral involvement is not uncommon. The middle ear infection is felt to result from infection via the eustachian tube at the time of or following a pharyngitis (bacterial or viral).

In general, otitis media is managed medically. However, at times tissue is removed for histopathologic examination. The pathologic alterations are generally straightforward but secondary changes such as glandular metaplasia of the surface epithelium, the result of chronic infection, may occur that might be confused with a true gland-forming neoplasm.

The histologic changes in chronic otitis media include a variable amount of chronic inflammatory cells consisting of lymphocytes, histiocytes, plasma cells, and eosinophils. Multinucleated giant cells and foamy histiocytes may be present. The middle ear low-cuboidal epithelium may or may not be seen. However, glandular metaplasia, a response of the middle ear epithelium to the infectious process, may be present (Fig. 13.43). The glands tend to be more common in nonsuppurative otitis media than in suppurative otitis media. The metaplastic glands are unevenly distributed in the tissue specimens, are variably shaped and are separated by abundant stromal tissue. The glands are lined by a columnar-to-cuboidal epithelium with or without cilia or goblet cell metaplasia. Glandular secretions may or may not be present so that the glands may appear empty or contain varying secretions, including thin (serous) or thick (mucoid) fluid content. The identification of cilia is confirmatory of middle ear glandular metaplasia and is a feature that is not found in association with middle ear adenomas (36). Further, the haphazard arrangement of the glands in the background of changes of chronic otitis media should allow for differentiating metaplastic glands from neoplastic glands. Acute inflammatory cells may be superimposed by those of chronic otitis media.

In addition to the inflammatory cell infiltrate and glandular metaplasia, other histopathologic findings can be seen in association with chronic otitis media (or represent sequelae of chronic otitis media) and include fibrosis, granulation tissue, tympanosclerosis, cholesterol granulomas, and reactive bone formation. Due to the presence of scar tissue, the middle ear ossicles may be destroyed (partial

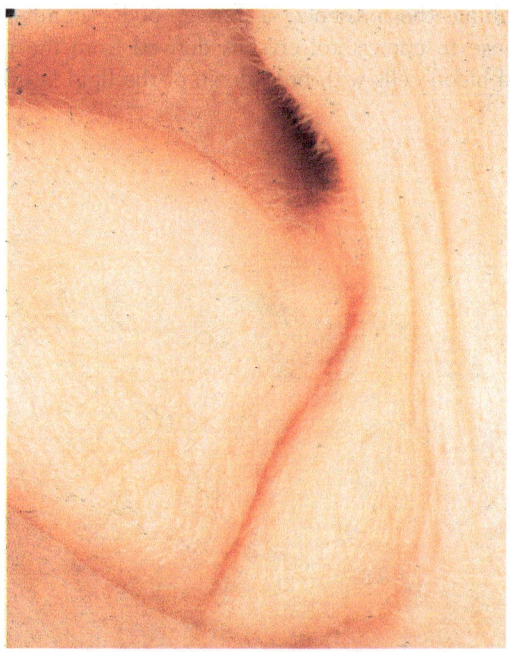

FIGURE 13.42 Individual with a grade 3 earlobe crease represented by a deep crease along 100% of the earlobe. This person had similar earlobe crease on the opposite ear. Bilateral grade 2 and 3 creases are associated with a significantly higher risk of death from atherosclerosis and myocardial infarction.

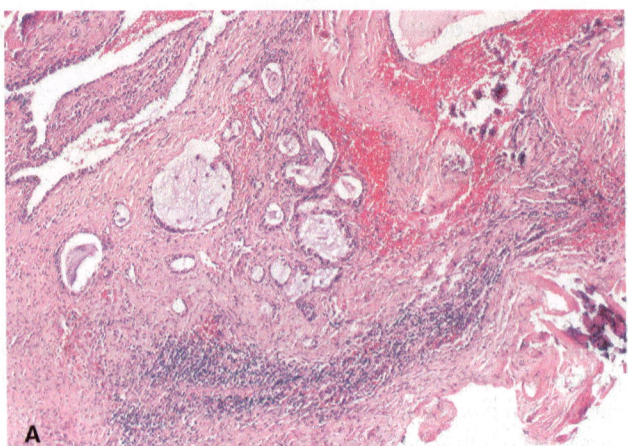 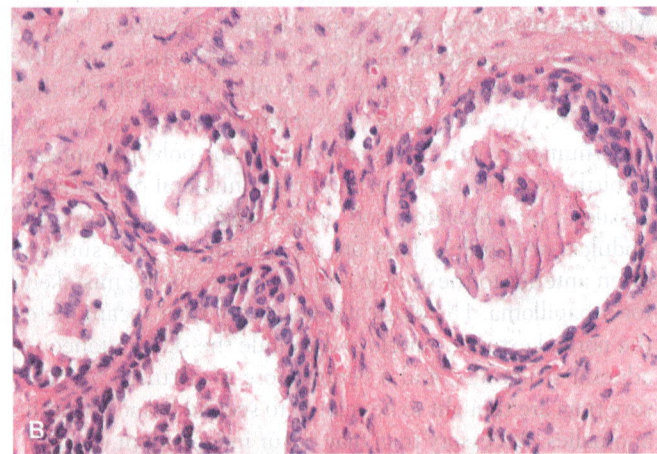

FIGURE 13.43 Under normal conditions glands are not identified in the middle ear space. However, glandular metaplasia can be found in the setting of otitis media. **A:** Otitis media showing chronic inflammation, fibrosis, glandular metaplasia, and foci of calcifications (*lower right*); residual normal cuboidal epithelium of the middle ear is seen in the upper left. **B:** Higher magnification showing glandular metaplasia is the setting of chronic otitis media.

or total) or may become immobilized. Perforation of the tympanic membrane pars tensa may occur with resulting ingrowth of squamous epithelium potentially leading to the development of cholesteatoma (see below).

Tympanosclerosis represents dystrophic mineralization (calcification or ossification) of the tympanic membrane or middle ear that is associated with recurrent episodes of otitis media (42). The incidence of tympanosclerosis in otitis media varies from 3% to 33% (42). Tympanosclerosis of the tympanic membrane can be seen in children following myringotomy and tube insertion. In this setting, the tympanosclerotic foci may or may not be permanent. Tympanosclerosis of the middle ear typically affects older patients, represents irreversible accumulation of mineralized material and is associated with conductive hearing loss (43,44).

On gross examination, tympanosclerotic foci may be localized or diffuse and appear as white nodules or plaques (Fig. 13.44). Histologically, dense "clumps" of mineralized calcified or ossified material or debris can be seen within the stromal tissues or in the middle (connective tissue) aspect of the tympanic membrane (Fig. 13.45). Tympanosclerosis may cause scarring and ossicular fixation.

Cholesterol granuloma is a histologic designation describing the presence a foreign-body granulomatous response to cholesterol crystals derived from the rupture of red blood cells with breakdown of the lipid layer of the

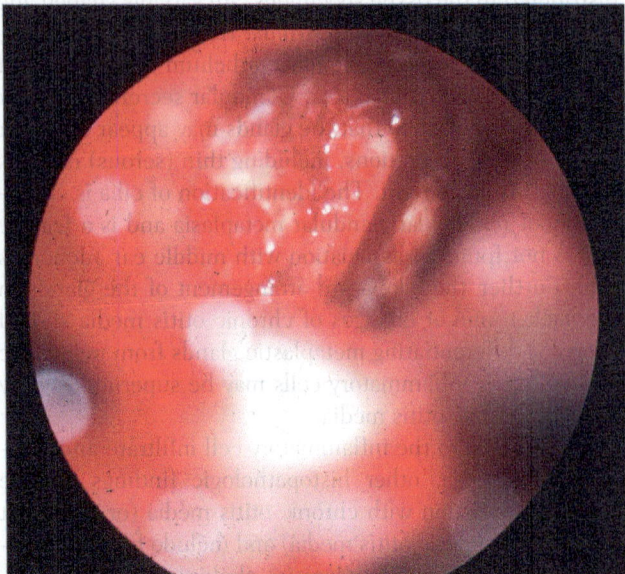

FIGURE 13.44 Tympanic membrane in tympanosclerosis showing calcified plaque on the tympanic membrane.

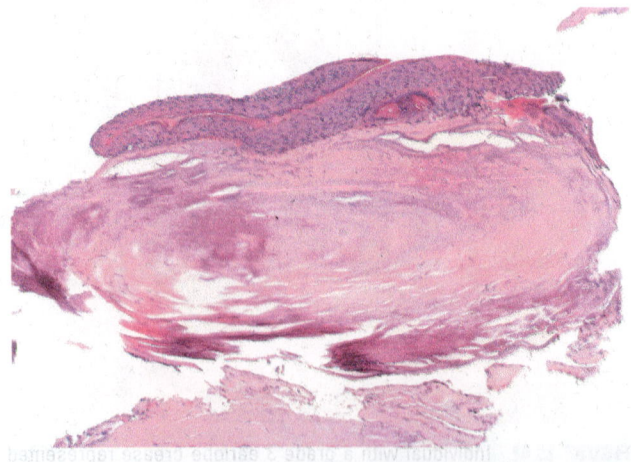

FIGURE 13.45 Tympanosclerosis. The tympanic membrane is thickened and calcified and covered on its external (external auditory canal) aspect by keratinizing the squamous epithelium (*top*) and internal (tympanic cavity) aspect by the cuboidal epithelium (*bottom right*).

erythrocyte cell membrane. Cholesterol granulomas arise in the middle ear and mastoid in any condition in which there is hemorrhage combined with interference in drainage and ventilation of the middle ear space (45). Cholesterol granuloma of the middle ear may present as idiopathic hemotympanum; patients may also complain of hearing loss and tinnitus. Most of the cholesterol granulomas in the middle ear and temporal bone have an indolent biologic behavior and cause no significant bone resorption (45).

In contrast to cholesterol granulomas of the middle ear and temporal bone, cholesterol granulomas of the petrous apex may behave aggressively producing a large tumor-like mass with expansion of the cyst and erosion/destruction of adjacent structures that may clinically mimic a neoplasm (e.g., jugulotympanic paraganglioma, endolymphatic sac papillary tumor) (46). Depending on the direction of expansion, apical cholesterol granulomas may invade into the cochlea, cerebellopontine angle, jugular foramen, cranial nerves V to XI, brain stem, and cerebellum producing life-threatening symptoms (47). Involvement of the petrous apex is more likely to be associated with sensorineural hearing loss; additional signs and symptoms may include headaches, cranial nerve deficits (e.g., facial paralysis), and bone erosion with involvement of the posterior or middle cranial fossa has been reported (7, 46,48). On axial computed tomography, apical cholesterol granulomas appear as round to ovoid to irregular-appearing cysts with smooth margins and evidence of bone remodeling.

The histology of cholesterol granulomas is the same irrespective of location and includes the presence of irregular-shaped clear-appearing spaces surrounded by histiocytes and/or multinucleated giant cells (foreign-body granuloma) (Fig. 13.46). Cholesterol granulomas are not related to cholesteatomas but may occur in association with or independent of a cholesteatoma.

Cholesteatoma (Keratoma)

Cholesteatoma is a pseudoneoplastic lesion of the middle ear characterized by the presence of stratified squamous epithelium that forms a sac-like accumulation of keratin within the middle ear space (akin to an epidermal inclusion cyst). Despite their invasive growth, cholesteatomas are not considered to be true neoplasms. The term cholesteatoma is a misnomer in that it is not a neoplasm nor does it contain cholesterol. Perhaps the designation of keratoma would be more accurate but the term cholesteatoma is entrenched in the literature. In the middle ear and the inner ear, cholesteatomas take three forms: acquired cholesteatoma, congenital cholesteatoma, and cholesteatoma of the petrous apex. Depending on the site of origin in the tympanic membrane, each of these cholesteatomas may be subdivided into pars flaccida (Shrapnell membrane) and pars tensa cholesteatomas.

Acquired Cholesteatoma

Acquired cholesteatoma is the most common type of cholesteatoma. It tends to be more common in men than in women and occur in older children and young adults. Acquired cholesteatoma is derived from entry of external ear canal epidermis into the middle ear. The latter may arise in one of several ways: via perforation of the tympanic membrane, following localized retraction of the tympanic membrane with epithelial invagination or ingrowth of a band of stratified squamous epithelium into the middle ear, via entrapment of squamous epithelium following surgery and/or trauma or via squamous metaplasia of the middle ear

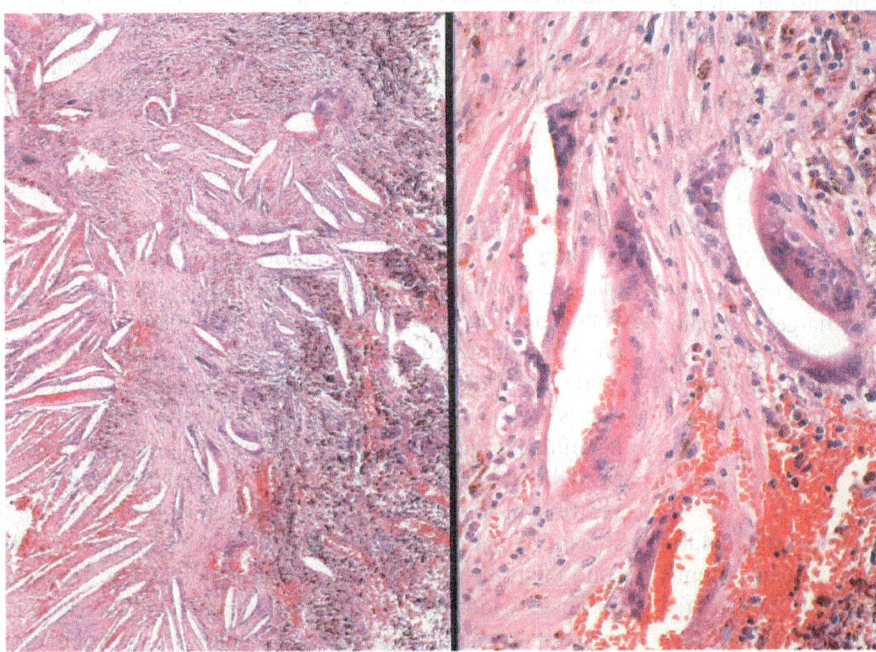

FIGURE 13.46 Cholesterol granuloma appears as empty, irregularly shaped clefts or spaces surrounded by histiocytes and multinucleated giant cells. Fresh hemorrhage and hemosiderin pigment are readily apparent.

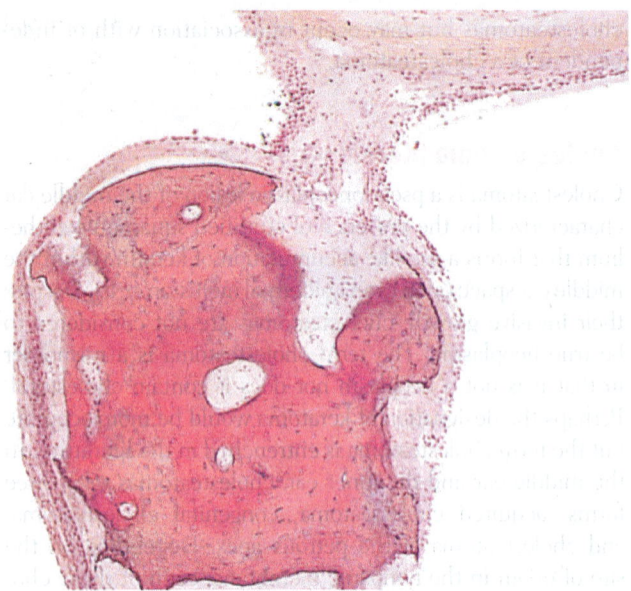

FIGURE 13.47 Section of malleus from an adult ear with a retraction pocket of the tympanic membrane at autopsy. There is a thin layer of stratified squamous epithelium between the bone and middle ear epithelium. This was found on serial section to be an ingrowth of the stratified squamous epithelium from the outer epithelial covering of the retraction pocket.

mucosa (49). A decrease in middle ear pressure can induce retraction of certain regions of the tympanic membrane in the pars flaccida, pars tensa, or both (49). Retraction pockets are felt to represent the precursors for the development of cholesteatoma (Fig. 13.47) (50,51). Dysfunction of the eustachian tube leading to chronic (recurrent) otitis media is felt to represent a causative factor (49). The triggers for cholesteatoma onset are diverse, and may involve tympanic membrane trauma (i.e., perforation, displacement, retraction, or invagination), tympanic membrane disease, and/or tympanic cavity mucosa disease. Research has revealed that cell migration is replaced under inflammatory conditions by hyperplasia, which is felt to be the trigger for the onset of cholesteatoma (52). Diseased mucosa can contribute to the development of retraction pockets and cholesteatoma (53).

The upper posterior part of the middle ear space is the most common site of acquired cholesteatomas (49). Initially, cholesteatomas may remain clinically silent until extensive invasion of the middle ear space and mastoid occurs. Symptoms include hearing loss, malodorous discharge, and pain and may be associated with a polyp arising in the attic of the middle ear or perforation of the tympanic membrane. Otoscopic examination may reveal the presence of white debris within the middle ear, which is considered diagnostic.

Congenital Cholesteatoma

Congenital cholesteatoma is a cholesteatoma of the middle ear that exists in the presence of an intact tympanic membrane presumably occurring in the absence of chronic otitis media that may result in perforation or retraction of the tympanic membrane. Congenital cholesteatomas are found in infants and young children. Small colonies of epidermoid cells referred to as epidermoid formations are found on the lateral anterior superior surface of the middle ear in temporal bones after 15 weeks of gestation (53). During the first postpartum year, the epidermoid colonies disappear; however, if the epidermoid cells do not disappear but continue to grow, they will become a congenital cholesteatoma. The latter have also been referred to as epidermoid cysts (54). In most of the cases, congenital cholesteatomas are found in the anterosuperior part of the middle ear. In early lesions, there are no symptoms and are discovered by otoscopic examination. In later lesions, the signs and symptoms may be the same as acquired cholesteatoma.

Congenital cholesteatoma is believed to have a different pathophysiology than acquired cholesteatoma in that these patients rarely have eustachian tube dysfunction (55). The absence of eustachian tube dysfunction likely accounts for their reasonable preoperative hearing and their lack of complications or recurrences postoperatively (55). The most important factor is early detection. Treatment remains surgical removal.

Dornelles et al. (56) attempted to evaluate the quantification of angiogenesis and matrix metalloproteinases (MMP) as markers of aggressiveness in cholesteatoma (56). These authors compared expression of CD31, MMP2, and MMP9 in pediatric and adult patients. The authors found that pediatric cholesteatomas presented a more exacerbated inflammatory degree and produced more MMP representing factors, that when combined, could characterize pediatric cholesteatomas as more aggressive than adult cholesteatomas (56).

Cholesteatoma of the Petrous Apex

Cholesteatoma of the petrous apex is an epidermoid cyst of this location and bears no relation to cholesteatoma of the middle ear. It is likely of congenital origin but no cell rests have been discovered that may explain the origin of these lesions. Symptoms usually relate to involvement of the VII and VIII cranial nerves in the cerebellopontine angle (54).

Pathology

Cholesteatomas irrespective of whether acquired or congenital appear as cystic, white to pearly appearing mass of varying size containing creamy or waxy granular material. The histologic diagnosis of cholesteatoma is made in the presence of a stratified keratinizing squamous epithelium, subepithelial fibroconnective or granulation tissue, and keratin debris (Fig. 13.48). The essential diagnostic feature is the keratinizing squamous epithelium and the presence of keratin debris alone is not diagnostic of a cholesteatoma. The keratinizing squamous epithelium is cytologically bland and shows cellular maturation without evidence of dysplasia. In spite of its benign histology, cholesteatomas are "invasive" and have widespread destructive capabilities. The destructive properties of cholesteatomas result from a combination

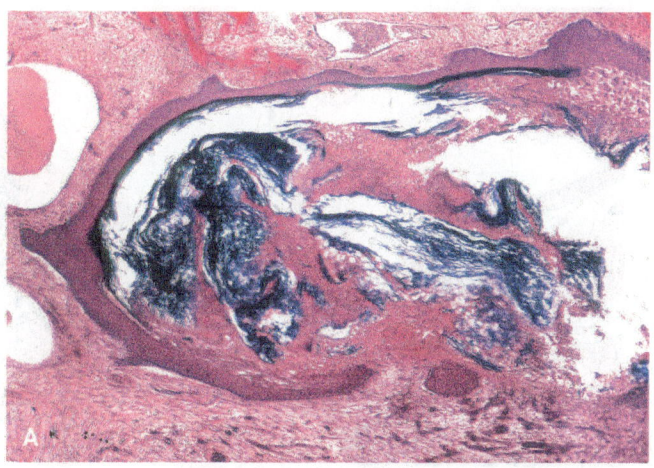 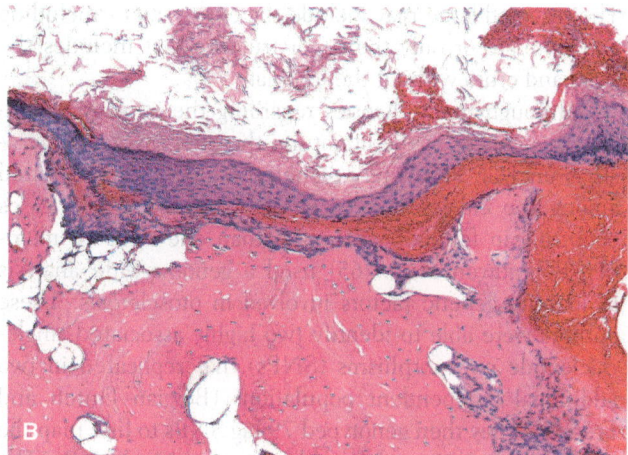

FIGURE 13.48 Cholesteatoma of the middle ear. **A:** The histologic diagnosis of cholesteatoma is based on the presence of finding keratinizing squamous epithelium within the middle ear space. **B:** Osseous involvement.

of interrelated reasons, including mass effect with pressure erosion of surrounding structures from the cholesteatoma, the production of collagenase, which has osteodestructive capabilities by its resorption of bony structures and bone resorption. Collagenase is produced by both the squamous epithelial and the fibrous tissue components of the cholesteatoma. This local aggressive behavior is the result of the continuing accumulation of the cholesteatomatous material with progressive erosion of surrounding structures. Depending on the location and extent of the cholesteatoma, erosion may include the lateral wall of the attic, the middle ear ossicles, the tegmental bone over the attic and antrum, and the mastoid cortex (49). Less frequent progression includes erosion of the lateral sinus and jugular bulb, the vestibular and cochlear capsules, the fallopian canal, the dura of the middle and posterior cranial fossa, the semicircular canals, and the facial nerve (49). Sequela of such erosions may include semicircular canal fistulas, exposed tympanic facial nerve, or brain herniation through the tegmen. The histologic diagnosis of cholesteatomas is relatively straightforward in the presence of keratinizing squamous epithelium. Cholesterol granuloma is not synonymous with cholesteatoma. These entities are distinctly different pathologic entities and should not be confused with one another.

Park et al. (57) evaluated differential expression of p63 and survivin in human middle ear cholesteatoma epithelium. p63 is a p53 homologue and a marker expressed in replicating keratinocytes; survivin is an inhibitor of apoptosis protein that is abundantly expressed in most solid and hematologic malignancies. Expression of p63 protein was diffusely observed in entire samples of cholesteatoma, especially in acquired cholesteatoma, compared with the control group. Congenital cholesteatoma showed variable p63 reactivity in a basal cell-like pattern. Primary and recurrent cholesteatomas showed no significant difference in p63 expression. Survivin was detected in 31 of the 40 cholesteatoma samples. Acquired cholesteatomas showed especially increased survivin expression compared with congenital cases. These findings indicate a putative role of p63 and survivin in the development of acquired cholesteatomas. Genetic alterations including upregulation of EGFR, TGF-α, and metalloproteinases as well as downregulation of tumor suppressor genes and altered expression of proto-oncogenes have been reported in cholesteatomas (58,59) but the mechanisms in the development of cholesteatomas remain unclear (60).

In contrast to cholesteatomas, squamous cell carcinoma shows dysplastic or overtly malignant cytologic features with a prominent desmoplastic stromal response to its infiltrative growth. Cholesteatomas do not transform into squamous cell carcinomas. In an attempt to determine whether cholesteatomas were low-grade squamous carcinomas, Desloge et al. (61) performed DNA analysis on human cholesteatomas to determine whether ploidy abnormalities were present. In ten cases with interpretable data, nine were euploid and one was aneuploid. These authors concluded that due to a lack of overt genetic instability, cholesteatomas could not be considered to be malignant neoplasms.

Otosclerosis

Otosclerosis is a disorder of the bony labyrinth and stapedial footplate that exclusively occurs in humans. Otosclerosis means hardening of the ear and is derived from Greek (ous, ear; skleros, hard; osis, condition); osseous ankylosis (Greek: ankoulon, to stiffen); chronic metaplastic osteitis; progressive otospongiosis. Otosclerosis primarily causes conductive hearing loss that usually begins in the second and third decades of life and is slowly progressive. The extent of the hearing loss directly correlates with the degree of stapedial footplate fixation. It is not uncommon for patients with otosclerosis to also have vestibular disturbances (62,63). Otosclerosis usually involves both ears; however, unilateral disease can occur up to 15% of cases (64). Surgical management of the conductive hearing loss caused by stapes fixation (stapedectomy) is the treatment of choice with replacement of the fixed stapes by prosthesis.

The resected bone may include the entire stapes including the footplate or only the superstructure that includes the head and crura without the footplate.

Although many theories regarding the etiology of otosclerosis appear in the literature, the etiology of otosclerosis is unclear. Hereditary (genetic) factors are often cited among the causes of otosclerosis with half of all cases occurring in families with more than one affected member. Schrauwen et al. (65) used a genome-wide analysis to identify genetic factors involved in otosclerosis. These authors were able to identify two highly associated single-nucleotide polymorphisms (SNPs) that replicated in two additional independent populations (Belgian–Dutch and French). They then genotyped 79 tag SNPs to fine map the two genomic regions defined by the associated SNPs. The region with the strongest association signal, was on chromosome 7q22.1 spanning intron 1 to intron 4 of reelin (RELN), a gene known for its role in neuronal migration. Expression of RELN was confirmed in the inner ear and in stapes footplate specimens. The authors provided evidence that implicates RELN in the pathogenesis of otosclerosis. Subsequently, the authors completed a replication study that includes four additional populations from Europe (1,141 total samples) (66). Several SNPs in this region replicated in these populations separately. While the power to detect significant association in each population is small, when all the four populations are combined, six of the seven SNPs replicated and showed an effect in the same direction as in the previous populations. The authors also confirmed the presence of allelic heterogeneity in this region. These data further implicate RELN in the pathogenesis of otosclerosis.

Environmental factors are potentially linked to the development of otosclerosis. Environmental factors include fluoride and viral factors, particularly measles. There is compelling evidence that measles virus may play a role in some cases as measles virus RNA has been detected in stapes footplate samples (67) and molecular detection of measles virus has been reported in primary cell cultures of otosclerotic tissue (68).

Michaels and Soucek (69) reported on the origin and growth of otosclerosis. These authors found that the main plaque of otosclerosis is a histologic replica of the external layer of the otic capsule and seems to arise from similar cells in the periosteum and to follow a defined invasive course into the footplate of the stapes, the basal coil of the cochlea and the saccule. This process most often begins from the adjacent temporal bone (anterior to the oval window) eventually involving the footplate of the stapes moving across the annulus fibrosus or the stapediovestibular joint (Fig. 13.49). Stapedial involvement causes fixation of the stapes with inability to transmit sound waves resulting in conductive hearing loss. While the otosclerotic changes can be seen in the resected stapedial footplate, even when the footplate is removed intact, it may be free of otosclerotic changes as fixation results via pressure on the nonotosclerotic footplate from swelling of the otosclerotic process in

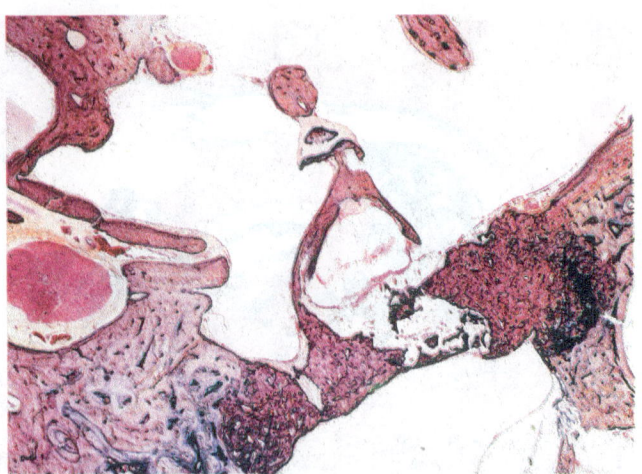

FIGURE 13.49 Otosclerosis of the temporal bone (anterior to the oval window) involving the footplate of the stapes moving across the annulus fibrosus or the stapediovestibular joint. Stapedial involvement causes fixation of the stapes with the inability to transmit sound waves resulting in conductive hearing loss.

the adjacent temporal bone (7). On the basis of its invasive growth into preexisting normal structures with replacement of these structures, including the cochlear and vestibular otic capsules, Michaels and Soucek (70) introduced the notion that otosclerosis represents an invasive (low-grade) osseous neoplasm.

INNER EAR

Presbycusis and Other Hearing Loss

Hearing loss may include conductive hearing loss and sensorineural hearing loss. There are many causes for conductive and sensorineural hearing loss, respectively (Figs. 13.50 and 13.51). Hearing loss that occurs with increasing age is referred to as presbycusis. There is still controversy as to the underlying electrophysiologic and histopathologic alterations associated with the development of presbycusis. Degenerative alterations within various microanatomic structures of the cochlea, including the hair cells, spiral ganglion cells, stria vascularis, and basilar membrane have been invoked as the cause of presbycusis (71). Alternatively, damage to the outer hair cells alone has been invoked as the cause of presbycusis (72,73). As Soucek et al. have shown in their studies of aged ears (72,73), the histopathologic changes include scanty to absent outer hair cells of the third row (Fig. 13.52) with complete loss of both inner and outer hair cells of all rows at the extreme lower end of the basal coil. In contrast to these aforementioned sites, Soucek et al. found that the inner hair cells sustained minimal loss, the first row of outer hair cells had greater loss, and the second row more loss but not to the extent seen in the third row of outer hair cells or at the extreme lower end of the basal coil (72,73). In addition, these authors also

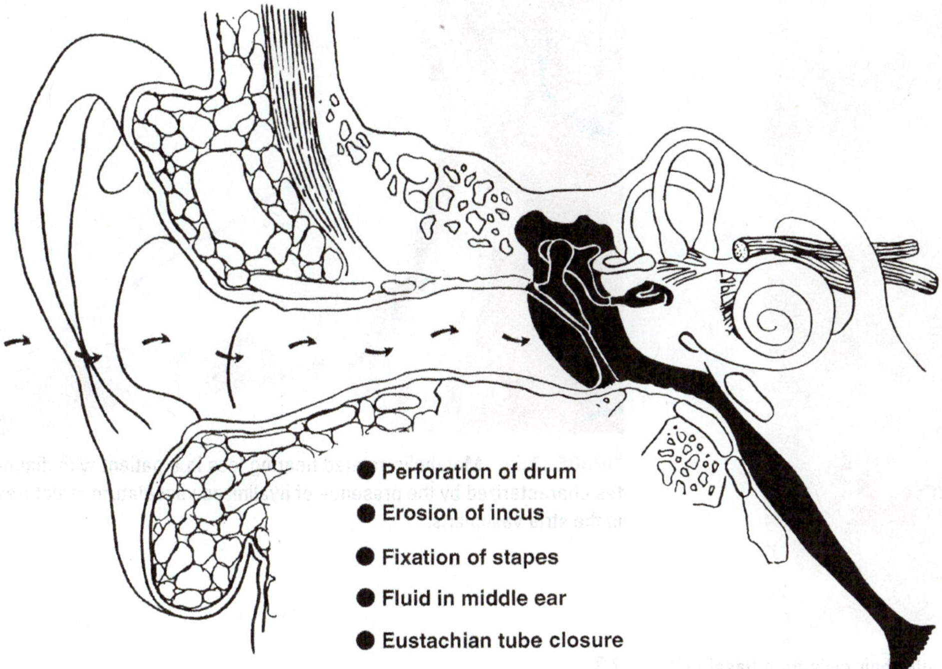

FIGURE 13.50 Causes of conductive hearing loss.

- Perforation of drum
- Erosion of incus
- Fixation of stapes
- Fluid in middle ear
- Eustachian tube closure

found the presence of enormously lengthened and thickened stereocilia and giant stereocilia which they felt contribute to the development of presbycusis. Degenerative alterations within various microanatomic structures of the membranous labyrinth resulting in sensorineural hearing loss may occur secondary to infectious disease (Fig. 13.53), metabolic abnormalities (Fig. 13.54), trauma (Fig. 13.55), sensory presbycusis (Fig. 13.56), and secondary to use of certain medications including cisplatin, diuretic agents, and other drugs (Figs. 13.57 and 13.58).

Ménière Disease

Ménière disease is an idiopathic disorder of the inner ear associated with a symptom complex of spontaneous, episodic attacks of vertigo, sensorineural hearing loss,

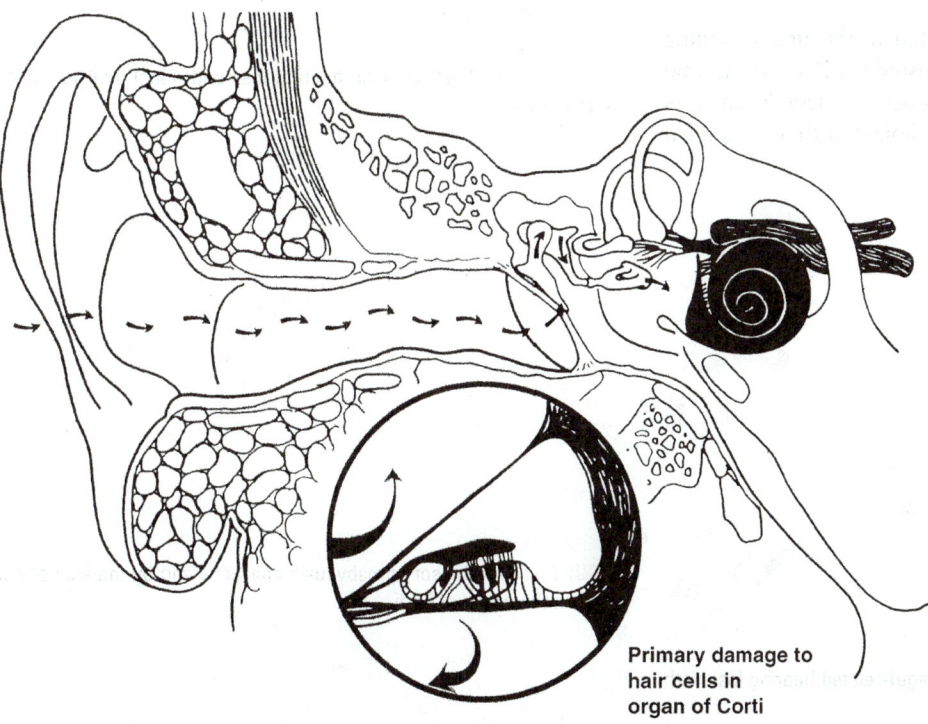

FIGURE 13.51 Cause of sensorineural hearing loss.

Primary damage to hair cells in organ of Corti

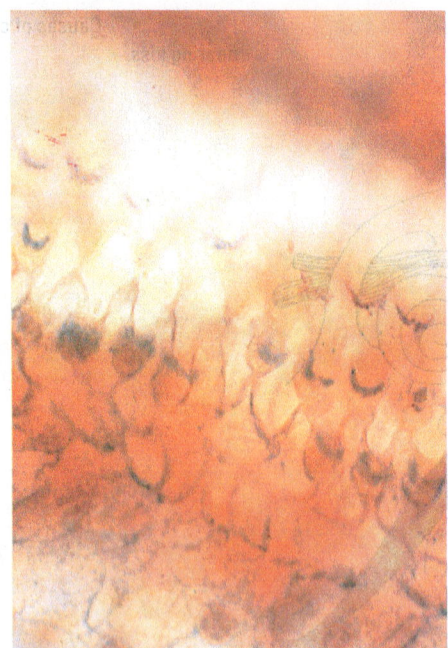

FIGURE 13.52 Surface preparation of outer hair cells from basal coil of cochlea of an elderly man. There are many gaps among the hair cells of the first two rows. Osmic acid, alcian blue, and phloxine eosin (oil immersion).

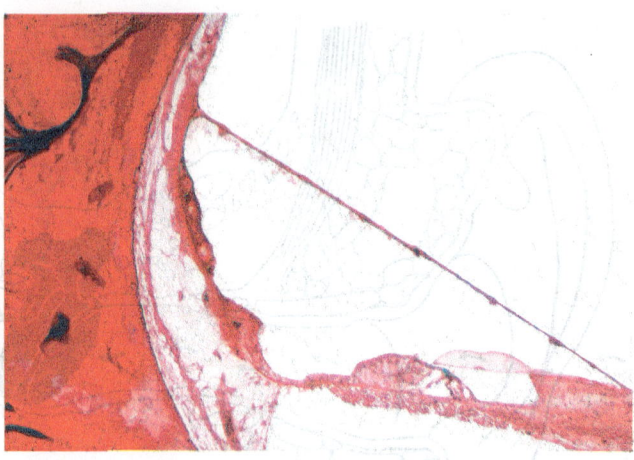

FIGURE 13.54 Metabolic-related hearing loss in a patient with diabetes characterized by the presence of hyalinized vasculature structures in the stria vascularis.

tinnitus, and a sensation of aural fullness. Ménière disease is characterized by a set of symptoms including fluctuating sensorineural hearing loss, episodes of vertigo, tinnitus, and pressure sensation in the ear. The onset of vertigo is frequently sudden reaching maximum intensity within a few minutes lasting for an hour or more and either subsiding completely or continuing as a sensation of unsteadiness for hours to days.

Genetic studies have contributed to the understanding of the genetic basis of vestibular disorders. Recently, exome sequencing has identified three single nucleotide variants in PRKCB, DPT, and SEMA3D linked with the familial

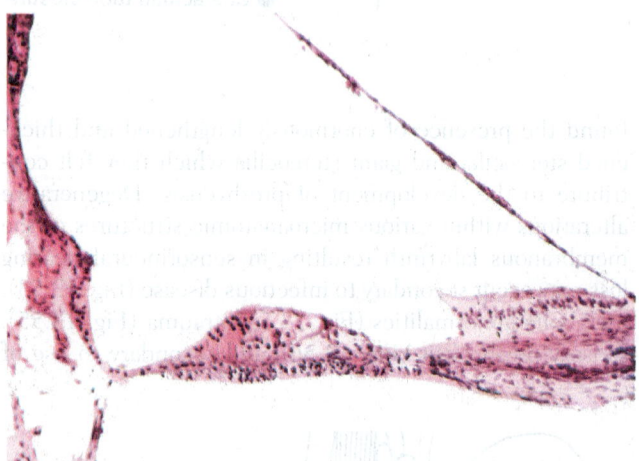

FIGURE 13.55 Posttraumatic hearing loss with focal avulsion of the organ of Corti.

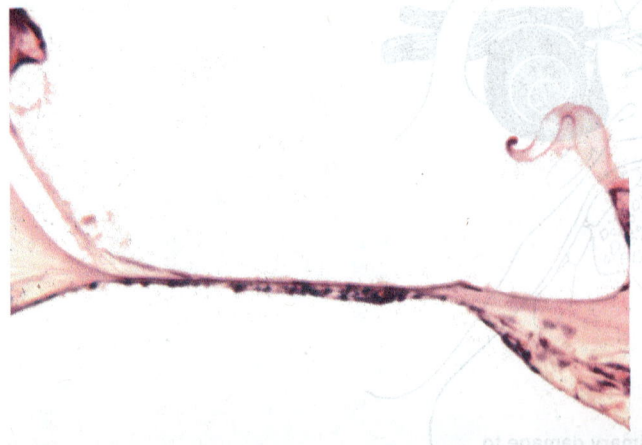

FIGURE 13.53 Viral labyrinthitis (end stage)-related hearing loss with total degeneration of the organ of Corti.

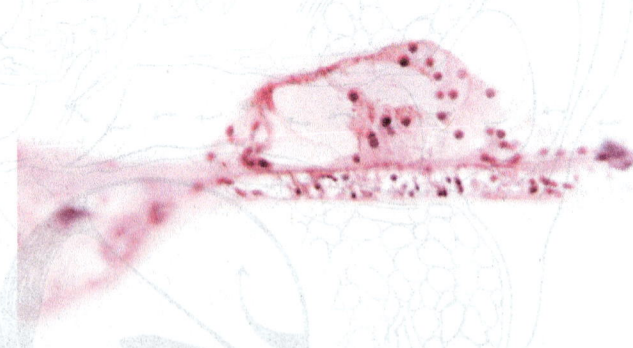

FIGURE 13.56 Sensory presbycusis characterized by the loss of hair cells in the organ of Corti.

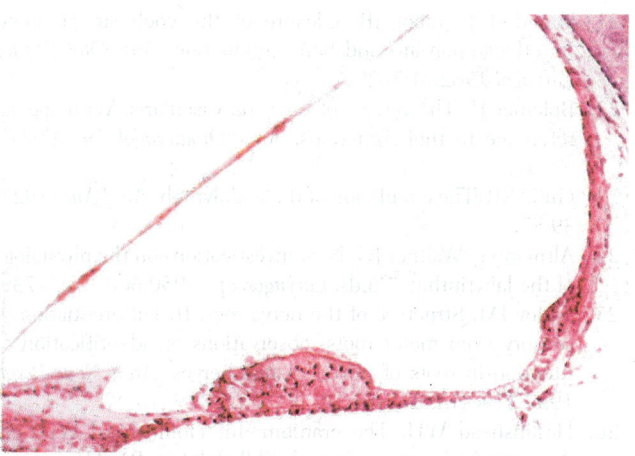

FIGURE 13.57 Strial presbycusis secondary to the ototoxic effect caused by cisplatin therapy with strial atrophy.

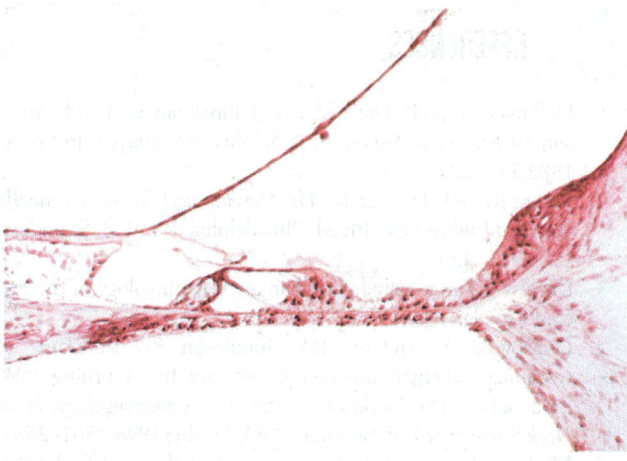

FIGURE 13.58 Kanamycin ototoxic effects on the organ of Corti with loss of hair cells.

Ménière disease further supporting the genetic background for most episodic or progressive vestibular-related syndromes, including the Ménière disease (74). With continued progress in the understanding of the disease mechanisms of vestibular-related syndromes improvements in medical treatment might be achievable. The pathogenesis of the Ménière disease is distortion of the membranous labyrinth defined as changes in the microanatomy of the membranous labyrinth as a consequence of the overaccumulation of endolymph (endolymphatic hydrops) and at the expense of the perilymphatic space (75,76). Endolymph which is produced by the stria vascularis in the cochlea and by cells in the vestibular labyrinth circulates in a radial and longitudinal fashion. In patients with Ménière disease, it is believed that there is inadequate absorption of endolymph by the endolymphatic sac (76).

In the early stages of the disease, endolymphatic hydrops primarily involves the cochlear duct and the saccule but in the later stages, the entire endolymphatic system is involved. Alterations of the membranous labyrinth include dilatation, outpouching, rupture, and collapse (Fig. 13.59). Fistulae (unhealed ruptures) may occur. Severe cytoarchitectural and atrophic changes may occur in the sense organs with loss of neurons in the cochlea.

Michaels and Soucek (77) described a thin highly vascular layer of bone (the vestibular arch) surrounding most of the intravestibular endolymphatic duct. In the normal ear, this contains osteoblasts, some of which are in apoptosis, which may help to control the potassium composition of the endolymph. These authors found that in Ménière disease, there is widespread death of vascular and other structures in the arch, probably by apoptosis (77–79). Such alterations may lead to hyperkalemia in the nearby endolymph and provoke hydrops and the symptoms of Ménière disease.

TEMPORAL BONE DISSECTION

For a detailed discussion of proper postmortem removal, sectioning, and processing for microscopic evaluation of the temporal bone, the reader may refer to other texts (7,80).

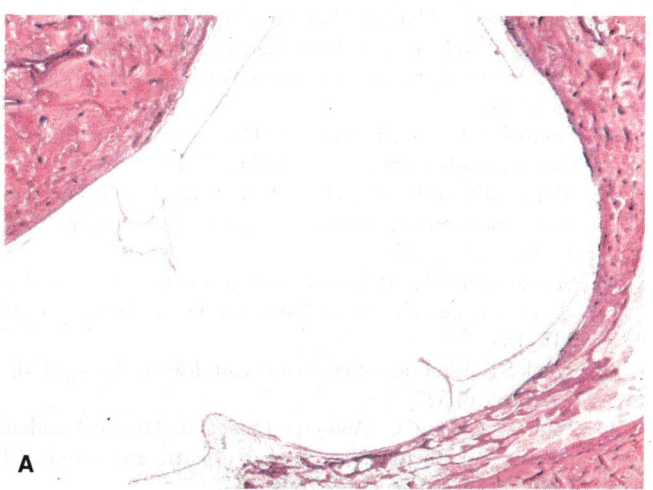
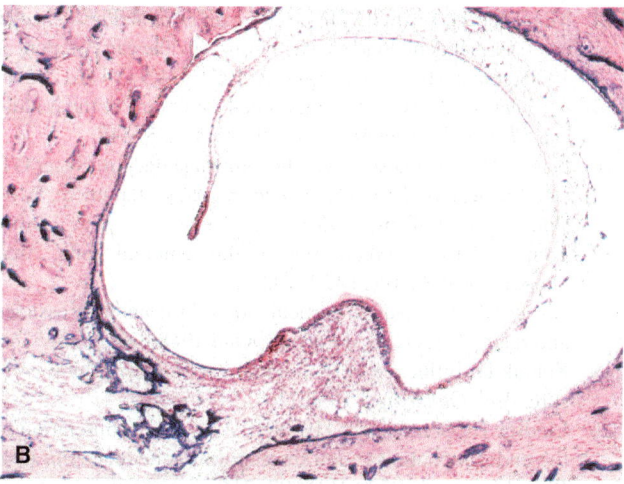

FIGURE 13.59 The Ménière disease. **A:** Dilatation. **B:** Rupture of the membranous labyrinth.

REFERENCES

1. Hollinshead WH. The ear. In: Hollinshead WH, ed. *Anatomy for Surgeons*. 3rd ed. Philadelphia, PA: Harper and Row; 1982:159–221.
2. Moore KL, ed. The ear. In: *The Developing Human: Clinically Oriented Embryology*. 4th ed. Philadelphia, PA: W.B. Saunders; 1988:412–420.
3. Dayal VS, Farkashidy J, Kokshanian A. Embryology of the ear. *Can J Otolaryngol* 1973;2:136–142.
4. Lysakowski A, McCrea RA, Tomlinson RD. Anatomy of vestibular end organs and neural pathways. In: Cummings CW, Frederickson JM, Harker LA, et al., eds. *Otolaryngology: Head Neck Surgery*. 3rd ed. St. Louis, MO: Mosby; 1998:2561–2583.
5. Michaels L, Soucek S. Development of the stratified squamous epithelium of the tympanic membrane and external canal: The origin of auditory epithelial migration. *Am J Anat* 1989;184(4):334–344.
6. Michaels L, Soucek S. Stratified squamous epithelium in relation to the tympanic membrane: Its development and kinetics. *Int J Pediatr Otorhinolaryngol* 1991;22(2):135–149.
7. Michaels L. The ear. In: Sternberg SS, ed. *Histology for Pathologists*. 2nd ed. Philadelphia, PA: Lippincott-Raven; 1997:337–366.
8. Michaels L, Soucek S. Auditory epithelial migration on the human tympanic membrane: II. The existence of two discrete migratory pathways and their embryologic correlates. *Am J Anat* 1990;189:189–200.
9. Nager GT. Anatomy of the membranous cochlea and vestibular labyrinth. In: Nager GT, ed. *Pathology of the Ear and Temporal Bone*. Baltimore, MD: Williams and Wilkins; 1993:3–48.
10. Schuknecht HF, ed. Anatomy. In: *Pathology of the Ear*. 2nd ed. Philadelphia, PA: Lea & Febiger; 1993:31–74.
11. Maybaum JL, Goldman JL. Primary jugular bulb thrombosis. A study of twenty cases. *Arch Otolaryngol* 1933;17(1):70–84.
12. Kamerer DB. Electromyographic correlation of tensor tympani and tensor veli palatini muscles in man. *Laryngoscope* 1978;88(4):651–662.
13. Graves GO, Edwards LF. The eustachian tube: A review of its descriptive, microscopic, topographic and clinical anatomy. *Arch Otolaryngol* 1944;39(5):359–397.
14. Moreano EH, Paparella MM, Zelterman D, et al. Prevalence of carotid canal dehiscence in the human middle ear: A report of 1000 temporal bones. *Laryngoscope* 1994;104(5 Pt 1):612–618.
15. Michaels L, Wells M. Squamous cell carcinoma of the middle ear. *Clin Otolaryngol Allied Sci* 1980;5(4):235–248.
16. Nager GT. Pneumatization of the temporal bone. In: Nager GT, ed. *Pathology of the Ear and Temporal Bone*. Baltimore, MD: Williams and Wilkins; 1993:53–62.
17. Tremble GE. Pneumatization of the temporal bone. *Arch Otolaryngol* 1934;19(2):172–182.
18. Davies DV. A note on the articulations of the auditory ossicles and related structures. *J Laryngol Otol* 1948;62(8):533–536.
19. Kobrak H. Influence of the middle ear on labyrinthine pressure. *Arch Otolaryngol* 1935;21(5):547–560.
20. Lindsey JR, Schuknecht HF, Neff WD, et al. Obliteration of the endolymphatic sac and the cochlear aqueduct. *Ann Otol Rhinol Laryngol* 1952;61(3):697–716, discussion, 738.
21. Tonndorf J, Tabor JR. Closure of the cochlear windows: Its effect upon air- and bone-conduction. *Ann Otol Rhinol Laryngol* 1962;71:5–29.
22. Belemer JJ. The vessels of the stria vascularis: With special reference to their functions. *Arch Otolaryngol* 1936;23(1):93–97.
23. Guild SR. The circulation of the endolymph. *Am J Anat* 1927;39:57.
24. Altmann F, Waltner JG. New investigations on the physiology of the labyrinthine fluids. *Laryngoscope* 1950;60(8):727–739.
25. Tarlov IM. Structure of the nerve root. II. Differentiation of sensory from motor roots; observations on identification of function in roots of mixed cranial nerves. *Arch Neur Psych* 1937;37(6):1338–1355.
26. Hollinshead WH. The cranium. In: Hollinshead WH, ed. *Anatomy for Surgeons*. 3rd ed. Philadelphia, PA: Harper and Row; 1982:26–27.
27. Hyams VJ, Batsakis JG, Michaels L. Acoustic neuroma. In: Hartmann WH, Sobin LH, eds. *Tumors of the Upper Respiratory Tract and Ear. Atlas of Tumor Pathology, Fascicle 25, Second Series*. Washington, DC: Armed Forces Institute of Pathology; 1988:323–326.
28. Heffner DK. Low-grade adenocarcinoma of probable endolymphatic sac origin. A clinicopathologic study of 20 cases. *Cancer* 1989;64(11):2292–2302.
29. Wenig BM, Heffner DK. Endolymphatic sac tumors: Fact or fiction? *Adv Anat Pathol* 1996;3:378–387.
30. Thompson LDR, Magliocca K, Stelow E, et al. CAIX and PAX8 are commonly immunoreactive in endolymphatic sac tumors: Differential with renal cell carcinoma in von-Hippel-Lindau patients. *Modern Pathol* 2018;98(Suppl):487–488.
31. Megerian CA, McKenna MJ, Nuss RC, et al. Endolymphatic sac tumors: Histopathologic confirmation, clinical characterization, and implication in von Hippel–Lindau disease. *Laryngoscope* 1995;105(8 Pt 1):801–808.
32. Sgambati MT, Stolle C, Choyke PL, et al. Mosaicism in von Hippel–Lindau disease: Lessons from kindreds with germline mutations identified in offspring with mosaic parents. *Am J Hum Genet* 2000;66(1):84–91.
33. Findeis-Hosey JJ, McMahon KQ, Findeis SK. Von Hippel-Lindau disease. *J Pediatr Genet* 2016;5(2):116–123.
34. Schnack DT, Kiss K, Hansen S, et al. Sporadic endolymphatic sac tumor-a very rare cause of hearing loss, tinnitus, and dizziness. *J Int Adv Otol* 2017;13(2):289–291.
35. Jegannathan D, Kathirvelu G, Mahalingam A. Three sporadic cases of endolymphatic sac tumor. *Neurol India* 2016;64(6):1336–1339.
36. Smith CA, Lowry OH, Wu ML. The electrolytes of the labyrinthine fluids. *Laryngoscope* 1954;64(3):141–153.
37. Møller MN, Kirkeby S, Vikeså J, et al. The human endolymphatic sac expresses natriuretic peptides. *Laryngoscope* 2017;127(6):E201–E208.
38. Schuknecht HF, ed. Developmental defects. In: *Pathology of the Ear*. 2nd ed. Philadelphia, PA: Lea & Febiger; 1993:115–189.
39. Frank ST. Aural sign of coronary heart disease. *N Engl J Med* 1973;289(6):327–328.
40. Patel V, Champ C, Andrews PS, et al. Diagonal earlobe creases and atheromatous disease: a postmortem study. *J R Coll Physicians Lond* 1992;26(3):274–277.

41. Wenig BM. Otitis media. In: Wenig BM, ed. *Atlas of Head and Neck Pathology*. 3rd ed. Philadelphia, PA: Saunders Elsevier; 2016:1108–1113.
42. Bhaya MH, Scachern PA, Morizono T, et al. Pathogenesis of tympanosclerosis. *Otolaryngol Head Neck Surg* 1993;109(3 Pt 1):413–420.
43. Gibb AG, Pang YT. Current considerations in the etiology and diagnosis of tympanosclerosis. *Eur Arch Otorhinolaryngol* 1994;251(8):439–451.
44. Nager GT, Vanderveen TS. Cholesterol granuloma involving the temporal bone. *Ann Otol Rhinol Laryngol* 1976;85(2 Pt 1):204–209.
45. Nager GT. Cholesterol granulomas. In: Nager GT, ed. *Pathology of the Ear and Temporal Bone*. Baltimore, MD: Williams & Wilkins; 1994:914–939.
46. Olcott C, Strasnick B. A blue middle ear mass: Cholesterol granuloma mimicking a glomus tumor and endolymphatic sac tumor. *Am J Otolaryngol* 2017;38(1):100–102.
47. Thedinger BA, Nadol JB Jr, Montgomery WW, et al. Radiographic diagnosis, surgical treatment, and long-term follow-up of cholesterol granulomas of the petrous apex. *Laryngoscope* 1989;99(9):896–907.
48. Nager GT. Cholesteatomas of the middle ear. In: Nager GT, ed. *Pathology of the Ear and Temporal Bone*. Baltimore, MD: Williams & Wilkins; 1994:298–350.
49. Michaels L. The biology of cholesteatoma. *Otolaryngol Clin North Am* 1989;22(5):869–881.
50. Wells M, Michaels L. Role of retraction pockets in cholesteatoma formation. *Clin Otolaryngol Allied Sci* 1983;8(1):39–45.
51. Schuknecht HF. Cholesteatoma. In: *Pathology of the Ear*. 2nd ed. Philadelphia, PA: Lea & Febiger; 1993:204–206.
52. Louw L. Acquired cholesteatoma pathogenesis: Stepwise explanations. *J Laryngol Otol* 2010;124(6):587–593.
53. Michaels L. Origin of congenital cholesteatoma from a normally occurring epidermoid rest in the developing middle ear. *Int J Pediatr Otorhinolaryngol* 1988;15(1):51–65.
54. de Souza CD, Sperling NM, da Costa SS, et al. Congenital cholesteatomas of the cerebellopontine angle. *Am J Otol* 1989;10(5):358–363.
55. Bennett M, Warren F, Jackson GC, et al. Congenital cholesteatoma: Theories, facts and 53 patients. *Otolaryngol Clin North Am* 2006;39(6):1081–1094.
56. Dornelles Cde C, da Costa SS, Neurer L, et al. Comparison of acquired cholesteatoma between pediatric and adult patients. *Eur Arch Otorhinolaryngol* 2009;266(10):1553–1561.
57. Park HR, Min SK, Min K, et al. Increased expression of p63 and surviving in cholesteatomas. *Acta Otolaryngol* 2009;129(3):268–272.
58. Kuo CL, Shiao AS, Yung M, et al. Updates and knowledge gaps in cholesteatoma research. *Biomed Res Int* 2015;2015:854024.
59. Kuo CL. Etiopathogenesis of acquired cholesteatoma: prominent theories and recent advances in biomolecular research. *Laryngoscope* 2015;125(1):234–240.
60. Sanderson A. Cholesteatoma. In: El-Naggar AK, Chan JKC, Grandis JR, Takata T, Slootweg PJ, eds. *WHO Classification of Head and Neck Tumours*. 4th ed. Lyon, France: IARC; 2017:269–270.
61. Desloge RB, Carew JF, Finstad CL, et al. DNA analysis of human cholesteatomas. *Am J Otol* 1997;18(2):155–159.
62. Cody DT, Baker HL Jr. Otosclerosis: Vestibular symptoms and sensorineural hearing loss. *Ann Otol Rhinol Laryngol* 1978;87(6 Pt 1):778–796.
63. Morales-Garcia C. Cochleo-vestibular involvement in otosclerosis. *Acta Otolaryngol* 1972;73(6):484–492.
64. Schuknecht HF, ed. Otosclerosis. In: *Pathology of the Ear*. 2nd ed. Philadelphia, PA: Lea & Febiger; 1993:365–379.
65. Schrauwen I, Ealy M, Huentelman MJ, et al. A genome-wide analysis identified variants in the RELN gene associated with otosclerosis. *Am J Hum Genet* 2009;84(3):328–338.
66. Schrauwen I, Ealy M, Fransen E, et al. Genetic variants in RELN gene are associated with otosclerosis in multiple European populations. *Hum Genet* 2010;127(2):155–162.
67. Karosi T, Kónya J, Szabó LZ, et al. Measles virus prevalence in otosclerotic stapes footplate samples. *Otol Neurotol* 2004;25(4):451–456.
68. Gantumur T, Niedermeyer HP, Neubert WJ, et al. Molecular detection of measles virus in primary cell cultures of otosclerotic tissue. *Acta Otolaryngol* 2006;126(8):811–816.
69. Michaels L, Soucek S. Origin and growth of otosclerosis. *Acta Otolaryngol* 2011;131(5):460–468.
70. Michaels L, Soucek S. Atypical mature bone in the otosclerotic otic capsule as the differentiated zone of an invasive osseous neoplasm. *Acta Otolaryngol* 2014;134(2):118–123.
71. Schuknecht HF, ed. Disorders of growth, metabolism, and aging. In: *Pathology of the Ear*. 2nd ed. Philadelphia, PA: Lea & Febiger; 1993.
72. Soucek S, Michaels L, Frohlich A. Pathological changes in the organ of Corti in presbycusis as revealed in microslicing and staining. *Acta Otolaryngol Suppl* 1987;436:93–102.
73. Soucek S, Michaels L, Frohlich A. Evidence of hair cell degeneration as the primary lesion in hearing loss of the elderly. *J Otolaryngol* 1986;15(3):175–183.
74. Roman-Naranjo P, Gallego-Martinez A, Lopez Escamez JA. Genetics of vestibular syndromes. *Curr Opin Neurol* 2018;31(1):105–110.
75. Paparella MM. The cause (multifactorial inheritance) and pathogenesis (endolymphatic malabsorption) of Ménière's disease and its symptoms (mechanical and chemical). *Acta Otolaryngol* 1985;99(3–4):445–451.
76. Klis SFL, Buijs J, Smoorenburg GF. Quantification of the relationship between electrophysiologic and morphologic changes in experimental endolymphatic hydrops. *Ann Otol Rhinol Laryngol* 1990;99(7 Pt 1):566–570.
77. Michaels L, Soucek S, Linthicum F. The intravestibular source of the vestibular aqueduct: Is structure and pathology in Ménière's disease. *Acta Otolaryngol* 2009;129(6):592–601.
78. Michaels L, Soucek S. The intravestibular source of the vestibular aqueduct: III. Osseous pathology of Ménière's disease, clarified by a developmental study of the intraskeletal channels of the otic capsule. *Acta Otolaryngol* 2010;130(7):793–798.
79. Michaels L, Soucek S, Linthicum F. The intravestibular source of the vestibular aqueduct. II: Its structure and function clarified by a developmental study of the intraskeletal channels of the otic capsule. *Acta Otolaryngol* 2010;130(4):420–428.
80. Schuknecht HF, ed. Histological method. In: *Pathology of the Ear*. 2nd ed. Philadelphia, PA: Lea & Febiger; 1993.

14

Mouth, Nose, and Paranasal Sinuses

Liron Pantanowitz ■ Karoly Balogh

EMBRYOLOGY AND PRENATAL CHANGES 396
GROSS ANATOMY 398
Jawbone 399
Nose 399
Paranasal Sinuses 399
Blood Vessels 400
Nerves 400
Lymph Nodes 400

Lymphatics 401
Tonsils 401
MICROSCOPY 402
Mouth 402
Nose and Paranasal Sinuses 416
REFERENCES 420

EMBRYOLOGY AND PRENATAL CHANGES

Development of the highly specialized part of the head is restricted to structures of importance to the surgical pathologist. For details, the reader is referred to other sources (1,2).

The oral region develops from an ectodermal depression, the stomodeum. The deep oral cavity is formed by the forward growth of structures about the margins of the stomodeum, giving rise to superficial parts of the face and jaws, as well as the walls of the oral cavity. The stomodeal prominence is surrounded bilaterally by the maxillary and mandibular processes and rostrally by the unpaired frontal prominence. The upper lip, maxilla, and nose are derived from structures surrounding the stomodeum. The caudal boundary of the oral cavity is formed by the paired mandibular processes, which, during the second year of life, fuse in the midline to form the mandible. The paired maxillary processes likewise meet in the midline, crowding the nasal elevation to ultimately form the maxilla and, by fusion in the midline, the palate. The contours of the face change with the rapid growth of the nose and jaws (2). The nose is formed on either side of the frontonasal elevation by an invagination of ectoderm into the mesoderm to form two nasal pits that gradually converge toward the midline, where they merge with each other. The underlying mesenchyme develops into bone, cartilage, and skeletal muscle.

At the end of the 2nd month of fetal life, the formation of the bony structures begins; the maxilla is one of the first bones to calcify. Simultaneously, the nasal pits become progressively deeper and extend downward toward the oral cavity. Later, elevations appear on the lateral walls of the right and left nasal cavity that will become the scroll-like nasal turbinates (conchae). The nasal cavities communicate with chambers in the adjacent bones known as paranasal sinuses. Named for the bones in which they lie, they comprise the frontal, maxillary, sphenoidal, and ethmoidal sinuses. The paranasal sinuses can be first identified around the 4th month of fetal life, but most of their expansion occurs after birth, and they attain full size many years later. The mucosa lining the nasal cavities invaginates into the surrounding bone, thereby lining the expanding sinus. While the palate has been taking shape from the roof of the mouth, the tongue has been forming in the floor. The posterior part of the tongue (behind the sulcus terminalis) is derived from the midventral areas of branchial arches II, III, and IV.

The tonsils first develop as endodermal epithelial buds that arise from the lining of the primitive oronasal cavity and grow into the subjacent mesenchyme to eventually give rise to the tonsillar crypts. Crypt formation may be simple, as in the lingual tonsil, or more complex, as in the palatine tonsils. Lymphoid tissue begins to accumulate and organize around the crypts at around the time when secondary budding of the crypts takes place. This development occurs in close association with mucous glands, which explains the close anatomic proximity of such glands to the tonsils.

Tooth development (odontogenesis) is of considerable importance to an understanding of the pathogenesis of

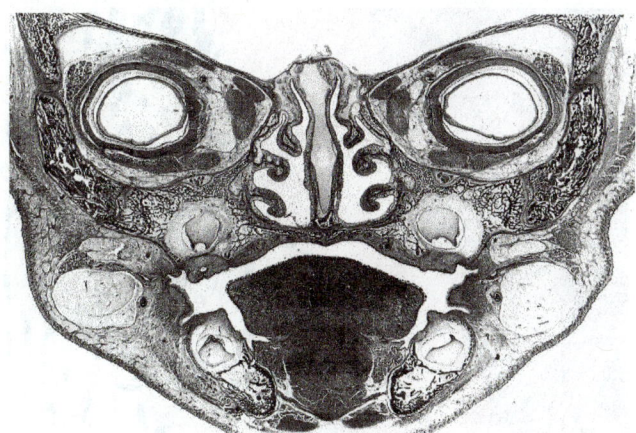

FIGURE 14.1 Coronal section of the head of a human fetus about 30 weeks of age (284-mm crown-rump length). The bell-shaped enamel organs are present in each quadrant. The tongue is relatively large. The paranasal sinuses are not yet discernible at this stage of fetal development.

odontogenic tumors and cysts. Odontogenesis is a highly coordinated and complex process that relies upon several genes, growth factors, structural proteins (e.g., amelogenin, tuftelin, predentin, cementum, enamelin), and extracellular matrix molecules being expressed in temporal- and space-specific patterns (3). The teeth begin to develop inside the gums of the upper and lower jaw (Fig. 14.1). Such regulatory interactions occur during the early stages of morphogenesis, particularly when the dental epithelium induces the condensation of mesenchymal cells around the epithelial bud. Teeth pass through three stages of development: growth, mineralization, and eruption. The growth period is further subdivided into the bud, cap, and bell stages.

Initially, the oral epithelium shows definite thickening and begins to grow into the subjacent mesenchyme around the entire arc of each jaw. The free margin of this epithelial band gives rise to two invaginating processes. The outer process (vestibular lamina) will form the vestibule that demarcates the cheeks and lips. From the inner horseshoe-shaped process (dental lamina), tooth buds (bud stage) arise at the site of each future tooth. Thus, the primordia for the temporary deciduous (primary) teeth are formed. Shortly afterward, the primordia of the succedaneous (permanent) teeth develop in the same way. The permanent tooth germs lie in a hollow of the alveolar sockets on the lingual side of the deciduous teeth. The developing enamel organ of each tooth takes the shape of a goblet with the dental lamina as its stem. As the dental lamina disintegrates, the inner lining cells (inner enamel epithelium) of the enamel organ differentiate to become columnar epithelial cells called ameloblasts, whereas the outer layer of cells (outer enamel epithelium) flatten into a layer of closely packed cells. Between the ameloblasts and the outer enamel epithelium is the loosely arranged epithelium of the stellate reticulum. Inside the goblet-shaped enamel organ, the mesenchymal cells proliferate to form a dense aggregate, the dental papilla (cap stage).

The dental papilla will form the dentin, cementum, and pulp. The dentin is the internal layer of the tooth, the cementum is the bony tissue covering the root of the tooth, and the pulp is the soft inner part of the tooth. More peripherally, the condensing mesenchymal cells extend around the enamel organ as the dental follicle. Dental follicle stem cells have been isolated and grown in culture for use in periodontal and bone regeneration work (4). The cells of the dental follicle eventually produce alveolar bone and collagen fibers of the periodontium. In the final (bell) stage of growth, the epithelium of the cap will form the enamel. During this stage, the outer and inner enamel epithelium meet at their apical ends, where they proliferate to form Hertwig's epithelial root sheath, which initiates the differentiation of the outermost cells of the papilla to become arranged in a row of single columnar cells to form the odontoblasts (Figs. 14.2 and 14.3). Nerves and blood vessels in the dental papilla begin to form the primitive dental pulp. The dental papilla grows toward the gum, crowding in on the enamel organ, which by then has lost its connection with the oral epithelium. During dentinogenesis nonmineralized predentin is produced by the odontoblasts against the inner surface of the enamel organ. As the odontoblasts produce predentin, their cell bodies recede toward the center of the tooth, so that each odontoblast leaves behind a thin process (Tomes' fiber) that occupies a dentinal tubule. The organic matrix of the predentin eventually mineralizes to become dentin, which is arranged in the shape of tubules running from the pulp chamber toward the periphery. Meanwhile the enamel cap of the tooth is being formed (amelogenesis) by the ameloblasts (5). The formation of dentin and enamel

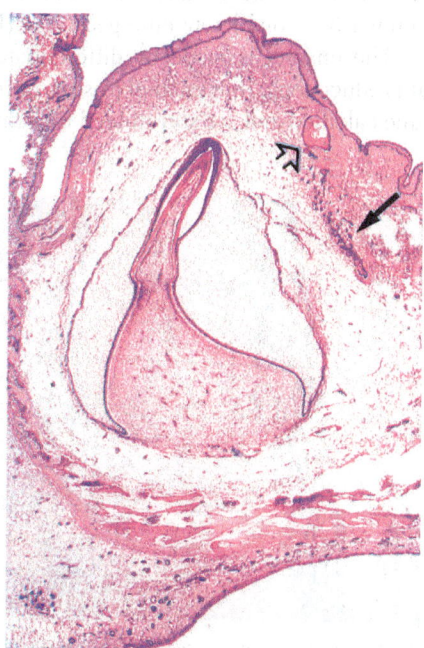

FIGURE 14.2 Enamel organ of deciduous tooth. Formation of enamel and dentin has begun at the crown area of the tooth. (*Arrow*, remnants of dental lamina; *arrowhead*, a small epithelial cyst [rest of Serres].)

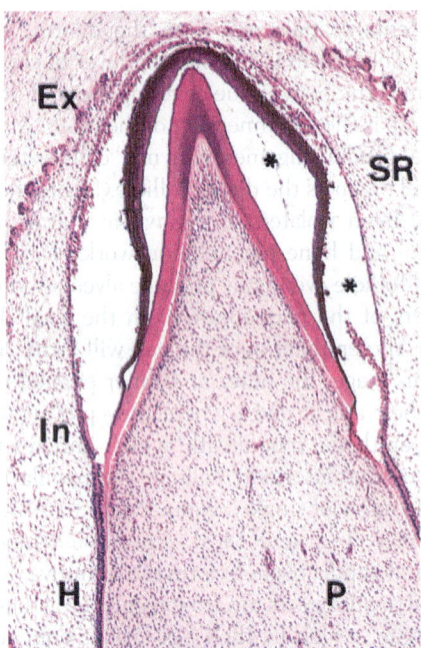

FIGURE 14.3 Enamel organ. Amelogenesis and dentinogenesis progress from crown to root. Early enamel and dentin appear as black bands, widest at the crown area and become thinner toward the root. (*Ex*, external enamel epithelium; *In*, inner enamel epithelium; *SR*, stellate reticulum; *H*, Hertwig's epithelial root sheath; *P*, dental papilla; *, artifact [separation].)

begins at the tip of the crown and progresses toward the root of the tooth (6). As the developing root increases in length, the previously formed crown moves closer to the surface of the gum. Even when the crown of the tooth begins to erupt, the root is still incomplete and continues growing until the crown has completely emerged (7,8) (Figs. 14.4 and 14.5). The enamel is made by differentiated ameloblasts that produce long, thin enamel prisms, or rods; these rods become calcified and are surrounded by a thin organic

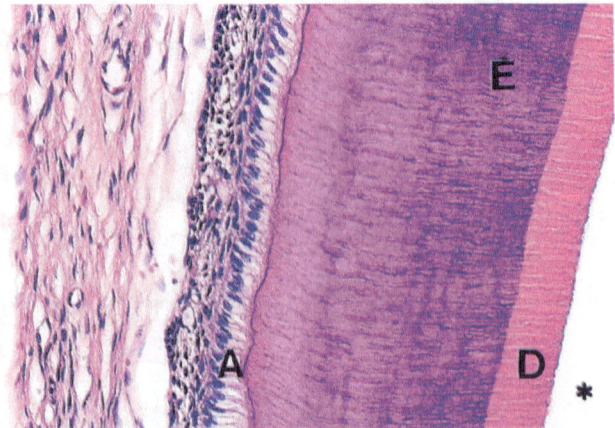

FIGURE 14.4 Developing tooth, sagittal section. Ameloblasts (A) line the surface of the enamel matrix (E) which is partly mineralized. Dentin (D) is not mineralized (predentin) and has been separated by an artifact (*) from pulp (missing).

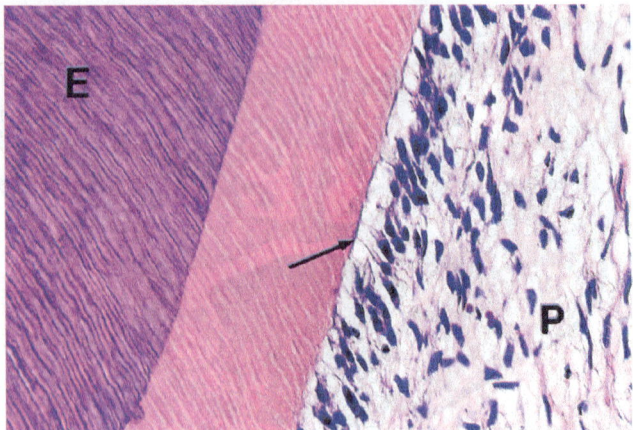

FIGURE 14.5 Developing tooth. Layer of polarized odontoblasts with Tomes' fibers (*arrow*) extending into tubules of predentin. Fibroblasts of pulp (P) are loosely arranged. (E, enamel matrix.)

matrix. Enamel production is completed when the crown is mineralized and its final size attained (9). At this point in time, the flattened ameloblasts and remainder of the cells of the enamel organ form a cuticle on the surface of the enamel; this membrane is then shed (10).

After the root has attained its full length and definitive position in the jaw, a bone-like hard substance, cement, is deposited on it (cementogenesis). Cement is produced by the mesenchymal cells adjacent to the root. These cells become differentiated into a cementoblast layer that resembles the osteogenic (cambial) layer of the periosteum (11,12). Fibers from the rest of the dental sac form the periodontal ligament, which firmly attaches the tooth in the bony alveolar socket (13).

As the jaws approach their adult size, the latent primordia of the permanent teeth follow the same developmental process as did the deciduous teeth (14) (Fig. 14.6). When a developing permanent tooth increases in size, the root of the corresponding deciduous tooth is partly resorbed by osteoclastic activity (Fig. 14.7). Thus, the anchorage of the deciduous tooth becomes weakened and the tooth is shed, permitting the underlying permanent tooth to erupt.

The minor salivary glands in the mouth develop following a pattern of epithelial–mesenchymal interactions between the outgrowth of an ectodermal bud from the lining of the stomodeum and the underlying mesenchyme. The proliferation, differentiation, and morphogenesis of these glands depend on intrinsic (programmed pattern of cell-specific gene expression) and extrinsic factors. The extrinsic factors include cell–cell and cell–matrix interactions, as well as growth factors (15).

GROSS ANATOMY

In this chapter we will consider only those features that are important for the surgical pathologist.

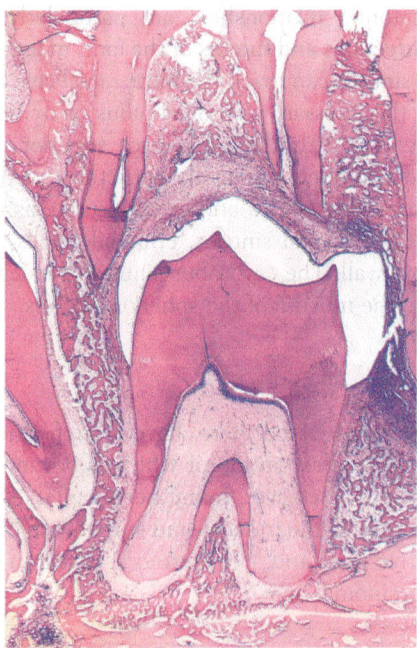

FIGURE 14.6 Deciduous and unerupted permanent teeth in a 10-year-old child. Perpendicular section through the roots of two deciduous teeth with underlying permanent molar tooth. Empty space was left by enamel that was dissolved by decalcification. Note the relationship between teeth and bone, respectively.

Jawbone

The mandible is a horseshoe-shaped bone; its horizontal part forms the body, which is continuous with the vertical parts of the two sides, the rami. The bone of the body has a thick cortex, and the compact shell contains plates of cancellous bone arranged along the trajectories. The upper part of the body is hollowed into sockets that carry eight teeth on each side. Each ramus is a nearly vertical, flattened, oblong plate of bone surmounted by two processes. The posterior articular process ends in the condyle, articulating with the articular disk of the temporomandibular joint. The anterior (coronoid) process serves for the insertion of the temporal muscle.

The right and left maxillae jointly form the upper jaw; they participate in forming boundaries of four cavities: the roof of the mouth, the floor and lateral wall of the nose, the floor of the maxillary sinus, and the floor of the orbit. The alveolar processes of the maxillae together form the alveolar arch.

Nose

The external nose and nasal septum are partly composed of hyalin cartilage and bone. The two orifices of the external nose, the nares (nostrils), are separated from each other by the median vertical soft tissue columella. The columella is attached posteriorly to the nasal septum, which forms the medial wall of the two approximately symmetrical chambers, the right and left nasal cavities. The nasal cavity extends from the nares anteriorly to the choanae posteriorly. Just behind the nares, the nasal cavity widens to form the vestibule. A ridge (limen nasi) on the lateral nasal wall separates the vestibule from the rest of the nasal cavity proper. In each nasal fossa is an olfactory region that occupies the superior part of the nasal cavity. The rest of the nasal fossa consists of the respiratory region. On the lateral wall of each nasal fossa are the superior, middle, and inferior turbinates. Rarely, turbinates may be bifid or trifurcate, and there may even be an anomalous accessory middle turbinate present. A fourth supreme turbinate may be present at the uppermost portion of the lateral nasal wall. The scroll-shaped turbinates hang over the corresponding funnel-shaped nasal passages, or meatuses, into which the various paranasal sinuses open. The concha bullosa (pneumatized turbinate) is a normal anatomic variant in around 50% of people. It may be associated with nasal deviation and sinusitis. The nasal mucosa is in continuity with the mucosa of these sinuses through their corresponding openings. The nasal mucous membrane is most vascular and thickest over the turbinates and is also relatively thick over the nasal septum.

Paranasal Sinuses

The air-filled paranasal cavities (sinuses) are located in the bones around the nasal cavity (Fig. 14.8). The maxillary and frontal sinuses open into the middle meatus of the nose. The sphenoidal sinus opens into the sphenoethmoidal recess above the superior turbinate. There are numerous ethmoidal sinuses that form small communicating cavities, also called ethmoid air cells (or ethmoid labyrinth). The ethmoid air cells have thin bony walls. According to their location, the ethmoidal sinuses can be divided into three groups: the anterior and middle ethmoidal sinuses, which open into the middle meatus, and the posterior ethmoidal sinus, which opens into the superior meatus of the nose. The most posterior sphenoethmoidal cell is known as the

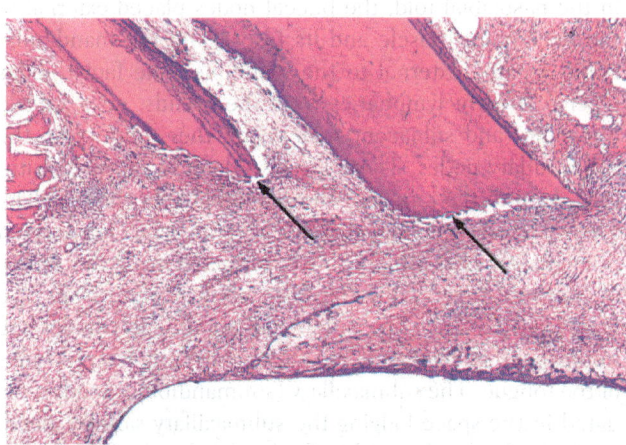

FIGURE 14.7 Roots of deciduous molar tooth before shedding. Resorption of dentin is indicated by numerous Howship lacunae and osteoclasts (*arrows*). The thin band (*bottom*) is the reduced internal enamel epithelium that covered the crown of the underlying permanent tooth; the enamel dissolved with decalcification.

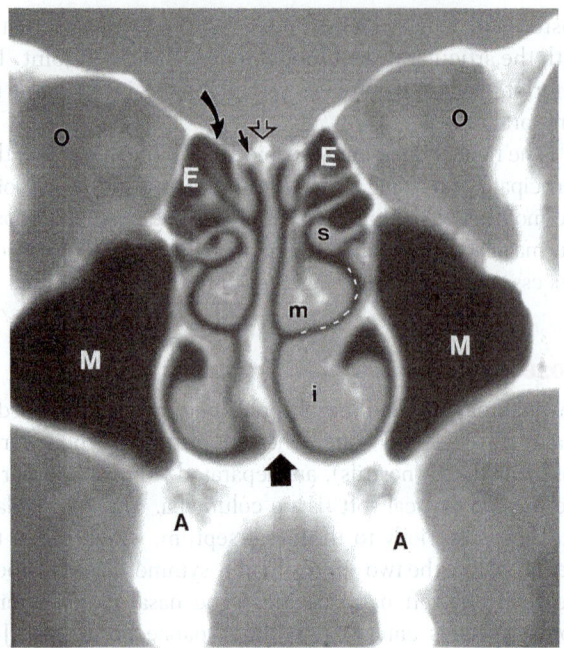

FIGURE 14.8 Coronal computed tomography (CT) image through the mid-portion of the paranasal sinuses, just behind the globes. The *large arrow* indicates the bottom of the nasal septum, the *open arrow* indicates the crista galli, *small arrow* the cribiform plate, and the *curved arrow* shows the fovea ethmoidalis (roof of the ethmoid sinus). The *dotted line* highlights the middle meatus. (*M*, maxillary sinus; *A*, alveolar ridge; *O*, orbit; *E*, ethmoid sinus; *i*, inferior turbinate; *m*, middle turbinate; *s*, superior turbinate.)

Onodi air cell, after the Hungarian Adolf Onodi. Its importance is related to the fact that it may get damaged during endoscopy. There are many variations in size, shape, and location of all paranasal sinuses (16). One or more of them may even be underdeveloped or absent.

Blood Vessels

The nasal cavity has an extraordinarily rich blood supply. The anterior and posterior ethmoidal branches of the ophthalmic artery supply the frontal and ethmoidal sinuses, as well as the roof of the nasal cavity. The sphenopalatine branch of the maxillary artery supplies the mucosa of the turbinates, meatuses, and the nasal septum. The mucosa of the maxillary sinus is supplied by branches of the maxillary artery and the sphenoidal sinus by the pharyngeal artery. The branches of all these vessels form a plexiform network in and below the mucous membrane. The veins of the nasal mucosa are well developed, particularly in the inferior turbinate and in the posterior part of the nasal fossa, where they form a cavernous plexus. The veins of the lower jaw drain via the inferior central vein into the pterygoid plexus. Blood from the upper jaw and facial structures drains in two directions: the more anterior parts into the anterior facial vein and the more posterior parts into the pterygoid plexus. The pterygoid plexus drains the teeth, soft palate, fauces, and pharynx.

These anatomic relationships are particularly important because infections and tumors of the face, mouth, nose, and paranasal sinuses can reach the intracranial cavernous sinus either via the emissary vein of Vesalius or by way of veins communicating with the inferior or superior ophthalmic veins. The latter veins drain the structures of the anterior face, such as lips, cheek, and external nose, as well as the mucosa of the frontal sinuses, ethmoidal cells, and upper lateral nasal wall. The cavernous sinus also receives venous blood from the mucosa of the sphenoidal sinus.

Nerves

The regions discussed here have a rich and complex innervation, the description of which is beyond the scope of this chapter. However, many nerves of the head lie in close proximity to the mucosa and submucosa of the upper aerodigestive tract and are, therefore, prone to early invasion by carcinoma.

Lymph Nodes

Lymph nodes of the head and neck are abundant and can be divided into 10 groups: the occipital, mastoid, parotid, facial, sublingual, submaxillary, submental, retropharyngeal, anterior cervical, and lateral cervical nodes. Only those lymph nodes related to the regions covered in this chapter are discussed here. There are three principal parotid lymph node groups: superficial (suprafascial or preauricular) nodes; subfascial (extraglandular) nodes contained in the parotid sheath; and deep intraglandular nodes. The parotid lymph nodes drain the parotid gland, external ear, frontotemporal facial region, eyelids, upper lip, root of the nose, floor of the nasal cavity, soft palate, and buccal mucosa. Their efferents pass into the superior deep cervical nodes.

The small superficial group of facial nodes includes, from rostral to caudal, the infraorbital (nasolabial) nodes situated in the nasolabial fold, the buccal nodes placed external to the buccinator muscle and its fascia, and the mandibular nodes located external to the mandible. The facial nodes receive afferent lymphatics from the eyelids, nose, cheek, upper lip, and subjacent nodes, and they empty into the submaxillary nodes. There are also deep facial nodes situated deep to the ramus of the mandible near the maxillary artery. Heterotopic buccal nodes may rarely be encountered immediately beneath the buccal mucosa near the orifice of Stensen duct, giving the false clinical impression of a neoplasm (17,18). The sublingual (or lingual) nodes are intercalated along the course of the collecting lymph trunks of the tongue. The submaxillary (submandibular) nodes, situated in the space lodging the submaxillary salivary gland, are located around or within the fascial sheath of this gland. They receive lymph vessels from the chin, lips, cheeks, nose (including the anterior nasal cavity), gums, teeth, floor of the mouth, hard palate, tongue, and other nearby nodes. The submental nodes receive lymphatics from similar regions.

Their afferent vessels connect partly with the submaxillary and internal jugular nodes. The retropharyngeal nodes, which lie between the posterior wall of the pharynx and prevertebral fascia, may project anteriorly onto the soft palate and, therefore, may be mistaken for palatine tonsils. The more lateral retropharyngeal nodes atrophy with age. These nodes drain the nasal cavities, palate, middle ear, nasopharynx, and orophrynx. They send efferent vessels to the internal jugular chain of nodes.

Lymphatics

For a detailed description of the lympahtic system draining the head and neck, the reader is referred to the compendium by Tobias, which is a translation of the original work by Rouvière (19). Lymphatics arising from the upper lip terminate in the parotid, submental, and submaxillary lymph nodes. Central lymphatics from the lower lip drain into the submental node, while those originating more laterally empty into the submaxillary nodes. Lymphatics arising from the mucosa of the cheeks traverse the buccinator muscle to eventually terminate in the submaxillary nodes. Their course may be interrupted by the buccinator nodes. Cutaneous lymphatics of the cheek end in the submaxillary, submental, and parotid nodes. The lymphatic network of the tongue is divided into a superficial and deep (muscular) set. They drain to the lingual and submaxillary nodes but end mainly in the deep cervical lymph nodes. The node at the bifurcation of the common carotid artery is considered to be the principal lymph node of the tongue (20). Lymphatics in the region of the tongue may cross the midline to reach nodes of the opposite side. The gingiva contains a similar superficial and deep anastomosing lymphatic network that drains into the sublingual, submental, submaxillary, internal jugular, and occasionally the retropharyngeal nodes. Lymphatic vessels that exit from the dental pulp of the teeth are in direct communication with those of the gingiva. Lymphatics from the floor of the mouth are continuous with those from the tongue and gums. Afferent lymphatics from the floor of the mouth drain into the sublingual, submental, and deep cervical nodes, while those from the posterolateral region terminate in the submaxillary and deep cervical nodes. The draining lymphatics of the palate, which are continuous with those of the gums and palatine tonsils, reach the submaxillary, retropharyngeal, and deep nodes of the neck.

The cutaneous lymphatics of the nose terminate in the submaxillary lymph nodes. Lymph from the nasal vestibule goes to the parotid and submaxillary nodes. Lymphatics originating from the anterior nasal cavities drain to the submental nodes, while those from the posterior cavities pass to the retropharyngeal and deep superior cervical nodes. The lymphatics from the olfactory region do not communicate with those of the respiratory region (20). Lymphatics arising from the olfactory region communicate to the subarachnoid space of the brain via small canaliculi passing through the foramina of the cribriform plate along with the olfactory nerve filaments. The lower aspect of the inferior turbinate drains to the internal jugular lymph nodes. The upper portion of the inferior turbinate, along with lymphatics from the middle turbinate, drains into the retropharyngeal and internal jugular lymph nodes. The superior turbinates drain to the retropharyngeal and deep cervical nodes. Lymphatics from the frontal and maxillary sinuses, along with the anterior and medial group of ethmoidal sinuses, drain to the submaxillary nodes. The posterior ethmoidal group and sphenoidal sinuses drain lymph into the retropharyngeal nodes.

Tonsils

Nonencapsulated lymphoid tissue present in the oropharynx is normally organized into epithelial-covered lymphoid aggregates termed *tonsils*. Tonsils are typically softer than lymph nodes on palpation because they lack a fibrous capsule or trabeculae. The word *tonsil* has also been used to refer to the palatine tonsils. Waldeyer ring, described by the 19th century anatomist Wilhelm von Waldeyer, refers to the circular collection of submucosal lymphoid tissue that guards the opening into the upper aerodigestive tract (21). Waldeyer ring is comprised of the palatine, pharyngeal, tubal, and lingual tonsils, as well as the lateral pharyngeal lymphoid bands and intervening isolated lymphoid follicles (pharyngeal granulations) (21,22). The pharyngeal bands are located on the posterolateral wall of the oropharynx, just behind the posterior tonsillar pillar. The oval-shaped palatine (faucial) tonsils are situated laterally in the oropharynx within the triangular tonsillar fossa, which is bound by the palatoglossal arch anteriorly and palatopharyngeal arch posteriorly. Their tonsillar crypts usually become occupied with desquamated epithelium, debris, and microorganisms that are grossly visible on the surface as white spots (follicles). Such crypt plugs may calcify. Such concretions have been referred to as tonsilloliths. The palatine tonsils are the only tonsils with a partial capsule, which is formed by compressed connective tissue on their attached side. This capsule separates the tonsils from the underlying musculature of the pharyngeal wall. The tonsils are largest in early childhood; after about 4 years of age, they begin to gradually atrophy. Following puberty, the tonsils become increasingly fibrotic. Bilateral enlargement of the tonsils may be seen with obesity, obstructive sleep apnea, Down syndrome, and because of disease affecting the tonsils. Unilateral enlargement of the tonsil is usually because of a pathologic condition. The pharyngeal tonsil (adenoid, or tonsil of Luschka) is a single pyramidal-shaped aggregate of lymphoid tissue located superiorly in the midline of the nasopharyngeal wall. Unlike the other tonsils, the adenoid does not have typical crypts, but rather numerous surface folds extending from the tonsillar base anterolaterally. The surface of the pharyngeal tonsil also forms a median recess known as the pharyngeal bursa. The tubal tonsil (eustachian tonsil or Gerlach tonsil) is that small portion of the pharyngeal tonsil that is located behind the pharyngeal opening of the eustachian tube. The lingual tonsil is situated on the dorsum of the tongue posteriorly, between the sulcus terminalis and the valleculae. In most individuals the median glossoepiglottic ligament divides the lingual tonsil into bilateral lobes.

Additional tonsillar structures may also be found in the normal human oropharynx. These include the so-called oral tonsils, which are structurally similar to the palatine tonsils (23). Oral tonsils occur chiefly in the palate, floor of the mouth, and on the ventral surface of the tongue. They are small (1 to 3 mm in diameter), firm, circumscribed, mobile lymphoid aggregates present under intact oral mucosa. Oral tonsils contain a single central crypt. It has been proposed by some authors that intraoral lymphoepithelial cysts originate from occluded crypts of oral tonsils (24,25). Reactive tonsillar tissue has also been noted in the region of the pyriform sinus, palate, and lateral surface of the tongue (26,27).

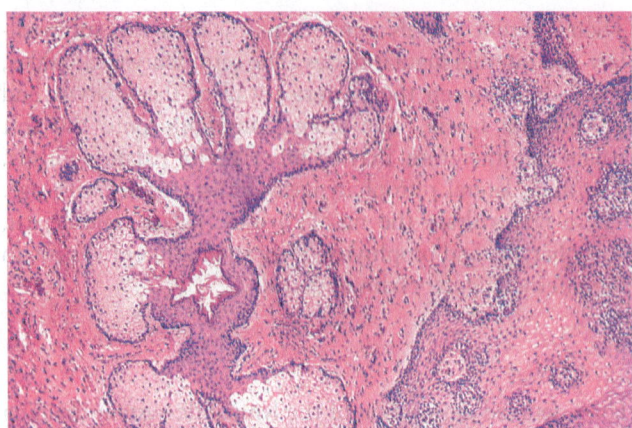

FIGURE 14.9 Ectopic sebaceous glands in the vermilion border (Fox–Fordyce granule).

MICROSCOPY

Mouth

Lips and Vermilion Border

The entrance to the digestive tract is surrounded by two fleshy folds of skin, the lips. They are partly covered by skin that bears hairs, sweat glands, and sebaceous glands and is richly endowed with sensory nerves. The inner surface of the lips is covered by the oral mucosa and forms a part of the wall of the oral cavity. Between the external integument and the oral mucosa are the orbicularis oris muscle, the labial vessels, nerves, and adipose tissue with numerous minor salivary glands. The latter are easily accessible for biopsies to diagnose Sjögren syndrome. The junction between the skin and oral mucosa is known as the vermilion border, where the keratinized squamous epithelium of the skin changes to the mucous membrane of the oral cavity. The squamous epithelium of the vermilion border is thin, and the tall connective tissue papillae are close to the surface. The blood in the rich capillary network shows through the thin epithelium, accounting for the redness of the lips. The transition zone has no hairs. In adults, ectopic sebaceous glands are commonly observed in the vermilion border, at the corners of the mouth, or in the buccal mucosa; these are termed Fordyce spots (or Fox–Fordyce granules) and increase with age, so that 70% to 80% of elderly persons have them. These ectopic sebaceous glands are considered normal (Fig. 14.9) (28,29). Like the skin, the vermilion border is exposed to physical forces and chemical agents. For this reason, actinic keratosis and solar elastosis can be seen on the vermilion border. The squamous epithelium of the transitional zone imperceptibly merges with the stratified squamous epithelium of the oral mucosa.

Oral Mucosa and Submucosa

The oral mucosa consists of an epithelial layer and an underlying layer of connective tissue, the lamina propria (Fig. 14.10). The mucosa of the oral cavity shows regional modifications in structure and cytokeratin expression that correspond to functional requirements. The stratified squamous epithelium of the oral mucosa has three functional types: the lining mucosa, masticatory mucosa, and specialized mucosa (30). Most of the oral mucosa is lined by nonkeratinized squamous epithelium, representing the lining mucosa. The palate, gingiva, and dorsum of the tongue are exposed to the forces of mastication and are covered by keratinized epithelium of the masticatory mucosa type. The mucosa of the palate is orthokeratinized, whereas the epithelium of the gingiva is often parakeratinized. Details of the specialized mucosa are described with the tongue. The masticatory mucosa has longer rete ridges, likely related to pressure associated with mastication (31). Throughout the oral cavity the epithelium is worn off by mastication and speaking; hence, exfoliated epithelial cells are a normal constituent of the saliva and are frequently encountered by the pathologist in sputum or as "contaminants" in bronchoscopic specimens. Squamous cells of the buccal mucosa have also

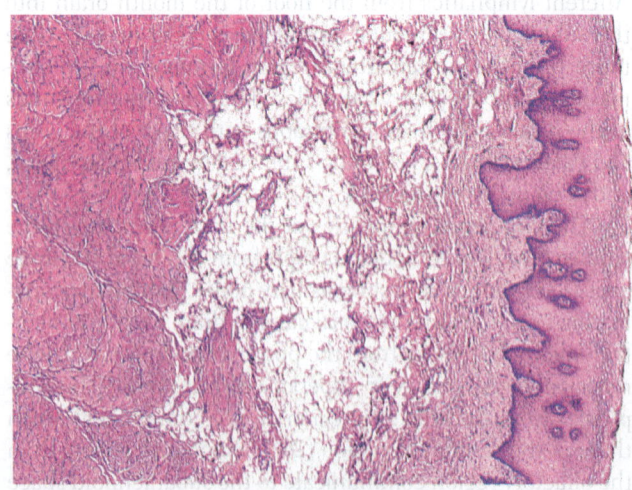

FIGURE 14.10 Inner aspect of cheek, cross section. *Left* to *right*: cross-striated muscle, adipose tissue, lamina propria, buccal mucosa.

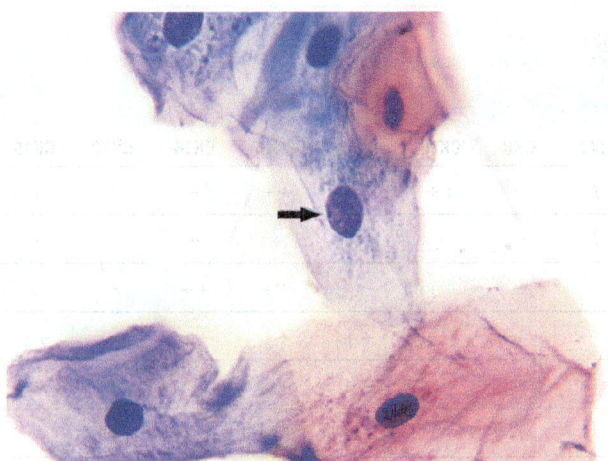

FIGURE 14.11 Cytologic image of a scraping of the buccal mucosa. Intermediate squamous cell with sex chromatin body (Barr body) (*arrow*) lying against the inner nuclear membrane (Papanicolaou stain).

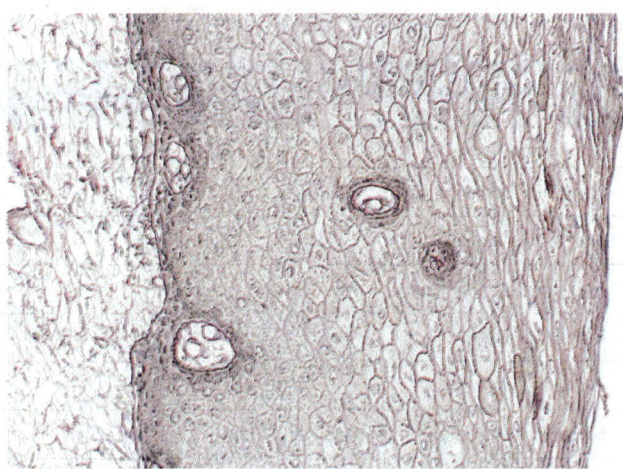

FIGURE 14.12 Buccal mucosa. Reticulin stain delineates the cell membrane of nonkeratinized squamous epithelial cells and the delicate basement membrane. Papillae of the lamina propria contain blood vessels.

been a convenient source for the microscopic demonstration of the sex chromosome (Barr body) (Fig. 14.11). The shed epithelial cells are replaced by the basal cells, which divide and then migrate to the surface and are themselves eventually worn off. The renewal of the oral mucosa takes about 12 days (32). As the name implies, the squamous epithelium of the mucosa is kept moist and glistening by mucus that is secreted by the numerous minor and paired major salivary glands. This thin film of mucus covers and protects all intraoral structures, including the teeth, which are bathed by saliva. Saliva rinses away bacteria, provides buffering agents (e.g., phosphate and bicarbonate) that neutralize acids created by bacteria that inhabit dental plaques, contains antibacterial agents, and minerals required for tooth remineralization. Hence, xerostomia promotes tooth decay.

The interface of the epithelium and lamina propria is delineated by the basal lamina, or basement membrane. In hematoxylin and eosin (H&E)-stained sections, it is sometimes hard to see the basal lamina, but special stains (e.g., reticulin) demonstrate it well (Fig. 14.12). The basal lamina is secreted by the epithelial cells and serves supportive and filtering functions. It also regulates differentiation, migration, and polarity of the epithelial cells. The basal lamina is composed of type IV collagen and heparan sulfate, as well as the two glycoproteins, laminin and entactin, that interact with other components of the extracellular matrix. A single layer of basal cells rests on the basal lamina. The basal cells continuously divide, and the new cells push the overlying ones toward the surface. During this process of differentiation, the small cuboidal basal cells become polyhedral and larger, forming the stratum spinosum. These cells contain abundant intracytoplasmic fibrils (tonofilaments) that attach to desmosomes, connecting the squamous epithelial cells with each other. Toward the superficial layers the cells gradually become flat. The nonkeratinized squamous epithelium lacks a stratum granulosum and stratum corneum. The surface cells may retain their nuclei, and their cytoplasm does not contain keratin filaments (Fig. 14.13) (33). In keratinizing epithelium, the cells form a stratum granulosum, which is a prominent layer three to five cells thick. The cells of this layer have numerous intracytoplasmic granules, called keratohyalin granules, which stain with hematoxylin. As the process of keratinization advances, the nucleus and cytoplasmic organelles become disrupted and disappear while the cell becomes filled with an intracellular protein, keratin. Thus, the surface layer, the stratum corneum, is formed.

All oral epithelia show expression of cytokeratin 5 and 14 (CK5 and CK14, respectively), the keratin pair typically expressed by basal cells of stratifying epithelium. The oral mucosa from various sites exhibits striking differences in cytokeratin synthesis (Table 14.1) (34,35). Such differences usually appear in the fetus by 23 weeks. The differences in

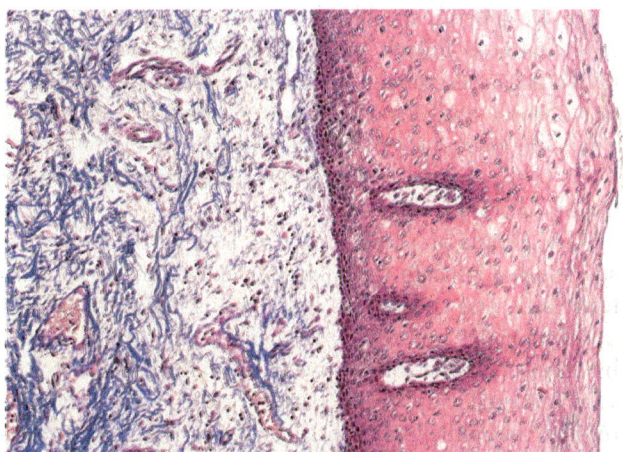

FIGURE 14.13 Buccal mucosa showing maturation of squamous epithelium: there is a row of small basal cells, larger cells of stratum spinosum, and parallel arranged flat surface cells. No keratinization is seen. Lamina propria shows delicate strands of connective tissue, blood vessels, and a few lymphocytes (Mallory trichrome).

TABLE 14.1
Cytokeratin Expression Profiles of Different Oral Epithelia, as Determined by Immunohistochemical and Electrophoretic Studies

Cytokeratin Type	CK1	CK4	CK5	CK6	CK7	CK8	CK10	CK13	CK14	CK16	CK18	CK19
Epidermis (for comparison)	++	/	++	+	/	–	++	/	++	+	/	/
Oral lining mucosa	/	++	++	+	/	–	–	++	+	–	–	+
Oral gingival epithelium	++	+	++	+	–	–	++	+	++	++	–	+
Epithelium of oral sulcus	–	++	++	/	–	+	–	++	++	++	+	++
Junctional epithelium	–	–	++	/	–	+	–	++	++	+	+	++
Masticatory mucosa (e.g., hard palate)	++	/	++	/	/	/	/	/	++	++	/	/
Epithelia of enamel organ	/	–	++	/	+	+	–	–	/	/	–	++
Rests of Malassez	/	–	++	/	–	–	–	–	+	–	–	++

+, weak or occasional expression; ++, strong expression; –, expression absent; /, no data.
(Modified from Mackenzie IC, Rittman G, Gao Z, et al. Patterns of cytokeratin expression in human gingival epithelia. *J Periodontal Res* 1991;26:468–478.)

the distribution of these cytoskeletal proteins reflect the relationship between morphology and function of these epithelia (36). The gingiva expresses a great complexity of cytokeratins, similar to that of the epidermis. For example, gingival epithelia are immunoreactive for CK1 and CK10 (differentiation that is associated with epithelial properties of toughness and rigidity), as well as CK4 and CK13 (differentiation associated with epithelial properties of flexibility and elasticity). In contrast, the lining mucosa shows a paucity of cytokeratins, resembling stratified nonkeratinizing squamous epithelium of the esophagus. Malignant transformation is often associated with alterations in the cytokeratin pattern.

Normal oral mucosal epithelial cells, even in the fetus, express the ABO blood group antigens (37). In fact, the oral mucosa has become a model for studying cellular glycosylation. In general, the blood group antigen expression on epithelial cells follows the general phenotype of the host individual as determined by routine serologic methods. The loss of these antigens on malignant epithelial cells may be a valuable marker for primary carcinoma. All epithelial cell layers of the enamel organ, however, are normally devoid of the blood group antigens.

The lamina propria is a delicate layer of connective tissue situated beneath the squamous epithelium. It contains few elastic and collagenous fibers and is rich in blood vessels, lymphatics, and nerves. The nerves belong to the sensory branches of the trigeminal nerve. The lamina propria also contains scattered lymphocytes, which are often found migrating through the epithelium. Consequently, few lymphocytes are a normal constituent of the saliva (salivary corpuscles).

The submucosa under the lining mucosa is composed of fairly loosely arranged connective tissue, which contains larger blood vessels, lymphatics, nerves, adipose tissue, and numerous minor salivary glands. Lymphatics in the oral submucosa are more numerous and of larger caliber than those in the lamina propria. This lymphatic network increases progressively from normal tissue to precancerous lesions and tumor tissue. Where the mucosa is in close proximity to the underlying bone (e.g., the hard palate), there is no submucosa and the fibers of the lamina propria are directly and tightly attached to bone. In these areas, the mucosa, lamina propria, and periosteum are joined together as one membrane and are generally referred to as a mucoperiosteum.

Palate and Uvula

The roof of the oral cavity is formed by the palate; the anterior two-thirds consist of the hard palate, and the posterior one-third is comprised of the soft palate. The palate separates the oral and nasal cavities. Anteriorly and laterally, the palate is bounded by the alveolar arches and gums; posteriorly, it is continuous with the soft palate. The hard palate is covered by masticatory mucosa, which has a series of ridges (palatal rugae) running across, but not crossing, the midline. The ridges are easily seen and palpated and can be felt with the tongue. The supporting dense connective tissue fibers of these ridges pass directly from the papillary layer of the lamina propria into the underlying bone. In the anterior lateral regions of the hard palate, the submucosa contains fat tissue, whereas more posteriorly its lateral regions contain minor salivary glands (palatine glands), which are pure mucous glands (Fig. 14.14).

The soft palate is the mobile portion. With no bony support, it is suspended from the posterior border of the hard palate like a curtain. Its oral surface is covered by lining mucosa, and its nasal surface, which is continuous with the floor of the nasal cavity, is mostly lined by ciliated respiratory epithelium. The soft palate contains fibers of striated muscle, blood vessels, and nerves (Fig. 14.15). The striated

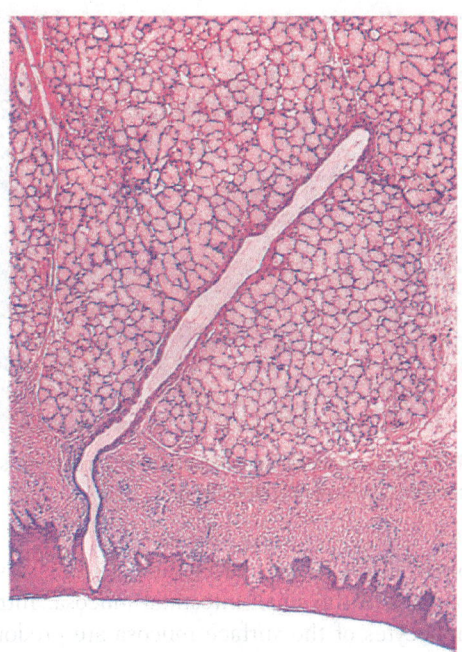

FIGURE 14.14 Hard palate with pure mucous minor salivary glands and duct. Note dense connective tissue of lamina propria (H&E).

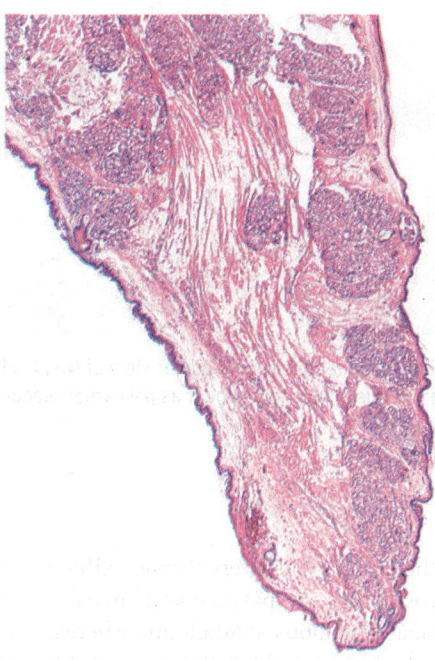

FIGURE 14.16 Sagittal section of uvula with numerous mucous glands and bundles of cross-striated muscle. More glands are seen near the oral surface (*right*).

muscle of the palate has a different cytoskeletal structure to limb muscles, and they accordingly may lack or have minimal desmin positivity (38). Larger mucous glands underlie the oral epithelium of the soft palate, whereas smaller groups of mixed glands are present on the nasal surface under the respiratory epithelium. From the middle of the posterior border of the soft palate hangs a small, conical process of soft tissue, the uvula. The uvula is microscopically similar to the soft palate (Fig. 14.16). It contains predominantly mucous glands and muscle fibers that become more sparse from the proximal to the distal end. The musculus uvulae muscle inserts into the actual mucosa of the uvula. Mast cells, usually located around blood vessels, are a frequent finding (39).

Floor of the Mouth

The mucous membrane of the floor of the mouth is thin and loosely attached to the underlying structures. The rete ridges are short. The submucosa contains some adipose tissue and numerous minor salivary glands (sublingual mucous glands). This is the anatomic site where ranulas (extravasation mucocele) may present. This is because they arise from the sublingual glands or ducts. They may present intraorally (simple ranulas) or plunge downward (deep ranulas) into the soft tissues of the neck.

Tonsils

The tonsils are organized aggregates of lymphoid tissue covered on their luminal surface by a mucous membrane. The close proximity of lymphocytes to the surface epithelium facilitates the direct internal transport of foreign material from the exterior. Epithelial-lined crypts and folds further aid in trapping foreign material. Tonsils normally lack a prominent fibrous capsule. This is in contrast to lymph nodes, which have a capsule and subcapsular sinus that

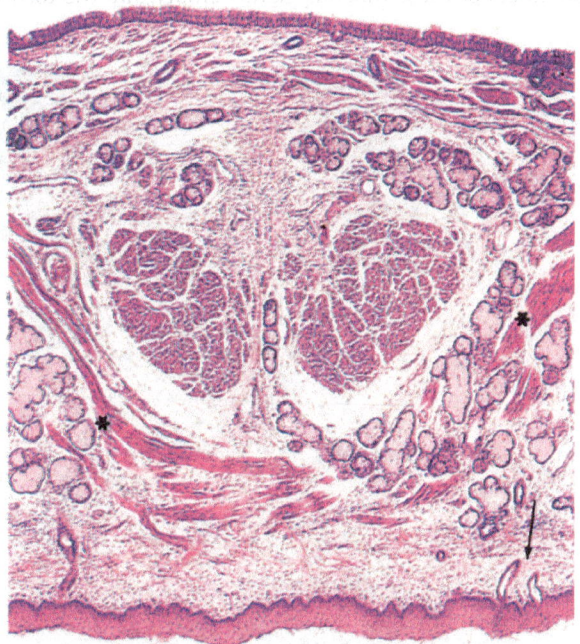

FIGURE 14.15 Soft palate sectioned in the coronal plane. Nasal respiratory mucosa (*top*), oral squamous mucosa (*bottom*). Fascicles of pharyngopalatine muscle are to the right and left of the midline. Fibers of levator veli palatini muscle (*) are obliquely descending. Ducts of minor salivary glands are near the oral mucosa (*arrow*).

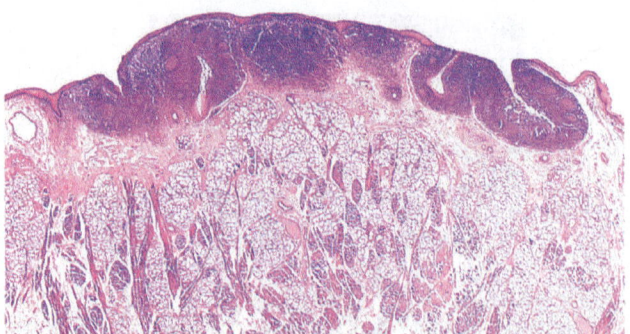

FIGURE 14.17 Lingual tonsil. Low-power view of lymphoid tissue and underlying mucous glands that appear as pale areas among bundles of skeletal muscle.

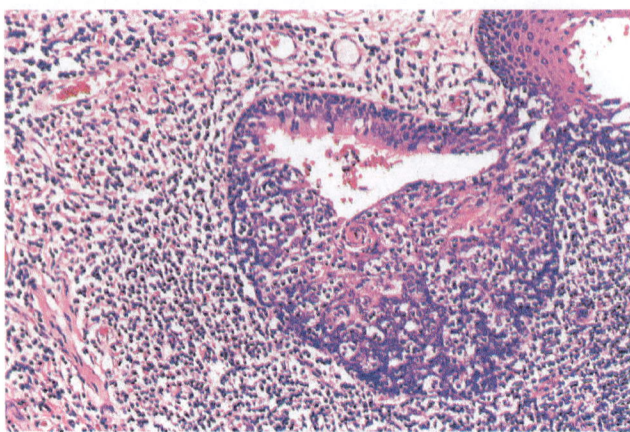

FIGURE 14.19 Lingual tonsil. Squamous epithelium of crypt is disrupted by lymphocytes that have migrated into it.

reflects the antigenic delivery through afferent lymphatics. The mucosa lining the palatine and lingual tonsils consists of stratified squamous epithelium, whereas the mucosa overlying the pharyngeal tonsil is a pseudostratified ciliated respiratory-type epithelium that contains occasional goblet cells. The epithelium lining the crypts or folds represents an extension of the regional surface epithelium. However, the epithelial lining of some crypts in the palatine tonsil may occasionally consist of respiratory mucosa. The palatine tonsil contains 10 to 30 crypts that may extend to the deep juxtacapsular region. In the lingual tonsil (Fig. 14.17) and pharyngeal tonsil, the lining epithelium forms only shallow folds 0.5- to 1.0-cm deep. Sulfur granules comprised of *Actinomyces* and other *Actinomyces*-like oral flora are a frequent finding within tonsillar crypts. As in lymph nodes, the lymphoid component may contain lymphoid follicles, some with active germinal centers. Intraepithelial lymphocytes within the surface and crypt-lining epithelium (called lymphoepithelium) are commonly observed (Figs. 14.18 and 14.19) and merely reflect the normal passage of lymphocytes. Sometimes the epithelium is so heavily infiltrated by lymphocytes that it is scarcely distinguishable. Intraepithelial lymphocyte trafficking primarily overlies subepithelial lymphoid follicles (Figs. 14.20 and 14.21), resembling Peyer patches of the small intestinal mucosa. Intraepithelial lymphocytes of the surface mucosa are predominantly T cells (CD3+, CD5+, CD7+, and CD8+), whereas those present within the crypt epithelium include both T cells and B cells (40). The epithelial cells of lymphoepithelium (known as M cells) exhibit numerous surface microvilli and microfolds. At the ultrastructural level, intraepithelial lymphocytes have been shown to be located within intracytoplasmic compartments that communicate with each other to form an intraepithelial network of channels (41).

Tonsils are normally found in close association with minor salivary glands (Fig. 14.22). Frequently, the excretory ducts of these mucous glands empty into the tonsillar

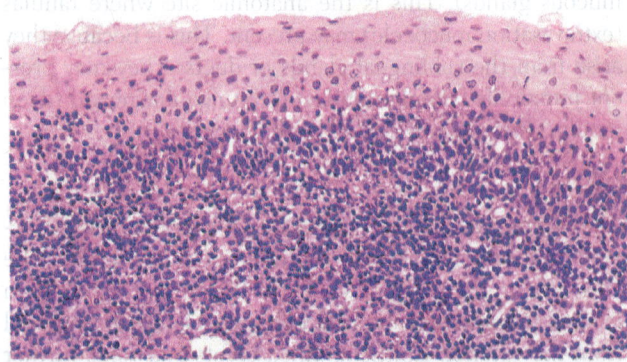

FIGURE 14.18 Lingual tonsil. The mucosa (nonkeratinized stratified squamous epithelium) is infiltrated with numerous lymphocytes that obscure the basement membrane.

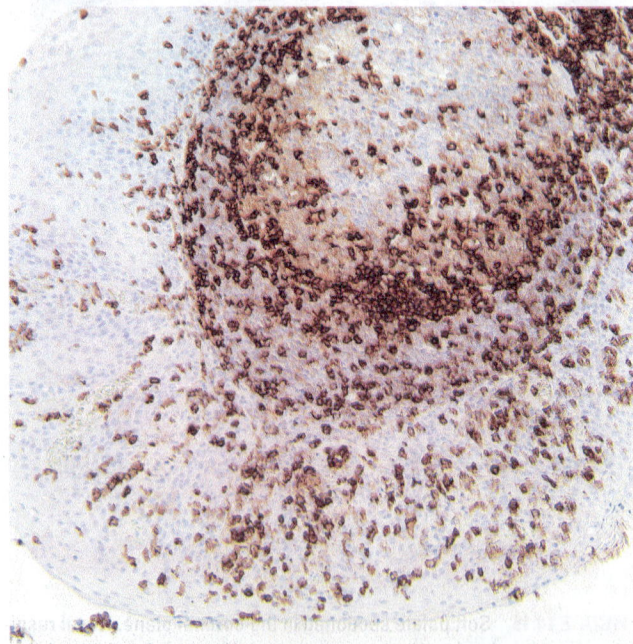

FIGURE 14.20 Tonsil lymphoepithelium overlying a secondary lymphoid follicle with a germinal center. The CD3 (T-cell marker) immunostain highlights abundant T-cells trafficking through the epithelium.

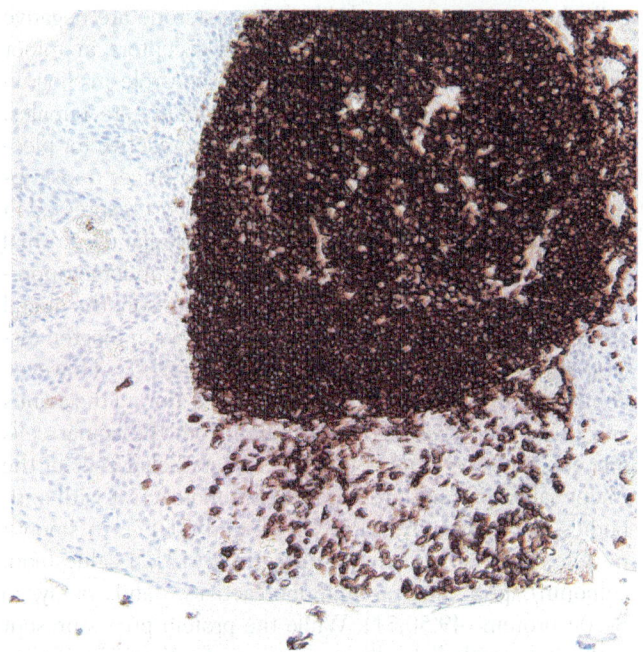

FIGURE 14.21 Tonsil showing CD20 (B-cell marker) immunoreactive lymphocytes located within a lymphoid follicle. B cells focally pass through the lymphoepithelium.

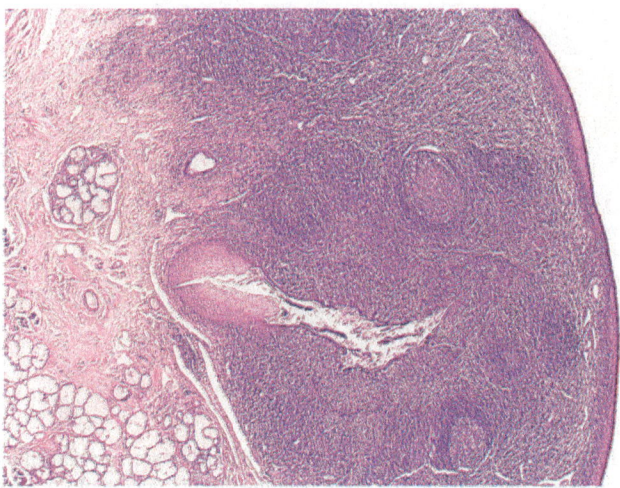

FIGURE 14.22 Lingual tonsil. Lymphoid tissue with follicles under mucosa and around its infolding (crypt). Note mucous glands and ducts.

crypts. The minor salivary glands (Weber glands) adjacent to the palatine tonsils are thought to be a putative reservoir of pathogenic bacteria and, therefore, should be removed along with the tonsil during a tonsillectomy. Small foci of hyalin cartilage and even bone may be present close to the fibrous capsule of the palatine tonsil, which has been proposed by some authors to represent metaplasia or heterotopia (42) but more than likely is an embryologic remnant of Reichert cartilage that originates from the second branchial arch.

Minor Salivary Glands

Numerous small salivary glands are scattered throughout the submucosa of the oral cavity, nose, and paranasal sinuses, as well as adjacent to the palatine and pharyngeal tonsils. These glands are not encapsulated and are named by their location. They can be classified as mucous, serous, and mixed seromucinous types (Table 14.2). These glands produce secretions similar to those of the major salivary glands, which empty onto the mucosal surface through numerous small excretory ducts. The secretory activity of

TABLE 14.2 Minor Salivary Glands of the Mouth, Nose, and Paranasal Sinuses

Name	Location	Type of Acini
Labial (superior and inferior)	Lips	Mixed (predominantly mucous)
Buccal	Cheek	Mixed (predominantly mucous)
Glossopalatine	Anterior faucial pillar Glossopalatine fold	Pure mucous
Palatine	Hard palate Soft palate Uvula	Pure mucous (mixed in uvula) Mixed (predominantly mucous)
Palatine tonsil (Weber glands)	Subjacent to tonsil capsule	Pure mucous
Sublingual	Floor of mouth	Mixed (predominantly mucous)
Lingual (glands of Blandin and Nuhn)	Anterior tongue	Mixed (predominantly mucous)
Tongue (Ebner glands)	Circumvallate papillae	Pure serous
Lingual tonsil	Base of tongue	Pure mucous
Nasal and paranasal	Nose and sinuses	Mixed

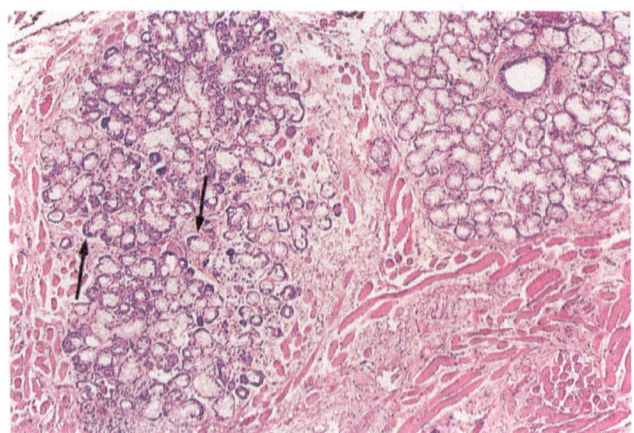

FIGURE 14.23 Minor salivary glands in the uvula are surrounded by cross-striated muscle. The gland with the distinct duct is of the pure mucous type. The other gland is seromucinous, with the serous cells forming darker-staining crescents (*arrows*).

these glands appears to be continuous, although they can respond to specific local chemical or physical stimuli.

Structurally, the minor salivary glands are compound tubular or tubuloacinar glands. Their secretory portions are the acini that are designated according to their secretion as mucous, serous, or mixed. Within mixed acini, the mucous cells are nearest to the excretory duct, whereas the serous cells are at the cul-de-sac of the acini and appear as crescents, called the demilunes of Giannuzzi (Figs. 14.23, 14.24 and 14.46). The mucous acini are more tubular than those of the serous type. The mucous cells are also larger, and their flattened nuclei are present at the cell bases. The mucous cells have a pale-appearing cytoplasm in H&E-stained sections (Fig. 14.14) and will also stain with Alcian blue, periodic acid–Schiff (PAS), or mucicarmine (43,44). The smaller serous cells have more rounded basal nuclei and have an eosinophilic cytoplasm that contains zymogen granules. Normal acinar and ductal cells express androgen receptor (45). In women, however, estradiol is positive in ductal epithelial cells, but testosterone and dihydrotestosterone are negative (46). This sex difference of hormonal receptors in minor salivary gland epithelia is thought to play a role in Sjögren disease, where approximately 90% of patients are females. Normal salivary gland tissue is not immunoreactive for pleomorphic adenoma gene 1 (PLAG1), a zinc finger transcription factor gene consistently rearranged and overexpressed in human pleomorphic adenomas of the salivary glands. Normal minor salivary glands also do not appear to undergo appreciable proliferation and apoptosis. By comparison, the ductal epithelial and acinar cells of salivary glands from Sjögren disease patients do exhibit increased apoptosis (47). However, contractile myoepithelial cells are wrapped around the acinus and assist by squeezing the secretion from the acinar cells into the excretory ducts (48). The myoepithelial cells of the minor salivary glands are variably immunoreactive with antibodies to cytokeratin (CK5, CK14, and CK17), to smooth muscle markers (smooth muscle actin [SMA], h-caldesmon, calponin), p63 (nuclear immunoreactivity), and, rarely, to S-100 protein (49,50,51). While the protein p63 is present within myoepithelial cells in all stages of salivary gland morphogenesis from initial bud to terminal bud stage, calponin is only detected increasingly as a salivary gland structure matures. Evidence for a neuroectodermal phenotype (S-100, GFAP, NSE) has not been observed in myoepithelial cells of salivary glands (50,51). It should be noted that melanocytes may be found in a small proportion (<2%) of minor salivary glands (52).

It is important to note that the minor salivary glands, wherever they occur in the mouth, nose, or paranasal sinuses, can become involved by the same pathologic processes as the major salivary glands. This is especially true for neoplasms, which arise from various cellular components of the minor salivary glands. Excess adipose tissue in association with these glands may represent a sialolipoma (53).

The surgical pathologist must be well aware of the fact that squamous metaplasia can occur in the excretory ducts and acini of minor salivary glands. For instance, epithelial regeneration after injury of various types may lead to squamous metaplasia that can mimic squamous cell carcinoma. A good example of this is seen in necrotizing sialometaplasia or in irradiated salivary glands. In the latter case, the diagnostic dilemma is usually compounded by the possibility of a recurrence of previous squamous cell carcinoma. Oncocytic cells may be found in minor salivary glands in varying numbers and distribution patterns (Fig. 14.25). Oncocytes ("swollen cells") are large, cuboidal, or columnar epithelial cells with a finely granular eosinophilic cytoplasm that have been identified in many exocrine or endocrine glands (54). Up to 60% of their cytoplasm is usually occupied by mitochondria that can be visualized after long-term (48 hours) staining with phosphotungstic acid–hematoxylin or on fresh-frozen sections incubated for the histochemical demonstration of mitochondrial enzyme activity, by means of immunohistochemistry (e.g., antimitochondrial antibody), or by electron

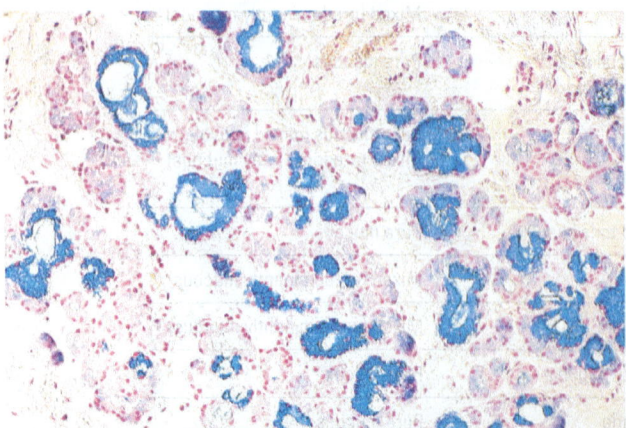

FIGURE 14.24 Mixed minor salivary gland of the uvula. Acid mucopolysaccharides in mucous cells are stained turquoise (Alcian blue at pH 2.6).

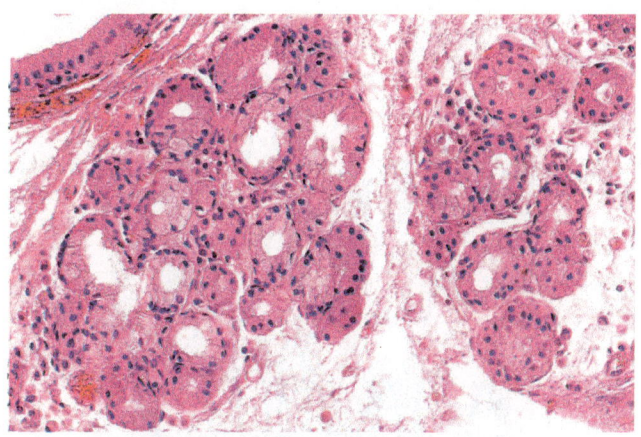

FIGURE 14.25 Oncocytes in minor salivary gland appear as cuboidal swollen cells with a finely granular oxyphilic cytoplasm.

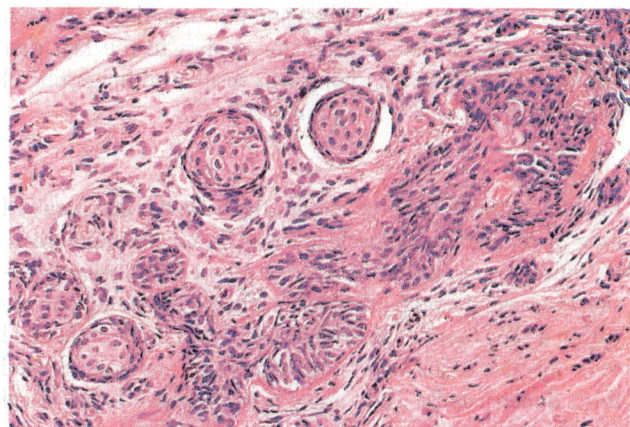

FIGURE 14.26 Juxtaoral organ of Chievitz. Small nests of nonkeratinized squamous epithelial cells are delineated by basement membrane. The elongated cells outside the epithelial islands are fibroblasts and Schwann cells. Nerve is seen below and to the right.

microscopy. Oncocytes are benign cells that occur with increasing frequency in older persons. They develop because of metaplasia of ductal and acinar epithelium. However, the etiology and functional significance of oncocytic metaplasia is not clear. In the minor salivary glands, oncocytes can be seen in nodular or diffuse oncocytosis, oncocytoma (55,56), and even oncocytic carcinomas (57).

Cheeks

The skin of the cheek is part of the facial skin. The inner surface of the cheeks is covered by squamous lining mucosa. The submucosa contains some fat cells and many minor salivary glands of the mixed type, embedded in loose connective tissue. The mucosa and submucosa are bound to the underlying buccal musculature by connective tissue fibers (Fig. 14.13).

Juxtaoral Organ of Chievitz

Deep in the wall of the cheeks overlying the angle of the mandible sits an anatomically well-defined small fusiform structure, the juxtaoral organ (JOO) of Chievitz, which is normally present in the buccotemporal space (51,52,58,59). In adults, it measures 0.7 to 1.7 cm in length and 0.1 to 0.2 cm in diameter and persists throughout life. It is multilobulated, has a dense fibrous capsule, and consists of round or elongate nests of nonkeratinizing squamous-like epithelial cells embedded in an organized connective tissue stroma that is rich in small nerves and sensory receptors innervated by two to four branches of the buccal nerve (60). The connective tissue envelope is divided into a thin inner stratum fibrosum internum, middle stratum nervosum, and outer stratum fibrosum externum. These nests of epithelial cells appear in a cluster on histologic sections, but serial sectioning shows them to be small sprouts and folds in continuity with a mass of epithelium. Thus, cross sections through different portions of the JOO can show considerable variation in number and shape of epithelial sprouts (Fig. 14.26). The larger nests of epithelium are composed of cells with a clear PAS-positive cytoplasm and round or oval nuclei, forming "light centers." Intercellular bridges can be seen toward the center of the cell nests. The cells in the smaller nests can show a whorl-like or concentric arrangement. Occasionally, a gland-like lumen or a follicle filled with colloid-like mucin-negative material is encountered. Melanin pigmentation has been reported in the JOO (61). The central epithelial cells of the JOO appear to be immunoreactive for cytokeratins, whereas the outer more basaloid cells are usually keratin negative. The cell nests are also positive for vimentin and epithelial membrane antigen (EMA) but are negative for S-100 protein, glial fibrillary acidic protein (GFAP), neuron-specific enolase (NSE), synaptophysin, and chromogranin (62,63).

The seemingly esoteric and minute JOO has considerable importance for the surgical pathologist because the presence of squamous epithelial nests intimately admixed with numerous small nerves may be misinterpreted as perineural invasion by squamous cell carcinoma (64). On the other hand, astute pathologists aware of this pitfall have, in a case of a mucoepidermoid carcinoma with lymphatic spread in the retromolar region, correctly recognized this finding as the epithelial nests of the JOO (65). Such cases unequivocally demonstrate the importance of awareness of this small organ. Cases of clinically enlarged (66) and hyperplastic JOOs have been described (67), but so far no carcinoma originating from it has been reported. The function of the JOO is unknown. Since Johan Henrik Chievitz, a Danish anatomist, described this structure in 1885 in a 10-week-old human embryo (68) it has been widely believed that the organ of Chievitz is a rudimentary structure, representing an abortive salivary gland anlage. More recently, the possibility of a neurosecretory and receptor function of the organ has been raised (69). The JOO has been shown to contain pacinian corpuscles (70), supporting its mechanosensory function. For a thorough review of the literature, the reader is referred to the small monograph by

Zenker (60) or review paper by Pantanowitz and Balogh (69). Finally, we would like to alert our readers to the fact that similar benign epithelial islands may reside within peripheral nerves in the maxilla (71) and mandible (72).

Tongue

Situated in the floor of the mouth, the tongue is an organized mass of cross-striated muscle invested by mucous membrane. Its muscles are partly extrinsic (i.e., have their origins outside the tongue) and partly intrinsic, being contained entirely within it. The bundles of cross-striated muscle are embedded in connective tissue with some adipocytes and are arranged three dimensionally. The tongue is well-supplied with blood vessels that form numerous anastomoses. Changes related to ageing include lingual varicosities, glossitis, and atrophy of the taste papillae. The tongue is richly endowed with myelinated and nonmyelinated nerves containing motor, sensory, and vegetative nerve fibers, some with ganglion cells. The ventral (under) surface of the tongue is covered by smooth lining mucosa that has short, blunt rete ridges (Fig. 14.27). Its submucosa merges with the connective tissue that intersects with the ventral muscle bundles of the tongue.

The dorsal (upper) surface of the tongue is divided into an anterior and posterior part by a V-shaped shallow groove, the sulcus terminalis. The anterior two-thirds of the dorsum of the tongue are lined by specialized mucosa, which is bound by connective tissue fibers to the underlying skeletal muscle of the tongue. This specialized mucosa is modified keratinized squamous epithelium covered with small projections (papillae) that are visible to the naked eye. The pathologist has to be aware of these papillae so as not to mistake them for papillary epithelial hyperplasia, papillomas, or oral hairy leukoplakia. According to their shape, the papillae can be filiform, fungiform, foliate, or circumvallate. The great majority are filiform papillae, conical projections of the keratinized epithelium (Fig. 14.28). Among these are scattered the fungiform papillae, which are rounded elevations above the surface

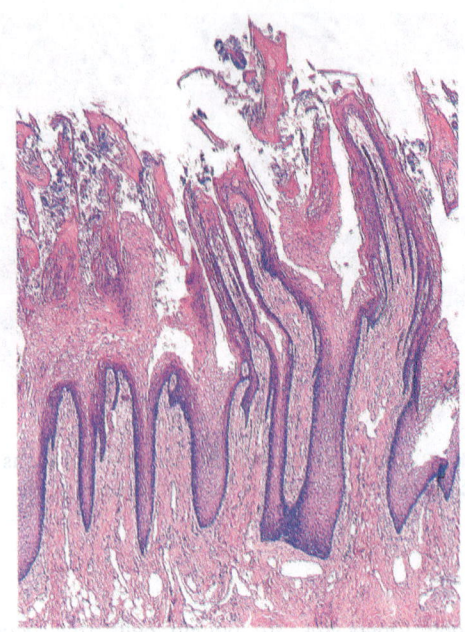

FIGURE 14.28 Dorsal surface of tongue. Filiform papillae have a connective tissue core beset with secondary papillae with pointed ends. The superficial squamous cells are keratinized. Note the slender, pointed rete ridges.

of the tongue; their surface is not keratinized (Fig. 14.29). Clinically, fungiform papillae appear as small red nodules because the thin epithelium does not mask the underlying vascular connective tissue. Microscopically, fungiform papillae should not be misinterpreted as denture-induced fibrous hyperplasia or small traumatic fibromas. The foliate papillae are located posteriorly along the sides of the tongue. At the junction of the anterior two-thirds and the posterior one-third of the tongue are the circumvallate papillae. These are the largest papillae, measuring 0.1 to 0.2 cm in diameter and are arranged in a V-shape immediately anterior to the sulcus terminalis. The circumvallate papillae number 6 to 12.

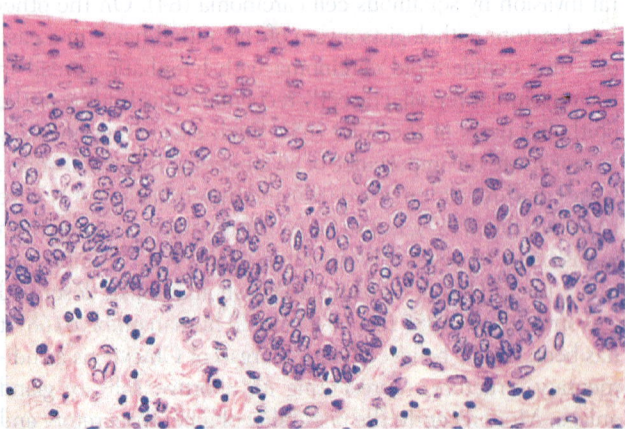

FIGURE 14.27 Ventral surface of tongue. The stratified nonkeratinized squamous epithelium of the lining mucosa has a slightly wavy interface with the lamina propria. A few scattered lymphocytes are seen in the lamina propria and in the epithelium.

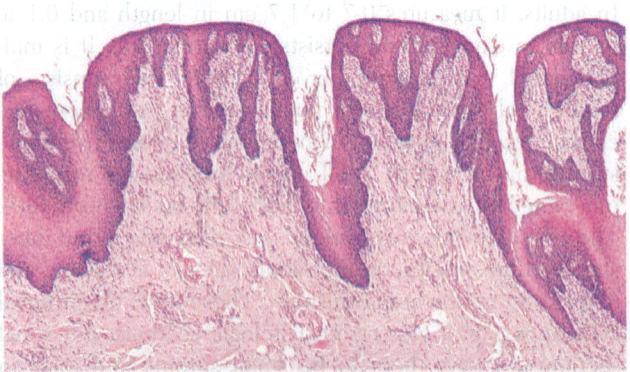

FIGURE 14.29 Fungiform papillae. Slightly rounded, elevated structures with a larger connective tissue core. Smaller intervening connective tissue papillae project into the base of the surface epithelium.

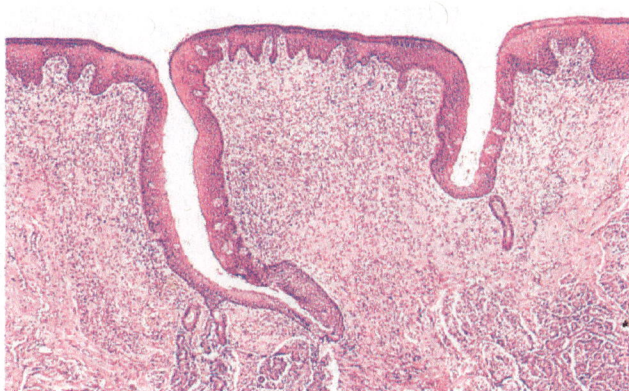

FIGURE 14.30 Circumvallate papilla. Numerous taste buds are on the lateral walls of the papilla and on the epithelium facing the papilla within the furrow. Ducts of serous glands open into the furrow surrounding the circumvallate papilla.

A small, ring-shaped furrow surrounds each circumvallate papilla and separates it from a circular, palisade-like mucosal elevation (vallum), which is the outer border of the circumvallate papilla (Fig. 14.30). Occasionally, there may be a round or rhomboid-shaped midline patch of smooth mucosa on the dorsal surface of the tongue that lacks both papillae and taste buds (called median rhomboid glossitis). This benign disorder is thought to arise from an embryologic defect.

Taste buds are present in large numbers on the side of the circumvallate papillae and in lesser numbers on the fungiform and foliate papillae, as well as elsewhere on the dorsal and lateral aspects of the tongue. These small epithelial organs stain lighter than the surrounding epithelium. Like other simple epithelia, taste buds express low–molecular-weight keratins such as CK18, and, accordingly, they are immunoreactive with the antibody CAM5.2 (Fig. 14.31). Numerous small serous glands (Ebner glands) are located under the circumvallate papillae. The ducts of these glands empty their secretion into the small furrow around each papilla; this serous secretion flushes out the furrows, thus facilitating perception of new tastes. The taste buds are

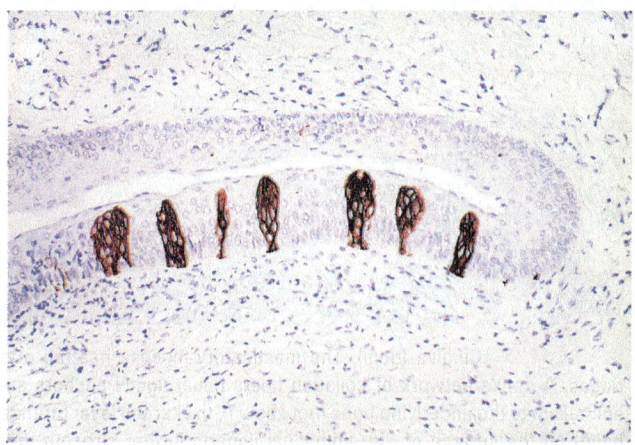

FIGURE 14.31 Taste buds showing immunoreactivity for CAM 5.2.

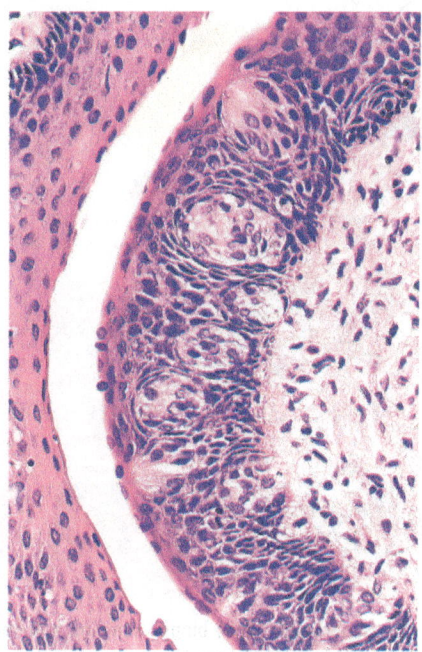

FIGURE 14.32 Taste buds on the side of a circumvallate papilla. The cells of the intraepithelial taste buds are spindle-shaped and oriented at a right angle to the surface. The cell nuclei are elongated and are situated mainly in the basal half of the buds. Nerve fibers ending on the sensory (gustatory) cells cannot be seen with H&E stain.

barrel-shaped intramucosal sensory receptors that occupy the full thickness of the mucosa and communicate with the surface through a small opening, the gustatory pore (Fig. 14.32). The taste buds are composed of three types of cells: (a) gustatory or taste cells; (b) supporting, or sustentacular, cells; and (c) basal cells. The taste cells are crescent shaped, have lightly staining cytoplasm, and possess numerous fine microvilli that protrude through the taste pore as gustatory hairs. The basal end of the taste cells has intimate contact with many fine nerve terminals that leave through the basement membrane and become myelinated outside the taste bud. The supporting cells are likewise crescentic, extending between the basement membrane and the surface; they form a shell for the taste bud and are also scattered between the gustatory cells. The supporting cells have a dark cytoplasm and possess microvilli that also protrude through the taste pore. The small basal cells, situated between the bases of the other cells, give rise to the other cells of the taste bud (73,74).

In the posterolateral region of the tongue one may normally encounter biphasic neuroepithelial structures similar to the JOO of Chievitz. The term "subgemmal nerve plexus" or "subgemmal neurogenous plaque (SNP)" has been used interchangeably in the literature for this structure (75–78). In this superficial region one may find clusters of squamous epithelial cells with bland cytomorphology in close association with the circumscribed subepithelial nerve plexus (Fig. 14.33). In many cases they may be associated with lymphoid tissue with reactive germinal centers (78).

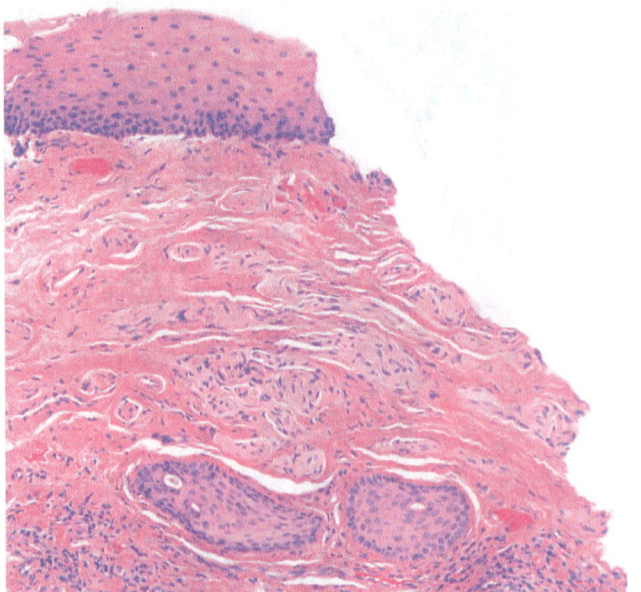

FIGURE 14.33 Superficial tongue biopsy showing a subgemmal neurogenous plaque comprised of superficial nerves in close proximity to bland squamous cell nests.

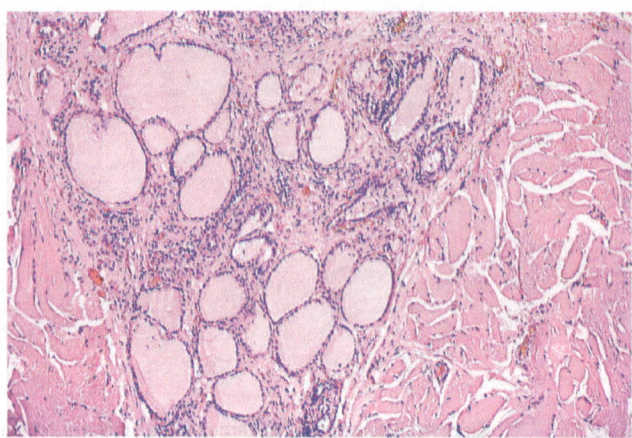

FIGURE 14.34 Lingual thyroid. The glandular parenchyma is embedded in skeletal muscle. The thyroid tissue is not encapsulated, and care should be taken to avoid mistaking it for invasive growth.

Immunohistochemical evaluation shows that the epithelium is positive for cytokeratin and CAM5.2 while the nerve fibers show positivity for S-100, CD56 and synaptophysin (77). The exact origin and function of these neuroepithelial structures and their association with this nerve plexus of taste buds has yet to be completely elucidated. The intimate association of epithelial remnants with peripheral nerves is a potential diagnostic pitfall for pathologists as they may be mistaken for a neural lesion or squamous cell carcinoma with perineural invasion.

The apex of the V-shaped sulcus terminalis projects backward and is marked by a small pit, the foramen cecum, which is an embryologic remnant indicating the upper end of the thyroglossal duct. Correspondingly, ectopic thyroid tissue can occur at the base of the tongue (lingual thyroid) or anywhere along the tract of the thyroglossal duct caudally (Fig. 14.34). Microscopically, ectopic thyroid resembles normal thyroid tissue. However, the surgical pathologist should be aware that the presence of thyroid glands within muscle may mimic carcinoma. Ectopic thyroid tissue may undergo all the physiologic and pathologic changes of the thyroid gland proper.

Gingiva

The gingiva (gum) is that portion of the oral mucosa that surrounds the neck of the teeth like a collar. Masticatory mucosa (i.e., parakeratinized or keratinized stratified squamous epithelium) covers the gum. There is no submucosal layer. Instead, the connective tissue of the lamina propria contains collagenous fibers that bind the epithelium tightly to the underlying alveolar periosteum and bone. The gingival epithelium interdigitates with the underlying connective tissue, forming long, interconnected rete ridges that are separated by connective tissue plates and papillae (Figs. 14.35 and 14.36). The gingival epithelium is divided anatomically into oral gingival, oral sulcular, and junctional epithelia. The cytokeratin expression profile of gingival epithelium corresponds to this anatomical division (Table 14.1). Oral gingival epithelium that extends onto the oral surface of the gum best fits the general pattern of masticatory mucosa. The short portion of gingiva apposed to the tooth (sulcular gingiva) differs from the rest of gingival epithelium in that it is thinner, lacks the characteristic rete ridges, and is not keratinizing (79,80).

The gingiva is highly vascular; its vessels originate in the periodontium and extend into the lamina propria, forming

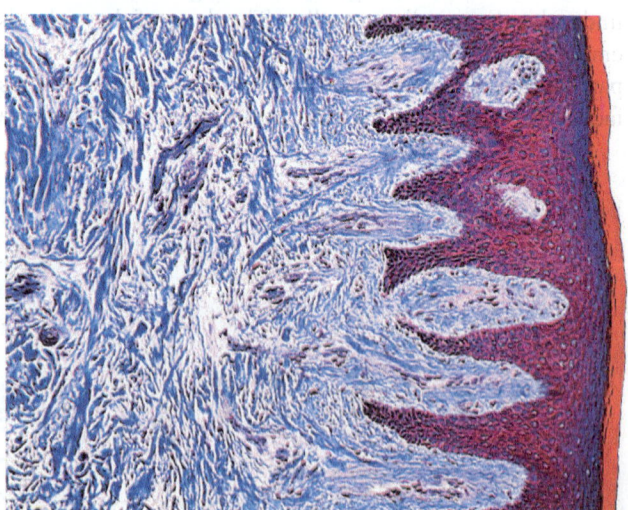

FIGURE 14.35 Gingiva (gum). The masticatory mucosa has tall rete ridges. A dense network of collagen fibers (blue) tightly anchors the epithelium to the underlying bone (not shown); the keratin layer (orange band) on the surface of the epithelium imparts further strength to it (Mallory trichrome).

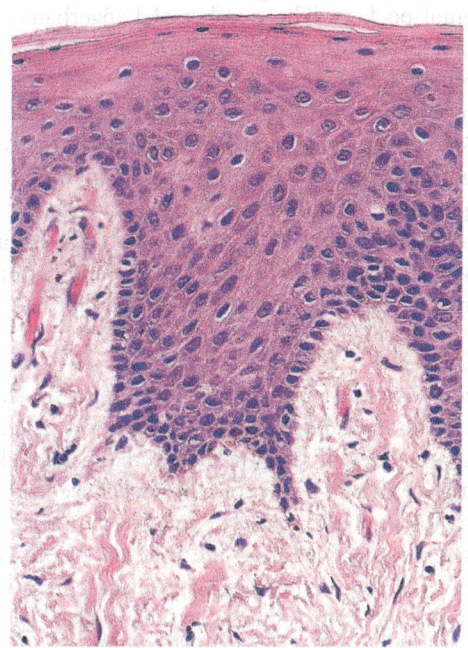

FIGURE 14.36 Gingiva. Tall rete ridges and dense lamina propria with blood vessels in papillae.

well-organized capillary loops. Occasionally random biopsies of gingiva have been performed to support the diagnosis of systemic diseases (e.g., amyloidosis).

Intraepithelial Nonkeratinocytes

Four different nonepithelial cell types normally occur in the oral mucosa: melanocytes, Merkel cells, Langerhans cells, and lymphocytes.

Melanocytes are found mainly in a basal location in the oral mucosa; they are more common in people with darker complexions (81,82). Small areas of melanin pigmentation, mostly <10 mm in diameter, may occur. They are most common on the gingiva but are also seen in the lips, palate, and buccal mucosa and are called mucosal melanosis (melanotic macules) (83) (Fig. 14.37). Melanin pigment

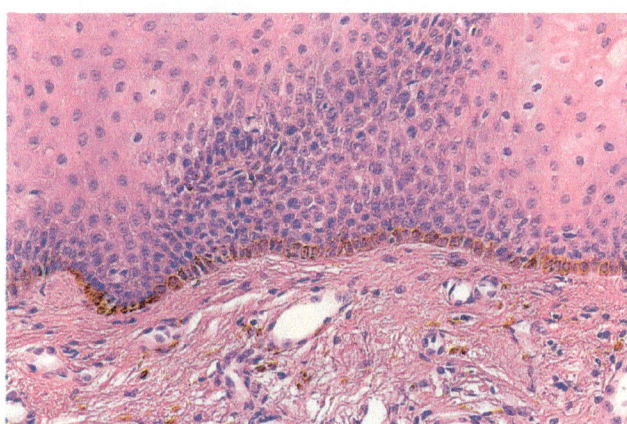

FIGURE 14.37 Mucosal melanosis of the lip. Numerous melanocytes above the basal lamina appear as a brown ribbon.

formed by melanocytes in the basal layer is transferred to adjacent epithelial cells. Such changes can sometimes occur after inflammatory reactions, in smokers, with Peutz–Jeghers syndrome and Addison disease, or secondary to drugs and human immunodeficiency virus (HIV) infection. Melanocytic hyperplasia (lentigo) and pigmented nevi may also occur in the oral mucosa but less commonly than on the skin (84–87). Histologically, a lentigo shows increased melanin pigmentation in the basal cell layer without an increase in the number of melanocytes. Intramucosal nevi, similar to intradermal nevi, are the most common type of nevus. Other types of nevi, such as compound nevi, junctional nevi, blue nevi, and combined forms can be observed on the vermilion border, cheek mucosa, gingiva, palate, and tongue. Understandably, primary malignant melanomas can arise anywhere from the oral mucosa (88).

Merkel cells also occur in the basal layer of the oral epithelium, either individually or in clusters (89). Clusters (named Merkel complexes) are preferentially located in masticatory mucosa in close contact with the tongue and with sensory nerves, which supports the notion that they have a mechanoreceptor function. They tend to be conspicuous on the mandibular lingual gingiva where they are believed to play a role in the proprioceptive positioning of the tongue. On routine H&E-stained sections, their cytoplasm appears lighter than that of the surrounding basal cells. These neuroendocrine cells are morphologically and functionally identical to those in the skin. They are immunoreactive with antibodies to S-100 protein, chromogranin, synaptophysin, NSE, CK20, and villin (90). Apart from marking Merkel cells in the oral mucosa, CK20 shows specificity for only lingual taste buds. Their ultrastructure is characterized by many intracytoplasmic dense-core, membrane-bound granules, 80 to 100 μm in diameter (Fig. 14.38). Merkel cells of the oral region differ from those found in the skin because they express S-100, and at the ultrastructural level also contain a nuclear rodlet. There is a higher prevalence of oral Merkel cells in edentulous subjects, and they may also increase as a consequence of tissue injury.

Langerhans cells, mostly located suprabasally, are microscopically similar to melanocytes and cannot be distinguished with certainty in routine H&E-stained sections. In the gingiva, the Langerhans cells are structurally and functionally similar to those in the skin (91,92). Their cytoplasm appears clear, and their small indented ("coffee bean") nucleus stains heavily with hematoxylin. Their dendritic processes, spread among the cells of the stratum spinosum, can be seen well with the immunohistochemical stain for S-100 protein (Fig. 14.39), as well as CD1a, the MHC class II molecules (e.g., HLA-DR), and various adhesion molecules (93). Electron microscopy shows characteristic Birbeck granules in their cytoplasm and a lack of tonofilaments and desmosomes. The frequency of oral mucosal Langerhans cells varies inversely with the degree of keratinization. They are quantitatively lowest in the floor of the mouth and do not occur around the basal portion of the taste buds and in epithelium lining

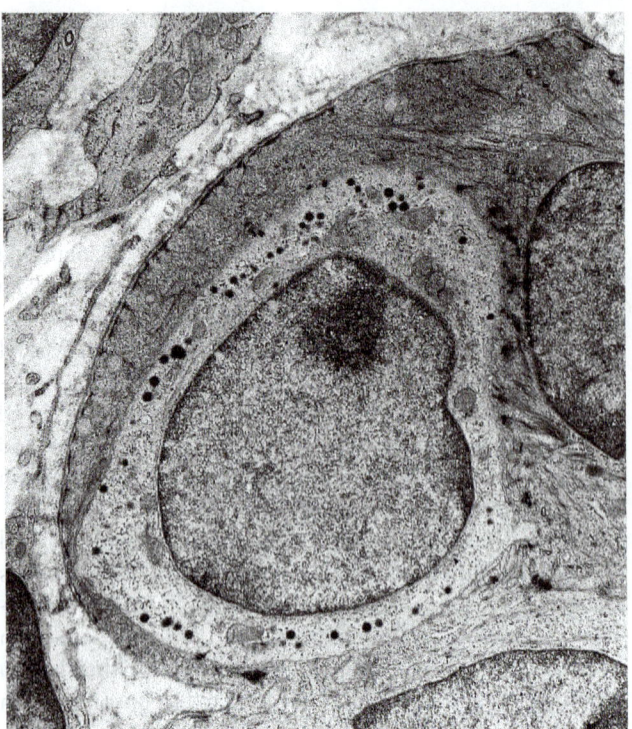

FIGURE 14.38 Merkel cell surrounded by keratinocytes in the basal layer. Transmission electron micrograph shows the lighter-staining cytoplasm with characteristic and subplasmalemmal, membrane-bound, dense-core granules. The nucleus has no fibrous lamina, unlike melanocytes. The adjacent dermis contains fibroblasts. (Original magnification ×11,500.)

periodontal pockets. The number of Langerhans cells is a significant prognostic factor for head and neck squamous cell carcinoma (94).

Langerhans cells play an important role in the immune response, being involved in the processing and presentation of antigens to subjacent lymphocytes. An increased number of Langerhans cells is seen in biopsy samples of the oral mucosa in oral lichen planus, associated with dental caries, with tobacco and alcohol consumption, and in tumor epithelium of invasive oral squamous cell carcinoma.

Teeth and Supporting Structures

The deciduous and permanent teeth have a similar microscopic appearance. The teeth are set in bony sockets on the alveolar processes of the maxillae and the mandible. The part of the tooth that lies within the socket is called the root; there may be multiple roots. The tip of each root is called the apex. The alveolar processes are covered by the gum, and the crowns of the teeth project above the gums. The roots of the teeth are held securely in their sockets by bundles of collagen fibers called the periodontal ligament (periodontal membrane) (12). The periodontium includes the tissues investing and supporting the teeth: the cementum, periodontal membrane, alveolar bone, and gingiva (Figs. 14.40 and 14.41). The center of each tooth has a pulp chamber, or pulp cavity, that is filled with dental pulp containing loosely arranged fibroblasts, nerves, blood vessels, and lymphatics (95) (Fig. 14.42). The pulp chamber narrows toward the root and becomes the root canal. The vessels and postganglionic

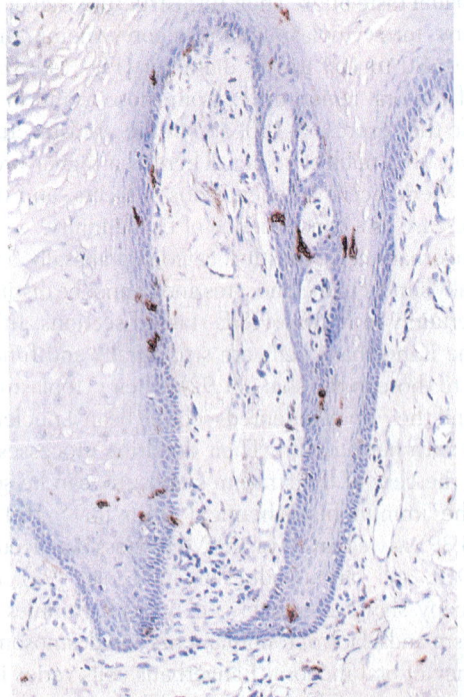

FIGURE 14.39 Langerhans cells in mucosa of tongue. Dendritic cells in the suprabasal epidermis demonstrate immunoreactivity for S-100 protein.

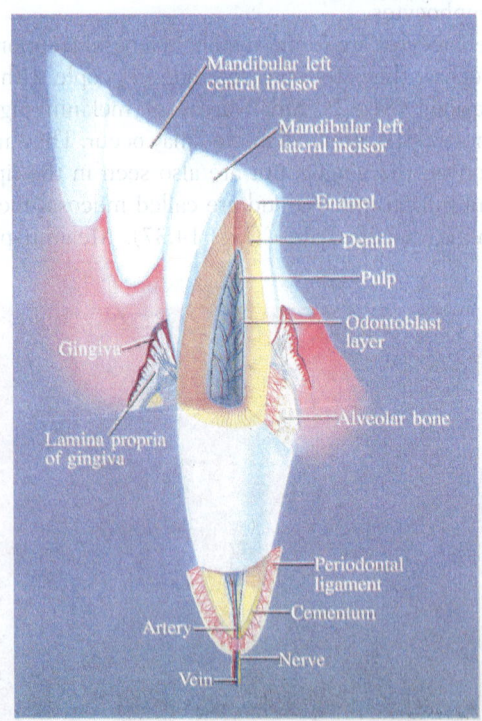

FIGURE 14.40 Schematic drawing depicts the periodontium including the gingiva, alveolar bone, periodontal ligament, and cementum.

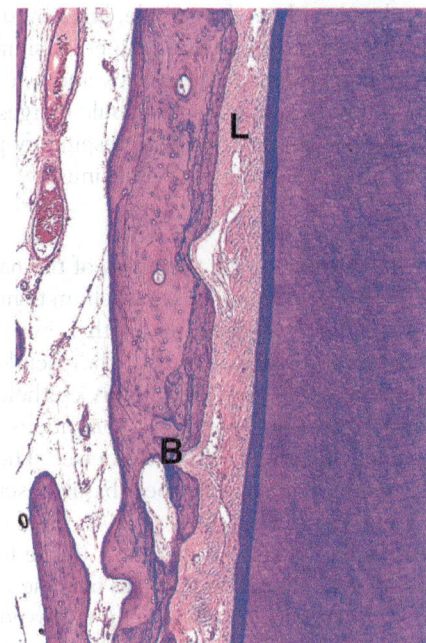

FIGURE 14.41 Root of tooth and supporting structures, perpendicular section. Dentin is covered by a thin layer of cementum (appearing as a blue band). The periodontal ligament (L) holds the tooth in the bony socket of the alveolar process (B).

sympathetic and sensory nerve fibers enter and leave the root canal through a small opening, the apical foramen. The pulp chamber of the growing tooth is lined by a single continuous layer of odontoblasts, which are tall columnar cells with oval nuclei. An elongated cell process, also known as Tomes' fiber, reaches from each odontoblast into the extracellular matrix secreted by them (Fig. 14.5). The matrix around the odontoblastic process eventually mineralizes, so that Tomes' fiber comes to lie within a dentinal tubule (96,97). Besides the odontoblastic process, the tubules also contain 200-μm long unmyelinated nerve fibers, which account for the well-known sensitivity of dentin. Dentin is arranged in the

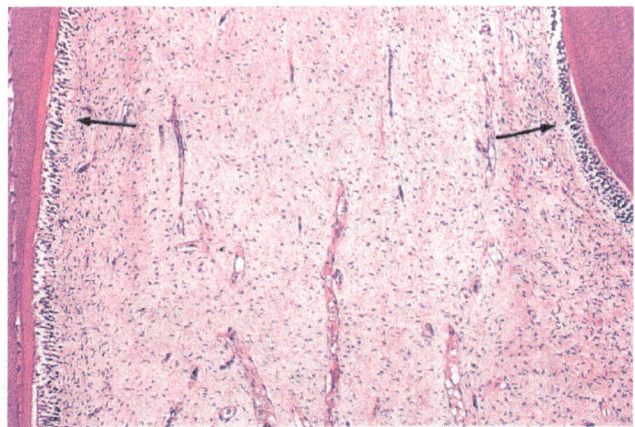

FIGURE 14.42 Pulp of developing tooth. Odontoblasts (*arrows*) line dentin. The pulp consists mostly of loosely arranged fibroblasts. Note the delicate wall of blood vessels.

shape of tubules running from the pulp chamber toward the periphery. The dentinal tubules and the meshwork of collagen between them are embedded in hydroxyapatite crystals. On a weight basis, 80% of dentin consists of inorganic calcium salts and 20% of organic material. It is harder than bone but softer than enamel. Dentin makes up most of the wall of the tooth. In the mature tooth, many odontoblasts become inactive, but some continue producing predentin at a reduced rate throughout the life of the tooth. In response to physiologic or pathologic stimuli, odontoblasts can upregulate their protein synthetic activity.

As the dental pulp ages, the number of fibroblasts decreases and, concomitantly, the number and size of collagen fibers increases. Pulp stones (denticles) are commonly observed in the dental pulp of aging individuals. True denticles contain dentinal tubules within a mineralized matrix and are surrounded by odontoblasts. False denticles are composed of a mineralized matrix arranged in concentric lamellae. Most denticles are asymptomatic.

Enamel covers the crown of the tooth. It is the hardest material found in the body and consists of 99.5% apatite crystals (98). Mature enamel is made up of long thin rods that dissolve during decalcification and are, therefore, not seen on conventional histologic sections. Enamel proteins such as amelogenin, enamelin, and the basement membrane-type proteoglycan perlecan are immunolocalized in particular odontogenic tumors such as ameloblastomas (99). Perlecan is found mainly in the intercellular spaces of the enamel organ, as well as in the dental papilla/pulp and dental follicle. The dentin–enamel junction lies at the former interface between the inner enamel epithelium and dental mesenchyme. Coronal dentin is covered with enamel, and radicular dentin is covered with cementum. Thus, cementum covers the root of the tooth. A slight indentation (cervical line) encircles the tooth and marks the junction of the crown with the root. The cementum joins the enamel at this junction (cementoenamel junction). Cementum is similar in structure and composition to bone but has fewer cells, called cementocytes, that occupy lacunae (11,12). It is composed of 55% organic material (mainly calcium) and 45% inorganic material. Cementum is attached by the periodontal ligament to the surrounding bone (Fig. 14.41). In older persons, many cementocytes die, and only the surface layer appears viable. Another aging phenomenon is cementicles, which are small round calcified bodies on or in the cementum and in the periodontal ligament. Cementicles are of no clinical significance.

From the pathologist's point of view, it is noteworthy that examination of teeth involved in neoplastic growth in most cases shows tumor invading the periodontal ligament and the alveolar bone, destroying these structures. The roots of the teeth may remain intact or may undergo resorption. However, the dental pulp is rarely invaded by neoplasm.

Odontogenic epithelium changes over time. Before tooth eruption, it consists of the external enamel epithelium, inner enamel epithelium, stellate reticulum, Hertwig's epithelial root sheath, and dental lamina; after complete tooth formation, it comprises the epithelial rests of Malassez. Most odontogenic epithelia express cytokeratins 5, 8, and 19 (100). In addition, the external enamel epithelium and stellate reticulum also express cytokeratins 7, 13, 14, 17, and 18; the inner enamel epithelium, cytokeratins 14 and 18; dental lamina, cytokeratins 7, 13, and 14; and epithelial rests of Malassez, cytokeratins 14 and 19. During odontogenesis, CK14 expression in ameloblasts is gradually replaced by CK19. Odontogenic epithelium is the source of odontogenic cysts and some neoplasms, which explains why CK19 is present in almost all epithelial cells of odontogenic cysts.

Pathologic Correlates of the Rests of Serres and Rests of Malassez

Developmental remnants of the dental lamina, called the rests of Serres, commonly occur under the gum as small nests of squamous epithelium (11,15) (Figs. 14.2 and 14.43). These epithelial islands may proliferate and undergo cystic degeneration, which leads to the formation of gingival cysts. Similarly, epithelial remnants of Hertwig's root sheath, called the rests of Malassez, are universally present in the periodontal membrane and, exceptionally, even in the bone of the alveolar ridge. When dental caries causes a bacterial infection and necrosis of the pulp, the infection usually spreads toward the apical foramen, and a periapical granuloma may develop. As a result of the inflammatory stimulus, the nearby epithelium of the rests of Malassez begins to proliferate and forms an epithelial lining in these apical granulomas (Fig. 14.43). It is also assumed that the rests of Serres and the rests of Malassez are potential sources of ameloblastomas and odontogenic cysts.

Nose and Paranasal Sinuses

External Nose and Nasal Vestibule

The external nose is covered by skin that is rich in sebaceous glands, sweat glands, and small hairs. The anterior skin of the nares and widened nasal vestibule, lined by skin that is continuous with the integument of the nose, similarly contains many hair follicles and sebaceous and sweat glands. The squamous epithelium of the vestibule merges with the respiratory mucosa, which covers the respiratory portion of the nasal cavity and all of the paranasal sinuses.

Nasal Mucosa

At the level of the limen nasi, the lining of the nasal cavity gradually changes from squamous epithelium to nonciliated cuboidal or columnar epithelium. Farther into the nasal cavity, this becomes continuous with the pseudostratified ciliated columnar epithelium (respiratory epithelium). The mucosa of the respiratory portion is continuous with that of the ostia and contiguous paranasal sinuses. The mucosal lining contains three main cell types: basal (reserve) cells, goblet cells, and ciliated cells (Fig. 14.44). Basal cells, confined to the vicinity of the basal lamina, divide to produce new daughter cells that differentiate to become mucous or ciliated cells. Interestingly, it has been observed that not just the surface cells have cilia, but so do some of the basal cells (101). The mucous cells rest on the basement membrane with a slender stem, and the cytoplasm of their apical portion contains varying amounts of mucus. As these cells fill up with mucus, they resemble a goblet with a foot and a stem. The cells discharge their contents to form a blanket of mucus that covers the surface of the respiratory epithelium. When the mucosa is irritated, for example, in allergic rhinitis, the number of goblet cells increases. Another source of this mucous coat is the secretion from the seromucinous glands in the lamina propria.

The majority of the cells of the respiratory epithelium are normally made up of ciliated cells bearing small finger-like cell processes, the cilia, which project into the lumen. Each cell has over 200 cilia, each about 5- to 7-μm long. Ultrastructurally, on cross section the ciliary shafts show a highly characteristic circular arrangement of nine pairs of microtubules (doublets), which are arranged symmetrically around two central microtubules (Fig. 14.45). Longitudinal

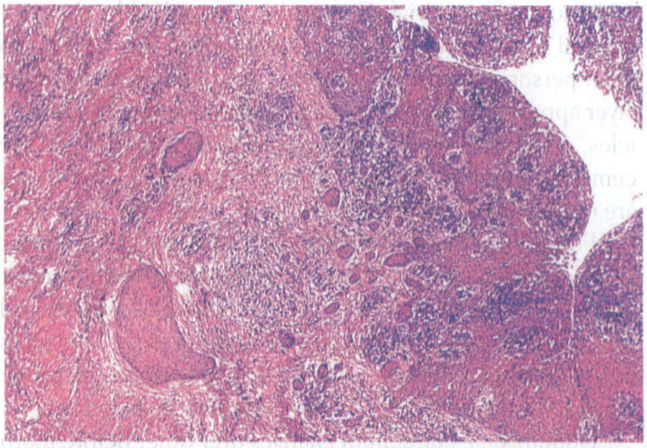

FIGURE 14.43 Rests of Malassez in periodontium near the apical granuloma.

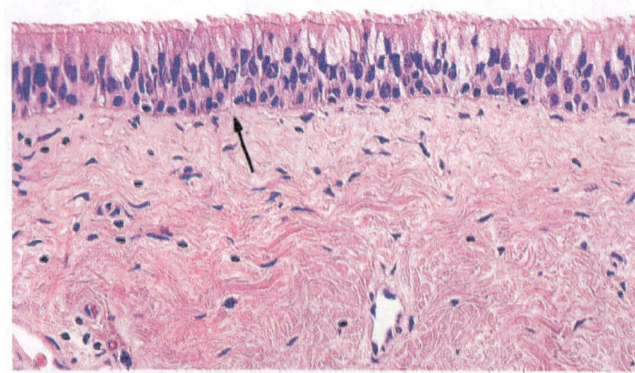

FIGURE 14.44 Pseudostratified respiratory mucosa of the nose with predominantly ciliated cells. Goblet cells have clear cytoplasm. The basal cells (*arrow*) are lying on thin basal lamina.

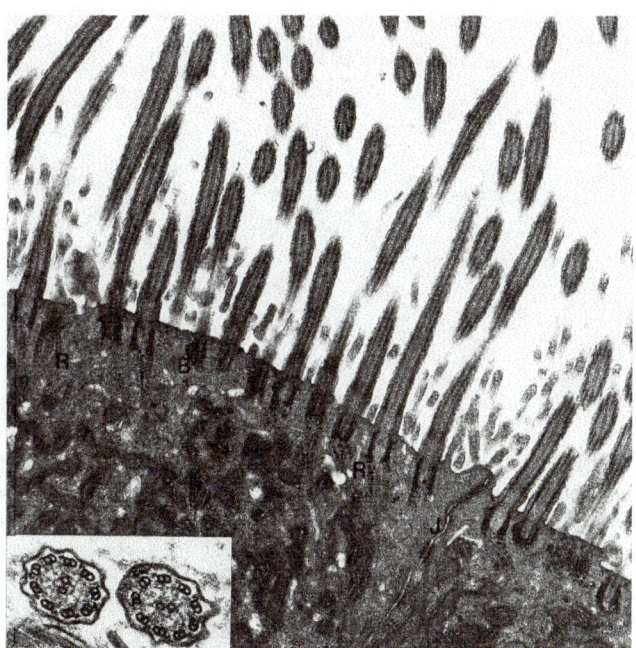

FIGURE 14.45 Transmission electron micrograph of nasal mucosa. Vertical section shows ciliated epithelial cells extending to the surface. The shafts of the slender long cilia have peripheral and central microtubules that appear as darker linear structures extending from the kinetosome (basal body) (*B*). Cross-banded filamentous rootlets (*R*) are associated with kinetosomes. Note junctional complexes (*J*). *Inset.* Cross section of the shaft of two cilia. Note the symmetrically arranged nine peripheral doublets and the central pair of single microtubules. (Original magnification ×25,000; *inset*, original magnification ×87,500.)

sections of the cilia show that the ciliary shaft ends in a basal body (kinetosome), from which it is derived (102). The nasal mucosa is a convenient site to biopsy when ultrastructural abnormalities of cilia are suspected, such as in immotile cilia syndrome (103,104). The function of the ciliated cells in the nose is to constantly move the protective mucous blanket by the coordinated sweeping motion of the cilia toward the pharynx. In order to perform this function, the cilia beat at 10 to 20 cycles/second. They have an effective whip-like stroke forward and a recovery stroke backward. The propulsive forward phase is much faster and more vigorous than the recovery phase (105). Ciliary activity is optimal at the normal nasal temperature of about 30°C. However, cilia are hardy and persist under unfavorable conditions, including under extreme cold and heat. They will also beat normally and forcefully in a pus-filled cavity. When injured or destroyed by an acute infection, they regenerate rapidly. They do not, however, tolerate excessive drying. Accordingly, they are dependent always upon a coating of moisture for their activity and preservation. The blanket of mucus covering the nasal mucosa and paranasal sinuses forms a conveyor of the bacteria and other foreign matter. The nasal mucociliary layer is the first line of defense against bacterial invasion in this location.

Melanocytes are also present in the normal mucosa of the upper airways. In the nasal cavity they can be seen in the respiratory epithelium and nasal glands. Melanocytes are commonly encountered in the lamina propria of the septum and turbinates, particularly in dark-skinned adults (106). This explains why primary malignant melanomas are well-known to arise in the nose and paranasal sinuses (107).

Intraepithelial lymphocytes are diffusely scattered throughout the nasal mucosa. These are uniformly CD8+ T cells (40). These T cells coexist with a population of dendritic cells that lack CD1a expression. The nasal mucosa and subepithelial tissue contain virtually no B cells. This finding may explain why most primary nasal lymphomas are of CD8+ T-cell derivation.

Beneath the mucous membrane is the lamina (or tunica) propria, containing numerous small mucous and serous glands that discharge their secretion through lobular ducts onto the surface (Fig. 14.46). These glands are embedded in vascular fibroconnective tissue, which is rich in elastic fibers and is firmly attached to the perichondrium and periosteum of the cartilages and bones forming the nasal cavity (108–110). Nasal seromucinous hamartoma (microglandular adenosis of the nose) is a rare tumor that may be encountered in the nasal cavity (111). These tumors are characterized by a disordered arrangement of small serous tubules, ducts and glands that lack a myoepithelial layer. They may resemble an inflammatory nasal polyp, respiratory epithelial adenomatoid hamartoma (REAH) or low-grade sinonasal adenocarcinoma.

The turbinates are somewhat curved structures that are supported by an osseous axis enveloped by relatively thick mucosa (Figs. 14.1 and 14.47). Their convex surface protrudes toward the nasal cavity. Located beneath their mucosa is a tunica propria or stroma that attaches the mucosa to the underlying structures. Their tunica propria is of variable thickness, being thickest in the areas more exposed to inhaled and exhaled air (i.e., over the nasal septum and medial aspects of the inferior and middle turbinates). In these areas, the epithelium contains many goblet cells and the basement membrane is prominent (112).

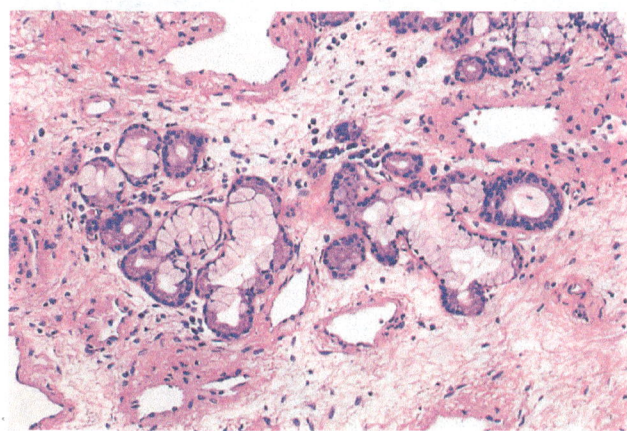

FIGURE 14.46 Nasal seromucinous gland with duct. Serous cells with darker-staining cytoplasm are at the periphery of tubuloacinar glands and form the demilunes of Giannuzzi.

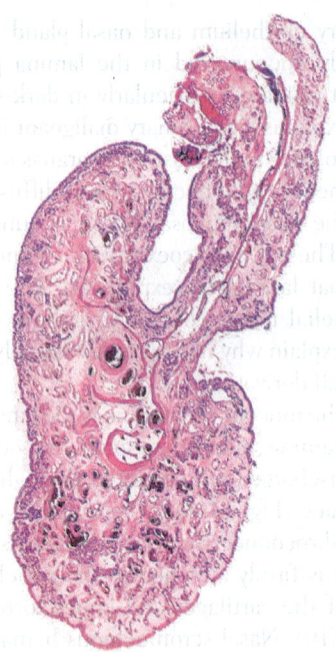

FIGURE 14.47 Middle turbinate, coronal section. Bone in the axis of the turbinate appears as a delicate, curled structure. The covering mucous membrane and tunica propria are rich in blood vessels and mucous glands, particularly on the convexity and inferior border of the turbinate, areas that are most exposed to the airstream in the nasal cavity. (Low-power view.)

These areas also have abundant blood vessels and clusters of mixed seromucinous glands (6 to 10 glands/mm^2) (Fig. 14.48). The glands vary from simple straight tubules lined with goblet cells to tubuloalveolar glands. The chief ducts of the latter open onto the mucosal surface by minute orifices. The glands tend to be at a level between the mucosa and the underlying bone.

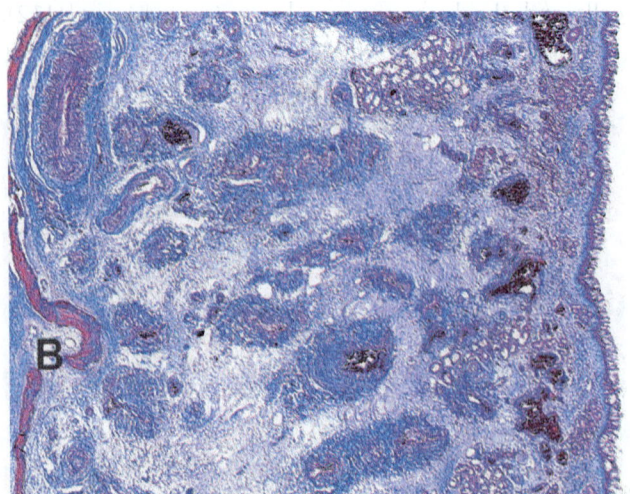

FIGURE 14.48 Turbinate, coronal section. Mucosal blood vessels are surrounded by a thick sheath of connective tissue (*blue*); note the large artery near the bone (*B*) (Mallory trichrome).

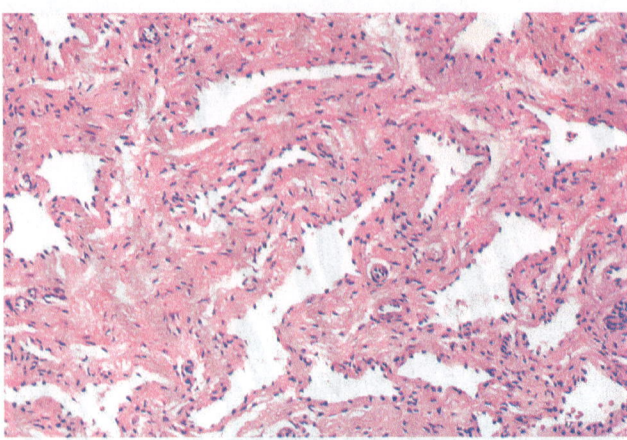

FIGURE 14.49 Inferior turbinate. Numerous larger blood vessels of variable size and shape are closely packed and form a sponge-like vascular system resembling erectile tissue. The endothelial cells are evenly distributed. Capillaries are lacking.

The turbinates and the lower part of the septum are rich in venous sinuses, which are of variable size and shape, forming a dense network of large veins that resemble erectile tissue (Fig. 14.49). These blood vessels are of irregular shape, have muscular walls, and can rapidly dilate and constrict, thereby permitting fast adjustments of mucosal temperature and secretion to climatic changes. It is important for the surgical pathologist to know about the normal rich vascular anatomy of the turbinates in order to avoid mistaking them for a hemangioma, angiofibroma, or angioleiomyoma. The stroma of the nasal mucosa also contains lymphatics, small nerves, and a sprinkling of lymphocytes and plasma cells but no lymphoid aggregates. A few mast cells and eosinophils are normally also present.

The osseous portion of the turbinates consists of thin, interconnecting laminae of lamellar bone, forming a continuous shell that is interconnected with bone trabeculae. The interosseous spaces contain numerous large veins, arteries, and some nerves. In contrast to the submucosal veins, the intraosseous veins have a rather large round or oval lumen on cross section and have proportionately thin walls. Occasional adipocytes, but no hematopoietic marrow, are seen in turbinated bone. The presence of prominent hematopoiesis in the facial and nasal bones or the paranasal sinuses is abnormal and may be observed in conditions such as thalassemia major.

The nasal septum consists of a large cartilaginous plate and four small osseous plates, all of which firmly unite with sutures (Fig. 14.50). The nasal mucosa is closely apposed to the underlying structures of the nasal septum. The periosteum and perichondrium of the nasal septum attach so closely to the overlying submucosa as to constitute one membrane, called the mucoperiosteum. A common site of nosebleed is Little's area (or Kiesselbach area) on the anterior part of the cartilaginous nasal septum above the intermaxillary line (113). The submucosa of this area is richly supplied with thin-walled dilated blood vessels (Fig. 14.51).

CHAPTER 14: Mouth, Nose, and Paranasal Sinuses

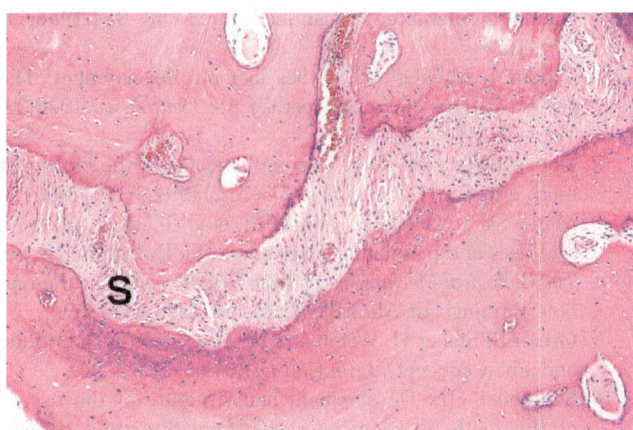

FIGURE 14.50 Suture (*S*) in the nasal septum. Parallel edges of the vomer (*top*) and maxilla are connected by parallel, densely arranged collagen fibers that are anchored in the bones.

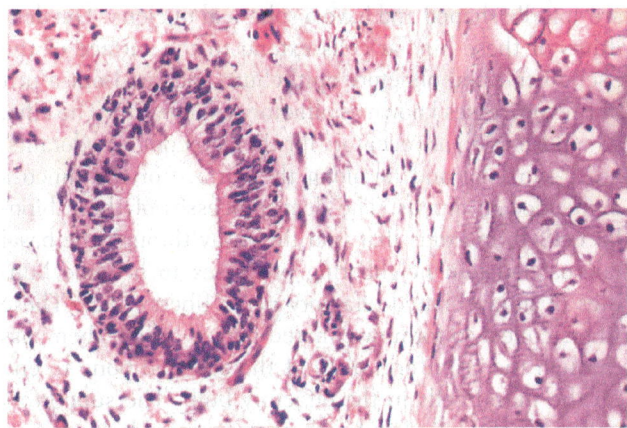

FIGURE 14.52 Vomeronasal organ of Jacobson in a 22-week-old embryo (180-mm crown-rump length), including a cross section of the tubular structure adjacent to vomeronasal cartilage. In humans the columnar epithelium has microvilli but no sensory epithelium.

Although rarely seen in surgical specimens, Little's area should not be mistaken for a pyogenic granuloma, which frequently occurs in this location.

Vomeronasal Organ of Jacobson

The vestigial remains of a paired embryonic structure, the vomeronasal organ of Jacobson, are situated under the mucosa of the lower anterior side of the nasal septum covering an area of 0.2 to 0.6 cm. In adults, it consists of a small tubular sac lined by columnar epithelium with microvilli, but it has no sensory cells with cilia and lacks other well-differentiated olfactory structures (Fig. 14.52). The duct-like organ is surrounded by numerous exocrine glands (114). The organ is best developed in the 20th week of embryonic life, after which regressive changes occur and it becomes rudimentary. In humans it has no known function and is of no pathologic significance (115). In many vertebrates, Jacobson organ is highly developed, particularly in animals of keen olfactory sensibility (116–118).

Olfactory Mucosa

The roof of the nasal cavity and contiguous portions of the nasal septum and superior turbinate form the olfactory region (119). Here, the ciliated columnar epithelium of the nasal mucosa is modified by liberally scattered cells of the sensory organ of smell. The nasal anatomy in detailed relation to olfactory function is dealt with by Hummel and Welge-Lüssen in their update on *Taste and Smell* (120) The olfactory epithelium consists of three types of cells: (a) olfactory nerve cells; (b) supporting, or sustentacular, cells; and (c) basal cells that lie on the basal lamina (121,122) (Fig. 14.53). The olfactory nerve cells

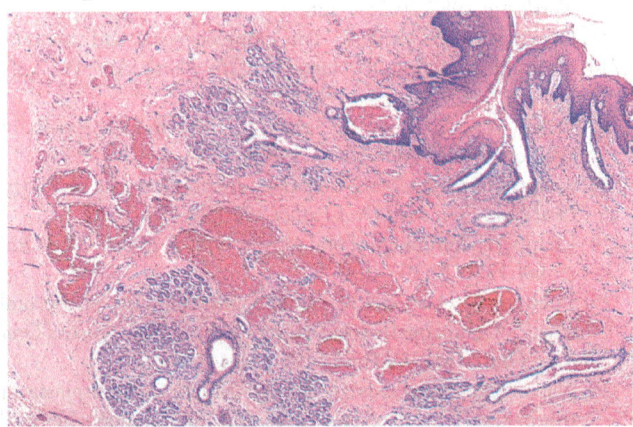

FIGURE 14.51 Little's area. Teleangiectatic, thin-walled blood vessels are clustered under the epithelium in the anterior portion of the nasal septum. This area is above the level of mucous glands.

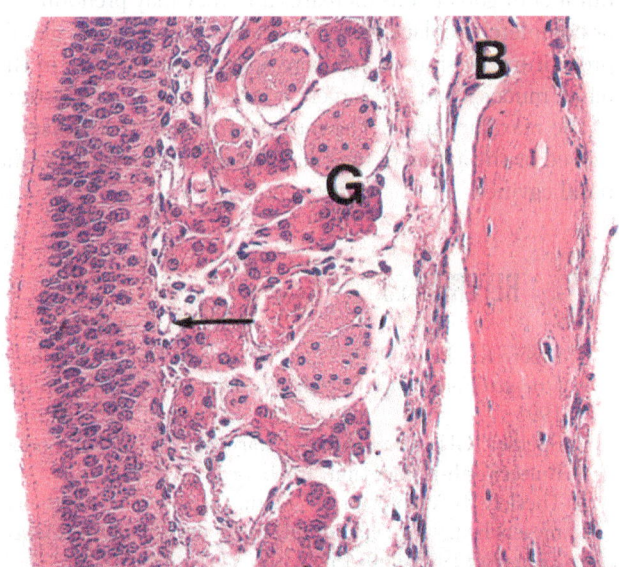

FIGURE 14.53 Olfactory mucosa. The population of olfactory nerve cells and supporting cells forms a pseudostratified columnar epithelium with distinct microvilli. Basal cells lie on basal lamina (*arrow*). Bowman glands (*G*) with excretory ducts and nerves are between the epithelium and bone of nasal septum (*B*).

are spindle shaped and have a spherical nucleus. The dendrites of these bipolar cells extend to the surface of the pseudostratified olfactory epithelium and send out a tuft of fine processes known as olfactory cilia (hairs). The cilia, which function as receptors for the detection of odorants, are 2-μm long and lie along the surface of the mucosa embedded in mucus. The deep processes of these bipolar cells form axons that find their way through the basal lamina and join neighboring processes to become bundles of unmyelinated olfactory nerve fibers (122). These fibers collect to form myelinated nerves, which then pass through the cribriform plate of the ethmoid bone to end on the mitral cells in the olfactory bulb. The supporting cells are tall, cylindrical cells that in the elderly contain lipofuscin, giving the yellow hue characteristic of the olfactory mucous membrane. The free surface of these cells possesses many slender microvilli that protrude into the covering mucus. The basal cells are small and conical, lying with their base on the basement membrane. They are believed to represent stem cells that can give rise to new supporting and sensory cells. Under the mucosa is the lamina propria, composed of loose connective tissue in which are found the olfactory glands of Bowman (123). The secretion of these tubuloalveolar glands is carried to the surface of the mucosa by narrow ducts.

Paranasal Sinuses

The sinuses are lined with a mucous membrane that is continuous with the nasal mucosa. The mucosa is, therefore, similar to that of the nasal cavity. However, the epithelium (schneiderian epithelium) and lamina propria are thinner and less vascular. In case of prolonged irritation of the mucosa, for example, in chronic allergic sinusitis, the number of goblet cells increases and they may predominate or completely replace the ciliated cells. Seromucous glands present in the sinuses are more sparse compared to in the nasal mucosa and are largely concentrated at the ostium of the maxillary sinus. The mucus formed in the sinuses is moved by the action of the cilia through the apertures to the nasal cavities.

REFERENCES

1. Moore KL, Persaud TVN. *The Developing Human: Clinically Oriented Embryology*. 5th ed. Philadelphia, PA: WB Saunders; 1993.
2. Sperber GH. *Craniofacial Embryology*. 4th ed. London: Butterworth-Heinemann; 1989.
3. Thesleff I, Vaahtokari A, Kettunen P, et al. Epithelial-mesenchymal signaling during tooth development. *Connect Tissue Res* 1995;32:9–15.
4. Honda MJ, Imaizumi M, Tsuchiya S, et al. Dental follicle stem cells and tissue engineering. *J Oral Sci* 2010;52:541–552.
5. Listgarten MA. Phase-contrast and electron microscopic study of the junction between reduced enamel epithelium and enamel in unerupted human teeth. *Arch Oral Biol* 1966;11:999–1016.
6. Schour I, Massler M. Studies in tooth development: The growth pattern of human teeth. *J Am Dent Assoc* 1940;27:1918–1931.
7. Gorski JP, Marks SC Jr. Current concepts of the biology of tooth eruption. *Crit Rev Oral Biol Med* 1992;3:185–206.
8. Marks SC Jr, Gorski JP, Cahill DR, et al. Tooth eruption—a synthesis of experimental observations. In: Davidovitch Z, ed. *The Biological Mechanisms of Tooth Eruption and Root Resorption*. Birmingham, AL: EBSCO Media; 1988:161–169.
9. Orban B, Sicher H, Weinmann JP. Amelogenesis (a critique and a new concept). *J Am Coll Dent* 1943;10:13–22.
10. Schroeder HE. Development and structure of the tissues of the tooth. In: Schroeder HE. *Oral Structural Biology*. New York: Thieme Medical; 1986:4–184.
11. Bhaskar SN, Orban BJ, eds. *Orban's Oral Histology and Embryology*. 11th ed. St. Louis, MO: CV Mosby Year Book; 1990.
12. Held AJ. Cementogenesis and the normal and pathologic structure of cementum. *Oral Surg Oral Med Oral Pathol* 1951;4:53–67.
13. Smukler H, Dreyer CJ. Principal fibres of the periodontium. *J Periodont Res* 1969;4:19–25.
14. Logan WHG, Kronfeld R. Development of the human jaws and surrounding structures from birth to the age of fifteen years. *J Am Dent Assoc* 1933;20:379–427.
15. Schroeder H. *Oral Structure Biology: Embryology, Structure and Function of Normal Hard and Soft Tissues of the Oral Cavity and the Temporomandibular Joints*. New York: Thieme; 1991.
16. Vaid S, Vaid N. Normal anatomy and anatomic variants of the paranasal sinuses on computed tomography. *Neuroimaging Clin N Am* 2015;25:527–548.
17. Gorlin RJ. Heterotopic lymphoid tissue: A diagnostic problem. *Oral Surg Oral Med Oral Pathol* 1957;10:87–89.
18. Sadeghi EM, Ashrafi MH. Heterotopic lymph node of the buccal mucosa simulating a tumor: A clinicopathological appraisal. *ASDC J Dent Child* 1982;49:304–306.
19. Tobias MJ. *Anatomy of the Human Lymphatic System*. Ann Arbor, MI: Edwards Brothers, Inc.; 1938.
20. Richtsmeier WJ, Shikhani AH. The physiology and immunology of the pharyngeal lymphoid tissue. *Otolaryngol Clin North Am* 1987;20:219–228.
21. Goeringer GC, Vidic B. The embryogenesis and anatomy of Waldeyer's ring. *Otolaryngol Clin North Am* 1987;20:207–217.
22. Dolen WK, Spofford B, Selner JC. The hidden tonsils of Waldeyer's ring. *Ann Allergy* 1990;65:244–248.
23. Knapp MJ. Oral tonsils: Location, distribution, and histology. *Oral Surg Oral Med Oral Pathol* 1970;29:155–161.
24. Knapp MJ. Pathology of oral tonsils. *Oral Surg Oral Med Oral Pathol* 1970;29:295–304.
25. Buchner A, Hansen LS. Lymphoepithelial cysts of the oral cavity. A clinicopathologic study of thirty-eight cases. *Oral Surg Oral Med Oral Pathol* 1980;50:441–449.
26. Napier SS, Newlands C. Benign lymphoid hyperplasia of the palate: Report of two cases and immunohistochemical profile. *J Oral Pathol Med* 1990;19:221–225.
27. Simpson HE. Lymphoid hyperplasia in foliate papillitis. *J Oral Surg Anesth Hosp Dent Serv* 1964;22:209–214.

28. Miles AEW. Sebaceous glands in the lip and cheek mucosa of man. *Br Dent J* 1958;105:235–248.
29. Sewerin I. The sebaceous glands in the vermilion border of the lips and in the oral mucosa of man. *Acta Odontol Scand* 1975;33(Suppl 68):13–226.
30. Meyer J, Squier CA, Gerson SJ, eds. *The Structure and Function of the Oral Mucosa*. New York: Pergamon Press; 1984.
31. Wu T, Xiong X, Zhang W, et al. Morphogenesis of rete ridges in human oral mucosa: A pioneering morphological and immunohistochemical study. *Cells Tissues Organs* 2013;197: 239–248.
32. Skougaard MR. Cell renewal, with special reference to the gingival epithelium. *Adv Oral Biol* 1970;4:261–288.
33. Squier CA, Finkelstein MW. Oral mucosa. In: Ten Cate AR, ed. *Oral Histology, Development, Structure and Function*. St. Louis, MO: CV Mosby; 1989:341–382.
34. Mackenzie IC, Rittman G, Gao Z, et al. Patterns of cytokeratin expression in human gingival epithelia. *J Periodontal Res* 1991;26:468–478.
35. Sawaf MH, Ouhayoun JP, Forest N. Cytokeratin profiles in oral epithelial: A review and a new classification. *J Biol Buccale* 1991;19:187–198.
36. Ouhayoun JP, Gosselin F, Forest N, et al. Cytokeratin patterns of human oral epithelia: Differences in cytokeratin synthesis in gingival epithelium and the adjacent alveolar mucosa. *Differentiation* 1985;30:123–129.
37. Mandel U. Carbohydrates in oral epithelia and secretions: Variation with cellular differentiation. *APMIS Suppl* 1992;27:119–129.
38. Shah F, Berggren D, Holmlund T, et al. Unique expression of cytoskeletal proteins in human soft palate muscles. *J Anat* 2016;228:487–494.
39. Olofsson K, Mattsson C, Hammarstrom ML, et al. Structure of the human uvula. *Acta Otolaryngol* 1999;119:712–717.
40. Graeme-Cook F, Bhan AK, Harris NL. Immunohistochemical characterization of intraepithelial and subepithelial mononuclear cells of the upper airways. *Am J Pathol* 1993; 143:1416–1422.
41. Winther B, Innes DJ. The human adenoid. A morphologic study. *Arch Otolaryngol Head Neck Surg* 1994;120:144–149.
42. Bhargava D, Raman R, Khalfan Al Abri R, et al. Heterotopia of the tonsil. *J Laryngol Otol* 1996;110:611–612.
43. Eversole LR. The histochemistry of mucosubstances in human minor salivary glands. *Arch Oral Biol* 1972;17: 1225–1239.
44. Munger BL. Histochemical studies on seromucous- and mucous-secreting cells of human salivary glands. *Am J Anat* 1964;115:411–429.
45. Laine M, Bläuer M, Ylikomi T, et al. Immunohistochemical demonstration of androgen receptors in human salivary glands. *Arch Oral Biol* 1993;38:299–302.
46. Kumagami H, Onitsuka T. Estradiol and testosterone in minor salivary glands of Sjögren's syndrome. *Auris Nasus Larynx* 1993;20:137–143.
47. Herrera-Esparza R, Bollain-y-Goytia J, Ruvalcaba C, et al. Apoptosis and cell proliferation: The paradox of salivary glands in Sjögren's disease. *Acta Reumatol Port* 2008;33: 299–303.
48. Tandler B, Denning CR, Mandel ID, et al. Ultrastructure of human labial salivary glands. 3. Myoepithelium and ducts. *J Morphol* 1970;130:227–245.
49. Ogawa Y. Immunocytochemistry of myoepithelial cells in the salivary glands. *Prog Histochem Cytochem* 2003;38: 343–426.
50. Grandi D, Campanini N, Becchi G, et al. On the myoepithelium of human salivary glands. An immunocytochemical study. *Eur J Morphol* 2000;38:249–255.
51. Ianez RF, Buim ME, Coutinho-Camillo CM, et al. Human salivary gland morphogenesis: Myoepithelial cell maturation assessed by immunohistochemical markers. *Histopathology* 2010;57:410–417.
52. Takeda Y. Existence and distribution of melanocytes and HMB-45-positive cells in the human minor salivary glands. *Pathol Int* 2000;50:15–19.
53. Nonaka CF, Pereira KM, de Andrade Santos PP, et al. Sialolipoma of minor salivary glands. *Ann Diagn Pathol* 2011; 15:6–11.
54. Hamperl H. Über das Vorkommen von Onkocyten in verschiedenen Organen und ihren Geschwülsten: (Mundspeicheldrüsen, Bauchspeicheldrüse, Epithelkörperchen, Hypophyse, Schilddrüse, Eileiter). *Virchows Arch A* 1936;298:327–375.
55. Chang A, Harawi SJ. Oncocytes, oncocytosis and oncocytic tumors. *Pathol Annu* 1992;27:263–304.
56. Balogh K Jr, Roth SI. Histochemical and electron microscopic studies of eosinophilic granular cells (oncocytes) in tumors of the parotid gland. *Lab Invest* 1965;14:310–320.
57. Goode RK, Corio RL. Oncocytic adenocarcinoma of salivary glands. *Oral Surg Oral Med Oral Pathol* 1988;65:61–66.
58. Tschen JA, Fechner RE. The juxtaoral organ of Chievitz. *Am J Surg Pathol* 1979;3:147–150.
59. Pantanowitz L, Tschen JA. Organ of Chievitz. *Ear Nose Throat J* 2004;83:230.
60. Zenker W. *Juxtaoral Organ (Chievitz' Organ). Morphology and Clinical Aspects*. Baltimore, MD: Urban & Schwarzenberg; 1982.
61. Ide F, Mishima K, Saito I. Melanin pigmentation in the juxtaoral organ of Chievitz. *Pathol Int* 2003;53:262–263.
62. Pantanowitz L, Tschen JA, Balogh K. The juxtaoral organ of Chievitz. *Int J Surg Pathol* 2003;11:37.
63. Pantanowitz L. Immunophenotype of the juxtaoral organ. *Int J Oral Maxillofac Surg* 2004;33:113.
64. Lutman GB. Epithelial nests in intraoral sensory nerve endings simulating perineural invasion in patients with oral carcinoma. *Am J Clin Pathol* 1974;61:275–284.
65. Mikó T, Molnár P. The juxtaoral organ—a pitfall for pathologists. *J Pathol* 1981;133:17–23.
66. Soucy P, Cimone G, Carpenter B. An unusual intraoral mass in a child: The organ of Chievitz. *J Pediatr Surg* 1990;25:1200.
67. Leibl W, Pflüger H, Kerjaschki D. A case of nodular hyperplasia of the juxtaoral organ in man. *Virchows Arch A Pathol Anat Histol* 1976;371:389–391.
68. Chievitz JH. Beiträge zur Entwicklungsgeschichte der Speicheldrüsen. *Arch Anat Physiol* 1885;9:401–436.
69. Pantanowitz L, Balogh K. Significance of the juxtaoral organ (of Chievitz). *Head Neck* 2003;25:400–405.
70. Ide F, Mishima K, Saito I. Pacinian corpuscle in the juxtaoral organ of Chievitz. *J Oral Pathol Med* 2004;33:443–444.
71. Eversole LR, Leider AS. Maxillary intraosseous neuroepithelial structures resembling those seen in the organ of Chievitz. *Oral Surg Oral Med Oral Pathol* 1978;46:555–558.
72. Jensen JL, Wuerker RB, Correll RW, et al. Epithelial islands associated with mandibular nerves. Report of two cases in the

walls of mandibular cysts. *Oral Surg Oral Med Oral Pathol* 1979; 48:226–230.
73. Kruger L, Mantyh PW. Gustatory and related chemosensory systems. In: Björklund A, Hökfelt T, Swanson LW, eds. *Handbook of Chemical Neuroanatomy. Vol. 7. Integrated Systems of the CNS Part II*. New York: Elsevier; 1989:323–411.
74. Oakley B. Neuronal–epithelial interactions in mammalian gustatory epithelium. In: Bock GR, ed. *Regeneration of Vertebrate Sensory Receptor Cells*. Chichester: Wiley; 1991:277–287.
75. McDaniel RK. Subepithelial nerve plexus (with ganglion cells) associated with taste buds. *Oral Surg Oral Med Oral Pathol Oral Radiol Endod* 1999;87:605–609.
76. Triantafyllou A, Coulter P. Structural organization of subgemmal neurogenous plaques in foliate papillae of tongue. *Hum Pathol* 2004;35:991–999.
77. Palazzolo MJ, Fowler CB, Magliocca KR, et al. Neuroepithelial structures associated with the subepithelial nerve plexus of taste buds: A fortuitous finding resembling the juxtaoral organ of Chievitz. *Oral Surg Oral Med Oral Pathol Oral Radiol* 2014;117:497–501.
78. Pellicioli AC, Fonseca FP, Silva RN, et al. Histomorphometric characterization of subgemmal neurogenous plaques. *Oral Surg Oral Med Oral Pathol Oral Radiol* 2017;123:477–481.
79. Ainamo J, Loe H. Anatomical characteristics of gingiva. A clinical and microscopic study of the free and attached gingiva. *J Periodontol* 1966;37:5–13.
80. Melcher AH, Bowen WH, eds. *Biology of the Periodontium*. New York: Academic Press; 1969.
81. Squier CA, Waterhouse JP. The ultrastructure of the melanocyte in human gingival epithelium. *Arch Oral Biol* 1967;12: 119–129.
82. Schroeder HE. Melanin containing organelles in cells of the human gingiva. *J Periodont Res* 1969;4:1–18.
83. Kaugars GE, Heise AP, Riley WT, et al. Oral melanotic macules. A review of 353 cases. *Oral Surg Oral Med Oral Pathol* 1993;76:59–61.
84. Buchner A, Merrell PW, Hansen LS, et al. Melanocytic hyperplasia of the oral mucosa. *Oral Surg Oral Med Oral Pathol* 1991;71:58–62.
85. Buchner A, Ledier AS, Merrell PW, et al. Melanocytic nevi of oral mucosa: A clinicopathologic study of 130 cases from northern California. *J Oral Pathol Med* 1990;19:197–201.
86. Buchner A, Hansen LS. Pigmented nevi of the oral mucosa: A clinicopathologic study of 36 new cases and review of 155 cases from the literature. Part I: a clinicopathologic study of 36 new cases. *Oral Surg Oral Med Oral Pathol* 1987;63: 566–572.
87. Buchner A, Hansen LS. Pigmented nevi of the oral mucosa: A clinicopathologic study of 36 new cases and review of 155 cases from the literature. Part II: analysis of 191 cases. *Oral Surg Oral Med Oral Pathol* 1987;63:676–682.
88. Trodahl JN, Sprague WG. Benign and malignant melanocytic lesions of the oral mucosa. An analysis of 135 cases. *Cancer* 1970;25:812–823.
89. Hashimoto K. Fine structure of Merkel cell in human oral mucosa. *J Invest Dermatol* 1972;58:381–387.
90. Mahomed F. Neuroendocrine cells and associated malignancies of the oral mucosa: A review. *J Oral Pathol Med* 2010;39: 121–127.
91. Waterhouse JP, Squier CA. The Langerhans cell in human gingival epithelium. *Arch Oral Biol* 1967;12:341–348.
92. Chou JM, Daniels TE. Langerhans cells expressing HLA-DQ, HLA-DR and T6 antigens in normal oral mucosa and lichen planus. *J Oral Pathol Med* 1989;18:573–576.
93. Barrett AW, Cruchley AT, Williams DM. Oral mucosal Langerhans' cells. *Crit Rev Oral Biol Med* 1996;7:36–58.
94. Kindt N, Descamps G, Seminerio I, et al. Langerhans cell number is a strong and independent prognostic factor for head and neck squamous cell carcinomas. *Oral Oncol* 2016;62:1–10.
95. Baume LJ. The biology of pulp and dentine. A historic terminologic-taxonomic, histologic-biochemical, embryonic and clinical survey. *Monogr Oral Sci* 1980;8:1–220.
96. Holland GR. The odontoblast process: Form and function. *J Dent Res* 1985;64:499–514.
97. Thomas HF. The dentin-predentin complex and its permeability: Anatomical review. *J Dent Res* 1985;64:607–612.
98. Nylen UM, Termine JD. Tooth enamel III. Its development, structure, and composition. *J Dent Res* 1979;58:675–1031.
99. Ida-Yonemochi H, Ikarashi T, Nagata M, et al. The basement membrane-type heparan sulfate proteoglycan (perlecan) in ameloblastomas: Its intercellular localization in stellate reticulum-like foci and biosynthesis by tumor cells in culture. *Virchows Arch* 2002;441:165–173.
100. Domingues MG, Jaeger MM, Araujo VC, et al. Expression of cytokeratins in human enamel organ. *Eur J Oral Sci* 2000;108: 43–47.
101. Joiner AM, Green WW, McIntyre JC, et al. Primary cilia on horizontal basal cells regulate regeneration of the olfactory epithelium. *J Neurosci* 2015;35:13761–13772.
102. Fawcett DW, Porter KR. A study of the fine structure of ciliated epithelium. *J Morphol* 1954;94:221–281.
103. Afzelius BA. The immotile-cilia syndrome and other ciliary diseases. *Int Rev Exp Pathol* 1979;19:1–43.
104. Howell JT, Schochet SS Jr, Goldman AS. Ultrastructural defects of respiratory tract cilia associated with chronic infections. *Arch Pathol Lab Med* 1980;104:52–55.
105. Sleigh MA, Blake JR, Liron N. The propulsion of mucus by cilia. *Am Rev Respir Dis* 1988;137:726–741.
106. Zak FG, Lawson W. The presence of melanocytes in the nasal cavity. *Ann Otol Rhinol Laryngol* 1974;83:515–519.
107. Cove H. Melanosis, melanocytic hyperplasia, and primary malignant melanoma of the nasal cavity. *Cancer* 1979;44:1424–1433.
108. Rhys-Evans PH. Anatomy of the nose and paranasal sinuses. In: Kerr AG, Groves J, Scott-Brown WG, eds. *Scott-Brown's Otolaryngology*. 5th ed. Vol I. London: Butterworth; 1987: 138–161.
109. Drake-Lee AB. Physiology of the nose and paranasal sinus. In: Kerr AG, Groves J, Scott-Brown WG, eds. *Scott-Brown's Otolaryngology*. 5th ed. Vol I. London: Butterworth; 1987:162–182.
110. Ballenger JJ. The clinical anatomy and physiology of the nose and accessory sinuses. In: Ballenger JJ, ed. *Diseases of the Nose, Throat, Ear, Head and Neck*. 14th ed. Malvern, PA: Lea & Febiger; 1991:3–22.
111. Ambrosini-Spaltro A, Morandi L, Spagnolo DV, et al. Nasal seromucinous hamartoma (microglandular adenosis of the nose): A morphological and molecular study of five cases. *Virchows Arch* 2010;457:727–734.
112. Trotter CM, Hall GH, Salter DM, et al. Histology of the mucous membrane of the human inferior nasal concha. *Clin Anat* 1990;3:307–316.
113. MacArthur FJ, McGarry GW. The arterial supply of the nasal cavity. *Eur Arch Otorhinolaryngol* 2017;274:809–815.

114. Jahnke V, Merker HJ. Electron microscopic and functional aspects of the human vomeronasal organ. *Am J Rhinol* 2000; 14:63–67.
115. Zuckerkandl E. Das Jacobsonsche organ. *Erg Anat Entwicklungsgesch* 1910;18:801–843.
116. Pearlman SJ. Jacobson's organ (Organon vomeronasale Jacobsoni): Its anatomy, gross, microscopic and comparative, with some observations as well on its function. *Ann Otol Rhinol Laryngol* 1934;43:739–768.
117. Negus VE. The organ of Jacobson. *J Anat* 1956;90:515–519.
118. Seifert K. Licht- und elektronenmikroskopische Untersuchungen am Jacobsonschen Organ (Organon vomeronasale) der Katze. *Arch Klin Exp Ohr Nas Kehlk Heilk* 1971;200: 223–251.
119. Naessen R. The identification and topographical localization of the olfactory epithelium in man and other mammals. *Acta Otolaryngol* 1970;70:51–57.
120. Hummel T, Welge-Lüssen A. *Taste and Smell. An update*. Basel, Switzerland: Karger; 2006.
121. Schneider RA. The sense of smell in man–its physiologic basis. *N Engl J Med* 1967;277:299–303.
122. Palay SL. The general architecture of sensory neuroepithelia. In: Bock GR, ed. *Regeneration of Vertebrate Sensory Receptor Cells*. Chichester: Wiley; 1991:3–24.
123. Seifert K. Licht- und elektronenmikroskopische Untersuchungen der Bowman-Drüsen in der Riechschleimhaut makrosmatischer Säuger. *Arch Klin Exp Ohren Nasen Kehlkopfheilkd* 1971;200:252–274.

15

Larynx and Pharynx

Stacey E. Mills

LARYNX 424
    Definition and Boundaries 424
    Embryology 424
    Gross and Functional Anatomy 424
    Microscopic Anatomy 426
    Neural, Vascular, and Lymphatic Components 432

PHARYNX 433
    Definition and Boundaries 433
    Embryology 434
    Gross Anatomy 434
    Microscopic Anatomy 435
    Neural, Vascular, and Lymphatic Components 437

REFERENCES 438

LARYNX

Definition and Boundaries

The larynx is a complex organ with numerous connective tissue elements and a variety of epithelia. The superior border of the larynx is the tip of the epiglottis and the aryepiglottic folds. The inferior limit is the inferior rim of the cricoid cartilage. The anterior boundary is composed of the lingual surface of the epiglottis, the thyroid cartilage, the anterior arch of the cricoid cartilage, the thyrohyoid membrane, and the cricothyroid membrane. The posterior boundary is the cricoid cartilage and the arytenoid region. The piriform fossa is frequently, and erroneously, considered to be a part of the larynx. In reality, it is a pouch of the hypopharynx that passes on each side of the larynx. It is, thus, a conduit for food and water, not air.

Although not part of the larynx per se, the pre-epiglottic space is an important area for the spread of carcinoma. This more or less triangular space is filled with fat and loose connective tissue. It is bounded posteriorly by the epiglottis, anteriorly by the thyroid cartilage and thyrohyoid membrane, and superiorly by the hyoepiglottic ligament.

Embryology

The supraglottic portion of the larynx is derived from the third and fourth branchial arches and is, therefore, related to the development of the oral cavity and oropharynx. The glottis and subglottis arise from the sixth branchial arch, which also give rise to the trachea and lungs. Bocca et al. have demonstrated that the larynx virtually consists of two hemilarynges (superior and inferior), each of them with their own different derivations and their own largely independent lymphatic circulations (1). These authors also discuss the importance of this embryologic derivation with respect to the origin and spread of laryngeal carcinoma. Each of these hemilarynges may become invaded by cancer independent of one another. The extension of cancer is often limited within the boundaries of this embryologic demarcation (1).

The first embryologic appearance of the respiratory apparatus occurs at approximately 21 days in the 3-mm embryo. At this time, an evagination, or groove, forms adjacent to the superior portion of the foregut, above the fourth branchial arch. The inferior portion of this evagination is the pulmonary anlage. The first portion of the larynx to develop is the epiglottis, but this does not appear as a definitively formed structure until approximately the 5th week of intrauterine development.

The outline of the larynx is recognizable in the 6-mm embryo. At this time, the respiratory groove described previously begins to close; this closure is completed with the formation of the arytenoid cartilages. By 60 to 70 days, at the stage of the 30-mm embryo, the vocal cords begin to differentiate. The embryonic development of the larynx is complex, and it is not surprising that at least 30 different congenital malformations have been described (2).

Gross and Functional Anatomy

The larynx is composed of an elastic cone, cartilages, intrinsic and extrinsic muscles, submucosa, and an overlying mucous

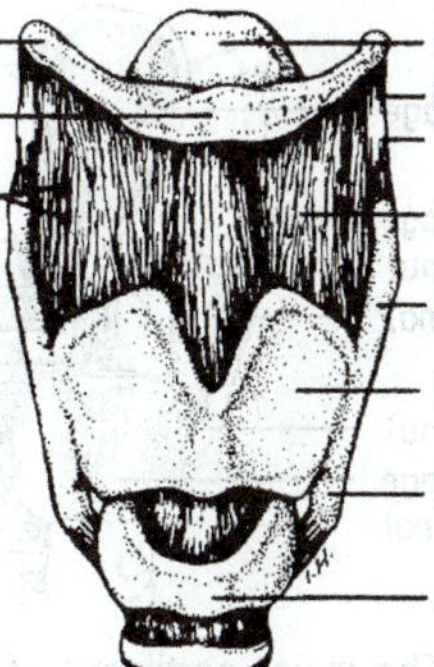

FIGURE 15.1 Anterior view of an unopened larynx shows the lamina of the thyroid cartilage, the arch of the cricoid cartilage, and the hyothyroid membrane as the major structures that define the anterior external surface of the larynx. (Reprinted with permission from Mills SE, Fechner RE. *Pathology of the Larynx. Atlas of Head and Neck Pathology Series*. Chicago, IL: American Society of Clinical Pathologists Press; 1985.)

membrane (Figs. 15.1 to 15.3). The elastic cone provides most of the structural strength to support the true vocal cords. The elastic tissue is thickened just under the mucosa of the free edge of the cord. This portion of the elastic cone is referred to as the vocal ligament. It is visible grossly as a white band beneath the mucous membrane (Fig. 15.3). The vocal ligament inserts on the thyroid cartilage anteriorly and the vocal process of the arytenoid cartilage posteriorly (Fig. 15.4).

The major cartilages of the larynx are the cricoid, the thyroid, and the paired arytenoid cartilage (Fig. 15.5). These major structural cartilages are all of hyalin type. The epiglottis, in contrast, is composed of elastic cartilage containing numerous fenestrations. Calcification of the thyroid and cricoid cartilages begins during the second decade of life in males and somewhat later in females. In older individuals, the thyroid cartilage is frequently ossified, replete with fibrofatty and hematopoietic bone marrow elements. The ossification of the thyroid cartilage is important in regard to the spread of laryngeal carcinoma. This cartilage is involved by continuous or metastatic carcinoma only when ossified. Hyalin cartilage, perhaps because of its elaboration of angiogenesis inhibiting factors, is remarkably resistant to the spread of neoplasia.

The cricoid and thyroid cartilages articulate with one another, but their motion is limited by several dense ligaments that anchor the cartilages together. The arytenoid cartilages articulate with the cricoid cartilage. Both the cricothyroid and cricoarytenoid joints are diarthrodial and lined by flattened synovial cells. These tiny joints are susceptible to conditions such as gout and rheumatoid arthritis, that more commonly affect larger synovial-lined spaces.

Each arytenoid cartilage has a protrusion, the vocal process, which is the posterior point of insertion of the vocal ligament, and the thyroarytenoid muscle. The position of the arytenoid cartilage determines the tension of the vocal ligament. During adduction of the cords, the arytenoid cartilages move medially along the facets of the cricoid cartilage; they also pivot or rock (Fig. 15.4). The rocking motion causes the vocal processes to move downward and toward the midline to complete the adduction of the vocal cords.

The muscles of the larynx can be divided into two groups. The extrinsic muscles originate from neighboring structures outside the larynx and insert on the thyroid, cricoid, or hyoid cartilages. These muscles include the omohyoid, sternohyoid, sternothyroid, and thyrohyoid muscles; they act as a whole upon the larynx during swallowing.

The principle intrinsic muscles of the larynx are the cricothyroid, posterior cricoarytenoid, lateral cricoarytenoid, and thyroarytenoid. There are also small strands of muscle that are in continuity with the thyroarytenoid muscle and insert along the length of the vocal ligaments. This is frequently referred to as the vocalis muscle. It should be remembered that the vocalis muscle is actually a component of the thyroarytenoid muscle, and some authors use these names interchangeably.

The lateral cricoarytenoid muscle adducts the vocal cord, and the posterior cricoarytenoid muscle abducts the cord. During phonation, the thyroarytenoid muscle slightly moves the thyroid cartilage. The degree of contraction of

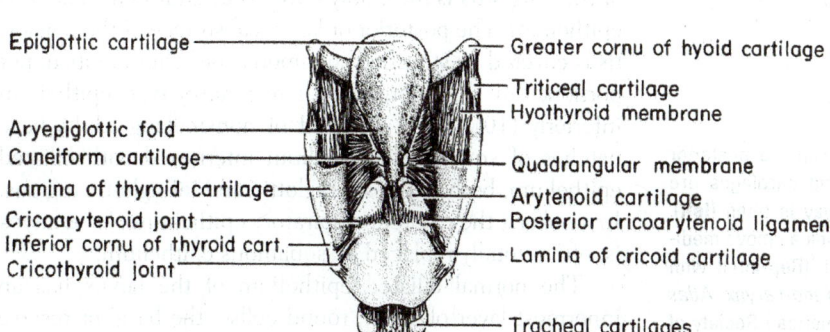

FIGURE 15.2 Posterior view of an unopened larynx emphasizes the position of the arytenoid cartilages. Major support and posterior definition of the larynx are provided by the lamina of the cricoid cartilage. (Reprinted with permission from Mills SE, Fechner RE. *Pathology of the Larynx. Atlas of Head and Neck Pathology Series*. Chicago, IL: American Society of Clinical Pathologists Press; 1985.)

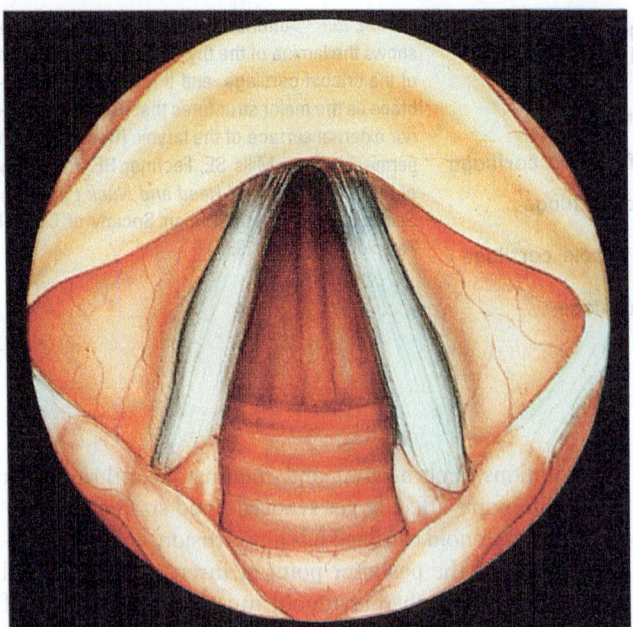

FIGURE 15.3 Larynx as viewed endoscopically from above. The elastic cone is visible through the mucosa of the true cord as a gray-to-white zone. False cords are loose folds of mucosa without further distinguishing features.

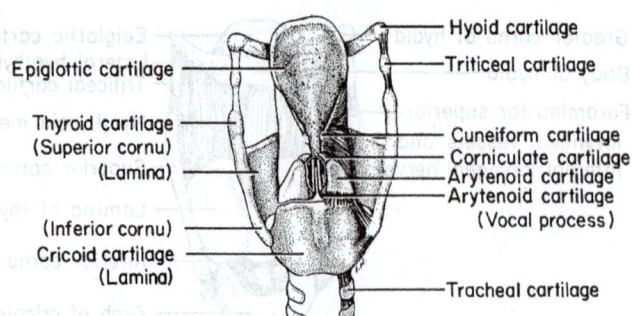

FIGURE 15.5 The major cartilages of the larynx are better seen in this drawing that deletes the associated soft tissues. (Reprinted with permission from Mills SE, Fechner RE. *Pathology of the Larynx. Atlas of Head and Neck Pathology Series.* Chicago, IL: American Society of Clinical Pathologists Press; 1985.)

the thyroarytenoid muscle determines the length and tension of the vocal cord.

The larynx can be divided into three major compartments (supraglottic, glottic, and subglottic) for purposes of discussing its submucosal and mucosal components. The supraglottic larynx extends from the tip of the epiglottis to the true cord (3). This portion of the larynx also includes the arytenoepiglottic (aryepiglottic) folds, false vocal cords, and

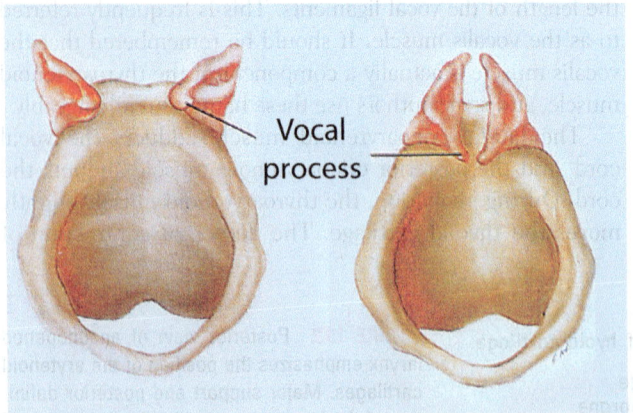

FIGURE 15.4 The arytenoid cartilage articulates with the posterior lamina of the cricoid cartilage. When the arytenoid cartilages are abducted, they are widely separated and the airway is open (**left**). When adducted, the arytenoid cartilages pivot, as well as move medially, thus bringing the vocal cords together (**right**). (Reprinted with permission from Mills SE, Fechner RE. *Pathology of the Larynx. Atlas of Head and Neck Pathology Series.* Chicago, IL: American Society of Clinical Pathologists Press; 1985.)

ventricles. The arytenoepiglottic folds run posteriorly from the base of the epiglottis to the region of the arytenoid cartilages. The false vocal cords are soft, rounded protrusions of the mucous membrane that lie superior to the true cords. The ventricles form the lower boundary of the false cords and separate them from the inferiorly located true cords. The ventricles extend upward behind the false cords as elliptical pouches. The greatest extension of the ventricles is slightly forward, where they end as dilated, blind pouches called saccules. Involvement of the ventricle is a frequent route of superior spread by glottic carcinoma, and this spread may be difficult to detect clinically.

The glottic compartment consists of the true vocal cords and the narrow band of mucous membrane called the anterior commissure, which bridges the vocal cords anteriorly (4,5). The subglottic compartment is the area between the lower border of the true vocal cords, where the squamous epithelium normally ends, and the first tracheal cartilage (6).

Microscopic Anatomy

Studies of larynges from newborns have shown that, initially, the larynx is lined by ciliated epithelium, except for the true vocal cords (7) (Figs. 15.6 and 15.7). Squamous epithelium begins to appear on the false vocal cords by about 6 months of age, but does not necessarily completely replace the ciliated respiratory mucosa (8,9). The lingual or anterior surface of the epiglottis is invariably covered by stratified squamous epithelium. The posterior or laryngeal surface of the epiglottis is covered by stratified squamous epithelium in its upper portion, but this merges with respiratory-type epithelium inferiorly (10). About one-half of nonsmoking adults have patches of squamous epithelium intermixed with ciliated epithelium, both in the supraglottic and infraglottic regions. In smokers, the ciliated, respiratory epithelium of the larynx is, often, totally replaced by squamous epithelium.

The normal ciliated epithelium of the larynx has an innermost layer of small, round cells—the basal or reserve cell layer. This single cell layer of basal cells is overlaid by a

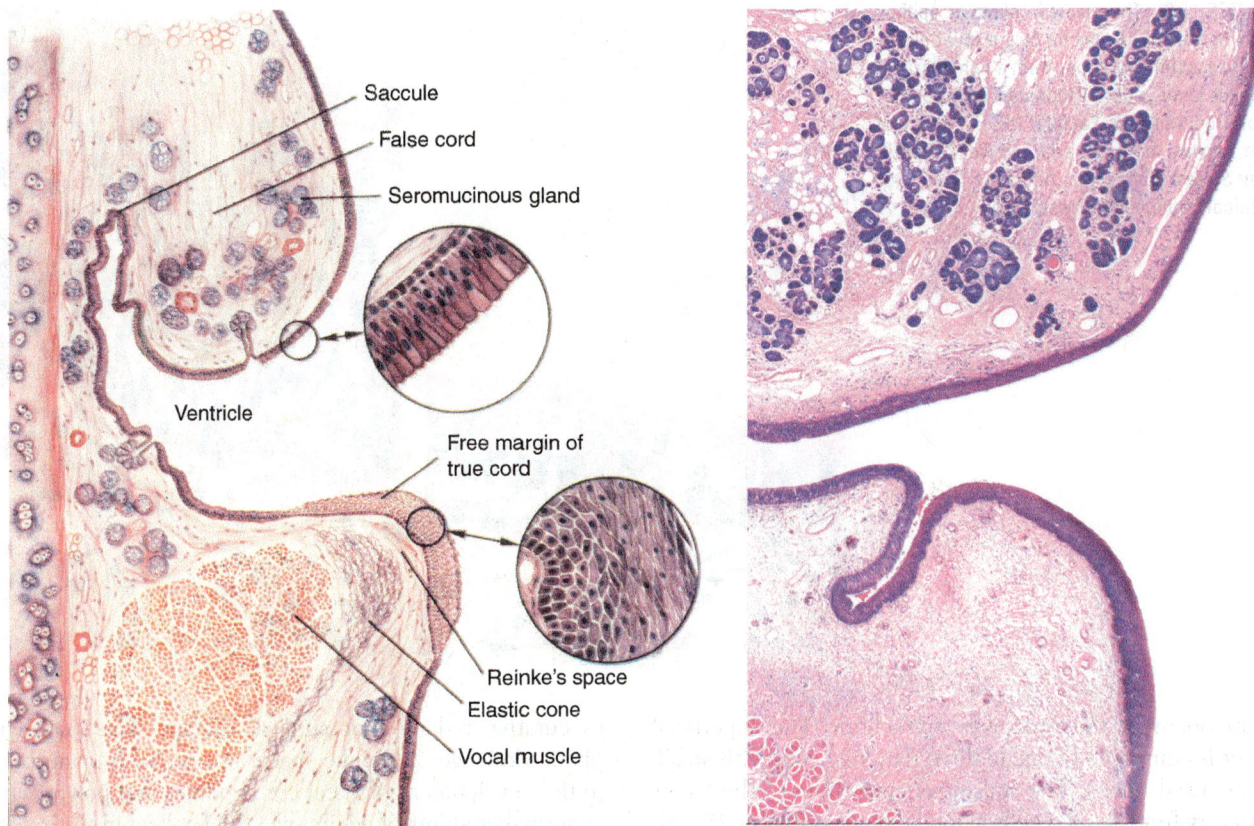

FIGURE 15.6 Drawing of the normal microscopic anatomy of the larynx on the left and a corresponding coronal section of the larynx on the right. Seromucinous glands are prominent in the false cord, and this cord is lined by ciliated columnar epithelium at birth. The vocalic muscle, elastic cone, and Reinke space are also visualized in the true cord (**left**). (Left image reprinted with permission from Mills SE, Fechner RE. *Pathology of the Larynx. Atlas of Head and Neck Pathology Series*. Chicago, IL: American Society of Clinical Pathologists Press; 1985.)

second row of ciliated columnar cells. Variation in the position of the nuclei within the columnar cell layer imparts a pseudostratified appearance to the epithelium. The ciliated layer may vary considerably in thickness (Fig. 15.8). Mucus-secreting cells may be numerous or rare. When there is abundant mucin, the cells assume a goblet configuration and may be located either within the middle portion of the epithelium, or near the surface (Fig. 15.9). Other mucus-secreting cells are barely recognizable and have only a few faintly discernible vacuoles within otherwise eosinophilic columnar cells.

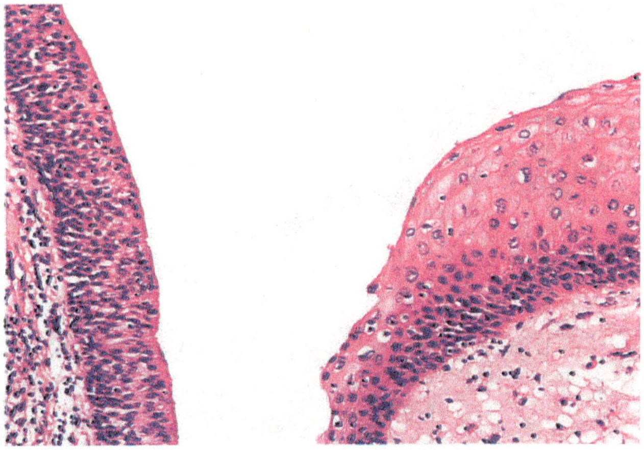

The squamous epithelium of the larynx has a basal layer of small cells with scant cytoplasm and ovoid nuclei that are typically oriented perpendicular to the surface. Mitotic figures are normally confined to this layer. Dendritic melanocytes may be present in the basal layer, especially in African Americans (11,12). The frequency with which this melanocytic change is observed, and whether it represents a congenital or acquired process, remains unclear. Rare laryngeal malignant melanomas presumably arise in such foci.

As the squamous cells in laryngeal mucosa mature and migrate toward the lumen, the nuclei enlarge, assume a more spherical shape, and have a more vesicular chromatin. The eosinophilic cytoplasm becomes abundant and slight cell shrinkage during fixation produces numerous, thin strands of cytoplasm from adjacent cells that remain attached by desmosomes. Because of these thin cytoplasmic strands between cells, the term "prickle cell layer" (malpighian layer) has been applied to this zone. This is the broadest

FIGURE 15.7 Section through ventricle discloses squamous epithelium lining true cord (**right**) and ciliated columnar-to-intermediate epithelium lining false cord (**left**).

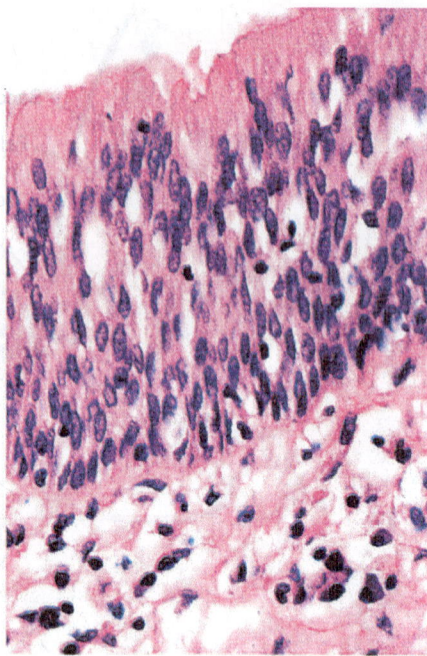

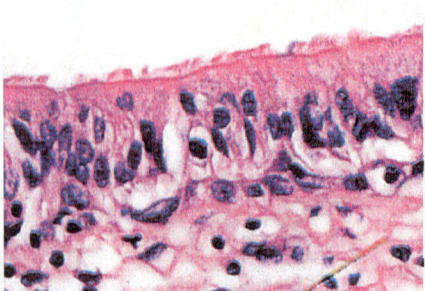

FIGURE 15.8 The ciliated columnar epithelium of the larynx may be only a few cells in thickness (**left**), or it may form a considerably thicker layer (**right**). (Reprinted with permission from Mills SE, Fechner RE. *Pathology of the Larynx. Atlas of Head and Neck Pathology Series*. Chicago, IL: American Society of Clinical Pathologists Press; 1985.)

component of the squamous epithelium. The superficial layer is composed of one to three flattened cells with small, condensed nuclei. The squamous epithelium of the larynx can vary from about 5 cells in total thickness to over 25 cells (Fig. 15.10). Normally, the larynx lacks a layer of parakeratotic surface cells. Continued exposure to irritants, such as cigarette smoke, may lead to foci of parakeratosis that may also be associated with orthokeratin formation.

The lamina propria of the true vocal cord is loose or dense connective tissue that lies between the vocal ligament and the squamous epithelium (Reinke space) (Fig. 15.11). Reinke space contains a few capillaries but lacks lymphatics, and only rarely has sparse seromucinous glands. As a result of this limited vascular access, carcinomas confined to the true vocal cords tend to remain localized, and are amenable to curative radiation or surgical therapy. The poor lymphatic drainage of Reinke space also probably contributes to the development of vocal cord nodules and polyps when abnormal amounts of edema-like fluid collect in this region. Likewise, vocal abuse or upper respiratory tract infections frequently producing edema in this region manifest clinically as hoarseness or dysphonia. The anterior commissure, unlike the true cords, contains more abundant capillaries, lymphatics, and seromucinous glands.

The junction between the ciliated columnar epithelium, inferior and superior to the squamous epithelium of the true vocal cords, may be abrupt, but usually there is a transitional zone that varies from several cells to a width of 1 to 2 mm. The transitional zone consists of columnar cells that are gradually replaced by small, basaloid or immature

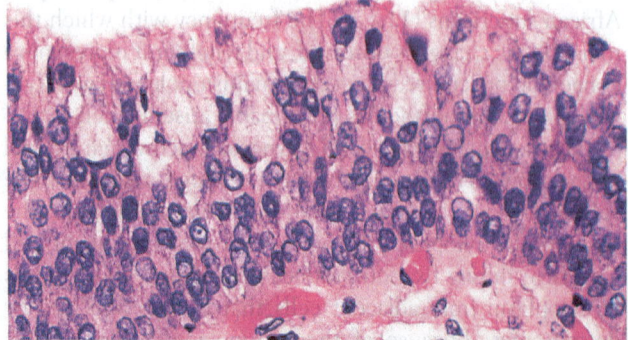

FIGURE 15.9 Goblet cells and columnar mucinous cells may be present in variable numbers within the nonsquamous epithelium of the larynx.

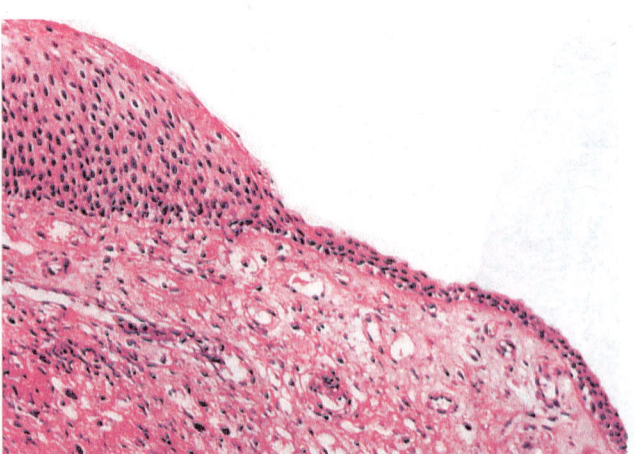

FIGURE 15.10 The squamous epithelium of the larynx can vary from approximately 5 cells in total thickness to over 25 cells in thickness, even within the same larynx.

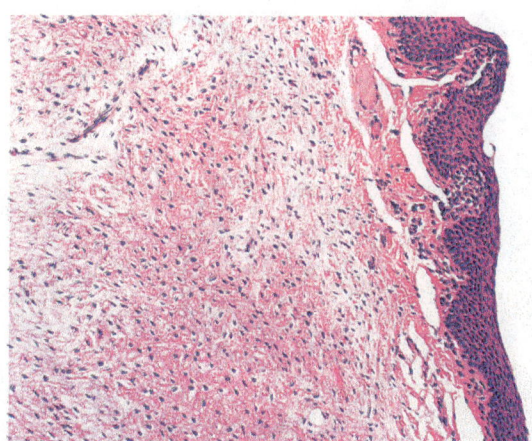

FIGURE 15.11 The true vocal cord is lined by squamous epithelium. A narrow, sparsely vascular zone (Reinke space) lies between the squamous epithelium and the underlying vocal ligament.

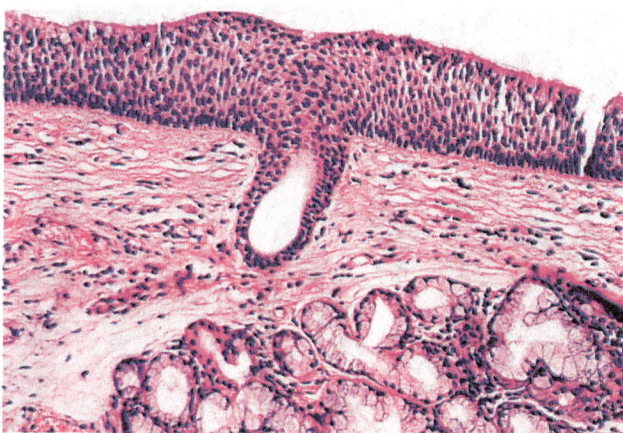

FIGURE 15.13 Seromucinous glands in the false cord drain into a duct that enters the overlying ciliated columnar epithelium. (Reprinted with permission from Mills SE, Fechner RE. *Pathology of the Larynx. Atlas of Head and Neck Pathology Series*. Chicago, IL: American Society of Clinical Pathologists Press; 1985.)

squamous cells (Fig. 15.12). In effect, this is a zone of immature squamous metaplasia in which the cells become progressively larger until they reach the size of the fully mature squamous epithelium that lines the true vocal cord.

The transitional zone often has a microscopically disorganized appearance when compared to the adjacent squamous and ciliated epithelia (Fig. 15.12). Furthermore, the epithelium in this zone may be thickened and consists predominantly of basaloid cells. The latter cells have uniform nuclei with mitotic figures confined to the basal-most cell layer. This normal pattern can easily be confused with dysplasia or so-called carcinoma in situ, particularly in frozen sections or otherwise suboptimal preparations. Awareness of this transitional zone and attention to cytologic detail will avoid confusion.

Human papillomavirus (HPV) subtypes have been implicated in the pathogenesis of a variety of squamous proliferations in the larynx. Using sensitive polymerase chain reaction (PCR) techniques, studies are beginning to document some HPV subtypes, such as type 11 in approximately 25% of light microscopically normal laryngeal specimens (13). Thus, the finding of this HPV subtype adjacent to a laryngeal carcinoma cannot be assumed to represent a causative association. HPV subtypes more commonly associated with malignancy (HPV 16, 18) have not yet been demonstrated in light microscopically normal laryngeal mucosa (14).

Seromucinous glands are present throughout most of the larynx and communicate with the surface epithelium by ducts that are lined either by squamous cells, columnar epithelium (Figs. 15.13 and 15.14), or a mixture of the

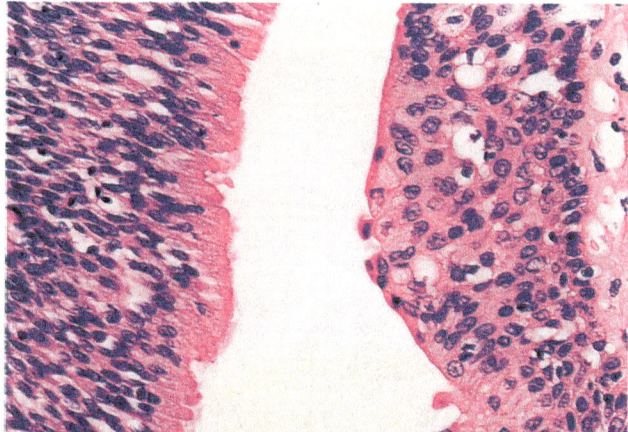

FIGURE 15.12 Ciliated columnar epithelium lines the false cord on the left. A transitional zone is seen on the true cord on the right. This zone of immature squamous metaplasia has a disorganized appearance that should not be confused with dysplasia. (Reprinted with permission from Mills SE, Fechner RE. *Pathology of the Larynx. Atlas of Head and Neck Pathology Series*. Chicago, IL: American Society of Clinical Pathologists Press; 1985.)

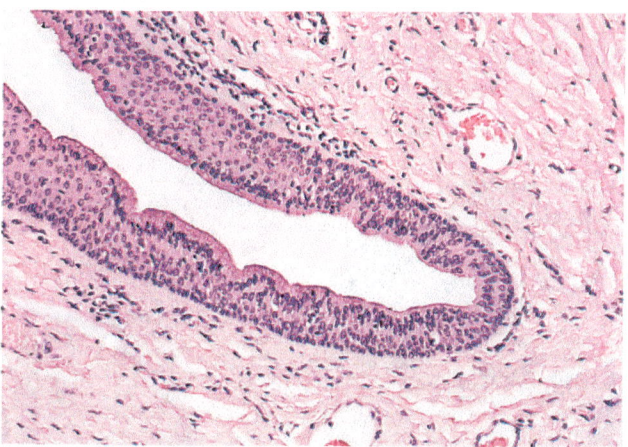

FIGURE 15.14 Ducts from seromucinous glands may be lined by squamous cells, ciliated columnar epithelium, or a mixture of the two.

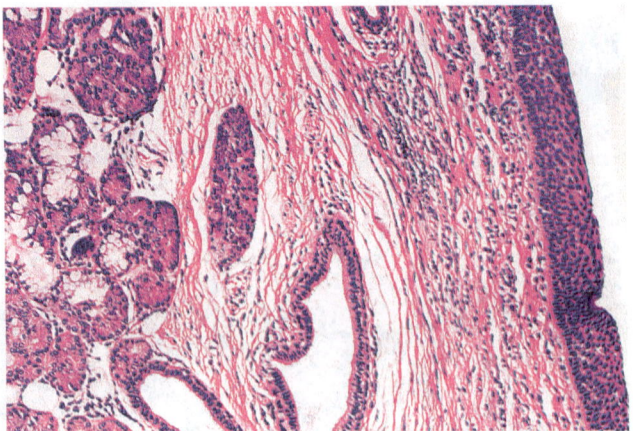

FIGURE 15.15 Seromucinous glands and their ducts are most prominent in the false cord.

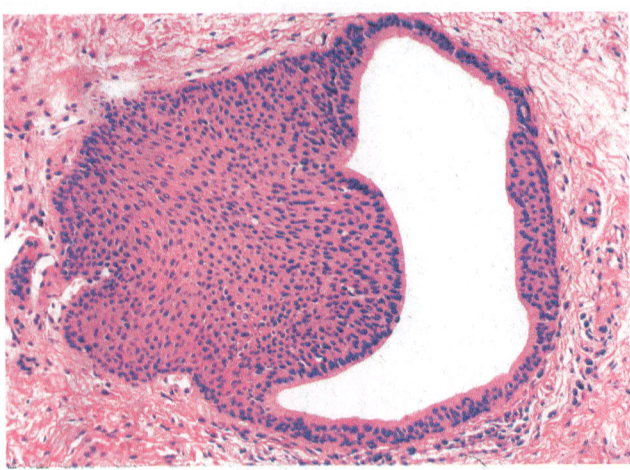

FIGURE 15.17 This seromucinous gland duct is associated with a large aggregate of metaplastic, nonkeratinizing squamous cells.

two (15). The columnar epithelial component may or may not be ciliated. The glands are most abundant in the false cords (Fig. 15.15), and there is also an extensive group of seromucinous glands just below the anterior commissure. Just superior to the anterior commissure is a narrow zone devoid of glands. In most cases, no glands are found beneath the squamous epithelium lining the free edge of the true vocal cords. Glands are present, however, beginning immediately at the squamocolumnar junction, both above and below the squamous epithelium of the true cords. Occasionally, there are glands in the stroma of the true vocal cord, and glands may be present in the underlying vocalis muscle (Fig. 15.16). The fenestration in the elastic cartilage of the epiglottis is filled with abundant seromucinous glands. These glands penetrate completely through the cartilage and afford a ready path for the spread of supraglottic carcinoma.

Laryngeal biopsies, particularly from the region of the false cords, will often contain seromucinous gland ducts lined by squamous epithelium and located deep beneath the surface mucosa (Fig. 15.17). Because of tangential sectioning, these ducts may appear as seemingly isolated squamous nests. Distinction from infiltrating carcinoma should not be a problem in adequately prepared sections. However, changes of basal cell hyperplasia or dysplasia also can involve these ducts. Fortuitous sections of such ducts may then result in seemingly isolated nests of basaloid or overtly dysplastic epithelium that are much more likely to be mistaken for invasive carcinoma (Fig. 15.18).

Oncocytic metaplasia of ductal and acinar cells in the seromucinous glands of the larynx is a common, age-related change. Oncocytes are not seen in the seromucinous glands of individuals younger than 18 years of age, but oncocytes are present in these glands in approximately 80% of people

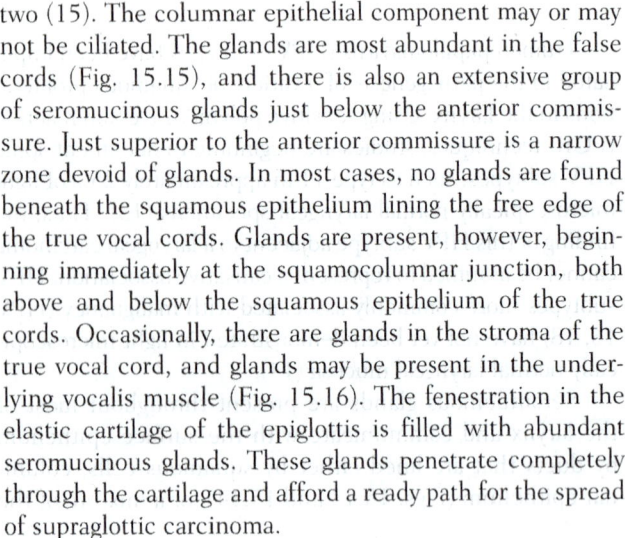

FIGURE 15.16 Seromucinous glands are occasionally located deep within the vocalis muscle.

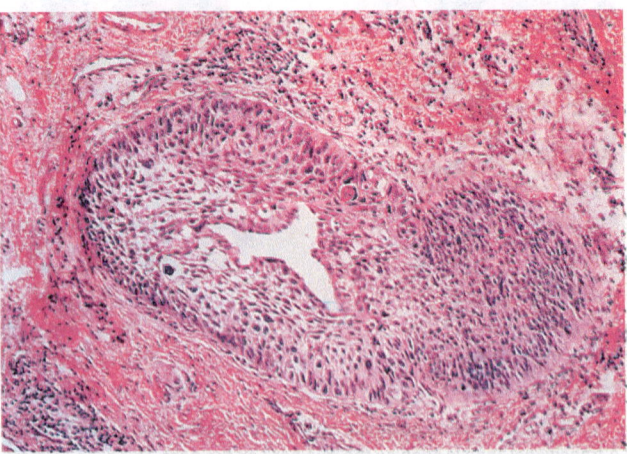

FIGURE 15.18 When ducts are involved with cytologically atypical squamous epithelium resembling surface dysplastic changes, they should not be misinterpreted as invasive carcinoma. In this example, the inner columnar cell lining is retained.

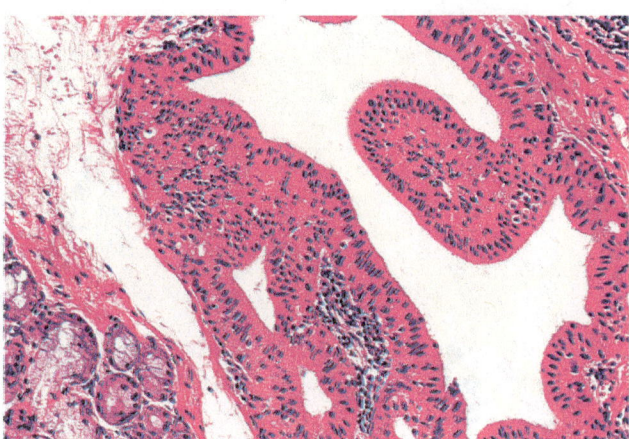

FIGURE 15.19 Oncocytic transformation of seromucinous epithelium can result in cystic structures.

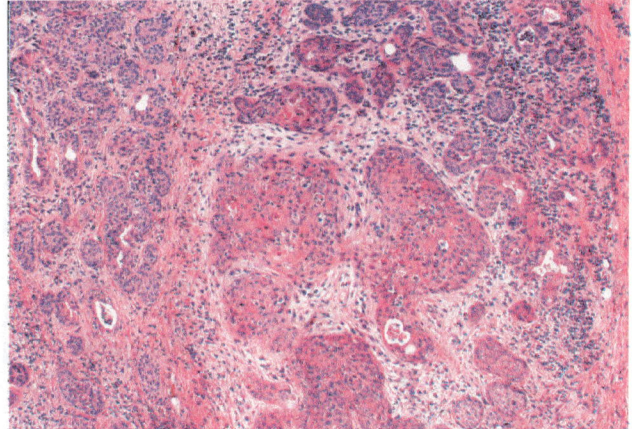

FIGURE 15.21 Higher magnification of necrotizing sialometaplasia shows replacement of the seromucinous lobules by aggregates of squamous cells with associated inflammation.

older than the age of 50 (16,17). Uncomplicated oncocytic metaplasia is asymptomatic, but, occasionally, oncocytic metaplasia may become cystic (Fig. 15.19) and, if sufficiently large, produce symptoms.

The seromucinous glands of the larynx may also undergo infarction and associated squamous metaplasia (Figs. 15.20 and 15.21). The resultant process, termed necrotizing sialometaplasia, is much more common in the oral cavity, and probably results from a traumatic or spontaneous ischemic event (18). The islands of metaplastic cells may be mitotically active and exhibit mild-to-moderate nuclear atypia. Confusion with mucoepidermoid or squamous cell carcinoma is common, particularly in frozen section specimens. At low-power magnification, the preservation of the acinar pattern, in association with infarction, inflammation, and extravasation of mucin, will aid in the correct diagnosis.

If the external surface of the larynx is carefully sampled, it is not unusual to find microscopic islands of normal thyroid tissue within the fibrous capsule of the larynx and trachea, just external to the cricothyroid membrane or embedded in the associated musculature (Fig. 15.22) (19). The thyroid follicles are small and appear normal, with well-formed colloid. Continuity with the main thyroid gland is not usually demonstrable (20). Less commonly, microscopic foci of thyroid tissue will be encountered internal to the cartilage of the larynx and trachea, usually at the junction of the cricoid cartilage and the first tracheal ring (19,21). These isolated foci of extrathyroidal thyroid tissue probably lose their connection to the main portion of the thyroid gland during embryologic development (19). Awareness of this phenomenon and attention to the microscopic features will avoid confusion with invasive or metastatic thyroid carcinoma.

The normal larynx contains at least two pairs of paraganglia (Fig. 15.23). The superior, supraglottic paraganglia are sharply localized to the upper, anterior third of the false cords, in close approximation to the margin of the thyroid

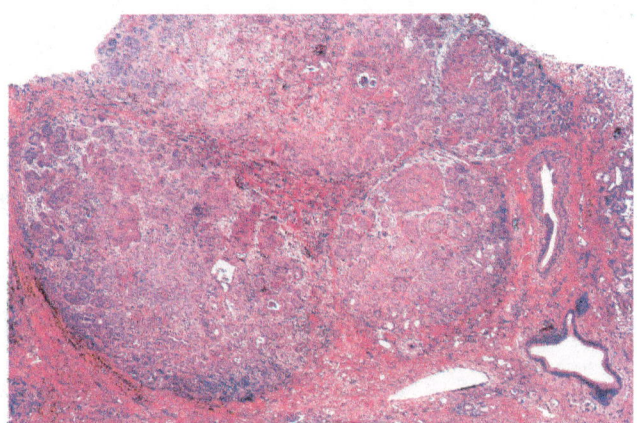

FIGURE 15.20 This low-power example of necrotizing sialometaplasia shows preservation of the pre-existing lobular architecture of the seromucinous glands.

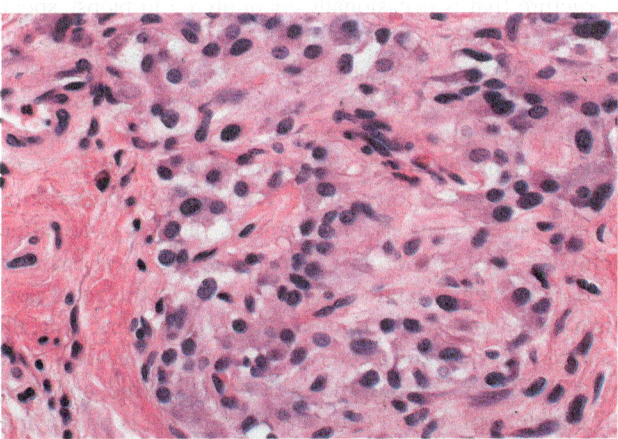

FIGURE 15.22 Larynx_paraganglion. A nest of normal paraganglion cells from the lateral supraglottic larynx. Such nests should not be confused with the insular growth pattern of a well-differentiated neuroendocrine carcinoma.

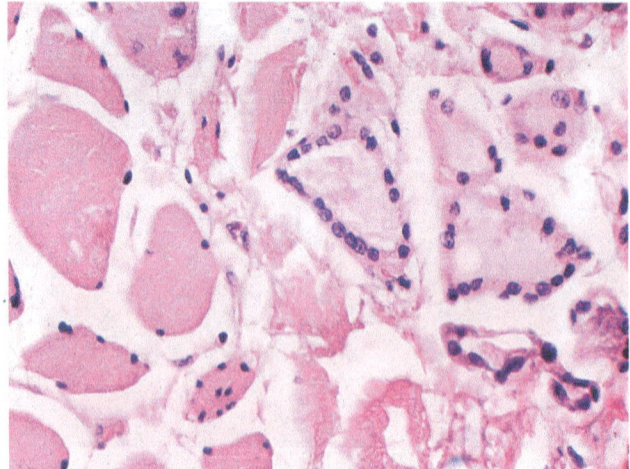

FIGURE 15.23 Thyroid_in_muscle. Small nests of normal thyroid follicles may be found in the soft tissue or skeletal muscle immediately external to the laryngeal cartilages.

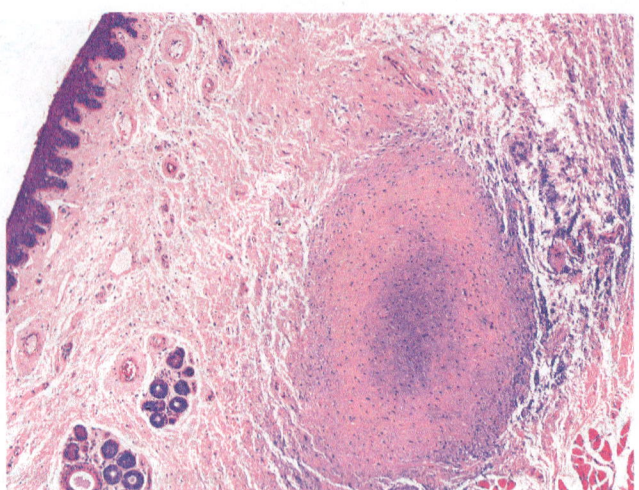

FIGURE 15.24 The vocal process of the arytenoid cartilage may appear in a laryngeal biopsy as a sharply circumscribed nodule of elastic-type cartilage. It should not be mistaken for a cartilaginous neoplasm.

cartilage and the internal branch of the superior laryngeal nerves (22,23). The paired inferior paraganglia are more variably situated, and may be found between the thyroid and cricoid cartilages or just below the cricoid cartilage (22,23). They are closely associated with the inferior laryngeal nerves. Aberrant or ectopic paraganglia have been described in various sites throughout the larynx. Laryngeal paraganglia are minute, neuroendocrine structures (0.1 to 0.4 mm) of unknown physiologic activity. Their close association with neurovascular bundles suggests chemoreceptor function, but this has not been proved. Laryngeal paraganglia presumably give rise to the rare paragangliomas of the larynx. It is important not to confuse a laryngeal paraganglioma with a more common and very similar appearing well-differentiated neuroendocrine carcinoma (carcinoid tumor). Paragangliomas should be cytokeratin negative and the cells nests are typically surrounded by S100-positive sustentacular cells.

The vocal process of the arytenoid cartilage is a normal structure that is occasionally encountered in biopsy specimens from the posterior portion of the true cord. It is a sharply circumscribed nodule of uniformly mature, elastic-type cartilage (Fig. 15.24). Its elastic nature, demonstrable with appropriate elastin stains, allows distinction from cartilaginous neoplasms of the larynx, all of which are composed of hyalin-type cartilage. The sharp circumscription of the cartilaginous arytenoid process allows it to be differentiated from chondroid metaplasia of the vocal ligament described below. Chondroid metaplasia of the vocal cord is a common, usually asymptomatic, finding that typically affects the mid and posterior portions of the vocal cord (24,25). The margins of the cartilage are blurred, and there is a peripheral zone of connective tissue that is rich in acid mucopolysaccharides (Fig. 15.25) (25). The metaplastic nodules contain dense aggregates of elastic fibers throughout the lesion. The multilobular pattern, typical of cartilaginous neoplasms, is absent. Chondroid metaplasia can occur in other soft tissues of the larynx, particularly in the region of the false cord. In one study, foci of chondroid metaplasia were found in 1% to 2% of larynges at autopsy (24).

Neural, Vascular, and Lymphatic Components

The intrinsic laryngeal muscles are innervated by branches of the vagus nerve. The cricothyroid muscle is supplied by the superior laryngeal branch of the vagus, and the remainder of the intrinsic musculature has been conventionally viewed as being innervated by the recurrent laryngeal branch of the vagus nerve. The terminal portion of the recurrent laryngeal nerve is referred to as the "inferior laryngeal nerve" (26). More recently, it has been shown that branches of the superior and recurrent laryngeal nerves form anastomoses, most commonly

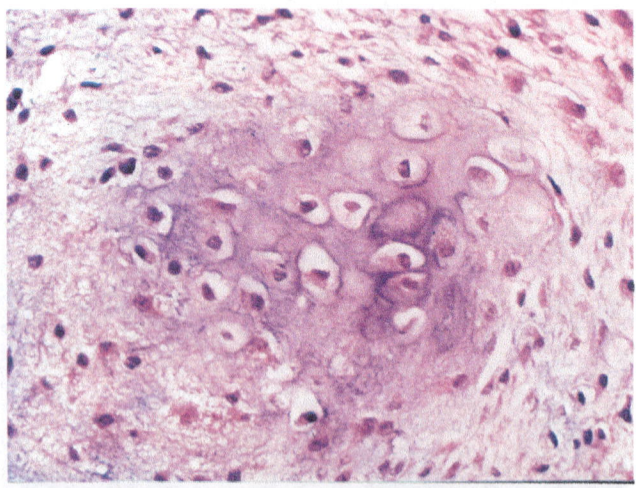

FIGURE 15.25 Chondroid metaplasia of the larynx has ill-defined margins. (Reprinted with permission from Mills SE, Fechner RE. *Pathology of the Larynx. Atlas of Head and Neck Pathology Series*. Chicago, IL: American Society of Clinical Pathologists Press; 1985.)

within the interarytenoid muscle, but less consistently in the piriform sinus. Branches from the superior laryngeal nerve, referred to as the "communicating nerve," may pass through the cricothyroid muscle to partially innervate the vocalis muscle (27,28). It has been suggested that the communicating nerve may be the nerve of the elusive fifth branchial arch (28).

The lower portions of the larynx are supplied with blood from the inferior laryngeal artery, a small branch of the inferior thyroid artery that accompanies the inferior laryngeal nerve. The inferior laryngeal artery has anastomoses with the larger superior laryngeal artery, derived from the superior thyroid artery. The laryngeal arteries are accompanied by similarly named veins. The superior laryngeal vein joins the superior thyroid vein and drains into the internal jugular vein (26). The inferior laryngeal vein joins the inferior thyroid vein. Numerous anastomoses across the front of the trachea between the left and right inferior laryngeal veins may lead to contralateral venous return (26).

The lymphatics of the larynx tend to drain along with the vasculature. Therefore, supraglottic lymphatics drain superiorly, and subglottic lymphatics drain inferiorly (1,26). As discussed earlier, lymphatics are scarce in the glottis. Some of the laryngeal lymphatics end in very small lymph nodes on the thyrohyoid membrane, cricotracheal ligament, or superior trachea (26). These nodes, however, drain into the deep cervical nodes (26). Lymphatics in the supraglottic larynx are prominent and, typically, terminate in the anterior jugular chain (29). Subglottic lymphatics terminate in the midline pretracheal nodes or, less commonly, in the lower cervical lymph nodes (29).

PHARYNX

Definition and Boundaries

The pharynx has three functionally and structurally disperse subparts—the nasopharynx, oropharynx, and hypopharynx (Fig. 15.26). The nasopharynx is the portion of the pharynx that lies above the soft palate. It has anterior, posterior, and lateral walls. The anterior wall is perforated by the posterior nares (choanae). The posterior wall is an arch that includes the roof of the nasopharynx, as well as the posterior portion against the base of the skull. The posterior wall extends inferiorly and, at the level of the horizontal projection of the soft palate, continues inferiorly as the posterior wall of the oropharynx. The anterior and posterior walls are connected by the lateral walls into which the eustachian tubes empty.

The oropharynx lies between the soft palate and the tip of the epiglottis. By definition, its superior boundary is a horizontal projection of the soft palate. Anteriorly, it is bounded by the fauces or opening from the mouth and, below this, the posterior aspect of the dorsum of the tongue. It should be noted that the lingual and palatine tonsils, although located anteriorly in the oropharynx are part of this region and are not part of the oral cavity. The inferior margin of the anterior portion of the oropharynx is marked by the opening of the piriform recess at the level of the tip of the epiglottis. A horizontal projection posteriorly from this point marks the posterior aspect of the inferior margin, which is continuous with the hypopharynx.

The hypopharynx is the portion of the pharynx below the tip of the epiglottis and extending downward to the beginning of the esophagus. The hypopharynx is wide superiorly, but rapidly narrows as it approaches the level of the cricoid cartilage and becomes continuous with the esophagus. The hypopharynx partially surrounds the larynx laterally, and is separated from it by the aryepiglottic folds. The latter extend from the upper posterior border of the larynx to the side of the epiglottis. The lateral extensions of the hypopharynx are called "piriform recesses" or sinuses (26) (Fig. 15.27).

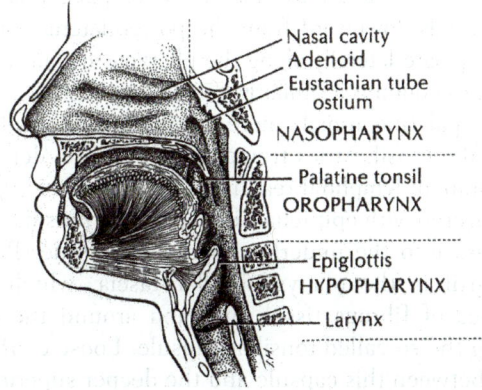

FIGURE 15.26 This sagittal section delineates the boundaries of the nasopharynx, oropharynx, and hypopharynx.

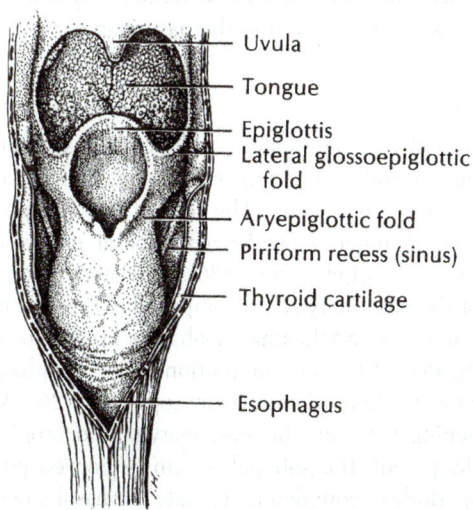

FIGURE 15.27 The piriform sinuses are a conduit between the oropharynx and the opening of the esophagus. They surround the larynx laterally.

Embryology

The embryologic pharynx is of endodermal derivation and, at its cephalic end, is in direct continuity with the ectoderm forming the stomodeum. Recent observations have suggested that the development of the roof of the pharynx is highly dependent on the closely adjacent notochord (30). The stomodeum and pharynx are separated by the buccopharyngeal membrane, which is lined on its external surface by ectoderm, and, internally, by endoderm. At the end of the 3rd week of embryologic development, the buccopharyngeal membrane ruptures, establishing contact between the stomodeum and the primitive pharyngeal portion of the foregut (30,31). Superiorly, the buccopharyngeal membrane corresponds to approximately the level of the nasal choanae. In the subsequent 5th through 7th weeks of gestation, the primitive nasal cavity forms and enlarges, with formation and later rupture of the bucconasal membrane, establishing the final connection between the nasal cavity and pharynx (30). In the 8th through 10th gestational weeks, the secondary palate develops behind the primary palate, ending the formation of the basic pharyngeal structures. At this point, however, the pharynx is proportionally quite small and after the 10th week of gestation, remarkable growth in this region occurs with enlargement of the pharynx and downward movement of the palate and tongue (30).

Thus, the lining of the nasal cavity and paranasal sinuses is of ectodermal origin and constitutes the so-called schneiderian membrane. The nasopharynx, oropharynx, and hypopharynx are, at least in large part, of endodermal origin. The sharp demarcation between endoderm and ectoderm at the level of the nasal cavity, is of considerable practical importance. Certain neoplasms, such as angiofibromas and lymphoepitheliomas, are virtually confined to the endodermally derived nasopharynx. In contrast, schneiderian papillomas and intestinal-type adenocarcinomas arise from the ectodermally derived lining of the nasal cavity and paranasal sinuses; they do not occur in the nasopharynx.

Gross Anatomy

By nature of their boundaries and lack of resectability, the nasopharynx and oropharynx are practically never encountered as gross specimens. The roof of the nasopharynx is composed of mucosa overlying the basal portions of the sphenoid and occipital bones (26). The lateral and posterior walls of the nasopharynx are composed of the superior constrictor muscles and the pharyngobasilar fascia. The soft palate is the floor of the anterior portion of the nasopharynx, the only truly mobile portion of the nasopharynx (26). Although the opening between the nasopharynx and oropharynx is normally patent, the soft palate can be moved posteriorly and superiorly to completely separate the nasal and oral segments. This is important as a component of proper speech, and to keep food and water out of the nasal region while eating and drinking.

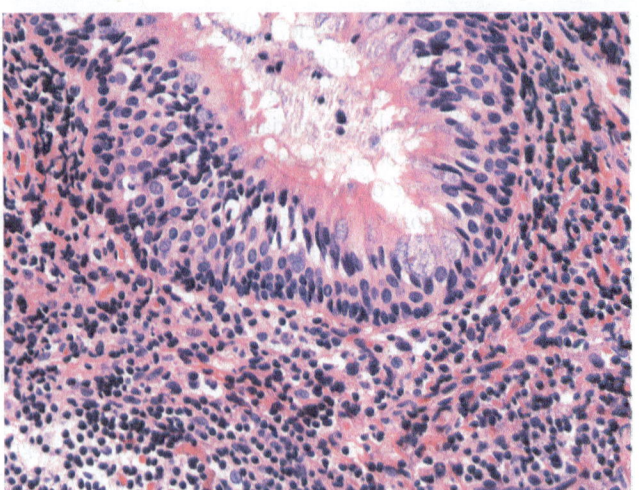

FIGURE 15.28 The (naso)pharyngeal tonsil or "adenoids" is typically composed, at least partially, of epithelial crypts lined by ciliated respiratory-type mucosa unlike the exclusively squamous-lined crypts of the palatine tonsils. Also unlike the palatine tonsils, the adenoids tend to atrophy after childhood.

The most important gross features of the nasopharynx encountered by pathologists are the pharyngeal tonsil (Fig. 15.28), Rosenmüller fossa, and the eustachian tube openings. The pharyngeal tonsil or adenoids is a prominent, convoluted mass in the roof of the nasopharynx in children. It typically atrophies in adults. The pharyngeal recess or Rosenmüller fossa is a mucosa-lined depression in the posterolateral portion of the nasopharynx. Just anterior to the recess, located in the lateral wall, is the ostium of the eustachian tube. This opening is surrounded on its superior and posterior aspects by mucosa-covered cartilage, the tubal torus, from the eustachian tube wall (26).

The superior portion of the anterior oropharynx is bounded by the fauces or opening of the mouth into the oropharynx. The lateral walls of the fauces are composed, on each side, of the two tonsillar pillars, between which lies the palatine tonsil in the tonsillar fossa. The anterior tonsillar pillar is the palatoglossal arch. This structure curves downward and forward, from the soft palate to the tongue. The posterior tonsillar pillar or palatopharyngeal arch extends downward from the posterolateral border of the soft palate laterally along the pharyngeal wall. Each of the arches contains a similarly named muscle (26).

The palatine tonsil, more commonly referred to as simply the tonsil, varies tremendously in size, depending on its state of lymphoid reactivity. The surface of the tonsil is covered with epithelial-lined pits, the tonsillar crypts that pass into the underlying lymphoid tissue. Beneath the tonsil is the pharyngobasilar fascia, which sends branches of fibrous tissue into and around the tonsil, forming the so-called tonsillar capsule. Loose connective tissue between this capsule and the deeper superior constrictor muscle forms a plane of cleavage that facilitates surgical removal (26).

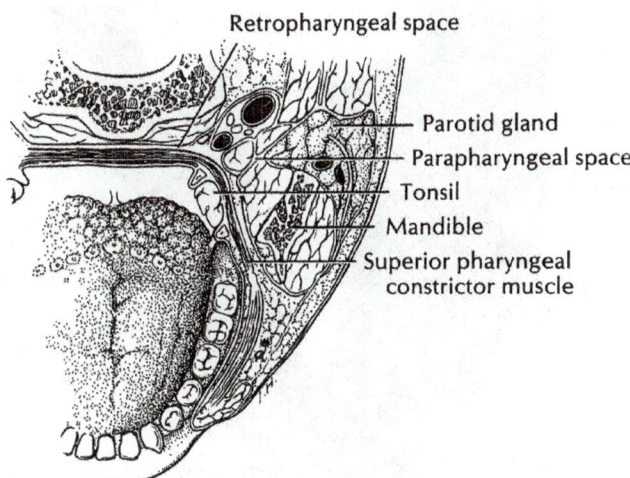

FIGURE 15.29 The lateral pharyngeal space lies deep to the tonsil and contains several vital structures. It is in continuity, posteriorly, with the retropharyngeal space.

The parapharyngeal or lateral pharyngeal space is an important zone of loose connective tissue lying deep to the tonsil and lateral to the pharynx (Fig. 15.29). This space is roughly pyramidal, with the base of the skull forming the base of the pyramid superiorly (19,26). Inferiorly, the apex is formed by the attachment of the cervical fascia to the hyoid bone. Medially is the superior constrictor muscle of the pharynx and laterally, the pterygoid lamina, inner surface of the mandibular ramus, and the deep lobe of the parotid gland (19). Contained within the peripharyngeal space are the internal carotid artery, internal jugular vein, cranial nerves IX to XII, the cervical sympathetic chain, vagal and carotid bodies, and multiple lymph nodes (19). Mass-producing lesions involving any of these structures may cause medial displacement of the tonsil and lateral pharyngeal wall. Tonsillar abscesses or other sources of infection may also involve and rapidly spread throughout this space. Posteriorly, the parapharyngeal space is in direct continuity with loose connective tissue behind the pharynx and anterior to the prevertebral fascia of the vertebral column (26). This has been referred to as the retropharyngeal space (Fig. 15.29).

Inferior to the fauces, the oropharynx is bounded anteriorly by the posterior aspect of the immobile portion of the tongue. The base of the tongue contains abundant submucosal lymphoid tissues that constitute the lingual tonsil. This structure, along with the palatine and pharyngeal tonsils, forms an oblique wreath of lymphoid tissues, encompassing the oropharynx and nasopharynx that is often referred to as Waldeyer ring.

The most important structures in the hypopharynx are the piriform sinuses (Fig. 15.26). These elongated, pear-shaped gutters extend laterally along both sides of the larynx, and posteriorly from the pharyngoepiglottic fold to the opening of the esophagus (29). Laterally, the piriform sinus lies against the thyroid cartilage. Medially, it is separated from the laryngeal ventricle by a thin layer of muscles derived from the aryepiglottic fold and the opening of the esophagus (29). Just posterior and lateral to the piriform sinus is the common carotid artery. Because of their close association, tumors arising in the hypopharynx often invade the larynx secondarily. These tumors should be distinguished from primary laryngeal neoplasms because of their poorer prognosis.

Microscopic Anatomy

The nasopharyngeal mucosa in the adult has a surface area of about 50 cm^2. Most of it is lined by stratified squamous epithelium and about 40% is covered by respiratory-type columnar epithelium (32). Squamous epithelium predominantly lines the lower portion of the anterior and posterior nasopharyngeal walls, as well as the anterior half of the lateral walls. Ciliated respiratory epithelium predominantly carpets the region of the posterior nares (choanae) and the roof of the posterior wall. The remainder of the nasopharynx, including the posterior lateral walls and the middle-third of the posterior wall, has alternating islands of squamous and respiratory epithelia.

The junction between squamous and respiratory epithelia may be sharp, or there may be zones of transitional or intermediate epithelia as previously described in the Larynx. We prefer the term "intermediate epithelium," as opposed to "transitional epithelium," because these cells lack the ultrastructural features of urinary tract epithelium. Intermediate epithelium primarily forms a wavy ring at the junction of the nasopharynx and oropharynx. The intermediate cells may be basaloid with minimal cytoplasm, and they typically have a cuboidal or round configuration. As discussed under Larynx, biopsy specimens containing intermediate epithelium must not be overly interpreted as areas of dysplasia or carcinoma in situ. This is most likely to be a problem when this zone is encountered in a frozen section.

In addition to the pharyngeal tonsil, less-prominent collections of lymphoid follicles may be present submucosally throughout the nasopharynx (Fig. 15.30). These follicles

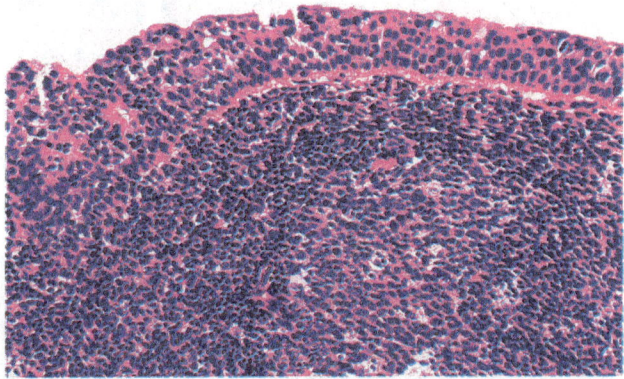

FIGURE 15.30 Submucosal lymphoid aggregates are present normally throughout the nasopharynx and should not be overly interpreted as severe chronic inflammation.

are particularly abundant in the rim of the eustachian tube opening (Gerlach tonsil), but they are also present under the mucosa of the lateral and posterior walls of the nasopharynx, as well as on the nasopharyngeal surface of the soft palate (29). Thus, a submucosal follicular lymphoid infiltrate is normal in nasopharyngeal biopsies and should not be overinterpreted as a pathologic inflammatory process.

Throughout the nasopharynx there are numerous submucosal seromucinous glands that produce predominantly mucin. These glands are particularly numerous in the region of the eustachian tube opening. As with the laryngeal seromucinous glands, oncocytic metaplasia in the glandular and ductal epithelium becomes increasingly frequent with advancing age (33,34).

The anterior portion of the pituitary gland forms from an intracranial invagination of epithelium in the form of Rathke pouch. Microscopic remnants of Rathke pouch epithelium are present in the roof of the nasopharynx in 95% to 100% of individuals (35–37). In most instances, this so-called pharyngeal pituitary is located in the midline, in the region of the vomerosphenoidal articulation. The nests of epithelial cells measure 0.2 mm to approximately 6 mm in greatest dimension. They are located deep in the mucosa or in the underlying periosteum (35). Most of the epithelial cells appear undifferentiated, but occasional basophilic and eosinophilic cells may be present (Fig. 15.31). Although it is not entirely clear, the pharyngeal pituitary may not have any physiologic function. Most pituitary adenomas that involve the nasopharynx reach this location by invasion from the pituitary fossa. Occasionally, however, apparently ectopic pituitary adenomas present in the nasopharynx, and it is tempting to speculate that such lesions arise from the pharyngeal pituitary (38,39).

The pharyngeal bursa is a normal embryonic structure situated posterior to Rathke pouch. Remnants of this bursa may be found in approximately 3% of normal adults (40,41). Cysts derived from this structure may be found in all ages, occasionally as an incidental finding, and occur in the regions of the adenoid (42). The cysts are separated from

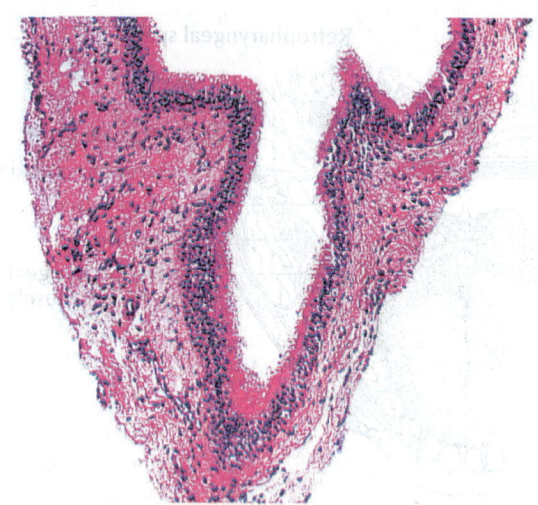

FIGURE 15.32 Nasopharyngeal cysts are rimmed by fibrous tissue and lined by ciliated columnar epithelium.

the adenoid by a fibrous membrane and will not be removed with routine adenoidectomy specimens (Fig. 15.32) (10). The median pharyngeal recess is a shallow depression formed normally in association with the pharyngeal tonsil. Unlike cysts derived from the pharyngeal bursa, those formed from the median pharyngeal recess are located within the adenoid and will be removed with it (10).

The cranial end of the embryonic notochord is closely associated with the roof of the developing nasopharynx (43). Although most of the notochord degenerates during embryonic and fetal development, notochordal remnants have been demonstrated in the submucosa of the nasopharynx and other closely adjacent locations (10,44). Most chordomas involving the nasopharynx are down growths of craniooccipital tumors, but rare primary nasopharyngeal tumors presumably arise from these nasopharyngeal notochord remnants (43,44).

Both the oropharynx and hypopharynx are lined continuously by stratified squamous epithelium. This mucus is typically nonkeratinizing, although areas of parakeratin or orthokeratin may be seen secondary to chronic irritation. As in the nasopharynx, the submucosa of the oropharynx and hypopharynx contains scattered lymphoid aggregates, as well as prominent submucosal seromucinous glands.

The stratified squamous epithelium covering the tonsils extends into the tonsillar crypts for considerable distances. As these cords of epithelium merge with the underlying lymphoid tissue, the epithelial cells assume a more basaloid appearance and have uniform, but vesicular nuclei. The junction between the lymphoid cells and the islands of squamous cells is often blurred (Fig. 15.33). Apparently, isolated irregular nests of basaloid focally keratinized squamous cells, often with vesicular nuclei, are common deep within the tonsil (Fig. 15.34), and such nests must not be confused with carcinoma. Attention to the low-power architecture will confirm that these nests are closely approximated to tonsillar crypts and are a normal finding.

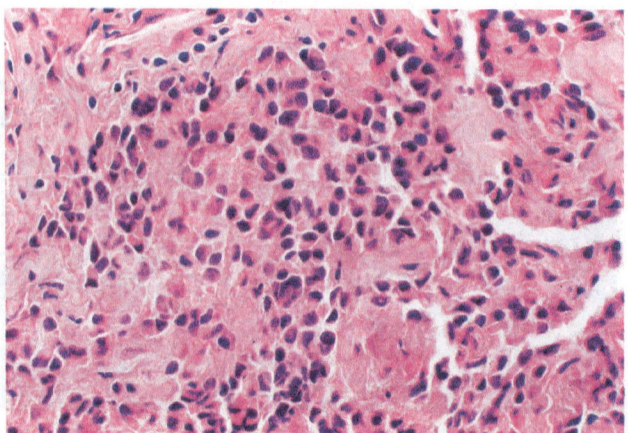

FIGURE 15.31 Nests of ectopic pituitary cells present in the superior portion of the nasopharynx.

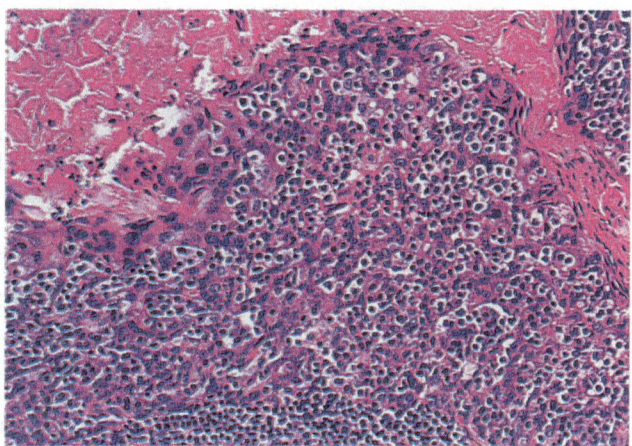

FIGURE 15.33 The junction between lymphoid tissue and the squamous cells lining the tonsillar crypts is often blurred.

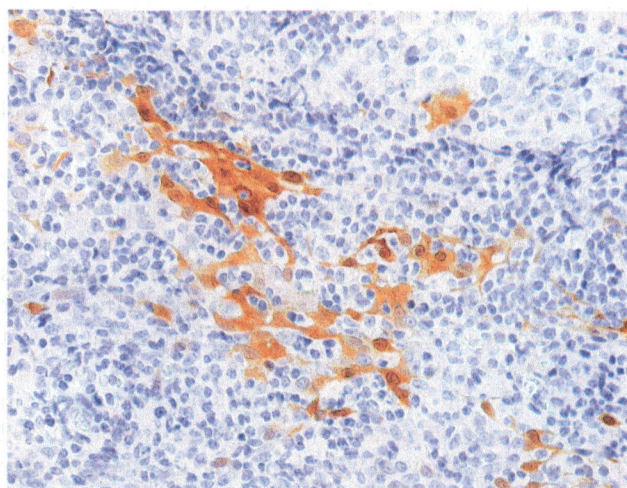

FIGURE 15.35 The normal crypt epithelium of the palatine tonsils will show strong positivity for p16, which should not be interpreted as evidence of HPV-related dysplasia or neoplasia.

The basaloid epithelium of the tonsillar crypts has been shown to be, like the transformation zone of the uterine cervix, particularly sensitive to infection by high-risk HPV. It is now recognized that HPV-associated squamous cell carcinomas in the head and neck, which are occurring with increasing frequency, almost entirely arise from the crypt epithelium of the lingual and palatine tonsils, both of which lie within the oropharynx. Unlike the uterine cervix, however, immunohistochemical staining for p16 cannot be used as a marker for HPV-associated dysplasia in this area, as normal crypt epithelium is often strongly p16 positive (45) (Fig. 15.35).

Occasionally, islands of metaplastic cartilage and bone are encountered within or immediately adjacent to the tonsils (19,46). This presumably represents a secondary reactive change to prior inflammation. Eggston and Wolff described this change in about one-fifth of all resected tonsils (46). These authors noted that patients with this change had an average age of 24 years and, therefore, were older than most individuals undergoing tonsillectomy (46).

Neural, Vascular, and Lymphatic Components

The nerves supplying the constrictor muscles of the pharynx, the stylopharyngeus muscle, and the muscles of the soft palate are derived almost entirely from the pharyngeal plexus. The latter structure is formed by the union of the pharyngeal branches of the glossopharyngeal and vagus nerves. The inferior constrictor muscle may receive a portion of its innervation from the external laryngeal nerve, a separate branch of the vagus that primarily supplies the larynx (26).

The blood supply to the superior portion of the pharynx is from the ascending pharyngeal artery, which runs upward along the posterior lateral wall of the pharynx (26) (Fig. 15.36). The inferior portion of the pharynx is supplied

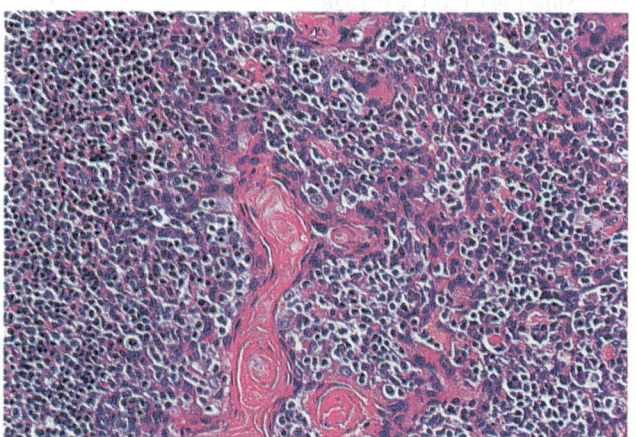

FIGURE 15.34 Irregular nests of epithelium are frequently present deep within the tonsil. These are closely approximated to tonsillar crypts and are a normal finding not to be misinterpreted as carcinoma.

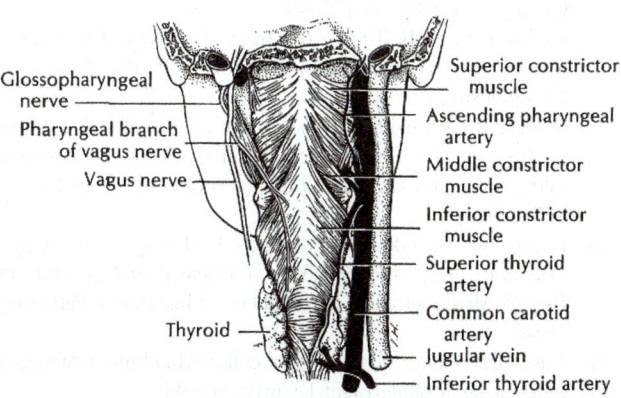

FIGURE 15.36 Posterior view of the pharynx with emphasis on vascular and neural components.

by branches from the superior and inferior thyroid arteries. The veins draining the pharynx merge posteriorly to form the pharyngeal plexus, which in turn drains at irregular intervals into the pterygoid plexus and the superior and inferior thyroid veins (26).

The lymphatics from the roof and posterior wall of the nasopharynx join in the midline and pass through the pharyngeal fascia. They then split to the right or left retropharyngeal lymph nodes. Some of the nasopharyngeal lymphatics terminate in the highest lymph nodes of the internal jugular and spinal chains (29). Most of the lymphatics from the soft palate converge at a group of lymph nodes located below the anterior belly of the digastric muscle, immediately in front of the jugular chain (29). Lymphatics from the tonsil pass through the lateral wall of the pharynx, and terminate in subdigastric nodes located anterior to the jugular chain (29). The hypopharynx is rich in lymphatics. These converge at an orifice in the thyrohyoid membrane, through which also passes the superior laryngeal artery. After exiting the thyrohyoid membrane, the lymphatics ramify into several trunks that terminate in lymph nodes of the internal jugular chain (29).

REFERENCES

1. Bocca E, Pignataro O, Mosciaro O. Supraglottic surgery of the larynx. *Ann Otol Rhinol Laryngol* 1968;77:1005–1026.
2. Cotton A, Reilly JS. Congenital malformations of the larynx. In: Bluestone CD, Stool SE, eds. *Pediatric Otolaryngology*. Philadelphia, PA: WB Saunders; 1983:1215–1224.
3. Stell PM, Gudrun R, Watt J. Morphology of the human larynx. III. The supraglottis. *Clin Otolaryngol Allied Sci* 1981;6:389–393.
4. Stell PM, Gregory I, Watt J. Morphometry of the epithelial lining of the human larynx. I. The glottis. *Clin Otolaryngol Allied Sci* 1978;3:13–20.
5. Andrea M, Guerrier Y. The anterior commissure of the larynx. *Clin Otolaryngol Allied Sci* 1981;6:259–264.
6. Stell PM, Gregory I, Watt J. Morphology of the human larynx. II. The subglottis. *Clin Otolaryngol Allied Sci* 1980;5:389–395.
7. Hopp ES. The development of the epithelium of the larynx. *Laryngoscope* 1955;65:475–499.
8. Tucker J, Vidic B, Tucker GF Jr, et al. Survey of the development of laryngeal epithelium. *Ann Otol Rhinol Laryngol* 1976;85(Suppl 30):1–16.
9. Scott GB. A quantitative study of microscopical changes in the epithelium and subepithelial tissue of the laryngeal folds, sinus, and saccule. *Clin Otolaryngol Allied Sci* 1976;1:257–264.
10. Hyams VJ, Batsakis JG, Michaels L. *Tumors of the Upper Respiratory Tract and Ear. Atlas of Tumor Pathology, 2nd Ser, Fasc 25*. Washington, DC: Armed Forces Institute of Pathology; 1988.
11. Busuttil A. Dendritic pigmented cells within human laryngeal mucosa. *Arch Otolaryngol* 1976;102:43–44.
12. Goldman JL, Lawson W, Zak FG, et al. The presence of melanocytes in the human larynx. *Laryngoscope* 1972;82:824–835.
13. Nunez DA, Astley SM, Lewis FA, et al. Human papillomaviruses: A study of their prevalence in the normal larynx. *J Laryngol Otol* 1994;108:319–320.
14. Morshed K, Polz-Dacewicz M, Szymanski M, et al. Short-fragment PCR assay for highly sensitive broad-spectrum detection of human papillomaviruses in laryngeal squamous cell carcinoma and normal mucosa: Clinicopathologic evaluation. *Eur Arch Otorhinolaryngol* 2008;265(Suppl 1):S89–S96.
15. Nassar VH, Bridger GP. Topography of the laryngeal mucous glands. *Arch Otolaryngol* 1971;94:490–498.
16. Lundgren J, Olofsson J, Hellquist H. Oncocytic lesions of the larynx. *Acta Otolaryngol* 1982;94:335–344.
17. Gallagher JC, Puzon BQ. Oncocytic lesions of the larynx. *Ann Otol Rhinol Laryngol* 1969;78:307–318.
18. Wenig BM. Necrotizing sialometaplasia of the larynx. A report of two cases and a review of the literature. *Am J Clin Pathol* 1995;103:609–613.
19. Michaels L. *Ear, Nose, and Throat Histopathology*. New York: Springer-Verlag; 1987.
20. Richardson GM, Assor D. Thyroid tissue within the larynx. Case report. *Laryngoscope* 1971;81:120–125.
21. Bone RC, Biller HF, Irwin TM. Intralaryngotracheal thyroid. *Ann Otol Rhinol Laryngol* 1972;81:424–428.
22. Lawson W, Zak FG. The glomus bodies (paraganglia) of the human larynx. *Laryngoscope* 1974;84:98–111.
23. Kleinsasser O. The inferior laryngeal glomus. A nonchromaffin paraganglion, unknown so far, of the structure of the so-called carotid gland in human larynx. *Arch Ohr Nas Kehlkopfheilk* 1964;184:214–224.
24. Hill MJ, Taylor CL, Scott GBD. Chondromatous metaplasia in the human larynx. *Histopathology* 1980;4:205–214.
25. Iyer PV, Rajagopalan PV. Cartilaginous metaplasia of the soft tissues of the larynx. Case report and literature review. *Arch Otolaryngol* 1981;107:573–575.
26. Hollinshead WH. *Textbook of Anatomy*. 2nd ed. New York: Harper & Row; 1984.
27. Sanders I, Wu BL, Mu L, et al. The innervation of the human larynx. *Arch Otolaryngol Head Neck Surg* 1993;119:934–939.
28. Wu BL, Sanders I, Mu L, et al. The human communicating nerve. An extension of the external superior laryngeal nerve that innervates the vocal cord. *Arch Otolaryngol Head Neck Surg* 1994;120:1321–1328.
29. del Regato JA, Spjut HJ, Cox JD. *Ackerman and del Regato's Cancer: Diagnosis, Treatment, and Prognosis*. 6th ed. St. Louis, MO: Mosby; 1985.
30. Sumida S, Masuda Y, Watanabe S, et al. Development of the pharynx in normal and malformed fetuses. *Acta Otolaryngol Suppl* 1994;517:21–26.
31. Langman J. *Medical Embryology*. 2nd ed. Baltimore, MD: Williams & Wilkins; 1969.
32. Ali MY. Histology of the human nasopharyngeal mucosa. *J Anat* 1965;99:657–672.
33. Morin GV, Shank EC, Burgess LP, et al. Oncocytic metaplasia of the pharynx. *Otolaryngol Head Neck Surg* 1991;105:86–91.
34. Benke TT, Zitsch RP 3rd, Nashelsky MB. Bilateral oncocytic cysts of the nasopharynx. *Otolaryngol Head Neck Surg* 1995;112:321–324.
35. Melchionna RH, Moore RA. The pharyngeal pituitary gland. *Am J Pathol* 1938;14:763–772.

36. Boyd JD. Observations on the human pharyngeal hypophysis. *J Endocrinol* 1956;14:66–77.
37. McGrath P. Extrasellar adenohypophyseal tissue in the female. *Australas Radiol* 1970;14:241–247.
38. Langford L, Batsakis JG. Pituitary gland involvement of the sinonasal tract. *Ann Otol Rhinol Laryngol* 1995;104:167–169.
39. Kikuchi K, Kowada M, Sasaki J, et al. Large pituitary adenoma of the sphenoid sinus and nasopharynx: Report of a case with ultrastructural evaluations. *Surg Neurol* 1994;42:330–334.
40. Hollender AR. The nasopharynx. A study of 140 autopsy specimens. *Laryngoscope* 1946;56:282–304.
41. Toomey JM. Cysts and tumors of the pharynx. In: Paparella MM, Shumrick DA, eds. *Otolaryngology*. Philadelphia, PA: WB Saunders; 1980.
42. Nicolai P, Luzzago F, Maroldi R, et al. Nasopharyngeal cysts. Report of seven cases with review of the literature. *Arch Otolaryngol Head Neck Surg* 1989;115:860–864.
43. Binkhorst CD, Schierbeek P, Petten GJ. Neoplasms of the notochord. Report of a case of basilar chordoma with nasal and bilateral orbital involvement. *Acta Otolaryngol* 1957;47:10–20.
44. Batsakis JG. *Tumors of the Head and Neck: Clinical and Pathological Considerations*. 2nd ed. Baltimore, MD: Williams & Wilkins; 1979.
45. Begum S, Cao D, Gillison M, et al. Tissue distribution of human papillomavirus 16 DNA integration in patients with tonsillar carcinoma. *Clin Cancer Res* 2005;11:5694–5699.
46. Eggston AE, Wolff D. *Histopathology of the Ear, Nose and Throat*. Baltimore, MD: Williams & Wilkins; 1947.

16

Major Salivary Glands

Fernando Martínez-Madrigal

EMBRYOLOGIC AND POSTNATAL DEVELOPMENTAL CHANGES 440	**HETEROTOPIC SALIVARY TISSUE AND ITS SIGNIFICANCE** 451
Parotid Gland 440	**AGING CHANGES** 453
Submandibular Gland 442	Oncocytes 453
Sublingual Gland 442	Fatty Infiltration 454
LIGHT MICROSCOPY 443	**REACTIVE CHANGES** 454
SECRETORY UNITS 443	Metaplasia 454
Acini 443	Hyperplasia 454
Ducts 444	Atrophy 455
SEBACEOUS GLANDS 446	Regeneration 455
MYOEPITHELIAL CELLS 448	Artifacts 456
THE ROLE OF MYOEPITHELIAL CELLS IN SALIVARY GLAND TUMORS 449	**CORRELATIVE NORMAL AND NEOPLASTIC HISTOLOGY** 456
	IMMUNOHISTOCHEMISTRY 458
LYMPHOID TISSUE 451	**SPECIMEN HANDLING** 459
	REFERENCES 460

The primary function of the salivary glands is to moisten the mucous membranes of the upper aerodigestive tract. In humans this function is fulfilled by the continuous exocrine secretion of numerous minor salivary glands. These glands are located in the submucosa throughout the oral cavity, pharynx, and upper airways. In developed species, most of the saliva is elaborated by three pairs of major glands or salivary glands named by their location: the parotid, the submaxillary or submandibular, and the sublingual gland. They are connected symmetrically to the oral cavity, where they empty their secretion only under specific stimuli. The saliva produced by these glands (750 to 1,000 mL per 24 hours) plays an important role in preparing food for digestion, as well as in controlling the bacterial flora of the mouth. In recent years endocrine secretions in saliva have come to the attention of endocrinologists; these secretions include androgens, epidermal growth factor, transforming growth factor alpha, melatonin, cytokines,

and other peptides which act as immunoregulatory and anti-inflammatory agents (1,2). The quality of the saliva produced by the major glands is variable and depends on both the stimuli and the predominant participating gland. The stimuli may be hormonal or sympathetic and parasympathetic.

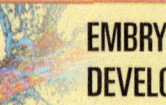

EMBRYOLOGIC AND POSTNATAL DEVELOPMENTAL CHANGES

Parotid Gland

During embryologic life, the parotid is the first of the three major glands to appear and is seen by the 6th week. It derives from the ectoderm as an epithelial bud from the primitive oral epithelium at the angle between the maxillary process and the mandibular arch (3). At the origin, the gland is formed by interactions among stem cells and progenitor cells. As the primordia grow, they ramify into a bush-like system surrounded by mesenchymal tissue. This mesenchyma

---

This chapter is an update of a previous version authored by Jaques Bosq and Odile Casiraghi.

and particularly, the basal lamina play an important role in the lobular organization of the gland. A protein called ectodysplasin plays a critical role in branching morphogenesis. Mutations of this protein result in X-linked hypohydrotic ectodermal dysplasia which may be associated with hypoplastic teeth, hair, and several exocrine glands including salivary glands (4). In the primitive gland the participation of fibroblastic growth factors/receptor signaling pathway are also essential. In transgenic mice that have, both copies of these genes deleted, the embryos do not develop salivary glands. In humans, the mutations may result in rare syndromes such as aplasia of lacrimal and salivary glands, and lacrimo-auriculo-dento-digital syndrome (5). Several studies have shown expression of fibronectin, laminin, gamma 2, and TIMP-3 in developing ducts; these proteins participate in epithelial morphogenesis, and probably in vascular and neural development (6–10). Apoptosis seems to play an important role in lumen formation. During the midstages of morphogenesis, apoptotic cells are detectable in developing salivary ducts at the site where lumina are formed (11). The lumina may be seen at day 14.5 with cytokeratin 7 (12,13). By the 7th week, the primitive gland moves in a dorsal and a lateral direction and reaches the preauricular region. Development of the facial nerve divides the gland by approximately the 10th week into superficial and deep portions.

By the 3rd month, the gland has attained its general pattern of organization. The epithelial structures are arranged in lobules, limited by a capsule of loose connective tissue (Fig. 16.1A). The mesenchyma is then colonized by numerous lymphocytes that later develop into intraglandular and extraglandular lymph nodes. By the 6th month, the epithelial cords are canalized and exhibit a double-cell ciliated cover. Cell differentiation begins in the excretory ducts with the progressive transformation of ciliated cells to columnar, squamous, and goblet cells (Fig. 16.1B) (14). Intralobular duct and acinar differentiation, including myoepithelial cell formation, begins at about the 8th month

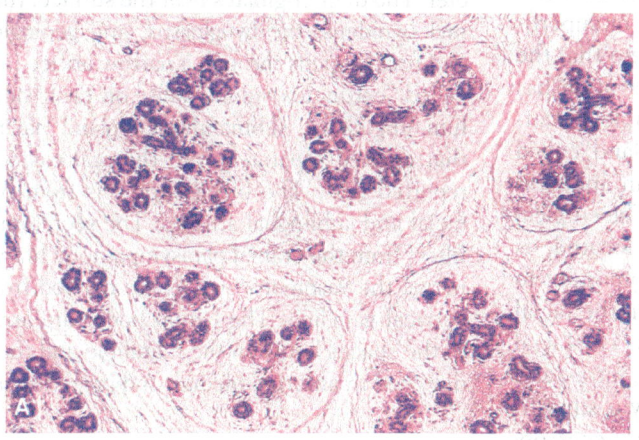
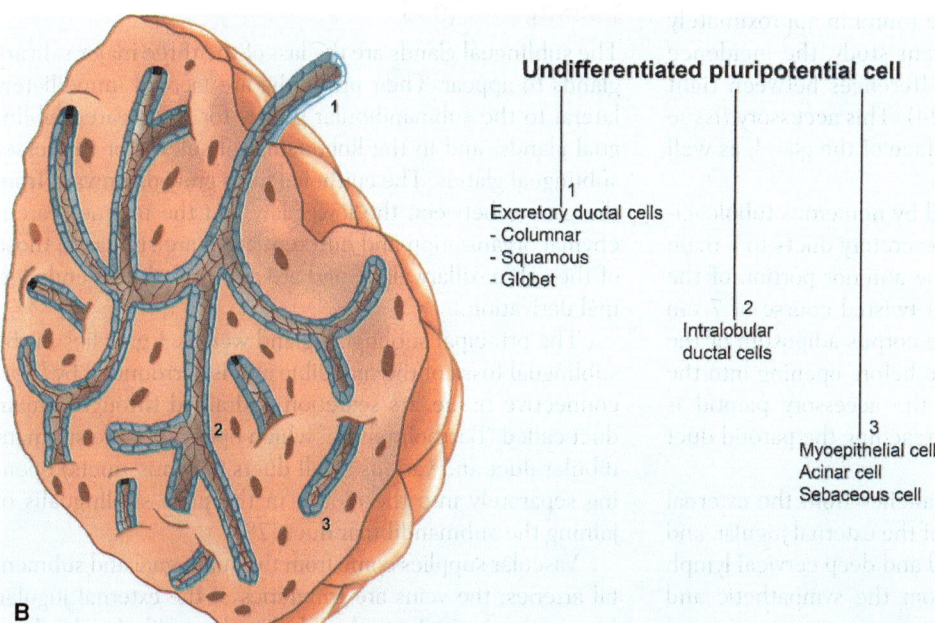

FIGURE 16.1 Development and histogenesis of the epithelial constituents of the salivary gland. **A:** Fetal parotid gland at 4 months; a lobular architecture is present. **B:** Schematic representation of the gland showing excretory ducts: (*1*) secretory ducts; (*2*) intralobular ducts; (*3*) and acini; the cellular lines of differentiation.

and myoepithelial cell differentiation by the 19th- to 24th-week period. These cells, arranged in the basal portions of the acini and intercalated ducts, appear as clear cells by electron microscopy. Between 25 and 32 weeks the myoepithelial cells become flattened and show cytoplasmic prolongations; myoepithelial markers may be detected by immunohistochemical methods at the earliest stages of development. These markers include smooth muscle actin, calponin, S-100 protein, and p63 protein (15,16). Saliva production starts at this time as a mucinous liquid, but several studies in rodents suggest that full maturation is completed only after birth (17–21).

The definitive location of the parotid is behind the inferior facial nerve, maxillary branch, below and in front of the external ear. It is enclosed within a fibroadipose capsule in a depression, whose anterior limit is the masseter muscle. Its superior limit is the zygomatic arch, the posterior limit is the tragus, and the inferior limit is the anterior border of the sternocleidomastoid muscle. The adult parotid is the largest of the three major salivary glands and weighs between 14 and 28 g. The gland is surrounded by a fine, poorly formed capsule and is divided into two portions by the facial nerve. The main portion, or superficial lobe, is flattened and quadrilateral; it is here that the majority of salivary tumors develop. This observation has permitted the development of conservative surgical treatment of many parotid tumors. The rest of the gland, called the deep lobe, is an irregular wedge shaped in anatomical relationship to the parapharyngeal space. The surgical anatomic area, where the parotid gland is located, is called the parotid region. In this region it is important to keep in mind the anatomical relations between the facial nerve, the gland, and the subcutaneous planes. The facial nerve has four parts designated as retro-, inter-, intra-, and preglandular. The parotid gland is covered by a superficial musculoaponeurosis and the skin (22,23). Accessory parotid tissue has been said to be found in approximately 20% of cases. However, in a recent study, the incidence was found to be 56% with no differences between right and left sides or between sexes (24). This accessory tissue may be found on the anterior surface of the gland, as well as along the parotid duct (25).

The parotid gland is composed by numerous tubuloacinar units connected through the excretory ducts to a main duct (Stensen duct) located in the anterior portion of the gland. The parotid duct follows a twisted course of 7 cm crossing the masseter muscle, the corpus adiposum of the cheek, and the buccinator muscle before opening into the oral vestibule. The secretion of the accessory parotid is emptied by an independent duct reaching the parotid duct in the masseter portion.

Blood supply is by arterial branches from the external carotid. The veins are tributaries of the external jugular, and the lymphatics join the superficial and deep cervical lymph nodes. Innervation is derived from the sympathetic and auriculotemporal nerves.

Submandibular Gland

The submandibular (submaxillary) gland, primordia appear at the end of the 6th week and, unlike the parotid, are probably of endodermal derivation (26). However, a recent study suggests that the sublingual process of the submandibular gland originates from a lateral ectodermal bud of the anlage of the submandibular gland. The epithelial bud appears in the groove between the lower jaw and tongue, at one side of the midplane. Extension of the glandular tissue in the mesenchyma goes backward beneath the lower jaw. Subsequent maturation and cell differentiation are similar to those of the parotid gland except for the lymphoid tissue, which is less obvious than in the parotid. Consequently, there is no lymph node formation inside the gland. The submandibular gland is finely encapsulated; it lies inside the submandibular triangle, an osteofibrous cavity, from which it takes the form of a triangular prism. This gland weighs approximately 7 to 8 g and, like the other major salivary glands, is organized in lobules connected to a main excretory duct—the submandibular duct (Wharton duct)—which measures 5 cm in length and 2 to 3 mm in diameter. The duct originates near the surface; runs between the mylohyoideus, the hyoglossus, and genioglossus muscles; and finally opens through a narrow orifice in a small papilla called "caruncula sublingualis" on each side of the frenulum linguae. A submandibular gland having three ducts that opened separately into the oral cavity has also been reported (27). The blood supply is from branches of the facial and sublingual arteries. The secretomotor nerves are fibers from the cranial parasympathetic branch of the facial nerve; the vasomotor nerves are derived from the superior cervical ganglion. The lymph nodes are arranged in a row in the spaces between the mandible and the gland, and are disposed in anterior, medial, and posterior groups.

Sublingual Gland

The sublingual glands are the last of the three major salivary glands to appear. Their primordia are located immediately lateral to the submandibular glands for the greater sublingual glands, and in the linguogingival sulcus for the lesser sublingual glands. The epithelial buds grow downward from the groove between the lower jaw and the tongue. Parenchymal organization and differentiation are similar to those of the submaxillary gland and are also probably of endodermal derivation.

The principal sublingual gland weighs 3 g. It lies in the sublingual fossa of the mandible and is surrounded by loose connective tissue. Its secretion is drained through a main duct called "Bartholin duct," which opens into the submandibular duct and various small ducts (Rivinus' ducts) opening separately into the mouth in the plica sublingualis or joining the submandibular duct (28).

Vascular supplies come from the sublingual and submental arteries; the veins are tributaries of the external jugular. Innervation is similar to that of the submandibular gland.

LIGHT MICROSCOPY

The salivary glands are compound exocrine tubuloacinar glands characterized by the aggregation of numerous secretory units. These units consist of acini where secretion is produced and a duct system that carries the secretion to the oral cavity and regulates the concentration of water and electrolytes. There are three types of salivary secretory units: the serous ones that contain amylase; the mucous ones where sialomucins are secreted; and mixed units made up of mucous and serous cells. According to the predominance of these types of secretory units, the salivary glands may be classified into three categories: serous, mucous, and mixed glands.

With the exception of rare mucous units, the parotid gland is of the serous type. The submandibular and the sublingual gland are mixed with a predominance of serous units in the first and a mucous predominance in the second. In accessory parotid gland, mixed secretory units can be found (29).

The lobular architecture of the glands is well defined by the anastomosed connective tissue trabeculae carrying the vascular and neural branches, as well as the excretory ducts.

SECRETORY UNITS

Acini

Serous acini consist of pear-shaped groups of epithelial cells surrounded by a distinct basement membrane. The epithelial cells have a basal nucleus and dense cytoplasm packed with basophilic (periodic acid–Schiff [PAS]-positive) zymogen granules. They vary in number depending on the different phases of the secretory cycle (Fig. 16.2) (30). The primary enzyme present in the zymogen granules is amylase or ptyalin, which splits starch into smaller water-soluble carbohydrates. However, there are other proteins in these granules including agglutinin, proline-rich proteins, and histatins (31). Other enzymes such as nonspecific antibacterial lysozyme, lactoferrin, trypsin and chymotrypsin-like proteases, lysyl endopeptidase, and histidine peptidase also have been detected in the cytoplasm of acinar cells (32–35). The acini have a central lumen, rarely visible by light microscopy, through which the secretion drains into the intercalated ducts. Ultrastructurally, acinar cells possess abundant endoplasmic reticulum, Golgi vesicles, mitochondria, and

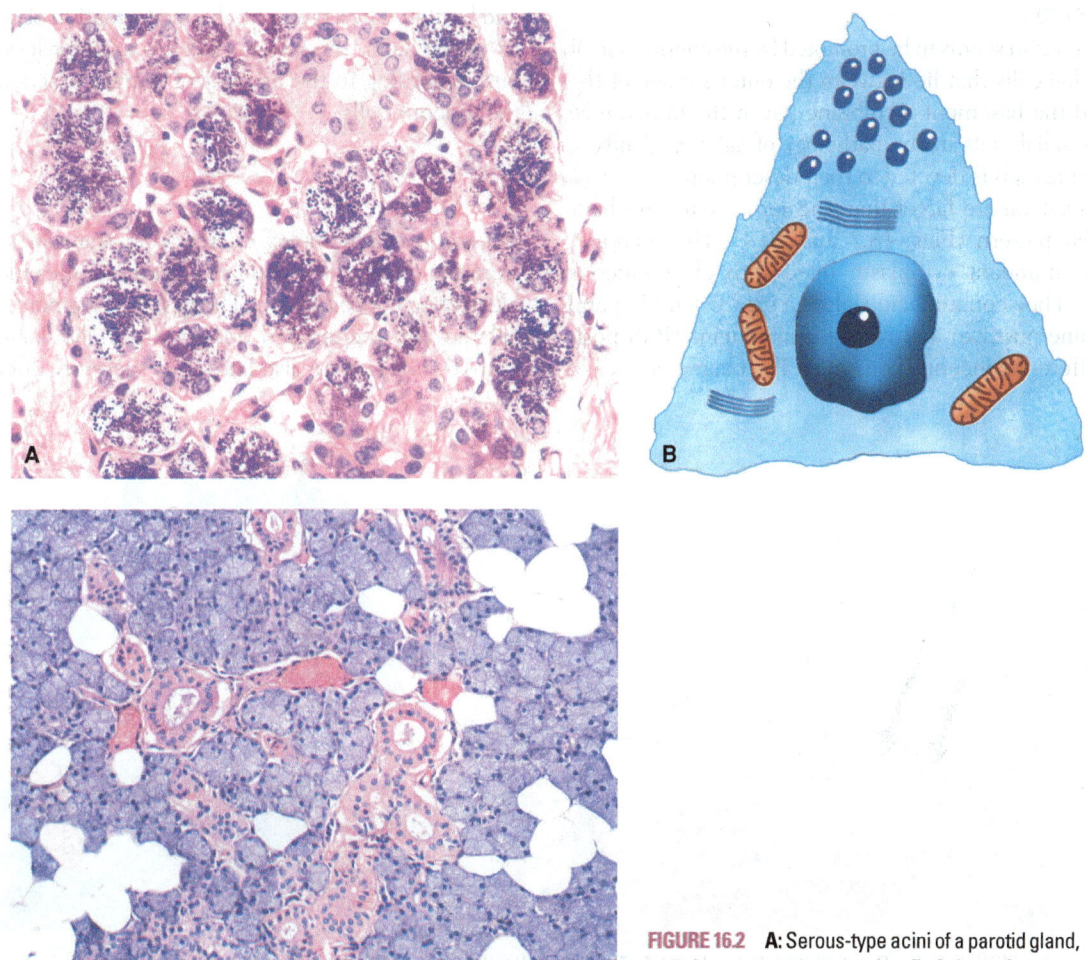

FIGURE 16.2 **A:** Serous-type acini of a parotid gland, with dense secretory granules. **B:** Schematic representation of an acinar cell. **C:** Acini after secretion.

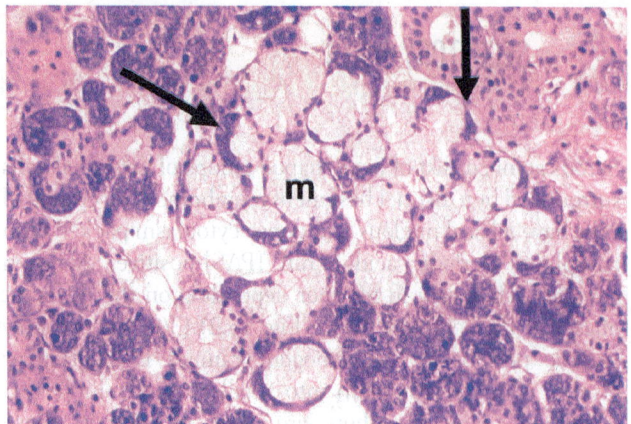

FIGURE 16.3 Histologic section of a submandibular gland. In mixed units (*arrows*) serous cells are grouped in a crescent-shaped formation on the periphery of the acini, whereas the mucous cells (*m*) are in direct contact with the duct system.

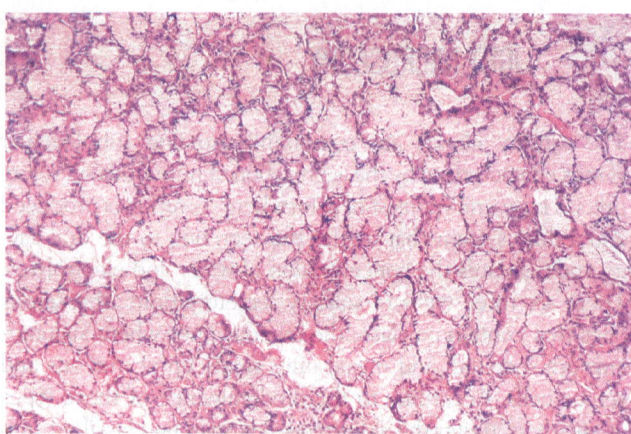

FIGURE 16.4 Mucous-type acini of the sublingual gland, larger and more irregular than the serous and mixed types. Note an inconspicuous duct system.

secretory granules. At the apical pole, the secretory cells are joined by an adhesive zone, whereas the basal side is adhered by desmosomes. Between the junctions, virtual spaces form the secretory capillaries, which are in continuation with the acinar lumen. Numerous microvilli protrude into the capillary lumen (30).

The excretion seems to be promoted by the contraction of myoepithelial cells that lie between the outer surface of the acinus and the basement membrane (given the importance of myoepithelial cells in the pathology of salivary glands, a separate paragraph is devoted to their description).

Mucous acini are larger than the serous type and have an irregular pattern (Figs. 16.3 and 16.4). The secretory cells have abundant cytoplasm filled with clear mucous substance. They contain acid sialomucins (alcian blue and mucicarmine positive) and neutral sialomucins (PAS positive) in different concentrations (36). The characteristics of these sialomucins also differ between submandibular and sublingual glands (37).

Mixed acini (Fig. 16.3) are typically found in the submandibular gland. These structures are characterized by the concentration of mucous cells near the intercalated duct and bordered by a crescent-shaped formation of serous cells. In mixed acini, the serous cells are more or less conspicuous, according to the amount of secretion accumulated in the mucous cells.

Ducts

A functionally complex duct system transports the saliva from the gland to the oral cavity, and modifies its water and electrolyte concentration. The first two segments, the intercalated and the striated duct, are intralobular (Figs. 16.5 and 16.6). They are also known as secretory ducts because

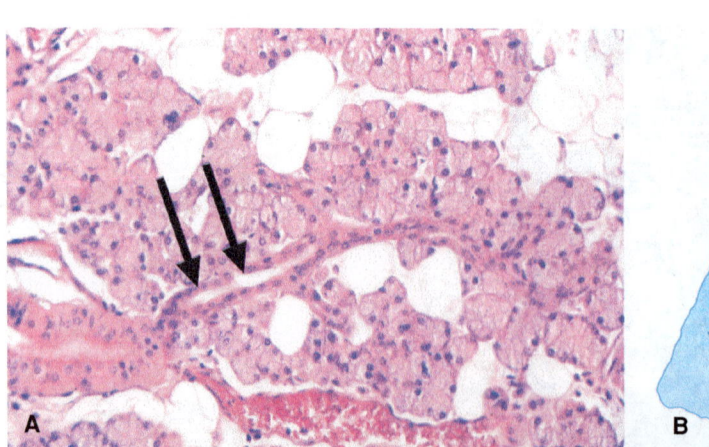
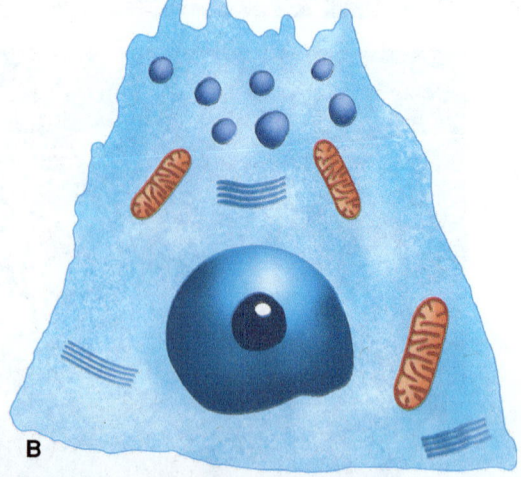

FIGURE 16.5 Parotid intralobular ducts. **A:** The intercalated ducts (*arrows*) (sectioned longitudinally) lie in contact with the acinus. **B:** Schematic representation of epithelial cell of the intercalated duct.

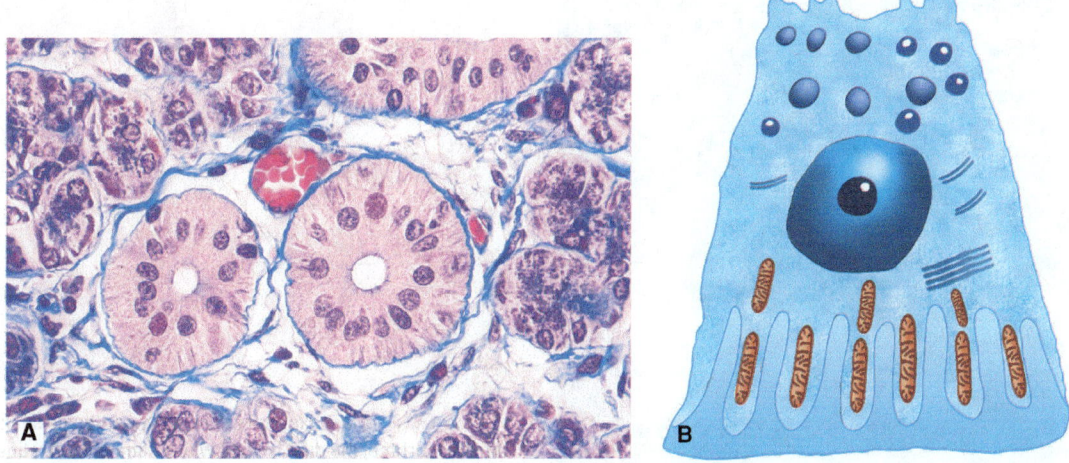

FIGURE 16.6 (A) Striated ducts are lined with a columnar epithelium of basal-striated appearance. (B) Schematic representation of a columnar cell of the striated duct.

of their metabolic activity. In salivary glands of rodents a granular duct is present between the intercalated and the striated duct (38). The other segments are interlobular and are called excretory ducts (39).

The intercalated duct lies directly in contact with the acinus. It is lined with a single layer of cuboidal epithelium and an irregular layer of myoepithelial cells (Fig. 16.5). The epithelial cells show a progressive transformation between the secretory and ductal cells and a high cytoplasmic content of lactoferrin and lysozyme (40). The lengths of the intercalated ducts are variable in the three major glands (Fig. 16.7). In the parotid gland, since the ducts are relatively long, they are easy to recognize in histologic sections (Fig. 16.5A). In contrast, they are short in the submandibular gland and hardly visible in the sublingual gland (Fig. 16.4). Undifferentiated cells exist on the basal side of the intercalated and striated ducts (41). These cells are positive for cytokeratins 5/6, 13, 16, and p63 on immunohistochemical staining (42,43) (Fig. 16.8).

The striated ducts are obvious in routine sections, particularly in the submandibular gland, where they are relatively longer (Figs. 16.3 and 16.7). The epithelial lining is simple columnar. On the basal side, it has characteristic parallel striations caused by the deep cell membrane invaginations and mitochondria (Fig. 16.6B). This structure represents a specialized surface on the epithelia involved in the transport of water and electrolytes. The numerous mitochondria are correlated with the strong eosinophilia

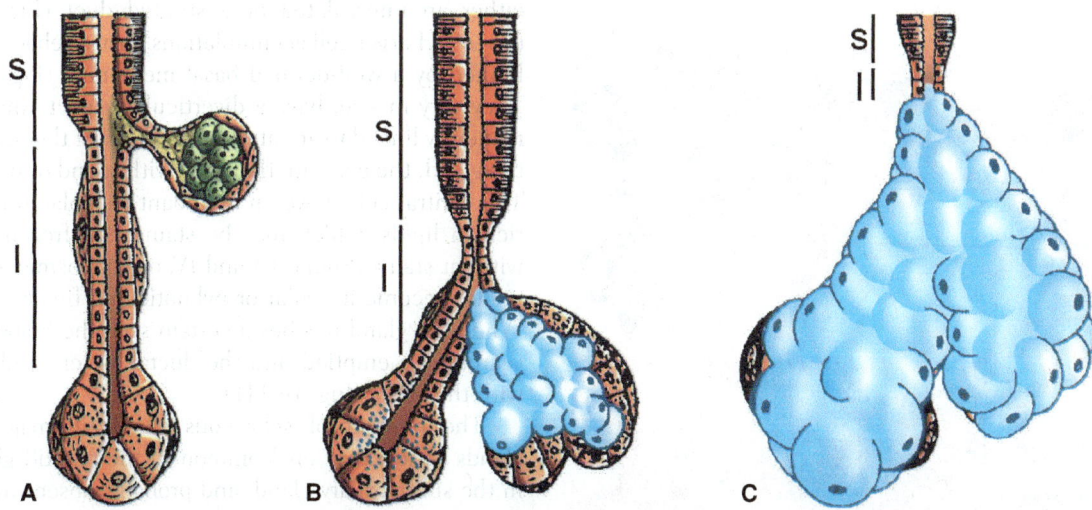

FIGURE 16.7 The morphology of the major salivary glands is characterized by three types of secretory units. In the parotid (**A**) the intercalated duct (*I*) is longer than in the submandibular (**B**) and sublingual glands (**C**). In contrast, the striated duct (*S*) is longer in the submandibular gland. Sebaceous glands are more frequent in the parotid gland; in the sublingual gland the intralobular ducts are inconspicuous.

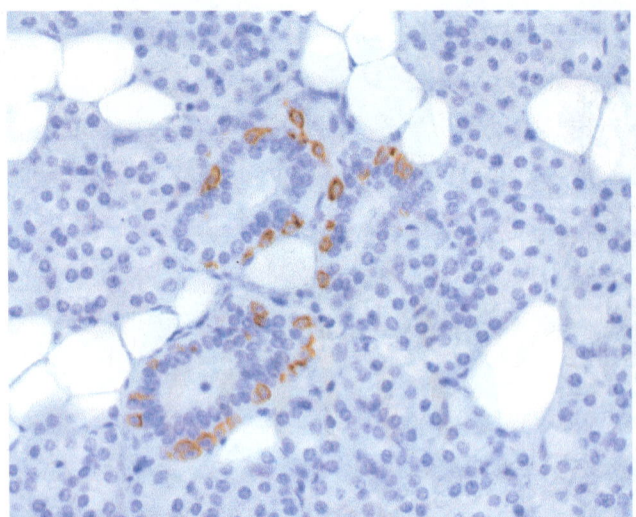

FIGURE 16.8 Basal cells stained with cytokeratin 5/6.

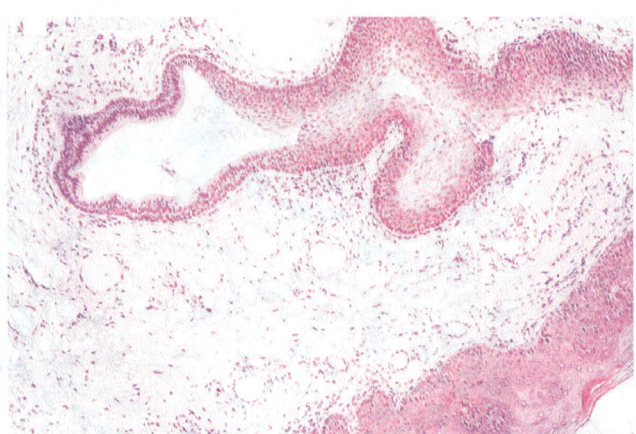

FIGURE 16.10 Main excretory duct in the caruncula sublingualis. Near the oral surface, the duct is lined with a squamous stratified epithelium.

of the duct. Various enzymes such as adenosine triphosphatase (ATPase), succinate dehydrogenase, and carbonic anhydrase (44) are present in the cytoplasm of the striated ducts and provide them with a metabolic energy system capable of concentrating some of the elements present in the saliva.

The striated ducts are connected with the interlobular ducts located in the septal connective tissue. These ducts are lined with a columnar pseudostratified epithelium with sparse goblet cells (Fig. 16.9). They become progressively larger before joining the principal duct. The principal function of interlobular ducts is to transport saliva, but their role in regeneration is proposed by means of the hypothetical undifferentiated pluripotential cells. In theory, these cells may follow the same cellular lines as in embryonic development, and are perhaps implicated in the metaplastic and neoplastic alterations of salivary glands (44) which are more frequent in these ducts. Whether these cells function as pluripotent cells is still a topic of discussion.

The principal duct consists of a thick external fibrous coat of collagen (similar to dermal collagen), and elastic fiber bundles. The epithelium is columnar stratified and becomes squamous stratified near the opening in the mucous membrane (Fig. 16.10).

SEBACEOUS GLANDS

In 1931, Hamperl (45) described the presence of sebaceous glands histologically similar to those of the cutaneous adnexa. Other authors have indeed recognized such structures which appear as isolated cells in the wall of either an intercalated or a striated duct (Fig. 16.11A) (46–49). Larger cell accumulations form a sebaceous gland limited by a well-defined basal membrane (Fig. 16.11B). They vary in size, have a diverticular aspect, and are permanently linked to an interlobular duct. At the periphery of the gland, the cells are flattened with round or oval nuclei. The central cells have an abundant vacuolated cytoplasm rich in lipids, which may be stained, in frozen sections, with fat stains (Sudan III and IV, oil red, osmic acid). The nuclei become irregular or pyknotic and finally disappear. When the gland reaches a certain size, the holocrine-type secretion is emptied into the ductal system and is mixed with the saliva (Fig. 16.11D).

The number of sebaceous glands in major salivary glands varies; they are common in the parotid gland, rare in the submaxillary gland, and probably absent in the sublingual gland. They are diffusely scattered throughout the parenchyma, where their numbers also vary greatly. Their presence or absence in the different lobules is not related to either age or sex (49).

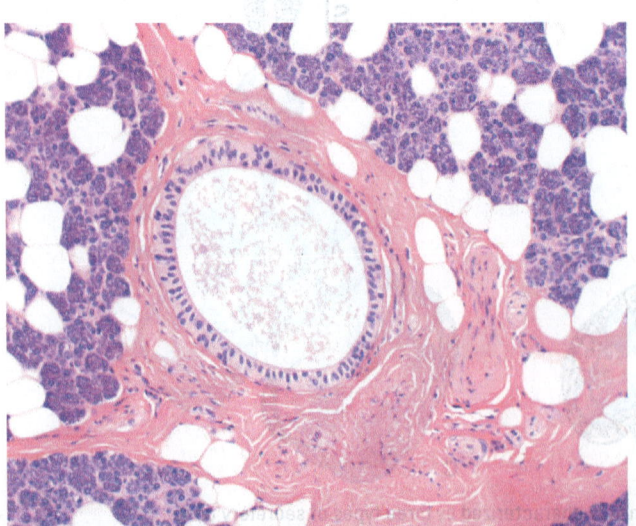

FIGURE 16.9 Interlobular duct adjacent to vessels in the septal connective tissue.

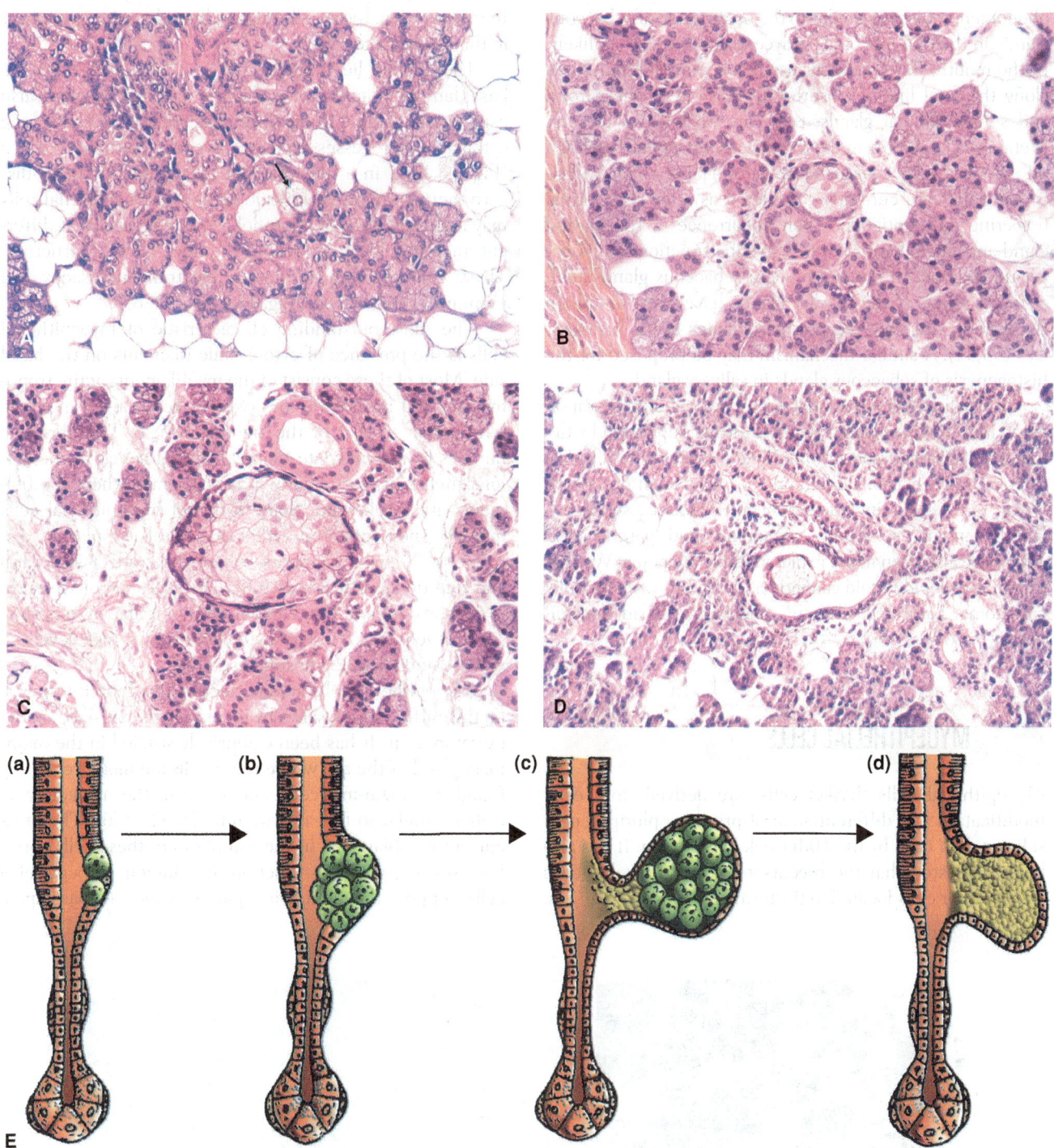

FIGURE 16.11 Sebaceous elements in a parotid gland. Isolated sebaceous cells can be seen in the duct wall (*arrows*) (**A**). They proliferate to form a well-defined gland (**B, C**); secretion is present in the lumen of the duct (**D**). Drawing (**E**) illustrates the above features.

In a review of 100 parotid glands selected at random from our material, we found sebaceous glands in 42% of cases. They were also found in 5% of 100 submandibular glands. These findings are in agreement with other authors. Thus, we conclude that their incidence in the parotid gland is more frequent than imagined. The more sections that are examined, the more sebaceous glands are found; it is, therefore, merely a question of looking for them. If the entire parotid gland were examined meticulously, it would be difficult not to find a sebaceous gland (49).

The presence of sebaceous glands in the salivary tissue has not been satisfactorily explained. A heterotopic phenomenon (48,49) similar to the occurrence of sebaceous glands in the oral mucosa (Fordyce disease) seems unlikely. In the mouth, this condition may result from aberrant buds along the fetal line of closure (50–52); but in the parotid and submandibular glands, there are no lines of closure. Metaplasia beginning in the ducts does not explain the high frequency of sebaceous glands in parotid parenchyma. Sebaceous glands are currently considered as a form of normal holocrine differentiation. Their occurrence in the parotid gland appears to be related to a specific function that is not yet understood. In the oral mucosa sebaceous glands analogous to those of the salivary glands have been found. In the former, androgen receptor participates in the histogenesis (53,54). A similar mechanism may be proposed for the histogenesis of sebaceous glands in salivary glands.

The belief that a potential for sebaceous differentiation exists in the salivary parenchyma is further supported by the fact that salivary tumors or tumor-like conditions with partial or complete sebaceous differentiation have been described. These rare lesions include sebaceous adenoma, sebaceous lymphadenoma, sebaceous carcinoma, and parotid cyst. They have also been noted in pleomorphic adenoma, Warthin tumor, mucoepidermoid carcinoma, epithelial–myoepithelial carcinoma, basal cell adenoma, and basal cell adenocarcinoma (55–61).

MYOEPITHELIAL CELLS

Myoepithelial cells (basket cells) are derived from early modification and differentiation of primitive pluripotential salivary duct cells by the 10th week of gestation. It has also been suggested that the precursors of myoepithelial cells are the clear cells located in the terminal and striated ducts. In regeneration, these cells migrate from the acinar periphery to the duct–acinar region.

These cells lie between the epithelial cells and the basal lamina of acini, intercalated ducts, and probably also exist in the striated ducts. The cells are flat and have long cytoplasmic processes extending over the epithelial surface (Fig. 16.12A) in a network that makes it difficult to discern them in routine histologic sections. Myoepithelial cells may assume, however, morphologic modifications at different anatomic locations within the ductal acinar structure. These cells are best studied by electron microscopy and immunohistochemistry (Fig. 16.12B) (62–65).

The most outstanding characteristic of myoepithelial cells is the presence of cytoplasmic filaments on the basal side. Most of these consist of the myofilaments actin, tropomyosin, and myosin (66,67), which are arranged in a pattern similar to that of the smooth muscle. Tonofibril-like bundles of intermediate filaments are attached to the cellular junctions, particularly in desmosomes where the filaments are cytokeratin. Some forms of myoepithelial cells may also show scattered, rather than basal, cytoplasmic distribution of these filaments, which may reflect structural and functional differences (68). The presence of vimentin is not constant and the filament desmin is absent in normal myoepithelium (69). The cytoplasm shows high levels of ATPase and alkaline phosphatase (70).

Myoepithelial cells are contractile; this function speeds up the outflow of the saliva by increasing the pressure on the excretory unit. It has been extensively studied in the mammary gland of the rat, where these cells are more frequently found. Oxytocin-induced contraction in the myoepithelial cells is similar to that of true muscle cells (70). The presence of myofilaments in the cytoplasm of these cells correlates strongly with this function. In addition, myoepithelial cells support the underlying parenchyma and participate

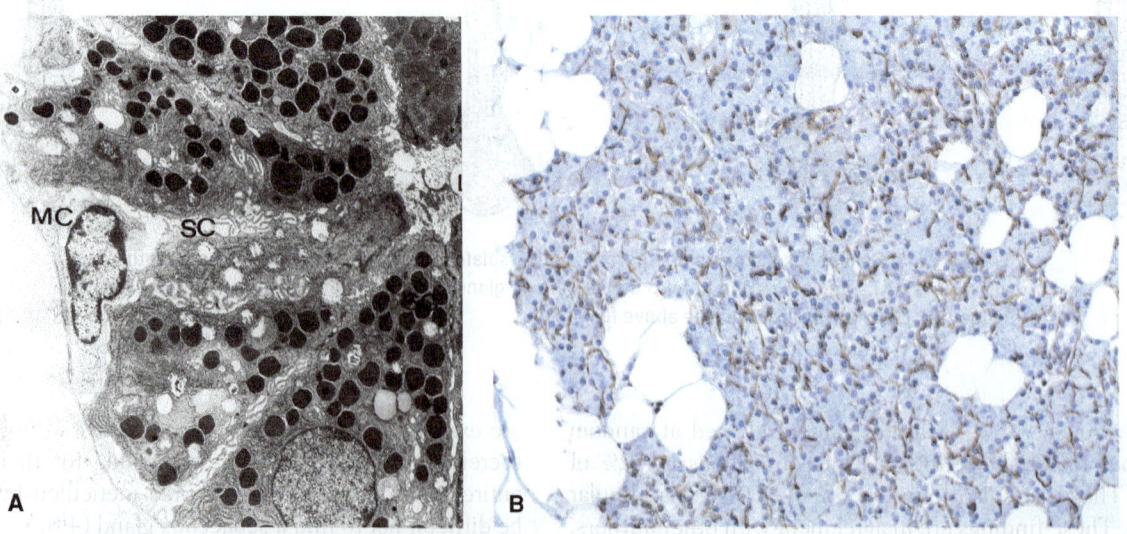

FIGURE 16.12 A: Ultrastructure of myoepithelial cell (MC) between epithelial secretory cells and secretory capillaries (SC) (×6000). **B:** Immunostaining of myoepithelial cells for muscular actin.

in the elaboration of the basal lamina. This last function is important in some hyperplastic and neoplastic alterations, where the myoepithelial cells produce fibronectin, laminin, and type III collagen (71–78). All these proteins are constituents of the basal lamina. In addition, myoepithelial cells are also involved in the production of tenascin, an extracellular matrix glycoprotein (79).

The myoepithelial cells share an epithelial and mesenchymal structure and function. Altered myoepithelial cells may manifest (in neoplastic proliferation) one or both characteristics. These cells are now considered a key factor in the morphology of many salivary neoplasms and in the morphologic variability of some tumors (80).

THE ROLE OF MYOEPITHELIAL CELLS IN SALIVARY GLAND TUMORS

The presence of myoepithelial cells in different histologic types of salivary gland tumors is well documented, as is the role of these cells in biologic behavior (Table 16.1).

The role of myoepithelial cells in the pleomorphic adenoma has been extensively studied. This tumor, sometimes called "mixed tumor" because of the epithelial and mesenchymal mixture of tissues, is the most frequent neoplasm of the major salivary glands (81,82). It is now accepted that myoepithelial cells play a crucial role in the neoplastic process by forming both epithelial and mesenchymal structures in most pleomorphic adenomas (83–90). The participation of the contractile elements is also accepted in epithelial–myoepithelial carcinoma, a malignant tumor that mimics the normal structure of the intercalated duct (91–96), and myoepithelioma including malignant cases, in which the myoepithelial cells are the only tumoral element showing different cellular forms (97–103). They also have been demonstrated in polymorphous low-grade adenocarcinoma (PLGA) (104,105), basal cell adenoma (106–110), adenoid cystic carcinoma (111,112), and basal cell adenocarcinoma (113). Myoepithelial cell participation is also present in congenital tumors of salivary gland origin such as sialoblastoma (114) and salivary gland anlage tumor (115). Although there are rare reports of myoepithelial cells in mucoepidermoid carcinoma (116) most studies have failed to show these cells.

Several morphologic types of modified myoepithelial cells are currently recognized (Fig. 16.13):

1. Stellate or myxoid cells, which are typically present in chondromyxoid areas of pleomorphic adenoma.

2. Spindle-shaped or myoid cells, which can be identified in pleomorphic adenoma and some types of myoepithelioma.

3. Hyalin or plasmacytoid cells (117), which can be seen in pleomorphic adenomas and can be present in myoepitheliomas also called plasmacytoid myoepitheliomas. These cells show abundant cytoplasmic filaments that give a hyalin eosinophilic aspect.

4. Clear cells, which are found in many salivary tumors on the external surface of ducts or duct-like structures. These are also characteristic in epithelial–myoepithelial carcinoma.

5. Lipoid cells, which are present in pleomorphic adenomas with extensive lipometaplasia (118).

6. Oncocytic cells, which are recognized in some types of epithelial–myoepithelial carcinoma of oncocytic type, pleomorphic adenoma and in oncocytic myoepithelioma (119,120).

7. Osteoblastic and myoepithelial cells are responsible for bone formation in cases of pleomorphic adenoma (121).

8. Squamous cells, which are present in pleomorphic adenomas (122).

Bidirectional differentiation of the modified myoepithelium has been well documented. Myoepithelial cells with mesenchymal characteristics secrete mesenchymal mucins such as the acid glycosaminoglycans (hyaluronic acid, heparin sulfate, chondroitin-4-sulfate, and chondroitin-6-sulfate) (123,124), basement membrane constituents, elastin (85,86), and tenascin (79). In addition to contractile filaments (actin and myosin) and related proteins such as calponin, vimentin becomes strongly positive, particularly in the spindle-shaped form (125,126). S-100 protein, which is a common marker used for myoepithelium, enhances its positivity in chondroid, myxoid, and stellate cells, particularly if they are associated with a myxoid stroma (127,128). Plasmacytoid myoepithelial cells may be negative for the muscular markers (129). Myoepithelial cells are a central element in the histologic formation and organization of different salivary gland tumors. The cytomorphologic features and the variability of the extracellular products account for the morphologic heterogeneity of these lesions. The presence of these cells varies widely, from minimal as in basal cell adenomas to

TABLE 16.1
Salivary Gland Tumors with Myoepithelial Cell Participation

Benign tumors	Myoepitheliomas Pleomorphic adenoma Basaloid adenomas
Malignant tumors	Epithelial–myoepithelial carcinoma Adenoid cystic carcinoma Polymorphous low grade adenocarcinoma Basaloid carcinoma
Congenital tumors	Sialoblastoma Salivary gland anlage tumor

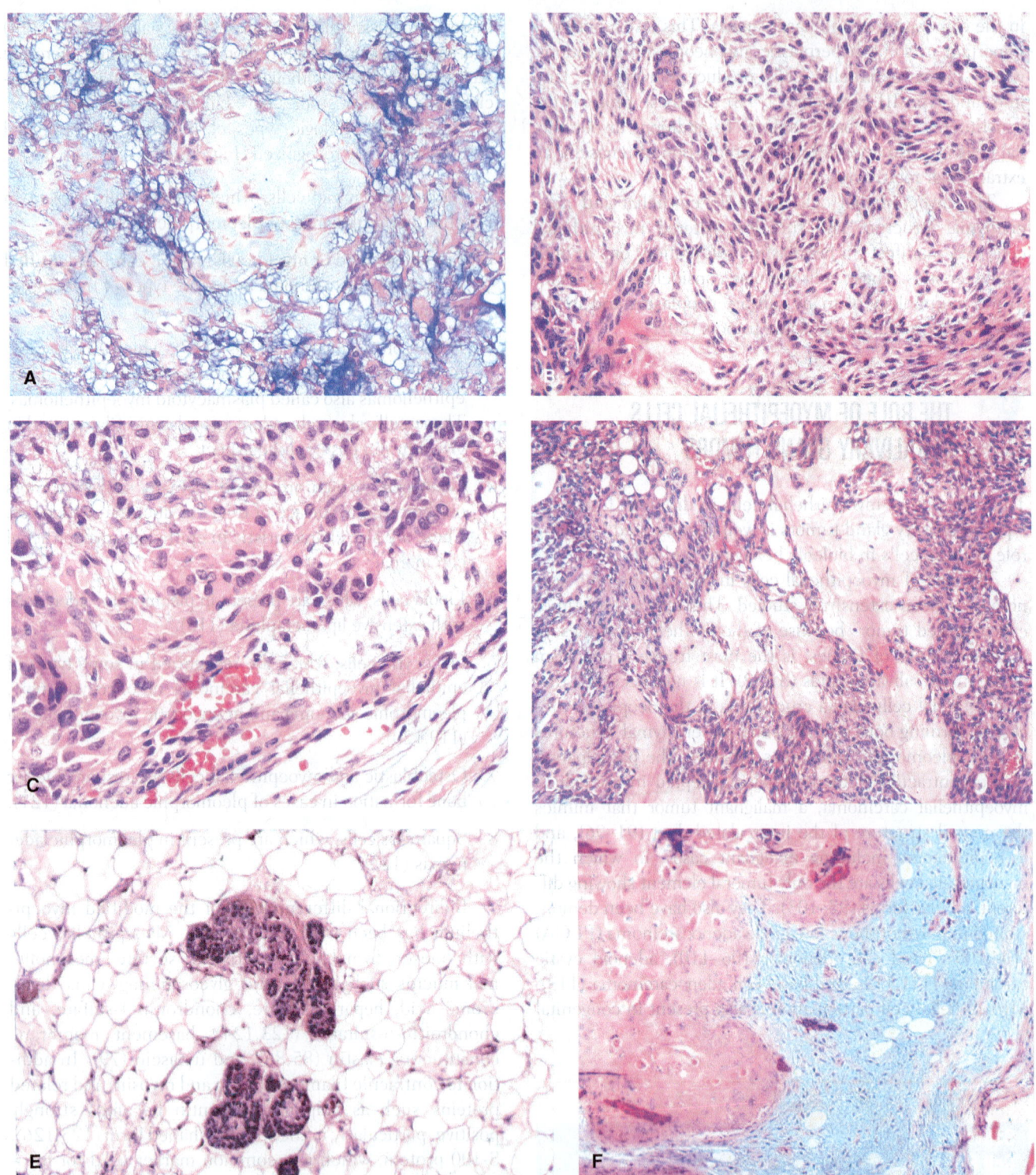

FIGURE 16.13 Some types of modified myoepithelial cells in pleomorphic adenomas (**A**) chondromyxoid, (**B**) spindle shaped, (**C**) hyalin or plasmacytoid, (**D**) osteoblastic, (**E**) lipoid, and (**F**) squamous.

marked, as in myoepitheliomas. Evidence of the protective effect of myoepithelial cells in malignant tumors is growing. Protease inhibitors like maspin, alpha-1-antitrypsin, TIMP-1, and nexin II are anti-invasive factors produced by myoepithelial cells (130,131). Malignant tumors with an important myoepithelial cell component often behave less aggressively. Myoepithelial carcinomas tend to be lobulated tumors rather than infiltrating and have a better survival. In addition there is evidence that myoepithelial cells may inhibit angiogenesis (132,133).

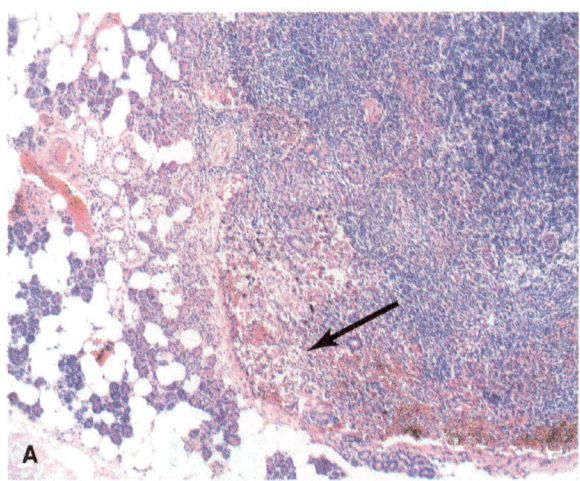
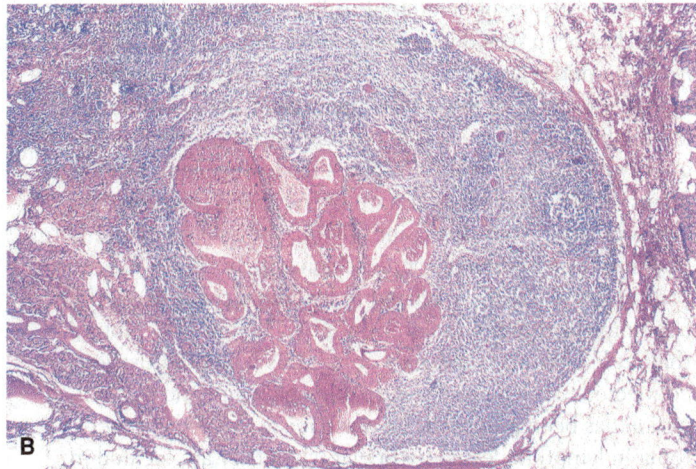

FIGURE 16.14 Lymph node of the parotid gland. **A:** Presence of glandular ducts in the medullary region (*arrow*). **B:** Duct dilatation and oncocytic transformation in another lymph node of the same patient.

LYMPHOID TISSUE

The immune system of salivary glands comprises of two elements of the mucosa-associated immune system. One is the secretory component, a glycoprotein receptor for dimeric IgA and pentameric IgM that is produced by epithelial cells in the acini, intercalated ducts, and striated ducts (134,135). The other element is lymphoid tissue, which is either distributed diffusely, or organized into lymph nodes. Isolated lymphoid cells are present in the connective tissue near the acini and ducts. They are variable in number in the different glands and yield principally IgA, (nearly 80% of the immunoglobulins in saliva), along with a lesser quantity of IgG and IgM (116). Small lymph nodes are usually present near the surface of the parotid gland, but not in the other salivary glands. Nevertheless, lymphoid cell aggregates are present in fetal submandibular and sublingual glands (136). These nodes usually contain salivary ducts and acini in the medullary region (Fig. 16.14A), a phenomenon probably due to the close relationship between developing gland and lymphoid tissue during embryonic life.

Lymph nodes are thought to participate in the histogenesis of Warthin tumor. Although they have been pinpointed as the origin of the lymphoid tissue that characterizes this neoplasm, the theory is still under debate. Different mechanisms have been proposed, but the most widely accepted theory states that the lesion originates from the ducts inside lymph nodes within or adjacent to the parotid gland (137–139). According to this concept, the epithelial component of the tumor corresponds to altered ducts inside a lymph node and the lymphatic component is, in fact, a lymph node. The following arguments support this theory: salivary tissue is frequently present in intraparotid or periparotid lymph nodes (Fig. 16.14A); with the exception of a few cases, this tumor is exclusive to the parotid region; it is common to find early stages of oncocytic and papillary transformations in lymph nodes of the parotid region (Fig. 16.14B); and finally, tumors identical to the epithelial structure of Warthin tumor occur outside the lymph nodes, but without lymphocytic components (140,141).

The diffuse lymphoid tissue may increase in chronic sialadenitis, particularly in immunologic reactions such as the benign lymphoepithelial lesion associated with Sjögren syndrome and the immunoglobulin G4-related disease. In these instances, the lymphoid tissue may obscure the glandular parenchyma in a diffuse or nodular manner, and epimyoepithelial islands may be formed (142,143). The polyclonal character of the lymphoid cells is a useful criterion in the differential diagnosis of malignant lymphoma, which can occur in a pre-existing benign lymphoepithelial lesion.

HETEROTOPIC SALIVARY TISSUE AND ITS SIGNIFICANCE

The presence of salivary tissue outside the major salivary glands and the oral cavity, pharynx, and upper airways is considered a heterotopia. This heterotopia may be classified as intranodal and extranodal in a number of locations in the head, neck, and other sites.

Heterotopia is common in the lymph nodes near the parotid gland, but is much less frequent in the submandibular region and in other upper cervical nodes (144,145). The glandular elements are either normal or atrophic; they consist mainly of ducts, but acini are also found. They are localized in the medullary region and comprise a variable proportion of lymphoid and salivary tissues. Although all types of secretory units are found, serous ones are predominant. The histologic architecture is similar to a normal gland. The lymph nodes exhibit a normal structure or some degree of lymphoreticular hyperplasia.

The incidence of heterotopic salivary tissue in the lymph nodes has been well documented (146). It is typically found in the parotid region of fetuses during various stages of development, usually in more than one lymph node. In adults, although the incidence is not constant, it is nonetheless frequent (147). In most of the reports, the histogenetic mechanisms of this phenomenon have been related to embryonic development. From this point of view, the salivary tissue is trapped during embryologic development. In the fetus, the parotid gland is closely related to lymphoid tissue from the beginning of the 2nd month. Moreover, Bairati (147) found that, at least in the first years of life, this lymphoid tissue is connected to the parotid gland. Although lymphatic dissemination has been proposed as a mechanism of salivary heterotopia in lymph nodes, in particular when they are located in the lower neck, this theory is only speculative (148).

Extralymphatic heterotopias are rare and often latent, but may be responsible for symptomatology. Heterotopic salivary tissue has been described in several sites including head and neck, thorax, and abdomen (Table 16.2). In the head and neck, heterotopia is limited to the mandible, ear, palatine tonsil, mylohyoid muscle, pituitary gland, and cerebellopontine angle (149–151). All these sites, with the exception of the last, may be related to the embryonic migration of the salivary glands. Rare salivary gland heterotopia may be found in the base of the neck, particularly around the sternoclavicular joint, in the thyroid gland and parathyroid glands, pulmonary hilar lymph nodes, anterior chest wall, and rectum (Fig. 16.15) (152–157).

Most examples of salivary heterotopia are explained in relation to lines of migration of the parotid and submandibular

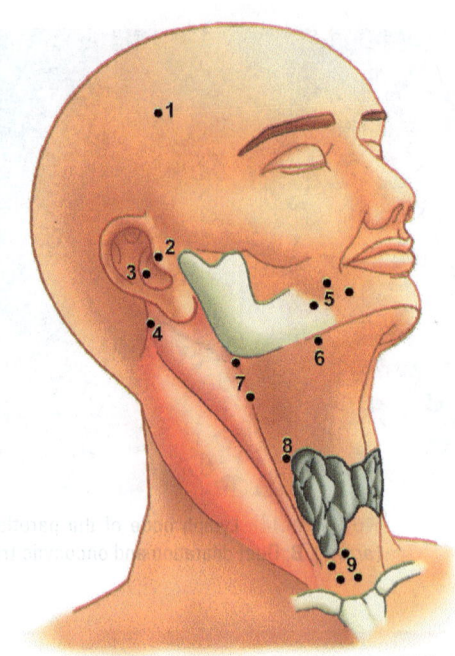

FIGURE 16.15 Extranodal salivary heterotopias. Pituitary gland (*1*), middle ear (*2*), external auditory canal (*3*), cerebellopontine angle (*4*), mandible (*5*), oropharynx (*6*), cervical superior (*7*), thyroid capsule (*8*), and lower anterolateral neck (*9*).

TABLE 16.2
Salivary Gland Heterotopias
Lacrimal gland
Pituitary gland
External auditory canal
Middle ear
Cerebellopontine angle
Upper neck
Thyroglossal duct
Thyroid gland
Parathyroid gland
Mediastinum
Stomach
Rectum
Prostate gland

glands. In the mandible the presence of salivary heterotopia may be related to a bone cavity and usually contains submandibular gland tissue. These inclusions are most common in the posterior lower jaw, near the angle. Originally described in 1942 by Stafne, they are often considered as heterotopias (158). This defect may be found in the anterior position. A recent study showed that heterotopic salivary tissue was present in 0.3% of maxillofacial marrow samples. The origin of this tissue is a matter of debate but the most accepted hypothesis is metaplasia of the odontogenic epithelium (159). In the lower neck, an association with cysts and sinuses is frequent. This condition, along with the topographic presentation, has been related to the branchial apparatus (160) and, in particular, to a defective closure of the precervical His' sinus. The different abnormalities related to this defect correspond embryologically to topographic distribution through the neck from the ear to the clavicle. When this defect occurs, the salivary tissue is the result of abnormal tissue differentiation (heteroplasia). Willis (159) has argued that this is the mechanism of heterotopia. This mechanism may also account for the salivary tissue in remnants of Rathke pouch (150) and the thyroglossal duct.

Neoplastic transformation in heterotopic salivary tissue may pose a problem in differential diagnosis of metastasis in a cervical lymph node (144). Excluding Warthin tumor, pleomorphic adenoma, mucoepidermoid carcinoma, and adenoid cystic carcinoma are the most frequent tumors arising in heterotopic salivary tissue. In fact, heterotopia is an explanation for many aberrant salivary tumors (148,160,161) and some cervical lymph node metastases

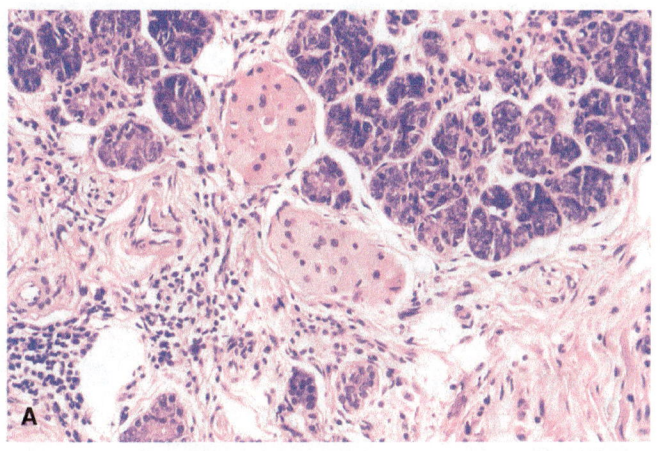
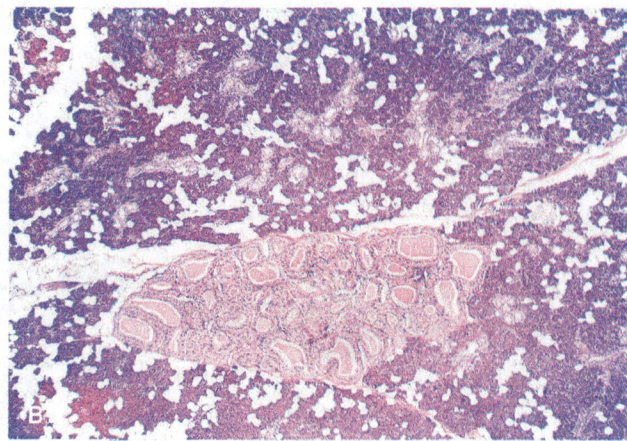
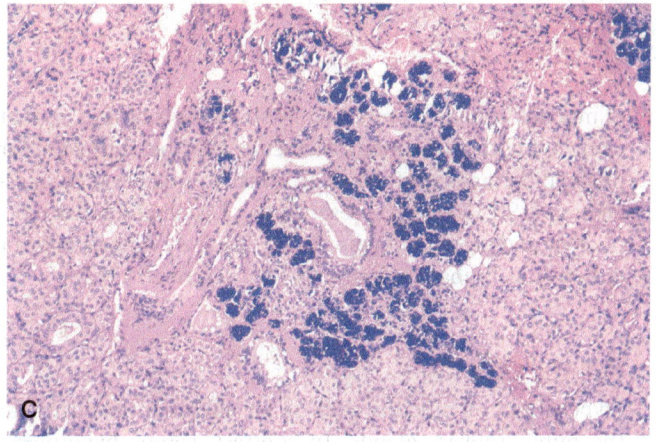

FIGURE 16.16 A: Oncocytes in intralobular ducts of a normal submandibular gland. Note the abundant and granulated cytoplasm. **B:** Nodular oncocytic hyperplasia, and **(C)** diffuse oncocytosis.

which are thought to be metastases of an unknown primary. Primary salivary tumors of the mandible may originate in this aberrant tissue (162).

AGING CHANGES

Oncocytes

The oncocyte is an altered swollen cell characterized by an abundant eosinophilic granular cytoplasm rich in altered mitochondria and enzymes (Fig. 16.16A) (163). This cell is frequently present in interlobular ducts and is less frequent in acinar cells. Oncocytes are more common in the parotid gland. They are rare before 50 years of age, increase in frequency with advancing years, and become constant after 70 years (164). Although seldom necessary, oncocytes may be detected by histochemical methods using acid phosphotungstic hematoxylin or more specifically by immunohistochemical methods with antibodies to human mitochondria (165).

Oncocytic proliferations are a common finding in organs with endocrine function or endocrine dependence (166). Numerous researchers are presently interested in the production of various peptides with endocrine function in the intralobular ducts of rodent salivary glands (167–170). Other workers are investigating the presence of neuroendocrine peptides such as the substance P-like, beta-endorphin–like and a calcitonin-related peptide. In addition, neuroendocrine regulation of inflammation by the submandibular gland has been explained by immunoneuroendocrine communication controlled by cervical sympathetic nerves (171–173).

The proliferation of oncocytes is called oncocytosis or oncocytic metaplasia when it is diffuse and generally without pathologic significance. In other cases, this proliferation presents a nodular pattern known as nodular hyperplasia or present as a diffuse oncocytosis (174–176). Histologically, it is easy to distinguish in the salivary parenchyma as one or several small foci of oncocytes that are well circumscribed, but not encapsulated. The cells may be arranged in solid cords or ductal structures and in rare cases may replace most of the gland (Fig. 16.16 B and C). Oncocytes participate in various salivary gland tumors in approximately 10% of cases (176). The most common is Warthin tumor, and they are also observed in basal cell adenoma, pleomorphic adenoma, myoepithelioma, PLGA, mucoepidermoid carcinoma, acinic cell carcinoma, and epithelial–myoepitelial carcinoma (177–179). Pure oncocytomas and oncocytic carcinomas occasionally occur in salivary glands (180,181) and the rare oncocytic lipoadenoma and oncocytic cystadenoma (141,182,183). An interesting observation shows that oncocytic differentiation in epithelial–myoepithelial carcinoma

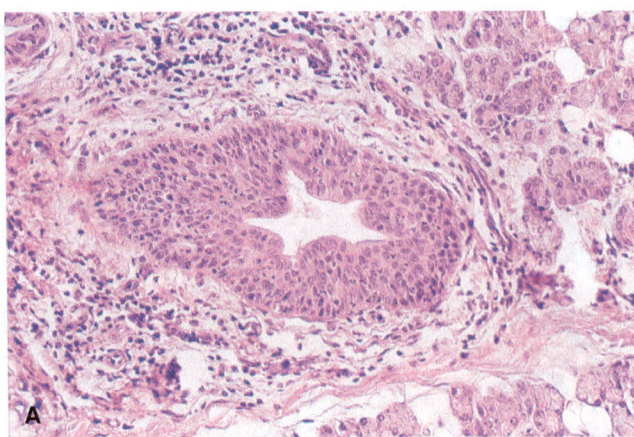 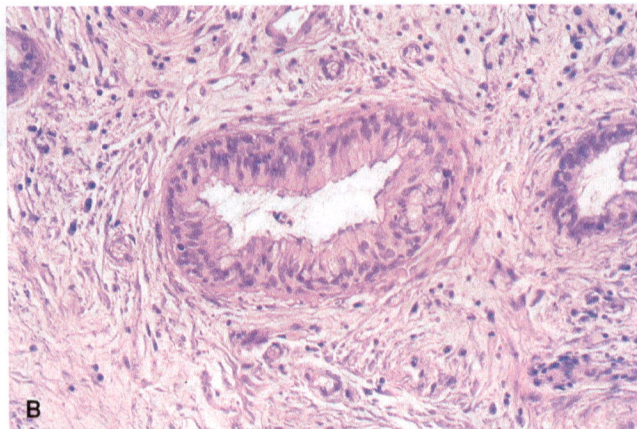

FIGURE 16.17 Metaplasia of excretory ducts. Squamous (**A**) and mucous metaplasia (**B**) showing ciliated cells simulating respiratory epithelium.

appears in patients 10 years older than the average age of patients with these neoplasms, as if an aging phenomenon also occurs in tumors (184).

Fatty Infiltration

Normally, some adipose cells are present in the areolar connective tissue of the salivary glands. This fatty tissue increases in adults; in the elderly, it forms an important proportion of salivary gland tissue. Fatty infiltration may reach huge proportions, especially in alcoholics and the malnourished (185).

REACTIVE CHANGES

Metaplasia

Squamous metaplasia may be present in larger salivary ducts in chronic inflammatory processes, particularly when associated with calculi (Fig. 16.17A) (186). (Remember that where the major salivary ducts open into the oral cavity, they are lined with a stratified squamous epithelium.) Metaplastic squamous transformation is also present in intralobular ducts and acini in ischemia and radiation injury. Light and electron micrographs show that the principal portion of salivary gland tissue undergoing squamous metaplasia is the acinar-intercalated duct cell complex (187).

Mucous metaplasia is found on interlobular ducts, and less frequently in intralobular ducts in cases of obstructive and postradiotherapy forms of sialadenitis (188). Proliferation of mucous goblet cells is accompanied by prominent ciliated cells mimicking the respiratory epithelium (Fig. 16.17B). Necrotizing sialometaplasia is a type of metaplasia peculiar to salivary tissue, but it is exceptional in major salivary glands (Fig. 16.18) (189). It consists of ischemic lobular infarction or necrosis of some acini, accompanied by extensive squamous metaplasia of salivary gland ducts and acini. Severe inflammation and granulation tissues are present. Necrosis of mucous acini is represented by small pools of mucin, that along with the squamous elements may be mistaken for mucoepidermoid carcinoma or invasive squamous cell carcinoma (190,191). The preservation of general lobular morphology and prominent granulation tissue are criteria in favor of benignity. Subacute forms are also described (192).

Hyperplasia

Hyperplasia of mucous acini is an alteration exclusive to the minor salivary glands. In contrast, serous hyperplasia occurs in parotid and, rarely, in submandibular and sublingual glands; it is called sialadenosis (193). This hyperplasia is associated with a number of metabolic, nutritional, and endocrine conditions or follows the ingestion of chemicals and drugs or chronic alcohol consumption (194–196). In most cases, a bilateral swelling of the glands is caused by enlarged acini and an accumulation of secretory granules

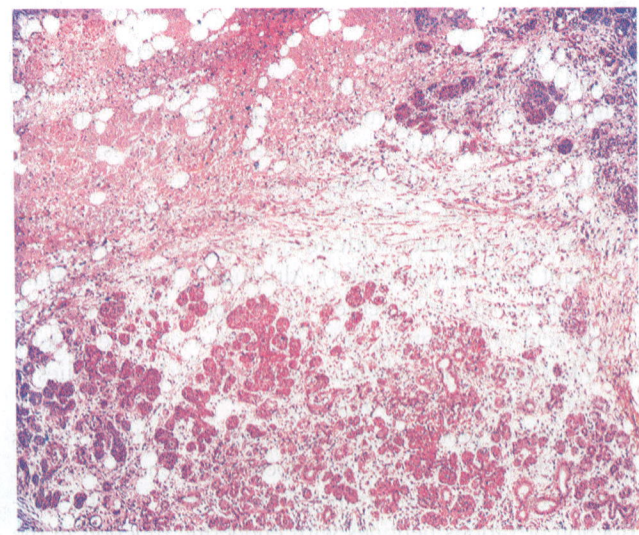

FIGURE 16.18 Necrotizing sialometaplasia of submandibular gland.

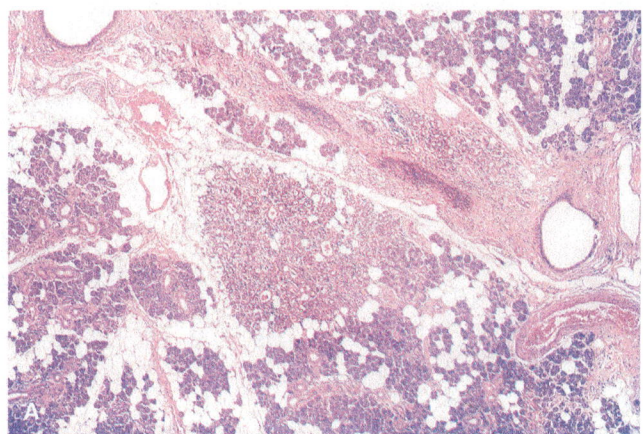
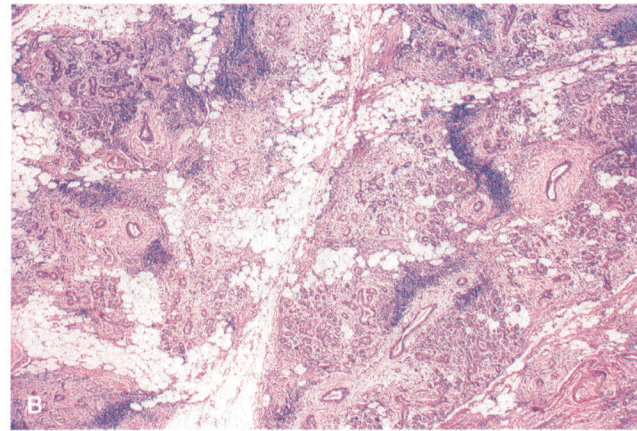

FIGURE 16.19 Atrophy of the salivary parenchyma. **A:** Focal atrophy in the vicinity of a parotid tumor; note the duct dilatation. **B:** Diffuse atrophy in chronic sialadenitis showing prominent periductal sclerosis.

in the cytoplasm. In other cases, granulation is lost and the cytoplasm looks vacuolated. The myoepithelial cells may show nuclear pyknosis or cytoplasmic vacuolation. Loss and thinning of the myofilaments in the myoepithelial cells, which results in loss of mechanical support for the acini and accumulation of intracellular granules with the consequent enlargement of acinar cells has been demonstrated (197). Adenomatoid salivary gland hyperplasia should be distinguished from true tumors (198,199). These cases may be misdiagnosed as true adenomas. Adenomatoid hyperplasia contains clusters or lobules of mucous or serous glands with normal or enlarged appearance, whereas adenomatous ductal proliferations show not only prominent ductal proliferation with some acinar cell complexes but also the normal lobular pattern is preserved. Such lesions contain epithelial and myoepithelial cells resembling intercalated ducts and are viewed as precursors of basal cell adenomas or epithelial–myoepithelial carcinoma (200).

Atrophy

Atrophy of one or more lobules of salivary tissue is a common finding in surgical specimens of tumoral salivary glands. This atrophy is caused by partial or total obstruction of an excretory duct. Accordingly, secretory units distal to the obstructed duct are dilated, and the acinar lumina become visible. The secretory cells lose their granules and have a similar appearance to that of the intercalated duct. The atrophic lobule has an inflammatory component; the cells gradually disappear and the parenchyma is replaced by adipose tissue and collagen fibers (Fig. 16.19A). The extent of atrophy depends on the size of the affected duct. It is generally greater in lithiasic obstruction. The atrophy present in terminal stage chronic sialadenitis shows a diffuse pattern with prominent periductal sclerosis and dense inflammatory infiltration (Fig. 16.19B). In the submandibular gland, diffuse atrophy is frequent after radiotherapy and the gland has a firm consistency that may be clinically mistaken for a submandibular neoplasm (188). Atypical cells are often found in postradiotherapy atrophy. Dilated ducts lose cell polarity and exhibit hyperchromatic nuclei and prominent myoepithelium. In addition, interlobular ducts lose their continuity and the interstitium is densely infiltrated with plasma cells. In experimental models atrophy occurs after ligation of the main salivary duct. Ducts cells persist in contrast to the disappearance of most acinar cells, which are depleted by apoptosis (201).

Regeneration

The parenchyma of salivary glands has a capacity for regeneration. It is particularly notable in the salivary gland a few weeks after partial resection. In general, regenerating tissue follows an embryonic pattern, showing solid buds and branching columns of undifferentiated cells that eventually form excretory units (Fig. 16.20A) (202). Regeneration may appear as duct-like structures, however these formations are frequently seen in atrophic glands and also in older patients. Whether this phenomenon is due to atrophy or regeneration or even a kind of metaplasia is still debated (203). In recent studies it has been shown that no regenerative activity is present in duct-like structures (204). These formations are certainly more frequent in older patients but are not an exclusive phenomenon of senescence. In some cases, such regenerating tissue exhibits an atypical appearance even in duct-like structures. Proliferating solid buds of undifferentiated cells may simulate basal cell adenoma or other basal cell neoplasms (Fig. 16.20B) (205). However, unlike neoplasms, the regenerating tissue preserves the lobular architecture characteristic of the normal salivary gland (Fig. 16.20B). Regeneration after atrophy due to duct obstruction is completed from residual parotid ducts that differentiate to form acinar cells (206), probably by stem cells that reside in ducts. The pattern is similar to the high proliferative activity of the terminal tubule, proacinar, and acinar cells during normal embryonic development of the rat submandibular gland (207). Regeneration of salivary tissue is obtained from bone marrow–derived cells in the treatment of xerostomia (208).

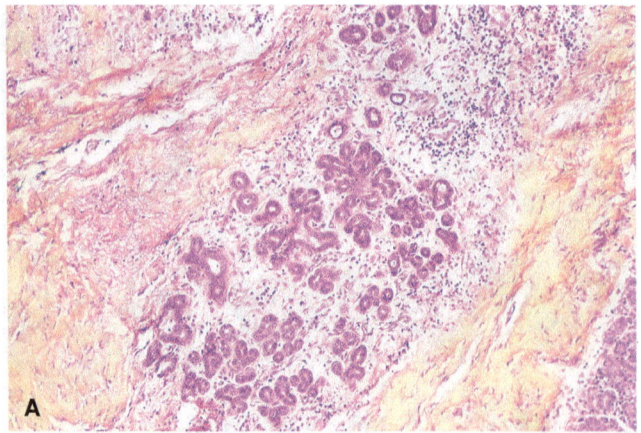
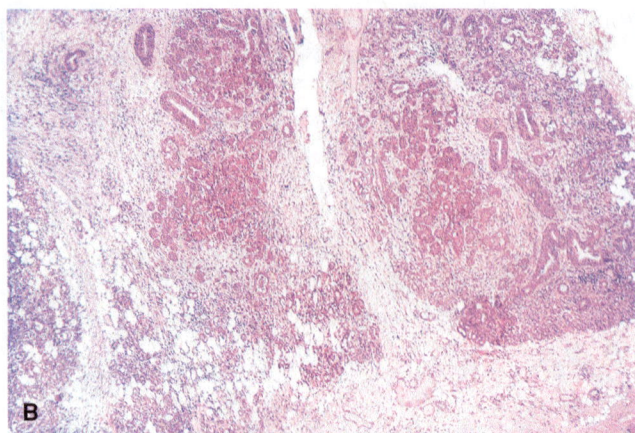
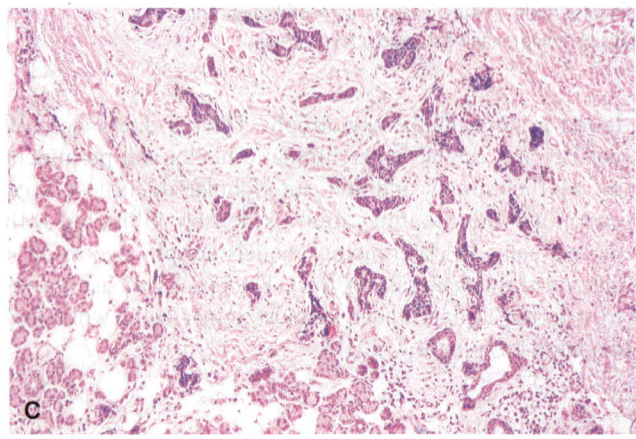

FIGURE 16.20 Regenerating salivary tissue of parotid gland. **A:** Formation of secretory units with an embryonic pattern. **B:** Atypical regenerating tissue; the lobular pattern is preserved. **C:** Infiltrating residual adenoid cystic carcinoma in a parotid gland. Solid buds consist of undifferentiated cells without lobular arrangement.

Artifacts

Artifactual changes in salivary gland surgical specimens are seen in cases of electrocautery and fine needle aspiration. Oncocytoid artifact is an interesting change that may be seen in parotid surgical specimens resected by elecrocautery. The acinar cells show large size with coarse granular eosinophilic cytoplasm, distinct cell borders and basal nuclei. These changes are sometimes misdiagnosed as oncocytoma (209). Patients with previous fine needle aspiration for diagnosis may show vascular implants of tumor cells in benign tumors such as pleomorphic adenoma; this phenomenon should not be misdiagnosed as a malignant tumor with lymphatic permeation (210).

CORRELATIVE NORMAL AND NEOPLASTIC HISTOLOGY

A characteristic of salivary glands is the ability to give rise to a large number of histologically distinct tumors. The histogenetic origin of these neoplasms is an interesting topic, but the numerous mechanisms that have been proposed remain hypothetical. The most attractive theories attempt to relate this phenomenon to embryonic development and, particularly, to the presence of ductal reserve cells (211–215).

A conjectural role of these reserve cells is the regeneration of salivary parenchyma, as well as the development of metaplastic tissue in reactive conditions. Batsakis et al. theorized two stem cell progenitors located at proximal and distal regions of the duct system, which are related to tumors mimicking the terminal ductoacinar complex and the excretory ducts system, respectively (213). The presence of basal cells with undifferentiated features in salivary ducts does not prove that they act as reserve cells. Conversely, experimental evidence exists for the proliferative capacity of differentiated acinar and myoepithelial cells (216–218).

A correlation between the normal structure of the salivary gland and the histologic appearance of salivary tumors can help us to understand morphologic classifications. Nevertheless, we must realize that this histologic similarity does not necessarily imply that a particular tumor arises from the structure that it mimics (214).

The intercalated duct represents the most important segment of the salivary gland in the morphologic organization of many salivary tumors. Many distinctive tumors have been related to it, including pleomorphic adenoma, adenoid cystic carcinoma, basal cell adenoma, epithelial–myoepithelial carcinoma, PLGA, basal cell carcinoma, and embryonic tumors (Fig. 16.21). These tumors show both epithelial and myoepithelial cell differentiation (219), as does the normal intercalated duct. According to Batsakis (213), these

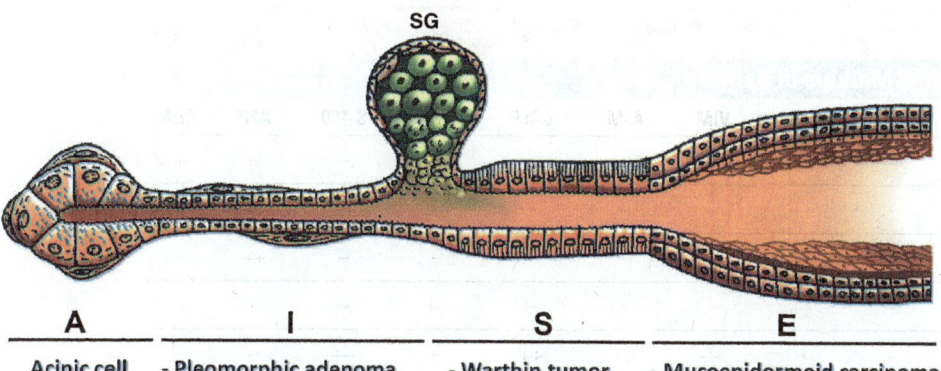

FIGURE 16.21 Morphologic similarity of some salivary tumors and the different epithelial structures of the salivary gland: acinus (*A*); intercalated duct (*I*); striated duct (*S*); sebaceous gland (*SG*); and excretory ducts (*E*). Not necessarily related to histogenesis.

A	I	S	E
Acinic cell carcinoma	- Pleomorphic adenoma - Adenoid cystic carcinoma - Monomorphic adenoma - Epithelial myoepithelial carcinoma - P L G A (polymorphous low grade adenocarcinoma)	- Warthin tumor - Oncocytoma	- Mucoepidermoid carcinoma - Ductal adenocarcinoma - Epidermoid carcinoma - Papilloma

tumors develop from "intercalated duct reserve cells" that follow the same direction as the embryonic terminal tubular cell. Statistically, approximately 80% of salivary tumors develop in the parotid gland where the intercalated ducts are relatively long (Fig. 16.7). In contrast, in the sublingual gland, which gives rise to less than 1% of salivary tumors, intercalated ducts are hardly visible.

A similar morphologic link exists between the acini, the most differentiated structure of the gland, and the acinic cell tumor, a well-differentiated neoplasm (Fig. 16.22A–C) (220);

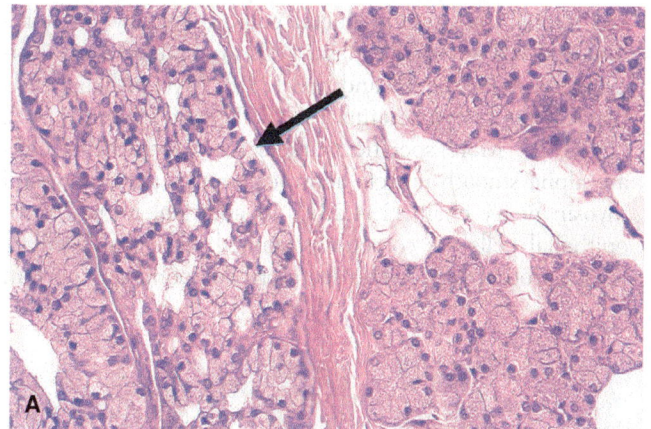
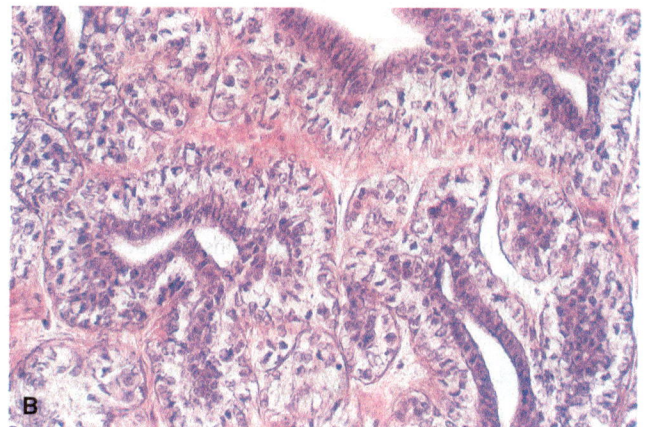
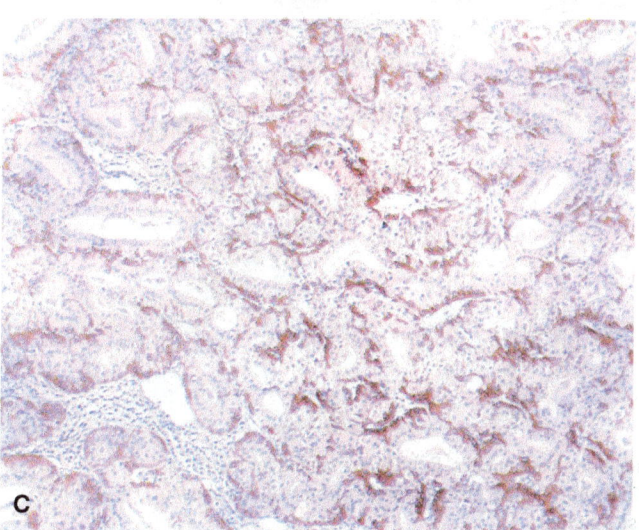

FIGURE 16.22 **A:** Acinic cell carcinoma of the parotid gland (*arrow*) mimicking the normal gland. **B:** Epithelial–myoepithelial carcinoma of the parotid gland showing both epithelial and myoepithelial cells of the intercalated duct. **C:** Immunostaining for muscular actin of an epithelial–myoepithelial carcinoma.

TABLE 16.3 Immunohistochemical Markers of Salivary Glands

Structure	LMK	HMK	VIM	A-M	CALP	EMA	S-100	AFP	CEA
Acinus	++	+	–	–	–	–	–	–	+
Intercalated duct	–	++	–	–	–	++	++	++	+
Striated duct	–	++	–	–	–	–	–	++	–
Excretory duct	–	++	–	–	–	++	–	–	–
Myoepithelial cell	+	–	+/–	++	++	–	++	–	–
Basal cell	++	–	–	–	–	–	–	–	–

LMK, low–molecular-weight keratin; HMK, high–molecular-weight keratin; VIM, vimentin; A-M, actin, myosin; CALP, calponin; EMA, epithelial membrane antigen; AFP, alpha-fetoprotein; S-100, S-100 protein; CEA, carcinoembryonic antigen.

between the mitochondria-rich cells of the striated duct, Warthin tumor, and oncocytomas (163),(164); and between the sebaceous glands and sebaceous tumors (48). A morphologic analogy may also be found between the larger excretory ducts and mucoepidermoid carcinoma, salivary duct adenocarcinoma, epidermoid carcinoma, adenosquamous carcinoma, and papillary tumors (Fig. 16.21) (221–229).

IMMUNOHISTOCHEMISTRY

An important aspect of cytodifferentiation in normal and neoplastic salivary tissues is the expression of different intermediate filaments, enzymes, immunologic components, and other proteins. These proteins may be stained by immunohistochemical methods.

In normal salivary glands, the immunohistochemistry may be summarized as follows (Table 16.3): the expression of cytokeratin varies according to individual cell types of the secretory unit. Acinar cells are stained by several types of lower-weight cytokeratins such as CK 7, 8, and 19. In addition these cells may be marked by their enzymes usually present in the normal acinus such as amylase and lysozyme. Cytokeratins 6 and 12 are weakly positive in acinar cells, but strongly positive in ductal cells, especially in excretory ducts (Fig. 16.23). Basal cells are stained with anticytokeratin 19 and 18 and p63 (230). Myoepithelial cells may coexpress cytokeratins 14, 17, 19, and vimentin (42), (131,133). More specific markers for myoepithelial cells are alpha smooth muscle actin, calponin, caldesmon, and myosin heavy chain (134,231). In addition, normal myoepithelial cells are sometimes stained with glial fibrillary acidic protein (232). The secretory component is present

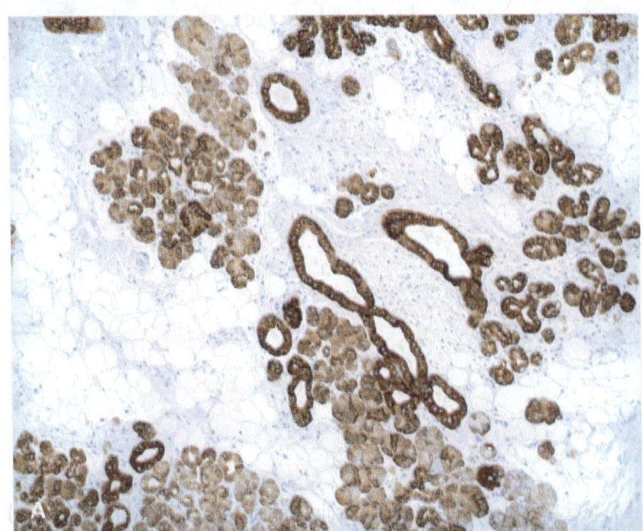
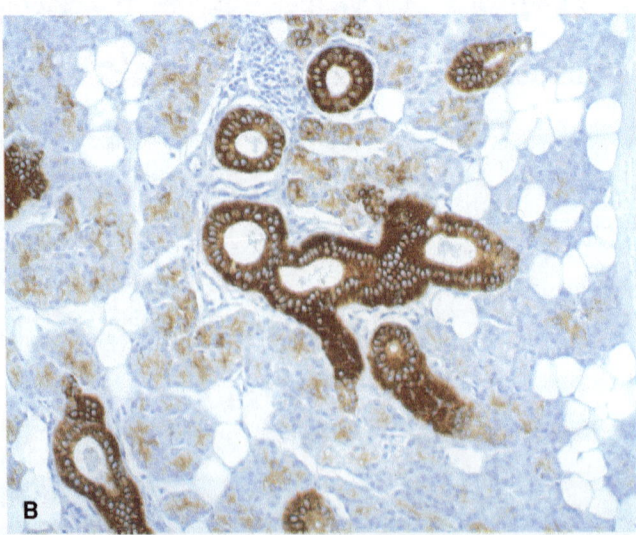

FIGURE 16.23 **A:** Immunostaining for cytokeratin 7 in acinar and ducts cells. **B:** Immunostaining for cytokeratin AE1–AE3 in a parotid gland. The acini are unstained but intercalated, striated, and excretory ducts show a progressive immunoreaction (peroxidase–antiperoxidase method).

in acinar cells, as well as intercalated and striated duct cells, except for the mucous units (233). Carcinoembryonic antigen (CEA) is present in acinar and intercalated duct cells; it is strongly positive in inflamed glands (234). Basal cells are stained with CK 14, 17, and p63 (231). Ductal epithelial cells of intercalated, striated, and interlobular ducts are strongly positive for epithelial membrane antigen (EMA) (235). Recently, the presence of alpha-fetoprotein in the human submandibular gland has been documented (236). When used as functional markers, the following enzymes may be stained: amylase and lactoferrin in serous acinar cells (237), lysozyme in intercalated ducts (31,32), and alkaline phosphatase and ATPase in myoepithelial cells (68). When used as histologic markers, all these proteins have proven useful in surgical pathology.

SPECIMEN HANDLING

The parotid gland is the most common location of major salivary gland tumors. Since most of them are benign and located on the superficial lobe, partial parotidectomy of the superficial lobe (lateral lobectomy) is the most common treatment. Superficial parotidectomy also suffices for small, well-differentiated, low-grade malignant neoplasms that have not compromised the facial nerve (238). The specimen should be sectioned horizontally and the relationship between the tumor and the gland should be stated (Fig. 16.24). The surgical limits should be described even in benign tumors (Fig. 16.25). Total parotidectomy with preservation of the facial nerve is usually indicated in recurrent or multiple benign tumors and large benign tumors of the isthmus and deep lobe.

Total parotidectomy including facial nerve resection (radical parotidectomy) is indicated in aggressive malignant tumors, malignant tumors situated in the deep lobe, or those that have compromised the facial nerve. All these specimens should be sectioned on their major axis to evaluate periparotid tissue infiltration (Fig. 16.26). Intraparotid and periparotid lymph nodes should be identified, and when radical parotidectomy includes neck dissection, the lymph nodes should be separated according to the different anatomical regions.

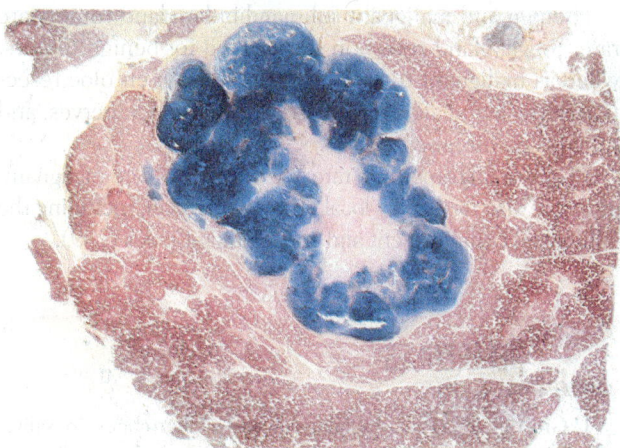

FIGURE 16.25 Superficial parotidectomy for a pleomorphic adenoma. Note that the tumor is well delimited within the normal gland.

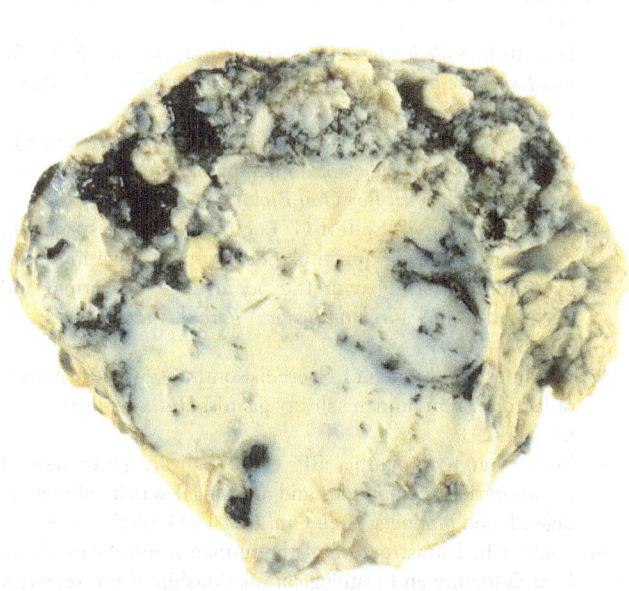

FIGURE 16.24 Histologic section of a parotid gland showing a pleomorphic adenoma. The tumor is apparently well delimited; tumoral buds may be found separate from the principal tumor.

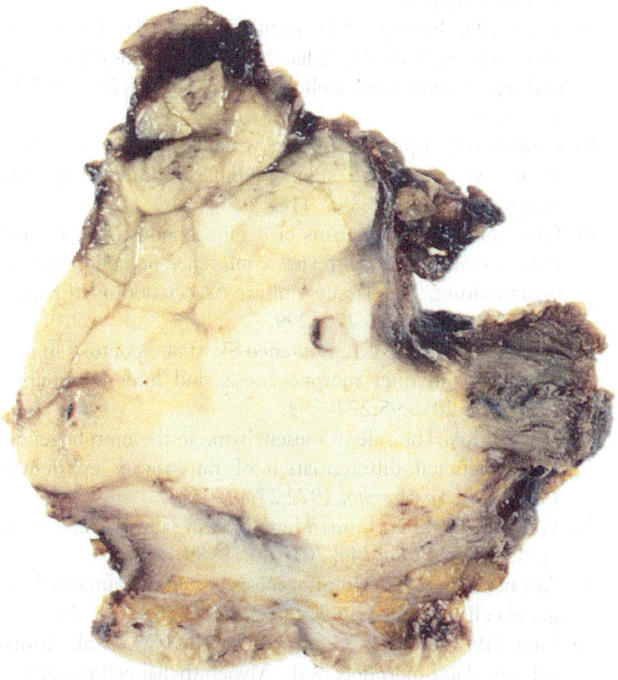

FIGURE 16.26 Radical parotidectomy for a high-grade mucoepidermoid carcinoma. Note the infiltration of the periparotid tissues.

Benign and malignant submandibular gland tumors are rare. Single gland resection is indicated for benign tumors, whereas malignant tumors are treated by an en bloc resection of the gland along with associated muscles, nerves, and mucous membrane.

Sublingual tumors are rare and most (80%) are malignant. They are also treated by local en bloc resection, including the sublingual compartment and surrounding tissues (239).

REFERENCES

1. Gröschl M. The physiological role of hormones in saliva. *Bioessays* 2009;31:843–852.
2. Mathison RD, Davison JS, Befus AD, et al. Salivary gland derived peptides as a new class of anti-inflammatory agents: Review of preclinical pharmacology of C-terminal peptides of SMR1 protein. *J Inflamm (Lond)* 2010;7:49.
3. Arey LB. *Developmental Anatomy*. Philadelphia, PA: WB Saunders; 1974.
4. Melnick M, Phair RD, Lipidot SA, et al. Salivary gland branching morphogenesis: A quantitative systems analysis of the Eda/Edar/NFkappaB paradigm. *BMC Dev Biol* 2009;9:32.
5. Lombaert IM, Knox SM, Hoffman MP. Salivary gland progenitor cell biology provides a rationale for therapeutic salivary gland regeneration. *Oral Dis* 2011;17:445–449.
6. Miletich I. Introduction to salivary glands: Structure, function and embryonic development. *Front Oral Biol* 2010;14:1–20.
7. Sequeira SJ, Larsen M, DeVine T. Extracellular matrix and growth factors in salivary gland development. *Front Oral Biol* 2010;14:48–77.
8. Sakai T. Epithelial branching morphogenesis of salivary gland: exploration of new functional regulators. *J Med Invest* 2009;56(Suppl):234–238.
9. Cohn RH. Banerjee SD, Bernfield MR. Basal lamina of embryonic salivary epithelia. Nature of glycosaminoglycan and organization of extracellular materials. *J Cell Biol* 1977;73:464–478.
10. Grobstein C. Epithelio-mesenchymal specificity in the morphogenesis of mouse submandibular rudiments in vitro. *J Exp Zool* 1953;124:383–413.
11. Grobstein C. Mechanisms of organogenetic tissue interaction. Second decennial review conference on cell tissue and organ culture. The Tissue Culture Association. *Natl Cancer Inst Monogr* 1967;26:279–299.
12. Teshima TH, Wells KL, Lourenco SV, et al. Apoptosis in early salivary gland duct morphogenesis and lumen formation. *J Dent Res* 2016;95:277–283.
13. Lawson KA. The role of mesenchyme in the morphogenesis and functional differentiation of rat salivary epithelium. *J Embryol Exp Morphol* 1972;27:497–513.
14. Wells KL, Patel N. Lumen formation in salivary gland development. *Front Oral Biol* 2010;14:78–89.
15. Azuma M, Sato M. Morphogenesis of normal human salivary gland cells in vitro. *Histol Histopathol* 1994;9:781–790.
16. Ianez RF. Buim ME, Coutinho-Camillo CM, et al. Human salivary gland morphogenesis: Myoepithelial cell maturation assessed by immunohistochemical markers. *Histopathology* 2010;57:410–417.
17. Lee SK, Hwang Jo, Chi JG, et al. Prenatal development of myoepithelial cell of human submandibular gland observed by immunohistochemistry of smooth muscle actin and rhodamine-phalloidin fluorescence. *Pathol Res Pract* 1993;189:332–341.
18. Adi MM, Chisholm DM, Waterhouse JP. Stereological and immunohistochemical study of development of human fetal labial salivary glands and their S-100 protein reactivity. *J Oral Pathol Med* 1994;23:36–40.
19. Lee SK, Kim EC, Chi JG, et al. Immunohistochemical detection of S-100, S-100 alpha, S-100 beta proteins, glial fibrillary acidic protein, and neuron specific enolase in the prenatal and adult human salivary glands. *Pathol Res Pract* 1993;189:1036–1043.
20. Line SE, Archer FL. The postnatal development of myoepithelial cell in the rat submandibular gland. An immunohistochemical study. *Virchows Arch B Cell Pathol* 1972;10:253–262.
21. Gresik EW. Postnatal developmental changes in submandibular glands of rat and mice. *J Histochem Cytochem* 1980;28:860–870.
22. Gasser RF. The early development of the parotid gland around the facial nerve and its branches in man. *Anat Rec* 1970;167:63–78.
23. Mayo GCh. *Gray's Anatomy*. Philadelphia, PA: Lea & Febiger; 1973.
24. Toh H, Kodama J, Fukuda J, et al. Incidence and histology of human accessory parotid glands. *Anat Rec* 1993;236:586–590.
25. Frommer J. The human accessory parotid gland: its incidence, nature, and significance. *Oral Surg Oral Med Oral Pathol* 1977;43:671–676.
26. Hamilton WJ, Boyd DJ, Mossman HW. *Human Embryology, Prenatal Development of Form and Function*. London: Williams & Wilkins; 1972.
27. Bloom W, Fawcett DW. *A Textbook of Histology*. 10th ed. Philadelphia, PA: WB Saunders; 1986.
28. Testut L. *Traité d'Anatomie Humaine*: Paris: Octave Doin; 1901.
29. Donath K. *Sialadenose der Parotis. Ultrastruktirelle, Klinische und Experimentelle Befunde zur Sekretiospathologie*. Stuttgart: Fischer; 1976.
30. Takano K, Malamud D, Bennick A, et al. Localization of salivary proteins in granules of human parotid and submandibular acinar cells. *Crit Rev Oral Biol Med* 1993;4:399–405.
31. Caselitz J, Jaup T, Seifert G. Lactoferrin and lysozyme in carcinomas of the parotid gland. A comparative immunocytochemical study with the occurrence in normal and inflamed tissue. *Virchows Arch A Pathol Anat Histol* 1981;394:61–73.
32. Reitamo S, Kontinnen YT, Sgerber-Kontinnen M. Distribution of lactoferrin in human salivary glands. *Histochemistry* 1980;66:285–291.
33. Xu L, Lal K, Santarpia RP, et al. Salivary proteolysis of histidine-rich polypeptides and antifungal activity of peptide degradation products. *Arch Oral Biol* 1993;38:277–283.
34. Tandler B. Ultrastructure of the human submaxillary gland. I. Architecture and histological relationship of the secretory cells. *Am J Anat* 1962;111:287–307.
35. Quinatrelli G. Histochemical identification of salivary mucins. *Ann NY Acad Sci* 1963;106:339–363.

36. Reddy MS, Bobek LA, Haraszthy GG, et al. Structural features of the low-molecular-mass human salivary mucin. *Biochem J* 1992;287:639–643.
37. Greep RO, Weiss L. *Histology*. New York: McGraw-Hill; 1973.
38. Amano O, Mizobe K, Bando Y, et al. Anatomy and histology of rodent and human major salivary glands: Overview of the Japan salivary gland society-sponsored workshop. *Acta Histochem Cytochem* 2012;45:241–250.
39. Korsrud FR, Brandtzaeg P. Characterization of epithelial elements in human major salivary glands by functional markers: Localization of amylase, lactoferrin, lysozyme, secretory component, and secretory immunoglobulins by paired immunofluorescence staining. *J Histochem Cytochem* 1982;30:657–666.
40. Riva A, Serra GP, Proto E, et al. The myoepithelial and basal cells of ducts of human major salivary glands: a SEM study. *Arch Histol Cytol* 1992;55(Suppl):115–124.
41. Born A, Schwechheimer K, Maier H, et al. Cytokeratin expression in normal salivary glands and in cystadenolymphomas demonstrated by monoclonal antibodies against selective cytokeratin polypeptides. *Virchows Arch A Pathol Anat Histopathol* 1987;411:583–589.
42. Burns BF, Dardick I, Parks WR. Intermediate filament expression in normal salivary glands and in pleomorphic adenomas. *Virchows Arch A Pathol Anat Histopathol* 1988;413:103–112.
43. Seifert GA, Miehlke A, Hanubrich J, et al. *Diseases of the Salivary Glands: Pathology, Diagnosis, Treatment, Facial Nerve Surgery*. Stuttgart: Georg Thiem 1986.
44. Regezi JA, Batsakis JG. Histogenesis of salivary gland neoplasms. *Otolaryngol Clin North Am* 1977;10:297–307.
45. Hamperl H. Beitraäge zur normalen und pathologischen histologic menschlicher speicheldrüsen. *Z Mikrosk Anat Forsch* 1931;27:1–55.
46. Hartz PH. Development of sebaceous glands from intralobular ducts of the parotid gland. *Arch Pathol (Chic)* 1946;41:651–654.
47. Lee CM. Intraparotid sebaceous glands. *Ann Surg* 1949;129:152–155.
48. Meza-Chavez L. Sebaceous glands in normal and neoplastic parotid glands: Possible significance of sebaceous glands in respect to the origin of tumors of the salivary glands. *Am J Pathol* 1949;25:627–645.
49. Micheau C. Les glandes dites sébacées de la parotide et de la sousmaxillaire. *Ann Anat Pathol* 1969;14:119–126.
50. Patey D, Thackray AC. The treatment of parotid tumors in the light of a pathological study of parotidectomy material. *Br J Surg* 1958;45:477–487.
51. Margolies A, Weidman F. Statistical and histologic studies of Fordyce's disease. *Arch Dermatol Syphilol* 1921;3:723–742.
52. Whitaker SB, Vigneswaran N, Singh BB. Androgen receptor status of the oral sebaceous glands. *Am J Dermatopathol* 1997;19:415–418.
53. Laine M, Blauer M, Ylikomi T, et al. Immunohistochemical demonstration of androgen receptors in human salivary glands. *Arch Oral Biol* 1993;38:299–302.
54. de VicenteRodríguez JC V, FresnoForcelledo MF F, González-García M, et al. Sebaceous adenoma of the parotid gland. *Med Oral Patol Oral Cir Bucal* 2006;1:E446–E448.
55. Ahn SH, Park SY. Sebaceous lymphadenocarcinoma of parotid gland. *Eur Arch Otorhinolaryngol* 2006;263:940–942.
56. Assor D. Sebaceous lymphadenoma of the parotid gland: a case report. *Am J Clin Pathol* 1970;53:100–103.
57. Seifert G, Bull HG, Donath K. Histologic subclassification of the cystadenolymphoma of the parotid gland. Analysis of 275 cases. *Virchows Arch A Pathol Anat Histol* 1980;388:13–38.
58. Martínez-Madrigal F, Casiraghi O, Khattech A, et al. Hypopharyngeal sebaceous carcinoma: A case report. *Hum Pathol* 1991;22:929–931.
59. Gnepp DR, Sporck FT. Benign lymphoepithelial parotid cyst with sebaceous differentiation—cystic sebaceous lymphadenoma. *Am J Clin Pathol* 1980;74:683–687.
60. Gnepp DR. My journey into the world of salivary gland sebaceous neoplasms. *Head Neck Pathol* 2012;6:101–110.
61. Stalhammer G, Elmberger G. Sebaseous epithelial-myoepithelial carcinoma of the parotid gland: A case report of a new histologic variant. *Ann Diagn Pathol* 2014;18:248–252.
62. Chaudry AP, Cutler LS, Yamane GM, et al. Ultrastructure of normal human parotid gland with special emphasis on myoepithelial distribution. *J Anat* 1987;152:1–11.
63. Cutler LS, Chaudhry A, Innes DJ. Ultrastructure of the parotid duct. Cytochemical studies of the striated duct and papillary cystadenoma lymphomatosum of the human parotid gland. *Arch Pathol Lab Med* 1977;101:420–424.
64. Drenckhan DU, Gröschel-Stewart U, Unsicker K. Immunofluorescence-microscopic demonstration of myosin and actin in salivary glands and exocrine pancreas of the rat. *Cell Tissue Res* 1977;183:273–279.
65. Tandler B. Ultrastructure of the human submaxillary gland. III. Myoepithelium. *Z Zell Forsch Mikrosk Anat* 1965;68:852–863.
66. Franke WW, Schmid E, Freudenstein C, et al. Intermediate-sized filaments of the prekeratin type in myoepithelial cells. *J Cell Biol* 1980;84:633–654.
67. Norberg L. Dardick I, Leung R, et al. Immunogold localization of actin and cytokeratin filaments in myoepithelium of human parotid salivary gland. *Ultrastruct Pathol* 1992;16:555–568.
68. Hamperl H. The myoepithelia (myoepithelial cells). Normal state; regressive changes; hyperplasia; tumors. *Curr Top Pathol* 1970;53:161–220.
69. Shear M. The structure and function of myoepithelial cells in salivary glands. *Arch Oral Biol* 1966;11:769–780.
70. Garrett JR, Emmelin N. Activities of salivary myoepithelial cells: A review. *Med Biol* 1979;57:1–28.
71. D'Ardenne AJ, Kirkpatrick P, Wells CA, et al. Laminin and fibronectin in adenoid cystic carcinoma. *J Clin Pathol* 1986;39:138–144.
72. Donath K, Seifert G. Ultrastruktur and Pathogenese der myoepithelialen Sialadenitis. Über das Vorkommen von Myoepithelzellen bei der benignen lymphoepithelialen Läsion. *Virchows Arch A Pathol Anat Histopathol* 1972;356:315–329.
73. Kallioinen M. Immunoelectron microscope demonstration of the basement membrane components laminin and type IV collagen in the dermal cylindroma. *J Pathol* 1985;147:97–102.
74. Orenstein JM, Dardick I, van Nostrand AW. Ultrastructural similarities of adenoid cystic carcinoma and pleomorphic adenoma. *Histopathology* 1985;9:623–638.
75. Seifert G, Donath K. Classification of the pathology of diseases of the salivary glands. Review of 2,600 cases in the salivary gland register. *Beitr Pathol* 1976;159:1–32.

76. Skalova A, Leivo I. Extracellular collagenous spherules in salivary gland tumors. Immunohistochemical analysis of laminin and various types of collagen. *Arch Pathol Lab Med* 1992;116: 649–653.
77. Skalova A. Leivo I. Basement membrane proteins in salivary gland tumors. Distribution of type IV collagen and laminin. *Virchows Arch A Pathol Anat Histopathol* 1992;420: 425–431.
78. Laurie GW, Leblond CP, Martin GR. Localization of type IV collagen, laminin, heparan sulfate proteoglycan and fibronectin to the basal lamina of basement membranes. *J Cell Biol* 1982;95:340–344.
79. Sunardhi-Widyaputra S, Van Damme B. Immunohistochemical expression of tenascin in normal human salivary glands and in pleomorphic adenomas. *Pathol Res Pract* 1993; 189:138–143.
80. Savera AT, Zarbo RJ. Defining the role of myoepithelium in salivary gland neoplasia. *Ad Anat Pathol* 2004;11:69–85.
81. Eneroth CM. Salivary gland tumors in the parotid gland, submandibular gland and the palate region. *Cancer* 1971;27: 1415–1418.
82. Thackray AC, Sabin LH. *Histological Typing of Salivary Gland Tumors. In: International Histological Classification of Tumors, No. 7.* Geneva: World Health Organization; 1972.
83. Dardick I, van Nostrand AW, Jeans MT, et al. Pleomorphic adenoma. I. Ultrastructural organization of "epithelial" regions. *Hum Pathol* 1983;14:780–797.
84. Dardick I, Van Nostrand AW, Phillips MJ. Histogenesis of salivary gland pleomorphic adenoma (mixed tumor) with an evaluation of the role of the myoepithelial cell. *Hum Pathol* 1982;13:62–75.
85. David R, Buchner A. Elastosis in benign and malignant salivary gland tumors. A histochemical and ultrastructural study. *Cancer* 1980;45:2301–2310.
86. Erlandson RA, Cardon-Cardo C, Higgins PJ. Histogenesis of benign pleomorphic adenoma (mixed tumor) of the major salivary glands. An ultrastructural and immunohistochemical study. *Am J Surg Pathol* 1984;8:803–820.
87. Hubner G, Klein HJ, Kleinsasser O, et al. Role of myoepithelial cells in the development of salivary gland tumors. *Cancer* 1971;27:1255–1261.
88. Seifert G, Langrock I, Donath K. Pathomorphologische Subklassifikation der pleomorphen Speicheldrüsenadenome. Analyse von 310 pleomorphen Parotisadenomen. *HNO* 1976; 24:415–426.
89. Shirasuna K, Sato M, Miyazaki T. A myoepithelial cell line established from a human pleomorphic adenoma arising in a minor salivary gland. *Cancer* 1980;45:297–305.
90. Gallo O, Bani D, Toccafondi G, et al. Characterization of a novel cell line from pleomorphic adenoma of the parotid gland with myoepithelial phenotype and producing interlenkin-6 as an autocrine growth factor. *Cancer* 1992; 70:559–568.
91. Corio RL, Sciubba JJ, Brannon RB, et al. Epithelial-myoepithelial carcinoma of intercalated duct origin. A clinicopathological and ultrastructural assessment of sixteen cases. *Oral Surg Oral Med Oral Pathol* 1982;53:280–287.
92. Angiero F, Sozzi D, Seramondi R, et al. Epithelial-myoepithelial carcinoma of the minor salivary glands: Immunohistochemical and morphological features. *Anticancer Res* 2009;29(11): 4703–4709.
93. Luna MA, Ordonez NG, Mackay B, et al. Salivary epithelial-myoepithelial carcinomas of intercalated ducts: a clinical, electron microscopic and immunocytochemical study. *Oral Surg Oral Med Oral Pathol* 1985;59:482–490.
94. Batsakis JG, el-Naggar AK, Luna MA. Epithelial-myoepithelial carcinoma of salivary glands. *Ann Otol Rhinol Laryngol* 1992; 101:540–542.
95. Seethala RR, Barnes EL, Hunt JL. Epithelial-myoepithelial carcinoma: a review of the clinicopathologic spectrum and immunophenotypic characteristics in 61 tumors of the salivary glands and upper aerodigestive tract. *Am J Surg Pathol* 2007;31:44–57.
96. Palmer RM. Epithelial-myoepithelial carcinoma: an immunocytochemical study. *Oral Surg Oral Med Oral Pathol* 1985; 59:511–515.
97. Crissman JD, Wirman JA, Harris A. Malignant myoepithelioma of the parotid gland. *Cancer* 1977;40:3042–3049.
98. Leifer C, Miller AS, Putong PB, et al. Myoepithelioma of the parotid gland. *Arch Pathol* 1974;98:312–319.
99. Luna MA, Mackay B, Gamez-Araujo J. Myoepithelioma of the palate. Report of a case with histochemical and electron microscopic observations. *Cancer* 1973;32:1429–1435.
100. Sciubba JJ, Brannon RB. Myoepithelioma of the salivary glands: report of 23 cases. *Cancer* 1982;49:562–572.
101. Dardick I, Cavell S, Boivin M, et al. Salivary gland myoepithelioma variants. Histological, ultrastructural, and immunocytological features. *Virchows Arch A Pathol Anat Histolpathol* 1989;416:25–42.
102. Martínez-Madrigal F, Santiago Payan H, Meneses A, et al. Plasmacytoid myoepithelioma of the laryngeal region: a case report. *Hum Pathol* 1995;26:802–804.
103. Nagao T, Sugano I, Ishida Y, et al. Salivary gland malignant myoepithelioma: A clinicopathologic and immunohistochemical study of ten cases. *Cancer* 1998;83:1292–1299.
104. Frierson HR, Mills SE, Garland TA. Terminal duct carcinoma of minor salivary glands. A nonpapillary subtype of polymorphous low-grade adenocarcinoma. *Am J Clin Pathol* 1985;84:8–14.
105. Gnepp D, Chen CH, Warren C. Polymorphous low-grade adenocarcinoma of minor salivary gland. An immunohistochemical and clinicopathologic study. *Am J Surg Pathol* 1984; 8:367–374.
106. Dardick I, Kahn HJ, Van Nostrand AW, et al. Salivary gland monomorphic adenoma. Ultrastructural, immunoperoxidase and histogenetic aspects. *Am J Pathol* 1984;115:334–348.
107. Dardick I, van Nostrand AW. Myoepithelial cells in salivary gland tumors—revisited. *Head Neck Surg* 1985;7:395–408.
108. Hoa W, Kech PC, Swerdlow MA. Ultrastructure of the basal cell adenoma of parotid gland. *Cancer* 1976;37:1322–1333.
109. Kahn HJ, Baumal R, Marks A, et al. Myoepithelial cells in salivary gland tumors: An immunohistochemical study. *Arch Pathol Lab Med* 1985;109:190–195.
110. Batsakis JG, Luna MA, el-Naggar AK. Basaloid monomorphic adenomas. *Ann Otol Rhinol Laryngol* 1991;100: 687–690.
111. Chaudhry AP, Leifer C, Cutle LS, et al. Histogenesis of adenoid cystic carcinoma of the salivary glands. Light and electron microscopic study. *Cancer* 1986;58:72–82.
112. Chen JC, Gnepp DR, Bedrossian CW. Adenoid cystic carcinoma of the salivary glands: An immunohistochemical analysis. *Oral Surg Oral Med Oral Pathol* 1988;65:316–326.

113. Williams SB, Ellis GL, Auclair PL. Immunohistochemical analysis of basal cell adenocarcinoma. *Oral Surg Oral Med Oral Pathol* 1993;75:64–69.
114. Hsueh C, Gonzalez-Crussi F. Sialoblastoma: a case report and review of the literature on congenital tumors of salivary glands origin. *Pediatr Pathol* 1992;12:205–214.
115. Dehner LP, Valbuena L, Perez-Atayde A, et al. Salivary gland anlage tumor ("congenital pleomorphic adenoma"). A clinicopathologic, immunohistochemical and structural study of nine cases. *Am J Surg Pathol* 1994;18:25–36.
116. Dardick I, Daya D, Hardie J, et al. Mucoepidermoid carcinoma: Ultrastructural and histogenetic aspects. *J Oral Pathol* 1984;13:342–358.
117. Lomax-Smith JD, Azzopardi JG. The hyaline cell: a distinctive feature of "mixed" salivary tumors. *Histopathology* 1978;2:77–92.
118. Haskell HD, Butt KM, Woo SB. Pleomorphic adenoma with extensive lipometaplasia: Report of three cases. *Am J Surg Pathol* 2005;29:1389–1393.
119. Seethala RR, Richmond JA, Hoschar AP, et al. New variants of epithelial-myoepithelial carcinoma: Oncocytic-sebaceous and apocrine. *Arch Pathol Lab Med* 2009;133:950–959.
120. Skálova A, Michal M, Ryska A, et al. Oncocytic myoepithelioma and pleomorphic adenoma of the salivary glands. *Virchows Arch* 1999;434:537–546.
121. Nakano K, Watanabe T, Shimizu T, et al. Immunohistochemical characteristics of bone forming cells in pleomorphic adenoma. *Int J Med Sci* 2007;4:264–266.
122. Dardick I, Jeans MT, Sinnott NM, et al. Salivary gland components involved in the formation of squamous metaplasia. *Am J Pathol* 1985;119:33–43.
123. Quintarelli G, Robinson L. The glycosaminoglycans of salivary gland tumors: A histochemical characterization and a critical evaluation. *Am J Pathol* 1967;51:19–37.
124. Takeuchi J, Sobue M, Yoshida M, et al, Pleomorphic adenoma of the salivary gland. With special reference to histochemical and electron microscopic studies and biochemical analysis of glycosaminoglycans in vivo and in vitro. *Cancer* 1975;36:1771–1789.
125. Caselitz J, Osborn M, Seifert G, et al. Intermediate-sized filament proteins (prekeratin, vimentin, desmin), in the normal parotid gland and parotid gland tumors: immunofluorescence study. *Virchows Arch A Pathol Anat Histopathol* 1981;393:273–286.
126. Savera AT, Gown AM, Zarbo RJ. Immunolocalization of three novel smooth muscle-specific proteins in salivary gland pleomorphic adenoma: assessment of the morphogenetic role of myoepithelium. *Mod Pathol* 1997;10:1093–1100.
127. Caselitz J, Osborn M, Wustrow J, et al. The expression of different intermediate-sized filaments in human salivary gland and their tumors. *Pathol Res Pract* 1982;175:266–278.
128. Morinaga S, Nakajima T, Shimosato Y. Normal and neoplastic myoepithelial cells in salivary glands. An immunohistochemical study. *Hum Pathol* 1987;18:1218–1226.
129. Hara K, Ito M, Takeuchi J, et al. Distribution of S-100b protein in normal salivary glands and salivary gland tumors. *Virchows Arch A Pathol Anat Histopathol* 1983;401:237–249.
130. Franquemont DW, Mills SE. Plasmacytoid monomorphic adenoma of salivary glands. Absence of myogenous differentiation and comparison to spindle cell myoepithelioma. *Am J Surg Pathol* 1993;17:146–153.
131. Sternlicht MD, Safarians S, Rivera SP, et al. Characterizations of the extracellular matrix and proteinase inhibitor content of human myoepithelial tumors. *Lab Invest* 1996;74:781–796.
132. Sternlicht MD, Barsky SH. The myoepithelial defense: a host defense against cancer. *Med Hypotheses* 1997;48:37–46.
133. Savera AT, Sloman A, Huvos AG, et al. Myoepithelial carcinoma of the salivary glands: A clinicopathologic study of 25 patients. *Am J Surg Pathol* 2000;24:761–774.
134. Brandtzaeg P. Mucosal and glandular distribution of immunoglobulin components. Immunohistochemistry with a cold ethanol-fixation technique. *Immunology* 1974;26:1101–1114.
135. Brandtzaeg P. Mucosal and glandular distribution of immunoglobulin components: differential localization of free and bound SC in secretory epithelial cells. *J Immunol* 1974;112:1553–1559.
136. Korsrud FR, Brandtzaeg P. Quantitative immunohistochemistry of immunoglobulin and J-chain-producing cells in human parotid and submandibular salivary glands. *Immunology* 1980;39:129–140.
137. Lee SK, Lim CY, Chi JG, et al. Immunohistochemical study of lymphoid tissue in human fetal salivary gland. *J Oral Pathol Med* 1993;22:23–29.
138. Bernier JL. Bhaskar SN. Lymphoepithelial lesions of salivary glands; histogenesis and classification based on 186 cases. *Cancer* 1958;11:1156–1179.
139. Hsu SM, Hsu PL, Nayak RN. Warthin's tumor: an immunohistochemical study of its lymphoid stroma. *Hum Pathol* 1981;12:251–257.
140. Thompson AS; Bryant HC. Histogenesis of papillary cystadenoma lymphomatosum (Warthin's tumor) of the parotid gland. *Am J Pathol* 1950;26:807–829.
141. Chin S, Kyung K, Kwak JJ, Oncocytic papillary cystadenoma of the major salivary glands: Three rare cases with diverse cytologic features. *J Cytol* 2014;31:221–223.
142. Azzopardi JG, Evans DJ. Malignant lymphoma of parotid associated with Mikulicz disease (benign lymphoepithelial lesion). *J Clin Pathol* 1971;24:744–752.
143. Yamada K, Yamamoto M, Saeki T, et al. New clues to the nature of immunoglobulin G4-related disease: A retrospective Japanese multicenter study of baseline clinical features of 334 cases. *Arthritis Res Ther* 2017;19:262.
144. Brown RB, Gaillard RA, Turner JA. The significance of aberrant or heterotopic parotid gland tissue in lymph nodes. *Ann Surg* 1953;138:850–856.
145. Micheau C. Les ectopies salivaires. *Arch Anat Cytol Pathol (Paris)* 1969;17:179–186.
146. Neisse R. Über den Einschluss von Parotisläppen in Lymphknoten. *Anat Hefte. (Wisbaden)* 1898;10(1):289–306.
147. Bairati A. Constate concrescenza fra noduli linfatici ed adenomeri delle ghiandole salivari nel'úomo durante lo sviluppo e nell'adulto. *Arch Biol. (Paris)* 1932;43:415–450.
148. Youngs LA. Scofield HH. Heterotopic salivary gland tissue in the lower neck. *Arch Pathol* 1967;83:550–556.
149. Curry B, Taylor CW, Fisher AW. Salivary gland heterotopia. A unique cerebellopontine angle tumor. *Arch Pathol Lab Med* 1982;106:35–38.
150. Schochet JR, McCormick WF, Halmi NS, Salivary gland rests in the human pituitary: light and electron microscopical study. *Arch Pathol* 1974;98:193–200.
151. Jernstrom P, Prietto C. Accessory parotid gland tissue at base of neck. *Arch Pathol* 1962;73:473–480.

152. Bouquot JE, Gnnepp DR, Dardick I, et al. Intraosseous salivary tissue: Jawbone examples of choristomas, hamartomas, embryonic rests and inflammatory entrapment. Another histogenetic source for intraosseous adenocarcinoma. *Oral Surg Oral Med Oral Pathol Radiol Endod* 2000;90:205–217.
153. de Courten A, Küffer R, Samson J, et al. Anterior lingual mandibular salivary gland defect (Stafne defect) presenting as a residual cyst. *Oral Surg Oral Med Oral Pathol Oral Radiol and Endod* 2002;94:460–464.
154. Carney JA. Salivary heterotopia, cysts, and the parathyroid gland: branchial pouch derivates and remnants. *Am J Surg Pathol* 2000;24:837–845
155. Lewis AL, Truong LD, Cagle P, et al. Benign salivary gland tissue inclusion in a pulmonary hiliar lymph node from a patient with invasive well-differentiated adenocarcinoma of the lung: a potential misinterpretation for the staging of carcinoma. *In J Surg Pathol* 2011;19:382–385.
156. Aby JL, Patel M, Sundram U, et al. Salivary gland choristoma (heterotopic salivary gland tissue) on the anterior chest wall of a newborn. *Pediatr Dermatol* 2014;31:e36–e37.
157. Downs-Kelly E, Hoschar AP, Prayson RA. Salivary gland heterotopia in the rectum. *Ann Diag Pathol* 2003;7:124–126.
158. Willis RA. *The Borderline of Embryology and Pathology*. London: Butterworth; 1962.
159. Willis RA. Some unusual developmental heterotopias. *Br Med J* 1968;3:267–272.
160. Dhawan IK, Bhargava S, Nayak NC, et al. Central salivary gland tumors of jaws. *Cancer* 1970;26:211–217.
161. Singer MI, Appelbaum EL, Loy KD, Heterotopic salivary tissue in the neck. *Laryngoscope* 1979;89:1772–1778.
162. Martínez-Madrigal F, Pineda-Daboin K, Casiraghi O, et al. Salivary gland tumors of the mandible. *Ann Diagn Pathol* 2000;347–353.
163. Micheau C, Riou G. Oncocytes et oncocytomes. Histoenzymologie, ultrastructure et description de l' ADN mitochondrial. *Arch Anat Pathol (Paris)* 1975;23:123–132.
164. Meza-Chavez L. Oxyphilic granular cell adenoma of the parotid gland (oncocytoma). Report of five cases and study of oxyphilic granular cells (oncocytes) in normal parotid gland. *Am J Pathol* 1949;25:523–547.
165. Shintaku M, Honda T. Identification of oncocyte lesions of salivary glands by anti-mitochondrial immunohistochemistry. *Histopathology* 1997;31:408–411.
166. Schramm U, Dahm HH. The ultrastructure of epithelial and myoepithelial oncocytes in human parotid gland. *Eur J Cell Biol* 1979;19:227–230.
167. Barka T. Biologically active polypeptides in submandibular glands. *J Histochem Cytochem* 1980;28:836–859.
168. Bing J, Poulsen K, Hackenthal E, et al. Renin in the submaxillary gland: A review. *J Histochem Cytochem* 1980;28:874–880.
169. Murphy RA, Watson AY, Metz J, et al. The mouse submandibular gland: an exocrine organ for growth factors. *J Histochem Cytochem* 1980;28:890–902.
170. Whitley BD, Ferguson JW, Harris AJ, et al. Immunohistochemical localization of substance P in human parotid gland. *Int J Oral Maxillofac Surg* 1992;21:54–58.
171. Pikula DL, Harris EF, Desiderio DM, et al. Methionine enkephalin-like, substance P-like, and beta-endorphin-like immunoreactivity in human parotid saliva. *Arch Oral Biol* 1992;37:705–709.

172. Salo A, Ylikoski J, Uusitalo H. Distribution of calcitonin gene-related peptide immunoreactive nerve fibers in the human submandibular gland. *Neurosci Lett* 1993;19:137–140.
173. Mathison R, Davison JS, Befus AD. Neuroendocrine regulation of inflammation and tissue repair by submandibular gland factors. *Immunol Today* 1994;15:527–532.
174. Blanck C, Eneroth CM, Jakobsson PA. Oncocytoma of the parotid gland: neoplasm or nodular hyperplasia. *Cancer* 1970;25:919–925.
175. Rooper LM, Onenerk M, Siddiqui MT, et al. Nodular oncocytic hyperplasia: Can cytomorphology alow for the preoperative diagnosis of a nonneoplastic salivary disease?. *Cancer Cytopathol* 2017;125:627–634.
176. Kontaxis A, Zanarotti U, Kainz J, et al. Diffuse hyperplastic oncocytosis of the parotid gland. *Laryngorhinootologie* 2004;83:185–188.
177. Dardick I, Bireck C, Lingen M, Differentiation and the cytomorphology of salivary gland tumors with specific reference to oncocytic metaplasia. *Oral Surg Oral Med Oral Pathol Oral Radiol Endod* 1999;88:691–701.
178. Ferreiro JA, Stylopoulos N. Oncocytic differentiation in salivary gland tumors. *J Laryngol Otol* 1995;109:569–571.
179. Chang A, Harawi SJ. Oncocytes, oncocytosis, and oncocytic tumors. *Pathol Annu* 1992;27:263–304.
180. Palmer TJ, Gleeson MJ, Eveson JW, et al. Oncocytic adenomas and oncocytic hyperplasia of salivary glands: A clinicopathologic study of 26 cases. *Histopathology* 1990;16:487–493.
181. Gray SR, Cornog JL, Seo IS. Oncocytic neoplasms of salivary glands. A report of fifteen cases including two malignant oncocytomas. *Cancer* 1976;38:1306–1317.
182. Xiao H, Wen T, Liu X. Submandibular oncocytic carcinoma. A case report and literature review. *Medicine (Baltimore)* 2016;95:e4897.
183. Lau SK, Thomson LD. Oncocytic lipoadenoma of the salivary gland: A clinicopathologic analysis of 7 cases and review of the literature. *Head Neck Pathol* 2015;9:39–46.
184. Seethala RR. Oncocytic and apocrine epithelial myoepithelial carcinoma: Novel variants of a challenging tumor. *Head Neck Pathol* 2013;7:S77–S84.
185. Hemenway WG, Allen GW. Chronic enlargement of the parotid gland. Hypertrophy and fatty infiltration. *Laryngoscope* 1959;69:1508–1523.
186. Isacsson G, Lundquist PG. Salivary calculi as an aetiological factor in chronic sialadenitis of the submandibular gland. *Clin Otolaryngol Allied Sci* 1982;7:231–236.
187. Dardick I, Jeans MT, Sinnott NM, et al. Salivary gland components involved in the formation of squamous metaplasia. *Am J Pathol* 1985;119:33–43.
188. Fajardo LF, Berthrong M. Radiation injury in surgical pathology. Part III. Salivary glands, pancreas and skin. *Am J Surg Pathol* 1981;5:279–296.
189. Beer GM, Neuwirth A. Nekrotisierende Sialometaplasie (Speicheldrüseninfarkt) der Glandula submandibularis. *Laryngol Rhinol Otol. (Stuttg)* 1983;62:468–470.
190. Abrams AM, Melrose RT, Howell FV. Necrotizing sialometaplasia. A disease simulating malignancy. *Cancer* 1973;32:130–135.
191. Carlson DL. Necrotizing sialometaplasia: a practical approach to diagnosis. *Arch Pathol Lab Med* 2009;133:692–698.

192. Fowler B, Brannon RB. Subacute necrotizing sialadenitis: report of 7 cases and review of the literature. *Oral Surg Oral Med Oral Patholo Oral Radiol Endod* 2000;89: 600–609.
193. Seifert G, Donath K. Die Sialadenose der Parotis. *Dtsch Med Wochenschr* 1975;100:1545–1548.
194. Mandel L, Baurmash H. Parotid enlargment due to alcoholism. *J Am Dent Assoc* 1971;82:369–373.
195. Campos LA. Hyperplasia of the sublingual glands in adult patients. *Oral Surg Oral Med Oral Pathol Oral Radiol Endod* 1996;81:584–585.
196. Yu YH, Park YS, Kim SH, et al. Sialadenosis in a patient with alcoholic fatty liver developing after heavy alcohol drinking. *Korean J Gastroenterol* 2009;54:50–54.
197. Ihrler S, Rath C, Zengel P, et al. Pathogenesis of sialadenosis: possible role of functionally deficient myoepithelial cells. *Oral Surg Oral Med Oral Pathol Oral Radiol Endod* 2010;110:218–223.
198. Yu GY, Donath K. Adenomatous ductal proliferation of the salivary gland. *Oral Surg Oral Med Oral Pathol Oral Radiol Endod* 2001;91:215–221.
199. Luna MA. Salivary gland hyperplasia. *Adv Anat Pathol* 2002; 9:251–255.
200. Weinreb I, Seethala RR, Hunt JL, et al. Intercalated duct lesions of the salivary gland. A morphologic spectrum from hyperplasia to adenoma. *Am J Surg Pathol* 2009;33: 1322–1329.
201. Walker NI, Gobé GC. Cell death and cell proliferation during atrophy of the rat parotid gland induced by duct obstruction. *J Pathol* 1987;153:333–344.
202. Carpenter GH, Cotroneo E. Salivary gland regeneration. *Front Oral Biol* 2010;14:107–128.
203. Ihrler S, Zietz C, Sendelhofert A, et al. A morphogenetic concept of salivary duct regeneration and metaplasia. *Virchows Arch* 2002;440:519–526.
204. Tolentino Ede S, Teixeira CS, Azevedo-Alanis LR, et al. Phenotype and cell proliferation activity of duct-like structures in human sublingual glands: a histological and immunohistochemical study. *J Appl Oral Sci* 2015;23:255–264.
205. Daley TD, Dardick I. An unusual parotid tumor with histogenetic implications for salivary gland neoplasms. *Oral Surg Oral Med Oral Pathol* 1983;55:374–381.
206. Takahashi S, Schoch E, Walker N. Origin of acinar cell regeneration after atrophy of the rat parotid induced by duct obstruction. *Int J Exp Pathol* 1998;79:293–301.
207. Alvares EP, Sesso A. Cell proliferation, differentiation and transformation in the rat submandibular gland during early postnatal growth. A quantitative and morphological study. *Arch Histol Jpn* 1975;38:177–208.
208. Tran SD, Sumita Y, Khalili S. Bone marrow-derived cells: a potential approach for the treatment of xerostomia. *Int J Biochem Cell Biol* 2011;43:5–9.
209. Shick PC, Brannon RB. Oncocytoid artifact of the parotid gland: a newly reported artifact. *Oral Surg Oral Med Oral Pathol Oral Radiol Endod* 1998;86:720–722.
210. Li S, Baloch ZW, Tomaszewski JE, et al. Worrisome histologic alterations following fine-needle aspiration of benign parotid lesiones. *Arch Pathol Lab Med* 2000;124:87–91.
211. Ellis GL, Auclair PL. *Tumors of the Salivary Glands in: Atlas of Tumors, Ser 4, Fasc 9*. Washington, DC: Armed Forces Institute of Pathology; 2008.
212. Eversole LR, Histogenic classification of salivary tumors. *Arch Pathol Lab Med* 1971;92:433–443.
213. Batsakis JG. Salivary gland neoplasia: an outcome of modified morphogenesis and cytodifferentiation. *Oral Surg Oral Med Oral Pathol* 1980;49:229–232.
214. Dardick I, van Nostrand AW. Morphogenesis of salivary gland tumors. A prerequisite to improving classification. *Pathol Annu* 1987;22:1–53.
215. Dardick I, Dardick AM, Aackay AJ, et al. Pathobiology of salivary glands. IV. Histogenetic concepts and cycling cells in human parotid and submandibular glands cultured in floating collagen gels. *Oral Surg Oral Med Oral Pathol* 1993;76: 307–318.
216. Burgess KL, Dardick I, Cummins MM, et al. Myoepithelial cells actively proliferate during atrophy of the rat parotid gland. *Oral Surg Oral Med Oral Pathol Oral Radiol Endod* 1996;82:674–680.
217. Zarbo R. Salivary gland neoplasia: A review for the practicing pathologist. *Mod Pathol* 2002;15:298–323.
218. Dardick I, Burford-Mason AP. Current status of the histogenetic and morphogenetic concepts of salivary gland tumorigenesis. *Crit Rev Oral Biol Med* 1993;4:639–677.
219. Dardick I, Van Nostrand AW, Jeans MT, et al. Pleomorphic adenoma. II. Ultrastructural organization of "stromal" regions. *Hum Pathol* 1983;14:798–809.
220. Micheau C, Lacour J. Epithelioma acineux de la parotide. *Ann Anat Pathol* 1971;16:173–188.
221. Mills SE, Garland TA, Allen MS Jr. Low-grade papillary adenocarcinoma of palatal salivary gland origin. *Am J Surg Pathol* 1984;8:367–374.
222. Garland TA, Innes DJ, Fechner RE. Salivary duct carcinoma: an analysis of four cases with review of the literature. *Am J Clin Pathol* 1984;81:436–441.
223. Chen KTK, Hafez GR. Infiltrating salivary duct carcinoma. A clinicopathologic study of five cases. *Arch Otolaryngol* 1981;107:37–39.
224. Allen MS Jr, Fitz-Hugh GS, Marsh WL Jr. Low-grade papillary adenocarcinoma of the palate. *Cancer* 1974;33: 153–158.
225. Batsakis JG, McClatchey KD, Johns M, et al. Primary squamous cell carcinoma of the parotid gland. *Arch Otolaryngol* 1976;102:355–357.
226. Martínez-Madrigal F, Baden E, Casiraghi O, et al. Oral and pharyngeal adenosquamous carcinoma. A report of four cases with immunohistochemical studies. *Eur Arch Otorhinolaryngol* 1991;248:255–258.
227. Luna MA, Batsakis JG, Ordonez NG, et al. Salivary gland adenocarcinomas: A clinicopathologic analysis of three distinctive types. *Semin Diagn Pathol* 1987;4:117–135.
228. Micheau C, Lacour J, Genin J, et al. Tumeurs mucoépidermoïdes de la parotide et de la cavité buccale. *Ann Anat Pathol (Paris)* 1972;17:59–71.
229. White DK, Miller AS, McDaniel RK, et al. Inverted ductal papilloma: a distinctive lesion of minor salivary gland. *Cancer* 1982;49:519–524.
230. Foshini MP, Eusebi V. Value of immunohistochemistry in the diagnosis of salivary gland tumors. *Pathol Case Rev* 2004;9:270–275.
231. Foschini MP, Scarpellini F, Gown AM, et al. Differential expression of myoepithelial markers in salivary, sweat and mammary glands. *Int J Surg Pathol* 2000;8:29–37.

232. Zarbo RJ, Haffield JS, Trojanowski JQ, et al. Immunoreactive glial fibrillary acidic protein in normal and neoplastic salivary glands: a combined immunohistochemical and immunoblot study. *Surg Pathol* 1988;I:55–63.
233. Fantasia JE, Lally ET. Localization of free secretory component in pleomorphic adenomas of minor salivary gland origin. *Cancer* 1984;53:1786–1789.
234. Caselitz J, Jaup T, Seifert G. Immunohistochemical detection of carcinoembryonic antigen (CEA) in parotid gland carcinomas. Analysis of 52 cases. *Virchows Arch A Pathol Anat Histopathol* 1981;394:49–60.
235. Gusterson BA, Lucas RB, Ormerod MG. Distribution of epithelial membrane antigen in benign and malignant lesions of the salivary glands. *Virchows Arch A Pathol Anat Histol* 1982;397:227–233.
236. Tsuji. T, Nagai N. Production of alpha-fetoprotein by human submandibular gland. *Int J Dev Biol* 1993;37:497–498.
237. Caselitz J, Seifert G, Grenner G, et al. Amylase as an additional marker of salivary gland neoplasms. An immunoperoxidase study. *Pathol Res Pract* 1983;176:276–283.
238. Conley J, Baker DC. *Cancer of the Salivary Glands in Cancer of the Head and Neck*. New York: Churchill Livingstone; 1981.
239. Rankow RM, Mignogna F. Cancer of the sublingual salivary gland. *Am J Surg* 1969;118:790–795.

SECTION VI

Thorax and Serous Membranes

Lungs

Humberto E. Trejo Bittar ■ Samuel A. Yousem

NORMAL STRUCTURE AND HISTOLOGY 469
    General 469
    Airways 470
    Lobule and Acinus 475
    Vasculature 478
    Lymphatics and Lymphoid Tissue 478
    Pleura 479
	ARTIFACTS SEEN IN LUNG BIOPSY AND RESECTION MATERIAL 484

	INCIDENTAL FINDINGS IN LUNG BIOPSY AND RESECTION TISSUE 488
	INCIDENTAL FINDINGS IN TRANSBRONCHIAL BIOPSIES 499
	EFFECTS OF AGING 500
SPECIAL STAINS AND THE EVALUATION OF LUNG HISTOLOGY 480	THE BIOPSY THAT LOOKS NORMAL AT FIRST GLANCE 500
PATTERN RECOGNITION BASED ON NORMAL ANATOMIC LANDMARKS 480	IMMUNOHISTOCHEMISTRY 501
	REFERENCES 503
SITE-RELATED CHANGES COMMONLY SEEN IN SURGICAL PATHOLOGY MATERIAL 481	

NORMAL STRUCTURE AND HISTOLOGY

The following review is based on several standard references (1–16).

General

The lungs are paired intrathoracic organs that are divided into lobes (three on the right—right upper lobe, right middle lobe, right lower lobe; two on the left—left upper lobe, left lower lobe). The lingula is a rudimentary appendage arising from the left upper lobe and is analogous to the middle lobe on the right. The lobes are further divided into bronchopulmonary segments (Table 17.1).

The segmental anatomy of the lung is important for radiologists, bronchoscopists, and pathologists in defining the location of lesions. The lobes are divided by fissures, each with their own pleural investments, although occasionally these fissures are incomplete or poorly developed. The segments are not separated by fissures and do not normally have separate pleural investments, although they are recognizable on the basis of their supplying bronchi (segmental bronchi).

The primordial lungs arise as a ventral bud off of the foregut extending caudally into the primitive thoracic mesenchyme. The bud elongates and bifurcates to form the right and left main bronchi. Bronchial cartilage, smooth muscle, and other connective tissues are derived from the surrounding mesenchyme. The right and left main bronchial buds elongate into their respective thoracic cavities, branching repeatedly until the bronchial tree is complete. The phases of airway and lung parenchymal development are summarized in Table 17.2.

As the lung progresses through successive phases of development, a complex series of epithelial–mesenchymal reactions occur, modified by physiologic mechanical forces and humoral factors. These events are overseen by master genes (such as homeobox genes), nuclear transcription factors, hormones, and other soluble mediators such as growth factors, chemokines, and cytokines (17,18). Some of these mediators and their relationship to lung development are shown in Table 17.3.

This chapter is an update of a previous version authored by Kevin O. Leslie, Samuel A. Yousem, and Thomas V. Colby.

TABLE 17.1	
Bronchopulmonary Segments[a]	

Right upper lobe
  1. Apical
  2. Posterior
  3. Anterior
Right middle lobe
  4. Lateral
  5. Medial
Right lower lobe
  6. Superior
  7. Medial basal
  8. Anterior basal
  9. Lateral basal
  10. Posterior basal
	Left upper lobe
	  1, 2. Apical posterior
	  3. Anterior
	Lingula
	  4. Superior
	  5. Inferior
	Left lower lobe
	  6. Superior
	  7. Anterior-medial basal
	  8. Lateral basal
	  9. Posterior basal

[a]Modified from Kuhn C III. Ultrastructure and cellular function in the distal lung. In: Thurlbeck WM, Abell MR, eds. *The Lung*. Baltimore, MD: Williams & Wilkins; 1978.

Airways

The airways serve as conduits for air traveling to and from the alveoli; remove inhaled foreign material via the mucociliary escalator; and play import roles in immune surveillance, and air-moisturizing and air-warming functions.

The airways arise by unequal dichotomous branching of the bronchial buds. In a normal individual, there are approximately 20 generations (range: approximately 10 to 30 divisions), extending from the trachea to the respiratory bronchioles. In histologic sections from normal lungs, the diameter of an airway is approximately the same as its accompanying artery (and vice versa) (19). Disparities in size (of either airway or artery) suggest a pathologic condition. From a radiologic and clinical standpoint, airways have been divided into "large" and "small" types. Arbitrarily small airways are those with an internal diameter of less than 2 mm (20). From a histologic standpoint, airways are defined as follows:

TABLE 17.2		
Phases of Lung Development		
Phase	Gestation (approx. weeks)	Major Events
Embryonic	3½–6	Development of major airways and pleura
Pseudoglandular	6–16	Development of airways to terminal bronchioles and parts of prospective lung parenchyma including the beginning of the development of the acinus
Canalicular	16–28	Completion of the branching morphogenesis. Further development of the acinus and its vascularization. Earliest alveolocapillary barrier formation. Beginning of surfactant production
Saccular	28–36	Subdivision of saccules by secondary crests
Alveolar	36 weeks to term (and up to 21 years of age)	Acquisition of alveoli

Modified from Schitny JC. Development of the lung. *Cell Tissue Res* 2017;367:427–444.

- *Bronchi* are cartilaginous airways and are usually more than 2 mm in diameter (Fig. 17.1). They are conducting airways, and the cartilage plates in their walls help prevent complete collapse during bronchial constriction and expiration. Submucosal glands are a characteristic landmark of bronchi. The external wall also contains a circular layer of smooth muscle. The cartilage plates may calcify and ossify with aging.

TABLE 17.3		
Lung Development and Regulatory Factors[a]		
Phase of Lung Development	Events	Major Molecular Mediators
Embryonic	Outgrowth of trachea, right and left main bronchi, and major airways	HNF-3β, Wnt, TTF-1, RA, RAR, Shh, Ptch, Gli2, Gli3, FGF-8, FGF-10, NHF-4, N-cadherin, activin-β-r, IIa, lefty-1/2, nodal, Pitx-2
Pseudoglandular	Formation of bronchial tree up to a preacinar level	GATA-6, Nkx2.1, Foxa1/2, N-myc, PDGF, PDGF-R, EGF, EGF-R, FGF, TGF-β, Shh, Ptch, VEGF, BMP-4, RA, RAR, Sox2, Sox9
Canalicular	Formation of the pulmonary acinus and of the future air–blood barrier; increase of capillary bed; epithelial differentiation; first appearance of surfactant	GATA-6, TTF-1, HNF-3β, Wnt/β-catenin, Mash-1, VEGF
Saccular	Formation of transitory airspaces	HNF-3β, TTF-1, NF1, VEGF, VEGF-R
Alveolar	Alveolarization by forming of secondary septa	PDGF, PDGF-R, FGF, FGF-R, VEGF, VEGF-R, angiopoietins, ephrins, RA, RAR
Microvascular maturation (birth—3 years)	Thinning of interalveolar walls; fusion of the capillary bilayer to a single layered network	VEGF, VEGF-R, PDGF, PDGF-R, angiopoietins, ephrins

[a]Modified from Roth-Kleiner M, Post M. Genetic control of lung development. *Biol Neonate* 2003;84:83–88; Schitny JC. Development of the lung. *Cell Tissue Res* 2017;367:427–444.

- *Bronchioles* are membranous airways that are usually less than 2 mm in diameter; they lack cartilage and submucosal glands and normally have few goblet cells (Fig. 17.2).
- *Nonrespiratory bronchioles* represent all bronchioles proximal to respiratory bronchioles.
- *Terminal bronchioles* are nonrespiratory bronchioles just proximal to respiratory bronchioles.
- *Respiratory bronchioles* are airways that have alveoli budding from their walls.

In the large bronchi, the surface epithelium rests on a basement membrane, below which there is an elastin-rich layer of connective tissue; together these elements comprise the *bronchial mucosa*. Beneath the bronchial mucosa lies the *submucosa*, in which submucosal glands, cartilage, nerves, ganglia, and branches of the bronchial arteries may be found. There is no clear histologic boundary between the mucosa and submucosa; however, the basement membrane can be used as an arbitrary boundary. Outside the submucosa, there is a peribronchial sheath of loose connective tissue, which is continuous with that of the accompanying pulmonary artery. The bronchial epithelium is a pseudostratified columnar epithelium composed primarily of ciliated columnar cells

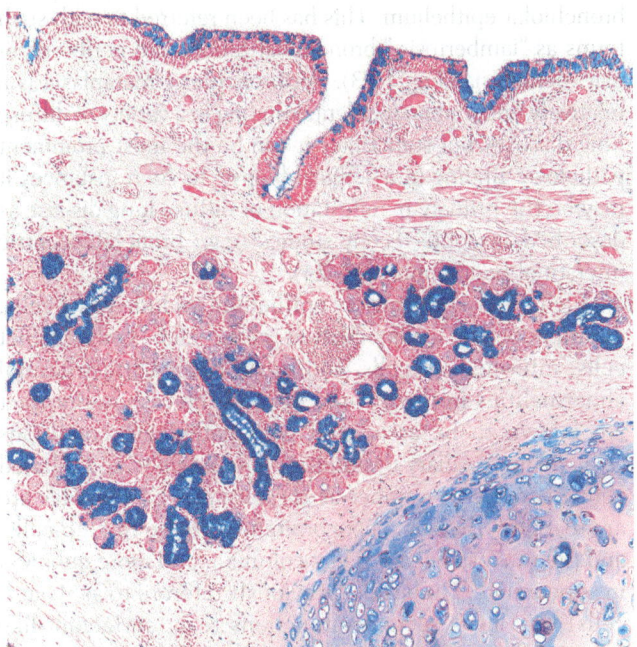

FIGURE 17.1 Bronchus. Alcian blue staining of the bronchus highlights the presence of goblet cells in the mucosa (slightly increased in this case), as well as the bronchial submucosal glands. Beneath the epithelial basement membrane, there is a vascularized layer of connective tissue with wisps of smooth muscle above the submucosal glands.

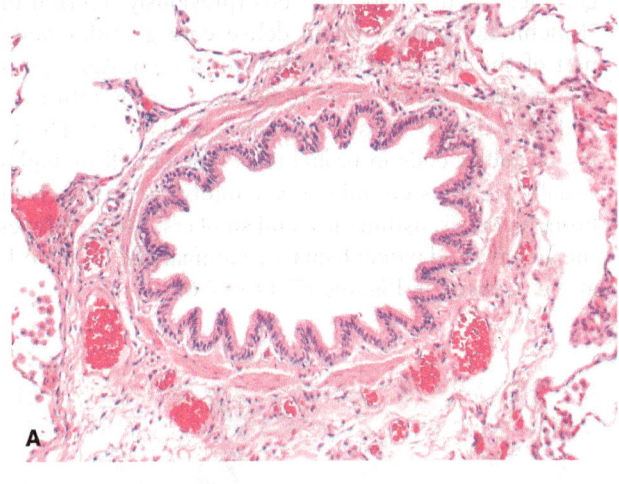
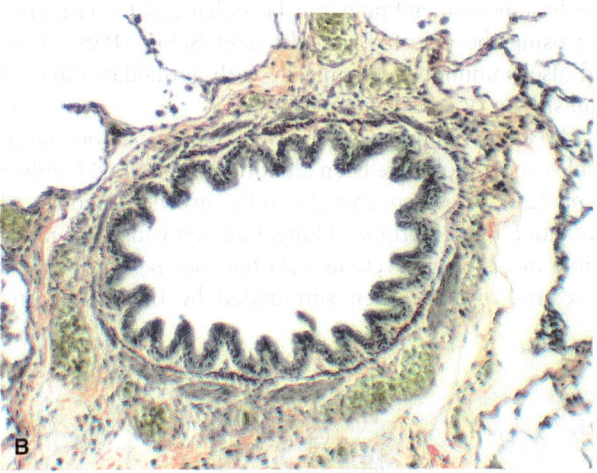
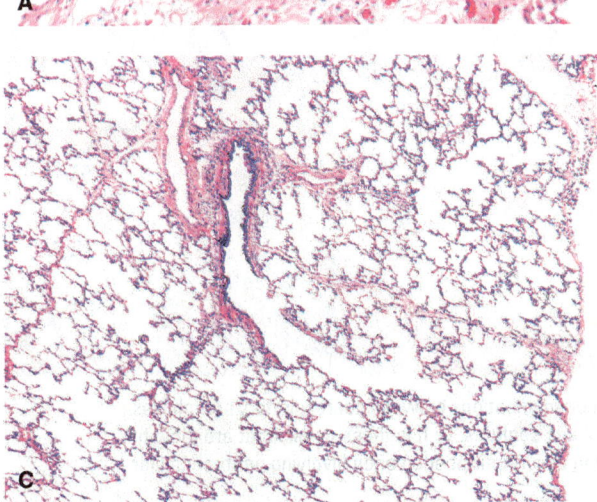

FIGURE 17.2 Bronchioles. Hematoxylin and eosin (**A**) and elastic tissue stains (**B**) illustrate normal bronchioles with a thin layer of connective tissue just beneath the epithelium overlying the elastica (**B**) and the smooth muscle investiture. The mucosa is low columnar, and there is no thickening of the subepithelial region. The smooth muscle is circumferential and is surrounded by an adventitial layer. **C:** A terminal bronchiole is continuous with the respiratory bronchiole, which extends into the alveolar ducts and ultimately the alveoli.

with interspersed mucous (goblet) cells. Lesser numbers of neuroendocrine cells, basal cells, brush cells, and migratory inflammatory cells are also normally present (see later). The height of the pseudostratified columnar epithelium decreases with progressive branching.

The walls of bronchioles are normally much thinner than those of the bronchi. The surface epithelium rests on a basement membrane, which overlies a thin layer of loose elastin-rich connective tissue. This is surrounded by a muscle layer (muscularis), which is in turn invested by a peribronchiolar connective tissue sheath continuous with that of the adjacent artery. The distinction of the mucosa from the submucosa in bronchioles is arbitrary, and sometimes the tissue beneath the basement membrane is referred to as the submucosal or submembranous connective tissue.

The airway basement membrane consists of three layers. The lamina lucida and lamina densa, together referred to as the true basement membrane (basal lamina), are composed of type IV collagen, laminin, and other fibrillary proteins. The basal lamina is very thin (0.1 μm thick) and cannot be visualized under light microscopy. Underneath the basal lamina is the lamina reticularis, composed of very fine fibrillary collagen (usually types I and III collagen). It is only found in adults and is not technically part of the basement membrane. The lamina reticularis is thickened in asthma and other inflammatory airway conditions. The basement membrane can be enhanced for visualization using the digested periodic acid–Schiff (PAS) stain, and also immunohistochemically with antibodies directed against type IV collagen and laminin.

Direct communications between nonrespiratory bronchioles and alveoli have been identified and termed *Lambert canals* (21). These are thought to be involved in collateral ventilation in the peripheral lung. Lambert canals are rarely visible in histologic sections (21) but may be conspicuous in scarred airways when surrounded by the metaplastic bronchiolar epithelium. This has been referred to with such terms as "lambertosis," bronchiolarization, and peribronchiolar metaplasia (Fig. 17.3). Peribronchiolar metaplasia is a relatively uncommon incidental finding in a variety of diffuse lung diseases but sometimes it can be the most prominent pathologic finding in a surgical biopsy. In such instances it may be the primary manifestation of diffuse lung disease as described in some recent studies (e.g., bronchiolocentric interstitial pneumonia) (22–24).

Cell types of the airway epithelium include basal cells, neuroendocrine cells, ciliated cells, club cells, goblet cells, intermediate cells, and brush cells. Ultrastructural abnormalities in the ciliated cells of the respiratory tract are known to be associated with pathologic conditions (e.g., primary ciliary dyskinesia). Goblet cells and ciliated cells decrease in number as the terminal bronchioles are approached; there is a concomitant increase in club cells, and the mucosa becomes less columnar and more cuboidal in appearance. Club cells (previously referred to as "Clara" cells) (25) have secretory functions (e.g., surfactant-like material, a protein believed to help in the stabilization of surfactant) and also act as progenitor cells for reconstituting the epithelium after bronchiolar injury. Club cell differentiation in tumors of the lung may be appreciated by the presence of apical PAS-positive, diastase-resistant granules, as well as ultrastructurally by their apical dense granules. Neuroendocrine cells (previously referred to as "Kulchitsky" cells) contain dense core granules and are part of the diffuse neuroendocrine system. Aggregates of neuroepithelial cells tend to occur at airway bifurcations and are referred to as "neuroepithelial bodies." The finding of goblet cells in bronchioles (goblet cell metaplasia) usually signifies chronic airway injury, as can be seen in bronchiectasis, asthmatics, and smokers. The cell types in the airways and parenchyma are summarized in Table 17.4 and illustrated in Figures 17.4 to 17.6.

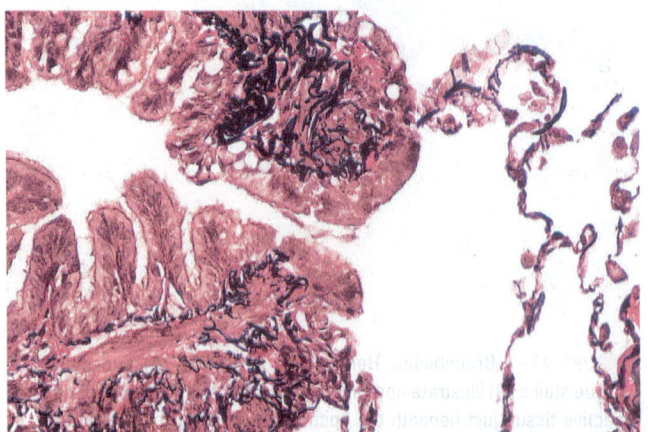
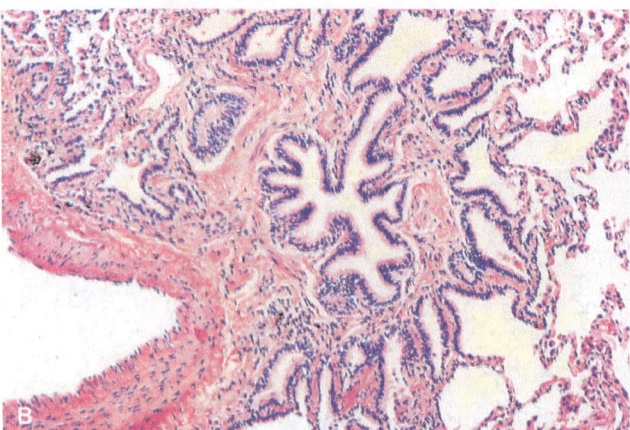

FIGURE 17.3 Lambert canals. **A:** These canals represent communications between nonrespiratory bronchioles and adjacent alveoli and are only rarely observed in histologic sections. **B:** It is these canals that are thought to be the origin of peribronchiolar metaplasia, which is seen as a repair phenomenon involving peribronchiolar alveoli after bronchiolar injury.

TABLE 17.4
Major Cell Types of the Lower Respiratory Tract[a]

Cell Type	Features	Function(s)	Location	Histochemical and/or Immunohistochemical Staining
Ciliated	Columnar, cuboidal, ciliated bronchial lining cells; each cell has approximately 250 cilia at the apical surface, and each cilium is approximately 6 μm long	Proximal transport of mucous stream (mucociliary escalator)	Bronchi and bronchioles	Epithelial markers,[b] tubulin
Goblet	Columnar mucus-secreting cells; contain mucous glycoprotein, which discharges apically	Contribute to airway mucous mucin content	Bronchi (more numerous proximally); small numbers in bronchioles	Epithelial markers,[b] histochemical mucin stains, MUC5AC
Basal	Short cells with relatively little cytoplasm; oriented along the basement membrane; do not reach the luminal surface of the epithelium	Precursor cell of ciliated and goblet cells	Bronchi; rare in bronchioles	Epithelial markers[b]
Neuroendocrine (Kulchitsky or K cells)	Basal-oriented cells with numerous dense-core (neurosecretory) granules; single or in groups (neuroepithelial bodies), the latter near sites of airway bifurcation	Specific functions not known; considered part of the diffuse neuroendocrine system. Believed to be involved in oxygen sensing, smooth muscle tonus, and immune responses	Bronchi; rare in bronchioles	Chromogranin-A, synaptophysin, CD56, NCAM
Brush	Found infrequently at all levels of the airways; some have termed these type III pneumocytes; they are named for a brush border of microvilli approximately 2 μm in length	Thought to be involved in fluid absorption or chemoreceptor function	All airways	Ultrastructurally identified
Serous	Identical to serous cells in the minor salivary gland tissues	Produce secretion of lower viscosity than that from mucous cells	Primarily bronchioles	Lysozyme
Neuroendocrine bodies	Clusters of 4–10 neuroendocrine cells adjacent to the subepithelial basement membrane	Unknown; hypotheses include chemoreceptor, tactile receptor, vasoconstrictive functions	Bronchi, bronchioles, and alveoli	Chromogranin-A, synaptophysin, CD56, calcitonin
Oncocytic	Eosinophilic mitochondria-rich cells in submucosal gland ducts	Ion secretory functions	Submucosal glands	Epithelial markers[b]
Squamous	Stratified squamous epithelium is an abnormal metaplastic replacement of normal pseudostratified respiratory epithelium	Protective, reparative	Bronchi, bronchioles, and occasionally alveoli	Epithelial markers,[b] desmoglein-3
Club	Cuboidal, nonciliated, nonmucous bronchiolar cells; protuberant apical cytoplasm with large, ovoid electron-dense granules; comprise the majority of nonciliated distal bronchiolar cells	Secretory functions of proteins of the extracellular lining fluid in distal airways, regulating its content; progenitor for other bronchiolar cells; role in protection of surfactant; metabolism of toxic substances; regulate the pulmonary immune system	Predominantly in bronchioles	CC10, CC16, diastase-resistant PAS-positive apical granules
Type I alveolar pneumocyte	Large, flat, squamous alveolar lining cells; cover some 93% of alveolar surface area; incapable of division	Provide a thin air–blood interface for gas transfer	Alveoli	Epithelial markers,[b] caveolin, and aquaporin

(continued)

TABLE 17.4
Major Cell Types of the Lower Respiratory Tract[a] (Continued)

Cell Type	Features	Function(s)	Location	Histochemical and/or Immunohistochemical Staining
Type II alveolar pneumocyte	Columnar alveolar lining cells; microvillous surface; synthesize and secrete surfactant (lamellar ultrastructural inclusions); capable of division	Maintain alveolar stability; progenitor for type I pneumocytes	Alveoli	Epithelial markers,[b] surfactant protein C, TTF-1, Napsin-A
Minor salivary tissue: serous, mucous, ductal cells	Submucosal minor salivary glands identical to other sites with serous and mucinous acinar cells that secrete into the ducts, which empty at the mucosal surface	Secretion and contribution to airway mucous stream	Bronchial submucosa	Epithelial markers,[b] histochemical stains for mucin, Alcian blue/PAS
Smooth muscle	Bundled smooth muscle surrounds the conducting airways to the level of the alveolar ducts	Contraction of the airway	Peripheral in the airway and external to the cartilage in bronchi	Muscle-specific actin, smooth muscle actin, desmin, vimentin
Other cells[c]				

[a] Table is modified from Castranova V, Rabovsky J, Tucker JH, et al. The alveolar type II epithelial cell: a multifunctional pneumocyte. *Toxicol Appl Pharmacol* 1988;93:472–483; Colby TV, Koss MN, Travis WD. Tumors of the lower respiratory tract. In: Rosai J, ed. *Atlas of Tumor Pathology*. 3rd series, Fascicle 13. Washington, DC: Armed Forces Institute of Pathology; 1995:465–471; Corrin B. *Pathology of the Lungs*. London: Churchill Livingstone; 2000.; Kasper M, Reimann T, Hempel U, et al. Loss of caveolin expression in type I pneumocyte as an indicator of subcellular alterations during lung fibrogenesis. *Histochem Cell Biol* 1998;109:41–48; Kreda SM, Gynn MC, Fenstermacher DA, et al. Expression and localization of epithelial aquaporins in the adult human lung. *Am J Respir Cell Mol Biol* 2001;24:224–234; Lou YP, Takeyama K, Grattan KM, et al. Platelet-activating factor induces goblet cell hyperplasia and mucin gene expression in airways. *Am J Respir Crit Care Med* 1998;157(pt 1):1927–1934; Rogers AV, Dewar A, Corrin B, et al. Identification of serous-like cells in the surface epithelium of human bronchioles. *Eur Respir J* 1995;6:498–504; Ryerse JS, Hoffmann JW, Mahmoud S, et al. Immunolocalization of CC10 in Clara cells in mouse and human lung. *Histochem Cell Biol* 2001;115:325–332; Branchfield K, Nantie L, Verheyden JM, et al. Pulmonary neuroendocrine cells function as airway sensors to control lung immune response. *Science* 2016;351(6274):707–710; Rokicki W, Rokicki M, Wojtacha J, et al. The role and importance of club cells (Clara cells) in the pathogenesis of some respiratory diseases. *Kardiochir Torakochirurgia Pol* 2016;13(1):26–30.
[b] For example, pancytokeratin (AE1/AE3, OSCAR), CAM5.2, epithelial membrane antigen, cytokeratin 5/6, others.
[c] Endothelial cells and pericytes; interstitial fibrocytes, fibroblasts, and myofibroblasts; macrophages; lymphoid cells, including Langerhans cells; mast cells; mesothelial pleural lining; cartilage and bone; smooth muscle; peripheral nerves; and myoepithelial cells.

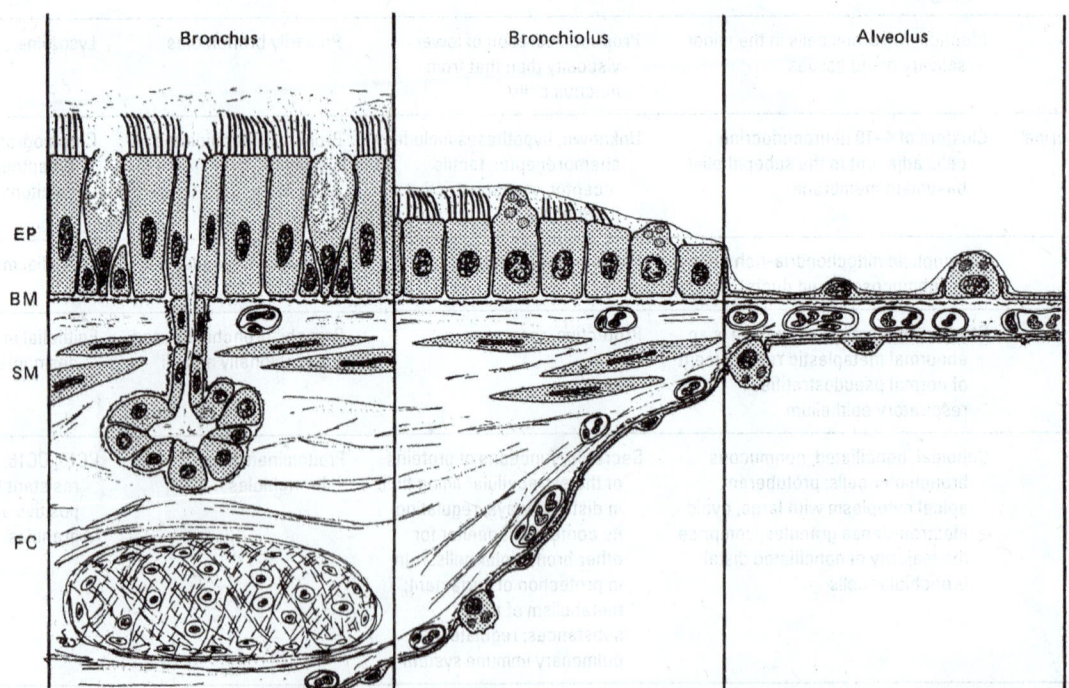

FIGURE 17.4 Respiratory tract epithelia. There is a progression of pseudostratified columnar epithelium in the large airways, to a more cuboidal epithelium in the small airways, to squamous-type epithelial cells (type I pneumocytes) in the alveoli. The epithelium in the large airways is designed for maintaining and moving the mucous stream, whereas the squamous pneumocytes in the airspaces facilitate gas transfer. (Reprinted with permission from Weibel ER, Taylor CR. Functional design of the human lung for gas exchange. In: Fishman AP, ed. *Pulmonary Diseases and Disorders*. Vol. 1. 3rd ed. New York: McGraw-Hill; 1988:21–61.)

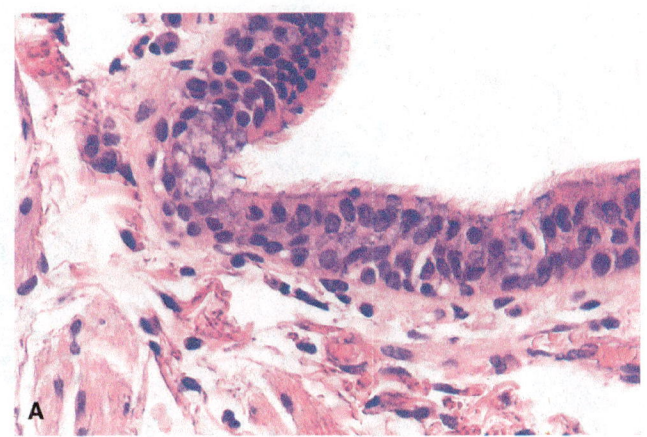

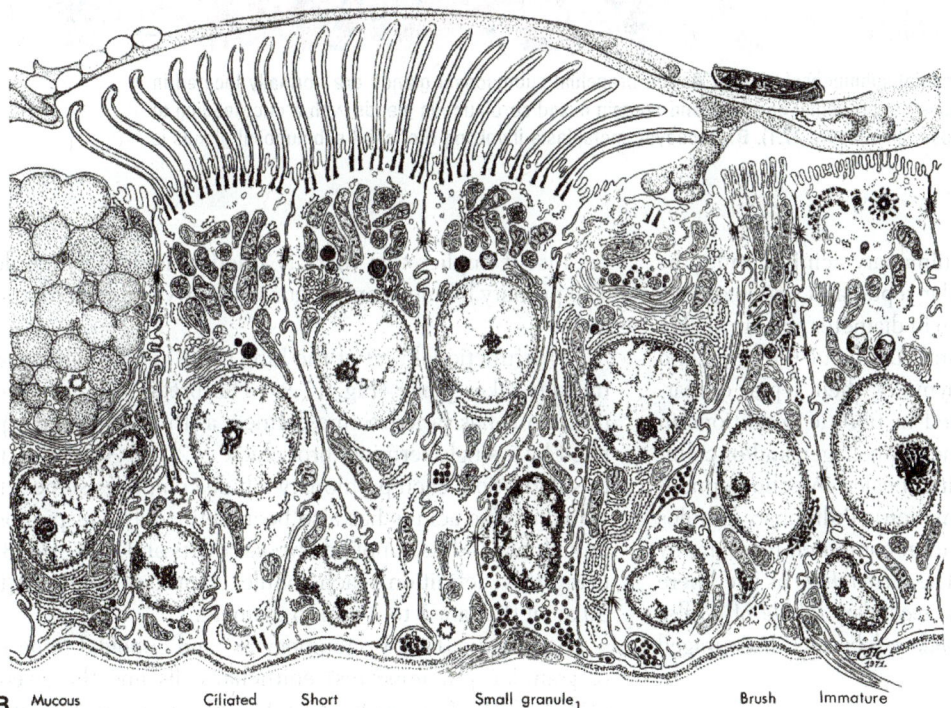

FIGURE 17.5 Bronchial epithelium. **A:** Normal bronchial epithelium is pseudostratified and columnar, with numerous ciliated cells and scattered basophilic and flocculent-appearing goblet cells. **B:** This ultrastructural schematic of bronchial epithelium shows the various cell types present. (Reprinted with permission from Sorokin SP. The respiratory system. In: Weiss L, ed. *Cell and Tissue Biology: A Textbook of Histology*. 6th ed. Baltimore, MD: Williams & Wilkins; 1988:769.)

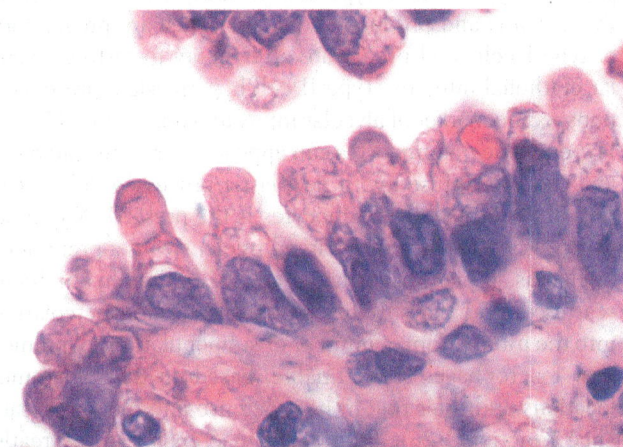

FIGURE 17.6 Club cells. Although club cells sometimes can be identified in bronchioles, these are better seen in neoplasms such as this lepidic adenocarcinoma. The apical snouting and increased cytoplasmic density are apparent.

Airway smooth muscle plays an important functional role in regulating airflow in the lungs. Smooth muscle is arranged in a complex spiral pattern around the airways and becomes progressively less prominent in the distal conducting airways. This muscle receives nutrition from the bronchial arteries. At the level of the alveolar ducts, bundles of airway smooth muscle can be seen, interrupted by alveolar openings and associated with increased lamellae of elastic fibers. In cross section, these may appear as isolated round or oblong aggregates.

Submucosal salivary-type glands containing both serous and mucous cells are found in the larger bronchi. In older individuals, oncocytic metaplasia can be seen in these glands (Fig. 17.7). Within the walls of the large airways, ganglia, nerves, and bronchial arteries are found.

Lobule and Acinus

Macroscopically, the lungs are divided into lobes, segments, and lobules. The smallest of these subdivisions is

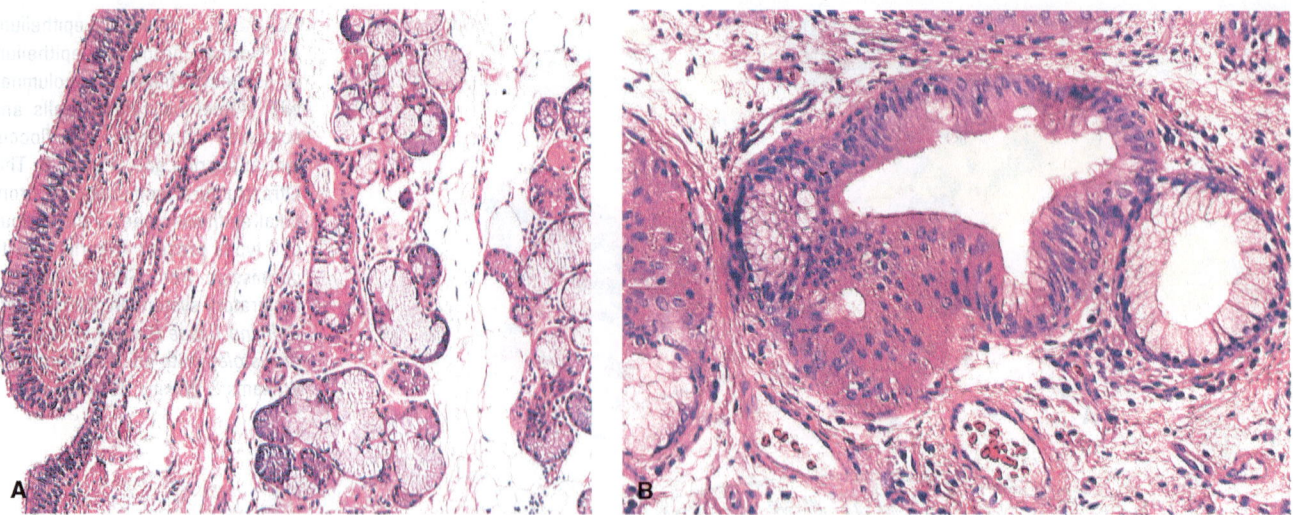

FIGURE 17.7 Bronchial submucosal glands. **A:** The bronchial submucosal glands are normally located in the submucosa above the bronchial cartilage and contain mixed seromucous glands with a duct leading to the bronchial mucosa (also Figure 17.1). **B:** Oncocytic metaplasia involving bronchial submucosal glands is relatively common.

the lobule, an aggregation of pulmonary acini bounded by connective tissue (the interlobular septa) and visible grossly (Fig. 17.8). Lobules are 1 to 2 cm in diameter and are visible to the naked eye from the pleural surface of the lung, and on cut surfaces of the parenchyma by their septal demarcations. Lobules are accentuated in fibrotic conditions in which the septa become thickened by collagen and/or cellular infiltrates (e.g., honeycombing, healed infectious pneumonia, chronic pleural inflammation). Pulmonary lobules are identifiable with high-resolution computed tomography (HRCT) scanning of the lung. The term *lobule* as used here has also been referred to as the *secondary lobule* of Miller (12). The use of the term *secondary lobule* is discouraged because it implies that there is a definable primary lobule. The primary lobule is only inconsistently visible microscopically.

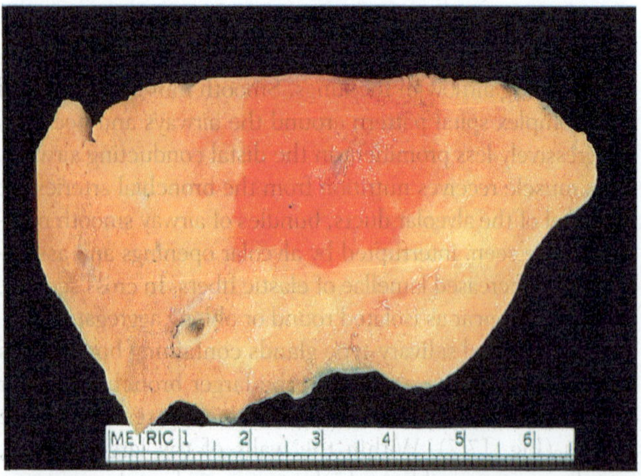

The functional unit of the lung is the acinus, where gas transfer takes place (Fig. 17.9). The precise definition of the acinus has varied. Some define it as the lung tissue supplied by a single terminal bronchiole (12,15). According to this definition, each pulmonary lobule comprises some 3 to 10 acini. The acinus has also been defined as a respiratory bronchiole and its supplied alveolar ducts and sacs (10,13); using this definition, each lobule comprises some 20 to 30 acini that are 1 to 2 mm in diameter.

Squamous (type I pneumocytes) and cuboidal (type II, or granular, pneumocytes) epithelial cells line the alveoli (Table 17.4). Gas exchange takes place across the cytoplasm of type I cells. Type II cells are present sparsely in the alveolus and produce surfactant. They are progenitors of type I cells and proliferate after injury to restore alveolar epithelial integrity. Type II cell hyperplasia represents a nonspecific marker of alveolar injury and repair (Fig. 17.10). Hyperplastic pneumocytes can appear very reactive/atypical and can be confused with neoplastic processes. A key feature of hyperplastic pneumocytes is the preserve N:C ratio despite the presence of enlarged nucleus with a prominent nucleolus. Macrophages are a normal finding in the lung, scattered over the surfaces of the alveoli and percolating into the interstitium; a number of subpopulations of pulmonary macrophages are definable, based on their anatomic locations and their role in host defense and mucous clearance functions (26). Pulmonary macrophages are greatly increased in cigarette smokers. Increased Langerhans cells are also found in the bronchiolar epithelium of smokers, but their accurate recognition requires special stains (e.g., S100 protein, CD1a, langerin).

FIGURE 17.8 Pulmonary lobule. This cut section of normal lung tissue shows focal hemorrhage highlighting a pulmonary lobule. The hemorrhage stops abruptly at the interlobular septa and, centrally, a bronchovascular bundle can be appreciated. The lobule is approximately 2 cm in diameter.

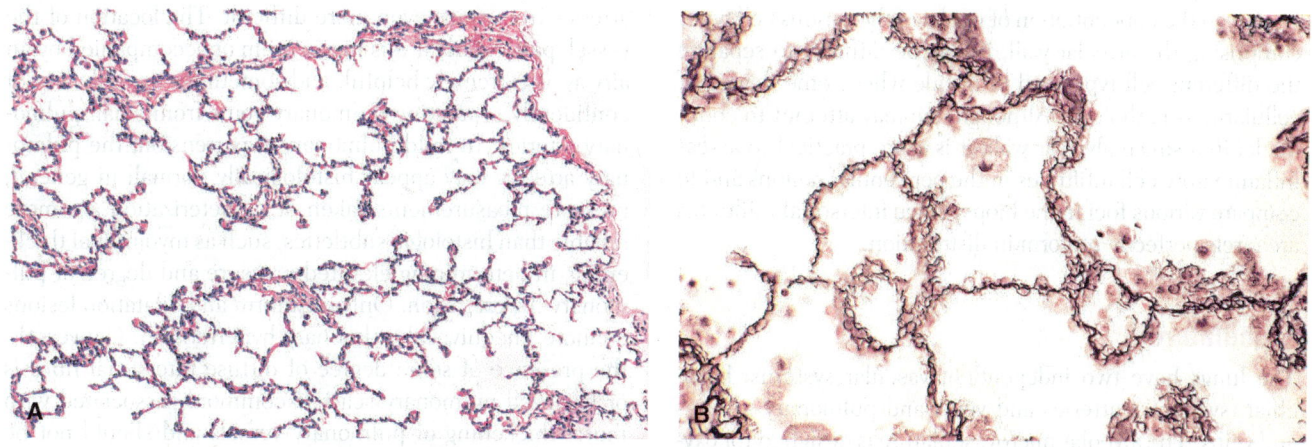

FIGURE 17.9 Distal lung parenchyma. The acinus is the functional unit of the lung where gas transfer takes place. **A:** An alveolar duct extends from the left to right and communicates directly with alveolar spaces; a small interlobular septum (*top*) and the pleura (*right*) are present (from the case illustrated in Fig. 17.2C). **B:** Reticulin stain highlights the vasculature of the alveolar septum, showing pulmonary capillaries winding around the access of the alveolar wall to maximize gas transfer surface area. A foamy macrophage is present (*upper center*), a normal finding in lung parenchyma.

The epithelial and capillary basement membranes in the alveolar septum are irregularly fused. Gas transfer takes place across the alveolar–capillary membrane, which includes the attenuated cytoplasm of the type I cell, the endothelial cell cytoplasm, and their fused basement membranes. Pores of Kohn represent direct communications between adjacent alveoli through a "pore" in the alveolar wall. They are thought to be involved in collateral ventilation. Pores of Kohn are rarely visible with the light microscope.

The lung is invested with a rich framework of connective tissue coursing throughout the interstitium. It is well developed and easily visible along bronchovascular sheaths and in the septa that delimit lobules. This framework is continuous from the hilum to the pleura and encompasses the interstitial compartment of the lung down to the level of the alveolar wall and perivascular areas. Within the alveolar walls, collagen, elastic fibers, mesenchymal cells, and a few inflammatory cells can be identified ultrastructurally. This alveolar interstitial space is normally inconspicuous by light microscopy in adults. In children (up to approximately age 4), some interstitial widening and increased cellularity are normal histologic findings.

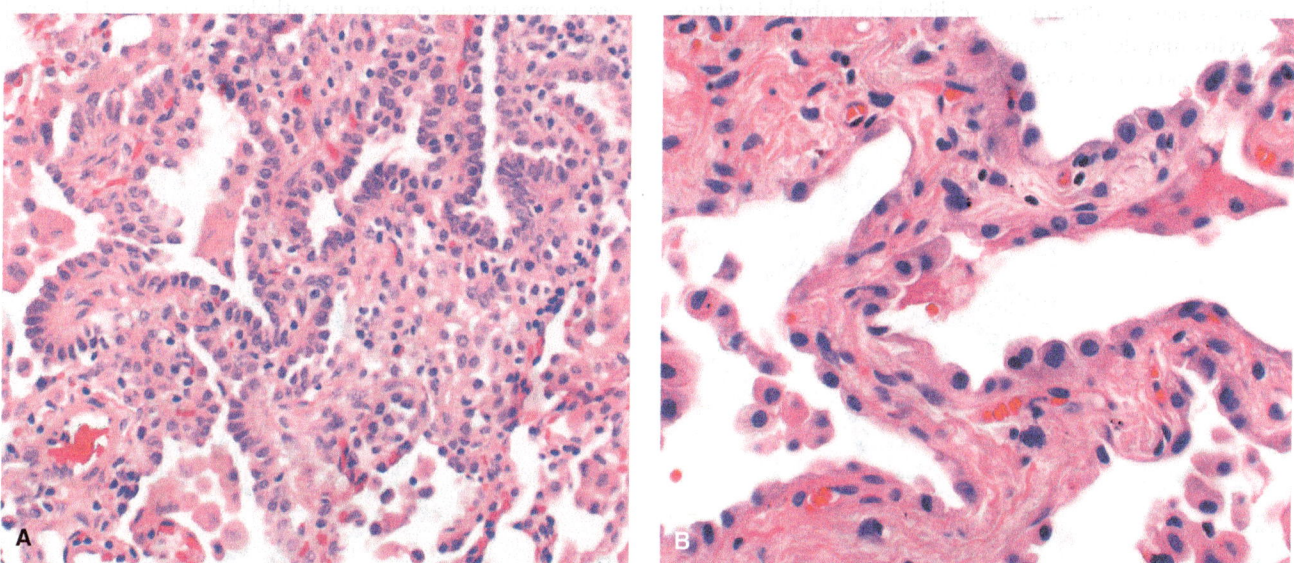

FIGURE 17.10 Reactive alveolar cell hyperplasia. **A:** A reactive proliferation of type II pneumocytes (alveolar cell hyperplasia) is common after injury. This case illustrates how this appears as a single row of cells protruding from the alveolar surface. **B:** Significant cytologic atypia is lacking. The interstitium underlying this process may show edema, inflammatory cells, and some fibrinous exudate consistent with recent lung injury.

Given the concentration of nuclei of the various cell types comprising the alveolar wall, it may be difficult to separate the different cell types and to decide when some degree of cellularity is pathologic. Although one may attempt to count nuclei in a single alveolar wall, it is more practical to assess inflammatory cell infiltrates in the perivenular regions and to compare various foci in the biopsy since interstitial infiltrates are rarely perfectly uniform in distribution.

Vasculature

The lungs have two independent vascular systems: bronchial (systemic) arteries and veins and pulmonary arteries and veins. The alveolar microvasculature is designed for oxygenation of venous blood derived from the pulmonary arteries. Large (elastic) pulmonary arteries in infants are similar to the aorta in structure; the elastic fiber lamellae become more irregular, fragmented, and less compact in adulthood. Elastic tissue remains relatively prominent in the pulmonary arterial tree to approximately the point where bronchi become bronchioles. At this juncture, the pulmonary arteries become primarily muscular arteries. The muscular pulmonary arteries and arterioles have an internal and external elastic membrane (Fig. 17.11A); pulmonary veins have only a lamellated single (outer) elastica (Fig. 17.11B). Small intra-acinar pulmonary veins merge into larger veins in the interlobular septa. The bronchial arteries in the walls of bronchi are part of the systemic circulation and have pressures similar to systemic arterial pressures. The pulmonary circulation is a low-pressure system with a normal mean pressure of approximately 10 mmHg (it is somewhat higher at higher elevations above sea level).

It may be difficult to separate small pulmonary arteries from venules, especially since a single elastic lamina forms as arteries diminish in caliber. In pathologic states, the veins may develop muscular hypertrophy and increased mural thickness (arterialization), making the distinction of arteries from veins even more difficult. The location of the vessel, particularly if it is in a septum or accompanied by an airway, is extremely helpful, and sometimes the only way of confidently separating pulmonary veins from small pulmonary arteries. In mild pulmonary hypertension, the pulmonary arteries may appear histologically normal; in general, pressure measurements taken at catheterization are more reliable than histologic subtleties, such as myointimal thickening, in determining elevated pressure and degree of pulmonary hypertension. Only plexiform and dilatation lesions connote unequivocal pulmonary hypertension. Conversely, the presence of some degree of diffuse interstitial fibrosis or localized pulmonary scars is commonly associated with mural thickening of pulmonary vessels and should not be interpreted as evidence of pulmonary hypertension.

Lymphatics and Lymphoid Tissue

The lung is invested with a rich supply of lymphatics and lymphoid tissue. Lymphatic drainage proceeds toward the hilum of the lung. Lymph fluid from the lower lobes tends to drain to mediastinal lymph nodes, with lymph fluid from the remaining portions of the lung draining to tracheobronchial lymph nodes. On the left side, the lymph fluid drains into the thoracic duct; and, on the right side, it drains into the right bronchomediastinal trunk. Both of these ultimately drain into the left and right subclavian veins, respectively. Lymphatic channels are found along bronchovascular structures, interlobular septae, and within the pleura, while pulmonary veins can be identified in the alveolar septae, interlobular septae, and pleura. Valves may be apparent in some sections. Lymphatics do not extend into alveolar walls so interstitial water is "pumped" out by lymphatics present either centrally in the lobule or at the lobule periphery. The lymphatic vessels are inconspicuous except in pathologic states, such as pulmonary edema or lymphangitic carcinoma. Lymphoreticular infiltrates and some pneumoconioses tend to be distributed

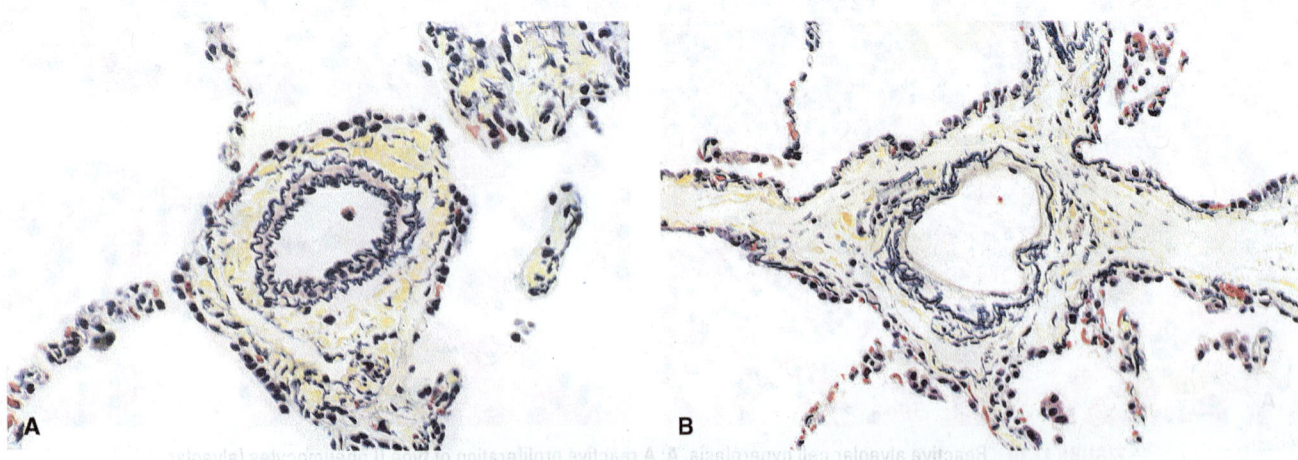

FIGURE 17.11 Pulmonary vasculature (elastic stains). Normal pulmonary arteries contain two elastic lamina (**A**), whereas veins have a single elastic lamina (**B**). The location of a vein within a septum (**B**) is also very helpful in identifying it as a vein.

along the lymphatic routes, but the lymphatic vessels themselves may not be prominent (such infiltrates are referred to as *perilymphatic/lymphangitic* radiologically).

Lymphoid tissue may be seen as small collections of lymphocytes along the lymphatic routes, especially branch points of the bronchovascular bundles; lymphoid tissue is generally absent or inconspicuous except in pathologic states. Lymphoid tissue along the airways is part of the diffuse mucosa-associated lymphoid tissue (MALT) and in the lung is referred to as bronchus-associated lymphoid tissue (BALT). Submucosal lymphoid tissue in the intermediate and small airways is associated with flattening and attenuation of the overlying respiratory mucosa (lymphoepithelium), which has increased HLA class II antigens. At these sites, B-lymphocyte emperipolesis is common and is thought to reflect active antigen processing by the BALT. BALT displays the same reactions observed in the lymphoid tissue at other sites; for example, reactive hyperplasia and immunoblastic proliferation, which can be confused with lymphoreticular malignancies.

Immunophenotypically the lymphoid tissue of BALT has four identifiable compartments, including B-cell–rich follicles, B-cell follicular mantle and marginal zones, and T-cell–rich interfollicular regions. A follicular dendritic cell network is present. Polyclonal plasma cells are identified in the perifollicular tissue. The finer details of the immunoarchitecture and the immunophenotypic characterization of these cells are beyond the scope of this chapter. The follicles tend to be polarized into a darker side and a paler side, with the latter oriented toward the epithelial surface; BALT also shares features of MALT as seen at other sites. In normal adult lungs, BALT is rarely present, and its presence correlates with some form of chronic antigenic stimulation (27–29). According to Tschernig et al. (29), BALT is not present at birth but is found normally with increasing age, probably as a result of exposure to environmental antigens, this is referred to as inducible BALT. After the individual has been exposed to most of the common antigens, the inducible BALT regresses and dendritic cells in the airways assume the role of antigen uptake and presentation. Its reappearance in adults follows chronic antigen stimuli, such as chronic infection allergens, response to tumors, or in autoimmunity (30).

As currently defined, BALT refers only to lymphoid tissue along the airways (31) and not to the lymphoid tissue that may be seen in the pleura and septa as part of the diffuse lymphoid system in the lung. The lymphoid tissue is normally present in the lung at the bifurcation of lymphatics and such aggregates often consist of small round lymphocytes, Langerhans cells, and pigmented macrophages with cytoplasmic anthracosilicotic material. These aggregates are distinct from BALT. Hyperplasia of BALT is frequently accompanied by lymphoid hyperplasia at other sites.

Intrapulmonary peribronchial lymph nodes are a normal finding, but peripheral intraparenchymal lymph nodes are less common; however, in smokers and others with high dust exposure, they are increasingly recognized (and biopsied) with current imaging techniques (32). Intrapulmonary lymph nodes are usually septal or subpleural in location (see later). Anthracosis and small amounts of silica and silicates in these nodes are common and nonspecific.

Pleura

The visceral pleura is composed of connective tissue, elastic tissue, and an outer mesothelial layer (Fig. 17.12). Two elastic tissue laminae may be seen but these are not sharply defined. In disease, particularly pleural fibrosis and

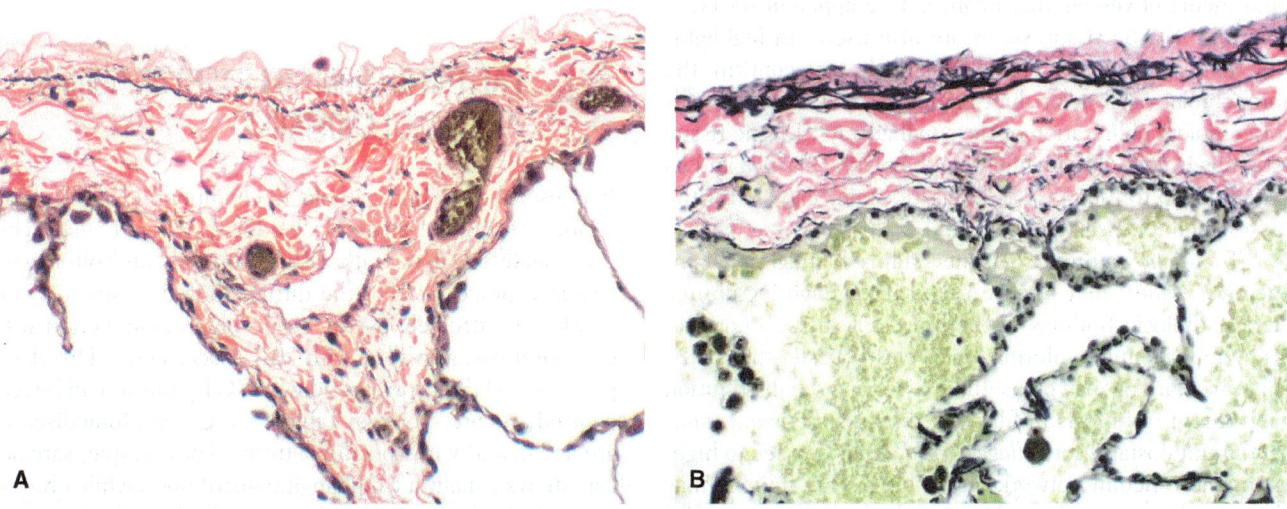

FIGURE 17.12 Pleural elastic tissue (elastic stains). The pleura contains an elastic tissue membrane, which may appear as a single thin layer of elastic tissue (**A**) or as a richer network with occasional elastic fibers distributed through the thickness of the visceral pleura (**B**). The field illustrated in (**A**) shows a normal lymphatic at the juncture between an interlobular septum and the visceral pleura.

adhesions, several layers may be apparent and the elastic tissue may greatly increase. Elastic tissue stains are useful in assessing whether a given pathologic process, such as carcinoma, has transgressed the visceral pleura (33), but interpretation is difficult when the pleura is fibrotic and the elastic tissue is increased. Pleural involvement has been shown to be important in staging non–small-cell lung cancer. When the internal elastic fibers are transgressed, small tumors (less than 3 cm), that by size alone would be staged as T1, are upstaged to T2. If the tumor invades the parietal pleura (e.g., chest wall), the minimum T descriptor is T3, regardless of the tumor size (33,34). Lymphatic vessels that are continuous with those in the interlobular septa are also identifiable in the pleura. When the pleura is fibrotic and where pleural adhesions are present, vessels may be thick and sclerotic or even pseudoangiomatous in appearance. Fatty metaplasia is often striking in the foci of pleural and subpleural scarring. The visceral pleura often remains viable over pulmonary infarcts because it has a separate vascular supply. Submesothelial fibroblasts may undergo mesothelial metaplasia (and become cytokeratin-positive) in inflammatory conditions of the pleura.

SPECIAL STAINS AND THE EVALUATION OF LUNG HISTOLOGY

While most diagnostic work in lung histopathology can be performed with routine *hematoxylin and eosin (H&E) staining*, there are a number of special stains that aid interpretation and may highlight findings. *Elastic tissue staining* is helpful in evaluating the pulmonary vasculature, airways, and pleura. Smaller arteries and veins often can be distinguished from each other with elastic tissue staining. Elastic tissue staining may highlight damage to the intima and media of vessels that might not be apparent on H&E staining. Elastic tissue stains are also useful in highlighting abnormalities of bronchioles and may confirm the bronchiolar or alveolar duct origin of small scars in cases of complete obliteration of the small airways. Elastic tissue staining is helpful in highlighting the pleural elastica and its relationship to tumors. Lastly, elastic stains can aid for the assessment of vascular invasion.

Trichrome staining (or other stains highlighting connective tissues) may also be useful in highlighting normal and pathologic findings in the lung, but they do not provide quite as much information as elastic tissue stains. Trichrome staining may be useful in assessing the distribution and extent of fibrosis in fibrosing diseases. *Reticulin stains* and immunostains for *collagen type IV* may be used to highlight the reticulin network of the lung. This staining may be useful in research studies, in which they are a useful indicator of invasion, and in highlighting normal histology but is not generally useful in diagnostic surgical pathology of the lung.

Immunostains for epithelial markers (such as EMA and cytokeratin stains) may be beneficial in atelectatic or fibrotic lung when it is difficult to appreciate the architectural features on H&E staining. Comparing these stains with stains for endothelial cells (such as CD31 or CD34) may provide an additional aid in assessing lung architecture and structural relationships. The use of CD31 may be somewhat confusing in cases where alveolar macrophages are abundant since alveolar macrophages frequently show prominent staining. The lymphoid tissue in the lung is assessed with the panoply of lymphoid markers used at other sites. Both CD3 and CD20 are often useful to check the proportion and distribution of T and B cells, respectively. In general, most inflammatory conditions have a preponderance of T cells as the diffuse component of the infiltrates, with scattered B-cell follicles. The presence of a dense diffuse population of CD20-positive B cells in lung parenchyma should be considered lymphoma until proven otherwise, and might be an indication for additional immunohistochemical and molecular studies (e.g., B- or T-cell receptor PCR rearrangement studies). In lymphoproliferative conditions, cytokeratin staining highlights lymphoepithelial lesions. Both S100 and CD1a are useful in identifying Langerhans cells; the latter stain is much more specific.

Normal mesothelial cells lining the pleura can stain with calretinin (nuclear and cytoplasmic), cytokeratin 5/6, D2-40, and WT-1 (nuclear positivity), especially when mesothelial reactive changes or hyperplasia are present. In some cases, separation of mesothelial hyperplasia from mesothelioma can be very challenging. In reactive conditions, mesothelial cells assume a myofibroblastic phenotype and may express smooth muscle actin, desmin, and other myogenic-type proteins. Lastly, FISH studies for *CDKN2A* (p16 protein) gene deletion and BAP1 nuclear expression loss by immunohistochemistry might be of help (35).

PATTERN RECOGNITION BASED ON NORMAL ANATOMIC LANDMARKS

It is useful to define pathologic conditions in the lung in relation to normal anatomic landmarks (Fig. 17.13). This can usually be done with diffuse diseases and often with localized processes. For the diffuse lung diseases this correlation is extremely useful, especially in conjunction with gross findings, as well as with HRCT scans (36). Histologic patterns and their corresponding HRCT patterns can be recognized and are shown in Table 17.5. Certain lung diseases are associated with specific patterns. For example, sarcoidosis shows usually a lymphangitic distribution while chronic hypersensitivity pneumonitis is usually bronchiolocentric. Idiopathic usual interstitial pneumonia demonstrates the classic subpleural and paraseptal distribution with more or less sparing of the center of the lobule.

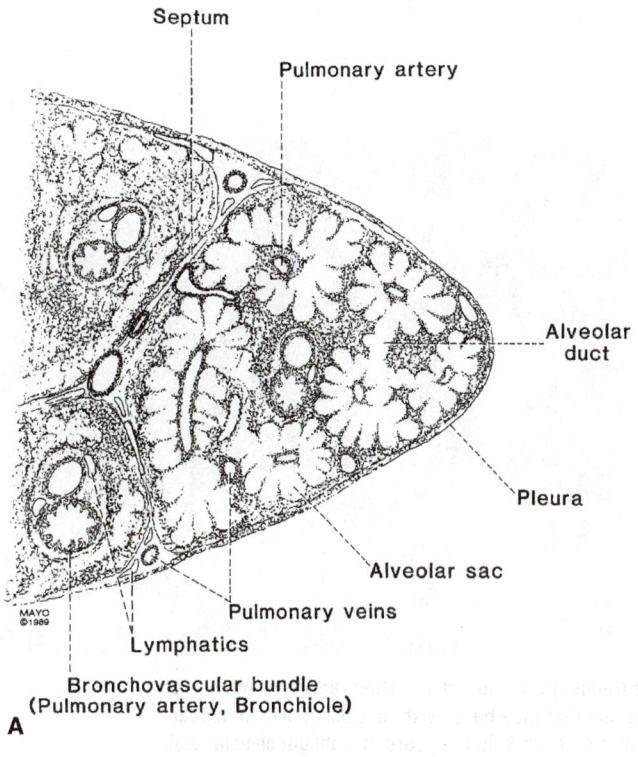

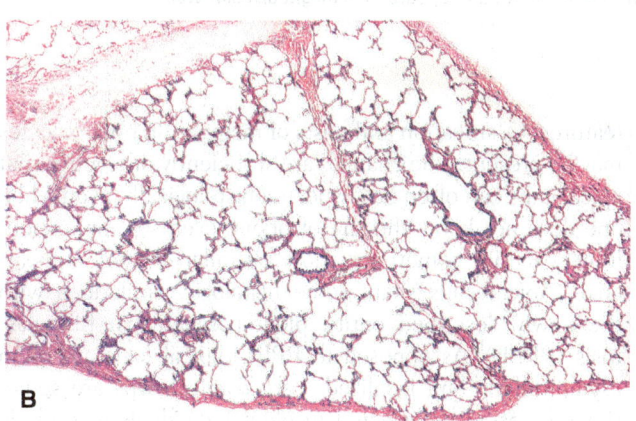

FIGURE 17.13 Wedge lung biopsy. **A:** This stylized diagram is used to depict anatomic landmarks. Structures depicted in (**A**) can be appreciated in an actual wedge biopsy specimen (**B**).

It is apparent that there is close correlation (but not a 1:1 relationship) between histology and HRCT. With some communication between the pathologist and the radiologist, there is a significant mutual appreciation for the similarity of the abnormalities seen. In this regard, the pathologist may be significantly aided by HRCT findings, which may suggest distributions that might not be apparent in biopsy material because of such things as the size of the biopsy (e.g., transbronchial biopsy) or sampling issues (nonrepresentative biopsies). Since 2002, it has been extensively demonstrated that the classification of difficult interstitial lung diseases is better achieved based on a multidisciplinary discussion, rather than on histologic grounds alone (37).

TABLE 17.5
Corresponding Histologic and Radiologic Patterns[a]

Histologic	Radiologic (HRCT)
Broncho/bronchiolocentric	Centrilobular Bronchovascular Nodular
Angiocentric	Bronchovascular (arterial) Interlobular septal (venous)
Pleural/subpleural	Pleural/subpleural
Lymphatic	Bronchovascular Interlobular septal Pleural
Peripheral acinar	Subpleural peripheral distribution (paraseptal)
Septal	Septal
Random nodular	Random nodular
Parenchymal consolidation	Consolidation, ground glass
Diffuse interstitial	Diffuse interstitial, ground glass
Mixed and unclassified	Mixed/unclassifiable

[a]Modified from Colby TV, Swensen SJ. Anatomic distribution and histopathologic pattern in diffuse lung disease: Correlation with HRCT. *J Thorac Imaging* 1996;11:1–26.

SITE-RELATED CHANGES COMMONLY SEEN IN SURGICAL PATHOLOGY MATERIAL

Site-specific changes that may be primary lesions or incidental findings in surgical material are shown in Table 17.6.

Biopsies from lobar tips, particularly from the lingula or right middle lobe, may show incidental inflammatory and fibrotic changes (38), including interstitial fibrosis, epithelial metaplasia, and even focal honeycombing—all of which may not be representative of a diffuse process. Myointimal proliferation is common in the arteries and veins of these biopsies. The airspaces may contain aggregates of macrophages and neutrophils. Because of their accessibility, these sites were often biopsied in the era of open lung biopsy. Incidental changes in lobar tips are usually obvious as such, since the more proximal lung tissue is either not affected

TABLE 17.6
Site-Specific Changes in Lung Tissue

- Inflammatory changes at lobar tips, especially lingula and right middle lobe
- Apical caps: Pleural and subpleural fibrosis in the apex and the upper lobes and superior segments of the lower lobes
- Upper lobe centriacinar emphysema
- Visceral pleural/subpleural fibrosis ("subpleural bulla")

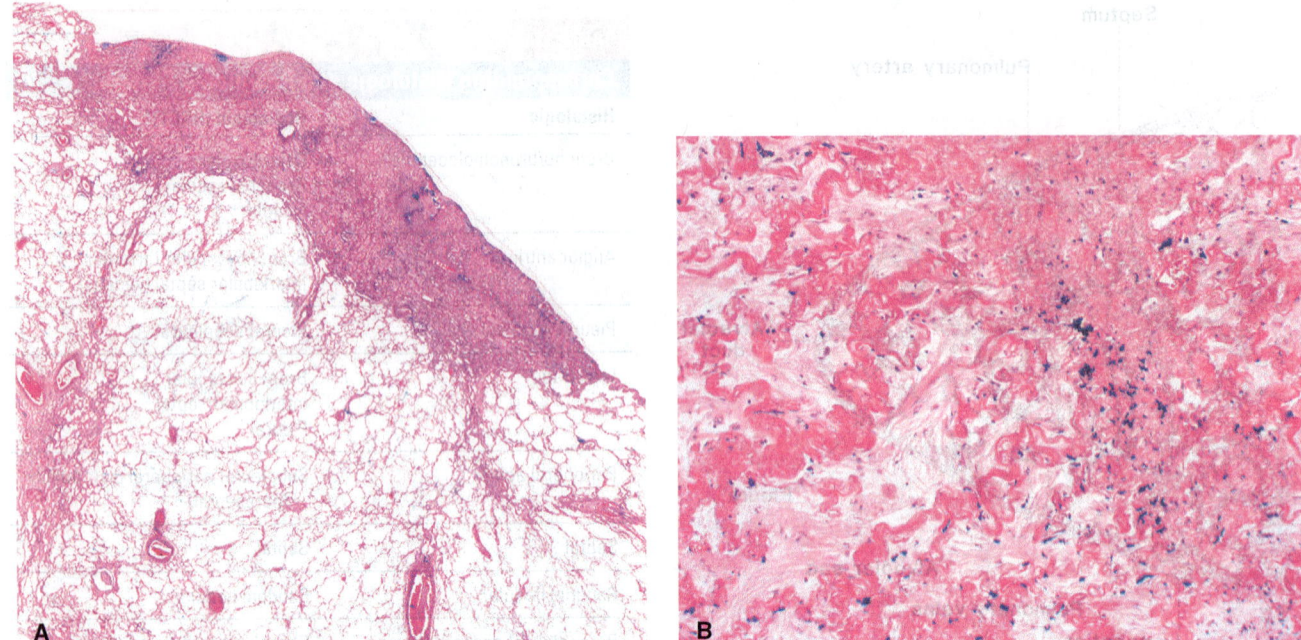

FIGURE 17.14 Apical cap. **A:** Apical caps occur most frequently in the apices. They represent regions of pleural and subpleural thickening by elastotic fibrous tissue that may be grayish or eosinophilic in appearance. **B:** Higher power sometimes shows a rich elastic tissue network that appears to highlight alveolar wall structure; some anthracotic pigmented is also noted.

or significantly less affected. Thus, in evaluation of lobar tip wedge biopsies, the findings of greatest significance are often in the more proximal portions of the specimen. Nonspecific inflammatory changes in lobar tips become a problem in small wedge biopsies, particularly those that are 2 cm or less in greatest dimension. Since lobar tips are so readily accessible to the surgeon, it is difficult to discourage surgeons from biopsying them. If possible, such biopsies should be at least 3 cm deep into the underlying parenchyma often corresponding to a 5 cm in greatest dimension biopsy. The possibility of middle lobe syndrome (which may affect the lingula, the right middle lobe, or both) (39,40) should be considered for persistent infiltrates in these sites. Today, the majority of surgical lung biopsies are performed by video thoracoscopy. The video-assisted thoracoscopic surgery (VATS) biopsy is performed with the lung deflated and nearly all sites are accessible.

Apical caps (Fig. 17.14) were once thought to be the result of healed tuberculosis, but they are common in patients who have never had tuberculosis; they are now thought to be an ischemic alteration related to the intrinsic physiologic underperfusion of their apical location (41–43). Apical caps occur most frequently in the apex of the upper lobes, but they are also encountered in the upper regions of the lower lobes (44). Apical caps are regions of fibrosis in the pleura and subpleural lung parenchyma that are rich in thickened elastic fibers; the background structure of collapsed alveolar walls and interposed eosinophilic collagen can often be discerned in the tissue; elastic tissue stains enhance these features. Ossification and nests of metaplastic pneumocytes may be present. The changes are sufficiently distinctive that apical caps can often be suspected histologically, even when one does not know the site of origin; even so, any ancient lung scar may sometimes show a similar elastotic appearance. Apical caps share some histologic similarities with the newly described entity, pleuroparenchymal fibroelastosis (PPFE). As opposed to PPFE, apical caps are often asymptomatic and localized. Larger apical caps are sometimes biopsied or resected in older individuals to exclude a carcinoma or a visceral pleural tumor (44). In the era of HRCT scans and imaging surveillance of smokers, more often smaller apical caps are also being biopsied. In addition, they can be PET-avid secondary to infection and can show remarkable cytologic atypia of pneumocytes and they should not be confused with invasive carcinoma.

Centriacinar (centrilobular) emphysema is a pathologic abnormality that is more common and more severe in the upper lobes (45); it is found predominantly in cigarette smokers and is a common finding in lobes resected for bronchogenic carcinoma. Emphysematous changes are frequently accompanied by some degree of fibrosis, particularly when a bullous change is present. The fibrosis tends to appear as strands of dense, hypocellular, brightly eosinophilic collagenous septa traversing the emphysematous spaces. Anthracosis is also a common finding in smokers and urban dwellers. Focal pleural and subpleural fibrosis (Fig. 17.15) is extremely common, especially as an incidental microscopic finding in lobar resections from smokers

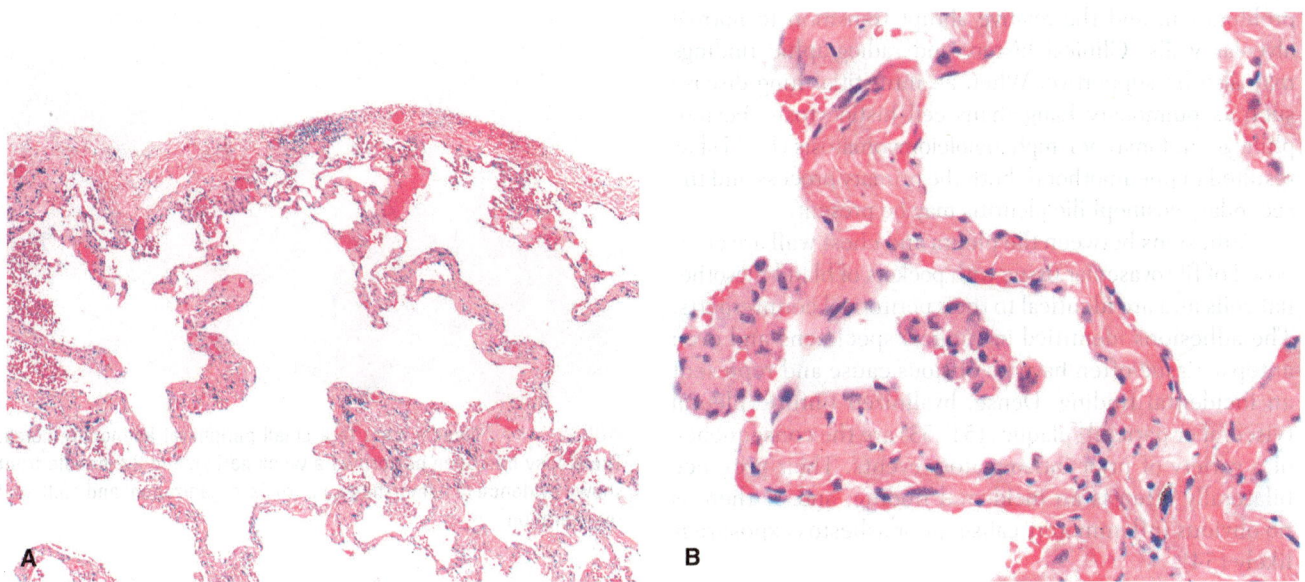

FIGURE 17.15 Subpleural emphysematous change in smoking. **A:** There is simplification of airspaces. **B:** Some of the alveolar walls show mild fibrosis with hyaline appearing collagen. Occasional clusters of pigmented alveolar macrophages (can also be referred to as smoker's macrophages) are also noted.

(46); abnormal airspaces formed by irregular fibrous septa are accompanied by smooth muscle hyperplasia, mucostasis, and bronchiolar metaplasia.

Subpleural bullous change (Fig. 17.16) can be the only pathologic change found in patients with recurrent pneumothoraces and who do not have diffuse lung disease (47). These are typically evident in the upper lobes. By convention, *blebs* are defined as being <1 cm in diameter and some are derived from air dissection into the visceral pleura, *bullae* are any emphysematous sharply demarcated air-containing spaces 1 cm or greater in diameter with lung parenchyma lined by TTF1-positive pneumocytes (48,49). Their rupture introduces air into the pleural space, inciting a mesothelial proliferation with numerous macrophages, giant cells, and eosinophils (referred to as eosinophilic pleuritis), and this reaction may accompany any condition that is associated with pneumothorax (50). Collections of interstitial air in the lung tissue, with or without giant cell and/or eosinophilic reaction, may be an accompanying finding. Focal subpleural scarring can usually be distinguished from chronic fibrosing interstitial pneumonias by its restriction to the subpleural region, lack of active fibroblastic

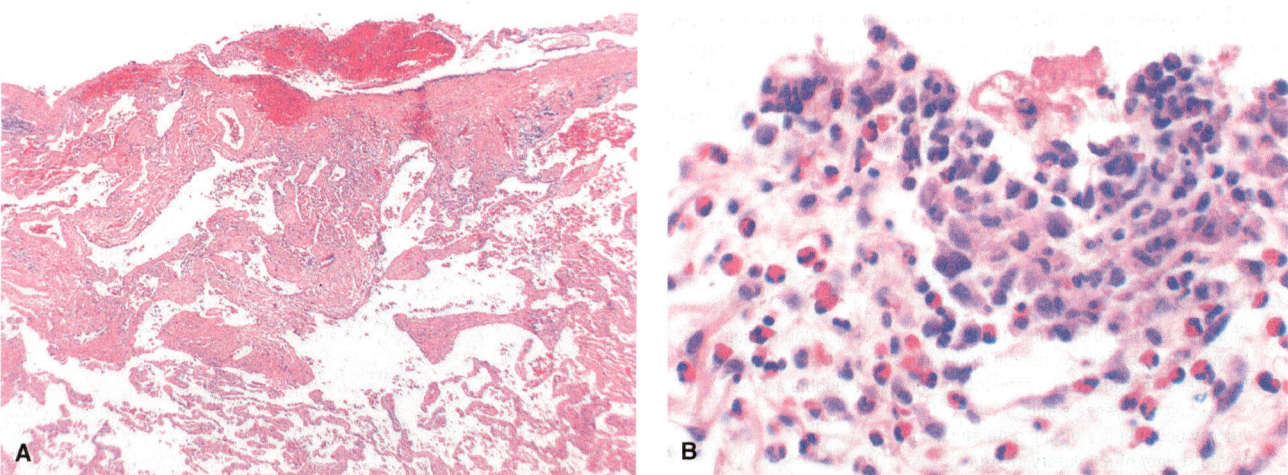

FIGURE 17.16 Pneumothorax. **A:** The so-called "subpleural blebs" are thought to predispose to pneumothorax. These are regions of pleural and subpleural scarring with abnormal airspaces somewhat reminiscent to smoking-related changes (also Fig. 17.15). **B:** Pneumothorax is often associated with a pleural reaction (*top*), which has been labeled eosinophilic pleuritis because of the association of eosinophil infiltrate and mesothelial and macrophage reaction on the pleural surface.

proliferation, and the relative abrupt transition to normal alveolar walls. Clinical history and radiographic findings may also be supportive. When an interstitial lung disease such as pulmonary Langerhans cell histiocytosis (eosinophilic granuloma) or lymphangioleiomyomatosis (LAM) has resulted in pneumothorax, both the primary process and the secondary eosinophilic pleuritis may be present.

Adhesions between the pleura and chest wall are composed of fibrovascular tissue with pockets of bland mesothelial cells and are identical to their peritoneal counterparts. The adhesions identified in surgical specimens and even autopsy tissue often have no obvious cause and represent an incidental finding. Dense, hyalinized fibrotic pleural (visceral or parietal) plaques (51–53) are the consequence of a variety of prior inflammatory events. Their presence bilaterally often is an incidental finding; and, if there is no obvious inflammatory cause, prior asbestos exposure is likely (54).

ARTIFACTS SEEN IN LUNG BIOPSY AND RESECTION MATERIAL

Artifacts related to lung biopsy or prior procedures are described in Table 17.7.

Knowledge of the clinical course of events prior to lung biopsy usually allows the pathologist to avoid misinterpreting changes of prior instrumentation. Previous bronchial biopsies may cause hemorrhage, airway inflammation, ulceration, granulation tissue reaction, and fibrous scarring. Strips of epithelium may be dislodged by mechanical trauma and embedded in inspissated mucus; residual basal cells may be all that is left adherent to the basement membrane. Bronchoalveolar lavage can produce vacuolation of alveolar pneumocytes and macrophages. Previous needle biopsies may induce necrosis and hemorrhage in the parenchyma, followed by organization and reactive epithelial atypia (Fig. 17.17). Patients who have been on positive-pressure ventilation (Fig. 17.18) may have disproportional bronchiolar and alveolar duct distension, especially when

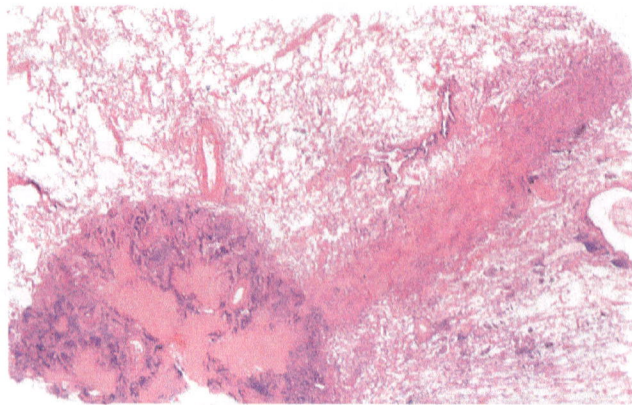

FIGURE 17.17 Needle tract to a small peripheral adenocarcinoma. The biopsy had been performed a week earlier, and the needle tract shows evidence of hemorrhage, necrosis, organization, and epithelial regeneration.

high inspiratory pressures are used in the acute respiratory distress syndrome (ARDS). Some associated acute inflammatory exudate in the lumen is common, often with relative absence of associated inflammation in the airway wall or surrounding alveolar spaces. Occasionally, one can find exogenous thrombotic foreign material in bronchial arteries when patients have been treated with bronchial artery embolization for persistent hemoptysis.

Compression of the lung tissue, particularly in transbronchial biopsies, may produce rounded spaces in the alveoli that resemble fat vacuoles and can easily be mistaken for exogenous lipoid pneumonia (Fig. 17.19A, B). This artifactual change, often called "bubble artifact" (55,56), can be recognized because there are no associated macrophages or giant cells with small or large distending intracytoplasmic lipid vacuoles (all the vacuoles are extracellular), and there is usually little fibrosis, which is a constant feature of chronic exogenous lipoid pneumonia.

TABLE 17.7
Artifacts Seen in Lung Biopsies and Resections

- Changes related to prior instrumentation including bronchoscopy, bronchoalveolar lavage, needle aspiration, and ventilatory assistance
- Compression/atelectasis; pseudolipoid change ("bubble artifact")
- Telescoping of vessels and airways
- Airway epithelium sloughing/detachment
- Hemorrhage/inflammatory changes
- Septal edema; lymphatic dilatation
- Material from surgical gloves (e.g., talc and starch)
- Inflation-induced alveolar distension resembling emphysema and patchy atelectasis in underinflated zones
- Sponge artifact

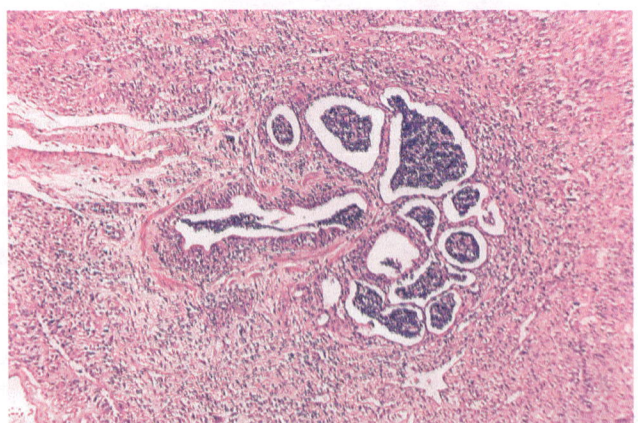

FIGURE 17.18 Ventilator-associated injury. Common changes in the setting of positive-pressure ventilator therapy include distension of bronchioles, flattening of their epithelium, and an acute inflammatory exudate in the lumen with minimal change in the surrounding alveolar wall.

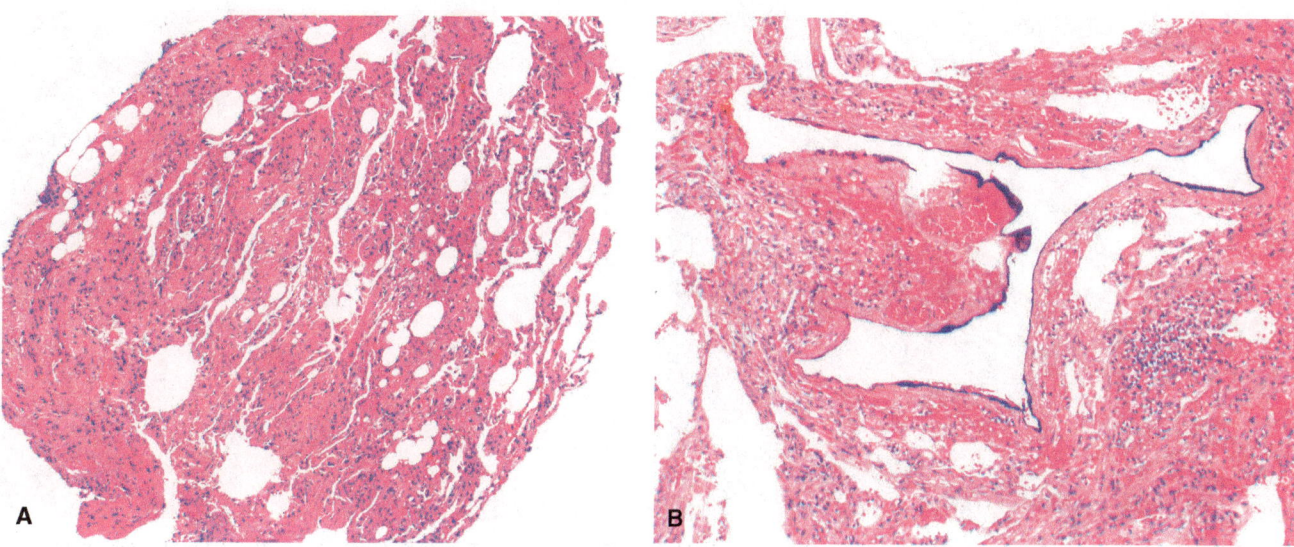

FIGURE 17.19 Bubble artifact. **A:** This fragment from a transbronchial biopsy shows compression and atelectasis (*left*) with some recognizable alveolar walls (*right*). The rounded spaces represent bubble artifact, which is common in such compressed biopsies. **B:** Sponge artifact is illustrated. Note the marked irregularity of the space corresponding to the irregular surface of sponges used in cassettes.

Compression of airways produces crinkling and telescoping of the epithelium, similar to that seen in endometrial biopsies. Sometimes entire strips of mucosa are displaced into the bronchiolar or alveolar spaces. Similarly, procedural telescoping of the endothelium can be seen in small vessels, mimicking the appearance of intimal thickening or organizing/recanalized thrombus (Fig. 17.20).

Compression-induced nuclear smearing artifact can be produced in any cellular tumor and even in reactive lymphoid tissue in the bronchial mucosa or biopsies of hilar or mediastinal nodes. The resulting changes may suggest small cell carcinoma. Reactive lymphoid follicles, lymphomas, and carcinoid tumors may be extremely difficult to distinguish from small cell carcinoma when this phenomenon is present. Recognition of these diagnostic pitfalls, examining multiple levels (especially at the periphery), and enlisting the aid of concomitant cytology specimens and immunohistochemistry allows resolution of most cases. In rare instances, rebiopsy may be necessary.

Procedural atelectasis may be encountered in all types of lung biopsies since lung tissue is soft and readily compressible (55,56). It is particularly common in VATS wedge biopsies because this procedure is typically performed with the lung collapsed and samples may become further compressed during retrieval through a small hole in the chest wall (57). In small biopsies, the use of forceps by the surgeon or pathology assistant can also compress the parenchyma. Atelectasis may be misinterpreted as interstitial pneumonia or interstitial fibrosis because the apposition of alveolar walls produces apparent scarring and hypercellularity (Fig. 17.21). With experience, this change can be recognized on routine H&E sections; connective tissue stains show an absence of scarring and a normal background of supporting fibrous tissue along vessels and in septa. In an atelectatic lung, the vessels and septa may appear to have more collagen than normal and to be thickened because they are contracted and shortened. Careful assessment of the nuclei in the atelectatic lung shows that most are endothelial or epithelial in origin, rather than inflammatory. Leukocyte common antigen (CD45) immunostaining and immunohistochemical stains for other lymphoid markers may be useful in this setting. It is also unusual in surgical biopsies (and larger specimens) for the entire specimen to be uniformly atelectatic; and, therefore, a low-power survey of the entire pattern generally helps one

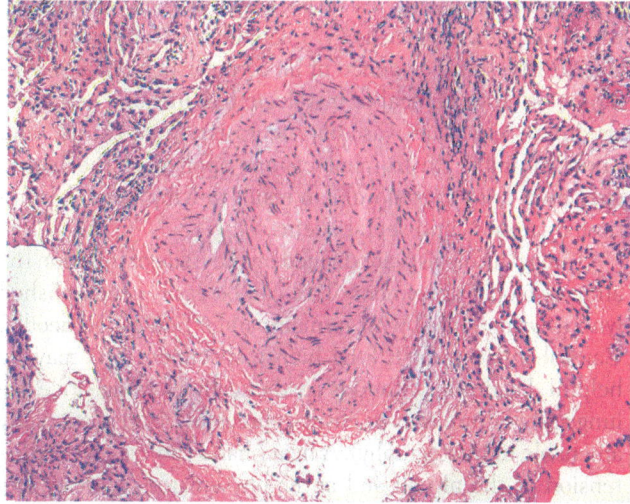

FIGURE 17.20 Telescoping of vessels. This vessel has the artifactual appearance of showing intimal thickening or thrombosis. This common artifact occurs secondary to intussusception of the wall of the vessel into the lumen.

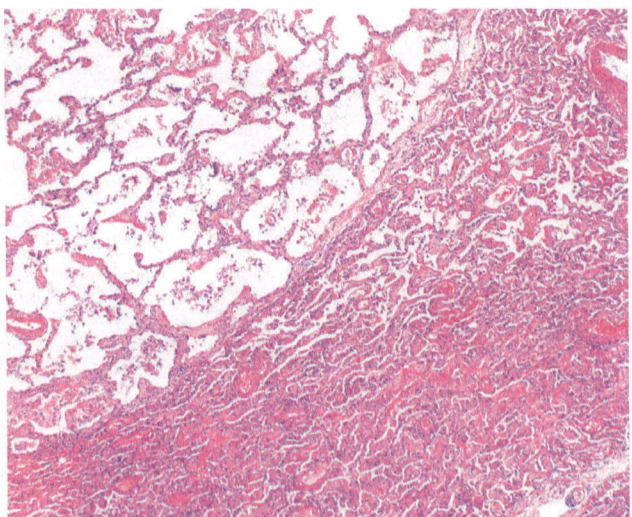 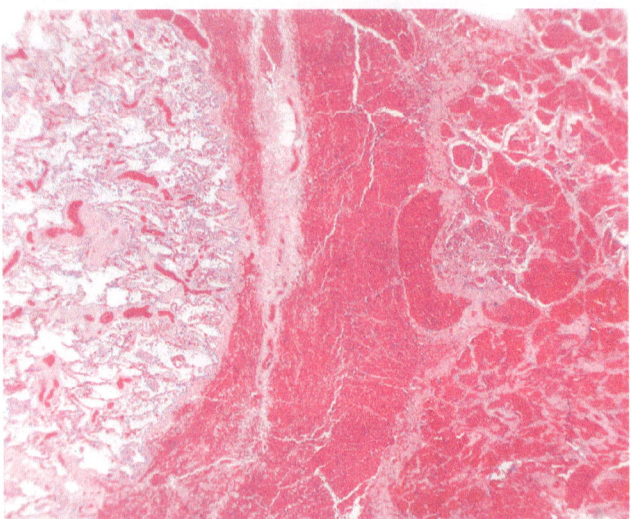

FIGURE 17.21 Atelectasis. Careful examination shows that recognizable alveolar walls can be traced into the region of atelectasis (*lower right*) and that the process stops somewhat abruptly at an interlobular septum that courses diagonally across the field (*lower left to upper right*).

FIGURE 17.22 Traumatic hemorrhage. The right side of the field shows extensive hemorrhage into alveolar spaces, whereas the tissue on the left shows a complete absence of hemorrhage. There is also dissection of red blood cells into the interlobular septal region (*center*). Such a well-demarcated focus of hemorrhage and dissection of red blood cells into the connective tissue would be very unusual in a diffuse alveolar hemorrhage syndrome. The findings are typical of traumatic/procedural hemorrhage.

appreciate atelectasis merging with a more normal lung. In fact, when significant fibrosis is present (usually associated with foci of honeycombing), atelectasis is rarely a problem because the more rigid fibrotic lung tissue tends to retain its inflated configuration. If atelectasis is a consistent problem, injecting the lung tissue with formalin can be preventive. Also, after slicing the biopsy, agitating the slices in a formalin container can expand the lung significantly.

Fresh intra-alveolar hemorrhage and fibrin deposition because of the trauma of surgery is extremely common in biopsy material and should not be overinterpreted as pathologic (Fig. 17.22). In fact, hemorrhage related to the trauma of the procedure is the most common cause of fresh blood in alveolar spaces. One can approach this problem from three points of view: the statistical, histologic, and clinical. Statistically, the vast majority of cases of fresh alveolar hemorrhage are traumatic since pathologic alveolar hemorrhage is relatively uncommon; thus, in any given case, acute hemorrhage is unlikely to be significant. When pathologic hemorrhage is present, there is usually (but not always) an associated fibrinous exudate, hyaline membranes, microfoci of organizing pneumonia, obvious distension of alveoli with blood, and evidence of prior hemorrhage manifested by hemosiderin-filled macrophages in the interstitium or airspaces. This last finding is not a reliable histologic criterion in patients who have been smokers and those with venous obstruction or chronic passive congestion. Lastly, correlation with the clinical history is essential. Suspected clinical diagnosis of hemoptysis, alveolar hemorrhage, or vasculitis should prompt careful interpretation of the morphologic finding of intra-alveolar hemorrhage. The clinician can usually confirm whether an alveolar hemorrhage syndrome or alveolar hemorrhage because of some other cause (e.g., cardiac) is in the realm of possibility in any given patient.

The most common cause of macrophages staining positively with iron stains is respiratory bronchiolitis in smokers (Fig. 17.23). The hemosiderin in smoker's macrophages is finely granular, in contrast to the coarse, dark blue staining in chronic hemorrhage as highlighted by the Prussian blue histochemical stain for iron. Nevertheless, it is surprising how many darkly staining Prussian blue–positive macrophages can be seen in the lungs of smokers.

Prolonged surgical manipulation of the lung, and even multiple transbronchial biopsies, can lead to margination of neutrophils in capillaries (especially those in the pleura), which mimics capillaritis (57). Capillaritis is usually associated with some evidence of an alveolar hemorrhage syndrome or other clinical or histologic features of a vasculitic syndrome (such as vascular necrosis, karyorrhexis, and fibrin thrombi). Instrument clamps applied to the biopsy specimen prior to removal can result in lymphatic obstruction, dilatation, and septal edema.

Lung pathologists are divided on the issue of inflation fixation of biopsy specimens. This can be easily accomplished with a syringe filled with formalin and a fine gauge needle. Careful inflation of a lung biopsy specimen (58) may be helpful diagnostically and is aesthetically pleasing since the lung architecture is more easily appreciated (and particularly amenable to photography). A heavy hand can create overdistension of the alveoli and an emphysematous appearance. If this occurs, clinical correlation may be required to assess whether emphysema is actually a clinical consideration. Patchy atelectatic (uninflated) portions of lung tissue are common in biopsies that have been nonuniformly inflated.

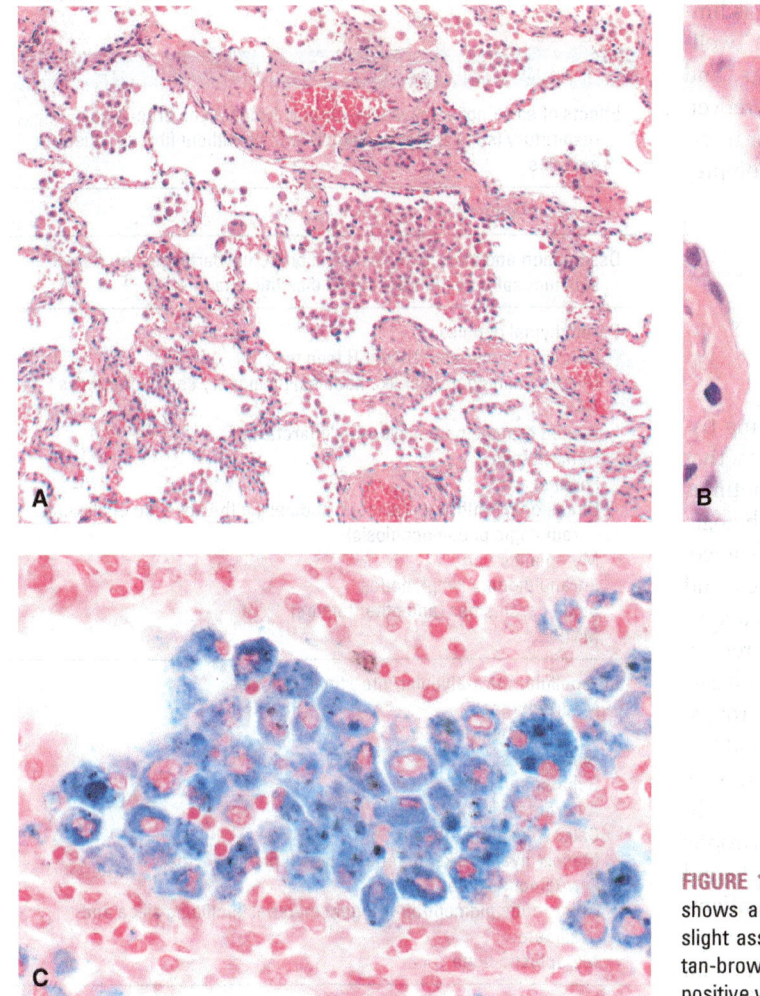
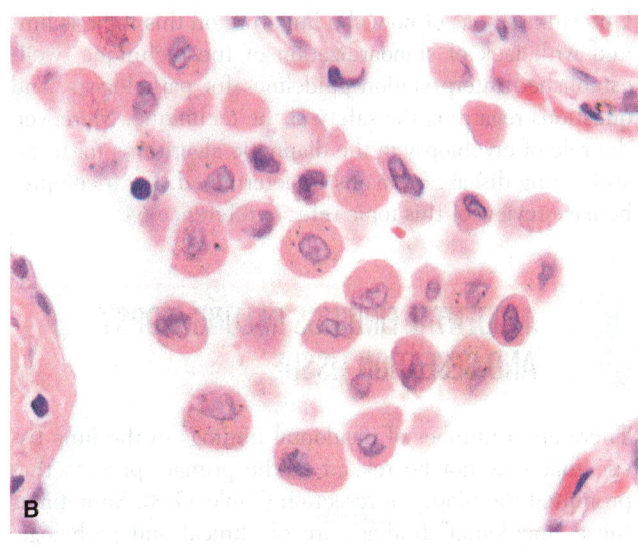

FIGURE 17.23 Respiratory bronchiolitis. A respiratory bronchiole (**A**) shows an accumulation of pigmented macrophages in the lung with slight associated interstitial widening. The macrophages have a slight tan-brown appearance, contain flecks of dark material (**B**), and stain positive with Prussian blue staining (**C**) with a fine granularity.

One problem that may be encountered in inflated biopsies is that cells and fluid may be "washed out" of the airspaces. This is especially true of smoker's (respiratory) bronchiolitis, which may be quite subtle in inflated specimens.

Plastic sponges are sometimes put in processing cassettes by pathology staff to ensure that small specimens are not lost during processing. Sponge artifact, with triangular "holes" in the tissue, is a well-known artifact in any tissue that is processed this way, particularly if it is placed on the sponges prior to complete formalin fixation (56).

As mentioned earlier, VATS lung biopsies (thoracoscopic biopsies) have largely replaced traditional open lung biopsy as the diagnostic procedure for obtaining wedge biopsies of lung tissue for histologic evaluation. Although there are minor disadvantages in comparison to traditional open lung biopsy, diagnostic accuracy does not appear to be compromised (57,59–61). Allowing for the fact that bimanual palpation is not as feasible with VATS biopsies, and that the tissue is forcibly pulled through a small hole in the chest wall, it is remarkable that sampling error and specimen artifacts are only a minor problem. The specimen size approaches that achieved with traditional open lung biopsy, and the minor degrees of hemorrhage, atelectasis/overinflation, and neutrophil margination represent artifactual changes that do not compromise diagnostic accuracy (57,59–61). Moreover, VATS lung biopsies provide excellent sampling of the peripheral/distal lung parenchyma, which cannot not be usually sampled with a transbronchial biopsy approach. This becomes very important for the diagnosis of pathologies like usual interstitial pneumonia or even some types of asthma (62).

The use of transbronchial biopsy with a cryoprobe, referred to as cryobiopsy, has recently emerged as an alternative to forceps and open lung biopsies for the sampling of the peripheral lung parenchyma. In this technique, the flexible cryoprobe, inserted via a bronchoscopic approach, rapidly freezes an area of peripheral lung parenchyma which is then extracted as a cryobiopsy. Specimens procured using this technique are larger than those obtained using forceps and arguably demonstrate less crush and compression artifact, resulting in the better appreciation of the histology and the morphologic features. Cryobiopsies have been reported to be of use for the diagnosis of diffuse parenchymal lung disease, with a 70% to 80% diagnostic yield (63).

Unfortunately, as of now, the literature on this topic is limited with lack of standardization of the technique, well-established interpretation guidelines for pathologists, and questions regarding the safety of the technique. Moreover, the role of cryobiopsy in the diagnotic algorithms for interstitial lung diseases remains undetermined. For a comprehensive review of this topic refer to reference 64.

INCIDENTAL FINDINGS IN LUNG BIOPSY AND RESECTION TISSUE

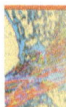

There are a number of incidental findings in the lung tissue that may not be related to the primary process that prompted the biopsy or resection (Table 17.8). Sometimes these "incidental" findings are of clinical and pathologic significance, and other times they are of no significance. Correlation of the individual finding(s) with the clinical and radiologic presentation helps determine their significance.

Findings related to smoking and emphysema are extremely common, especially in lungs resected for non–small-cell carcinoma (46). They may be divided into three broad groups: large airway changes, small airway lesions, and abnormalities of the alveolar parenchyma. In the large airways, one sees goblet cell hyperplasia, squamous metaplasia (with or without dysplasia), basement membrane thickening, hypertrophy and hyperplasia of bronchial glands with dilated ducts and mucostasis, and, often, a mild submucosal chronic inflammatory infiltrate (45,48). The changes in the small airways may be quite dramatic and may mimic or even produce an interstitial lung disease (46,65,66). Smoking-induced respiratory bronchiolitis (Fig. 17.23) includes goblet cell metaplasia, a mild inflammatory infiltrate in the airway walls, metaplasia of type II cells in the surrounding alveoli, mild peribronchiolar fibrosis, and prominent accumulations of pigmented macrophages in the adjacent airspace and the bronchiolar lumen. The pigmented macrophages (smokers' macrophages) contain phagocytosed debris from inhaled cigarette smoke and have prominent secondary lysosomes in their cytoplasm. This results in a dirty granular tan or brown appearance to the cytoplasm. They contain PAS-positive (lysosomes) and finely granular Prussian blue–positive (hemosiderin) material, as well as tiny, irregular flecks of brown-black material.

Smoking-related changes in the most distal pulmonary parenchyma usually manifest as centriacinar emphysema with airspace enlargement and loss of alveolar walls (45,48). Histologic quantification of emphysema on biopsy material is difficult, although one can often determine whether it is present and subjectively quantify it. Bullous emphysema (with abnormal airspaces >1 cm in diameter) is more common in the upper lobes and is usually associated with some fibrosis in the septa of the bullae and adjacent alveolar walls. The fibrosis is relatively acellular, noninflammatory, eosinophilic, and poorly vascularized. Metaplasia or ulceration

TABLE 17.8 Incidental Findings in Lung Tissue

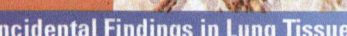

Effects of smoking: emphysema, chronic lymphocytic bronchitis, respiratory (smoker's) bronchiolitis with or without fibrosis, dust macules
Changes of asthma
Ossification and marrow formation in bronchial cartilages, bronchial submucosal fatty infiltration, and elastotic changes

Parenchymal nodules
  Carcinoid tumorlets; DIPNECH (see text)
  Minute (meningothelial-like nodules) pulmonary chemodectomas
  AAH
  Healed granulomatous disease, infarcts, etc.
  Hamartomas
  Focal scars
  Occasional (anthraco-) silicotic nodules (in the absence of clinical/radiologic pneumoconiosis)
  Metaplastic bone
  Intrapulmonary lymph nodes
  Small carcinomas (and other tumors)
  MMPH

Intracellular/intra-alveolar/interstitial structures
  Macrophages
  Corpora amylacea
  Blue bodies
  Schaumann bodies
  Asteroid bodies
  Calcium oxalate crystals
  Mallory hyaline-like material in type II pneumocytes
  Ferruginous bodies
  Anthracotic pigment/birefringent material (including silica and silicates)
  Metaplastic bone

Epithelioid and/or cholesterol granulomas, giant cells, lipogranulomas

Intravascular/vascular
  Megakaryocytes
  Thrombi (mimic emboli)
  Bone marrow emboli
  Calcification and iron encrustation of the elastic tissue
  Senile amyloid
  Foreign material (e.g., intravascular talcosis)

Interstitial air in the lung parenchyma

Hilar/peribronchial lymph nodes
  Sinus and paracortical histiocytes (may simulate granulomas)
  Occasional silicotic or anthracosilicotic nodules
  Anthracosis/birefringent material
  Hamazaki–Wesenberg bodies

Pleural adhesions; hyaline pleural plaques

AAH, atypical adenomatous hyperplasia; MMPH, multifocal micronodular pneumocyte hyperplasia.

of the epithelium and interstitial dissection of air occur in bullae and may induce a distinctive giant cell reaction analogous to that seen in persistent interstitial emphysema. Respiratory bronchiolitis with fibrosis (67), also referred to as smoking-related interstitial fibrosis (SRIF) (68), is a distinctive type of fibrosing interstitial lung disease seen in

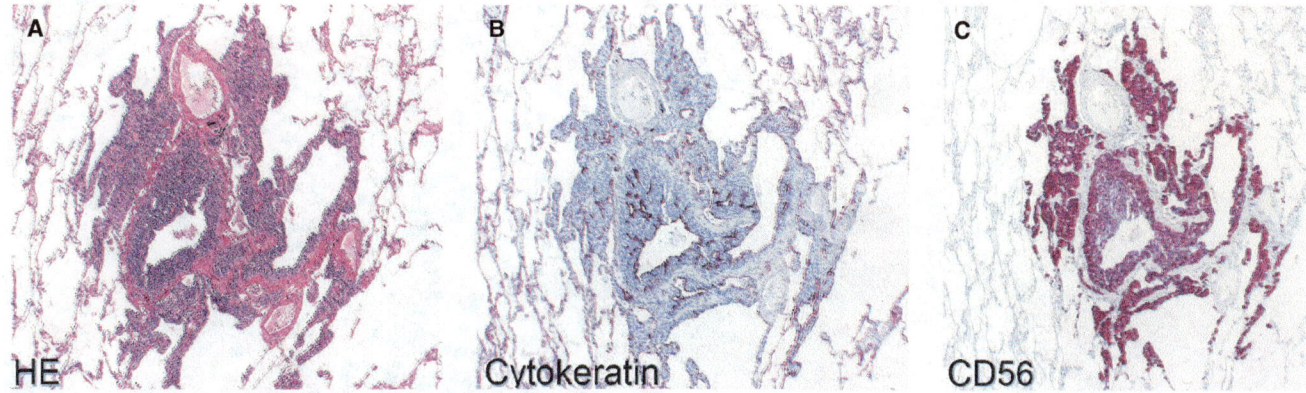

FIGURE 17.24 Tumorlet. **A:** Tumorlets are typically discrete nodules that are bronchiolocentric. The bronchiole is not apparent in (**A**) because it has been overrun by the proliferation, but the adjacent pulmonary artery is identifiable. **B:** Cytologically, tumorlets have a neuroendocrine appearance with nests of cells with granular chromatin and absence of necrosis and significant mitotic activity. The nests are often embedded in a fibrous stroma, and some of them may appear to float freely in airspaces or spaces that resemble lymphatics. **C:** Neuroendocrine markers, such as chromogranin, are strongly positive.

smokers. It is characterized by the presence of diffuse or patchy pauciinflammatory alveolar septal widening by eosinophilic hyalinizing collagenous fibrosis. It normally occurs in close relationship with areas of emphysema and respiratory bronchiolitis, and it can also be associated with areas of smooth muscle hyperplasia.

Asthmatics are predisposed to a number of lung conditions that may lead to lung biopsy, although the asthmatic changes themselves may not be the dominant lesion. These airway changes include goblet cell hyperplasia/metaplasia in the airway epithelium, thickening of the basement membrane and submembranous region, smooth muscle hypertrophy and hyperplasia, lymphoid hyperplasia, and a variable infiltrate of eosinophils, mast cells, lymphocytes, and a few neutrophils, and fibrous tissue in the wall (45,48,69). Mucostasis (including Curschmann spirals) may be an accompanying feature; but, when mucostasis is extensive and is associated with sloughing of epithelial fragments into the airways (creola bodies), one should suspect that the asthma itself is the main lesion. Such an appearance is typical of status asthmaticus. Some distal atelectasis with a few airspace macrophages and eosinophils may also be seen. Rare and poorly formed nonnecrotizing granulomas might be seen in specimen from severe asthmatics with clinical correlate asthmatic granulomatosis (70,71). In patients with quiescent asthma or past history of asthma, the airways may be entirely normal or show only minor inflammatory or fibrotic changes.

Metaplastic bone, including bone marrow and calcification, is an aging change that is occasionally seen in bronchial cartilages (72). Metaplastic bone may also be seen in regions of scarring (dystrophic ossification), particularly in apical caps. Small bony nodules may also be seen with no apparent associated pathologic changes. In some older individuals with chronic bronchitis, the bronchial submucosa may have a gray elastotic appearance, particularly in bronchoscopic biopsies, representing calcification of elastic fibers in the submucosa and basal lamina.

Carcinoid tumorlets (73–76), also referred to simply as tumorlets, and minute pulmonary meningothelial-like nodules (76–78) are nodular proliferations that are quite common. They may be mistaken for each other, other lesions, or even metastases. Tumorlets (Fig. 17.24) represent well-circumscribed proliferations of neuroendocrine cells that usually occur around and within the walls of small airways, particularly in scarred or bronchiectatic airways, and in a small number of patients with unexplained airflow destruction. They lack mitotic figures and necrosis. While there is a superficial resemblance to small cell carcinoma, they are actually more similar to spindle cell carcinoid tumors. In frozen sections, tumorlets may be mistaken for other lesions, particularly metastases. This confusion is compounded by the fact that sometimes tumorlets have cellular clusters at the periphery that retract from the surrounding stroma, simulating lymphatic or airspace invasion.

Tumorlets are often multiple; in aggregation some may become large enough to be recognized radiographically (especially when they occur in areas of bronchiectasis) and to be removed to exclude carcinoma. Exactly where one draws the line between a carcinoid tumorlet and a carcinoid tumor, particularly in cases with multiple lesions, is a bit arbitrary, although a cutoff point of 0.5 cm diameter or larger for carcinoid tumor is reasonable (40,76). Importantly, this measurement cutoff does not apply to tumorlets that may extend for >5 mm along the length of an airway, while maintaining a <5 mm width or thickness. Diffuse idiopathic pulmonary neuroendocrine cell hyperplasia (DIPNECH) is closely related to tumorlets, and the two often coexist (76). According to the World Health Organization (WHO), DIPNECH is defined as "a generalized proliferation of pulmonary neuroendocrine cells (PNCs) that may be confined to the mucosa of airways (with or

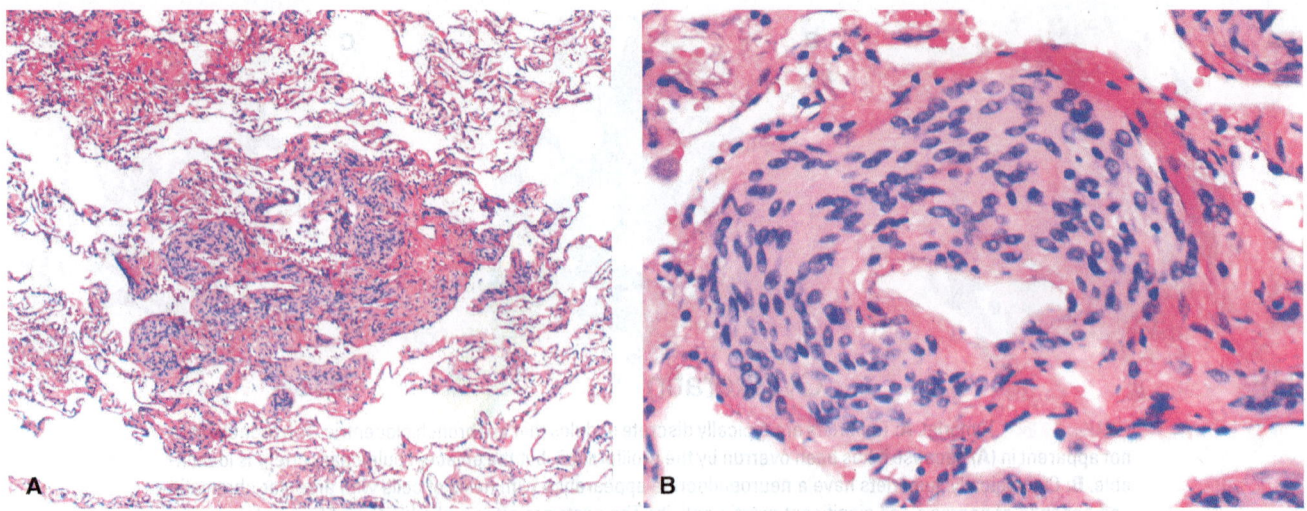

FIGURE 17.25 Minute pulmonary meningothelial-like nodule. These small parenchymal nodules are sometimes associated with pulmonary veins. **A:** They are associated with syncytial appearing cells in a collagenous stroma. **B:** Cytologically, they bear a distinct resemblance to meningothelial cells.

without luminal protrusion), may invade locally to form of tumorlets, or may develop into carcinoid tumors" (76). When this proliferation expands and invades the bronchiolar submucosa, the designation of tumorlet is appropriate. When DIPNECH is encountered, usually multiple airways are involved, and the patients typically have evidence of airflow obstruction (76). Similarly, the presence of multiple tumorlets (and multiple carcinoid tumors) should prompt one to search for evidence of DIPNECH and to consider the possibility of clinical evidence of airflow obstruction (e.g., cough and wheezing) (79).

Minute pulmonary meningothelial-like nodules (formerly called minute pulmonary chemodectomas) (Fig. 17.25) were originally thought to represent an intrapulmonary proliferation of perivenular chemoreceptor cells (76–78). However, the accumulated evidence suggests that the cellular constituents are more closely related to meningothelial cells (76–78). A study by Ionescu et al. (80) showed that meningothelial-like nodules were almost uniformly positive for vimentin, about one-third stain for EMA, and they are negative with cytokeratin and synaptophysin by immunohistochemistry. In a genotypic study, some loss of heterozygosity was demonstrated by the same authors, and this was more common and affected more loci in cases of multiple meningothelial-like nodules in comparison to cases with solitary meningothelial-like nodules (80). The authors concluded that isolated meningothelial-like nodules were probably reactive, that cases of multiple meningothelial-like nodules might represent a transition from a reactive to a neoplastic proliferation, and that meningothelial-like nodules were different from meningiomas based on the major molecular events and their formation and progression (80). Minute pulmonary meningothelial-like nodules are composed of interstitial clusters of fusiform cells with pale eosinophilic cytoplasm, forming small stellate nodules (rarely grossly appreciable) within the alveolated parenchyma. Like meningioma cells, meningothelial-like nodules also express progesterone receptor and they are distinctively negative for vascular, melanoma, and muscle markers. They are largely negative for neuroendocrine markers synaptophysin and chromogranin but they can show some CD56 positivity. In certain occasions, differentiation between meningothelial-like nodules and tumorlets can be a challenge. In such cases, the very characteristic location within the alveolar septae, as opposed to the airway-centered location of tumorlets favors meningothelial-like nodules. They are regarded as an incidental finding and they are largely asymptomatic. Meningothelial-like nodules have been reported to occur in 4.9% of autopsies and up to 9.5% on cancer resections. In extensively sampled resections, they can be seen in up to 47% of cases. In recent years, due to the use of HRCT scans, these lesions can come to clinical attention and might be resected. In rare occasions, they can present as multiple bilateral micronodules, a phenomenon referred to as *diffuse pulmonary meningotheliomatosis*.

Atypical adenomatous hyperplasia (AAH) is a proliferative epithelial process occurring as small nodular lesions in the lung parenchyma (Fig. 17.26). These were first recognized in resection specimens for carcinoma and named bronchioloalveolar cell adenomas (81). Miller found these lesions in 23 (10.74%) of 247 consecutive resection specimens for carcinoma (81). They are most easily recognized grossly in cases that are inflated with the Bouin fixative. The WHO defines AAH as "a small (usually less or equal to 0.5 cm), localized proliferation of mild to moderately atypical type II pneumocytes and/or club cells lining alveolar walls and sometimes respiratory bronchioles" (76). The lesions are considered a preinvasive lesion (slow-growing tumors without angiolymphatic invasion or distant metastasis) to some nonmucinous adenocarcinomas; and the evidence supporting this is epidemiologic, morphologic, morphometric,

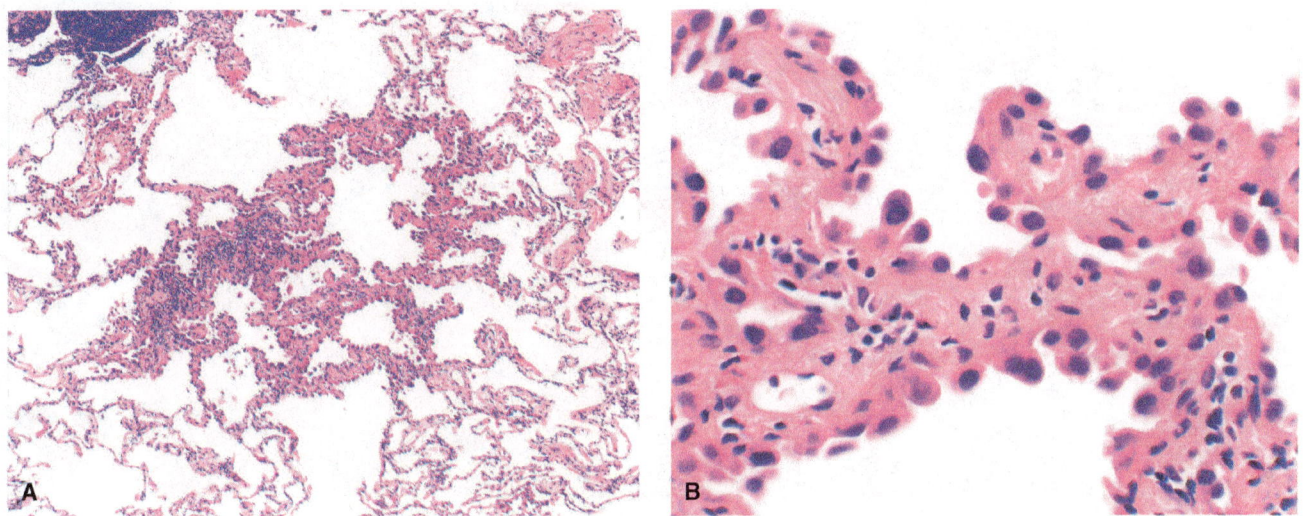

FIGURE 17.26 Atypical adenomatous hyperplasia (AAH). **A:** In this well-inflated specimen, a 2- to 3-mm diameter lesion is apparent as slight alveolar septal thickening and a proliferation of knob-shaped cells along alveolar walls. **B:** Cytologically, the cells lining the alveoli have mild-to-moderate atypia but lack the crowding and marked atypia associated with adenocarcinoma in situ. Some nuclear inclusions characteristic of type II pneumocytes are also apparent (*lower left*).

cytofluorometric, and genetic. AAH generally represents an incidental histologic finding (rare cases have been identified radiologically) and is found in 2% to 4% of routine autopsies of non–cancer-bearing patients and up to 35% of lobectomies for adenocarcinoma of the lung. AAH occurs close to respiratory bronchioles, in areas lacking significant inflammation or fibrosis, and demonstrates no more than moderate atypia. The presence of cytoplasmic snouts suggests a club cell origin. Inconspicuous pseudopapillae can be seen and should not be confused with invasive carcinoma. In general, we advocate a conservative approach to these lesions, since (a) there are many causes of type II cell proliferation, and many of them are reactive; and (b) while some studies support the concept that AAH is a direct precursor of lung adenocarcinomas (mainly based on the presence in AAH of similar *KRAS* and *EGFR* driver mutations seen in adenocarcinoma), there are no unequivocal histologic/pathologic studies documenting the progression of AAH to adenocarcinoma. Moreover, no studies exist showing what percent of lesions of AAH might progress to adenocarcinoma. AAH should not be confused with in situ adenocarcinoma, which is usually larger, with a more monotonous proliferative cell population and with a greater degree of cytologic atypia.

Focal scars (see following), healed granulomatous disease, and organized infarcts are among other incidental nodular lesions occasionally encountered in the lung. Early infarcts have a wedge shape with hemorrhagic necrosis, and the overlying pleura is viable with a fibrinous pleuritis. They often also have a peripheral rim of granulation tissue. Older infarcts are often rounded and have a rim of fibrous tissue; they can even be mistaken for healed granulomas. Necrotic tumor nodules sometimes mimic infarcts. Squamous metaplasia is common in the airspaces adjacent to organizing infarcts and around bronchioles. It may be sufficiently exuberant to be mistaken for a neoplastic process. A single anthracosilicotic nodule is an occasional finding that may be accepted as incidental and insignificant if there is no clinical or radiologic evidence of pneumoconiosis. When anthracosilicotic nodules are multiple, the occupational history and the possibility of pneumoconiosis should be explored.

Although extensive parenchymal scarring is usually a pathologic process, focal scars a few millimeters in diameter are a common incidental finding in biopsy material. One distinctive form of scar that is frequently observed (and may be identifiable as 2- to 3-mm centrilobular nodules in CT scans) consists of scars centered on alveolar ducts in the periphery of the lung, particularly common in (ex-) smokers (Fig. 17.27). They are round or somewhat stellate in character and have numerous fascicles of smooth muscle—and thus sometimes have been confused with primary muscle proliferations such as LAM. There are a number of histologic changes that accompany pulmonary scarring, regardless of cause. These include vascular intimal and medial thickening, sometimes to the point of luminal occlusion (endarteritis obliterans); smooth muscle and myofibroblastic hyperplasia in the interstitium; metaplasia and hyperplasia of type II cells or bronchiolar-type epithelium (peribronchiolar metaplasia); accumulations of intra-alveolar macrophages and mucostasis; carcinoid tumorlets (particularly along scarred small airways); dystrophic calcification or ossification; microscopic pericicatricial emphysema; and metaplastic adipose tissue in the pleural and peribronchial regions. The proliferation of type II cells associated with scars may be confused with adenocarcinoma. Adenocarcinoma generally has uniform dense cellularity and cellular crowding with abrupt transition to

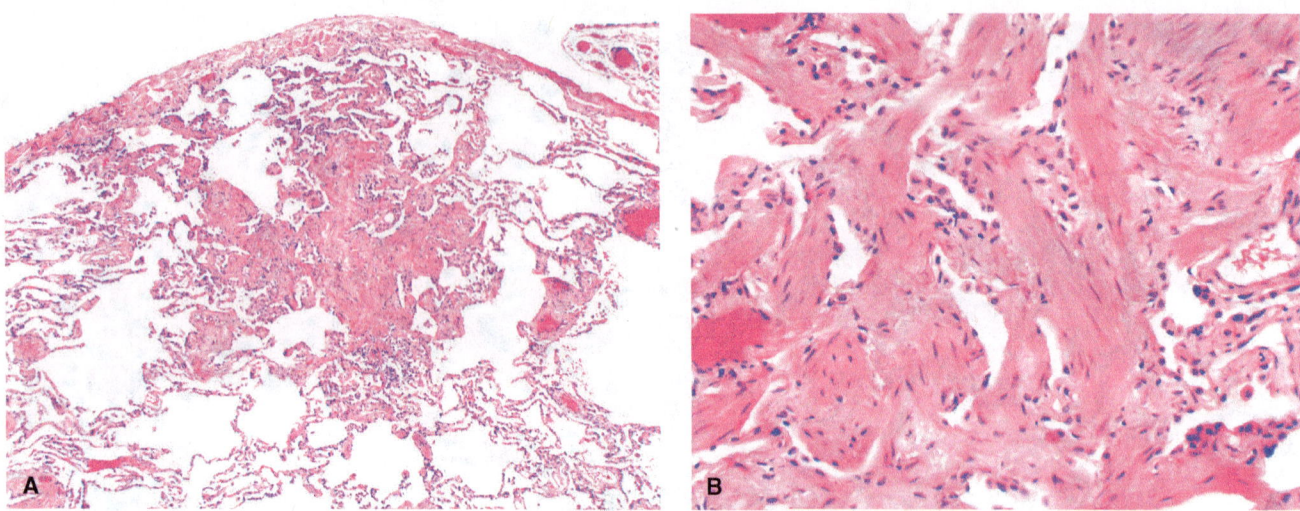

FIGURE 17.27 Incidental parenchymal scar. These are typically subpleural and appear to center on alveolar ducts (**A**) and commonly have fascicles of normal appearing smooth muscle (**B**).

normal alveolar walls, significant cytologic atypia, and lack of ciliated cells. Although AAH tends to have relatively little interstitial widening and fibrosis, AAH enters into the differential diagnosis in this situation. Of note, both proliferations would be TTF-1 and Napsin-A-positive.

In rare instances, mature bone is observed in normal alveoli; it may represent the residue of an organized airspace exudate, from chronic passive congestion of mitral stenosis or an ancient organized pneumonia (82). Extensive dystrophic ossification (and rarely calcification) occasionally accompanies lesions with diffuse pulmonary fibrosis (Fig. 17.28) (83). Focal dystrophic ossification is a common finding in focal lung scar, regardless of cause.

Intrapulmonary lymph nodes (Fig. 17.29) are not uncommonly encountered in wedge biopsies for pulmonary nodules. They vary from loosely organized microscopic foci of lymphoid tissue to fully developed lymph nodes identified grossly or radiologically.

Micronodular pneumocyte hyperplasia (MNPH) is a multifocal micronodular proliferation of type II pneumocytes with mild thickening of the interstitium (Fig. 17.30) (84). This condition is rare and generally an incidental finding in a biopsy taken for another lesion, usually LAM, given the association of MNPH with tuberous sclerosis. Rarely, MNPH is the sole lesion present, and the lesions may be sufficiently large to be identifiable on CT scans as multiple small nodules.

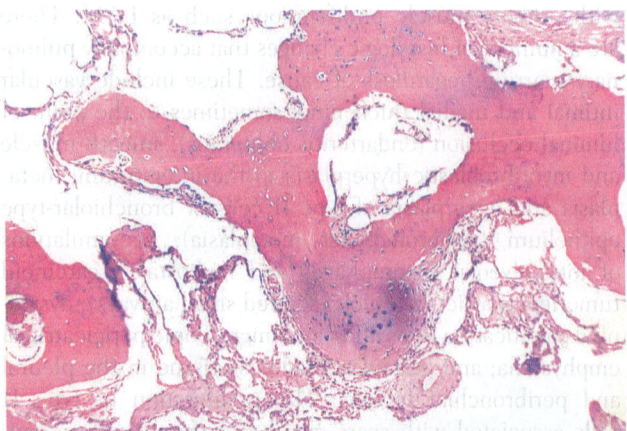

FIGURE 17.28 Ossification. An incidental focus of pulmonary ossification is noted; tissue is from a patient with usual interstitial pneumonia.

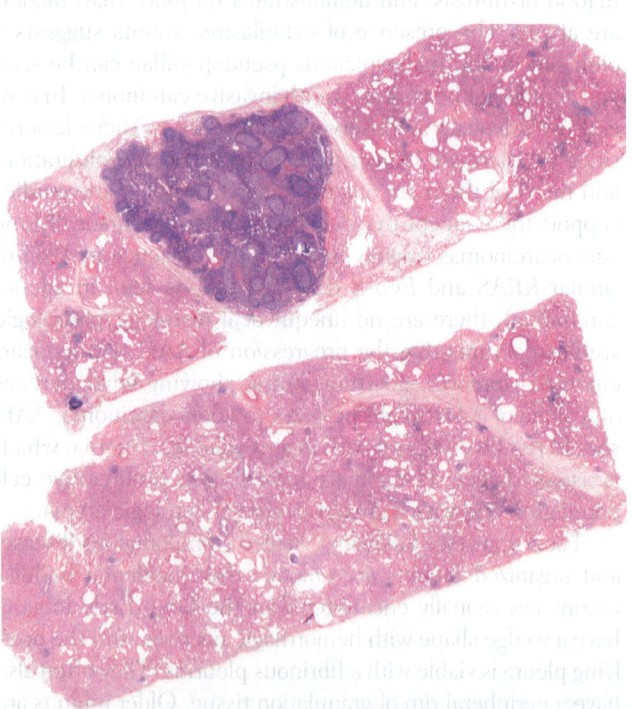

FIGURE 17.29 Intrapulmonary lymph node. There is a relatively large lymph node that appears to be within or adjacent to an interlobular septum in a wedge biopsy from the peripheral lung. Reactive follicles are apparent even at scanning power microscopy.

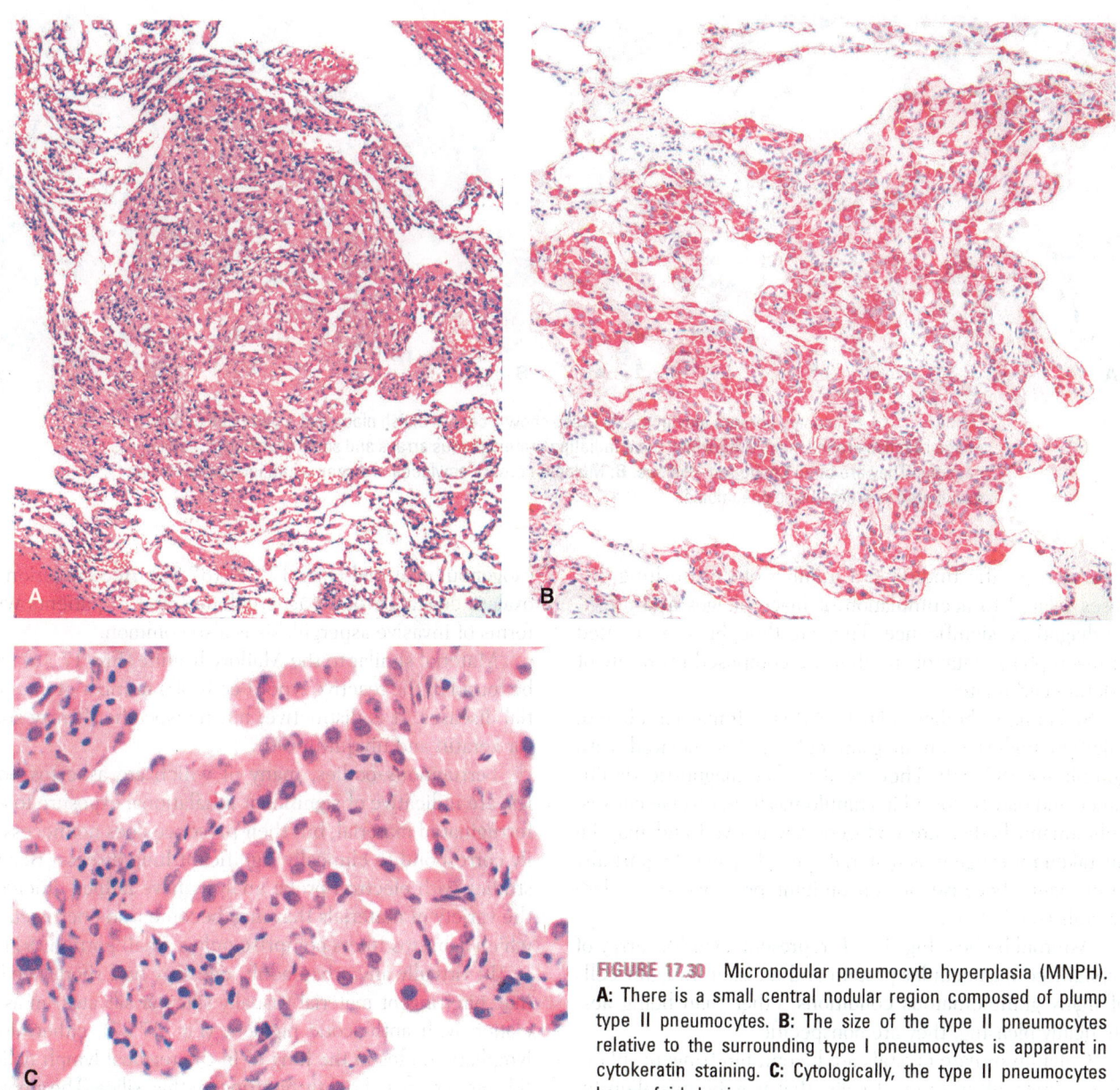

FIGURE 17.30 Micronodular pneumocyte hyperplasia (MNPH). **A:** There is a small central nodular region composed of plump type II pneumocytes. **B:** The size of the type II pneumocytes relative to the surrounding type I pneumocytes is apparent in cytokeratin staining. **C:** Cytologically, the type II pneumocytes have a fairly benign appearance.

The lesions are typically >5 mm in size. They can usually be distinguished from AAH and other causes of alveolar cell hyperplasia by their distinct rounded nodular character at scanning microscopy, the large plump eosinophilic type II cells lacking significant atypia, the slight interstitial collagen deposition within the lesions, and the presence of airspace histiocytes in the regions of the nodules.

A number of intra-alveolar and intracellular structures are seen in the lung. Small numbers of intra-alveolar macrophages are a normal finding, and an increase in their numbers is nonspecific and a common reaction in smokers (42). Focal desquamative interstitial pneumonia-like reactions are seen in many pathologic conditions, especially in smokers and in conditions with fibrosis and architectural disorganization (46,85). When hemosiderin is present, causes for alveolar hemorrhage (both primary and secondary) should be excluded.

Corpora amylacea (86,87) are eosinophilic, rounded, slightly lamellated proteinaceous bodies (Fig. 17.31) that stain positively with PAS stains and faintly with Congo red stain; they are more common in the lungs of older individuals. Sometimes there is a blue-gray, calcified, or polarizable crystalline particulate body in the center and a macrophage or giant cell response around them. The exact nature and cause of corpora are unclear, but they are of no clinical significance and should not be confused with aspirated exogenous material or food particles.

Blue bodies (Fig. 17.32) are intra-alveolar, lamellated, basophilic, calcified structures found in airspaces associated with alveolar macrophages and giant cells (87). They

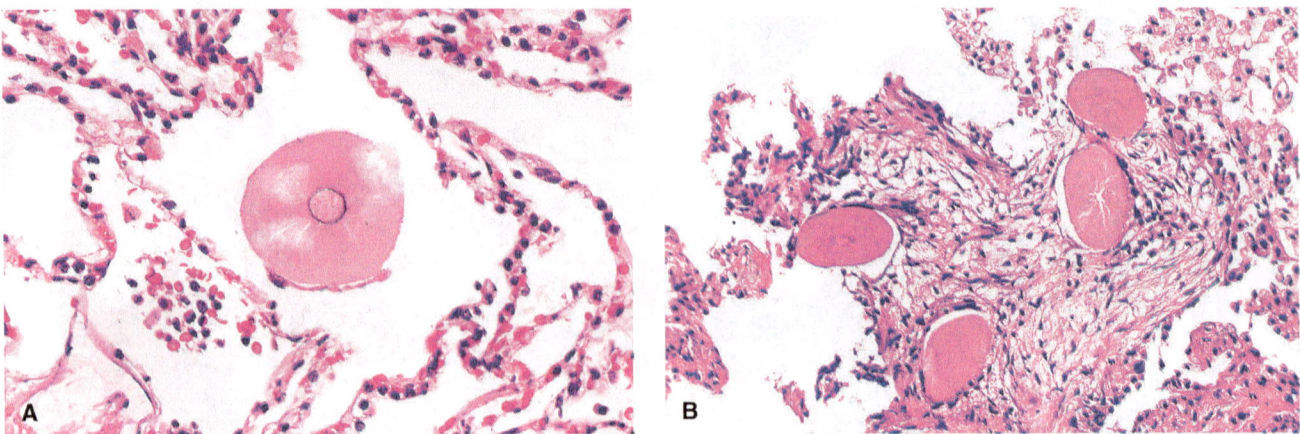

FIGURE 17.31 Pulmonary corpora amylacea. **A:** These show a central bluish nidus and a giant cell or macrophage reaction around them. Others may have radiating proteinaceous arrays and show cracking in histologic sections. They are often Congo red–positive. **B:** Multiple corpora amylacea are seen as an incidental finding associated with organizing pneumonia.

are a nonspecific finding in a number of diffuse lung diseases related to accumulation of macrophages and are of no diagnostic significance. They are thought to be related to macrophage catabolism; they are composed primarily of calcium carbonate.

Schaumann bodies (Fig. 17.33) are similar lamellated, calcified bodies seen in giant cells and associated with granulomas (87–89). They are also of no diagnostic significance and may be found in granulomas from diverse causes. Schaumann bodies are endogenously derived and may be mistaken for exogenous material since they may be partially birefringent because of concomitant presence of oxalate crystals (see below).

Asteroid bodies (Fig. 17.34) represent a starlike array of crystallized intracellular protein and are seen in giant cells of many granulomatous conditions; other than being aesthetically pleasing, they are nonspecific.

Calcium oxalate crystals are lucent, birefringent, plate-like crystals, often in giant cells, that may be mistaken for exogenous material (Fig. 17.35) (87,88). Accumulation of oxalate crystals around aspergillomas and in patients with forms of invasive aspergillosis is also common.

Material similar to the Mallory hyaline (Fig. 17.36) may be found in the reactive type II cells of a number of interstitial diseases. It is distinctive, but nonspecific. It may stain for keratin and ubiquitin (90).

Ferruginous bodies, many of which are asbestos bodies, are indicative of significant inhalational exposure to the ferruginated material, but their presence does not necessarily correspond to clinically significant lung disease. Recent studies with electron-probe analysis have helped elucidate the variety of materials that may become iron encrusted, of which asbestos fibers comprise only a small portion (91).

In virtually any urban adult, one may find short, needle-like, birefringent material (usually silica or silicates) in association with anthracotic pigment (Fig. 17.37), either along lymphatic routes in the lung or in the regional lymph nodes. Silicates are more brightly birefringent than silica. The amount

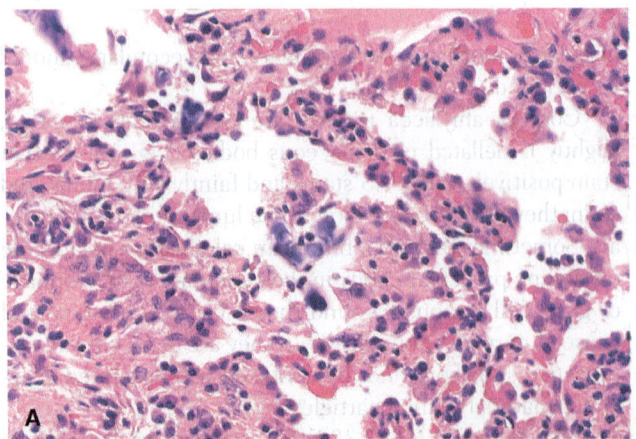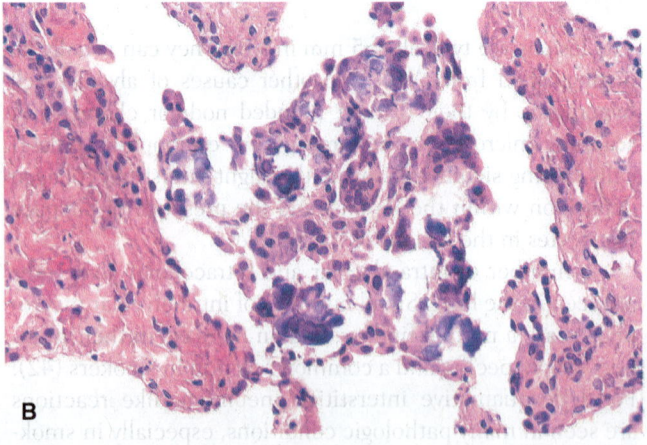

FIGURE 17.32 Blue bodies. **A, B:** Blue bodies are gray or blue, intra-alveolar, calcified, lamellated structures often associated with clusters of macrophages, including giant cells.

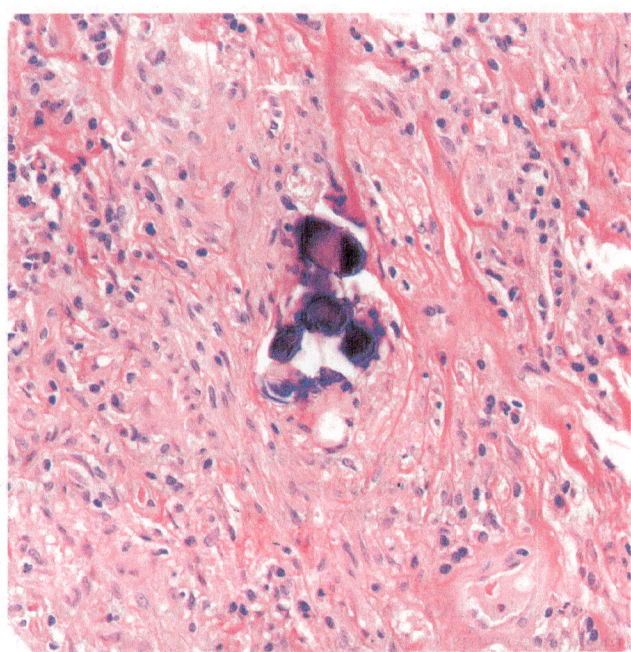

FIGURE 17.33 Schaumann body. There is a bluish calcified structure associated with the surrounding granulomatous inflammation. A lamellated appearance similar to a psammoma body is focally apparent. The pale zones in this case represent loosened oxalate crystals that would be birefringent (see Fig. 17.35).

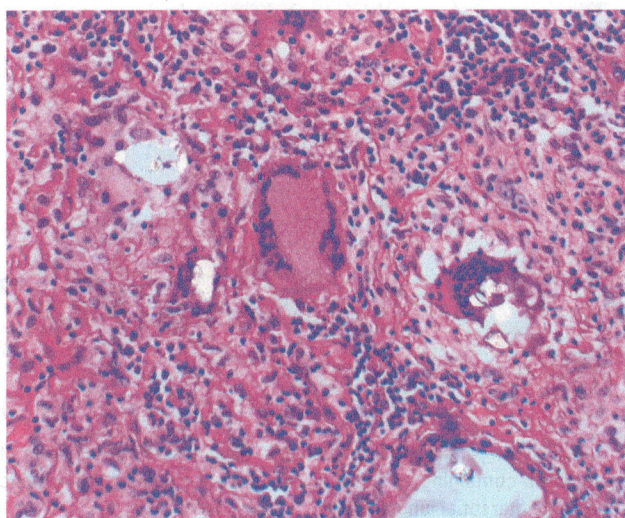

FIGURE 17.35 Calcium oxalate crystals. Calcium oxalate crystals are commonly associated with Schaumann bodies and granulomatous inflammation and show bright birefringence, as noted in this partially polarized photomicrograph. The association with giant cells is characteristic.

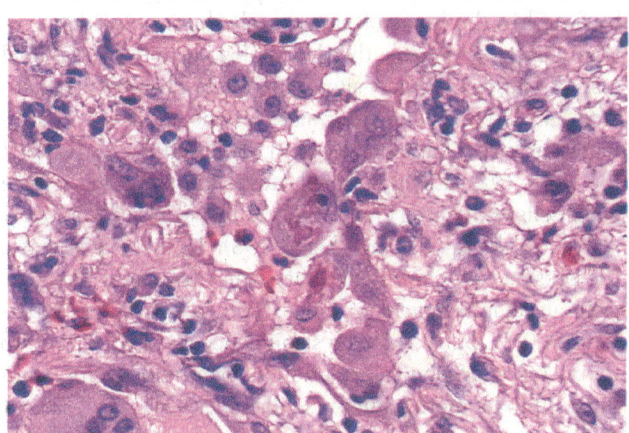

FIGURE 17.36 Hyaline material resembling Mallory hyaline may be seen in reactive type II pneumocytes in a number of acute and chronic conditions.

of birefringent material may be quite impressive in individuals (particularly smokers) who have no significant occupational exposure. This material should be distinguished from the formalin pigment, as well as from surgical glove talc or starch; the latter is limited to handled surfaces and often demonstrate a Maltese-cross configuration with polarization. The diagnosis of silicosis (and silicatosis) is not based solely on the presence of birefringent material; it requires clinicopathologic correlations: appropriate imaging findings and parenchymal silicotic nodules or masses of histiocytes (within which early fibrotic nodules may be seen to form) along lymphatic routes. Precise

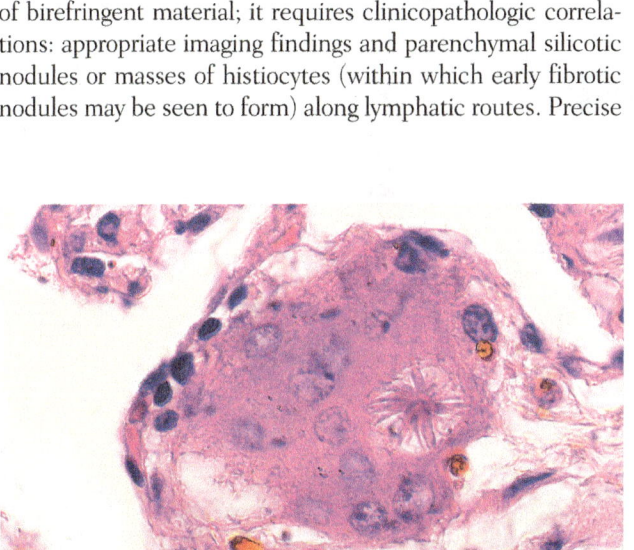

FIGURE 17.34 Asteroid body. An asteroid body in a giant cell is illustrated from a case of sarcoidosis.

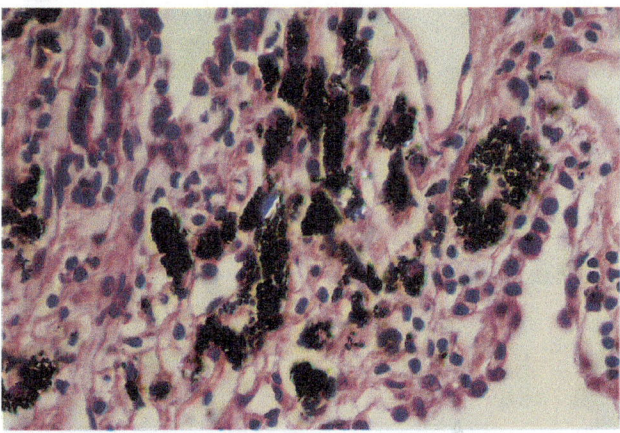

FIGURE 17.37 Silica and silicates in the normal lung. Birefringent silica and silicate particles are a common nonspecific finding in and around the anthracotic pigment that is so commonly seen in urban adults and smokers.

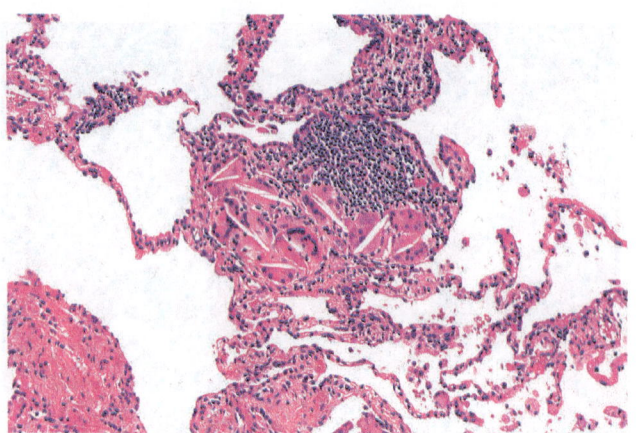

FIGURE 17.38 Cholesterol granulomas. Granulomas and clusters of giant cells containing cholesterol clefts are a frequent nonspecific finding in interstitial lung disease.

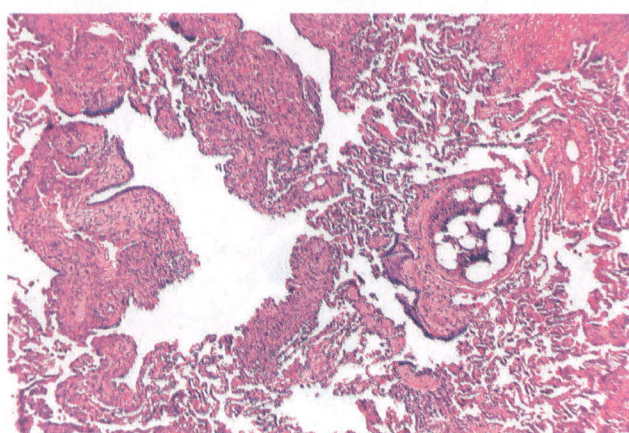

FIGURE 17.40 Bone marrow embolus. An incidental bone marrow embolus (*right center*) identified in a pulmonary artery in a biopsy from a patient with lymphangioleiomyomatosis (*left*).

characterization of any material identified requires special techniques such as electron-probe analysis.

An occasional nonnecrotizing epithelioid granuloma may be found in the lungs of patients who have no evidence of granulomatous disease; they are analogous to the occasional granuloma seen at many sites in the body. Hung et al. evaluated 347 lung resections for mass lesions and found granulomatous inflammation away from the lesion in only 7.8% of the cases (92). Likewise, cholesterol granulomas or single giant cells containing cholesterol clefts may also be an occasional incidental finding (Fig. 17.38). In some instances, the presence of cholesterol granulomas has been linked to prior alveolar hemorrhage, mucostasis, or pulmonary hypertension (93), but usually no significance can be ascribed to them. Lipogranulomas are an occasional nonspecific finding, said to be more common in diabetics (94).

An interesting finding is the presence of scattered megakaryocytes in alveolar walls (Fig. 17.39), predominantly within alveolar capillaries. Large numbers can be seen, particularly during sepsis. They are of no diagnostic significance but should not be overinterpreted as malignant or virally infected cells. Along with the bone marrow and spleen, the lung acts as a major reservoir for megakaryocytes (95).

Bone marrow emboli, common in autopsy material, are also seen in biopsy specimens (Fig. 17.40). Rarely correlated with any clinically significant process, they may be a consequence of bony trauma, excision of ribs or secondary to strenuous CPR. In some cases, however, such as thoracoscopic biopsies, bony trauma cannot be implicated, and the marrow emboli are an unexplained incidental finding.

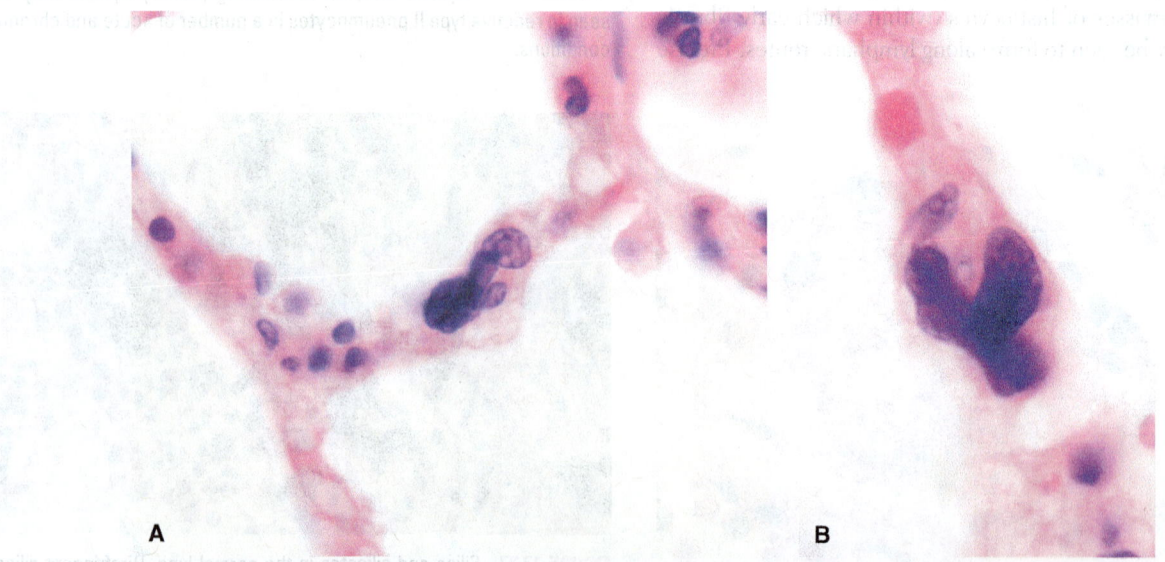

FIGURE 17.39 Megakaryocytes. **A, B:** Megakaryocytes are a common finding in normal lung, often present within alveolar capillaries.

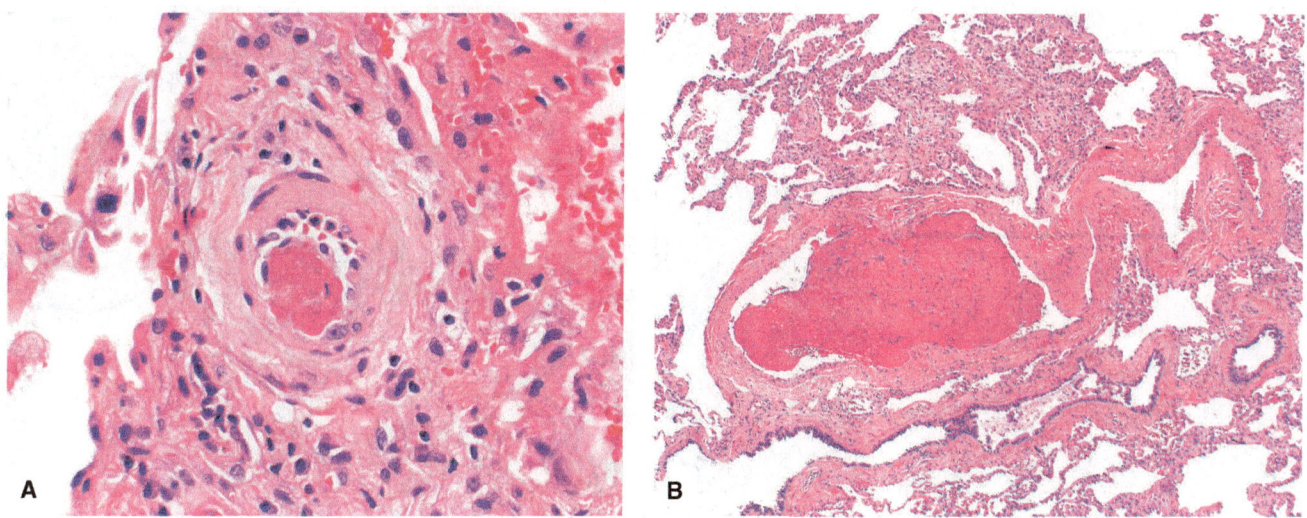

FIGURE 17.41 Thromboemboli in acute lung injury. Small (**A**) or even somewhat large (**B**) fibrin thrombi are commonly present in biopsies showing extensive acute lung injury. Hyaline membranes are apparent adjacent to the artery in (**A**), and organization is apparent at the top of the field in (**B**).

Recent intravascular thrombi (probably formed in situ) are a relatively common accompanying finding in any severe acute inflammatory lung disease (Fig. 17.41), and they should not be considered as evidence of pulmonary emboli without corroborating clinical information.

In patients with chronic hemorrhagic, chronic pulmonary congestion (as in congestive heart failure), or metabolic abnormalities, calcification and iron encrustation of the pulmonary elastic tissue may occur and even elicit a giant cell reaction (Fig. 17.42). This phenomenon has been inappropriately labeled endogenous pneumoconiosis (96).

Intravascular foreign material is usually birefringent and may have a giant cell reaction. While it usually occurs in intravenous drug abuse (intravascular talcosis), occasional fragments of foreign material are seen in patients without a history of drug abuse, perhaps related to intravenous lines during hospitalization or surgery.

The finding of interstitial air, either localized or diffuse, is well known to pediatric lung pathologists and may be an incidental finding in adults who have been on ventilators. Interstitial air can occur as an incidental finding in a region of subpleural fibrosis but also be a significant pathologic finding in its own right (Fig. 17.43) (97). The abnormal air-filled spaces resemble honeycombing; however, they lack the expected bronchiolar metaplastic epithelial lining and careful inspection shows either a complete lack of a cellular lining or a histiocytic and giant cell reaction lining the spaces. Interstitial air presenting in this way may be encountered in patients with interstitial lung disease, in patients with a history of pneumothorax, and in and around bullae and blebs. As in ventilated children, interstitial air may be encountered in adults on assisted ventilation and sometimes may be completely missed, being interpreted as tissue tearing.

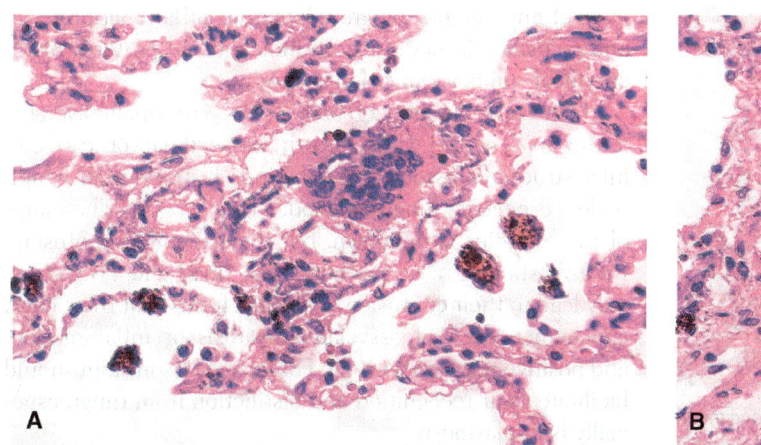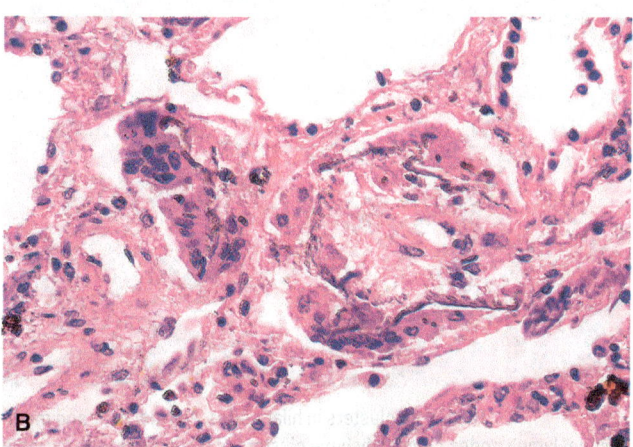

FIGURE 17.42 Iron deposition on elastic tissue. **A, B:** Chronic hemorrhage, in this case because of severe chronic passive congestion, may result in encrustation of interstitial and vascular elastic fibers by hemosiderin. A giant cell reaction is a frequent accompanying finding.

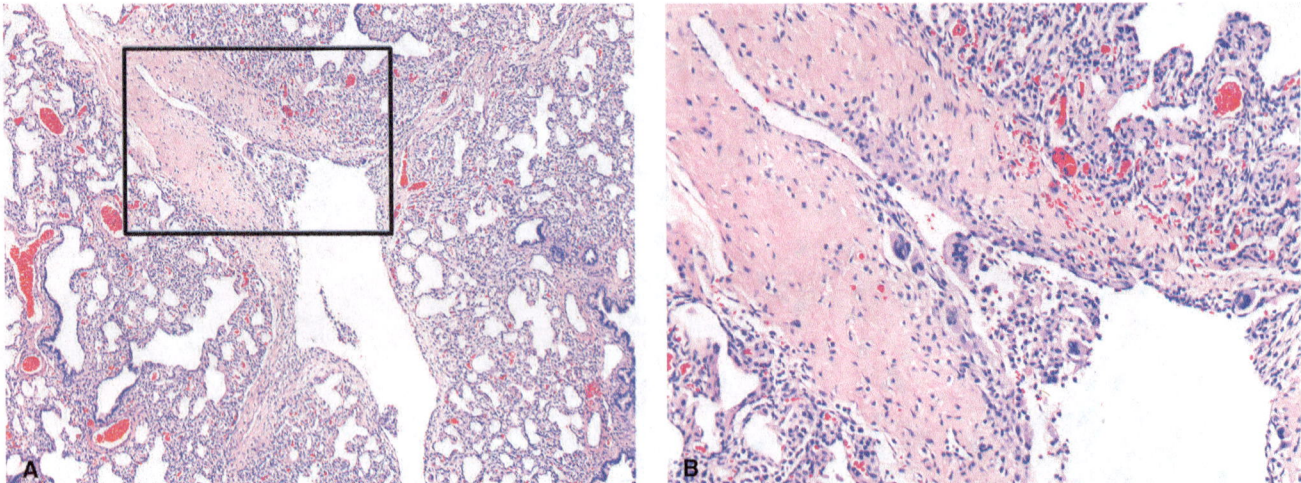

FIGURE 17.43 Interstitial air. When air dissects into the lung interstitium and becomes persistent (typically during positive end-expiratory pressure ventilation) peculiarly shaped airspaces (**A**) may be seen within interlobular septa in the peripheral lung. These artificial spaces represent interstitial air and become lined by giant cells (**B**-*box* from **A**). In children on ventilator support this process is referred to as persistent interstitial pulmonary emphysema (PIPE). The case illustrated is from a child with PIPE.

Hilar and peribronchial lymph nodes are rarely carefully examined beyond the evaluation for metastatic carcinoma. Nevertheless, they frequently exhibit a number of characteristic changes. Clusters of dust-filled macrophages in the sinuses and paracortical areas may resemble small granulomas (Fig. 17.44). Silicotic or anthracosilicotic nodules, old healed infectious granulomas, and sinus histiocytosis are also common. When sarcoidosis is a consideration, one may have difficulty distinguishing the normal histiocytosis of hilar nodes from the granulomas of sarcoidosis. In general, this problem can be approached by maintaining a high threshold for granulomas, requiring well-formed, rounded granulomatous masses (particularly with accumulations of intergranulomatous fibrinoid or hyalinized material), giant cells, and careful clinicopathologic correlation.

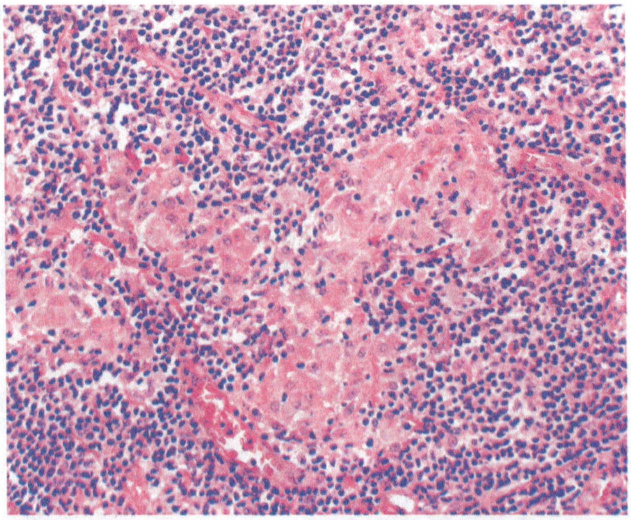

Although multiple intraparenchymal anthracosilicotic nodules should make one suspect the possibility of pneumoconiosis, anthracosilicotic nodules in hilar and intraparenchymal nodes are quite common in the absence of pneumoconiosis. The nodules are composed of concentric whorled and layered hyalinized collagen and are usually surrounded by a nonpalisaded rim of dust-filled macrophages that contain birefringent material when examined with polarized light. Central degenerative changes may be evident. Anthracosilicotic nodules should be distinguished from old/healed granulomatous disease. Of note, anthracosilicotic nodules can be secondarily infected, particularly with mycobacterial organisms (silicotuberculosis). Presence of any necrotizing granulomatous inflammation in an anthracosilicotic nodule is an indication to perform histochemical stains for microorganisms.

Hamazaki–Wesenberg bodies (98) are small (average: 5 μm in length), yellow-brown intracellular or extracellular structures associated with sinus histiocytes in lymph nodes, especially lung hilar nodes (Fig. 17.45). The cause of these bodies is unknown, but they resemble lipofuscin. Positive staining with methenamine silver and PAS stains may lead to their confusion with yeast forms, but their H&E appearance, lack of associated necrosis or inflammation, and positive reaction with the Fontana–Masson stain should facilitate their recognition and distinction from fungi, especially histoplasmosis.

Changes in the pleura in wedge biopsies may be incidental or part of the underlying pathologic process, and their significance needs to be assessed on an individual case basis.

FIGURE 17.44 Histiocyte clusters in hilar nodes. Normal hilar and mediastinal lymph nodes commonly have clusters of histiocytes with variable amounts of dust particles/anthracotic pigment in them. Sometimes they may appear somewhat granulomatous and may be difficult to distinguish from a true granulomatous reaction.

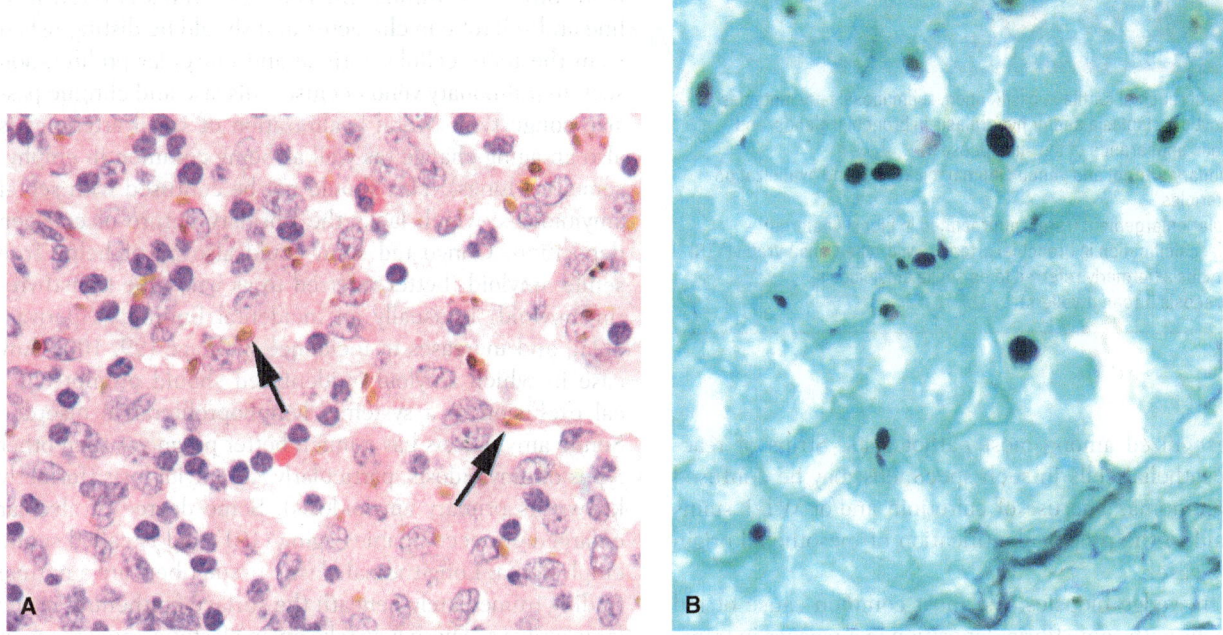

FIGURE 17.45 Hamazaki–Wesenberg bodies. **A:** Hamazaki–Wesenberg bodies represent yellow-brown oval structures associated with histiocytes, occasionally encountered in hilar and mediastinal lymph nodes (*arrows*). **B:** Their positive staining with silver stains sometimes leads to confusion with fungi.

INCIDENTAL FINDINGS IN TRANSBRONCHIAL BIOPSIES

The major artifacts or incidental findings in transbronchial biopsies that lead to misinterpretation include atelectasis (misinterpreted as interstitial pneumonia), bubble artifact (misinterpreted as lipoid/aspiration pneumonia), and portions of the pleura (either entirely missed or misinterpreted as neoplastic or suspicious for being neoplastic) (55,56). Such portions of pleura may even include some pleural fat, a particularly common finding in fibrosing interstitial pneumonias. The finding of pleural tissue in transbronchial biopsies (Fig. 17.46) is not uncommon but also is not

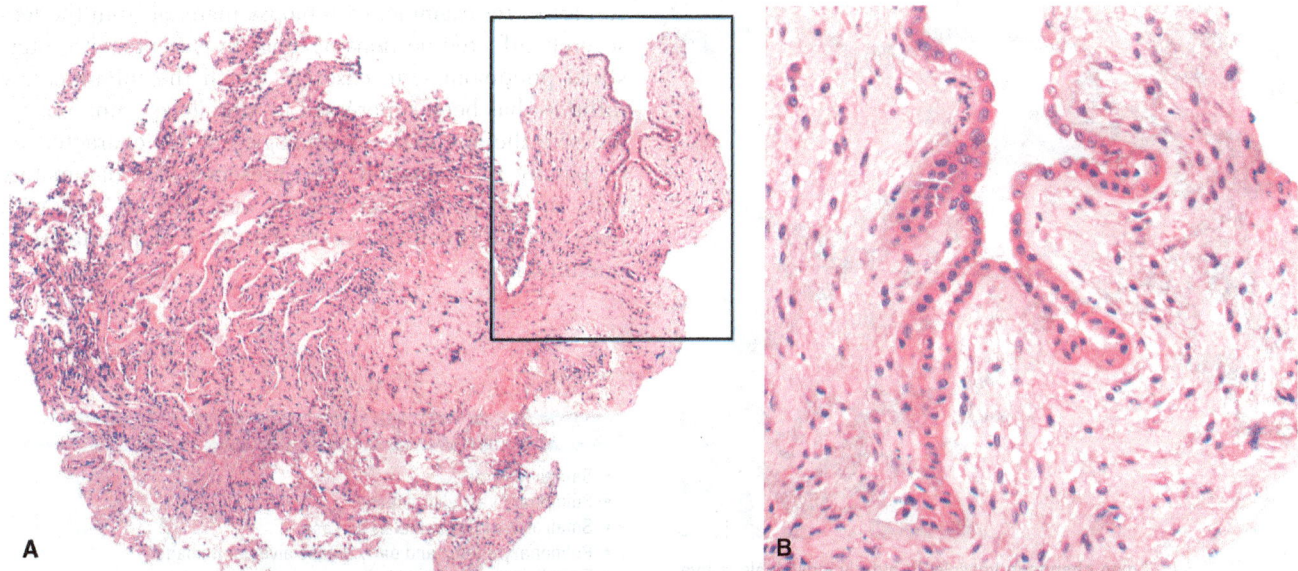

FIGURE 17.46 Visceral pleura in transbronchial biopsies. Transbronchial biopsies directed toward the periphery of the lung may sample portions of the visceral pleura (**A**, ***Box***; and **B**). These may lead to misdiagnosis, particularly if there is an associated reactive pleuritis.

> **TABLE 17.9**
> **Effects of Aging Seen in Lung Biopsies**
>
> - Tracheobronchial cartilage ossification, submucosal fatty metaplasia, oncocytic metaplasia and/or hyperplasia in bronchial glands, and elastotic appearance of the submucosa
> - Pulmonary arterial and venous intimal thickening and hyalinization of arterioles
> - Alveolar enlargement (rarely appreciated in biopsy material)
> - Medial calcification in bronchial arteries, wild-type transthyretin (TTR) amyloidosis (formerly referred to as senile amyloidosis)
> - Anthracosis (urban dwellers)

well recognized among most pathologists. Strips of reactive mesothelial cells in such specimens may be confused with carcinoma. The use of calretinin and/or WT-1 stains could aid in the proper identification of mesothelial origin in these cases.

As in wedge biopsies, the most common cause of red blood cells with some fibrin deposition in airspaces in transbronchial biopsies is trauma related to the procedure of the biopsy rather than an alveolar hemorrhage syndrome.

EFFECTS OF AGING

Some of the effects of aging on the lung are shown in Table 17.9. Calcification and ossification of cartilages in the large airways may be seen. Intimal thickening/atherosclerosis can be an age-related change in pulmonary arteries and veins (Fig. 17.47), and apical pulmonary arteries are affected more often (2). Intimal thickening of veins is often hyaline and sclerotic in character, and should be distinguished from the more cellular intimal and muscular proliferation seen in pulmonary veno-occlusive disease and chronic passive congestion. Mural hyalinization of small arterioles is also an aging change (as well as being common in emphysematous lungs). This should not be confused with septal amyloidosis, which lacks the fibrillary nature of collagen deposition. Congo red stain could also be of help. True senile amyloid (better referred to as wild-type transthyretin amyloid) is usually an incidental finding, is perivascular, and increases in incidence with age (99, 100). Any case in which amyloid is identified should prompt clinical exclusion of a systemic lymphoproliferative disorder. Senile amyloidosis has a much better prognosis than other types of amyloidosis, particularly AL amyloidosis (formerly known as primary amyloidosis). Some degree of alveolar enlargement accompanies aging (101) and is called senile emphysema. Longitudinal elastic tissue fibers are a normal finding immediately beneath the surface epithelium in the large airways. These may take on an elastotic appearance in the lungs of older individuals.

THE BIOPSY THAT LOOKS NORMAL AT FIRST GLANCE

When a lung biopsy for presumed diffuse lung disease initially appears normal, a number of possibilities should be considered (Table 17.10), especially pulmonary edema (Fig. 17.48).

Although one can argue that interstitial infiltrates that are so subtle as to be overlooked are probably not clinically significant, their recognition is necessary. This situation can arise, for example, with biopsy material from the less severely affected portions of lungs in patients with interstitial pneumonias, in cases in which the inflammatory infiltrate has been suppressed by steroids or immunosuppressive therapy, and in pathologic entities characterized by patchy inflammation. The presence of inflammatory cells in the perivenular regions and alveolar wall with reactive type II cells is usually indicative of an interstitial pneumonia.

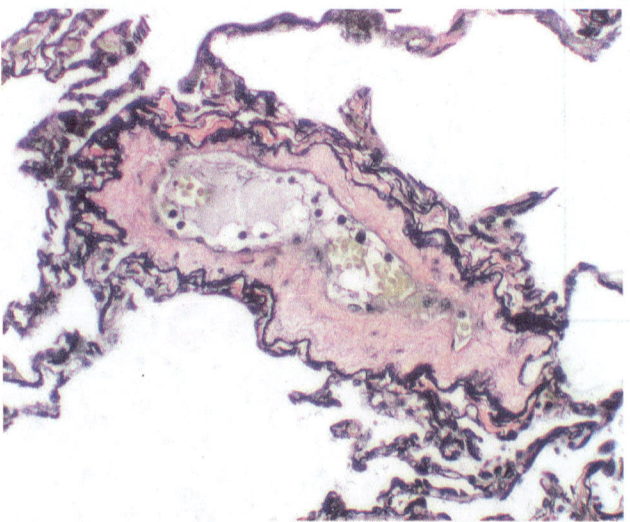

FIGURE 17.47 Aging change in vessels. In elderly individuals, a hyaline thickening of the intima may be encountered as an incidental finding. Clinical correlation is suggested, since this feature may also be encountered in the setting of pulmonary hypertension.

> **TABLE 17.10**
> **Situations in Which a Lung Biopsy may Appear Normal**
>
> - Sampling error
> - Pulmonary vascular disease
> - Small airway (bronchiolar) disease
> - Pulmonary edema and early diffuse alveolar damage
> - Emboli, including fat emboli
> - A very subtle interstitial infiltrate
> - Cardiac disease with secondary pulmonary abnormalities

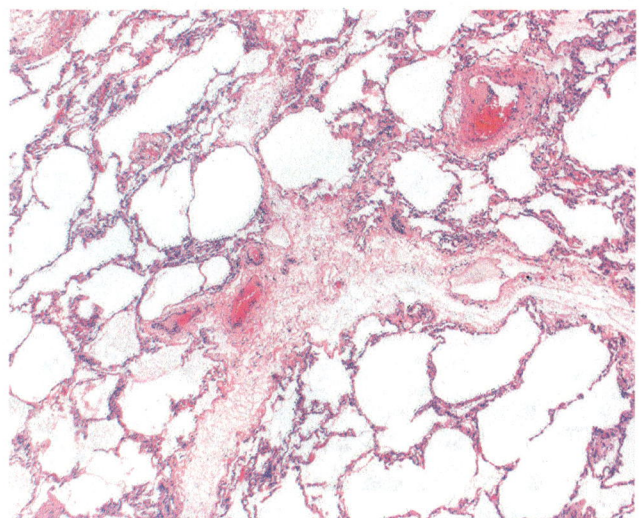

FIGURE 17.48 Pulmonary edema. Pulmonary edema may produce a deceptively normal appearance in a biopsy. Attention to septal widening, as noted in the accompanying text, and faint flocculent material in airspaces may be a clue to the diagnosis.

IMMUNOHISTOCHEMISTRY

Immunohistochemistry is applied frequently to the study of primary and metastatic neoplasms in the lung. Knowledge of the expected immunoreactivity of normal lung and pleura is helpful in these situations and such knowledge can be put to good use in the study of certain nonneoplastic disorders where lung histology may be obscured by a disease process. The immunostaining pattern of normal lung cells is summarized in Table 17.4.

Some examples of lung tissue stained with several commonly employed antibodies are presented in Figures 17.49 to 17.51 (102–107). The most frequent immunostains used on pulmonary pathology are summarized in Table 17.11. When applying immunostains for the diagnosis of lung malignancies, it is important to recognize staining of the uninvolved underlying benign lung architecture. For example, one should be aware of TTF-1/Napsin-A positivity of entrapped pneumocytes in otherwise solid tumors. Likewise, lepidic spreading tumors show TTF-1/Napsin-A positivity of the underlying benign alveolated parenchyma. This positivity should not be confused as evidence of adenocarcinoma. Also, the lung contains large amounts of airspace macrophages, and many times these macrophages can show nonspecific staining, particularly with Napsin-A antibodies. Of note, p63 immunostain is not a specific marker of squamous cell carcinoma. The WHO recommends the use of p40 as the most specific marker of squamous differentiation (76). Importantly, the lung is a common site of metastases. It is imperative to recognize that certain immunostains, otherwise considered to be relatively specific of an organ of origin can be expressed in primary lung malignancies. For example, GCDFP15, estrogen and progesterone receptor, and GATA3 immunostains can be positive in a percentage of lung non–small-cell carcinomas (108–111). In that same sense, CDX2 is often expressed in primary mucin-producing adenocarcinomas of the lung (112). Likewise, TTF-1 is expressed by other malignancies besides lung primary ones, most notoriously in almost all thyroid neoplasms (except

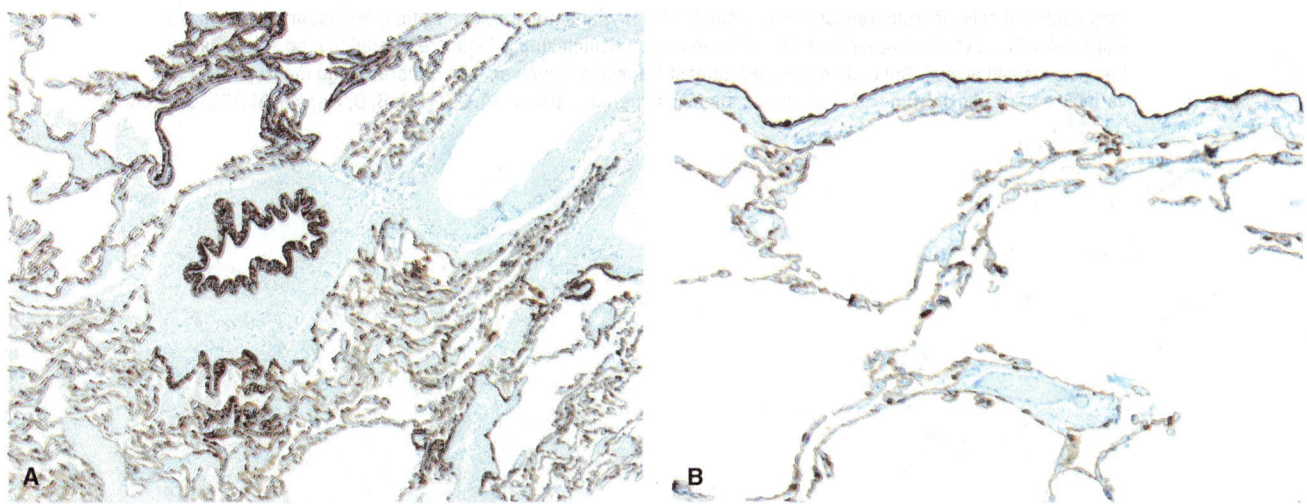

FIGURE 17.49 Pancytokeratin (CAM5.2). Cytokeratin immunoreactivity in normal peripheral lung varies somewhat by the molecular weight of the target cytokeratin peptide against which the antibody is directed (1,2). Broad-spectrum antibodies to cytokeratin stain all lung epithelial and pleural mesothelial cells, similar to the epithelial membrane antigen (EMA). **A:** Note the intense immunoreactivity of CAM5.2 in bronchiolar epithelium and the surrounding alveolar lining cells. **B:** Normal mesothelial cells can be better and more consistently visualized with broad-spectrum antibodies as compared to more targeted cocktails of specific cytokeratin polypeptides (e.g., CK5/6) used for characterizing mesothelioma (102,103).

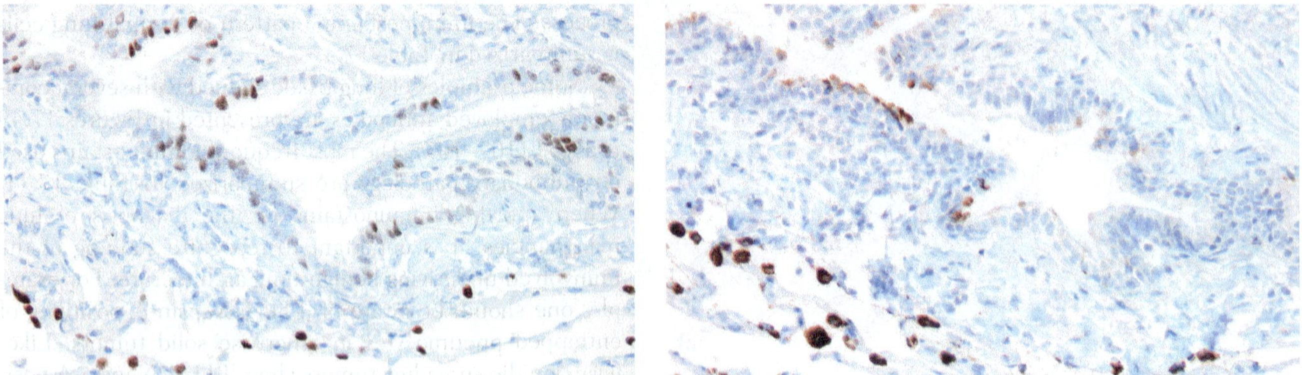

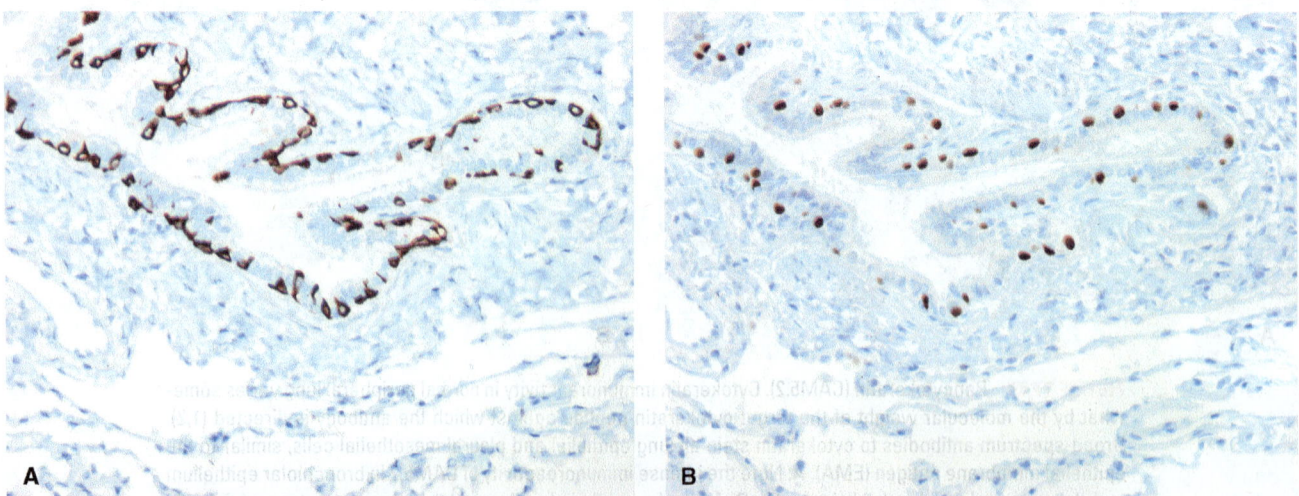

FIGURE 17.50 TTF-1 and Napsin-A. These two antibody targets are useful in narrowing potential origins for carcinomas in lung or present in the setting of the metastatic disease of unknown origin (3, 4). Both stain lung epithelial cells; thyroid transcription factor-1 (TTF-1) with a nuclear localization, the aspartic proteinase Napsin-A with a cytoplasmic localization. TTF-1 in a normal adult lung is highly restricted to lung epithelium of the airways and alveoli. Antibodies directed against Napsin-A, however, also decorate lung macrophages to variable extent, and produce more abundant staining in peripheral lung. (**A, C, TTF-1; B, D, Napsin-A**) (104,105).

FIGURE 17.51 Cytokeratin 5/6 and p63. These antibodies are useful markers for basal-type epithelial and myoepithelial cells in many organs (5). In the lung tissue, both show immunoreactivity in peripheral airway epithelium but not alveolar epithelial cells (106). (**A, Cytokeratin 5/6; B, p63**)

TABLE 17.11 Immunostains Commonly Used for the Diagnosis of Lung Primary Neoplasms

Adenocarcinoma	Squamous Cell Carcinoma	Neuroendocrine Neoplasms
TTF-1	p40 (highest specificity)	Synaptophysin
Napsin-A	p63	Chromogranin-A
Surfactant protein C (rarely used)	Cytokeratin 5/6 (lowest specificity)	CD56

anaplastic thyroid carcinomas), while it is also expressed in small percentage of ovarian serous carcinomas, endometrial and endocervical adenocarcinomas, and colonic adenocarcinomas. Napsin-A can be expressed in a large proportion of papillary renal cell carcinomas and in some clear cell carcinomas of the gynecologic tract (107). Lastly, negativity for TTF-1 and Napsin-A does not exclude lung adenocarcinoma. In such cases, pathologists still rely on the use of histochemical stains for mucin (e.g., mucicarmine, PASD) to demonstrate glandular differentiation.

In the era of personalized medicine, immunohistochemistry in pulmonary pathology now also includes certain immunostains used for prognostic purposes. Some of these stains include ALK and PD-L1 immunostains. A detailed used of these stains is out of the scope of this chapter. Recent review on the use of these stains in lung cancer prognosis can be found in reference 113.

REFERENCES

1. Nagaishi C. *Functional Anatomy and Histology of the Lung*. Baltimore, MD: University Park Press; 1972.
2. Wagenvoort CA, Wagenvoort N. *Pathology of Pulmonary Hypertension*. New York: John Wiley; 1977.
3. Kuhn C 3rd. Ultrastructure and cellular function in the distal lung. In: Thurlbeck WM, Abell MR, eds. *The Lung*. Baltimore, MD: Williams & Wilkins; 1978.
4. Scadding JG, Cumming G, eds. *Scientific Foundations of Respiratory Medicine*. Philadelphia, PA: WB Saunders; 1981.
5. Gail DB, Lenfant CJ. Cells of the lung: Biology and clinical implications. *Am Rev Respir Dis* 1983;127:366–387.
6. Bienenstock J, Befus AD. Gut-and-bronchus-associated lymphoid tissue. *Am J Anat* 1984;170:437–445.
7. Langston C, Kida K, Reed M, et al. Human lung growth in late gestation and in the neonate. *Am Rev Respir Dis* 1984; 129:607–613.
8. Murray JF. *The Normal Lung*. 2nd ed. Philadelphia, PA: WB Saunders; 1986.
9. Fawcett DW, Bloom W, Raviola E. *A Textbook of Histology*. 12th ed. New York: Chapman and Hall; 1994.
10. Coalson JJ. The adult lung: Structure and function. In: Saldana MJ, ed. *Pathology of Pulmonary Disease*. Philadelphia, PA: JB Lippincott: 1994:3–14.
11. Wang NS. Anatomy. In: Dail DH, Hammar SP, eds. *Pulmonary Pathology*. 2nd ed. New York: Springer-Verlag; 1994:21–44.
12. Kuhn C III. Normal anatomy and histology. In: Thurlbeck WM, Churg AM, eds. *Pathology of the Lung*. 2nd ed. New York: Thieme Medical Publishers; 1995:1–36.
13. Weibel ER, Taylor CR. Functional design of the human lung for gas exchange. In: Fishman AP, ed. *Pulmonary Diseases and Disorders*. Vol 1. 3rd ed. New York: McGraw-Hill; 1998:21–61.
14. Albertine KH, Williams MC, Hyde DM. Anatomy of the lungs. In: Murray JF, Nadel JA, eds. *Textbook of Respiratory Medicine*. 3rd ed. Philadelphia, PA: WB Saunders; 2000:3–33.
15. Corrin B. *Pathology of the Lungs*. London: Churchill Livingstone; 2000.
16. Leslie KO, Wick MR. Lung anatomy. In: Leslie KO, Wick MR, eds. *Practical Pulmonary Pathology*. Philadelphia, PA: Churchill Livingstone; 2005:1–18.
17. Chinoy MR. Lung growth and development frontiers. *Bioscience* 2003;8:392–415.
18. Roth-Kleiner M, Post M. Genetic control of lung development. *Biol Neonate* 2003;84:83–88.
19. Yaegashi H, Takahashi T. The airway dimension in ordinary human lung. A standardized morphometry of lung sections. *Arch Pathol Lab Med* 1994;118:969–974.
20. Hansell DM. Small airways diseases: Detection and insights with computed tomography. *Eur Respir J* 2001;17(6): 1294–1313.
21. Lambert MW. Accessory bronchiolealveolar communications. *J Pathol Bacteriol* 1955;70:311–314.
22. Yousem SA, Dacic S. Idiopathic bronchiolocentric interstitial pneumonia. *Mod Pathol* 2002;15:1148–1153.
23. Churg A, Meyers J, Suarez T, et al. Airway-centered interstitial fibrosis: A distinct form of aggressive diffuse lung disease. *Am J Surg Pathol* 2004;28:62–68.
24. Fukuoka J, Franks TJ, Colby TV, et al. Peribronchiolar metaplasia: A common histologic lesion in diffuse lung disease and a rare cause of interstitial lung disease; clinicopathologic features of 15 cases. *Am J Surg Pathol*. 2005;29(7):948–954.
25. Winkelmann A, Noack T. The Clara cell: A "Third Reich eponym." *Eur Respir J* 2010;36(4):722–727.
26. Lehnert BE. Pulmonary and thoracic macrophage subpopulations and clearance of particles from the lung. *Environ Health Perspect* 1992;97:17–46.
27. Gould SJ, Isaacson PG. Bronchus-associated lymphoid tissue (BALT) in human fetal and infant lung. *J Pathol* 1993;169: 229–234.
28. Richmond J, Pritchard GE, Ashcroft T, et al. Bronchus associated lymphoid tissue (BALT) in human lung: Its distribution in smokers and non-smokers. *Thorax* 1993;48:1130–1134.
29. Tschernig T, Kleemann WJ, Pabst R. Bronchus-associated lymphoid tissue (BALT) in the lungs of children who had died from sudden infant death syndrome and other causes. *Thorax* 1995;50:658–660.
30. Randall TD. Bronchus-associated lymphoid tissue (BALT) structure and function. *Adv Immunol* 2010;107:187–241.
31. Bienenstock J. Bronchus-associated lymphoid tissue. *Int Arch Allergy Appl Immunol* 1985;76(suppl 1):62–69.
32. Kradin RL, Spirn PW, Mark EJ. Intrapulmonary lymph nodes. Clinical, radiologic, and pathologic features. *Chest* 1985;87: 662–667.
33. Gallagher B, Urbanski SJ. The significance of pleural elastica invasion by lung carcinomas. *Hum Pathol* 1990;21:512–517.

34. Amin MB, Edge SB, Greene FL, et al., eds. *AJCC Cancer Staging Manual*. 8th ed. New York: Springer, 2017.
35. Sheffield BS, Hwang HC, Lee AF, et al. BAP1 immunohistochemistry and p16 FISH to separate benign from malignant mesothelial proliferations. *Am J Surg Pathol* 2015;39(7): 977–982.
36. Colby TV, Swensen SJ. Anatomic distribution and histopathologic pattern in diffuse lung disease: Correlation with HRCT. *J Thorac Imaging* 1996;11:1–26.
37. Travis WD, Cotabel U, Hansell DM, et al. An official American Thoracic Society/European Respiratory Society statement: Update of the International Multidisciplinary Classification of the Idiopathic Interstitial Pneumonias. *Am J Respir Crit Care Med* 2013;188(6):733–748.
38. Newman SL, Michael RP, Wang NS. Lingular lung biopsy: is it representative? *Am Rev Respir Dis* 1985;132:1084–1086.
39. Albo RJ, Grimes OF. The middle lobe syndrome: A clinical study. *Dis Chest* 1966;50:509–518.
40. Kwon KY, Myers JL, Swensen SJ, et al. Middle lobe syndrome: A clinicopathological study of 21 patients. *Hum Pathol* 1995;26:302–307.
41. Renner RR, Markarian B, Pernice NJ, et al. The apical cap. *Radiology* 1974;110:569–573.
42. McCloud TC, Isler RJ, Novelline RA, et al. The apical cap. *AJR* 1981;137:299–306.
43. Lagstein A. Pulmonary apical cap-what's old is new again. *Arch Pathol Lab Med* 2015;139(10):1258–1262.
44. Yousem SA. Pulmonary apical cap: A distinctive but poorly recognized lesion in pulmonary surgical pathology. *Am J Surg Pathol* 2001;25:679–683.
45. Thurlbeck WM, Wright JL. *Thurlbeck's Chronic Airflow Obstruction*. 2nd ed. Hamilton, ON: BC Decker; 1999.
46. Fraig M, Shreesa U, Savici D, et al. Respiratory bronchiolitis: A clinicopathologic study in current smokers, ex-smokers and never-smokers. *Am J Surg Pathol* 2002;26:647–653.
47. Lichter I, Gwynne JF. Spontaneous pneumothorax in young subjects: A clinical and pathological study. *Thorax* 1971;26: 409–417.
48. Thurlbeck WM. *Chronic Airflow Obstruction in Lung Disease*. Philadelphia, PA: WB Saunders; 1976.
49. Ryu JH, Swensen SJ. Cystic and cavitary lung diseases: Focal and diffuse. *Mayo Clin Proc* 2003;78(6):744–752.
50. Askin FB, McCann BG, Kuhn C. Reactive eosinophilic pleuritis: A lesion to be distinguished from pulmonary eosinophilic granuloma. *Arch Pathol Lab Med* 1977;101:187–191.
51. Churg A. Asbestos fibers and pleural plaques in a general autopsy population. *Am J Pathol* 1982;109:88–96.
52. Meurman L. Asbestos bodies and pleural plaques in a Finnish series of autopsy cases. *Acta Pathol Microbiol Immunol Scand* 1966;181:1–107.
53. Roberts GH. The pathology of parietal pleural plaques. *J Clin Pathol* 1971;24:348–353.
54. Hillerdal G. Pleural plaques and risk for bronchial carcinoma and mesothelioma. A prospective study. *Chest* 1994;105: 144–150.
55. Katzenstein ALA. *Katzenstein and Askin's Surgical Pathology of Non-neoplastic Lung Disease*. 3rd ed. Philadelphia, PA: WB Saunders; 1997.
56. Kendall DM, Gal AA. Interpretation of tissue artifacts in transbronchial lung biopsy specimens. *Ann Diagn Pathol* 2003;7:20–24.
57. Kadokura M, Colby TV, Myers JL, et al. Pathologic comparison of video-assisted thoracic surgical lung biopsy with traditional open lung biopsy. *J Thorac Cardiovasc Surg* 1995; 109:494–498.
58. Churg A. An inflation procedure for open lung biopsies. *Am J Surg Pathol* 1983;7:69–71.
59. Bensard DD, McIntyre RC Jr, Waring BJ, et al. Comparison of video thoracoscopic lung biopsy to open lung biopsy in the diagnosis of interstitial lung disease. *Chest* 1993;103: 765–770.
60. Ferson PF, Landreneau RJ, Dowling RD, et al. Comparison of open versus thoracoscopic lung biopsy for diffuse infiltrative pulmonary disease. *J Thorac Cardiovasc Surg* 1993;106: 194–199.
61. Carnochan FM, Walker WS, Cameron EW. Efficacy of video-assisted thoracoscopic lung biopsy: An historical comparison with open lung biopsy. *Thorax* 1994;49:361–363.
62. Doberer D, Trejo Bittar HE, Wenzel SE. Should lung biopsies be performed in patients with severe asthma? *Eur Respir Rev* 2015;24(137):525–539.
63. Ravaglia C, Bonifazi M, Wells AU, et al. Safety and diagnostic yield of transbronchial lung cryobiopsy in diffuse parenchymal lung diseases: A comparative study versus video-assisted thoracoscopic lung biopsy and a systematic review of the literature. *Respiration* 2016;91:215–227.
64. Lentz RJ, Argento AC, Colby TV, et al. Transbronchial cryobiopsy for diffuse parenchymal lung disease: A state-of-the-art review of procedural techniques, current evidence, and future challenges. *J Thorac Dis* 2017;9(7):2186–2203.
65. Niewoehner DE, Kleinerman J, Rice DB. Pathologic changes in the peripheral airways of young cigarette smokers. *N Engl J Med* 1974;291:755–758.
66. Myers JL, Veal CF Jr, Shin MS, et al. Respiratory bronchiolitis causing interstitial lung disease. A clinicopathologic study of six cases. *Am Rev Respir Dis* 1987;135:880–884.
67. Yousem SA. Respiratory bronchiolitis-associated interstitial lung disease with fibrosis is a lesion distinct from fibrotic nonspecific interstitial pneumonia: A proposal. *Mod Pathol* 2006;19(11):1474–1479.
68. Katzenstein AL, Mukhopadhyay S, Zanardi C, et al. Clinically occult interstitial fibrosis in smokers: Classification and significance of a surprisingly common finding in lobectomy specimens. *Hum Pathol* 2010;41(3):316–325.
69. Trejo Bittar HE, Yousem SA, Wenzel SE. Pathobiology of severe asthma. *Annu Rev Pathol* 2015;10:511–545.
70. Wenzel SE, Vitari CA, Shende M, et al. Asthmatic granulomatosis: A novel disease with asthmatic and granulomatous features. *Am J Respir Crit Care Med* 2012;186(6):501–507.
71. Trejo Bittar HE, Doberer D, Mehrad M, et al. Histologic findings of severe/therapy-resistant asthma from video-assisted thoracoscopic surgery biopsies. *Am J Surg Pathol* 2017;41(2): 182–188.
72. Ashley DJ. Bony metaplasia in trachea and bronchi. *J Pathol* 1970;102:186–188.
73. Churg A, Warnock ML. Pulmonary tumorlet. A form of peripheral carcinoid. *Cancer* 1976;37:1469–1477.
74. Gould VE, Linnoila RI, Memoli VA, et al. Neuroendocrine components of the bronchopulmonary tract: Hyperplasias, dysplasias, and neoplasms. *Lab Invest* 1983;49:519–537.
75. Ranchod M. The histogenesis and development of pulmonary tumorlets. *Cancer* 1977;39:1135–1145.

76. Travis W, Brambilla E, Burke AP, et al., eds. *World Health Organization Classification of Tumours of the Lung, Pleura, Thymus and Heart.* 4th ed. Lyon, France: IARC Press, 2015.
77. Kuhn C 3rd, Askin FB. The fine structure of so-called minute pulmonary chemodectomas. *Hum Pathol* 1975;6:681–691.
78. Gaffey MJ, Mills SE, Askin FB. Minute pulmonary meningothelial-like nodules. A clinicopathologic study of so-called minute pulmonary chemodectoma. *Am J Surg Pathol* 1988;12:167–175.
79. Miller RR, Muller NL. Neuroendocrine cell hyperplasia and obliterative bronchiolitis in patients with peripheral carcinoid tumors. *Am J Surg Pathol* 1995;19:653–658.
80. Ionescu DN, Sasatomi E, Aldeeb D, et al. Pulmonary meningothelial-like nodules: A genotypic comparison with meningiomas. *Am J Surg Pathol* 2004;28:207–214.
81. Miller RR. Bronchioloalveolar cell adenomas. *Am J Surg Pathol* 1990;14:904–912.
82. Elkeles A, Glynn LE. Disseminated parenchymatous ossification in the lungs in association with mitral stenosis. *J Pathol Bacteriol* 1946;58:517–522.
83. Green JD, Harle TS, Greenberg SD, et al. Disseminated pulmonary ossification. A case report with demonstration of electron-microscopic features. *Am Rev Respir Dis* 1970;101:293–298.
84. Muir TE, Leslie KO, Popper H, et al. Micronodular pneumocyte hyperplasia. *Am J Surg Pathol* 1998;22:465–472.
85. Bedrossian CW, Kuhn C 3rd, Luna MA, et al. Desquamative interstitial pneumonia-like reaction accompanying pulmonary lesions. *Chest* 1977;72:166–169.
86. Hollander DH, Hutchins GM. Central spherules in pulmonary corpora amylacea. *Arch Pathol Lab Med* 1978;102:629–630.
87. Koss MN, Johnson FB, Hochholzer L. Pulmonary blue bodies. *Hum Pathol* 1981;12:258–266.
88. Visscher D, Churg A, Katzenstein AL. Significance of crystalline inclusions in lung granulomas. *Mod Pathol* 1988;1:415–419.
89. Schaumann J. On the nature of certain peculiar corpuscles present in the tissue of lymphogranulomatosis benigna. *Acta Med Scand* 1941;106:239–253.
90. Warnock ML, Press M, Churg A. Further observations on cytoplasmic hyaline in the lung. *Hum Pathol* 1980;11:59–65.
91. Churg A, Warnock ML. Asbestos and other ferruginous bodies: their formation and clinical significance. *Am J Pathol* 1981;102:447–456.
92. Hung Y, Hunninghake G, Putman RK, et al. Non-neoplastic pulmonary parenchymal findings in patients undergoing lung resection for mass lesions. *Mod Pathol* 2016;29:472A.
93. Glancy DL, Frazier PD, Roberts WC. Pulmonary parenchymal cholesterol-ester granulomas in patients with pulmonary hypertension. *Am J Med* 1968;45:198–210.
94. Reinila A. Perivascular xanthogranulomatosis in the lungs of diabetic patients. *Arch Pathol Lab Med* 1976;100:542–543.
95. Borges I, Sena I, Azevedo P. Lung as a niche for hematopoietic progenitors. *Stem Cell Rev* 2017;13(5):567–574.
96. Walford RL, Kaplan L. Pulmonary fibrosis and giant-cell reaction with altered elastic tissue: Endogenous pneumoconiosis. *AMA Arch Pathol* 1957;63:75–90.
97. Unger JM, England DM, Bogust GA. Interstitial emphysema in adults: Recognition and prognostic implications. *J Thorac Imaging* 1989;4:86–94.
98. Ro JY, Luna MA, Mackay B, et al. Yellow-brown (Hamazaki-Wesenberg) bodies mimicking fungal yeasts. *Arch Pathol Lab Med* 1987;111:555–559.
99. Kunze WP. Senile pulmonary amyloidosis. *Pathol Res Pract* 1979;164:413–422.
100. Khoor A, Colby TV. Amyloidosis of the lung. *Arch Pathol Lab Med* 2017;141(2):247–254.
101. Gillooly M, Lamb D. Airspace size in lungs of lifelong nonsmokers: Effect of age and sex. *Thorax* 1993;48:39–43.
102. Blobel GA, Moll R, Franke WW, et al. Cytokeratins in normal lung and lung carcinomas. I. Adenocarcinomas, squamous cell carcinomas and cultured cell lines. *Virchows Arch B Cell Pathol Incl Mol Pathol* 1984;45(4):407–429.
103. Moll R, Divo M, Langbein L. The human keratins: biology and pathology. *Histochem Cell Biol* 2008;129(6):705–733.
104. Chuman Y, Bergman A, Ueno T, et al. Napsin A, a member of the aspartic protease family, is abundantly expressed in normal lung and kidney tissue and is expressed in lung adenocarcinomas. *FEBS Lett* 1999;462(1-2):129–134.
105. Nakamura N, Miyagi E, Murata S, et al. Expression of thyroid transcription factor-1 in normal and neoplastic lung tissues. *Mod Pathol* 2002;15(10):1058–1067.
106. Saad RS, Liu YL, Silverman JF. Distribution of basal/myoepithelial markers in benign and malignant bronchioloalveolar proliferations of the lung. *Appl Immunohistochem Mol Morphol* 2010;18(3):219–225.
107. Woo JS, Reddy OL, Koo M, et al. Application of immunohistochemistry in the diagnosis of pulmonary and pleural neoplasms. *Arch Pathol Lab Med* 2017;141(9):1195–1213.
108. Wang LJ, Greaves WO, Sabo E. GCDFP-15 positive and TTF-1 negative primary lung neoplasms: A tissue microarray study of 381 primary lung tumors. *Appl Immunohistochem Mol Morphol* 2009;17(6):505–511.
109. Striebel JM, Dacic S, Yousem SA. Gross cystic disease fluid protein-(GCDFP-15): Expression in primary lung adenocarcinoma. *Am J Surg Pathol* 2008;32(3):426–432.
110. Su JM, Hsu HK, Chang H, et al. Expression of estrogen and progesterone receptors in non-small-cell lung cancer: Immunohistochemical study. *Anticancer Res* 1996;16(6B):3803–3806.
111. Berg KB, Churg A. GATA3 Immunohistochemistry for distinguishing sarcomatoid and desmoplastic mesothelioma from sarcomatoid carcinoma of the lung. *Am J Surg Pathol* 2017;41(9):1221–1225.
112. Cowan ML, Li QK, Illei PB. CDX-2 expression in primary lung adenocarcinoma. *Appl Immunohistochem Mol Morphol* 2016;24(1):16–19.
113. Mino-Kenudson M. Immunohistochemistry for predictive biomarkers in non-small cell lung cancer. *Transl Lung Cancer Res* 2017;6(5):570–587.

18

Thymus

David Suster ■ Saul Suster

EMBRYOLOGY 506	IMMUNOHISTOCHEMISTRY 514
DEVELOPMENTAL ABNORMALITIES 507	Thymic Epithelial Cells 514
	Thymic Lymphocytes 515
APOPTOSIS 508	MOLECULAR BIOLOGY 516
ANATOMY 508	FUNCTION 516
HISTOLOGY 509	AGE-RELATED AND OTHER TROPHIC CHANGES 517
Epithelial Cells 510	Thymic Involution 517
Hassall Corpuscles 510	Thymic Hyperplasia 517
Thymic Lymphocytes (Thymocytes) 510	
Other Cell Types 510	ARTIFACTS AND OTHER POTENTIAL PITFALLS IN DIFFERENTIAL DIAGNOSIS 518
ULTRASTRUCTURE 513	REFERENCES 523

The thymus is a prototypical lymphoepithelial organ. As such, it is composed of intimately admixed epithelial and lymphoid elements that act in concert to perform their assigned roles. In addition, the thymus harbors other cellular constituents, such as a variety of mesenchymal-derived elements, scattered neuroendocrine cells, and presumably germ cells, all of which may take part in the development of neoplastic and nonneoplastic processes of this organ. Although much progress has been made in the immunohistochemical characterization of the cellular components of the thymus, the diagnosis of thymic lesions remains largely dependent on the light microscopic interpretation of the findings by the pathologist.

EMBRYOLOGY

The thymus is derived from the third and, to a lesser extent, the fourth pharyngeal pouches, which contain elements derived from all the three germinal layers. During the 6th week of gestation, the endodermal lining of the ventral wing of the third pharyngeal pouch forms a pronounced saccule, which subsequently detaches from the pharyngeal wall, giving rise to the thymic primordia (1,2). It is postulated that, at approximately the same time, the cervical sinus (an ectodermal structure that results from the fusion of the second, third, and fourth branchial clefts) attaches to the thymic primordia, investing them with a layer of ectodermal cells (1,3). As development continues, the thymic primordia migrate in a caudal and a medial direction along with the lower parathyroid glands. During the 8th week, these primordia enlarge toward their lower ends, forming two epithelial bars that fuse along the midline to occupy their definitive position within the antero-superior mediastinum. During this descent, the tail portion of the organ becomes thin and elongated and breaks up into small fragments that usually disappear but that may persist in the soft tissues of the neck, often in intimate connection with the lower parathyroid gland and sometimes embedded within the thyroid gland (see the section on Developmental Abnormalities) (1,4).

Once migration has been completed, the thymic endodermal-derived epithelial cells develop into a reticular

---

This chapter is an update of a previous version authored by Saul Suster and Juan Rosai.

network of cells. The surrounding mesenchymal elements form a capsule around it; and, as a result of ingrowth of the capsule, trabeculae form that divide the organ into numerous lobules. By the 10th week, small lymphoid cells originating in the fetal liver and bone marrow populate the thymus, and the organ differentiates into a cortex and a medulla (5). Small tubular structures composed of epithelial cells (sometimes referred to as medullary duct epithelium) also make their appearance at this stage that will later give rise to Hassall corpuscles (6). The thymus progressively enlarges until puberty and from then on and thereafter begins to involute, although persisting in an atrophic state into old age.

DEVELOPMENTAL ABNORMALITIES

Disturbances in the embryologic development of the thymus may give rise to a series of congenital anomalies. One of the anomalies most frequently encountered is the presence of parathyroid gland tissue within the thymus (Fig. 18.1) (7). Such ectopically located tissue is most frequently encountered within the thymic capsule or in close proximity to it (8). This abnormality is easily explained by the close developmental relationship that exists between the two organs, as described in the section on embryology. The thymus itself also may be found in ectopic locations; this usually results from failure of the organ to migrate to its final destination during embryonic development. Undescended thymuses are most often located in the lateral neck, in close association with or even buried within the parathyroid or thyroid glands (9). The thymic rests tend to undergo cystic changes (9). They also may give rise to thymomas, ectopic examples of which have been described in submandibular (10), paratracheal (11,12), and intratracheal locations (13), as well as within the thyroid gland (14,15). A morphologically distinctive lesion of the thymus displaying combined features of neoplasia and hamartoma occurring in the lower neck has also been recognized (16). Ectopic nodules composed of thymic tissue have been reported in several other locations, including the base of the skull (17) and the pulmonary hilus at the root of the bronchus (18). Given that thymomas can also occur within lung parenchyma and in the pleura away from the mediastinum, it is logical to assume that thymic rests may also be present in such locations. The lungs and pleura, however, develop much earlier than the thymus during embryogenesis, making the misplacement of thymic tissue during embryologic migration unlikely as an explanation for the development of these tumors in pulmonary and pleural locations. Some authors have postulated origin from uncommitted pluripotential stem cells for such tumors (19). Ectopic thymomas have also been identified in the middle and posterior mediastinum; although rare, it has been postulated that such

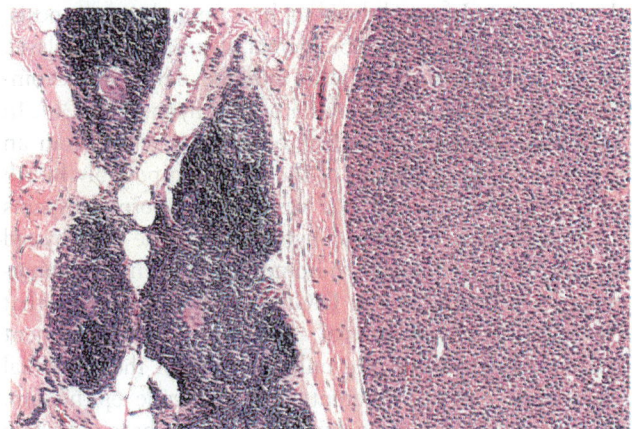

FIGURE 18.1 Ectopic parathyroid tissue adjacent to the normal thymus.

tumors may have had a direct connection to the thymic gland or its surrounding adipose tissue (20).

Ectopic sebaceous glands have been reported in the thymus (21) and are felt to be related to the contribution of the ectodermally derived cervical sinus to the developing thymus. Mature-appearing salivary gland tissue also may be present in the thymus (Fig. 18.2) and has been reported as a component of an intrathoracic cyst that contained normal thymus and parathyroid tissue within its walls (22). It was postulated that this finding could be related to a developmental malformation whereby salivary gland anlage had been incorporated into the uppermost portion of the third pharyngeal pouch during embryogenesis.

Morphologic abnormalities of the thymus characterized by an embryonal appearance, with a predominance of small spindle epithelial cells adopting a lobular configuration and lacking small lymphocytes and Hassall corpuscles, have been observed in association with combined immunodeficiency syndromes and T-cell defects (23). Such morphologic alterations have been termed thymic dysplasia and are believed to represent disturbances of normal

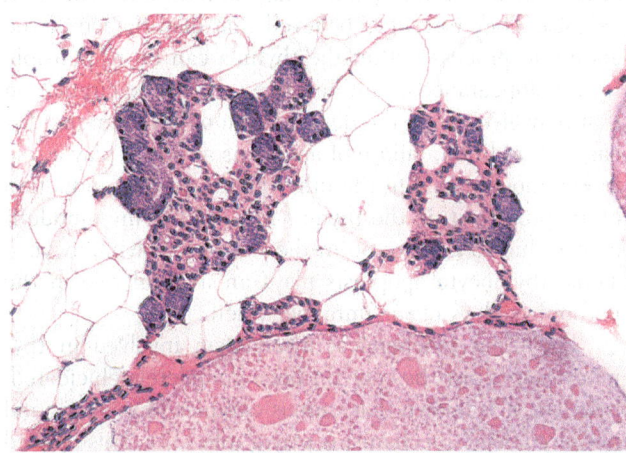

FIGURE 18.2 Mature-appearing salivary gland acini are seen adjacent to cystically dilated Hassall corpuscle.

development. In conditions such as reticular dysgenesis, Swiss-type hypogammaglobulinemia, thymic alymphoplasia, and ataxia–telangiectasia, the immune deficit is accompanied by aplasia or hypoplasia of the thymus (24–26). In DiGeorge syndrome, which is believed to result from an arrest in the development of the third and possibly fourth branchial arches, there is a vestigial but normal thymus associated with absence or hypoplasia of the parathyroid glands (27). In Nezelof syndrome (28), the thymic abnormality is similar to that of DiGeorge syndrome except that the parathyroids are normal. The failure of development is thus thought to involve only that part of the branchial endoderm that will differentiate into thymic epithelium. Histologic changes in the thymus similar to those of thymic dysplasia of primary immunodeficiency disease have been observed in infants as a consequence of graft versus host disease after blood transfusions (29). A case of congenital aplasia of the parathyroid glands and thymus in the newborn also has been described (30). The term *thymic dysplasia* in the setting of immunodeficiency conditions may be misleading because of its currently accepted connotation as a preneoplastic condition. The alterations in such conditions are unrelated to neoplastic etiology.

APOPTOSIS

Apoptosis is the name that has been given to the process of physiologic (programmed) cell death. Most thymic lymphocytes die in situ by such a process. During T-cell ontogeny in the thymus, the T cells (T lymphocytes) may undergo a process of positive or negative selection. The accumulated evidence appears to support that apoptosis plays a major role in the process of negative selection and that the majority of cortical thymocytes die by this mechanism. Autoreactive thymocytes or harmful cells in the thymus with injured DNA or alterations of their metabolism are also thought to be eliminated by the process of apoptosis at a specific stage of their differentiation (31,32). Therefore, it is believed that disturbance of the apoptotic process within the thymus can be responsible for the appearance of autoreactive cells in the circulation that may give rise to the development of autoimmune disease. In addition, failure of apoptosis also may play a role in carcinogenesis. On the other hand, massive induction of apoptosis within the thymus may lead to immunodeficiency due to a decrease in the number of lymphocytes. Thus, thymocyte apoptosis plays an integral role in the pathophysiology of the immune system.

The exact biochemical mechanism involved in thymocyte apoptosis has not yet been completely elucidated; however, it is known that various complex physiologic and nonphysiologic mechanisms play a role (33). This has led many investigators to seek the genes and their products that are necessary for apoptosis. Several groups have noted that messenger RNA (mRNA) levels for various proteins are increased early in thymocytes after treatment with glucocorticoids or radiation, two agents known to induce massive apoptosis of cortical thymocytes (34,35). Several genes also have been identified whose expression is increased in cells undergoing apoptosis. Among them, three proto-oncogene products have been shown to act as important regulators of the apoptotic process in mammals: c-myc, bcl-2, and p53. In thymocytes, bcl-2 mRNA is present in the surviving mature thymocytes of the medulla and also in most immature ($CD4^+/CD8^+$) thymocytes, although the majority of cortical thymocytes (most of which die by apoptosis) display no bcl-2, suggesting that this oncogene may be involved in the preservation of T cells (36). Alterations of the p53 gene also have been shown to play a role in the process of thymocyte apoptosis. Malfunction of the tumor suppressor gene p53 may promote carcinogenesis by permitting mutated cells to duplicate their DNA before it is repaired. In mice, p53-deficient thymocytes have been shown to display drastic resistance to the apoptotic effects of radiation (37). The latter observation suggests that the integrity of the p53 gene, whose product is known to arrest cell proliferation, may be necessary for the normal apoptotic process in the thymus.

Another pathway of thymocyte apoptosis that has been the object of scrutiny is the role of the T-cell receptor (TCR)/CD3 complex. During thymocyte development, rearrangement of TCR genes leads to expression of unique, clonally expressed TCRs. Potentially autoreactive thymocytes bearing TCRs with high avidity for self will undergo TCR-mediated, activation-induced apoptosis (negative selection), whereas thymocytes with TCRs of low avidity survive (positive selection) (38,39). Recent experiments have demonstrated that the activation of the TCR/CD3 complex leads to the preferential elimination of immature ($CD4^+/CD8^+$) thymocytes (40). These and other studies have demonstrated that TCR-mediated signals are involved in apoptosis, and this phenomenon is strongly related to the mechanism of negative selection, although the precise in situ mechanism of apoptosis has not yet been elucidated (41,42).

ANATOMY

The fully mature human thymus is an encapsulated midline structure predominantly located in the anterosuperior mediastinum and composed of two lobules joined in the midline by loose connective tissue and thymic parenchyma. The base of the organ lies on the pericardium and great vessels. The upper poles of each lobe extend into the lower neck and are closely applied to the trachea. The lower poles extend down over the pericardium for a variable distance, generally up to the level of the fourth costal cartilage. The anterior border of the gland is made up by the cervical fascia, strap muscles of the neck, sternum, costal cartilages, and intercostal muscles, and the lateral borders are covered by reflections of the parietal pleura.

The size and weight of the gland may vary considerably depending on the age of the person, although wide variations among individuals in the same age group have been observed (43). The mean weight at birth is about 20 g. The organ exhibits a continuous growth in size until puberty, then it reaches a mean weight of approximately 35 to 50 g; thereafter, it undergoes atrophy, as manifested by a decrease in weight and volume and progressive fatty replacement of the parenchyma.

The blood supply of the organ is derived from the internal mammary, superior and inferior thyroid arteries, and, to a lesser degree, the pericardiophrenic arteries. The arterial branches course along fibrous septa to the region near the corticomedullary junction, where they branch into the cortex and the medulla. The capillaries descend from the outer cortex toward the medulla to form postcapillary venules, and they exit the thymus through the septa as interlobular veins. The venous system drains into the left brachiocephalic, internal thoracic, and inferior thyroid veins. There are no true thymic intraparenchymatous afferent lymphatics. Lymph vessels arise in the interstitium of the lobular septa and merge to form large lymph vessels that course alongside the arteries in the septa. The innervation of the organ is derived from branches of the vagus nerve and the cervical sympathetic nerves.

HISTOLOGY

The basic structural unit of the thymus is the lobule. Each lobule is composed of two morphologically distinctive areas, the cortex and the medulla, both of which are largely composed of varying proportions of epithelial cells and thymic lymphocytes (thymocytes) (Fig. 18.3). In the cortex, the sparse epithelial cells present are overshadowed by the numerous, closely packed small lymphocytes. The medulla, in contrast, contains a larger number of epithelial cells and fewer lymphocytes. The cortex and the medulla combined correspond to the thymic epithelial compartment, which is the site of T-cell maturation within this organ. Another important anatomic compartment of the thymus is the perivascular space. In the mature infant thymus, the perivascular space represents a virtual space containing thymic blood vessels and corresponding to a portion of tissue that is contained within the capsule but outside of the thymic epithelial network (44). The perivascular space becomes more prominent with aging and in pathologic processes such as thymoma, and eventually it is replaced with fat and lymphocytes in the involuted thymus of the adult (45). In addition to the epithelial and perivascular space compartments, there is also a stromal compartment that harbors a variety of other cell types. A thin fibrous capsule is generally present surrounding the entire gland. The interplay of these various cellular elements and compartments contributes to define the various organotypical features of the normal thymus.

One of the problems involved in defining the "normal" thymus is that the histologic appearance of the organ changes over time, depending on its stage of maturation or involution. Thus, the "normal" thymus of the adult will look quite different from the "normal" thymus in a child or adolescent. Studies by Hale (45) have shown that the thymus gland does not actually decrease in size or alter its shape over time with the normal process of involution. While the overall size and shape of the gland are retained throughout adulthood into old age, the various cellular constituents are replaced as the normal process of functional involution takes place. Thus, in the thymus of the adult and old age, the normal thymopoietic elements represented by the epithelial compartment become reduced and progressively disappear, being gradually replaced by mature adipose tissue. Residual epithelial elements, however, always remain and generally undergo a process of atrophy that results in a change in the shape of the cells from large, round cells with vesicular nuclei and abundant cytoplasm to small, oval- to spindle-shaped cells with hyperchromatic nuclei and scant cytoplasm (46). Small, microscopic, thymopoietic remnants of thymic epithelium can also be found, which usually retain the normal architecture and appearance of the mature cortex in childhood. Other involutional changes include the formation of cystic structures, usually resulting from dilatation of residual Hassall corpuscles, and the formation of small, abortive glandular or epithelial rosette-like structures within the lymphopoietic islands.

The most distinctive organotypical features of the mature thymus of childhood and adolescence thus include a fibrous capsule, a lobular architecture with sharp separation between the cortex and the medulla, a dual cell population characterized by an admixture of large, round thymic

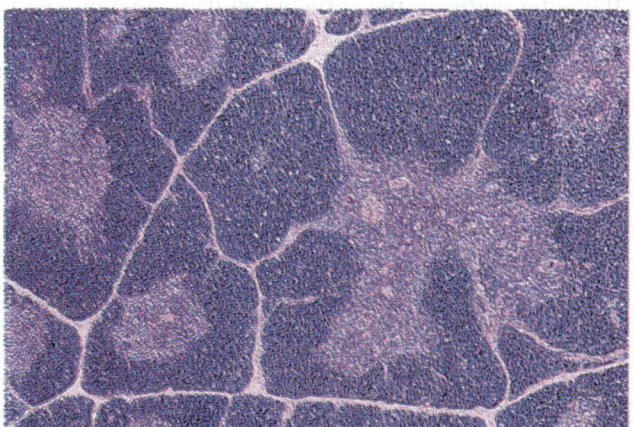

FIGURE 18.3 Normal lobular architecture of the thymus demonstrating clear separation between the cortex and medulla.

epithelial cells with immature T cells, and perivascular spaces. The organotypical features of the "normal" involuted thymus of the adult, on the other hand, include the presence of small, spindle-shaped thymic epithelial cells, abundant cystic structures and rosette-like epithelial structures, and the paucity of immature T cells. These features represent a continuum that will be manifested in various proportions depending on the age, functional status of the organ, various physiologic conditions, and disease states affecting the thymus.

Epithelial Cells

The epithelial cells of the thymus have traditionally been divided into cortical and medullary; some of the latter are arranged in round keratinized structures known as Hassall corpuscles. In the active thymus of infancy, most epithelial cells are plump, with round or oval nuclei. Their cytoplasm (particularly in the case of the cortical cells) is endowed with numerous prolongations that join with those of adjacent cells to form a veritable network or reticulum. This feature (rather than the relationship with reticulin fibers or presumptive embryologic origin) has led to the previous designation of "reticuloepithelial cells." These various epithelial elements play an active role in promoting T-cell maturation in the thymus, either through the action of their humoral substances or through direct contact with thymocytes (47).

A subset of thymic epithelial cells that are predominantly localized to the cortex has been designated as nurse cells. They are characterized by having an abundant cytoplasm within which are engulfed numerous mature T cells. A ring-like staining pattern has been observed in these cells with antibodies against epithelial cells by immunohistochemistry on sections of human thymus (48). It has been postulated that nurse cells may provide a specialized microenvironment for T-cell maturation, differentiation, and selection in the thymus (48,49).

Hassall Corpuscles

Hassall corpuscles constitute the most readily identifiable feature of the thymus at the light microscopic level. They are restricted to the medulla and are characterized by a concentric pattern of keratinization, the keratin formed being of high–molecular-weight (epidermal) type (Fig. 18.4). These structures may show much variation in their morphologic appearance, mainly as a result of reactive changes secondary to inflammation. This includes cystic degeneration with accumulation of cellular debris, dystrophic calcification, and infiltration by lymphocytes, foamy macrophages, and eosinophils (Fig. 18.5). The thymic lesions known as Dubois microabscesses and traditionally ascribed to congenital syphilis (50) represent an exaggeration of the cystic changes in Hassall corpuscles as a result of infection. We believe that most so-called multilocular thymic cysts are

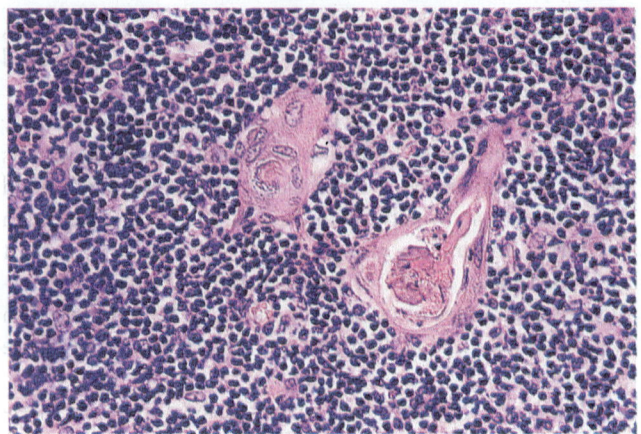

FIGURE 18.4 Normal Hassall corpuscles showing characteristic concentric arrangement of keratinizing epithelial cells.

not congenital abnormalities but rather the result of cystic enlargement of Hassall corpuscles secondary to acquired inflammatory changes in this organ (51). An additional feature that can be seen in relation to cystic Hassall corpuscles is the presence of glandular elements, as manifested by the appearance of columnar epithelium (sometimes ciliated- or of goblet-cell type) and the secretion of sulfated acid mucopolysaccharides in the lumen (52). It is likely that these glandular changes are related to the embryologic origin of Hassall corpuscles (6).

Thymic Lymphocytes (Thymocytes)

The predominant cell population of the thymic cortex is made up of lymphocytes that may be large, medium, or small. Large, mitotically active lymphoblasts comprise about 15% of the lymphoid cells and are found predominantly in the subcapsular portion of the outer cortex (53). These lymphocytes have a round or oval (occasionally convoluted) nucleus, one or two prominent nucleoli, and relatively abundant, strongly basophilic cytoplasm. A gradient of smaller, less mitotically active cells occurs from the outer cortex to the corticomedullary junction and to a lesser degree into the medulla of the normal thymus (Fig. 18.6). In the capsular region and deep cortex, most of the thymic lymphocytes are short lived and die in situ (54). This results in lympholysis and active phagocytosis, features that impart these areas with a prominent "starry sky" appearance and that become particularly prominent in accidental (stress) thymic involution but can also be seen in neoplastic conditions such as thymoma and lymphoblastic lymphoma (see the section on Thymic Involution) (Fig. 18.7).

Other Cell Types

In addition to epithelial cells and lymphocytes of T-cell lineage, the thymus contains an array of additional cell types.

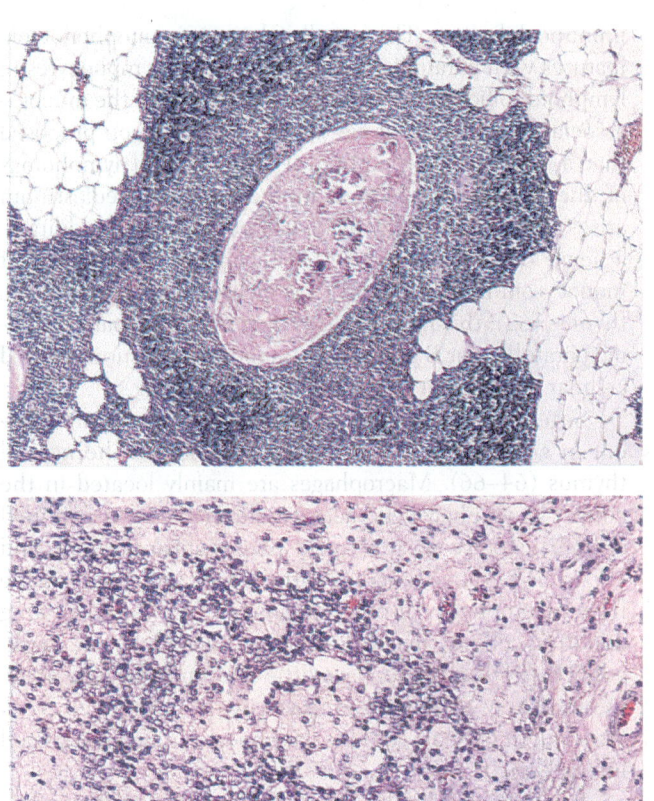

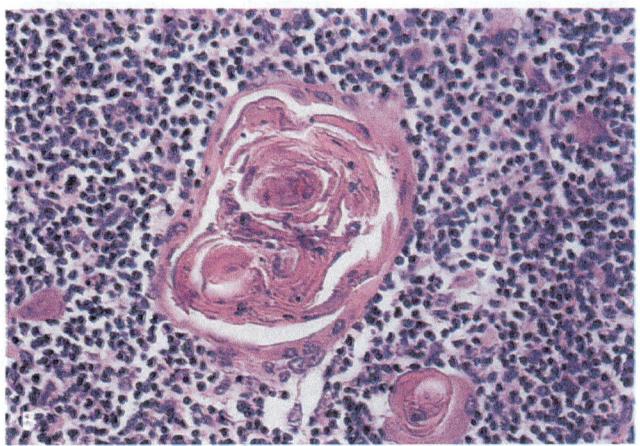

FIGURE 18.5 Hassall corpuscles showing (**A**) cystic dilatation with accumulation of cellular debris, (**B**) dystrophic calcification, and (**C**) accumulation of foamy macrophages.

The first of these, B cells (B lymphocytes), can be found aggregated as lymphoid follicles or scattered as individual cells. Lymphoid follicles with active germinal centers may be found in otherwise normal thymuses, especially in children and adolescents (Fig. 18.8) (54,55). The presence of such B-cell structures would seem difficult to reconcile with the fact that the thymus constitutes a predominantly T-cell organ. However, ultrastructural studies have indicated that germinal centers in the thymus arise within perivascular spaces, the latter being clearly separated from the thymic parenchyma by

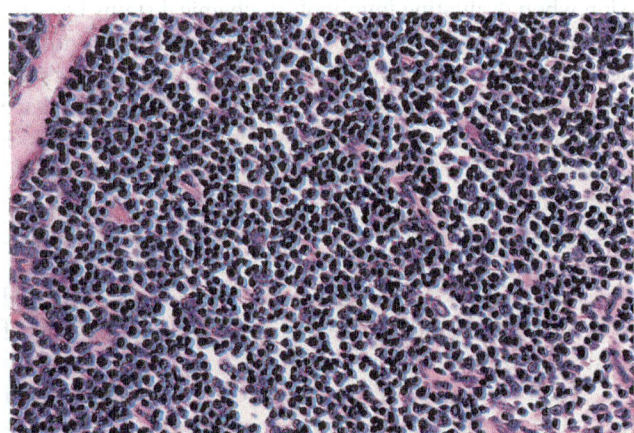

FIGURE 18.6 Normal thymic cortex. There are numerous cortical thymocytes, most of which have small nuclei with densely packed chromatin.

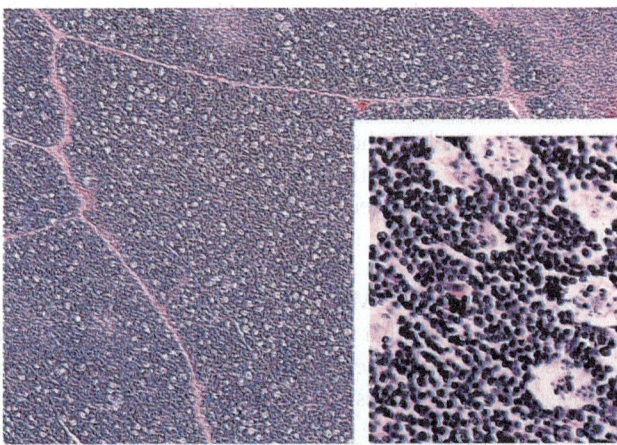

FIGURE 18.7 Prominent starry sky appearance in the deep cortex of a patient with accidental thymic involution. Note the abundance of tingible body macrophages (*inset*).

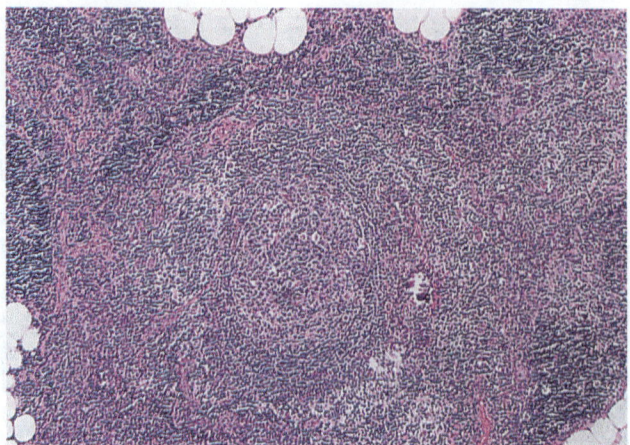

FIGURE 18.8 Lymphoid follicle with germinal center in the normal thymus.

a basal lamina (56). This observation led to the proposal that the thymus may be divided into two major functional compartments: (a) the cortex and the medulla (which constitute the true thymic parenchyma) and (b) the extraparenchymal compartment composed of perivascular spaces (57). Germinal centers in the thymus could thus be explained as being derived from pre-existing perivascular B cells in the extraparenchymal compartment. Germinal centers are well known to be prominent in patients with myasthenia gravis and other immune-mediated diseases (see the section on Thymic Hyperplasia) (9), but their presence in an otherwise normal thymus should not necessarily be taken as an indicator of an underlying immune disorder. The incidence of germinal centers in the thymus of normal individuals without septicemia or disease of a presumed autoimmune cause has varied in published studies from 2.1% (55) to 40% (56). This wide variation may be related to a sampling factor or to the age of the patients; germinal centers would be expected to be less frequent in the older age groups. Also, stress has been shown to be a factor responsible for the decrease in the number of these structures (58). Determination of the incidence and number of germinal centers in normal human thymus glands still remains an unsettled issue.

Isolated B cells are found in both fetal and normal adult thymuses distributed along the septa and in close proximity to small vessels at the corticomedullary junction and in the medulla (59). Intrathymic B cells have been found to be significantly increased in patients with myasthenia gravis, a finding that some investigators consider to be a more specific change for this disorder than the presence of germinal centers (59,60). More recently, a population of intramedullary B cells with a tendency to cluster around Hassall corpuscles has been identified in the thymus gland from fetuses, newborn babies, children, and adults; these lymphocytes show evidence of activation and bear a distinctive immunophenotype (61). Unlike B cells of germinal centers and surrounding mantle zones, the medullary B cells are negative for CD21 and do not express surface/cytoplasmic immunoglobulins. These cells share immunophenotypic features with parafollicular marginal zone B lymphocytes in lymphoid follicles and are believed to be part of the mucosa-associated lymphoid tissue (MALT). It has been proposed that a significant proportion of non-Hodgkin lymphomas of the B-cell type located in the anterior mediastinum arises from this intrathymic B-cell population. In addition, a newly described type of MALT lymphoma composed of monocytoid B cells recently was identified arising from the thymus (62); this finding raises the possibility that extranodal parafollicular B cells may be another as yet unidentified cellular constituent of the normal thymus (63).

Several other types of hematolymphoid cells are present in small number but constant fashion in the normal thymus (64–66). Macrophages are mainly located in the cortex, show phagocytic activity, are markedly α-naphthyl acetate esterase positive, acid phosphatase positive, and HLA-DR negative, and are antigenically indistinguishable from macrophages of other organs (47,66). Interdigitating dendritic cells are mainly located in the medulla, are markedly HLA-DR positive, have little lysosomal enzyme activity, and show S100 protein reactivity (67). Both cell types are thought to be involved in lymphocyte and epithelial cell interaction.

Langerhans cells also have been identified in the thymic medulla; both interdigitating dendritic cells and Langerhans cells are said to be increased in the thymuses of patients with myasthenia gravis (68). The latter cells provide the anatomic substrate for the development of Langerhans cell histiocytosis within the thymus (69). Eosinophils are usually present in the thymus of children, sometimes in large numbers (70). They appear in fetal life and persist until puberty, after which they become infrequent. They are found mainly in the connective tissue septa or within the medulla and occasionally may be present within Hassall corpuscles.

Mast cells are also normally present in human thymuses. They are usually found within and scattered parallel to the connective tissue septa, often in a perivascular location. The presence of mast cells can be a source of confusion when evaluating immunohistochemical stains because of their propensity to react with a wide variety of antibodies; they are easily identified by the use of metachromatic stains. Increased numbers of mast cells in the thymus have been observed in patients with severe combined immunodeficiency and thymic alymphoplasia (71), but the significance of this finding is not understood. Plasma cells are rare in the normal thymus; they are usually located in the connective tissue septa or, more rarely, in the medulla (72). Plasma cells may be numerous in the involuting thymus and may also be present in increased numbers in the thymus of patients with myasthenia gravis (73).

Neuroendocrine cells are now accepted as being a minor but constant component of the normal thymus (74). Peptide- and amine-producing neuroendocrine cells have been identified in the thymus glands of reptiles and birds (75–77) and, to a lesser degree, in mammalian (including human) thymuses. It has been postulated that some of these cells may be embryologically and functionally analogous to C cells of thyroid (78). The physiologic role of these various neuroendocrine elements in the thymus is not yet understood, but their presence has been offered as the probable substrate for the development of neuroendocrine tumors and other neuroendocrine neoplasms in this organ, including calcitonin-positive medullary carcinomas (79,80).

Myoid cells can be found in the thymic medulla. They are common in reptilian and avian thymuses but also can be found (albeit with some difficulty) in human thymuses, particularly in infants. They have microscopic, immunohistochemical, and ultrastructural features of striated muscle cells (81,82). Their histogenesis remains a subject of debate, some studies pointing toward a derivation from the neural crest (83) and others showing the existence of shared epitopes with thymic epithelial cells (84). Myoid cells have been said to be increased in the thymus of patients with myasthenia gravis (59,85) and in patients with true thymic hyperplasia (86), suggesting that these cells may play a role in immunoregulatory mechanisms. Thymic neoplasms thought to harbor the neoplastic counterpart of myoid cells also have been described (87).

Germ cells are another cellular element thought to be normally present in the thymus. It has been proposed that scattered germ cells reach the thymus during ontogenesis and that some of them persist into adult life. However, direct evidence of their presence in the normal thymus gland has never been demonstrated, and the only presumptive evidence of their occurrence is the fact that nearly all mediastinal germ cell tumors arise within the thymus (9). Rosai et al. (88) have recently proposed that germ cells in the thymus may develop into somatic cells, thus making their detection and identification difficult by conventional means. They further hypothesized that thymic myoid cells may be of germ cell origin and thus provide indirect evidence for the existence of the latter in this organ (88).

Connective tissue elements of the thymus include vessels, fibrous tissue, nerves, and fat. The vasculature of the thymus arises from arteries that enter the organ via fibrous trabeculae from the capsule. In contrast to other major lymphoid organs, the thymus lacks a hilus. The thymic vessels are ensheathed by a layer of thymic epithelial cells. This anatomic configuration, plus the failure of the thymus to produce antibodies against circulating antigen led to the concept of the blood–thymus barrier (89). Raviola and Karnovsky (90), in an elaborate study using electron-opaque tracers of different molecular dimensions, demonstrated convincingly that, although some bloodborne macromolecules do penetrate the thymus, their distribution was limited to the medulla, thus pointing to the existence of a blood–thymus barrier operating at the level of the cortex. However, more recent studies have challenged the concept of the blood–thymus barrier by showing that the thymic cortex also may be permeable to immunoglobulin molecules present in the extravascular compartment (91).

The presence of a distinct anatomic compartment bound by the vessel wall and the sheath of epithelial cells has been postulated. It has further been suggested that it is through these perivascular spaces that the mature T cells exit the thymus to colonize peripheral lymphoid organs once their maturation process is complete. The spaces are inconspicuous in the normal thymus; they may appear dilated in atrophic and involuting organs, but they acquire their greatest prominence in some thymomas (9).

ULTRASTRUCTURE

Ultrastructurally, very elongated cytoplasmic processes can be appreciated in the epithelial cells of the thymic cortex, which are also covered by basal lamina material (92–94). Medullary epithelial cells are more densely packed and have blunted cytoplasmic projections. A consistent feature of medullary epithelial cells is the greater frequency of desmosomes and the presence of dense tonofilaments that often insert into desmosomes. This feature is particularly obvious in Hassall corpuscles. Cortical epithelial cells may display a range of ultrastructural appearances depending on the electron density of their cytoplasm, including pale cells with electron-lucent cytoplasm, intermediate cells with variable electron density, and dark cells with electron-dense cytoplasm. The same range may be observed in medullary epithelial cells; in addition, the medulla contains undifferentiated epithelial cells with sparse cytoplasm (95).

Thymic myoid cells display ultrastructural features of skeletal muscle, including myofilaments with dense patches (Fig. 18.9). Some investigators have identified cells displaying both tonofilaments and myofilaments by electron microscopy, and in some instances myoid cells

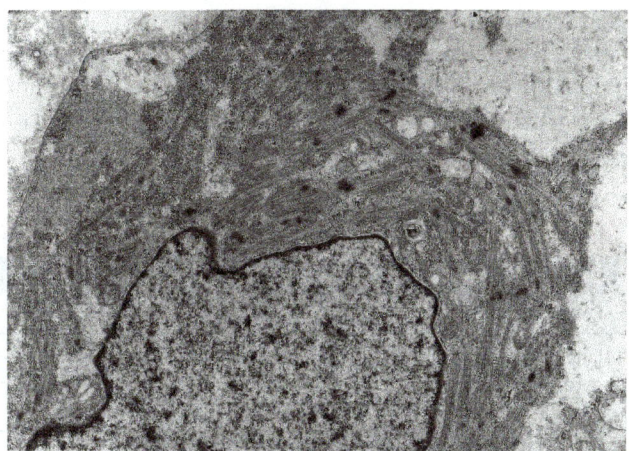

FIGURE 18.9 Ultrastructural appearance of myoid cell in the thymus. Note the bundles of actin and myosin myofilaments with clearly discernible Z lines in the cytoplasm.

have been observed to display desmosomal connections with epithelial cells (73).

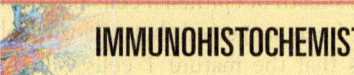

IMMUNOHISTOCHEMISTRY

Thymic Epithelial Cells

Immunohistochemical studies have demonstrated that thymic epithelial cells may express a variety of distinctive differentiation antigens. Currently, at least four antigenically distinctive types of epithelial cells are recognized in the normal thymus: subcapsular cortical, inner cortical, medullary, and the cells of Hassall corpuscles (Table 18.1) (96–99). Inner cortical epithelium, in addition to exhibiting keratin positivity, strongly reacts with TE-3, a murine monoclonal antibody raised against human thymic stroma (100). Subcapsular cortical epithelial cells and medullary epithelial cells react strongly with TE-4 monoclonal antibody. Both cells also label with A2B5, a monoclonal antibody directed against a complex neuronal ganglioside found on the cell surface of neurons and neuroendocrine cells (101).

Another marker of subcapsular cortical epithelium and medullary epithelium in normal thymus is that detected with anti-p19, an antibody that defines the structural core protein of the human T-cell lymphoma virus and that is believed to be acquired during normal thymic ontogeny. In the normal human thymus, the antigen defined by anti-p19 is found to parallel the reactivity of A2B5 antibody in epithelial cells (102). Interestingly, a recent study on thymomas has demonstrated that the expression of the p19 antigen is lost with malignant transformation (103).

Subcapsular cortical, inner cortical, and medullary epithelial cells also have been found to express class I and class II major histocompatibility antigens (98,104). However, recent studies using double immunolabeling have shown that HLA-DR expression is absent in medullary epithelial cells and that the positivity reported in previous studies may have been the result of diffusion of the stain from surrounding interdigitating dendritic cells (68). A recent study has demonstrated that the epithelial cells in the normal thymus and in thymomas also express epithelium-associated glycoprotein H (tissue blood group O antigen),

peanut agglutinin receptor antigen (PNA-r), and Sophora japonica agglutinin receptor antigen (SJA-r), which are detectable by lectin binding (105). Recent studies also have demonstrated expression of the epidermal growth factor receptor and transforming growth factor alpha in subcapsular, cortical, and medullary epithelial cells, suggesting that this substance plays a role in the growth and differentiation of these cells (106). Subcortical epithelial cells lining the boundaries between the thymic parenchyma and its surrounding fibrous tissue also demonstrate positivity for Leu-7, a differentiation antigen found in human null/killer cells and neuroendocrine cells (107). The cells of Hassall corpuscles show the strongest keratin positivity of all thymic epithelial cells and react particularly strongly with the high–molecular-weight keratin AE2 antibody, which is considered a marker of terminal epithelial maturation (108). Conversely, they are unreactive for the other antigens mentioned above.

In a diagnostic setting, there are no reliable or distinctive markers that may help separate thymic epithelial cells from other types of epithelial cells. Thymic epithelial neoplasms, as a group, are usually immunoreactive with pan-cytokeratin antibodies and react with a wide variety of specific cytokeratin subsets. The most common subset of cytokeratins expressed in thymoma are CK8/CK18 low–molecular-weight cytokeratins (CAM5.2), CK19, and CK5/6 (109). Broad-spectrum cytokeratin and cytokeratin cocktails such as AE1/AE3 are also helpful for labeling the epithelial cells in these tumors. Another marker that has been recently shown to strongly label thymic epithelial cells is p63 (110). Virtually 100% of all thymic epithelial cells in all types of thymomas show strong nuclear expression for this marker. In the appropriate context, p63 positivity may serve as an aid for the diagnosis of thymoma; however, this marker is not specific for these tumors and may also be seen in squamous cell carcinomas, urothelial and myoepithelial neoplasms, and other tumors. More specific markers of squamous differentiation such as p40 and desmoglein-3 have been recently shown to be expressed in normal thymic tissue as well as in thymomas and thymic carcinoma (111). Their role for diagnosis, however, is quite limited. Other markers that may also react to a more limited extent with epithelial cells in thymomas include EMA, MUC1, bcl-2, and CD57.

TABLE 18.1 Summary of Main Antigenic Determinants Found in Epithelial Cells of the Normal Thymus

Cells	Keratin	TE-3	TE-4	A2B5	Anti-p19	Antithymosin α1	Antithymopoietin	HLA/Ia
Inner cortical epithelium	+	+	−	−	−	−	−	+
Subcapsular cortical epithelium	+	−	+	+	+	+	+	+
Medullary epithelium	+	−	+	−	+	+	−	−
Hassall corpuscles	++	−	−	−	−	−	−	−

Thymic Lymphocytes

The normal lymphoid population of the thymus has been shown to exhibit marked immunophenotypic heterogeneity, reflective of their functional status. The very term *thymocyte*, which was originally introduced to designate all thymic lymphocytes, has acquired a more specific immunologic meaning and is now restricted to immature thymic lymphocytes of T-cell lineage (with the exclusion of pre–T-cell lymphocytes). Thymocytes can be divided into three types in accordance with their different stages of intrathymic maturation (21,112–114). The earliest stage of differentiation is found in subcapsular thymocytes, which are characterized by a Leu-1$^+$ (T1), Leu-2a$^+$ (T8), Leu-3a$^+$ (T4), Leu-4$^+$ (T3), Leu-5$^+$ (T11), Leu-6$^+$ (T6), Leu-9$^+$ (T2), TdT$^+$, and T200$^+$ phenotype (Fig. 18.10A). The next stage in maturation is seen in cortical thymocytes, which comprise the majority of thymic lymphocytes (60% to 70%) and are characterized by a Leu-1$^+$ (T1), Leu-2a$^+$ (T8), Leu-3a$^+$ (T4), Leu-4$^+$ (T3), Leu-5$^+$ (T1-1), Leu-6$^+$ (T6), Leu-9$^+$ (T2), Leu-M3, OKT10 (T10), TdT$^+$, and T200$^+$ phenotype. The last stage of intrathymic maturation is seen in medullary thymocytes, which show a Leu-1$^+$ (T1), Leu-4$^+$ (T3), Leu-5$^+$ (T11), Leu-9$^+$ (T2), and T200$^+$ phenotype (Fig. 18.10B).

Antigens Leu-2a and Leu-3a are present in only one-third to two-thirds of these cells, respectively (59,112). Of the above markers, the ones that may distinguish specifically between cortical and medullary thymocytes are CD1, CD14, CD38, and TdT. Recent studies on thymomas have attempted to correlate the degree of T-cell maturation with the morphologic appearance of the tumor (107,115–117). It has been well established that the lymphoid cell population in thymomas is made up of immature T cells (116,118,119). In lymphocyte-rich thymomas, the lymphocytes have the phenotypic markers of cortical thymocytes; it has, therefore, been proposed that these tumors are attempting to recapitulate the structure and function of the cortical compartment of the normal thymus (117,120,60). In the better-differentiated examples, the analogy with the normal thymus is accentuated by the presence of foci of medullary differentiation. These findings support the originally proposed theory that, in thymomas, prothymocytes from the stem cell compartment undergo a series of maturational events induced by the neoplastic thymic epithelial cells analogous to those that take place in the normal thymus, the lymphoid elements in these tumors thus being an environmental component rather than a neoplastic component (9). This contention, which was initially based solely on light microscopic observations of thymomas, has recently gained support from studies with DNA hybridization for TCR genes that showed that the lymphoid elements in thymomas lacked gene rearrangements that would denote a clonal proliferation of T cells (121). As already indicated, such an interaction is thought to be mediated by thymic hormones produced by thymic epithelial cells.

The use of lymphoid markers is of very limited value in the setting of histopathologic diagnosis for the identification or subclassification of thymic epithelial neoplasms. In general terms, however, identification of immature T lymphocytes admixed with the neoplastic epithelial cells in the appropriate context may be helpful for supporting the diagnosis of thymoma. The best markers in this setting are CD1a, CD3, and

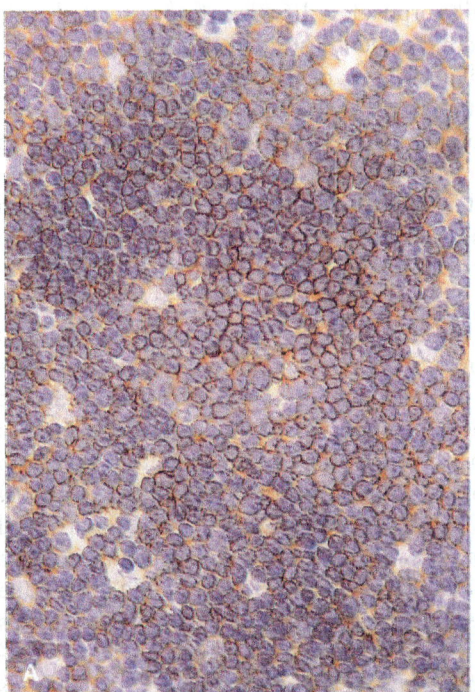
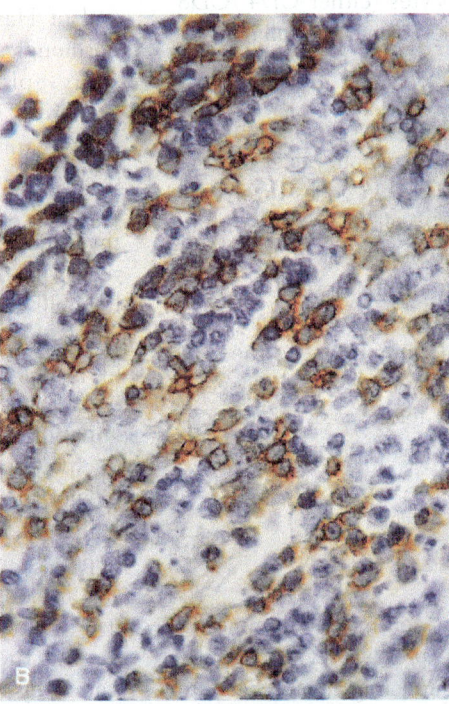

FIGURE 18.10 A: Immunoperoxidase stain of cortical thymocytes on fresh-frozen tissue with CD5 antibody. **B:** Medullary thymocytes showing focal CD4 positivity on fresh-frozen tissue.

nuclear expression of TdT. Another marker that strongly labels immature T lymphoblasts in thymoma is CD99 (122).

MOLECULAR BIOLOGY

Molecular studies have demonstrated the presence of rearrangement and expression of T-cell antigen receptors (TCRs) in thymic lymphocytes. Expression of the TCR represents a critical step in the development of T cells in the thymus (123,124). The TCR molecules are heterodimeric proteins analogous in structure to the immunoglobulin molecules. Rearrangement and expression of the TCRs are needed for the T cell to recognize antigen in association with self-major histocompatibility complex (MHC) antigens. There are two major types of TCRs: one type contains α- and β-polypeptide chains and the other contains γ- and δ-chains. The α-β-TCR is expressed in nearly all T cells, whereas the γ-δ-TCR is expressed in only about 2% of T cells. Immature thymic lymphocytes ($CD4^-/CD8^-$) have been shown to contain mRNA only for the β-chain of the TCR. Mature thymic lymphocytes ($CD4/CD8^+$), on the other hand, contain mRNA for both β- and α-chains (125).

As immature thymocytes begin to undergo TCR gene rearrangements, they first acquire cytoplasmic then cell surface expression of CD3, CD4, and CD8. The $CD4^+/CD8^+$ (i.e., "double-positive") lymphocytes are located within the thymic cortex and also express CD1a surface marker, as well as strong positivity for the Ki-67 nuclear proliferation antigen (45). As double-positive thymocytes complete their TCR gene rearrangement and undergo positive and negative selection, they progressively lose their expression of CD1a, Ki-67, and either CD4 or CD8. The resulting "single-positive" thymocytes (either $CD4^+/CD8^-$ or $CD4^-/CD8^+$) migrate into the thymic medulla, where they complete their maturation before they are released into the circulation.

The genetic mechanisms that promote lineage commitment in the thymus are not well understood. Recent studies have suggested that there are at least 25 genes involved in the segregation of the different T-cell lineages. Commitment to the CD4 lineage appears to be controlled by the upregulation of the genes associated with increased survival followed by expression of genes that regulate nucleosome remodeling and TCR signaling. Commitment to the CD8 lineage appears to be influenced by upregulation of genes that regulate lymphocyte homing followed by suppression of genes that inhibit apoptosis (126).

FUNCTION

The thymus plays a central role in cell-mediated immunity. In early embryonic development, prothymocytes enter the thymus from the bone marrow and migrate to the outer cortex where they undergo a process of maturation. Mature thymocytes move from the outer cortex to the medulla and then migrate into the peripheral circulation, where they function as mature T cells. During their sojourn in the thymus, T cells learn to distinguish self from nonself and acquire the ability to recognize antigens bound to cell surface molecules encoded by the MHC. Circulating helper ($CD4^+$) and suppressor ($CD8^+$) thymus-derived T cells play a variety of roles in cell-mediated immunity, including the induction of cytotoxicity, delayed-type hypersensitivity reactions, and transplant rejection.

A controversial aspect of thymic function is that related to the production of thymic hormones, which are thought to play a role in the induction of differentiation of early T-cell precursors in the thymus. Four distinct types of thymic hormones have been identified: thymopoietin, thymosin, thymulin (formerly known as facteur thymique serique), and thymic humoral factor (125,127,128). Thymopoietin and thymulin are said to be produced only by thymic epithelium, whereas thymosins are a family of peptides that are synthesized in many organs. The production of thymic hormones by thymic epithelial cells has been an extremely interesting but a highly contested subject. At the immunohistochemical level, studies using polyclonal and monoclonal antibodies claim to have demonstrated the presence of thymulin, thymosin α1, and thymopoietin in the cytoplasm of murine and human thymic epithelial cells (128–131). In some studies, hormone localization has been found to be restricted to $A2B5^+$ cells, that is, subcapsular cortical and medullary epithelial cells (132). This finding has led to the suggestion that these two cell subtypes represent the functional (secretory or endocrine) portion of the thymus, as contrasted with the nonsecretory epithelium of the inner cortical region and of Hassall corpuscles. In a murine system, thymic hormones also have been described in a subtype of medullary epithelial cell characterized ultrastructurally by numerous cytoplasmic membrane-bound vacuoles containing amorphous material (133). A study by Hirokawa et al. (134), using rabbit antisera against synthetic thymosin α1 and bovine thymosin β3 in 45 cases of human thymomas and normal thymus of newborns, described reactivity of the tumor cells and normal thymic epithelial cells with these antibodies in 80% and 89% of cases, respectively. The thymosin-containing cells were said to be predominantly localized to the medulla and the subcapsular cortex, and the reaction was most intense in the lymphocyte-rich thymomas. These reactions appeared to be specific for thymic tumors because neither thymosin α1 nor thymosin β3 could be detected in other epithelial malignancies tested, including gastric, pulmonary, and hepatic carcinomas. So far, however, sufficiently reliable specific antibodies have not become available for routine use in diagnostic pathology. In general, thymic hormones have as their main role to induce in situ T-cell differentiation by direct, cell-to-cell, receptor-based interactions as well as by in situ paracrine information in the thymic microenvironment. More recently, the use of thymic hormones as immunostimulants for enhancing the reactivity of humoral immunity in patients with cancer has been employed. Thymosin fraction 5, thymic humoral factor γ2, thymosin α1, and thymopentin have been utilized in several clinical immunotherapeutic protocols as an adjunct to treatment of various cancers (135).

In addition to thymic hormones, thymic epithelial cells may contain a wide variety of neuropeptides such as oxytocin, vasopressin, β-endorphin, somatostatin, and other anterior pituitary hormones (136–138), as well as produce various cytokines and growth factors, including interleukin (IL)-1, IL-6, and granulocyte–monocyte colony-stimulating factor (139,140).

The spectrum of biologic effects of cytokines in the thymus is determined by the expression of cytokine receptors on the thymic cell surface. Thymic cytokines may act by autocrine or paracrine mechanisms. Examples of paracrine thymic cytokines are IL-7, which induces thymocyte growth and differentiation, and interferon (IFN)-γ (produced by thymocytes), which induces thymic epithelial cell activation. An example of an autocrine factor is IL-2, for which the producers and targets are thymocytes. The ability of thymocytes to produce cytokines and express cytokine receptors is gradually reduced as they mature from the stage of precursor cells to cortical thymocytes. After the completion of the selection process of maturation, the ability of thymocytes to produce cytokines and respond to their action is restored (141). The role and function of cytokines in the thymus are different from that of cytokines in the peripheral compartments of the immune system; in the thymus they are involved with the migration and the development of thymocytes and autoregulation of thymocytes cell numbers, while in the periphery they are mainly involved in the regulation of inducible processes such as inflammation, immune response, etc.

AGE-RELATED AND OTHER TROPHIC CHANGES

Thymic Involution

The thymus undergoes a slow physiologic process of involution with age. This process starts at puberty, at which time the organ reaches its maximum absolute weight. From then on, it undergoes gradual and progressive atrophic changes (142–144). This process of aging, also known as physiologic involution, is accompanied by gradual changes in thymocyte populations relative to different rates of involution of the cortical and the medullary epithelium. In its early stages, the changes consist primarily of a decrease in the number of cortical thymocytes with relative sparing of the epithelial elements (145). In the more advanced stages, the parenchyma of the thymus reverts to a more primitive appearance and is replaced by islands of epithelial cells depleted of lymphocytes, with partly cystic, closely aggregated Hassall corpuscles and abundant intervening adipose tissue (146). It should be realized that, while thymic involution can proceed to a point where no thymic tissue can be appreciated grossly, microscopic thymic remnants are probably always present. The best way to locate them is to examine microscopically the pre-epicardial fat in a serial fashion. Recent studies have suggested that the process of involution in the thymus may be quantitative rather than qualitative. It has been demonstrated that thymopoiesis continues to occur in the thymus of adult humans late into life and that thymic activity and function appear to be well maintained into old age and may be indispensable for T-cell reconstitution in different immunologic settings (147–149).

A type of change not related to senescence that must be distinguished from the normal physiologic type of involution is accidental or stress involution. This condition results from the dramatic response of the thymus gland to episodes of severe stress, in which the sudden release of corticosteroids from the adrenal cortex leads to rapid depletion of thymic cortical lymphocytes (150). Microscopically, there is prominent karyorrhexis of lymphocytes with active phagocytosis by macrophages, which creates a prominent starry sky appearance characteristically confined to the cortex. If the stimulus persists, a loss of corticomedullary distinction ensues, with accentuation of the epithelial elements, cystic dilatation of Hassall corpuscles, and the emergence of elongated, epithelium-lined cystic spaces that recapitulate the early stages of Hassall corpuscle formation. With further loss of thymocytes, the lobular architecture collapses and fibrosis ensues. The thymus is thus transformed into a mass of adipose tissue containing scattered islands of parenchyma with a few lymphocytes.

Acute thymic involution in infancy and childhood has been observed to significantly correlate with the duration of acute illness. It has been proposed that morphologic parameters such as the presence of abundant macrophages in the cortex, increase of interlobular fibrous tissue, and lymphoid depletion of the cortex may enable the pathologist to estimate the duration of acute disease before death (151). A precocious type of thymic involution manifested by epithelial injury also has been observed in both children and adult patients with acquired immunodeficiency syndrome (AIDS) (152,153). These changes have been interpreted by some as an indication that the thymus may constitute a primary target organ in human immunodeficiency virus infection (154), whereas others have considered these changes as an expression of stress involution (153,155).

Thymic Hyperplasia

True thymic hyperplasia is defined as an enlargement of the thymus gland (as determined by weight or volume) beyond that considered as the upper limit of normal for any given age group (156). The existence of true thymic hyperplasia has been questioned in the past, largely

TABLE 18.2 Weight and Volume of Normal Human Thymuses

N	Age (Years)	Weight (g)[a]	Volume (cm³)[a]
6	0–1	27.3 ± 16.4	26.8 ± 16.1
4	1–4	28.0 ± 19.3	27.9 ± 10.4
7	5–9	22.1 ± 9.2	21.5 ± 8.8
5	10–14	21.5 ± 6.1	21.1 ± 6.4
9	15–19	20.2 ± 10.3	19.3 ± 10.1
18	20–24	21.6 ± 9.5	23.0 ± 10.6
9	25–29	23.1 ± 11.8	23.7 ± 11.9
5	30–34	25.5 ± 9.9	27.6 ± 11.2
17	35–44	21.9 ± 9.2	22.2 ± 10.5
14	45–54	24.8 ± 12.8	26.5 ± 12.4
15	55–64	21.3 ± 9.5	23.5 ± 10.4
17	65–84	23.8 ± 16.1	25.6 ± 17.0
5	85–90	18.2 ± 5.4	20.4 ± 6.8
5	91–107	12.4 ± 6.9	13.4 ± 7.2
136	Total	22.8 ± 12.5	23.4 ± 11.9

[a]Values are means ± SD.
Reprinted from Le PT, Lazorick S, Whichard LP, et al. Human thymic epithelial cells produce IL-6, granulocyte-monocyte-CSF, and leukemia inhibitory factor. *J Immunol* 1990;145:3310–3315.

because of the diagnostic excesses committed with the much abused concept of status thymicolymphaticus. The latter is probably a myth, but true thymic hyperplasia is currently accepted as a distinct entity (157–159).

In the past, to establish a diagnosis of true thymic hyperplasia, reference was made to standard weight charts of normal thymus glands for comparison. Hammar, in 1906 (160), made the first extensive study on the normal weights of the thymus in fresh autopsy specimens. More recently, several workers have updated these studies; the most comprehensive of these is that of Steinman (144), who examined the weight and volume of human thymuses in 136 healthy individuals (Table 18.2). He concluded that determination of the volume of the gland, as measured by the displacement of a physiologic saline solution, was more reliable than weighing the gland and constitutes the optimal parameter for this type of evaluation. In practice, determination of the volume of the gland may not be easy to accomplish in the setting of standard processing of specimens in surgical pathology laboratories. A diagnosis of "consistent with thymic hyperplasia" is therefore acceptable in the setting of a histologically normal thymus when the clinical imaging studies indicate the presence of a mediastinal "mass" or otherwise obvious enlargement of the thymus gland.

Thymic hyperplasia has been recognized as a complication of chemotherapy for Hodgkin disease in children (161,162) and germ cell tumors in adults (163,164) and has been interpreted as the expression of an immunologic rebound phenomenon. A similar enlargement of the thymus also has been observed in children recovering from thermal burns (165) and after cessation of administration of corticosteroids in infants (166). Marked enlargement of the thymus has also been observed in the setting of thymic reconstitution after chemotherapy (167) or after the institution of antiretroviral therapy in HIV-infected patients (168).

True thymic hyperplasia must be distinguished from lymphoid hyperplasia. In the latter condition, the term *hyperplasia* refers to an increased number of lymphoid follicles in the medullary region of the gland. This is the result of increased migration of mature T-cells and B-cells into the perivascular space, adjacent to but outside of the thymic epithelial meshwork. The problem in establishing the presence of lymphoid hyperplasia vis-à-vis the occurrence of lymphoid follicles in the normal thymus has already been discussed. Lymphoid hyperplasia of the thymus most commonly has been associated with myasthenia gravis but also has been observed in several other immune-mediated disorders, including systemic lupus erythematosus, rheumatoid arthritis, scleroderma, allergic vasculitis, and thyrotoxicosis.

ARTIFACTS AND OTHER POTENTIAL PITFALLS IN DIFFERENTIAL DIAGNOSIS

Microscopic changes related to involution may be a source of considerable confusion in the interpretation of thymic biopsies. Such changes are primarily related to the distribution, architectural arrangement, and cytologic appearance of the epithelial cells (Fig. 18.11). Some of these cells may acquire a spindle, atrophic appearance, whereas others can arrange themselves in rosette-like formations devoid of central lumina (Fig. 18.12). The fact that these appearances also are found with some frequency in thymic dysplasia and thymoma (but not in the normal active gland of infancy) suggests that they represent regressive and functionally inactive states of the epithelial cells (9). Another distinctive appearance of involuting thymic epithelial cells is as thin, elongated, and sometimes serpiginous strands of oval to spindle thymic epithelial cells admixed with occasional small lymphocytes that course through the mediastinal fat (Fig. 18.13A). The epithelial cells can be nicely highlighted by p63 immunostaining (Fig. 18.13B). These strands of epithelial cells can sometimes be traced back to solid nests of involuting thymic remnants. Microscopic clusters containing oval to spindle epithelial cells with dense chromatin and scant eosinophilic cytoplasm admixed with a few small lymphocytes can also be seen, and may give rise to the diagnosis of metastatic malignancy (Fig. 18.13C,D). Similar clusters can be observed in association with cystic

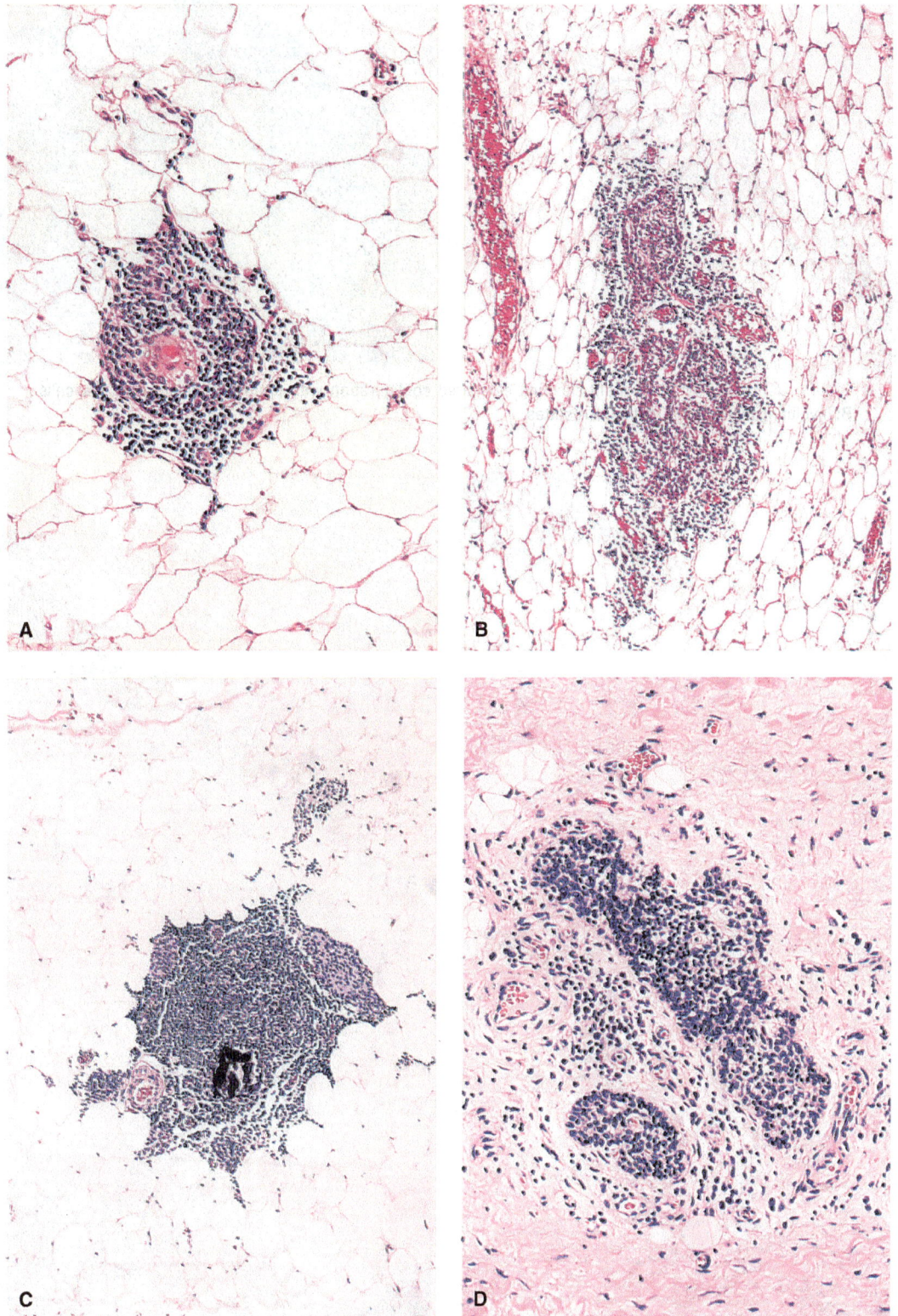

FIGURE 18.11 Epithelial remnants in involuting thymus. **A:** Abortive Hassall corpuscle surrounded by small lymphocytes and scattered epithelial cells. **B:** Anastomosing strands of epithelial cells surrounded by small lymphocytes embedded within the pre-epicardial fat. **C:** Residual thymic island with predominance of lymphocytes, small solid epithelial cell clusters at the periphery, and calcified Hassall corpuscle. **D:** Anastomosing strands of epithelial cells admixed with small lymphocytes embedded within a collagenized stroma.

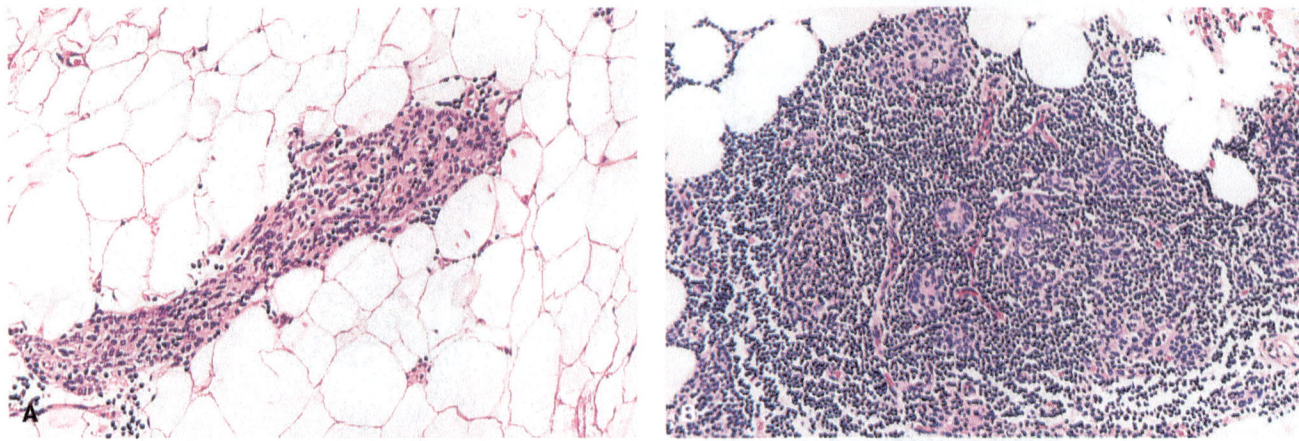

FIGURE 18.12 A: Thymic remnant showing elongated configuration with prominent spindling of the cells. **B:** Involuting thymus with epithelial rosettes.

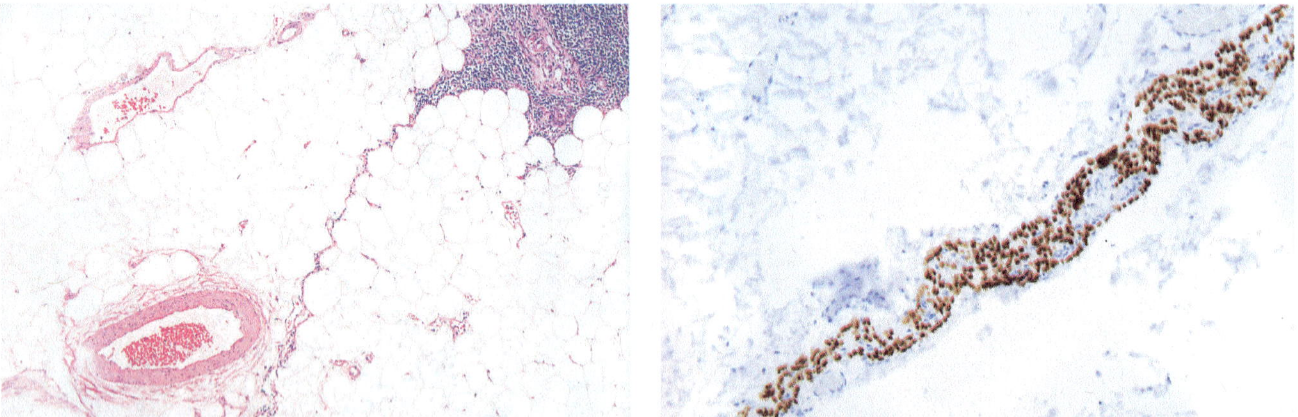

FIGURE 18.13 A: A slender, thin, serpiginous strand of atrophic thymic epithelium admixed with scant lymphocytes is seen coursing through the fat and originating from a small island of involuting thymus (*top right*). **B:** Immunohistochemical stain for p63 at higher magnification shows strong nuclear positivity in the thymic epithelial cells. **C:** Microscopic island of involuting thymic epithelium is present in the fat which is composed of oval to spindle epithelial cells with eosinophilic cytoplasm and a sprinkling of small lymphocytes. **D:** Another microscopic island of involuting thymic epithelium is shown composed of atrophic and tightly packed spindle cells admixed with scattered small lymphocytes.

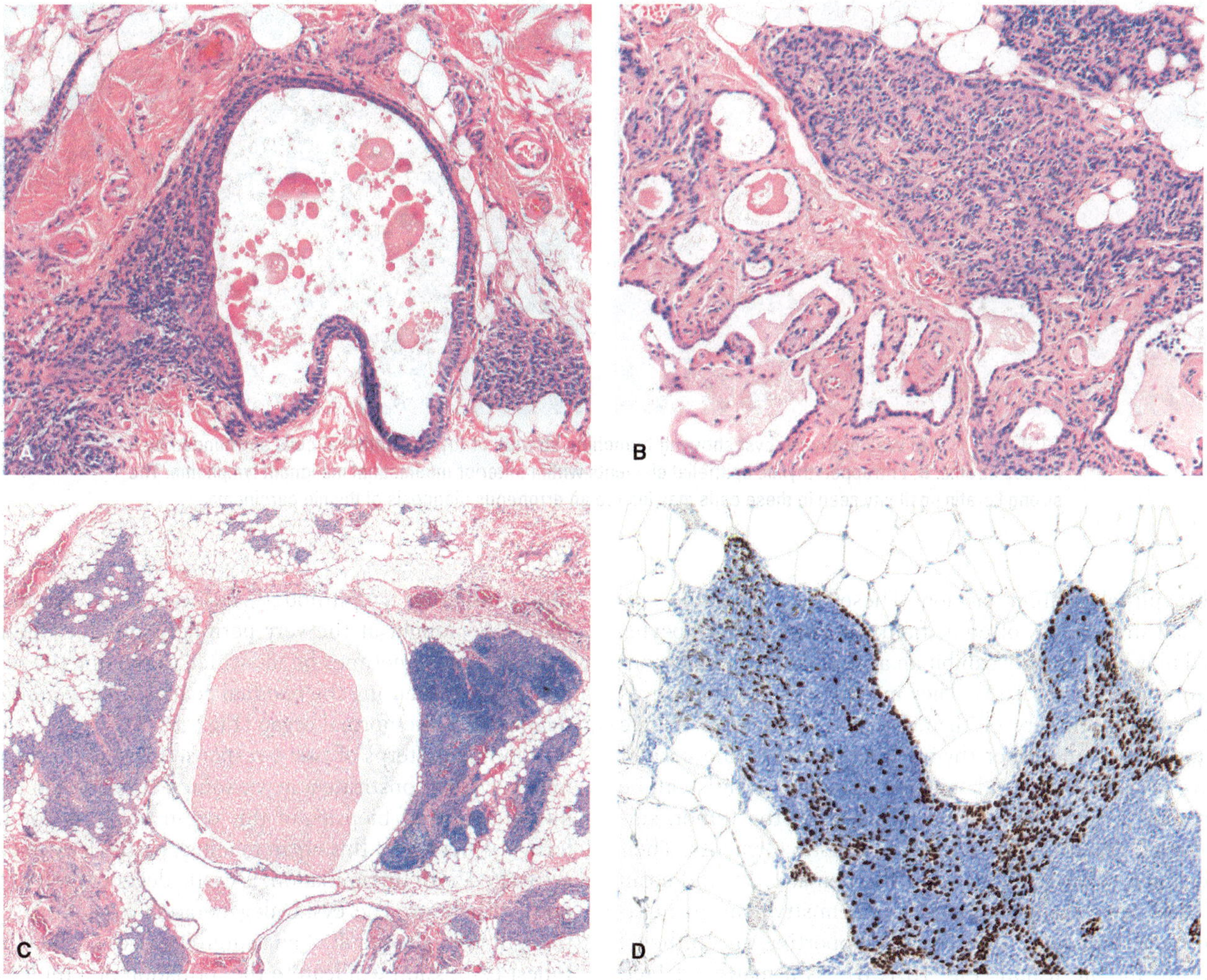

FIGURE 18.14 **A:** Focus of involuting thymic epithelium showing cystic dilatation. The cells lining the cyst range from flat- to cuboidal- to columnar-ciliated epithelium. **B:** Another focus of involuting thymic epithelium shows cystically dilated spaces lined by a layer of cuboidal epithelial cells simulating glandular structures. **C:** Large, cystically dilated spaces are seen flanked by islands of involuting thymic epithelium. The island on the left shows the typical appearance of involuted thymus in adults; the island on the right simulates a lymph node. **D:** Immunostaining for p63 in the solid nodule resembling a lymph node highlights numerous scattered involuting thymic epithelial cells with strong nuclear positivity.

and glandular structures (Fig. 18.14A,B). Some of the cystic spaces may be seen adjacent to dense lymphoid collections that resemble lymph nodes; immunostaining for p63 will highlight the thymic epithelial cells scattered throughout these structures, identifying them as involuting thymic elements (Fig. 18.14C,D). Tissues showing the above features are a frequent finding in the fat submitted for central lymph node dissection in patients undergoing surgery for thyroid carcinoma.

Sometimes thymic remnants are almost exclusively formed of epithelial elements, arranged in well-defined round nests that may simulate neuroendocrine growths (Fig. 18.15) (169). A particularly distinctive appearance is that of thin, elongated strands of thymic epithelium composed of a single or double cell layer, surrounded by or circumscribing dense connective tissue in a

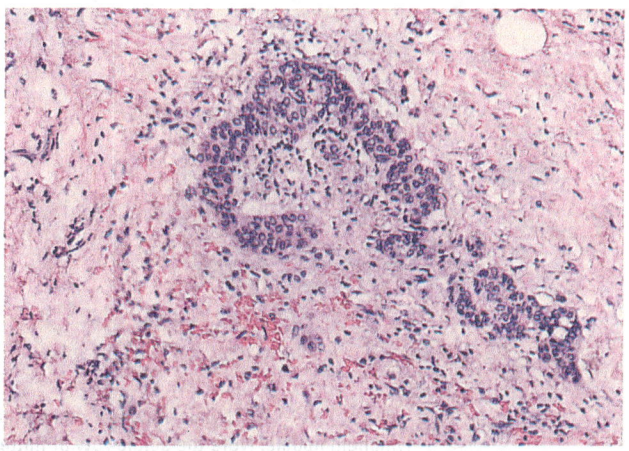

FIGURE 18.15 Strands of residual thymic epithelium arranged in small nests resembling neuroendocrine growths.

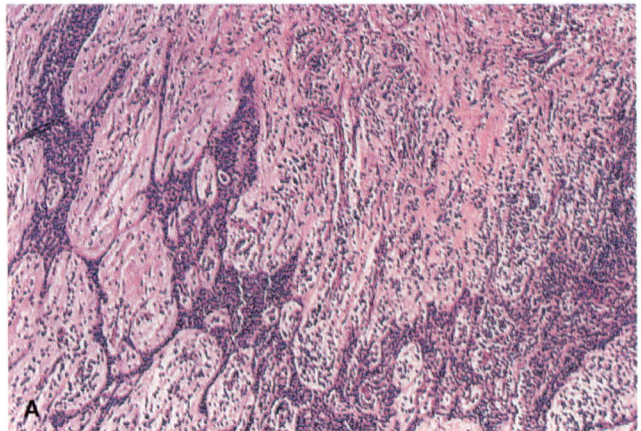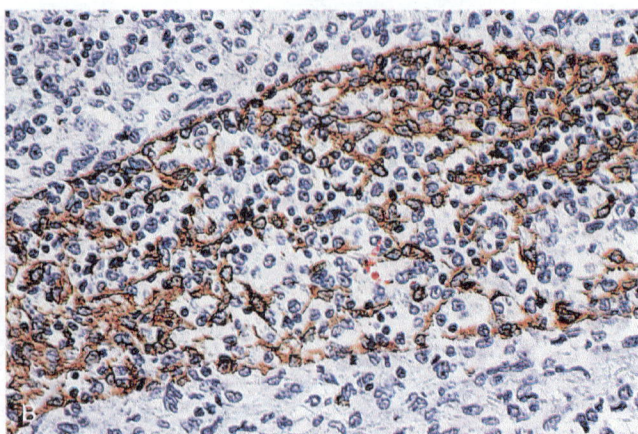

FIGURE 18.16 **A:** Wall of thymic cyst showing branching strands of thymic epithelial cells surrounded by a fibrous stroma. **B:** Entrapped thymic epithelial elements within anterior mediastinal malignant lymphoma. The strong keratin positivity seen in these cells may lead to an erroneous diagnosis of thymic carcinoma.

fibroepitheliomatous fashion. These thin, elongated epithelial strands may often be flanked by small lymphocytes and may occasionally exhibit an antler-like branching configuration (Fig. 18.16A). They may be seen by themselves or at the periphery of thymic cysts, thymomas, thymic lymphomas, and other thymic neoplasms. In the case of thymic lymphomas and seminomas, these strands can be present not only around but also within the tumor, surrounded and infiltrated by the neoplastic elements. Their presence, whether detected at the hematoxylin and eosin (H&E) level or by immunohistochemistry, can be interpreted erroneously as evidence supporting an epithelial nature for the lesion (Fig. 18.16B). As a matter of fact, these structures constitute the single most important cause of misdiagnosis in cases of large cell lymphoma of the thymus. Conversely, some thymic remnants (perhaps the majority) are made up almost exclusively of lymphocytes, thus simulating lymph nodes. A clue to their real nature should be sought at the very periphery, in which epithelial cells can sometimes be identified encircling the nests, perhaps representing the residual coat of subcapsular cortical cells of the normal organ (Fig. 18.17).

Certain patterns of tissue response to injury in the thymus may also constitute a major source of confusion in the interpretation of biopsies of this organ (170). A common form of response of this organ to injury, particularly in cases associated with inflammation, is cystic degeneration of thymic epithelium. The cystic degeneration in such cases is thought to be the result of an acquired process, which in its fullest expression will lead to the formation of a multilocular thymic cyst (51). The main histologic features of such cysts include the creation of large cavities lined by squamous, columnar, or cuboidal epithelium, often in continuity with remnants of normal thymic epithelium within the

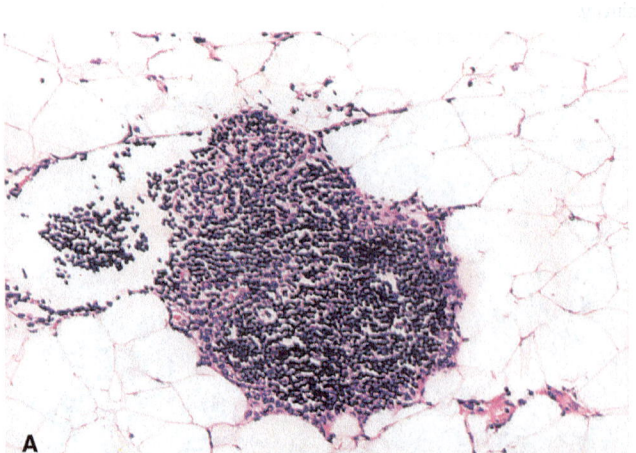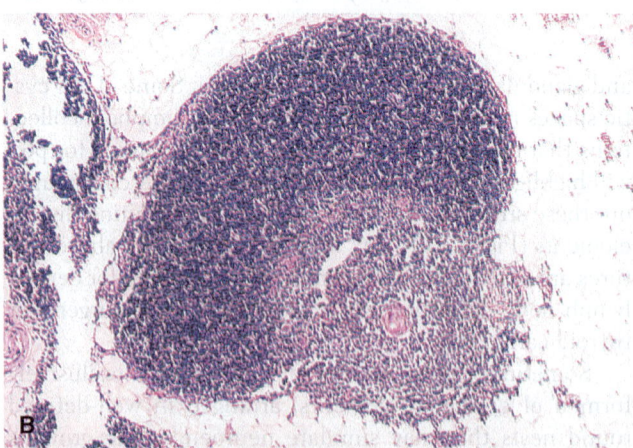

FIGURE 18.17 **A:** Thymic remnant composed predominantly of small lymphocytes simulating a lymphoid nodule. Note the single row of flattened epithelial cells at the periphery. **B:** Thymic remnant composed of cortical and medullary portion, the latter containing a small Hassall corpuscle (*bottom half*).

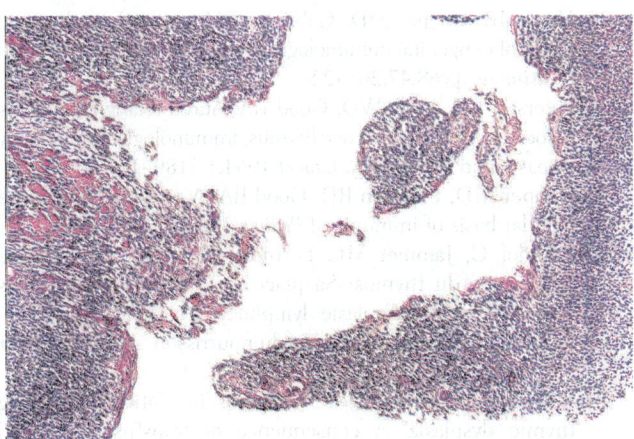

FIGURE 18.18 Cystic dilatation of Hassall corpuscles is seen in an acquired multilocular thymic cyst. Note the cyst lining is in continuity with Hassall corpuscles, and the walls of the cysts contain abundant inflammatory infiltrate.

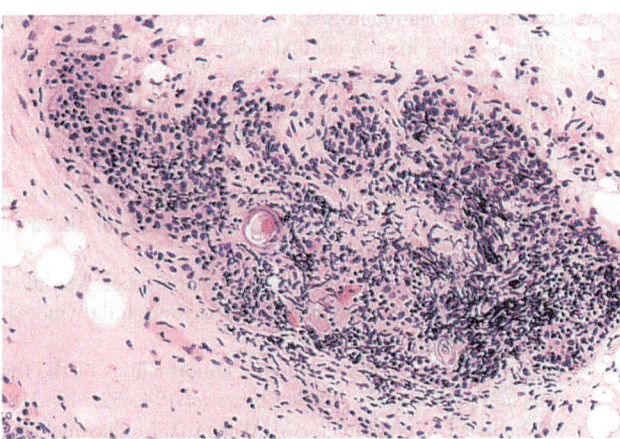

FIGURE 18.19 Extensive crush artifact is seen in this thymic remnant obtained through mediastinoscopic biopsy.

cyst walls; severe acute and chronic inflammation accompanied by fibrovascular proliferation, necrosis, hemorrhage, and cholesterol granulomas; and reactive lymphoid hyperplasia with prominent germinal centers. In some instances, the cyst lining may show a moderate degree of cytologic atypia with features of pseudoepitheliomatous hyperplasia that can be easily misinterpreted for malignancy (171). In most of the cases, the cystic structures are closely associated with Hassall corpuscles, many of which show marked dilatation and may be found to be in continuity with the lining of the cystic cavities (Fig. 18.18). We believe that this type of reaction is the result of an exaggerated response of medullary duct epithelium-derived structures of the thymus to an underlying inflammatory process (51). However, it is important to point out that seemingly identical changes may take place in uninvolved thymic parenchyma in cases of Hodgkin disease, mediastinal seminoma, and (less commonly) thymoma, to the extent that the neoplastic elements may be overshadowed by the cystic/inflammatory process (172,173). Other primary thymic neoplasms, which also may be closely associated with prominent cystic changes, although to a lesser extent, include basaloid carcinoma and mucoepidermoid carcinoma (174,175). Careful search and extensive sampling must therefore be undertaken in cystic mediastinal lesions for proper identification of the diagnostic neoplastic areas.

Another form of tissue response to injury of the thymus that may introduce difficulties for diagnosis is that of stromal fibrosis. Fibrous overgrowth of the stroma may be the result of various mechanisms in a variety of nonneoplastic conditions (including a specific stimulus such as ionizing radiation or fungal infection [176,177]) or of undetermined etiology (such as in idiopathic sclerosing mediastinitis [178,179]). In addition, a variety of malignant conditions of this organ also may be accompanied by prominent fibrous changes of the stroma, including primary diffuse large cell lymphoma of the mediastinum, Hodgkin disease, and thymic seminoma (170). In many such instances, the gland may show extensive sclerosis with entrapment of a few scattered foci harboring the diagnostic atypical cells. Such cases may prove literally impossible to diagnose in small mediastinoscopic biopsies and will require extensive sampling of the mass to identify the diagnostic areas. The surgeon must be informed of the need for obtaining additional tissue for diagnosis at the time of frozen section examination.

Another potential pitfall for diagnosis is given by the high cellularity, immaturity, and mitotic activity of the normal thymic cortex, which can pose great diagnostic difficulties in mediastinoscopic biopsies and result in a mistaken diagnosis of malignant lymphoma, particularly of the lymphoblastic type. The paucity or absence of cells with convoluted nuclei and the identification (morphologically or immunohistochemically) of epithelial cells regularly scattered throughout the lymphoid population should point toward the correct interpretation. Finally, an additional source of difficulty for diagnosis lies in the presence of biopsy-induced artifacts, one of the most common being the crush artifact, leading to marked nuclear elongation reminiscent of that seen in small cell carcinoma (Fig. 18.19).

REFERENCES

1. Norris EH. The morphogenesis and histogenesis of the thymus gland in man: In which the origin of the Hassall's corpuscles of the human thymus is discovered. *Contrib Embryol Carnegie Inst* 1938;27:193–207.
2. Weller GL Jr. Development of the thyroid, parathyroid and thymus glands in man. *Contrib Embryol Carnegie Inst* 1933;24:93–139.

3. Cordier AC, Haumont SM. Development of thymus, parathyroids and ultimo-branchial bodies in NMRI and nude mice. *Am J Anat* 1980;157:227–263.
4. Gilmour JR. The embryology of parathyroid glands: the thymus and certain associated rudiments. *J Pathol Bacteriol* 1937;45:507–522.
5. Jotereau FV, Houssaint E, Le Douarin NM. Lymphoid stem cell homing to the early thymic primordium of the avian embryo. *Eur J Immunol* 1980;10:620–627.
6. Shier KJ. The thymus according to Schambacher: Medullary ducts and reticular epithelium of the thymus and thymomas. *Cancer* 1981;48:1183–1199.
7. Gilmour JR. Some developmental abnormalities of the thymus and parathyroids. *J Pathol Bacteriol* 1941;52:213–218.
8. Nathaniels EK, Nathaniels AM, Wang CA. Mediastinal parathyroid tumors: A clinical and pathological study of 84 cases. *Ann Surg* 1970;171:165–170.
9. Rosai J, Levine GD. Tumors of the thymus. In: *Atlas of Tumor Pathology. 2nd series, fascicle 13*. Washington, DC: Armed Forces Institute of Pathology; 1976.
10. Domaniewski J, Ukleja Z, Rejmanowski T. Problemy immunologiczne i kliniczne w grasiczakach ektopicznych. *Otolaringol Pol* 1975;29:579–585.
11. Martin JM, Rundhawa G, Temple WJ. Cervical thymoma. *Arch Pathol Lab Med* 1986;110:345–357.
12. Yamashita H, Murakami N, Noguchi S, et al. Cervical thymoma and incidence of cervical thymus. *Acta Pathol Jpn* 1983;33:189–194.
13. Wadon A. Thymoma intratracheale. *Zentralbl Allg Pathol Anat* 1934;60:308–312.
14. Harach HR, Saravia Day E, Fransilla KO. Thyroid spindle-cell tumor with mucous cysts. An intrathyroid thymoma? *Am J Surg Pathol* 1985;9:525–530.
15. Miyauchi A, Kuma K, Matsuzuka F, et al. Intrathyroidal epithelial thymoma: An entity distinct from squamous cell carcinoma of the thyroid. *World J Surg* 1985;9:128–135.
16. Rosai J, Limas C, Husband EM. Ectopic hamartomatous thymoma: A distinctive benign lesion of the lower neck. *Am J Surg Pathol* 1984;8:501–513.
17. Gagens EW. Malformation of the auditory apparatus in the newborn associated with ectopic thymus. *Arch Otolaryngol* 1932;15:671–680.
18. Castleman B. Tumors of the thymus gland. In: *Atlas of Tumor Pathology. 1st series, fascicle 19*. Washington, DC: Armed Forces Institute of Pathology; 1955.
19. Marchevski AM. Lung tumors derived from ectopic tissues. *Semin Diagn Pathol* 1995;12:172–184.
20. Weissferdt A, Moran CA. The spectrum of ectopic thymomas. *Virchows Archiv* 2016;469:245–254.
21. Wolff M, Rosai J, Wright DH. Sebaceous glands within the thymus: Report of three cases. *Hum Pathol* 1984;15:341–343.
22. Breckler IA, Johnston DG. Choristoma of the thymus. *AMA J Dis Child* 1956;92:175–178.
23. Landing B, Yutuc I, Swanson V. Clinicopathologic correlation in immunologic deficiency diseases of children, with emphasis on thymic histologic patterns. In: *Proceedings of the International Symposium on Immunodeficiency*. Tokyo: Tokyo University Press; 1976:3–33.
24. Blackburn WR, Gordon DS. The thymic remnant in thymic alymphoplasia. Light and electron microscopic studies. *Arch Pathol* 1967;84:363–375.
25. Hoyer JR, Cooper MD, Gabrielsen AE, et al. Lymphopenic forms of congenital immunologic deficiency diseases. *Medicine (Baltimore)* 1968;47:201–226.
26. Peterson RD, Kelly WD, Good RA. Ataxia-telangiectasia. Its association with a defective thymus, immunological-deficiency disease, and malignancy. *Lancet* 1964;1:1189–1193.
27. Cooper MD, Petersen RD, Good RA. A new concept of the cellular basis of immunity. *J Pediatr* 1965;67:907–908.
28. Nezelof C, Jammet ML, Lortholary P, et al. L'hypoplasie hereditaire du thymus: Sa place et sa responsabilite dans une observation d'aplasie lymphocytaire, normoplasmocytaire et normoglobulinemique du nourrisson. *Arch Fr Pediatr* 1964;21:897–920.
29. Seemayer TA, Bolande RP. Thymus involution mimicking thymic dysplasia: A consequence of transfusion-induced graft versus host disease in a premature infant. *Arch Pathol Lab Med* 1980;104:141–144.
30. Huber J, Cholnoky P, Zoethout HE. Congenital aplasia of parathyroid glands and thymus. *Arch Dis Child* 1967;42:190–192.
31. Fowlkes BJ, Pardoll DM. Molecular and cellular events of T cell development. *Adv Immunol* 1989;44:207–264.
32. MacDonald HR, Lees RK. Programmed death of autoreactive thymocytes. *Nature* 1990;343:642–644.
33. Kizaki H, Tadakuma T. Thymocyte apoptosis. *Microbiol Immunol* 1993;37:917–925.
34. Colbert RA, Young DA. Glucocorticoid-induced messenger ribonucleic acids in rat thymic lymphocytes: Rapid primary effects specific for glucocorticoids. *Endocrinology (Baltimore)* 1986;119:2598–2605.
35. Domashenko AD, Nazarova LF, Umansky SR. Comparison of the spectra of proteins synthesized in mouse thymocytes after irradiation or hydrocortisone treatment. *Int J Radiat Biol* 1990;57:315–329.
36. Korsmeyer SJ. Bcl-2: A repressor of lymphocyte death. *Immunol Today* 1992;13:285–288.
37. Lowe SW, Schmitt EM, Smith SW, et al. p53 is required for radiation-induced apoptosis in mouse thymocytes. *Nature* 1993;362:847–849.
38. Smith CA, Williams GT, Kinsgton R, et al. Antibodies to CD3/T-cell receptor complex induce death by apoptosis in immature T cells in thymic cultures. *Nature* 1989;337:181–184.
39. von Boehmer H. Positive selection of lymphocytes. *Cell* 1994;76:219–228.
40. Shi YF, Bissonnette RP, Parfrey N, et al. In vivo administration of monoclonal antibodies to the CD3 T cell receptor complex induces cell death (apoptosis) in immature thymocytes. *J Immunol* 1991;146:3340–3346.
41. Blackman M, Kappler J, Marrack P. The role of the T cell receptor in positive and negative selection of developing T cells. *Science* 1990;248:1335–1341.
42. Mountz JD, Zhou T, Wu J, et al. Regulation of apoptosis in immune cells. *J Clin Immunol* 1995;15:1–16.
43. Hammar JA. Die Menschen thymus in Gesundheit und krankheit. *Z Mikrosk Anat Forsch* 1926;6(suppl):107–208.
44. Flores KG, Li J, Sempowski GD, et al. Analysis of the human thymic perivascular space during aging. *J Clin Invest* 1999;104:1031–1039.
45. Hale LP. Histologic and molecular assessment of human thymus. *Ann Diagn Pathol* 2004;8:50–60.

46. Suster S, Moran CA. Thymoma, atypical thymoma, and thymic carcinoma. A novel conceptual approach to the classification of thymic epithelial neoplasms. *Am J Clin Pathol* 1999; 111:826–833.
47. Lobach DF, Haynes BF. Ontogeny of the human thymus during fetal development. *J Clin Immunol* 1987;7:81–97.
48. Dipasquale B, Tridente G. Immunohistochemical characterization of nurse cells in normal human thymus. *Histochemistry* 1991;96:499–503.
49. von Gaudecker B. Functional histology of the human thymus. *Anat Embryol (Berl)* 1991;183:1–15.
50. Rippert H. Die Entwicklungsstörung der Thymusdrüse bei kongenitaler Lues. *Frankfurt Z Pathol* 1912;11:209–218.
51. Suster S, Rosai J. Multilocular thymic cyst: An acquired reactive process. Study of 18 cases. *Am J Surg Pathol* 1991;15:388–398.
52. Henry K. Mucin secretion and striated muscle in the human thymus. *Lancet* 1966;1:183–185.
53. Cantor H, Weissman I. Development and function of subpopulations of thymocytes and T lymphocytes. *Prog Allergy* 1976;20:1–64.
54. Everett NB, Tyler RW. Lymphopoiesis in the thymus and other tissues: Functional implications. *Int Rev Cytol* 1967;22:205–237.
55. Middleton G. The incidence of follicular structures in the human thymus at autopsy. *Aust J Exp Biol Med Sci* 1967;45:189–199.
56. Vetters JM, Barclay RS. The incidence of germinal centres in thymus glands of patients with congenital heart disease. *J Clin Pathol* 1973;26:583–591.
57. Levine GD, Rosai J. Light and electron microscopy of the human fetal thymus. In: Johannessen JV, ed. *Electron Microscopy in Human Medicine*. Vol. 5. New York: McGraw-Hill; 1980.
58. Goldstein G, Mackay IR. The thymus in systemic lupus erythematosus: A quantitative histopathological analysis and comparison with stress involution. *Br Med J* 1967;2:475–478.
59. Palestro G, Tridente G, Botto Micca F, et al. Immunohistochemical and enzyme histochemical contributions to the problem concerning the role of the thymus in the pathogenesis of myasthenia gravis. *Virchows Arch B Cell Pathol Incl Mol Pathol* 1983;44:173–186.
60. Shirai T, Miyata M, Nakase A, et al. Lymphocyte subpopulation in neoplastic and non-neoplastic thymus and in blood of patients with myasthenia gravis. *Clin Exp Immunol* 1976;26:118–123.
61. Isaacson PG, Norton AJ, Addis BJ. The human thymus contains a novel population of B lymphocytes. *Lancet* 1987;2:1488–1491.
62. Isaacson PG, Chan JK, Tang C, et al. Low-grade B-cell lymphoma of mucosa-associated lymphoid tissue arising in the thymus. A thymic lymphoma mimicking myoepithelial sialadenitis. *Am J Surg Pathol* 1990;14:342–351.
63. Cardoso De Almeida P, Harris NH, Bhan AK. Characterization of immature sinus histiocytes (monocytoid cells) in reactive lymph nodes by use of monoclonal antibodies. *Hum Pathol* 1984;15:330–335.
64. Duijvestijn AM, Schutte R, Köhler YG, et al. Characterization of the population of phagocytic cells in thymic cell suspensions. A morphological and cytochemical study. *Cell Tissue Res* 1983;231:313–323.
65. Kaiserling E, Stein H, Muller-Hermelink HK. Interdigitating reticulum cells in the human thymus. *Cell Tissue Res* 1974;155:47–55.
66. Ruco LP, Rosati S, Monardo F, et al. Macrophages and interdigitating reticulum cells in normal thymus and in thymoma: An immunohistochemical study. *Histopathology* 1989;14:37–45.
67. Lauriola L, Michetti F, Stolfi VM, et al. Detection by S-100 immunolabelling of interdigitating reticulum cells in human thymomas. *Virchows Arch B Cell Pathol Incl Mol Pathol* 1984;45:187–195.
68. Bofill M, Janossy G, Willcox N, et al. Microenvironments in the normal thymus and the thymus in myasthenia gravis. *Am J Pathol* 1985;119:462–473.
69. Siegal GP, Dehner LP, Rosai J. Histiocytosis X (Langerhans' cell granulomatosis) of the thymus. A clinicopathologic study of four childhood cases. *Am J Surg Pathol* 1985;9:117–124.
70. Bhathal PS, Campbell PE. Eosinophil leucocytes in the child's thymus. *Australas Ann Med* 1965;14:210–213.
71. Wise WS, Still WJ, Joshi VV. Severe combined immunodeficiency with thymic mast cell hyperplasia. *Arch Pathol Lab Med* 1976;100:283–286.
72. Goldstein G. Plasma cells in the human thymus. *Aust J Exp Biol Med Sci* 1966;44:695–699.
73. Henry K. The human thymus in disease with particular emphasis on thymitis and thymoma. In: Kendall MD, ed. *The Thymus Gland*. London: Academic Press; 1981:85–111.
74. Moll UM, Lane BL, Robert F, et al. The neuroendocrine thymus. Abundant occurrence of oxytocin-, vasopressin-, and neurophysin-like peptides in epithelial cells. *Histochemistry* 1988;89:385–390.
75. Ciaccio C. Contributo all'istochimica delle cellule cromaffini. II. Cellule cromaffini del timo di gallum domesticus. *Bull Soc Ital Biol Sper* 1942;17:619–620.
76. Håkanson R, Larsson LI, Sundler F. Peptide and amine producing endocrine-like cells in the chicken thymus. A chemical, histochemical and electron microscopic study. *Histochemistry* 1974;39:25–34.
77. Vialli M, Casati C. Sulla presenza di cellule enterocromaffini nel timo dei rettili. *Riv Istochim Norm Patol* 1958;4:343.
78. Vialli M. Elementi del sistema delle cellule enterocromaffinie cellule C nel timo. *Ann Histochem* 1973;18:3–7.
79. Rosai J, Higa E. Mediastinal endocrine neoplasm, of probable thymic origin, related to carcinoid tumor: Clinicopathologic study of 8 cases. *Cancer* 1972;29:1061–1074.
80. Wick MR, Rosai J. Neuroendocrine neoplasms of the thymus. *Pathol Res Pract* 1988;183:188–199.
81. Drenckhahn D, von Gaudecker B, Muller-Hermelink HK, et al. Myosin and actin containing cells in the human postnatal thymus: Ultrastructural and immunohistochemical findings in normal thymus and in myasthenia gravis. *Virchows Arch B Cell Pathol Incl Mol Pathol* 1979;32:33–45.
82. Hayward AR. Myoid cells in the human fetal thymus. *J Pathol* 1972;106:45–48.
83. Nakamura H, Ayer-Le Lièvre C. Neural crest and thymic myoid cells. *Curr Top Dev Biol* 1986;20:111–115.
84. Dardenne M, Savino W, Bach JF. Thymomatous epithelial cells and skeletal muscle share a common epitope defined by a monoclonal antibody. *Am J Pathol* 1987;126:194–198.
85. Van de Velde RL, Friedman NB. Thymic myoid cells and myasthenia gravis. *Am J Pathol* 1970;59:347–368.

86. Judd RL, Welch SL. Myoid cell differentiation in true thymic hyperplasia and lymphoid hyperplasia. *Arch Pathol Lab Med* 1988;112:1140–1144.
87. Murakami S, Shamoto M, Miura K, et al. A thymic tumor with massive proliferation of myoid cells. *Acta Pathol Jpn* 1984;34:1375–1383.
88. Rosai J, Parkash V, Reuter VE. On the origin of mediastinal germ cell tumors in men. *Int J Surg Pathol* 1995;2:73–78.
89. Marshall AH, White RG. The immunological reactivity of the thymus. *Br J Exp Pathol* 1961;42:379–385.
90. Raviola E, Karnovsky MJ. Evidence for a blood–thymus barrier using electron-opaque tracers. *J Exp Med* 1972;136:466–498.
91. Stet RJ, Wagenaar-Hilbers JP, Nieuwenhuis P. Thymus localization of monoclonal antibodies circumventing the blood-thymus barrier. *Scand J Immunol* 1987;25:441–446.
92. Bearman RM, Levine GD, Bensch KG. The ultrastructure of the normal human thymus. A study of 36 cases. *Anat Rec* 1978;190:755–781.
93. Hirokawa K. Electron microscopic observation of the human thymus of the fetus and the newborn. *Acta Pathol Jpn* 1969;19:1–13.
94. Pinkel D. Ultrastructure of the human fetal thymus. *Am J Dis Child* 1968;115:222–238.
95. van de Wijngaert FP, Kendall MD, Schuurman HJ, et al. Heterogeneity of epithelial cells in human thymus. An ultrastructural study. *Cell Tissue Res* 1984;237:227–237.
96. de Maagd RA, MacKenzie WA, Schuurman HJ, et al. The human thymus microenvironment: Heterogeneity detected by monoclonal anti-epithelial cell antibodies. *Immunology* 1985;54:745–754.
97. Haynes BF. The human thymic microenvironment. *Adv Immunol* 1984;36:87–142.
98. Janossy G, Thomas JA, Bollum FJ, et al. The human thymic microenvironment. An immunohistologic study. *J Immunol* 1980;125:202–212.
99. Van Ewijk W. Immunohistology of lymphoid and non-lymphoid cells in the thymus in relation to T lymphocyte differentiation. *Am J Anat* 1984;170:330–331.
100. McFarland EJ, Scearce RM, Haynes BF. The human thymic microenvironment: cortical thymic epithelium is an antigenically distinct region of the thymic microenvironment. *J Immunol* 1984;133:1241–1249.
101. Eisenbarth GS, Shimizu K, Bowring MA, et al. Expression of receptors for tetanus toxin and monoclonal antibody A2B5 by pancreatic islet cells. *Proc Natl Acad Sci USA* 1982;79:5066–5070.
102. Haynes BF, Robert-Guroff M, Metzgar RS, et al. Monoclonal antibodies against human T cell leukemia virus p19 defines a human thymic epithelial antigen acquired during ontogeny. *J Exp Med* 1983;157:907–920.
103. Savino W, Berrih S, Dardenne M. Thymic epithelial antigen, acquired during ontogeny and defined by the anti-p19 monoclonal antibody, is lost in thymomas. *Lab Invest* 1984;51:292–296.
104. Bhan AK, Reinherz EL, Poppema S, et al. Location of T cell and major histocompatibility complex antigens in the human thymus. *J Exp Med* 1980;152:771–782.
105. Wiley EL, Nosal JM, Freeman RG. Immunohistochemical demonstration of H antigen, peanut agglutinin receptor, and Sophora japonica receptor expression in infant thymuses and thymic neoplasias. *Am J Clin Pathol* 1990;93:44–48.
106. Le PT, Lazorick S, Whichard LP, et al. Regulation of cytokine production in the human thymus: Epidermal growth factor and transforming growth factor alpha regulate mRNA levels of interleukin 1 alpha (IL-1 alpha), IL-1 beta, and IL-6 in human thymic epithelial cells at a post-transcriptional level. *J Exp Med* 1991;174:1147–1157.
107. Chan WC, Zaatari GS, Tabei S, et al. Thymoma: An immunohistochemical study. *Am J Clin Pathol* 1984;82:160–166.
108. Lobach DF, Scearce RM, Haynes BF. The human thymic microenvironment. Phenotypic characterization of Hassall's bodies with the use of monoclonal antibodies. *J Immunol* 1985;134:250–257.
109. Chu PG, Weiss LM. Expression of cytokeratin 5/6 in epithelial neoplasms: An immunohistochemical study of 509 cases. *Mod Pathol* 2002;15:6–10.
110. Dotto J, Pelosi G, Rosai J. Expression of p63 in thymomas and normal thymus. *Am J Clin Pathol* 2007;127:415–420.
111. Walts AE, Hiroshima K, Marchevski AM. Desmoglein 3 and p40 immunoreactivity in neoplastic and nonneoplastic thymus: A potential adjunct to help resolve selected diagnostic and staging problems. *Ann Diagn Pathol* 2015;19:216–220.
112. Hsu SM, Jaffe ES. Phenotypic expression of T lymphocytes in thymus and peripheral lymphoid tissues. *Am J Pathol* 1985;121:69–78.
113. Janossy G, Bofill M, Trejdosiewicz LK, et al. Cellular differentiation of lymphoid subpopulations and their microenvironments in the human thymus. In: Muller-Hermelink HK, ed. *The Human Thymus: Histophysiology and Pathology.* Berlin: Springer-Verlag; 1986:89–125.
114. Tidman N, Janossy C, Bodger M, et al. Delineation of human thymocyte differentiation pathways utilizing double-staining techniques with monoclonal antibodies. *Clin Exp Immunol* 1981;45:457–467.
115. Chilosi M, Iannucci AM, Pizzolo G, et al. Immunohistochemical analysis of thymoma. Evidence of medullary origin of epithelial cells. *Am J Surg Pathol* 1984;8:309–318.
116. Mokhtar N, Hsu SM, Lad RP, et al. Thymoma: Lymphoid and epithelial components mirror the phenotype of normal thymus. *Hum Pathol* 1984;15:378–384.
117. Sato Y, Watanabe S, Mukai K, et al. An immunohistochemical study of thymic epithelial tumors. II. Lymphoid component. *Am J Surg Pathol* 1986;10:862–870.
118. Lauriola L, Maggiano N, Marino M, et al. Human thymoma: Immunologic characteristics of the lymphocytic component. *Cancer* 1981;48:1992–1995.
119. van der Kwast TH, van Vliet E, Cristen E, et al. An immunohistologic study of the epithelial and lymphoid components of six thymomas. *Hum Pathol* 1985;16:1001–1008.
120. Eimoto T, Teshima K, Shirakusa T, et al. Heterogeneity of epithelial cells and reactive components in thymomas: An ultrastructural and immunohistochemical study. *Ultrastruct Pathol* 1986;10:157–173.
121. Katzin WE, Fishleder AJ, Linden MD, et al. Immunoglobulin and T-cell receptor genes in thymomas: Genotypic evidence supporting the nonneoplastic nature of the lymphocytic component. *Hum Pathol* 1988;19:323–328.
122. Robertson PB, Neiman RS, Worapongoaiboon S, et al. 013 (CD99) positivity in hematologic proliferations correlated with TdT positivity. *Hum Pathol* 1997;10:277–282.

123. Swerdlow SH, Angermeier PA, Hartman AL. Intrathymic ontogeny of the T cell receptor associated CD3 (T3) antigen. *Lab Invest* 1988;58:421–427.
124. Nikolic-Zugic J. Phenotypic and functional stages in the intrathymic development of alpha beta T cells. *Immunol Today* 1991;12:65–70.
125. Bach JF, Dardenne M, Pleau JM, et al. Biochemical characteristics of a serum thymic factor. *Nature* 1976;266:55–56.
126. McCarty N, Shinohara ML, Lu L, et al. Detailed analysis of gene expression during development of T cell lineages in the thymus. *Proc Natl Acad Sci USA* 2004;101:9339–9344.
127. Goldstein AL, Low TLK, McAdoo M, et al. Thymosin alpha 1. Isolation and sequential analysis of an immunologically active thymic polypeptide. *Proc Natl Acad Sci USA* 1977;74:725–729.
128. Goldstein G. The isolation of thymopoietin (thymin). *Ann NY Acad Sci* 1975;249:177–185.
129. Fabien N, Auger C, Monier JC. Immunolocalization of thymosin alpha 1, thymopoietin and thymulin in mouse thymic epithelial cells at different stages of culture: A light and electron microscopic study. *Immunology* 1988;63:721–727.
130. Jambon B, Montague P, Bene MC, et al. Immunohistologic localization of "facteur thymique serique" (FTS) in human thymic epithelium. *J Immunol* 1981;127:2055–2059.
131. Savino W, Dardenne M. Thymic hormone-containing cells. VI. Immunohistologic evidence for the simultaneous presence of thymulin, thymopoietin and thymosin alpha 1 in normal and pathological human thymuses. *Eur J Immunol* 1984;14:987–991.
132. Haynes BF, Warren RW, Buckley RH, et al. Demonstration of abnormalities in expression of thymic epithelial surface antigens in severe cellular immunodeficiency diseases. *J Immunol* 1983;130:1182–1188.
133. Clark SL Jr. The thymus in mice of strain 129/J, studied with the electron microscope. *Am J Anat* 1963;112:1–33.
134. Hirokawa K, Utsuyama M, Moriizumi E, et al. Immunohistochemical studies in human thymomas. Localization of thymosin and various cell markers. *Virchows Arch B Cell Pathol Incl Mol Pathol* 1988;55:371–380.
135. Bodey B, Bodey B Jr, Siegel SE, et al. Review of thymic hormones in cancer diagnosis and treatment. *Int J Immunopharmacol* 2000;22:261–273.
136. Geenen V, Robert F, Defresne MP, et al. Neuroendocrinology of the thymus. *Horm Res* 1989;31:81–84.
137. Jevremovic M, Terzic M, Kartaljevic G, et al. The determination of immunoreactive beta-endorphin concentration in the human fetal and neonatal thymus. *Horm Metab Res* 1991;23:623–624.
138. Batanero E, de Leeuw FE, Jansen GH, et al. The neural and neuroendocrine components of the human thymus. II. Hormone immunoreactivity. *Brain Behav Immun* 1992;6:249–264.
139. Le PT, Lazorick S, Whichard LP, et al. Human thymic epithelial cells produce IL-6, granulocyte-monocyte-CSF, and leukemia inhibitory factor. *J Immunol* 1990;145:3310–3315.
140. Wainberg MA, Numazaki K, Destephano L, et al. Infection of human thymic epithelial cells by human cytomegalovirus and other viruses: Effect on secretion of interleukin 1–like activity. *Clin Exp Immunol* 1988;72:415–421.
141. Yarilin AA, Belyakov IM. Cytokines in the thymus: Production and biological effects. *Curr Med Chem* 2004;11:447–464.
142. Hirokawa K. Age-related changes of thymus. Morphological and functional aspects. *Acta Pathol Jpn* 1978;28:843–857.
143. Simpson JG, Gray ES, Beck JS. Age involution in the normal adult thymus. *Clin Exp Immunol* 1975;19:261–265.
144. Steinman GG. Changes in the human thymus during aging. In: Muller-Hermelink HK, ed. *The Human Thymus. Histophysiology and Pathology*. Berlin: Springer-Verlag; 1986:43–88.
145. Steinmann GG, Klaus B, Muller-Hermelink HK. The involution of the aging human thymic epithelium is independent of puberty. A morphometric study. *Scand J Immunol* 1985;22:563–575.
146. Smith SM, Ossa-Gomez LJ. A quantitative histologic comparison of the thymus in 100 healthy and diseased adults. *Am J Clin Pathol* 1981;76:657–665.
147. Jamieson BD, Douek DC, Killian S, et al. Generation of functional thymocytes in the human adult. *Immunity* 1999;10:569–575.
148. Bertho JM, Demarquay C, Moulian N, et al. Phenotypic and immunohistological analyses of the human adult thymus: Evidence for an active thymus during adult life. *Cell Immunol* 1997;179:30–40.
149. Shanker A. Is thymus redundant after adulthood? *Immunol Lett* 2004;15:79–86.
150. Selye H. Thymus and adrenals in the response of the organism to injuries and intoxications. *Br J Exp Pathol* 1936;17:234–248.
151. van Baarlen J, Schuurman HJ, Huber J. Acute thymus involution in infancy and childhood: A reliable marker for duration of acute illness. *Hum Pathol* 1988;19:1155–1160.
152. Joshi VV, Oleske JM, Saad S, et al. Thymus biopsy in children with acquired immunodeficiency syndrome. *Arch Pathol Lab Med* 1986;110:837–842.
153. Seemayer TA, Laroche AC, Russo P, et al. Precocious thymic involution manifest by epithelial injury in the acquired immune deficiency syndrome. *Hum Pathol* 1984;15:469–474.
154. Grody WW, Fligiel S, Naeim F. Thymus involution in the acquired immunodeficiency syndrome. *Am J Clin Pathol* 1985;84:85–95.
155. Schuurman HJ, Krone WJ, Broekhuizen R, et al. The thymus in acquired immune deficiency syndrome. Comparison with other types of immunodeficiency diseases, and presence of components of human immunodeficiency virus type 1. *Am J Pathol* 1989;134:1329–1338.
156. Kendall MD, Johnson HR, Singh J. The weight of the human thymus gland at necropsy. *J Anat* 1980;131(pt 3):485–497.
157. Lack EE. Thymic hyperplasia with massive enlargement: Report of two cases with review of diagnostic criteria. *J Thorac Cardiovasc Surg* 1981;81:741–746.
158. Katz SM, Chatten J, Bishop HC, et al. Massive thymic enlargement. Report of a case of gross thymic hyperplasia in a child. *Am J Clin Pathol* 1977;68:786–790.
159. Judd RL. Massive thymic hyperplasia with myoid cell differentiation. *Hum Pathol* 1987;18:1180–1183.
160. Hammar JA. Uber Gewicht, Involution und Persistenz der Thymus im Postfotalleben der Menschen. *Arch Anat Physiol Anat Abt* 1906;(suppl):91–182.
161. Durkin W, Durant J. Benign mass lesions after therapy for Hodgkin's disease. *Arch Intern Med* 1979;139:333–336.
162. Shin M, Ho K. Diffuse thymic hyperplasia following chemotherapy for nodular sclerosing Hodgkin's disease. An immunologic rebound phenomenon? *Cancer* 1983;51:30–33.

163. Carmosino L, DiBenedetto A, Feffer S. Thymic hyperplasia following successful chemotherapy. A report of two cases and review of the literature. *Cancer* 1985;56:1526–1528.
164. Due W, Dieckmann KP, Stein H. Thymic hyperplasia following chemotherapy of a testicular germ cell tumor. Immunohistological evidence for a simple rebound phenomenon. *Cancer* 1989;63:446–449.
165. Gelfand DW, Goldman AS, Law AJ. Thymic hyperplasia in children recovering from thermal burns. *J Trauma* 1972;12: 813–817.
166. Caffey J, Silbey R. Regrowth and overgrowth of the thymus after atrophy induced by the oral administration of adrenocorticosteroids to human infants. *Pediatrics* 1960;26:762–770.
167. Mackall CL, Fleisher TA, Brown MR, et al. Age, thymopoiesis, and $CD4^+$ T-lymphocyte regeneration after intensive chemotherapy. *N Engl J Med* 1995;332:143–149.
168. Markert ML, Alvarez-McLeod AP, Sempowski GD, et al. Thymopoiesis in HIV-infected adults after highly active antiretroviral therapy. *AIDS Res Hum Retroviruses* 2001;17:1635–1643.
169. Croxatto OC. Cordones epiteliales con aspecto endocrino observado en restos timicos del adulto. *Medicina (B Aires)* 1972;32:203–208.
170. Suster S, Moran CA. Malignant thymic neoplasms that may mimic benign conditions. *Semin Diagn Pathol* 1995;12:98–104.
171. Suster S, Barbuto D, Carlson G, et al. Multilocular thymic cysts with pseudoepitheliomatous hyperplasia. *Hum Pathol* 1991;22:455–460.
172. Suster S, Rosai J. Cystic thymomas. A clinicopathologic study of ten cases. *Cancer* 1992;69:92–97.
173. Moran CA, Suster S. Mediastinal seminomas with prominent cystic changes. A clinicopathologic study of 10 cases. *Am J Surg Pathol* 1995;19:1047–1053.
174. Suster S, Rosai J. Thymic carcinoma. A clinicopathologic study of 60 cases. *Cancer* 1991;67:1025–1032.
175. Moran CA, Suster S. Mucoepidermoid carcinomas of the thymus. A clinicopathologic study of six cases. *Am J Surg Pathol* 1995;19:826–834.
176. Penn CR, Hope-Stone HF. The role of radiotherapy in the management of malignant thymoma. *Br J Surg* 1972;59: 533–539.
177. Goodwin RA, Nickell JA, Des Prez RM. Mediastinal fibrosis complicating healed primary histoplasmosis and tuberculosis. *Medicine (Baltimore)* 1972;51:227–246.
178. Light AM. Idiopathic fibrosis of the mediastinum: A discussion of three cases and review of the literature. *J Clin Pathol* 1978;31:78–88.
179. Sobrinho-Simoes MA, Vaz Saleiro JV, Wagenvoort CA. Mediastinal and hilar fibrosis. *Histopathology* 1981;5:53–60.

Heart

Gerald J. Berry

HEART WEIGHTS 530	Atrioventricular Valves 539
PRENATAL FETAL CIRCULATION 530	Chordae Tendineae 540
POSTNATAL CIRCULATION 531	Applied Anatomy of Intracardiac Valves 540
PERICARDIUM 531	Aging Changes of Intracardiac Valves 541
Applied Anatomy 532	PAPILLARY MUSCLES 541
CARDIAC SKELETON 532	CONDUCTION SYSTEM 542
Applied Anatomy 532	Sinoatrial Node 542
INTERNAL STRUCTURE OF THE HEART WALL 532	Atrioventricular Node 542
INTERATRIAL SEPTUM 534	Aging Changes in the Human Conduction System 545
Applied Anatomy 535	CARDIAC INNERVATION 545
RIGHT ATRIUM 535	Autonomic Nerves 545
LEFT ATRIUM 535	LYMPHATICS 545
RIGHT VENTRICLE 536	SMALL INTRAMURAL CORONARY ARTERIES 546
Applied Anatomy 538	VEINS AND VENULES 546
LEFT VENTRICLE 538	THE ENDOMYOCARDIAL BIOPSY 546
Applied Anatomy 538	Tissue Handling and Processing 547
CARDIAC VALVES 538	Biopsy Limitations and Tissue Artifacts 547
Semilunar Valves 538	SUMMARY 549
	REFERENCES 549

This chapter was originally authored by Dr. Margaret Billingham. Previous editions were revised by the two of us. Dr. Billingham died on July 14, 2009. She was Professor of Pathology, emerita, and the former Director of Cardiac Pathology at Stanford University. Dr. Billingham made innumerable contributions to the fields of cardiovascular pathology and cardiovascular medicine, including cardiac transplant pathology, myocarditis, anthracycline cardiotoxicity, and cardiomyopathies. She was a founding member of the Society of Cardiovascular Pathology and was awarded its Distinguished Achievement Award in 2001. She was a member of the Society of Heart and Lung Transplantation and served as its president in 1990. She published over 500 peer-reviewed articles, abstracts, and book chapters and directed numerous teaching workshops on the endomyocardial biopsy in transplant and nontransplant pathology. Dr. Billingham is warmly remembered for the impact that her teaching, friendship, and mentorship had on scores of residents, fellows, and colleagues around the world. It is an honor to update her work for this edition.

With the introduction of the cardiopulmonary bypass technique into clinical practice over 60 years ago, pathologists found themselves examining cardiac specimens in the surgical pathology laboratory for the first time. For many years the specimens consisted of excised valves, pericardiectomy specimens, ventricular aneurysmectomy excisions, and interventricular myomectomy specimens. It was not until cardiac transplantation began in the late 1960s that surgical pathologists began handling entire heart specimens. Currently, more than 140,000 heart and combined heart–lung transplant procedures in adults have been recorded in the registries of the International Society of Heart and Lung Transplantation (1,2). Thoracic transplantation in the pediatric age group ranging from neonates to adolescents is now commonly performed, and close to 15,000 heart and combined heart–lung cases have been recorded (3,4). The explanted hearts from infants and children often have complicated congenital lesions that have undergone one or more corrective surgical interventions. Surgical pathologists need to have expertise in the morphologic evaluation of end-stage heart disease of all types. Since the early 1970s, endomyocardial biopsies for the assessment of allograft rejection, infiltrative lesions, and inflammatory disorders are performed routinely. Today many institutions have ventricular assist device (VAD), and total artificial heart programs and ventricular apical specimens are routinely submitted. Like other biopsy specimens, these fall under the auspices of the surgical pathologist. Further, the introduction of complex electrophysiologic mapping techniques and imaging modalities such as transesophageal and 3D echocardiography, intravascular ultrasound, multidetector-row computed tomography (MDCT) imaging and coronary CT angiography (CCTA), and magnetic resonance imaging (MRI) have renewed interest in structural–functional correlations (5,6). Pathologists assume a critical role in the clinical evaluation and application of these technologies.

The purpose of this chapter is to review normal cardiac anatomy and histology. The histology of the great vessels is described elsewhere in this book. For the most part, adult histology is described, but where important differences exist, the histology in infants and children is also addressed. Furthermore, the purpose is not intended to be encyclopedic. Rather, we highlight those areas that are of practical importance to the surgical pathologist to enable the distinction between normal changes and subtle cardiac pathology. As each of the major anatomic divisions of the heart is described, relevant aspects of aging, gender changes, and/or applied anatomy are mentioned. We have also included recommendations for handling endomyocardial biopsy specimens and common artifactual alterations in this discussion.

HEART WEIGHTS

The weight of the normal adult heart is generally achieved by the end of the second decade of life. Heart weight in infants and children is related to age and body size, and tables are readily available (7,8). A variety of approaches to estimating the weight of the adult heart have been used in clinical practice. These differ in complexity and accuracy; for example, the practical guidelines for unfixed adult heart weights published by Hudson in 1965 (9) propose that the male heart weighs 0.45% of the body weight (325 ± 75 g; average 300 g) and the female heart weighs 0.40% of the body weight (275 ± 75 g; average 250 g). Heart weight varies with age, sex, and body height and weight. Using this type of approach, the heart weight in young athletic adults may approach or exceed the upper limits of normal by up to 25%, whereas in the elderly it may approach or be slightly below the lower limits of normal.

Kitzman et al. from the Mayo Clinic (10) proposed a more comprehensive approach that predicts the normal heart weight of a formalin-fixed specimen based on body weight or height. In their study, body height as a predictor proved less accurate than body weight. The impact of formalin fixation on the weight of the heart has been addressed with conflicting findings. In one study heart weight increased by 5% after fixation, although considerable individual variation—ranging from weight loss to weight gain—was reported (11). Descriptive tables of normal ventricular wall thickness, chamber size, valvular orifice measurements and techniques for specimen handling and dissection are available in textbooks and postmortem dissection manuals (8,12–14).

PRENATAL FETAL CIRCULATION

It is beyond the scope of this chapter to discuss cardiac embryology. Developmental molecular biology has provided many new insights into cardiogenesis and the developmental genetics of congenital heart defects, some of which have radically altered previously held tenets (15–21). The human heart begins to beat spontaneously after the 2nd week of gestation (GW) and is fully formed by the 8th to 9th GW. Well-oxygenated blood leaves the placenta via the umbilical vein, a portion of which passes through the hepatic sinusoids, and the remainder bypasses the liver by way of the ductus venosus to enter the inferior vena cava (IVC). Caval blood enters the right atrium together with an admixture of deoxygenated blood from the lower body. Approximately one-third of this blood is diverted through the interatrial septum (ostium secundum) into the left atrium, where it mixes with the small amount of deoxygenated blood returning from the lungs. The blood then passes into the left ventricle and exits into the ascending aorta to supply the coronary arteries, brain, and upper limbs. Approximately 50% of the blood is returned to the placenta for reoxygenation via the umbilical arteries. The remainder of the blood supplies the lower half of the body. Blood returning to the heart from the upper body reaches the right atrium through the superior vena cava (SVC). It mixes with the residual two-thirds of the blood from the IVC and enters the right ventricle. A small portion is distributed to the lungs, but the majority is diverted across the ductus arteriosus to the descending aorta. Blood is returned to the placenta with only a small amount reaching the lower body of the fetus.

POSTNATAL CIRCULATION

At birth, a series of anatomic and physiologic changes occur, beginning with the infant's first respiratory efforts. Circulation of fetal blood through the placenta ceases and the infant's lungs expand. As alveoli become aerated, the pulmonary vascular bed dilates causing an increase in pulmonary blood flow and abrupt decline in pulmonary vascular resistance. Additionally, active remodeling of the pulmonary vasculature begins and continues over a period of a few weeks. This consists primarily in the reduction of the muscular medial layer of arterioles and small arteries. Increased blood return to the left atrium by way of the pulmonary veins results in slightly higher left atrial pressures compared with the right atrium. This causes the flap covering the foramen ovale to seal, creating an indentation called the fossa ovale. By the end of the 1st month after birth, the significant differences in ventricular hemodynamic load result in thickening of the left ventricular wall and thinning of the right ventricular wall. The ductus arteriosus, located between the left pulmonary artery and the aortic arch, functionally closes within 15 hours after birth, and the umbilical veins begin to constrict.

PERICARDIUM

The pericardium surrounds the heart and consists of a fibrous and a serous sac. The fibrous, or parietal pericardium envelops the heart and is reflected off the ascending aorta, the pulmonary arterial trunk, the terminal 2 to 4 cm of the SVC, the distal segment of the IVC, and the pulmonary veins. In addition to its protective function as a physical barrier between the heart and pulmonary and mediastinal processes, it provides immunologic and essential mechanical and geomechanical functions (22,23). In the normal state, the fibrous pericardium surrounding the heart remains unattached to the serous (visceral) pericardium except at the pericardial reflections. The parietal pericardium is composed predominantly of collagenous fibrous tissue (fibrosa layer) intermixed with occasional elastic fibers, lymphatic and other small vessels (Fig. 19.1). Its inelastic tendencies account for the development of cardiac tamponade when it is acutely stretched with more than 250 mL of fluid. It can contain variable amounts of adipose tissue, particularly toward the apex of the heart. A thin layer of mesothelial cells on its inner surface lines the parietal pericardium. It

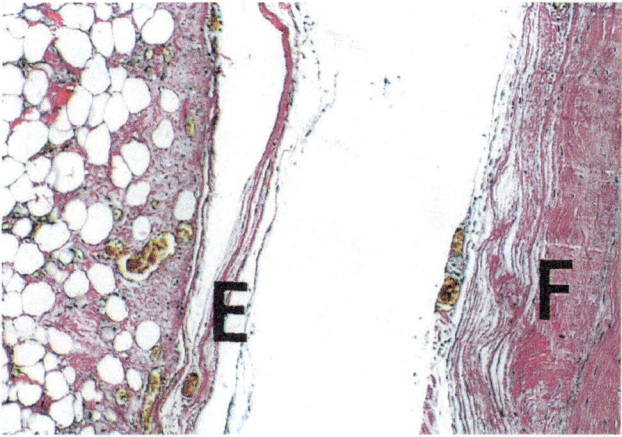

FIGURE 19.1 Section showing fibrous pericardium (*F*) separated from the thinner epicardium (*E*) (elastic van Gieson).

is normally less than 1 mm in thickness, although there can be some variation in thickness over different regions of the heart and great vessels. Both CT and MRI imaging provide enhanced resolution of the parietal pericardium and are routinely used to assess for developmental, posttraumatic, inflammatory, and neoplastic conditions (24,25). Heterotopic tissues within this layer can include thyroid and thymic elements. Neoplastic and hyperplastic alterations have been described, including intracardiac thyroid in the right ventricular outflow tract (26).

The serous or visceral pericardium is also called the epicardium of the heart. It is a single layer of mesothelium that envelops the heart and is in continuity with the fibrous pericardium at the pericardial reflections at the great vessels (Fig. 19.2). This delicate membrane covering the heart contains a fibroconnective submesothelial layer and variable amounts of adipose tissue within which are embedded the coronary arteries and veins, lymphatic vessels, nerves,

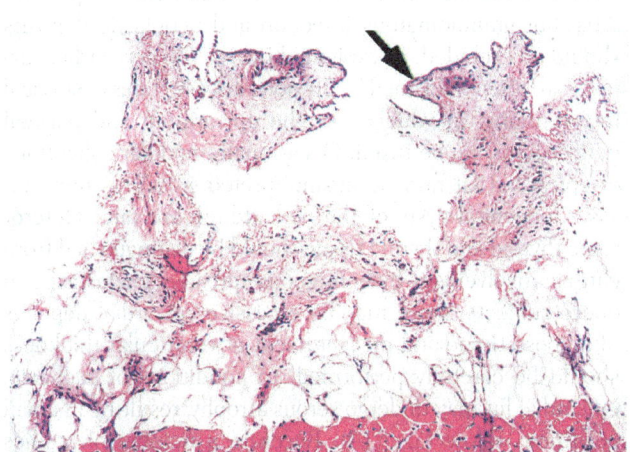

FIGURE 19.2 Section showing the epicardium lined by mesothelial cells (*arrow*) and covering the subepicardial adipose tissue and myocardium (H&E).

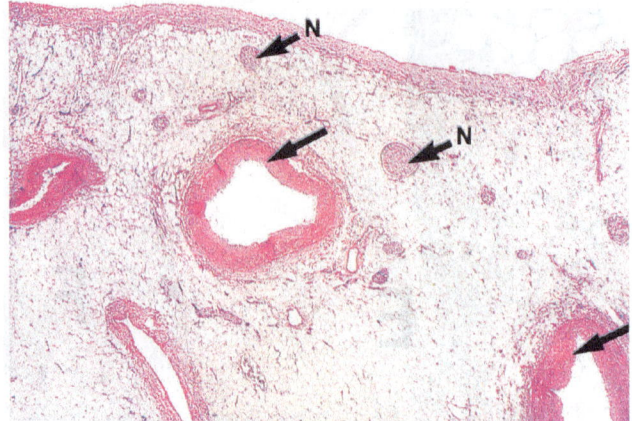

FIGURE 19.3 Section of the epicardium showing the relationship of coronary vessels (*arrows*) and nerves (*N*) to the epicardium (H&E).

fibroblasts, and macrophages (Fig. 19.3). The normal epicardium often has small aggregates of lymphocytes that are present from birth.

Between the two mesothelial layers of the parietal and visceral pericardium is a potential space containing up to 50 mL of straw-colored fluid that allows the surfaces to glide over one another in the normal state. The histologic composition of the two layers of the pericardium does not alter with age and is similar in infants, children, and adults.

Applied Anatomy

Awareness of the anatomy of the pericardium and its normal variants is important for cardiac surgeons and radiologists. Two sinuses (the transverse and oblique sinuses) and various recesses are found at the points of reflection of the parietal and the visceral pericardium near the great vessels and atria. The transverse sinus provides access to the left atrium and the mitral valve (27). Surgical pathologists may receive pericardiectomy specimens in cases of constrictive pericarditis, recurrent effusions, or tamponade. Nonspecific fibrosis and chronic inflammation are observed in constrictive pericarditis, but granulomatous infection and neoplastic deposits should be excluded. In explanted hearts, the pericardial surfaces are often thickened by previous disease states or surgical interventions, in which case the epicardium and parietal pericardium can be fused. Occasionally, nodular collections of epicardial fat may be misinterpreted grossly as metastases. Congenital cysts of the pericardium are rare. Heterotopic thyroid and thymic tissue should be distinguished from cardiac involvement by contiguous spread or metastasis. In obese subjects, there may be excessive epicardial deposits of adipose tissue and measurement of ventricular thickness should be carefully performed. In conditions of cachexia, epicardial fat may undergo serous atrophy, resulting in small gelatinous tissue tags (14). Recently, a number of studies have shown a relationship between epicardial fat deposits and the severity of atrial fibrillation, metabolic syndrome, and coronary artery disease (28,29).

CARDIAC SKELETON

The cardiac skeleton at the base of the heart is the central supporting structure to which most of the fibers of the myocardium are attached and into which the atrioventricular (AV) and aortic valves are anchored. A separate mass of fibrous tissue (the conus ligament) joins the pulmonary ring to the aortic ring. It also serves to separate the atrial and ventricular chambers. It is composed of the right and left fibrous trigones, membranous septum of the interventricular septum, and the fibrous annuli of the AV foramina (30). The fibrous skeleton is composed of layers of dense collagenous connective tissue admixed with small numbers of elastic fibers and, on occasion, small aggregates of adipose tissue. The fibrous tissue of the mitral and aortic valve rings is more substantial than the right-sided valves, and the right and left trigones create the direct mitral–aortic continuity (31). The right trigone and membranous septum form the central fibrous body within which the AV bundle is embedded. Bone or cartilage is not normally found in the fibrous skeleton of human hearts, although they have been described in some animal species.

Applied Anatomy

Portions of the cardiac skeleton may be seen in explanted valves. The close proximity of the fibrous skeleton to the conduction system and valvular leaflets is an important consideration for surgeons. Embryologic variations and surgical alterations can significantly affect the functional outcomes of all these components.

INTERNAL STRUCTURE OF THE HEART WALL

The wall of the heart in all chambers consists of three main layers: (a) the endocardium, (b) the intermediate or central muscular portion or myocardium, and (c) the external portion or epicardium. Most investigators believe that the endocardium is homologous with the tunica intima of blood vessels, the myocardium with the smooth muscle media, and the external epicardium with the adventitial layer. The endocardium consists of a single layer of endothelial cells (Figs. 19.4 and 19.5) with a subendothelial portion containing a loose elastic framework and collagen bundles, as well as nerves and delicate blood vessels (Fig. 19.6). In the atria the subendothelial layer is situated between the endothelial layer and the prominent elastic layer. A more detailed discussion of the myoarchitecture of the heart, its relationship to its supporting fibrous matrix, and the controversies surrounding the configuration of myocytes has been published (32). This has importance in ventricular remodeling during systolic heart failure, as dilatation results in alteration of the normal helical fiber orientation. For example, the oblique

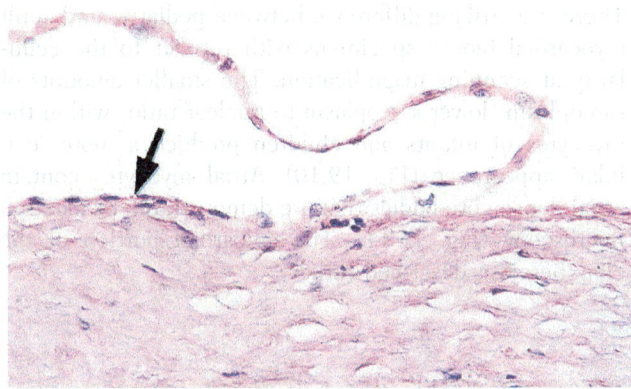

FIGURE 19.4 Section showing a single layer of endothelial cells covering the myocardium (*arrow*) (H&E).

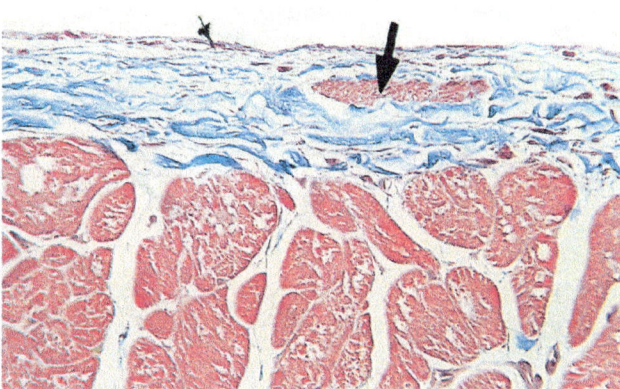

FIGURE 19.7 Section of the endocardium showing smooth muscle bundle (*arrow*) (Masson trichrome).

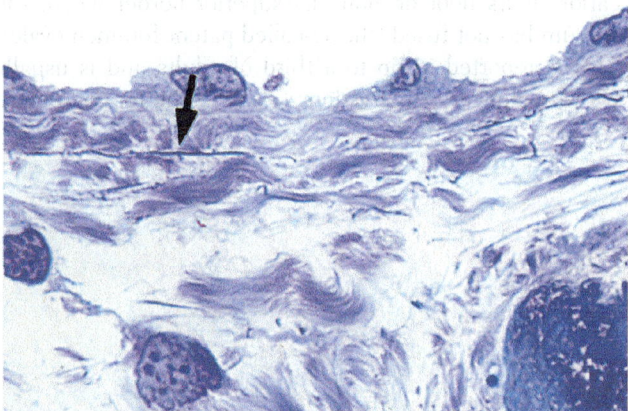

FIGURE 19.5 A 1-μm thick section (plastic embedded) of the endothelium covering the fenestrated elastic fibers (*arrow*) and collagen fibers of the subendocardium (toluidine blue).

fibers transition to a transverse alignment contributing to diminished ejection fraction (33).

While the chambers of the heart are composed of these three layers, there can be variation in the thickness of one or more components. A rudimentary layer of smooth muscle is often found in the endocardium of both atria and the ventricles (Fig. 19.7). The endocardium of the atria is thicker than the ventricles. Small bundles of smooth muscle are often found but are of questionable functional significance. The myocardium is composed of bundles of myocytes separated by fibrous bands or fibrovascular structures (Fig. 19.8). The individual myocytes form a syncytium with end-to-end junctions (called intercalated discs) and sometimes side-to-side junctions. Individual myocytes contain a central ovoid nucleus with a clear zone at the poles (Fig. 19.9). The normal cardiac myocyte contains

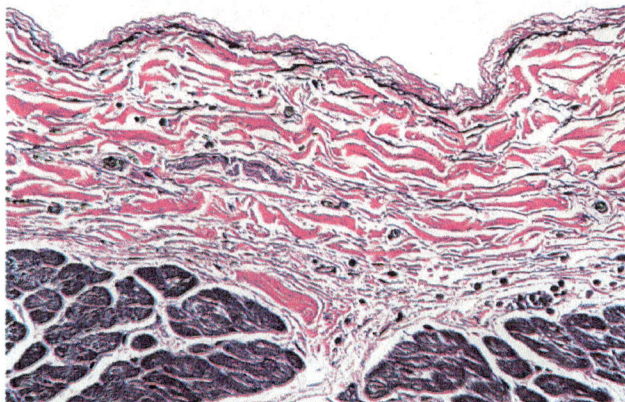

FIGURE 19.6 Section of the endocardium showing the distribution of the elastic fibers (*black*) and the collagen bundles (*red*), as well as vessels and nerves in the subendocardial layer.

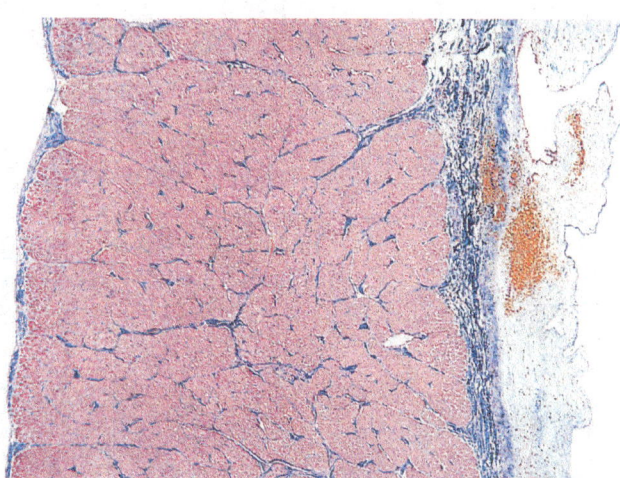

FIGURE 19.8 Section through the right ventricular wall showing the distribution of collagen from the endocardium (*left*) through the myocardium and to the epicardium (*right*) in the normal heart (Masson trichrome).

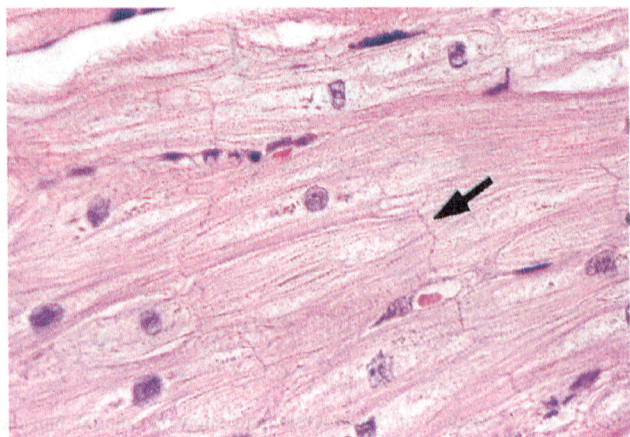

FIGURE 19.9 Section of myocardium showing ovoid nuclei and intercalated discs (*arrow*) (H&E).

small amounts of lipofuscin granules (lysosomes), which increase with age and are found in large quantities in a variety of acquired myocardial disorders. The myocytes are filled with contractile myofibrils (actin and myosin).

There is a striking difference between pediatric and adult myocardial biopsy specimens with respect to the cellularity at scanning magnification. The smaller amounts of sarcoplasm (lower sarcoplasm to nuclear ratio) within the myocytes of infants and children produce a more "cellular" appearance (Fig. 19.10). Atrial myocytes contain atrial dense-core bodies that are demonstrable by electron microscopy (Fig. 19.11). The epicardial portion of the chambers was described earlier.

INTERATRIAL SEPTUM

The interatrial septum separates the right and left atrial chambers. In the normal state this separation is complete, although the foramen ovale may retain a small communication at its floor or along its superior border where the septum has not fused (the so-called patent foramen ovale). This is reported in up to a third of adults and is usually without clinical complications (34,35). The foramen ovale

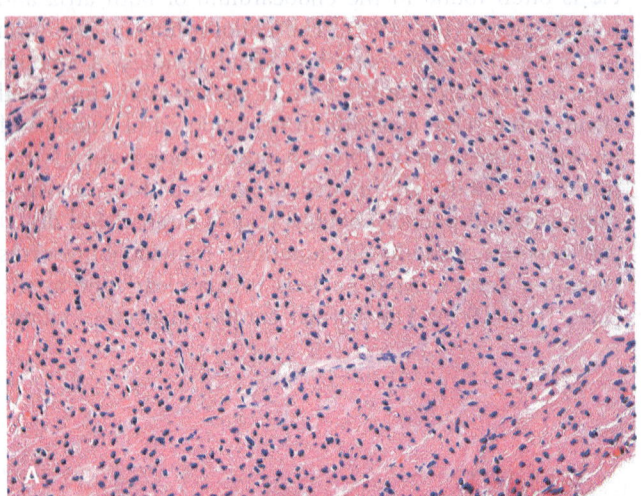

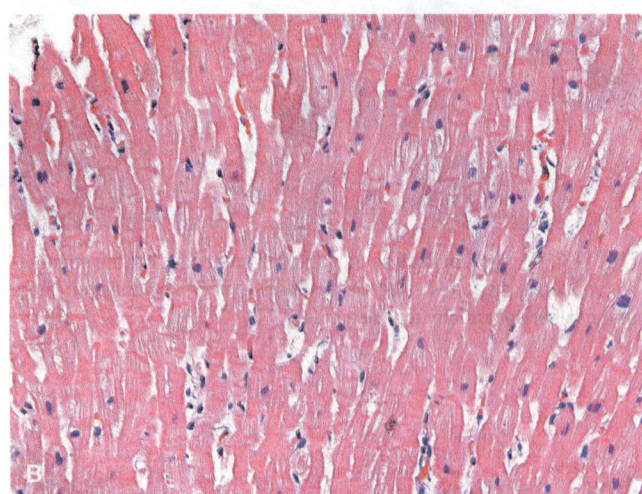

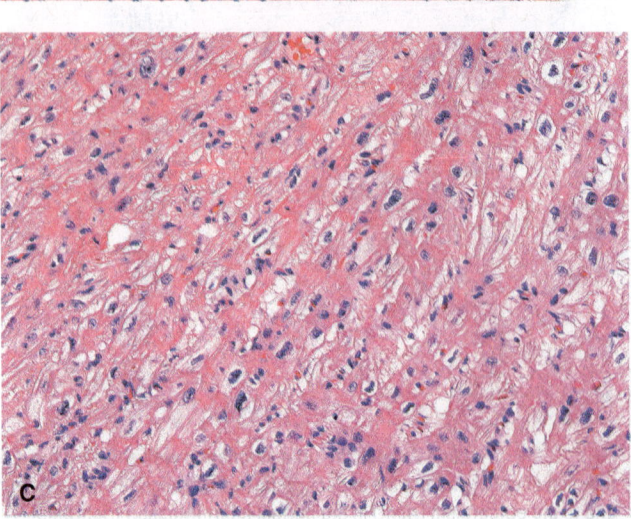

FIGURE 19.10 Pediatric and adult myocardium. Normal pediatric myocardium (**A**) compared to normal adult myocardium (**B**) at same magnification. **C:** Right ventricular biopsy from an infant with idiopathic dilated cardiomyopathy (IDCM) compared to adult biopsy with IDCM (**D**). Note: Same magnification utilized for all 4 panels.

Applied Anatomy

Lipomatous hypertrophy of the interatrial septum is characterized by accumulations of adipose tissue within the U-shaped lip, or limbus, of the oval fossa and may produce bulging of the interatrial septum. In some patients, the patent foramen ovale can cause interatrial shunting and paradoxical embolism.

RIGHT ATRIUM

Venous return to the heart occurs via the IVC and SVC into the right atrium. The right atrium forms the right lateral cardiac border and is located anterior to the left atrium and to the right of it. Anteromedially, the right atrial appendage protrudes from the right atrium and overlaps the aortic root (31). The atrium is composed of the auricular appendage, the smooth-walled venous sinus that contains the openings of the cavae and coronary sinus, the septal component, and the portion near the opening of the tricuspid valve (36,37). Extending between the right sides of the openings of both cavae is a prominent muscular ridge called the terminal crest, which underlies the sulcus terminalis. The broad-based triangular appendage defines the morphologic right atrium. The interior surface of this appendage is trabeculated by muscular bands called pectinate muscles. The portion of the right atrium lateral to the terminal crest is smooth walled and is derived embryologically from the sinus venosus (Fig. 19.12). The right atrial wall measures 2 mm in thickness.

The orifice of the SVC is valveless. The opening of the IVC has an inconstant, rudimentary valve called the eustachian valve. It forms a crescentic fold over the anterior border of the IVC orifice and serves to direct blood toward the foramen ovale and into the left atrium during fetal life. The opening of the coronary sinus has a rudimentary crescent-shaped flap of tissue called the thebesian valve; these valves vary greatly in size and may be fenestrated or absent. Chiari network, usually appearing as a lacelike veil of tissue, represents the remnant of the right sinus venosus valve and is occasionally found in normal hearts (Fig. 19.13). A fascinating review of the historical figures that have produced eponyms in cardiac anatomy is noteworthy (38). The right atrial chamber is covered by endocardium. In the subendocardium, elastic fibers pass into a typical fenestrated elastic membrane that contains blood vessels, nerves, and branches of the conducting system. In the spaces between the muscle bundles of the atria, the wall is so thin that the connective tissue of the endocardium blends with the epicardium. The epicardial surface of the atrium is rich in nerves and ganglia (Fig. 19.14).

LEFT ATRIUM

Like the right atrium, this chamber consists of an appendage, a venous component containing the ostia of the four pulmonary veins, a septal component, and a region near the

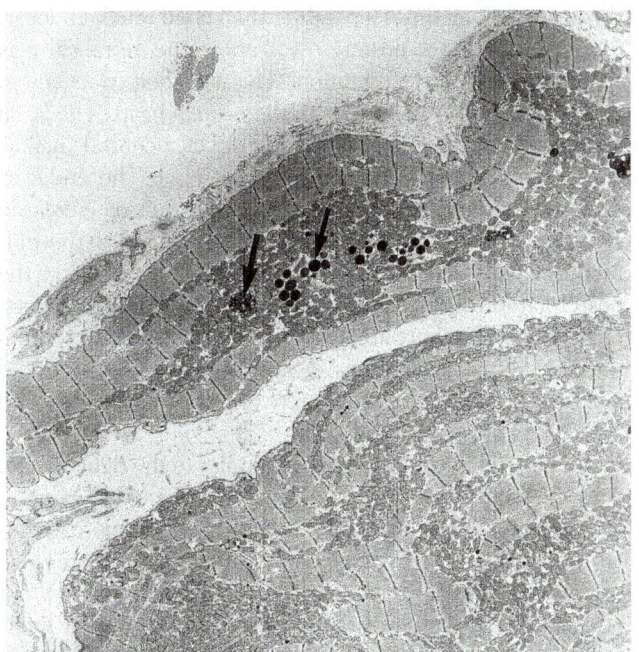

FIGURE 19.11 Electron micrograph of atrial dense-core granules (*small arrow*) that can be differentiated from the lipofuscin granules (*large arrow*).

is closed by the septum to form the circular, dime-sized oval fossa or fossa ovalis. This represents the true interatrial septum, with the remainder of the anatomic structure comprising caval or pulmonary venous infoldings and the muscular and membranous components of the AV region (31). The membrane covering the oval fossa is a paper-thin, translucent layer early in life that becomes fibrotic, opaque, and thickened with age, measuring up to 2 mm in thickness. The histology of the septum displays variable amounts of atrial muscle, fibrous tissue, mature adipose tissue, and, on occasion, brown fat (Fig. 19.12). The thickness of the atrial septum varies considerably.

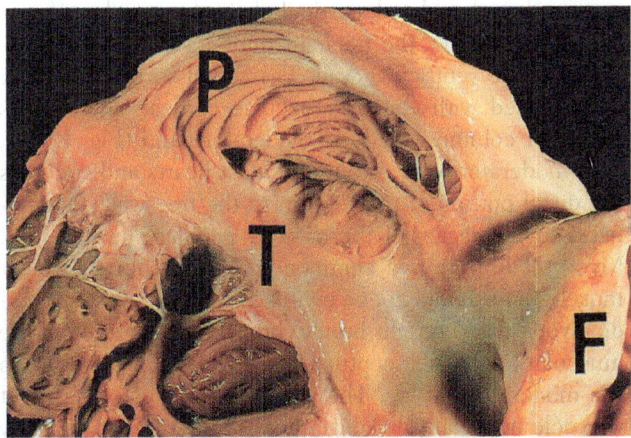

FIGURE 19.12 The right atrium showing the pectinate muscles (*P*), the crista terminalis (*T*), and the interatrial septal fat (*F*).

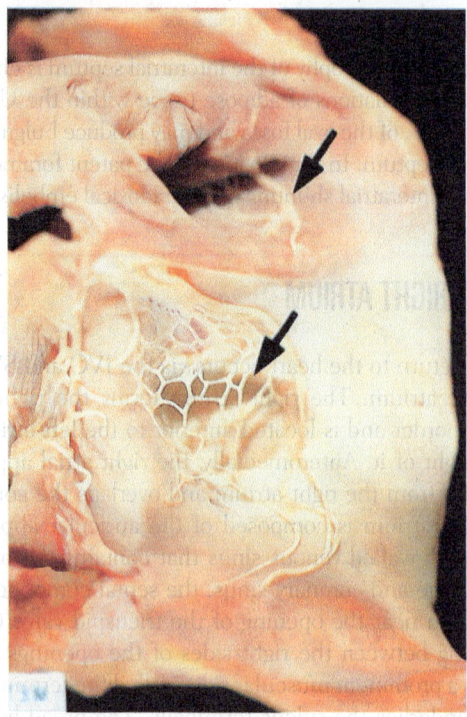

FIGURE 19.13 Picture of Chiari network (*arrows*), or lacelike pattern of the remnants of the thebesian valve, in the IVC opening into the right atrium.

mitral valve orifice. On average, the wall of the left atrium is 3 mm in thickness. The septal surface is smooth. The four pulmonary veins open into the left atrium in the posterior wall. The atrial appendage has a narrow, angulated tubular shape resembling a hockey stick (although there can be some variation in appearance) and is lined by pectinate muscles. At its interface with the venous portion of the atrium, it lacks a terminal crest. The endocardial layer is thicker and more opaque than the right side, due in part to the higher pressures of the pulmonary veins emptying into

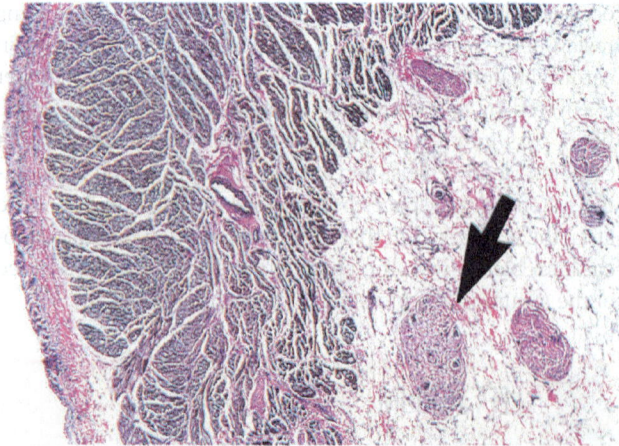

FIGURE 19.14 Section through the right atrium showing the nerves and ganglion cells (*arrow*) in the overlying subepicardial adipose tissue (elastic van Gieson).

the atrium. Sometimes a patch of thickened rough endocardium is seen on the posterior wall above the mitral valve as a result of mitral regurgitation. This is called MacCallum patch but is not usually seen in the normal heart. The atrial septum is smooth on the left side but has a central shallow depression corresponding to the oval fossa. The endocardium of the left atrium is thicker as a result of increased collagen layers, particularly near the openings of the pulmonary veins. The two left pulmonary veins enter on the posterolateral surface, and the right veins enter on the posteromedial side; there are no true valves at the venous–atrial junction. Small collections of atrial muscle can be found within the walls of the pulmonary veins at this junction and may act as physiologic valves.

In general, the composition is similar to the right atrium. Anderson and Cook emphasized two differences (39). Firstly, the myocytes of the left atrium are arranged in a more irregular fashion than the right atrium and secondly, the presence of sleeves of myocardium are in continuity between the roof of the atrium and the distal pulmonary veins at their interface. These pulmonary venous sleeves are sites of development of atrial fibrillation and targets for ablation techniques. MR imaging is routinely utilized to assess the morphology of the LA and pulmonary veins and to evaluate for postablation stenosis (40).

RIGHT VENTRICLE

The right ventricle, in both healthy and diseased states, has become the recent subject of intensive investigation (41–43). This includes techniques for morphologic and functional assessment and targeted therapeutic interventions. The morphologic right ventricle lies anterior to the other heart chambers. It has an inflow portion (sinus), an apical trabecular component, and an outflow portion (infundibulum [conus]) (44). The outflow tract is separated anatomically from the inflow tract by a muscular arch called the crista supraventricularis. The endocardial surface is coarsely trabeculated, particularly in the apical region.

On sectioning, the trabeculations form the inner two-thirds of the ventricular wall. The septal surface is deeply trabeculated with coarse trabeculae carneae and a thick muscular column called the moderator band (Fig. 19.15). This moderator band is found in most hearts and connects the distal portion of the septum to the free wall. It terminates in the region of the anterior papillary muscle (45). Myocyte disarray is a common finding within trabecular muscles and should not be confused with hypertrophic cardiomyopathy. The right bundle branch travels through the muscular ventricular septum and courses down to end in the moderator muscle. The papillary muscles of the right ventricle are relatively constant, with an anterior papillary muscle located on the anterior wall near its junction with the septum and a small posterior papillary muscle arising

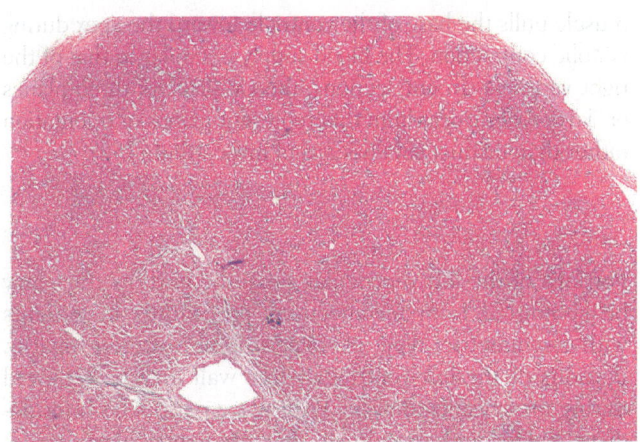

FIGURE 19.15 A section of trabeculae carneae from the normal right ventricle.

under the crista supraventricularis at the inferior border of the right ventricular outflow tract. In addition, there is an inconstant group of posterior papillary muscles that can arise from the diaphragmatic wall of the right ventricle.

The histology of the right ventricle consists of a thin endocardial layer. The thickness of myocardial wall in normal human adults is about one-third the left ventricle and measures up to 5 mm. The endocardium is similar to the other chambers, except it has more variability from region to region, with the thickest area found in the septum. The subendocardial space includes a fenestrated elastic membrane and, on occasion, bundles of smooth muscle, particularly in the interventricular septum (Fig. 19.8). The interventricular septum also contains blood vessels, nerves, and the left bundle branch of the conduction system. The ventricular free wall has numerous vascular channels consisting of intertrabecular channels that lead into myocardial sinusoids and thebesian veins. Myocardial sinusoids are also found within the trabeculae. Arterioluminal vessels, leading directly from the systemic coronary circulation into the capillary beds, empty into the myocardial sinusoids. The myocardium is richly supplied with small vascular channels that form an intramural circulation (46). There is an extensive web of capillaries that course among the cardiac muscle fibers, are fed by branches of the coronary arteries, and are drained, in part, by the coronary veins. They are also directed to the intramyocardial sinusoids and then into the lumen of the heart. Deep within the myocardial musculature is found, in addition to the capillary bed, a richly anastomosing network of irregular channels that have been called myocardial sinusoids. These sinusoids receive vessels from the coronary arteries and the capillaries and communicate with coronary veins. The connections between the coronary arteries and the cardiac chambers are called arterioluminal vessels (Fig. 19.16). Within the myocardium, variable amounts of adipose tissue can be found, particularly in the outer half of the free wall. When extensive, it is called fatty infiltration of the right ventricle and represents a metaplastic change. It should not be confused with arrhythmogenic right ventricular dysplasia/cardiomyopathy (ARVD/CMP).

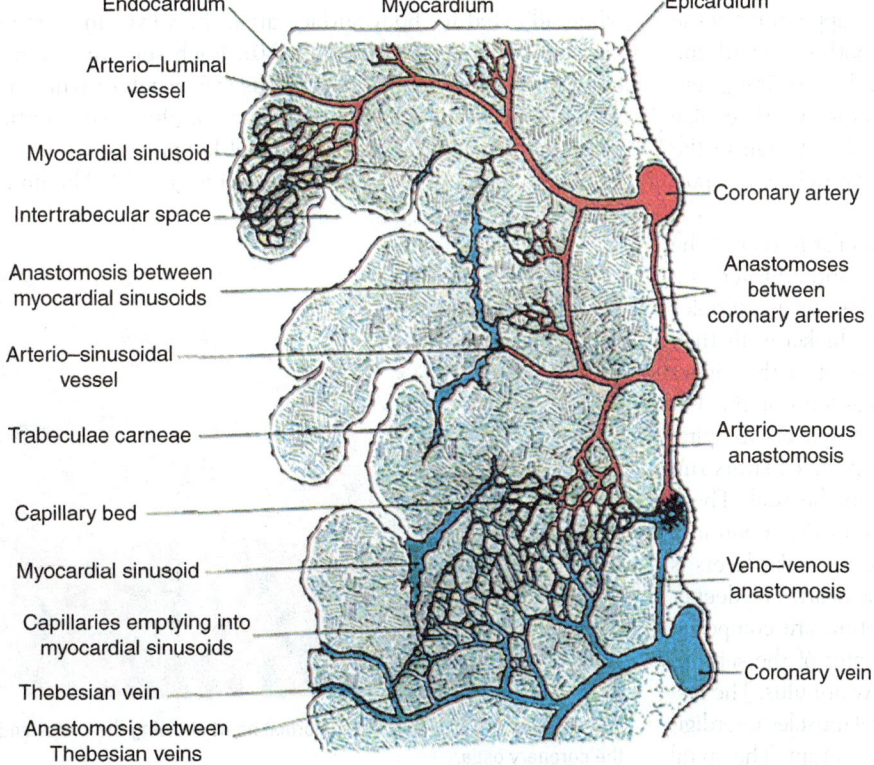

FIGURE 19.16 Diagrammatic representation of the various intramural vascular channels. (Reprinted with permission from Barry A, Patten B. The structure of the adult heart. In: Gould SE, ed. *Pathology of the Heart and Blood Vessels*. Springfield, IL: Charles C Thomas; 1968:104–105.)

Applied Anatomy

The importance of recognizing the presence of myocyte disarray and adipose tissue as common findings within the trabeculated musculature of the right ventricle of the normal adult heart has been discussed. The distinction of "physiologic adipose tissue" from ARVD/CMP is problematic and clinical, molecular, and morphologic criteria have been enumerated (47–49). Currently, CT and MR imaging are being evaluated to aid in this distinction (50). The apical trabecular region is also the site of pacemaker wire placement and endomyocardial biopsy sampling.

LEFT VENTRICLE

The left ventricle receives blood from the left atrium during ventricular diastole and ejects blood into the systemic arterial circulation across the aortic valve during ventricular systole. The left ventricle is somewhat bullet- or triangular-shaped, with the blunt tip directed anteriorly and inferiorly and to the left (51). Like the right ventricle, it is composed of inflow, septal or apical, and outflow components. It lacks the moderator band and septomarginal trabeculations of the right ventricle (36). The left ventricular chamber is surrounded by a thick muscular wall measuring up to 15 mm in thickness (*Note*: the papillary muscles are not included in the measurement). The medial wall of the left ventricle is the interventricular septum, which is shared with the right ventricle. The septum is roughly triangular in shape, with the base of the triangle at the level of the aortic cusps; it is entirely muscular, except for the small membranous septum located just below the right coronary and posterior cusps. The upper third of the septum, or outflow tract, is lined by smooth endocardium. The inferior two-thirds of the septum and the remaining ventricular walls are composed of the crisscrossing trabeculae carneae, which are thinner and less prominent than in the right ventricle. The free wall of the left ventricle is the portion that is exclusive of the septum.

The histology of the left ventricle is similar to that of the right side, although the endocardium is slightly thicker as a result of higher hemodynamic pressures. The small arterioles adjacent to the endocardium have slightly thicker walls than those of the right ventricle, likely on account of the higher pressure in the left ventricle. The myocardium of the left ventricle is arranged in such a way that it appears to spiral inward from the superficial layers. The superficial layers run at right angles to the layers deeper within the wall. These layers are intimately interdigitated to prevent dissection into lamina structures. The attachment of the muscular layers is from the fibrous skeleton at the base of the heart. The deeper muscle layers of the interventricular septum are composed of the deep bulbospiral muscle in the center of the septum originating from the septal portion of the AV annulus. The fascicles of the deep bulbospiral and sinospiral muscles interdigitate within the muscular interventricular septum. The spiral muscle pulls the base of the ventricle toward the apex during systolic contraction. The blood supply is similar to that of the right ventricle. In cut sections, the LV displays three planes or "layers" of myocardium that represent planes of orientation rather than distinct subdivisions of myocardium (52).

Applied Anatomy

Portions of the left ventricular subaortic outflow tract may be submitted from myomectomy procedures in patients with asymmetric type of hypertrophic cardiomyopathy. Portions of the left ventricular free wall may be removed during aneurysmectomy or VAD placement. The intermediate bulbospiral muscle of the interventricular septum is primarily involved in idiopathic hypertrophic subaortic stenosis (IHSS). Since it lies deep within the septum, the disarray associated with IHSS may not always be seen in the superficial myomectomy specimen. The mechanisms of myocyte replacement, senescence, and apoptosis in the normal aging heart and the role of human cardiac stem cells are currently under investigation (53).

CARDIAC VALVES

Semilunar Valves

The semilunar valves consist of the pulmonic and aortic valves. The normal valve circumference for the aortic valve is 5.7 to 7.9 cm for women and 6.0 to 8.5 cm for men. The normal pulmonic valve circumference is 5.7 to 7.4 cm for women and 9.2 to 9.9 cm for men (54). Interestingly, when adjusted for body surface area, the valves in women are slightly larger than in men (10). Each semilunar valve consists of three semicircular cusps (55), each of which is attached by its semicircular border, or annulus, to the aortic or pulmonic ring. The three points of lateral attachment of adjacent cusps are the commissures (Fig. 19.17). The lines

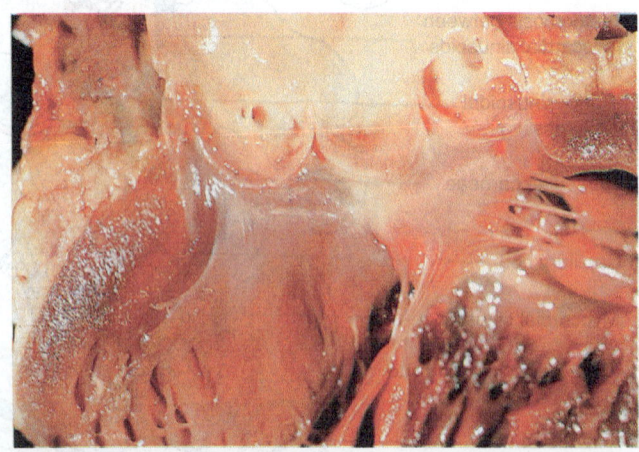

FIGURE 19.17 Aortic valve from normal heart showing the cusps and the coronary ostia.

of cusp apposition are not at the free margin but are angulated lines extending from well below the point of attachment in the commissure to just below the midpoint of the free edge. In the aortic valve, these lines (the linea alba) and the central nodules (the noduli arantii) can be seen (55). In the pulmonic valve, these landmarks are less obvious because of the lower right-sided pressures. The lunulae are thin, delicate areas of cusp between the linea alba and the free edge.

The semilunar aortic and pulmonic valves are similar in configuration, except that the aortic cusps are slightly thicker and contain coronary ostia. They are situated at the summit at the outflow tract of their corresponding ventricle, the pulmonic valve being anterior, superior, and slightly to the left of the aortic valve in the normal heart. The cusps, which are often slightly unequal in width, circle the inside of the respective vessel root (e.g., pulmonary artery trunk or aortic root). Behind each cusp, the vessel wall bulges outward, creating a pouch-like dilatation known as the sinus of Valsalva. The portion of the cusp adjacent to the rim is thin and may contain small perforations in the normal situation. The noduli arantii meet in the center and contribute to the support of the leaflets. Since the plane of the aortic valve is oblique with the right posterior side lower than the left anterior side, the origin of the left coronary artery is slightly superior to that of the right coronary artery. The ostia of coronary arteries are located in the upper third of their respective sinuses and measure from 3 to 4 mm in diameter (the left ostium is slightly wider than the right ostium). The right coronary artery passes anteriorly and to the left. In some hearts, there is a separate ostium in the right coronary sinus for the conus artery, sometimes called the third coronary artery (51).

The molecular mechanisms of valvular development during embryogenesis have been further clarified in recent studies (56). The histology of the semilunar valves is that of a well-defined multilayered structure. Three distinct layers are recognizable: the fibrosa, the spongiosa, and the ventricularis. The fibrosa is a layer of dense collagen that constitutes the major structural component of the cusp and extends to its free edge (52). The densely packed collagen bundles blend into the collagen of the valvular ring in the region of the commissures. Some fibroblasts are present in this layer, as are some very fine elastic fibers. The spongiosa is adjacent to the fibrosa and occupies a central position in the thickness of the cusp (Fig. 19.18). It is best developed in the basal third of the cusp. It does not extend to the free edge, which is composed only of fibrosa and ventricularis layers. The spongiosa is composed of large amounts of proteoglycans and glycosaminoglycans, loosely arranged collagen fibrils, scattered fibroblasts, and mesenchymal cells and serves as a "shock absorber" for the valve (57). The ventricularis is adjacent to the spongiosa and is in direct contact with the endothelial layer of the inflow surface of the cusp (i.e., closest to the ventricular surface). It is distinguished from the fibrosa by its abundance of elastic fibers.

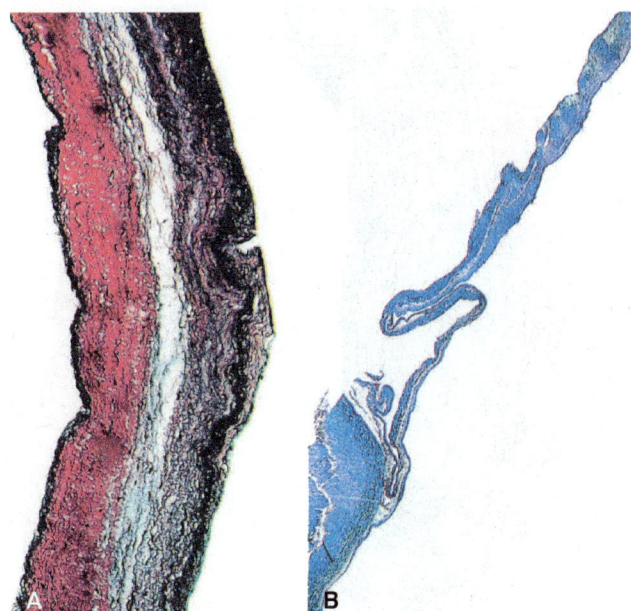

FIGURE 19.18 High- (**A**) and low-power (**B**) views of a section of the aortic cusp showing the three distinct layers as described in the text.

This feature is often helpful in orienting and identifying the layers of excised aortic valvular cusps. The surface lining of the cusps consists of a single layer of endothelial cells. At the base of the cusp, a superficial accumulation of elastic fibers called the atrialis is present, which some authors consider a fourth layer in the semilunar valve apparatus. The surface topography of the aortic cusp varies according to its state of stress. The bundles are wavy and the inflow surface is smoother in the stressed state and rougher in the relaxed state (57).

Atrioventricular Valves

The AV valves consist of the mitral valve and the tricuspid valve. The normal circumference of the tricuspid valve is 10 to 11.1 cm in women and 11.2 to 11.8 cm in men. The normal circumference of the mitral valve is 8.2 to 9.1 cm in women and 9.2 to 9.9 cm in men (54). The valvular apparatus is made up of the annulus, commissures, leaflets, chordae tendineae, and papillary muscles. The annulus is composed of a ring of circumferentially oriented collagen and elastic fibers with extensions into the ventricle and the atrium. Currently, a number of different descriptors are used in clinical practice to distinguish the two leaflets of the mitral valve (58). The smaller but broader leaflet is designated as the anterior or aortic leaflet and comprises a third of the circumference. It is arbitrarily divided into three segments (A1, A2, A3). The posterior or mural leaflet is likewise separated into three segments, beginning near the anterolateral commissure (P1) and ending near the posteromedial commissure (P3). The central segment (P2) can vary considerably in size (59).

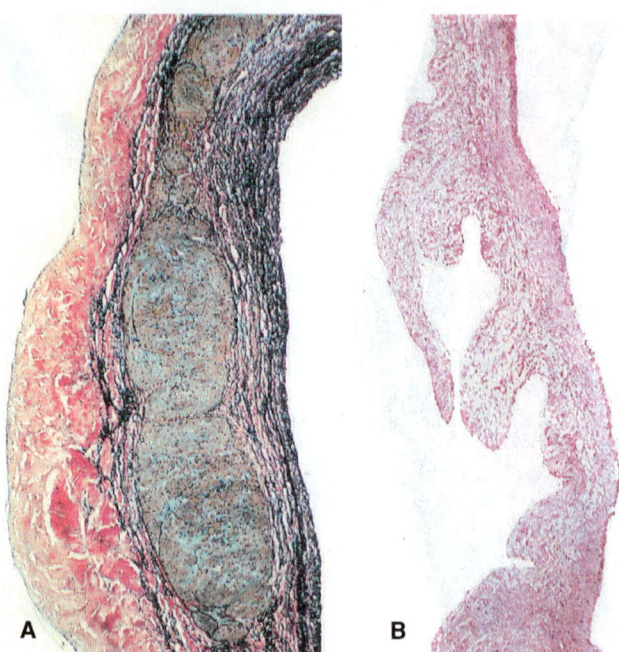

FIGURE 19.19 High- (**A**) and low-power (**B**) views of a section of the mitral leaflet showing the three distinct layers with muscle in the central portion near the base of the valve.

The AV valves have four histologic layers (atrialis/auricularis, spongiosa, fibrosa, and ventricularis) (Fig. 19.19). As in the semilunar valves, all layers contain valve interstitial cells which are essential for extracellular matrix remodeling and maintaining structural integrity (60). There is an abundance of collagen fibers and the different types include type I (74%), type III (24%), and type V (2%) (54). The collagen bundles of the annulus spread down into the majority of the cusps of the mitral valve (except at the free edge of the leaflet) and are known as the fibrosa. They continue into the chordae tendineae and finally spread out into a network that covers the tip of the papillary muscles (Fig. 19.20). Adjacent to the fibrosa layer on the ventricular side of the valve is the ventricularis. The ventricularis contains many elastic and collagen fibers and is covered by endothelium. Some of the elastic fibers extend into the chordae tendineae, but in general, this layer is incomplete, as it does not extend to the free edge of the leaflet. The spongiosa is situated on the atrial side of the fibrosa layer. Like the semilunar valves, it has a rich matrix of proteoglycans and glycosaminoglycans and a few elastic fibers, collagen fibrils, and connective tissue cells such as interstitial fibroblasts (57,59). This layer, along with the fibrosa layer, extends throughout the entire length of the leaflet. The spongiosa in the anterior and posterior mitral leaflets can contain cardiac myocytes that are a direct extension of the left atrial myocardium but not in continuity (Fig. 19.19). In the anterior mitral leaflet, this layer extends into the middle third, whereas in the posterior leaflet it only extends into its proximal third. Neural elements and lymphatics can be found in the leaflets. The atrial aspect of the spongiosa (i.e., layer closest to the atrium) is covered by the atrialis or auricularis, which in turn has a continuous endothelial lining. The auricularis contains collagen and elastic fibers and smooth muscle cells. It is prominent near the annulus but thins out in the distal third of the leaflet such that the most distal aspect of the valves is composed only of spongiosa and fibrosa. The endothelial cells on the atrial aspect of the AV valves are plump and have irregular nuclei compared with the flatter endothelial cells on the ventricular aspect.

The architecture of the tricuspid valve apparatus and the layered arrangements of its leaflets are similar to those in the mitral valve; however, the individual layers are thinner in the tricuspid valve. Cardiac muscle bundles insert fairly low into the base of the tricuspid leaflets but do not extend into the leaflet substance. In the posterior and septal leaflets, the auricularis is thicker and contains more abundant smooth muscle cells.

Chordae Tendineae

The chordae tendineae in the normal state are thin fibrous cords that emanate in a fan-like manner from the broad leaflets of the AV valves and insert into the papillary muscles (Fig. 19.20). The central cores of the chordae are composed of longitudinally oriented collagen fibrils. The core is surrounded more peripherally by loosely arranged collagen fibrils and elastic fibers and is embedded in proteoglycan-rich matrix (Fig. 19.21) (57,59). Some chordae contain a small central core of muscle known as chordae muscularis (Fig. 19.22), although others contain blood vessels and collagen in variable amounts and appear fleshier in color (Fig. 19.23). The endothelial cells on the chordae resemble the flattened ovoid nuclei of the ventricular surface of the leaflets.

Applied Anatomy of Intracardiac Valves

Semilunar and AV valves are frequently encountered in the surgical pathology laboratory. Indications for valvular

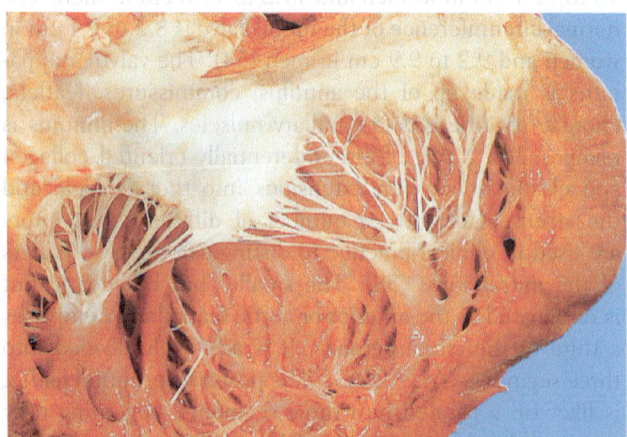

FIGURE 19.20 A normal mitral valve with chordae tendineae inserting into the papillary muscles.

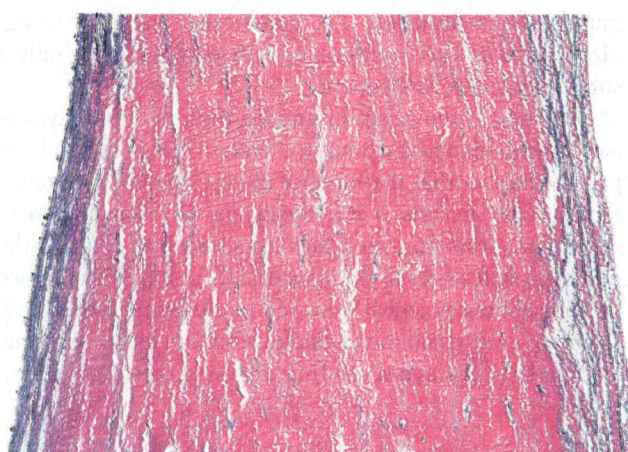

FIGURE 19.21 Longitudinal section of chordae tendineae showing the relationships of elastic fibers on the surface and collagen in the center (elastic van Gieson).

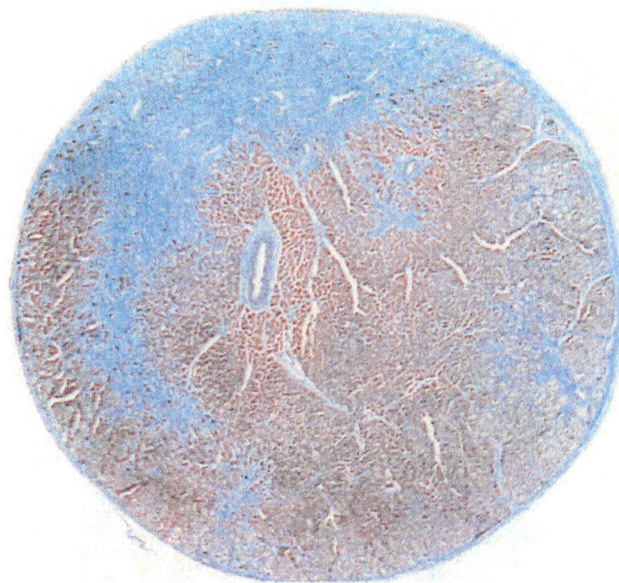

FIGURE 19.23 Transverse section of a muscular chorda showing fibrous tissue, muscle, and small vessel within the chorda (Masson trichrome).

replacement or repair include a variety of congenital, infectious, inflammatory, degenerative, and paraneoplastic causes. In many cases, the chordae and portions of papillary muscle may be attached. In the setting of myocardial infarction, infection, or valvular prolapse, ruptured papillary muscles may become surgical specimens. Lambl excrescences and fibrous nodules are papillary projections along the lines of closure or free edge of the valve, respectively.

Aging Changes of Intracardiac Valves

With age, all the cardiac valves become thicker, more opaque, and less pliable, particularly left-sided valves. The increase in collagen content may account for the loss of plasticity, and calcifications or lipid accumulations may be present—the so-called aortic valve sclerosis. Small windows or fenestrations may be found above the lines of closure but these do not affect valvular function. The anterior leaflet of the mitral valve often shows yellow atheromatous alteration or atheromatosis due to lipid deposition, while the posterior leaflet may become more opaque. Mild myxomatous degeneration is also more common in the mitral valve leaflets of the elderly. The mitral valve annulus (the so-called mitral annular calcification) may become calcified with age. Age-related changes in the pulmonic valve can include opacification of the leaflets, central nodular thickening along the edge of cusps (nodules of Morgagni), Lambl excrescences, and fenestrations. Myxomatous degeneration can occur in the tricuspid valve. Leaflets that contact pacemaker wires can become thickened and nodular. The valvular circumferences of all valves increase with age (10).

PAPILLARY MUSCLES

The two papillary muscles of the right ventricle (anterior and conal) are relatively constant. There is also a group of inconstant posterior papillary muscles on the inferior wall. In the left ventricle, there are two constant papillary muscles: the anterolateral and posteromedial. The papillary muscles receive the chordae. They are variable in shape and width and on occasion may have multiple heads (Fig. 19.20).

The histology of the papillary muscles includes the fibrous cap, into which the chordae insert (Fig. 19.24). This is a normal constituent and should not be interpreted as abnormal fibrosis. The small arteries and arterioles in the papillary muscle are notable for their wall thickness and irregularity in comparison to other intracardiac small vessels

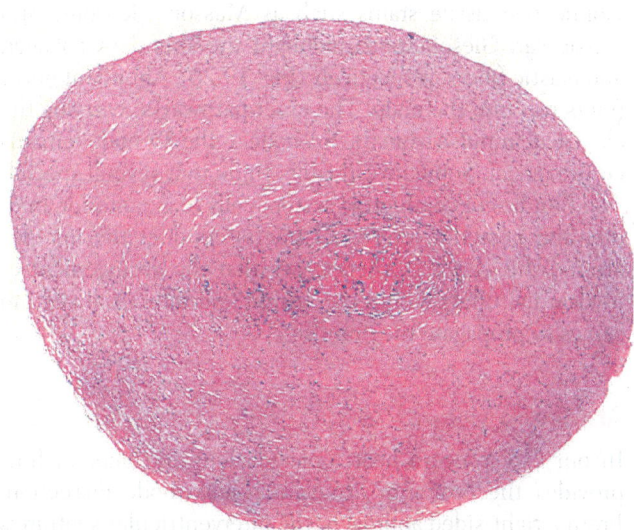

FIGURE 19.22 Transverse section of chordae tendineae showing central core of muscle (H&E).

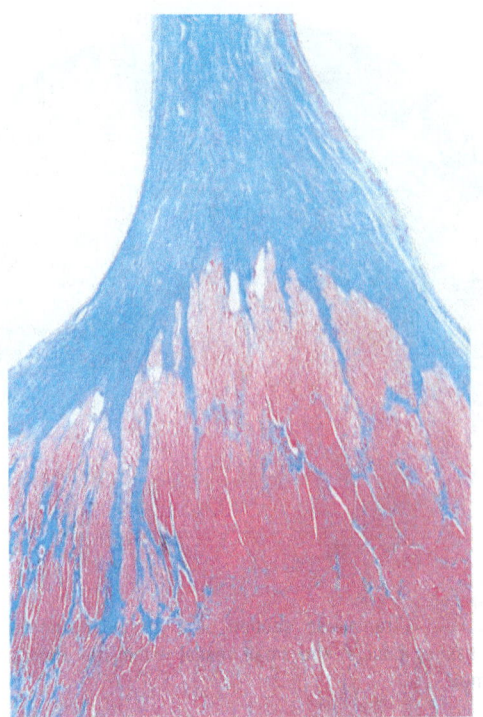

FIGURE 19.24 Longitudinal section of papillary muscle showing the fibrous cap of the insertion of the chordae tendineae (Masson trichrome).

(Fig. 19.25). The myocardium and the endocardial covering are similar to their counterparts described elsewhere. In marked ventricular dilatation, the papillary muscles may become thinned and flattened.

CONDUCTION SYSTEM

Myocardial fibers are delineated along two functional pathways in humans: (a) contractile fibers and (b) myocardial fibers specialized for the initiation and propagation of an impulse for contraction. The conduction system is recognized to be myogenic in origin, with nerves playing only a subsidiary controlling function.

For most pathologists, examining the conduction system is often regarded as a daunting exercise. This is due in large part to the fact that the number of cases requiring detailed morphologic analysis is infrequent and is often limited to specific requests from clinicians. In addition to detailing the microscopic features of the sinoatrial (SA) and AV nodes, we will present our practical approach to the dissection of these structures. We recommend careful attention to key anatomic landmarks to ensure successful retrieval of these structures.

Sinoatrial Node

The SA node has the highest intrinsic rate and is recognized as the primary pacemaker of the heart. This node is situated within the terminal groove at the junction of the SVC and the lateral border of the right atrium (Fig. 19.26). Its position is constant and is marked by the apex of the crest of the atrial appendage. It is ovoid or cigar shaped in most hearts, but cases of horseshoe-shaped SA nodes that extend into the interatrial groove are reported. Removal of a rectangular block of tissue that includes the distal SVC and atrium on either side of the terminal groove is recommended. Serial sectioning in a longitudinal plane parallel to the terminal groove at 2-mm intervals is recommended, and all the tissue slices can be accommodated in two tissue cassettes. Grossly identifying the SA nodal artery is also helpful in procuring the node (Fig. 19.26). This is a branch of the right coronary artery that is found in slightly more than half of the general population. Microscopically, the node is arranged around a central artery adjacent to the epicardial adipose tissue. The node is composed of dense connective tissue within which the small muscle fibers are embedded. The muscle fibers contain sparse myofibrils, the striations are not prominent, and the whole mass has a pseudosyncytial appearance. Connective tissue stains such as Masson trichrome and elastic van Gieson stains highlight the abundant collagen and elastic fibers, respectively (Fig. 19.26). Abundant nerve fibers run into the node. The exact pathway(s) carrying the electrical impulse from the SA node to the AV node remains controversial. Some investigators think that several specialized bundles of conducting system cells (e.g., anterior, middle, and posterior internodal tracts) conduct the impulse around the atrium. Others argue that the arrangement of myocardial fibers within the atrium and interatrial septum serves to propagate the impulse (16).

Atrioventricular Node

In our experience a heart opened along the lines of flow provides the optimum exposure for AV node dissection. From a right-sided approach, the interventricular septum is oriented with the tip of the apex pointing downward. The important landmarks include the oval fossa, ostium of the

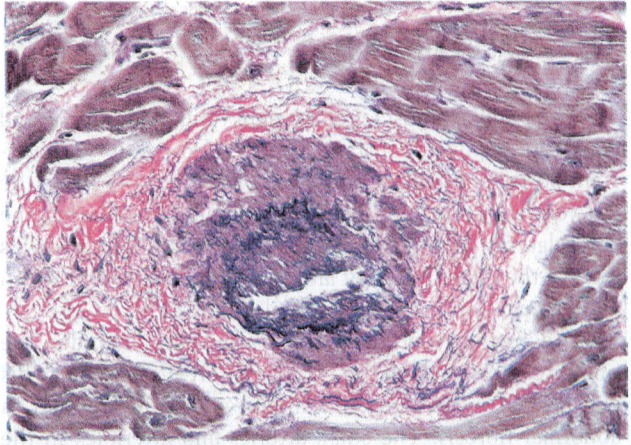

FIGURE 19.25 Section of abnormally thickened arteriole within a papillary muscle (elastic van Gieson).

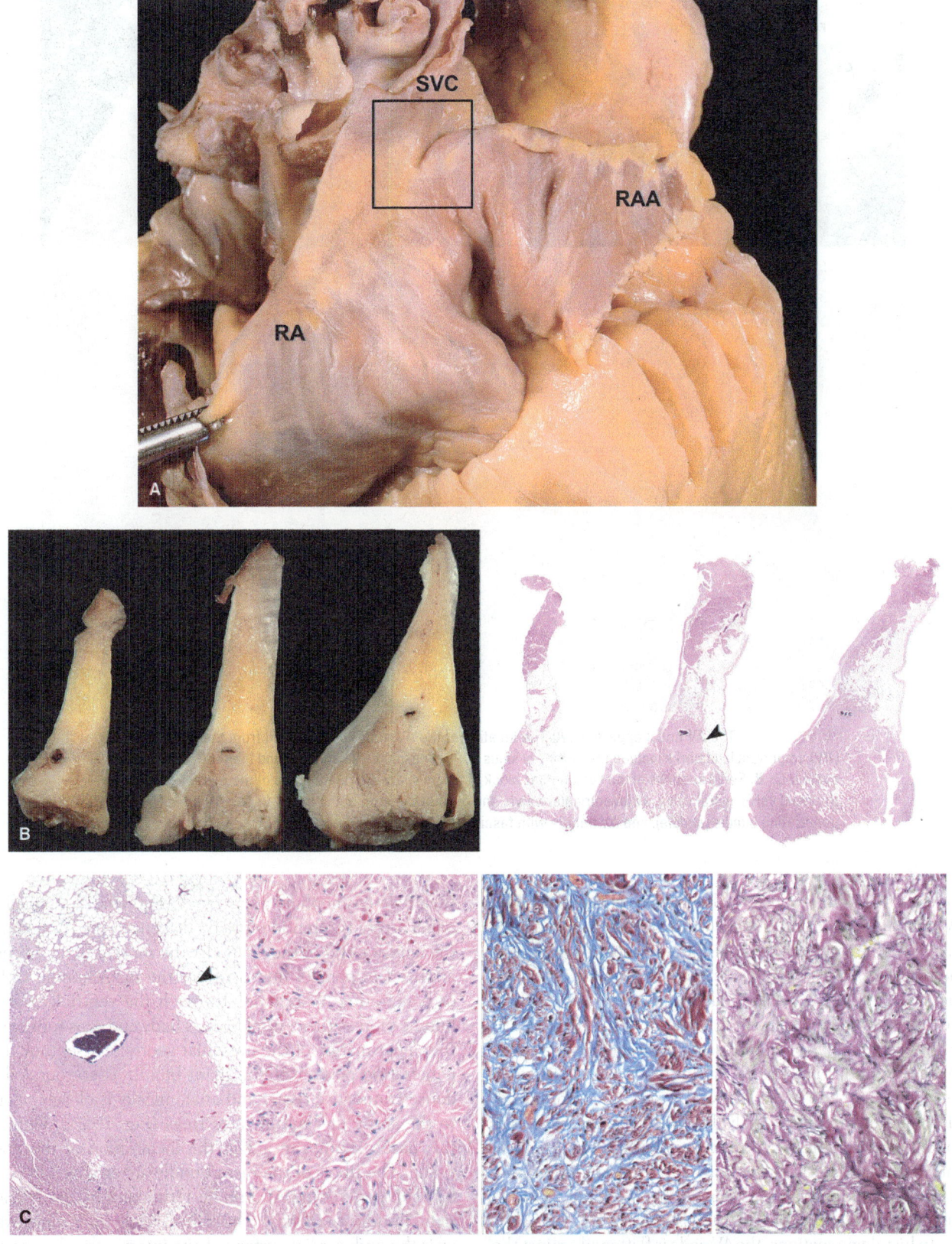

FIGURE 19.26 The SA node. **A:** The location of the SA node within the terminal groove at the junction of the superior vena cava (*SVC*) and crest of the atrial appendage (*box*). RA, right atrium; RAA, right atrial appendage. **B:** Macroscopic and low-power magnification of serial sections of nodal tissue. Note the nodal artery that is adjacent to the SA node. **C:** High-power magnification of the SA node showing the specialized fibers embedded within collagen and elastic tissue (H&E, trichrome, and elastic van Gieson stains).

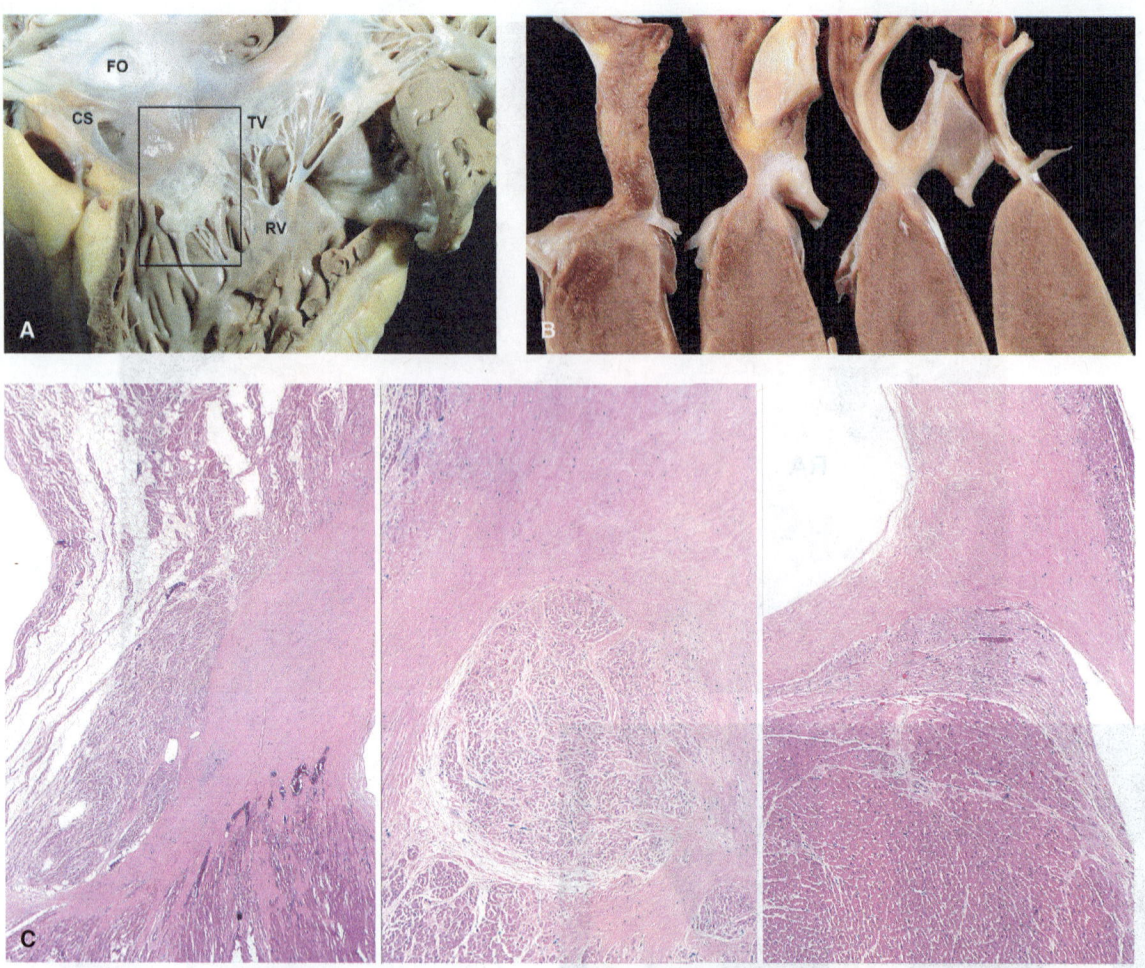

FIGURE 19.27 The AV nodal apparatus. **A:** The location of the AV node (*box*) viewed from the right ventricle (*RV*). Important landmarks include the coronary sinus (*CS*), tricuspid valve annulus and leaflet (*TV*), and fossa ovale (*FO*). **B:** Serial sections of the rectangular block of tissue show the relationship of the nodal tissue to the tricuspid valve, mitral valve, atrioventricular valve, and fibrous skeleton of the heart. **C:** The AV node (*left*), AV penetrating bundle (*middle*), and AV bundle with fascicle (*right*) are shown.

coronary sinus, and tricuspid valve annulus and leaflets. The AV node lies within the subendocardial tissues on the right side of the interatrial septum just anterior to the opening of the coronary sinus, posterior to the membranous interventricular septum (tendon of Todaro), and above the tricuspid valve annulus within the triangle of Koch (Fig. 19.27) (61). A rectangular block of tissue, beginning with a vertical incision adjacent to the ostium of the coronary sinus and extending 1 to 2 cm below the annulus, is removed. After careful trimming of valvular structures, the block will contain components of the tricuspid valve (septal leaflet) and mitral and aortic valves (Fig. 19.27). Serial sectioning at 2- to 3-mm intervals and sequential placement in tissue cassettes yield a total of 8 to 10 cassettes.

In histologic sections, the AV node is flattened against the central fibrous body and is composed of a network of muscle fibers, with the superficial zone having fibers arranged in a parallel manner. These specialized fibers retain their intercalated discs and striations but are characterized by their pale eosinophilic appearance (Fig. 19.27). A small AV nodal artery is often identified adjacent to the AV node. At the anterior end of the AV node, the muscle fibers become arranged in parallel lines to form the main bundle of His or penetrating AV bundle. To reach the ventricle, the AV bundle pierces the central fibrous body and runs forward on the upper margin of the muscular ventricular septum. This penetrating portion of the main bundle is surrounded by dense connective tissue and anatomically is closely related to the aortic and mitral valve rings (Fig. 19.27). Connective tissue stains can aid in the localization of the nodal tissue. The fibers of the main bundle are arranged in parallel. The penetrating AV bundle terminates as the left and right bundle branches. The left fascicle runs downward over the endocardial surface of the interventricular septum to the base of the anterior papillary muscle, and the right fascicle ends in the moderator band of the right ventricle. Direct connection of both bundle branches to a complex ramifying system of subendocardial conduction fibers can

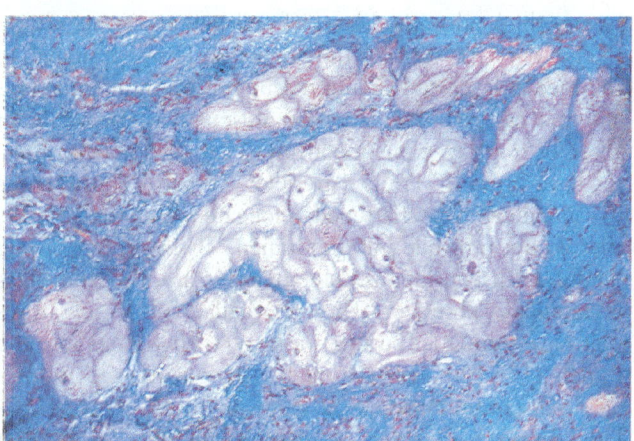

FIGURE 19.28 Section showing the pale cells of the mammalian conducting system. These cells contain glycogen and only sparse myofibrils (Masson trichrome).

be demonstrated in mammalian hearts. Light microscopy shows the fibers in the bundle of His and the conduction bundles to be small and contain few myofibrils (Fig. 19.28).

Aging Changes in the Human Conduction System

With advancing age, the SA node displays progressive increase in fibrous and adipose tissues and reduction of constituent nodal cells, while the AV node remains relatively unchanged comparatively except for minimal increases in adipose tissue or elastic fibers. Similarly, fibrous tissue increases in the upper portion of the interventricular septum. These changes are associated with a loss of conduction fibers in the region of the left bundle branch. Up to 50% of the left bundle origin may be lost in people over 60 years of age (62).

CARDIAC INNERVATION

The nerve supply of the heart is autonomic, including both the sympathetic and parasympathetic supply via both the efferent and afferent fibers. Histologically, large nerves can be seen in the epicardium and adjacent to the coronary blood vessels. Small nerves within the myocardium are hard to identify unless special stains are used. Myocardial nerves are best viewed using electron microscopic examination, by which the autonomic nerves can be distinguished. Cardiac ganglia (parasympathetic) can be found over the surface of the atria and in the AV groove (Fig. 19.14).

Autonomic Nerves

Axonal varicosities occur at irregular intervals along autonomic fibers, and their morphology is considered useful in determining whether the nerve is adrenergic or cholinergic (57). In cholinergic nerves, the varicosities contain accumulations of agranular vesicles and a few mitochondria. In

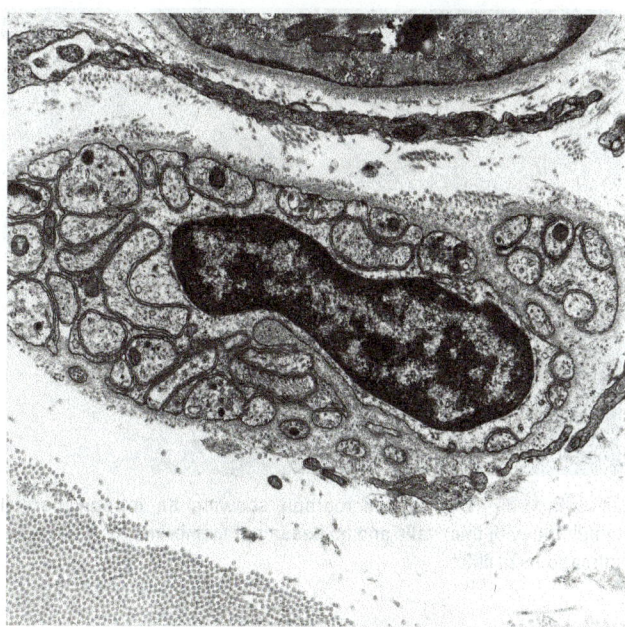

FIGURE 19.29 Electron micrograph of sympathetic nerve showing dense-core granules in the myocardium (original magnification ×22,500).

adrenergic nerves, the varicosities contain vesicles rich in electron-dense cores. Each of these cores is separated from the limiting membrane of the vesicle by an electron-lucent zone (Fig. 19.29). Presumptive sensory nerve terminals have large diameters and contain numerous mitochondria. They are located in perivascular regions and are surrounded by Schwann cells. A given Schwann cell may enclose adrenergic and cholinergic axons together with sensory axons (57). Autonomic ganglia are found in the subepicardial tissue of the atria and atrial appendages and at the root of the great vessels, along the interatrial and AV grooves in the atrial septum, and in the vicinity of the SA and AV nodes. Large nerves can be seen in the subepicardial layer adjacent to the epicardial coronary arteries.

LYMPHATICS

There are two networks of lymphatics in the heart: (a) in the endocardium and (b) in the epicardium. The route of drainage of the endocardial network is through channels in the myocardium into the epicardial lymphatics. The epicardial meshwork of channels, containing many valves, drains toward the AV sulcus by means of several longitudinal channels that run for the most part parallel to the coronary veins in the anterior and posterior longitudinal sulci of the ventricles (57). Lymphatics leave the pericardial cavity to empty into one of the pulmonary hilar lymph nodes and join the lymphatic drainage system of the mediastinum or into the thoracic duct. Lymphatics are also found in the myocardial valves and lie within the grooves of the coronary blood vessels.

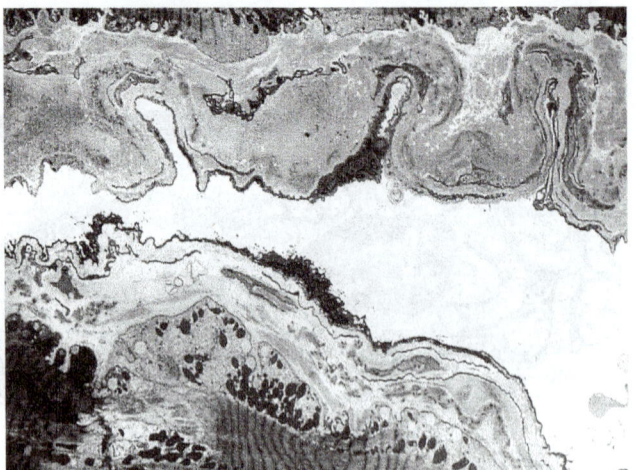

FIGURE 19.30 Electron micrograph showing an intramyocardial lymphatic with thin walls and no basement membrane (original magnification ×20,000).

The lymph capillaries and larger lymphatic vessels accompany blood vessels in the myocardial interstitium. The walls of the myocardial lymphatics consist of extremely thin endothelial cells, the nuclei of which bulge into the lumen (Fig. 19.30). In contrast to endothelial cells of blood capillaries, those of the lymphatic capillaries do not have a well-defined external basal lamina. The larger lymphatics are confined to the outer third of the myocardial wall and occasionally contain valves. These flap-like structures contain a core of collagen embedded in microfibrils and are covered by endothelia.

SMALL INTRAMURAL CORONARY ARTERIES

The structure of the intramural coronary arteries and the larger coronary arteries is similar and consists of the endothelium (intima), spirally aligned smooth muscle (media), and adventitia (Fig. 19.31). Of note, muscular arteries have a thick adventitial layer of collagen and some elastic fibers. The thickness of the adventitia is often similar to the medial layer and should not be misinterpreted as perivascular fibrosis. The smallest muscular arteries contain three or four layers of smooth muscles, while larger arteries have up to 40 layers. Arterioles (vessels <100 microns in diameter) have flattened, elongated endothelial cells that do not protrude into the lumen. Their internal elastic lamina is discontinuous. Metarterioles are also known as precapillary sphincters. The endothelial cells in metarterioles have numerous surface projections that bulge into the lumen (57). Although the medial smooth muscles form a single discontinuous layer, it gradually disappears as capillaries begin. Capillaries are distinguished by the fact that their walls are composed of only a single layer of endothelial cells. They do not have smooth muscle cells but may have closely associated pericytes (57). Capillary endothelial cells may have microvilli and cytoplasmic processes (filopodia). The myocardium has a rich network of capillaries. These branches undergo anastomosis and eventually become thin-walled venules measuring up to 100 μm in diameter.

VEINS AND VENULES

Venules have thin, flat endothelial cells and characteristically contain a large amount of connective tissue in the vicinity of their external surface; they contain collagen fibrils that approach the endothelial layer and are anchored on its outer surface (57). Venules gradually increase in size to become veins. Veins have larger lumens but thinner walls than their arterial counterparts.

Veins have three layers: intima, media, and adventitia. The intima is thin, lacks smooth muscle cells, and has a poorly defined internal elastic lamina. The media is also thin and contains few smooth muscle cells and elastic fibers. The adventitia is thick with abundant collagen and elastic fibers. Cardiac veins drain blood into either the coronary sinus or directly into the chambers (thebesian veins).

THE ENDOMYOCARDIAL BIOPSY

The transvenous endomyocardial biopsy is currently utilized for the diagnosis of allograft rejection and a variety of inflammatory, metabolic, and neoplastic conditions that affect the heart. Introduced in the early 1960s, the bioptome and the technique have undergone modifications that now permit clinicians the opportunity to obtain cardiac tissue in a safe outpatient setting (63). The right internal jugular vein or femoral vein approaches are commonly used. Complications are uncommon and include local problems (such as hematomas and nerve injury) and cardiac problems (such as arrhythmias, tricuspid valve apparatus damage, and ventricular perforation).

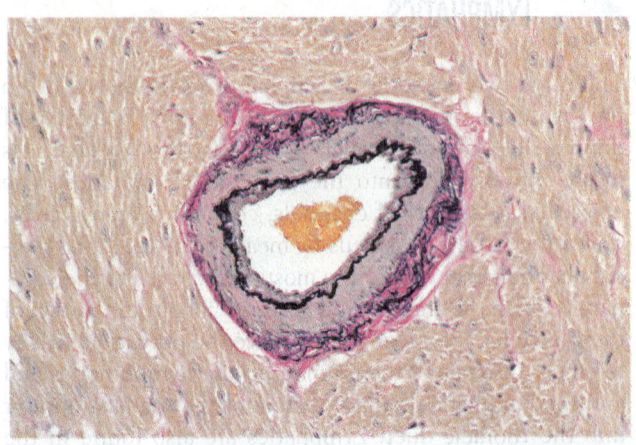

FIGURE 19.31 Transverse section of intramyocardial arteriole (elastic van Gieson).

Tissue Handling and Processing

Proper tissue procurement and handling are critical for optimal diagnostic evaluation (64). Biopsy specimens should be gently extracted from the bioptome with a needle tip to limit crush artifactual distortion. The clinical indications for the biopsy determine, in large part, the method of tissue handling. For example, for standard light microscopy, the tissue should immediately be placed in a standard fixative such as 10% neutral buffered formalin. To demonstrate the type of amyloid fibril in cardiac amyloidosis by immunofluorescence (e.g., AL, AA, or transthyretin), one or two pieces should be received in saline or Zeus medium and then snap frozen in a plastic BEEM capsule containing an embedding medium. The diagnosis of chronic anthracycline cardiotoxicity requires that *all* the biopsy pieces (minimum of three to five pieces) be submitted in fixative for transmission electron microscopy (e.g., 2.5% glutaraldehyde with 2% paraformaldehyde in 0.1M sodium cacodylate buffer, pH 7.2).

For routine diagnostic evaluation, overnight processing and paraffin embedding are sufficient. For emergent cases, a 60- to 90-minute rapid ("ultra") processing cycle is available, and microscopic slides can be prepared within 3 to 4 hours. All the biopsy pieces should be embedded in the same block. We recommend that a minimum of three slides be prepared, with each sectioned at 4 to 5 μm thickness from various depths within the paraffin block. Multiple fragments, or "ribbons," are placed on each slide.

We routinely stain with hematoxylin and eosin (H&E) and use stains such as Masson trichrome to confirm the presence of myocyte damage or fibrosis, Congo red stain for amyloid fibrils, and the Prussian blue stain for iron deposition. Immunohistochemical, immunofluorescent, and molecular studies are utilized for specific indications. Paraffin-section immunohistochemistry is used to evaluate for the presence of infectious myocarditis (e.g., cytomegalovirus [CMV] or toxoplasmic myocarditis), posttransplant lymphoproliferative disorders (PTLD) (B-cell clonality, Epstein–Barr virus [EBV] latent membrane proteins, anomalous coexpression of B-cell and T-cell antigens), or acute antibody-mediated rejection (intravascular collections of CD68+ histiocytes and deposition of C4d on the microvasculature). In situ hybridization is helpful to demonstrate the presence of EBV or other viral genome or light chain restriction in PTLD.

Biopsy Limitations and Tissue Artifacts

Sampling error in the diagnosis of rejection, myocarditis, and infection remains a major consideration in the clinical management of patients and the evaluation of new noninvasive diagnostic modalities. In general, the false-negative rate is low, particularly when four or more pieces of tissue are submitted. The issue of how many lymphocytes are normally found in the myocardium has been addressed in a number of studies. In an endomyocardial biopsy study, the mean number of lymphocytes reported is fewer than 5 per high-power field (65). Tazelaar and Billingham reported foci of mononuclear inflammatory cells in 9.3% of cases in which biopsy samples were obtained from donor hearts just before transplant. These foci ranged from 6 to at least 50 cells in number (66). In an autopsy study of young men who died from acute traumatic injury, focal collections of at least 100 mononuclear cells were found in 5% of cases. The study predated the Dallas criteria and the term "focal myocarditis" was utilized (67). These studies support the concept that small clusters of mononuclear cells, including lymphocytes and macrophages, are normal within the myocardium and should not be indiscriminately classified as myocarditis.

A variety of artifacts occur in endomyocardial biopsy specimens that may mimic pathologic lesions. The surgical pathologist must be aware of these patterns to avoid a misdiagnosis that could lead to unnecessary therapeutic interventions. These have been reviewed in detail in a recent publication and only selected topics will be briefly reviewed (68). The most common biopsy artifact is the presence of contraction bands in myocytes (Fig. 19.32A). They are identical to the linear bands observed in acute ischemic necrosis and catecholamine ("pressor") effect. These changes are induced by the biopsy procedure itself and can be diminished by using fixatives stored at room temperature. In ischemic injury, the nuclei of surrounding myocytes are usually pyknotic (Fig. 19.32B), while in artifactually induced contraction bands, the nuclei remain normal in appearance.

Another frequent artifact is intussusception, or "telescoping," of small arteries that has been confused with luminal occlusion by thrombus and transplant-related arteriosclerosis. Connective tissue stains such as Masson trichrome or elastic van Gieson highlight the internal elastic membranes of both vessel segments (Fig. 19.32C). Intramyocardial accumulations of mature adipose tissue can simulate the epicardial tissue, especially if associated with vessels of relatively large caliber (Fig. 19.32D). Both can be found in the right ventricular apical region, and adipose tissue is found not uncommonly in woman and elderly patients. This should not be confused with arrhythmogenic right ventricular cardiomyopathy; clinical–pathologic correlation is essential for this purpose.

Ventricular perforation is identified by the presence of mesothelial cells (Fig. 19.32E). Accumulations of fresh platelet- and fibrin-rich thrombus may be identified along the endocardial surface of biopsy fragments (Fig. 19.32F). These form as a result of the repetitive placement of the bioptome along the endocardial surface and do not indicate chronic mural thrombi. A number of patterns of bioptome-induced tissue distortion or crush artifact can be observed in biopsy samples. The "hour-glass" or "Victorian waistband" effect is caused by central constriction of the tissue by the bioptome mechanism (Fig. 19.32G). A more problematic artifact is the smearing of cytoplasmic and nuclear components of cells that yields strands of basophilic material (Fig. 19.32H). In this setting, it may not be possible to distinguish the cell types (lymphocytes, endothelial cells, histiocytes, myocytes), and we do not attempt to evaluate

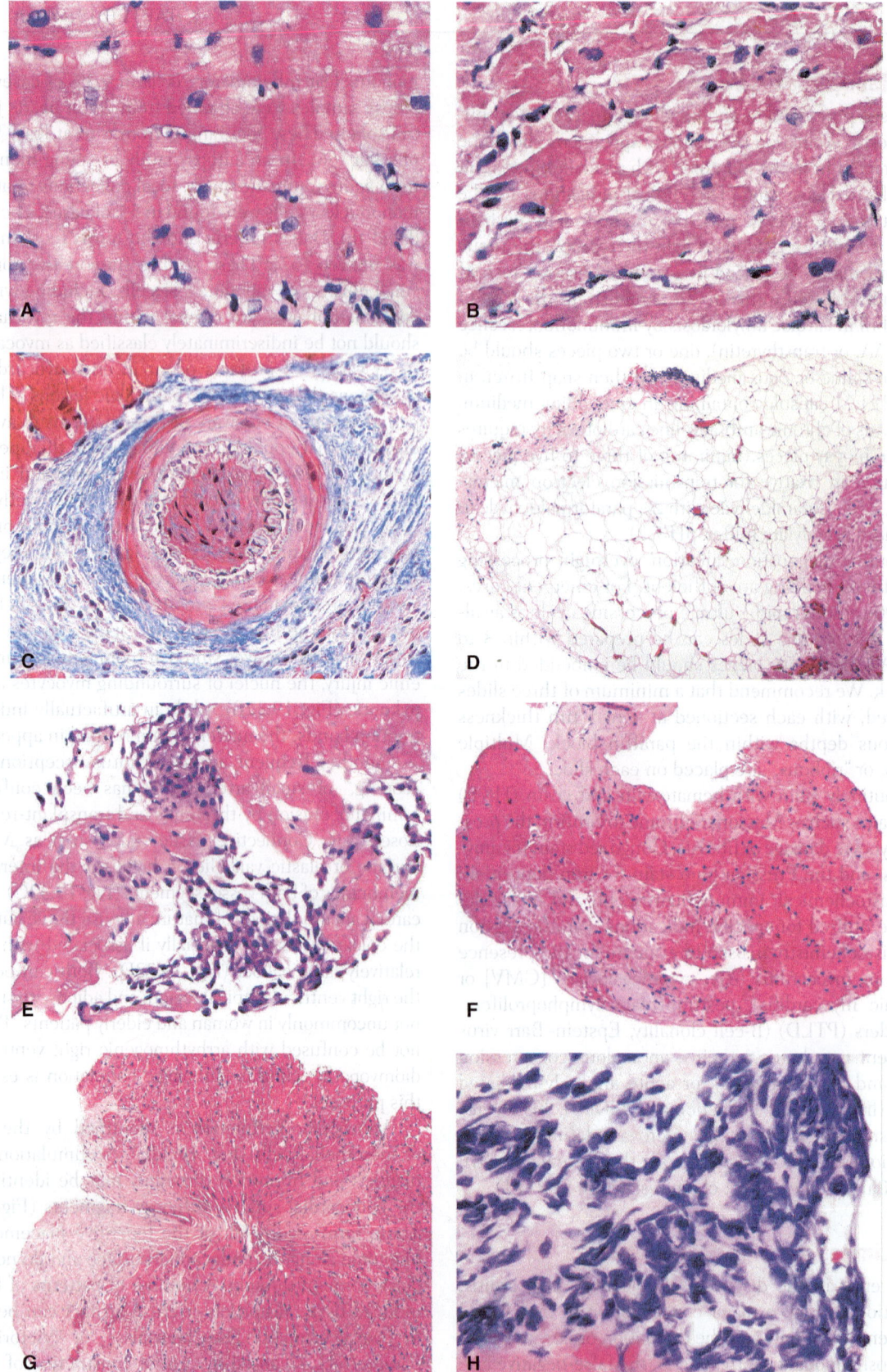

FIGURE 19.32 Artifacts of endomyocardial biopsy specimens. **A:** Contraction band artifact (H&E); note the normal appearance of myocyte nuclei. **B:** Contraction band necrosis with hyperchromatic pyknotic nuclei and eosinophilic cytoplasm. The changes are contrasted with the common contraction band artifact in **A**. **C:** Telescoping of intramyocardial artery is highlighted by a trichrome stain. **D:** Intramyocardial adipose tissue. The presence of fat does not imply epicardial localization or perforation. **E:** Mesothelial cells admixed with fibrin indicative of ventricular perforation. **F:** Thrombus without attached myocardial tissue. **G:** Bioptome-induced "Victorian waistband" artifact. **H:** Crush artifactual distortion of cells.

these foci for allograft rejection or myocarditis. In some cases, procurement of additional leveled H&E-stained sections can provide less distorted foci in the deeper aspects of the biopsy sample. In our experience, immunohistochemical stains have not been consistent or helpful.

SUMMARY

Because of the unique structural–functional nature of cardiac disease, the surgical pathologist should have a working knowledge of anatomy, histology, and physiology. Moreover, the alterations produced by the endomyocardial biopsy and the bioptome require familiarity with the myriad of tissue artifacts. With a practical understanding of these points, the evaluation of specimens ranging from endomyocardial samples to explanted hearts will enhance the diagnostic information provided to clinicians and patients.

REFERENCES

1. Lund LH, Khush KK, Cherikh WS, et al. The Registry of the International Society for Heart and Lung Transplantation: Thirty-Fourth Adult Heart Transplantation Report-2017; Focus Theme: Allograft ischemic time. *J Heart Lung Transplant* 2017;36:1037–1046.
2. Chambers DC, Yusen RD, Cherikh WS, et al. The Registry of the International Society for Heart and Lung Transplantation: Thirty-Fourth Adult Lung and Heart-Lung Transplantation Report-2017; Focus Theme: Allograft ischemic time. *J Heart Lung Transplant* 2017;36:1047–1059.
3. Rossano JW, Cherikh WS, Chambers DC, et al. The Registry of the International Society for Heart and Lung Transplantation: Twentieth Pediatric Heart Transplantation Report-2017; Focus Theme: Allograft ischemic time. *J Heart Lung Transplant* 2017;36:1060–1069.
4. Goldfarb SB, Levvey BJ, Cherikh WS, et al. The Registry of the International Society for Heart and Lung Transplantation: Twentieth Pediatric Lung and Heart-Lung Transplantation Report-2017; Focus Theme: Allograft ischemic time. *J Heart Lung Transplant* 2017;36:1070–1079.
5. Jacobs JE. Computed tomographic evaluation of the normal cardiac anatomy. *Radiol Clin North Am* 2010;48:701–710.
6. Surkova E, Muraru D, Aruta P, et al. Current clinical applications of three-dimensional echocardiography: When the technique makes the difference. *Curr Cardiol Rep* 2016;18:109.
7. Scholz DG, Kitzman DW, Hagen PT, et al. Age-related changes in normal human hearts during the first 10 decades of life. Part I (growth): A quantitative anatomic study of 200 specimens from subjects from birth to 19 years old. *Mayo Clin Proc* 1988;63:126–136.
8. Ludwig J, ed. *Handbook of Autopsy Practice*. 3rd ed. Totowa, NJ: Humana Press; 2002.
9. Hudson R. Structure and function of the heart. In: Hudson R, ed. *Cardiovascular Pathology*. Vol. 1. London: Edward Arnold; 1965:12–23.
10. Kitzman DW, Scholz DG, Hagen PT, et al. Age-related changes in normal human hearts during the first 10 decades of life. Part II (maturity): A quantitative anatomic study of 765 specimens from subjects 20 to 99 years old. *Mayo Clin Proc* 1988;63:137–146.
11. Hutchins GM, Anaya OA. Measurements of cardiac size, chamber volumes and valve orifices at autopsy. *Johns Hopkins Med J* 1973;133:96–106.
12. Sheaff MT, Hopster DJ. Organ dissection—cardiovascular system. In: Sheaff MT, Hopster DJ, eds. *Post Mortem Technique Handbook*. London: Springer; 2001.
13. Maleszewski JJ, Lai CK, Veinot JP. Anatomic considerations and examination of cardiovascular specimens (excluding devices). In: Buja LM, Butany J, eds. *Cardiovascular Pathology*. 4th ed. New York: Elsevier; 2016:1–56.
14. Edwards WD. Applied anatomy of the heart. In: Brandenberg RO, Fuster V, Guiliani ER, McGoon ER, eds. *Cardiology: Fundamentals and Practice*. Chicago, IL: Year Book Medical; 1987:47–112.
15. Cook AC, Yates RW, Anderson RH. Normal and abnormal fetal cardiac anatomy. *Prenat Diagn* 2004;24:1032–1048.
16. Bruneau BG. The developmental genetics of congenital heart disease. *Nature* 2008;451:943–948.
17. Bajolle F, Zaffran S, Bonnet D. Genetics and embryological mechanisms of congenital heart diseases. *Arch Cardiovasc Dis* 2009;102:59–63.
18. Huang JB, Liu YL, Sun PW, et al. Molecular mechanisms of congenital heart disease. *Cardiovasc Pathol* 2010;19:e183–e193.
19. Gittenberger-de Groot AC, Bartelings MM, Poelmann RE, et al. Embryology of the heart and its impact on understanding fetal and neonatal heart disease. *Semin Fetal Neonatal Med* 2013;18:237–244.
20. Schleich JM, Abdulla T, Summers R, et al. An overview of cardiac morphogenesis. *Arch Cardiovasc Dis* 2013;106:612–623.
21. Andres-Delgado L, Mercader N. Interplay between cardiac function and heart development. *Biochim Biophys Acta* 2016;1863:1707–1716.
22. Klein AL, Abbara S, Agler DA, et al. American Society of Echocardiography clinical recommendations for multimodality cardiovascular imaging of patients with pericardial disease: Endorsed by the Society for Cardiovascular Magnetic Resonance and Society for Cardiovascular Computed Tomography. *J Am Soc Echocardiogr* 2013;26:965–1012.
23. Rodriguez ER, Tan CD. Structure and Anatomy of the human pericardium. *Prog Cardiovasc Dis* 2017;59:327–340.
24. Cummings KW, Green D, Johnson WR, et al. Imaging of pericardial diseases. *Semin Ultrasound CT MR* 2016;37:238–254.
25. O'Leary SM, Williams PL, Edwards MP, et al. Imaging the pericardium: Appearances on ECG-gated 64-detector row cardiac computed tomography. *Br J Radiol* 2010;83:194–205.
26. Burke A, Virmani R. Tumors of the heart and great vessels. In: *Atlas of Tumor Pathology*. 3rd series, fascicle 16. Washington, DC: Armed Forces Institute of Pathology; 1996:127–170.
27. Wilcox BR, Cook AC, Anderson RH. *Surgical Anatomy of the Heart*. Cambridge: Cambridge University Press; 2004.
28. Wong CX, Abed HS, Molaee P, et al. Pericardial fat is associated with atrial fibrillation severity and ablation outcome. *J Am Coll Cardiol* 2011;57:1745–1751.

29. Bertaso AG, Bertol D, Duncan BB, et al. Epicardial fat: definition, measurements and systematic review of main outcomes. *Arq Bras Cardiol* 2013;101:e18–e28.
30. Anderson RH, Becker AE. *The Heart: Structure in Health and Disease*. London: Gower Medical Publishing; 1992.
31. Malouf JF, Edwards WD, Tajik AJ, et al. Functional anatomy of the heart. In: Fuster V, Alexander RW, O'Rouke RA, eds. *Hurst's the Heart*. 11th ed. New York: McGraw-Hill; 2004:45–86.
32. Anderson RH, Smerup M, Sanchez-Quintana D, et al. Three-dimensional arrangement of the myocytes in the ventricular walls. *Clin Anat* 2009;22:64–76.
33. Buckberg G, Hoffman JI, Mahajan A, et al. Cardiac mechanics revisited: the relationship of cardiac architecture to ventricular function. *Circulation* 2008;118:2571–2587.
34. Sweeney LJ, Rosenquist GC. The normal anatomy of the atrial septum in the human heart. *Am Heart J* 1979;98:194–199.
35. Calvert PA, Rana BS, Kydd AC, et al. Patent foramen ovale: anatomy, outcomes, and closure. *Nat Rev Cardiol* 2011;8:148–160.
36. Sheppard M, Davies MJ. *Practical Cardiovascular Pathology*. London: Arnold Publishers; 1998.
37. Corradi D, Maestri R, Macchi E, et al. The atria: From morphology to function. *J Cardiovasc Electrophysiol* 2011;22:223–235.
38. Conti AA. Calling the heart by name: Distinguished eponyms in the history of cardiac anatomy. *Heart Surg Forum* 2011;14:e183–e187.
39. Anderson RH, Cook AC. The structure and components of the atrial chambers. *Europace* 2007;9:vi3–vi9.
40. Hauser TH, Peters DC, Wylie JV, et al. Evaluating the left atrium by magnetic resonance imaging. *Europace* 2008;10:iii22–iii27.
41. Giusca S, Jurcut R, Ginghina C, et al. The right ventricle: Anatomy, physiology and functional assessment. *Acta Cardiol* 2010;65:67–77.
42. Banerjee D, Haddad F, Zamanian RT, et al. Right ventricular failure: A novel era of targeted therapy. *Curr Heart Fail Rep* 2010;7:202–211.
43. Walker LA, Buttrick PM. The right ventricle: biologic insights and response to disease: Updated. *Curr Cardiol Rev* 2013;9:73–81.
44. Davies MJ. Introduction to normal cardiac anatomy. In: Davies MJ, Mann JM, eds. *The Cardiovascular System. Part B: Acquired Diseases of the Heart*. New York: Churchill Livingstone; 1995:1–6.
45. Ho SY, Nihoyannopoulos P. Anatomy, echocardiography, and normal right ventricular dimensions. *Heart* 2006;92(Suppl 1):i2–i13.
46. Barry A, Patten B. The structure of the adult heart. In: Gould SE, ed. *Pathology of the Heart and Blood Vessels*. Springfield, IL: Charles C Thomas; 1968:104–105.
47. Marcus FI, McKenna WJ, Sherrill D, et al. Diagnosis of arrhythmogenic right ventricular cardiomyopathy/dysplasia. *Eur Heart J* 2010;31:806–814.
48. Corrado D, Link MS, Calkins H. Arrhythmogenic right ventricular cardiomyopathy. *N Engl J Med* 2017;376:61–72.
49. Saffitz JE. Molecular mechanisms in the pathogenesis of arrhythmogenic cardiomyopathy. *Cardiovasc Pathol* 2017;28:51–58.
50. Kimura F, Matsuo Y, Nakajima T, et al. Myocardial fat at cardiac imaging: How can we differentiate pathologic from physiologic fatty infiltration. *Radiographics* 2010;30:1587–1602.
51. James TN, Sherf L, Schlant RC, et al. Anatomy of the heart. In: Hurst JW, Logue RB, Rackley CE, et al., eds. *The Heart*. 5th ed. New York: McGraw-Hill; 1982:22–74.
52. Ho SY. Anatomy and myoarchitecture of the left ventricular wall in normal and in disease. *Eur J Echocardiogr* 2009;10:iii3–iii7.
53. Kajstura J, Gurusamy N, Ogórek B, et al. Myocyte turnover in the aging human heart. *Circ Res* 2010;107:1374–1386.
54. Silver MM, Freedom RM. Gross examination and structure of the heart. In: Silver MD, ed. *Cardiovascular Pathology*. Vol. 1. 2nd ed. New York: Churchill Livingstone; 1991:1–42.
55. Davies MJ, Pomerance A, Lamb D. Techniques in examination and anatomy of the heart. In: Pomerance A, Davies MJ, eds. *Pathology of the Heart*. Oxford: Blackwell Scientific; 1975:1–48.
56. Combs MD, Yutzey KE. Heart valve development: regulatory networks in development and disease. *Circ Res* 2009;105:408–421.
57. Ferrans VJ, Rodríguez ER. Ultrastructure of the normal heart. In: Silver MD, ed. *Cardiovascular Pathology*. 2nd ed. New York: Churchill Livingstone; 1991:43–101.
58. Carpentier A, Brancgini B, Cour JC, et al. Congenital malformations of the mitral valve. Pathology and surgical treatment. *J Thorac Cardiovasc Surg* 1976;72:854–866.
59. McCarthy KP, Ring L, Rana BS. Anatomy of the mitral valve: understanding the mitral valve complex in mitral regurgitation. *Eur J Echocardiogr* 2010;11:i3–i9.
60. Liu AC, Joag VR, Gotlieb AI. The emerging role of valve interstitial cell phenotypes in regulating heart valve pathobiology. *Am J Pathol* 2007;171:1407–1418.
61. Edwards WD. Cardiovascular system. In: Ludwig J, ed. *Handbook of Autopsy Practice*. 3rd ed. Totowa, NJ: Humana Press; 2002:21–44.
62. Davies MJ, Anderson RH. The pathology of the conduction system. In: Pomerance A, Davies MJ, eds. *The Pathology of the Heart*. Oxford: Blackwell Scientific; 1975:367–412.
63. Baughman KL. History and current techniques of endomyocardial biopsy. In: Baumgartner WA, Reitz B, Kasper E, Theodore J, eds. *Heart and Lung Transplantation*. 2nd ed. Philadelphia, PA: WB Saunders; 2002:267–281.
64. Berry GJ, Billingham ME. The pathology of human cardiac transplantation. In: Baumgartner WA, Reitz B, Kasper E, Theodore J, eds. *Heart and Lung Transplantation*. Philadelphia, PA: WB Saunders; 2002:286–306.
65. Edwards WD, Holmes DR Jr, Reeder GS. Diagnosis of active lymphocytic myocarditis by endomyocardial biopsy: Quantitative criteria for light microscopy. *Mayo Clin Proc* 1982;57:419–425.
66. Tazelaar HD, Billingham ME. Myocardial lymphocytes: Fact, fancy or myocarditis? *Am J Cardiovasc Pathol* 1986;1:47–50.
67. Stevens PJ, Ground KEU. Occurrence and significance of myocarditis in trauma. *Aerosp Med* 1970;41:776–780.
68. Hauck AJ, Edwards WD. Histopathologic examination of tissues obtained by endomyocardial biopsy. In: Fowles RE, ed. *Cardiac Biopsy*. Mount Kisco, NY: Futura Publishing; 1992:95–153.

Serous Membranes

Darryl Carter ■ Lawrence True ■ Christopher N. Otis

ANATOMY 551	Interactions of Mesothelial and Submesothelial Cells 561
FUNCTIONAL ANATOMY 552	REACTIVE MESOTHELIUM 561
MESOTHELIAL CELLS 554	Fibrous Pleurisy 562
Morphology 554	Reactive Mesothelium versus Mesothelioma 562
Histochemistry 555	Reactive Mesothelium versus Carcinoma 563
Immunohistochemistry 557	Endosalpingiosis and Endometriosis 564
Ultrastructure 558	Multilocular Peritoneal Inclusion Cyst 565
SUBMESOTHELIAL LAYER 559	REFERENCES 566
Histochemistry 559	
Immunohistochemistry 561	

ANATOMY

The serous membranes are derived from the mesoderm and line the pleural, pericardial, and peritoneal cavities with mesothelial cells, which normally appear as a simple or cuboidal epithelium. The parietal and visceral mesothelia are separated by a thin layer of fluid and supported by a fibrous submesothelial layer, which becomes continuous with the outer layer of invested organs and the chest or abdominal walls. The serous membranes show functional differentiation according to their location and are capable of a great variety of reactive changes, which may mask or mimic neoplastic changes.

The pleura is a continuous membrane that covers the chest wall and the lungs. The visceral pleura coats the entire pulmonary surface, including the major and minor fissures that divide the lungs into lobes, whereas the parietal pleura extends over the ribs, sternum, and supporting structures and is reflected over the mediastinal structures on both right and left. In the posterior mediastinum, the two layers of parietal pleura are separated by a thin band of fibrovascular connective tissue. Superiorly, the cervical pleura is reflected into the retroclavicular area over the apex of the lung and is coated by a thickened layer of fibrous tissue and skeletal muscle; inferiorly, the diaphragmatic pleura represents its caudal extent. Anteriorly, the pleura is reflected over part of the pericardium. The posterior visceral pleura becomes continuous with the diaphragmatic pleura over the pulmonary ligament. The heart and great vessels lie in the pericardium, which is lined by a continuous layer of mesothelium. The visceral (epicardial) side is connected to the myocardium, and the parietal (pericardial) layer rests on a dense fibrous tissue layer containing branches of the internal mammary and musculophrenic vessels, descending aorta, and branches of the vagus, phrenic, and sympathetic nerves. The thoracic surface of the pericardium is coated with parietal pleura.

The peritoneum is a nearly continuous membrane lining the potential space between the intra-abdominal viscera and the abdominal wall. In females, it is normally interrupted by the lumina of the fallopian tubes. Anatomically, it is more complex than either the pleura or the pericardium. The parietal layer covers the abdominal wall, diaphragm, anterior surfaces of the retroperitoneal viscera, and the pelvis. The visceral peritoneum invests the intestines and other intra-abdominal viscera. The elongated structures in which the parietal and visceral layers come together are the mesentery, which contains blood vessels, lymphatics, lymph nodes, and nerves.

The greater omentum is a double sheet with four layers of mesothelium between which there are numerous blood vessels and adipose tissue, which may be abundant; lymphatics and lymph nodes are less prominent than in the mesentery. The peritoneal cavity is grossly divided into the greater sac, over the intestines, the retrogastric lesser sac, the right and left retrocolic areas, and the pelvis. Outpouchings of peritoneum are often seen as pathology specimens. Inguinal hernia sacs are pouches of parietal peritoneum, often invested with the fibrous tissue and occasionally with the skeletal muscle, which have been pushed through the abdominal musculature into the inguinal canal. Umbilical or ventral hernias are also outpouchings of peritoneum, but the specimens received by pathologists after surgical repair are usually the preperitoneal fibroadipose tissue pushed ahead of the parietal peritoneum rather than the mesothelial sac itself.

The scrotum acquires a lining of parietal mesothelium, the processus vaginalis, into which the testes descend during the seventh month of gestation. A mesothelial layer forms the surface of the tunica vaginalis. Distention of this mesothelial sac on the tunica vaginalis results in a hydrocele—communicating with the peritoneal cavity when congenital but noncommunicating in acquired hydroceles. The sac of an inguinal hernia communicates with the peritoneal cavity but not with the mesothelium-lined space of the scrotum. Both the hernia and hydrocele sacs are capable of a wide range of reactive changes.

FUNCTIONAL ANATOMY

Sahn (1) and Pistolesi et al. (2) described the functional anatomy of the pleura, which is a continuous membrane surrounding a space that normally contains approximately 10 mL of clear colorless fluid. The surface is lined by a single layer of mesothelial cells anchored to a basement membrane that lies on layers of collagen and elastic tissues containing vascular and lymphatic vessels. The lining mesothelial cells are 16 to 40 μm in diameter, have rounded nuclei, which usually display a nucleolus, and a relatively large amount of cytoplasm. Although the visceral and parietal pleurae are opposing parts of the same continuous membrane, there are major functional differences between them.

The human visceral pleura is similar to that of horses, cattle, sheep, and pigs (3), which have been studied experimentally. It has an arterial blood supply from the bronchial arteries, with a venous return that passes first into the pulmonary veins and then into the left atrium except for certain hilar regions that are drained by bronchial veins into the right atrium. The lymphatics that pass through the visceral pleura are the superficial layer of pulmonary lymphatics, which are intersegmental, especially in the lower lobes (4). There are extensive connections to the peribronchial, perivascular, and interlobular lymphatic spaces and the lymphoid tissue (5). Blood and lymphatic vessels are invested by two layers of collagen and elastic fibers. An external elastic lamina supports the mesothelial cells and an internal layer invests the

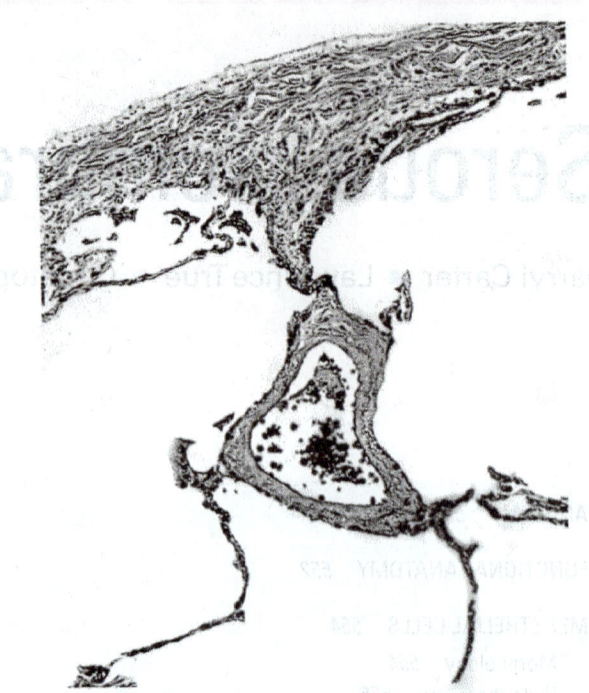

FIGURE 20.1 Visceral pleura. The mesothelial cells on the surface are flattened and, when viewed in profile, so thin as to be barely evident. On the posterior surface of the left lower lobe, the dense submesothelial layer is composed of collagen and elastin, and extends into the adjacent pulmonary interstitium and around pulmonary vessels.

vessels and becomes continuous with the pulmonary interstitium (Figs. 20.1 and 20.2).

Histologic identification of integrity of the visceral pleural elastin is considered clinically important in determining

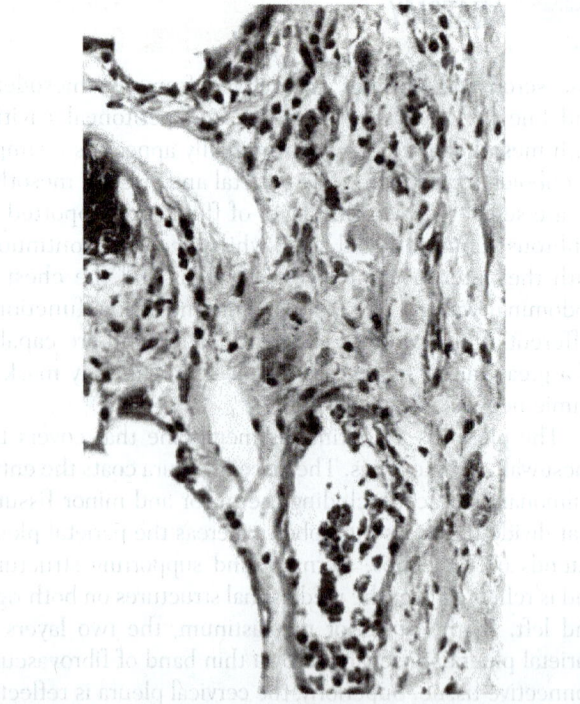

FIGURE 20.2 Visceral pleura. Capillaries are prominent, the lymphatics are dilated, deeply placed, and entirely invested by the submesothelial layer.

pleural invasion by primary lung cancer, and is significant for staging (6). However, the elastin layer of the visceral pleura is also interrupted in nonneoplastic conditions of the lung that extend to the pleura. In sheep, and probably in humans, the thickness of the external layer increases in both the craniocaudal and ventrodorsal directions, perhaps because of postural reasons (7). The visceral pleura is innervated by branches of the vagus nerves and sympathetic nerve trunks.

The parietal pleura is anatomically, histologically, and functionally different. Although the single layer of mesothelial cells that lie on the surface of the parietal pleura are cytologically similar to those that form the continuous membrane over the visceral pleura, this surface is interrupted by stomata which range in size from 2 to 12 μm in diameter. Li (8) described the stomata on the human diaphragmatic pleura as usually penetrating deep through connective tissue with apparent communication between the pleural cavity and the underlying lymphatic lacunae. In some areas, stomata are covered with great microvilli (longer and with a denser network of filaments) on the surfaces of the surrounding mesothelial cells. The underlying lymphatics drain directly into intercostal lymphatics and then into the mediastinum, where they are particularly dense along the retrocardiac surface (9–16).

Fluid and particulate matter extravasated from the lung are collected in these lymphatics and passed into the mediastinum, where the mesothelium covers collections of macrophages called Kampmeier foci (17). Boutin et al. (18) showed the concentration of asbestos fibers in these areas, which are also termed "black spots" when there is a concentration of carbon in individuals who have inhaled coal dust. Miserocchi et al. (19) described asbestos-fiber accumulation in "black spots" corresponding to the stomata.

The arterial and venous blood supply to the parietal pleura is from the intercostal vessels. The thickness of the fibroelastic layer investing the parietal pleural lymphatics is relatively constant and considerably less than that of most of the visceral pleura, suggesting that it serves as a membrane across which fluid may diffuse. The parietal pleura is innervated by branches of the intercostal nerves, which are responsible for the pain associated with pleurisy.

Wassilev et al. (20) described stomata on the peritoneum of the abdominal wall, omentum, mesentery, ovaries, and pelvis, as well as on the underside of the diaphragm. They found variation in the structure of the stomata according to the location. The parietal stomata were clustered, oval in shape, and delimited by flattened mesothelial cells, whereas the hepatic stomata were deeper gaps in adjacent cuboidal mesothelial cells and were covered or occluded by the microvilli on the surface of mesothelial cells. Li and Yu (21) found that the diaphragmatic stomata were approximately 10 μm² in size, among cuboidal but not flattened mesothelial cells, and opened into submesothelial connective tissue with a rich plexus of lymphatics, which they suggested carried away peritoneal fluid and particles.

Milky spots on the peritoneum and especially the omentum have been described as a glomerular-like capillary network of blood vessels, which enables fluid exchange between the peritoneal cavity, blood stream, and surrounding omental tissue. They lie directly beneath the stomata and are associated with macrophages, T and B lymphocytes, and plasma cells. They are said to be a preferred site for implantation of cancer cells in peritoneal carcinomatosis (22).

The serous membranes serve as a selective barrier for fluid and cells. A small volume of fluid is required for capillary action to facilitate adherence of visceral and parietal pleurae as the lungs and chest wall expand and contract. Elements of the serous membranes regulate fluid interchange to keep this fluid at a minimal level to prevent compromise of the lung volumes. Control appears to be at the capillary level because fluid is freely diffusible through the visceral mesothelium and is collected in parietal lymphatics via stomata in the parietal mesothelium. The bushy, elongated microvilli, which are the diagnostic hallmark of mesothelial cells, are sometimes enlarged where associated with stomata. Another level of control results from the relatively low protein content (1.0 to 1.5 g/dL) of pleural fluid. The point of protein regulation is unknown, although there is speculation that it occurs at the level of mesothelial microvilli (21). In the thoracic cavity, the direction of flow appears to be via diffusion from capillaries of both visceral and parietal pleurae, with resorption primarily through parietal pleural capillaries. Turnover is estimated at 0.7 mL/hr (Fig. 20.3) (21). Small molecules (less than 4 nm in diameter) diffuse through the intercellular spaces and junctions between mesothelial cells. Loss of control results in serous effusions such as those seen in congestive heart failure.

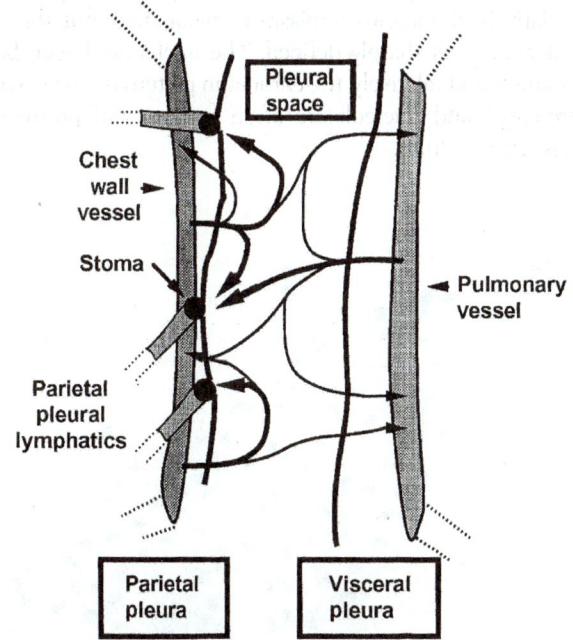

FIGURE 20.3 Model of the dynamics of pleural fluid formation. A transudate from capillaries in visceral and parietal pleurae is partly reabsorbed by those capillaries and the rest diffuses into the pleural space, where it is resorbed via stomata into parietal pleural lymphatics.

Larger molecules, up to 50 nm in diameter, are transferred across the mesothelium by pinocytotic uptake and transcellular transport. Larger structures, such as cells in bloody effusions, are transported via the stomata and "crevices." Loss of control of these mechanisms results in accumulation of exudative pleural fluid. Mesothelial cells express the secretory component of IgA, which is otherwise limited to surfaces with direct environmental contact (23). The glycoprotein-rich pleural fluid acts as a lubricant to minimize friction between visceral and parietal pleurae. The site of synthesis and mechanisms of control of the carbohydrate-rich fractions of the pleural fluid are unknown. The submesothelial connective tissue distributes mechanical forces from the pleura uniformly throughout the lungs. Such a redistribution of forces is not required of the abdominal serosa. Both mesothelial cells and fibroblasts contribute to collagen synthesis.

MESOTHELIAL CELLS

Morphology

Cross sections of normal mesothelial cells are thin and barely apparent in histologic sections but defoliated sheets of normal mesothelial cells may be evident in cytologic preparations of peritoneal washes taken during a laparotomy (Fig. 20.4). When thus visualized, they have abundant clear cytoplasm with crisply defined cell borders, small and centrally placed nuclei with a homogeneous chromatin pattern, and are usually without a nucleolus (Fig. 20.5).

In a variety of reactive processes, the mesothelial cells undergo markedly proliferative and hyperplastic changes. A relatively abundant cytoplasm is maintained, but the cell borders are less sharply defined. The nuclei are larger, both absolutely and relatively, the chromatin pattern is more hyperchromatic, and nucleoli are often present and prominent (Figs. 20.6 to 20.9).

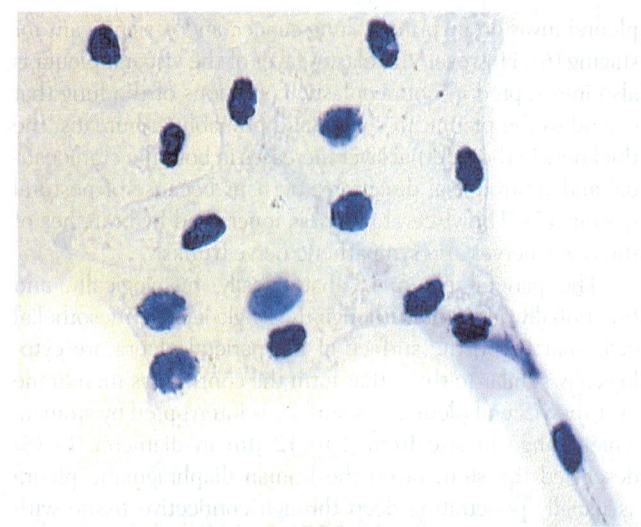

FIGURE 20.5 At higher magnification, a sheet of relatively normal mesothelial cells with abundant, clear cytoplasm and crisply defined cell borders. The centrally placed nuclei are small and have a homogeneous chromatin.

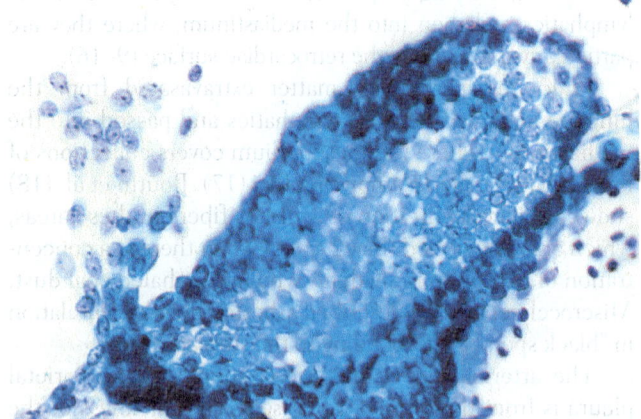

FIGURE 20.6 This detached fragment of reactive mesothelium shows an intact mesothelial layer with cells in two phases of the reactive process shown in Figures 20.7 and 20.8.

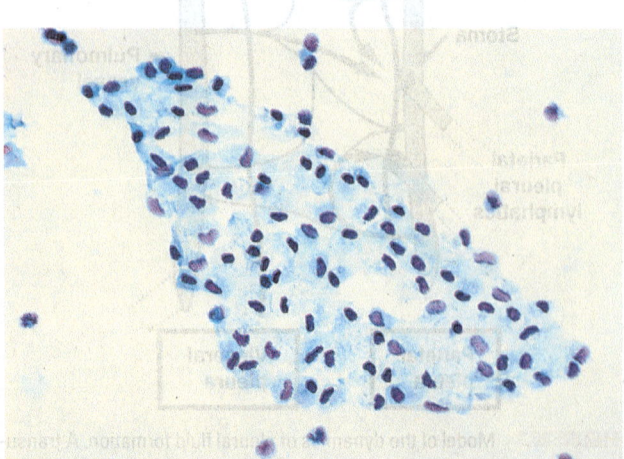

FIGURE 20.4 In this peritoneal wash specimen, a sheet of normal mesothelial cells has been detached.

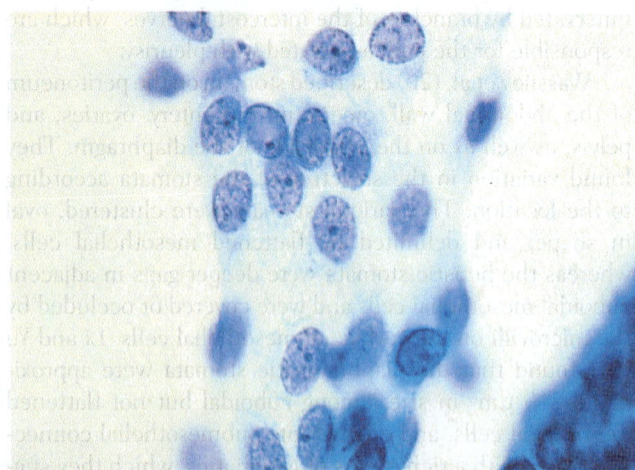

FIGURE 20.7 The reactive mesothelial cells from the left side of Figure 20.6 have abundant cytoplasm, and the nuclei are larger with a more vesicular chromatin pattern. Nucleoli are present but not prominent.

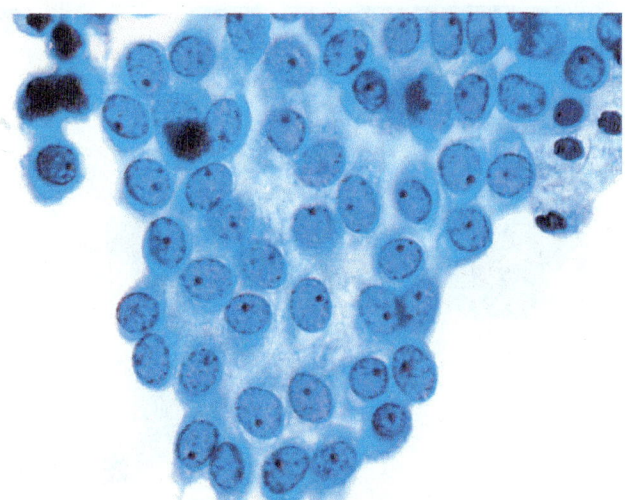

FIGURE 20.8 The more reactive mesothelial cells from the right side of Figure 20.6 have less cytoplasm, larger nuclei with a more vesicular chromatin pattern, and more prominent nucleoli.

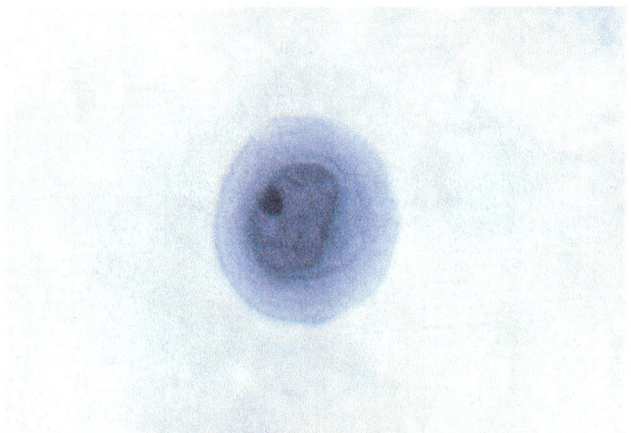

FIGURE 20.10 This individual reactive mesothelial cell has a limited amount of cytoplasm and a relatively large nucleus with a nucleolus. The cell border is highly irregular and fuzzy, consistent with the presence of the numerous elongated microvilli, which are evident on electron microscopy (see Fig. 20.24). The cytoplasm is divided into an outer less dense layer and an inner denser layer, which, ultrastructurally, corresponds to the presence of intermediate filaments with the characteristics of keratin (see Fig. 20.25).

As the hyperplastic changes in the reactive mesothelial cells progress, cell groups become smaller, and individual cells predominate. When clustered, reactive mesothelial cells present an irregular outside border. The nucleus, and especially the nucleolus, may enlarge dramatically, but the nuclei are similar in size, shape, and pattern from cell to cell. Normal mitotic figures may be seen. The cytoplasm may become multivacuolated as the cells degenerate and imbibe fluid (Figs. 20.10 to 20.17).

Histochemistry

Mesothelial positivity for histochemical stains that detect negative groups, such as the positively charged dye Alcian blue, is evidence of their content of acid mucoproteins. That the intensity of staining reactions for acid mucosubstances is diminished by preincubating the tissue sections in hyaluronidase is evidence that at least some of the terminal hexose groups of the mucosubstances are either hyaluronic acid or chondroitin sulfate. Furthermore, the fact that histochemical mucin is decreased, but not abolished, by incubating cells in neuraminidase before histochemical staining is evidence that some of the terminal carbohydrate groups are sialated (24). MacDougall et al. (25) have documented that neoplastic mesothelial cells may stain with mucicarmine. Negativity for the periodic acid–Schiff (PAS) reaction after sialidase digestion is evidence that mesothelial cells lack significant quantities of neutral mucoproteins.

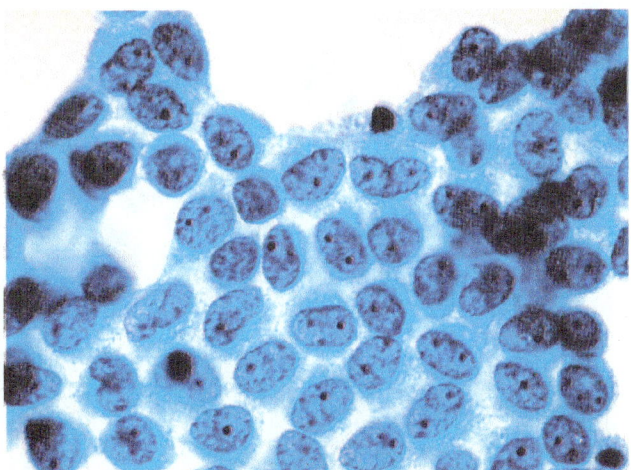

FIGURE 20.9 In this sheet of reactive mesothelial cells, the cytoplasm is smaller and the nuclei are relatively larger and have a more irregular chromatin pattern.

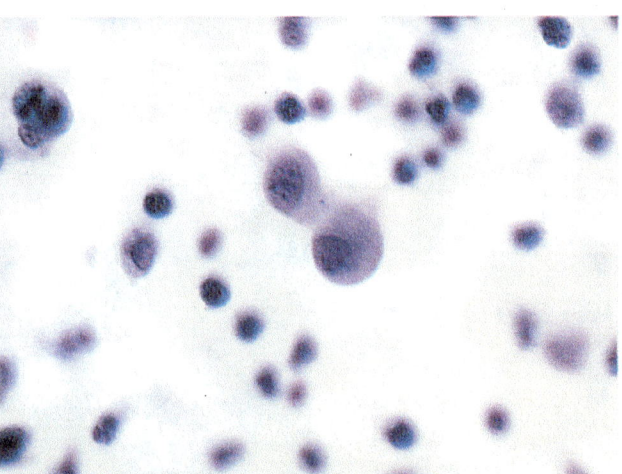

FIGURE 20.11 Mesothelial reaction is frequently associated with inflammatory cells. These reactive mesothelial cells, which are several times the size of either neutrophils or lymphocytes, are joined as a pair.

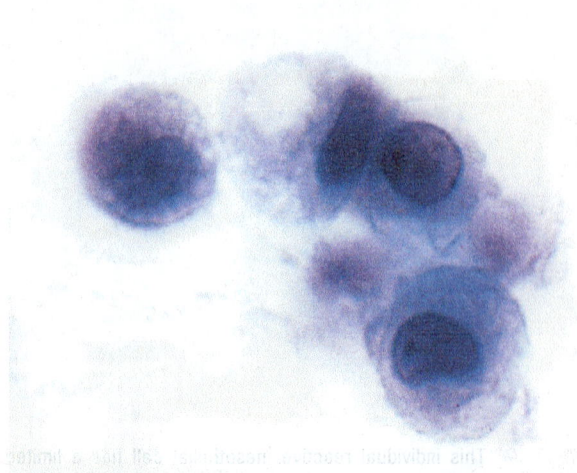

FIGURE 20.12 These reactive mesothelial cells are loosely joined together. The uppermost cell has a vacuole in the cytoplasm, which could be either a vesicle or an intracytoplasmic lumen.

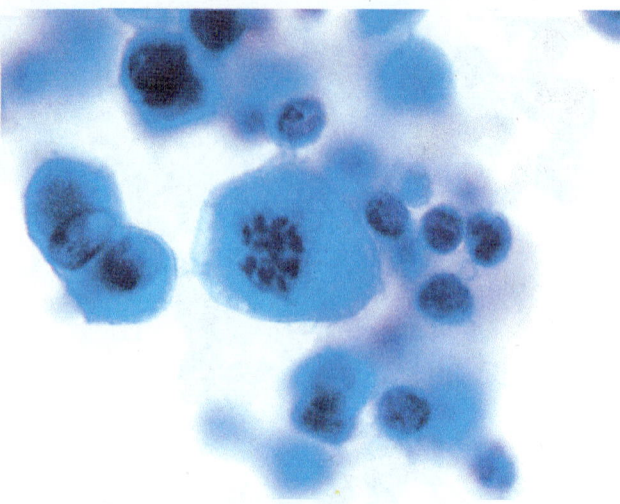

FIGURE 20.15 Normal mitotic figures may be seen in the proliferating cells of reactive mesothelium.

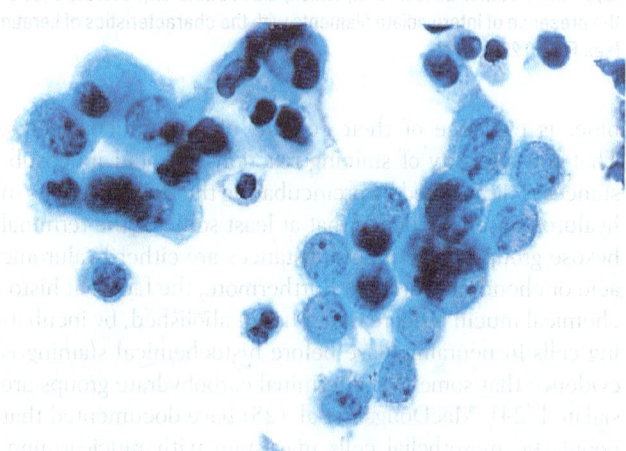

FIGURE 20.13 When reactive mesothelial cells are in groups, an irregular or "knobby" outside border is formed, whereas acini form a smooth outer border. Note the "fuzzy" border on the mesothelial cell.

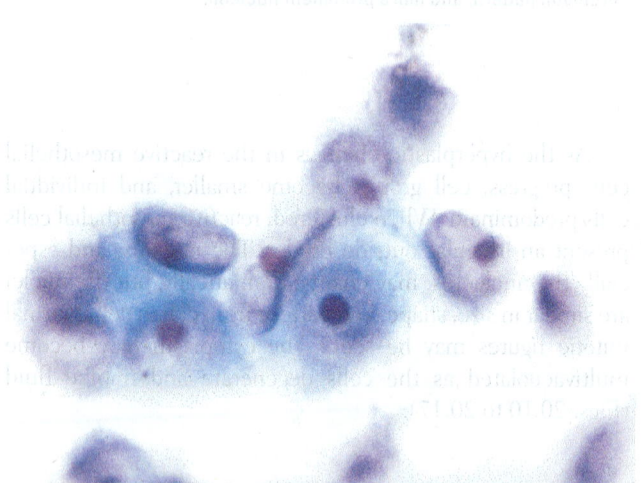

FIGURE 20.16 The nucleoli of reactive mesothelial cells may be prominent.

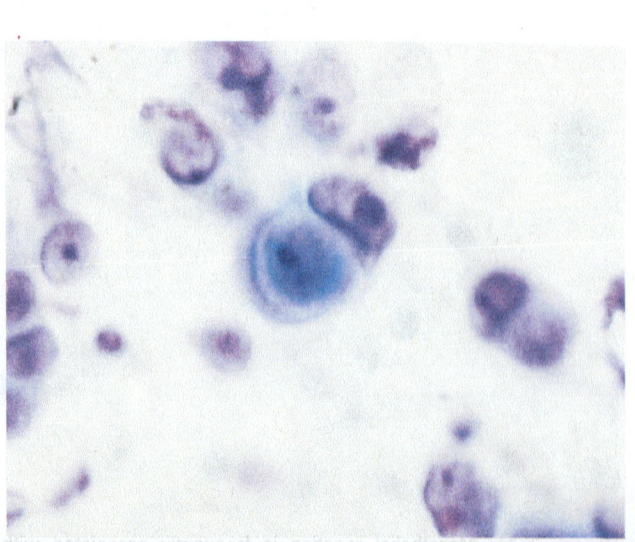

FIGURE 20.14 Occasionally, very reactive mesothelial cells may show cellular interactions similar to those of a keratin pearl.

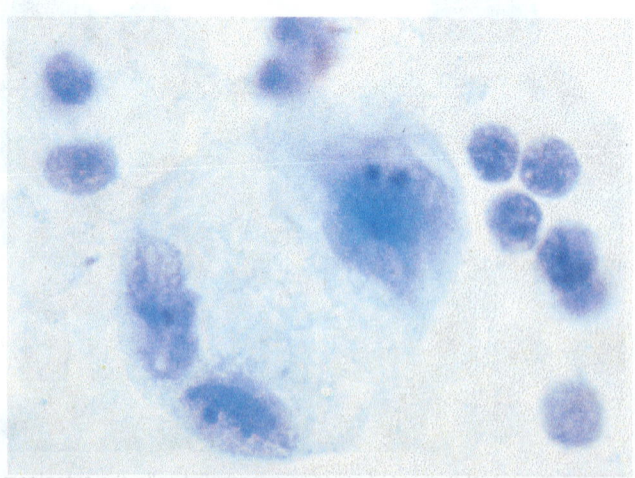

FIGURE 20.17 Reactive mesothelial cells may degenerate and swell. These three cells have abundant multivacuolated cytoplasm and large nuclei with prominent nucleoli.

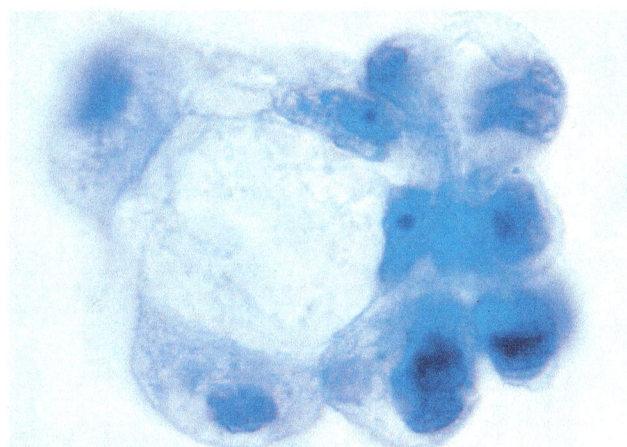

FIGURE 20.18 When markedly reactive mesothelial cells form irregular groups and combine with degenerating forms, they may mimic the appearance of mucin-producing adenocarcinoma.

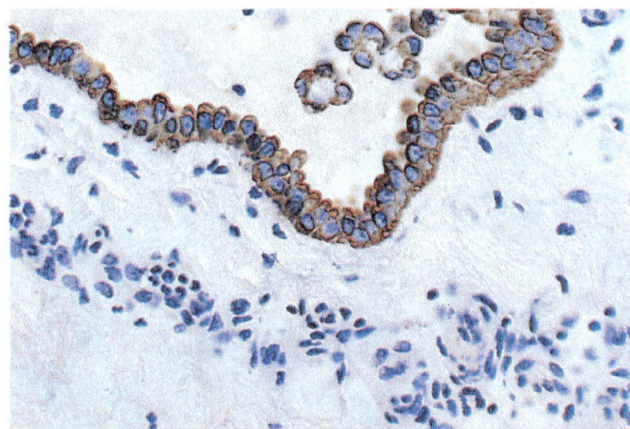

FIGURE 20.19 Keratin expression in the mesothelium and detached mesothelial cells, stained with a cocktail of monoclonal antibodies (AE1/AE3).

The types of terminal carbohydrate groups of membrane proteins and lipids can also be characterized with lectins, which have specific and discrete ranges of sugar group affinities. Concanavalin A mesothelial cell reactivity indicates the presence of terminal groups that are either mannose or glucose.

Immunohistochemistry

Immunohistochemical studies of serous membranes have shown that the mesothelium expresses a complex and varied phenotype with overlap of other normal tissues and many malignancies. The great majority of benign mesothelial proliferations express several keratins, especially AE1/AE3, CK8/18 (Cam5.2), CK19, CK5/6, and CK7 that can be detected with monoclonal antibodies immunoreactive with the small, acidic, type I keratins (Fig. 20.18) (26). The mesothelium does not express CK20 (27). Ovarian epithelial tumors express a spectrum of keratins similar to that of the mesothelium (28).

Mesothelial cells, benign and malignant, frequently and preferentially express calretinin, podoplanin, WT-1, HBME-1 and thrombomodulin. Vimentin and desmin are also expressed by reactive mesothelium, especially when in spindle form.

Calretinin, a calcium-binding protein of 29 kDa similar to S-100 protein, is found in the nucleus and the cytoplasm of reactive and neoplastic mesothelia and is very useful in the identification of mesothelial differentiation. However, it may also be expressed in some adenocarcinomas (Fig. 20.19) (29–32). Cytokeratin 5/6 is found in the cytoplasm of most mesothelial cells and squamous cell carcinomas, but few adenocarcinomas (33). WT-1, a product of Wilms tumor gene, is found in the nucleus of reactive and neoplastic mesothelia and in ovarian surface epithelium and tumors derived therefrom (Fig. 20.20) (34). D2-40, an antigen originally identified as characteristic of lymphatic endothelium, is also expressed by mesothelial cells with a high level of sensitivity (Fig. 20.21), but it also marks ovarian serous carcinoma (35).

The mesothelium less frequently and less reliably expresses other antigens, including thrombomodulin, a transmembrane glycoprotein, which is expressed in cell membranes in about half the mesotheliomas but also some adenocarcinomas. Mesothelin, N-cadherin, E-cadherin, epithelial membrane antigen (EMA), Her2/Neu, and EGFR are also expressed (36).

The diagnosis of mesothelioma in situ requires demonstration of invasive mesothelioma elsewhere in the same specimen or in a subsequent specimen.

The plasticity of the immunophenotype of mesothelial cells is demonstrable in abnormal states. Reactive mesothelial cells can express the muscle cell cytoskeleton proteins,

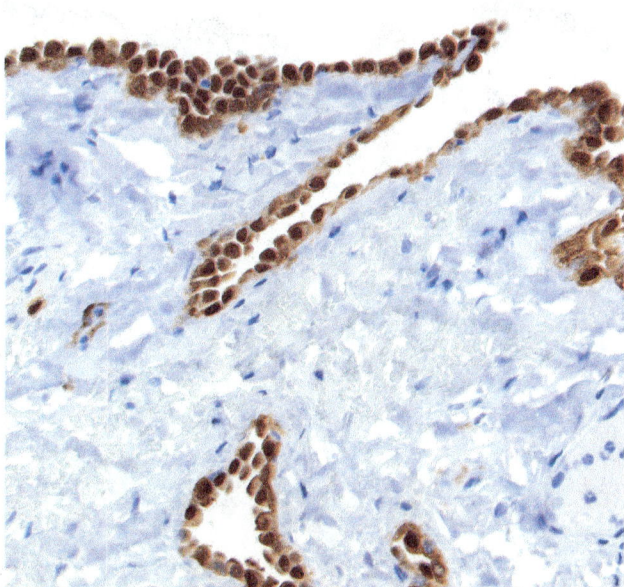

FIGURE 20.20 Calretinin immunohistochemical staining of both nucleus and cytoplasm in benign mesothelial cells.

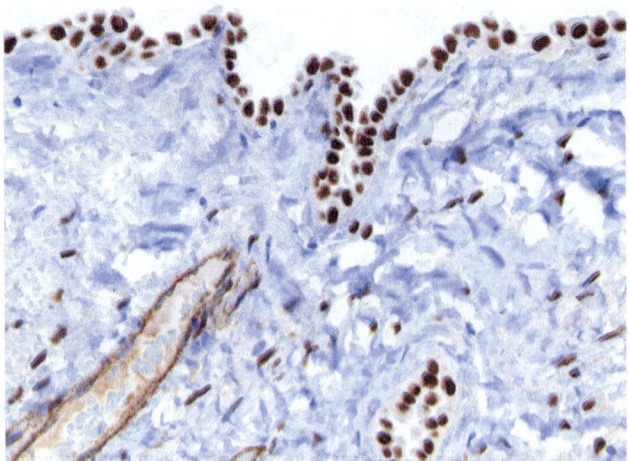

FIGURE 20.21 WT-1 immunoreactivity in benign mesothelium is nuclear (original magnification 40×).

desmin and muscle-specific actin (37). There is experimental evidence that the pattern of intermediate filament expression by mesothelial cells is dependent on the shape and cell–cell interaction. Induction of spindle morphology inhibits keratin synthesis. In contrast, induction of an epithelioid morphology (e.g., with retinoids) stimulates keratin synthesis and inhibits vimentin synthesis; the ability of cells to respond in this manner also depends on the presence of cell–cell interactions (Figs. 20.22 to 20.25) (38).

Ultrastructure

The most characteristic morphologic feature of mesothelial cells is the presence of numerous long and slender

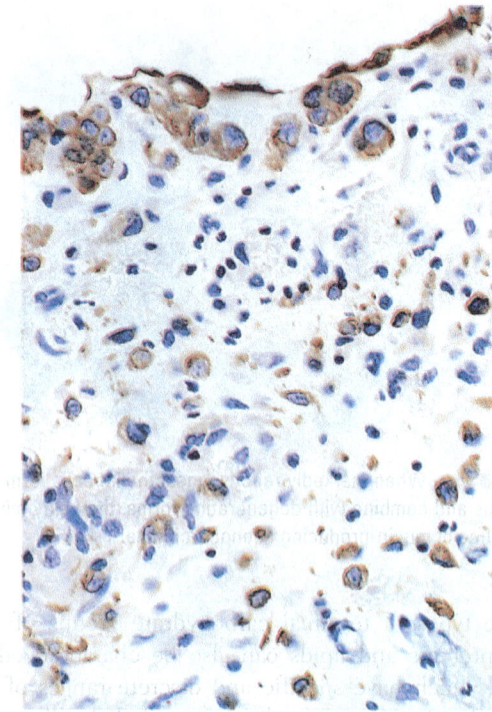

FIGURE 20.23 Keratin (AE1/AE3) immunoreactivity of proliferating submesothelial spindle cells.

microvilli (Figs. 20.26 and 20.27), measuring up to 3 μm in length and 0.1 μm in diameter. They are more numerous in caudal portions of the parietal pleura and in the visceral pleura. Other organelles are not specific for mesothelial cells. Multiple types of junctions are found—tight junctions that serve as a barrier to certain molecules, gap

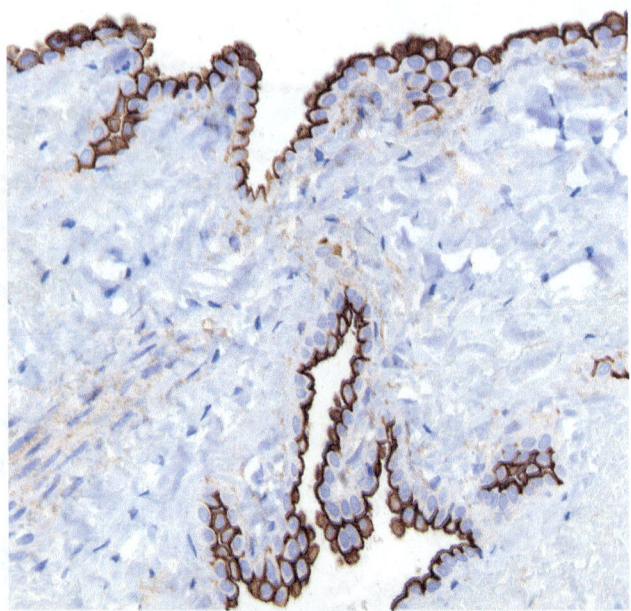

FIGURE 20.22 D2-40 immunoreactivity in benign mesothelium is predominantly membranous.

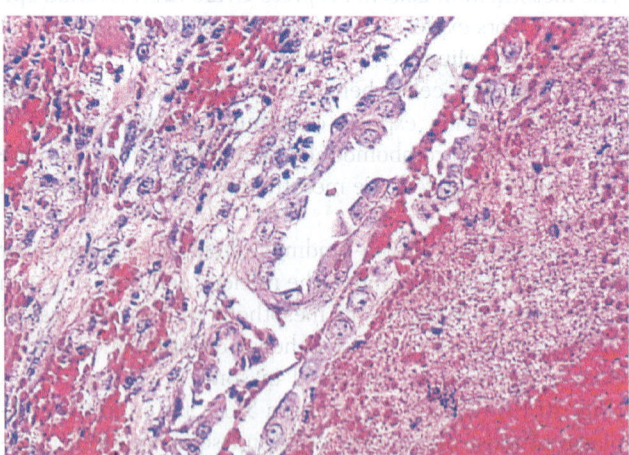

FIGURE 20.24 A patient with severe rheumatoid arthritis and pleural effusion with florid reactive mesothelial hyperplasia of the pleura, which may be difficult to distinguish from neoplastic proliferation. The proliferating mesothelial cells may become entrapped in the fibrous tissue of organization and may mimic invasion.

CHAPTER 20: Serous Membranes

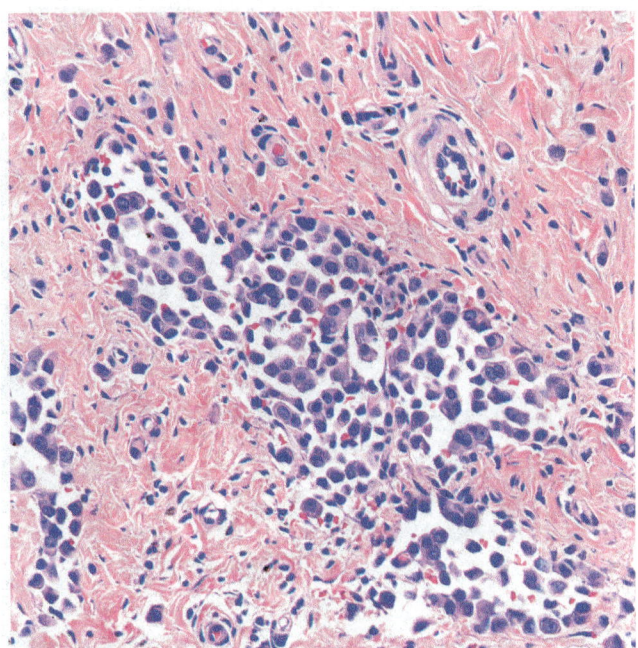

FIGURE 20.25 The reactive mesothelium in this photomicrograph is from a hernia sac of an 18-month-old boy. It is composed of proliferating epithelioid cells on the surface and subjacent spindle-shaped cells that give the impression of proliferating fibroblasts.

SUBMESOTHELIAL LAYER

Much of the submesothelial layer is composed of collagen, elastin, and other extracellular proteins. Normally, the submesothelial layer contains few cells, and most of these are fibroblasts, but during reactive processes, the submesothelial layer may become much more prominent as myofibroblasts, inflammatory cells, and capillaries proliferate there. Deciduoid reaction in the submesothelium of the peritoneum may especially mimic an infiltrating neoplasm (Fig. 20.30). The term "visceral fasciae" has been used to describe the fascia lying immediately beneath the mesothelium and surrounding the viscera. It varies in thickness from about 134 microns around the lung, to 792 microns around the heart, and 987 microns around the abdominal viscera. Elastic fibers form a well-defined layer, corresponding to the elastic lamina, in the pleura and peritoneum. Beneath them, collagen fibers are arranged in parallel bundles separated by loose connective tissue rich in elastic fibers (39).

Histochemistry

The main constituents of the submesothelial tissue are elastic fibers, staining with Verhoeff van Gieson; collagen, staining with Masson trichrome; and glycosylated proteins, including glycosaminoglycans, staining with alcian blue. The majority of the carbohydrate groups are negatively charged (as a result of an abundance of hyaluronic acid and other acidic groups), and stain as acidic mucoproteins. Staining intensity can be diminished by pretreating with hyaluronidase showing that hyaluronic acid groups are responsible, in large part, for the intensity of staining.

junctions for cell–cell transport, and desmosomes for cell–cell adherence. Intermediate filaments are often prominent and are often arranged in a perinuclear, circumferential distribution, although they do not aggregate into bundles (Figs. 20.28 and 20.29).

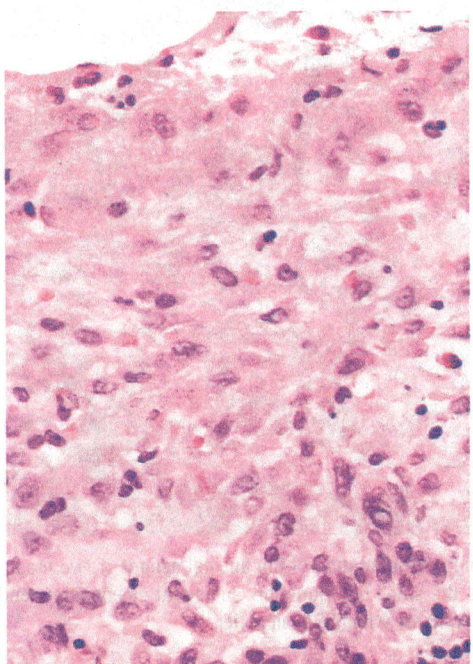
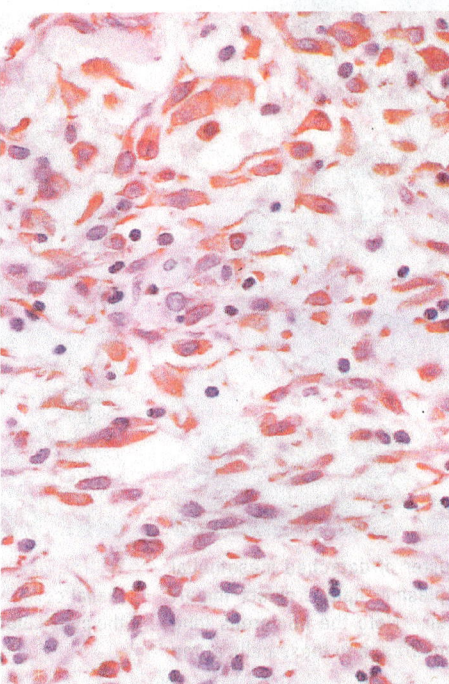

FIGURE 20.26 The reactive peritoneum shown in Figure 20.25 is shown at higher magnification in H&E on the left. On the right, immunohistochemical stain for keratin (AE1/AE3) illustrates that both the epithelioid and spindle cells are keratin positive, indicative of their mesothelial differentiation.

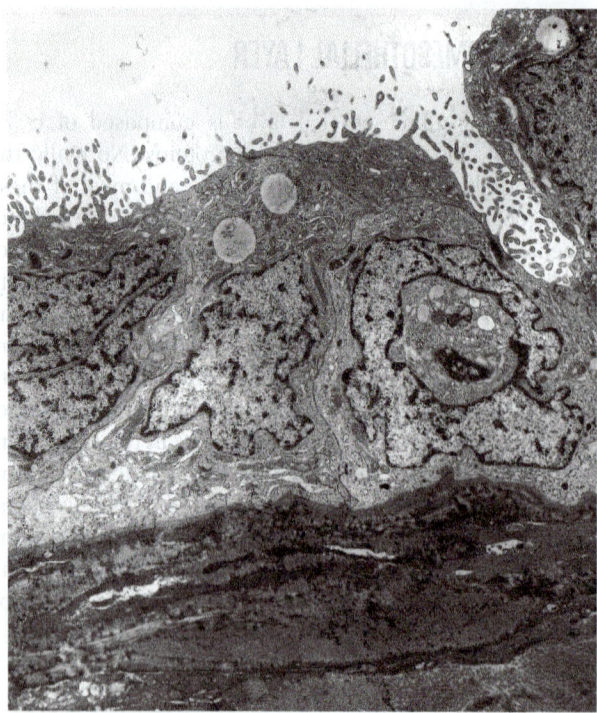

FIGURE 20.27 Mesothelial cells with their elongated microvilli, cover the surface of the serosa. The subjacent stroma is composed of collagen and fibroblasts.

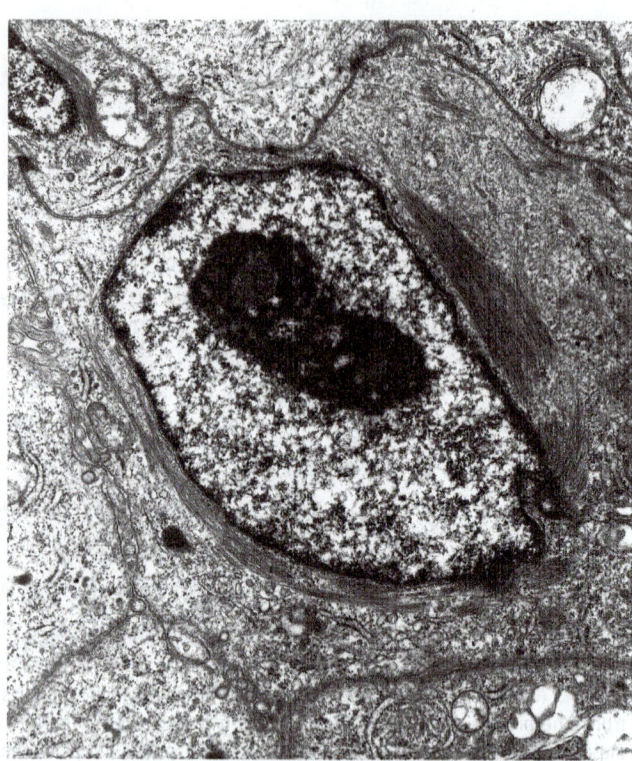

FIGURE 20.29 Ultrastructure of a mesothelial cell. Intermediate filaments are arranged in a perinuclear distribution.

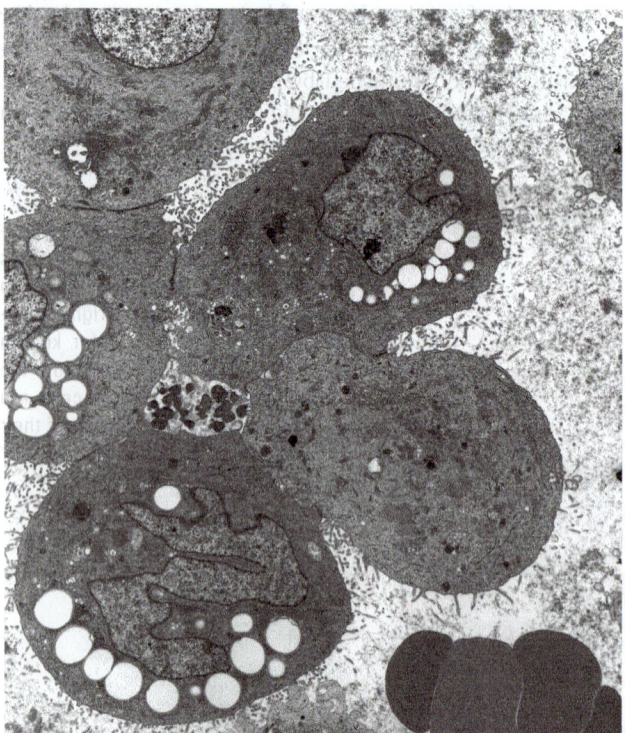

FIGURE 20.28 Ultrastructure of a cluster of detached mesothelial cells within a pleural effusion. Cytoplasmic lipid droplets impart a vacuolated appearance to some cells. Note the numerous long microvilli, which impart the "fuzzy" appearance to these cells at the light microscopic level.

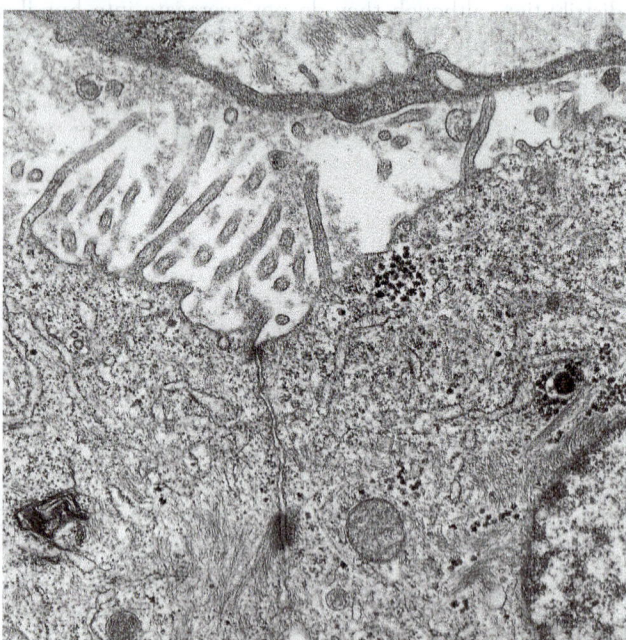

FIGURE 20.30 High magnification of the luminal aspect of two mesothelial cells. Note the small tight junction, subjacent desmosome, and the cytoskeletal filaments within the microvilli.

Immunohistochemistry

The antigens of the submesothelial layer can be categorized into matrix constituents and antigens of the mesenchymal cells. The extracellular matrix materials are those typical of most connective tissues. Types I and III collagen and fibronectin are abundant. Elastin fibers are plentiful and basement membrane proteins, including type IV collagen and laminin, are found at the mesothelial cell–stromal interface. Proteoglycans are plentiful. The pattern of intermediate filament expression by the submesothelial stromal cells varies with their state of excitation; quiescent cells express only vimentin, but stromal cells in regions of injury or inflammation also synthesize keratin detectable with antibodies to type I keratins (38).

Interactions of Mesothelial and Submesothelial Cells

The submesothelial mesenchymal cell population serves as the anchoring substratum for the mesothelium. Both mesothelial and submesothelial cells contribute to the extracellular proteins that comprise the matrix. Up to 3% of the total protein synthesized by mesothelial cells are collagens and laminin.

Whether submesothelial cells serve as a source of mesothelial cell renewal, either in normal development, or in conditions of rapid mesothelial cell turnover, is a controversial topic. Earlier ultrastructural and kinetics studies, using thymidine incorporation, suggested that stromal cells contribute to the repopulation of denuded mesothelium (40,41). This notion is consistent with the observation that submesothelial cells, when stimulated to proliferate, synthesize keratin and assume a more epithelioid morphology. However, later studies have demonstrated that healing of injured serosa is usually accomplished by multiplication and migration of surface mesothelial cells at the edges of the wounded area (42).

REACTIVE MESOTHELIUM

The capacity for mesothelial and submesothelial cellular elements to react and proliferate to produce morphologic patterns mimicking neoplasia is well known and is frequently a source of diagnostic confusion with malignancy. The process may be diffuse or localized. Mesothelial hyperplasia in the hernia sac or hydrocele specimens is well described (43) and may be nodular, demonstrates nuclear atypia and frequent mitotic figures, and be accompanied by proliferating spindle cell elements. Amin (44) reviewed the differential diagnosis of paratesticular mesothelial hyperplasia, adenomatoid tumors, and other histologically similar lesions. Bolen, Hammar, and McNutt (45) showed that normal surface mesothelium expressed high– and low–molecular weight cytokeratins and scattered submesothelial

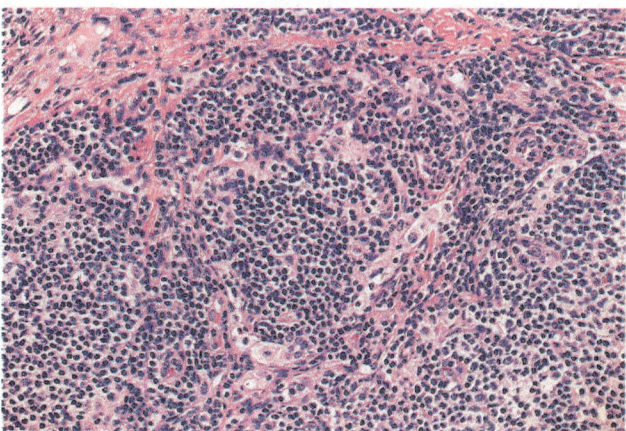

FIGURE 20.31 Internal mammary lymph node with large epithelioid cells in the sinuses found during coronary artery bypass graft surgery in a 61-year-old man. No pleural lesion was present.

cells expressed vimentin, but not keratin. However, reactive, nonneoplastic submesothelial cells coexpressed low–molecular-weight cytokeratin and vimentin.

Reactive mesothelial cells have been found in mediastinal lymph nodes (Figs. 20.31 and 20.32) by Brooks et al. (46), Parkash et al. (47), and Argani and Rosai (48), but the mechanisms by which they enter lymphatics and survive in the sinuses of nodes are not known. This rare event may produce a difficult differential diagnosis. Clear demonstration of the mesothelial phenotype of these cells excludes metastatic carcinoma, but not mesothelioma. Sussman and Rosai (49) showed that mesothelioma may present as a lymph node metastasis. Therefore, clinical presentation and close follow-up may be the only way to distinguish "misplaced" reactive mesothelial cells from mesothelioma.

An uncommon manifestation of mesothelial proliferation is the psammoma body—a laminated calcified structure that most likely arises through concentric calcification

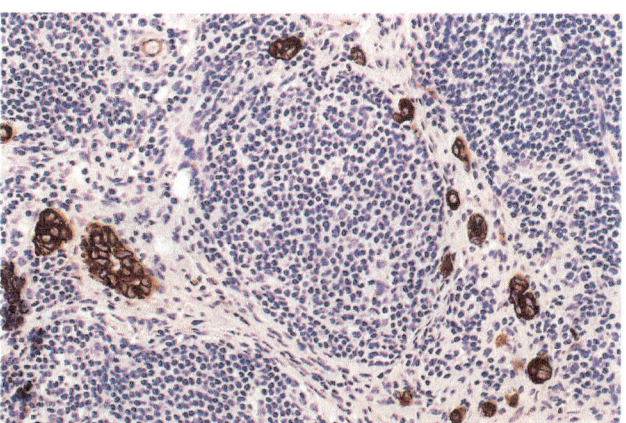

FIGURE 20.32 Immunohistochemical stain for keratin (AE1/AE3) demonstrates the epithelioid cells singly and in groups. They were negative for CEA, Leu-M1, BER-EP4, and B72.3 and hence were considered reactive mesothelial cells.

of dead cells. Psammoma bodies are nonspecific because they may be observed in inflammatory processes accompanied by mesothelial hyperplasia, and malignant mesothelial or epithelial neoplasia.

Fibrous Pleurisy

Fibrous pleurisy is a benign reactive process that usually occurs in the setting of organizing pleural effusions. The differential diagnosis of fibrous pleurisy and desmoplastic mesothelioma may be extremely difficult. Both may have regions of increased cellularity in a predominantly fibrous background containing spindle cells that are immunoreactive to keratin antibodies. Fibrous pleurisy tends to have a higher cellularity immediately beneath the fibrinous exudative surface of the pleura and demonstrates "layering" of spindle cells parallel to the fibrosis with intervening zones of fibrinous exudate. This organization imparts a histologic sense of order to the reactive process that may assist in its recognition (Fig. 20.33). Desmoplastic mesothelioma is characterized by the invasion of normal structures, notably fat, by spindle cells. The invasion may be subtle and often requires immunohistochemical stains for keratin for identification. Bland necrosis, a vaguely storiform pattern and small but overtly sarcomatous foci are characteristics of desmoplastic mesothelioma and are not seen in fibrous pleurisy (50).

Reactive Mesothelium versus Mesothelioma

Because most mesotheliomas are very well differentiated and of low nuclear grade, reactive mesothelium may mimic mesothelioma and malignant mesothelioma may masquerade as reactive mesothelium. Husain et al. (51) recently described the characteristics which best allow for differential diagnosis. Reactive mesothelium shows zonation with the most cellular and atypical proliferation adjacent to the surface and proliferation of capillaries perpendicular to the pleural surface in a "sunburst" pattern, whereas mesotheliomas most often

TABLE 20.1 Reactive Mesothelium versus Mesothelioma

	Reaction	Mesothelioma
Proliferation	Zonal	Diffuse
Capillaries	"Sunburst"	Random
Stromal expansion	Flat	Nodular
Necrosis	No	Often
Spread	Confined to pleura	Invades normal stroma

show nodular expansion of the stroma, tumor necrosis, sarcomatous foci and, most significantly, invasion of stroma; see Table 20.1. They concluded that invasion of normal structures, most often fat in the chest wall, was the most reliable feature to diagnose mesothelioma.

However, there is a need for distinguishing reaction from mesothelioma on cytologic or small biopsy samples, where invasion cannot be determined. There are numerous reports of immunostains, singly and in combination, which have been used for this purpose. Wu et al. (52) described the use of antibodies to XIAP, an X-linked inhibitor of apoptosis protein, and reported no staining on normal mesothelium, but staining on 8% of reactive mesothelium and 80% of mesotheliomas; staining was also observed on other malignancies, especially ovarian carcinomas in which 100% staining was observed. Sato et al. (53), used two antibodies to CD146, a cell adhesion molecule, on effusions and found immunocytochemical staining on all 23 mesotheliomas with one or the other antibody, but no staining on reactive cases. Hasteh et al. (54) reported that immunocytochemical staining with a panel of antibodies staining positively for EMA, p53, and GLUT-1 and negatively for desmin was associated with mesothelioma; the reverse was true for reactive mesothelium. Kato et al. (55) used immunohistochemistry for the identification of GLUT-1, a protein from a family of glucose transporters, with immunostaining of the plasma membranes in a linear pattern in 40 mesotheliomas, and none in the reactive mesothelial cases. Kuperman et al. (56) found GLUT-1 and EMA useful in the distinction between reactive and neoplastic mesothelial cells in effusions. However, there is overlap between reactive and neoplastic mesothelium in immunohistochemical profiles and panels of antibodies are needed to attempt to resolve the differential diagnosis without a demonstration of invasion.

Recently, two tests have been used to distinguish the mesothelium from reaction.

Monaco et al. (57) used fluorescence in situ hybridization (FISH) testing for p16 deletion and reported it to be more sensitive and specific for mesothelioma than GLUT-1 immunostaining. The p16 gene, which encodes the cyclin-dependent kinase 4 inhibitor, CDKN2A, is deleted in most mesotheliomas. The use of FISH to detect this deletion has

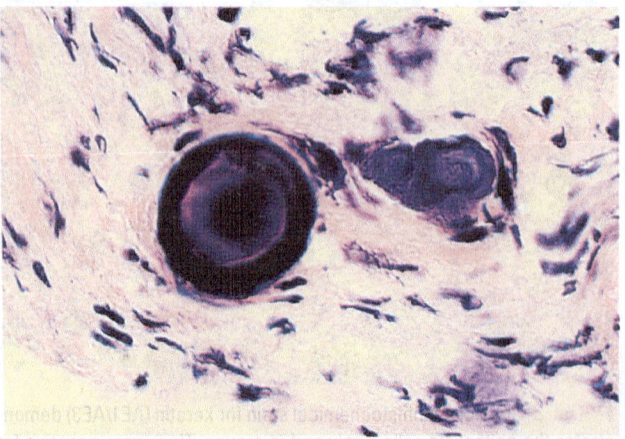

FIGURE 20.33 Psammoma bodies in the left pelvic peritoneum of a 58-year-old female.

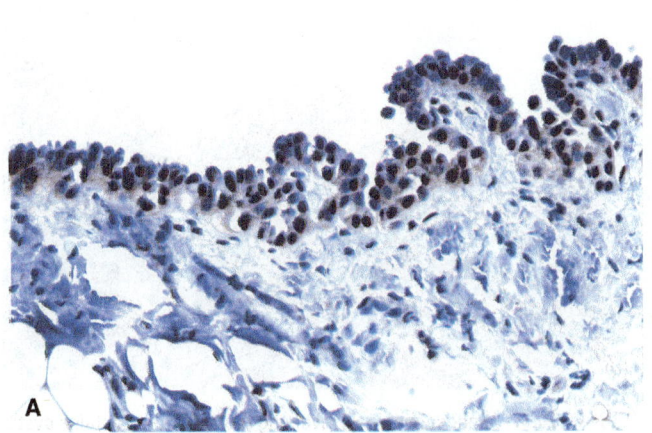 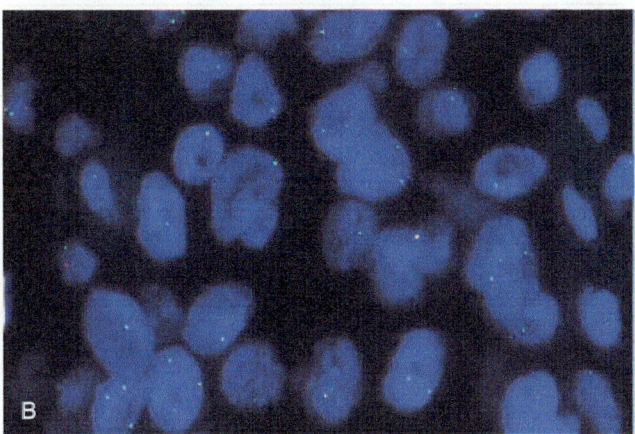

FIGURE 20.34 **A:** Immunoperoxidase stain for BAP-1 stains the nuclei of normal mesothelial cells in this section of pleura. Immunostaining is lost with BAP-1 mutation in mesothelioma. **B:** Fluorescence in situ hybridization (FISH) analysis with CDKN2A (*red signal*) and CEN-9 (*green signal*) dual color probe set demonstrates homozygous deletion of the CDKN2A gene (0 *red signals*, 1–2 *green signals*). Homozygous deletion of the CDKN2A gene, which encodes for the protein p16, is useful to distinguish malignant mesothelioma from reactive mesothelial hyperplasia.

been exploited in pleural fluid and formalin-fixed, paraffin-embedded tissues to distinguish mesothelioma from normal, benign and/or reactive mesothelium, in which p16 deletion is not observed. Illei et al. (58) reported p16 deletions in 12 of 13 mesothelioma-containing pleural fluids, but none of the benign fluids. Chiosea et al. (59) found p16 deletions in paraffin-embedded sections in 67% of pleural mesotheliomas (but only 25% of peritoneal mesotheliomas) and none in reactive mesothelium. They also immunostained for p16 product expression but found a lack of correlation between deletion and lack of expression. Takeda et al. (60) reported p16 deletions in 35 of 40 mesotheliomas and none in adenomatoid tumors, benign cystic mesotheliomas or reactive mesothelium, and Chung et al. (61) detected p16 deletions in 60% of malignant pleural mesotheliomas but not in reactive mesothelium. It should be noted that p16 deletions occur in other types of malignancies and are not mesothelioma specific.

Germline deletion of BAP-1, which is the BRCA-1–associated protein and a tumor suppressor gene with cell cycle regulatory functions, DNA damage repair, and signaling functions, is associated with predisposition for development of mesothelioma and melanoma, as well as renal cell carcinoma and other malignancies (62). Cignotti et al. (63) found BAP-1 expression by immunohistochemistry in all benign and reactive mesothelial proliferations studied (see Fig. 20.34A), but loss of expression was found in 66% of epithelioid and biphasic mesotheliomas studied. However, loss of BAP-1 expression was found in only 15% of sarcomatoid or desmoplastic mesotheliomas.

The combination of BAP-1 loss by immunohistochemistry and p16 deletion by FISH is highly specific for mesothelioma (see Fig. 20.34B), but is not highly sensitive and negative results were not found to exclude mesothelioma (64). Hwang et al. (65) found the combination of BAP-1 immunohistochemistry and p16 FISH deletion analysis useful in the interpretation of pleural effusions and epithelioid mesothelioma, but p16 deletion was not useful in the differential diagnosis of sarcomatoid mesothelioma (see Table 20.2) (66).

Reactive Mesothelium versus Carcinoma

The distinction of metastatic carcinoma from reactive mesothelium is facilitated by immunohistochemistry, because the antigenic makeup of mesothelial and epithelial cells is fundamentally different. Mesothelial cells usually lack the glycoproteins detected by antibodies to CEA, MOC-31, and BER-EP4 and the determinant detected by Leu-M1

TABLE 20.2

Differentiation of Reactive From Neoplastic Mesothelium by Immunohistochemistry and FISH

Assay	Reactive	Mesothelioma
BAP-1: IPOX	Present	Absent
P16: FISH	Present	Deleted
Desmin: IPOX	Present	Absent
GLUT-1: IPOX	Absent	Present
IMP3: IPOX	Absent	Present
XIAP: IPOX	Absent	Present
CD146: IPOX	Absent	Present
EMA: IPOX	Absent	Present
P53: IPOX	Absent	Present

TABLE 20.3 Immunohistochemical Marker Useful in the Distinction of Mesothelium From Adenocarcinoma	
Mesothelium	Adenocarcinoma
Calretinin	CEA
CK5/6	MOC-31
WT-1	B72.3
D240	Claudin 4

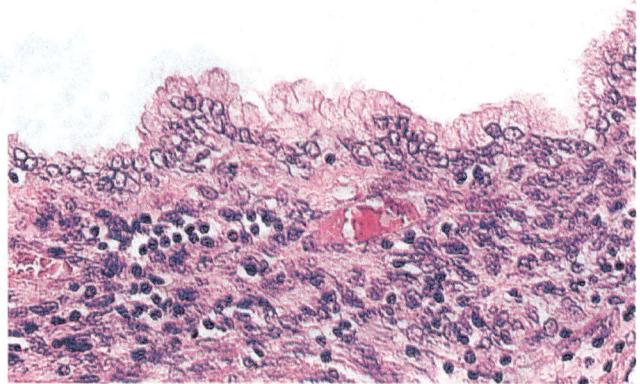

FIGURE 20.35 Endosalpingiosis involving the omentum contains cystic glands lined by mucinous epithelium with basally oriented nuclei and apical cytoplasm. Periglandular stroma contains mononuclear inflammatory cells.

(CD15) (67–70). Latza et al. (71) and Sheibani et al. (72) reported that BER-EP4 was useful to distinguish malignant epithelium (adenocarcinoma) from malignant mesothelioma, but Gaffey et al. (73) and Otis (74) reported BER-EP4 immunoreactivity in high proportions of both benign and malignant mesothelial tumors, as well as adenocarcinomas.

Antibodies chosen for the diagnostic profiles are based on the metastatic malignancy considered in the differential diagnosis. Differentiation from adenocarcinoma of the lungs is based on its characteristic expression of TTF-1, CEA, Napsin-A, MOC-31, BER-EP4, or B72.3 and their absence in reactive mesothelium (51). Claudin 4 is a tight junction protein expressed in most epithelial cells, but absent in mesothelial cells (75). The tissue-specific nuclear transcription protein TTF-1 is important in the embryogenesis of thyroid and lungs and is found in the nuclei of pneumocytes and many adenocarcinomas of the lung, but not in the mesothelium (76). Because of variations in sensitivity and specificity in these antibodies, combinations of two or more mesothelial and two or more epithelial markers are recommended (77). PAX8 has been found useful in distinguishing ovarian lesions from mesothelial lesions (see Table 20.3) (78).

Endosalpingiosis and Endometriosis

Epithelial elements may be observed in glandular arrangements throughout the peritoneum, omentum, and within lymph nodes. Such glandular structures were recognized in the early 1900s and misinterpreted by some as metastatic carcinoma, a mistake that is unfortunately still committed today. Endometriosis and endosalpingiosis were discussed by Sampson (79–81) earlier, with reference to mechanisms of pathogenesis that are still debated.

Endosalpingiosis refers to glandular spaces lined by epithelium similar to fallopian tube epithelium, with three cell types (ciliated, secretory, and intercalated) (Fig. 20.35) (82). On occasion, psammoma bodies are present. Periglandular stroma containing chronic inflammatory cells is separated from the epithelium by PAS-positive basement membrane. Endosalpingiosis may be differentiated from endometriosis by the lack of endometrial stroma or evidence of stromal hemorrhage associated with endometriosis (83–85). This condition is seen exclusively in women and has been reported in 12.5% of omenta removed during surgery in females. A large proportion of these women have coexisting benign disease of the fallopian tube. The origin of the glandular inclusions is debated but is most likely either related to the influence of müllerian development on the peritoneal mesothelium (coelomic lining) or is a sequela of disease within the tube resulting in extratubal growth of displaced tubal epithelium. Although definitive evidence of neoplasia arising in endosalpingiosis has not been documented, considerable difficulty may be encountered when differentiating extraovarian tumor implants removed in the setting of common epithelial ovarian tumors from endosalpingiosis with cellular atypia. Evaluation of the severity of epithelial atypia, mitotic activity, the presence of ciliated cells, and the presence of invasive characteristics may aid in establishing a diagnosis of malignancy in this setting. Metaplasia in endosalpingiosis may also be a source of diagnostic difficulty—particularly mucinous metaplasia, which may be mistaken for metastatic mucinous adenocarcinoma (Figs. 20.36 and 20.37).

Endometriosis is defined by the presence of glands lined by endometrial-type epithelium surrounded by endometrial

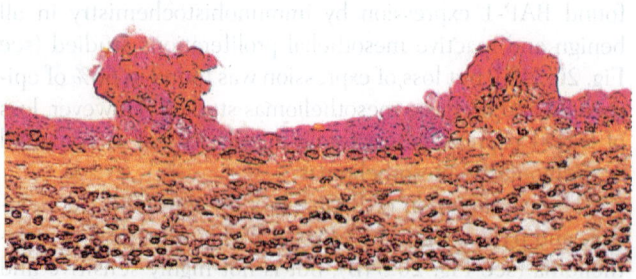

FIGURE 20.36 Mucicarmine stain of mucinous change in endosalpingiosis demonstrates intracytoplasmic mucin in apical cytoplasm.

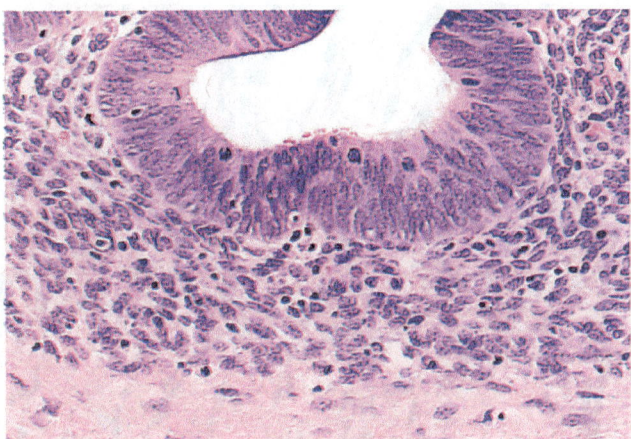

FIGURE 20.37 Endometriosis involving the peritoneum with extension into the soft tissue of the anterior abdominal wall of a 23-year-old woman. Endometrial glands and stroma are present.

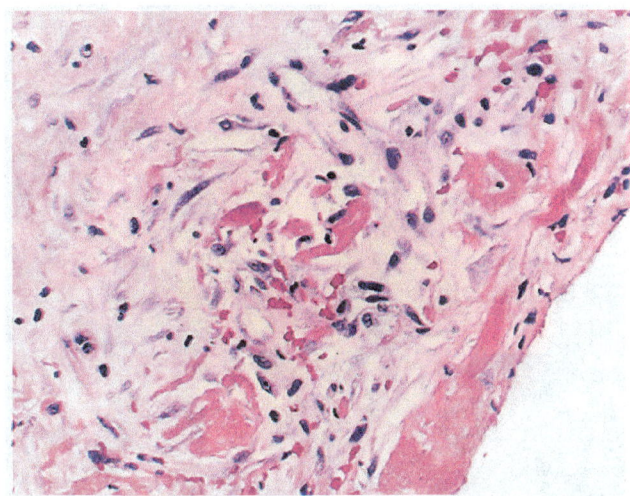

FIGURE 20.39 The histologic appearance of fibrous pleurisy reflects its inflammatory nature, with granulation tissue, fibrin, and a zonal pattern ranging from active inflammation to quiescent dense fibrosis.

stroma, outside the uterine endometrial mucosa and myometrium (86). The condition occurs most frequently in women of childbearing age. It may occur in a variety of body sites, ranging from the pelvic peritoneum to distant organs such as lungs, kidney, and skin, but the most frequent site is the peritoneal lining of the pelvic organs (Fig. 20.38). Although the histogenesis of endometriosis remains unclear, two general theories have been proposed: ectopic growth of endometrial elements displacement of endometrial tissue, through local means (such as entry of endometrium into the pelvis through the uterine tubes) or via vascular routes to distant organs (81,82) versus metaplastic change of the pelvic peritoneum along müllerian lines of differentiation (87,88). Although the mesothelium normally lacks sex steroid receptors, reactive mesothelium adjacent to endometriosis expresses focal immunoreactivity for estrogen and progesterone receptors (89). Both mechanisms may play a role in the histogenesis of endometriosis.

Endometriosis may appear as brown–maroon foci on the peritoneal surfaces and may be accompanied by fibrosis or adhesions. Microscopically, endometrial stroma surrounding endometrial epithelium is present. Response to hormonal influences is often seen and may be synchronous with intrauterine endometrium. Metaplasia occurs in both epithelial and stromal elements, similar to metaplasias encountered in the endometrium of the uterus. The presence of hemosiderin-laden macrophages and fibrosis may be the only evidence that endometriosis had once been present. However, a definitive diagnosis of endometriosis may not be rendered unless both endometrial glands and stroma are seen.

Another common type of metaplasia, more frequently observed in pregnancy, is a decidual change. Although usually encountered in the submesothelial layer of pelvic peritoneal surfaces, decidual changes may be seen in distant sites including the serosal surfaces of the liver, spleen and diaphragm, and within lymph nodes. In these locations, decidual changes may be mistaken for metastatic carcinoma or malignant mesothelioma (Fig. 20.39) (90).

Multilocular Peritoneal Inclusion Cyst

Multilocular peritoneal inclusion cyst (MPIC) is a mesothelial-lined multilocular lesion that occurs almost exclusively in women. The lesion usually involves the pelvis, although it may occur in other abdominal locations, including the omentum and mesentery. Usually MPIC is mass-forming and may attain diameters up to 20 cm. Grossly, it is composed of multiple cysts, some of which may be thin walled and translucent (Fig. 20.39). Histologically, the septa range from thin and delicate to thickened and inflamed. The mesothelial lining ranges from single flattened cells to hobnail-type cells. Squamous metaplasia of the lining mesothelium may be present. Some regions may resemble the cellular pattern of an adenomatoid tumor (Figs. 20.40–20.42) (91).

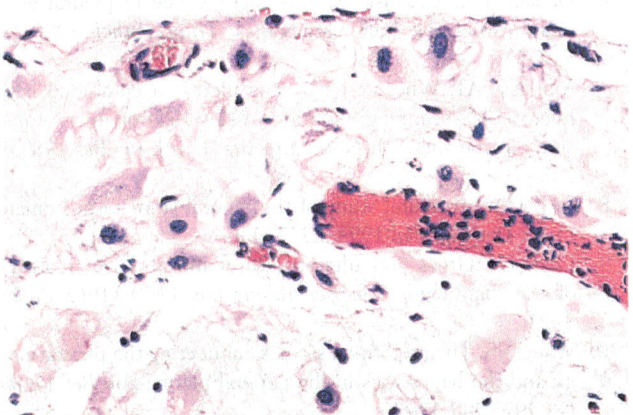

FIGURE 20.38 Decidual change in the pelvis during pregnancy is seen in the subserosal tissue. Loosely cohesive cells with abundant eosinophilic cytoplasm are present.

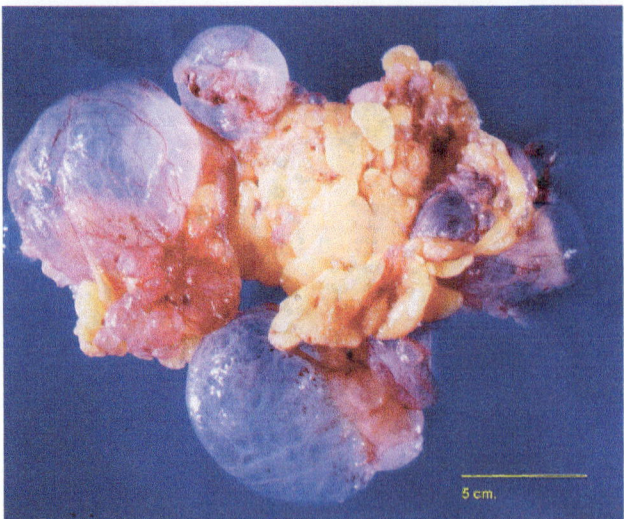

FIGURE 20.40 MPIC in the omentum of a 73-year-old patient discovered incidentally at surgery for urogynecologic repair procedure. The cysts vary in size, some being translucent while others are fibrotic, particularly toward the center of the mass.

The true nature of MPIC remains somewhat controversial, with some authors maintaining that it is a neoplasm while others assert it is a reactive lesion that develops in response to injury or even endometriosis. The original designation of *multicystic mesothelioma* reflects the notion that the lesion is neoplastic. Recurrences are frequent, although MPIC-related deaths probably do not occur.

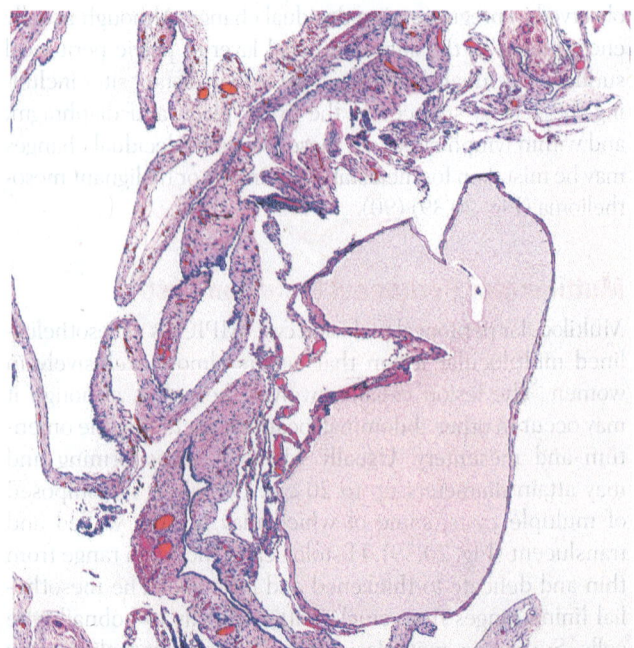

FIGURE 20.41 Histologically, MPICs reflect the gross features, with septae that vary in thickness and cysts that vary in size.

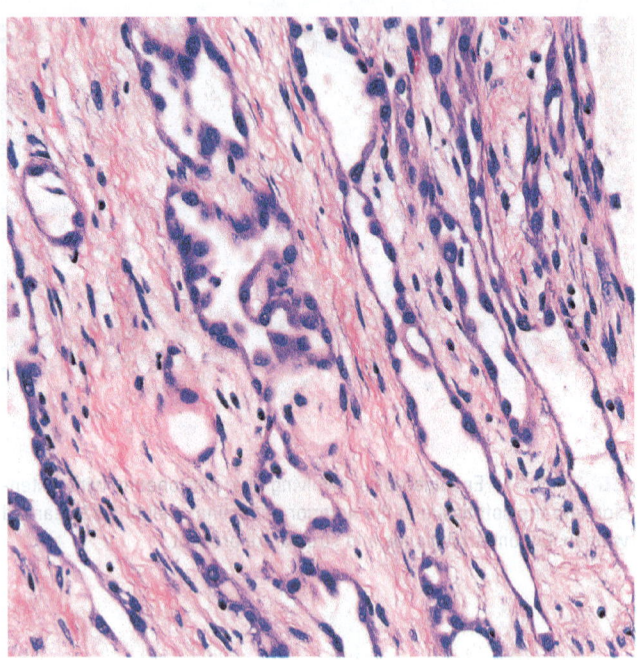

FIGURE 20.42 Some regions in MPICs may contain mesothelial proliferations that closely resemble an adenomatoid tumor.

REFERENCES

1. Sahn SA. State of the art. The pleura. *Am Rev Respir Dis* 1988;138:184–234.
2. Pistolesi M, Miniati M, Giuntini C. Pleural liquid and solute exchanges. *Am Rev Respir Dis* 1989;140:825–847.
3. Albertine KH, Wiener-Kronish JP, Roos PJ, et al. Structure, blood supply, and lymphatic vessels of the sheep's visceral pleura. *Am J Anat* 1982;165:227–294.
4. Fourdrain A, Lafitte S, Iquille J, et al. Lymphatic drainage of lung segments in the visceral pleura: a cadaveric study. *Surg Radiol Anat* 2017;10:276–317.
5. Grant T, Levin B. Lymphangiographic visualization of pleural and pulmonary lymphatics in a patient without a chylothorax. *Radiology* 1974;113:49–50.
6. Gallagher B, Urbanski SJ. The significance of pleural elastica invasion by lung carcinomas. *Hum Pathol* 1990;21:512–517.
7. Mariassy AT, Wheeldon EB. The pleura: a combined light microscopic, scanning, and transmission electron microscopic study in the sheep. I. Normal pleura. *Exp Lung Res* 1983;4:293–314.
8. Li J. Ultrastructural study of the pleural stomata in human. *Funct Dev Morphol* 1993;3:277–280.
9. Leak LV. Gross and ultrastructural morphologic features of the diaphragm. *Am Rev Respir Dis* 1979;119(2 Pt 2):3–21.
10. Wang NS. The preformed stomas connecting the pleural cavity and the lymphatics in the parietal pleura. *Am Rev Respir Dis* 1975;111:12–20.
11. Wang NS. Morphological data of pleura. Normal conditions. In: Chretien J, Hirsch A, eds. *Diseases of the Pleura*. New York: Masson; 1983:10–24.

12. Wang NS. Anatomy and physiology of the pleural space. *Clin Chest Med* 1985;6:3–16.
13. Bernaudin JF, Fleury J. Anatomy of the blood and lymphatic circulation of the pleural serosa. In: Chretien J, Bignon J, Hirsch A, eds. *The Pleura in Health and Disease*. Vol. 30. New York: Marcel Dekker; 1985:101–124.
14. Li J, Zhao Z, Zhao J, et al. A study of the three dimensional organization of the human diaphragmatic lymphatic lacunae and lymphatic drainage units. *Ann Anat* 1996;178:537–544.
15. Lee KF, Olak J. Anatomy and physiology of the pleural space. *Chest Surg Clin N Am* 1994;4:391–403.
16. Staub NC, Wiener-Kronish JP, Albertine KH. Transport through the pleura. Physiology of normal liquid and solute exchange in the pleural space. In: Chretien J, Bignon J, Hirsch A, eds. *The Pleura in Health and Disease*. New York: Marcel Dekker; 1985:169–193.
17. Kampmeier OF. Concerning certain mesothelial thickenings and vascular plexuses of the mediastinal pleura associated with histiocyte and fat-cell production, in the human newborn. *Anat Rec* 1928;39:201–208.
18. Boutin C, Dumortier P, Rey F, et al. Black spots concentrate oncogenic asbestos fibers in the parietal pleura. Thoracoscopic and mineralogic study. *Am J Respir Crit Care Med* 1996;153:444–449.
19. Miserocchi G, Sancini G, Mantegazza F, et al. Translocation pathways for inhaled asbestos fibers. *Environ Health* 2008;7:4.
20. Wassilev W, Wedel T, Michailova K, et al. A scanning electron microscopy study of peritoneal stomata in different peritoneal regions. *Ann Anat* 1998;180:137–143.
21. Li JC, Yu SM. Study of the ultrastructure of the peritoneal stomata in humans. *Acta Anat* 1991;141:28–30.
22. Liu J, Geng X, Li Y. Milky spots: omental functional units and hotbeds for peritoneal cancer metastases. *Tumour Biol* 2016;37:5715–5726.
23. Ernst CS, Brooks JJ. Immunoperoxidase localization of secretory component in reactive mesothelium and mesotheliomas. *J Histochem Cytochem* 1981;29:1102–1104.
24. Roth J. Ultrahistochemical demonstration of saccharide components of complex carbohydrates at the alveolar cell surface and at the mesothelial cell surface of the pleura visceralis of mice by means of concanavalin A. *Exp Pathol (Jena)* 1973;8:157–167.
25. MacDougall DB, Wang SE, Zidar BL. Mucin-positive epithelial mesothelioma. *Arch Pathol Lab Med* 1992;116:874–880.
26. Wu YJ, Parker LM, Binder NE, et al. The mesothelial keratins: a new family of cytoskeletal proteins identified in cultured mesothelial cells and nonkeratinizing epithelia. *Cell* 1982;31(3 Pt 2):693–703.
27. Moll R, Lowe A, Laufer J, et al. Cytokeratin 20 in human carcinomas. A new histodiagnostic marker detected by monoclonal antibodies. *Am J Pathol* 1992;140:427–447.
28. Moll R, Franke WW, Schiller DL, et al. The catalog of human cytokeratins: patterns of expression in normal epithelia, tumors, and cultured cells. *Cell* 1982;31:11–24.
29. Doglioni C, Tos AP, Laurino L, et al. Calretinin: a novel immunocytochemical marker for mesothelioma. *Am J Surg Pathol* 1996;20:1037–1046.
30. Nagel H, Hemmerlein B, Ruschenburg I, et al. The value of anti-calretinin antibody in the differential diagnosis of normal and reactive mesothelia versus metastatic tumors in effusion cytology. *Pathol Res Pract* 1998;194:759–764.
31. Oates J, Edwards C. HBME-1, MOC-31, WT1 and calretinin: an assessment of recently described markers for mesothelioma and adenocarcinoma. *Histopathology* 2000;36:341–347.
32. Ordonez NG. Value of calretinin immunostaining in diagnostic pathology: a review and update. *Appl Immunohistochem Mol Morphol* 2014;22:401–415.
33. Chu PG, Weiss LM. Expression of cytokeratin 5/6 in epithelial neoplasms: an immunohistochemical study of 509 cases. *Mod Pathol* 2002;15:6–10.
34. Hecht JL, Lee BH, Pinkus JL, et al. The value of Wilms tumor susceptibility gene 1 in cytologic preparations as a marker for malignant mesothelioma. *Cancer* 2002;96:105–109.
35. Chu AY, Litzky LA, Pasha TL, et al. Utility of D2-40, a novel mesothelial marker, in the diagnosis of malignant mesothelioma. *Mod Pathol* 2005;18:105–110.
36. Ordonez NG. The immunohistochemical diagnosis of mesothelioma: a comparative study of epithelioid mesothelioma and lung adenocarcinoma. *Am J Surg Pathol* 2003;27:1031–1051.
37. Pitt MA, Haboubi NY. Serosal reaction in chronic gastric ulcers: an immunohistochemical and ultrastructural study. *J Clin Pathol* 1995;48:226–228.
38. Bolen JW, Hammer SP, McNutt MA. Reactive and neoplastic serosal tissue. A light-microscopic, ultrastructural, and immunocytochemical study. *Am J Surg Pathol* 1986;10:34–47.
39. Stecco C, Sfriso MM, Porzionato A, et al. Microscopic anatomy of the visceral fasciae. *J Anat* 2017;231:121–128.
40. Raftery AT. Regeneration of parietal and visceral peritoneum in the immature animal: a light and electron microscopical study. *Br J Surg* 1973;60:969–975.
41. Raftery AT. Regeneration of parietal and visceral peritoneum: an electron microscopical study. *J Anat* 1984;115(Pt 3):375–392.
42. Whitaker D, Papadimitriou JM. Mesothelial healing: morphological and kinetic investigations. *J Pathol* 1985;145:159–175.
43. Rosai J, Dehner LP. Nodular mesothelial hyperplasia in hernia sacs: a benign reactive condition simulating a neoplastic process. *Cancer* 1975;35:165–175.
44. Amin MB. Selected other problematic testicular and paratesticular lesions: rete testis neoplasms and pseudotumors, mesothelial lesions and secondary tumors. *Mod Pathol* 2005;18(Suppl 2):S131–S145.
45. Bolen JW, Hammar SP, McNutt MA. Serosal tissue: reactive tissue as a model for understanding mesotheliomas. *Ultrastruct Pathol* 1987;11:251–262.
46. Brooks JS, LiVolsi VA, Pietra GG. Mesothelial cell inclusions in mediastinal lymph nodes mimicking metastatic carcinoma. *Am J Clin Pathol* 1990;93:741–748.
47. Parkash V, Vidwans M, Carter D. Benign mesothelial cells in mediastinal lymph nodes. *Am J Surg Pathol* 1999;23:1264–1269.
48. Argani P, Rosai J. Hyperplastic mesothelial cells in lymph nodes: report of six cases of a benign process that can simulate metastatic involvement by mesothelioma or carcinoma. *Hum Pathol* 1998;29:339–346.

49. Sussman J, Rosai J. Lymph node metastasis as the initial manifestation of malignant mesothelioma: report of six cases. *Am J Surg Pathol* 1990;14:819–828.
50. Husain AN, Colby T, Ordonez N, et al. Guidelines for the pathologic diagnosis of malignant mesothelioma: 2012 update of the consensus statement from the International Mesothelioma Interest Group. *Arch Pathol Lab Med* 2013;137:647–667.
51. Husain AN, Colby T, Ordonez N. Guidelines for the pathologic diagnosis of malignant mesothelioma: 2017 update of the consensus statement from the International Mesothelioma Interest Group. *Arch Pathol Lab Med* 2018;142:89–108.
52. Wu M, Sun Y, Li G, et al. Immunohistochemical detection of XIAP in mesothelioma and mesothelial lesions. *Am J Clin Pathol* 2007;128:783–787.
53. Sato A, Torii I, Okamura Y, et al. Immunohistochemistry of CD146 is useful to discriminate between malignant pleural mesothelioma and reactive mesothelium. *Mod Pathol* 2010;23:1458–1466.
54. Hasteh F, Lin GY, Weidner N, et al. The use of immunohistochemistry to distinguish reactive mesothelial cells from malignant mesothelioma in cytologic effusions. *Cancer Cytopathol* 2010;118:90–96.
55. Kato Y, Tsuta K, Seki K, et al. Immunohistochemical detection of GLUT-1 can discriminate between reactive mesothelium and malignant mesothelioma. *Mod Pathol* 2007;20:215–220.
56. Kuperman M, Florence RR, Pantanowitz L, et al. Distinguishing benign from malignant mesothelial cells by Glut-1, EMA and Desmin expression: an evidence-based approach. *Diagn Cytopathol* 2013;41:131–140.
57. Monaco SE, Shuai Y, Bansal M, et al. The diagnostic utility of p16 FISH and GLUT-1 immunohistochemical analysis in mesothelial proliferations. *Am J Clin Pathol* 2011;135:619–627.
58. Illei PB, Ladanyi M, Rusch VW, et al. The use of CDKN2A deletion as a diagnostic marker for malignant mesothelioma in body cavity fluids. *Cancer* 2003;99:51–56.
59. Chiosea S, Krasinskas A, Cagle PT, et al. Diagnostic importance of 9p21 homozygous deletion in malignant mesothelioma. *Mod Pathol* 2008;21:742–747.
60. Takeda M, Kasai T, Enomoto Y, et al. 9p21 deletion in the diagnosis of malignant mesothelioma, using fluorescent in situ hybridization analysis. *Pathol Int* 2010;60:395–399.
61. Chung CT, Santos GC, Hwang DM, et al. FISH assay development for the detection of p16/CDKN2A deletion in malignant mesotheliomas. *J Clin Pathol* 2010;63:630–634.
62. Testa JR, Cheung M, Pei J, et al. Germline BAP-1 mutations predispose to malignant mesothelioma. *Nat Genet* 2011;43:1022–1025.
63. Cignognetti M, Lonardi S, Fisogni S, et al. BAP-1 (BRCA1-associated protein 1) is a highly specific marker for differentiating mesothelioma from reactive mesothelial proliferations. *Mod Pathol* 2015;28:1043–1057.
64. Sheffield BS, Hwang HC, Lee AF, et al. BAP-1 immunohistochemistry and p16 FISH to separate benign from malignant mesothelial proliferations. *Am J Surg Pathol* 2016;39:977–982.
65. Hwang HC, Sheffield BS, Rodriguez S, et al. Utility of BAP-1 immunohistochemistry and p16(CDKN2A) FISH in the diagnosis of malignant mesothelioma in effusion cytology specimens. *Am J Surg Pathol* 2016;40:120–126.
66. Hwang HC, Pyott S, Rodriguez S, et al. BAP-1 immunohistochemistry and p16 FISH in the diagnosis of sarcomatous and desmoplastic mesothelioma. *Am J Surg Pathol* 2016;40:714–718.
67. Otis CN, Carter D, Cole S, et al. Immunohistochemical evaluation of pleural mesothelioma and pulmonary adenocarcinoma. A bi-institutional study of 47 cases. *Am J Surg Pathol* 1987;11:445–456.
68. Sheibani K, Battifora H, Burke JS, et al. Leu-M1 antigen in human neoplasms: an immunohistologic study of 400 cases. *Am J Surg Pathol* 1986;10:227–236.
69. Sheibani K, Esteban JM, Bailey A, et al. Immunopathologic and molecular studies as an aid to the diagnosis of malignant mesothelioma. *Hum Pathol* 1992;23:107–116.
70. Sheibani K. Immunopathology of malignant mesothelioma. *Hum Pathol* 1994;25:219–220.
71. Latza U, Niedobitek G, Schwarting R, et al. Ber-EP4: new monoclonal antibody which distinguishes epithelia from mesothelia. *J Clin Pathol* 1990;43:213–219.
72. Sheibani K, Shin SS, Kezirian J, et al. Ber-EP4 antibody as a discriminant in the differential diagnosis of malignant mesothelioma versus adenocarcinoma. *Am J Surg Pathol* 1991;15:779–784.
73. Gaffey MJ, Mills SE, Swanson PE, et al. Immunoreactivity for Ber-EP4 in adenocarcinomas, adenomatoid tumors, and malignant mesotheliomas. *Am J Surg Pathol* 1992;16:593–599.
74. Otis CN. Uterine adenomatoid tumors: immunohistochemical characteristics with emphasis on Ber-EP4 immunoreactivity and distinction from adenocarcinoma. *Int J Gynecol Pathol* 1996;15:146–151.
75. Ordonez NG. Value of claudin-4 immunostaining in the diagnosis of mesothelioma. *Am J Clin Pathol* 2013;139:611–619.
76. Ordonez NG. Value of thyroid transcription factor-1, E-cadherin, BG8, WT1 and CD44S immunostaining in distinguishing epithelial pleural mesothelioma from pulmonary and nonpulmonary adenocarcinoma. *Am J Surg Pathol* 2000;24:598–606.
77. Yaziji H, Battifora H, Barry TS, et al. Evaluation of 12 antibodies for distinguishing epithelioid mesothelioma from adenocarcinoma: Identification of a three antibody immunohistochemical panel with maximal sensitivity and specificity. *Mod Pathol* 2006;19:514–523.
78. Laury AR, Hornick JL, Perets R, et al. PAX8 reliably distinguishes ovarian serous tumors from malignant mesothelioma. *Am J Surg Pathol* 2010;34:627–635.
79. Sampson JA. Heterotopic or misplaced endometrial tissue. *Am J Obstet Gynecol* 1925;10:649–664.
80. Sampson JA. Postsalpingectomy endometriosis (endosalpingiosis). *Am J Obstet Gynecol* 1930;20:443–480.
81. Sampson JA. The pathogenesis of postsalpingectomy endometriosis in laparotomy scars. *Am J Obstet Gynecol* 1946;50:597–620.
82. Zinsser KR, Wheeler JE. Endosalpingiosis in the omentum: a study of autopsy and surgical material. *Am J Surg Pathol* 1982;6:109–117.
83. Hsu YK, Parmley TH, Rosenshein NB, et al. Neoplastic and non-neoplastic mesothelial proliferations in pelvic lymph nodes. *Obstet Gynecol* 1980;55:83–88.

84. Horn LC, Bilek K. Frequency and histogenesis of pelvic retroperitoneal lymph node inclusions of the female genital tract. An immunohistochemical study of 34 cases. *Pathol Res Pract* 1995;191:991–996.
85. Schnurr RC, Delgado G, Chun B. Benign glandular inclusions in para-aortic lymph nodes in women undergoing lymphadenectomies. *Am J Obstet Gynecol* 1978;130:813–816.
86. Clement PB. Endometriosis, lesions of the secondary müllerian system, and pelvic mesothelial proliferations. In: Kurman RJ, ed. *Blaustein's Pathology of the Female Genital Tract*. 3rd ed. New York: Springer-Verlag; 1987:517–559.
87. Ferguson BR, Bennington JL, Haber SL. Histochemistry of mucosubstances and histology of mixed müllerian pelvic lymph node glandular inclusions: evidence for histogenesis by müllerian metaplasia on coelomic epithelium. *Obstet Gynecol* 1969;33:617–625.
88. Lauchlan SC. The secondary müllerian system. *Obstet Gynecol Surv* 1972;27:133–146.
89. Nakayama K, Masuzawa H, Li S, et al. Immunohistochemical analysis of the peritoneum adjacent to endometriotic lesions using antibodies for Ber-EP4 antigen, estrogen receptors, and progesterone receptors: implication of peritoneal metaplasia in the pathogenesis of endometriosis. *Int J Gynecol Pathol* 1994;13:348–358.
90. Clement PB. Reactive tumor-like lesions of the peritoneum. *Am J Clin Pathol* 1995;103:673–676.
91. Weiss SW, Tavassoli FA. Multicystic mesothelioma. An analysis of pathologic findings and biologic behavior in 37 cases. *Am J Surg Pathol* 1988;12:737–746.

SECTION VII

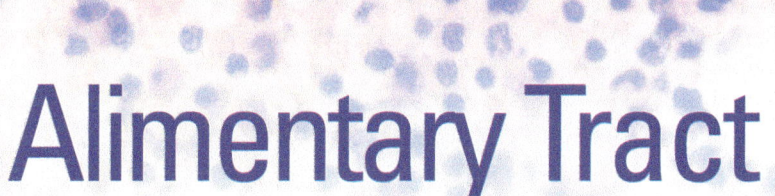

Alimentary Tract

Esophagus

James R. Conner ▪ Hala El-Zimaity ▪ Robert H. Riddell

EMBRYOLOGY 573	VENOUS DRAINAGE 590
Esophageal Atresia 574	LYMPHATIC DRAINAGE 590
Esophageal Duplication 574	INNERVATION (NERVES AND INTERSTITIAL CELLS OF CAJAL) 590
Lower Esophageal Rings and Webs 575	
TOPOGRAPHY AND RELATIONS 576	
MACROSCOPIC/ENDOSCOPIC FEATURES 578	DIAGNOSTIC CONSIDERATIONS 591
Glycogenic Acanthosis 578	Barrett Esophagus 591
Heterotopias 578	Gastroesophageal Reflux Disease 593
Esophageal Musculature 579	Eosinophilic Esophagitis 595
Lower Esophageal Sphincter 581	Lymphocytic Esophagitis 595
Gastroesophageal Junction 581	Exfoliative (Sloughing) Esophagitis (Esophagitis Dissecans Superficialis) 595
HISTOLOGY 582	Acute Necrotizing Esophagitis 595
Mucosa 583	Adenocarcinomas of the Gastroesophageal Region 596
Submucosa 586	ACKNOWLEDGMENT 596
Muscularis Propria 588	REFERENCES 596
Serosa 589	
ARTERIAL SUPPLY 589	

EMBRYOLOGY

In the early stages of development, the notochord induces the formation of the foregut from endoderm (1). At about 21 days' gestation, septa arise from the lateral walls of the foregut, fuse, and divide the foregut into the esophagus and trachea. This process of septation begins at the carina and extends cephalad, being completed by 5 to 6 weeks' gestation (Fig. 21.1).

The esophagus is initially lined by a thin layer of stratified columnar epithelium, which proliferates to almost occlude the lumen (2). New vacuoles appear in the luminal cells of the foregut and coalesce to form a single esophageal lumen with a superficial layer of ciliated epithelial cells (Fig. 21.2) (2). As early as 8 weeks' gestation, and beginning in the middle third of the esophagus, ciliated cells appear. These extend cephalad and caudally to almost cover the entire stratified columnar epithelium (2–4). At approximately 10 weeks, a single layer of columnar cells populates the proximal and distal ends of the esophagus (2). At approximately 4 months' gestation, the esophageal cardiac-type glands form as a result of the downward growth of these columnar cells into the lamina propria with subsequent proliferation and differentiation (3,5). They go distally as far as the oxyntic mucosa, so that similar glands can be found in the cardia. Some have used this to argue that the cardia is therefore intrinsically a part of the esophagus, (6) although it could just as easily be interpreted that they are just present in all mucosae proximal to oxyntic mucosa.

At approximately 5 months' gestation, stratified squamous epithelium initially appears in the middle one-third of the esophagus and extends cephalad and caudally, replacing the ciliated epithelium (Fig. 21.3) (3,4). The upper esophagus is the last area to be replaced by squamous epithelium; and, if this process of squamous replacement is not completed at birth, there may be persistence of ciliated cells in the

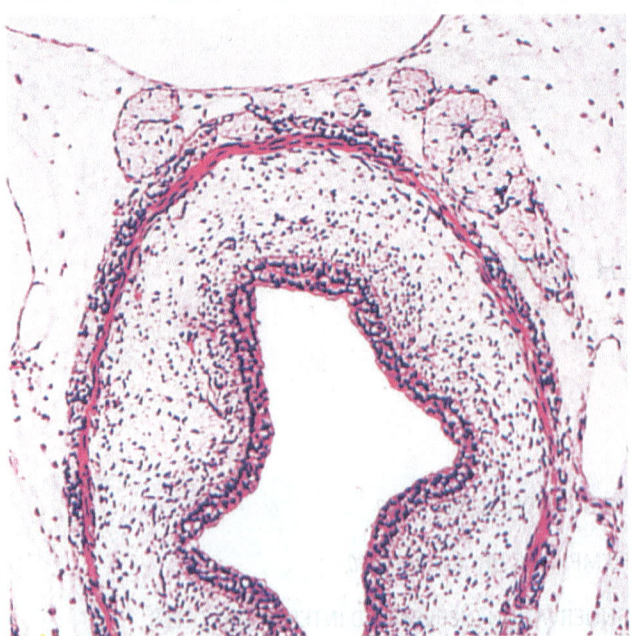

FIGURE 21.1 Fetal esophagus (late first trimester). Transverse section overview of the esophagus demonstrating inner mucosal layer, middle submucosal layer, and thin outer muscle layer. Note the vagus nerves lying over the esophagus.

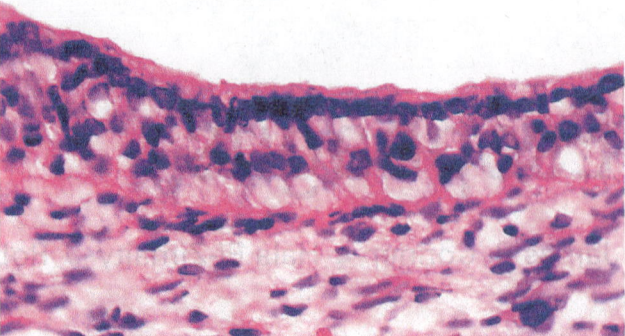

FIGURE 21.2 Fetal esophagus (late first trimester). The epithelial layer is composed of stratified columnar epithelium. Note the lack of muscularis mucosae.

upper esophagus (2,4). This may progress to gastric differentiation resulting in the so-called "inlet patch" (discussed subsequently). Interestingly, the mucosa of the fetal upper esophagus lacks a muscularis mucosae (Fig. 21.3).

These residual cells are usually short lived, being replaced by squamous epithelium within 2 to 3 days postpartum (4,7). However, in some patients they either persist into adult life or there is metaplasia back to ciliated cells (8). The single layer of columnar cells is also replaced by squamous epithelium, although some cells may persist at birth, usually located over the esophageal cardiac glands. The submucosal glands develop after the appearance of the squamous epithelium and are likely derived from this squamous epithelial layer (4,7).

Development of the gastrointestinal neuromuscular system begins at 4 weeks with neural crest cells entering the foregut and migrating rostrocaudally. The myenteric plexus develops first, followed by formation of the submucosal plexus 2 to 3 weeks later. At about 6 weeks' gestation, the circular muscle layer develops, followed by the development of the longitudinal layer at approximately 9 weeks' gestation. Initially, the muscularis propria consists entirely of smooth muscles, after which striated muscles gradually develop in the upper esophagus so that by 5 months, the normal ratio and arrangement of both muscle types are established (4). Interstitial cells of Cajal (ICC) appear at week 9 and become closely associated with the myenteric plexus (9). By week 14, the fetal gut has a mature appearance (9).

Developmental defects of the esophagus can be attributed to errors in this morphogenetic sequence. This includes esophageal atresia with or without tracheoesophageal fistula, congenital esophageal stenosis, congenital esophageal duplication and duplication cyst, congenital esophageal rings, and congenital esophageal webs.

Esophageal Atresia

Esophageal atresia with or without tracheoesophageal fistula is the most common significant esophageal malformation, with an incidence of approximately 1 in 3,500 live births. This anomaly is caused by a failure of the primitive gut to recanalize in week 8 (10). Likewise, congenital esophageal stenosis results from incomplete esophageal recanalization during the 8th week of human embryologic development (10). Congenital esophageal stenosis can be located at any level of the esophagus, but is more frequent in the distal third. It appears either as a web (membranous diaphragm) or a long segment of esophagus with a thread-like lumen (fibromuscular stenosis). As there are often inclusions of cartilage or respiratory glands embedded in the wall of the esophagus in the region of the stricture, this anomaly may also represent an incomplete separation of the respiratory bud in some cases (10). The incidence of esophageal stenosis is low, occurring once in every 25,000 live births (11).

Esophageal Duplication

The notochord can induce the formation of the neural tube, gastrointestinal tract, and other organ systems. It has been shown experimentally that a split notochord can result in the duplication of any region of the gastrointestinal tract (1), which may include duplications of the esophagus ranging from the more common cysts to esophagus segments of variable length (1,12,13). As a consequence of this ability to induce development of more than one organ system, any patient presenting with duplications, segmental or cystic, should undergo radiologic evaluation that specifically explores for axial skeletal defects. Occurrence of abnormalities during the phase of foregut septation is one proposed mechanism for the formation of tracheoesophageal fistulas

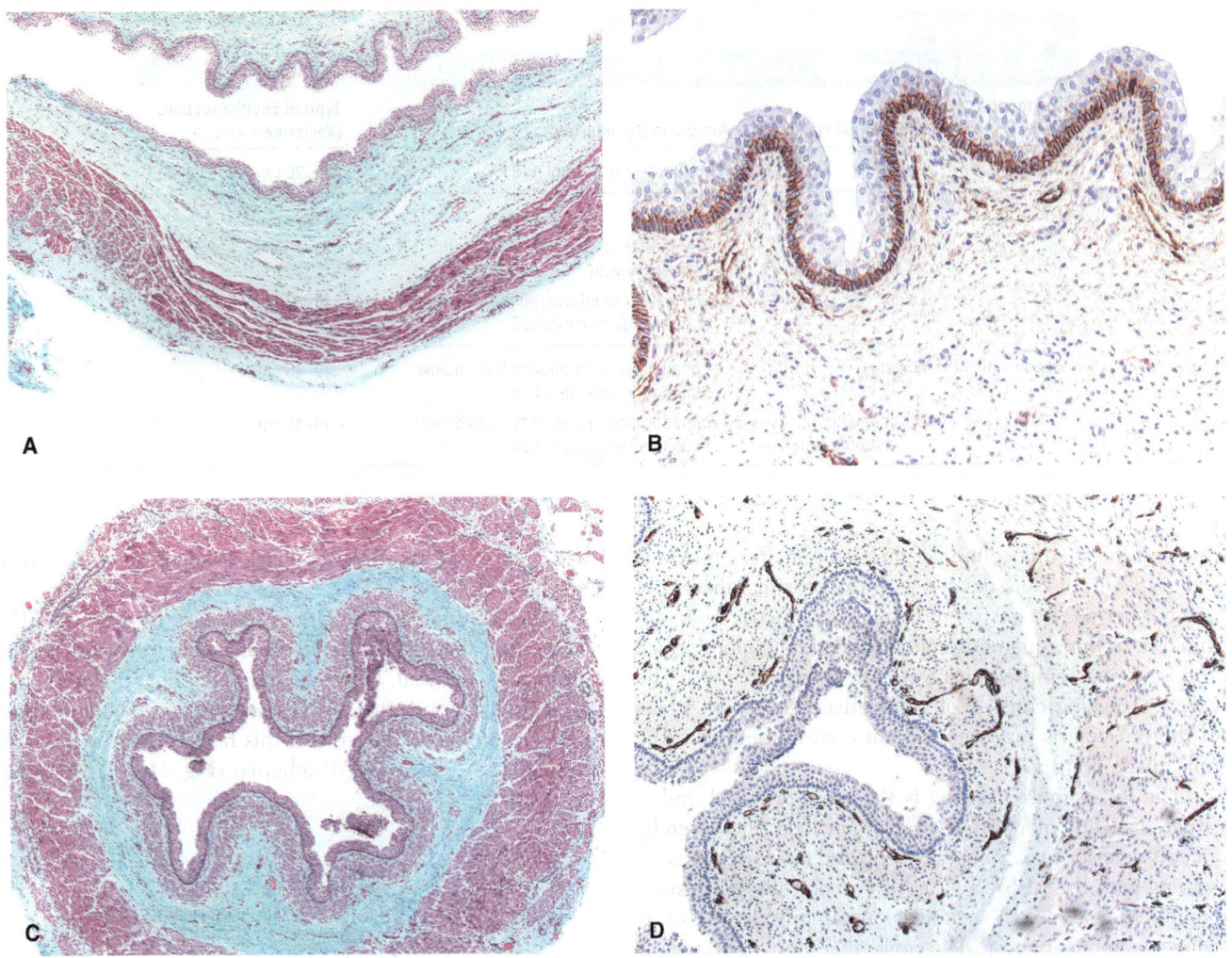

FIGURE 21.3 **A:** Fetal esophagus (third trimester - at 33 weeks). Fig 22.3A. Upper esophagus. The epithelial layer at this stage consists of stratified squamous mucosa but note the lack of a muscularis mucosae (trichrome stain). **B:** Third trimester mucosa showing mature nonkeratinized squamous mucosa, here illustrated with D2-40 that highlights both the basal layer and the relatively paucity of subepithelial lymphatics. A mild condensation of stromal cells immediately beneath the epithelium shows the location of the future muscularis mucosae. **C:** Transverse section of mid-esophagus (same esophagus as "**A**") showing a well formed muscularis mucosae. Note also the individual smooth muscle cells of developing muscularis mucosae. (trichome stain). **D:** Muscularis mucosae of mid-esophagus showing the anastomosing plexus of capillaries on both sides of the muscularis mucosae (CD31).

(with or without atresia) or of mediastinal cysts of bronchogenic or esophageal origin (14,15). It has been suggested that esophageal duplications also may occur as a result of segments of fused vacuoles formed during the vacuolization phase persisting and differentiating toward esophageal structures (1).

Lower Esophageal Rings and Webs

Congenital esophageal rings and esophageal webs are thought to result from incomplete vacuolization of the esophageal columnar epithelium during early embryonic life. The congenital esophageal ring is a concentric extension of the normal esophageal tissue, usually consisting of different anatomic layers including mucosa, submucosa, and sometimes muscles. The location is variable, but most are found in the distal esophagus (16).

Esophageal rings may originate from incomplete vacuolization of the esophageal columnar epithelium during early embryonic life. However, they are also associated with inflammatory conditions such as scleroderma, (17) and gastroesophageal reflux (18). Schatzki ring is the most common esophageal ring and is found in 6% to 14% of subjects undergoing an upper gastrointestinal series. Schatzki ring is a mucosal ring located at the squamocolumnar junction. Since it is difficult to exactly localize the squamocolumnar junction and the lower esophageal sphincter (LES), the exact anatomic relationship between Schatzki

TABLE 21.1 Regions of the Esophagus, Their Boundaries and Approximate Distances From the Incisors

Anatomic Name	Esophageal Name	Anatomic Boundaries	Typical Esophagectomy (Variation ++)
Cervical	Upper	Hypopharynx to sternal notch	15–<20 cm
Thoracic	Upper	Sternal notch to azygos vein	20–<25 cm
	Middle	Lower border of azygos vein to inferior pulmonary vein	<25–<30 cm
	Lower	Lower border of inferior pulmonary vein to esophagogastric junction	<30–<40 cm
Abdominal	Lower	Esophagogastric junction to 5 cm below esophagogastric junction	<40–45 cm
	Esophagogastric junction/cardia	Esophagogastric junction to 5 cm below esophagogastric junction	<40–45 cm

ring and the squamocolumnar junction remains controversial. Typically, it is associated with the proximal margin of a hiatal hernia. It consists of two layers, mucosa and submucosa, having squamous epithelium on its upper surface and columnar epithelium on its lower surface (19). The core of the ring consists of connective tissue plus fibers of the muscularis mucosae without contribution from the muscularis propria.

The lower muscular ring is the most proximal and is situated slightly more proximal than Schatzki ring, often by a centimeter or two. Some have equated the lower muscular ring with the LES (20,21). Microscopically, this ring is composed of a thickened circular smooth muscle with overlying squamous mucosa. The congenital esophageal web is a thin, usually eccentric, transverse membrane covered by normal squamous epithelium (16). These rings are usually asymptomatic but may be associated with intermittent dysphagia, sometimes becoming progressive or associated with attacks of sudden dysphagia (22).

TOPOGRAPHY AND RELATIONS

The adult human esophagus has cervical, thoracic, and abdominal parts. The esophagus begins in the neck at the cricoid cartilage, passes through the thorax within the posterior mediastinum, and extends for several centimeters past the diaphragm to its junction with the stomach. The overall length varies with trunk length, but in adults, the average length is approximately 23 to 25 cm. In practice, endoscopic distances are measured from the incisor teeth; and, in the average male, the junction of the esophagus and stomach is generally considered to be approximately 40 cm from the incisors. This length may vary from approximately 38 to 43 cm. Although convenient and commonly used in practice, the use of this distance is a crude and unreliable measurement for locating the gastroesophageal junction. It has been found that the esophageal length correlates with height in children (23).

The International Classification of Diseases (ICD) recognized three anatomic compartments traversed by the esophagus: cervical, thoracic, and abdominal (Table 21.1). ICD also arbitrarily divides the esophagus into equal thirds: upper, middle, and lower, and this has formed the basis of the UICC/AJCC and CAP schemas (Fig. 21.4) (24). Using

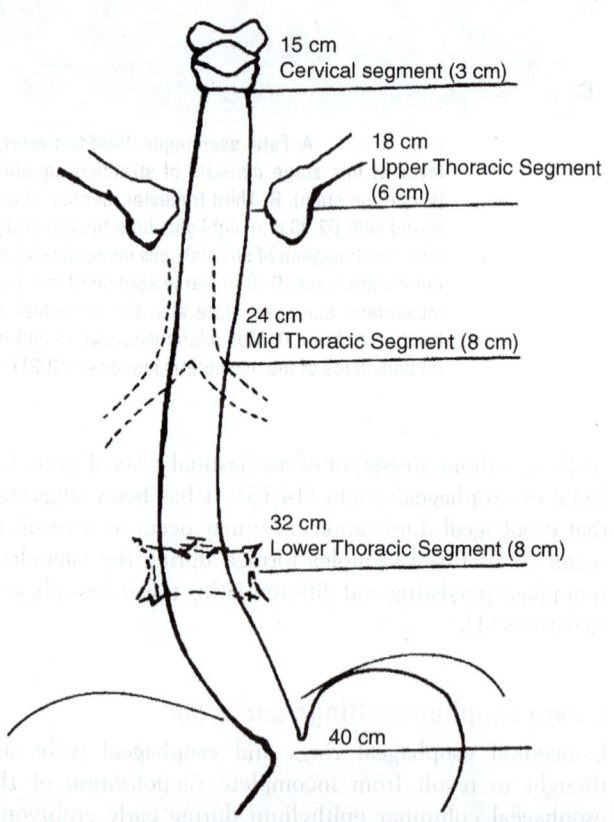

FIGURE 21.4 Esophageal segments with approximate lengths and distances from the incisors.

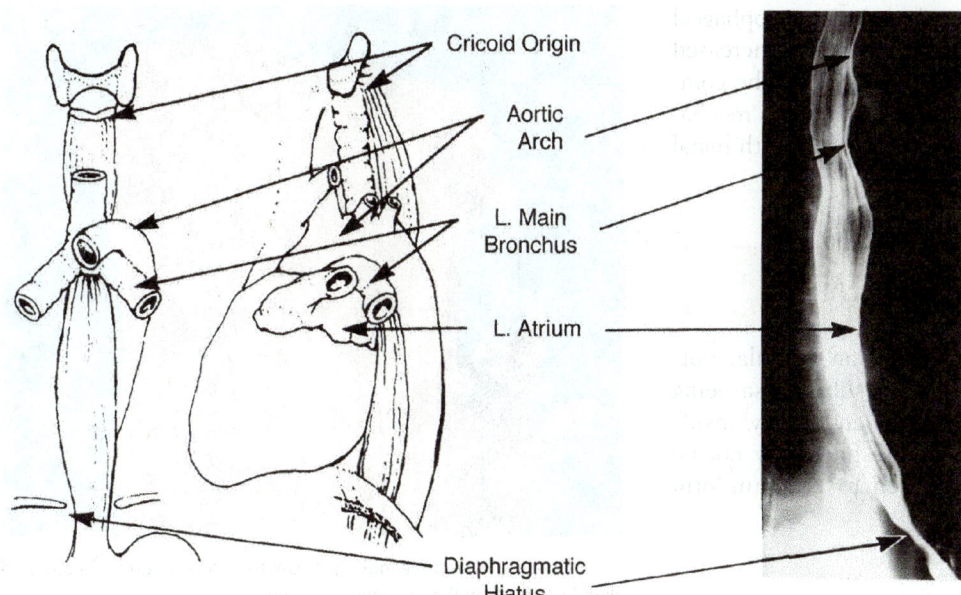

FIGURE 21.5 Relationship of the esophagus with normal esophageal constrictions. Barium swallow of the normal esophagus (*right*) demonstrates narrowing of the lumen at the sites of constriction.

the anatomic boundaries is far more logical than "typical esophagectomy" which depend on the length of the esophagus, which depends largely on the patients' height. Where we are in the esophagus at 35 cm is likely very different in Danny DeVito and Shaquille O'Neil!

Along its course, the normal esophagus has several points of constriction (Fig. 21.5). These occur at the cricoid origin of the esophagus, along the left side of the esophagus at the aortic arch, at the crossing of the left main bronchus and left atrium, and where the esophagus passes through the diaphragm. These constrictions may become clinically significant if food or pills become lodged at these sites of luminal narrowing, with the possibility of contact mucosal injury. The most common sites for lodgment are at the level of the aortic arch and left atrium, where, especially in patients with left atrial enlargement, compression may become significant (25–27).

Knowledge of the relationships of the esophagus with other anatomic structures is important because these relationships may be directly affected by esophageal diseases such as carcinoma or diverticula. Disease of adjacent structures may cause local compression of the esophagus, resulting in dysphagia or lodgment of food or pills.

The **cervical portion** of the esophagus is in relation, *in front*, with the trachea; and at the common carotid artery (especially the left, as it inclines to that side), and parts of the lobes of the thyroid gland; the recurrent laryngeal nerves ascend between it and the trachea; to its left side is the thoracic duct.

In the **thoracic segment**, the esophagus continues posterior to the trachea to the level of bifurcation, a site for the formation of the rare midesophageal diverticula secondary to traction from inflamed mediastinal lymph nodes (28). The esophagus courses posterior to the left atrium. The azygos veins ascend on either side of the thoracic segment. Initially, the right and left vagus nerves run lateral to the esophagus, giving branches that form plexi on the posterior and anterior esophageal surfaces. At variable sites in the lower thoracic segment, the left and right nerves course onto the anterior and posterior surfaces of the esophagus, respectively, divide to form the anterior and posterior plexuses, and then reunite to form the anterior and posterior vagal trunks that course down to the stomach. An awareness that variations of this pattern exist is most important for the surgeon performing the now rare operation of vagotomy.

The **abdominal portion** of the esophagus lies in the esophageal groove on the posterior surface of the left lobe of the liver. It is short and only measures about 1.25 cm in length, and only its front and left aspects are covered by the peritoneum. The esophagus enters the abdomen by passing through the esophageal hiatus, which is formed by muscles of the diaphragm and contains the phrenoesophageal ligament. In most cases, the muscle sling encircling the esophagus is formed entirely from the right diaphragmatic crus, (20,22) although variations of this pattern do occur. The phrenoesophageal ligament arises from the fascia of the abdominal diaphragm and divides into an ascending and a descending leaf. The former passes up through the hiatus to insert approximately 2 to 3 cm above the hiatus, whereas the descending leaf has a variable insertion at or below the gastroesophageal junction or even into the gastric fundus (29). The liver forms an impression on the anterior aspect of the esophagus. On the right side the junction with the stomach is smooth, whereas on the left the junction forms a sharp angle known as the incisura or angle of His.

The proposed functions of the phrenoesophageal ligament include: (a) assisting in maintaining the pressure differential between the thorax and the abdomen; (b) providing fixation mechanisms with maintenance of the gastroesophageal junction within the abdomen during episodes of increased intraabdominal pressure; and (c) contributing to the competence of the LES, thus representing a possible mechanism for the absence of reflux in some patients with hiatal hernias (29–31).

MACROSCOPIC/ENDOSCOPIC FEATURES

In the empty state, the esophagus has an irregular outline as a result of the mucosa and the submucosa being thrown into longitudinal folds. During endoscopy, insufflation causes distension so that these folds may not be appreciated, and the mucosa is seen to be a uniform white-pink.

Glycogenic Acanthosis

Glycogenic acanthosis can be seen in up to 25% of the population with the combined use of endoscopy and even barium studies (32–34). Macroscopically, glycogenic acanthosis interrupts the uniformity of the mucosa and presents as white nodules or small plaques on the mucosal folds, primarily in the distal one-third of the esophagus. These lesions vary in size, may be up to 1 cm in diameter, and, if extensive, may coalesce to larger plaques. Microscopically, glycogenic acanthosis consists of hyperplasia of the cells of the prickle layer containing abundant glycogen. Glycogenic acanthosis may resemble, and thus may be confused macroscopically with, monilial plaques or leukoplakia. Glycogenic acanthosis should be considered a variant of normal with as yet no defined relationship to infection or malignancy. However, there is an association with Cowden syndrome.

Heterotopias

Heterotopias are defined as normal tissue occurring in sites not expected for that tissue. In the literature, structures accepted as esophageal heterotopias are inconsistently defined. Esophageal cardiac-type glands and ciliated epithelium have been considered as heterotopias (7,8,35,36) or as embryologic remnants (4) by some investigators. The categorization of melanocytes, Merkel cells, and endocrine cells presents a similar problem because these cells have not been regularly found in the esophagus (37,38). Melanosis has also been described (39–41).

Gastric-type mucosa occurring in the upper one-third of the esophagus within 3 cm of the upper esophageal sphincter is designated as the "inlet patch" (Fig. 21.6) (4,7,35). Macroscopically, the inlet patch typically has a deep pink, velvety appearance, (35) and presents either as a single patch or, less commonly, as multiple patches of gastric mucosa situated just below the upper esophageal sphincter. Microscopically,

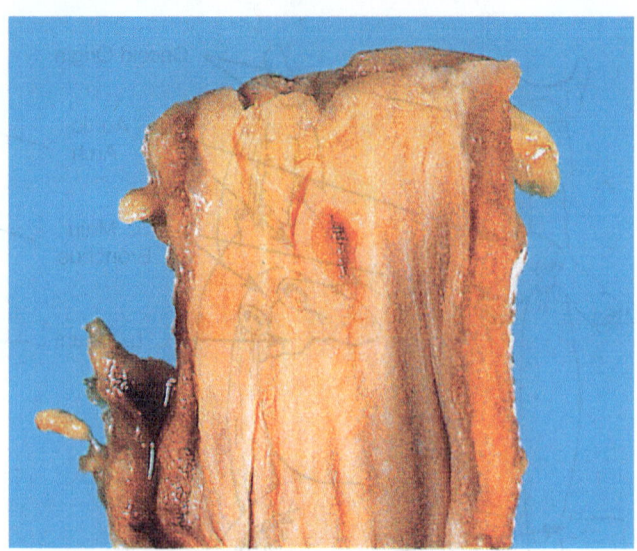

FIGURE 21.6 Proximal esophagus. Gastric body heterotopia situated slightly distal from the esophageal origin.

the patch can be lined with either cardiac-type glands or gastric oxyntic mucosa. *Helicobacter* with a variable chronic inflammatory cell infiltrate is common in infected patients and reflux may facilitate their colonization (Fig. 21.7) (42). Inlet patches have been found in approximately 2% to 4% of esophagi (some figures are even higher), and can be found at all ages (43,44). Nonetheless, they are often overlooked at endoscopy as they are typically small, and looking for them is often not a high priority. Most patients have no symptoms referable to the inlet patch, but, the patch can be quite large and, if parietal cells are present, can become the site of small peptic erosions, ulcers, stenosis, fistula, intestinal metaplasia, (45) high-grade dysplasia, (46,47) and adenocarcinoma (48,49).

Theories for the origin of these heterotopias include a metaplastic change in pre-existing cardiac-type glands, cell arrest where cells destined to become body mucosa remain in the esophagus rather than descend to the site of the future stomach, persistence of embryologic columnar mucosa with gastric differentiation, similar to that occurring distally, or otherwise unexplained heterotopia (4,35).

Sebaceous glands are occasionally found in the esophagus (Fig. 21.8) and are accepted as heterotopias (50,51). Thyroid tissue also has been described as heterotopic tissue in the esophagus (52). Pancreatic metaplasia is probably the most common form of metaplasia in the cardia, usually close to the Z line, although it may also be found in Barrett esophagus and in an inlet patch (Fig. 21.9) (53–55). While it has no known significance, if it secretes activated pancreatic juice, then it may well potentiate Barrett esophagus, as it is a normal constituent of duodenal juice, the regurgitation of which into the esophagus is involved in its pathogenesis. Endocrine tissue can be observed in pancreatic metaplasia (personal observation) but is vanishingly rare.

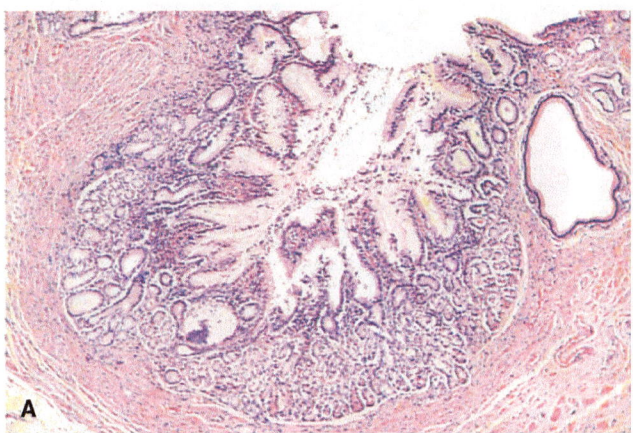
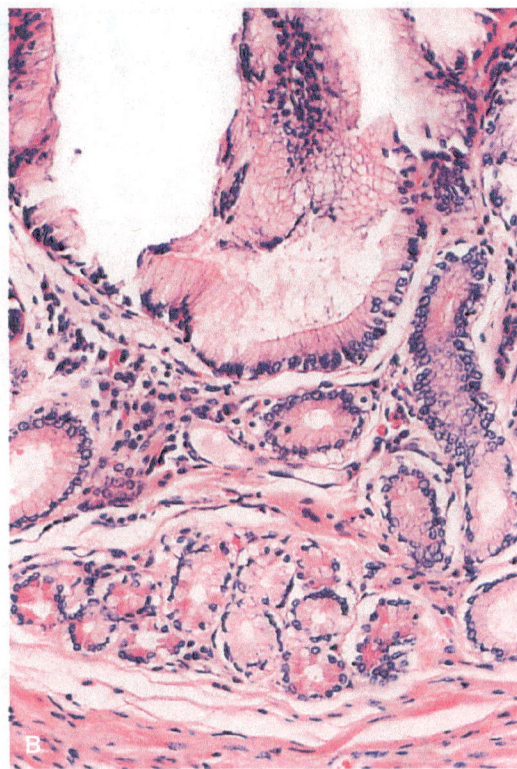

FIGURE 21.7 A: Proximal esophagus. Gastric heterotopia composed of cardiac-type mucosa with scattered chief cells and a mild chronic inflammatory cell infiltrate. **B:** Detail of Fig 21.7A.

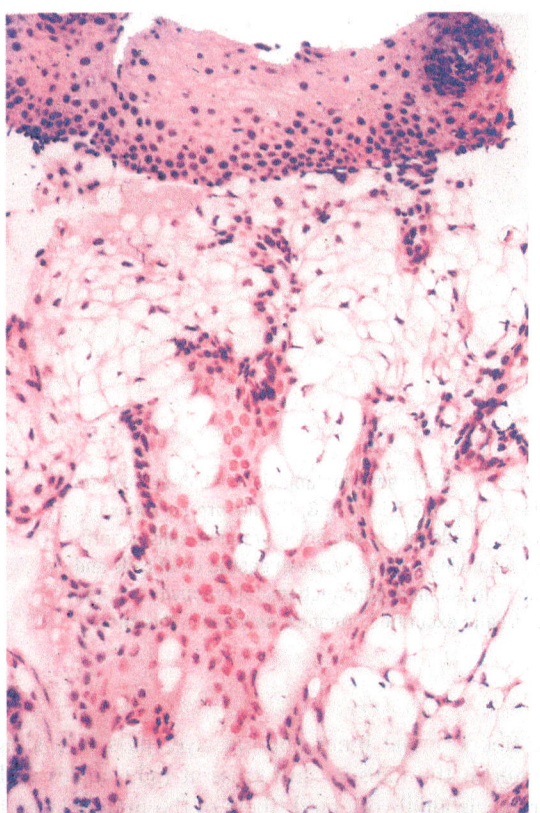

FIGURE 21.8 Sebaceous glands that in this case formed a nodule that was examined via biopsy.

Esophageal Musculature

The muscularis propria of the esophagus consists of an outer longitudinal and inner circular layer. The esophageal entrance is bounded superiorly by the cricopharyngeal and inferior pharyngeal constrictor muscles, both of which contribute muscle fibers to the esophageal musculature (30,31). Horizontal fibers from both these muscles form the upper esophageal sphincter, which manometrically is a localized zone of increased pressure measuring 2 to 4.5 cm in length (20,22,56). Together, these muscle groups act in tandem to initiate and control swallowing.

The longitudinal layer originates as two bands from its origin at the cricoid cartilage. The muscles sweep dorsally where they incompletely interdigitate, leaving a bare V-shaped area (area of Laimer) exposing the underlying circular layer. This area represents an area of potential weakness where a posterior pulsion diverticulum (Zenker diverticulum) may form. Theories regarding Zenker diverticulum center upon a structural or physiologic abnormality of the cricopharyngeus muscle (57). The circular layer of the esophagus is slightly thinner than the longitudinal layer, a pattern that is reversed from the remainder of the gastrointestinal tract (30,31). In the upper third, the external longitudinal layer consists of striated muscle that is readily visible on both H&E stain, and/or a variety of histochemical or immunohistochemical stains but their number diminishes and finally disappear around the junction of the upper and middle thirds (31).

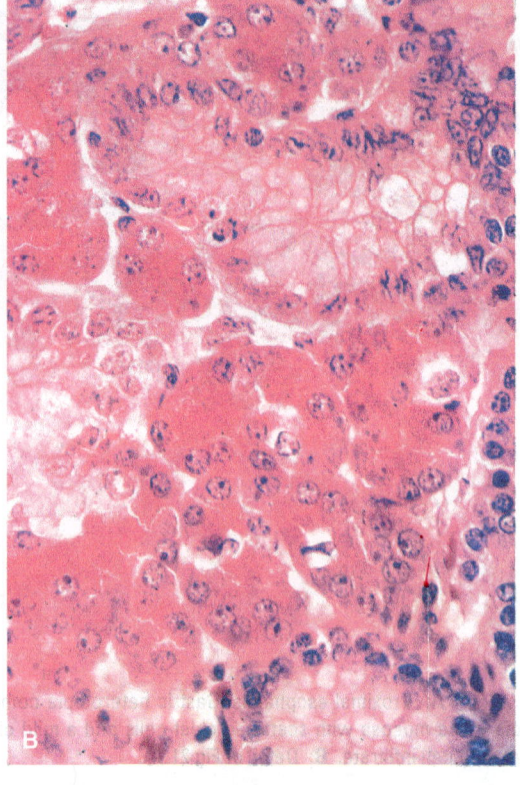

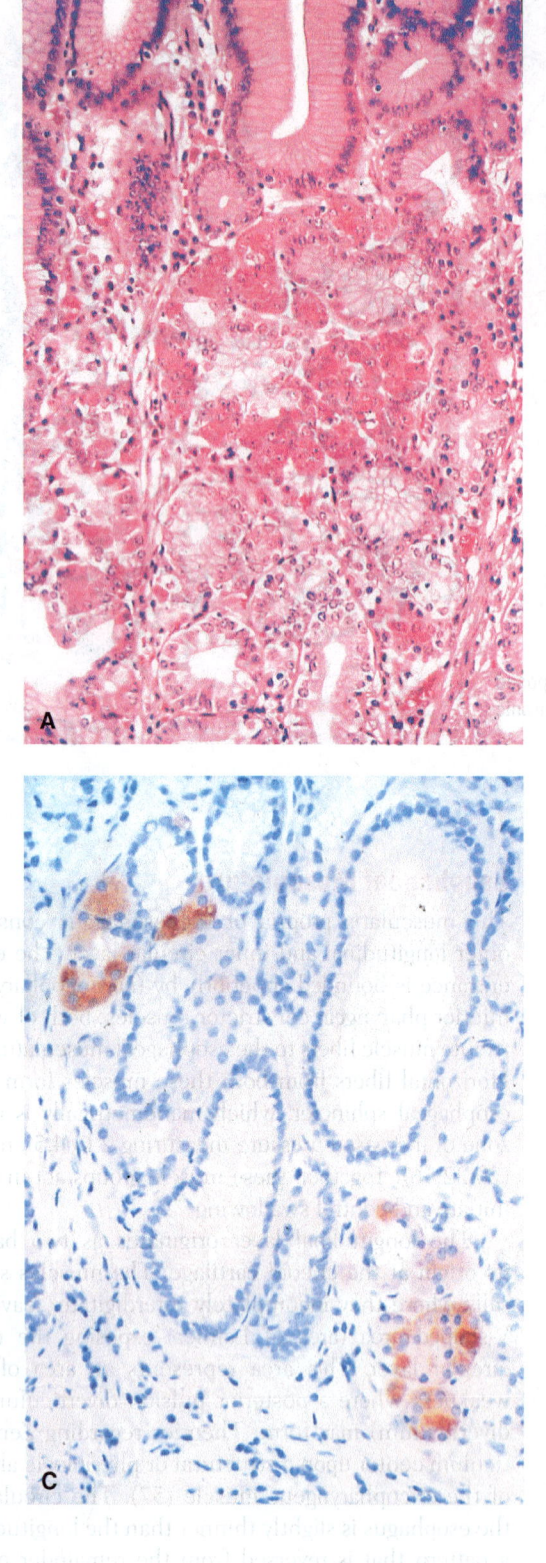

FIGURE 21.9 Pancreatic metaplasia in a biopsy from the cardiac side of the Z line. **A, B**: Glands are an admixture of mucus glands and eosinophilic granular cells superficially resembling a cross between gastric chief cells and Paneth cells. **C**: Immunohistochemical reactivity is found in pancreatic exocrine hormones, amylase in this case.

At the gastroesophageal junction, the esophageal longitudinal layer is continuous with the outer longitudinal layer of the stomach. The circular layer continues over the stomach, dividing in the region of the cardia to form the middle circular and inner oblique muscle layers of the stomach. The fibers of the inner oblique layer pass in a sling-like manner at the incisura and cross at right angles with the more horizontally oriented fibers of the middle layer, forming a muscular ring to which a possible sphincter function has been ascribed (30,31).

Lower Esophageal Sphincter

The LES is best defined manometrically, where it presents as a 2- to 4-cm zone of pressure that is higher than intragastric or intraesophageal pressure. The distal end of the LES defines the muscular component of the gastroesophageal junction (56). At rest, the sphincter maintains an average pressure of 20 mm Hg (range: 10 to 26) (22). The function of the LES is to keep the lumen closed during rest, thus preventing reflux, and to relax during swallowing, thereby allowing food to pass through. Physiologically, a competent sphincter exists, and various changes in the musculature of the distal esophagus thought to represent such a sphincter have been described (20,58–60).

Gastroesophageal Junction

The gastroesophageal junction can be defined physiologically, anatomically, microscopically, or endoscopically (depending on one's viewpoint), and can be considered as being either muscular or mucosal in nature. The muscular gastroesophageal junction is most accurately defined physiologically by manometric studies in which the distal segment of the LES defines the junction (56). Unfortunately, in disease states such as severe gastroesophageal reflux disease (GERD) or Barrett esophagus, the pressure may be so low as to not allow for localization by these means.

Anatomical landmarks that can be used to define the gastroesophageal junction include the peritoneal reflection from the stomach onto the diaphragm or the incisura (angle of His) (30,31); however, their use is limited to those carrying out dissections or resected surgical specimens.

The upper margin of the diaphragmatic indentation has been used as a guide to define the gastroesophageal junction; however, in the presence of hiatal hernia, this demonstrates variable movement (30,31).

The mucosal gastroesophageal junction does not correspond to the muscular gastroesophageal junction as defined above; and, particularly if the mucosa is red and inflamed, it may not even be visible, but may also be the site of Schatzki ring. However there has been a shift in definitions. The mucosal junction was considered to lie normally within the LES and at one point used to be considered to be within 2 cm of the muscular junction as defined by the proximal edge of the gastric folds (61); thus, it was considered that the distal 2 cm of the tubular esophagus could be lined by gastric cardia-type mucosa, and it was this that led to Barrett esophagus originally being defined as 3 cm or more of glandular mucosa within the tubular esophagus, as it ensured that at least 1 cm of mucosa should be Barrett mucosa. Indeed, some of these tongues of Barrett esophagus fail to reveal goblet cells on initial sampling, but in one study, 23% of these patients had goblet cells in these tongues when rebiopsied (62).

Practically, while the endoscopic definition of the gastroesophageal junction differs worldwide, and all have advantages and disadvantages, (63) the most important definition is that in which **the gastroesophageal junction is defined as the upper limit of the proximal gastric folds**. This is used almost everywhere with the exception of Japan, but is affected by respiration, gut motor activity, and the degree of distension of the esophagus and stomach, all of which can vary with the moment.

The proximal margin of the gastric folds has been shown to closely approximate the muscular gastroesophageal junction and thus may provide a fixed and reasonably reproducible anatomic landmark for the muscular gastroesophageal junction (61). The squamocolumnar junction should, therefore, approximate these when the esophagus is partially distended by gas. The mucosal squamocolumnar junction is seen macroscopically and endoscopically as a serrated line of contrast known as the Z line or ora serrata (Fig. 21.10). The Z line consists of small projections of red gastric epithelium, up to 5-mm long and 3-mm wide, extending upward into the squamous epithelium. Sometimes the Z line is accompanied by a ring (Schatzki ring) (Fig. 21.11) that has squamous mucosa above and glandular mucosa distally, (64,65) which is sometimes associated with dysphagia. Although extension of this gastric mucosa

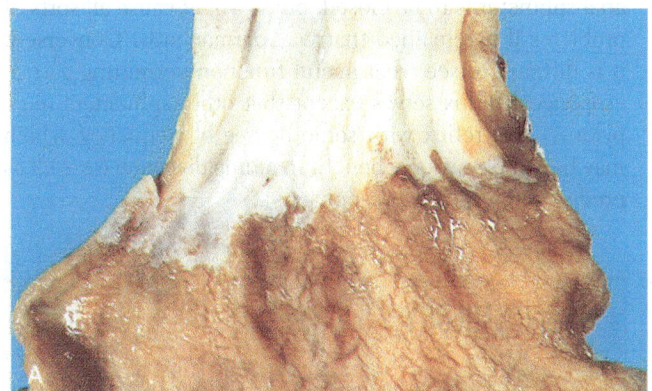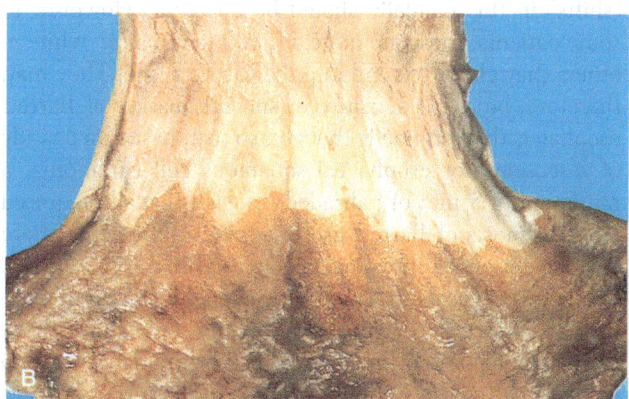

FIGURE 21.10 Gastroesophageal region. Formalin-fixed specimen demonstrates the variation of the normal squamocolumnar junction (Z line).

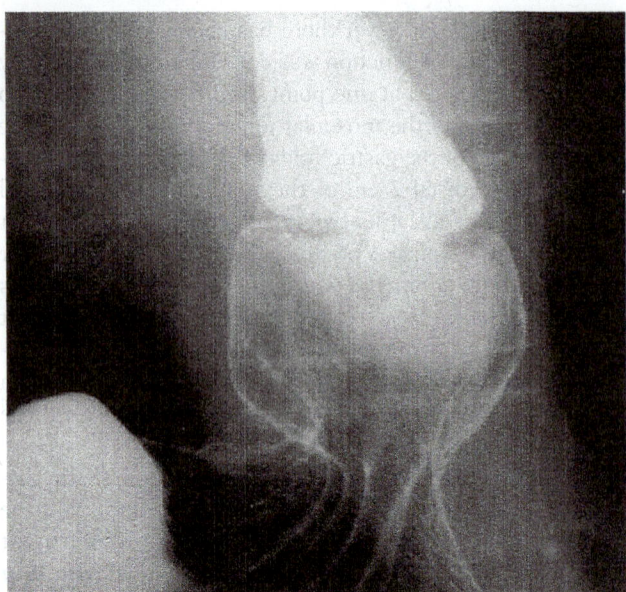

FIGURE 21.11 Lower esophageal mucosal ring (Schatzki ring). The mucosal ring is outlined by the column of barium.

may be circumferentially symmetric, it is often asymmetric. The mucosal gastroesophageal junction may be straight rather than serrated, this occurring most often in the presence of a lower mucosal (Schatzki's) ring.

In Japan and parts of Asia, the gastroesophageal junction is defined by the distal end of esophageal palisade vessels (66,67). However, this is an approximation, as the end of these vessels can be present above, at and even below the Z line in normal individuals, and can also be obscured by inflammation. The two most commonly used landmarks are, therefore, both dubious scientifically.

In the lower esophagus, the submucosal vessels of the distal esophagus are connected to the gastric submucosal vessels at the first gastric folds by a series of vessels referred to as longitudinal (vertical) vessels. These vessels, present in the lamina propria, are about 2 to 4 cm in length and can be often seen through the squamous or columnar mucosa (66,68). Their lower visible limit is also supposed to mark the original site of the gastroesophageal junction so that "shifts" in this caudally should be apparent. However, in some patients, these are quite difficult to visualize, while in others they clearly extend into the gastric rugae. They may, therefore, be a less sensitive or specific marker of Barrett esophagus than originally thought, so that, based on a study of resections for esophageal squamous cell carcinoma, a minimum of 5 mm of palisaded vessels is usually required for a diagnosis of Barrett esophagus (69). Note that there is no mention of intestinal metaplasia in this definition. While this suggests that great care should be taken in making an endoscopic diagnosis of Barrett esophagus without the usual biopsy confirmation, there have (to date) been no studies relating this minimum criteria for Barrett esophagus with biopsies. It is, therefore, unclear if patients with minimum criteria were biopsies, what proportion of these would

have goblet cells: we suspect very few. Even in the studies cited, the endoscopic diagnosis was not confirmed histologically so that the sensitivity and other characteristics of this technique are still unclear.

Microscopically, the gastroesophageal junction is the squamocolumnar junction, but it is also clear that without the endoscopic correlation, there is no way of knowing whether any biopsy that contains both squamous and glandular mucosa, the latter with or without goblet cells in the glandular mucosa, is normal or pathologic.

The most distal esophagus immediately below the squamous mucosa is normally lined by cardiac-type mucosa that varies from a millimeter to about a centimeter. The old view that this extended for 2 to 3 cm is clearly wrong, but in some patients, there is a direct transition from squamous to oxyntic mucosa. The view that the length of the cardiac mucosa may be dependent on the degree of reflux is not unreasonable. Some studies have demonstrated that the length of cardiac or oxyntocardiac mucosa correlates with the severity of acid reflux suggesting that this metaplastic epithelium results from acid reflux (reflux carditis) (70,71). Because reflux is physiologic, the issue of where physiology stops and pathology starts is the issue. While one can use definitions such as time the lower esophagus remains at pH 4 or less, it may be relative changes within the same patient that are critical.

In both autopsy- and endoscopy-based studies (35,54,70,72,73) that included pediatric patients, columnar/cardiac mucosa was either not identified in up to 65% of cases, present as a short segment of less than 1 cm., combined with oxyntic or oxyntocardiac mucosa, or demonstrated considerable circumferential variation within individuals. The authors suggest either that: (a) cardiac mucosa of the gastroesophageal junction is not normal (but rather acquired) and that only squamous (esophageal) and oxyntic (stomach) mucosa are normal for this region; or (b) it is a physiologic response to gastroesophageal reflux; but, either way it develops in response to a stimulus that includes some degree of acid reflux. So again it becomes a matter of semantics as to whether one regards reflux as pathologic or physiologic. One could also argue that the normal physiologic position of the anal sphincter is to be closed, but it would cause all sorts of problems if it remained that way permanently! Conversely, it is difficult to see what useful function permitting gastroesophageal reflux serves except that other sphincters (e.g., pylorus) also reflux with some degree of frequency, which may have a physiologic benefit in aiding digestion (as well as predisposing to Barrett esophagus).

HISTOLOGY

The wall of the esophagus consists of four layers: mucosa, submucosa, muscularis propria, and adventitia. Unlike other areas of the gastrointestinal tract, the esophagus does

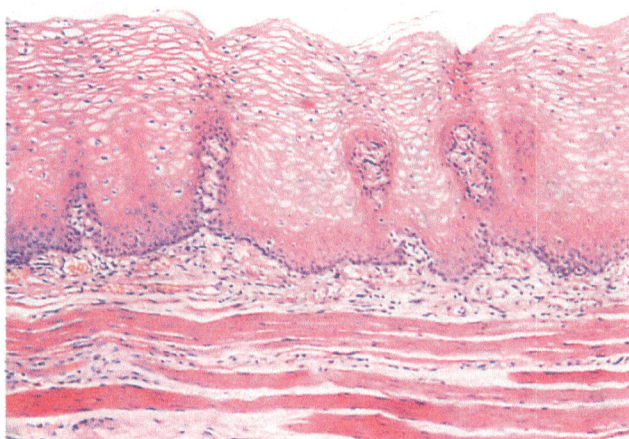

FIGURE 21.12 Midesophagus. The esophageal mucosa consists of a surface epithelial layer, middle lamina propria, and lower muscularis mucosae, which consists of longitudinally oriented smooth muscle bundles.

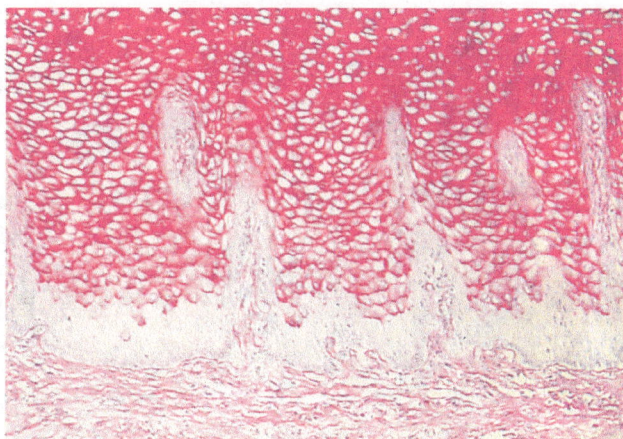

FIGURE 21.13 Midesophagus. The basal cell layer of the esophageal epithelium shows lack of glycogen, allowing for ready distinction from the overlying glycogen-rich cells (PAS).

not have a distinct serosal covering. This allows esophageal tumors to spread more easily and make them harder to treat surgically (74). The missing serosal layer also makes luminal disruptions more challenging to repair.

Mucosa

The mucosa consists of a nonkeratinizing, stratified squamous epithelium, lamina propria, and muscularis mucosae (Fig. 21.12).

Epithelium

The squamous epithelium can be divided into basal, prickle, and superficial cell layers. The basal layer occupies approximately 5% to 15% of the epithelium, being one to three cells thick; however, in the distal 3 cm, approximately 60% of normal individuals without objective or subjective evidence of gastroesophageal reflux may show basal cell hyperplasia of greater than 15% (75,76). The upper extent of the basal zone has been arbitrarily defined as the level where the nuclei are separated by a distance equal to their diameter (77). Periodic acid–Schiff (PAS) stain may be used to demonstrate the upper extent of the glycogen-poor basal cells (Fig. 21.13). Above the basal cell layer, the prickle and superficial cell layers consist of glycogen-rich cells that become progressively flatter toward the surface. The glandular mucosa of the distal esophagus is typical cardiac mucosa with variable numbers of specialized gastric cells and cardiac glands.

Within the squamous mucosa a variety of other cell types exist. These include:

Melanocytes, likely originally reported as argentaffin or argyrophil cells, have been reported in between 3% and 8% of esophagi (39,78,79). Clinically these can form aggregates and be visible as "melanosis esophagi" (80). The presence of melanocytes, referred to as melanosis, (39,40,81) accounts for the occurrence of primary melanoma of the esophagus (82,83) and one possible blue nevus (78).

Merkel cells have not only both endocrine markers (chromogranin A, synaptophysin, etc) but also immunoreactivity with CK20 and CAM5.2. However, the evidence that these cells exist at all is very limited. CK20 immunoreactive cells were not found in the developing esophagus in one study (84) while in one small systematic study they were found to be most concentrated in the midesophagus; CK20 immunoreactive cells were also found in 2/6 small cell carcinomas, perhaps not surprisingly (37). Argyrophilic positive endocrine cells are almost certainly melanocytes or Merkel cells, (37,38) although the rare occurrence of pure small cell carcinoma may arise from these cells (85).

Endocrine cells. Cells that were originally described to be endocrine because of their argyrophilia, were almost certainly melanocytes, while those with endocrine markers immunohistochemically were likely Merkel cells (v.s.). There appears to be no good data to support endocrine cells being present normally in the esophagus.

Intraepithelial inflammatory cells. While it is traditional to think of intraepithelial lymphocytes (IELs) as being part of the normal esophageal physiology, antigen-presenting cells are also present. In addition, occasional mast cells can be found in the epithelium close to and in the lamina propria (86). Intraepithelial antigen-presenting cells can be demonstrated using S100 or MHC2. IELs are CD8+ and are normal, but it is virtually impossible to distinguish IELs and APCs in routine sections, and they are therefore collectively perhaps best called intraepithelial mononuclear cells.

Occasional lymphocytes are a normal finding in the epithelium and are usually located in a suprabasal location (87–89). As they interdigitate between the epithelial cells, their nuclei become convoluted and may be confused with the nuclei of neutrophils. The term *squiggle cell*, or *intraepithelial cells with irregular nuclear contours*, is used to describe this appearance (Fig. 21.14). As in the rest of the gastrointestinal tract, IELs are CD3+/CD8+, indicating suppressor/cytotoxic function. Langerhans cells, which are

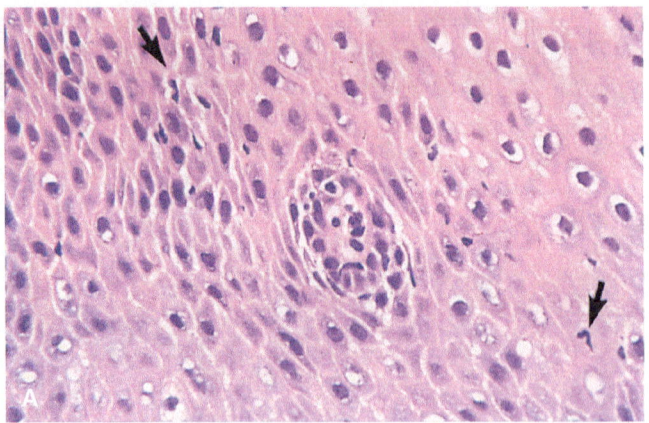
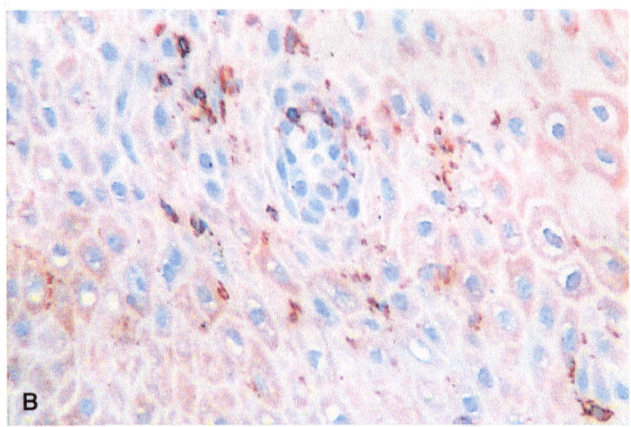

FIGURE 21.14 **A:** Numerous lymphocytes within the esophageal epithelium, some of which have a "squiggle" appearance (*arrows*). In addition, the intercellular spaces are dilated causing very prominent prickles, while some of these have formed small "bubbles" primarily at the junction between epithelial cells (best seen in the upper right quadrant). Care needs to be taken not to include perinuclear vacuolization/cytoplasmic retraction or paranuclear vacuoles as dilated intercellular spaces. **B:** Intraepithelial lymphocytes are of T-cell origin, as demonstrated using T-cell markers, and are primarily suppressor (CD3+, CD8+) cells.

S100+, CD6+, and CD1a+, also are located in a suprabasal location (Fig. 21.15); they function as antigen-presenting cells, similar to Langerhans cells of the skin (87,88).

Cytology specimens of the esophagus have stratified squamous epithelium, gastric-type epithelium representing the distal 1 to 2 cm, and contaminants from the oropharynx, respiratory tract, and foreign materials such as food particles.

Squamous epithelium in cytologic material consists predominantly of superficial and intermediate squamous cells, with the deeper parabasal cells or squamous "pearls" occasionally observed. Gastric-type epithelium from the lower 1 to 2 cm of the esophagus is brushed as cohesive fragments of uniform cells displaying a honeycomb arrangement. The peripheral cells of the cluster are flattened. The nuclei are regular and paracentrally situated and contain a few granules of chromatin and occasionally a small nucleolus.

The electron microscopic appearance of the epithelial layer demonstrates similarities to nonkeratinizing squamous epithelium elsewhere (Fig. 21.16). The cuboidal basal cells are attached to the basement membrane by hemidesmosomes. Progressing superficially, the epithelial cells become more flattened and the nuclei more pyknotic (87). Cell processes and desmosomes are most extensive in the prickle

FIGURE 21.15 Langerhans cell (*arrow*) in a suprabasal position (S100).

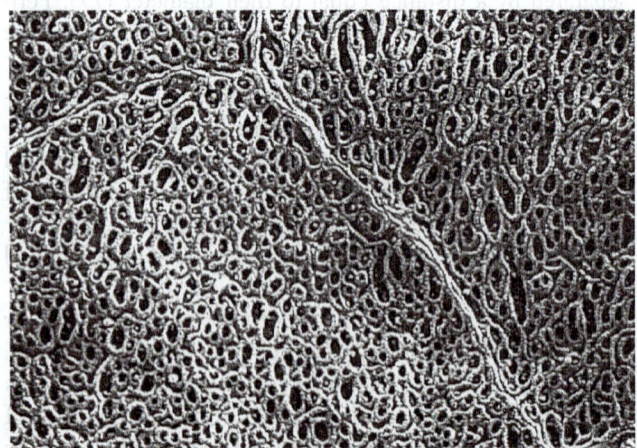

FIGURE 21.16 Scanning electron micrograph of the surface esophageal mucosa in which intercellular junctions are readily appreciated.

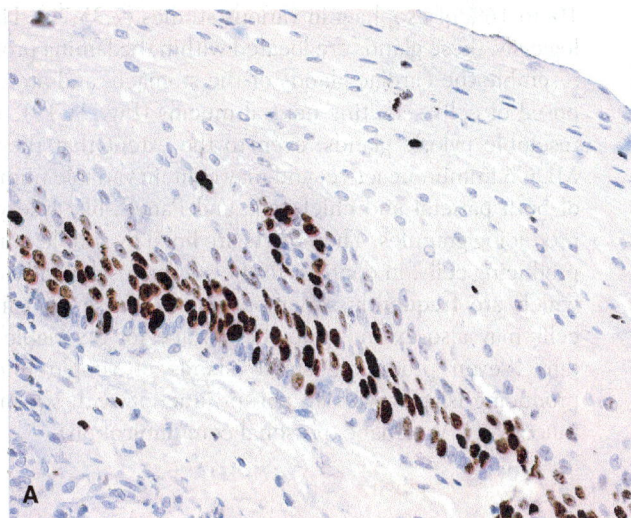
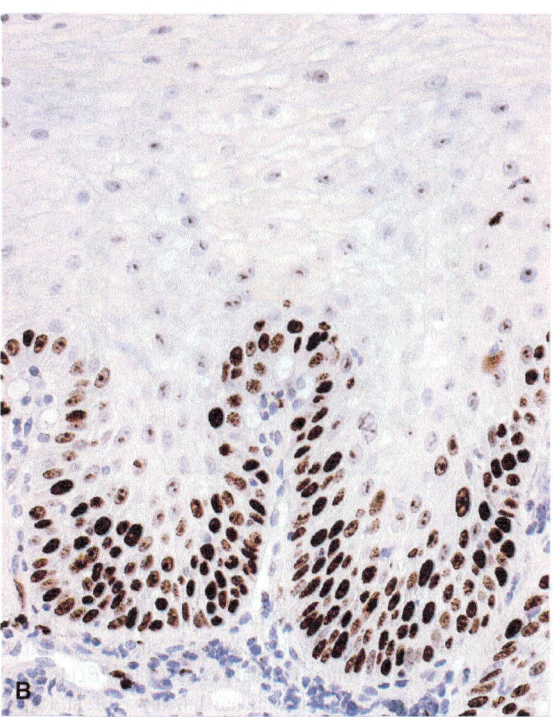

FIGURE 21.17 Basal layer of esophagus immunostained with MIB-1. **A:** The basal cell layer is relatively thin and unstimulated, consisting of only about three cell layers. Many of the cells in the basal layer are completely unstained, therefore, representing likely stem cells, while the proliferating cells with black nuclei are in the cell layer immediately above. **B:** In this biopsy, the basal layer is much thicker and, therefore, more proliferative, and there are fewer noncycling stem cells in the basal layer.

cell layer, becoming fewer and more simplified superficially (90). Membrane-bound, acid phosphatase–containing structures measuring 200 to 300 nm in diameter are identified within the epithelial cells and are postulated to have a lysosomal function, possibly involved in the digestion of cell junctions necessary for epithelial sloughing (90,91).

Cell kinetics of the human esophagus have not been studied extensively. The basal cells are responsible for epithelial regeneration; and, although data on human esophageal mucosal renewal are not available, epithelial turnover in the esophagus is slower than that in the small bowel (92). In mice, basal cell proliferation has been shown to have a circadian rhythm, (93) and the epithelial turnover time in the normal rat esophagus is approximately 7 days (94). In patients with GERD, there is an increased proliferative activity of the basal cells, resulting in basal cell hyperplasia (95).

Stem cells in the esophagus consist of a single basal layer of cells attached to the basement membrane that lie between the papillae (interpapillary basal cells) and have a low proliferative activity, being almost entirely Ki-67 negative (Fig. 21.17). In animal models, when these cells divide, one remains attached to the basement membrane, while the other migrates and differentiates. They, therefore, have a high proliferative capacity, divide relatively infrequently in vivo, and are phenotypically "primitive." Under experimental conditions, such stem cells "home" to damaged esophagus, while it can also be shown that bone marrow–derived cells can also home to the esophagus and differentiate into esophageal stem cells, including squamous epithelium (96). As such, basally situated stem cells do not show differentiation characteristics, possessing a different immunophenotype from the more differentiated cells in being CK13 immunoreactive; CK13 is expressed at high levels in the cells of both the papillary basal layer (PBL) and epibasal layers but is absent from the keratinocytes of the interpapillary basal layer (IBL). In addition, CK14 and CK15 are patchy in the IBL, which contrast with the high levels of expression in the PBL and epibasal layers. Also, mRNA for the differentiation marker CK4 is detectable in the papillary region from the second epibasal layer onward but does not appear in the interpapillary region until the third epibasal layer (97,98). Therefore, IBL cells appear to be the least differentiated cell type in the tissue (98). Suprabasal integrin expression is a consistent finding at the tips of the esophageal papillae, so PBL cells probably migrate to this site (99). This concept is illustrated in Figure 21.18.

Lamina Propria

The lamina propria is the nonepithelial portion of the mucosa above the muscularis mucosae; it consists of areolar connective tissue and contains vascular structures, scattered inflammatory cells, and mucus-secreting glands. In adults, the presence of scattered inflammatory cells, including lymphocytes and plasma cells, is considered a

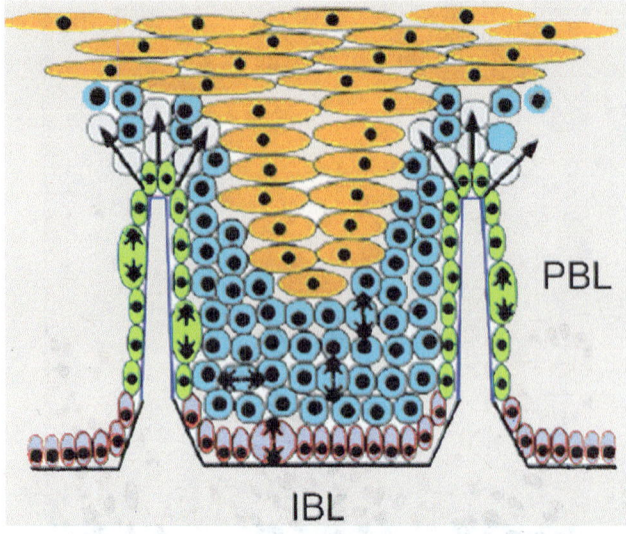

FIGURE 21.18 A model of the cellular organization in the esophageal epithelium. The interpapillary basal layer (*IBL*) cells (blue-grey) constitute the epithelial stem cell compartment. IBL cells proliferate infrequently and asymmetrically. Proliferating cells reside in the epibasal (suprabasal) layers (blue). Papillary basal cells (*PBL*) (green) are proliferative and intermediate in behavior between IBL and epibasal cells (see text). Differentiated squamous cells are shown in orange. (Modified with permission from Seery JP, Watt FM. Asymmetric stem-cell divisions define the architecture of human oesophageal epithelium. *Curr Biol* 2000;10:1447–1450.)

normal finding and does not correlate with acid reflux (77). Lymphocytes identified in the lamina propria are both CD4+ and CD8+, with the T4 population predominating (87). Immunoglobulin (Ig)A-producing B cells (plasma cells) predominate with a smaller population of IgG- and IgM-producing B cells (plasma cells) (87). Finger-like extensions of lamina propria, termed papillae, extend into the epithelium, with the maximum depth of extension allowable in the normal esophagus varying from 50% (100) to 75% (100,101). Practically, it is easy to use the "rule of thirds" when examining biopsies, in which papillae should not extend into the upper one-third, and basal cells should not get higher than half way up the basal one-third (adapted from: Ismail-Beigi et al. (76)). In the distal 3 cm of the esophagus, up to 60% of individuals without objective evidence of reflux demonstrate papillary lengths that may exceed these values (75). Conversely, increasing basal cell hyperplasia and papillary height does correlate with increasing severity of reflux (102).

Esophageal cardiac-type glands are diffusely scattered in the lamina propria through all levels of the esophagus, predominating in the distal and proximal regions (4,35). While they have been variably considered as heterotopias, (7,35) normal constituents, or embryologic remnants, there is little doubt that they perform a lubricating function and are physiologically necessary to facilitate bolus passage. However, their number is highly variable, and they are not always identified in the esophagus, having been found in 1% to 16% of esophagi in various studies (7,35,79). Histologically, these glands are located within the lamina propria, resemble the cardiac glands of the stomach, and are composed of cells secreting neutral mucins (Fig. 21.19). They resemble pyloric glands, even to the extent that they are MUC6 immunoreactive, and may contain variable numbers of both parietal and chief cells and Paneth-like lysozyme-producing granules. Their ducts are lined by simple mucus-producing cells, in contrast to the submucosal gland ducts, which are frequently squamous lined. These duct-lining cells may also extend onto the surface for a variable distance, even producing small islands of simple mucus-producing islands with an abrupt junction with squamous mucosa (H. Watanabe, personal communication).

Muscularis Mucosae

The muscularis mucosae is composed of smooth muscle bundles oriented longitudinally, (56) rather than having both a circular and a longitudinal arrangement as in the stomach and intestines. (Fig. 21.3C) The muscularis mucosae begin at the cricoid cartilage of the pharynx and become thicker distally. At the gastroesophageal junction, the esophageal muscularis mucosae is thicker than that of the stomach and may be so thick as to be mistaken for muscularis propria on biopsy (Fig. 21.20). This thicker appearance, along with the longitudinal arrangement, is used sometimes to indicate an esophageal origin for the biopsy, and the differences between the muscularis mucosae of the stomach and esophagus can be used to identify the muscular gastroesophageal junction. Following ulceration of the mucosa, the epithelium and muscularis mucosae both regenerate forming a double muscularis mucosae that is so characteristic of Barrett esophagus. In late fetal life the upper esophagus is still devoid of a muscularis mucosae, which forms later (Fig. 21.3A, B)

Submucosa

The submucosa consists of loose connective tissue containing vessels, nerve fibers (including Meissner's plexus), lymphatics, and submucosal glands (Fig. 21.21). The submucosal glands are considered to be a continuation of the minor salivary glands of the oropharynx and are scattered throughout the entire esophagus, but they are more concentrated in the upper and lower regions (4).

Submucosal glands consist of mucous cells, with or without a minor serous component, and produce acid mucins (Fig. 21.22), as well as bicarbonate, which may have a local protective effect. The glands are drained by ducts, initially lined by a single layer of cuboidal epithelium, becoming stratified squamous in type, which penetrate the muscularis mucosae and epithelium to open into the esophageal lumen. This duct epithelium has been immunohistochemically shown to be CK14+/CK19+/CK7+/CK8/18+/variable CK20+ (103). This profile is similar to normal esophageal squamous epithelium and multilayered epithelium (MLE),

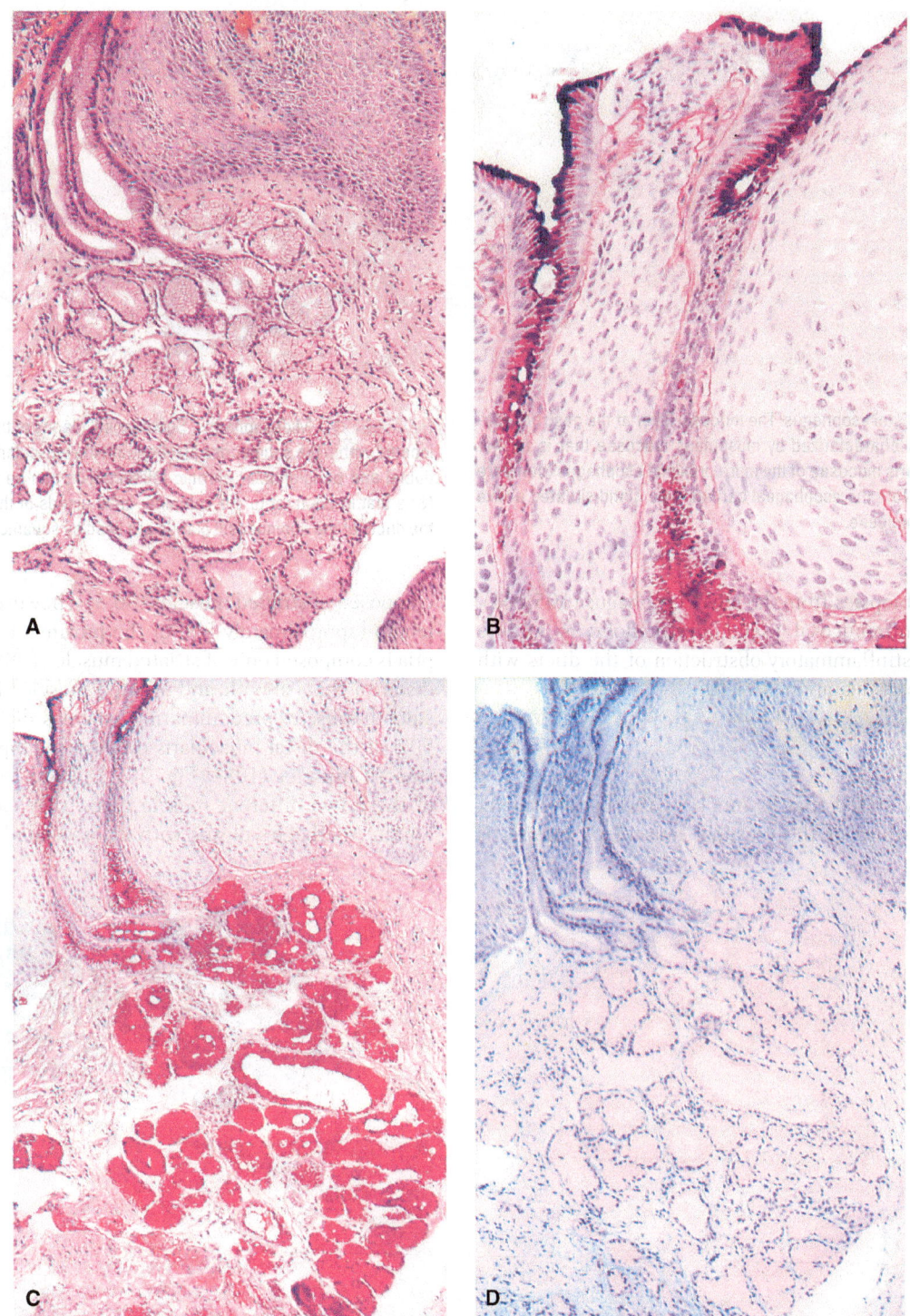

FIGURE 21.19 Midesophagus. **A:** Esophageal cardiac-type glands are located within the lamina propria. The ducts are lined by gastric foveolar–like cells. **B:** The duct-lining cells may extend over the stratified squamous epithelium for variable distances (PAS-D). **C,D:** The glands stained PAS-D positive and Alcian blue at pH 2.5 negative, characteristic of neutral mucins.

the latter representing a possible intermediate or early stage of Barrett esophagus (103). Microscopic periductal aggregates of chronic inflammatory cells and duct dilatation are not uncommon findings in the normal esophagus (104). The presence of submucosal glands is indicative of an esophageal origin because these glands are not present in the stomach; unfortunately, submucosal glands are almost never present in mucosal biopsy specimens. However, the ducts of the glands may be seen in the lamina propria of mucosal biopsies but are still only demonstrable in

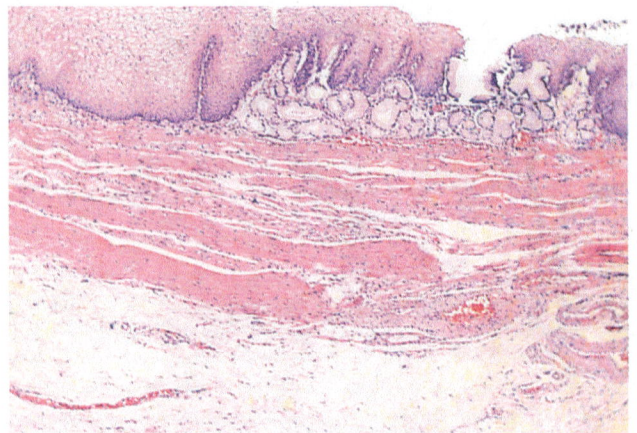

FIGURE 21.20 Distal esophagus. The mucosal layer at the gastroesophageal junction is characterized by muscularis mucosae that is thicker than the muscularis mucosae of the more proximal esophagus (compare with Fig. 21.12). Note the esophageal cardiac-type gland situated above the muscularis mucosae.

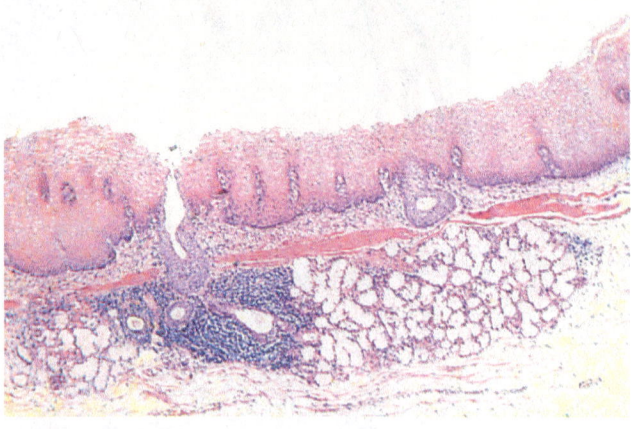

FIGURE 21.21 Midesophagus. Submucosal glands of the esophagus are located within the submucosa just beneath the muscularis mucosae. Periductal and periglandular chronic inflammation can be a normal finding. Note that in contrast to the columnar-lined glands of the lamina propria, the ducts of the submucosal glands are lined by squamous epithelium.

up to 14% of biopsies from the lower esophagus (105,106). Esophageal intramucosal pseudodiverticulosis is said to arise from postinflammatory obstruction of the ducts with subsequent duct dilatation (104,107).

Muscularis Propria

It is generally stated that as much as the upper quarter to upper one-third of the proximal muscularis propria is composed of striated muscles (30,31); however, only a short length (approximately 5%) of the proximal muscularis propria is composed only of striated muscle (108). Immediately distal to this, smooth and striated muscles intermix, with smooth muscles predominating, whereas slightly more than 50% of the distal muscularis propria is composed solely of smooth muscles (108) (Fig. 21.23). Despite the presence of these two different muscle types, they can function as a unit. Auerbach's plexus with its associated ICC is found

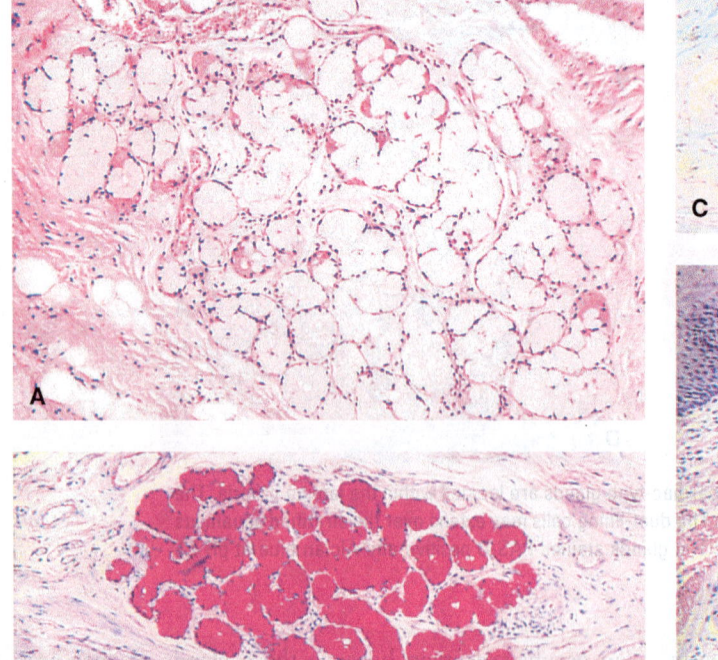

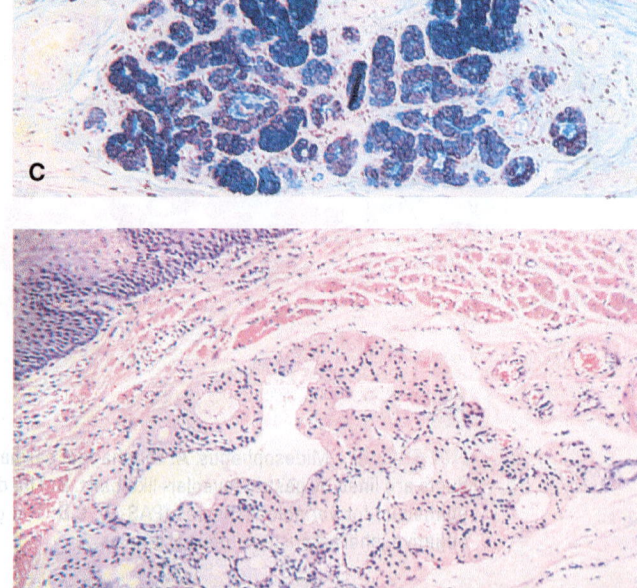

FIGURE 21.22 Midesophagus. **A:** The submucosal glands are composed predominantly of mucus-secreting cells with a variable serous component. **B,C:** The submucosal glands stained positive with PAS-D and Alcian blue at pH 2.5, a characteristic of acid mucins. **D:** Submucosal glands may demonstrate oncocytic metaplasia.

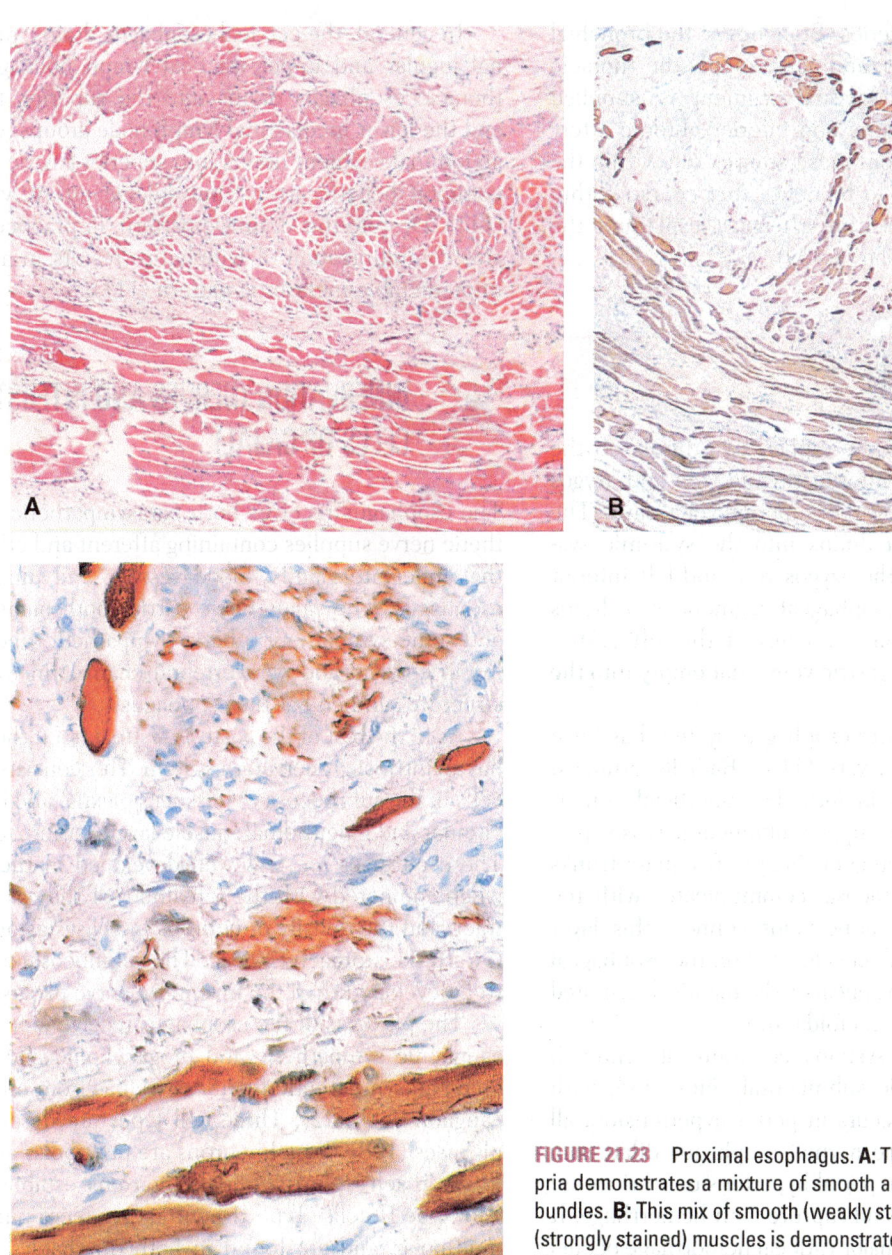

FIGURE 21.23 Proximal esophagus. **A:** The muscularis propria demonstrates a mixture of smooth and striated muscle bundles. **B:** This mix of smooth (weakly stained) and striated (strongly stained) muscles is demonstrated using a myoglobin antibody. **C:** Detailed photomicrographs of myoglobin-stained section demonstrates peripherally located nuclei typical of striated muscle.

between the two muscle layers, while the interstital cells are also present in the muscularis propria. Disease processes may preferentially involve only one of the muscular layers, as in scleroderma (in which atrophy predominantly involves the circular layer) or in achalasia (in which the circular layer may become hypertrophied) (4).

Serosa

Only short segments of the thoracic and intraabdominal esophagus are lined by serosa derived from the pleura and peritoneum, respectively (4). The majority of the esophagus is surrounded by fascia, which condenses around the esophagus, forming a sheath-like structure. In the upper mediastinum, the esophagus is given support as this fascial tissue extends out to surround and form a similar sheath-like arrangement around adjacent structures (30,31).

ARTERIAL SUPPLY

The cervical portion of the esophagus is supplied by branches of the inferior thyroid artery with contribution from various intercostal arteries. Branches of the bronchial arteries, intercostal arteries, and aorta supply the thoracic segment, whereas the abdominal segment is supplied by branches of the left gastric and inferior phrenic artery (4,30,31,109). Branches from these arteries run within the muscular layer, giving rise to branches that course within the submucosa. Anastomoses are extensive, explaining the rarity of esophageal infarction (4,109).

VENOUS DRAINAGE

The venous return from the upper two-thirds of the esophagus drains into the inferior thyroid vein and azygos system, eventually reaching the superior vena cava. The lower esophageal segment drains into the systemic system through branches of the azygos vein and left inferior phrenic vein. The lower esophageal segment also drains into the portal system from branches of the left gastric vein and through the short gastric veins that empty into the splenic vein (4,30,31,109).

The anatomy of the lower esophageal system has been shown to consist of four layers (110). Radially arranged intraepithelial channels drain into the superficial venous plexus, which is found in the upper submucosa. This superficial venous plexus, consisting of three to five main trunks located in the lower submucosa, communicates with the deep intrinsic veins. Perforating veins connect this layer with the adventitial layer of veins located on the esophageal surface. The venous system appears to be mainly distributed within the esophageal mucosal folds (67).

The portal and caval systems communicate through the esophageal and gastric submucosal veins; and, with increased blood flow, as occurs in portal hypertension, all the venous channels of the normal esophagus dilate and are referred to as varices. In portal hypertension, varices are complicated by ulceration and rupture with hemorrhage. It has been suggested that a major variceal hemorrhage occurs as a result of rupture of a varix of the deep intrinsic veins, whereas minor variceal hemorrhages occur as a result of rupture of a varix in the superficial venous plexus or even from the intraepithelial channels (110).

LYMPHATIC DRAINAGE

A rich network of lymphatics in the lamina propria and submucosa connects with lymphatics in the muscular and adventitial layers. Lymphatics in the muscular layer are predominantly oriented in a longitudinal direction (4). In view of this longitudinal arrangement, extensive intramucosal and submucosal spread beyond a grossly visible tumor is not uncommon. This becomes an important consideration when assessing resection margins at frozen section.

In general, the cervical esophagus drains into the internal jugular and upper tracheal lymph node groups. The thoracic esophagus drains into the superior, the middle, and the lower mediastinal lymph node groups, whereas the abdominal segment drains into superior gastric, celiac axis, common hepatic artery, and splenic artery lymph nodes (111). Despite this drainage pattern, in practice the extensive communication of lymphatics results in a varied and unpredictable metastatic pattern (111).

INNERVATION (NERVES AND INTERSTITIAL CELLS OF CAJAL)

The esophagus receives both parasympathetic and sympathetic nerve supplies containing afferent and efferent fibers that innervate glands, blood vessels, and muscles of the esophagus. The vagus nerve carries both parasympathetic and some sympathetic fibers. Sympathetic fibers originating in cervical and paravertebral chains run with vascular structures and end at the esophagus.

As in the rest of the gastrointestinal tract, the esophagus has an intrinsic innervation system. This consists of ganglion cells in the submucosa (Meissner's plexus) and between the circular and longitudinal muscle layers (Auerbach's plexus). These plexuses are less well developed in the esophagus when compared with the remainder of the gastrointestinal tract, and the density of neurons increases as one proceeds toward the stomach (30,31). The submucosal plexus is less well developed than the myenteric nerve plexus.

The plexuses of the esophagus receive input from postganglionic sympathetic and preganglionic and postganglionic parasympathetic fibers, as well as from other intrinsic ganglion cells (22). Three cell types are described in the plexuses (108). Type I neurons are multipolar and confined to Auerbach's plexus, and their axons establish synapses with type II cells. Type II neurons are more numerous, are multipolar, and are found in both Auerbach's and Meissner's plexuses. These cells supply the muscularis propria and muscularis mucosae and stimulate secretory activity.

ICC are widely distributed within the submucosal, intramuscular, and intermuscular layers associated with the terminal networks of sympathetic nerves. In the few studies that have examined the distribution of ICCs in the esophagus, they have been identified in the distal one-third of the esophagus in close association with smooth muscles, as well as in the middle one-third associated with both smooth and striated muscles (112). Gastrointestinal stromal tumors (GISTs), including those of esophageal origin, originate from these ICCs. When compared to the rest of the gastrointestinal tract, esophageal stromal tumors are more frequently benign leiomyomas rather than GISTs (113). However, leiomyomas have a readily identifiable subpopulation of ICCs, so are more likely hamartomas than neoplasms.

Regulatory peptides identified within nerve fibers and around smooth muscle bundles include vasoactive intestinal peptide (VIP), substance P, enkephalin, and neuropeptide Y (NPY) (114,115). Nerve fibers containing VIP and NPY are the most abundant types present in the esophagus, and the pattern of innervation by these peptide-containing neurons differs from that in the stomach and small intestine (116). Cholecystokinin (CCK) receptors are found in both the mucosa and nerves of the cardia (117).

DIAGNOSTIC CONSIDERATIONS

The most common indications for endoscopic biopsy of the esophagus include Barrett esophagus, reflux esophagitis, eosinophilic esophagitis (EOE), and dysplasia/cancer diagnosis.

Barrett Esophagus

In North America, and much of the rest of the world, the diagnosis of Barrett requires two components:

a. An endoscopic demonstration of a proximal shift in the Z line (i.e., an abnormal endoscopic appearance)

b. The presence of glandular mucosa with intestinal metaplasia on biopsy

In the United Kingdom, the diagnosis can be made irrespective of the presence of intestinal metaplasia, primarily on the assumption that all cases with true endoscopic evidence of Barrett have goblet cells somewhere, and are all likely to be predisposed to carcinoma (118). In practice there is likely a subgroup of patients with columnar-lined esophagus without goblet cells, who may be at lower (not no) risk of carcinoma.

Endoscopic Appearance

Barrett esophagus demonstrates a red velvety ("salmon colored") mucosa corresponding to the columnar epithelium, with an apparent focal or diffuse cephalad migration of the Z line relative to the previous normal mucosal gastroesophageal junction (Fig. 21.24). When well-formed this is straightforward, and may be in the form of tongues, a circumferential proximal migration, or a combination of both. Indeed both of these components form part of the Prague system in which the circumferential measurement from the upper end of the gastric folds is measured (the "C" measurement) and the most proximal limit, the maximum "M" measurement. So a patient with a total of 5-cm Barrett esophagus of which the lower 3 cm is circumferential is a C3M5 Barrett's (119). Barrett mucosa merges imperceptibly with the gastric mucosa distally. The junction with the esophageal squamous epithelium may appear as a symmetric or asymmetric Z line (as at the normal gastroesophageal junction) or as islands of columnar mucosa alternating with the squamous epithelium

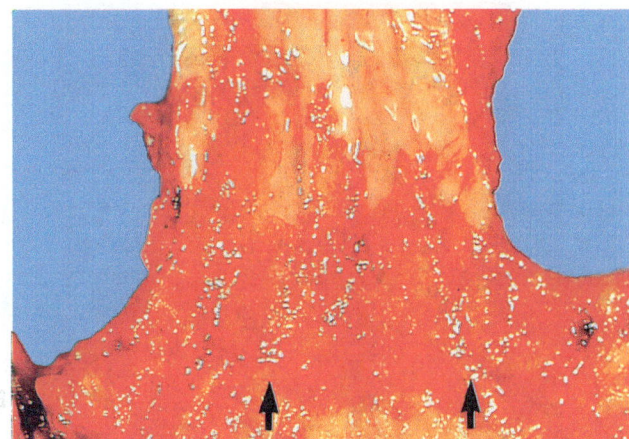

FIGURE 21.24 Gastroesophageal region. Barrett esophagus, demonstrating proximal extension of columnar-lined mucosa well into the tubular esophagus. This columnar-lined mucosa extends more than 2 cm from the proximal gastric folds (*arrows*).

("island pattern"). Foci of squamous epithelium are occasionally identified within Barrett mucosa. Inflamed squamous mucosa may be indistinguishable from Barrett mucosa endoscopically, and, therefore, also from the squamo-Barrett junction, when both are present.

Historically Barrett esophagus is subdivided into long (>3 cm) and short segments (1 to 3 cm). Some also consider columnar mucosa <1 cm to represent an ultrashort form of Barrett's, while others require at least 1 cm for the diagnosis. Practice variation in segments <1 cm is due to both technical and philosophical differences in determining where an irregular Z line stops and Barrett esophagus starts. In one study it was clear that while endoscopists looking at videos had good interobserver variability for BE overall, that when the length of BE was less than 1 cm, there was little agreement (119). This interpretation can have major implications for future surveillance. Dysplasia cannot be ignored regardless of the disease in which it is arising, but intestinal metaplasia could just as easily represent metaplasia in the gastric cardia (as a result of gastritis), which may or may not be grounds for follow-up. Practically therefore, while ultrashort Barrett esophagus has to exist, it is almost impossible to diagnose due to lack of reproducibility of the endoscopic criteria. In line with this view, the American College of Gastroenterology guidelines (2016) require endoscopic evidence of Barrett mucosa extending >1 cm proximally from the gastroesophageal junction to make the diagnosis (120).

Histologic Appearances and Integration with Endoscopic Appearance

Multiple definitions have been used for what defines Barrett's histologically (63). Barrett esophagus is defined (2016) in the United States as "extension of salmon-colored mucosa into the tubular esophagus extending ≥1 cm proximal to the gastroesophageal junction with biopsy confirmation of IM" (Fig. 21.25) (120). As discussed above, this does

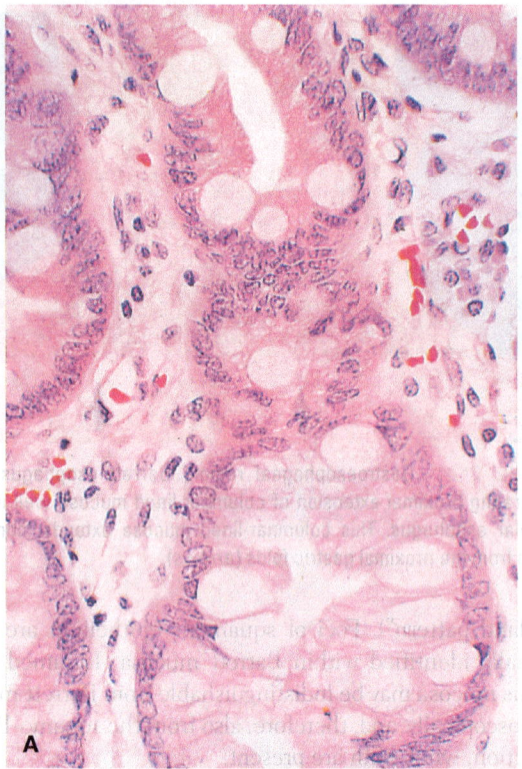
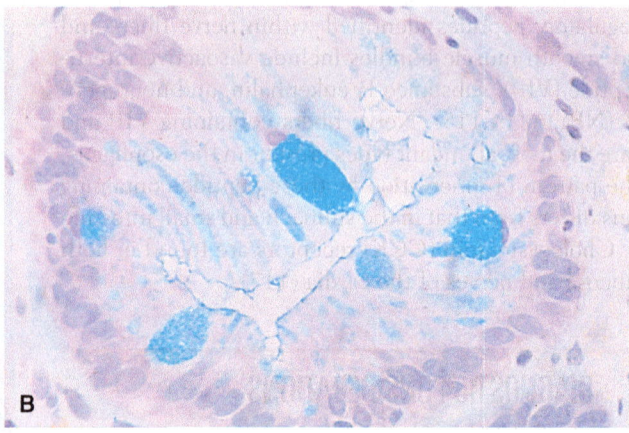

FIGURE 21.25 Barrett esophagus. **A:** Intestinal metaplasia is recognized by the presence of goblet cells. Incomplete intestinal metaplasia (lower half of gland) is characterized by goblet cells associated with gastric foveolar–like columnar cells, whereas complete intestinal metaplasia (upper half of the gland) is characterized by goblet cells associated with small intestinal, absorptive-like columnar cells. **B:** Goblet cells in intestinal metaplasia stain positive with Alcian blue at pH 2.5. It is not recommended to do this either routinely or for diagnostic purposes.

not parallel the definition in the United Kingdom where, the presence of columnar metaplasia alone in the distal esophagus of a patient with the typical endoscopic abnormality defines Barrett esophagus, the assumption being that all columnar mucosae have goblet cells somewhere (118). The presence or absence of goblet cells is nonetheless still noted in pathology reports from the United Kingdom; this simply is not required for the diagnosis (118). With both definitions, the diagnosis of Barrett esophagus is, therefore, primarily endoscopic, biopsy being used to confirm the diagnosis and to ensure as far as possible that dysplasia or carcinoma is not already present. Indeed, in many countries, including much of North America and Europe, clinicians and pathologists are uncomfortable with the United Kingdom definition, (121) but are much more confident in making the diagnosis if goblet cells are present.

Underlying the diagnostic requirement for goblet cells in North America, is the requirement of intestinal metaplasia. This is perceived as the only type of columnar epithelium that clearly predisposes to malignancy. The evidence is less strong for non-intestinal columnar epithelium. It has been argued that the inclusion of patients with cardia-type epithelium under the rubric of "Barrett esophagus" would substantially increase the number of patients with that disorder, and would substantially increase treatment costs, (63) an odd reason for justifying a definition. The definition also suggests that while nonintestinalized mucosa cannot be called Barrett esophagus, it offers no alternative, so that "columnar-lined esophagus" may be the best alternative.

The importance of noting the presence of "columnar-lined esophagus" is that patients with apparent non-goblet cell Barrett esophagus are likely also at some increased risk of adenocarcinoma, so should not be lost to surveillance or follow-up, (8,122–125). While there is little in the way of detailed North American guidelines for surveillance in this setting, some surveillance, perhaps at less frequent intervals than is used in patients with goblet cells, makes sense. The presence and extent of columnar-lined epithelium in biopsies should, therefore, be stated for completeness, in addition to the presence or absence of goblet cells. The first (diagnostic) endoscopy is, in practice, the first surveillance endoscopy, so appropriate biopsies are required, even before histologic confirmation of goblet cells is made.

In some biopsies, metaplastic esophageal columnar–lined epithelium (with or without goblet cells) cannot easily be distinguished from mucosa arising from the "normal" gastric cardia. Although not present in every case, there are some morphologic features that can be helpful in making this distinction (126–130). Biopsies taken from the esophagus are more likely to show crypt atrophy and disarray, (126,128) and are analogous to a typical biopsy with crypt architectural distortion seen in ulcerative colitis. In contrast, cardiac mucosa tends to exist in regular islands rather than diffuse atrophy. The lamina propria in esophageal (Barrett's) epithelium has larger spaces between glands and/or more atrophy and inflammation than that encountered in the cardia (128). The most reliable clue to esophageal origin is the presence of submucosal esophageal glands or their ducts,

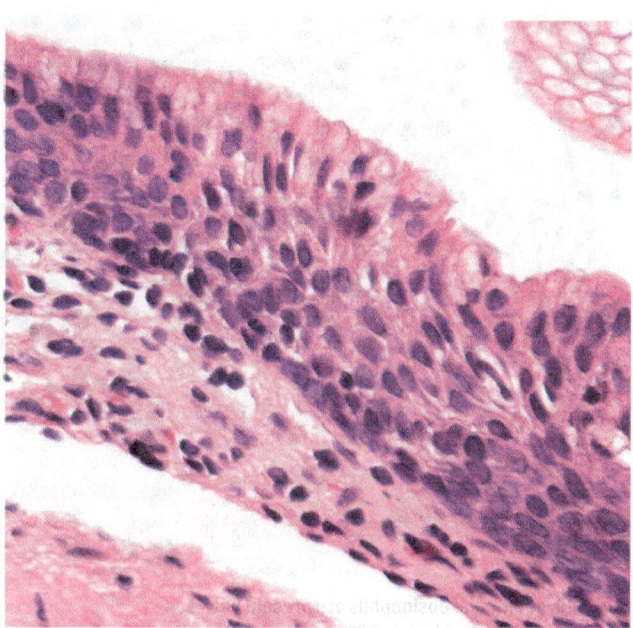

FIGURE 21.26 Multilayered epithelium, in which there is apical mucin production at the luminal surface (*top*), but the remainder of the epithelium appears squamous with intercellular bridges.

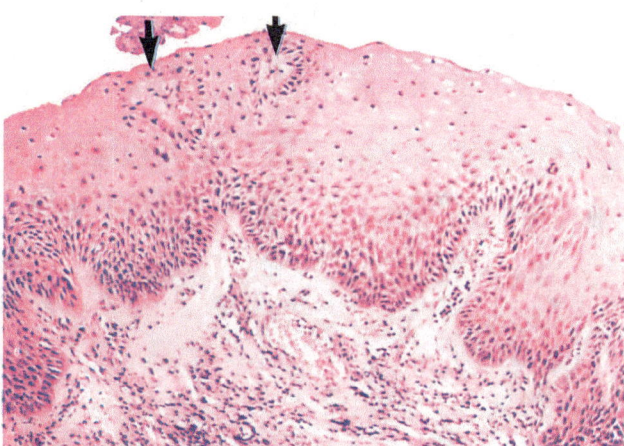

FIGURE 21.27 Reflux esophagitis. Basal cell hyperplasia and lengthening of the papillae are present. The papillae have extended almost to the surface of the mucosa (*arrows*).

as generally these are not present in the cardia (130). Also, the muscularis mucosae is much thicker in the esophagus and is separated from the basal epithelium in the esophagus by an epithelium-free layer of lamina propria (130). Intestinal metaplasia in Barrett's is usually extensive with a villiform surface, a pattern rarely seen in the cardia (130). Finally, Barrett epithelium with intestinal metaplasia is usually characterized by an absence of enterochromaffin cells although pancreatic metaplasia may be seen (130).

MLE is a distinctive type of epithelium histologically characterized by multiple layers of basaloid cells with an overlying layer of columnar epithelium (Fig. 21.26). This epithelium has been shown to have mucin and immunohistochemical qualities similar to normal squamous epithelium, duct gland epithelium, and Barrett epithelium (103); and it is associated with reflux-induced injury (131) and intestinal metaplasia in patients with Barrett disease (132). As such, it is postulated that MLE may represent an early/transitional phase of columnar metaplasia in Barrett esophagus, although some believe that this is ciliated ultrastructurally and, therefore, represents simple metaplasia or persistent fetal epithelium (36,133).

Gastroesophageal Reflux Disease

The problems encountered in GERD are related to squamous epithelial changes in the distal 3 cm of the esophagus and to the significance of intraepithelial inflammatory cells.

Reactive Squamous Hyperplasia

Reflux-associated squamous hyperplasia (RASH) consists of basal cell hyperplasia of greater than 15% total epithelial thickness and extension of the papillae into the upper one-third of the epithelium (Fig. 21.27) (76). Practically, in well-oriented biopsy samples, the esophageal mucosa can be divided into thirds; the papillae should not be seen extending into the upper one-third, and the basal cell layer should not extend more than half way into the lower one-third. This is operatively a simple and rapid technique for assessing the presence and degree of RASH. However, it should be remembered that squamous hyperplasia is a reaction to any form of esophageal injury and needs to be interpreted in light of the clinical context. Along these lines, RASH-like changes have been described in the distal 3 cm of the esophagus in approximately 60% of patients without objective or subjective evidence of acid reflux (75); thus, if present in biopsy samples originating from this zone, such hyperplastic changes should be considered normal, despite the fact that these changes are much more likely to be found in patients with GERD and nonerosive reflux disease (NERD) (102). Changes of RASH are a much more specific indicator of reflux if the biopsy samples are taken above the distal 3 cm of the esophagus (75,77).

Dilated Intercellular Spaces

Apart from squamous hyperplasia, dilatation of the intercellular spaces of the squamous epithelium as a result of gastroesophageal reflux has been demonstrated at both the electron and the light microscopic level (Fig. 21.14) (134–136). This early epithelial damage is morphologically characterized by irregular dilatation of the intercellular spaces of the basal and prickle cell layers in both erosive and nonerosive esophagitis. Using ultrastructural measurement, it seems that dilatation of more than 2.4 µm is highly suggestive of GERD (136). This is approximately half the diameter of an IEL. Further, patients with NERD have a dilated intercellular spaces (DIS) measurement of approximately half of this at 1.5 µm, which is still about three times the normal value of 0.45 to 0.5 µm (137). Readers will no

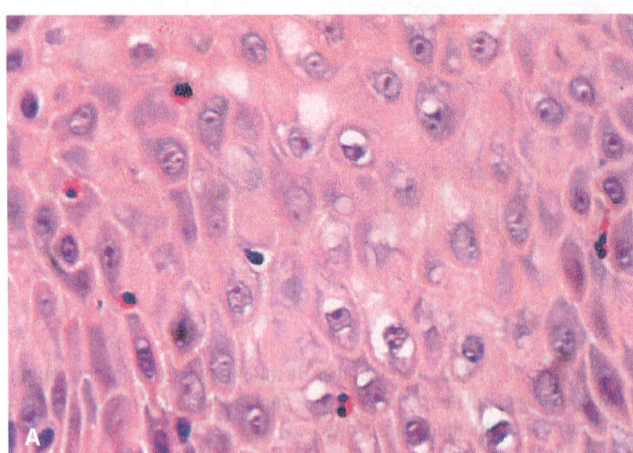
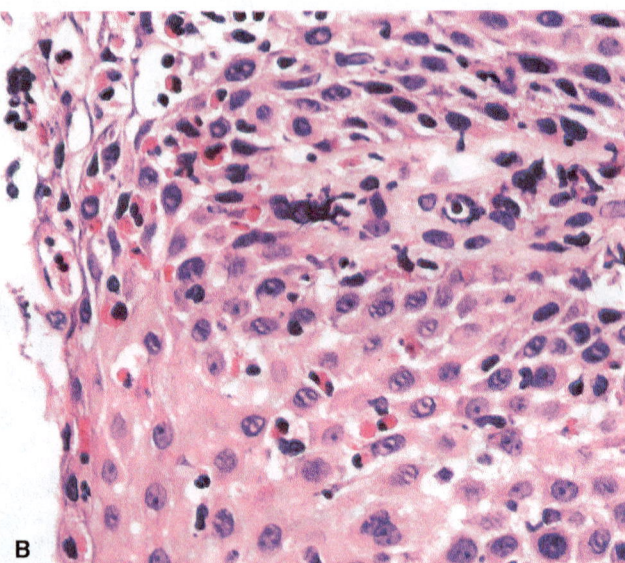

FIGURE 21.28 Eosinophilic esophagitis. **A:** Reflux esophagitis. Intraepithelial eosinophils are present between the epithelial cells. **B:** Allergic esophagitis (feline esophagus). There is marked basal cell hyperplasia, spongiosis with dilated intercellular spaces, and numerous eosinophils.

doubt be pleased to know that these measurements were made ultrastructurally! Treatment with omeprazole results in complete recovery of DIS (138). DIS have also been shown to be one of the histologic changes (along with basal cell hyperplasia) seen in biopsies from endoscopic lesions referred to as "red streaks," (139) along with newly reepithelialized lesions or granulation tissue beneath squamous epithelium. Its utility as a marker of GERD when unaccompanied by other morphologic features of reflux disease has yet to be fully determined.

Intraepithelial Inflammatory Cells and Eosinophilic Esophagitis

Intraepithelial eosinophils (IEEs) and intraepithelial neutrophils (IENs) are generally not considered to be normal constituents of the epithelium throughout its entire length, although rare IEEs in the distal 3 cm of approximately one-third of adult patients are considered normal (77). The presence of IEEs and/or IENs are considered relatively sensitive indicators of reflux esophagitis, (77,101,140) as one or both of these inflammatory cell types are present in the vast majority of cases. However, neither is particularly specific. Neutrophils can be found in the setting of erosion or ulceration of any cause, including infectious and medication-associated ("pill") esophagitis, although reflux is by far the most common cause of neutrophils in the distal esophagus. When present, IENs are frequently, but not always, accompanied by the other histologic features of esophagitis. Eosinophils are often present in reflux esophagitis, but EOE (see below) should always be carefully considered, especially when the inflammatory infiltrate is composed exclusively of eosinophils (Fig. 21.28A,B).

Other Reflux Associated Findings

Vascular changes such as dilated capillaries and extravasated red blood cells in the lamina propria should not be considered as criteria for GERD, (76,77) although some have been impressed by its usefulness (141). Increased vascularization in the lamina propria, thought of as indicative of RASH is not considered a diagnostic criterion (142). The presence of intraepithelial mononuclear cells (squiggle cells) is associated with GERD but rarely used as the sole criterion (102,143,144).

Appropriate Biopsy and Tissue Handling Protocols for Reflux Esophagitis

In the assessment of biopsy tissues for RASH, well-oriented biopsy specimens of full epithelial thickness are necessary. Quite often biopsy samples are taken with small pinch forceps, resulting in a specimen that is small, superficial, and difficult to orient. If endoscopy is being performed to obtain a tissue diagnosis, an appropriate endoscope with large particle grasp forceps should be used. Changes of GERD may have a patchy distribution; thus, multiple biopsies are recommended. It is important to avoid the use of picric acid–containing dyes and fixatives (such as Bouin's solution) because this interferes with the staining of the eosinophil granules, thus preventing their recognition.

Inflammatory Changes on the Cardiac Side of the Z Line

Because of the increasing use of biopsy samples immediately on the squamous side of the Z line to detect inflammatory cells, some biopsy samples inevitably contained cardiac mucosa immediately distal to the Z line. Some of these specimens contained an excess of chronic and sometimes acute inflammatory changes, which were not only unaccompanied by inflammatory changes elsewhere in the stomach, as might be expected with *Helicobacter pylori* gastritis, but also inflammation appeared to be completely limited to the gastric cardia and, therefore, was appropriately termed gastric carditis (145). However, it appears to be a more sensitive marker for GERD than inflammatory changes in the squamous mucosa, as judged by correlation with 24-hour pH studies, (71,146–148) the proviso being that *Helicobacter* infection (gastritis) is not present as this also causes carditis (145,149,150).

Eosinophilic Esophagitis

IEEs have been described in esophagitis due to acid reflux, alkaline reflux, and infections (101) and are thus not a specific finding. However, when eosinophils are the predominant inflammatory cell type and >15 eosinophils are present in at least one high-power field, the possibility of EOE should be raised (Fig. 21.28B). EOE is an allergic syndrome, unrelated to GERD, that can be seen in both adults and children. The primary symptom is most often dysphagia, although other patients present with nausea, vomiting, reflux-like symptoms, or acute food impaction. It tends to occur in younger males, and when fully developed is characterized endoscopically by rings, leading to the endoscopic terms feline esophagus, ringed esophagus, or trachealization of the esophagus. Some patients also present with white patches in the esophagus and, importantly, some have normal (or extremely subtle) endoscopic exams despite having relatively advanced disease histologically. The esophagus is fragile and can perforate if dilatation of areas of narrowing is attempted. Histologically, the diagnostic feature is increased eosinophils; >15 in a single high-power field is required for the diagnosis, (151) although as discussed above increased IEEs may also be seen in reflux esophagitis, so histology is not entirely specific. Other features that can be used to favor EOE over reflux esophagitis include marked basal cell hyperplasia and spongiosis, and involvement of the superficial epithelial layers, to include eosinophilic microabscesses and surface epithelial injury. Patients often have other evidence of allergies and may respond to orally administered steroids such as fluticazone or allergen withdrawal, including an elemental diet (152–156). Some patients respond to PPI therapy and this can be initial therapy in many patients. PPIs have long been known to have anti-inflammatory properties, so patients are sometimes divided into PPI responsive and non–PPI-responsive despite clinical, endoscopic, histologic, and molecular features strongly supporting EOE over reflux esophagitis (157).

Lymphocytic Esophagitis

Lymphocytic esophagitis is an ill-defined entity (158) with an excess of IELs, and appears to have numerous causes. Further, the exact nature of the cells present is still an issue, as there are several different cell types including lymphocytes that, unlike other parts of eth GI tract, can be helper (CD3+, CD4+, CD*–), suppressor cells (CD3+, CD4–, CD8+), antigen-presenting cells (S100+), and mast cells (CD117 or mast cell tryptase+). The most common cause is likely reflux disease, and is limited largely to the lower esophagus. The relation to an esophageal contact dermatitis–like reaction has been postulated, (159) as has an association with motility disorders, (160) Crohn disease, (161) and other esophageal diseases. Some patients with clinical features of EOE prove to have a lymphocytic infiltrate, but it is unclear how these differing responses are related. No gender or age prevalence has been identified so far except where the underlying disease has been identified when it reflects that population. Typically peripapillary and parabasal intraepithelial infiltrates of CD3+ lymphocytes are seen. A diffuse dilatation of intercellular spaces is observed in almost all cases. The number of lymphocytes range from few up to more than 100 per HPF. The normal mid- and upper esophagus rarely shows more than occasional lymphocytes per HPF. Thus, all overt intraepithelial infiltrates by lymphocytes in the upper, and likely mid-esophagus, can be regarded as "lymphocytic esophagitis." An effort to identify the underlying disease should always be made, and specific therapy is directed at the underlying disease, if treatment is required at all.

Exfoliative (Sloughing) Esophagitis (Esophagitis Dissecans Superficialis)

Exfoliative esophagitis was first described in 1890 (162) by Reichmann but is frequently unrecognized or misinterpreted (163). In this condition, the superficial esophageal mucosa separates from the underlying squamous mucosa. The desquamated epithelium can be expectorated. Patients often complain of severe pain, are often elderly, have other debilitating illnesses, and are taking multiple medications (164). However, the actual etiology is unknown. Malignant transformation has not been described, and the esophagus seems to heal without complications. The desquamated epithelium has a surprisingly normal appearance, so the diagnosis is easily missed. It depends on identifying (165) the split in the superficial part of the epithelium; this can usually only be appreciated if the junction where the separation is occurring is included (Fig. 21.29). Medications are always suspected, and patients with this were found to be taking multiple medications and have more debilitating illness than the control population.

Acute Necrotizing Esophagitis

In the English literature, this disease has been described as "black esophagus" and is caused by prior severe ischemia. Endoscopically, the involved esophageal segments appear black; it has, therefore, been called "black esophagus" (166–168). Microscopically, instead of the usual epithelium, necrosis with numerous neutrophils is seen. Epithelium most often cannot be detected.

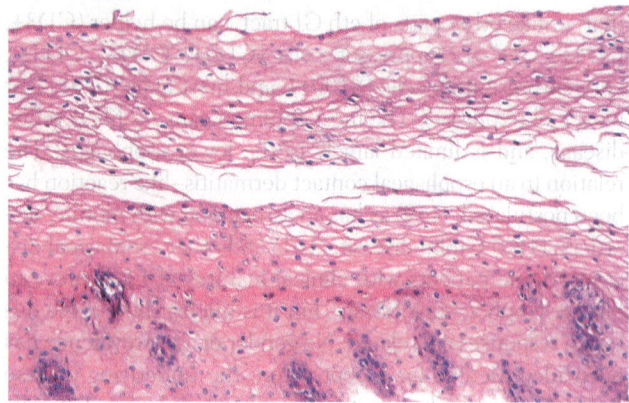

FIGURE 21.29 Sloughing esophagitis. Notice the split in the epithelium which may or may not be accompanied by vacuolization and edema. Sometimes just the superficial part is included in biopsies, so its appearance is well worth recognizing. (Courtesy of Dr M Vieth, Bayreuth.)

Adenocarcinomas of the Gastroesophageal Region

Adenocarcinomas arising in the gastroesophageal region may have their origin from the gastric cardia, from Barrett mucosa, or theoretically from the gastric cardiac-type mucosa present in the distal 2 cm of the esophagus. Gastric cardiac adenocarcinomas can be defined macroscopically as those occurring at or below the gastroesophageal junction, with the bulk of the tumor found in the gastric cardia and not involving the body or distal stomach (166). The presence of premalignant changes in the adjacent cardiac epithelium, such as a villous adenoma or dysplasia, would be confirmatory. Adenocarcinomas arising from Barrett esophagus are predominantly located in the esophagus and are usually associated with demonstrable Barrett mucosa histologically. Those arising from the gastric epithelium of the distal 2 cm of the esophagus can be classified with those of the gastric cardia unless associated with Barrett mucosa. Occasionally, an adenocarcinoma may involve both the lower esophagus and gastric cardia equally, with obliteration of the landmarks of the gastroesophageal junction and any premalignant mucosa. In these cases, identification of the site of origin may be impossible; however, from a practical viewpoint, this distinction may not be important because their clinical behaviors are similar (169–171).

ACKNOWLEDGMENT

We thank Dr. G. W. Stevenson for the radiographic material.

REFERENCES

1. Vaage S, Knutrud O. Congenital duplications of the alimentary tract with special regard to their embryogenesis. A follow-up study in surgically corrected cases. *Prog Pediatr Surg* 1974;7:103–123.
2. Johns BA. Developmental changes in the oesophageal epithelium in man. *J Anat* 1952;86(4):431–442.
3. Berardi RS, Devaiah KA. Barrett's esophagus. *Surg Gynecol Obstet* 1983;156(4):521–538.
4. Enterline H, Thompson J. *Pathology of the Esophagus*. New York: Springer-Verlag; 1984.
5. Borrelli O, Hassall E, D'Armiento F, et al. Inflammation of the gastric cardia in children with symptoms of acid peptic disease. *J Pediatr* 2003;143(4):520–524.
6. Chandrasoma P, Makarewicz K, Wickramasinghe K, et al. A proposal for a new validated histological definition of the gastroesophageal junction. *Hum Pathol* 2006;37(1):40–47.
7. Rector LE, Connerley ML. Aberrant mucosa in the esophagus in infants and in children. *Arch Pathol* 1941;31:285–294.
8. Takubo K, Vieth M, Honma N, et al. Ciliated surface in the esophagogastric junction zone: A precursor of Barrett's mucosa or ciliated pseudostratified metaplasia?. *Am J Surg Pathol* 2005;29(2):211–217.
9. Wallace AS, Burns AJ. Development of the enteric nervous system, smooth muscle and interstitial cells of Cajal in the human gastrointestinal tract. *Cell Tissue Res* 2005;319(3):367–382.
10. El-Gohary Y, Gittes GK, Tovar JA. Congenital anomalies of the esophagus. *Semin Pediatr Surg* 2010;19(3):186–193.
11. Katzka DA, Levine MS, Ginsberg GG, et al. Congenital esophageal stenosis in adults. *Am J Gastroenterol* 2000;95(1):32–36.
12. Le Roux BT. Intrathoracic duplication of the foregut. *Thorax* 1962;17:357–362.
13. Tarnay TJ, Chang CH, Nugent RG, et al. Esophageal duplication (foregut cyst) with spinal malformation. *J Thorac Cardiovasc Surg* 1970;59(2):293–298.
14. Abell MR. Mediastinal cysts. *AMA Arch Pathol.* 1956;61:360–379.
15. Rosenthal AH. Congenital atresia of the esophagus with tracheoesophageal fistula. Report of eight cases. *Arch Pathol* 1931;12:756–772.
16. Tobin RW. Esophageal rings, webs, and diverticula. *J Clin Gastroenterol* 1998;27(4):285–295.
17. Lovy MR, Levine JS, Steigerwald JC. Lower esophageal rings as a cause of dysphagia in progressive systemic sclerosis–coincidence or consequence?. *Dig Dis Sci* 1983;28(9):780–783.
18. Marshall JB, Kretschmar JM, Diaz-Arias AA. Gastroesophageal reflux as a pathogenic factor in the development of symptomatic lower esophageal rings. *Arch Intern Med* 1990;150(8):1669–1672.
19. Varadarajulu S, Noone T. Symptomatic lower esophageal muscular ring: Response to botox. *Dig Dis Sci* 2003;48(11):2132–2134.
20. Goyal RK. The lower esophageal sphincter. *Viewp Dig Dis* 1976;8:1–4.
21. Goyal RK, Bauer JL, Spiro HM. The nature and location of lower esophageal ring. *N Engl J Med* 1971;284(21):1175–1180.
22. Feldman M, Friedman LS, Sleisinger MS. In: Sleisinger MS, Fordtran JS, eds. *Sleisenger and Fordtran's Gastrointestinal and Liver Disease: Pathophysiology, Diagnosis and Management.* 7th ed. Philadelphia, PA: WB Saunders; 2002:549–671.
23. Strobel CT, Byrne WJ, Ament ME, et al. Correlation of esophageal lengths in children with height: Application to the Tuttle test without prior esophageal manometry. *J Pediatr* 1979;94(1):81–84.

24. Esophagus. In: Greene FL, Page DL, Fleming ID, et al., eds. *AJCC Cancer Staging Manual*. New York: Springer; 2002: 91–95.
25. Abid S, Mumtaz K, Jafri W, et al. Pill-induced esophageal injury: Endoscopic features and clinical outcomes. *Endoscopy* 2005;37(8):740–744.
26. Gulsen MT, Buyukberber NM, Karaca M, et al. Cyproterone acetate and ethinylestradiol-induced pill oesophagitis: A case report. *Int J Clin Pract Suppl* 2005;(147):79–81.
27. McCullough RW, Afzal ZA, Saifuddin TN, et al. Pill-induced esophagitis complicated by multiple esophageal septa. *Gastrointest Endosc* 2004;59(1):150–152.
28. Marshall JB, Singh R, Demmy TL, et al. Mediastinal histoplasmosis presenting with esophageal involvement and dysphagia: Case study. *Dysphagia* 1995;10(1):53–58.
29. Bombeck CT, Dillard DH, Nyhus LM. Muscular anatomy of the gastroesophageal junction and role of phrenoesophageal ligament; autopsy study of sphincter mechanism. *Ann Surg* 1966;164(4):643–654.
30. Netter FH. Upper Digestive Tract. Digestive System. Part I of CIBA Collection of Medical Illustrations. Summit, NJ: CIBA-Geigy; 1957.
31. Netter FH. *Atlas of Human Anatomy*. St. Louis, MO: ICDH Learning/Elsevier; 2003.
32. Katagiri A, Kaneko K, Konishi K, et al. Lugol staining pattern in background epithelium of patients with esophageal squamous cell carcinoma. *Hepatogastroenterology* 2004;51(57): 713–717.
33. McGarrity TJ, Wagner Baker MJ, Ruggiero FM, et al. GI polyposis and glycogenic acanthosis of the esophagus associated with PTEN mutation positive Cowden syndrome in the absence of cutaneous manifestations. *Am J Gastroenterol* 2003;98(6):1429–1434.
34. Vadva MD, Triadafilopoulos G. Glycogenic acanthosis of the esophagus and gastroesophageal reflux. *J Clin Gastroenterol* 1993;17(1):79–83.
35. Tang P, McKinley MJ, Sporrer M, et al. Inlet patch: Prevalence, histologic type, and association with esophagitis, Barrett esophagus, and antritis. *Arch Pathol Lab Med* 2004;128(4): 444–447.
36. Takubo K, Honma N, Arai T. Multilayered epithelium in Barrett's esophagus. *Am J Surg Pathol* 2001;25(11): 1460–1461.
37. Harmse JL, Carey FA, Baird AR, et al. Merkel cells in the human oesophagus. *J Pathol* 1999;189(2):176–179.
38. Tateishi R, Taniguchi K, Horai T, et al. Argyrophil cell carcinoma (apudoma) of the esophagus. A histopathologic entity. *Virchows Arch A Pathol Anat Histol* 1976;371(4):283–294.
39. Ohashi K, Kato Y, Kanno J, et al. Melanocytes and melanosis of the oesophagus in Japanese subjects—analysis of factors affecting their increase. *Virchows Arch A Pathol Anat Histopathol* 1990;417(2):137–143.
40. Bogomoletz WV, Lecat M, Amoros F. Melanosis of the oesophagus in a Western patient. *Histopathology* 1997;30(5): 498–499.
41. Yamazaki K, Ohmori T, Kumagai Y, et al. Ultrastructure of oesophageal melanocytosis. *Virchows Arch A Pathol Anat Histopathol* 1991;418(6):515–522.
42. Gutierrez O, Akamatsu T, Cardona H, et al. Helicobacter pylori and heterotopic gastric mucosa in the upper esophagus (the inlet patch). *Am J Gastroenterol* 2003;98(6):1266–1270.
43. Jacobs E, Dehou MF. Heterotopic gastric mucosa in the upper esophagus: A prospective study of 33 cases and review of literature. *Endoscopy* 1997;29(8):710–715.
44. Borhan-Manesh F, Farnum JB. Incidence of heterotopic gastric mucosa in the upper oesophagus. *Gut* 1991;32(9):968–972.
45. Avidan B, Sonnenberg A, Chejfec G, et al. Is there a link between cervical inlet patch and Barrett's esophagus?. *Gastrointest Endosc* 2001;53(7):717–721.
46. Klaase JM, Lemaire LC, Rauws EA, et al. Heterotopic gastric mucosa of the cervical esophagus: A case of high-grade dysplasia treated with argon plasma coagulation and a case of adenocarcinoma. *Gastrointest Endosc* 2001;53(1):101–104.
47. Mion F, Lambert R, Partensky C, et al. High-grade dysplasia in an adenoma of the upper esophagus developing on heterotopic gastric mucosa. *Endoscopy* 1996;28(7):633–635.
48. Abe T, Hosokawa M, Kusumi T, et al. Adenocarcinoma arising from ectopic gastric mucosa in the cervical esophagus. *Am J Clin Oncol* 2004;27(6):644–645.
49. Hirayama N, Arima M, Miyazaki S, et al. Endoscopic mucosal resection of adenocarcinoma arising in ectopic gastric mucosa in the cervical esophagus: Case report. *Gastrointest Endosc* 2003;57(2):263–266.
50. Nakanishi Y, Ochiai A, Shimoda T, et al. Heterotopic sebaceous glands in the esophagus: Histopathological and immunohistochemical study of a resected esophagus. *Pathol Int* 1999; 49(4):364–368.
51. Kushima R, von Hinuber G, Lessel W, et al. Sebaceous gland metaplasia in cardiac-type mucosa of the oesophago-gastric junction. *Virchows Arch* 1996;428(4–5):297–299.
52. Postlethwait RW, Detmer DE. Ectopic thyroid nodule in the esophagus. *Ann Thorac Surg* 1975;19(1):98–100.
53. Polkowski W, van Lanschot JJ, ten Kate FJ, et al. Intestinal and pancreatic metaplasia at the esophagogastric junction in patients without Barrett's esophagus. *Am J Gastroenterol* 2000;95(3):617–625.
54. Popiolek D, Kahn E, Markowitz J, et al. Prevalence and pathogenesis of pancreatic acinar tissue at the gastroesophageal junction in children and young adults. *Arch Pathol Lab Med* 2000;124(8):1165–1167.
55. Krishnamurthy S, Dayal Y. Pancreatic metaplasia in Barrett's esophagus. An immunohistochemical study. *Am J Surg Pathol* 1995;19(10):1172–1180.
56. Goyal RK. Columnar cell-lined (Barrett's) esophagus. A historical perspective. In: Spechler SJ, Goyal RK, eds. *Barrett's Esophagus*. New York: Elsevier; 1985:1–17.
57. van Overbeek JJ. Pathogenesis and methods of treatment of Zenker's diverticulum. *Ann Otol Rhinol Laryngol* 2003;112(7):583–593.
58. Theisen J, Oberg S, Peters JH, et al. Gastro-esophageal reflux disease confined to the sphincter. *Dis Esophagus* 2001; 14(3–4):235–238.
59. Wolf C, Timmer R, Breumelhof R, et al. Prolonged measurement of lower oesophageal sphincter function in patients with intestinal metaplasia at the oesophagogastric junction. *Gut* 2001;49(3):354–358.
60. Liebermann-Meffert D, Allgower M, Schmid P, et al. Muscular equivalent of the lower esophageal sphincter. *Gastroenterology* 1979;76(1):31–38.
61. McClave SA, Boyce HW, Jr., Gottfried MR. Early diagnosis of columnar-lined esophagus: A new endoscopic diagnostic criterion. *Gastrointest Endosc* 1987;33(6):413–416.

62. Jones TF, Sharma P, Daaboul B, et al. Yield of intestinal metaplasia in patients with suspected short-segment Barrett's esophagus (SSBE) on repeat endoscopy. *Dig Dis Sci* 2002; 47(9):2108–2111.
63. Spechler SJ, Sharma P, Souza RF, et al. American Gastroenterological Association medical position statement on the management of Barrett's esophagus. *Gastroenterology* 2011;140(3):1084–1091.
64. Jamieson J, Hinder RA, DeMeester TR, et al. Analysis of thirty-two patients with Schatzki's ring. *Am J Surg* 1989; 158(6):563–566.
65. Mitre MC, Katzka DA, Brensinger CM, et al. Schatzki ring and Barrett's esophagus: Do they occur together?. *Dig Dis Sci* 2004;49(5):770–773.
66. Choi DW, Oh SN, Baek SJ, et al. Endoscopically observed lower esophageal capillary patterns. *Korean J Intern Med* 2002;17(4):245–248.
67. Vianna A, Hayes PC, Moscoso G, et al. Normal venous circulation of the gastroesophageal junction. A route to understanding varices. *Gastroenterology* 1987;93(4):876–889.
68. Hoshihara Y, Kogure T, Yamamoto T, et al. Endoscopic diagnosis of Barrett's esophagus. *Nihon Rinsho* 2005;63(8): 1394–1398.
69. Ogiya K, Kawano T, Ito E, et al. Lower esophageal palisade vessels and the definition of Barrett's esophagus. *Dis Esophagus* 2008;21(7):645–649.
70. Chandrasoma PT, Lokuhetty DM, Demeester TR, et al. Definition of histopathologic changes in gastroesophageal reflux disease. *Am J Surg Pathol* 2000;24(3):344–351.
71. Der R, Tsao-Wei DD, Demeester T, et al. Carditis: A manifestation of gastroesophageal reflux disease. *Am J Surg Pathol* 2001;25(2):245–252.
72. Chandrasoma P. Histopathology of the gastroesophageal junction: A study on 36 operation specimens. *Am J Surg Pathol* 2003;27(2):277–278.
73. Zhou H, Greco MA, Daum F, et al. Origin of cardiac mucosa: Ontogenic consideration. *Pediatr Dev Pathol* 2001;4(4): 358–363.
74. Boyce HB, Boyce GA. Esophagus: Anatomy and structural anomalies. Yamada T, Alpers DH, Kaplowitz N, et al., eds. *Textbook of Gastroenterology*. 4th ed. Philadelphia, PA: Lippincott Williams & Wilkins; 2003.
75. Weinstein WM, Bogoch ER, Bowes KL. The normal human esophageal mucosa: A histological reappraisal. *Gastroenterology* 1975;68(1):40–44.
76. Ismail-Beigi F, Horton PF, Pope CE, 2nd. Histological consequences of gastroesophageal reflux in man. *Gastroenterology* 1970;58(2):163–174.
77. Groben PA, Siegal GP, Shub MD, et al. Gastroesophageal reflux and esophagitis in infants and children. *Perspect Pediatr Pathol* 1987;11:124–151.
78. Lam KY, Law S, Chan GS. Esophageal blue nevus: An isolated endoscopic finding. *Head Neck* 2001;23(6):506–509.
79. De La Pava S, Nigogosyan G, Pickren JW, et al. Melanosis of the esophagus. *Cancer* 1963;16:48–50.
80. Chang F, Deere H. Esophageal melanocytosis morphologic features and review of the literature. *Arch Pathol Lab Med* 2006;130(4):552–557.
81. Sharma SS, Venkateswaran S, Chacko A, et al. Melanosis of the esophagus. An endoscopic, histochemical, and ultrastructural study. *Gastroenterology* 1991;100(1):13–16.
82. Awsare M, Friedberg JS, Coben R. Primary malignant melanoma of the esophagus. *Clin Gastroenterol Hepatol* 2005;3(7):xxvii.
83. Suzuki Y, Aoyama N, Minamide J, et al. Amelanotic malignant melanoma of the esophagus: Report of a patient with recurrence successfully treated with chemoendocrine therapy. *Int J Clin Oncol* 2005;10(3):204–207.
84. Botta MC, Ambu R, Liguori C, et al. CK20 expression in the gastrointestinal tract of the embryo and fetus. *Pathologica* 2001;93(6):640–644.
85. Saint Martin MC, Chejfec G. Barrett esophagus-associated small cell carcinoma. *Arch Pathol Lab Med* 1999;123(11): 1123.
86. Collins MH. Histopathologic features of eosinophilic esophagitis. *Gastrointest Endosc Clin N Am* 2008;18(1):59–71; viii–ix.
87. Seefeld U, Krejs GJ, Siebenmann RE, et al. Esophageal histology in gastroesophageal reflux. Morphometric findings in suction biopsies. *Am J Dig Dis* 1977;22(11):956–964.
88. Geboes K, De Wolf-Peeters C, Rutgeerts P, et al. Lymphocytes and Langerhans cells in the human oesophageal epithelium. *Virchows Arch A Pathol Anat Histopathol* 1983;401(1): 45–55.
89. Geboes K, Haot J, Mebis J, et al. The histopathology of reflux esophagitis. *Acta Chir Belg* 1983;83(6):444–448.
90. Hopwood D, Logan KR, Bouchier IA. The electron microscopy of normal human oesophageal epithelium. *Virchows Arch B Cell Pathol* 1978;26(4):345–358.
91. Geboes K, Desmet V. Histology of the esophagus. *Front Gastrointest Res* 1978;3:1–17.
92. Bell B, Almy TP, Lipkin M. Cell proliferation kinetics in the gastrointestinal tract of man. 3. Cell renewal in esophagus, stomach, and jejunum of a patient with treated pernicious anemia. *J Natl Cancer Inst* 1967;38(5):615–628.
93. Burns ER, Scheving LE, Fawcett DF, et al. Circadian influence on the frequency of labeled mitoses method in the stratified squamous epithelium of the mouse esophagus and tongue. *Anat Rec* 1976;184(3):265–273.
94. Eastwood GL. Gastrointestinal epithelial renewal. *Gastroenterology* 1977;72(5 Pt 1):962–975.
95. Livstone EM, Sheahan DG, Behar J. Studies of esophageal epithelial cell proliferation in patients with reflux esophagitis. *Gastroenterology* 1977;73(6):1315–1319.
96. Epperly MW, Guo H, Shen H, et al. Bone marrow origin of cells with capacity for homing and differentiation to esophageal squamous epithelium. *Radiat Res* 2004;162(3): 233–240.
97. Viaene AI, Baert JH. Expression of cytokeratin mRNAs in normal human esophageal epithelium. *Anat Rec* 1995;241(1): 88–98.
98. Seery JP. Stem cells of the oesophageal epithelium. *J Cell Sci* 2002;115(Pt 9):1783–1789.
99. Seery JP, Watt FM. Asymmetric stem-cell divisions define the architecture of human oesophageal epithelium. *Curr Biol* 2000;10(22):1447–1450.
100. Goldman H, Antonioli DA. Mucosal biopsy of the esophagus, stomach, and proximal duodenum. *Hum Pathol* 1982;13(5): 423–448.
101. Brown LF, Goldman H, Antonioli DA. Intraepithelial eosinophils in endoscopic biopsies of adults with reflux esophagitis. *Am J Surg Pathol* 1984;8(12):899–905.

102. Vieth M, Peitz U, Labenz J, et al. What parameters are relevant for the histological diagnosis of gastroesophageal reflux disease without Barrett's mucosa? *Dig Dis* 2004;22(2): 196–201.
103. Brien TP, Farraye FA, Odze RD. Gastric dysplasia-like epithelial atypia associated with chemoradiotherapy for esophageal cancer: A clinicopathologic and immunohistochemical study of 15 cases. *Mod Pathol* 2001;14(5):389–396.
104. Muhletaler CA, Lams PM, Johnson AC. Occurrence of oesophageal intramural pseudodiverticulosis in patients with pre-existing benign oesophageal stricture. *Br J Radiol* 1980; 53(628):299–303.
105. Vieth M, Seitz G. 50 years of Barrett esophagus. Current diagnostic possibilities in pathology. *Pathologe* 2001;22(1):62–71.
106. Kuramochi H, Vallbohmer D, Uchida K, et al. Quantitative, tissue-specific analysis of cyclooxygenase gene expression in the pathogenesis of Barrett's adenocarcinoma. *J Gastrointest Surg* 2004;8(8):1007–1016; discussion 16–17.
107. Medeiros LJ, Doos WG, Balogh K. Esophageal intramural pseudodiverticulosis: A report of two cases with analysis of similar, less extensive changes in "normal" autopsy esophagi. *Hum Pathol* 1988;19(8):928–931.
108. Meyer GW, Austin RM, Brady CE 3rd, et al. Muscle anatomy of the human esophagus. *J Clin Gastroenterol* 1986;8(2): 131–134.
109. Geboes K, Geboes KP, Maleux G. Vascular anatomy of the gastrointestinal tract. *Best Pract Res Clin Gastroenterol* 2001;15(1):1–14.
110. Kitano S, Terblanche J, Kahn D, et al. Venous anatomy of the lower oesophagus in portal hypertension: Practical implications. *Br J Surg* 1986;73(7):525–531.
111. Akiyama H, Tsurumaru M, Kawamura T, et al. Principles of surgical treatment for carcinoma of the esophagus: Analysis of lymph node involvement. *Ann Surg* 1981;194(4):438–446.
112. Faussone-Pellegrini MS, Cortesini C. Ultrastructure of striated muscle fibers in the middle third of the human esophagus. *Histol Histopathol* 1986;1(2):119–128.
113. Miettinen M, Sarlomo-Rikala M, Sobin LH, et al. Esophageal stromal tumors: A clinicopathologic, immunohistochemical, and molecular genetic study of 17 cases and comparison with esophageal leiomyomas and leiomyosarcomas. *Am J Surg Pathol* 2000;24(2):211–222.
114. Aggestrup S, Uddman R, Jensen SL, et al. Regulatory peptides in the lower esophageal sphincter of man. *Regul Pept* 1985;10(2–3):167–178.
115. Aggestrup S, Uddman R, Sundler F, et al. Lack of vasoactive intestinal polypeptide nerves in esophageal achalasia. *Gastroenterology* 1983;84(5 Pt 1):924–927.
116. Wattchow DA, Furness JB, Costa M. Distribution and coexistence of peptides in nerve fibers of the external muscle of the human gastrointestinal tract. *Gastroenterology* 1988;95(1):32–41.
117. Mantyh CR, Pappas TN, Vigna SR. Localization of cholecystokinin A and cholecystokinin B/gastrin receptors in the canine upper gastrointestinal tract. *Gastroenterology* 1994;107(4):1019–1030.
118. Playford RJ. New British Society of Gastroenterology (BSG) guidelines for the diagnosis and management of Barrett's oesophagus. *Gut* 2006;55(4):442.
119. Sharma P, Dent J, Armstrong D, et al. The development and validation of an endoscopic grading system for Barrett's esophagus: The Prague C & M criteria. *Gastroenterology* 2006; 131(5):1392–1399.
120. Shaheen NJ, Falk GW, Iyer PG, et al, ACG clinical guideline: Diagnosis and management of Barrett's esophagus. *Am J Gastroenterol* 2016;111(1):30–50.
121. Chua YC, Aziz Q. Perception of gastro-oesophageal reflux. *Best Pract Res Clin Gastroenterol* 2010;24(6):883–891.
122. Edebo A, Vieth M, Tam W, et al. Circumferential and axial distribution of esophageal mucosal damage in reflux disease. *Dis Esophagus* 2007;20(3):232–238.
123. Riddell RH, Odze RD. Definition of Barrett's esophagus: Time for a rethink—is intestinal metaplasia dead? *Am J Gastroenterol* 2009;104(10):2588–2594.
124. Liu W, Hahn H, Odze RD, et al. Metaplastic esophageal columnar epithelium without goblet cells shows DNA content abnormalities similar to goblet cell-containing epithelium. *AM J gastroenterol* 2009;104(4):816–824.
125. Vieth M, Barr H. Editorial: Defining a bad Barrett's segment: Is it dependent on goblet cells? *AM J Gastroenterology* 2009;104(4):825–827.
126. Srivastava A, Odze RD, Lauwers GY, et al. Morphologic features are useful in distinguishing Barrett esophagus from carditis with intestinal metaplasia. *Am J Surg Pathol* 2007; 31(11):1733–1741.
127. El-Zimaity HM, Graham DY. Cytokeratin subsets for distinguishing Barrett's esophagus from intestinal metaplasia in the cardia using endoscopic biopsy specimens. *AM J Gastroenterol* 2001;96(5):1378–1382.
128. Petras RE, Sivak MV Jr, Rice TW. Barrett's esophagus. A review of the pathologist's role in diagnosis and management. *Pathol Annu* 1991;26 Pt 2:1–32.
129. Krause WJ, Ivey KJ, Baskin WN, et al. Morphological observations on the normal human cardiac glands. *Anat Rec* 1978; 192(1):59–71.
130. Appelman HD, Kalish RJ, Clancy PE, et al. Distinguishing features of adenocarcinoma in Barrett's esophagus and in the gastric cardia. In: Spechler SJ, Goyal RK, eds. *Barrett's Esophagus: Pathophysiology, Diagnosis and Management.* New York: Elsevier; 1985:167–187.
131. Wieczorek TJ, Wang HH, Antonioli DA, et al. Pathologic features of reflux and Helicobacter pylori-associated carditis: A comparative study. *Am J Surg Pathol* 2003;27(7):960–968.
132. Shields HM, Rosenberg SJ, Zwas FR, et al. Prospective evaluation of multilayered epithelium in Barrett's esophagus. *Am J Gastroenterol* 2001;96(12):3268–3273.
133. Takubo K, Vieth M, Aryal G, et al. Islands of squamous epithelium and their surrounding mucosa in columnar-lined esophagus: A pathognomonic feature of Barrett's esophagus? *Hum Pathol* 2005;36(3):269–274.
134. Solcia E, Villani L, Luinetti O, et al. Altered intercellular glycoconjugates and dilated intercellular spaces of esophageal epithelium in reflux disease. *Virchows Arch* 2000;436(3): 207–216.
135. Bove M, Vieth M, Casselbrant A, et al. Acid challenge to the esophageal mucosa: effects on local nitric oxide formation and its relation to epithelial functions. *Dig Dis Sci* 2005;50(4): 640–648.
136. Tobey NA, Hosseini SS, Argote CM, et al. Dilated intercellular spaces and shunt permeability in nonerosive acid-damaged esophageal epithelium. *Am J Gastroenterol* 2004; 99(1):13–22.

137. Caviglia R, Ribolsi M, Maggiano N, et al. Dilated intercellular spaces of esophageal epithelium in nonerosive reflux disease patients with physiological esophageal acid exposure. *Am J Gastroenterol* 2005;100(3):543–548.
138. Calabrese C, Bortolotti M, Fabbri A, et al. Reversibility of GERD ultrastructural alterations and relief of symptoms after omeprazole treatment. *Am J Gastroenterol* 2005;100(3):537–542.
139. Vieth M, Haringsma J, Delarive J, et al. Red streaks in the oesophagus in patients with reflux disease: Is there a histomorphological correlate? *Scand J Gastroenterol* 2001;36(11):1123–1127.
140. Winter HS, Madara JL, Stafford RJ, et al. Intraepithelial eosinophils: A new diagnostic criterion for reflux esophagitis. *Gastroenterology* 1982;83(4):818–823.
141. Straumann A, Spichtin HP, Grize L, et al. Natural history of primary eosinophilic esophagitis: A follow-up of 30 adult patients for up to 11.5 years. *Gastroenterology* 2003;125(6):1660–1669.
142. Onbasi K, Sin AZ, Doganavsargil B, et al. Eosinophil infiltration of the oesophageal mucosa in patients with pollen allergy during the season. *Clin Exp Allergy* 2005;35(11):1423–1431.
143. Kobayashi S, Kasugai T. Endoscopic and biopsy criteria for the diagnosis of esophagitis with a fiberoptic esophagoscope. *Am J Dig Dis* 1974;19(4):345–352.
144. Cucchiara S, D'Armiento F, Alfieri E, et al. Intraepithelial cells with irregular nuclear contours as a marker of esophagitis in children with gastroesophageal reflux disease. *Dig Dis Sci* 1995;40(11):2305–2311.
145. Voutilainen M, Farkkila M, Mecklin JP, et al. Chronic inflammation at the gastroesophageal junction (carditis) appears to be a specific finding related to Helicobacter pylori infection and gastroesophageal reflux disease. The Central Finland Endoscopy Study Group. *Am J Gastroenterol* 1999;94(11):3175–3180.
146. Esposito S, Valente G, Zavallone A, et al. Histological score for cells with irregular nuclear contours for the diagnosis of reflux esophagitis in children. *Hum Pathol* 2004;35(1):96–101.
147. Riddell RH. The biopsy diagnosis of gastroesophageal reflux disease, "carditis," and Barrett's esophagus, and sequelae of therapy. *Am J Surg Pathol* 1996;20 Suppl 1:S31–S50.
148. Csendes A, Smok G, Burdiles P, et al. "Carditis": An objective histological marker for pathologic gastroesophageal reflux disease. *Dis Esophagus* 1998;11(2):101–105.
149. Lembo T, Ippoliti AF, Ramers C, et al. Inflammation of the gastro-oesophageal junction (carditis) in patients with symptomatic gastro-oesophageal reflux disease: A prospective study. *Gut* 1999;45(4):484–488.
150. Gulmann C, Rathore O, Grace A, et al. "Cardiac-type" (mucinous) mucosa and carditis are both associated with Helicobacter pylori-related gastritis. *Eur J Gastroenterol Hepatol* 2004;16(1):69–74.
151. Dellon ES, Gonsalves N, Hirano I, et al. ACG clinical guideline: Evidenced based approach to the diagnosis and management of esophageal eosinophilia and eosinophilic esophagitis (EoE). *Am J Gastroenterol* 2013;108(5):679–692.
152. Straumann A, Spichtin HP, Bucher KA, et al. Eosinophilic esophagitis: Red on microscopy, white on endoscopy. *Digestion* 2004;70(2):109–116.
153. Sant'Anna AM, Rolland S, Fournet JC, et al. Eosinophilic esophagitis in children: Symptoms, histology and pH probe results. *J Pediatr Gastroenterol Nutr* 2004;39(4):373–377.
154. Parfitt JR, Gregor JC, Suskin NG, et al. Eosinophilic esophagitis in adults: Distinguishing features from gastroesophageal reflux disease: A study of 41 patients. *Mod Pathol* 2006;19(1):90–96.
155. Sgouros SN, Bergele C, Mantides A. Eosinophilic esophagitis in adults: A systematic review. *Eur J Gastroenterol Hepatol* 2006;18(2):211–217.
156. Spergel J, Rothenberg ME, Fogg M. Eliminating eosinophilic esophagitis. *Clin Immunol* 2005;115(2):131–132.
157. Molina-Infante J, Gonzalez-Cordero PL, Lucendo AJ. Proton pump inhibitor-responsive esophageal eosinophilia: Still a valid diagnosis? *Curr Opin Gastroenterol* 2017;33(4):285-92.
158. Rubio CA, Sjodahl K, Lagergren J. Lymphocytic esophagitis: A histologic subset of chronic esophagitis. *Am J Clin Pathol* 2006;125(3):432–437.
159. Purdy JK, Appelman HD, Golembeski CP, et al. Lymphocytic esophagitis: A chronic or recurring pattern of esophagitis resembling allergic contact dermatitis. *Am J Clin Pathol* 2008;130(4):508–513.
160. Putra J, Muller KE, Hussain ZH, et al. Lymphocytic esophagitis in nonachalasia primary esophageal motility disorders: Improved criteria, prevalence, strength of association, and natural history. *Am J Surg Pathol* 2016;40(12):1679–1685.
161. Oberhuber G. Histology of Crohn disease type lesions in the upper gastrointestinal tract. *Pathologe* 2001;22(2):91–96.
162. Takubo K. *Pathology of the Esophagus.* 2007.
163. Patterson T. A simple superficial oesophageal cast. (oesophagitis exfoliativa: Oesophagitis dissecans superficialis). *J Path Bact* 1935;40:559–569.
164. Purdy JK, Appelman HD, McKenna BJ. Sloughing esophagitis is associated with chronic debilitation and medications that injury the esophageal mucosa. *Mod Pathol* 2012;25(5):767–775.
165. Carmack SW, Vemulapalli R, Spechler SJ, et al. Esophagitis dissecans superficialis ("sloughing esophagitis"): A clinicopathologic study of 12 cases. *Am J Surg Pathol* 2009;33(12):1789–1794.
166. Obermeyer R, Kasirajan K, Erzurum V, et al. Necrotizing esophagitis presenting as a black esophagus. *Surg Endosc* 1998;12(12):1430–1433.
167. Goldenberg SP, Wain SL, Marignani P. Acute necrotizing esophagitis. *Gastroenterology* 1990;98(2):493–496.
168. Augusto F, Fernandes V, Cremers MI, et al. Acute necrotizing esophagitis: A large retrospective case series. *Endoscopy* 2004;36(5):411–415.
169. Marsman WA, Tytgat GN, Ten Kate FJ, et al. Differences and similarities of adenocarcinomas of the esophagus and esophagogastric junction. *J Surg Oncol* 2005;92(3):160–168.
170. Sabel MS, Pastore K, Toon H, et al. Adenocarcinoma of the esophagus with and without Barrett mucosa. *Arch Surg* 2000;135(7):831–835; discussion 6.
171. Di Martino N, Izzo G, Cosenza A, et al. Adenocarcinoma of gastric cardia in the elderly: Surgical problems and prognostic factors. *World J Gastroenterol* 2005;11(33):5123–5128.

Stomach

David A. Owen

EMBRYOLOGY AND POSTNATAL DEVELOPMENT 601	ULTRASTRUCTURE 608
GROSS MORPHOLOGIC FEATURES 601	GASTRIC FUNCTION 608
Blood Supply 602	SPECIAL TECHNIQUES AND PROCEDURES 609
Nerve Supply 602	AGE CHANGES 609
Lymphatics 603	ARTIFACTS 609
GENERAL HISTOLOGIC FEATURES 603	DIFFERENTIAL DIAGNOSIS 609
Surface Epithelium 604	Metaplasia 612
Cardiac and Pyloric Mucosa 604	SPECIMEN HANDLING 613
Oxyntic Gland Mucosa 605	REFERENCES 613
Endocrine Cells 606	
Lamina Propria 607	
Submucosa 607	
Muscular Components 607	

EMBRYOLOGY AND POSTNATAL DEVELOPMENT

The stomach develops as a fusiform dilatation of the foregut caudal to the esophagus. This occurs first when the embryo is 7 mm in length. Initially, it is attached to the back of the abdomen by the dorsal mesogastrium and to the septum transversum (diaphragm) by the ventral mesogastrium. As the stomach enlarges, the dorsal mesogastrium becomes the greater omentum and the ventral mesogastrium becomes the lesser omentum.

The stomach is derived from endoderm, and early glandular differentiation of the mucosal lining occurs first at the 80-mm stage of fetal development. Enzyme and acid production first occur at the 4th month of fetal life and are well established by the time of birth. The newborn stomach is fully developed and similar to that of the adult.

GROSS MORPHOLOGIC FEATURES

The stomach is a flattened J-shaped organ located in the left upper quadrant of the abdomen. At its upper end, it joins the esophagus several centimeters below the level of the diaphragm. At its distal end, it merges with the duodenum, just to the right of the midline. The stomach is extremely distensible, and its size varies depending on the volume of food present.

For the purposes of gross description, the stomach can be divided into four regions: cardia, fundus, corpus (or body), and antrum (Fig. 22.1) (1,2). The superomedial margin is termed the lesser curvature, and the inferolateral margin is termed the greater curvature. The gastroesophageal junction (GEJ) is defined anatomically as the point where the tubular esophagus becomes the saccular stomach. It is present approximately 40 cm distal to the incisor teeth, although this distance varies depending on the height of the individual. Generally, this is the same level where the flat squamous esophageal mucosa is replaced by gastric mucosal folds (rugae). The cardia is found just distal to the lower end of the esophagus. It is a small and ill-defined area, extending 1 to 3 cm from the GEJ. The fundus is the portion of the stomach that lies above the GEJ, just below the left hemidiaphragm. The antrum comprises the distal third of the stomach, proximal to the pyloric sphincter (pylorus), with the remainder of the stomach referred to as the corpus (body). Since they have the same type of mucosa, some authors do not distinguish between the corpus and the fundus and designate both these parts of the stomach as fundus. This is acceptable when discussing

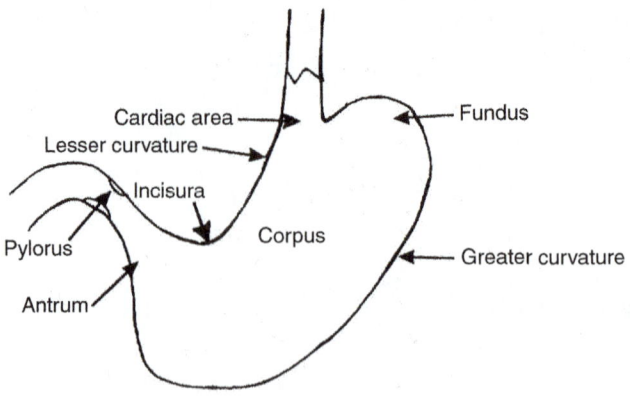

FIGURE 22.1 Gross anatomical zones of the stomach.

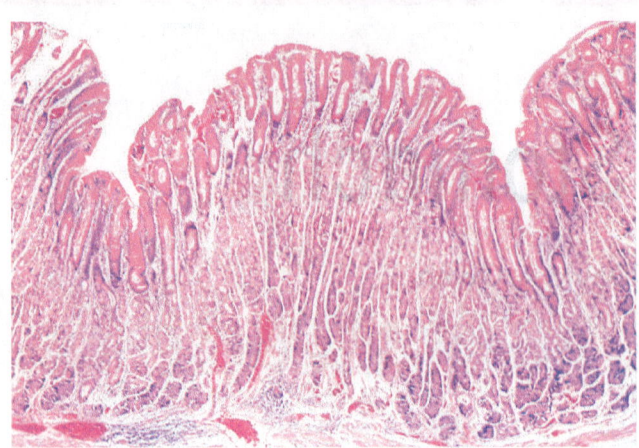

FIGURE 22.3 Low-power view of the gastric oxyntic mucosa. The grooves in the mucosa are fixed anatomical features called areae gastricae.

mucosal diseases but causes confusion when describing gross anatomy. The junction between the antrum and the corpus is poorly demarcated. By external examination, it comprises the portion of the stomach distal to the incisura, a notch on the lesser curvature (1). Internally, the gastric mucosa is usually thrown into coarse folds called rugae. These are prominent when the stomach is empty but flattened out when the organ is distended. The rugae are most prominent in the corpus and fundus because this is where the major dilatation to accommodate food occurs. The antrum is characterized by mucosa that is flatter and more firmly anchored to the underlying submucosa (Fig. 22.2).

The wall of the stomach has four layers: mucosa, submucosa, muscularis propria, and subserosa. Apart from the mucosa, these layers are structurally similar to the bowel wall elsewhere in the gastrointestinal tract. When viewed close up, the surface of the mucosa is dissected by thin shallow grooves termed areae gastricae (3). These are structurally fixed and do not flatten out when the stomach is distended. They are best seen when the mucosa is viewed en face with a hand lens. *Areae gastricae* may be demonstrated radiologically via double-contrast barium examination but also can be recognized on histologic sections, particularly from gastrectomy specimens, where they appear as shallow depressions on an otherwise monotonously smooth surface (Fig. 22.3).

Blood Supply

Five arteries supply blood to the stomach. The left gastric artery arises directly from the celiac axis and supplies the cardiac region. The right gastric artery (which supplies the lesser curve) and the right gastroepiploic artery (which supplies the greater curve) arise from the hepatic artery. The left gastroepiploic and the short gastric arteries arise from the splenic artery and also supply the greater curvature. All these vessels anastomose freely, both on the subserosal layer of the stomach and in the muscularis propria, with extensive true plexus formation present within the submucosa. This richness of blood supply explains why it is so unusual to see gastric infarcts. The mucosal arteries are derived from this submucosal plexus but are end arteries that supply an area of mucosa that is largely independent of the adjacent mucosal arteries (4).

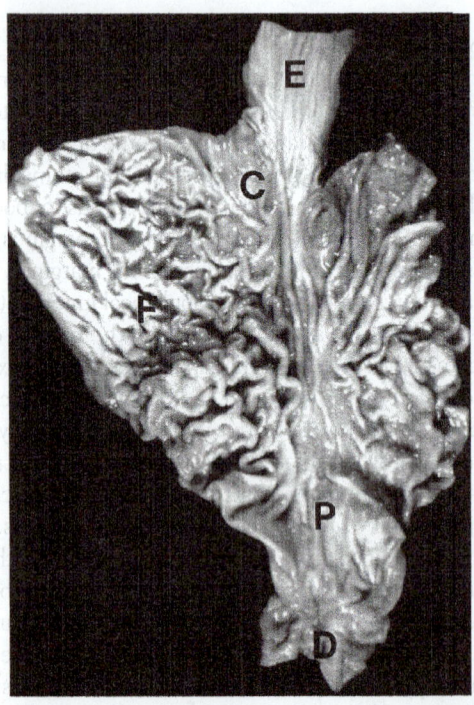

FIGURE 22.2 Mucosal zones of the stomach. The cardiac mucosa (*C*) is present distal to the lower end of the esophagus (*E*). The pyloric mucosa (*P*) occupies a triangular zone proximal to the duodenum (*D*). Elsewhere, the oxyntic mucosa (*F*) shows prominent rugal folds.

Nerve Supply

The sympathetic nerve supply to the stomach is derived from the celiac plexus via nerves that follow the gastric and gastroepiploic arteries. Branches also are received from the left and right phrenic nerves. The parasympathetic supply is the vagus nerve via the main anterior and posterior trunks that lie adjacent to the esophagogastric junction. Shortly after entering the abdomen, the anterior vagus nerve gives off a hepatic branch, and the posterior vagus nerve gives off a celiac branch. Therefore, truncal vagotomy above these branches results in denervation of not only the stomach but also the entire intestinal tract. Sectioning below these nerves results only in gastric denervation. A highly selective vagotomy (gastric corpus denervation) is achieved by sectioning lateral branches as the two main gastric nerves pass along the lesser curvature, with preservation of the terminal portions of the vagi that supply the antrum. No true nerve plexuses occur on either subserosal layer of the stomach but instead are concentrated in Meissner plexus in the submucosa and Auerbach plexus between the circular and longitudinal fibers of the muscularis propria.

Lymphatics

Recent studies (5,6) have disproved the former view that lymphatic channels are present at all levels of the lamina propria. By using careful ultrastructural techniques, lymphatics have been shown to be limited to the portion of the lamina propria immediately superficial to the muscularis mucosae. From there, efferents penetrate the muscle and communicate with larger lymphatic channels running in the submucosa. This arrangement implies that gastric cancer may have lymph node metastases, even though the primary tumor is entirely superficial to the muscularis mucosae.

The lymphatic trunks of the stomach generally follow the main arteries and veins. Four areas of drainage can be identified, each with its own group of nodes. The largest area comprises the lower end of the esophagus and most of the lesser curvature, which drains alongside the left gastric artery to the left gastric nodes. From the immediate region of the pylorus, on the lesser curvature, drainage is to the right gastric and hepatic nodes. The proximal portion of the greater curvature drains to pancreaticosplenic nodes in the hilum of the spleen, and the distal portion of the greater curvature drains to the right gastroepiploic nodes in the greater omentum and to pyloric nodes at the head of the pancreas. Efferents from all four groups ultimately pass to celiac nodes around the main celiac axis.

Pathologists need to be aware of the location of different groups of lymph nodes and their nomenclature. A system based on location has been devised by the Japanese Gastric Cancer Association (7) and recognizes the following stations: perigastric along the greater curvature, perigastric along the lesser curvature, right and left paracardial (cardioesophageal), suprapyloric, infrapyloric, left gastric artery, celiac artery, common hepatic artery, hepatoduodenal (portal), splenic artery, and splenic hilum. Nodes at these locations are regarded as regional and if positive are counted in the N category of the TNM system. However, at the present time, the TNM system does not require the location of the nodes to be recorded in order to derive the pathologic stage of a neoplasm (8). This is still based on the number of positive nodes.

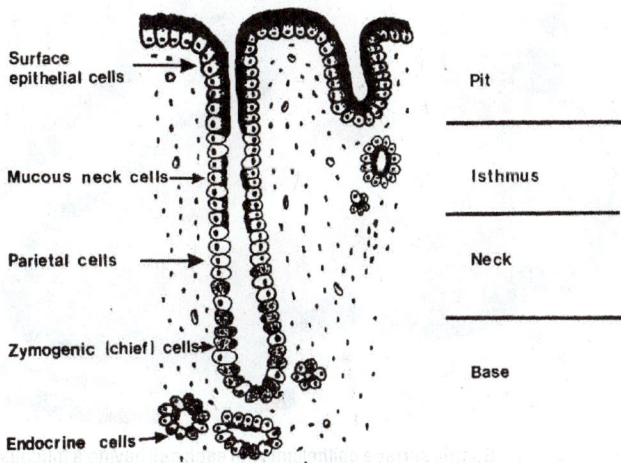

FIGURE 22.4 Diagrammatic representation of gastric oxyntic mucosa. Zymogenic (chief) cells are seen mainly in the basal portion of the glands and parietal cells mainly in the isthmic portion. The neck portion contains zymogenic cells, parietal cells, and mucous neck cells. A small number of endocrine cells are present in the basal zone.

GENERAL HISTOLOGIC FEATURES

Histologically, the mucosa has a similar pattern throughout the stomach. It consists of a superficial layer containing foveolae (pits), which represent invaginations of the surface epithelium, and a deep layer consisting of coiled glands that empty into the base of the foveolae (Fig. 22.4). The glandular layer differs in structure and function in different zones of the stomach that correspond roughly, but not precisely, to the gross anatomic regions (Fig. 22.1).

Adjacent to the GEJ is the cardiac mucosa, where the glands are mucus secreting. Extending proximally from the pylorus is the pyloric mucosa (sometimes called the antral mucosa), where the glands are also mucus secreting. This zone is triangular, extending much further (5 to 7 cm) proximally along the lesser curvature than it does along the greater curvature (3 to 4 cm). The pyloric mucosal zone is not identical to the antral region, although some accounts use these terms interchangeably. Also, contrary to what is implied in some descriptions, the incisura has no fixed relationship to the proximal margin of the pyloric mucosal zone. Elsewhere within the stomach (corpus and fundus), the mucosa is specialized to secrete acid and pepsin (oxyntic mucosa).

Histologic transition between pyloric and oxyntic mucosae is gradual rather than abrupt, with intervening junctional mucosae (1 to 2 cm in width) having a mixed histologic appearance. A broad mucosal transition zone is also present at the pylorus itself, where gastric and duodenal mucosae merge. However, at the lower end of the normal esophagus, the change from nonkeratinizing squamous epithelium to columnar epithelium is abrupt, both grossly and microscopically. The position of this squamocolumnar junction is variable and may not always coincide precisely with the

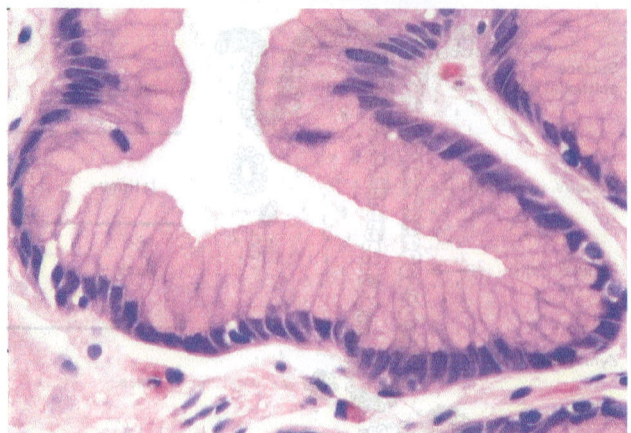

FIGURE 22.5 Gastric surface epithelium with each cell having a mucous globule in the superficial cytoplasm. Intraepithelial lymphocytes are present. These are surrounded by a clear halo (formalin fixation artifact).

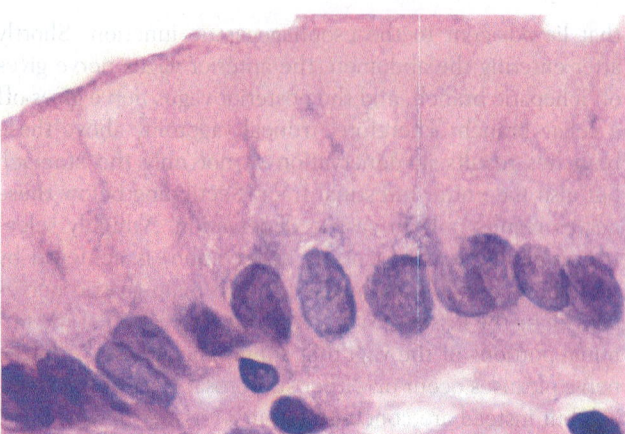

FIGURE 22.7 Gastric surface epithelium showing cytoplasmic mucus present in multiple small vacuoles.

strict anatomic esophagogastric junction. This is also the point where the gastric mucosal folds begin. Columnar epithelium that is present in flat mucosa proximal to the mucosal folds is considered to be within the anatomic esophagus and metaplastic in origin. In some individuals, the mucosal junction is located 0.5 to 2.5 cm proximal to the anatomic junction and may be serrated, rather than being a regular circumferential line (Z line).

Surface Epithelium

Histologically, the gastric mucosa is covered by tall, columnar, mucus-secreting cells with intervening foveolae that are lined by a similar epithelium (Fig. 22.5). The surface and foveolar lining cells are similar throughout all the mucosal zones of the stomach. The gastric glands empty into the base of the foveolae. Separating the foveolae and the glands is the lamina propria. In the cardiac and pyloric mucosal zones, the foveolae are wider than in other areas, sometimes giving the mucosa a slightly villous appearance (Fig. 22.6).

The cells of the surface epithelium and foveolae are tall and columnar with basally situated nuclei and superficial cytoplasm that is almost entirely filled with mucus (Fig. 22.7). The nuclei have an even distribution of chromatin, with single inconspicuous nucleoli. On hematoxylin and eosin (H&E)-stained sections, the appearance of the mucus varies, depending on the exact type of stain used. For example, with alcoholic eosin, the mucus appears as a single vacuole that is clear or lightly eosinophilic. With aqueous eosin, the mucus is more heavily eosinophilic and is seen to be present in numerous, small, closely aggregated vacuoles. Histochemically, the foveolar mucus is all neutral, periodic acid–Schiff (PAS) positive, but Alcian blue negative at pH 2.5 and lower (9).

Cardiac and Pyloric Mucosa

In the cardiac and pyloric zones, the foveolae occupy approximately one-half of the mucosal thickness (Fig. 22.6). Both the cardiac and pyloric glands are mucus secreting and are loosely packed with abundant intervening lamina propria (Fig. 22.8).

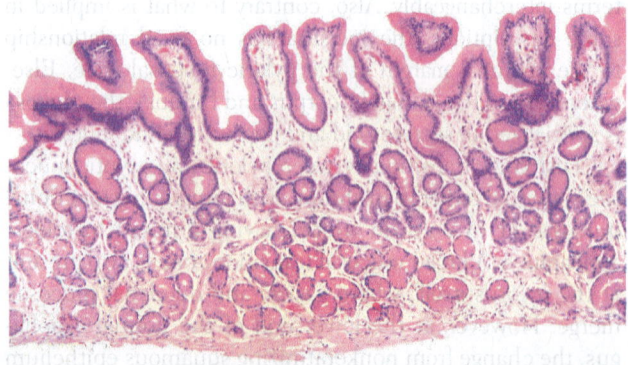

FIGURE 22.6 Gastric pyloric mucosa. Note that the glands are loosely packed and occupy about half the mucosal thickness. The surface epithelium appears slightly villous.

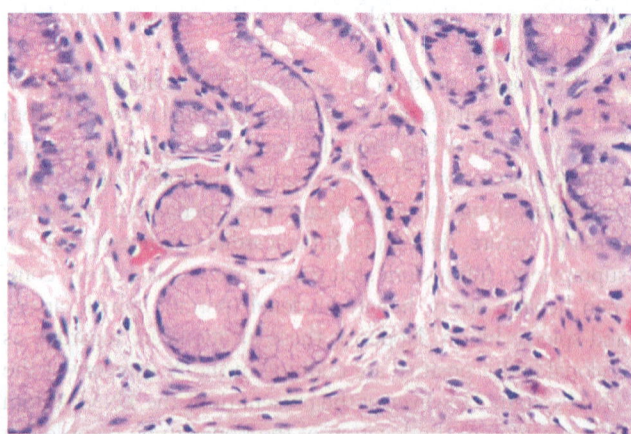

FIGURE 22.8 Pyloric glands containing cells with a bubbly, foamy appearance.

Occasional cystic glands may be found in the cardiac mucosa but usually are not encountered in the pyloric mucosa. The cells of the mucus glands have ill-defined borders and a bubbly cytoplasm that is different from the foveolar and surface epithelia. They resemble Brunner glands of the duodenum. Isolated parietal cells are not infrequently found either singly or in small groups, particularly in the pyloric mucosa and especially at the junctional zone, where it meets the oxyntic mucosa (1). However, it is uncommon for zymogenic (chief) cells to be present outside of the oxyntic mucosa and junctional area. The pyloric glands secrete neutral mucin only. The cardiac glands secrete predominantly neutral mucin with small amounts of sialomucin (9).

The extent of the cardiac mucosa and even its existence as a component of the normal GEJ have been disputed. Chandrasoma et al. (10) studied the gastroesophageal region in unselected adult autopsies. They found that when one histologic section was taken through this region, only 27% of cases had a zone of pure cardiac mucosa, 44% of cases had a zone of cardiofundic mucosa (glands containing a mixture of mucus-secreting cells and parietal cells), and 29% of cases had only pure oxyntic mucosa. When the entire GEJs from a selected group of adult autopsies were examined, all cases had cardiofundic mucosa present, but only 44% had a zone of pure cardiac mucosa. They also found that the zones of pure cardiac and cardiofundic mucosae were incomplete so that in some sections the esophageal squamous epithelium was present immediately adjacent to pure oxyntic mucosa. The average length of the cardiac and cardiofundic mucosae was 5 mm, and it never extended beyond 15 mm from the lower margin of the squamous esophageal epithelium. Other investigators have obtained similar results (11). In contrast, Kilgore et al. (12) and Zhou et al. (13) examined autopsy material from fetuses, infants, and young children. They found that pure cardiac mucosa was present in every case and measured 1.0 to 4.0 mm in length (average 1.8 mm). In 38% of cases, there was an abrupt transition from cardiac to oxyntic glands and in the remainder of cases, an additional zone of cardiofundic mucosa was present that generally measured less than 1.0 mm in length. In all instances where cardiofundic mucosa was present, it was in addition to a zone of pure cardiac mucosa. These findings suggest that pure cardiac mucosa and cardiofundic mucosa are normal findings but the extent of the mucus-secreting mucosa is less than was previously thought. However, note that the term cardia refers to a loosely defined gross anatomical zone. The cardia is therefore larger than the zone of pure cardiac mucosa and may contain cardiofundic and pure oxyntic mucosa.

Cardiac mucosal abnormalities may occur when there is gastroesophageal reflux or when the stomach is infected by *Helicobacter pylori*. The changes may include inflammatory nuclear atypia, intestinal metaplasia (IM), and the presence of hybrid mucosa (14). Hybrid mucosa is multilayered, with squamous cells at the base of the mucosa and columnar epithelium on the surface. With the development of these inflammatory changes, it may be difficult or even

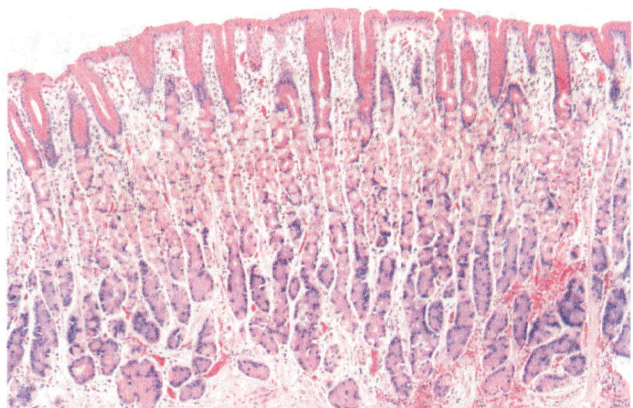

FIGURE 22.9 Gastric oxyntic mucosa. Note the short foveolae and the tightly packed glands. Purplish zymogenic cells predominate at the base, and pinkish parietal cells predominate in the upper part of the glands.

impossible to distinguish between damaged cardiac mucosa and glandular metaplasia of esophageal squamous epithelium (Barrett esophagus). Reference to specialized pathology texts is required (15). This distinction has a practical importance because at the present time it appears that Barrett esophagus carries a higher potential for malignant change than does metaplastic cardiac mucosa (16).

Oxyntic Gland Mucosa

The oxyntic gland mucosa has foveolae that occupy less than one-quarter of the mucosal thickness. In contrast to the cardiac and pyloric mucosae, the glands are tightly packed and are straight rather than coiled (Fig. 22.9). For descriptive purposes, they can be divided into three portions: base, neck, and isthmus. The basal portion consists mainly of zymogenic cells (pepsinogen secreting). These are cuboidal and have a basally situated nucleus, which typically contains one or more small nucleoli and cytoplasm that usually stains pale blue–gray (basophilic) with some variation, depending on the type of hematoxylin used (Fig. 22.10). The bluish color of the cytoplasm is due to the presence of rough endoplasmic

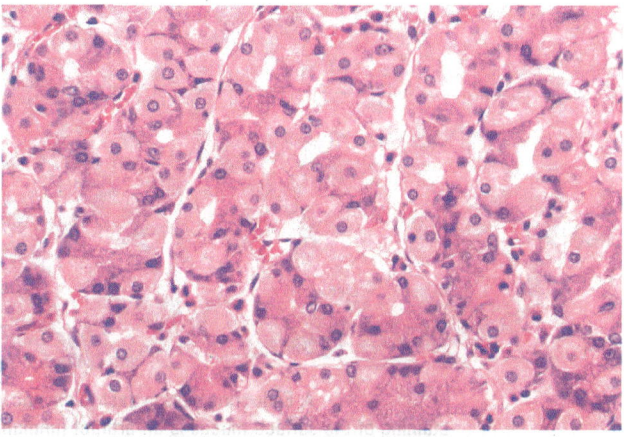

FIGURE 22.10 Oxyntic glands, showing parietal cell cytoplasm staining light pink and zymogenic cell cytoplasm staining purplish (H&E).

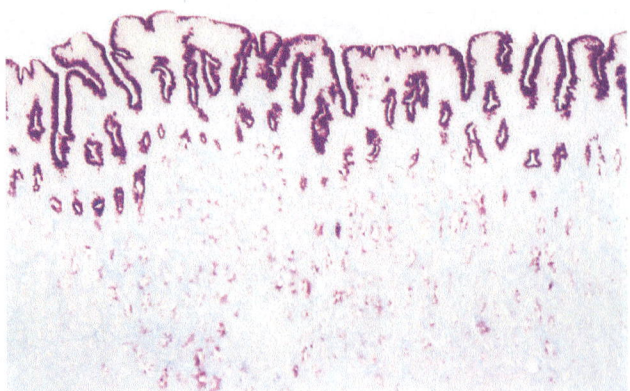

FIGURE 22.11 Oxyntic mucosa. The surface and foveolar lining epithelia are intensely positive. Paler-staining mucous neck cells are present within the glands (PAS).

reticulum containing ribosomal ribonucleic acid (RNA). The isthmic (most superficial) portion of the glands contains predominantly parietal cells (acid and intrinsic factor secreting). These are roughly triangular, with their base along the basement membrane. The nuclei are centrally placed with evenly distributed chromatin, and the cytoplasm stains a deep pink (acidophilic) on well-differentiated H&E-stained sections (Fig. 22.10). This staining property of the parietal cell cytoplasm reflects the presence of abundant microcanaliculi that consist entirely of protein. The neck (middle) portion of the fundic glands contains a mixture of zymogenic and parietal cells, together with a third type, mucous neck cells (Fig. 22.11). Mucous neck cells are difficult to recognize on an H&E stain but are easily identified using a PAS stain, where they are seen to resemble the mucus-secreting cells of the cardiac and pyloric glands. These cells produce neutral and acidic mucin, especially sialomucin, which stains positively with PAS/diastase and with Alcian blue at pH 2.5 (17). Mucous neck cells are found in lesser numbers in the isthmic portion of the glands, and occasional parietal cells can be encountered in the basal portion of the glands. Mucous neck cells are also present in the pyloric mucosa.

Studies indicate that the mucous neck cells located in glands from all areas of the stomach have proliferation and mucosal regeneration as their major functions. These undifferentiated cells act as stem cells and may migrate upward to renew parietal cells, foveolar and surface epithelia or downward to renew zymogenic or neuroendocrine cells (18). It has been estimated that, in humans, the gastric surface epithelium is normally replaced every 4 to 8 days. The parietal and zymogenic cells turn over much more slowly, likely every 1 to 3 years.

Endocrine Cells

The stomach contains a wide variety of hormone-producing cells. In the pyloric mucosa, about 50% of the whole endocrine cell population is G cells (gastrin producing), 30% are enterochromaffin (EC) cells (serotonin producing), and 15% are D cells (somatostatin producing). In the oxyntic mucosa, however, a major portion of the endocrine cells are enterochromaffin like (ECL) and secrete histamine. Small numbers of X cells (secretion product unknown) and EC cells are also present. In the oxyntic mucosa, the cells secreting these hormones are mostly located in the glands, particularly toward the base. They are inconspicuous and are difficult to detect without the use of special stains. Their numbers are variable but generally there are less than 20 cells per gland, with most glands containing less than 10 cells (Fig. 22.12A). In the pyloric mucosa, endocrine cells are most common in the neck region. On routine sections, they are rounded

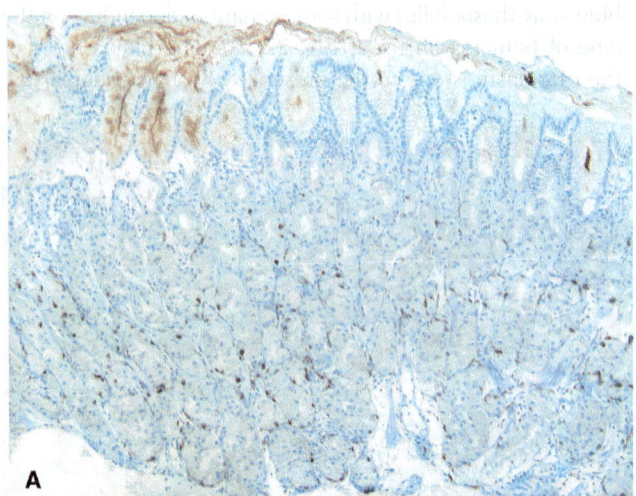
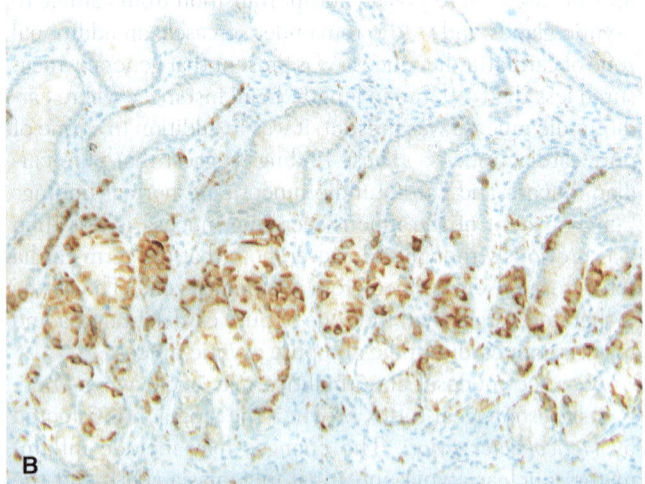

FIGURE 22.12 **A:** Endocrine cells in gastric oxyntic glands. Only scanty numbers of cells are present. The brown staining of the surface mucus is an artifact (immunostain for synaptophysin). **B:** Endocrine cells in the gastric pyloric mucosa. The cells are numerous and located predominately in the mucous neck region (immunostain for synaptophysin).

with regular nuclei, with an even distribution and clear cytoplasm (a fixation artifact). In pyloric mucosa, the cells are more numerous with between 20 and 50 cells per crypt (Fig. 22.12B). This wide range makes it difficult to assess mucosal biopsies for the presence of G-cell hyperplasia. Hormones from the endocrine cells either enter the blood or modulate other locally situated cells (paracrine effect).

The EC cells and some of the ECL cells have argentaffin granules, which can be stained by Fontana, Masson, or the diazo technique. Other cells are argyrophilic but not argentaffinic and may be stained by the Grimelius technique (19). Silver stains have now been replaced by more sensitive immunologic techniques (synaptophysin and chromogranin) (20). Individual hormones, for example, gastrin and somatostatin, may be demonstrated by specific antibodies. In addition to the presence of hormones in epithelial cells, some hormones also are found in neurons and nerve endings present in the stomach wall and mucosa. It is generally believed that vasoactive intestinal peptide is predominant in neural tissue and that catecholamines, bombesin, substance P, enkephalins, and possibly gastrin are also found at these sites. When hyperplasia of G cells occurs, it is generally linear. Overgrowth of ECL cells in the fundic mucosa occurs secondary to hypergastrinemia, arising as a consequence of pernicious anemia which causes destruction of parietal cells and loss of gastric acidity. ECL cell hyperplasia has been divided into five growth patterns: pseudohyperplasia, hyperplasia, dysplasia, microinfiltration, and neoplasia (21).

Lamina Propria

The epithelial cells of the surface, foveolae, and glands all rest on a basement membrane, which is similar to that seen elsewhere in the intestinal tract. Within the mucosa is a well-developed lamina propria that provides structural support, consisting of a fine meshwork of reticulin with occasional collagen and elastic fibers that are condensed underneath the basement membrane (Fig. 22.13). The lamina propria is more abundant in the superficial portion of the mucosa between the foveolae, especially in the pyloric mucosa. It contains numerous cell types, including fibroblasts, histiocytes, plasma cells, and lymphocytes. It is also normal to find occasional polymorphs and mast cells. As mentioned, the lamina propria contains capillaries, arterioles, and nonmyelinated nerve fibers. A few fibers of smooth muscle may extend upward from the muscularis mucosa into the lamina propria, occasionally reaching the superficial portion of the mucosa, especially in the distal antrum.

The lymphoid tissue of the stomach has not been studied as extensively as that of the small bowel. The isolated lymphocytes and plasma cells in the lamina propria are predominantly of B-cell lineage and are immunoglobulin A (IgA) secreting. Intraepithelial lymphocytes are present in the stomach but are much less frequent than in the small bowel. They are commonly surrounded by a clear halo, which represents a formalin fixation artifact. These lymphocytes, as well as small numbers of lamina propria lymphocytes, are of T-cell origin.

Recently it has been shown that small numbers of primary lymphoid follicles (aggregates of small lymphocytes) can be found in the normal stomach (22). However, secondary lymphoid follicles (follicles with germinal centers) are found only in gastritis, usually secondary to infection with *H. pylori*.

Submucosa

The submucosa is located between the muscularis mucosae and the muscularis propria and also forms the cores of the gastric rugae. It consists of loose connective tissue, in which many elastic fibers are found. The autonomic nerve plexus of Meissner is found in the submucosa, as are plexuses of veins, arteries, and lymphatics.

Muscular Components

In classical anatomy texts (23,24), the main muscle mass of the stomach is referred to as the muscularis externa. In North America, however, the alternative name, muscularis propria, is widely used and preferred. This is because the term *muscularis externa* is ambiguous, as it is sometimes not clear whether it refers to the whole of the main muscle mass or only its external layer.

Three layers of fibers can be recognized in the muscularis propria: outer longitudinal, inner circular, and innermost oblique. The external fibers are continuous with the longitudinal muscle of the esophagus. The inner circular layer is aggregated into a definite sphincter mass at the pylorus, where it is sharply separated from the circular fibers of the duodenum by a connective tissue septum. The oblique muscular fibers are an incomplete layer present interior to the circular fibers and are most obvious in the cardiac area. Evidence for the presence of a circular sphincter at the cardia is controversial (25). Histologic examination is not conclusive, and although radiologic techniques show arrest of swallowed food at this level, this may be due to external compression from the adjacent crura of the diaphragm.

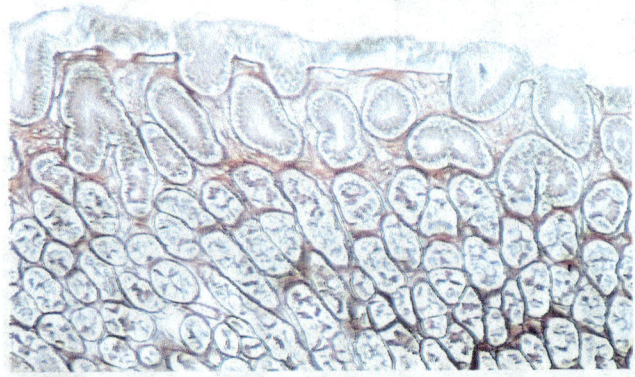

FIGURE 22.13 Normal gastric oxyntic mucosa (reticulin).

The muscularis mucosae consist of two layers, the inner circular and outer longitudinal, together with some elastic fibers. Thin bundles of smooth muscles also penetrate into the lamina propria, where they terminate in the basement membrane of the epithelium. This is most obvious in the antral area.

ULTRASTRUCTURE

The surface and foveolar lining epithelial cells are ultrastructurally similar. They are characterized by multiple rounded, electron-dense mucous vacuoles in the superficial cytoplasm and stubby microvilli projecting from the luminal surface. The basal cytoplasm contains moderate amounts of rough endoplasmic reticulum and some mitochondria. Adjacent epithelial cells are joined by tight junctions (zonula occludens) at their luminal aspect and by adherence junctions along the rest of the cell interfaces. These tight junctions are considered to play an important role in maintaining mucosal integrity and the gastric mucosal barrier.

Parietal cells are unique ultrastructurally (Fig. 22.14) (26). In the unstimulated state, the cytoplasm contains an apical crescent-shaped canaliculus lined by stubby microvilli (Fig. 22.14). Between the microvilli are elongated membrane invaginations termed microtubules. Upon stimulation, the microtubules disappear, to be replaced by a dense meshwork of intracellular canaliculi (27). The canalicular system is considered essential for the formation of hydrochloric acid. This is achieved by active transport of hydrogen ions across the canalicular membrane. Since this process has high energy requirements, most of the remainder of the parietal cell cytoplasm is occupied by mitochondria.

The zymogenic cells (chief cells) are similar to protein-secreting exocrine cells elsewhere in the body. They have rough-surfaced vesicles in the superficial cytoplasm and abundant rough endoplasmic reticulum in the remainder of the cell.

GASTRIC FUNCTION

The function of the stomach is to act as a reservoir and mixer of food and to initiate the digestive process. Gastric secretion of acid, pepsin, and electrolytes is partly under nervous control by the vagus and partly under the control of gastrin, produced by G cells in the antrum. Gastrin release from the G cells may occur either as a result of distention of the antrum or by direct stimulation from ingested food, particularly amino acids and peptides. Hydrochloric acid is produced by the active transport of hydrogen ions across the cell membrane. High concentrations of hydrochloric acid are achieved so that most ingested microorganisms are killed and the contents of the stomach are normally sterile.

Gastric mucus is secreted in two forms: a soluble fraction produced by the gastric glands and an insoluble form produced by the surface and foveolar lining cells. Biochemically, the mucus is a complex glycoprotein consisting of a protein core with branched carbohydrate side chains. Histochemically, gastric mucin is almost entirely neutral, although the mucous neck cells secrete small amounts of sulfomucin and sialomucin (17). By immunohistochemistry,

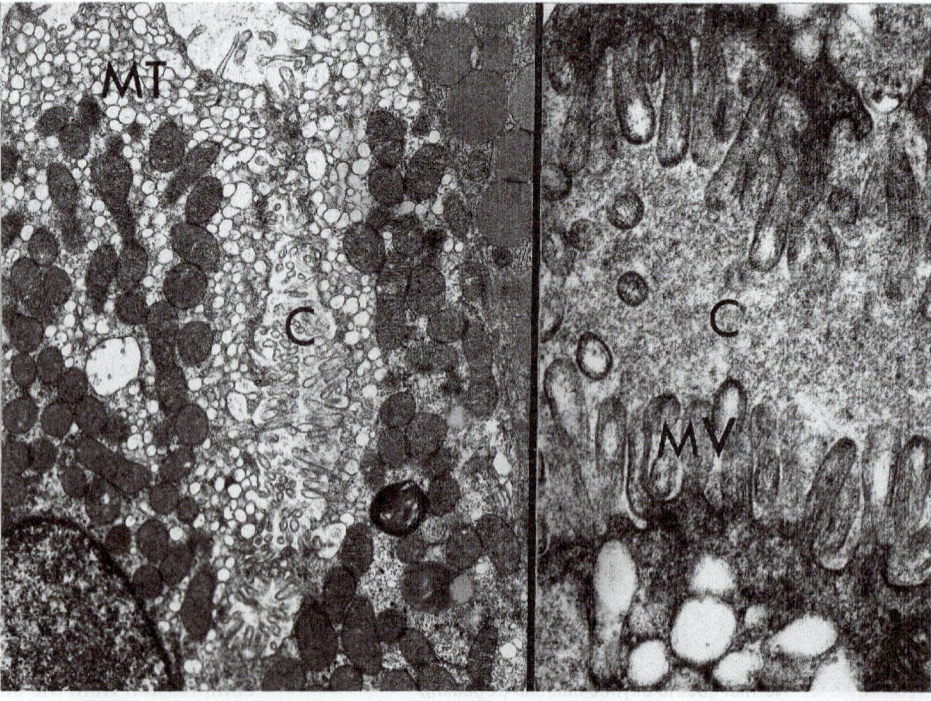

FIGURE 22.14 Ultrastructural appearances of the parietal cell canaliculus (C). Note the fingerlike microvilli (MV) and the microtubular invaginations (MT). (Original magnifications: left, ×9,000; right, ×41,000.)

mucins MUC5AC, MUC1, and MUC6 are detected in the normal stomach (28). Typically, MUC5AC is present in foveolar epithelium and mucus neck cells. MUC1 is present in the foveolar epithelium, chief and parietal cells. MUC6 is present in the antral glands and mucous neck cells. The exact physiologic role of gastric mucin is not determined, although the soluble mucin likely plays a role in lubrication. The mucin forms a surface coating with alternating layers of MUC5AC and MUC6 mucin proteins (29). This forms a barrier that, together with bicarbonate secreted by the superficial epithelial cells, prevents back diffusion of acid and gastric autodigestion. The actual structural barrier is formed by the continuous layer of luminal mucosal cells and the tight junctions between adjacent cells. This process is likely modulated by prostaglandins which promote mucosal blood flow.

SPECIAL TECHNIQUES AND PROCEDURES

Relatively few special techniques are applicable to routine diagnosis. Stains that demonstrate the carbohydrate composition of mucin are the most widely used, and the combined PAS/Alcian blue is the most versatile. This combination stains neutral mucin magenta, acid mucin light blue, and combinations purple. The combined stain is preferred over a straight PAS because the mucus in some gastric carcinomas is PAS negative. A mucicarmine stain is not recommended because it does not permit identification of the mucin type and is also negative with some types of acid mucin. Sialomucin and sulfomucin may be distinguished by a combined high-iron diamine and Alcian blue stain, which stains sulfomucin black and sialomucin light blue. At the present time, however, this distinction is of limited diagnostic utility.

Usually, there is no difficulty in distinguishing chief and parietal cells on a good H&E stain (Fig. 22.10). If necessary, special stains, such as a Maxwell stain (30), can aid this distinction. Parietal cells can be recognized and quantified by use of a human milk fat globulin antibody (31).

At the present time, the use of cytokeratin 7 and cytokeratin 20 immunostains to distinguish metaplastic gastric cardiac mucosa from the mucosa of Barrett esophagus is controversial. Different results have been obtained by different observers, so this methodology cannot be recommended for routine use (15).

AGE CHANGES

Many older adults have a reduced gastric acid output. Histologically, this is characterized by a reduction in the area of oxyntic mucosa with expansion of the zone of pyloric mucosa. This results in proximal displacement of the fundo-pyloric junction, a change termed pyloric (or pseudopyloric) metaplasia. Recently it has become recognized that hypochlorhydria of the elderly is not simply the result of aging but may also be secondary to chronic gastritis (32).

ARTIFACTS

A variety of artifacts may occur in gastric biopsy specimens (Fig. 22.15). Most of these artifacts relate to rough handling of the specimen, either at the time the biopsy sample is taken or when it is removed from the forceps. Crushing is common and can result in compression of the lamina propria, leading to a false impression of an inflammatory infiltrate. Crush artifact also produces telescoping of the foveolar lining cells. Stretching of the mucosa results in separation of the pits and glands, leading to an impression of edema. Hemorrhage into the lamina propria is also common in gastric biopsy samples and has to be distinguished from hemorrhagic gastritis. This can be difficult in small biopsy samples, but usually the microscopic appearances of hemorrhagic gastritis are characteristic. They include superficial epithelial damage and erosions.

DIFFERENTIAL DIAGNOSIS

One of the problems for pathologists examining gastric biopsy samples is determining whether the specimen is normal or shows minor degrees of gastritis. It is therefore appropriate to review briefly certain aspects of the classification and diagnosis of gastritis. Specific types of gastritis, for example, acute hemorrhagic gastritis or granulomatous gastritis, are usually so distinct that confusion with a normal stomach is unlikely (33). On the other hand, *H. pylori* gastritis may be patchy and may be associated with atrophy. In the early stage of *H. pylori* gastritis (chronic superficial gastritis), an infiltrate of inflammatory cells is observed in the superficial portion of the mucosa, particularly in the lamina propria between the gastric pits (Fig. 22.16). Later, the inflammation spreads deeply to involve the whole thickness of the mucosa and is accompanied by atrophy of gastric glands (chronic atrophic gastritis). Ultimately, the inflammation may burn itself out and all glands are destroyed, leaving only a thinned mucosa containing foveolar structures (gastric atrophy) (33).

The superficial gastric lamina propria normally contains some chronic inflammatory cells. It is often a matter of judgment whether these are considered normal or increased in number because there is no simple satisfactory method of objective measurement. In actual practice, it may be even more difficult to evaluate these cells because the gastric biopsy samples obtained by endoscopists are frequently distorted by crushing or stretching. In assessing possible minor degrees of inflammation, therefore, study should also be made of the superficial and foveolar lining

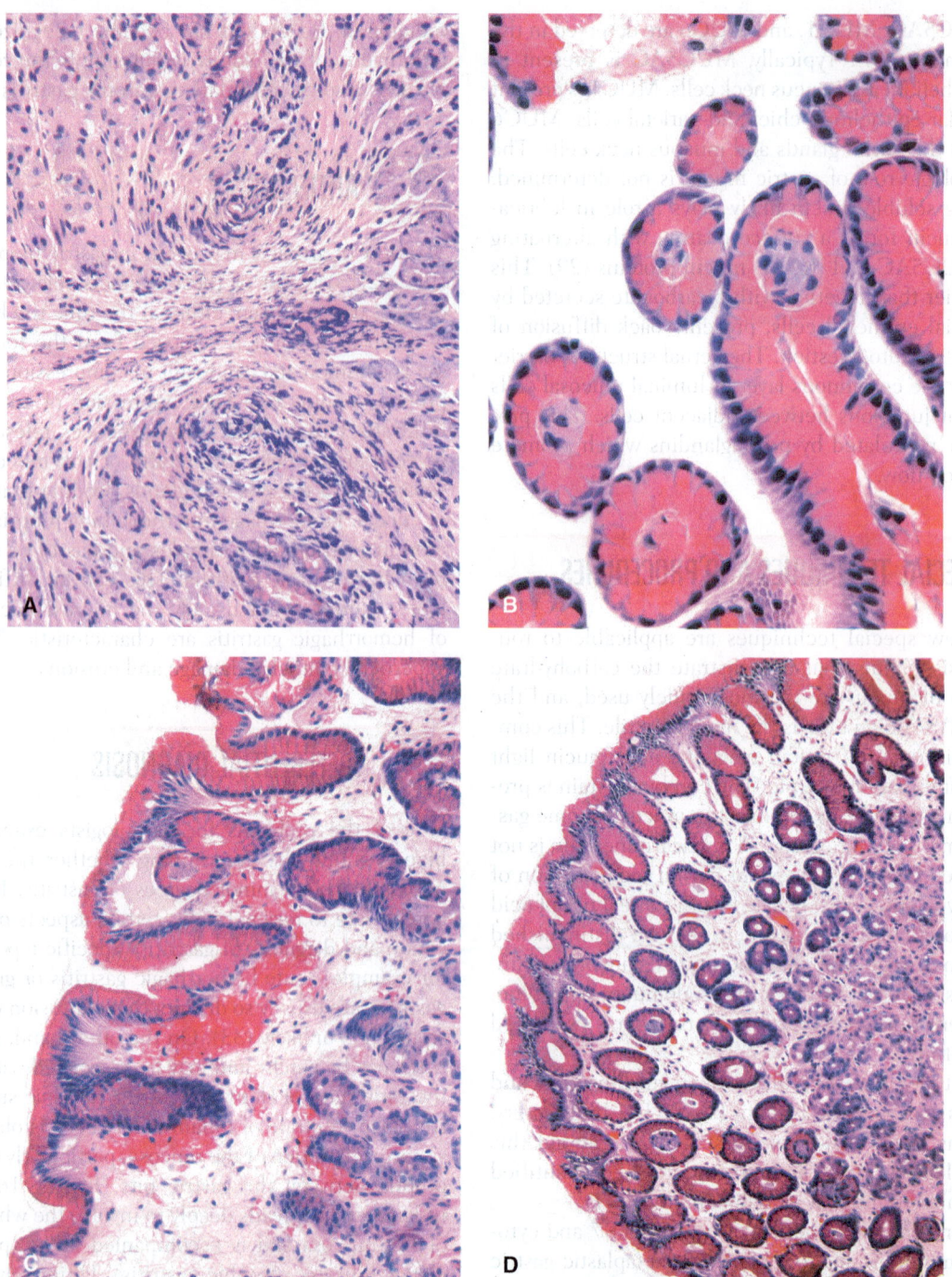

FIGURE 22.15 Biopsy artifacts: crushing, producing an apparent lamina propria infiltrate (**A**); crushing, resulting in displacement (telescoping) of cells into pit lumen (**B**); biopsy-induced hemorrhage (**C**); and stretching, producing an appearance of superficial edema (**D**).

epithelia, where a number of useful diagnostic features may be identified, depending on the degree of activity of the inflammation. The earliest changes seen are a reduction in the mucin content of the cytoplasm, an increase in nuclear size, and the presence of one or more prominent nucleoli (Fig. 22.17). At the base of the foveolae, there may be increased numbers of mitoses, reflecting a more rapid cell turnover. These findings are features of epithelial damage and regeneration and are common to all forms of gastritis and to reactive gastropathy (chemical gastritis). In severe active *H. pylori*–related inflammation, the epithelium and the lamina propria are infiltrated by acute inflammatory cells (Fig. 22.18), and organisms may be seen on the mucosal surface (Fig. 22.19). Optimum recognition of organisms is enhanced by using special stains (Giemsa, methylene blue, immunohistochemical stains).

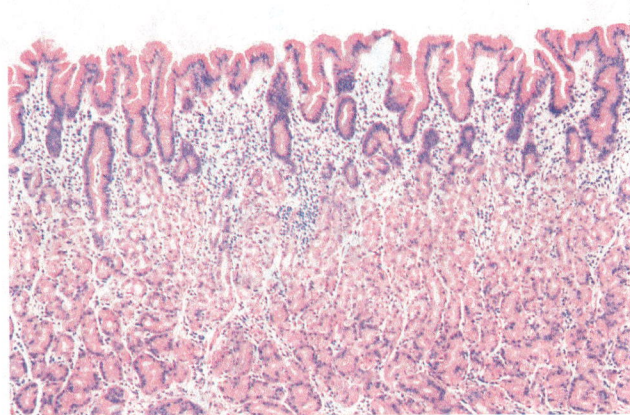

FIGURE 22.16 Mild chronic superficial gastritis with chronic inflammatory cells present in the superficial lamina propria in excess of normal. This is a borderline biopsy sample and illustrates the least number of cells acceptable for a diagnosis of gastritis.

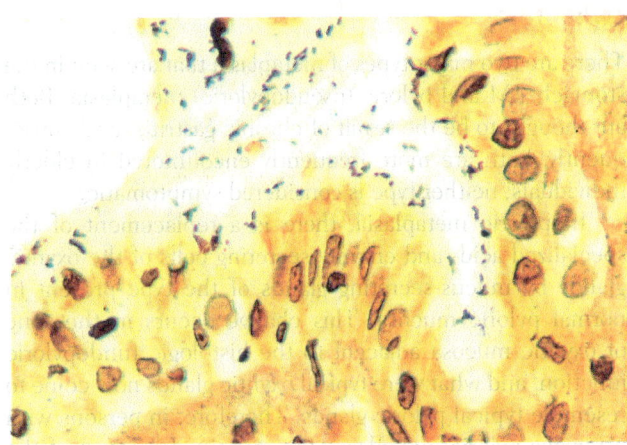

FIGURE 22.19 *Helicobacter pylori* organisms present in the mucous layer on the gastric mucosal surface.

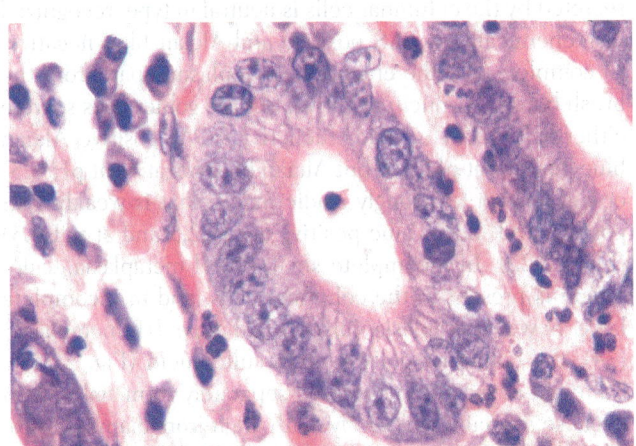

FIGURE 22.17 Gastritis showing cytoplasmic mucin loss with enlarged nuclei that contain prominent nucleoli.

Where gastritis has been present for some time, there may be atrophy of the mucosal glands, which can be accompanied by an increase in inflammatory cells in the deeper layers of the mucosa. On an H&E section, this is seen as a separation of the glands with increased intervening lamina propria. However, minor degrees of atrophy may be difficult to distinguish, particularly if there is biopsy artifact. In these instances, a reticulin stain can be useful in confirming atrophy by demonstrating coarse condensation of fibers in the lamina propria (Fig. 22.20).

Reactive gastropathy occurs when there is increased exfoliation of cells from the mucosal surface. Chemical agents, especially refluxed bile and nonsteroidal anti-inflammatory drugs, are common causes. The gastric surface and foveolar epithelia show regenerative changes as described above, but the mucosa is not infiltrated by inflammatory cells. The more severe examples of reactive gastropathy may be characterized by a "corkscrew" appearance of the foveolae.

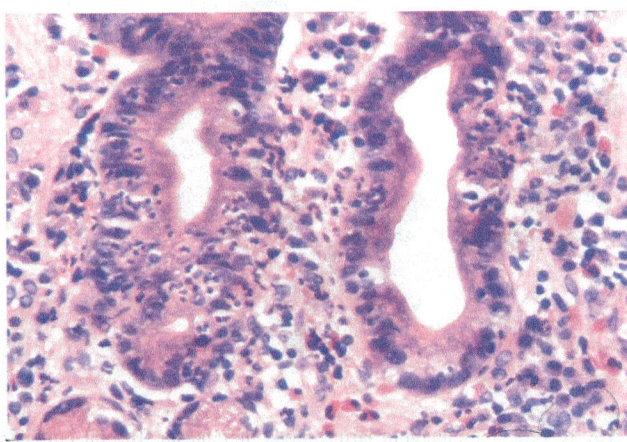

FIGURE 22.18 Gastric pits infiltrated by neutrophils in a case of *Helicobacter pylori* gastritis.

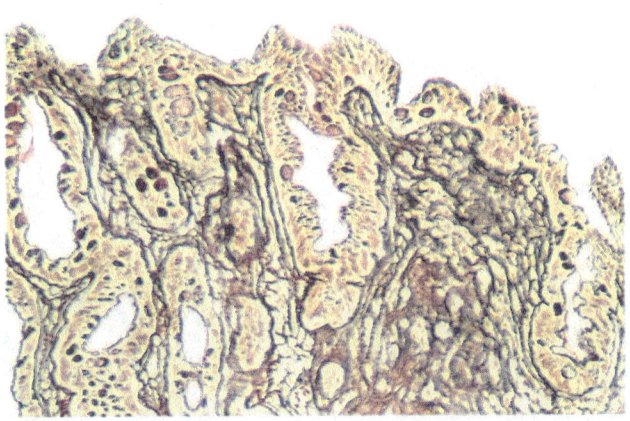

FIGURE 22.20 Coarse condensation of mucosal fibers in atrophic gastritis (reticulin).

Metaplasia

There are two major types of metaplasia that are seen in the stomach: IM and pyloric (pseudopyloric) metaplasia. Both are thought to be the result of chronic gastritis, and consequently, both are more frequently encountered in elderly individuals; neither type is considered symptomatic.

In pyloric metaplasia, there is a replacement of the specialized acid- and enzyme-secreting cells of the oxyntic glands by mucus-secreting glands of the type present in normal pyloric mucosa. This change occurs in the zone of oxyntic mucosa adjacent to the histologic fundopyloric junction, and what were typical oxyntic glands now come to resemble typical pyloric glands. Therefore, in persons with extensive pyloric metaplasia, the oxyntic gland area of the stomach contracts, the pyloric gland area expands, and the junctional zone is moved proximally toward the cardia (30). Unless the site of biopsy is known with accuracy, pyloric metaplasia cannot be diagnosed on routine H&E sections. However, although the fundic glands lose zymogenic and parietal cells, they still retain pepsinogen I activity. This can be demonstrated by immunohistochemical methods (34).

In IM, there is a change in the cells of the surface and pit epithelia so that morphologically and histochemically they come to resemble the cells of either the small or large bowel; IM may be complete (type I) or incomplete (type II) (33,34). In complete small bowel IM, the gastric mucosa changes to resemble normal small bowel epithelium, characterized by fully developed goblet cells and enterocytes with a brush border (Fig. 22.21). In advanced cases, the contour of the mucosa changes with the development of villi and crypts. Paneth cells may be present in the base of the crypts. In incomplete metaplasia, recognizable absorptive cells are not seen. The epithelium consists of a mixture of intestinal-type goblet cells and columnar mucus-secreting cells, morphologically resembling those of the normal gastric epithelium.

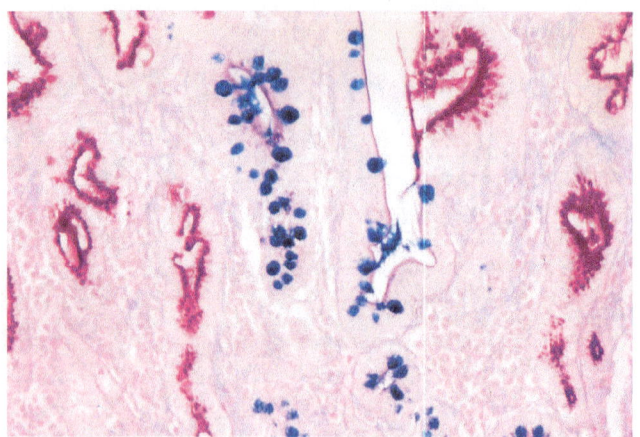

FIGURE 22.22 Complete intestinal metaplasia (PAS/Alcian blue).

Histochemical changes detected in the carbohydrate composition of mucus in the various types of IM are interesting and complex (17,35). In the normal stomach, mucus secreted by the columnar cells is neutral in type, recognized histochemically as PAS positive and Alcian blue negative. In complete IM, the enterocyte cytoplasm, apart from the brush border, is mucin negative, but the goblet cells secrete either sialomucin (an acid mucin that is PAS positive, Alcian blue positive at pH 2.5, but Alcian blue negative at pH 0.5) or sulfomucin (a strongly acidic mucin that is weakly PAS positive and Alcian blue positive at pH 2.5 and at pH 0.5) (Fig. 22.22). In incomplete small bowel metaplasia, sialomucin is present in the columnar cells, and in incomplete large bowel metaplasia (also called type III metaplasia) (34), the columnar cells contain sulfomucin (Fig. 22.23). Sulfomucin may be recognized separately from sialomucin because it stains positively with high-iron diamine (36). The details of these methods are well described in standard textbooks of histochemistry (37).

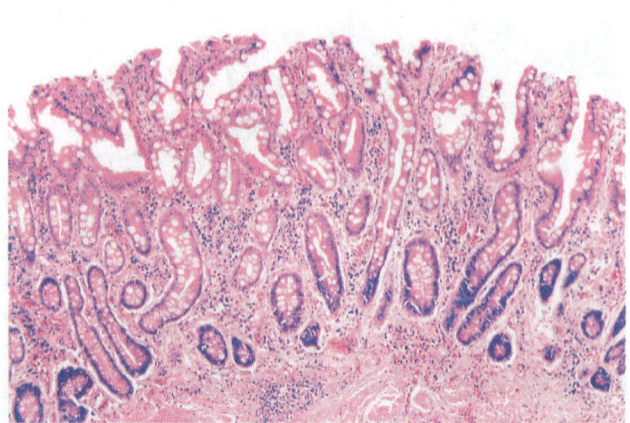

FIGURE 22.21 Complete intestinal metaplasia (IM).

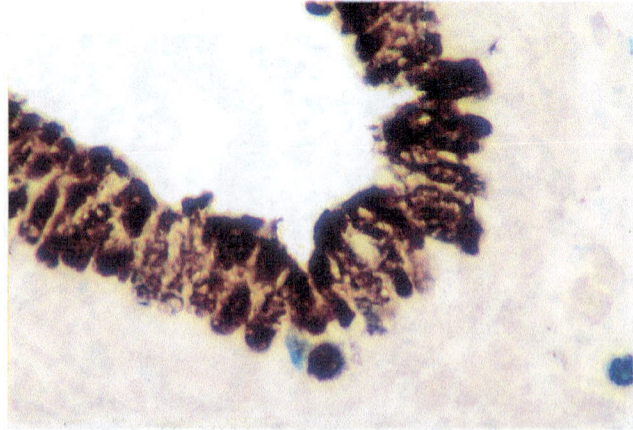

FIGURE 22.23 Incomplete large bowel metaplasia. The pit contains columnar cells with cytoplasmic sulfomucin (high-iron diamine and Alcian blue).

IM also shows changes in mucin core peptide expression. Normally, the gastric surface epithelium expresses MUC5AC and smaller amounts of MUC1. In complete IM of the stomach, this expression is lost and the goblet cells stain for intestinal mucin (MUC2). Incomplete metaplasia may express mixtures of all types of mucin core peptides. There are also differences in mucin core protein expression between gastric cardiac metaplasia and Barrett metaplasia, but these are inconsistent and not particularly helpful for diagnostic purposes (26).

Minor degrees of gastric IM are relatively common in persons in North America and elsewhere. The variants described above rarely exist as a pure entity, and mixtures of the various types within the same gastric foveola are encountered frequently. However, IM should never be considered normal and almost always reflects some degree of gastric damage, usually from chronic gastritis.

Less commonly encountered forms of metaplasia include subnuclear vacuolation (38) and ciliated metaplasia (39). These changes all involve the pyloric mucus glands. Subnuclear vacuolation is not strictly a metaplastic change because it does not simulate the appearance of any other type of normal cells and probably represents a degenerative change secondary to gastritis or duodenal reflux. The vacuoles are clear on H&E sections and indent the nucleus. Ultrastructurally, they consist of a membrane-lined space derived either from endoplasmic reticulum or Golgi and probably contain nonglycoconjugated mucus core protein (40). Ciliated cells are found at the base of antral glands where there is superficial IM (37). The cause and significance of this change is not known.

Pancreatic acinar metaplasia (41) may be present in up to 1.2% of gastric biopsy samples or 13% of gastrectomy specimens. The cells, which are indistinguishable from normal acinar cells, also produce lipase and trypsinogen. Seventy-five percent of cases are positive for amylase. Cells are present in nests and variably sized lobules scattered among the cardiac and oxyntic mucosae. Islets are not present.

SPECIMEN HANDLING

Gastric mucosa is delicate and should be handled with care. Tissue should be gently removed from the biopsy forceps and oriented before being placed flat on a supportive mesh, such as filter paper or Gelfoam. A variety of fixatives are suitable, depending on personal preferences, although routine formalin is suitable for most purposes. Sections are cut in ribbons, usually at two or three levels.

For the best results, it is suggested that gastrectomy specimens be opened and pinned out on a corkboard or wax platform before being immersed in formalin and fixed overnight. If sections are taken directly from a fresh specimen, they almost invariably curl up, resulting in irregular orientation of the final slide.

REFERENCES

1. Lewin KJ, Riddell RH, Weinstein WM. Normal structure of the stomach. In: Lewin KJ, Riddell RH, Weinstein WM, eds. *Gastrointestinal Pathology and its Clinical Implications*. New York: Igaku-Shoin; 1992:496–505.
2. Jacobson BC, Crawford JM, Farraye FA. GI tract endoscopic and tissue processing techniques and normal histology. In: Odze RD, Goldblum JR, eds. *Surgical Pathology of the GI Tract Liver and Pancreas*. 2nd ed. Philadelphia, PA: WB Saunders; 2009:3–30.
3. Mackintosh CE, Kreel L. Anatomy and radiology of the areae gastricae. *Gut* 1977;18:855–864.
4. Piasecki C. Blood supply to the human gastroduodenal mucosa with special reference to the ulcer-bearing areas. *J Anat* 1974;118(Pt 2):295–335.
5. Lehnert T, Erlandson RA, Decosse JJ. Lymph and blood capillaries in the human gastric mucosa. A morphologic basis for metastasis in early gastric carcinoma. *Gastroenterology* 1985;89:939–950.
6. Listrom MB, Fenoglio-Preiser CM. Lymphatic distribution of the stomach in normal, inflammatory, hyperplastic, and neoplastic tissue. *Gastroenterology* 1987;93:506–514.
7. Schmidt B, Yoon SS. D1 versus D2 lymphadenectomy for gastric cancer. *J Surg Oncol* 2013;107:259–264.
8. Ajani JA, In H, Sano T, et al. Stomach. In: Amin M, ed. *AJCC Cancer Staging Manual*. 8th ed. Chicago, IL: American Joint Committee on Cancer; 2017:259–264.
9. Filipe MI. Mucins in the human gastrointestinal epithelium: A review. *Invest Cell Pathol* 1979;2:195–216.
10. Chandrasoma PT, Der R, Ma Y, et al. Histology of the gastroesophageal junction: An autopsy study. *Am J Surg Pathol* 2000;24:402–409.
11. Sarbia M, Donner A, Gabbert HE. Histopathology of the gastroesophageal junction: A study on 36 operation specimens. *Am J Surg Pathol* 2002;26:1207–1212.
12. Kilgore SP, Ormsby AH, Gramlich TL, et al. The gastric cardia: Fact or fiction? *Am J Gastroenterol* 2000;95:921–924.
13. Zhou H, Greco MA, Daum F, et al. Origin of cardiac mucosa: Ontogenic consideration. *Pediatr Dev Pathol* 2001;4:358–363.
14. Glickman JN, Chen YY, Wang HH, et al. Phenotypic characteristics of a distinctive multilayered epithelium suggests that it is a precursor in the development of Barrett's esophagus. *Am J Surg Pathol* 2001;25:569–578.
15. Lash RH, Lauwers G, Odze RD, et al. Inflammatory disorders of the stomach. In: Odze RD, Goldblum JR, eds. *Surgical Pathology of the GI Tract, Liver, Biliary Tract and Pancreas*. 2nd ed. Philadelphia, PA: WB Saunders; 2009:269–320.
16. Goldblum JR. Inflammation and intestinal metaplasia of the gastric cardia: Helicobacter pylori, gastroesophageal reflux disease or both. *Dig Dis* 2000;18:14–19.
17. Goldman H, Ming SC. Mucins in normal and neoplastic gastrointestinal epithelium. Histochemical distribution. *Arch Pathol* 1968;85:580–586.
18. Matsuyama M, Suzuki H. Differentiation of immature mucous cells into parietal, argyrophil, and chief cells in stomach grafts. *Science* 1970;169:385–387.
19. Grimelius L. A silver stain for alpha-2 cells in human pancreatic islets. *Acta Soc Med Ups* 1968;73:243–270.

20. Rindi G, Buffa R, Sessa F, et al. Chromogranin A, B and C immunoreactivities of mammalian endocrine cells. Distribution, distinction from costored hormones/prohormones and relationship with the argyrophil component of secretory granules. *Histochemistry* 1986;85:19–28.
21. Solcia E, Fiocca R, Villani L, et al. Hyperplastic, dysplastic, and neoplastic enterochromaffin-like cell proliferations of the gastric mucosa. Classification and histogenesis. *Am J Surg Pathol* 1995;19(Suppl 1):S1–S7.
22. Genta RM, Hamner HW, Graham DY. Gastric lymphoid follicles in Helicobacter pylori infection: Frequency, distribution, and response to triple therapy. *Hum Pathol* 1993;24:577–583.
23. Cormack DH. The digestive system. In: Cormack DH, ed. *Ham's Histology*. 9th ed. Philadelphia, PA: JB Lippincott; 1987:495–517.
24. Fawcett DW. The esophagus and stomach. In: Fawcett DW, ed. *Bloom and Fawcett: A Textbook of Histology*. 12th ed. New York: Chapman & Hall; 1994:593–616.
25. Bowden RE, El-Ramli HA. The anatomy of the esophageal hiatus. *Br J Surg* 1967;54:983–989.
26. Rubin W, Ross LL, Sleisenger MH, et al. The normal human gastric epithelia. A fine structural study. *Lab Invest* 1968;19:598–626.
27. Forte JG, Forte TM, Black JA, et al. Correlation of parietal cell structure and function. *J Clin Gastroenterol* 1983;5(Suppl 1):17–27.
28. Glickman JN, Shahsafaei A, Odze RD. Mucin core peptide expression can help differentiate Barrett's esophagus from intestinal metaplasia of the stomach. *Am J Surg Pathol* 2003;27:1357–1365.
29. Ho SB, Takaura K, Anway R, et al. The adherent gastric mucous layer is composed of alternating layers of MUC5AC and MUC6 proteins. *Dig Dis Sci* 2004;49:1598–1606.
30. Maxwell A. The alcian dyes applied to the gastric mucosa. *Stain Technol* 1963;38:286–287.
31. Walker MM, Smolka A, Waller JM, et al. Identification of parietal cells in gastric body mucosa with HMFG-2 monoclonal antibody. *J Clin Pathol* 1995;48:832–834.
32. Kekki M, Samloff IM, Ihamaki T, et al. Age- and sex-related behavior of gastric acid secretion at the population level. *Scand J Gastroenterol* 1982;17:737–743.
33. Owen DA. The stomach. In: Mills SE, ed. *Sternberg's Diagnostic Surgical Pathology*. 5th ed. Philadelphia, PA: Lippincott Williams & Wilkins; 2010:1279–1312.
34. Dixon MF, Genta RM, Yardley JH, et al. Classification and grading of gastritis. The updated Sydney System. International Workshop on the Histopathology of Gastritis, Houston 1994. *Am J Surg Pathol* 1996;20:1161–1181.
35. Jass JR, Filipe MI. The mucin profiles of normal gastric mucosa, intestinal metaplasia and its variants and gastric carcinoma. *Histochem J* 1981;13:931–939.
36. Filipe MI, Potet F, Bogomoletz WV, et al. Incomplete sulphomucin-secreting intestinal metaplasia for gastric cancer. Preliminary data from a prospective study from three centres. *Gut* 1985;26:1319–1326.
37. Filipe MI, Lake BD. *Histochemistry in Pathology*. Edinburgh: Churchill Livingstone; 1983:310–313.
38. Rubio CA, Slezak P. Foveolar cell vacuolization in operated stomachs. *Am J Surg Pathol* 1988;12:773–776.
39. Rubio C, Hayashi T, Stemmerman G. Ciliated gastric cells: A study of their phenotypic characteristics. *Mod Pathol* 1990;3:720–723.
40. Thompson IW, Day DW, Wright NA. Subnuclear vacuolated mucous cells: A novel abnormality of simple mucin-secreting cells of non-specialized gastric mucosa and Brunner's glands. *Histopathology* 1987;11:1067–1081.
41. Doglioni C, Laurino L, Dei Tos AP, et al. Pancreatic (acinar) metaplasia of the gastric mucosa. Histology, ultrastructure, immunocytochemistry and clinicopathologic correlations of 101 cases. *Am J Surg Pathol* 1993;17:1134–1143.

Small Intestine

Megan G. Lockyer ■ Robert E. Petras

GROSS ANATOMY AND SURGICAL PERSPECTIVE 615	**SPECIAL CONSIDERATIONS** 631
PHYSIOLOGY 616	Geographic, Age-Related, and Dietary Factors 631
HISTOLOGY 616	Metaplastic and Heterotopic Tissues 631
Mucosa 617	Lymphoid Proliferations 631
Submucosa 623	Morphologic Changes Associated with Ileal Diversion and Continence-Restoring Procedures 632
Muscularis Externa 624	**MUCOSAL BIOPSY SPECIMEN EVALUATION IN SUSPECTED MALABSORPTION** 633
Serosa and Subserosal Region 625	Specimen Procurement and Processing 633
DISTINCTIVE REGIONAL CHARACTERISTICS OF THE SMALL BOWEL 626	Specimen Interpretation and Common Artifacts 633
Duodenum 626	**ACKNOWLEDGMENT** 635
Jejunum 628	**REFERENCES** 635
Ileum 629	

GROSS ANATOMY AND SURGICAL PERSPECTIVE

The small intestine, located within the abdominal cavity, is a multiple-coiled tubular organ that extends from the gastric pylorus to the junction of the cecum and ascending colon. Its average length in human adults is 6 to 7 m (1). Three subdivisions—the duodenum, jejunum, and ileum—are defined and characterized by various anatomic relationships. The duodenum is the most proximal portion of the small intestine; it measures about 12 in (20 to 25 cm) in length and extends from the pylorus to the duodenojejunal flexure. The duodenum, excluding the most proximal several centimeters, is a fixed, retroperitoneal structure that forms a C or U shape around the head of the pancreas (2). Four subdivisions of the duodenum have been described: (a) the first portion, also known as the duodenal cap or bulb, is the most proximal and superior segment; (b) the descending or second portion, into which the common bile duct and major and minor pancreatic ducts empty into their respective papillae; (c) the horizontal or third portion; and (d) the ascending or fourth portion, which veers forward at the level of the second lumbar vertebra, just left of midline, to become continuous with the remainder of the small bowel (2).

The origin of the jejunum is marked by a strip of fibromuscular tissue, the so-called ligament of Treitz, which anchors the terminal duodenum and the duodenojejunal flexure to the posterior abdominal wall (3). Distal to the ligament of Treitz, the remainder of the small bowel is arbitrarily subdivided into the jejunum (the proximal two-fifths) and the ileum (the distal three-fifths, terminating at the ileocecal junction within the right iliac fossa) (2).

Although a discrete point demarcating jejunum from ileum does not exist, several relatively distinctive features become gradually more apparent from proximal to distal; these features help surgeons isolate specific segments of the small bowel. For example, the proximal jejunum has a thicker wall and is about twice the diameter of the distal ileum. In addition, jejunal segments have more prominent permanent circular folds (plicae circulares, also known as valvulae conniventes) that can be palpated externally at surgery (1,4). The quantity of mesenteric adipose tissue is greater in the ileum, thus imparting a dense opaque appearance that contrasts with the less fatty, translucent mesentery

---

This chapter is an update of a previous version authored by William E. Katzin and Robert E. Petras.

of the jejunum. Finally, most of the jejunum lies within the upper abdominal cavity, whereas most of the ileum lies within the lower abdominal cavity and pelvis (4).

The arterial vascular supply of the small bowel originates from two major aortic axes: the celiac and superior mesenteric trunks (5). The duodenum is supplied by branches and interanastomosing arcades of both trunks, and its blood supply is intimately associated with that of the pancreatic head. The jejunum and ileum receive their blood from more distal branches of the superior mesenteric artery (5). The lymphatic and venous drainage systems follow the arterial supply and flow into regional lymphatics and lymph nodes or the portal venous system, respectively. Capillaries and lymphatic lacteals traverse the villi. It is usually impossible to distinguish one from the other with routine staining except after a fat-containing meal, in which case the lacteal will dilate. Lymphatic endothelium can be selectively immunostained using D2-40 antibody. Lacteals of adjacent villi interconnect and in the lower portion of the villi fuse to form a wider sinus that eventually drains into the lymphatic network of the submucosa (6,7).

Sympathetic neural input to the small bowel is carried by the celiac and superior mesenteric plexuses, whereas the parasympathetic supply is derived from distal branches of the vagus nerve; both of these closely follow the arterial paths into the bowel wall.

PHYSIOLOGY

The small intestine has several functional roles, the most important of which is the breakdown and absorption of ingested nutrients. Salivary gland, gastric, and pancreatic enzymes act on the larger ingested carbohydrates and proteins to produce more appropriately sized molecules for further digestion in the small intestine. The brush border created by the numerous apical microvilli on absorptive epithelial cells offers an array of aminopeptidases and di- and oligosaccharidases which act as key enzymes in completing the process of peptide and carbohydrate hydrolysis (8–10). The resulting monosaccharides, free amino acids, and di- and tripeptides are subsequently absorbed across the epithelial layer, and most pass into the portal venous system for storage or systemic distribution (11).

Fat digestion is initiated by lingual lipase, produced by glands in the tongue, and gastric lipase. Fat digestion is mostly catalyzed by pancreatic lipases in the lumen of the small intestine, which act on emulsified droplets of dietary fat admixed with bile salts. The products of digestion, including free fatty acids and monoglycerides are then able to diffuse across the lipid bilayer membrane of enterocytes (12). Most undergo intracytoplasmic resynthesis to form triglycerides which eventually are combined with cholesterol, phospholipids, and apoproteins to form chylomicrons. Mature chylomicrons exit the Golgi complex for exocytosis across the basolateral enterocyte membrane and subsequent entry into regional lymphatics (11,13).

Water and electrolytes, vitamins, minerals, and various drugs also are absorbed at points along the mucosa of the small bowel (14). Therefore, the structural integrity of this viscus is critical to the maintenance of nutritional status, as well as in appropriate drug handling. There are regional differences in absorption that are important clinically. For example, iron is absorbed proximally whereas vitamin B_{12} (cobalamin) is preferentially absorbed in the ileum. Deficiencies in these substances should prompt investigation for celiac sprue and Crohn disease.

The small intestine also functions to propel and segmentally mix both newly accepted gastric contents and the residual material left after initial digestive efforts. Although a number of factors influence gut motility, the most basic contractile activity is initiated at the level of the individual smooth muscle cells within the wall (15). Important functional differences exist, based on whether an individual is feeding or fasting. With feeding, a distended bowel segment initiates peristalsis, a forward propulsive motion that is mediated through the enteric nervous system; the intrinsic neurons of the myenteric plexus of Auerbach are most important in this regard (15,16). In contrast, during fasting or between meals, a slow yet continually recurring set of contractions attempts to clear the enteric lumen of any residual debris. The hormone motilin is believed to be important in the generation of these migratory motor complexes (16). Other endocrine influences, as well as the autonomic and central nervous systems, play a modulatory role in these intrinsic activities.

A variety of hormones can be detected within individual cells lining the small intestinal mucosa (17). Although the precise physiologic role of most of these cells and their secretory products remains to be determined, some are thought to exert a modulatory effect on gut motility or to influence the function of nearby epithelial cells (16,18).

The gut in general and the small bowel in particular have a crucial function in mucosal immunity. The mucosa/gut-associated lymphoid tissues, which are discussed in detail later in this chapter, are important in the local defense against mucosally encountered microorganisms and generate the initial immunologic responses to these various agents (19). In addition, these tissues are the breeding ground for various reactive and neoplastic pathologic conditions.

HISTOLOGY

Although regional histologic differences exist within the small intestine, the general microscopic structure is similar throughout its length. The wall of the small bowel can be divided into four basic layers: mucosa, submucosa, muscularis externa or propria, and serosa.

Mucosa

Mucosal Architecture and Design

Since the principal function of the small intestine is absorption of ingested nutrients, the mucosa, which is the layer in contact with luminal contents, is specifically designed for this purpose. Several architectural adaptations augment the otherwise limited surface area of the small intestine (20). One of these, the grossly evident permanent circular folds (plicae circulares), courses perpendicular to the longitudinal axis of the bowel (Fig. 23.1) (20,21). These mucosa-covered folds contain submucosal cores and traverse nearly the entire circumference of the bowel lumen before overlapping with adjacent permanent folds. In addition to enhancing the surface area, they act as partial barriers that attenuate the forward flow of intraluminal contents, thus increasing the time of contact with absorptive surfaces.

The mucosa is composed of an epithelial component, a lamina propria, and muscularis mucosae. The surface epithelium and lamina propria form intraluminal projections called villi. These microscopic fingerlike and leaflike projections cover the entire luminal surface of the small bowel and are the most important morphologic modification responsible for enhancing the surface area (Figs. 23.2 and 23.3) (20,22,23). Each villous surface is covered by a single layer of epithelium consisting of various cell types. Beneath this epithelial layer lies a core of lamina propria that contains a centrally located,

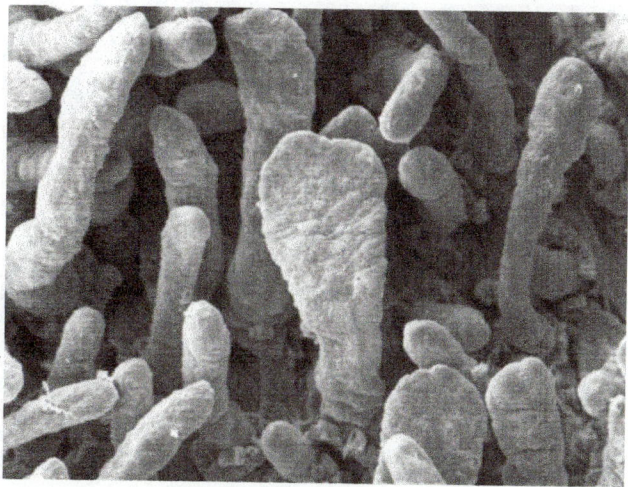

FIGURE 23.2 Scanning electron micrograph of small intestinal mucosa discloses the fingerlike and leaflike appearance of villi. Fingerlike villi predominate in the more distal segments of small bowel (jejunum and ileum), whereas leaflike villi are more common in the duodenum. Mixed populations, as in this micrograph, are considered normal.

blind-ended lymphatic channel (lacteal), an arteriovenous capillary network, and an abundant migratory cell population (Fig. 23.4) (24,25).

In the intervening regions and beneath the villi lie the crypts of Lieberkühn. These tubular intestinal glands open between the villi and extend down to the muscularis mucosae (Fig. 23.3). The crypts are depressions of the surface epithelium, whereas the villi are extensions above it. However, these mucosal compartments are contiguous in that the lamina propria forming the villous cores also surrounds the crypts. The ratio of villous length to crypt length in normal small bowel varies from about 3:1 to 5:1 (Fig. 23.3) (20). The crypts and surrounding lamina propria lie upon

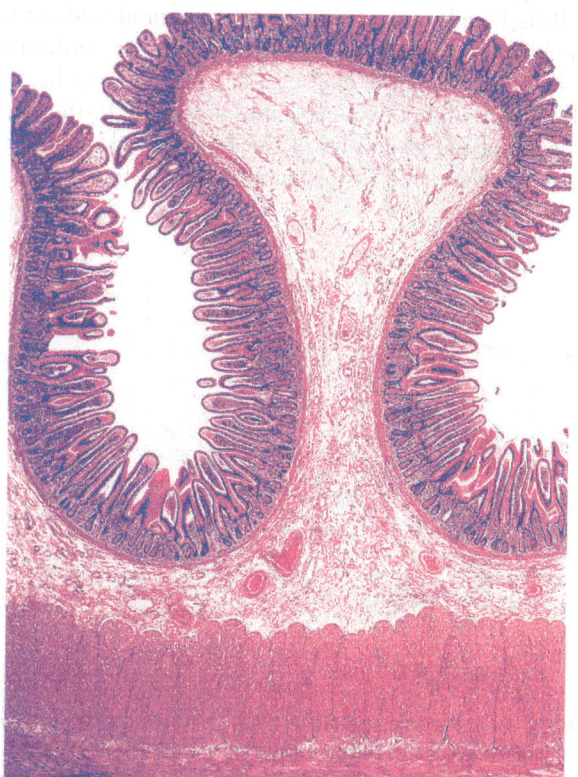

FIGURE 23.1 A single plica, or permanent circular fold, with its submucosal core and mucosal surface. The absorptive surface area is further augmented by intraluminal mucosal projections (villi).

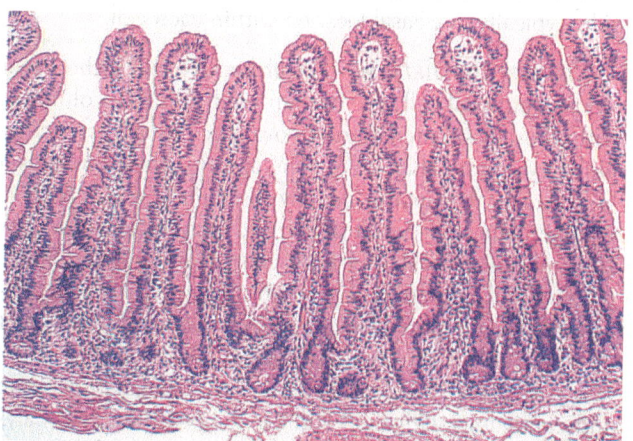

FIGURE 23.3 Normal jejunal villi. These villi are long and slender mucosal projections with a core of lamina propria covered by a luminal epithelial layer. A single row of intestinal glands (crypts) is found at the base of the mucosa. These crypts lie between adjacent villi and are surrounded by the same lamina propria that forms the villous cores.

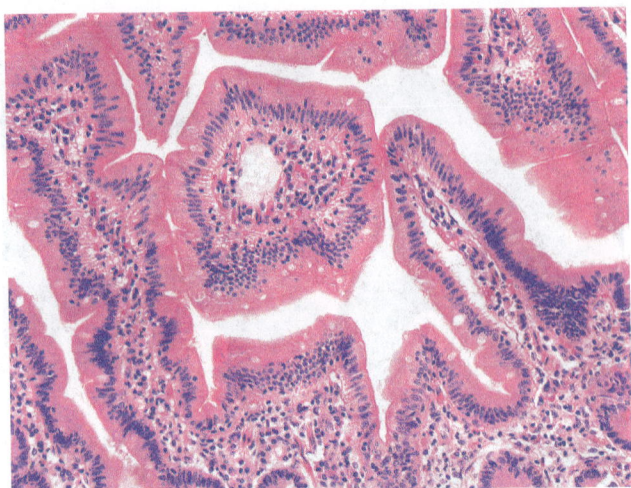

FIGURE 23.4 The duodenal villous surface is covered by a single layer of tall columnar epithelial cells. The underlying lamina propria core contains lymphoid and plasma cells and a connective tissue framework, including a lymphatic vessel (lacteal) and a subepithelial capillary network.

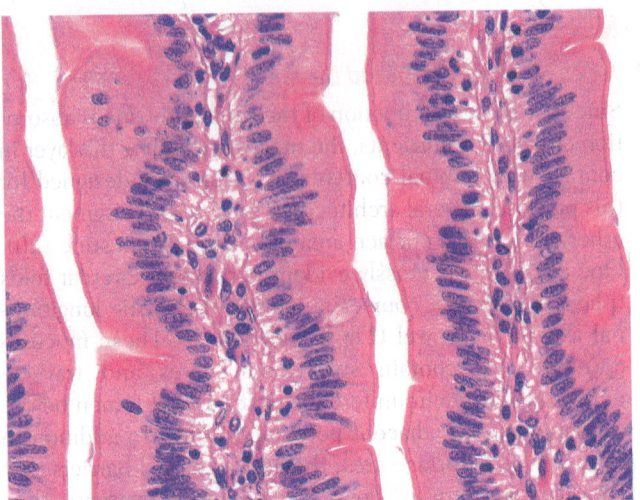

FIGURE 23.5 High-magnification view of a jejunal villi disclosing the general features of villous morphology. Both columnar absorptive cells and goblet cells (with apical clear vacuole) cover the villous surfaces; each cell type has a basally situated oval-to-round nucleus. Microvilli (brush border) are seen extending from the columnar absorptive cell surface. Note the intraepithelial lymphocytes scattered among and between the epithelial cells.

the muscularis mucosae, a thin fibromuscular layer that separates the mucosa from the underlying submucosa. The smooth muscle of the muscularis mucosae and that of the muscularis externa can be distinguished using smoothelin immunoreactivity; the muscularis externa demonstrates robust positivity, whereas the muscularis mucosae typically shows absent or weak staining (26).

Mucosal Components and Their Composition

> **EPITHELIUM** The mucosal epithelium is divided into the villous and crypt compartments. Although similar in appearance, the cell types differ somewhat, and their basic functions are distinct. Common to both, however, is a basic polarity of cellular organization, with nuclei aligned side by side, typically in a basal location within each cell.

> **VILLOUS EPITHELIUM** The absorptive cell is the major villous epithelial cell type encountered. It is tall, columnar, with a basally situated round-to-oval nucleus and an eosinophilic cytoplasm (Fig. 23.5). The apical surface contains a brush border that appears densely eosinophilic, stains positive with periodic acid–Schiff (PAS), and is composed of microvilli and the glycocalyx, or fuzzy coat (Figs. 23.5 and 23.6). Microvilli, which are best seen on ultrastructural examination, are evenly spaced surface projections that also augment the mucosal surface area of the small intestine (Fig. 23.7) (27). Multiple filamentous structures emanating from and contiguous with their surface comprise the glycocalyx (24). The microvillus membrane–glycocalyx complex houses important enzymes—peptidases and disaccharidases—that function in terminal digestive processes. This layer also acts as a physical barrier to microorganisms and other foreign matter (28). The small intestine has a single mucus layer composed predominantly of MUC2 mucin (29,30), a gel-forming mucin. MUC2 and other components forming the glycocalyx are continually synthesized within the absorptive cell and transported to the surface to replace the preexisting coat in a dynamic fashion (24,28,31). The inclusion of Paneth cell products with enterocyte produced antibacterial proteins in the mucus layer creates an antibacterial gradient shielding the epithelial cell surface from bacteria. Although its functional capacities are under further study, absence of the glycocalyx of the small bowel mucosa was the sole detectable histologic abnormality found in some

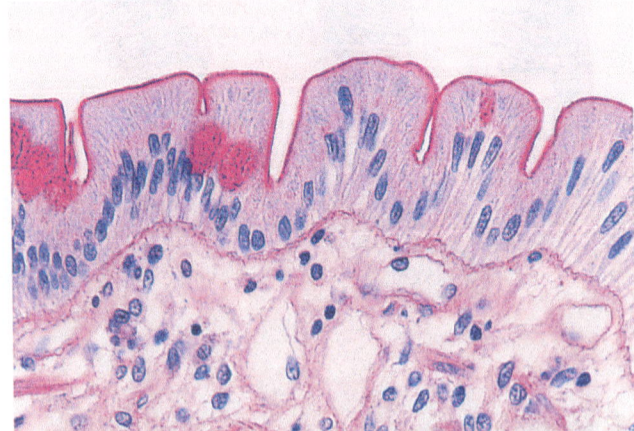

FIGURE 23.6 Periodic acid–Schiff (PAS) stain highlights the microvillus membrane–glycocalyx complex along the apical surface of the absorptive cells. The thin subepithelial basement membrane that separates the lamina propria from the epithelial compartment also stains with PAS but to a lesser degree. The neutral subgroup of mucins contained within the goblet cells are PAS positive as well.

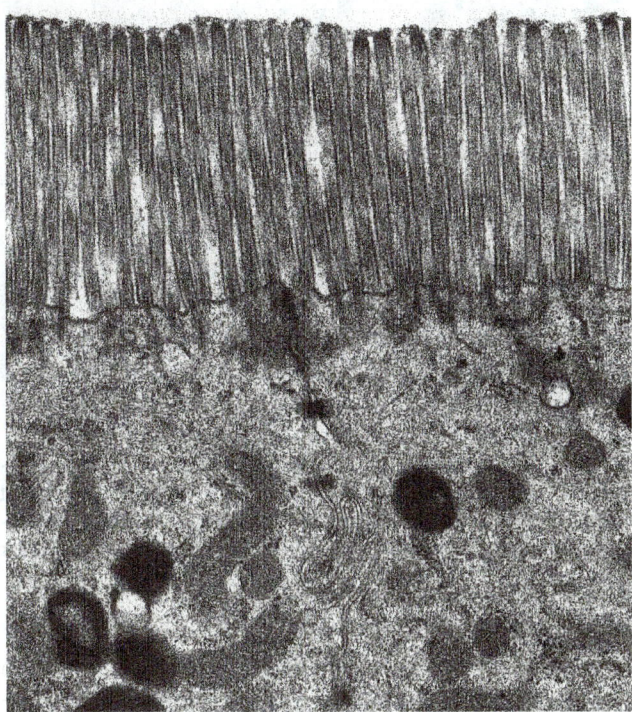

FIGURE 23.7 Transmission electron micrograph of microvilli emanating from the absorptive columnar cell surfaces. The glycocalyx component is the filamentous layer overlying the microvilli, but most of this has been artifactually removed during processing.

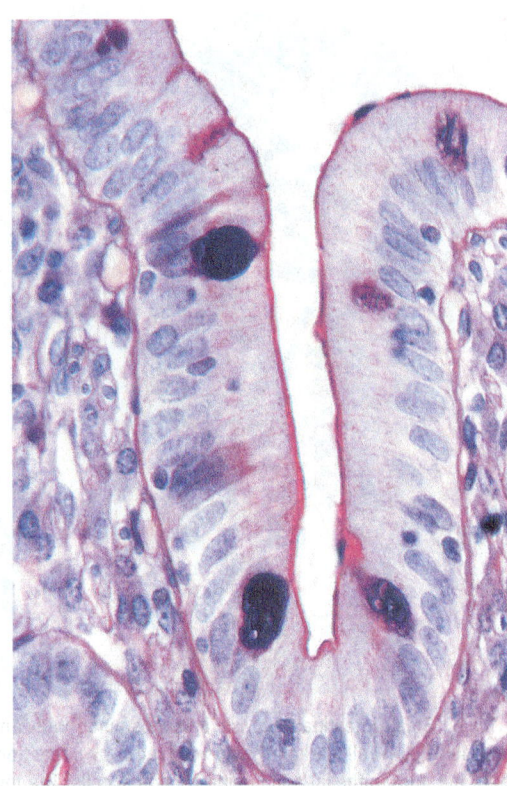

FIGURE 23.8 Alcian blue/PAS combination stain showing characteristic blue-purple apical mucin droplet of intestinal goblet cells. The heterogeneous composition (neutral and acid mucins) allows both stains to be incorporated into the droplet, imparting this distinctive color.

children with allergic enteropathy (i.e., cow's milk allergy) (28). In addition, fewer goblet ells and decreased mucus production as has been documented in premature infants may produce a poorly developed mucus secretion system, and, therefore, a decreased ability to secrete mucus as a response to infection resulting in serious diseases like necrotizing enterocolitis (30).

Interspersed among the absorptive cells are goblet cells, which have a characteristic apical mucin droplet and an attenuated, basally situated, bland nucleus (Fig. 23.5). They contain both neutral and acid mucins and function as secretory cells, sustaining a moist viscid environment within the lumen (27). Further examination of goblet cell function has revealed a possible gate-keeping role with antigen presentation via endocytosis at the rim of the goblet cell theca resulting in controlled secretion and an immunomodulatory response (30). In a combined Alcian blue/PAS stain, the droplets usually appear blue-purple (Fig. 23.8). The acid mucins of the small intestine are primarily sialomucins, in contrast to the colonic goblet cell, which contains predominantly acid sulfomucins (32,33). The number of goblet cells increases with distal progression along the small bowel constituting 4%, 6%, and 12% in the duodenum, jejunum, and ileum, respectively (27,29). Scattered endocrine cells are present within the villous epithelium, but they are more abundant within the crypts.

Intraepithelial lymphocytes are scattered among and lie between individual epithelial cells, usually just above the basement membrane; normally there is about one lymphocyte for every four or five epithelial cells in the proximal small intestine (Fig. 23.5) (34–36). Intraepithelial lymphocytes are CD3-positive T cells (Fig. 23.9), and most express CD8 (37–39). Approximately 5% to 30% bear a $\gamma\delta$ T-cell receptor and are either CD4-negative/CD8-negative or are CD8-positive (40). CD4-negative/CD8-negative intraepithelial lymphocytes are more common in the ileal mucosa (40) where intraepithelial lymphocyte counts are far less (less than 5 per 100 enterocytes) (41). $\gamma\delta$ T cells act as mediators of host-microbial homeostasis by stimulating goblet cell function and regulating mucin expression and glycosylation (42). An increase in the number of intraepithelial lymphocytes is characteristic of several disorders, including gluten-sensitive enteropathy (celiac sprue), tropical sprue, giardiasis, lymphocytic colitis, and collagenous colitis (41–44).

> **CRYPT EPITHELIUM** The crypt epithelium primarily functions in epithelial cell renewal (27); and as a consequence of this regenerative function, mitoses are seen frequently within the crypts (normal range: 1 to 12 mitoses/crypt) (45). The crypt also contains goblet cells and columnar cells, some of which are undifferentiated or stem cells (46). The four major epithelial cell types of the mucosa

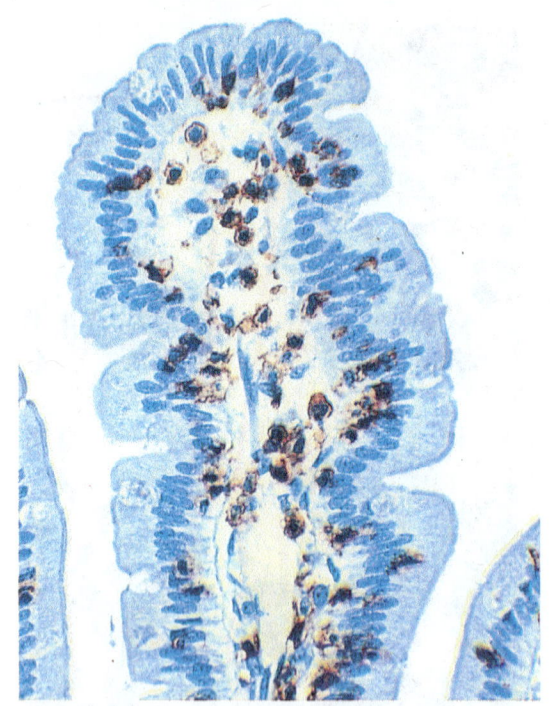

FIGURE 23.9 Small intestinal mucosa immunostained with antibody UCHL1 (CD45RO), a T-cell marker. The positive red-brown reaction highlights both the intraepithelial and lamina propria T cells. The intraepithelial cells are predominantly CD8 positive, whereas most T cells in the lamina propria are CD4 positive.

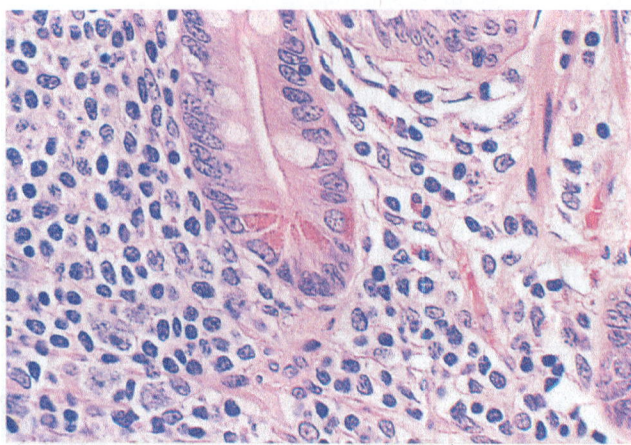

FIGURE 23.10 A single crypt surrounded by normal cellular lamina propria with abundant migratory cells. Both absorptive columnar and goblet cells are seen lining the crypt. In addition, an endocrine cell (infranuclear eosinophilic granules) and several Paneth cells (supranuclear granules) are clearly evident.

At least 16 distinct types of endocrine cells have been described along the gut (53,56) and each has a characteristic regional distribution and composition. Individual cells containing cholecystokinin, secretin, gastric inhibitory polypeptide, and motilin populate more proximal segments of the small bowel, whereas enteroglucagon-, substance P–,

(absorptive, goblet, endocrine, and Paneth cells) arise from this stem cell. Differentiation and maturation occur in about 4 to 6 days as the cells migrate from the crypt depths to the villous tips, where they are subsequently sloughed into the lumen presumably through apoptosis (46–50); however, the Paneth cell remains within the crypt base (44,48). Complex molecular pathways, especially Wnt signaling, play key roles in this proliferation and differentiation (51).

Endocrine cells are relatively abundant in the crypts, occurring as single cells or in discontinuous groupings along the intestinal tract (17). They are of two morphologic types. The "open" type have a pyramidal shape that tapers toward the glandular lumen with which they communicate, whereas "closed" cells are spindle shaped and have no luminal connection (17). The former are the most frequent type found in the small bowel. Some endocrine cells disclose eosinophilic basal (infranuclear) granules on hematoxylin and eosin (H&E) staining so that they are easily identified on routine preparations (Fig. 23.10); however, not all enteroendocrine cells have such a quality. Identification is more readily accomplished using immunohistology for nonspecific markers of endocrine cells (e.g., chromogranin and synaptophysin) (Fig. 23.11) or by precise identification of specific endocrine chemical content (52–54). Specific hormonal content immunostaining may have diagnostic value in studying neuroendocrine tumors (55). Electron microscopy also can be used to identify cytoplasmic neurosecretory granules but is rarely used clinically.

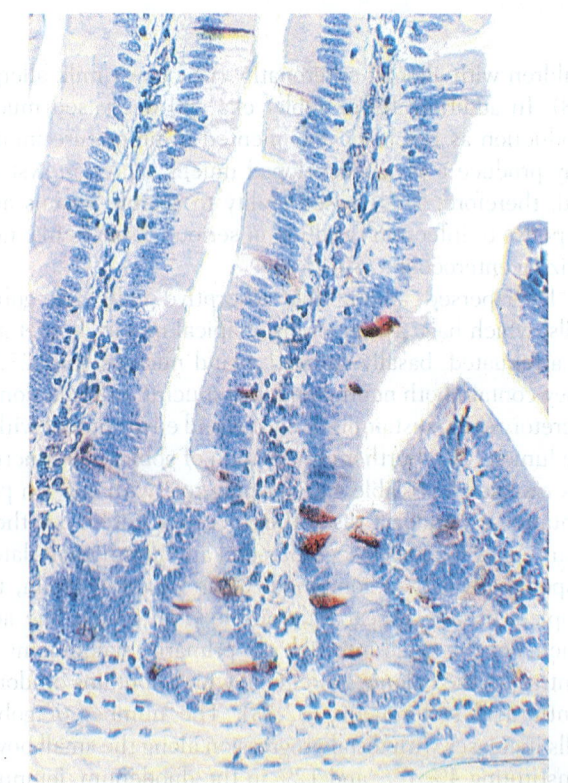

FIGURE 23.11 Immunostain for chromogranin shows numerous endocrine cells within the crypts and several scattered along the villous surface.

and neurotensin-storing cells are seen in greater frequency in the ileum. Serotonin- and somatostatin-containing cells are not so regionalized and are found throughout the gastrointestinal tract (54). Some of these endocrine cells are known to play key roles in daily gastrointestinal activity. For example, secretin and cholecystokinin are released in response to various foodstuffs and modulate pancreatic secretion and gallbladder function, respectively. Most other gut endocrine cells are still of uncertain or unknown physiologic significance (56).

Paneth cells, normally found only in the crypt, comprise most of the base of individual crypts throughout the entire small intestine (57). They are also encountered to a lesser degree in the appendix, cecum, and ascending colon (58). Paneth cells have a pyramidal shape with their apices pointing toward the lumen. Their cytoplasm contains characteristic supranuclear, intensely eosinophilic granules that are easily visualized in H&E-stained sections (Fig. 23.10). Interestingly, fixatives containing picric acid (e.g., Hollande, Bouin) mask the eosinophilic staining of these granules, often disclosing only unstained cytoplasmic vacuoles (Fig. 23.12) (57). Their round nuclei often contain a prominent nucleolus. These cells contain lysozyme, defensins, and immunoglobulins and appear capable of phagocytosis. Paneth cell alpha-defensin HD-5 is active against bacteria and can be localized to the cell with immunohistochemistry and in situ hybridization (Fig. 23.13) (59,60). Their cellular content and location suggest that they may function as a protector of the stem cell and help regulate intestinal microbials (59,60).

The crypt epithelium also contains intraepithelial lymphocytes that are predominantly CD8-positive T cells (61). Other inflammatory cell types, such as the neutrophil or the

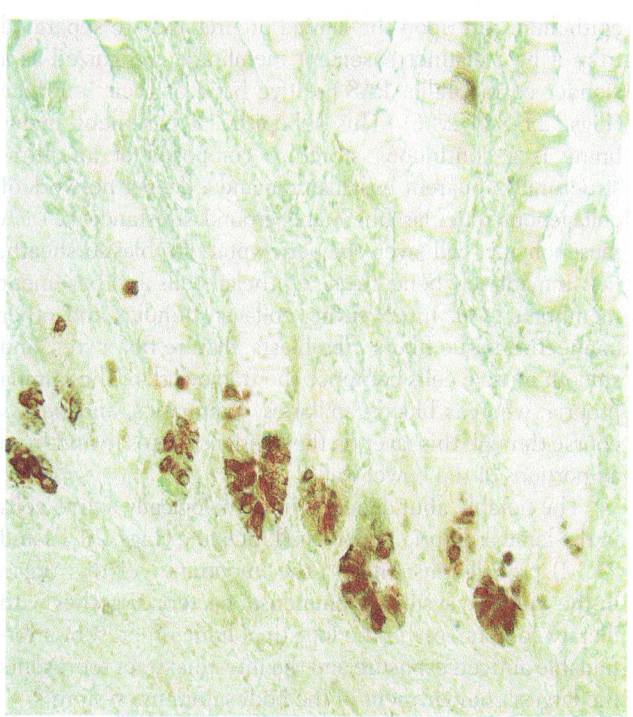

FIGURE 23.13 Immunostain for defensin HD5 highlights Paneth cells at the base of the crypts.

plasma cell, are not normally present within either the crypt or villous epithelial compartments; their presence would indicate a pathologic state (43).

> ***IMMUNOSTAINING PATTERNS OF THE EPITHELIUM*** Carcinoembryonic antigen (CEA) and CD10 are present on the apical surfaces of cells covering the villi and lining the crypts, and have been shown to localize to the glycocalyx surface component (62,63). In addition, the mucin droplets of goblet cells contain an abundance of CEA and consequently mark intensely with polyclonal anti-CEA. However, no intracytoplasmic immunostaining for CEA is evident in the normal small bowel (62). CEA and CD10 immunohistochemistry can be used to demonstrate pathologic conditions such as the microvillus inclusion disease (63,64).

Human leukocyte antigen (HLA)-DR–like antigens have been shown to be present in a scattered, focal distribution on the apices of small intestinal columnar-shaped cells (65). Immunostaining with anti–HLA-DR discloses a diminishing intensity of reactivity from the villous surfaces to the crypt bases. Immune-related cells such as lymphocytes (mostly B cells) and macrophages along with the walls of capillaries in the lamina propria also show immunoreactivity for HLA-DR (65).

> ***LAMINA PROPRIA*** The lamina propria, the intermediate layer of the mucosa, functions both structurally and immunologically. It rests upon the muscularis mucosae, surrounds the crypts, and extends upward as the cores of the intestinal villi. The crypt epithelium and the villous

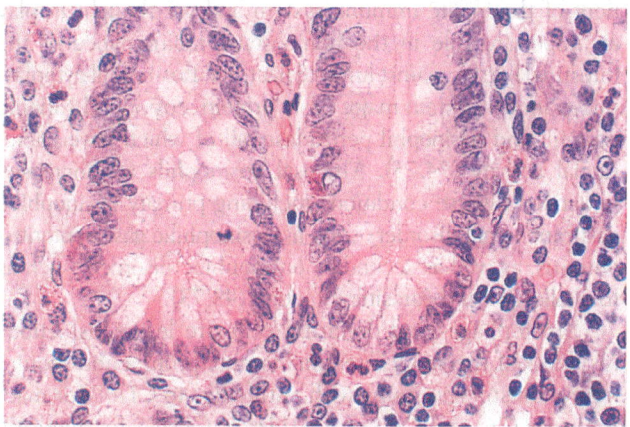

FIGURE 23.12 Although Hollande and other picric acid–containing fixatives are superior preservers of cytomorphologic detail, the characteristic supranuclear eosinophilic granules of Paneth cells are not as easily visualized when compared with the appearance in 4% formaldehyde solution (see Fig. 23.10). Clear vacuoles replace the distinct eosinophilic granules within Paneth cells (along the crypt bases). Note that the single endocrine cell in this crypt maintains its infranuclear granular staining quality.

epithelium rest upon the lamina propria and are separated from it by a distinct basement membrane recognized as a slender eosinophilic, PAS-positive band at their interface (Figs. 23.4 to 23.6). This subepithelial basement membrane is a continuous structure composed of an ultrastructurally apparent basal lamina and a deeper network of collagenous/reticular fibers and ground substance (24). A mesenchymal cell layer, the pericryptal fibroblastic sheath, lies immediately beneath the epithelial cells and basement membrane (66). Interweaving collagen bundles and other connective tissue fibers, fibroblasts, mature fibrocytes, and smooth muscle cells comprise the framework of the lamina propria, whereas blood capillaries, lymphatics, and nerves course through this layer on their various routes to and from all portions of the bowel wall.

The notable abundance of immunologically active cells in the lamina propria of the small intestine (Figs. 23.10 and 23.12) provides insight into the importance of this organ in the immune system. Commensal bacteria together with dietary components in the intestinal lumen represent a formidable antigen exposure and the intestinal tract represents the largest compartment of the body's immune system.

In simplified terms, the intestinal immune system can be divided into dispersed and organized components. The dispersed elements include the immunocompetent and inflammatory cells within the lamina propria, as well as intraepithelial lymphocytes seen throughout the small intestine. Organized intestinal lymphoid tissue includes Peyer patches and isolated lymphoid follicles. From an immunologic perspective, organized lymphoid tissue in the small intestine is primarily the site of induction of B- and T-cell responses, whereas the dispersed lymphoid tissue within the lamina propria mostly has an effector function.

The lamina propria of the small intestine contains numerous plasma cells, lymphocytes, and eosinophils, as well as a smaller number of macrophages/histiocytes, dendritic cells, and mast cells. Plasma cells are the most abundant cellular constituents of the lamina propria and most contain cytoplasmic IgA (Fig. 23.14). The jejunum is estimated to harbor more than 2.5×10^{10} IgA-secreting plasma cells, more plasma cells than those contained in the bone marrow, lymph nodes, and spleen combined (67). Intraluminal secretion of IgA requires active participation by intestinal surface epithelial cells. Polymeric IgA first binds to receptors on the epithelial basolateral membrane where it undergoes receptor-mediated endocytosis. Following directed transport across the cytoplasm, luminal secretion occurs following fusion of the vesicles with the luminal membrane. IgM is secreted into the intestinal lumen in a similar manner. In contrast to nonmucosal sites, IgG-expressing plasma cells are infrequent in the intestine (68,69).

The lymphoid population of the lamina propria consists mostly of CD3-positive/CD4-positive T cells (Fig. 23.9) (37,67,70). This population includes Th2 cells that release B-cell growth factor supporting the production of IgA, and Treg cells that can counteract inflammatory responses (71,72).

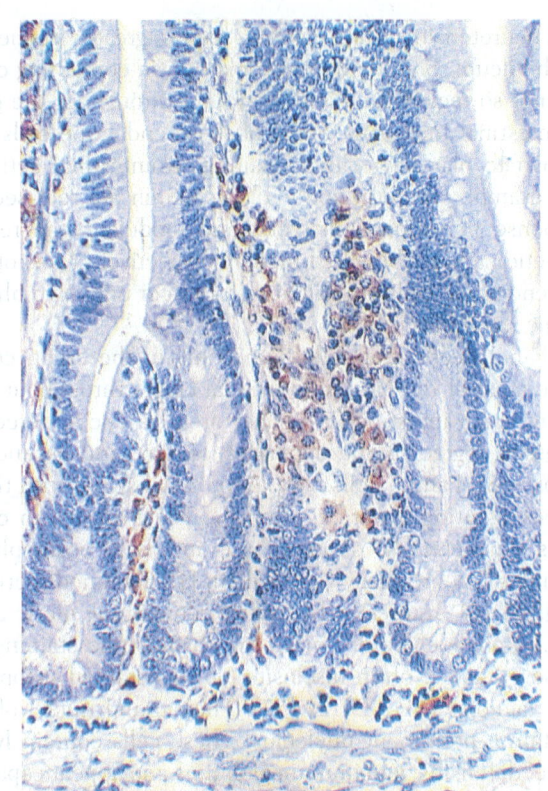

FIGURE 23.14 Numerous IgA-containing plasma cells (red-brown cytoplasmic staining) within the lamina propria of normal small intestine, immunostained for α-heavy chain. Note that, in contrast to T cells (see Fig. 23.9), the plasma cells localize to the lamina propria and are not normally found in the epithelium.

Eosinophils, are generated in the bone marrow, primarily home to mucosal sites, the principal target being gastrointestinal lamina propria are found in significant numbers even in healthy individuals (73). Eosinophils are an essential component of the innate immune system and are thought to play an important role in the homeostatic maintenance of the intestinal barrier against luminal bacteria. Eosinophil cytoplasmic granules contain major basic protein, eosinophil cationic protein, and eosinophil peroxidase, all of which have bactericidal activity (74,75). Mucosal eosinophils are increased in various disease conditions including primary eosinophilic gastrointestinal disorders such as eosinophilic gastroenteritis/enteritis, as well as secondary eosinophilic disorders such as food allergies and parasitic infection (43,73).

Macrophages and dendritic cells are less conspicuous residents of the small intestinal lamina propria and require immunohistologic stains with antibodies to CD68 for macrophages (76) and CD11b, CD11c, or CD209 for dendritic cells (77,78) for their visualization. In addition to the phagocytic and bactericidal activities of macrophages, these cells are regulators of mucosal immunity, playing an important role in antigen presentation to T cells (79). Dendritic cells may also play an active role in the extrathymic generation of Treg cells in the intestinal tract (80). In the small intestine, macrophages are mostly located in the lamina propria just below the surface epithelium, often concentrated near the tips of the villi (38,81). In contrast to blood monocytes, intestinal macrophages appear to be maintained in a state of only partial activation and fail to produce the levels of pro-inflammatory cytokines and reactive oxygen and nitrogen intermediates characteristic of conventional macrophages and monocytes. This state of refractoriness may be critical for mucosal homeostasis, in which macrophages function in the uptake and killing of microbes without initiating a potentially injurious inflammatory cascade. A dramatic expression of the phagocytic capacity of macrophages in the small intestine can be seen in cases of disseminated *Mycobacterium avium–intracellulare* complex infection and in the Whipple disease, where the lamina propria becomes filled with engorged macrophages (43,82,83).

Mast cells are also relatively inconspicuous in sections of the small intestine when viewed in routine H&E-stained sections. However, with histochemical stains such as toluidine blue or giemsa, or with immunohistologic stains using antibodies to c-kit (CD117) or mast cell tryptase, lamina propria mast cells are readily seen. That said, estimates of normal mucosal mast cell counts vary widely in the literature. In the duodenum, mast cells in healthy individuals can average over 50 per high-magnification field (84). Mast cells have surface receptors for IgE and can participate in hypersensitivity reactions. Cytoplasmic granules of mast cells contain histamine and serotonin, which together with other factors from eosinophils can lead to both nerve stimulation and smooth muscle contraction. Activated mast cells also release various cytokines, leukotrienes, and prostaglandins. Given their potent armament, activation of gastrointestinal mast cells, for example, in the setting of protein allergy, can have local effects including abdominal pain, diarrhea, and vomiting, as well as distant effects including cutaneous hypersensitivity reactions (hives) or asthma. A potential role for mast cells in the pathogenesis of irritable bowel syndrome may be related to their proximity to enteric nerve fibers (73).

Rarely, subepithelial (lamina propria) endocrine cells may be found in the small bowel; however, these are much more prominent in the vermiform appendix (85). Occasionally, in apparently healthy individuals and in certain disease states (e.g., Crohn disease), ganglion cells are found in the lamina propria of the small bowel. These could potentially be confused with cytomegalovirus infection–induced cellular changes.

> **MUSCULARIS MUCOSAE** The muscularis mucosae, which is the outermost layer or limit of the mucosa, is a slender band of tissue composed of elastic fibers and smooth muscle arranged in an outer longitudinal and an inner circular layer (Fig. 23.15). However, these layers are usually not well delineated on routine light microscopy. As stated above, absent or weak immunostaining for smoothelin is characteristic of this layer (26). Tufts of smooth muscle radiate from the muscularis mucosae into the lamina propria and extend

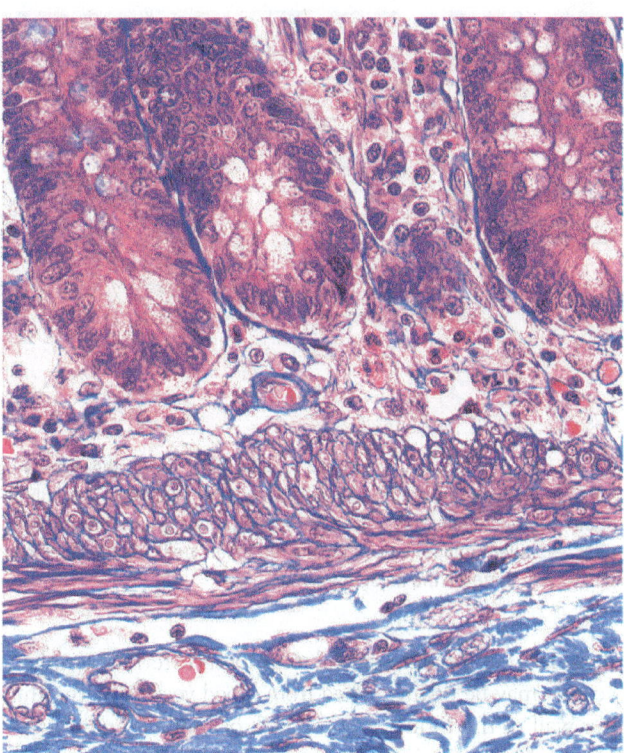

FIGURE 23.15 High-magnification photomicrograph disclosing inner circular and outer longitudinal smooth muscle bands of the muscularis mucosae; this layering is often inconspicuous on hematoxylin and eosin preparations, where the muscularis mucosae appears as a thin eosinophilic strip between the lamina propria and underlying submucosa (Masson trichrome).

into the villi. The muscularis mucosae provides an important structural foundation for the mucosa, and its absence in some biopsy specimens can cause a loss of villous orientation, an artifact that may interfere with optimal evaluation (86). The muscularis mucosae may not be distinct in all places, especially in the duodenum in areas of Brunner glands and adjacent to mucosal lymphoid aggregates.

Submucosa

Between the muscularis mucosae and muscularis externa is the submucosa, a loose, paucicellular layer composed of a regular, honeycomb-like arrangement (at the ultrastructural level) of collagenous and elastic fibers and related fibroblasts. The submucosa also may contain scattered, rather inconspicuous migratory cells (e.g., histiocytes, lymphoid and plasma cells, and mast cells) and adipose tissue. Its histologic appearance and principal role in maintaining the structural integrity of the small bowel are similar throughout the gastrointestinal tract (87). The submucosa is a major focus of vascular routing and related distribution of regional blood and lymphatic flow. Relatively large caliber arterioles, venules, and lymphatic vessels form extensive individual plexuses and networks within this layer (Fig. 23.16). From this "vascular center," numerous penetrating capillary vessels supply and

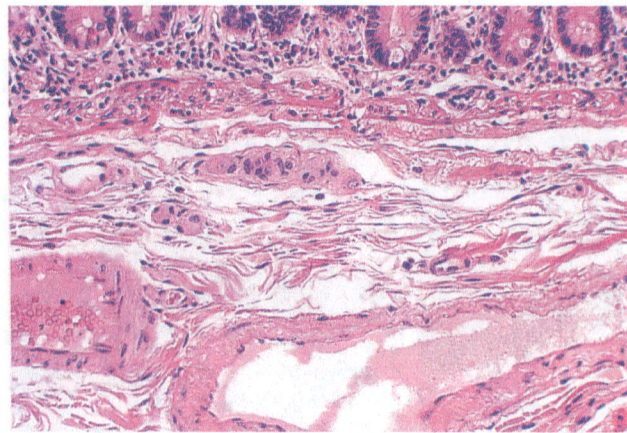

FIGURE 23.16 Normal submucosa separated from the overlying mucosa by the eosinophilic-staining muscularis mucosae. The submucosa is paucicellular, disclosing fibrocollagenous tissue and a prominent vascular component. Note the ganglion cells of the Meissner plexus just beneath the muscularis mucosae.

drain most of the mucosa and muscularis externa. Lymphatic vessels may be distinguished from blood vessels by the thinner wall of the former and the lack of luminal erythrocytes. However, certain immunohistologic patterns and electron microscopic characteristics are more helpful for definitive identification (25,88,89). Specifically, the endothelial cells of blood capillaries immunostain for PAL-E and factor VIII–related antigen, whereas lymphatic capillary endothelia typically lack these antigenic sites and remain unstained with such antibody preparations (88,89). In addition, blood capillaries as seen by ultrastructural analysis have a continuous basal lamina, endothelial fenestrations, and ensheathing pericytes. However, lymphatic capillaries have a discontinuous basal lamina and lack both fenestrations and surrounding pericytes (24,25). Although small lymphatic vessels are a conspicuous submucosal component, prominent dilated lymphatic structures in this layer, as well as in the mucosa, can be seen in pathologic states such as intestinal lymphangiectasia or Crohn disease (43,90).

Neural structures are also prominent in the submucosa. The submucosal Meissner plexus forms one of the two major integrative centers of the enteric nervous system. It consists of a network of ganglia that interconnect through neural processes (91). The ganglia contain compact aggregates of neurons (ganglion cells) routinely identified on H&E preparations by their characteristic large oval shape, abundant pink cytoplasm, vesicular nucleus, and single prominent, often eosinophilic nucleolus (Fig. 23.16). Abundant S100-positive Schwann cells, gliallike cells, and neural processes are also present in the Meissner plexus. The entire plexus, including the ganglia, contains no connective tissue elements or vascular structures in the normal state (91–93). The plexus is also normally devoid of inflammatory cells; therefore, if these are seen, an injury pattern specific to the neural plexus (such as an inflammatory neuropathy) should be considered, as long as primary inflammatory bowel disease can be excluded (92). Neural interconnections exist between the Meissner plexus and the myenteric plexus of Auerbach (discussed below), as well as with extrinsic (autonomic) neural processes.

Muscularis Externa

The muscularis externa (or muscularis propria) is the thick outer smooth muscle layer that surrounds the submucosa. It is covered externally by subserosal connective tissue and, in most places, by a serosa. Its two distinct muscular layers, oriented perpendicular to each other, are arranged as an outer longitudinally running muscle fiber layer and an inner circular muscle band (Fig. 23.17) and stain prominently with immunostains such as smooth muscle actin and smoothelin (26). Blood vessels, lymphatics, and nerves course through the muscularis externa and slender collagenous septa surround groups of smooth muscle cells, creating characteristic bundles and packets of muscle (Fig. 23.17). However, fibrous tissue in this layer is minimal in the normal small bowel (89) so even slight fibrous alterations or collagen deposition may be significant. Moreover, the fact that only a few disease entities (including ischemia, irradiation, familial visceral myopathy, scleroderma, and mycobacterial infection) are associated with fibrosis of the muscularis propria aids in narrowing a broad differential diagnosis (43).

The myenteric plexus of Auerbach, the other major neural plexus of the enteric nervous system, lies between the outer longitudinal and inner circular muscle layers (Figs. 23.17 to 23.19). The Auerbach plexus is similar in composition to the submucosal plexus, although it typically has larger ganglia, a greater number of neurons, and a more compact plexus network (92). As a consequence of these features,

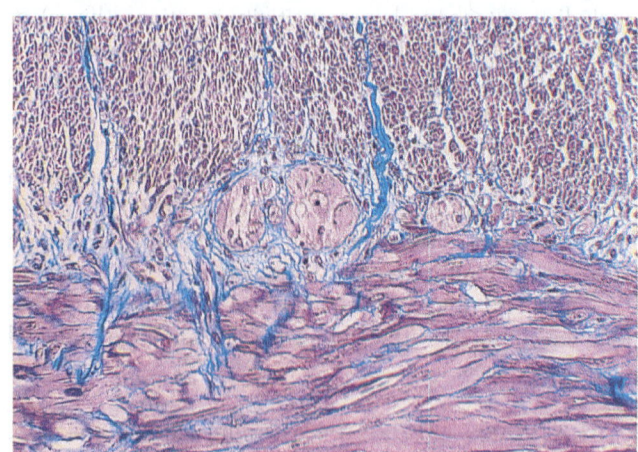

FIGURE 23.17 The Masson trichrome stain clearly delineates the inner circular (*above*) from the outer longitudinal (*below*) smooth muscle bands of the muscularis externa. The prominent muscular component (*red*) is partitioned into bundles of varying size by delicate collagenous fibers (*blue*). Note the ganglia of the myenteric plexus of Auerbach, characteristically located between the two muscle bands. Fibrous tissue is minimal within the muscularis externa and is also not normally part of the plexus.

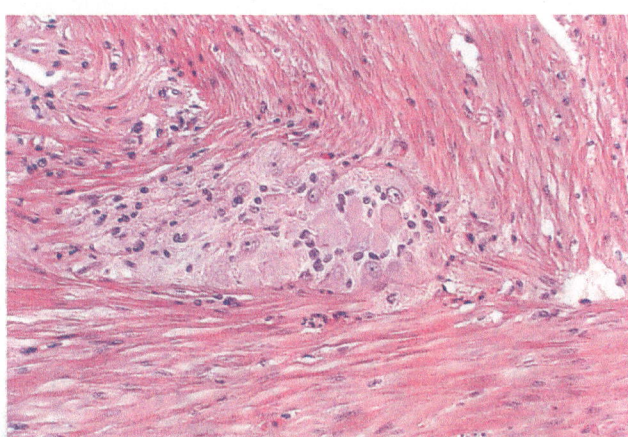

FIGURE 23.18 A single ganglion of the myenteric plexus of Auerbach located at the interface of the inner (*above*) and outer (*below*) smooth muscle layers of the muscularis externa. Ganglion cells (neuronal cell bodies) are evident and characterized by a polygonal shape, abundant pink cytoplasm, and an eccentric nucleus; spindled neural projections and Schwann cells are also intermixed.

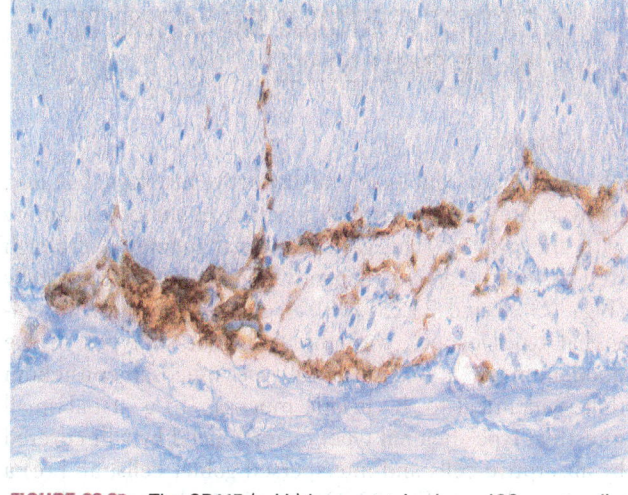

FIGURE 23.20 The CD117 (c-kit) immunostain shows ICC surrounding the myenteric plexus of Auerbach.

it is best to evaluate the myenteric plexus for specific disease processes involving the enteric nervous system, such as the various visceral neuropathies. Since routine processing allows only a small portion of the plexus to be visualized and because many of these conditions cause no detectable changes on routine H&E-stained sections, special preparations of thicker, larger, and silver-stained sections cut en face are currently necessary to diagnose many of these disorders (92). Finally, although of lesser importance, a deep muscular, subserous plexus and several mucosal plexuses are also present within the small bowel (94). Interstitial cells of Cajal (ICC) form a meshwork around the Auerbach plexus and in septa between circular muscle lamellae (Fig. 23.20). These "pacemaker cells" require special staining (e.g., CD117 and CD34 immunostaining) for visualization and play an essential role in intestinal motility (95–97).

Serosa and Subserosal Region

The serosa is the covering that envelops most of the external surface of the small bowel. Its outermost layer consists of a single row of cuboidal mesothelial cells, under which lies a thin band of loose connective tissue. A subserosal zone of connective tissue lying between this mesothelial covering and the muscularis externa also contains ramifying branches of blood vessels, lymphatics, and nerves (Fig. 23.21).

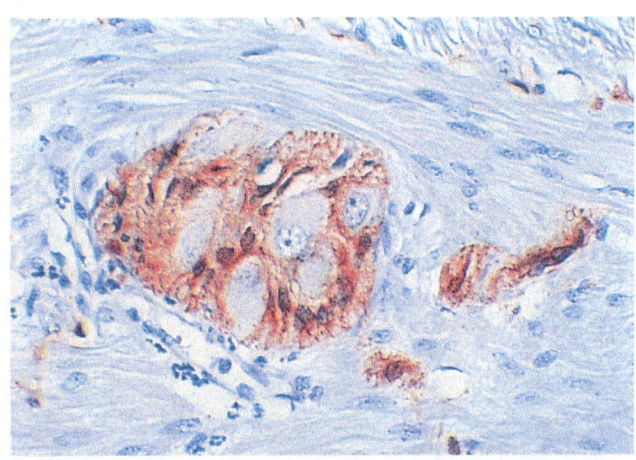

FIGURE 23.19 This S-100 immunostain highlights the otherwise inconspicuous spindled Schwann cell component of the ganglion. It also marks the Schwann cells accompanying the neural projections that interconnect these ganglia to one another within the plexus system. Note that the ganglion cells show no such immunoreactivity.

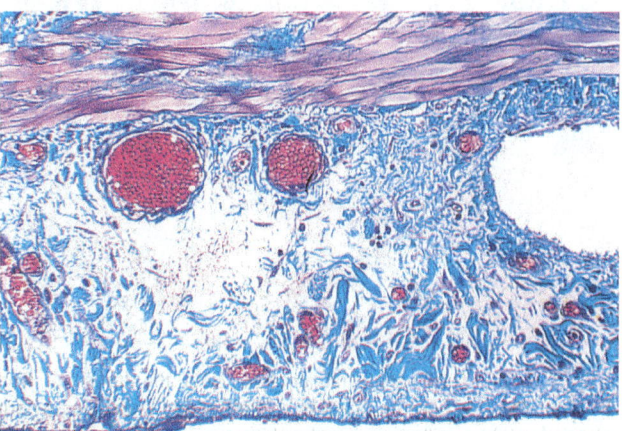

FIGURE 23.21 The subserosal region contains a delicate fibrocollagenous network, blood vessels, lymphatics, and nerves. The serosa consists of a thin fibrous layer (*blue* and *bottom*) covered by a single layer of mesothelial cells; however, the mesothelium is often denuded in surgical specimens. A portion of the outer layer of the muscularis externa is also present in this field (*top*) (Masson trichrome).

DISTINCTIVE REGIONAL CHARACTERISTICS OF THE SMALL BOWEL

Duodenum

The duodenum exhibits several distinctive histologic features, many related to its proximal location in direct continuity with the pylorus. The gastroduodenal junction, although well delineated grossly, is poorly demarcated histologically (Figs. 23.22 and 23.23) (98). A gradual transition in epithelial types occurs, with three distinct subtypes in the duodenum (99): (a) an antral-type mucosal epithelium that is identical to the pyloric mucosa; (b) a "usual small intestinal type" (jejunal type) characterized by villi covered by absorptive cells and interspersed goblet cells; and (c) a transitional type (Fig. 23.23), in which the same villus is covered by epithelium having features of both antral-type and usual small intestinal-type epithelia. In the region of the gastroduodenal junction, irregular undulating slips of antral-type mucosa extend about 1 to 2 mm into the anatomic duodenum, which then abuts a 2- to 3-mm segment of transitional-type epithelium (99). Distal to this, only the usual small intestinal–type mucosa is found (99). The transitional-type epithelium occurring in more distal aspects of the duodenum and in the rest of the small intestine is termed gastric metaplasia (43).

Although the duodenal mucosa may demonstrate long villi with a villous-to-crypt length ratio on the order of 3:1 to 5:1, more commonly, particularly in the first portion (the duodenal cap or bulb), the villi are shorter and broader with occasional branching extensions (Fig. 23.24) (100). They often have a leaflike shape with few fingerlike forms when

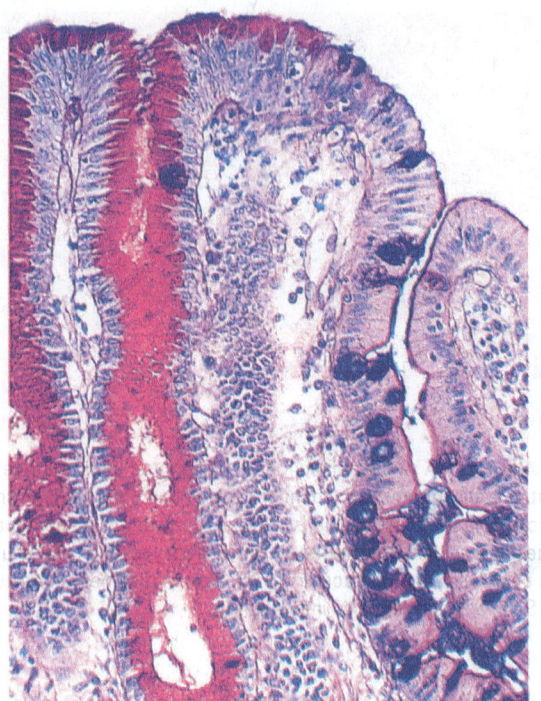

FIGURE 23.23 Several villi within the confines of the gastroduodenal junction disclosing both "usual small intestinal-type" epithelium and antral-type, PAS-positive, foveolar epithelium. This transitional-type epithelium is a characteristic hybrid found in this region. At more distal small intestinal sites, this transitional-type epithelium is termed gastric metaplasia (Alcian blue/PAS).

viewed under a scanning electron or dissecting microscope (Fig. 23.25) (27,100,101). Also, the number of mononuclear cells within the lamina propria is increased in the duodenum when compared with the rest of the proximal

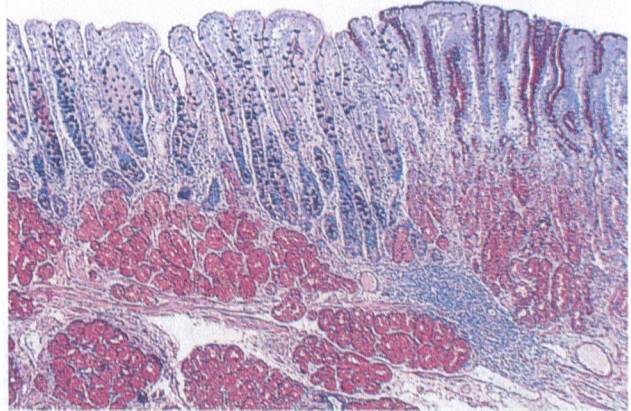

FIGURE 23.22 Gastroduodenal junction. Note the transition from PAS-positive (*red*) gastric foveolar epithelium and underlying pyloric glands (*right*) to a villous mucosal architecture of the duodenum (*left*) lined predominantly by Alcian blue/PAS-positive (*blue-purple*) goblet cells and absorptive cells. Note that both pyloric (*right*) and Brunner glands (*left*) are composed predominantly of cells containing only neutral, PAS-positive mucin. Brunner glands, however, are predominantly submucosal in location, while pyloric glands are an intramucosal structure (Alcian blue/PAS).

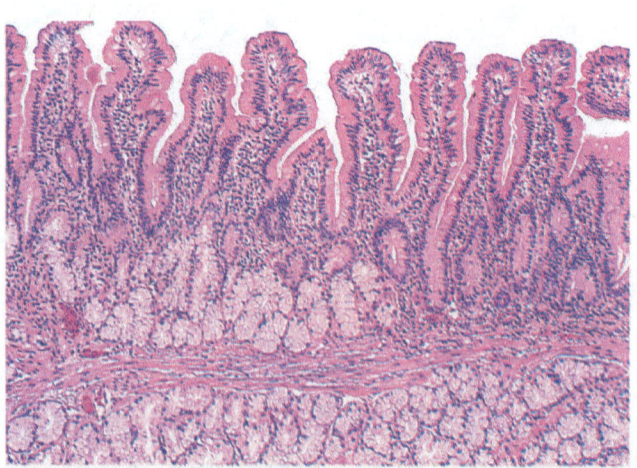

FIGURE 23.24 Short, slightly broader villi predominate in the duodenum. The underlying submucosal Brunner glands are a distinctive feature of this portion of the small bowel. Note that a fair portion of Brunner glands normally occurs above the muscularis mucosae.

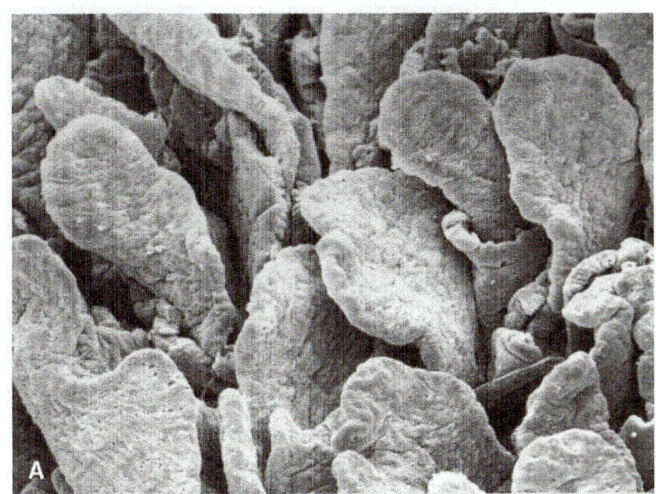
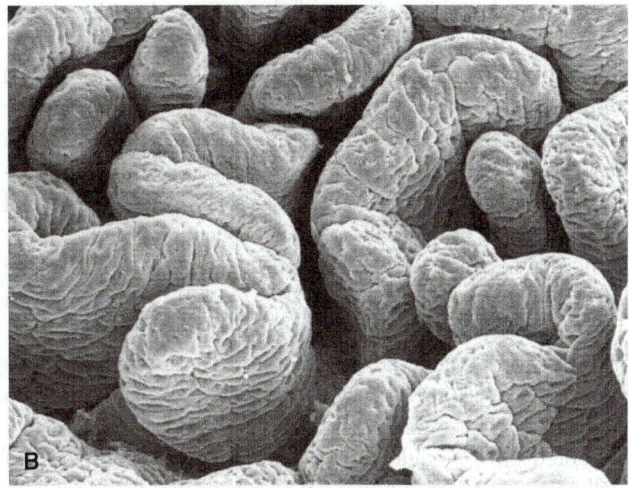

FIGURE 23.25 Two views of duodenal mucosa using scanning electron microscopy: Leaflike **(A)** and ridge-shaped **(B)** villi predominate in these normal duodenal specimens.

small intestine (100,101). This varied constellation of findings is considered normal and is probably a consequence of the effect of acidic gastric contents on this most proximal intestinal site (58,101).

The submucosa of the gastrointestinal tract lacks glands except at two sites: the esophagus and the duodenum. The submucosal Brunner glands are the type localized to the duodenum. Indeed, these glands are typically used by the pathologist to identify histologically a segment of small intestine as duodenum. Brunner glands, which begin just distal to the gastroduodenal junction, are most concentrated in this region and gradually decrease in quantity along the duodenum (102). Beyond the entrance of the ampulla of Vater, only scattered groups can be found. In rare instances, Brunner glands extend beyond the duodenojejunal flexure for a short distance (103–105).

Brunner glands are lobular collections of tubuloalveolar glands predominantly located within the submucosa; however, they often extend through the muscularis mucosae into the deep portions of mucosa beneath the crypts of Lieberkühn (Figs. 23.24 and 23.26). On average, about one-third of the gland population resides within the mucosa (103). Brunner glands are lined by cuboidal-to-columnar cells with pale, uniform cytoplasm and an oval, basally situated nucleus. Their cytoplasm contains neutral mucins that are PAS positive and diastase resistant (Fig. 23.22). Occasionally, mucus cells with apically concentrated mucin and perinuclear vacuolization or clearing are seen. Although opinions vary, these changes are thought to represent the secretory phase of the gland (i.e., recently fed state) (106,107). The glands empty by way of ducts lined by similar epithelium, which are often seen passing through slips of muscularis mucosae (Fig. 23.26). These ducts drain into the crypts at varying levels (105). Brunner glands and their ducts can be distinguished from surrounding crypts by the absence of goblet cells and by their diffuse cytoplasmic PAS positivity (105).

Although most of the lining epithelial cells of Brunner glands are of the mucus type, scattered endocrine cells and Paneth cells are present as well. Many can be detected on routine H&E-stained sections because of their eosinophilic granulated cytoplasm (108). By using immunohistologic methods, some have been shown to contain somatostatin, gastrin, and peptide YY (109). However, the ducts that drain Brunner glands are devoid of endocrine cells (109).

Peptidergic neural fibers, predominantly those with immunoreactivity for vasoactive intestinal peptide and substance P, course within and between individual Brunner glands. These neuroendocrine substances are probably important in local regulation of acinar secretion, although this function has been verified only for vasoactive intestinal peptide (109). The function of Brunner glands has not been fully elucidated, but their mucus is felt to be of prime importance for protection of the duodenal mucosa from the

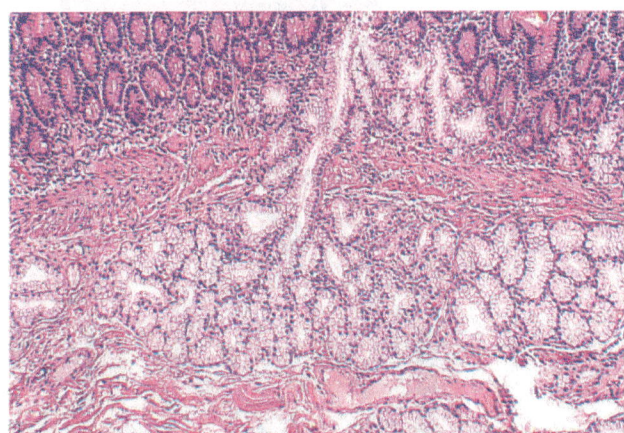

FIGURE 23.26 The submucosal Brunner gland lobule with draining duct extending through muscularis mucosae. Note the stark contrast between the crypt epithelium and that of Brunner glands and their ducts.

potentially damaging effects of the delivered acidic gastric contents (104).

Hyperplasia of Brunner glands exists in three forms: (a) diffuse glandular proliferation, imparting a coarse nodularity to most of the duodenum; (b) isolated discrete nodules in the proximal duodenum; and (c) a solitary nodule, often designated as an "adenoma" of Brunner glands (103,110,111). All the three types are typically composed of an increased quantity of normal-appearing Brunner glands, accompanied by variable proportions of smooth muscle (Fig. 23.27). The distinction between adenoma and hyperplasia is arbitrary, and no substantial evidence exists to suggest that any of these proliferations are truly neoplastic (110). Moreover, carcinoma arising from a population of Brunner glands has yet to be convincingly documented (43). Nodules or polypoid structures composed of collections of these submucosal glands in the duodenum are probably best termed Brunner gland nodules (43).

Pseudomelanosis duodeni, or brown-black pigment, located primarily within lamina propria macrophages, rarely may be observed in the proximal duodenum (Fig. 23.28) (112). Lipomelanin, ceroid, iron, sulfide, and hemosiderin have been identified in these deposits. Most reported patients were hypertensive and also suffered from upper gastrointestinal bleeding, chronic renal failure, or diabetes mellitus (112).

Jejunum

The jejunum is the least distinctive segment of the small bowel; and, as such, its histologic features are most similar to those described for the small bowel in general. However, a characteristic feature is the prominent development of the plicae circulares, or permanent circular folds, also termed valves of Kerckring and valvulae conniventes (Fig. 23.1). These folds are tallest and most numerous (i.e., closely

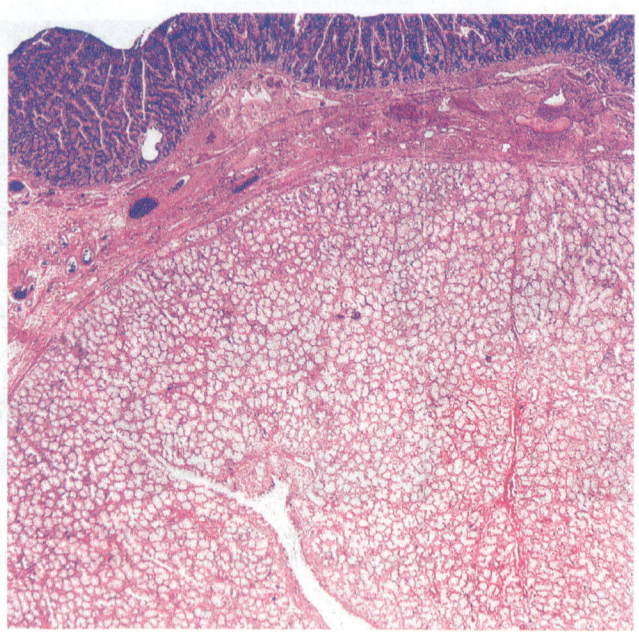

FIGURE 23.27 The Brunner gland nodule disclosing abundant normal-appearing submucosal Brunner glands intermixed with smooth muscle, underlying an unremarkable duodenal mucosal villous surface.

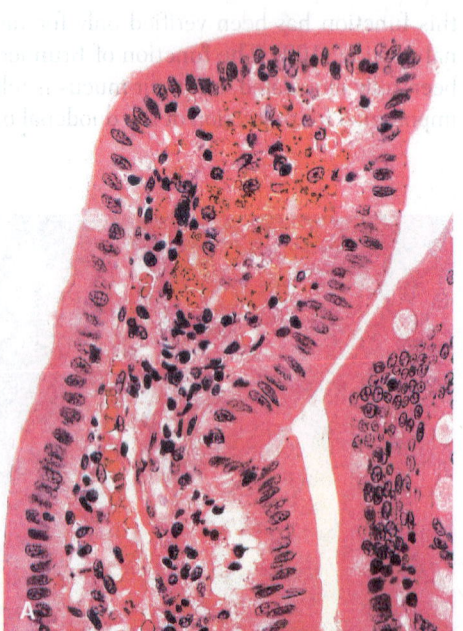 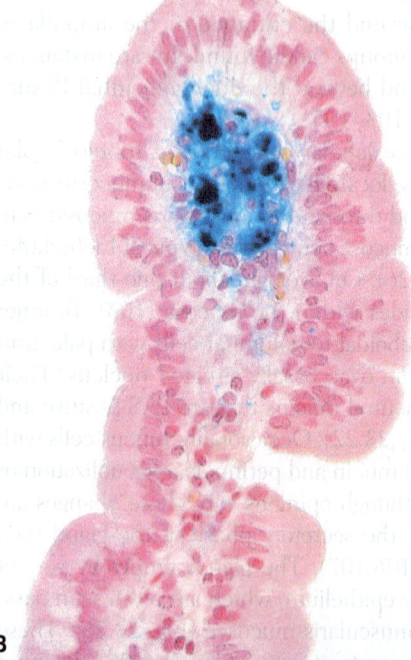

FIGURE 23.28 **A:** Macrophages containing granular brown-black pigment within the lamina propria of the duodenum, a characteristic of pseudomelanosis duodeni. **B:** Prussian blue stain disclosing the prominent iron content of the pigment.

spaced) in this portion of the small bowel (27). Histologically, the jejunal villi are tall with a villous-to-crypt ratio on the order of 3:1 to 5:1. Most jejunal villi are slender and fingerlike (Figs. 23.2 and 23.3), in contrast to the slightly shorter villi of the ileum and to the leaflike, occasionally branched and blunted villi of the proximal duodenum (27,57). These morphologic transitions are gradual, particularly in the mobile small intestine, where the separation between jejunum and ileum is arbitrarily defined.

Ileum

The ileum has a number of distinctive features, including its unique junction with the large intestine, a high concentration of lymphoid tissue, and deposits of pigment. The ileum protrudes approximately 2 to 3 cm into the large intestine at the junction of the cecum and ascending colon. This nipple-like extension of the terminal ileum is encircled by large bowel mucosa and has been likened to the relationship of the uterine cervix with the vagina (113). A muscular sphincter at this site, along with the external ligamentous support, is responsible for modifying its function in order to prevent reflux and to allow forward passage of ileal contents (113,114). Histologically, the mucosal transition demonstrates a gradual loss of villi occurring at variable lengths along the short intracecal ileal segment; the ileal mucosa blends rather with the mucosa of the large bowel (Fig. 23.29). The ileocecal region normally can contain abundant fat within its submucosa, diffusely distributed and proportional to adipose content in the rest of the abdominal cavity (Fig. 23.29) (115). In fact, on rare occasions, a distinct mass of fat is evident. This benign entity, the so-called lipohyperplasia of the ileocecal region, reportedly can cause variable symptoms, including abdominal pain and lower gastrointestinal bleeding (115).

The distinctive mucosal characteristics of the ileum, when compared with both jejunum and duodenum, include shorter and fewer plicae circulares and an increased proportion of goblet cells within the epithelium (Fig. 23.30).

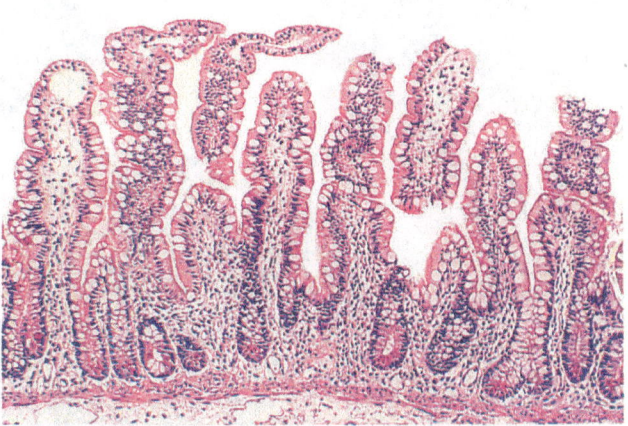

FIGURE 23.30 Characteristic ileal mucosa with slender, relatively short villi (compared with jejunal villi in Figure 23.3) lined by abundant goblet cells with a lesser number of absorptive columnar cells.

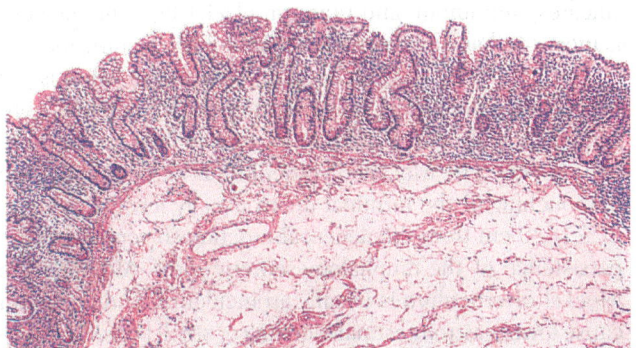

FIGURE 23.29 Transition from the villous mucosal surface of the ileum (*left*) to the flat mucosa of the large intestine (*right*) at the ileocecal junction. Note the prominent submucosal adipose tissue characteristic of this region.

The villi are typically shorter and show less serration than at more proximal sites and often have a predominantly fingerlike shape (27). The villi are less straight causing tangential cuts to appear even in normal samples (116). These features become gradually more apparent along the length of the small intestine and are most evident in the distal ileum.

The ileum contains prominent organized lymphoid tissue including Peyer patches and isolated lymphoid follicles (27). Peyer patches are distributed mostly along the antimesenteric border of the small intestine, with the greatest density in the terminal ileum. Peyer patches first emerge in humans at 19 weeks of gestation (117). Their number and size reach a maximum at puberty (117,118), after which they regress but persist throughout life in most individuals (119). Larger Peyer patches are grossly and endoscopically visible. The lymphoid tissue in Peyer patches can become hyperplastic and this florid lymphoid hyperplasia has been linked to more than one-third of childhood cases of idiopathic intussusception in the region of the ileocecal valve (120–122).

Peyer patches occupy the mucosa and a variable portion of the submucosa. The villi over these lymphoid aggregates are often poorly formed or absent. From an immunologic perspective, organized lymphoid tissue in the small intestine can be regarded as primarily sites of immune induction of B- and T-cell responses. Structurally and functionally the Peyer patch can be divided into four distinct compartments including the follicle, the subepithelial dome, the interfollicular zone, and the follicle-associated epithelium (123). Lymphoid follicles within Peyer patches can vary from as few as five to as many as several hundreds. Like their counterpart in lymph nodes, the follicles within Peyer patches contain a predominance of B cells together with follicular dendritic cells, and macrophages. Most follicles contain a germinal center with CD10-positive and BCL-2–negative B cells, where under the influence of CD4-positive T_h cells, dendritic cells, and macrophages, immunoglobulin class-switching occurs, resulting in the production of

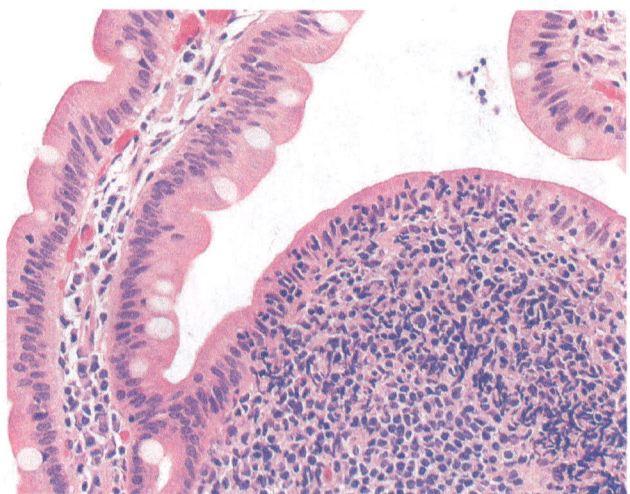

FIGURE 23.31 High magnification of surface epithelium above a lymphoid nodule within the Peyer patch. The polymorphous germinal center (*below*) is surrounded by monotonous, small, round lymphocytes that comprise the nodule's mantle zone. Above this lies the subepithelial dome region with lymphocytes, plasma cells, and macrophages. The follicle-associated epithelium characteristically has few, if any, goblet cells; ultrastructurally and phenotypically, most of these epithelial cells would be identified as M cells.

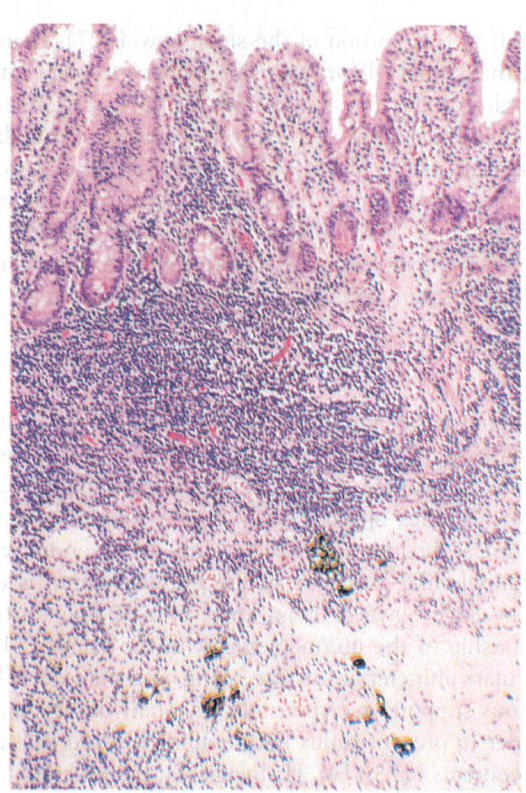

FIGURE 23.32 Dense brown-black granular pigment within the depths of the Peyer patch of the ileum. The pigment is typically confined to macrophages.

IgA-expressing B cells (124,125). The germinal center is surrounded by a mantle zone of small IgD-positive, IgM-positive B cells. The subepithelial dome, situated between the lymphoid follicle and the overlying follicle-associated surface epithelium, contains a heterogeneous population of cells including B cells, macrophages, dendritic cells, and plasma cells (Fig. 23.31) (119). The interfollicular zone, a T-cell–rich zone absent in isolated lymphoid follicles, is a site of interaction between antigen-loaded dendritic cells and T cells resulting in T-cell priming (126).

In contrast to lymph nodes that receive antigen via afferent lymphatics, luminal antigens from within the small intestine are transported to Peyer patches, as well as to isolated lymphoid follicles, via the follicle-associated epithelium. Specialized antigen-transporting epithelial cells called M (membrane or microfold) cells sample the intestinal lumen and transport antigens to the underlying lymphoid tissue for processing and initiation of immune responses (127–130). M cells have distinctive morphologic features including a poorly organized brush border, short, irregular villi, and a thinner glycocalyx compared to adjacent enterocytes (127). M cells also do not produce enzymes with digestive activity, and absence of alkaline phosphatase and sucrase-isomaltase, typical for absorptive enterocytes, therefore can be used as a negative marker for their identification (131). At their basolateral surface, M cells have a large intraepithelial invagination that contains B and T cells, as well as macrophages and dendritic cells (132). This architecture facilitates interaction between antigens derived from the intestinal lumen with cells of the adaptive immune system. On activation by antigen, M cells can recruit dendritic cells to the subepithelial dome (125). Dendritic cells play an important role in the uptake of antigens that have been transported across the follicle-associated epithelium. In addition to capturing soluble antigens, dendritic cells are also able to take up apoptotic epithelial cells (133).

Irregularly distributed deposits of granular brown-black pigment can commonly be found in the deep portions of Peyer patches in adults (Fig. 23.32) (134). Although its origin is controversial, atmospheric or dietary sources are most probable (134,135). Accumulating principally within macrophages, this pigment has been shown by x-ray spectroscopy to contain a distinct mineral composition that includes silicates, aluminum, and titanium (134,135). The pigment is inert and has no known clinicopathologic significance.

A final distinctive feature often seen in the ileum is the Meckel diverticulum; it is the most common intestinal congenital anomaly and is found in 1% to 2% of the general population (43). The Meckel diverticulum is an antimesenteric outpouching of the terminal ileum usually located approximately 20 cm from the ileocecal junction. It represents the persistence of the omphalomesenteric duct. Although the Meckel diverticulum is usually an incidental finding, it can cause lower gastrointestinal bleeding or small bowel obstruction (136,137). Histologically, small intestinal mucosa alone lines the diverticulum in about 50% to 70% of cases. Ectopic gastric or pancreatic tissues are found in the remainder, typically encountered at the distalmost aspect (137).

SPECIAL CONSIDERATIONS

Geographic, Age-Related, and Dietary Factors

Since geographic and local environmental factors can affect small bowel morphology, historical data about the residence or recent travel of an individual are essential to evaluate histologic material accurately. Specimens from individuals residing in, or visiting at length, certain less-developed tropical locations such as Africa, southern India, and Thailand show a distinctly different villous appearance from those of individuals who live in temperate climate zones (43,138–141). The morphologic alterations seen in individuals from such tropical areas include leaflike villi predominating over fingerlike forms in jejunal segments examined via biopsy and an increased number of lamina propria mononuclear cells (142). This difference in the villous population is reflected histologically as stubby villi with a pyramidal shape (i.e., a broader base than apex) and occasional branched and fused villous tips (138,139). Interestingly, although the villi are shorter, the villous-to-crypt length ratio usually remains constant in all geographic settings (139). Such alterations should probably be considered a normal variant because these individuals are typically asymptomatic and otherwise healthy (138). The cause of these morphologic changes is uncertain, but environmental factors, particularly regional enteric flora, presumably play a role (138). Similar mucosal changes are seen in normal individuals in temperate environments, but only in proximal portions of the duodenum. Therefore, these particular mucosal alterations must be analyzed in the context of both the patient's residence and the site within the small intestine in order to prevent misinterpretation as a pathologic change, such as tropical sprue.

Aging also modifies small bowel mucosal architecture. Although the literature on humans is limited, it has been shown that specimens from elderly individuals generally have shorter and broader villi than those from younger individuals (143). Moreover, lower animal and human fetuses have been documented as having fingerlike villi exclusively, suggesting that exposure to the environment or aging itself modifies villous architecture (143,144). However, the functional significance of these changes is uncertain (143).

Diet alters villous architecture in laboratory animals. A diet high in fiber results in broad and fused villi, whereas a fiber-free diet seems to prevent the formation of leaflike forms (24). If this finding is valid in humans, it may be one factor related to the presence of stubby, leaflike villi seen in patients in less-developed countries where high-fiber diets are common.

Metaplastic and Heterotopic Tissues

Gastric-type mucosa is not an unusual finding in the small intestine. A distinction can be made between metaplasia, an acquired alteration, and heterotopia, thought to be congenital in origin. Gastric metaplasia characteristically consists solely of antral-type, PAS-positive, foveolar columnar cells lying along the surface epithelium (Fig. 23.23). This change is focal and often in direct continuity with usual columnar absorptive epithelium on the same villus (101). Gastric metaplasia may be encountered in more than 60% of healthy asymptomatic individuals in the duodenal bulb, where it can be regarded as within normal limits (101). More distally, however, it is less commonly seen in the asymptomatic person but rather frequently is associated with duodenitis or mucosal ulceration (101,145). Scattered chief and parietal cells without any organized arrangement are also associated with this type of metaplasia or with reparative processes (145).

In contrast, gastric heterotopia is usually a grossly evident mucosal polyp that contains all cellular elements encountered in the normal gastric fundic mucosa. Characteristically, mucus foveolar epithelium overlies an organized arrangement of glands lined by chief and parietal cells; this is typically well-demarcated from the surrounding usual intestinal villous epithelium. Gastric heterotopia is also fairly common, being reported in up to 2% of the population (146); it may be found anywhere along the gastrointestinal tract (145). Gastric heterotopia is a well-defined entity in the proximal duodenum and usually presents as a mucosal nodule on the anterior wall. Although they are usually of no clinical significance, larger ones may cause obstructive symptoms (146). In contrast, gastric heterotopia distal to the ligament of Treitz is usually symptomatic and often causes intussusception (147). This relationship with clinical symptoms may derive from patient selection bias because asymptomatic gastric heterotopias at a distal site would not be routinely detectable.

Heterotopic pancreas tissue also can be found anywhere along the small intestine but most commonly is found in the duodenum and jejunum (148,149). It can form submucosal, intramural, or serosal nodules and is composed of various admixtures of pancreatic acini, ducts, and islets of Langerhans (Fig. 23.33). Isolated ductal structures admixed with smooth muscle may be the predominant or exclusive component, and in these instances the alternative term adenomyoma has been used (43,149). Nodules of pancreatic tissue within the small intestine are usually asymptomatic, although larger lesions (greater than 1.5 cm) with prominent mucosal involvement may become clinically significant (149,150). Combined submucosal pancreatic heterotopia with overlying gastric-type mucosa in the duodenal bulb has been reported (151).

Lymphoid Proliferations

Lymphoid tissue is a prominent feature of the small bowel. The gut-associated lymphoid tissue in this region, as in the entire gastrointestinal tract, includes intraepithelial lymphocytes, lamina propria mononuclear cells, isolated lymphoid follicles, and Peyer patches (152). The normal appearance and immunologic composition of these distinct lymphoid

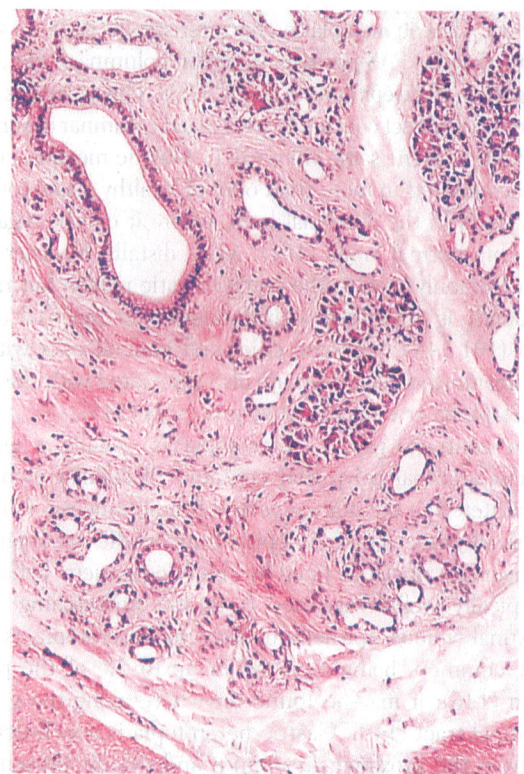

FIGURE 23.33 Heterotopic pancreas in the duodenum characterized in this instance by variably sized ducts, acini, and abundant smooth muscle.

populations have been detailed earlier in the chapter. All these compartments participate at some level in mucosal immune responses, but they also provide the milieu for various hyperplastic and neoplastic proliferations, as well as for certain immunodeficiency states. Some of these disorders have histologic features that deviate only slightly from a normal appearance and from one another. In addition, some are believed to be preneoplastic.

Lymphoid hyperplasias are divided into two broad categories: focal and diffuse forms (153). Focal lymphoid hyperplasia is a localized, well-circumscribed proliferation of benign lymphoid tissue characterized by a polymorphic infiltrate of lymphocytes within which numerous benign follicles with reactive germinal centers are dispersed. These proliferations often involve only the mucosa and submucosa, but they may extend through the entire bowel wall (153). Focal lymphoid hyperplasia is predominantly found in the terminal ileum of children or adolescents who present either with ileocecal intussusception or with a clinical syndrome mimicking appendicitis (120,122,153).

Diffuse or nodular lymphoid hyperplasia is a distinct entity in which multiple nodules composed of aggregates of benign lymphoid follicles disfigure the mucosa and submucosa along extensive lengths of the small intestine and can involve the colon (153–155). It is usually asymptomatic and incidentally encountered (153). However, this pattern may also be associated with common variable immunodeficiency or selective IgA deficiency, often with giardiasis-related diarrhea. Histologically these patients have greatly diminished or absent plasma cells in the nearby lamina propria (153,156). Nodular lymphoid hyperplasia, with or without immunodeficiency, has also been associated with an increased risk for the development of various malignancies (e.g., malignant lymphoma, carcinoma) (153–157).

Differentiation of these benign lymphoid lesions from malignant lymphoma may require careful evaluation of morphologic, phenotypic, and molecular features. The lack of a reactive follicular architecture (e.g., a germinal center with surrounding mantle cell zone) or the presence of mucosal ulceration, favor the diagnosis of lymphoma (153,158–160). Most small bowel malignant lymphomas are of B-cell lineage (160), and therefore demonstration of light-chain restriction by immunohistology or flow cytometry, or detection of clonal immunoglobulin gene rearrangements by PCR can aid in the diagnosis of a neoplastic process (161–163). Some malignant lymphomas, including marginal zone lymphoma (MALT lymphoma) or mantle cell lymphoma, typically consist of small cytologically bland cells that are distinguished by their monotonous appearance. High-grade lymphomas including diffuse large B-cell lymphoma and Burkitt lymphoma are distinguished by their atypical cytologic features and destructive growth. T-cell receptor gene rearrangement analysis may be necessary in some cases, particularly when the patient has a history of celiac disease, to rule out the possibility of enteropathy-associated T-cell lymphoma.

Morphologic Changes Associated with Ileal Diversion and Continence-Restoring Procedures

With the increasing number of diversion and continence-restoring procedures being performed after total colectomy, it has become common to see biopsy and revision specimens after such operations. As a consequence, familiarity with the altered yet "normal" morphology within these ileal creations must be appreciated in order to evaluate them optimally. The expected mucosal changes include villous shortening and crypt lengthening (approximate 1:1 to 2:1 ratio), increased numbers of goblet cells and lymphoid follicles, and a denser mononuclear cell infiltrate within the lamina propria (43,164,165). These alterations are similar after either colectomy with conventional ileostomy or after ileoanal anastomosis with ileal reservoir formation (e.g., pouch) (165–167). However, ileostomy stomas in particular show additional changes of mucosal prolapse exemplified by fibromuscular obliteration of the lamina propria and superficial erosions and microhemorrhages (43). In addition, goblet cell mucin alterations have been seen in nearly 50% of pouches examined, with conversion to predominantly sulfomucins (i.e., colonic epithelial mucin) (167). However, another group of investigators saw no change in goblet cell mucins from the typical small bowel acid sialomucins in ileal segments after either ileoanal anastomosis with pouch formation or conventional ileostomy (165).

Nonetheless, all these changes should be interpreted as "normal" because more definitive and specific criteria need to be met to establish persistent, recurrent, or novel disease in these specimens.

MUCOSAL BIOPSY SPECIMEN EVALUATION IN SUSPECTED MALABSORPTION

Specimen Procurement and Processing

The usefulness of small bowel mucosal biopsy is unquestioned (168), particularly in the evaluation of malabsorptive states. In the past, up to four biopsy samples were usually obtained from the area of the ligament of Treitz via a suction biopsy device attached to a long tube (169). Currently, a standard upper endoscope has been used, and comparable specimens have been procured (102,170). Since this technique is performed under direct visualization, many more biopsy specimens can be obtained. Regardless of the biopsy technique used, the most critical part of the procedure is proper orientation of the specimen. Ideally, specimens are immediately mounted mucosa-side up on a solid substance such as filter paper or plastic mesh and then placed into the fixative. After processing, the histotechnologist embeds the tissue perpendicular to the mounting material. Alternatively, biopsy specimens may be placed unmounted into the fixative immediately. The tissue can then be properly oriented after processing at the time of embedding. Since the specimen will naturally curl, some tangential sectioning can be expected. Proper specimen evaluation requires examination of optimally oriented intestinal villi obtained from the central region of the biopsy specimen. Although serial sectioning has been advocated by some (142), step sectioning (three to seven levels) is a reasonable alternative.

Our standard small bowel biopsy procedure consists of obtaining four to six endoscopic biopsy specimens (43). One can be used to make a touch preparation that is then fixed in alcohol and stained via the Giemsa technique. The other tissue samples are placed in the fixative and routinely processed. Step-section slides are obtained: two are stained with H&E and one with Alcian blue/PAS. The PAS stain is a useful screen for Whipple disease and *M. avium–intracellulare* complex infection. A trichrome stain is optional but can be used to confirm collagen deposition seen in ischemia or collagenous sprue. In addition, the iron hematoxylin counterstain used in the trichrome technique makes it easier to identify giardiasis.

Specimen Interpretation and Common Artifacts

With appropriate specimen procurement, the mucosa with muscularis mucosae and a small portion of upper submucosa should be available for histologic examination. These specimens should be evaluated in a systematic fashion, including assessment of (a) villous architecture, (b) surface and crypt epithelia, (c) lamina propria constituents, and (d) submucosal structures (86). A well-oriented specimen is essential for optimal evaluation. However, it must be remembered that villi vary in length and shape, particularly in the proximal duodenum, and that villous apices bend and twist in various planes to create unusual forms; these variations should not be misinterpreted as a villous abnormality (43,57,86). In general, if four normal villi in a row are observed, the villous architecture of the entire specimen is probably normal (86,142). This does not mean that specimens with fewer than four well-aligned normal villi should be considered inadequate because even one normal intestinal villus in a proximal small bowel biopsy specimen rules out untreated celiac sprue (43). Conversely, identification of four normal villi in a row does not necessarily exclude focal lesions, although it almost always does (142). The pathologist must be wary of certain common artifacts that may lead to erroneous interpretations. Careful attention to certain features (described below) within the various mucosal compartments will aid in their recognition.

Tangential Sectioning

Inappropriate orientation of the specimen, occurring at any point during processing, will lead to various tangential cuts or sections. The mucosa must be sectioned perpendicular to its long axis, or a distorted pattern disclosing apparently short and broad villi and an expanded lamina propria compartment will be observed. However, several features aid in recognizing an oblique cut: (a) numerous elliptically shaped glands, (b) a multilayered arrangement of the crypts (Fig. 23.34), or (c) a multilayered surface epithelium (Fig. 23.35) (86). If any of these features are present, the villous architecture must be interpreted with caution.

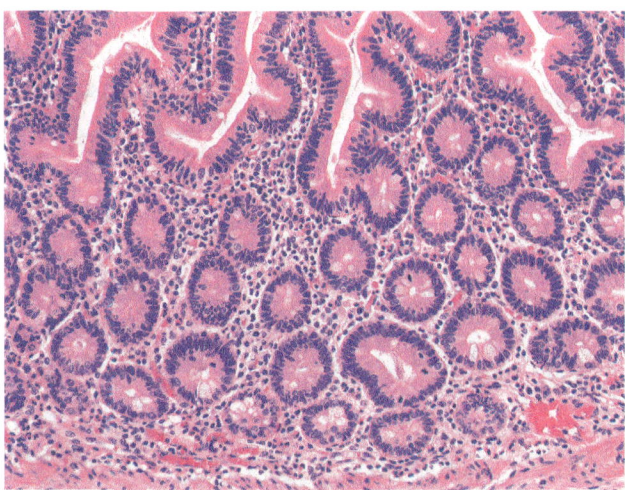

FIGURE 23.34 Multilayering of crypts indicates a tangential or oblique section of small intestine. The villous architecture overlying the crypts is normal, albeit unusual in appearance; this is also a product of malorientation of the biopsy specimen.

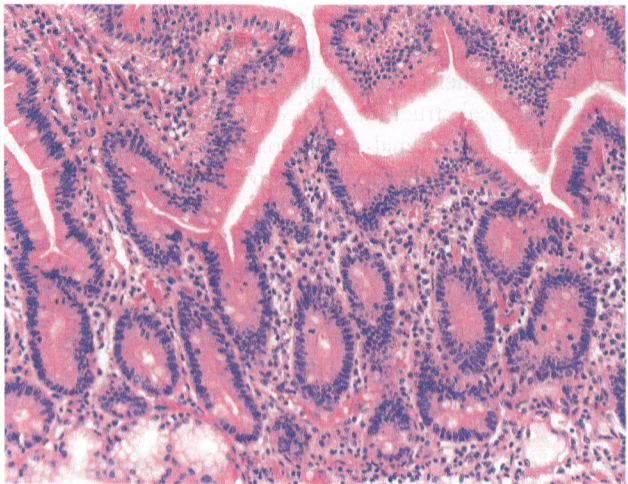

FIGURE 23.35 Another clue in identifying a tangential cut is multilayering, or "stratification," of the surface epithelium (*left portion of central villus*). The normal surface layer is one-cell thick. This broad and short villous appearance is a consequence of malorientation and should be interpreted accordingly.

Brunner Gland–Related Artifact

Brunner glands have an inconsistent effect on villous architecture (43). Occasionally, normal-length villi can be encountered overlying Brunner glands (Fig. 23.36), but more commonly the villi appear distorted, short, broad, and stubby (Fig. 23.24) (43,57). To minimize the potential effects of this artifact on interpretation, biopsy specimens of the small bowel for evaluation of malabsorptive states are routinely obtained as distally as possible in the duodenum or from the proximal jejunum (i.e., near the ligament of Treitz) (102,170). Occasionally, however, more proximal small bowel biopsies are necessary for evaluation of duodenitis or ulcer disease.

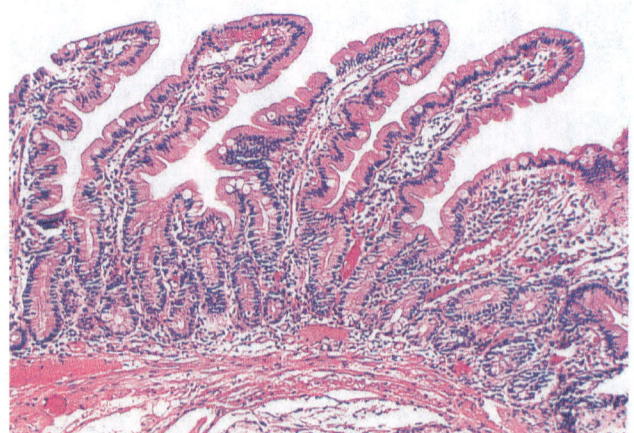

FIGURE 23.36 Occasionally, long slender villi, similar to those seen in the jejunum, are found overlying Brunner glands. However, villi associated with Brunner glands are more commonly shorter and broader (see Fig. 23.24).

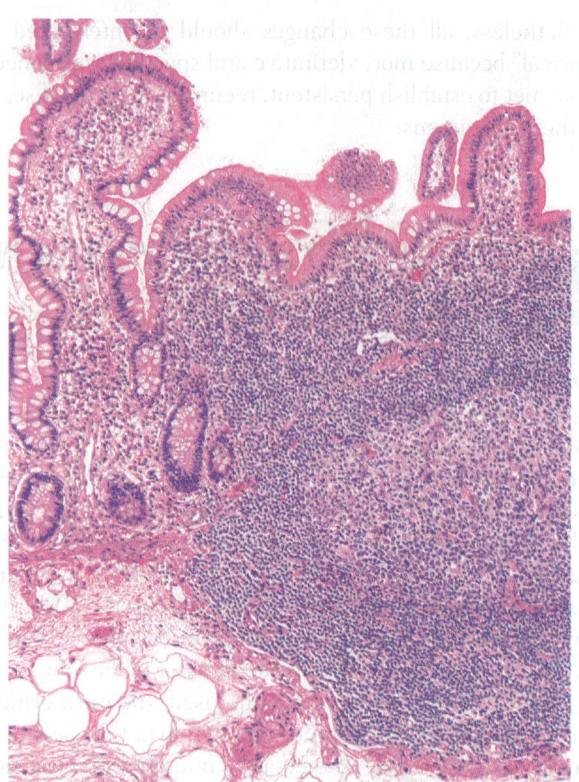

FIGURE 23.37 Lamina propria lymphoid aggregates of the Peyer patch. This organized lymphoid tissue typically extends into the underlying submucosa. The four components of the Peyer patch are seen and include a lymphoid follicle with prominent germinal center, an overlying flattened follicle-associated epithelium, an intervening pale-staining subepithelial dome region, and the T-cell–rich interfollicular zone.

Lymphoid Aggregate–Related Artifact

Mucosal lymphoid aggregates, or nodules, are scattered along the small bowel and often distort the villous architecture. Villi are usually absent over lymphoid aggregates, and nearby villous forms may be distorted, short, and stubby (Fig. 23.37) (86). Therefore, when a lymphoid aggregate is seen below an isolated flat portion of the surface epithelium, it should not be misinterpreted as a severe villous abnormality.

Absence of Muscularis Mucosae

As mentioned earlier, the muscularis mucosae is an important structural component of the mucosa. In its absence (for instance, in a very superficial mucosal biopsy specimen), the tissues tend to spread laterally, resulting in villi becoming more widely spaced and appearing short and broad (Fig. 23.38) (86,171).

Biopsy Trauma–Related Artifacts

As a direct result of the traumatic pinch or suction biopsy procedures, certain alterations of normal mucosa can be seen. Separation of the villous surface epithelium from the underlying lamina propria or focally denuded epithelium are not unusual (86,171). The lack of acute erosive changes

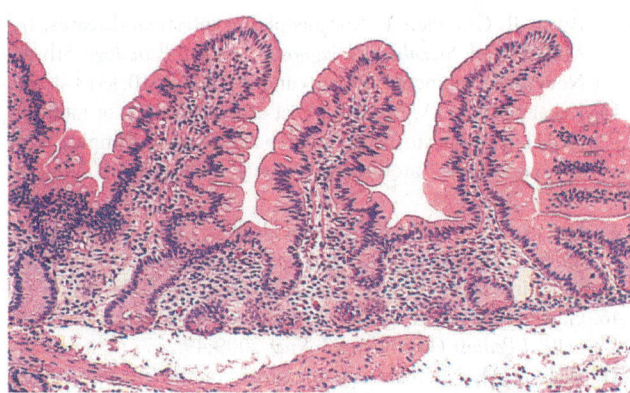

FIGURE 23.38 Absence of muscularis mucosae in a small bowel biopsy specimen, resulting in shorter- and broader-appearing villi that are widely spaced.

(e.g., neutrophilic infiltrate, cellular necrosis) or evidence of chronic ulceration (e.g., granulation tissue, regenerative epithelium) allows this alteration to be recognized as biopsy related. In addition, focal hemorrhage and scattered polymorphonuclear leukocytes may be observed in the lamina propria as a consequence of the biopsy procedure. Crush or compression artifact can occur at the site of closure of the endoscopic forceps, resulting in a condensation of the lymphoplasmacytic component that can be misinterpreted as increased chronic inflammation (170). In addition, the connective tissue may be altered in such a way that it appears more tightly packed, mimicking fibrosis or excessive collagen deposition (172).

Fixative-Related Artifacts

Certain fixatives other than formalin (4% formaldehyde solution) can cause interpretive problems. Although the Hollande fixative better preserves cytologic and nuclear detail, several artifacts may interfere with evaluation. The brightly eosinophilic granules of Paneth cells and sometimes eosinophilic leukocytes seen readily in formalin-fixed tissue are not as well preserved by the Hollande fixative. In addition, suboptimal clearing of the Hollande fixative from the specimens before paraffin embedding can result in residual minute, round, basophilic structures that resemble yeast forms or parasites (e.g., cryptosporidium, *Giardia lamblia*) (172).

ACKNOWLEDGMENT

We thank James T. McMahon, PhD, for the electron micrographs.

REFERENCES

1. Hirsch J, Ahrens EH, Blankenhorn DH. Measurement of human intestinal length in vivo and some causes of variation. *Gastroenterology* 1956;31:274–284.
2. Thorek P. *Anatomy and Surgery*. 3rd ed. New York: Springer-Verlag; 1985.
3. Costacurta L. Anatomical and functional aspects of the human suspensory muscle of the duodenum. *Acta Anat (Basel)* 1972; 82:34–46.
4. Kahn E, Daum F. Anatomy, histology and developmental anomalies of the small intestine and colon. In: Feldman M, Friedman LS, Brandt LJ, eds. *Sleisenger and Fordtran's Gastrointestinal and Liver Disease: Pathophysiology/Diagnosis/Management*. 9th ed. Philadelphia, PA: Saunders Elsevier; 2010:1615–1641.
5. Parks DA, Jacobson ED. Physiology of the splanchnic circulation. *Arch Intern Med* 1985;145:1278–1281.
6. Granger DN, Barrowman JA. Microcirculation of the alimentary tract. II. Pathophysiology of edema. *Gastroenterology* 1983; 84:1035–1049.
7. Ohtani O, Ohtani Y. Organization and developmental aspects of lymphatic vessels. *Arch Histol Cytol* 2008;71:1–22.
8. Alpers DH. Digestion and absorption of carbohydrates and proteins. In: Johnson LR, ed. *Physiology of the Gastrointestinal Tract*. 2nd ed. New York: Raven Press; 1987:1469–1487.
9. Feracci H, Bernadac A, Gorvel JP, et al. Localization by immunofluorescence and histochemical labelling of a aminopeptidase N in relation to its biosynthesis in rabbit and pig enterocytes. *Gastroenterology* 1982;82:317–324.
10. Lojda Z. The histochemical demonstration of brush border endopeptidase. *Histochemistry* 1979;64:205–221.
11. Goodman BE. Insights into digestion and absorption of major nutrients in humans. *Adv Physiol Educ* 2010;34:44–53.
12. Davenport HW. *Physiology of the Digestive Tract*. 5th ed. Chicago, IL: Year Book Medical; 1982.
13. Glickman RM. Fat absorption and malabsorption. *Clin Gastroenterol* 1983;12:323.
14. Farrell JJ. Digestion and absorption of nutrients and vitamins. In: Feldman M, Friedman LS, Brandt LJ, eds. *Sleisenger and Fordtran's Gastrointestinal and Liver Disease*. 9th ed. Philadelphia, PA: Saunders Elsevier; 2011:1695–1734.
15. Quigley EM. Small intestinal motor activity—its role in gut homeostasis and disease. *Q J Med* 1987;65:799–810.
16. Fiorenza V, Yee YS, Zfass AM. Small intestinal motility: Normal and abnormal function. *Am J Gastroenterol* 1987;82: 1111–1114.
17. Lewin KJ. The endocrine cells of the gastrointestinal tract: The normal endocrine cells and their hyperplasias. In: Sommers SC, Rosen PP, Fechner RE, eds. *Pathology Annual. Part 1*. Norwalk, CT: Appleton-Century-Crofts; 1986:1–27.
18. Solcia E, Capella C, Buffa R, et al. Endocrine cells of the digestive system. In: Johnson LR, ed. *Physiology of the Gastrointestinal Tract*. 2nd ed. New York: Raven Press; 1987: 111–130.
19. Elson CO, Kagnoff MF, Fiocchi C, et al. Intestinal immunity and inflammation: Recent progress. *Gastroenterology* 1986;91: 746–768.
20. Rubin W. The epithelial "membrane" of the small intestine. *Am J Clin Nutr* 1971;24:45–64.
21. Wilson JP. Surface area of the small intestine in man. *Gut* 1967;8:618–621.
22. Holmes R, Hourihane DO, Booth CC. The mucosa of the small intestine. *Postgrad Med J* 1961;37:717–724.
23. Toner PG, Carr KE. The use of scanning electron microscopy in the study of the intestinal villi. *J Pathol* 1969;97:611–617.

24. Trier JS, Madara JL. Functional morphology of the mucosa of the small intestine. In: Johnson LR, ed. *Physiology of the Gastrointestinal Tract*. 2nd ed. New York: Raven Press; 1987: 1209–1249.
25. Dobbins WO. The intestinal mucosal lymphatic in man. A light and electron microscopic study. *Gastroenterology* 1966; 51:994–1003.
26. Montani M, Thiesler T, Kristiansen G. Smoothelin is a specific and robust marker for distinction of muscularis propria and muscularis mucosae in the gastrointestinal tract. *Histopathology* 2010;57:244–249.
27. Neutra MR, Padykula HK. The gastrointestinal tract. In: Weiss L, ed. *Modern Concepts of Gastrointestinal Histology*. New York: Elsevier; 1984:658–706.
28. Poley JR. Loss of the glycocalyx of enterocytes in small intestine: A feature detected by scanning electron microscopy in children with gastrointestinal intolerance to dietary protein. *J Pediatr Gastroenterol Nutr* 1988;7:386–394.
29. Ermund A, Schutte A, Johansson MEV, et al. Studies of mucus in mouse stomach, small intestine, and colon. Gastrointestinal mucus layers have different properties depending on location as well as over Peyer's patches. *Am J Physiol Gastrointest Liver Physiol* 2013;305:G341–G347.
30. Pelaseyed T, Bergstrom JH, Gustafsson JK, et al. The mucus and mucins of the goblet cells and enterocytes provide the first defense line of the gastrointestinal tract and interact with the immune system. *Immunol Rev* 2014;260:8–20.
31. Trier JS. The surface coat of gastrointestinal epithelial cells. *Gastroenterology* 1969;56:618–622.
32. Dawson IMP. Atlas of gastrointestinal pathology as seen on biopsy. In: Gresham GA, ed. *Current Histopathology*. Vol 6. Philadelphia, PA: JB Lippincott; 1983:63–67.
33. Filipe MI. Mucins in the human gastrointestinal epithelium: A review. *Invest Cell Pathol* 1979;2:195–216.
34. Dobbins WO III. Human intestinal intraepithelial lymphocytes. *Gut* 1986;27:972–985.
35. Ferguson A, Murray D. Quantitation of intraepithelial lymphocytes in human jejunum. *Gut* 1971;12:988–994.
36. Hayat M, Cairns A, Dixon MF, et al. Quantitation of intraepithelial lymphocytes in human duodenum: What is normal? *J Clin Pathol* 2002;55:363–395.
37. Selby WS, Janossy G, Bofill M, et al. Lymphocyte subpopulations in the human small intestine: The findings in normal mucosa and in the mucosa of patients with adult coeliac disease. *Clin Exp Immunol* 1983;52:219–228.
38. Cerf-Bensussan N, Schneeberger EE, Bhan AK. Immunohistologic and immunoelectron microscopic characterization of the mucosal lymphocytes of human small intestine by the use of monoclonal antibodies. *J Immunol* 1983;130:2615–2622.
39. Greenwood JH, Austin LL, Dobbins WO III. In vitro characterization of human intestinal intraepithelial lymphocytes. *Gastroenterology* 1983;85:1023–1035.
40. Wittig BM, Zeitz M. The gut as an organ of immunology. *Int J Colorectal Dis* 2003;18:181–187.
41. Sapp H, Ithamukkala S, Brien TP, et al. The terminal ileum is affected in patients with lymphocytic or collagenous colitis. *Am J Surg Pathol* 2002;26:1484–1492.
42. Kober OI, Ahl D, Pin C, et al. γδ T-cell-deficient mice show alterations in mucin expression, glycosylation, and goblet cells but maintain an intact mucus layer. *Am J Physiol Gastrointest Liver Physiol* 2014;306:G582–G593.
43. Petras R, Gramlich T. Non-neoplastic intestinal diseases. In: Mills SE, ed. *Sternberg's Diagnostic Surgical Pathology*. 5th ed. New York: Lippincott Williams and Wilkins; 2010:1313–1323.
44. Kakar S, Nehra V, Murray JA, et al. Significance of intraepithelial lymphocytosis in small bowel biopsy samples with normal mucosal architecture. *Am J Gastroenterol* 2003;98: 2027–2033.
45. Ferguson A, Sutherland A, MacDonald TT, et al. Technique for microdissection and measurement in biopsies of human small intestine. *J Clin Pathol* 1977;30:1068–1073.
46. Garrison AP, Helmrath MA, Dekaney CM. Intestinal stem cells. *J Pediatr Gastroenterol Nutr* 2009;49:2–7.
47. Watson AJ. Necrosis and apoptosis in the gastrointestinal tract. *Gut* 1995;37:165–167.
48. de Santa Barbara P, van den Brink GR, Roberts DJ. Development and differentiation of the intestinal epithelium. *Cell Mol Life Sci* 2003;60:1322–1332.
49. Reed JC. Mechanisms of apoptosis. *Am J Pathol* 2000;157: 1415–1430.
50. Williamson RC. Intestinal adaptation (first of two parts). Structural, functional, and cytokinetic changes. *N Engl J Med* 1978;298:1393–1402.
51. Ahuja V, Dieckgraefe BK, Anant S. Molecular biology of the small intestine. *Curr Opin Gastroenterol* 2006;22:90–94.
52. Facer P, Bishop AE, Lloyd RV, et al. Chromogranin: A newly recognized marker for endocrine cells of the human gastrointestinal tract. *Gastroenterology* 1985;89:1366–1373.
53. Sjolund K, Sanden G, Hakanson R, et al. Endocrine cells in human intestine: An immunocytochemical study. *Gastroenterology* 1983;85:1120–1130.
54. Buffa R, Rindi G, Sessa F, et al. Synaptophysin immunoreactivity and small clear vesicles in neuroendocrine cells and related tumours. *Mol Cell Probes* 1987;1:367–381.
55. Albrecht S, Gardiner GW, Kovacs K, et al. Duodenal somatostatinoma with psammoma bodies. *Arch Pathol Lab Med* 1989;113:517–520.
56. Liddle RA. Gastrointestinal hormones and neurotransmitters. In: Feldman M, Friedman LS, Brandt LJ, eds. *Sleisenger and Fordtran's Gastrointestinal and Liver Disease*. 9th ed. Philadelphia, PA: Saunders Elsevier; 2010:3–20.
57. Goldman H, Antonioli DA. Mucosal biopsy of the esophagus, stomach, and proximal duodenum. *Hum Pathol* 1982;13: 423–448.
58. Sandow MJ, Whitehead R. The Paneth cell. *Gut* 1979;20: 420–431.
59. Wehkamp J, Fellermann K, Herrlinger KR, et al. Mechanisms of disease: Defensins in gastrointestinal diseases. *Nat Clin Pract Gastroenterol Hepatol* 2005;2:406–415.
60. Wehkamp J, Salzman NH, Porter E, et al. Reduced paneth cell alpha-defensins in ileal Crohn's disease. *Proc Natl Acad Sci USA* 2005;102:18129–18134.
61. Jenkins D, Goodall A, Scott BB. T-lymphocyte populations in normal and coeliac small intestinal mucosa defined by monoclonal antibodies. *Gut* 1986;27:1330–1337.
62. Isaacson P, Judd MA. Carcinoembryonic antigen (CEA) in the normal human small intestine: A light and electron microscopic study. *Gut* 1977;18:786–791.
63. Groisman GM, Amar M, Livne E. CD10: A valuable tool for the light microscopic diagnosis of microvillus inclusion disease (familial microvillus atrophy). *Am J Surg Pathol* 2002; 26:902–907.

64. Groisman GM, Ben-Izhak O, Schwersenz A, et al. The value of polyclonal carcinoembryonic antigen immunostaining in the diagnosis of microvillus inclusion disease. *Hum Pathol* 1993;24:1232–1237.
65. Scott H, Solheim BG, Brandtzaeg P, et al. HLA-DR-like antigens in the epithelium of the human small intestine. *Scand J Immunol* 1980;12:77–82.
66. Parker FG, Barnes EN, Kaye GI. The pericryptal fibroblast sheath. IV. Replication, migration and differentiation of the subepithelial fibroblasts of the crypt and villus of the rabbit jejunum. *Gastroenterology* 1974;67:607–621.
67. Kindt TJ, Goldsby RA, Osborne BA. Antigens and antibodies. In: Kuby J. ed. *Kuby Immunology*. 6th ed. New York: W.H. Freeman and Company; 2007:99.
68. Chiba M, Ohta H, Nagasaki A, et al. Lymphoid cell subsets in normal human small intestine. *Gastroenterol Jpn* 1986;21: 336–343.
69. Kingston D, Pearson JR, Penna FJ. Plasma cell counts of human jejunal biopsy specimens examined by immunofluorescence and immunoperoxidase techniques; a comparative study. *J Clin Pathol* 1981;34:381–385.
70. Brandtzaeg P, Halstensen TS, Kett K, et al. Immunobiology and immunopathology of human gut mucosa: Humoral immunity and intraepithelial lymphocytes. *Gastroenterology* 1989;97:1562–1584.
71. Rescigno M, DiSabatino A. Dendritic cells in intestinal homeostasis and disease. *J Clin Invest* 2009;119:2441–2450.
72. Izcue A, Powrie F. Special regulatory T-cell review: Regulatory T cells and the intestinal tract–patrolling the frontier. *Immunology* 2008;123:6–10.
73. Powell N, Walker MM, Nicholas JT. Gastrointestinal eosinophils in health, disease, and functional disorders. *Nat Rev Gastroenterol Hepatol* 2010;7:146–156.
74. Lehrer RI, Szklarek D, Barton A, et al. Antibacterial properties of eosinophil major basic protein and eosinophil cationic protein. *J Immunol* 1989;142:4428–4434.
75. Persson T, Andersson P, Bodelsson M, et al. Bactericidal activity of human eosinophilic granulocytes against *Escherichia coli*. *Infect Immun* 2001;69:3591–3596.
76. Schneider EN, Smoller BR, Lamps L. Histiocytic subpopulations in the gastrointestinal tract: Distribution and possible relationship to function. *Appl Immunohistochem Mol Morphol* 2004;12:356–359.
77. Kelsall B. Recent progress in understanding the phenotype and function of intestinal dendritic cells and macrophages. *Mucosal Immunol* 2008;1:460–469.
78. Kamada N, Hisamatsu T, Honda H, et al. Human CD14+ macrophages in intestinal lamina propria exhibit potent antigen-presenting ability. *J Immunol* 2009;183:1724–1731.
79. Fries PN, Giebel PJ. Mucosal dendritic cell diversity in the gastrointestinal tract. *Cell Tissue Res* 2011;343:33–41.
80. Kretschmer K, Apostolou I, Hawiger D, et al. Inducing and expanding regulatory T cell populations by foreign antigen. *Nat Immunol* 2005;6:1219–1227.
81. Platt AM, Mowat AM. Mucosal macrophages and the regulation of immune responses in the intestine. *Immunol Lett* 2008;119:22–31.
82. Comer GM, Brandt LJ, Abissi CJ. Whipple's disease: A review. *Am J Gastroenterol* 1983;78:107–114.
83. Roth RI, Owen RL, Keren DF, et al. Intestinal infection with Mycobacterium avium in acquired immune deficiency syndrome (AIDS). Histological and clinical comparison with Whipple's disease. *Dig Dis Sci* 1985;30:497–504.
84. Siegert SI, Diebold J, Ludolph-Hauser D, et al. Are gastrointestinal mucosal mast cells increased in patients with systemic mastocytosis? *Am J Clin Pathol* 2004;122:560–565.
85. Lundqvist M, Wilander E. Subepithelial neuroendocrine cells and carcinoid tumors of the human small intestine and appendix. A comparative immunohistochemical study with regard to serotonin, neuron-specific enolase and S-100 protein reactivity. *J Pathol* 1986;148:141–147.
86. Perera DR, Weinstein WM, Rubin CE. Symposium on pathology of the gastrointestinal tract- Part II. Small intestinal biopsy. *Hum Pathol* 1975;6:157–217.
87. Lord MG, Valies P, Broughton AC. A morphologic study of the submucosa of the large intestine. *Surg Gynecol Obstet* 1977;145:55–60.
88. Lee AK, DeLellis RA, Silverman ML, et al. Lymphatic and blood vessel invasion in breast carcinoma: A useful prognostic indicator? *Hum Pathol* 1986;17:984–987.
89. Schlingemann RO, Dingjan GM, Emeis JJ, et al. Monoclonal antibody PAL-E specific for endothelium. *Lab Invest* 1985;52: 71–76.
90. Vardy PA, Lebenthal E, Shwachman H. Intestinal lymphangiectasia: A reappraisal. *Pediatrics* 1975;55:842–851.
91. Gershon MD, Erde SM. The nervous system of the gut. *Gastroenterology* 1981;80:1571–1594.
92. Krishnamurthy S, Schuffler MD. Pathology of neuromuscular disorders of the small intestine and colon. *Gastroenterology* 1987;93:610–639.
93. Ferri GL, Probert L, Cocchia D, et al. Evidence for the presence of S-100 protein in the glial component of the human enteric nervous system. *Nature* 1982;297:409–410.
94. Goyal RK, Crist JR. Neurology of the gut. In: Sleisenger MH, Fordtran JS, eds. *Gastrointestinal Disease*. 4th ed. Philadelphia, PA: WB Saunders; 1989:21–52.
95. Streutker CJ, Huizinga JD, Driman DK, et al. Interstitial cells of Cajal in health and disease. Part I: Normal ICC structure and function with associated motility disorders. *Histopathology* 2007;50:176–189.
96. Farrugia G. Interstitial cells of Cajal in health and disease. *Neurogastroenterol Motil* 2008;20(Suppl 1):54–63.
97. Hagger R, Finlayson C, Jeffrey I, et al. Role of the interstitial cells of Cajal in the control of gut motility. *Br J Surg* 1997;84:445–450.
98. Lawson HH. The duodenal mucosa in health and disease. A clinical and experimental study. *Surg Annu* 1989;21:157–180.
99. Lawson HH. Definition of the gastroduodenal junction in healthy subjects. *J Clin Pathol* 1988;41:393–396.
100. Korn ER, Foroozan P. Endoscopic biopsies of normal duodenal mucosa. *Gastrointest Endosc* 1974;21:51–54.
101. Kreuning J, Bosman FT, Kuiper G, et al. Gastric and duodenal mucosa in "healthy" individuals. An endoscopic and histopathological study of 50 volunteers. *J Clin Pathol* 1978; 31:69–77.
102. Dandalides SM, Carey WD, Petras RE, et al. Endoscopic small bowel mucosal biopsy: A controlled trial evaluating forceps size and biopsy location in the diagnosis of normal and abnormal mucosal architecture. *Gastrointest Endosc* 1989;35: 197–200.
103. Robertson HE. The pathology of Brunner's glands. *Arch Pathol* 1941;31:112–130.

104. Lang IM, Tansy MF. Brunner's glands. In: Young JA, ed. *Gastrointestinal Physiology. IV. International Review of Physiology*. Vol 28. Baltimore, MD: University Park Press; 1983:85–102.
105. Treasure T. The ducts of Brunner's glands. *J Anat* 1978;127:299–304.
106. Leeson TS, Leeson RC. The fine structure of Brunner's glands. *J Anat* 1968;103:263–276.
107. Thompson IW, Day DW, Wright NA. Subnuclear vacuolated mucous cells: A novel abnormality of simple mucin-secreting cells of non-specialized gastric mucosa and Brunner's glands. *Histopathology* 1987;11:1067–1081.
108. Kamiya R. Basal-granulated cells in human Brunner's glands. *Arch Histol Jpn* 1983;46:87–101.
109. Bosshard A, Chery-Croze S, Cuber JC, et al. Immunocytochemical study of peptidergic structures in Brunner's glands. *Gastroenterology* 1989;97:1382–1388.
110. Silverman L, Waugh JM, Huizenga KA, et al. Large adenomatous polyp of Brunner's glands. *Am J Clin Pathol* 1961;36:438–443.
111. Franzin G, Musola R, Ghidini O, et al. Nodular hyperplasia of Brunner's glands. *Gastrointest Endosc* 1985;31:374–378.
112. West B. Pseudomelanosis duodeni. *J Clin Gastroenterol* 1988;10:127–129.
113. Rosenberg JC, Didio LJ. Anatomic and clinical aspects of the junction of the ileum with the large intestine. *Dis Colon Rectum* 1970;13:220–224.
114. Kumar D, Phillips SF. The contribution of external ligamentous attachments to function of the ileocecal junction. *Dis Colon Rectum* 1987;30:410–416.
115. Axelsson C, Andersen JA. Lipohyperplasia of the ileocaecal region. *Acta Chir Scand* 1974;140:649–654.
116. Cuvelier C, Demetter P, Mielants H, et al. Interpretation of ileal biopsies: Morphological features in normal and diseased mucosa. *Histopathology* 2001;38:1–12.
117. Spencer J, MacDonald TT, Finn T, et al. The development of gut associated lymphoid tissue in the terminal ileum of fetal human intestine. *Clin Exp Immunol* 1986;64:536–543.
118. Cornes JS. Number, size, and distribution of Peyer's patches in the human small intestine: Part I The development of Peyer's patches. *Gut* 1965;6:225–229.
119. Cornes JS. Number, size, and distribution of Peyer's patches in the human small intestine: Part II The effect of age on Peyer's patches. *Gut* 1965;6:225–233.
120. Pang LC. Intussusception revisited: Clinicopathologic analysis of 261 cases with emphasis on pathogenesis. *South Med J* 1989;82:215–228.
121. Schenken JR, Kruger RL, Schultz L. Papillary lymphoid hyperplasia of the terminal ileum: An unusual cause of intussusception and gastrointestinal bleeding in childhood. *J Pediatr Surg* 1975;10:259–265.
122. Fieber SS, Schaefer HJ. Lymphoid hyperplasia of the terminal ileum–a clinical entity? *Gastroenterology* 1966;50:83–98.
123. Bjerke K, Brandtzaeg P, Fausa O. T cell distribution is different in follicle-associated epithelium of human Peyer's patches and villous epithelium. *Clin Exp Immunol* 1988;74:270–275.
124. Spencer J, Finn T, Isaacson PG. Human Peyer's patches: An immunohistochemical study. *Gut* 1986;27:405–410.
125. Finke D. Induction of intestinal lymphoid tissue formation by intrinsic and extrinsic signals. *Semin Immunopathol* 2009;31:151–169.
126. Shreedhar VK, Kelsall BL, Neutra MR. Cholera toxin induces migration of dendritic cells from the subepithelial dome region to T- and B-cells areas of Peyer's patches. *Infect Immun* 2003;71:504–509.
127. Corr SC, Gahan CC, Hill C. M-cells: Origin, morphology and role in mucosal immunity and microbial pathogenesis. *FEMS Immunol Med Microbiol* 2008;52:2–12.
128. Kraehenbuhl JP, Neutra MR. Molecular and cellular basis of immune protection of mucosal surfaces. *Physiol Rev* 1992;72:853–879.
129. Neutra MR, Frey A, Kraehenbuhl JP. Epithelial M-cells: Gateways for mucosal infection and immunization. *Cell* 1996;86:345–348.
130. Neutra MR, Pringault E, Kraehenbuhl JP. Antigen sampling across epithelial barriers and induction of mucosal immune responses. *Annu Rev Immunol* 1996;14:275–300.
131. Gebert A, Rothkotter HJ, Pabst R. M cells in Peyer's patches of the intestine. *Int Rev Cytol* 1996;167:91–159.
132. Trier JS. Structure and function of intestinal M-cells. *Gastroenterol Clin North Am* 1991;20:531–547.
133. Fleeton MN, Contractor N, Leon F, et al. Peyer's patch dendritic cells process viral antigen from apoptotic epithelial cells in the intestine of reovirus-infected mice. *J Exp Med* 2004;200:235–245.
134. Shepherd NA, Crocker PR, Smith AP, et al. Exogenous pigment in Peyer's patches. *Hum Pathol* 1987;18:50–54.
135. Urbanski SJ, Arsenault AL, Green FH, et al. Pigment resembling atmospheric dust in Peyer's patches. *Mod Pathol* 1989;2:222–226.
136. Mackey WC, Dineen P. A fifty year experience with Meckel's diverticulum. *Surg Gynecol Obstet* 1983;156:56–64.
137. Artigas V, Calabuig R, Badia F, et al. Meckel's diverticulum: Value of ectopic tissue. *Am J Surg* 1986;151:631–634.
138. Bennett MK, Sachdev GK, Jewell DP, et al. Jejunal mucosal morphology in healthy north Indian subjects. *J Clin Pathol* 1985;38:368–371.
139. Cook GC, Kajubi SK, Lee FD. Jejunal morphology of the African in Uganda. *J Pathol* 1969;98:157–169.
140. Lindenbaum J, Gerson CD, Kent TH. Recovery of small-intestinal structure and function after residence in the tropics. I. Studies in Peace Corps volunteers. *Ann Intern Med* 1971;74:218–222.
141. Gerson CD, Kent TH, Saha JR, et al. Recovery of small-intestinal structure and function after residence in the tropics. II. Studies in Indians and Pakistanis living in New York City. *Ann Intern Med* 1971;75:41–48.
142. Dobbins WO III. Small bowel biopsy in malabsorptive states. In: Norris HT, ed. *Pathology of the Colon, Small Intestine, and Anus*. New York: Churchill Livingstone; 1983:121–167.
143. Webster SG, Leeming JT. The appearance of the small bowel mucosa in old age. *Age Ageing* 1975;4:168–174.
144. Chacko CJ, Paulson KA, Mathan VI, et al. The villus architecture of the small intestine in the tropics: A necropsy study. *J Pathol* 1969;98:146–151.
145. Wolff M. Heterotopic gastric epithelium in the rectum: A report of three new cases with a review of 87 cases of gastric heterotopia in the alimentary canal. *Am J Clin Pathol* 1971;55:604–616.
146. Lessells AM, Martin DF. Heterotopic gastric mucosa in the duodenum. *J Clin Pathol* 1982;35:591–595.

147. Tsubone M, Kozuka S, Taki T, et al. Heterotopic gastric mucosa in the small intestine. *Acta Pathol Jpn* 1984;34: 1425–1431.
148. Lai EC, Tompkins RK. Heterotopic pancreas. Review of a 26 year experience. *Am J Surg* 1986;151:697–700.
149. Dolan RV, ReMine WH, Dockerty MB. The fate of heterotopic pancreatic tissue. A study of 212 cases. *Arch Surg* 1974; 109:762–765.
150. Armstrong CP, King PM, Dixon JM, et al. The clinical significance of heterotopic pancreas in the gastrointestinal tract. *Br J Surg* 1981;68:384–387.
151. Tanemura H, Uno S, Suzuki M, et al. Heterotopic gastric mucosa accompanied by aberrant pancreas in the duodenum. *Am J Gastroenterol* 1987;82:685–688.
152. Tomasi TB Jr. Mechanisms of immune regulation at mucosal surfaces. *Rev Infect Dis* 1983;5(Suppl 4):S784–S792.
153. Ranchod M, Lewin KJ, Dorfman RF. Lymphoid hyperplasia of the gastrointestinal tract: A study of 26 cases and review of the literature. *Am J Surg Pathol* 1978;2:383–400.
154. Rambaud JC, De Saint-Louvent P, Marti R, et al. Diffuse follicular lymphoid hyperplasia of the small intestine without primary immunoglobulin deficiency. *Am J Med* 1982;73: 125–132.
155. Matuchansky C, Touchard G, Lemaire M, et al. Malignant lymphoma of the small bowel associated with diffuse nodular lymphoid hyperplasia. *N Engl J Med* 1985;313:166–171.
156. Daniels JA, Lederman HM, Maitra A, et al. Gastrointestinal tract pathology in patients with common variable immunodeficiency (CVID): A clinicopathologic study and review. *Am J Surg Pathol* 2007;31:1800–1812.
157. Hermans PE, Diaz-Buxo JA, Stobo JD. Idiopathic late-onset immunoglobulin deficiency: Clinical observations in 50 patients. *Am J Med* 1976;61:221–237.
158. Lewin KJ, Kahn LB, Novis BH. Primary intestinal lymphoma of "Western" and "Mediterranean" type, alpha chain disease and massive plasma cell infiltration: A comparative study of 37 cases. *Cancer* 1976;38:2511–2528.
159. Lewin KJ, Ranchod M, Dorfman RF. Lymphomas of the gastrointestinal tract: A study of 117 cases presenting with gastrointestinal disease. *Cancer* 1978;42:693–707.
160. Grody WW, Magidson JG, Weiss LM, et al. Gastrointestinal lymphomas: Immunohistochemical studies on the cell of origin. *Am J Surg Pathol* 1985;9:328–337.
161. Tubbs RR, Sheibani K. Immunohistology of lymphoproliferative disorders. *Semin Diagn Pathol* 1984;1:272–284.
162. Little JV, Foucar K, Horvath A, et al. Flow cytometric analysis of lymphoma and lymphoma-like disorders. *Semin Diagn Pathol* 1989;6:37–54.
163. Grody WW, Gatti RA, Naiem F. Diagnostic molecular pathology. *Mod Pathol* 1989;2:553–568.
164. Goldman H, Antonioli DA. Mucosal biopsy of the rectum, colon, and distal ileum. *Hum Pathol* 1982;13:981–1012.
165. Bechi P, Romagnoli P, Cortesini C. Ileal mucosal morphology after total colectomy in man. *Histopathology* 1981;5:667–678.
166. Philipson B, Brandberg A, Jagenburg R, et al. Mucosal morphology, bacteriology, and absorption in intra-abdominal ileostomy reservoir. *Scand J Gastroenterol* 1975;10:145–153.
167. Shepherd NA, Jass JR, Duval I, et al. Restorative proctocolectomy with ileal reservoir: Pathological and histochemical study of mucosal biopsy specimens. *J Clin Pathol* 1987;40: 601–607.
168. Trier JS. Diagnostic value of peroral biopsy of the proximal small intestine. *N Engl J Med* 1971;285:1470–1473.
169. Brandborg LL, Rubin GE, Quinton WE. A multipurpose instrument for suction biopsy of the esophagus, stomach, small bowel, and colon. *Gastroenterology* 1959;37:1–16.
170. Achkar E, Carey WD, Petras R, et al. Comparison of suction capsule and endoscopic biopsy of small bowel mucosa. *Gastrointest Endosc* 1986;32:278–281.
171. Whitehead R. Mucosal biopsy of the gastrointestinal tract. In: Bennington JL, ed. *Major Problems in Pathology*. Vol 3. 3rd ed. Philadelphia, PA: WB Saunders; 1985.
172. Haggitt RC. Handling of gastrointestinal biopsies in the surgical pathology laboratory. *Lab Med* 1982;13:272–278.

24

Colon

Maria Westerhoff ■ Joel K. Greenson

EMBRYOLOGY 640	EFFECTS OF PREPARATION AND ARTIFACTS 654
ANATOMIC CONSIDERATIONS 641	Bowel Preparation Effects 654
FUNCTION 642	Incorrect Tissue Orientation and Tangential Sectioning 654
LIGHT MICROSCOPY 642	Tissue Trauma 655
Mucosa 642	ACKNOWLEDGMENTS 656
Submucosa 652	REFERENCES 656
Muscularis Externa, Subserosal Zone, and Serosa 653	

EMBRYOLOGY

The gastrointestinal tract is a remarkably complex organ system derived from a simple tubal structure composed of all three germ layers (endoderm, mesoderm, and ectoderm). The end result is a large and highly specialized organ that, albeit deep inside the body, interfaces constantly with the environment in more than just food absorption. Early in development, the gut is patterned into four asymmetrical axes—anterior–posterior (AP), dorsoventral (DV), left–right (LR), and radial (RAD). This is the result of critical developmental pathways directed by reciprocal mesodermal (mesenchymal) to endodermal (epithelial) cell–cell interactions and endodermal to endodermal cell–cell interactions (1–8). The fifth axis of embryologic development is the functional axis of developmental immunologic programming; it forms the intercellular and humoral environment for the colonization of the gastrointestinal tract by resident flora (9–11). Because gut epithelium is a constitutively developing tissue, that is, it is constantly differentiating from a stem cell in a progenitor pool throughout adult life, these pathways, axes of development, and cell–cell "cross talk" continue to be important in the adult intestinal epithelium (7,8,12–14).

Development and differentiation along the AP axis gives rise to the foregut, midgut, and hindgut, resulting in regionally specific differentiation from mouth to anus. The right colon: cecum, appendix, ascending colon, and proximal two-thirds of the transverse colon, arise from the midgut. The hindgut gives rise to the left colon: descending colon, sigmoid colon, and rectum (15,16). The significant variation in patterns of gene expression, physiologic function, disease distribution, and even histologic appearance between the right and left colon reflects the midgut and hindgut derivation (7,17–32).

The LR axis is manifested in the colon by characteristic turning and looping of the gut, resulting in portions of colon with varying mesentery and fixation within the abdominal cavity (15).

The fundamental axis maintained in the adult is the radial (crypt to surface) axis, which is dependent upon colonization of the large intestine by successive consortia of bacterial species to form the microbiome (the complete set of genes within the microbiotica) (10–12). Homeostasis of intestinal epithelium occurs throughout life along the radial axis, with the epithelial and mesenchymal progenitor/proliferative cells being deeper in the radial axis than the differentiated functional cells and the apoptotic cells that are more luminal (13,33–35). In other words, the proliferative zone of the colonic mucosa is in the bases of the crypts and apoptosis is not a normal finding in this area. On top of this are mucosa-associated bacteria within or adherent to the cells. The microbiome is critical for the normal structure, development, and optimal function of not only the large intestine, but also of the mucosal immune system (10,12,36,37). In fact, there are studies suggesting that even disrupted maternal gut microbiota can lead to altered infant gut development and resident microbiota, and subsequently can have consequences on future disease risks such as obesity (38).

This chapter is an update of a previous version authored by Julia Dahl and Joel K. Greenson.

Overall, once the primitive gut tube subdivides into fore-, mid-, and hindgut around the 4th developmental week, the midgut is at this stage midline in the embryo; however, it remains open to the yolk sac (39). Around the 6th week, the midgut is pushed out into the extraembryonic coelom as the growing liver is taking up space within the abdominal cavity as well. It is thought that the first rotation of the gut takes place at this time, with the small intestine to the right and the colon to the left. The umbilical (extraembryonic) portion of the gut then elongates, but the growth of the intra-abdominal portion is minimal, understandably due to the space occupied by the liver. The gut returns to the intra-abdominal position around the 10th week. Traditionally, it is thought that the small bowel enters first, followed by the cecum, but recent reports observe in animal studies that the ileal loops may actually be last to enter. There is then a 180-degree rotation causing the cecum to be placed into the right upper side of the abdomen. This is followed by the descent of the cecum into the right iliac fossa. In regards to hindgut, the descending colon becomes fixed and retroperitoneal when the mesentery fuses with the peritoneum of the left dorsal part of the abdominal wall (40). The sigmoid mesocolon, however, persists. The terminal aspect of the hindgut enters the cloaca (hence the anus is derived from both hindgut and the posterior part of the cloaca).

Abnormalities of any of the developmental pathways or along any axis during organogenesis may result in gross morphologic malformations. This includes diverticula, rotational malformations, atresias, duplications and aganglionic segments (15,16,41–45). Perturbations of developmental pathways used for organ homeostasis may result in metaplasias, polyposis syndromes, and malignant transformation (12,46–50). Recent studies have implicated the microbiome as being important in a vast array of diseases both within the gastrointestinal tract and systemically. The influence of the microbiome on drug toxicity, as well as irritable bowel syndrome, inflammatory bowel disease (IBD), allergy, and obesity is an area of emerging research (51–59). Interestingly, microbiota also play a role in gut motility by having an effect on the development of enteric glial cells and the enteric nervous system as a whole (60,61).

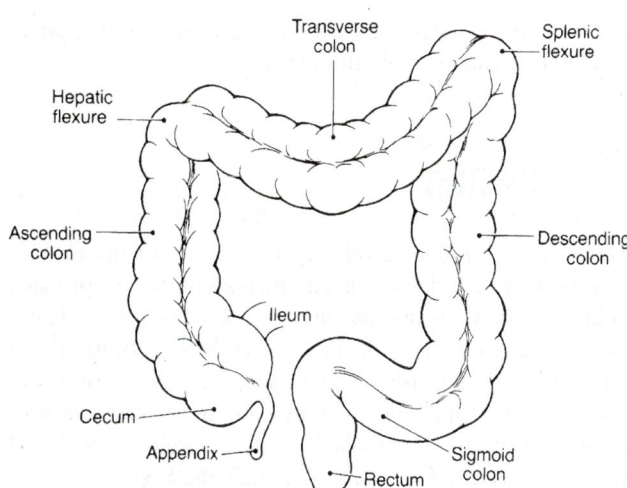

FIGURE 24.1 Major regions of the colon.

ANATOMIC CONSIDERATIONS

The colon is the terminal 1.0 to 1.5 m segment of the gastrointestinal tract, following the periphery of the abdominal peritoneal cavity, with the rectum extending into the pelvis and concluding at the anal canal (Fig. 24.1) (62,63). Typically, the cecum is entirely covered by peritoneum, while the ascending colon is retroperitoneal, with peritoneum on the lateral and anterior surfaces. The transverse colon has a mesentery and is completely surrounded by peritoneum. The descending colon is also retroperitoneal and thus lacks serosa on the posterior aspect. The sigmoid is intraperitoneal with a mesentery. The rectum is divided into thirds, with the upper having peritoneum on the anterior and lateral surfaces, middle third having peritoneum only on the anterior aspect, and the lower third having no peritoneal covering at all. There is considerable anatomic variation in the position of the colon segments, mesenteric coverings, and attachments to the posterior abdominal wall (63,64). Nonetheless, the vascular supply, venous drainage, and innervation pattern for the two primary (right and left) colon segments along the embryologic AP (midgut/hindgut) axis are consistent. The right colon receives its blood supply from the superior mesenteric artery, its parasympathetic nervous innervation from the vagus nerve, and sympathetic innervation from the superior mesenteric ganglia. The left colon receives its blood supply from the inferior mesenteric artery, parasympathetic innervation from sacral nerves S2, S3, and S4 through the nervi erigentes (pelvic splanchnic nerves); and sympathetic innervation from the inferior mesenteric ganglia. Venous drainage is predominantly portal. The rectum receives blood from the middle and inferior rectal arteries, parasympathetic innervation from the nervi erigentes, and sympathetic innervation through the hypogastric plexus through lumbar spinal segments L1, L2, and L3 (21,62–64).

Unique external features of the colon include the teniae coli and haustra, visible through the investing serosa and subserosal tissue. The muscular layers of the large intestine are composed of both longitudinally and circularly arranged fibers. The longitudinal fibers are present circumferentially through the length of the colon but are primarily concentrated into three flat bands called the teniae coli (62–64).

From the luminal perspective, various landmarks are recognized by the endoscopist. The cecum is readily identified by the ileocecal valve, the appendiceal orifice, and blind-ended, saclike appearance. The subjacent portal vasculature imparts a blue hue to the mucosa at the hepatic flexure. Orientation of the teniae coli within the transverse colon results in a T-shaped lumen, ending in a slitlike orifice and acute angle of the splenic flexure. Although the descending and sigmoid colon may have thickened mucosal folds and diverticular orifices, calibration marks on the colonoscope are more reliable means of approximating the location within this region.

FUNCTION

There have been considerable recent advancements characterizing the vast and interrelated functions of the two primary, unique colon segments: the right and left colon (17,21,65). Not only do they have distinct embryologic derivation, the right and left colon display segment-specific arrays of physiologic functions including motility patterns, commensal bacterial populations, metabolic activity, as well as local and systemic immune functions (17,23,25,26,28,31,32,66–71). These varied functions are reflected in differing patterns of gene, lectin, and surface marker expression, distributions of disease involvement, as well as the rates and sequences involved in neoplastic transformation (25,26,30,31,65). Subtle regional variations of the colonic mucosa as a result of the segmental nature of the right and left colon have been well recognized by gastrointestinal pathologists (17,22,24) and are described in the following sections.

In regards to its role in immunity, the intestinal mucosa is the largest immune organ of the body (11,69,72–75). The plasma cells within the mucosa represent 80% of the antibody-producing cells within the entire body and produce antibodies than any other part of the body (69,72,73,75). The process of antigen sampling (commensal bacterial and dietary antigens) across specialized regions of the colon results in "gut priming" and routinely confers protection from potential infection locally and in other mucosal tissues (systemic immunization) (36,37,41,52,54,76–83). At baseline, the gut immune system is highly activated in response to normal flora—the so-called physiologic inflammation—in which the intestinal microflora and the intestinal immunologic mechanisms influence each other locally and systemically, forming an interdependent mutualistic ecosystem, the balance of which is required for maintenance of health and prevention of disease (36,37,41,77,79,80,84,85).

Beginning at birth, or even possibly in utero, colonization of the human gut is characterized by a succession of microbial consortia, the composition of which is influenced by host genome, maternal factors prior to and during pregnancy, diet, and environmental exposures (10,11,12,54,57,69). There are an estimated 400 to 1,000 microbial species (bacteria, fungi, and a few protozoa) forming complex ecosystems from the terminal ileum to the rectum (54,57,69,70,86–89). The diversity of the microbiota varies from person to person, is considered relatively stable once adulthood is reached, but remains pliable to alteration via diet or disease (11,57,69). Bacterial cells outnumber human cells roughly 1,000:1, with highest concentration in the cecum and decreasing gradient and varying composition proceeding distally. Locally, the colonic epithelium and commensal flora serve as important barriers to infection via tight junctions and secretion of antimicrobial substances, as well as competition for nutrient substrates (74–77,90).

The colon participates in several integral metabolic processes that include absorption, secretion, fermentation, and oxidation unique to the colonic epithelium or in concert with the commensal bacteria. The commensal microbiota are integral in the formation of short-chain fatty acids, metabolic intermediates and vitamins, detoxification or biotransformation of bile acids, as well as phosphate and oxalate excretion (31,86,87,89,91–93). Fermentation of carbohydrates to form short-chain fatty acids, particularly butyrate, serves as a major source of energy for colonocytes, and butyrate plays a crucial role in colonocyte growth and differentiation (89,92,94–96). Nearly equal to the activity observed in the liver, colonocytes have the capacity to mediate biotransformation of bile salts, drugs, and xenobiotics (77,96). Many of these processes are segment-specific to either the right or the left colon.

The well-recognized function of the colon is absorption of water and storage of the feces, with a stool output of 200 to 500 g daily. The cecum receives 1.3 to 1.8 L of electrolyte-rich ileal effluent daily and is a high-capacity absorptive surface. It effectively absorbs 80% of the chylous water (and sodium ions, Na^+) during prolonged mucosal exposure to the luminal contents made possible by the retrograde peristalsis unique to the cecum (23,28,29,32). Bulk absorption of water and sodium occurs via electroneutral sodium chloride (NaCl) transport, which occurs at the surface and in the superficial portions of the crypts (23,32,97). Within the left colon, low-capacity electrogenic absorption via luminal sodium channels that are regulated by aldosterone and angiotensin, serve in further absorption of water from the fecal contents, as well as sodium preservation (23,32,98,99). Additionally, another mechanism for water absorption unique to the left colon has been observed; it involves the formation of a hyperosmolar (Na^+) compartment between the colonocytes and pericrypt myofibroblasts and may be vital in extracting water from the osmotically dense feces, allowing final stool compaction (29,72,73). Lubricating the increasingly dense feces with various mucins is an additional important function of the left mucosa.

LIGHT MICROSCOPY

The colon contains four histologically distinct compartments: (a) mucosa, (b) submucosa, (c) muscularis propria, and (d) serosa. The enteric nervous system spans all four compartments with ganglia and plexus in both the submucosa and muscularis propria extending processes throughout the lamina propria, submucosa, and muscular layers.

Mucosa

The luminal colonic mucosa is the most metabolically and immunologically active compartment of the colon. The luminal surface is covered by glycocalyx (glycans, enzymes, lectins, and mucin), facilitating formation of the commensal

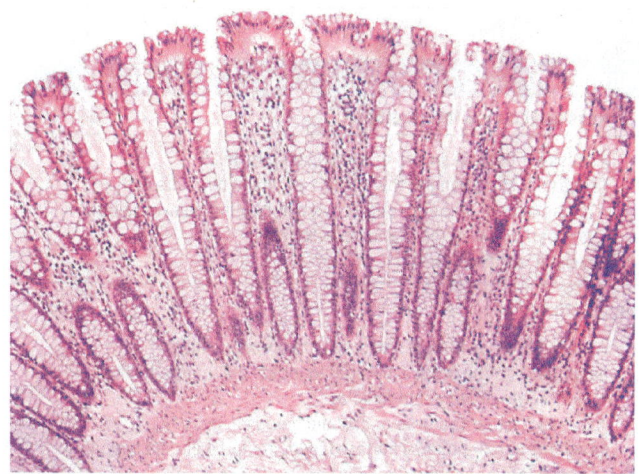

FIGURE 24.2 Normal colonic mucosa. The histologic section of this endoscopic mucosal biopsy specimen is oriented so the simple columnar surface epithelium facing the lumen is at the top of the figure and the cut surface of the specimen is at the bottom. The mucosal crypts are lined up in parallel, and they open to the lumen. The lamina propria consists of the stromal elements investing the crypts and extend from the surface epithelium to the smooth muscle cells of the muscularis mucosae at the bottom.

microbial ecosystem and serving as an integral barrier function (100–102). Beneath this, the columnar epithelium lines regularly spaced crypts that span the depth of the lamina propria. The crypts are aligned perpendicular to and extend to the muscularis mucosae, imparting the well-known "rack of test tubes" appearance (Fig. 24.2). Although some variation in space between crypts is expected in normal individuals, irregularly oriented or bifurcated crypts are considered abnormal (see Regional Variation in Histologic Features, below).

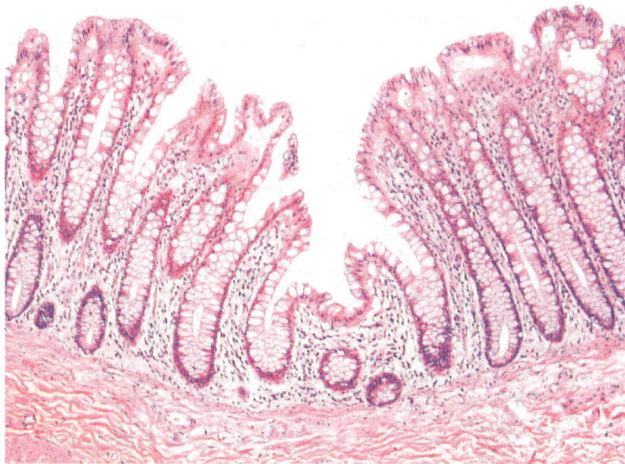

FIGURE 24.3 Innominate grooves of colonic mucosa. Multiple crypts open in a "mirror image" across a common crypt lumen at the groove, with the common crypt lumen opening to the colonic lumen. This normal finding is not a true branching of the crypts and should not be misinterpreted as architectural distortion indicative of chronic mucosal injury (i.e., inflammatory bowel disease). The innominate groove common lumen is generally within the superficial one-third of the mucosa.

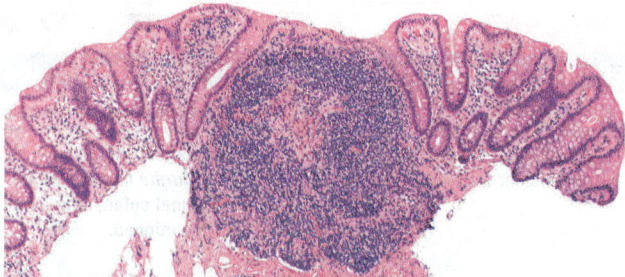

FIGURE 24.4 Colonic lymphoid aggregate. This lymphoid aggregate splays the adjacent crypts, which appear in a diagonal or near horizontal axis (rather than vertical), and mimics basal lymphoplasmacytosis at the crypt/lymphoid aggregate margin, resembling minor architectural disarray. Goblet cells are absent in the crypt epithelium adjacent to the follicle, while retained on the opposite side of the crypt. These normal features of colonic lymphoid aggregates should not be misinterpreted as architectural distortion indicative of chronic mucosal injury (i.e., inflammatory bowel disease) (see Table 24.2). These aggregates may contain well-formed germinal centers and appear as small polyps endoscopically.

There are regularly occurring folds in the mucosa; additional variations from the normal pattern of colonic mucosa are seen innominate grooves adjacent to lymphoid follicles, with lymphoglandular complexes, and with ridges created by muscularis mucosae contraction (Figs. 24.3 to 24.5). These normal variations must be distinguished from the histologic changes of chronic mucosal injury (as in IBD) (Table 24.1).

Advances in immunohistochemistry and development of new antibodies has allowed further classification of cell types, with utility in assessing both normal and pathologic histologic patterns and providing useful adjuncts to standard histochemical stains (Table 24.2) (75,103–143).

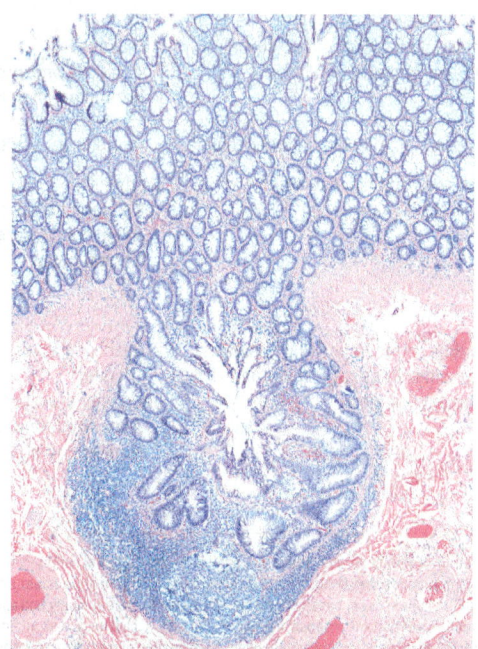

FIGURE 24.5 Lymphoglandular complex. Crypt epithelium is present within a lymphoid follicle that extends from the mucosa through the muscularis mucosae into the submucosa.

TABLE 24.1
Common Artifacts and Variants: A Guide to Evaluation and Interpretation

Histologic Feature	Common Misinterpretation	Keys to Accurate Interpretation
Mucosa with regular eosinophilic subnuclear material	Collagenous colitis **Accurate Interpretation:** Normal colon, tangentially sectioned.	Assess for other features of microscopic colitis.[a] Tangential sectioning of the surface epithelium results in the cytoplasm of adjacent enterocytes appearing below the basally aligned nuclei of "in plane" enterocytes. Levels or a trichrome stain.
Normal colon—histologic features seen in association with adjacent lymphoid aggregates or follicles:		
Focally increased surface intraepithelial lymphocytes with otherwise normal architecture.	Lymphocytic colitis **Accurate Interpretation:** Normal colon	Assess for other features of the microscopic colitides.[a] Level through the biopsy material to locate the adjacent lymphoid aggregate or lymphoid follicle.
Focal "architectural distortion" in association with numerous lamina propria mononuclear cells. Other biopsy fragments appear normal.	Nonspecific colitis IBD: Ulcerative colitis (UC), indeterminate colitis (IDC), Crohn disease **Accurate Interpretation:** Normal colon	Assess for other features of chronic mucosal injury.[b] Level through the biopsy material to locate the adjacent lymphoid aggregate or lymphoid follicle.
Normal colon—histologic features mimicking chronic colitis (IBD):		
Biopsy contains horizontal and unusually oriented crypts.	IBD (either UC or IDC). **Accurate Interpretation:** Normal colon	Biopsy material evulsed without the muscularis mucosae frequently contains unusually oriented crypts. Assess crypt morphology only in areas in which the muscularis mucosae is present, "tethering" the crypts. Examine other tissue fragments; levels when necessary. Assess for other features of chronic mucosal injury.[b]
Right (or ascending) colon biopsy with numerous lamina propria mononuclear cells	Nonspecific colitis IBD (either UC or IDC) **Accurate Interpretation:** Normal proximal (right) colon	Ensure site of biopsy Determine extent of mononuclear expansion, if any. The right colon contains significantly more lamina propria inflammatory cells than the left colon. Assess for other features of chronic mucosal injury.[b]
Deeply eosinophilic granular cells at the base of crypts in the right colon (Paneth cells), could this mean chronic mucosal injury?	Nonspecific colitis UC, IDC, or Crohn's **Accurate Interpretation:** Normal colon	Assess for other features of chronic mucosal injury.[b] Endocrine cells have apical (luminal) nuclei and fine basal granules and are normal throughout the colon. Paneth cells have basal nuclei; coarse luminal granules are normal in the right colon and pathologic in the left.
Bifurcated crypts in sigmoid colon and/or rectum, without other findings	Inactive IBD **Accurate Interpretation:** Normal colon or rectum	One to two bifurcated crypts within the sigmoid colon or rectum is acceptable. Assess for other features of chronic mucosal injury.[b]
Normal colon—histologic features commonly encountered resulting from bowel preparation effects:		
Widely spaced crypts, without other findings	Edema Nonspecific colitis **Accurate Interpretation:** Normal colon	Water content/edema is not a reproducible finding. Review clinical history for type of bowel preparation, sodium phosphate enemas frequently cause edema. Ensure biopsy fragment contains muscularis mucosa. If other features suggest (i.e., lamina propria pallor [reduced mononuclear cells] and crypt distortion), consider treated IBD.
Basal and/or surface epithelial apoptosis with or without reactive-appearing surface enterocytes.	Resolving acute self-limited colitis Antibiotic-associated colitis **Accurate Interpretation:** Normal colon	Review the clinical history to determine bowel preparation used (oral sodium phosphate frequently causes basal apoptosis, while sodium phosphate enemas may cause surface or basal apoptosis bowel preparation effect). Alert clinical colleagues that sodium phosphate causes bowel preparation effect and is ill advised in the evaluation of diarrhea or GVHD patients.

[a]Histologic features of microscopic colitis: (a) increased intraepithelial lymphocytes; (b) accompanying damage to surface epithelium (reactive appearance, epithelial sloughing); (c) superficially dense mononuclear inflammatory infiltrate; and with or without (d) thickening or irregularity of the subepithelial basement membrane collagen table (usually entraps superficial capillaries).
[b]Histologic features of chronic mucosal injury (chronic colitis, also known as inflammatory bowel disease, or IBD): (a) mononuclear expansion of lamina propria, displacing crypts and resulting in (b) basal plasmacytosis; (c) crypt architectural distortion (bifurcated or irregularly oriented crypts; crypt "dropout"); and (d) Paneth cell (left colon only) or pyloric metaplasia.
GVHD, graft-versus-host disease; IBD, inflammatory bowel disease; IDC, indeterminate colitis; UC, ulcerative colitis.

TABLE 24.2
Predominant Immunohistochemical and Histochemical Staining Patterns of Many of the Normal Cell Types Present in the Human Colon (54,88–128)

Cell Type	Immunohistochemical Profile Positive	Negative	Histochemical Stain
Colonic enterocyte	CK20, pCEA, mCEA, villin, Cdx2, AE1/AE3, SATB2	CK7, EGFR (extremely low expression)	AB2.5—patchy apical blush
Goblet cell (S, surface; C, crypts)	MUC1 (S/C), MUC2 (S/C), MUC3 (S), MUC4 (S/C), MUC5B (C), MUC11 (S/C), MUC12 (S/C)	MUC3 (C), MUC5A (S/C), MUC5B (S)	+AB2.5, mucicarmine, PAS, PAS-D
Enteroendocrine cell	Chromo-A, Chromo-B, synaptophysin, NSE, specific peptides; AE1/AE3	—	Grimelius
Paneth cell	HL-5, HL-6 (R); AE1/AE3	—	Autofluorescent with eosin
M cell	No known definitive differentiating stains	—	No known definitive differentiating stains
Intraepithelial lymphocytes (surface)	CD3 TCRαβ, CD3 TCRγδ	CD10, CD43, CD138	—
Intraepithelial lymphocytes (M cell)	CD3, CD45 RO, CD45 RA (rare), CD20 (rare)	CD138	—
Lymphoid aggregate (follicle center)	CD19, CD20, CD10, CD68, occasional CD20, occasional S100, scattered CD45 RO/CD3	Bcl-2	—
Lymphoid aggregate (periphery/paracortex)	CD3, CD5, CD20 (rare), S100 (IDC, occasional)	CD138	—
LP plasma cells	CD79a, CD138	CD20, CD3, CD123	—
LP lymphocytes	CD3 (CD4+/CD8+ varying ratio) CD5 (occasional)	Keratin, S100	—
Eosinophils	CD15	—	Autofluorescent with eosin
Mast cells	Tryptase, CD117 (c-kit)	CD34	Giemsa, toluidine blue
Macrophages	CD68, HAM56, MAC387, lysozyme, α1 anti-trypsin	LCA, keratin	Iron (hemosiderin and anthracene pigment of melanosis coli)
Dendritic macrophages	CD11b (subepithelial dome), CD123	α-SMA, keratin	—
Muciphages	CD68, HAM56	—	AB2.5; PAS-D
Pericrypt myofibroblasts	Vimentin, HHF35, SMMHC, α-SMA	Desmin	MT–mixed blue and red
Subepithelial myofibroblasts	Vimentin, α-SMA	Desmin	MT–mixed blue and red
Basement membrane	Collagen IV, tenascin (minimal)	Tenascin (thick)	MT–blue; saffron–deep red; eosin–autofluorescence
Muscularis mucosa	Vimentin, HHF35, α-SMA, desmin	—	MT–red
Arterioles, capillaries, veins	*Luminal:* CD31, CD34, vimentin, vWF, factor XIII *Wall:* α-SMA	α-SMA, HHF-35	MT–red; elastin
Lymphatic vessels	CD34, vimentin, D2-40 (R)®	vWF	MT–red
Enteric glia and ganglia	Synaptophysin, PDGFR-α(R), NSE	α-SMA	—
Schwann cells	S100, vimentin	α-SMA	—
Interstitial cells of Cajal	CD34, CD117 (c-kit)	S100, CD31	—
Submucosal adipose	S100	—	Oil red O
SM lymphocytes	CD3, scattered CD138 plasma cells	—	—
Muscularis propria	α-SMA, desmin, vimentin	—	MT–deep red
Serosal mesothelium	Calretinin, vimentin, AE1/AE3, CK7	pCEA	—

—, no information; AB2.5, Alcian blue 2.5; AE1/AE3, pan-cytokeratin; C, crypts; Chromo-A, chromogranin A; Chromo-B, chromogranin B; CK20, cytokeratin 20; DGFR, epidermal growth factor; IDC, interdigitating dendritic cells; LCA, leukocyte common antigen; LP, lamina propria; mCEA, monoclonal carcinoembryonic antigen; MT, Masson trichrome; MUC, mucin gene; NSE, neuron-specific enolase; PAS, periodic acid–Schiff; PAS-D, periodic acid–Schiff with diastase digestion; pCEA, polyclonal carcinoembryonic antigen; PDGFR-α(R), platelet-derived growth factor receptor alpha; R, research; S, surface; SM, submucosa; SMMHC, smooth muscle myosin heavy chain; vWF, von Willebrand factor.

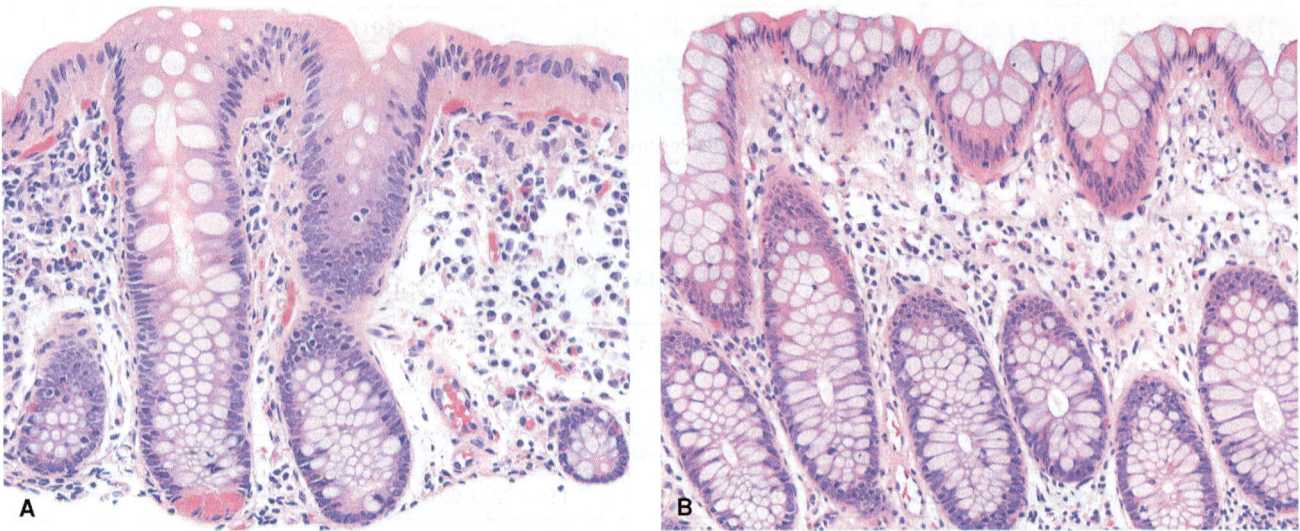

FIGURE 24.6 Normal mucosa from the cecum (**A**) and rectum (**B**). **A:** The mucosa in the cecum has more absorptive cells and fewer goblet cells compared to the rectum. The lamina propria is more cellular, with greater density of plasma cells, eosinophils, and lymphoid aggregates in the cecum as compared to the rectum. Paneth cells are normally present, residing at the base of the crypts. **B:** The rectal mucosa has a higher ratio of goblet cells to absorptive cells, with a less dense lamina propria and more easily identified muciphages. Paneth cells are not normally seen within the rectum.

Regional Variation in Histologic Features

Although the overall mucosal architecture as described above is maintained, the right and left colon do display important histologic differences. This includes where the presence of Paneth cells are considered normal and the density of lamina propria mononuclear cells as will be described below (Fig. 24.6). These differences make it essential to dissuade our clinical colleagues from pooling biopsies and simply labeling them *colon*. We encourage gastroenterologists and surgeons to uniformly separate and appropriately label biopsy material from the right and left colon, whether it be for evaluation of diarrhea or classification of polyps; this is because the range of what is considered "normal" differs significantly depending on location (17,22,24) and neoplastic sequence and progression varies within the right and left colon (21,30,119).

Reflecting a dominant function in absorption and antigen processing, the right colon displays a higher absorptive cell (colonocyte) to goblet cell ratio (roughly 5:1) as compared to the left colon (Fig. 24.6). Proceeding distally, an increase in goblet cells is apparent, with a ratio of 3 or 4:1 for colonocyte to goblet cell. This reflects the increased formation of mucin in the descending and sigmoid colon necessary for consolidation and transit of stool (17,28,29,144). Paneth cells are normally present at the base of crypts within the midgut-derived right colon; however, importantly they are indicative of metaplasia secondary to chronic mucosal injury starting from the distal one-third of the transverse colon (Fig. 24.6).

Surface intraepithelial lymphocytes (IELs) are seen in greater concentrations in the right colon than the left and can be particularly marked overlying lymphoid aggregates (22,24,145–147). Similarly, lamina propria mononuclear cell density is also greater in the right colon than the left (descending and sigmoid colon), as are organized lymphoid aggregates, possibly related to the higher concentration of commensal microorganisms and resultant antigen sampling activities (24). Distally, as goblet cell concentration and mucin increases, lamina propria macrophages that are specifically scavenging mucin (muciphages) are increasingly observed. In the sigmoid colon and rectum, most gastrointestinal pathologists will accept a few bifurcated crypts as being within the range of normal (22), although this has not been systematically studied nor reported.

Epithelium

The colonic mucosa is composed of a single layer of columnar cells making test tube–like invaginations to form millions of crypts (28,148). These are invested in basement membrane, surrounded by lamina propria (22,145,147), and separated from the submucosa by the muscularis mucosae.

The mucosal crypt architecture shows remarkable consistency despite the high epithelial turnover rate and variety of specialized cell types (149,150). Mucosal renewal is generally attributed to stem cells located near the base of the intestinal crypts and maintained within a mesenchymal niche (15,33,34,148,149,151–154). Multipotent stem cells divide and give rise to a transient population of progenitor cells in this maturation process that starts from the base of the crypt and toward the luminal surface (33,148,154). The granule-containing epithelial cell types appear to ignore the direction of luminal migration during maturation; that is, Paneth cells migrate down toward the crypt base and enteroendocrine cells home toward the mid and deeper regions of the crypts (Fig. 24.7) (15,17,157).

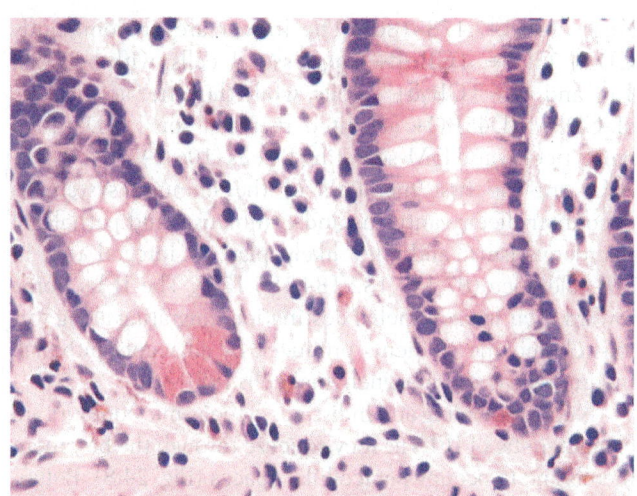

FIGURE 24.7 Normal right colon with Paneth cells and an endocrine cell. Within the crypt on the left are three Paneth cells at the base of the crypt. Note the basal nucleus and coarse, luminal-facing granules that empty into the crypt lumen. Within the crypt on the right is an endocrine cell at the base of the crypt. The endocrine cell is smaller, has a luminal nucleus and fine, basally facing granules that empty into the pericrypt myofibroblast sheath and adjacent vasculature.

During migration toward the luminal surface, dividing transit cells commit and differentiate to one of five distinct epithelial cell types: absorptive colonocyte, mucus-secreting goblet cell, enteroendocrine cell, Paneth cell, or M cell. At any given time, 75% to 80% of all colonocytes are associated with the crypts, and only 10% to 15% of colonocytes form the surface epithelium (intercrypt table) (146,150). Epithelial cell turnover is brisk; besides stem cells, most cells are replaced within a week.

> **ABSORPTIVE COLONOCYTES** Absorptive colonocytes compose the majority of the surface epithelium (100,102,158). The luminal surface is characterized by rigid, tightly packed apical microvilli (15,150), the tips of which contain integral membrane mucinlike glycoproteins that form a brush border glycocalyx (159) visible as a striate luminal border. Absorptive colonocyte cytoplasm is lightly eosinophilic, with small apical vesicles containing mucin (of different composition than goblet cell mucin) positioned for luminal release (23,82,109,119). The apical poles of columnar cells fan out over the "flask" of the goblet cells, such that only the apexes of goblet cells contact the lumen (150). Basally aligned colonocyte nuclei are oval, uniformly sized, and aligned with the long axis parallel to the long axes of the cells.

> **GOBLET CELLS** Goblet cells are dispersed throughout the surface epithelium and crypts. Although their "wine goblet" shape makes them distinctive and appear numerous, they are outnumbered by absorptive colonocytes. The large number of mucous granules takes up most of the cytoplasm and the nucleus is depressed at the base of the cell. Mucin composition varies regionally along the length of the colon due to differential synthesis of the several known secreted and membrane-bound mucins (17). This variation is reflected in the differential histochemical staining patterns commonly observed (119,160,161). Goblet cell cytoplasm is relatively clear with standard hematoxylin and eosin (H&E) stains; however, mucin granules become distinct with mucicarmine, Alcian blue pH 2.5, and periodic acid–Schiff stains (17). Goblet cell nuclei, when compared to adjacent absorptive colonocytes, appear hyperchromatic, dense, and irregular (150).

> **ENDOCRINE CELLS** Endocrine cells within the gut epithelium represent the largest population of hormone-producing cells in the body (148,157,162,163), comprising approximately 1% of the individual cells lining the intestinal lumen, predominantly located in the crypts and, rarely, scattered within the lamina propria (15,17,30,142,150,162,164,165). More than 30 peptide hormone genes are known to be expressed throughout the digestive tract, in a regionally and spatially distinct pattern (162,166). Enteroendocrine cells contain basally oriented, small, but distinct, deeply eosinophilic granules (157,162). The round, smoothly contoured nuclei of enteroendocrine cells are pushed towards the lumen, with opposite polarity to the other epithelial cell types (Fig. 24.7). This opposite nuclear polarity can be a useful feature; for example, enteroendocrine [amine precursor uptake decarboxylase] can be mistaken for Paneth cells due to their eosinophilic granules. The luminal, rather than basal, location of the APUD cell nuclei is one feature that helps distinguish them from Paneth cells.

Enteroendocrine cells may be further identified by their histochemical silver staining properties and may also be identified immunohistochemically with varying immunoreactivity to chromogranin A, synaptophysin, neuron-specific enolase, and specific antibodies to the putative peptide hormone of the cell or cell proliferation (i.e., carcinoid tumor) (Table 24.1).

> **PANETH CELLS** Paneth cells disregard the rule of luminal migration; they are normally encountered at the base of the crypts within the midgut-derived right colon (15,74,134,148,155). Hence, they are not a sign of chronic injury when present in the cecum, ascending colon, and proximal two-thirds of the transverse colon. Nevertheless, it has been reported that Paneth cells can be present in the rectum of the pediatric population without being associated with IBD (167). These pyramidal-shaped cells have basally aligned oval nuclei and apical coarse, densely eosinophilic cytoplasmic granules (Figs. 24.6B and 24.7) (15,74). Granule and cellular contents include: α-defensins, β-defensins, NOD2, lysozyme, phospholipase A2, secretory leukocyte inhibitor, monomer IgA, TNF-α, heavy metal ions, zinc-binding protein, trypsin and trypsinogen, EGF, osteopontin, FAS ligand (CD95L), CD44v6, CD15, REG protein, and numerous others (74,148,155,168,169). The diverse Paneth cell contents reflect their significant role in innate immunity. Additionally putative roles in regulation of cell matrix interactions, apoptosis, and cellular immunity, as well as stem-cell niche maintenance, have been proposed (74,148,155,168,170).

In addition to characteristic granule staining with H&E stains, granules are conspicuously stained by periodic acid–Schiff, and phloxine-tartrazine (74); and, interestingly, Paneth cell autofluorescence is elicited by eosin stain (Table 24.2) (134).

M Cells and Follicle-Associated Epithelium

Membranous (M) cells occur in the dome region of organized lymphoid follicles. They are associated with both the immunologic cells and variants of absorptive colonocytes (the follicle-associated epithelium) unique to the dome region (88,146,148,171,172). Estimates of M cells in human colon vary widely, reported from "rare" to approximately 10% of surface epithelial cells (146,172–176). Light microscopy has insufficient magnification to distinguish the unique features of M cells. On electron microscopy, they show reduced and irregular microvilli, apical microfolds, absence of thick brush borders, and the presence of a cell surface–amplifying basolateral membrane subdomain that also forms an intraepithelial pocket. The M-cell intraepithelial pocket provides a docking site for special populations of intraepithelial B and T lymphocytes and immediately overlies the dome region of lymphoid follicles (146,171–174). These unique features provide openings in the epithelial barrier through which M cells sample the contents of the lumen and transfer antigens to antigen-presenting cells via a specialized method of transcytosis (76,80,171,177). The follicle-associated crypts contain few or no goblet cells, enteroendocrine cells or Paneth cells (173,175). These closely apposed columnar enterocytes may mimic features of adenoma, particularly with distortion of the crypt architecture generally produced by the adjacent lymphoid aggregate.

Intraepithelial Inflammatory Cells

IELs occur in two compartments: within the paracellular spaces of the colonocytes. They are in highest density near lymphoid aggregates within M-cell pockets (Fig. 24.8), hence, lymphocytic colitis should not be diagnosed based on these areas (145,147,178–180). The former are predominantly CD3+, CD8+, TCRαβ+ suppressor T cells, with between 15% and 40% TCRγδ+ T cells, while the latter are mixture of CD3+/CD45RO+ activated memory, some CD45RA+ naive T cells, and IgM-secreting B cells (106,147,181–183). IELs are the first members of the immune system to encounter dietary antigens and commensal and pathologic microorganisms, and they likely play an integral role in oral tolerance (87,179,182,184,185,177). The IELs home toward their intraepithelial destination, migrating along various chemokine gradients produced by adjacent epithelial, inflammatory, and mesenchymal cells (88,186).

Nuclear molding and indistinct cytoplasmic contours are characteristic of IELs as they squeeze through the basement membrane to occupy paracellular spaces (Fig. 24.8). Retention of the classic lymphocyte with its round nucleus and thin rim of cytoplasm is more common in IELs overlying aggregates. Normal IEL density ranges from 1 to 5 lymphocytes per 100 colonocytes, except in follicle-associated epithelium, where M-cell–associated IELs are normally abundant (183). In general, 20 or greater lymphocytes per 100 colonocytes are considered pathologic (82,145,147,187). The number of IELs decreases from the ascending colon to rectum, with highest concentration in the lymphoid aggregate and commensal bacteria–rich cecum (145,146). This is why it is imperative to ascertain the site of each colon biopsy to avoid misinterpreting the normal IEL density in right colon biopsies as lymphocytic colitis (Table 24.2).

Intraepithelial eosinophils may occasionally be seen in the normal colon, although at much lower numbers than lymphocytes (187–189). In general, ascending colon epithelium can have more eosinophils in the epithelium than descending colon. Several studies mention that normal colons do not have aggregates of eosinophils within the colonic crypts (eosinophilic crypt abscesses) and that infiltration of eosinophils into the surface epithelium is rare (190,191).

Stem and Dividing Transit Cells

It is estimated that between four and six stem cells are present per crypt. In addition, some dividing transit cells are apparently able to be "recruited" to serve as stem cells following injury with stem cell loss (33). These proliferative and undifferentiated cells are morphologically indistinct; however, they appear to have a large nucleus with diffuse chromatin and scant cytoplasm with few small organelles (15,148). Mitotic activity is frequently encountered in the basal one-fifth of the crypt, and apoptosis may rarely also be seen (149,151,154).

Apoptosis

The epithelial cells of the colon have remarkably short life spans (Table 24.3), during which they mature, migrate, and function (15,23,35,67,151,154,192). Programmed cell death (apoptosis) is the conclusion of the normal process of colonocyte turnover. It is recognizable histologically by apoptotic bodies predominantly in the surface epithelium, where they are generally found in the basal aspect of the epithelium

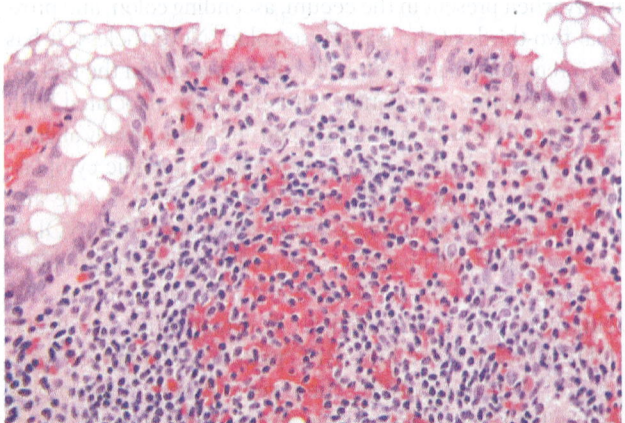

FIGURE 24.8 Intraepithelial lymphocytes (IELs) overlying a lymphoid follicle. Large numbers of IELs are typically seen overlying lymphoid aggregates. This should not be misinterpreted as lymphocytic colitis.

TABLE 24.3
The Life Span of the Various Colon Epithelial Cells and Number of Replacements Per Average Human Life Span Vary Between Cell Types. Despite the High Rate of Turnover, Preservation of Genetic Information is the Rule Rather Than the Exception

Cell Type	Life Span	Number of Replacements/Life
Absorptive Colonocyte	4–8 days	3,285–6,570
Goblet Cell	3–4 days	6,570–8,760
Enteroendocrine Cell	10–15 days	1,750–2,630
Paneth Cell	20 days	1,300
M Cell	Unknown	Unknown
Stem Cell Lineage/Niche	8.2 years	9–10

near the basement membrane (Fig. 24.9). Apoptotic bodies consist of vacuoles containing pyknotic nuclear debris surrounded by free space (25,152,154,193–200). Lamina propria inflammatory cells similarly undergo apoptosis, but this is frequently overlooked histologically (195,201,202). Sodium phosphate bowel preparations transiently increase the rate of apoptosis (see Bowel Preparation Effects, below); similar effects are seen with other physical and chemical agents. Increased apoptosis (both surface and/or crypt) may also be seen in several disease states, including graft-versus-host disease, autoimmune enteropathies, systemic autoimmune disorders, and with certain medications (79,203,204). Altered apoptosis (increased, decreased, and abnormal localization) is seen in neoplastic progression (205).

Basement Membrane

In well-oriented sections, the normal basement membrane is between 3 and 5 μm thick, regular, and stains with connective tissue stains (Masson trichrome, saffron, eosin von Gieson elastin) (Fig. 24.10) (206,207). Basement membrane thickness greater than 10 mm is considered pathologic, particularly also if there is entrapment of superficial lamina propria capillaries (135,206).

The basement membrane complex anchors the various epithelial cells to the underlying myofibroblast network and lamina propria. This fenestrated extracellular support matrix is produced collaboratively by epithelial and mesenchymal cells (118,146,149,208). In addition to allowing IELs to traverse the basement membrane, the fenestrations allow epithelial, mesenchymal, and dendritic cell processes to sample and/or present antigens. They also have functional implications in water and ion transport (23,34,149).

Lamina Propria

The lamina propria invests the colonic crypts, extending from the fenestrated basement membrane complex to the muscularis mucosae. The various lamina propria inflammatory and mesenchymal cells each perform integral immunologic, metabolic, and proliferative, functions.

> **LAMINA PROPRIA INFLAMMATORY CELLS** The lamina propria houses localized antigen-sampling and processing factories. This includes over 30,000 discrete lymphoid aggregates, with highest concentration within the cecum and distributed along the length of the colon (209,210). In addition to lymphoid aggregates, the normal colonic lamina propria contains mature B lymphocytes, plasma cells, T lymphocytes, eosinophils, mast cells, and macrophages, filling between 30% and 50% of the "free" lamina propria space (24). T cells include helper, suppressor, and lymphokine-activated killer (LAK) cells, but natural killer (NK) cells are unlikely to be encountered. Normally, there is a decreasing inflammatory cell gradient from lumen to muscularis mucosae; there are more inflammatory cells near the luminal surface and less as one gets deeper near the muscularis

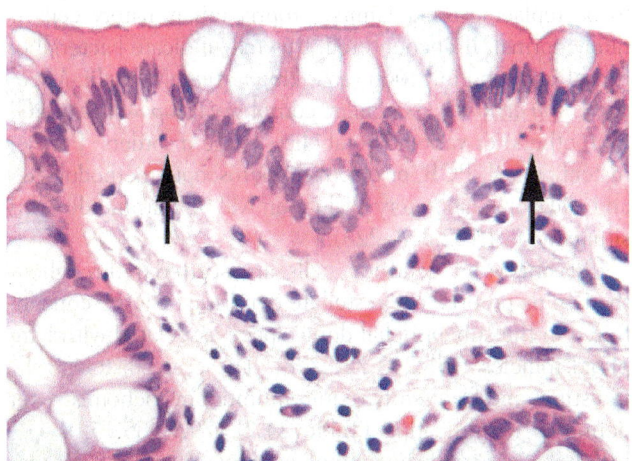

FIGURE 24.9 Apoptosis. Two apoptotic bodies are seen within the surface epithelium (*arrows*).

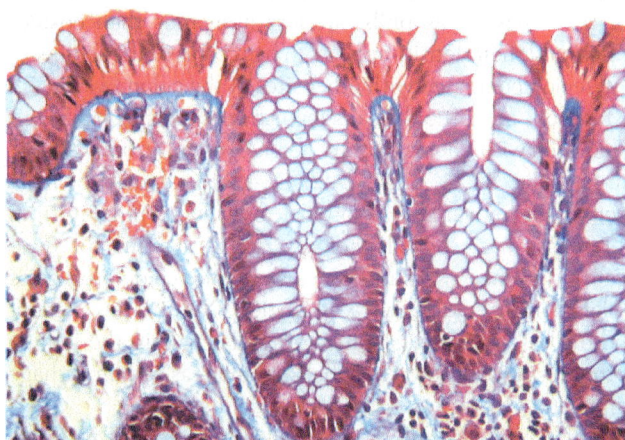

FIGURE 24.10 Normal basement membrane. The normal basement membrane is 3 to 5 μm thick and has a crisp, delicate, and regular lower border; it blends into the crypt sheath imperceptibly (trichrome stain).

mucosa. The lamina propria loose connective tissue in turn is obscured by the density of inflammatory cells near the luminal aspect of the mucosa, but becomes visible approaching the muscularis mucosa due to less occupation by inflammatory cells in the deep lamina propria (211). The predominant cell type of the lamina propria is the IgA-secreting plasma cell, with much smaller proportions of IgM-, IgE-, and IgG-secreting plasma cells also present (201,212). Secreted IgA and IgM are transported luminally, providing humoral immune protection (158,201,212). The distinct "cartwheel" nucleus, perinuclear Golgi zone, and amphophilic cytoplasm characteristic of plasma cells observed in other tissues are retained in colonic plasma cells. Of the remaining lamina propria lymphocytes, more than 90% of the lymphocytes were CD3+ T cells, with fewer than 50% also CD8+ (146,147,180). There are also CD20-positive B lymphocytes present within and adjacent to lymphoid follicles (80,85,158,213,209).

Myeloid cells that normally reside in the lamina propria include eosinophils and mast cells. In the normal colon, the number of eosinophils is highly variable, dependent upon both the region of colon sampled (187–189,192,193,214) and the geographic residence of the patient (215). A range of normal eosinophil counts in the lamina propria has been reported as 0 to 8 per high-power field (hpf); however, the eosinophil concentration should be interpreted on the basis of the "company it keeps" (i.e., other features of colitis vs. otherwise normal) (209). Higher mean eosinophil concentration is seen in biopsies of patients from the southern United States, compared to the northern United States, with a rather extreme degree of variability (215). Although eosinophils are increased in parasitic and allergic disease, collagenous colitis, ulcerative colitis, Crohn disease, and other pathologic conditions, consideration of the geographic residence and site of biopsy are integral before considering increased eosinophils (as an isolated histologic finding) to be pathologic (189,215). As expected, eosinophils are generally more numerous in the lamina propria of the ascending colon compared to that of the descending colon (190). Mast cells, or tissue-based basophils, are less numerous than eosinophils, and their density appears to be increased in the ileocecal region compared with other sites of the colon (216,217). Mast cells are difficult to distinguish with routine H&E, but stain well with Giemsa, toluidine blue, tryptase, and CD117 (c-kit) (Fig. 24.11, Table 24.2) (214). The density of mast cells is highly variable in normal individuals, ranging from 11 to 55 in an hpf. Therefore, routine staining for mast cells is not necessary in normal-appearing colonic biopsies taken for chronic diarrhea evaluation. Neutrophils are not normally seen in any significant number within the lamina propria, although they may be seen in areas of hemorrhage and within blood vessels (218).

Macrophages are commonly seen scattered throughout the lamina propria and are occasionally concentrated at the basal aspect of the crypts (79,219–222) (Fig. 24.12). While macrophages are generally difficult to see with H&E,

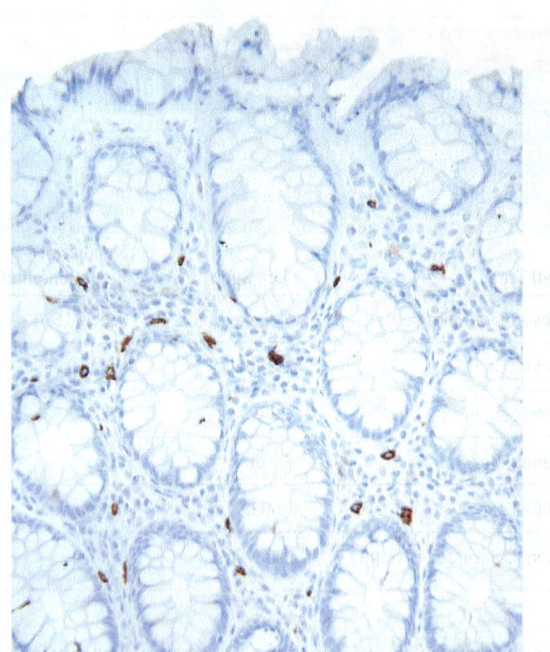

FIGURE 24.11 Mucosal mast cells. Although difficult to discern on H&E-stained sections, mucosal mast cells are easily identified with CD117. Mucosal mast cells serve well as an internal control when evaluating CD117 stains of gastrointestinal tract mesenchymal tumors. (Anti-CD117 stain.)

visualization may be enhanced by specific histochemical stains that detect the variety of materials they scavenge and store: apoptotic debris, microbes, lipofuscin, cholesterol esters, gangliosides, mucolipids, glycogen, mucopolysaccharides, and others (Fig. 24.12, Table 24.2) (220,221). Muciphages are the most commonly recognized macrophages. They ingest mucin that has exuded from adjacent goblet cells (and to a lesser extent enterocytes). As normal constituents of the lamina propria, muciphages have increased concentration within the left colon, in keeping with the increased number of goblet cells present in this location. Distention of the lamina propria by muciphages to the point that they appear to be replacing other lamina propria inflammatory cells is rarely normal. If encountered, this may indicate bacterial or fungal ingestion/infection (e.g., *Tropheryma whippelii*, *Mycobacterium avium-intracellulare* complex, *Histoplasma capsulatum*, others) or various metabolic storage disorders. Further histochemical, PCR, or electron microscopic methodologies and additional laboratory evaluation will be warranted in this situation (114,122,223–226).

Plasmacytoid dendritic cells are scattered throughout the lamina propria, while stellate dendritic cells are concentrated in the subepithelial dome space associated with lymphoid follicles (158,213,227,228). These are histologically indistinct and frequently require immunohistochemistry for definitive identification (Table 24.2) (79,90,85,158). The former have recently been implicated in allergic and autoimmune disorders (108), while the latter are integral in antigen presentation (79,82,229).

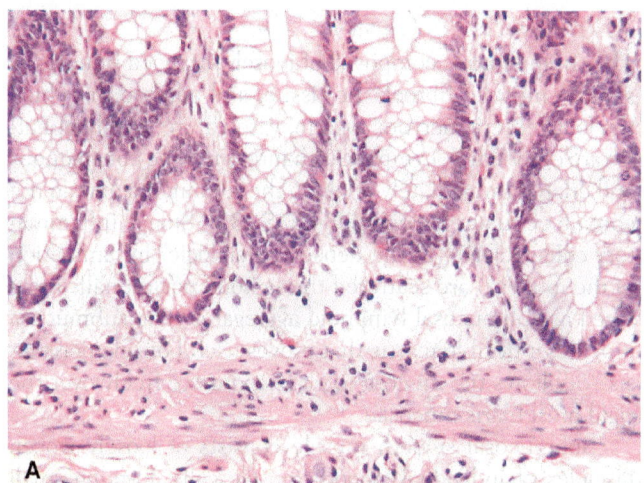 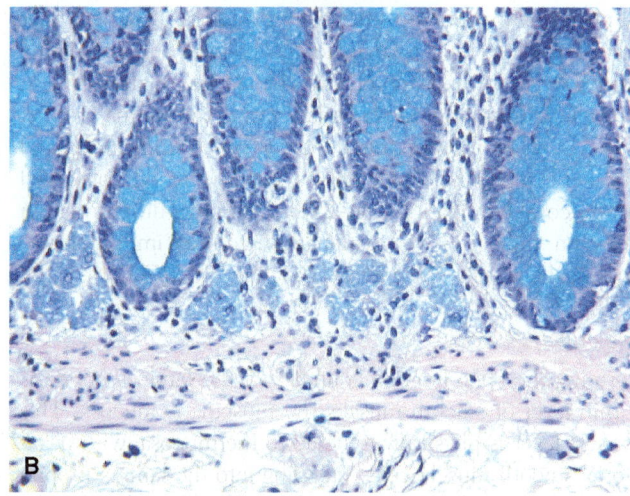

FIGURE 24.12 Lamina propria muciphages. **A:** These pale macrophages at the base of the mucosa are stuffed with mucins. This finding is not infrequent and does not generally correlate with disease. **B:** The same area stained with Alcian blue pH 2.5; the muciphages show strong cytoplasmic staining. Similar findings are seen with PAS with diastase digestion. Of note, bacteria-laden macrophages in Whipple disease are generally negative when stained with Alcian blue pH 2.5 but densely stain with PAS with diastase.

Myofibroblasts (Pericrypt Myofibroblast Sheath and Lamina Propria Myofibroblasts)

The lamina propria contains two distinct populations of myofibroblasts: the pericrypt myofibroblast sheath and the subepithelial myofibroblast (SEM) syncytia. Interacting closely with the epithelium, lamina propria inflammatory cells, and the muscularis mucosa, myofibroblasts function in absorption, ion and mucin secretion, immune regulation, and differentiation (maintenance of stem cell niche) (5,23,144,230). The rim of fusiform cells organized in close apposition to each colonic crypt was originally designated the pericryptal fibroblastic sheath (Fig. 24.13) (208,230). This specialized population of mesenchymal cells is now known to be a syncytium (both anatomically and functionally) of cells that surrounds the crypts and extends into the lamina propria, forming a reticular network within the extracellular matrix, attaching to one another with both gap and adherens junctions (103,112,208,230,231), and displaying distinct immunophenotypes (Table 24.2).

In the region of the crypts, the myofibroblasts are oval and scaphoid and appear to overlap like shingles on a roof. The SEMs exist in two distinct morphologic states: (a) the activated myofibroblast and (b) the stellate-transformed myofibroblast (208,230). Myofibroblasts often are surrounded by an incomplete basal lamina and embedded in a subepithelial sheet of reticular fibers that also contains fenestrae through which lymphocytes and macrophages traverse. Gap junctions couple some myofibroblasts to the tissue smooth muscle, and the cells are commonly in close apposition to terminals of nerve fibers; however, it has not been determined whether the interstitial cell of Cajal (ICC) network is physically connected to the SEM network (208,230,232).

Vasculature and Lymphatics in the Lamina Propria

Capillaries and high endothelial venules are scattered throughout the lamina propria, as well as lymphatic channels that are immediately superficial to the muscularis mucosa (233,234). Capillaries are composed of a circumferential endothelial lining and may contain red blood cells, as well as inflammatory cells. Irregularly shaped, distorted, and engorged capillaries frequently indicate prolapse of the mucosa. In addition

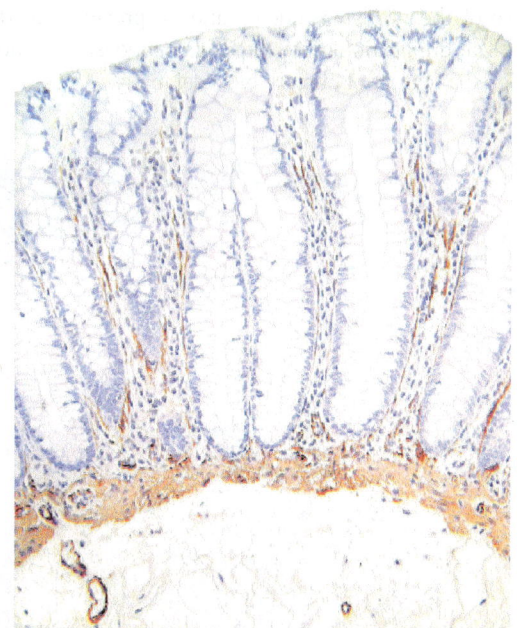

FIGURE 24.13 Lamina propria myofibroblasts, antimuscle-specific actin (MSA) stain. This stain for muscle-specific actin highlights the pericryptal myofibroblast sheath, muscularis mucosae, and submucosal blood vessels.

to providing oxygen and nutrients to mucosal cells, vascular adhesion molecules participate in "homing" of circulating lymphocytes to their appropriate colonic microenvironment. Lymphatic tributaries rarely initiate within the lamina propria; however, when present, they appear to have thinner walls and cross the muscularis mucosae to join the readily observed submucosal lymphatics (234–238). Definitive differentiation between capillaries and lymphatics requires immunohistochemical analysis (Table 24.2) (104,114,120,237).

Muscularis Mucosa

Forming the deep-limiting boundary of the lamina propria is a thin layer of smooth muscle, the muscularis mucosa. This muscle layer is physically tethered to the mucosa, with occasional smooth muscle cells extending into the lamina propria or coalescing with the pericryptal myofibroblast sheath. The muscularis mucosa receives innervation via the submucosal plexus (112,238,239). Because the colonic glands are tethered to the muscularis mucosa, this structure is valuable in evaluating crypt architecture in endoscopic biopsies. Biopsies that do not contain muscularis mucosae may resemble architectural distortion, with glands adopting horizontal or curved configurations. This is particularly relevant in assessing for IBD and sessile serrated adenomas, where crypt architectural distortions are key components of making the histologic diagnoses. Careful examination of other biopsy fragments that have muscularis mucosae, as well as assessment for other features of mucosal injury (Table 24.1), may allow an accurate diagnosis. The muscularis mucosa is normally traversed by lymphoglandular complexes (Fig. 24.5), vascular channels, and neural twiglets. It participates in absorptive, secretory, proliferative, and possibly motility functions. Isolated thickening may occur with prolapse of the overlying mucosa and, in proximity to diverticuli. Clear duplication of the muscularis mucosae is generally considered a feature of chronic mucosal injury.

Submucosa

The submucosa is composed of loosely arranged bundles of smooth muscle, fibroelastic tissue, and adipose, in which the local enteric nervous system, vasculature, and lymphatics are embedded. Lymphatic channels may be conspicuous and dilated immediately beneath the submucosa and do not contain cellular elements (234,235,237). Sparse inflammatory cells (relative to the dense "physiologic" inflammation of the mucosa) are scattered throughout, occasionally organized as submucosal lymphoid aggregates. The submucosa provides a flexible matrix that proves useful during peristalsis—it allows the mucosa to glide and move freely over the rigid muscularis mucosae.

Submucosal smooth muscle consists of loosely woven fascicles of individual smooth muscle cells, forming small bundles. These smooth muscle collections are closely apposed to ICCs, which in turn are immediately adjacent to nerve varicosities—forming the neuroeffector junctions that receive, transmit, and integrate central, parasympathetic, and sympathetic nervous system commands (232,240,241). The two submucosal neural plexuses are the submucosal plexus of Meissner (located immediately beneath the muscularis mucosae) and Henle's deep submucosal plexus (lying on the inner aspect of the muscularis propria). Neural plexuses are composed of neurons, glial cells, and stromal elements (242–244). Ganglion cells are unique in their histologic appearance with round or oval nuclei, a prominent (often eosinophilic) nucleolus, and ample basophilic cytoplasm stippled with Nissl substance (Fig. 24.14). Ganglion cells characteristically cluster together and may mimic giant cells, epithelioid cells, or granulomas. When present conspicuously in the mucosa, ganglion cells may reflect chronic damage, such as in the context of diverticular disease or IBD. Nerve axons are fibrillar and distinguishing these axons from fibroblasts or their elastofibrotic products may require

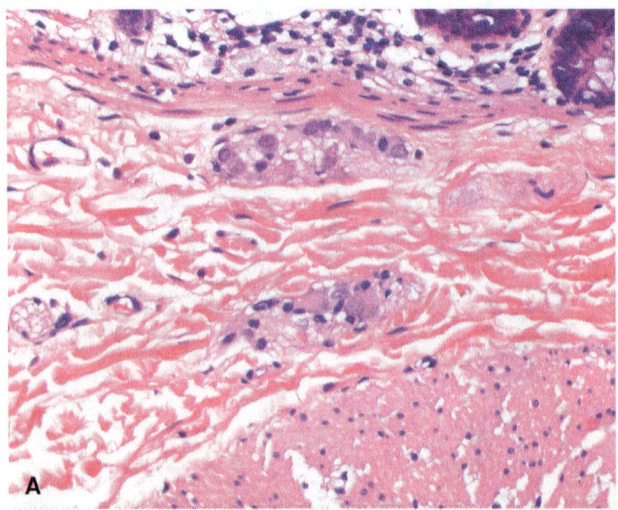
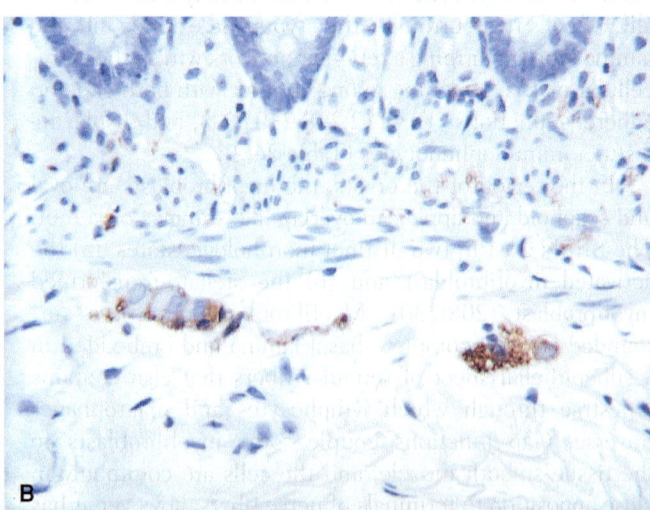

FIGURE 24.14 Ganglion cells of Meissner plexus. **A:** Submucosal nerve twigs and clusters of ganglion cells comprising Meissner plexus. (H&E stain, ×20). **B:** Same area stained with S100 (hematoxylin counterstain), highlighting the Schwann cells. The ganglion cells on the left are conspicuously negative with S100 (also ×20).

the use of histochemical or immunohistochemical stains (Fig. 24.14B, Table 24.2) (62,132,241,242,244–247).

ICCs are modified myofibroblasts. Histologic features evident with routine H&E stain include a fusiform cell body and large oval nucleus; silver stain or immunohistochemical evaluation will reveal two or more dendritic processes, connecting ICCs to one another, to ganglion cells, or to an adjacent smooth muscle (231,241,245,248,249). These intriguing cells are thought to play an important role in the control of gut motor activity (231,250,251). The normal ICC density within the submucosa is substantially less than that seen surrounding the myenteric plexus (see below) (241,250–252). In regards to vasculature, arterioles (from the superior and inferior mesenteric arteries), venules, and lymphatics are present throughout the submucosa (Fig. 24.15). These vessels in histologic sections are frequently distended by red blood cells and appear tortuous.

The amount of adipose within the submucosa varies substantially between the right and left colon and among patients. Of note, the ileocecal valve and cecum submucosa may appear particularly expanded by mature adipocytes, resembling a lipoma. However, in the absence of the submucosal adipose forming a discrete, lobulated mass, this abundant adipose tissue is within the range of normal.

Muscularis Externa, Subserosal Zone, and Serosa

The muscularis propria or external smooth muscle layers of the colon consist of an inner circular layer and an outer longitudinal layer (Fig. 24.16) (253,254). Structural variations of the muscularis propria have been identified, which may reflect

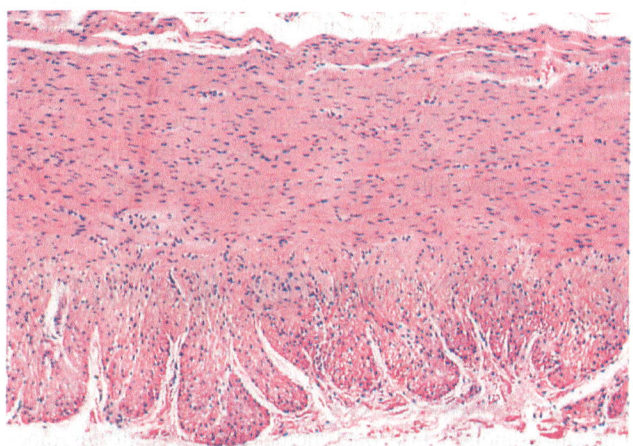

FIGURE 24.16 Muscularis propria and subserosal tissue. Both layers of the muscularis propria can be seen with the neural tissue of Auerbach plexus. Below the muscle layers is the fibrovascular adipose tissue of the subserosa.

different motility and storage functions of various regions of the colon (245,248). Smoothelin, a cytoskeletal protein that is expressed in terminally differentiated contractile smooth muscle cells, may serve a role in the contractile apparatus of these cells. One recent study shows that a marked reduction in smoothelin expression can be seen in the outer longitudinal muscle layer of some cases of colonic inertia (255). Auerbach plexus lies between the two muscle layers and resembles Meissner plexus histologically. The ICCs, the putative pacemaker cells of the gut that drive peristalsis, can be identified throughout the muscularis propria with immunizations for CD117 and CD34 (Fig. 24.17) (131,256,257).

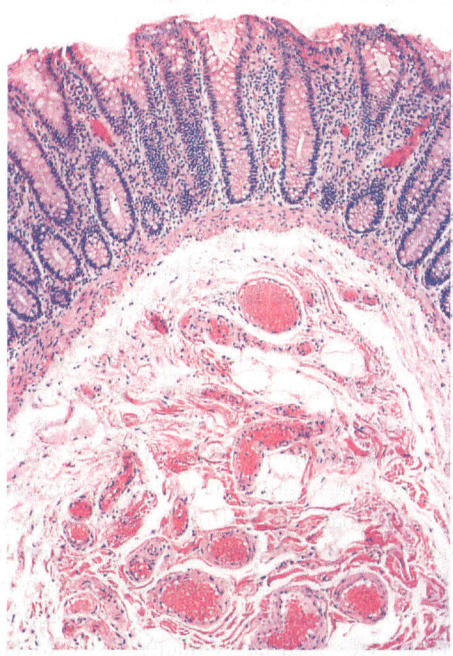

FIGURE 24.15 Colonic submucosal vasculature. Most of the blood vessels in this section contain erythrocytes.

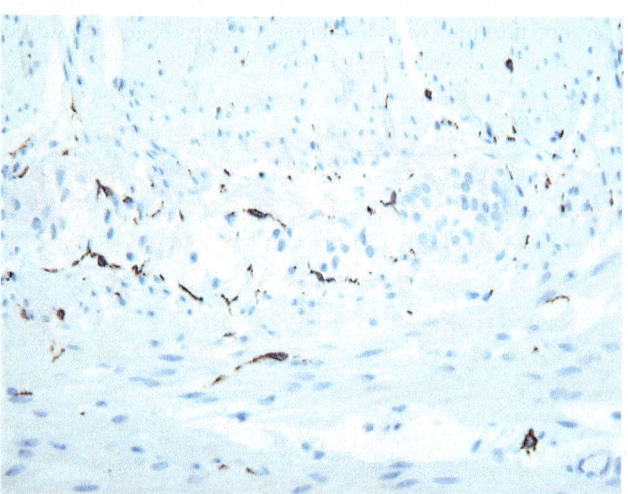

FIGURE 24.17 Interstitial cells of Cajal (ICC). The CD117 strongly positive, dendritic-appearing cells between the muscle layers and surrounding Auerbach plexus are the ICCs. These cells are considered to be the pacemaker cell of the gut and perform other functions in gut motility. (Anti-CD117 stain.)

Patients with motility disorders may have decreased numbers of these cells within their bowel walls (251,254). The muscularis is perforated by blood and lymphatic vessels and is encased in a subserosal zone of fibroadipose tissue. Strictly speaking, the serosa is limited to the mesothelial lining and immediately adjacent fibroelastic tissue.

EFFECTS OF PREPARATION AND ARTIFACTS

Bowel Preparation Effects

Commonly used bowel preparations for colonoscopy (sodium phosphate enemas, bisacodyl enemas and suppositories, dioctyl sodium sulfosuccinate, soapsuds enemas) can produce abnormalities of the mucosa that mimic or obscure inflammatory conditions and impart an edematous or hyperemic appearance of the mucosa to the endoscopist (258–260). Histologic features suggesting bowel preparation include: flattening of the absorptive colonocytes to a cuboidal shape, reduction in goblet cell mucus (due to increased mucus secretion), detached surface epithelium leaving an exposed basement membrane, focal surface epithelial and crypt neutrophilic infiltrate, accentuated red blood cell extravasation within the lamina propria, and increase in crypt or surface epithelial apoptosis (Fig. 24.18). Oral sodium phosphate incites exaggeration of the previously described features of bowel preparation. Endoscopically visible aphthous erosions, erosions, and uncommonly frank ulcers have been reported. Histologically, neutrophilic cryptitis and increased basal apoptosis may be seen in addition to other common features of bowel preparation (Fig. 24.19) (258,261,262). This basal apoptosis is histologically identical to low-grade graft-versus-host disease. Hence, oral sodium phosphate bowel preparations should not be used in bone marrow transplant patients. Although bowel preparation histologic changes may not interfere with rendering a polyp diagnosis, subtle inflammatory changes may be overlooked in the midst of various bowel preparation changes or alternately misdiagnosed as a pathologic condition. In the evaluation of patients for reasons other than colorectal cancer screening, bowel preparation with polyethylene glycol is suggested, as it appears to incite minimal histologic alterations (263,264). Nonetheless, polyethylene glycol preparation has also been reported in randomized trials to result in superficial mucus loss, epithelial cell loss, lymphocyte and neutrophil infiltration, and rarely aphthous erosions (265).

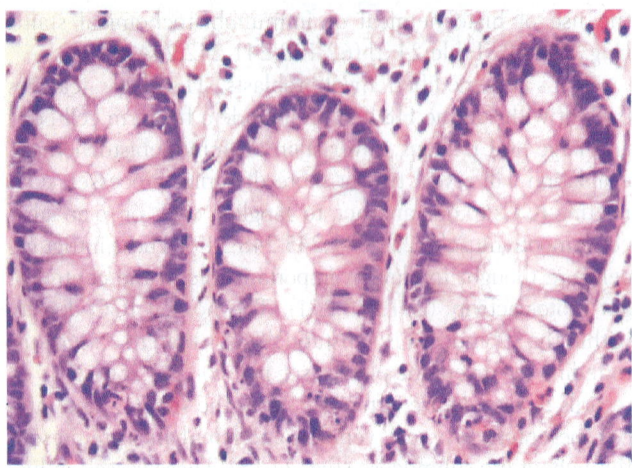

FIGURE 24.19 Oral sodium phosphate bowel preparation effect. Colonic crypts with apoptotic bodies and neutrophils are secondary to the effects of bowel preparation. Such changes could easily be interpreted as representing infectious colitis or graft-versus-host disease (GVHD) in the right clinical setting.

Incorrect Tissue Orientation and Tangential Sectioning

Difficulties with proper tissue orientation are most common to endoscopically procured biopsy specimens, owing to their small size. In both endoscopic biopsies and surgical resections, the most accurate interpretation is possible when the tissue is sectioned perpendicular to the plane of the surface epithelium. Evaluation of crypt architecture, inflammatory cell gradient, and thickness and regularity of the subepithelial collagen band may be hindered significantly by tangential sectioning (Table 24.1) (266). The appearance of acini (doughnuts) rather than "test tubes" within the lamina propria is a clear indication of tangential sectioning. Features of chronic mucosal injury may not be sampled in tangential sections that contain only the most superficial aspects of the mucosa. Cytoplasm of adjacent colonocytes in tangentially sectioned tissue may mimic a thickened (but regular) collagen band, risking a misinterpretation of collagenous colitis (Fig. 24.20). Tangential sections with exaggerated samples of the basal portions of colonic crypts show cross sections of less mature colonocytes with larger nuclei, less cytoplasm, and without adjacent goblet cells, thus mimicking the features of a tubular adenoma.

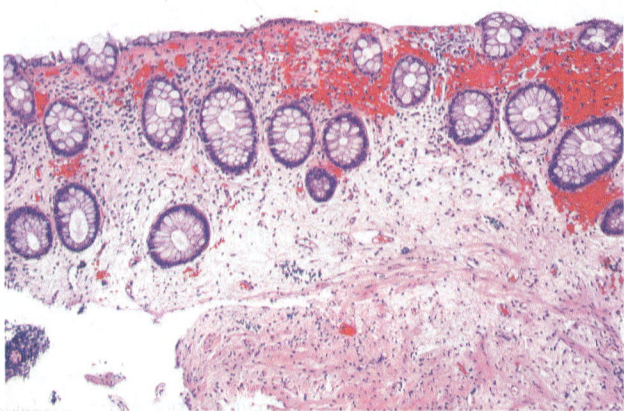

FIGURE 24.18 Enema effect. There is edema with extravasation and lysis of red blood cells (hemorrhage) within the lamina propria. The surface epithelium is largely denuded. Mucin depletion due to induced goblet cell secretion and increased apoptosis may also be seen.

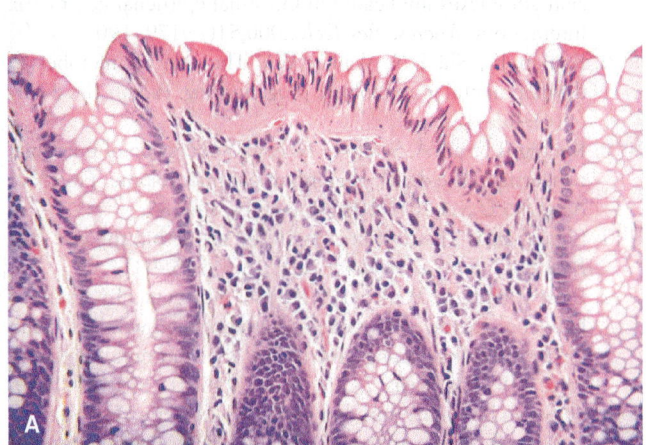
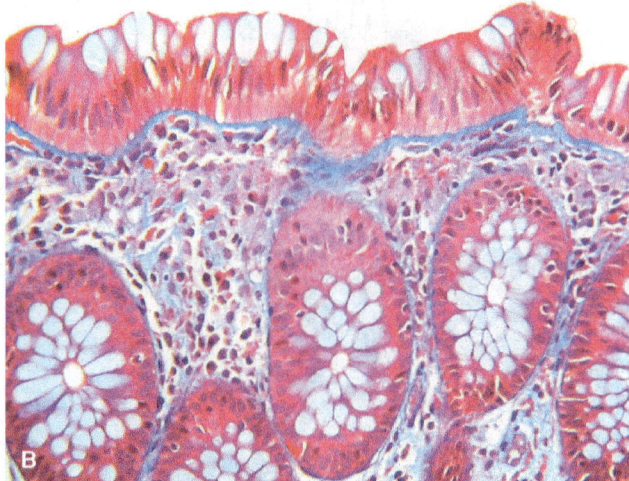

FIGURE 24.20 Normal colon mimicking collagenous colitis. **A:** This normal mucosa shows blending of the colonocyte cytoplasm with the basement membrane to give the illusion of a thickened subepithelial collagen table. Note that there is no surface damage or colitis present. **B:** This trichrome-stained section shows focal thickening in an area where the crypt sheath joins the surface tangentially. Care must be taken when evaluating tangential sections. Again note the lack of colitis or surface damage.

Tissue Trauma

Tissue trauma occurs with avulsion of the mucosa during forceps biopsy or in improper handling in the pathology gross room. The former may produce endoscopically visible edema, petechiae, friability, tears, and hemorrhage (264,266), and there may be histologic features of "crush" artifact. Biopsy samples may contain what appears to be an acellular lamina propria resembling edema, as well as extravasated red blood cells primarily in the luminal portion of the lamina propria. In the absence of other features of mucosal inflammation (i.e., neutrophilic inflammation or epithelial damage), these features should not be considered pathologic. Polyfoam pads may cause triangular artifacts in biopsy material and are not recommended (267). Despite relative fixation, crush artifact may occur with pressure applied to the biopsy material with rigid forceps. Use of a plastic pipette with large bore opening (i.e., cutting the tip off of a disposable pipette) to transfer biopsy material to the cassette avoids crush artifact. Crushing of the tissue results in crowding of glands and epithelial cells and is accompanied by stripping of the surface epithelium that then dislodges into the lumen.

Pseudolipomatosis

Pseudolipomatosis is characterized by vacuolated, unlined spaces in the lamina propria and mucosa that resemble loosely arranged adipocytes (Fig. 24.21). These lesions are due to air trapping from insufflation of the colon during endoscopy (268).

Electrocautery

Endoscopic removal of polyps with electrocautery ("hot" biopsy, or snare) frequently results in thermodesiccation of the tissue, compressing crypts together and altering the nuclear features. Characteristically, the crypts are closely apposed, with elongated, pyknotic and distorted nuclei (Fig. 24.22). These features may be difficult or impossible to distinguish from a tubular adenoma. Prolonged electrodesiccation may result in loss of both overall architecture and nuclear detail.

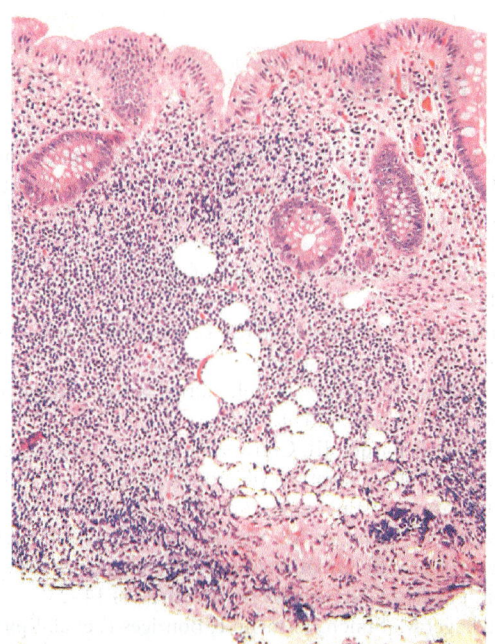

FIGURE 24.21 Pseudolipomatosis. The clear spaces within this lymphoid aggregate represent air bubbles due to insufflation during endoscopy. This artifact is frequently misinterpreted as adipose tissue/lipoma.

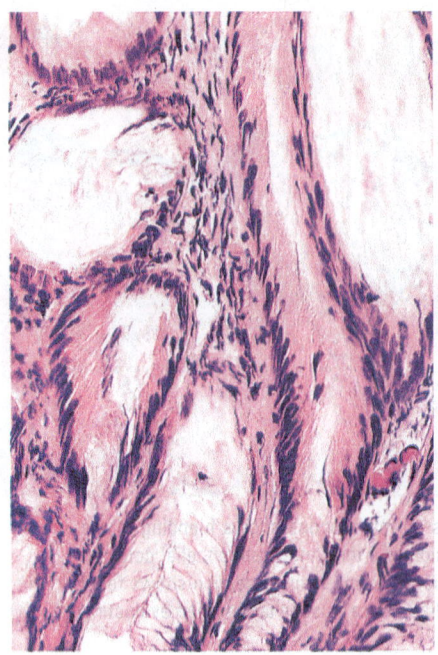

FIGURE 24.22 Electrodesiccation and compression artifact in the bases of adjacent crypts in normal colonic mucosa produced by an endoscopic electrocautery snare. Affected nuclei are pyknotic and elongated. Colonic crypts distorted by this artifact may be difficult or impossible to differentiate from the tubules of an adenoma.

ACKNOWLEDGMENTS

The authors are grateful for the continuing influence of the late Dr. Rodger C. Haggitt in the preparation of this manuscript.

REFERENCES

1. Batlle E, Henderson JT, Beghtel H, et al. Beta-catenin and TCF mediate cell positioning in the intestinal epithelium by controlling the expression of EphB/ephrinB. *Cell* 2002; 111(2):251–263.
2. Beck F. Homeobox genes in gut development. *Gut* 2002; 51(3):450–454.
3. Bonhomme C, Duluc I, Martin E, et al. The Cdx2 homeobox gene has a tumour suppressor function in the distal colon in addition to a homeotic role during gut development. *Gut* 2003;52(10):1465–1471.
4. Chailler P, Basque JR, Corriveau L, et al. Functional characterization of the keratinocyte growth factor system in human fetal gastrointestinal tract. *Pediatr Res* 2000;48(4):504–510.
5. Haffen K, Kedinger M, Simon-Assmann P. Mesenchyme-dependent differentiation of epithelial progenitor cells in the gut. *J Pediatr Gastroenterol Nutr* 1987;6(1):14–23.
6. Kedinger M, Simon-Assmann P, Bouziges F, et al. Epithelial-mesenchymal interactions in intestinal epithelial differentiation. *Scand J Gastoenterol Suppl* 1988;151:62–69.
7. Roberts DJ. Molecular mechanisms of development of the gastrointestinal tract. *Dev Dyn* 2000;219(2):109–120.
8. Stutzmann J, Bellissent-Waydelich A, Fontao L, et al. Adhesion complexes implicated in intestinal epithelial cell-matrix interactions. *Microsc Res Tech* 2000;51(2):179–190.
9. Kaplan JL, Shi HN, Walker WA. The role of microbes in developmental immunologic programming. *Pediatr Res* 2011; 69(6):465–472.
10. Koenig JE, Spor A, Scalfone N, et al. Succession of microbial consortia in the developing infant gut microbiome. *Proc Natl Acad Sci U S A* 2011;108 Suppl 1:4578–4585.
11. Shanahan F. The host-microbe interface within the gut. *Best Prac Res Clin Gastroenterol* 2002;16(6):915–931.
12. Bajaj-Elliott M, Poulsom R, Pender SL, et al. Interactions between stromal cell–derived keratinocyte growth factor and epithelial transforming growth factor in immune-mediated crypt cell hyperplasia. *J Clin Invest* 1998;102(8):1473–1480.
13. de Santa Barbara P, van den Brink GR, Roberts DJ. Development and differentiation of the intestinal epithelium. *Cell Mol Life Sci* 2003;60(7):1322–1332.
14. Karam SM. Lineage commitment and maturation of epithelial cells in the gut. *Front Biosci* 1999;4:D286–D298.
15. de Santa Barbara P, van den Brink GR, Roberts DJ. Molecular etiology of gut malformations and diseases. *Am J Med Genet* 2002;115(4):221–230.
16. Moore KL, Persaud TVN. The digestive system. In: Moore KL, Persaud TVN, eds. *The Developing Human: Clinically Oriented Embryology*. 7th ed. Philadelphia, PA: WB Saunders; 2003:266–284.
17. Arai T, Kino I. Morphometrical and cell kinetic studies of normal human colorectal mucosa. Comparison between the proximal and the distal large intestine. *Acta Pathol Jpn* 1989; 39(11):725–730.
18. Baker K, Zhang Y, Jin C, et al. Proximal versus distal hyperplastic polyps of the colorectum: Different lesions or a biological spectrum? *J Clin Pathol* 2004;57(10):1089–1093.
19. Birkenkam-Demtroder K, Olesen SH, Sørensen FB, et al. Differential gene expression in colon cancer of the caecum versus the sigmoid and rectosigmoid. *Gut* 2005;54(3): 374–384.
20. Calam J, Ghatei MA, Domin J, et al. Regional differences in concentrations of regulatory peptides in human colon mucosal biopsy. *Dig Dis Sci* 1989;34(8):1193–1198.
21. Gervaz P, Bucher P, Morel P. Two colons-two cancers: Paradigm shift and clinical implications. *J Surg Onc* 2004;88(4): 261–266.
22. Greenson JK, Odze RD. Inflammatory bowel disease of the large intestine. In: Odze RD, Goldblum JR, Crawford JM, eds. *Surgical Pathology of the GI Tract, Liver, Biliary Tract and Pancreas*. Philadelphia, PA: WB Saunders; 2004;213–214.
23. Kunzelmann K, Mall M. Electrolyte transport in the mammalian colon: Mechanisms and implications for disease. *Physiol Rev* 2002;82(1):245–289.
24. Lee E, Schiller LR, Fordtran JS. Quantification of colonic lamina propria cells by means of a morphometric point-counting method. *Gastroenterology* 1988;94(2):409–418.
25. Liu LU, Holt PR, Krivosheyev V, et al. Human right and left colon differ in epithelial cell apoptosis and in expression of Bak, a pro-apoptotic Bcl-2 homologue. *Gut* 1999;45(1): 45–50.
26. Macfarlane GT, Gibson GR, Cummings JH. Comparison of fermentation reactions in different regions of the human colon. *J Appl Bacteriol* 1992;72(1):57–64.

27. Moskaluk CA, Zhang H, Powell SM, et al. Cdx2 protein expression in normal and malignant human tissues: An immunohistochemical survey using tissue microarrays. *Mod Pathol* 2003;16(9):913–919.
28. Naftalin RJ, Zammit PS, Pedley KC. Regional differences in rat large intestinal crypt function in relation to dehydrating capacity in vivo. *J Physiol* 1999;514(pt 1):201–210.
29. Naftalin RJ. The dehydrating function of the descending colon in relationship to crypt function. *Physiol Res* 1994;43(2):65–73.
30. Paluszkiewicz P, Berbeć H, Pawlowska-Wakowicz B, et al. p53 protein accumulation in colorectal cancer tissue has prognostic value only in left-sided colon tumours. *Cancer Detect Prev* 2004;28(4):252–259.
31. Priebe MG, Vonk RJ, Sun X, et al. The physiology of colonic metabolism. Possibilities for interventions with pre- and probiotics. *Eur J Nutr* 2002;41(suppl 1):I2–I10.
32. Sandle GI. Salt and water absorption in the human colon: A modern appraisal. *Gut* 1998;43(2):294–299.
33. Booth C, Potten CS. Gut instincts: Thoughts on intestinal epithelial stem cells. *J Clin Invest* 2000;105(11):1493–1499.
34. Marshman E, Booth C, Potten CS. The intestinal epithelial stem cell. *Bioessays* 2002;24(1):91–98.
35. Seidelin JB. Colonic epithelial cell turnover: Possible implications for ulcerative colitis and cancer initiation. *Scand J Gastroenterol* 2004;39(3):201–211.
36. Atarashi K, Tanoue T, Shima T, et al. Induction of colonic regulatory T cells by indigenous Clostridium species. *Science* 2011;331(6015):337–341.
37. Ishikawa H, Tanaka K, Maeda Y, et al. Effect of intestinal microbiota on the induction of regulatory CD25+ CD4+ T cells. *Clin Exp Immunol* 2008;153(1):127–135.
38. Collado MC, Isolauri E, Laitinen K, et al. Effect of mother's weight on infant's microbiota acquisition, composition, and activity during early infancy: A prospective follow-up study initiated in early pregnancy. *Am J Clin Nutr* 2010;92(5):1023–1030.
39. Metzger R, Metzger U, Fiegel HC, et al. Embryology of the midgut. *Semin Pediatr Surg* 2011;20(3):145–151.
40. Kluth D, Fiegel HC, Metzger R. Embryology of the hindgut. *Semin Pediatr Surg* 2011;20(3):152–160.
41. Wang Y, Devkota S, Musch MW, et al. Regional mucosa-associated microbiota determine physiological expression of TLR2 and TLR4 in murine colon. *PLoS ONE* 2010;5(10):e13607.
42. Bajpai M, Mathur M. Duplications of the alimentary tract: Clues to the missing links. *J Pediatr Surg* 1994;29(10):1361–1365.
43. Bossard P, Zaret KS. Repressive and restrictive mesodermal interactions with gut endoderm: Possible relation to Meckel's diverticulum. *Development* 2000;127(22):4915–4923.
44. Martinez-Frias ML, Bermejo E, Rodrigues-Pinilla E. Anal atresia, vertebral, genital, and urinary tract anomalies: A primary polytopic developmental field defect identified through an epidemiological analysis of associations. *Am J Med Genet* 2000;95(2):169–173.
45. Robertson K, Mason I, Hall S. Hirschsprung's disease: Genetic mutations in mice and men. *Gut* 1997;41(4):436–441.
46. Houlston R, Bevan S, Williams A, et al. Mutations in DPC4 (SMAD4) cause juvenile polyposis syndrome, but only account for a minority of cases. *Hum Mol Genet* 1998;7(12):1907–1912.
47. Howe JR, Roth S, Ringold JC, et al. Mutations in the SMAD4/DPC4 gene in juvenile polyposis. *Science* 1998;280(5366):1086–1088.
48. Howe JR, Bair JL, Sayed MG, et al. Germline mutations of the gene encoding bone morphogenetic protein receptor 1A in juvenile polyposis. *Nat Genet* 2001;28(2):184–187.
49. Roth S, Sistonen P, Salovaara R, et al. SMAD genes in juvenile polyposis. *Genes Chromosomes Cancer* 1999;26(1):54–61.
50. Ruiz i Altaba A. Gli proteins and Hedgehog signaling: Development and cancer. *Trends Genet* 1999;15(10):418–425.
51. Arora T, Sharma R. Fermentation potential of the gut microbiome: Implications for energy homeostasis and weight management. *Nutr Rev* 2011;69(2):99–106.
52. Chow J, Lee SM, Shen Y, et al. Host-bacterial symbiosis in health and disease. *Adv Immunol* 2010;107:243–274.
53. Collins SM, Denou E, Verdu EF, et al. The putative role of the intestinal microbiota in the irritable bowel syndrome. *Dig Liver Dis* 2009;41(12):850–853.
54. Kinross JM, Darzi AW, Nicholson JK. Gut microbiome-host interactions in health and disease. *Genome Med* 2011;3(3):14.
55. Li-Wan-Po A, Farndon P. Barking up the wrong genome—we are not alone. *J Clin Pharm and Ther* 2011;36(2):125–127.
56. McGarr SE, Ridlon JM, Hylemon PB. Diet anaerobic bacterial metabolism, and colon cancer: A review of the literature. *J Clin Gastroenterol* 2005;39(2):98–109.
57. Spor A, Koren O, Ley R. Unravelling the effects of the environment and host genotype on the gut microbiome. *Nat Rev Microbiol* 2011;9(4):279–290.
58. Taleb S, Tedgui A, Mallat Z. Regulatory T-cell immunity and its relevance to atherosclerosis. *J Intern Med* 2008;263(5):489–499.
59. Turnbaugh PJ, Bäckhed F, Fulton L, et al. Diet-induced obesity is linked to marked but reversible alterations in the mouse distal gut microbiome. *Cell Host Microbe* 2008;3(4):213–223.
60. Gohir W, Ratcliffe EM, Sloboda DM. Of the bugs that shape us: Maternal obesity, the gut microbiome, and long-term disease risk. *Pediatr Res* 2015;77(1–2):196–204.
61. Obata Y, Pachnis V. The effect of microbiota and the immune system on the development and organization of the enteric nervous system. *Gastroenterology* 2016;151(5):836–844.
62. Guyton, AC. The digestive and metabolic systems. In: Guyton AC, ed. *Anatomy and Physiology*. Philadelphia, PA: WB Saunders; 1984:643–700.
63. Smith ME, Morton DG. The colon. In: Smith ME, Morton DG, eds. *The Digestive System*. Edinburgh: Churchill Livingstone; 2001:175–186.
64. Netter FH. Abdomen. In: Netter FH, Colacino S, eds. *Atlas of Human Anatomy*. Summit, NJ: Ciba-Geigy Corp; 1989:251–256, 264–268.
65. Glebov OK, Rodriguez LM, Nakahara K, et al. Distinguishing right from left colon by the pattern of gene expression. *Cancer Epidemiol Biomarkers Prev* 2003;12(8):755–762.
66. Wood JD, Alpers DH, Andrews PL. Fundamentals of neurogastroenterology. *Gut* 1999;45(suppl 2):II6–II16.
67. Howell SJ, Wilk D, Yadav SP, et al. Antimicrobial polypeptides of the human colonic epithelium. *Peptides* 2003;24(11):1763–1770.

68. Fihn BM, Jodal M. Permeability of the proximal and distal rat colon crypt and surface epithelium to hydrophilic molecules. *Pflugers Arch* 2001;441(5):656–662.
69. Eckburg PB, Bik EM, Bernstein CN, et al. Diversity of the human instestinal microbial flora. *Science* 2005;308(5728):1635–1638.
70. Gosalbes MJ, Durbán A, Pignatelli M, et al. Metatranscriptomic approach to analyze the functional human gut microbiota. *PLoS ONE* 2011;6(3):e17447.
71. Wang Y, Antonopoulous DA, Zhu X, et al. Laser capture microdissection and metagenomic analysis of intact mucosa-associated microbial communities of human colon. *Appl Microbiol Biotechnol* 2010;88(6):1333–1342.
72. Thiagarajah JR, Pedley KC, Naftalin RJ. Evidence of amiloride-sensitive fluid absorption in rat descending colonic crypts from fluorescence recovery of FITC-labelled dextran after photobleaching. *J Physiol (Lond)* 2001;536(Pt 2):541–553.
73. Hopkins MJ, Sharp R, Macfarlane GT. Age and disease related changes in intestinal bacterial populations assessed by cell culture, 16S rRNA abundance, and community cellular fatty acid profiles. *Gut* 2001;48(2):198–205.
74. Porter EM, Bevins CL, Ghosh D, et al. The multifaceted Paneth cell. *Cell Mol Life Sci* 2002;59(1):156–170.
75. Boman HG. Antibacterial peptides: Basic facts and emerging concepts. *J Intern Med* 2003;254(3):197–215.
76. Köhler H, McCormick BA, Walker WA. Bacterial-enterocyte crosstalk: Cellular mechanisms in health and disease. *J Pediatr Gastroenterol Nutr* 2003;36(2):175–185.
77. Lu L, Walker WA. Pathologic and physiologic interactions of bacteria with the gastrointestinal epithelium. *Am J Clin Nutr* 2001;73(6):1124S–1130S.
78. Zuercher AW, Jiang HQ, Thurnheer MC, et al. Distinct mechanisms for cross-protection of the upper versus lower respiratory tract through intestinal priming. *J Immunol* 2002;169(7):3920–3925.
79. Demetter P, De Vos M, Van Huysse JA, et al. Colon mucosa of patients both with spondyloarthritis and Crohn's disease is enriched with macrophages expressing the scavenger receptor CD163. *Ann Rheum Dis* 2005;64(2):321–324.
80. Didierlaurent A, Sirard JC, Kraehenbuhl JP, et al. How the gut senses its content. *Cell Microbiol* 2002;4(2):61–72.
81. Girardin SE, Hugot JP, Sansonetti PJ. Lessons from Nod2 studies: Towards a link between Crohn's disease and bacterial sensing. *Trends Immunol* 2003;24(12):652–658.
82. Hershberg RM, Mayer LF. Antigen processing and presentation by intestinal epithelial cells—polarity and complexity. *Immunol Today* 2000;21(3):123–128.
83. Neutra MR. Current concepts in mucosal immunity. V. Role of M cells in transepithelial transport of antigens and pathogens to the mucosal immune system. *Am J Physiol* 1998;274(5 pt 1):G785–G791.
84. Noverr MC, Huffnagle GB. Does the microbiota regulate immune responses outside the gut? *Trends Microbiol* 2004;12(12):562–568.
85. Spahn TW, Kucharzik T. Modulating the intestinal immune system: The role of lymphotoxin and GALT organs. *Gut* 2004;53(3):456–465.
86. Mai V, Morris JG Jr. Colonic bacterial flora: Changing understandings in the molecular age. *J Nutr* 2004;134(2):459–464.
87. Ouwehand A, Isolauri E, Salminen S. The role of the intestinal microflora for the development of the immune system in early childhood. *Eur J Nutr* 2002;41(supp 1):I32–I37.
88. Pickard KM, Bremner AR, Gordon JN, et al. Microbial-gut interactions in health and disease. Immune responses. *Best Pract Res Clin Gastroenterol* 2004;18(2):271–285.
89. Pryde SE, Duncan SH, Hold GL, et al. The microbiology of butyrate formation in the human colon. *FEMS Microbiol Lett* 2002;217(2):133–139.
90. Berkes J, Viswanathan VK, Savkovic SD, et al. Intestinal epithelial responses to enteric pathogens: Effects on the tight junction barrier, ion transport, and inflammation. *Gut* 2003;52(3):439–451.
91. Roediger WE, Babidge W. Human colonocyte detoxification. *Gut* 1997;41(6):731–734.
92. Macfarlane GT, Macfarlane S. Human colonic microbiota: Ecology, physiology and metabolic potential of intestinal bacteria. *Scand J Gastroenterol Suppl* 1997;222:3–9.
93. Zaharia V, Varzescu M, Djavadi I, et al. Effects of short chain fatty acids on colonic Na+ absorption and enzyme activity. *Comp Biochem Physiol A Mol Integr Phsiol* 2001;128(2):335–347.
94. Topping DL, Clifton PM. Short-chain fatty acids and human colonic function: Roles of resistant starch and nonstarch polysaccharides. *Physiol Rev* 2001;81(3):1031–1064.
95. Grieg ER, Boot-Handford RP, Mani V, et al. Decreased expression of apical Na+ channels and basolateral Na+, K+-ATPase in ulcerative colitis. *J Pathol* 2004;204(1):84–92.
96. Willemsen LE, Koetsier MA, van Deventer SJ, et al. Short chain fatty acids stimulate epithelial mucin 2 expression through differential effects on prostaglandin E1 and E2 production by intestinal myofibroblasts. *Gut* 2003;52(10):1442–1447.
97. Naftalin RJ, Pedley KC. Regional crypt function in rat large intestine in relation to fluid absorption and growth of the pericryptal sheath. *J Physiol* 1999;514(pt 1):211–227.
98. Hirasawa K, Sato Y, Hosoda Y, et al. Immunohistochemical localization of angiotensin II receptor and local renin-angiotensin system in human colonic mucosa. *J Histochem Cytochem* 2002;50(2):275–282.
99. Thiagarajah JR, Griffiths NM, Pedley KC, et al. Evidence for modulation of pericryptal sheath myofibroblasts in rat descending colon by transforming growth factor beta and angiotensin II. *BMC Gastroenterol* 2002;2:4.
100. Anderson JM, Van Itallie CM. Tight junctions and the molecular basis for regulation of paracellular permeability. *Am J Physiol* 1995;269(4 pt 1):G467–G475.
101. Kucharzik T, Walsh SV, Chen J, et al. Neutrophil transmigration in inflammatory bowel disease is associated with differential expression of epithelial intercellular junction proteins. *Am J Pathol* 2001;159(6):2001–2009.
102. Walsh SV, Hopkins AM, Nusrat A. Modulation of tight junction structure and function by cytokines. *Adv Drug Deliv Rev* 2000;41(3):303–313.
103. Adegboyega PA, Mifflin RC, DiMari JF, et al. Immunohistochemical study of myofibroblasts in normal colonic mucosa, hyperplastic polyps, and adenomatous colorectal polyps. *Arch Pathol Lab Med* 2002;126(7):829–836.
104. Akishima Y, Ito K, Zhang L, et al. Immunohistochemical detection of human small lymphatic vessels under normal and pathological conditions using the LYVE-1 antibody. *Virchows Arch* 2004;444(2):153–157.

105. Aldenborg F, Enerbäck L. The immunohistochemical demonstration of chymase and tryptase in human intestinal mast cells. *Histochem J* 1994;26(7):587–596.
106. Brandtzaeg P, Farstad IN, Helgeland L. Phenotypes of T cells in the gut. *Chem Immunol* 1998;71:1–26.
107. Buffa R, Marè P, Gini A, et al. Chromogranins A and B and secretogranin II in hormonally identified endocrine cells of the gut and the pancreas. *Basic Appl Histochem* 1988;32(4):471–484.
108. Castellaneta A, Abe M, Morelli AE, et al. Identification and characterization of intestinal Peyer's patch interferon-alpha producing (plasmacytoid) dendritic cells. *Hum Immunol* 2004;65(2):104–113.
109. Corfield AP, Myerscough N, Longman R, et al. Mucins and mucosal protection in the gastrointestinal tract: New prospects for mucins in the pathology of gastrointestinal disease. *Gut* 2000;47(4):589–594.
110. Ferri GL, Probert L, Cocchia D, et al. Evidence for the presence of S-100 protein in the glial component of the human enteric nervous system. *Nature* 1982;297(5865):409–410.
111. Frängsmyr L, Baranov V, Hammarström S. Four carcinoembryonic antigen subfamily members, CEA, NCA, BGP and CGM2, selectively expressed in the normal human colonic epithelium are integral components of the fuzzy coat. *Tumour Biol* 1999;20(5):277–292.
112. Fulcheri E, Cantino D, Bussolati G. Presence of intra-mucosal smooth muscle cells in normal human and rat colon. *Basic Appl Histochem* 1985;29(4):337–344.
113. Fujisaki J, Shimoda T. Expression of cytokeratin subtypes in colorectal mucosa, adenoma, and carcinoma. *Gastroenterol Jpn* 1993;28(5):647–656.
114. Gabbiani G, Schmid E, Winter S, et al. Vascular smooth muscle cells differ from other smooth muscle cells: Predominance of vimentin filaments and specific alpha-type actin. *Proc Natl Acad Sci U S A* 1981;78(1):298–302.
115. Galli SJ, Tsai M, Wershil BK. The c-kit receptor, stem cell factor, and mast cells. What each is teaching us about the others. *Am J Pathol* 1993;142(4):965–974.
116. Grimelius L. Silver stains demonstrating neuroendocrine cells. *Biotech Histochem* 2004;79(1):37–44.
117. Hamrock D, Azmi FH, O'Donnell E, et al. Infection by Rhodococcus equi in a patient with AIDS: Histological appearance mimicking Whipple's disease and Mycobacterium avium-intracellulare infection. *J Clin Pathol* 1999;52(1):68–71.
118. Higaki S, Tada M, Nishiaki M, et al. Immunohistological study to determine the presence of pericryptal myofibroblasts and basement membrane in colorectal epithelial tumors. *J Gastroenterol* 1999;34(2):215–220.
119. Jass JR. Mucin core proteins as differentiation markers in the gastrointestinal tract. *Histopathology* 2000;37(6):561–564.
120. Jones TR, Kao KJ, Pizzo SV, et al. Endothelial cell surface expression and binding of factor VIII/von Willebrand factor. *Am J Pathol* 1981;103(2):304–308.
121. Kato H, Yamamoto T, Yamamoto H, et al. Immunocytochemical characterization of supporting cells in the enteric nervous system in Hirschsprung's disease. *J Pediatr Surg* 1990;25(5):514–519.
122. Kawana T, Nada O, Ikeda K. An immunohistochemical study of glial fibrillary acidic (GFA) protein and S-100 protein in the colon affected by Hirschsprung's disease. *Acta Neuropathol (Berl)* 1988;76(2):159–165.
123. Kende AI, Carr NJ, Sobin LH. Expression of cytokeratins 7 and 20 in carcinomas of the gastrointestinal tract. *Histopathology* 2003;42(2):137–140.
124. Kurki P, Virtanen I. The detection of smooth muscle antibodies reacting with intermediate filaments of desmin type. *J Immunol Methods* 1985;76(2):329–335.
125. Lamps LW, Molina CP, West AB, et al. The pathologic spectrum of gastrointestinal and hepatic histoplasmosis. *Am J Clin Pathol* 2000;113(1):64–72.
126. Lee MJ, Lee HS, Kim WH, et al. Expression of mucins and cytokeratins in primary carcinomas of the digestive system. *Mod Pathol* 2003;16(5):403–410.
127. Meyer T, Brinck U. Differential distribution of serotonin and tryptophan hydroxylase in the human gastrointestinal tract. *Digestion* 1999;60(1):63–68.
128. Moll R, Lowe A, Laufer J, et al. Cytokeratin 20 in human carcinomas. A new histodiagnostic marker detected by monoclonal antibodies. *Am J Pathol* 1992;140(2):427–447.
129. O'Connell FP, Pinkus JL, Pinkus GS. CD138 (syndecan-1), a plasma cell marker immunohistochemical profile in hematopoietic and nonhematopoietic neoplasms. *Am J Clin Pathol* 2004;121(2):254–263.
130. Ozğul C, Karaöz E, Erdoğan D, et al. Expression of epidermal growth factor receptor in normal colonic mucosa and in adenocarcinomas of the colon. *Acta Physiol Hung* 1997–1998;85(2):121–128.
131. Park HJ, Kamm MA, Abbasi AM, et al. Immunohistochemical study of the colonic muscle and innervation in idiopathic chronic constipation. *Dis Colon Rectum* 1995;38(5):509–513.
132. Petchasuwan C, Pintong J. Immunohistochemistry for intestinal ganglion cells and nerve fibers: Aid in the diagnosis of Hirschsprung's disease. *J Med Assoc Thai* 2000;83(11):1402–1409.
133. Qualtrough D, Hinoi T, Fearon E, et al. Expression of CDX2 in normal and neoplastic human colon tissue and during differentiation of an in vitro model system. *Gut* 2002;51(2):184–190.
134. Rubio CA, Nesi G. A simple method to demonstrate normal and metaplastic Paneth cells in tissue sections. *In Vivo* 2003;17(1):67–71.
135. Rubio CA, Slezak P. The subepithelial band in collagenous colitis is autofluorescent. A study in H&E stained sections. *In Vivo* 2002;16(2):123–126.
136. Sarsfield P, Rinne A, Jones DB, et al. Accessory cells in physiological lymphoid tissue from the intestine: An immunohistochemical study. *Histopathology* 1996;28(3):205–211.
137. Sartore S, De Marzo N, Borrione AC, et al. Myosin heavy-chain isoforms in human smooth muscle. *Eur J Biochem* 1989;179(1):79–85.
138. Smithson JE, Warren BF, Young S. et al. Heterogeneous expression of carcinoembryonic antigen in the normal colon and upregulation in active ulcerative colitis. *J Pathol* 1996;180(2):146–151.
139. Truong LD, Rangdaeng S, Cagle P, et al. The diagnostic utility of desmin. A study of 584 cases and review of the literature. *Am J Clin Pathol* 1990;93(3):305–314.
140. Werling RW, Yaziji H, Bacchi CE, et al. CDX2, a highly sensitive and specific marker of adenocarcinomas of intestinal origin: An immunohistochemical survey of 476 primary and metastatic carcinomas. *Am J Surg Pathol* 2003;27(3):303–310.

141. West AB, Isaac CA, Carboni JM, et al. Localization of villin, a cytoskeletal protein specific to microvilli, in human ileum and colon and in colonic neoplasms. *Gastroenterology* 1988;94(2):343–352.
142. Wiedenmann B, Waldherr R, Buhr H, et al. Identification of gastroenteropancreatic neuroendocrine cells in normal and neoplastic human tissue with antibodies against synaptophysin, chromogranin A, secretogranin I (chromogranin B), and secretogranin II. *Gastroenterology* 1988;95(5):1364–1374.
143. Wong NA, Herriot M, Rae F. An immunohistochemical study and review of potential markers of human intestinal M cells. *Eur J Histochem* 2003;47(2):143–150.
144. Thiagarajah JR, Gourmelon P, Griffiths NM, et al. Radiation induced cytochrome c release causes loss of rat colonic fluid absorption by damage to crypts and pericryptal myofibroblasts. *Gut* 2000;47(5):675–684.
145. Kirby JA, Bone M, Robertson H, et al. The number of intraepithelial T cells decreases from ascending colon to rectum. *J Clin Pathol* 2003;56(2):158.
146. Kraehenbuhl JP, Neutra MR. Epithelial M cells: Differentiation and function. *Annu Rev Cell Dev Biol* 2000;16:301–332.
147. Sapp H, Ithamukkala S, Brien TP, et al. The terminal ileum is affected in patients with lymphocytic or collagenous colitis. *Am J Surg Pathol* 2002;26(11):1484–1492.
148. Brittan M, Wright NA. The gastrointestinal stem cell. *Cell Prolif* 2004;37(1):35–53.
149. Bleuming SA, Peppelenbosch MP, Roberts, DJ, et al. Homeostasis of the adult colonic epithelium: A role for morphogens. *Scand J Gastroenterol* 2004;39(2):93–98.
150. Halm DR, Halm ST. Secretagogue response of goblet cells and columnar cells in human colonic crypts. *Am J Physiol Cell Physiol* 2000;278(1):C212–C233.
151. Kim KM, Shibata D. Methylation reveals a niche: Stem cell succession in human colon crypts. *Oncogene* 2002;21(35):5441–5449.
152. Potten CS. Epithelial cell growth and differentiation. II. Intestinal apoptosis. *Am J Physiol* 1997;273(2 pt 1):G253–G257.
153. Potten CS, Booth C, Tudor GL, et al. Identification of a putative intestinal stem cell and early lineage marker; musashi-1. *Differentiation* 2003;71(1):28–41.
154. Sancho E, Batlle E, Clevers H. Live and let die in the intestinal epithelium. *Curr Opin Cell Biol* 2003;15(6):763–770.
155. Ayabe T, Ashida T, Kohgo Y, et al. The role of Paneth cells and their antimicrobial peptides in innate host defense. *Trends Microbiol* 2004;12(8):394–398.
156. Ouellette AJ. IV. Paneth cell antimicrobial peptides and the biology of the mucosal barrier. *Am J Physiol* 1999;277(2Pt 1):G257–G261.
157. Schonhoff SE, Giel-Moloney M, Leiter AB. Minireview: Development and differentiation of gut endocrine cells. *Endocrinology* 2004;145(6):2639–2644.
158. Neutra MR, Mantis NJ, Kraehenbuhl JP. Collaboration of epithelial cells with organized mucosal lymphoid tissues. *Nat Immunol* 2001;2(11):1004–1009.
159. Corfield AP, Wiggins R, Edwards C, et al. A sweet coating—how bacteria deal with sugars. *Adv Exp Med Biol* 2003;535:3–15.
160. Filipe MI. Mucins in the human gastrointestinal epithelium: A review. *Invest Cell Pathol* 1979;2(3):195–216.
161. Culling CF, Reid PE, Dunn WL, et al. The relevance of the histochemistry of colonic mucins based upon their PAS reactivity. *Histochem J* 1981;13(6):889–903.
162. Rehfeld JF. The new biology of gastrointestinal hormones. *Physiol Rev* 1998;78(4):1087–1108.
163. Skipper M, Lewis J. Getting to the guts of enteroendocrine differentiation. *Nat Genet* 2000;24(1):3–4.
164. Hirschowitz L, Rode J. Changes in neurons, neuroendocrine cells and nerve fibers in the lamina propria of irradiated bowel. *Virchows Arch A Pathol Anat Histopathol* 1991;418(2):163–168.
165. Qian J, Hickey WF, Angeletti RH. Neuroendocrine cells in intestinal lamina propria. Detection with antibodies to chromogranin A. *J Neuroimmunol* 1988;17(2):159–165.
166. Roth KA, Gordon JI. Spatial differentiation of the intestinal epithelium: Analysis of enteroendocrine cells containing immunoreactive serotonin, secretin, and substance P in normal and transgenic mice. *Proc Natl Aca Sci U S A* 1990;87(16):6408–6412.
167. Pezhouh MK, Cheng E, Weinberg AG, et al. Significance of Paneth cells in histologically unremarkable rectal mucosa. *Am J Surg Pathol* 2016;40(7):968–971.
168. Lala S, Ogura Y, Osborne C, et al. Crohn's disease and the NOD2 gene: A role for Paneth cells. *Gastroenterology* 2003;125(1):47–57.
169. Ogura Y, Lala S, Xin W, et al. Expression of NOD2 in Paneth cells: A possible link to Crohn's ileitis. *Gut* 2003;52(11):1591–1597.
170. Lin PW, Simon PO Jr, Gerwitz AT, et al. Paneth cell cryptidins act in vitro as apical paracrine regulators of the innate inflammatory response. *J Biol Chem* 2004;279(19):19902–19907.
171. Baranov V, Hammarstrom S. Carcinoembryonic antigen (CEA) and CEA-related cell adhesion molecule 1 (CEACAM1), apically expressed on human colonic M cells, are potential receptors for microbial adhesion. *Histochem Cell Biol* 2004;121(2):83–89.
172. Sierro F, Pringault E, Simon-Assmann P, et al. Transient expression of M-cell phenotype by enterocyte-like cells of the follicle-associated epithelium of mouse Peyer's patches. *Gastroenterology* 2000;119(3):734–743.
173. Neutra MR, Mantis NJ, Frey A, et al. The composition and function of M cell apical membranes: Implications for microbial pathogenesis. *Semin Immunol* 1999;11(3):171–181.
174. Cetin Y, Muller-Koppel L, Aunis D, et al. Chromogranin A (CgA) in the gastro-entero-pancreatic (GEP) endocrine system. II. CgA in mammalian entero-endocrine cells. *Histochemistry* 1989;92(4):265–275.
175. Gebert A, Fassbender S, Werner K, et al. The development of M cells in Peyer's patches is restricted to specialized dome-associated crypts. *Am J Pathol* 1999;154(5):1573–1582.
176. Jepson MA, Clark MA, Hirst BH. M cell targeting by lectins: A strategy for mucosal vaccination and drug delivery. *Adv Drug Deliv Rev* 2004;56(4):511–525.
177. Melgar S, Hammarström S, Oberg A, et al. Cytolytic capabilities of lamina propria and intraepithelial lymphocytes in normal and chronically inflamed human intestine. *Scan J Immunol* 2004;60(1–2):167–177.
178. Farstad IN, Lundin KE. Gastrointestinal intraepithelial lymphocytes and T cell lymphomas. *Gut* 2003;52(2):163–164.

179. Helgeland L, Dissen E, Dai KZ, et al. Microbial colonization induces oligoclonal expansions of intraepithelial CD8 T cells in the gut. *Eur J Immunol* 2004;34(12):3389–3400.
180. MacDonald TT, Bajaj-Elliot M, Pender SL. T cells orchestrate intestinal mucosal shape and integrity. *Immunol Today* 1999;20(11):505–510.
181. Brandtzaeg P. Development and basic mechanisms of human gut immunity. *Nutr Rev* 1998;56(pt 2):S5–S18.
182. Ebert EC. Interleukin-12 up-regulates perforin- and Fas-mediated lymphokine-activated killer activity by intestinal intraepithelial lymphocytes. *Clin Exp Immunol* 2004;138(2):259–265.
183. Kagnoff MF. Current concepts in mucosal immunity. III. Ontogeny and function of gamma delta T cells in the intestine. *Am J Physiol* 1998;274(3 Pt 1):G455–G458.
184. Chen Y, Chou K, Fuchs E, et al. Protection of the intestinal mucosa by intraepithelial gamma delta T cells. *Proc Nat Acad Sci U S A* 2002;99(22):14338–14343.
185. Lin T, Yoshida H, Matsuzaki G, et al. Autospecific gamma delta thymocytes that escape negative selection find sanctuary in the intestine. *J Clin Invest* 1999;104(9):1297–1305.
186. Shibahara T, Wilcox JN, Couse, T, et al. Characterization of epithelial chemoattractants for human intestinal lymphocytes. *Gastroenterology* 2001;120(1):60–70.
187. Rothenberg ME, Mishra A, Brandt EB, et al. Gastrointestinal eosinophils. *Immunol Rev* 2001;179:139–155.
188. Bochner BS, Schleimer RP. Mast cells, basophils, and eosinophils: Distinct but overlapping pathways for recruitment. *Immunol Rev* 2001;179:5–15.
189. Levy AM, Yamazaki K, Van Keulen VP, et al. Increased eosinophil infiltration and degranulation in colonic tissue from patients with collagenous colitis. *Am J Gastroenterol* 2001;96(5):1522–1528.
190. Polydorides AD, Banner BF, Hannaway PJ, et al. Evaluation of site-specific and seasonal variation in colonic mucosal eosinophils. *Hum Pathol* 2008;39(6):832–836.
191. Turner KO, Sinkre RA, Neumann WL, et al. Primary colonic eosinophilia and eosinophilic colitis in adults. *Am J Surg Pathol* 2017;41(2):225–233.
192. Harnois C, Demers MJ, Bouchard V, et al. Human intestinal epithelial crypt cell survival and death: Complex modulations of Bcl-2 homologs by Fak, PI3-K/Akt-1, MEK/Erk, and p38 signaling pathways. *J Cell Physiol* 2004;198(2):209–222.
193. Barkla DH, Gibson PR. The fate of epithelial cells in the human large intestine. *Pathology* 1999;31(3):230–238.
194. Gomez-Angelats M, Bortner CD, Cidlowski JA. Cell volume regulation in immune cell apoptosis. *Cell Tissue Res* 2000;301(1):33–42.
195. Gupta S. Molecular signaling in death receptor and mitochondrial pathways of apoptosis (Review). *Int J Oncol* 2003;22(1):15–20.
196. Huppertz B, Frank HG, Kaufmann P. The apoptosis cascade—morphological and immunohistochemical methods for its visualization. *Anat Embryol (Berl)* 1999;200(1):1–18.
197. Luciano L, Groos S, Busche R, et al. Massive apoptosis of colonocytes induced by butyrate deprivation overloads resident macrophages and promotes the recruitment of circulating monocytes. *Cell Tissue Res* 2002;309(3):393–407.
198. Schuster N, Krieglstein K. Mechanisms of TGF-beta-mediated apoptosis. *Cell Tissue Res* 2002;307(1):1–14.
199. Watson AJ. Apoptosis and colorectal cancer. *Gut* 2004;53(11):1701–1709.
200. Xiao ZQ, Moragoda L, Jaszewski R, et al. Aging is associated with increased proliferation and decreased apoptosis in the colonic mucosa. *Mech Ageing Dev* 2001;122(15):1849–1864.
201. Medina F, Segundo C, Campos-Caro A, et al. Isolation, maturational level, and functional capacity of human colon lamina propria plasma cells. *Gut* 2003;52(3):383–389.
202. Simon HU. Regulation of eosinophil and neutrophil apoptosis—similarities and differences. *Immunol Rev* 2001;179:156–162.
203. Iqbal N, Salzman D, Lazenby AJ, et al. Diagnosis of gastrointestinal graft-versus-host disease. *Am J Gastroenterol* 2000;95(11):3034–3038.
204. Iwamoto M, Koji T, Makiyama K, et al. Apoptosis of crypt epithelial cells in ulcerative colitis. *J Pathol* 1996;180(2):152–159.
205. Backus HH, Van Groeningen CJ, Vos W, et al. Differential expression of cell cycle and apoptosis related proteins in colorectal mucosa, primary colon tumours, and liver metastases. *J Clin Pathol* 2002;55(3):206–211.
206. Anagnostopoulos I, Schuppan D, Riecken EO, et al. Tenascin labelling in colorectal biopsies: A useful marker in the diagnosis of collagenous colitis. *Histopathology* 1999;34(5):425–431.
207. Gledhill A, Cole FM. Significance of basement membrane thickening in the human colon. *Gut* 1984;25(10):1085–1088.
208. Powell DW, Mifflin RC, Valentich JD, et al. Myofibroblasts. II. Intestinal subepithelial myofibroblasts. *Am J Physiol* 1999;277(2 pt 1):C183–C201.
209. Azzali G. Structure, lymphatic vascularization and lymphocyte migration in mucosa-associated lymphoid tissue. *Immunol Rev* 2003;195:178–189.
210. Brandtzaeg P, Johansen FE, Baekkevold ES, et al. The traffic of mucosal lymphocytes to extraintestinal sites. *J Pediatr Gastroenterol Nutr* 2004;39(suppl. 3):S725–S726.
211. Goldstein NS, Bhanot P. Paucicellular and asymptomatic lymphocytic colitis. Expanding the clinicopathologic spectrum of lymphocytic colitis. *Am J Clin Pathol* 2004;122(3):405–411.
212. Fischer M, Kuppers R. Human IgA- and IgM-secreting intestinal plasma cells carry heavily mutated VH region genes. *Eur J Immunol* 1998;28(9):2971–2977.
213. Brandtzaeg P, Pabst R. Let's go mucosal: Communication on slippery ground. *Trends Immunol* 2004;25(11):570–577.
214. Nishida Y, Murase K, Isomoto H, et al. Different distribution of mast cells and macrophages in colonic mucosa of patients with collagenous colitis and inflammatory bowel disease. *Hepatogastroenterology* 2002;49(45):678–682.
215. Pascal RR, Gramlich TL, Parker KM, et al. Geographic variations in eosinophil concentration in normal colonic mucosa. *Mod Pathol* 1997;10(4):363–365.
216. Barbara G, Stanghellini V, DeGiorgio R, et al. Activated mast cells in proximity to colonic nerves correlate with abdominal pain in irritable bowel syndrome. *Gastroenterology* 2004;126(3):693–702.
217. Boyce JA. Mast cells: Beyond IgE. *J Allergy Clin Immunol* 2003;111(1):24–32, quiz 33.
218. Doyle LA, Sepehr GJ, Hamilton MJ, et al. A clinicopathologic study of 24 cases of systemic mastocytosis involving the gastrointestinal tract and assessment of mucosal mast cell density in irritable bowel syndrome and asymptomatic patients. *Am J Surg Pathol* 2014;38(6):832–843.

219. Mayer L. Current concepts in mucosal immunity. I. Antigen presentation in the intestine: New rules and regulations. *Am J Physiol* 1998;274(1 pt 1):G7–G9.
220. Rubio CA. Rectal muciphages are rich in lysozymes: A novel source of antimicrobial mucosal defense? *Scand J Gastroenterol* 2002;37(6):743–744.
221. Salto-Tellez M, Price AB. What is the significance of muciphages in colorectal biopsies? The significance of muciphages in otherwise normal colorectal biopsies. *Histopathology* 2000;36(6):556–569.
222. Schenk M, Bouchon A, Birrer S, et al. Macrophages expressing triggering receptor expressed on myeloid cells-1 are underrepresented in the human intestine. *J Immunol* 2005;174(1):517–524.
223. Alkan S, Beals TF, Schnitzer B. Primary diagnosis of Whipple disease manifesting as lymphadenopathy: Use of polymerase chain reaction for detection of Tropheryma whippelii. *Am J Clin Pathol* 2001;116(6):898–904.
224. Dobbins WO 3rd, Weinstein WM. Electron microscopy of the intestine and rectum in acquired immunodeficiency syndrome. *Gastroenterology* 1985;88(3):738–749.
225. Lee SH, Barnes WG, Hodges GR, et al. Perforated granulomatous colitis caused by Histoplasma capsulatum. *Dis Colon Rectum* 1985;28(3):171–176.
226. Nguyen HN, Frank D, Handt S, et al. Severe gastrointestinal hemorrhage due to Mycobacterium avium complex in a patient receiving immunosuppressive therapy. *Am J Gastroenterol* 1999;94(1):232–235.
227. Hart AL, Lammers K, Brigidi P, et al. Modulation of human dendritic cell phenotype and function by probiotic bacteria. *Gut* 2004;53(11):1602–1609.
228. Zareie M, Singh PK, Irvine EJ, et al. Monocyte/macrophage activation by normal bacteria and bacterial products: Implications for altered epithelial function in Crohn's disease. *Am J Pathol* 2001;158(3):1101–1109.
229. Bodey B, Siegel SE, Kaiser HE. Antigen presentation by dendritic cells and their significance in antineoplastic immunotherapy. *In Vivo* 2004;18(1):81–100.
230. Powell DW, Mifflin RC, Valentich JD, et al. Myofibroblasts. I. Paracrine cells important in health and disease. *Am J Physiol* 1999;277(1 pt 1):C1–C9.
231. Skalli O, Schurch W, Seemayer T, et al. Myofibroblasts from diverse pathologic settings are heterogeneous in their content of actin isoforms and intermediate filament proteins. *Lab Invest* 1989;60(2):275–285.
232. Ward SM, Sanders KM, Hirst GD. Role of interstitial cells of Cajal in neural control of gastrointestinal smooth muscles. *Neurogastroenterol Motil* 2004;16(suppl 1):112–117.
233. Biberthaler P, Langer S. Comparison of the new OPS imaging technique with intravital microscopy: Analysis of the colon microcirculation. *Eur Surg Res* 2002;34(1–2):124–128.
234. Fenoglio CM, Kay GI, Lane N. Distribution of human colonic lymphatics in normal, hyperplastic, and adenomatous tissue. Its relationship to metastasis from small carcinomas in pedunculated adenomas, with two case reports. *Gastroenterology* 1973;64(1):51–66.
235. Dobbins WO 3rd. The intestinal mucosal lymphatics in man. A light and electron microscopic study. *Gastroenterology* 1966;51(6):994–1003.
236. Fogt F, Zimmerman RL, Ross HM, et al. Identification of lymphatic vessels in malignant, adenomatous and normal colonic mucosa using the novel immunostain D2-40. *Oncol Rep* 2004;11(1):47–50.
237. Fogt F, Pascha TL, Zhang PJ, et al. Proliferation of D2-40-expressing intestinal lymphatic vessels in the lamina propria in inflammatory bowel disease. *Int J Mol Med* 2004;13(2):211–214.
238. Percy WH, Fromm TH, Wangsness CE. Muscularis mucosae contraction evokes colonic secretion via prostaglandin synthesis and nerve stimulation. *Am J Physiol Gastrointest Liver Physiol* 2003;284(2):G213–G220.
239. Percy WH, Brunz JT, Burgers RE, et al. Interrelationship between colonic muscularis mucosae activity and changes in transmucosal potential difference. *Am J Physiol Gastrointest Liver Physiol* 2001;281(2):G479–G489.
240. Daniel EE, Wang YF. Gap junctions in intestinal smooth muscle and interstitial cells of Cajal. *Microsc Res Tech* 1999;47(5):309–320.
241. Hagger R, Gharaie S, Finlayson C, et al. Regional and transmural density of interstitial cells of Cajal in human colon and rectum. *Am J Physiol* 1998;275(6 pt 1):G1309–G1316.
242. Coerdt W, Michel JS, Rippin G, et al. Quantitative morphometric analysis of the submucous plexus in age-related control groups. *Virchows Arch* 2004;444(3):239–246.
243. Wedel T, Spiegler J, Soellner S, et al. Enteric nerves and interstitial cells of Cajal are altered in patients with slow-transit constipation and megacolon. *Gastroenterology* 2002;123(5):1459–1467.
244. Wilder-Smith CH, Talbot IC, Merki HS, et al. Morphometric quantification of normal submucous plexus in the distal rectum of adult healthy volunteers. *Eur J Gastroenterol Hepatol* 2002;14(12):1339–1342.
245. Faussone-Pellegrini MS, Pantalone D, Cortesini C. Smooth muscle cells, interstitial cells of Cajal and myenteric plexus interrelationships in the human colon. *Acta Anat (Basel)* 1990;139(1):31–44.
246. Tunru-Dinh V, Wu ML. Intramucosal ganglion cells in normal adult colorectal mucosa. *Int J Surg Pathol* 2007;15(1):31–37.
247. Oh HE, Chetty R. Intramucosal ganglion cells are common in diverticular disease. *Pathology* 2008;40(5):470–474.
248. Faussone-Pellegrini MS, Cortesini C, Pantalone D. Neuromuscular structures specific to the submucosal border of the human colonic circular muscle layer. *Can J Physiol Pharmacol* 1990;68(11):1437–1446.
249. Mazzia C, Porcher C, Jule Y, et al. Ultrastructural study of relationships between c-kit immunoreactive interstitial cells and other cellular elements in the human colon. *Histochem Cell Biol* 2000;113(5):401–411.
250. Rumessen JJ, Peters S, Thuneberg L. Light and electron microscopical studies of interstitial cells of Cajal and muscle cells at the submucosal border of human colon. *Lab Invest* 1993;68(4):481–495.
251. Ward SM, Sanders KM. Interstitial cells of Cajal: Primary targets of enteric motor innervation. *Anat Rec* 2001;262(1):125–135.
252. Takayama I, Horiguchi K, Daigo Y, et al. The interstitial cells of Cajal and a gastroenteric pacemaker system. *Arch Histol Cytol* 2002;65(1):1–26.
253. Krishnamurthy S, Schuffler MD. Pathology of neuromuscular disorders of the small intestine and colon. *Gastroenterology* 1987;93(3):610–639.

254. Fraser ID, Condon RE, Schulte WJ, et al. Longitudinal muscle of muscularis externa in human and nonhuman primate colon. *Arch Surg* 1981;116(1):61–63.
255. Chan OT, Chiles L, Levy M, et al. Smoothelin expression in the gastrointestinal tract: Implication in colonic inertia. *Appl Immunohistochem Mol Morphol* 2013;21(5):452–459.
256. Hirota S, Isozaki K, Moriyama Y, et al. Gain-of-function mutations of c-kit in human gastrointestinal stromal tumors. *Science* 1998;279(5350):577–580.
257. Kindblom LG, Remotti HE, Aldenborg F, et al. Gastrointestinal pacemaker cell tumor (GIPACT): Gastrointestinal stromal tumors show phenotypic characteristics of the interstitial cells of Cajal. *Am J Pathol* 1998;152(5):1259–1269.
258. Driman DK, Preiksaitis HG. Colorectal inflammation and increased cell proliferation associated with oral sodium phosphate bowel preparation solution. *Hum Pathol* 1998;29(9):972–978.
259. Levine DS. Proctitis following colonoscopy. *Gastrointest Endosc* 1988;34(3):269–272.
260. Pockros PJ, Foroozan P. Golytely lavage versus a standard colonoscopy preparation: Effect on normal colonic mucosal histology. *Gastroenterology* 1985;88(2):545–548.
261. Rejchrt S, Bures J, Siroký M, et al. A prospective, observational study of colonic mucosal abnormalities associated with orally administered sodium phosphate for colon cleansing before colonoscopy. *Gastrointest Endosc* 2004;59(6):651–654.
262. Wong NA, Penman ID, Campbell S, et al. Microscopic focal cryptitis associated with sodium phosphate bowel preparation. *Histopathology* 2000;36(5):476–478.
263. Fa-Si-Oen PR, Penninckx F. The effect of mechanical bowel preparation on human colonic tissue in elective open colon surgery. *Dis Colon Rectum* 2004;47(6):948–949.
264. Allen TV, Achord JL. The pickle of proper bowel biopsy orientation. *Gastroenterology* 1977;72(4 pt 1):774–775.
265. Bucher P, Gervaz, P, Egger JF, et al. Morphologic alterations associated with mechanical bowel preparation before elective colorectal surgery: A randomized trial. *Dis Colon Rectum* 2006;49(1):109–112.
266. Haggitt RC. Handling of gastrointestinal biopsies in the surgical pathology laboratory. *Lab Med* 1982;13:272–278.
267. Carson FL. Polyfoam pads—a source of artifact. *J Histotechnol* 1981;4:33–34.
268. Snover DC, Sandstad J, Hutton S. Mucosal pseudolipomatosis of the colon. *Am J Clin Pathol* 1985;84(5):575–580.

25

Appendix

Megan G. Lockyer ■ Robert E. Petras

GROSS ANATOMY/SURGICAL PERSPECTIVE 664	SPECIAL CONSIDERATIONS 672
Development of the Vermiform Appendix and Congenital Anomalies 665	Normal Variation of Mucosal Inflammation Versus Acute Appendicitis 672
FUNCTION 665	Obliteration of the Appendiceal Lumen (Appendiceal Neuromas) 672
NORMAL HISTOLOGY OF THE APPENDIX 665	Mucocele of the Appendix 674
Mucosal Architecture and Design 665	Dissection and Processing Techniques 674
Submucosa 671	REFERENCES 674
Muscularis Externa, Subserosal Region, and the Serosa 672	

GROSS ANATOMY/SURGICAL PERSPECTIVE

The vermiform (worm-like) appendix is a slender tubular extension of the posteromedial aspect of the cecum originating below, and within 1 to 3 cm of, the ileocecal junction. Although the appendix has a relatively constant relationship with the cecum at the appendiceal base, the remainder of its length can be found in a variable number of positions, including retrocecal, subcecal, pelvic, and juxtaileal (1–3). A retrocecal position occurs most commonly, being present in nearly 70% of the population (3,4). Unusual locations, including a vermiform appendix buried within the cecal wall, have been documented (5). Although the appendix itself lacks taeniae, the base of the vermiform appendix lies at the convergence of the three cecal/ascending colon taeniae. These aid in locating the appendix when it is not readily apparent; the prominent anterior taenia is most easily traced for this purpose (1,6).

Vermiform appendices can vary remarkably in length, but an average of 7 to 10 cm (2,4). The peritoneum covers almost all its external surface. The mesoappendix (mesentery of the appendix), a fold of peritoneum contiguous with the mesentery of the terminal ileum, extends along its length, terminating just proximal to the tip (1).

The appendiceal vascular supply courses within the mesoappendix; and with distal progression, these vessels gradually rest nearer to the appendiceal muscular wall. In the proximity of the tip where there is no mesoappendix, blood vessels lie essentially "unprotected" on its external surface (1). The appendicular artery, a derivative of the inferior branch of the ileocolic artery of the superior mesenteric trunk, provides the majority of blood to the appendix (4,7). However, a variable supply with accessory arterial contributions is not unusual (8). Branches of the ileocolic vein drain the appendiceal venous network into the superior mesenteric vein and eventually into the portal circulation, whereas lymphatic vessels drain into regional (e.g., ileocolic) lymph nodes (6). Innervation is derived from branches of the vagus nerve (parasympathetic) and superior mesenteric plexus (sympathetic). Venous, lymphatic, and neural components closely follow the arterial vasculature (6).

Grossly, the external surface of the vermiform appendix appears smooth, pink-tan or gray, and glistening. The appendiceal diameter typically measures 5 to 8 mm. The wall is tan-white and the mucosal lining is light yellow, often disclosing a nodular appearance imparted by the characteristic and prominent lymphoid component (9). Because of these lymphoid aggregates, the central lumen on cross section is often irregular (stellate) rather than round. The normal luminal diameter measures 1 to 3 mm; however, in one study a luminal diameter of 1.2 cm or more was arbitrarily defined as dilatation (10). Focal occlusions of the appendiceal lumen are not uncommon (9).

This chapter is an update of a previous version authored by William E. Katzin and Robert E. Petras.

Development of the Vermiform Appendix and Congenital Anomalies

The vermiform appendix originates from the primordial structure termed the cecal diverticulum (5,11). First apparent during the 6th week of fetal life, this blind-ended sac progressively develops. Its most proximal portion, in continuity with the remainder of the large bowel, enlarges and expands, forming the cecum proper, whereas its distal aspect or apex simply elongates, remains narrow, and becomes the vermiform appendix (11). Continued growth through infancy and childhood leads to differing cecoappendiceal relationships over this period. For example, the "infantile" cecoappendiceal junction lacks a conspicuous transition; the appendix arises from the inferior aspect of the cecum in this age group. In contrast, an abrupt, easily recognizable junction on the posteromedial cecum is observed in the adult (2).

Abnormal embryologic development can result in agenesis, hypoplasia, and various duplications or even triplication of the appendix (5,9,12–14). Duplication of the appendix can mimic cecal duplication. In general, appendiceal duplication is recognized by the presence of complete and separate inner circular and outer longitudinal muscle bands and the presence of a prominent lymphoid component (12).

Duplications have been well described and categorized and can be associated with other complex and life-threatening congenital anomalies. The classification of appendiceal duplications includes type A, an appendix with a common base, single cecum, and bifurcated distal portion; type B, two separate appendices with distinct bases arising from a single cecum; and type C, two cecal structures, each with its own single appendix (12,13). The type C anomaly is always associated with other organ duplications and often necessitates extensive operative correction in infancy; a type B variant is also associated with other systemic anomalies (12). However, the majority of type B and all type A duplications are found incidentally or during operation for suspected appendicitis in older children and adults. Horseshoe appendix, an extremely rare abnormality with only six cases reported, has also been attributed to abnormal embryologic development though more cases and further studies are required (15,16).

FUNCTION

The exact role of the appendix is uncertain. However, rather than simply representing a vestigial, functionless structure, the abundant quantity of organized lymphoid tissue suggests involvement in mucosal immunity (17). It has been suggested that B lymphocytes derived from the appendix migrate and populate distant sites of the gastrointestinal tract lamina propria and evolve in these widespread foci into functional immunoglobulin (Ig)A-secreting plasma cells (17,18). In this role, the appendix can both attenuate potentially harmful immunoglobulin responses and enhance regional mucosal immunity (18). It has also been proposed that the appendix may function as a "safe house" for commensal bacteria, providing a reservoir of beneficial organisms to repopulate the gut in the event that its contents are purged following infection with a pathogen (19). The appendiceal biofilm, a layer of loose mucin and commensal gut bacteria adjacent to the lumen, is actively shed from the mucosal surface, and is accelerated through an increased turnover of enterocytes during diarrheal-inducing infection. In addition, diarrheal-inducing infectious agents have been shown to enhance mucin gene expression in the mucus layers overlying the mucosa possibly in response to disruption of these mucus layers secondary to bacterial invasion (20).

NORMAL HISTOLOGY OF THE APPENDIX

The histologic composition of the appendix is similar to that of the large bowel. The four layers, from its luminal to external surface, include the mucosa, submucosa, muscularis externa (or propria), and serosa. The distinctive features of the appendix are emphasized.

Mucosal Architecture and Design

A single layer of surface epithelium covers the luminal aspect of the appendiceal mucosa. This overlies the lamina propria within which crypts, or intestinal glands, contiguous with the surface epithelial cells are irregularly dispersed (Fig. 25.1). The lamina propria is a cellular layer with an abundant migratory cell component and prominent, often confluent, lymphoid aggregates. In contrast to the scattered lymphoid nodules within the large bowel proper, the appendix, particularly in young individuals, contains abundant and organized lymphoid structures spread around its

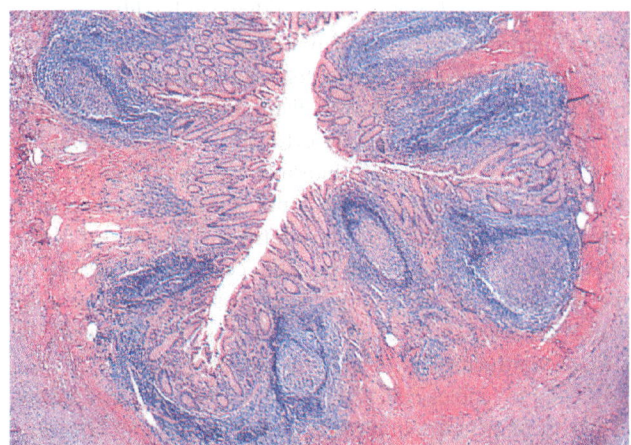

FIGURE 25.1 Low-magnification view of a cross section of the vermiform appendix. The irregular (stellate) lumen is lined by a single layer of surface epithelium. The remainder of the mucosa (crypts, surrounding lamina propria, and the rather inconspicuous muscularis mucosae) surrounds this surface epithelial layer. Note the characteristic lymphoid nodules within the lamina propria that also extend into the submucosa.

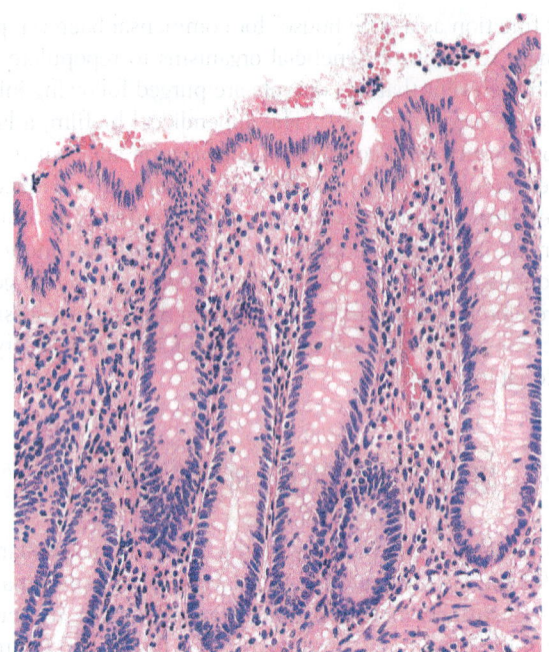

FIGURE 25.2 The surface epithelium is composed of a single layer of predominantly columnar cells with rare interspersed goblet cells. The crypt linings have a similar cellular composition but contain more goblet cells.

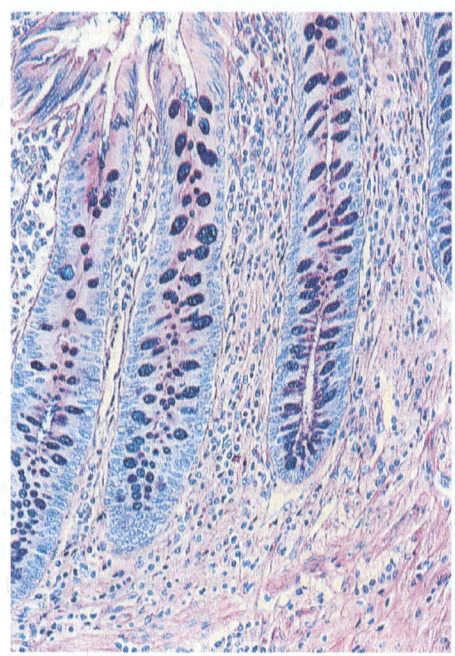

FIGURE 25.3 Since goblet cells contain both neutral and acid mucopolysaccharides, their apical mucin droplets stain blue-purple with the mixed Alcian blue/PAS preparation.

entire luminal circumference. These lymphoid nodules often distort the luminal contour (9,21). The outermost component and limit of the mucosa is the muscularis mucosae. This slender fibromuscular band is poorly developed in the appendix and often focally deficient.

Surface Epithelium

Several different cell types comprise the surface epithelium. A prominent cell that can be identified at the light microscopic level is tall and columnar with eosinophilic cytoplasm, and it has a round, basally located nucleus (Fig. 25.2). These cells represent several distinct cell types that can be differentiated at the ultrastructural level, including "senescent" mucous cells, the so-called absorptive cells, and membranous or M cells (22–25). Goblet cells with distinctive apical mucin droplets surrounded by eosinophilic cytoplasm and undermined by an attenuated basal nucleus intermix with the columnar cells (Fig. 25.2). The goblet cell apical mucin droplet contains both periodic acid–Schiff (PAS) positive neutral mucin and Alcian blue–positive acid sulfomucin. This combination results in the formation of a blue-purple color in a mixed Alcian blue/PAS stain (Fig. 25.3) (23,26). The mucus layer overlying the surface epithelium is composed predominantly of MUC2 produced by goblet cells. This mucus lining has two layers, unlike its intestinal counterpart which has only one. The inner mucus layer is firm and acts as a barrier to bacteria while the outer mucus layer is looser and contains commensal bacteria forming the biofilm (20,27). Overlying lymphoid aggregates, as in other portions of the small and the large bowel, is a specialized or follicle-associated epithelium that is distinct from the surrounding surface epithelium. It characteristically has fewer goblet cells, and many of the columnar cells are of the M (membrane or microfold) cell type (Fig. 25.4) (26). The M cell, a specialized epithelial cell, assists in luminal transport of antigens into the epithelium for appropriate immunologic

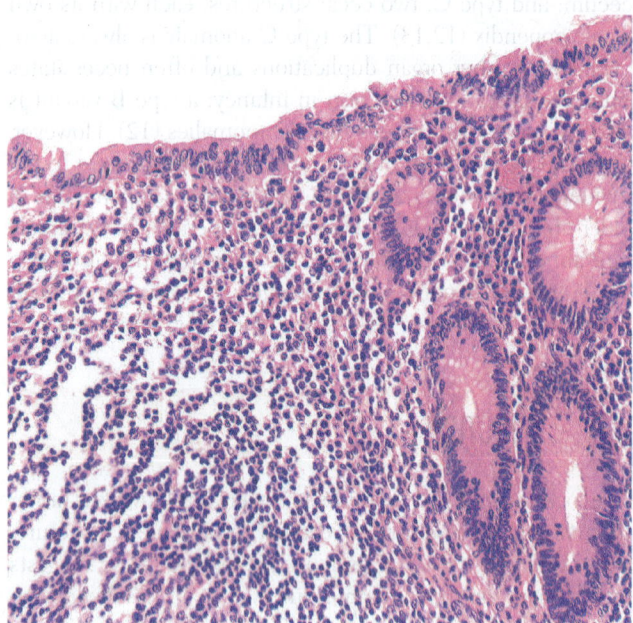

FIGURE 25.4 Surface epithelium overlying a lymphoid aggregate composed solely of tall columnar cells without intermixed goblet cells. Ultrastructurally, most of these would be classified as membranous or M cells. Note the increased numbers of intraepithelial lymphocytes between the individual columnar cells. Directly beneath the epithelium is the dome region of the lymphoid nodule. The apical portion of the germinal center with surrounding mantle zone is present near the bottom of the micrograph.

processing (28,29). M cells are columnar in shape with an attenuated brush border; several lymphocytes are often seen deforming their dependent cytoplasm. Definitive characterization rests on ultrastructural examination, which shows apical cytoplasmic vesicles and shortened microvilli or microfolds (25,28). Since circumferentially distributed organized lymphoid aggregates and lymphoid tissue are prominent in the normal appendix, the specialized follicle-associated epithelium often lines the majority of the appendiceal lumen. Thus, functionally, the surface epithelium is probably primarily involved in antigen processing, as well as in forming a barrier to luminal contents. The luminal surface is also the site where senescent cells are sloughed into the lumen (23,24). Scattered endocrine cells can be seen within the surface epithelium but are more abundant in the underlying crypts. Migratory T and B lymphocytes can be found anywhere within the surface epithelium (30,31), but are more abundant in the follicle-associated epithelium (Fig. 25.4).

Crypt Epithelium

In contrast to the colon, where crypts line up evenly like test tubes in a rack, appendiceal crypts are more irregular in shape, length, and distribution (32). In areas with abundant lymphoid tissue or lymphoid aggregates, crypts are typically absent (Fig. 25.5) (33).

Several different cell types line the crypts. The goblet and columnar cell variants discussed above are the most abundant (Figs. 25.2 and 25.6). Undifferentiated stem cells

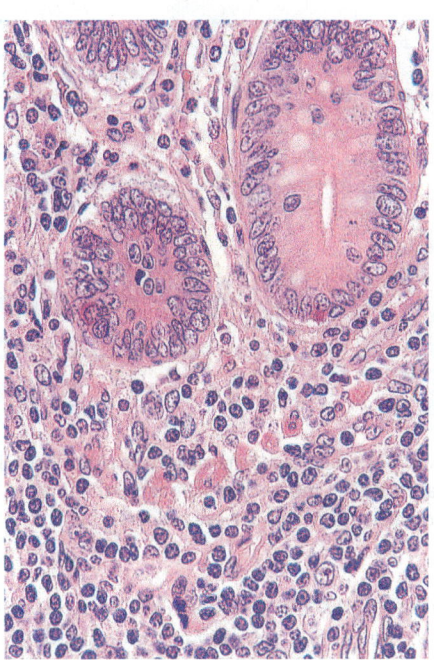

FIGURE 25.6 Crypts lying within a normocellular lamina propria. The round or ovoid crypts are lined predominantly by eosinophilic columnar cells and goblet cells. A single endocrine cell (containing infranuclear eosinophilic granules) is present at the base of each crypt. The lamina propria contains plasma cells, lymphocytes, and scattered eosinophils. Note the polygonal cells with abundant eosinophilic cytoplasm within the lamina propria. These are the subepithelial (laminal propria) endocrine cells that are often found near the crypt bases.

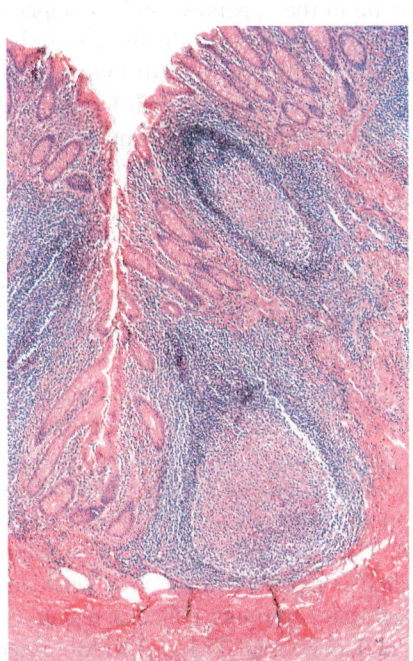

FIGURE 25.5 Lymphoid aggregates are often a prominent component within the appendiceal mucosa. Note the absence of crypts in the region of the lymphoid nodules and the distortion of surrounding crypts. This is a normal finding in the appendix and is similar to the alteration associated with isolated lymphoid aggregates in the colon.

are scattered about, but are inconspicuous. These are typically located at the crypt base, rest on the basement membrane, and do not extend to the crypt lumen; they are best identified by ultrastructural means (23). Isolated or clustered endocrine cells are seen along the crypt epithelium. Their appearance varies from a flask-shaped cell with a narrow strip of apical cytoplasm contiguous with the surface to a spindle-shaped cell with no luminal connection (34,35). Although some endocrine cells can be recognized on hematoxylin and eosin (H&E)-stained sections by their eosinophilic, infranuclear granules (Fig. 25.6) (36), definitive identification rests on immunohistologic analysis for chromogranin (or other pan-reactive neuroendocrine markers) (Fig. 25.7) or ultrastructural analysis, which discloses neurosecretory granules within their cytoplasm. More specific immunohistologic methods show that endocrine cells within the appendiceal epithelium contain a variety of amine and polypeptide substances, including serotonin, substance P, somatostatin, and enteroglucagon (37). Paneth cells also can be found in the crypt bases within the normal appendix in nearly 96% of specimens (38–40). This cell has a basally situated round nucleus with a conspicuous nucleolus and abundant eosinophilic supranuclear granules (Fig. 25.8). Paneth cells contain lysozyme, defensins, immunoglobulins and appear capable of phagocytosis. Paneth cell

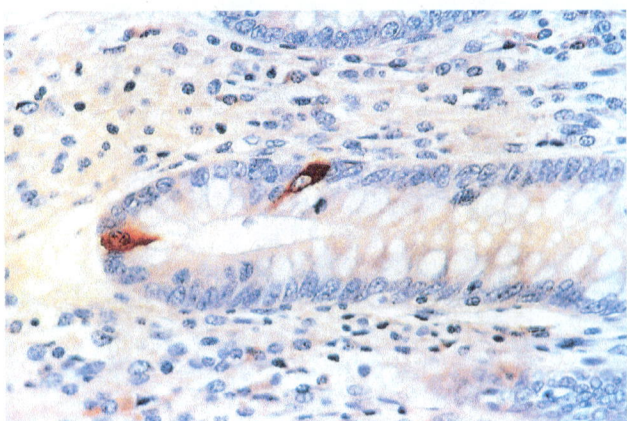

FIGURE 25.7 Scattered endocrine cells within the epithelium of an appendiceal crypt highlighted with antichromogranin. Intense red-brown cytoplasmic staining is evident in these endocrine cells.

alpha-defensin HD-5 is active against bacteria and can be localized to the cytoplasm using immunohistology or in-situ hybridization technique. Their cellular content and their localization near stem cells suggest that Paneth cells may protect the stem cell from damage by luminal contents and help regulate intestinal microbials (41,42).

Intraepithelial lymphocytes occur within the crypt epithelium (43,44), but neutrophils and plasma cells are not normal constituents of either epithelial compartment. Rarely, gastric, ileal, or esophageal squamous-type mucosa can be seen interrupting the normal appendiceal lining; some recognize these as true heterotopias (45–47).

The crypt functions in cell production and renewal because all cells of both epithelial compartments originate from the crypt's stem cells. Most of these cells travel to the surface epithelium, where they are subsequently sloughed intraluminally; the exception (Paneth cell) remains in the crypt base (43,44). It is believed that apoptosis within the crypt functions to regulate cell migration toward the surface; however, it is uncertain whether this type of cell death is responsible for epithelial cell loss into the lumen (48).

Subepithelial Basement Membrane

A slender zone separates the epithelial compartments from the lamina propria and is composed of collagen and other matrix components (49). The subepithelial basement membrane stabilizes the epithelial layers. A PAS stain can be used to highlight this layer, which measures only the microns in thickness (Fig. 25.3) (24,49).

Lamina Propria

The lamina propria, the central layer of the mucosa, surrounds the crypts and forms a connective tissue framework around them. Its structural components are collagen and elastic fibers and associated fibroblasts intermingled with blood capillaries, lymphatics, and nerve fibers (22–24). As in large bowel lymphoid tissue, its migratory cell component consists primarily of plasma cells and T cells, along with scattered B cells, macrophages, dendritic cells, eosinophils, and mast cells (22,31,50). (Figs. 25.6 and 25.8). However, depending on an individual's age, a varying number of organized lymphoid structures distort the lamina proprial architecture. These lymphoid aggregates can extend beneath the muscularis mucosae into the underlying submucosa (Figs. 25.1 and 25.5), are often confluent, and appear similar in composition and function to Peyer patches of the small bowel (25). As in Peyer patches (see Chapter 23), this organized lymphoid tissue in the appendix can be compartmentalized into: (a) the lymphoid follicle; (b) the subepithelial dome; (c) the interfollicular region; and (d) follicle-associated epithelium (Fig. 25.9) (51–53). The follicle has, in most cases, a mitotically active germinal center containing a polymorphic population of follicular center B cells, CD4(+) Th cells, and tingible body macrophages (Fig. 25.10) (17,50–54). Immediately surrounding the germinal center is the mantle zone, a darkly staining cuff of small B cells that express IgM and IgD. Overlying the lymphoid aggregate is the subepithelial dome region that harbors a heterogeneous population of cells including B and T cells, macrophages, dendritic cells, and occasional plasma cells (25,53). A prominent collagenous network and closely associated lymphatic vessels surround and define the lymphoid nodule (18). This collagenous/fibrous border is contiguous with the connective tissue framework of the interfollicular zones and adjacent lamina propria (18). The zone surrounding a single lymphoid nodule (parafollicular region) and the area between confluent lymphoid aggregates (the interfollicular region) consist predominantly of T cells (Fig. 25.11) (53). Moreover, the ratio of CD4-positive T cells to CD8-positive T cells is normally about 8:1 in these areas (53). Finally, as detailed previously, the follicle-associated epithelium is specialized and morphologically distinct from the adjacent absorptive-type surface epithelium.

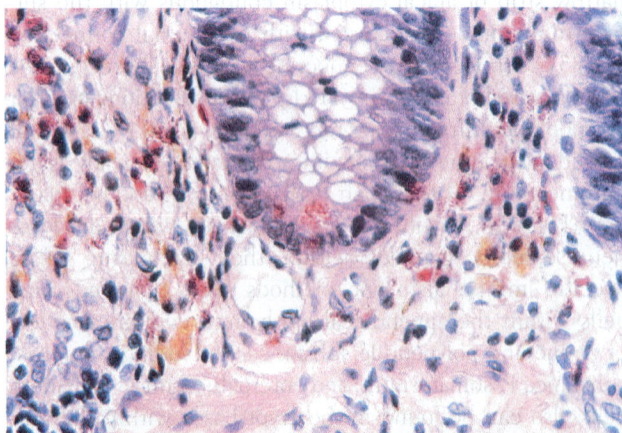

FIGURE 25.8 Appendiceal crypt disclosing Paneth cell (at its base) with characteristic supranuclear eosinophilic granules. The surrounding lamina propria has a conspicuous, albeit normal, quantity of eosinophils. Also, note the golden brown, granular pigment within the macrophages, which is characteristic of melanosis.

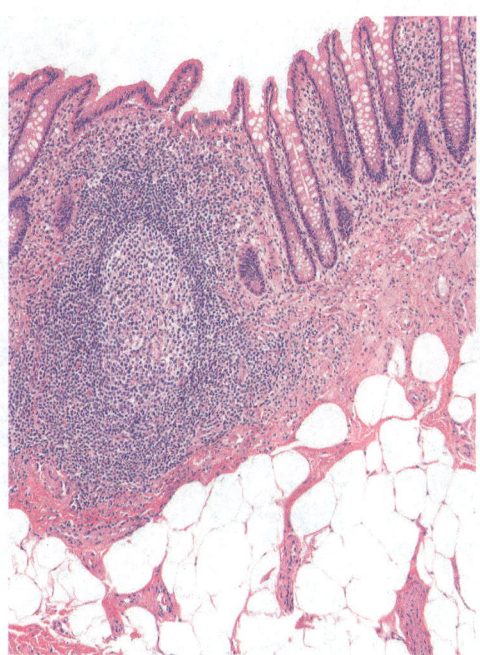

FIGURE 25.9 Characteristic lymphoid nodule within lamina propria of appendix. A germinal center forms the "core" of the follicle and is surrounded, at least in part, by a mantle zone of small round lymphocytes. Between the overlying epithelium and the mantle is the dome, which contains a mixed cellular population of lymphocytes, plasma cells, and macrophages. A portion of the parafollicular area (T lymphocyte zone) is seen. Lymphatic and blood vessels are seen beneath the lymphoid nodule in the underlying superficial submucosa.

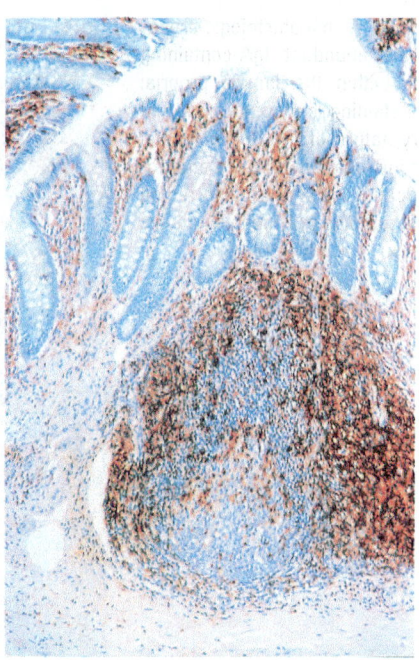

FIGURE 25.11 A pan–T-cell immunomarker, Leu-22 (CD43), disclosing the characteristic T lymphocyte distribution within the appendiceal mucosa. The lamina propria and interfollicular regions (between lymphoid follicles) are normally populated by numerous T lymphocytes. There is a sprinkling of T lymphocytes within the germinal center; these are predominantly CD4+ T lymphocytes.

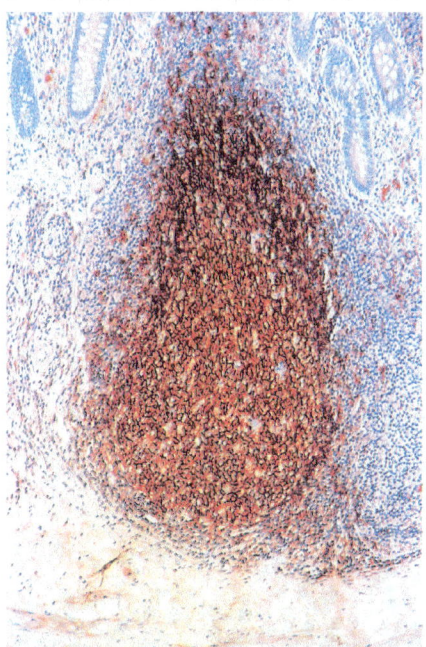

FIGURE 25.10 The germinal center and the mantle zone contain predominantly B lymphocytes. A pan–B-lymphocyte immunomarker, L26 (CD20), discloses this characteristic immunophenotype. Scattered macrophages and occasional T lymphocytes (see Fig. 25.11) are also normally found within the germinal center. Only scattered B-lymphocytes are present within the interfollicular zone and adjacent lamina propria.

The phenotype of the mononuclear cell population within the appendiceal mucosa is different from the colon. Although the quantity of B cells and plasma cells containing IgA and IgM is similar in both, IgG-containing cells are more abundant in the appendix (Fig. 25.12) (17,53). In fact, nearly 50% of the B cells in the subepithelial dome region are IgG immunoreactive (17). In addition T cells express more of the integrin subunit β_7 compared to T cells throughout the gut. Integrin $\alpha_4\beta_7$ is primarily on T cells between the lamina propria and epithelium, and is involved in the "tethering and rolling" or "homing" step in attracting lymphocytes which may promote antigen processing (20).

Lymphoid tissue, although a characteristic feature of the appendix, varies in quantity with age. The newborn's appendix contains scant or no lymphoid tissue. With increasing age the lymphoid nodules accumulate, peaking in the first decade (21,55). Lymphoid aggregates then steadily diminish in quantity throughout the remainder of life. However, appendices excised incidentally from middle-aged adults can still occasionally show a prominent organized lymphoid component (10). In contrast, lymphoid nodules and associated lymphocytes can be scant in the central obliterative form of appendiceal neuroma (fibrous obliteration of the appendiceal lumen) and occasionally in appendices removed from normal patients at any age (10). Thus, a great range of normal variation exists in the appendix with respect to its lymphoid content.

FIGURE 25.12 A: Immunohistologic preparation showing abundant IgA-containing plasma cells within the lamina propria; the epithelial staining is a consequence of the secretory nature of the IgA molecule. **B:** Abundant IgG-bearing cells are characteristically located within the dome region and along the margins of lymphoid nodules in the appendix.

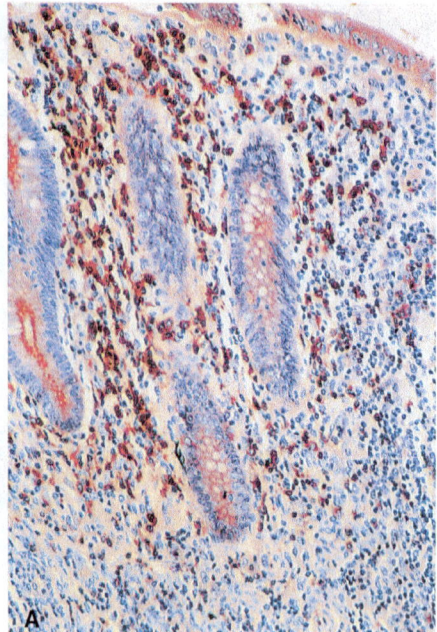
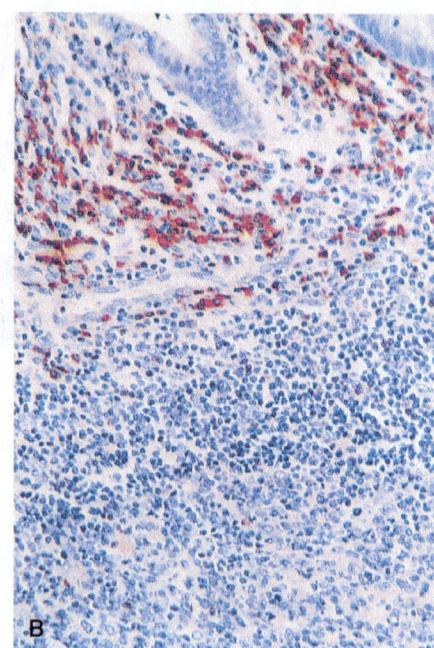

Macrophages with intracellular golden-brown pigment (lipofuscin), not infrequently observed in the colonic mucosa, can also be found in the appendiceal lamina propria; this alteration results from anthracene-containing laxative abuse and has been termed melanosis coli when seen in the colon proper (Fig. 25.8) (9,56). Interestingly, this pigmentation is a result of apoptosis induced by anthraquinones (48).

The lamina propria of the appendix contains a well-developed mucosal nervous plexus that is different from the more prominent submucosal and myenteric plexuses. Although all contain neurons (ganglion cells), Schwann cells, and neural processes (axons and neuropil), only the mucosal plexus contains endocrine (neurosecretory) cells. As a consequence, this network has been termed the mucosal neuroendocrine complex (57). These complexes, located just beneath the crypts, are composed of collections of endocrine cells and seen on H&E-stained preparations as polygonal cells with pale granular cytoplasm (Fig. 25.6), often intimately associated with spindled Schwann cells, neural processes, and occasional neurons. These collections, or neuroendocrine ganglia, are interconnected by neural fibers that can be highlighted immunohistologically with antibody preparations to neuron-specific enolase and, in a subset, to substance P (37); anti-S100 also can outline this network as it marks the accompanying Schwann cells. The mucosal plexus also communicates with other neural networks of the enteric nervous system (57–60). The subepithelial endocrine cells are not always conspicuous but can be highlighted using general neuroendocrine immunomarkers, such as antichromogranin (Fig. 25.13), antisynaptophysin, and anti-neuron-specific enolase, or by using electron microscopy (61,62). Most of these cells have been shown by specific immunohistologic analysis to contain serotonin (58,62). The mucosal neuroendocrine complex is believed to modulate neural communication, through serotonin mediators, between the epithelium and the deeper submucosal and intermuscular plexuses (62). Interestingly, because most appendiceal carcinoids are biphasic, consisting of an admixture of endocrine cells and S100+ Schwann cells (similar to the architecture of the mucosal neuroendocrine complex), the majority of

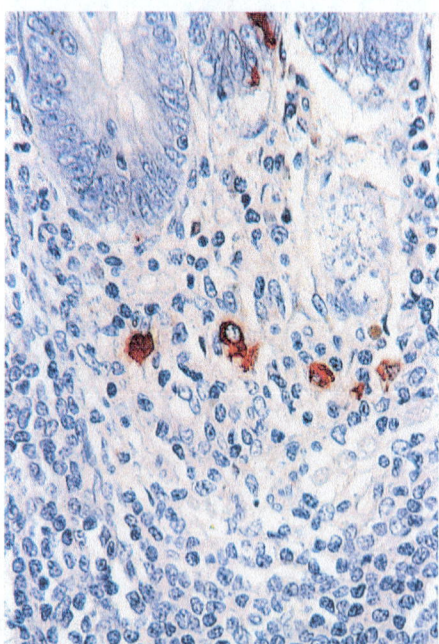

FIGURE 25.13 Antichromogranin highlights the subepithelial (lamina propria) endocrine cells beneath the crypts. These are more prominent and abundant in the appendix than in any other portion of gastrointestinal tract. Note also the epithelial-based endocrine cell in the overlying crypt.

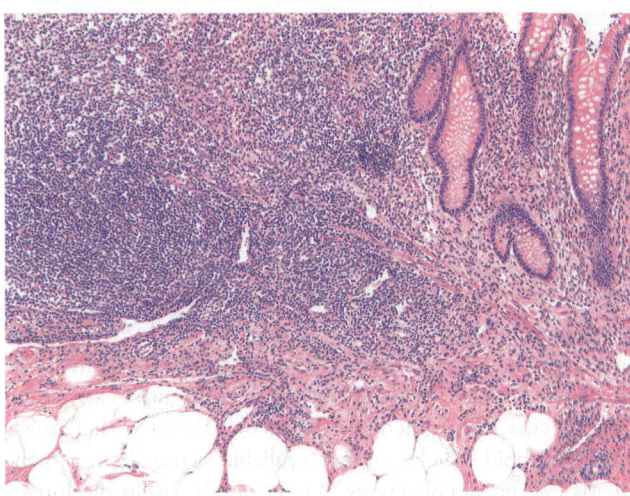

FIGURE 25.14 Characteristic focal deficiency of muscularis mucosae in region of lymphoid nodule. There is adipose tissue within the submucosa; this is a normal finding.

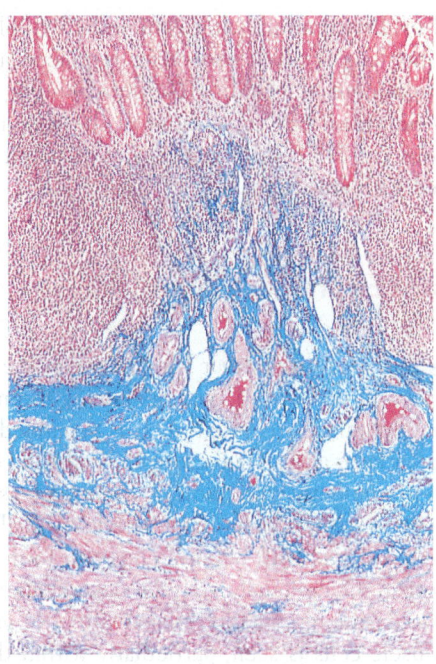

FIGURE 25.15 Normal appendiceal submucosa outlined in blue, highlighting its prominent collagenous framework. Numerous vascular spaces are also present within this layer. The mucosa (crypts) is *above* and the inner circular layer of the muscularis externa is *below* (Masson trichrome).

these appendiceal neoplasms are believed to be derived from these lamina propria endocrine cells rather than from the epithelium-based ones (58).

Muscularis Mucosae

The muscularis mucosae is a thin band of fibromuscular tissue separating the lamina propria and mucosal epithelium from the underlying submucosa. It characteristically forms a continuous layer in the large bowel (22); but in the appendix, the muscularis mucosae is attenuated, poorly developed, and often focally absent, particularly in the region of penetrating lymphoid aggregates (Fig. 25.14) (33,63). In these areas, the muscularis mucosae may exist solely as isolated smooth muscle cells in the underlying submucosa (63). Smooth muscle fibers of the muscularis mucosae can be distinguished from those making up the muscularis externa by differential immunostaining with smoothelin (64). The muscularis mucosae demonstrates weak or absent staining whereas the muscularis externa shows robust diffuse positive staining.

Submucosa

The submucosa separates the mucosa from the muscularis externa. Its loose architectural framework contains a meshwork of collagenous and elastic fibers and associated fibroblasts (Fig. 25.15). The submucosa can also contain inconspicuous migratory cells, such as macrophages, lymphoid and plasma cells, and mast cells, along with adipose tissue (Fig. 25.14) (21,65). The morphologic appearance of the appendiceal submucosa and its primary role in maintaining structure are similar throughout the gastrointestinal tract (65). Arterioles, venules, blood capillaries, and lymphatic vessels are a prominent component of the submucosa (Fig. 25.15) (7,22). Lymphatic vessels (or sinuses) are most prominent just beneath the bases of lymphoid aggregates (18). Neural structures, particularly Meissner plexus, are also conspicuous (Fig. 25.16). This plexus consists of ganglia, collections of neurons (ganglion cells) with associated neuronal processes, and Schwann cells that interconnect, creating a neural network throughout the submucosal layer (66,67). The ganglion cell is

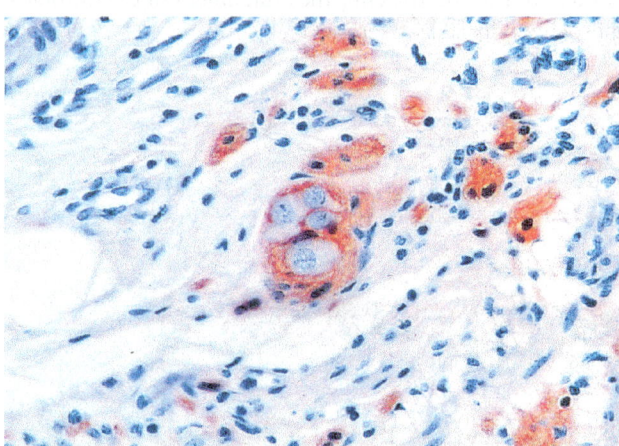

FIGURE 25.16 Submucosal neural network outlined with anti-S100. A single ganglion of Meissner plexus is at the center; the ganglion cells (neurons) have abundant pale cytoplasm, a large eccentric nucleus, and show no immunoreactivity. The Schwann cells of the ganglion and those ensheathing the neuronal processes of the remainder of the plexus are highlighted.

large and oval with abundant eosinophilic cytoplasm; its vesicular nucleus is often eccentrically placed and contains a prominent nucleolus. The surrounding spindle and wavy Schwann cell component of the ganglia is less conspicuous on H&E-stained preparations, but can be highlighted with anti-S100 (Fig. 25.16).

Muscularis Externa, Subserosal Region, and the Serosa

The thick smooth muscle layer lying between the submucosa and serosal portions of the appendix is the muscularis externa (or muscularis propria). It is separated into an inner circular layer and an outer longitudinal band (33) and both stain prominently with immunostains such as smooth muscle actin and smoothelin (64). The individual smooth muscle cells are oval with blunted ends and form bundles of varying sizes. Occasionally, granular degeneration (eosinophilic cytoplasmic granularity) of individual or groups of smooth muscle cells is seen, particularly within the inner circular layer (63,68). Between the two muscle bands lies the myenteric (Auerbach) plexus, which is morphologically and functionally similar to the previously described submucosal plexus of Meissner (Fig. 25.17) (67). Similarly to small intestine and colon, interstitial cells of Cajal form a meshwork around Auerbach plexus and in septa around smooth muscle cells. These cells which are involved in motility require special staining (e.g., CD117 immunostaining) for visualization. In addition, blood and lymphatic vessels and nerve fibers course through this muscular layer (18,69). Just external to the outer longitudinal smooth muscle layer is the subserosal region, consisting of loose connective tissue and ramifying blood vessels, lymphatics, and nerves. The outermost surface, or serosa, is lined by a single layer of cuboidal mesothelial cells that overlies a slender band of fibrous tissue. Only the attachment of the fibrofatty mesoappendix lacks a serosa (1).

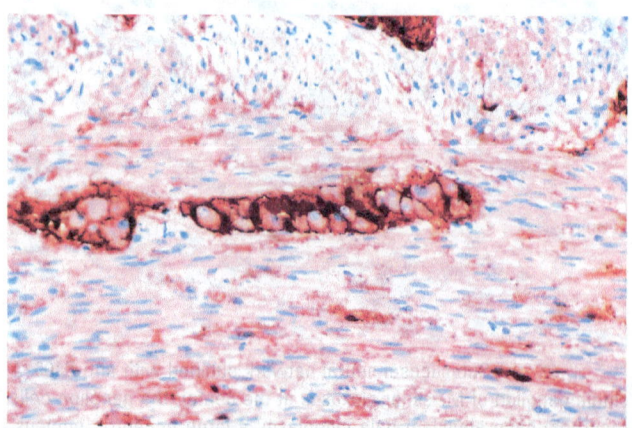

FIGURE 25.17 Anti-S100 highlighting Schwann cells of the neural network of the muscularis externa and a ganglion of the myenteric (Auerbach) plexus.

SPECIAL CONSIDERATIONS

Normal Variation of Mucosal Inflammation Versus Acute Appendicitis

Acute appendicitis is usually characterized by an abundant neutrophilic and eosinophilic infiltrate within the mucosa, submucosa, and often muscularis externa with at least focal mucosal ulceration; frequently suppurative inflammation extends into and through the appendiceal wall (9,10). However, the changes seen in early appendicitis can be quite minimal, and criteria considered sufficient to diagnose early acute appendicitis have varied (9,10,70–76). We agree that "reactive" lymphoid follicles are not a reliable sign of acute appendicitis (9). Focal collections of neutrophils within the lumen and lamina propria have been considered nondiagnostic by some investigators because many "incidental" appendectomy specimens contain these changes (9,10,73–75). However, we believe that if care is taken to recognize marginating neutrophils and early mucosal migration of these acute inflammatory cells (i.e., a result of the operative procedure alone), then other collections of neutrophils within the mucosa or intraluminal pus reflect stasis, infection, and changes of early appendicitis (71–73). Whether acute appendicitis becomes chronic or whether it can be recognized in a chronic state has long been debated (72). Fibrous obliteration of the appendiceal lumen is probably not a sequelae of acute appendicitis (60). However, prominent fibrosis, a marked chronic inflammatory cell infiltrate within the wall, and granulation tissue are abnormal and suggest an organizing appendicitis (9). Occasional specimens exhibit infiltration of the appendiceal wall by eosinophilic leukocytes with no other apparent abnormality (10). This change could reflect appendicitis elsewhere in the specimen that was not sampled; however, it remains possible that an infiltrate composed predominantly of eosinophils could represent appendicitis in a resolving phase or be a manifestation of eosinophilic gastroenteritis (71,77,78).

Obliteration of the Appendiceal Lumen (Appendiceal Neuromas)

Obliteration of the appendiceal lumen with the absence of the lining mucosa and underlying crypts frequently occurs and has a prevalence in surgical specimens of nearly 30% (9,60). This process usually affects the distal aspect or just the tip, but occasionally the entire lumen is obliterated. This process is often termed fibrous obliteration; however, some studies have shown that in many cases the occlusive proliferation appears to be predominantly neurogenic (37,60,79). Other diagnostic terms have been proposed, including neurogenic appendicopathy and appendiceal neuroma. The typical appendiceal neuroma, or the central obliterative form, is composed of a collection of spindle cells in a loose myxoid background with varying amounts of collagen, fat, and chronic inflammatory cells (Figs. 25.18 and 25.19).

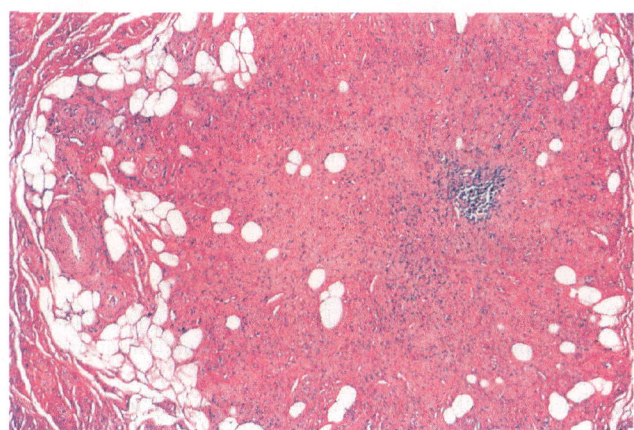

FIGURE 25.18 Obliteration of appendiceal lumen. The occlusive proliferation is composed of spindled cells within a collagenous and myxoid background, along with scattered adipocytes. A focus of chronic inflammatory cells is also present.

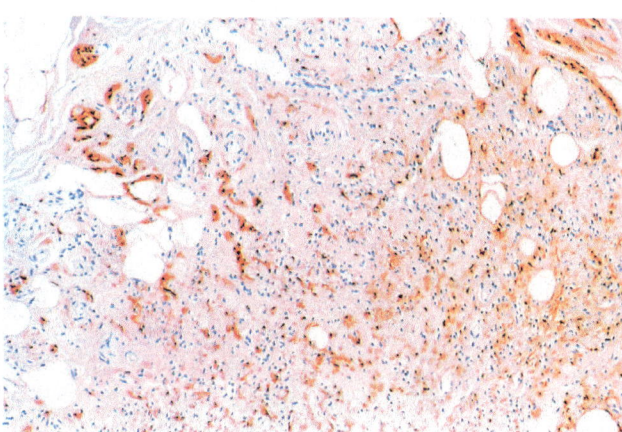

FIGURE 25.20 Prominent neurogenic (Schwann cell) component highlighted by anti-S100 within the obliterated lumen.

This typically occludes the lumen and blends imperceptibly with the surrounding submucosa (60). The involved segment usually lacks a mucosa and lymphoid follicles are typically not seen (24). Immunostaining for neuron-specific enolase and S100 highlights the spindle cells and identifies their neuronal (axons) and perineuronal (Schwann cell) nature, respectively (37,60) (Fig. 25.20). Moreover, endocrine cells visualized with anti-neuron-specific enolase and antichromogranin (Fig. 25.21) occur in many of the cases, usually intermingled with the other elements; serotonin and somatostatin have been identified in some of these endocrine cells by immunohistologic methods (37,60). Ultrastructural analysis discloses neuronal processes, Schwann cells, and cells with neurosecretory granules (endocrine cells) corroborating the immunostaining results (60).

Another variant of this entity, the intramucosal appendiceal neuroma, primarily affects the mucosa, causing no luminal obliteration. Although morphologically similar to the central obliterative form, this intramucosal variant deceptively expands the lamina propria, separates the crypts, and replaces the usual prominent migratory cell population (Fig. 25.22) (58). Immunostaining with S100 can be helpful in visualizing these more subtle changes.

Both of these entities are believed to be proliferative rather than involutional, progressing through consecutive stages of growth, regression, and finally an end-stage with fibrosis (60,80). Overlapping features are therefore expected with varied admixtures of neurogenic components, collagen, and fat. It is hypothesized that associated endocrine cell hyperplasia, often found in adjacent uninvolved appendiceal segments, may be responsible for painful stimuli mimicking typical acute appendicitis (60). However, appendiceal neuromas are often found in specimens removed at incidental appendectomy.

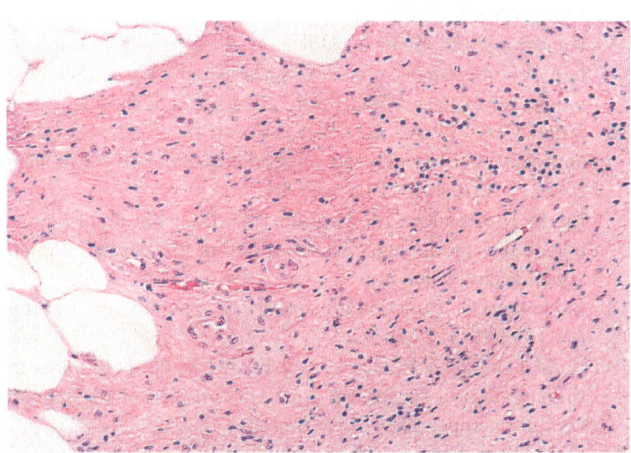

FIGURE 25.19 High magnification of Figure 25.18 showing spindled cell proliferation in an eosinophilic, fibromyxoid background.

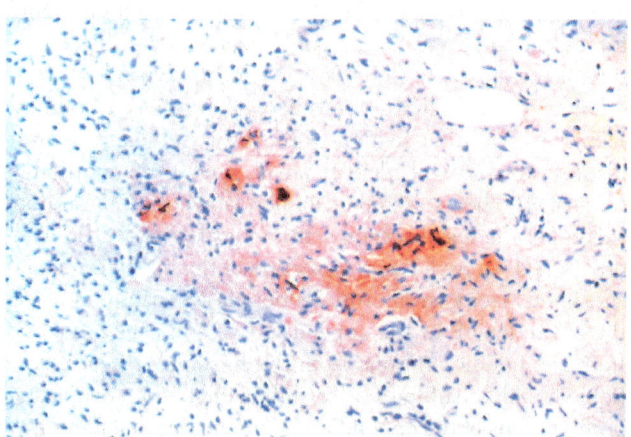

FIGURE 25.21 Scattered endocrine (neurosecretory) cells are evident within the obliterative luminal proliferation as highlighted by antichromogranin; specific immunomarkers show some of these to contain serotonin or somatostatin.

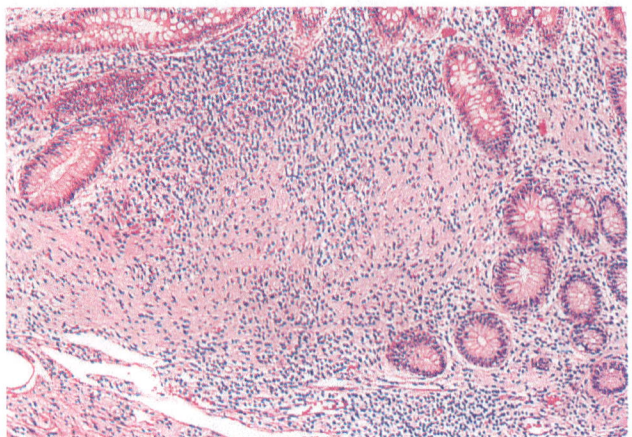

FIGURE 25.22 Intramucosal variant of appendiceal neuroma. The characteristic subtle spindle cell (schwannian) proliferation expands the lamina propria and separates the crypts. A diminished number of migratory cells are evident in this area.

Mucocele of the Appendix

The term *mucocele* has been used to describe a dilated appendiceal lumen filled with mucin (81). *Mucocele*, however, should not be used as a specific diagnostic term because the condition is almost always caused by a neoplastic proliferation including mucinous cystadenoma, low- or high-grade appendiceal mucinous neoplasm or mucinous cystadenocarcinoma (72,81–84). Characteristic architectural and cytologic features should permit identification of these entities.

Dissection and Processing Techniques

Gross dissection and processing of the appendix are generally straightforward. Routine description of size, appearance, and any unusual lesions should be recorded. Luminal patency should be assessed (i.e., obliteration or dilatation) along with the focality and regional distribution of any changes. The tip should be closely inspected for carcinoid tumors because these commonly occur in the distal portion of the appendix (9,83,85). When grossly evident, they often appear as bulbous, tan-yellow expansions, or nodules. However, a routine section of the tip is standard at most institutions and will identify small, grossly unidentifiable tumors (9). The common recommendation of a longitudinal section of the distal several centimeters is often difficult to orient, and we prefer a cross section of the tip. In the usual specimen, 1-cm serial cross-sectioning is performed along the entire length of the appendix. Two cross sections, one from the middle and one from the proximal line of resection, should be submitted for embedding. Since neoplastic proliferations of the appendix (e.g., mucinous cystadenoma/cystadenocarcinoma, carcinoid tumor and its variants) are not infrequently discovered incidentally during microscopic evaluation of the specimen, we recommend routinely sampling the margin of resection. Otherwise, it could be difficult to reconstruct the gross specimen in an attempt to assess the adequacy of excision. The choice of a fixative is not crucial and routine 4% formaldehyde solution is adequate. Modifications of dissection and processing may be necessary in certain situations.

REFERENCES

1. Williams PL, Warwick R, Dyson M, eds. *Gray's Anatomy of the Human Body*. 37th ed. New York: Churchill Livingstone; 1989.
2. Buschard K, Kjaeldgaard A. Investigation and analysis of the position, fixation, length, and embryology of the vermiform appendix. *Acta Chir Scand* 1973;139(3):293–298.
3. Wakeley CP. The position of the vermiform appendix as ascertained by an analysis of 10,000 cases. *J Anat* 1933;67(Pt 2): 277–283.
4. Thorek P. *Anatomy and Surgery*. 3rd ed. New York: Springer-Verlag; 1985.
5. Abramson DJ. Vermiform appendix located within the cecal wall. Anomalies and bizarre locations. *Dis Colon Rectum* 1983;26(6):386–389.
6. Hollinshead WH, Rosse C. *Textbook of Anatomy*. 4th ed. New York: Harper & Row; 1985.
7. Parks DA, Jacobson ED. Physiology of the splanchnic circulation. *Arch Intern Med* 1985;145(7):1278–1281.
8. Solanke TF. The blood supply of the vermiform appendix in Nigerians. *J Anat* 1968;102(pt 2):353–361.
9. Gray GF Jr, Wackym PA. Surgical pathology of the vermiform appendix. In: Sommers SC, Rosen PP, Fechner RE, eds. *Pathology Annual. Part 2*. Norwalk, CT: Appleton-Century-Croft; 1986:111–144.
10. Butler C. Surgical pathology of acute appendicitis. *Hum Pathol* 1981;12(10):870–878.
11. Moore KL. *The Developing Human: Clinically Oriented Embryology*. 3rd ed. Philadelphia, PA: WB Saunders; 1982.
12. Bluett MK, Halter SA, Salhany KE, et al. Duplication of the appendix mimicking adenocarcinoma of the colon. *Arch Surg* 1987;122(7):817–820.
13. Wallbridge PH. Double appendix. *Br J Surg* 1962;50:346–347.
14. Tinckler LF. Triple appendix vermiformis—A unique case. *Br J Surg* 1968;55(1):79–81.
15. Nageswaran H, Khan U, Hill F, et al. Appendiceal duplication: A comprehensive review of published cases and clinical recommendations. *World J Surg* 2018;42(2):574–581.
16. Singh ChG, Nyuwi KT, Rangaswamy R, et al. Horseshoe appendix: An extremely rare appendiceal anomaly. *J Clin Diag Research* 2016;10(3):PD25–PD26.
17. Bjerke K, Brandtzaeg P, Rognum TO. Distribution of immunoglobulin producing cells is different in normal human appendix and colon mucosa. *Gut* 1986;27(6):667–674.
18. Bockman DE. Functional histology of appendix. *Arch Histol Jpn* 1983;46(3):271–292.
19. Randal Bollinger R, Barbas AS, Bush EL, et al. Biofilms in the large bowel suggest an apparent function of the human vermiform appendix. *J Theor Biol* 2007;249(4):826–831.
20. Kooij IA, Sahami S, Meijer SL, et al. The immunology of the vermiform appendix: A review of the literature. *Clin Exp Immuno* 2016;186(1):1–9.

21. Hwang JMS, Krumbhaar EB. The amount of lymphoid tissue of the human appendix and its weight at different age periods. *Am J Med Sci* 1940;199:75–83.
22. Hamilton SR. Structure of the colon. *Scand J Gastroenterol Suppl* 1984;93:13–23.
23. Shamsuddin AM, Phelps PC, Trump BF. Human large intestinal epithelium: Light microscopy, histochemistry, and ultrastructure. *Hum Pathol* 1982;13(9):790–803.
24. Levine DS, Haggitt RC. Normal histology of the colon. *Am J Surg Pathol* 1989;13(11):966–984.
25. Bockman DE, Cooper MD. Early lymphoepithelial relationships in human appendix: A combined light- and electron-microscopic study. *Gastroenterology* 1975;68(5 Pt 1):1160–1168.
26. Filipe MI. Mucins in the human gastrointestinal epithelium: A review. *Invest Cell Pathol* 1979;2(3):195–216.
27. Ermund A, Schutte A, Johansson ME, et al. Studies of mucus in mouse stomach, small intestine and colon. I. Gastrointestinal mucus layers have different properties depending on location as well as over the Peyer's patches. *Am J Physiol Gastrointest Liver Physiol* 2013;305(5):G341–G347.
28. Owen RL, Jones AL. Epithelial cell specialization within human Peyer's patches: An ultrastructural study of intestinal lymphoid follicles. *Gastroenterology* 1974;66(2):189–203.
29. Wolf JL, Bye WA. The membranous epithelial (M) cell and the mucosal immune system. *Annu Rev Med* 1984;35:95–112.
30. Dobbins WO 3rd. Human intestinal intraepithelial lymphocytes. *Gut* 1986;27(8):972–985.
31. Bartnik W, ReMine SG, Chiba M, et al. Isolation and characterization of colonic intraepithelial and lamina proprial lymphocytes. *Gastroenterology* 1980;78(5 pt 1):976–985.
32. Fawcett DW. *Bloom and Fawcett: A Textbook of Histology*. 11th ed. Philadelphia, PA: WB Saunders; 1986.
33. Neutra MR, Padykula HA. The gastrointestinal tract. In: Weiss L, ed. *Modern Concepts of Gastrointestinal Histology*. New York: Elsevier; 1984:658–706.
34. Lewin KJ. The endocrine cells of the gastrointestinal tract. The normal endocrine cells and their hyperplasias. Part 1. In: Sommers SC, Rosen PP, Fechner RE, eds. *Pathology Annual*. Norwalk, CT: Appleton-Century-Croft; 1986:1–27.
35. Sjolund K, Sanden G, Hakanson R, et al. Endocrine cells in human intestine: An immunocytochemical study. *Gastroenterology* 1983;85(5):1120–1130.
36. Millikin PD. Eosinophilic argentaffin cells in the human appendix. *Arch Pathol* 1974;98(6):393–395.
37. Hofler H, Kasper M, Heitz PU. The neuroendocrine system of normal human appendix, ileum and colon, and in neurogenic appendicopathy. *Virchows Arch A Pathol Anat Histopathol* 1983;399(2):127–140.
38. Sandow MJ, Whitehead R. The Paneth cell. *Gut* 1979;20(5):420–431.
39. Geller SA, Thung SN. Morphologic unity of Paneth cells. *Arch Pathol Lab Med* 1983;107(9):476–479.
40. Vestfrid MA, Suarez JE. Paneth's cells in the human appendix. A statistical study. *Acta Anat (Basel)* 1977;97(3):347–350.
41. Wehkamp J, Fellermann K, Herrlinger KR, et al. Mechanisms of disease: Defensins in gastrointestinal diseases. *Nat Clin Pract Gastroenterol Hepatol* 2005;2(9):406–415.
42. Wehkamp J, Salzman NH, Porter E, et al. Reduced Paneth cell alpha-defensins in ileal Crohn's disease. *Proc Natl Acad Sci USA* 2005;102(50):18129–18134.
43. Eastwood GL. Gastrointestinal epithelial renewal. *Gastroenterology* 1977;72(5 pt 1):962–975.
44. Lipkin M. Proliferation and differentiation of normal and diseased gastrointestinal cells. In: Johnson LR, ed. *Physiology of the Gastrointestinal Tract*. 2nd ed. New York: Raven Press; 1987:255–284.
45. Aubrey DA. Gastric heterotopia in the vermiform appendix. *Arch Surg* 1970;101(5):628–629.
46. Ashley DJ. Aberrant mucosa in the vermiform appendix. *Br J Surg* 1958;45(192):372–373.
47. Droga BW, Levine S, Baber JJ. Heterotopic gastric and esophageal tissue in the vermiform appendix. *Am J Clin Pathol* 1963;40:190–193.
48. Watson AJ. Necrosis and apoptosis in the gastrointestinal tract. *Gut* 1995;37(2):165–167.
49. Gledhill A, Cole FM. Significance of basement membrane thickening in the human colon. *Gut* 1984;25(10):1085–1088.
50. Heatley RV. The gastrointestinal mast cell. *Scand J Gastroenterol* 1983;18(4):449–453.
51. Tomasi TB Jr. Mechanisms of immune regulation at mucosal surfaces. *Rev Infect Dis* 1983;5(Suppl 4):S784–S792.
52. Dotan I, Mayer L. Mucosal immunity. In: Feldman M, Friedman LS, Brandt LJ, eds. *Sleisenger and Fordtran's Gastrointestinal and Liver Disease*. 9th ed. Philadelphia, PA: Saunders Elsevier; 2010:21–30.
53. Spencer J, Finn T, Isaacson PG. Gut associated lymphoid tissue: A morphological and immunocytochemical study of the human appendix. *Gut* 1985;26(7):672–679.
54. van der Valk P, Meijer CJ. The histology of reactive lymph nodes. *Am J Surg Pathol* 1987;11(11):866–882.
55. Berry RJ, Lack LA. The vermiform appendix of man, and the structural changes therein coincident with age. *J Anat Physiol* 1906;40(Pt 3):247–256.
56. Walker NI, Bennett RE, Axelsen RA. Melanosis coli. A consequence of anthraquinone-induced apoptosis of colonic epithelial cells. *Am J Pathol* 1988;131(3):465–476.
57. Papadaki L, Rode J, Dhillon AP, et al. Fine structure of a neuroendocrine complex in the mucosa of the appendix. *Gastroenterology* 1983;84(3):490–497.
58. Lundqvist M, Wilander E. Subepithelial neuroendocrine cells and carcinoid tumours of the human small intestine and appendix. A comparative immunohistochemical study with regard to serotonin, neuron-specific enolase and S-100 protein reactivity. *J Pathol* 1986;148(2):141–147.
59. Millikin PD. Extraepithelial enterochromaffin cells and Schwann cells in the human appendix. *Arch Pathol Lab Med* 1983;107(4):189–194.
60. Stanley MW, Cherwitz D, Hagen K, et al. Neuromas of the appendix. A light-microscopic, immunohistochemical and electron-microscopic study of 20 cases. *Am J Surg Pathol* 1986;10(11):801–815.
61. Facer P, Bishop AE, Lloyd RV, et al. Chromogranin: A newly recognized marker of endocrine cells in the human gastrointestinal tract. *Gastroenterology* 1985;89(6):1366–1373.
62. Rode J, Dhillon AP, Papadaki L. Serotonin-immunoreactive cells in the lamina propria plexus of the appendix. *Hum Pathol* 1983;14(5):464–469.
63. Sobel HJ, Marquet E, Schwarz R. Granular degeneration of appendiceal smooth muscle. *Arch Pathol* 1971;92(6):427–432.

64. Montani M, Thiesler T, Kristiansen G. Smoothelin is a specific and robust marker for distinction of muscularis propria and muscularis mucosae in the gastrointestinal tract. *Histopathology* 2010;57(2):244–249.
65. Lord MG, Valies P, Broughton AC. A morphologic study of the submucosa of the large intestine. *Surg Gynecol Obstet* 1977;145(1):55–60.
66. Gershon MD, Erde SM. The nervous system of the gut. *Gastroenterology* 1981;80(6):1571–1594.
67. Krishnamurthy S, Schuffler MD. Pathology of neuromuscular disorders of the small intestine and colon. *Gastroenterology* 1987;93(3):610–639.
68. Hausman R. Granular cells in musculature of the appendix. *Arch Pathol* 1963;75:360–372.
69. Richter A, Wit C, Vanderwinden JM, et al. Interstitial cells of Cajal in the vermiform appendix in childhood. *Eur J Pediatr Surg* 2009;19(1):30–33.
70. Pieper R, Kager L, Nasman P. Clinical significance of mucosal inflammation of the vermiform appendix. *Ann Surg* 1983;197(3):368–374.
71. Petras R, Gramlich T. Non-neoplastic intestinal diseases. In: Mills SE, ed. *Sternberg's Diagnostic Surgical Pathology*. 5th ed. New York: Lippincott Williams & Wilkins; 2010:1313–1367.
72. Morson BC, Dawson IMP, Day DW, et al. *Morson and Dawson's Gastrointestinal Pathology*. 3rd ed. Oxford: Blackwell Scientific; 1990.
73. Schenken JR, Anderson TR, Coleman FC. Acute focal appendicitis. *Am J Clin Pathol* 1956;26(4):352–359.
74. Campbell JS, Fournier P, Da Silva T. When is the appendix normal? A study of acute inflammations of the appendix apparent only upon histologic examination. *Can Med Assoc J* 1961;85:1155–1157.
75. Touloukian RJ, Trainer TD. Significance of focal inflammation of the appendix. *Surgery* 1964;56:942–944.
76. Miller SM, Narasimhan RA, Schmalz PF, et al. Distribution of interstitial cells of Cajal and nitrergic neurons in normal and diabetic human appendix. *Neurogastroenterol Motil* 2008;20(4):349–357.
77. Johnstone JM, Morson BC. Eosinophilic gastroenteritis. *Histopathology* 1978;2(5):335–348.
78. Klein NC, Hargrove RL, Sleisenger MH, et al. Eosinophilic gastroenteritis. *Medicine (Baltimore)* 1970;49(4):299–319.
79. Aubock L, Ratzenhofer M. "Extraepithelial enterochromaffin cell—nerve-fibre complexes" in the normal human appendix, and in neurogenic appendicopathy. *J Pathol* 1982;136(3):217–226.
80. Olsen BS, Holck S. Neurogenous hyperplasia leading to appendiceal obliteration: An immunohistochemical study of 237 cases. *Histopathology* 1987;11(8):843–849.
81. Qizilbash AH. Mucoceles of the appendix: Their relationship to hyperplastic polyps, mucinous cystadenomas, and cystadenocarcinomas. *Arch Pathol* 1975;99(10):548–555.
82. Higa E, Rosai J, Pizzimbono CA, et al. Mucosal hyperplasia, mucinous cystadenoma, and mucinous cystadenocarcinoma of the appendix: A re-evaluation of appendiceal "mucocele." *Cancer* 1973;32(6):1525–1541.
83. Riddell RH, Petras RE, Williams GT, et al. Tumors of the intestines. In: Rosai J, Sobin LH, eds. *Atlas of Tumor Pathology. Third Series Fascicle #32*. Washington, DC: Armed Forces Institute of Pathology; 2003.
84. Carr NJ, Cecil TD, Mohamed F, et al; Peritoneal Surface Oncology Group International. A consensus for classification and pathologic reporting of pseudomyxoma peritonei and associated appendiceal neoplasia: The Results of the Peritoneal Surface Oncology Group International (PSOGI) Modified Delphi Process. *Am J Surg Pathol* 2016;40(1):14–26.
85. Glasser CM, Bhagavan BS. Carcinoid tumors of the appendix. *Arch Pathol Lab Med* 1980;104(5):272–275.

Anal Canal

Meredith E. Pittman ■ Rhonda K. Yantiss

DEFINITION AND BOUNDARIES 677	LIGHT MICROSCOPY 681
EMBRYOLOGY 677	Mucosa 682
	Submucosa 684
GROSS AND FUNCTIONAL ANATOMY 679	Muscles 686
Musculature 680	DIAGNOSTIC CONSIDERATIONS 687
Innervation 680	Epithelial Metaplasia and Heterotopia 687
Vasculature 681	Inflammatory Conditions 687
	Neoplasia 687
	REFERENCES 689

The anal canal is a small but complex structure where various muscle groups, vascular plexuses, and epithelial cell types converge and create a functional barrier between the digestive tract and the external world. The purpose of this chapter is to describe the embryologic, gross, and histologic features that are important to understanding anatomy and distinguishing normal variants from potential pathologic mimics that occur in this region.

DEFINITION AND BOUNDARIES

The anal canal can be described as an epithelium-lined cylinder that is pinched closed at both ends and surrounded by an intricate meshwork of vasculature and muscle. The anatomic structures and length included in its definition depend on the discipline queried. The embryologic anal canal measures approximately two centimeters and encompasses the area between the anal verge distally and the dentate line proximally (1). The surgical anal canal is the more commonly referenced and practical representation; it is defined as a nearly four-centimeter segment that extends from the anal verge past the dentate line to the anorectal ring (Fig. 26.1) (2,3). In both the embryologic and surgical definitions, the anal canal is bordered posteriorly by the coccyx, anteriorly by the urethra in men and the perineal body and posterior vaginal wall in women, and laterally by the ischiorectal fossae (1). The World Health Organization and the TNM system use the surgical definition of the anal canal for tumor classification and staging (4,5).

EMBRYOLOGY

The anatomic complexity of the anal canal and supporting structures reflects the origins of different components in the embryo: the hindgut, the cloaca, and the proctodeum (6). The primitive gut is a blind-ended tube that forms during cephalocaudal and lateral embryonic folding (7). The caudal portion of this tube is the hindgut, which is recognizable by the 4th week of development and ultimately gives rise to the left third of the transverse colon, the descending colon, sigmoid colon, rectum, and proximal anal canal (8).

Below the level of the pubococcygeal line, the hindgut expands into the cloaca, an endoderm-lined space in continuity with the ventral urachal allantois. The cloaca has a ventrocaudal membrane (the blind end of the hindgut) that separates the endoderm from ectoderm (8–10). During the 6th week of gestation, a layer of mesoderm known as the urorectal septum begins to divide the cloaca into a ventral urogenital cavity and a dorsal hindgut/rectal cavity.

This chapter is an update of a previous version authored by Claus Fenger.

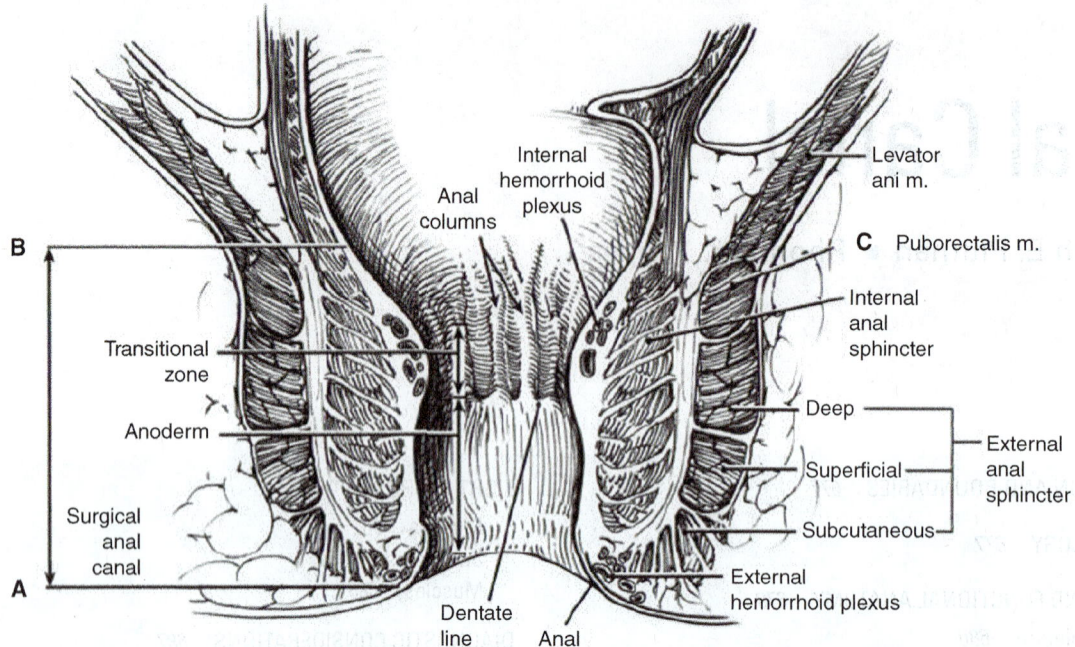

FIGURE 26.1 A coronal view of the major structures of the anal canal. The surgical anal canal extends from the anal verge (**A**) in the cephalic direction to the anorectal ring (**B**), a physiologic boundary formed by the puborectalis muscle (**C**). Reprinted with permission from: Pescatori M, Regadas FSP, Murad Regadas SM, et al. *Imaging Atlas of the Pelvic Floor and Anorectal Diseases*. Italy: Springer-Verlag; 2008.

The septum is complete by the 10th week of gestation, fully dividing the rectum and urogenital cavity (Fig. 26.2). Most developmental abnormalities of the anorectum presumably arise from the anomalous growth and/or positioning of the urorectal septum at 6 to 10 weeks of gestation (7,11–13).

The cloacal membrane ruptures by the end of the 7th gestational week to create an anal opening, thereby providing continuity between the endoderm and proctodeum. Proliferation and invagination of proctodeum during this time causes the cloacal membrane to migrate dorsally prior to rupture. As a result, the lower third of the anal canal is derived from the ectoderm, while the upper two-thirds are derived from the endoderm. The vasculature and innervation of the anal region reflect derivation from the endoderm

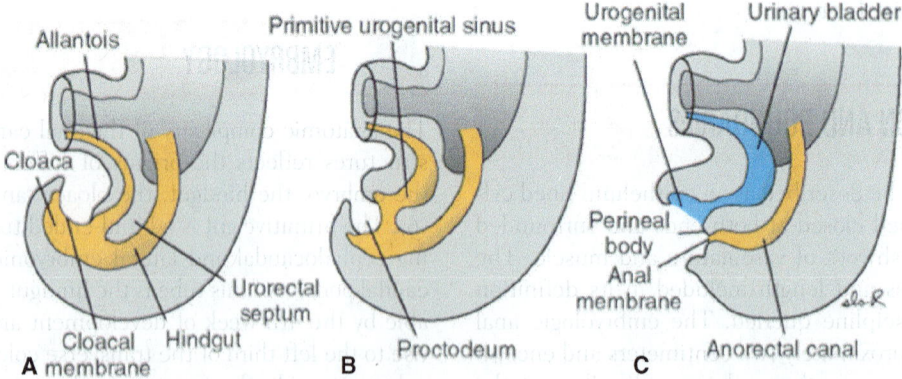

FIGURE 26.2 Embryologic development of the anal canal. The cloaca is an expansion of the primitive hindgut and the urachal allantois (**A**). The cloacal membrane is the blind ending of the hindgut. During the 6th and 7th weeks of gestation, the urorectal septum lengthens and migrates closer to the cloacal membrane (**B**). At the same time, the proctodeum invaginates and causes the cloacal membrane to move in a dorsocephalic direction. The cloacal membrane ruptures at the end of the 7th week of gestation, and by the 10th week of development the urorectal septum has provided complete separation of the hindgut dorsally and the urogenital sinus ventrally (**C**). Reprinted with permission from: Sadler TW, Langman J. *Langman's Medical Embryology*. Philadelphia, PA: Wolters Kluwer Health/Lippincott Williams & Wilkins; 2012.

and proctodeum: inferior mesenteric artery branches and autonomic nerves supply hindgut derivatives, but internal pudendal artery and inferior rectal nerve branches supply ectoderm derivatives.(6,8,10)

The external and internal anal sphincters develop during the 10th and 12th gestational weeks, respectively. Similar to other layers of the anal canal wall, they are derived from splanchnic mesenchyme (14). The anatomic orientation and development of the gut tube and associated mesenchyme is directed in part by expression of sonic hedgehog (Shh) genes. In the hindgut and cloaca, sonic hedgehog signaling induces site-specific expression of Hoxd13, a transcription factor known to be essential for appropriate endodermal differentiation to anorectal type epithelium (15,16).

GROSS AND FUNCTIONAL ANATOMY

The tubular anal canal consists of mucosa supported by submucosa and surrounded by a network of overlapping muscles. The internal surface has three grossly distinct regions. The proximal mucosa has a smooth, somewhat granular appearance that gives rise to 8 to 12 longitudinal mucosal folds known as the anal columns of Morgagni (3). Each longitudinal fold terminates at an anal valve created by a semilunar fold of tissue; each valve links two anal columns (17). The semilunar valves enclose small anal sinuses, or anal crypts, a subset of which contain openings to anal glands (18–20). The anal glands penetrate the submucosa and terminate within the internal anal sphincter muscle, or in the intersphincteric space proximal to the external anal sphincter (21,22). The functional role of the anal glands is unknown.

The mucosa at the level of the anal valves is pale with a circumferential undulating appearance; this boundary is the dentate, or pectinate, line. The mucosa distal to the dentate line is the pectin. It is a smooth, squamous-lined region terminating at the anal verge. Mucosa at the anal verge is wrinkled and slightly pigmented; this circumferential ring of tissue marks the end of the smooth anoderm and the beginning of perianal skin (1,3,23).

The dentate line corresponds to the site where proximal anorectal-type mucosa meets distal anodermal mucosa in fetuses and young children, but these two types of mucosae are separated by the anal transition zone in many adults (Figs. 26.3 and 26.4). The length of the anal transition zone varies from person to person but generally extends only a few millimeters above and below the dentate line. Visualization of the anal transition zone in a gross specimen requires special techniques, such as staining with alcian blue or green to differentiate between regional epithelial mucins (Fig. 26.5) (24).

The submucosa of the anal canal contains fibroelastic connective tissue and loosely dispersed smooth muscle cells. The connective tissue is particularly rich in venules

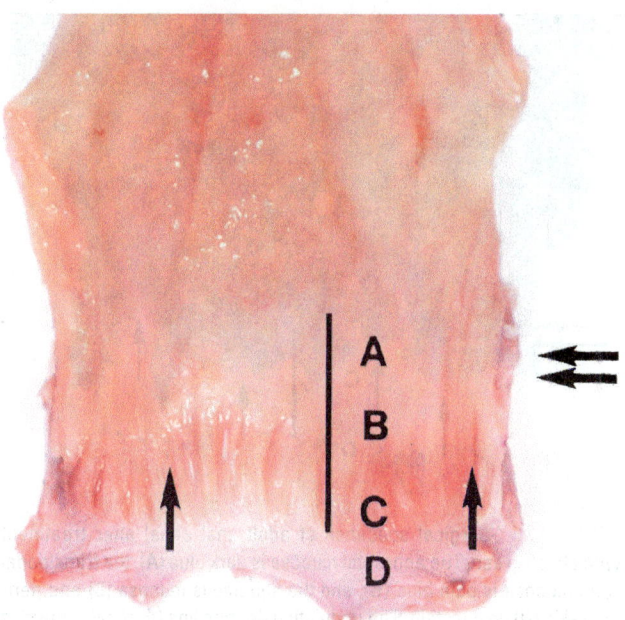

FIGURE 26.3 The simplest way to visualize the internal surface and structures of the anal canal is to cut longitudinally along one side of the cylinder and open the canal, in essence making a tubular structure into a flat rectangular piece of tissue, as seen in this surgical specimen. This autopsy specimen from the lower rectum and anal canal of an infant demonstrates well-formed anal columns (*single black arrows*). Anal valves are not apparent, and there is only a thin rim of perianal skin at the bottom. The *black vertical line* indicates the extent of the surgical anal canal and includes the anorectal zone (**A**), a small transition zone (**B**), the squamous mucosa (pecten, **C**), and the anal verge (**D**).

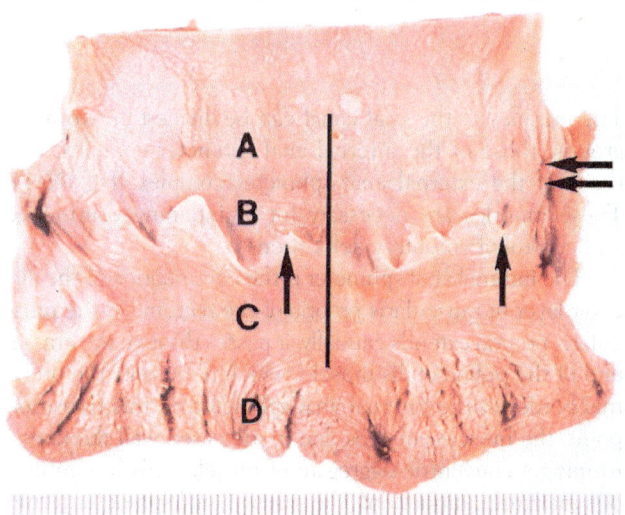

FIGURE 26.4 This autopsy specimen is from an adult. The anal columns are less apparent, but the anal valves are well formed. The *single black arrows* show the undulating dentate line, which roughly follows the base of the anal columns/valves. The extent of the surgical anal canal is marked by the *vertical black line* and includes the anorectal zone (**A**), the transition zone (**B**), the squamous mucosa (pecten, **C**), and the wrinkled perianal skin of the anal verge (**D**).

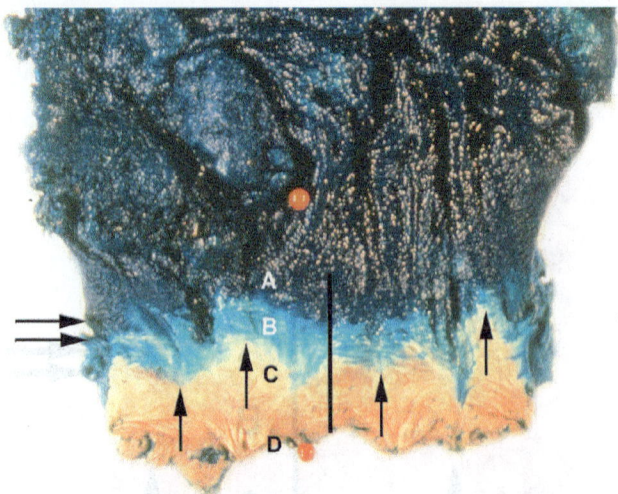

FIGURE 26.5 Surgical specimen of adult anal canal after treatment with alcian green. The anorectal mucosa is dark blue (**A**), the transitional zone mucosa is pale blue (**B**), and the squamous mucosa (**C**) and perianal skin (**D**) do not stain. The undulating dentate line (*vertical arrows*) is highlighted by this stain. The extent of the surgical anal canal is depicted by the *vertical black line*.

from the hemorrhoidal vessels in the right anterior, right posterior, and left lateral positions. These anal cushions provide nearly 20% of the resting anal pressure at the level of the internal anal sphincter, and are best visualized in vivo. Viewed from the external surface during anoscopy, the anal orifice is compressed by the anal cushions, resulting in a "Y-shaped" cutaneous slit oriented anteroposteriorly. It often has a corrugated appearance in vivo due to the presence of tonically contracted intersphincteric longitudinal fibers that insert into the dermis of the perianal skin (25–27).

Musculature

The muscles of the anal canal can be divided in two main groups, those of the internal anal sphincter complex, and those of the external anal sphincter complex (Fig. 26.1). These muscles are necessary for maintaining continence and control of voluntary defecation.

The internal anal sphincter is the continuation of the circular layer of muscularis propria of the rectum. As the muscularis propria extends caudally, it passes through the cranial end of the puborectalis muscle, which represents the proximal border of the internal anal sphincter. At this transition point, the muscle enlarges due to increased wall thickness, forming a concentric aggregate of muscle cells in continuous maximal contraction. The internal anal sphincter terminates abruptly at a site proximal to the anal verge, although its precise location varies from person to person (28,29).

The external anal sphincter is anatomically complicated; it is composed of striated skeletal muscles and is vaguely elliptical in shape (1,11). It surrounds the entirety of the internal anal sphincter and continues caudally to terminate approximately 1-cm distal to the internal anal sphincter (3).

The muscular divisions of the external anal sphincter are not entirely understood. It is widely viewed as a tripartite structure with deep, subcutaneous, and superficial regions (19). The deep external sphincter muscle is ring-like and fused with the puborectalis muscle. The subcutaneous portion of the external sphincter is similarly ring-like in orientation. The superficial division runs between the deep and subcutaneous portions. Here, the skeletal muscle fibers are arranged with an elliptical orientation from the perineal body anteriorly to the coccyx posteriorly.

Some anatomists have suggested the external anal sphincter contains only deep and superficial layers, whereas others hypothesize that the sphincter consists of a single aggregate of fibers in continuity with the puborectalis muscle (30,31). Regardless of its precise nature, the striated muscles have increased resting tone through the tonic contractile activity of type 1 skeletal muscle fibers, thereby maintaining continence.

A potential intersphincteric space lies between the internal and external anal sphincters. This space contains the longitudinal anal muscle, which represents a continuation of the external/longitudinal smooth muscle layer of the muscularis propria (32). Skeletal muscle fibers from the levator ani, puborectalis, and pubococcygeus muscles can also be found in this area; histologic sections of the intersphincteric space contain a combination of smooth and skeletal type muscle fibers (33). At the distal end of the longitudinal anal muscle, fibroelastic septa extend through the external sphincter into the perianal dermis. These strands are known as the corrugator cutis ani muscle and cause the characteristic folding of perianal skin (34).

The levator ani, puborectalis, and pubococcygeus muscles comprise the pelvic diaphragm, the muscular structure that largely defines the pelvic floor and separates the pelvic cavity from the perineum. These striated muscles consist of predominantly slow/tonic motor units (35,36). The puborectalis muscle is especially relevant to discussions of the anal canal because it forms the anorectal ring that defines the proximal limit of the surgical anal canal (19). The puborectalis muscle is fixed anteriorly to the pubis, producing a U-shaped loop of muscle and providing the ventral kink that serves as the division between the rectum and the anal canal. Muscles of the pelvic floor play a crucial role in maintaining both fecal and urinary continence (35,37).

Innervation

Sensory and motor nerves innervate the anal canal. The sensory components are important for voluntary control of defecation, although sensation does not appear to be necessary for involuntary control (38). The upper anal canal is rich in pressure sensitive nerve endings carried by the inferior rectal branch of the pudendal nerve (39). Sensory pain fibers are present below, but not above, the dentate line. The perianal skin of the anal verge receives somatic sensation from S4 in a dermatomal distribution (40).

Motor control is more complex, and different nerves supply various muscles of the anal sphincters. The internal anal sphincter has both intrinsic myogenic neuronal function, as well as innervation from extrinsic autonomic nerves (29). The intrinsic enteric nervous system (myenteric plexus) facilitates spontaneous, rhythmic contractions of the sphincter muscle, even in absence of extrinsic nerve control (41). Extrinsic autonomic control is derived from the hypogastric pelvic nerve plexus, which includes nerve L5 and is predominately made up of sympathetic neurons. Sympathetic control allows for continuous excitatory signals and tonic contraction of the sphincter. Opposing parasympathetic fibers are carried from S2, S3, and S4 (42).

The external anal sphincter receives motor control from the inferior rectal branch of the pudendal nerve and the perineal branch of S4. Like the internal sphincter, these nerve fibers are predominately sympathetic in nature and provide tonic contraction. However, the skeletal component of this muscle is imparted with neural motor control, which can promote further contraction of this sphincter. When under voluntary control, the fibers of the external sphincter and the puborectalis muscle function as a unit (43).

The pelvic diaphragm, which includes the puborectalis and levator ani, are also supplied by S2–S4, which provide for sympathetic tonic contraction, as well as the ability for voluntary control. Fecal incontinence can result from damage to nerve fibers within the pelvic diaphragm, either from a specific event (e.g., childbirth) or as a consequence of aging (36,44).

Vasculature

The vascular supply of the anal canal reflects its embryologic origins. The routes described below seem straightforward in this writing; however, the actual vasculature of the anal canal consists of dense anastomosing arteriovenous networks that are important for surgical management of this area.

The anal canal above the dentate line is a derivative of the hindgut and, thus, it is supplied by branches of the inferior mesenteric artery. The inferior mesenteric artery gives rise to the left colic artery, which in turn gives rise to the superior hemorrhoidal (rectal) artery. The superior hemorrhoidal artery bifurcates and runs through the rectal submucosa where branches ramify to supply the anal canal. Draining venules coalesce into rich, saccular venous plexuses in the right posterior, right anterior, and left lateral anal canal. These regions correspond to physiologic anal cushions and are the sites of pathologic internal hemorrhoidal varices (Fig. 26.1) (23,26,45).

The anorectum above the dentate line has venous drainage primarily to the inferior vena cava. Blood from the middle and inferior hemorrhoidal veins flows to the internal iliac vein and then to the inferior vena cava. The lymphatic vessels above the dentate line drain to inferior mesenteric and internal iliac lymph nodes (46).

Below the dentate line, the vascular and lymphatic routes correspond to those that supply the proctodeum in the embryo. The internal iliac arteries give rise to the internal pudendal artery, which give rise to inferior hemorrhoidal arteries. The middle hemorrhoidal artery also arises from the anterior division of the internal iliac and serves this region. Superficial capillaries and veins from the internal and middle hemorrhoidal systems are the nidus for pathologic external hemorrhoids. Venous drainage from this area is predominantly to the portal venous system via the inferior mesenteric vein. Lymph flows primarily along inferior rectal lymphatic channels to the superficial inguinal lymph nodes. Because lymph also drains to perirectal and internal iliac lymph nodes, these are considered "regional" in the staging of anal cancer (5,47).

LIGHT MICROSCOPY

The microscopic anatomy of the anal canal varies by anatomic region: the anorectum above the dentate line, the anal transition zone, the anal canal below the dentate line, and the anal verge (Fig. 26.6). Each region is

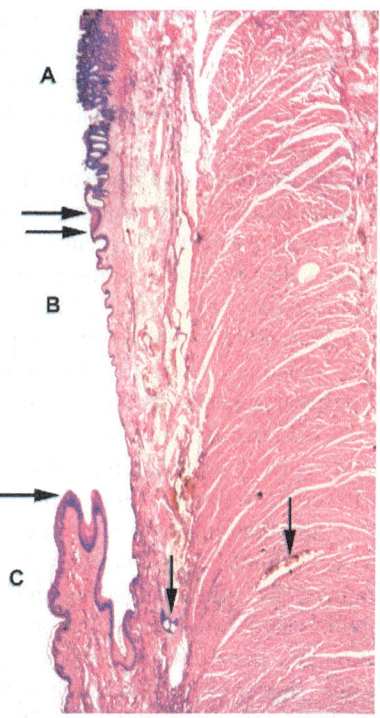

FIGURE 26.6 A longitudinal section of the anal canal demonstrates the anorectal zone (**A**), anal transition zone (**B**), and squamous mucosa (**C**). The anal transition zone extends into an anal sinus with a valve. The *vertical black arrows* indicate anal glands in the submucosa and internal sphincter. The *single horizontal arrow* indicates the dentate line; the *double horizontal arrow* marks the proximal border of the anal transition zone (H&E).

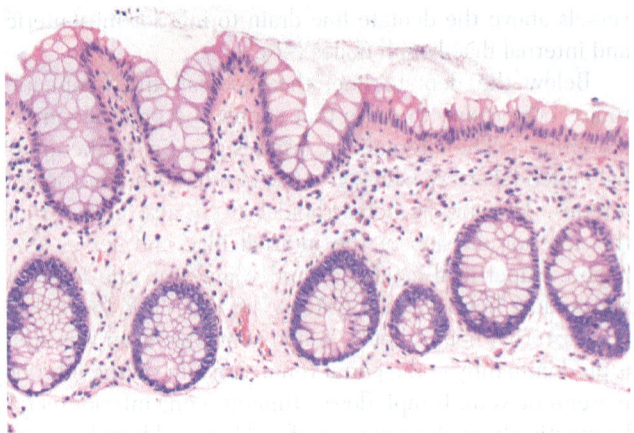

FIGURE 26.7 The mucosa in the upper anorectum is histologically similar to that of the colorectum. The epithelium contains mucin-filled goblet cells and eosinophilic absorptive colonocytes. Loose mesenchyme and occasional inflammatory cells comprise the lamina propria, which supports the epithelium.

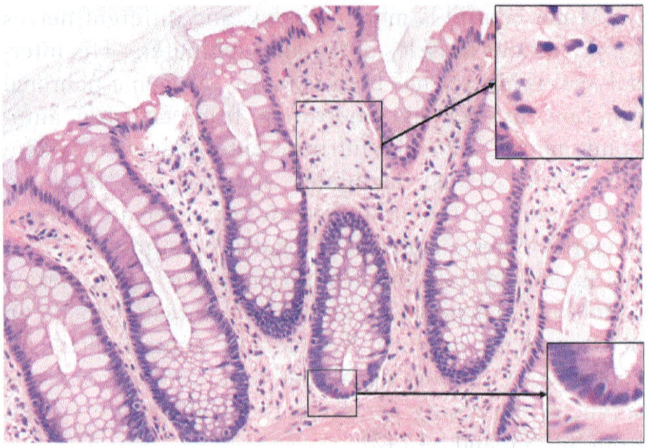

FIGURE 26.8 Scattered endocrine cells (bottom inset) usually contain brightly granular eosinophilic cytoplasm and round nuclei. Aggregates of muciphages (upper inset) are commonly present. Thin fascicles of smooth muscle cells comprise the muscularis mucosae, which runs longitudinally under the crypts.

made up of mucosa, submucosa, and muscle, which will be described below.

Mucosa

The term "mucosa" collectively refers to the superficial layers of epithelium, lamina propria, and muscularis mucosae of the gastrointestinal tract. The lamina propria consists of delicate mesenchyme that supports the epithelium, and the muscularis mucosae is a thin, discontinuous band of smooth muscle cells running longitudinally between the lamina propria and submucosa.

The anorectal junction is an anatomic landmark that denotes the proximal end of the surgical anal canal; the mucosa in this region is virtually identical to colorectal mucosa. Goblet cells, absorptive colonocytes, and endocrine cells comprise the epithelial lining in order of decreasing abundance (Fig. 26.7). Goblet cells are necessary for lubricating the mucosa. They contain abundant mucin-filled cytoplasm that appears almost clear in hematoxylin and eosin (H&E)-stained sections; these cells also contain small, flattened nuclei near the basement membrane. Colonocytes are fewer in the anorectum than the abdominal colon, and they are often inconspicuous due to high numbers of goblet cells. Similar to colonocytes elsewhere, they are tall columnar cells with faintly eosinophilic cytoplasm, microvilli, and basally located nuclei that are rounder and less hyperchromatic than those of adjacent goblet cells. Endocrine cells, are small, cuboidal cells that contain densely packed, brightly eosinophilic granules and nuclei that are luminally oriented in the crypts (Fig. 26.8).

The epithelium of the anorectum grows as a single cell layer along a basement membrane; tubular crypts increase the surface area (11,48). Crypts of the abdominal colon are often described as "test tubes in a rack" to invoke their regular architectural appearance; they are oriented parallel to one another and perpendicular to the muscularis mucosae. The crypts of the anorectum have a slightly less uniform appearance and are often irregularly dispersed in the lamina propria. They may be shortened, angulated, or occasionally branching, especially toward the surface (49). These subtle architectural changes are considered within the range of normal.

The lamina propria contains scattered lymphocytes, plasma cells, and loosely arranged collagen fibrils, as well as scattered capillaries. Mucin-filled macrophages (i.e., muciphages) can be numerous, especially under the surface epithelium (Fig. 26.8). The muscularis mucosae is thin and parallel to the luminal surface epithelium. Mucosal prolapse-type changes are common in the anorectum. In this situation, thin bundles of smooth muscle cells emanate from the muscularis mucosae vertically into the lamina propria between and parallel to the tubular crypts. Epithelial changes, such as mucin depletion, crypt serration, and erosions may also be present.

The anorectal mucosa and that of the anal transition zone merge between 3 and 20 mm proximal to the dentate line in adults, whereas transitional epithelium is absent in the fetus and newborn (50). The epithelial lining of the anal transition zone is stratified and contains four to nine cell layers. The basal layers consist of polarized cuboidal cells, whereas the surface cells display variable morphology and may be flat, cuboidal, columnar with apical mucin, or polygonal, similar to umbrella cells of the urothelium (Figs. 26.9 to 26.11) (49). The layers between the deepest and most superficial epithelial cell layers can be oriented perpendicular to the basement membrane with elongated nuclei that impart a streaming appearance, or their long axes may be parallel to the basement membrane, reminiscent of stratified squamous epithelium. Mucin is sparse in the anal

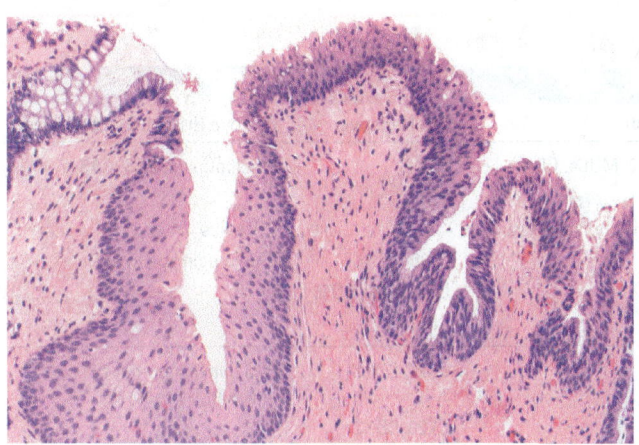

FIGURE 26.9 The anorectal mucosa and anal transition zone merge above the dentate line in adults. Goblet cell-rich epithelium gives way to transitional epithelium, which contains several layers of small basal cells with slightly hyperchromatic nuclei.

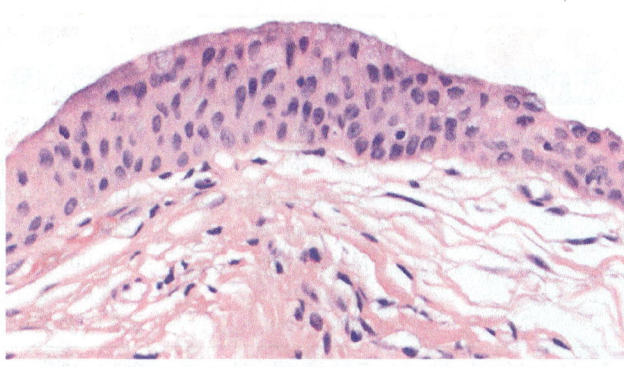

FIGURE 26.10 Superficial cells in the anal transitional zone are short columnar cells with a small amount of acid mucin that imparts blue discoloration to the cytoplasm.

transition zone and generally has a basophilic appearance when present; histochemical stains demonstrate a predominance of sialomucins rather than the sulphomucins more common in the colon (Table 26.1) (24,51).

Between 6 and 12 anal glands arise from the anal crypts (crypts of Morgagni). These glands extend into the submucosa, and at least half penetrate the internal sphincter. The glandular epithelium varies according to the location along the gland: squamous cells are numerous at the gland orifice on the luminal surface, the neck region is lined by transitional-type epithelium, and columnar cells are present in the deep regions where the glands extend into the submucosa (Fig. 26.12) (20). Inflamed anal glands may participate in the pathogenesis of anal fistulae (fistula-in-ano) and rarely give rise to adenocarcinomas of the anal canal (Table 26.2) (21,61).

The anal transition zone epithelium merges with the smooth, nonkeratinizing stratified squamous epithelium at, or below, the dentate line. Again, the basal cell layer is composed of uniform, cuboidal cells with basophilic cytoplasm, whereas superficial cells are flattened with eosinophilic cytoplasm and small, round, or slightly elongated nuclei with dense chromatin (Fig. 26.13). Melanocytes, Langerhans cells, intraepithelial lymphocytes, and Merkel cells are present in small numbers in this region (Fig. 26.14) (52,62,63).

The stratified squamous mucosa transitions to keratinized perianal skin at the level of the anal verge. It displays a superficial granular cell layer with keratohyalin granules and a cornified layer of basket-weave keratin (Fig. 26.15). Dermal papillae are well formed, and hair follicles and other adnexal structures are present (Fig. 26.16).

The transitions between epithelial regions of the anal canal are gradual and irregular in some cases, resulting in map-like configurations that can be appreciated with alcian green histochemical stains performed on the gross

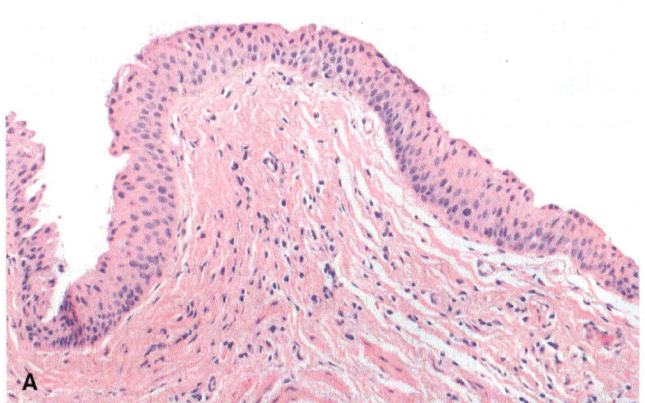
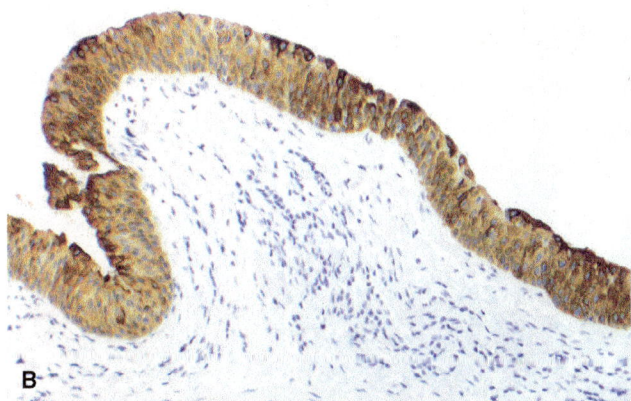

FIGURE 26.11 Surface cells in the transitional mucosa may be flattened and contain eosinophilic cytoplasm reminiscent of squamous cells (**A**). Transitional zone epithelium shows strong, diffuse immunostaining for cytokeratin 7, unlike squamous mucosa of the anus (**B**).

TABLE 26.1
Cell Types of the Anorectum and Their Staining Patterns (50–60)

	Cell Type	IHC Positive (Selected)	IHC Negative	Positive Histochemical Stains
Anorectal mucosa	Goblet cell	AE1/AE3, MUC1, MUC2, MUC4, CEA	CK7	Mucicarmine, PAS, PAS-d
	Colonic absorptive cell	AE1/AE3, CK20, CDX2	CK7	
	Endocrine cell	AE1/AE3, chromogranin, synaptophysin		Grimelius
	Macrophage	CD68, CD163	S100	PAS (mucin positive)
	Plasma cell	CD19, CD138	CD3, CD20, CD56	
	Lymphocyte	CD3, CD20, CD45	CD138	
Anal transitional zone	Transitional epithelium	CK7, CK19	CK20, CDX2	PAS (luminal border of columnar cells)
	Anal glands	CK7, CK19, CK5/6, p63	CK20, CDX2	
	Endocrine cell	AE1/AE3, chromogranin, synaptophysin, serotonin		Grimelius
Anal mucosa	Keratinocyte	CK5/6, p63, p40		
	Melanocyte	S100, melan-A	AE1/AE3	Fontana–Masson
	Merkel cell	CK20, NSE	CK7	
	Langerhans cell	S100, CD1a		ATPase
	Lymphocyte	CD3, CD20, CD45		
Anal verge/perianal skin	Keratinocyte	CK5/6, p63, p40		
	Melanocyte	S100, melan-A	AE1/AE3	Fontana–Masson
	Adnexal structures	Variable: 34Be12, EMA, aSMA, calponin		PAS, PAS-d
	Mast cell	CD117, tryptase		Toluidine blue
	Macrophage	CD68, CD163	S100	
Submucosa	Endothelial cells	CD34, CD31		
	Fibroblasts	vimentin		
	Collagen			Masson trichrome
	Adipose tissue	vimentin, S100		Oil red O (frozen)
	Lymphatic vessels	CD31, D2-40	CD34	
	Peripheral nerves	S100		

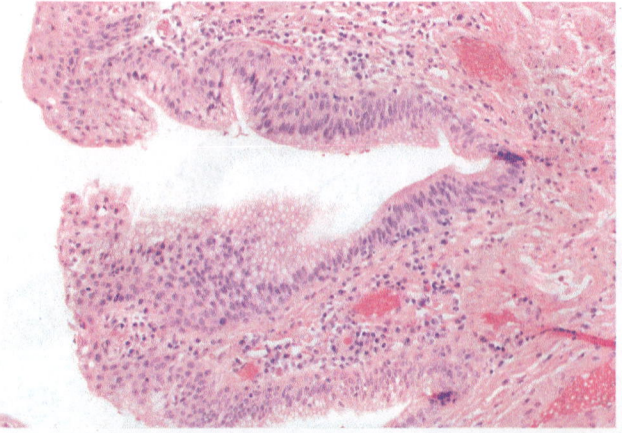

FIGURE 26.12 Anal glands are normally present in the transition zone. They are usually lined by transitional-type epithelium and scattered goblet cells. This gland opens onto the surface within an anal crypt.

specimen. The proximal anal canal stains a deep blue-green, corresponding to mucins of the anorectal mucosa. The distal anal canal is lined by squamous epithelium, which does not pick up the stain. The middle transitional region has a pale turquoise hue (Fig. 26.6) (49).

Submucosa

The submucosa displays regional variations along the length of the anal canal. Above the dentate line, it consists of loosely arranged collagen fibrils, fibroblasts, and extracellular matrix, in which the anal vascular cushions are embedded (Fig. 26.17) (44). The connective tissue scaffolding around the hemorrhoidal vessels loosens with advanced age, allowing veins and venules to progressively engorge under the forces of gravity, resulting in hemorrhoidal varices and/or

TABLE 26.2
Pathologic Processes That Occur in Different Components of the Anal Canal

Normal Structures	Pathologic Disorders
Anorectal mucosa	Colorectal carcinoma (Neuro)endocrine tumors
Anal transition zone	HPV-related squamous intraepithelial neoplasia Squamous cell carcinoma
Anal glands	Anal fistulae Adenocarcinoma, anal gland subtype
Anal squamous mucosa	Squamous cell carcinoma Benign melanocytic nevus Malignant melanoma
Perianal skin	Squamous cell carcinoma Basal cell carcinoma Extramammary Paget disease Benign melanocytic nevus Malignant melanoma
Venous plexuses	Hemorrhoids Anal fissure
Perianal hair follicles	Pilonidal cysts
Muscular sphincters	Incontinence Prolapse

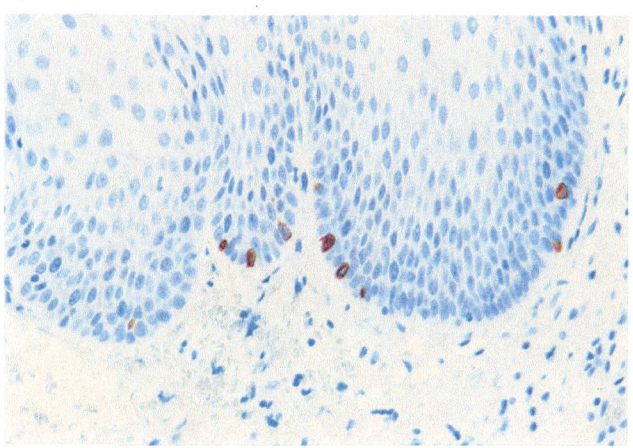

FIGURE 26.14 Scattered Merkel cells in the basal layer of the squamous mucosa are highlighted by an immunostain for CK20.

thrombosis (Fig. 26.18) (Table 26.2) (64). Multinucleated stromal cells can be identified in the lamina propria and submucosa of the anal canal; these are benign fibroblast-type cells of no clinical consequence (Fig. 26.19) (65,66).

The pectin below the dentate line contains a submucosa rich in elastic tissue and collagen fibrils that tether the mucosa to the underlying muscle. Elastic fibers are most prominent at the anal verge underlying the transition from anal mucosa to perianal skin (Fig. 26.20) (23).

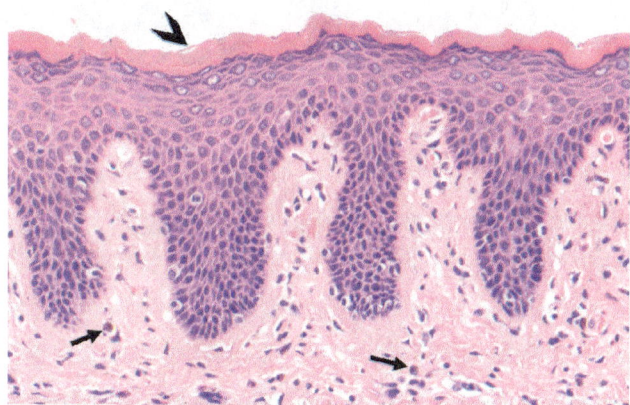

FIGURE 26.15 Perianal skin has well-formed dermal papillae, a superficial granular layer, and keratinization with a compact or basket-weave layer of brightly eosinophilic keratin at the surface (*arrowhead*). Pigmented dermal macrophages (*black arrow*) are frequently present.

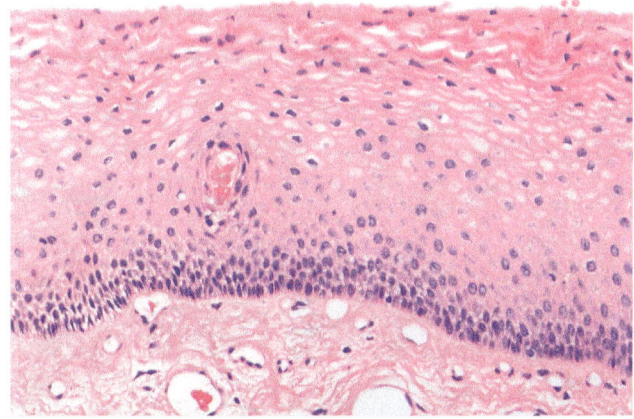

FIGURE 26.13 The mucosa of the pecten, the distal anal canal, consists of stratified squamous epithelium without papillae or surface keratinization.

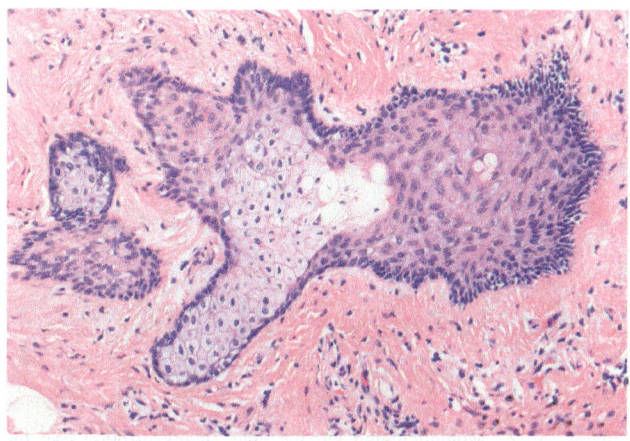

FIGURE 26.16 A sebaceous gland located in the dermis of the perianal skin.

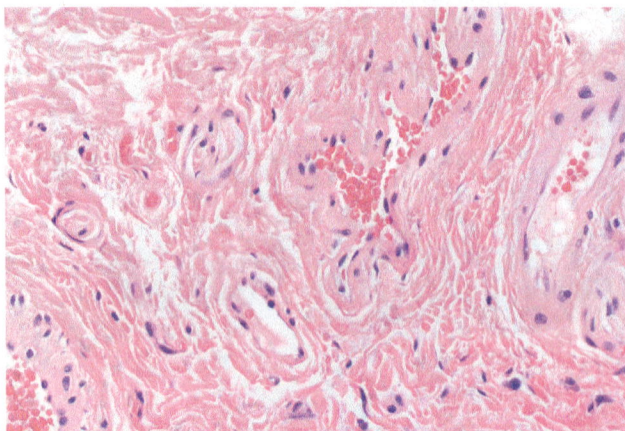

FIGURE 26.17 The vascular cushions of the anal canal represent a rich venous network within the submucosa.

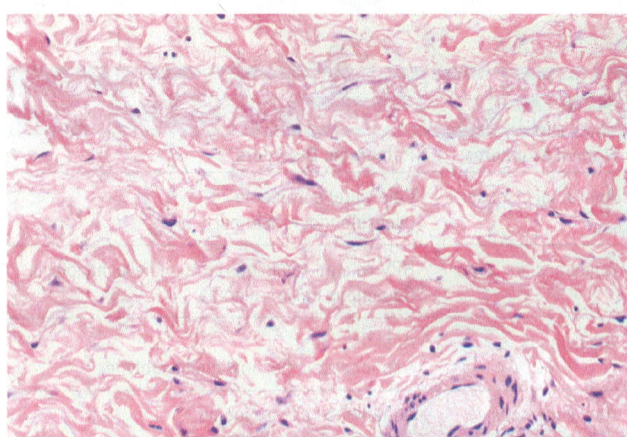

FIGURE 26.20 The submucosa of the distal anus contains increased amounts of gray-blue elastic fibers, especially near the perianal skin.

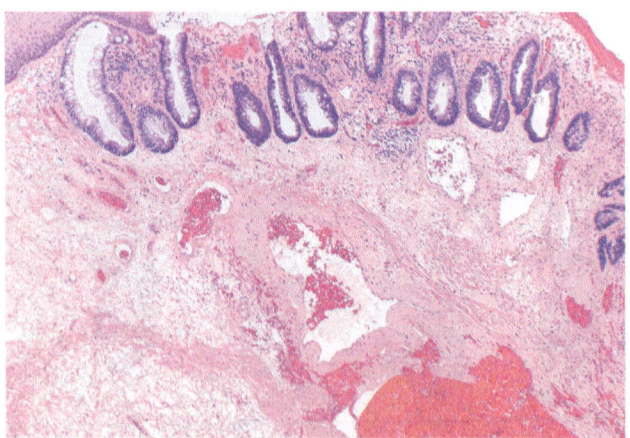

FIGURE 26.18 Pathologic hemorrhoids occur as the submucosal fibers around the plexus loosen, and veins become progressively engorged. Dilated veins fill the submucosa at the junction between anorectal and transitional epithelium in the anal canal.

Muscles

There are two features to keep in mind when observing the muscular layers of the anal canal. First, a full thickness section through the anal wall that includes sphincter muscle will show a mixture of smooth and striated muscle (35). Smooth muscle cells are thin and are arranged in bundles parallel to one another (Fig. 26.21). Each smooth muscle cell contains a single nucleus. Skeletal muscle cells are polygonal and multinucleated, features that are best seen when cut in cross section. The sarcomere pattern of striations can be appreciated in longitudinally sectioned fibers (Fig. 26.22).

Second, the muscle layers of the anal canal are intricately associated with each other. Unlike the inner and outer layers of the colonic muscularis propria, the muscles of the anal canal can be arranged in parallel, longitudinal, perpendicular, radial, or circumferential aggregates depending on their location in the sphincter and the method of tissue sampling. The net effect is a rather haphazard-appearing arrangement of

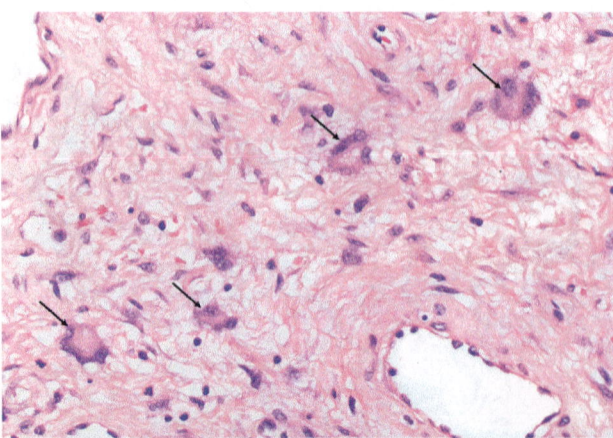

FIGURE 26.19 Multinucleated stromal cells (*black arrows*) can be found in the lamina propria and submucosa of the anal canal. They probably represent activated fibroblasts.

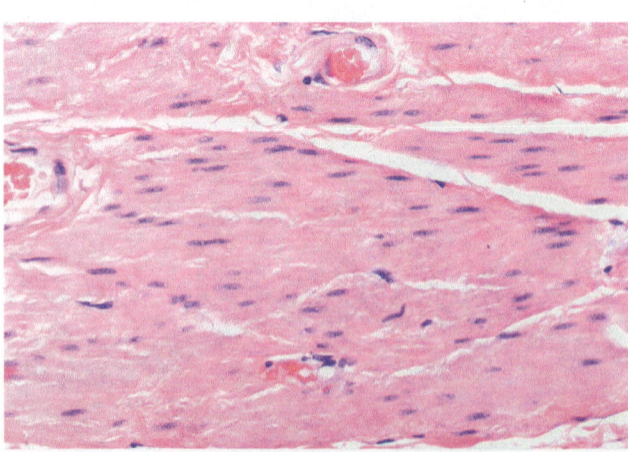

FIGURE 26.21 Tight fascicles of slender smooth muscle cells comprise the internal anal sphincter and longitudinal anal muscle.

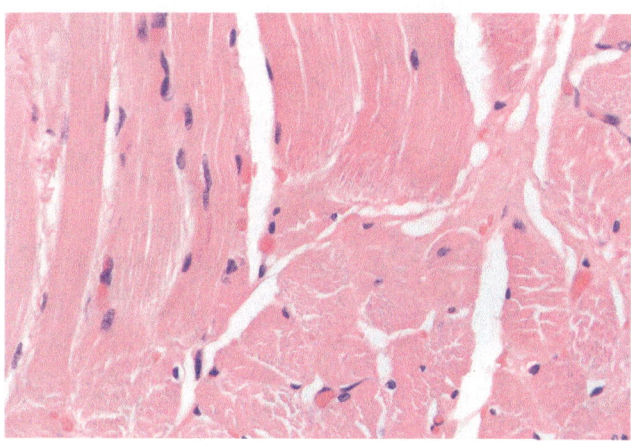

FIGURE 26.22 Brightly eosinophilic skeletal muscle fibers are multinucleated and contain cytoplasmic striations. Skeletal muscle is found in the external anal sphincter, longitudinal anal muscle, and pelvic diaphragm.

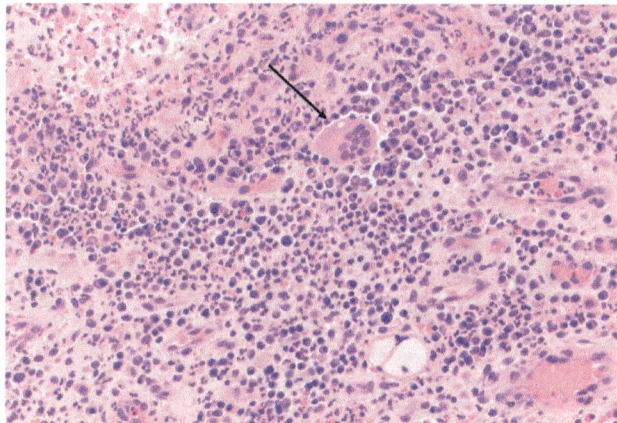

FIGURE 26.23 Granulation tissue from a fistula tract contains scattered multinucleated giant cells (*arrow*), neutrophils, plasma cells, and small capillaries.

irregularly intersecting fascicles. Fortunately, clear demarcation between muscle groups is not relevant to clinical practice in most situations.

DIAGNOSTIC CONSIDERATIONS

Pathologists receive anal resection or anal biopsy specimens for evaluation of disease. Brief mention will be made here of the more common abnormalities encountered and how they differ from the normal histology described above.

Epithelial Metaplasia and Heterotopia

Epithelial cell types other than those previously described can be identified in sections taken from the anal canal. Patients who have longstanding colorectal disease, such as inflammatory bowel disease, may have metaplasia of anorectal epithelium as a result of chronic mucosal injury. Paneth cell metaplasia and pseudopyloric metaplasia are the most common altered cell types in anorectal injury. Rarely, heterotopic aggregates of gastric oxyntic glands can be found in the anal canal, similar to islands of gastric oxyntic mucosa of the proximal esophagus, duodenum, and intestines. This abnormality may produce the impression of a polyp, but is otherwise of no clinical significance (67,68).

Inflammatory Conditions

Anal fissures are linear erosions that can ulcerate, causing painful, nonhealing wounds. Men and women are equally affected. Potential inciting factors include constipation and hard stool, diarrhea from frequent stooling, or other underlying inflammatory or infectious conditions involving the anal canal. Fissures most commonly occur in the posterior midline, followed by the anterior midline (69). It is possible that the posterior wall is more susceptible to fissures because it is less perfused than other parts of the anus; increased anal pressure due to straining further reduces blood flow, leading to ischemia, erosion, and ultimately fissure formation (29,70,71). The microscopic findings of a sampled fissure are nonspecific and demonstrate inflamed and ulcerated anal mucosa.

Anal fistulae are defined as inflammatory tracts leading from the epithelialized anal canal to another epithelialized surface, usually the skin. Anal fistulae are probably due to anal gland infection (21,72). The "cryptoglandular theory" of fistulous disease is supported by autopsy data confirming similarities between the locations and growth patterns of anal glands and those of anal fistulae. Modern classification schemes allow for more than a dozen types of fistulae; treatment is multimodal but almost always requires a surgical approach (73). Histologic features include inflamed epithelium, granulation tissue, fibrotic submucosa, and, in some cases, a giant cell reaction to fecal material (Fig. 26.23). Anal fistulae are commonly seen in patients with Crohn disease (74).

Infection is another cause of anal inflammatory changes. Most commonly, herpes simplex virus infection causes ulcers with diagnostic cytologic changes in epithelial cells at the ulcer edge. These include multinucleation, margination of chromatin, and nuclear molding, often accompanied by dense cytoplasmic eosinophilia (Fig. 26.24). Other sexually transmitted diseases, specifically chlamydia and syphilis, may manifest as dense submucosal chronic inflammation with numerous plasma cells (Fig. 26.25) (75). Although immunohistochemical stains for spirochetes exist, definitive clinical diagnosis is usually confirmed with serologic testing or nucleic acid–amplification testing (76).

Neoplasia

The most common form of neoplastic disease in the anal canal is that of squamous epithelial dysplasia and/or

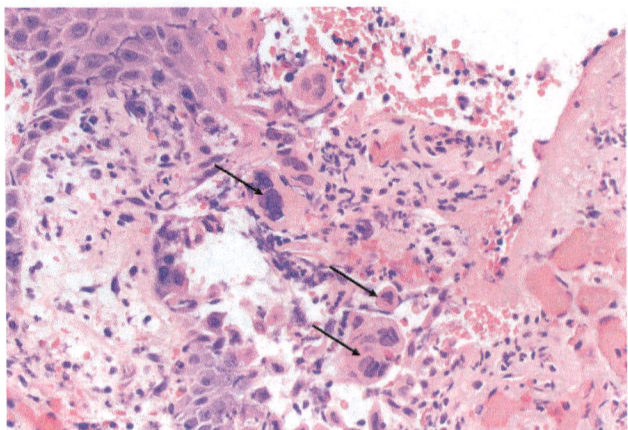

FIGURE 26.24 Herpesvirus infection induces nuclear abnormalities in squamous epithelial cells; multinucleation with hypereosinophilia (*arrows*) are accompanied by macrophage-rich ulcer debris. Infected nuclei have a "glassy" appearance with marginated chromatin and nuclear molding.

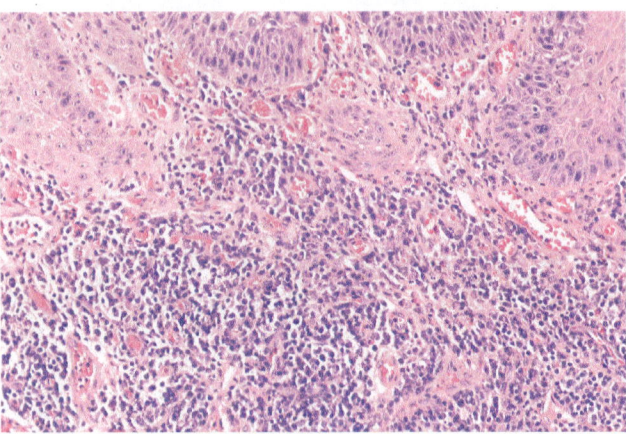

FIGURE 26.25 The hallmark of *Treponema pallidum* infection is the presence of dense subepithelial lymphoplasmacytic inflammation. *Chlamydia trachomatis* (lymphogranuloma venereum) elicits similar inflammatory changes and cannot be distinguished based on morphologic features alone.

squamous cell carcinoma (77). Similar to the transformation zone of the uterine cervix, the epithelium of the anal transitional zone is particularly susceptible to infection with human papilloma virus and, thus, is prone to squamous dysplasia. The dysplasia may be low or high grade and appear as a flat plaque or verrucous growth. Distinguishing dysplasia from reactive cytologic abnormalities in the transitional zone epithelium can be challenging. Features of low-grade dysplasia include dysmaturation and disorganization of squamous cells in the lower one-third of the epithelium, often accompanied by superficial koilocytosis (Fig. 26.26). High-grade dysplastic lesions show dysmaturation and mitotic figures at all levels of the epithelium (Fig. 26.27) (78). Immunohistochemical stains for p16 typically show diffuse "block-like" positivity in areas of high-grade dysplasia (79,80).

Other forms of neoplasia that can be seen in this area include primary extramammary Paget disease (Fig. 26.28), secondary Paget disease due to colonization of the squamous epithelium by occult rectal adenocarcinoma, squamous cell carcinoma of the perianal skin, adenocarcinoma derived from anal glands, and malignant melanoma. All of these tumors can share histologic features, that is, single atypical cells with abundant cytoplasm dispersed in benign squamous epithelium. In some cases, the clinical history may be helpful, whereas others require immunohistochemical stains to correctly classify disease (81,53). Of note, reactive squamous epithelial cells can show cytoplasmic clearing, but their nuclear features are essentially normal (82).

Hidradenoma papilliferum (i.e., papillary hidradenoma, papillary apocrine adenoma) is the most common benign

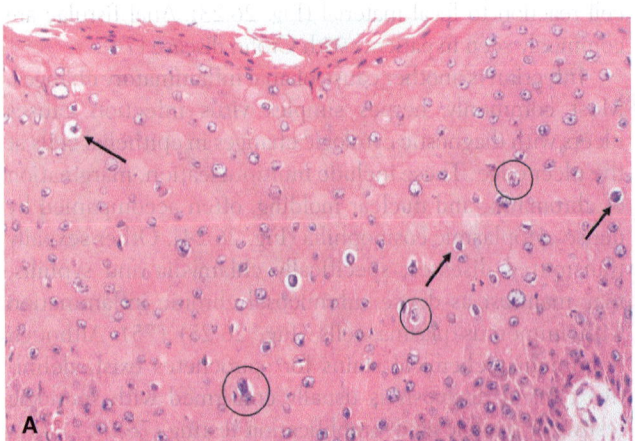
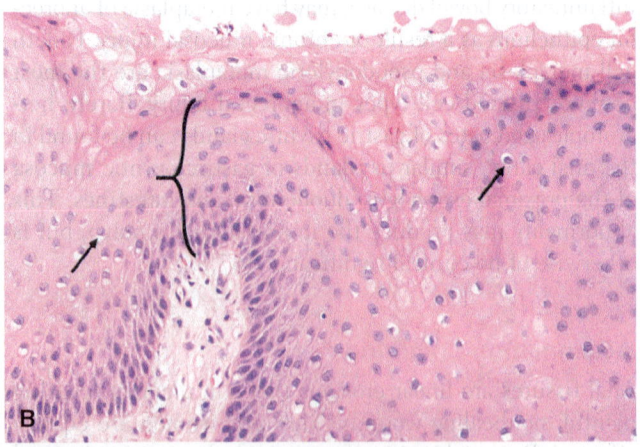

FIGURE 26.26 Human papilloma virus infection causes disorganization of squamous epithelium with binucleated keratinocytes (*black circles*) and koilocytosis (**A**, *black arrows*). Reactive changes in squamous mucosa can mimic HPV infection, but normal maturation is present (*bracket*) and cytoplasmic halos are unassociated with nuclear abnormalities (*arrow*). Superficial keratinocytes contain uniform pale cytoplasm, which may be related to surface trauma (**B**).

adnexal neoplasm of perianal skin. This lesion usually presents as a well-circumscribed dermal nodule in perianal or, more commonly, vulvar skin (83). Tumors are composed of papillary fronds–lined luminal cuboidal cells and basal myoepithelial cells, often in densely collagenous stroma (Fig. 26.29).

REFERENCES

1. Garza A, Beart RW Jr. Anatomy and Embryology of the Anus, Rectum, and Colon. In: *Corman's Colon and Rectal Surgery*. 6th ed. Philadelphia, PA: Wolters Kluwer Health/Lippincott Williams & Wilkins; 2013:1–26.
2. Symington J. The Rectum and Anus. *J Anat Physiol* 1888; 23(Pt 1):106–115.
3. Halligan S, Stoker J. Imaging of fistula in ano. *Radiology* 2006; 239(1):18–33.
4. Welton ML, Lambert R, Bosman FT. Tumours of the anal canal. In WHO classification of tumours of the digestive system. In: *WHO Classification of Tumours of the Digestive System*. 4th ed. Lyon, France: IARC Press; 2010:183–194.
5. Welton ML, Steele SR, Goodman, KA, et al. Anus. In: *AJCC Cancer Staging Manual*. 8th ed. Switzerland: Springer; 2017: 275–284.
6. Schoenwolf GC, Bleyl SB, Brauer PR, et al. Development of the Gastrointestinal Tract. In: *Larsen's Human Embryology*. 5th ed. Philadelphia, PA: Elsevier/Churchill Livingstone; 2015: 341–374. Available at: https://www.clinicalkey.com/#!/content/book/3-s2.0-B978145570684600014X. Accessed January 18, 2018.
7. Nievelstein RA, van der Werff JF, Verbeek FJ, et al. Normal and abnormal embryonic development of the anorectum in human embryos. *Teratology* 1998;57(2):70–78.
8. Coalson RE, Tomasek JJ. Digestive System and Mesenteries. In: *Embryology*. New York: Springer; 1992:78–85.
9. Kluth D, Fiegel HC, Metzger R. Embryology of the hindgut. *Semin Pediatr Surg* 2011;20(3):152–160.
10. Sadler TW, Langman J. *Langman's Medical Embryology*. 12th ed. Philadelphia, PA: Wolters Kluwer Health/Lippincott Williams & Wilkins; 2012.
11. Schizas AMP, Williams AB. The Normal Anus. In: *Anus*. London: Springer; 2014:1–12.
12. Matsumaru D, Murashima A, Fukushima J, et al. Systematic stereoscopic analyses for cloacal development: The origin of anorectal malformations. *Sci Rep* 2015;5:13943.
13. van der Putte SC. The development of the human anorectum. *Anat Rec (Hoboken)* 2009;292(7):951–954.
14. Moore KL, Persaud TVN, Torchia MG. Alimentary System. In: *The Developing Human*. 10th ed. Philadelphia, PA: Elsevier; 2016:209–240. Available at: https://www.clinicalkey.com/#!/content/book/3-s2.0-B978032331338400011X?scrollTo=%23hl0001186. Accessed January 18, 2018.
15. Le Guen L, Marchal S, Faure S, et al. Mesenchymal-epithelial interactions during digestive tract development and epithelial stem cell regeneration. *Cell. Mol. Life Sci* 2015;72(20): 3883–3896.
16. Mao J, Kim BM, Rajurkar M, et al. Hedgehog signaling controls mesenchymal growth in the developing mammalian digestive tract. *Development* 2010;137(10):1721–1729.

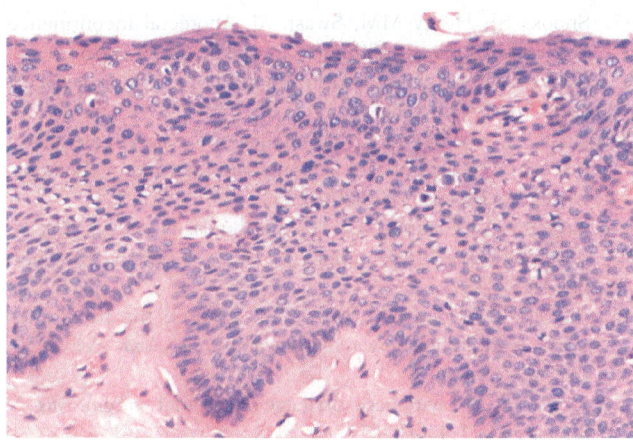

FIGURE 26.27 High-grade squamous intraepithelial neoplasia is characterized by immature, basaloid cells with hyperchromatic nuclei in the upper two-thirds of the squamous epithelium. Mitotic figures and dyskeratotic cells are also present.

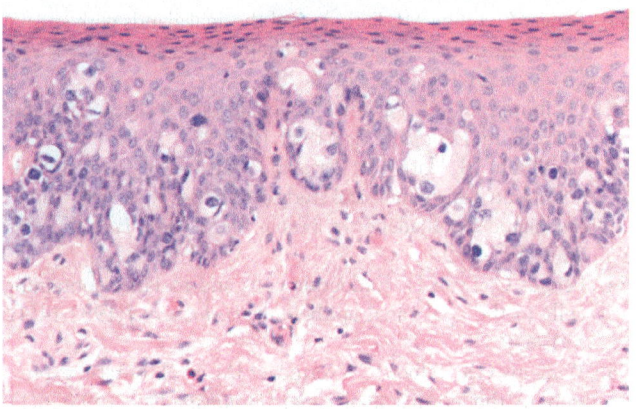

FIGURE 26.28 Extrammamary Paget disease displays clustered cells with pale cytoplasm and enlarged, hyperchromatic nuclei, predominantly in the basal third of the squamous epithelium. These malignant cells contain mucin and are immunopositive for cytokeratin 7.

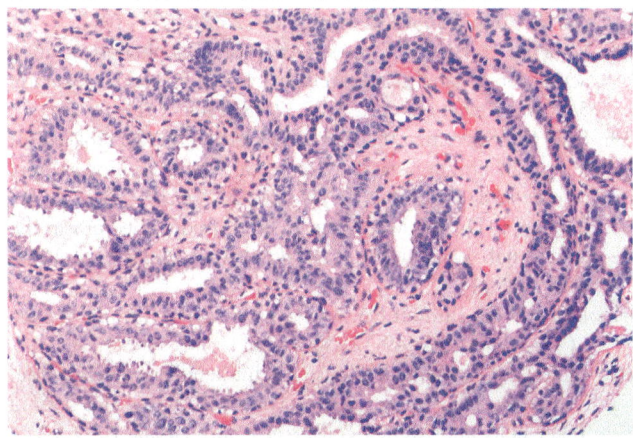

FIGURE 26.29 Hidradenoma papilliferum is a benign neoplasm that arises in perianal and vulvar skin. Its complex architecture can simulate features of adenocarcinoma. The double layer of luminal columnar cells and basal myoepithelial cells is a clue to a benign diagnosis.

17. Glisson F. Tractatus de ventriculo et intestinis. In: *Bibliotheca Anatomica Sive Thesaurus. Vol 1*. 2nd ed. Geneva: Chouet et Ritter; 1699.
18. Morgagni GB. *Adversaria Anatomica Omnia. Advers III, Animadv. VI.* Patavii, Italy: Josephus Cominus; 1717.
19. Milligan ETC, Morgan CN. Surgical anatomy of the anal canal: with special reference to anorectal fistulæ. *The Lancet* 1934;224:1150–1156.
20. McColl I. The comparative anatomy and pathology of anal glands. Arris and Gale lecture delivered at the Royal College of Surgeons of England on 25th February 1965. *Ann R Coll Surg Engl* 1967;40(1):36–67.
21. Parks AG. Pathogenesis and treatment of fistula-in-ano. *Br Med J* 1961;1(5224):463–469.
22. Seow-Choen F, Ho JM. Histoanatomy of anal glands. *Dis. Colon Rectum* 1994;37(12):1215–1218.
23. Saraswati R, Novelli M. Surgical Treatment and Pathology: Normal Histology. In: *Anus*. London: Springer; 2014:43–47.
24. Fenger C. The anal transitional zone. *Acta Pathol Microbiol Immunol Scand Suppl* 1987;289:1–42.
25. Lestar B, Penninckx F, Kerremans R. The composition of anal basal pressure. An in vivo and in vitro study in man. *Int J Colorectal Dis* 1989;4(2):118–122.
26. Thomson WH. The nature of haemorrhoids. *Br J Surg* 1975;62(7):542–552.
27. Thomson H. The anal cushions—a fresh concept in diagnosis. *Postgrad Med J* 1979;55(644):403–405.
28. Goligher JC, Leacock AG, Brossy JJ. The surgical anatomy of the anal canal. *Br J Surg* 1955;43(177):51–61.
29. Lund JN, Scholefield JH. Aetiology and treatment of anal fissure. *Br J Surg* 1996;83(10):1335–1344.
30. Oh C, Kark AE. Anatomy of the external anal sphincter. *Br J Surg* 1972;59(9):717–723.
31. Parks AG. Modern concepts of the anatomy of the anorectal region. *Postgrad Med J* 1958;34(393):360–366.
32. Macchi V, Porzionato A, Stecco C, et al. Histotopographic study of the longitudinal anal muscle. *Clin Anat* 2008;21(5):447–452.
33. Lawson JO. Pelvic anatomy. II. Anal canal and associated sphincters. *Ann R Coll Surg Engl* 1974;54(6):288–300.
34. Lunniss PJ, Phillips RK. Anatomy and function of the anal longitudinal muscle. *Br J Surg* 1992;79(9):882–884.
35. Dickinson VA. Maintenance of anal continence: a review of pelvic floor physiology. *Gut* 1978;19(12):1163–1174.
36. Parks AG, Swash M, Urich H. Sphincter denervation in anorectal incontinence and rectal prolapse. *Gut* 1977;18(8):656–665.
37. Felt-Bersma RJF. Physiology of the Rectum and Anus. In: *Colon, Rectum and Anus: Anatomic, Physiologic and Diagnostic Bases for Disease Management*. Cham: Springer; 2017:55–69.
38. Read MG, Read NW. Role of anorectal sensation in preserving continence. *Gut* 1982;23(4):345–347.
39. Duthie HL, Gairns FW. Sensory nerve-endings and sensation in the anal region of man. *Br J Surg* 1960;47:585–595.
40. Cuming T, Bailey AC, Sashidharan PN. Perianal Skin Conditions. In: *Anus*. London: Springer; 2014:253–274.
41. Penninckx F, Kerremans R, Beckers J. Pharmacological characteristics of the non-striated anorectal musculature in cats. *Gut* 1973;14(5):393–398.
42. Frenckner B, Ihre T. Influence of autonomic nerves on the internal and sphincter in man. *Gut* 1976;17(4):306–312.
43. Snooks SJ, Henry MM, Swash M. Anorectal incontinence and rectal prolapse: differential assessment of the innervation to puborectalis and external anal sphincter muscles. *Gut* 1985;26(5):470–476.
44. Haas PA, Fox TA Jr. The importance of the perianal connective tissue in the surgical anatomy and function of the anus. *Dis Colon Rectum* 1977;20(4):303–313.
45. Noorani A, Carapeti E. Haemorrhoids: Anatomy, Pathophysiology and Presentation. In: *Anus*. London: Springer; 2014:157–167.
46. Blair JB, Holyoke EA, Best RR. A note on the lymphatics of the middle and lower rectum and anus. *Anat Rec* 1950;108(4):635–644.
47. Hardy KJ. The lymphatic drainage of the anal margin. *Aust N Z J Surg* 1971;40(4):367–369.
48. Walls EW. Observations on the microscopic anatomy of the human anal canal. *Br J Surg* 1958;45(193):504–512.
49. Fenger C. Histology of the anal canal. *Am J Surg Pathol* 1988;12(1):41–55.
50. Fenger C, Filipe MI. Mucin histochemistry of the anal canal epithelium. Studies of normal anal mucosa and mucosa adjacent to carcinoma. *Histochem. J.* 1981;13(6):921–930.
51. Fenger C, Filipe MI. Pathology of the anal glands with special reference to their mucin histochemistry. *Acta Pathol Microbiol Scand A* 1977;85(3):273–285.
52. Clemmensen OJ, Fenger C. Melanocytes in the anal canal epithelium. *Histopathology* 1991;18(3):237–241.
53. Goldblum JR, Hart WR. Perianal Paget's disease: A histologic and immunohistochemical study of 11 cases with and without associated rectal adenocarcinoma. *Am. J. Surg. Pathol.* 1998;22(2):170–179.
54. Fenger C, Lyon H. Endocrine cells and melanin-containing cells in the anal canal epithelium. *Histochem J* 1982;14(4):631–639.
55. Williams GR, Talbot IC, Northover JM, et al. Keratin expression in the normal anal canal. *Histopathology* 1995;26(1):39–44.
56. Williams GR, Talbot IC, Leigh IM. Keratin expression in anal carcinoma: an immunohistochemical study. *Histopathology* 1997;30(5):443–450.
57. Ramalingam P, Hart WR, Goldblum JR. Cytokeratin subset immunostaining in rectal adenocarcinoma and normal anal glands. *Arch Pathol Lab Med* 2001;125(8):1074–1077.
58. Lisovsky M, Patel K, Cymes K, et al. Immunophenotypic characterization of anal gland carcinoma: loss of p63 and cytokeratin 5/6. *Arch Pathol Lab Med* 2007;131(8):1304–1311.
59. Saad RS, Silverman JF, Khalifa MA, et al. CDX2, cytokeratins 7 and 20 immunoreactivity in rectal adenocarcinoma. *Appl Immunohistochem Mol Morphol* 2009;17(3):196–201.
60. Fetissof F, Dubois MP, Assan R, et al. Endocrine cells in the anal canal. *Virchows Arch A Pathol Anat Histopathol* 1984;404(1):39–47.
61. Behan WM, Burnett RA. Adenocarcinoma of the anal glands. *J Clin Pathol* 1996;49(12):1009–1011.
62. Lundquist K, Kohler S, Rouse RV. Intraepidermal cytokeratin 7 expression is not restricted to Paget cells but is also seen in Toker cells and Merkel cells. *Am J Surg Pathol* 1999;23(2):212–219.
63. Gervaz E, Dauge-Geffroy MD, Sobhani I, et al. Quantitative analysis of the immune cells in the anal mucosa. *Pathol Res Pract* 1995;191(11):1067–1071.

64. Loder PB, Kamm MA, Nicholls RJ, et al. Haemorrhoids: pathology, pathophysiology and aetiology. *Br J Surg* 1994;81(7): 946–954.
65. Groisman GM, Amar M, Polak-Charcon S. Multinucleated stromal cells of the anal mucosa: a common finding. *Histopathology* 2000;36(3):224–228.
66. Pitt MA, Roberts IS, Agbamu DA, et al. The nature of atypical multinucleated stromal cells: a study of 37 cases from different sites. *Histopathology* 1993;23(2):137–145.
67. Rifat Mannan AA, Kahvic M, Bharadwaj S, et al. Gastric heterotopia of the anus: report of two rare cases and review of the literature. *Indian J Pathol Microbiol* 2008;51(2):240–241.
68. Steele SR, Mullenix PS, Martin MJ, et al. Heterotopic gastric mucosa of the anus: a case report and review of the literature. *Am Surg* 2004;70(8):715–719.
69. Stewart DB, Gaertner W, Glasgow S, et al. Clinical practice guideline for the management of anal fissures. *Dis Colon Rectum* 2017;60(1):7–14.
70. Schouten WR, Briel JW, Auwerda JJ. Relationship between anal pressure and anodermal blood flow. The vascular pathogenesis of anal fissures. *Dis Colon Rectum* 1994;37(7):664–669.
71. Klosterhalfen B, Vogel P, Rixen H, et al. Topography of the inferior rectal artery: a possible cause of chronic, primary anal fissure. *Dis Colon Rectum* 1989;32(1):43–52.
72. Robinson AM, DeNobile JW. Anorectal abscess and fistula-in-ano. *J Natl Med Assoc* 1988;80(11):1209–1213.
73. Parks AG, Gordon PH, Hardcastle JD. A classification of fistula-in-ano. *Br J Surg* 1976;63(1):1–12.
74. Panés J, Rimola J. Perianal fistulizing Crohn's disease: pathogenesis, diagnosis and therapy. *Nat Rev Gastroenterol Hepatol* 2017;14(11):652–664.
75. Arnold CA, Limketkai BN, Illei PB, et al. Syphilitic and lymphogranuloma venereum (LGV) proctocolitis: clues to a frequently missed diagnosis. *Am J Surg Pathol* 2013;37(1): 38–46.
76. de Vries HJ, Zingoni A, White JA, et al. 2013 European Guideline on the management of proctitis, proctocolitis and enteritis caused by sexually transmissible pathogens. *Int J STD AIDS* 2014;25(7):465–474.
77. Fléjou JF. An update on anal neoplasia. *Histopathology* 2015; 66(1):147–160.
78. Darragh TM, Colgan TJ, Cox JT, et al; Members of LAST Project Work Groups. The lower anogenital squamous terminology standardization project for HPV-associated lesions: background and consensus recommendations from the College of American Pathologists and the American Society for Colposcopy and Cervical Pathology. *Arch. Pathol. Lab. Med.* 2012;136(10):1266–1297.
79. Pirog EC, Quint KD, Yantiss RK. P16/CDKN2A and Ki-67 enhance the detection of anal intraepithelial neoplasia and condyloma and correlate with human papillomavirus detection by polymerase chain reaction. *Am J Surg Pathol* 2010; 34(10):1449–1455.
80. Walts AE, Lechago J, Bose S. P16 and Ki67 immunostaining is a useful adjunct in the assessment of biopsies for HPV-associated anal intraepithelial neoplasia. *Am J Surg Pathol* 2006;30(7):795–801.
81. Dawson H, Serra S. Tumours and inflammatory lesions of the anal canal and perianal skin revisited: An update and practical approach. *J Clin Pathol* 2015;68(12):971–981.
82. Val-Bernal JF, Pinto J. Pagetoid dyskeratosis is a frequent incidental finding in hemorrhoidal disease. *Arch Pathol Lab Med* 2001;125(8):1058–1062.
83. Baker GM, Selim MA, Hoang MP. Vulvar adnexal lesions: a 32-year, single-institution review from Massachusetts General Hospital. *Arch Pathol Lab Med* 2013;137(9):1237–1246.

27 Liver

Arief A. Suriawinata ■ Swan N. Thung

EMBRYOLOGY 693

GROSS MORPHOLOGY 694

HISTOLOGY 694
- Structural Organization 694
- Hepatocytes 695
- Bile Canaliculi 699
- Sinusoidal Lining Cells 699
- Portal Tracts 701
- Blood Supply and Drainage 702
- Lymphatics 704
- Bile Ducts 704
- Nerve Supply and Innervation 706

EXTRACELLULAR MATRIX 706

AGING CHANGES 706

METHODOLOGY 707
- Liver Biopsy 707
- Specimen Handling 707
- Special Stains 707
- Immunohistologic Studies 708
- Electron Microscopy 710
- Molecular Studies 710

FREQUENT HISTOLOGIC CHANGES OF LITTLE SIGNIFICANCE 710
- The Liver at Autopsy 710
- Surgical Liver Biopsy Specimens 711

MINOR BUT SIGNIFICANT HEPATIC ALTERATIONS 711
- Nonspecific Reactive Hepatitis 712
- Mild Acute Hepatitis and Residual Hepatitis 712
- Sinusoidal Dilatation 712
- Nodular Regenerative Hyperplasia 713
- Hepatoportal Sclerosis 714
- Vicinity of Space-Occupying Lesions 714

BROWN PIGMENTS 714
- Lipofuscin 715
- Dubin–Johnson Pigment 715
- Hemosiderin 715
- Copper-Associated Protein 716
- Bile 716

ACKNOWLEDGMENTS 716

REFERENCES 716

The embryology, gross morphology, normal histology, and minor pathologic alterations of the human liver—the single largest organ in the human body—are described in this chapter. The knowledge of normal liver parenchyma provides the basis of the interpretation of liver resection and biopsy specimens, in which deviation from normal is suspected. Some morphologic changes, particularly in needle biopsy specimens, are frequently subtle but may be of diagnostic importance. The pathologist should be familiar with these histologic variations of and from the normal liver. Therefore, this chapter also discusses minor histopathologic alterations that are not readily appreciated, but the clinical findings are significant. In addition, this chapter also describes nonspecific histologic alterations that are rather frequently encountered, may even be prominent in surgical and autopsy liver specimens, but often have little clinical significance. Brown pigments that are often encountered in the interpretation of liver specimens are discussed toward the end of this chapter.

Part of this chapter is also dedicated to handling and processing of liver biopsy specimens in order to obtain optimal sections for routine histologic evaluation and immunohistochemistry, and to preserve the submitted tissue for ancillary tests including molecular tests and electron microscopy studies. Immunohistochemistry is routinely performed on liver tissue nowadays, particularly in the diagnosis of primary and metastatic liver tumors.

EMBRYOLOGY

Liver is one of the first organs to develop, and rapidly becomes the largest organ during embryogenesis. It arises as hepatic diverticulum from the endodermal layer of the most distal portion of the foregut during the 3rd to 4th week of gestation. The endoderm also gives rise to lungs, pancreas, thyroid, and gastrointestinal tract. When embryo reaches 4 to 5 mm in length, the hepatic diverticulum differentiates cranially into proliferating hepatic cords and caudally into the gallbladder and extrahepatic bile ducts. The anastomosing cords of hepatoblasts grow into the mesenchyme of the septum transversum. As the hepatic cords extend outward during the 5th week of gestation, they are penetrated by the inwardly growing capillary plexus, which arises from the vitelline veins in the outer margins of the septum transversum and forms the primitive hepatic sinusoids.

Scattered mesenchymal cells derived from the septum transversum lie between the endothelial walls of the sinusoids and the hepatic cords, forming the connective tissue elements of the hepatic stroma, as well as the liver capsule. Hematopoietic tissue and Kupffer cells are also derived from splanchnic mesenchyme of the septum transversum. Once these structures are established, the liver grows rapidly to fill most of the embryonal abdominal cavity and by 9 weeks of gestation accounts for approximately 10% of the total weight of the embryo. The bile canaliculi appear in the 10-mm embryo as intercellular spaces between hepatoblasts.

The extrahepatic biliary tree arises directly from the endoderm, while the epithelium of the intrahepatic bile ducts arises from the proximal part of the primitive hepatic cords. This process is largely determined by the progressive development and branching of the portal vein with its surrounding mesenchyme. First, the hepatoblasts in direct contact with the mesenchyme around the portal vein transforms into bile duct–type cells. Then a second layer transforms into bile duct epithelial cells, resulting in a circular cleft in the shape of a cylinder around the portal vein and its enveloping mesenchyme (Fig. 27.1). These cells can be identified by their positivity of cytokeratin 19. This primitive channel duct in the 8-mm embryo (5 to 6 weeks of gestation) is referred as the ductal plate (1), which then undergoes gradual remodeling to form the normal anastomosing system of bile ducts in the portal tracts (2). Failure of remodeling of the ductal plate results in excess of bile duct structures retaining a fetal configuration (Fig. 27.2) (3). In patients with ductal plate malformation such as congenital hepatic fibrosis, ductal plate remnants, which should be absent at birth, are seen throughout the liver. Occasionally, ductal plate remnants can be seen embedded in fibrous stroma of the portal tracts in an otherwise normal liver.

The differentiation of intrahepatic ducts occurs in embryos of 22 to 30 mm. Despite the common ancestry of hepatocytes and bile duct cells, each cell type is structurally and functionally distinct. The walls of the terminal twigs of the biliary tree, the canals of Hering, which connect bile canaliculi to bile ducts, include both typical hepatocytes and bile duct cells, without intermediate forms.

Intrahepatic hematopoiesis begins during the 6th week, hepatocyte bile formation by the 12th week, and excretion of bile into the duodenum by the 16th week. Hematopoiesis is among the most important functions of fetal liver. The third trimester marks the cessation of hematopoiesis with a concomitant decrease in liver growth so that the liver accounts for approximately 5% of the newborn's body weight. An increased extramedullary hematopoiesis or myelopoiesis in the liver beyond the third trimester suggests the presence of an active fetal response to intrauterine ascending infection (4).

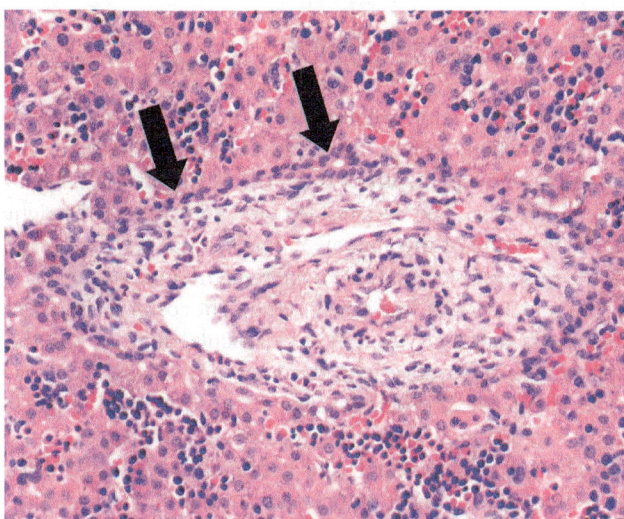

FIGURE 27.1 Ductal plate (*arrows*) developing around the portal vein mesenchyme in the liver of a 10-week-old embryo. There is extramedullary hematopoiesis in the sinusoids.

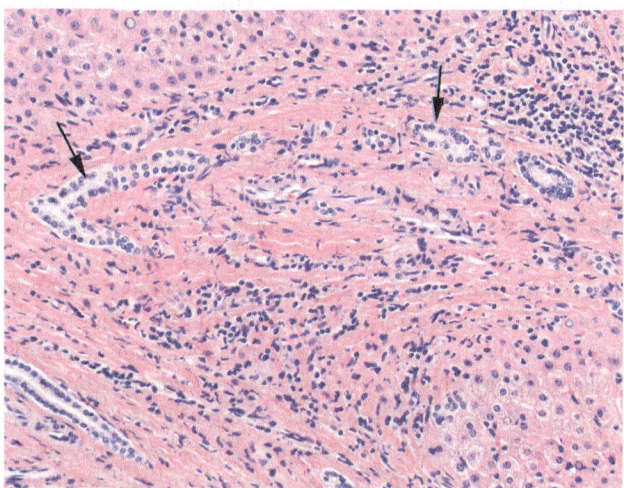

FIGURE 27.2 Ductal plate remnant (*arrows*) in portal tract stroma, similar to that seen in liver of an embryo, can occasionally be encountered in an otherwise normal liver.

GROSS MORPHOLOGY

The liver of an adult weighs 1,400 to 1,600 g, comprising 2.5% of the body weight. It is relatively larger in infancy, representing one-eighteenth of the birth weight, mainly due to a large left lobe. The liver resides predominantly in the right upper quadrant of the abdomen and is completely protected by the rib cage. It extends from the right 5th intercostal space in the midclavicular line down to the right costal margin and to the left as far as the left midclavicular line. It has the appearance of a wedge with the base to the right and measures about 10 cm in vertical span, 12 to 15 cm in thickness, and 15 to 20 cm in its greatest transverse diameter.

The superior, anterior, and lateral surfaces of the liver are smooth and almost completely covered by peritoneum, except for a small triangular area—the "bare area" below the diaphragm—which is surrounded by the reflections of the peritoneum forming the coronary ligaments. A thin layer of fibrous connective tissue, the Glisson capsule, surrounds the liver and extends into the parenchyma to form extensions that support arterial and biliary structures. Anteriorly, the falciform and round ligaments, which during fetal life conducted the left umbilical vein, connect the liver to the abdominal wall. Through the posterior surface of the liver at the base of the bare area runs the inferior vena cava, to which two to four hepatic veins connect. The fossa of the gallbladder and the round ligament separate the quadrate lobe from the right and left liver lobes, respectively. The fossa of the ductus venosus (i.e., the connection of the left umbilical vein to the inferior vena cava) and the inferior vena cava separate the caudate lobe from the left and right lobes of the liver. The horizontal portal fissure (or porta hepatis), which joins the upper ends of the gallbladder fossa and the groove of the round ligament, contains the branches of the hepatic artery, the portal vein, the hepatic nerve plexus, the hepatic ducts, and lymph vessels.

The liver is divided by deep grooves into two large lobes—the right (lateral to falciform ligament) and left (medial to falciform ligament)—and two smaller lobes, the caudate and quadrate lobes. This traditional division is only of topographical significance. Functionally, the division into eight segments based on either Couinaud or Bismuth segmental classification (5–7), which does not correspond to the anatomical division into lobes, is more important. Each segment is served by its own vascular inflow, outflow, and biliary drainage. The center of each segment contains branch of hepatic artery, portal vein, and bile duct, while hepatic veins are located in the periphery of each segment. This segmental division is of critical importance, particularly when dissecting small space-occupying lesions from these areas or when removing segments of liver for transplantation (8). Each segment can be resected without damaging those remaining. For the liver to remain viable, resections must be performed along vessels that define the peripheries of these segments, which mean that resection lines should be parallel to the hepatic veins. Anatomical and functional variations occur not infrequently, particularly in the right liver. Imaging studies, including magnetic resonance imaging or computed tomography, can provide detailed insight into the individual segmental anatomy (9).

HISTOLOGY

Structural Organization

The structural organization of the liver into parenchymal, interstitial, vascular, and ductal elements is based on its many functions and its position between the digestive tract and the rest of the body. The functional unit of the liver is represented by the hepatic lobule or rather, as defined by Rappaport, the hepatic acinus (Fig. 27.3) (10,11). The latter is a regular three-dimensional structure in which blood flows from the central axis, formed by the terminal portal venule and terminal hepatic arteriole in the portal tract, into the acinar sinusoids and empties into several terminal hepatic venules at the periphery of the acinus (Fig. 27.4).

In contrast, the hepatic lobule consists of an efferent central venule with cords of hepatocytes radiating to several peripheral portal tracts (Fig. 27.5). Therefore, in a two-dimensional view, the acinus occupies parts of several adjacent lobules. The acini measure 560 to 1,050 μm in length and 300 to 600 μm in width. The division of the hepatic parenchyma into the classic lobules, with changes described as being centrilobular, midzonal, and periportal, is still used as a convenient landmark. However, Rappaport acinus has now come to be more generally accepted. The acinus is subdivided into zones 1, 2, and 3 with decreasing

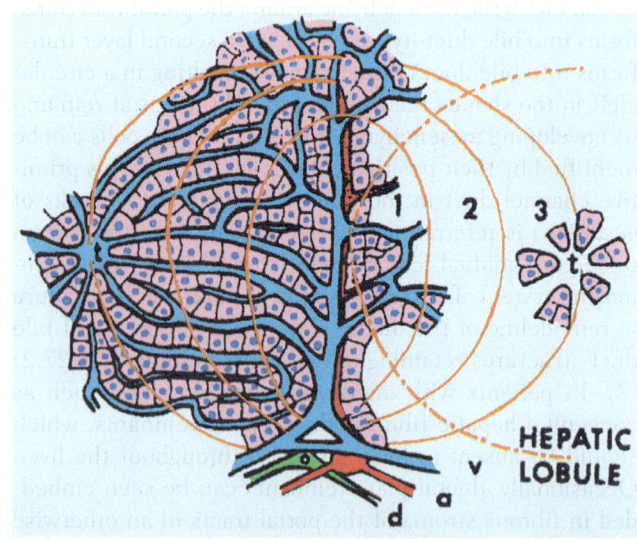

FIGURE 27.3 Diagram comparing the hepatic acinus with zones *1*, *2*, and *3* to the hepatic lobule (*dash-dotted line*). Portal tract contains portal venule (*v*), hepatic arteriole (*a*), and hepatic duct (*d*). *t,* terminal hepatic venule.

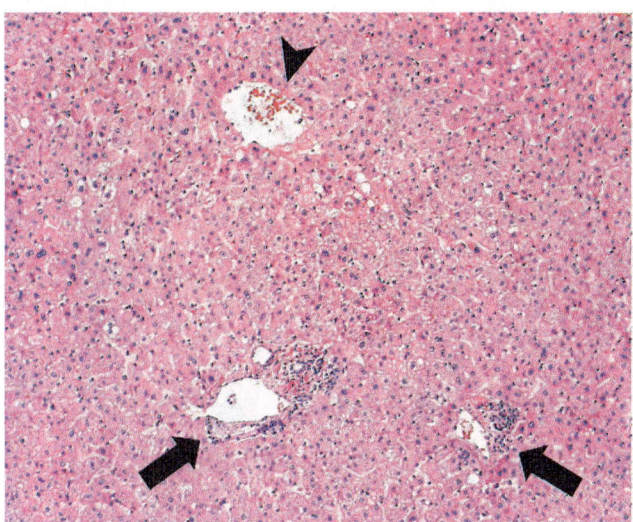

FIGURE 27.4 Normal human liver showing two portal tracts (*arrows*) and one terminal hepatic venule (*arrowhead*).

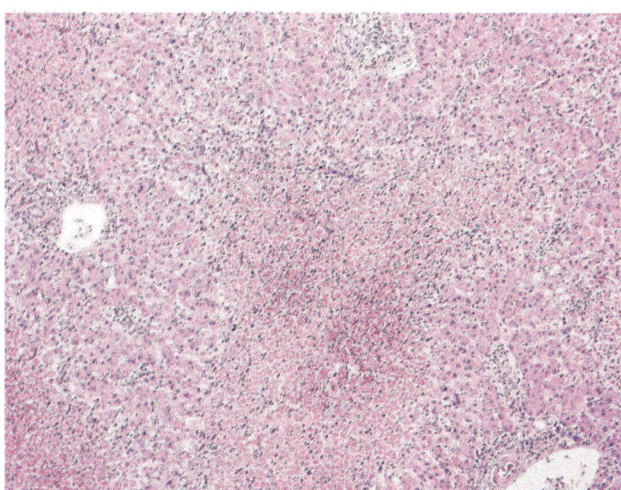

FIGURE 27.6 Centrilobular and midzonal geographic coagulative necrosis in acetaminophen-induced toxicity.

oxygenation and increasing susceptibility to ischemia and toxic or drug-induced injury. The hepatocytes in zone 1 are nearest to portal tracts and correspond to the periportal area of the classic lobule. Zone 2 corresponds roughly to the midzonal area of a classic lobule, and zone 3 corresponds to parts of several centrilobular areas.

The terminal vascular branches, which bring substances for nutrition and metabolism into the acinus, run along the terminal bile ducts that drain the secretory products of the same acinus. These vessels form a vascular plexus around the bile ducts (12). Thus, as a result of the sinusoidal blood flow, structural, secretory, and functional unity is established in the acinus. The oxygen gradient, metabolic heterogeneity, and differential distribution of enzymes across the three zones of the acinus explain the zonal distribution of liver damage due to ischemia and toxic substances, with zone 3 being the most susceptible zone to ischemic and toxic injury (13). The periportal hepatocytes contain carbamoyl phosphate synthetase and glucose-6-phosphatase enzymes, whereas the predominant enzymes in perivenular hepatocytes are glutamine synthetase and NADPH-cytochrome (14). In clinical practice, one may be able to corroborate the suspicious offending agent with histologic zonal pattern of injury. Alcoholic liver disease and drug-induced injury commonly produce centrilobular or zone 3 hepatocyte injury, because the centrilobular area is populated by hepatocytes with a high level of cytochrome P-450 activity for drug metabolism (15). A long list of drugs (13), classically acetaminophen (16), can cause centrilobular hepatocyte coagulative necrosis, which may extend to midzonal areas resulting in geographic pattern of hepatocyte necrosis (Fig. 27.6). In rare instances, one may see exclusively midzonal necrosis, such as in furosemide toxicity; or periportal necrosis, such as in cocaine toxicity (17).

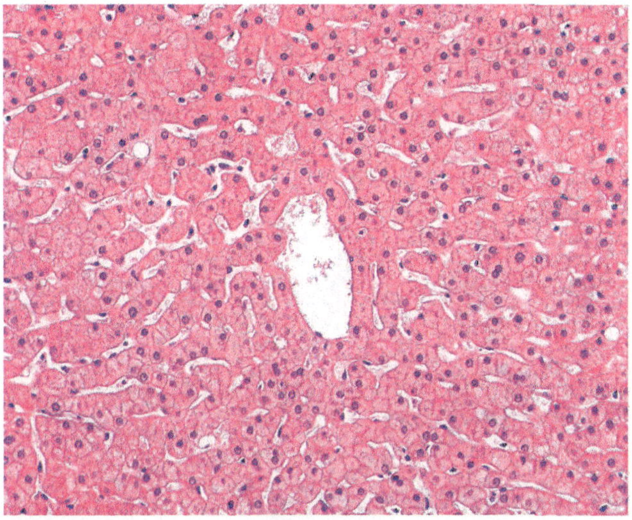

Hepatocytes

The hepatocytes are arranged in sponge-like plates that are normally one-cell-layer thick in the adult, and are separated by sinusoids along which blood flows from portal tracts to terminal hepatic venules (Fig. 27.7). Surrounding the terminal hepatic venules, the hepatocytes exhibit a more regular radial pattern. Away from the perivenular area, the liver cell plates are arranged less regularly without distinct radial arrangement. The hepatocytes in the periportal area are closely packed and smaller than other parenchymal cells with more intense nuclear staining and more basophilic cytoplasm (Fig. 27.8). The periportal area is also the regenerative compartment of the liver parenchyma. The hepatocytes bordering the portal tracts are joined together and form

FIGURE 27.5 Terminal hepatic venule surrounded by converging hepatocyte plates and sinusoids.

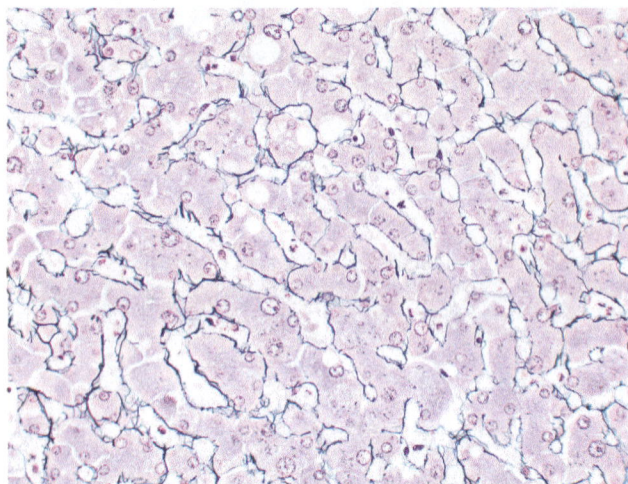

FIGURE 27.7 Normal adult liver parenchyma composed of one-cell-thick hepatocyte plates, each lined by reticulin fibers (reticulin stain).

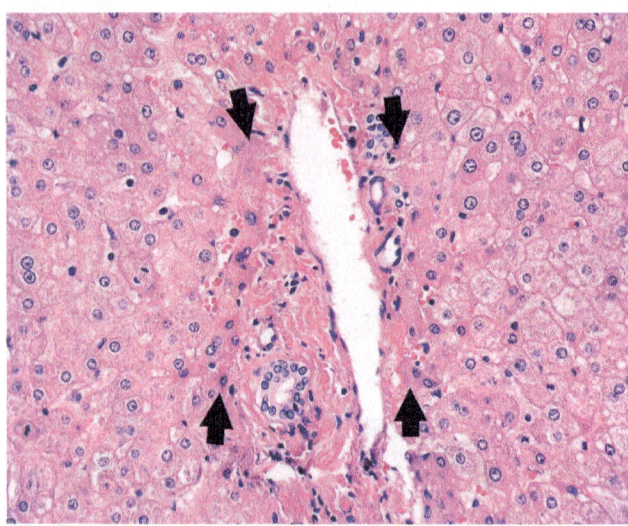

FIGURE 27.9 Normal portal tract with bile duct, hepatic arteriole, portal venule, and clearly defined limiting plate (*arrows*).

a distinct row called the limiting plate (Fig. 27.9). Destruction of this limiting plate by necroinflammation and/or apoptosis is a hallmark of chronic hepatitis (piecemeal necrosis or interface hepatitis) (Fig. 27.10).

In children up to 5 or 6 years of age, the liver cells are uniform and arranged in two-cell-thick plates (Fig. 27.11) (18). In adults, the presence of two-cell-thick plates, the formation of rosettes, hepatocyte buds, and the increase of mitotic activity indicate parenchymal regeneration.

The individual hepatocyte is a polygonal epithelial cell approximately 25 μm in diameter with a well-defined plasma membrane that is differentiated into three specialized regions or domains: basolateral (70% of total surface area), which faces the sinusoid; bile canalicular (15%), bounding part of the intercellular space that constitutes the bile canaliculi; and lateral (15%), facing the rest of the intercellular space. Each domain has different molecular, chemical, and antigenic compositions and functions.

The nucleus is centrally located, round, and contains one or more nucleoli. At birth, all but a rare few hepatocytes are mononuclear. In adults, although binucleate forms are not uncommon (up to 25% of cells), mitotic activity is rare. Nuclei vary in size in the adult, and the great majority is diploid (19). Some nuclei are larger than others, indicating polyploidy, particularly in individuals over 60 years (Fig. 27.12). The significance of polyploidy is unknown and is usually more marked in the midzonal area. It may represent the mechanism to generate genetic diversity and permits adaptation of hepatocytes to xenobiotic or nutritional injury (20). Since cell size is proportional to cell ploidy,

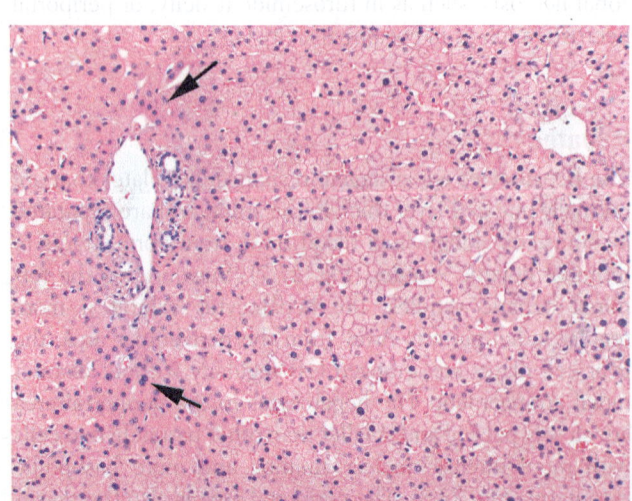

FIGURE 27.8 The periportal regenerative compartment of hepatic lobule contains smaller and more basophilic hepatocytes (*arrows*).

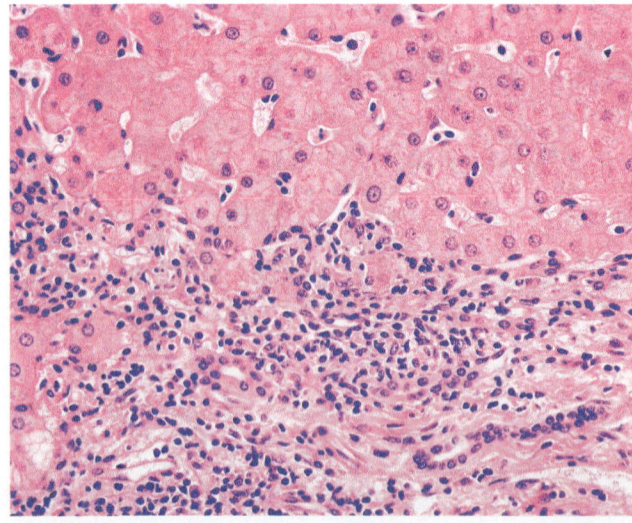

FIGURE 27.10 Interface hepatitis causing destruction of limiting plate in chronic viral hepatitis.

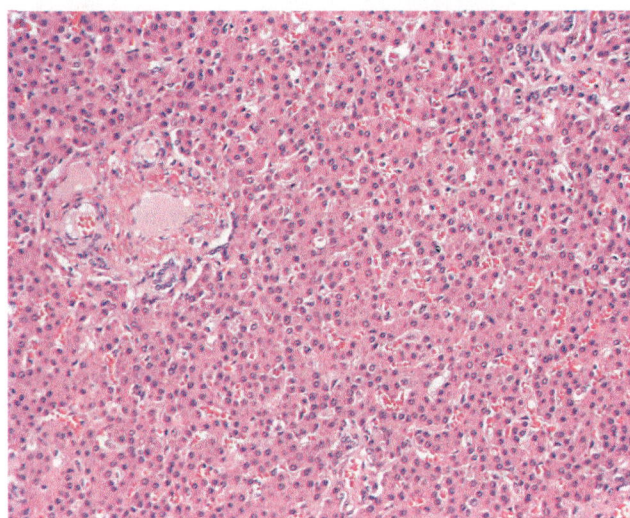

FIGURE 27.11 Liver of a child showing small uniform hepatocytes that are arranged in two-cell–thick plates.

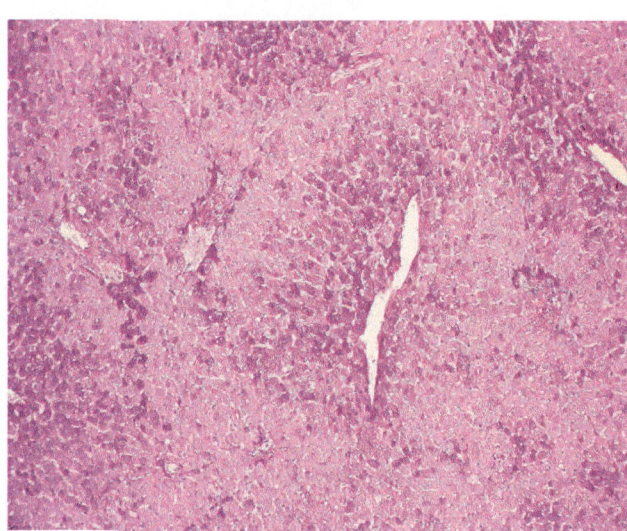

FIGURE 27.13 PAS reaction shows irregular distribution of cytoplasmic glycogen (darker color) in the hepatocytes.

polyploidy does not provide an increased quantity of genetic material per unit volume of cytoplasm, that is, nuclear to cytoplasmic ratio remains low.

The cytoplasm of the hepatocytes is eosinophilic due to numerous mitochondria and it also contains fine basophilic granules, which represent rough endoplasmic reticulum. The hepatocytes contain abundant cytoplasmic glycogen, which after proper fixation is stainable with periodic acid–Schiff (PAS) reagent (Fig. 27.13). On hematoxylin and eosin (H&E) preparations, glycogen gives a fine, reticulated, foamy appearance to the cytoplasm (Fig. 27.14). The quantity and distribution of cytoplasmic glycogen reflect diurnal and diet-related variations. An irregular distribution pattern may sometimes be found in biopsies and is not of diagnostic significance (Fig. 27.13). Glycogen accumulation in hepatocyte nuclei around portal tracts produces a vacuolated appearance and is common in adolescents and young adults (Fig. 27.15). In adults, such an appearance may be conspicuous in conditions such as glucose intolerance, diabetes mellitus, Wilson disease, and pancreatic carcinoma (21).

Isolated acidophilic bodies and rare apoptotic bodies represent normal turnover of hepatocytes (Fig. 27.16). Occasional focal necroses where chronic inflammatory cells replace a few necrotic hepatocytes are not unusual in otherwise apparently normal liver.

Hepatocyte Regeneration

Liver is the only human organ that is capable of natural regeneration. Regeneration may be rapid as seen after partial hepatectomy (22). This is predominantly due to the

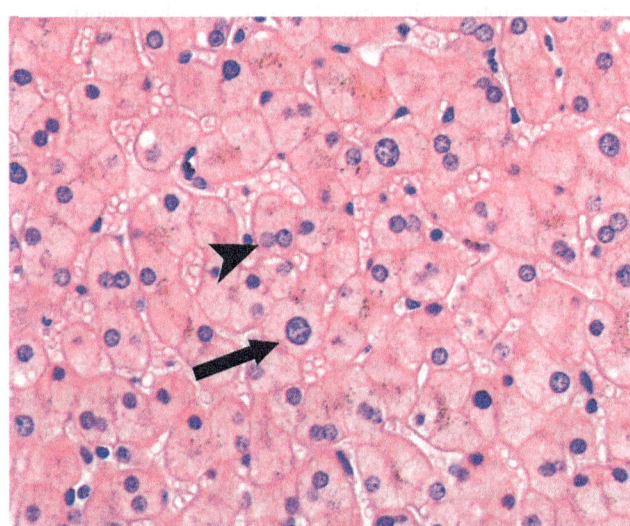

FIGURE 27.12 Liver of a 65-year-old patient showing significant polyploidy of hepatocyte nuclei (*arrow*) and binucleate forms (*arrowhead*).

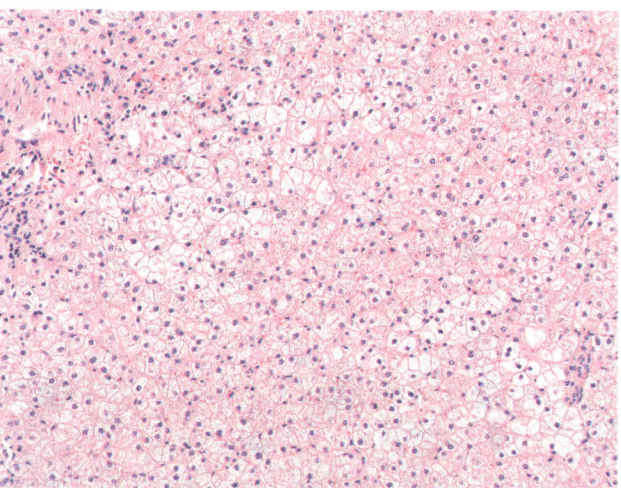

FIGURE 27.14 Irregular distribution of cytoplasmic glycogen, producing patchy collection of hepatocytes with clear cytoplasm, is of no clinical significance in the absence of other histopathologic findings.

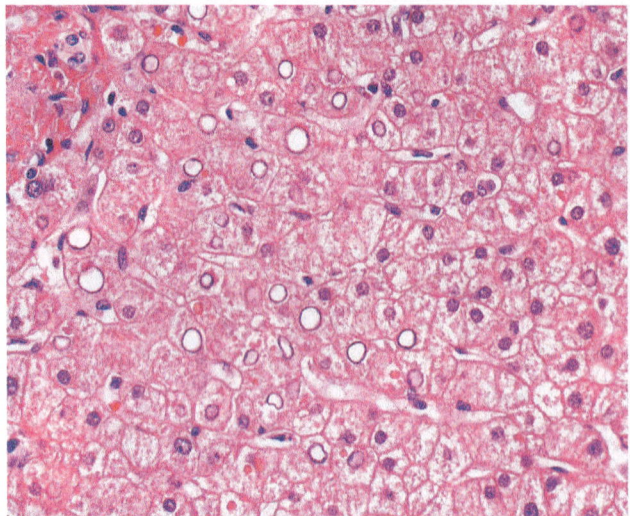

FIGURE 27.15 Glycogen accumulation in hepatocyte nuclei resulting in clear, empty appearance.

hepatocytes reentering the cell cycle: quiescent cells stimulated by mediators including cytokines, move into a primed state (G0 to G1) when growth factors can stimulate DNA synthesis and cellular replication.

In the event of injury, regeneration is observed predominantly in the periportal hepatocytes in mild injury or throughout the hepatic parenchyma in severe injury. It is manifested by mitoses, multinucleation, and crowding of the periportal cell plates by small, uniform, darkly stained, or basophilic hepatocytes. Liver cell plates in the periportal region become irregularly thickened and occasional hepatocellular rosettes may appear. Nuclear displacement to the sinusoidal pole with hyperchromasia is a cytologic indication of regenerative activity. All of these changes impart a darkened periportal region under low magnification, which is often the only remarkable change in mild acute hepatitis or in residual hepatitis as a reaction to recent injury. In severe hepatocellular injury or hepatitis, the feature of regeneration may be overwhelmed by the amount of ballooning degeneration, cytolytic necrosis, apoptosis, bridging necrosis, and inflammatory infiltrate.

The degree of hepatocyte regeneration often correlates with the degree of necroinflammatory activity in chronic hepatitis, particularly when interface hepatitis is the predominant process.

If hepatocytes are extensively damaged, such as in massive hepatic necrosis, the conventional hepatocyte regeneration is impaired. Hepatocytes may be derived from bipotential progenitor cells, the so-called oval cells, residing in the canals of Hering (22). These cells can differentiate into either hepatocytes or cholangiocytes.

Hepatocyte Degeneration and Death

In general there are two types of cell death that can be distinguished by morphologic features, apoptosis, and cytolytic necrosis, although it is likely that these are two ends of a spectrum with possible intermediate forms.

Apoptosis occurs at all stages during fetal growth and development of ductal plates and hepatoblasts. There is a good correlation between the proliferative and apoptotic activities in the ductal plate, depending on the remodeling process. Involution of liver and neoplasia is also controlled by apoptosis, which is induced by transforming growth factor β1. In these involuting livers or regressing tumors, scattered apoptotic bodies, rather than massive cytolytic necrosis, are observed. In viral infections such as cytomegalovirus and herpes hepatitis, apoptosis has been proposed as a mechanism of cell death. Similarly, viral hepatitis C leads to increased apoptosis in hepatocytes (23). In viral hepatitis B and C, however, cell death may be mediated directly by the virus or by the host immune system through the release of cytokines such as tumor necrosis factor α to the infected cells (24,25). In normal liver tissue, although rare, individual apoptotic bodies may be seen, which suggests that apoptosis is a physiologic process in the liver. Apoptosis involves shrinkage, nuclear disassembly, and fragmentation of the cell into discrete bodies with intact plasma membranes, which are then rapidly phagocytosed by neighboring Kupffer cells (Fig. 27.17).

Cytolytic necrosis is manifested histologically by ballooning degeneration, and the hepatocytes become swollen and pale staining as the result mainly from dilatation of the endoplasmic reticulum (Fig. 27.18). This is a consequence of loss of mitochondrial function and resultant ATP depletion, leading to loss of ion homeostasis and plasma membrane integrity. The cytoplasm is partially rarefied, particularly along the cellular periphery, and the cytoplasmic remnants clump around the nucleus; cell membranes are frequently indistinct. Ballooned hepatocytes undergo lytic necrosis which is not visible, but the occurrence can be inferred to small foci of stromal collapse that are accompanied by collections of lymphocytes and Kupffer cells, that

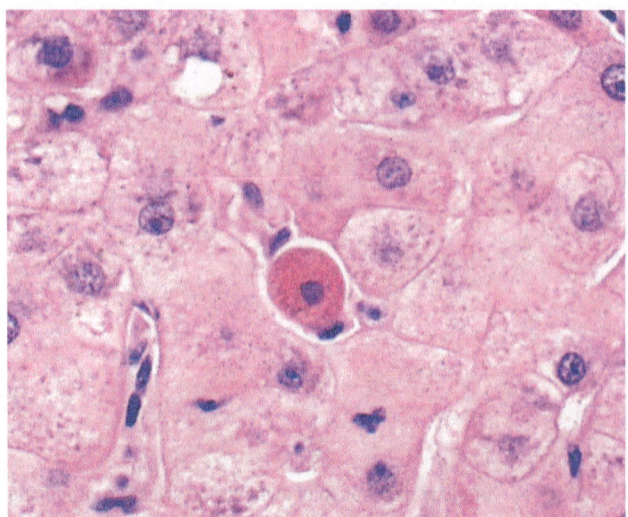

FIGURE 27.16 A hepatocyte undergoing apoptosis.

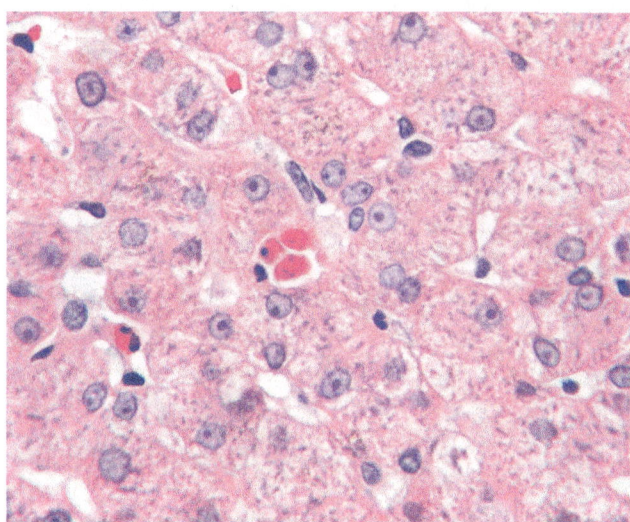

FIGURE 27.17 Acidophilic and apoptotic bodies.

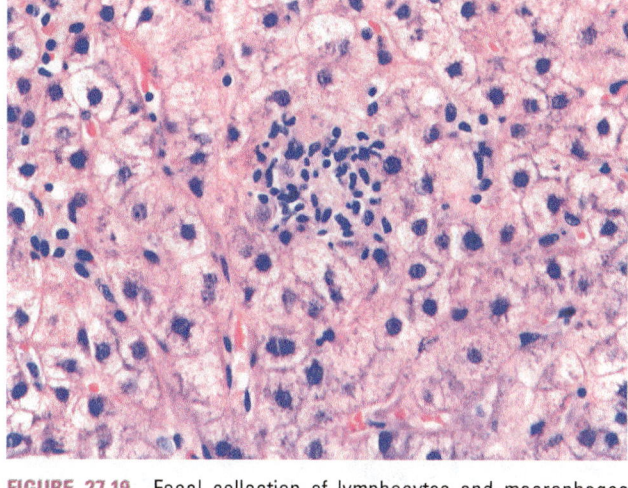

FIGURE 27.19 Focal collection of lymphocytes and macrophages surround hepatocyte with lytic necrosis.

is, spotty necrosis (Fig. 27.19). The degree of ballooning degeneration varies across the lobule, although classically the centrilobular region is the most severely affected. In addition to hepatocyte injury and regeneration, there are varying degrees of cholestasis, Kupffer cell activation, ductular reaction, and bile duct damage.

Bile Canaliculi

The bile canaliculus is an intercellular space with a diameter of approximately 1 μm, formed by the apposition of the edges of gutter-like hemicanals on adjacent surfaces of two or three neighboring hepatocytes. Bile canaliculi are not readily recognized under the light microscope unless distended in conditions causing parenchymal cholestasis, which is accompanied by pseudoglandular formation of hepatocytes (Fig. 27.20). Bile canaliculi form a chicken wire–like network in the center of the hepatic plates and can be demonstrated immunohistochemically with polyclonal anticarcinoembryonic antigen (pCEA) or CD10 (Fig. 27.21) (26).

The canalicular membrane of the hepatocytes is host to a number of biliary proteins that are responsible for the formation and flow of bile in the liver. Inherited defect of these proteins lead to heterogeneous intrahepatic cholestatic syndromes, which are known as progressive familial intrahepatic cholestasis (27).

Sinusoidal Lining Cells

In normal liver biopsy specimens, the hepatic sinusoids are slit-like spaces that contain a few blood cells. The periportal sinusoids are more tortuous than the perivenular ones.

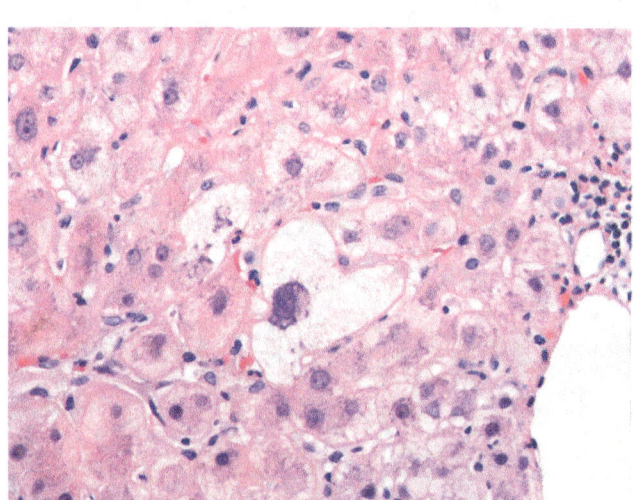

FIGURE 27.18 Ballooning degeneration of the hepatocytes.

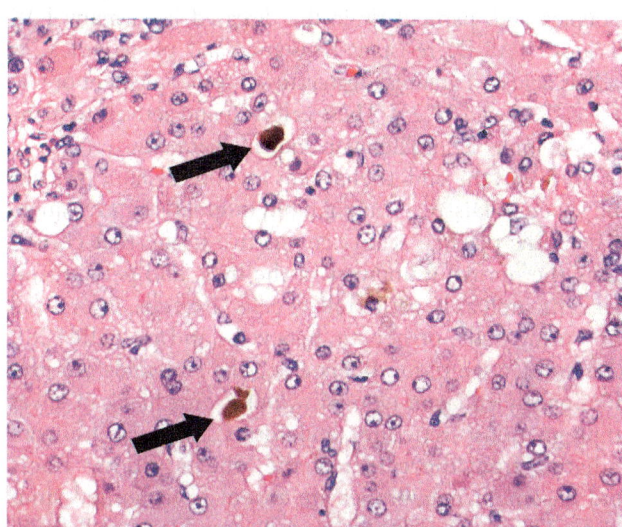

FIGURE 27.20 Canalicular bile thrombi (*arrows*) in zone 3 of the acinus.

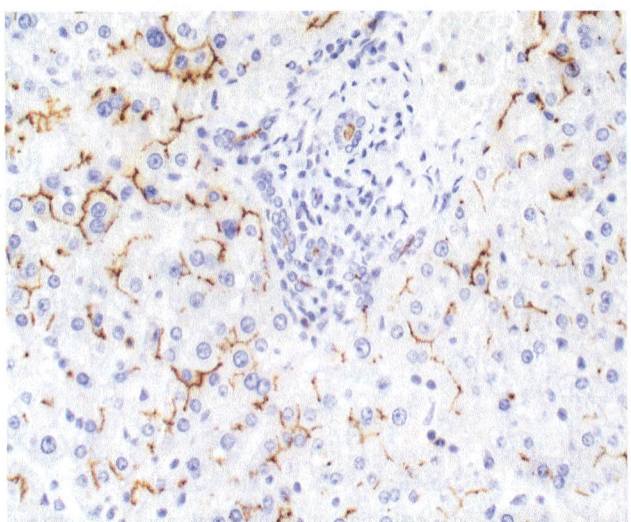

FIGURE 27.21 CD10 immunostaining delineates the twig-like structures of bile canaliculi, as well as the lumen of bile ducts and ductules.

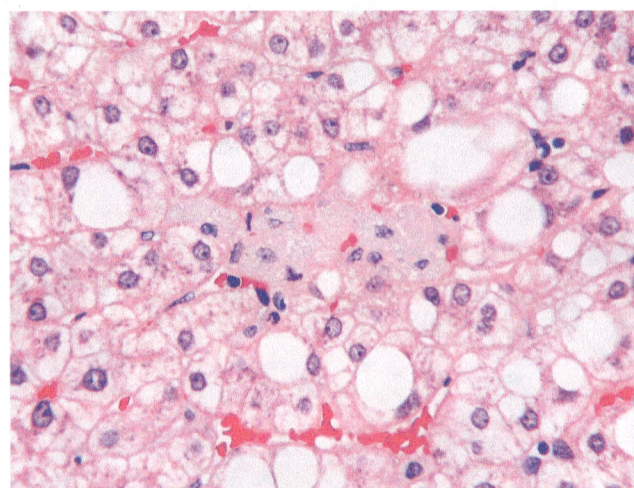

FIGURE 27.22 Collection of ceroid-containing macrophages signifying a focus of recent hepatocyte drop out.

Hepatic sinusoids separate cords of hepatocytes and are lined by sinusoidal lining cells supported by reticulin fibers (Fig. 27.7). Sinusoidal lining cells, which include endothelial and Kupffer cells, constitute a coordinated defense system (28). They are rather inconspicuous in normal biopsy specimens. The endothelial cells have thin, indistinct cytoplasm and small, elongated, darkly stained nuclei without nucleoli. The sieve-like plates of the endothelial cytoplasm and the absence of a structurally defined basement membrane (in contrast to capillaries) facilitate exchange between blood and hepatocytes.

The Kupffer cells have a bean-shaped nucleus and plump cytoplasm with star-shaped extensions. They are more numerous near the portal tracts. They belong to the mononuclear phagocytic system and are derived in part from the bone marrow. The Kupffer cells represent up to 90% of the resident macrophages in the liver and account for approximately 15% of the total liver cell population. They contain vacuoles and, particularly in the diseased liver, many PAS diastase (PAS-D) resistant lysosomes and phagosomes, as well as acid-fast granular aggregates of ceroid pigment or bile (Figs. 27.22 and 27.23). These cells respond actively to many types of injury by proliferation and enlargement.

Between the endothelial cells and the hepatocytes lies the space of Disse, a zone of rapid intercellular exchange. It contains plasma, scanty connective tissue that constitutes the normal framework of the liver, and perisinusoidal cells such as hepatic stellate cells (Ito cells, interstitial fat-storing cells, or hepatic lipocytes) and pit cells (28). The connective tissue fibers along the sinusoids are predominantly collagen type III, which stains black in silver impregnations (reticulin) and forms a regular network radiating from the center of the lobules. Elastic fibers and basement membranes are absent from normal sinusoids. The space of Disse is not discernible in well-fixed, normal liver biopsy material; but in postmortem liver, the hepatocytes shrink, pericellular edema develops, and the space becomes more conspicuous (Fig. 27.24). Extravasation of red blood cells into the space of Disse occurs in hepatic vein outflow obstruction.

On light microscopy of normal liver, hepatic stellate cells are quiescent and difficult to differentiate from sinusoidal lining cells. They are modified resting fibroblasts that can store fat and vitamin A, and produce hepatocyte growth factor and collagen (29). Hepatic stellate cells are the main fibrogenic cell type in injured liver (30). When loaded with fat, such as in hypervitaminosis A (31), they may be recognized due to cytoplasmic fat droplets of rather uniform size with scalloping of the elongated nucleus (Fig. 27.25). Hepatic stellate cells are highly responsive to stimuli released during inflammation, such as oxidative stress and

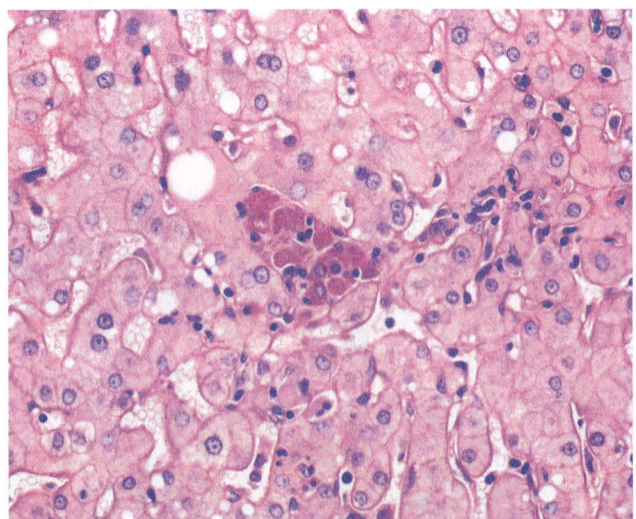

FIGURE 27.23 Ceroid pigment in macrophages as an indicator of previous hepatocyte injury/necrosis (PAS-D).

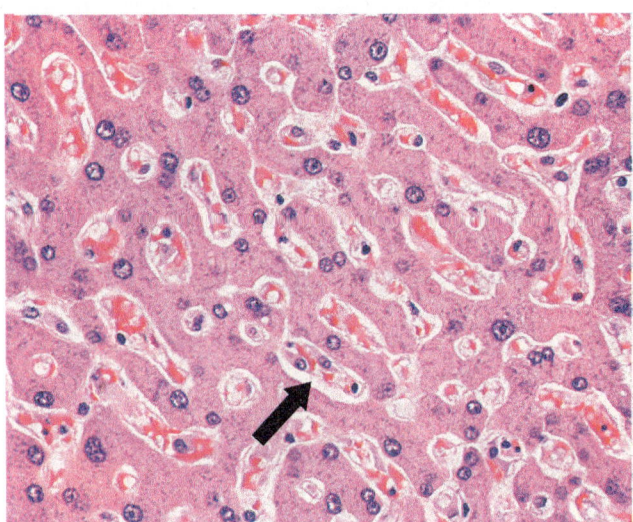

FIGURE 27.24 Autopsy liver specimen exhibiting dilatation of sinusoids and space of Disse (*arrow*) with prominent sinusoidal lining cells including endothelial and Kupffer cells.

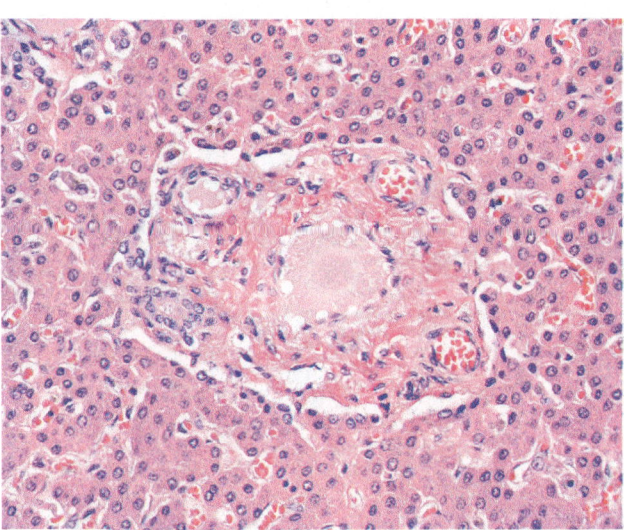

FIGURE 27.26 Normal portal tract in a newborn with bile ducts and their corresponding hepatic arteries of approximately the same diameter.

proinflammaotry cytokines that promote their transdifferentiation into myofibroblasts. When activated, these cells contain stainable desmin and actin in their cytoplasm, justifying their designation as myofibroblasts.

Pit cells have not been characterized by light microscopy. Under the electron microscope, they have neurosecretory-like electron-dense granules and rod-cored vesicles. However, recent evidence indicates that pit cells are not endocrine cells, but correspond to the large granular lymphocytes and have natural killer cell activity (32,33).

Occasional inflammatory cells, lymphocytes, or polymorphonuclear leukocytes may be present in the hepatic sinusoids. During the first few weeks after birth, the presence of foci of extramedullary hematopoietic cells in the sinusoids and wall of terminal hepatic venules is a normal feature.

Portal Tracts

Each portal tract contains a bile duct and several bile ductules, a hepatic artery branch, a portal vein branch, and lymphatic channels embedded in connective tissue (Fig. 27.26). The amount of connective tissue and the size of the intraportal structures depend on the size of the portal tract. Nerve fibers, both sympathetic and parasympathetic for innervation of blood vessels and bile ducts, can be seen in large portal tracts. The larger portal tracts are round or triangular, the smaller ones are triangular or branching, and the smallest terminal divisions are round or oval. The size of a portal tract is approximately three to four times the diameter of the hepatic artery branch.

The portal tracts normally contain a few lymphocytes, macrophages, and mast cells, but no polymorphonuclear leukocytes or plasma cells. The number of inflammatory cells increases with age. However, their density varies from one portal tract to the next.

The portal tracts also contain portal fibroblasts. Portal fibroblasts and hepatic stellate cells are profibrogenic cells and the main resident of mesenchymal cells in normal liver. The connective tissue of the portal tracts consists mainly of collagen type I, which is seen as thick, deep blue fibers on the trichrome stain (Fig. 27.27). Newly formed collagen type III appears as fine, light blue fibers. In the subcapsular region of the liver, large portal tracts are often encountered, containing more and denser connective tissue (Fig. 27.28). Irregular extensions of fibrous tissue from the Glisson capsule into the parenchyma, sometimes connecting adjacent portal tracts, must not be interpreted as bridging fibrous

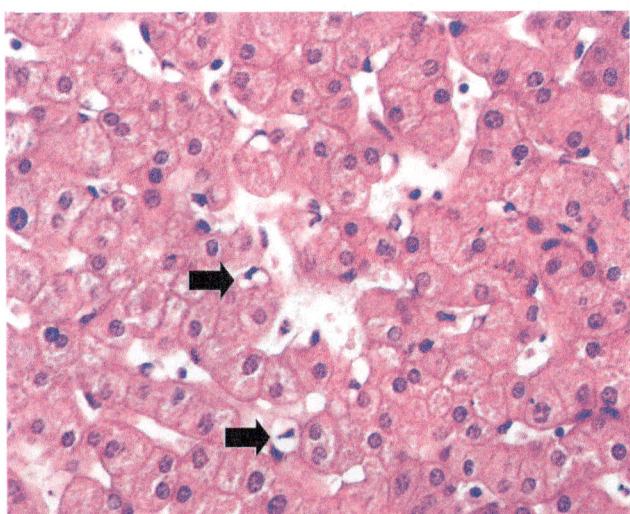

FIGURE 27.25 Prominent hepatic stellate cells (Ito cells) in the liver biopsy specimen of a patient with hypervitaminosis A. The nuclei of the hepatic stellate cells are scalloped (*arrows*) due to fat droplets in cytoplasm.

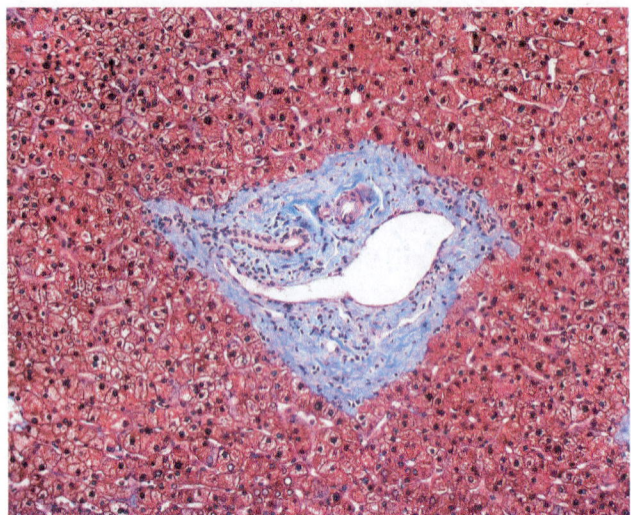

FIGURE 27.27 The connective tissue of portal tracts consists mainly collagen type I, which appears as thick, deep blue fibers on trichrome stain.

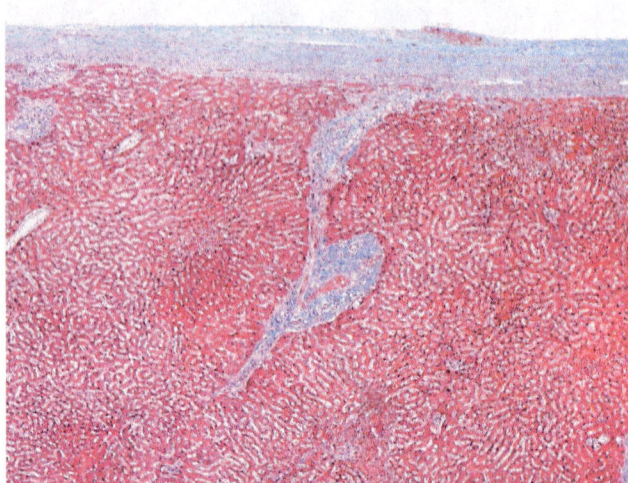

FIGURE 27.29 Subcapsular liver parenchyma with extension of the Glisson capsule into the parenchyma which may be mistaken for bridging fibrosis (trichrome stain).

septa or cirrhosis in wedge or superficial biopsy specimens of subcapsular parenchyma (Fig. 27.29) (34).

Blood Supply and Drainage

The liver is nourished by a dual blood supply, approximately three-fourths via the portal vein and the remainder via the hepatic arteries. The portal vein carries nutrient-rich venous blood from the alimentary tract including the pancreas, whereas the hepatic artery supplies oxygen-rich arterial blood from the celiac axis for liver and biliary tree survival.

The right, middle, and left hepatic veins provide venous outflow. The right hepatic vein drains the right lobe, the middle hepatic vein drains primarily the middle portion of the left lobe and a variable portion of the right, and the left hepatic vein provides the principal drainage of the left lateral lobe. The middle and the left hepatic vein often join together to form a common trunk before entering the vena cava. In addition, there are short venous segments that drain the posterior surface of the liver directly into the inferior vena cava.

Portal Vein

Portal veins are the largest vessels in portal tracts and produce venules that empty into periportal sinusoids (Fig. 27.30). Portal vein may be absent in up to 30% of portal tracts without any clinical significance. An increase of profiles of the portal veins is commonly seen in cirrhotic liver as the result of portal hypertension.

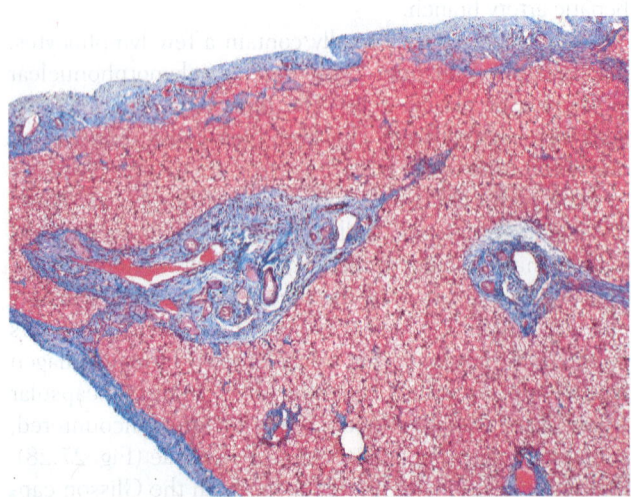

FIGURE 27.28 Subcapsular liver parenchyma containing large portal tracts (trichrome stain).

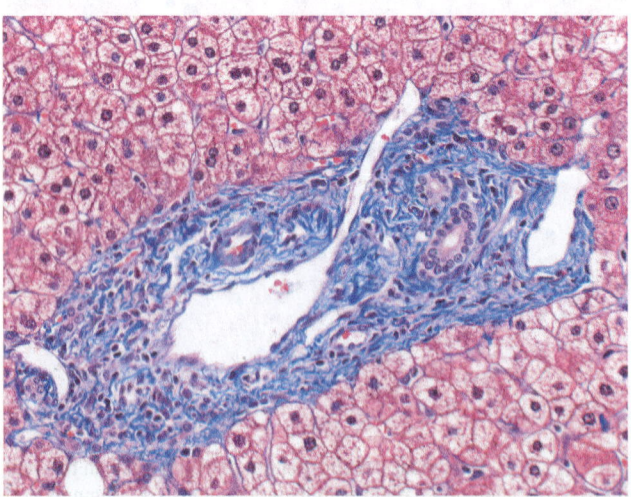

FIGURE 27.30 Portal venule empties into the periportal sinusoids (trichrome stain).

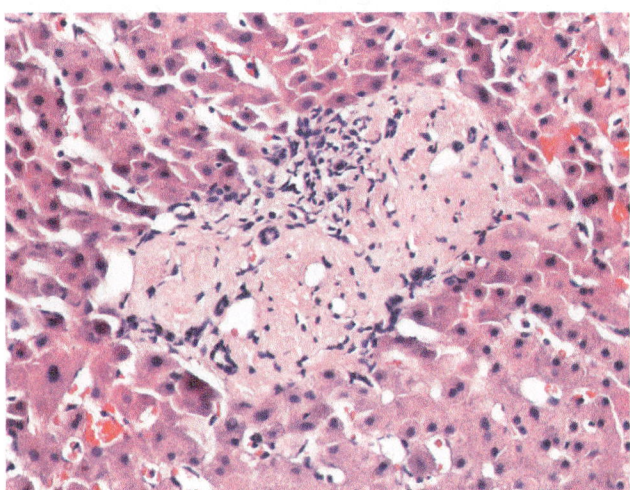

FIGURE 27.31 Luminal obliteration of portal vein in hepatoportal sclerosis.

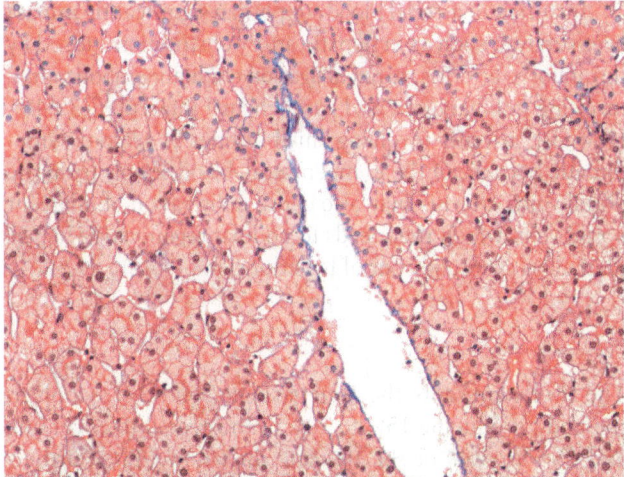

FIGURE 27.32 Normal hepatic venule has a thin fibrous wall (trichrome stain).

Thrombosis of portal vein occurs secondary to cirrhosis, tumor in the hepatic hilum or pancreas, or hypercoagulable states (12,35,36). Portal vein thrombosis in noncirrhotic liver often causes lobar atrophy of the liver, frequently the left lobe, and portal hypertension with venous collaterals (cavernous transformation). In portal thrombosis, portal vein may be absent or shows recanalization.

Obstruction confined to the small portal veins rarely causes portal hypertension, but there are conditions such as hepatoportal sclerosis or obstructive portal venopathy, congenital hepatic fibrosis, and chronic schistosomiasis that may cause clinically significant portal hypertension (37,38). In hepatoportal sclerosis, portal vein wall is thickened and hyalinized, resulting in narrowing and occasional luminal obliteration and alternates with some that are dilated and herniated into the hepatic lobule (Fig. 27.31).

Hepatic Vein

The intrahepatic course of the valveless hepatic veins, which are embedded in a thin sheath of connective tissue, is straight to the inferior vena cava. There is a defined spatial relationship between the terminal hepatic venules and the branches of the portal vein and hepatic artery in the portal tracts, which interdigitate but do not directly connect in the three-dimensional space. The distance between two terminal hepatic venules represents the size of an acinus.

The smaller branches (or sublobular veins) and the smallest efferent veins (or terminal hepatic venules) are in direct contact with the hepatic parenchyma. The terminal hepatic venules have a very thin wall lined by endothelial cells, which is readily demonstrable after staining with trichrome for collagen or Victoria blue for elastic fibers, but they do not have an adventitia around their wall (Fig. 27.32).

Thickening of the wall of terminal hepatic venules is often part of pericellular fibrosis and central hyaline sclerosis in alcoholic liver disease. In patients with a history of fatty liver disease, the findings of perivenular and pericellular fibrosis confirm previous episodes of steatohepatitis. Embedded small clusters of hepatocytes in the wall of hepatic venules usually seen in liver with significant or higher stage of fibrosis. It should be noted, however, that mild perivenular fibrosis may be seen focally in apparently normal individuals, as well as in children up to 2 years of age.

Hepatic Artery

The hepatic artery branches are intimately related to the corresponding portal veins. They may show thickening and hyalinization of the wall in older individuals or more significantly in hypertensive individuals, although these changes are usually milder than in other organs (Fig. 27.33). The terminal hepatic arterioles regulate the parenchymal blood supply with their muscular sphincter, whereas the portal venous supply is controlled by mesenteric venous blood flow.

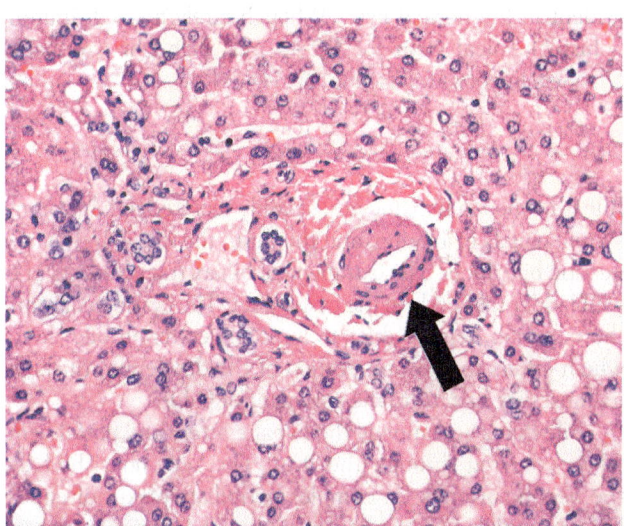

FIGURE 27.33 Thickened hepatic artery in an older individual (*arrow*).

Insufficient arterial blood supply can significantly impact liver survival, such as in hepatic artery obstruction caused by thrombosis, arteritis, surgical ligation or chemoembolization, resulting in biliary tree and parenchymal infarction (39,40). However, arteritis involving small arteries is seldom symptomatic because of the compensatory blood supply from the portal vein. Arteritis may also cause obliteration of adjacent portal vein, which then leads to nodular regenerative hyperplasia and eventually portal hypertension (41,42).

Lymphatics

The liver represents the largest single source of lymph in the body, producing 15% to 20% of the overall total volume and 25% to 50% of the thoracic duct flow (43). Furthermore, hepatic lymph has an unusually high protein content, about 85% to 95% of that in plasma, and a high content of lymphocytes. Most of the hepatic lymphatics leave the liver at the porta hepatis and drain into hepatic nodes along the hepatic artery and into the celiac nodes. Other important efferent routes are via the falciform ligament and the superior epigastric vessels to the parasternal nodes, from the bare area to posterior mediastinal nodes, and from the visceral surface to the left gastric nodes.

The capsule and the stroma of the liver are rich in lymphatic structures. The lymphatic plexus found in the capsule forms anastomoses with the intrahepatic lymphatics. The significance of these anastomoses is evident when hepatic venous pressure is increased, resulting in exudation of excess lymph from the capsular plexus that forms protein-rich ascitic fluid. The intrahepatic lymphatic system exists as a fine, valved plexus associated with branches of hepatic artery in portal tracts. Hepatic lymph is most likely formed in the interstitial space of Disse and the lymphatic channels in portal tracts drain the space of Disse. The lymph flows in the same direction as the bile, opposite to that of the blood. Lymphatic channels are readily identified in the fibrous bands, portal tracts, and the capsule of cirrhotic liver, but are less evident in the normal liver. Although rarely needed, immunohistochemical stain for D2-40 may highlight lymphatic channels in portal tracts (Fig. 27.34) (44).

Bile Ducts

Bile is formed in hepatocytes, steadily secreted into bile canaliculi, canals of Hering, and then into the intra- and extrahepatic bile ducts. The extrahepatic biliary tract consists of a gallbladder that ends in the cystic duct. The cystic duct joins the common hepatic duct to form the common bile duct, which enters the second portion of the duodenum through its muscular structure, the sphincter of Oddi.

Bile ducts accompany the hepatic artery and portal vein while coursing through the liver. They are nourished by the hepatic arteries via complex peribiliary plexus of capillaries, supplying all structures within the portal tracts. In transplanted liver, in the absence of anastomosing plexus

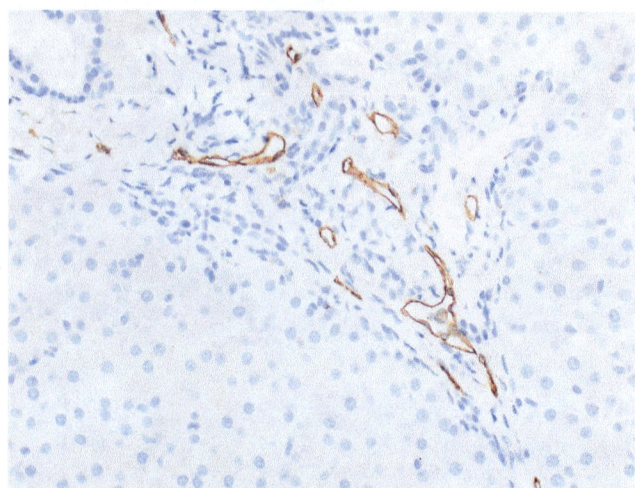

FIGURE 27.34 D2-40 immunostain highlights lymphatic channels in a cirrhotic liver.

of capillaries of the native liver, survival of the biliary tree relies solely on arterial supply from an intact hepatic artery. Thrombosis to hepatic artery leads to ischemia of the bile ducts, bile leaks, and parenchymal necrosis.

The larger intrahepatic or septal bile ducts are lined by tall columnar epithelial cells measuring about 10 mm in diameter with basally situated, pale, oval nuclei and light eosinophilic cytoplasm (Fig. 27.35). They have an internal diameter greater than 100 μm and a distinct basement membrane stainable with PAS-D. Lymphocytes may occasionally be present within the lining epithelium. The larger bile ducts are located in the central part of the portal tracts and have more periductal fibrous tissue than the smaller ones. The collagen fibers are arranged in an irregular and circumferential—but not concentric—manner as may be seen in chronic biliary tract diseases such as primary sclerosing cholangitis and as a sequel of chronic cholecystitis.

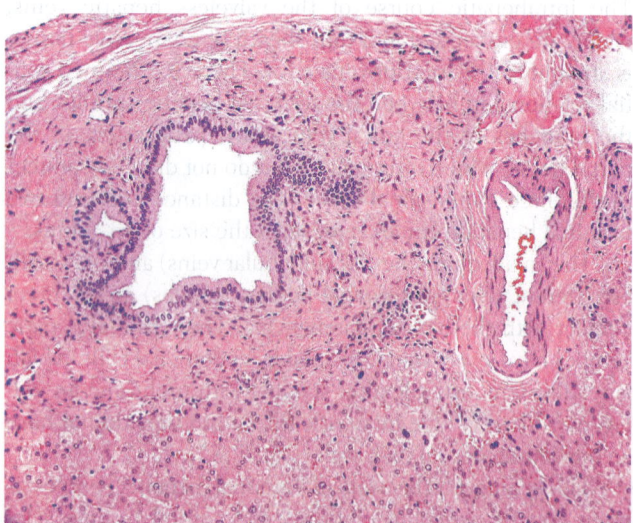

FIGURE 27.35 A large portal tract containing an artery and a bile duct lined by columnar epithelial cells.

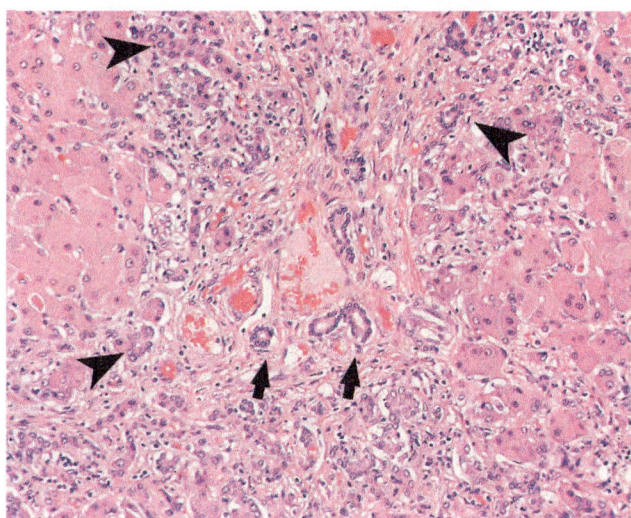

FIGURE 27.36 Bile ductules (*arrowheads*) are located in the peripheral zone of the portal tract and are smaller than the bile ducts (*arrows*).

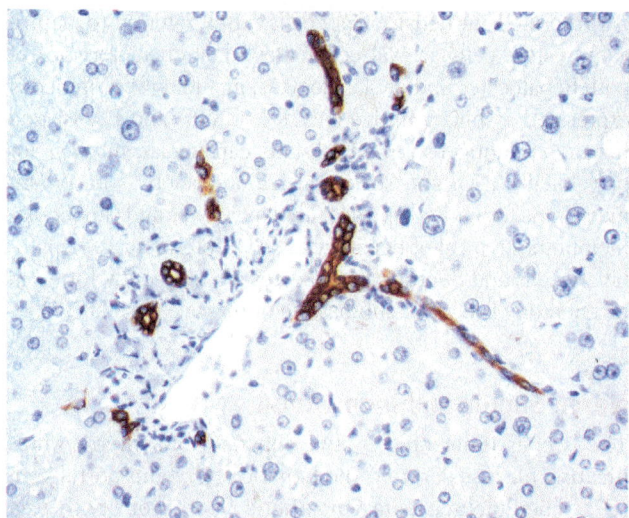

FIGURE 27.37 CK7 immunostaining of bile duct, bile ductules, and canals of Hering.

The smaller or interlobular bile ducts are lined by cuboidal or low columnar epithelium (Fig. 27.26). They have a basement membrane and a small amount of periductal connective tissue. One or more interlobular ducts may be present in a portal tract. Bile ducts are always accompanied by a hepatic artery (45), which has approximately the same diameter as the bile duct (external caliber ratio of bile duct to artery is 0.7:0.8). In normal liver, the absence of bile duct and hepatic artery should not exceed 10% of the portal tracts. The bile ducts are connected to the bile canaliculi by bile ductules and canals of Hering.

Bile ductules are located in the peripheral zone of the portal tracts and are smaller (lumen of less than 20 μm) than the interlobular bile ducts (Fig. 27.36) (46). Bile ductules link canals of Hering and the interlobular bile ducts. Bile ductules may be observed at the edge of the portal tract stroma or may transverse the limiting plate, in which case it will have an "intralobular" as well as an "intraportal" segment. They have a basement membrane, are lined by cuboidal cholangiocytes, and are accompanied by a portal vein but not by a hepatic artery branch. Canals of Hering, which are the physiologic link between hepatocyte canaliculi and the biliary tree, are not discernible on routine sections of normal liver. They are lined partly by cholangiocytes and partly by hepatocytes. Canals of Hering can be demonstrated by staining for high–molecular-weight biliary cytokeratins (CK7, CK19), which are prominent in all cells of ductal origin (Fig. 27.37) (47). Isolated progenitor cells (equivalent to oval cells in rodent models, not visible under light microscopy examination) with CK7, CK19, and NCAM/CD56 immunophenotype may be identified in canals of Hering (48).

In diseased liver, a unifying term "ductular reaction" is used for proliferative reaction of ductular phenotype, encompassing proliferating bile ductules, ductular hepatocytes, intermediate hepatobiliary cells, and cells possibly deriving from circulation including from the bone marrow (46). Ductular reaction occurs in a variety of chronic liver diseases and can be so extensive as to raise the question of adenocarcinoma. In chronic liver diseases, ductular reaction involves not only ductular cells and stem cells, but also inflammatory cells, stroma, and other structures leading to progressive fibrosis (49,50).

Proliferating bile ductules demonstrate structural features typical of cholangiocytes, such as basement membrane formation and lumen. Proliferating bile ductules are invariably accompanied by inflammatory cell infiltrates (predominantly neutrophils). Proliferating bile ductules are typically found in large duct obstruction or chronic cholestatic diseases, such as primary biliary cholangitis and primary sclerosing cholangitis. Proliferating bile ductules can be differentiated from ductular hepatocytes that lack basement membrane and are seen abundantly in zone 1 of the liver acini in massive hepatic necrosis (Fig. 27.38).

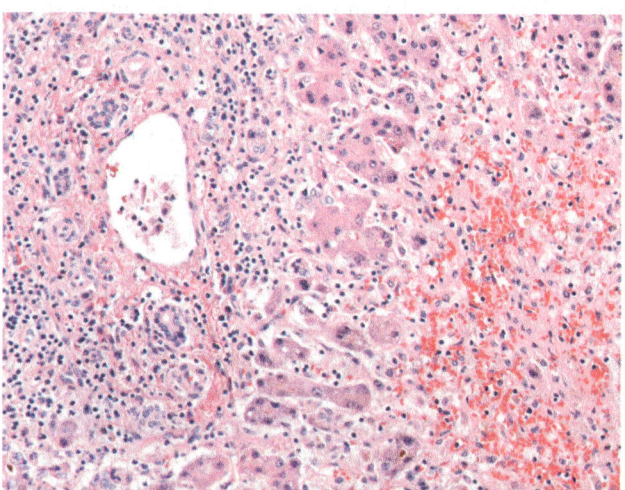

FIGURE 27.38 Ductular hepatocytes in acinar zone 1 in massive hepatic necrosis.

Intermediate hepatobiliary cells (often referred to as progenitor/stem cells or oval cells) show dual characteristics of both hepatocytes and cholangiocytes, including simultaneous expression of biliary antigens (CK7, CK19, and OV-6) and hepatocyte antigens (HepPar1 and canalicular staining for polyclonal CEA), and structural features such as basement membrane formation typical of cholangiocytes and canalicular membranes typical of hepatocytes (48). Intermediate hepatobiliary cells and ductular hepatocytes are frequently found in regenerating liver after submassive or massive necrosis (51).

Nerve Supply and Innervation

The liver is innervated by two separate, but intercommunicating plexuses around the hepatic artery and portal vein (52). They include parasympathetic fibers from both vagi and sympathetic fibers, which receive their preganglionic connections from spinal segments T7 to T10. The hilar plexuses also include afferent visceral and phrenic fibers. Besides their presence around vascular structures in portal tracts, nerve fibers (mostly sympathetic) are present in the parenchyma along the sinusoids. Release of neurotransmitter from the intrasinusoidal fibers modulates hepatocyte and perisinusoidal cell function. It controls in part carbohydrate and lipid metabolism and induces contraction of perisinusoidal cells, thereby regulating intrasinusoidal blood flow (26). However, neural mechanisms may have only a minor regulatory role because limited reinnervation in liver allografts does not seem to impair their function. Denervation probably explains the impaired normal response of the liver to ischemia and sinusoidal dilatation in liver allografts (53), and impaired metabolic function in cirrhosis (54).

EXTRACELLULAR MATRIX

Both interstitial and basement membrane collagens are present in the liver and play an important role, not only as structural elements but also in hepatic function. Collagen I—the main component of the dense, birefringent connective tissue fibers—is seen mainly in portal tracts and walls of hepatic veins and rarely in the normal parenchyma, whereas collagens III and IV are present along the sinusoids. Collagen I can be demonstrated with connective tissue stains; collagen III can be seen with silver impregnation for reticulin. Collagen II, characteristic of cartilage, is absent from the liver. Collagens IV and V, the basement membrane collagens, and laminin are seen in the basement membrane of vessels, bile ducts, and bile ductules, but (except for some collagen IV) not along the sinusoids of normal human liver. Distribution of elastic fibers in the liver, as demonstrated by orcein, resorcin, or Victoria blue stains, seems to follow that of collagen I. Fibronectin, an extracellular matrix glycoprotein, is present diffusely along the sinusoidal surface of hepatocytes and in portal tracts together with the other collagens. All components of the extracellular matrix are visualized best by immunohistochemical staining using specific antibodies.

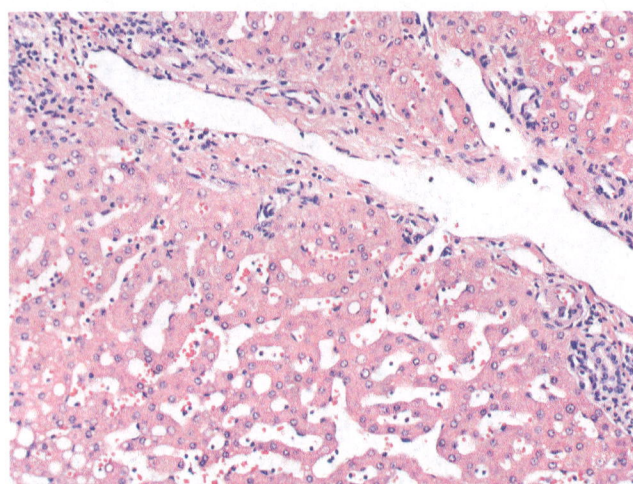

FIGURE 27.39 Hepatocyte atrophy causing sinusoidal dilatation in older individuals.

AGING CHANGES

There are several changes in the liver related to aging. These changes are more commonly seen in individuals 60 years of age and older. There is increased variation of the size of the hepatocytes and their nuclei, similar to that seen in patients on methotrexate, due to increased polyploid cells (55). With aging, the liver cell cords become atrophic and there may be apparent dilatation of sinusoids (Fig. 27.39). More abundant lipofuscin deposition is present in the centrilobular hepatocytes (Fig. 27.40), and sometimes there are some iron pigments in the periportal hepatocytes. The portal tracts contain

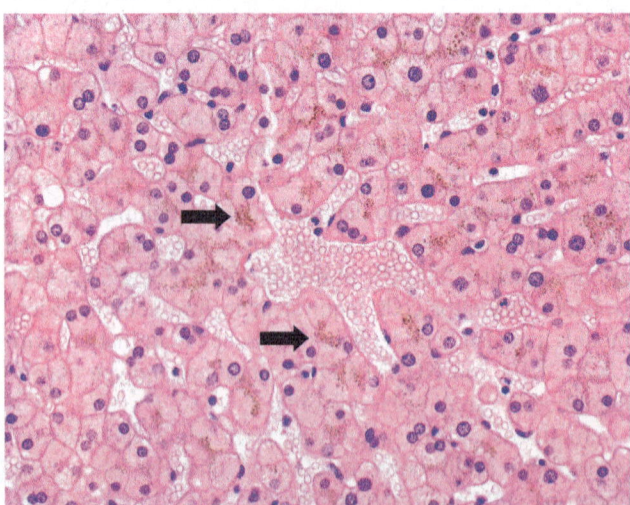

FIGURE 27.40 Marked lipofuscin pigment deposition in older individuals (*arrows*).

denser collagen and may exhibit a higher number of mononuclear inflammatory cells than in younger subjects. The arteries may have thickened walls (Fig. 27.33), even in normotensive individuals. These histologic changes of aging need to be kept in mind because they are often present in viable donors for which frozen sections are requested and should not be interpreted as pathologic. These aging-related findings are accompanied by alteration in the metabolic function of the liver, including the metabolism of toxins and drugs, and therefore may increase the susceptibility of the liver to hypovolemia and drug-induced injury, decrease its capacity for regeneration and shorter post transplantation survival (56).

METHODOLOGY

Liver Biopsy

The role of liver biopsy continues to evolve over time (57). Historically, liver biopsy was used almost exclusively as a diagnostic tool. However, as the result not only of new natural history data and the introduction of many new therapies for patients with liver disease, liver biopsy and histologic assessment of the liver has now taken on an important role in clinical management. Currently, liver biopsy has three major roles: (a) for diagnosis; (b) for assessment of prognosis (disease staging and grading); and/or (c) to assist in making therapeutic management decisions (58).

In order to justify the inherent risk in the procedure, it is essential that the resulting liver biopsy specimen is adequate to allow detailed interpretation. At the times of the biopsy procedure, the needle liver biopsy specimen is immediately examined for adequacy. It should be at least 1.5 cm in total length for many liver diseases (59); otherwise, another pass is recommended. Adequate size of the specimen minimizes sampling error, improves architectural assessment and increases accuracy of staging and grading in chronic hepatitis. Studies in patients with viral hepatitis have shown that grading and staging accuracy is reduced in biopsies less than 2.0 or 2.5 cm in length (59,60). It has been proposed that the adequate number of portal tracts for grading and staging of chronic liver disease should be greater than 11. Short specimens may lead to the failure to recognize cirrhosis in up to 20% of cases. It should also be noted that the size of the sample is proportional to the method and size of the needle used for sampling. Sampling error, particularly in focally or irregularly distributed disease processes, always must be taken into consideration.

Squeezing of tissue during the biopsy procedure results in distortion of cells and elongation of nuclei, which makes cytologic evaluation of the specimen difficult.

Specimen Handling

After the biopsy procedure, the liver specimen should be handled as little as possible and with utmost care to avoid squeezing and drying artifacts. If the case so indicates, small pieces of liver tissue may be frozen for histochemistry, immunohistochemistry, chemical analysis, molecular studies, or fixed in glutaraldehyde for electron microscopy. If infectious disease is suspected, cultures should be taken. Then the tissue should be transferred quickly into the appropriate fixative solution, usually 10% buffered formalin. Physiologic saline should not be used as it may cause distortion and dissociation of the hepatocytes on frozen section and routine histologic examination.

Needle biopsy specimens may be arranged on a piece of card to prevent distortion and fragmentation. At this stage, the gross appearance of the liver specimen is noted. Particular attention should be paid to fragmentation, which suggests cirrhosis, and to the number, size, shape, and color of the fragments. Tumors or granulomas can be recognized as white areas in an otherwise reddish-brown normal liver parenchyma. Gray-black discoloration is seen in Dubin–Johnson syndrome, rusty brown in hemochromatosis, green in cholestasis, yellow in fatty liver, and brown in older individuals from the lipofuscin deposition.

Needle biopsy specimens are fixed for at least three hours at room temperature, whereas wedge biopsy specimens, after sectioning into 2-mm thick slices, need longer fixation. Formalin penetrates most tissues at about 0.5 mm per hour at room temperature. In order to avoid shrinkage and hardening of the tissue, it is important to process liver specimens separately from other tissues and on a more rapid schedule in the automated tissue processor. Rush liver biopsy specimens can be manually processed to shorten the time schedule to meet the needs of critically ill patients. More than 10 consecutive sections, 3 to 5 μm in thickness, can be cut without artifact from well-embedded specimens. Usually paraffin is used for embedding, but plastic embedding may be used to obtain thinner sections.

It should be emphasized that an adequate and properly processed liver specimen without artifacts is an important prerequisite for the accurate evaluation by an experienced histopathologist, who should be supplied with all relevant clinical and laboratory data.

Microscopic examination should conform to a routine and include all tissue fragments and all structures of the liver (architecture, portal triads, limiting plate, hepatocytes, sinusoidal cells, and terminal hepatic venules). We usually start with careful examination of zone 3 of the acinus because many changes are found here (congestion, fat, necrosis, cholestasis, pigments, endophlebitis) and then move to the remainder of the parenchyma and portal tracts.

Special Stains

The tissue is routinely stained with H&E. Masson trichrome, Sirius red, or chromotrope-aniline blue stains are used for fibrous tissue; Victoria blue or orcein is used for hepatitis B surface antigen (HBsAg), elastic fibers, lipofuscin, ceroid, and copper-binding protein; PAS-D is used for gly-

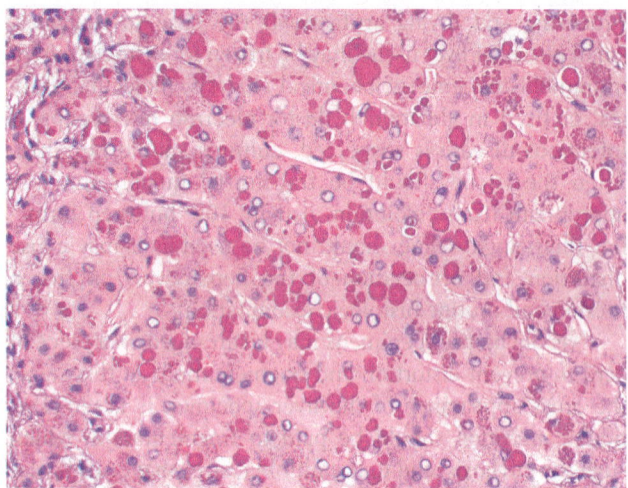

FIGURE 27.41 Alpha-1-antitrypsin granules and globules in hepatocytes (PAS-D).

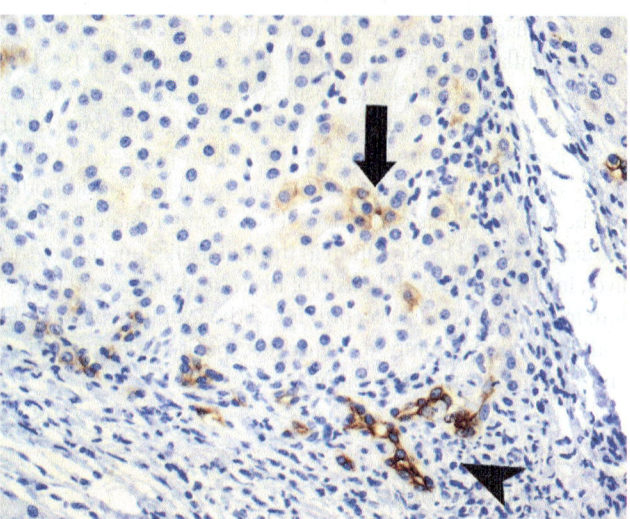

FIGURE 27.42 Proliferating bile ductules (*arrowhead*) and hepatocytes undergoing ductular metaplasia (*arrow*) in chronic cholestasis are positive for CK7.

coproteins, including α1-antitrypsin inclusions (Fig. 27.41), ceroid in macrophages, chronic passive congestion inclusions, basement membranes of bile ducts, cytoplasmic inclusions of cytomegalovirus, and *Mycobacterium avium-intracellulare*. Stains for reticulin and iron are also important. If it is not possible to perform all these stains, at a minimum, a special stain for connective tissue, such as Masson trichrome, and/or reticulin should be obtained in order to assess the lobular architecture and to facilitate the diagnosis of cirrhosis.

Immunohistologic Studies

The development of monoclonal antibodies and highly sensitive immunohistochemical staining procedures (peroxidase–antiperoxidase and avidin–biotin–peroxidase complex methods), has made it possible to demonstrate many antigens in routinely processed (i.e., formalin-fixed and paraffin-embedded) tissue sections. Blocking of biotin is often required prior to the application of primary antibodies because hepatocytes contain large amount of endogenous biotin, which can give a false positive reaction; such a false positive is even more pronounced with the use of antigen retrievals.

Normal Liver and Nonneoplastic Diseases

Cytokeratins (CK) are the intermediate filaments of epithelial cells and are present in hepatocytes and, in greater amounts, in the bile duct epithelium. Different as well as similar cytokeratins are expressed by hepatocytes and bile ducts. Embryonal hepatocytes contain CK8, CK18, and CK19. The expression of CK19 in hepatocytes disappears by the 10th week of gestation. Mature hepatocytes in the normal liver contain only CK8 and CK18, and therefore, stain diffusely with keratin CAM 5.2. Cytokeratin staining of hepatocytes is usually more intense in the acinar zone 1. Most hepatocytes also stain with keratin 35βH11, which reacts with CK8 only. Hepatocytes do not stain with vimentin, epithelial membrane antigen, CK7, and CK19. Periportal hepatocytes in cholestatic disease may, however, stain for CK7 (Fig. 27.42). Hepatocyte paraffin-1 (HepPar1) and thyroid transcription factor-1 (TTF1) stain hepatocytes in a diffuse, granular, cytoplasmic pattern (Fig. 27.43) (61,62). Arginase-1 stains hepatocytes in cytoplasmic and nuclear pattern (63). Normal hepatocytes do not stain with AFP, but hepatocytes in cirrhotic nodules may occasionally show focal positive staining. Glypican-3 stains hepatocellular carcinoma, but not normal hepatocytes (64).

Cytokeratin polypeptides may be altered in specific liver diseases, such as alcoholic hepatitis, chronic cholestasis, and

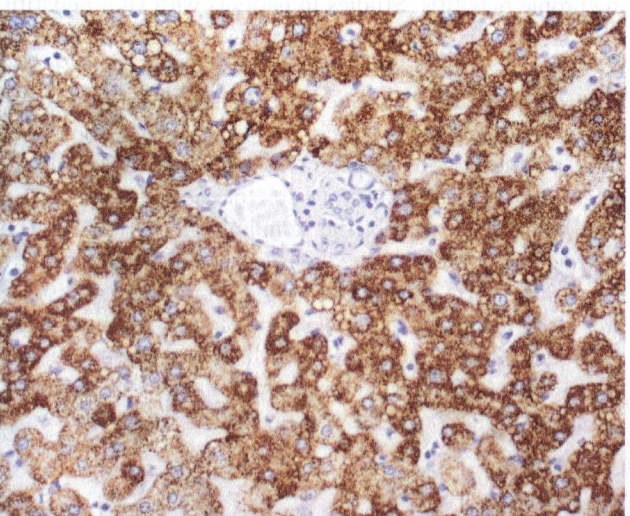

FIGURE 27.43 Granular staining of hepatocytes using HepPar1 antibody excludes other cells and all structures in the portal tract.

Wilson disease, with formation of Mallory–Denk hyalins. Mallory–Denk hyalins are composed of heterogeneous cytokeratin filament and usually react strongly with antibody to CK8, CK18, 34βE12, CAM 5.2, p62, and ubiquitin (65). They also occasionally react with CK7 and CK19.

Bile canaliculi can be demonstrated using pCEA and CD10 (66) (Fig. 27.21).

Sinusoidal endothelial cells show phenotypic differences with vascular endothelium. Normally, they do not bind the lectin ulex europaeus; they do not express factor VIII–related antigen or contain other molecules found in vascular endothelium, such as CD34 and CD31. They, however, assume these phenotypic properties in chronic liver diseases, in cirrhosis, and in hepatocellular carcinoma. In normal liver, positive staining for CD31 and CD34 are limited to vascular endothelium of portal tract vessels and periportal sinusoids.

Several markers of neural/neuroectodermal differentiation have been found in hepatic stellate cells. These are synaptophysin, glial fibrillary acidic protein (GFAP), and neural cell adhesion molecule (NCAM), which can be used to identify resting stellate cells. When activated, these cells show expression of vimentin, desmin, and smooth muscle actin, which suggests myofibroblastic differentiation (67).

Bile ducts and ductules are readily revealed by immunostaining for bile duct–type CK7 and CK19 (Figs. 27.37 and 27.42). Bile ducts also stain with CK8, CK18, AE1/AE3, 35βH11, and 34βE12 antibodies.

Immunohistochemistry in nonneoplastic liver diseases is commonly performed for: (a) localization of hepatotropic and nonhepatotropic viral antigens; (b) identification of biliary epithelium; and (c) identification of inclusion bodies in storage and hereditary diseases.

The presence or absence and distribution pattern of viral antigens are helpful in the diagnostic and prognostic evaluation of viral hepatitis, particularly hepatitis B surface and core antigens (Figs. 27.44 and 27.45) in hepatitis B

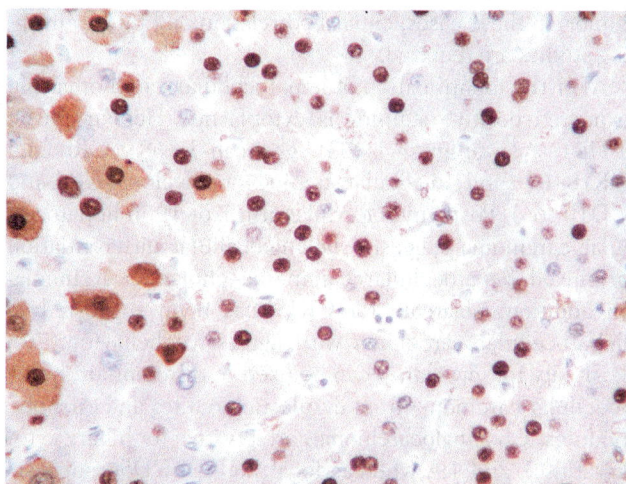

FIGURE 27.45 Immunostaining of hepatitis B core antigen (HBcAg) in numerous nuclei and cytoplasm of hepatocytes in an immunosuppressed patient with high viral replication.

virus (HBV) or in dual HBV and hepatitis C virus (HCV) infection. The detection of hepatitis A, C, and delta (D) antigens and of herpes virus antigens (cytomegalovirus, herpes simplex virus, and Epstein–Barr virus) confirms the cause of acute or chronic hepatitis. Since the cloning and sequencing of the HCV genome in 1989, there have been a number of studies for the detection of HCV antigens in the liver. However, the reports are conflicting and there is no reliable HCV antibody available. The detection rate of positive cases varied, which may be related to tissue sampling and differences in sensitivity of various methods and specificity and/or avidity of the antibodies. Immunohistochemical studies on frozen sections appeared to demonstrate HCV antigens more reliably than on formalin-fixed, paraffin-embedded sections.

Cytokeratin 7 or 19 immunostain is performed for identification and counting of bile duct when bile duct loss/ductopenia, graft-versus-host disease or chronic allograft rejection is suspected. In addition, both CKs can be used to evaluate the degree of ductular reaction in biliary diseases and chronic viral hepatitis. In chronic viral hepatitis, a higher degree of ductular reaction correlates with a higher degree of interface hepatitis and fibrosis progression. CK7 staining of periportal cholestatic hepatocytes confirms longstanding cholestasis.

Alpha-1-antitrypsin and fibrinogen immunostains are performed to identify intracytoplasmic inclusion bodies in α1-antitrypsin deficiency and fibrinogen storage disease respectively.

Neoplastic Diseases

The most common use of immunohistochemistry for liver specimen is for identification, immunophenotyping, classification, and prognostication of primary or metastatic tumors to the liver (57). Primary or metastatic poorly/undifferentiated tumors may lose their organ-specific antigenicity, and immunohistochemistry may fail to pinpoint organ of origin of the

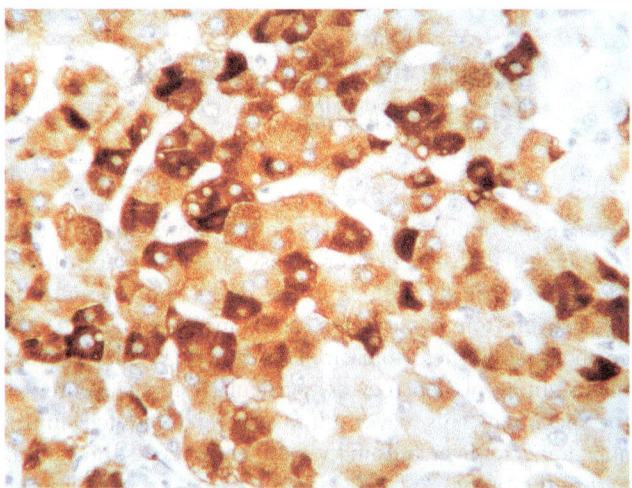

FIGURE 27.44 HBsAg immunostain demonstrates cytoplasmic hepatitis B surface antigen deposition in a patient with chronic hepatitis B.

tumor. In these cases, clinical correlation and further imaging studies are required.

For the identification of hepatocellular carcinoma, the expected positive staining is cytoplasmic HepPar1 (61), TTF-1 (62), arginase-1 (63), glypican-3 (68), CK8 and CK18 (69); and canalicular staining for polyclonal CEA and CD10 (66). Positivity for cytokeratin 7 or 19 in hepatocellular carcinoma suggests cholangiocellular differentiation or mixed hepatocellular carcinoma–cholangiocarcinoma. In addition, positivity for CK19 has been suggested in hepatocellular carcinoma with aggressive behavior (70). Positivity for glypican-3 can be used to differentiate hepatocellular carcinoma from dysplastic nodules and cirrhotic nodules. Cholangiocarcinomas are positive for biliary cytokeratins 7 and 19; whereas focal NCAM/CD56 suggests cholangiolocellular component (71). Nuclear p53 positivity is common in high-grade biliary intraepithelial neoplasia and cholangiocarcinoma (72). Cholangiocarcinoma may also lose Smad4 protein expression similar to pancreatic adenocarcinoma (73).

In benign hepatocellular tumors, serum amyloid A, C-reactive protein, glutamine synthetase, β-catenin, CK7, and Ki67 play an important role in differentiating these lesions (74). Focal nodular hyperplasia shows positivity for CK7 in the ductules and map-like staining pattern for glutamine synthetase. Inflammatory hepatocellular adenoma shows positive staining for serum amyloid A and C-reactive protein, and occasional CK7 staining in ductular structures. Conventional hepatocellular adenoma shows diffuse or patchy (not map-like) positivity for glutamine synthetase, and negative for CK7 and serum amyloid A. In addition, higher rate of Ki67, diffuse strong positivity for glutamine synthetase, and nuclear positivity for β-catenin are seen in hepatocellular adenoma with high risk of transformation to well-differentiated hepatocellular carcinoma.

Workup for metastatic tumors involves various antibodies, including establishing a line of differentiation (epithelial, stromal, or melanoma) and organ of origin. For epithelial tumor or adenocarcinoma, CK7 and 20 immunostaining profile and additional organ-specific antibodies (TTF-1, CDX-2, etc.) are required (75).

Electron Microscopy

Electron microscopy has a limited but a well-defined role in: (a) investigating hereditary and metabolic liver diseases; (b) viral infection not otherwise identified by light microscopy or serology; (c) tumors of unknown histogenesis; (d) certain drug-induced liver injuries; and (e) diseases of unclear etiology (57). Tissue obtained for electron microscopic study should be fixed in 3% glutaraldehyde.

Molecular Studies

The majority of routine molecular diagnostic applications in liver diseases are geared toward the assessment of hepatitis B and C (57). Molecular technologies have been developed for the qualitative and quantitative detection and genotyping of these viruses, providing prognostic indicator and treatment guidance.

In regard to neoplastic diseases of the liver, molecular assays are currently used in investigational studies to understand the pathogenesis of benign hepatocellular tumors, preneoplastic nodules, hepatocellular carcinoma, and cholangiocarcinoma; which can provide better surveillance, diagnosis, treatment, and prognostication of these lesions (57).

In situ hybridization (ISH) employs radioactive/fluorescent/antigen-labeled complementary DNA or RNA sequences to localize a specific DNA or RNA sequence in tissue. ISH may be performed on formalin-fixed and paraffin-embedded tissue sections. ISH has been applied to liver tissue for the identification of hepatitis A, B, C, and D viruses, cytomegalovirus and Epstein–Barr virus. ISH can be used to identify albumin mRNA which is highly specific for normal hepatocytes and hepatocellular tumors.

Polymerase chain reaction (PCR) is a technique to amplify exponentially a single or few copies of DNA sequence, employing DNA polymerase and generating thousands to millions copies of the particular DNA sequence. Reverse transcription PCR allows the identification of RNA. Currently, these techniques are the most sensitive and specific method to demonstrate HBV DNA, HCV RNA, and their genotypes in the blood and liver tissue. In addition, PCR can be used to identify infectious organisms or specific genetic mutations.

Microarray analysis provides an arrayed series of thousands of DNA sequences. Each may contain a specific DNA sequence, the relative abundance of which is determined by chemiluminescence-labeled targets. It can be used to measure changes in expression levels, to detect single nucleotide polymorphisms, and for comparative studies in neoplastic and nonneoplastic liver diseases.

FREQUENT HISTOLOGIC CHANGES OF LITTLE SIGNIFICANCE

The Liver at Autopsy

Liver tissue obtained at autopsy often shows changes that are not usually seen in liver biopsy specimens and therefore may cause difficulties in the evaluation. Agonal loss of glycogen from hepatocytes causes increased density and eosinophilia of the cytoplasm. Poor fixation results in irregular staining of hepatocytes, particularly in the center of the specimen. This may result in striking differences in the appearance of liver cells in the peripheral versus the central part of the tissue.

Agonal necrosis, particularly of hepatocytes in zone 3 in patients with shock or heart failure, may not be reflected in

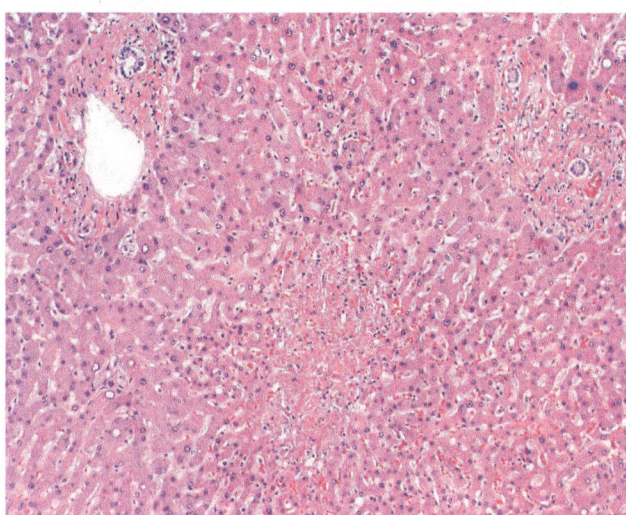

FIGURE 27.46 Agonal necrosis of centrilobular hepatocytes in autopsy liver.

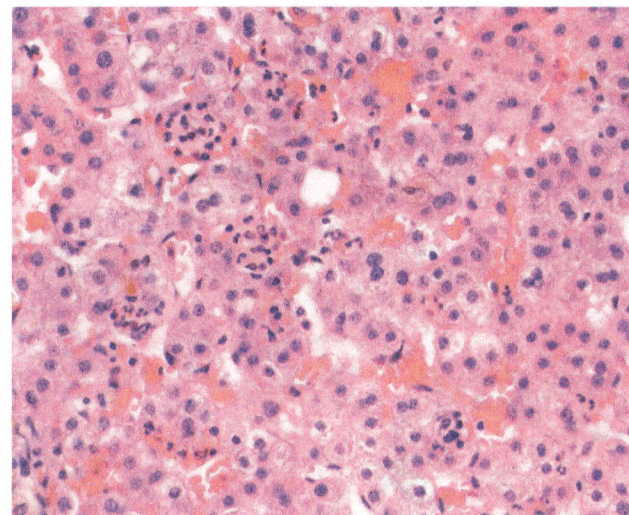

FIGURE 27.47 Surgical biopsy specimen showing clusters of polymorphonuclear neutrophils in sinusoids resembling microabscesses (surgical hepatitis).

elevated aminotransferase levels (Fig. 27.46). Its terminal nature is recognized from the lack of any inflammatory response. Autolysis of hepatocytes, particularly in hepatitis and cholestasis resulting in loss of cellular detail and prominent sinusoidal lining cells, is often more pronounced than in other tissues because the liver is rich in proteolytic enzymes. Loss of inflammatory cells by autolysis may make the diagnosis of hepatitis in postmortem specimens difficult. Trichrome stain assists greatly in the identification of portal tracts and central venules (and thus the appreciation of lobular architecture) and, by demonstrating the fibrous septa, the chronicity of the condition.

Dilatation of the sinusoidal and perisinusoidal spaces of Disse is of little significance in postmortem liver tissues as opposed to similar changes in well-preserved biopsy specimens. Mild accumulation of lymphocytes in some portal tracts is frequently seen in autopsy livers and does not justify the diagnosis of chronic hepatitis. Large tissue sections obtained at autopsy often include many large triangular portal tracts with abundant connective tissue that can be distinguished from true portal fibrosis by evaluation of the size of the intraportal structures. In addition, increased fibrous tissue in portal tracts and parenchyma is a normal phenomenon in older individuals.

Surgical Liver Biopsy Specimens

Surgical biopsy specimens may have several features not seen in needle biopsy specimens that may cause diagnostic difficulties. If the surgeon removes a small, superficial wedge of liver tissue from the inferior margin, the triangular tissue fragment is covered on two sides by the Glisson capsule. The fibrous connections between the superficial portal tracts and the capsule may imitate cirrhosis (Fig. 27.29). However, these changes usually do not extend more than 2 mm into the liver parenchyma. Large portal tracts can be occasionally encountered in subcapsular liver parenchyma (Fig. 27.28).

In biopsy specimens removed at the end of a long surgical procedure, clusters of polymorphonuclear neutrophils are seen in or under the capsule, in sinusoids, around terminal hepatic venules, in portal tracts, and in areas of small focal necroses resembling microabscesses, probably as a result of minor trauma (Fig. 27.47). This characteristic lesion must be distinguished from inflammatory liver diseases such as cholangitis. Other "innocent" hepatic lesions include focal steatosis involving small groups of hepatocytes (<5%), lipogranulomas from mineral oil deposition in perivenular areas and in portal tracts in the absence of significant steatosis; and unexplained mitoses of hepatocytes that normally have a life span of many years.

MINOR BUT SIGNIFICANT HEPATIC ALTERATIONS

There are minor alterations in hepatic parenchyma that are often dismissed on histopathologic examination of the liver. These minor alterations are frequently clinically significant, may explain the abnormalities that the patients have and justify the indications for liver biopsies. They include mild inflammation in the liver parenchyma such as in nonspecific reactive hepatitis, mild acute hepatitis, and residual hepatitis; subtle alterations of hepatic parenchyma caused by abnormal vascularity such as chronic venous congestion, nodular regenerative hyperplasia and hepatoportal sclerosis; or subtle alterations of hepatic parenchyma in the vicinity of a space-occupying lesion in a missed targeted liver biopsy. They require a close inspection of the liver biopsy itself and

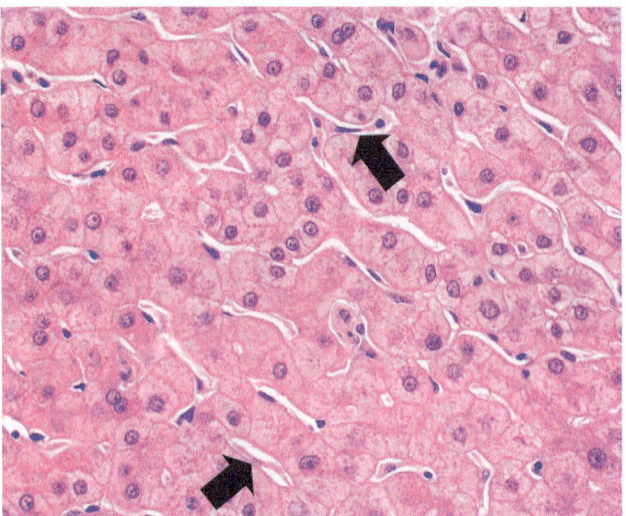

FIGURE 27.48 Nonspecific reactive hepatitis characterized by activation of sinusoidal lining cells (*arrows*).

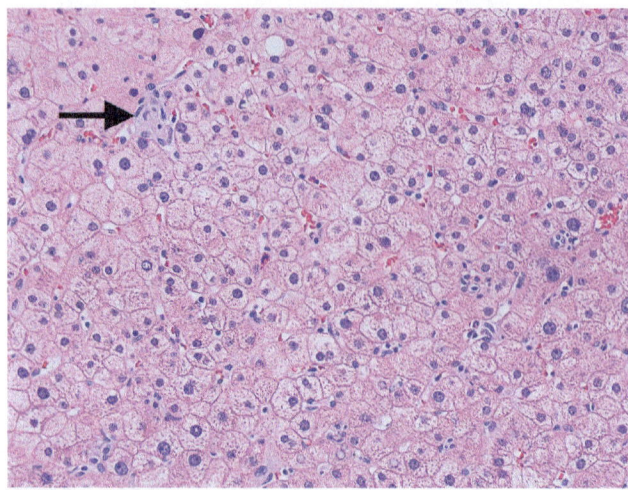

FIGURE 27.49 Cluster of macrophages (*arrow*) containing debris of necrotic hepatocyte in residual hepatitis

often with the aid of special stains such as reticulin stain and PAS-D stain; and most importantly the knowledge of normal liver structures and lobular architecture to identify minor and subtle alterations.

Nonspecific Reactive Hepatitis

This poorly defined histologic change represents a reaction of the liver to a variety of extrahepatic or systemic diseases, particularly infectious diseases, autoimmune diseases, connective tissue diseases, gastrointestinal diseases, and acquired immunodeficiency syndrome (AIDS) (76,77). Nonspecific reactive hepatitis must be differentiated from primary liver diseases, such as mild chronic hepatitis and residual stages of acute viral hepatitis and drug-induced injury. The alterations consist of activation of sinusoidal lining cells with prominent Kupffer cells, foci of isolated hepatocyte necrosis with accumulation of macrophages and other inflammatory cells, and mild infiltration of some portal tracts by mononuclear cells without interface hepatitis (Fig. 27.48). Scattered hepatocytes may also contain microvesicular or macrovesicular fat droplets.

Mild Acute Hepatitis and Residual Hepatitis

Mild acute hepatitis is a mild diffuse hepatocellular injury due to hepatitis viruses, drugs or other causes, resulting in gastrointestinal and influenza-like symptoms. Aminotransferase and other liver enzyme activities are mildly elevated and the disease usually resolves in a few months. Mild acute hepatitis requires no specific treatment. Mild acute hepatitis is characterized by subtle, but diffuse changes, including panlobular disarray with degeneration and regeneration of the hepatocytes, accompanied by activation of sinusoidal lining cells and diffuse infiltration of sinusoids and portal tracts by inflammatory cells, primarily lymphocytes and macrophages and some plasma cells. Cholestasis or bridging necrosis is not seen in mild acute hepatitis.

The term residual or prolonged hepatitis is used to describe changes in liver biopsies taken late in the course of acute hepatitis with residual abnormalities in liver enzyme activities (57). Since most of hepatocellular injury has occurred, the prognosis of residual hepatitis is good and does not require further treatment when the cause of injury has been identified. The features of typical acute hepatitis, which include diffuse hepatocellular damage and inflammation have subsided, with mild pleomorphism of the hepatocytes, irregular cell plates with a few foci of lobular necrosis and mild inflammation. Clusters of PAS-D-resistant macrophages, which contain debris of necrotic or apoptotic hepatocyte or ceroid pigment and may be iron positive, are observed predominantly in the centrilobular area and portal tracts (Figs. 27.23 and 27.49). Focal reticulin fiber condensation may be seen as a result of hepatocyte loss. The portal tracts may be expanded with mild lymphocytic infiltrate and mild fibrosis or with thin fibrous septa.

Sinusoidal Dilatation

Acute or chronic venous congestion with dilatation of sinusoids in Rappaport acinus zone 3 and of terminal hepatic venules is frequently seen at autopsy but also in biopsy specimens; it is usually a consequence of right-sided congestive heart failure, whereas irregular necrosis of hepatocytes in zone 3 is often caused by left-sided heart failure or shock.

Chronic venous congestion causes stasis and increase of hepatic venous pressure, dilatation of sinusoids in zone 3, followed by extravasation of red blood cells to the perisinusoidal spaces of Disse and atrophy of hepatocytes around the terminal hepatic venules (Fig. 27.50). The latter may falsely produce the impression of reverse lobulation mimicking

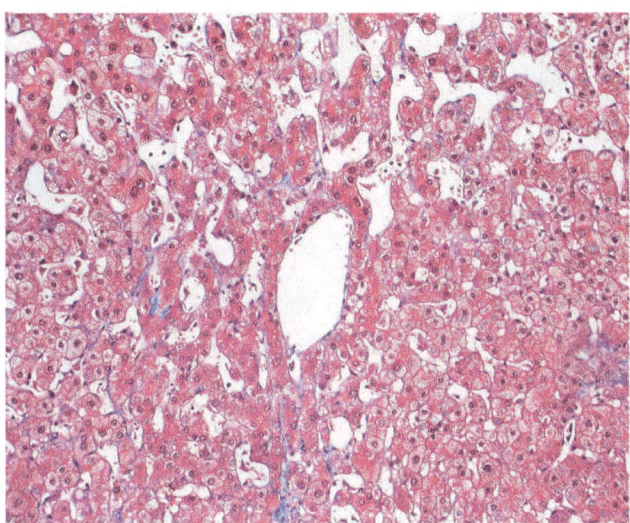

FIGURE 27.50 Dilated central venule and zone 3 sinusoids accompanied by atrophy of hepatocytes in chronic venous congestion.

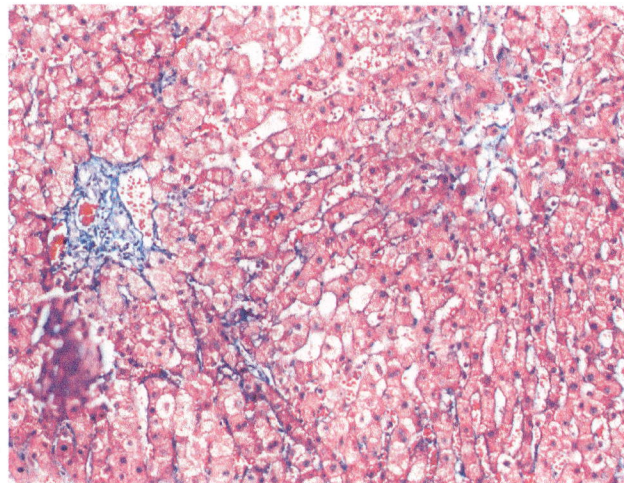

FIGURE 27.51 Dilatation of zone 1 sinusoids in contraceptive steroids injury.

that of nodular regenerative hyperplasia (nodular regenerative hyperplasia-like change). In contrast to chronic venous congestion, nodular regenerative hyperplasia shows regenerative hyperplasia of periportal hepatocytes, collapse of zone 3 sinusoids, and compressed zone 3 hepatocytes; producing true reverse lobulation. In more severe chronic venous congestion cases, there is also atrophy of hepatocytes with increased lipofuscin accumulation, scattered small droplet fat vacuoles, extravasation of red blood cells to the perisinusoidal space of Disse, intracytoplasmic eosinophilic globules in centrilobular hepatocytes, enlargement of Kupffer cells containing ceroid pigment, focal cholestasis, and progressive fibrosis in the periphery of the acinus (rather than concentric around the central venules). Special stains for iron may demonstrate iron deposition in centrilobular Kupffer cells. Engorgement of sinusoids around terminal hepatic venules is also observed in other conditions such as Budd–Chiari syndrome, veno-occlusive disease, sepsis, malignant tumors, collagen diseases, granulomatous diseases, Crohn disease, and in patients with AIDS.

In contrast, dilatation of sinusoids in Rappaport acinus zone 1 has been observed in pregnancy, in renal transplant patients, after exposure to anabolic/androgenic or contraceptive steroids (Fig. 27.51), and near space-occupying lesions. After exposure to vinyl chloride, thorotrast, arsenicals, and oral contraceptives, sinusoidal dilatation may be accompanied by hepatocellular and sinusoidal cell hypertrophy, hyperplasia, and dysplasia, increased reticulin fibers along sinusoids and portal fibrosis.

Nodular Regenerative Hyperplasia

Nodular regenerative hyperplasia is a diffuse nodular regeneration of the hepatocytes, associated with various disorders, such as autoimmune diseases (rheumatoid arthritis, systemic sclerosis, systemic lupus erythematosus), primary biliary cholangitis, primary sclerosing cholangitis, hematologic malignancies, endocrine or metabolic disorders, or drugs (41,78–80). In majority of the cases, the proposed pathogenesis is either obliteration of small portal veins or arteritis.

Nodular regenerative hyperplasia occurs in both sexes at any age, but most frequently between the ages of 40 and 70. Many patients are asymptomatic, but they may develop portal hypertension as in cirrhosis, and rarely hepatic failure, ascites, or rupture of liver with massive hemorrhage.

The liver parenchyma shows widely scattered parenchymal nodules varying in diameter from 1 to 4 mm. The capsular surface of the liver often reveals minimal shallow irregularities that may be mistaken for cirrhosis. The nodules either replace almost the entire parenchyma or confined to one portion of the liver. The nodules in nodular regenerative hyperplasia are not surrounded by fibrous septa; therefore they are ill defined and soft, distinct from those found in cirrhosis. The nodules consist of hyperplastic hepatocytes arranged in plates more than one-cell-layer thick, particularly adjacent or surrounding the portal tracts. The surrounding centrilobular parenchyma is compressed and atrophic and the sinusoids are congested (the so-called linear congestion). Reticulin stain shows condensation of reticulin framework around the expanding nodules and the irregular thickened hepatocyte plates within the nodules, but dense septa as in cirrhosis are not seen (Fig. 27.52). There is little if any pericellular fibrosis. The hyperplastic hepatocytes are slightly larger and more variable than normal, and arranged in two-cell-thick plates with occasional binucleation. Obliteration of small portal veins is often seen.

Because of the subtle alterations of the lobular architecture, the diagnosis is often difficult in needle biopsy specimen and sometimes may require an open liver biopsy. Alternating areas of hyperplastic hepatocytes and atrophic hepatocytes with linear congestion on needle biopsy should lead to a reticulin stain to confirm nodular regenerative hyperplasia.

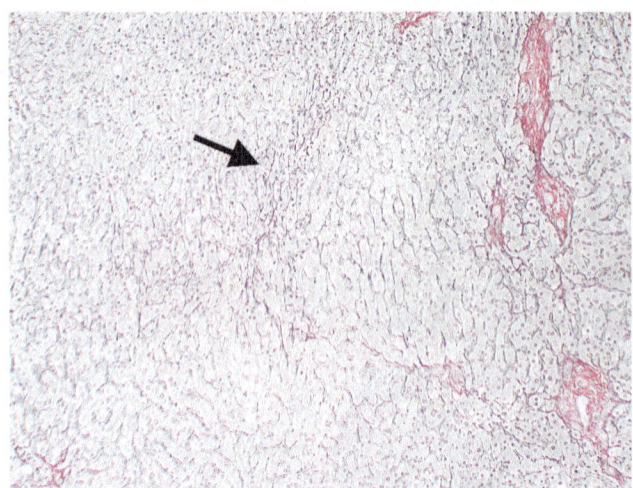

FIGURE 27.52 Compression and atrophy of centrilobular parenchyma resulting in condensation of reticulin framework (*arrow*) in nodular regenerative hyperplasia.

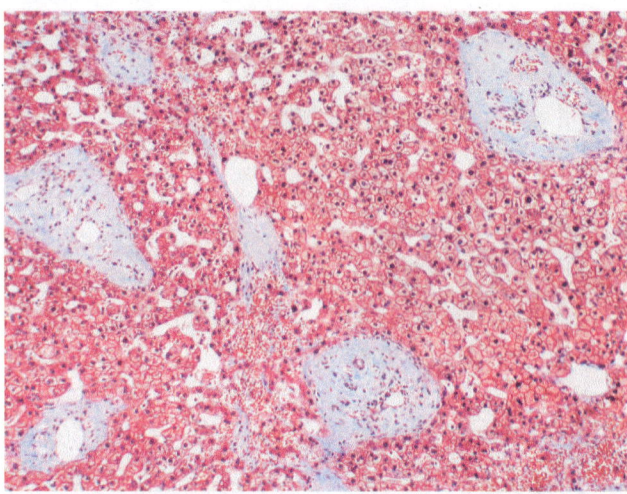

FIGURE 27.53 Hepatoportal sclerosis showing atrophy of liver parenchyma resulting in close proximation of densely fibrotic portal tracts.

Hepatoportal Sclerosis

Hepatoportal sclerosis, also known as idiopathic portal hypertension, noncirrhotic portal hypertension, or obliterative portal venopathy, is a condition consisting of portal hypertension, splenomegaly, and anemia secondary to hypersplenism characterized by dense portal tract thrombosis and obliteration of portal veins in noncirrhotic patients. Hepatoportal sclerosis is a term used by Mikkelsen et al. in 1965 (81) to describe noncirrhotic sclerosis of intrahepatic portal veins, similar to the condition described by Banti in the early 20th century to describe portal hypertension, splenomegaly, and anemia not associated with hematologic disease (Banti disease). Other terms, noncirrhotic or idiopathic portal hypertension with histologic features of obliterative portovenopathy, also coined in the 1960s to describe noncirrhotic intrahepatic portal vein sclerosis with more favorable prognosis than patients with cirrhosis.

Although the etiology in the majority of cases is unknown, there are several known causes of hepatoportal sclerosis such as chronic exposure to copper, arsenic, and vinyl chloride (81,82). Per definition, portal hypertension that is caused by parasitic infection, myeloproliferative disease, and portal thrombosis should be excluded from hepatoportal sclerosis.

The liver is either of normal size or more often mildly atrophic with wrinkled capsule. Atrophy may not be uniformly distributed; therefore, the liver lobes may be disproportionate in their sizes when compared to normal liver. Portal tracts are round and densely fibrotic with fibrous obliteration of larger portal veins and/or with numerous dilated small portal vein branches (Figs. 27.31 and 27.53). Some of the dilated small portal vein branches may dilate or herniate into the periportal liver parenchyma. Bile ducts may show periductal fibrosis. While the lobular architecture is fairly well-maintained, occasional portal-to-portal or portal-to-central bridging fibrosis may be present. The centrilobular hepatocytes become atrophic causing dilatation of sinusoids, reverse lobulation and close proximation of the portal tracts. The subtle histologic alterations in hepatoportal sclerosis can be underappreciated.

Vicinity of Space-Occupying Lesions

Nonspecific reactive changes are also seen in patients with space-occupying lesions in the liver (57). Although the biopsy specimen may not include the neoplasm, the abscess, or the cyst, a characteristic histologic triad is often observed in the adjacent liver (83). The histologic changes are the result of local obstruction of blood and bile flow by the expanding mass. These changes consist of proliferating and distorted bile ductules with irregular and even atypical epithelium accompanied by neutrophils in edematous portal tracts, and focal sinusoidal dilatation and congestion (Fig. 27.54). The changes may be subtle and are usually focal, involving adjacent small portal tracts. The liver cell plates may be compressed and distorted with atrophy of hepatocytes. In contrast to large bile duct obstruction and other biliary tract diseases such as primary sclerosing cholangitis, cholestasis is usually absent. The described triad is characteristic for the vicinity of a space-occupying lesion, and its recognition in a liver specimen should lead to continued search for a neoplasm, cyst, or abscess.

BROWN PIGMENTS

There are several pigments that can cause brown discoloration of the liver parenchyma. In normal condition, the only brown pigment that can be encountered is lipofuscin (57).

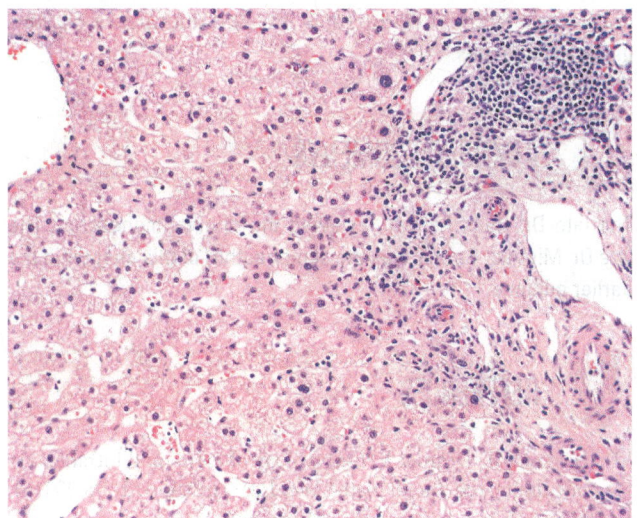

FIGURE 27.54 Liver biopsy specimen of a patient with metastatic carcinoma showing dilatation of sinusoids in zone 2, as well as ductular reaction and infiltration of portal tract by neutrophils. The specimen does not contain metastatic carcinoma, but the histologic changes are consistent with the vicinity of a space-occupying lesion.

Hemosiderin and copper are abundant in the cytoplasm of hepatocytes during the first week of life, then gradually disappear and should be absent at the age of 6 to 9 months. Therefore, brown cytoplasmic pigments representing hemosiderin and copper should not be seen in normal children and adult livers. It should be noted however, that small quantities of stainable iron are common in normal hepatocytes, particularly in older individuals.

Lipofuscin

Lipofuscin, the "wear and tear" or "aging" pigment (84), is commonly seen in varying quantities as fine, well-delineated, light brown, PAS-D-resistant, partly acid-fast–positive granules in the cytoplasm of hepatocytes in zone 3, particularly at the canalicular pole (Fig. 27.40). Lipofuscin is produced by lysosomal oxidation of lipids. Under the electron microscope, lipofuscin granules appear as secondary lysosomes in pericanalicular location that contain irregular and lobulated electron-dense granules, lipid droplets, and a heterogeneous matrix.

Lipofuscin has no functional or clinical significance (57). There is a progressive increase of its amount in individual hepatocytes and in the number of cells involved in older individuals (84). An increase of lipofuscin pigment also occurs in atrophic liver, starvation, chronic wasting diseases, and malignancies, producing brown discoloration of the liver on gross examination. Lipofuscin is not found in recently regenerated hepatocytes. It may be difficult to distinguish lipofuscin from the pigment that accumulates in hepatocytes in large amounts in Dubin–Johnson syndrome.

In contrast to lipofuscin, iron and copper are coarser, birefringent, and usually deposited in periportal hepatocytes. Intracellular bile is poorly defined and less granular than the other pigments and often forms thrombi in bile canaliculi in zone 3.

Dubin–Johnson Pigment

Dubin–Johnson syndrome is an autosomal recessive familial disorder of bilirubin metabolism characterized by chronic or intermittent benign jaundice due to the defect in hepatocellular excretion of organic anions into bile (85). Dubin–Johnson syndrome results in black to dark-green discoloration of the liver that can be recognized macroscopically even on a needle biopsy specimen (86). Otherwise the liver is grossly normal. Abundant dark-brown coarse pigment in the pericanalicular cytoplasm of centrilobular hepatocytes is noted. In contrast to lipofuscin, the granules are darker and more variable in size and extend into the midlobular and periportal hepatocytes. Electron microscope demonstrates distinctive oval or irregularly shaped, pleomorphic electron-dense lysosomes. They contain very dense bodies frequently associated with lipid droplets, in a finely granular background and lack the typical lobulation of lipofuscin granules. Other liver abnormalities and particularly cholestasis are not seen.

Hemosiderin

Iron can accumulate in the liver in a variety of conditions, including hereditary hemochromatosis and secondary iron overload conditions associated with systemic macrophage iron accumulation (transfusions, hemolytic conditions, anemia of chronic disease, etc.), hepatitides (hepatitis C, alcoholic liver disease, porphyria cutanea tarda), and liver-specific iron accumulation of uncertain pathogenesis in cirrhosis (87).

In the early stages, hereditary hemochromatosis and secondary iron overload result in distinct pattern of hemosiderin deposition; but as the disease progresses, the histologic distinction between them becomes less clear. Hereditary hemochromatosis causes preferential hemosiderin deposition in periportal hepatocytes of homozygotic patients in the early stages and heterozygotic patients throughout life. In the early stages of hereditary hemochromatosis, Kupffer cells do not contain excess iron and other liver abnormalities are not observed. With increasing age, continued iron deposition in hepatocytes leads to hepatocellular damage and fibrosis that is directly related to the iron content of the liver. Iron is deposited in all hepatocytes throughout the hepatic lobules, as well as in Kupffer cells, portal macrophages, and bile ducts and ductules (Fig. 27.55). Iron in bile ducts and ductules is typical, but not pathognomonic for hereditary hemochromatosis.

Secondary iron overload results in hemosiderin deposition primarily in Kupffer cells, distributed evenly throughout the liver lobules without any zonal preference. In severe cases of secondary iron overload, coarse uneven hemosiderin deposition is also seen in hepatocytes throughout the

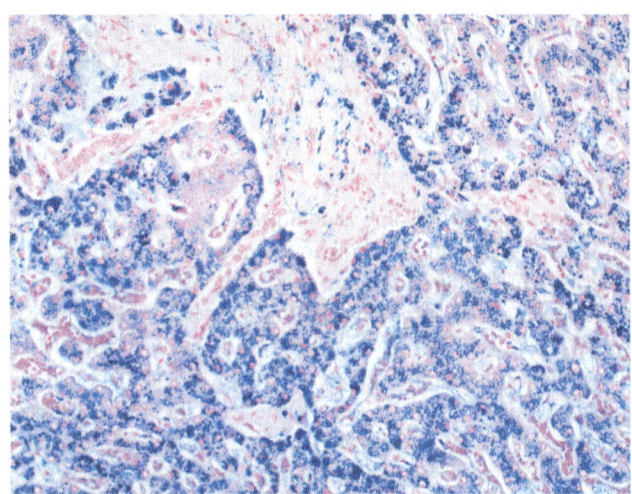

FIGURE 27.55 Severe hemosiderin deposition in hepatocytes, Kupffer cells, and portal macrophages in hereditary hemochromatosis (Perl iron stain).

hepatic lobule. Fibrosis or cirrhosis is usually absent. However, in sideroblastic anemia and thalassemia major, the severe secondary iron overload mimics that of hereditary hemochromatosis. It can also cause fibrosis and cirrhosis, but with more iron in clustered macrophages and Kupffer cells. Other causes of secondary iron overload include alcoholic liver disease and blood transfusion. Secondary iron overload from excessive ingestion or peripheral hemolysis (such as caused by Ribavirin) results in hemosiderin deposition in hepatocytes.

Copper-Associated Protein

Copper-associated protein is usually found in periportal hepatocytes or, in cirrhosis, in hepatocytes at the periphery of nodules. Copper itself is also demonstrable in the same location. Increase in copper deposition is seen in chronic cholestasis/cholate-stasis and Wilson disease (88). In chronic cholestasis, the periportal and periseptal hepatocytes have rarefied cytoplasm, usually accompanied by ductular reaction and in biliary cirrhosis by biliary halo. In Wilson disease, copper-associated protein is distributed in hepatocytes throughout the acinus or the cirrhotic nodule, in contrast to the periportal or periseptal deposition in chronic cholestasis.

Bile

In normal condition, bile in liver parenchyma is invisible (57). Bile can be visualized only in pathologic conditions, referred generally as cholestasis. Bile can accumulate in the cytoplasm of hepatocytes, bile canalicular spaces (Fig. 27.20), Kupffer cells, bile ducts and ductules. Accumulation in the cytoplasm of hepatocytes is called hepatocytic or parenchymal cholestasis, in canalicular spaces is called canalicular cholestasis, and in bile ductules is called ductular or cholangiolar cholestasis.

ACKNOWLEDGMENTS

The late Dr. Hans Popper reviewed the original manuscript. The late Dr. Michael Gerber was the senior author of this chapter in the earlier editions.

REFERENCES

1. Roskams T, Desmet V. Embryology of extra- and intrahepatic bile ducts, the ductal plate. *Anat Rec (Hoboken)* 2008;291(6): 628–635.
2. Desmet VJ. Intrahepatic bile ducts under the lens. *J Hepatol* 1985;1(5):545–559.
3. Desmet VJ. Ludwig symposium on biliary disorders–part I. Pathogenesis of ductal plate abnormalities. *Mayo Clin Proc* 1998;73(1):80–89.
4. Miranda RN, Omurtag K, Castellani WJ, et al. Myelopoiesis in the liver of stillborns with evidence of intrauterine infection. *Arch Pathol Lab Med* 2006;130(12):1786–1791.
5. Bismuth H. Surgical anatomy and anatomical surgery of the liver. *World J Surg* 1982;6(1):3–9.
6. Couinaud C. Dorsal sector of the liver. *Chirurgie* 1998;123(1): 8–15.
7. Rutkauskas S, Gedrimas V, Pundzius J, et al. Clinical and anatomical basis for the classification of the structural parts of liver. *Medicina (Kaunas)* 2006;42(2):98–106.
8. Reichert PR, Renz JF, D'Albuquerque LA, et al. Surgical anatomy of the left lateral segment as applied to living-donor and split-liver transplantation: A clinicopathologic study. *Ann Surg* 2000;232(5):658–664.
9. van Leeuwen MS, Noordzij J, Hennipman A, et al. Planning of liver surgery using three dimensional imaging techniques. *Eur J Cancer* 1995;31A(7–8):1212–1215.
10. Rappaport AM. Hepatic blood flow: Morphologic aspects and physiologic regulation. *Int Rev Physiol* 1980;21:1–63.
11. Rappaport AM. The structural and functional unit in the human liver (liver acinus). *Anat Rec* 1958;130(4):673–689.
12. Wanless IR, Wong F, Blendis LM, et al. Hepatic and portal vein thrombosis in cirrhosis: Possible role in development of parenchymal extinction and portal hypertension. *Hepatology* 1995;21(5):1238–1247.
13. Kleiner DE. The pathology of drug-induced liver injury. *Semin Liver Dis* 2009;29(4):364–372.
14. Lamers WH, Hilberts A, Furt E, et al. Hepatic enzymic zonation: A reevaluation of the concept of the liver acinus. *Hepatology* 1989;10(1):72–76.
15. Nelson DR, Koymans L, Kamataki T, et al. P450 superfamily: Update on new sequences, gene mapping, accession numbers and nomenclature. *Pharmacogenetics* 1996;6(1):1–42.
16. Larson AM. Acetaminophen hepatotoxicity. *Clin Liver Dis* 2007;11(3):525–548, vi.
17. Wanless IR, Dore S, Gopinath N, et al. Histopathology of cocaine hepatotoxicity. Report of four patients. *Gastroenterology* 1990;98(2):497–501.

18. Morgan JD, Hartroft WS. Juvenile liver. Age at which one-cell-thick plates predominate in the human liver. *Arch Pathol* 1961;71:86–88.
19. Feldmann G. Liver ploidy. *J Hepatol* 1992;16(1–2):7–10.
20. Duncan AW, Taylor MH, Hickey RD, et al. The ploidy conveyor of mature hepatocytes as a source of genetic variation. *Nature* 2010;467(7316):707–710.
21. Seeff LB, Zimmerman HJ. Relationship between hepatic and pancreatic disease. *Prog Liver Dis* 1976;5:590–608.
22. Fausto N, Campbell JS. The role of hepatocytes and oval cells in liver regeneration and repopulation. *Mech Dev* 2003;120(1):117–130.
23. Thomas DL, Seeff LB. Natural history of hepatitis C. *Clin Liver Dis* 2005;9(3):383–398, vi.
24. Locarnini S. Molecular virology of hepatitis B virus. *Semin Liver Dis* 2004;24(Suppl 1):3–10.
25. Lee JY, Locarnini S. Hepatitis B virus: Pathogenesis, viral intermediates, and viral replication. *Clin Liver Dis* 2004;8(2):301–320.
26. Loke SL, Leung CY, Chiu KY, et al. Localisation of CD10 to biliary canaliculi by immunoelectron microscopical examination. *J Clin Pathol* 1990;43(8):654–656.
27. Morotti RA, Suchy FJ, Magid MS. Progressive familial intrahepatic cholestasis (PFIC) type 1, 2, and 3: A review of the liver pathology findings. *Semin Liver Dis* 2011;31(1):3–10.
28. Wisse E, Braet F, Luo D, et al. Structure and function of sinusoidal lining cells in the liver. *Toxicol Pathol* 1996;24(1):100–111.
29. Hautekeete ML, Geerts A. The hepatic stellate (Ito) cell: Its role in human liver disease. *Virchows Arch* 1997;430(3):195–207.
30. Wallace K, Burt AD, Wright MC. Liver fibrosis. *Biochem J* 2008;411(1):1–18.
31. Nollevaux MC, Guiot Y, Horsmans Y, et al. Hypervitaminosis A-induced liver fibrosis: Stellate cell activation and daily dose consumption. *Liver Int* 2006;26(2):182–186.
32. Nakatani K, Kaneda K, Seki S, et al. Pit cells as liver-associated natural killer cells: Morphology and function. *Med Electron Microsc* 2004;37(1):29–36.
33. Luo DZ, Vermijlen D, Ahishali B, et al. On the cell biology of pit cells, the liver-specific NK cells. *World J Gastroenterol* 2000;6(1):1–11.
34. Petrelli M, Scheuer PJ. Variation in subcapsular liver structure and its significance in the interpretation of wedge biopsies. *J Clin Pathol* 1967;20(5):743–748.
35. Amitrano L, Guardascione MA, Ames PR. Coagulation abnormalities in cirrhotic patients with portal vein thrombosis. *Clin Lab* 2007;53(9–12):583–589.
36. Amitrano L, Ames PR, Guardascione MA, et al. Antiphospholipid antibodies and antiphospholipid syndrome: Role in portal vein thrombosis in patients with and without liver cirrhosis. *Clin Appl Thromb Hemost* 2011;17(4):367–370.
37. Bioulac-Sage P, Le Bail B, Bernard PH, et al. Hepatoportal sclerosis. *Semin Liver Dis* 1995;15(4):329–339.
38. Okuda K. Non-cirrhotic portal hypertension versus idiopathic portal hypertension. *J Gastroenterol Hepatol* 2002;17(Suppl 3):S204–S213.
39. Chuang CH, Chen CY, Tsai HM. Hepatic infarction and hepatic artery pseudoaneurysm with peritoneal bleeding after radiofrequency ablation for hepatoma. *Clin Gastroenterol Hepatol* 2005;3(11):A23.
40. Chen V, Hamilton J, Qizilbash A. Hepatic infarction. A clinicopathologic study of seven cases. *Arch Pathol Lab Med* 1976;100(1):32–36.
41. Reynolds WJ, Wanless IR. Nodular regenerative hyperplasia of the liver in a patient with rheumatoid vasculitis: A morphometric study suggesting a role for hepatic arteritis in the pathogenesis. *J Rheumatol* 1984;11(6):838–842.
42. Kuramochi S, Tashiro Y, Torikata C, et al. Systemic lupus erythematosus associated with multiple nodular hyperplasia of the liver. *Acta Pathol Jpn* 1982;32(3):547–560.
43. Ohtani O, Ohtani Y. Lymph circulation in the liver. *Anat Rec (Hoboken)* 2008;291(6):643–652.
44. Yokomori H, Oda M, Kaneko F, et al. Lymphatic marker podoplanin/D2-40 in human advanced cirrhotic liver–re-evaluations of microlymphatic abnormalities. *BMC Gastroenterol* 2010;10:131.
45. Crawford AR, Lin XZ, Crawford JM. The normal adult human liver biopsy: A quantitative reference standard. *Hepatology* 1998;28(2):323–331.
46. Roskams TA, Theise ND, Balabaud C, et al. Nomenclature of the finer branches of the biliary tree: Canals, ductules, and ductular reactions in human livers. *Hepatology* 2004;39(6):1739–1745.
47. Saxena R, Theise N. Canals of Hering: Recent insights and current knowledge. *Semin Liver Dis* 2004;24(1):43–48.
48. Theise ND, Saxena R, Portmann BC, et al. The canals of Hering and hepatic stem cells in humans. *Hepatology* 1999;30(6):1425–1433.
49. Richardson MM, Jonsson JR, Powell EE, et al. Progressive fibrosis in nonalcoholic steatohepatitis: Association with altered regeneration and a ductular reaction. *Gastroenterology* 2007;133(1):80–90.
50. Clouston AD, Powell EE, Walsh MJ, et al. Fibrosis correlates with a ductular reaction in hepatitis C: Roles of impaired replication, progenitor cells and steatosis. *Hepatology* 2005;41(4):809–818.
51. Craig CE, Quaglia A, Selden C, et al. The histopathology of regeneration in massive hepatic necrosis. *Semin Liver Dis* 2004;24(1):49–64.
52. Tiniakos DG, Lee JA, Burt AD. Innervation of the liver: morphology and function. *Liver* 1996;16(3):151–160.
53. Dhillon AP, Sankey EA, Wang JH, et al. Immunohistochemical studies on the innervation of human transplanted liver. *J Pathol* 1992;167(2):211–216.
54. Lee JA, Ahmed Q, Hines JE, et al. Disappearance of hepatic parenchymal nerves in human liver cirrhosis. *Gut* 1992;33(1):87–91.
55. Gupta S. Hepatic polyploidy and liver growth control. *Semin Cancer Biol* 2000;10(3):161–171.
56. Schmucker DL. Age-related changes in liver structure and function: Implications for disease? *Exp Gerontol* 2005;40(8–9):650–659.
57. Suriawinata A, Thung NS. *Liver Pathology: An Atlas and Concise Guide*. 1st ed. New York: Demos Medical Publishing; 2011.
58. Rockey DC, Caldwell SH, Goodman ZD, et al. Liver biopsy. *Hepatology* 2009;49(3):1017–1044.
59. Colloedo G, Guido M, Sonzogni A, et al. Impact of liver biopsy size on histological evaluation of chronic viral hepatitis: The smaller the sample, the milder the disease. *J Hepatol* 2003;39(2):239–244.

60. Schiano TD, Azeem S, Bodian CA, et al. Importance of specimen size in accurate needle liver biopsy evaluation of patients with chronic hepatitis C. *Clin Gastroenterol Hepatol* 2005;3(9):930–935.
61. Wennerberg AE, Nalesnik MA, Coleman WB. Hepatocyte paraffin 1: A monoclonal antibody that reacts with hepatocytes and can be used for differential diagnosis of hepatic tumors. *Am J Pathol* 1993;143(4):1050–1054.
62. Gu K, Shah V, Ma C, et al. Cytoplasmic immunoreactivity of thyroid transcription factor-1 (clone 8G7G3/1) in hepatocytes: True positivity or cross-reaction? *Am J Clin Pathol* 2007;128(3):382–388.
63. Yan BC, Gong C, Song J, et al. Arginase-1: A new immunohistochemical marker of hepatocytes and hepatocellular neoplasms. *Am J Surg Pathol* 2010;34(8):1147–1154.
64. Capurro M, Wanless IR, Sherman M, et al. Glypican-3: A novel serum and histochemical marker for hepatocellular carcinoma. *Gastroenterology* 2003;125(1):89–97.
65. Zatloukal K, French SW, Stumptner C, et al. From mallory to mallory–denk bodies: What, how and why? *Exp Cell Res* 2007;313(10):2033–2049.
66. Morrison C, Marsh W Jr, Frankel WL. A comparison of CD10 to pCEA, MOC-31, and hepatocyte for the distinction of malignant tumors in the liver. *Mod Pathol* 2002;15(12):1279–1287.
67. Cassiman D, Libbrecht L, Desmet V, et al. Hepatic stellate cell/myofibroblast subpopulations in fibrotic human and rat livers. *J Hepatol* 2002;36(2):200–209.
68. Libbrecht L, Severi T, Cassiman D, et al. Glypican-3 expression distinguishes small hepatocellular carcinomas from cirrhosis, dysplastic nodules, and focal nodular hyperplasia-like nodules. *Am J Surg Pathol* 2006;30(11):1405–1411.
69. Van Eyken P, Sciot R, Paterson A, et al. Cytokeratin expression in hepatocellular carcinoma: An immunohistochemical study. *Hum Pathol* 1988;19(5):562–568.
70. Durnez A, Verslype C, Nevens F, et al. The clinicopathological and prognostic relevance of cytokeratin 7 and 19 expression in hepatocellular carcinoma. A possible progenitor cell origin. *Histopathology* 2006;49(2):138–151.
71. Sempoux C, Fan C, Singh P, et al. Cholangiolocellular carcinoma: An innocent-looking malignant liver tumor mimicking ductular reaction. *Semin Liver Dis* 2011;31(1):104–110.
72. Batheja N, Suriawinata A, Saxena R, et al. Expression of p53 and PCNA in cholangiocarcinoma and primary sclerosing cholangitis. *Mod Pathol* 2000;13(12):1265–1268.
73. Kang YK, Kim WH, Jang JJ. Expression of G1-S modulators (p53, p16, p27, cyclin D1, Rb) and Smad4/Dpc4 in intrahepatic cholangiocarcinoma. *Hum Pathol* 2002;33(9):877–883.
74. Bioulac-Sage P, Cubel G, Balabaud C, et al. Revisiting the pathology of resected benign hepatocellular nodules using new immunohistochemical markers. *Semin Liver Dis* 2011;31(1):91–103.
75. Maeda T, Kajiyama K, Adachi E, et al. The expression of cytokeratins 7, 19, and 20 in primary and metastatic carcinomas of the liver. *Mod Pathol* 1996;9(9):901–909.
76. Volta U. Pathogenesis and clinical significance of liver injury in celiac disease. *Clin Rev Allergy Immunol* 2009;36(1):62–70.
77. Daniels JA, Torbenson M, Vivekanandan P, et al. Hepatitis in common variable immunodeficiency. *Hum Pathol* 2009;40(4):484–488.
78. Wanless IR, Solt LC, Kortan P, et al. Nodular regenerative hyperplasia of the liver associated with macroglobulinemia. A clue to the pathogenesis. *Am J Med* 1981;70(6):1203–1209.
79. Wanless IR. Micronodular transformation (nodular regenerative hyperplasia) of the liver: A report of 64 cases among 2,500 autopsies and a new classification of benign hepatocellular nodules. *Hepatology* 1990;11(5):787–797.
80. Youssef WI, Tavill AS. Connective tissue diseases and the liver. *J Clin Gastroenterol* 2002;35(4):345–349.
81. Mikkelsen WP, Edmondson HA, Peters RL, et al. Extra- and intrahepatic portal hypertension without cirrhosis (hepatoportal sclerosis). *Ann Surg* 1965;162(4):602–620.
82. Centeno JA, Mullick FG, Martinez L, et al. Pathology related to chronic arsenic exposure. *Environ Health Perspect* 2002;110(Suppl 5):883–886.
83. Gerber MA, Thung SN, Bodenheimer HC Jr, et al. Characteristic histologic triad in liver adjacent to metastatic neoplasm. *Liver* 1986;6(2):85–88.
84. Hohn A, Jung T, Grimm S, et al. Lipofuscin-bound iron is a major intracellular source of oxidants: Role in senescent cells. *Free Radic Biol Med* 2010;48(8):1100–1108.
85. Nisa AU, Ahmad Z. Dubin–Johnson syndrome. *J Coll Physicians Surg Pak* 2008;18(3):188–189.
86. Arias IM, Blumberg W. The pigment in Dubin–Johnson syndrome. *Gastroenterology* 1979;77(4 pt 1):820–821.
87. Batts KP. Iron overload syndromes and the liver. *Mod Pathol* 2007;20(Suppl 1):S31–S39.
88. Ludwig J, Moyer TP, Rakela J. The liver biopsy diagnosis of Wilson's disease. Methods in pathology. *Am J Clin Pathol* 1994;102(4):443–446.

Gallbladder and Extrahepatic Biliary System

Edward B. Stelow ■ Seung-Mo Hong

- GALLBLADDER 719
  - Gross Anatomy 719
  - Physiology 720
  - Blood Supply and Lymphatic Drainage 720
  - Nerve Supply 721
  - Histology 721
  - Ultrastructure 724
- CYSTIC DUCT 725
- RIGHT AND LEFT HEPATIC DUCTS, COMMON HEPATIC DUCT, AND COMMON BILE DUCT 726
  - Gross Anatomy 726
  - Arterial Supply, Venous Drainage, and Relationship to Bile Ducts 726
  - Lymphatic Drainage 726
  - Nerve Supply 727
  - Histology 727
- VATERIAN SYSTEM AND MINOR PAPILLA 728
  - Gross Anatomy 728
  - Vascular and Nerve Supply and Lymphatic Drainage 730
  - Histology 730
- BILIARY INTRAEPITHELIAL NEOPLASIA 733
- REFERENCES 734

The gallbladder, extrahepatic biliary sytem, liver, and dorsal pancreas all develop from the hepatic diverticulum of the midgut that appears in the 4th week of embryonic life (1). The cranial bud of the diverticulum extends outward to form the common duct and, eventually, the liver. The lumen of the common duct extends into the cystic duct and gallbladder which remains solid until the 12th week of life. Uncommonly the gallbladder does not develop or, conversely, two or more gallbladders may develop (2–4).

The gallbladder is one of the most common surgical pathology specimens. It is most often resected because of stones or inflammatory disease and is only rarely resected because of neoplasia. Somewhat uncommonly, grossly and microscopically "normal" gallbladders are removed incidentally during surgery for other reasons, for example, liver transplantation. At most institutions these specimens are rarely seen. The situation is quite different with the extrahepatic bile ducts and ampullae of Vater. These sites are infrequently sampled by biopsy only when neoplasia is suspected, especially cholangiocarcinoma or ampullary adenocarcinoma. The distal common bile duct and ampulla can be studied in the occasional pancreatoduodenectomy specimen but will often be abnormal due to the effects of an ampullary or periampullary neoplasm. The remaining extrahepatic bile duct is rarely resected. The complete biliary system and ampulla can be only studied with autopsy material, however, due in some part to the toxicity of bile, significant autolysis is usually present in these specimens.

This chapter discusses the gross anatomy, physiology, histology, immunohistochemistry, and ultrastructure of the normal gallbladder, extrahepatic bile ducts, ampulla of Vater, and minor papilla.

GALLBLADDER

Gross Anatomy

The gallbladder is a piriform bladder that is attached to the extrahepatic biliary system via the cystic duct and rests in a shallow depression located on the inferior surface of the posterior right lobe of the liver. It measures up to 10-cm long and 3- to 4-cm wide in normal adults, and its wall is approximately 1- to 2-mm thick, varying due to the degree of muscular contraction. The serosal surface of the liver extends to cover the gallbladder while interlobular connective tissue of the liver merges with the subserosal connective tissue of the gallbladder. The gallbladder is anatomically divided

---

This chapter is an update of a previous version authored by Henry F. Frierson Jr.

into a blindly ending fundus, a large central body, and a narrow neck that joins the cystic duct. The tapered area of the body that joins the neck is considered the infundibulum. It is here that a peritoneal fold, the cholecystoduodenal ligament, attaches the gallbladder to the first portion of the duodenum. Hartmann pouch, a small bulge at the infundibulum, is probably not normal and may be the result from chronic inflammation or stone impaction (5). The neck is somewhat serpentine, measures 5- to 7-mm long, and narrows as it connects with the cystic duct (6).

Physiology

The gallbladder concentrates, stores, and releases bile. Approximately 800 to 1,000 mL of bile flow daily into the gallbladder from the liver (7). Its filling results from complex neural and hormonal stimulations that result in its relaxation and the contraction and closing of the sphincter of Oddi. When the sphincter is closed, the intraluminal pressure of the bile ducts will increase as bile is continuously produced by the liver; bile will then flow into the gallbladder. When relaxed the gallbladder can store only 40 to 70 mL of bile and retains a constant intraluminal pressure (7). A much larger volume, however, is handled as the gallbladder concentrates bile via a sodium-coupled transport of chloride, mediated by NaK-ATPase (8). The active transport of electrolyte into the lateral intercellular space creates an osmotic gradient, and water ultimately flows through the basement membrane into the capillaries of the lamina propria. The gallbladder also has a secretory role, liberating mucosubstances from the surface epithelial cells and neck mucous glands.

Contraction of the gallbladder is also mediated by complex neural and humoral mechanisms and occurs both after and between meals (9). Cholecystokinin, released from the mucosa of the proximal duodenum after fatty meals, is the most important hormone that promotes gallbladder contraction (10). Motilin aids in interdigestive gallbladder contraction which occurs in tandem with giant migratory complexes of the intestines every two hours or so (9,11). Other peptides including pancreatic polypeptide and somatostatin may affect gallbladder motility (9,11–13). The vagal system may also play a role both directly and indirectly in gallbladder contraction (14). The complicated balance of humoral and neural mechanisms involved in the working of the gallbladder is sometimes disrupted and many disease states including gallstone disease have been implicated in the development of gallbladder dysmotility (15). Dysmotility may, in turn, result in gallbladder pathology (16).

Blood Supply and Lymphatic Drainage

The arterial supply of the gallbladder varies both in its anatomy and in its relationship to the extrahepatic biliary system. The cystic artery supplies the gallbladder and usually arises from the proximal portion of the right hepatic artery. Indeed, 72% of all cystic arteries in a study by Moosman

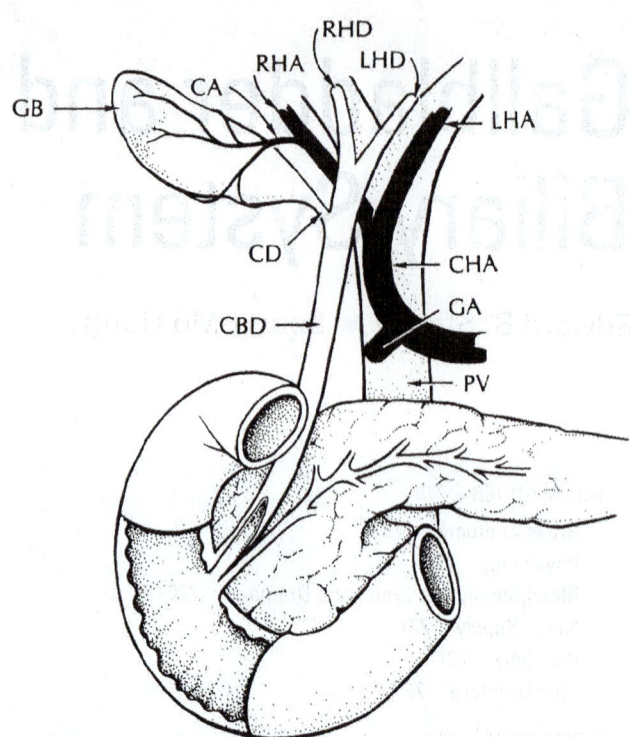

FIGURE 28.1 Although variations are common, this diagram depicts the "usual" relationships of the extrahepatic bile ducts, portal vein, and branches of the common hepatic artery. *PV*, portal vein; *GA*, gastroduodenal artery; *CHA*, common hepatic artery; *LHA*, left hepatic artery; *LHD*, left hepatic duct; *RHD*, right hepatic duct; *RHA*, right hepatic artery; *GB*, gallbladder; *CA*, cystic artery; *CD*, cystic duct; *CBD*, common bile duct.

and Coller arose from the right hepatic artery, whereas 13% arose from the superior mesenteric artery; the remainder originated from the common hepatic artery, left hepatic artery, gastroduodenal artery, celiac artery, or aorta (17). Most commonly, the artery is located superior to the cystic duct (Fig. 28.1). In Moosman's study, 70% of all cystic arteries coursed to the right of the common hepatic duct, and 17% traveled anterior to the common hepatic duct; the remainder of the cystic arteries passed posterior to the common hepatic duct, anterior or posterior to the common bile duct, to the right and inferior to the cystic duct, or posterior to both hepatic ducts (17). The cystic artery branches to form superficial channels that lie over the gallbladder serosa and deep channels that lie between the gallbladder and its hepatic bed (6). One of the more common anatomic variations noted is the double cystic artery. In their study of the extrahepatic biliary tree in 250 cadavers, Moosman and Coller noted a double cystic artery in 14% of their cases (17). Michels found double cystic arteries in one-quarter of 200 cadavers (18).

A single large cystic vein does not exist (6). The venous drainage consists, in part, of small venous channels on the hepatic side of the gallbladder that lead directly into the liver. Other small veins flow toward the cystic duct and merge with channels from the common bile duct before terminating in the portal venous system.

The lymphatic system of the gallbladder has been investigated by anatomic and physiologic studies and by studies of gallbladder malignancy (19,20). The lymphatics of the gallbladder drain first into lymph nodes at the gallbladder neck or cystic duct. Following this, drainage may proceed to retropancreatic, celiac, or mesenteric lymph nodes. These pathways appear to all converge at abdominal aortic lymph nodes located at the superior mesenteric artery (19). In a study in which dye was injected directly into lymphatic vessels of the gallbladder, the dye flowed initially into the cystic node and pericholedochal nodes, then into lymph nodes posterior to the pancreas, portal vein, and common hepatic artery, and finally into interaortocaval nodes near the left renal vein (20). Ascending lymph flow to the hepatic hilum does not usually occur, however retrograde flow to the hepatic hilum may occur when there is blockage of lymphatic channels by cancer, inflammation, or surgical ligation (20).

Nerve Supply

Nerve branches from the left trunk of the vagus join the hepatic plexus. The hepatic plexus then supplies the gallbladder with sympathetic, parasympathetic, and possibly afferent nerve fibers (6). Vagal stimulation, both directly and indirectly, may then stimulate interdigestive periodic contractions of gallbladder smooth muscle (14). Neuropeptide Y nerve fibers, which may also participate in gallbladder smooth muscle contraction, are found in all layers of the gallbladder. They form a particularly dense network in the lamina propria, running near the epithelium and paralleling the muscle bundles (21).

Histology

The layers of the gallbladder include the mucosa (surface epithelium and lamina propria), smooth muscle, perimuscular subserosal connective tissue, and serosa. A muscularis mucosa and submucosa are not present. The luminal folds are lined by a single layer of columnar epithelium and have cores of lamina propria. The height and width of the folds are variable, and branching is characteristic (Fig. 28.2). The columnar epithelial cells have lightly eosinophilic cytoplasm with occasional small apical vacuoles (Fig. 28.3). Nuclei are aligned at the cell base or slightly more centrally. They are oval and uniform and have fine chromatin and smooth membranes. Nucleoli are absent or very small and inconspicuous. Occasional columnar cells are narrow with dark eosinophilic cytoplasm (5). These cells, dignified with the appellation "pencil-like" cells, appear to be little more than contracted columnar cells, although they reportedly have a few ultrastructural and enzymatic properties which differ from those of the usual columnar cells. Basal cells are inconspicuous and have nuclei that lie just above and parallel to the basement membrane.

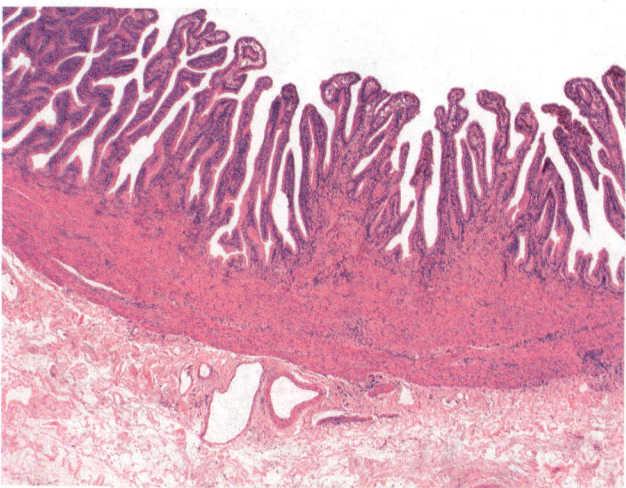

FIGURE 28.2 The luminal folds of the gallbladder vary in height and contain a delicate core of lamina propria above the bundles of smooth muscle.

Tubuloalveolar mucous glands are located only in the neck of the gallbladder (22). They have cuboid or low columnar cells with abundant clear to lightly basophilic cytoplasm and round, basally oriented nuclei (Fig. 28.4). Their lectin-binding profile is dissimilar to that of the surface epithelial cells (23). The neck mucous glands also differ morphologically and histochemically from the antral-type metaplastic glands found in the fundus, body, or neck

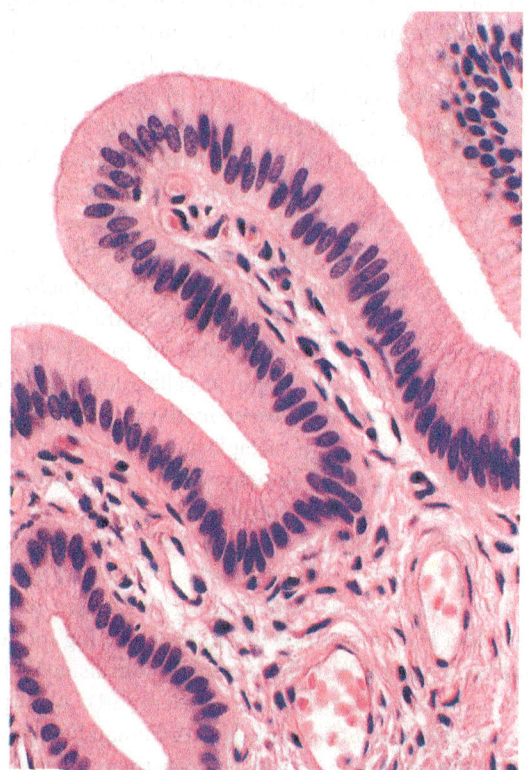

FIGURE 28.3 The gallbladder is lined by a single layer of tall columnar cells with basally oriented nuclei.

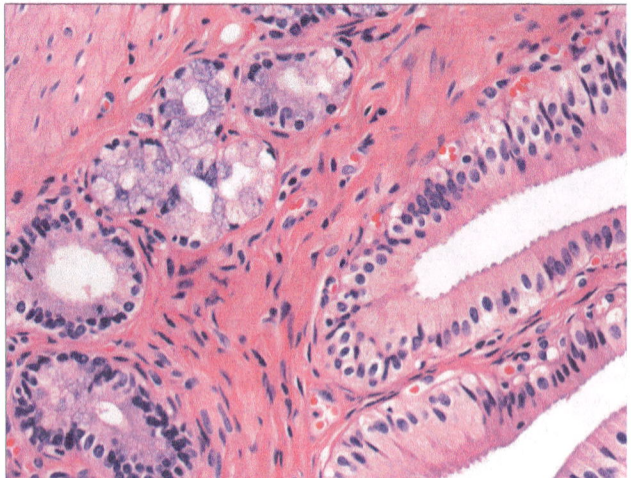

FIGURE 28.4 Mucous glands are present only in the neck of the normal gallbladder.

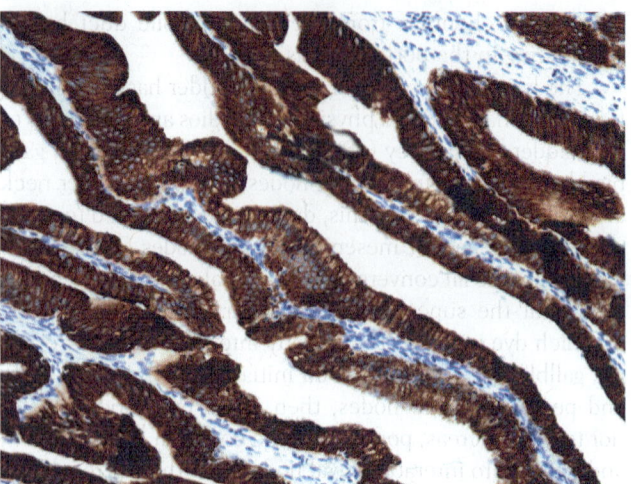

FIGURE 28.5 The epithelial lining of the gallbladder reacts strongly with anitbodies directed against cytokeratin 7 (immunoperoxidase technique).

of chronically inflamed gallbladders or those that contain gallstones (22). Rare endocrine cells can be found here but are otherwise absent in the normal gallbladder (24,25). Gastric metaplasia (foveolar-type epithelium or antral-type glands) and "intestinal" metaplasia (absorptive cells with prominent brush borders, endocrine cells, goblet cells, and Paneth cells) are not observed in the normal gallbladder but commonly occur in chronic cholecystitis and cholelithiasis (5,22,26–30). Squamous metaplasia, rarely found in diseased gallbladders, is also absent in normal gallbladders (5). Melanocytes are not found in the normal epithelial lining. However, a few small lymphocytes are often seen between the surface columnar cells.

Gallbladder epithelial cells contain chiefly sulfated acid mucin with very small quantities of nonsulfated acid mucin (22). In contrast, metaplastic cells (goblet cells, superficial gastric-type cells, antral-type glands) contain nonsulfated acid mucin and neutral mucin, but little sulfated acid mucin. By immunohistochemistry, the epithelial cells express MUC5AC and MUC6, akin to gastric epithelium, however, pepsinogens I and II, present in pyloric gland metaplasia, are not seen in normal gallbladder epithelium (29,31). Lysozyme is also absent in the normal columnar cells but may be found in metaplastic glands (32). Alpha-1-antitrypsin and alpha-1-antichymotrypsin are present in both normal and metaplastic epithelia (32).

Immunohistochemical staining for carcinoembryonic antigen (CEA) (polyclonal; unabsorbed) of normal gallbladders shows focal weak staining along the apices of some lining cells (33). In contrast to the results using monoclonal antibodies to CEA, inflamed epithelium usually shows immunostaining with polyclonal antisera (34). Absorption of at least one polyclonal antibody with human liver powder abolishes the immunoreactivity because there is removal of the CEA-related glycoproteins nonspecific cross-reacting antigen (NCA) and biliary glycoprotein (BGP) (34). The surface epithelium and neck mucous glands are strongly immunoreactive for epithelial membrane antigen and low–molecular-weight keratin (CAM5.2 antibody). The CAM5.2 antibody also stains some smooth muscle fibers in the gallbladder wall. Normal gallbladder epithelium also reacts with antibodies directed against cytokeratin (CK)7 and carbohydrate antigen (CA)19.9 and does not react with antibodies directed against CK20, MUC2, and CDX2 (Fig. 28.5) (35–38). Because endocrine cells are not found in the normal epithelium of the fundus or body, immunohistochemical staining for neuron-specific enolase and chromogranin A is absent (24). A few argentaffin (enterochromaffin) cells are present in the mucous glands of the neck; these cells are readily detected by an antibody to chromogranin A (24). Normal gallbladder mucosa lacks immunoreactivity for estrogen receptor, whereas in 6 of 31 cases of cholelithiasis, a few immunoreactive cells were observed chiefly in metaplastic mucous glands (pseudopyloric glands) (39). Adhesion molecules expressed by normal gallbladder epithelial cells include alpha-catenin, beta-catenin, gamma-catenin, CD44, CD99, and E-cadherin (40).

The lamina propria contains loose connective tissue, elastic fibers, nerve fibers, small blood vessels, and lymphatic channels. Mast cells and macrophages may be seen in small numbers, and it has been noted that these cells are more numerous in normal or minimally inflamed gallbladders than in those with overt chronic cholecystitis (Fig. 28.6) (41). Polymorphonuclear leukocytes normally are not present in the lamina propria, but small numbers of lymphocytes and plasma cells are usual. Plasma cells that contain immunoglobulin (Ig)A occur chiefly in the lamina propria, whereas IgM-containing cells are more frequent in the smooth muscle layer (42). A few IgG-containing plasma cells also may be present.

The smooth muscle consists of loosely arranged bundles of circular, longitudinal, and oblique fibers that do

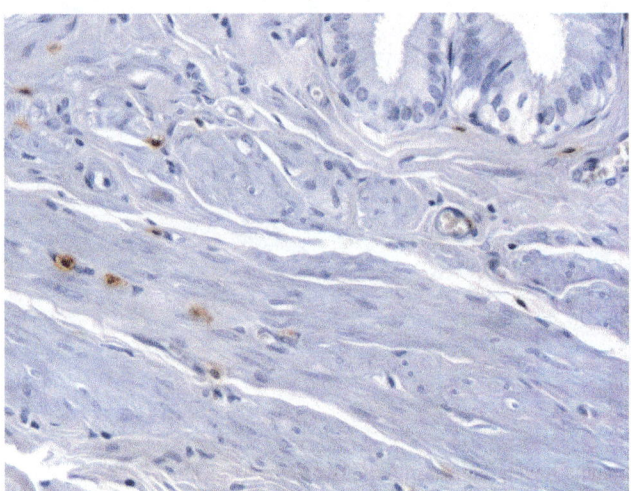

FIGURE 28.6 Occasional mast cells are identified within the gallbladder by kit-immunostaining. No interstitial cells of Cajal were identified (immunoperoxidase technique).

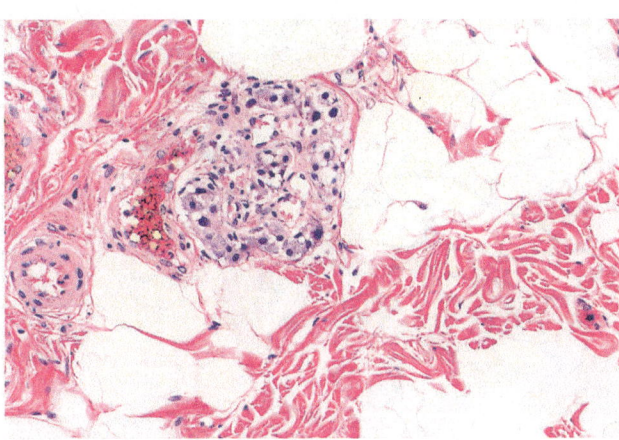

FIGURE 28.8 Paraganglia are located in the subserosal connective tissue of the normal gallbladder.

not form well-developed layers like they do in the luminal gut. Fibrovascular connective tissue focally separates the muscle bundles. The muscle fibers sometimes extend high into the lamina propria to just beneath the epithelial basement membrane. The thickness of the muscle layer is quite variable which may simply reflect variable contractile states of the specimen. Ganglion cells are found in the lamina propria, between smooth muscle bundles, and in the subserosal connective tissue (Fig. 28.7). Smooth muscle fibers are typically immunoreactive with antibodies to smoothelin and desmin consistent with a contractile muscularis propria (43). We have been unable to identify interstitial cells of Cajal, although they have been rarely noted by other authors and rare gastrointestinal stromal tumors of the gallbladder have been reported (5,44).

The subserosal tissue contains loose collagen fibers, fibroblasts, elastic fibers, adipocytes, blood vessels, nerves, and lymphatics. Small aggregates of lymphocytes may occur around vessels. Uncommonly, a lymph node is found in the subserosal connective tissue (45). Paraganglia, infrequently seen in routine sections, are found adjacent to blood vessels and small nerves (Fig. 28.8). Examining serial blocks and subserial sections of gallbladders, the investigators of one study found one to five paraganglia in the subserosal tissue of nine of ten cholecystectomy specimens (46).

Rokitansky–Aschoff sinuses represent herniations of epithelium into the lamina propria, smooth muscle, or subserosal connective tissue (Fig. 28.9). Although these are commonly considered a feature of chronic cholecystitis, they are often present in histologically normal gallbladders albeit more superficially. In a series of 125 cholecystectomy specimens that were inflamed or contained gallstones, 86% had Rokitansky–Aschoff sinuses, almost 90% of which penetrated into or through the smooth muscle (47). The sinuses were also observed in 42% of 112 normal gallbladders examined at autopsy (48). When present in normal

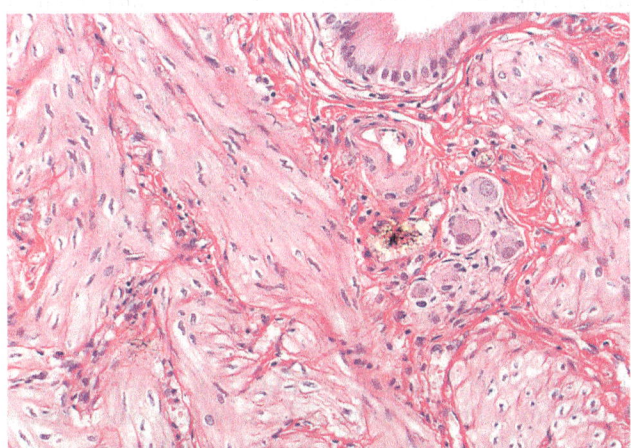

FIGURE 28.7 Ganglion cells are readily seen in the connective tissue layers of the gallbladder.

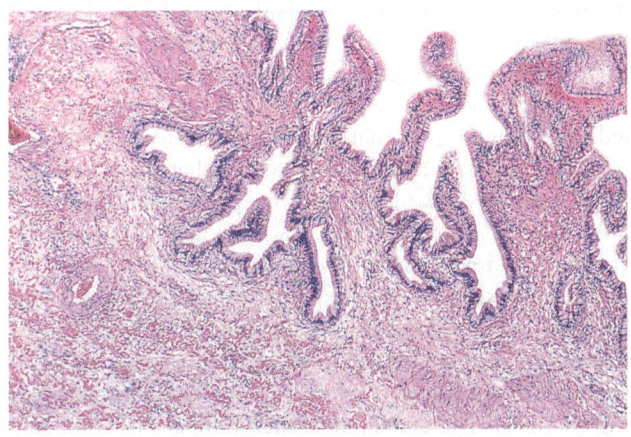

FIGURE 28.9 Rokitansky–Aschoff sinuses occur in the normal gallbladder but uncommonly penetrate through the smooth muscle bundles.

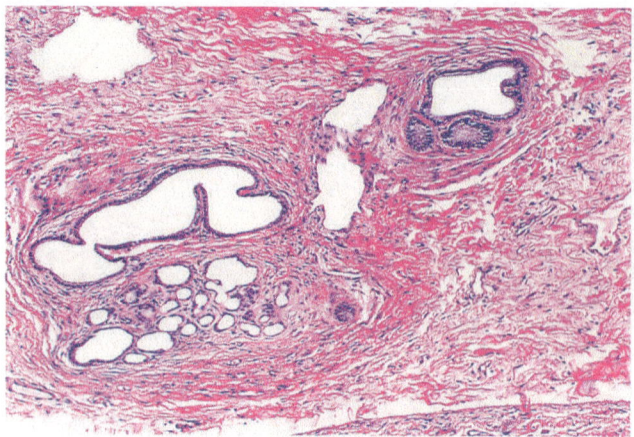 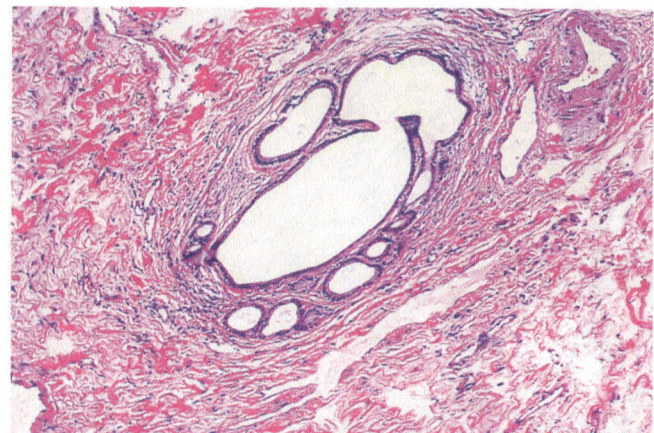

FIGURE 28.10 Luschka ducts consist of groups of small ducts having lumina of various caliber. They are surrounded by condensed connective tissue.

gallbladders, they were generally confined to the lamina propria, with infrequent penetration of the smooth muscle. The sinuses are not found in gallbladders from fetuses, but a few superficial outpouchings may be observed in organs from infants (49). The diameters of the sinuses are variable, and flask-shaped formations are usual. Although the exact mechanism for their formation is unknown, herniation of the epithelium may result from over distention (with increased intraluminal pressure) and extreme contractions of the gallbladder with subsequent weakening of its wall (49). The sinuses are uncommonly involved by intraepithelial neoplasia and when this happens careful attention showed be paid to distinguish the changes from invasive adenocarcinoma (50). The recognition of non-neoplastic epithelium, bile within the dilatations and lack of desmoplasia all point to noninvasive disease.

Luschka ducts are small, usually microscopic, bile ducts that lie in the subserosal connective tissue most commonly on the hepatic side of the gallbladder (Fig. 28.10). Occasionally, a few ducts are present in the subserosal connective tissue on the peritoneal side. The ducts have been found in 10% to 12% of routine sections from cholecystectomy specimens, occurring in both normal and diseased organs (48,49). They have been observed in gallbladders from infants, adolescents, and adults and may represent embryonic remnants. Reports of their drainage sites are varied. Most have argued that they communicate with intrahepatic bile ducts, but some have argued that those beneath the serosa possibly drain into the peritoneal cavity and others, rarely, have suggested that they may drain into the gallbladder lumen, especially within its neck (47,49,51).

The ducts are solitary or multiple but are usually present in small groups surrounded by a distinctive ring of connective tissue and may be adjacent to blood vessels. In serial sections, they sometimes are seen as a system of anastomosing channels. The diameters of their lumina vary from several microns up to a few millimeters. The ducts are lined by cells similar to those of the intrahepatic bile ducts. In some instances, small foci of hepatic parenchyma are located adjacent to the ducts (49). Luschka ducts are distinct from Rokitansky–Aschoff sinuses and the two should not communicate. It should be noted that the term "Luschka duct" has been used somewhat indiscriminately and has been used to refer to entities ranging from Rokitansky–Aschoff sinuses to true accessory ducts.

At surgery and by cholangiography, larger accessory ducts (up to several millimeters long) sometimes are seen in the gallbladder bed. They may be mistaken grossly for small veins or thin strands of fibrous tissue (52). If these ducts are not ligated during surgery, a bile leak may develop which typically ceases spontaneously. In one study, 9% of 204 patients with randomly selected cholecystectomies had bile leaks from the drain tube; some of these were considered to be due to a divided subvesical duct (53). Although these ducts lie in the gallbladder wall, they usually do not drain into the lumen of the fundus but communicate with the cystic or hepatic ducts (54,55). In a study of 20 autopsy dissections from patients without biliary disease, six subvesical ducts were found, five of which were placed centrally in the gallbladder bed and one in the lateral peritoneal reflection (53). Five led to the right hepatic duct, and one entered the common hepatic duct.

Ectopic hepatic, pancreatic, adrenal, gastric, and thyroid tissues, as well as foregut cysts have been reported in the gallbladder (56–65). Ectopic hepatic and adrenal tissues are typically incidental findings, whereas ectopic pancreatic or gastric tissues may lead to symptoms related to their secretions (56).

Ultrastructure

The surface columnar cells measure 15 to 25 μm in height and 2.5 to 7.0 μm in width and rest on a basement membrane (66). These cells have numerous apical microvilli with filamentous glycocalyx and core rootlets (Fig. 28.11). The microvilli are shorter and more variable in size and density

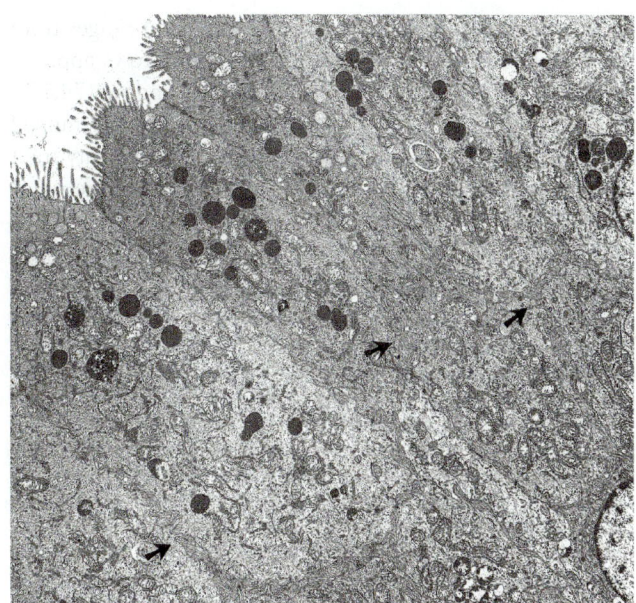

FIGURE 28.11 Ultrastructurally, the apical portion of the columnar cells of the gallbladder contains abundant microvilli with core rootlets, mitochondria, Golgi apparatus, mucous granules, lysosomes, and a few strands of rough endoplasmic reticulum. The lateral cell membranes form complex interdigitations (*arrows*).

than those of the intestinal epithelium. Pinocytotic vesicles are formed from the intervillous portions of the cell membrane. The lateral cell membranes are straight at the apex and connected by junctional complexes. Below this boundary, the cell membranes have complex interdigitations that surround lateral intercellular spaces (Fig. 28.11). The diameter of the intercellular space varies depending on the state of fluid transport (67). It is collapsed when there is no water transport but is distended during influx of electrolytes and water. The nuclei are oval, have prominent euchromatin, and occasional small nucleoli. The cytoplasm contains rough endoplasmic reticulum, mitochondria, glycogen, filaments, Golgi apparatus, mucous granules, vesicles, and lysosomes.

Pencil cells have slender outlines, narrow nuclei, and dense cytoplasm that are packed with organelles. At the base of the pencil cell, cytoplasmic extensions project into the basement membrane, unlike that of the typical columnar cell (68). However, microvilli and lateral membrane interdigitations are similar for the pencil cell.

The basal cell measures 10 to 15 μm in diameter, has an irregular nucleus, and has cytoplasmic organelles that include rough and smooth endoplasmic reticulum, mitochondria, vacuoles, and ring-shaped osmiophilic inclusions (66,68). They have a cytoplasmic extension that runs parallel to the basement membrane, changes direction to run perpendicularly, and then branches toward the lumen (66). The branches are variable in length, delicate, and complex. Throughout the lining epithelium there are intraepithelial nerve endings that originate from the nerve submucosal plexus and are associated with the small basal cells (66).

Capillaries are found just below the epithelial basement membrane, and their lumina change in size according to the state of fluid transport. The epithelial cells of the glands in the gallbladder neck have a few short microvilli, relatively even lateral membranes, rare secretory granules, and round nuclei (69).

CYSTIC DUCT

The cystic duct is located at the right free edge of the lesser omentum and usually joins the right lateral portion of the common hepatic duct approximately 2 cm distal to the union of the right and left hepatic ducts. In one study, the mean length of the cystic duct was 30 mm and ranged in size from 4 to 65 mm (17). The mean collapsed diameter was 4 mm. Connection and drainage into the common hepatic duct varies. Anatomic studies have found that most cystic ducts drain laterally at an acute angle into the common bile duct (17,70). In some cases, it may form an angular junction with either the anterior or posterior aspect of the common hepatic duct. A short cystic duct parallel to the common hepatic duct may be present, and a long cystic duct has been rarely noted. Rarely, the cystic duct may spiral and join the common hepatic duct anteriorly or posteriorly. In a cholangiographic study involving large numbers of patients, however, the cystic duct drained laterally at an acute angle into the common bile duct in only 17% of the cases, whereas in 35% it drained in a spiral form, in 41% posteriorly, and in 7% it first ran parallel to the common hepatic duct (70). In rare instances, the cystic duct may join the right and left hepatic ducts, forming a trifurcation. The cystic duct usually passes inferiorly to the cystic artery and to the right of the right hepatic artery.

The lining of the cystic duct is pleated, and in some areas there are short folds of varying width and height. The surface cells are identical microscopically and immunohistochemically to those of the gallbladder (71). Groups of mucous glands are embedded in the dense, collagenous lamina propria. Lectin-binding patterns of the lining cells are similar to those for the surface epithelial cells of the gallbladder body and neck, and the lectin-binding profiles for the mucous glands of the cystic duct are indistinguishable from those of the glands at the gallbladder neck (23). Enterochromaffin cells containing serotonin have been described in cystic ducts from patients with pancreaticobiliary disease (72). In this same group of patients, a few intramural gland cells have shown immunoreactivity for somatostatin.

The connective tissue of the large, oblique folds, grossly visible in the cystic duct at the junction with the gallbladder neck, contains thin groups of smooth muscle fibers (spiral valve of Heister) (Fig. 28.12). The smooth muscle is believed to prevent both overdistention and collapse of the cystic duct when it is subjected to changes in pressure (6). These cells show no or only limited immunoreactivity with antibodies to

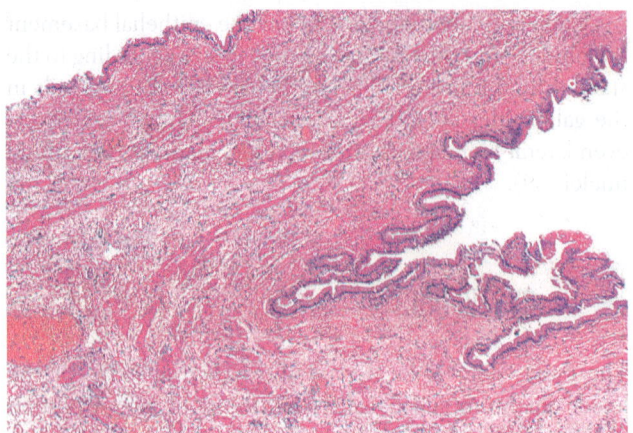

FIGURE 28.12 The stroma of the spiral valve of Heister contains thin strands of smooth muscle fibers.

smoothelin (43). Abundant collagen and some elastic fibers, nerve fibers, and ganglion cells are intermixed with the smooth muscle. Nerve fibers showing immunoreactivity for vasoactive intestinal peptide (VIP) and other peptides have been described in the wall (13,72). The loose subserosal connective tissue contains adipose tissue, nerves with occasional ganglion cells, large blood vessels, and lymphatic channels. Lymphocytes and plasma cells are sparse or absent.

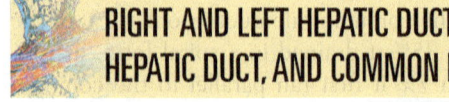

RIGHT AND LEFT HEPATIC DUCTS, COMMON HEPATIC DUCT, AND COMMON BILE DUCT

Gross Anatomy

The right and left hepatic ducts, common hepatic duct, and common bile duct are embedded between the serous layers of the hepatoduodenal ligament (the right free border of the lesser omentum). The hepatic ducts emerge from the liver and, in most instances, unite in the hilum approximately 1 cm from the liver to form the common hepatic duct. In 10% to 30% of cases, two large segmental ducts drain the right hepatic lobe and join separately with the left hepatic duct, common hepatic duct, or cystic duct; it is incorrect to label one of these ducts the right hepatic duct and the other "accessory" (73). In a dissection of 100 autopsy specimens, the mean length of the right hepatic duct was 0.8 cm (range 0.2 to 2.5) and that of the left hepatic duct 1.0 cm (range 0.2 to 3.5) (74) The usual diameter of each hepatic duct was 3 to 4 mm and the length of the common hepatic duct ranged from 0.8 to 5.2 cm (mean 2.0) (74). Its diameter ranged from 0.4 to 2.5 cm (75). The diameter of the common hepatic duct and its number of elastic fibers increase with age (75). The common bile duct, resulting from the union of the cystic duct and common hepatic duct, can be divided into supraduodenal, retroduodenal, pancreatic, and intraduodenal segments. It is usually about 1-mm thick and 5-cm long, but its length is quite variable (range 1.5 to 15.0 cm) (74,76). The diameter at its midpoint ranges from 0.4 to 1.4 cm (mean 0.66), and its lumen narrows approximately 50% after entering the duodenal window (74,77). In an autopsy study of 100 selected subjects who ranged in age from 15 to 102 years, lacked a history of biliary tract disease, and had completely intact biliary tracts, the outer diameters of the upper portions of the common bile ducts ranged from 0.4 to 1.2 cm (mean 0.74) (78). The outer diameters increased with age but were not related to body weight or length (78). The pits in the surface epithelium (sacculi of Beale) are conspicuous in the extraduodenal portion of the common bile duct and the hepatic ducts. At approximately 2 mm from the duodenal wall, the wall of the common bile duct thickens (due to an increase in muscle), resulting in the abrupt narrowing of the duct's lumen.

Arterial Supply, Venous Drainage, and Relationship to Bile Ducts

The common hepatic artery arises from the celiac trunk and divides into right and left hepatic branches (Fig. 28.1). Variations in the origins of the right and left hepatic arteries and their relationships to the extrahepatic bile ducts are typical (79). In one study, almost 42% of 200 cadavers had "aberrant" hepatic arteries (either replaced or accessory) (18). Most often, the right hepatic artery is dorsal to the common hepatic duct and right hepatic duct. The common hepatic and left hepatic arteries lie to the left of the extrahepatic bile ducts and ventral to the portal vein. The gastroduodenal artery lies to the left of the common bile duct, and a branch, the superior pancreaticoduodenal, traverses the duct either dorsally or ventrally (6).

The extrahepatic bile ducts are supplied by numerous arteries. The major arteries that supply branches to the common hepatic duct and the common bile duct include the retroduodenal, right and left hepatic, posterior superior and anterior superior pancreaticoduodenal, common hepatic, cystic, gastroduodenal, and retroportal arteries (80). The most important branches travel along the lateral borders of the common bile duct (81).

The portal vein, formed by the union of the splenic and superior mesenteric veins, lies dorsal to the bile ducts (Fig. 28.1). The mean length is 6.4 cm (range 4.8 to 8.8) and its mean diameter is 0.9 cm (range 0.64 to 1.21) (82). Venous channels that drain the superior portion of the common bile duct and common hepatic duct drain into marginal vessels that then enter the liver directly (83). Vessels from the inferior portion of the common bile duct lead to the portal vein.

Lymphatic Drainage

Lymphatic channels from the common bile duct drain into lymph nodes located along the hepatoduodenal ligament or within the posterior pancreaticoduodenal area. Drainage then proceeds to lymph nodes at the superior mesenteric artery, aorta, and common hepatic duct (84,85).

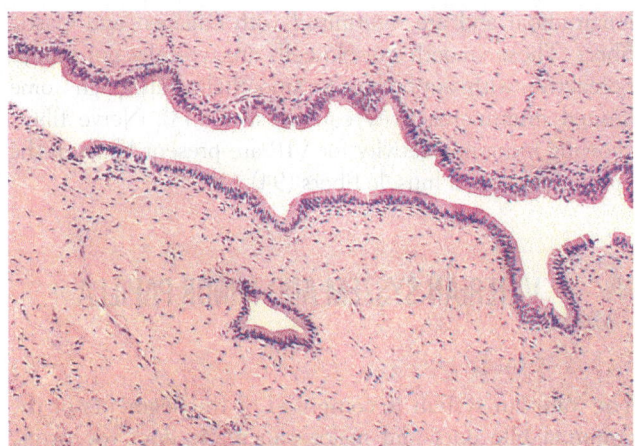

FIGURE 28.13 Intrapancreatic segment of common bile duct. The extrahepatic bile ducts are lined by a single layer of tall columnar cells overlying dense, collagenous connective tissue. In segments of the common bile duct away from the duodenum, a few small groups of smooth muscle fibers are sometimes found in the outer half of the wall.

Nerve Supply

The nerve supply to the cystic and hepatic ducts derives from the anterior portion of the hepatic plexus, whereas nerves that supply the common bile duct arise from the posterior segment of the hepatic plexus. The nerve of the common bile duct, lying dorsally, is the right portion of the posterior hepatic plexus. Smaller branches from the posterior hepatic plexus travel inferiorly along the common bile duct and accompany the duct to the major duodenal papilla (6). Neuropeptide Y–containing nerve fibers have the same pattern of distribution in the common bile duct as in the gallbladder (21).

Histology

The extrahepatic bile ducts, serving as conduits for the flow of bile, are lined by a single layer of tall columnar cells surrounded by a dense connective tissue layer (Fig. 28.13). The surface of the epithelium is relatively flat or pleated. The columnar cells have basally oriented nuclei that are oval and uniform. Nucleoli are absent or very small. Goblet cells are absent in normal epithelium. The epithelium dips into the stroma to form shallow depressions or deeper pits—the sacculi of Beale. In some sections, the deeper sacculi appear isolated from the surface epithelium, but deeper sections will often show their connections. Surrounding the sacculi are unevenly distributed lobules of glands that empty into the sacculi (Fig. 28.14). These glands have been termed diverticula, crypts, parietal sacculi, deep glands, biliary glands, periductal glands, and extrahepatic peribiliary glands (86). When located in the more peripheral connective tissue, the glands are encircled by condensed stroma. The peribiliary tubular glands are branched or, occasionally, simple and tubular (86). Although they are found in all parts of the extrahepatic bile duct system, they are less

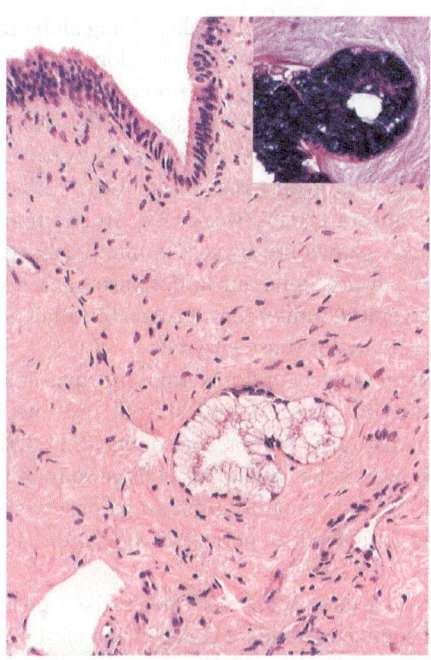

FIGURE 28.14 Glands embedded in the subepithelial collagenous stroma of the extrahepatic bile ducts typically contain cells with mucin-filled cytoplasm. (*Inset:* Alcian blue–periodic acid–Schiff (PAS) stain from the same field).

frequent in the central portion of the common bile duct and in the intrapancreatic portion than around the bile duct at the ampulla. They are lined by low columnar or cuboid cells, many of which are filled with mucus (Fig. 28.14). With inflammation and fibrosis, the sacculi and peribiliary glands may be distorted, mimicking well-differentiated adenocarcinoma with desmoplastic stroma. In small biopsy specimens and especially frozen sections, the distinction between adenocarcinoma and distorted benign glands may be impossible. The lack of a lobular arrangement and the presence of marked nuclear atypia and perineural invasion are diagnostic of adenocarcinoma (87). Hence, a haphazard growth pattern and cells whose nuclei vary in size and have irregular nuclear membranes are characteristic of adenocarcinoma. Benign glands of the extrahepatic bile ducts have not been reported to invade nerves.

The surface epithelial cells contain smaller quantities of mucin than the cells that line the gallbladder (88). The former also contain sulfated acid mucin, whereas metaplastic and dysplastic cells primarily contain nonsulfated acid mucin and smaller quantities of sulfated and neutral mucins. The normal lining epithelium stains similarly to that of the gallbladder for epithelial membrane antigen and low–molecular-weight keratin (CAM5.2 antibody). Cytokeratin 7 is consistently expressed in normal epithelium, while cytokeratin 20 expression depends on the condition of the epithelial cells. In normal cells, expression of cytokeratin 20 is usually absent, however, it may be expressed when metaplasia, hyperplasia, or carcinoma are present (35,89). CEA immunoreactivity may be absent (using absorbed polyclonal antibody) or appear as focal weak staining along the apices of some cells (using unabsorbed polyclonal antibody) (90). Cytoplasmic staining using either polyclonal or monoclonal anti-CEA antibodies is typically absent (91). Immunoreactivity for lysozyme has been found in the cytoplasm of the cells in the glands, whereas staining of the surface epithelial cells is absent or very weak (90). In addition, cells of the peribiliary glands are usually immunoreactive for pancreatic and salivary alpha-amylase, trypsin, and lipase (86). The surface epithelium of the common bile duct also shows immunoreactivity for these enzymes.

Gastric metaplasia and intestinal metaplasia are sometimes found in inflamed and fibrotic extrahepatic bile ducts that may also harbor carcinoma (28,88,92). Scattered endocrine cells, including cells immunoreactive for chromogranin and somatostatin, can be observed between mucin-containing cells in normal, as well as diseased biliary epithelium (72,92–94).

The stroma directly beneath the surface epithelium is dense and contains abundant collagen and elastic fibers and some small vessels (Fig. 28.13). Lymphocytes are sparse. Pancreatic acini and ducts may be seen in the wall of the intrapancreatic portion of the common bile duct (95). Small pancreatic ducts sometimes empty into this segment of the duct. The peripheral stroma of the common bile duct is less dense than the inner connective tissue and contains large blood vessels, lymphatics, nerves and ganglion cells, elastic fibers, and smooth muscle fibers (96). This stroma merges with the connective tissue of the hepatoduodenal ligament. The distribution of smooth muscle fibers varies throughout the bile duct. Scattered muscle fibers or no muscle fibers are present of the upper third of the bile duct, whereas a continuous or interrupted pattern of thick smooth muscle bundles is present throughout the lower third of the bile duct (Fig. 28.15) (97). The muscle fibers are more frequently longitudinal and are intermixed with collagen and elastic fibers. These smooth muscle cells are typically not immunoreactive with antibodies to smoothelin, although some limited immunoreactivity can be seen (43). Nerve fibers showing immunoreactivity for VIP are present beneath the epithelium and in muscle fibers (94).

VATERIAN SYSTEM AND MINOR PAPILLA

Gross Anatomy

The Vaterian system is composed of the segments of the common bile duct and major pancreatic duct (occurring either separately or as a common channel) at the duodenum, major papilla, and the sphincteric musculature. It also includes the extraduodenal portion of the common bile duct and major pancreatic duct that join to form a common channel outside the duodenal wall (74). It is a complex structural unit composed of a highly developed mucosa, musculature, and nerve supply that regulates the flow of bile and pancreatic secretions. Its sphincteric function (sphincter of Oddi) is a part of the overall gastrointestinal motility system and is subject to regulation by myogenic, neural, and gastrointestinal hormonal elements (13,98).

The major pancreatic duct of Wirsung drains many small channels in its course from the tail of the pancreas to the duodenal ostium. It typically inserts into the duodenal window caudal or a little lateral to the common bile duct. Its lumen narrows at the duodenal wall. The minor duct of Santorini, usually present, joins the major pancreatic duct at a variety of angles and locations within the pancreas. Uncommonly, the duct of Wirsung is smaller than the duct of Santorini and the latter may be the chief conduit for drainage of the pancreas (99). The duct of Santorini leads into the minor papilla but also may end blindly in 10% to 20% of cases (99,100). The luminal pressure of the major pancreatic duct is nearly always higher than that of the common bile duct except when the gallbladder empties (101).

The relationship of the common bile duct and duct of Wirsung at the papilla is complex and variable. The ducts may have separate openings into the duodenum, an interposed septum, or a common channel (sometimes forming an ampulla) (Fig. 28.16). The ampulla, defined strictly, is a dilated, jug-like conduit resulting from the union of the common bile duct and major pancreatic duct. In various studies of the pancreaticoduodenal junction, the frequency for separate openings into the duodenal lumen ranged from 12% to 54% and for a common channel from 46% to 88% (73,99,100,102–106). In most studies, more than two-thirds of the patients had a common channel. In a detailed gross and radiographic study, DiMagno et al. examined 390 pancreaticoduodenal specimens at autopsy and found that 74% of the patients had a common channel, 19% had separate openings for the

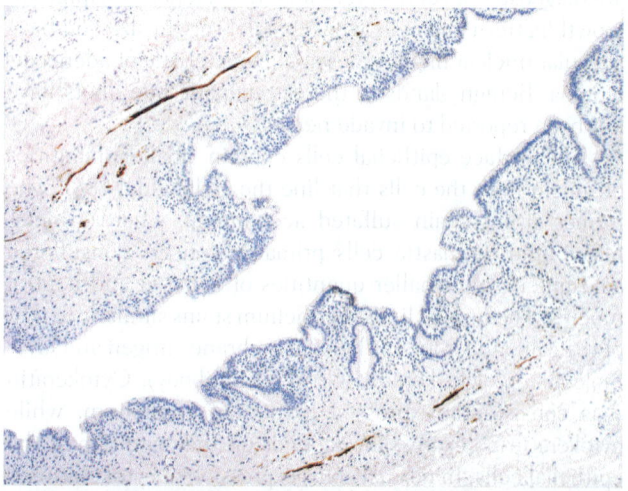

FIGURE 28.15 Occasional strands of smooth muscle are demonstrated in the upper portion of the common bile duct reacting with antibodies directed against desmin (immunoperoxidase technique).

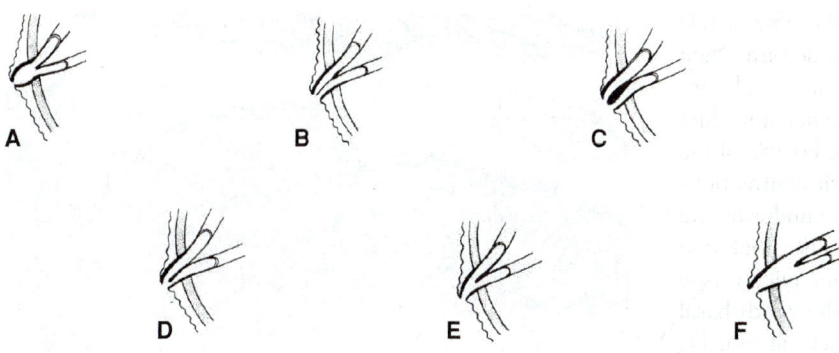

FIGURE 28.16 Relationship of the common bile duct and duct of Wirsung at the major papilla: **(A)** ampulla; **(B)** interposed septum; **(C)** separate openings; **(D)** short common channel; **(E)** long common channel; and **(F)** extended common channel.

pancreatic duct and common bile duct, and 7% had an interposed septum (102). Twenty-five percent of their specimens had a well-defined ampulla, 18% had a long common channel (defined as a channel greater than 3 mm long in the absence of an ampulla), and 31% had a short common channel (defined as a channel less than 3 mm in length) (102). For those specimens with an interposed septum, the two ducts emptied together at the ostium of the papilla. For the ducts that opened separately into the duodenal lumen, their ostia were located from 1 mm to several centimeters apart. On occasion, the ducts will unite before the duodenal wall is breached, forming an extended common channel. In one study, the length of the extended common channel ranged from 0.9 to 3.3 cm (mean 2.2) (107). This lengthy common channel occurred in 13.8% of patients with carcinoma of the biliary tract (18 of 130 cases) and in those with congenital biliary dilatation (four of four cases) but was absent in a control group of 30 cases (107). This confluence of the pancreatic and bile ducts outside of the duodenal wall has been increasingly described in association with congenital dilatation of the bile duct, choledochal cyst, and cholangiocarcinoma of the extrahepatic bile ducts and gallbladder (108–110).

The major papilla, a cylindrical protuberance housing the terminations of the common bile duct and major pancreatic duct or a common channel, is situated medially at the midportion of the second part of the duodenum. It is usually completely or partially covered by a triangular fold of duodenal mucosa; a longitudinal mucosal fold projects from the caudal portion of its base, forming a frenulum, which was absent in about one-quarter of the cases in one study (111). In one series, the papilla had a mean length of 11.7 mm and a mean width of 5.2 mm (104). Rarely, the major papilla is located at or just below the level of the duodenal mucosa or is absent. Mucosal reduplications (valves of Santorini) at the ostium of the major papilla consist of columnar-shaped protrusions and traverse leaf-like flaps of ductal mucosa (112,113). In one study, the columnar-shaped projections which arose from the terminal common bile duct numbered one to four per specimen and ranged from 1 to 5 mm in length (113). They were found in approximately one-third of adults but were not observed in fetuses. Leaf-like flaps were present in the caudal wall of the common channel in over 90% of fetuses and adults and were separated by small cul-de-sacs of varying size and depth. The flaps sometimes extended into the major pancreatic duct. In cases in which a common channel was absent, the leaf-like flaps were found only at the orifice of the duct of Wirsung. It was postulated by the authors that the flaps may flatten during the flow of pancreatic juice into the duodenum; when the cul-de-sacs are filled, the ostium is blocked and regurgitation is prevented (113).

The sphincter of Oddi consists of the intrinsic circular and longitudinal musculature of the Vaterian system. It is embryologically and functionally distinct from the musculature of the duodenal wall. However, the muscle fibers from the duodenal wall aid in anchoring the Vaterian system in place in the duodenal window. In a study of the structure of the dense connective tissue around the major duodenal papilla, the papilla and duodenal wall were noted to form both a morphologic and a functional unit (114). Connective tissue fibers spread from the papilla orifice to the circular duodenal musculature and cross at different angles from the orifice to the distal common bile duct. The arrangement and amount of muscle bundles that form the sphincter are highly complex and variable. Important fibers are those around the intrapancreatic (near the duodenal wall) and intraduodenal portions of the common bile duct (sphincter choledochus) (115). In one study, accumulation of circular muscle fibers extended up the common bile duct to a mean distance of 13.6 mm from the pore of the papilla (111). Smooth muscle fibers are also present in the wall of the common channel, around the duct of Wirsung, and near the ostium of the papilla. It is controversial whether the smooth muscle bundles around the pancreatic duct above the common channel have important sphincteric function, but the finding of a sustained pancreatic duct high-pressure zone with phasic contractions after sphincterotomy may be evidence that the sphincter of Oddi extends above the common channel to include portions of the pancreatic duct (115–117). Muscle fibers have been found to extend up the pancreatic duct a mean of 7.3 mm from the papillary pore (111). The tunica muscularis of the duodenum may not have a primary role in managing the flow of bile and pancreatic juice at the choledochoduodenal junction.

The sphincter of Oddi serves to inhibit the flow of bile into the duodenum, pumps bile into the duodenum when necessary, and likely precludes the entry of duodenal contents into the common bile duct or major pancreatic duct (98). Manometric studies have shown that the control of the flow of bile during fasting results from the phasic contractions of the sphincter of Oddi that may primarily be under neural control (118,119). These contractions result in the liberation of small volumes of bile. The flow of pancreatic juice is also regulated. The contractions are in addition to the steady basal pressure of the sphincter of Oddi, which is several mm Hg higher than that for the common bile and pancreatic ducts (120). The high-pressure zone measures 4 to 6 mm long, and the phasic contractions may be antegrade, retrograde, or simultaneous (117). Cholecystokinin has been found to inhibit the phasic contractions of the sphincter and decrease the basal pressure, allowing the flow of large quantities of bile into the duodenum (118). Manometric and contractility studies of the effects of various hormones on the sphincter of Oddi in humans and animals have been summarized (98,117). Glucagon-like cholecystokinin decreases sphincteric pressure, whereas gastrin and secretin elevate basal pressure (117). The phasic contractions and basal tone of the sphincter can be increased or decreased by exogenous drugs. For instance, most narcotics increase sphincteric pressure, whereas atropine decreases it (117).

The minor papilla is nearly always present but may be difficult to locate grossly (100). Its size is variable. It is usually situated 2 cm proximal to the major papilla (100,121).

Vascular and Nerve Supply and Lymphatic Drainage

The intraduodenal portion of the common bile duct is supplied by vessels from the anterior and posterior superior pancreaticoduodenal arteries (6). Venous drainage occurs via small veins that lead to the portal vein. The fine venous architecture of the major papilla has been described in detail (122). Lymphatic drainage is variable but generally lymphatics from the pancreaticoduodenal junction drain into the anterior and posterior pancreaticoduodenal lymph nodes and then to the nodes at the inferior pancreaticoduodenal artery (123). The Vaterian system is innervated extrinsically by parasympathetic nerve fibers in the vagal nerve and by sympathetic nerve fibers in the splanchnic nerves (13, 98). Although little is known regarding the role of these nerve fibers in regulating the motility of the sphincter of Oddi, some evidence indicates that its motility is inhibited by vagal activation (98,124). Three separate ganglia cell groups provide intrinsic innervation. These are found at the base of the papilla in the duodenal wall, within the musculature of the papilla, and within the submucosa (98). This intrinsic innervation appears to provide tonic inhibition and is similar to that for other gastrointestinal sphincters, including the lower esophageal, pyloric, and internal anal sphincters.

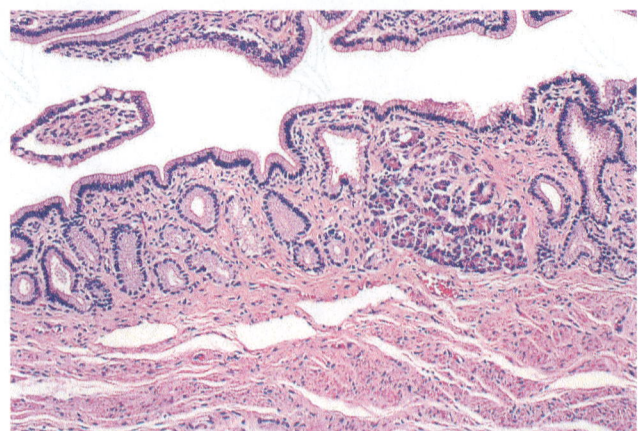

FIGURE 28.17 The duct of Wirsung at the papilla of Vater is lined by a single layer of tall columnar cells with occasional interspersed goblet cells. Accessory pancreatic ducts and acini are also observed.

Histology

The epithelial lining of the duct of Wirsung is identical to that of the common bile duct. The cytoplasm of the columnar cells also contains sulfated acid mucin (125). The epithelium may undergo hyperplastic, metaplastic, or dysplastic changes. Surrounding the normal epithelium is a dense fibrous layer with abundant collagen and elastic fibers. A few ganglion cells may be seen in the outer half of the fibrous wall. Small pancreatic ducts draining acini traverse the dense fibrous layer. At the orifice of the papilla, the epithelium of Wirsung duct is thrown into folds (mucosal reduplications) that have cores of fibrovascular stroma. Goblet cells are found interspersed between the columnar lining cells within the papilla. Numerous small accessory pancreatic ducts drain into the ductal lumen near the ostium, and pancreatic acini are sometimes present just beneath the lining of the duct (Fig. 28.17). A few lymphocytes may be seen within the ductal epithelium, and lymphocytes, plasma cells, and mast cells sparsely populate the fibrovascular cores. Circular smooth muscle bundles are present around the duct as it penetrates the duodenal wall (121).

The epithelium of the terminal portion of the common bile duct and common channel (if present) covers long, slender papillary fronds or valvules that in some respects resemble the fimbriae of the fallopian tube (Fig. 28.18). They correspond to the mucosal reduplications seen grossly. These papillary formations are considerably larger than the duodenal villi, which are few or absent at the surface of the papilla. The valvules may branch and sometimes project beyond the ostium of the papilla, shorter fronds at the periphery, and longer ones centrally (77,126,127). The columnar lining cells have eosinophilic cytoplasm and basal nuclei. Interspersed goblet cells are more numerous near the ostium. The stroma forming the cores of the fronds contains a few lymphocytes, mast cells, and plasma cells. Muscle fibers, present at the base of the fronds, are occasionally found in the stroma of the fronds. The smooth muscle,

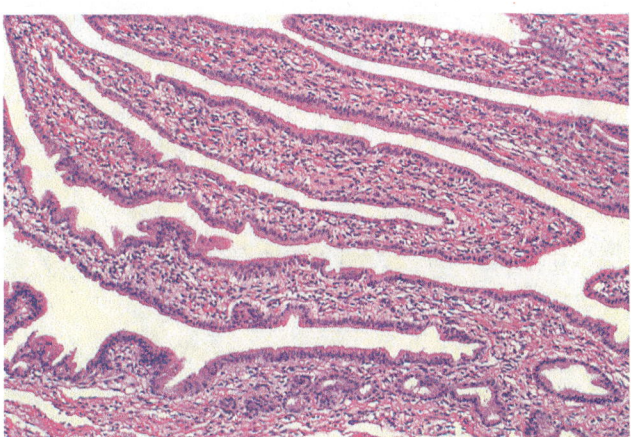

FIGURE 28.18 Near the ostium of the major papilla, the epithelium of the common bile duct lines prominent papillary fronds (valvules).

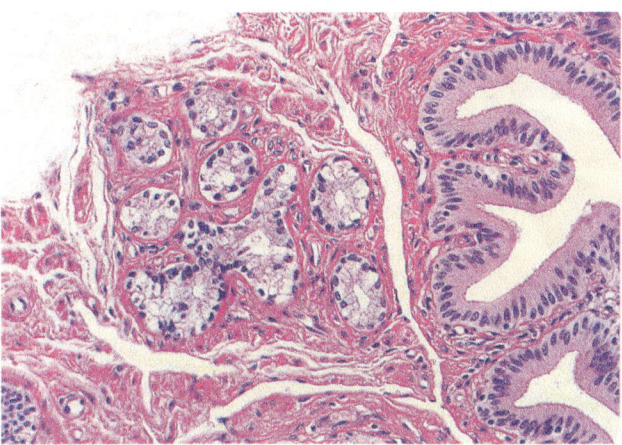

FIGURE 28.19 Mucous glands are present around the common bile duct at the papilla and drain into recesses between the papillary fronds.

forming the sphincter choledochus, becomes apparent in the wall of the duct several millimeters before the duct enters the duodenal window. About 5 mm from the duodenal wall, longitudinal muscle fibers are present around two-thirds of the common bile duct; at 2 mm from the duodenal musculature, circular muscle fibers increase and completely surround the duct (121). These intrinsic muscle fibers are separated from the muscularis propria of the duodenum by connective tissue and, at times, pancreatic tissue (121). Variable amounts of circular and longitudinal muscle fibers also surround the common channel. Before forming a common channel, the common bile duct is set apart from the pancreatic duct by a septum that eventually loses its muscle fibers, becoming a thin connective tissue membrane (121). Interspersed between areas of smooth muscle around the common bile duct or common channel are collagen, elastic fibers, small nerves, and ganglion cells. When the common bile duct and duct of Wirsung are separate within the papilla, they are distinguishable by light microscopy because the common bile duct is larger, has more prominent fronds, a greater amount of enveloping smooth muscle, and bile in its lumen.

A bewildering assortment of peribiliary glands and ducts of various caliber surround the common bile duct at the papilla. Frequently, it is only possible to distinguish mucous glands from the terminations of accessory pancreatic ducts by studying serial sections (95). Mucous glands drain into the shallow or deep recesses between the papillary fronds (Fig. 28.19). The number of these glands and their distribution are variable. Glands near the surface of the papilla may be distended with mucus and some may even represent dilated accessory pancreatic ducts (126). The number and distribution of accessory pancreatic ducts within the major papilla are also inconstant. These small accessory pancreatic channels, having been studied in serial sections and by camera lucida drawings, empty into the common bile duct (Fig. 28.20), duct of Wirsung, common channel, surface of papilla, or through the duodenal mucosa near the papilla

(95,128). They are sometimes numerous and may cause obstruction of the common bile duct, duct of Wirsung, or common channel. In such instances, a diagnosis of accessory duct hyperplasia may be appropriate (although some may use terms such as "pancreatic heterotopia" or "adenomyosis") (126). In an autopsy study, accessory pancreatic ducts were absent in only 2 of 100 major papillae (128). The ducts drain small lobules of pancreatic acini located within or, more often, near the papilla. In one study, pancreatic acini were found in 8% of 145 major papillae, whereas pancreatic islets were not seen in any of the major papillae (129). The ducts appear as packets of multiple lumens of small caliber encircled by a cellular fibrovascular stroma

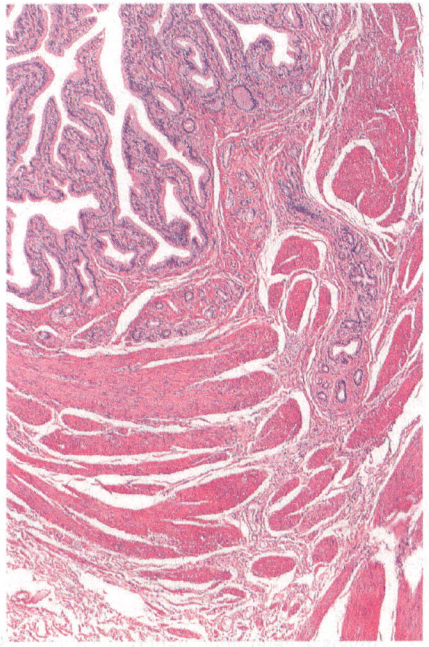

FIGURE 28.20 Accessory pancreatic ducts pierce the large smooth muscle bundles to empty into the lumen of the common bile duct.

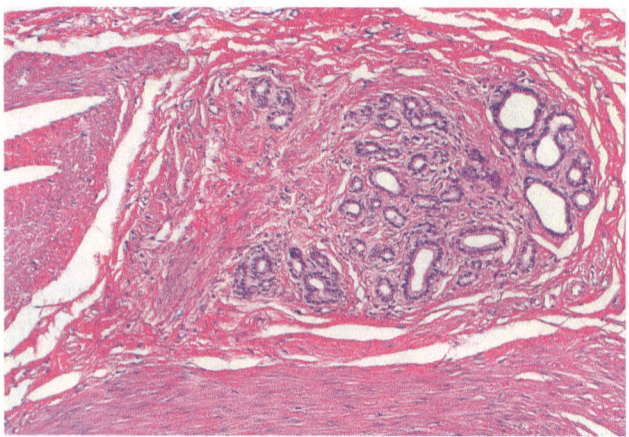

FIGURE 28.21 Accessory pancreatic ducts that penetrate the smooth muscle bundles at the choledochoduodenal junction are surrounded by a fibrovascular stroma.

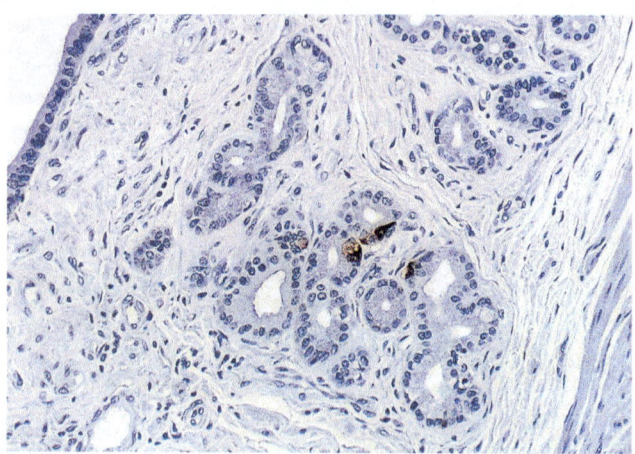

FIGURE 28.23 Some of the small ducts around the duct of Wirsung at the major papilla contain a few cells that are immunoreactive for chromogranin A (immunoperoxidase technique).

(Fig. 28.21). Within a group of ducts, the larger central duct is surrounded by smaller branches. Groups of ducts are sometimes seen penetrating the duodenal smooth muscle. Small groups of heterotopic pancreatic acini and ducts also occur in the submucosa of the duodenum away from the major papilla (Fig. 28.22).

Immunohistochemically, the cells lining the common bile duct and the duct of Wirsung at the papilla are positive for low–molecular-weight keratin (CAM5.2 antibody), cytokeratin 7, and epithelial membrane antigen. There may be linear apical staining for CEA (unabsorbed polyclonal antibody). The adjacent mucous glands and accessory pancreatic ducts have the same immunoreactivity for keratin and epithelial membrane antigen. A few scattered cells lining the large ducts within the pancreas are positive for neuron-specific enolase, chromogranin A, insulin, and glucagon (130). Chromogranin-positive cells are sometimes located in the lining epithelium of the duct of Wirsung and common bile duct within the papilla. Mucous glands and accessory pancreatic ducts also contain scattered cells immunoreactive for neuron-specific enolase and chromogranin A (Fig. 28.23). In patients with pancreaticobiliary disease, a few cells lining the lumen of the papilla and in adjacent mucous glands have been found to be immunoreactive for somatostatin (72). Although usually absent, endocrine cell micronests may be scattered singly or are grouped in the stroma adjacent to pancreatic ducts, ductules, or accessory glands but not around the common bile duct (129). They have been found in about 3% of major papillae. They consist of round, oval, trabecular, or ribbon-like groups of cells that immunohistochemically are distinct from those of pancreatic islets. They are typically scattered, rarely nodular, and immunohistochemically stain for somatostatin and pancreatic polypepide. It is unclear whether they are a normal finding or represent a metaplastic or hyperplastic condition. The functional role of these endocrine cells in the papilla of Vater is unknown.

At the minor papilla, the pancreatic duct of Santorini contains papillary fronds that are lined by simple columnar epithelium with some goblet cells (Figs. 28.24 and 28.25). Small pancreatic ducts open into the lumen of the duct of Santorini at the minor papilla or separately into the duodenum (100). Small lobules of pancreatic acini may be present within the connective tissue of the minor papilla and were seen in 77% of 167 minor papillae in a study by Noda et al., who noted that 14% of the papillae also contained well-formed pancreatic islets (129). Atrophic or poorly formed islets are present uncommonly. Smooth

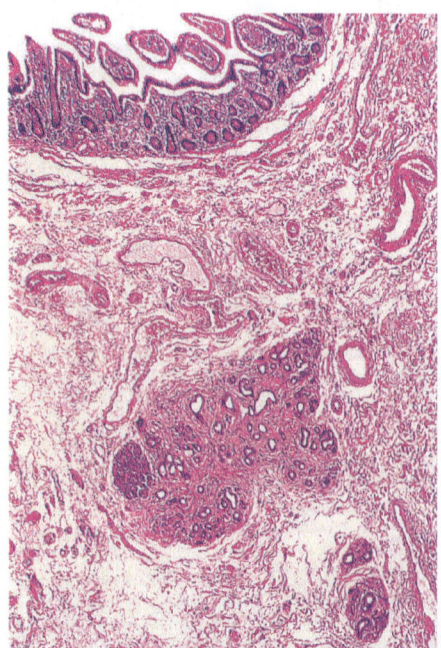

FIGURE 28.22 Groups of heterotopic pancreatic ducts and acini may be seen in the submucosa of the duodenum away from the papilla of Vater.

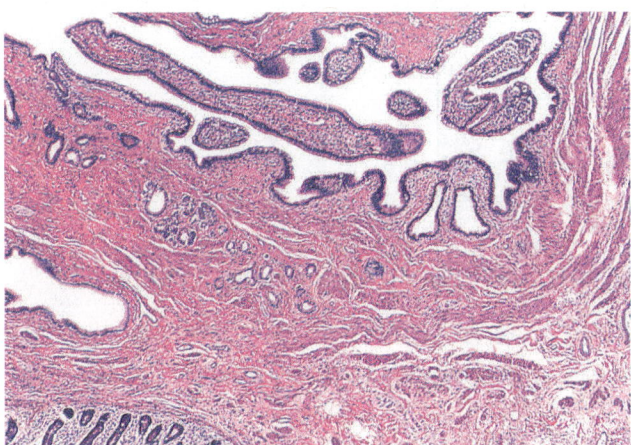

FIGURE 28.24 The duct of Santorini at the minor papilla contains papillary fronds and is surrounded by muscle bundles.

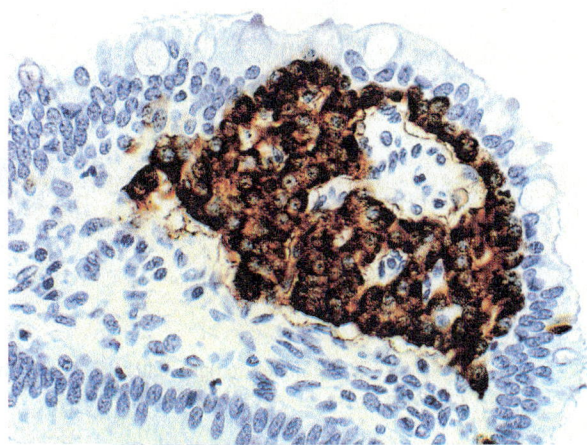

FIGURE 28.27 A group of cells below the lining epithelium of the duct of Santorini at the minor papilla is immunoreactive for chromogranin A (immunoperoxidase technique).

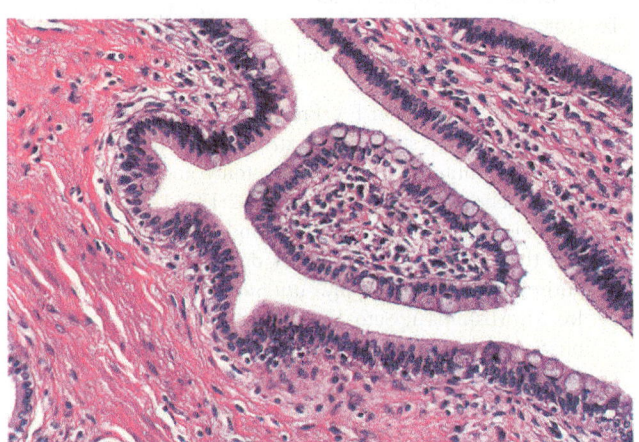

FIGURE 28.25 The duct of Santorini at the minor papilla is lined by tall columnar cells with interspersed goblet cells.

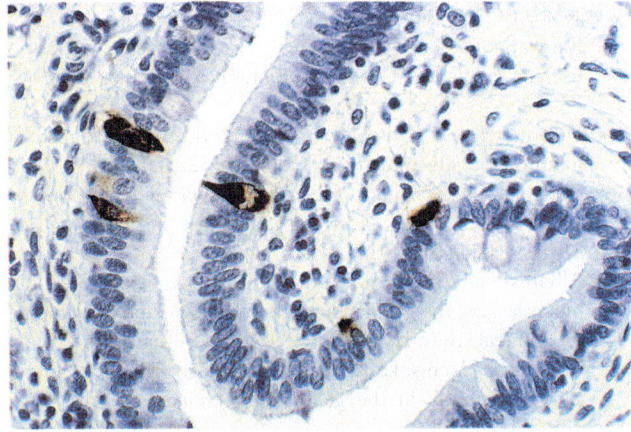

FIGURE 28.26 A few cells that line the duct of Santorini at the minor papilla are flask shaped and immunoreactive for chromogranin A (immunoperoxidase technique).

muscle bundles separated by collagen, small nerves, and ganglion cells surround the duct. The bundles of muscle occasionally are continuous with those of the muscularis mucosae of the duodenum, but in many instances the continuity between the groups of muscle fibers is lacking (100). The lining epithelial cells and those of the small pancreatic ducts stain strongly for low–molecular-weight keratin (CAM5.2 antibody), cytokeratin 7, and weakly for CEA (unabsorbed polyclonal antibody). A few cells within small ducts and some that line the lumen of the duct of Santorini are flask shaped and immunoreactive for neuron-specific enolase and chromogranin A (Fig. 28.26). Small groups of neuroendocrine cells may extend below the epithelial lining (Fig. 28.27). In the abovementioned study of 167 minor papillae, 16% contained endocrine "micronests," which were predominantly scattered and rarely nodular (129). They were usually immunoreactive for somatostatin and pancreatic polypeptide and lacked staining for insulin and glucagon. It is possible that some of these micronests represent metaplasia/hyperplasia or neoplasia.

BILIARY INTRAEPITHELIAL NEOPLASIA

Biliary intraepithelial neoplasia (BilIN) represents a progressive neoplastic transformation of normal or metaplastic epithelium to adenocarcinoma corresponding to the accumulation of progressive genetic abnormalities (Fig. 28.28) (131,132). It can be graded either within a three-tiered system (BilIN 1, BilIN 2, and BilIN 3) or a two-tiered system (low- and high-grade intraepithelial neoplasia). The lesions may be flat, pseudopapillary or papillary, usually intestinal or pancreatobilliary in phenotype, and are graded based on the degree of nuclear and cytologic atypia. BilIN 1 lesions have an abundant cytoplasmic mucin and little nuclear and cytologic atypia. BilIN 2 lesions have obvious nuclear and

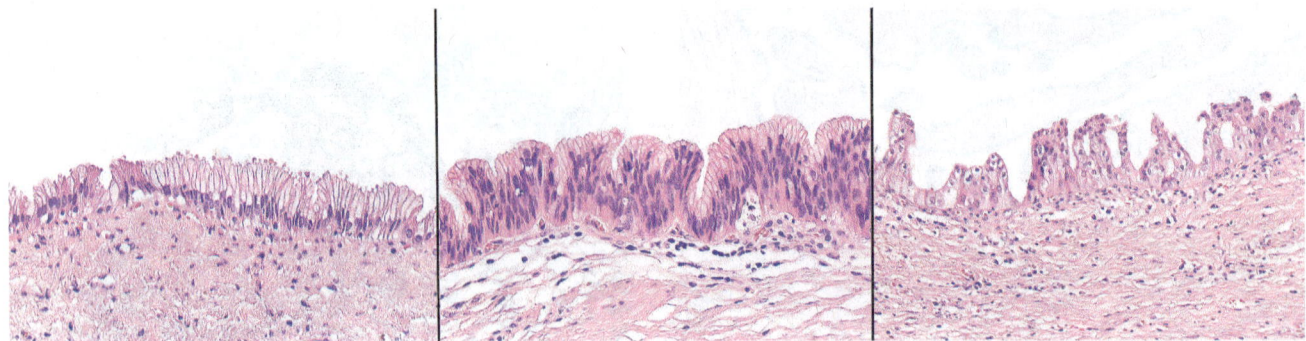

FIGURE 28.28 From left to right, BilIN 1, 2, and 3. The neoplastic epithelium shows progressive nuclear and cytologic atypia.

cytologic atypia but the atypia is not as severe as that seen with adenocarcioma. BilIN 3 lesions have nuclear and cytologic features of adenocarcinoma.

REFERENCES

1. Ando H. Embryology of the biliary tract. *Dig Surg* 2010;27: 87–89.
2. Frey C, Bizer L, Ernst C. Agenesis of the gallbladder. *Am J Surg* 1967;114:917–926.
3. Malde S. Gallbladder agenesis diagnosed intra-operatively: A case report. *J Med Case Reports* 2010;4:285.
4. Kurzweg FT, Cole PA. Triplication of the gallbladder: Review of literature and report of a case. *Am Surg* 1979;45: 410–412.
5. Albores-Saavedra J, Henson DE, Klimstra DS. *Normal anatomy. Tumors of the Gallbladder, Extrahepatic Bile Ducts, and Ampulla of Vater.* 3rd ed. Washington, DC: Armed Forces Institute of Pathology; 2000:1–16.
6. Lindner HH. Embryology and anatomy of the biliary tree. In: Way LW, Pellegrini CA, eds. *Surgery of the Gallbladder and Bile Ducts.* Philadelphia, PA: WB Saunders; 1987:3–22.
7. Guyton AC. The liver and biliary system. *Textbook of Medical Physiology.* Philadelphia, PA: WB Saunders; 1976: 936–944.
8. Frizzell RA, Heintze K. Transport functions of the gallbladder. In: Javitt NB, ed. *Liver and Biliary Tract Physiology.* Baltimore, MD: University Park Press; 1980:221–247.
9. Shaffer EA. Review article: Control of gall-bladder motor function. *Aliment Pharmacol Ther* 2000;14(Suppl 2):2–8.
10. Rehfeld JF. Clinical endocrinology and metabolism. Cholecystokinin. *Best Pract Res Clin Endocrinol Metab* 2004;18: 569–586.
11. Pomeranz IS, Davison JS, Shaffer EA. In vitro effects of pancreatic polypeptide and motilin on contractility of human gallbladder. *Dig Dis Sci* 1983;28:539–544.
12. Fisher RS, Rock E, Levin G, et al. Effects of somatostatin on gallbladder emptying. *Gastroenterology* 1987;92:885–890.
13. Balemba OB, Salter MJ, Mawe GM. Innervation of the extrahepatic biliary tract. *Anat Rec* 2004;280A:836–847.
14. Magee DF, Naruse S, Pap A. Vagal control of gall-bladder contraction. *J Physiol* 1984;355:65–70.
15. Lavoie B, Balemba OB, Godfrey C, et al. Hydrophobic bile salts inhibit gallbladder smooth muscle function via stimulation of GPBAR1 receptors and activation of KATP channels. *J Physiol* 2010;588:3295–3305.
16. Colecchia A, Sandri L, Staniscia T, et al. Gallbladder motility and functional gastrointestinal disorders. *Dig Liver Dis* 2003; 35(Suppl 3):S30–S4.
17. Moosman DA, Collier FA. Prevention of traumatic injury to the bile ducts; a study of the structures of the cystohepatic angle encountered in cholecystectomy and supraduodenal choledochostomy. *Am J Surg* 1951;82:132–143.
18. Michels NA. The hepatic, cystic and retroduodenal arteries and their relations to the biliary ducts with samples of the entire celiacal blood supply. *Ann Surg* 1951;133:503–524.
19. Ito M, Mishima Y, Sato T. An anatomical study of the lymphatic drainage of the gallbladder. *Surg Radiol Anat* 1991; 13:89–104.
20. Shirai Y, Yoshida K, Tsukada K, et al. Identification of the regional lymphatic system of the gallbladder by vital staining. *Br J Surg* 1992;79:659–662.
21. Ding WG, Fujimura M, Mori A, et al. Light and electron microscopy of neuropeptide Y-containing nerves in human liver, gallbladder, and pancreas. *Gastroenterology* 1991;101: 1054–1059.
22. Laitio M. Morphology and histochemistry of nontumorous gallbladder epithelium. A series of 103 cases. *Pathol Res Pract* 1980;167:335–345.
23. Karayannopoulou G, Damjanov I: Lectin binding sites in the human gallbladder and cystic duct. *Histochemistry* 1987;88: 75–83.
24. Delaquerriere L, Tremblay G, Riopelle JL. Argentaffine cells in chronic cholecystitis. *Arch Pathol* 1962;74:142–151.
25. Yamamoto M, Nakajo S, Tahara E. Endocrine cells and lysozyme immunoreactivity in the gallbladder. *Arch Pathol Lab Med* 1986;110:920–927.
26. Albores-Saavedra J, Nadji M, Henson DE, et al. Intestinal metaplasia of the gallbladder: A morphologic and immunocytochemical study. *Hum Pathol* 1986;17:614–620.
27. Kozuka S, Hachisuka K. Incidence by age and sex of intestinal metaplasia in the gallbladder. *Hum Pathol* 1984;15: 779–784.
28. Kozuka S, Kurashina M, Tsubone M, et al. Significance of intestinal metaplasia for the evolution of cancer in the biliary tract. *Cancer* 1984;54:2277–2285.

29. Tatematsu M, Furihata C, Miki K. Complete and incomplete pyloric gland metaplasia of human gallbladder. *Acta Pathol Jpn* 1987;37:39–46.
30. Tsutsumi Y, Nagura H, Osamura Y, et al. Histochemical studies of metaplastic lesions in the human gallbladder. *Arch Pathol Lab Med* 1984;108:917–921.
31. Chang HJ, Kim SW, Lee BL, et al. Phenotypic alterations of mucins and cytokeratins during gallbladder carcinogenesis. *Pathol Int* 2004;54:576–584.
32. Aroni K, Kittas C, Papadimitriou CS, et al. An immunocytochemical study of the distribution of lysozyme, a1-antitrypsin and a1-antichymotrypsin in the normal and pathological gall bladder. *Virchows Arch A Pathol Anat Histopathol* 1984;403:281–289.
33. Albores-Saavedra J, Nadji M, Morales AR, et al. Carcinoembryonic antigen in normal, preneoplastic and neoplastic gallbladder epithelium. *Cancer* 1983;52:1069–1072.
34. Maxwell P, Davis RI, Sloan JM. Carcinoembryonic antigen (CEA) in benign and malignant epithelium of the gall bladder, extrahepatic bile ducts, and ampulla of Vater. *J Pathol* 1993;170:73–76.
35. Cabibi D, Licata A, Barresi E, et al. Expression of cytokeratin 7 and 20 in pathological conditions of the bile tract. *Pathol Res Pract* 2003;199:65–70.
36. Sakamoto H, Mutoh H, Ido K, et al. A close relationship between intestinal metaplasia and Cdx2 expression in human gallbladders with cholelithiasis. *Hum Pathol* 2007;38:66–71.
37. Osawa H, Kita H, Satoh K, et al. Aberrant expression of CDX2 in the metaplastic epithelium and inflammatory mucosa of the gallbladder. *Am J Surg Pathol* 2004;28:1253–1254.
38. Agrawal V, Goel A, Krishnani N, et al. p53, carcinoembryonic antigen and carbohydrate antigen 19.9 expression in gall bladder cancer, precursor epithelial lesions and xanthogranulomatous cholecystitis. *J Postgrad Med* 2010;56:262–266.
39. Yamamoto M, Nakajo S, Tahara E. Immunohistochemical analysis of estrogen receptors in human gallbladder. *Acta Pathol Jpn* 1990;40:14–21.
40. Choi YL, Xuan YH, Shin YK, et al. An immunohistochemical study of the expression of adhesion molecules in gallbladder lesions. *J Histochem Cytochem* 2004;52:591–601.
41. Hudson I, Hopwood D. Macrophages and mast cells in chronic cholecystitis and "normal" gall bladders. *J Clin Pathol* 1986;39:1082–1087.
42. Green FH, Fox H. An immunofluorescent study of the distribution of immunoglobulin-containing cells in the normal and the inflamed human gall bladder. *Gut* 1972;13:379–384.
43. Raparia K, Zhai QJ, Schwartz MR, et al. Muscularis mucosae versus muscularis propria in gallbladder, cystic duct, and common bile duct: smoothelin and desmin immunohistochemical study. *Ann Diagn Pathol* 2010;14:408–412.
44. Mendoza-Marin M, Hoang MP, Albores-Saavedra J. Malignant stromal tumor of the gallbladder with interstitial cells of Cajal phenotype. *Arch Pathol Lab Med* 2002;126:481–483.
45. Weedon D. *Pathology of the Gallbladder*. New York: Masson; 1984.
46. Fine G, Raju UB. Paraganglia in the human gallbladder. *Arch Pathol Lab Med* 1980;104:265–268.
47. Elfving G. Crypts and ducts in the gallbladder wall. *Acta Pathol Microbiol Scand* 1960;49(Suppl 135):1–45.
48. Robertson HE, Ferguson WJ. The diverticula (Luschka's crypts) of the gallbladder. *Arch Pathol Lab Med* 1945;40:312–333.
49. Halpert B. Morphological studies on the gall-bladder. II. The "true Luschka ducts" and the "Rokitansky-Aschoff sinuses" of the human gallbladder. *Bull Johns Hopkins* 1927;41:77–103.
50. Albores-Saavedra J, Shukla D, Carrick K, et al. In situ and invasive adenocarcinomas of the gallbladder extending into or arising from Rokitansky-Aschoff sinuses: A clinicopathologic study of 49 cases. *Am J Surg Pathol* 2004;28:621–628.
51. Beilby JO. Diverticulosis of the gall bladder. The fundal adenoma. *Br J Exp Pathol* 1967;48:455–461.
52. Moosman DA. Accessory bile ducts: Their significance during cholecystectomy. *J Mich State Med Soc* 1964;63:355–358.
53. Foster JH, Wayson EE. Surgical significance of aberrant bile ducts. *Am J Surg* 1962;104:14–19.
54. McQuillan T, Manolas SG, Hayman JA, et al. Surgical significance of the bile duct of Luschka. *Br J Surg* 1989;76:696–698.
55. Goor DA, Ebert PA. Anomalies of the biliary tree. Report of a repair of an accessory bile duct and review of the literature. *Arch Surg* 1972;104:302–309.
56. Tejada E, Danielson C. Ectopic or heterotopic liver (choristoma) associated with the gallbladder. *Arch Pathol Lab Med* 1989;113:950–952.
57. Mutschmann PN. Aberrant pancreatic tissue in the gallbladder wall. *Am J Surg* 1946;72:282–283.
58. Busuttil A. Ectopic adrenal within the gall-bladder wall. *J Pathol* 1974;113:231–233.
59. Curtis LE, Sheahan DG. Heterotopic tissues in the gallbladder. *Arch Pathol* 1969;88:677–683.
60. Bulut AS, Karayalcin K. Ciliated foregut cyst of the gallbladder: Report of a case and review of literature. *Patholog Res Int* 2010;2010:193535.
61. Cassol CA, Noria D, Asa SL. Ectopic thyroid tissue within the gall bladder: Case report and brief review of the literature. *Endocr Pathol* 2010;21:263–265.
62. Liang K, Liu JF, Wang YH, et al. Ectopic thyroid presenting as a gallbladder mass. *Ann R Coll Surg Engl* 2010;92:W4–W6.
63. Al-Shraim M, Rabie ME, Elhakeem H, et al. Pancreatic heterotopia in the gallbladder associated with chronic cholecystitis: A rare combination. *JOP* 2010;11:464–466.
64. Hayama S, Suzuki Y, Takahashi M, et al. Heterotopic gastric mucosa in the gallbladder: Report of two cases. *Surg Today* 2010;40:783–787.
65. Mrak K, Eberl T, Tschmelitsch J, et al. Heterotopic pancreatic tissue in the cystic duct: Complicating factor or coexisting pathology. *South Med J* 2010;103:471–473.
66. Gilloteaux J, Pomerants B, Kelly TR. Human gallbladder mucosa ultrastructure: Evidence of intraepithelial nerve structures. *Am J Anat* 1989;184:321–333.
67. Kaye GI, Wheeler HO, Whitlock RT, et al. Fluid transport in the rabbit gallbladder. A combined physiological and electron microscopic study. *J Cell Biol* 1966;30:237–268.
68. Evett RD, Higgins JA, Brown AL Jr. The fine structure of normal mucosa in human gall bladder. *Gastroenterology* 1964;47:49–60.
69. Laitio M, Nevalainen T. Gland ultrastructure in human gall bladder. *J Anat* 1975;120:105–112.

70. Berci G. Biliary ductal anatomy and anomalies. The role of intraoperative cholangiography during laparoscopic cholecystectomy. *Surg Clin North Am* 1992;72:1069–1075.
71. Repassy G, Schaff Z, Lapis K, et al. Mucosa of the Heister valve in cholelithiasis: Transmission and scanning electron microscopic study. *Arch Pathol Lab Med* 1978; 102:403–405.
72. Dancygier H, Klein U, Leuschner U, et al. Somatostatin-containing cells in the extrahepatic biliary tract of humans. *Gastroenterology* 1984;86:892–896.
73. Northover JMA, Terblanche. J. Applied surgical anatomy of the biliary tree. In: Blumgart LH, ed. *The Biliary Tract Clinical surgery International*. Vol 5. Edinburgh: Churchill Livingstone; 1982:1–16.
74. Dowdy GS Jr., Waldron GW, Brown WG. Surgical anatomy of the pancreatobiliary ductal system. Observations. *Arch Surg* 1962;84:229–246.
75. Takahashi Y, Takahashi T, Takahashi W, et al. Morphometrical evaluation of extrahepatic bile ducts in reference to their structural changes with aging. *Tohoku J Exp Med* 1985;147:301–309.
76. Blidaru D, Blidaru M, Pop C, et al. The common bile duct: size, course, relations. *Rom J Morphol Embryol* 2010;51:141–144.
77. Baggenstoss AH. Major duodenal papilla. Variations of pathologic interest and lesions of the mucosa. *Arch Pathol Lab Med* 1938;26:853–868.
78. Mahour GH, Wakim KG, Ferris DO. The common bile duct in man: its diameter and circumference. *Ann Surg* 1967;165:415–419.
79. Benson EA, Page RE. A practical reappraisal of the anatomy of the extrahepatic bile ducts and arteries. *Br J Surg* 1976;63:853–860.
80. Chen WJ, Ying DJ, Liu ZJ, et al. Analysis of the arterial supply of the extrahepatic bile ducts and its clinical significance. *Clin Anat* 1999;12:245–249.
81. Northover JM, Terblanche J. A new look at the arterial supply of the bile duct in man and its surgical implications. *Br J Surg* 1979;66:379–384.
82. Douglass BE, Baggenstoss AH, Hollinshead WH. The anatomy of the portal vein and its tributaries. *Surg Gynecol Obstet* 1950;91:562–576.
83. Vellar ID. Preliminary study of the anatomy of the venous drainage of the intrahepatic and extrahepatic bile ducts and its relevance to the practice of hepatobiliary surgery. *ANZ J Surg* 2001;71:418–422.
84. Yoshida T, Shibata K, Yokoyama H, et al. Patterns of lymph node metastasis in carcinoma of the distal bile duct. *Hepatogastroenterology* 1999;46:1595–1598.
85. Yoshida T, Matsumoto T, Sasaki A, et al. Lymphatic spread differs according to tumor location in extrahepatic bile duct cancer. *Hepatogastroenterology* 2003;50:17–20.
86. Terada T, Kida T, Nakanuma Y. Extrahepatic peribiliary glands express alpha-amylase isozymes, trypsin and pancreatic lipase: An immunohistochemical analysis. *Hepatology* 1993;18:803–808.
87. Qualman SJ, Haupt HM, Bauer TW, et al. Adenocarcinoma of the hepatic duct junction. A reappraisal of the histologic criteria of malignancy. *Cancer* 1984;53:1545–1551.
88. Laitio M. Carcinoma of extrahepatic bile ducts. A histopathologic study. *Pathol Res Pract* 1983;178:67–72.
89. Rullier A, Le Bail B, Fawaz R, et al. Cytokeratin 7 and 20 expression in cholangiocarcinomas varies along the biliary tract but still differs from that in colorectal carcinoma metastasis. *Am J Surg Pathol* 2000;24:870–876.
90. Nagura H, Tsutsumi Y, Watanabe K, et al. Immunohistochemistry of carcinoembryonic antigen, secretory component and lysozyme in benign and malignant common bile duct tissues. *Virchows Arch A Pathol Anat Histopathol* 1984;403:271–280.
91. Davis RI, Sloan JM, Hood JM, et al. Carcinoma of the extrahepatic biliary tract: A clinicopathological and immunohistochemical study. *Histopathology* 1988;12:623–631.
92. Hoang MP, Murakata LA, Padilla-Rodriguez AL, et al. Metaplastic lesions of the extrahepatic bile ducts: A morphologic and immunohistochemical study. *Mod Pathol* 2001;14:1119–1125.
93. Yamamoto M, Nakajo S, Tahara E, et al. Endocrine cell carcinoma of extrahepatic bile duct. *Acta Pathol Jpn* 1986;36:587–593.
94. Dancygier H. Endoscopic transpapillary biopsy (ETPB) of human extrahepatic bile ducts–light and electron microscopic findings, clinical significance. *Endoscopy* 1989;21 Suppl 1:312–320.
95. Cross KR. Accessory pancreatic ducts; special reference to the intrapancreatic portion of the common duct. *AMA Arch Pathol* 1956;61:434–440.
96. Hong SM, Presley AE, Stelow EB, et al. Reconsideration of the histologic definitions used in the pathologic staging of extrahepatic bile duct carcinoma. *Am J Surg Pathol* 2006;30:744–749.
97. Hong SM, Kang GH, Lee HY, et al. Smooth muscle distribution in the extrahepatic bile duct: Histologic and immunohistochemical studies of 122 cases. *Am J Surg Pathol* 2000;24:660–667.
98. Allescher HD. Papilla of Vater: Structure and function. *Endoscopy* 1989;21 Suppl 1:324–329.
99. Millbourn E. On the excretory ducts of the pancreas in man, with special reference to their relations to each other, to the common bile duct and to the duodenum. *Acta Anat (Basel)* 1950;9:1–34.
100. Baldwin WM. The pancreatic ducts in man, together with a study of the microscopical structure of the minor duodenal papilla. *Anat Rec* 1911;5:197–228.
101. Parry EW, Hallenbeck GA, Grindlay JH. Pressures in the pancreatic and common ducts; values during fasting, after various meals, and after sphincterotomy; an experimental study. *AMA Arch Surg* 1955;70:757–765.
102. DiMagno EP, Shorter RG, Taylor WF, et al. Relationships between pancreaticobiliary ductal anatomy and pancreatic ductal and parenchymal histology. *Cancer* 1982;49:361–368.
103. Howard J, Jones R. The anatomy of the pancreatic ducts. The etiology of acute pancreatitis. *Am J Med Sci* 1947;214:617–622.
104. Newman HF, Weinberg SB, Newman EB, et al. The papilla of Vater and distal portions of the common bile duct and duct of Wirsung. *Surg Gynecol Obstet* 1958;106:687–694.
105. Stamm BH. Incidence and diagnostic significance of minor pathologic changes in the adult pancreas at autopsy: A systematic study of 112 autopsies in patients without known pancreatic disease. *Hum Pathol* 1984;15:677–683.
106. Sterling JA. The common channel for bile and pancreatic ducts. *Surg Gynecol Obstet* 1954;98:420–424.

107. Suda K, Matsumoto Y, Miyano T. An extended common channel in patients with biliary tract carcinoma and congenital biliary dilatation. *Surg Pathol* 1988;1:65–69.
108. Okada A, Nakamura T, Higaki J, et al. Congenital dilatation of the bile duct in 100 instances and its relationship with anomalous junction. *Surg Gynecol Obstet* 1990;171:291–298.
109. Hara H, Morita S, Sako S, et al. Relationship between types of common channel and development of biliary tract cancer in pancreaticobiliary maljunction. *Hepatogastroenterology* 2002;49:322–325.
110. Kamisawa T, Suyama M, Fujita N, et al. Pancreatobiliary reflux and the length of a common channel. *J Hepatobiliary Pancreat Sci* 2010;17:865–870.
111. Flati G, Flati D, Porowska B, et al. Surgical anatomy of the papilla of Vater and biliopancreatic ducts. *Am Surg* 1994;60:712–718.
112. Suarez CV. The Santorini valves. *Mt Sanai J Med* 1981;48:149–157.
113. Brown JO, Echenberg RJ. Mucosal reduplications associated with the ampullary portion of the major duodenal papilla in humans. *Anat Rec* 1964;150:293–302.
114. Dziwisch L, Lierse W. Three-dimensional arrangement of dense connective tissue around the human major duodenal papilla. Including the ampullary region and the distal choledochal duct. *Acta Anat (Basel)* 1989;135:231–235.
115. Boyden EA. The anatomy of the choledochoduodenal junction in man. *Surg Gynecol Obstet* 1957;104:641–652.
116. Suarez CV. Structure of the major duodenal papilla. *Mt Sinai J Med* 1982;49:31–37.
117. Goff JS. The human sphincter of Oddi. Physiology and pathophysiology. *Arch Intern Med* 1988;148:2673–2677.
118. Toouli J, Hogan WJ, Geenen JE, et al. Action of cholecystokinin-octapeptide on sphincter of Oddi basal pressure and phasic wave activity in humans. *Surgery* 1982;92:497–503.
119. Tanaka M. Function and dysfunction of the sphincter of Oddi. *Dig Surg* 2010;27:94–99.
120. Coelho JC, Moody FG. Certain aspects of normal and abnormal motility of sphincter of Oddi. *Dig Dis Sci* 1987;32:86–94.
121. Hand BH. An anatomical study of the choledochoduodenal area. *Br J Surg* 1963;50:486–494.
122. Biazotto W. The fine venous architecture of the major duodenal papilla in human beings. *Anat Anz* 1990;171:105–108.
123. Shirai Y, Ohtani T, Tsukada K, et al. Patterns of lymphatic spread of carcinoma of the ampulla of Vater. *Br J Surg* 1997;84:1012–1016.
124. Smirnov VM, Lychkova AE. Mechanism of synergism between sympathetic and parasympathetic autonomic nervous systems in the regulation of motility of the stomach and sphincter of Oddi. *Bull Exp Biol Med* 2003;135:327–329.
125. Kozuka S, Sassa R, Taki T, et al. Relation of pancreatic duct hyperplasia to carcinoma. *Cancer* 1979;43:1418–1428.
126. Edmondson HA. *Tumors of the gallbladder and extrahepatic bile ducts. Atlas of Tumor Pathology Fascicle 26.* Washington, DC: Armed Forces Institute of Pathology; 1967:121–167.
127. Suda K, Ootaka M, Yamasaki S, et al. Distended glands or overreplacement of ampullary mucosa at the papilla of Vater. *J Hepatobiliary Pancreat Surg* 2004;11:260–265.
128. Loquvam GS, Russell WO. Accessory pancreatic ducts of the major duodenal papilla. Normal structures to be differentiated from cancer. *Am J Clin Pathol* 1950;20:305–313.
129. Noda Y, Watanabe H, Iwafuchi M, et al. Carcinoids and endocrine cell micronests of the minor and major duodenal papillae. Their incidence and characteristics. *Cancer* 1992;70:1825–1833.
130. Alpert LC, Truong LD, Bossart MI, et al. Microcystic adenoma (serous cystadenoma) of the pancreas. A study of 14 cases with immunohistochemical and electron-microscopic correlation. *Am J Surg Pathol* 1988;12:251–263.
131. Nakanishi Y, Zen Y, Kondo S, et al. Expression of cell cycle-related molecules in biliary premalignant lesions: Biliary intraepithelial neoplasia and biliary intraductal papillary neoplasm. *Hum Pathol* 2008;39:1153–1161.
132. Zen Y, Adsay NV, Bardadin K, et al. Biliary intraepithelial neoplasia: An international interobserver agreement study and proposal for diagnostic criteria. *Mod Pathol* 2007;20:701–709.

Pancreas

Carlie S. Sigel ■ Ralph H. Hruban ■ Günter Klöppel ■ David S. Klimstra

ANATOMIC CONSIDERATIONS 738	Extrainsular Neuroendocrine Cells 757
Location and Relationship to Other Structures 738	Connective Tissues 757
Gross Anatomy 741	Cytologic Features 758
DEVELOPMENT 742	MINOR ALTERATIONS 759
Organogenesis 742	Acinar Cells 760
Cytogenesis 743	Ductal Cells 761
Developmental Anomalies and Heterotopia 744	Islet Cells 765
MICROSCOPIC FEATURES 746	CHRONIC PANCREATITIS, ATROPHY, AND FIBROSIS 768
Acini 746	REFERENCES 772
Ducts 749	
Islets of Langerhans 753	

The pancreas is an unpaired organ located in the left superior retroperitoneum. It is principally an epithelial organ that includes both exocrine elements (acini and ducts) and neuroendocrine elements (islets of Langerhans). The stroma is sparse in the normal gland, although areas of fibrosis commonly develop as individuals age. There are relatively few opportunities for pathologists to observe the normal histology of the pancreas because normal pancreatic tissue is rarely resected, the gland quickly autolyzes, and the nonneoplastic parenchyma adjacent to the resected neoplasms usually has substantial obstructive changes. For this reason, normal histology and minor variations may be unfamiliar to practicing pathologists.

ANATOMIC CONSIDERATIONS

Location and Relationship to Other Structures

The pancreas is located in the retroperitoneum posterior to the omental bursa at the level of the second and third lumbar vertebrae, and it extends from the duodenal loop at the right of the midline to the left across the posterior abdominal wall toward the hilum of the spleen (Fig. 29.1) (1). Four continuous anatomic areas of the pancreas are defined by the adjacent organs and vessels. The **head** of the gland is cupped within the C-shaped second and third portions of the duodenum. The distal portion of the common bile duct passes through the posterosuperior head of the pancreas to enter the duodenum at the ampulla of Vater. The left lobe of the liver lies anterior to the head. The **neck** of the gland is the slender area of the pancreas anterior to the mesenteric vessels. It lies just inferior to the pylorus. The **body** of the pancreas extends from the neck lateral to the left border of the aorta. The posterior wall of the gastric antrum usually overlies the body, and the proximal jejunum immediately distal to the ligament of Treitz passes inferior to the body. The posterior aspect of the body approaches the left adrenal gland and the left kidney (2). The **tail** of the pancreas extends from the left border of the aorta laterally and gradually tapers to a blunt end within several centimeters of the hilum of the spleen. In most individuals, the tail is located either centrally (50%) or inferiorly (42%) within the splenic hilum; rarely (8%) it is in the superior hilum (3,4). The anterior aspect of the pancreas as well as the superior surfaces of the neck, body, and tail are covered by the peritoneal surface of the posterior aspect of the lesser sac (5). The remaining surfaces of the gland are retroperitoneal.

Because of the proximity of the pancreas to several organs and other anatomic structures, the origin of neoplasms of

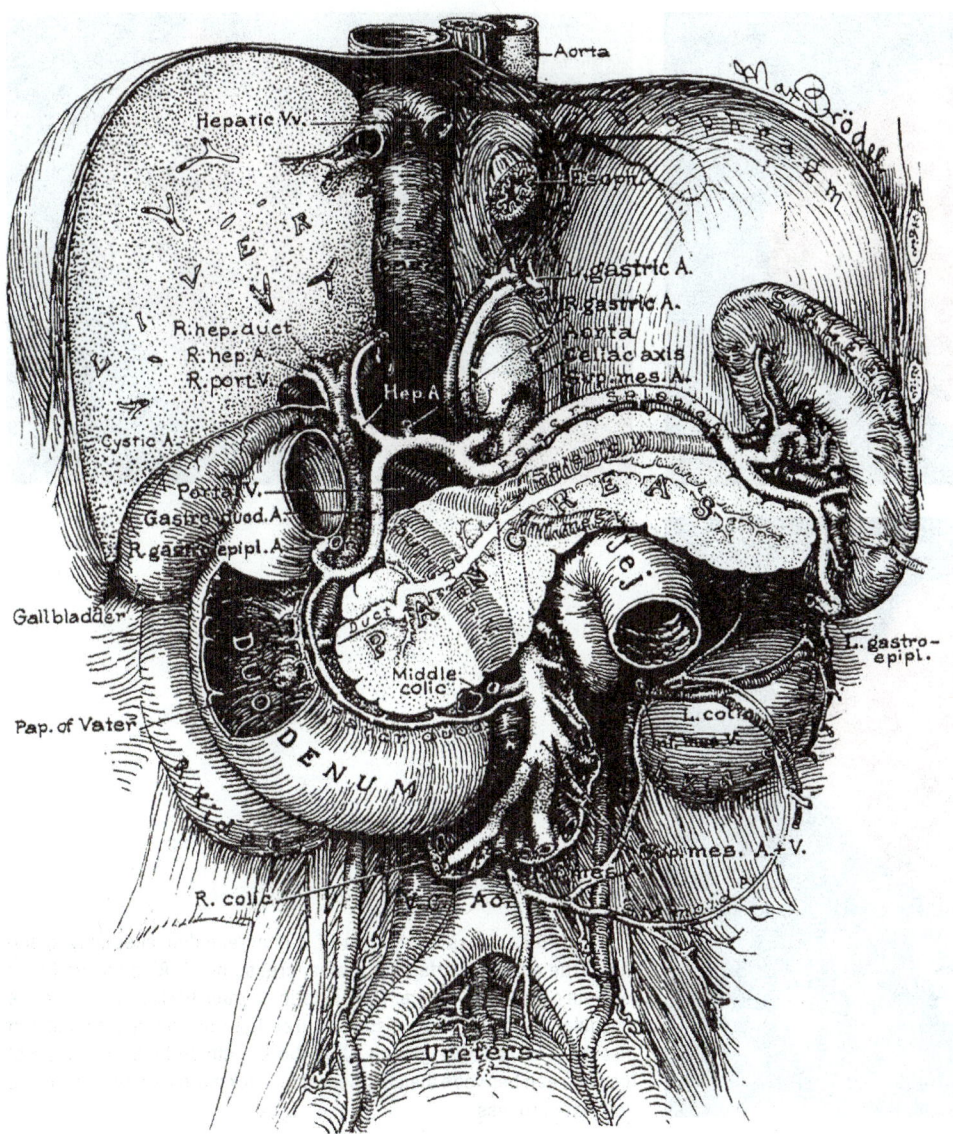

FIGURE 29.1 Anatomic relationships of the pancreas. The anterior aspect of the upper abdominal viscerae is shown after removal of the stomach and omentum. Note the close relationship of the pancreas to the duodenum, jejunum, spleen, and major vessels. Drawing by M. Brodell. Reprinted with permission from Fawcett DW. *Bloom and Fawcett: A Textbook of Histology.* 12th ed. New York: Chapman and Hall; 1994.

these sites may be difficult to define radiographically. Pancreatic masses and cysts may be confused with neoplasms of the duodenum, the ampulla of Vater, the distal bile duct, the left adrenal gland, the superior poles of either kidney, the spleen, the left lobe of the liver, the greater curve of the stomach, the root of the mesentery, and the superior retroperitoneum.

A number of major blood vessels are closely related to the pancreas (5,6). The body of the pancreas rests on the aorta. The celiac trunk arises from the aorta superior to the neck of the pancreas and gives off the hepatic artery as well as the tortuous splenic artery, which runs superior to the pancreatic tail. The superior mesenteric artery arises posterior to the junction of the neck and body, and the adjacent superior mesenteric vein passes through a groove between the head and the neck, with a portion of the head (the uncinate process) extending around the superior mesenteric vessels to lie anterior to the aorta. This vascular groove constitutes an important surgical margin in pancreatoduodenectomy specimens, and its proper identification and evaluation is therefore critical (Fig. 29.2) (7). The head of the gland also rests on the inferior vena cava, the right renal vessels, and the left renal vein. These major vessels all lie posterior to the pancreas, allowing for safe surgical access to the gland from the anterior aspect (8). The splenic vein accompanies the splenic artery along the superior aspect of the tail, joining the superior mesenteric vein to form the portal vein near the posterosuperior border of the head.

The arteries supplying the pancreas are primarily branches of the celiac trunk and the superior mesenteric artery (2,4). The arterial supply has many anastomoses between the different vessels, and numerous anatomic variations exist (9–12). The pancreatic head is supplied by the anterior and posterior pancreatoduodenal arteries, which form arcades in the pancreatoduodenal sulcus. The anterior

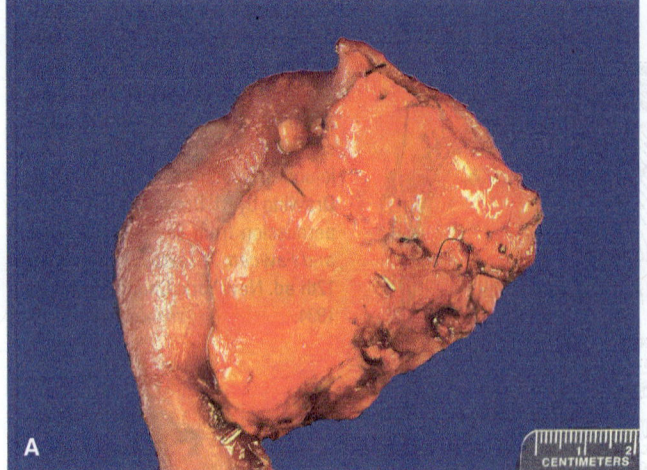
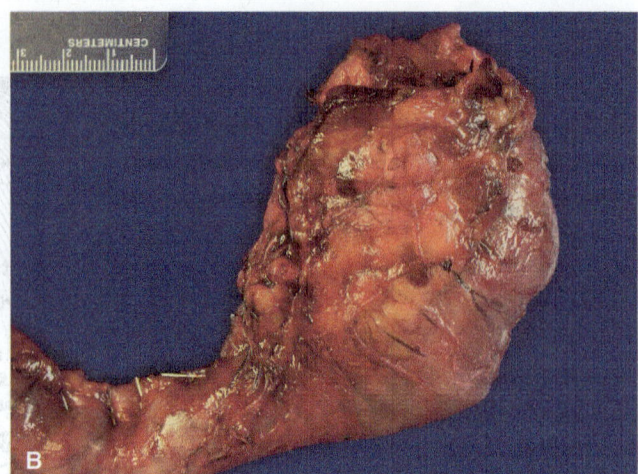
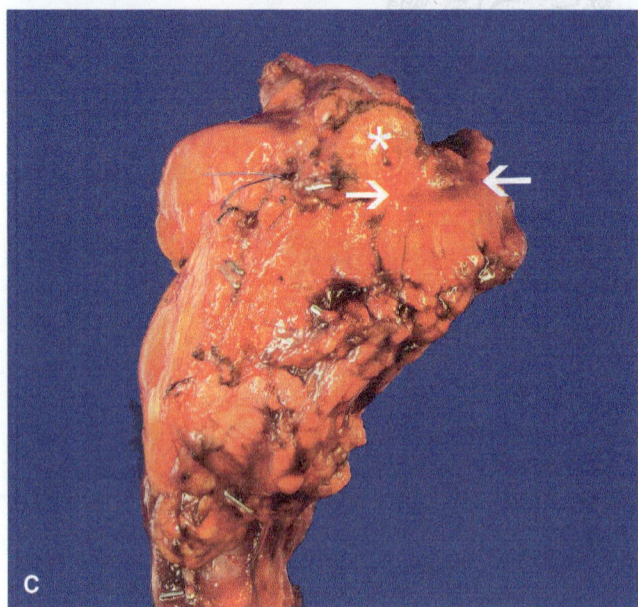

FIGURE 29.2 Gross orientation of a pancreatoduodenectomy specimen. The anterior surface of the pancreatic head (**A**) is covered by a smooth peritoneal surface. The posterior surface (**B**) is somewhat more irregular, as it has been dissected free from the retroperitoneal soft tissues. The vascular groove (**C**) is the smooth surface (*arrows*) that can be seen between the cut pancreatic neck margin (*asterisk*) and the uncinate process.

or prepancreatic arcade is formed from the anterior superior pancreatoduodenal artery (a branch of the gastroduodenal artery) and the anterior inferior pancreatoduodenal artery (a branch of the superior mesenteric artery). The posterior arcade is formed from the posterior superior pancreatoduodenal artery (from the gastroduodenal artery) and the posterior inferior pancreatoduodenal artery (from the superior mesenteric artery). Venous drainage is by the pancreaticoduodenal veins, tributaries of the splenic and superior mesenteric vein.

The body and tail of the gland are supplied by the dorsal, inferior, and caudal pancreatic arteries and are drained by the inferior and left pancreatic veins. The dorsal pancreatic artery, also known as the superior pancreatic artery, has various origins, including the first 2 cm of the splenic artery, the hepatic artery, the celiac trunk, or the superior mesenteric artery. The right branch of the dorsal pancreatic artery extends across the pancreatic head and supplies the neck of the pancreas, joining the anterior pancreatic arcade. The left branch, known as the inferior pancreatic artery, runs along the inferior body of the pancreas.

Within the pancreas, a large branch of the splenic artery known as the great pancreatic artery, or pancreatica magna, provides left and right branches that course parallel to the main pancreatic duct. The right branch joins the inferior or dorsal pancreatic arteries, and the left branch joins the caudal pancreatic artery. Branches of these pancreatic arteries supply interlobular arteries, and one intralobular artery supplies each lobule.

Major lymphatic vessels follow the course of the blood vessels. Approximately 55% of interlobular lymphatics are closely related to the accompanying artery and vein, 25% are separated from other structures by connective tissue, and 20% are closely related to acinar cells. Only 2% border the ductal system (13). The interlobular lymphatics drain toward the surface of the pancreas and enter a surface network, sometimes referred to as collecting vessels, and converge toward the lymph nodes.

There are two major systems of lymph nodes draining the pancreas: one rings the pancreas and the other surrounds the aorta from the level of the celiac trunk to the origin of the superior mesenteric artery. Lymph nodes may be closely opposed to the periphery of the gland or even embedded within its substance, especially along the inferior and superior borders and in the anterior and posterior pancreatoduodenal regions. Lymph nodes are also found around the celiac axis, adjacent to the common bile duct, and at the splenic hilus (14). Several classification systems exist for these lymph nodes although from the standpoint of involvement by carcinoma, the location of regional lymph node metastases does not appear to have clinical significance.

Innervation of the pancreas is from the vagus nerve (parasympathetic) and the splanchnic nerves (sympathetic) via the celiac and superior mesenteric plexi (2,5). The course of the nerves accompanies the vasculature (4).

Gross Anatomy

In adults the pancreas usually measures 15 to 20 cm in length and weighs 85 to 120 g. It is slightly larger in men than in women (6,15). The pancreas weighs 2 to 3 g in the newborn, and reaches 7 g at 1 year of age (16). The weight of the gland gradually decreases after age 40 to a mean of 70 g in the ninth decade of life (15,17).

The four anatomic regions of the pancreas (the head, neck, body, and tail) are grossly indistinct (Fig. 29.3). The bulk of the organ is composed of the head, including the uncinate process, which develops separately and may be anatomically separate in some individuals (see below). The uncinate process, from the Latin "uncus" or hook, extends inferiorly and posteriorly from the head of the gland and lies behind the pancreatic neck and the superior mesenteric vessels. These vessels frequently indent the uncinate process, producing the hook shape. The neck of the pancreas is the short constricted area that rests anterior to the mesenteric vessels. The neck and body are somewhat triangular in cross section, whereas the tail flattens out as it approaches the spleen (2).

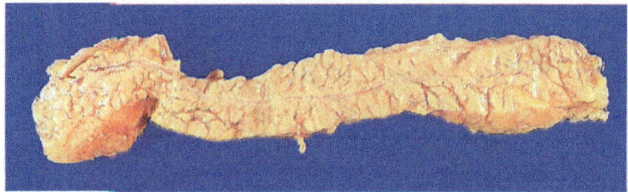

FIGURE 29.3 Gross appearance of the normal pancreas. The bulbous head (*left*) is connected to the neck, body, and tail, which merge imperceptibly. The parenchyma consists of distinctly lobulated pink–tan fleshy tissue. The pancreatic duct (opened longitudinally) is thin and smooth throughout its course.

The normal pancreas is pink-tan to yellow and uniformly lobulated. The anterior surface is smooth and covered by a layer of peritoneum; the remaining surfaces are invested by a thin layer of loose fibroconnective tissue. No discrete capsule is present, and when there is significant parenchymal fat or fibrosis, the interface with the surrounding retroperitoneal adipose tissue is usually indistinct.

Cut sections of the pancreas reveal arborizing thin-walled white ducts extending into the well-demarcated lobules. The main pancreatic duct of Wirsung averages 2 to 3 mm (ranging from 1.8 to 9 mm) in diameter (18), gradually enlarging to 4.5 mm near the ampulla of Vater, through which it drains into the duodenum. The main duct is narrower in the tail. The diameter is greater in older individuals by about 1 mm in each region of the gland. Main ducts greater than 10 mm in diameter are considered pathologically dilated. Up to 50 secondary (or branch) ducts drain into the main duct (19,20), entering alternately from either side in a herringbone pattern (Fig. 29.4) (6,21). The course of the major ducts varies depending on the pattern of fusion and atrophy of ducts that occurs during development. In general, the main pancreatic duct of Wirsung begins in the tail, collecting tributaries as it passes through the body and neck toward the head. The duct makes an acute turn

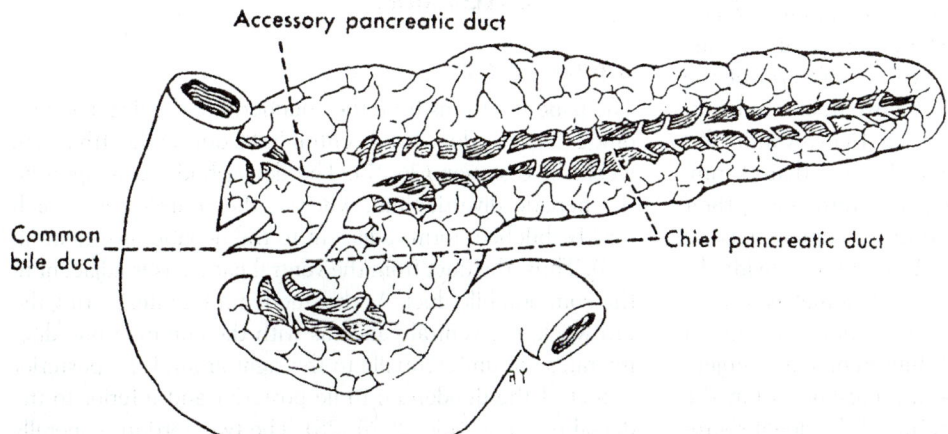

FIGURE 29.4 Schematic diagram of the pancreas showing the pattern of the major ducts and their tributaries. In this example the accessory duct is patent at the duodenum through the minor papilla. Reprinted with permission from Cubilla AL, Fitzgerald PJ. Tumors of the exocrine pancreas. In: Hartmann WH, Sobin LH, eds. *Atlas of Tumor Pathology*. 2nd series, Fascicle 19. Washington, DC: Armed Forces Institute of Pathology; 1984.

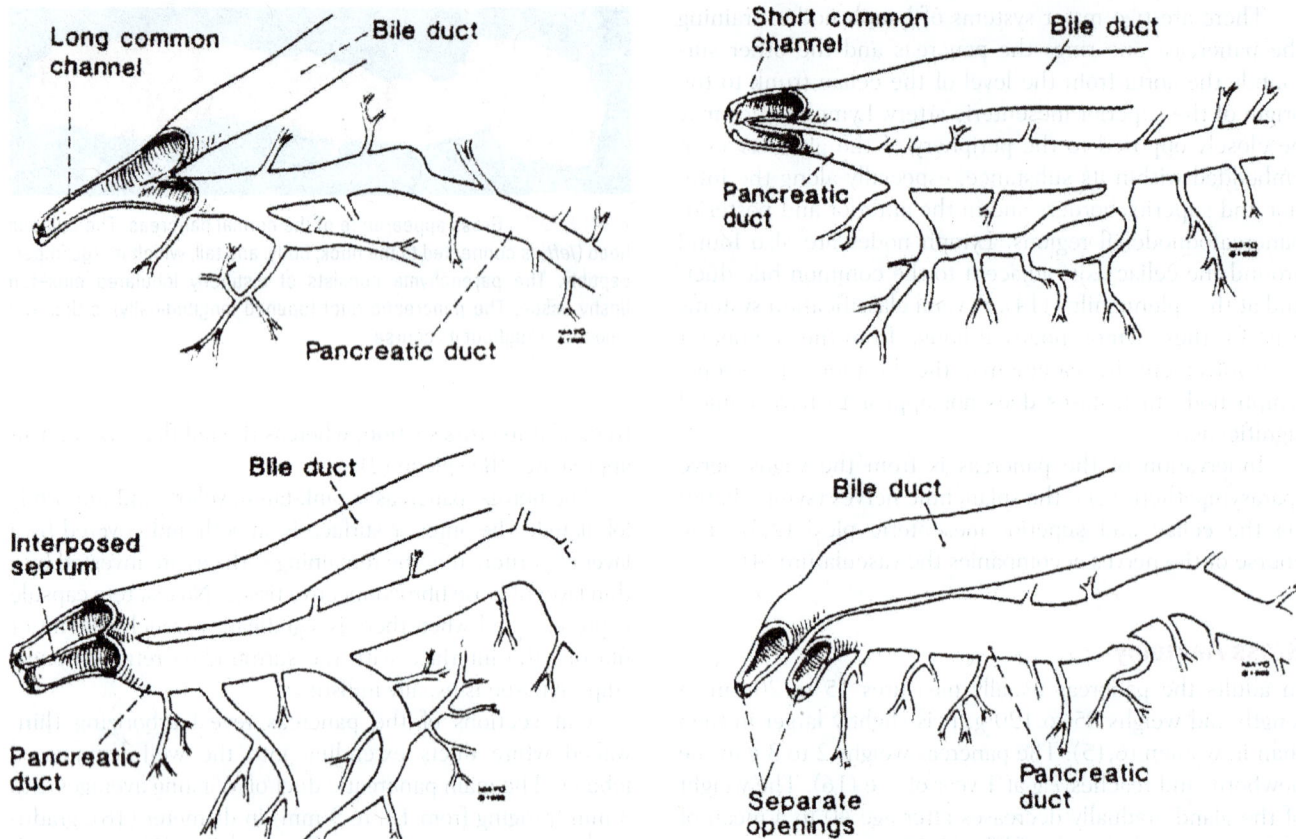

FIGURE 29.5 Anatomic variations in the paths of the pancreatic and biliary ducts at the ampulla. A long common channel (the prototypical ampulla) is only present in some individuals. In others, the ducts fuse within only a few millimeters of the duodenum, resulting in a short common channel, or the two ducts enter separately. Reprinted with permission from DiMagno EP, Shorter RG, Taylor WF, et al. Relationships between pancreaticobiliary ductal anatomy and pancreatic ductal and parenchymal histology. *Cancer* 1982;49(2):361–368.

inferiorly in the head of the gland, where it is joined by the accessory duct of Santorini from the superior head as well as the major duct from the uncinate process, ultimately exiting through the ampulla at the major papilla. The accessory duct generally does not communicate separately with the duodenum, although retention of embryonic patency through the minor duodenal papilla is not uncommon.

The relationship of the main duct to the distal common bile duct is also highly variable. The prototypical ampulla is a flask-shaped common channel within the wall of the duodenum formed by the fusion of the two ducts. In truth, a significant common channel is unusual. In many individuals, the length of the common channel is less than 3 mm. In others, the two ducts remain separate throughout their course, entering side by side at the major papilla or completely separately (Fig. 29.5) (4,15,22). In these individuals, a common channel does not exist or is extremely short. In one study only 43% of individuals had a common channel greater than 3 mm in length (23). Villiform mucosal projections known as valves of Santorini are present within the distal ducts and may prevent the reflux of duodenal secretions (24,25). The intraduodenal portions of the pancreatic and bile ducts are surrounded by thin fascicles of smooth muscle (the sphincter of Oddi), which are continuous with both the muscularis mucosae and the muscularis propria of the surrounding duodenum.

DEVELOPMENT

Organogenesis

The pancreas forms from the endoderm of the distal embryonic foregut as dorsal and ventral buds during the 4th to 5th weeks of gestation (26,27). The dorsal bud forms opposite the hepatic diverticulum, whereas the ventral bud, which may be bilobed, forms adjacent to the hepatic diverticulum (20). Thus, the duct from the ventral pancreas is adjacent to the common bile duct. As the duodenum rotates during the 6th week, the ventral pancreas with the common bile duct migrates circumferentially to the right around the posterior aspect of the duodenum to lie posterior and inferior to the dorsal pancreas (Fig. 29.6) (28). The two portions generally fuse during the 7th week. The dorsal portion makes up the

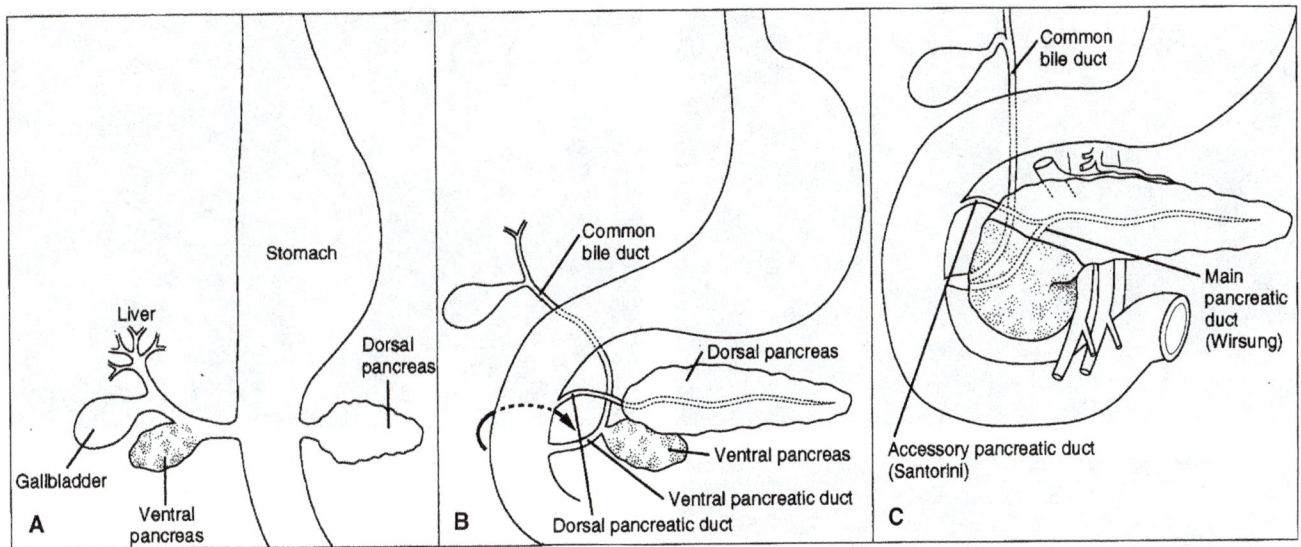

FIGURE 29.6 Development of the pancreas. The dorsal and ventral buds form on opposite sides of the duodenum (**A**). During the 6th week, the ventral pancreas migrates posteriorly around the duodenum (**B**) to lie inferior to the dorsal pancreas, where it comprises much of the head of the gland (**C**). Reprinted with permission from Skandalakis LJ, Rowe JS Jr, Gray SW, et al. Surgical embryology and anatomy of the pancreas. *Surg Clin North Am* 1993;73(4):661–697.

superior head as well as the entire neck, body, and tail of the adult gland, and the ventral portion becomes the remainder of the head, including the uncinate process (27). The ductal systems of the two lobes also normally fuse, with connection of the dorsal duct to the duodenum at the minor papilla being lost and the ventral duct providing the drainage for the exocrine secretions. Thus, the distal two-thirds of the main pancreatic duct (of Wirsung) develop from the embryonic dorsal duct, whereas the proximal third forms from the ventral duct. The remaining proximal portion of the dorsal embryonic duct becomes the accessory duct of Santorini. The complicated union of these ducts accounts for the tortuous nature of the main pancreatic duct in adults. The ampulla of Vater develops during the 8th week.

Cytogenesis

The complex events required for normal cellular development of the pancreas have three overlapping components (29,30). First, as described above, the foregut endoderm becomes patterned to form the dorsal and ventral pancreatic buds which are composed of multipotent progenitor cells. Second, the cells in the buds undergo lineage commitment to either neuroendocrine or exocrine cell fates. Third, pancreatic morphogenesis occurs by way of extensive growth and branching resulting in the mature organ. Complex gene regulatory networks and epigenetic factors control these events, and it is important to note that tissue specification, lineage commitment, and growth are highly interdependent and have considerable spatial and temporal overlap.

Many transcription factors are required for pancreas specification (26,30). Prior to and during budding, the pancreatic primordium expresses the homeodomain protein PDX1 (also known as IPF1) (29) and PDX1-positive progenitors give rise to all three epithelial cell lines (31,32). The developing ductal epithelium retains uniform PDX1 expression, but as the organ matures, PDX1 expression is lost in the ductal cells, being primarily restricted to the islet cells, with low levels detectable in some acinar cells.

Additional key transcriptional factors involved in pancreatic morphogenesis include SOX9, SOX17, MNX1, GATA4, GATA6, HLXB9, ISL1, and PTF1A (33). Transcription factors with a significant role in directing neuroendocrine fate include, but are not limited to NGN3, NEUROD/Beta2, NKX2.2, and NKX6.1 (32,34). Less is known about exocrine determination, but important transcription factors for this component include PDX1, NKX6.1, SOX9, HNF6, and HNF1β.

Pancreatic development is also regulated by cell fate determining signals from developmental patterning pathways, such as the Notch and Hedgehog signaling pathways. Notch signals are required for ductal branching and normal neuroendocrine and exocrine lineage commitment (33,35–37). Of the three hedgehog genes essential for mammalian embryogenesis (sonic hedgehog [Shh], Indian hedgehog [Ihh] and desert hedgehog [Dhh]), Shh expression in midgestational embryos is critical for proper foregut and gastrointestinal development. In contrast, Shh is excluded from the developing pancreas, and repression of Shh permits appropriate transcriptional activation of pancreatic genes (38).

The ductal network develops from expansion and remodeling of the epithelium in the pancreatic buds in a process called "branching morphogenesis." As the ducts branch progressively, lumina are formed (39). Simultaneously, cells of

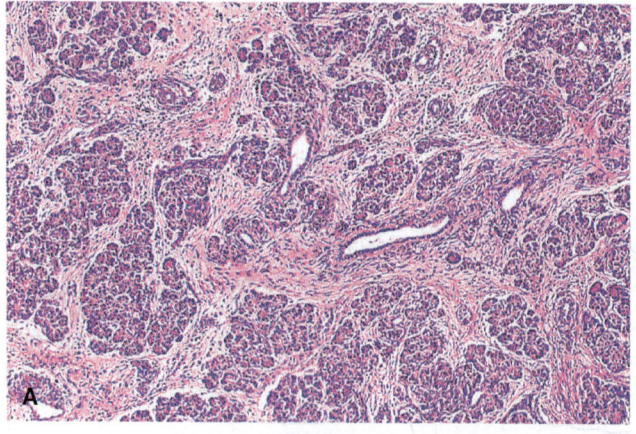
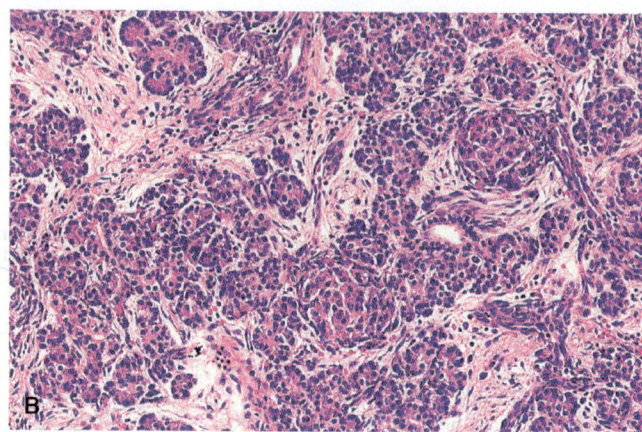
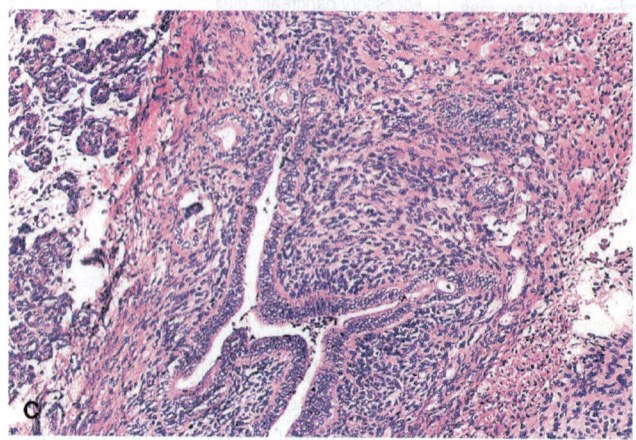

FIGURE 29.7 The fetal pancreas at 18 to 20 weeks of gestation exhibits a well-developed lobular architecture (**A**). The loose connective tissue between the lobules is relatively abundant. Both acinar and neuroendocrine elements are well developed (**B**) and are functioning at this stage. The mesenchyme surrounding the ducts is highly cellular (**C**), resembling the so-called ovarian-like stroma of mucinous cystic neoplasms.

the acinar fate segregate into the tips of the ductal network while future neuroendocrine and ductal cells are allocated to the trunk domain (39,40). The pancreatic lobules are formed by the accumulation of acinar units around ductular branches that are separated by layers of mesenchyme. By the 4th month the acinar cells contain zymogen granules (16). Ultrastructurally, the earliest granules identified in acinar cells are elongated and angular, with a fibrillary internal matrix. These granules, along with small spherical granules, may be detected at 15 to 20 weeks gestation (41–43). By 20 weeks, the granules resemble the zymogen granules of the adult pancreas and the elongate granules disappear. The nature of the elongate granules remains unclear, and enzymes have yet to be detected in them. However, it is interesting that similar "irregular fibrillary granules" have been repeatedly detected in pancreatic neoplasms with acinar differentiation (42,44–48).

Islet cells also develop from the ducts at 8 to 10 weeks gestation, delaminating from the ductal epithelium into the surrounding mesenchyme, and later forming clusters (49). Insulin-expressing cells appear first, and over several weeks other cells emerge that express glucagon, somatostatin, and pancreatic polypeptides (50). In even the earliest developing islets, differentiated alpha and beta cells can be recognized (51–53). At 16 weeks the alpha and beta cells segregate to opposite ends of the islets; these bipolar islets are gradually replaced between 18 and 20 weeks by mantle islets having a central core of beta cells surrounded by a rim of alpha cells (52–54). Maturity of the islets is reached in late gestation and the early postnatal period (55). Although the microscopic architecture of the mature adult islets is more complex, the peripheral location of the alpha cells is roughly maintained in mature islets.

During the 3rd to 4th months the pancreatic tissue becomes increasingly organized around the branching ductal structures to form lobules (Fig. 29.7A,B). The characteristics of the ductal lining cells specific to their level within the ductal system become established during this period. The mesenchymal elements of the early pancreas are prominent. The early periductal stroma is highly cellular (Fig. 29.7C), resembling the ovarian-like subepithelial stroma that characterizes mucinous cystic neoplasms (56,57). As the pancreas develops, the mesenchyme becomes increasingly less abundant and less cellular, ultimately constituting a relatively minimal component of the adult gland.

Developmental Anomalies and Heterotopia

Complete or partial pancreatic agenesis is rare. Complete agenesis can be isolated or part of a congenital syndrome such as polysplenia/heterotaxy syndrome (58). Pancreatic agenesis can results from germline abnormalities in genes that code for key transcription factors in pancreatic development, including *PDX1*, *PTF1A*, and *GATA6*. Most individuals with partial pancreatic agenesis survive, but depending upon the amount of pancreatic tissue that develops, they may have diabetes mellitus.

Pancreatic hypoplasia, also referred to as congenital short pancreas, is more common than pancreatic agenesis. This condition may be a component of a congenital syndrome or present as an isolated anomaly (58). Germline mutations in *HNF1B* are associated with pancreatic hypoplasia. These individuals may also show exocrine dysfunction, maturity-onset diabetes, and anomalies of the renal and genital tract (59,60). The pancreas appears shortened but otherwise retains the normal appearing lobular architecture. Pancreatic hypoplasia can be asymptomatic or associated with hypofunction (61–64).

Annular or ring pancreas is an extremely rare developmental anomaly in which there is partial or complete encircling of the second part of the duodenum by pancreatic tissue (Fig. 29.8). Pancreas divisum usually accompanies annular pancreas (65), and the condition affects only 0.015% of the population. Possibly it is the failure of one of the lobes of the ventral embryonic bud to regress, causing it to encircle the duodenum during the normal rotation of the duodenum. Annular pancreas commonly causes duodenal obstruction which varies in severity and age of onset, depending on the extent of luminal constriction. Some cases are also associated with duodenal atresia (66). The band of pancreatic tissue partially or completely encircling the duodenum is flattened and may be embedded within the muscularis propria. Histologically, the annular tissue contains all of the normal parenchymal elements intermixed with smooth muscle. Because the portion of pancreas encircling the duodenum is derived from the ventral pancreas, it is rich in pancreatic polypeptide–containing islets (67).

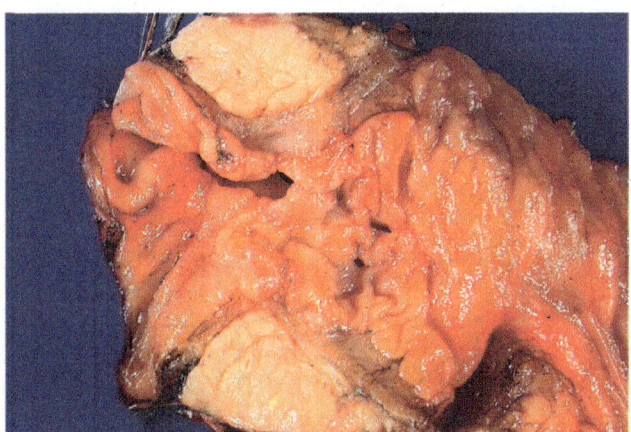

FIGURE 29.8 Annular pancreas. The pancreatic tissue completely encircles the duodenum, which is opened longitudinally to. Reprinted with permission from Hruban RH, Pitman MB, Klimstra DS. Tumors of the pancreas. In: Silverberg SG, Sobin LH, eds. *Atlas of Tumor Pathology*. 4th ed. Washington, DC: American Registry of Pathology; 2006.

There are many variations in the anatomy of the pancreatic duct system and in its relationship to the common bile duct (20,66,68,69). The embryonic communication between the dorsal pancreatic duct and the duodenum fails to obliterate in up to 50% of adults resulting in a patent accessory duct (of Santorini) at the minor papilla, about 2 cm proximal to the opening of the main duct and bile duct at the major papilla. In a minority of such instances (4%) the dorsal duct may provide the main route of drainage for the gland and may be much larger in diameter than the ventral duct (69). This condition appears to be more prevalent in children, suggesting that obliteration of the accessory duct opening may continue to occur in adulthood (70). Also, the ducts of the dorsal and ventral buds may also fail to fuse entirely, resulting in two separate ductal systems, a condition known as pancreas divisum. This anomaly occurs in 5% to 10% of individuals. The pancreatic parenchyma of the two lobes is usually fused in individuals with pancreas divisum, so the abnormality may not be detected unless a careful study of the ductal system is performed. There are three types of pancreas divisum: type 1 or classical pancreas divisum involves total failure of the ducts to fuse, causing most of the pancreatic secretions to drain through the duct of Santorini at the diminutive minor papilla, with the duct of Wirsung draining only the inferior head of the pancreas through the major papilla; type 2 involves dominant dorsal drainage in which the ventral duct regresses completely, leaving the single dorsal duct at the minor papilla as the only means of egress for exocrine secretions; and type 3 involves incomplete pancreas divisum, where a small communicating branch of the ventral duct remains. Although hotly debated, pancreas divisum is probably not associated with acute or chronic pancreatitis (69,71,72).

Anomalous junction of the main pancreatic duct with the distal common bile duct may occur within the head of the pancreas more than 2 cm proximal to the duodenum (20,66). This abnormality may be associated with choledochal cysts and carcinomas of the extrahepatic bile ducts or gallbladder (20,73,74). In a rare abnormality of the pancreatic duct, bifid pancreas, the main pancreatic duct bifurcates within the body of the pancreas (75).

Pancreatic heterotopia is defined as pancreatic tissue located outside of the normal anatomic position of the gland (66). Heterotopic pancreatic tissue is found in portions of the upper gastrointestinal tract and its appendages in up to 1.5% of individuals at autopsy. The surgical or endoscopic incidence, however, is only 0.1% to 0.2%. Twenty-five to 50% of the cases detected during life are symptomatic (76–78). Although it is presumed to be congenital in origin, most symptomatic cases are detected in adulthood (76). The stomach and duodenum are the most common locations of pancreatic heterotopia, most duodenal cases occurring in the second portion several centimeters proximal to the ampulla of Vater. Often the tissue is found in the submucosa beneath the minor duodenal papilla and represents remnants of the embryonic dorsal ductal system. Pancreatic heterotopia also may occur elsewhere in the duodenum and may involve the ampulla of

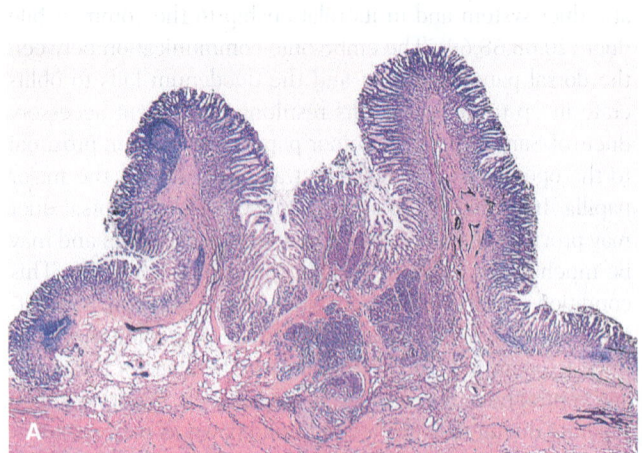
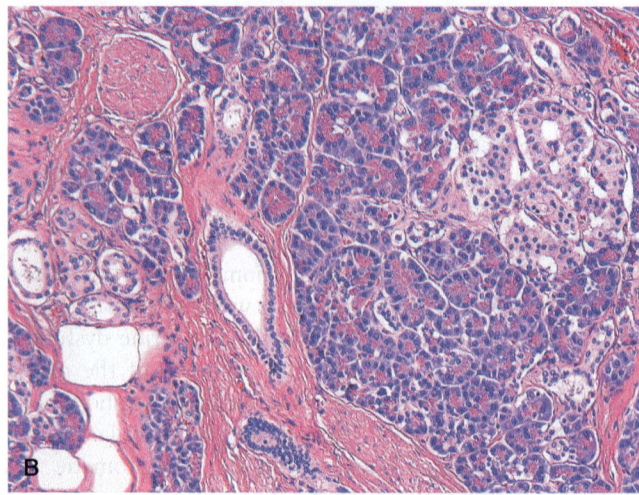

FIGURE 29.9 Heterotopic pancreatic tissue in the stomach. At low power, a submucosal nodule of pancreatic tissue results in an umbilicated appearance (**A**). In this example there are acini, ducts, and islets arranged in a disorganized pattern, with interspersed bundles of smooth muscle (**B**).

Vater (79,80). Other sites of pancreatic heterotopia include the jejunum, Meckel diverticulum, the large bowel, spleen, gallbladder, mesentery, and the liver, where it is generally located around the bile ducts (81,82). In the tubular gastrointestinal tract, heterotopic pancreas appears as lobulated submucosal nodules of yellow to white firm tissue ranging from several millimeters to several centimeters in size. The overlying mucosa may be umbilicated in larger examples but appears otherwise unremarkable (Fig. 29.9A). Rarely heterotopic pancreatic tissue is present on the serosal surface or in perigastric fat. Microscopically the type and amount of the different pancreatic cell types varies. Most cases have acini and ducts. Pancreatic heterotopia with only ducts can be surrounded by interlacing smooth muscle fascicles appearing as an "adenomyoma" (Fig. 29.9B). All three elements, including ducts, acini, and islets, are present in 12% of cases (82). Some duodenal foci of heterotopic pancreas exhibit acini with the features of Brunner glands, emphasizing the embryologic relationship these glands have with the pancreas (19). One of the important reasons to recognize heterotopic pancreas is to avoid misinterpretation of these ductules as carcinoma; however, any process that involves pancreas can arise in these foci, including adenocarcinoma (83–85). Benign processes such as chronic pancreatitis and pseudocysts can arise and rarely, other pancreatic neoplasms have arisen in heterotopic pancreas, including pancreatic intraepithelial neoplasia (PanIN), intraductal papillary mucinous neoplasm (IPMN), acinar cell carcinoma, and pancreatic neuroendocrine tumor (86–89).

Heterotopic tissues also may be found within the pancreas. Accessory splenic tissue may be found in the tail of the pancreas or more rarely in the head (90). In most cases the splenic tissue is small (less than 2 cm), dark red, and spherical. Intrapancreatic adrenal cortical tissue has also been described (91). Developmental cysts such as foregut cysts can also occur in the pancreas, where they can mimic pancreatic cystic neoplasms (Fig. 29.10).

MICROSCOPIC FEATURES

Microscopically the pancreas is arranged in 1- to 10-mm lobules (Fig. 29.11). The parenchyma within the lobules consists almost entirely of the epithelial elements, including the acini, the ducts, and the islets of Langerhans. There is minimal intralobular connective tissue, but fibroconnective tissue containing vessels and nerves separates the lobules.

Acini

Acinar cells make up approximately 85% of the mass of the pancreas and constitute the main exocrine secretory component of the gland. The prototypical architecture of the acinus in routine histologic sections appears to be a single layer of polygonal cells surrounding a minute central lumen,

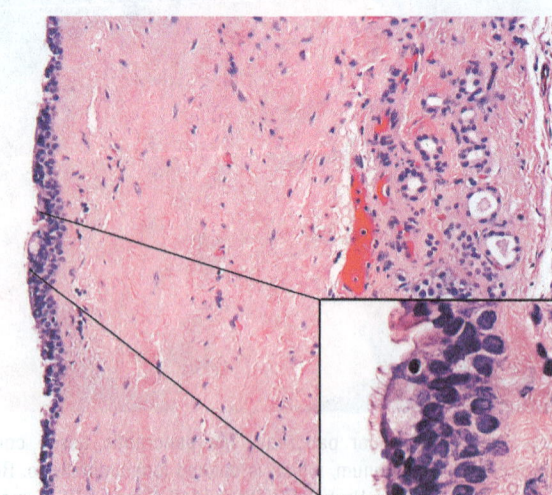

FIGURE 29.10 A rare pancreatic foregut cyst is lined by a single layer of ciliated columnar epithelial cells (*inset*).

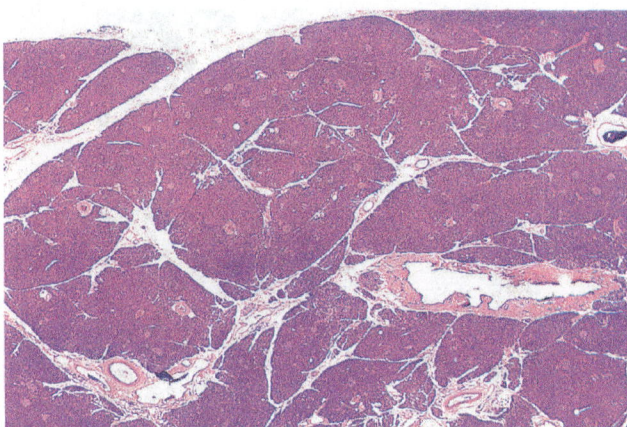

FIGURE 29.11 At low power, the normal pancreas has a well-developed lobular arrangement of highly cellular glandular tissue.

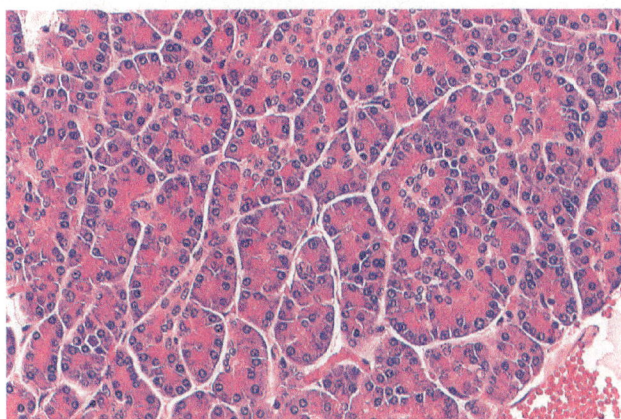

FIGURE 29.13 Other acini have tubular configurations and exhibit interanastomosing loops when studied by serial sectioning.

suggesting a spherical configuration (Fig. 29.12); however, the three-dimensional architecture of the pancreatic acini is much more complex (92). In fact, tubular acini are commonly detected in histologic sections (Fig. 29.13). Also, not all acini are located at the terminal end of ductules. Some acini bud from the sides of the ductules or are situated between two ductules. Anastomosing loops of acini also may be found (92). Thus, the secretions of a given acinus may pass through a number of different pathways to reach the ductal system.

Individual acinar cells are polarized, with basally situated round nuclei and apical granular eosinophilic cytoplasm. The eosinophilia of the apical cytoplasm reflects the accumulation of numerous zymogen granules (Fig. 29.12), which contrast with the basophilic zymogen granules of salivary serous acini. The zymogen granule content is highly dynamic, depending on the secretory state of the pancreas, which is regulated by digestive hormones (1). The basal cytoplasm of the acinar cells is basophilic due to the abundant rough endoplasmic reticulum (RER), with its high concentration of ribonucleoproteins. There may be a clear cytoplasmic zone on the luminal side of the nucleus that contains the Golgi apparatus. The nuclei are uniform and frequently contain small but distinct central nucleoli; clumps of chromatin are generally present beneath the nuclear membrane. The acinar cells sit directly upon the basement membrane; in contrast to salivary acini, there are no myoepithelial cells surrounding the pancreatic acini.

Although the acinar cells from different regions of the pancreas are all morphologically and functionally similar, there are subtle differences in the size and zymogen granule content in the acinar cells immediately adjacent to islets compared with those distant from islets, perhaps as a reflection of regional variations in islet hormone levels (93,94).

Zymogen granules stain positively with periodic acid–Schiff (PAS) stain, and the staining is resistant to diastase digestion (Fig. 29.14). Acinar cells also can be demonstrated using stains for butyrate esterase, which is positive in the

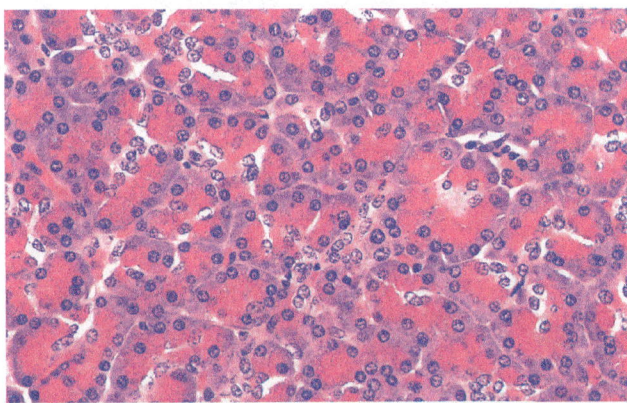

FIGURE 29.12 Acinar cells contain abundant granular eosinophilic cytoplasm in the apical aspect, with basophilic basal cytoplasm. The nuclei are also basally located. Most acini consist of spherically arranged individual acinar cells.

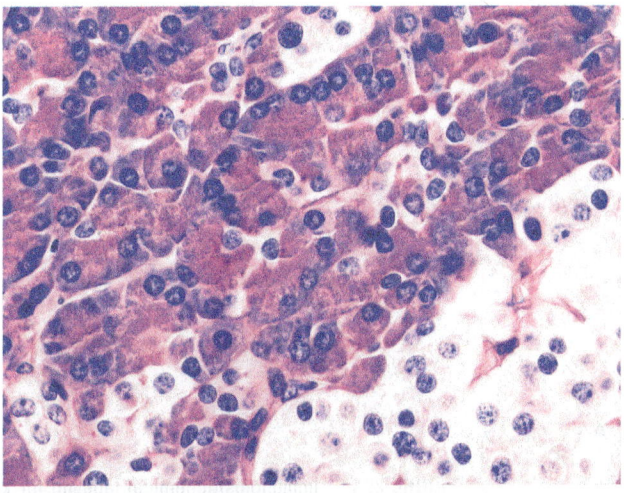

FIGURE 29.14 Zymogen granules are positive with periodic acid–Schiff stain with diastase pretreatment. Islet cells (*lower right*) are negative.

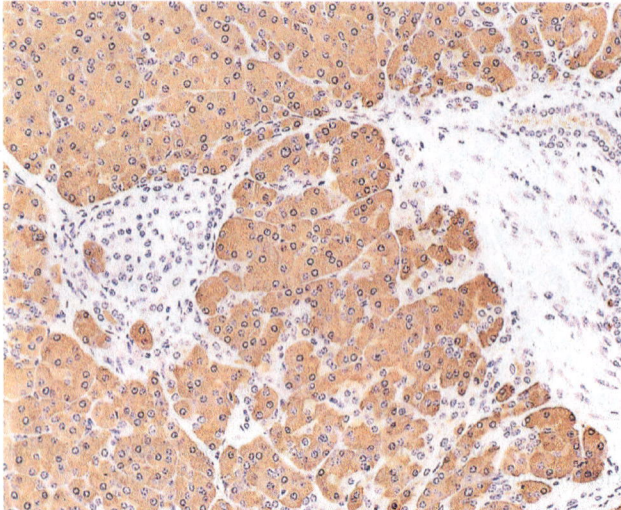

FIGURE 29.15 Immunohistochemical staining for trypsin results in intense labeling of acinar cells but not ductal and islet cells. Faint luminal labeling of ductal cells may be seen due to deposition of luminal enzymatic secretions on the apical cell surfaces (*upper right*).

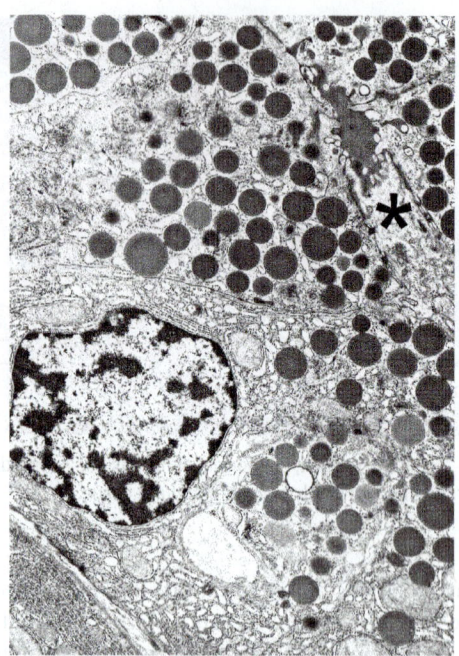

FIGURE 29.17 The ultrastructural appearance of acinar cells. These polarized cells have abundant parallel stacks of rough endoplasmic reticulum with interspersed mitochondria in the basal cytoplasm. Homogeneous electron-dense zymogen granules are concentrated in the apical cytoplasm underlying the lumina. The luminal spaces are lined by short microvilli. Adjacent acinar cells are joined to one another and to the centroacinar cells (*asterisk*) by apical junctional complexes. The centroacinar cells have lucent cytoplasm devoid of secretory granules.

presence of enzymatically active lipase (45). Immunohistochemical labeling for pancreatic enzymes such as trypsin, chymotrypsin, lipase, amylase, and elastase is positive in acinar cells (Fig. 29.15) and with the exception of amylase, these stains are also sensitive markers for acinar differentiation in pancreatic neoplasms (45–47,95) Antibodies directed against the C-terminal of BCL10 also detect acinar differentiation due to homology between BCL10 and the digestive enzyme carboxyl ester hydrolase (96). Each individual zymogen granule contains all of the various digestive enzymes, usually in a proenzyme form (97,98). Keratins detected by the CAM5.2 antibody (cytokeratin 8 and cytokeratin 18) are present in acinar cells; however, the AE1 antibody and antibodies against cytokeratins 7, 19, and 20 do not label normal acinar cells (Fig. 29.16). Mucins are not produced, and immunohistochemical labeling for glycoproteins such as DUPAN-2, CEA, CA19.9, and MUC proteins is negative. Finally, neuroendocrine specific antibodies such as chromogranin and synaptophysin are negative as well.

Ultrastructural examination shows features characteristic of active exocrine secretion. The RER is arranged in parallel stacks and fills the basal cytoplasm (Fig. 29.17).

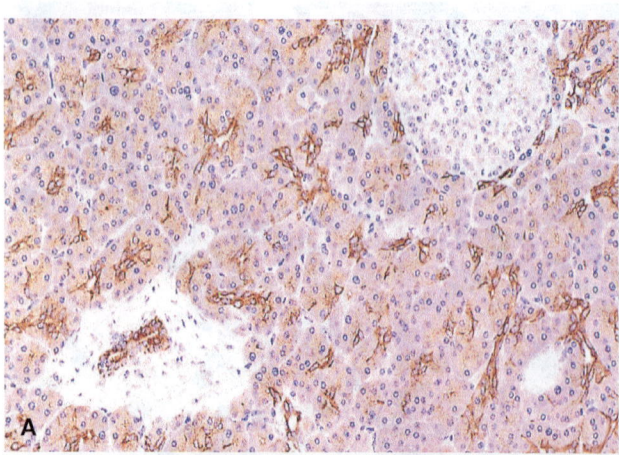
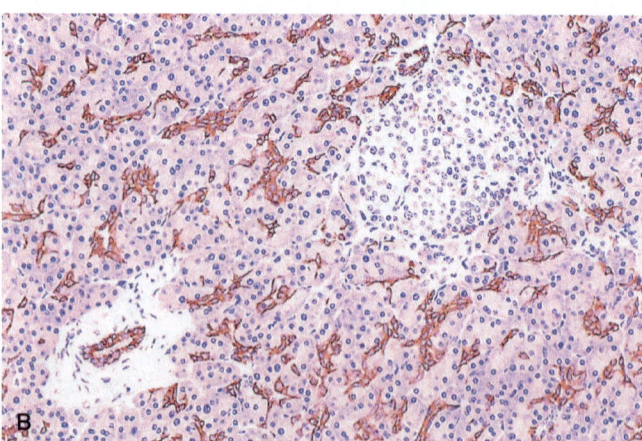

FIGURE 29.16 Immunohistochemical labeling for keratins. The CAM5.2 antibody shows diffuse labeling of acinar cells and ductal cells, the latter being more intensely positive (**A**). The AE1/AE3 antibodies label only ductal cells (**B**). Islet cells show only focal faint labeling with these antibodies.

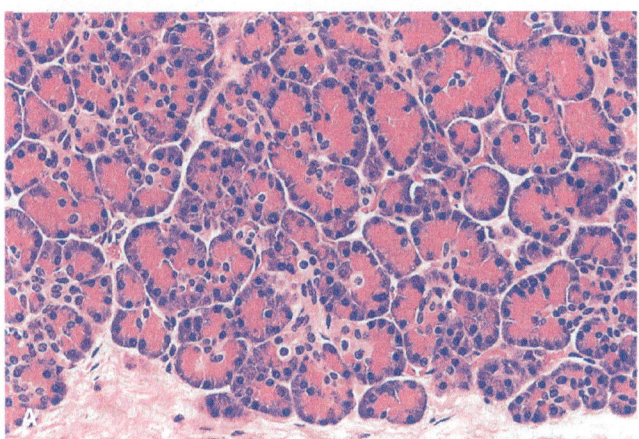 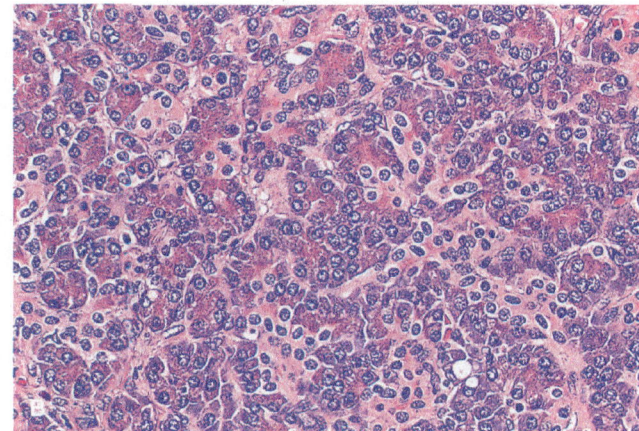

FIGURE 29.18 Most centroacinar cells are inconspicuous small cells with minimal cytoplasm and oval nuclei situated in the center of the acini (**A**). In other regions the centroacinar cells may be more prominent, with more abundant lightly eosinophilic cytoplasm (**B**). Centroacinar cells constitute the beginning of the ductal system and convey the secretions of acinar cells to the intercalated ducts.

Scattered mitochondria and free polyribosomes are present between RER cisternae (99). The Golgi apparatus is situated in the central region of the cytoplasm near the nucleus. Immature electron-dense zymogen granules emanate from the *trans* side of the Golgi apparatus. Larger round, homogeneous mature zymogen granules are present within the apical cytoplasm. They measure 250 to 1,000 nm and have dense secretory content with closely opposed limiting membranes. Upon stimulation, the membranes of the secretory granules fuse with the apical plasma membrane, expelling the contents into the lumen; the excess cell membranes are then recycled to the Golgi apparatus (100,101). Accumulated secretions are often present within the lumina, sometimes with crystal formation. The luminal membranes have sparse, short microvilli containing inner microfilaments that are continuous with the terminal web of filaments beneath the apical membrane (99). Adjacent acinar cells are joined by apical junctional complexes composed of zonula occludens- and zonula adherens-type junctions, whereas desmosomes (macula adherens junctions) join cells along the basal aspects of their lateral membranes (16,99). Each acinus is surrounded by a continuous basement membrane.

Ducts

The ductal system of the pancreas has diverse structure and function along its course. The ductal epithelial cells secrete approximately two liters of fluid per day composed of water, chloride, and bicarbonate via transmembrane electrolyte and fluid transporters. Ductal fluid buffers the acidity of the pancreatic juices, transports acinar secretions, and stabilizes the proenzymes secreted by acini until they become activated within the duodenum (102). The ductal system is subdivided into five continuous segments: centroacinar cells; intercalated ducts; intralobular ducts; interlobular ducts (large and small); and main ducts (103). The ductal system begins with the centroacinar cells, which are small, relatively inconspicuous, flat to cuboidal cells with pale or lightly eosinophilic cytoplasm and central oval nuclei (Fig. 29.18). Centroacinar cells are located in the middle of the acini, where they partially border the acinar lumina along with the acinar cells, to which they are joined by tight junctions. Ultrastructurally the centroacinar cells have cytoplasms largely devoid of organelles, with only scattered mitochondria; no zymogen, neurosecretory, or mucigen granules are present. Relative to the acinar cells, the cytoplasm is less dense and RER is minimal. The cell surfaces contain scattered short microvilli similar to those on the adjacent acinar cells. Adjacent cells are joined by abundant junctional complexes, and there are often complex interdigitations between them. Some centroacinar cells have more abundant granular oncocytic cytoplasm (Fig. 29.19)

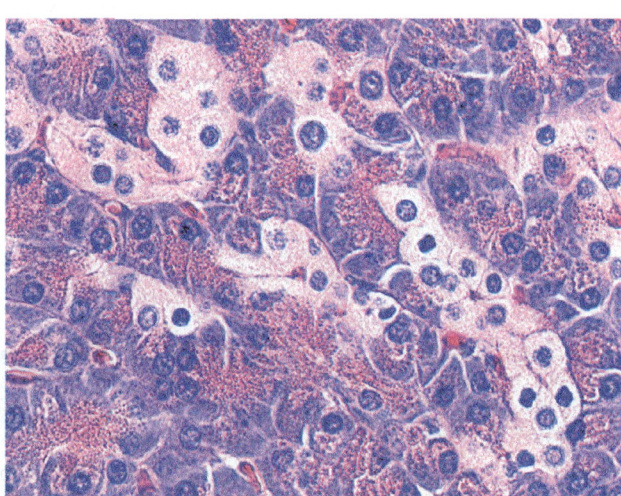

FIGURE 29.19 Some centroacinar cells are enlarged and have oncocytic cytoplasm, a variation of uncertain significance.

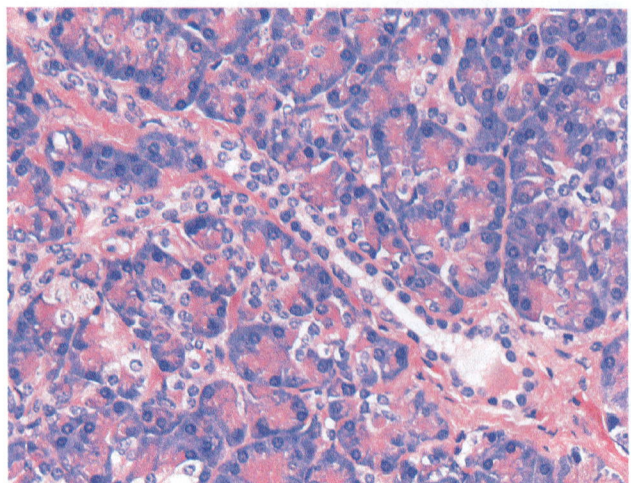

FIGURE 29.20 The ductal system within the lobules consists of innumerable intercalated ducts that fuse to form intralobular ducts. The cytologic appearance of the intercalated and intralobular ductal cells resembles that of the centroacinar cells, and the transition from one to the next is imperceptible. Only minimal collagenized stroma surrounds the intralobular ducts (*lower right*).

that reflects numerous mitochondria (103,104); the significance of this variation is unknown.

The lumen surrounded by acinar and centroacinar cells drains into the intercalated ducts, which are the smallest ducts outside the acini but supply most of the fluid secreted by the pancreas via aquaporin water channels (Fig. 29.20) (105,106). The cells lining the intercalated ducts resemble the centroacinar cells. They are cuboidal and have central oval nuclei with indistinct nucleoli. Mucins are not detected with alcian blue or mucicarmine stains in centroacinar or intercalated duct cells. The intercalated ducts fuse to form the intralobular ducts, and the transition is imperceptible. The cells lining the intralobular ducts are essentially identical to those of the intercalated ducts, although the nuclei are round rather than oval (Fig. 29.20). Neither intercalated nor intralobular ducts have a significant collagenous matrix surrounding them. The ductal cells rest directly on the basement membrane and lack both myoepithelial and basal cells; thus, in contrast to several other organs, the presence or absence of these cells cannot be used to help distinguish benign ducts from invasive pancreatic ductal adenocarcinoma.

Once the ducts leave the lobules, they become enveloped by a variably thick rim of collagen and are termed interlobular ducts (Fig. 29.21). The interlobular ductal cells have slightly more cytoplasm than those of the intralobular ducts and assume a low columnar shape in the larger ducts. As in the smaller ducts, cytoplasmic mucin is not detectable by routine histology in intralobular or interlobular ductal cells; mucinous cytoplasm visible by routine histology is considered a pathologic change signifying neoplastic transforamtion (see below). However, some cytoplasmic mucin may be found using special stains. As the interlobular ducts approach the main pancreatic ducts (of Wirsung or Santorini), they develop an increasingly thick collagenous wall within which lobular aggregates of small ductules may be seen, resembling the ductules of Beale that surround the major bile ducts (Fig. 29.22).

The main pancreatic ducts receive numerous tributaries of interlobular ducts (Fig. 29.23). The lining epithelium remains flat, without papillary projections, except in the very distal duct within the ampulla, where simple papillae are found (Fig. 29.24). The cells are low columnar with basal round nuclei. In these large ducts, there may be apical cytoplasmic clearing, reflecting mucin, but tall columnar cells with obvious abundant mucin are not normally found, and special stains are often needed to identify the mucin (103). The mucins of the intralobular and smaller interlobular ductal cells are predominantly sulphomucins and stain positively with alcian blue at pH 1.0 (Fig. 29.25)

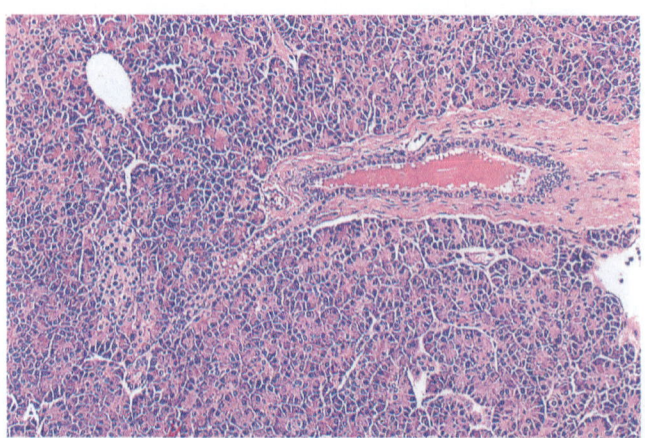
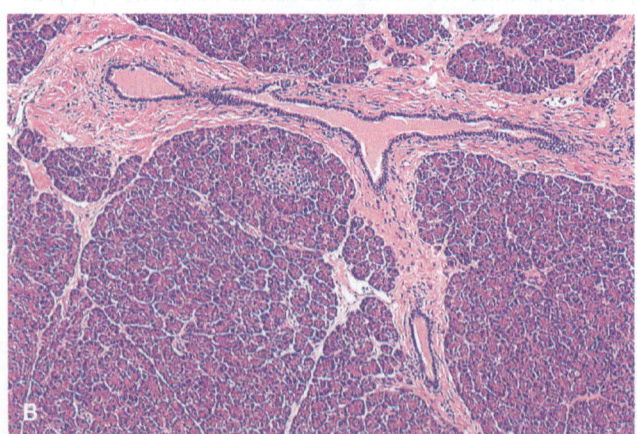

FIGURE 29.21 Intralobular ducts come together to form interlobular ducts (**A**). The interlobular ducts are surrounded by a variably thick rim of dense fibrous tissue and carry the pancreatic secretions to the major ducts, receiving tributaries of small interlobular ducts as they pass through the connective tissue septa of the gland (**B**).

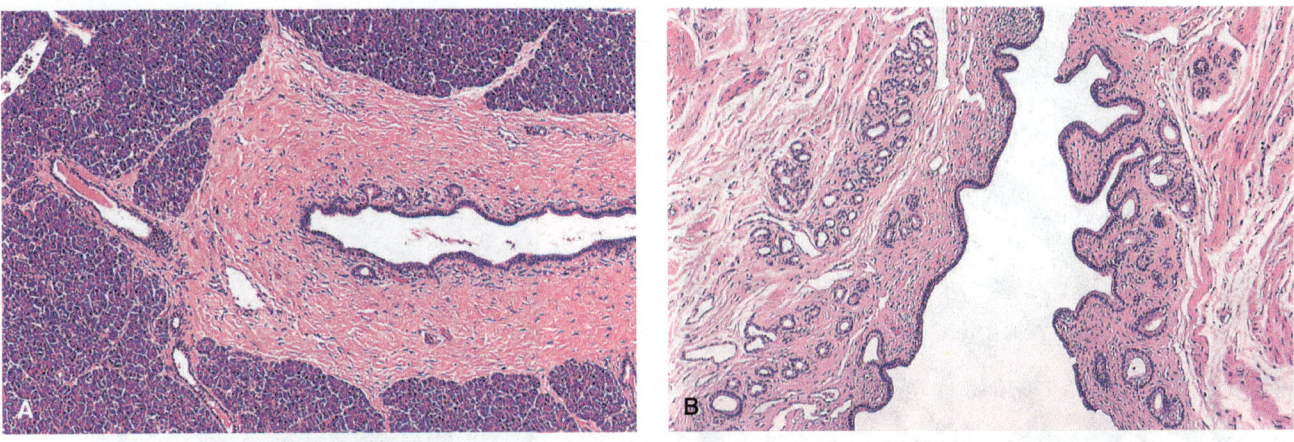

FIGURE 29.22 The largest interlobular ducts are surrounded by a thick rim of collagen (**A**). Small lobular aggregates of ductules are present within the wall of the larger ducts (**B**).

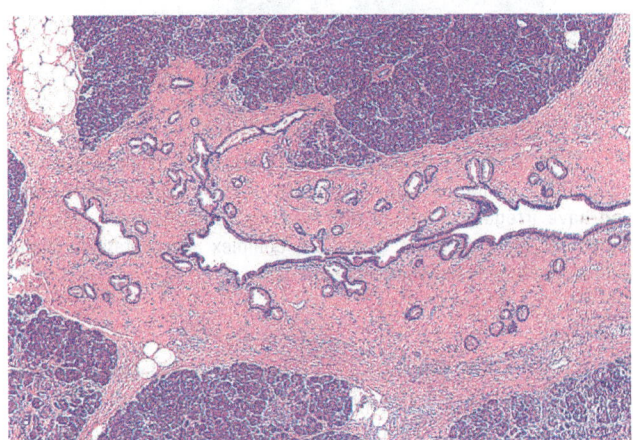

FIGURE 29.23 Numerous interlobular ducts join the main pancreatic duct along its course.

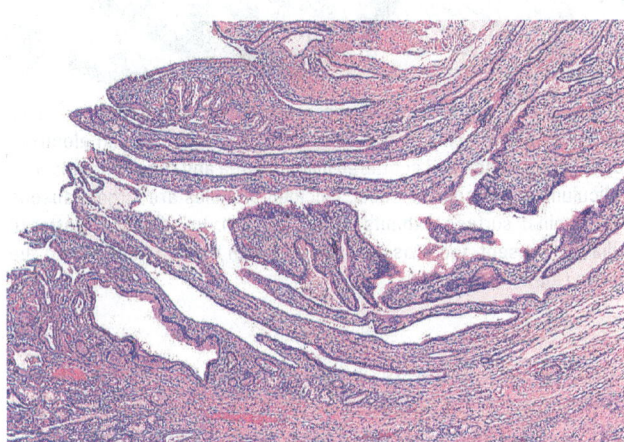

FIGURE 29.24 As the main pancreatic duct enters the ampulla of Vater, the ductal epithelium forms broad, simple papillae known as the valves of Santorini.

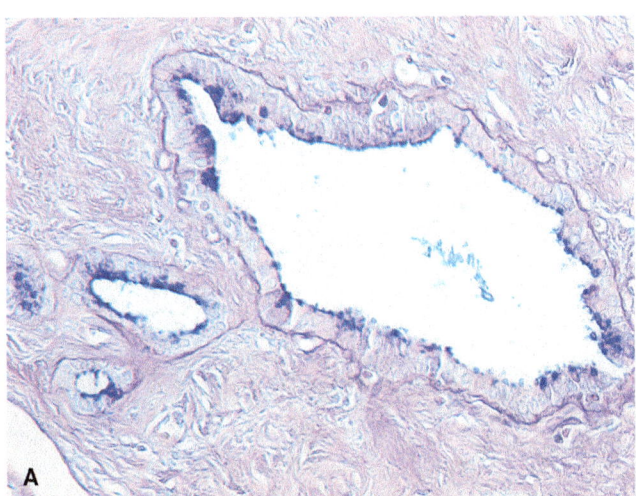
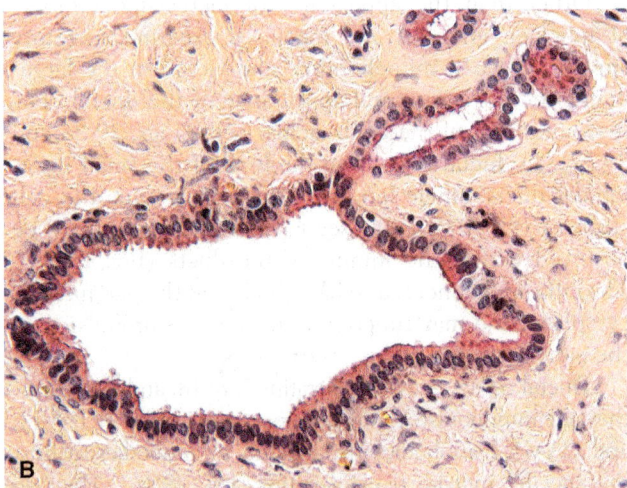

FIGURE 29.25 The cells of the intralobular and smaller interlobular ducts contain mucin in the apical cytoplasm that stains positively with Alcian blue/PAS (**A**). Staining with mucicarmine shows a similar distribution of mucin (**B**).

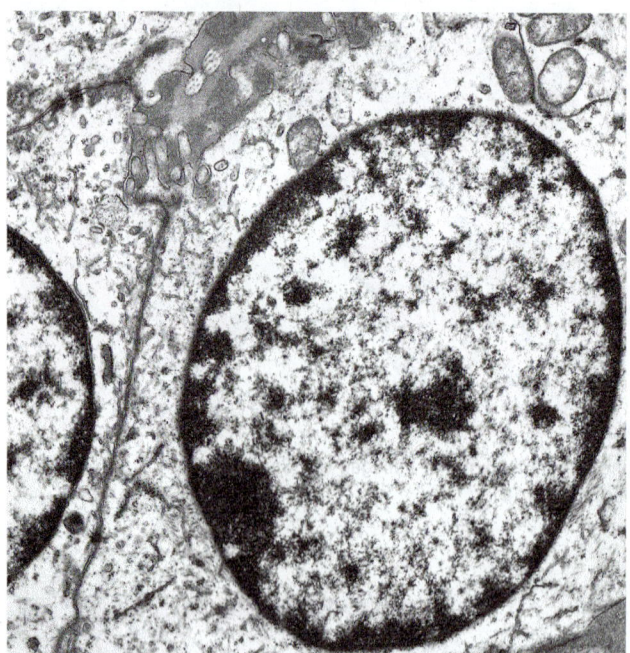

FIGURE 29.26 Ultrastructural appearance of intralobular ductal cells. The cytoplasm resembles that of centroacinar cells, with an electron-lucent appearance and scattered mitochondria and rough endoplasmic reticulum. In the smaller ducts, mucigen granules are largely absent. The luminal surface exhibits short microvilli. In addition, scattered cilia are present, the cross section of which may be seen within the lumen (*top*).

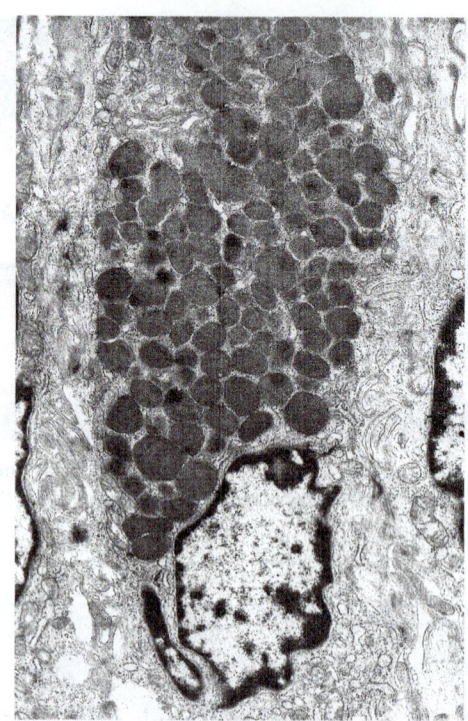

FIGURE 29.27 In the larger ducts, more abundant mucigen granules accumulate within the apical cytoplasm. These granules vary in size and have irregular contours and heterogeneous, variably electron-dense secretory contents. There are complex interdigitations of the lateral membranes between adjacent cells.

(107,108). In the cells of the larger ducts there are fewer sulphomucins and more neutral mucins and sialomucins (107). There is relatively frequent cell exfoliation in the main duct, perhaps reflecting a high turnover rate due to injury; degenerating cells may be observed within the epithelium by electron microscopy (99). The thick connective tissue wall contains numerous periductal ductules, as well as fascicles of smooth muscle (1).

Other than the appearance of increasing numbers of mucigen granules and increased exocrine secretory apparatus (RER, mitochondria, and Golgi) in the larger ducts, the ultrastructural appearance of the ductal cells resembles that of the centroacinar cells (Figs. 29.26 and 29.27). In ductal cells from the level of the small interlobular ducts, single long kinocilia project from the cell surfaces (99,103); cross sections of these cilia may be observed within the lumina of the ducts (Fig. 29.26). The cilia are connected to basal bodies in the paranuclear cytoplasm and may function in mixing and propulsion of the pancreatic secretions (109).

Ductal cells express cytokeratins 7, 8, 18, and 19; hence, they are immunohistochemically reactive with the AE1, AE3, and CAM5.2 antibodies, in addition to antibodies against the specific individual cytokeratins (Fig. 29.16). They do not normally express cytokeratin 20. Exocrine enzyme and neuroendocrine markers are also negative in the ductal cells themselves, although individual neuroendocrine cells can be found within the larger ducts (see below), and enzyme markers often label the apical surface of ductal cells due to precipitation of luminal enzymatic contents. Carbonic anhydrase is detectable in ductal cells, reflecting their role in fluid and ion transport (110); most is detected in intercalated and intralobular ducts (111), although ducts of larger caliber may weakly express this enzyme (Fig. 29.28). Other

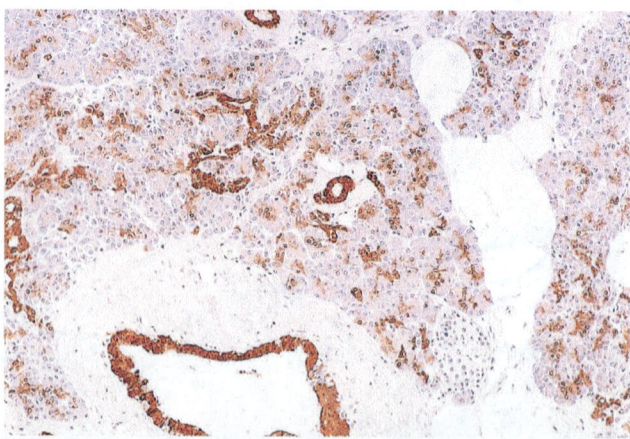

FIGURE 29.28 Immunohistochemical staining for carbonic anhydrase. In this preparation, there is staining of ductal cells of all sizes, including centroacinar, intercalated duct, as well as intralobular and interlobular ductal cells.

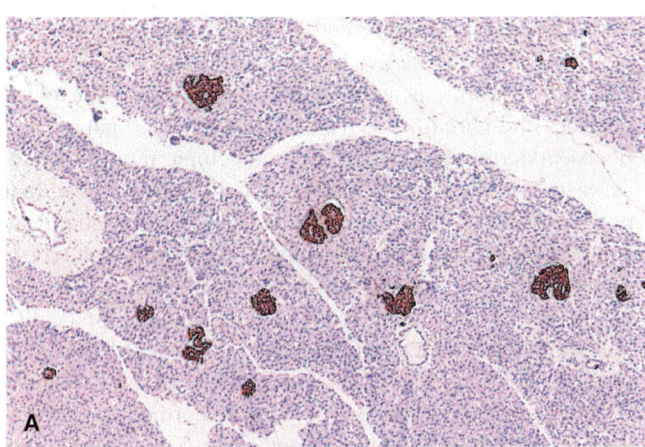 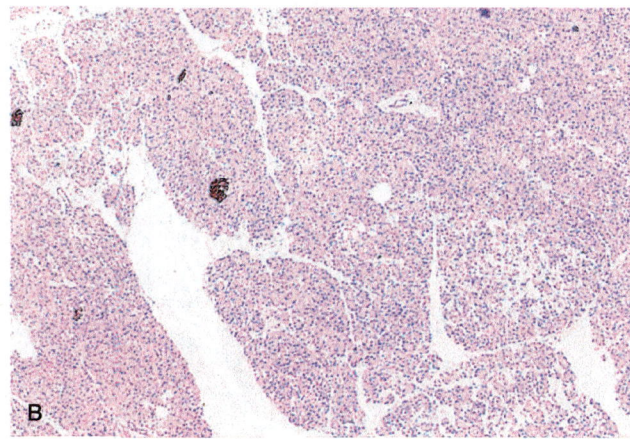

FIGURE 29.29 As highlighted by immunohistochemical labeling for chromogranin, the concentration of islets varies considerably from one lobule (**A**) to the next (**B**).

markers of ductal cells include antibodies against CA19-9, DUPAN-2, cystic fibrosis transmembrane conductance regulator (CFTR), N-terminal gastrin-releasing peptide (N-GRP), and transcription factors such as HNF1β, HNF6, and SOX9 (112–117). Normal ducts do not label with antibodies to carcinoembryonic antigen when monoclonal antisera are used (118) and also fail to label for B72.3 and CA125. Members of the MUC family of glycoproteins are variably expressed; MUC1 is present in smaller intralobular and intercalated ducts and MUC6 is expressed in centroacinar cells and intercalated ducts; MUC2, MUC4, and MUC5AC are not normally expressed (119–121).

Islets of Langerhans

The neuroendocrine component of the pancreas constitutes only 1% to 2% of the volume of the gland in adults (1,94) but about 10% in the newborn (108,122). The vast majority of neuroendocrine cells are found in the over one million islets of Langerhans, first described by Paul Langerhans in 1869. Although islets are distributed throughout the pancreas, they are somewhat more numerous in the tail (123,124). Apparently random variations in islet concentration may occur from one lobule to the next, resulting in the appearance of plentiful islets in one area and sparse islets in an adjacent region (Fig. 29.29).

The apparent volume of islets observed in histologic sections also varies with the age of the individual and the presence and extent of exocrine atrophy, as commonly occurs in chronic pancreatitis (125). In the fetus and neonate the relative volume of neuroendocrine cells far outmeasures that of the adult, especially in the portions derived from the dorsal lobe (Fig. 29.30) (126).

Two types of islets are found. Most (90%) are the compact islets: sharply circumscribed nests usually measuring 75 to 225 μm, although islets as small as 50 μm or as large as 280 μm also may be found (127). Compact islets are found predominantly in the body and tail of the gland, with fewer in the head. The second type of islet, the diffuse islet, is essentially restricted to the posteroinferior head of the gland derived from the embryonic ventral lobe (128,129). These islets are much less numerous than the compact islets and may measure up to 450 μm.

Despite the circumscribed appearance of the compact islets, they are actually composed of interdigitating trabecula that appears as small lobules in cross section (127). Most cells of the compact islets have uniform round nuclei with coarsely clumped chromatin and inconspicuous nucleoli (Fig. 29.31). The cytoplasm is pale and amphophilic. Occasional islet cells have nuclei two to four times the size of their neighbors, although no irregularities of shape or chromatin pattern are present. These nuclei have a 4n or 8n DNA content and have been shown to occur exclusively in beta cells (130); they do not have any pathologic significance. Mitotic figures are extremely rare in normal islets (131). The islets contain numerous small vessels, although these capillary-sized vessels are almost inapparent

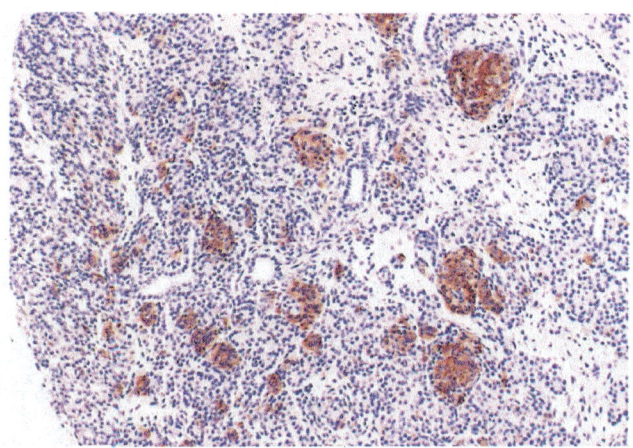

FIGURE 29.30 A fetal pancreas stained immunohistochemically for chromogranin. Note the abundance of neuroendocrine cells relative to acinar cells at this stage of development.

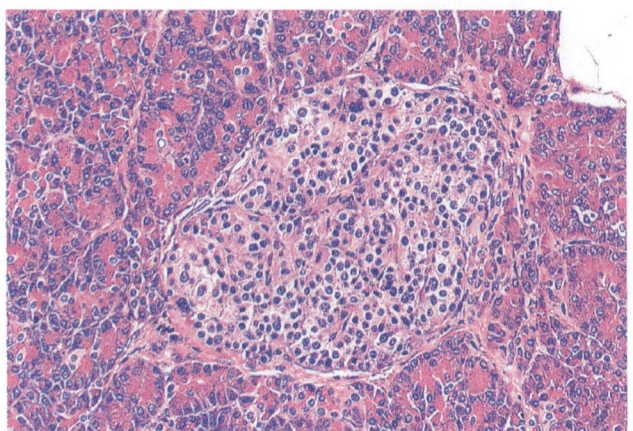

FIGURE 29.31 Compact islets consist of round to oval, generally circumscribed collections of neuroendocrine cells. Small capillaries separate the islet into lobules. The nuclei have a stippled chromatin pattern and there is moderate amphophilic cytoplasm. Some islet cells contain enlarged nuclei several times the size of those in the neighboring cells.

by light microscopy. Essentially all of the islet cells contact the vasculature (132). In contrast to those supplying the acinar tissue, the capillaries of the islets have a fenestrated endothelium (1). A thin layer of connective tissue separates the compact islets from the surrounding acinar tissue, but they are not truly encapsulated.

Diffuse islets have a trabecular appearance, with winding cords of cells intermingled among acini (Fig. 29.32A). Compared to compact islets, they are composed of more columnar shaped cells. The cytoplasm is basophilic, the nuclei are somewhat hyperchromatic, and there may be more prominent nucleoli than in the compact islets (Fig. 29.32B). Because they are less commonly encountered and have a pseudoinfiltrative appearance, diffuse islets may be mistakenly regarded as neoplastic, especially in the setting of chronic pancreatitis.

Each neuroendocrine cell produces only one specific peptide hormone. The five major peptides produced by islet cells are insulin, glucagon, somatostatin, pancreatic polypeptide, and ghrelin (133,134). Although some pancreatic neuroendocrine neoplasms produce ectopic peptides such as gastrin or vasoactive intestinal polypeptide, these are not expressed in normal islet cells. Classical histochemical staining can be used to distinguish the different cell types. Aldehyde-fuchsin stains insulin-secreting beta cells, the Grimelius silver stain labels glucagon-secreting alpha cells, and the Hellerstrom–Hellman silver stain identifies somatostatin-secreting delta cells. Immunohistochemical labeling with antibodies against the peptide hormones provides a more specific method to distinguish the cell types. There is a fairly consistent distribution of the cell types within the compact islets. The beta cells are more centrally located, whereas the alpha cells populate the periphery of the islet lobules (Fig. 29.33). Beta cells constitute 60% to 70% and alpha cells make up 15% to 20% of the compact islets, whereas the delta (5% to 10%) and ghrelin secreting epsilon (~1%) cells are much less numerous (127,135). Alpha cells are generally found in close contact with delta cells (136). PP cells are rare in the compact islets, being concentrated in the diffuse islets where they constitute the majority (70%) of the cells (Fig. 29.34) (137–139). The remaining cells of the diffuse islets are largely beta cells (20%), with minor amounts of alpha and delta cells (5% of each). The difference in proportion of cell types between the compact and diffuse islets reflects their different embryologic origins (128,129). The relative proportion of the different peptide-producing cells also varies with age; for instance, the ratio of beta to delta cells in the compact islets is manyfold higher in adults than in infants, in whom delta cells constitute one-third of the islet cell population (122,140). All of the islet cells also express general neuroendocrine markers such as neuron-specific enolase, CD56 (neural cell adhesion molecule), synaptophysin, and chromogranin

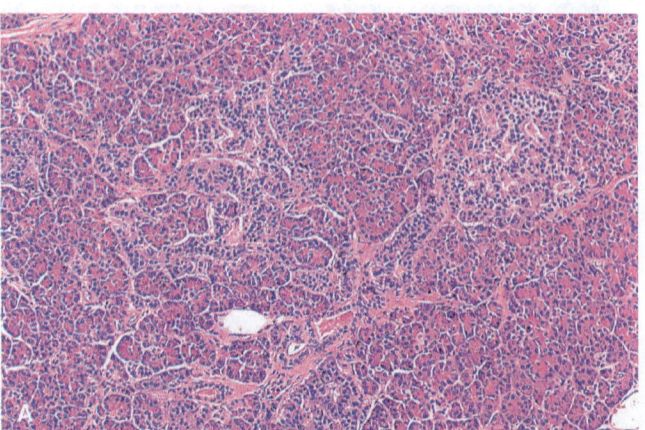 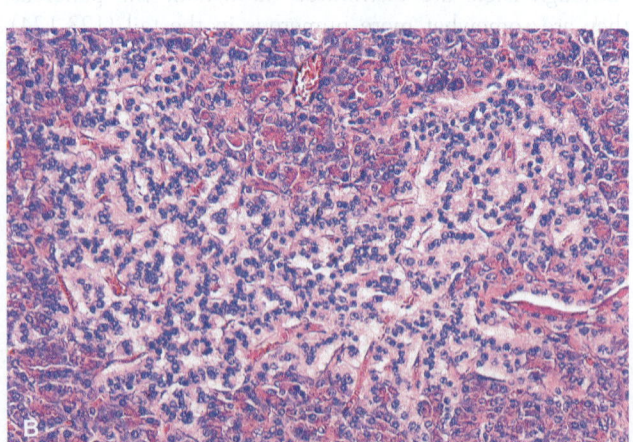

FIGURE 29.32 Diffuse islets are composed of trabeculae of neuroendocrine cells interspersed between adjacent acini (**A**). The borders of the diffuse islets are ill defined (**B**). The cells have somewhat basophilic cytoplasm.

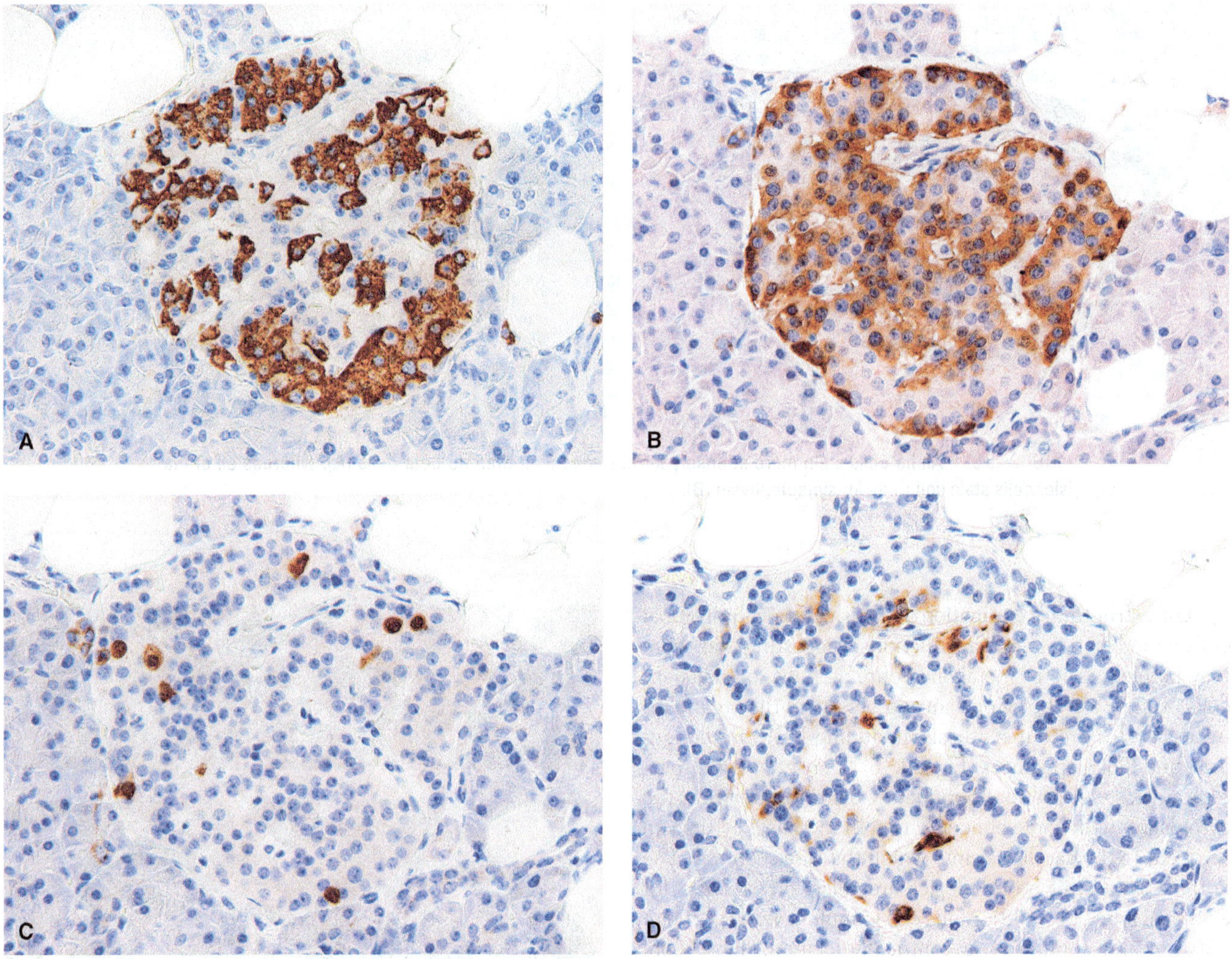

FIGURE 29.33 The distribution of the different peptide-producing cells within the islets of Langerhans. Beta cells (labeled for insulin) are the most numerous (**A**) and are situated in the central regions of the islet. Alpha cells (labeled for glucagon) are generally arranged around the periphery (**B**). Delta cells (labeled for somatostatin) (**C**) and PP cells (labeled for pancreatic polypeptide) (**D**) are much less numerous and do not display an obvious pattern of arrangement.

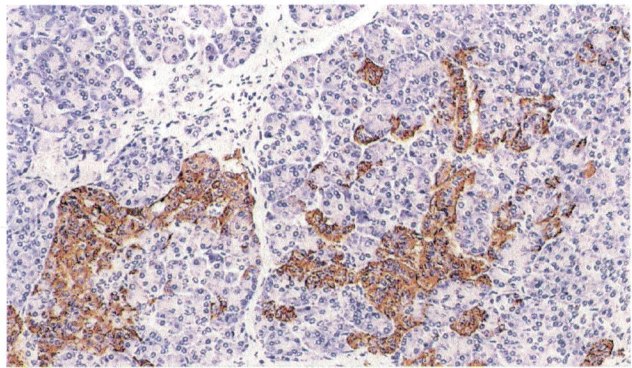

FIGURE 29.34 Immunohistochemistry for pancreatic polypeptide shows positive staining in most of the cells in the diffuse islets.

(Fig. 29.35). The last marker is expressed more intensely in alpha cells than in beta cells, and the pattern of labeling also reflects the characteristic distribution of the cell types in the compact islets.

Keratins generally are not detected in islet cells by immunohistochemistry, although there may be some faint labeling with CAM5.2. Acinar enzymes also are not detectable. CD99 and progesterone receptors are expressed in normal islets, as well as some pancreatic neuroendocrine neoplasms (141–143). The homeodomain protein PDX1, a transcription factor important in pancreatic development, is also expressed in adult islet cells (144), as is ISL1 (145), which has been used diagnostically as a marker of pancreatic origin in well-differentiated neuroendocrine tumors (146).

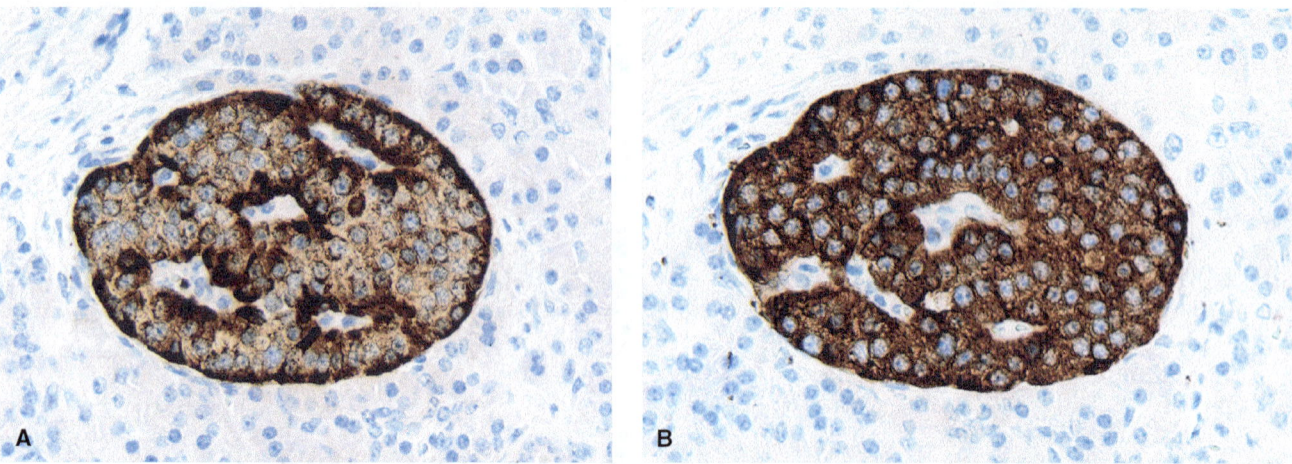

FIGURE 29.35 Alpha cells stain more intensely for chromogranin than do beta cells (**A**), whereas all of the islet cells stain uniformly for synaptophysin (**B**).

Ultrastructural examination of the islets shows polygonal cells joined by tight and gap junctions, suggesting that there may be electronic or metabolic coupling between adjacent cells (127,136). The cytoplasm contains all of the organelles necessary for protein synthesis, including RER, mitochondria, and Golgi apparatus (Fig. 29.36). Dense-core neurosecretory granules are found randomly distributed within the cytoplasm, with some concentration in the basal cytoplasm adjacent to the capillaries into which they are secreted. The granule sizes and morphologies are relatively specific for each cell type (147,148). Alpha cell granules measure 200 to 300 nm and contain an eccentrically located, dense core within a less dense outer region that is separated from the limiting membrane by a thin halo (Fig. 29.37A). Beta cells contain 225- to 375-nm granules with either a finely granular or a crystalline core surrounded by a wide halo underlying the limiting membrane (Fig. 29.37B). Cytoplasmic lipid inclusions (or ceroid bodies) are often found in beta cells

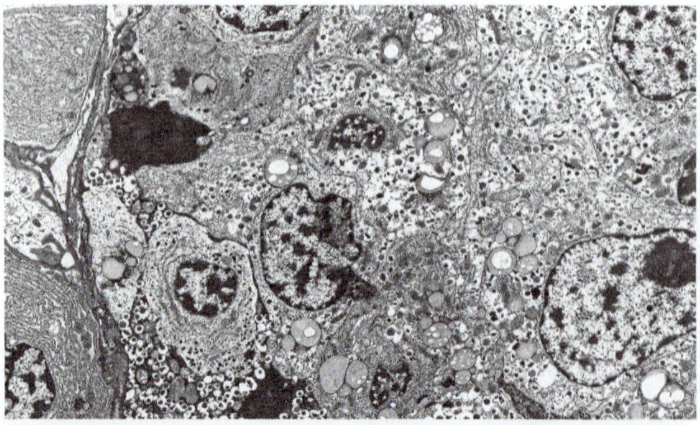

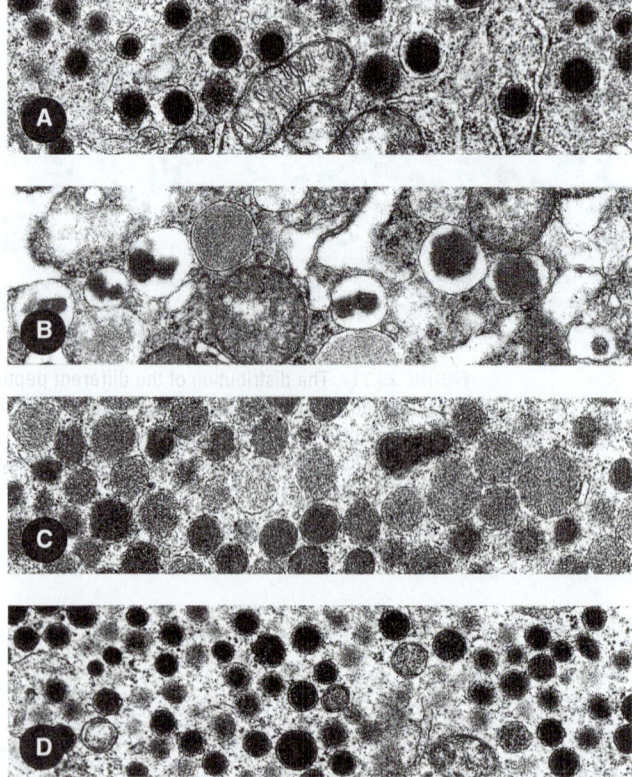

FIGURE 29.36 Ultrastructural appearance of islets of Langerhans. The islets are circumscribed and separated from the adjacent acinar cells (*left*). The peptide granules are randomly distributed within the cytoplasm. Lipid inclusions (ceroid bodies) are found within the beta cells

FIGURE 29.37 Ultrastructural appearance of islet cell granules. Alpha cell granules (**A**) are round and contain an eccentric electron-dense core within a less dense peripheral region. There is a thin halo beneath the limiting membrane. Beta cell granules (**B**) are polymorphous and contain crystalline cores with a wide halo beneath the limiting membrane. Delta cell granules (**C**) are round with a moderately dense core surrounded by a very thin halo. The granules of PP cells (**D**) are smaller and have homogeneous hyperdense cores. Reprinted with permission from Bommer G, Friedl U, Heitz PU, et al. Pancreatic PP cell distribution and hyperplasia. Immunocytochemical morphology in the normal human pancreas, in chronic pancreatitis and pancreatic carcinoma. *Virchows Arch A Pathol Anat Histol* 1980;387(3):319–331.

(Fig. 29.36) (136). Delta cell granules are slightly smaller (170 to 220 nm) than alpha cell granules and have a uniformly dense core (Fig. 29.37C). Delta cells have cytoplasmic processes extending toward the alpha and beta cells, presumably allowing local paracrine release of somatostatin in addition to systemic release into the bloodstream (127). The PP cells of the ventrally derived portion of the pancreas have 180- to 220-nm granules of variable shape and density, whereas the PP cell granules of the remainder of the pancreas are smaller (120 to 150 nm) and more homogeneous (Fig. 29.37D) (108). The cells are separated from the fenestrated endothelial cells of the capillaries only by the basement membranes of both cells and minimal interstitial material (136).

Extrainsular Neuroendocrine Cells

In addition to the neuroendocrine cells of the islets of Langerhans, there are small numbers of individual neuroendocrine cells within the ducts and scattered among the acini (Fig. 29.38). These extrainsular neuroendocrine cells are especially abundant during infancy, but they constitute less than 10% of the total pancreatic neuroendocrine cell population in the adult (108). The ductal neuroendocrine cells are most commonly detected in the main and larger interlobular ducts and are rare in the smaller ducts (103,149). Some of them border the lumina and are joined to neighboring ductal cells by tight junctions (150), whereas others are situated between the ductal cells and the basement membrane. They may secrete peptides directly into the pancreatic ducts, accounting for the detection of neuroendocrine peptides in pancreatic juice (150). Specific peptides may be found, especially insulin, somatostatin, and pancreatic polypeptide (149,151). Some of the extrainsular neuroendocrine cells in the larger ducts also produce serotonin

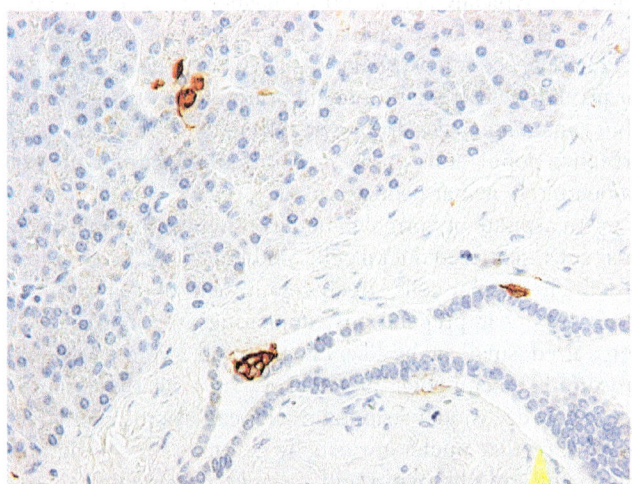

FIGURE 29.38 Extrainsular neuroendocrine cells within the ducts and between the acini are only detectable with immunohistochemical labeling for chromogranin.

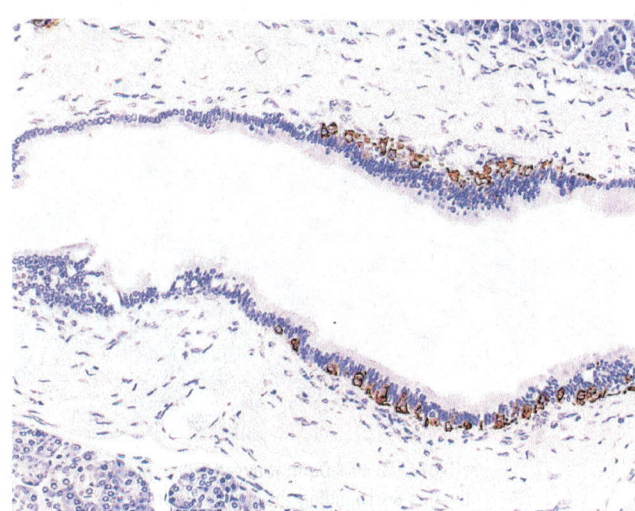

FIGURE 29.39 The number of ductal neuroendocrine cells is increased in areas showing proliferation (low-grade PanIN) of the ductal epithelium (*right*).

(151); these cells may be the origin of the extremely rare true carcinoid tumors (serotonin-producing pancreatic neuroendocrine tumors) of the pancreas, which can occur adjacent to major pancreatic ducts that become obstructed by the neoplasm (152–154). The number of ductal neuroendocrine cells appears to increase in the presence of PanIN (Fig. 29.39) (149).

Connective Tissues

In the normal adult pancreas there is little connective tissue between the lobules and almost none within them. In the neonatal pancreas, mesenchymal tissue comprises nearly 30% of the volume of the gland (Fig. 29.7A); it gradually decreases during infancy (122). The acini are surrounded by basement membranes, but very little other collagen is present (Fig. 29.40).

Small portal vessels exist that deliver hormonal secretions from the islets directly to the exocrine elements of the gland (93,94,155,156). A complex capillary network surrounds the acini, and accompanying nerve fibers may be found. The acini and ducts are innervated by bundles of unmyelinated nerves that travel through the interlobular connective tissues. In most cases the nerve endings are separated from the acinar or ductal cells by the basement membrane, although in some cases direct contact with the basal cell membrane of acinar cells may be seen (103). Islets are innervated by both sympathetic and parasympathetic fibers; in addition, there are peptidergic fibers from the autonomic ganglia. Some of the periacinar nerves produce neuropeptide Y, whereas vasoactive intestinal polypeptide-containing nerves are found within islets and adjacent to ducts (157). Other peptides found in pancreatic nerves include substance P, cholecystokinin, and calcitonin gene–related peptide (157). Small autonomic

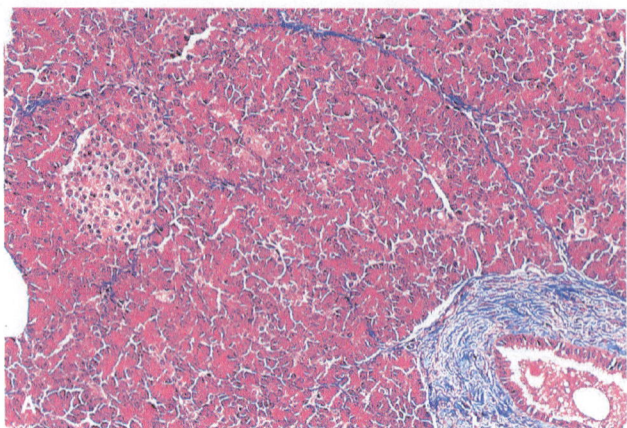
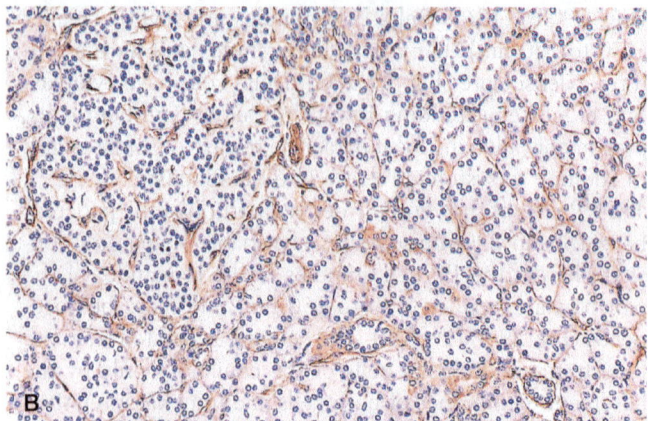

FIGURE 29.40 Connective tissues are minimal within the pancreas. Collagen is largely restricted to the tissues surrounding the interlobular ducts, with only thin bands extending into the lobules, as demonstrated with a trichrome stain (**A**). Immunohistochemical staining for type IV collagen (**B**) shows that an extensive network of basement membranes surrounds each acinus and duct and accompanies the capillaries within the islets (*upper left*).

ganglia are located between clusters of acini (Fig. 29.41). Paraganglia also may be found occasionally in the peripancreatic tissues and presumably represent the origin of peripancreatic paragangliomas (158). The muscular arteries run in the interlobular connective tissue, away from the centrally located pancreatic ducts. This separation of the ducts and muscular arteries is maintained in chronic pancreatitis, and the presence of a gland close to a muscular artery suggests that the gland is malignant (159).

In almost every individual there are some adipocytes within the pancreas (Fig. 29.23). The proportion of the gland composed of fat varies from 3% to 20% (6). The amount of adipose tissue in the pancreas varies with the nutritional state and the age of the individual, older and overweight individuals having more intrapancreatic fat (160). The portions of the gland derived from the dorsal lobe may have more intraparenchymal fat than those from the ventral lobe (161,162).

Recently a population of vitamin A–storing fibroblast-like stromal cell has been described (163,164). These pancreatic "stellate cells" are biologically and morphologically similar to hepatic stellate (or Ito) cells, and activation of these cells appears to play a major role in the production of extracellular matrix proteins during the development of fibrosis in chronic pancreatitis (163,165). Another recently described stromal cell type is the interstitial cell of Cajal. Pancreatic interstitial cells of Cajal have the same morphologic and immunophenotypic properties as do those in the tubular gastrointestinal tract, including immunohistochemical labeling for CD117 (166).

Cytologic Features

Normal pancreatic cells are most commonly a minor component of fine needle aspirations of the pancreas because biopsy is typically performed to diagnose a suspected neoplasm. Since reactive cellular changes, fibrosis, and atrophy commonly occur in the pancreas adjacent to neoplasms, the expected yield from the neighboring benign tissue is low but can create major diagnostic difficulty when cellular and reactive populations mimic well-differentiated ductal and, albeit rarely, acinar neoplasms.

An aspirate of normal pancreas produces abundant acinar cells, scattered ductal cells, and few if any recognizable islet cells. Acinar cells largely retain their lobular architecture in smear preparations, appearing as cohesive, well organized small grape-like clusters and two-dimensional rosette-like acini (Fig. 29.42) (167–169). Scattered single cells and occasional stripped nuclei can also be seen. The round, regular nuclei are usually central to eccentric and have uniform chromatin and variably prominent nucleoli. The pyramidal to polygonal cells have abundant finely granular cytoplasm. The clarity and hue of the zymogen granules is preparation dependent, staining blue-green with the

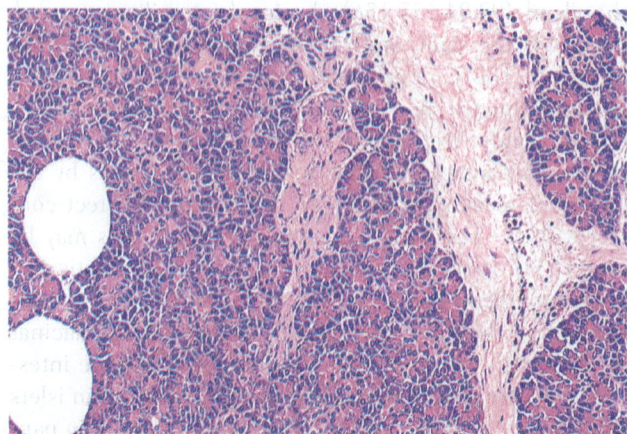

FIGURE 29.41 Small autonomic ganglia are located within lobules of acinar tissue.

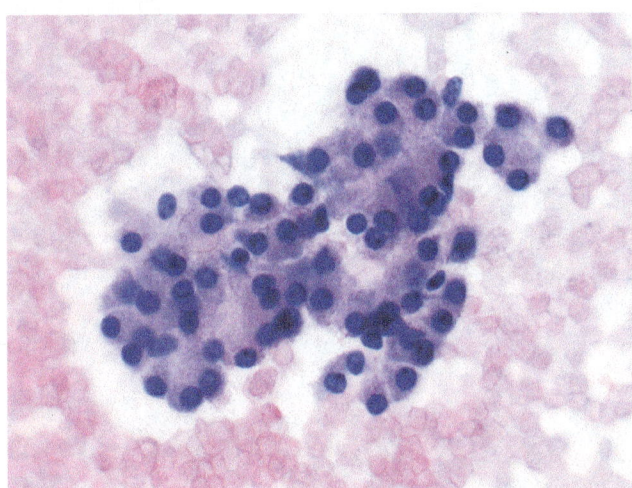

FIGURE 29.42 Cytology of normal acinar cells on hematoxylin and eosin stain. The cells are organized in acini. The cytoplasm has a pyramidal shape with round basal nuclei, small nucleoli, and apical eosinophilic zymogen granules.

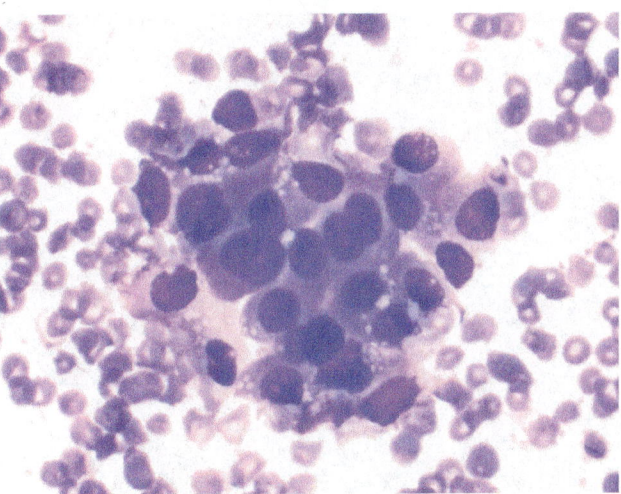

FIGURE 29.44 Cytology of normal islet cells on Diff-Quik stain. Polygonal to plasmacytoid islet cells are loosely arranged with round nuclei and amphophilic cytoplasm.

standard Papanicolaou stain, eosinophilic with hematoxylin and eosin stains (Fig. 29.42), and light purple with the Romanowsky stain and its variants such as Diff-Quik or Giemsa. Scattered small cytoplasmic vacuoles are sometimes seen on Romanowsky type stains. The architectural arrangement of the cells is key to differentiating benign acinar cells from an acinar neoplasm, the latter generally forming large crowded aggregates and irregular clusters in contrast to the small, uniform grape-like clusters of benign acini (169).

Smearing normal ductal epithelium produces flat cohesive sheets or tubules of epithelium containing round, uniform, polarized, and evenly spaced nuclei; this appearance has been commonly regarded as a honeycomb-like (Fig. 29.43) (167,168). The apical cytoplasm and basal nuclear polarity can best be seen when the epithelium is present in strips or at the edges of sheets. Ductal cells have round to oval nuclei with even chromatin and generally small, inconspicuous nucleoli. The dense, nongranular and nonvacuolated cytoplasm stains aqua blue with the Papanicolaou stain and more indigo blue to purple with Romanowsky type stains. Reactive ductal epithelial cells remain cohesive, with mild to moderate variation in nuclear size and organization. Chromatin is fine and nuclear membranes are smooth with only minor irregularities. When abundant apical mucin and crowded nuclei appear in sheets of ductal cells, low-grade PanIN, mucinous cystic neoplasm, IPMN, or adenocarcinoma become considerations, prompting close inspection for nuclear abnormalities and cytologic atypia.

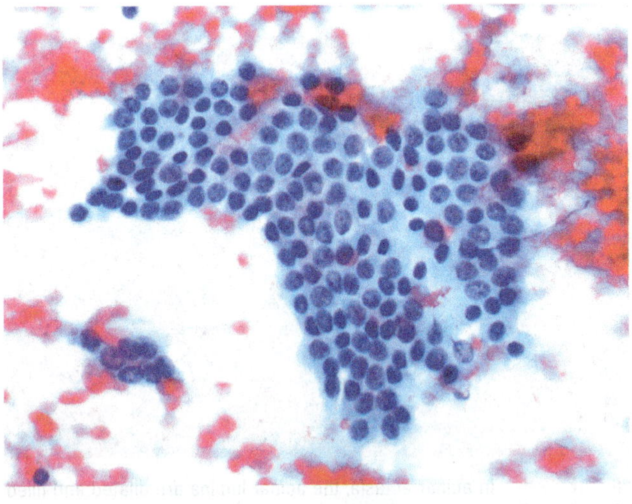

Islet cells are rarely appreciable in aspirate smears but can be distinguished from acinar cells by their relatively larger nuclei, denser chromatin, polygonal to plasmacytoid shape, and pale amphophilic cytoplasm (Fig. 29.44). Mild nuclear size variation as can be seen in neuroendocrine cells of other organs is not unusual.

MINOR ALTERATIONS

A number of minor alterations may affect various components of the pancreas due to physiologic changes, response to injury, or aging. Some of these changes are so subtle that they may be overlooked, but others may be confused for a neoplastic process. Recognition of these potential diagnostic pitfalls is essential for the accurate interpretation of biopsies and is complicated by the fact that many of these alterations may accompany pancreatic neoplasms.

FIGURE 29.43 Cytology of normal ductal cells on hematoxylin and eosin stain. The flat sheet of cells has evenly spaced, round, and uniform nuclei.

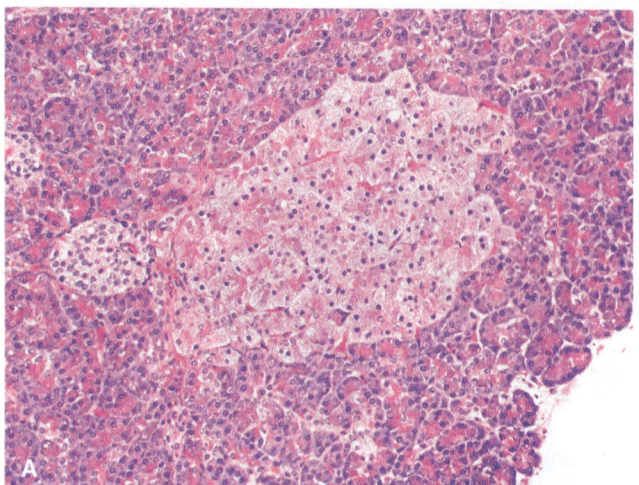
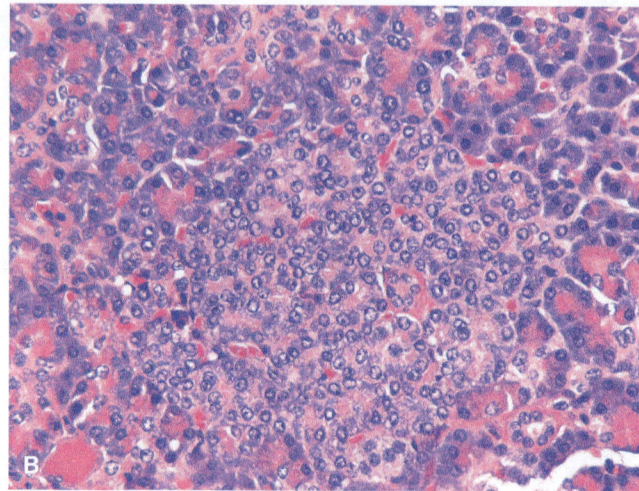

FIGURE 29.45 Atypical acinar cell nodules. The eosinophilic type (**A**) is more common and consists of a collection of acini showing loss of basophilia in the basal cytoplasm and hyperchromasia of the nuclei. The eosinophilic granules within the apical cytoplasm are maintained. An islet of Langerhans, with which these lesions may be confused, is present at the *lower right*. The basophilic type of atypical acinar cell nodule (**B**) exhibits an increased nucleus to cytoplasm ratio with loss of eosinophilic granularity of the apical cytoplasm. Some degree of nuclear atypia is also present.

Acinar Cells

Acinar cell nodules are common incidental findings that consist of circumscribed clusters of acini showing cytoplasmic or nuclear differences from the surrounding acini (170–172). Alternative terms include "pale acinar nodule," "atypical acinar cell nodule," "focal acinar transformation," "eosinophilic degeneration," and "focal acinar cell dysplasia" (15,108,173,174). The last term suggests the lesion may be preneoplastic, but there is no proof of neoplastic alterations in acinar cell nodules in humans, where they are found in nearly half of nontumorous pancreata (175). The lesions are more prevalent in adults, suggesting that they are acquired (173). Acinar cell nodules are often similar in size to compact islets or they can be larger, so they may be confused for islets of small neuroendocrine neoplasms (neuroendocrine microadenomas). Two types of acinar cell nodules exist (171). The more common is the eosinophilic type, which appears as an abnormally pale, eosinophilic cluster of acini (Fig. 29.45A). At high power, the cells are larger than the adjacent normal acinar cells, and the deep basophilia of the basal cytoplasm is lacking. The cytoplasm also may be vacuolated. The nuclei appear normal or hyperchromatic. This change is due to dilatation of the RER or paucity of zymogen granules (172,176) and may be a result of localized hypoxia or other degenerative phenomena. The other less common type of acinar cell nodule, the basophilic type, exhibits loss of the eosinophilic zymogen granules from the apical cytoplasm, as well as an increased nucleus-to-cytoplasm ratio (Fig. 29.45B). Nuclear enlargement, mild atypia, and prominent nucleoli also may be seen. The reason for such localized depletion of zymogen granules is unclear.

Acinar ectasia refers to the dilatation of acini that may occur during active secretion (1) or may be due to ductal obstruction (174). Acinar ectasia is also a relatively common finding at autopsy, where it is associated with premortem uremia, septicemia, and dehydration (15,177,178). Acinar ectasia often involves an entire lobular unit. The ectatic acini resemble small ductules, with flattened lining cells, but some of the cells are still recognizable as acinar cells that have lost most of their zymogen granules (Fig. 29.46). Centroacinar cells also line the dilated lumina and may proliferate (178). The dilated lumina often contain retained eosinophilic secretions.

Metaplastic changes less commonly involve the acini than the ducts; they include replacement by mucinous

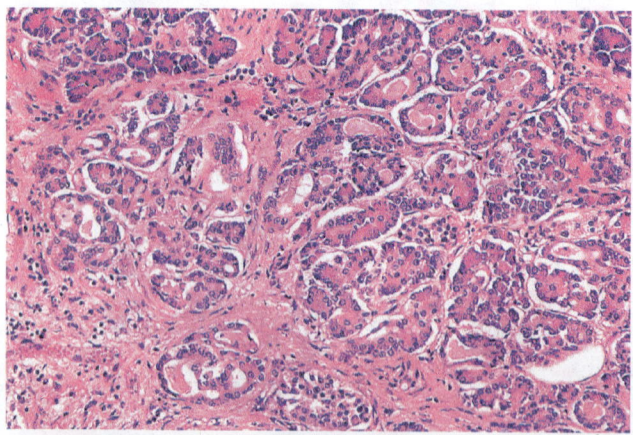

FIGURE 29.46 In acinar ectasia, the acinar lumina are dilated and filled with eosinophilic secretions. The lining cells have a flattened appearance, often resembling small ductules cells more than acinar cells.

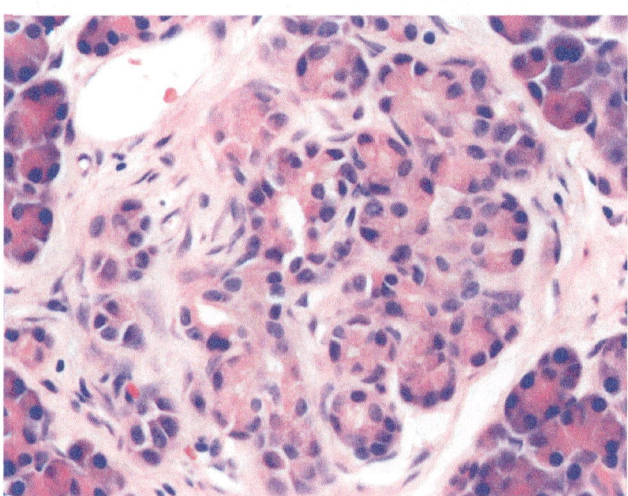

FIGURE 29.47 The apparent replacement of acinar cells by centroacinar or ductular cells has been designated "acinar to ductal metaplasia."

cells or squamous cells (179). Proliferating centroacinar cells may appear to replace the acinar cells, especially in the presence of early atrophy (174). The possibility that acinar cells may transform into centroacinar or ductular cells ("acinar to ductal metaplasia") has been suggested, especially in animal models of pancreatic neoplasia. (180,181). In humans, lesions morphologically similar to those found in animal models have been observed (Fig. 29.47) (182,183), and some investigators have also utilized the term acinar to ductal metaplasia for them (184). However, it remains speculative whether the appearance of prominent tubular glands within the acinar lobules indicates that the ductal cells arose via metaplasia from acinar cells, versus a process of acinar atrophy with resulting prominence of the remaining centroacinar cells and small ductules. Only when the ductules in these lesions exhibit PanIN are molecular alterations characteristic of ductal neoplasia (such as *KRAS* mutations) observed (185).

Ductal Cells

Many metaplastic changes may affect the pancreatic ducts, including squamous, oncocytic, goblet cell (intestinal), and acinar metaplasia. However, the most common alteration in ductal cells, especially those of the medium-sized and large pancreatic ducts, is the replacement of the cuboidal, nonmucinous epithelium with tall columnar cells containing abundant luminal mucin, resembling gastric foveolar or pyloric gland cells, which is easily appreciable on routinely stained slides (Figs. 29.48 and 29.49) (186–188). For many years this alteration was regarded as mucinous metaplasia (or mucous cell hypertrophy or pyloric gland metaplasia). However, these mucinous changes in the ductal epithelium share some of the genetic alterations of invasive carcinomas (such as activating mutations in codon 12 of the *KRAS* oncogene and telomere shortening (189–194) and it is clear that they form the beginning of a spectrum of preinvasive neoplasia that also includes ductal lesions with increased degrees of cytoarchitectural atypia (186,187,195,196). Thus, the lesions previously designated as mucinous metaplasia are now regarded to be the earliest stage of PanIN, termed low-grade PanIN (197–199). The ductal epithelium in low-grade PanIN may remain flat (Fig. 29.48A), or there may be micropapillae or true papillae with fibrovascular cores (Fig. 29.48B). Nuclear abnormalities including early loss of polarity with full-thickness nuclear pseudostratification as well as nuclear crowding, enlargement, and hyperchromasia may also be seen (Fig. 29.50). Mitoses are found rarely in low-grade PanIN, and when present are basal and morphologically normal. These proliferations with low to intermediate grade cytologic features appear to have a very low risk of progression to invasive cancer (200–202).

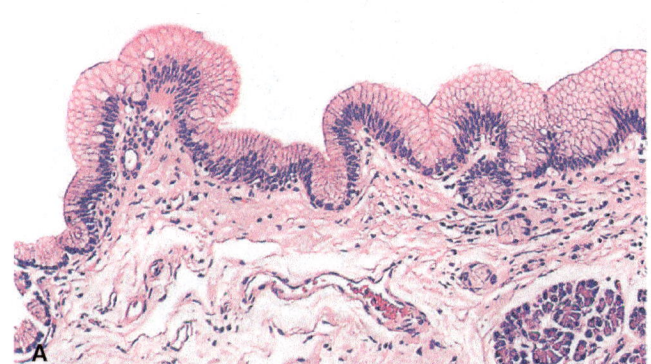
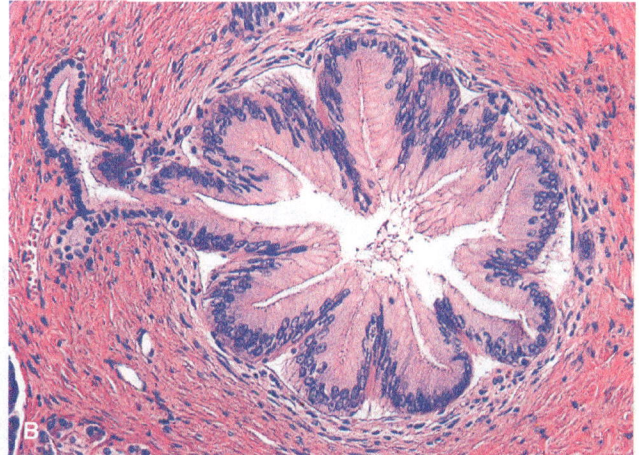

FIGURE 29.48 Low-grade pancreatic intraepithelial neoplasia (PanIN). The normal cuboidal to low columnar ductal epithelial cells are replaced by tall columnar cells containing abundant apical mucin (**A**); in this example with no papilla formation (previously termed PanIN-1A). The nuclei remain basally located and show minimal pseudostratification. Another lesion (**B**) has similar cytologic features but demonstrates papilla formation (previously termed PanIN-1B). Note the transition to normal ductal epithelium (*left*)

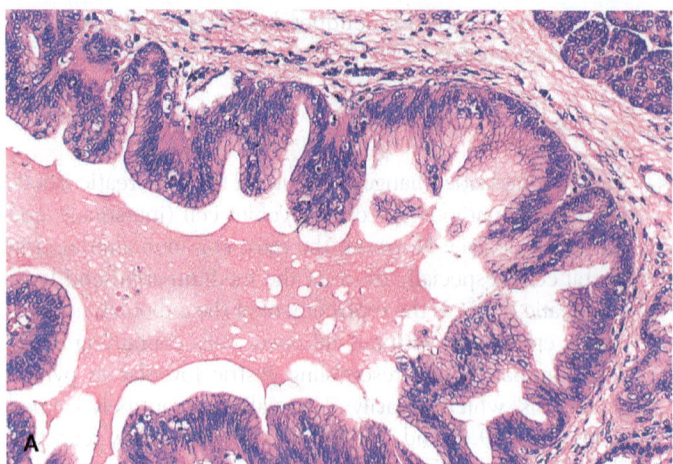 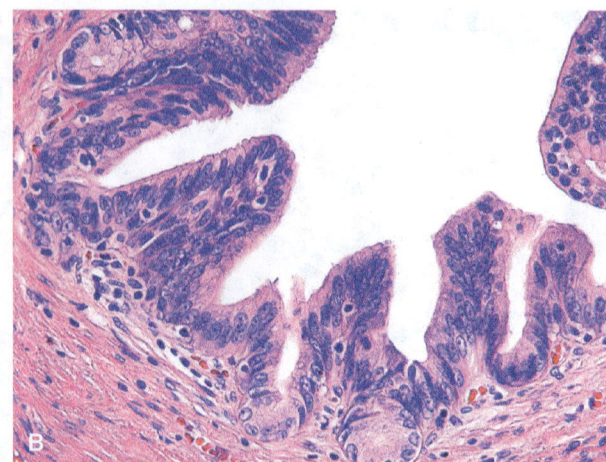

FIGURE 29.49 Low-grade PanIN may also show pseudostratified nuclei with focal loss polarity (**A**). At higher power (**B**) the nuclei are enlarged, moderately atypical, and overlapping. This moderate level of atypia was previously termed PanIN-2.

By recent consensus, low-grade PanIN currently refers to lesions with up to intermediate/moderate levels of atypia, which have been previously categorized as PanIN-1A, 1B, and 2 (199). PanIN may involve a single ductal profile, may extend into clusters of ductules adjacent to larger ducts, and may occur multifocally throughout the pancreas (Fig. 29.49). Low-grade PanIN is present in up to half of nontumorous pancreata (15,19,174,187,196) and is usually more prevalent in the head of the gland and as we age. Although low-grade PanIN commonly exhibits *KRAS* mutation—a finding supporting its classification as a neoplastic alteration—the other common mutations of invasive ductal adenocarcinoma are absent (203).

Ductal proliferative lesions with greater degrees of cytoarchitectural atypia are considered high-grade PanIN (previously designated "PanIN-3," "carcinoma *in situ*," or "severe dysplasia") (199). High-grade PanIN demonstrates more significant architectural and cytologic atypia (Fig. 29.51). These lesions are usually papillary or micropapillary, although rarely they may be flat. Cribriforming, budding of clusters of cells into the lumen, and luminal necrosis may occur. Also, the nuclei show complete loss of polarity and are enlarged, hyperchromatic, and irregular. The nucleus to cytoplasm ratio is increased. Nucleoli can be prominent, and mitoses are usually identifiable, sometimes including atypical forms (197,198). High-grade PanIN contains more of the mutations of invasive carcinomas, although mutations in genes other than *KRAS* occur at low frequency. Inactivating mutations in *p16/CDKN2A*, *TP53*, *ARID1A*, *PIK3CA*, *TGFBR2,* and *BRCA2* can occur, although mutations in *SMAD4* are not found in high-grade PanIN from cases lacking an associated invasive carcinoma component (203). Mutations in *RNF43* and *GNAS*, genes implicated in mucinous cystic neoplasm and IPMN rather than conventional

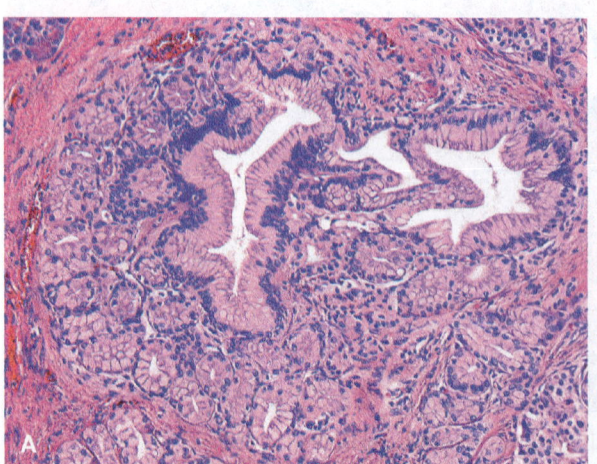 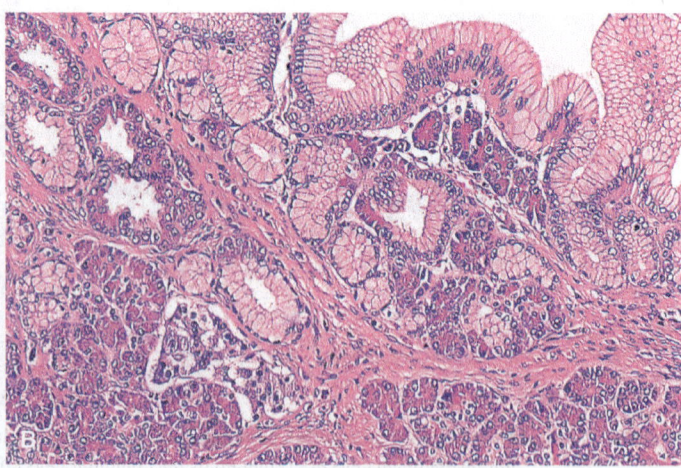

FIGURE 29.50 Low-grade PanIN may involve aggregates of small ductules around larger ducts, resulting in clusters of mucinous glands (**A**). Because the smallest components of the ductal system are involved, cells with low-grade PanIN may abut adjacent acinar cells (**B**).

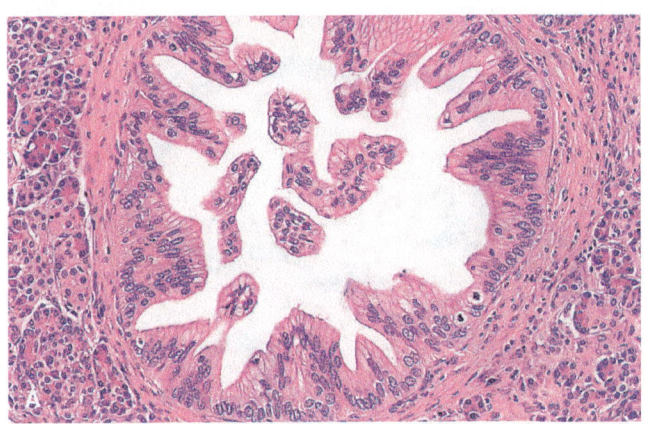
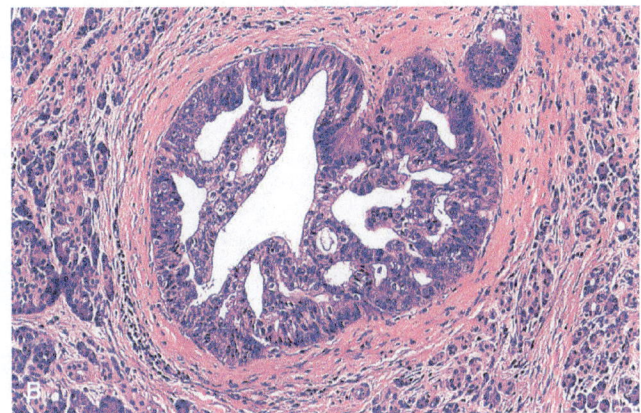

FIGURE 29.51 In high-grade PanIN there is complete loss of polarity, with budding of disorganized cellular clusters into the ductal lumen. The nuclei are markedly irregular and vary in morphology between adjacent cells. Increased mitoses are present (**A**). In another focus (**B**), architectural abnormalities include cribriforming, and there is extreme nuclear atypia.

invasive ductal adenocarcinoma, may also occur in high-grade PanIN (203). Also, promoter methylation of the *ppENK, TSLC1,* and *p16* genes has been demonstrated in PanINs, the prevalence increasing from low to high grade (204,205) (189–194). The proliferation rate, as measured by immunohistochemical labeling for Ki-67, increases with increasing grades of PanIN (206).

Low- and high-grade PanIN often coexist within the same pancreas, with transitions from one to the next. Low- and high-grade PanINs are associated with invasive ductal adenocarcinomas (115,186,187), and high-grade PanIN is usually only found in pancreata also harboring an invasive ductal adenocarcinoma (186,187), although it can rarely occur in a pancreas without invasive carcinoma (200,203). Along with the genetic data, these observations support the concept that PanINs progress to invasive carcinoma, but the frequency and time course of progression is unknown and in the case of low-grade PanIN, the frequency appears to be very low and the interval is likely prolonged.

The cells in foci of PanIN produce largely neutral mucins and sialomucins; sulphomucins are less abundant than in normal ductal cells (108). The histochemical and immunohistochemical profiles of the mucins in these cells resemble those of the superficial gastric mucosa in some cases or of the pyloric glands in others (116,188). Because there is little morphologic difference between these two mucin-producing cells types, pyloric gland differentiation may not be distinguishable from gastric foveolar differentiation by routine microscopy. The morphologic progression from low- to high-grade PanIN is also accompanied by increasingly abnormal expression of tumor-associated glycoproteins such as CEA, B72.3, and CA125 (115).

Up to one-third of pancreata exhibit squamous metaplasia (19,174). Although squamous metaplasia may occur in the larger interlobular and main ducts, it is most common in the intralobular and intercalated ducts, and metaplastic cells may extend into the center of the acini (Fig. 29.52). It is exceptional for squamous metaplasia to exhibit keratinization

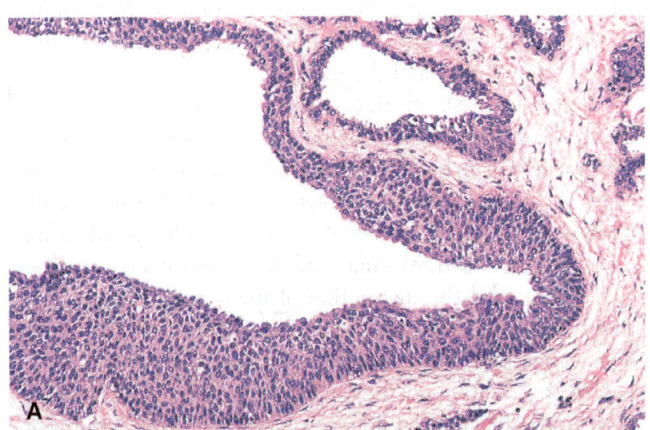
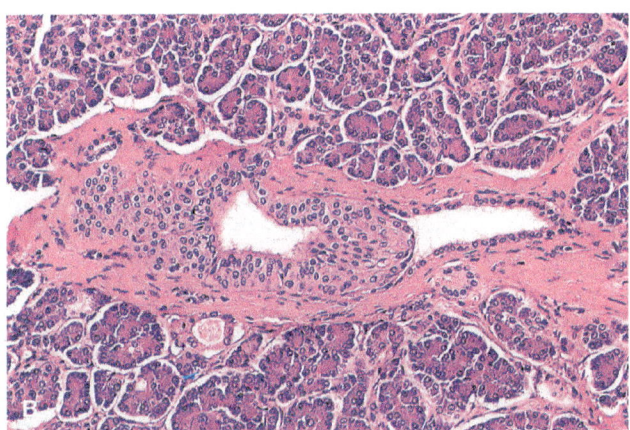

FIGURE 29.52 Squamous metaplasia of the ducts. There are multiple layers of immature-appearing squamous cells without keratinization. The process may involve larger ducts (**A**). In this example (**B**) there is partial involvement of a small interlobular duct.

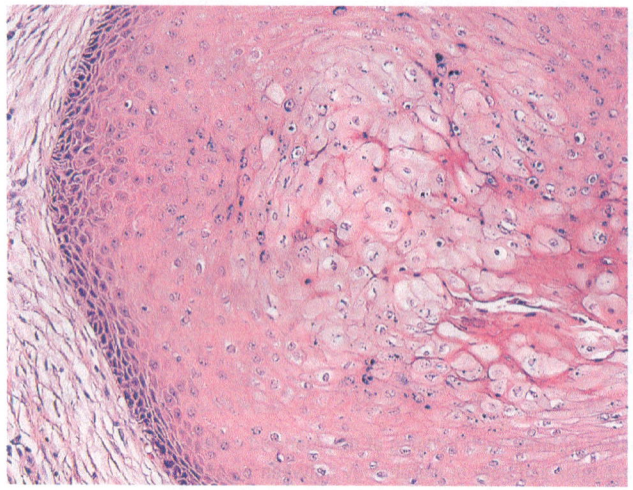

FIGURE 29.53 Squamous metaplasia of the ducts with keratinization, an uncommon finding.

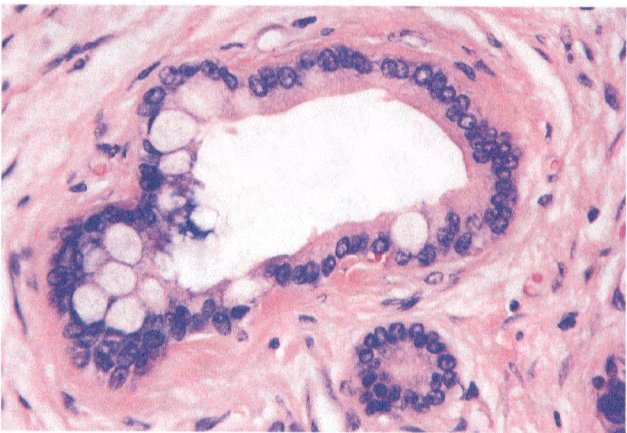

FIGURE 29.55 Goblet cell metaplasia involving a small duct. Flask-shaped goblet cells are distinct from the mucinous columnar cells of low-grade PanIN.

or a granular cell layer, which occurs most commonly in the setting of advanced chronic pancreatitis (Fig. 29.53). For this reason, the terms "multilayered metaplasia" and "transitional metaplasia" have been suggested for this lesion (174). Histologically, the stratified squamous epithelium appears immature, with only minimal flattening of the superficial layers. There may be retention of a luminal mucinous cell layer. In the smaller ducts and ductules, the metaplastic epithelium may fill the lumen, virtually obliterating it. In most instances squamous metaplasia is associated with chronic pancreatitis; there is no known preneoplastic significance. A grossly cystic lesion of the pancreas lined by similar epithelium is designated as "squamoid cyst of pancreatic ducts" (207).

Oncocytic changes are common in centroacinar cells, and oncocytic metaplasia may affect intercalated and intralobular ducts as well (104,208,209). The oncocytic cells have abundant granular eosinophilic cytoplasms (reflecting the accumulation of mitochondria), and the nuclei may be enlarged and contain prominent nucleoli (Fig. 29.54). Involvement of clusters of small ductules may occur. Like mucinous and squamous metaplasia, oncocytic metaplasia may be associated with chronic inflammatory processes or it may occur in the absence of other specific abnormalities (19,210). It has been suggested that oncocytic changes in the ducts may be a preneoplastic alteration (211), but molecular genetic abnormalities have yet to be identified in this lesion.

Goblet cells may be found within the ductal epithelium, especially in the main ducts near the ampulla of Vater (1,107). In addition, isolated goblet cells may appear in smaller ducts, presumably as a metaplastic change (Fig. 29.55) (174,179). In contrast to low-grade PanIN, the mucin-containing goblet cells occur singly and are more flask shaped. Presumably they reflect an intestinal metaplastic phenotype rather than the gastric phenotype of PanIN. Replacement of the ductal epithelium with mucinous cells having all of the histologic and immunohistochemical features of intestinal epithelium has been described (211) but appears to be rare. True intestinal-type epithelium, with pseudostratified cells having elongate nuclei and expressing MUC2 and CDX2 by immunohistochemistry, is commonly found in IPMN (212,213), which may extend into smaller ducts, but this phenomenon is neoplastic and therefore must be distinguished from intestinal metaplasia of the ducts.

Sometimes small ducts may demonstrate partial or complete replacement by acinar cells. When this process is very localized, it has been referred to as acinar metaplasia (214,3). However, larger lesions composed of cysts lined by benign acinar cells, designated "acinar cell cystadenoma" or "acinar cystic tranformation," have also been described (215–217), and the distinction of microscopic examples of this lesion from acinar metaplasia is somewhat arbitrary. In acinar metaplasia the acinar cells occur singly or in clusters within the ducts, and they exhibit the same appearance as their normally situated counterparts (Fig. 29.56). Immunohistochemical labeling for trypsin, chymotrypsin, or BCL10 facilitates identification of acinar metaplasia, although the granular apical cytoplasmic staining of true acinar cells must

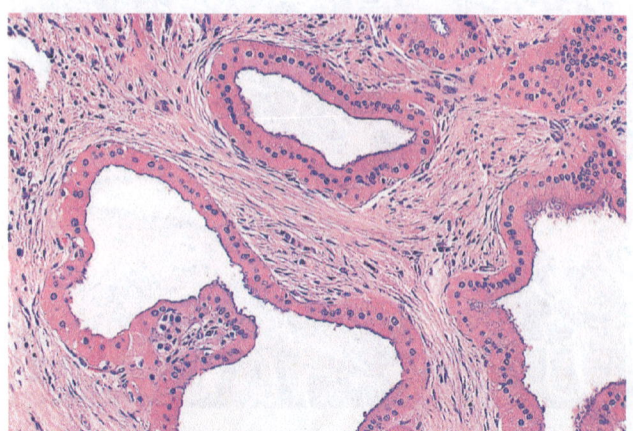

FIGURE 29.54 Oncocytic changes involving small ducts. In this example there is associated fibrosing pancreatitis.

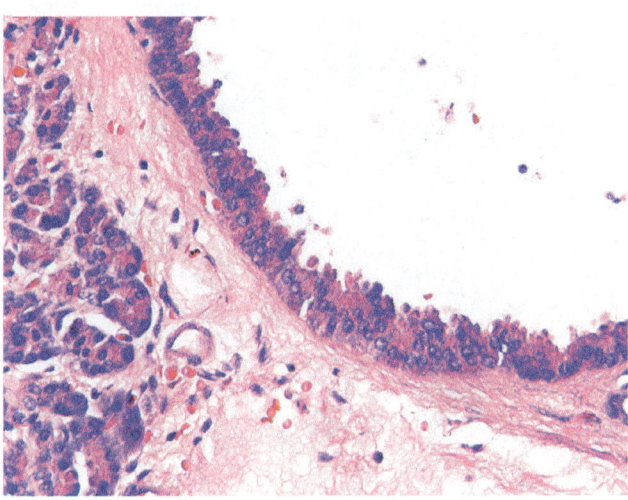

FIGURE 29.56 This small interlobular duct shows acinar metaplasia, with slightly enlarged acinar cells replacing the normal cuboidal ductal epithelium.

be distinguished from the labeling of deposited intraluminal enzyme secretions on the surface of ductal cells (Fig. 29.15).

Another frequent alteration of the ducts is ectasia. Ectatic ducts are generally (but not invariably) found in association with chronic pancreatitis in older patients (15,19,218), often due to ductal obstruction. The ectatic ducts range up to several millimeters in size and occasionally are recognizable grossly. Dilatation of the main pancreatic duct to more than 4 mm is found in 16% of patients at autopsy (15). Because ectatic ducts are often tortuous and the dilatation may be localized, they may appear as single or multiple small cysts (retention cysts) in cross section (Fig. 29.57A). Careful study of serial sections shows the continuity with the ductal system. Retention cysts are usually grossly evident, are mostly unilocular, have no apparent communication with the main duct, and may reach several centimeters in diameter. The lining epithelium may harbor PanIN, usually low grade but sometimes high grade, as well (Fig.29.57B). Simple cysts with PanIN may be difficult to distinguish from IPMNs (219–224), and attempts have been made to reach a consensus on diagnostic criteria (198,199). In general, multicystic lesions with micropapillae or true papillae and lacking ovarian-type stroma are regarded as IPMNs, whereas solitary cysts >1 cm with flat epithelium are designated "simple mucinous cysts."

Islet Cells

Islet hyperplasia is defined as an absolute increase in the size or number of islets relative to the normal islet volume at a given age. Individual compact islets larger than 250 microns in diameter are regarded to be hyperplastic (225). However, making an assessment that there is an increase in the total volume of islet tissue in the pancreas is difficult. There are a number of conditions, most associated with pancreatic atrophy, that can result in the appearance of increased numbers of islets when in fact the islet volume is not increased, but rather the volume of exocrine elements has decreased (see below). Plus, the density of islets varies in different regions of the pancreas. Thus, some objective assessment of islet volume must be made for a diagnosis of islet hyperplasia, rather than simply a casual observation of "numerous" islets. Conditions associated with islet hyperplasia in infancy include Beckwith–Wiedemann syndrome, maternal diabetes, erythroblastosis fetalis, and hyperinsulinemic hypoglycemia (108); cases have also been described in adults with hyperinsulinism (226). Islet hyperplasia may occur either by proliferation of islet cells or by neoformation of islet cells from uncommitted progenitors (136). The distribution of the different peptide cell types is usually maintained, although there may be a relative increase in the number of beta cells, some of which may show hypertrophy.

Nesidioblastosis is a descriptor of the morphologic findings accompanying functional disorders of beta cells

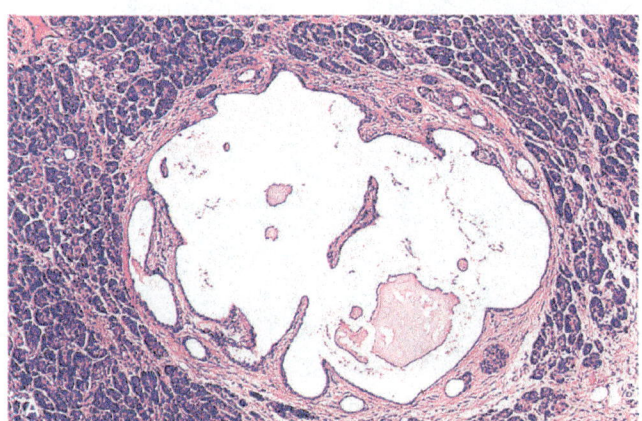 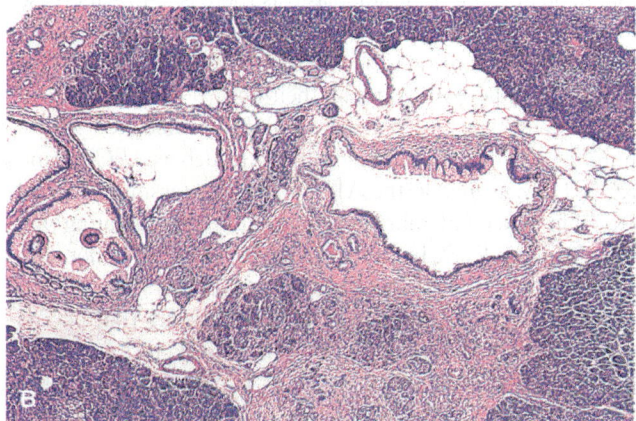

FIGURE 29.57 Duct ectasia. The dilated ducts may be lined by a flattened cuboidal epithelium resembling normal ductal epithelium (**A**) or there may be involvement by PanIN (**B**). In the latter circumstance, the lesion merges morphologically with intraductal papillary mucinous neoplasm and simple mucinous cyst.

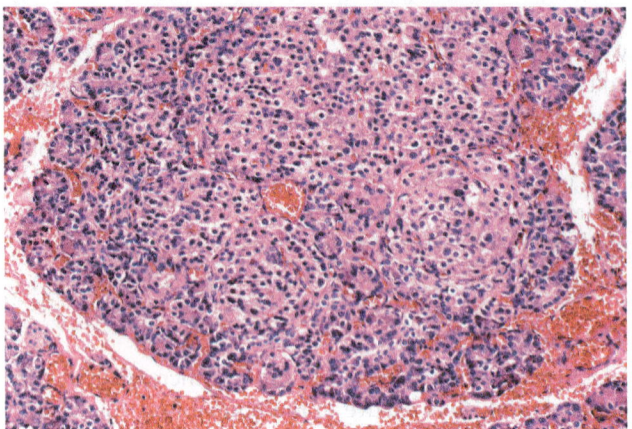

FIGURE 29.58 The pancreas from an infant with persistent neonatal hyperinsulinemic hypoglycemia shows the focal form of nesidioblastosis. There is localized aggregation of islets separated by thin bands of acini.

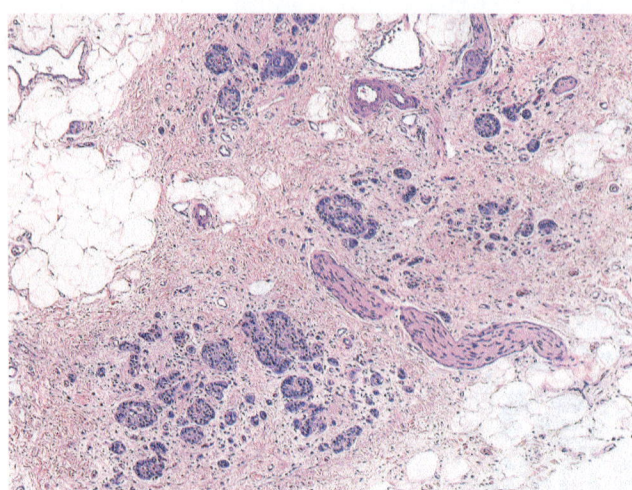

FIGURE 29.59 Islet aggregation involving compact islets. With extreme atrophy, there is complete loss of exocrine elements, leaving the clustered islets embedded in fibrous stroma.

associated with hyperinsulinemic hypoglycemia in the absence of an insulinoma (227–231). This condition generally occurs in neonates and infants, where it is known as persistent neonatal hyperinsulinemic hypoglycemia (PNHH); rarely a similar condition occurs in adults. Morphologic abnormalities include hypertrophic beta cells within the islets and, particularly in neonates, close association of islet cells with small pancreatic ducts (ductuloinsular complexes), and abnormal aggregation of islets. Both focal and diffuse types are described (227). In focal nesidioblastosis there is a localized nodular lesion that may resemble an insulinoma, but more often there is simply an aggregate of ill-formed islet-like clusters associated with small ductules (Fig. 29.58). Some of the nuclei within the lesion are enlarged. The islets in the remaining pancreas are normal. The diffuse form of nesidioblastosis shows islet abnormalities throughout the gland without discrete localized aggregation of islets. The principal finding is the presence of enlarged, hyperchromatic beta cell nuclei. The size of nuclei in β cells varies somewhat in normal neonates, but in nesidioblastosis there is a 40% increase in nuclear volume compared with age-matched controls. By immunohistochemistry, the islets in both focal and diffuse types of nesidioblastosis retain their normal complements of peptide cell types. Genetically, PNHH is associated with a number of different mutations in genes such as *ABCC8* and *KCNJ11* that encode the ATP-sensitive potassium channel (K_{ATP}) in the cell membrane of beta cells, demonstrating that this disorder clearly has a functional basis and does not simply reflect an increase in beta cell mass (232–235).

The apparent increase in number of islets that occurs secondary to exocrine atrophy has been termed "islet aggregation" and is *not* a result of hyperplasia. With the progressive atrophy that occurs in chronic pancreatitis, eventually most of the acini and many of the ducts disappear, leaving only residual islets embedded in fibrous or adipose tissue (Fig. 29.59) (182). This phenomenon may be widespread in patients with significant chronic pancreatitis or it may only involve one lobule of the gland. This islet aggregation, which is usually associated with an overall loss of neuroendocrine cells, should be distinguished from true islet cell hyperplasia. The clustering of islets in regions of severe atrophy may resemble a solid tumor-like process with a nesting pattern, reminiscent of a pancreatic neuroendocrine tumor (Fig. 29.60). Individual islets may be found in the peripancreatic adipose tissue. The appearance of infiltrative growth is even more marked when the process involves the regions of the head of the pancreas containing the diffuse islets; these islets lack the insular arrangement of the compact islets from the tail, appearing as small clusters, trabeculae, and individual cells when the exocrine elements undergo atrophy (Fig. 29.61). In contrast to most pancreatic neuroendocrine tumors, the border

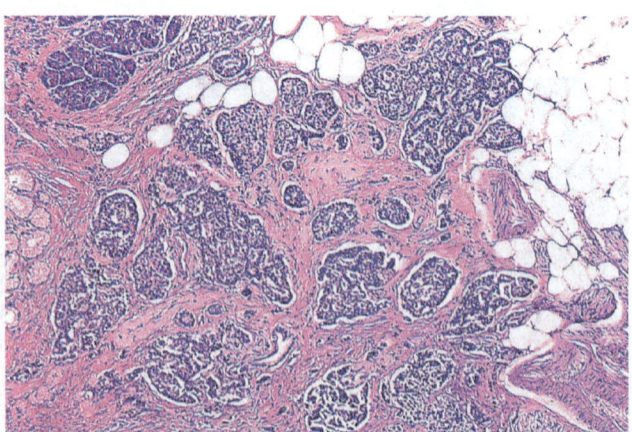

FIGURE 29.60 When advanced atrophy of exocrine elements occurs, aggregation of the remaining neuroendocrine elements may simulate a neoplasm. The nests of cells may be poorly circumscribed and separated by bands of fibrous tissue, with extension into peripancreatic adipose tissue.

of foci of islet aggregation is ill defined. The surrounding pancreas often exhibits areas of pancreatitis that are less advanced, with incomplete acinar atrophy. In problematic cases, immunohistochemical labeling for the specific peptides may be helpful. In islet aggregation, the normal peptide cell types are present, in roughly normal numbers and distribution, although the relative proportions of alpha and PP cells may be increased (135,236). Although more than one peptide may be expressed in neuroendocrine tumors, it is exceptional for all of the normal peptides to be found in normal numbers, and there may be expression of peptides not found in normal islets (vasoactive intestinal polypeptide or gastrin). Bear in mind that the diffuse islets have a different normal peptide cell constitution (abundance of PP cells) from that of the compact islets (Fig. 29.62). Another

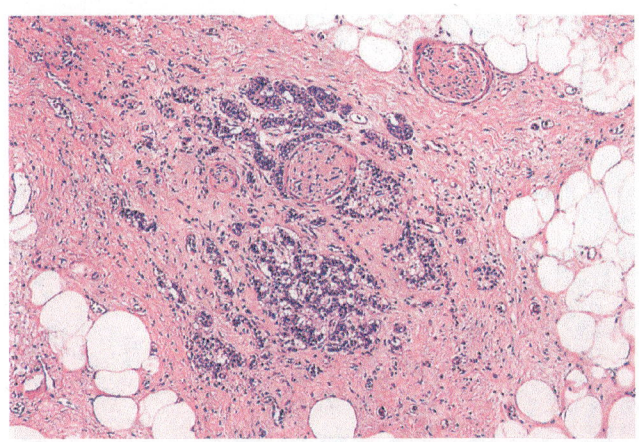

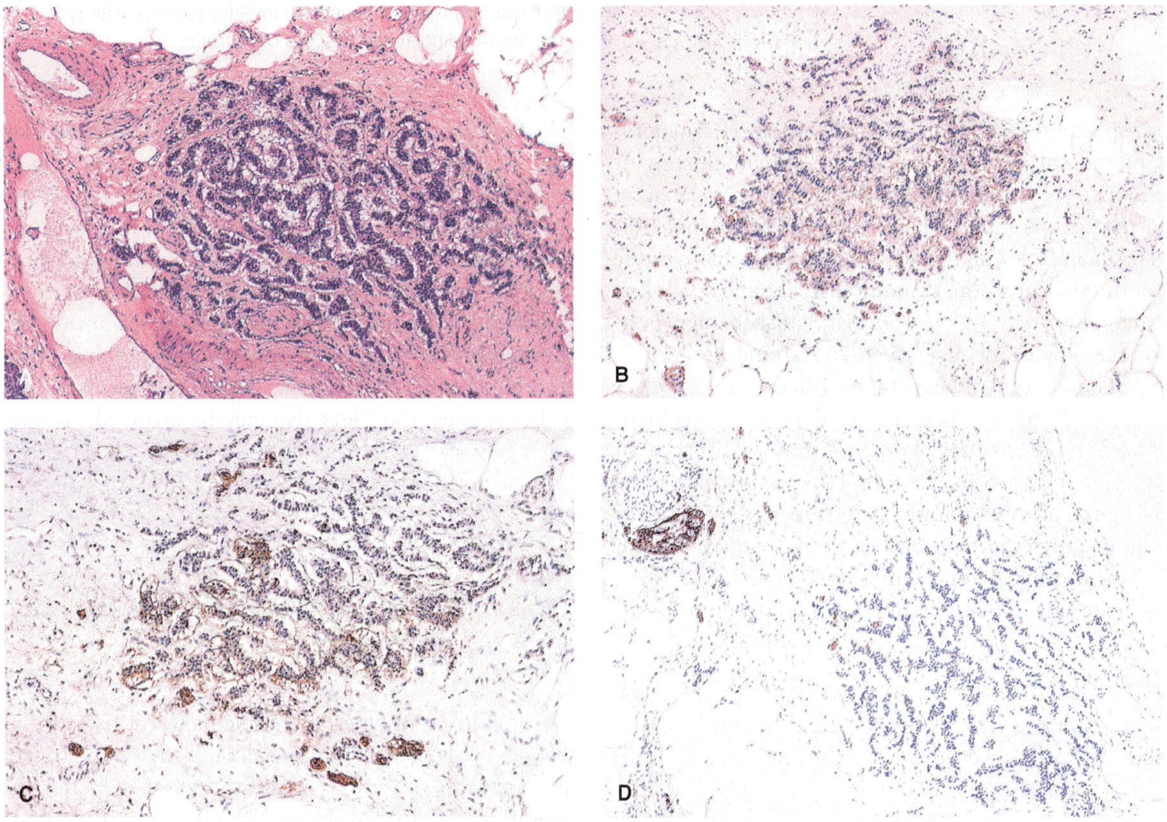

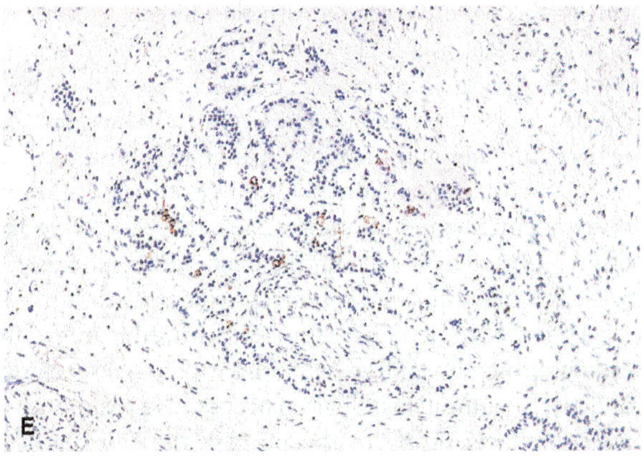

FIGURE 29.61 Exocrine atrophy in areas containing diffuse-type islets results in a pseudoinfiltrative pattern of individual cells and trabeculae.

FIGURE 29.62 Immunohistochemistry may be helpful for distinguishing foci of islet aggregation from a neuroendocrine tumor. In this focus (**A**) with a trabecular and infiltrative pattern, there is an abundance of PP cells (**B**) and beta cells (**C**), with smaller numbers of alpha (**D**) and delta (**E**) cells, a composition typical of nonneoplastic diffuse-type islets.

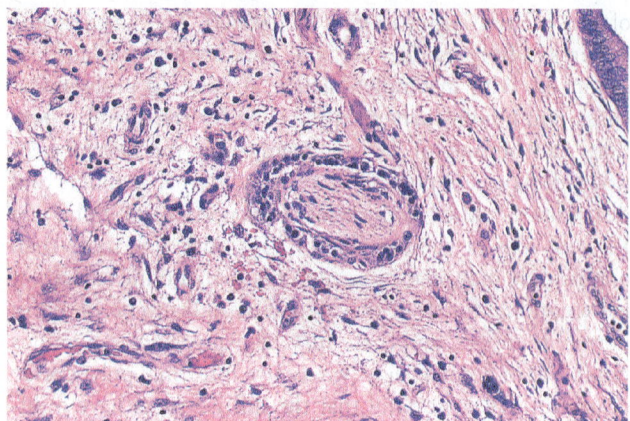

FIGURE 29.63 Perineural invasion by islet cells in chronic pancreatitis may simulate carcinoma.

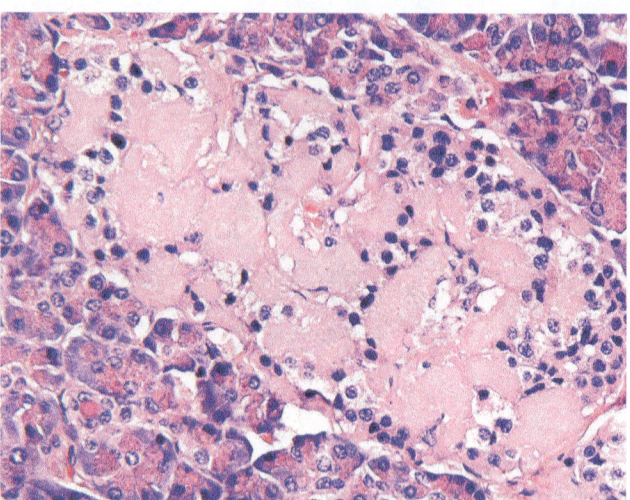

FIGURE 29.65 Amyloid-like hyalinization of the perivascular tissue may be seen in the islets, especially in older patients with type II diabetes. The surrounding acinar tissue is not fibrotic.

pseudoneoplastic property of islet cells in chronic pancreatitis is perineural invasion (Fig. 29.63). Small clusters of islet cells may surround nerves, simulating the perineural invasion that is common in pancreatic ductal adenocarcinoma. Fortunately, benign glands only exceptionally rarely exhibit perineural invasion. Immunohistochemical labeling for chromogranin may be used to distinguish benign perineural invasion by islet cells from adenocarcinoma.

The appearance of dilated blood-filled spaces within the islets (Fig. 29.64) has been referred to as peliosis insulis. Although reported in a pancreas from a patient with multiple endocrine neoplasia-1 (MEN-1) also harboring multiple pancreatic neuroendocrine tumors (237), peliosis insulis usually occurs in otherwise normal pancreata. It is of unclear etiology and significance. The blood-filled spaces are not observed to be lined by endothelium ultrastructurally.

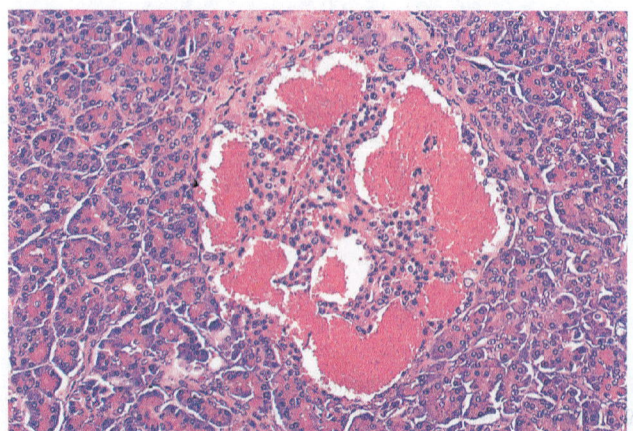

FIGURE 29.64 The appearance of dilated, blood-filled spaces within the islets has been called peliosis insulis. It is probably of no clinical significance.

Perivascular deposition of amyloid or amyloid-like material may be seen in islets of older individuals (Fig. 29.65), especially in association with non–insulin-dependent (type II) diabetes mellitus (238,239). Insular amyloid is biochemically different from systemic amyloid, and there is no association between insular amyloidosis and systemic amyloidosis. In insular amyloidosis, the hyalinized stroma is limited to the islets. In patients with generalized fibrosis of the pancreatic parenchyma due to chronic pancreatitis or other causes, the islets also may be involved (insular fibrosis); however, the hyalinized stroma in these cases lacks ultrastructural features of amyloid (239).

CHRONIC PANCREATITIS, ATROPHY, AND FIBROSIS

Several different types of chronic pancreatitis exist, with etiologies ranging from chronic alcoholism, ductal obstruction, autoimmune disorders, malnutrition, to genetic predisposition (240–246). Although the distribution of the disease within the pancreas varies with the different etiologies, the histologic features of most types (except for autoimmune pancreatitis) are similar, especially at the end stages when fibrosis and atrophy are prominent (19). In fact, microscopic foci of fibrosis and atrophy (histologic chronic pancreatitis) are common incidental findings in pancreatic resection specimens and at autopsy, and the pathologic findings often reported as "focal chronic pancreatitis" are only loosely related to the clinical disease of chronic pancreatitis.

When chronic pancreatitis is localized it may clinically, radiographically, and grossly mimic pancreatic carcinoma, and the resultant histologic patterns also frequently simulate neoplasia. Early in the process the fibrosis is largely

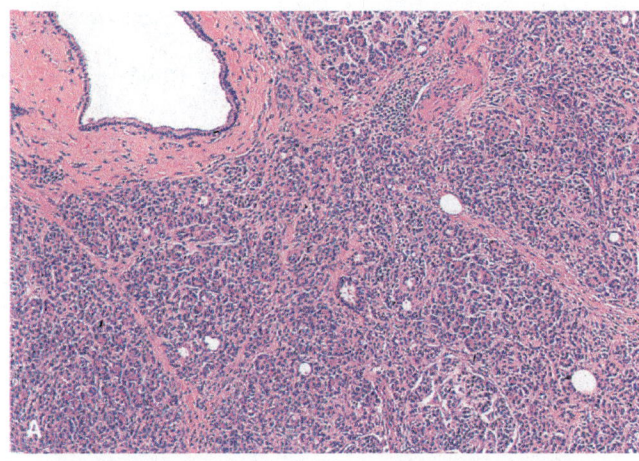
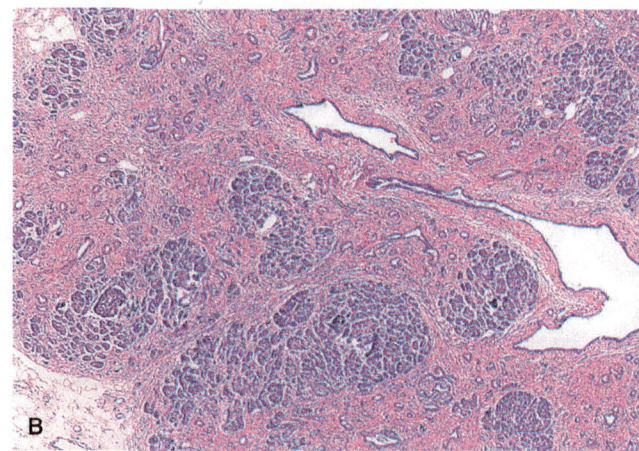
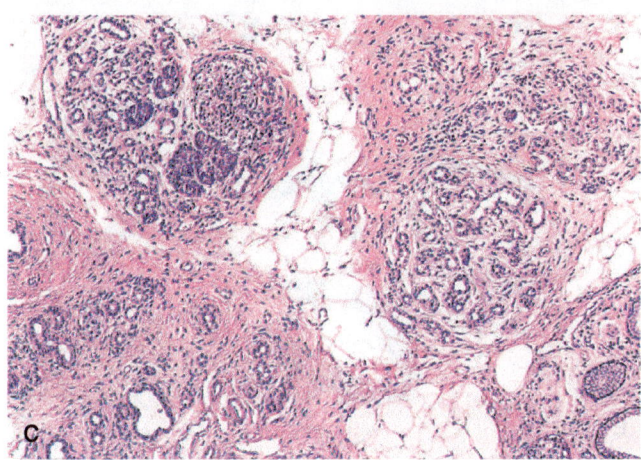

FIGURE 29.66 Progressive changes in chronic pancreatitis. In the early stages (**A**) the fibrosis is largely limited to the periductal and septal areas of the gland. The lobules show prominence of ductules. There are scattered aggregates of chronic inflammatory cells. As the pancreatitis progresses (**B**), the amount of fibrosis is increased, entrapping small lobules of residual acinar tissue. The ducts are ectatic. In the terminal stages (**C**), most of the acinar tissue is atrophic, leaving lobular aggregates of small ductules and islets within a fibrotic and fatty stroma.

around the periphery of the lobules, there is minimal acinar atrophy, and chronic inflammatory cells are evident (Fig. 29.66A). However, as chronic pancreatitis progresses, the fibrosis involves the entire lobule, with marked distortion of the architecture of the gland. There is progressive exocrine atrophy, with eventual complete loss of acinar elements. The ducts become ectatic and irregularly shaped (Fig. 29.66B). Ultimately, in some cases even the ducts are lost, leaving only the islets embedded in fat or fibrous connective tissue. In experimental pancreatitis induced by duct ligation, acinar atrophy occurs by necrosis and apoptosis (247,248), resulting in closely packed lobules of ductular structures. Small ductules and islets remaining after acinar atrophy become encircled and distorted by the fibrous tissue (Fig. 29.66C), often acquiring a pseudoinfiltrative appearance. Ductuloinsular complexes may be found (Fig. 29.67). As the gland is replaced by fibrous tissue, it decreases in size and acquires a hard consistency. Inflammatory cells are sparse at this stage and may be aggregated around small nerves (174). Duct ectasia, calcification, and intraductal calculi may occur (249), especially in pancreatitis of alcoholic etiology. Although chronic pancreatitis is common in the background of invasive adenocarcinoma most of the chronic pancreatitis commonly accompanying ductal adenocarcinoma is secondary to ductal obstruction by the neoplasm rather than representing a pre-existing condition. In fact, study of patients with a hereditary increased risk of pancreatic carcinoma has revealed discrete regions of chronic pancreatitis ("lobular atrophy") associated with ducts involved by PanIN; these foci can even be identified radiographically in some cases (250).

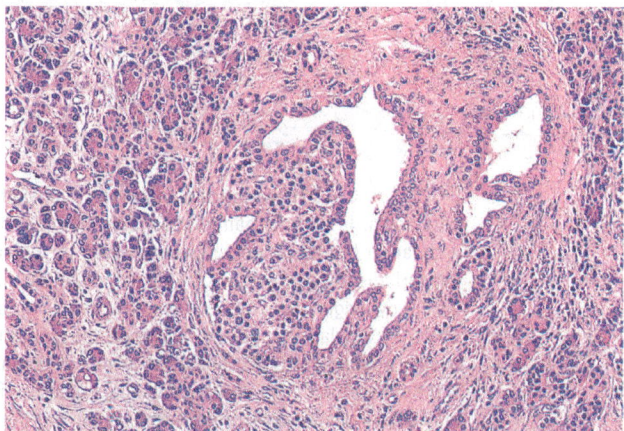

FIGURE 29.67 A ductuloinsular complex in an adult with mild chronic pancreatitis. Small ductules are surrounded by nests of neuroendocrine cells, a finding that does not necessarily reflect true islet cell hyperplasia.

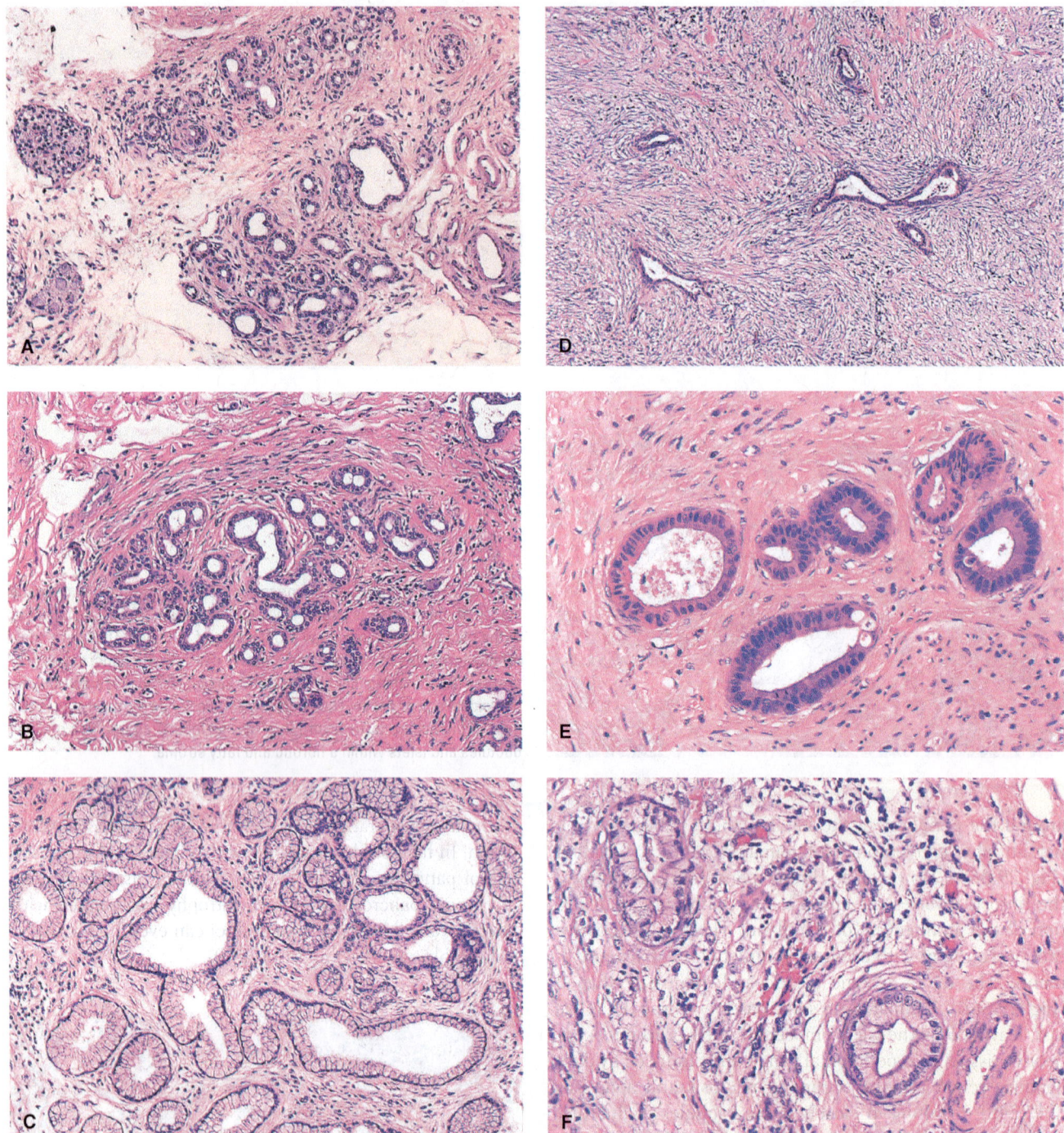

FIGURE 29.68 Comparison of ductules in atrophic chronic pancreatitis with well-differentiated ductal adenocarcinoma. In chronic pancreatitis, there is preservation of the lobular arrangement of small ductules (**A**) with larger branching ductules surrounded by collections of smaller tubular glands. Some residual islets of Langerhans are also present. At higher power (**B**) the cells are generally uniform, with round nuclei having a similar cytologic appearance from cell to cell. In areas showing mucinous metaplasia (**C**), there may not be as obvious a lobular arrangement. However, the glands retain a benign cytologic appearance and have uniformly basally oriented nuclei. In infiltrating adenocarcinoma (**D**), the lobular arrangement of the glands is lost. There is a haphazard configuration of angulated glands within a desmoplastic stroma. In some instances (**E**) there may not be significant stromal desmoplasia and the glands may retain rounded contours. However, there is variability in cytologic appearance from one cell to the next, with occasional macronucleoli, loss of polarity, and mitotic figures. Some individual glands of infiltrating carcinoma may be almost impossible to distinguish from benign ductules (**F**). This remarkably well-differentiated gland (*lower right*) contrasts with an adjacent gland showing marked loss of nuclear polarity. The abnormal location of the gland adjacent to a muscular artery is another clue that it is malignant.

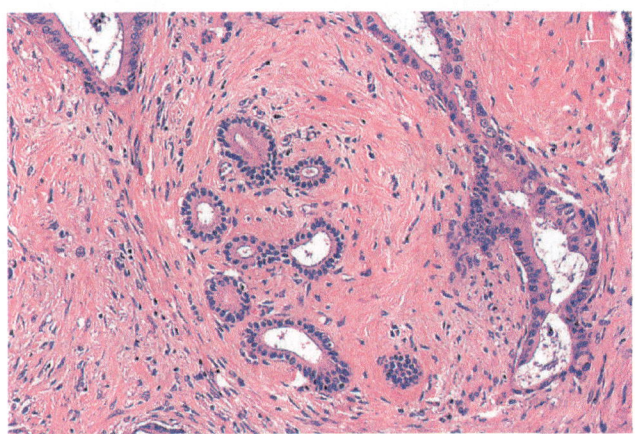

FIGURE 29.69 It is helpful to identify two populations of cells in specimens harboring an infiltrating adenocarcinoma. In this example, a lobular collection of benign ductules contrasts with irregularly shaped glands of adenocarcinoma.

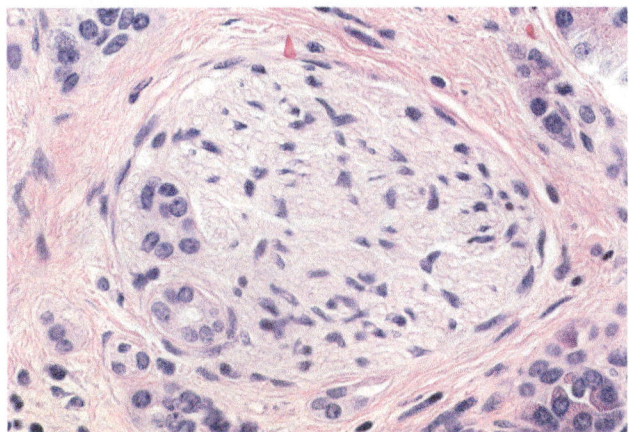

FIGURE 29.70 A rare example of a benign perineural gland in a region of chronic pancreatitis. Reprinted with permission from Hruban RH, Pitman MB, Klimstra DS. Tumors of the pancreas. In: Silverberg SG, Sobin LH, eds. *Atlas of Tumor Pathology*. 4th ed. Washington, DC: American Registry of Pathology; 2006.

The distinction of chronic pancreatitis from infiltrating ductal adenocarcinoma on small biopsies can be very challenging (251). The distorted ducts and ductules in areas of fibrosis closely resemble the pattern of ductal adenocarcinoma, and the fibrotic stroma may simulate the desmoplastic stroma often accompanying carcinoma. Features that support the interpretation of chronic pancreatitis include a retention of the lobular arrangement of the small collections of ductules, normal location of the glands, and uniformity of nuclear morphology from one cell to the next (Fig. 29.68A–C). Features that conversely favor the diagnosis of carcinoma include haphazardly arranged individual angulated glands infiltrating the stroma, glands in abnormal locations (adjacent to muscular arteries (159), in the perineurium, within vessels, or immediately apposed to adipocytes), significant cytologic abnormalities (variation in shape and size of nuclei from one cell to the next, macronucleoli, loss of nuclear polarity), and individual cells or small cell clusters in the stroma (Figs. 29.68D–F and 29.69). Perineural invasion by glandular cells is a highly specific finding for a diagnosis of carcinoma, with the caveat that extremely rare examples of perineural benign glands have been documented (Fig. 29.70). In addition, one must not mistake perineural nonneoplastic islet cells for carcinoma. It is helpful when two cytologically distinct populations of cells are found in the biopsy, since some of the nuclear features of well-differentiated carcinomas are very subtle unless compared with a second population of clearly benign glands. Unfortunately, biopsy samples of the pancreas are frequently small, and it is uncommon for all of the characteristic features to be present. Even if carcinoma is present, it may only be represented by two or three glands. Furthermore, needle biopsy samples are sometimes subjected to frozen section examination, which may introduce artifacts complicating the interpretation. Even for the experienced observer, there may be cases having rare atypical glands that cannot be confidently diagnosed as benign or malignant. Producing deeper sections sometimes reveals additional diagnostic features. In addition, immunohistochemistry can be useful to document some of the abnormalities characteristic of carcinoma. Most benign glands do not express CEA, B72.3, CA125, or p53 at immunohistochemically detectable levels (115), and they will all show normal intact labeling for the Dpc4 protein. By contrast, most pancreatic cancers express CEA diffusely in the cytoplasm, 75% label for B72.3, 50% to 75% for p53, 45% for CA125, and 55% show complete loss of Dpc4 expression (Fig. 29.71) (252). Expression of mesothelin also supports a diagnosis of carcinoma..

Atrophy of pancreatic parenchyma due to long-standing ductal obstruction is often associated with infiltration by

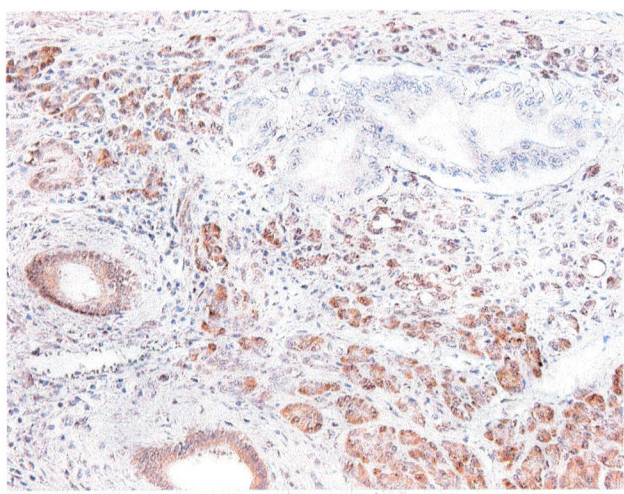

FIGURE 29.71 Immunohistochemisty for Dpc4 shows both nuclear and cytoplasmic labeling in normal acini and ducts, whereas the invasive carcinoma has complete absence of labeling.

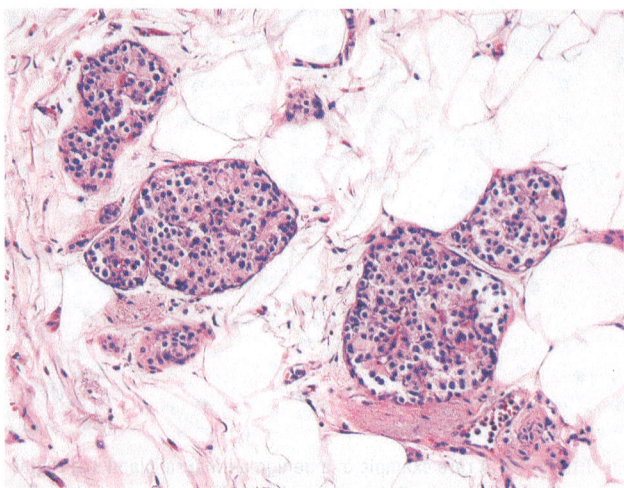

FIGURE 29.72 With extreme atrophy, the residual islets of Langerhans may be completely surrounded by adipose tissue.

adipose tissue. Only rare islets may be found between lobules of fat in extreme cases (Fig. 29.72). One primary form of fatty infiltration is Shwachman syndrome, an extremely rare autosomal recessive syndrome affecting the pancreas, bone marrow, and skeleton (253). An enlarged gland may result, but the amount of parenchymal tissue is reduced and exocrine insufficiency is present (19). The terms "lipomatosis" or "lipomatous pseudohypertrophy" have been applied to pancreata containing more than 25% adipose tissue (Fig. 29.73). The distribution of the adipose tissue is generally not uniform and, when localized, it can simulate a pancreatic neoplasm radiographically (254) Lipomatosis is usually associated with parenchymal atrophy and is more common in older individuals (15). Other associations include adult-under diabetes and generalized atherosclerosis, conditions that are also more prevalent in the elderly.

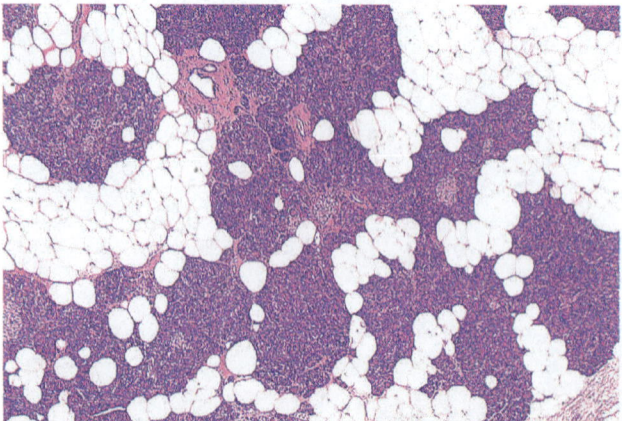

FIGURE 29.73 In pancreatic lipomatosis, adipose tissue comprises more than 25% of the volume of the gland. As in this case, the remaining parenchyma may not necessarily show changes of atrophic chronic pancreatitis.

Pancreatic lipomatosis is not necessarily associated with generalized obesity (15).

REFERENCES

1. Fawcett DW. *Bloom and Fawcett: A Textbook of Histology.* 12th ed. New York: Chapman and Hall; 1994.
2. Moore K, Dalley AF, Agur AMR. *Clinically Oriented Anatomy.* 8th ed. Philadelphia, PA: LWW; 2017.
3. Lack EE. *Pathology of the Pancreas, Gallbladder, Extrahepatic Biliary Tract, and Ampullary Region.* New York: Oxford University Press, Inc; 2003.
4. Skandalakis LJ, Rowe JS Jr., Gray SW, et al. Surgical embryology and anatomy of the pancreas. *Surg Clin North Am* 1993; 73(4):661–697.
5. Pansky B. Anatomy of the pancreas. Emphasis on blood supply and lymphatic drainage. *Int J Pancreatol* 1990;7(1-3): 101–108.
6. Bockman DE. Anatomy of the pancreas. In: Go VL, Brooks FP, DiMagno EP, et al, eds. *The Exocrine Pancreas. Biology, Pathobiology, and Diseases.* New York: Raven Press; 1986:1–7.
7. Verbeke CS. Resection margins and R1 rates in pancreatic cancer—are we there yet? *Histopathology* 2008;52(7): 787–796.
8. Ibukuro K. Vascular anatomy of the pancreas and clinical applications. *Int J Gastrointest Cancer* 2001;30(1-2):87–104.
9. Okahara M, Mori H, Kiyosue H, et al. Arterial supply to the pancreas; variations and cross-sectional anatomy. *Abdom Imaging* 2010;35(2):134–142.
10. Bertelli E, Di Gregorio F, Bertelli L, et al. The arterial blood supply of the pancreas: A review. IV. The anterior inferior and posterior pancreaticoduodenal aa., and minor sources of blood supply for the head of the pancreas. An anatomical review and radiologic study. *Surg Radiol Anat* 1997;19(4):203–212.
11. Bertelli E, Di Gregorio F, Bertelli L, et al. The arterial blood supply of the pancreas: A review. II. The posterior superior pancreaticoduodenal artery. An anatomical and radiological study. *Surg Radiol Anat* 1996;18(1):1–9.
12. Bertelli E, Di Gregorio F, Bertelli L, et al. The arterial blood supply of the pancreas: A review. I. The superior pancreaticoduodenal and the anterior superior pancreaticoduodenal arteries. An anatomical and radiological study. *Surg Radiol Anat* 1995;17(2):97–106, 101–103.
13. Navas V, O'Morchoe PJ, O'Morchoe CC. Lymphatic system of the rat pancreas. *Lymphology* 1995;28(1):4–20.
14. Cubilla AL, Fortner J, Fitzgerald PJ. Lymph node involvement in carcinoma of the head of the pancreas area. *Cancer* 1978; 41(3):880–887.
15. Stamm BH. Incidence and diagnostic significance of minor pathologic changes in the adult pancreas at autopsy: A systematic study of 112 autopsies in patients without known pancreatic disease. *Hum Pathol* 1984;15(7):677–683.
16. Heitz PU, Beglinger C, Gyr K. Anatomy and physiology of the exocrine pancreas. In: Kloppel G, Heitz PU, eds. *Pancreatic Pathology.* New York: Churchill-Livingstone; 1984:3–21.
17. Saisho Y, Butler AE, Meier JJ, et al. Pancreas volumes in humans from birth to age one hundred taking into account sex, obesity, and presence of type-2 diabetes. *Clin Anat* 2007; 20(8):933–942.

18. Birnstingl M. A study of pancreatography. *Br J Surg* 1959; 47:128–139.
19. Cubilla AL, Fitzgerald PJ. Tumors of the exocrine pancreas. In: Hartmann WH, Sobin LH, eds. *Atlas of Tumor Pathology. 2nd Series, Fascicle 19*. Washington, DC: Armed Forces Institute of Pathology; 1984.
20. Kozu T, Suda K, Toki F. Pancreatic development and anatomical variation. *Gastrointest Endosc Clin N Am* 1995;5(1):1–30.
21. Noe M, Rezaee N, Asrani K, et al. Immunolabeling of cleared human pancreata provides insights into three-dimensional pancreatic anatomy and pathology. *Am J Pathol* 2018;188(7):1530–1535.
22. Baggenstoss AH. Major duodenal papilla. Variations of pathologic interest and lesions of the mucosa. *Arch Pathol* 1938;26:853–868.
23. DiMagno EP, Shorter RG, Taylor WF, et al. Relationships between pancreaticobiliary ductal anatomy and pancreatic ductal and parenchymal histology. *Cancer* 1982;49(2):361–368.
24. Flati G, Flati D, Porowska B, et al. Surgical anatomy of the papilla of Vater and biliopancreatic ducts. *Am Surg* 1994;60(9):712–718.
25. Frierson HF Jr. The gross anatomy and histology of the gallbladder, extrahepatic bile ducts, Vaterian system, and minor papilla. *Am J Surg Pathol* 1989;13(2):146–162.
26. Larsen HL, Grapin-Botton A. The molecular and morphogenetic basis of pancreas organogenesis. *Semin Cell Dev Biol* 2017;66:51–68.
27. Jennings RE, Berry AA, Strutt JP, et al. Human pancreas development. *Development* 2015;142(18):3126–3137.
28. Watt AJ, Zhao R, Li J, et al. Development of the mammalian liver and ventral pancreas is dependent on GATA4. *BMC Dev Biol* 2007;7:37.
29. Edlund H. Pancreas: How to get there from the gut? *Curr Opin Cell Biol* 1999;11(6):663–668.
30. Dassaye R, Naidoo S, Cerf ME. Transcription factor regulation of pancreatic organogenesis, differentiation and maturation. *Islets* 2016;8(1):13–34.
31. Burlison JS, Long Q, Fujitani Y, et al. Pdx-1 and Ptf1a concurrently determine fate specification of pancreatic multipotent progenitor cells. *Dev Biol* 2008;316(1):74–86.
32. Gu G, Dubauskaite J, Melton DA. Direct evidence for the pancreatic lineage: NGN3+ cells are islet progenitors and are distinct from duct progenitors. *Development* 2002;129(10):2447–2457.
33. Bastidas-Ponce A, Scheibner K, Lickert H, et al. Cellular and molecular mechanisms coordinating pancreas development. *Development* 2017;144(16):2873–2888.
34. Bechard ME, Bankaitis ED, Hipkens SB, et al. Precommitment low-level Neurog3 expression defines a long-lived mitotic endocrine-biased progenitor pool that drives production of endocrine-committed cells. *Genes Dev* 2016;30(16):1852–1865.
35. Murtaugh LC, Stanger BZ, Kwan KM, et al. Notch signaling controls multiple steps of pancreatic differentiation. *Proc Natl Acad Sci U S A* 2003;100(25):14920–14925.
36. Afelik S, Jensen J. Notch signaling in the pancreas: Patterning and cell fate specification. *Wiley Interdiscip Rev Dev Biol* 2013;2(4):531–544.
37. Qu X, Afelik S, Jensen JN, et al. Notch-mediated post-translational control of Ngn3 protein stability regulates pancreatic patterning and cell fate commitment. *Dev Biol* 2013;376(1):1–12.
38. Hebrok M. Hedgehog signaling in pancreas development. *Mech Dev* 2003;120(1):45–57.
39. Villasenor A, Chong DC, Henkemeyer M, et al. Epithelial dynamics of pancreatic branching morphogenesis. *Development* 2010;137(24):4295–4305.
40. Zhou Q, Law AC, Rajagopal J, et al. A multipotent progenitor domain guides pancreatic organogenesis. *Dev Cell* 2007;13(1):103–114.
41. Chong JM, Fukayama M, Shiozawa Y, et al. Fibrillary inclusions in neoplastic and fetal acinar cells of the pancreas. *Virchows Arch* 1996;428(4-5):261–266.
42. Laitio M, Lev R, Orlic D. The developing human fetal pancreas: An ultrastructural and histochemical study with special reference to exocrine cells. *J Anat* 1974;117(Pt 3):619–634.
43. Lebenthal E, Lev R, Lee PC. Prenatal and postnatal development of the human exocrine pancreas. In: Go VL, Brooks FP, DiMagno EP, et al., eds. *The Exocrine Pancreas. Biology, Pathobiology, and Diseases*. New York: Raven Press; 1986:33–43.
44. Hassan MO, Gogate PA. Malignant mixed exocrine-endocrine tumor of the pancreas with unusual intracytoplasmic inclusions. *Ultrastruct Pathol* 1993;17(5):483–493.
45. Klimstra DS, Heffess CS, Oertel JE, et al. Acinar cell carcinoma of the pancreas. A clinicopathologic study of 28 cases. *Am J Surg Pathol* 1992;16(9):815–837.
46. Klimstra DS, Rosai J, Heffess CS. Mixed acinar-endocrine carcinomas of the pancreas. *Am J Surg Pathol* 1994;18(8):765–778.
47. Klimstra DS, Wenig BM, Adair CF, et al. Pancreatoblastoma. A clinicopathologic study and review of the literature. *Am J Surg Pathol* 1995;19(12):1371–1389.
48. Tucker JA, Shelburne JD, Benning TL, et al. Filamentous inclusions in acinar cell carcinoma of the pancreas. *Ultrastruct Pathol* 1994;18(1-2):279–286.
49. Gouzi M, Kim YH, Katsumoto K, et al. Neurogenin3 initiates stepwise delamination of differentiating endocrine cells during pancreas development. *Dev Dyn* 2011;240(3):589–604.
50. Jeon J, Correa-Medina M, Ricordi C, et al. Endocrine cell clustering during human pancreas development. *J Histochem Cytochem* 2009;57(9):811–824.
51. Clark A, Grant AM. Quantitative morphology of endocrine cells in human fetal pancreas. *Diabetologia* 1983;25(1):31–35.
52. Grasso S, Palumbo G, Fallucca F, et al. The development and function of the endocrine pancreas of fetuses and infants born to normal and diabetic mothers. *Acta Endocrinol Suppl (Copenh)* 1986;277:130–135.
53. Robb P. The development of the islets of Langerhans in the human foetus. *Q J Exp Physiol Cogn Med Sci* 1961;46:335–343.
54. Conklin JL. Cytogenesis of the human fetal pancreas. *Am J Anat* 1962;111:181–193.
55. Puri S, Hebrok M. Dynamics of embryonic pancreas development using real-time imaging. *Dev Biol* 2007;306(1):82–93.
56. Albores-Saavedra J, Gould EW, Angeles-Angeles A, et al. Cystic tumors of the pancreas. *Pathol Annu* 1990;25(Pt 2):19–50.

57. Compagno J, Oertel JE. Mucinous cystic neoplasms of the pancreas with overt and latent malignancy (cystadenocarcinoma and cystadenoma). A clinicopathologic study of 41 cases. *Am J Clin Pathol* 1978;69(6):573–580.
58. Khan N, Dandan W, Al Hassani N, et al. A newly-discovered mutation in the RFX6 gene of the rare Mitchell–Riley syndrome. *J Clin Res Pediatr Endocrinol* 2016;8(2):246–249.
59. Duval H, Michel-Calemard L, Gonzales M, et al. Fetal anomalies associated with HNF1B mutations: Report of 20 autopsy cases. *Prenat Diagn* 2016;36(8):744–751.
60. Haldorsen IS, Vesterhus M, Raeder H, et al. Lack of pancreatic body and tail in HNF1B mutation carriers. *Diabet Med* 2008;25(7):782–787.
61. Balasubramanian M, Shield JP, Acerini CL, et al. Pancreatic hypoplasia presenting with neonatal diabetes mellitus in association with congenital heart defect and developmental delay. *Am J Med Genet A* 2010;152A(2):340–346.
62. Schnedl WJ, Piswanger-Soelkner C, Wallner SJ, et al. Agenesis of the dorsal pancreas and associated diseases. *Dig Dis Sci* 2009;54(3):481–487.
63. Klein WA, Dabezies MA, Friedman AC, et al. Agenesis of dorsal pancreas in a patient with weight loss and diabetes mellitus. *Dig Dis Sci* 1994;39(8):1708–1713.
64. Wang JT, Lin JT, Chuang CN, et al. Complete agenesis of the dorsal pancreas—a case report and review of the literature. *Pancreas* 1990;5(4):493–497.
65. England RE, Newcomer MK, Leung JW, et al. Case report: Annular pancreas divisum—a report of two cases and review of the literature. *Br J Radiol* 1995;68(807):324–328.
66. Newman BM, Lebenthal E. Congenital abnormalities of the exocrine pancreas. In: Go VL, Brooks FP, DiMagno EP, et al., eds. *The Exocrine Pancreas. Biology, Pathobiology, and Diseases*. New York: Raven Press; 1986:773–782.
67. Dowsett JF, Rode J, Russell RC. Annular pancreas: A clinical, endoscopic, and immunohistochemical study. *Gut* 1989;30(1):130–135.
68. Dimitriou I, Katsourakis A, Nikolaidou E, Noussios G. The main anatomical variations of the pancreatic duct system: Review of the literature and its importance in surgical practice. *J Clin Med Res* 2018;10(5):370–375.
69. Adibelli ZH, Adatepe M, Imamoglu C, et al. Anatomic variations of the pancreatic duct and their relevance with the Cambridge classification system: MRCP findings of 1158 consecutive patients. *Radiol Oncol* 2016;50(4):370–377.
70. Dawson W, Langman J. An anatomical-radiological study on the pancreatic duct pattern in man. *Anat Rec* 1961;139:59–68.
71. Pezzilli R. Pancreas divisum and acute or chronic pancreatitis. *JOP* 2012;13(1):118–119.
72. Bertin C, Pelletier AL, Vullierme MP, et al. Pancreas divisum is not a cause of pancreatitis by itself but acts as a partner of genetic mutations. *Am J Gastroenterol* 2012;107(2):311–317.
73. Kimura K, Ohto M, Saisho H, et al. Association of gallbladder carcinoma and anomalous pancreaticobiliary ductal union. *Gastroenterology* 1985;89(6):1258–1265.
74. Kinoshita H, Nagata E, Hirohashi K, et al. Carcinoma of the gallbladder with an anomalous connection between the choledochus and the pancreatic duct. Report of 10 cases and review of the literature in Japan. *Cancer* 1984;54(4):762–769.
75. Krishnamurty VS, Rajendran S, Korsten MA. Bifid pancreas. An unusual anomaly associated with acute pancreatitis. *Int J Pancreatol* 1994;16(2-3):179–181.
76. Lai EC, Tompkins RK. Heterotopic pancreas. Review of a 26 year experience. *Am J Surg* 1986;151(6):697–700.
77. Pang LC. Pancreatic heterotopia: A reappraisal and clinicopathologic analysis of 32 cases. *South Med J* 1988;81(10):1264–1275.
78. Tanaka K, Tsunoda T, Eto T, et al. Diagnosis and management of heterotopic pancreas. *Int Surg* 1993;78(1):32–35.
79. Laughlin EH, Keown ME, Jackson JE. Heterotopic pancreas obstructing the ampulla of Vater. *Arch Surg* 1983;118(8):979–980.
80. Tsunoda T, Eto T, Yamada M, et al. Heterotopic pancreas: A rare cause of bile duct dilatation—report of a case and review of the literature. *Jpn J Surg* 1990;20(2):217–220.
81. Seifert G. Congenital anomalies. In: Kloppel G, Heitz PU, eds. *Pancreatic Pathology*. New York: Churchill-Livingstone; 1984:22–26.
82. Zhang Y, Sun X, Gold JS, et al. Heterotopic pancreas: A clinicopathological study of 184 cases from a single high-volume medical center in China. *Hum Pathol* 2016;55:135–142.
83. Persson GE, Boiesen PT. Cancer of aberrant pancreas in jejunum. Case report. *Acta Chir Scand* 1988;154(10):599–601.
84. Tanimura A, Yamamoto H, Shibata H, et al. Carcinoma in heterotopic gastric pancreas. *Acta Pathol Jpn* 1979;29(2):251–257.
85. Goodarzi M, Rashid A, Maru D. Invasive ductal adenocarcinoma arising from pancreatic heterotopia in rectum: Case report and review of literature. *Hum Pathol* 2010;41(12):1809–1813.
86. Tsapralis D, Charalabopoulos A, Karamitopoulou E, et al. Pancreatic intraductal papillary mucinous neoplasm with concomitant heterotopic pancreatic cystic neoplasia of the stomach: a case report and review of the literature. *Diagn Pathol* 2010;5:4.
87. Ma C, Gocke CD, Hruban RH, et al. Mutational spectrum of intraepithelial neoplasia in pancreatic heterotopia. *Hum Pathol* 2016;48:117–121.
88. Sun Y, Wasserman PG. Acinar cell carcinoma arising in the stomach: A case report with literature review. *Hum Pathol* 2004;35(2):263–265.
89. Chetty R, Weinreb I. Gastric neuroendocrine carcinoma arising from heterotopic pancreatic tissue. *J Clin pathol* 2004;57(3):314–317.
90. Landry ML, Sarma DP. Accessory spleen in the head of the pancreas. *Hum Pathol* 1989;20(5):497.
91. Albores-Saavedra J. The Pseudometastasis. *Patologia* 1994;32:63–71.
92. Akao S, Bockman DE, Lechene de la Porte P, et al. Three-dimensional pattern of ductuloacinar associations in normal and pathological human pancreas. *Gastroenterology* 1986;90(3):661–668.
93. Henderson JR, Daniel PM, Fraser PA. The pancreas as a single organ: The influence of the endocrine upon the exocrine part of the gland. *Gut* 1981;22(2):158–167.
94. Williams JA, Goldfine ID. The insulin–acinar relationship. In: Go VL, Brooks FP, DiMagno EP, et al., eds. *The Exocrine Pancreas. Biology, Pathobiology, and Diseases*. New York: Raven Press; 1986:347–360.

95. Hoorens A, Lemoine NR, McLellan E, et al. Pancreatic acinar cell carcinoma. An analysis of cell lineage markers, p53 expression, and Ki-ras mutation. *Am J Pathol* 1993;143(3): 685–698.
96. La Rosa S, Franzi F, Marchet S, et al. The monoclonal anti-BCL10 antibody (clone 331.1) is a sensitive and specific marker of pancreatic acinar cell carcinoma and pancreatic metaplasia. *Virchows Arch* 2009;454(2):133–142.
97. Bendayan M, Roth J, Perrelet A, et al. Quantitative immunocytochemical localization of pancreatic secretory proteins in subcellular compartments of the rat acinar cell. *J Histochem Cytochem* 1980;28(2):149–160.
98. Kraehenbuhl JP, Racine L, Jamieson JD. Immunocytochemical localization of secretory proteins in bovine pancreatic exocrine cells. *J Cell Biol* 1977;72(2):406–423.
99. Kern HF. Fine structure of the human exocrine pancreas. In: Go VL, Brooks FP, DiMagno EP, et al., eds. *The Exocrine Pancreas. Biology, Pathobiology, and Diseases.* New York: Raven Press; 1986:9–19.
100. Palade G. Intracellular aspects of the process of protein synthesis. *Science* 1975;189(4200):347–358.
101. Romagnoli P. Increases in apical plasma membrane surface paralleling enzyme secretion from exocrine pancreatic acinar cells. *Pancreas* 1988;3(2):189–192.
102. Pallagi P, Hegyi P, Rakonczay Z Jr. The physiology and pathophysiology of pancreatic ductal secretion: The background for clinicians. *Pancreas* 2015;44(8):1211–1233.
103. Kodama T. A light and electron microscopic study on the pancreatic ductal system. *Acta Pathol Jpn* 1983;33(2): 297–321.
104. Greider MH. Oxyphil cells of the human pancreas. *Anat Rec* 1967;157:251.
105. Delporte C. Aquaporins and gland secretion. *Adv Exp Med Biol* 2017;969:63–79.
106. Burghardt B, Nielsen S, Steward MC. The role of aquaporin water channels in fluid secretion by the exocrine pancreas. *J Membr Biol* 2006;210(2):143–153.
107. Roberts PF, Burns J. A histochemical study of mucins in normal and neoplastic human pancreatic tissue. *J Pathol* 1972;107(2):87–94.
108. Solcia E, Capella C, Kloppel G. Tumors of the pancreas. In: Rosai J, Sobin LH, eds. *Atlas of Tumor Pathology. 3rd Series, Fascicle 20.* Washington, DC: Armed Forces Institute of Pathology; 1996.
109. diIorio P, Rittenhouse AR, Bortell R, et al. Role of cilia in normal pancreas function and in diseased states. *Birth Defects Res C Embryo Today* 2014;102(2):126–138.
110. Schulz I. Electrolyte and fluid secretion in the exocrine pancreas. In: Johnson LR, ed. *Physiology of the Gastrointestinal Tract.* New York: Raven Press; 1981:795–819.
111. Spicer SS, Sens MA, Tashian RE. Immunocytochemical demonstration of carbonic anhydrase in human epithelial cells. *J Histochem Cytochem* 1982;30:864–873.
112. Atkinson BF, Ernst CS, Herlyn M, et al. Gastrointestinal cancer-associated antigen in immunoperoxidase assay. *Cancer Res* 1982;42(11):4820–4823.
113. Borowitz MJ, Tuck FL, Sindelar WF, et al. Monoclonal antibodies against human pancreatic adenocarcinoma: Distribution of DU-PAN-2 antigen on glandular epithelia and adenocarcinomas. *J Natl Cancer Inst* 1984;72(5): 999–1005.
114. Haglund C, Lindgren J, Roberts PJ, et al. Gastrointestinal cancer-associated antigen CA 19-9 in histological specimens of pancreatic tumours and pancreatitis. *Br J Cancer* 1986;53(2): 189–195.
115. Klimstra DS, Hameed MR, Marrero AM, et al. Ductal proliferative lesion associated with infiltrating ductal adenocarcinoma of the pancreas. *Int J Pancreatol* 1994;16:224–225.
116. Sessa F, Bonato M, Frigerio B, et al. Ductal cancers of the pancreas frequently express markers of gastrointestinal epithelial cells. *Gastroenterology* 1990;98(6):1655–1665.
117. Furuhata A, Minamiguchi S, Shirahase H, et al. Immunohistochemical antibody panel for the differential diagnosis of pancreatic ductal carcinoma from gastrointestinal contamination and benign pancreatic duct epithelium in endoscopic ultrasound-guided fine-needle aspiration. *Pancreas* 2017;46(4): 531–538.
118. Kim JH, Ho SB, Montgomery CK, et al. Cell lineage markers in human pancreatic cancer. *Cancer* 1990;66(10): 2134–2143.
119. Balague C, Gambus G, Carrato C, et al. Altered expression of MUC2, MUC4, and MUC5 mucin genes in pancreas tissues and cancer cell lines. *Gastroenterology* 1994;106(4): 1054–1061.
120. Terada T, Ohta T, Sasaki M, et al. Expression of MUC apomucins in normal pancreas and pancreatic tumours. *J Pathol* 1996;180(2):160–165.
121. Moschovis D, Bamias G, Delladetsima I. Mucins in neoplasms of pancreas, ampulla of Vater and biliary system. *World J Gastrointest Oncol* 2016;8(10):725–734.
122. Rahier J, Wallon J, Henquin JC. Cell populations in the endocrine pancreas of human neonates and infants. *Diabetologia* 1981;20(5):540–546.
123. Wittingen J, Frey CF. Islet concentration in the head, body, tail and uncinate process of the pancreas. *Ann Surg* 1974; 179(4):412–414.
124. Wang X, Misawa R, Zielinski MC, et al. Regional differences in islet distribution in the human pancreas–preferential beta-cell loss in the head region in patients with type 2 diabetes. *PloS one* 2013;8(6):e67454.
125. Fowler JL, Lee SS, Wesner ZC, et al. Three-dimensional analysis of the human pancreas. *Endocrinology* 2018;159(3): 1393–1400.
126. Stefan Y, Grasso S, Perrelet A, et al. A quantitative immunofluorescent study of the endocrine cell populations in the developing human pancreas. *Diabetes* 1983;32(4):293–301.
127. Grube D, Bohn R. The microanatomy of human islets of Langerhans, with special reference to somatostatin (D-) cells. *Arch Histol Jpn* 1983;46(3):327–353.
128. Malaisse-Lagae F, Stefan Y, Cox J, et al. Identification of a lobe in the adult human pancreas rich in pancreatic polypeptide. *Diabetologia* 1979;17(6):361–365.
129. Stefan Y, Grasso S, Perrelet A, et al. The pancreatic polypeptide-rich lobe of the human pancreas: Definitive identification of its derivation from the ventral pancreatic primordium. *Diabetologia* 1982;23(2):141–142.
130. Ehrie MG, Swartz FJ. Diploid, tetraploid and octaploid beta cells in the islets of Langerhans of the normal human pancreas. *Diabetes* 1974;23(7):583–588.
131. Lecompte PM, Merriam JC Jr. Mitotic figures and enlarged nuclei in the Islands of Langerhans in man. *Diabetes* 1962;11: 35–39.

132. El-Gohary Y, Sims-Lucas S, Lath N, et al. Three-dimensional analysis of the islet vasculature. *Anat Rec (Hoboken)* 2012;295(9):1473–1481.
133. Wierup N, Sundler F, Heller RS. The islet ghrelin cell. *J Mol Endocrinol* 2014;52(1):R35–R49.
134. Pisania A, Weir GC, O'Neil JJ, et al. Quantitative analysis of cell composition and purity of human pancreatic islet preparations. *Lab Invest* 2010;90(11):1661–1675.
135. Bommer G, Friedl U, Heitz PU, et al. Pancreatic PP cell distribution and hyperplasia. Immunocytochemical morphology in the normal human pancreas, in chronic pancreatitis and pancreatic carcinoma. *Virchows Arch A Pathol Anat Histol* 1980;387(3):319–331.
136. Kloppel G, Lenzen S. Anatomy and physiology of the endocrine pancreas. In: Kloppel G, Heitz PU, eds. *Pancreatic Pathology*. New York: Churchill-Livingstone; 1984: 133–153.
137. Orci L, Baetens D, Ravazzola M, et al. Pancreatic polypeptide and glucagon: non-random distribution in pancreatic islets. *Life Sci* 1976;19(12):1811–1815.
138. Orci L, Malaisse-Lagae F, Baetens D, et al. Pancreatic-polypeptide-rich regions in human pancreas. *Lancet* 1978; 2(8101):1200–1201.
139. Wang X, Zielinski MC, Misawa R, et al. Quantitative analysis of pancreatic polypeptide cell distribution in the human pancreas. *PloS one* 2013;8(1):e55501.
140. Orci L, Stefan Y, Malaisse-Lagae F, et al. Instability of pancreatic endocrine cell populations throughout life. *Lancet* 1979;1(8116):615–616.
141. Fellinger EJ, Garin-Chesa P, Triche TJ, et al. Immunohistochemical analysis of Ewing's sarcoma cell surface antigen p30/32MIC2. *Am J Pathol* 1991;139(2):317–325.
142. Hochwald SN, Zee S, Conlon KC, et al. Prognostic factors in pancreatic endocrine neoplasms: An analysis of 136 cases with a proposal for low-grade and intermediate-grade groups. *J Clin Oncol* 2002;20(11):2633–2642.
143. Weidner N, Tjoe J. Immunohistochemical profile of monoclonal antibody O13: Antibody that recognizes glycoprotein p30/32MIC2 and is useful in diagnosing Ewing's sarcoma and peripheral neuroepithelioma. *Am J Surg Pathol* 1994;18(5):486–494.
144. Park JY, Hong SM, Klimstra DS, et al. Pdx1 expression in pancreatic precursor lesions and neoplasms. *Appl Immunohistochem Mol Morphol* 2011;19(5):444–449.
145. Jensen J. Gene regulatory factors in pancreatic development. *Dev Dyn* 2004;229(1):176–200.
146. Hermann G, Konukiewitz B, Schmitt A, et al. Hormonally defined pancreatic and duodenal neuroendocrine tumors differ in their transcription factor signatures: Expression of ISL1, PDX1, NGN3, and CDX2. *Virchows Arch* 2011;459(2):147–154.
147. Kloppel G. Endokrines pankreas und diabetes mellitus. In: Doerr W, Seifert G, eds. *Spezielle Pathologische Anatomie*. Vol. 14. Berlin: Springer; 1981.
148. Pelletier G. Identification of four cell types in the human endocrine pancreas by immunoelectron microscopy. *Diabetes* 1977;26(8):749–756.
149. Chen J, Baithun SI, Pollock DJ, et al. Argyrophilic and hormone immunoreactive cells in normal and hyperplastic pancreatic ducts and exocrine pancreatic carcinoma. *Virchows Arch A Pathol Anat Histopathol* 1988;413(5):399–405.
150. Bendayan M. Presence of endocrine cells in pancreatic ducts. *Pancreas* 1987;2(4):393–397.
151. Oertel JE, Heffess CS, Oertel YC. Pancreas. In: Sternberg SS, ed. *Histology for Pathologists*. New York: Raven Press; 1992: 657–668.
152. Patchefsky AS, Solit R, Phillips LD, et al. Hydroxyindole-producing tumors of the pancreas. Carcinoid-islet cell tumor and oat cell carcinoma. *Ann Intern Med* 1972;77(1): 53–61.
153. Wilson RW, Gal AA, Cohen C, et al. Serotonin immunoreactivity in pancreatic endocrine neoplasms (carcinoid tumors). *Mod Pathol* 1991;4(6):727–732.
154. McCall CM, Shi C, Klein AP, et al. Serotonin expression in pancreatic neuroendocrine tumors correlates with a trabecular histologic pattern and large duct involvement. *Hum Pathol* 2012;43(8):1169–1176.
155. Chey WY. Hormonal control of pancreatic exocrine secretion. In: Go VL, Brooks FP, DiMagno EP, et al, eds. *The Exocrine Pancreas. Biology, Pathobiology, and Diseases*. New York: Raven Press; 1986:301–313.
156. Henderson JR, Daniel PM. A comparative study of the portal vessels connecting the endocrine and exocrine pancreas, with a discussion of some functional implications. *Q J Exp Physiol Cogn Med Sci* 1979;64(4):267–275.
157. Adeghate E, Donath T. Distribution of neuropeptide Y and vasoactive intestinal polypeptide immunoreactive nerves in normal and transplanted pancreatic tissue. *Peptides* 1990; 11(6):1087–1092.
158. Zhang Y, Nose V. Endocrine tumors as part of inherited tumor syndromes. *Adv Anat Pathol* 2011;18(3):206–218.
159. Sharma S, Green KB. The pancreatic duct and its arteriovenous relationship: An underutilized aid in the diagnosis and distinction of pancreatic adenocarcinoma from pancreatic intraepithelial neoplasia. A study of 126 pancreatectomy specimens. *Am J Surg Pathol* 2004;28(5):613–620.
160. Olsen TS. Lipomatosis of the pancreas in autopsy material and its relation to age and overweight. *Acta Pathol Microbiol Scand A* 1978;86A(5):367–373.
161. Orci L, Stefan Y, Malaisse-Lagae F, et al. Pancreatic fat. *N Engl J Med* 1979;301(23):1292.
162. Suda K, Mizuguchi K, Hoshino A. Differences of the ventral and dorsal anlagen of pancreas after fusion. *Acta Pathol Jpn* 1981;31(4):583–589.
163. Jaster R. Molecular regulation of pancreatic stellate cell function. *Mol Cancer* 2004;3:26.
164. Haqq J, Howells LM, Garcea G, et al. Pancreatic stellate cells and pancreas cancer: Current perspectives and future strategies. *Eur J Cancer* 2014;50(15):2570–2582.
165. Masamune A, Watanabe T, Kikuta K, et al. Roles of pancreatic stellate cells in pancreatic inflammation and fibrosis. *Clin Gastroenterol Hepatol* 2009;7(Suppl 11):S48–S54.
166. Popescu LM, Hinescu ME, Ionescu N, et al. Interstitial cells of Cajal in pancreas. *J Cell Mol Med* 2005;9(1):169–190.
167. Centeno BA, Pitman MB. Fine needle aspiration biopsy of the pancreas. In: Centeno BA, Pitman MB, eds. *Neoplasms of the Exocrine and Endocrine Pancreas*. Boston: Butterworth-Heinemann; 1999:109–160.
168. Hruban RH, Pitman MB, Klimstra DS. Tumors of the pancreas. In: Silverberg SG, Sobin LH, eds. *Atlas of Tumor Pathology*. 4th ed. Washington, DC: American Registry of Pathology; 2006.

169. Sigel CS, Klimstra DS. Cytomorphologic and immunophenotypical features of acinar cell neoplasms of the pancreas. *Cancer Cytopathol* 2013;121(8):459–470.
170. Shinozuka H, Lee RE, Dunn JL, et al. Multiple atypical acinar cell nodules of the pancreas. *Hum Pathol* 1980;11(4):389–391.
171. Tanaka T, Mori H, Williams GM. Atypical and neoplastic acinar cell lesions of the pancreas in an autopsy study of Japanese patients. *Cancer* 1988;61(11):2278–2285.
172. Troxell ML, Drachenberg C. Allograft pancreas: pale acinar nodules. *Hum Pathol* 2016;54:127–133.
173. Longnecker DS, Hashida Y, Shinozuka H. Relationship of age to prevalence of focal acinar cell dysplasia in the human pancreas. *J Natl Cancer Inst* 1980;65(1):63–66.
174. Oertel JE. The pancreas. Nonneoplastic alterations. *Am J Surg Pathol* 1989;13 Suppl 1:50–65.
175. Longnecker DS, Shinozuka H, Dekker A. Focal acinar cell dysplasia in human pancreas. *Cancer* 1980;45(3):534–540.
176. Kodama T, Mori W. Atypical acinar cell nodules of the human pancreas. *Acta Pathol Jpn* 1983;33(4):701–714.
177. Baggenstoss AH. The pancreas in uremia: A histopathologic study. *Am J Pathol* 1948;24:1003–1017.
178. Walters MN. Studies on the exocrine pancreas. I. Nonspecific pancreatic ductular ectasia. *Am J Pathol* 1964;44:973–981.
179. Walters MN. Goblet-cell metaplasia in ductules and acini of the exocrine pancreas. *J Pathol Bacteriol* 1965;89:569–572.
180. Schmid RM. Acinar-to-ductal metaplasia in pancreatic cancer development. *J Clin Invest* 2002;109(11):1403–1404.
181. Hruban RH, Adsay NV, Albores-Saavedra J, et al. Pathology of genetically engineered mouse models of pancreatic exocrine cancer: Consensus report and recommendations. *Cancer Res* 2006;66(1):95–106.
182. Bockman DE, Boydston WR, Anderson MC. Origin of tubular complexes in human chronic pancreatitis. *Am J Surg* 1982;144(2):243–249.
183. Aichler M, Seiler C, Tost M, et al. Origin of pancreatic ductal adenocarcinoma from atypical flat lesions: A comparative study in transgenic mice and human tissues. *J Pathol* 2012;226(5):723–734.
184. Hong SM, Heaphy CM, Shi C, et al. Telomeres are shortened in acinar-to-ductal metaplasia lesions associated with pancreatic intraepithelial neoplasia but not in isolated acinar-to-ductal metaplasias. *Mod Pathol* 2011;24(2):256–266.
185. Shi C, Hong SM, Lim P, et al. KRAS2 mutations in human pancreatic acinar-ductal metaplastic lesions are limited to those with PanIN: Implications for the human pancreatic cancer cell of origin. *Mol Cancer Res* 2009;7(2):230–236.
186. Cubilla AL, Fitzgerald PJ. Morphological lesions associated with human primary invasive nonendocrine pancreas cancer. *Cancer Res* 1976;36(7 Pt 2):2690–2698.
187. Kloppel G, Bommer G, Ruckert K, et al. Intraductal proliferation in the pancreas and its relationship to human and experimental carcinogenesis. *Virchows Arch A Pathol Anat Histol* 1980;387(2):221–233.
188. Roberts PF. Pyloric gland metaplasia of the human pancreas. A comparative histochemical study. *Arch Pathol* 1974;97(2):92–95.
189. Brat DJ, Lillemoe KD, Yeo CJ, et al. Progression of pancreatic intraductal neoplasias to infiltrating adenocarcinoma of the pancreas. *Am J Surg Pathol* 1998;22(2):163–169.
190. Goggins M, Hruban RH, Kern SE. BRCA2 is inactivated late in the development of pancreatic intraepithelial neoplasia: Evidence and implications. *Am J Pathol* 2000;156(5):1767–1771.
191. Maitra A, Adsay NV, Argani P, et al. Multicomponent analysis of the pancreatic adenocarcinoma progression model using a pancreatic intraepithelial neoplasia tissue microarray. *Mod Pathol* 2003;16(9):902–912.
192. Moskaluk CA, Hruban RH, Kern SE. p16 and K-ras gene mutations in the intraductal precursors of human pancreatic adenocarcinoma. *Cancer Res* 1997;57(11):2140–2143.
193. van Heek NT, Meeker AK, Kern SE, et al. Telomere shortening is nearly universal in pancreatic intraepithelial neoplasia. *Am J Pathol* 2002;161(5):1541–1547.
194. Wilentz RE, Iacobuzio-Donahue CA, Argani P, et al. Loss of expression of Dpc4 in pancreatic intraepithelial neoplasia: Evidence that DPC4 inactivation occurs late in neoplastic progression. *Cancer Res* 2000;60(7):2002–2006.
195. Klimstra DS, Longnecker DS. K-ras mutations in pancreatic ductal proliferative lesions. *Am J Pathol* 1994;145(6):1547–1550.
196. Mukada T, Yamada S. Dysplasia and carcinoma in situ of the exocrine pancreas. *Tohoku J Exp Med* 1982;137(2):115–124.
197. Hruban RH, Adsay NV, Albores-Saavedra J, et al. Pancreatic intraepithelial neoplasia: A new nomenclature and classification system for pancreatic duct lesions. *Am J Surg Pathol* 2001;25(5):579–586.
198. Hruban RH, Takaori K, Klimstra DS, et al. An illustrated consensus on the classification of pancreatic intraepithelial neoplasia and intraductal papillary mucinous neoplasms. *Am J Surg Pathol* 2004;28(8):977–987.
199. Basturk O, Hong SM, Wood LD, et al. A revised classification system and recommendations from the Baltimore consensus meeting for neoplastic precursor lesions in the pancreas. *Am J Surg Pathol* 2015;39(12):1730–1741.
200. Konstantinidis IT, Vinuela EF, Tang LH, et al. Incidentally discovered pancreatic intraepithelial neoplasia: What is its clinical significance? *Annals of Surgical Oncology*. 2013;20(11):3643–3647.
201. Gaujoux S, Brennan MF, Gonen M, et al. Cystic lesions of the pancreas: Changes in the presentation and management of 1,424 patients at a single institution over a 15-year time period. *J Am Coll Surg*. 2011;212(4):590–600; discussion 600–603.
202. Allen PJ, D'Angelica M, Gonen M, et al. A selective approach to the resection of cystic lesions of the pancreas: Results from 539 consecutive patients. *Annals of surgery* 2006;244(4):572–582.
203. Hosoda W, Chianchiano P, Griffin JF, et al. Genetic analyses of isolated high-grade pancreatic intraepithelial neoplasia (HG-PanIN) reveal paucity of alterations in TP53 and SMAD4. *J Pathol* 2017;242(1):16–23.
204. Hong SM, Park JY, Hruban RH, et al. Molecular signatures of pancreatic cancer. *Arch Pathol Lab Med* 2011;135(6):716–727.
205. Scarlett CJ, Salisbury EL, Biankin AV, et al. Precursor lesions in pancreatic cancer: Morphological and molecular pathology. *Pathology* 2011;43(3):183–200.
206. Klein WM, Hruban RH, Klein-Szanto AJ, et al. Direct correlation between proliferative activity and dysplasia in

207. Othman M, Basturk O, Groisman G, et al. Squamoid cyst of pancreatic ducts: A distinct type of cystic lesion in the pancreas. *Am J Surg Pathol* 2007;31(2):291–297.
208. Tasso F, Picard D. Sur les oncocytes du pancréas humain. *C R Soc Biol (Paris)* 1969;163:1855–1858.
209. Tasso F, Sarles H. Canalicular cells and oncocytes in the human pancreas. Comparative study on the normal condition and in chronic pancreatitis. *Ann Anat Pathol (Paris)*. 1973;18:277–300.
210. Frexinos J, Ribet A. Oncocytes in human chronic pancreatitis. *Digestion* 1972;7(5):294–301.
211. Albores-Saavedra J, Wu J, Crook T, et al. Intestinal and oncocytic variants of pancreatic intraepithelial neoplasia. A morphological and immunohistochemical study. *Ann Diagn Pathol* 2005;9(2):69–76.
212. Adsay NV, Merati K, Andea A, et al. The dichotomy in the preinvasive neoplasia to invasive carcinoma sequence in the pancreas: Differential expression of MUC1 and MUC2 supports the existence of two separate pathways of carcinogenesis. *Mod Pathol* 2002;15(10):1087–1095.
213. Adsay NV, Merati K, Basturk O, et al. Pathologically and biologically distinct types of epithelium in intraductal papillary mucinous neoplasms: Delineation of an "intestinal" pathway of carcinogenesis in the pancreas. *Am J Surg Pathol* 2004;28(7):839–848.
214. Klimstra D, Hruban R, Pitman M. Pancreas. In: Mills SE, ed. *Histology for Pathologists*. Philadelphia, PA: Lippincott, Williams and Wilkins; 2006:723–760.
215. Zamboni G, Terris B, Scarpa A, et al. Acinar cell cystadenoma of the pancreas: A new entity? *Am J Surg Pathol* 2002;26(6):698–704.
216. Singhi AD, Norwood S, Liu TC, et al. Acinar cell cystadenoma of the pancreas: A benign neoplasm or non-neoplastic ballooning of acinar and ductal epithelium? *Am J Surg Pathol* 2013;37(9):1329–1335.
217. Khor TS, Badizadegan K, Ferrone C, et al. Acinar cystadenoma of the pancreas: a clinicopathologic study of 10 cases including multilocular lesions with mural nodules. *Am J Surg Pathol* 2012;36(11):1579–1591.
218. Komatsu K. Pancreatographical and histopathological study of dilations of the pancreatic ductules with special references to cystic dilatation. *Juntendoo Med J* 1974;19:250–269.
219. Agostini S, Choux R, Payan MJ, et al. Mucinous pancreatic duct ectasia in the body of the pancreas. *Radiology* 1989;170(3 Pt 1):815–816.
220. Nagai E, Ueki T, Chijiiwa K, et al. Intraductal papillary mucinous neoplasms of the pancreas associated with so-called "mucinous ductal ectasia." Histochemical and immunohistochemical analysis of 29 cases. *Am J Surg Pathol* 1995;19(5):576–589.
221. Nishihara K, Fukuda T, Tsuneyoshi M, et al. Intraductal papillary neoplasm of the pancreas. *Cancer* 1993;72(3):689–696.
222. Sessa F, Solcia E, Capella C, et al. Intraductal papillary-mucinous tumours represent a distinct group of pancreatic neoplasms: an investigation of tumour cell differentiation and K-ras, p53 and c-erbB-2 abnormalities in 26 patients. *Virchows Arch* 1994;425(4):357–367.
223. Tian FZ, Myles J, Howard JM. Mucinous pancreatic ductal ectasia of latent malignancy: An emerging clinicopathologic entity. *Surgery* 1992;111(1):109–113.
224. Krasinskas AM, Oakley GJ, Bagci P, et al. "Simple mucinous cyst" of the pancreas: A clinicopathologic analysis of 39 examples of a diagnostically challenging entity distinct from intraductal papillary mucinous neoplasms and mucinous cystic neoplasms. *Am J Surg Pathol* 2017;41(1):121–127.
225. Solicia E, Capella C, Kloppel G. Tumors of the endocrine pancreas. In: *Atlas of Tumor Pathology of the Pancreas*. Washington, DC: Armed Forces Institute of Pathology; 1997:145–196.
226. Weidenheim KM, Hinchey WW, Campbell WG Jr. Hyperinsulinemic hypoglycemia in adults with islet-cell hyperplasia and degranulation of exocrine cells of the pancreas. *Am J Clin Pathol* 1983;79(1):14–24.
227. Goossens A, Gepts W, Saudubray JM, et al. Diffuse and focal nesidioblastosis. A clinicopathological study of 24 patients with persistent neonatal hyperinsulinemic hypoglycemia. *Am J Surg Pathol* 1989;13(9):766–775.
228. Stanley CA, Thornton PS, Ganguly A, et al. Preoperative evaluation of infants with focal or diffuse congenital hyperinsulinism by intravenous acute insulin response tests and selective pancreatic arterial calcium stimulation. *J Clin Endocrinol Metab* 2004;89(1):288–296.
229. Suchi M, MacMullen C, Thornton PS, et al. Histopathology of congenital hyperinsulinism: Retrospective study with genotype correlations. *Pediatr Dev Pathol* 2003;6(4):322–333.
230. Thomas PM, Cote GJ, Wohllk N, et al. Mutations in the sulfonylurea receptor gene in familial persistent hyperinsulinemic hypoglycemia of infancy. *Science* 1995;268(5209):426–429.
231. Kloppel G, Anlauf M, Raffel A, et al. Adult diffuse nesidioblastosis: genetically or environmentally induced? *Hum Pathol* 2008;39(1):3–8.
232. Clayton PT, Eaton S, Aynsley-Green A, et al. Hyperinsulinism in short-chain L-3-hydroxyacyl-CoA dehydrogenase deficiency reveals the importance of beta-oxidation in insulin secretion. *J Clin Invest* 2001;108(3):457–465.
233. Glaser B, Kesavan P, Heyman M, et al. Familial hyperinsulinism caused by an activating glucokinase mutation. *N Engl J Med* 1998;338(4):226–230.
234. Reinecke-Luthge A, Koschoreck F, Kloppel G. The molecular basis of persistent hyperinsulinemic hypoglycemia of infancy and its pathologic substrates. *Virchows Arch* 2000;436(1):1–5.
235. Stanley CA, Lieu YK, Hsu BY, et al. Hyperinsulinism and hyperammonemia in infants with regulatory mutations of the glutamate dehydrogenase gene. *N Engl J Med* 1998;338(19):1352–1357.
236. Bartow SA, Mukai K, Rosai J. Pseudoneoplastic proliferation of endocrine cells in pancreatic fibrosis. *Cancer* 1981;47(11):2627-2633.
237. Kovacs K, Horvath E, Asa SL, et al. Microscopic peliosis of pancreatic islets in a woman with MEN-1 syndrome. *Arch Pathol Lab Med* 1986;110(7):607–610.
238. Westermark P. Amyloid in the islets of Langerhans: Thoughts and some historical aspects. *Ups J Med Sci* 2011;116(2):81–89.
239. Kloppel G. Islet histopathology in diabetes mellitus. In: Kloppel G, Heitz PU, eds. *Pancreatic Pathology*. New York: Churchill-Livingstone; 1984:154-192.

240. Castellani C, Bonizzato A, Rolfini R, et al. Increased prevalence of mutations of the cystic fibrosis gene in idiopathic chronic and recurrent pancreatitis. *Am J Gastroenterol* 1999; 94(7):1993–1995.
241. Gorry MC, Gabbaizedeh D, Furey W, et al. Mutations in the cationic trypsinogen gene are associated with recurrent acute and chronic pancreatitis. *Gastroenterology* 1997; 113(4):1063–1068.
242. Ito T, Nakano I, Koyanagi S, et al. Autoimmune pancreatitis as a new clinical entity. Three cases of autoimmune pancreatitis with effective steroid therapy. *Dig Dis Sci* 1997; 42(7):1458–1468.
243. Kloppel G, Maillet B. Pathology of acute and chronic pancreatitis. *Pancreas* 1993;8(6):659–670.
244. Lilja P, Evander A, Ihse I. Hereditary pancreatitis-a report on two kindreds. *Acta Chir Scand* 1978;144(1):35–37.
245. Whitcomb DC, Gorry MC, Preston RA, et al. Hereditary pancreatitis is caused by a mutation in the cationic trypsinogen gene. *Nat Genet* 1996;14(2):141–145.
246. Yoshida K, Toki F, Takeuchi T, et al. Chronic pancreatitis caused by an autoimmune abnormality. Proposal of the concept of autoimmune pancreatitis. *Dig Dis Sci* 1995;40(7):1561–1568.
247. Abe K, Watanabe S. Apoptosis of mouse pancreatic acinar cells after duct ligation. *Arch Histol Cytol* 1995;58(2):221–229.
248. Walker NI. Ultrastructure of the rat pancreas after experimental duct ligation. I. The role of apoptosis and intraepithelial macrophages in acinar cell deletion. *Am J Pathol* 1987;126(3):439–451.
249. Gyr K, Heitz PU, Beglinger C. Pancreatitis. In: Kloppel G, Heitz PU, eds. *Pancreatic Pathology*. New York: Churchill-Livingstone; 1984:44–72.
250. Brune K, Abe T, Canto M, et al. Multifocal neoplastic precursor lesions associated with lobular atrophy of the pancreas in patients having a strong family history of pancreatic cancer. *Am J Surg Pathol* 2006;30(9):1067–1076.
251. Hruban R, Pitman M, Klimstra D. *Tumors of the Pancreas*. Washington, DC: American Registry of Pathology; 2006.
252. Tascilar M, Offerhaus GJ, Altink R, et al. Immunohistochemical labeling for the Dpc4 gene product is a specific marker for adenocarcinoma in biopsy specimens of the pancreas and bile duct. *Am J Clin Pathol* 2001;116(6): 831–837.
253. Seifert G. Lipomatous atrophy and other forms. In: Kloppel G, Heitz PU, eds. *Pancreatic Pathology*. New York: Churchill-Livingstone; 1984:27–31.
254. Altinel D, Basturk O, Sarmiento JM, et al. Lipomatous pseudohypertrophy of the pancreas: A clinicopathologically distinct entity. *Pancreas* 2010;39(3):392–397.

SECTION VIII

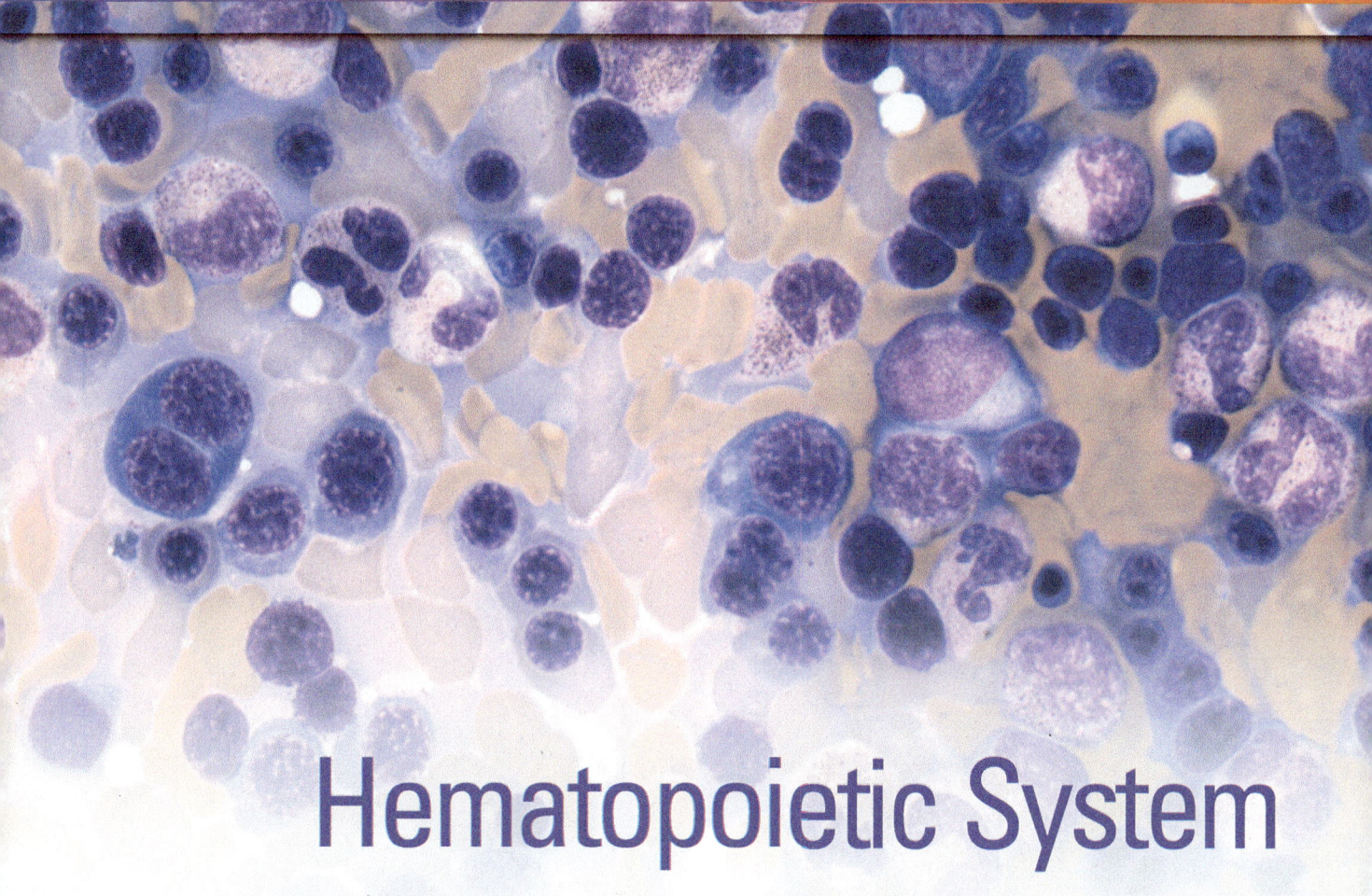

Hematopoietic System

Lymph Nodes

Paul van der Valk

- EMBRYOLOGY/DEVELOPMENTAL CHANGES 784
- GROSS FEATURES 784
- ANATOMY 784
  - Blood Supply 784
  - Lymphatics 784
- LIGHT MICROSCOPY: THE DIFFERENT COMPARTMENTS, HISTOLOGY, AND FUNCTION 784
  - The Follicle 786
  - Follicular Dendritic Cells 786
  - Lymphoid Cells 786
  - Tingible Body Macrophages 787
  - The Medullary Cords 788
  - Lymphoid Cells 788
  - Macrophages 789
  - Other Cell Types 789
  - The Paracortex 789
  - Epitheloid (or Postcapillary or High Endothelial) Venules 789
  - Interdigitating Dendritic Cells 790
  - Lymphoid Cells 790
  - Other Cell Types 790
  - The Sinuses 791
  - Function 792
- CHANGES IN COMPARTMENTS: BENIGN VERSUS MALIGNANT 792
  - Follicular Changes 793
  - Changes in the Medullary Cords 793
  - Changes in the Paracortex 794
  - Sinusoidal Changes 794
  - Combined Patterns 794
- ARTIFACTS 795
  - Technical Artifacts 795
  - Intrinsic Artifacts 795
- HANDLING OF LYMPH NODE SPECIMENS 795
- SPECIAL TECHNIQUES AND PROCEDURES 795
- REFERENCES 796

The lymph nodes are part of the immune system, a complex system whose job is to adequately deal with foreign substances (1). "Dealing with" here is taken in the broadest sense: it can mean either ignoring an antigen entirely, that is, tolerance, or mount a destructive reaction to it, clearing it from the system. In certain areas an effective elimination is of course vitally important. This certainly goes for the lymph nodes where (foreign) antigens serve no purpose or are downright detrimental and are therefore best eliminated (unlike the gastrointestinal tract where reactivity against food antigens is not always advantageous and tolerance is often the better response). As the lymph nodes are to deal with antigens, their histology reflects the (re)activity of the immune system; the nature of the antigen determines whether a reaction will be mounted against it, but also determines what effector cells will be employed. This will be reflected in the morphology of the lymph nodes, as we will see later.

As the entire body is continually confronted with antigen, lymph nodes are required throughout the body and are concentrated in areas draining organs with environmental contact. Of course, the skin has numerous draining lymph nodes, partly grouped in areas where lymphatics converge, such as the axillary, cervical, and inguinal regions. Also, the gastrointestinal tract and the airways have small collections of lymphoid cells in their mucosal surfaces (the so-called mucosa-associated lymphoid tissue or MALT), including draining lymph nodes, the mesenteric, and mediastinal and hilar lymph nodes (2–5). Drainage from extra-abdominal areas is through the parailiacal and paraaortal nodes. All these systems converge on a single lymphatic channel, the thoracic duct, that returns the lymphatic fluid to the bloodstream. The only organ where no lymphatics are found is the brain, that drains its extracellular fluid via the cerebrospinal fluid or the extraparenchymatous Virchow–Robin space.

Under antigenic pressure lymph nodes can "appear" where they are usually not found. Whether this appearance is actually an enlargement of very small lymph nodes already present or de novo formation of a lymph node is uncertain.

EMBRYOLOGY/DEVELOPMENTAL CHANGES

Relatively little is known of the development of the lymph nodes during the embryonic period. They seem to arise from the lymphatic sacs, which in turn develop from the venous system. From the sacs, a lymphatic plexus forms and as early as in the first trimester small collections of lymphoblasts can be found in association with this plexus (6). In the second trimester a differentiation in cortex and medulla begins to take place, gradually forming the familiar compartmentalized structure of the lymph node parenchyma, probably also under the influence of nonlymphoid cells, such as macrophages and interdigitating dendritic cells (IDCs), and mesenchymally derived cells such as follicular dendritic cells (FDCs) and may be fibroblastic reticulum cells (FRCs). After the compartmentalization is completed no other changes take place than those that follow antigenic challenge.

GROSS FEATURES

Reactive lymph nodes are mostly small structures, round or reniform in shape. When detectable they are usually enlarged through stimulation of some degree. Normally they do not exceed a diameter of 1 cm, but during immune reactions they can become much larger. However, a diameter of more than 3 cm is unusual in benign lymph nodes (though not unheard of) and should raise the suspicion of malignancy. The cut surface is a pinkish-brown color and homogeneous. A white (fish meat) aspect or distinct nodularity is suspicious. Often in lymph node dissection specimens the lymph node consists of a small rim of parenchyma enclosing fatty tissue and they can be difficult to find; in those cases their resistance to the palpating finger gives them away.

ANATOMY

Blood Supply
Arterioles enter the lymph node at the hilus, branch, and rapidly form a plexus of capillaries in the parenchyma. Subtle differences exist on the level of the basement membranes of the capillaries of the follicles and of the paracortex, with laminin 5 found exclusively in the basement membranes of the follicular compartment, for instance (7). It has become clear that the expression of surface markers, such as chemokine receptors, guide migration of lymphocytes to and through compartments of the lymphoid tissues and thus plays a role in the positioning of lymphocytes in the different compartments (8–10).

Venous drainage accompanies the arteriolar route. The postcapillary venules in the lymph nodes are special, as they are the main route of entrance of lymphocytes homing to the lymph nodes. They will be discussed in more detail later.

Lymphatics
The lymph node is positioned in the lymphatic system. The afferent lymphatics enter the lymph node through the capsule, draining into the subcapsular sinus. This sinus is lined by endothelial cells, but the system of branching sinuses arising from it no longer have an endothelial lining. Further discussion of the different cell types in the sinuses follows below.

LIGHT MICROSCOPY: THE DIFFERENT COMPARTMENTS, HISTOLOGY, AND FUNCTION

Examination of a sectioned lymph node at low power reveals more or less clearly defined areas or compartments (Fig. 30.1A); most obvious are the follicles, round(ish) structures with pale centers and a dark rim. The centers often show a mottled appearance. These areas are mostly present in the cortical area, that is, the outer area of the lymph node just below the capsule. Occasionally follicles are found in the deeper areas. Between the follicles, and extending to the deeper parenchyma is an ill-defined area, the paracortex or paracortical area, recognizable by their rather pronounced vessels, the epithelioid or high endothelial venules, the specialized postcapillary venules mentioned earlier. On occasion, this area shows a mottling not unlike that of the follicles (Fig. 30.1B). In the medullary region of the lymph node, if present in the specimen, low-power view shows dark areas separated by lighter staining ones often in a somewhat reticular pattern. The dark areas are the medullary cords, where plasma cells are found and, in the appropriate stains, mast cells. The lighter areas in between these sheets of dark-staining small lymphocytes are the sinuses, filled with histiocytes, whose ample pale cytoplasm causes the light aspect of this area. The sinuses run through the entire parenchyma, but are especially well visible in the medullar area and are directly subcapsular.

These different areas can be easily recognized on low-power microscopy (Fig. 30.1A), but it must be stressed that their representation varies in different specimens; often, for instance, the medullary cords are not found.

As we are in constant contact with antigens a lymph node is virtually always stimulated to some degree and the increase in one area caused by this stimulation will often be at the cost of the volume of the other compartments (Fig. 30.2). Such stimulation will not only increase the size of the compartment (and decrease or increase the size of

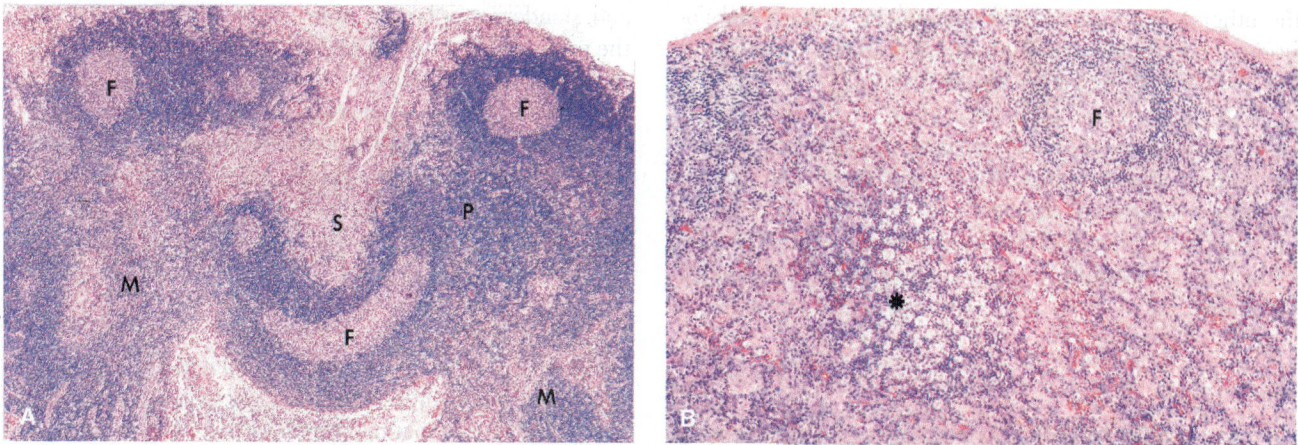

FIGURE 30.1 **A:** Low-power view of lymph node (periodic acid–Schiff stained, paraffin-embedded section). This "smiling" picture illustrates the four different compartments of the lymph node. In the upper corners and in the middle of the bottom ("the eyes and mouth") the follicles (*F*) are seen. The paracortical area (*P*) here is fairly small; usually there is more paracortex present. The less sharply defined sections where light and dark areas are juxtaposed represent the medullary cords (*M*, *dark*) and sinuses (*S, light*). **B:** Low-power view of another lymph node (hematoxylin and eosin [H&E]-stained, paraffin-embedded section). In the *upper right* there is a follicle (*F*) which is recognizable. The rest of the picture shows paracortical area, with considerable influx of macrophages and IDCs. In the center the typical mottling of the paracortex is seen (*asterisk*).

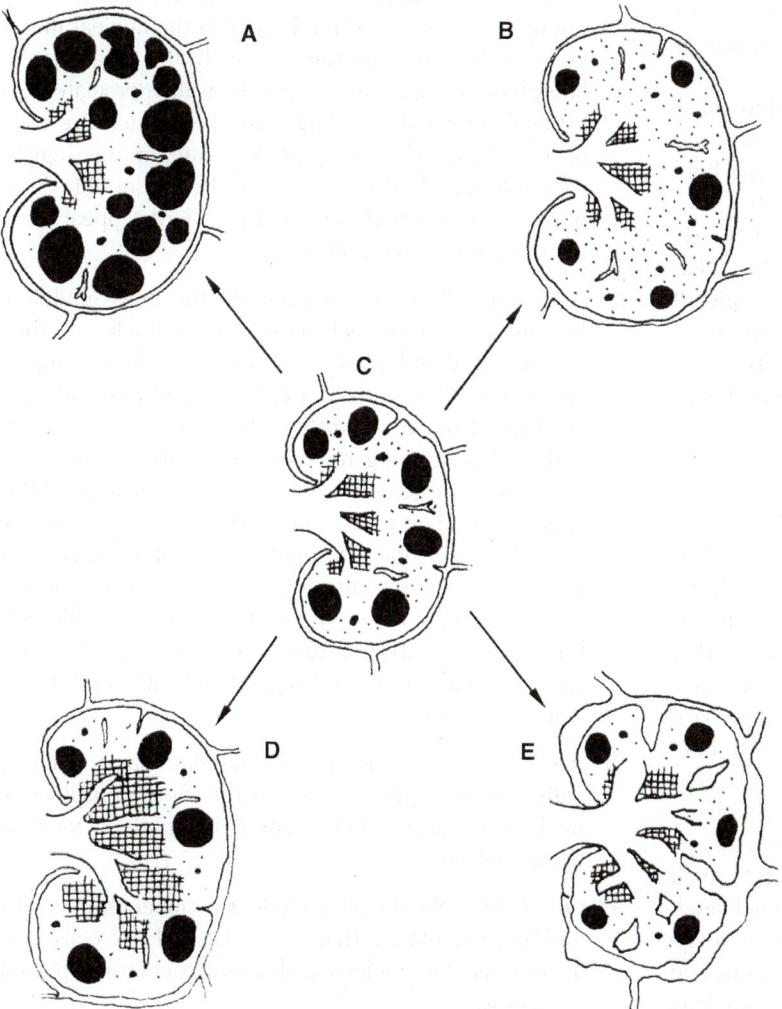

FIGURE 30.2 Schematic representation of the lymph node with enlargement of the four different compartments, respectively the follicular (*A*), the paracortical (*B*), the medullary (*D*) and the sinusoidal (*E*) compartments. (*C*) represents an "unstimulated" lymph node.

the others), but also cause a shift in the cellular composition. This usually means an increase in the proliferative fraction of each compartment, the blast cells (11).

This adaptability to the constantly changing antigenic challenges explains the variety in "normal" lymph node histology: Almost all lymph nodes that come under the microscope are stimulated to some degree.

Each of the four different compartments, follicle, paracortical area, medullary cords, and sinuses, is discussed separately.

The Follicle

Distinction must be made between *primary* and *secondary* follicles. Primary follicles are aggregates of small, dark-staining lymphoid cells. In these primary follicles a germinal center can develop, turning them into secondary follicles. Thus, the mantle zone around the follicle center has the same characteristics as the primary follicle. The outer zone of the mantle zone is somewhat less densely packed as the inner layer. This outer rim is sometimes called the marginal zone (12), largely based on a very loose resemblance with the splenic marginal zone and on the fact that marginal zone lymphomas tend to localize perifollicularly. However, if the marginal zone exists in the lymph node, it is difficult to distinguish, except when it is expanded in benign or lymphomatous proliferations (13).

In the follicle center an immunologic reaction takes place, that is called, after its location, the follicle center cell reaction. It requires the cooperation of FDCs, lymphoid cells, and tingible body macrophages (TBM) (Fig. 30.3A,B).

The function of the reaction is the generation of B cells that have been affinity-selected against an antigen (i.e., that produce an antibody with the best possible fit to the antigen) and that can function either as a direct precursor for antibody-producing plasma cells or as (long-term) memory cells.

The cellular composition of both the lymphoid and nonlymphoid cells will now be described.

Follicular Dendritic Cells

FDCs (previously called dendritic reticulum cells) trap antigens on their surface and present them to B cells (14,15). Since these cells can retain antigen on their surface it was postulated they can provide a long-lasting reaction to that antigen, which may be important for immune memory (16); however, this is controversial and other functions have been proposed (17). FDCs are difficult to recognize in light microscopic sections, they were first described by electron microscopy and later by enzyme and immunohistochemistry (15,18–21). They have a large, but inconspicuous nucleus with a very fine, almost vesicular chromatin with a small nucleolus. Not infrequently, they are or appear binucleated, with the nuclei pressed together. The cytoplasm is invisible with the light microscope, but in ultrathin sections and with immunohistochemistry they appear to have many long and slender cytoplasmic protrusions. These are linked to the protrusions of other FDCs via (hemi)desmosomes, thus forming a round network with a fingerprint-like configuration. In this way, they are responsible for the shape of the follicle. Their origin is still a matter of debate; a derivation from the mononuclear phagocyte system was proposed (21), as was an origin in the perivascular mesenchyme, possibly via a circulating mesenchymal stem cell (22,23).

Lymphoid Cells

The lymphoid cells of the primary follicle and the mantle zone have small, slightly irregular nuclei, with condensed, dark-staining chromatin. They have scanty cytoplasm and consequently, they are packed closely together. The outer rim of the mantle zone, the marginal zone equivalent of the lymph node, houses cells that are slightly bigger and less densely packed, but they have the same dark nuclei (12). All these cells are B cells, staining with antibodies to CD20, 22, and 24 and the transcription factor Pax5. They also express IgM on their surface and the mantle zone cells also express IgD simultaneously (20,24,25). In the germinal center, distinctive B cells can be found:

1. Blast cells with large vesicular nuclei and several small, but distinct nucleoli, often located at the nuclear membrane. When they are round, they have a small rim of basophilic cytoplasm, especially well-appreciated in cytologic preparations. These are the proliferative cells of the follicle; where they predominate, mitotic figures are easily found. Also, because of their basophilic cytoplasm, areas where they are in the majority appear dark: the dark zone of the follicle.

2. After this phase of proliferation, the cells gradually become smaller and get more irregular nuclei. As they get smaller they lose their nucleoli and the chromatin condenses. This leads to a cell that is almost indistinguishable from the mantle cells, a small irregular cell with a dark-staining nucleus and a virtually invisible cytoplasm. These cells are less densely packed and the area where they predominate appears a little lighter than the dark zone: the light zone. Naturally, cells in transition between large round to small irregular are frequent, giving rise to a particularly polymorphic cellular picture, with a mixture of cells, large, medium sized, or small, round or irregular and with vesicular or condensed chromatin.

3. A smaller part of the cells are medium sized to large, with a finely dispersed chromatin and inconspicuous nucleoli and scanty, but intensely basophilic cytoplasm (lymphoblasts).

4. Other B-lymphoid cells include occasional plasma cells and "immunoblasts," that is, very large blastic cells with a big vesicular nucleus and a single centrally placed nucleolus.

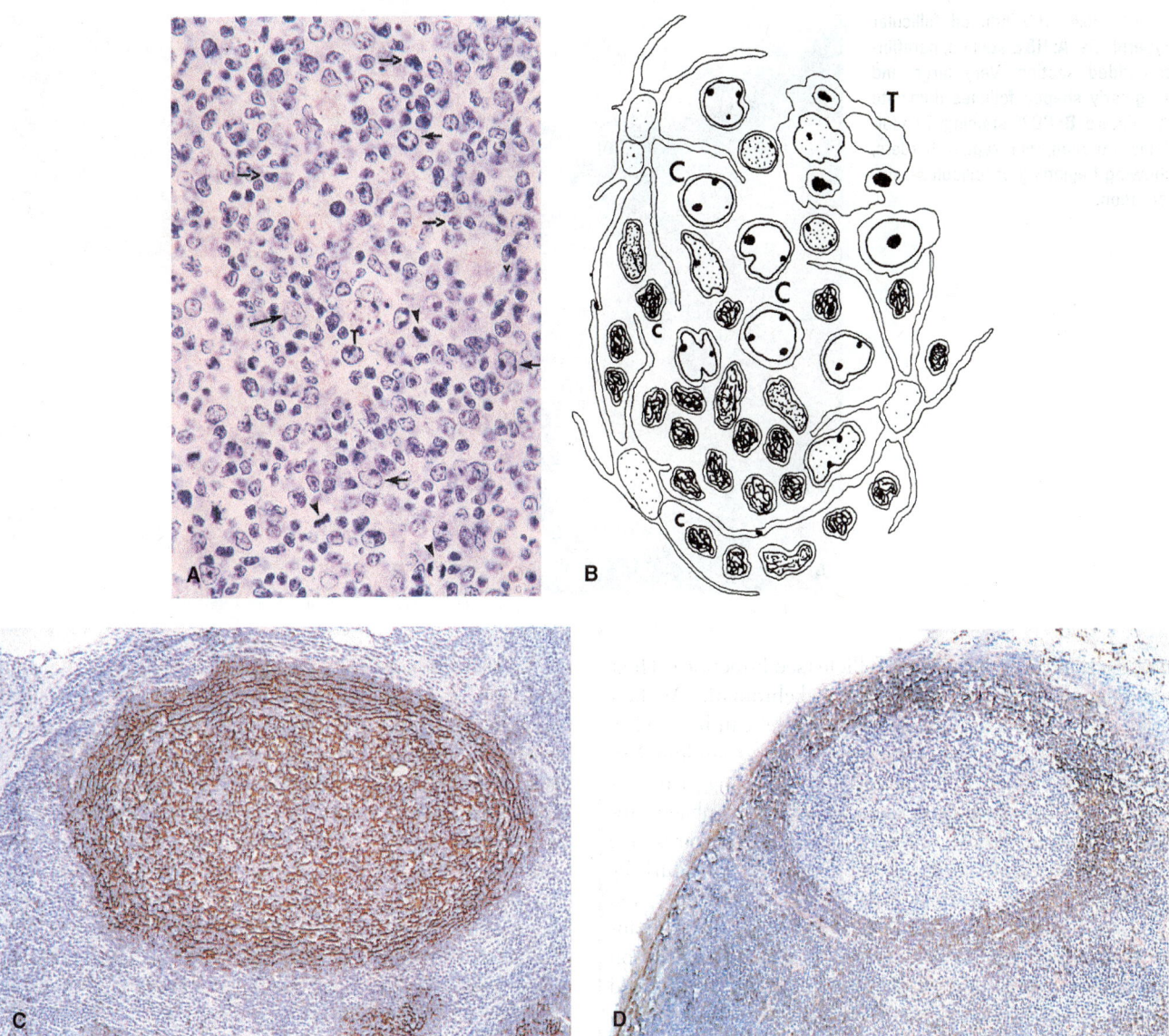

FIGURE 30.3 The follicular compartment. **A:** Giemsa-stained, plastic-embedded section, showing the pleomorphism of the follicle center. All typical elements are present: mitotic figures (*arrowheads*), a tingible body macrophage (*T*) with phagocytized debris, staining intensely black, blastic cells (*short arrows*), small follicle center cells (*open arrows*), and an FDC (*long arrow*). **B:** Diagrammatic representation of a follicle, stressing the FDC morphology. Other elements are tingible body macrophage (*T*) and blastic (*C*) and small (*c*) lymphoid cells. **C:** Frozen section stained with a CD35 antibody against the C3b-receptor on FDCs. Note the somewhat fingerprint-like pattern of FDC lattice. **D:** Frozen section stained for IgD. The mantle cells are positive, the cells in the center are not.

5. In addition there is a variable number of small, dark-staining lymphocytes (a little smaller than the small follicle center cells themselves), probably representing T lymphocytes. These cells have a typical phenotype, expressing among others CD4 and PD-1, and function to regulate the formation of the follicles and guide the B cells through their follicle center phase (26). The number of these various cells varies considerably. On occasion, plasma cells can be quite numerous; also, sometimes T lymphocytes can outnumber the B lymphocytes in the follicle.

As these cells are B cells too, they react with the same markers as mentioned for the mantle and marginal zone cells (with the exception of IgD). In addition, they are mostly positive with the markers CD10 and Bcl-6, considered markers of follicle center cells (25).

Tingible Body Macrophages

TBM are large cells with abundant, pale cytoplasm, that contains phagocytized debris and apoptotic bodies from surrounding lymphocytes that have died in the selection

FIGURE 30.4 HIV-induced follicular hyperplasia. **A:** H&E-stained, paraffin-embedded section. Very large and irregularly shaped follicles dominate the picture. **B:** CD20-staining. Two follicles are seen, with ragged borders, showing beginning of follicular disintegration.

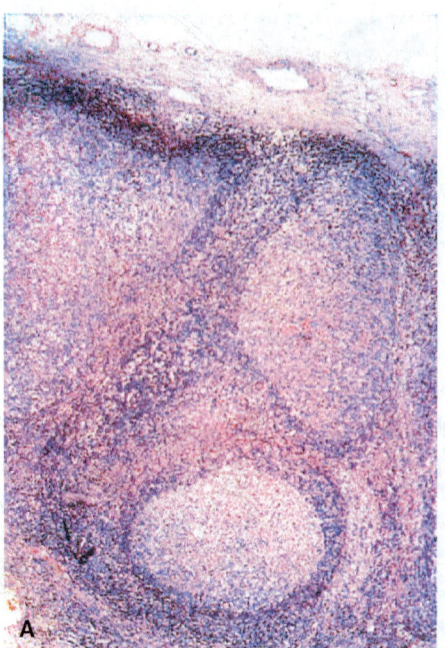
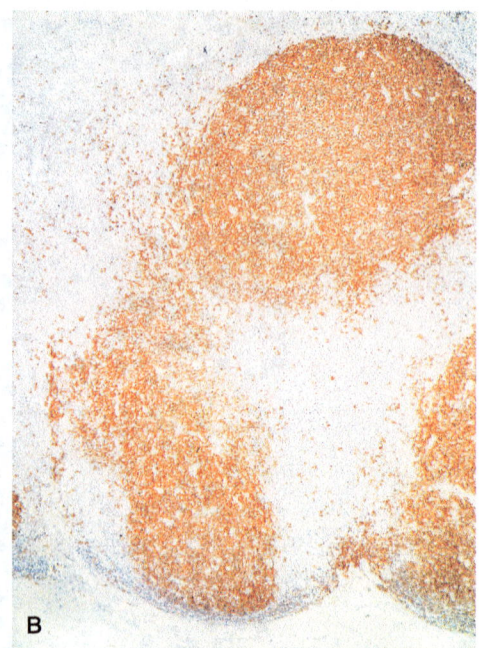

process that takes place in the follicle (see Function). Their nuclei are large, with a finely dispersed chromatin. As their nuclear size is fairly constant, these nuclei can be used to measure the size of the nuclear size of the surrounding lymphocytes, especially in lymphomas (as big or bigger means a large-cell lymphoma). Because of their avid phagocytosis their cytoplasm often is very clear and their presence causes white spots in the tissue, a mottling colourfully described as the "starry sky" pattern. It should be noted that this highly characteristic feature, often used to distinguish between benign and malignant, is in fact a fixation artifact; the phagosomes in the cytoplasma are exaggerated by the shrinking during the fixation process in formalin. In some fixatives, such as sublimate-formaldehyde or B5, and in frozen sections(!) this starry sky pattern is not or not easily seen!

Variations of the Follicular Pattern

From the above a characteristic pattern for the morphology of the follicle emerges. A more or less round or oval area, with a dark outer edge (the mantle zone) and a lighter center, that shows mottling and upon closer inspection a very polymorphic cytologic picture and many mitotic figures. Sometimes zonation is seen, with the dark zone directed inward (i.e., toward the hilus of the lymph node), the light zone directed more to the capsule of the node. As it is very dependent on how the follicle is cut in the section, this zonation is often not seen (18,27).

Variations occur in the shape of the follicles and in their composition. An important cause for variation is time; the pattern described above takes time to evolve. In the beginning the follicle consists largely of blasts, with smaller follicle center cells appearing as the follicle center cell reaction runs its cause (27).

In reactive conditions sometimes follicles can become very large and coalesce; HIV lymphadenopathy is a good example (Fig. 30.4) (28–30). Their composition can also vary somewhat. Changes that occur with malignancy are discussed later. With involution of the follicle they can become hyalinized and atrophic or they can be overrun by T lymphocytes, a phenomenon that is called progressive transformation of the germinal center (18,31) and can make the follicle difficult to recognize. It is only by their remnant round shape that they then are recognized as follicles (and by special stains for FDCs). Fortunately, this somewhat alarming appearing feature usually involves only a few follicles at the same time, so the presence of normal follicles is reassuring.

The Medullary Cords

The medullary cords are found in the hilar region of the lymph node, between the sinuses. The cellular composition of this compartment is described next (Fig. 30.5).

Lymphoid Cells

Small lymphocytes make up the majority of cells in the medullary cords. They have small, more or less round nuclei and a scant-to-moderate amount of cytoplasm. In some cells, the chromatin is clumped and peripherally distributed in the nucleus, similar to the plasma cell nucleus, though the typical "clock-face" chromatin is not seen. Cells with this kind of chromatin tend to have more cytoplasm and sometimes even a perinuclear hof, clearly indicative of plasmacytoid differentiation. They are called lymphoplasmacytoid or lymphoplasmacytic cells. Immunologically, the cells can be identified with CD20 and, even better with CD79a, general B-cell markers. Staining for immunoglobulins can

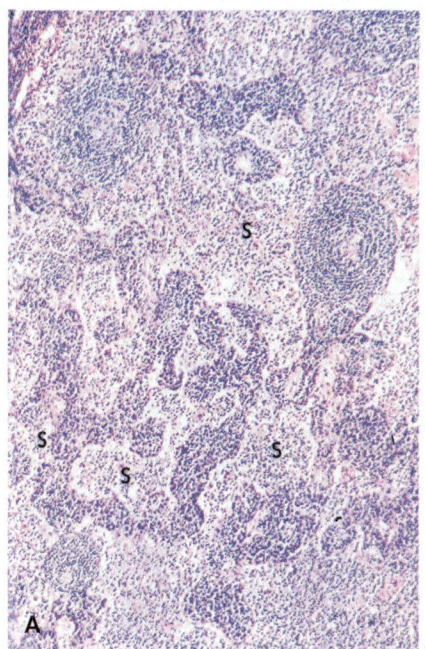 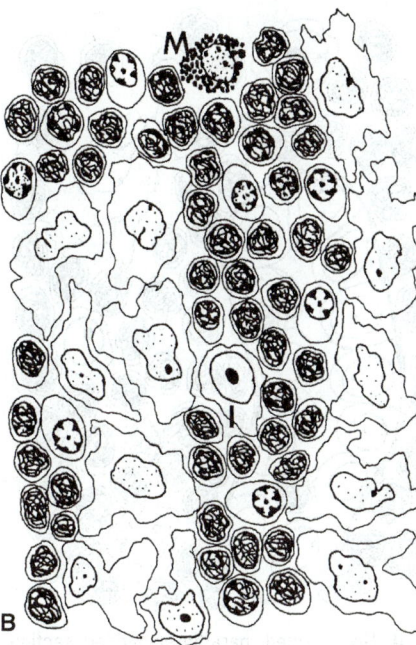

FIGURE 30.5 Medullary cords. **A:** H&E-stained, paraffin-embedded section. The sheets and ribbons of dark-staining cells are the medullary cords, containing small lymphocytes and plasma cells; they are separated by the lighter staining areas, the sinuses (*S*). **B:** Schematic representation, also depicting an immunoblast (*I*) and a mast cell (*M*).

sometimes show cytoplasmic IgM and light chains. Many of the cells with less cytoplasm and irregular nuclei are T lymphocytes (CD2, 3, 5, and 7 positive), necessary to modulate or drive the process of antibody formation that takes place in the medullary cords. The blast cells of this process, the immunoblasts, are striking, though infrequent. They have large vesicular nuclei with a large, centrally located nucleolus and abundant basophilic cytoplasm. Plasma cells are also present, but in varying number. They are distinctive cells, with their small round nuclei with its clock-face chromatin, small clumps of dark chromatin at the nuclear membrane, like the numbers on a dial. The nucleus is eccentrically located in the cytoplasm and a perinuclear hof, a clearing of the cytoplasm next to the nucleus is present. The outer rim of the cytoplasm is deeply basophilic. Under some conditions, plasma cells accumulate immunoglobulins in their cytoplasm, the so-called Russell bodies, globular structures that stain positive with PAS and that can indent the nucleus if they reach sufficient size. Plasma cells are CD20 negative, but retain their CD79a and are, of course, positive for cytoplasmic immunoglobulins and CD138.

Macrophages

Macrophages are fairly scarce here. They have medium-sized to large irregular nuclei and abundant cytoplasm. They are not as avidly phagocytic as TBM from the follicle center, perhaps because they are geared more toward antigen handling and presentation than toward phagocytosis.

Other Cell Types

T lymphocytes were already mentioned. The mast cell is the other cell type that can be found especially in the medullary cords, easily demonstrated with a metachromatic dye as Giemsa, where their characteristic purple granulation allows their recognition. The granules generally obscure the nucleus.

The Paracortex

The paracortex or paracortical area was the last compartment to be described and named (32,33), probably because its boundaries are indistinct and the area is best appreciated in not routinely used fixatives, such as Zenker's or sublimate-formaldehyde. Nevertheless, it has some typical structural elements that allow easy recognition—the epithelioid venules and the IDC (Fig. 30.6).

Epitheloid (or Postcapillary or High Endothelial) Venules

These highly distinct vessels are found only in the paracortex; they are lined with plump, cuboidal, or even cylindrical endothelial cells with a fairly large oval nucleus, with vesicular chromatin and indistinct nucleoli. Sometimes the lumina of these vessels appear to be obliterated by the endothelium. These vessels have long since been recognized as the port of entrance for blood-borne lymphocytes to the lymph node parenchyma (33,34). Therefore they play a crucial role in recirculation, distribution, and homing of lymphocytes in different lymphoid organs, a process mediated by specific homing receptors on the lymphocyte surface, that react with organ-specific ligands (or vascular addressins) on the endothelial cell surface (Fig. 30.7) (35–38). In this process of positioning of lymphoid cells and thus optimizing immune responses chemokines also play an important role (38–40), as was already mentioned above.

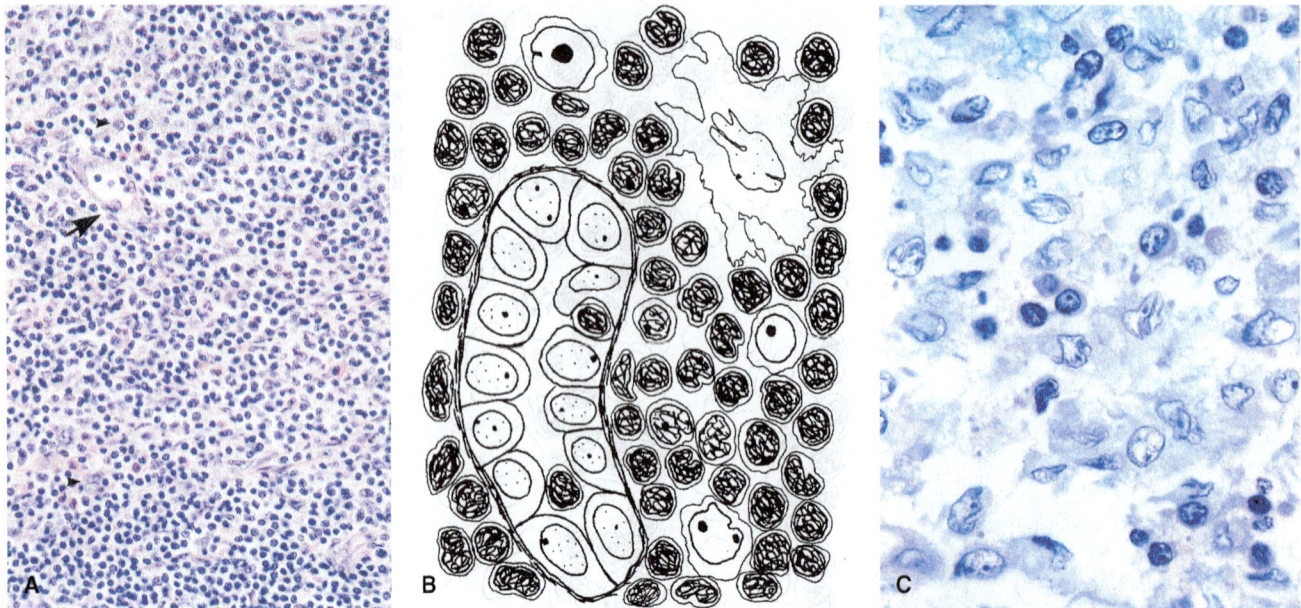

FIGURE 30.6 The paracortex. **A:** H&E-stained, paraffin-embedded section. An epithelioid venule is seen (*arrow*); small lymphocytes dominate the picture, with an occasional blast present. IDCs, with their markedly irregular, grooved, and pale nuclei are scattered throughout the area (*arrowheads*). **B:** Schematic representation. Note the typical IDC. **C:** Giemsa-stained, plastic-embedded section. Demonstrating an increase in IDCs, characteristically displaying their irregular pale nuclei and abundant cytoplasm (lymph node with dermatopathic lymphadenopathy).

Interdigitating Dendritic Cells

IDCs are large cells with a large and bizarre nucleus with deep clefts and folds. The chromatin pattern is delicate, almost transparent, and nucleoli are inconspicuous. The cytoplasm is abundant, pale, and with ill-defined borders (Fig. 30.6C). Electron microscopy shows protrusions, broad and veil-like, in contrast to the thin processes of the FDC. Also, contact places are lacking. Furthermore, they have a typical organelle of undetermined function: the tubulovesicular system (18). When present in large numbers IDCs cause a mottling of the paracortex.

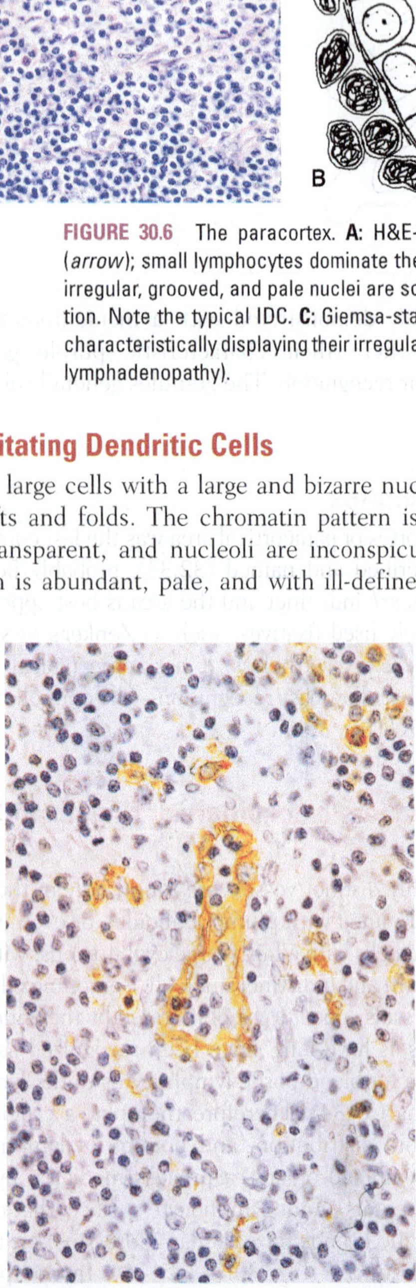

The IDC is a bone marrow–derived cell, intimately related to the Langerhans cell of the skin, which it closely resembles, both morphologically and functionally (41–44). Both are antigen-presenting cells to T lymphocytes, important to initiate and/or maintain immune responses. Immunologically, these cells are best demonstrated in stains for S100 protein, or by HLA-DR, among the class II–negative T lymphocytes (Fig. 30.8).

Lymphoid Cells

The cytology of the paracortex is somewhat variable, but in most cases small T lymphocytes predominate. They have small, irregular nuclei with coarse chromatin and little cytoplasm. They are demonstrated with stains for CD2, 3 (Fig. 30.8), 5, and 7 and are either CD4 or CD8 positive, with the CD4 outnumbering the CD8. Blast cells are present in varying numbers; they are large cells with vesicular nuclei of a varying shape.

Other Cell Types

The only other cell type worth mentioning is the FRC, because it is often found at the edge of the paracortex (18).

FIGURE 30.7 HECA 452 staining. Paracortical area with a highlighted epithelioid venule. Lymphocytes are seen adhering to the endothelium and passing through the vessel wall.

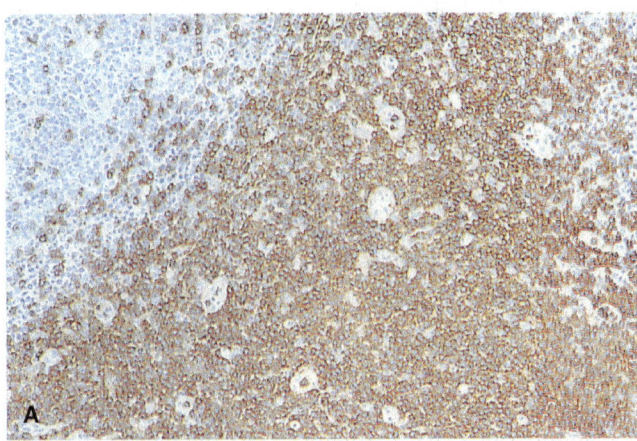
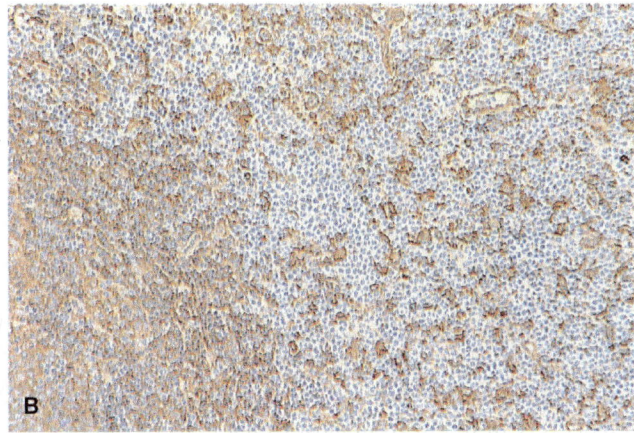

FIGURE 30.8 Immunohistochemistry of paracortex. **A:** Frozen section stained with CD3. Most cells in the paracortex are positive. In the *upper left* corner a segment of a follicle (B-cell area) is seen. **B:** HLA-DR–stained frozen section. Here the IDCs stain positive: They are larger and show more cytoplasm than the group of follicular (B) cells on the *left*.

It is a somewhat enigmatic cell, that forms reticulin fibers that are involved in the transport of cytokines and/or antigens through the parenchyma, the so-called FRC conduit system; this is an effective means of spreading important activating molecules through the entire node (45).

The Sinuses

The sinuses are the structures carrying the lymphatic fluid from the afferent lymphatics through the lymph node to the efferent lymph vessels. The afferent lymph vessels drain into the subcapsular sinus, a structure at least partly lined by endothelium. As the sinuses traverse through the lymph node, they lose their endothelial lining and acquire a "lining" of macrophages (46). The macrophages in the sinuses are similar to macrophages elsewhere: large cells with a medium-sized to large, irregular, and vesicular nucleus; a low nucleus-to-cytoplasm ratio; and signs of phagocytic activity.

Apart from the macrophages, that look the same here as anywhere else in the lymph node, small lymphocytes are also found in the sinuses (Figs. 30.5A and 30.9A). In addition, occasionally neutrophils or eosinophils can be found here as well.

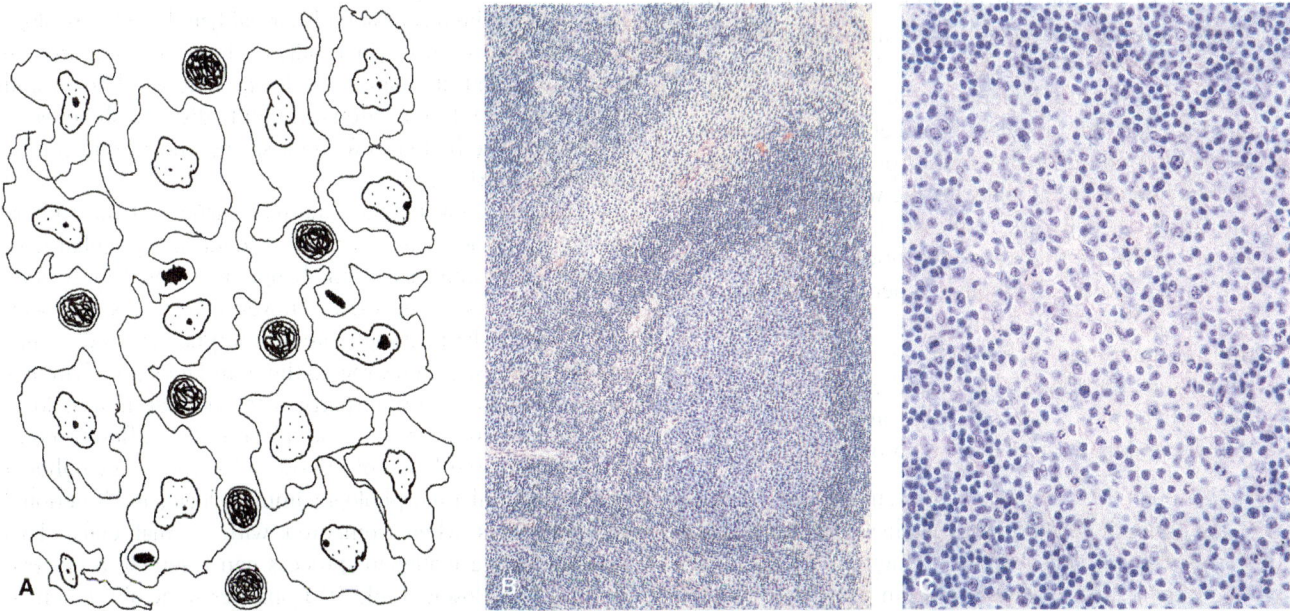

FIGURE 30.9 The sinuses. **A:** Schematic representation with predominance of macrophages and some lymphocytes. **B:** Low-power view of immature sinus histiocytosis, recognizable as the pale area to the upper left of the central follicle. **C:** Detail of **B**, showing the cells to be somewhat larger than the dark, small lymphocytes and having fairly abundant cytoplasm.

Mention must be made of two other cell types. The first is the so-called sinus-lining cell, an ill-defined cell type that is primarily recognized in immune stains for keratins. It is found in the area of the subcapsular sinus and has a coarsely dendritic morphology (47). Its nature is unclear, though they are probably a specialized form of FRCs, characterized by the expression of low–molecular-weight keratins (42), but in evaluating lymph node sections for metastatic tumor it is important to be aware of these cells and not confuse them with metastatic tumor cells. With the sentinel node procedure coming to the fore more and more (48), this is a point of considerable importance. Fortunately, the appearance of the sinus-lining cells is very different from most tumor cells or tumor cell deposits.

The second is the immature sinus histiocyte, a misnomer, for it concerns B lymphocytes (Fig. 30.9B,C). These cells are primarily seen in certain reactive conditions in which they can partially fill the sinuses. They have small, more lymphoid appearing nuclei, but have ample cytoplasm. Also called monocytoid B cells (another unfortunate name!), they are indeed B lymphocytes, probably marginal zone cells (49,50).

Function

Each of the above-described compartments has a specific function, housing its own immunologic reaction; together these reactions make up the individual's immunologic integrity.

1. In the follicle, the follicle center cell reaction takes place. In this reaction the naïve B lymphocytes are exposed to antigen (on the FDC surface) and they adapt their antigen receptor (the immunoglobulin) to make a perfect fit to the presented antigen, by a process called somatic hypermutation. This involves rearranging their immunoglobulin receptor genes and has a certain amount of trial-and-error to it. Thus, some of the changes are actually for the worse and decrease the fit. Such cells are ruthlessly eliminated through apoptosis (hence the many apoptotic cells in this compartment). Eventually though, a perfect fit is achieved and the cell is rescued from elimination by expressing the anti-apoptotic Bcl-2 molecule. Normal follicles, where selection takes place, are therefore negative for Bcl-2. In general, several clones are developing in a follicle, making it an oligoclonal proliferation (51).
    a. Through this complicated molecular biologic process of antibody selection the follicle center cell reaction results in B cells, expressing high-avidity antibodies on their surface. These cells can recirculate through the body as memory cells, spreading immune competence through the entire body and waiting for another encounter with the antigen; others go to the medullary cords or to the bone marrow to enter the plasma cell reaction and develop into plasma cells that produce antibodies for secretion.
2. In the medullary cords the plasma cell reaction takes place. As mentioned above it leads to the formation of plasma cells and the secretion of antibodies. The antibody production in the lymph node does not substantially contribute to the level of circulating antibodies, but it may be locally important, for instance for fixing antibodies on FDCs.
3. In the paracortex we find the specific cellular response, that generates antigen-specific effector T lymphocytes of the various subsets: helper cells, suppressor cells, regulatory cells, memory cells, and maybe more (35). The cellular processes here are still poorly understood. It is likely that T-cell memory, cytokine production, and a number of other reactions take place in the paracortex, but little is known about this. Its role in the delayed-type contact hypersensitivity is well-recognized (32).
4. The sinuses, with their abundant macrophages, are a filtering system, clearing foreign substances from the lymph. Given their ability to handle antigens a function in antigen presenting might be plausible, but little is known about this.

CHANGES IN COMPARTMENTS: BENIGN VERSUS MALIGNANT

The differential diagnosis of benign and malignant lesions is important in the discussion of normal lymph node histology for two reasons: (a) it is naturally of the utmost importance for the surgical pathologist to decide between benign and malignant; and (b) it is often difficult to distinguish between these two. The first goes without saying, the second can be somewhat clarified.

Though a link between normal tissue and the tumors arising from them has been self-evident for epithelial neoplasms, the same insight for lymphomas and lymph node structure was slow to arrive. However, now this has been firmly established through careful morphologic and immunologic studies. We now regard the (non-Hodgkin's) lymphomas as malignant counterparts of the normal immunologic reactions to antigens that take place in the different compartments of the lymphoid tissues (18,52–54). Lymphoma cells have similar morphologic, immunologic, and functional characteristics when compared with normal cells. This explains why a malignant process can resemble a reactive condition so closely. Table 30.1 opposes some of the benign variations in normal histology to malignant counterparts. As this chapter deals with normal histology and many excellent texts have been written on lymphomas we will discuss this matter only briefly.

TABLE 30.1 Benign Compartmental Enlargement and Their Malignant Counterparts

Compartment	Benign	Malignant
Follicle	Follicular hyperplasia	Follicular lymphomas
Paracortex	Paracortical hyperplasia Dermatopathic lymphadenopathy	T-NHL Mycosis fungoides
Medullary cords	Medullary hyperplasia Reactive plasmocytosis	Lymphoplasmacytic lymphoma Plasmacytoma
Sinuses	Sinus histiocytosis	Malignant histiocytosis

T-NHL, T-cell non-Hodgkin lymphoma.

Follicular Changes

The most important here is the distinction between follicular hyperplasia and follicular lymphoma. The term follicular hyperplasia covers a large number of conditions, mostly difficult to differentiate from each other on morphology. Thus, it occurs in: (a) lymph nodes in the vicinity of a (bacterial) inflammation (e.g., tonsillitis, but also in syphilis (55)); (b) in autoimmune diseases, such as rheumatoid arthritis and systemic lupus erythematosus (30,56); (c) viral infections, such as HIV (22,23); and (d) in a number of idiopathic conditions, such as Castleman disease, multicentric angiofollicular hyperplasia, reactive lymph node hyperplasia with giant follicles (57–61) (it is by no means clear if these are all separate entities). Sometimes special stains can help in elucidating an etiology (spirochetal stains, p24 for HIV). In essence the follicles are all more or less the same so they are taken together here.

The most important morphologic criteria arguing for a benign lesion, mentioned in the literature (18,30,62–65) are:

1. Cellular pleomorphism of the follicle center
2. Presence of TBM
3. High number of mitotic figures
4. Well-defined mantle zone
5. Differences in size and shape of the follicles
6. Low number of follicles per surface area and predominant cortical localization
7. Well-developed and intact FDC networks in the follicle center
8. Zonation of the follicles, with clearly distinguishable dark and light zones

Despite this impressive list of criteria it may not be possible in all cases, even by an experienced pathologist, to distinguish reliably between benign and malignant pathology on morphology alone. Therefore, there are some additional arguments from immunohistochemistry and molecular biology (66): (a) demonstration of light chain restriction by immunohistochemistry (expression of either kappa or lambda light chain by follicular lesions is considered proof of malignancy); (b) expression of Bcl-2 by follicle center cells; (c) demonstration of clonality by detection of rearrangement of immunoglobulin genes, either by Southern blotting or by polymerase chain reaction (PCR) analysis; (d) demonstration of a t(14; 18) translocation (perhaps not 100% proof, but a very strong argument). All these criteria argue for malignancy, of course.

Even with these additional techniques it is not always possible to diagnose all cases with certainty. It is good to realize that the majority of the lymph nodes pathologists see are quickly scanned and judged (dissection specimens!) and this rarely yields problems. However, a high index of suspicion is probably a good general attitude, simply because of the occasional treacherous similarities between benign and malignant follicular processes.

Changes in the Medullary Cords

Here, two distinctions can be important. The first is reactive plasmacytosis (Fig. 30.10) versus plasmacytoma. Mostly, a preserved lymph node architecture and the presence of plasma cell precursors strongly favor the diagnosis of a reactive condition (18). In rare doubtful cases, immunohistochemistry can clinch the diagnosis, by demonstrating light chain restriction. Secondly, expansion of the medullary cords, a rare event in itself can be mimicked by a lymphoplasmacytic lymphoma. In rare instances, this lymphoma does not efface the architecture but expands the medullary cords. If the expansion is sufficient to arouse suspicion, marker studies can settle this easily, again by showing light chain restriction. It is good to realize that demonstrating clonality in paraffin sections may be difficult, due to diffusion artifacts. The intercellular fluid is rich in immunoglobulins and these can diffuse into the cells of a specimen if fixation is delayed.

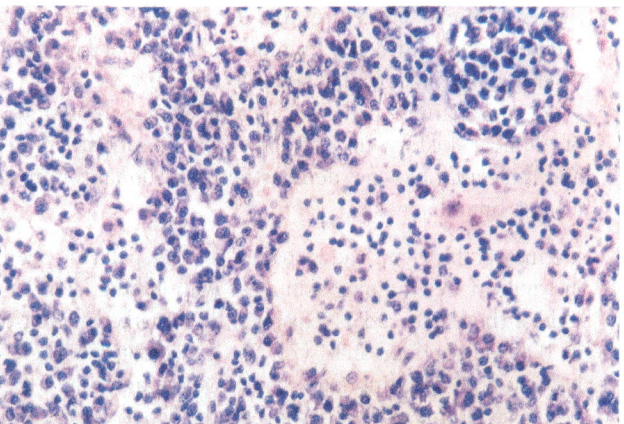

FIGURE 30.10 H&E-stained, paraffin-embedded section. Reactive plasmacytosis. The medullary cords here consist almost entirely of plasma cells. Sinuses are patent, sign of preserved lymph node structure.

Subsequent fixation will trap the polyclonal immunoglobulins inside the cells, potentially obscuring monoclonality. In practice when a lesion is clearly monoclonal, this will be demonstrable; however, caution must always be taken in interpreting immunoglobulin stains.

Changes in the Paracortex

Paracortical hyperplasia can take three forms, each with their own differential diagnostic considerations.

1. Expansion of the paracortex by predominantly small lymphocytes, usually with increase of epithelioid venules. Distinctive features, suggestive of malignancy are cellular monotony and destruction of lymph node architecture by the proliferation. Immunohistochemical features that may be supportive are: (a) demonstration of an aberrant phenotype (for instance strong predominance of CD4 or CD8, or loss of markers, normally present, such as CD7 or CD5, or expression of markers normally not expressed by lymph node T cells, such as CD1); (b) demonstration of clonality by molecular biology, that is, Southern blotting or PCR analysis of the T-cell receptor chains (67,68).

2. Expansion with an increase of blasts. This can be seen in viral infections or vaccinations and in some cases of drug reactions (the antiepileptic drugs feature prominent here) (30,63,69) and can be histologically very frightening. In some conditions, even necrosis can occur, such as in Kikuchi's histiocytic necrotizing lymphadenitis (70). On occasion, the changes can exhibit a nodular pattern (71). In such cases a preserved architecture should raise the possibility of a benign condition, no matter the histologic picture. Simple analysis with immunohistochemistry will reveal blasts of B-cell origin next to blasts of T-cell origin; also mitotic cells labeled by both B-cell and T-cell markers argue strongly for a benign proliferation and against a peripheral T-cell lymphoma. A differential diagnosis with Hodgkin disease also sometimes is a consideration; Reed–Sternberg cells can be found in reactive conditions. Therefore, this differential can be very problematical. But keep in mind that cases of Hodgkin disease with intact lymph node architecture are rare. In short, this pattern can be a headbreaker; combination of clinical history, morphology, immunophenotyping, and molecular biology (demonstration of clonality) must bring a final diagnosis.

3. Dermatopathic lymphadenopathy. In this pattern, seen in lymph nodes draining skin areas with itching skin disorders, the paracortex is expanded by a marked increase in IDCs/Langerhans cells (72,73). It is mentioned here, because the skin lymphomas, mycosis fungoides, and the Sézary syndrome, when they involve the lymph nodes, will do so in the background of a dermatopathic lymphadenopathy. This problem will thus arise only in the setting of a patient known to suffer from one of these skin lymphomas.

That does not make the problem easier in itself. The only way to settle this is to make a careful search for the diagnostic large cerebriform mononuclear cells, that can be rather scanty (74,75). Their demonstration is clinically very relevant (76). Immunohistochemistry and molecular biology unfortunately are not helpful here (77).

Sinusoidal Changes

Sinusoidal changes are very common in lymph node specimens. Lymph nodes draining tumors or inflammatory areas often show sinus histiocytosis. Typical condition showing a sinusoidal pattern includes sinus histiocytosis with massive lymphadenopathy (78,79) and Langerhans cell histiocytosis (63,80). The former condition is a peculiar clinicopathologic entity in which the histiocytes seem to engulf large numbers of lymphocytes in their cytoplasm without destroying them, a phenomenon dubbed emperipolesis. It is a highly characteristic picture. The latter can also cause a (mostly but not always benign) sinus histiocytosis. The typical features of Langerhans cells, with their deeply grooved nuclei and the admixture with eosinophils are important clues. Immunohistochemistry with CD1 (and S100) will prove the true nature of the cells. Malignant conditions in the sinuses are almost always easily recognized on histology as frankly malignant. Metastatic carcinoma or melanoma, anaplastic large-cell lymphoma (81), and malignant histiocytosis (82) all can be difficult to distinguish from one another, but doubts about their malignancy are rare.

As mentioned earlier the sinuses can be filled with immature sinus histiocytes or monocytoid B cells. A malignant equivalent is a malignant lymphoma, nodal marginal zone B-cell lymphoma (83). A predominant sinusoidal localization of such a lymphoma is rare, but can occur. Demonstration of clonality is helpful and necessary in such cases.

Finally a particular sinusoidal pattern involving a proliferation of small vessels can be seen on occasion, often as a reaction of the lymph node to ischemia or irradiation. This pattern is called vascular transformation of the sinuses and can show some histologic variation, from a delicate vascular pattern to a more spindle-cell proliferation resembling Kaposi sarcoma (84).

Combined Patterns

Follicular, medullary, paracortical, and sinusoidal patterns often occur simultaneously and any combination is possible. As combined patterns are extremely rare in lymphomas any combination argues for a benign condition. For example, Toxoplasma and Epstein–Barr virus infections often cause combined patterns. If suspicion of a malignancy arises, the same criteria as mentioned for the single patterns apply.

In addition a number of other patterns may occur, such as granulomatous patterns. As this chapter cannot aspire to completeness and this is not a treatise on benign conditions of the lymph node, they will not be discussed further.

ARTIFACTS

A number of extrinsic and intrinsic factors can influence lymph node histology. Though they are not patterns they can cause considerable difficulties in evaluating histology and are therefore mentioned here.

Technical Artifacts

Lymph node tissue is vulnerable and easily damaged in processing. Undue pressure on a specimen during dissection can cause considerable crushing artifacts, to the point of obliterating morphology completely. *Specimens with extensive crushing artifacts should best not be evaluated.* Differences are already subtle and no chance should be taken with poor material.

Another disturbing artifact is fixation related. It occurs especially in large specimens or if processing is too quick. If the fixation time in formalin is too short, only the outer edge of the specimen is fixed. The central part will not be reached by the formalin and will be fixed in the alcohol of the dehydrating series. This causes a marked difference in the aspect of outer and inner segments. The inner segment shows loss of cohesion, and cells appear more shrunken and hyperchromatic (Fig. 30.11). Great care should be taken in evaluating such specimens.

Intrinsic Artifacts

Though the above described architecture is found in all nodes throughout the body, in some areas typical features can be found, mostly the result of repeated inflammation or reactions. It is most often seen in inguinal nodes and takes the form of depositions of fibrotic material that can distort the normal architecture. This should be kept in mind in evaluating such a specimen. Similarly, in retroperitoneal lymph nodes hyalinization can be found.

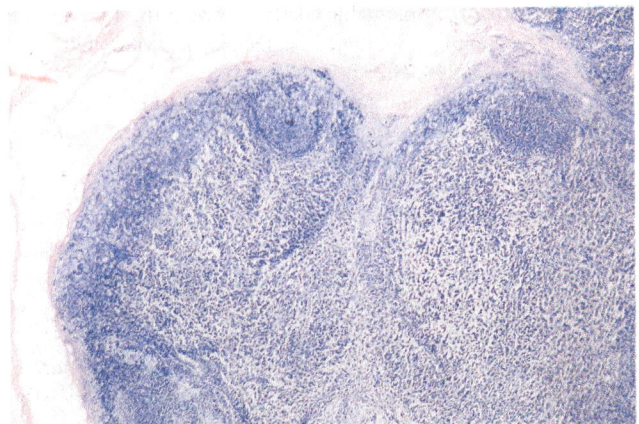

FIGURE 30.11 Fixation artifact. Edge of the specimen is properly fixed, the center, fixed in alcohol during the dehydration procedure, shows loss of tissue structure.

HANDLING OF LYMPH NODE SPECIMENS

In an area where morphologic differences are (very) subtle, additional techniques can be decisive in making a diagnosis. In the earlier days this meant having snap-frozen material available to do marker studies and/or molecular biology. However, the situation at the moment is that all commonly used markers in characterizing lymphoid tissues and its tumors are applicable on formalin-fixed, paraffin-embedded material. In addition, PCR analysis with multiple primers is a good alternative for molecular biologic evaluation of gene rearrangements and translocations. Nevertheless, it is still good policy to ask clinicians to send in lymph node specimens fresh and to snap-freeze a part of the specimen (20). It is no longer necessary to use a special fixative for immunohistochemistry (Bouin's fixative, sublimate-formaldehyde, B5, Sensofix, zinc-containing fixatives, among others); most of these are toxic and they also damage DNA to such a degree that molecular biologic analysis becomes impossible. It can be helpful to make touch imprints, by *carefully* pressing the cut surface of a specimen against a slide. The cytologic picture can be helpful, especially in cases where the histology is not so good.

Electron microscopy is not particularly helpful in diagnosing lymphoid lesions, benign or malignant. For very rare lesions, tumors of dendritic cells for instance, this may be of assistance and it is a small effort to slice off a very small and thin fragment for fixation in glutaraldehyde. However, and this is a general principle, *if a specimen is small any manipulation is a risk of damaging the cells in the lesion severely and should be kept to a minimum or even avoided altogether.*

If circumstances so dictate, consider sending a piece of tissue to the microbiology department for culture.

For research purposes, and if the size of the specimen allows it, a cell suspension can be made. Routine use of cell suspensions to perform marker analysis is not to be encouraged. One loses the morphologic control on the lesion and its cells, which is extremely important.

SPECIAL TECHNIQUES AND PROCEDURES

Immunohistochemistry can hardly be described as a very special technique, given its omnipresence in pathologic diagnostics. It is, however, not always used properly. Therefore, we will stress the basic rules for this important additional technique here once again.

1. Use positive and negative controls. Given the various problems (endogenous peroxidase, alkaline phosphatase, or nonspecific binding of antibodies through their Fc fragment: the very real possibility of technical mistakes), they are absolutely essential.

2. Use panels of antibodies. As no single antibody is absolutely specific for one molecule and cross-reactions can be very confusing, it is a sound policy to use a well-constructed panel in which individual staining results will confirm each other. Panels for classification of lymphoid lesions have been reported (85,86); they are primarily in use for classification of lymphoma, but are also useful for benign lymphoid lesions, as in lymphoid lesions it usually concerns the differential diagnosis between benign and malignant.

3. Use the morphology. Immunohistochemistry is an additional technique; one should always be extremely cautious if morphology and immunohistochemistry are not at odds. Also, morphology can direct the interpretation of the immunohistochemistry, for instance by looking at the immunophenotype of those cells that are considered the tumor cells. In lymphoid lesions there are always a lot of admixed cells, that are also of lymphoid origin. The best example is that of a paracortical expansion where the blasts proved to be of B-cell origin with the immunohistochemistry, a strong argument for a benign process.

4. Use your common sense. This goes without saying. It is curious, however, how often this essential piece of advice is ignored!

By and large, similar advice goes for molecular biology in the evaluation of lymphoid lesions. Controls, common sense, and the use of multiple primer pairs or techniques to confirm test results are equally important as for immunohistochemistry. Here, the demonstration of clonality must be considered a (strong) argument for malignancy, however, not all clonal lesions are malignant and certainly will not behave in a malignant fashion, the obvious example being monoclonal gammopathy of undetermined significance (87). Again, the data must be interpreted in their entire context.

Another point is the lineage determination, for instance by demonstration of immunoglobulin and T-cell receptor rearrangement. The terms lineage infidelity and lineage promiscuity already suggest that there are exceptions to the rule that only B cells rearrange immunoglobulin genes and only T cells rearrange T-cell receptor genes (88–92).

Obviously, additional techniques are invaluable in the analysis of lymphoid lesions, but only if they are properly used!

REFERENCES

1. Hall JG. The functional anatomy of lymph nodes. In: Stansfeld AG, ed. *Lymph Node Biopsy Interpretation*. Edinburgh: Churchill Livingstone; 1985:1–25.
2. Parrott DMV. The gut as a lymphoid organ. *Clin Gastroenterol* 1976;5:211–228.
3. McDermott MR, Bienenstock J. Evidence for a common mucosal immunologic system. I. Migration of B-immunoblasts into intestinal, respiratory and genital tissues. *J Immunol* 1979;122:1892–1898.
4. Sminia T, Plesch BE. An immunohistochemical study of cells with surface and cytoplasmic immunoglobulins in situ in Peyer's patches and lamina propria of rat small intestine. *Virchows Arch B Cell Pathol Incl Mol Pathol* 1982;40:181–189.
5. Azzali G. Structure, lymphatic vascularization and lymphocyte migration in mucosa-associated lymphoid tissue. *Immunol Rev* 2003;195:178–189.
6. Hoorweg K, Cupedo T. Development of human lymph nodes and Peyer's patches. *Semin Immunol* 2008;20:164–170.
7. Jaspars LJ, van der Linden JC, Scheffer GL, et al. Monoclonal antibody 4C7 recognizes an endothelial basement membrane component that is selectively expressed in capillaries of lymphoid follicles. *J Pathol* 1993;170:121–128.
8. Schaerli P, Willimann K, Lang AB, et al. Cxc chemokine receptor 5 expression defines follicular homing T-cells with B cell helper function. *J Exp Med* 2000;192:1553–1573.
9. Stein JV, Nombela-Arrieta C. Chemokine control of lymphocyte trafficking: A general overview. *Immunol* 2005;116:1–12.
10. Campbell DJ, Koch MA. Phenotypical and functional specialization of FoxP3+ regulatory T cells. *Nat Rev Immunol* 2011;11:119–130.
11. Taylor CR. Classification of lymphoma. *Arch Pathol Lab Med* 1978;102:549–554.
12. van den Oord JJ, de Wolf-Peeters C, Desmet VJ. The marginal zone of the human reactive lymph node. *Am J Clin Pathol* 1986;86:475–479.
13. Nathwani BN, Hernandez AM, Drachenberg MR. Chapter 14: Diagnostic significance of morphologic patterns of lymphoid proliferations in lymph nodes. In: Knowles DM, ed. *Neoplastic Hematopathology*. 2nd ed. Philadelphia, PA: Lippincott Williams & Wilkins; 2001:507–536.
14. Nossal GJV, Abbot A, Mitchell J, et al. Antigens in immunity. XV. Ultrastructural features of antigen capture primary and secondary follicles. *J Exp Med* 1968;127:277–290.
15. Park CS, Choi YS. How do follicular dendritic cells interact intimately with B-cells in the germinal centre? *Immunology* 2005;114:2–10.
16. Aguzzi A, Krautler NJ. Characterizing follicular dendritic cells: A progress report. *Eur J Immunol* 2010;40:2134–2138.
17. Haberman AM, Shlomchik SJ. Reassessing the function of immune-complex retention by follicular dendritic cells. *Nat Rev Immunol* 2003;3:757–764.
18. Lennert K. Malignant lymphomas, other than Hodgkin's disease. In: *Handbuch der speziellen pathologischen Anatomie und Histologie I/3/B*. Berlin: Springer-Verlag; 1978.
19. Van der Valk P, van der Loo EM, Jansen J, et al. Analysis of lymphoid and dendritic cells in human lymph node, tonsil and spleen. A study using monoclonal and heterologous antibodies. *Virchows Arch B Cell Pathol Incl Mol Pathol* 1984;45:169–185.
20. Ellis DW, Eaton M, Fox RM, et al. Diagnostic pathology of lymphoproliferative disorders. *Pathology* 2005;37:434–456.
21. Petrasch S, Brittinger G, Wacker HH, et al. Follicular dendritic cells in non-Hodgkin lymphomas. *Leuk Lymphoma* 1994;15:33–43.
22. Cyster JG, Ansel KM, Reif K, et al. Follicular stromal cells and lymphocyte homing to follicles. *Immunol Rev* 2000;176:181–193.

23. Allen CD, Cyster JG. Follicular dendritic cell networks of primary follicles and germinal centers: Phenotype and function. *Semin Immunol* 2008;20:14–25.
24. Stein H, Bonk A, Tolksdorf G, et al. Immunohistologic analysis of the organization of normal lymphoid tissue and non-Hodgkin's lymphomas. *J Histochem Cytochem* 1980;28:746–760.
25. Knowles DM. Immunophenotypic markers useful in the diagnosis and classification of hematopoietic neoplasms. In: Knowles DM, ed. *Neoplastic Hematopathology*. 2nd ed. Philadelphia, PA: Lippincott Williams & Wilkins; 2001: 93–226.
26. Crotty S. Follicular helper CD4 T-cells (TFH). *Annu Rev Immunol* 2011;29:621–663.
27. Schwickert TA, Lindquist RL, Shakhar G, et al. In vivo imaging of germinal centres reveals a dynamic open structure. *Nature* 2007;446:83–87.
28. Ewing EP, Chandler GW, Spira TJ, et al. Primary lymph node pathology in AIDS and AIDS-related lymphadenopathy. *Arch Pathol Lab Med* 1985;109:977–981.
29. Chadburn A, Metroka C, Mouradian J. Progressive lymph node histology and its prognostic value in patients with acquired immunodeficiency syndrome and AIDS-related complex. *Hum Pathol* 1989;20:579–587.
30. Ioachim HL, Ratech H. *Ioachim's Lymph Node Pathology*. 3rd ed. Philadelphia, PA: Lippincott Williams & Wilkins; 2002.
31. Chang CC, Osipov V, Wheaton S, et al. Follicular hyperplasia, follicular lysis, and progressive transformation of germinal centers. A sequential spectrum of morphologic evolution in lymphoid hyperplasia. *Am J Clin Pathol* 2003;120: 322–326.
32. Oort J, Turk JL. A histological and autoradiographic study of lymph nodes during the development of contact sensitivity in the guinea pig. *Br J Exp Pathol* 1964;46:147–154.
33. Worbs T, Föster R. T-cell migration dynamics within lymph nodes during steady state: An overview of extracellular in intracellular factors influencing the basal intranodal T-cell motility. *Curr Top Microbiol Immunol* 2009;334:71–105.
34. Denucci CC, Mitchell JS, Shimizu Y. Integrin function in T-cell homing to lymphoid and nonlymphoid sites: Getting there and staying there. *Crit Rev Immunol* 2009;29:87–109.
35. Stevens SK, Weismann IL, Butcher EC. Differences in the migration of B and T lymphocytes: organ-selective localization in vivo and the role of lymphocyte-endothelial cell regonition. *J Immunol* 1982;128:844–851.
36. Arata-Kawai H, Singer MS, Bistrup A, et al. Functional contributions of N- and O-glycans to L-selectin ligands in murine and human lymphoid organs. *Am J Pathol* 2011;178:423–433.
37. Pals ST, Kraal G, Horst E, et al. Human lymphocyte-high endothelial venule interaction: Organ selective binding of T and B lymphocyte populations to high endothelium. *J Immunol* 1986;137:760–763.
38. Wiedle G, Dunon D, Imhof BA. Current concepts in lymphocyte homing and recirculation. *Crit Rev Clin Lab Sci* 2001; 38:1–31.
39. Lopez-Giral S, Quintana NE, Cabrerizo M, et al. Chemokine receptors that mediate B-cell homing to secondary lymphoid tissues are highly expressed in B-cell chronic lymphocytic leukemia and non-Hodgkin's lymphomas with widespread nodular dissemination. *J Leukoc Biol* 2004;76:462–471.
40. Schaerli P, Moser B. Chemokines: Control of primary and memory T-cell traffic. *Immunol Res* 2005;31:57–74.
41. Thorbecke GJ, Silberberg-Sinakin I, Flotte TH. Langerhans cells as macrophages in skin and lymphoid organs. *J Invest Dermatol* 1980;75:32–43.
42. Willard-Mack CL. Normal structure, function, and histology of lymph nodes. *Toxicol Pathol* 2006;34:409–424.
43. Bousso P. T-cell activation by dendritic cells in the lymph node: Lessons from the movies. *Nat Rev Immunol* 2008;8:675–684.
44. Shklovskaya E, Roediger B, Fazekas de St Groth B. Epidermal and dermal dendritic cells display differential activation and migratory behaviour while sharing the ability to stimulate CD4+ T cell proliferation in vivo. *J Immunol* 2008;181: 418–430.
45. Roozendaal R, Mebius RE, Kraal G. The conduit system of the lymph node. *Int Immunol* 2008;20:1483–1487.
46. Forkert PG, Thliveris JA, Bertalanfy FD. Structure of sinuses in the human lymph node. *Cell Tissue Res* 1997;183: 115–130.
47. Wacker HH, Frahm SO, Heidebrecht HJ, et al. Sinus-lining cells of the lymph nodes recognized as a dendritic cell type by the new monoclonal antibody Ki-M9. *Am J Pathol* 1997;151: 423–434.
48. Turner RR, Giuliano AE, Hoon DS, et al. Pathologic examination of sentinel lymph node for breast cancer. *World J Surg* 2001;25:798–805.
49. Sheibani K, Fritz RM, Winberg CD, et al. "Monocytoid" cells in reactive follicular hyperplasia with and without multifocal histiocytic reactions: An immunohistochemical study of 21 cases including suspected cases of toxoplasmic lymphadenitis. *Am J Clin Pathol* 1984;81:453–458.
50. Kurtin PJ. Marginal zone B cells, monocytoid B cells, and the follicular microenvironment. Determinants of morphologic features in a subset of low-grade B-cell lymphomas. *Am J Clin Pathol* 2000;114:505–508.
51. Gatto D, Brink R. The germinal center reaction. *J Allergy Clin Immunol* 2010;126:898–907.
52. Lukes RJ, Collins RD. A functional approach to the classification of malignant lymphomas. *Recent Results Cancer Res* 1974;46:18–30.
53. Mann RB, Jaffe ES, Bernard CW. Malignant lymphomas—a conceptual understanding of morphologic diversity. *Am J Pathol* 1979;94:104–191.
54. Jaffe ES, Harris NL, Stein H, et al. Introduction: An overview of the classification of the lymphoid neoplasms. In: Swerdlow SH, Campo E, Harris NL, et al., eds. *WHO Classification of Tumours of Hematopoietic and Lymphoid Tissues*. Lyon: IARC; 2008:158–166.
55. Evans N. Lymphadenitis of secondary syphilis: Its resemblance to giant follicular lymphadenopathy. *Arch Pathol* 1944;37: 175–179.
56. Nosanchuk JS, Schnitzer B. Follicular hyperplasia in lymph nodes from patients with rheumatoid arthritis. *Cancer* 1969; 24:334–354.
57. Keller AR, Holchholzer L, Castleman B. Hyaline-vascular and plasma cell types of giant lymph node hyperplasia of the mediastinum and other locations. *Cancer* 1972;29:670–683.
58. Osborne BM, Butler JJ, Variakojis D, et al. Reactive lymph node hyperplasia with giant follicles. *Am J Clin Pathol* 1982;78: 493–499.
59. Martino G, Cariati S, Tintisona O, et al. Atypical lymphoproliferative disorders: Castleman's disease. Case report and review of the literature. *Tumori* 2004;90:352–355.

60. Newlon JL, Couch M, Brennan J. Castleman's disease: Three case reports and a review of the literature. *Ear Nose Throat J* 2007;86:414–418.
61. Schnitzer B. Reactive lymphoid hyperplasia. In: Jaffe ES, ed. *Surgical Pathology of the Lymph Nodes and Related Organs*. Philadelphia, PA: WB Saunders; 1995:98–132.
62. Rappaport H. Tumors of the hematopoietic system. In: *Atlas of Tumor Pathology. 3rd series. Fascicle 8*. Washington, DC: Armed Forces Institute of Tumor Pathology; 1966.
63. Dorfman RF, Warnke R. Lymphadenopathy simulating the malignant lymphomas. *Hum Pathol* 1974;5:519–550.
64. Nathwani BN, Winberg CD, Diamond LW, et al. Morphologic criteria for the differentiation of follicular lymphoma from florid reactive follicular hyperplasia. A study of 80 cases. *Cancer* 1981;48:1794–1806.
65. Mann RB. Follicular lymphoma and lymphocytic lymphoma of intermediate differentiation. In: Jaffe ES, ed. *Surgical Pathology of the Lymph Nodes and Related Organs*. Philadelphia, PA: WB Saunders; 1985:165–202.
66. Harris NL, Ferry JA. Follicular lymphoma and related disorders (germinal center lymphomas). In: Knowles DM, ed. *Neoplastic Haematology*. Baltimore, MD: Lippincott Williams & Wilkins; 2001:823–853.
67. O'Leary H, Savage KJ. The spectrum of peripheral T-cell lymphomas. *Curr Opin Hematol* 2009;16:292–298.
68. Catovsky D, Ralfkiaer E, Muller-Hermelink HK. T-cell prolymphocytic leukaemia. In: Swerdlow SH, Campo E, Harris NL, et al., eds. *WHO Classification of Tumours of Haemotopoietic and Lymphoid Tissues*. Lyon: IARC Press; 2008:270–271.
69. Vittorio C, Muglia J. Anticonvulsant hypersensitivity syndrome. *Arch Intern Med* 1995;155:2285–2290.
70. Kuo T. Kikuchi's disease (histiocytic necrotizing lymphadenitis): A clinicopathologic study of 79 cases with an analysis of histologic subtypes, immunohistology, and DNA ploidy. *Am J Surg Pathol* 1995;20:798–809.
71. van den Oord JJ, de Wolf-Peeters C, Desmet VJ, et al. Nodular alteration of the paracortical area. An in situ immunohistochemical analysis of primary, secondary and tertiary T nodules. *Am J Pathol* 1985;120:55–66.
72. van den Oord JJ, de Wolf-Peeters C, de Vos R, et al. The cortical area in dermatopathic lymphadenitis and other reactive conditions of the lymph node. *Virchows Arch B* 1984;45:289–299.
73. Good DJ, Gascoyne RD. Atypical lymphoid hyperplasia mimicking lymphoma. *Hematol Oncol Clin North Am* 2009;23:729–745.
74. Scheffer E, Meijer CJ, Van Vloten WA. Dermatopathic lymphadenopathy and lymph node involvement in mycosis fungoides. *Cancer* 1980;45:137–148.
75. Willemze R, Scheffer E, Meijer CJ. Immunohistochemical studies using monoclonal antibodies on lymph nodes from patients with mycosis fungoides and Sézary's syndrome. *Am J Pathol* 1986;120:46–54.
76. van Doorn R, van Haselen CW, van Voorst Vader P, et al. Mycosis fungoides: Disease evolution and prognosis of 309 Dutch patients. *Arch Dermatol* 2000;136:504–510.
77. Ralfkiaer E, Cerroni L, Sander CA, et al. Mycosis fungoides. In: Swerdlow SH, Campo E, Harris NL, et al., eds. *WHO Classification of Tumours of Haemotopoietic and Lymphoid Tissues*. Lyon: IARC Press; 2008:296–298.
78. Rosai J, Dorfman RF. Sinus histiocytosis with massive lymphadenopathy: Pseudolymphomatous benign disorder. Analysis of 34 cases. *Cancer* 1972;30:1174–1180.
79. McClain KL, Natkunam Y, Swerdlow SH. Atypical cellular disorders. *Hematology Am Soc Hematol Educ Program* 2004;1:283–296.
80. Callihan TR. Langerhans' cell histiocytosis (histiocytosis X). In: Jaffe ES, ed. *Surgical Pathology of the Lymph Nodes and Related Organs*. Philadelphia, PA: WB Saunders; 1995:537–559.
81. Delsol G, Falini B, Müler-Hermelink HK, et al. Anaplastic large cell lymphoma. In: Swerdlow SH, Campo E, Harris NL, et al., eds. *WHO Classification of Tumours of Haemotopoietic and Lymphoid Tissues*. Lyon: IARC Press; 2008:312–316.
82. Pileri SA, Grogan TM, Harris NL, et al. Tumours of histiocytes and accessory dendritic cells: An immunohistochemical approach to classification from the International Lymphoma Study Group based on 61 cases. *Histopathology* 2002;41:1–29.
83. Dallenbach FE, Coupland SE, Stein H. Marginal zone lymphomas: Extranodal MALT type, nodal and splenic. *Pathologe* 2000;21:162–177.
84. Samet A, Gilbey P, Talmon Y, et al. Vascular transformation of the lymph node sinuses. *J Laryngol Otol* 2001;115:760–762.
85. Oudejans JJ, van der Valk P. Immunohistochemical classification of T cell and NK cell neoplasms. *J Clin Pathol* 2002;55:892.
86. Oudejans JJ, van der Valk P. Immunohistochemical classification of B cell neoplasms. *J Clin Pathol* 2003;56:193.
87. McKenna RW, Kyle RA, Kuehl WM, et al. Plasma cell neoplasms. In: Swerdlow SH, Campo E, Harris NL, et al., eds. *WHO Classification of Tumours of Haemotopoietic and Lymphoid Tissues*. Lyon: IARC Press; 2008:200–213.
88. Adriaansen HJ, Soeting PW, Wolvers-Tettero IL, et al. Immunoglobulin and T-cell receptor gene rearrangements in acute non-lymphocytic leukemias. Analysis of 54 cases and a review of the literature. *Leukemia* 1991;5:744–751.
89. Waldmann TA, Davis MA, Bongiovanni KF, et al. Rearrangement of genes for the antigen receptor on T-cells as markers of lineage and clonality in human lymphoid neoplasms. *N Engl J Med* 1985;313:776–783.
90. Asou N, Matsuoka M, Hattori T, et al. T-cell gamma gene rearrangements in hematologic neoplasms. *Blood* 1987;69:968–970.
91. Zuniga M, D'Eustachio P, Ruddle NH. Immunoglobulin heavy chain gene rearrangement and transcription in murine T-cell hybrids and T-lymphomas. *Proc Natl Acad Sci USA* 1982;79:3015–3019.
92. Schmidt CA, Przybylski GK. What can we learn from leukaemia as for the process of lineage commitment in hematopoiesis? *Int Rev Immunol* 2001;20:107–115.

Spleen

J. Han J.M. van Krieken ■ Attilio Orazi

INTRODUCTION 799	ULTRASTRUCTURE 807
PRENATAL AND DEVELOPMENTAL CHANGES 800	FUNCTION 807
APOPTOSIS 801	Filter Function 808
	Immunologic Function 808
GROSS FEATURES/ORGAN WEIGHT 802	Hematopoiesis 809
ANATOMY 802	Reservoir Function 809
Blood Supply 802	AGING DIFFERENCES 809
Nerves 802	DIFFERENTIAL DIAGNOSIS 809
Lymphatics 802	SPECIMEN HANDLING 810
LIGHT MICROSCOPY 802	HISTOLOGIC TECHNIQUE 810
Vascular Tree 802	SPECIAL PROCEDURES 810
Red Pulp 804	CONCLUSION 811
White Pulp 805	REFERENCES 811
Perifollicular Zone 807	
FLOW CYTOMETRY 807	

INTRODUCTION

Since antiquity, a variety of ideas on the physiology and anatomy of the spleen have been developed (1). As producer of black bile, the spleen was seen as the origin of melancholy and as such used in poetry, even nowadays. Galen (131–201 AD) called the human spleen an enigmatic organ, a notion that has persisted for a long time. In the 17th century, Malpighi described, macroscopically, the splenic lymphoid tissue as white pulp against a background of red pulp. In 1857, Billroth published one of the first histology studies of the human spleen in which he divided the red pulp into cord tissue and venous sinuses. Still, until the second half of the 20th century, the spleen was considered a rather useless reservoir for blood cells and was hardly studied. In the 1970s, by using electron microscopy, Weiss was able to elucidate the ultrastructure of the organ, which gave insights into the red pulp function (2). Knowledge on the organization of the white pulp started to arise also in the 70s and is still increasing as of today (3–5).

Nevertheless, many pathologists still lack a clear understanding of the normal histology and functions of the human spleen. This is due to several reasons. The organ is extremely vulnerable to autolysis, which often makes histologic findings in postmortem specimens difficult to interpret and of limited teaching value. Surgically removed spleens are suitable, if processed without delay. However, since the number of splenectomies performed in most institutions is relatively scarce, it is not surprising that pathologists may feel uncomfortable when interpreting splenic pathology as a result of a lack of familiarity with splenic histologic features. For this reason, collaboration was initiated: the International Spleen Consortium (6).

A substantial source of confusion with respect to the structure and function of the human spleen lies in the terminology and definitions applied to this organ, because they are partially based on studies of animal spleens. The human

TABLE 31.1 Summary of Splenic Histology, Function, and Relationship to Lymph Node Compartments

Spleen Compartment	Description	Function/Composition	Equivalent in Lymph Node
White Pulp			
T-cell area	Irregular area of small lymphocytes containing lymph vessels bordering arteries	Predominant CD4 lymphocytes	Paracortex
B-cell follicle	Round area of small lymphocytes surrounded by medium-sized lymphocytes (a germinal center may be present)	Production of Ig-producing cells and probably memory cells	Follicle
Perifollicular zone	Area between white and red pulp containing many erythrocytes and lacking a normal sinusoidal structure	Place of retarded blood flow with interaction of blood cells, cells, antigens, and antibodies	Medulla (?)
Red Pulp			
Sinuses/cord tissue with sheathed capillaries	Tissue containing a meshwork of sinuses (with interrupted basement membrane) and capillaries, partly sheathed	Removal of particles from blood cells. Possible place of interaction of new antigens with reticulum cells	Sinus: Partly high endothelial venule Sheathed capillary: Medullary sinus
Nonfiltering area	Area of red pulp tissue lacking capillaries and containing lymphocytes	Probably place of onset of immune reaction	Medulla or compartment of primary follicles
Perivascular rim	Small area along the vessel tree containing lymphocytes and plasma cells	Probably connected to lymphatics	Medulla (?)

and animal spleens do not have an identical architecture; for example, in the human spleen, the marginal sinus as described in rodent spleens is not present. Furthermore, certain definitions (e.g., of the marginal zone) vary widely from author to author (7–10).

The next problem is the large variation that occurs in the "normal" spleen. The spleen is a compartmentalized organ (Table 31.1). Stimulation of one of the many functions of the spleen can lead to morphologic changes in the compartment that is mainly responsible for that function. The normal spleen, therefore, can show wide variation. As one of us has shown, it is essential to define a normal control population if one undertakes histologic studies in the spleen in specific disorders (11). For example, a morphometric analysis showed that spleens removed incidentally during abdominal surgery (i.e., for highly selective vagotomy or early gastric cancer) differed from traumatically ruptured spleens; we therefore excluded the latter from our "normal" group. These issues make it difficult to differentiate physiologic from pathologic changes.

PRENATAL AND DEVELOPMENTAL CHANGES

During embryogenesis, the spleen can be recognized from about the 5th week of gestation, and blood vessels appear in it by the 9th week. Red and white pulp cannot be distinguished until the 9th month. The functional role of the spleen during prenatal development varies widely from that of the adult spleen, and this is reflected in the microscopic anatomy of the organ. Hematopoiesis was considered to take place in the fetal spleen (and liver) and to contribute largely to blood cell formation in the fetus until the 6th month of gestation, but it has been shown that, in fact, the spleen is not a stem cell niche for hematopoiesis but functions as a site of maturation for hematopoietic precursors derived from the bone marrow through the peripheral blood (12,13). In adults, one may see foci of hematopoietic cells (extramedullary hematopoiesis) in the spleen in many reactive conditions (e.g., sepsis), as well as in disorders of the bone marrow associated with myelofibrosis. Extramedullary hematopoiesis as seen in the spleen is also referred to as myeloid metaplasia.

The immune system develops during fetal growth, and this development continues after birth (14). This functional maturation is reflected by the morphology: until birth the splenic white pulp does not contain follicles and marginal zones. There are immature B cells in clusters and T cells scattered throughout the organ. Their numbers increase with the developmental age of the fetus; and, from the end of the second semester onward, B- and T-cell areas can be recognized (15,16). Phagocytosis can be demonstrated at the 12th week of gestation (12).

Developmental anomalies of the spleen are very familiar (17). The presence of accessory spleens (the so-called spleniculi, small extra pieces of spleen tissue with the complete and normal histology of the red and white pulp) can be found in at least 25% of autopsies. In disorders being treated with splenectomy, these spleniculi may lead to recurrence of the disease.

Rare but well known is the polysplenia associated with immotile cilia syndrome (18). In this syndrome, left–right orientation of thoracic and abdominal organs may be abnormal and the spleen at the right side is often divided into many small pieces, generally having normal function. This is not to be confused with acquired splenosis, in which many small fragments of spleen are present after trauma. Congenital asplenia, which is exceedingly rare, is associated with abnormalities of the cardiovascular system. Splenogonadal

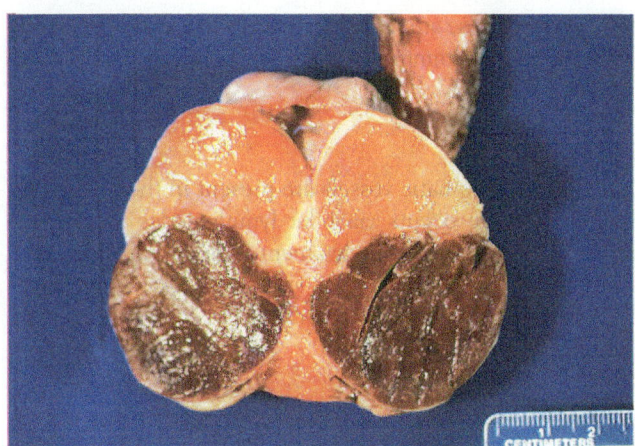

FIGURE 31.1 Gross appearance of splenogonadal fusion. Note ectopic splenic tissue within the testis.

fusion is a rare developmental anomaly (Fig. 31.1). There are approximately 120 cases reported since the first description of this entity in 1883 by Bostroem. Close proximity of the spleen and gonad during early embryologic development allows fusion, whether continuous or discontinuous, of these seemingly unrelated organs. A testicular or scrotal mass is its usual clinical presentation (19).

APOPTOSIS

In the development of the spleen, apoptosis does not seem to play an important role, but the lymphoid compartment, as in other lymphoid tissues, shows extensive apoptosis, especially in the germinal centers of the B-cell follicles. This is illustrated in Figure 31.2, where the "starry-sky" phenomenon can be observed. The starry-sky cells are macrophages that phagocytose remnants of lymphocytes that are dying through apoptosis, generally because they have an unsuccessful gene rearrangement of the antigen receptor or because of the fact that the produced immunoglobulin recognizes autoantigen. This physiologic process is important in the protection against autoimmune diseases. The Bcl-2 protein that protects against certain forms of apoptosis (see Chapter 1), which is expressed in most B and T cells, is lacking in germinal center B cells, rendering them susceptible for apoptosis. In follicular lymphoma, the t(14;18) translocation leads to aberrant expression of Bcl-2 in the tumor cells. This is sometimes deceptive in the recognition of follicular lymphoma in the spleen for the following reasons. Since the spleens of patients over about 20 years of age only rarely contain active germinal centers, the distinction between a primary follicle and a follicular lymphoma can be difficult. The mere absence of a Bcl2 negative germinal center is therefore not indicative of follicular lymphoma: the presence of the t(14;18) needs to be proven by for instance fluorescent in-situ hybridization. Furthermore, the involvement of the spleen by follicular lymphoma is often nodular but does not lead to the disturbance of the architecture that is so noticeable in the lymph nodes involved by follicular lymphoma (20).

Apoptosis also plays an important role in maintaining a normal number and function of T cells. In cases of autoimmune lymphoproliferative syndrome (a pediatric disorder due to a genetic defect of FAS or Fas ligand that is associated with splenomegaly and autoimmunity), a decreased rate of apoptosis in T lymphocytes is responsible for the marked degree of lymphoid hyperplasia seen in the T-cell–rich areas of the spleen (21).

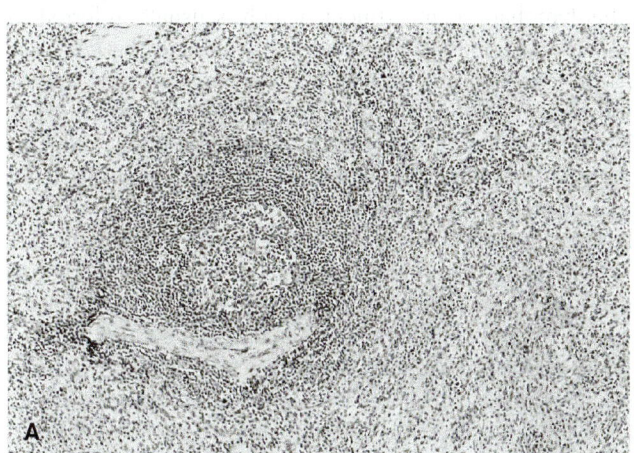
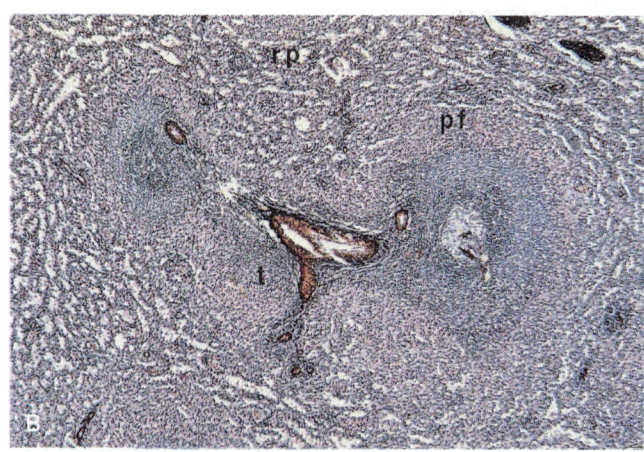

FIGURE 31.2 Spleen removed in idiopathic thrombocytopenic purpura. **A:** Formalin-fixed paraffin embedding (H&E, original magnification ×40). **B:** Methylmethacrylate embedding (methenamine-silver/H&E, original magnification ×40). Overview of red and white pulp showing central arteriole with T-cell area, a primary follicle, and a secondary follicle containing a germinal center. Note the absence of the marginal zone around the T-cell area and the presence of the erythrocyte-rich (pink) perifollicular zone surrounding both the T- and B-cell compartments of the white pulp. Note the lack of detail on the structure of the red pulp and the difficult discernible perifollicular zone in standard H&E section (*rp*, red pulp; *pf*, perifollicular zone; *t*, T-cell area).

GROSS FEATURES/ORGAN WEIGHT

The human spleen is a bean-shaped organ surrounded by a smooth capsule covered by the peritoneum. In contrast to several species, the capsule does not contain smooth muscle fibers and, therefore, does not have the capability of undergoing contraction in response to acute blood loss. The spleen in animals such as dogs and cats has an important red blood cell reservoir function. By undergoing rapid contraction, the spleen can squeeze out its red blood cell reservoir and, by doing so, produce a rapid increase in the amount of circulating blood. Recently, it has been shown, however, that evolution in Homo sapiens is ongoing. Divers from Bajau, the so-called sea nomads, have acquired a mutation in the PDE10A gene resulting in extraordinary breath-holding ability, thanks to splenic contraction (22).

The surface of the spleen may be covered with fibrotic or even calcified plaques, the cause of which is unknown. It is not uncommon to find several grooves at the outer surface that have no clinical significance. The weight of the spleen is highly variable (23). In adults, the spleen generally weighs 150 to 250 g; but, in the elderly, the spleen is often substantially smaller, even when there is no apparent hypofunction. A recent finding indicates that in a proportion of stroke patients, the volume of the spleen decreases together with an increase of cytokine levels (24).

On the cut surface, the red and white pulp can be discerned, the latter consisting of small (less than or equal to 2 mm) nodules. It is important to realize that involvement of the spleen in malignant lymphoma often is observed foremost in the white pulp, which becomes enlarged but often not to a great extent.

ANATOMY

Blood Supply

Blood reaches the spleen via the splenic artery, a large branch of the celiac artery, and enters the spleen through four to six branches; their number and location is, however, highly variable. Venous outflow occurs via four to six venous branches. These combine within the lienorenal ligament to form the splenic vein, which drains into the portal vein. This is why portal hypertension can produce "congestive" splenomegaly. The blood flow within the spleen is highly specialized and relates to the different functions of the spleen.

Nerves

The spleen is innervated by nonmyelinated fibers from the major splanchnic nerves and the celiac plexus. These nerve fibers run along the splenic artery. Innervation in human spleens is less extensive than in cat and dog spleens, and this might be related to the more important reservoir function of the spleen in these animals, as previously mentioned. An interesting role in the immune response is recently discussed (25).

Lymphatics

No afferent lymphatic vessels are present in the spleen. Its lymph drainage occurs via hilar lymph nodes and lymph nodes in the gastrosplenic ligament. The lymph then flows through lymphatics along the splenic artery to the celiac lymph nodes along the celiac artery. The lymphatics in the spleen are described below.

LIGHT MICROSCOPY

Vascular Tree

After entering at the hilus, the splenic artery branches like a tree. Within the splenic parenchyma, these arterial branches, called trabecular arteries, are accompanied by veins and lymph vessels and surrounded by collagenous fibers. These vessels containing fibrous structures are usually referred to as trabeculae or septa, a term which is inappropriate to describe what in essence perivascular collagen cuffs are. Real, albeit short, true septa are also present in the spleen. These are connected to the capsule, lack inside vessels, and only extend for a short length into the splenic tissue. Foci of condensed reticular fibers devoid of vessels are found throughout the red pulp. The condensed reticulum appears to be in direct continuity with the reticular meshwork of the surrounding red pulp; it may represent areas of collapse or involution of the red pulp tissue.

Trabecular arteries branch to form central arteries and arterioles that are no longer accompanied by veins and are surrounded not by a collagenous cuff but rather by lymphatic tissue predominantly composed of T lymphocytes. This lymphatic compartment, which is usually referred to as periarterial or periarteriolar lymphoid sheath (PALS) is present around the vessels and becomes smaller toward the capillary ending. The arterioles are usually described as branching into penicillar arterioles, which run in parallel. In humans, however, this phenomenon seems to be restricted to involuted specimens in which the disappearance of tissue between arterioles has left them lying close to each other.

Branching of arterioles and capillaries often occurs at right angles, as can frequently be seen in sections. Reconstructions based on serial sections have shown that the terminal end of the capillary forms a peculiar and specifically splenic structure (7) (Figs. 31.3 and 31.4). These structures are known by several names, determined partly by the species in which they have been studied, for example, sheathed capillaries, Hülsekapillaren, ellipsoids, or periarteriolar macrophage sheaths. In humans, they are present in the red pulp and the perifollicular zone (PFZ) and are generally referred to as sheathed capillaries. The sheathed capillary is surrounded by a "sheath" of mononuclear phagocytes and rare reticulum cells. Since autolysis is so rapid, visualization of the sheathed

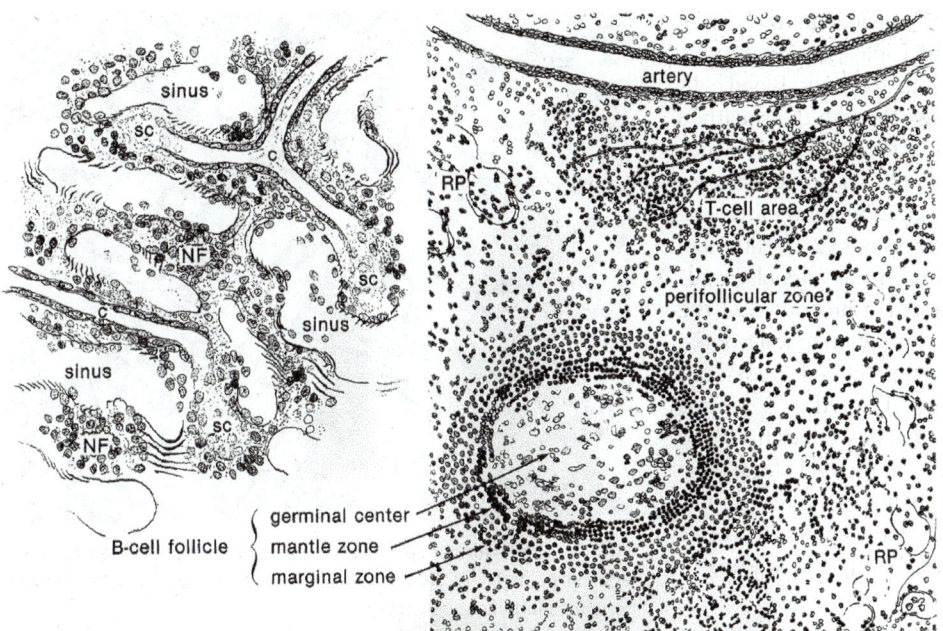

FIGURE 31.3 Schematic impression of red (*left*) and white (*right*) pulp, showing the main compartments and structures of the human spleen. The capillaries (*c*) end as sheathed capillaries (*sc*) without direct communication with the sinuses. The nonfiltering areas (*NF*) are bordered by sinuses and are devoid of (sheathed) capillaries. The perifollicular zone surrounds the white pulp (follicle and T-cell area) and lacks fully developed sinuses. Note the zoning in the B cell but not in the T-cell compartment. The T-cell area contains a lymphatic plexus (*Left*, original magnification ×250; *right*, original magnification ×100).

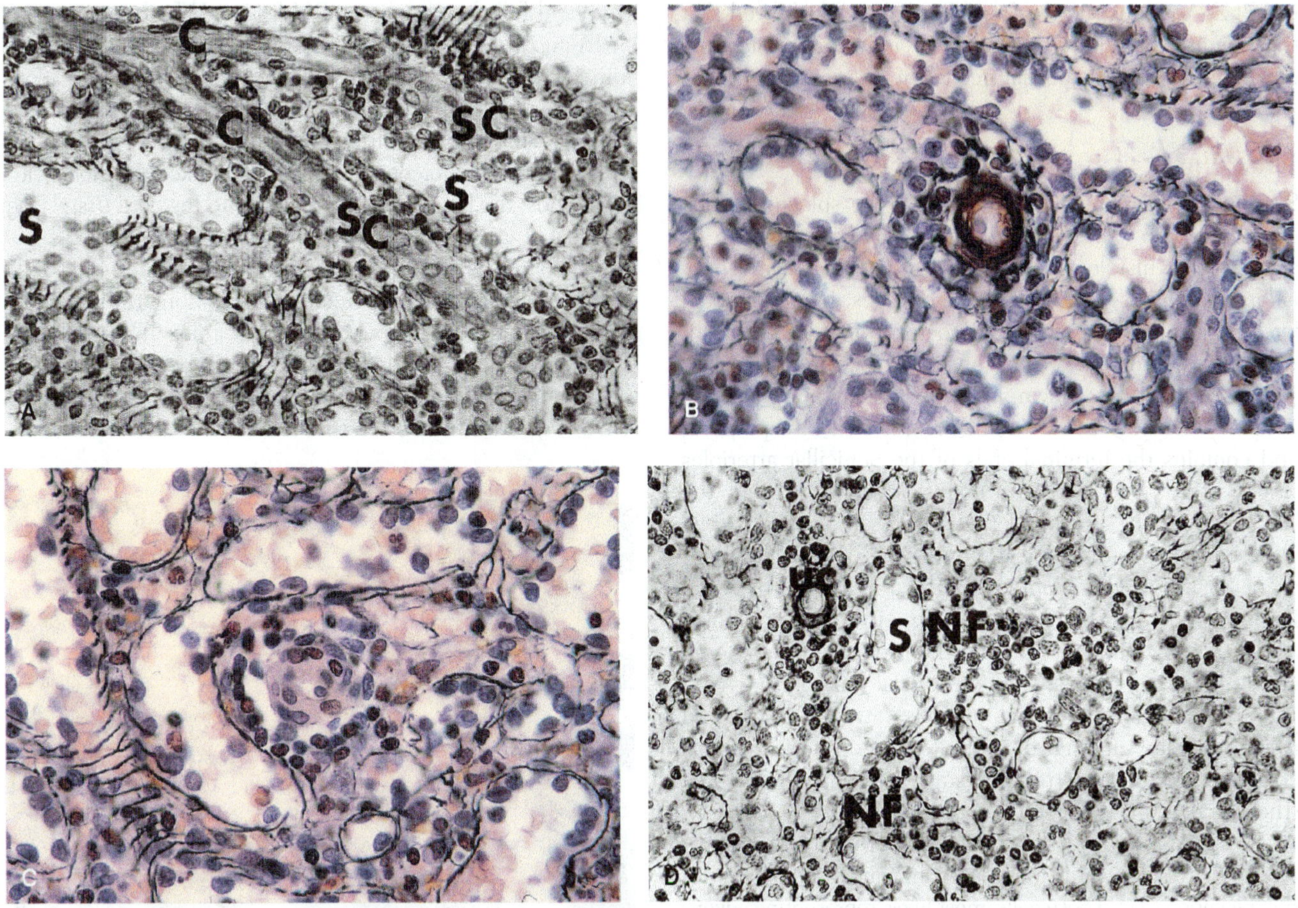

FIGURE 31.4 A: Traumatically ruptured spleen. Methylmethacrylate embedding (methenamine-silver/H&E, original magnification ×400). Capillary transitioning into sheathed capillary. Note the proximity to, but lack of connection with, the sinuses (*C*, capillary [unsheathed]; *SC*, sheathed capillary; *S*, sinus). **B:** Same specimen as in (**A**) (original magnification ×1,000). Detail of unsheathed capillary. **C:** Same specimen as in (**A**) (original magnification ×1,000). Detail of sheathed capillary. **D:** Same specimen as in (**A**) (original magnification ×250). Detail of the red pulp showing sinuses in cord tissue. Note the nonfiltering areas devoid of capillaries and completely surrounded by sinuses (*Uc*, unsheathed capillary; *S*, sinus; *NF*, nonfiltering area).

capillaries in particular is dependent on adequate tissue processing. The endothelial lining of the capillary ends abruptly in a string of concentrically arranged macrophages. Blood cells coming from an arteriole have to pass through the sheathed capillary on their way to the lumen of the sinus, which they reach by slowly percolating through the cord macrophages and red pulp stroma (open circulation; 26), and then via the slits in the basement membrane of the sinus (2,7). Although no direct anatomic connection between the arteriolar ends and the sinuses has been demonstrated, a proportion of the arteriolar branches may end in close opposition to walls of the sinuses, allowing a more rapid circulation (closed circulation) of at least a portion of the blood flow. The red pulp sinuses are considered as the first part of the splenic venous tree. The localization of the sheathed capillaries at the end of the arterial tree seems perfect for their functioning as a filtering unit.

Within the sinusoidal meshwork, there are large sinuses that open directly into veins running along the arteries in the collagenous cuff.

Small efferent lymph vessels can be found in the T-lymphocyte compartment of the white pulp in about two-thirds of the spleens. They are not seen in the surrounding PFZ. A reconstruction from serial sections showed that these lymph vessels form a network around arterioles and eventually follow the arterial tree to the hilar region (7).

Red Pulp

Seventy-five percent of the volume of the spleen is made up of red pulp (7). The two-dimensional picture given by conventional histology sections suggests that the red pulp is largely composed of cordal macrophages, interconnected by their cytoplasmic processes to form a reticular meshwork that provides structural support to the venous sinuses. Serial sections have shown, however, that the red pulp also contains a loose reticular framework, is rich in capillaries, and contains the terminal ends of the penicillar arterioles (Fig. 31.4D). The sinuses account for about 30% of the red pulp (7). The sinus endothelial cells are surrounded by almost circular strands of discontinuous basement membrane that is predominantly composed of collagen IV and laminin, known as the ring fibers (Fig. 31.5). The ring fibers are both interconnected among themselves and anchored to the dendritic processes of the cordal macrophages and splenic (fibroblastic) reticulum cells. Stromal fibers and reticulum cells running throughout the red pulp cords also contribute to provide structural support to this splenic area (the reticular meshwork of the red pulp).

A subpopulation of reticulum cells that express nerve growth factor receptor is found predominantly in the periarteriolar location (27). These cells, most likely representing adventitial reticulum cells similar to those present in the adventitia of blood vessels, also have been observed within the stroma of bone marrow and lymph nodes (28). Myoid reticulum cells (smooth muscle actin positive, or SMA positive) are found scattered throughout the red pulp. These cells are, however,

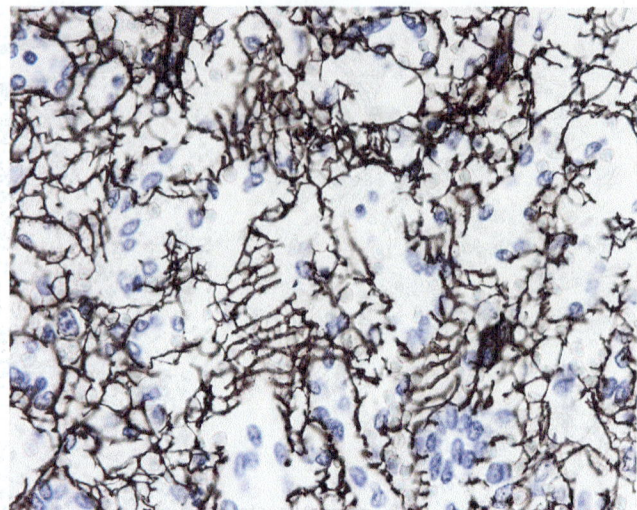

FIGURE 31.5 Normal spleen with red pulp stained with an antibody against collagen IV showing the ring fibers surrounding the sinuses (original magnification ×250).

much more concentrated within the marginal zone of the lymphoid follicles and in the PALS (29). Whether or not the SMA-positive red pulp cells correspond to fibroblastic reticulum cells that have undergone myofibroblastic differentiation, or are a truly separate population, is unclear at this time. The red pulp sinuses themselves form a complex network of their own with many interconnections and bulblike extensions with blind ends, the latter of which project into the cord tissue (see Figure 4 of van Krieken et al. (7).

The sinuses are lined by elongated, flat endothelial cells with typical bean-shaped nuclei having a longitudinal cleft; these cells are also known as littoral cells. Immunohistochemistry has shown that these cells are positive for endothelial markers and unique among other endothelial cells to CD8 (Fig. 31.6) and often to CD68 and CD21.

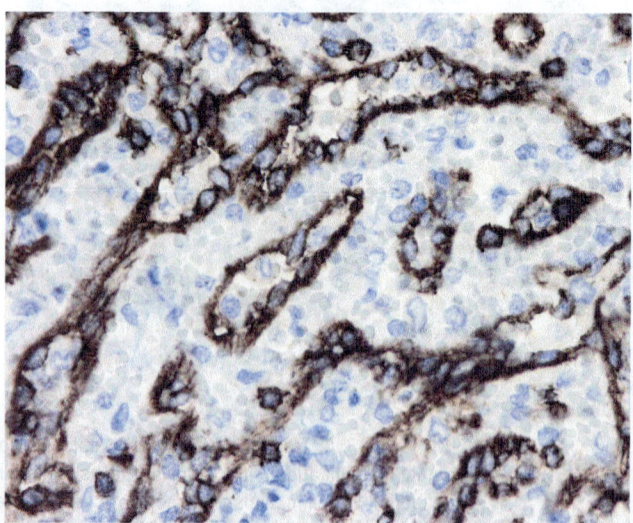

FIGURE 31.6 Normal spleen, red pulp stained with anti-CD8 showing the positive sinus endothelial cells (original magnification ×400).

The preponderant function of red pulp is blood filtration. However, in serial sections, one might notice that a fair amount of the red pulp tissue does not include capillary endings, including sheathed capillaries, and that these areas are surrounded only by sinuses. Small aggregates of lymphocytes (both B and T) and mononuclear phagocytes are present (Fig. 31.4), which means that these nonfiltering areas of the red pulp should be regarded as a splenic lymphoid compartment in addition to the white pulp. Morphometrically, the size of this lymphoid, nonfiltering red pulp compartment seems to be comparable to that of the white pulp (30). Newly formed white pulp follicles might originate from the small lymphoid aggregates of these nonfiltering areas. Studies into mice spleen resulted in the recognition of a subpopulation of cordal macrophages which have an immune regulatory function (31). In addition, at least in rodents, the presence of large numbers of splenic monocytes assembled in clusters in the cords of the subcapsular red pulp. These reserve monocytes which can be quickly released from the spleen are thought to represent an important "rapid deployment force" involved in the regulation of tissue inflammatory responses, including atherosclerosis (32,33).

Blood cells can only reach these areas by passing through large stretches of red pulp tissue or, which seems more likely, via influx from the sinus by passing through the sinus endothelium. A retrograde return of lymphocytes from the venous sinus lumen back into the splenic tissue is known for the rat spleen, where lymphocytes migrate through the walls of what is called the marginal sinus into the white pulp. This type of sinus is histologically not discernible in the white pulp of the human spleen. In humans, the role played in the rat by the marginal sinus in the exchange of lymphocytes between the sinusoidal circulation and the splenic lymphoid compartment might be played by the previously described blind-ended bulblike extensions of the red pulp sinuses, representing a splenic endothelial component with high endothelial venule-like characteristics. This hypothesis is supported by the observation that in humans, splenic follicles are surrounded by a PFZ, a distinct splenic compartment containing erythrocyte-filled vascular spaces (7,9,10). The PFZ sinuses differ from the typical red pulp sinuses in their enhanced expression of CD34. Recent evidence has suggested that this zone may represent the entry compartment for recirculating lymphocytes into the white pulp since it is capable of supporting influx and local proliferation of lymphoreticular cells, particularly CD4-positive T lymphocytes (9). It has been suggested that the entry of these cells may be dependent on the presence in the perifollicular area of specialized reticulum cells with an endothelial-like phenotype secreting lymphokines and guiding the T cells into the PALS (9).

White Pulp

The white pulp consists of B- and T-cell lymphoid compartments (Fig. 31.2). The B-cell compartment mainly consists

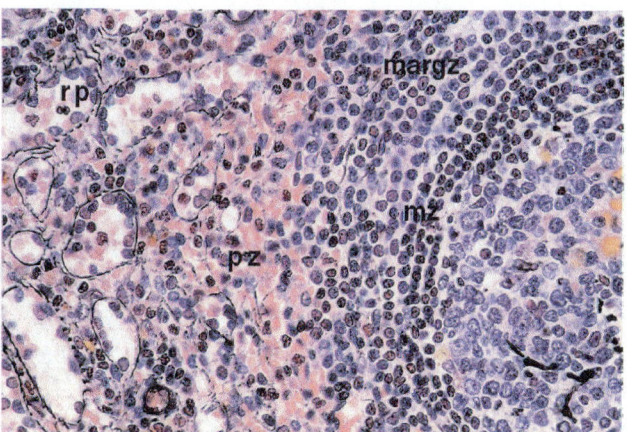

FIGURE 31.7 Same specimen as in Figure 31.3. A secondary follicle (germinal center to the right) borders the red pulp (*mz*, mantle zone; *margz*, marginal zone; *pz*, perifollicular zone; *rp*, red pulp; original magnification ×100).

of the splenic lymphoid follicles. These are composed of a germinal center (only found in secondary follicles) directly surrounded by a ring of small lymphocytes, called the mantle zone or corona, which in turn is surrounded by the marginal zone that contains medium-sized lymphocytes (Fig. 31.7). The germinal centers have similar features to those found in other lymphoid organs. They are formed by a scaffold of follicular dendritic cells that express CD21, CD23, CD35, and the low-affinity nerve growth factor receptor. The B cells of the germinal centers express CD20, CD19, CD10, and CD79a but not CD5. They have a high proliferation activity with Ki-67 and do not express Bcl-2. The T lymphocytes present within the germinal centers are predominantly CD4 positive; tingible-body macrophages are CD68 positive. Mantle zones consist predominantly of CD5-positive small lymphocytes that are IgM-, IgD-, and DBA.44-positive and alkaline phosphatase–negative (Fig. 31.8). The most important difference in relation to the lymphoid follicles found in peripheral lymphoid is that the splenic follicles have a remarkable unique structure surrounding the mantle zone: the splenic marginal zone. The marginal zone lymphocytes which form this anatomical structure are B-lymphocytes that, in contrast to mantle cells, are positive with alkaline phosphatase and are IgD-, and DBA.44-negative (34).

The marginal zone also contains a population of macrophages functionally distinct from the cord histiocytes of the red pulp. At least in animal models, marginal zone macrophages seem to be important in maintaining the anatomic structure of the marginal zone by attracting newly differentiated marginal zone B lymphocytes into it. These cells move into the marginal zone area from the germinal center, where they derive from a common follicular/marginal zone precursor B cell (35); they are also considered to be part of the recirculating pool of B-lymphocytes (36).

The reticulin framework of the marginal zone is characterized by the presence of numerous SMA-positive

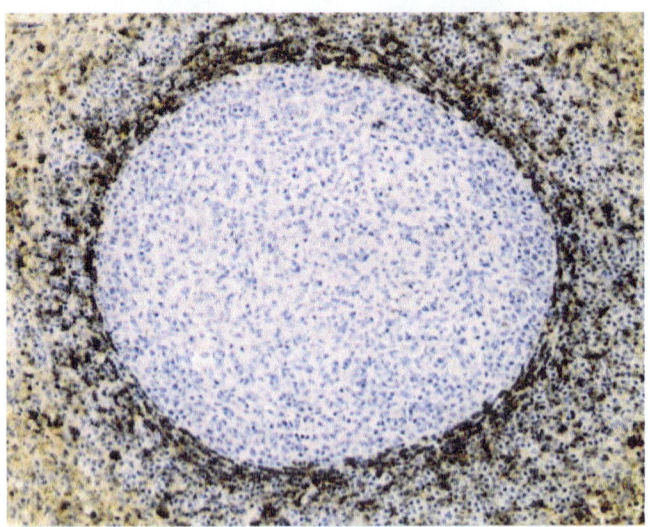 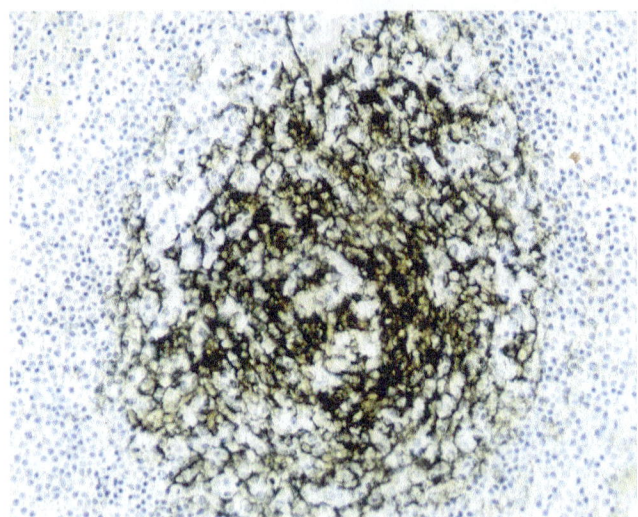

FIGURE 31.8 Normal spleen showing the positive mantle zone cells for DBA.44 (*left*, original magnification ×40) and the dendritic cells stained for CD21 (*right*, original magnification ×40).

reticulum cells arranged in a concentric meshwork pattern. The marginal zone SMA-positive cells continue into the T-cell zones, where reticulum cells, exhibiting the same immunophenotype, form the reticular framework of the PALS. Cells with SMA positivity are also seen, although less frequently, in the PFZ and scattered throughout the red pulp. These cells become more prominent in the presence of red pulp congestion, such as seen in cases of fibrocongestive splenomegaly (Fig. 31.9) (8).

In the rat spleen, the mantle and marginal zones are separated by a marginal sinus that can easily be seen by light microscopic examination. It plays an essential role in the splenic immune function as the site of entry of lymphocytes and antigens (37). This dividing sinus is not discernible in humans, at least by light microscopy. By using electron microscopy, a marginal sinus-like structure was described (38), although, surprisingly, it seems to be absent in active follicles (39). However, neither the exact location nor functional properties of this structure are known.

The light microscopic differences with rodent spleens have led to confusion in the definition of follicular structures of the human spleen. The term *marginal zone* has been used with different meanings (7,9–12,40,41). Some investigators use the term to refer to the ring of medium-sized lymphocytes that surrounds the outer border of the mantle zone; few others have included the mantle zone, still others only the bordering area between the red and the white pulp, and sometimes even the zone surrounding the T-cell areas (PALS). We prefer to reserve the term *marginal zone* for the unique splenic structure that encases from the outside the IgD- and IgM-positive small lymphocytes of the mantle zone (in the secondary follicle) or of the primary follicle. We refer to the bordering area between the red and the white pulp as the PFZ. The same definitions are used in the extensive Japanese literature on the histology of the human spleen. However, the Japanese investigators call our marginal zone the inner marginal zone and refer to the PFZ as the outer marginal zone. Because of the totally different architecture and cell population of these two structures, we find it preferable to use different names.

The T-cell areas lie around arterioles but are not as regularly arranged as in the PALS seen in the rodent spleen (Fig. 31.10). The arterioles are not constantly covered by these cylindrical lymphoid cuffs; they can be seen "naked" traversing follicles and even germinal centers (12,42).

In humans, the PALS are rather irregular aggregates of small polymorphic T lymphocytes, most of which express CD4. They represent a complex organizational structure of various subsets of T-cells (43). The T-cell areas are surrounded by a perifollicular-like zone as well. The follicles sometimes border T-cell areas, with which they share a common PFZ.

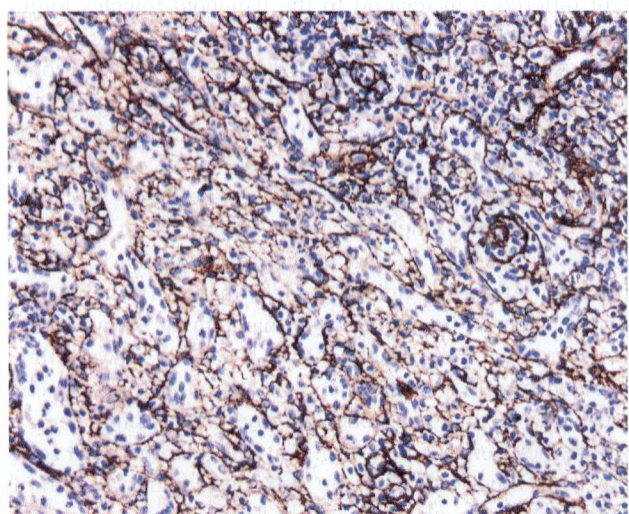

FIGURE 31.9 Spleen in fibrocongestive splenomegaly showing increased expression for smooth muscle actin (original magnification ×100).

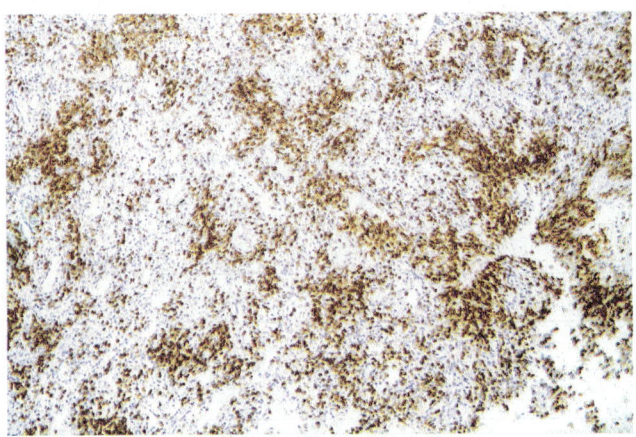

FIGURE 31.10 Normal spleen stained with anti-CD3 antibody (original magnification ×40) showing the somewhat loosely organized T-cell compartment.

Perifollicular Zone

PFZ is a specialized compartment of the red pulp that is associated with its own reticular stroma; PFZ is found both at the outside of the white pulp marginal zone (in the follicles) and at the periphery of the T-cell areas (PALS). In the PFZ, the reticular fibers are more widely spaced than in the rest of the red pulp (Figs. 31.3 and 31.7). In silver-stained plastic sections, the PFZ can be identified by the paucity of basal membrane strands and by the presence of a vascular pattern that is different from the one seen in the rest of the red pulp. At the outer border of this area, red pulp sinuses are more widely spaced than elsewhere, and a rich network of capillaries, including sheathed capillaries, is present. The PFZ contains a considerable number of erythrocytes and leukocytes (7,9,10).

The PFZ zone at the outside of the white pulp stands out in silver-stained sections but may be poorly visible in routine hematoxylin and eosin (H&E)-stained sections. However, since the PFZ contains a large number of erythrocytes, it can be recognized by its deeply congested appearance around the densely packed lymphocytes of the T- and B-cell areas (Fig. 31.2A). The erythrocytes are seen more regularly in PFZ than in the red pulp sinuses; the red pulp sinuses outside the PFZ often appear to be less filled with these cells than the cord tissue.

The PFZ, which makes up about 8% of the spleen, contains a mixture of blood cells comparable with that of the peripheral blood. It has been suggested that this area is responsible for the passage of about 10% of the splenic blood, which is known to have a retarded flow. In humans, weakly expressed sialoadhesin-positive macrophages are present in the PFZ and in the red pulp. In some specimens, sialoadhesin is however strongly expressed by a large number of dispersed perifollicular macrophages. Interestingly, in striking contrast to rats, the human marginal zone does not contain sialoadhesin-positive macrophages and marginal metallophilic macrophages are also absent in humans. Thus, sialoadhesin-positive macrophages and IgM(+) IgD(−) memory B lymphocytes both share the marginal zone as a common compartment in rats, while they occupy different compartments in humans (10).

FLOW CYTOMETRY

The spleen has been only rarely investigated by flow cytometry, but there are reference values for lymphocyte cells in normal and reactive spleens (44). These are generally comparable to those seen in other lymphoid organs, but there are a few differences (Table 31.2). In contrast to the thymus and bone marrow, the spleen contains only very rare TdT-positive lymphoid precursors. Within the B-cell subsets, the spleen shows a frequency of CD19-positive/CD20-negative B cells that is higher than in the peripheral blood or lymph node. This corresponds to the presence, in the spleen, of a sizable proportion of early plasma cells (CD138 negative), as well as more mature plasma cells. Other findings included a significant population of CD20/CD5-positive B cells, accounting for approximately 10% of the B lymphocytes; the presence of CD4/CD8 ratio of 1.2:1 (lower than in the blood but similar to the one seen in the lymph node) and a mean number of γ/δ-positive T cells (of all CD3-positive cells) of 6% in normal and 10% in reactive spleens. While in the peripheral blood, NK/T cells account for less than 6% of the CD3-positive circulating lymphocytes, there is a relatively high frequency of these cells in the spleen.

ULTRASTRUCTURE

Electron microscopy (especially scanning electron microscopy), including the use of microcasts from the vasculature, has elucidated largely the functional microanatomy of the spleen. These studies have shown the routes that blood cells take through the spleen and have also clearly illustrated the pitting function of the spleen (removal of inclusions in erythrocytes) exerted by the sinusoids. In spleens examined in a diagnostic-oriented setting, however, there is hardly, if ever, the necessity of using ultrastructural studies.

FUNCTION

The human spleen has several important functions. However, splenectomy in general does not lead to impaired health, except for an increased risk of overwhelming postsplenectomy infections caused by encapsulated bacteria (e.g., pneumococci). The reason for this is that many functions of the spleen, at least in adults, can be taken over by other organs.

In humans, the spleen is involved in the primary immune response to blood-borne antigens and polysaccharide antigens; it also acts as a regulator of immune reactions elsewhere in the body. It contains a specific environment that facilitates the binding of antibodies and antigens; cells or microorganisms

TABLE 31.2 Expression of Surface and Intracellular Markers by Human Spleen Lymphocytes

Cell Marker	Normal (Cadaveric) Spleen		Reactive (Nonmalignant) Spleen		P-value[a]
	N	Mean ± sd (%)	N	Mean ± sd (%)	
CD2	14	38±10	12	50±14	0.015
CD3		31±9		43±14	0.009
CD4		17±8		23±7	NS
CD5		32±8		42±13	0.028
CD7		37±11		44±12	NS
CD8		14±5		19±7	0.028
CD4/CD8 ratio		1.2±3		1.2±0.2	NS
CD10		1±1		1±1	NS
CD11c		28±10		25±10	NS
CD13		1±1		1±1	NS
CD16/56+CD3−		15±7		12±5	NS
CD16/56+CD3+		5±2		5±4	NS
CD19		55±11		45±14	0.04
CD20		49±9		42±12	NS
CD20+CD5+		8±6		11±7	NS
CD23		34±13		35±12	NS
CD30		1±1		1±1	NS

[a]NS, not significant ($P > 0.05$).

covered by antibodies are trapped and destroyed in the spleen, as are erythrocytes that have decreased flexibility and lowered osmotic resistance. Each of these functions takes place in a specific splenic compartment, which is capable of undergoing rapid changes in its size and composition, even under physiologic conditions. Therefore, the main splenic functions to be considered include blood filtering, immunologic function, hematopoiesis, and reservoir.

Filter Function

The location and specialized anatomy of the spleen is especially suitable for its function as a filter of the blood. Normal blood cells are capable of traversing the barrier of macrophages of the sheathed capillary, the red pulp cord macrophages, and the sinus endothelium (collectively, the filtering unit of the spleen) at a speed comparable to that of the blood in the capillary bed of other organs. However, in cases in which the flexibility of the red blood cell is diminished (e.g., by aging, intoxication, or congenital defects), the macrophages of the splenic filtering unit can eliminate the abnormal cell by ingesting it, a process that was nicely modeled (45). The filtering function includes a process known as pitting, a term which is used to describe the removal of inclusions, such as nuclear remnants known as Howell–Jolly (H–J) bodies, from erythrocytes without destroying the cell. The presence of H–J bodies in circulating erythrocytes in the peripheral blood indicates the presence of splenic hypofunction (e.g., in splenectomized patients).

In addition to red blood cells, the macrophages of the spleen can readily take up bacteria, antigens, and immune complexes. The spleen is capable of filtering out reticulocytes, platelets, hematopoietic stem cells, lymphocytes, and dendritic cells from the blood and providing the proper microambient conditions for their further differentiation. Also, it sequesters monocytes from the blood and facilitates their transformation into splenic macrophages.

Immunologic Function

The spleen plays a more important role in the development of the immune system, but even in adults the spleen is still involved in B- and T-lymphocyte production and differentiation (4,43). The spleen receives B and T cells from the recirculating lymphocyte pool and sorts them into dedicated compartments such as the follicles and the PALS, where they can interact with antigens and antigen-presenting cells and become capable of mounting effective immune responses.

The marginal zone is a component of the B-cell follicle and is a remarkably larger compartment in the spleen than elsewhere (e.g., the tonsils). Although the exact physiologic function(s) of the marginal zone is still unclear, its main immunologic role relates to the thymus-independent rapid response to blood-borne microorganisms; since these are rapidly trapped in the spleen and brought directly into contact with numerous immunocompetent cells, the spleen is well situated for this task.

Hematopoiesis

In rodents, the spleen has a large hematopoietic function, but this is not the case in humans. As described above, the hematopoietic function is only present in the fetal spleen; in the adult spleen, hematopoiesis does not occur. Hematopoietic cells encountered in the adult spleen originate from circulating, marrow-derived, progenitors/early precursors that become entrapped in the spleen and are capable of undergoing further differentiation. When this "physiologic" phenomenon reaches pathologic relevance by causing splenomegaly, it is termed splenic myeloid metaplasia or extramedullary hematopoiesis. Although splenic myeloid metaplasia can be seen in many different conditions, the most striking examples of this condition can be observed in patients with primary myelofibrosis.

Reservoir Function

The human spleen contains about 300 mL of blood. This is a relatively small amount in contrast to that seen in a dog or cat. In these animals, the spleen functions as an important blood reservoir; and in situations where more blood is needed, its rapid contraction can increase substantially the amount of circulating blood cells. It is highly doubtful that this function occurs at all in humans, whose splenic capsule lacks a significant component of smooth muscle fibers. The aforementioned "sea nomads" are the exception (22). The spleen, however, does function as a reservoir for factor VIII of the clotting system, platelets, granulocytes, and iron. Although described in rodents, it is uncertain whether the human spleen may serve as a reservoir for "rapid deployment" monocytes (see Red Pulp section).

AGING DIFFERENCES

In infancy and childhood, the immune system is not yet fully developed, and this is also reflected in the histology of the spleen (46). The marginal zone is observed as a separate compartment only after 4 months of age; moreover, the marginal zone B cells in the spleen of infants have a different phenotype (lack CD21; IgD- and IgM positive) compared with adult marginal zone B cells. An important age difference, in our experience, is the regular occurrence of germinal centers in the white pulp of normal spleens in patients younger than 20 years; older patients have been shown to have only rare secondary follicles (30). The often-mentioned age-dependent atrophic change has only been documented in patients in their 8th decade of life (30). However, recent evidence in mice has suggested an age-related alteration in marginal zone microarchitecture and function (47). It is unclear whether a selective loss of marginal zone function can also occur in humans.

Hyalinization of vessels in the spleen is seen frequently, even in very young children and, therefore, does not represent a pathologic finding (48).

In infants, the elastic fibers of the splenic capsule are homogeneously intermingled with collagen fibers, an arrangement that stabilizes the capsule during spleen growth and enlargement. With aging, collagen fibers predominate in the outer capsular surface over elastic fibers with the latter more evident in the deep lamina of the splenic capsule. In elderly individuals, the elastic fibers shorten, fragment, and thicken. The progressive decrease in the amount of elastic fibers in the splenic capsule with aging may restrict splenic distention and contribute to involution of the spleen as one grows older (49).

DIFFERENTIAL DIAGNOSIS

In the spleen, compartmentalized lymphoid tissue (white pulp) is interwoven by the filtering red pulp. Each splenic compartment reacts to external stimuli with physiologic changes in its composition and histology. As in the lymph node, the line between pathologic and impressive but essential physiologic reactions is vague. The amount of white pulp, for instance, varied from 5% to 22% of the total splenic tissue in a normal control group (30).

As previously mentioned, normal blood cells can pass undamaged through the barrier of macrophages of the sheathed capillary and the red pulp cord tissue, as well as the sinus endothelium (i.e., the filtering unit of the spleen) at a speed comparable with that of the blood flow in the capillary bed of other organs. However, when the flexibility of the blood cells is diminished (e.g., by aging, intoxication, or congenital defects), the red pulp macrophages can ingest the abnormal cells. In this process, the sheathed capillaries seem to lose their macrophages, which spread out into the surrounding red pulp or enter the sinuses to be transported to the liver. In cases characterized by chronic stimulation of the filtering function, it can be demonstrated that the amount and length of the capillaries increase in parallel with the hypertrophy of the red pulp, whereas the sheathed capillaries are less readily seen in the sections. In idiopathic thrombocytopenic purpura (ITP), remnants of phagocytosed thrombocytes can be seen as periodic acid–Schiff (PAS)-positive fragments in cord macrophages. If blood cells are covered by immunoglobulins or immunocomplexes, parts of the cell membrane can be removed by the sinus endothelium by "pitting and culling," giving rise to a spherocyte. This happens in a fashion similar to the removal of nuclear remnants, as previously described.

In septicemia, the filtering compartment may show morphologic findings (activation and hyperplasia of macrophages) indistinguishable from those seen in cases of acute or chronic hemolysis; these changes are most likely induced by the presence of circulating immunocomplexes, fragmented cells, or antibody-coated cells. In these conditions, postmortem autolysis of the activated macrophages can lead to early disintegration of the red pulp cells and stroma. The septic spleen at autopsy thus probably represents an artifact that can be the result of, but is not specific for, sepsis; it, especially, should not be diagnosed as splenitis. In septic spleens, there is a significant depletion of B- and T-areas, accompanied by a reactive germinal center hyperplasia regardless of the type of bacteria responsible. However, depletion of splenic B areas was shown to be significantly pronounced in the setting of premortal enterococcemia in comparison with a panel of gram-negative flagellated bacteria (50).

True splenitis, in which the spleen contains an inflammatory response to a local noxious agent such as in typhoid fever or tropical diseases, is rare in the Western hemisphere. Lymphoplasmacytoid cells and plasma cells normally rim arteries and arterioles and extend along red pulp capillaries. This perivascular cellular rim also may contain some macrophages or small epithelioid granulomas, the significance of which is unclear. The perivascular presence of plasma cells is a normal finding and by no means justifies a diagnosis of splenitis, nor is the diffuse influx of granulocytes throughout the red pulp in specimens resected during prolonged surgery.

The effects of chronic venous congestion are not clear. In our preliminary studies in patients dying with chronic cardiac disease, the so-called effect of chronic cardiac congestion on the lymphoid and filtering compartments appears more likely to be the effect of concomitant infections or is therapy mediated. In chronic venous congestion due to portal hypertension, the sinuses are normal in size but contain fewer buds and appear rigid. The amount of cord tissue and the number of capillaries are both decreased; in the cord tissue, an increase of reticular fibers (fibrocongestive splenomegaly) and increased expression of smooth muscle actin in reticulum cells are seen. Infarcts in the splenic tissue are microscopically more irregularly defined and poorly demarcated than could be expected macroscopically due to the intricate distribution of the splenic vessels. In three-dimensional reconstructions, capillaries from different arterioles are seen to cross each other with overlapping territories.

Primary tumors of the spleen are rare. Metastatic carcinoma seems specially to occur in neuroendocrine tumors, including small-cell carcinoma of the lung, with a conspicuous tendency for intrasinusoidal spread. Malignant lymphomas exhibit a homing pattern to specific splenic compartments dependent on the type of lymphoma, similar to that observed in other lymphoid organs (51). In non-lymphomatous hematopoietic malignancies involving the spleen, their distribution pattern is similar to that observed in the bone marrow: Extramedullary erythropoiesis and megakaryopoiesis are found primarily along and within the sinuses of the red pulp, whereas myelopoiesis is found in proximity of the capillaries within the cord tissue. Blastic infiltration seen in cases of acute leukemia can be found anywhere in the spleen.

SPECIMEN HANDLING

The spleen is quite vulnerable and, due to the large numbers of macrophages and granulocytes, may undergo rapid autolysis. Proper and rapid fixation is therefore important, and this goal is not reached when the entire organ is put into formalin. For proper handling, the specimen has to be received fresh, and handling has to be rapid. An appropriate protocol is given by the International Spleen Consortium (6). The organ is weighed and the surface examined. After that, the organ is cut into small slices of 0.5 cm. Then the cut surface is inspected carefully for nodules larger than normal white pulp. Ideally, pieces should be submitted for flow cytometry, and snap frozen for cryostat section immunohistochemistry or molecular techniques. When no abnormalities are seen, at least three or four blocks are taken out randomly and processed for microscopic examination.

HISTOLOGIC TECHNIQUE

Routine paraffin embedding leads to shrinkage and loss of cellular detail. Since routine H&E staining often does not yield sufficient information, methenamine-silver/H&E stain, or at least, PAS and Gomori reticulin stains are necessary for an adequate morphologic analysis of the splenic microarchitecture (Fig. 31.11).

SPECIAL PROCEDURES

The spleen is only rarely removed for diagnostic purposes. Staging laparotomy is no longer part of the required diagnostic workup of a patient with Hodgkin disease. Therefore,

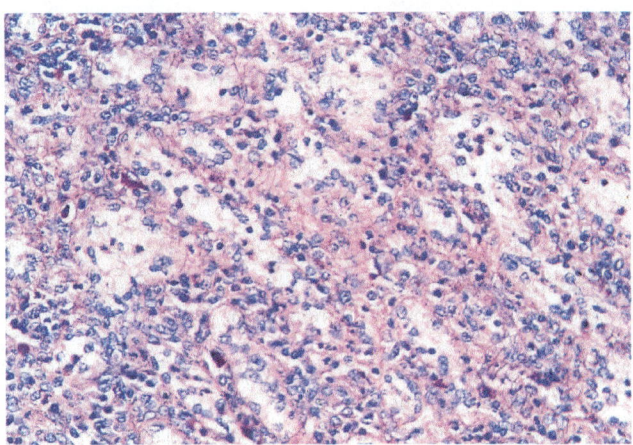

FIGURE 31.11 Same specimen as in Figure 31.1. Detail of red pulp showing with some difficulty, the structure of the sinuses (PAS stain, paraffin-embedded, original magnification ×200).

splenic pathology may be seen as an unsuspected incidental finding in a patient splenectomized for other reasons (e.g., chronic idiopathic thrombocytopenia, trauma). Not uncommonly, splenic lymphoma may be discovered as an incidental finding. A high degree of suspiciousness of the grossing pathologist is necessary in these cases since, for optimal lymphoma diagnosis, it is often necessary to apply techniques that require fresh/frozen tissue, such as flow cytometry, frozen tissue immunohistochemistry, molecular analysis, and/or cytogenetics (Fig. 31.9).

In view of the frequent lack of fresh specimens, clonality assessment in a spleen is usually done by immunohistochemistry applied to paraffin-embedded tissue, looking for a restricted pattern of immunoglobulin light chain expression in B cells. This is one of the most important "special techniques" used in routine diagnostic laboratories. In addition, clonality can also be established by using a polymerase chain reaction–based technique for detecting immunoglobulin gene rearrangement, which can also be successfully applied to paraffin-embedded tissue (52).

Immunohistochemistry can also be necessary to characterize other hematopoietic and nonhematopoietic tumors, the latter primary or metastatic, which can occur (although infrequently) in the spleen. In storage disorders such as Gaucher disease, electron microscopy can be of additional value, although biochemical analysis is considered by most experts as the most practical and specific approach.

CONCLUSION

The human spleen has always been a somewhat enigmatic organ. Studies of its histology must be based on carefully selected, surgically excised "normal" spleens. The organ should be processed immediately and appropriately for optimal results.

Previous studies by one of us of a large series of spleens with adequate histologic techniques and with reconstruction based on serial sections have shown that the spleen is a highly compartmentalized organ (Table 31.1). Each compartment has its own structure and cell populations and often a separate function. The old division into red and white pulp is probably oversimplified and should be expanded.

Human and animal spleens are different in many important structural aspects; data extrapolation from animal studies to humans is therefore problematic and often unwarranted.

REFERENCES

1. Paraskevas GK, Koutsouflianiotis KN, Nitsa Z, et al. Knowledge of the anatomy and physiology of the spleen throughout Antiquity and the Early Middle Ages. *Anat Sci Int* 2016;91: 43–55.
2. Chen L, Weiss L. Electron microscopy of the red pulp of human spleen. *Am J Anat* 1972;134:425–458.
3. Neely HR, Flajnik MF. Emergence and evolution of secondary lymphoid organs. *Annu Rev Cell Dev Biol* 2016;32:693–711.
4. Rodríguez-Perea AL, Arcia ED, Rueda CM, et al. Phenotypical characterization of regulatory T cells in humans and rodents. *Clin Exp Immunol* 2016;185:281–291.
5. Meng W, Zhang B, Schwartz GW, et al. An atlas of B-cell clonal distribution in the human body. *Nat Biotechnol* 2017; 35:879–884.
6. O'Malley DP, Louissaint A Jr, Vasef MA, et al; International Spleen Consortium. Recommendations for gross examination and sampling of surgical specimens of the spleen. *Ann Diagn Pathol* 2015;19(5):288–295.
7. van Krieken JH, Te Velde J, Hermans J, et al. The splenic red pulp; a histomorphometrical study in splenectomy specimens embedded in methylmethacrylate. *Histopathology* 1985; 9:401–416.
8. Kraus MD. Splenic histology and histopathology: an update. *Semin Diagn Pathol* 2003;20:84–93.
9. Steiniger B, Barth P, Hellinger A. The perifollicular and marginal zones of the human splenic white pulp: do fibroblasts guide lymphocyte immigration? *Am J Pathol* 2001;159:501–512.
10. Steiniger B, Barth P, Herbst B, et al. The species-specific structure of microanatomical compartments in the human spleen: strongly sialoadhesin-positive macrophages occur in the perifollicular zone, but not in the marginal zone. *Immunology* 1997;92:307–316.
11. van Krieken JH, te Velde J, Kleiverda K, et al. The human spleen: a histological study in splenectomy specimens embedded in methylmethacrylate. *Histopathology* 1985;9:571–585.
12. Wolf BC, Luevano E, Neiman RS. Evidence to suggest that the human fetal spleen is not a hematopoietic organ. *Am J Clin Pathol* 1983;80:140–144.
13. Yamamoto K, Miwa Y, Abe-Suzuki S, et al. Extramedullary hematopoiesis: elucidating the function of the hematopoietic stem cell niche. *Mol Med Rep* 2016;13:587–591.
14. Timens W, Rozeboom T, Poppema S. Fetal and neonatal development of human spleen: an immunohistological study. *Immunology* 1987;60:603–609.

15. Jones JF. Development of the spleen. *Lymphology* 1983;16:83–89.
16. Namikawa R, Mizuno T, Matsuoka H, et al. Ontogenic development of T and B cells and non-lymphoid cells in the white pulp of human spleen. *Immunology* 1986;57:61–69.
17. Varga I, Galfiova P, Adamkov M, et al. Congenital anomalies of the spleen from an embryological point of view. *Med Sci Monit* 2009;12:RA269–RA276.
18. Moller JH, Nakib A, Anderson RC, et al. Congenital cardiac disease associated with polysplenia. A developmental complex of bilateral "left-sidedness." *Circulation* 1967;36:789–799.
19. Khairat AB, Ismail AM. Splenogonadal fusion: case presentation and literature review. *J Pediatr Surg* 2005;40:1357–1360.
20. Howard MT, Dufresne S, Swerdlow SH, et al. Follicular lymphoma of the spleen: multiparameter analysis of 16 cases. *Am J Clin Pathol* 2009;131:656–662.
21. Oren H, Ozkal S, Gülen H, et al. Autoimmune lymphoproliferative syndrome: report of two cases and review of the literature. *Ann Hematol* 2002;81:651–653.
22. Ilardo MA, Moltke I, Korneliussen TS, et al. Physiological and genetic adaptations to diving in sea nomads. *Cell* 2018;173:569–580.e15.
23. Myers J, Segal RJ. Weight of the spleen. I. Range of normal in a nonhospital population. *Arch Pathol* 1974;98:33–35.
24. Vahidy FS, Parsha KN, Rahbar MH, et al. Acute splenic responses in patients with ischemic stroke and intracerebral hemorrhage. *J Cereb Blood Flow Metab* 2016;36:1012–1021.
25. Jung WC, Levesque JP, Ruitenberg MJ. It takes nerve to fight back: the significance of neural innervation of the bone marrow and spleen for immune function. *Semin Cell Dev Biol* 2017;61:60–70.
26. Steiniger B, Stachniss V, Schwarzbach H, et al. Phenotypic differences between red pulp capillary and sinusoidal endothelia help localizing the open splenic circulation in humans. *Histochem Cell Biol* 2007;128:391–398.
27. Cattoretti G, Schiro R, Orazi A, et al. Bone marrow stroma in humans: anti-nerve growth factor receptor antibodies selectively stain reticular cells in vivo and in vitro. *Blood* 1993;81:1726–1738.
28. Orazi A, O'Malley DP, Thomas JL, et al. Stromal changes in reactive and malignant disorders of the spleen. *Mod Pathol* 2004;17:264A.
29. Pinkus GS, Warhol MJ, O'Connor EM, et al. Immunohistochemical localization of smooth muscle myosin in human spleen, lymph node, and other lymphoid tissues. Unique staining patterns in splenic white pulp and sinuses, lymphoid follicles, and certain vasculature, with ultrastructural correlations. *Am J Pathol* 1986;123:440–453.
30. van Krieken JH, te Velde J, Hermans J, et al. The amount of white pulp in the spleen: a morphometrical study done in methacrylate-embedded splenectomy specimens. *Histopathology* 1983;7:767–782.
31. Kurotaki D, Kon S, Bae K, et al. CSF-1-dependent red pulp macrophages regulate CD4 T cell responses. *J Immunol* 2011;186:2229–2237.
32. Swirski FK, Nahrendorf M, Etzrodt M, et al. Identification of splenic reservoir monocytes and their deployment to inflammatory sites. *Science* 2009;325:612–616.
33. Potteaux S, Ait-Oufella H, Mallat Z. Role of splenic monocytes in atherosclerosis. *Curr Opin Lipidol* 2015;26:457–463.
34. van Krieken JH, von Schilling C, Kluin PM, et al. Splenic marginal zone lymphocytes and related cells in the lymph node: a morphologic and immunohistochemical study. *Hum Pathol* 1989;20:320–325.
35. Pillai S, Cariappa A, Moran ST. Marginal Zone B lymphocytes. *Annu Rev Immunol* 2005;23:161–196.
36. Steiniger B, Timphus EM, Barth PJ. The splenic marginal zone in humans and rodents: an enigmatic compartment and its inhabitants. *Histochem Cell Biol* 2006;126:641–648.
37. Sasou S, Satodate R, Katsura S. The marginal sinus in the perifollicular region of the rat spleen. *Cell Tissue Res* 1976;172:195–203.
38. Schmidt EE, MacDonald IC, Groom AC. Microcirculatory pathways in normal human spleen, demonstrated by scanning electron microscopy of corrosion casts. *Am J Anat* 1988;181:253–266.
39. Schmidt EE, MacDonald IC, Groom AC. Changes in splenic microcirculatory pathways in chronic idiopathic thrombocytopenic purpura. *Blood* 1991;78:1485–1489.
40. Takasaki S. Light microscopic, scanning and transmission electron microscopic, and enzyme histochemical observations on the boundary zone between the red pulp and its surroundings in human spleens. *Tokyo Yikekai Med J* 1979;94:553–568.
41. Kraal G. Cells in the marginal zone of the spleen. *Int Rec Cytol* 1992;132:31–74.
42. Steiniger B, Ruttinger L, Barth PJ. The three-dimensional structure of human splenic white pulp compartments. *J Histoch Cytochem* 2003;51:655–663.
43. Woon HG, Braun A, Li J, et al. Compartmentalization of total and virus-specific tissue-resident memory CD8+ T cells in human lymphoid organs. *PLoS Pathog* 2016;12:e1005799.
44. Colovai AI, Giatzikis C, Ho EK, et al. Flow cytometric analysis of normal and reactive spleen. *Mod Pathol* 2004;17:918–927.
45. Pivkin IV, Peng Z, Karniadakis GE, et al. Biomechanics of red blood cells in human spleen and consequences for physiology and disease. *Proc Natl Acad Sci U S A* 2016;113:7804–7809.
46. Timens W, Boes A, Rozeboom-Uiterwijk T, et al. Immaturity of the human splenic marginal zone in infancy. Possible contribution to the deficient infant immune response. *J Immunol* 1989;143:3200–3206.
47. Birjandi SZ, Ippolito JA, Ramadorai AK, et al. Alterations in marginal zone macrophages and marginal zone B cells in old mice. *J Immunol* 2011;186:3441–3451.
48. Lindley RP. Splenic arteriolar hyalin in children. *J Pathol* 1986;148:321–325.
49. Rodrigues CJ, Sacchetti JCL, Rodrigues AJ. Age-related changes in the elastic fiber network of the human splenic capsule. *Lymphology* 1999;32:64–69.
50. Gunia S, Albrecht K, May M, et al. The white pulp in the setting of the septic spleen caused by different bacteria: a comparative morphometric study. *APMIS* 2005;113:675–682.
51. van Krieken JH, Feller AC, te Velde J. The distribution of non-Hodgkin's lymphoma in the lymphoid compartments of the human spleen. *Am J Surg Pathol* 1989;13:757–765.
52. van Krieken JH, Langerak AW, Macintyre EA, et al. Improved reliability of lymphoma diagnostics via PCR-based clonality testing: report of the BIOMED-2 Concerted Action BHM4-CT98-3936. *Leukemia* 2007;21:201–206.

Bone Marrow

S.H. Kroft

- TECHNIQUES FOR STUDYING THE MARROW 813
- GENERAL FEATURES OF HEMATOPOIESIS 815
- REGULATION OF HEMATOPOIESIS 816
- HEMATOPOIESIS IN THE EMBRYO AND FETUS: DEVELOPMENT OF THE BONE MARROW 817
- POSTNATAL CHANGES IN THE DISTRIBUTION OF RED MARROW AND IN THE TYPE OF HEMOGLOBIN 818
- STRUCTURAL ORGANIZATION OF HEMATOPOIETIC MARROW 818
  - Blood Supply 818
  - Nerve Supply 819
- Extracellular Matrix (Connective Tissue) 819
- Stromal Cells 820
- HEMATOPOIETIC CELLS 826
  - Neutrophil Precursors 826
  - Eosinophil and Basophil Precursors 831
  - Monocyte Precursors 832
  - Red Cell Precursors 835
  - Megakaryocytes 840
  - Lymphocytes and Plasma Cells 843
- CELLULARITY OF THE MARROW 847
- MARROW DIFFERENTIAL COUNT 848
- REFERENCES 849

The bone marrow is a large and complex organ that is distributed throughout the cavities of the skeleton. The total mass of the bone marrow of an adult has been estimated to be 1,600 to 3,700 g, exceeding that of the liver. About half of this mass consists of hematopoietically inactive fatty marrow (which appears yellow) and the remainder of hematopoietically active marrow (which appears red). Although essentially hematopoietically inactive, even fatty marrow contains a few scattered microscopic foci of hematopoietic cells. The functions of hematopoietic marrow include: (a) the formation and release of various types of blood cells (hematopoiesis), mast cells, osteoclasts, and some endothelial progenitor cells; (b) the phagocytosis and degradation of circulating particulate material such as microorganisms and abnormal or senescent red cells and leukocytes; and (c) antibody production. In addition to hematopoietic stem cells, the marrow contains mesenchymal stem cells that can differentiate under appropriate conditions into adipocytes, hepatocytes, osteoblasts and osteocytes, chondrocytes, skeletal and cardiac muscle cells, kidney cells, and neural cell lineages (1). The nonhematopoietic marrow serves as a large store of reserve lipids. The various functions of hematopoietic marrow are based on a high degree of structural organization. However, this organization is labile, altering rapidly in response to many stimuli.

TECHNIQUES FOR STUDYING THE MARROW

Thorough microscopic evaluation of bone marrow requires examination of both aspirate smear and trephine (core) biopsy preparations. Many consider peripheral blood smears to also be an essential part of a complete marrow evaluation; however, peripheral blood morphology is not addressed in this chapter. Aspirate smear preparations provide superior assessment of cytologic detail of hematopoietic cells, whereas trephine biopsies provide information related to architecture, cellularity, focal lesions (e.g., lymphoid aggregates, granulomas, amyloidosis), fibrosis, or necrosis (2–6).

In adults, marrow is aspirated from the posterior superior iliac spine or the anterior iliac crest (2,4). Sternal aspirates may be obtained in certain situations, as well. In children, marrow is usually aspirated from the posterior superior iliac spine and, in the case of patients less than 1 year of age, also from the upper end of the medial surface of the tibia just below and medial to the tibial tuberosity. Smears of bone marrow aspirate material may be prepared in a variety of ways, including particle crush preparations, direct smears, and buffy coat smears; each technique carries certain advantages and disadvantages (4,6). The marrow smears are air dried and stained using one of several Romanowsky-type stains, including May–Grünwald–Giemsa (MGG) or Wright–Giemsa (4,7). Aspirate smears will also often be stained using a Prussian blue stain for iron (Perls' acid ferrocyanide method). Touch imprints of trephine biopsies may also be air dried and treated in a similar fashion as aspirate smears.

Trephine biopsies are generally obtained from the posterior superior iliac spine or anterior iliac crest. This provides a core of bone and associated marrow. The biopsy specimen is commonly fixed in 10% neutral buffered formalin for 6 hours, but may be fixed in a variety of other solutions for varying lengths of time, including but not limited to acetic acid zinc formalin (AZF), B5 (mercuric acid and formalin), Bouin's fixative (picric acid, acetic acid, and formalin), or Zenker's solution (mercuric chloride, potassium dichromate, sodium sulfate, water, acetic acid). The fixed specimen is then decalcified by one of a variety of methods, including EDTA, formic acid, picric acid, nitric acid, or proprietary, commercially available decalcifying solutions, and then embedded in paraffin. Decalcification and paraffin embedding result in some shrinkage of marrow tissue, loss of activity of cellular enzymes, and variable loss of cytologic detail. In addition, certain decalcification procedures cause leaching of the iron stores (i.e., of the hemosiderin present within macrophages). Although decalcification may affect antigenic integrity, the immunoreactivity of many antigens is retained in trephine biopsy specimens. Histologic studies also can be performed on clot sections of aspirated marrow. In general, this involves concentration of particles in a liquid aspirate, induction of clotting, fixation, and paraffin embedding (4,6). Clot sections, having not been decalcified, exhibit better retention of immunoreactivity and better integrity of nucleic acids for molecular studies. Methods for embedding undecalcified trephine biopsies in methyl methacrylate are also available. Semithin sections of such specimens provide superior cytologic detail, but these plastic-embedding methods are technically demanding and not in wide use (4).

Sections of paraffin-embedded marrow fragments or decalcified bone cores are optimally cut to a thickness of 2 to 3 μm and are routinely stained with hematoxylin and eosin (H&E). A reticulin stain (by a silver impregnation method) and a Giemsa stain may also be routinely applied, although practice patterns vary regionally. Various other cytochemical stains may be performed on marrow sections in specific circumstances, including periodic acid–Schiff (PAS) reaction for glycogen or glycoprotein, Leder's stain for chloroacetate esterase, and a trichrome stain for collagen fibrosis.

Recent years have seen a dramatic increase in the number of commercially available immunohistochemistry antibodies suitable for use in paraffin-embedded tissue sections. While the decalcification process and the wide variety of fixatives in use for bone marrow trephines has historically limited the application of immunohistochemistry in trephine biopsies, improvements in commercial reagents, antigen retrieval techniques, and decalcification processes now enable the routine use of a large number of immunohistochemical stains in bone marrow cores, although procedures often need to be modified for optimal results (8). Immunohistochemistry may now be used to characterize a wide variety of normal and abnormal marrow cell populations in marrow trephines (and clot sections) (8–13). While an exhaustive list of available antibodies used in diagnosis of pathologic processes in bone marrow sections is beyond the scope of this chapter, a list of antibodies commonly used for identifying various cell lineages is provided in Table 32.1. Certain antibodies may also be applied using immunocytochemical techniques to fixed bone marrow smears, as well, although this is no longer common practice. It is important to note that, because of the wide variability in preanalytical and analytical procedures, immunohistochemical findings may differ considerably from laboratory to laboratory; recommendations for improving standardization have recently been published (14).

TABLE 32.1 Lineage Antigens Commonly Assessed in Bone Marrow Sections Using Immunohistochemistry

Cell Lineage	Antigens
Leukocytes	CD45
Immature cells (blasts)	CD34, CD117 (myeloid), TdT (lymphoid)
B cells	CD10 (immature and germinal center), CD19, CD20, CD22, CD79a, Bcl-6 (germinal center), Pax-5, MUM-1/4 (postgerminal center)
Plasma cells	CD138, kappa and lambda light chains
T cells	CD2, CD3, CD4, CD5, CD7, CD8
NK cells	CD2, CD7, CD56, CD57, TIA-1, granzyme-B
Maturing granulocytes	CD10 (mature), CD15, CD33, CD117 (early promyelocytes), lysozyme, myeloperoxidase
Monocytes/Macrophages	CD4, CD15, CD33, CD68, CD163, lysozyme
Erythroid Precursors	CD71, CD117 (pronormoblasts), E-cadherin (pronormoblasts), CD235a (glycophorin A), hemoglobin A
Megakaryocytes	CD31, CD41, CD42, CD61, factor VIII–related antigen (von Willebrand factor)
Mast Cells	CD117, mast cell tryptase
Endothelial cells	CD31, CD34
Osteoblasts	CD56

Due to advances in immunophenotyping (by both flow cytometry and immunohistochemistry), electron microscopy is uncommonly used in the modern bone marrow pathology practice, although it is still useful in specialized situations. If electron microscopic studies are to be performed, an aliquot of a marrow aspirate is mixed with heparinized Hanks' solution. A few marrow fragments are then removed without delay and placed in a solution of 2.5% to 4% glutaraldehyde in 0.1 M phosphate buffer (pH 7.3). Alternatively, 1-mm pieces of the trephine biopsy core are fixed in glutaraldehyde for 1 hour, after which the marrow is gently teased out of the bone using a dissecting microscope.

In this chapter, unless otherwise stated, the descriptions of cells in marrow smears apply to smears stained by a Romanowsky method. The electron microscopic data relate to ultrathin sections stained with uranyl acetate and lead citrate. Such sections are prepared from marrow fragments that were fixed in glutaraldehyde and postfixed in osmium tetroxide.

GENERAL FEATURES OF HEMATOPOIESIS

Blood cells are produced in the embryo and fetus and throughout postnatal life. In the developing fetus and growing child, the total number of hematopoietic cells and blood cells increases progressively with time. By contrast, the hematopoietic systems of healthy adults are examples of steady-state cell renewal systems. In such systems, a relatively constant rate of loss of mature blood cells from the circulation is balanced by the production of new blood cells at the same rate. The number of hematopoietic cells and blood cells therefore remains constant.

New blood cells are eventually derived from a small number of hematopoietic stem cells, estimated at 2×10^4 total cells (15). These cells have two properties: (a) the ability to mature into all types of blood cells; and (b) an extensive capacity to generate new stem cells and thus to maintain their own number (self-renewal). In humans, the existence of pluripotent hematopoietic stem cells with both the above properties has been demonstrated by the success of bone marrow transplantation. These hematopoietic stem cells differentiate into progenitor cells that are committed to one or more lineages; these committed progenitor cells do not have the capacity for self-renewal or to sustain long-term hematopoiesis. As these committed progenitors branch and mature, they have more and more restricted differentiation potential. One putative model of hematopoietic differentiation is illustrated in Figure 32.1, although others have been proposed (16). In the illustrated scheme, the pluripotent stem cells give rise to lymphoid stem cells and multipotent

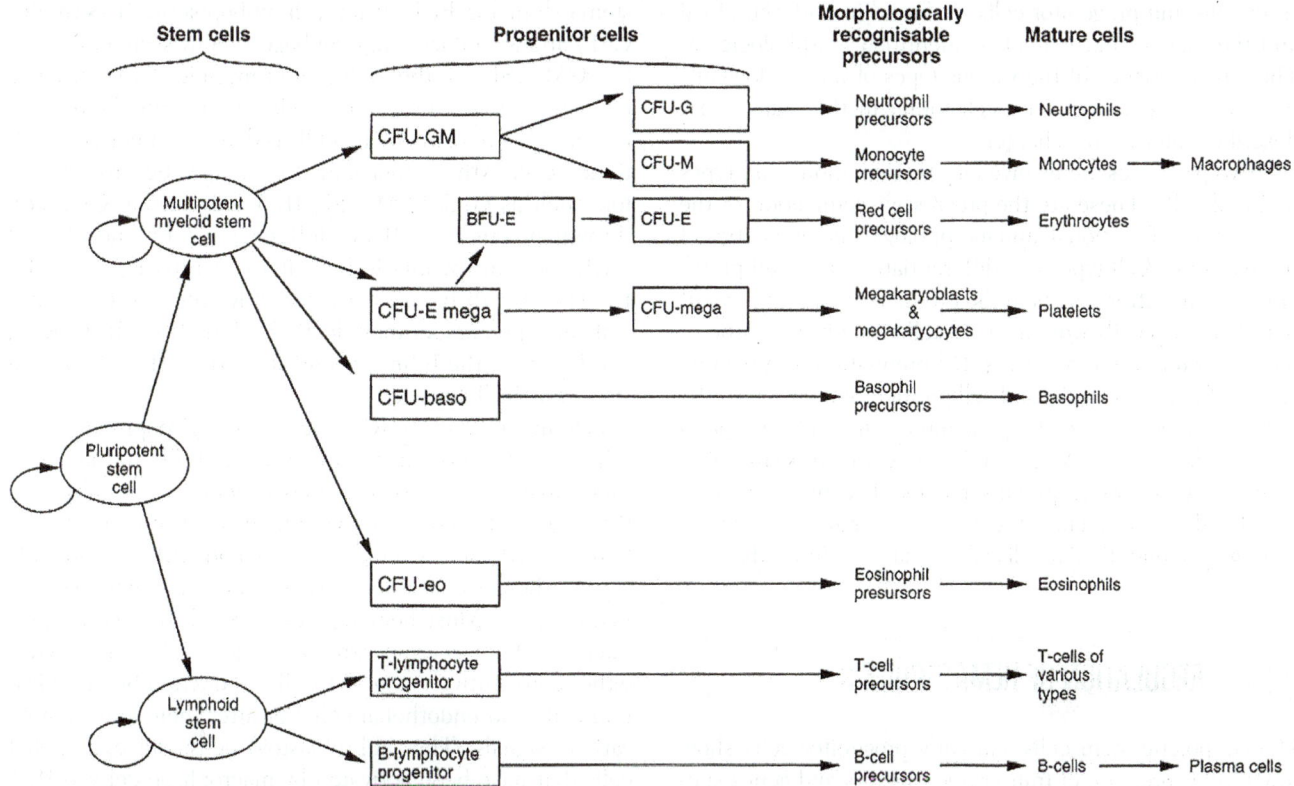

FIGURE 32.1 Model of hematopoiesis showing the relationships between the various types of stem cells, progenitor cells, and morphologically recognizable precursor cells. *BFU*-E, erythroid burst-forming units; *CFU*, colony-forming units; *E*, erythroblasts; *GM*, granulocytes and macrophages; *eo*, eosinophil granulocyes; *baso*, basophil granulocytes; *mega*, megakaryocytes; *G*, neutrophil granulocytes; *M*, macrophages.

myeloid stem cells (17–20). They may also give rise to endothelial cells (21). The lymphoid stem cells mature into all types of lymphocytes. The myeloid stem cells mature into neutrophil, eosinophil, and basophil granulocytes, monocytes, erythrocytes, platelets, mast cells, and osteoclasts.

Hematopoietic progenitor cells have been identified and characterized by their ability to form colonies containing cells of one or more hematopoietic lineages in vitro and are therefore called colony-forming units (CFUs) or colony-forming cells (CFC). These generate colonies containing a mixture of granulocytes, erythroblasts, macrophages, and megakaryocytes and are, therefore, termed CFU-GEMM. Bipotent hematopoietic progenitor cells that give rise to colonies containing granulocytes and macrophages are termed CFU-GM. There are also bipotent progenitor cell-generating colonies containing a mixture of erythroblasts and megakaryocytes (CFU-E mega). The unipotent progenitor cells that give rise to neutrophil granulocytes, eosinophil granulocytes, basophil granulocytes, macrophages, erythroblasts, and megakaryocytes are described as CFU-G, CFU-eo, CFU-baso, CFU-M, CFU-E, and CFU-mega, respectively. These develop into the most immature of the morphologically recognizable blood cell precursors in the marrow. Thus, CFU-G develops into myeloblasts, CFU-eo into eosinophil promyelocytes, CFU-baso into basophil promyelocytes, CFU-M into monoblasts, CFU-E into pronormoblasts, and CFU-mega into megakaryoblasts. The stem cells and progenitor cells are found in both the blood and the marrow but cannot be identified morphologically. The characteristics of the various types of morphologically recognizable hematopoietic cell found in the marrow are described later in this chapter.

Two processes are involved in the formation of all types of blood cells. These are the progressive acquisition of the biochemical, functional, and morphologic characteristics of the particular cell type (i.e., differentiation) and cell proliferation. The latter results in the production of a large number of mature cells from a single cell committed to one or more differentiation pathways. Differentiation occurs at all stages of hematopoiesis, and cell proliferation occurs in the hematopoietic stem cells, progenitor cells and, except in the megakaryocytic lineage, in the more immature morphologically recognizable precursor cells. The nearly mature blood cells seem to enter the circulation mainly by passing through the endothelial cells of the marrow sinusoids.

REGULATION OF HEMATOPOIESIS

Hematopoietic stem cells and early progenitor cells show low-level expression of transcription factors and genes specific to several hematopoietic lineages (multilineage priming). Commitment to a single lineage involves enhancement of transcription factors controlling the gene expression programs specific to that lineage and permanent silencing by those transcription factors of gene programs required for differentiation down other lineages (20).

The mechanisms underlying the commitment of a stem cell to differentiate are not yet fully understood (20,22). According to one model, the probability of a stem cell undergoing self-renewal or differentiation is a stochastic process. Environmental signals (soluble factors, cell–cell and cell–extracellular matrix interactions) mediated by specific receptor–ligand interactions operate only by influencing stem cell and progenitor cell apoptosis (and, thus, survival) and proliferation. Another model proposes that all decisions taken by stem cells and progenitor cells are determined by environmental signals. Bone marrow stromal cells (e.g., macrophages, nonphagocytic reticular or fibroblastoid cells, adipocytes, endothelial cells) play a major role in generating such signals; they provide niches for the attachment of stem cells and their progeny, are a source of the extracellular matrix involved in such attachment, and secrete various membrane-bound and soluble stimulatory hematopoietic growth factors and inhibitory cytokines (23,24). It is likely that elements of both mechanisms are operative (20).

Stem cells and early hematopoietic progenitor cells interact via specific cell surface receptors with multilineage hematopoietic growth factors (20,22). The latter include stem cell factor (steel factor, kit ligand), FLT3 ligand, interleukin-1 (IL-1) and IL-6 for the pluripotent stem cells, and stem cell factor, FLT3 ligand, thrombopoietin, IL-3 (multi-CSF) and granulocyte-macrophage–colony stimulating factor (GM-CSF) for the multipotent myeloid stem cells. The regulation of later progenitor cells and the morphologically recognizable hematopoietic cells is dependent both on multilineage growth factors and lineage-specific growth factors such as G-CSF, M-CSF, IL-5 (influencing CFU-eo), thrombopoietin and IL11 (influencing CFU-mega), and erythropoietin (mainly influencing late BFU-E and CFU-E). The growth factors influencing lymphocyte progenitor cells and precursors include IL-2, IL-4, IL-5, IL-6, IL-7, and IL-11 for the B lineage and IL-2, IL-3, IL-4, IL-7, and IL-10 for the T lineage.

Hematopoietic growth factors are glycoproteins and influence the survival, proliferation, and differentiation of their target cells via second messengers. In their absence, the target cells undergo programmed cell death (apoptosis). Some growth factors such as G-CSF and GM-CSF not only regulate hematopoiesis but also enhance the function of the mature cells. Most hematopoietic growth factors are produced by bone marrow stromal cells and T lymphocytes, either constitutively (e.g., M-CSF production by fibroblastoid cells and endothelial cells) or after their activation by various signals. Thus, fibroblastoid cells and endothelial cells that have been activated by macrophage-derived IL-1 or tumor necrosis factor (TNF) and endotoxin-stimulated macrophages produce M-CSF, GM-CSF, G-CSF, IL-6, and stem cell factor. Antigen- or IL-1– activated T cells produce IL-3, IL-5, and GM-CSF.

The main organ of erythropoietin production in postnatal life is the kidney, and the probable site of synthesis appears to be peritubular cells. About 10% of the erythropoietin is produced in the liver, which is the main organ of synthesis in the fetus. There is an oxygen sensor in the peritubular cells of the kidney, and the production of erythropoietin is inversely proportional to the degree of oxygenation of renal tissue. A limited amount of data suggests that there also may be paracrine or autocrine erythropoietin production in the bone marrow. The erythropoietin receptor is upregulated at the late BFU-E and CFU-E stages, and signaling through this receptor is required to prevent apoptosis.

In addition to the stimulatory cytokines mentioned above, inhibitors (negative regulators) of hematopoiesis are produced by macrophages, fibroblastoid cells, and endothelial cells. These include transforming growth factor-β1 (TGF-β1), which inhibits multilineage progenitor cells, early erythroid progenitors, and megakaryocytes; TNF-α, which inhibits the proliferation of granulocyte precursors; interferon-α, which inhibits megakaryocyte progenitors; and macrophage inflammatory protein-1α (MIP-1α), which inhibits the proliferation of stem cells.

Recombinant forms of a number of growth factors, or alternatively agonists for their receptors, are used therapeutically to manage patients with cytopenias, and these produce predictable morphologic changes in the marrow related to their physiologic roles.

HEMATOPOIESIS IN THE EMBRYO AND FETUS: DEVELOPMENT OF THE BONE MARROW

Studies in experimental animals have shown that hematopoietic stem cells responsible for embryonic (primitive) hematopoiesis develop in the yolk sac. Those responsible for fetal and postnatal (definitive) hematopoiesis are considered to arise in the aorto-gonad-mesonephros region by some investigators and the yolk sac by others (25–27). The stem cells migrate through the blood stream to colonize the fetal liver and other fetal tissues.

In the human embryo, erythropoietic cells first appear within the blood islands of the yolk sac about 19 days after fertilization (28,29). A few megakaryocytes are found in these blood islands during the 6th and 7th weeks of gestation. Yolk sac erythropoiesis is megaloblastic and results in the production of nucleated red cells (Fig. 32.2) that contain three embryonic hemoglobins: hemoglobins Gower I ($\zeta_2\varepsilon_2$), Gower II ($\alpha_2\varepsilon_2$), and Portland I ($\zeta_2\gamma_2$), and, in later embryos, hemoglobin F ($\alpha_2\gamma_2$) (30).

Hematopoietic foci develop in the hepatic cords during the 6th week of gestation, and the liver becomes the major site of erythropoiesis in the middle trimester of pregnancy (31,32). During this period, about half the nucleated cells of the liver consist of erythropoietic cells (Fig. 32.3). A few granulocyte precursors and megakaryocytes also are found in this organ. Fetal hepatic erythropoiesis is normoblastic and gives rise to nonnucleated red cells containing hemoglobin F. These red cells are considerably larger than the red cells of adults. The number of erythropoietic cells in the liver decreases progressively after the 7th month of gestation; a few cells persist until the end of the 1st postnatal week.

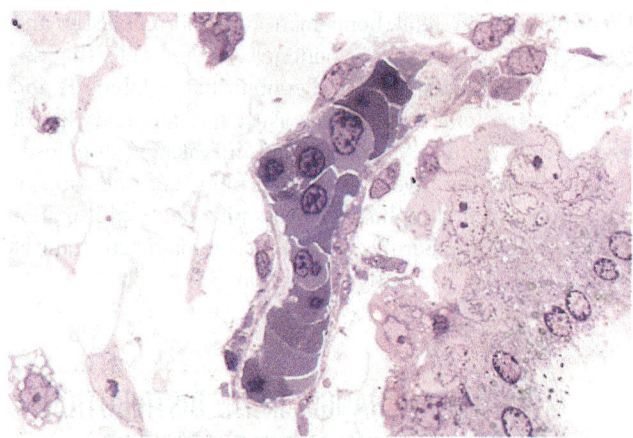

FIGURE 32.2 Semithin section of a plastic-embedded chorionic villus biopsy sample obtained at 7 weeks of gestation, showing a blood vessel containing nucleated embryonic red cells (toluidine blue).

Marrow cavities are formed as a result of the erosion of bone or calcified cartilage by blood vessels and cells from the periosteum (28). The first marrow cavity to develop is that of the clavicle (at about 2 months gestational age). After the formation of the marrow cavities, the vascular connective tissue present within them becomes colonized by circulating hematopoietic stem cells. The latter generate erythropoietic cells during the 3rd and 4th months of gestation, the order of appearance of erythropoietic cells being the same as the order of formation of the marrow cavities. After the 6th month, the bone marrow becomes the major site of hematopoiesis (33).

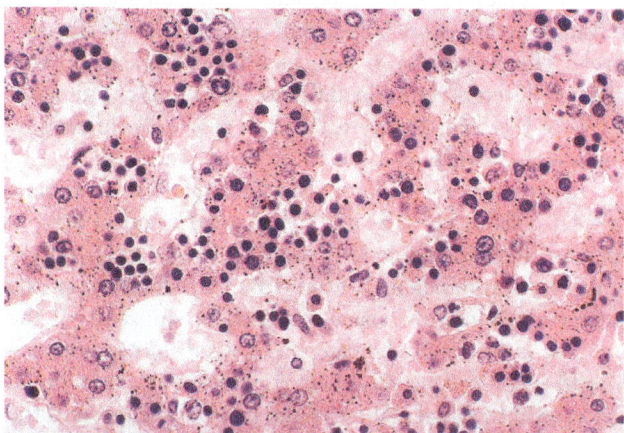

FIGURE 32.3 Fetal liver tissue obtained postmortem showing erythropoietic activity. The erythroblasts (identifiable by their darkly staining, round nuclei) are found extravascularly, both within the hepatic cords and between the cords and the sinusoidal endothelial cells. The brown material within hepatocytes is formalin pigment, a common postmortem fixation artifact (H&E).

Erythropoiesis in fetal bone marrow is normoblastic and results in the production of nonnucleated red cells that are larger than adult red cells and contain hemoglobins F and A ($\alpha_2\beta_2$). The fetal bone marrow is the predominant site of intrauterine granulocytopoiesis and megakaryocytopoiesis. In this tissue, the myeloid/erythroid ratio (i.e., the ratio of the number of neutrophil precursors plus neutrophil granulocytes to the number of erythroblasts) remains constant at about 1:4 after 6.5 months of gestation (33).

POSTNATAL CHANGES IN THE DISTRIBUTION OF RED MARROW AND IN THE TYPE OF HEMOGLOBIN

At birth, all the marrow cavities contain red, hematopoietic marrow. Furthermore, the red marrow contains only a few fat cells. After the first 4 years of life, an increasing number of fat cells appear between the hematopoietic cells, particularly in certain regions of the marrow, and these regions eventually become yellow and virtually devoid of hematopoietic cells (34,35). Zones of yellow, fatty marrow are found just below the middle of the shafts of the long bones between the ages of 10 and 14 years and, subsequently, extend in both directions, distal spread being more rapid than proximal spread. By the age of about 25 years, hematopoietic marrow is confined to the proximal quarters of the shafts of the femora and humeri, the skull bones, ribs, sternum, scapulae, clavicles, vertebrae, pelvis, and the upper half of the sacrum. Although the distribution of hematopoietic marrow remains essentially unaltered throughout adult life, its fat cell content increases slightly with increasing age and more substantially after the age of 70 years, in association with a gradual expansion of the volume of the marrow cavities.

The percentages of hemoglobins F and A in the blood of full-term neonates are 50% to 85% and 15% to 50%, respectively. The proportion of hemoglobin F decreases postnatally at different rates in different individuals, but adult levels of less than 1% are reached in nearly all children by the age of 2.5 years.

Because young children have red marrow containing few fat cells in virtually all their marrow cavities, a rapid increase in hematopoietic tissue in this age group is presumably accommodated mainly by a reduction in the proportion of marrow space occupied by sinusoids. If the increase in the rate of hematopoiesis is substantial and prolonged (e.g., in congenital hemolytic anemias), there is an increase in the total volume of the marrow cavities and the reestablishment of extramedullary hematopoiesis in organs such as the liver, spleen, and lymph nodes (36). The expansion of the marrow cavities leads to skeletal abnormalities, such as frontal and parietal bossing, dental deformities, and malocclusion of the teeth. It also causes thinning of the cortex, which may lead to fractures after minor trauma. In adults, increased hematopoiesis is initially associated with the replacement of fat cells in red marrow by hematopoietic cells and also with the spread of red marrow into marrow cavities normally containing yellow marrow (36). If the increase in hematopoiesis is marked, extramedullary hematopoiesis may develop.

STRUCTURAL ORGANIZATION OF HEMATOPOIETIC MARROW

The marrow cavities of most bones contain trabeculae of cancellous bone. The inner surface of the cortex and the outer surfaces of the trabeculae are lined by the endosteum, which consists of a single layer of cells supported on a delicate layer of reticular connective tissue. In most areas of the endosteum, the cells consist of very flat bone-lining cells (endosteal lining cells), but in some areas they consist of osteoblasts or osteoclasts. The marrow, which is located between the trabeculae, is supplied with an extensive microvasculature and some myelinated and nonmyelinated nerve fibers. It does not have a lymphatic drainage (37). The space between the small blood vessels contains a few reticulin fibers and a variety of cell types. The latter include fat cells, precursors of red cells, granulocytes, monocytes and platelets, lymphocytes, plasma cells, macrophages (phagocytic reticular cells), nonphagocytic reticular cells, and mast cells (38,39).

Blood Supply

One or more nutrient canals penetrate the shafts of the long bones obliquely. Each canal contains a nutrient artery and one or two nutrient veins. After entering the marrow, the nutrient artery divides into ascending and descending branches, which coil around the central longitudinal vein, the main venous channel of the marrow. The ascending and descending arteries give off numerous arterioles and capillaries that travel radially toward the endosteum and often open into a plexus of sinusoids (19). The sinusoids drain through a system of collecting venules and larger venous channels into the central longitudinal vein, which in turn drains mainly into the nutrient veins. In the diaphyses of long bones containing yellow fatty marrow, the nutrient artery gives off relatively few branches until it reaches the lower edge of the red marrow, where it breaks up into numerous vessels that penetrate the hematopoietic tissue. Many blood vessels of various sizes supply the marrow within flat and cuboidal bones, entering the marrow cavity via one or more large nutrient canals, as well as through numerous smaller canals.

There are interconnections between the blood supply of the bone marrow and bone through an endosteal network of blood vessels. This network communicates both with the periosteal vessels via fine veins passing through the bone and with branches of the nutrient artery. Furthermore, studies in experimental animals have shown that many capillaries derived from the nutrient artery enter Haversian canals but swing back into the marrow and open into sinusoids or venules (40–43). There has been much speculation as to whether blood reaching the marrow from the bone contains one or more hematopoietic factors derived from the bone or endosteal cells.

The sinusoids of human bone marrow have thin walls consisting of an inner complete layer of flattened endothelial cells with little or no underlying basement membrane and an outer incomplete layer of adventitial cells (44). The endothelial cells are characterized by the presence of numerous small pinocytotic vesicles along both their luminal and abluminal surfaces (Fig. 32.4). The nucleus is flattened and contains moderate quantities of nuclear membrane–associated condensed chromatin. The cytoplasm also contains ribosomes, rough endoplasmic reticulum (RER), mitochondria, some microfilaments, a few lysosomes, and occasional fat droplets. Adjacent endothelial cells overlap and may interdigitate extensively. These areas of contact are characterized by: (a) a strictly parallel alignment of the membranes of the interacting cells with a narrow gap between the opposing membranes; and (b) short stretches in which the membranes fuse together, forming tight junctions (not true desmosomes). There is an increased electron density of the cytoplasm immediately adjacent to and on both sides of the tight junctions (Fig. 32.4). Some endothelial cells show alkaline phosphatase activity. Endothelial cells contain no stainable iron except when the iron stores are increased.

They produce extracellular matrix, stem cell factor, IL6, GM-CSF, IL-1α, IL-11, and G-CSF, and are thus intimately involved with the regulation of hematopoiesis. Endothelial cells of the sinusoids allow the bidirectional migration of progenitor cells and hematopoietic stem cells through them by a mechanism involving specific binding molecules.

Adventitial cells project long peripheral cytoplasmic processes, which may be closely associated with some extracellular reticulin fibers. Some of these processes lie along the sinusoidal surface, and others protrude outward between hematopoietic cells. Thus, adventitial cells are a type of reticular cell (i.e., form part of the cytoplasmic network or reticulum of the marrow stroma). The cytoplasm of adventitial cells contains ribosomes, RER, some pinocytotic vesicles, a few electron-dense lysosomes, occasional fat globules, and numerous microfilaments that are often arranged in bands. The latter are usually situated within the peripheral cytoplasmic processes. The cytoplasm of some adventitial cells appears very electron lucent. Adventitial cells stain strongly for alkaline phosphatase.

Nerve Supply

In the case of a long bone, the nerve supply enters the bone marrow mainly via the nutrient canal but also through a number of epiphyseal and metaphyseal foramina. Bundles of nerve fibers travel together with the nutrient artery and its branches and supply the smooth muscle in such vessels or, occasionally, terminate between hematopoietic cells (45).

Extracellular Matrix (Connective Tissue)

Normal marrow contains a scanty incomplete network of fine branching reticulin (type III collagen) fibers between the parenchymal cells (Fig. 32.5). A higher concentration of

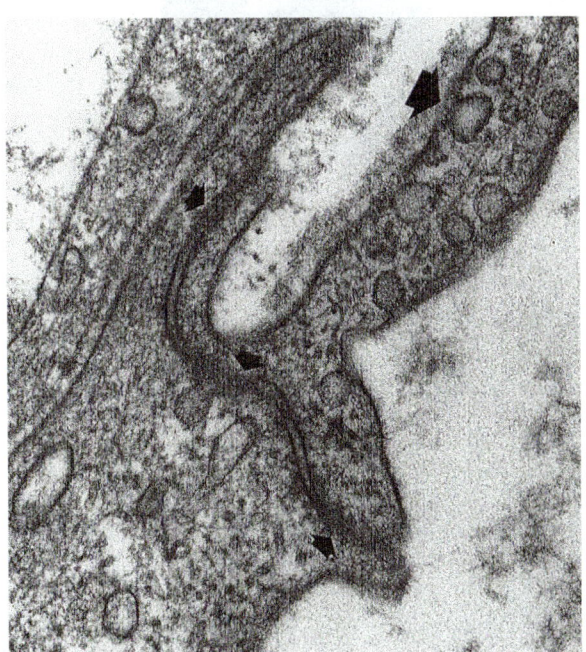

FIGURE 32.4 Electron micrograph of part of the wall of a sinusoid from normal bone marrow. There are three tight junctions (*small arrows*) at the area of contact between two adjacent endothelial cells. Several pinocytotic vesicles (*large arrow*) are present both at the luminal and abluminal surface of one of the endothelial cells, and a single pinocytotic vesicle is present at the outer surface of the adventitial cell.

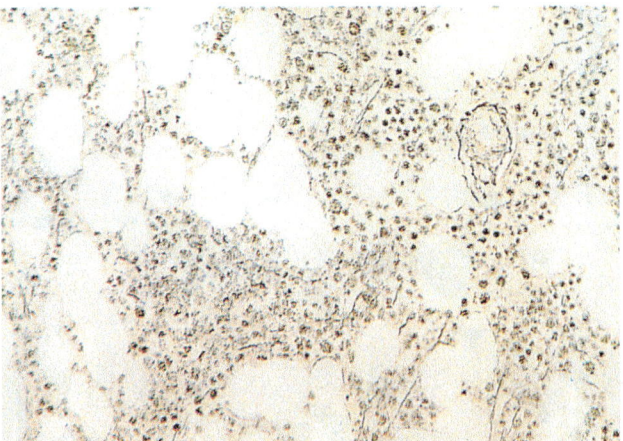

FIGURE 32.5 Section of a decalcified, paraffin-embedded trephine biopsy core from a hematologically normal adult, showing a scant network of fine reticulin fibers. The upper right-hand quadrant of the photomicrograph shows a circular arrangement of fibers associated with a blood vessel. (Silver impregnation of reticulin.)

thicker fibers is found in and around the walls of the larger arteries and near the endosteum; such fibers are continuous with the fibers in the parenchyma. Other extracellular matrix components produced by stromal cells include fibronectin, vascular cell adhesion molecule (VCAM)-1, vitronectin, thrombospondin, and proteoglycans such as heparan sulphate and chondroitin sulphate.

Stromal Cells

The stromal cells comprise: (a) osteoblasts, bone marrow fat cells (adipocytes), and nonphagocytic reticular cells (including myofibroblasts), all of which are derived from mesenchymal stem cells within the marrow; (b) osteoclasts, macrophages, and mast cells that are derived from the myeloid hematopoietic stem cell; and (c) endothelial cells (discussed above) that are derived either from the hematopoietic stem cell or a more primitive marrow cell that also gives rise to hematopoietic stem cells (21). Some stromal cells are intimately involved in the regulation of hematopoiesis.

Osteoblasts and Osteoclasts

Osteoblasts are present in the endosteum in areas of deposition of osseous matrix (osteoid). Osteoblasts are frequently found in a continuous layer, usually one or two cells thick, and appear like an area of epithelium. They become surrounded by the osteoid they produce and thus eventually become osteocytes. Osteoclasts are large multinucleate cells involved in bone resorption. Osteoblasts arise from progenitor cells closely associated with the endosteal lining cells. Although it is usually considered that osteoblast progenitor cells are not derived from hematopoietic stem cells, studies in mice indicate that osteoblasts and hematopoietic cells arise from a common primitive marrow cell (46). Osteoblasts produce cytokines such as IL6, G-CSF, and GM-CSF that influence hemopoiesis (47). Osteoclasts originate from the myeloid hematopoietic stem cells. The relationship between the osteoclast progenitor cell and other hematopoietic progenitor cells (e.g., CFU-GEMM, CFU-GM, CFU-M) is not clear (48).

Romanowsky-stained normal marrow smears may contain groups of osteoblasts or individual osteoclasts. They are relatively commonly seen in the marrow aspirates of children, but are generally only seen in adults when there is increased bony remodeling activity. In aspirate smears, osteoblasts have an oval or elongated shape and are 20 to 50 μm in diameter (Fig. 32.6A). They have abundant basophilic cytoplasm, often with somewhat indistinct margins,

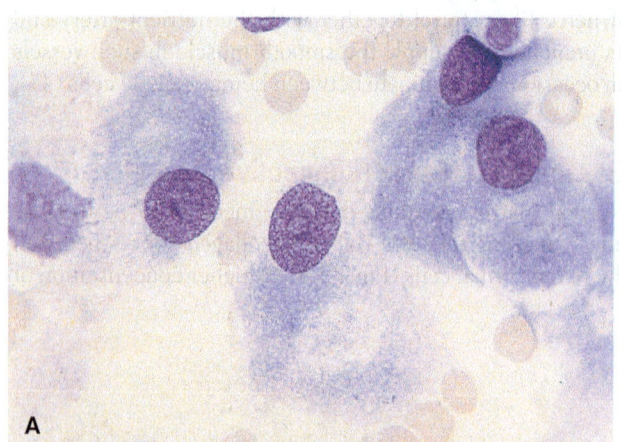

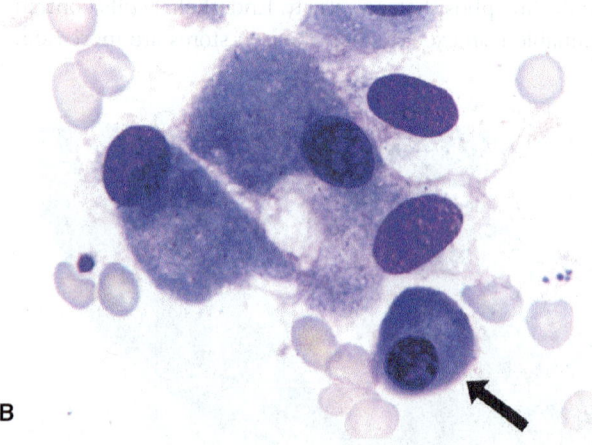

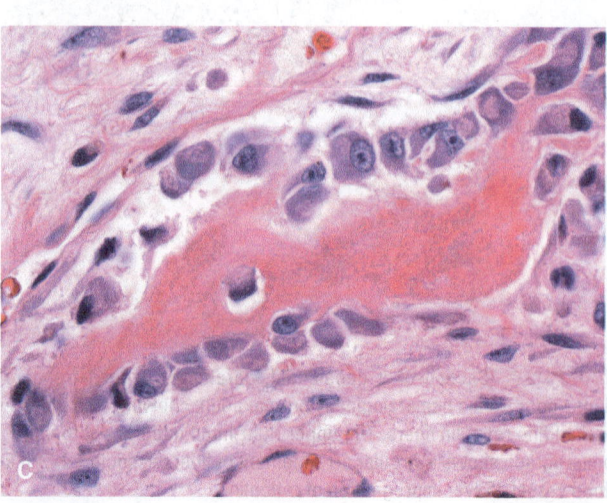

FIGURE 32.6 **A:** Group of osteoblasts from a May–Grünwald–Giemsa (MGG)–stained smear of normal bone marrow. **B:** Several osteoblasts, with an adjacent plasma cell for comparison (*arrow*) (Wright–Giemsa). **C:** Exuberant osteoblastic proliferation in a marrow trephine due to repair following a previous trephine biopsy at this site (H&E).

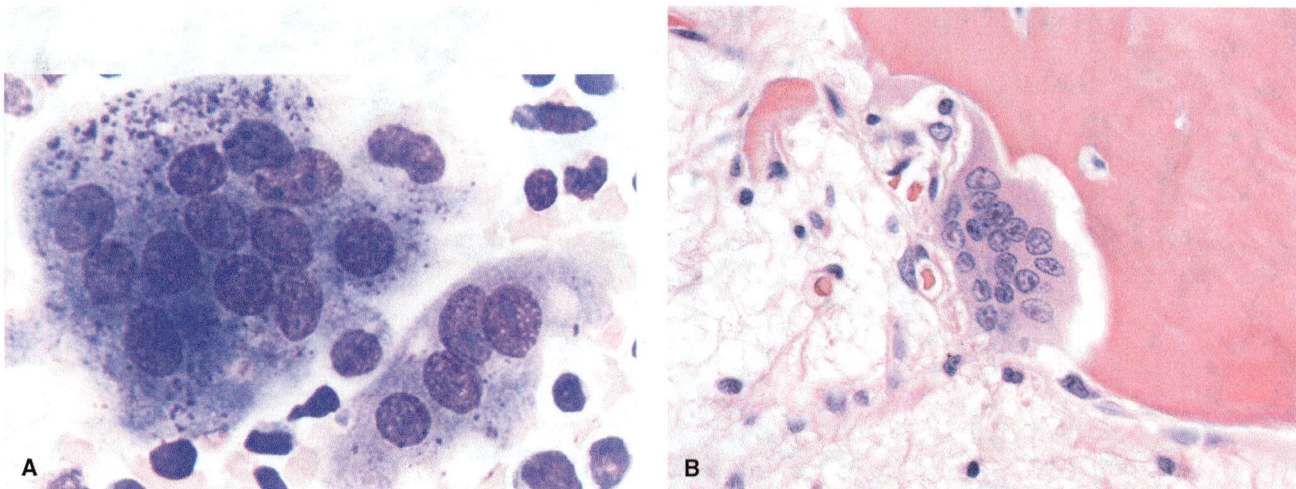

FIGURE 32.7 A: Two multinucleate osteoclasts from an aspirate smear of normal bone marrow with increased bony remodeling (Wright–Giemsa). **B:** A multinucleated osteoclast residing in a pit on the surface of a bone trabeculum (Howship lacuna or resorption lacuna) (H&E).

and a single small eccentric nucleus that often appears to be extruding from the cytoplasm. The chromatin has a reticular quality, and one to three nucleoli are present. The cytoplasm contains a rounded pale area corresponding to the Golgi apparatus, which often is situated some distance from the nucleus. Osteoblasts superficially resemble plasma cells, but the latter are smaller, contain heavily stained clumped chromatin, generally lack nucleoli, and have a Golgi zone situated immediately adjacent to the nucleus (Fig. 32.6B). Osteoblasts stain positively for alkaline phosphatase activity. In histologic sections, osteoblasts are cuboidal or pyramidal and have eccentric nuclei, distinct nucleoli, and dense, eosinophilic cytoplasm (Fig. 32.6C). Osteoclasts appear in aspirate smears as giant, multinucleate cells with abundant pale blue cytoplasm containing many azurophilic (purple-red) granules (Fig. 32.7A). The individual nuclei are rounded in outline, uniform in size, contain a single distinct nucleolus, and do not overlap. In marrow sections, osteoclasts characteristically reside in depressions or pits in the bony trabeculae, known as a Howship lacunae or resorption lacunae (Fig. 32.7B). Osteoclasts are strongly acid phosphatase positive. They must be distinguished from the other polyploid giant cells in the marrow, the megakaryocytes. These are usually not multinucleate but contain a single, large lobulated nucleus.

Fat Cells

The number of fat cells in hematopoietic bone marrow varies markedly with age, generally increasing with increasing age (49,50). In normal adults, 30% to 70% of the area of a histologic section of hematopoietic marrow consists of fat cells (Fig. 32.8). Fat cells are the largest cells in the marrow, and sections of such cells have average diameters of about 85 μm. Ultrastructural studies show that these cells have a single large fat globule at their center and a narrow rim of cytoplasm at their periphery. This cytoplasmic rim contains a flattened nucleus, several small lipid droplets, ribosomes, strands of endoplasmic reticulum, and several mitochondria. The fat cells of the bone marrow only have small quantities of reticulin and collagen fibers around them. They are in intimate contact with vascular channels, macrophages, and all types of hematopoietic cells. Marrow fat cells seem to be formed by the accumulation of lipid within adventitial cells, other nonphagocytic reticular cells, and, possibly, sinus endothelial cells. Whenever there is an increase or decrease in the number of hematopoietic cells in bone marrow, there is a corresponding decrease or increase, respectively, of the number of fat cells so that the intersinusoidal space within marrow cavities is fully occupied by cells. The mechanisms underlying this inverse relationship

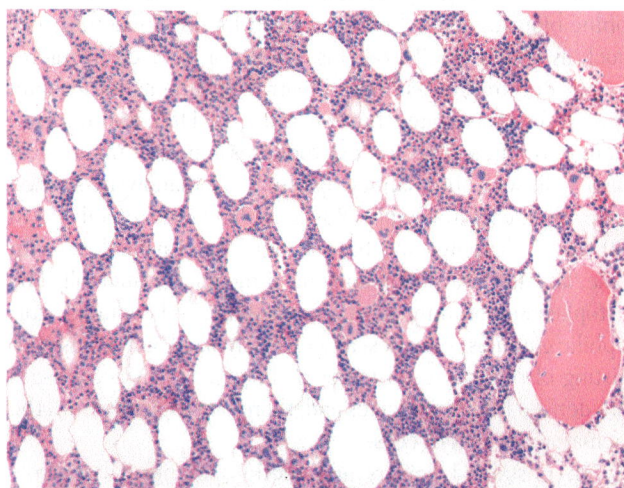

FIGURE 32.8 Section of a decalcified, paraffin-embedded trephine biopsy core from a hematologically normal adult. About 60% of the area of marrow tissue in this photomicrograph is occupied by fat cells. There may be a substantial variation in cellularity in different parts of the same section (H&E).

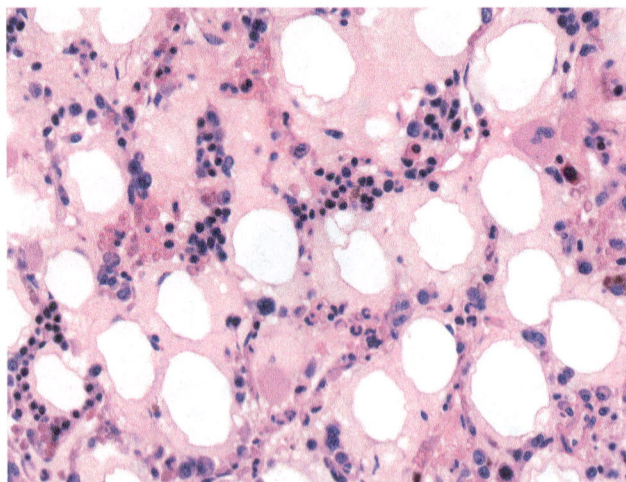

FIGURE 32.9 Bone marrow biopsy from patient with cachexia due to advanced AIDS demonstrating gelatinous transformation, also known as serous fat atrophy. There is an accumulation of homogeneous, pink mucopolysaccharide material in the interstitium, preferentially located around adipocytes.

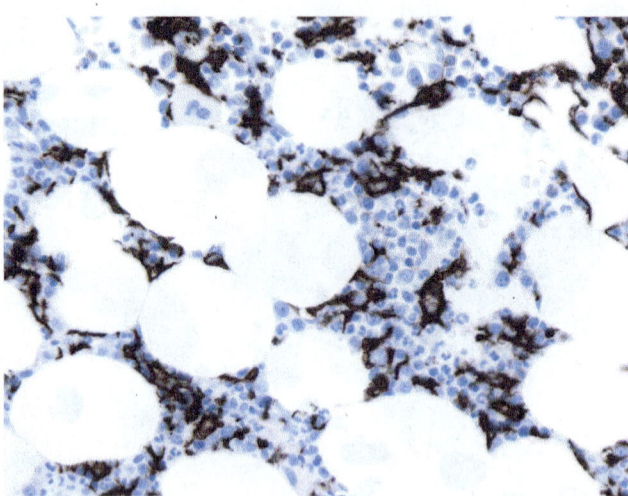

FIGURE 32.10 Immunohistochemical demonstration of macrophages in a section of a paraffin-embedded trephine biopsy core from a hematologically normal subject with anti-CD163. Note the abundant dendritic processes highlighted by the reaction.

between the mass of fat cells and hematopoietic cells in the marrow are uncertain. In severe anorexia nervosa or cachexia secondary to chronic disorders, such as tuberculosis or various malignancies, there is a marked reduction in fat cells, often together with a reduction in hematopoietic tissue. In these conditions, the space normally occupied by cells is filled with a gelatinous extracellular substance composed of acid mucopolysaccharide (Fig. 32.9)(51). This "gelatinous transformation" or "serous fat atrophy" may be associated with decreased cell counts in the blood.

Macrophages (Phagocytic Reticular Cells)

The bone marrow contains many macrophages. The frequency of this cell type is best appreciated in sections of trephine biopsies stained for an antigen found in macrophages such as CD68 or CD163 (Fig. 32.10) or in electron micrographs of ultrathin sections of marrow fragments rather than in smears of aspirated bone marrow. In H&E-stained sections of trephine biopsies, macrophages appear as moderately large cells with abundant cytoplasm. In Romanowsky-stained marrow smears, they appear as irregularly shaped cells 20 to 30 μm in diameter and have a round or oval nucleus with pale, lace-like chromatin and one or more large nucleoli. The cytoplasm is voluminous, stains pale blue, and contains azurophilic granules, vacuoles, and variously sized inclusions consisting of phagocytosed material (Fig. 32.11). Macrophages are derived from monocytes and, therefore originally from the hematopoietic stem cells.

In unstained smears and sections of normal marrow and in Giemsa- or H&E-stained sections, macrophages may show refractile yellow-brown hemosiderin-containing intracytoplasmic inclusions, which vary between 0.5 and 4 μm in diameter. These appear as blue or blue-black granules when stained by Perls' acid ferrocyanide method. This stain also may color the entire cytoplasm a diffuse pale blue (Fig. 32.12). The amount of iron-positive granules within the marrow fragments on a marrow smear (Fig. 32.13) or the amount in a histologic section of a trephine biopsy sample may be assessed semiquantitatively and is a useful guide to the total iron stores in the body (52). Stainable storage iron is absent in iron deficiency (with or without anemia) and increased in conditions such as hereditary hemochromatosis or transfusion-induced iron overload. Patients who have received therapeutic parenteral iron may show a unique pattern of iron deposition, consisting of curvilinear arrangements of uniformly sized granules (Fig. 32.14) (53). Iron deposited in this form may not be bioavailable (54). Macrophages contain PAS-positive material and are strongly positive for α-naphthyl acetate esterase and acid

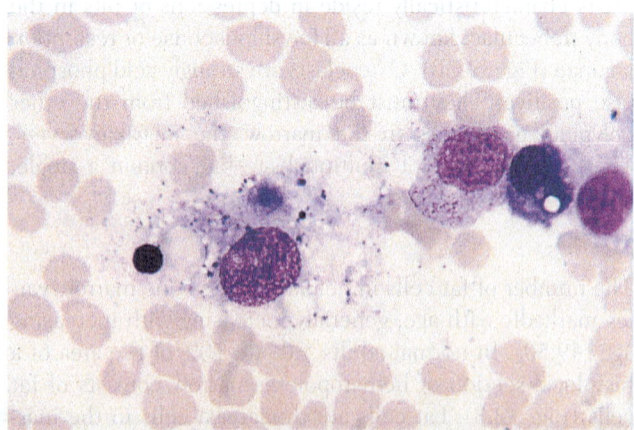

FIGURE 32.11 Macrophage from a normal marrow containing a dark extruded erythroblast nucleus and several intracytoplasmic inclusions of various shapes, sizes, and staining characteristics. The large pale rounded inclusions may represent degraded red cells (MGG).

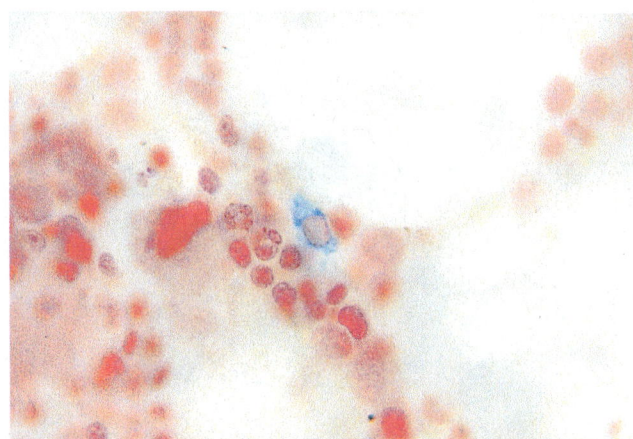

FIGURE 32.12 Section of a paraffin-embedded normal marrow fragment (*clot section*). The macrophage in the center shows blue hemosiderin-containing intracytoplasmic granules and a diffuse bluish coloration of the cytoplasm (Perls' acid ferrocyanide reaction).

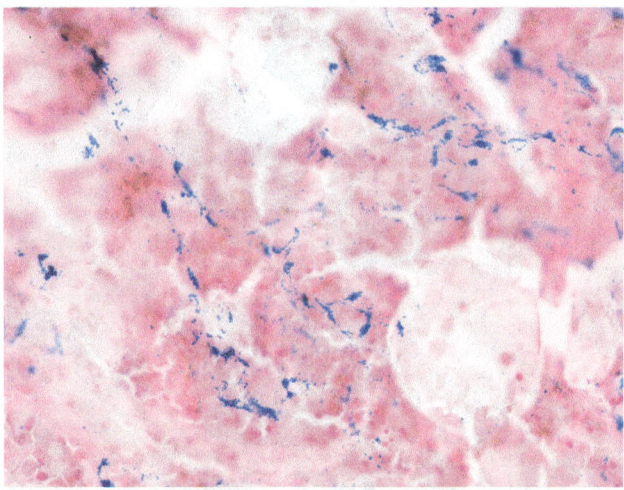

FIGURE 32.14 This iron stain demonstrates the distinct curvilinear arrays of iron granules seen following parenteral iron administration.

phosphatase. They do not stain for α-naphthol AS-D chloroacetate esterase activity (42), and most do not stain with Sudan black. Some macrophages appear to stain positively for alkaline phosphatase activity.

Ultrastructural studies of marrow fragments show that macrophages form long cytoplasmic processes at their periphery and that such processes extend for considerable distances between various types of hematopoietic cells (Fig. 32.15). Some cytoplasmic processes protrude through the endothelial cell layer into the sinusoidal lumen (Fig. 32.16) and appear to be involved in recognizing and phagocytosing circulating microorganisms and senescent or damaged erythrocytes and granulocytes. The nucleus often has an irregular outline and contains small to moderate quantities of nuclear membrane–associated condensed chromatin. The cytoplasm has many strands of RER, scattered ferritin molecules, a well-developed Golgi apparatus, several mitochondria, a number of small or medium-sized homogeneous electron-dense primary lysosomes of variable shape, and a number of large inclusions. Some of the latter have a complex ultrastructure with both electron-dense and electron-lucent areas and myelin figures and may contain numerous ferritin and hemosiderin molecules; these appear to represent secondary lysosomes with residual material from phagocytosed cells (Fig. 32.17). Other large inclusions can be recognized readily as granulocytes, extruded erythroblast nuclei, and erythrocytes at various stages of degradation. A few reticulin fibers may be found in contact with parts of the cell surface.

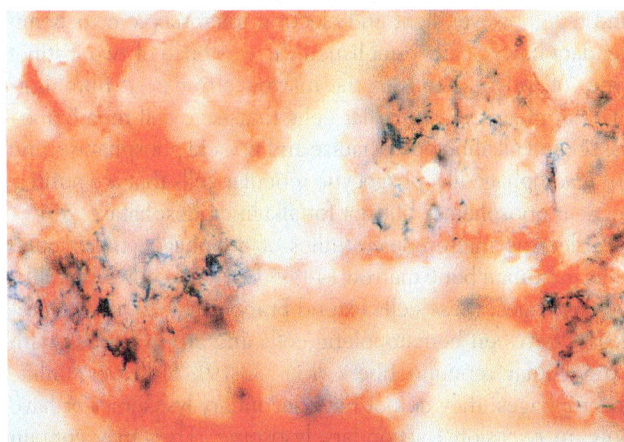

FIGURE 32.13 Marrow fragment from a normal marrow smear stained by Perls' acid ferrocyanide reaction. The dark blue granular material represents hemosiderin within macrophages.

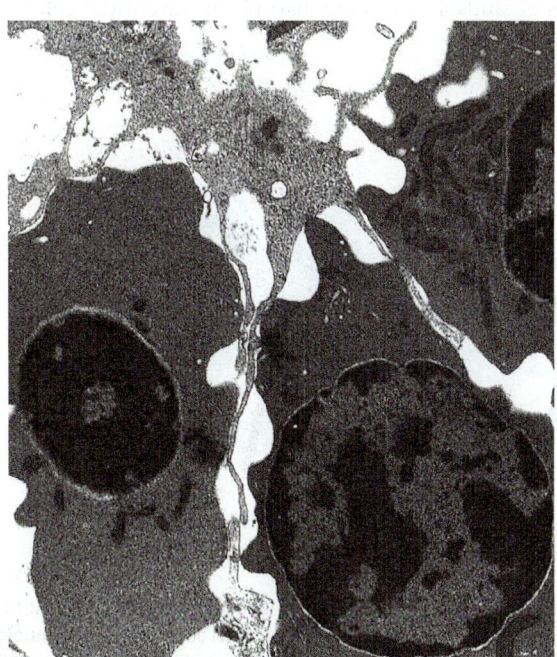

FIGURE 32.15 Electron micrograph of three erythroblasts from a normal marrow showing fine processes of macrophage cytoplasm extending between the cells.

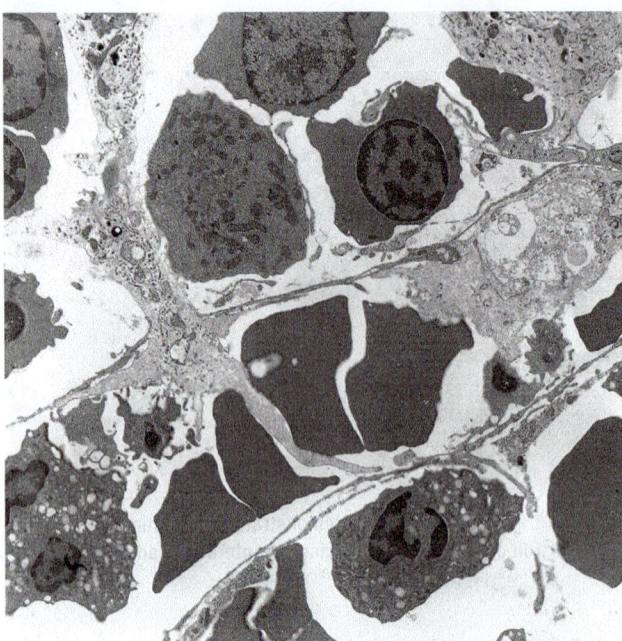

FIGURE 32.16 Electron micrograph of a sinusoid from a normal bone marrow. A process of macrophage cytoplasm is seen protruding through the lining endothelial cell into the sinusoidal lumen. Serial sectioning of this sinusoid showed that the mass of macrophage cytoplasm occupying the right-hand side of the sinusoidal lumen connected transendothelially with a second extrasinusoidal cytoplasmic process. Both processes arose from the same macrophage.

Macrophages are present within erythroblastic islands (Fig. 32.18), plasma cell islands, and lymphoid nodules but also may occur elsewhere in the marrow parenchyma. Some are found immediately adjacent to the endothelial cells of sinusoids, forming part of the adventitial cell layer.

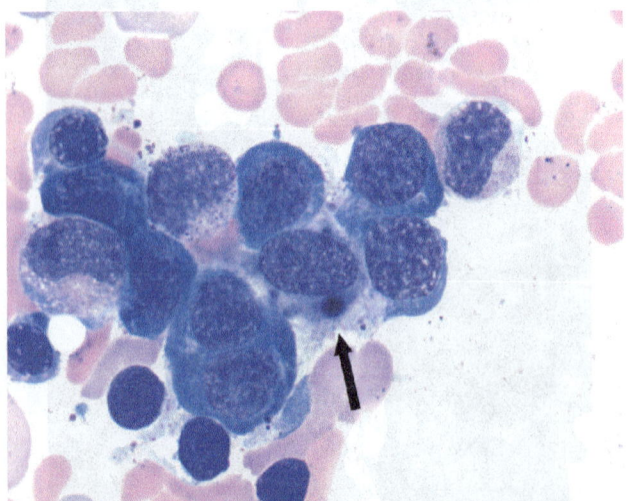

FIGURE 32.17 Electron micrograph of a macrophage lying next to an early polychromatic erythroblast in a normal bone marrow. The nucleus of the macrophage is irregular in outline, and its cytoplasm contains several inclusions and vacuoles. Some of the inclusions are utrastructurally complex and probably represent secondary lysosomes. There are some reticulin fibers (*arrow*) near the macrophage.

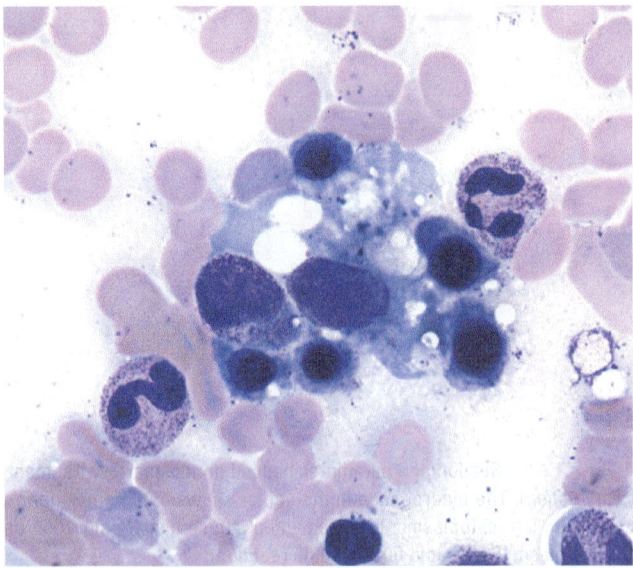

FIGURE 32.18 Several erythroid precursors intimately associated with a macrophage containing debris.

Bone marrow macrophages not only function as phagocytic cells but also generate various hematopoietic growth factors (e.g., c-kit ligand or stem cell factor, M-CSF, IL-1, and G-CSF) and are thus involved in short-range regulation of lymphopoiesis and myelopoiesis. They presumably also are involved in antigen processing.

Nonphagocytic Reticular Cells

In Romanowsky-stained marrow smears, nonphagocytic reticular cells have an irregular or spindle shape and resemble macrophages, except that they lack large intracytoplasmic inclusions. Light microscope cytochemical and histochemical data indicate that these cells are PAS negative, strongly positive for alkaline phosphatase, negative for acid phosphatase, negative or only weakly positive for α-naphthyl acetate esterase, and negative for stainable iron. Thus, there seems to be some overlap between the cytochemical characteristics of nonphagocytic reticular cells and macrophages (42,43). In the case of mice and rats, however, light and electron microscopic cytochemical data have clearly established the existence of two distinct types of reticular cells in the marrow stroma: (a) fibroblast-like nonphagocytic reticular cells that have cell membrane–associated alkaline phosphatase and no acid phosphatase; and (b) macrophage-like phagocytic reticular cells that are positive for acid phosphatase but not for alkaline phosphatase (55).

Electron microscopic studies of nonphagocytic reticular cells in human bone marrow (44,56,57) have shown that, like macrophages, these cells extend branching cytoplasmic processes between hematopoietic cells and are in contact with extracellular reticulin fibers (Fig. 32.19). However, unlike macrophages, they do not have secondary lysosomes or have only an occasional secondary lysosome. They may contain variable numbers of filaments or a few small fat globules in their cytoplasm. The intracytoplasmic filaments sometime occur in bundles, and the cells are then ultrastructurally

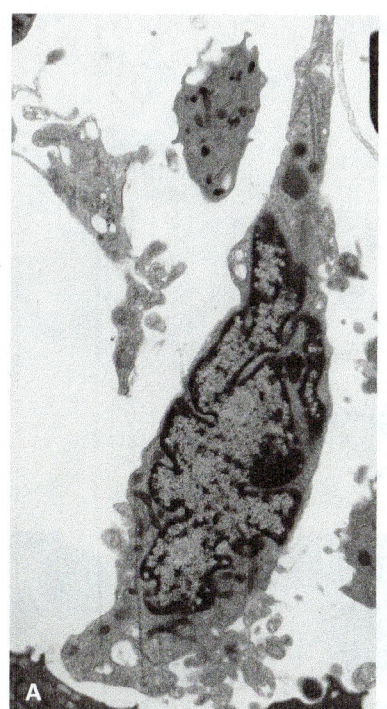 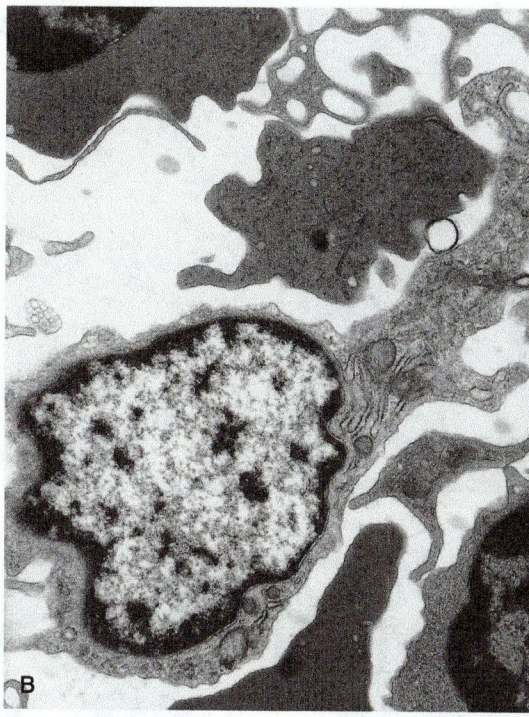

FIGURE 32.19 Electron micrographs of two nonphagocytic reticular cells from normal bone marrow. The nuclear outline of one of these cells (**A**) shows several deep clefts and that of the other (**B**) is less irregular.

indistinguishable from adventitial cells. It is possible that the nonphagocytic reticular cells comprise a number of different cell types including fibroblasts or myofibroblasts, adventitial cells, and cells whose functions have not yet been defined. Myeloid cell and B-lymphoid progenitors are located adjacent to myofibroblasts.

At least some of the nonphagocytic reticular cells arise from a mesenchymal stem cell capable of giving rise to colonies of fibroblast-like or myofibroblast-like cells in vitro. As mentioned earlier, nonphagocytic reticular cells appear to play an important role in the microenvironmental regulation of hematopoiesis, both by binding to primitive hematopoietic cells (58) and by producing certain hematopoietic growth factors both constitutively and in response to stimulation by monokines (59). In mice and presumably also in humans, they synthesize collagen (types I and III) and fibronectin.

Mast Cells

Mast cells tend to be found in association with the periphery of lymphoid follicles and the adventitia of small arteries and adjacent to the endosteal cells of bone trabeculae and the endothelial cells of sinusoids.

Hematopoietic stem cells generate morphologically unrecognizable progenitors of mast cells within the bone marrow (60), and the most mature of these cells enter the blood (61,62). The circulating cells, which still lack mast cell granules, migrate into the tissues, where they proliferate and mature into mast cells. Although mast cells and basophils show morphologic similarities and functional overlap, their relationship in the myeloid developmental pathways remains controversial (63).

Unlike the granules of basophils, which are very water soluble, those of mast cells are much less so. Nevertheless, mast cells are not easily recognized in sections of marrow stained with H&E, in which their granules are pale and refractile appearing (Fig. 32.20A). By contrast, they are readily identified in sections stained with the Giemsa stain. In such sections, mast cells have round or oval outlines and many dark purple cytoplasmic granules. The nucleus is often oval and may be situated eccentrically. A small minority of normal mast cells have a spindled shape. Mast cells are easily highlighted in sections using immunohistochemistry for mast cell tryptase (Fig. 32.20B) or CD117, where they are seen as scattered, single cells. In marrow aspirate smears, mast cells are primarily concentrated in particles (Fig. 32.20C). In Romanowsky-stained smears, mast cells vary between 5 and 25 μm in their long axis and usually have a round or ovoid appearance (Fig. 32.20D). The cytoplasm is packed with uniform, coarse purple-black granules; in contrast to basophils, the granules in mast cells generally don't overlie the nucleus. The nucleus is small, round or oval, and either centrally or eccentrically located. It contains less condensed chromatin than that of a basophil granulocyte. The granules of mast cells are rich in heparin and stain metachromatically with toluidine blue. Mast cells are also peroxidase negative, PAS positive, acid phosphatase positive, and α-naphthol AS-D chloroacetate esterase positive. Unlike basophil granulocytes, mast cells are capable of mitosis.

Ultrastructurally, the granules of mast cells vary considerably in appearance. They may be homogeneously electron dense, have areas of increased electron density at their centers, or contain parallel arrangements, whorls, or scrolls

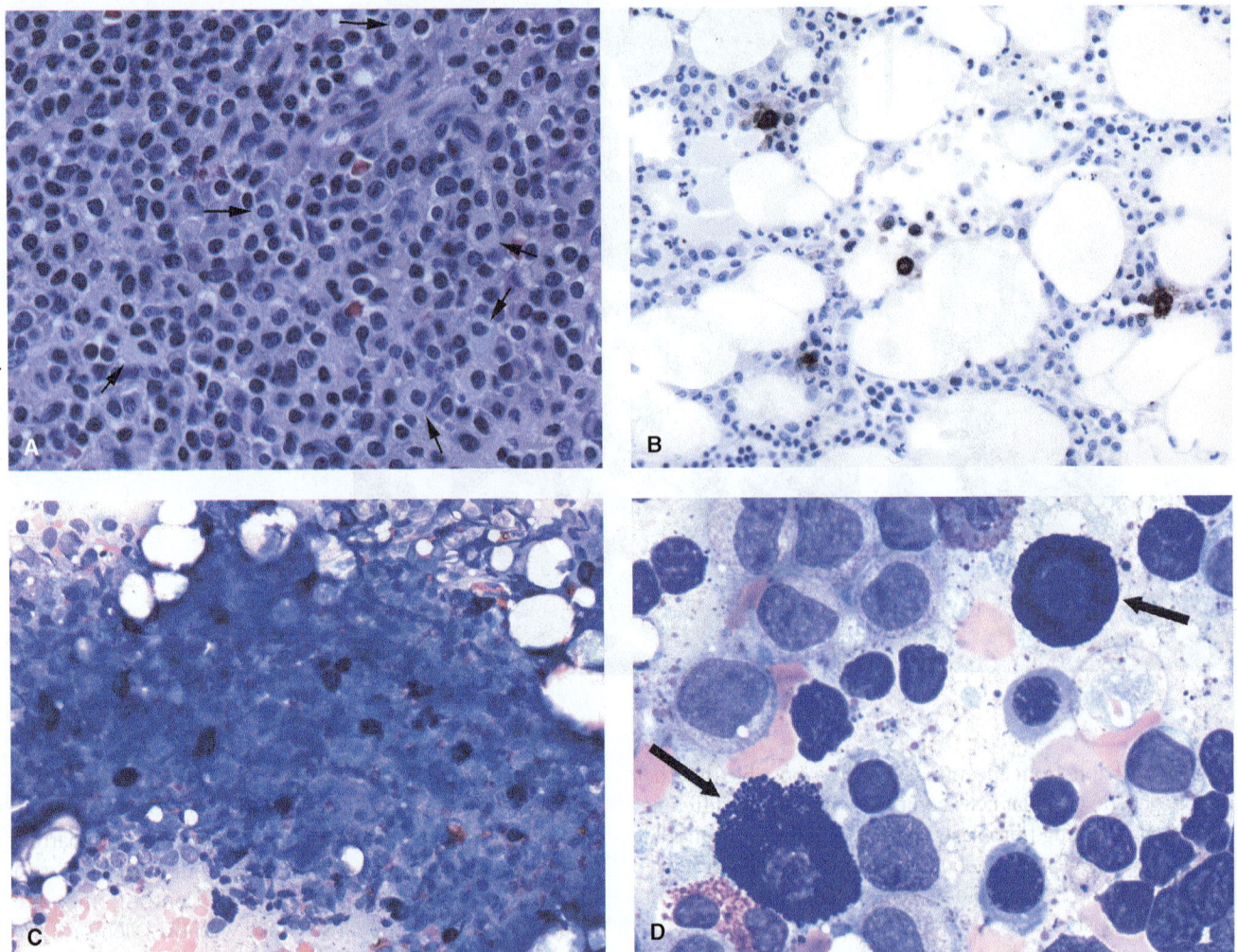

FIGURE 32.20 **A:** This lymphoid infiltrate in a bone marrow trephine biopsy contains multiple mast cells (*arrows*). These are polygonal cells with moderately abundant cytoplasm containing pale, refractile granules. **B:** Immunohistochemistry for mast cell tryptase in a normal marrow highlighting several, scattered mast cells. **C:** This marrow particle in a Wright–Giemsa-stained marrow smear with mast cell hyperplasia contains multiple, darkly staining mast cells. **D:** Two mast cells (*arrows*) in a Wright–Giemsa-stained bone marrow smear.

of a crystalline or fibrillar structure (Figs. 32.21A,B). The nucleus contains moderate quantities of condensed chromatin. In addition to the numerous granules, the cytoplasm contains some mitochondria, a few short strands of endoplasmic reticulum, occasional lipid droplets, and some fibrils.

HEMATOPOIETIC CELLS

Neutrophil Precursors

Aspirate Smears

The earliest morphologically recognizable neutrophil precursor is termed the myeloblast. The successive cytologic classes through which myeloblasts mature into circulating neutrophil granulocytes are termed neutrophil promyelocytes, neutrophil myelocytes, neutrophil metamyelocytes, neutrophil bands, and segmented neutrophils (Fig. 32.22).

Cell division occurs in myeloblasts, promyelocytes, and myelocytes but not in more mature cells.

A myeloblast is 10 to 20 μm in diameter. It has a large, rounded nucleus with finely dispersed chromatin and two to five nucleoli. The nucleus-to-cytoplasm ratio is moderately high, and the cytoplasm is basophilic and either nongranular or contains a few, fine granules. It is likely that only some myeloblasts mature into neutrophil promyelocytes and that others mature into eosinophil or basophil promyelocytes.

Neutrophil promyelocytes are larger than myeloblasts and have more abundant basophilic cytoplasm containing a few to many purple-red (azurophilic) granules. Early promyelocytes resemble myeloblasts—they are medium in size with a high nuclear to cytoplasmic ratio and fine chromatin—but have overtly granulated cytoplasm. More mature promyelocytes are larger, with more abundant, heavily granulated, and often eccentrically distributed cytoplasm. A paranuclear clearing corresponding to the Golgi apparatus may be evident

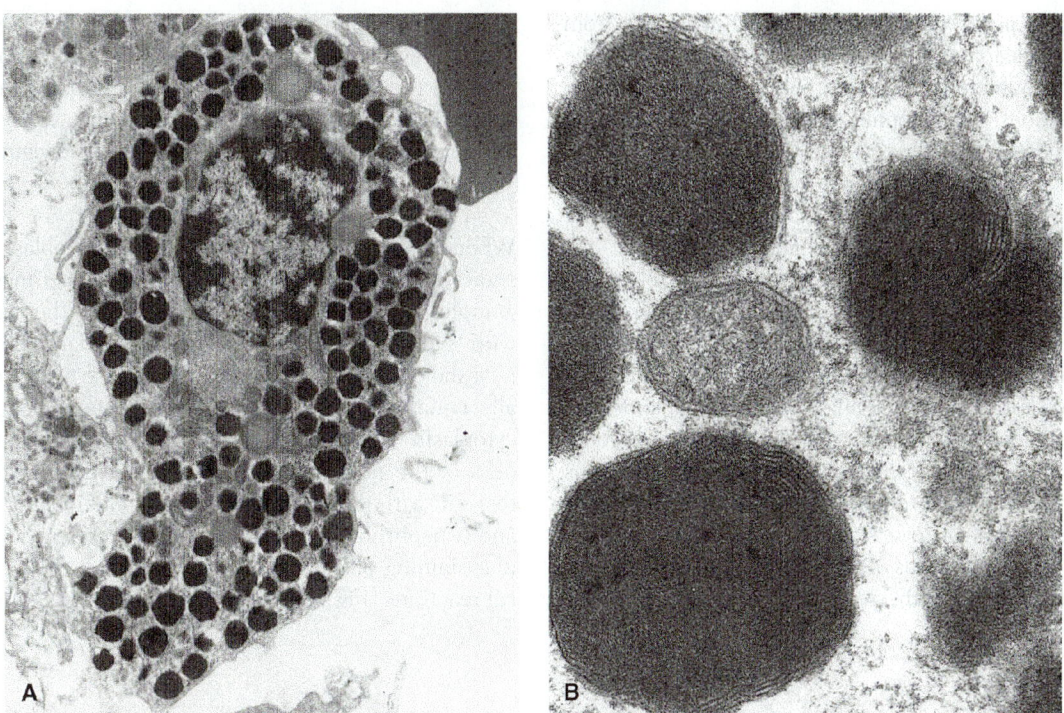

FIGURE 32.21 Electron micrographs of mast cells from normal bone marrow. **A:** The cytoplasm is packed with characteristic granules and contains four lipid droplets. **B:** Granules from a mast cell at high magnification showing parallel lamellae.

in late promyelocytes, as well. Nucleoli may be prominent. Neutrophil myelocytes are characterized by a lower nuclear to cytoplasmic ratio than promyelocytes; eccentric, round or oval nuclei; and the presence in their cytoplasm of fine light pink or pale orange (neutrophilic or "specific") granules. Early myelocytes are large, have prominent residual azurophilic granules in addition to relatively few neutrophilic granules, and have relatively immature chromatin, and often distinct nucleoli. Late myelocytes are smaller, have abundant secondary granules with few or no residual azurophilic granules, have distinctly coarser chromatin, and indistinct or absent nucleoli. The neutrophil metamyelocyte has an indented nucleus, with

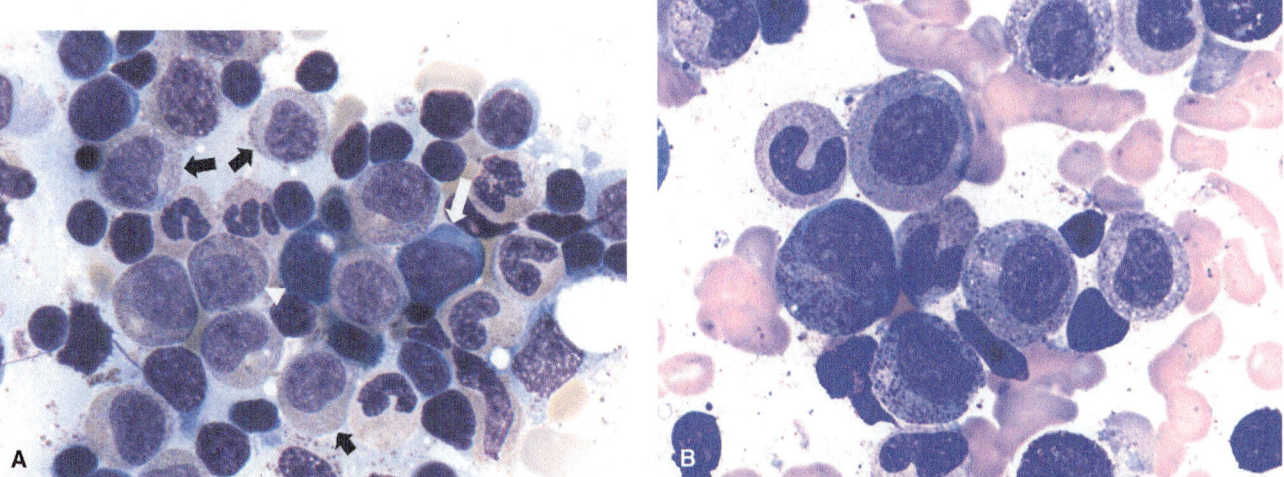

FIGURE 32.22 Neutrophil precursors from a Wright–Giemsa-stained normal marrow smear. **A:** A blast is indicated by the *white arrow*. Immediately adjacent to the blasts are five neutrophilic granulocytes. Beginning at three o'clock and proceeding clockwise: Band, late metamyelocyte, myelocyte, myelocyte, segmented neutrophil. A myelocyte is indicated by the white arrowhead. This is surrounded by four neutrophilic granulocytes. From 6 o'clock moving clockwise: Metamyelocyte, myelocyte, band, and segmented neutrophil. Several additional metamyelocytes are indicated by *black arrows*. Also note a hematogone in the upper left corner of the field. **B:** Left to right, top to bottom: Band, myelocyte, promyelocyte, late metamyelocyte, myelocyte, early metamyelocyte, myelocyte.

the indentation penetrating less than half the distance from the farthest nuclear margin (64). The cytoplasm is acidophilic and contains numerous fine neutrophilic granules. Under normal conditions, no azurophilic granules are present at the metamylocyte stage and beyond, but they may be present in reactive states, such as in bacterial infections or administration of recombinant granulocyte colony stimulating factor. Neutrophil bands (also called juvenile neutrophils or stab forms) have U-shaped or long, relatively narrow, band-like nuclei that are often twisted into various configurations. Early band forms are distinguished from metamyelocytes based on an indentation that penetrates greater than half the distance from the furthest nuclear margin. The nuclei contain large clumps of condensed chromatin and may show one or more partial constrictions along their length. These constrictions still contain recognizable chromatin structure. These constrictions become progressively more complete and eventually develop into fine strands or filaments that lack chromatin structure, at which point the cell is considered a segmented neutrophil. Most segmented neutrophils have two to five nuclear segments that are joined together by such filaments. Some of the neutrophil granulocytes of females have a drumstick-like nuclear appendage (representing an inactivated X chromosome) attached to one of the nuclear segments.

Cytochemistry

When stained by the PAS reaction, myeloblast cytoplasm shows a diffuse, pale red-purple tinge, sometimes with fine granules of the same color. Myeloblasts either do not stain with Sudan black or show a few small sudanophilic granules near the nucleus. They are also peroxidase negative and, usually, α-naphthol AS-D chloroacetate esterase negative. The cytoplasm of neutrophil promyelocytes and more mature cells of the neutrophil series stain positively with the PAS reagent, with Sudan black, and with reactions for peroxidase and α-naphthol AS-D chloroacetate esterase activity. A granular staining pattern is produced with all these cytochemical reactions (Fig. 32.23). The intensity of staining increases

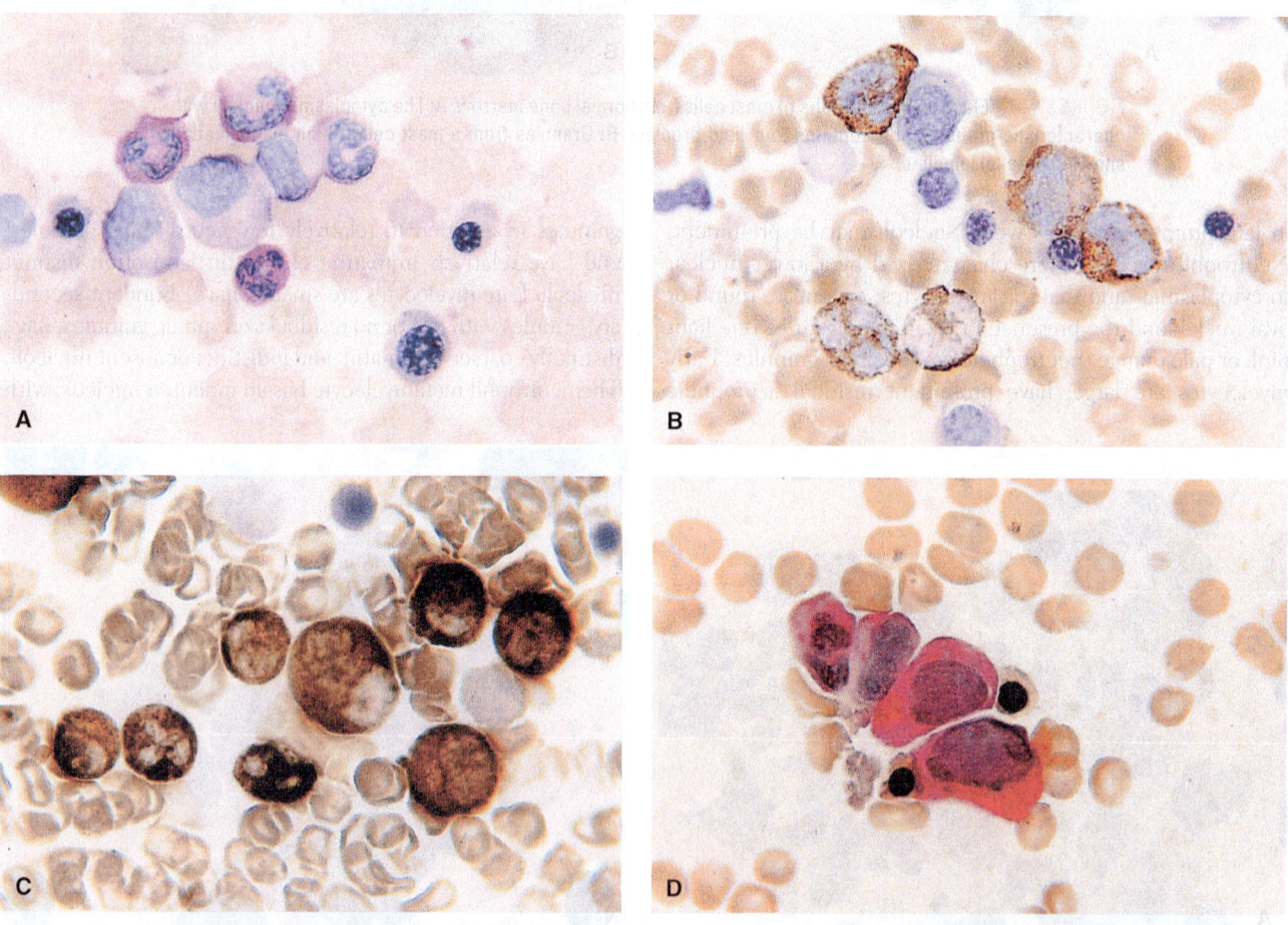

FIGURE 32.23 Cytochemical reactions of neutrophil precursors and neutrophil granulocytes. **A:** Faint PAS positivity in neutrophil myelocytes and stronger positivity in neutrophil granulocytes. The three erythroblasts are PAS negative. **B:** Sudan black positivity in two neutrophil myelocytes, one eosinophil myelocyte, a neutrophil metamyelocyte, and a neutrophil granulocyte. The lymphocytes and erythroblasts are sudanophobic. **C:** Strong peroxidase positivity in neutrophil myelocytes and granulocytes; p-phenylene diamine and catechol were used as the substrate. **D:** Alpha-naphthol AS-D chloroacetate esterase positivity in three neutrophil myelocytes and a neutrophil granulocyte. The two erythroblasts have not stained. The diazonium salt of fast violet-red LB was used as the capture agent.

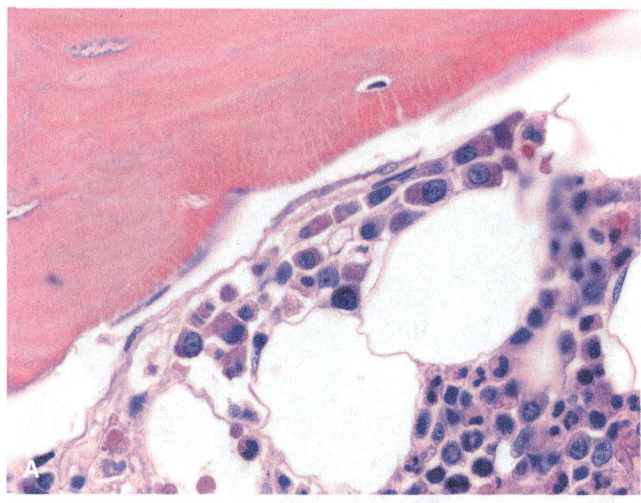
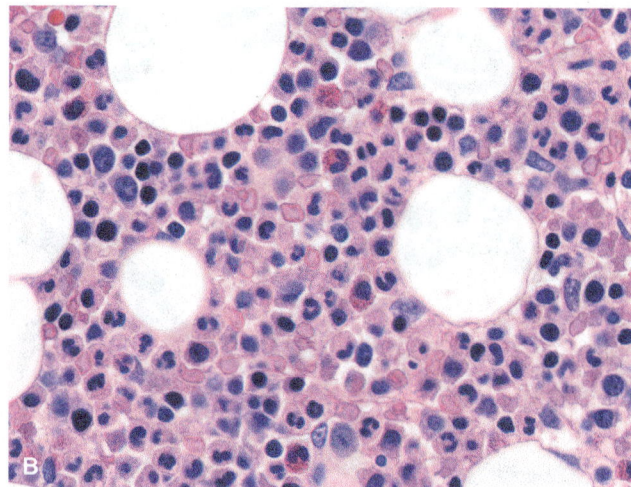
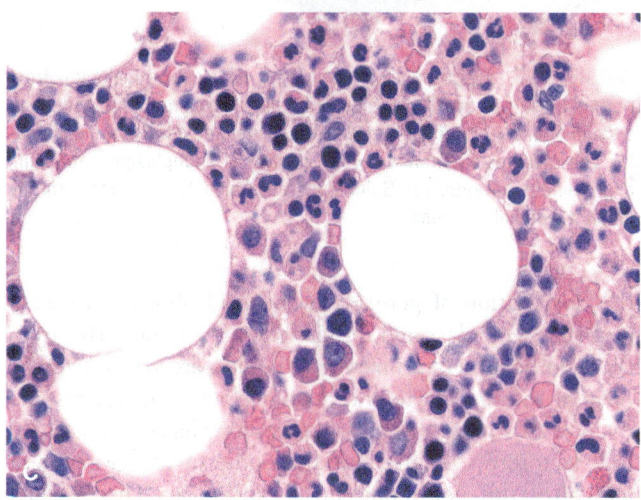

FIGURE 32.24 **A:** Early granulocyte precursors (promyelocyes and myelocytes) immediately adjacent to a bony trabeculum in a marrow trephine section. **B:** Intertrabecular area containing a mixture of neutrophil granulocytes in the more mature stages of maturation (metamyelocytes, bands, and segmented neutrophils) with scattered late-stage erythroid precursors (identifiable by their dense, round nuclei). Several eosinophils are easily distinguished based on their bright red granules. **C:** A few early granulocytes (promyelocytes and myelocytes) are present in the lower center area of this intertrabecular field (H&E).

in cell classes of increasing maturity with the PAS reaction and, to a lesser extent, with Sudan black. Promyelocytes and neutrophil myelocytes, but not neutrophil granulocytes, stain for α-naphthyl acetate esterase activity and, more weakly, for α-naphthyl butyrate esterase activity. Acid phosphatase activity is present in cells at and after the promyelocyte stage; this activity is strongest in the immature cells and weak in neutrophil granulocytes. A few neutrophil metamyelocytes stain weakly for alkaline phosphatase activity, and segmented neutrophil granulocytes stain with a variable intensity (weak to strong) (65–68). Immunocytochemical studies indicate that both lysozyme (muramidase) and elastase are present in promyelocytes and all of the more mature cells of the neutrophil series, and that lactoferrin is present in neutrophil myelocytes, metamyelocytes, and granulocytes.

Biopsy Sections

In marrow sections, early granulocytopoietic cells (myeloblasts and promyelocytes) mainly are found near the endosteum of bone trabeculae and the adventitial aspects of arterioles (Fig. 32.24A). Maturing granulocyte precursors radiate outward from these sites, and the neutrophil granulocytes often are found in the center of intertrabecular areas (Fig. 32.24B), adjacent to sinusoids. A few promyelocytes and myelocytes are present singly or in small clusters at sites away from bone trabeculae and blood vessels (Fig. 32.23C).

Myeloblasts are not identifiable in H&E-stained sections of normal bone marrows. More mature granulocyte precursors are identifiable based on their moderately abundant, granular, eosinophilic cytoplasm (Fig. 32.24). Promyelocytes have round or oval, often eccentric nuclei, finely stippled chromatin, and one to several small, regular nucleoli. Myelocytes are cytologically similar, but have more clumped chromatin and indistinct or absent nucleoli. More mature granulocytic elements are easily identifiable based on their characteristic nuclear conformation, although in histologic sections the fine chromatin strands that join the nuclear lobes of granulocytes usually are not seen. Maturing granulocytic elements may be highlighted by immunohistochemistry for myeloperoxidase (Fig. 32.25).

Ultrastructure

Myeloblasts show no special ultrastructural features (69–72). The nucleus has one or more well-developed nucleoli

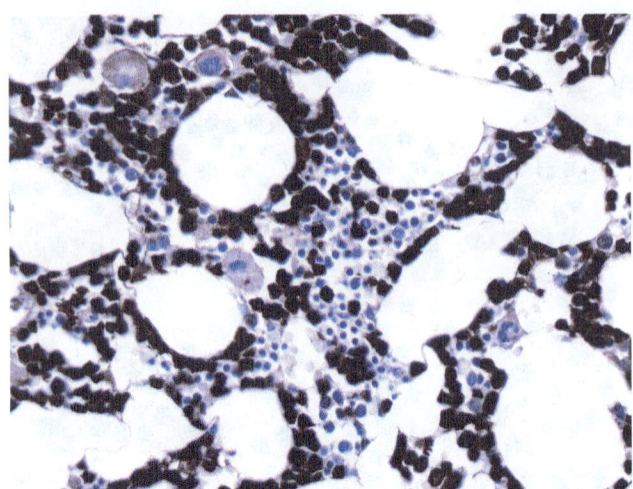

FIGURE 32.25 Immunohistochemistry for myeloperoxidase in a normal marrow section. The maturing granulocytes stain dark brown.

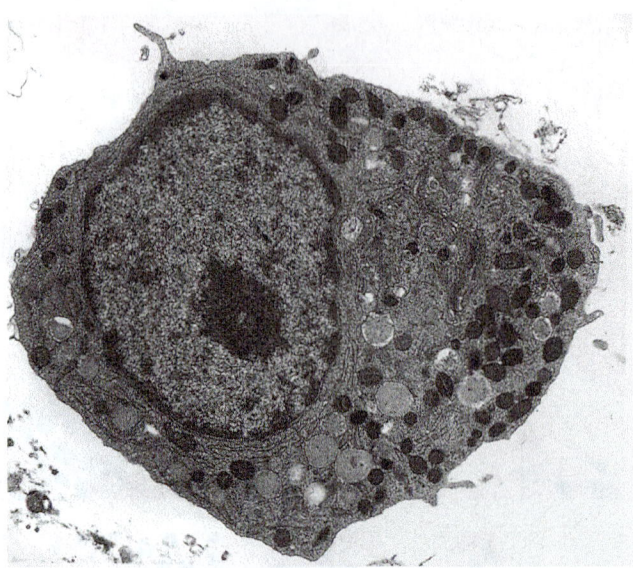

FIGURE 32.26 Electron micrograph of a neutrophil myelocyte from normal bone marrow. The nucleus contains a prominent nucleolus and a small quantity of nuclear membrane–associated condensed chromatin. The cytoplasm contains several strands of endoplasmic reticulum, a prominent paranuclear Golgi apparatus, and two ultrastructurally distinct types of granules.

and shows only slight peripheral chromatin condensation. The cytoplasm contains many ribosomes but only a few strands of endoplasmic reticulum and a poorly developed Golgi apparatus. By contrast, the cytoplasm of a promyelocyte is much more complex, being rich in ribosomes, RER, and mitochondria. It also contains a highly developed Golgi apparatus. During the maturation of a promyelocyte to a neutrophil granulocyte, there is a progressive increase in the degree of condensation of chromatin; a progressive reduction in the quantity of ribosomes, RER, and mitochondria; a diminution of the Golgi apparatus after the myelocyte stage; and the accumulation of large quantities of glycogen at the metamyelocyte and granulocyte stages. The cytoplasm of a promyelocyte characteristically contains variable numbers of immature and mature primary granules. Mature primary granules are elliptical, measure 0.5 to 1.0 μm in their long axis, are electron dense, and contain peroxidase, lysozyme, elastase, α1-antitrypsin, and sulphated mucosubstances. Some have a core with a linear periodic substructure. Ultrastructurally different granules, the secondary granules, are found in addition to primary granules at the neutrophil myelocyte stage (Figs. 32.26 and 32.27). Secondary granules are larger and less electron dense than primary granules, have rounded outlines, tend to undergo a variable degree of extraction, and are only peroxidase positive if a high concentration of diaminobenzidine is used as alkaline pH. They contain lysozyme and vitamin B_{12}–binding protein. Another variety of granule, known as tertiary granules, is present at and after the metamyelocyte stage. These granules are small (0.2 to 0.5 μm in their long axis), pleomorphic (including rounded, elongated, or dumbbell-shaped forms), and peroxidase negative. Their electron density is usually between that of primary and secondary granules (Fig. 32.28). Other electron microscopic cytochemical studies have shown that acid phosphatase is present in primary granules but not in secondary or tertiary granules. The above data on the distribution of peroxidase and acid phosphatase suggest that secondary and tertiary granules do not arise from the modification of primary granules but are synthesized de novo at the myelocyte and metamyelocyte stages, respectively (72). Immunoelectron microscopy has demonstrated that lactoferrin is only found in some of the granules at and after the neutrophil myelocyte stage. The alkaline

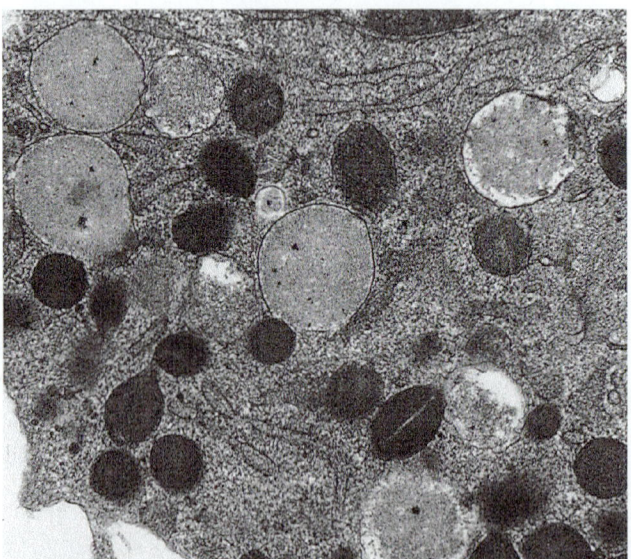

FIGURE 32.27 Part of the cytoplasm of the cell in Figure 32.26 at higher magnification. Two types of granules can be clearly recognized. These are: (a) rounded or elliptical, very electron-dense primary granules (formed at the promyelocyte stage); and (b) larger, rounded, less electron-dense secondary granules (formed at the myelocyte stage).

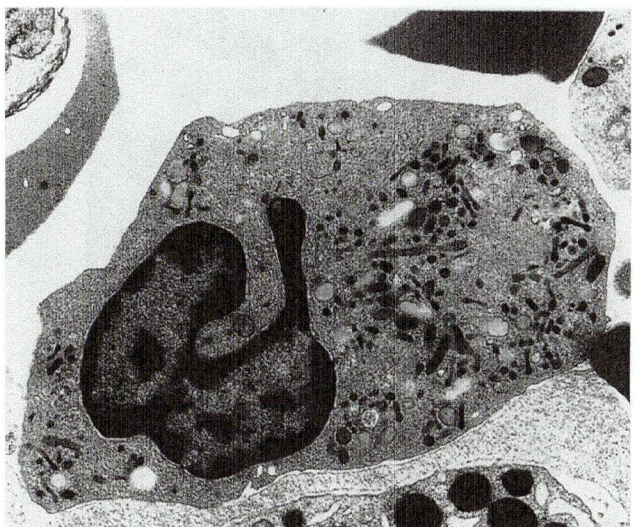

FIGURE 32.28 Electron micrograph of a neutrophil granulocyte from a normal bone marrow. In addition to some primary and secondary granules, the cytoplasm contains several small pleomorphic tertiary granules.

phosphatase activity in neutrophil granulocytes is present within small membrane-bound intracytoplasmic vesicles called phosphosomes.

The primary granules observed with the electron microscope correspond to the azurophilic granules seen in Romanowsky-stained smears, and the secondary and tertiary granules correspond to the neutrophilic or specific granules. Although primary granules are present in all granule-containing cells of the neutrophil series, they lose their azurophilic property and are therefore not detectable by light microscopy at and after the metamyelocyte stage.

Eosinophil and Basophil Precursors

Aspirate Smears

The eosinophil and basophil granulocytes develop through stages that are essentially similar to those through which the neutrophil granulocytes develop. The earliest morphologically recognizable precursors are cells in which a few eosinophil or basophil granules have formed, that is, the eosinophil promyelocytes and basophil promyelocytes. Eosinophil promyelocytes have rounded nuclei with dispersed chromatin and nucleoli and contain two types of granules: large red-orange (eosinophilic) granules and large, dark purple granules (Fig. 32.29A). Eosinophil myelocytes have smaller nuclei with more clumped chromatin, a lower nuclear to cytoplasmic ratio, and predominantly eosinophilic granules with few or no basophilic granules (Fig. 32.29A). Eosinophil metamyelocytes, and granulocytes have only large eosinophilic granules (Fig. 32.29B). Basophil myelocytes, metamyelocytes, and granulocytes are characterized by the presence of large, round, deeply basophilic granules that often overlie the nucleus (Fig. 32.30); the more mature granules stain metachromatically with toluidine blue. The majority of circulating eosinophil and basophil granulocytes have two nuclear segments.

Cytochemistry

The granules of eosinophil and basophil granulocytes and their precursors do not stain by the PAS reaction (68,73). However, PAS-positive deposits are found between the specific granules in both cell lineages. The periphery of the eosinophil granules of all cells of the eosinophil series stains strongly with Sudan black, and the core stains weakly or not at all. Basophil granules are strongly sudanophilic in basophil promyelocytes and myelocytes, but the degree of sudanophilia decreases with increasing maturity; in mature

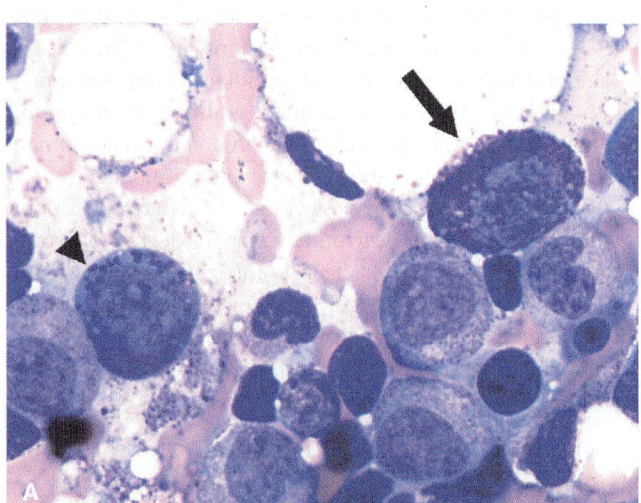
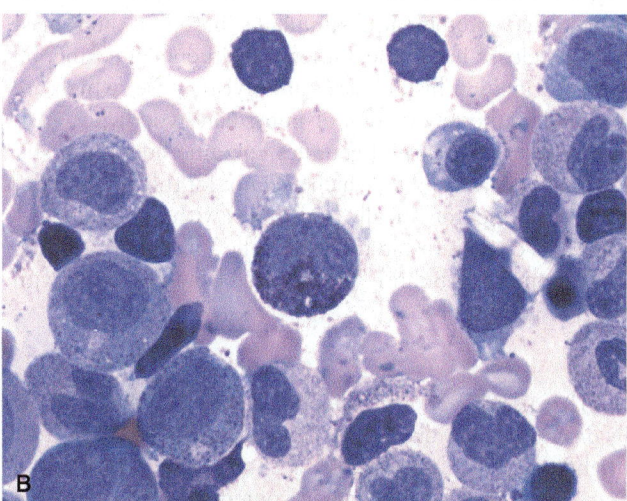

FIGURE 32.29 **A:** An eosinophil promyelocyte (*arrowhead*) and an eosinophil myelocyte (*arrow*) in in a normal Wright–Giemsa-stained bone marrow aspirate smear. Note the presence of both eosinophilic granules and dark basophilic granules in the eosinophil promyelocytes. **B:** An eosinophil metamyelocyte (*center*).

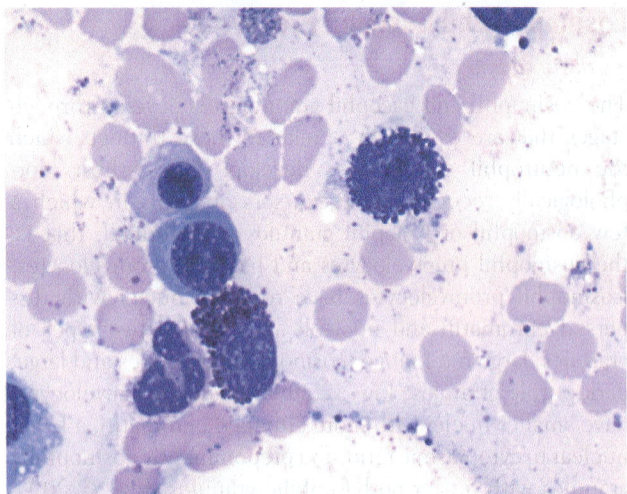

FIGURE 32.30 A basophil metamyelocyte from a Wright–Giemsa-stained normal marrow smear (*upper right*). A late eosinophil myelocyte is also present (*lower left*).

basophils, the granules either do not stain or stain metachromatically (reddish). Peroxidase and acid phosphatase, but not lysozyme, are demonstrable in the eosinophil granules in all eosinophil precursors and eosinophils. Human eosinophil peroxidase is biochemically and immunochemically distinct from myeloperoxidase, the type of peroxidase present in the neutrophil series. In the basophil series, the granules are strongly positive for peroxidase in basophil promyelocytes and myelocytes, weakly positive in basophil metamyelocytes, and almost negative in basophil granulocytes. Basophil granules stain positively for acid phosphatase. Basophil and eosinophil granulocytes are essentially negative for α-naphthol AS-D chloroacetate esterase and α-naphthyl butyrate esterase.

Eosinophil granules contain eosinophil cationic proteins and an arginine- and zinc-rich major basic protein that are involved in the killing of metazoan parasites. The major basic protein also stimulates basophils and mast cells to release histamine. Other constituents of eosinophil granules include histaminase and arylsulfatase, which are involved in the modulation of immediate-type hypersensitivity reactions. Basophil granules contain chondroitin sulfate and heparin sulfate, which account for their property of staining metachromatically (red-violet) with toluidine blue. They also contain histamine, one of the substances released when immunoglobulin E (IgE)-coated basophils react with specific antigen.

Biopsy Sections

In H&E tissue sections, eosinophils and precursors are easily discriminated from other cellular elements based on their bright red, refractile granules (Fig. 32.24B). Because basophil granules are water soluble, their contents become extracted during routine fixation for histologic studies. Consequently, basophil granulocytes cannot be seen in histologic sections processed in the usual way.

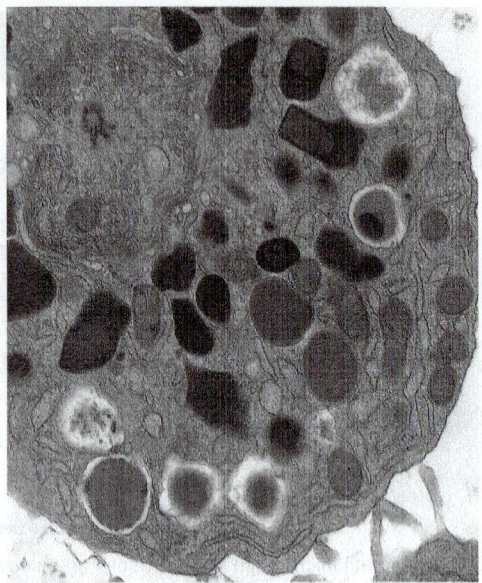

FIGURE 32.31 Electron micrograph of part of the cytoplasm of an early eosinophil myelocyte. A centriole surrounded by well-developed Golgi saccules, several strands of rough endoplasmic reticulum, and a number of large granules are seen. Some of the granules are homogeneously electron dense (primary granules), but others have a central crystalloid (secondary granules).

Ultrastructure

On the basis of their electron microscopic features, two types of eosinophil granules, termed primary and secondary granules, are recognized (69,74). Primary granules are large, rounded, homogeneous, and electron dense, and secondary granules contain a central electron-dense crystalloid inclusion consisting largely of polymerized major basic protein. It is generally held that the primary granules mature into secondary granules. Early eosinophil promyelocytes contain only primary granules, but more mature promyelocytes contain many primary and a few secondary granules. Eosinophil myelocytes contain some primary and several secondary granules (Fig. 32.31). By contrast, the majority of the granules in eosinophil metamyelocytes and granulocytes are secondary granules (Fig. 32.32). The primary granules of eosinophil promyelocytes are larger and more rounded than the primary granules of neutrophil promyelocytes and promonocytes.

Cells of the basophil series contain characteristic basophil granules, which are prone to undergo varying degrees of extraction during processing for electron microscopy (Fig. 32.33). Basophil granules are made up of numerous, closely packed, fine rounded particles (Fig. 32.34); the particles are about 20 nm in diameter in mature basophils and slightly smaller in basophil promyelocytes and myelocytes.

Monocyte Precursors

Aspirate Smears

Immature monocytic cells are often designated as "monoblasts" and "promonocytes." However, it is worth noting that

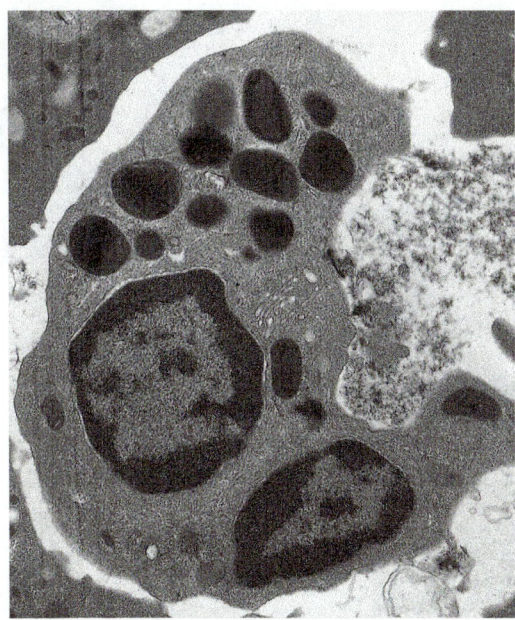

FIGURE 32.32 Electron micrograph of an eosinophil granulocyte from normal bone marrow. The majority of the cytoplasmic granules are crystalloid-containing secondary granules. Note that the uppermost granule is unusual in that its crystalloid stains more lightly than the surrounding granule matrix.

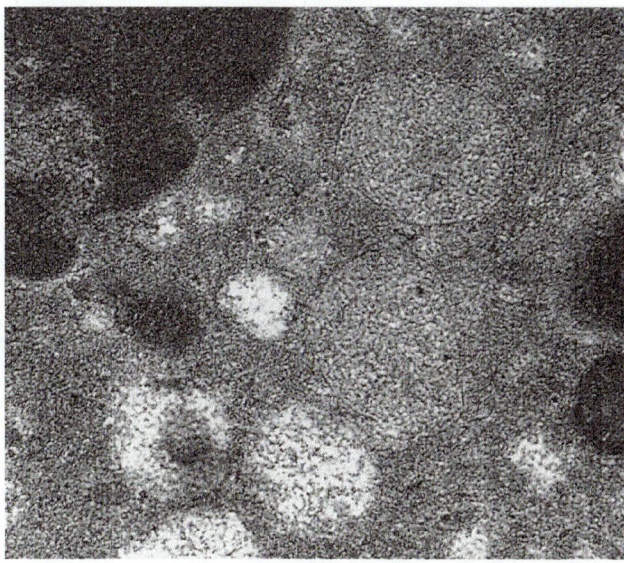

FIGURE 32.34 Electron micrograph illustrating the particulate ultrastructure of basophil granules at high magnification.

the monoblasts and promonocytes seen in acute myeloid leukemias do not closely resemble any normal marrow precursor, and thus the use of these terms to describe monocytic precursors in normal marrows may be misleading. Blood monocytes are not end cells but develop further in the tissues to become macrophages. Certain data suggest that macrophages and osteoclasts have a common progenitor. All these cells are considered to constitute the mononuclear phagocyte system.

In normal marrows, monocytes (and immature monocytes) are inconspicuous, but they may increase in number in reactive and regenerative states. Monoblasts are not identifiable with certainty in Romanowky-stained marrow smears, although blastic cells exhibiting monocytic differentiation may be identified with cytochemical stains (Fig. 32.35). The most immature identifiable monocytes in marrow smears are large cells with mildly indented nuclei, slightly coarse chromatin, small or inconspicuous nucleoli, and small amounts of moderately basophilic cytoplasm containing few or no identifiable granules (Fig. 32.36). As

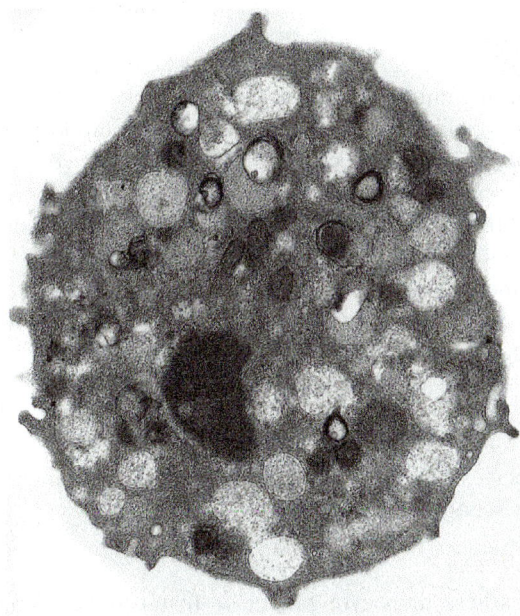

FIGURE 32.33 Electron micrograph of a basophil granulocyte from a normal bone marrow. The granules have been markedly extracted during processing, but the characteristic closely packed rounded particles can still be recognized in several of the granules.

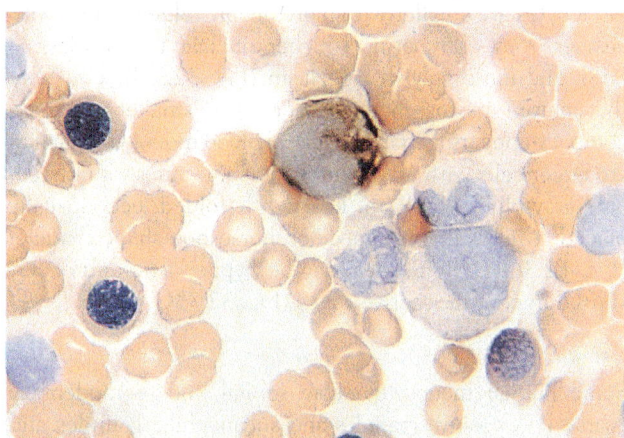

FIGURE 32.35 A cell with strong α-naphthyl acetate esterase activity from a normal marrow smear (the diazonium salt of fast blue BB was used as the capture agent). This cell has a slightly convoluted nucleus and relatively little cytoplasm and is most probably a monoblast or early promonocyte.

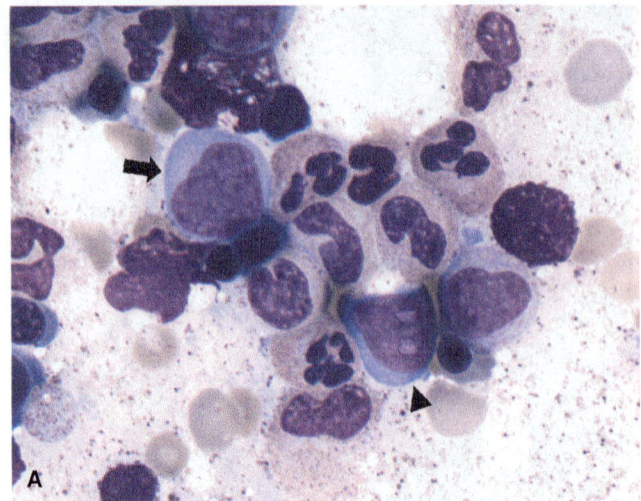
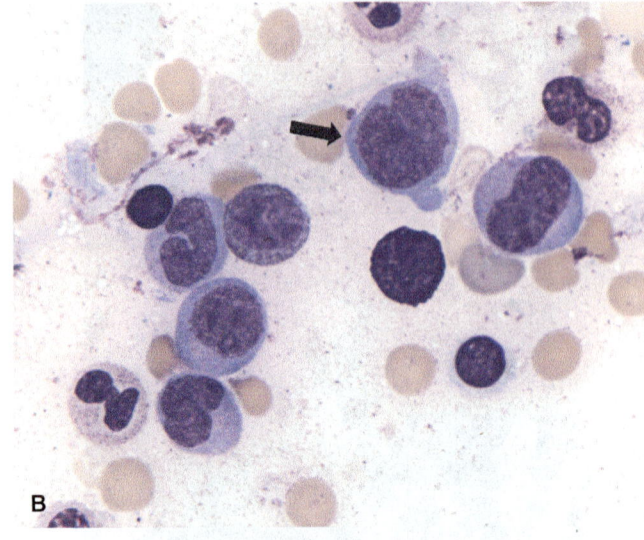
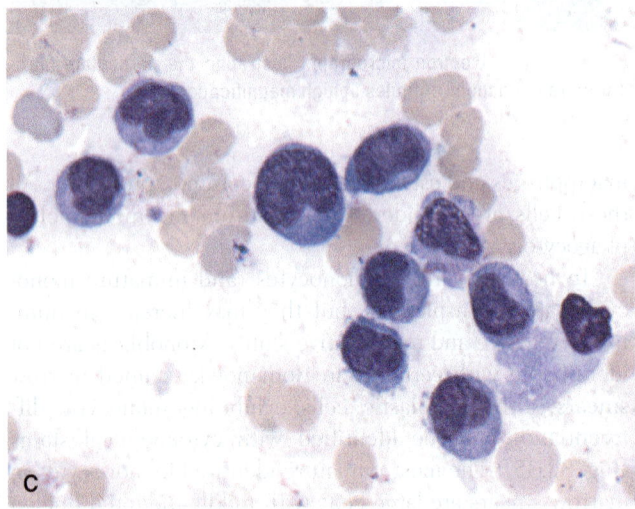

FIGURE 32.36 Monocyte maturation (Wright–Giemsa). **A:** An early monocyte precursor (*arrow*). Compare to the myeloblast also in the field (*arrowhead*) **B:** Immature monocyte (*arrow*), with a more mature form to the right and slightly below. A vertical array of monocytic cells is also evident in the left part of the field. From bottom to top: Mature marrow monocytes, immature monocyte, blood monocyte. **C:** An immature monocyte, accompanied by an array of mature marrow monocytes in this example of marrow monocyte hyperplasia.

they mature, the nuclei become more obviously indented; the cytoplasm remains basophilic, but is more abundant with more obvious granularity (Fig. 32.36). Mature marrow monocytes are smaller with more deeply folded nuclei with coarser, ropy chromatin, a higher nuclear to cytoplasmic ratio, and more grayish cytoplasm (Fig. 32.36B, C). Note that mature marrow monocytes are often smaller and more compact-appearing than peripheral blood monocytes, which are larger cells with more abundant, sometimes vacuolated, pale gray-blue cytoplasm, less tightly folded, eccentrically placed, oval, kidney-shaped, or horseshoe-shaped nuclei (Fig. 32.36B). Monocytes may be hyperplastic and/or left shifted in certain reactive states (Fig. 32.36C) (75).

Cytochemistry

Some normal monocytes show several fine or moderately coarse PAS-positive granules and sudanophilic granules and a few peroxidase-positive granules scattered in their cytoplasm (65,68,76). Monocytes do not stain for alkaline phosphatase, but stain strongly for acid phosphatase. They contain lysozyme.

Monocytes are α-naphthol AS-D chloroacetate esterase negative but are α-naphthyl acetate esterase (nonspecific esterase) positive. Alpha-naphthyl acetate esterase activity is present not only in monocytes and macrophages, but also in other myeloid cells, including neutrophil promyelocytes and myelocytes, megakaryocytes, and immature red cell precursors. Alpha-naphthyl butyrate esterase activity is stronger than α-naphthyl acetate esterase activity in monocytes and macrophages and is much weaker in the other types of myeloid cells mentioned above. Both the α-naphthyl acetate and the α-naphthyl butyrate esterase activities of monocytes are inhibited by fluoride; in granulocytes and their precursors, these enzyme activities are fluoride insensitive.

Biopsy Sections

Monocytes are not identifiable with certainty in normal biopsy sections.

Ultrastructure

The earliest monocyte precursor that can be identified on ultrastructural criteria (69,72) is the promonocyte. The nucleus of this cell has only small quantities of nuclear membrane–associated condensed chromatin, and has one or more nucleoli. The cytoplasm contains many ribosomes, a moderate number of mitochondria, several strands of RER, bundles of fibrils, a prominent Golgi apparatus, and a few characteristic cytoplasmic granules. The strands of endoplasmic reticulum are shorter and less abundant than in neutrophil promyelocytes. Two types of cytoplasmic granules are seen in promonocytes: (a) immature granules, which have a central zone of flocculent electron-dense material and a clear peripheral zone; and (b) mature granules, which are smaller than the immature granules, vary considerably in size and shape, and are homogeneously electron dense. The maturation of promonocytes first into marrow monocytes and then into blood monocytes is associated with some increase in the quantity of condensed chromatin in the nucleus, a progressive reduction in the number of ribosomes, RER, and fibrils in the cytoplasm, and an increase in the number of cytoplasmic granules. Most or all of the granules of marrow monocytes and all the granules of blood monocytes are of the mature type. Ultrastructural cytochemical studies have shown that some large round granules have acid phosphatase activity and that such granules are more frequent in promonocytes than monocytes. All the promonocyte granules and some of the monocyte granules are peroxidase positive.

Red Cell Precursors

Aspirate Smears

In this chapter, the term *erythroblast* is used to describe any nucleated red cell precursor, normal or pathologic, and the term *normoblast* to describe all cells that have the morphologic characteristics of the erythroblasts found in normal bone marrow. The terms used to describe various classes of normal red cell precursor are, in order of increasing maturity, pronormoblast, basophilic normoblast, early polychromatic normoblast, late polychromatic normoblast, marrow reticulocyte, and blood reticulocyte (Fig. 32.37). Cell division occurs only in the first three of these cytologic classes.

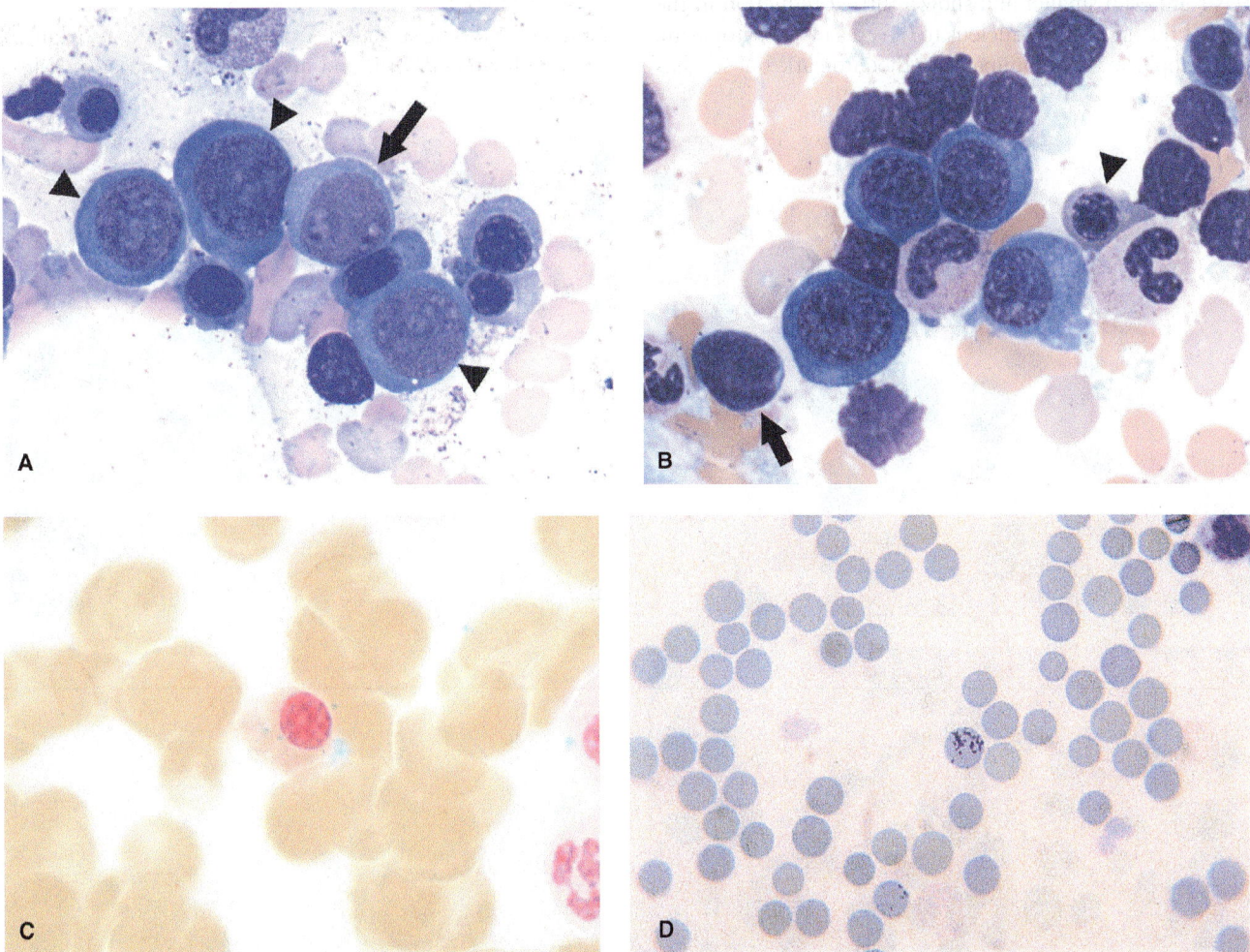

FIGURE 32.37 Red cell precursors from a normal Wright-Giemsa-stained bone marrow smear (**A–C**) and a reticulocyte from normal peripheral blood (**D**). **A:** Three pronormoblasts (*arrowheads*) and five polychromatophilic normoblasts. A myeloblast (*arrow*) is also present. **B:** Four basophilic normoblasts and a late polychromatic normoblast (*arrowhead*). Also present is a hematogone (maturing B-cell precursor, *arrow*) **C:** A sideroblast showing two fine, blue siderotic granules. (**A** and **B**, Wright–Giemsa stain; **C**, Perls' acid ferrocyanide reaction; **D**, supravital staining with brilliant cresyl blue.)

Marrow samples containing normoblasts are said to show normoblastic erythropoiesis.

Pronormoblasts are large cells with a diameter of 12 to 20 μm. They have distinctly round nuclei and have moderate amounts of deeply basophilic, agranular cytoplasm distributed as an even rim around the nucleus. The chromatin has a finely stippled appearance, and there are one or more prominent, irregular nucleoli. The basophilic normoblasts resemble pronormoblasts except that their chromatin is slightly more condensed and consequently has a coarsely granular appearance. The early polychromatic normoblasts are smaller than basophilic normoblasts and have a smaller nucleus and a lower nucleus-to-cytoplasm ratio. The cytoplasm is polychromatic and agranular, and the nucleus contains several medium-sized clumps of condensed chromatin, particularly adjacent to the nuclear membrane. The polychromasia results from the presence of moderate quantities of cytoplasmic RNA (which stains blue), as well as of hemoglobin (which stains red). Late polychromatic normoblasts are even smaller and show a further reduction in the ratio of the area of the nucleus to the area of the cytoplasm. The cytoplasm is predominantly orthochromatic but still has a grayish tinge (i.e., is faintly polychromatic). The nucleus is small and eccentric and contains large clumps of condensed chromatin. The nuclear diameter is less than about 6.5 μm. When mature, late polychromatic normoblasts extrude their nuclei and become marrow reticulocytes; the extruded nuclei are rapidly phagocytosed and degraded by adjacent macrophages. The marrow reticulocyte is irregular in outline and has faintly polychromatic cytoplasm. It is motile and soon enters the marrow sinusoids. When marrow and blood reticulocytes are stained supravitally with brilliant cresyl blue, the ribosomal RNA responsible for their polychromasia precipitates into a basophilic reticulum (hence the term *reticulocyte*). Reticulocytes circulate in the blood for 1 to 2 days before becoming mature red cells. The average volume of blood reticulocytes is 20% larger than that of red cells. The latter are circular, biconcave, and acidophilic (i.e., stain red) and, in dried fixed smears, have an average diameter of 7.2 μm (range: 6.7 to 7.7 μm).

Cytochemistry

Normal erythroblasts are PAS negative. They also fail to stain with Sudan black and are peroxidase negative. Most

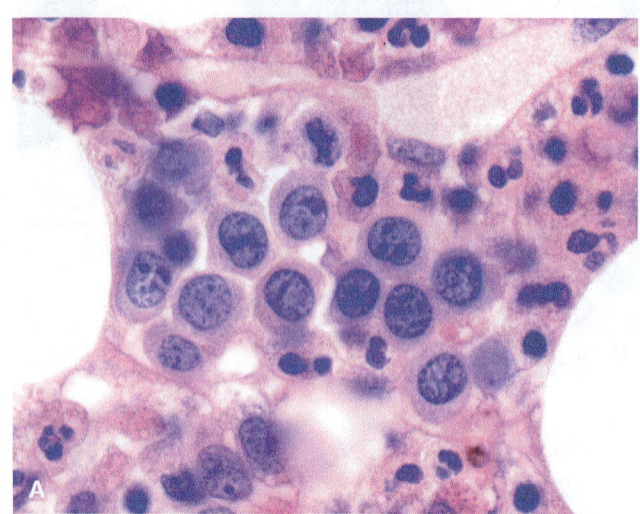
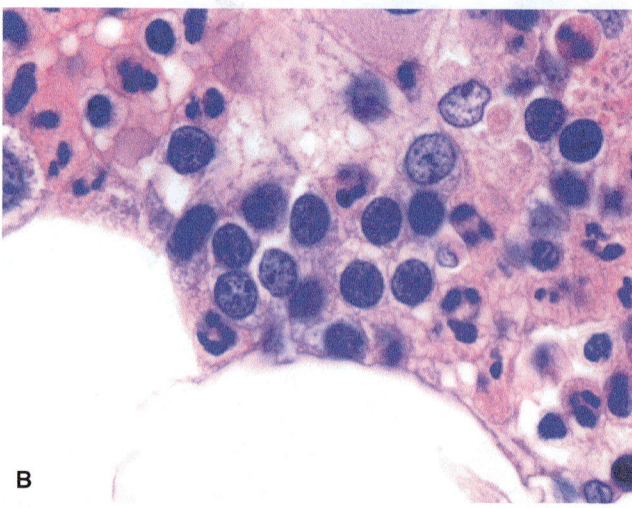
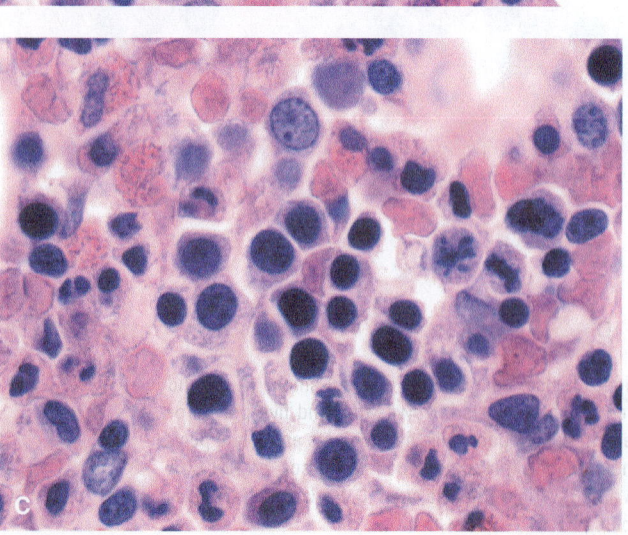

FIGURE 32.38 Erythroid islands in a marrow trephine section. Early (**A**), intermediate (**B**), and intermediate-to late (**C**) erythroid precursors.

nucleated red cells are α-naphthol AS-D chloroacetate esterase negative, but occasional cells show a few positive granules. A few α-naphthol butyrate esterase positive granules are seen in some nucleated red cells of all degrees of maturity; the positive granules are sometimes seen at the nuclear margin. Coarse acid phosphatase–positive paranuclear granules are frequently present in all types of erythroblasts.

In normal bone marrow smears stained by Perls' acid ferrocyanide method, 30% to 50% of the polychromatic erythroblasts contain one to five small blue granules that are usually just visible at high magnification (Fig. 32.37C). These iron-containing (siderotic) granules are randomly distributed within the cytoplasm and correspond to the siderosomes seen under the electron microscope. Erythroblasts containing siderotic granules are termed *sideroblasts*. In iron deficiency anemia and anemia of chronic disease (anemia of inflammation), the percentage of sideroblasts is decreased, or sideroblasts may be altogether absent. In conditions associated with an increased percentage saturation of transferrin (e.g., hemolytic anemias), the percentage of sideroblasts, the average number of siderotic granules per cell, and the average size of such granules are increased.

Biopsy Sections

In marrow sections, erythroblasts of varying degrees of maturity are found in aggregates or islands (Fig. 32.38). Pronormoblasts and basophilic normoblasts are large cells with round nuclei with sharp nuclear membranes, distinctly stippled chromatin and irregular nucleoli. Their cytoplasm is densely amphophilic, in contrast to the granular eosinophilic appearance of early granulocyte precursors. The late erythroblasts contain round, heavily stained nuclei showing little structural detail, and have moderate quantities of poorly staining cytoplasm, usually with a distinct cytoplasmic membrane. Intermediate to late erythroblasts can be reliably identified by immunohistochemical staining for glycophorin A or hemoglobin A (Table 32.1, Fig. 32.39).

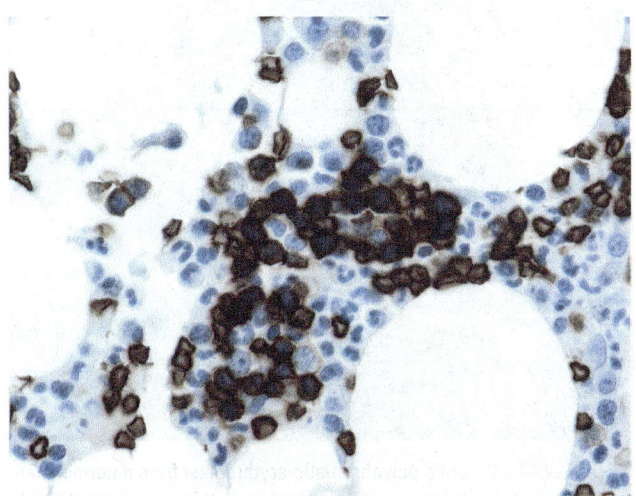

FIGURE 32.39 Immunohistochemistry for glycophorin A highlighting both maturing normoblasts and mature erythrocytes.

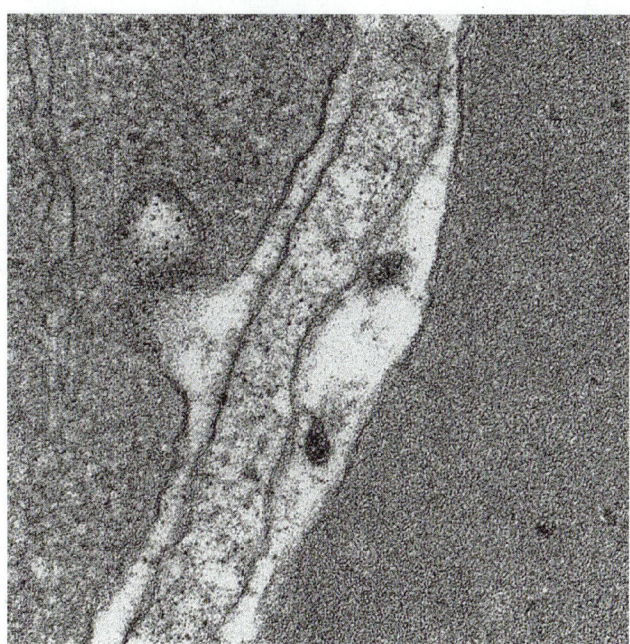

FIGURE 32.40 Part of an early polychromatic erythroblast showing a rhopheocytotic surface invagination with a few adherent ferritin molecules. A rhopheocytotic vesicle containing several ferritin molecules is closely apposed to the surface invagination. A narrow process of ferritin-containing macrophage cytoplasm is present between the erythroblast displaying rhopheocytosis and the adjacent cell.

Normal pronormoblasts should lack both of these antigens, but are positive for E-cadherin, which is absent in more mature forms (77). CD71 may be used to identify all stages of erythroblasts (78).

Ultrastructure

All nucleated red cell precursors are characterized by the presence of small surface invaginations that develop into intracytoplasmic vesicles (rhopheocytotic vesicles) (69) (Fig. 32.40). The nucleus of the pronormoblast has a small quantity of nuclear membrane–associated condensed chromatin (Fig. 32.41). The cytoplasm is of low-electron density and contains numerous ribosomes, a moderately well-developed Golgi apparatus, several mitochondria, some strands of endoplasmic reticulum, and small numbers of scattered ferritin molecules. It also contains a few pleomorphic electron-dense acid phosphatase–positive lysosomal granules, which are usually arranged in a group near the Golgi saccules. During the maturation of a pronormoblast into a late polychromatic normoblast (Fig. 32.42), the following changes are seen: (a) a steady increase in the quantity of condensed chromatin; (b) a gradual increase in the electron density of the cytoplasmic matrix due to the synthesis of increasing quantities of hemoglobin; (c) a progressive reduction in the number of ribosomes in the cytoplasm; (d) a reduction in the number and size of the mitochondria; and (e) an increasing tendency for some of the intracytoplasmic ferritin molecules to aggregate and form siderosomes (Figs. 32.43 and 32.44). Small autophagic vacuoles are

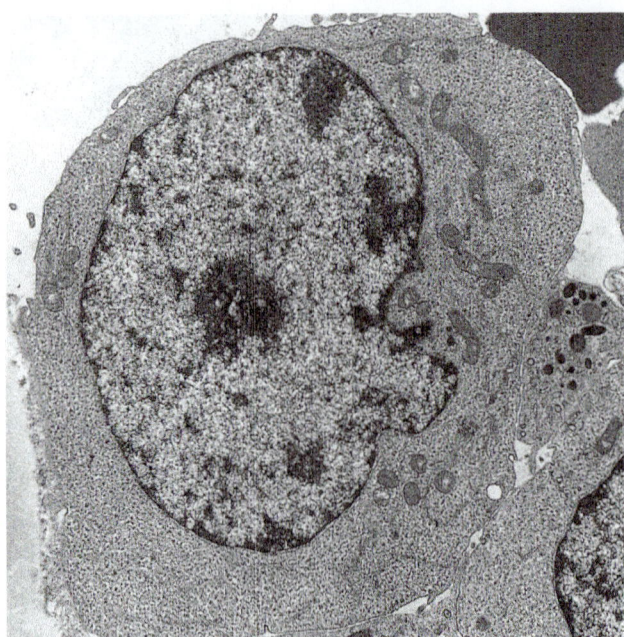

FIGURE 32.41 Electron micrograph of a pronormoblast from normal bone marrow. The nucleus contains very small quantities of condensed chromatin and has a prominent nucleolus. The cytoplasm is relatively electron lucent and rich in polyribosomes.

found in 22% and slight to substantial degrees of myelinization of the nuclear membrane in 12% of erythroblast profiles (79). Other data shown by electron microscopic studies of the erythron are that: (a) part of the cell's cytoplasmic membrane and a narrow rim of hemoglobin-containing cytoplasm completely surrounds the extruded erythroblast nucleus (Fig. 32.45); (b) the marrow reticulocytes enter the sinusoids by passing through, rather than between, endothelial cells; and (c) whereas reticulocytes contain ribosomes and mitochondria, mature red cells do not.

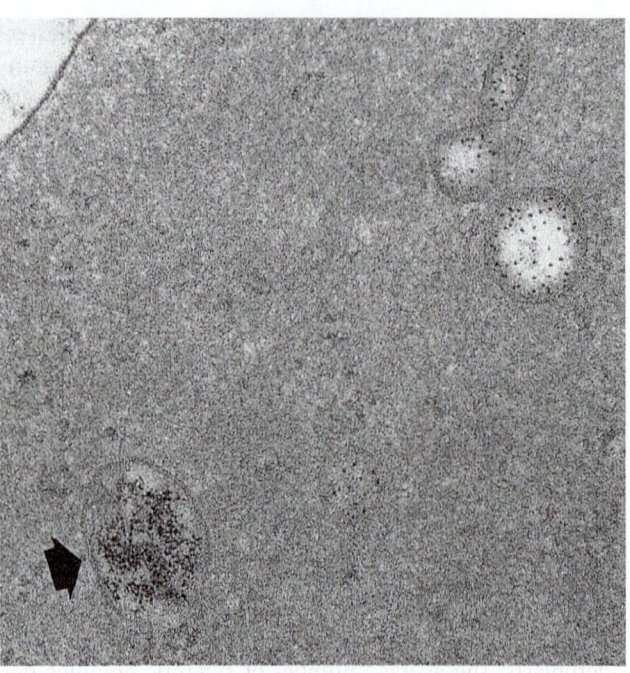

FIGURE 32.43 Electron micrograph of part of the cytoplasm of a polychromatic erythroblast from normal bone marrow. The cytoplasm shows a membrane-bound accumulation of ferritin and hemosiderin (siderosome) (*arrow*) and a few ferritin-containing rhopheocytotic vesicles.

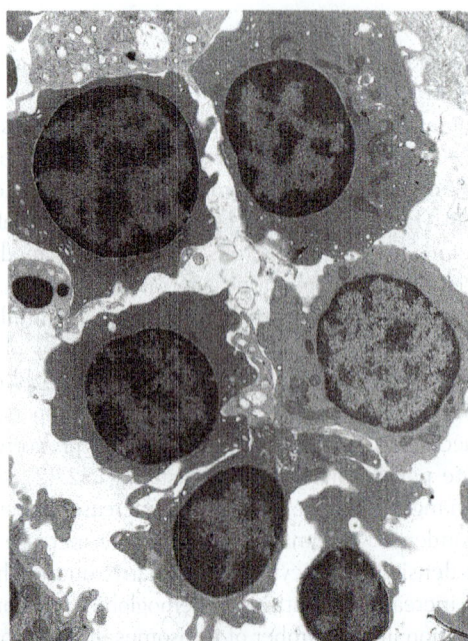

FIGURE 32.42 Electron micrograph of a group of six erythroblasts at various stages of maturation. Note that maturation is associated with an increase in the electron density of the cytoplasm. The lowermost cell is a late erythroblast about to extrude its nucleus.

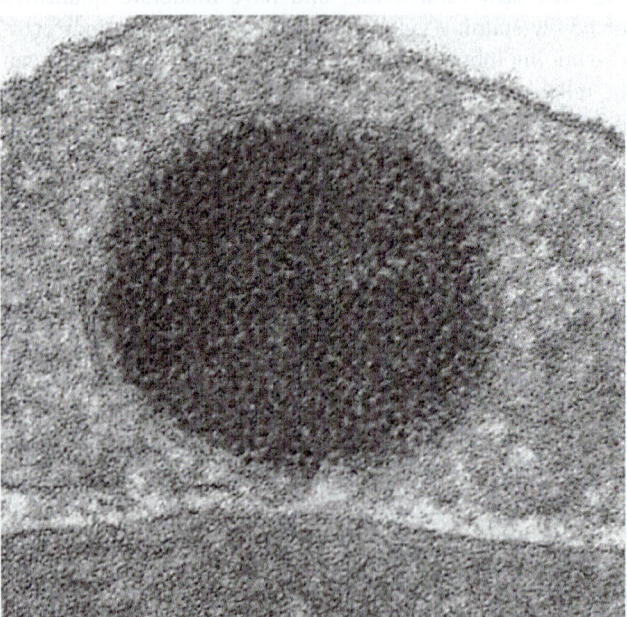

FIGURE 32.44 Part of a polychromatic erythroblast from a normal marrow showing a membrane-bound siderosome that is much more densely packed with ferritin and hemosiderin molecules than the siderosome in Figure 32.43.

CHAPTER 32: Bone Marrow

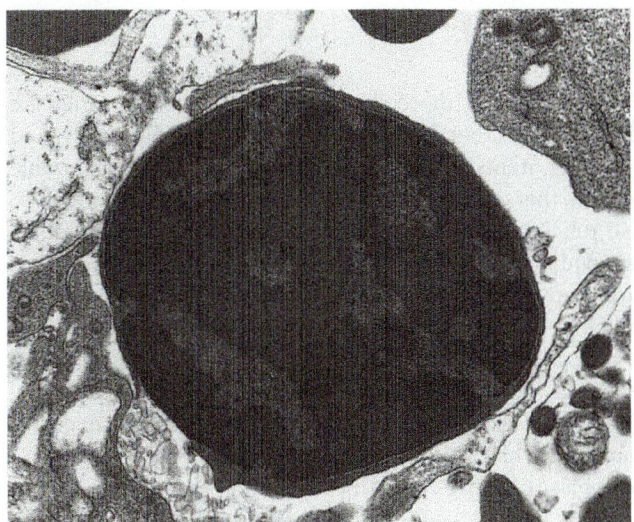

FIGURE 32.45 Electron micrograph of an extruded erythroblast nucleus. Note that the nucleus is surrounded by a rim of hemoglobin-containing cytoplasm and lies in close contact with processes of macrophage cytoplasm.

Dyserythropoiesis and Ineffective Erythropoiesis

Most of the erythroblasts in normal bone marrow are uninucleate and do not display any unusual morphologic features. However, when 400 to 1,000 consecutive erythroblasts (excluding mitoses) were studied in bone marrow smears from each of 10 healthy volunteers with stainable iron in the bone marrow, 0% to 0.57% (mean: 0.31%) were found to be binucleate, 0.7% to 4.8% (mean: 2.4%) showed intererythroblastic cytoplasmic bridges, 0% to 0.9% (mean: 0.24%) showed cytoplasmic stippling, and 0% to 0.7% (mean: 0.39%) showed cytoplasmic vacuolation. In addition, 0% to 0.55% (mean: 0.22%) had markedly irregular nuclear outlines or karyorrhectic nuclei, and 0% to 0.39% (mean: 0.18%) contained Howell–Jolly bodies (micronuclei), a marker of chromosome breaks (Fig. 32.46) (80). In another study of 15 healthy males in which 5,000 erythroid cells (including mitoses) were assessed per subject, 0.14% ± 0.04 (SD) were found to be binucleate or multinucleate cells or to be pluripolar mitoses (81). When there is increased erythropoietin (either endogenously or exogenously), in addition to an expansion of the number of erythroid precursors, there may be a shift toward

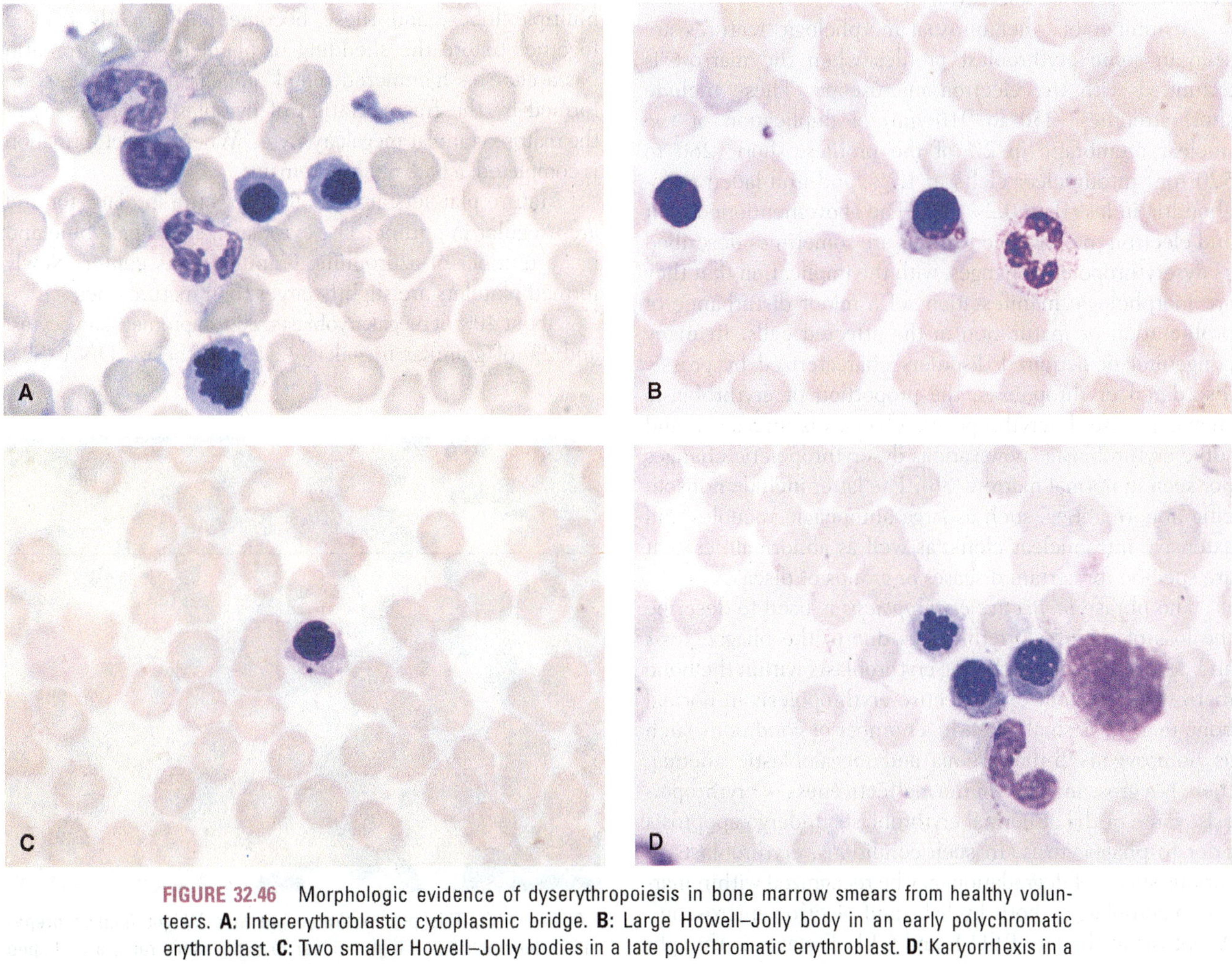

FIGURE 32.46 Morphologic evidence of dyserythropoiesis in bone marrow smears from healthy volunteers. **A:** Intererythroblastic cytoplasmic bridge. **B:** Large Howell–Jolly body in an early polychromatic erythroblast. **C:** Two smaller Howell–Jolly bodies in a late polychromatic erythroblast. **D:** Karyorrhexis in a late polychromatic erythroblast.

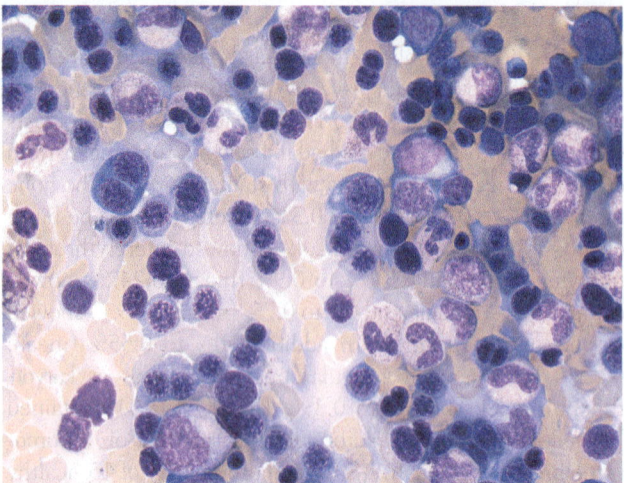

FIGURE 32.47 Erythroid hyperplasia in a patient with hemolytic anemia. There are multiple binucleate erythroid precursors and one with nuclear irregularity (*center*).

immaturity, increased binucleation, megaloblastoid change (dyssynchrony between nuclear and cytoplasmic maturation), and nuclear irregularity of the late-stage nucleated red cells (terminal dyserythropoiesis)(Fig. 32.47).

A number of other unusual morphologic features are seen in some erythroblast profiles when the marrow is examined with the electron microscope. These include short stretches (250 to 910 nm) of duplication of the nuclear membrane in 2% of the profiles, short (260 to 520 nm) intranuclear clefts in 1.7%, and iron-laden mitochondria in less than 0.2% (79). The abovementioned light and electron microscopic features are sometimes described as dyserythropoietic changes, with the implication that they are morphologic manifestations of a minor disturbance of proliferation or maturation in the affected cells. In many congenital or acquired disorders characterized by grossly disordered erythropoiesis, the proportion of erythroblasts showing these dyserythropoietic changes is increased, and some erythroblasts show various dyserythropoietic changes not seen in normal marrow (36). The latter include nonspecific abnormalities, such as large autophagic vacuoles and extensive intranuclear clefts, as well as abnormalities that are specific for certain diseases or groups of diseases.

The phrase *ineffective erythropoiesis* is used to describe the loss of potential erythrocytes due to the phagocytosis and destruction of developing erythroblasts within the bone marrow. The extent of ineffective erythropoiesis in normal bone marrow is small (19). In a number of conditions such as homozygous β-thalassemia and megaloblastic anemia, there is a gross increase in the ineffectiveness of erythropoiesis; some of the abnormal erythroblasts undergo apoptosis prior to phagocytosis. In such conditions, erythroblasts at various stages of degradation may be recognized within marrow macrophages, both by light and electron microscopy. Apoptosis at the late BFU-E and CFU-E stages is thought to be a major factor controlling the rate of erythropoiesis.

Megakaryocytes

Aspirate Smears

The majority of the cells of the megakaryocyte series are larger than other hematopoietic cells and have polyploid DNA contents. The earliest morphologically recognizable cells in this series are called megakaryoblasts. These are 20 to 30 μm in diameter and have a single large, oval, kidney-shaped, or lobed nucleus that is surrounded by a narrow rim of intensely basophilic agranular cytoplasm. The nucleus contains several nucleoli. Megakaryoblasts (group I megakaryocytes) mature into promegakaryocytes (group II megakaryocytes), which in turn develop into granular megakaryocytes (group III megakaryocytes). Promegakaryocytes are larger than megakaryoblasts and have a larger volume of cytoplasm relative to that of the nucleus (Fig. 32.48). They possess a single large multilobed nucleus with the overlapping lobes arranged in a C-shaped formation. The cytoplasm is less basophilic than that of megakaryoblasts and contains a few azurophilic granules that are usually grouped within the concavity formed by the overlapping nuclear lobes. The granular megakaryocytes (Fig. 32.49) are up to 100 μm in diameter and have abundant pale-staining cytoplasm containing many lavender-colored granules. The nucleus has multiple lobes, and these become fairly tightly packed together before the shedding of platelets. The chromatin has a coarse, "hammered metal" appearance. Platelets are formed by the fragmentation of cytoplasmic processes of the mature granular megakaryocytes. When platelet formation is completed, a bare nucleus remains.

Mature platelets are usually 2 to 3 μm in diameter and are irregular in outline. The cytoplasm stains pale blue and has a number of azurophilic granules at its center. Newly formed platelets are slightly larger than mature ones.

About 40% of megakaryoblasts, 20% of promegakaryocytes, and 2% of granular megakaryocytes synthesize DNA (82).

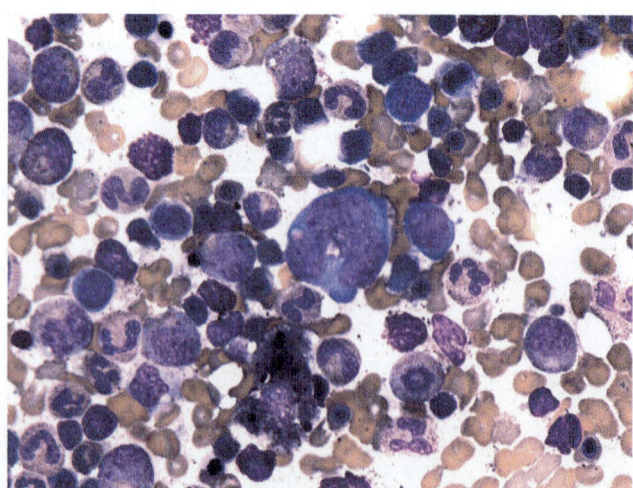

FIGURE 32.48 This promegakaryocyte in a Wright–Giemsa preparation demonstrates a high nuclear to cytoplasmic ratio, a C-shaped nucleus, and basophilic cytoplasm devoid of lavender granulation.

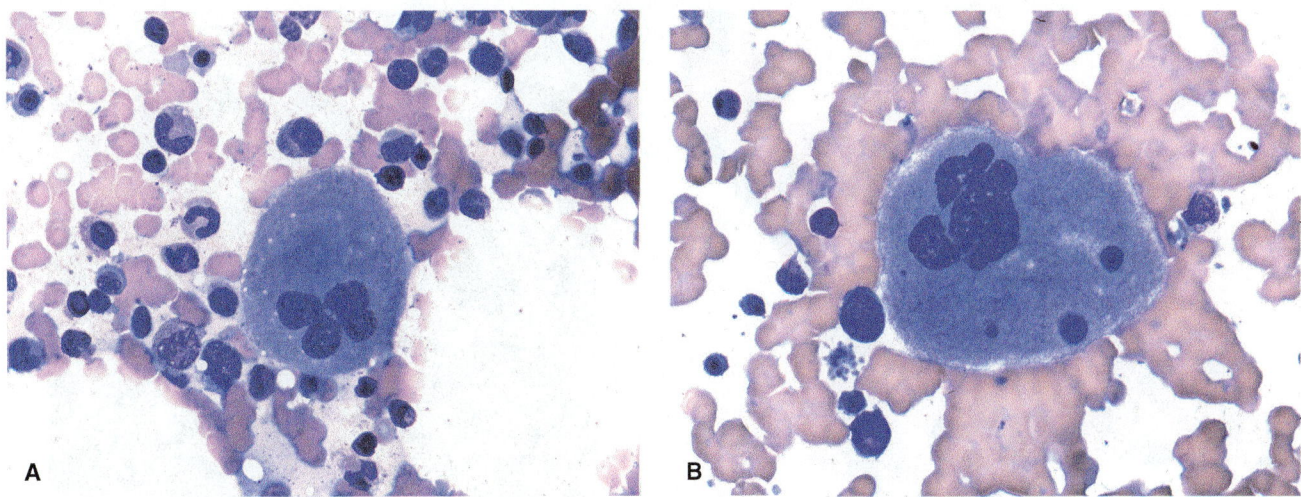

FIGURE 32.49 Two granular megakaryocytes from a Wright–Giemsa-stained bone marrow smear. The megakaryocyte on the right has two lymphocytes in its cytoplasm (emperipoloesis, see Figure 32.53).

However, cell division is probably uncommon in megakaryoblasts and is not seen in the other two cell types. The occurrence of cycles of DNA replication without cytokinesis results in the characteristic polyploidy of these cells. The total DNA content of megakaryoblasts ranges between 4c and 32c and of promegakaryocytes and granular megakaryocytes between 8c and 64c (1c = the haploid DNA content). There is a positive correlation between the nuclear area and DNA content of megakaryocytes.

Cytochemistry

When stained by the PAS reaction, megakaryocytes show a diffuse and finely granular positivity over both the nucleus and the perinuclear and intermediate zones of the cytoplasm (65–68). A narrow peripheral zone of the cytoplasm is often PAS negative, and this may be surrounded by clumps of positive granules within attached platelets. Within platelets, PAS-positive material appears as scattered, lightly staining fine granules at the periphery and as clumps of darkly staining coarse granules at the center. Megakaryocytes and platelets are usually unstained by Sudan black, but occasional megakaryocytes may show a diffuse positivity with fine positive granules scattered both in the cytoplasm and over the nucleus. Megakaryocytes and platelets display strong acid phosphatase activity.

Peroxidase activity cannot be demonstrated in megakaryocytes by light microscopy but can be demonstrated in a characteristic distribution using the electron microscope.

Megakaryocytes show no α-naphthol AS-D chloroacetate esterase activity. However, they have substantial α-naphthyl acetate esterase activity and weaker α-naphthyl butyrate esterase activity; the latter generates many coarse or fine positive granules in the cytoplasm and over the nucleus.

Biopsy Sections

Megakaryocytes are readily recognized by their large size, dense, light or dark pink cytoplasm, and lobulated nucleus in sections stained either with H&E (Fig. 32.50) or Giemsa. In sections of normal bone marrow they are singly scattered or in loose clusters of two to five cells, and are usually not found in a paratrabecular location. Small numbers of small megakaryocytes with tightly convoluted, hyperchromatic nuclei and minimal or no cytoplasm may also be seen (senescent megakaryocytes) (Fig. 32.51). These should not be confused with dysplastic megakaryocytes.

Megakaryocytes and megakaryoblasts may be identified immunohistochemically using antibodies directed to a variety of antigens, including CD31, CD41 (platelet glycoprotein IIb), CD42 (platelet glycoprotein Ib), CD61 (platelet glycoprotein IIIa), and factor VIII-related antigen (von Willebrand factor) (Fig. 32.52). Using a CD61 antibody, the mean value for the total number of megakaryocytes and megakaryoblasts in 15 normal subjects was 24/mm^2 (range: 14 to 38) and for megakaryoblasts alone it was 2.8/mm^2 (range: 1.2 to 4.9) (83).

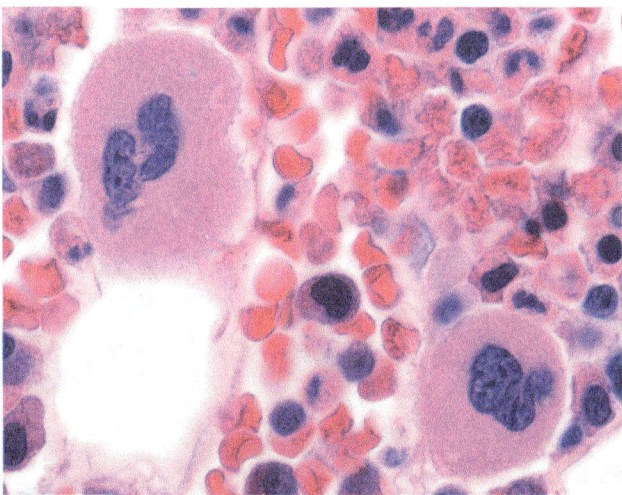

FIGURE 32.50 Two megakaryocytes in a normal bone marrow trephine section (H&E).

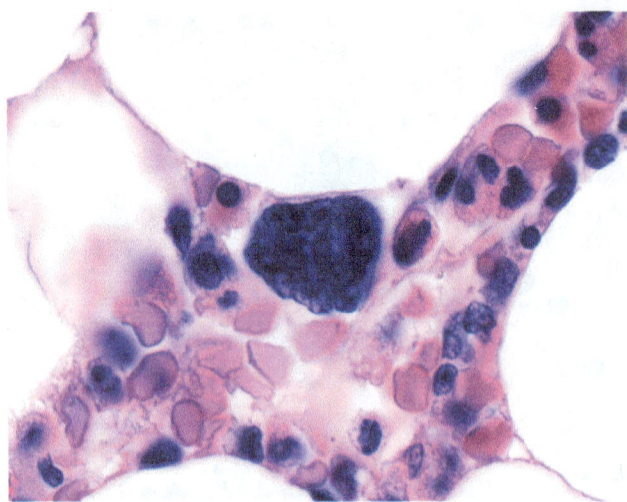

FIGURE 32.51 Hyperchromatic, hyperconvoluted megakaryocyte "nucleus" in a normal bone marrow trephine section (H&E).

Ultrastructure

The nucleus of a megakaryoblast has two or more lobes, very little condensed chromatin, and prominent nucleoli (69,84,85). The cytoplasm contains large numbers of ribosomes, scattered RER, several mitochondria, and a few membrane-lined vesicles representing the beginning of the demarcation membrane system (DMS). The cytoplasm also contains a well-developed Golgi apparatus within a deep nuclear indentation. A few immature α granules and a few lysosomal vesicles containing acid phosphatase and arylsulfatase are present near the Golgi apparatus. The maturation of megakaryoblasts into promegakaryocytes and granular megakaryocytes (Fig. 32.53) is accompanied by a progressive increase in the quantity of nuclear membrane–associated condensed chromatin, an increase in the number of α granules, a progressive development of the DMS, and a reduction in the number of ribosomes, RER, and mitochondria. Megakaryocyte maturation also is accompanied

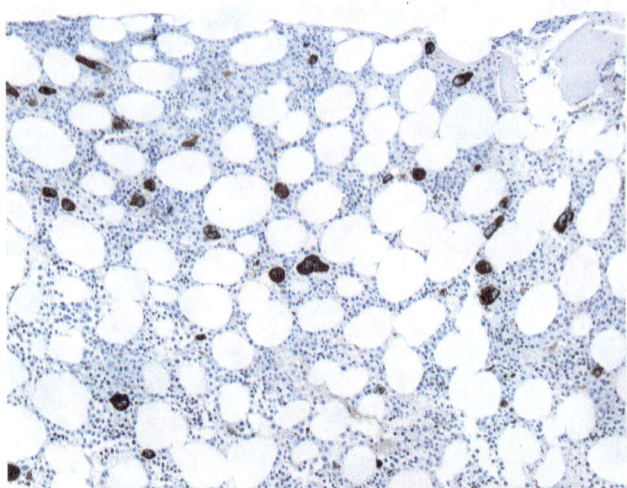

FIGURE 32.52 Normal bone marrow trephine stained with an antibody to factor VIII-related antigen (von Willebrand factor).

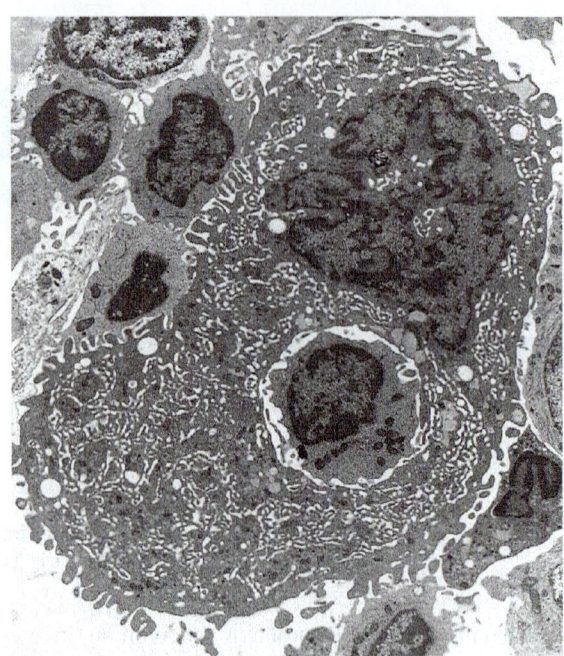

FIGURE 32.53 Electron micrograph of a granular megakaryocyte from normal bone marrow. The cytoplasm contains a lymphocyte that appears to be traveling through the megakaryocyte (emperipolesis).

by the formation of increasing quantities of glycogen in the cytoplasm; the glycogen particles often are found in large clumps. The DMS is an extensive system of membrane-lined cytoplasmic sacs, which arises as invaginations of the surface membrane; it demarcates areas of cytoplasm that eventually become platelets (Fig. 32.54).

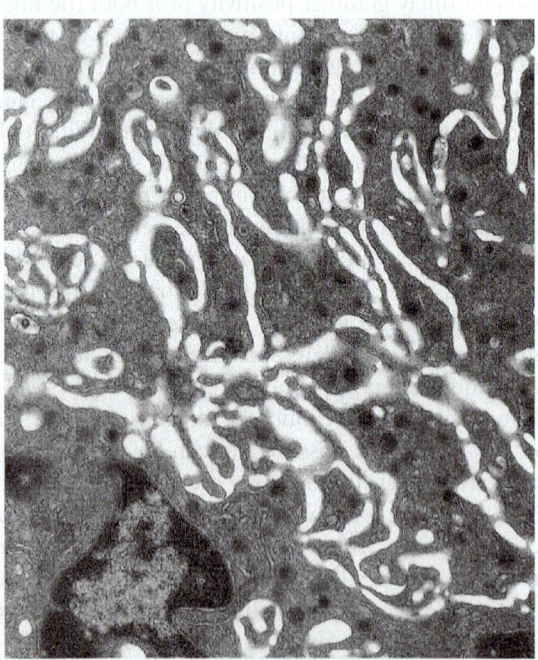

FIGURE 32.54 Electron micrograph of a part of the intermediate zone of the cytoplasm of a granular megakaryocyte, showing the extensive demarcation membrane system, demarcating granule-containing future platelet areas.

Three zones can be recognized in the extensive cytoplasm of a granular megakaryocyte (Fig. 32.53): (a) a narrow perinuclear zone containing the Golgi apparatus and some of the ribosomes, RER, and mitochondria; (b) a wide intermediate zone containing many ovoid, electron-dense alpha granules, numerous sacs of the DMS, lysosomal vesicles, ribosomes, RER, and mitochondria; and (c) a narrow outer zone that is devoid of organelles. Mature granular megakaryocytes protrude cytoplasmic processes that lie near to or within marrow sinusoids. Platelets are formed by the fragmentation of these processes, the platelet membranes being made up of membranes of the DMS.

Ultrastructural cytochemical studies of the oxidation of 3,3'-diaminobenzidine have demonstrated a platelet peroxidase (PPO) in the endoplasmic reticulum and perinuclear space but not in the Golgi apparatus of megakaryoblasts and megakaryocytes and in the dense bodies and dense tubular system of platelets (86). A few small rounded cells present in normal marrow also have PPO activity in the endoplasmic reticulum and perinuclear space and have been identified as promegakaryoblasts (87). PPO appears to be distinct from myeloperoxidase.

Some normal megakaryocytes display the phenomenon of emperipolesis (88,89). This term is used to describe the movement of one cell type within the cytoplasm of another. The cytoplasm of an affected megakaryocyte may contain one or more cells of a number of types, including neutrophil and eosinophil granulocytes and their precursors, lymphocytes, erythroblasts, and red cells (Figs. 32.49 and 32.53). The physiologic relevance of megakaryocyte emperipolesis is uncertain; one suggestion has been that certain marrow cells may enter the circulation via the processes of megakaryocyte cytoplasm that protrude into marrow sinusoids.

Nonactivated platelets are biconvex and have a smooth surface. Their shape is maintained by an equatorial bundle of microtubules situated below the cell membrane, as well as by microfilaments found between various organelles. Other structures found in the cytoplasm include various types of granules, mitochondria, a surface-connected canalicular system, the dense tubular system, and many glycogen particles, which may occur singly or in clumps (Fig. 32.55).

Four types of cytoplasmic granules are recognized, namely, the α granules, λ granules (lysosomal granules), δ granules, and peroxisomes (69,90,91). The α and λ granules are moderately electron dense and can be distinguished from each other only by ultrastructural cytochemistry; for example, λ granules have acid phosphatase activity and α granules do not. Substances present in α granules include β-thromboglobulin, platelet factor 4, platelet-derived growth factor, fibrinogen, fibronectin, von Willebrand factor, and thrombospondin. In addition to acid phosphatase, the λ granules contain β-glucuronidase and arylsulfatase. The δ granules (dense granules) are smaller and much more electron dense than α granules and often have a peripheral electron-lucent zone, which gives them a bull's-eye appearance. They contain serotonin, calcium, and the storage pool of ADP and

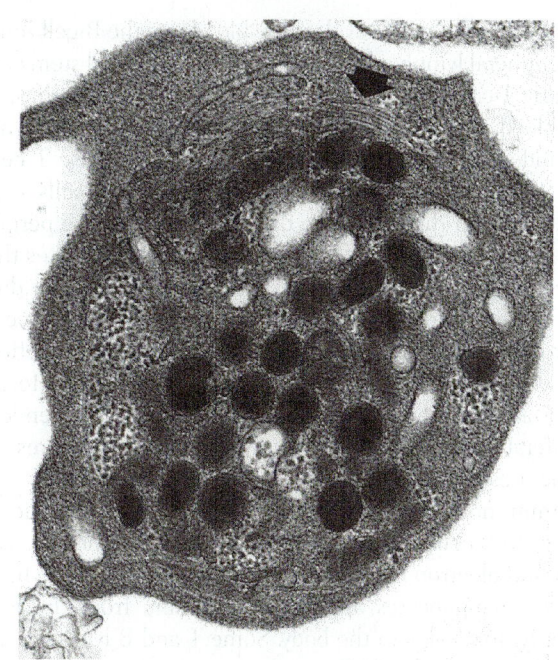

FIGURE 32.55 Electron micrograph of a platelet from normal blood. The platelet has been sectioned near, rather than at, the equatorial plane and, consequently, shows only part of the circumferential band of microtubules (*arrow*). The section also shows the electron-lucent vesicles of the surface-connected canalicular system, several platelet granules, a few mitochondria, and numerous clumps of glycogen molecules.

ATP. The peroxisomes are smaller than the α and λ granules; they are moderately electron dense and contain catalase.

The surface-connected canalicular system is an extensive system of electron-lucent intracytoplasmic canaliculi and saccules that open to the exterior at multiple sites on the cell membrane. This canalicular system provides a large surface through which various substances, including granule contents, can be discharged extracellularly. The channels of the dense tubular system are shorter and narrower than those of the surface-connected canalicular system and contain material with an electron density similar to that of the cytoplasm. The dense tubular system contains PPO and seems to be derived from the endoplasmic reticulum of megakaryocytes. It is an important site of synthesis of thromboxane A_2, which is involved in the release of granule contents. It is also rich in calcium and may regulate various calcium-dependent reversible reactions such as the activation of actomyosin and the polymerization of tubulin.

Lymphocytes and Plasma Cells

All lymphocytes are eventually derived from the lymphoid stem cells present in the marrow, which are in turn derived from the pluripotent hematopoietic stem cells. The lymphoid stem cells generate both B-cell progenitors and T-cell progenitors. The former mature through a number of antigen-independent intermediate stages into B cells; this maturation occurs within the microenvironment of the marrow. The newly formed B cells travel via the blood into the B-cell zones of peripheral lymphoid tissue. Either the lymphoid stem cells or early T-cell progenitors migrate from the marrow through the blood into the thymus. Here, these cells undergo antigen-independent maturation into T cells, and those T cells that recognize self are deleted. The mature T cells then travel through the blood into the T-cell zones of the peripheral lymphoid organs. The mature B and T lymphocytes that enter the peripheral lymphoid tissue are triggered into division when they react with specific antigen in the presence of appropriate accessory cells. Their progeny develop into effector cells or memory cells. In the case of B cells, the effector cell is an antibody-secreting plasma cell. Antigen-dependent proliferation of B cells occurs in normal marrow and results in the presence of plasma cells in this tissue.

Immunohistochemical studies show that the ratio of T cells to B cells in normal adult marrow is around 3:1. The light and electron microscopic appearances of mature bone marrow lymphocytes are indistinguishable from those of other lymphocytes in the body. Some T and B lymphocytes have fine or coarse PAS-positive granules arranged in one to four (usually one or two) rings around the nucleus, and occasional cells have large clumps of PAS-positive material. Lymphocytes are peroxidase negative and α-naphthol AS-D chloroacetate esterase negative, and over 99% of cells are alkaline phosphatase negative. Some lymphocytes show a positive paranuclear dot when stained for α-naphthyl butyrate esterase; this staining is unaffected by fluoride. A substantial proportion of normal lymphocytes show either a paranuclear dot or diffuse granular positivity when stained for acid phosphatase. A paranuclear dot is found in both T cells and B cells but more frequently in T cells.

In the majority of normal marrow trephine sections, mature lymphocytes are distributed inconspicuously through the interstitium among maturing hematopoietic elements. In a minority of otherwise normal marrows, discrete lymphoid aggregates are present, and the frequency of such aggregates increases with increasing age (92). Focal benign lymphoid aggregates are typically small, only rarely exceeding 1 mm in diameter, and round. They are typically well circumscribed, with little infiltration into the surrounding interstices. They are composed predominantly of small, bland lymphocytes with regular to mildly irregular nuclei, clumped chromatin, and scanty cytoplasm (Fig. 32.56).

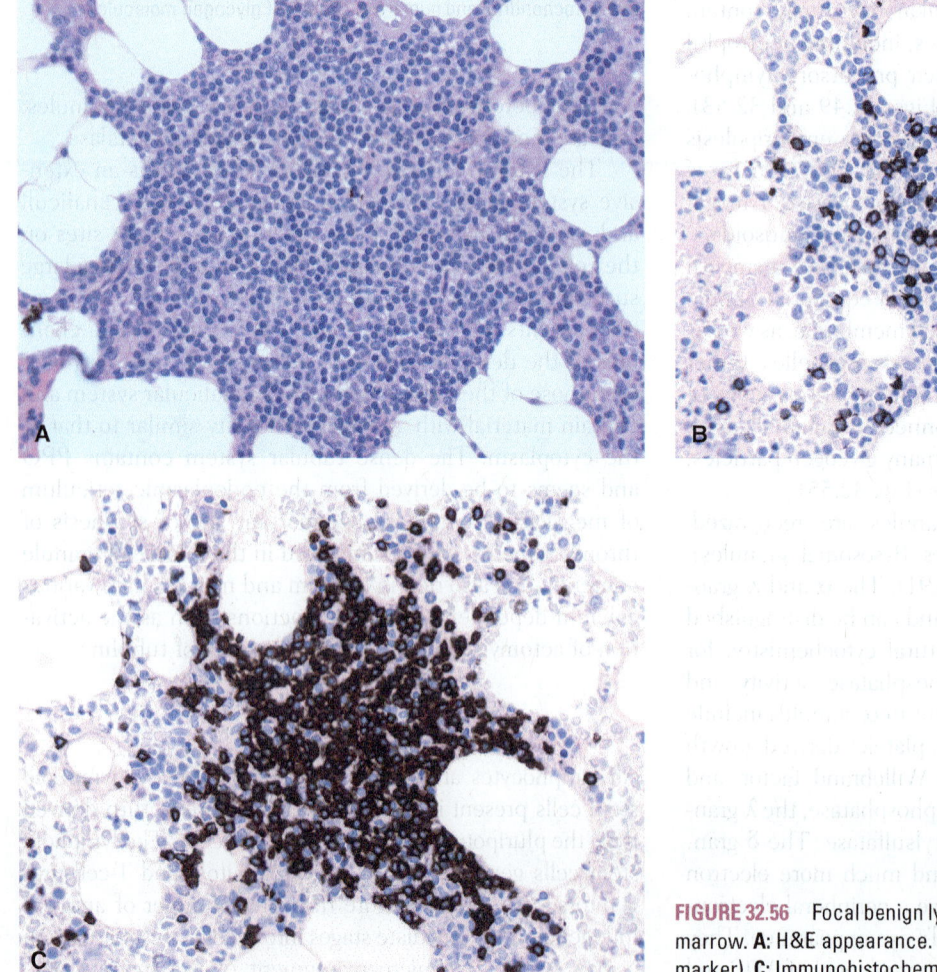

FIGURE 32.56 Focal benign lymphoid aggregate in an otherwise normal marrow. **A:** H&E appearance. **B:** Immunohistochemistry for CD20 (B-cell marker). **C:** Immunohistochemistry for CD3 (T-cell marker).

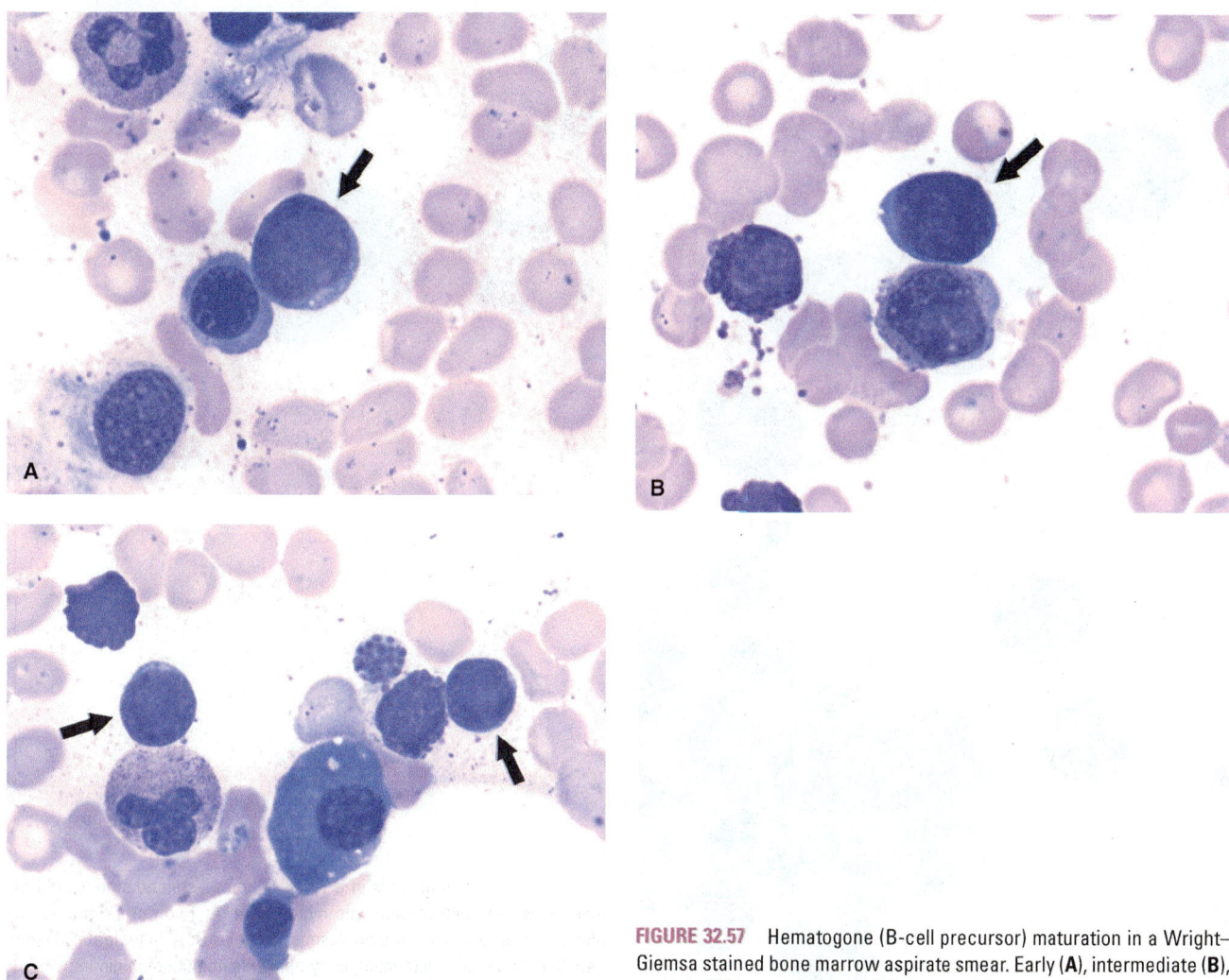

FIGURE 32.57 Hematogone (B-cell precursor) maturation in a Wright–Giemsa stained bone marrow aspirate smear. Early (**A**), intermediate (**B**), and late (**C**) hematogones (all designated by *arrows*).

A few admixed histiocytes are often present, and they may contain one or more small blood vessels. Focal benign lymphoid aggregates virtually never occupy a paratrabecular location; paratrabecular lymphoid aggregates exhibiting an intimate association with bony trabeculae almost always represent lymphomatous infiltrates. Immunohistochemistry of focal benign lymphoid aggregates typically reveals an admixture of T cells and B cells, usually with a predominance of the former (Fig. 32.56) (93). B-cell–predominant lymphoid aggregates are more likely to represent lymphomatous infiltrates (94).

Small numbers of maturing B-cell precursors (colloquially known as "hematogones") are detectable in small numbers (usually less than 1%) by flow cytometry in most marrows from children and adults (95). However, they may be hyperplastic in some reactive and regenerative states, particularly in younger patients, rarely comprising up to 70% of nucleated bone marrow cells. In Romanowsky-type smears, hematogones show a spectrum of maturation (Fig. 32.57). The most immature hematogones are medium to large in size, with regular or mildly indented nuclei, dense, evenly distributed chromatin, inconspicuous or absent nuclei, and narrow rim of pale basophilic, agranular cytoplasm. These may be confused with myeloblasts, but may be differentiated based on denser chromatin, less conspicuous nucleoli, and scantier cytoplasm. As hematogones mature, they become smaller and their chromatin becomes denser, although it remains evenly distributed (rather than clumped, as in mature lymphocytes). These more mature hematogones are also distinguished by their very scanty cytoplasm, with the nucleus appearing to form the cell border for a large proportion of the circumference of the cell. In marrow sections, hyperplastic hematogones form interstitial concentrations without distorting the normal marrow architecture. Cytologically they resemble mature lymphocytes, but show slightly more open, granular chromatin.

Plasma Cells

Plasma cells in smears of normal bone marrow vary somewhat in size and appearance (Fig. 32.58). Most are 14 to 20 μm in diameter and have deep blue cytoplasm. The

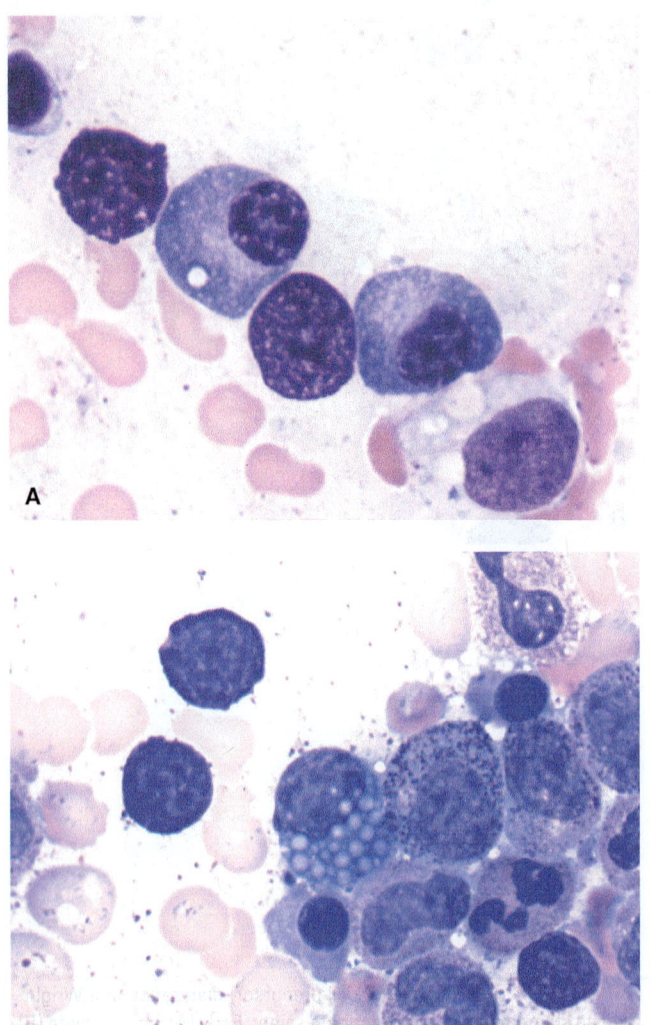
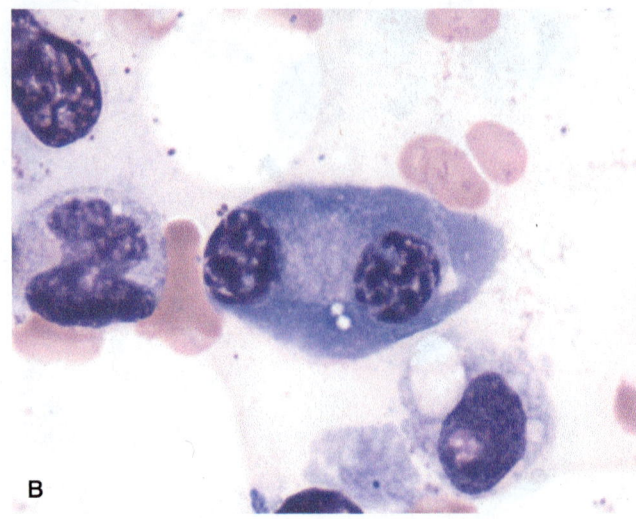

FIGURE 32.58 Plasma cells in a Wright–Giemsa-stained smear of bone marrow with a mild plasmacytic hyperplasia. **A:** Two normal appearing plasma cells, one with a cytoplasmic vacuole. **B:** A binucleate plasma cell. **C:** Plasma cells with multiple cytoplasmic immunoglobulin inclusions (Mott cell).

cytoplasm has a pale paranuclear area corresponding to the Golgi apparatus and may contain one or more vacuoles. The nucleus is small relative to the volume of cytoplasm, contains moderate quantities of condensed chromatin, and is eccentrically located. Although most plasma cells are uninucleate, a few are binucleate (Fig. 32.58B) or multinucleate. Some normal plasma cells have other features. For example, occasional cells may contain one or a few large, round acidophilic, PAS-positive cytoplasmic inclusions (Russell bodies), or multiple smaller, slightly basophilic round inclusions (Mott cells, grape cells, or morular cells)(Fig. 32.58C). Rare plasma cells have many pleomorphic cytoplasmic inclusions and, consequently, appear reticulated. Others have eosinophilic cytoplasms, usually at the periphery, but sometimes in the entire cell (flaming cell); when the eosinophilia is confined to the periphery, it contrasts markedly with the intense basophilia of the rest of the cytoplasm. Occasional plasma cells have azurophilic rods that resemble Auer rods present in acute myeloid leukemia, but that are PAS, Sudan black, and peroxidase negative. Plasma cells show strong acid phosphatase activity, particularly around the nucleus and over the Golgi zone. They do not stain for α-naphthol AS-D chloroacetate esterase.

In trephine sections, plasma cells are often located in intimate association with small blood vessels that lack a smooth muscle layer (Fig. 32.59) (96), although they may also be seen as single cells scattered throughout the interstitium. Occasionally, an intact blood vessel with adherent plasma cells will be present in bone marrow aspirate smears, as well (Fig. 32.59B). In marrow sections, plasma cells exhibit characteristic features: eccentric nucleus with distinctly, often peripherally clumped chromatin and moderately abundant, densely amphophilic cytoplasm with a paranuclear clearing. Immunohistochemistry or in situ hybridization for kappa and lambda will demonstrate an admixture of kappa- and lambda-expressing plasma cells, usually with a slight excess of the former (Fig. 32.60).

The electron microscope shows that the eccentric rounded nucleus of a plasma cell contains a variable quantity of condensed chromatin (Fig. 32.61). The presence of moderately large clumps of nuclear membrane–associated condensed chromatin gives the nuclei of mature plasma cells a cartwheel or clock face appearance in histologic sections (but not in marrow smears). The cytoplasm contains numerous long flattened sacs of RER that are arranged either parallel

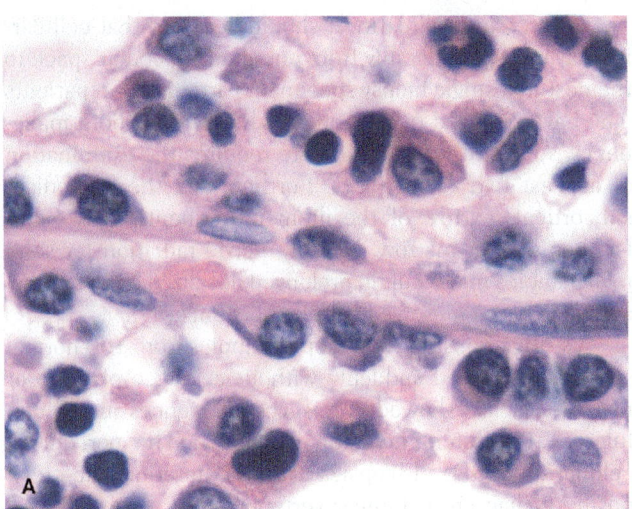
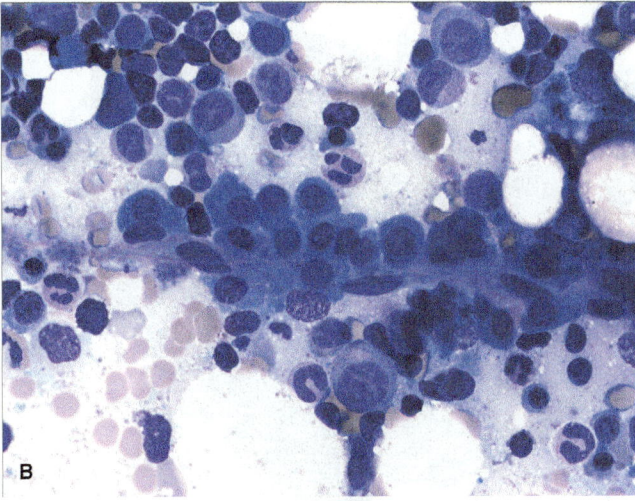

FIGURE 32.59 **A:** Normal perivascular localization of plasma cells in a marrow trephine section (left and right—longitudinal and cross sectional profiles of vessels, respectively) (H&E). **B:** An aspirated blood vessel in a Wright-Giemsa stained aspirate smear demonstrating adhesion of plasma cells to the vessel.

to each other (Fig. 32.61), concentrically, or spirally; the sacs are distended to varying extents with a granular, moderately electron-dense material, consisting mostly of immunoglobulin. The cytoplasm also contains mitochondria, a large Golgi apparatus situated immediately adjacent to the nuclear membrane (Fig. 32.62), and a few small- or medium-sized membrane-bound electron-dense granules. The latter are often found near the Golgi complex, contain acid phosphatase, and appear to be primary lysosomes. Occasional cells contain larger cytoplasmic inclusions that vary markedly in size, electron density, and shape and are often lined by RER. Many of these inclusions are rounded, elliptical, or irregular in outline, but a few are rhomboidal or needle-like and have a crystalline structure. Thus, the various types of cytoplasmic inclusion seen under the light microscope appear to be formed by the accumulation of unusually large quantities of immunoglobulin within regions of the RER.

CELLULARITY OF THE MARROW

The term *marrow cellularity* is usually defined as the proportion of the area of a histologic section excluding bone occupied by hematopoietic cells (by cells other than fat cells). Cellularity may be assessed by point counting using an eyepiece with a graticule (histomorphometry) or, more accurately, by computerized image analysis (97). However, crude estimation serves for clinical purposes. The shrinkage of tissue subjected to decalcification and paraffin embedding

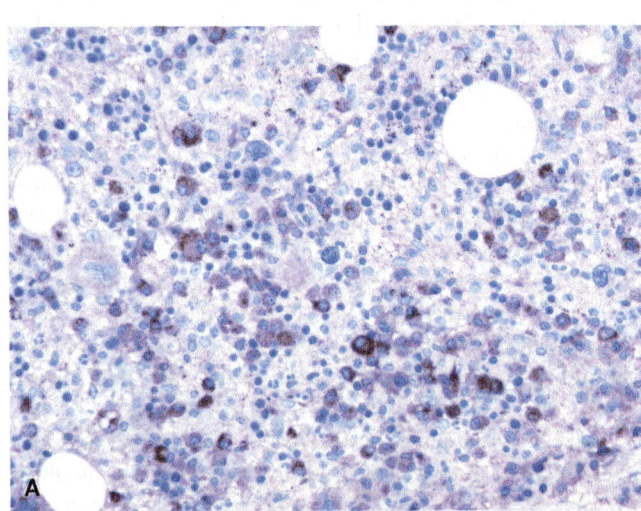
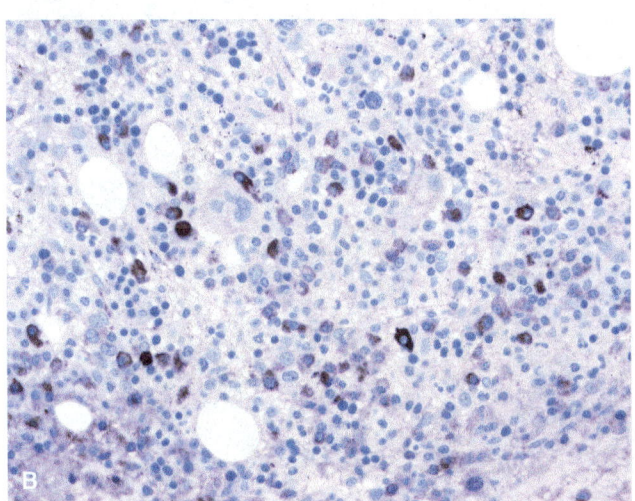

FIGURE 32.60 Light chain immunohistochemistry in an aspirate clot section from a patient with reactive plasmacytosis. **A:** Kappa light chain. **B:** Lamda light chain.

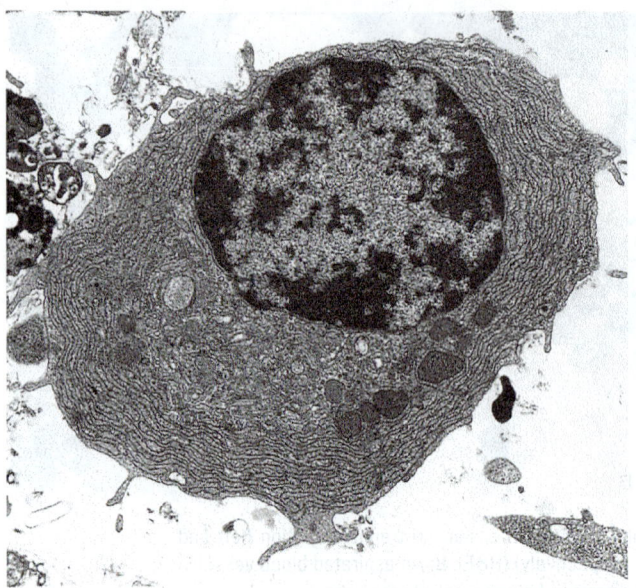

FIGURE 32.61 Electron micrograph of a plasma cell from a normal bone marrow showing numerous parallel sacs of rough endoplasmic reticulum and a very prominent Golgi apparatus immediately adjacent to the nucleus. The nucleus has moderate quantities of condensed chromatin.

results in the cellularity of paraffin-embedded sections being about 5% lower than in plastic-embedded sections (98).

In healthy subjects, cellularity varies with age (49,50). In neonates, there are very few fat cells in the marrow, and the cellularity approaches 100%. Cellularity decreases steadily in the first three decades and stabilizes at 30% to 70% between the ages of 30 and 70 years. During the eighth decade of life, cellularity decreases further and may be less than 20%; this reduction is largely caused by a reduction in bone volume and a consequent increase in the volume of the marrow cavities.

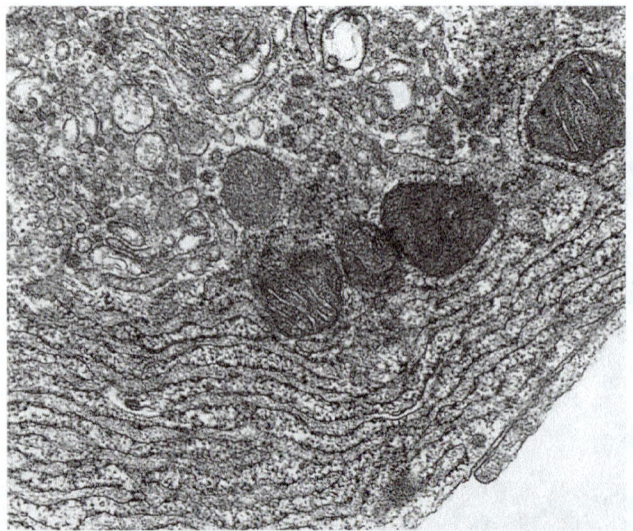

FIGURE 32.62 Electron micrograph showing part of the Golgi apparatus and some of the sacs of RER from the plasma cell in Figure 32.61, at higher magnification. Four mitochondria are also present.

In assessing cellularity, it should be noted that cellularity may vary considerably from one intertrabecular space to the next in a single biopsy specimen, particularly in patients who have received treatment for a hematolymphoid malignancy, so that a reliable estimate requires the examination of at least five such spaces. Furthermore, the immediate subcortical marrow of the ilium is frequently less cellular than deeper marrow. Notably, pelvic radiation for solid malignancies may result in prolonged, localized bone marrow aplasia, despite preserved peripheral counts (99).

A study of postmortem biopsy samples from 100 normal subjects who died suddenly without evidence of bone or marrow disease showed only slight differences in the cellularity at different hematopoietic sites. The percentage cellularity ($\pm$ SD) in biopsies from the anterior iliac crest, posterior iliac crest, lumbar vertebrae, and sternum were, 60 ± 6, 62 ± 7, 64 ± 7, and 61 ± 8, respectively (94).

MARROW DIFFERENTIAL COUNT

During the first day of life, the erythroblasts account for 18.5% to 65% (mean: 40%) of the nucleated cells in a marrow smear. Over the next 8 to 10 days, this figure decreases progressively to 0% to 20.5% (mean: 8%). After a period of erythroblastopenia lasting about 3 weeks, the percentage of erythroblasts increases again, reaching values of 6.5% to 31.5% (mean: 16%) at the age of 3 months (100). These changes are caused by an increase in arterial oxygen saturation soon after birth and the consequent suppression of erythropoietin production. Erythropoietin production increases again 6 to 13 weeks later when the hemoglobin concentration in the blood decreases to about 11 g/dL. The proportion of granulocytes and their precursors ranges between 20% and 73% (mean: 46%) of the nucleated marrow cells on the first day of life (100), increases during the next 3 weeks, and then decreases again to reach a stable value of about 55% after the 2nd month. The average value for the proportion of lymphocytes in the marrow increases from 12% during the first 2 days of life, to 33% at 7 to 10 days, and 47% at 1 month. The lymphocyte percentage then remains stable until the end of the 1st year, after which it decreases slowly to 19% at 4 to 4.5 years, which is only slightly higher than the adult value of 15% (100–103). Plasma cells are infrequent in the neonate, accounting for up to 0.4% (mean: 0.016%) of nucleated marrow cells (104). They gradually increase in number to reach a mean value of 0.386% at the age of 12 to 15 years (5,000 cell differential count). Plasma cells in healthy adults comprise 0.4% to 2.0% of marrow aspirate cells.

The differential count on 2,000 consecutive nucleated cells in bone marrow smears from normal adults is given in Table 32.2 (105). The mean and range for the myeloid/erythroid ratio in healthy adults are 3.1 and 2.0:8.3, respectively (106).

TABLE 32.2

Differential Counts[a] on Marrow Smears From 28 Healthy Adults Aged Between 20 and 29 Years

Cell Type	Percentages		
	Mean	95% Confidence Limits	Observed Range
Myeloblasts	1.21	0.75–1.67	0.75–1.80
Promyelocytes	2.49	0.99–3.99	1.00–3.75
Myelocytes			
Neutrophil	17.36	11.54–23.18	12.25–22.65
Eosinophil	1.37	0–2.85	0.25–3.45
Basophil	0.08	0–0.21	0.00–0.25
Metamyelocytes			
Neutrophil	16.92	11.40–22.44	11.45–23.60
Eosinophil	0.63	0.07–1.19	0.25–1.30
Juvenile neutrophil granulocytes (stab forms)	8.70	3.58–13.82	4.85–13.95
Granulocytes			
Neutrophil	13.42	4.32–22.52	8.70–8.95
Eosinophil	0.93	0.21–1.65	0.45–1.55
Basophil	0.20	0–0.48	0.05–0.50
Monocytes	1.04	0.36–1.72	0.65–2.10
Plasma cells	0.46	0–0.96	0.10–0.95[b]
Lymphocytes	14.60	6.66–22.54	9.35–25.05
Basophilic erythropoietic cells	0.92	0.40–1.44	0.50–1.60
Early polychromatic normoblasts	6.76	2.56–10.96	3.30–12.20
Late polychromatic normoblasts	11.58	6.16–17.0	7.85–19.55
Reticular cells	0.24	0–0.54	0.05–0.65

[a]2,000 cells were studied in each individual.
[b]The observed range in 63 cases, aged 20–93 years, was 0.10–2.00%.
From Jacobson KM. Untersuchungen über das knochenmarkspunktat bei normalen individuen verschiedener altersklassen. *Acta Med Scand* 1941;106:417–446.

REFERENCES

1. Chamberlain G, Fox J, Ashton B, et al. Concise review: Mesenchymal stem cells: Their phenotype, differentiation capacity, immunological features, and potential for homing. *Stem Cells* 2007;25:2739–2749.
2. Bain BJ. Bone marrow aspiration. *J Clin Pathol* 2001;54:657–663.
3. Brynes RK, McKenna RW, Sundberg RD. Bone marrow aspiration and trephine biopsy. An approach to a thorough study. *Am J Clin Pathol* 1978;70:753–759.
4. Lee SH, Erber WN, Porwit A, et al. ICSH guidelines for the standardization of bone marrow specimens and reports. *Int J Lab Hematol* 2008;30:349–364.
5. Bain BJ. Bone marrow trephine biopsy. *J Clin Pathol* 2001;54:737–742.
6. Foucar K. Procurement and indications for bone marrow examination. In: Foucar K, Reichard K, Czuchlewski D, eds. *Bone Marrow Pathology*, 3rd ed. Chicago: ASCP Press; 2010. 53–65.
7. Woronzoff-Dashkoff KP. The ehrlich-chenzinsky-plehn-malachowski-romanowsky-nocht-jenner-may-grunwald-leishman-reuter-wright-giemsa-lillie-roe-wilcox stain. The mystery unfolds. *Clin Lab Med* 1993;13:759–771.
8. Fend F, Tzankov A, Bink K, et al. Modern techniques for the diagnostic evaluation of the trephine bone marrow biopsy: Methodological aspects and applications. *Prog Histochem Cytochem* 2008;42:203–252.
9. Reichard K. Specialized techniques in bone marrow evaluation. In: Foucar K, Reichard K, Czuchlewski D, eds. *Bone Marrow Pathology*. Chicago: ASCP Press; 2010. 67–83.
10. Olsen RJ, Chang CC, Herrick JL, et al. Acute leukemia immunohistochemistry: A systematic diagnostic approach. *Arch Pathol Lab Med* 2008;132:462–475.
11. Pileri SA, Ascani S, Milani M, et al. Acute leukaemia immunophenotyping in bone-marrow routine sections. *Br J Haematol* 1999;105:394–401.
12. Kremer M, Quintanilla-Martinez L, Nahrig J, et al. Immunohistochemistry in bone marrow pathology: A useful adjunct for morphologic diagnosis. *Virchows Arch* 2005;447:920–937.
13. Pileri SA, Roncador G, Ceccarelli C, et al. Immunohistochemistry of bone-marrow biopsy. *Leuk Lymphoma* 1997;26 Suppl 1:69–75.
14. Torlakovic EE, Brynes RK, Hyjek E, et al; International Council for Standardization in Haematology. ICSH guidelines for the standardization of bone marrow immunohistochemistry. *Int J Lab Hematol* 2015;37:431–449.
15. Abkowitz JL, Catlin SN, McCallie MT, et al. Evidence that the number of hematopoietic stem cells per animal is conserved in mammals. *Blood* 2002;100:2665–2667.
16. Ceredig R, Rolink AG, Brown G. Models of haematopoiesis: Seeing the wood for the trees. *Nat Rev Immunol* 2009;9:293–300.
17. Ogawa M. Hematopoiesis. *J Allergy Clin Immunol* 1994;94:645–650.
18. Gordon MY. Human haemopoietic stem cell assays. *Blood Rev* 1993;7:190–197.
19. Wickramasinghe SN. *Human Bone Marrow*. Oxford: Blackwell Scientific; 1975.
20. Kaushansky K. Hematopoietic stem cells, progenitors, and cytokines. In: Kaushansky K, Lichtman MA, Prchal JT, et al., eds. *Williams Hematology*. New York: McGraw Hill; 2016. 257–277.
21. Loges S, Fehse B, Brockmann MA, et al. Identification of the adult human hemangioblast. *Stem Cells Dev* 2004;13:229–242.
22. Chow A, Frenette PS. Origin and development of blood cells. In: Greer JP, Arber DA, Glader B, et al., eds. *Wintrobe's Clinical Hematology*. Philadelphia, PA: Wolters Kluwer/Lippincott Williams & Wilkins; 2014. 65–81.

23. Verfaillie C. Regulation of hematopoiesis. In: Wichramasinghe SN, McCullough J, eds. *Blood and Bone Marrow Pathology*. Edinburgh: Churchill Livingstone; 2003. 71–85.
24. Koury MJ, Mahmud N, Rhodes MM. Origin and development of blood cells. In: Greer JP, Foerster J, Rodgers G.M, et al., eds. *Wintrobe's Clinical Hematology*. Philadelphia, PA: Wolters Luwer/Lippincott Williams & Wilkins; 2009. 79–105.
25. Palis J, Robertson S, Kennedy M, et al. Development of erythroid and myeloid progenitors in the yolk sac and embryo proper of the mouse. *Development* 1999;126:5073–5084.
26. Moore MA, Metcalf D. Ontogeny of the haemopoietic system: Yolk sac origin of in vivo and in vitro colony forming cells in the developing mouse embryo. *Br J Haematol* 1970;18:279–296.
27. Dzierzak E, Medvinsky A, de Bruijn M. Qualitative and quantitative aspects of haematopoietic cell development in the mammalian embryo. *Immunol Today* 1998;19:228–236.
28. Kelemen E, Calvo W, Fliedner TM. *Atlas of Human Hematopoietic Development*. Berlin: Springer-Verlag; 1979.
29. Bloom W, Bartelmez GW. Hematopoiesis in young human embryos. *Am J Anat* 1940;67:21–53.
30. Steinberg MH, Nagel RL. Hemoglobins of the embryo, fetus, and adult. In: Steinberg MH, Forget BG, Higgs DR, et al., eds. *Disorder of Hemoglobin Genetics, Pathophysiology, and Clinical Management*. Cambridge: Cambridge University Press; 2009. 119–135.
31. Emura I, Sekiya M, Ohnishi Y. Two types of immature erythrocytic series in the human fetal liver. *Arch Histol Jpn* 1983;46:631–643.
32. Gilmour JR. Normal haemopoiesis in intrauterine and neonatal life. *J Pathol Bacteriol* 1941;52:25–55.
33. Kalpaktsoglou PK, Emery JL. Human bone marrow during the last three months of intrauterine life. A histological study. *Acta Haematol* 1965;34:228–238.
34. Piney A. The anatomy of the bone marrow with special reference to the distribution of the red marrow. *Br Med J* 1922;2:792–795.
35. Custer RP, Ahlfeldt FE. Studies on the structure and function of bone marrow. II. Variations in cellularity in various bones with advancing *J Lab Clin Med* 1932;17:960–962.
36. Wickramasinghe SN, McCullough J. *Blood and Bone Marrow Pathology*. Edinburgh: Churchill Livingstone; 2003.
37. Munka V, Gregor A. Lymphatics and bone marrow. *Folia Morphol (Praha)* 1965;13:404–412.
38. Bain BJ, Clark DM, Lampert IA, et al. *Bone Marrow Pathology*. Oxford: Blackwell Science; 2001.
39. Bartl R, Frisch B. Normal bone marrow: Histology, histochemistry and immunohistochemistry. In: Wickramasinghe SN, McCullough J, eds. *Blood and Bone Marrow Pathology*. Edinburgh: Churchill Livingstone; 2003.
40. De Bruyn PP, Breen PC, Thomas TB. The microcirculation of the bone marrow. *Anat Rec* 1970;168:55–68.
41. Branemark PI. Bone marrow microvascular structure and function. *Adv Microbiol* 1968;1:1–65.
42. Trubowitz S, Masek B. A histochemical study of the reticuloendothelial system of human marrow—its possible transport role. *Blood* 1968;32:610–628.
43. Burgio VL, Magrini U, Ciardelli L, et al. An enzyme-histochemical approach to the study of the human bone-marrow stroma. *Acta Haematol* 1984;71:73–80.
44. Wickramasinghe SN. Observations on the ultrastructure of sinusoids and reticular cells in human bone marrow. *Clin Lab Haematol* 1991;13:263–278.
45. Miller MR, Kasahara M. Observations on the innervation of human long bones. *Anat Rec* 1963;145:13–17.
46. Dominici M, Pritchard C, Garlits JE, et al. Hematopoietic cells and osteoblasts are derived from a common marrow progenitor after bone marrow transplantation. *Proc Natl Acad Sci U S A* 2004;101:11761–11766.
47. Benayahu D, Horowitz M, Zipori D, et al. Hemopoietic functions of marrow-derived osteogenic cells. *Calcif Tissue Int* 1992;51:195-201.
48. Chambers TJ. Regulation of osteoclast development and function. In: Rifkin BR, Gay CV, eds. *Biology and Physiology of the Osteoclast*. Boca Raton: CRC Press; 1992. 105–128.
49. Hartsock RJ, Smith EB, Petty CS. Normal variations with aging of the amount of hematopoietic tissue in bone marrow from the anterior iliac crest. A study made from 177 cases of sudden death examined by necropsy. *Am J Clin Pathol* 1965;43:326–331.
50. Sturgeon P. Volumetric and microscopic pattern of bone marrow in normal infants and children. III. Histologic pattern. *Pediatrics* 1951;7:774–781.
51. Bohm J. Gelatinous transformation of the bone marrow: The spectrum of underlying diseases. *Am J Surg Pathol* 2000;24:56–65.
52. Gale E, Torrance J, Bothwell T. The quantitative estimation of total iron stores in human bone marrow. *J Clin Invest* 1963;42:1076–1082.
53. Thomason RW, Lavelle J, Nelson D, et al. Parenteral iron therapy is associated with a characteristic pattern of iron staining on bone marrow aspirate smears. *Am J Clin Pathol* 2007;128:590–593.
54. Thomason RW, Almiski MS. Evidence that stainable bone marrow iron following parenteral iron therapy does not correlate with serum iron studies and may not represent readily available storage iron. *Am J Clin Pathol* 2009;131:580–585.
55. Westen H, Bainton DF. Association of alkaline-phosphatase-positive reticulum cells in bone marrow with granulocytic precursors. *J Exp Med* 1979;150:919–937.
56. Biermann A, Graf von Keyserlingk D. Ultrastructure of reticulum cells in the bone marrow. *Acta Anat (Basel)* 1978;100:34–43.
57. Tanaka Y. An electron microscopic study of non-phagocytic reticulum cells in human bone marrow. I. Cells with intracytoplasmic fibrils. *Nihon Ketsueki Gakkai Zasshi* 1969;32:275–286.
58. Tsai S, Patel V, Beaumont E, et al. Differential binding of erythroid and myeloid progenitors to fibroblasts and fibronectin. *Blood* 1987;69:1587–1594.
59. Broudy VC, Zuckerman KS, Jetmalani S, et al. Monocytes stimulate fibroblastoid bone marrow stromal cells to produce multilineage hematopoietic growth factors. *Blood* 1986;68:530–534.
60. Kirshenbaum AS, Kessler SW, Goff JP, et al. Demonstration of the origin of human mast cells from CD34+ bone marrow progenitor cells. *J Immunol* 1991;146:1410–1415.

61. Denburg JA, Richardson M, Telizyn S, et al. Basophil/mast cell precursors in human peripheral blood. *Blood* 1983;61: 775–780.
62. Zucker-Franklin D, Grusky G, Hirayama N, et al. The presence of mast cell precursors in rat peripheral blood. *Blood* 1981; 58:544–551.
63. Dahlin JS, Hallgren J. Mast cell progenitors: Origin, development and migration to tissues. *Mol Immunol* 2015;63: 9–17.
64. Glassy EF. *Color Atlas of Hematology*. Northfield: College of American Pathologists; 1998. 80–85.
65. Rozenszajn L, Leibovich M, Shoham D, et al. The esterase activity in megaloblasts, leukaemic and normal haemopoietic cells. *Br J Haematol* 1968;14:605–610.
66. Gibb RP, Stowell RE. Glycogen in human blood cells. *Blood* 1949;4:569–579.
67. Rheingold JJ, Wislocki GB. Histochemical methods applied to hematology. *Bull New Engl Med Cent* 1948;10: 133–137.
68. Hayhoe FGJ, Quaglino D. *Haematological Cytochemistry*. Edinburgh: Churchill Livingstone; 1988.
69. Bessis M. *Living Blood Cells and Their Ultrastructure*. Berlin: Springer-Verlag; 1973.
70. Cawley JC, Hayhoe FGJ. *Ultrastructure of Haemic Cells. A Cytologic Atlas of Normal and Leukaemic Blood and Bone Marrow*. London: WB Saunders; 1973.
71. Bainton DF, Ullyot JL, Farquhar MG. The development of neutrophilic polymorphonuclear leukocytes in human bone marrow. *J Exp Med* 1971;134:907–934.
72. Scott RE, Horn RG. Ultrastructural aspects of neutrophil granulocyte development in humans. *Lab Invest* 1970;23: 202–215.
73. Parwaresch MR. *The Human Blood Basophil*. Berlin: Springer-Verlag; 1976.
74. Scott RE, Horn RG. Fine structural features of eosinophile granulocyte development in human bone marrow. Evidence for granule secretion. *J Ultrastruct Res* 1970;33:16–28.
75. Hintzke M, Harrington AM, Olteanu H, et al. Bone marrow monocytosis: A survey of 150 cases. *Am J Clin Pathol* 2015; 144:A150.
76. Leder LD. The origin of blood monocytes and macrophages. A review. *Blut* 1967;16:86–98.
77. Ohgami RS, Chisholm KM, Ma L, et al. E-cadherin is a specific marker for erythroid differentiation and has utility, in combination with CD117 and CD34, for enumerating myeloblasts in hematopoietic neoplasms. *Am J Clin Pathol* 2014;141:656–664.
78. Marsee DK, Pinkus GS, Yu H. CD71 (transferrin receptor): An effective marker for erythroid precursors in bone marrow biopsy specimens. *Am J Clin Pathol* 2010;134:429–435.
79. Wickramasinghe SN, Hughes M. Globin chain precipitation, deranged iron metabolism and dyserythropoiesis in some thalassaemia syndromes. *Haematologia (Budap)* 1984;17:35–55.
80. Wickramasinghe SN, Lee MJ, Furukawa T, et al. Composition of the intra-erythroblastic precipitates in thalassaemia and congenital dyserythropoietic anaemia (CDA): Identification of a new type of CDA with intra-erythroblastic precipitates not reacting with monoclonal antibodies to alpha- and beta-globin chains. *Br J Haematol* 1996;93:576–585.
81. Nemec J, Polak H. Erythropoietic polyploidy. I. The morphology of polyploid erythroid elements and their incidence in healthy subjects. *Folia Haematol Int Mag Klin Morphol Blutforsch* 1965;84:24–40.
82. Queisser U, Queisser W, Spiertz B. Polyploidization of megakaryocytes in normal humans, in patients with idiopathic thrombocytopenia and with pernicious anaemia. *Br J Haematol* 1971;20:489–501.
83. Thiele J, Wagner S, Weuste R, et al. An immunomorphometric study on megakaryocyte precursor cells in bone marrow tissue from patients with chronic myeloid leukemia (CML). *Eur J Haematol* 1990;44:63–70.
84. Jean G, Lambertenghi-Deliliers G, Ranzi T, Poirier-Bassetti M. The human bone marrow megakaryocyte. An ultrastructural study. *Haematologia (Budap)* 1971;5:253–264.
85. Breton-Gorius J, Reyes F. Ultrastructure of human bone marrow cell maturation. *Int Rev Cytol* 1976;46:251–321.
86. Breton-Gorius J. The value of cytochemical peroxidase reactions at the ultrastructural level in haematology. *Histochem J* 1980;12:127–137.
87. Breton-Gorius J, Gourdin MF, Reyes F. Ultrastructure of the leukemic cell. In: Catovsky D, ed. *The Leukemic Cell (Methods in Hematology)*. Edinburgh: Churchill-Livingstone; 1981; 85–128.
88. Rozman C, Vives-Corrons JL. On the alleged diagnostic significance of megakaryocytic 'phagocytosis' (emperipolesis). *Br J Haematol* 1981;48:510.
89. Larsen TE. Emperipolesis of granular leukocytes within megakaryocytes in human hemopoietic bone marrow. *Am J Clin Pathol* 1970;53:485–489.
90. Berndt MC, Castaldi PA, Gordon S, et al. Morphological and biochemical confirmation of gray platelet syndrome in two siblings. *Aust N Z J Med* 1983;13:387–390.
91. White JG. Current concepts of platelet structure. *Am J Clin Pathol* 1979;71:363–378.
92. Rywlin AM, Ortega RS, Dominguez CJ. Lymphoid nodules of bone marrow: Normal and abnormal. *Blood* 1974;43: 389–400.
93. Thiele J, Zirbes TK, Kvasnicka HM, et al. Focal lymphoid aggregates (nodules) in bone marrow biopsies: Differentiation between benign hyperplasia and malignant lymphoma—a practical guideline. *J Clin Pathol* 1999;52:294–300.
94. Naemi K, Brynes RK, Reisian N, et al. Benign lymphoid aggregates in the bone marrow: Distribution patterns of B and T lymphocytes. *Hum Pathol* 2013;44:512–520.
95. McKenna RW, Washington LT, Aquino DB, et al. Immunophenotypic analysis of hematogones (B-lymphocyte precursors) in 662 consecutive bone marrow specimens by 4-color flow cytometry. *Blood* 2001;98:2498–2507.
96. Kass L, Kapadia IH. Perivascular plasmacytosis: A light-microscopic and immunohistochemical study of 93 bone marrow biopsies. *Acta Haematol* 2001;105:57–63.
97. Al-Adhadh AN, Cavill I. Assessment of cellularity in bone marrow fragments. *J Clin Pathol* 1983;36:176–179.
98. Kerndrup G, Pallesen G, Melsen F, et al. Histomorphometrical determination of bone marrow cellularity in iliac crest biopsies. *Scand J Haematol* 1980;24:110–114.
99. Harrington AM, Hari P, Kroft SH. Utility of CD56 Immunohistochemical studies in follow-up of plasma cell myeloma. *Am J Clin Pathol* 2009;132:60–66.
100. Gairdner D, Marks J, Roscoe JD. Blood formation in infancy. Part I. The normal bone marrow. *Arch Dis Child* 1952;27: 128–133.

101. Rosse C, Kraemer MJ, Dillon TL, et al. Bone marrow cell populations of normal infants; the predominance of lymphocytes. *J Lab Clin Med* 1977;89:1225–1240.
102. Diwany M. Sternal marrow puncture in children. *Arch Dis Child* 1940;15:159–170.
103. Glaser K, Poncher HG, Limarzi LR. The cellular composition of the bone marrow in normal infants and children. *J Lab Clin Med* 1948;33:1639.
104. Steiner ML, Pearson HA. Bone marrow plasmacyte values in childhood. *J Pediatr* 1966;68:562–568.
105. Jacobsen KM. Untersuchungen uber das knochenmarkspunktat bei normalen individuen verschiedener altersklassen. *Acta Med Scand* 1941;106:417–446.
106. Young RH, Osgood EE. Sternal marrow aspirated during life. Cytology in health and disease. *Arch Intern Med* 1935;55:186–203.

SECTION IX

Genitourinary Tract

Kidney

William L. Clapp

33

- INTRODUCTION 856
- PEDIATRIC KIDNEY 856
- KIDNEY DEVELOPMENT 856
- EMBRYONIC KIDNEYS 856
    - Pronephros 856
    - Mesonephros 857
- METANEPHROS 857
    - Overview 857
    - Formation of the Renal Pelvis and Calyces 857
    - Formation of the Collecting System 858
    - Nephron Formation 859
- MOLECULAR REGULATION OF KIDNEY DEVELOPMENT 861
- INTERMEDIATE MESODERM SPECIFICATION 867
- NEPHRIC DUCT 867
- URETERIC BUD FORMATION 867
- URETERAL BRANCHING 868
    - Gdnf/Ret Signaling 868
    - Other Signaling Pathways 869
- URETERIC BRANCH GROWTH 871
- COLLECTING SYSTEM DIFFERENTIATION 871
    - Ureteral Tip and Trunk 871
    - Cell Types 872
- METANEPHRIC MESENCHYME 873
    - Specification 873
    - Nephron Progenitor Population 874
- PATTERNING OF THE NEPHRON 876
    - Early Events: Pretubular Aggregate and Renal Vesicle 876
    - Later Events: Proximal and Distal Tubules 877
- INTERSTITIUM 877
- GLOMERULOGENESIS 878
- VASCULATURE 879
- DEVELOPMENT OF THE JUXTAGLOMERULAR APPARATUS 880
- GROSS ANATOMY 880
    - Kidney Position and Blood Supply 880
    - Kidney Weight and Configuration 880
    - Fetal Lobations 881
- HISTOLOGY 882
- CORTICAL ARCHITECTURE 882
- NEPHRON NUMBER 884
- GLOMERULAR MATURATION AND GROWTH 884
    - Early Juxtamedullary Glomeruli 887
    - Glomerulosclerosis in Infants 887
    - Ectopic Glomeruli 888
- TUBULAR MATURATION AND GROWTH 889
- ADULT KIDNEY 889
- GROSS ANATOMY 889
- NEPHRON 892
- ARCHITECTURE 893
- PARENCHYMA 895
- GLOMERULUS 895
    - Overview 895
    - Endothelial Cells 897
    - Mesangial Cells 898
    - Glomerular Basement Membrane 899
    - Podocytes 901
    - Glomerular Filtration Barrier 905
    - Parietal Epithelial Cells 905
- JUXTAGLOMERULAR APPARATUS 906
- PROXIMAL TUBULE 908
- THIN LIMBS OF HENLE LOOP 913
- DISTAL TUBULE 915
    - Thick Ascending Limb 915
    - Distal Convoluted Tubule 916
- CONNECTING TUBULE 916
- COLLECTING DUCT 917
    - Cortical Collecting Duct 917
    - Outer Medullary Collecting Duct 920
    - Inner Medullary Collecting Duct 921
- PAPILLARY SURFACE EPITHELIUM 922
- INTERSTITIUM 922
- VASCULATURE 924
- LYMPHATICS 927
- NERVES 927
- ACKNOWLEDGMENTS 928
- REFERENCES 928

INTRODUCTION

The kidney has an intricate structure that underlies its diverse roles of excreting waste products, regulating body fluid and solute balance, regulating blood pressure, and secreting hormones. A familiarity with the basic structure of the kidney facilitates the evaluation and comprehension of diseases and functional disorders that can affect the kidney. The structure of the normal human kidney is considered in this chapter. Although the focus is on the human kidney, analogous renal structures in other mammalian species are discussed or illustrated when pertinent.

PEDIATRIC KIDNEY

Renal enthusiasts, especially developmental biologists and pathologists, have long been fascinated with how a kidney develops from primitive mesoderm into such a wondrously complex organ. A basic understanding of nephrogenesis provides a framework to enhance our knowledge of congenital kidney disease. The human kidney is structurally immature at the time of birth, and important morphologic changes occur during infancy and childhood. Pathologists not familiar with the histologic peculiarities of the pediatric kidney may mistake normal findings for abnormalities or fail to observe significant abnormalities of renal maturation. The following section covers the pediatric kidney, focusing first on kidney development prior to birth, and second, on the kidney after birth.

KIDNEY DEVELOPMENT

During development cells proliferate, migrate, differentiate, die, and interact with other cells to form tissues and organs. These different aspects of cell behavior are controlled by genes in a temporal and spatial manner. The kidney has long been considered an excellent model system for the study of organogenesis. However, it is not surprising that understanding the mechanisms of kidney development remains a considerable challenge, when one considers the elaborate architecture and heterogeneous cellular elements of the organ. Detailed reviews of the morphologic and molecular aspects of kidney development are available (1–12).

EMBRYONIC KIDNEYS

Organogenesis begins during the third week of human embryogenesis with the initial formation of the central nervous and cardiovascular systems. The urogenital system

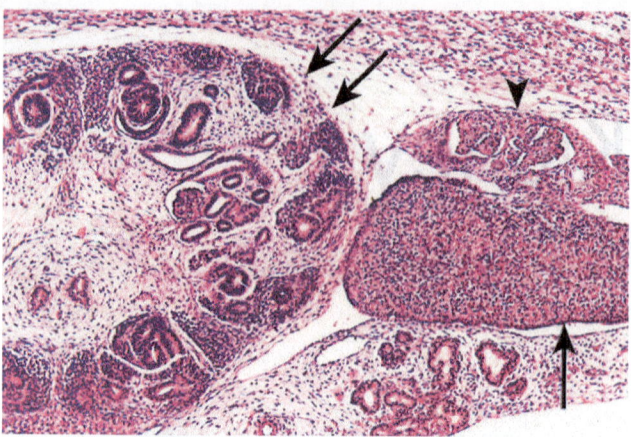

FIGURE 33.1 Mesonephros and metanephros. The mesonephros (*arrowhead*) contributes somatic cell lineages to the gonadal ridge (*single arrow*), which will develop into the gonad. Early nephron formation is present in the metanephros (*double arrows*), whose development is dependent on the presence of the mesonephros. (Reprinted with permission from Murphy WM, Grignon DJ, Perlman EJ. Tumors of the kidney, bladder, and related urinary structures. In: Silverberg SG, Sobin LH, eds. *Atlas of Tumor Pathology. 4th series, fascicle 1*. Washington, DC: Armed Forces Institute of Pathology; 2004.)

represents the last organ system to develop. Kidney development goes through three successive stages: pronephros, mesonephros, and metanephros. All three systems develop from the intermediate mesoderm (IM), located between the dorsal somites and lateral plate mesoderm (LPM), and extending from the cervical to the caudal regions of the embryo. The pronephros and mesonephros are transient structures in mammals. However, all three systems are essential with the formation of each subsequent organ dependent on the presence of the preceding structure. The mesonephros forms before the pronephros regresses and the metanephros develops before the mesonephros disappears (Fig. 33.1). This developmental scheme may be likened to a wave of nephrogenesis moving in a cervical to caudal direction through the IM. Some genes that regulate metanephric kidney development appear to be involved in forming the earlier embryonic kidneys.

Pronephros

The pronephros develops in the cervical region at the end of the third week of human gestation. However, most of our knowledge of the pronephros has come from the study of lower vertebrates. The zebrafish pronephric kidney has become a relevant model for studying the cell and molecular processes that are conserved in mammalian kidney development (13). The pronephros consists of a glomus (glomerulus-like structure), tubules, and a duct. The glomus, not physically connected to the tubules, projects into the coelomic cavity and filters blood. Ciliated tubules, called nephrostomes, open into the coelom and collect the filtrate. The nephrostomes connect to proximal tubules (PTs) which empty into a distal tubule that joins the pronephric duct. In humans, the pronephros is a rudimentary organ and does not function. As the pronephric duct extends caudally, the glomus and tubules regress. However, the pronephric duct persists and becomes the mesonephric duct.

Mesonephros

The human mesonephros develops in the middle of the fourth week of gestation as a thoracic organ, caudal to the pronephros. Considerable variation in structure and function of the mesonephros exists, even among mammalian species (14). Although 40 to 42 nephrons are formed in the human mesonephros, only 30 to 32 or less are present at any given time because the more cranial nephrons degenerate as the more caudal ones form (2). The mesonephric nephrons consist of glomeruli directly connected to tubules, with proximal and distal segments, some of which directly connect to the mesonephric duct (*wolffian* duct or simply the nephric duct [ND]). The distal mesonephric duct fuses with the cloaca, a precursor of the urinary bladder. In some mammals, such as the mouse, two sets of mesonephric tubules exist. The cranial tubules are connected to the mesonephric duct, whereas the more caudal tubules, representing the majority of the mesonephric nephrons, never fuse with the mesonephric duct. Elegant fate mapping studies have demonstrated that the mesonephric tubules largely derive from a mesenchymal-to-epithelial transition within the mesenchyme adjacent to the mesonephric duct (15). Moreover, numerous genes involved in the formation of the definitive mammalian kidney, the metanephros, are also expressed in the mesonephric tubule (16). For example, genes expressed in early structures (e.g., renal vesicle [RV]) of metanephric kidney development are expressed in early mesonephric tubules but not retained in more mature mesonephric tubules. Genes expressed in more differentiated metanephric structures, such as the early proximal tubule, are expressed in more mature mesonephric tubules. These findings support the notion that the mesonephros and metanephros share some common cell and molecular pathways of tubulogenesis. The excretory function of the human mesonephros is believed to be limited. As observed with the pronephros, the mesonephros undergoes apoptosis and degenerates. In the male, some mesonephric tubules form the efferent ducts of the epididymis, whereas the mesonephric duct gives rise to the duct of the epididymis, the vas deferens and the seminal vesicle. In females, the mesonephros undergoes dissolution, with the epoophoron, paroophoron, and Gartner duct remaining as vestigial structures. In both males and females, the mesonephric duct is involved in the formation of the paramesonephric duct (mullerian duct) (17). In males, the mullerian duct degenerates. In females, the mullerian duct forms the oviducts, uterine horns, cervix, and anterior vagina.

METANEPHROS

Overview

The metanephros, the definitive and permanent kidney, develops from a mutual inductive interaction between the mesonephric duct (nephric or wolffian duct) and a condensed area of mesenchymal cells in the caudal IM, called the metanephric mesenchyme (MM) or blastema. Although the nephric duct and MM are both formed from the IM, their respective epithelial and mesenchymal cell types provide for complex molecular signaling between each other. During around the fourth week of gestation, the first step in human metanephric development occurs. Factors expressed by the MM induce the ureteric bud (UB), a branch of the caudal nephric duct to grow dorsally until it encounters the mesenchyme. The ureteric bud undergoes iterative branching to form the renal pelvis, calyces, and collecting ducts. Induced by the ureteric bud, the MM differentiates into the glomeruli, proximal and distal tubules, and Henle loops. Thus, cells of the metanephric kidney originate from two different lineages to form the collecting ducts and nephrons. The reciprocal inductive interaction between the ureteric bud and the MM is the central process of kidney development. For detailed information, the reader is directed to the classic light microscopic (18–20), microdissection (2,3,21) and experimental (1,4) studies. The following outlines the morphologic features of renal organogenesis followed by the molecular aspects.

Formation of the Renal Pelvis and Calyces

Growing into the adjacent MM, the ureteric bud branches repeatedly while it also elongates. This complex three-dimensional branching pattern creates an elaborate renal architecture. The ureteric bud and its branches consist of a stalk or trunk portion, which elongates, and an actively growing ampullary tip. Two main categories of branching have been observed (2,3,21–24). The most common type is terminal branching of the ampullary tip. The most common form of terminal branching is bifid forming a "T" structure. However, asymmetric bifid branching forming an "L" structure and even trifid branching have been observed. Lateral branching from the stalk segment has been noted but is far less frequent. Experimental studies have demonstrated that ureteric bud stalks which have had their existing tips removed can branch and form new tips (25). Thus, the developing collecting duct system exhibits considerable developmental plasticity. The first three to five generations of ureteric bud branches form the renal pelvis, with more divisions occurring in the poles than in the midpolar region (Fig. 33.2). Urine production is accompanied by progressive dilatation and coalescence of the earlier branches to form the early pelvic-calyceal system by 11 to 12 weeks. Subsequent generations of branches form the calyces. Extensive tissue remodeling of the calyceal system occurs. By 11 to 14 weeks, the calyces become compressed between the expanding renal pelvis and

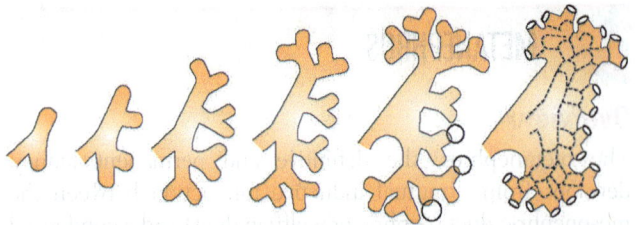

FIGURE 33.2 Diagram depicting early branches of ureteric bud that dilate and coalesce to form the renal pelvis. Examples of third-, fourth-, and fifth-generation branches are *circled*. (Modified with permission from Potter EL. *Normal and Abnormal Development of the Kidney*. Chicago: Year Book; 1972.)

the aggregation of nephrons induced by collecting ducts in the developing papillae. The minor calyces convert from a bulbous configuration to their definitive cup-like shape and the papillae become conical (Fig. 33.3). The fate of the very first nephrons formed, presumably induced by and attached to the first generations of the ureteric bud that form the pelvis and calyces, remains a question. They are believed to either degenerate or attach to a later generation branch that elongates eventually to reach the juxtamedullary cortex.

Formation of the Collecting System

At 8 weeks, the first nephrons can be observed attached to ureteric bud branches. The organogenetic processes of collecting duct branching and elongation, and nephron formation occur simultaneously. Collecting duct morphogenesis has been divided into four periods (2). In the first period, from the 5th to the 14th week of gestation, branching occurs from the ampullary tips and individual nephrons remain attached to their ampullae. In an iterative bifurcation model of branching, one of the two new ampullae retains the old nephron whereas the other induces the formation of a new one. The second period, weeks 14 to 22, is characterized by the formation of arcades. Ampullae rarely branch but single elongating tips repeatedly induce new nephrons while carrying attached older nephrons. As new nephrons are formed, the connecting tubule (CNT) of the older nephron merges its point of attachment away from the ampulla to the CNT of the newer nephron. Repetition of this process results in three to seven nephrons forming around a single ampulla, joined to one another in an arcade by their CNTs. Arcades are associated with juxtamedullary nephrons in the inner cortex of the fully developed kidney.

In the third period, weeks 20 to 36, the ampullae advance beyond the attachment point of the arcade, toward the outer surface. The ampullae do not branch but induce five to seven nephrons, each of which will have a direct connection to the developing collecting tubule. This type of nephron attachment predominates in the outer cortex of the mature kidney (Fig. 33.4). Since nephrons retain contact

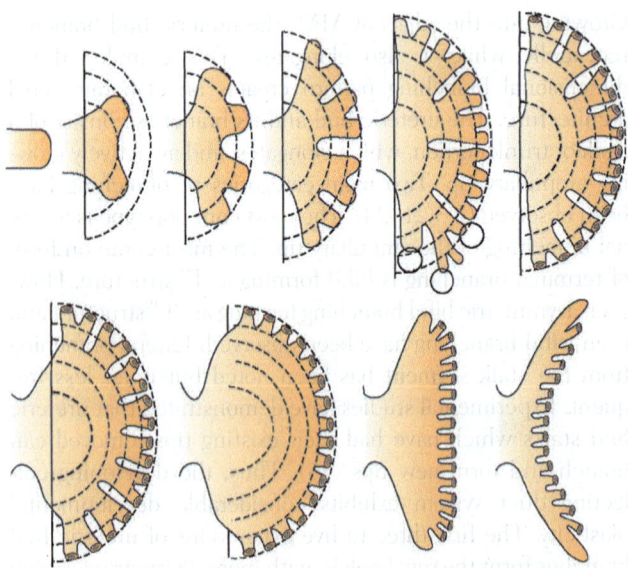

FIGURE 33.3 Diagram illustrating later branches of ureteric bud forming a minor calyx and papilla. *Circles* indicate generation branches that may expand to form part of the calyx or, if not expanding, form papillary ducts. The expanding pelvis and the peripheral zone of differentiating nephrons compress the original saccular cavity, producing the cup-like shape of the calyx and the conical configuration of the papilla. (Modified with permission from Potter EL. *Normal and Abnormal Development of the Kidney*. Chicago: Year Book; 1972.)

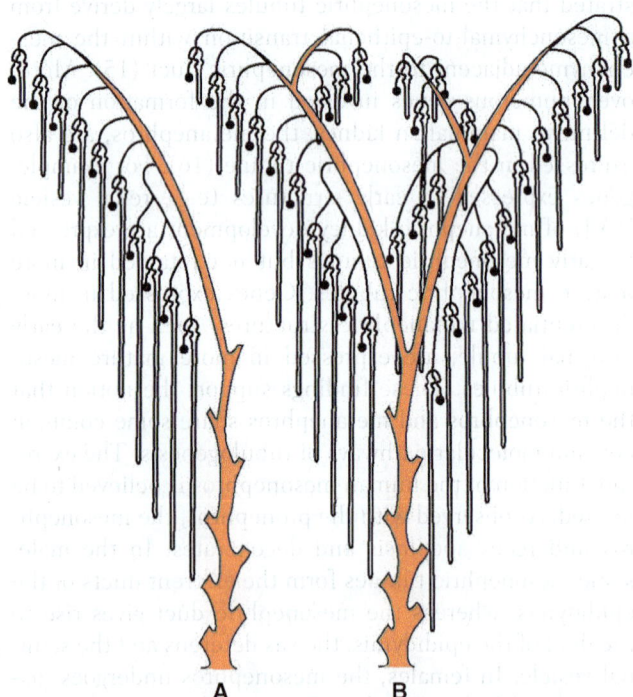

FIGURE 33.4 Diagram demonstrating the pattern of nephrons and collecting tubules at birth. **A:** The most common arrangement is for each collecting tubule to have a single arcade composed of three to five nephrons and five to seven nephrons individually attached. **B:** Depending on the division of the ampullary tips, other variations are possible. (Modified with permission from Potter EL. *Normal and Abnormal Development of the Kidney*. Chicago: Year Book; 1972.)

with their ampullae of origin, either through arcades or directly, the longitudinal growth of the collecting tubules positions the attached glomeruli in the cortex. In the fourth period, beginning at 32 to 36 weeks, the ampullae disappear and no new nephrons form. Normally, nephrogenesis does not occur beyond 36 weeks of gestation. The last nephrons formed are in the outer cortex with their glomeruli near the renal capsule.

Nephron Formation

Over 100 years ago, investigations by Herring and Huber provided a fairly accurate morphologic view of human nephron development (Fig. 33.5) (18,19). They were also prescient in regard to some mechanisms of nephrogenesis, for example, in the development of glomerular capillaries. From 8 weeks of gestation, the nephrons and collecting duct system develop together. The stages in individual nephron development do not vary and occur continuously throughout the periods of collecting duct formation. The formation of nephrons can be divided into two phases: the induction stage and the morphogenetic stage (4,26). In the induction stage, the mesenchyme condenses around the ampullary tips in response to inducing signals from the ureteric bud. Two types of mesenchymal condensates have been described to form in this induction stage prior to epithelial differentiation of the mesenchyme (27). The first condensate, called the *cap*, closely surrounds each ampullary tip.

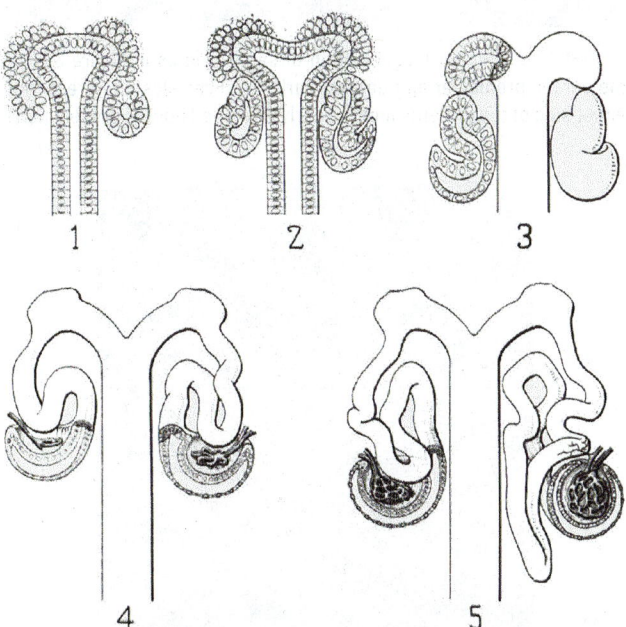

FIGURE 33.5 Huber's schematic drawings of nephron development. **1.** Condensation stage with the cap. A renal vesicle (*right*) is present. **2.** Comma-shaped body. **3.** S-shaped body. **4.** Early glomerular capillary development, Bowman capsule formation and tubule elongation. **5.** Glomerular and tubule maturation (*right*). (Reprinted from Huber GC. On the development and shape of uriniferous tubules of certain of the higher mammals. *Am J Anat* 1905;4(suppl):1–98.)

A short time later, another condensate, termed the *pretubular aggregate (PTA)*, forms at the lateral edges of the ampullary tip, below the cap. The cap mesenchyme (CM) is believed to regulate ureteric bud branching and contains the progenitor cells of the nephron epithelia, whereas the cells of the PTA having differentiated from the cap are believed to be committed to form the nephron elements.

The morphogenetic stage of nephron formation involves several complex phases (Fig. 33.5). First, the cells of the PTA undergo a mesenchyme-to-epithelium transition, characterized by expression of epithelial markers and synthesis of basement membrane matrix glycoproteins. The cells develop intercellular junctions, become polarized and surrounded by a basal lamina, forming a structure termed the renal *vesicle*. A central cavity may be observed in the vesicle. It may be difficult to distinguish between PTAs and renal vesicles in histologic sections. Soon after formation, the vesicle fuses to the ureteric duct epithelium and a continuous basal lamina surrounds both the vesicle and the duct. Opposite the area of fusion between the vesicle and the ureteric duct, a vascular cleft develops representing the site where the glomerular capillaries will emerge. The vesicle becomes a *comma*-shaped tubular structure. Another crevice forms near the fusion between the comma-structure and the ureteric duct. After elongation and folding, an S-shaped figure representing an early nephron forms (Fig. 33.6). At this stage, the S-shaped body is already compartmentalized into distinct cell types that are arranged into three areas. The vascular cleft lies below the upper and middle limbs of the S-shaped body, and above the lower limb. The lower limb, most distant from the ureteric bud, differentiates into the visceral epithelium (podocytes) and parietal epithelium (Bowman capsule) of the glomerulus. The midportion (limb) of the S-body forms the proximal tubule and the loop of Henle. The upper limb becomes the distal convoluted tubule (DCT) and fuses with the ureteric bud branches to form the CNT. Active nephron formation occurs across the developing renal cortex in a band, known as the *nephrogenic zone* (Figs. 33.7 to 33.9). After nephron formation ceases, generally by 36 weeks of gestation, the nephrogenic zone disappears (Fig. 33.10). The growth of the collecting ducts and the incremental formation of nephrons result in a centrifugal developmental pattern extending through the renal cortex. The earliest nephrons to form are found in the juxtamedullary zone of cortex, whereas the last nephrons to develop are in the outer cortex. This principle is fundamental to understanding postnatal structural changes in the kidney and is sometimes useful in the timing of developmental disturbances in the cortex. For example, a disturbance during the early months of development may result in an abnormality of the entire cortical thickness, whereas one that occurs in the last half of gestation may involve only the outermost layers of cortical nephrons. In summary, the coincident processes of ureteral-derived epithelial branching and nephron formation largely establish the basic architectural organization of the kidney.

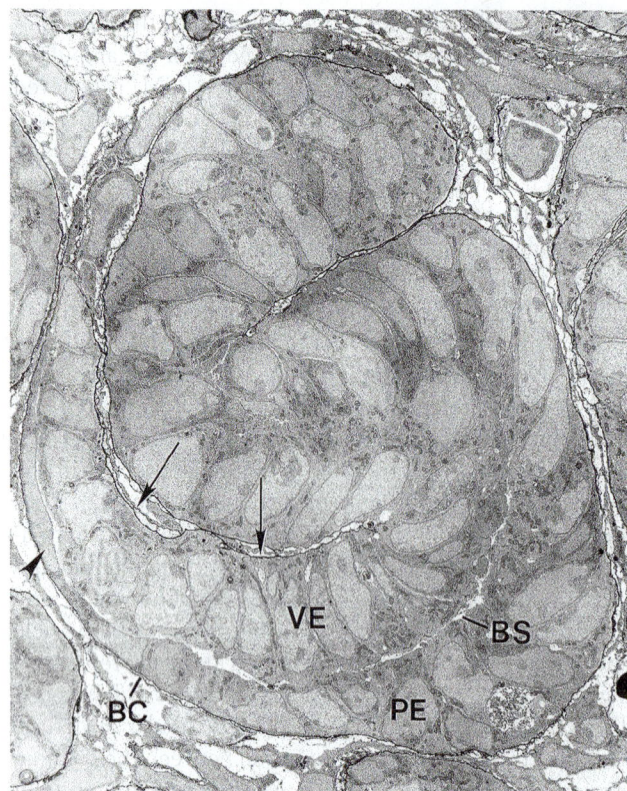

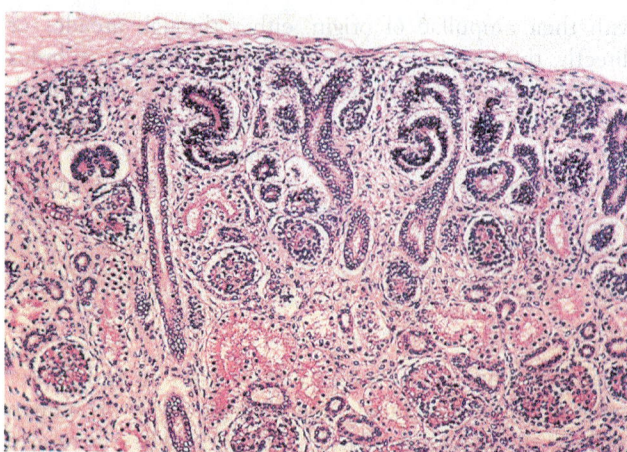

FIGURE 33.8 Nephrogenic zone from developing kidney at 26 weeks of gestation illustrating several stages of nephron formation.

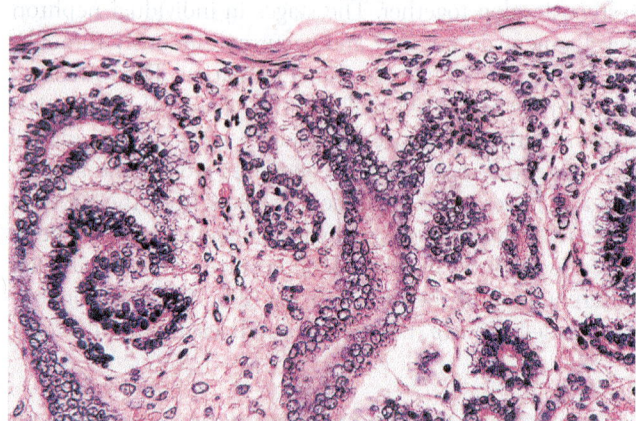

FIGURE 33.9 Higher magnification of same field as in Figure 33.7. In the center, pretubular aggregates (early renal vesicles) are present on either side of the ureteric duct. An early S-shaped body is present (*left*).

FIGURE 33.6 Electron micrograph of S-shaped figure from newborn mouse kidney. The basement membranes are rendered black by labeling with anti-laminin IgG conjugated to horseradish peroxidase. The vascular cleft (*arrows*), visceral epithelial cells (*VE*), Bowman space (*BS*), parietal epithelial cells (*PE*), and Bowman capsule (*BC*) can be seen. The visceral epithelial cells will differentiate into podocytes. Some parietal epithelial cells are becoming squamous (*arrowhead*) and will line Bowman capsule. The epithelial cells above the vascular cleft will give rise to the PTs, loops of Henle, and DCTs. (Magnification ×5,000.) (Modified with permission from Clapp WL, Abrahamson DR. Development and gross anatomy of the kidney. In: Tisher CC, Brenner BM, eds. *Renal Pathology*. 2nd ed. Philadelphia, PA: JB Lippincott; 1994:3–59.)

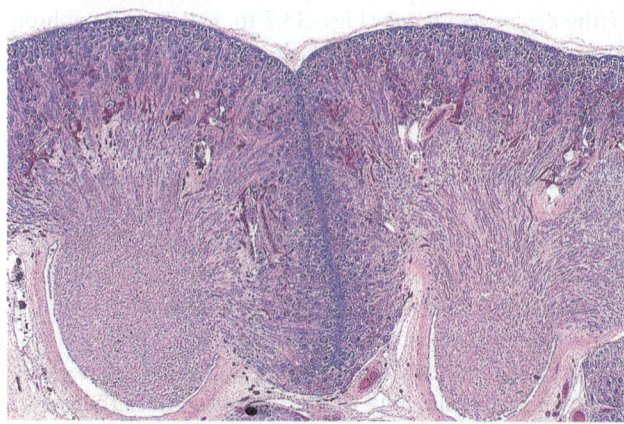

FIGURE 33.7 Developing kidney at 21 weeks of gestation showing two medullary pyramids with surrounding cortex. The nephrogenic zone represents a thin layer outlining the peripheral aspects of the lobes, both at the surface and in the midplane of the septa (column) of Bertin, between the two renal lobes.

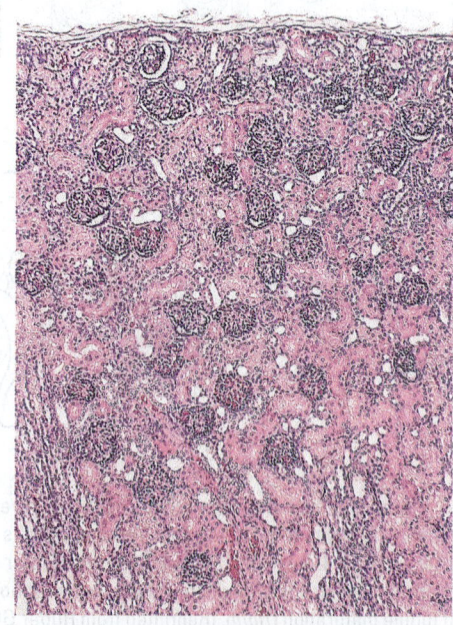

FIGURE 33.10 Newborn kidney (40 weeks of gestation). Note the absence of a nephrogenic zone. Some glomeruli are near the renal capsule.

MOLECULAR REGULATION OF KIDNEY DEVELOPMENT

To make a kidney requires an orchestration of numerous complex cellular and molecular events. Several experimental approaches and model systems have enhanced our understanding of kidney development. The mouse has been the most powerful model organism. However, as will be presented, cell and molecular studies of human kidney development are expanding. A variety of in vitro studies have been valuable, including organic culture of mouse metanephric rudiments, pioneered by Grobstein (1), and cell cultures of individual nephrogenic lineages. Gene targeting studies such as gene ablation in mice ("knockout" mice) have provided powerful in vivo evidence for the role of certain genes in renal organogenesis (Table 33.1). However, the generation of knockout mice using homologous recombination in embryonic stem cells may result in embryonic lethality, preventing an analysis of the significance of the target gene in kidney development. Moreover, since a gene may be expressed in different cell types, the knockout phenotype may be complex and difficult to understand. "Conditional" knockout mice with genes disrupted only in specific renal cell types can be created using site-specific DNA recombinase systems (e.g., Cre-loxP) (28). Using this approach with temporal control of gene expression (e.g., tetracycline-responsive promoter) allows for functional dissection of a gene in a specific renal cell at any developmental timepoint. Another approach is large-scale mouse mutagenesis using the chemical mutagen N-ethyl-N-nitrosourea (ENU). It represents an unbiased phenotype-driven strategy to identify genes responsible for renal developmental defects (29). This approach, associated with point mutations rather than gene deletions, leads to phenotypes that resemble human disorders more closely than conventional knockouts.

High-throughput global gene expression studies have led to a more detailed view of kidney development. Brunskill et al. used either laser capture microdissection (LCM) or fluorescence-activated cell sorting (FACS) to isolate cells from 15 distinct compartments of the developing mouse kidney (30). The compartment purification was facilitated by using green-fluorescent protein (GFP)-transgenic mice or specific lectin staining patterns. Microarrays were then employed to generate global gene (RNA) expression profiles for each compartment. In situ hybridizations (ISHs) validated the microarray data and in several cases revealed expression restricted to a subregion of a compartment. Interestingly, of over 7,000 genes showing differential expression, only 3% of the genes showed expression restricted to one compartment. Thus, most genes show quantitative rather than qualitative differences in expression from one developing compartment to the next. Some genes are expressed at low levels in early developmental compartments before their signature strong expression in a later related compartment. For example, the CM shows some weak ("anticipatory") expression of some genes which show strong expression in the subsequent renal vesicle. This work was established within the Genitourinary Developmental Molecular Anatomy Project (GUDMAP), an international consortium working to produce a high-resolution morphologic and molecular map of the developing urogenital tract (31). The GUDMAP database (http://www.gudmap.org) serves as a valuable interactive online resource for research in kidney development. For example, the GUDMAP database can be used with bioinformatic analysis to identify transcription factors that bind to conserved binding sites (cis-regulatory modules) in the promoters of genes highly expressed in a particular anatomic compartment (32). This type of analysis can provide insights into the genetic circuitry that controls, for example, the differentiation of the CM into the renal vesicle. Recent studies are increasing the limits of resolution by evaluating gene expression at the single-cell level in the developing kidney (33). Some single-cell progenitor cells of the MM co-express markers of both nephron epithelial and stromal lineages. Moreover, single cells of the renal vesicle co-express markers of both podocyte and proximal tubule lineages. These findings are consistent with "multilineage priming," whereby promiscuous multilineage gene expression in a single progenitor cell primes the cell for subsequent specific lineage commitment. Such studies will enhance our understanding of specific cell types and general cell differentiation (34).

Analysis of the GUDMAP database has been extended to identify kidney developmental "anchor" genes, defined as a gene whose expression is absolutely specific to one temporal–spatial anatomic compartment (35). Bioinformatic analysis followed by high-resolution ISH revealed a total of 37 anchor genes representing six anatomic compartments in the developing mid-gestation murine kidney. The 37 anchor genes included 5 genes restricted to the medullary collecting duct (MCD), 1 gene specific for the ureteric tip, 1 gene restricted to the renal vesicle, 3 genes marking the glomerular podocytes, 1 gene restricted to the juxtaglomerular (JG) arterioles, 1 gene specific for the loop of Henle, and 25 genes marking the early proximal tubule. No anchor genes were identified within the medullary or cortical interstitium, the S-shaped body or the cortical collecting duct (CCD). The lack of anchor genes within these compartments or structures may reflect their cellular and segmental heterogeneity, transient developmental stage, and/or the commonality of gene expression.

The 25 early proximal tubule anchor genes displayed specific patterns of expression which marked the early subdivision into S_1, S_2, and S_3 segments. Bioinformatic analysis of the promoters of the proximal tubule anchor genes identified binding sites for several transcription factors, which are expressed in the developing proximal tubule. Moreover, functional genetic network analysis reidentified some of these transcription factors and their relationship to the target anchor genes in the process of proximal tubule differentiation. These studies set the stage for the generation

TABLE 33.1 Genes Involved in Kidney Development

Developmental Process Gene (Human Syndrome)	Function	Expression in Normal Developing Kidney	Mutant Kidney Phenotype (Mouse)
Specification of the Nephrogenic Mesenchyme			
Lim1	Transcription factor	Intermediate mesoderm, nephric duct, mesonephros, ureteric bud, collecting ducts, pretubular aggregates, S-shaped bodies, podocytes	Absent pro-, meso-, and metanephros (Lim1 required at multiple steps of kidney development)
Eya1 (Mutations in branchiooto-renal [BOR] syndrome)	Transcription coactivator (interacts with Six1)	Intermediate mesoderm, uninduced and induced metanephric mesenchyme	Intact pro- and mesonephros, but absent metanephric blastema, renal agenesis
Six1 (Mutations in branchiooto-renal [BOR] syndrome)	Transcription factor (interacts with Eya1)	Uninduced and induced metanephric mesenchyme and collecting tubules	Ureteric bud forms but does not fully invade metanephric mesenchyme, which undergoes apoptosis, renal agenesis
Sall1 (Mutations in Townes–Brocks syndrome)	Transcription factor	Mesonephros, induced metanephric mesenchyme	Ureteric bud forms but does not fully invade metanephric mesenchyme, which undergoes apoptosis, renal hypoplasia, or agenesis
Hoxa11, Hoxd11	Transcription factors	Intermediate mesoderm, metanephric mesenchyme	Impaired ureteric bud branching, renal hypoplasia in Hoxa11/Hoxd11 double mutants
Pax2	Transcription factor	Intermediate mesoderm, nephric duct, mesonephros, ureteric bud, induced metanephric mesenchyme	Intact nephric duct but mesonephric tubules and ureteric bud fail to form, renal agenesis
WT1	Transcription factor	Intermediate mesoderm, mesonephros, uninduced and induced metanephric mesenchyme, comma- and S-shaped bodies, podocytes	Absent caudal mesonephros, ureteric bud fails to form, metanephric mesenchyme undergoes apoptosis, renal agenesis
Cell Survival			
BMP7	Growth factor	Mesonephric duct, ureteric bud, induced metanephric mesenchyme, distal tubules, comma- and S-shaped bodies, podocytes	Increased apoptosis in metanephric mesenchyme, decreased ureter bud branching, hydroureter, severe renal hypoplasia
FGF-8	Growth factor	Pretubular aggregates, vesicles, tubule progenitors in S-body	Increased apoptosis in S-body precursors, truncated nephrons, severe renal hypoplasia
Bcl-2	Antiapoptotic factor	Ureteric bud, induced metanephric mesenchyme, parietal epithelium of Bowman capsule, tubules, and collecting ducts	Increased apoptosis especially in metanephric mesenchyme, cysts in tubules and collecting ducts, severe renal hypoplasia
AP-2b	Transcription factor	Distal tubules and collecting ducts	Increased apoptosis and cyst formation in distal tubules and collecting ducts
Pax2 (Heterozygous mutations in renal-coloboma syndrome)	Transcription factor	Intermediate mesoderm, nephric duct, mesonephros, ureteric bud, induced metanephric mesenchyme	Heterozygous Pax-2 mutations result in increased apoptosis in collecting ducts, reduced ureteric branching, hypoplastic kidneys
Cell Proliferation			
FGF-7	Growth factor	Interstitial fibroblasts or stroma surrounding ureteric bud and developing collecting ducts	Decreased growth of ureteric bud and collecting ducts, decreased number of nephrons, renal hypoplasia
N-Myc	Transcription factor	Induced metanephric mesenchyme	Decreased cell proliferation, decreased ureteric bud tips and nephrons, renal hypoplasia
Glypican-3 (Mutations in Simpson–Golabi–Behmel syndrome)	Heparan sulfate proteoglycan	All metanephric mesenchyme and ureteric bud derivatives	Increased cell proliferation in cortical collecting ducts, increased apoptosis in medullary collecting ducts, renal medullary cystic dysplasia

TABLE 33.1
Genes Involved in Kidney Development (*Continued*)

Developmental Process Gene (Human Syndrome)	Function	Expression in Normal Developing Kidney	Mutant Kidney Phenotype (Mouse)
Branching of Ureteric Bud			
GDNF	Growth factor	Intermediate mesoderm, mesonephros, induced metanephric mesenchyme, pretubular aggregates	Ureteric bud fails to form or has abnormal branching, renal hypoplasia, or agenesis
c-ret	GF receptor (TK) (receptor for GDNF)	Mesonephric duct, ureteric bud, and tips of ureteric bud	Similar to GDNF-deficient mice
GFRa1	GF co-receptor (forms signaling complex with GDNF and c-ret)	Induced metanephric mesenchyme, pretubular aggregates, mesonephric duct, ureteric bud, and tips of ureteric bud	Similar to GDNF-deficient mice
GDF11	Growth factor	Mesonephric duct, uninduced and induced metanephric mesenchyme, ureteric bud and branches	No ureteric bud formation, metanephric mesenchyme undergoes apoptosis, renal hypoplasia, or agenesis
Sprouty1	Receptor (TK) antagonist	Mesonephric duct, ureteric bud, and tips of ureteric bud	Supernumerary ureteric buds, multiple ureters, multiplex kidneys
Emx2	Transcription factor	Intermediate mesoderm, mesonephric duct, mesonephros, ureteric bud, comma- and S-shaped bodies	Ureteric bud invades metanephric mesenchyme but fails to dilate or branch, no induction of mesenchyme, renal agenesis
RARa, RARb2	Transcription factors	RARa—ureteric bud, metanephric mesenchyme, stroma RARb2—stroma only	Decreased ureteric bud branching (defective stroma signaling) in RARa/b2 double mutants, renal hypoplasia
BMP4	Bone morphogenetic protein	Stromal mesenchymal cells around ureteric bud branches	Reduced and ectopic ureteral branching, ectopic ureterovesical junction, hydroureter, double collecting ducts, hypo/dysplastic kidneys (heterozygous BMP4 null mice)
Foxc1/2	Transcription factor	Intermediate mesoderm, mesonephros, uninduced and induced metanephric mesenchyme	Double ureters with one a hydroureter, duplex kidneys (Foxc1/Foxc2 compound heterozygous mutants similar to Foxc1 homozygous mutants)
Slit2	Secreted protein	Mesonephric duct, anterior intermediate mesoderm, ureteric bud tips	Supernumerary ureteric buds, hydroureter, fused multiple kidneys
Robo2	Transmembrane (receptor for Slit2)	Intermediate mesoderm, induced metanephric mesenchyme	Supernumerary ureteric buds, hydroureter, fused multiple kidneys
Pod1	Transcription factor	Induced metanephric mesenchyme, stromal cells, and podocytes	Decreased ureteric branching, arrest in tubular and glomerular differentiation, renal hypoplasia
Heparan sulfate 2-sulfotransferase	Enzyme (synthesis of heparan sulfate, a component of HS proteoglycan)	Mesonephric duct, transient in ureteric bud, metanephric mesenchyme	Ureteric bud outgrowth but no branching, no condensation of metanephric mesenchyme, renal agenesis
Integrin α8	Transmembrane adhesion receptor	Intermediate mesoderm, induced metanephric mesenchyme, pretubular aggregates	Limited ureteric bud invasion of metanephric mesenchyme, decreased ureteric branching, renal hypoplasia, or agenesis
Integrin α3b1	Transmembrane adhesion receptor	Ureteric bud, collecting ducts, podocytes	Decreased branching of medullary collecting ducts, microcystic proximal tubules, defective glomerulogenesis
Pbxl	Transcription factor	Induced metanephric mesenchyme and stromal cells	Decreased and irregular ureteric bud branching, large mesenchymal condensates, renal hypoplasia, or unilateral agenesis

(continued)

TABLE 33.1

Genes Involved in Kidney Development (*Continued*)

Developmental Process Gene (Human Syndrome)	Function	Expression in Normal Developing Kidney	Mutant Kidney Phenotype (Mouse)
Grem1	Bone morphogenetic protein (BMP) antagonist	Intermediate mesoderm, mesonephric duct, metanephric mesenchyme	Ureteric bud forms but fails to invade metanephric mesenchyme, which undergoes apoptosis, renal agenesis
Wnt11	Secreted glycoprotein	Ureteric bud tips	Loss of ureteric tips, reduced ureteric branching, renal hypoplasia
Formin (Mutations in mice cause the limb deformity syndrome)	Protein that regulates cytoskeleton function	Mesonephric duct, mesonephros, ureteric bud, metanephric mesenchyme	Decreased ureteric bud outgrowth, renal hypoplasia, unilateral, or bilateral renal agenesis
Angiotensinogen (*Agt*)	Renin substrate	Ureteric bud, stroma, S-shaped bodies, glomeruli, proximal tubules	Hypoplastic papillae, hydronephrosis, thickened blood vessels, reduced blood pressure
Renin	Enzyme (cleaves Agt to form angiotensin I)	Developing arcuate and interlobular arteries and afferent arterioles, restricted to juxtaglomerular apparatus with maturity	Hypoplastic papillae, hydronephrosis, thickened blood vessels, reduced blood pressure
Angiotensin-converting enzyme (*ACE*)	Enzyme (converts angiotensin I to angiotensin II)	Glomeruli, proximal tubules and collecting ducts, small arteries	Hypoplastic papillae, hydronephrosis, thickened blood vessels, reduced blood pressure
Angiotensin II receptor, type 1 (AT_1)	Angiotensin II receptor	Ureteric bud, stroma, S-shaped bodies, proximal tubules, collecting ducts	Hypoplastic papillae, hydronephrosis, thickened blood vessels, reduced blood pressure
Angiotensin II receptor, type 2 (AT_2)	Angiotensin II receptor	Stroma adjacent to ureteric bud stalk	3% have abnormalities, duplicated collecting system, and hydronephrotic upper pole
Mesenchymal-to-Epithelial Transition			
Wnt4	Secreted glycoprotein	Pretubular aggregates, comma-shaped body, distal S-shaped body	Ureteric bud branching occurs, no mesenchymal–epithelial transition, renal agenesis
Wnt9b	Secreted glycoprotein	Mesonephric duct, ureteric bud, and collecting ducts but not branching tips	No mesenchymal–epithelial transition, renal agenesis
Foxd1(BF2)	Transcription factor	Interstitial stroma cells	Decreased ureteric bud branching, large mesenchymal condensates, abnormal renal capsule, small fused pelvic kidneys
Pod1	Transcription factor	Induced metanephric mesenchyme, stromal cells, and podocytes	Increased size of induced mesenchymal condensates, arrest in tubular and glomerular differentiation, renal hypoplasia
Fras1 (Mutations in Fraser syndrome)	Extracellular matrix (ECM) protein	Basal side of ureteric ducts	Ureteric bud invades metanephric mesenchyme but decreased induction, apoptosis of mesenchyme, renal hypoplasia, or agenesis
Grip1	Cytoplasmic protein (interacts with *Fras1*)	Basal side of ureteric ducts	Similar abnormal phenotype as in *Fras1*-deficient mice
Cadherin-6 (*K-cadherin*)	Transmembrane adhesion protein	Renal vesicle, proximal end of comma- and S-shaped bodies, developing proximal tubules and Henle loops	Delayed fusion of some comma-shaped bodies to ureteric bud leading to loss of nephrons
Glomerulogenesis			
WT1 (Mutations in WAGR, Denys-Drash, and Frasier syndromes)	Transcription factor	Intermediate mesoderm, mesonephros, uninduced and induced metanephric mesenchyme, S-shaped body, podocytes	Disturbed podocyte differentiation, glomerulosclerosis

TABLE 33.1 Genes Involved in Kidney Development *(Continued)*

Developmental Process Gene (Human Syndrome)	Function	Expression in Normal Developing Kidney	Mutant Kidney Phenotype (Mouse)
PDGF-β	Growth factor	Glomerular endothelial cells and podocytes	Dilated glomerular capillaries with no mesangial cells
PDGFR-β	Growth factor receptor (receptor for *PDGF-β*)	Glomerular mesangial cells	Dilated glomerular capillaries with no mesangial cells
Notch2	Transmembrane receptor	Developing collecting ducts, comma- and S-shaped bodies, podocytes	Abnormal glomeruli arrested at capillary loop stage, with disorganized podocytes and no mesangial cells
VEGF-A	Growth factor	S-shaped bodies, podocytes, collecting ducts	Small glomeruli, lack capillary loops, few endothelial cells
Laminin α5	Basement membrane protein	Basement membranes of ureteric bud, developing tubules, and glomerular basement membrane (GBM)	Abnormal glomeruli with displaced endothelial and mesangial cells, and clustered podocytes
Laminin β2	Basement membrane protein	Glomerular basement membranes beginning at capillary loop stage	Absence of podocyte foot processes, proteinuria
Laminin α3b1	Transmembrane adhesion receptor	Ureteric bud, collecting ducts, podocytes	Glomerular capillary loops dilated and fewer in number, loss of podocyte foot processes, dual GBMs (failure of fusion)
Collagen IV α5 (Mutations in Alport syndrome)	Basement membrane protein	Forms heterodimer with α3 (IV) and α5 (IV) chains in GBM from capillary stage onward	Thinning and "basket-weave" thickening of GBMs
Nephrin (Mutations in congenital nephrotic syndrome of Finnish type)	Transmembrane protein	Podocyte filtration slit diaphragm	Foot process effacement, absent filtration slit diaphragms, proteinuria
CD2AP	Adapter protein (interacts with nephrin)	Podocyte filtration slit diaphragm domain	Irregular foot processes, absent filtration slit diaphragms, proteinuria
Podocin (Mutations in autosomal recessive steroid-resistant nephrotic syndrome)	Membrane protein (interacts with nephrin)	Podocyte filtration slit diaphragm domain	Irregular foot processes, absent filtration slit diaphragms, proteinuria
α-actinin (Mutations in autosomal dominant focal segmental glomerulosclerosis [FSGS])	Cross-links actin filaments	Podocyte filtration slit diaphragm domain	Foot process effacement, GBM duplication, proteinuria, and FSGS
TRPC6 (Mutations in autosomal dominant FSGS)	Cation-channel	Podocyte filtration slit diaphragm domain	Foot process effacement and FSGS (humans)
Neph1	Transmembrane protein (interacts with nephrin)	Podocyte filtration slit diaphragm	Foot process effacement, proteinuria
FAT1	Protocadherin	Podocyte filtration slit diaphragm	Foot process effacement
Lmx1b (Mutations in nail patella syndrome)	Transcription factor	Podocytes	Abnormal foot processes, absent filtration slit diaphragms
Podocalyxin	CD34-related transmembrane protein	Podocyte apical membrane domain	Abnormal podocytes, foot process effacement, absent filtration slit diaphragms, anuria

(continued)

TABLE 33.1
Genes Involved in Kidney Development (Continued)

Developmental Process Gene (Human Syndrome)	Function	Expression in Normal Developing Kidney	Mutant Kidney Phenotype (Mouse)
GLEPP1 (Ptpro)	Receptor tyrosine phosphatase	Podocyte apical membrane domain	Shortened and widened podocyte foot processes, reduced glomerular filtration rate
Kreisler (Krml1/MafB)	Transcription factor	Podocytes, initially at capillary loop stage	Abnormal podocyte differentiation with no foot processes
Tubular Differentiation			
PKD1 (polycystin-1) (Mutations in autosomal dominant polycystic kidney disease [ADPKD])	Transmembrane protein (adhesion receptor, in cilia, interacts with polycystin-2)	Developing nephron segments and collecting ducts	Renal cysts arising from developing nephron segments and collecting ducts
PKD2 (polycystin-2) (Mutations in autosomal dominant polycystic kidney disease [ADPKD])	Transmembrane protein (calcium channel, in cilia, interacts with polycystin-1)	Developing nephron segments and collecting ducts	Renal cysts arising from developing nephron segments and collecting ducts
Frem2 (Mutations in Fraser syndrome)	Extracellular matrix (ECM) protein	Mesonephros, ureteric bud especially at tips, tubule derivatives	Cysts of collecting ducts and thick ascending limbs
Cox-2 (Cyclooxygenase-2)	Enzyme (prostaglandin synthesis)	Developing collecting ducts, S-shaped bodies, macula densa, cortical thick ascending limb, medullary interstitial cells	Progressive postnatal outer cortical dysplasia, tubular cysts, and glomerular hypoplasia
EGFR	Growth factor receptor (TK)	Mesonephric duct, ureteric bud, collecting ducts	Dilatation of collecting ducts, uremia
Brnl	Transcription factor	Renal vesicle, comma- and S-shaped bodies, developing Henle loop (HL), distal convoluted tubule (DCT), macula densa (MD)	Disrupted differentiation of HLs, MD, and DCT
Psen1/Psen2	Presinilins- (transmembrane protein with γ-secretase activity)	Developing early nephron structures	Renal vesicles and pretubular aggregates form, but no comma- or S-shaped bodies; proximal tubules and glomeruli fail to form (Psen1/Psen2 double null mutant mice with human PSEN1 transgene)
Tensin	Adhesion protein (phosphoprotein, binds actin)	Proximal and distal tubules (adult kidney)	Hydronephrosis, cystic dilatation of proximal tubules
R-cadherin	Transmembrane adhesion protein	Induced metanephric mesenchyme, renal vesicle, comma- and S-shaped bodies	Dilatation and cytoplasmic vacuolization of proximal tubules

of anchor-gene driven transgenic reporter mice which will help dissect the mechanisms of kidney development. The following sections provide an overview of the molecular aspects of kidney development. Excellent comprehensive reviews are available (7–12).

Most of our understanding of the cell and molecular aspects of kidney development, and which is mainly resented in this chapter, has come from studies in mice. A series of landmark studies have explored human kidney development with modern cell and molecular methods. Based on examination of 135 human kidney specimens, Lindstrom et al. described the similarities and differences of human and mouse kidney organogenesis (36). They differ in nephrogenic zone organization, timing of nephron formation and molecular features, including the expression of anchor-gene markers. For example, in humans, the ureteric epithelium is initially bilayered, the first nephron structures appear at 37 to 41 days post-ovulation or Carneige stage 16 (CS16), the first connected S-shaped body occurs 3 to 14 days later, lobulation begins 48 to 51 days post-ovulation (CS19), and the ureteric tips and surrounding progenitor cells display a rosette-like architectural pattern.

INTERMEDIATE MESODERM SPECIFICATION

Both the mesonephric duct (nephric duct) and the MM form from the IM. The IM is a strip of tissue in the early embryo between the paraxial somatic mesoderm (PM) and the LPM. Little is known about how the IM becomes specified to develop into the kidney morphogenetic program of the pronephros, mesonephros, and finally the metanephros. The IM is specified along both the mediolateral and anteroposterior (AP) axes. The earliest known marker genes of the IM include *Osr1*, *Lhx1*, *Pax2*, and *Pax8*. Along the mediolateral axis and lateral to the IM, secreted factors of the bone morphogenetic protein (BMP) family, including BMP2 and their cognate receptor ALK3, activate the IM marker genes (37,38). Signals medial to the IM, including activin, a member of the transforming growth factor β (TGF-β) family activate the IM genes (39). It is not clear how these signals, lateral and medial to the IM, are integrated.

The progression of development of the transient kidneys (pronephros and mesonephros) and the permanent kidney (metanephros) in a cranial-caudal direction along the anteroposterior axis is striking. Is the IM differentially specified along the AP axis to direct either a pronephric, mesonephric, or metanephric gene program? The *Hox* genes are well known to determine the developmental fate of cells within distinct regions along the AP axis. Encoding homeodomain-containing transcription factors, the *Hox* genes are arranged into four chromosomal clusters, which are subdivided into 13 sets of paralogous genes. The *Hox* genes of paralog group 4, including *Hoxb4*, *Hoxc4*, and *Hoxd4* are involved in establishing the anterior border of the kidney morphogenetic field (40). Expression of the *Hox11* paralog group, *Hoxa11*, *Hoxc11*, and *Hoxd11*, is restricted in the IM to the posterior, metanephric level (15). Deletion of the *Hox11* paralog genes results in agenesis of the metanephros but not the mesonephros (40,41). Thus, specific patterns of Hox gene expression establish the anterior and posterior borders of the IM that will become the MM.

NEPHRIC DUCT

In the early embryo, the previously discussed signals along with the *Hox* gene expression domains induce the IM to form the nephric duct. Several genes including *Pax2*, *Pax8*, *Lhx1*, *Gata3*, and β-catenin (*Ctnnb1*) form a regulatory network essential for normal ND development (42–45). As the ND elongates caudally, it converts from a solid core of mesenchymal cells to an epithelial duct. It eventually contacts and fuses with the cloaca. Cellular extensions from the caudal tip of the ND participate in guiding the duct toward the cloaca. Insertion of the ND into the cloaca is regulated by *Ret* expression in the ND, which is dependent upon *Gata3* and retinoic acid (RA) signaling (46). Direct contact with the ND induces apoptosis in the cloaca which is necessary for fusion of the ND with the cloaca (47).

URETERIC BUD FORMATION

The first step in metanephric kidney development is the outgrowth of the ureteric bud (UB) from the nephric duct. Signals from the MM induce this budding and in turn, the UB induces the MM to form the epithelia of the nephron (nephrogenesis). Failure to form a UB results in renal agenesis and incorrect positioning of the UB leads to congenital anomalies of the kidney and urinary tract (CAKUT) (48,49). *Gdnf/Ret* signaling is a major pathway regulating UB formation (50). The glial-derived neurotrophic factor (GDNF) secreted by the MM interacts with RET, a proto-oncogene receptor tyrosine kinase and a co-receptor GFRα1, both expressed in the ND, to induce UB outgrowth.

The initial processes in UB morphogenesis have been described using chimeric mice, in which fluorescent reporter proteins (e.g., GFP) are expressed specifically in the ND–UB lineage (51). These elegant studies have allowed analysis of early UB cells with different gene activities on the basis of differential labeling (e.g., GFP, CFP). Prior to definitive UB outgrowth, a segment in the caudal ND thickens. Cells with elevated RET activity migrate within the ND and concentrate to form a RET-rich cellular domain that will become the initial budding tip. Simultaneously, this ND segment converts from a cuboidal to a pseudostratified epithelium. Unlike the cell migration, this epithelial reorganization occurs independent of RET signaling.

The dominant view is that UB formation is mainly dependent on *Gdnf/Ret* signaling (Fig. 33.11). The UB fails to form leading to renal agenesis in most embryos without *Gdnf* or without *Ret* (48). However, several activators and inhibitors influence the *Gdnf/Ret* pathway to coordinate normal UB outgrowth (52,53). Activators of *Gdnf* expression in the MM include *Pax2*, *Eya1*, *Hox11* paralogs, *Sall1*, *Grem1*, nephronectin, and integrin α8β1. Mutations of these genes result in defective UB formation and often renal agenesis. The opposite phenotype of supernumerary UBs and ureters results when genes that limit *Gdnf* expression are mutated. Examples of inhibitor genes include *Spry1*, *Bmp4*, *Robo2*, *Slit2*, and *Foxc2*. The proteins encoded by these various genes often interact in regulatory networks. For example, *Pax2*, *Eya1*, and *Hox11* paralog proteins interact in a complex (54) and integrin α8β1 interacts with its ligand nephronectin to activate *Gdnf* expression (55). SLIT2 in the ND interacts with its receptor ROBO2 in the MM to restrict *Gdnf* expression (56). Moreover, an activator may interact with an inhibitor to facilitate UB sprouting. For example, *Grem1*, a BMP antagonist, is upregulated in the mesenchyme surrounding the ND prior to initiation of UB outgrowth and reduces the activity of *Bmp4* which inhibits *Gdnf/Ret* signaling (57). In other words, the

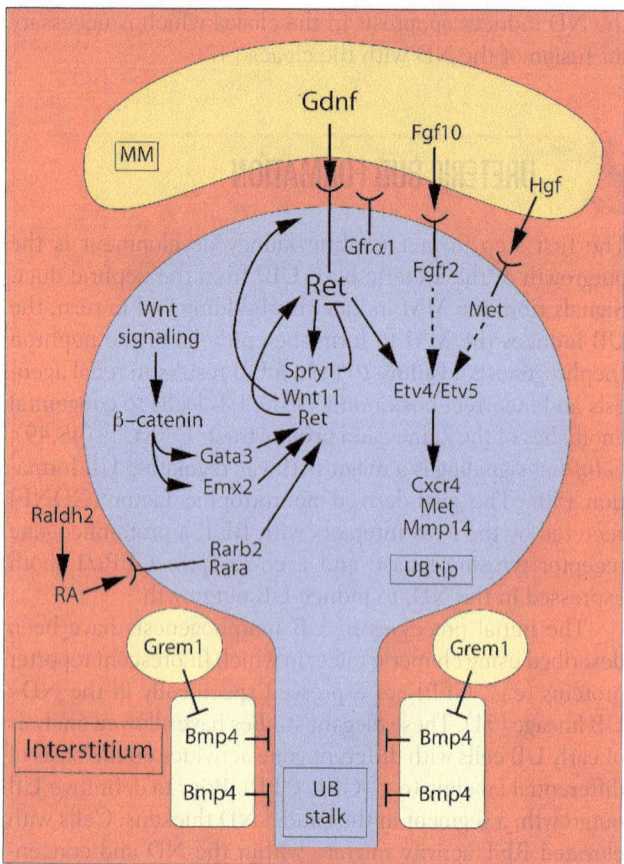

FIGURE 33.11 Schematic drawing of the genetic signaling networks controlling ureteric bud branching morphogenesis. The *Gdnf/Ret* pathway, restricted to the ureteric bud (UB) tip, involves GDNF from the metanephric mesenchyme (MM) binding to the RET receptor and GFRα1 co-receptor. *Gdnf/Ret* signaling activates the expression of W*nt11* and *Spry1*. In feedback loops, *Spry1* negatively regulates *Ret* signaling, *Wnt11* upregulates *Gdnf*, and *Ret* positively regulates its own expression. *Ret* expression is also controlled by canonical (β-catenin-dependent) Wnt signaling through *Gata3* and *Emx2* and by retinoic acid (RA), generated in the interstitium from retinaldehyde dehydrogenase 2 (*Raldh2*), acting through its receptors *Rarb2* and *Rara*. *Cxcr4*, *Met*, and *Mmp14*, involved in processes such as cell migration, are activated by *Etv4/Etv5*, which are downstream targets of *Gdnf/Ret*. *Etv4/Etv5* may also be regulated by *Fgf10/Fgfr2* and *Hgf/Met* signaling (dotted arrows). Along the UB stalk, the inhibition of ureteral branching by *Bmp4* in the surrounding mesenchyme is suppressed by *Grem1*. (Modified from Costantini F. GDNF/Ret signaling and renal branching morphogenesis. *Organogenesis* 2010;6:252–262.)

negative regulation of UB formation by *Bmp4* is suppressed by its antagonist *Grem1*.

Relatively less is known about the control of *Ret* expression in the UB. However, studies have provided support for RA, β-catenin and *Gata3* having important roles in the regulation of *Ret* expression. *Ret* expression in UB cells is activated by paracrine RA signaling between the stromal mesenchyme and the UB (58). Specifically, RA synthesized by retinaldehyde dehydrogenase 2 (*Raldh2*) in stromal cells is secreted and binds to RA receptors in UB cells, inducing *Ret* expression. The canonical Wnt/β-catenin pathway is involved in the positive regulation of *Ret* expression. Conditional inactivation of β-catenin in the nephric duct results in decreased *Ret* expression and aberrant and ectopic UB formation causing a range of renal defects, including dysplasia, duplex kidneys, and aplasia (44). Conditional inactivation of *Gata3* in the ND results in similar renal defects, thus phenocopying the β-catenin mutants (45). The expression of β-catenin is relatively unaffected in the *Gata3* mutants. These results suggest *Gata3* acts in a signaling cascade downstream of β-catenin, but upstream of *Ret*. Moreover, it is believed this cascade operates to maintain UB cells in an undifferentiated or precursor state and prevent premature differentiation and ectopic ureteric budding.

Although its expression is induced in the UB by *Gdnf/Ret* signaling, Sprouty1 (*Spry1*), an inhibitor of receptor tyrosine kinase signaling, acts in a feedback loop to negatively regulate *Gdnf/Ret* function (59). Mice deficient in *Gdnf* or *Ret* or *Spry1* have defective (or absent) ureters or kidneys (52,53). Surprisingly, the creation of double mutant kidneys by deleting *Spry1* in *Gdnf*-deficient or in *Ret*-deficient mice largely rescues UB formation and kidney development (60). In other words, the mice deficient in *Gdnf* and *Spry1* or the mice deficient in *Ret* and *Spry1* have largely normal kidneys. Thus, *Gdnf* and *Ret* become nonessential in the absence of *Spry1*. These results emphasize the necessity of balance between positive signaling via *Gdnf/Ret* and negative regulation by *Spry1*. This balance appears more important than the specific signaling role of *Gdnf/Ret*. Other signaling pathways must exist to maintain UB formation in the absence of *Gdnf*, *Ret*, and *Spry1*. Fibroblast growth factor 10 (FGF10), expressed in the MM and interacting with its receptor FGFR2 in the UB, proves to be representative of one alternative pathway. Deleting *fgf10* in the double mutant *Gdnf*-deficient, *Spry1*-deficient mice causes failure of UB outgrowth (60). These data indicate FGF10 can replace *Gdnf/Ret* signaling in promoting correct UB outgrowth when *Spry1* is absent. An important principle that emerges from these studies is that a correct balance between activating and inhibitory signals from different genes is more important for normal UB outgrowth and branching than the signals from a single gene.

URETERAL BRANCHING

Gdnf/Ret Signaling

Since nephron formation begins at the ampullary tip of the UB, the number of UB branches largely determines the final nephron numbers in the adult kidney. Molecular signals that regulate the UB outgrowth continue to play important roles in UB branching. Again, GDNF from the MM interacting with RET in the ureteric bud epithelium is a key signaling pathway (Fig. 33.11). After interacting with GDNF, RET, as a tyrosine kinase receptor, activates downstream signaling, including the Ras/Erk MAP kinase, P13 kinase-Akt, and protein kinase C (PKC) (61). The importance of these pathways in kidney development has been demonstrated in several studies. Inhibition of phosphatidylinositol 3-kinase (PI3K) activity blocks the UB outgrowth and branching (62). On the other hand, conditional UB deletion of *PTEN*, encoding a phosphatase which normally antagonizes the P13K pathway, results in disturbed UB branching characterized by ectopic budding (63).

Activation of RET causes autophosphorylation of several key tyrosine (Y) residues in the RET cytoplasmic domain (64). These residues serve as docking sites for intracellular adaptor molecules in the above pathways. Moreover, there are two major alternative splice isoforms of RET, RET9, and RET51, the latter being longer and containing an additional tyrosine docking site. The different tyrosines have specificity for certain intracellular adaptors which transduce the various signaling pathways. For example, recruitment of PLCγ to Y1015 (RET9 and RET51) activates the PKC pathway. RET Y1062 (RET9 and RET51) serves as a docking site for multiple adaptors. Recruitment of the GRB2-SOS complex to Y1062 activates Ras/Erk MAP kinase signaling, whereas recruitment of the GRB2-GAB1 complex to Y1062 activates the PI3K-AKT pathway. When mutated in mice, the RET tyrosine residues in the two RET isoforms display remarkable organotypic specificities (65–67). For example, mutation of RET51 Y1015 causes supernumerary ureters and hypodysplasia resembling a CAKUT (congenital anomalies of kidneys or urinary tract) phenotype, whereas mutation of RET9 Y1015 results in a CAKUT phenotype but also colon aganglionosis resembling Hirschsprung disease. Mutation of RET51 Y1062 results in Hirschsprung disease only, whereas mutation of RET9 Y1062 causes renal agenesis and Hirschsprung disease. Interestingly, the tyrosine phosphatase Shp2, as part of a larger complex, binds to RET Y1062 and mediates the downstream activation of Ras/Erk MAP kinases and PI3K-AKT pathways. Conditional deletion of Shp2 in the UB results in downregulation of *Ret* target genes and severe renal hypoplasia/dysgenesis (68). These findings indicate these key tyrosine docking sites linked to different signaling pathways downstream of *Ret* activation have distinct roles in organogenesis, for example, regulating enteric nerve development and/or renal branching morphogenesis. However, the molecular basis for this organotypic specificity remains unclear.

Microarray screening using RNA from UB cultures, grown with and without GDNF, identified several target genes of *Gdnf/Ret* signaling that participate in UB growth and branching (69) (Fig. 33.11). They included genes such as *Spry1* and *Wnt11* known to be upregulated by *Gdnf/Ret* but also additional genes such as *Etv4* and *Etv5*. Encoding two related transcription factors of the ETS family, *Etv4* and *Etv5* are strongly co-expressed in the UB tips. Mice deficient in both *Etv4* alleles and one *Etv5* allele (compound heterozygotes) have severe ureteric branching defects resulting in renal agenesis or hypoplasia, whereas mice lacking all *Etv4* and *Etv5* alleles (double homozygotes) never develop kidneys (69). Thus, *Etv4/Etv5* operate downstream of *Gdnf/Ret* signaling and are essential for ureteric branching.

The expression of several *Ret*-regulated genes including *Cxcr4*, *Myb*, *Met*, and *Mmp14* is severely reduced in *Etv4/Etv5* mutant kidneys suggesting they are downstream transcriptional targets of *Etv4/Etv5* (69). Cxcr4 is the receptor for the CXC chemokine ligand 12 (Cxcl 12). Inhibition of *Cxcr4* in embryonic kidney organ cultures impairs ureteric branching (70). Furthermore, an intact Cxcl 12–Cxcr4 interaction is required for the eventual development of the glomerular vasculature (71). *Met* encodes the receptor tyrosine kinase for hepatocyte growth factor (HGF). Mice with conditional deletion of *Met* in ureteric epithelium have ureteric branching defects (72). Normal kidney development depends upon a correct balance between extracellular matrix (ECM) synthesis and degradation. By degrading ECM components, mainly collagens and laminins, matrix metalloproteinases (MMP) play an important role. *Mmp14* encodes MMP14 (also called MT1-MMP), a membrane type MMP. Studies in *Mmp14*-null mice have revealed MMP14 has important roles in ureteric branching as well as cell migration (73). Thus, positively regulated by *Gdnf/Ret* signaling, *Etv4/Etv5* and their downstream targets *Cxcr4*, *Met*, and *Mmp14* represent a gene network controlling ureteral branching morphogenesis. Other pathways likely intersect this gene network. For example, *Sox9*, encoding a transcriptional regulator, is required for normal ureteric branching (74). Although *Sox9* neither activates *Ret* expression nor is regulated by *Gdnf/Ret* signaling, it is required for activation of *Etv4/Etv5*, which are essential effector genes of *Gdnf/Ret* signaling.

Other Signaling Pathways

Fibroblast Growth Factors

Several other signaling pathways are involved in ureteric branching. The following discussion includes some examples. FGF signaling is critical throughout kidney development (75). The ligands Fgf7, Fgf8, and Fgf10 and the Fgf receptors Fgfr1, Fgfr2, and Fgfl1 are the most relevant to renal development. Both Fgfr1 and Fgfr2 are receptor tyrosine kinases and alternative splicing results in each receptor having IIIb and IIIc isoforms. Although Fgrl1 binds to some Fgfs, it lacks a tyrosine kinases domain and may act as a decoy receptor, binding and sequestering Fgfs away from the other Fgfrs (76). Conditional gene deletion studies have demonstrated that both *Fgfr1* and *Fgfr2* (mainly the IIIc isoform) in the MM are vital for full formation of the MM and ureteric branching (77,78). Conditional deletion of the *Ffgrs* in the UB indicates that the Fgfr2 IIIb isoform (not Fgfr1), which is the receptor isoform for both Fgf7 and Fgf10 ligands, in the ureteric lineage is essential for normal ureteric branching (79,80). *Fgfrs* activate several downstream signaling pathways also activated by *Ret*. The FGF receptor substrate 2α (Frs2α) is a well-characterized adaptor that binds to Fgfrs and mediates the activation of these signaling pathways. However, ureteral gene deletion studies provide evidence that although Fgfr2 and Frs2α have important roles in regulating ureteral branching, they appear to act independently but also in an incremental manner (81).

Renin–Angiotensin System

The renin–angiotensin system plays a critical role in kidney development. Inactivation in mice of angiotensinogen, renin, angiotensin-converting enzyme, AT_1R or AT_2R, the two major receptors for angiotensin II (Ang II), causes severe collecting system defects reflecting aberrant ureteral branching (82). AT_1R and AT_2R are G protein-coupled receptors. However, stimulation of AT_1R by Ang II increases tyrosine phosphorylation of the epidermal growth factor receptor (EGFR) and Ret, promoting branching of the ureteric epithelium (83,84). These findings suggest molecular crosstalk cooperation between G-protein and receptor tyrosine kinase signaling pathways. In addition, AT_1R stimulation inhibits the expression of Spry1, which in turn normally inhibits Gdnf/Ret signaling (85). Culture studies have shown Ang II-stimulation of AT_1R and AT_2R leads to UB-cell proliferation and migration, important processes for branching (86,87).

Integrins

Integrins are heterodimeric transmembrane receptors consisting of associated α and β subunits (88). They are the primary cellular receptors for ECM proteins and are classified into collagen, laminin, and arginine-glycine-aspartic acid (RGB) binding integrins. Some integrins play a greater role in glomerular development than in ureteral branching morphogenesis. However, conditional deletion of the integrin β1 subunit in the UB results in severe ureteral branching defects and decreased nephron formation (89,90). The integrin β1 cytoplasmic tail contains a tyrosine residue (Y783) that is important for binding to the cytosolic protein talin, which provides a link to the actin cytoskeleton. Disruption of this interaction leads to defective ureteral branching (91). Integrin-linked kinase (ILK) is a cytoplasmic protein that binds β1- and β3-integrin cytoplasmic domains and regulates the actin cytoskeleton by recruiting actin-binding proteins such as α-parvin. ILK lacks functional kinase activity and thus is a pseudokinase. Mice with ILK mutations of the binding site for α-parvin die of renal agenesis (92). Conditional deletion of ILK in the ureteric epithelium results in decreased branching but also decreased p38 MAPK activity and intraluminal obstruction of the collecting system due to continued collecting duct cell proliferation (93). ILK is required to activate p38 MAPK which induces cell cycle arrest during normal tubulogenesis.

Laminins

Laminins are trimeric molecules that consist of an α, β, and γ chain. They play key roles in several different areas of renal development. Laminin-111 and laminin-511 are expressed in UB structure basement membranes (94). Conditional deletion of the Lamc1 gene, encoding the laminin γ1 subunit, in the ureteral epithelium causes failure of the UB outgrowth or defective ureteral branching (95). In addition, cultures of laminin γ1-deficient collecting duct cells reveal a decrease in mediators of β1-integrin signaling (95). Since several β1-integrins serve as laminin receptors, these findings indicate that a functional interaction between laminin γ1- and β1-integrin is important for ureteral morphogenesis.

Bone Morphogenetic Proteins

A fine regulatory balance exists between factors that promote and factors that inhibit ureteral branching. The BMPs, the largest family within the TGF-β superfamily of growth factors, generally inhibit ureteral branching (96). BMPs bind to a membrane heteromeric receptor complex composed of two types of serine/threonine kinase receptors, type I ALK and type II receptors. BMPs activate either the canonical Smad protein signaling pathway or the noncanonical mitogen-activated protein kinase (MAPK) family of signaling proteins (e.g., p38). The BMPs 2, 4, and 7 are the most studied in kidney development. Bmp2 is expressed in the condensed MM adjacent to the tips of the ureteral branches. Genetic studies in mice have provided evidence that BMP2 inhibits branching at the ureteral tips (97). Bmp4 is expressed in the MM surrounding the nephric duct, the nascent UB and in the mesenchyme adjacent to the ureteral trunks. Genetic evidence indicates Bmp4 inhibits ureteral branching but promotes ureteral trunk elongation (98,99). BMP2 and BMP4 bind to the type I receptor ALK3. Conditional deletion of Alk3 in the ureteric bud lineage reveals an inhibitory function for ALK3 during early ureteral branching (100). Bmp7 is expressed in both the MM and the UB branches. Recent studies implicate Bmp7 in inhibiting ureteric bud outgrowth and branching (101). GREM1 plays a role in this UB outgrowth and branching by antagonizing BMP7 (101) as well as BMP4 (57).

Semaphorins

Semaphorins are a large protein family involved in providing guidance cues in cellular processes, such as migration (102). They include secreted, transmembrane, and glycosylphosphatidylinositol (GPI)-linked proteins, many of which bind to plexin transmembrane receptors. Some secreted semaphorins bind to transmembrane co-receptors, such as neuropilin-1, which then assemble with a plexin to form a holo receptor complex. The intracellular pathways downstream of semaphorin/plexin signaling include Ras-specific GTPase activating proteins (GAPs), PI3-Akt, Rho-GTPases, and GSK-3β. These molecules are involved in the regulation of integrin-mediated adhesion, actin dynamics and microtubule organization (102). Both in vitro and in vivo studies have shown that both Sema3a-neuropilin1 (Npn1) and Sema4d-plexinB1 signaling inhibit ureteral branching (103,104). However, other semaphorins appear to have opposite functions. For example, Sema4c-plexinB2 signaling appears to stimulate ureteral branching (105).

Hippo Pathway

The Hippo pathway is a conserved kinase cascade that controls tissue growth in both *Drosophila* and vertebrates (106,107). It has multiple upstream inputs and multiple transcriptional outputs which also mediate crosstalk with other signaling pathways, including Wnt, BMP, and TGF-β pathways. Activation of the Hippo kinases Mst1/2 and Lats1/2 leads to phosphorylation of the transcriptional coactivators Yap and Taz, which excludes them from the nucleus. Loss of Hippo signaling (inhibition of Mst1/2 or Lats1/2) results in nuclear accumulation of Yap and Taz which promotes proliferation and inhibits apoptosis. Yap and Taz are required for normal ureteral branching (108) and also proper Ret-dependent nephric duct insertion into the cloaca (109).

URETERIC BRANCH GROWTH

The UB undergoes branching and growth to develop an elaborate collecting system. Morphometric studies in the developing murine kidney have shown extensive UB branching in the first half of metanephric development followed by a period of UB trunk segment growth by elongation, and finally a few rounds of terminal branching prior to birth (110). However, ureteral branching displays structural and temporal discontinuity rather than a continuous, reiterative process (111,112).

Studies focusing on Wnt signaling have provided insights into the molecular mechanisms underlying UB-derived collecting duct growth. Wnt signaling pathways have been broadly categorized as canonical, with utilization of β-catenin and noncanonical, which is β-catenin-independent (113). Signaling that controls planar cell polarity (PCP) is one type of a noncanonical pathway. PCP refers to the organization of cells in a plane perpendicular to the apical–basal cellular axis, which, in a renal tubule is the plane parallel to the basement membrane along the longitudinal axis (114). Genes in the PCP pathway are involved in regulating the lengthening and narrowing (*convergent extension*) of the developing collecting ducts. Convergent extension in development occurs by several mechanisms, including oriented cell division and cell intercalation. Studies have shown that the nuclear mitotic spindle is oriented along the longitudinal tubular axis of postnatal collecting ducts, reflecting an intrinsic planar cell polarization (115). Moreover, a disruption of PCP gene-directed oriented cell division has been documented in some models of polycystic kidney disease associated with shortened dilated collecting ducts (115–117). Thus, PCP-regulated oriented cell division results in lengthening of postnatal collecting ducts without a change in diameter. In other words, after oriented division, the two daughter cells are aligned along the longitudinal axis of the duct, which increases the length rather than the diameter of the duct. Signaling by *Wnt9b* regulates this oriented cell division in the postnatal collecting duct (118).

However, in the embryonic collecting ducts, cell division is not oriented. One would predict that unoriented cell division within a tubule structure would lead to an increase in the number of cells within the tubule wall and a subsequent increased tubule diameter. Unexpectedly, the number of cells within the collecting ducts decreases as the duct diameter decreases during the embryonic period. The cells within the embryonic collecting ducts have an elongated shape arrangement, perpendicular to the longitudinal duct axis (118). This cellular orientation is consistent with cell intercalation, a PCP-regulated mechanism where cells in adjacent rows along one axis move among each other to simultaneously lengthen and narrow the tissue (119). Embryonic collecting ducts deficient in *Wnt9b* generally lack this elongated shape arrangement and become shortened and dilated (118). A multicellular rosette mechanism of cell intercalation was found to control the convergent extension (120). Thus, the lengthening and narrowing of the collecting ducts during embryonic development appear to be regulated by *Wnt9b*-mediated cell intercalation. In summary, *Wnt9b* influences collecting duct growth in both embryonic and postnatal periods, through different PCP-linked mechanisms, cell intercalation, and oriented cell division, respectively.

Another Wnt gene, *Wnt7b*, is important for development of the renal inner medulla (papilla) (121). *Wnt7b* signaling to the interstitium via the canonical β-catenin-dependent Wnt pathway regulates elongation of developing MCDs and loops of Henle. In the absence of *Wnt7b*, these structures dilate and the renal medulla never forms. The absence of *Dkk1*, an antagonist of *Wnt7b*, leads to hypertrophy of the collecting ducts and overgrowth of the renal papilla (122). Thus, a correct balance of signaling by *Wnt7b* and its antagonist *Dkk1* is critical for collecting duct and loop of Henle morphogenesis and formation of the renal medulla. Finally, studies have implicated α3β1 integrin, a major laminin receptor, acting in concert with c-Met, the receptor for HGF, to positively regulate *Wnt7b* in the developing renal medulla (123).

COLLECTING SYSTEM DIFFERENTIATION

Ureteral Tip and Trunk

The ureteral branch consists of a trunk or stalk which elongates and an ampullary tip. It is the ureteral tip which induces the adjacent MM to form nephrons. Proliferating epithelial cells with elevated *Ret* expression driven by *Gdnf* signaling form the tips (124,125). The cellular processes underlying actual branching from the ureteral tip have not been established with certainty. On the basis of isolated ureteric bud cultures, one model proposes a "purse-string" mechanism, whereby contraction of actin microfilaments in the apical region changes the columnar cell shape from rectangular to more triangular (126). Subsequently, the epithelial monolayer of triangular or wedge-shaped cells with decreased apical surface area, pushes outward to form smooth outpouches with a continuous lumen. This possibility is supported by the findings that a functional actin-cytoskeleton (127) and the actin depolymerizing factors, cofilin1 and destrin (128), are required for ureteral branching.

Descendents of the tip cells eventually populate much of the trunk epithelium. Thus, there is increasing cell differentiation from the tip along to the trunk. For example, a trunk epithelial marker is the water channel protein aquaporin-2, which will also be expressed in the mature collecting duct. Tip markers include *Ret*, *Vsnl1*, and *Wnt11*. *Visinin like 1* (*Vsnl1*) encodes a calcium-sensor protein, and is a new marker for tip cells (129). *Wnt11*, expressed in the ureteral tips during all stages of kidney development, is required for ureteral branching morphogenesis (130). *Wnt11* expression in the tip is dependent upon *Gdnf/Ret* signaling, and reciprocally *Gdnf* expression in the MM is dependent upon a tip *Wnt11* signal. Thus, it has been proposed that *Gdnf*, *Ret*, and *Wnt11* function in a positive, autoregulatory feedback loop to drive ureteral branching (130). Both genetic studies in mice and cell culture findings have implicated the Wnt receptors frizzled 4 (*Fz4*) and frizzled 8 (*Fz8*) in mediating the actions of *Wnt11* (131). A rather unusual cellular mechanism associated with cell division has been noted in the tips of ureteral branches (132). Tip cells about to divide project out and undergo mitosis in the tubular lumen while still attached to the underlying basement membrane. Subsequently, one daughter cell remains still attached and retreats back into the epithelium whereas the other daughter cell remains in the lumen and eventually reenters the epithelium a few cell diameters away. The significance of this "mitosis-associated cell dispersal" process is unknown.

Cell Types

A clear understanding of the process by which specific cell types are established in the developing collecting system has been complicated by the diversity of cell types within the different duct segments. The collecting system epithelium consists of principal cells, responsible for vasopressin-regulated water reabsorption and aldosterone-regulated sodium reabsorption, and intercalated cells (ICs) which regulate acid–base homeostasis. The principal cells are more numerous than intercalated cells throughout the collecting system and are characterized by aquaporin-2 expression. The intercalated cells, which express carbonic anhydrase II, can be divided into three subtypes: type A, type B, and nonA–nonB cells. Type A ICs, expressing apical vacuolar H^+-ATPase and the basolateral exchanger AE1, secrete H^+ into the urine. Type B ICs, expressing the apical anion exchanger pendrin and basolateral H^+-ATPase, secrete HCO_3^- into the urine. The nonA–nonB ICs express apical H^+-ATPase and apical pendrin. Their function remains to be established. In the mature (adult) collecting system, the different intercalated cells have distinct distributions (133). Type A ICs are located in the CNT, CCD, outer medullary collecting duct (OMCD) and initial inner medullary collecting duct

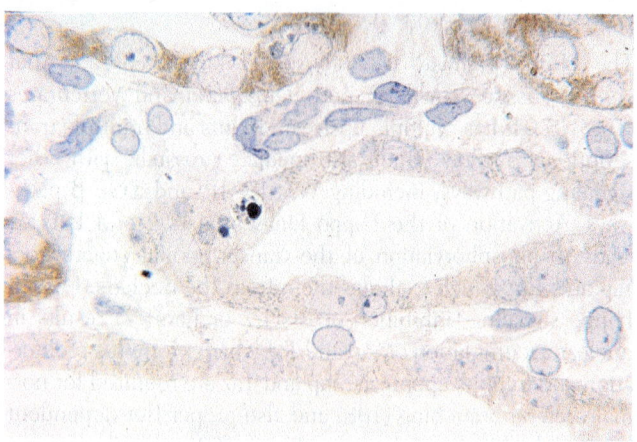

FIGURE 33.12 Developing MCD in a postnatal kidney. After etching with sodium methoxide, toluidine blue is removed from normal nuclei but remains in the nuclear fragments of apoptotic bodies (Epon, ×300; courtesy of Dr. Jin Kim).

(IMCDi), whereas type B and nonA–nonB ICs are primarily present in the CNT and the CCD.

During development of the collecting system, both in the embryonic and postnatal periods, there is considerable cellular remodeling (134,135). Although there are some specific differences, there are broad similarities between humans and rodents regarding the distribution of the various cell types. The principal cell or segment-specific cell types (e.g., CNT cells) remain by far the most numerous cell type in all segments. In the fetal kidney, intercalated cells initially appear in the CNT and MCD. Type A ICs remain the predominant IC subtype in these segments throughout development. After birth, the type A ICs increase significantly as a percentage of the total cells in each of the collecting system segments. Although some Type B cells are present in the fetal OMCD, they are removed by apoptosis after birth (136) (Figs. 33.12 and 33.13). In the postnatal period, intercalated cells increase dramatically in the CCD

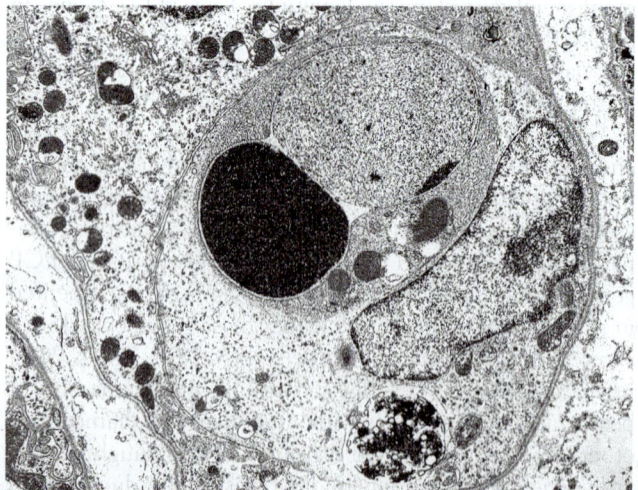

FIGURE 33.13 Electron micrograph of a postnatal MCD illustrating a phagocytosed apoptotic body composed of a nucleus with condensed chromatin and organelle remnants (×1,200; courtesy of Dr. Jin Kim).

with the type B ICs becoming the most abundant subtype in this duct segment. After birth, some nonA–nonB ICs are located in the CCD but more are situated in the CNT, where they are similar in abundance as the type B ICs but still less than the type A ICs.

A clear understanding of cell type differentiation in the collecting duct remains a challenge. It is not clear when commitment to a specific cell type occurs. Immunolocalization, lineage tracing and gene deletion studies indicate that a subset of ureteric bud tip cells expressing an amino-terminus truncated p63 (ΔNp63) serve as progenitors of intercalated cells (137). The expression of ΔNp63 is transient and ceases after birth. The forkhead gene *Foxi1* encodes a transcription factor that is expressed in both type A and type B ICs but not in principal cells (138). Mice lacking *Foxi1* fail to express the type A IC marker AE1 and also the type B IC marker pendrin. In these mutant mice, principal cells and intercalated cells in the collecting duct are replaced by a single cell type expressing both aquaporin-2 (PC cell marker) and carbonic anhydrase II (IC cell marker). These findings suggest principal cells and intercalated cells arise from a common progenitor cell and that activation of Foxi1 is necessary for differentiation of these precursor cells into intercalated cells. It has also been reported that mice lacking *Cp2l1*, a transcription factor of the grainy-head gene family, show defective maturation of the collecting ducts with a loss of both type A and type B intercalated cell marker genes (139). At least some precursor cells that give rise to intercalated cells have been reported to express aquaporin 2 (140). The transcription factor TFCP2L1 has been reported to induce the expression of intercalated cell–specific genes (141).

Notch signaling is a cell–cell communication pathway that is involved in cell fate determination and differentiation. After conditional inactivation of Notch signaling in the developing collecting duct, mice display increased urine production, decreased urine osmolality, sodium wasting, and a severe urinary concentrating defect compatible with nephrogenic diabetes insipidus (142). The collecting ducts show a prominent decrease in principal cells and an increase in intercalated cells, such that the latter abnormally outnumber the former. Transgenic overexpression of Notch signaling in the defective collecting ducts leads to a dramatic reversal in the cellular composition such that the entire duct is made up of principal cells. Other studies also show increased notch signaling confers a principal cell fate (143). Thus, Notch signaling appears critical for principal cell differentiation in the collecting duct. The transcription factor Elf5 has been reported to induce the expression of principal cell-specific genes (144).

METANEPHRIC MESENCHYME

Specification

Recent studies have provided insights into the specification of early cell lineages in the MM. *Osr1*, encoding a transcriptional regulator, is broadly expressed in the IM and the LPM. Most cell types in the developing metanephric kidney, including the ureteral epithelium, the MM and its nephron epithelial derivatives, the interstitium, vasculature, and smooth muscle arise from progenitor cells expressing *Osr1* (145). Prior to ureteric bud invasion of the MM, *Osr1* positive cells give rise to both epithelial (*Pax2/Six2*⁺) and interstitial cell (*Foxd1*⁺) lineages. However, after UB invasion, *Osr1* expression becomes restricted to the CM nephron progenitors (145). The following genes define the early nephron progenitor cells (NPCs) (Fig. 33.14). *Osr1* is the earliest known marker gene of the MM. Mice deficient in *Osr1* do not form an MM, and lack expression of other genes required for kidney formation, including *Eya1*, *Six2*, *Pax2*, *Sall1*, and *Gdnf*, resulting in renal agenesis (146). *Eya1* is another factor in the early lineage determination of the MM. *Eya1* regulates *Six1*, *Pax2*, and *Gdnf* expression and loss of *Eya1* leads to renal agenesis (147,148). Functioning as a transcriptional coactivator with phosphatase activity, *Eya1* interacts with *Six1*, converting the latter into a transcriptional activator (149). *Six1*, expressed in the MM, is required for ureteric bud invasion into the mesenchyme. Loss of *Six1* results in reduced expression of *Pax2*, *Sall1*, *Six2*, and *Gdnf* in the MM and renal agenesis (150).

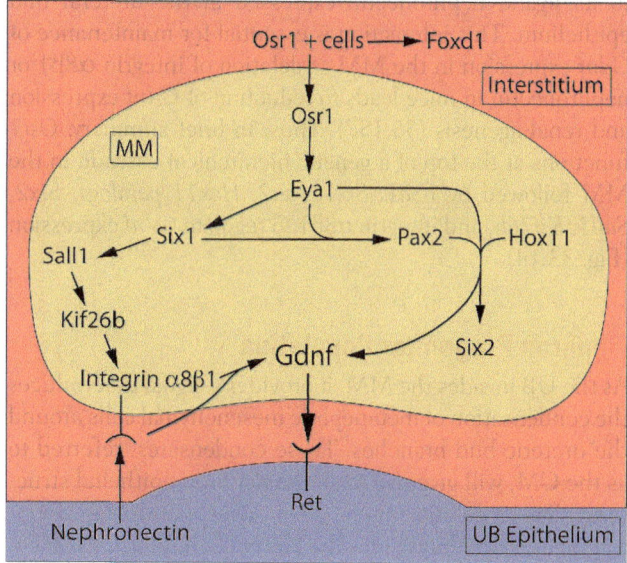

FIGURE 33.14 Schematic diagram illustrating a working model of the hierarchical cascade of transcription factors in the metanephric mesenchyme (MM) that defines the early nephron progenitor cells and leads to regulation of *Gdnf* expression. The earliest gene, *Osr1*, is expressed in cells that give rise to either nephron (*Pax2/Six2*⁺) or interstitial (*Foxd1*⁺) progenitors. *Eya1*, another early factor, regulates *Six1*, and an *Eya1/Six1* complex activates *Pax2*. A complex of *Eya1/Pax2/Hox11* upregulates *Six2*, which is required for nephron progenitor maintenance. The *Eya1/Pax2/Hox 11* complex also activates *Gdnf*. Downstream of *Six1*, *Sall1* upregulates *Kif26b*, which maintains expression of integrin α8β1. The binding of integrin α8β1 to nephronectin, expressed in the UB epithelium, is an interaction important for the maintenance of *Gdnf* expression.

Studies indicate *Six1* upregulates the expression of *Grem1* in the MM, which in turn, reduces the activity of *Bmp4*, an inhibitor of UB outgrowth, leading to the initiation of ureteral branching (151).

Pax2, encoding a transcription factor, is expressed in the nephric duct but also in the MM prior to induction. Mice deficient in *Pax2* exhibit renal agenesis, largely due to the critical roles of *Pax2* in ND maintenance (152) and the regulation of *Gdnf* expression in the MM (153). Moreover, Pax2 and Eya1 form a complex with the Hox11 paralogs (Hoxa11, Hoxc11, and Hoxd11) to activate the expression of *Gdnf* and *Six2* in the MM (54). *Sall1* encodes a transcription factor that is expressed in the MM and its deletion results in renal agenesis (154). Studies have revealed that in the absence of *Sall1* in the MM, *Wnt9b*, normally specifically expressed in the ureteral stalk, becomes ectopically expressed in the ureteral tips disrupting ureteral branching (155). Thus, *Sall1* in the MM normally downregulates *Wnt9b* expression in the ureteral tips, which normally express *Wnt11*, allowing for the initiation of ureteral branching. *Sall1* expression is absent in the MM of mice lacking *Six1*, suggesting *Sall1* is a transcriptional target of *Six1* (150). A kinesin family gene, *Kif26b*, is expressed in the MM and is a downstream target of *Sall1*. Deletion of *Kif26b* in mice leads to reduced expression of integrin α8β1 and *Gdnf* in the MM and renal agenesis (156). Integrin α8β1 expressed in the MM binds to its ligand nephronectin expressed in the ureteral bud epithelium. This interaction is essential for maintenance of *Gdnf* expression in the MM as deletion of integrin α8β1 or nephronectin in mice leads to reduction of *Gdnf* expression and renal agenesis (55,157). Thus, in brief summary, *Osr1* functions at the top of a genetic hierarchical cascade in the MM followed by *Eya1*, *Six1*, *Pax2*, *Hox11* paralogs, *Six2*, *Sall1*, *Kif26b*, and integrin α8β1 to regulate *Gdnf* expression (Fig. 33.14).

Nephron Progenitor Population

As the UB invades the MM, it provides a signal that induces the condensation of metanephric mesenchymal cells around the ureteric bud branches. These condensates, referred to as the CM, will give rise to all the nephron epithelial structures. These cellular interactions occur within the "nephron niche," which includes the ureteral ampulla, CM, PTA, renal vesicle, S-body, stroma, and endothelial progenitors (158). In recent years, our understanding of the nephron progenitor population in the CM has increased (159,160).

Although *Wnt11*, expressed at the UB tips, is required for ureteral branching and stimulates *Gdnf* expression (130), it is the *Wnt* gene *Wnt9b*, expressed throughout the ureteric bud epithelium, except at the very tips, that primarily induces the formation of the CM (161). Cell lineage tracing studies have identified a self-renewing cell population in the CM. Cells expressing *Six2* and *Cited1* seem to define a stem cell population capable of self-renewal and expansion of the CM but that also undergoes depletion as nephrogenesis ceases. In *Six2* knockout mice, there is premature and ectopic tubule differentiation and depletion of the CM resulting in hypoplastic kidneys (162). Thus, *Six2* normally inhibits precocious differentiation of the CM into nephron epithelia and maintains the progenitor cells in an undifferentiated state. In Six2 heterozygote mice, one would expect a phenotype intermediate between, wild-type and Six2 null mice, but paradoxically, there is an increase in ureteral branching and final nephron number, suggesting a unique dose response to the level of Six2 (163). The Six2-positive cells are multipotent giving rise to all epithelial components of the nephron, including podocytes and all tubule segments, except the collecting system (164). The critical importance of this population is shown by studies showing that decreasing the number of progenitor cells in the CM leads to a reduction in the number of nephrons generated (165). In human kidney, Six1 in addition to Six2, appears to have a regulatory role in nephron progenitors (166). The expression of *Cited1* in a subpopulation of the Six2-positive cells further defines this epithelial progenitor population (167). *Cited1* is not required for nephrogenesis but likely still contributes to the maintenance of this population (168). However, *Six2* has the specific and critical role in characterizing this population.

Gene expression studies have demonstrated that the CM is not a homogeneous compartment. The CM can be divided into three subdomains; the "inner capping mesenchyme" ($Six2^+$, $Cited1^+$), the "outer capping mesenchyme" ($Six2^+$, $Cited1^+$, $Eya1^+$, $Meox1^+$) and the "induced mesenchyme" ($Six2^+$, $Eya1^+$, $Wnt4^+$) (Fig. 33.15) (169). However, this spatial and molecular complexity of the CM is certainly not appreciated by light microscopy since the cells of the CM resemble mesenchymal "blastemal" cells. The inner and the outer capping mesenchyme contain the $Six2^+$, $Cited1^+$ cell population which appears to be true stem cells. These domains are not rigidly defined as time lapse imaging has demonstrated that cells move within and between the domains (170). Signaling mechanisms are required to prevent depletion of the CM. The survival of these progenitor cells is maintained by several other genes including *Fgf9*, *Fgf10*, *Frs2a*, *Bmp7*, *Sall1*, and *p53* (171–176). Moreover, *Osr1* and *Six2* interact synergistically to maintain the progenitor pool (177).

Metabolic programming also plays a role in NPC maintenance. Younger nephron progenitor cells use glycolysis to a significantly greater degree than older NPCs and inhibition of glycolysis in NPCs leads to accelerated differentiation and enhanced nephrogenesis in embryonic kidneys (178). Recent studies are exploring the role of epigenetics in kidney development and disease (179). For example, histone deacetylases 1 and 2 (HDAC1 and HDAC2) interact with Six2, Osr1, and Sall1 to maintain a correct balance of NPC self-renewal and differentiation into nephrons (180).

The cessation of nephrogenesis is associated with an accelerated wave of new nephron formation in the outer nephrogenic zone with an altered topology, such that multiple

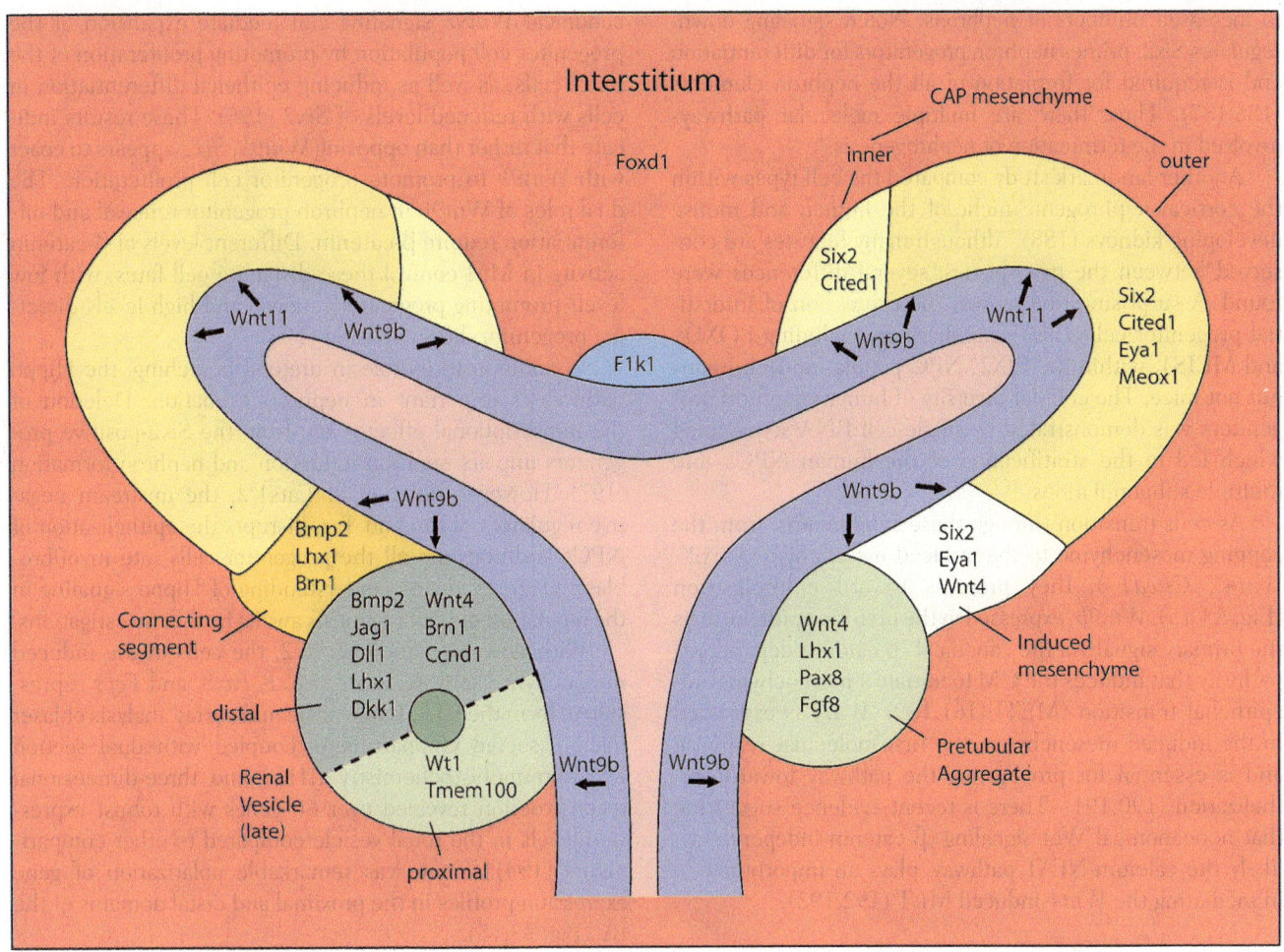

FIGURE 33.15 Schematic representation of the compartments and molecules involved in early nephrogenesis. *Wnt11*, expressed at the UB tips, is important for ureteral branching and *Gdnf* expression. However, *Wnt9b*, expressed throughout the ureteral epithelium except the very tips, primarily induces the formation of the cap mesenchyme (CM). The cap mesenchyme is divided into three subdomains: inner capping mesenchyme (*Six2, Cited1*⁺), outer capping mesenchyme (*Six2, Cited1, Eya1, Meox1*⁺) and induced mesenchyme (*Six2, Eya1, Wnt4*⁺). Cells positive for *Six2* and *Cited1* are the progenitors that give rise to all the epithelial elements of the nephron. Differentiation of the CM proceeds around and under the UB tips. *Wnt9b* is required for the formation of the PTA (*right*) which expresses *Wnt4, Lhx1, Pax8,* and *Fgf8*. *Wnt4* is necessary to transform the mesenchymal PTA to an epithelial renal vesicle (RV) (*left*). Within the RV, a proximal domain defined by *Wt1* and *Tmem100* expression, will give rise to the glomerular podocytes and PTs. A distal domain of the RV, characterized by numerous genes (*Bmp2, Jag1, Dll1, Lhx1, Dkk1, Wnt4, Brn1, Ccnd1*) will generate the loops of Henle and the distal tubule. The connecting segment (*Bmp2, Lhx1, Brn1*⁺), which joins the late RV to the UB tip, is formed from cells in the distal RV. Interstitial cells express *Foxd1*. Vascular endothelial cell progenitors are marked by *Flk1* expression. (Modified from Mugford JW, Yu J, Kobayashi A, et al. High-resolution gene expression analysis of the developing mouse kidney defines novel cellular compartments within the nephron progenitor population. *Dev Biol* 2009;333:312–323; Georgas K, Rumballe B, Valerius MT, et al. Analysis of early nephron patterning reveals a role for distal RV proliferation in fusion to the ureteric tip via a cap mesenchyme-derived connecting segment. *Dev Biol* 2009;332:273–286.)

new nephrons are attached to a single ureteral tip (181,182). There is coincident loss of the CM. The molecular mechanisms causing the cessation of nephrogenesis are not clear. However, studies have revealed that genes associated with cell proliferation are activated prior to genetic markers of cell differentiation, which in turn, are increased prior to the downregulation of *Six2* and *Cited1* (183). Intrinsic cell aging and cell–cell contact alterations within the CM progenitor populations appears to play a role in cessation of nephrogenesis (184). Hamartin, encoded by the tuberous sclerosis 1 gene, *Tsc1*, is an inhibitor of mammalian target of rapamycin (mTOR) and appears to regulate cessation of nephrogenesis in mice (185). Surprisingly, loss of one *Tsc1* allele in NPCs results in delayed cessation of nephrogenesis leading to increased numbers of nephrons. Notch signaling downregulates Six2, primes nephron progenitors for differentiation and is required for formation of all the nephron elements (186,187). Thus, there are multiple molecular pathways involved in the termination of nephrogenesis.

Another landmark study compared the cell types within the cortical nephrogenic niche of the human and mouse developing kidneys (188). Although many features are conserved between the two species, several differences were found. A surprising finding was the expression of interstitial progenitor cell (IPC) gene markers, including FOXD1 and MEIS1, within the SIX2+ NPC population in humans but not mice. The cellular diversity of human nephron progenitors was demonstrated by single-cell RNA sequencing which led to the stratification of the human NPCs into multiple subpopulations.

As cells transition through these subdomains, from the capping mesenchyme to the induced mesenchyme ($Six2^+$, $Wnt4^+$, $Cited1-$), they progress toward epithelization (Fig. 33.15). Wnt9b, expressed in the ureteric epithelium, is the primary signal via the canonical (β-catenin-dependent) pathway that induces the CM to initiate a mesenchymal-to-epithelial transition (MET) (161,189). Wnt4 is expressed in the induced mesenchyme as a first molecular response and is essential for propagating the pathway toward epithelization (190,191). There is recent evidence suggesting that noncanonical Wnt signaling (β-catenin-independent), likely the calcium/NFAT pathway, plays an important role in mediating the Wnt4-induced MET (192,193).

PATTERNING OF THE NEPHRON

Early Events: Pretubular Aggregate and Renal Vesicle

A group of cells within the induced mesenchyme forms a PTA in the curve ("armpit") beneath the UB tips. The PTA undergoes a MET to form a renal vesicle (RV), which develops a central lumen and becomes surrounded by a basement membrane. Thus, the PTA is the precursor to the RV. Cells transition through the compartments from the capping mesenchyme to the induced mesenchyme to the PTA and the RV with overlapping gene expression profiles (Fig. 33.15) (194). The MET of the CM to nephron epithelia is a "genetic switch" regulated by the balance between signals which favor stem cell maintenance and those signals driving epithelial differentiation. Deletion of Six2 results in depletion of the progenitor cells with accompanying massive differentiation of the CM (162,164). Wnt9b derived from the UB induces the CM to form the PTA, which expresses Wnt4. In the absence of Wnt9b, the PTA does not form (161). Wnt4 expression in the PTA is necessary for epithelization in forming the RV (190,191). A working model is that Six2 blocks MET by antagonizing the actions of Wnt9b. However, studies have provided evidence that canonical Wnt9b signaling can mediate expansion of the progenitor cell population by promoting proliferation of the $Six2^+$ cells, as well as inducing epithelial differentiation in cells with reduced levels of Six2 (195). These results indicate that rather than opposing Wnt9b, Six2 appears to coact with Wnt9b to promote progenitor cell proliferation. The dual roles of Wnt9b in nephron progenitor renewal and differentiation require β-catenin. Different levels of β-catenin activity in MM control these disparate cell fates, with low levels promoting progenitor renewal and high levels directing progenitor differentiation (196).

In addition to its role in ureteral branching, the Hippo pathway is important in nephron formation. Deletion of the transcriptional effector Yap from the Six2-positive progenitors impairs nephron induction and nephron formation (197). However, deletion of Lats1/2, the upstream negative regulators of Yap and Taz, disrupts the epithelization of NPCs and converts all the progenitor cells into myofibroblasts (198). A clearer understanding of Hippo signaling in the regulation of nephrogenesis awaits further investigations.

With downregulation of Six2, the cells in the induced mesenchyme activate Wnt4, Lhx1, Pax8, and Fgf8 expression to form the PTA. Large-scale microarray analysis of laser microdissected compartments coupled with dual section ISH/immunohistochemistry (IHC) and three-dimensional reconstruction revealed over 60 genes with robust expression levels in the renal vesicle compared to other compartments (194). There was remarkable polarization of gene expression profiles in the proximal and distal domains of the RV (Fig. 33.15).

The majority of polarized genes are expressed in the distal RV compared to the proximal RV. Proximal domain RV gene markers include Wt1 and Tmem100 which have continued restricted expression in successor structures, the glomerular podocytes and PTs, respectively. Wt1 tumor suppressor gene is actually expressed throughout the CM prior to PTA and RV development. The Wt1 gene encodes a zinc finger transcription factor that activates or represses target gene transcription depending on the developmental, cellular, or even promoter context. Wt1 is expressed in diverse developing tissues and often in cells undergoing MET (199). Wt1 has different roles in different structures during kidney development. Mice deficient in Wt1 die with several developmental defects involving the mesothelium, heart as well as renal agenesis (200). Wt1 has an essential function in mediating the MET from nephron progenitors to nephron epithelia. Isolated Wt1 mutant MM fails to differentiate when co-cultured with wild type UB (201). Studies using chromatin immunoprecipitation (ChIP) coupled to microarray analysis (ChIP-chip) revealed that Bmp7, Pax2, and Sall1 are Wt1 transcriptional targets in NPCs that likely play a role in the MET mediated by Wt1 (202). Wt1 activates Wnt4 expression in the kidney mesenchyme by binding to the Wnt4 gene promoter and altering the state of its chromatin to an active state (203). It is possible that during nephrogenesis, Wt1 represses *Wnt4* expression in other cell types by binding to the *Wnt4* promoter and switching the chromatin state ("chromatin flip-flop") to a repressive state.

Another Wilms tumor suppressor gene, *Wtx*, is mutated in up to 30% of Wilms tumors which is more than the 15% to 20% mutational incidence of *Wt1* in Wilms tumors (204). *Wtx* is expressed in the MM and early nephron epithelia similar to that of *Wt1*. Interestingly, *Wtx* appears to have a dual role as both an activator and an inhibitor of the Wnt signaling pathway (205,206). Deletion of Wtx in mice results in severe renal developmental defects, either agenesis or overgrowth, associated in both phenotypes with alterations in the MM (207).

The distal domain RV gene markers include those involved in BMP (*Bmp2*), Notch (*Jag1*, *Dll1*), and Wnt (*Wnt4*, *Dkk1*, *Ccnd1*) signaling pathways (Fig. 33.15) (194). The distal markers show continued restricted expression in the medial and distal limbs of the S-shaped body and later in the loop of Henle and distal tubule. They are not expressed in the developing glomeruli at any stage. A long-standing question is the cellular origin of the connecting segment (CS), which joins the late RV (or comma-shaped structure) to the tip of the UB. The distal RV markers *Bmp2*, *Lhx1*, and *Brn1* are also expressed in the early connecting segment, which does not express the UB marker *Calb1* (calbindin). "Fusion" of the RV with the UB creating the connecting segment involves loss of the UB basement membrane and penetration of cells, originally derived from the CM, but expressing distal RV markers into the UB tip (194). Thus, the evidence favors the connecting segment originating from the CM and not the ureteric epithelium.

Later Events: Proximal and Distal Tubules

The Notch signaling pathway is an evolutionarily conserved pathway that enables short-range communication between adjacent cells to determine their developmental fate (208). In mammals, there are four receptors, Notch1-4, and five different ligands, Delta-like 1(Dll1), Dll3, Dll4, Jagged 1 and 2. Signaling is initiated by the binding of a ligand on one cell to a receptor on an adjacent cell, followed by a series of proteolytic cleavages of the receptor. An extracellular domain of the Notch receptor is cleaved by metalloproteases and this extracellular domain bound to the ligand is endocytosed by the ligand-presenting cell. The transmembrane domain of the residual receptor is cleaved by γ-secretase and the resulting Notch intracellular domain (NICD) translocates to the nucleus, where it associates with a transcription complex leading to the activation of Notch target genes.

Notch1 and *Notch2* and genes encoding their ligands *Jag1* and *Dll1* are all expressed in the RV. Previous studies implicated Notch signaling in proximal tubule differentiation and repression of other nephron segments, including distal tubules (209–211). However, more recent investigations demonstrate Notch signaling downregulates Six2 and is required for the formation of all segments of the nephron (186,187).

Brn1, a POU-domain transcription factor, is expressed in the distal domain of the RV and also in the connecting segment. At later stages, *Brn1* is expressed in the developing Henle loop, DCT, and macula densa (MD) but not in the glomerulus, proximal tubule, or collecting duct (212). *Brn1*-deficient mice die after birth of renal failure due to disturbed development of Henle loop accompanied by increased apoptosis and defective differentiation of the DCT and MD. Thus, *Brn1* has an essential role in distal tubule patterning.

The Hox genes are master regulators during development. Although they are most known in general for their role in determining segment identity and in the kidney for defining the anterior and posterior kidney morphogenetic fields, they likely have multiple cellular functions. Studies of multiple Hox 9, 10, and 11 mutant mice resulted in several phenotypes, including reduced ureteral branching, depletion of nephron progenitors, and defective stroma development (213,214). However, the most surprising phenotype was "lineage infidelity" at the cellular level within tubules. Within individual tubules, cells expressed markers characteristic of another tubule segment or expressed genes associated with multiple tubule segments. For example, the most common lineage infidelity was the presence of cells with collecting duct markers (DBA lectin) within proximal tubules (LTA lectin). Thus Hox genes have an additional function at the cellular level, directing specific cell differentiation within tubule segments.

Another milestone study compared nephron patterning in human and mouse developing kidneys (215). Although significant conservation was observed between the two species, there were notable differences. For example, Lef1, a Wnt target, is an initial marker of the initiation of nephrogenesis and is expressed in the mouse PTA. In humans, Lef1 is expressed also in NPCs suggesting an earlier inductive response and commitment to nephrogenesis. Immunostaining for transcription factors revealed several cellular subdomains within the renal vesicle (six subdomains) and S-shaped body (9 subdomains) in both species. Thus, cellular heterogeneity in developing nephrons is greater than previously appreciated. Detailed studies in human kidneys indicate NPCs are progressively recruited over time from their niche into forming nephrons and that the timing predicts a proximal–distal cell fate (216).

INTERSTITIUM

Compared to other parenchymal components, there is far less known about the interstitium (stroma) in kidney development (217). It is generally believed that the MM is originally derived from the IM. A traditional view is that cells of the MM originally derived from the IM not induced by the ureteric bud will become interstitial cells. Although *Osr1* is expressed in the early MM, there is evidence that some *Osr1* positive cells, prior to UB invasion and induction, give rise to cells expressing *Foxd1*, the earliest known marker of interstitial cells (169). There are at least three distinct *Foxd1* stromal compartments: capsular, cortical, and medullary. Foxd1-expressing cortical stromal cells are maintained by self-renewal and as discussed before, a fraction of these cells reside in the Six2⁺ CM in early nephrogenesis (218). NPCs lacking Pax2 have been shown to differentiate into interstitial cells, thus Pax2 has a role in maintaining NPCs and repressing an interstitial differentiation pathway (219). Less is known about the medullary stroma. However, there is evidence that β-catenin is essential for the differentiation of stromal progenitors to form the medullary stroma (220). A question is what embryonic tissue do the interstitial precursor cells arise from? Cell lineage tracing studies suggest that most metanephric interstitial cells derive from the paraxial mesoderm (PM) and few originate from the IM (221). This may potentially explain why paraxial mesodermal derivatives, such as cartilage and muscle, may be ectopically present in renal dysplasia or Wilms tumor.

In addition to providing a structural framework around the other components, an emerging view is that the developing interstitium plays an essential role in nephron and collecting duct differentiation (217,222). The interstitial cell marker *Foxd1* encodes a forkhead transcription factor. Genetic ablation of *Foxd1* in mice leads to small kidneys with aberrant nephron differentiation and impaired ureteral branching emphasizing an important role of the stroma in nephrogenesis (223). The loss of *Foxd1* also results in renal capsule abnormalities that include the ectopic presence of *Bmp4* expressing cells, and fused kidneys that never ascend from the pelvis to the lumbar region (224). Studies implicate the *Hox10* genes in development of the interstitium and capsule as the defects observed in the *Foxd1* mutant kidneys are largely phenocopied in *Hox10* triple mutant kidneys (225). Foxd1 represses the expression of the proteoglycan decorin which inhibits Bmp-Smad signaling, which stimulates nephron progenitor differentiation (226). Stromal cells isolated from the cortical interstitium and capsule of human kidneys have been reported to be distinct mesenchymal stromal cell (MSC) populations (227,228).

FAT4, an atypical cadherin produced in the interstitium operates in the Hippo pathway, and its signaling allows the activation of β-catenin target genes that promote nephron progenitor differentiation (229). Loss of FAT4 or its ligands DCHS1/2 (Dachsous 1 and 2) results in expansion of the nephron progenitor pool (230). A model emerging from these studies is that FAT4 produced in the stroma binds to DCHS1/2 in the CM to restrict the nephron progenitors.

Hedgehog (HH) signaling is involved in diverse areas of developmental and cell biology (231). HH binding to the Patched (PTC) family of cell surface receptors alleviates the PTC inhibition of Smoothed (SMO), which in turn, results in the activation of the GLI transcriptional mediators. Within the cortical stroma, HH–SMO–GLI signaling has been demonstrated to control nephron formation with TGF-β2 playing a role in the signaling cascade (232).

Stromal cells express retinaldehyde dehydrogenase 2 (Raldh2) which synthesizes retinoic acid, which binds to its receptors in ureteral branch cells, inducing Ret expression and promoting branching (233). Moreover, stromal retinoic acid activates the expression of Ecm1, which downregulates Ret expression in the ureteral branch (234). Other stroma cell–expressed molecules include *Rara, Rarb2, Pod1, Fgf7, Bmp4,* and *Pbx1*. Thus, in brief summary the interstitium and renal capsule appear to provide signals that are critical for correct patterning of the nephron and ureteral components.

A loose stroma containing spindle-shaped cells surrounds the early ureteric bud branches and early nephrons and is known as the primary interstitium (or "clear-cell type stroma"). As nephrogenesis proceeds, a cortical interstitium and a medullary interstitium, each with distinct cellular phenotypes, forms. In the postnatal period, the interstitial cells resemble fibroblasts, dendritic cells or macrophages according to morphologic and immunophenotypical findings (235–237). Much remains to be learned about their origins and functions.

GLOMERULOGENESIS

To appreciate how some glomerular diseases arise or how the glomerulus responds to injury, an understanding of glomerular development is indispensable. For more detailed information of glomerulogenesis, readers are referred to several excellent reviews (238–241). Glomerular development proceeds through a sequence of structures described as vesicle, comma-shaped, S-shaped, capillary loop, and maturing glomerulus stages. The vesicle and comma-shaped stages were discussed previously. At the S-shaped stage, the lower limb beneath the vascular cleft separates into two layers (lips) divided by a narrow developing Bowman space (Fig. 33.6). Lining the upper, internal lip are the visceral epithelial cells, which will differentiate into podocytes. On the opposite side of Bowman space, the cells of the lower, outer lip will become the parietal epithelial cells (PECs) lining Bowman capsule.

During the S-shaped stage, microvessels can often be identified within the vascular cleft of the S-figure. Since this vascular cleft is the site where the glomerular capillaries emerge, the origin of the microvessels has generated considerable study. A long-standing question has been whether the glomerular endothelial cells have an *angiogenic* or a *vasculogenic* origin. Earlier evidence favored the process of angiogenesis, whereby endothelial cells sprout from external vessels that grow into the kidney. Other studies provide compelling evidence for a vasculogenic mechanism, whereby endothelial cells of the early glomerular capillaries originate from intrinsic angioblasts, likely derived from the MM (242,243). Release of growth factors, such as vascular endothelial growth factor (VEGF), from the immature podocytes may attract the angioblasts, expressing VEGF receptors (as Flk1) into the vascular clefts. Other signaling systems such as the angiopoietin (ligand)-Tie (receptor) axis also play a role in endothelial cell and vascular development (244). At this stage, the endothelial cells contain few fenestrae. The early podocytes are cuboidal or columnar, whereas the PECs are already flattening. Situated between the endothelial and podocyte layers are two basement membranes. The basement membrane beneath the podocytes is usually thicker and more continuous than the one underneath the endothelial cells.

During the capillary loop stage, the capillaries start to fill out into an expanding Bowman space. The endothelial cells flatten and develop numerous fenestrae. With maturation, the endothelial cells lose their diaphragms which bridge the fenestrae (245). This endothelial maturation depends on ADAM10, a regular of Notch signaling (246). The podocytes develop a complex cellular architecture as they become terminally differentiated and cease to undergo mitosis. They flatten and form cytoplasmic primary processes, which in turn, elaborate foot processes that interdigitate with those from adjacent podocytes and adhere to the developing glomerular basement membrane (GBM). Intercellular junctional complexes are present at the apical membranes between podocytes. With foot process development, these junctions migrate down the lateral surfaces of the emerging foot processes and disappear, when they are either replaced by or converted into the slit diaphragms. This cellular process has been elegantly demonstrated by block-face scanning electron microscopy (SEM) (247). Slit diaphragms, specialized intercellular junctions, bridge the space between adjacent foot processes. The slit diaphragm is connected to the podocyte cytoskeleton as part of a multifunctional protein complex, that includes nephrin, CD2-associated protein (CD2AP), and podocin (248). Nephrin is the protein encoded by the *NPHS1* gene that is mutated in congenital nephrotic syndrome of the Finnish type, which is associated with loss of the slit diaphragm, abnormal foot processes and massive proteinuria (249). Thus, the slit diaphragm is critical for maintaining podocyte architecture and the glomerular filtration barrier.

The dual GBM, synthesized by both the endothelium and podocytes, is still present but areas of fusion between the two membranes are found. Beginning during the capillary loop stage, a complex series of transitions in the GBM protein composition occurs. There is developmental switching of both type IV collagen and laminin isoforms in the GBM, events which are essential for forming normal glomerular capillaries. Whereas the immature GBMs of comma- and S-shaped nephrons contain laminin $\alpha1\beta1\gamma1$ (laminin 111), GBMs at later developmental stages and in adults contain laminin $\alpha5\beta2\gamma1$ (laminin 521) (239). Collagen type IV is made up of six distinct α chains ($\alpha1[IV]$ to $\alpha6[IV]$), which form different triple helical molecules called protomers. There are three types of protomers: $\alpha1.\alpha2.\alpha1(IV)$, $\alpha3.\alpha4.\alpha5(IV)$, and $\alpha5.\alpha6.\alpha5(IV)$. The immature GBMs of comma-, S-shaped, and early capillary loop stage glomeruli contain collagen $\alpha1.\alpha2.\alpha1(IV)$. Starting in capillary loop stages, this collagen network is replaced by $\alpha3.\alpha4.\alpha5(IV)$, which persists as the only collagen IV network normally present in the mature GBM. The mechanisms responsible for both laminin and collagen IV isoform switching in the developing GBM are not known. The laminin isoform switching process precedes the one for type IV collagen isoforms (250). Ultrastructural immunolabeling studies have demonstrated that whereas endothelial cells, mesangial cells, and podocytes synthesize collagen $\alpha1.\alpha2.\alpha1(IV)$, only podocytes make collagen $\alpha3.\alpha4.\alpha5(IV)$ (251).

Glomeruli in the maturing stage resemble adult glomeruli by histology but are smaller in diameter. The podocytes of the maturing glomeruli may have a cuboidal appearance. A single-fused GBM predominates and areas of dual unfused basement membranes are rarely seen. At this time, the synthesis of components for the GBM is largely by the podocytes. In areas where foot process interdigitation is continuing, irregular outpocketings of basement membrane are found beneath the podocytes. These outpockets or loops reflect newly synthesized GBM, which will be deposited into the existing GBM.

The development of the mesangium occurs relatively later in glomerulogenesis. Although the mesangial cells likely derive from the MM, their origin is not entirely clear. The mesangial cell precursors are believed to be distinct from the VEGF receptor expressing angioblasts that differentiate into the glomerular endothelial cells. However, the emergence of mesangial cells in the glomerulus is dependent on platelet-derived growth factor-β (PDGF-β), produced by podocytes and endothelial cells, and its receptor, PDGF receptor-β (PDGF-Rβ), expressed on mesangial cells (252,253). Mutant mice lacking PDGF-β or PDGF-Rβ have abnormal glomeruli with no mesangial cells.

VASCULATURE

There is less known about the development of the renal vasculature compared to other renal parenchymal components. However, recent studies are beginning to illuminate the field (254,255). Renal vascularization appears synchronized with nephrogenesis resulting in a complex network of vessels of variable size and containing several cell types. Several major morphogenetic processes are believed to underlie renal vascular development: vasculogenesis, angiogenesis, and hemovasculogenesis. In vasculogenesis, vessels originate from intrinsic cells. An example is endothelial cell precursors forming tubes followed by coating of vascular smooth muscle cells. Angiogenesis, the sprouting of new vessels from pre-existing vessels, occurs in branching from the renal artery and from juxtamedullary efferent arterioles to form the vasa recta. There is less known about hemovasculogenesis, which refers to the simultaneous formation of blood precursors and vessels. One concept is that vasculogenesis predominates during early nephrogenesis and vessel branching and elongation occurs later in kidney development and continues after birth. Whole mount three-dimensional analysis of early human embryos have shown in several tissues a phase of vasculogenesis preceding angiogenesis (256).

Within the interstitium there are vascular progenitor cells. *Foxd1*-positive stromal cells give rise to vascular smooth muscle cells, pericytes, renin-expressing cells, and mesangial cells (257). A subset of *Foxd1*-positive cells express the transcription factor Tbx18 differentiate into vascular smooth muscle cells, pericytes, and mesangial cells (258). A hemovascular progenitor expressing the stem cell leukemia/T-cell acute lymphoblastic protein 1 (SCL/Tal1) was shown to give rise to endothelial cells and also blood precursors (259). These studies also demonstrated that sphingosine-1-phosphate (S1P) and its receptor S1PR1, expressed in SCL/Tal1 derived blood cells and endothelial cells, operate in a signaling pathway to regulate renal vascular development. Endothelial cell precursors are heterogeneous. For example, a $CD146^+$ cell population, essential for development of the renal microvasculature, differentiates into $CD31^+$ endothelial cells (260). Another population, a subset of cortical stroma *Foxd1*-positive cells, expressing Flk1 (VEGFR2) is critical for forming peritubular capillaries (261).

Detailed anatomic spatiotemporal studies suggest that renal vascularization is mostly an angiogenic process whereby blood vessels initially wrap around the ureteric bud, migrate to the nephrogenic zone and form new polygonal vascular plexuses around ureteric bud tips and NPCs (262). The vascular networks contain red cells, are enclosed by a basement membrane and are connected to older blood vessels. This patterning of developing renal blood vessels has been corroborated by another study, which in addition showed prominent molecular heterogeneity of endothelial cells (263).

DEVELOPMENT OF THE JUXTAGLOMERULAR APPARATUS

In the human mesonephros a complete juxtaglomerular apparatus (JGA) has not been observed, although renin-expressing cells have been noted (264). Renin expression in the metanephric kidney has been detected as early as 8 weeks of gestation and renin mRNA levels are significantly higher in the developing kidney than in the adult organ (264,265). In the developing kidney, renin-expressing cells are found in intrarenal arteries including the arcuate and interlobular arteries. As development progresses, the distribution of renin-expressing cells shifts from the larger vessels to the JGA, primarily the terminal afferent arteriole, in the mature kidney (266,267). Within the afferent arterioles themselves, heterogeneous patterns of renin expression exist (268). The juxtaglomerular cell, as a cellular component of the mature JGA, is located in the wall of the terminal afferent arteriole close to the glomerulus. Renin progenitor cells differentiate into JG cells (269). Renin cells display a unique set of genes distinct from other cell types (270). The JG cells have a dual endocrine-contractile phenotype, which had been demonstrated to be maintained by RBP-J, a transcriptional mediator of the Notch pathway (271). The unique gene repertoire of renin cells affords them considerable plasticity to differentiate along different pathways. They can differentiate into non–renin-expressing cells, such as vascular smooth muscle cells and glomerular mesangial cells (269).

GROSS ANATOMY

Kidney Position and Blood Supply

Upon formation the metanephric kidneys are situated close to each other in the pelvis at the level of the upper sacrum. Between the sixth and ninth weeks of gestation, the kidneys are found further apart and at higher levels in the abdomen until they reach their final upper lumbar position (272). This "ascent" of the kidneys is believed to result largely from differential growth of the caudal part of the embryo away from the kidneys (273,274). However, others have argued that the cephalad movement of the kidneys is active and not caused by differential growth of the vertebral column (275). With this migration, the renal hilum, where the main vessels enter and exit, rotates from a ventral orientation to face anteromedially. Initially, the kidneys receive their blood supply from branches of the common iliac arteries. With their ascension, the kidneys are supplied by arteries originating from progressively higher levels of the distal aorta (272). The question of whether some of these vessels anastomose in a peri-aortic plexus is not well studied (276). As the ascending kidneys receive new branches from the aorta, the older, caudal branches undergo involution. Persistence of these inferior vessels may result in accessory renal arteries. The most cephalad branches arising from the abdominal aorta become the permanent main renal arteries.

Kidney Weight and Configuration

The various reference values reported for fetal and neonatal kidney weights correspond relatively closely, despite potential variability due to factors such as the social and economic status and the level of health care in a given population (277–282). Separate values from nonmacerated and macerated cases are available (282), as well as values using pre-fixation (255,256) and post-fixation weighing (281,282) of the kidneys. Data for the combined weight (right and left) of the kidneys during the second and third trimesters are shown in Figure 33.16. Different reference values published for combined kidney weights during infancy and childhood also favorably compare (277,283). The data of Emery and Mithal (277) are illustrated in Figure 33.17.

The newborn kidney has a shorter, more rounded configuration than that of the adult. The upper and lower poles

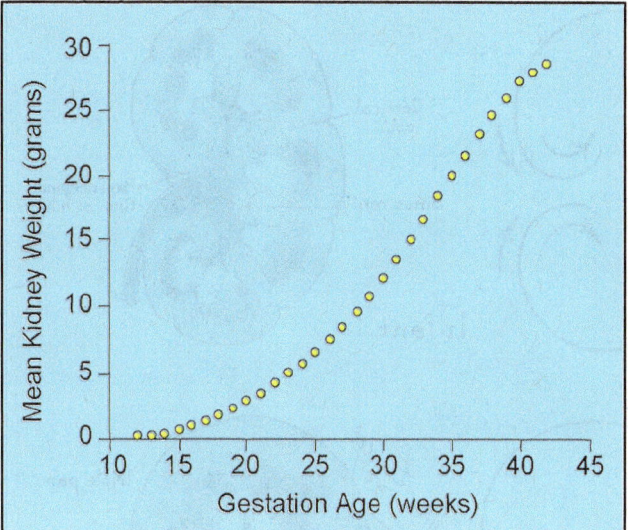

FIGURE 33.16 Mean combined (*right and left*) weight of kidneys from second and third trimester fetuses and neonates. (Modified with permission from Hansen K, Sung CJ, Huang C, et al. Reference values for second trimester fetal and neonatal organ weights and measurements. *Pediatr Dev Pathol* 2003;6:160–167.)

project further medially, so the renal sinus is relatively deeper in the infant (Figs. 33.18 and 33.19) (284). The renal sinus of infants contains much less fat and connective tissue than in the adult, and the cortical septa (columns) of Bertin approach much closer to the pelvic-calyceal system. Figure 33.19 illustrates the process of "unrolling" of the renal poles during childhood, as the kidney assumes the more elongated configuration observed in adults. This change in configuration

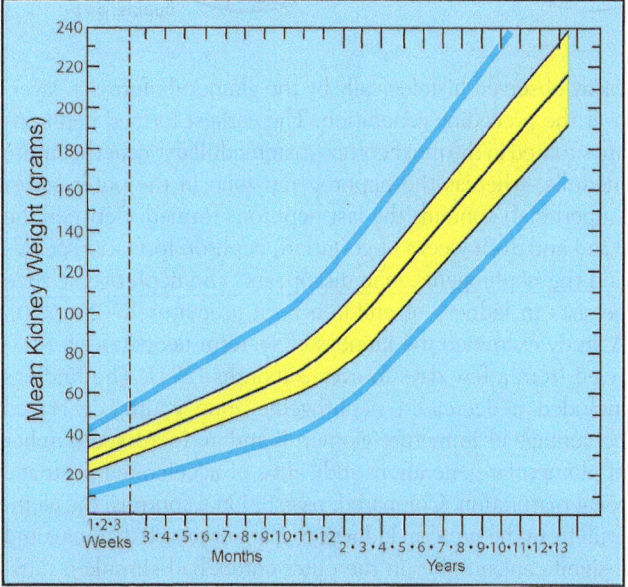

FIGURE 33.17 Mean combined (*right and left*) weight of kidneys at various postnatal ages. The middle black line represents the means. The 50th percentile (*yellow band*) and 95th percentile (*blue lines*) ranges are shown. (Modified with permission from Emery JL, Mithal A. The weights of kidneys in late intra-uterine life and childhood. *J Clin Pathol* 1960;13:490–493.)

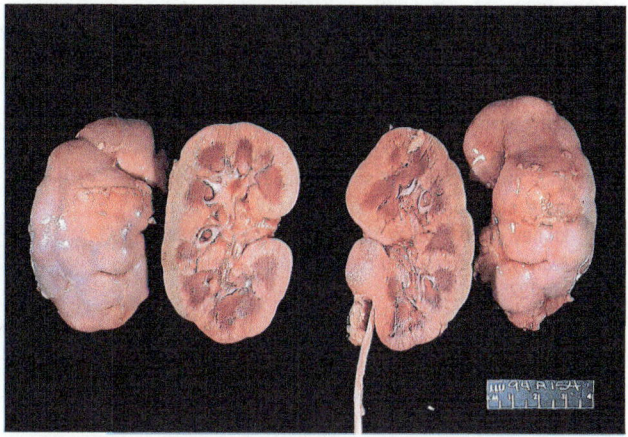

FIGURE 33.18 Gross appearance of newborn kidneys. The rounded configuration with a relatively deeper sinus, characteristic of the infantile kidney, is seen on the sectioned surface. Fetal lobations are prominent on the external surface.

produces a shallower renal sinus with partial exteriorization of the pelvis. As the pelvic-calyceal system assumes a more exterior position, it also becomes displaced further from the parenchyma lining the sinus. The additional space created between the pelvic-calyceal system and the cortical columns of Bertin is normally filled with fat, which increases in amount as the kidney approaches maturity.

Fetal Lobations

A renal lobe consists of a medullary pyramid and its surrounding cortical parenchyma (Figs. 33.7 and 33.18). The centrilobar cortex covers the base of a pyramid, whereas the septal cortex surrounds the sides of a pyramid. Thus, a column (septum) of Bertin represents the confluence of two layers of septal cortex from two adjacent lobes. Although a lobe does not represent a functional renal unit, it may be viewed as an anatomic organizational unit (285). Lobation begins in the human kidney at 6 to 7 weeks and proceeds to maximum development with an average of 14 lobes at 28 weeks of gestation (286,287). At this stage, generally 14 papillae and calyces are present corresponding with the same number of lobes. Deep clefts on the surface separate the lobes. After the 28th week, a process of variable lobar fusion decreases the number of surface fissures, papillae, and calyces. The degree of calyceal fusion is greater than papillae fusion. In full-term infant kidneys, the mean number reported for calyces is 9 and for papillae, it is 11 (287). Considerably more lobar fusion, creating compound papillae, occurs in the polar regions than in the midpolar region, where simple papillae are more likely to be retained.

The surface of the neonatal kidney is divided into polygons by prominent fissures that correspond roughly, although not precisely, to the lobar outlines (Fig. 33.18). These fetal lobations usually decrease in prominence with advancing age, persisting longer on the ventral surface than the dorsal surface of the organ. Although there is considerable individual variation in the chronology of their disappearance,

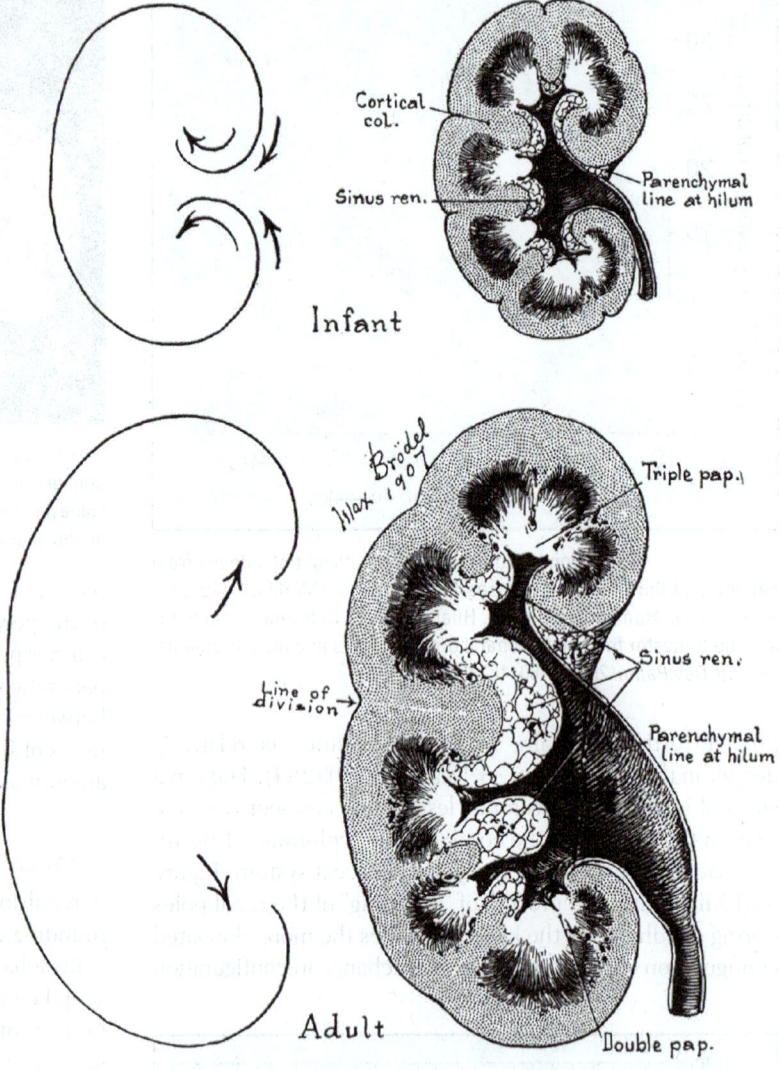

FIGURE 33.19 Max Brödel's classic illustration of the process of unrolling of the kidney in postnatal life. The rounded configuration of the infantile organ becomes elongated as the upper and lower poles diverge and pelvic-calyceal structures are partially everted from their original position within the renal sinus. The space thus created within the renal sinus is filled by fat, which is far more abundant in the adult kidney than in the infant kidney. (From Kelley HA, Burnam CF. *Diseases of the Kidneys, Ureters, and Bladder.* Vol. 1. New York: Appleton; 1925).

they are usually inconspicuous by 4 to 5 years of age (288). The only valid generalization is that fetal lobations usually diminish in number and prominence in the first few years of life, but they remain apparent, especially on the ventral surfaces, in a significant proportion of adult kidneys. In one study, one or more interlobar fissures were detected in up to 50% of adult kidneys (287). In older children and adults, it is important to distinguish persistent fetal lobations from cortical scars. Fetal lobation is a more accurate term than "fetal lobulation" because a lobule is an architectural feature of the cortex, primarily observed on the histologic level.

HISTOLOGY

CORTICAL ARCHITECTURE

The developing renal cortex has unique temporal and spatial features of organization. Each generation of nephrons, most easily observed histologically by the glomeruli, forms a "layer" over the preceding generation. The earliest formed nephrons are situated in the inner cortex (juxtamedullary) near the future medulla, whereas the nephrogenic zone in the outer cortex (superficial) contains the last nephrons formed. Between the 32nd and 36th weeks of gestation, nephron formation ceases and the nephrogenic zone disappears. The nephrogenic zone persists in kidneys of children born prematurely (289,290). A study examined the kidneys of preterm neonates who survived from a few days to over 2 months (291). The findings included a decreased nephrogenic zone width, decreased percentage of immature glomeruli and an increased number of glomerular generations indicative of accelerated postnatal renal maturation. Compared to gestational controls, the glomeruli from the preterm kidneys had an increased diameter and a significant number in the outer cortex had shrunken tufts. These findings suggest preterm infants may have an increased vulnerability to renal disease later in life.

The histologic features of the developing renal cortex have been used as an index of fetal maturation (290). The ratio of the width of the nephrogenic zone to the width of the remaining cortex decreases in a linear fashion as the birth weight increases (279,292). This approach has been used to detect infants with reduced intrauterine growth in whom this ratio is less than expected for the birth weight. Using glomeruli as representative of nephrons, studies have employed counting of the number of layers (or rows) of glomeruli from inner to outer cortex, as a method to evaluate nephrogenesis (293–295). Each successive layer is assumed to represent a new glomerular "generation." These estimates are performed on well-oriented sections that are orthogonal to the cortex and display a well-defined corticomedullary junction. The studies are in fair agreement between gestations of 24 to 36 weeks in which the average number of rows ("nephron generations") of glomeruli are as follows: 5 to 7 (24 weeks), 8 to 9 (28 weeks), 9 to 10 (32 weeks), and 10 to 14 (36 weeks). A comprehensive study of 71 infants generally confirmed these results and found the number of glomerular generations was directly proportional to gestational age, body weight, and kidney weight (296). However, there was considerable variability in the final number of glomerular generations, ranging from 8 to 12 per kidney. There was also some variation in the timing of cessation of nephrogenesis. Interestingly, the study revealed an increase in glomerular size from mid-gestation to term in females, whereas glomerular size in males remained constant over this period. The proportional number of podocytes and endothelial cells within mature glomeruli appeared to remain constant during gestation.

After the full complement of nephrons is attained by the normal fetus, subsequent renal growth reflects hypertrophy and maturation of the nephrons. As tubules elongate and increase in diameter, they become interposed between glomeruli. The glomeruli in the outer cortex of newborns are crowded together (Fig. 33.10), whereas the older, more mature glomeruli deeper in the cortex are more widely separated. This process of tubular growth not only separates glomeruli from one another, but it also tends to separate them from the cortical surface near where they originally developed. In a normal term newborn, one observes many glomeruli very close to the renal capsule (Fig. 33.10). By about 2 months of age, the process of nephron growth has begun to separate the outermost glomeruli and a narrow zone largely devoid of glomeruli develops beneath the renal capsule (Fig. 33.20). This latter zone has been termed the *cortex corticis* (297). The cortex corticis becomes progressively wider during childhood (Fig. 33.21). Although it is normal to find an occasional glomerulus adjacent to the capsular surface in normal infants and children, the presence of numerous very superficial glomeruli suggests defective renal growth during late fetal or early postnatal life. Abnormally crowded glomeruli also can be an important clue to defects in nephron growth and differentiation, which may involve only the outer cortex, or the entire cortical mantle. Thus, the cortical architecture may be viewed as a record of the developmental history of the kidney.

The cortex is subdivided into distinctly demarcated *lobules* by radially oriented groups of tubules termed *medullary*

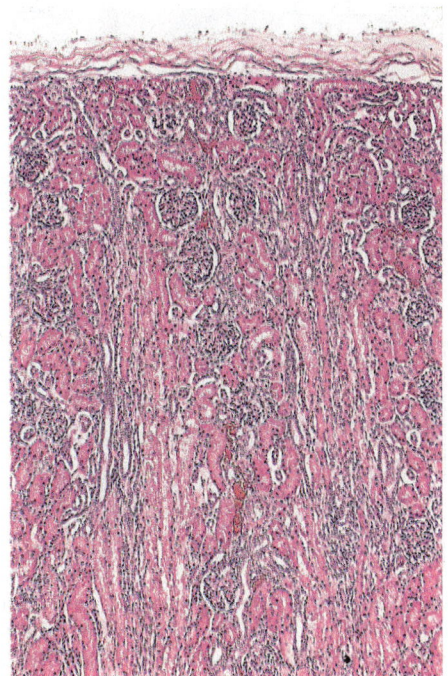

FIGURE 33.20 Renal cortex at 2 months of age. Glomeruli in the outer cortex are becoming more widely spaced due to tubular elongation. Superficial glomeruli are beginning to separate from the renal capsule, the first indication of the cortex corticis.

rays that extend from the base of the pyramids upward into the cortex (Fig. 33.22). A lobule is defined as the cortical domain surrounding a medullary ray. Despite their name, the medullary rays (of Ferrein) actually are part of the cortex and contain the straight segments of the proximal tubule, the thick ascending limbs (TALs), and the collecting ducts. Medullary rays usually extend to near the cortical surface in infants, but not in older children. The presence of complete medullary rays is a good indicator that the plane of a given

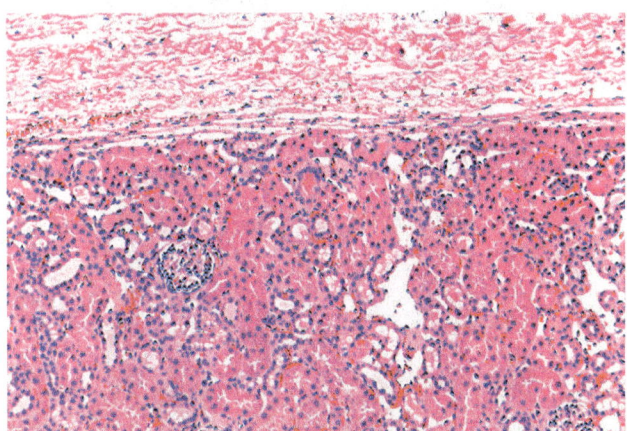

FIGURE 33.21 Micrograph of well-developed renal cortex corticis. The zone without glomeruli beneath the distinct renal capsule is evident. (Reprinted with permission from Murphy WM, Grignon DJ, Perlman EJ. Tumors of the kidney, bladder, and related urinary structures. In: Silverberg SG, Sobin LH, eds. *Atlas of Tumor Pathology. 4th series, fascicle 1.* Washington, DC: Armed Forces Institute of Pathology; 2004.)

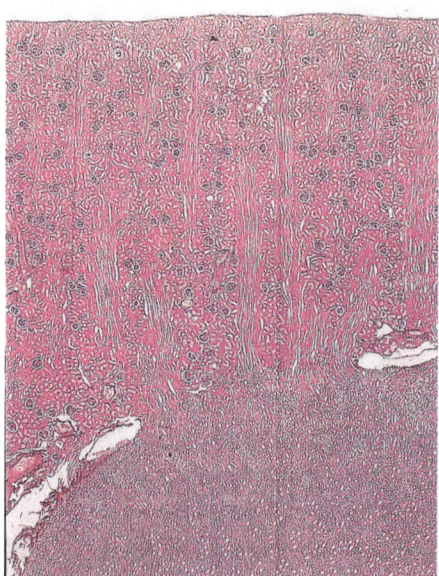

FIGURE 33.22 Kidney at 21 months of age. This perpendicularly oriented section illustrates the full length of several medullary rays that extend from the corticomedullary junction to a level near the cortex corticis. Each medullary ray marks the center of a cortical lobule.

section is perpendicular and reflective of the true thickness of the cortex. Medullary ray nodules are complex tangled tubular configurations commonly seen in the medullary rays of infants during the early months of life, being most prominent between 1 and 6 months of age (Fig. 33.23) (298). These structures apparently represent a normal transitory developmental phenomenon of variable prominence, which is pathologic only when extreme.

NEPHRON NUMBER

The number of nephrons in a kidney is determined in utero. The final number is dependent on gestational age and a favorable intrauterine environment. Unbiased, precise stereologic methods have been used to count glomeruli which serve as a surrogate for nephron number. One study of human intrauterine renal growth revealed the glomerular number increased from 15,000 at 15 weeks of gestation to 740,000 by 40 weeks (299). The greatest rate of nephron induction has been observed between 15 and 17 weeks of gestation, however, approximately 60% of the total nephrons are believed to form during the third trimester (299). Nephron number, inferred from glomerular number estimates in children and adults without renal disease, is strongly correlated with birth weight (300). Intrauterine growth retardation has been shown to impair nephron formation, as measured in fetuses and in infants dying within a year of birth (301,302).

It is apparent that a kidney having a quantitative abnormality, such as low nephron number, may not demonstrate an obvious defect of nephron spatial topography on histologic examination. However, studies have demonstrated an inverse correlation between the number of glomeruli and mean glomerular volume, suggesting glomeruli increase in size to compensate for an innate low nephron number (300,302). Large glomeruli may be susceptible to scarring. Glomerulomegaly has been used as an adverse factor to assess the risk of disease progression in childhood nephrotic syndrome (303). Thus, increased glomerular size (volume or area) may be useful as an indicator for nephron deficiency in individuals susceptible to renal disease.

Until a few years ago, each human kidney was believed to contain 1 million nephrons. It is now appreciated that there is a remarkably wide variation in total nephrons per kidney among "normal" adults, ranging from as low as 227,000 to over 2,000,000 (304–306). Nephron endowment is programmed in the perinatal period capping the nephron number in an individual's lifetime. Some time ago, Brenner et al. postulated that an inborn deficit of nephrons predisposes to acquired renal disease, including hypertension, in adults (307). A study showing that hypertensive individuals had fewer nephrons but a larger glomerular volume than age-matched normotensive controls supports this hypothesis (308). The endowment of nephrons from nephrogenesis and the developmental origins of renal disease are fertile areas for investigation.

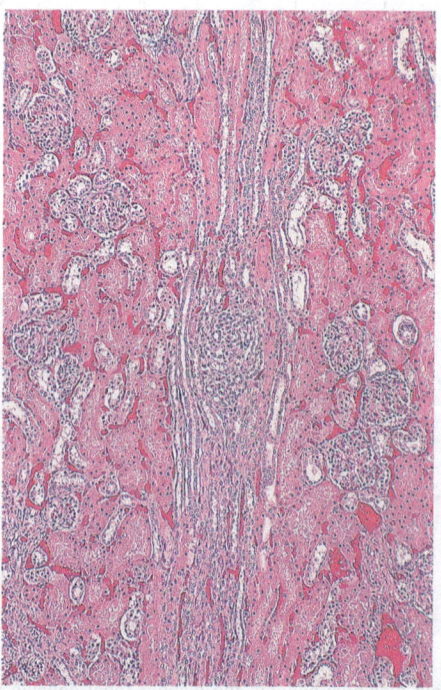

FIGURE 33.23 Medullary ray nodule. In the center of the micrograph, a tangled cluster of collecting ducts forms a nodule near the midportion of a medullary ray. This structure is usually transitory, being uncommon in the first month of life and extremely rare after 1 year of age.

GLOMERULAR MATURATION AND GROWTH

Newly formed glomeruli are structurally distinctive, and their evolution toward a mature form is a gradual process. Since the period of glomerular development spans a 6- to 7-month period of fetal life, a spectrum of maturational stages is normally present in infant kidneys. As mentioned before, this spectrum is organized in a temporal–spatial manner in the cortex. Familiarity with normal glomerular maturation can facilitate an assessment of the renal developmental status in infants.

Dramatic changes in glomerular structure and size occur through the early months and years of life. For convenience of study, several stages of glomerular development have been defined in studies. (309–312). Figure 33.24 shows representative glomeruli from the midcortical region of infants and children from birth to 9 years of age to illustrate the maturational changes. Figure 33.24A shows the characteristic appearance of recently formed glomeruli from a term newborn infant. In addition to their small size, the most obvious distinctions from mature glomeruli are

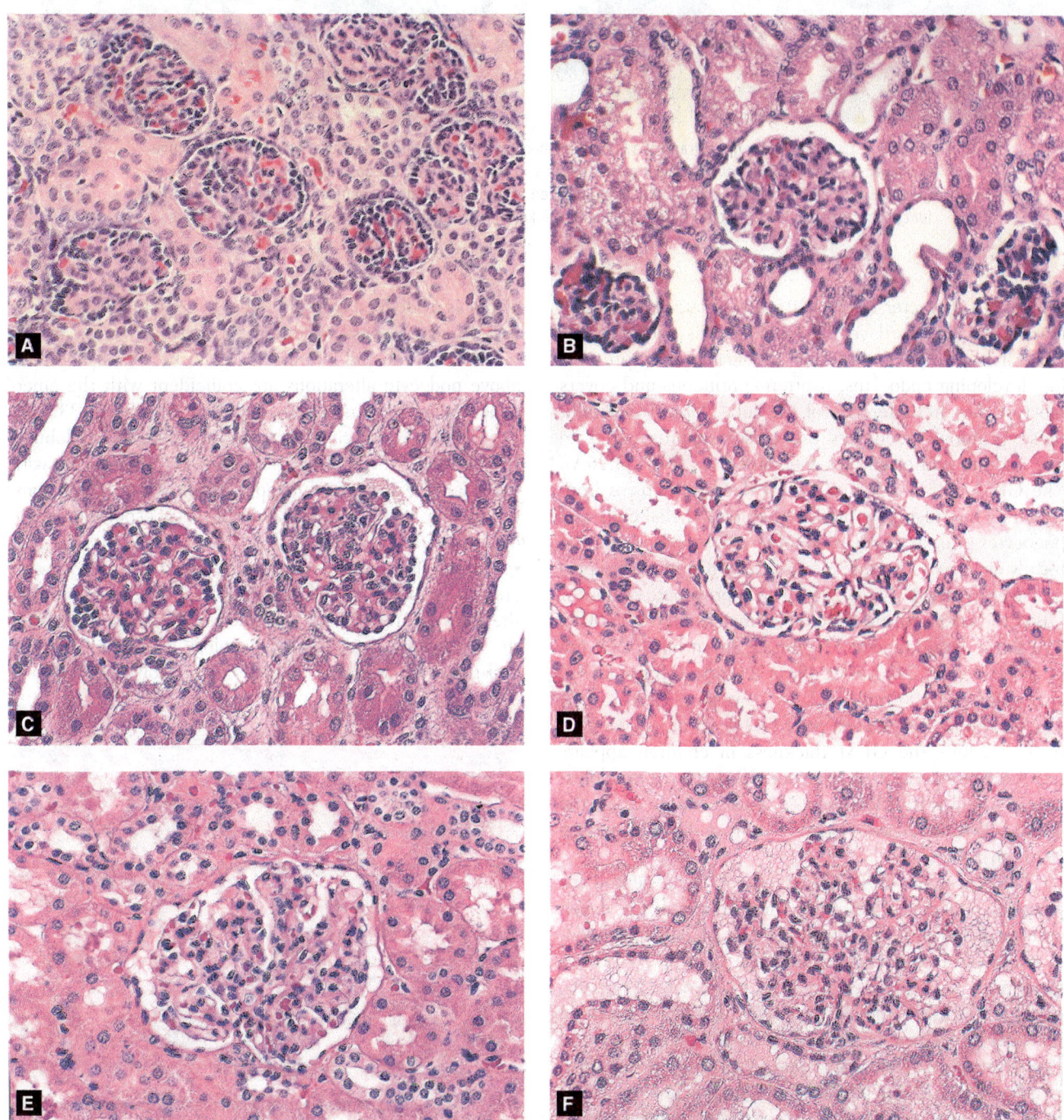

FIGURE 33.24 Normal midcortical glomeruli of six infants and children from birth to 9 years of age. All the micrographs were taken at the same magnification. **A:** Newborn. **B:** 6 months. **C:** 11 months. **D:** 21 months. **E:** 5 years. **F:** 9 years.

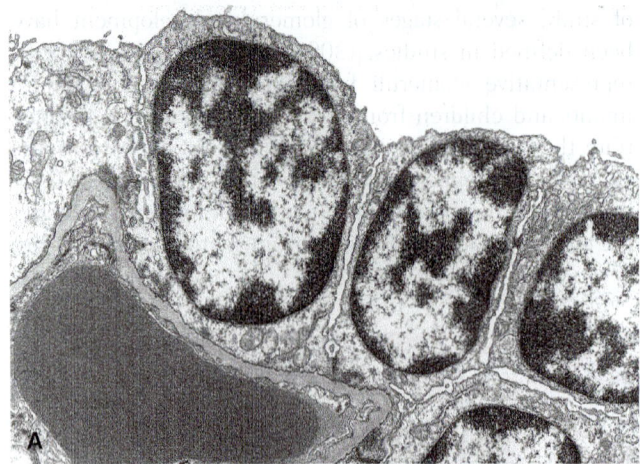 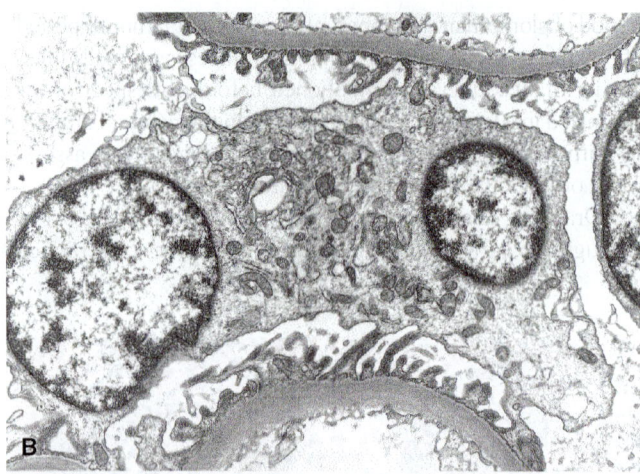

FIGURE 33.25 **A:** Electron micrograph of a normal glomerulus from an infant 2 months of age. Note the continuous layer of primitive podocytes lacking foot processes and the thin glomerular basement membrane. **B:** Mature glomerulus from a patient 16 years of age, photographed at the same magnification as in A. There is prominent foot process development, and the GBM is distinctly thicker than in the infant. (Courtesy of Dr. Gary W. Mierau.)

the simple character of the tufts with relatively few capillary loops and the layer of cuboidal cells surfacing the visceral layer of the tuft. This cuboidal layer, representing developing podocytes, is often continuous and covers most of the circumference of the tufts. Ultrastructurally, these primitive podocytes are closely approximated to one another and often lack foot processes (Fig. 33.25A). The GBM is thin and two lamina densa structures, representing basal laminae produced by endothelial cells and podocytes prior to their fusion into a single lamina, may be focally observed. The thickness of the GBM increases progressively with age (Fig. 33.25). The approximate values for GBM thickness during childhood range as follows: 100 to 130 nm in fetal kidneys, 170 nm ($\pm$ 30) at birth; 208 nm ($\pm$ 24) at 1 year; 245 nm ($\pm$ 49) at 2 years; 268 nm ($\pm$ 43) at 6 years; and 300 nm ($\pm$ 42) by 10 years (311,313,314). The growth rate is greatest prior to 2 years of age. In contrast to adults the GBM thickness in children appears less sex dependent (301). Further GBM growth in adolescence, which is less documented, must occur to reach the adult GBM thickness in men (373 nm $\pm$ 42) and women (326 nm $\pm$ 45) (315).

The continuous cuboidal layer of cells is transient as the maturing podocytes flatten over the surfaces of the developing capillaries. A few small clusters of cuboidal podocytes remain in infant glomeruli (Fig. 33.24B, C). After a glomerulus has been in existence for more than 12 months, remnants of the cuboidal layer are usually not seen in normally developed glomeruli. In 1940, Gruenwald and Popper suggested that some podocytes may be sloughed into Bowman space as part of the maturation process (309). In fact, several studies have demonstrated that podocytes are shed from the glomerulus and excreted in the urine in various glomerular diseases as well as healthy individuals (316,317). Moreover, most of the urinary podocytes are viable as evidenced by their ability to grow in culture under in vitro conditions. Whether podocyturia occurs in the normal neonate and infant remains to be established. The above podocyte alterations are coincident with the emergence of more conspicuous capillary loops (Fig. 33.24C, D). Eventually, the capillary loops are arranged into lobules (Fig. 33.24E, F). However, an occasional glomerulus with the small size and immature appearance of a neonatal glomerulus may be observed in older infants, especially in the outer third of the cortex (Fig. 33.26).

Glomerular growth during childhood has been evaluated in several investigations (318–322). In these studies, the source of renal tissue, postmortem or biopsy specimen; the observational technique, histology or microdissection; and the morphometric method varied. However, it is well

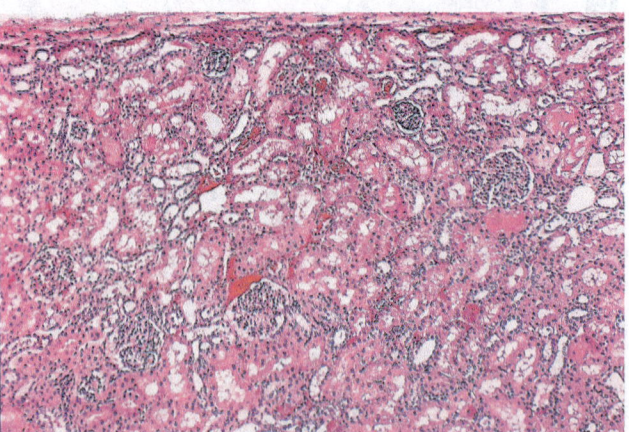

FIGURE 33.26 Persistent immature glomeruli at 12 months of age. Two miniature glomeruli with cuboidal cells at the periphery of the tuft are present near the renal capsule. Small numbers of defective glomeruli can be found in infant kidneys, but they are destined to undergo sclerosis and involution.

established that glomerular size increases from birth to adolescence. Souster and Emery reported that the midcortical and juxtamedullary mean glomerular area in fetuses actually decreased between 12 and 20 months of gestation (320). After this initial decrease, the glomeruli remained at the same size until birth, after which they steadily grew. Moore et al. observed that the mean glomerular diameter in normal children increased from 112 to 167 μm between birth and 15 years of age, averaging 3.6 μm per year during this period (321). Akaoka et al. found that the mean glomerular tuft area in children with minimal change nephrotic syndrome and recurrent hematuria, increased from 6,600 μm^2 to 11,000 μm^2 between 2 and 15 years of age (322). In the latter study, the glomerular capillary lumina area did not correlate with the glomerular tuft area, whereas the number of capillaries per glomerulus showed a positive correlation with the glomerular tuft area. Although some of the glomeruli were not normal in this study, the findings support the concept that glomerular growth occurs by an increase in the number or length of capillaries rather than by hemodynamic capillary dilatation.

Juxtamedullary glomeruli are larger than superficial glomeruli at birth and during infancy. However, some uncertainty exists regarding these regional differences in glomerular size in later childhood and young adults. Some authors have observed no size difference between juxtamedullary and superficial glomeruli by the 14th to 36th postnatal month (318,320), whereas others have found a size difference persists until at least 15 years of age (319,321). Methodologic differences in the studies or the wide variation in glomerular size existing among individuals (323) may account for these disparate findings.

Investigations using stereologic methods have provided estimates for the number of cells in glomeruli. Steffes et al. observed that the total number of cells per glomerulus increased along with the mean glomerular volume in comparing normal individuals under 20 years of age to those greater than 20 years (324). The number of endothelial cells and mesangial cells increased with age, whereas the number of podocytes remained unchanged with age. These results are consistent with the large amount of animal data indicating that mature podocytes are largely terminally differentiated and do not replicate. This concept is also supported by the expression pattern of cell cycle regulatory proteins during glomerulogenesis (325–327). The proliferation marker Ki-67 is expressed in podocyte precursors in comma- and S-shaped bodies but its expression is markedly reduced in podocytes of the glomerular capillary loop stage. The cyclin-dependent kinase (CDK) inhibitors p27 and p57 are absent in the comma- and S-shaped bodies but expressed in maturing podocytes of the capillary loop stage as well as mature podocytes in adult kidneys. These findings suggest the CDK inhibitors are involved with arresting the cell cycle of podocytes at the capillary loop stage and maintaining the fully mature podocytes in a quiescent differentiated state.

A stereologic approach combined with immunohistochemistry and confocal microscopy has provided an evaluation of podocyte number in both children and adults (328). Glomeruli from children, including some less than 3 years of age, contained the same number of podocytes (450 to 500 podocytes per glomerulus) as small- and medium-sized glomeruli from adults. However, large adult glomeruli contained more podocytes (800 podocytes per glomerulus). The postnatal origin of these additional podocytes is not clear. The large adult glomeruli had a lower podocyte density (podocyte number per glomerular tuft volume), thus resulting in relative podocyte depletion, which may make them more susceptible to glomerular injury.

Early Juxtamedullary Glomeruli

The maturational process in the very early generations of glomeruli may be accelerated because even in very young fetuses these juxtamedullary glomeruli rarely possess a cuboidal layer and are considerably larger than their immediate superficial neighbors. Attention was drawn to these large juxtamedullary glomeruli in humans by Kampmeier, who noted that they subsequently disappeared, suggesting that they were transient structures (329). Tsuda observed in human fetuses that the diameter of juxtamedullary glomeruli were nearly twice that of superficial glomeruli as early as 3 months of gestation (293). Emery and Macdonald noted that the disappearance of these large glomeruli, in the early months after birth, was associated with the presence of scarred glomeruli in the same region (330). These findings support Kampmeier's suggestion that they represent a transient population of nephrons. It is presumed that these precociously formed glomeruli are functionally important during fetal life and likely undergo involution early in the postnatal period. Relatively little study has been made of these interesting structures.

Glomerulosclerosis in Infants

Glomerulosclerosis in infantile kidneys is commonly observed. In most cases, it is a presumably normal phenomenon that must be distinguished from the pathologic changes of glomerular disease. In 1909, Herxheimer concluded that sclerotic glomeruli usually represented defective development of glomeruli in otherwise normal kidneys and were not manifestations of a disease process (331). Other investigators have suggested this context of glomerulosclerosis might result from excretion of toxic substances, renal infection, or have a vascular origin (332,333).

Emery and Macdonald conducted thorough studies of glomerulosclerosis in children's kidneys that were considered morphologically within normal limits (330). Their series of 475 cases included kidneys from fetuses at 24 weeks of gestation to children 15 years of age. The percentage of sclerotic glomeruli in each kidney was most often in the range of 1% to 2% (65% of cases), although higher percentages from 3% to 10% affected glomeruli (30% of cases) were observed. The proportion of infants having sclerotic glomeruli was age dependent. Scarred glomeruli occurred in 25% to 40% of kidneys from late fetuses and newborns. They were detected in 70% of kidneys by 2 months of age, remaining near this level throughout the first year. Afterward, their incidence steadily declined and was about 10% of children at 6 years of age.

Emery and Macdonald found that sclerotic glomeruli localized to two areas; the deep inner cortex (juxtamedullary zone near the arcuate vessels) and the superficial outer cortex (near the capsule). Sclerotic glomeruli in the juxtamedullary zone were more common in the first 6 months of life than in older children. Affected glomeruli in the outer cortex were most prominent in the first 2 years after birth. The presence of scarred glomeruli in the juxtamedullary zone coincided with the disappearance of the large glomeruli seen in this region during the months after birth, as discussed previously. Thus, it appears the sclerosing glomeruli in the juxtamedullary zone represent the involution of the large glomeruli that localize to this zone during nephrogenesis. The glomerular scarring in the outer cortex near the capsule likely reflects a different etiologic process, that if linked to nephrogenesis, is probably occurring relatively late. In a study of 800 infant kidneys, Thomas reported a similar distribution pattern of sclerotic glomeruli in the cortex (334). The general consensus is that these lesions are defects of development but without functional or clinical significance. A point of significance for pathologists is perhaps that they not be overinterpreted as evidence of glomerular disease, unless their number is considerably above the usual range (greater than 20%) mentioned above. Nevertheless, this area deserves further study. As previously mentioned, in the kidneys of preterm neonates, up to 13% of glomeruli in the outer cortex show tuft contraction within Bowman space, which may represent a stage toward glomerulosclerosis (291). Moreover, it is noteworthy that glomerular involution primarily in the outer cortex has been described as a special form of global sclerosis associated with relapsing minimal change nephritic syndrome (335).

A typical example of infantile glomerulosclerosis is illustrated in Figure 33.27. The scarred glomeruli may occur singly or in small groups. They are usually smaller than normal, immature in appearance, and variably hyalinized. The afferent arteriole is often thickened, and periglomerular fibrosis may be present as well as some chronic inflammatory cells in the interstitium. In later stages, only a small globule of hyaline material in a small focus of sclerosis without capillary lumens may be seen. The tubules associated with the sclerotic glomeruli often contain proteinaceous material and apparently disappear along with the glomeruli.

Ectopic Glomeruli

In the kidneys from fetuses and infants, glomeruli are often found outside the confines of the renal parenchyma, either in

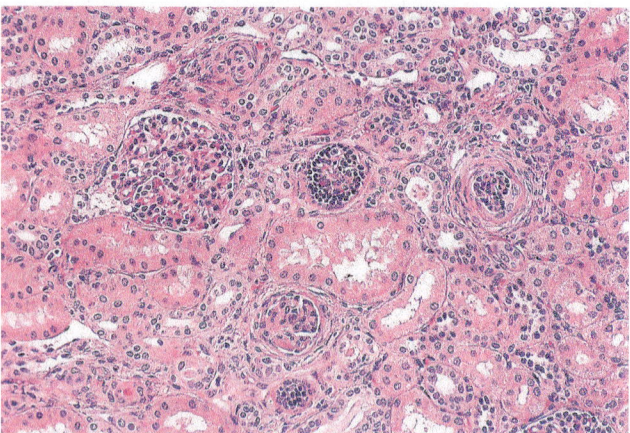

FIGURE 33.27 Infantile glomerulosclerosis at 9 months of age. One small, developmentally immature glomerulus is seen near the center, and two adjacent glomeruli are undergoing involutional sclerosis.

the renal sinus (Fig. 33.28) or in the connective tissue around interlobar vessels. These *ectopic* glomeruli occur in several mammalian species as well as in young humans (336). They appear to degenerate during postnatal life and are not found in adult human kidneys. It has been suggested that some vessels supplying the pelvic mucosa and medulla may be derived from degenerated ectopic glomeruli (336,337). The ectopic glomeruli may represent the early large juxtamedullary glomeruli, described by Kampmeier, that have persisted at least until infancy rather than degenerate.

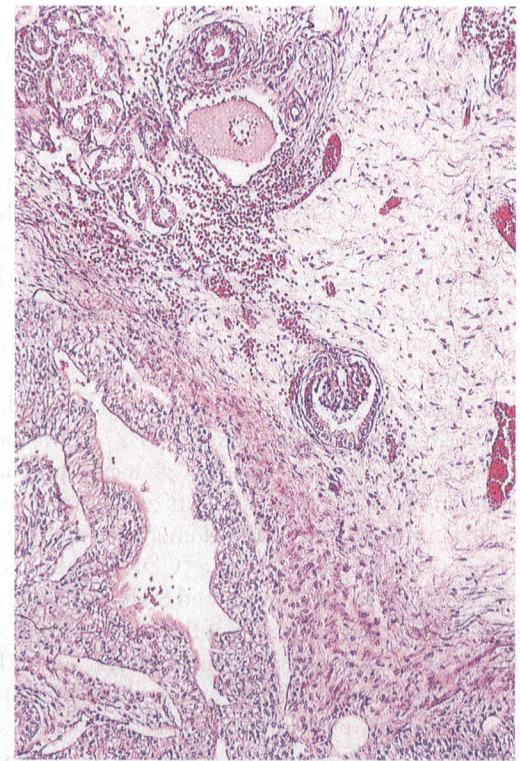

FIGURE 33.28 Ectopic glomerulus in the renal sinus.

TUBULAR MATURATION AND GROWTH

There is less known about the maturation and growth of tubules between birth and adulthood compared to glomeruli. Although all tubular segments increase in size during postnatal maturation, the proximal convoluted tubules undergo very prominent elongation and increased tortuosity (2). The results of microdissection studies reported from two laboratories were fairly similar (318,338). The mean lengths of PTs observed were: about 2 mm at birth, 3.5 mm at 3 months, 6.5 mm at 1 year of age, 7.7 mm at 2 years, and 12.0 mm at 12 years. The mean proximal tubular length of 20 mm in adult kidney indicates that proximal tubule elongation continues through adolescence and young adulthood.

PTs at birth are less uniform in size than glomeruli. PTs in the outer cortex of the newborn kidney were observed to be the shortest, those in the midcortex intermediate in length, and those from the juxtamedullary cortex the longest, consistent with a centrifugal pattern of development (318). These regional differences in PTs decreased significantly after 1 month of age and disappeared by 14 months. Whether tubular function, such as solute and volume reabsorption, of the maturing PTs from different cortical regions also follows a centrifugal pattern of maturation remains uncertain (339). It is interesting that in the adult kidney, the PTs from the outer cortex have been observed to be longer than those from the mid- and juxtamedullary cortex (318). The ratio of glomerular surface area to proximal tubular volume was proposed as a theoretical anatomic correlate of functional glomerulotubular balance, that is, the balance between the capacity of the glomerulus to filter and the tubule to reabsorb the filtrate (318). Values for this ratio; 28 in the term newborn kidney, 13 in the 3-month kidney, 6 in the 6-month kidney, and 3 in the adult kidney, suggested morphologic dominance of glomeruli over tubules early in life until the tubules, in effect, "grew up to their glomeruli" (318). However, it is difficult to correlate these morphologic ratios with experimental functional data indicating proportionate increases in glomerular filtration rate (GFR) and proximal tubule reabsorption after birth, consistent with maintenance of glomerulotubular balance during postnatal maturation (340).

During postnatal maturation the loops of Henle undergo striking elongation (2). The newborn kidney lacks a well-formed inner medulla and contains loops of Henle that are relatively short (2,19,21). At birth the loops of Henle are shortest in the younger nephrons, whereas longer loops belong to the older nephrons. As the kidney increases in size after birth, the loops of Henle elongate, the medullary interstitium increases, and the medulla becomes separated into outer and inner zones. From birth until full maturation, loops of Henle may increase in length as much as threefold. In the mature kidney, the location of the tips of the loops of Henle relates to the age of their associated nephrons. The loops of the last formed nephrons (outer cortex) reach the junction between the outer and inner medulla, and are known as short loops of Henle. In contrast, the loops of the earliest formed nephrons (juxtamedullary cortex) extend deep into the inner medulla near the tip of the papilla and are referred to as long loops of Henle. Prior to birth, thin portions of loops of Henle are only observed in the long loops of Henle. These thin portions are present in the *descending* limbs of the long loops of Henle and continue to lengthen after birth. *Descending* thin limbs (DTLs) are not seen in short loops of Henle until after birth. Only long loops of Henle develop *ascending* thin limbs (ATLs), which are derived from the TALs, likely by an ascending process of apoptotic remodeling (341,342).

ADULT KIDNEY

GROSS ANATOMY

The kidneys lie within the retroperitoneum and extend from the 12th thoracic to the 3rd lumbar vertebrae with the right kidney usually slightly more caudad. Craniocaudal movement of the kidneys during respiration may be up to 4 cm and they may be 2.5 cm lower in the erect than in the supine position. They are situated within the perirenal space, which contains abundant fat and is traversed by fine fibrous septae (343–345). Anterior and posterior layers of the renal fascia, known as Gerota fascia enclose the kidneys. Visualization of the renal fascia with radiologic procedures has been reported in normal individuals (346,347). Each kidney weighs 125 to 170 g in men and 115 to 155 g in women (348). If differences in body build are considered, kidney weight correlates best with body surface area, whereas age, sex, and race have less influence (349). Each kidney is 11 to 12 cm in length, 5 to 7.5 cm in width, and 2.5 to 3 cm in thickness. Magnetic resonance imaging (MRI) has shown mean kidney lengths of 12.4 +/− 0.9 cm for men and 11.6 +/− 1.1 cm for women and mean kidney volumes of 202 +/− 36 mL for men and 154 +/− 33 mL for women (350). However, the estimated renal volume may vary with changes in blood pressure and intravascular volume. The upper poles slant somewhat toward the midline and the posterior and the hilar aspect of each kidney has an anteromedial orientation. The anterior surface of each kidney is more convex compared to the flatter posterior surfaces. The left kidney tends to be slightly larger and may demonstrate irregularities of the lateral contour from compression by the spleen in up to 10% of normal individuals (351). A glistening tough fibroelastic capsule surrounds the kidney.

The aperture on the concave medial surface of each kidney is the hilum, through which pass the vessels, nerves, and ureter. In the hilum, the main renal artery branches to form anterior and posterior divisions (Fig. 33.29), which in turn divide into segmental arteries that supply the apical,

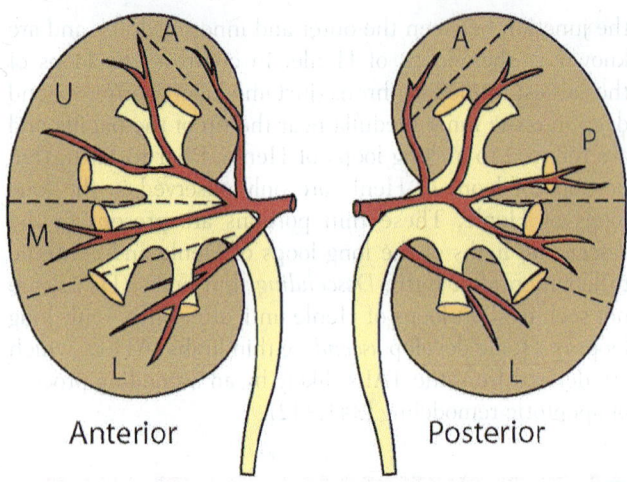

FIGURE 33.29 Diagram of the vascular supply of the human kidney. The anterior division of the renal artery divides into three segmental branches that supply the upper (U) and middle (M) segments of the anterior surface and most of the lower (L) segment. The small apical (A) segment is usually supplied by a branch from the anterior division. The posterior division of the renal artery supplies the posterior (P) segment, which represents more than half of the posterior surface of the kidney. (Modified with permission from Graves FT. The anatomy of the intrarenal arteries and its application to segmental resection of the kidney. Br J Surg 1954;42: 132–139. Copyright © 1954 British Journal of Surgery Society Ltd.)

upper, middle, lower, and posterior segmental regions of the parenchyma (352,353). However, most of the segmental arteries arise from the anterior division. No collateral circulation has been demonstrated between the segmental arteries. Thus, they may be considered end-arteries. Some of the so-called accessory arteries actually represent normal segmental arteries with an early origin from the main-stem renal artery or aorta (353). Therefore, ligation of such a segmental artery in the belief that it is an accessory vessel results in necrosis of the corresponding parenchymal segment. The intrarenal veins do not follow a segmental distribution, and there are numerous anastomoses of the veins throughout the kidney. There are variable drainage patterns of the large extrarenal veins which join to form the main renal vein (354). A relatively common occurrence is a posterior primary venous tributary, whose retropelvic position should be remembered during renal surgical intervention.

On the cut surface of a bisected kidney, the outer cortex and the striated inner region, the medulla, can be distinguished. The presence of glomeruli and convoluted tubules results in the cortex having a more granular appearance. The human kidney is a multipapillary type of mammalian kidney (355), with the medulla divided into 8 to 18 striated conical masses called pyramids (Fig. 33.30). The striated appearance reflects the parallel linear orientation of the loops of Henle and collecting ducts. The base of each pyramid is located at the corticomedullary junction, whereas the apex extends toward the renal pelvis, forming a papilla. The tip of each papilla, the area cribrosa, is perforated by 20 to 70 small openings (3) that represent the distal ends of the collecting ducts (of Bellini). The cortex is about 1 cm in thickness, encircles the base of each pyramid, and extends downward between pyramids to form the columns (septa) of Bertin.

Despite well-described radiologic features (356,357), an enlarged column of Bertin has on occasion been clinically mistaken for a renal tumor. Longitudinal striations extending from the base of the pyramids out into the cortex are termed the medullary rays (of Ferrein). Regardless of their name, they are actually part of the cortex and are formed by

FIGURE 33.30 Diagram of a bisected kidney illustrating major anatomic structures.

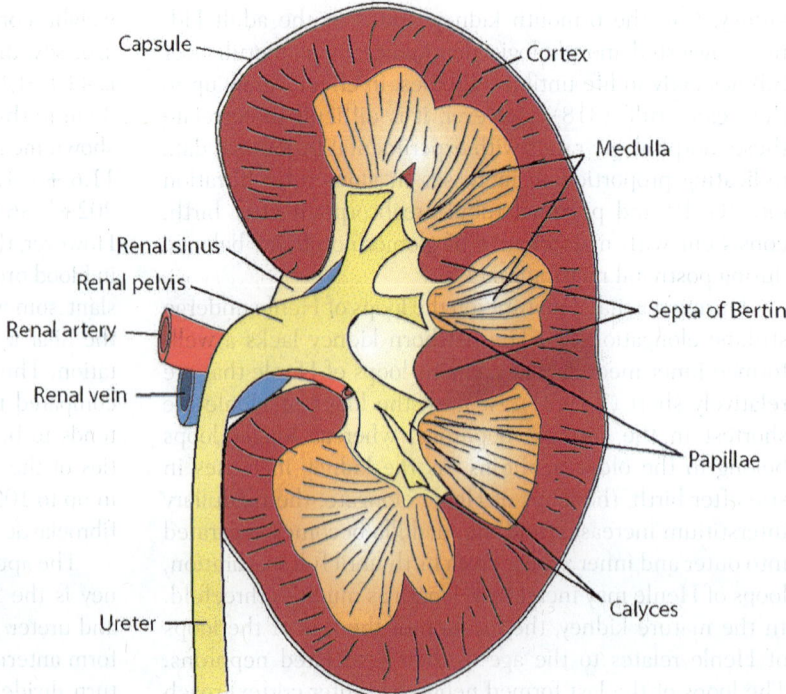

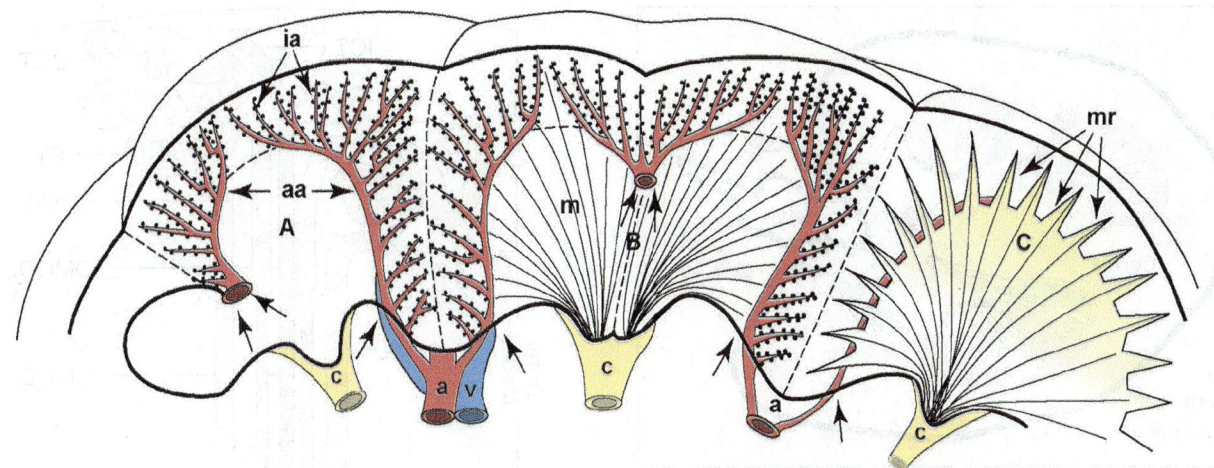

FIGURE 33.31 Diagram of three renal lobes. **A:** Arcuate (*aa*) and interlobular (*ia*) arteries. **B:** Cortex and medulla (*m*) are illustrated in a double lobe with fused double papillae. **C:** Lobe showing medullary rays (*mr*). A septum of Bertin represents the approximation of two layers of septal cortex from two adjacent lobes. (*Small double arrows* in A and B, subsidiary septal arteries; *single arrows*, location where arcuate vessels enter the renal parenchyma; *a*, interlobar arteries; *v*, interlobar vein; *c*, calyces). (Modified with permission from Hodson CJ. The renal parenchyma and its blood supply. *Curr Probl Diagn Radiol* 1978;7:1–32. Copyright © 1978 Elsevier.)

the straight segments of the PTs, the cortical TALs, and the CCDs. The medullary rays may be visualized during excretory urography in conditions with tubular fluid stasis (358).

A single pyramid with its surrounding cortical parenchyma constitutes a renal lobe (Fig. 33.31) (359). The human kidney has an average of 14 lobes. During development, variable lobar fusion leads to coalescence of some papillae and remodeling of the corresponding calyces gradually reducing the number of papillae and calyces. The mean number of calyces and papillae reported is 9 and 11, respectively (287). There is a greater degree of lobar fusion in the polar regions than in the midpolar region of the kidney. Although the mature kidney eventually develops a smooth outer surface, a degree of persistent fetal lobation may be observed in some adult kidneys.

There are two main types of renal papillae (360). Simple papillae drain only one lobe and have convex tips containing small, often slit-like orifices. Compound papillae drain two or more adjacent fused lobes and have flattened, ridged, or concave tips with round, often gaping orifices. The distribution of papillae types within the kidney is related to the embryologic pattern of fusion involving the lobes, papillae, and calyces (Fig. 33.32). It is believed that the more open orifices of compound papillae are less capable of preventing intrarenal reflux (361), which may be associated with an increase in intrapelvic pressure. This concept is supported by the observation that pyelonephritic scars associated with intrarenal reflux are present more commonly in the renal poles, where the compound papillae predominantly occur.

The renal pelvis is the sac-like expansion of the upper ureter. Two or three outpouchings or major calyces (infundibula) extend from the pelvis and divide into the minor calyces, into which the papillae protrude. In addition, elaborate leaf-like extensions, termed fornices, extend from the minor calyces into the medulla, and secondary pouches increase the pelvic surface area (362). The walls of the calyces, pelvis and ureters contain specialized cells which serve a pacemaker function to facilitate urine movement to the bladder.

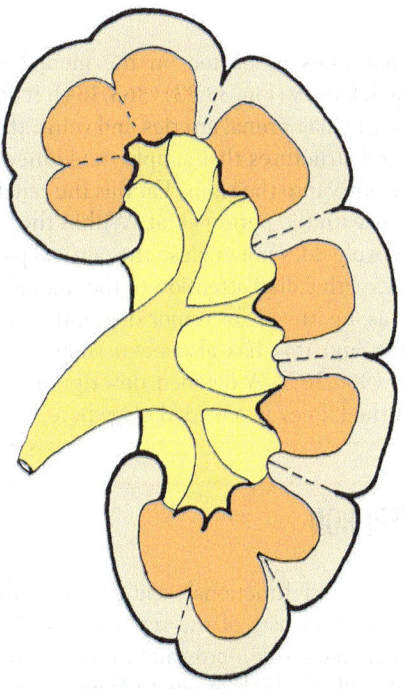

FIGURE 33.32 Schematic representation of the lobar architecture. In the polar regions, there is a greater degree of lobe fusion, resulting in the formation of compound papillae and calyces and the loss of septal cortex. The individual lobes tend to be retained in the midpolar region, and the septal cortex extends between renal pyramids, as septa of Bertin, to the renal sinus. (Modified with permission from Hodson CJ. The renal parenchyma and its blood supply. *Curr Probl Diagn Radiol* 1978;7:1–32.)

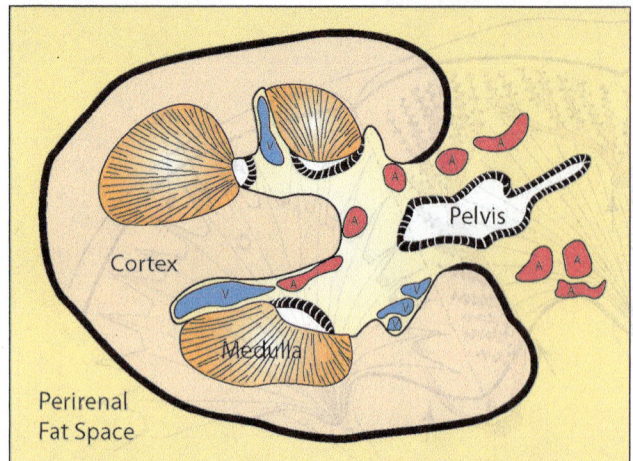

FIGURE 33.33 Diagram of kidney cross section, showing the renal sinus which is filled with fat (*yellow*). The renal sinus contains the pelvic-calyceal system and the major renal vessels. The renal capsule (*thick black line*) surrounds the convex surface of the kidney but disappears from the cortical surface as the latter enters the renal sinus. The cortical surfaces, including the septa of Bertin, facing the renal sinus lack a capsule. The capsule surrounding the pelvic-calyceal system is indicated by a cross-hatched thick black line. The capsule covering the calyces, appears to extend over the medullary pyramids on cross section, and it envelopes the renal pelvis as well. (Modified with permission from Murphy WM, Grignon DJ, Perlman EJ. Tumors of the kidney, bladder, and related urinary structures. In: Silverberg SG, Sobin LH, eds. *Atlas of Tumor Pathology*. 4th series, fascicle 1. Washington, DC: Armed Forces Institute of Pathology; 2004.)

The renal sinus is located on the medial or concave aspect of each kidney (Fig. 33.33) (363,364). It contains the renal pelvis, the major renal arteries and veins, the lymphatics and neural structures that supply the kidney. The renal hilum is the entry into the sinus. Fat fills the renal sinus and is contiguous with the perirenal fat. Within the renal sinus, the renal capsule does not enclose the cortical parenchymal surface. Beckwith called attention to the importance of the renal sinus as a pathway for tumor dissemination in Wilms tumor (365), and this has also been shown in renal cell carcinomas (366,367). A detailed description of the gross anatomy of the kidney is provided elsewhere (5).

NEPHRON

The structural and functional unit of the kidney is the nephron, which consists of the renal corpuscle (glomerulus and Bowman capsule), proximal tubule, thin limbs, and distal tubule, all of which originate from the metanephric blastema. The total number of nephrons in a human kidney varies markedly among normal individuals (368). A 10-fold variation in nephron number has been reported, from approximately 200,000 to more than 2.5 million nephrons per kidney. The usual range is about 600,000 to 1,200,000 nephrons per kidney.

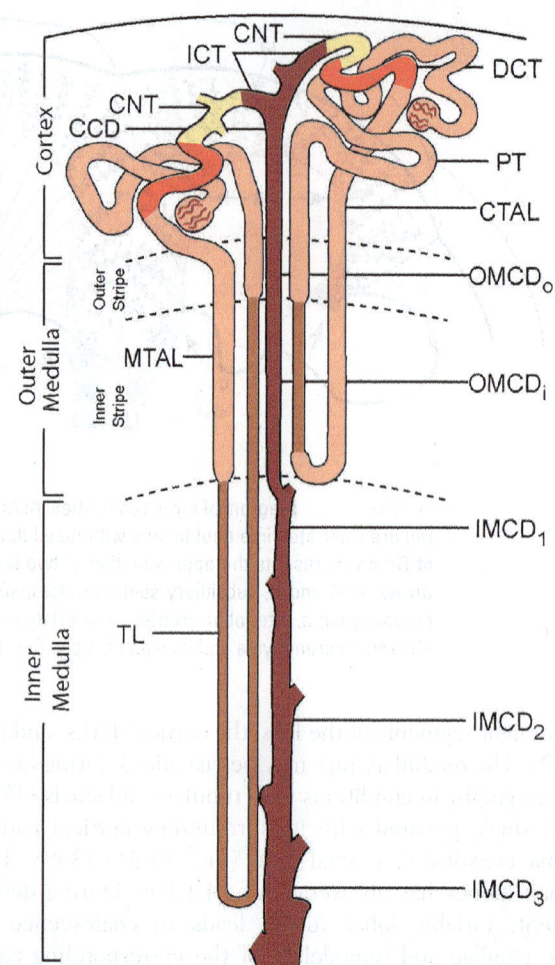

FIGURE 33.34 Diagram illustrating the segments of the nephron and the zones of the kidney. (*PT*, proximal tubule; *TL*, thin limb of Henle loop; *MTAL*, medullary thick ascending limb; *CTAL*, cortical thick ascending limb; *DCT*, distal convoluted tubule; *CNT*, connecting tubule; *ICT*, initial collecting tubule; *CCD*, cortical collecting duct; $OMCD_o$, collecting duct in outer stripe of outer medulla; $OMCD_i$, collecting duct in inner stripe of outer medulla; $IMCD_1$, outer third of inner medullary collecting duct; $IMCD_2$, middle third of inner medullary collecting duct; $IMCD_3$, inner third of inner medullary collecting duct. (Modified with permission from Madsen KM, Tisher CC. Structural-functional relationships along the distal nephron. *Am J Physiol* 1986;250 (pt 2):F1–F15. Copyright © 1986, The American Physiological Society.)

Nephrons can be classified according to the position of their glomeruli in the cortex or the length of their loop of Henle (Fig. 33.34). In the former scheme, superficial, midcortical, and juxtamedullary nephrons are distinguished. Superficial nephrons have glomeruli located in the outer cortex, and their efferent arterioles usually ascend to the cortical surface. The glomeruli of juxtamedullary nephrons are located immediately above the corticomedullary junction in the inner cortex, and their efferent arterioles form the descending vasa recta (DVR). The glomeruli of midcortical nephrons are situated in the midcortex above the juxtamedullary region, but below the superficial nephrons.

In the more commonly used classification there are two main populations of nephrons: those with a short loop of Henle and those with a long loop. The length of the loop of Henle is generally related to the location of its parent glomerulus in the cortex. The short loops generally form their bend at various levels within the inner stripe of the outer medulla, whereas the long loops of Henle enter and turn back within the inner medulla. In human kidneys, some nephrons have short loops of Henle which do not enter the medulla. Although there are numerous gradations between these two main types of nephrons, there are seven times more short than long loop nephrons in human kidneys (369). A correlation between the urinary concentrating ability and the relative length of the medulla has been established in several mammalian kidneys (370).

The connecting segment or tubule (CNT), which joins the nephron to the collecting duct system, is believed to originate from the metanephric blastema. The collecting duct system includes the initial collecting tubule (ICT), the CCD, the OMCD, and the inner medullary collecting duct (IMCD) (371,372). The collecting duct system has a different embryologic origin, the ureteric bud and also because it collects tubule fluid from different nephrons, it has not been classically considered a nephron component. Although not strictly correct in an anatomic sense, for practical considerations, the term nephron is commonly used to include the connecting segment and entire collecting duct.

Structural and functional heterogeneity exists along the nephron. Internephron heterogeneity refers to the differences between analogous segments in superficial and juxtamedullary nephrons. Intranephron or axial heterogeneity may be defined as the differences between early and successive later portions of an individual nephron segment.

ARCHITECTURE

The renal cortex can be divided into lobules. A renal lobule consists of a centrally positioned medullary ray and its surrounding cortical parenchyma containing all nephrons draining into the collecting ducts of the medullary ray. In contrast to lobules of other organs, renal lobules are not distinctly separated by fine connective tissue septa; therefore, they are difficult to distinguish histologically. Furthermore, because it has been difficult to establish any structural–functional significance, the concept of the renal lobule is not commonly used.

The nephron segments and blood vessels in the cortex and medulla have a specific geometric arrangement (373). This intricate architecture allows for integration (axial) of complex transport functions along the length of a specific nephron segment, as well as integration (regional) between different nephron segments in a specific region or zone (374).

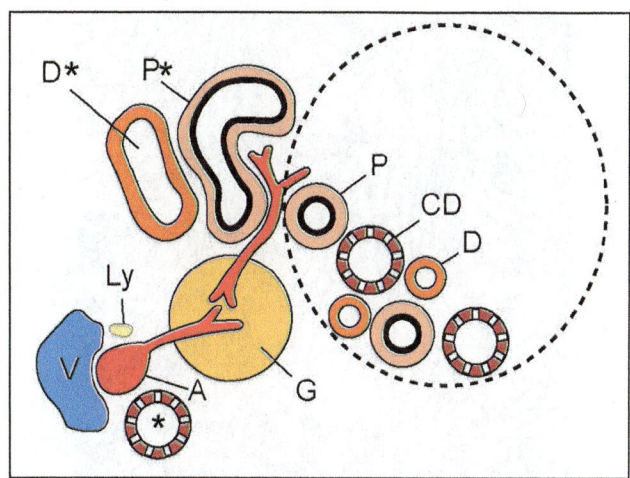

FIGURE 33.35 Diagram of architectural regions of the renal cortex. A medullary ray is encircled by the *dotted line*, and the cortical labyrinth is outside the *dotted line*. The proximal straight (*P*) and distal straight ascending limb (*D*) tubules and the collecting ducts (*CD*) are located in the medullary ray. The adjacent cortical labyrinth contains the interlobular vessels: Arteries (*A*), veins (*V*), and lymphatics (*Ly*); arcades (*) of CNTs; glomeruli (*G*); and the proximal (*P**) and distal (*D**) convoluted tubules. (Modified with permission from Kriz W, Kaissling B. Structural organization of the mammalian kidney. In: Seldin DW, Giebisch D, eds. *The Kidney: Physiology and Pathophysiology*. 3rd ed. Philadelphia, PA: Lippincott Williams & Wilkins; 2000:587–654.)

Two architectural regions of the renal cortex can be distinguished: the cortical labyrinth and the medullary rays (Fig. 33.35). The cortical labyrinth represents a continuous parenchymal zone that surrounds the regularly distributed medullary rays. Glomeruli, proximal and distal convoluted tubules, interlobular vessels (also termed cortical radial vessels), and a rich capillary network are situated in the cortical labyrinth. The large majority of convoluted tubular profiles are PTs. CNTs of juxtamedullary nephrons fuse and form the so-called arcades, which are adjacent to the interlobular vessels within the cortical labyrinth. Individual nephrons, with their interlobular vessels, glomeruli, and attached tubular segments, are difficult to distinguish in this complex topography by histology. Oriented longitudinal and/or cross sections often display this geometric topography. The medullary rays (Figs. 33.36 and 33.37) contain the proximal and distal straight tubules and collecting ducts, all of which enter into the medulla. The distal straight tubules are the TALs. Within an individual medullary ray, the straight tubules of superficial nephrons are situated centrally, the straight tubules of midcortical nephrons are localized peripherally, and the collecting ducts occupy a position between the two groups. The straight tubules of juxtamedullary nephrons descend directly into the medulla, never entering the medullary rays.

The tubules in the cortex have a compact back-to-back appearance with little intervening interstitium. Rarely, a discrete cortical scar consistent with a previous biopsy site may be observed (Fig. 33.38). Incidental tumors, benign or

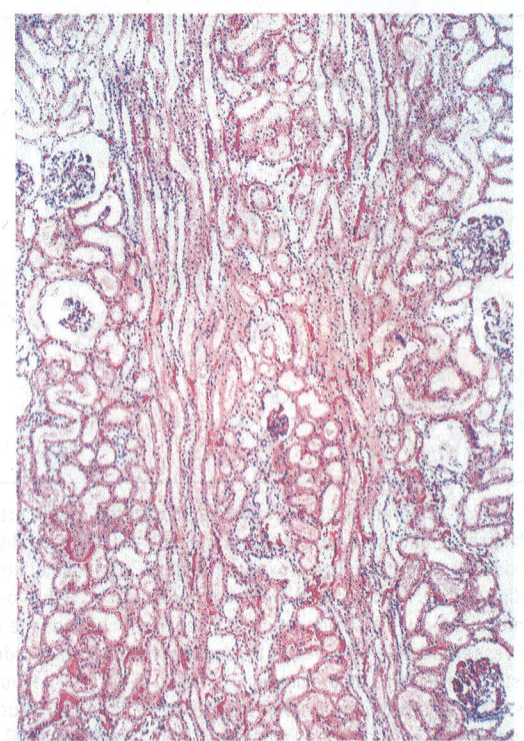

FIGURE 33.36 Longitudinal section of cortex demonstrating two linear aggregates of tubules representing medullary rays (H&E, ×50).

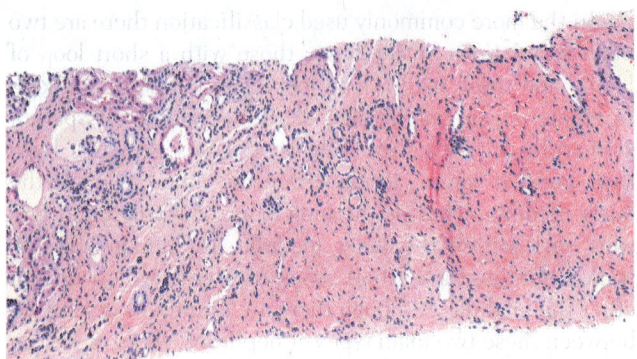

FIGURE 33.38 Focal fibrous scar, suggestive of previous biopsy site, situated in middle of renal cortex, which is otherwise intact (H&E, ×100).

malignant and, primary or metastatic, may be detected in a renal biopsy (Fig. 33.39).

The localization of specific segments of the nephrons at various levels in the medulla account for the division of the medulla into an outer and inner zone, with the former subdivided into an inner and outer stripe (Fig. 33.34). The relative tissue volumes for the cortex and the outer and inner medulla are 70%, 27%, and 3%, respectively (372). Glomeruli are not present in the medulla.

The outer stripe of the outer medulla is relatively thin. It contains the terminal portions of the proximal straight tubules, the TALs, and the collecting ducts. The outer stripe is also distinguished by the absence of thin limbs of Henle. In contrast to the outer stripe, the inner stripe of the outer medulla is thicker. It contains thin descending limbs, TALs, and collecting ducts. It is further characterized by the absence of the proximal straight tubules. Aggregations of descending and ascending vasa recta (DVR and AVR) known as vascular bundles develop in the outer stripe but are located predominantly in the inner stripe. Compared with the kidneys of some mammals with very high urine concentrating ability, the human kidney has a simple medulla (373). In contrast to the complex medulla, the vascular bundles of the simple medulla do not fuse to form larger vascular structures, and they do not incorporate the DTLs of short loops (Fig. 33.40). The inner medulla contains the thin descending and thin ascending limbs of long loops, as well as the collecting ducts. TALs are absent in the inner medulla.

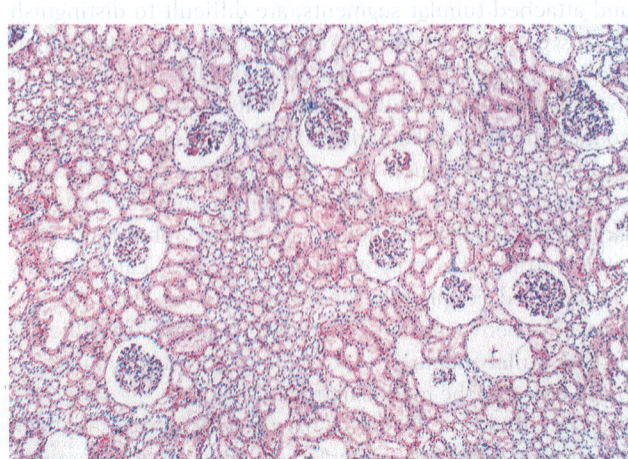

FIGURE 33.37 Cross section of cortex illustrating medullary rays that are regularly distributed within the cortical labyrinth (H&E, ×50).

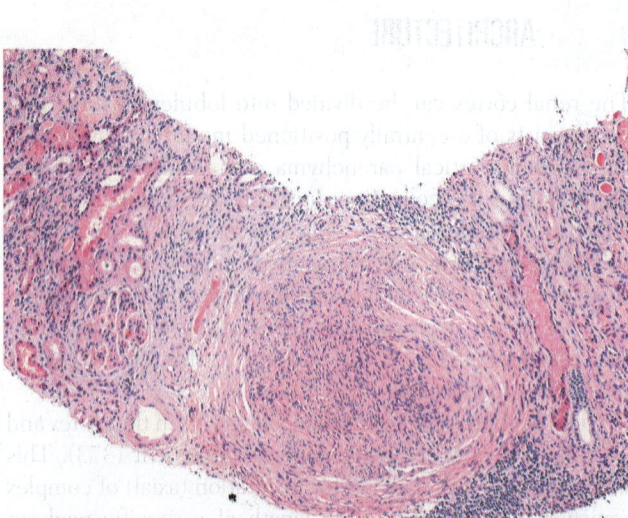

FIGURE 33.39 Circumscribed leiomyoma enclosed within a renal biopsy specimen (H&E, ×100).

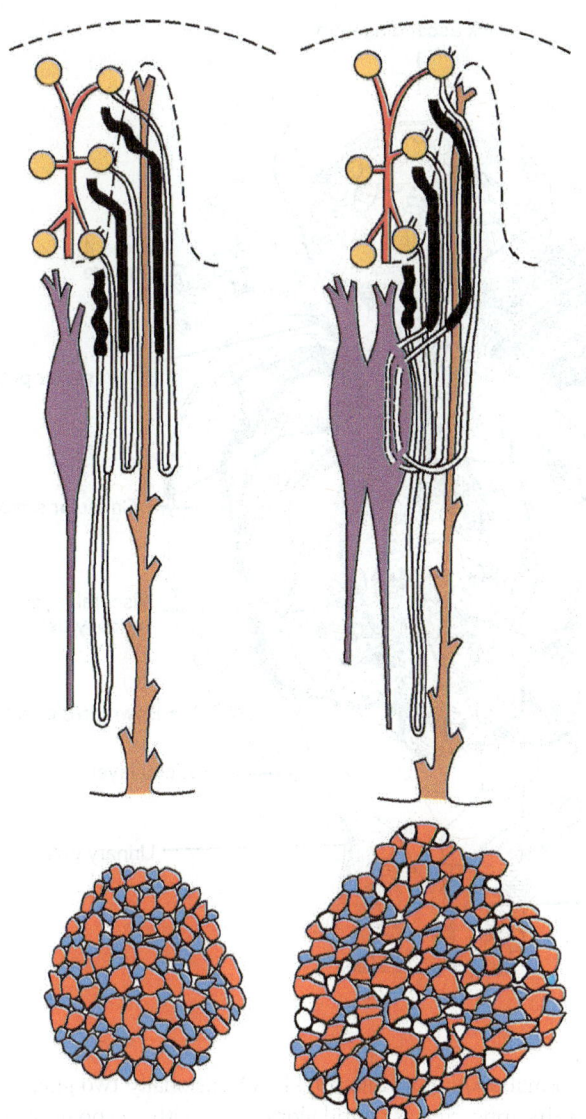

FIGURE 33.40 Schematic diagram demonstrating the simple and complex types of medulla. **Upper left**: In the simple medulla, the loops of Henle remain separate from the vascular bundle (*purple*). The vascular bundle itself (**lower left** cross section) contains only descending (*red*) and ascending (*blue*) vasa recta. **Upper right**: In the complex medulla, the DTLs of short loops of Henle descend within the vascular bundles (*purple*), which tend to fuse. Therefore, the complex bundles (**lower right** cross section) contain the DTLs of short loops (*white*) in addition to descending (*red*) and ascending (*blue*) vasa recta. (Modified with permission from Jamison RL, Kriz W. *Urinary Concentrating Mechanism: Structure and Function.* New York: Oxford University Press; 1982.)

PARENCHYMA

An accurate morphologic evaluation of the kidney requires a detailed systematic examination of the glomeruli, tubules, interstitium, and blood vessels of the renal parenchyma. A standard nomenclature for structures of the kidney exists (375). A detailed approach to the histopathologic evaluation of the kidney has been described (376) and technical guidelines for handling the renal biopsy are available (377,378). The following discussion emphasizes normal morphologic aspects and structural–functional relationships in the kidney. The reader is directed to detailed discussions for more information (373,379).

GLOMERULUS

Overview

In 1666, Malpighi first described the glomeruli and demonstrated their continuity with the renal vasculature (380). About 175 years later, Bowman elucidated in detail the capillary architecture of the glomerulus and the continuity between its surrounding capsule and the proximal tubule (381,382). The renal corpuscle consists of a tuft of interconnected capillaries and an enclosing capsule named after Bowman. The term "glomerulus" is commonly used to refer to the glomerular capillary tuft and Bowman capsule, although the term "renal corpuscle" is more accurate in a strict anatomic sense. The glomerulus does not simply represent a ball of capillaries. Providing structural support for the capillary tuft is a central region termed the mesangium, which contains cells and their surrounding matrix material. The capillaries are lined by a thin layer of endothelial cells, contain a basement membrane, and are covered by epithelial cells (called podocytes) that form the visceral layer of Bowman capsule. The parietal epithelium is continuous with the visceral epithelium at the vascular pole where the afferent arteriole enters the glomerulus and the efferent arteriole exits. The glomerulus somewhat resembles a blind-pouched extension (Bowman capsule) of the proximal tubule invaginated by a tuft of capillaries (Fig. 33.41) (383). The cavity situated between the two epithelial layers of Bowman capsule is called Bowman space or the urinary space. At the urinary pole, this space and the parietal layer of Bowman capsule continue into the lumen and epithelium of the proximal tubule. The glomerular tuft originates from the afferent arteriole, which enters the glomerulus at the vascular pole and divides into several lobules. Anastomoses are believed to exist between individual capillaries within a lobule as well as between lobules (373,384,385). The efferent arteriole is formed by rejoined capillaries and leaves the glomerulus at the vascular pole. In contrast to the afferent arteriole, the efferent arteriole has a more continuous intraglomerular segment. The glomerulus is responsible for the ultrafiltration of plasma. The glomerular filtration barrier consists of the fenestrated endothelium, the peripheral GBM, and the slit diaphragms between the podocyte foot processes.

The glomerulus has a round configuration and an average diameter of about 200 μm (373,379). Although the diameter of juxtamedullary glomeruli has been reported up to 20% to 50% greater than that of superficial glomeruli, especially in animals (373), others have found no significant size difference

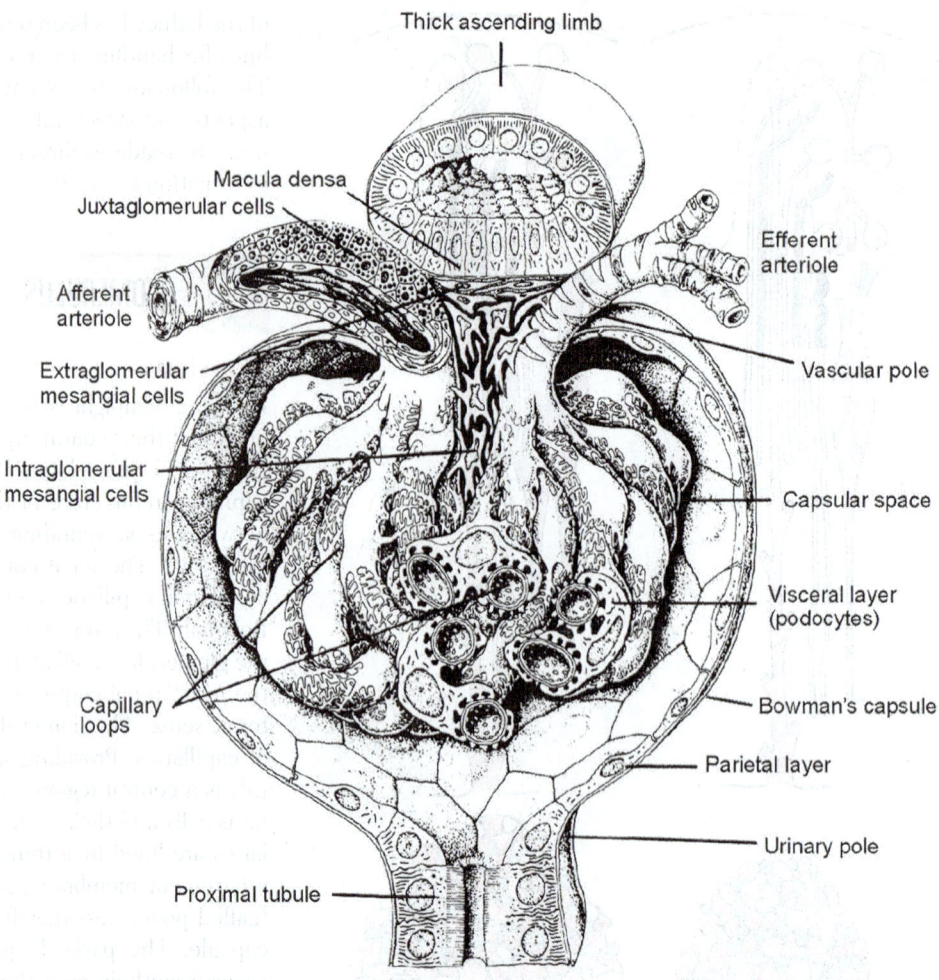

FIGURE 33.41 Schematic three-dimensional representation of the glomerulus. (Modified with permission from Geneser F. *Textbook of Histology.* Philadelphia, PA: Lea & Febiger; 1986.)

between these glomerular populations in the normal human adult kidney (386). It has been reported that the glomeruli in solitary functioning kidneys are significantly larger than those in control patients with two kidneys (387). In adults 50 to 70 years of age, the volume of normal appearing glomeruli in the superficial cortex has been reported to be 20% larger than those in the juxtamedullary cortex (323). This may reflect compensatory glomerular hypertrophy accompanying global glomerulosclerosis in the superficial cortex of these older patients. Although the glomerulus has a lobular architecture, the lobulation is often inconspicuous in light microscopic sections. An accentuated degree of lobulation may be more prominent in autopsy kidneys than in biopsy specimens. An apparent increase in the number of glomerular cells can be observed with an increased section thickness, therefore an accurate assessment of glomerular cellularity requires histologic sections 2 to 4 μm thick (Fig. 33.42). In general, the presence of more than three cells in a mesangial area away from the vascular pole constitutes hypercellularity. The delicate character of the glomerular capillary walls can be observed on thin histologic and frozen sections (Fig. 33.43) (388). A fortuitous tangential section may show a prominent lumen of a hilar arteriole which should not be mistaken for abnormal dilatation (Fig. 33.44). Occasionally, two glomerular tufts appearing as a bifid glomerulus with an apparent single vascular pole, can be observed (Fig. 33.45). Some renal biopsies have limited numbers of glomeruli. Moreover, in an occasional case, the glomeruli are displaced from the main

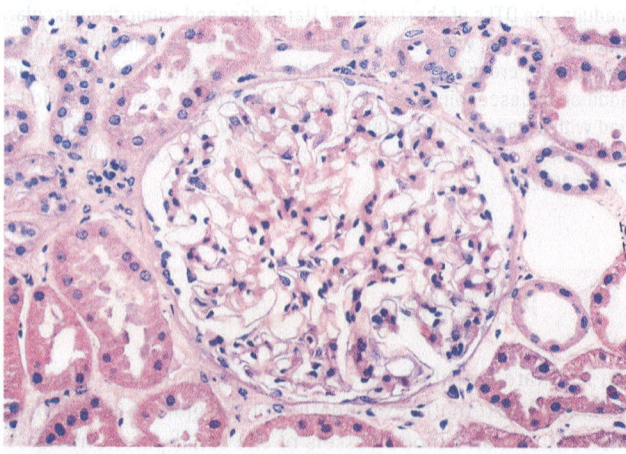

FIGURE 33.42 Glomerulus exhibiting round configuration and normal cellularity (H&E, ×250).

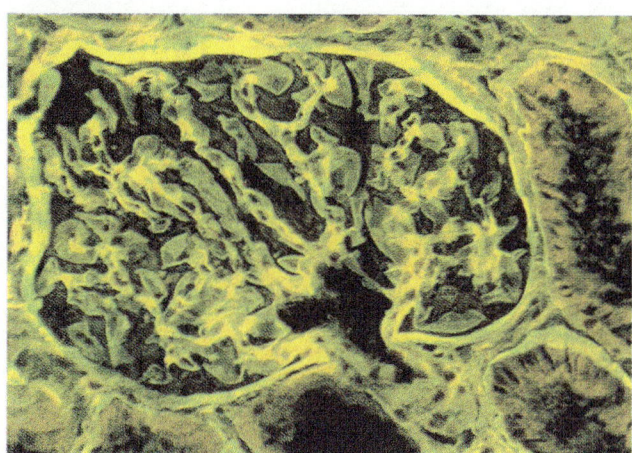

FIGURE 33.43 Fluorescent micrograph of an H&E-stained frozen section. Note the delicate character of the glomerular capillaries. (Courtesy of Dr. Stephen M. Bonsib.)

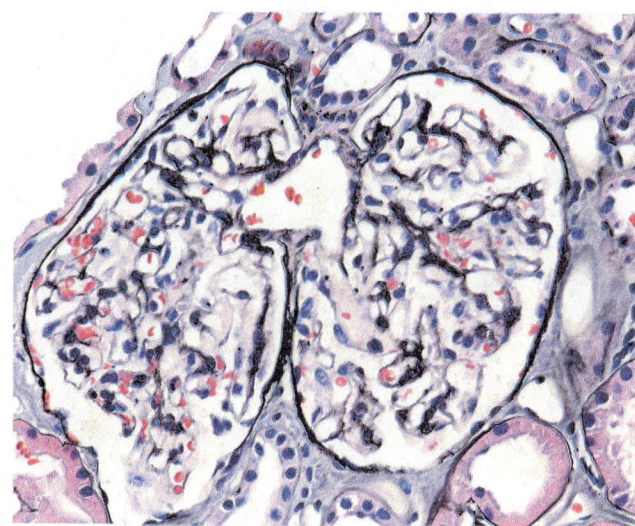

FIGURE 33.45 Bifid glomerulus with two capillary tufts sharing a hilar arteriole and even a juxtaglomerular apparatus (Jones silver stain, ×400).

tissue fragment and may be detected upon careful examination as single glomeruli isolated in space or in surrounding tissue (Fig. 33.46 A and B).

Global glomerulosclerosis may occur as part of aging, without renal disease. The mean percentage of global glomerulosclerosis in normal kidneys was reported as follows: less than 1% between 1 and 20 years of age, 2% between 20 and 40 years, 7% between 40 and 60 years, and 11% between 60 and 80 years (389–391). It has been suggested that the 90th percentile for global glomerulosclerosis may be generally estimated within a given patient by subtracting 10 from half the patient's age (391). More recent studies have examined the changes in human kidneys with aging (392). Kidney volume decreases after the age of 50 years (393), and simple renal cysts increase with age (394). In biopsies from over 2,000 ostensibly healthy living donor kidneys, the range of values for globally sclerotic glomeruli were reported (395). For example, in a biopsy section with 17 to 32 glomeruli, the 95th percentile (upper limit of normal) for the number of globally sclerotic glomeruli ranged from 1 glomerulus for a 20-year old to 5.5 glomeruli for a 70-year old. Another study of living donor kidneys showed a dramatic loss of intact glomeruli with aging (396). From the youngest age group (18 to 29 years) to the oldest age group (70 to 75 years), the number of nonsclerotic glomeruli was 48% lower and the number of globally sclerotic glomeruli increased by only 15%.

Endothelial Cells

A thin fenestrated endothelium lines the glomerular capillaries. By light microscopy, the endothelial cells have light eosinophilic cytoplasm and slightly oval nuclei. Their nuclei are present within the capillary lumina. The endothelial cells are extremely attenuated around the capillary lumen, and the thicker portions of the cells containing the nuclei lie adjacent to the mesangium away from the urinary space. The cytoplasm contains microtubules, microfilaments, and intermediate filaments (397). The attenuated portion of endothelial cytoplasm is perforated by fenestrae 70 to 100 nm in diameter (384). It has been argued that endothelial fenestrae do not simply arise from fusion of plasma membrane invaginations, called caveolae (398). As mentioned earlier, most investigations have indicated that adult glomerular endothelial cells lack diaphragms across the fenestrae, whereas they have been observed in the embryonic glomerulus.

The endothelial cell surface carries a negative charge because of the presence of polyanionic glycoproteins, including podocalyxin, a major sialoprotein of glomerular endothelial cells as well as of podocytes (399,400). The glomerular endothelial cells have a glycocalyx surface layer that fills the fenestrae forming "sieve plugs" (401,402). This

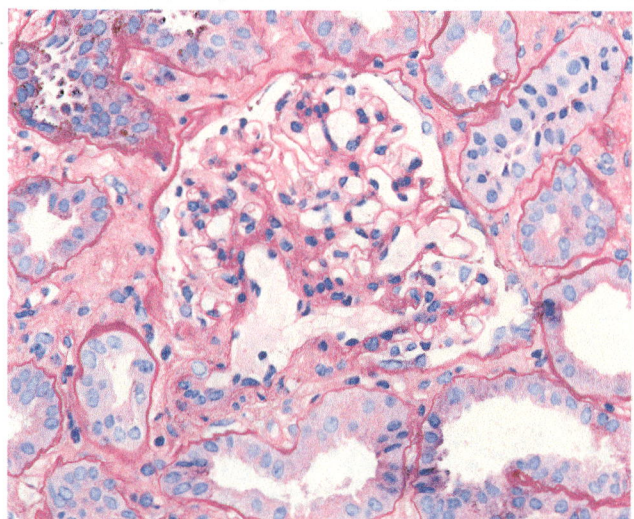

FIGURE 33.44 PAS-stained tangential section through a glomerular hilar arteriole (PAS, ×400).

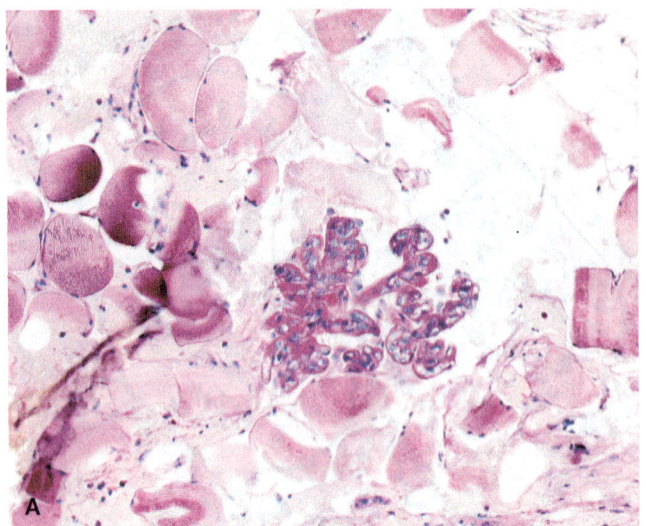
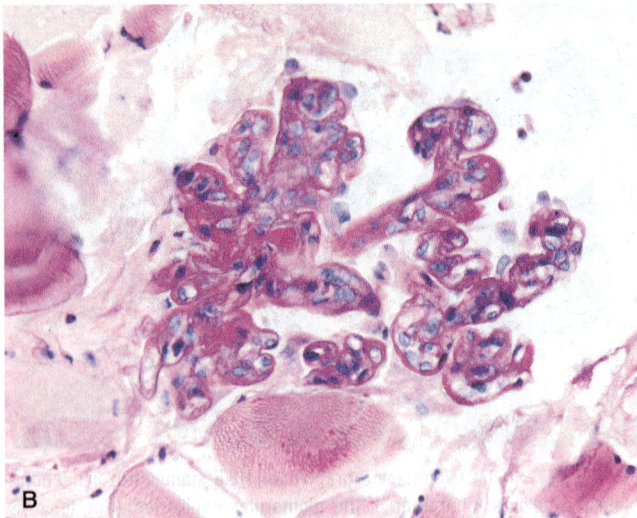

FIGURE 33.46 **A.** Isolated glomerulus, the only glomerulus present in a renal biopsy specimen, embedded within skeletal muscle (PAS, ×200). **B.** Higher magnification reveals glomerular hypercellularity and thickened capillary walls due to subendothelial deposits ("wire-loop" lesions) characteristic for lupus nephritis (PAS, ×400).

glycocalyx has been best visualized with special electron microscopic techniques using cationic dyes, lipid particles, or with high pressure freezing (403,404). The glycocalyx, consists of membrane-bound proteoglycans (syndecan and glypican), secreted glycoproteins (perlecan and versican), and secreted glycoaminoglycans (GAGs, hyaluronan). There is accumulated evidence that the glomerular endothelial glycocalyx is an important component of the glomerular filtration barrier (405–411).

VEGF, produced by podocytes, is an important regulator of glomerular endothelial cell function. VEGF induces fenestrae and increases permeability of endothelial cells, both in vivo and in vitro (412,413). VEGF-A is the best characterized growth factor produced by podocytes and its main receptor, VEGFR2, is expressed on endothelial cells. Deletion or inhibition of podocyte-derived VEGF-A leads to defective glomerular endothelial differentiation or injury (414,415). Thus, current evidence indicates that maintenance of glomerular endothelial differentiation appears dependent on podocyte-derived VEGF (416, 417). Glomerular endothelial cells synthesize nitric oxide (NO) and endothelin-1, a vasoconstrictor (418). There is strong expression of CD34 in glomerular endothelial cells (Fig. 33.47).

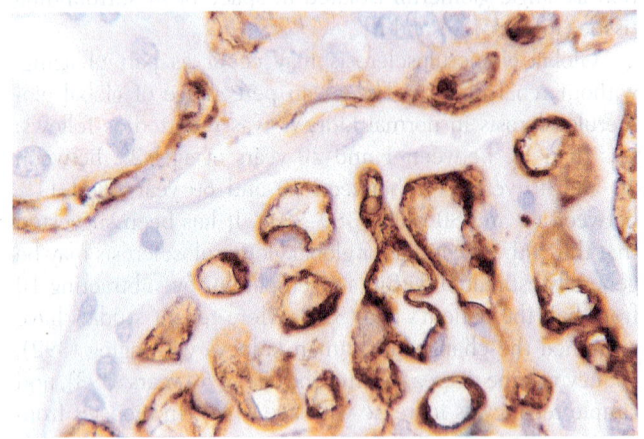

FIGURE 33.47 Glomerular endothelium showing immunoreactivity for CD34. Some peritubular capillaries show staining along the upper border. (CD34 immunohistochemistry, ×630.)

Mesangial Cells

The mesangium, composed of mesangial cells and their surrounding matrix, is observed as a periodic acid–Schiff (PAS)- and methenamine silver-positive structural support for the glomerular capillary loops (Fig. 33.48). By light microscopy, the mesangial cells usually can be distinguished by their mesangial location and dark-staining nuclei. Ultrastructurally, they are irregular in shape and have elongated thin cytoplasmic processes that may extend a short distance between

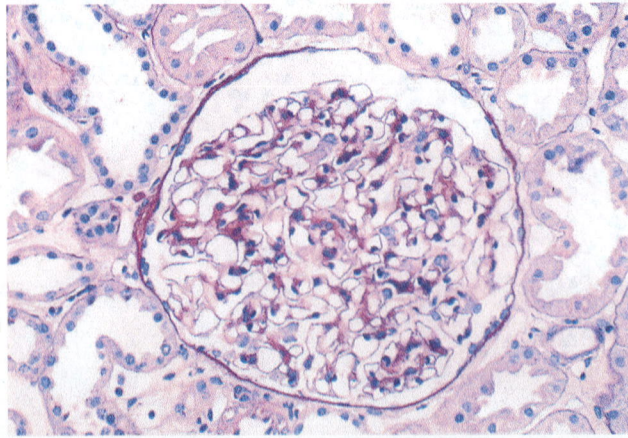

FIGURE 33.48 PAS-stained normal glomerulus illustrating the PAS-positive mesangium within the central regions of the glomerular capillaries (×250).

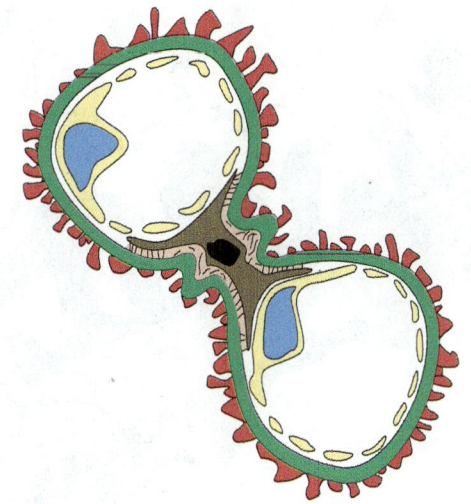

FIGURE 33.49 Schematic diagram illustrating the relationship between the mesangium and the glomerular capillaries. The visceral epithelial cell (podocyte) cytoplasm (*red*) and endothelial cell cytoplasm (*yellow*) are depicted. Note that the glomerular basement membrane (*green*) encloses the mesangium and its attached capillaries. The central mesangial cell is represented by *dark brown* cytoplasm and a *black* nucleus, and the mesangial matrix is represented by the *light brown* fibrillar texture. The cytoplasmic processes of mesangial cells are connected to the glomerular basement membrane directly or indirectly by microfibrils in the mesangial matrix.

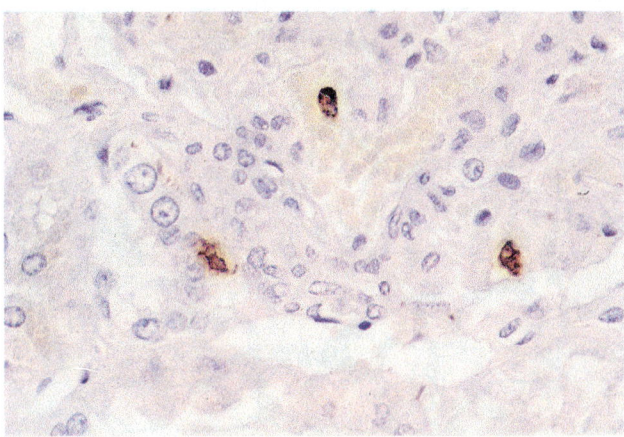

FIGURE 33.50 KP-1 immunohistochemical stain illustrating that a small percentage of cells in the mesangium label as tissue monocytes (KP-1 immunohistochemistry, ×630).

the endothelium and the GBM. The mesangial cell processes have microfilaments that contain actin, myosin, and α-actinin (419,420). With smooth muscle contractile properties, the mesangial cell has been proposed to be a specialized pericyte that likely modulates glomerular filtration (421). Whereas the endothelium forms a continuous layer around the inner circumference of the glomerular capillary, the basement membrane and the visceral epithelial cell layer do not completely encircle the capillary but enclose the mesangial matrix and cells between the capillaries (Fig. 33.49).

Mesangial cells are involved in the generation of the mesangial matrix. The mesangial matrix is similar but not identical to the GBM and contains several types of collagens (collagen type IV α1 and α2 chains, collagen V), various laminin isoforms, as well as fibronectin and proteoglycans (perlecan). The matrix is especially rich in microfibrils, unbranched, noncollagenous structures that contain fibrillins and microfibril-associated glycoproteins (MAGPs) (422,423). The presence of microfibril-mediated attachments between mesangial cell processes and the GBM suggests that the mesangial cell and the GBM represent a biomechanical functional unit (424–426). It has been proposed that the contractile apparatus of the mesangium appears to maintain the structure of the capillary walls by counteracting the distention caused by the intracapillary hydraulic pressure (427). Several molecules mediate interactions between mesangial cells and the surrounding matrix, other glomerular cells and the GBM (428). Afadin, a F-actin–binding protein, localizes to cell contacts between mesangial cells and endothelial cells (429). Integrin α3β1 and Lu/BCAM are mesangial receptors that mediate adhesion of mesangial cells to the laminin α5 chain in the GBM (430). Integrin α8β1 produced by mesangial cells binds to its ligand nephronectin in the GBM and this interaction is believed to regulate mesangial cell adhesion (431). The fibronectin receptor integrin α4β1 is also expressed on mesangial cells (432). These contacts serve in signaling pathways that regulate the production of ECM and the synthesis of growth factors, vasoactive mediators and cytokines.

The mesangial cell also has phagocytic capability and plays a role in the clearance of macromolecules and debris from the mesangium (433). Mesangial cells can respond to, as well as generate, a variety of molecules, including interleukin I, PDGF, and arachidonic acid metabolites, which may play a central role in the response to glomerular injury (434). PDGF-β, the main ligand for the receptor PDGFR, is a mitogen for mesangial cell proliferation and genetic deletion of PDGF-β and PDGFR leads to an absence of mesangial cells and the mesangium (435). It is recognized that a small subpopulation of cells in the mesangium are bone marrow–derived macrophages and play a role in immune responsiveness (Fig. 33.50) (436–438). Occasional leukocytes are observed in the normal glomerulus and label with leukocyte common antigen (CD45 and CD45RB) immunohistochemistry.

The mesangium is continuous with the extraglomerular mesangium, a component of the JGA, along the glomerular stalk. Interestingly, it has been demonstrated that renin lineage cells residing in the extraglomerular mesangial region may migrate and repopulate the intraglomerular mesangium upon glomerular injury (439,440).

Glomerular Basement Membrane

The GBM can be demonstrated on light microscopy by PAS and Jones silver stains (Fig. 33.51). The silver preparation

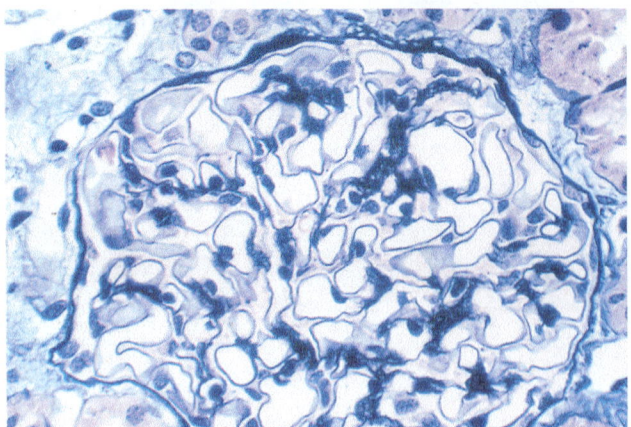

FIGURE 33.51 Jones silver-stained normal glomerulus illustrating the silver-positive GBM and positive basement membrane of Bowman capsule (×500).

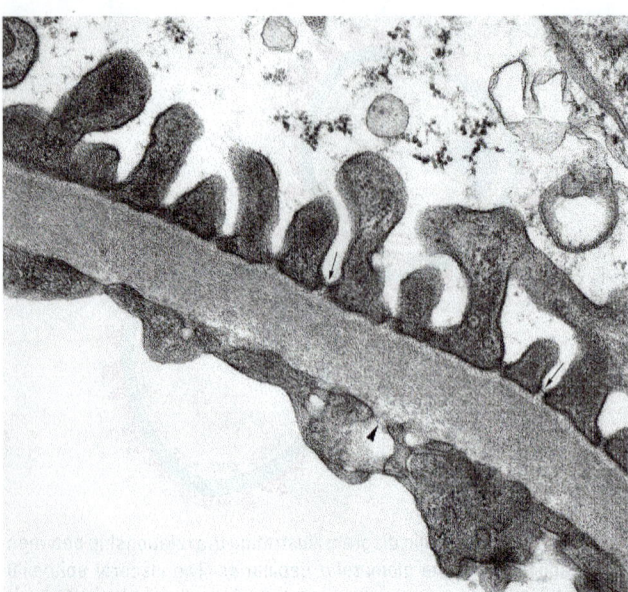

FIGURE 33.53 Transmission electron micrograph of a glomerulus. Bowman space is above and the capillary lumen is below the glomerular capillary wall. A fenestra or pore (*arrowhead*) in the endothelium is evident. Note the regular alignment of the foot processes of the podocytes. Filtration slit diaphragms (*arrows*) are present between individual foot processes. The GBM consists primarily of the lamina densa. The electron-lucent lamina rara interna and lamina rara externa are not prominent (×48,000).

is more specific for membranes and gives a distinct outline of the GBM. Examination of a normal peripheral capillary loop away from the vascular pole and the mesangium shows a delicate basement membrane (Fig. 33.52). Hematoxylin and eosin (H&E) and PAS preparations may stain capillary luminal contents and the cytoplasm of the endothelial and podocyte cell layers, resulting in an apparent thickening of the GBM. The basement membrane is situated between the endothelium and the podocytes in the glomerular capillary wall. On ultrastructural examination, the GBM completely surrounds the endothelium of the peripheral capillary loops and the mesangium between the loops. The GBM consists of a central dense layer, the lamina densa and two surrounding thinner electron-lucent layers, the lamina rara interna and the lamina rara externa. In comparison with laboratory animals, the electron-lucent layers appear less prominent in the human glomerulus (Fig. 33.53).

The adult GBM ranges between 310 and 380 nm in mean thickness (441–443). It is significantly thicker in men (mean 373 nm) than in women (mean 326 nm) and increases in width until the fourth decade of life (315). Quantitative data on the normal adult glomerular capillary structure include the following values: mean glomerular volume of 1.38×10^6 μm^3, average capillary diameter of 6.75 μm, and capillary filtration surface/glomerulus of 200×10^3 μm^2 (444). Proteomic analysis has identified at least 212 proteins in the normal human glomerular extracellular matrix (445,446). However, the major components of the GBM include type IV collagen, laminin, nidogen (entactin), and heparan sulfate proteoglycans (HSPGs) (447); collagen IV is the major constituent of the GBM. Six chains, α1(IV) to α6(IV), make up the collagen IV protein family (448). Three chains of collagen IV self-associate to form triple-helical molecules called protomers. Despite many possible combinations, the six chains of collagen IV form only three types of protomers, which are designated as α1.α2.α1(IV), α3.α4.α5(IV), and α5.α6.α5(IV). The triple helical protomers unite at the noncollagenous domain (NC1) at the carboxy terminus forming hexamers, which in turn, assemble to form a polymerized network which serves as a scaffold for integration of other GBM components. Three canonical sets of hexamers form three distinct networks in basement membranes: the α1.α2.α1 to α1.α2.α1 (IV), the α3.α4.α5(IV) to α3.α4.α5(IV), and the α1.α2.α1 to α5.α6.α5 (IV) networks (449). The α3.α4.α5(IV) to α3.α4.α5(IV) network predominates in the adult GBM and mutations of the genes encoding the α3, α4, and α5(IV) chains cause Alport syndrome (450). In Goodpasture syndrome, autoantibodies are targeted to the α3(IV) chain (450). The α1.α2.α1 to

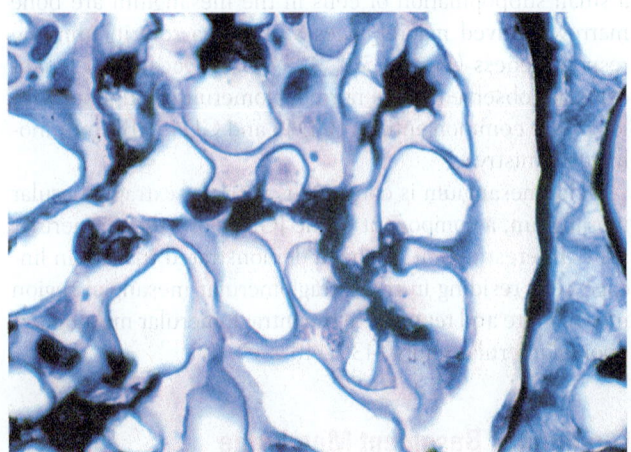

FIGURE 33.52 Higher magnification micrograph demonstrating thin regular GBMs of peripheral capillary loops. (Jones silver stain, ×1250.)

α5.α6.α5 (IV) network is found in Bowman capsule. The α1.α2.α1(IV) protomers are synthesized by both endothelial cells and podocytes but the α5.α6.α5 (IV) protomers are secreted only by podocytes (251).

Laminins are heterotrimers composed of three chains: α, β, and γ. Laminin-521, containing the α5, β2, and γ1 chains, is the major laminin isoform in the adult GBM (447). Laminin α5 and β2 are synthesized by both glomerular endothelial cells and podocytes (451). Mutations of laminin β2 result in a congenital nephrotic syndrome called Pierson syndrome in humans (452).

Nidogen (also called entactin) is a glycoprotein that binds to both collagen IV and laminin in the GBM (453) but does not appear essential for GBM formation (454). Proteoglycans consist of glycosaminoglycan (GAG) chains bound to a core protein (455). The GAG chains contain either heparan sulfate or chondroitin sulfate. HSPGs include agrin, perlecan, and collagen XVIII. They are primarily responsible for the negative charge of the GBM (456,457). Agrin is the major HSPG found in the GBM, whereas perlecan and collagen XVIII are present mainly in the mesangium matrix (458–460). Advanced microscopic methods, including stochastic optical reconstruction microscopy (STORM), have revealed a nanoscale organization of molecules within the GBM (461). The α3α4α5(IV) network is in the center of the GBM, whereas the α1α2α1(IV) network localizes near the endothelial side of the GBM. Laminin-521 maps to the central portion of the GBM but also in two layers near the endothelial and podocyte sides of the GBM. Agrin is situated in two layers along the endothelial and podocyte surfaces of the GBM with more detected near the podocytes.

Podocytes

The podocytes (visceral epithelial cells) are the largest cells in the glomerulus. By light microscopy, they are positioned on the outside of the glomerular capillary wall, often bulge into the urinary space, and have prominent nuclei and abundant light eosinophilic cytoplasm. SEM shows that the podocytes have a prominent cell body containing the nucleus and organelles and long cytoplasmic ramifications, the primary processes that surround the glomerular capillaries and divide into individual foot processes (Fig. 33.54) (462). The foot processes cover the capillary wall, contact the lamina rara externa of the GBM, and interdigitate with foot processes from different podocytes. Advanced microscopy methods, including serial block-face SEM (SBF-SEM) and focused ion beam SEM (FIB-SEM), have revealed that some foot processes arise directly from the podocyte cell body as well as from the elongated cytoplasmic processes (463,464). These studies also demonstrated tortuous ridge-like prominences along the basal surface of the cell body and the processes, from which the proximal portions of the foot processes emerge.

Three-dimensional electron microscopy reconstructions have revealed additional complex architectural features of

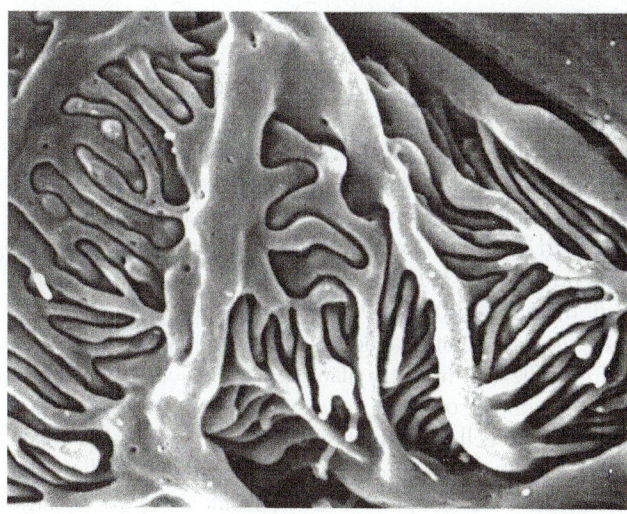

FIGURE 33.54 Scanning electron micrograph of glomerulus illustrating the primary processes of podocytes wrapping around the capillary loops. Note the interdigitation of the foot processes (×13,000; courtesy of Dr. Jill W. Verlander).

the podocyte layer. Neal et al. also demonstrated foot processes (termed anchoring processes) directly between the podocyte cell body and the GBM (465). Moreover, their study characterized three distinct compartments of Bowman space. The subpodocyte space (SPS), first described by Gautier in 1950 (466), exists as a restricted area under the podocyte cell body and is associated with a reported 60% of the glomerular filtration surface (465). The SPS has been reported to connect via narrow passages, called subpodocyte exit pores (SEPs), with the main Bowman space. The SPS is a higher-resistance pathway than the parallel pathway across the barrier surface not covered by the SPS (467). In addition, this resistance across the SPS may be regulated by alterations of the SEPs (468). The interpodocyte space (IPS) was characterized as a narrow anastomosing region interconnecting the SPS with the main peripheral Bowman space (465). SBF-SEM studies suggest that the SPS and IPS are not free-flowing urinary spaces (469). The physiologic role of these podocyte partitions of Bowman space remains to be clarified.

By transmission electron microscopy, the cells have abundant rough endoplasmic reticulum, a well-developed Golgi apparatus, and prominent lysosomes. Podocytes have an elaborate cytoskeleton which underlies their stability, shape, adhesion, and response to stress (470). There are numerous intermediate filaments, microtubules, and microfilaments in the cytoplasm (397). The intermediate filaments (vimentin) and microtubules predominate in the cell body and primary processes whereas, the foot processes contain a dense microfilament contractile apparatus (471–473). The latter, containing actin, myosin, α-actinin, talin, and vinculin, connects to the intermediate filaments and microtubules of the primary processes (474). Electron microscopic studies have demonstrated at least two distinct actin filament networks in podocyte foot processes (475). Bundles of actin filaments, containing α-actinin and synaptopodin, extend along the longitudinal axis of the foot processes. A second actin network containing cortactin is situated between the longitudinal network and the plasma membrane. In glomerular diseases with proteinuria, the podocyte cytoskeleton is disrupted leading to foot process effacement. It is known that most cells contain both contractile and noncontractile actin fibers (bundles of actin filaments). The former typically have both α-actinin and myosin (476). Super resolution microscopic studies have revealed additional details of the podocyte cytoskeleton (477). Whereas the actin filaments in the center of the foot process contain α-actinin and synaptopodin, the actin filaments in the cell body and primary processes contain myosin IIA but lack synaptopodin. These results suggest the actin filaments in the foot process are noncontractile, whereas the actin filaments in the cell body and primary processes are contractile. Moreover, in models of podocyte injury with foot process effacement, myosin IIA translocates to the cytoplasm adjacent to the GBM forming a mat of aggregated filaments. This ultrastructural arrangement of contractile proteins may allow the podocytes to play an active role in modifying the glomerular filtration surface area.

Using SBF-SEM, three-dimensional reconstruction studies have confirmed the complex geometry of podocytes and their foot processes (478). Podocyte cell body volumes range from 30% to 50% of the total cell volume and major or primary cell processes 30% to 50% of the cell volume. Although the foot processes account for only 20% of the cell volume, they constitute nearly 60% of the surface area. Based on the data, it was concluded that the foot processes are intrinsically fragile. Complex models of podocyte actin cytoskeletal dynamics have been constructed to further investigate podocyte function and response to injury.

Two structures in the foot processes, focal adhesions (FAs) and filtration slit diaphragms (SDs), interact with and control the actin cytoskeleton (479). Focal adhesions anchor the foot processes to the GBM. They consist of transmembrane protein complexes containing integrins and their interacting partners which link to the actin cytoskeleton (480). For example, α3β1 integrin interconnects laminin in the GBM with the talin, paxillin, vinculin adaptor cytoplasmic complex, which connects to the actin cytoskeleton. Mutations of the integrin α3 subunit in humans are associated with severe proteinuria (481). GTPases, several of which regulate FA maturation, control actin dynamics. These include the small GTPases, including RhoA, Rac1, and Cdc42 (482). and also the large GTPase protein dynamin (483).

The adjacent foot processes near the GBM are separated by a 30- to 40-nm space termed the filtration pore or slit, which is bridged by a thin extracellular structure called the filtration slit diaphragm. In addition to functioning as a critical barrier to filtration, the slit diaphragm regulates actin cytoskeletal dynamics in the foot processes (484). On ultrastructural examination, the slit diaphragm has always attracted the attention of pathologists. Over 30 years ago, on the basis of electron microscopy, Karnovsky and co-workers proposed an isoporous zipper-like structural model for the slit diaphragm (485–487). In this model, a central filament, corresponding to the central dot of the diaphragm on cross section, is connected to the adjacent foot processes by spaced cross-bridges, between which are rectangular pores. A three-dimensional reconstruction of the slit diaphragm by electron tomography has provided results that generally agree with the Karnovsky model (488). The study showed that the slit diaphragm consists of a network of winding strands, about 30 to 35 nm long, which merge centrally into a longitudinal density. The strands, creating a slit diaphragm thickness between 5 and 10 nm, surround pores the same size or smaller than albumin molecules. The pores appear more irregular than previously supposed. It was earlier proposed that the SD has a sheet-like rather than a zipper-like substructure based on a freeze-etching replica ultrastructural method (489). An investigation using enhanced SEM revealed variable shape pores in the center of the SD and no central filament (490). This finding favored the SD as a heteroporous structure rather than a zipper-like structure. High-resolution helium ion SEM studies have shown the SD with cross-bridging filaments and surrounding pores forming a ladder-like structure in the middle of the filtration slit, also without a distinct central midline, thus supporting the heteroporous model (491,492). Cryo-EM tomographic studies have revealed further molecular complexity of the SD (493). Bridging shorter strands in the lower part of the SD closest to the GBM consist of Neph1 whereas longer strands in the top part of the SD toward the apical side contain nephrin. This study supports the SD as a layered bipartite molecular assembly.

The slit diaphragm appears unique but shares similarities with tight and adherens junctions (494,495). It separates the different membrane surfaces of the podocyte. Podocytes, similar to other epithelial cells, are polarized with distinct membrane domains (Fig. 33.55) (496). The basal membrane domain and the apical membrane domain are located below and above, respectively, the slit diaphragm. The slit diaphragm area, including the bridging diaphragm as well as the adjacent podocyte foot process membrane and cytoplasm, may also be considered a surface domain, a very specialized one.

A major advance in our understanding of the podocyte was the identification of the protein nephrin, encoded by NPHS1, the gene mutated in congenital nephrotic syndrome of the Finnish type (248,249). Nephrin, a transmembrane adhesion protein of the immunoglobulin superfamily, localizes to strands of the slit diaphragm (497). Lack of nephrin in humans or animals leads to the loss of the slit diaphragm, foot process effacement, and massive proteinuria (249,498). An increasing number of other proteins localize to the slit diaphragm domain, where they interact with nephrin and other partners, forming a multifunctional complex (Fig. 33.56) (248,474,499). Some proteins are present in the actual slit diaphragm itself. For example, there is evidence that

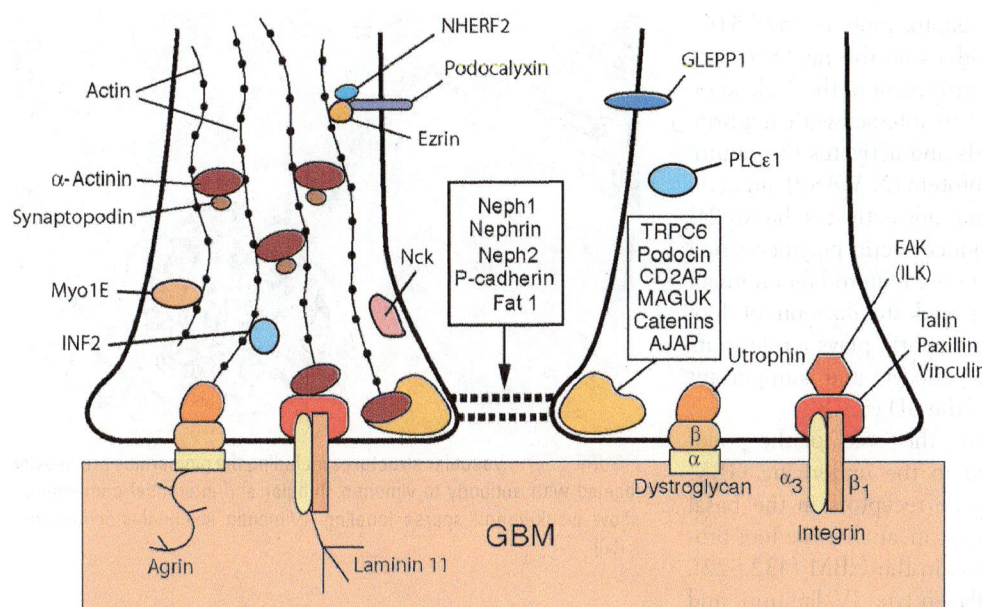

FIGURE 33.55 Schematic drawing of the membrane domains of the podocyte: The filtration slit diaphragm, basal membrane, and apical membrane domains. Molecular interactions within these domains of the podocyte foot processes are represented. See the text for further explanations. (Modified from Pavenstadt H, Kriz W, Kretzler M. Cell biology of the glomerular podocyte. *Physiol Rev* 2003;83: 253–307; Kerjaschki D. Caught flat-footed: podocyte damage and the molecular bases of focal glomerulosclerosis. *J Clin Invest* 2001;108: 1583–1587.)

nephrin and Neph1, a protein similar to nephrin, are present as molecular bilayer in the SD (493).

Other proteins are present in the podocyte cytoplasm or plasma membrane adjacent to the slit diaphragm. For example, members of the membrane-associated guanylate kinase (MAGUK) family of scaffolding proteins, including MAGI-1, MAGI-2, CASK, and ZO-1 localize adjacent to the slit diaphragm (500,501). These scaffolding proteins connect junctional membrane proteins to the actin cytoskeleton and signaling cascades. In addition, multiple adherens junction-associated proteins (AJAP), including α-actinin, IQGAP1, αII spectrin, and βII spectrin are also components of this expanding nephrin-associated multiprotein complex (500,501).

Mutations or deficiencies of genes encoding many of the proteins that comprise the slit diaphragm domain complex, including nephrin (249), Neph1 (502), Fat1 (503), podocin (504), CD2AP (505), α-actinin (506,507), TRPC6 (508,509), PLCE1 (510), INF2 (511), and MYO1E (512), (Fig. 33.51) cause glomerular diseases in humans and animals characterized by absent or defective slit diaphragms, foot process effacement and proteinuria. Focal segmental glomerulosclerosis (FSGS) is the pathologic lesion found in many of these disorders, which are often called the podocytopathies. As mentioned, the SD serves as a signaling center to control actin dynamics in the foot processes (513). For example, α-actinin, an important protein in the slit diaphragm domain interacts with synaptopodin, another actin-associated protein to facilitate the formation of long unbranched parallel actin filaments in differentiated podocytes (514). Nephrin plays a central role in signaling. One crucial pathway of nephrin influencing the actin

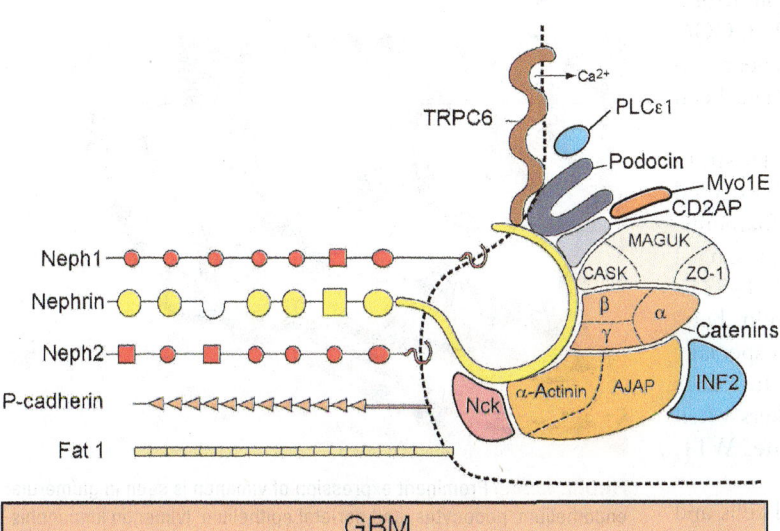

FIGURE 33.56 Schematic drawing of a working model of the podocyte filtration slit diaphragm domain. The *left* side portrays the molecular composition of the slit diaphragm itself, which spans between adjacent foot processes. The *right* side illustrates the molecular interactions of the nephrin-associated multiprotein complex within the podocyte foot process membrane and cytoplasm. See the text for further explanations. (Modified from Pavenstadt H, Kriz W, Kretzler M. Cell biology of the glomerular podocyte. *Physiol Rev* 2003;83:253–307; Kerjaschki D. Caught flat-footed: podocyte damage and the molecular bases of focal glomerulosclerosis. *J Clin Invest* 2001;108:1583–1587; Huber TB, Benzing T. The slit diaphragm: a signaling platform to regulate podocyte function. *Curr Opin Nephrol Hypertens* 2005;14:211–216; and Lehtonen S, Ryan JJ, Kudlicka K, et al. Cell junction-associated proteins IQGAP1, MAGI-2, CASK, spectrins, and alpha-actinin are components of the nephrin multiprotein complex. *Proc Natl Acad Sci USA* 2005;102:9814–9819.)

cytoskeleton involves the Nck adaptor proteins (515,516). Phosphorylation of tyrosine residues on the nephrin cytoplasmic domain results in the recruitment of the Nck adaptor proteins Nck1 and/or Nck2 to interact with nephrin. After this interaction, Nck binds and activates the neuronal Wiskott–Aldrich syndrome protein (N-WASP), an actin nucleation protein. N-WASP binds and activates the Arp2/3 multiprotein complex, which induces actin polymerization (517). Nck and N-WASP proteins are required for an intact filtration barrier foot processes and stabilization of foot processes (518–520). Moreover, nephrin plays a role in its endocytic trafficking within the podocyte and is important for turnover and maintenance of the SD (521).

The basal membrane domain, the "sole" of the podocyte foot process, is embedded in the underlying GBM (Fig. 33.55). Two types of surface receptors in the basal membrane, integrins and dystroglycan, anchor the foot processes by binding to their ligands in the GBM (432,522). The $\alpha3\beta1$ integrin binds to collagen type IV, laminin, and nidogen/entactin whereas, dystroglycan binds to laminin, agrin, and perlecan (474). Both integrins and dystroglycan are coupled by adapter molecules to the actin cytoskeleton. The integrins bind the talin, paxillin, vinculin complex (472), and dystroglycan binds utrophin (522). The induction of cellular responses from integrin–ligand interactions, known as "outside-in" signaling, is believed to be mediated by focal adhesion kinase (FAK) and ILK (474,523). Similar to the filtration slit domain, an intact basal membrane domain is required to maintain foot process integrity.

The apical membrane domain, above the slit diaphragm, has a prominent glycocalyx surface of negatively charged glycoproteins (Fig. 33.55) (524). These include podocalyxin (525) and GLEPP1 (526). Podocalyxin interacts with a complex composed of ezrin and NHERF2 (Na^+/H^+ exchanger-regulatory factor 2), which in turn, associates with the actin cytoskeleton (527,528). Genetic evidence exists indicating podocalyxin is important for foot process stability (529). Proteins within podocyte organelles are also important for podocyte function and intact filtration. Mutations of mitochondrial genes, including COQ2, COQ6, PDSS2, MT-TL1, and ADCK4 and defects of nuclear proteins WT1, PAX2, LMX1B, and SMARCAL1 have been associated with proteinuric syndromes (530).

The development of the glomerulus as a vascular structure distinct from the remainder of the nephron is reflected in the intrarenal distribution of intermediate filaments. Vimentin is present in glomerular endothelial and mesangial cells and podocytes (Figs. 33.57 and 33.58) (473,531–534).

Human podocytes often do not stain for desmin, however rat podocytes may show desmin expression, especially in response to injury (534,535). The glomerular tuft does not stain for cytokeratins. Other podocyte markers often demonstrated by immunohistochemistry include WT1, CD10, GLEPP1, podocalyxin, and nephrin.

Mature podocytes are terminally differentiated cells and generally do not replicate. They express the CDK inhibitors

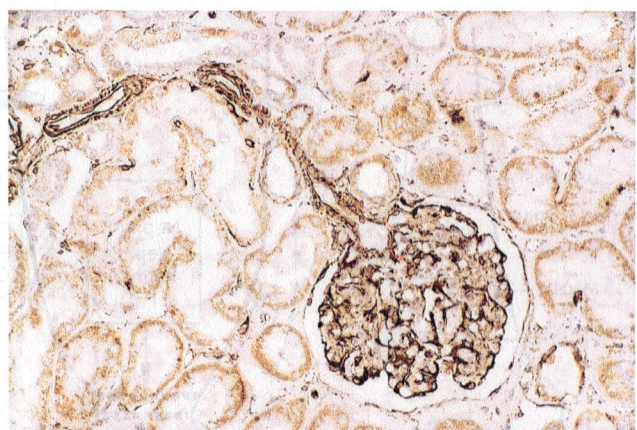

FIGURE 33.57 Vascular structures including the glomerulus are heavily labeled with antibody to vimentin. Tubular and interstitial components show weaker and sparse labeling. (Vimentin immunohistochemistry, ×100)

P27 and p57, which are involved in maintaining cell quiescence (536). The Wilms tumor suppressor gene, WT1, plays an indispensable role in the regulation of cell growth and differentiation during early nephrogenesis (199). Embryonic mice homologous for a targeted mutation of WT1 fail to develop kidneys (200). Striking evidence also exists for the importance of WT1 in glomerular podocyte differentiation. During kidney development, WT1 expression is detected in the MM and becomes stronger in the renal vesicle, but highest levels occur during glomerulus formation within the podocyte cell layer (537,538). Expression of the WT1 protein, a transcription factor, in the nuclei of podocytes does not disappear with glomerular maturation but persists in the adult kidney (Fig. 33.59). Greater than 95% of patients with the Denys–Drash syndrome (nephrotic syndrome and genital anomalies and/or Wilms tumor), characterized by shrunken glomeruli with hypertrophied podocytes, have point mutations affecting the zinc finger DNA-binding domain of WT1 (539). These

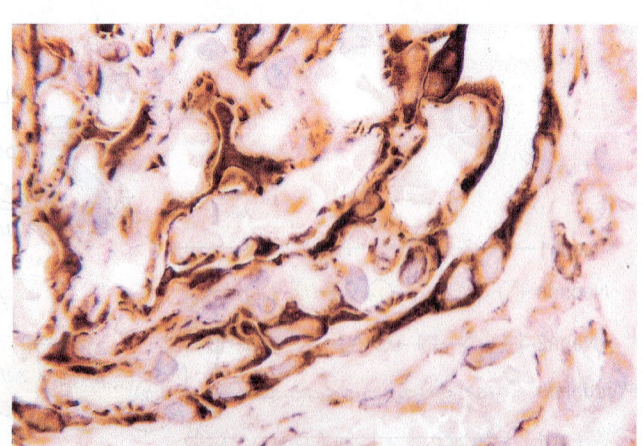

FIGURE 33.58 Prominent expression of vimentin is seen in glomerular endothelium, podocytes, and parietal epithelium (vimentin immunohistochemistry, ×630).

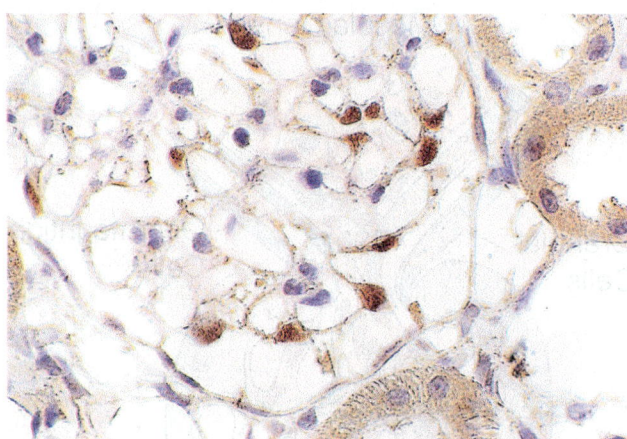

FIGURE 33.59 Light micrograph demonstrating expression of the WT1 protein in podocyte nuclei of an adult glomerulus (WT1 immunohistochemistry, ×400).

findings provide a functional link between a molecular defect of WT1 and podocyte pathology and indicate that WT1 has a major role in maintenance of podocyte structure and function in the mature kidney. As a master regulator, WT1 regulates the expression of other podocyte genes that are required for intact glomerular filtration (540,541). Studies using a multiomic integrative approach, including whole exome sequencing and mass spectrometry-based proteomics are identifying podocyte genes which will enhance our understanding of the role of podocytes in health and disease (542,543).

Glomerular Filtration Barrier

The glomerular capillary wall functions as a filter that is selective for the size and charge of molecules (544–546). To pass through the capillary wall, a molecule must journey along an extracellular pathway through the fenestrated endothelium, the GBM, and the filtration slit diaphragm.

Increasing evidence indicates the glomerular endothelial glycocalyx is an important layer of the glomerular filtration barrier (403,406). Historically, the GBM has been considered the main barrier to filtration. Over recent years, the role of the podocyte slit diaphragm has emerged.

The permeability of the glomerular capillary wall to water and small molecules is very high, whereas its permeability to molecules the size of albumin and larger is very low. Studies employing mathematical modeling have suggested that the GBM and filtration slits contribute equally to the total resistance to water filtration. A model incorporating ultrastructural data have shown that the slit diaphragm is the most restrictive part of the barrier to the filtration of macromolecules (547).

Mutations or deficiencies of genes encoding proteins of the filtration slit diaphragm domain, including nephrin and several of its interacting protein partners, result in massive proteinuria, providing genetic evidence for the crucial role of the slit diaphragm in glomerular permselectivity (499).

Although the protein networks within the GBM contribute to the size selectivity of the filtration barrier, the slit diaphragm appears to be the most important size-selective filter.

The GBM has been favored as the principal structure responsible for the charge-selective permeability of the glomerular capillary wall (544,545). This charge selectivity in the GBM has been associated with the presence of polyanionic molecules, such as HSPGs. Therefore, it was somewhat surprising that mice deficient for the heparan sulfate side chains of perlecan were found to have no morphologic GBM defects and exhibited no proteinuria (548).

Agrin is the major HSPG in the GBM and its removal led to a loss of GBM negative charge, but did not alter the filtration barrier function in mice (549). However, there is evidence that an intact GBM does serve as a major barrier to protein permeability. The deletion of the laminin β2 chain in the GBM leads to albuminuria in mice (model for the human disorder Pierson syndrome) that occurs before slit diaphragm abnormalities and foot process effacement (550). These results suggest that the GBM does serve as a barrier to protein and that an intact slit diaphragm alone is not sufficient to prevent proteinuria.

The "integrated view" of the glomerular filtration barrier is that the endothelium, the GBM, and the podocytes and their slit diaphragms do not act independently but are linked to one another in a functional unit. Each of these components are important for normal glomerular filtration.

Parietal Epithelial Cells

The parietal layer of Bowman capsule consists of relatively flat squamous epithelial cells, called PECs. They have prominent proliferative potential (551). Keratins, cadherins, the transcription factor Pax2, and claudin-1 are expressed in PECs (Fig. 33.60) (532–534,552). The cells are 0.1 to 0.3 μm

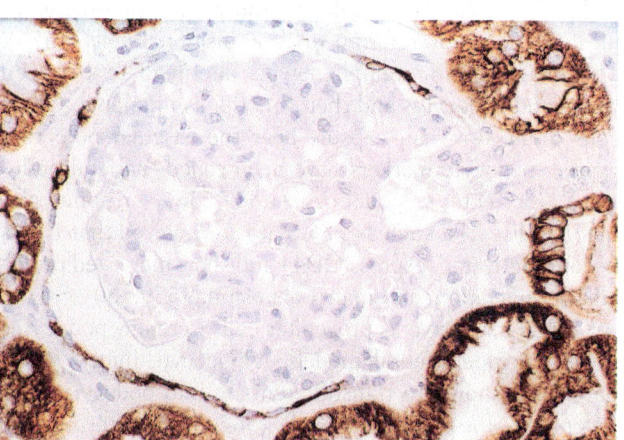

FIGURE 33.60 Keratin expression is not observed in the glomerular tuft, but immunoreactivity is seen in the parietal epithelial cells. The vascular pole is on the *right*. The macula densa (*far right center*) and other tubule segments are immunoreactive for keratin (CAM 5.2 immunohistochemistry, ×400).

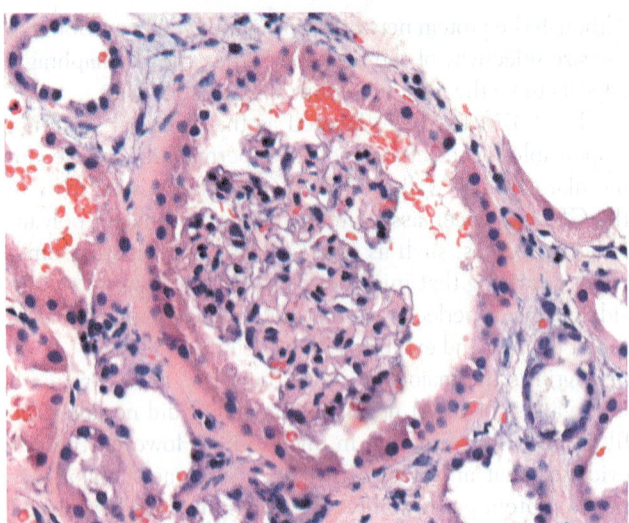

FIGURE 33.61 Glomerulus with circumferential tubular metaplasia of Bowman capsule (H&E, ×400).

in height but may increase to 2 to 3.5 μm at the nucleus. The epithelium rests on the basement membrane of Bowman capsule, which has a range from 1,200 to 1,500 nm in thickness and may have a lamellated appearance. In contrast to the GBM, the basement membrane of Bowman capsule expresses the α6 chain of type IV collagen, which is part of the α1.α2.α1(IV) to α5.α6.α5(IV) network (553). The PEC layer functions as a physical barrier for the glomerular ultrafiltrate. When this layer is experimentally compromised, macromolecules can leak into the periglomerular interstitial space (554). On occasion, the flat PEC layer may be replaced with proximal tubular epithelium. It is common in mice but such tubular metaplasia of Bowman capsule in humans has been noted in various condition, especially acute tubular injury (Fig. 33.61).

Different populations of PECs appear to exist (555). "Peripolar cells," situated at the vascular pole between PECs and podocytes and containing prominent cytoplasmic granules, are currently referred to as "transitional cells" (556). They have an immunophenotype intermediate between PECs and podocytes and their function is unknown. Other cells lining Bowman capsule near the vascular pole that express podocyte markers have been called "parietal podocytes" (or "ectopic podocytes") (557,558). In some glomerular diseases, such as FSGS, it is recognized that PECs become activated, express CD44 and show increased proliferation, migration, and matrix deposition (559,560).

PECs may serve as progenitor cells to renew podocytes (561). In experimental models of podocyte injury, PECs have been shown to transdifferentiate into podocytes and repopulate the glomerular tuft (562–565). Alternatively, in other models of glomerular injury, podocytes have been shown to migrate onto Bowman capsule and express PEC markers (566–568). The functional relevance of these apparent bidirectional movements of podocytes and PECs remains to be determined.

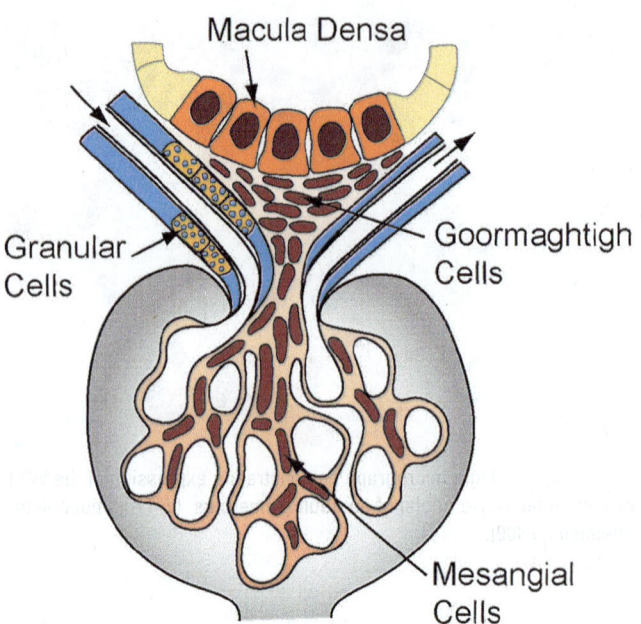

FIGURE 33.62 The basic components of the JGA. (Modified with permission from Kriz W, Kaissling B. Structural organization of the mammalian kidney. In: Seldin DW, Giebisch D, eds. *The Kidney: Physiology and Pathophysiology*. 3rd ed. Philadelphia, PA: Lippincott Williams & Wilkins; 2000:587–654.)

JUXTAGLOMERULAR APPARATUS

The JGA, discovered by Golgi, is situated at the vascular pole of the glomerulus and includes the afferent and efferent arterioles, extraglomerular mesangial region, and MD (Fig. 33.62). A prominent JGA may occasionally be observed in a normal glomerulus and should not be mistaken for a lesion such as segmental glomerulosclerosis (Fig. 33.63).

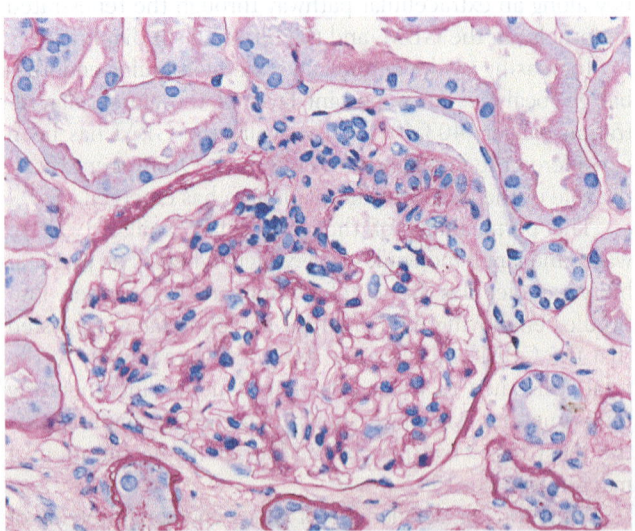

FIGURE 33.63 Glomerulus with prominent juxtaglomerular apparatus. Caution in interpretation is necessary in the evaluation of glomerular cellularity at the vascular pole because of the continuum of the extraglomerular and intraglomerular mesangial regions (PAS, ×400).

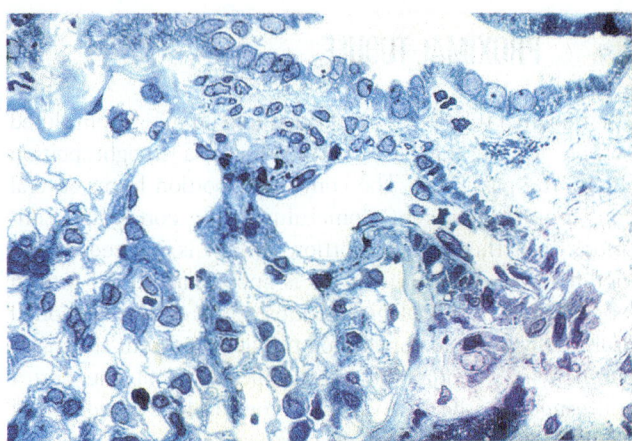

FIGURE 33.64 Light micrograph depicting the JGA. From the top to the bottom of the micrograph are the macula densa, extraglomerular mesangium, afferent arteriole, and glomerulus (×750; courtesy of Dr. Luciano Barajas). (Reprinted with permission from Barajas L, Salido EC, Smolens P, et al. Pathology of the juxtaglomerular apparatus including Bartter's syndrome. In: Tisher CC, Brenner BM, eds. *Renal Pathology with Clinical and Functional Correlations*. 2nd ed. Philadelphia, PA: JB Lippincott; 1994:948–978.)

The JGA is the major structural unit of the renin–angiotensin system. Although the general outline of this anatomical unit usually can be observed in light microscopic sections (Fig. 33.64), histochemical or immunocytochemical methods are usually required to demonstrate the distinctive juxtaglomerular granular cells. These cells tend to occur in clusters and are most abundant in the wall of the afferent arteriole but are also found in the wall of the efferent arteriole and the extraglomerular mesangial region (569–571). Ultrastructural analysis shows the presence of myofilaments, attachment bodies, a well-developed endoplasmic reticulum and Golgi apparatus, and numerous membrane-bound granules (Fig. 33.65). The granules are variable in shape and size. It is believed that the smaller, often rhomboid-shaped granules with a crystalline substructure, called protogranules, observed in the Golgi region represent mature granules. Renin and angiotensin II have been immunolocalized to the granules of these cells (572,573). Renin release occurs by exocytosis. It is believed to be modulated by adrenergic nerve activity (574,575).

In addition to the classical role of renin cells in blood pressure regulation, recent studies have revealed renin-expressing cells display considerable plasticity and have roles in regeneration and oxygen sensing (576). Several studies using genetic labeling techniques and experimental podocyte depletion have shown that cells of renin lineage (in addition to PECs as previously discussed) remarkably appear to serve as podocyte progenitors (577–581). Evidence for the endocrine plasticity of renin cells exists. Deletion of the von Hippel–Lindau (PVHL), which targets hypoxia inducible factor-2 (HIF-2) for degradation, in JG cells converts the cells from a renin-expressing to erythropoietin-producing cells, likely in response to HIF-2 stabilization (582–584).

The extraglomerular mesangium, also called lacis or cells of Goormaghtigh is located between the afferent and efferent arterioles and has extensive contact with the basal surface of the MD. This extraglomerular region is continuous with the intraglomerular mesangium and the Goormaghtigh cells are similar in ultrastructure to the mesangial cells. There are numerous gap junctions between the extraglomerular mesangial cells and the cells of the intraglomerular mesangium and glomerular arterioles (585,586). The gap junctions consist of connexin proteins, especially connexin 40 (587,588). These morphologic features and the central position within the JGA suggest that the extraglomerular mesangium may represent the structural–functional link between the MD and the glomerular arterioles and mesangium.

The MD represents a plaque of specialized tubular cells within the cortical thick ascending limb (CTAL) of Henle adjacent to the hilum of the glomerulus. The cells are low columnar and their apical situated nuclei may protrude into the tubular lumen (Fig. 33.66). By electron microscopy, they have cytoplasmic organelles largely lateral to and beneath the apical nuclei, and basal cellular processes that interdigitate with the extraglomerular mesangial cells. The lateral intercellular spaces between the MD cells vary in width but usually are more dilated compared with the lateral intercellular spaces of other nephron segments (589). In contrast with contiguous portions of the TAL, there is evidence that the MD lacks epidermal growth factor and Tamm–Horsfall protein but is water permeable (Fig. 33.67) (590–592). The anatomic arrangement of the JGA is suited for functional regulation of the adjacent structures. The MD plays a role in tubuloglomerular feedback, a mechanism whereby luminal concentrations of sodium and/or chloride are sensed by the MD leading to the transfer of a signal to the glomerular arterioles to regulate the GFR (593,594). Studies support

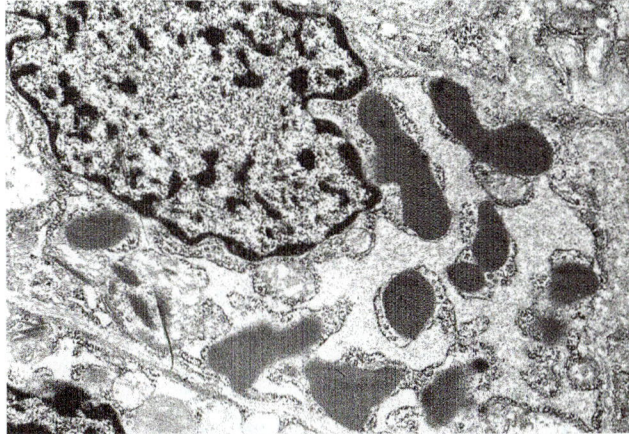

FIGURE 33.65 Electron micrograph of a juxtaglomerular granular cell. Note the prominent cytoplasmic membrane-bound granules (×19,000; courtesy of Dr. Luciano Barajas). (Reprinted with permission from Barajas L, Bloodworth JMB Jr, Hartroft PM. Endocrine pathology of the kidney. In: Bloodworth JMB Jr, ed. *Endocrine Pathology: General and Surgical*. 2nd ed. Baltimore, MD: Williams & Wilkins; 1982:723–766.)

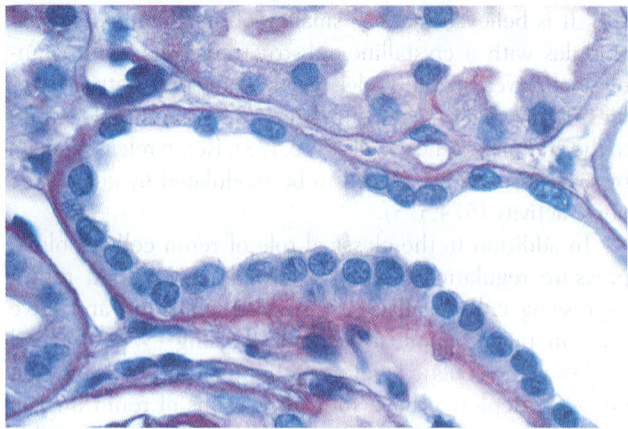

FIGURE 33.66 Macula densa characterized as a morphologically distinct plaque of low columnar cells with apically situated nuclei (PAS, ×750).

the following general sequence: increased sodium chloride concentration at the MD results in formation and release of ATP and adenosine; adenosine interacts with receptors on extraglomerular mesangial cells triggering an increase in cytosolic calcium; gap junctions transmit the calcium flux to the adjacent afferent arteriole resulting in vasoconstriction, inhibition of renin release, and decreased glomerular filtration. The neuronal isoform of nitric oxide synthase (nNOS) and the cyclooxygenase enzyme COX-2 immunolocalize to the MD (595–597). There is evidence that both NO and COX-2–generated prostaglandins play a role in the signaling between the MD and the renin-secreting cells in the afferent arteriole (598,599).

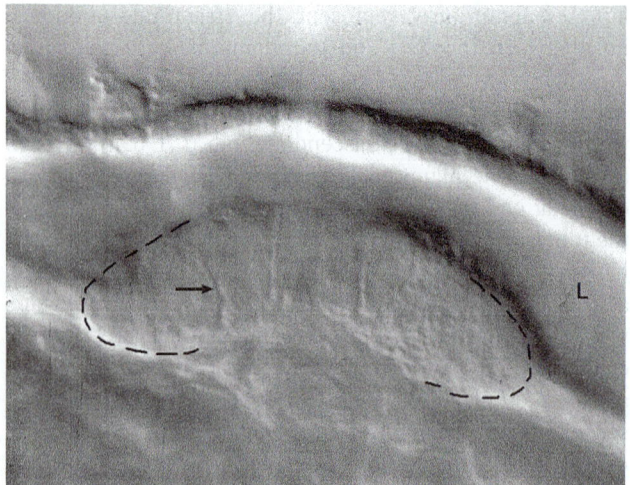

FIGURE 33.67 Differential interference contrast image of an isolated TAL segment perfused in vitro. The tubular lumen (*L*) and macula densa (*dashed lines* enclose the ends of the macula densa plaque) are observed. In response to a reduction in tubular luminal osmolality, there is dilatation of the lateral intercellular spaces (*arrow*) in the macula densa, suggesting increased water flow (×1250). (Modified with permission from Kirk KL, Bell PD, Barfuss DW, et al. Direct visualization of the isolated and perfused macula densa. *Am J Physiol* 1985;248(pt 2):F890–F894.)

PROXIMAL TUBULE

The proximal tubule (PT) is divided into an initial convoluted portion (PCT), the pars convoluta, and a straight portion (PST), the pars recta. The convoluted portion forms several coils around its parent glomerulus in the cortex and continues into the straight portion, which is located in the medullary ray. The human PT is approximately 14 mm in length (600). In histologic sections of the cortex, sectioned profiles of proximal convoluted tubules represent the major parenchymal component. The appearance of the cortex and especially the PTs varies, according to the method of fixation. A decrease in blood pressure results in decreased filtration and renal volume (601,602). After immersion fixation of excised pieces of renal tissue, the cortex has a more homogeneous compact appearance and there is collapse of the proximal tubular lumens (Fig. 33.68) (603). Free nuclei and vesicular membranous material may be observed in the proximal tubular lumens.

It is well known that renal parenchyma, especially the tubules, undergo significant postmortem autolysis and that these changes occur more rapidly than in other tissues, such as the liver, heart, and skeletal muscle (604,605). Within the kidney, PTs typically show greater autolytic changes including loss of cellular adhesion and nuclei (Figs. 33.69 and 33.70). In autopsy specimens, it may be difficult to distinguish acute tubular injury from autolysis and in a given case, both cellular lesions may be present. It may be extremely difficult in toxic forms of acute tubular injury. Most cases of ischemic-type acute tubular injury show a more patchy distribution of injured tubules which are often dilated with attenuated or sloughed epithelium, luminal casts and occasional mitotic figures. Further studies are needed to confirm the useful of reported particular tubular epithelial lesions as a feature of acute tubular injury in postmortem kidneys (606) and the value of immunohistochemical expression of KIM-1, a PT marker upregulated in acute kidney injury (607,608).

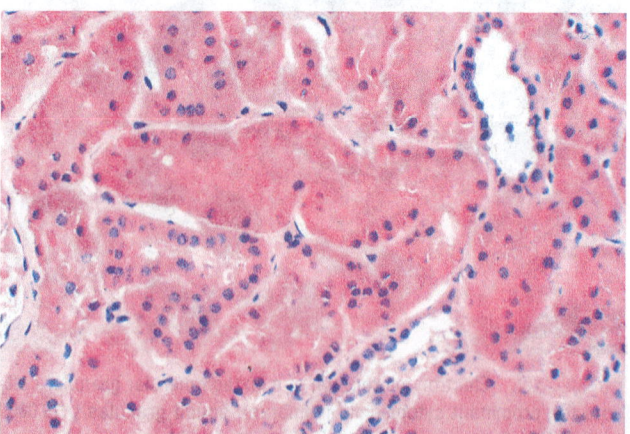

FIGURE 33.68 Immersion-fixed renal biopsy specimen demonstrating diffuse collapse of the proximal tubular lumens. Note the patent lumens of the distal nephron segments (H&E, ×250).

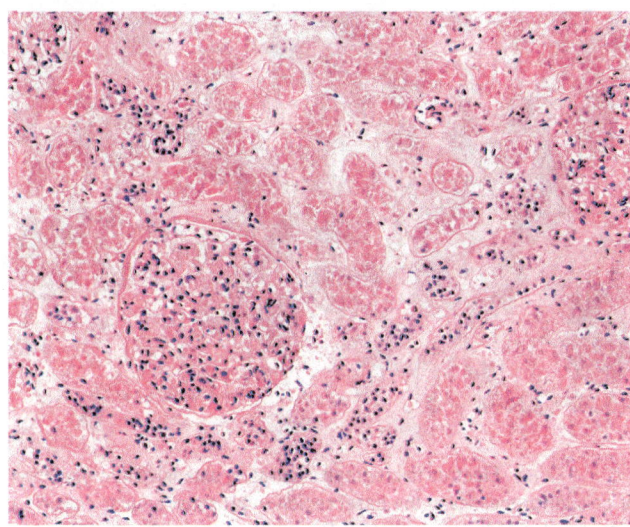

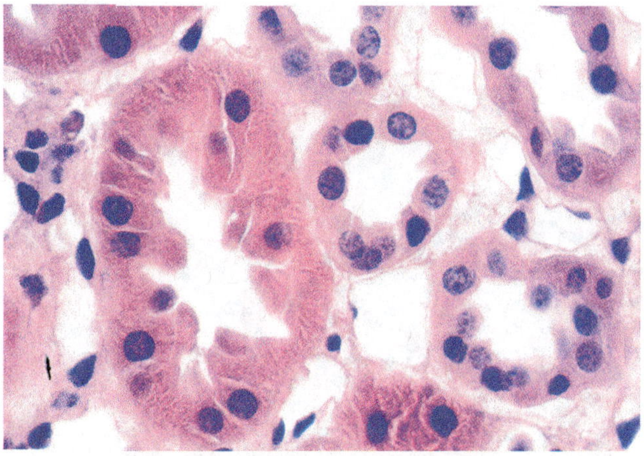

FIGURE 33.71 Cross section of a proximal tubule (*left* of *center*). The proximal tubular cells are taller and more eosinophilic than the cells of the distal nephron segments (*right*) (H&E, ×630).

FIGURE 33.69 Autolysis showing loss of cellular features including nuclei, especially in proximal tubules. Cellular degeneration is present in the distal tubules and glomeruli but their nuclei are still apparent (H&E, ×200).

Fixation of an experimental functioning kidney in situ by rapid freezing, dripping of fixative on the renal surface, or vascular perfusion results in more conspicuous intertubular interstitial spaces and widely open lumens of the PTs. The cells of the PT are cuboidal to low columnar with eosinophilic, often granular cytoplasm and round nuclei situated in the center or near the base of the cells (Fig. 33.71). Ex vivo perfusion (EVP) of donor organs by providing oxygen and nutrients and more suitable storage time are transforming organ transplantation. Donor kidneys perfused ex vivo display more patent and somewhat more dilated lumens in glomeruli, tubules, and peritubular capillaries on histologic examination (Figs. 33.72 to 33.74).

The lateral cell borders of the PTs are indistinct because of extensive interdigitations of lateral cellular processes from adjacent cells (Fig. 33.75). A complex intercellular space forms from these interdigitations. In the basal part of the cells there are vertical striations that represent numerous elongated mitochondria. Cytoplasmic apical vacuoles and granules correspond to a well-developed endocytic-lysosomal apparatus. There is a prominent PAS-positive luminal brush border composed of the numerous densely packed long microvilli (Fig. 33.76). Thin actin filaments, 6 nm in diameter, are inside each microvillus and extend into the apical cytoplasm. The brush border, apical cytoplasmic vacuoles, and basal striations are less prominent in

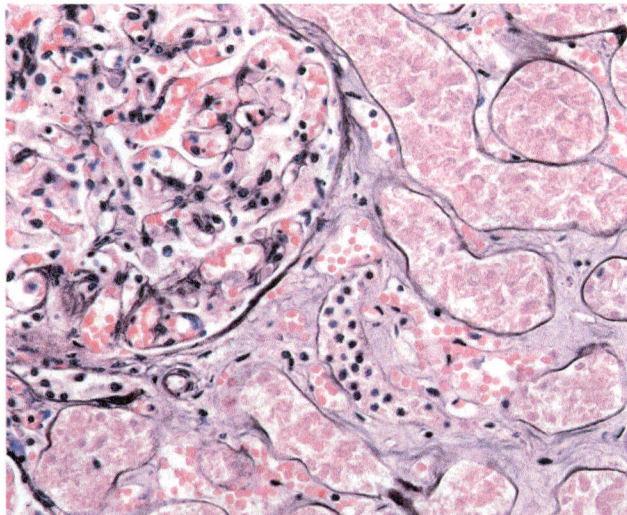

FIGURE 33.70 Silver stain illustrating autolysis. Proximal tubules are most affected. A few distal tubules are identified by their dark nuclei. The glomerular basement membranes, Bowman capsule and tubular basement membranes are still relatively intact (Jones silver stain, ×400).

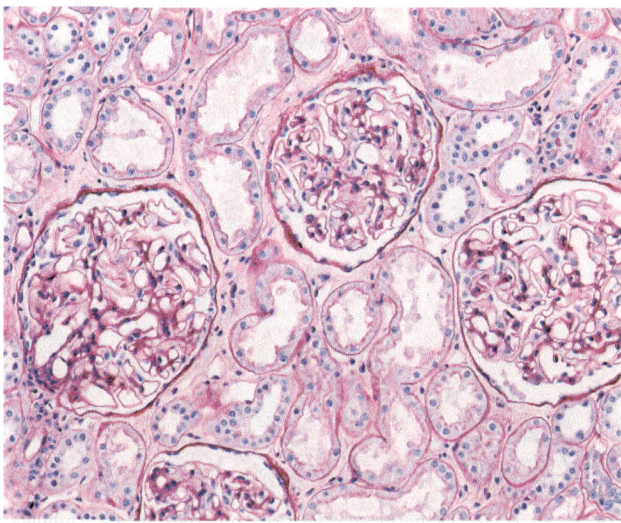

FIGURE 33.72 Ex vivo perfused kidney with intact architecture and patent and dilated lumens in glomeruli and tubules. (PAS, ×200).

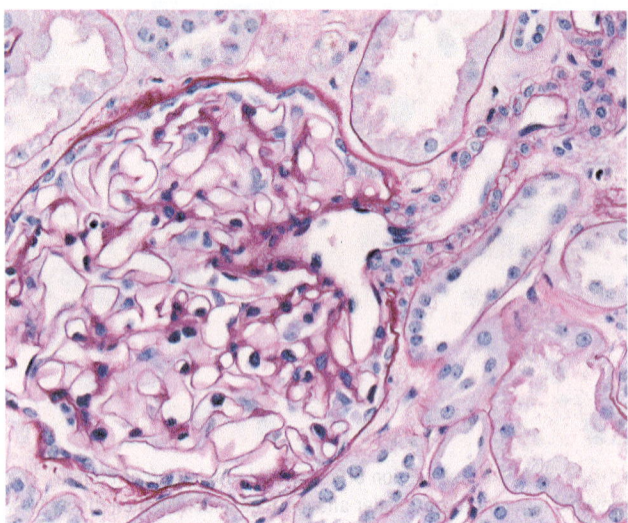

FIGURE 33.73 Ex vivo perfused kidney illustrating crisp cellular detail of a glomerulus, hilar arteriole, and proximal and distal tubules. The brush border of the proximal tubules is somewhat thinned (PAS, ×400).

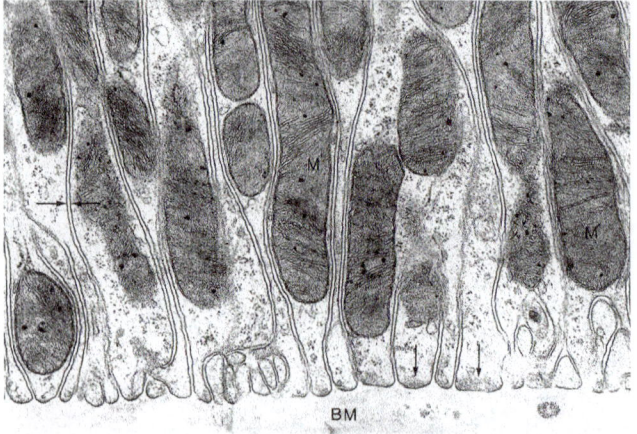

FIGURE 33.75 Electron micrograph illustrating extensive interdigitation of cellular processes in the basal region of proximal tubular cells. The mitochondria (*M*) are elongated. The width of the extracellular space (*opposing arrows*) is constant, and there are bundles of cytoplasmic filaments (*single arrows*) adjacent to the basement membrane (*BM*) (×40,000). (Reprinted with permission from Maunsbach AB, Christensen EI. Functional ultrastructure of the proximal tubule. In: Windhager EE, ed. *Handbook of Physiology. Renal Physiology.* New York: Oxford University Press; 1992:41–107.)

the pars recta. Beneath the microvilli in the apical cytoplasm is the terminal web, an arrangement of filaments containing spectrin and myosin (609). Lectins have been used as selective probes to delineate renal tubular segments (610–612). Although a certain degree of nonspecificity has been reported, the lectin *Lotus tetragonolobus* has been used as a marker of proximal tubular epithelium (Fig. 33.77). CD10, CD15, and CD138 (Fig. 33.78) are PT markers.

Keratins 8 and 18 are expressed in both the convoluted and straight portions of the PT, whereas keratin 19 is focally expressed in the straight portion (532,533,613). The specific expression of the cell adhesion protein cadherin-6 in the PT has been reported (614). Cytokeratins 7 and 34βE12 are absent in PTs.

In most mammals, distinct segments of the tubule portion of the nephron can be distinguished by structural and functional differences. However, species difference exist (615). The structural differences have been characterized mainly on the ultrastructural level (616). However, these tubule segments often can be detected on light microscopy because of their known distribution within specific zones of the kidney (Fig. 33.34). In general, the degree of tubule segmentation has not been characterized in detail in the human kidney.

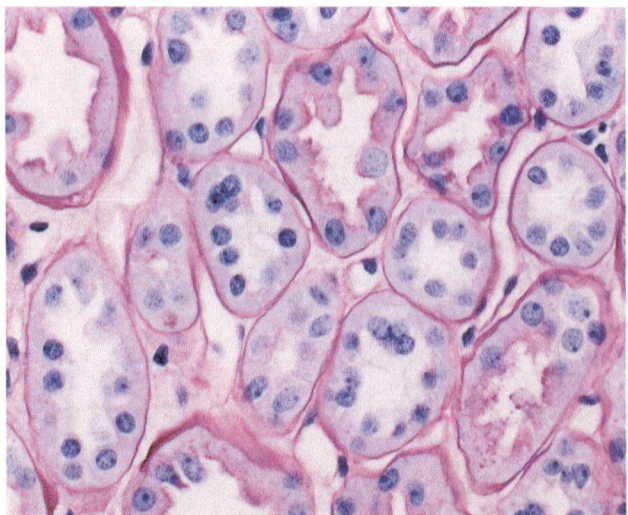

FIGURE 33.74 Ex vivo perfused kidney with proximal and distal tubules. The peritubular capillaries surrounding the tubules are easily identified and display flattened endothelial nuclei (PAS, ×630).

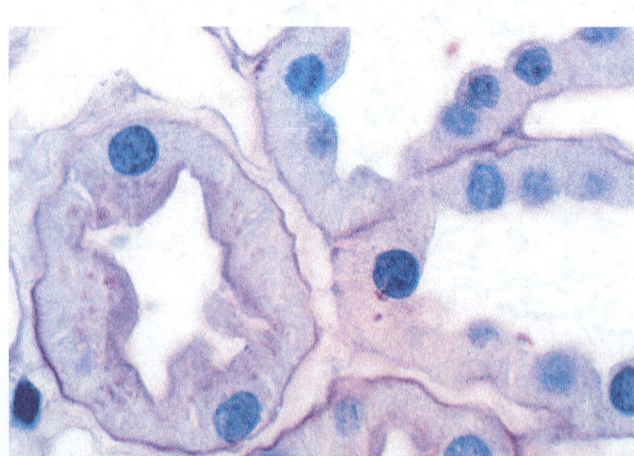

FIGURE 33.76 PAS-stained cross section of proximal tubule to the left of the center of the micrograph. Note the prominent PAS-positive brush border (PAS, ×1250).

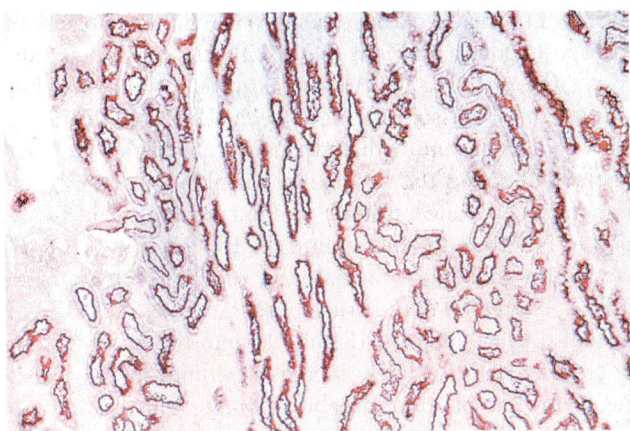

FIGURE 33.77 Staining of the brush border of the PTs with lectin *Lotus tetragonolobus*. The distal nephron segments and glomeruli are negative. (Courtesy of Dr. Randolf A. Hennigar.)

In several mammals, the PT can be divided into three morphologically distinct segments (Fig. 33.79) (616). In contrast to the rat and rabbit, no significant segmentation has been demonstrated in the mouse (617). There are also differences in the total length of PTs between species (618). The S_1 segment originates at the glomerulus and constitutes one-half to two-thirds of the pars convoluta. The S_2 segment represents the remainder of the pars convoluta and the initial part of the pars recta. The S_3 corresponds to the remainder of the pars recta and is located in the inner cortex and outer stripe of the outer medulla. Although a pars convoluta and a pars recta have been described in the human kidney (619), the segmentation of the PT into three divisions has not been closely examined.

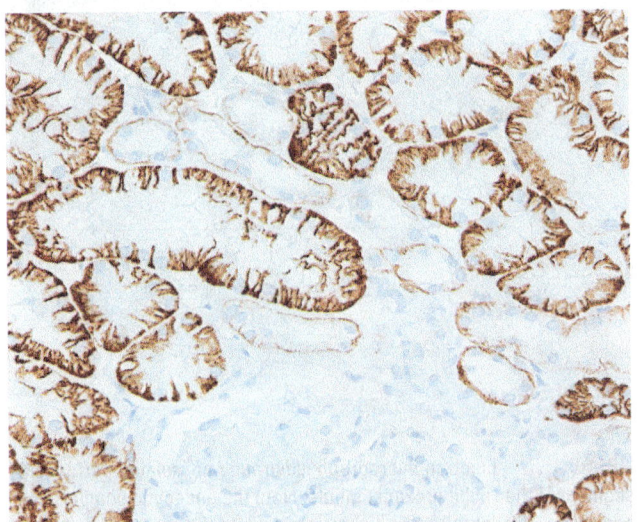

FIGURE 33.78 CD138 (syndecan-1) immunohistochemistry showing strong immunoreactivity in basolateral membranes and cytoplasm of proximal tubules and mild staining along basal aspects of distal tubules and collecting ducts. Glomeruli are negative (CD138 immunohistochemistry, ×400).

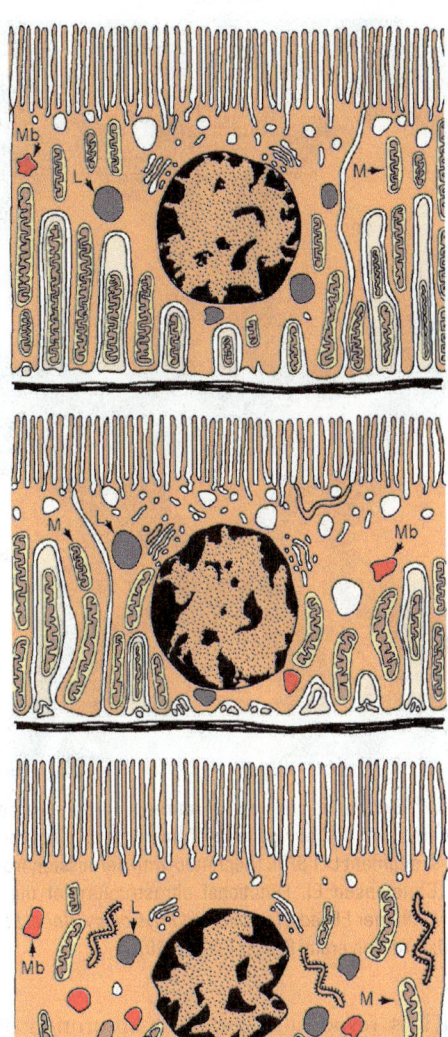

FIGURE 33.79 Schematic diagram of the three segments of the proximal tubule: **upper**, S_1; **middle**, S_2; **lower**, S_3. The prominent basolateral processes are lined with mitochondria. The interdigitating cellular processes that come from adjacent cells are shaded lighter (*Mb*, microbody; *M*, mitochondrion; *L*, lysosome). (Modified with permission from Maunsbach AB, Christensen EI. Functional ultrastructure of the proximal tubule. In: Windhager EE, ed. *Handbook of Physiology. Renal Physiology.* New York: Oxford University Press; 1992:41–107.)

The cells in the S_1 segment have a tall brush border, a well-developed endocytic lysosomal apparatus, numerous elongated mitochondria, and extensive basolateral invaginations and interdigitations. The cells in the S_2 segment are similar to those in the S_1 segment; however, the brush border is shorter, and the endocytic organelles, mitochondria, and basolateral invaginations and interdigitations are less prominent (Fig. 33.80). The cells in the S_3 segment are more cuboidal and have relatively fewer endocytic organelles, small mitochondria, and inconspicuous membrane invaginations and interdigitations. The length of the brush border in the S_3 segment varies among species, but it appears shorter in humans.

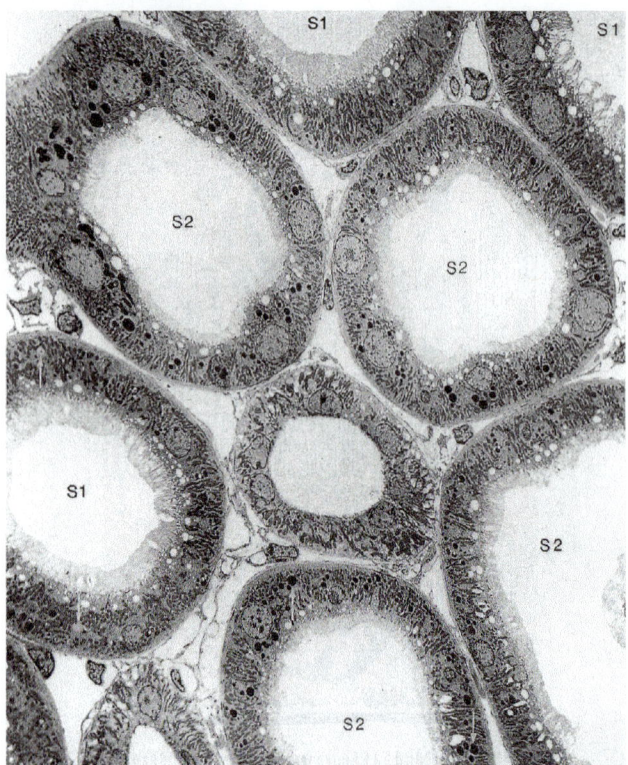

FIGURE 33.80 Electron micrograph of rat renal cortex. The cells in the S_1 segment are taller and have a more prominent brush border than the cells in the S_2 segment (×1,870). (Reprinted with permission from Maunsbach AB, Christensen EI. Functional ultrastructure of the proximal tubule. In: Windhager EE, ed. *Handbook of Physiology. Renal Physiology.* New York: Oxford University Press; 1992:41–107.)

The PT is responsible for the reabsorption of about 65% of the filtered water, sodium, chloride, potassium, and other solutes. The reabsorption of chloride, bicarbonate, glucose, amino acids, and fluid is coupled to the active transport of sodium (620). An excellent correlation exists along the length of the PT between the elaborately developed basolateral membrane expressed as surface area (Fig. 33.81), the high Na$^+$/K$^+$-ATPase activities that are localized to the basolateral membrane, and the capacity to transport sodium and ions (621,622). The α1β2 heterodimer is the main Na$^+$/K$^+$-ATPase isozyme of the kidney but the α2- and α3-isoforms have been detected (623,624). This sodium pump-mediated active transport of Na$^+$ out of the cell across the basolateral membrane establishes a lumen-to-cell concentration gradient for Na$^+$. The transport of Na$^+$ from the lumen into the PT cell, down its concentration gradient, is mediated by the Na$^+$/H$^+$ exchanger, NHE3, expressed in the brush border (625,626). NHE3 in response to angiotensin II traffics into the brush border microvilli, where it likely increases sodium intake (627). Reabsorption of chloride, bicarbonate, glucose, amino acids, and fluid is coupled to sodium transport. The numerous mitochondria located in close proximity to the plasma membrane provide a source for the cellular energy required for active transport. Although the mitochondria appear as isolated organelles, three-dimensional electron microscopic studies have demonstrated that they are actually connected with extensive branching (628). In general, the intrinsic rates at which fluid and solutes are transported decrease along the PT from S_1 to S_3. The discovery of the aquaporins, a family of water channel proteins, has enhanced our understanding of the kidney's role as the primary organ that regulates water balance (629,630). Aquaporin-1, AQP1, abundant in both the apical and basolateral membranes of the PT, mediates osmotic water permeability in this segment (631,632).

The well-developed endocytic-lysosomal apparatus in the PT (Fig. 33.82) plays an important role in reabsorption

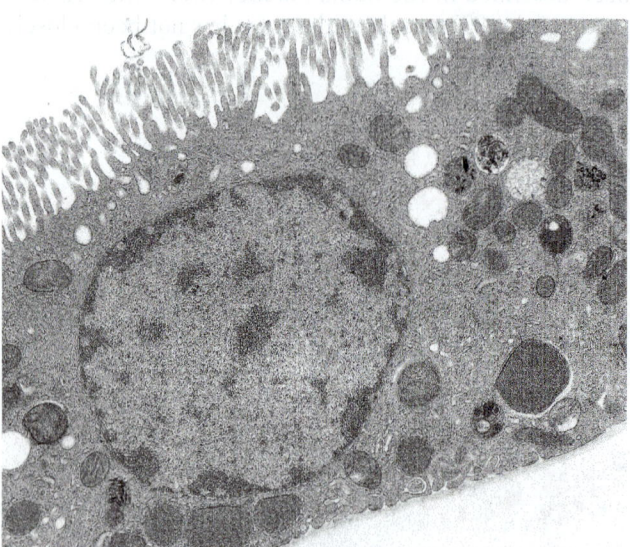

FIGURE 33.82 Electron micrograph illustrating an isolated perfused S_2 segment of the rabbit proximal tubule. Note the endocytic compartment consisting of coated pits and vesicles, apical tubules, small endocytic vesicles, and larger endocytic vacuoles. The lysosomes are heterogeneous and contain electron-dense material. The mitochondria are numerous (×15,000). (Reprinted with permission from Clapp WL, Park CH, Madsen KM, et al. Axial heterogeneity in the handling of albumin by the rabbit proximal tubule. *Lab Invest* 1988;58:549–558.)

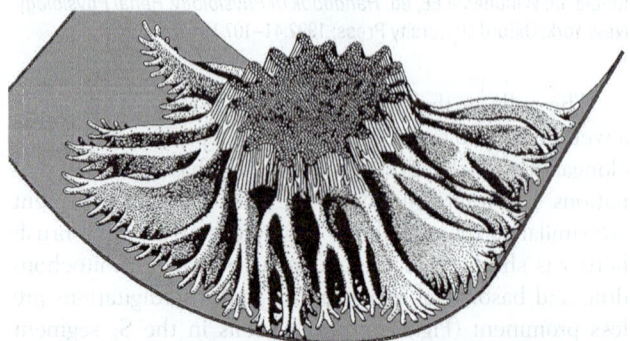

FIGURE 33.81 Three-dimensional schematic drawing of the proximal convoluted tubule illustrating the complex basal and lateral cellular processes that interdigitate with those from adjacent cells. (Modified with permission from Welling LW, Welling DJ. Shape of epithelial cells and intercellular channels in the rabbit proximal nephron. *Kidney Int* 1976;9:385–394.)

and degradation of albumin and low–molecular-weight proteins filtered by the glomerulus (633). This apparatus includes clathrin-coated pits, small vesicles, variable-sized endosomes, apical dense tubules, and lysosomes. Proteins are absorbed by endocytosis and transferred through the endosomal compartment to the lysosomes, where they are degraded. This is a selective process dependent upon the size and charge of the protein molecule (634–636). The capacity for protein degradation decreases from the S_1 to the S_3 segment (637). Upon exposure to an acidic environment in the endosomes (638), the internalized ligand–receptor complexes are segregated and the receptors are recycled back to the luminal membrane via small vacuolar structures, termed apical dense tubules (639). The apical dense tubules form an intricate anastomosing network in the apical cytoplasm. Megalin and cubilin are multiligand, endocytic receptors expressed throughout the endocytic apparatus of the PT (640). The receptors function independently but also interact as a dual complex to facilitate the uptake of albumin (641), as well as numerous ligands, including low–molecular-weight proteins, vitamin-binding proteins, hormones, lipoproteins, and drugs (642). Certain aspects of proximal tubular handling of albumin are controversial. These involve studies suggesting that normally, large amounts of filtered albumin undergo transcytosis in the PT and is recycled intact to the blood versus the pathway that normally small amounts of filtered albumin undergo megalin/cubilin mediated uptake leading to lysosomal degradation of albumin within the PT cells (643–645).

In autophagy, cytoplasmic material is sequestered in a double-membrane structure, the autophagosome, which fuses with lysosomes, resulting in degradation of the enclosed material.

Autophagic structures are often observed in proximal tubular cells and are important for normal tubule homeostasis. Moreover, studies indicate autophagy in PTs has a protective role against acute kidney injury (646).

The normal adult kidney has a relatively low rate of cell turnover with little proliferation (647–649). However, renal cell proliferation is accelerated during hypertrophy and following injury. Histologic assessment of cell proliferation can be made by determining a mitotic index or immunostaining with an antibody that detects proteins present during the cell cycle (650). During recovery after tubular injury, such as ischemia or toxin exposure, cell proliferation in tubular cells, especially in the PT, increases markedly (Fig. 33.83) (651,652). Recent studies have addressed whether reparative tubular cells arise from a pre-existing intratubular stem cell population or if fully differentiated tubular cells dedifferentiate and then proliferate to replace injured neighboring cells. A population of CD24- and CD133-positive cells have been described scattered throughout the PT (653). These scattered tubular cells (STCs) are not conspicuous, are smaller, have fewer mitochondria and no brush border compared to

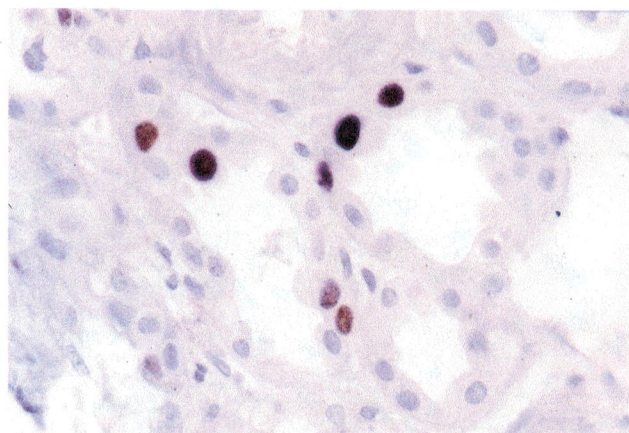

FIGURE 33.83 Biopsy of kidney allograft with cyclosporin A toxicity. Normally there is sparse labeling for Ki-67, a nuclear protein expressed by proliferating cells. In this example, there is a prominent increase in labeling of the tubular nuclei (Ki-67 immunohistochemistry, ×210).

surrounding cells. Experimental genetic labeling studies indicate that the STCs are not a fixed stem cell population but represent terminally differentiated cells that undergo dedifferentiation and express putative stem cell markers (654–656). Apoptosis has been documented in the adult kidney during the repair response to various forms of tubular injury, including ischemia, toxic insults, and hydronephrosis (Fig. 33.84) (657–660).

THIN LIMBS OF HENLE LOOP

The transition of the thin limbs of Henle loop with other nephron segments marks the borders between certain zones of the kidney (Fig. 33.34). Between the outer and inner stripes of the outer medulla, there is an abrupt transition from the PT to the DTL of Henle loop. Short-looped nephrons have only a short DTL located in the inner stripe of the

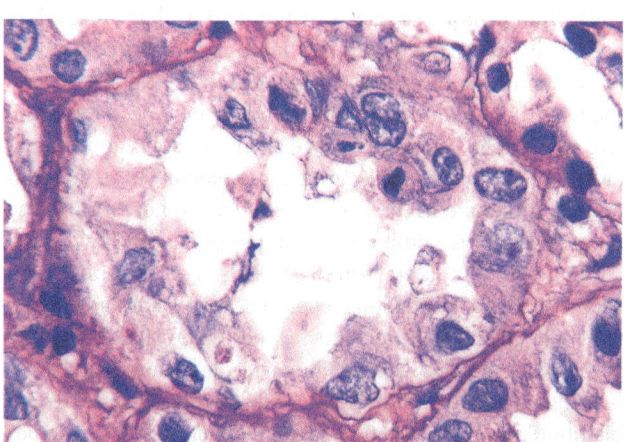

FIGURE 33.84 Micrograph from same case as in Figure 33.83. Several apoptotic nuclei are present (1 to 2 o'clock positions) in the tubular epithelium (PAS, ×400).

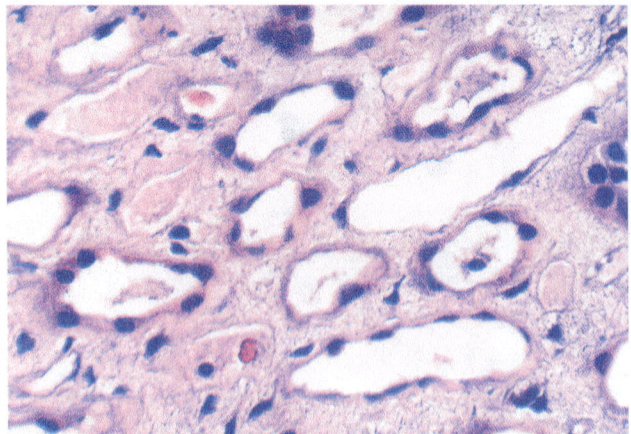

FIGURE 33.85 Several thin limbs of Henle are depicted in the center of the light micrograph. The lining epithelium is extremely attenuated, and the nuclei protrude into the lumens (H&E, ×200).

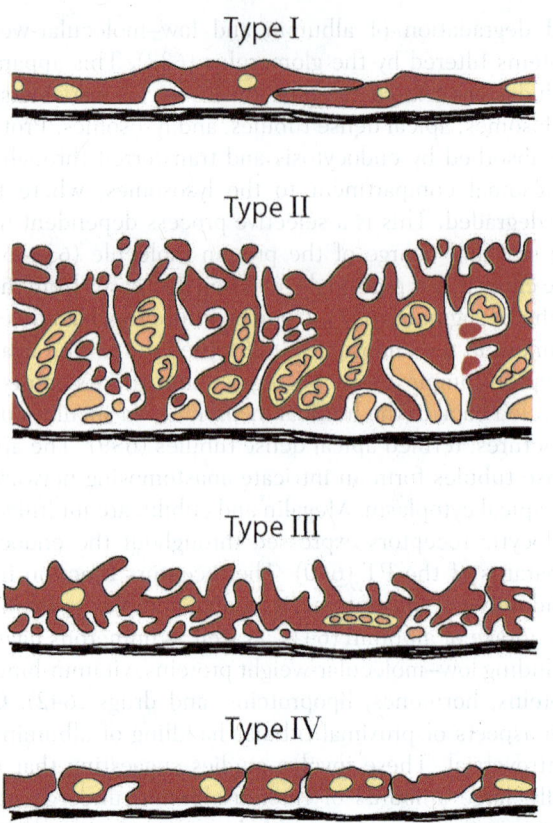

FIGURE 33.86 Schematic drawing of the four types of epithelium in the thin limbs of Henle loop. (The interdigitating cellular processes that come from adjacent cells are shaded lighter.) (Modified with permission from Madsen KM, Tisher CC. Anatomy of the kidney. In: Brenner BM, ed. *Brenner and Rector's The Kidney*. 7th ed. Philadelphia, PA: WB Saunders; 2004:3–72. Copyright © 2004 Elsevier.)

outer medulla. Near the hairpin turn of the short loop, the DTL continues into the TAL. Long-looped nephrons have both a long DTL and a long ATL. The long DTL traverses the inner stripe of the outer medulla and enters the inner medulla, whereas the long ATL resides entirely within the inner medulla. At the border between the outer and inner medulla, the long ATL continues into the TAL. Nephrons originating in the extreme outer cortex have short loops that remain in the cortex and do not reach the medulla.

By light microscopy, the thin limb is lined with a flat, simple epithelium about 1 to 2 μm thick (Fig. 33.85). The lenticularly shaped nucleus bulges slightly into the lumen. Four types of epithelium have been described in the thin limb in several mammals (Fig. 33.86) (372,661). It is not known if four types exist in humans, but at least two different types of epithelium have been demonstrated (662). Type I is present in the DTL of short-looped nephrons. It is an extremely thin, simple epithelium with few cellular interdigitations and cell organelles. Type II epithelium lines the initial part of the DTL of long-looped nephrons located in the outer medulla. This epithelium exhibits species variation and is characterized by taller cells, short microvilli, and more prominent cell organelles than in the other epithelial types. In the rat and mouse the type II epithelium is complex and characterized by extensive lateral interdigitations, whereas in the rabbit and human kidney the interdigitations are less prominent (372). Type III epithelium, found in the DTL of long-looped nephrons in the inner medulla, is composed of simple cells with few organelles and without lateral interdigitations. Type IV epithelium forms the bends of the long loops and lines the entire ATL in the inner medulla. It is characterized by low, flattened cells with few organelles and no microvilli, but abundant lateral interdigitations. In summary, these distinct epithelia types are distributed as follows: type I in the DTL of short loops, types II and III in the DTL of long loops, and type IV in the ATL of long loops. Thin limb epithelium has been reported to be immunoreactive for keratins 7, 8, 18, and 19 (532,533).

The thin limb of Henle loop plays an important role in urinary concentration, a complex process which is not yet fully understood. Physiologic studies have demonstrated that the DTL is permeable to water but has low permeability to sodium chloride, whereas the thin ascending limb is largely impermeable to water but has a high permeability to sodium chloride (372,663). These physiologic investigations are supported by immunohistochemical studies (631,664,665). The aquaporin water channel protein AQP1 mediates water permeability and is expressed in the DTL, primarily of long loops, but is absent in ATLs. The urea transporter UT-A2, which mediates urea secretion into the loop, is expressed in specific segmental patterns in DTLs. The kidney-specific chloride channel C1C-K1 is expressed exclusively in the ATL (666,667). Mice as well as humans lacking AQP1 (668,669) and mice deficient for C1C-K1 (670) have impaired urine concentrating ability. In the passive model proposed by Kokko and Rector (671) and Stephenson (672), a hypertonic medullary interstitium concentrates sodium chloride in the DTL by extraction of water. The fluid that then enters the ATL has a higher sodium chloride concentration, resulting in passive salt absorption and dilution of the fluid of the ATL. The morphologic features of a simple epithelium with few organelles in the ATL are consistent with the lack of demonstrable active transport in this segment. Urea secreted into the DTL is returned to the collecting ducts where it is reabsorbed. Thus, urea is recycled. Thus, the thin limb contributes to the maintenance of a hypertonic medullary interstitium and delivers a dilute fluid to more distal segments.

The inner stripe of the outer medulla and the outer aspect of the inner medulla display a complex tubulovascular organization (673–675). Both the outer medulla (inner stripe) and the inner medulla (outer) contain two distinct topographic regions: the vascular bundle and the collecting duct (CD) cluster regions. The vascular bundles, containing the DVR and AVR, surround the CD cluster region, which contain the collecting ducts, ATLs, some aquaporin-1 negative DTLs, and a peritubular capillary bed. Some aquaporin-1 positive DTLs enter the vascular bundle region of the inner medulla but not the outer medulla. A detailed understanding of the role of this complex architecture in supporting the steep corticomedullary osmolality gradient required for urinary concentration remains to be determined.

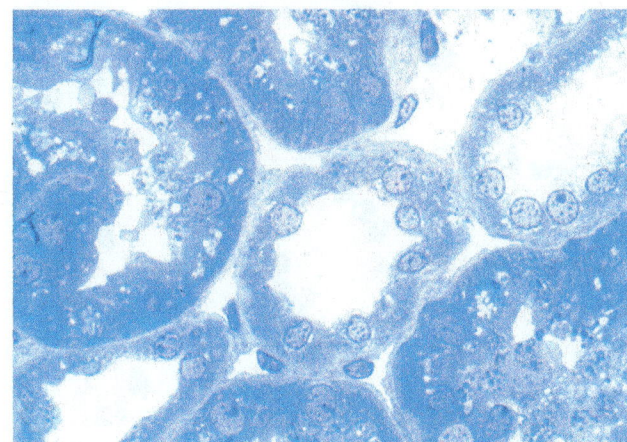

FIGURE 33.87 Light micrograph demonstrating a cross section of a TAL in the center. There is no brush border, and the cells are lower than the adjacent proximal tubular cells (toluidine blue-stained, 1-μm Epon section, ×750).

DISTAL TUBULE

The distal tubule consists of three distinct segments: The TAL of Henle loop, the MD, and the DCT (Fig. 33.34). The lengths of these three segments varies among species. The MD, as previously discussed (see JGA), is a specialized plaque of cells within the TAL. The TAL in the cortex extends beyond the MD before it joins the DCT. Sometimes, the term "distal tubules" is used informally and not precisely to refer to all nephron segments beyond the thin limbs of Henle loop.

Thick Ascending Limb

In short-looped nephrons, the transition from the DTL to the TAL occurs before the hairpin turn. In long-looped nephrons, the transition from the thin ascending limb to the TAL marks the border between the inner medulla and the inner stripe of the outer medulla. The TAL can be divided into a medullary (MTAL) and a cortical segment (CTAL). The ratio of medullary to cortical TAL for an individual nephron depends on the nephron origin. Juxtamedullary nephrons contain mainly MTALs, whereas superficial cortical nephrons contain mainly CTALs. The cells are eosinophilic and cuboidal, and the round nucleus tends to be located in the apical region and causes a bulge of the cell into the lumen (Fig. 33.87). Similar to the PT cells, the cells of the TAL have indistinct lateral cell borders because of elaborate basolateral membrane invaginations and interdigitations. They also have cytoplasmic basal striations because of elongated mitochondria. These morphologic features are characteristic for epithelial cells involved in active transport. However, in contrast to the PT, the cells are lower and less eosinophilic and there is no brush border in the TAL. As the TAL ascends into the cortex, there is a gradual decrease in cell height, basolateral membrane area, and size of the mitochondria (676). SEM has shown two luminal surface configurations of cells in the TAL (677). Cells with a relatively smooth surface are most commonly found in the medullary segment, whereas cells with a rough surface due to luminal microprojections and apical lateral membrane invaginations predominate in the cortical segment. The functional significance of these structural findings remains unexplained. The CTAL continues into the DCT just beyond the MD. The cells of the TAL synthesize Tamm–Horsfall protein and secrete it into the tubular lumen (591). This segment expresses keratins 8 and 18 (531,533,613), and also kidney-specific (Ksp)-cadherin (678).

An important function of the TAL is the active reabsorption of sodium chloride. There is a correlation between structure and function in the ascending limb. The basolateral membrane surface area, mitochondrial density, and the Na^+/K^+-ATPase activity are all greater in the medullary segment than in the cortical segment of the TAL (620,676,679). The reabsorption of sodium chloride in both the medullary and cortical segments of the TAL is driven by the basolateral Na^+/K^+-ATPase creating a favorable electrochemical gradient. Entry of sodium chloride across the apical membrane is mediated by the $Na^+/K^+/2Cl^-$ cotransporter (NKCC2), which localizes to the TAL apical plasma membrane (680). NKCC2 is the target of loop diuretics, such as furosemide. This reabsorption of salt coupled with the water impermeability of the TAL results in a hypertonic interstitium and delivery of a hypotonic fluid to more distal tubular segments.

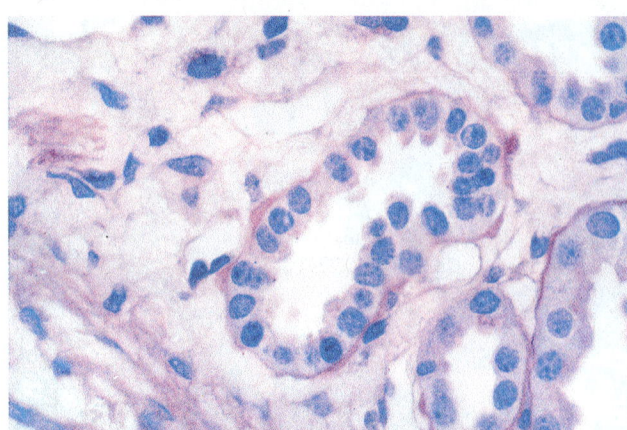

FIGURE 33.88 Light micrograph showing a DCT. Note the absence of a brush border and the nuclei situated close to the lumen (PAS, ×630).

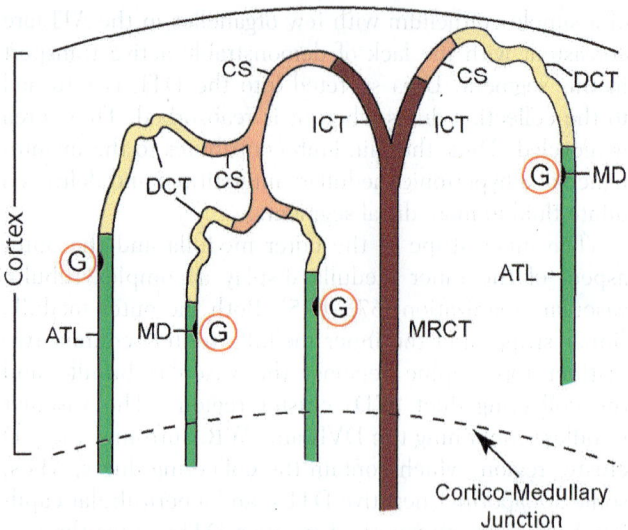

FIGURE 33.89 Diagram of the various anatomic arrangements of the distal tubule connecting to the cortical collecting duct in superficial, midcortical, and juxtamedullary nephrons. (*G*, glomerulus; *ATL*, ascending thick limb [of Henle]; *MD*, macula densa; *DCT*, distal convoluted tubule; *CS*, connecting segment; *ICT*, initial collecting tubule; *MRCT*, medullary ray collecting tubule).

Distal Convoluted Tubule

The DCT begins just beyond the MD in the cortex and represents the terminal part of the distal tubule. The cells of the DCT are similar to those of the TAL and contain numerous mitochondria. DCT cells contain prominent basolateral membrane infoldings. However, the DCT cells are taller, characteristically have nuclei closer to the lumen, and lack lateral interdigitations in the apical region between adjacent cells (Fig. 33.88). The cells have a single cilium and small microprojections on the luminal surface. In comparison with the PT, the cells of the DCT are lower and less eosinophilic, have a less prominent apical endocytic apparatus, and lack a brush border. More nuclei are observed in a cross section than in the PT, and the lumen is normally open. The epithelium of the DCT shows immunoreactivity for keratins 8, 18, and 19 (532,613), and Ksp-cadherin (678).

The DCT has a higher level of Na^+/K^+-ATPase activity than any other tubular segment (679) and this correlates with the high mitochondrial density. Basolateral membrane Na^+/K^+-ATPase in the DCT drives solute and water reabsorption. Apical membrane transport of NaCl is mediated by the cotransporter NCC, which is the target of thiazide diuretics (681,682). The NCC cotransporter is distinct from the furosemide-sensitive cotransporter NKCC2, presents in the TAL. The DCT, similar to the TAL, is relatively impermeable to water but is responsible for the reabsorption of sodium chloride (683–685). Altered transport activity of upstream tubular segments such as the TAL results in increased NCC expression and sodium reabsorption in the DCT (686).

CONNECTING TUBULE

The CNT is a transitional segment that connects the DCT with the collecting duct system. In superficial nephrons, the CNT continues directly into an ICT (Fig. 33.89). In contrast, the CNTs of juxtamedullary nephrons and of many midcortical nephrons join to form an arcade that ascends in the cortex before draining into an ICT. In humans, most nephrons empty individually into ICTs (372). Fourteen percent of the nephrons are connected to arcades, and each arcade consists of about three nephron attachments (3). Each cortical collecting tubule receives an average of 11 nephrons (3). In superficial nephrons, the CNT is situated adjacent to the afferent arteriole of its parent glomerulus (687). Physiologic studies have shown that increased sodium reabsorption in the CNT is associated with dilatation of the adjacent afferent arteriole (688). This functional link has been called "connecting tubule glomerular feedback" (CTGF). It results in an increase in renal blood flow and GFR which favors sodium excretion.

In most species, including humans, the CNT contains different cell types resulting from an intermixing of cells from the adjacent DCT and CCD (689). However, the CNT cell is the most characteristic cell type of this transitional segment. It occurs only in this segment. They display ultrastructural features intermediate between the DCT cells and the principal cells of the CCD, and contain true infoldings of the basal cell membrane (690). Various types of intercalated cells, similar to those in the CCD, are also present in the CS and are likely involved in tubular acid–base regulation. Three types of intercalated cells, type A, type B, and non A–non B are found in the CNT. In several species, the non A–non B intercalated cell is the most prevalent. The intercalated cells will be discussed further in the collecting duct section. The CNT is an important site of sodium reabsorption, potassium secretion, calcium reabsorption, and significant amounts of water transport. Proteins in the CNT mediating these transport function include the sodium channel, ENaC, potassium channel ROMK, Na+/Ca2+ exchanger, Ca2+-ATPase, calcium channel TRPV5, and aquaporin-2 (AQP2) (691–695).

COLLECTING DUCT

The collecting duct begins in the cortex and descends to the tip of the papilla, also called the area cribrosa, where the inner medullary segments terminate as the ducts of Bellini. These terminal collecting duct segments were apparently described by Eustachio nearly 100 years before the observation of Bellini (696). During its course, there is an increase in diameter from the cortical portion to the terminal segments at the area cribrosa. The collecting duct can be divided into the CCD, OMCD, and IMCD. Significant cellular heterogeneity exists along the collecting duct. Although there is a degree of nonspecificity, the lectins *Dolichos biflorus* and *Arachis hypogaea* have been used as markers for collecting duct epithelium (Fig. 33.90) (611). The distal tubules and collecting ducts show variable but generally more intense staining for keratins than the PTs (Figs. 33.91 and 33.92). Keratins 8, 18, and 19 are prominently expressed throughout the CCD and MCD (532,533,613). There is also staining for keratin 7. Scattered keratin 7- and 19-negative cells have been observed to be intercalated cells (532). Keratins 5/6, 17, and 20 as well as vimentin are restricted primarily to MCDs (613). GATA3, a transcription factor, is strongly expressed throughout the entire collecting duct system (Fig. 33.93). There is less immunoreactivity for Ksp-cadherin in collecting ducts compared to the TALs and DCTs (678).

Cortical Collecting Duct

The CCD can be subdivided further into the ICT and the medullary ray portion. The latter is the main segment and it runs in parallel with the cortical PST and TAL in the medullary

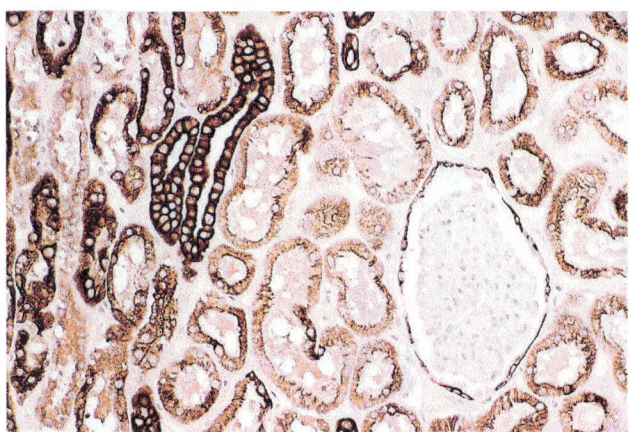

FIGURE 33.91 Distal tubules, collecting ducts, PTs, and parietal epithelium lining Bowman capsule showing expression of keratins. The distal tubules and collecting ducts label more intensely than do the PTs (CAM 5.2 immunohistochemistry, ×100).

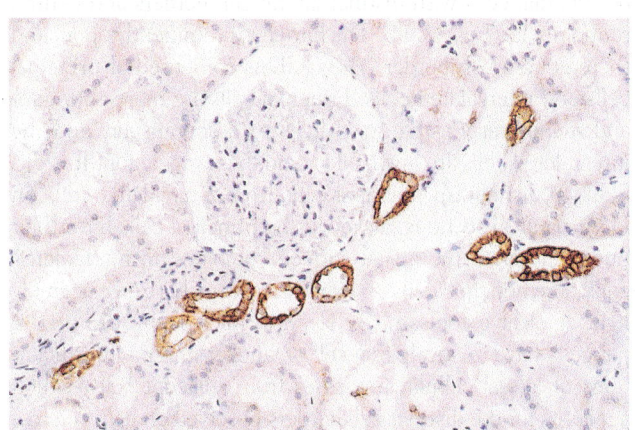

FIGURE 33.92 Detection of keratin expression varies depending on the specificity and dilution of the antibody. In this micrograph, there is prominent immunoreactivity of the distal tubules and collecting ducts (35βH11 immunoperoxidase, ×100).

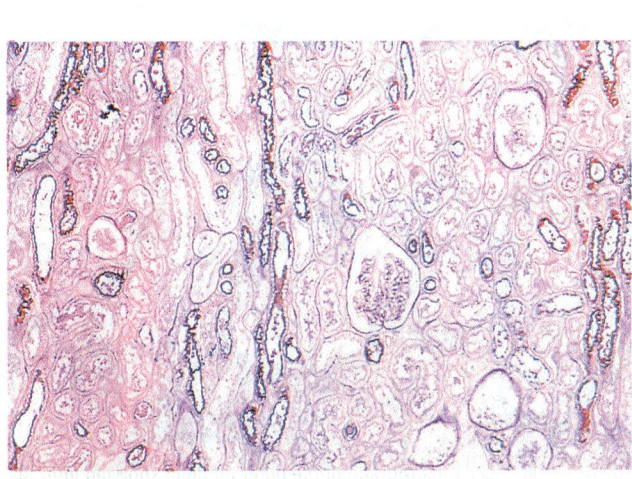

FIGURE 33.90 Staining of the collecting ducts and TALs with lectin *Arachis hypogaea*. The PTs and glomeruli are negative. (Courtesy of Dr. Randolf A. Hennigar.)

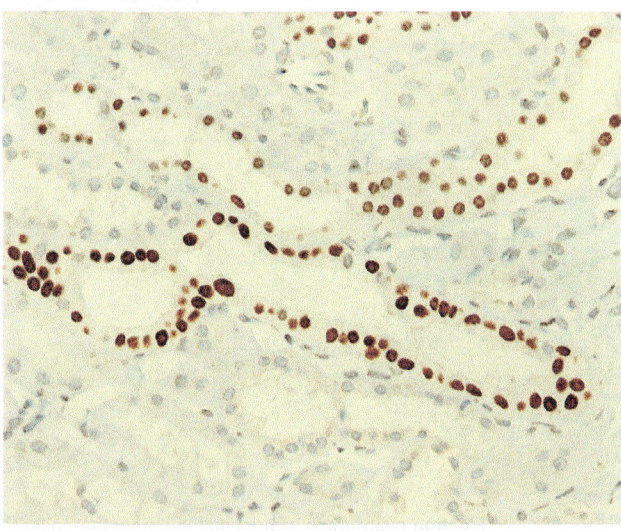

FIGURE 33.93 Elongated collecting ducts displaying positive nuclear immunoreactivity for GATA3. (GATA3 immunohistochemistry, ×400).

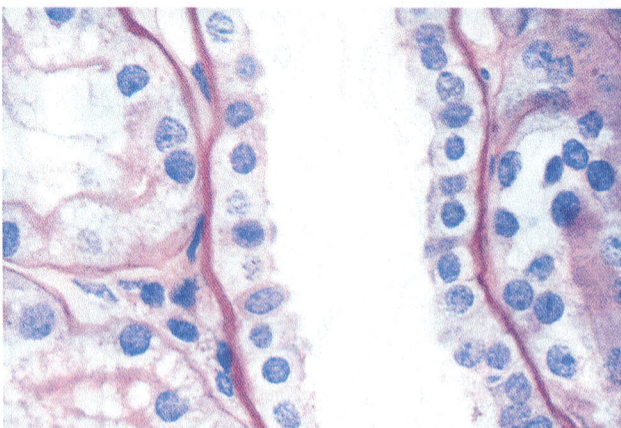

FIGURE 33.94 Micrograph illustrating a CCD. Note the distinct lateral cell orders (PAS, ×500).

ray. By light microscopy, the epithelium of the CCD consists of cuboidal cells with distinct lateral cell borders and central round nuclei (Fig. 33.94). The lumen is prominently open, and there is no brush border. The CCD is composed of principal cells and intercalated cells. Principal cells are more abundant and mainly responsible for salt and water transport and the intercalated cells are involved in acid–base regulation. It is difficult to distinguish principal cells from intercalated cells on H&E paraffin sections, although the principal cells have their nuclei closer to the apical surface compared to intercalated cells. The principal cells on light microscopy have an extremely light or clear cytoplasm. By electron microscopy, the principal cells have relatively few cell organelles and no interdigitations of lateral cellular processes from adjacent cells, which accounts for the distinct cell borders observed on light microscopy (Fig. 33.95). However, there are prominent infoldings of the basal plasma membrane, which gives the basal region an accentuated clear appearance on light microscopy (697). The principal cell has a fairly smooth luminal surface with short microvilli and a single cilium by SEM (see Fig. 33.104).

Principal cells are involved in sodium reabsorption and potassium secretion. Sodium reabsorption is mediated by the amiloride-sensitive sodium channel, ENaC, located in the apical membrane of principal cells throughout the entire collecting duct (698,699). Experimental conditions of dietary potassium loading or mineralocorticoid stimulation have shown increases in potassium secretion and Na^+/K^+-ATPase activity in the CCD along with an increase in the surface area of the basolateral membrane of the principal cells (700–704). These findings indicate that the principal cells are involved in potassium secretion in the CCD. Potassium secretion is mediated largely by the apical membrane potassium channel, ROMK. The entire collecting duct becomes permeable to water in the presence of the antidiuretic hormone vasopressin. After vasopressin binds to its receptor on the basolateral membrane of principal cells (705) small apical cytoplasmic tubulovesicles, called aggrephores, containing the water channel AQP2 are shuttled to the apical membrane, which markedly increases water permeability (706,707). The presence of the water channels AQP3 and AQP4 in the basolateral membranes of principal cells facilitate the final exit of water into the interstitium (708,709).

The intercalated or "dark cells" are interspersed in the lining epithelia of the collecting duct. Although intercalated cells usually represent the minority cell type in epithelia where they are found, they constitute 30% to 40% of the cells in the CCD in some mammals (371). They are also present in the connecting segment, the OMCD and the initial portion of the IMCD. Intercalated cells may be identified on 1-μm thick toluidine blue-stained Epon sections by their densely staining cytoplasm and their often convex luminal surface covered with numerous microprojections (Fig. 33.96). The darkly staining cytoplasm is due

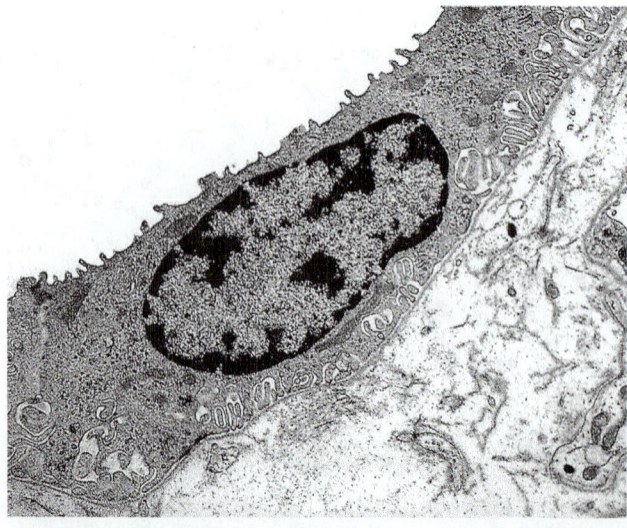

FIGURE 33.95 Electron micrograph of principal cell from the collecting duct. Note the relatively prominent infoldings of the basal plasma membrane (×12,500).

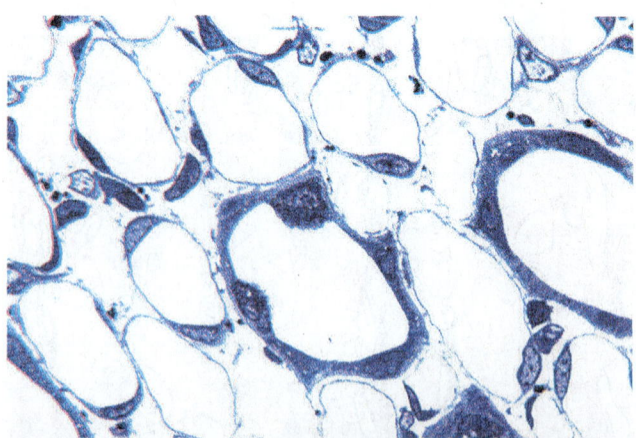

FIGURE 33.96 Light micrograph of the outer medulla showing intercalated cells in the collecting ducts. The intercalated cells exhibit a bulging apical surface covered with microprojections and dark-staining cytoplasm (1-μm toluidine blue-stained Epon section, ×160).

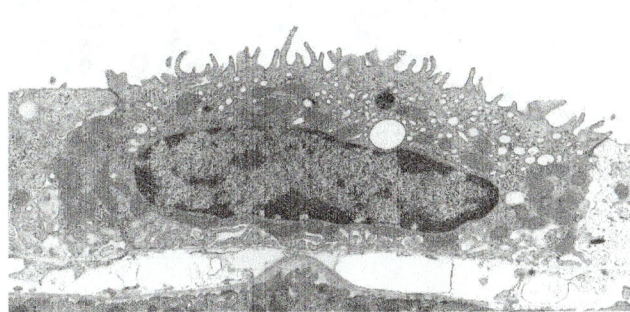

FIGURE 33.97 Electron micrograph of a type A intercalated cell in the CCD. Note the prominent tubulovesicular membrane compartment in the apical cytoplasm and the numerous microprojections on the luminal surface (×11,800; courtesy of Dr. Jill W. Verlander).

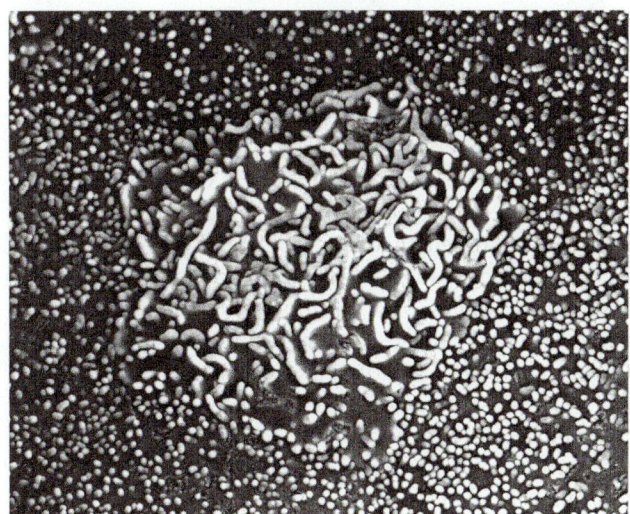

FIGURE 33.99 Scanning electron micrograph of the luminal surface of a type A intercalated cell in the CCD. The type A cell is well demarcated and has a large luminal surface covered primarily with microplicae but also microvilli (×15,000; courtesy of Dr. Jill W. Verlander).

in part to the presence of relative more organelles, especially mitochondria. Three distinct populations of intercalated cells, types A and B and non A–non B have been described in the CCD of mammals (710–713). On ultrastructural examination, the type A intercalated cells have prominent microprojections of the apical membrane and extensive tubulovesicular structures in the apical cytoplasm (Fig. 33.97). In comparison with the type A cells, the type B intercalated cells have a denser cytoplasm, more mitochondria, a smaller apical membrane area, a small number of microprojections on the apical surface, more spherical vesicular structures throughout the cytoplasm but fewer vesicles beneath the apical membrane, and a larger basolateral membrane surface area (Fig. 33.98). By SEM, the type A cells have a large convex luminal surface covered with numerous complex microprojections or small folds called microplicae (Fig. 33.99), whereas the type B cells display a small angular luminal surface with relatively small microvilli (Fig. 33.100) (711). The type B intercalated cells may be inconspicuous on SEM.

The non A–non B intercalated cells are primarily located in the CNT and the ICT. For example, they account for 40% to 50% of intercalated cells in the mouse connecting segment and initial collecting duct. The non A–non B intercalated cells are larger than type A and type B intercalated cells, have abundant mitochondria, and have prominent apical microprojections similar to those of type A cells. Compared to the type A and B intercalated cells, the nonA–nonB intercalated cells have been studied in fewer species, mainly the rat and the mouse. There are significant

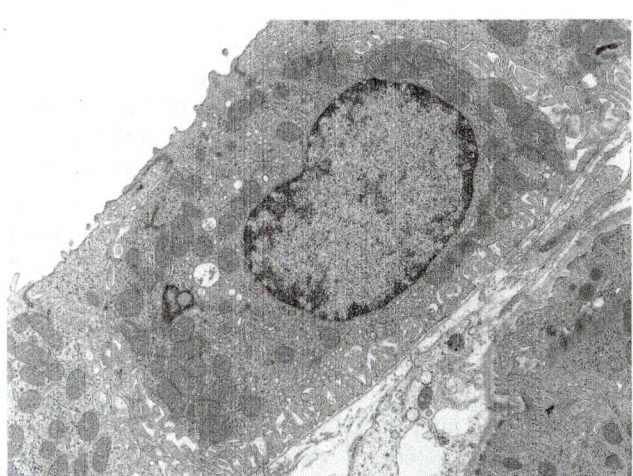

FIGURE 33.98 Electron micrograph of a type B intercalated cell in the CCD. There are numerous vesicles throughout the cytoplasm, and the basolateral membrane is prominent. Note the paucity of microprojections on the luminal surface. Compared to the type A intercalated cell, there are fewer vesicles beneath the apical membrane (×11,800; courtesy of Dr. Jill W. Verlander).

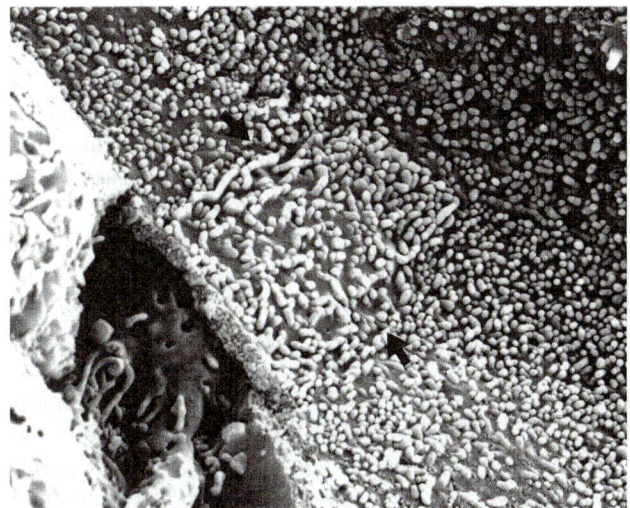

FIGURE 33.100 Scanning electron micrograph of the luminal surface of a CCD. A type B intercalated cell (arrows) displays a small angular luminal surface covered with short microprojections, mainly microvilli (×15,000; courtesy of Dr. Jill W. Verlander).

differences in the prevalence and distribution of the different types of intercalated cells throughout the connecting segment and CCD among mammalian species (371).

All intercalated cell subtypes are typified by their high levels of carbonic anhydrase type II, an enzyme that catalyzes the interconversion of CO_2 to HCO_3, consistent with their role in urine acidification (714). Physiologic studies have demonstrated that the CCD reabsorbs bicarbonate in acid-loaded animals (715) and secretes bicarbonate in alkali-loaded animals (716). In a study of experimental acute respiratory acidosis, there was a striking increase in the apical membrane surface area of the type A intercalated cells, whereas no morphologic changes were observed in the type B cells (711).

Studies have immunolocalized the vacuolar-type proton pump H^+-ATPase in the apical membrane (717–719) and the Cl^-/HCO_3^- exchanger, AE1, in the basolateral membrane (710,719–721) of type A intercalated cells. The AE1 protein is specific for the type A intercalated cell. Type A cells are responsible for H^+ secretion in the CCD. The immunolocalization of the H^+-ATPase to the basolateral membrane of type B intercalated cells (718,719) and the physiologic evidence for an apical Cl^-/HCO_3^- exchange in these cells (722) indicate that type B cells are involved in bicarbonate secretion. Apical Cl^-/HCO_3^- exchange in the type B cell is mediated by the protein pendrin, which immunolocalizes to the apical membrane and apical cytoplasmic vesicles of the B cell (133,723,724). Furthermore, the renal cortical expression of pendrin is increased in alkali-loaded animals and decreased in acid-loaded animals (725). Type B intercalated cells are most numerous in the CCD. Pendrin is not in the same protein family as AE1 (726). Mutations of the gene encoding pendrin result in Pendred syndrome, a disorder mainly associated with a thyroid goiter and deafness (727). The cell-specific ultrastructural features, distribution of the transporters and cell responses to physiologic changes have established that type A intercalated cells secrete acid whereas type B intercalated cells secrete base.

The non A–non B intercalated cells express pendrin in the apical membrane and cytoplasmic vesicles like type B intercalated cells but also express the H^+-ATPase in the apical membrane like type A intercalated cells (133,728). Thus, the types of intercalated cells may be defined by their cellular distribution of the H^+-ATPase and the presence or absence of the anion exchangers, AE1 and pendrin (729). Although the function of non A–non B intercalated cells is not well understood, they appear to have an important role in chloride reabsorption via pendrin-mediated apical Cl^-/HCO_3^- exchange (730,731). Pendrin expression in the CCD appears to be regulated by *Nedd4-2*, a E3 ubiquitin-protein ligase, which is highly expressed in type B and non A–non B cells (732).

Single-cell expression studies are increasing our understanding of the function of specific cell types. Single-cell RNA sequencing (scRNA-seq) has established thorough

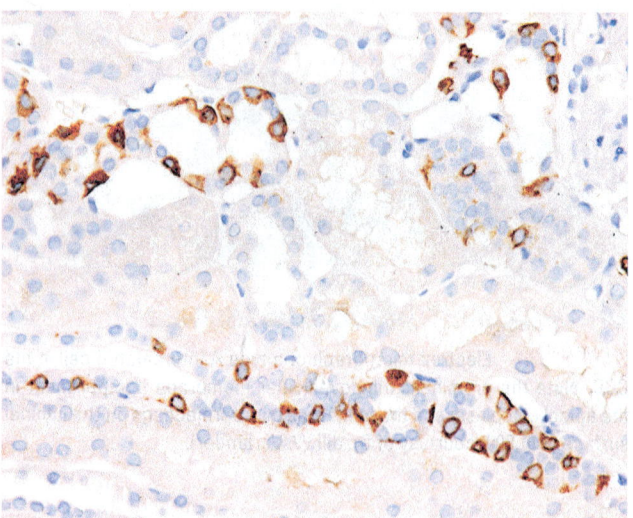

FIGURE 33.101 Type A intercalated cells along collecting ducts showing expression of c-Kit. (c-Kit immunohistochemistry ×400).

transcriptomes of type A and type B intercalated cells and principal cells in the mammalian collecting duct (733). In this study, the receptor tyrosine kinase c-Kit was expressed strongly in type A intercalated cells. This cell-specific expression of c-Kit can be demonstrated by immunohistochemistry (Fig. 33.101). Also, a small number of hybrid cells expressed both aquaporin-2 (principal cell marker) and either AE1 (type A intercalated cell marker) or pendrin (type B intercalated cell marker) were detected. Another single-cell expression investigation also found hybrid cells in the collecting duct expressing markers of both principal cells and intercalated cells (734). Moreover, it was shown that Notch signaling regulates a transition toward more principal cells and less intercalated cells, implying a phenotypic switch in the hybrid cells.

Outer Medullary Collecting Duct

The collecting duct traverses the outer medulla without receiving tributaries. Similar to the CCD, the OMCD contains principal cells and intercalated cells (Fig. 33.102). The principal cells in this segment are similar to those in the CCD but are taller and have fewer organelles and basal membrane infoldings. They also express apical membrane ENaC and AQP2 and basolateral Na^+/K^+-ATPase consistent with sodium and water reabsorption. The intercalated cells constitute 18% to 40% of the cells in the OMCD in some species and gradually decrease along this segment (735,736). The intercalated cells in the OMCD resemble the type A intercalated cells in the CCD but are taller and have a less dense cytoplasm. Type B and non A–non B intercalated cells are typically absent in the OMCD.

The OMCD plays a major role in urine acidification. An increase in the surface area of the apical plasma membrane of the type A intercalated cells in this segment has been demonstrated after hydrogen ion stimulation (737,738).

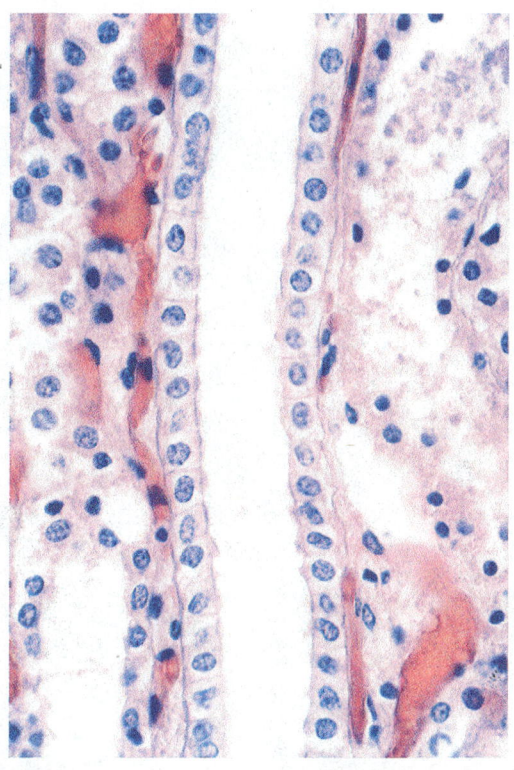

FIGURE 33.102 Light micrograph illustrating longitudinal section of an OMCD (H&E, ×250).

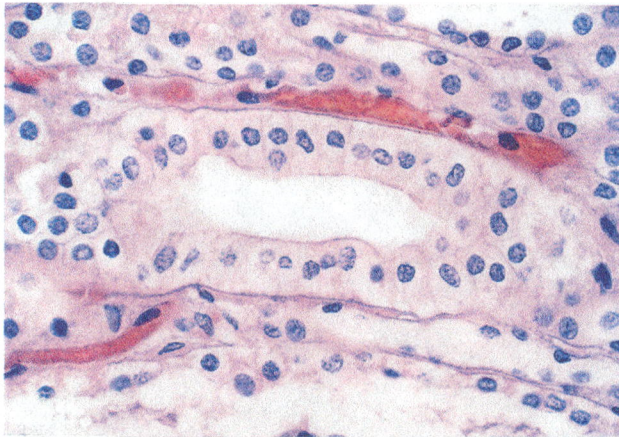

FIGURE 33.103 Micrograph illustrating columnar cells of the collecting duct in the inner medulla (H&E, ×500).

These type A cells with their apical and basolateral membranes containing the H^+-ATPase and the chloride/bicarbonate exchanger, AE1, respectively are responsible for hydrogen ion secretion (717,721). The OMCD is also an important segment for potassium reabsorption, especially during dietary potassium restriction. This is mediated by both the gastric H^+/K^+-ATPase α1 and colonic H^+/K^+-ATPase α2 isoforms in the apical membrane of the type A intercalated cells (739–743).

Ammonia metabolism plays an important role in acid–base homeostasis. Most of the ammonia secretion is handled by the collecting duct (744). Rhesus (Rh) transporters Rhbg and Rhcg, mainly expressed in type A intercalated cells throughout the collecting duct, mediate renal ammonia secretion. Type B intercalated cells do not express the Rh transporters.

Inner Medullary Collecting Duct

The IMCD represents the terminal portion of the collecting duct. Although the IMCD is often called the papillary collecting duct, only the inner two-thirds of the IMCD are located in the papilla. Descending through the inner medulla, the collecting ducts join in successive fusions, which result in an arborescent architectural arrangement. There is a significant increase in diameter and height of the epithelium as the ducts descend (745). The height of the cells increases gradually from cuboidal to columnar (Fig. 33.103). However, in the terminal portion of the human inner medulla there is often an abrupt transition between collecting ducts lined with cuboidal cells and the ducts of Bellini, which are composed of tall columnar cells.

Structural and functional heterogeneity exists along the IMCD (745). It can be subdivided arbitrarily into three portions: the outer third ($IMCD_1$), middle third ($IMCD_2$), and inner third ($IMCD_3$). However, there is physiologic evidence for the division of the IMCD into two functionally distinct segments, which are termed initial IMCD and terminal IMCD (746,747). The initial IMCD is the outer segment and mainly corresponds to the $IMCD_1$, whereas the terminal IMCD includes most of the $IMCD_2$ and the $IMCD_3$. The initial IMCD consists mainly of cells that are similar in structure to the principal cells in the OMCD. In the rat, intercalated cells, similar to the type A intercalated cells in the OMCD, comprise approximately 10% of the cells in the initial IMCD (Fig. 33.104) (748). Intercalated cells are rare to absent in the initial IMCD of the human (689) and rabbit (735). The terminal IMCD is composed of mainly one cell type, the IMCD cell. Compared with principal cells, the IMCD cells are taller and have small stubby apical microprojections, lighter staining cytoplasm containing numerous ribosomes, small lysosomes in the basal cytoplasm, fewer infoldings of the basal plasma membrane but prominent lateral membrane infoldings (Fig. 33.105) (749). By SEM, the IMCD cells display more numerous small microvilli and lack the central cilium characteristic of principal cells (Fig. 33.106). In fact, only two epithelia cells in the kidney, IMCD cells and intercalated cells, have no central cilium.

The IMCD has an important role in urinary concentration. The reabsorption of urea and water in this segment causes the formation of concentrated urine. Physiologic studies demonstrated that urea and water permeabilities are low in the initial IMCD and relatively high in the terminal IMCD (746,747). Water permeability is increased by

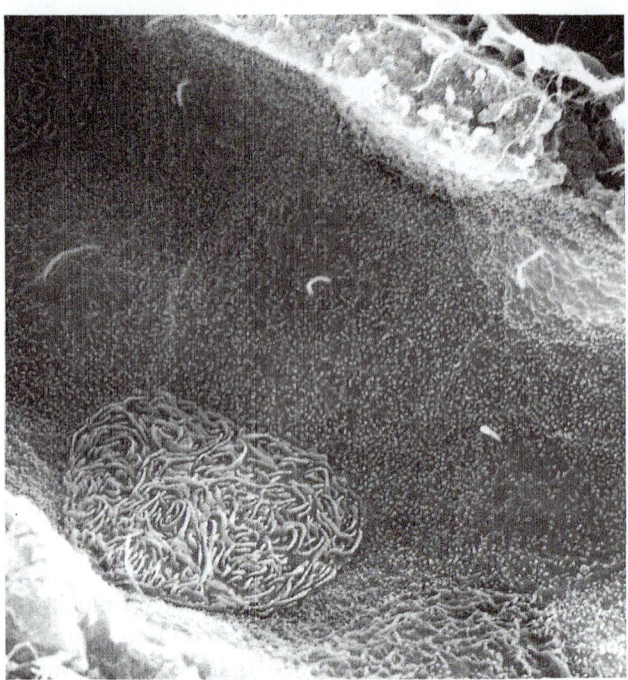

FIGURE 33.104 Scanning electron micrograph of the IMCD. The intercalated cell is round and exhibits a convex luminal surface covered with microplicae without cilia. The adjacent principal cells are characterized by short microvilli and a single central cilium on their luminal surface (×12,000). (Reprinted with permission from Clapp WL, Madsen KM, Verlander JW, et al. Morphologic heterogeneity along the rat inner medullary collecting duct. *Lab Invest* 1989;60:219–230.)

vasopressin in both subsegments and is mediated by the aquaporin water channel AQP2 present in the apical membrane of the IMCD cells (706). Vasopressin increases urea permeability only in the terminal IMCD. The urea transporters UT-A1 and UT-A3, present in IMCD cells (not in principal cells in the initial IMCD) mediate urea transport in the terminal IMCD (750–752). Although less studied, there is evidence that the IMCD is also involved in urine acidification. Acid secretion mediated by a H^+/K^+-ATPase has been demonstrated in isolated perfused segments from this region (753).

PAPILLARY SURFACE EPITHELIUM

A layer of cuboidal epithelium lines the external surface of the renal papilla. These cells have a relatively smooth surface but with glycocalyx, cytoplasmic vesicles, and few mitochondria. (754,755). They lack the luminal asymmetric unit membrane typical of transitional epithelium. Various proteins including UT-B1, H^+/K^+-ATPase, and osteopontin have been localized to the papillary surface epithelium, which support studies indicating urea transport, acid secretion, and inhibition of crystal deposition in this epithelium (756–758). In antidiuresis, widely dilated intercellular

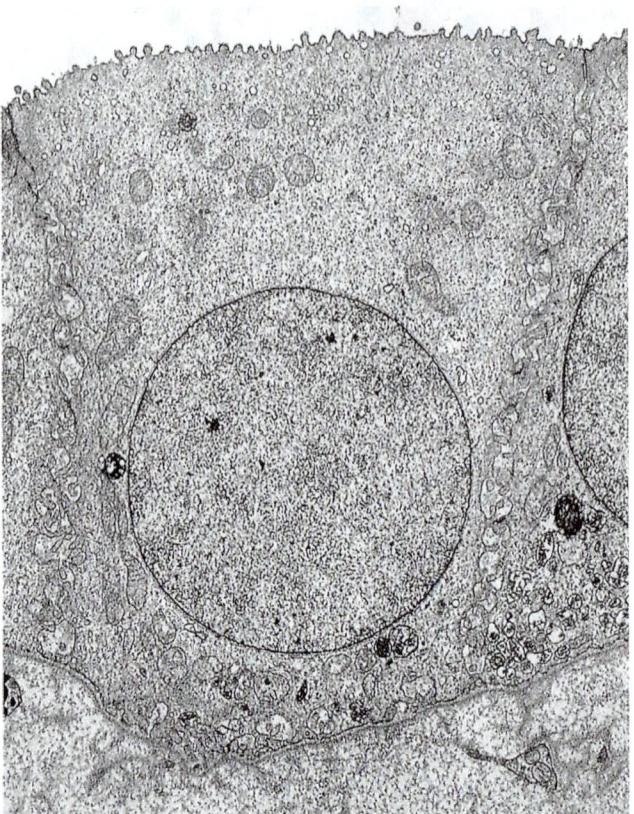

FIGURE 33.105 Electron micrograph of an IMCD cell. The cell is tall, has extensive lateral membranes, and exhibits small stubby microvilli. Infoldings of the basal plasma membrane are not prominent (×12,500). (Reprinted with permission from Clapp WL, Madsen KM, Verlander JW, et al. Morphologic heterogeneity along the rat inner medullary collecting duct. *Lab Invest* 1989;60:219–230.)

spaces have been observed in the papillary epithelium, suggesting significant fluid movement (759).

INTERSTITIUM

The renal interstitium, a complex space between the parenchymal components of both the cortex and medulla, includes extracellular matrix, several types of interstitial cells, lymphatics, and nerves (760,761). In humans, estimates of the relative cortical interstitial volume range from 5% to 20%, with a mean of 12% (390,762,763). A significant increase with age has been reported (763). The relative volume of the renal interstitium increases from the cortex to the tip of the papilla. The interstitial volume has been reported from 10% to 20% in the outer medulla to approximately 30% to 40% at the papillary tip in some species (764).

The interstitium in both the cortex and medulla may be divided into different compartments (760). The cortical interstitium includes the periarterial connective tissue and

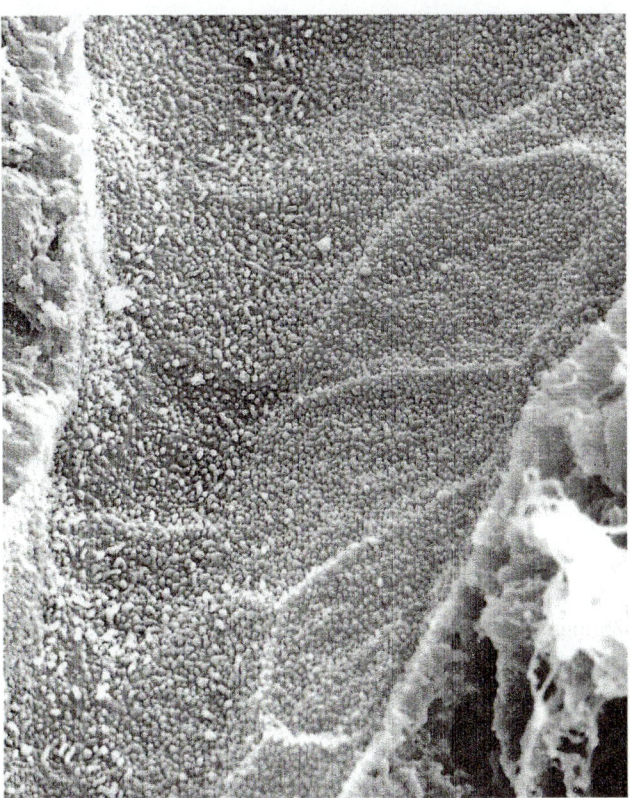

FIGURE 33.106 Scanning electron micrograph of the terminal IMCD. The entire luminal surface of the IMCD cells is covered with abundant short microvilli. There is an absence of cilia (×12,500). (Reprinted with permission from Clapp WL, Madsen KM, Verlander JW, et al. Morphologic heterogeneity along the rat inner medullary collecting duct. *Lab Invest* 1989;60:219–230.)

the peritubular interstitium. The periarterial connective tissue constitutes a loose sheath around the intrarenal arteries and contains the lymphatic vessels and nerves. The sheath communicates with the peritubular interstitium. It should not be overinterpreted as representing focal interstitial fibrosis in the cortex. The peritubular interstitium includes the spaces between the glomeruli, tubules, and peritubular capillaries. In the normal cortex, it is inconspicuous on light microscopy, and the tubules and capillaries often have a back-to-back architectural appearance (Fig. 33.107). In the medulla, interstitial spaces include a narrow zone in the outer stripe of the outer medulla, the interbundle region of the inner stripe, and the expansive inner medulla. This appreciable amount of interstitium in the medulla should not be mistaken for interstitial fibrosis by the pathologist. The extracellular matrix of the interstitium consists of fibrils within a ground substance (760,761,765). It contains sulfated and nonsulfated glycosaminoglycans, fibronectin, laminin, interstitial collagens (types I, III, VI), and microfibrils.

Various types of fibroblasts, pericytes, and immune cells, including dendritic cells, macrophages, and lymphocytes are within the interstitium (766–768). Cortical fibroblasts have a spindle shape but may have a stellate appearance. They have elongated cell processes rich in actin filaments, contain prominent endoplasmic reticulum and express the enzyme ecto-5-nucleotidase (5-NT). The strongest 5-NT expression is from fibroblasts in the deep inner cortex. Fibroblasts in the renal capsule or in the periarterial connective tissue show little 5-NT expression. Fibroblasts (5-NT–positive) in the deep inner cortex produce erythropoietin (769,770). Studies have indicated that some erythropoietin-(EPO) producing interstitial cells may have originated from migrating neural crest cells (771) whereas others have reported these cells derive from FoxD1-expressing stromal cells (772).

In organs, the perivascular region around microvessels contains a variety of cell types, including pericytes (773,774). Pericytes surround capillaries and display characteristic ultrastructural features. They have close contacts with endothelial cells through special membrane invaginations, called peg-sockets, which contain adherens junctions (775). They are present in the cortex and also in the medulla, especially surrounding the DVR, and are essential for kidney function (776). Evidence from numerous studies indicate kidney fibrosis results from a proliferation of resident renal cells transforming into myofibroblasts rather than tubular epithelial–mesenchymal transition (EMT) (777). Genetic fate tracing studies indicate pericytes are progenitors of myofibroblasts in renal injury (778). A population of mesenchymal stem cell (MSC)–like cells expressing Gli1 and localizing to the pericyte niche are reported to be a source of myofibroblasts in renal injury (779).

Complex networks of resident immune cells, including dendritic cells and macrophages, exist in the kidney (780). Moreover, there are different subsets of these cells. These cells have multiple immune roles and link innate and adaptive immunity. Dendritic cells are professional antigen-presenting cells. Multiple markers are necessary to distinguish renal dendritic and macrophages. In one study, $CD11c^+$, $MHC-II^+$,

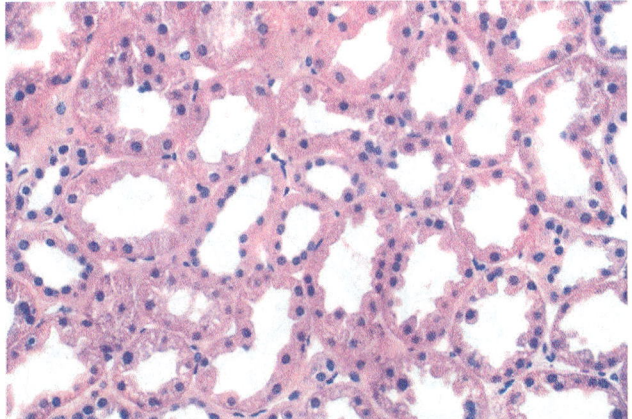

FIGURE 33.107 Biopsy specimen of the cortex of a kidney donated for transplantation. Note the compact arrangement of the tubules and the limited amount of interstitial tissue (H&E, ×250).

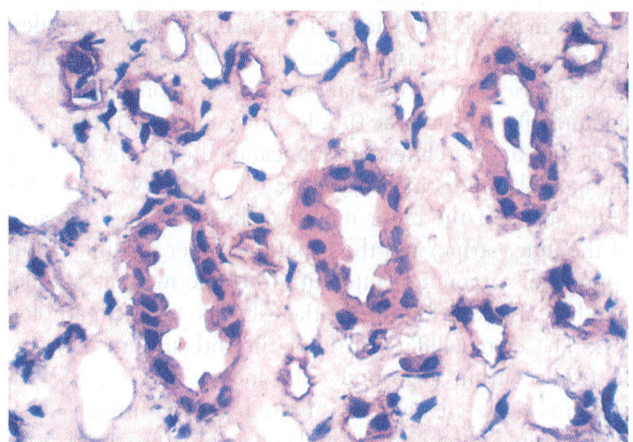

FIGURE 33.108 Renal biopsy specimen illustrating the inner medulla. Note the prominent amount of interstitium surrounding the tubules (H&E, ×500).

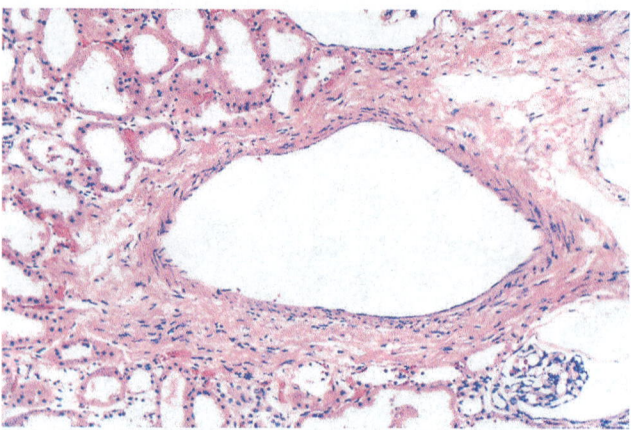

FIGURE 33.109 Micrograph of the corticomedullary junction illustrating an arcuate artery (H&E, ×125).

$F4/80^-$, $CD64^-$, $ZBTB46^+$ cells were designated as dendritic cells whereas $CD11c^+$, MHC-II$^+$, $F4/80^+$, $CD64^+$, $ZBTB46^-$ cells were called macrophages (781). Lymphocytes and granulocytes are uncommon in the kidney.

The medullary interstitium has a gelatinous appearance on light microscopy (Fig. 33.108). Several types of interstitial cells exist in the medulla, but the most distinctive are the lipid-laden cells, especially prominent in the inner medulla. These cells, called renomedullary interstitial cells, are often arranged in rows between the loop of Henle and the vasa recta, have irregular, long cytoplasmic processes, and contain lipid inclusions. These cells can be observed on 1-um thick toluidine blue-stained sections of the inner medulla. The lipid droplets contain mainly triglycerides that are rich in unsaturated fatty acids, including arachidonic acid, phospholipids, and cholesterol (760). The renomedullary interstitial cells are believed to exert an antihypertensive function of the renal medulla, largely attributed to the production of medullipin (782,783). These cells also express cyclooxygenase (COX-2) (784).

VASCULATURE

The intricate microvasculature of the kidney underlies its complex hemodynamic functions (373). The segmental arteries, originating from the anterior and posterior divisions of the main renal artery, divide to form the interlobar arteries, which course toward the cortex along the septa of Berlin between adjacent renal pyramids. At the corticomedullary junction, the interlobar arteries give rise to the arcuate arteries, which follow a gently curved course along the base of the pyramids parallel to the kidney surface (Fig. 33.109). The interlobular arteries branch sharply from the arcuate arteries and ascend in the cortex in a radial fashion toward the renal surface. Since the renal lobules cannot be clearly distinguished, it has been recommended that the interlobular arteries be called cortical radial arteries (373). Most afferent arterioles originate from the interlobular arteries, and each supplies a single glomerulus. The angle of origin of the afferent arterioles becomes less recurrent and more open as the interlobular arteries extend to the outer cortex (Fig. 33.110) (785). The length of the afferent arterioles is variable; average values of 170 to 280 μm have been reported (Fig. 33.111) (786,787). Some rare branches of the intrarenal arteries that do not terminate in glomeruli, the so-called aglomerular vessels, may result from degeneration of the connected glomeruli (785). Aglomerular arterioles near the corticomedullary junction have been observed to enter the medulla, and shunt arterioles between afferent and efferent arterioles have been reported (788–790). The wall structure of the intrarenal arteries and the proximal portion of the afferent arterioles resembles that of blood vessels of the same size elsewhere in the body. The endothelium stains for factor VIII–related

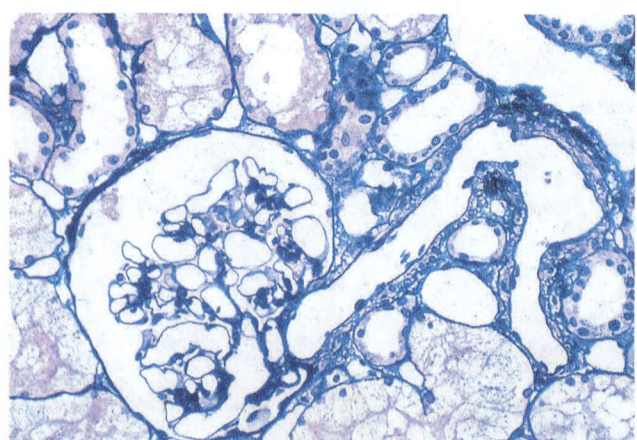

FIGURE 33.110 Juxtamedullary glomerulus with a connected hilar arteriole. Note the recurrent angle of the arteriole (Jones silver stain, ×250).

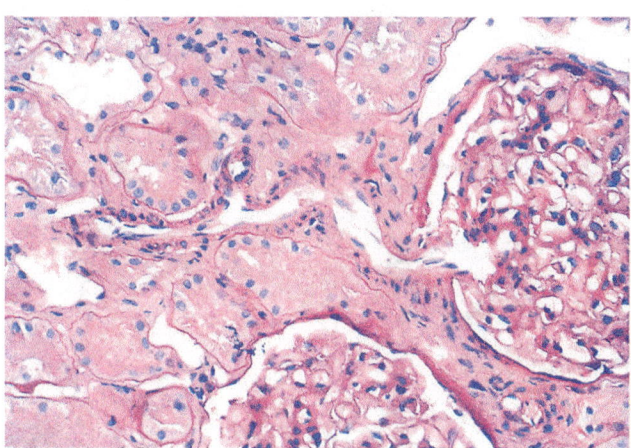

FIGURE 33.111 Micrograph depicting the transverse course of an afferent arteriole supplying a glomerulus (PAS, ×250).

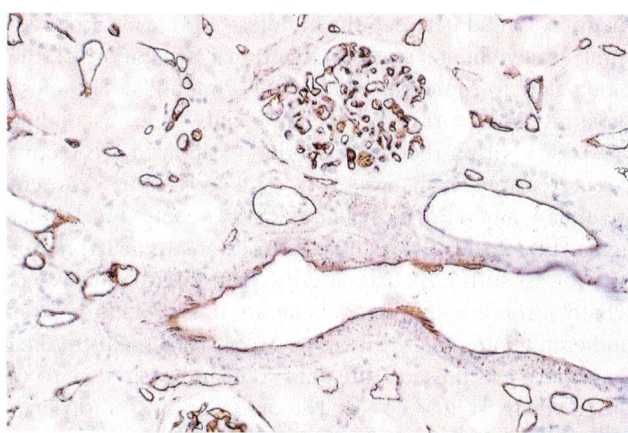

FIGURE 33.113 CD34 immunoperoxidase staining demonstrates a greater variety of vascular structures that label more intensely than with factor VIII. In the micrograph, arteries, veins, glomeruli, and peritubular capillaries are immunoreactive (CD34 immunohistochemistry, ×100).

antigen (Fig. 33.112) (791,792) and CD34 (Fig. 33.113) (793,794), whereas the muscularis stains for smooth muscle actin (Fig. 33.114) (795) and vimentin.

The efferent arterioles from the glomeruli branch to form a complex postglomerular microcirculation (Fig. 33.115). Although gradations exist, three basic types of efferent arterioles may be distinguished (796,797). The superficial or outer cortical efferent arterioles are fairly long and divide into extensive capillary networks that supply the convoluted tubules of the cortical labyrinth. These capillaries are readily identified by CD34 and smooth muscle actin staining (Figs. 33.114, 33.116, and 33.117).

The midcortical efferent arterioles are variable in length and supply the cortical labyrinth as well as the straight tubules of the medullary rays. With the exception of the outer cortex, there is dissociation between the tubule segments and the efferent arterioles of their parent glomeruli. In the midcortex and inner cortex, tubule segments are supplied by capillaries of efferent arterioles from other glomeruli (798,799). The efferent arterioles from juxtamedullary nephrons descend and supply the entire medulla. In contrast to the efferent arterioles of superficial and midcortical glomeruli (Fig. 33.118), those from juxtamedullary glomeruli are larger in diameter, display more layers of smooth muscle cells, and have more endothelial cells on cross sections (373). In the outer stripe of the outer medulla, the efferent arterioles of juxtamedullary nephrons divide to form the DVR that descend in the vascular bundles but at intervals leave the bundles to form capillary plexuses.

The ascending (or venous) vasa recta drain the renal medulla. The AVR from the inner medulla join the vascular bundles, whereas most from the inner stripe of the outer

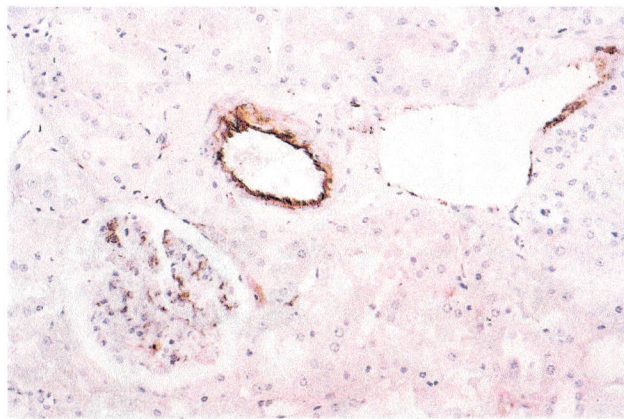

FIGURE 33.112 Factor VIII is produced by endothelium. The micrograph shows factor VIII immunoperoxidase staining of a medium-sized artery (*center*), vein (*right*), and glomerulus (*left*) (factor VIII immunohistochemistry, ×100).

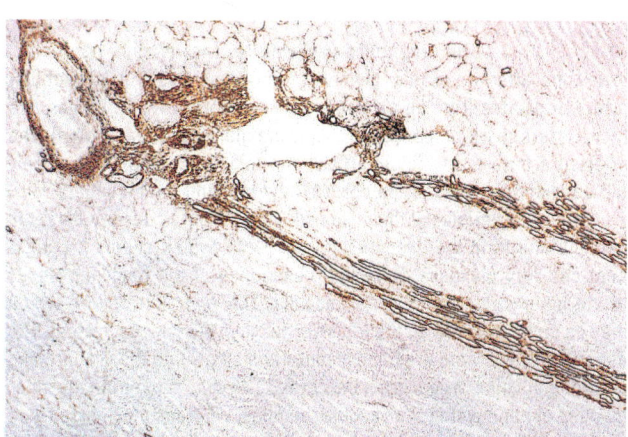

FIGURE 33.114 Smooth muscle actin immunoperoxidase stain illustrating a labeled large artery (*upper left*) and arterioles at the corticomedullary junction and two positive-stained columns of vasa recta (*midright*) penetrating the medulla. Two venous profiles (*upper center*) have minimal muscularis. (SMA immunohistochemistry, ×40)

medulla ascend between the bundles (373). This architectural arrangement creates a functional separation of the blood flow to the outer and the inner medulla. The close proximity of the arterial descending and venous ascending vasa recta within the vascular bundles allows for effective countercurrent exchange (373). The AVR at the corticomedullary junction empty into the arcuate and interlobular veins (Fig. 33.114), which do form extensive anastomoses in contrast to the arcuate arteries. The interlobular veins, which accompany the interlobular arteries, drain the cortex and empty into the arcuate veins. In sections the intrarenal veins have less musculature than comparably sized veins in other organs (Fig. 33.114). The arcuate veins empty into

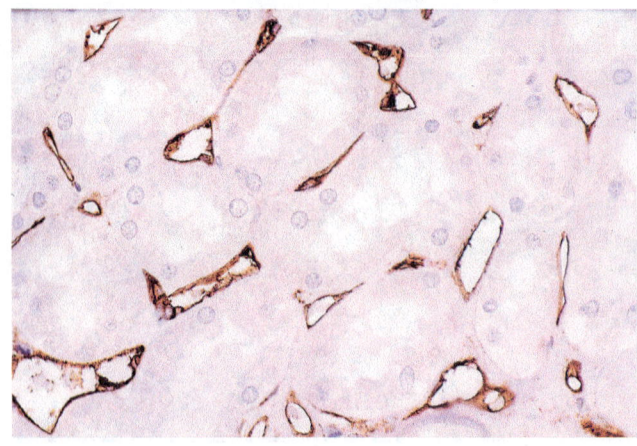

FIGURE 33.116 The extensive cortical peritubular capillary network is shown by endothelial labeling with CD34 antibody (CD34 immunohistochemistry, ×400).

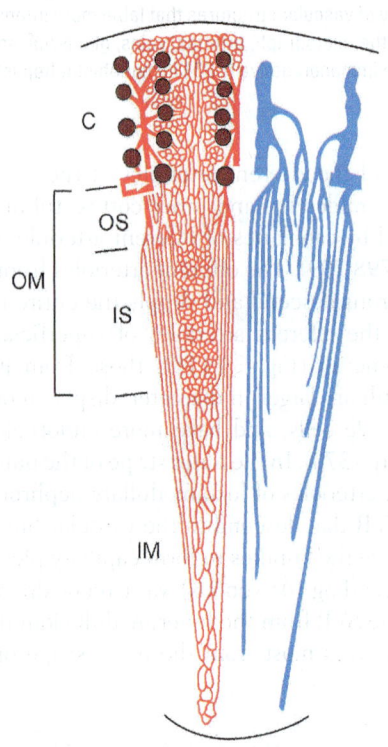

FIGURE 33.115 The renal microvasculature. The *left* side (*red*) illustrates the arterial vessels, glomeruli, and capillaries. An interlobular artery originates from an arcuate artery (*white arrow*) and gives rise to the afferent arterioles, which supply the glomeruli (*dark brown*). The efferent arterioles of the superficial and midcortical glomeruli supply the capillary plexuses of the cortical labyrinth and the medullary rays. The efferent arterioles of the juxtamedullary glomeruli descend into the medulla and form the descending vasa recta, which supply the adjacent capillary plexuses. Note the prominence of the capillary plexus in the inner stripe of the outer medulla. The *right* side (*blue*), which may be superimposed on the left side, displays the venous system. The ascending vasa recta drain the medulla and empty into the arcuate and interlobular veins, which drain the cortex. The vasa recta from the inner medulla ascend within the vascular bundles, whereas most vasa recta from the inner stripe ascend between the bundles (*C*, cortex; *OM*, outer medulla; *OS*, outer stripe; *IS*, inner stripe; *IM*, inner medulla). (Modified with permission from Kriz W, Kaissling B. Structural organization of the mammalian kidney. In: Seldin DW, Giebisch D, eds. *The Kidney: Physiology and Pathophysiology*. 3rd ed. Philadelphia, PA: Lippincott Williams & Wilkins; 2000:587–654.)

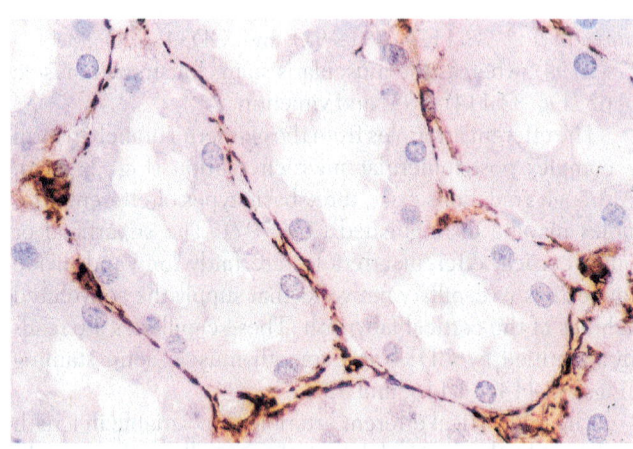

FIGURE 33.117 Smooth muscle actin expression complements and parallels the CD34 expression in documenting the cortical peritubular capillaries (SMA immunohistochemistry, ×400).

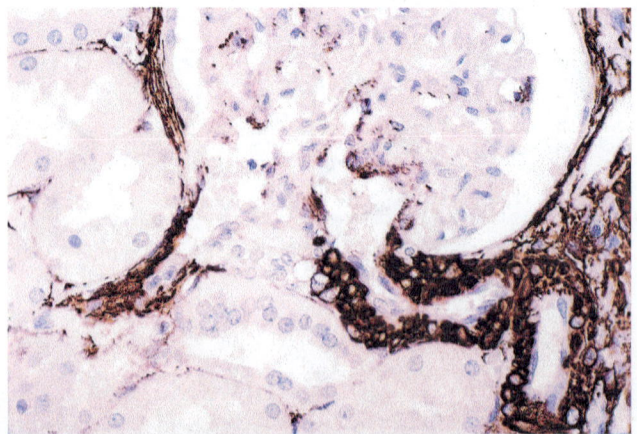

FIGURE 33.118 Smooth muscle actin immunoperoxidase of a superficial glomerulus delineating the more prominent smooth muscle investment of the afferent arteriole (*right*) compared with the efferent arteriole (*left*) (SMA immunohistochemistry, ×400).

the interlobar veins, which converge to form a single renal vein that exits at the hilum of the kidney.

LYMPHATICS

Lymphatic networks in the kidney include a deeper cortical system and less extensive capsular and subcapsular networks (800–802). The less prominent lymphatics within the capsule drain into the subcapsular lymphatic channels which appear to connect with the larger lymphatics in the cortex. The larger channels surround the interlobular arteries and empty into arcuate and interlobal lymphatics which finally drain into the larger lymph vessels at the hilum (Fig. 33.119). They are often more noticeable around interlobular veins than around interlobular arteries but are sporadic around glomeruli or between tubules (803). The interlobal and hilar lymphatics possess valves. Lymphatics are sparse to absent in the medulla of health kidneys (802,803). In the cortex, the lymphatics are embedded in the loose periarterial connective tissue but they are not conspicuous on routine histologic sections. They have a thin endothelial layer. It has been proposed that the periarterial spaces and the lymphatics may function as a unit to allow exchange with the venous system and serve as a route for the intrarenal distribution of hormones and inflammatory cells (804). Several markers of lymphatic endothelium are now available including: VEGFR-3 (receptor for VEGF-C), LYVE-1 (hyaluronate receptor), hyakuronate receptor, Prox-1 (lymphatic transcription factor), podoplanin (a membrane glycoprotein), and D2-40 (lymphatic endothelium-specific protein) (805,806). Interestingly, fenestrated AVR have been reported to express both endothelial and lymphatic markers, suggesting that they are specialized hybrid vessels (807).

NERVES

The nerve supply to the kidney derives from postganglionic fibers primarily from the celiac plexus (808). The nerve fibers generally accompany the arteries and arterioles in the cortex and the outer medulla (809). They generally lie within the perivascular interstitium but penetrate vessel walls to innervate the smooth muscle. On 1-µm thick toluidine blue–stained sections, a nerve often has a small round configuration but should not be mistaken for a small glomerulus (Fig. 33.120). Staining for myelin by S100 (Fig. 33.121) or for peripheral axons with antibodies against phosphoneurofilament (pNF) (Fig. 33.122) demonstrates the nerve fibers (810–813). There is prominent innervation of the JGA (Fig. 33.123) (814). The efferent arterioles and the DVR are accompanied by nerve fibers (815). Although there is innervation of the tubules, it is less extensive than of the vasculature (816,817). Relative to its length, the TAL

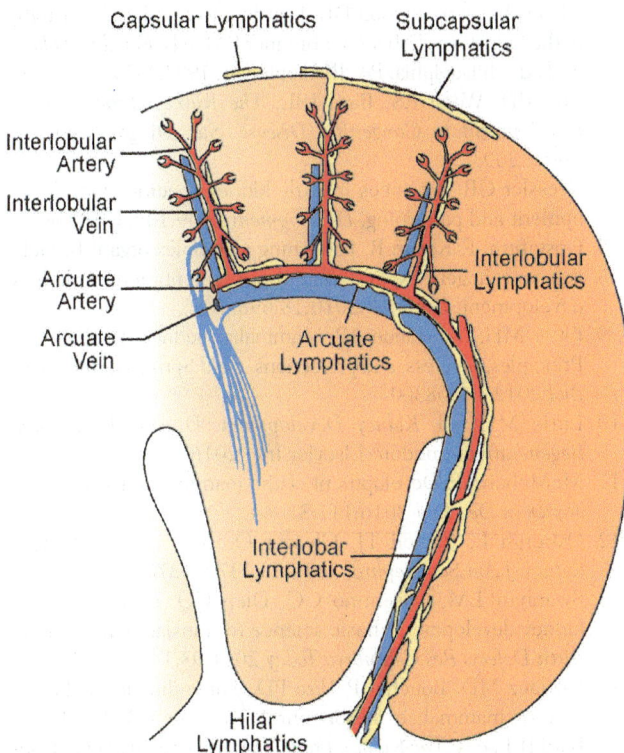

FIGURE 33.119 The lymphatic vessels of the kidney. The arteries (*red*), veins (*blue*), and lymphatics (*yellow*) are illustrated. The lymphatics are primarily distributed in the cortex, although a subcapsular network is also present. Note the absence of the lymphatics in the medulla. (Modified with permission from Madsen KM, Tisher CC. Anatomy of the kidney. In: Brenner BM, ed. *Brenner and Rector's The Kidney*. 7th ed. Philadelphia, PA: WB Saunders; 2004:3–72. Copyright © 2004 Elsevier.)

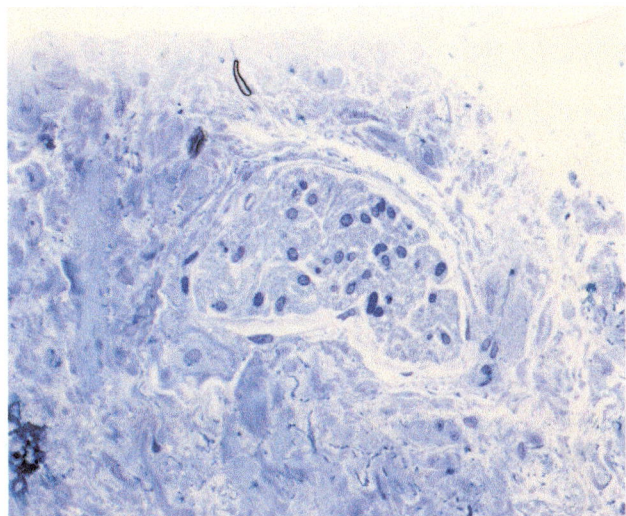

FIGURE 33.120 Light micrograph of renal cortex showing a small nerve. It has a circumscribed contour but in contrast to a glomerulus, lacks capillaries and their lumens and a Bowman capsule (1-µm thick toluidine blue–stained Epon section, ×630).

receives the largest nerve supply of any tubule segment (818). Studies using the efferent nerve marker tyrosine hydroxylase and the afferent nerve marker calcitonin-related peptide showed efferent fibers predominant along the renal artery (819).

ACKNOWLEDGMENTS

Portions of this chapter are adapted from contributions by Drs. Bruce Beckwith and Byron Croker in previous editions.

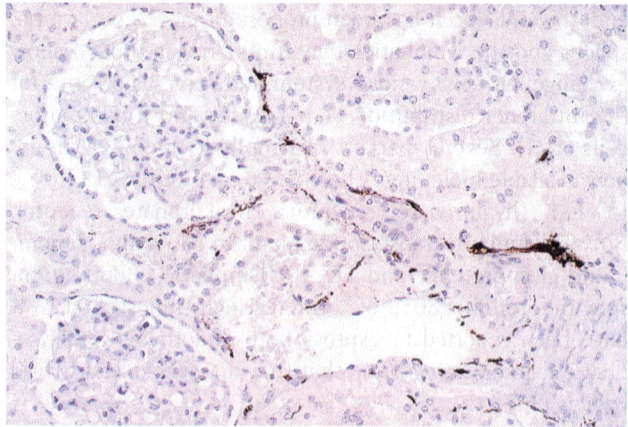

FIGURE 33.121 S100 immunohistochemical stain demonstrating nerves extending along the afferent arteriole to the vascular pole of the glomerulus (S100 immunohistochemistry, ×100).

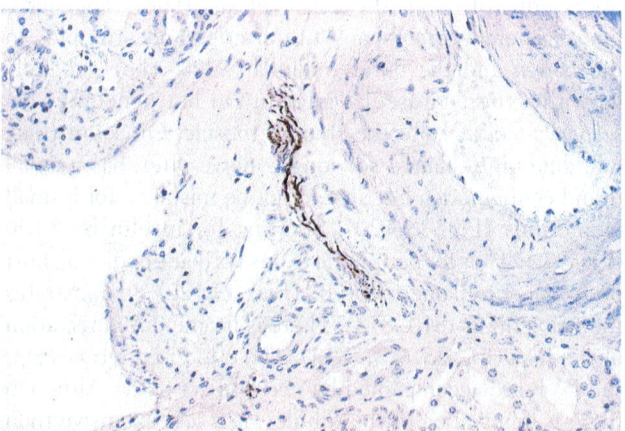

FIGURE 33.122 Phosphoneurofilament (pNF) immunohistochemical stain showing a nerve between an artery (*right*) and a vein (*left*) (pNF immunohistochemistry, ×100).

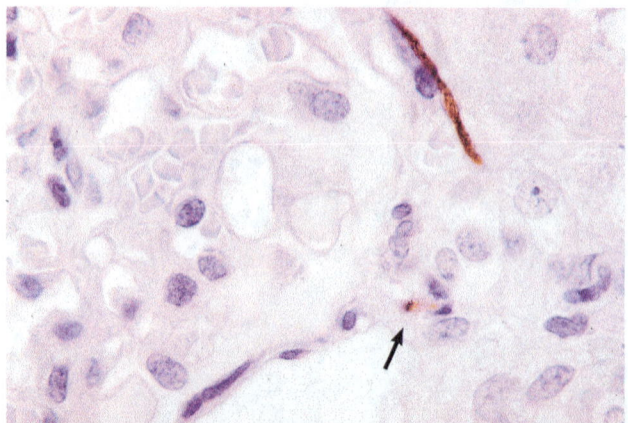

FIGURE 33.123 Two axons are demonstrated in this view of the vascular pole of a glomerulus (*center*). One axon has a longitudinal profile (*upper right*), and the other is observed in cross section as a dot (*arrow*) (pNF immunohistochemistry, ×630).

REFERENCES

1. Grobstein C. Inductive interaction in the development of the mouse metanephros. *J Exp Zool* 1955;130:319–340.
2. Potter EL. *Normal and Abnormal Development of the Kidney*. Chicago: Year Book Medical Publishers, Inc; 1972.
3. Oliver J. *Nephrons and Kidneys: A Quantitative Study of Development and Evolutionary Mammalian Renal Architectonics*. New York: Hoeber Medical Division, Harper & Row; 1968.
4. Saxen L. *Organogenesis of the Kidney*. Cambridge: Cambridge University Press; 1987.
5. Clapp WL, Abrahamson DR. Development and gross anatomy of the kidney. In: Tisher CC, Brenner BM, eds. *Renal Pathology*. 2nd ed. Philadelphia, PA: JB Lippincott; 1994;3–59.
6. Vize PD, Woolf AS, Bard JBL. *The Kidney: From Normal Development to Congenital Disease*. San Diego: Academic Press; 2003.
7. Dressler GR. Advances in early kidney specification, development and patterning. *Development* 2009;136:3863–3874.
8. Costantini F, Kopan R. Patterning a complex organ: Branching morphogenesis and nephron segmentation in kidney development. *Dev Cell* 2010;18:698–712.
9. Little MH, McMahon AP. Mammalian kidney development: Principles, progress, and projections. *Cold Spring Harb Perspect Biol* 2012;4:a008300.
10. Little MH, ed. *Kidney Development, Disease, Repair and Regeneration*. London: Elsevier Inc; 2016.
11. McMahon AP. Development of the mammalian kidney. *Curr Topics in Dev Biol* 2016;117:31–64.
12. Oxburgh L, Carroll TJ, Cleaver O, et al. (Re)Building a kidney. *J Am Soc Nephrol* 2017;28:1370–1378.
13. Swanhart LM, Cosentino CC, Diep CQ, et al. Zebrafish kidney development: Basic science to translational research. *Birth Defects Res C Embryo Today* 2011;93:141–156.
14. Vazquez MD, Bouchet P, Vize PD. Three-dimensional anatomy of mammalian mesonephroi. In: Vize PD, Woolf AS, Bard JBL, eds. *The Kidney. From Normal Development to Congenital Disease*. San Diego: Academic Press; 2003:87–92.
15. Mugford JW, Sipila P, Kobayashi A, et al. Hoxd11 specifies a program of metanephric kidney development within the intermediate mesoderm of the mouse kidney. *Dev Biol* 2008;319:396–405.
16. Georgas KM, Chiu HS, Rumballe BA, et al. Expression of metanephric nephron-patterning genes in differentiating mesonephric tubule. *Dev Dyn* 2011;240:1600–1612.

17. Masse J, Watrin T, Laurent A, et al. The developing female genital tract: From genetics to epigenetics. *Int J Dev Biol* 2009; 53:411–424.
18. Herring PT. The development of the Malpighian bodies of the kidney, and its relation to pathological changes which occur in them. *J Pathol Bacteriol* 1900;6:459–496.
19. Huber GC. On the development and shape of uriniferous tubules of certain of the higher mammals. *Am J Anat* 1905; 4(Suppl):1–98.
20. Felix W. The development of the urogenital organs. In: Kiebel F, Mall FP, eds. *Manual of Human Embryology*. Vol. 2. Philadelphia, PA: JB Lippincott; 1912:752–979.
21. Peter K. *Untersuchungen ueber Bau und Entwicklung der Niere*. Jena, Germany: Gustav Fischer; 1927.
22. Davies J. Development of the ureteric bud. In: Vize PD, Woolf AS, Bard JB, eds. *The Kidney: From Normal Development to Congenital Disease*. San Diego: Academic Press; 2003: 165–179.
23. Al-Awqati Q, Goldberg MR. Architectural patterns in branching morphogenesis in the kidney. *Kidney Int* 1998;54:1832–1842.
24. Watanabe T, Costantini F. Real-time analysis of ureteric bud branching morphogenesis in vitro. *Dev Biol* 2004;271:98–108.
25. Sweeny D, Lindstrom N, Davies JA. Developmental plasticity and regenerative capacity in the renal ureteric/collecting duct system. *Development* 2008;135:2505–2510.
26. Bard J. The metanephros. In: Vize PD, Woolf AS, Bard JB, eds. *The Kidney: From Normal Development to Congenital Disease*. San Diego: Academic Press; 2003:139–148.
27. Sariola H, Sainio K, Bard J. Fates of the metanephric mesenchyme. In: Vize PD, Woolf AS, Bard JB, eds. *The Kidney: From Normal Development to Congenital Disease*. San Diego: Academic Press; 2003:181–193.
28. Gawlik A, Quaggin SE. Conditional gene targeting in the kidney. *Curr Mol Med* 2005;5:527–536.
29. Ly JP, Onay T, Quaggin SE. Mouse models to study kidney development, function and disease. *Curr Opin Nephrol Hypertens* 2011;20:382–390.
30. Brunskill EW, Aronow BJ, Georgas K, et al. Atlas of gene expression in the developing kidney at microanatomic resolution. *Dev Cell* 2008;15:781–791.
31. Harding SD, Armit C, Armstrong J, et al. The GUDMAP database -an online resource for genitourinary research. *Development* 2011;138:2845–2853.
32. Potter SS, Brunskill EW, Patterson LT. Defining the genetic blueprint of kidney development. *Pediatr Nephrol* 2011;26: 1469–1478.
33. Brunskill EW, Park JS, Chung E, et al. Single cell-dissection of early kidney development: Multilineage priming. *Development* 2014;141:3093–3101.
34. Potter SS. Single-cell RNA sequencing for the study of development, physiology and disease. *Nat Rev Nephrol* 2018;14: 479–492.
35. Thiagarajan RD, Georgas KM, Rumballe BA, et al. Identification of anchor genes during kidney development defines ontological relationships, molecular subcompartments and regulatory pathways. *PLoS ONE* 2011;6:e17286.
36. Lindstrom NO, McMahon JA, Guo J, et al. Conserved and divergent features of human and mouse kidney organogenesis. *J Am Soc Nephrol* 2018;29:785–805.
37. James RG, Schultheiss TM. BMP signaling promotes intermediate mesoderm gene expression in a dose-dependent, cell-autonomous and translation-dependent manner. *Dev Biol* 2005;288:113–125.
38. Giovanni VD, Alday A, Chi L, et al. ALK3 controls nephron number and androgen production via lineage-specific effects in intermediate mesoderm. *Development* 2011;138:2717–2727.
39. Preger-Ben Noon E, Brak H, Guttmann-Raviv N, et al. Interplay between activin and Hox genes determines the formation of the kidney morphogenetic field. *Development* 2009;136:1995–2004.
40. Patterson LT, Pembaur M, Potter SS. Hoxa11 and Hoxd11 regulate branching morphogenesis of the ureteric bud in the developing kidney. *Development* 2001;128:2153–2161.
41. Wellik DM, Hawkes PJ, Capecchi MR. Hox11 paralogous genes are essential for metanephric kidney induction. *Genes Dev* 2002;16:1423–1432.
42. Bouchard M, Souabni A, Mandler M, et al. Nephric lineage specification by Pax2 and Pax8. *Genes Dev* 2002;16: 2958–2970.
43. Grote D, Souabni A, Busslinger M, et al. Pax2/8-regulated Gata 3 expression is necessary for morphogenesis and guidance of the nephric duct in the developing kidney. *Development* 2006;133:53–61.
44. Marose TD, Merkel CE, McMahon AP, et al. Beta-catenin is necessary to keep cells of ureteric bud/Wolffian duct epithelium in a precursor state. *Dev Biol* 2008;314:112–126.
45. Grote D, Boualia SK, Souabni A, et al. Gata3 acts downstream of beta-catenin signaling to prevent ectopic metanephric kidney induction. *PLoS Genet* 2008;4:e1000316.
46. Chia I, Grote D, Marcotte M, et al. Nephric duct insertion is a crucial step in urinary tract maturation that is regulated by a Gata3-Raldh2-Ret molecular network in mice. *Development* 2011;138:2089–2097.
47. Hoshi M, Reginensi A, Joens MS, et al. Reciprocal spatiotemporally controlled apoptosis regulates Wolffian duct cloaca fusion. *J Am Soc Nephrol* 2018;29:775–783.
48. Schedl A. Renal abnormalities and their developmental origin. *Nat Rev Genet* 2007;8:791–802.
49. Uetani N, Bouchard M. Plumbing in the embryo: Developmental defects of the urinary tract. *Clin Genet* 2009;75: 307–317.
50. Costantini F. GDNF/Ret signaling and renal branching morphogenesis: From mesenchymal signals to epithelial cell behaviors. *Organogenesis* 2010;6:252–262.
51. Chi X, Michos O, Shakya R, et al. Ret-dependent cell rearrangements in the Wolffian duct epithelium initiate ureteric bud morphogenesis. *Dev Cell* 2009;17:199–209.
52. Costantini F, Shakya R. GDNF/ret signaling and the development of the kidney. *Bioessays* 2006;28:117–127.
53. Boyle S, deCaestecker M. Role of transcriptional networks in coordinating early events during kidney development. *Am J Physiol Renal Physiol* 2006;291:F1–F8.
54. Gong KQ, Yallowitz AR, Sun H, et al. A Hox-Eya-Pax complex regulates early kidney developmental gene expression. *Mol Cell Biol* 2007;27:7661–7668.
55. Linton JM, Martin GR, Reichardt LF. The ECM protein nephronectin promotes kidney development via integrin α8β1-mediated stimulation of Gdnf expression. *Development* 2007;134:2501–2509.
56. Grieshammer U, Ma L, Plump AS, et al. SLIT2-mediated ROBO2 signaling restricts kidney induction to a single site. *Dev Cell* 2004;6:709–717.

57. Michos O, Goncalves A, Lopez-Rios J, et al. Reduction of BMP4 activity by gremlin1 enables ureteric bud outgrowth and GDNF/WNT11 feedback signaling during kidney branching morphogenesis. *Development* 2007;134:2397–2405.
58. Rosselot C, Spraggon L, Chia I, et al. Non-cell-autonomous retinoid signaling is crucial for renal development. *Development* 2010;137:283–292.
59. Basson MA, Akbulut S, Watson-Johnson J, et al. Sprouty 1 is a critical regulator of GDNF/RET-mediated kidney induction. *Dev Cell* 2005;8:229–239.
60. Michos O, Cebrian C, Hyink D, et al. Kidney development in the absence of Gdnf and Spry1 requires Fgf10. *PLoS Genet* 2010;6:e1000809.
61. Takahashi M. The GDNF/RET signaling pathway and human disease. *Cytokine Growth Factor Rev* 2001;12:361–373.
62. Tang MJ, Cai Y, Tsai SJ, et al. Ureteric bud outgrowth in response to RET activation is mediated by phophatidylinositol 3-kinase. *Dev Biol* 2002;243:128–136.
63. Kim D, Dressler GR. PTEN modulates GDNF/RET mediated chemotaxis and branching morphogenesis in the developing kidney. *Dev Biol* 2007;307:290–299.
64. Jain S. The many faces of RET dysfunction in the kidney. *Organogenesis* 2009;5:177–190.
65. Wong A, Bogni S, Kotka P, et al. Phosphotyrosine 1062 is critical for the in vivo activity of the Ret9 receptor tyrosine kinase isoform. *Mol Cell Biol* 2005;25:9661–9673.
66. Jain S, Encinas M, Johnson EM, et al. Critical and distinct roles for key RET tyrosine docking sites in renal development. *Genes Dev* 2006;20:321–333.
67. Jain S, Knoten A, Hoshi M, et al. Organotypic specificity of key RET adaptor-docking sites in the pathogenesis of neurocristopathies and renal malformations in mice. *J Clin Invest* 2010;120:778–790.
68. Willecke R, Heuberger J, Grossmann K, et al. The tyrosine phophatase Shp2 acts downstream of GDNF/Ret in branching morphogenesis of the developing mouse kidney. *Dev Biol* 2011;360:310–317.
69. Lu BC, Cebrian C, Chi X, et al. Etv4 and Etv5 are required downstream of GDNF and Ret for kidney branching morphogenesis. *Nat Genet* 2009;41:1295–1302.
70. Ueland J, Yuan A, Marlier A, et al. A novel role for the chemokine receptor Cxcr4 in kidney morphogenesis: An in vitro study. *Dev Dyn* 2009;238:1083–1091.
71. Takabatake Y, Sugiyama T, Kohara H, et al. The CXCL12 (SDF-1)/CXCR4 axis is essential for the development of renal vasculature. *J Am Soc Nephrol* 2009;20:1714–1723.
72. Ishibe S, Karihaloo A, Ma H, et al. Met and the epidermal growth factor receptor act cooperatively to regulate final nephron number and maintain collecting duct morphology. *Development* 2009;136:337–345.
73. Riggins KS, Mernaugh G, Su Y, et al. MT1-MMP-mediated basement membrane remodeling modulates renal development. *Exp Cell Res* 2010;316:2993–3005.
74. Reginensi A, Clarkson M, Neirijnck Y, et al. SOX9 controls epithelial branching by activating RET effector genes during kidney development. *Hum Mol Genet* 2011;20:1143–1153.
75. Bates CM. Role of fibroblast growth factor receptor signaling in kidney development. *Am J Physiol Renal Physiol* 2011;301: F245–F251.
76. Trueb B. Biology of FGFRL1, the fifth fibroblast growth factor receptor. *Cell Mol Life Sci* 2011;68:951–964.
77. Poladia DP, Kish K, Kutay B, et al. Role of fibroblast growth factor receptors 1 and 2 in the metanephric mesenchyme. *Dev Biol* 2006;291:325–339.
78. Sims-Lucas S, Cusack B, Baust J, et al. Fgfr1 and the IIIc isoform of Fgfr2 play critical roles in the metanephric mesenchyme mediating early inductive events in kidney development. *Dev Dyn* 2011;240:240–249.
79. Zhao H, Kegg H, Grady S, et al. Role of fibroblast growth factor receptors 1 and 2 in the ureteric bud. *Dev Biol* 2004; 276:403–415.
80. Sims-Lucas S, Argyropoulos C, Kish K, et al. Three-dimensional imaging reveals ureteric and mesenchymal defects in Fgfr2-mutant kidneys. *J Am Soc Nephrol* 2009;20:2525–2533.
81. Sims-Lucas S, Cusack B, Eswarakumar VP, et al. Independent roles of Fgfr2 and Frs2α in ureteric epithelium. *Development* 2011;138:1275–1280.
82. Yosypiv IV. Renin-angiotensin system in ureteric bud branching morphogenesis: Insights into the mechanism. *Pediatr Nephrol* 2011;26:1499–1512.
83. Yosypiv IV, Schroeder M, El-Dahr SS. Angiotensin II type I receptor-EGF receptor cross-talk regulates ureteric bud branching morphogenesis. *J Am Soc Nephrol* 2006;17:1005–1014.
84. Song R, Spera M, Garrett C, et al. Angiotensin II-induced activation of c-Ret signaling is critical in ureteric bud branching morphogenesis. *Mech Dev* 2010;127:21–27.
85. Yosypiv IV, Boh MK, Spera MA, et al. Downregulation of Spry-1, an inhibitor of GDNF/Ret, causes angiotensin II-induced ureteric bud branching. *Kidney Int* 2008;74:1287–1293.
86. Song R, Spera M, Garrett C, et al. Angiotensin II AT2 receptor regulates ureteric bud morphogenesis. *Am J Physiol Renal Physiol* 2010;298:F807–F817.
87. Song R, Preston G, Yosypiv IV. Angiotensin II stimulates in vitro branching morphogenesis of the isolated ureteric bud. *Mech Dev* 2011;128:359–367.
88. Matthew S, Chen X, Pozzi A, et al. Integrins in renal development. *Pediatr Nephrol* 2012;27:891–900.
89. Wu W, Kitamura S, Truong DM, et al. β1-integrin is required for kidney collecting duct morphogenesis and maintenance of renal function. *Am J Physiol Renal Physiol* 2009;297: F210–F217.
90. Zhang X, Mernaugh G, Yang DH, et al. β1 integrin is necessary for ureteric bud branching morphogenesis and maintenance of collecting duct structural integrity. *Development* 2009;136:3357–3366.
91. Mathew S, Palamuttam RJ, Mernaugh G, et al. Talin regulates integrin β1-dependent and –independent cell functions in ureteric bud development. *Development* 2017;144:4148–4158.
92. Lange A, Wickstrom SA, Jakobson M, et al. Integrin-linked kinase is an adaptor with essential functions during mouse development. *Nature* 2009;461:1002–1006.
93. Smeeton J, Zhang X, Bulus N, et al. Integrin-linked kinase regulates p38 MAPK-dependent cell cycle arrest in ureteric bud development. *Development* 2010;137:3233–3243.
94. Miner JH, Yurchenco PD. Laminin functions in tissue morphogenesis. *Annu Rev Cell Dev Biol* 2004;20:255–284.
95. Yang DH, McKee KK, Chen ZL, et al. Renal collecting system growth and function depend upon embryonic γ1 laminin expression. *Development* 2011;138:4535–4544.
96. Cain JE, Hartwig S, Bertram JF, et al. Bone morphogenetic protein signaling in the developing kidney: Present and future. *Differentiation* 2008;76:831–842.

97. Hartwig S, Hu MC, Cella C, et al. Glypican-3 modulates inhibitory Bmp2-Smad signaling to control renal development in vivo. *Mech Dev* 2005;122:928–938.
98. Miyazaki Y, Oshima K, Fogo A, et al. Bone morphogenetic protein 4 regulates the budding site and elongation of the mouse ureter. *J Clin Invest* 2000;105:863–873.
99. Cain JE, Bertram JF. Ureteric branching morphogenesis in BMP4 heterozygous mutant mice. *J Anat* 2006;209:745–755.
100. Hartwig S, Bridgewater D, Di Giovanni V, et al. BMP receptor ALK3 controls collecting system development. *J Am Soc Nephrol* 2008;19:117–124.
101. Goncalves A, Zeller R. Genetic analysis reveals an unexpected role of BMP7 in initiation of ureteric bud outgrowth in mouse embryos. *PLoS ONE* 2011;6:e19370.
102. Tran TS, Kolodkin AL, Bharadwaj R. Semaphorin regulation of cellular morphology. *Annu Rev Cell Dev Biol* 2007;23:263–292.
103. Tufro A, Teichman J, Woda C, et al. Semaphorin3a inhibits ureteric bud branching morphogenesis. *Mech Dev* 2008;125:558–568.
104. Korostylev A, Worzfeld T, Deng S, et al. A functional role for semaphorin 4D/plexin B1 interactions in epithelial branching morphogenesis during organogenesis. *Development* 2008;135:3333–3343.
105. Perala N, Jakobson M, Ola R, et al. Sema4C-Plexin B2 signaling modulates ureteric branching in developing kidney. *Differentiation* 2011;81:81–91.
106. Halder G, Johnson RL. Hippo signaling: Growth control and beyond. *Development* 2011;138:9–22.
107. Varelas X. The Hippo pathway effectors TAZ and YAP in development, homeostasis and disease. *Development* 2014;141:1614–1626.
108. Reginensi A, Enderle L, Gregorieff A, et al. A critical role for NF2 and the Hippo pathway in branching morphogenesis. *Nat Commun* 2017;7:12309.
109. Reginensi A, Hoshi M, Boualia SK, et al. Yap and Taz are required for Ret-dependent urinary tract morphogenesis. *Development* 2015;142:2696–2703.
110. Cebrian C, Borodo K, Charles N, et al. Morphometric index of the developing murine kidney. *Dev Dyn* 2004;231:601–608.
111. Short KM, Combes AN, Lefevre J, et al. Global quantification of tissue dynamics in the developing mouse kidney. *Dev Cell* 2014;29:188–202.
112. Sampogna RV, Schneider L, Al-Awqati Q. Developmental programming of branching morphogenesis in the kidney. *J Am Soc Nephrol* 2015;26:2414–2422.
113. McNeill H, Woodgett JR. When pathways collide: Collaboration and connivance among signaling proteins in development. *Nat Rev Mol Cell Biol* 2010;11:404–413.
114. McNeill H. Planar cell polarity and the kidney. *J Am Soc Nephrol* 2009;20:2104–2111.
115. Fischer E, Legue E, Doyen A, et al. Defective planar cell polarity in polycystic disease. *Nat Genet* 2006;38:21–23.
116. Saburi S, Hester I, Fischer E, et al. Loss of Fat4 disrupts PCP signaling and oriented cell division and leads to cystic kidney disease. *Nat Genet* 2008;40:1010–1015.
117. Luyten A, Su X, Gondela S, et al. Aberrant regulation of planar cell polarity in polycystic kidney disease. *J Am Soc Nephrol* 2010;21:1521–1532.
118. Karner CM, Chirumamilla R, Aoki S, et al. Wnt9b signaling regulates planar cell polarity and kidney tubule morphogenesis. *Nat Genet* 2009;41:793–799.
119. Keller R. Mechanisms of elongation in embryogenesis. *Development* 2006;133:2291–2302.
120. Lienkamp SS, Liu K, Karner CM, et al. Vertebrate kidney tubules elongate using a planar cell polarity-dependent, rosette-based mechanism of convergent extension. *Nat Genet* 2012;44:1382–1387.
121. Yu J, Carroll TJ, Rajagopal J, et al. A Wnt7b-dependent pathway regulates the orientation of epithelial cell division and establishes the cortico-medullary axis of the mammalian kidney. *Development* 2009;136:161–171.
122. Pietila I, Ellwanger K, Railo A, et al. Secreted Wnt antagonist Dickkopf-1 controls kidney papilla development coordinated by Wnt-7b signaling. *Dev Biol* 2011;353:50–60.
123. Liu Y, Chattopadhyay N, Qin S, et al. Coordinate integrin and c-Met signaling regulate Wnt gene expression during epithelial morphogenesis. *Development* 2009;136:843–853.
124. Michael L, Davies JA. Pattern and regulation of cell proliferation during murine ureteric bud development. *J Anat* 2004;204:241–255.
125. Shakya R, Watanabe T, Costantini F. The role of GDNF/Ret signaling in ureteric bud cell fate and branching morphogenesis. *Dev Cell* 2005;8:65–74.
126. Meyer TN, Schwesinger C, Bush KT, et al. Spatiotemporal regulation of morphogenetic molecules during in vitro branching of the isolated ureteric bud; toward a model of branching through budding in the developing kidney. *Dev Biol* 2004;275:44–67.
127. Michael L, Sweeney DE, Davies JA. A role for microfilament-based contraction in branching morphogenesis of the ureteric bud. *Kidney Int* 2005;68:2010–2018.
128. Kuure S, Cebrian C, Machingo Q, et al. Actin depolymerizing factors cofilin1 and destrin are required for ureteric bud branching morphogenesis. *PLoS Genet* 2010;6:e1001176.
129. Ola R, Jakobson M, Kvist J, et al. The GDNF target Vsnl1 marks the ureteric tip. *J Am Soc Nephrol* 2011;22:274–284.
130. Majumdar A, Vainio S, Kispert A, et al. Wnt11 and Ret/Gdnf pathways cooperate in regulating ureteric branching during metanephric kidney development. *Development* 2003;130:3175–3185.
131. Ye X, Wang Y, Rattner A, et al. Genetic mosaic analysis reveals a major role for frizzled 4 and frizzled 8 in controlling ureteric growth in the developing kidney. *Development* 2011;138:1161–1172.
132. Packard A, Georgas K, Michos O, et al. Luminal mitosis drives epithelial dispersal within the branching ureteric bud. *Dev Cell* 2013;27:319–330.
133. Kim YH, Kwon TH, Frische S, et al. Immunocytochemical localization of pendrin in intercalated cell subtypes in rat and mouse kidney. *Am J Physiol Renal Physiol* 2002;283:F744–F754.
134. Song HK, Kim WY, Lee HW, et al. Origin and fate of pendrin-positive intercalated cells in developing mouse kidney. *J Am Soc Nephrol* 2007;18:2672–2682.
135. Hiatt MJ, Ivanova L, Toran N, et al. Remodeling of the fetal collecting duct epithelium. *Am J Pathol* 2010;176:630–637.
136. Kim J, Cha H, Tisher CC, et al. Role of apoptotic and non-apoptotic cell death in removal of intercalated cells from developing rat kidney. *Am J Physiol Renal Physiol* 1996;270:F575–F592.
137. El-Dahr SS, Li Y, Gutierrez E, et al. p63+ ureteric bud tip cells are progenitors of intercalated cells. *JCI Insight* 2017;2:e89996.

138. Blomqvist SR, Vidarsson H, Fitzgerald S, et al. Distal renal tubular acidosis in mice that lack the forkhead transcription factor Foxi1. *J Clin Invest* 2004;113:1560–1570.
139. Yamaguchi Y, Yonemura S, Takada S. Grainyhead-related transcription factor is required for duct maturation in the salivary gland and the kidney of the mouse. *Development* 2006;133:4737–4748.
140. Wu H, Chen L, Zhou Q, et al. Aqp2-expressing cells give rise to renal intercalated cells. *J Am Soc Nephrol* 2013;24:243–252.
141. Werth M, Schmidtt-Ott KM, Leete T, et al. Transcription factor *TFCP2L1* patterns cells in the mouse kidney collecting duct. *ELife* 2017;6:e24265.
142. Jeong HW, Jeon US, Koo BK, et al. Inactivation of Notch signaling in the renal collecting duct causes nephrogenic diabetes insipidus in mice. *J Clin Invest* 2009;119:3290–3300.
143. Guo Q, Wang Y, Tripathi P, et al. Adam10 mediates the choice between principal cells and intercalated cells in the kidney. *J Am Soc Nephrol* 2015;26:149–159.
144. Grassmeyer J, Mukherjee M, deRiso J, et al. Elf5 is a principal lineage specific transcription factor in the kidney that contributes to Aqp2 and Avpr2 gene expression. *Dev Biol* 2017;424:77–89.
145. Mugford JW, Sipila P, McMahon JA, et al. Osr1 expression demarcates a multi-potent population of intermediate mesoderm that undergoes progressive restriction to an Osr1-dependent nephron progenitor compartment within the mammalian kidney. *Dev Biol* 2008;324:88–98.
146. James RG, Kamel CN, Wang Q, et al. Odd-skipped related 1 is required for development of the metanephric kidney and regulates formation and differentiation of kidney precursor cells. *Development* 2006;133:2995–3004.
147. Sajithlal G, Zou D, Silvius D, et al. Eya1 acta as a critical regulator for specifying the metanephric mesenchyme. *Dev Biol* 2005;284:323–336.
148. Xu PX, Adams J, Peters H, et al. Eya1-deficient mice lack ears and kidneys and show abnormal apoptosis of organ primordial. *Nat Genet* 1999;23:113–117.
149. Li X, Oghi KA, Zhang J, et al. Eya protein phosphatase activity regulates Six1-Dach-Eya transcriptional effects in mammalian organogenesis. *Nature* 2003;426:247–254.
150. Xu PX, Zhang W, Huang L, et al. Six1 is required for the early organogenesis of mammalian kidney. *Development* 2003;130:3085–3094.
151. Nie X, Xu J, El-Hashash A, et al. Six1 regulates Grem1 expression in the metanephric mesenchyme to initiate branching morphogenesis. *Dev Biol* 2011;352:141–151.
152. Torres M, Gomex-Pardo E, Dressler GR, et al. Pax-2 controls multiple steps of urogenital development. *Development* 1995;121:4057–4065.
153. Brophy PD, Ostrom L, Lang KM, et al. Regulation of ureteric bud outgrowth by Pax2-dependent activation of the glial derived neurotrophic factor gene. *Development* 2001;128:4747–4756.
154. Nishinakamura R, Matsumoto Y, Nakao K, et al. Murine homolog of SALL1 is essential for ureteric bud invasion in kidney development. *Development* 2001;128:3105–3115.
155. Kiefer SM, Robbins L, Stumpff KM, et al. Sall1-dependent signals affect Wnt signaling and ureter tip fate to initiate kidney development. *Development* 2010;137:3099–3106.
156. Uchiyama Y, Sakaguchi M, Terabayashi T, et al. Kif26b, a kinesin family gene, regulates adhesion of the embryonic kidney mesenchyme. *Proc Natl Acad Sci USA* 2010;107:9240–9245.
157. Muller U, Wang D, Denda S, et al. Integrin $\alpha 8\beta 1$ is critically important for epithelial-mesenchymal interactions during kidney development. *Cell* 1997;88:603–613.
158. Carroll TJ, Das A. Defining the signals that constitute the nephron progenitor niche. *J Am Soc Nephrol* 2013;24:873–876.
159. Kopan R, Chen S, Little N. Nephron progenitor cells: Shifting the balance of self-renewal and differentiation. *Curr Top Dev Biol* 2014;107:293–331.
160. O'Brien LL, McMahon AP. Induction and patterning of the metanephric nephron. *Semin Cell Dev Biol* 2014;36:31–38.
161. Carroll TJ, Park JS, Hayashi S, et al. Wnt9b plays a central role in the regulation of mesenchymal to epithelial transitions underlying organogenesis of the mammalian urogenital system. *Dev Cell* 2005;9:283–292.
162. Self M, Lagutin OV, Bowling B, et al. Six2 is required for suppression of nephrogenesis and progenitor renewal in the developing kidney. *EMBO J* 2006;25:5214–5228.
163. Combes AN, Wilson S, Phipson B, et al. Haploinsufficiency for the Six2 gene increases nephron progenitor proliferation promoting branching and nephron number. *Kidney Int* 2018;93:589–598.
164. Kobayashi A, Valerius MT, Mugford JW, et al. Six2 defines and regulates a multipotent self-renewing nephron progenitor population throughout mammalian kidney development. *Cell Stem Cell* 2008;3:169–181.
165. Cebrian C, Asai N, D'Agati VD, et al. The number of fetal nephron progenitor cells limits ureteric branching and adult nephron endowment. *Cell Reports* 2014;7:127–137.
166. O'Brien LL, Guo Q, Lee Y, et al. Differential regulation of mouse and human nephron progenitors by the Six family of transcriptional regulators. *Development* 2016;143:595–608.
167. Boyle S, Misfeldt A, Chandler KJ, et al. Fate mapping using Cited1-CreERT2 mice demonstrates that the cap mesenchyme contains self-renewing progenitor cells and gives rise exclusively to nephronic epithelia. *Dev Biol* 2008;313:234–245.
168. Boyle S, Shioda T, Perantoni AO, et al. Cited1 and Cited2 are differentially expressed in the developing kidney but are not required for nephrogenesis. *Dev Dyn* 2007;236:2321–2330.
169. Mugford JW, Yu J, Kobayashi A, et al. High-resolution gene expression analysis of the developing mouse kidney defines novel cellular compartments within the nephron progenitor population. *Dev Biol* 2009;333:312–323.
170. Combes AN, Lefevre JG, Wilson S, et al. Cap mesenchyme cell swarming during kidney development is influenced by attraction, repulsion and adhesion to the ureteric tip. *Dev Biol* 2016;418:297–306.
171. Barak H, Huh SH, Chen S, et al. FGF9 and FGF10 maintain the stemness of nephron progenitors in mice and man. *Dev Cell* 2012;22;1191–1207.
172. Giovanni VD, Walker KA, Bushnell D, et al. Fibroblast growth factor receptor-Frs2α signaling is critical for nephron progenitors. *Dev Biol* 2015;400:82–93.
173. Tomita M, Asada M, Asada N, et al. Bmp7 maintains undifferentiated kidney progenitor population and determines nephron numbers at birth. *PLOS ONE* 2013;8:e73554.
174. Brown AC, Muthukrishnan SD, Guay JA, et al. Role for compartmentalization in nephron progenitor differentiation. *Proc Natl Acad Sci USA* 2013;110:4640–4645.
175. Kanda S, Tanigawa S, Ohmori T, et al. Sall1 maintains nephron progenitors and nascent nephrons by acting as both an activator and a repressor. *J Am Soc Nephrol* 2014;25:2584–2595.

176. Li Y, Liu J, Li W, et al. p53 enables metabolic fitness and self renewal of nephron progenitors. *Development* 2015;142:1228–1241.
177. Xu J, Liu H, Park JS, et al. Osr1 acts downstream of and interacts synergistically with Six2 to maintain nephron progenitor cells during kidney organogenesis. *Development* 2014;141:1442–1452.
178. Liu J, Edgington-Giordano F, Dugas C, et al. Regulation of nephron progenitor cell self-renewal by intermediary metabolism. *J Am Soc Nephrol* 2017;28:3323–3335.
179. Hilliard SA, El-Dahr SS. Epigenetics of renal development and disease. *Yale J Biol Med* 2016;89:565–573.
180. Liu H, Chen S, Yao X, et al. Histone deacetylases 1 and 2 regulate the transcriptional programs of nephron progenitors and renal vesicles. *Development* 2018;145:dev153619.
181. Hartman HA, Lai HL, Patterson LT. Cessation of renal morphogenesis in mice. *Dev Biol* 2007;310:379–387.
182. Rumballe BA, Georgas KM, Combes AN, et al. Nephron formation adopts a novel spatial topology at cessation of nephrogenesis. *Dev Biol* 2011;360:110–122.
183. Brunskill EW, Lai HL, Jamison DC, et al. Microarrays and RNA-Seq identify molecular mechanisms driving the end of nephron production. *BMC Dev Biol* 2011;11:15.
184. Chen S, Brunskill EW, Potter SS, et al. Intrinsic age-dependent changes and cell-cell contacts regulate nephron progenitor lifespan. *Dev Cell* 2015;35:49–62.
185. Volovelsky O, Nguyen T, Jarmas AE, et al. Hamartin regulates cessation of mouse nephrogenesis independently of mTOR. *Proc Natl Acad Sci USA* 2018;115:5998–6003.
186. Chung E, Deacon P, Marable S, et al. Notch signaling promotes nephrogenesis by downregulating Six2. *Development* 2016;143:3907–3913.
187. Chung E, Deacon P, Park JS. Notch is required for the formation of all nephron segments and primes nephron progenitors for differentiation. *Development* 2017;144:4530–4539.
188. Linstrom NO, Guo J, Kim AD, et al. Conserved and divergent features of mesenchymal progenitor cell types within the cortical nephrogenic niche of the human and mouse kidney. *J Am Soc Nephrol* 2018;29:806–824.
189. Park JS, Valerius MT, McMahon AP. Wnt/(beta)-catenin signaling regulates nephron induction during mouse kidney development. *Development* 2007;134:1103–1108.
190. Stark K, Vainio S, Vasslleva G, et al. Epithelial transformation of metanephric mesenchyme in the developing kidney regulated by Wnt-4. *Nature* 1994;372:679–683.
191. Kispert A, Vainio S, McMahon AP. Wnt-4 is a mesenchymal signal for epithelial transformation of metanephric mesenchyme in the developing kidney. *Development* 1998;125:4225–4234.
192. Tanigawa S, Wang H, Yang Y, et al. Wnt4 induces nephronic tubules in metanephric mesenchyme by a non-canonical mechanism. *Dev Biol* 2011;352:58–69.
193. Burn SF, Webb A, Berry RL, et al. Calcium/NFAT signaling promotes early nephrogenesis. *Dev Biol* 2011;352:288–298.
194. Georgas K, Rumballe B, Valerius MT, et al. Analysis of early nephron patterning reveals a role for distal RV proliferation in fusion to the ureteric tip via a cap mesenchyme-derived connecting segment. *Dev Biol* 2009;332:273–286.
195. Karner CM, Das A, Ma Z, et al. Canonical Wnt9b signaling balances progenitor cell expansion and differentiation during kidney development. *Development* 2011;138:1247–1257.
196. Ramalingam H, Fessler AR, Das A, et al. Disparate levels of beta-catenin activity determine nephron progenitor cell fate. *Dev Biol* 2018;440:13–21.
197. Reginensi A, Scott RP, Gregorieff A, et al. Yap- and Cdc42-dependent nephrogenesis and morphogenesis during mouse kidney development. *PLoS Genet* 2013;9:e1003380.
198. McNeill H, Reginensi A. Lats1/2 regulate Yap/Taz to control nephron progenitor epithelization and inhibit myofibroblast formation. *J Am Soc Nephrol* 2017;28:852–861.
199. Hastie ND. Wilms tumor 1(WT1) in development, homeostasis and disease. *Development* 2017;144:2862–2872.
200. Kreidburg JA, Sariola H, Loring JM, et al. WT-1 is required for early kidney development. *Cell* 1993;74:679–691.
201. Donovan MJ, Natoli TA, Sainio K, et al. Initial differentiation of the metanephric mesenchyme is independent of WT1 and the ureteric bud. *Dev Genet* 1999;24:252–262.
202. Hartwig S, Ho J, Pandey P, et al. Genomic characterization of Wilms tumor suppressor 1 targets in nephron progenitor cells during kidney development. *Development* 2010;137:1189–1203.
203. Essafi A, Webb A, Berry RL, et al. A Wt1-controlled chromatin switching mechanism underpins tissue-specific Wnt4 activation and repression. *Dev Cell* 2011;21:559–574.
204. Rivera MN, Kim WJ, Wells J, et al. An X chromosome gene, WTX, is commonly inactivated in Wilms tumor. *Science* 2007;315:642–645.
205. Tannberger K, Pfister AS, Brauburger K, et al. Amer1/WTX couples Wnt-induced formation of Ptdins (4,5)P2 to LRP6 phosphorylation. *EMBO J* 2011;30:1433–1443.
206. Major MB, Camp ND, Berndt JD, et al. Wilms tumor suppressor WTX negatively regulates WNT/β-catenin signaling. *Science* 2007;316:1043–1046.
207. Moisan A, Rivera MN, Lotinun S, et al. The WTX tumor suppressor regulates mesenchymal progenitor cell fate specification. *Dev Cell* 2011;20:583–596.
208. Kopan R, Hagan MX. The canonical notch signaling pathway: Unfolding the activation mechanism. *Cell* 2009;137:216–233.
209. Cheng HT, Miner JH, Lin M, et al. Gamma-secretase activity is dispensable for mesenchyme-to-epithelium transition but required for podocyte and proximal tubule formation in developing mouse kidney. *Development* 2003;130:5031–5042.
210. Cheng HT, Kim M, Valerius MT, et al. Notch2, but not Notch1, is required for proximal fate acquisition in the mammalian nephron. *Development* 2007;134:801–811.
211. Surendran K, Botle S, Barak H, et al. The contribution of Notch1 to nephron segmentation in the developing kidney is revealed in a sensitized Notch2 background and can be augmented by reducing Mint dosage. *Dev Biol* 2010;337:386–395.
212. Nakai S, Sugitani Y, Sato H, et al. Crucial roles of Brn1 in distal tubule formation and function in mouse kidney. *Development* 2003;130:4751–4759.
213. Drake KA, Adam M, Mahoney R, et al. Disruption of Hox9, 10, 11 function results in cellular level lineage infidelity in the kidney. *Sci Rep* 2018;8:6306.
214. Magella B, Mahoney R, Adam M, et al. Reduced Abd-B Hox function during kidney development results in lineage infidelity. *Dev Biol* 2018;438:84–93.
215. Lindstrom NO, Tran T, Guo J, et al. Conserved and divergent molecular and anatomic features of human and mouse nephron patterning. *J Am Soc Nephrol* 2018;29:825–840.

216. Lindstrom NO, Brandine GD, Tran T, et al. Progressive recruitment of mesenchymal progenitors reveals a time-dependent process of cell fate acquisition in mouse and human nephrogenesis. *Dev Cell* 2018;45:651–660.
217. Li W, Hartwig S, Rosenblum ND. Developmental origins and functions of stromal cells in the normal and diseased mammalian kidney. *Dev Dyn* 2014;243:853–863.
218. Kobayashi A, Mugford JW, Krautzberger AM, et al. Identification of a multipotent self-renewing stromal progenitor population during mammalian kidney organogenesis. *Stem Cell Reports* 2014;3:650–662.
219. Naiman N, Fujioka K, Fujino M, et al. Repression of interstitial identity in nephron progenitor cells by Pax2 establishes the nephron-interstitium boundary during kidney development. *Dev Cell* 2017;41:349–365.
220. Boivin FJ, Bridgewater D. β-Catenin in stromal progenitors controls medullary stromal development. *Am J Physiol Renal Physiol* 2018;314:F1177–F1187.
221. Guillaume R, Bressan M, Herzlinger D. Paraxial mesoderm contributes stromal cells to the developing kidney. *Dev Biol* 2009;329:169–175.
222. Levinson R, Mendelsohn C. Stromal progenitors are important for patterning epithelial and mesenchymal cell types in the embryonic kidney. *Sem Dev Biol* 2003;14:225–231.
223. Hatini V, Huh SO, Herzlinger D, et al. Essential role of stromal mesenchyme in kidney morphogenesis revealed by targeted disruption of winged helix transcription factor BF-2. *Genes Dev* 1996;10:1467–1478.
224. Levinson RS, Batourina E, Choi C, et al. Foxd1-dependent signals control cellularity in the renal capsule, a structure required for normal renal development. *Development* 2005;132:529–539.
225. Yallowitz AR, Hrycaj SM, Short KM, et al. Hox10 genes function in kidney development in the differentiation and integration of the cortical stroma. *PLoS ONE* 2011;6:e23410.
226. Fetting JL, Guay JA, Karolak MJ, et al. FOXD1 promotes nephron progenitor differentiation by repressing decorin in the embryonic kidney. *Development* 2014;141:17–27.
227. Leuning DG, Reinders ME, Li J, et al. Clinical-grade isolated human kidney perivascular stromal cells as an organotypic cell source for kidney regenerative medicine. *Stem Cells Transl Med* 2017;6:405–418.
228. Leuning DG, Engelse MA, Lievers E, et al. The human kidney capsule contains a functionally distinct mesenchymal stromal cell population. *PLoS One* 2017;12:e0187118.
229. Das A, Tangigawa S, Karner CM, et al. Stromal-epithelial crosstalk regulates kidney progenitor cell differentiation. *Nature Cell Biol* 2013;15:1035–1044.
230. Bagherie-Lachidan M, Reginensi A, Pan Q, et al. Stromal Fat4 acts non-autonomously with Dchs1/2 to restrict the nephron progenitor pool. *Development* 2015;142:2564–2573.
231. Briscoe J, Therond PP. The mechanisms of Hedgehog signaling and its roles in development and disease. *Nat Rev Mol Cell Biol* 2013;14:416–429.
232. Rowan CJ, Li W, Martirosyan H, et al. Hedgehog-GLI signaling in *Foxd1*-positive stromal cells promotes nephrogenesis via TGFβ signaling. *Development* 2018;145:dev159947.
233. Rosselot C, Spraggon L, Chia I, et al. Non-cell-autonomous retinoid signaling is crucial for renal development. *Development* 2010;137:283–292.
234. Paroly SS, Wang F, Spraggon L, et al. Stromal protein Ecm1 regulates ureteric bud patterning and branching. *PLOS ONE* 2013;9:e84155.
235. Sundelin B, Bohman SO. Postnatal development of the interstitial tissue of the rat kidney. *Anat Embryol (Berl)* 1990;182:307–317.
236. Maric C, Ryan GB, Alcorn D. Embryonic and postnatal development of the rat renal interstitium. *Anat Embryol (Berl)* 1997;195:503–514.
237. Marxer-Meier A, Hegyi I, Loffing J, et al. Postnatal maturation of renal cortical peritubular fibroblasts in the rat. *Anat Embryol (Berl)* 1998;197:143–153.
238. Abrahamson DR, Wang R. Development of the glomerular capillary and its basement membrane. In: Vize PD, Woolf AS, Bard JBL, eds. *The Kidney: From Normal Development to Congenital Disease*. San Diego: Academic Press; 2003:221–249.
239. Miner JH, Abrahamson DR. Molecular and cellular mechanisms of glomerular capillary development. In: Alpern RJ, Moe OW, Caplan M, eds. *Seldin and Giebisch's The kidney: Physiology and Pathophysiology*. 5th ed. Amsterdam: Elsevier, Inc; 2013:891–910.
240. Quaggin SE, Kreidberg JA. Development of the renal glomerulus: good neighbors and good fences. *Development* 2008;135:609–620.
241. Miner JH. Organogenesis of the kidney glomerulus. *Organogenesis* 2011;7:75–82.
242. Robert B, St. John PL, Hyink DP, et al. Evidence that embryonic kidney cells expressing flk-1 are intrinsic, vasculogenic angioblasts. *Am J Physiol* 1996;271:F744–F753.
243. Robert B, St. John PL, Abrahamson DR. Direct visualization of renal vascular morphogenesis in Flk1 heterozygous mutant mice. *Am J Physiol* 1998;275:F164–F172.
244. Woolf AS, Yuan HT. Development of kidney blood vessels. In: Vize PD, Woolf AS, Bard JBL, eds. *The Kidney: From Normal Development to Congenital Disease*. San Diego: Academic Press; 2003:251–266.
245. Ichimura K, Stan RV, Kurihara H, et al. Glomerular endothelial cells form diaphragms during development and pathologic conditions. *J Am Soc Nephrol* 2008;19:1463–1471.
246. Farber G, Hurtado R, Loh S, et al. Glomerular endothelial maturation depends on ADAM10, a key regulator of notch signaling. *Angiogenesis* 2018;21:335–347.
247. Ichimura K, Kakuta S, Kawasaki Y, et al. Morphological process of podocyte development revealed by block-face scanning electron microscopy. *J Cell Sci* 2017;130:132–142.
248. Patrakka J, Tryggvason K. Nephrin—a unique structural and signaling protein of the kidney filter. *Trends Mol Med* 2007;13:396–403.
249. Kestila M, Lenkkeri U, Mannikko M, et al. Positionally cloned gene for a novel glomerular protein—nephrin—is mutated in congenital nephrotic syndrome. *Mol Cell* 1998;1:575–582.
250. Abrahamson DR, St. John PL, Stroganova L, et al. Laminin and type IV collagen isoform substitutions occur in temporally and spatially distinct patterns in developing kidney glomerular basement membranes. *J Histochem Cytochem* 2013;61:706–718.
251. Abrahamson DR, Hudson BG, Stroganova L, et al. Cellular origins of type IV collagen networks in developing glomeruli. *J Am Soc Nephrol* 2009;20:1471–1479.
252. Leveen P, Pekny M, Gebre-Medhin S, et al. Mice deficient for PDGF B show renal, cardiovascular, and hematological abnormalities. *Genes Dev* 1994;8:1875–1887.

253. Soriano P. Abnormal kidney development and hematological disorders in PDGF beta-receptor mutant mice. *Genes Dev* 1994;8:1888–1896.
254. Sequeira-Lopez MLS, Gomez RA. Development of the renal arterioles. *J Am Soc Nephrol* 2011;22:2156–2165.
255. Mohamed T, Sequeira-Lopez MLS. Development of the renal vasculature. *Semin Cell Dev Biol* 2018;pii:S1084-9521(17)30450-0.
256. Belle M, Godefroy D, Couly G, et al. Tridimensional visualization and analysis of early human development. *Cell* 2017; 169:161–173.
257. Sequeira-Lopez MLS, Lin EE, Li M, et al. The earliest metanephric arteriolar progenitors and their role in kidney vascular development. *Am J Physiol Regul Integr Comp Physiol* 2015; 308:R138–R149.
258. Xu, J, Nie X, Cai X, et al. Tbx18 is essential for normal development of vasculature network and glomerular mesangium in the mammalian kidney. *Dev Biol* 2014;391:17–31.
259. Hu Y, Li M, Gothert JR, et al. Hemovascular progenitors in the kidney require sphingosine-1-phosphate receptor for vascular development. *J Am Soc Nephrol* 2016;27:1984–1995.
260. Halt KJ, Parssinen HE, Junttila SM, et al. CD146+ cells are essential for kidney vasculature development. *Kidney Int* 2016;90:311–324.
261. Muherjee E, Maringer K, Papke E, et al. Endothelial marker-expressing stromal cells are critical for kidney formation. *Am J Physiol Renal Physiol* 2017;313:F611–F620.
262. Munro ADA, Hohenstein P, Davies JA. Cycles of vascular plexus formation within the nephrogenic zone of the developing mouse kidney. *Sci Rep* 2017;7;3273.
263. Daniel E, Azizoglu DB, Ryan AR, et al. Spatiotemporal heterogeneity and patterning of developing renal blood vessels. *Angiogenesis* 2018;21:617–634.
264. Celio MR, Groscurth P, Inagami T. Ontogeny of renin immunoreactive cells in the human kidney. *Anat Embryol (Berl)* 1985;173:149–155.
265. Gomez RA, Lynch KR, Chevalier RL, et al. Renin and angiotensinogen gene expression in maturing rat kidney. *Am J Physiol* 1988;254:F582–F587.
266. Minuth M, Hackenthal E, Poulsen K, et al. Renin immunocytochemistry of the differentiating juxtaglomerular apparatus. *Anat Embryol (Berl)* 1981;162:173–181.
267. Gomez RA, Lynch KR, Sturgill BC, et al. Distribution of renin mRNA and its protein in the developing kidney. *Am J Physiol* 1989;257:F850–F858.
268. Reddi V, Zaglul A, Pentz ES, et al. Renin-expressing cells are associated with branching of the developing kidney vasculature. *J Am Soc Nephrol* 1998;9:63–71.
269. Sequeira Lopez ML, Pentz ES, Nomasa T, et al. Renin cells are precursors for multiple cell types that switch to the renin phenotype when homeostasis is threatened. *Dev Cell* 2004;6:719–728.
270. Brunskill EW, Sequeira-Lopez MLS, Pentz ES, et al. Genes that confer the identity of the renincell. *J Am Soc Nephrol* 2011;22:2213–2225.
271. Castellanos-Rivera RM, Pentz ES, Lin E, et al. Recombination signal binding protein for Ig-κJ region regulates juxtaglomerular cell phenotype by activating the myo-endocrine program and suppressing ectopic gene expression. *J Am Soc Nephrol* 2015;26:67–80.
272. Moore KL, Persaud TVN. *The Developing Human; Clinically Oriented Embryology*. 7th ed. Philadelphia, PA: Saunders; 2003.
273. Gruenwald P. The normal changes in the position of the embryonic kidney. *Anat Rec* 1943;85:163–176.
274. Friedland GW, De Vries P. Renal ectopia and fusion. Embryologic basis. *Urology* 1975;5:698–706.
275. Muller F, O'Rahilly R. Somitic-vertebral correlation and vertebral levels in the human embryo. *Am J Anat* 1986;177: 3–19.
276. Bremer JL. The origin of the renal artery in mammals and its anomalies. *Am J Anat* 1915;18:179–200.
277. Emery JL, Mithal A. The weights of kidneys in late intrauterine life and childhood. *J Clin Pathol* 1960;13:490–493.
278. Gruenwald P, Minh HN. Evaluation of body and organ weights in perinatal pathology. *Am J Clin Pathol* 1960;34:247–253.
279. Singer DB, Sung CR, Wigglesworth JS. Fetal growth and maturation: With standards for body and organ development. In: Wigglesworth JS, Singer DB, eds. *Textbook of Fetal and Perinatal Pathology*. 2nd ed. Oxford: Blackwell; 1998:8–40.
280. Guihard-Costa AM, Menez F, Delezoide AL. Organ weights in human fetuses after formalin fixation: Standards by gestational age and body weight. *Pediatr Dev Pathol* 2002;5:559–578.
281. Hansen K, Sung CJ, Huang C, et al. Reference values for second trimester fetal and neonatal organ weights and measurements. *Pediatr Dev Pathol* 2003;6:160–167.
282. Maroun LL, Graem N. Autopsy standards of body parameters and fresh organ weights in nonmacerated and macerated human fetuses. *Pediatr Dev Pathol* 2005;8:204–217.
283. Coppoletta JM, Wolbach SB. Body length and organ weights of infants and children. *Am J Pathol* 1933;9:55–70.
284. Kelley HA, Burnam CF. *Diseases of the Kidneys, Ureters, and Bladder*. Vol. 1. New York: Appleton; 1925.
285. Hodson J. The lobar structure of the kidney. *Br J Urol* 1972;44:246–261.
286. Lofgren F. *Das Topographische System der Malpighischen Pyramiden der Menschenniere*. Lund: Hakan Ohlssons Boktryckeri; 1949.
287. Sykes D. The morphology of renal lobulations and calices, and their relationship to partial nephrectomy. *Br J Surg* 1964;51:294–304.
288. Crelin ES. *Functional Anatomy of the Newborn*. New Haven: Yale University Press; 1973.
289. Campos ES. Pathological changes in the kidney in congenital syphilis. *Johns Hopkins Hosp Bull* 1923;34:253–263.
290. Potter EL, Thierstein ST. Glomerular development in the kidney as an index of fetal maturity. *J Pediatr* 1943;22:695–706.
291. Sutherland MR, Gubhaju L, Moore L, et al. Accelerated maturation and abnormal morphology in the preterm neonatal kidney. *J Am Soc Nephrol* 2011;22:1365–1374.
292. Singer DB, Klish W. Morphometric studies of the renal glomerulogenic zone. *Am J Pathol* 1970;59:32a.
293. Tsuda S. Histologic investigation of the foetal kidney. *Jap J Obstet Gynecol* 1934;17:337–341.
294. Dorovini-Zis K, Dolman CL. Gestational development of brain. *Arch Pathol Lab Med* 1977;101:192–195.
295. Hinchliffe SA, Sargent PH, Chan YF, et al. "Medullary ray glomerular counting" as a method of assessment of human nephrogenesis. *Path Res Pract* 1992;188:775–782.
296. Ryan D, Sutherland MR, Flores TJ, et al. Development of the human fetal kidney from mid to late gestation in male and female infants. *EBioMedicine* 2018;27:275–283.

297. Peter K. Harnorgane. Organe Uropoietica. In: Peter K, Wetzel G, Heiderich F, eds. *Handbuch der Anatomie des Kindes*. Vol. 2. Munich: JF Bergmann; 1938:1–41.
298. Benjamin DR, Beckwith JB. Medullary ray nodules in infancy and childhood. *Arch Pathol* 1973;96:33–35.
299. Hinchliffe SA, Sargent PH, Howard CV, et al. Human intrauterine renal growth expressed in absolute number of glomeruli assessed by the disector method and Cavalieri principle. *Lab Invest* 1991;64:777–784.
300. Hughson M, Farris AB, Douglas-Denton R, et al. Glomerular number and size in autopsy kidneys: The relationship to birth weight. *Kidney Int* 2003;63:2113–2122.
301. Hinchliffe SA, Lynch MRJ, Sargent PH, et al. The effect of intrauterine growth retardation on the development of nephrons. *Br J Obstet Gynaecol* 1992;99:296–301.
302. Manalich R, Reyes L, Herrera M, et al. Relationship between weight at birth and the number and size of renal glomeruli in humans: A histomorphometric study. *Kidney Int* 2000;58:770–773.
303. Fogo A, Hawkins EP, Berry PL, et al. Glomerular hypertrophy in minimal change disease predicts subsequent progression to focal glomerulosclerosis. *Kidney Int* 1990;38:115–123.
304. Nyengaard JR, Bendtsen TF. Glomerular number and size in relation to age, kidney weight, and body surface in normal man. *Anat Rec* 1992;232:194–201.
305. Merlet-Benichou C, Gilbert T, Vilar J, et al. Nephron number: Variability is the rule. Causes and consequences. *Lab Invest* 1999;79:515–527.
306. Hoy WE, Hughson MD, Bertram JF, et al. Nephron number, hypertension, renal disease, and renal failure. *J Am Soc Nephrol* 2005;16:2557–2564.
307. Brenner BM, Garcia DL, Anderson S. Glomeruli and blood pressure: Less of one, more of the other? *Am J Hypertens* 1988;1:335–347.
308. Keller G, Zimmer G, Mall G, et al. Nephron number in patients with primary hypertension. *N Eng J Med* 2003;348:101–108.
309. Gruenwald P, Popper H. The histogenesis and physiology of the renal glomerulus in early postnatal life: Histological examinations. *J Urol* 1940;43:452–459.
310. Macdonald MS, Emery JL. The late intrauterine and postnatal development of human renal glomeruli. *J Anat* 1959;93:331–340.
311. Vernier RL, Birch-Andersen A. Studies of the human fetal kidney. I. Development of the glomerulus. *J Pediatr* 1962;60:754–768.
312. Thony HC, Luethy CM, Zimmermann A, et al. Histological features of glomerular immaturity in infants and small children with normal or altered tubular function. *Eur J Pediatr* 1995;154(Suppl 3):S65–S68.
313. Volger C, McAdams J, Homan SM. Glomerular basement membrane and lamina densa in infants and children: An ultrastructural evaluation. *Pediatr Pathol* 1987;7:527–534.
314. Ramage IJ, Howatson AG, McColl JH, et al. Glomerular basement membrane thickness in children: A stereologic assessment. *Kidney Int* 2002;62:895–900.
315. Steffes MW, Barbosa J, Basgen JM, et al. Quantitative glomerular morphology of the normal human kidney. *Lab Invest* 1983;49:82–86.
316. Vogelmann SU, Nelson WJ, Myers BD, et al. Urinary excretion of viable podocytes in health and renal disease. *Am J Physiol* 2003;285:F40–F48.
317. Petermann AT, Krofft R, Blonski M, et al. Podocytes that detach in experimental membranous nephropathy are viable. *Kidney Int* 2003;64:1222–1231.
318. Fetterman GH, Shuplock NA, Philipp FJ, et al. The growth and maturation of human glomeruli and proximal convolutions from term to adulthood. *Pediatrics* 1965;35:601–619.
319. Zolnai B, Palkovits M. Glomerulometrics III. Data referring to the growth of the glomeruli in man. *Acta Biol Hung* 1965;15:409–423.
320. Souster LP, Emery JL. The sizes of renal glomeruli in fetuses and infants. *J Anat* 1980;130:595–602.
321. Moore L, Williams R, Staples A. Glomerular dimensions in children under 16 years of age. *J Pathol* 1993;171:145–150.
322. Akaoka K, White RHR, Raafat F. Human glomerular growth during childhood: A morphometric study. *J Pathol* 1994;173:261–268.
323. Samuel T, Hoy WE, Douglas-Denton R, et al. Determinants of glomerular volume in different cortical zones of the human kidney. *J Am Soc Nephrol* 2005;16:3102–3109.
324. Steffes MW, Schmidt D, McCrery R, et al. Glomerular cell number in normal subjects and in type 1 diabetic patients. *Kidney Int* 2001;59:2104–2113.
325. Combs HL, Shankland SJ, Setzer SV, et al. Expression of the cyclin kinase inhibitor, $p27^{kip1}$, in developing and mature human kidney. *Kidney Int* 1998;53:892–896.
326. Nagata M, Nakayama K, Terada Y, et al. Cell cycle regulation and differentiation in the human podocyte lineage. *Am J Pathol* 1998;153:1511–1520.
327. Hiromura K, Haseley LA, Zhang P, et al. Podocyte expression of the CDK-inhibitor p57 during development and disease. *Kidney Int* 2001;60:2235–2246.
328. Puelles VG, Douglas-Denton RN, Cullen-McEwen LA, et al. Podocyte number in children and adults: Associations with glomerular size and numbers of other glomerular resident cells. *J Am Soc Nephrol* 2015;26:2277–2288.
329. Kampmeier OF. The metanephros or so-called permanent kidney in part provisional and vestigial. *Anat Rec* 1926;33:115–120.
330. Emery JL, Macdonald MS. Involuting and scarred glomeruli in the kidneys of infants. *Am J Pathol* 1960;36:713–723.
331. Herxheimer G. Uber hyaline Glomeruli der Neugeborenen und Sauglinge. *Frankfurt Ztschr Path* 1909;2:138–152.
332. Schwarz L. Weitere Beitrage zur Kenntnis der anatomischen Nierenveranderungen der nNeugeborenen und sauglinge. *Virchows Arch Path Anat* 1928;267:654–689.
333. Friedman HH, Grayzel DM, Lederer M. Kidney lesions in stillborn and newborn infants. "Congenital glomerulosclerosis." *Am J Pathol* 1942;18:699–713.
334. Thomas MA. Congenital glomerulosclerosis. *Pathology* 1969;1:105–112.
335. Dijkman HBPM, Wetzels JFM, Gemmink JH. Glomerular involution in children with frequently relapsing minimal change nephrotic syndrome: An unrecognized form of glomerulosclerosis? *Kidney Int* 2007;71:44–52.
336. Moffat DB, Fourman J. Ectopic glomeruli in the human and animal kidney. *Anat Rec* 1964;149:1–11.
337. MacCallum DB. The bearing of degenerating glomeruli on the problem of the vascular supply of the mammalian kidney. *Am J Anat* 1939;65:69–103.
338. Darmady EM, Offer J, Prince J, et al. The proximal convoluted tubule in the renal handling of water. *Lancet* 1964;2:1254–1257.

339. Evan AP, Larsson L. Morphologic development of the nephron. In: Edelmann CM Jr, Bernstein J, Meadow SR, et al., eds. *Pediatric Kidney Disease*. 2nd ed. Boston, MA: Little Brown & Co; 1992:19–48.
340. Satlin LM, Woda CB, Schwartz GJ. Development of function in the metanephric kidney. In: Vize PD, Woolf AS, Bard JBL, eds. *The Kidney: From Normal Development to Congenital Disease*. San Diego: Academic Press; 2003:267–325.
341. Kim J, Lee GS, Tisher CC, et al. Role of apoptosis in development of the ascending thin limb of Henle in rat kidney. *Am J Phsiol Renal Physiol* 1996;271:F831–F845.
342. Neiss WF. Histogenesis of the loop of Henle in the rat kidney. *Anat Embryol (Berl)* 1982;164:315–330.
343. Raptopoulos V, Kleinman PK, Mark S, et al. Renal fascial pathway; posterior extension of pancreatic effusions within the anterior pararenal space. *Radiology* 1986;158:367–374.
344. Tobin CE. The renal fascia and its relation to the transversalis fascia. *Anat Rec* 1944;89:295–311.
345. Kunin M. Bridging septa of the perinephric space: anatomic, pathologic, and diagnostic considerations. *Radiology* 1986;158:361–365.
346. Kochkodan EJ, Hagger AM. Visualization of the renal fascia: A normal finding in urography. *AJR Am J Roentgenol* 1983;140:1243–1244.
347. Parienty RA, Pradel J, Picard JD, et al. Visibility and thickening of the renal fascia on computed tomograms. *Radiology* 1981;139:119–124.
348. Wald H. The weight of normal adult human kidneys and its variability. *Arch Pathol Lab Med* 1937;23:493–500.
349. Kaisiske BL, Umen AJ. The influence of age, sex, race, and body habitus on kidney weight in humans. *Arch Pathol Lab Med* 1986;110:55–60.
350. Cheong B, Muthupillai R, Rubin MF. Normal values for renal length and volume as measured by magnetic resonance imaging. *Clin J Am Soc Nephrol* 2007;2:38–45.
351. Frimann-Dahl J. Normal variations of the left kidney. An anatomical and radiologic study. *Acta Radiol* 1961;55:207–216.
352. Graves FT. The anatomy of the intrarenal arteries and its application to segmental resection of the kidney. *Br J Surg* 1954;42:132–139.
353. Graves FT. *Anatomical Studies for Renal and Intrarenal Surgery*. Bristol, England: Wright; 1986.
354. Satyapal KS. Classification of the drainage patterns of the renal veins. *J Anat* 1995;186:329–333.
355. Sperber I. Studies on the mammalian kidney. *Zool Bidrag Uppsala* 1944;22:249–431.
356. Hodson CJ, Mariani S. Large cloisons. *AJR Am J Roentgenol* 1982;139:327–332.
357. Lafortune M, Constantin A, Breton G, et al. Sonography of the hypertrophied column of Bertin. *AJR Am J Roentgenol* 1986;146:53–56.
358. Bigongiari LR, Patel SK, Appelman H, et al. Medullary rays. Visualization during excretory urography. *AJR Am J Roentgenol* 1975;125:795–803.
359. Hodson CJ. The renal parenchyma and its blood supply. *Curr Probl Diagn Radiol* 1978;7:5–32.
360. Ransley PG, Risdon RA. Renal papillary morphology in infants and young children. *Urol Res* 1975;3:111–113.
361. Ransley PG. Intrarenal reflux. Anatomical, dynamic and radiologic studies–part I. *Urol Res* 1977;5:61–69.
362. Schmidt-Nielsen B. The renal pelvis. *Kidney Int* 1987;31:621–628.
363. Murphy WM, Grignon DJ, Perlman EJ. Tumors of the kidney, bladder, and related urinary structures. In: Silverberg SG, Sobin LH, eds. *Atlas of Tumor Pathology. 4th series 4, Fascicle 1*. Washington, DC: Armed Forces Institute of Pathology; 2004.
364. Amis ES, Cronan JJ. The renal sinus: An imaging review and proposed nomenclature for sinus cysts. *J Urol* 1988;139:1151–1159.
365. Beckwith JB. National Wilms tumor study: An update for pathologists. *Pediatr Dev Pathol* 1998;1:79–84.
366. Bonsib SM, Gibson D, Mhoon M, et al. Renal sinus involvement in renal cell carcinomas. *Am J Surg Pathol* 2000;24:451–458.
367. Bonsib SM. The renal sinus is the principal invasive pathway. A prospective study of 100 renal cell carcinomas. *Am J Surg Pathol* 2004;28:1594–1600.
368. Bertram JF, Douglas-Denton RN, Diouf B, et al. Human nephron number: Implications for health and disease. *Pediatr Nephrol* 2011; 26(9):1529–1533.
369. Oliver J. *Architecture of the Kidney in Chronic Bright's Disease*. New York: Harper & Row. Hoeber Medical Division; 1939.
370. Schmidt-Nielsen B, O'Dell R. Structure and concentrating mechanism in the mammalian kidney. *Am J Physiol* 1961;200:1119–1124.
371. Madsen KM, Tisher CC. Structural-functional relationships along the distal nephron. *Am J Physiol* 1986;250:F1–F15.
372. Jamison RL, Kriz W. *Urinary Concentrating Mechanism: Structure and Function*. New York: Oxford University Press; 1982.
373. Kriz W, Kaissling B. Structural organization of the mammalian kidney. In: Alpern RJ, Caplan MJ, Moe OW eds. *Seldin and Giebisch's The Kidney: Physiology and Pathophysiology*. 5th ed. Philadelphia, PA: Elsevier, Inc; 2013:595–691.
374. Knepper M, Burg M. Organization of nephron function. *Am J Physiol* 1983;244:F579–F589.
375. Kriz W, Bankir L. A standard nomenclature for structures of the kidney. *Kidney Int* 1988;33:1–7.
376. Zhou XJ, Laszik Z, Nadasdy T, et al., (eds). Algorithmic approach to the interpretation of renal biopsy. *Silva's Diagnostic Renal Pathology*. 2nd ed. Cambridge: Cambridge University Press; 2017: 69–91.
377. Pirani CL, Croker BP. Handling and processing of renal biopsy and nephrectomy specimens. In: Tisher CC, Brenner BM, eds. *Renal Pathology*. 2nd ed. Philadelphia, PA: JB Lippincott; 1994:1683–1694.
378. Walker PD, Cavallo T, Bonsib SM, et al. Practice guidelines for the renal biopsy. *Mod Pathol* 2004;17:1555–1563.
379. Fenton RA, Praetorius J. Anatomy of the kidney. In: Skorecki K, Chertow GM, Marsden PA, et al., eds. *Brenner and Rector's The Kidney*. 10th ed. Philadelphia, PA: Elsevier; 2016: 42–82.
380. Haymann JM Jr. Malpighi's "Concerning the structure of the kidneys." *Ann Med Hist* 1925;7:242–263.
381. Bowman W. On the structure and use of the Malpighian bodies of the kidney, with observations on the circulation through that gland. *Philos Trans R Soc Lond* 1842;132:57–80.
382. Fine LG. William Bowman's description of the glomerulus. *Am J Nephrol* 1985;5:437–440.
383. Geneser F. *Textbook of Histology*. Philadelphia, PA: Lea & Febiger; 1986.
384. Jorgensen F. *The Ultrastructure of the Normal Human Glomerulus*. Copenhagen: Munksgaard; 1966.

385. Tisher CC, Brenner BM. Structure and function of the glomerulus. In: Tisher CC, Brenner BM, eds. *Renal Pathology*. 2nd ed. Philadelphia, PA: JB Lippincott; 1994:143–161.
386. Newbold KM, Sandison A, Howie AJ. Comparison of size of juxtaglomerular and outer cortical glomeruli in normal adult kidney. *Virchows Archiv A Pathol Anat* 1992;420:127–129.
387. Newbold KM, Howie AJ, Koram A, et al. Assessment of glomerular size in renal biopsies including minimal change nephropathy and single kidneys. *J Pathol* 1990;160:255–258.
388. Bonsib SM, Reznicek MJ. A fluorescent study of hematoxylin and eosin-stained sections. *Mod Pathol* 1990;3:204–210.
389. Kaplan C, Pasternak B, Shah H, et al. Age-related incidence of sclerotic glomeruli in human kidneys. *Am J Pathol* 1975;80:227–234.
390. Kappel B, Olsen S. Cortical interstitial tissue and sclerosed glomeruli in the normal human kidney, related to age and sex. *Virchows Arch A Pathol Anat Histol* 1980;387:271–277.
391. Smith SM, Hoy WE, Cobb L. Low incidence of glomerulosclerosis in normal kidneys. *Arch Pathol Lab Med* 1989;113:1253–1255.
392. Hommos MS, Glassock RJ, Rule AD. Structural and functional changes in human kidneys with healthy aging. *J Am Soc Nephrol* 2017;28:2838–2844.
393. Wang X, Vrtiska TJ, Avula RT, et al. Age, kidney function, and risk factors associate differently with cortical and medullary volumes of the kidney. *Kidney Int* 2014;85:677–685.
394. Rule AD, Sasiwimonphan K, Lieske JC, et al. Characteristics of renal cystic and solid lesions based on contrast-enhanced computed tomography of potential kidney donors. *Am J Kidney Dis* 2012;59:611–618.
395. Kremers WK, Denic A, Lieske JC, et al. Distinguishing age-related from disease-related glomerulosclerosis on kidney biopsy: The Aging Kidney Anatomy study. *Nephrol Dail Transplant* 2015;30:2034–2039.
396. Denic A, Lieske JC, Chakkera HA, et al. The substantial loss of nephrons in healthy kidneys with aging. *J Am Soc Nephrol* 2017;28:313–320.
397. Vasmant D, Maurice M, Feldmann G. Cytoskeletal ultrastructure of podocytes and glomerular endothelial cells in man and in the rat. *Anat Rec* 1984;210:17–24.
398. Sorensson J, Fierlbeck W, Heider T, et al. Glomerular endothelial fenestrae in vivo are not formed from caveolae. *J Am Soc Nephrol* 2002;13:2639–2647.
399. Horvat R, Hovoka A, Dekan G, et al. Endothelial cell membranes contain podocalyxin—the major sialoprotein of visceral glomerular epithelial cells. *J Cell Biol* 1986;102:484–491.
400. Kerjaschki D, Sharkey DJ, Farquhar MG. Identification and characterization of podocalyxin—the major sialoprotein of the renal glomerular epithelial cell. *J Cell Biol* 1984;98:1591–1596.
401. Rostgaard J, Qvortrup K. Electron microscopic demonstrations of filamentous sieve plugs in capillary fenestrae. *Microvasc Res* 1997;53:1–13.
402. Rostgaard J, Qvortrup K. Sieve plugs in fenestrae of glomerular capillaries—site of the filtration barrier? *Cells Tissues Organs* 2002;170:132–138.
403. Dane MJC, van den Berg BM, Lee DH, et al. A microscopic view on the renal endothelial glycocalyx. *Am J Physiol Renal Physiol* 2015;308:F956–F966.
404. Hegermann J, Lunsdorf H, Ochs M, et al. Visualization of the glomerular endothelial glycocalyx by electron microscopy using cationic colloidal thorium dioxide. *Histochem Cell Biol* 2016;145:41–51.
405. Hjalmarsson C, Johansson BR, Haraldsson B. Electron microscopic evaluation of the endothelial surface layer of glomerular capillaries. *Microvas Res* 2004;67:9–17.
406. Satchell S. The role of the glomerular endothelium in albumin handling. *Nat Rev Nephrol* 2013;9:717–725.
407. Friden V, Oveland E, Tenstad O, et al. The glomerular endothelial coat is essential for glomerular filtration. *Kidney Int* 2011;79:1322–1330.
408. Dane MJ, Khairoun M, Lee DH, et al. Glomerular endothelial surface layer acts as a barrier against albumin filtration. *Am J Pathol* 2013;182:1532–1540.
409. Desideri S, Onions KL, Qiu Y, et al. A novel assay provides sensitive measurement of physiologically relevant changes in albumin permeability in isolated human and rodent glomeruli. *Kidney Int* 2018;93:1086–1097.
410. Ciarimboli G, Hjalmarsson C, Bokenkamp A, et al. Dynamic alterations of glomerular charge density in fixed rat kidneys suggest involvement of endothelial cell coat. *Am J Physiol* 2003;285:F722–F730.
411. Jeansson M, Haraldsson B. Morphological and functional evidence for an important role of the endothelial cell glycocalyx in the glomerular barrier. *Am J Physiol Renal Physiol* 2006;290:F111–F116.
412. Roberts WG, Palade GE. Increased microvascular permeability and endothelial fenestration induced by vascular endothelial growth factor. *J Cell Sci* 1995;108:2369–2379.
413. Esser S, Wolburg K, Wolburg H, et al. Vascular endothelial growth factor induces endothelial fenestrations in vitro. *J Cell Biol* 1998;140:947–959.
414. Ermina V, Sood M, Haigh J, et al. Glomerular-specific alterations of VEGF-A lead to distinct congenital and acquired renal diseases. *J Clin Invest* 2003;111:707–716.
415. Ermina V, Jefferson JA, Kowalewska J, et al. VEGF inhibition and renal thrombotic microangiopathy. *N Eng J Med* 2008;358:1129–1136.
416. Bartlett CS, Jeansson M, Quaggin SE. Vascular growth factors in glomerular disease. *Ann Rev Physiol* 2016;78:437–461.
417. Ballerman BJ. Glomerular endothelial cell differentiation. *Kidney Int* 2005;67:1668–1671.
418. Ballerman BJ, Marsden PA. Endothelium-derived vasoactive mediators and renal glomerular function. *Clin Invest Med* 1991;14:508–517.
419. Becker CG. Demonstration of actomyosin in mesangial cells of the renal glomerulus. *Am J Pathol* 1972;66:97–110.
420. Drenckhahn D, Schnittler H, Nobiling R, et al. Ultrastructural organization of contractile proteins in rat glomerular mesangial cells. *Am J Pathol* 1990;137:1343–1351.
421. Schlondorff D. The glomerular mesangial cell: An expanding role for a specialized pericyte. *FASEB J* 1987;1:272–281.
422. Sterzel RB, Hartner A, Schlotzer-Schrehardt U, et al. Elastic fiber proteins in the glomerular mesangium in vivo and in cell culture. *Kidney Int* 2000;58:1588–1602.
423. Schaefer L, Mihalik D, Babelova A, et al. Regulation of fibrillin-1 by biglycan and decorin is important for tissue preservation in the kidney during pressure-induced injury. *Am J Pathol* 2004;165:383–396.
424. Mundel P, Elger M, Sakai T, et al. Microfibrils are a major component of the mesangial matrix in the glomerulus of the rat kidney. *Cell Tissue Res* 1988;254:183–187.

425. Sakai T, Kriz W. The structural relationship between mesangial cells and basement membrane of the renal glomerulus. *Anat Embryol (Berl)* 1987;176:373–386.
426. Kriz W, Elger M, Lemley K, et al. Structure of the glomerular mesangium: A biomechanical interpretation. *Kidney Int* 1990;38(suppl 30):2–9.
427. Kriz W, Elger M, Mundel P, et al. Structure-stabilizing forces in the glomerular tuft. *J Am Soc Nephol* 1995;5:1731–1739.
428. Kurihara H, Sakai T. Cell biology of mesangial cells: The third cell that maintains the glomerular capillary. *Ana Sci Int* 2017;92:173–186.
429. Tsurumi H, Kurihara H, Miura K, et al. Afadin is localized at cell-cell contacts in mesangial cells and regulates migratory polarity. *Lab Invest* 2016;96:49–59.
430. Kikkawa Y, Virtanen I, Miner JH. Mesangial cells organize the glomerular capillaries by adhering to the G domain of laminin alpha5 in the glomerular basement membrane. *J Cell Biol* 2003;161:187–196.
431. Zimmerman SE, Hiremath C, Tsunezumi J, et al. Nephronectin regulates mesangial cell adhesion and behavior in glomeruli. *J Am Soc Nephrol* 2018;29:1128–1140.
432. Kerjaschki D, Ojha PP, Susani M, et al. A beta-1-integrin receptor for fibronectin in human kidney glomeruli. *Am J Pathol* 1989;134:481–489.
433. Michael AF, Keane WF, Raij L, et al. The glomerular mesangium. *Kidney Int* 1980;17:141–154.
434. Sterzel RB, Lovett DH. Interactions of inflammatory and glomerular cells in the response to glomerular injury. In: Wilson CB, Brenner BM, Stein JH, eds. *Immunopathology of Renal Disease*. New York: Churchill Livingstone; 1988:137–173.
435. Floege J, Eitner F, Alpers CE. A new look at platelet-derived growth factor in renal disease. *J Am Soc Nephrol* 2008;19:12–23.
436. Schreiner GF, Kiely JM, Cotran RS. Characterization of resident glomerular cells in the rat expressing Ia determinants and manifesting genetically restricted interactions with lymphocytes. *J Clin Invest* 1981;68:920–937.
437. Falini B, Flenghi L, Pileri S, et al. PG-M1: A new monoclonal antibody directed against a fixative-resistant epitope on the macrophage-restricted form of the CD689 molecule. *Am J Pathol* 1993;142:1359–1372.
438. Imasawa T, Utsunomiya Y, Kawamura T, et al. The potential of bone marrow-derived cells to differentiate to glomerular mesangial cells. *J Am Soc Nephrol* 2001;12:1401–1409.
439. Hugo C, Shankland SJ, Bowen-Pope DF, et al. Extraglomerular origin of the mesangial cell after injury. *J Clin Invest* 1997;100:786–794.
440. Starke C, Betz H, Hickmann L, et al. Renin lineage cells repopulate the glomerular mesangium after injury. *J Am Soc Nephrol* 2015;26:48–54.
441. Jorgensen F, Bentzon MW. The ultrastructure of the normal human glomerulus. Thickness of glomerular basement membranes. *Lab Invest* 1968;18:42–48.
442. Osawa G, Kimmelstiel P, Seling V. Thickness of glomerular basement membranes. *Am J Clin Pathol* 1966;45:7–20.
443. Osterby R. Morphometric studies of the peripheral glomerular basement membrane in early juvenile diabetes. Development of initial basement membrane thickening. *Diabetologica* 1972;8:84–92.
444. Ellis EN, Mauer M, Sutherland DER. Glomerular capillary morphology in normal humans. *Lab Invest* 1989;60:231–236.
445. Lennon R, Byron A, Humphries JD, et al. Global analysis reveals the complexity of the human glomerular extracellular matrix. *J Am Soc Nephrol* 2014;25:939–951.
446. Hobeika L, Barati MT, Caster DJ, et al. Characterization of glomerular extracellular matrix by proteomic analysis of laser-captured microdissected glomeruli. *Kidney Int* 2017;91:501–511.
447. Miner JH. The glomerular basement membrane. *Exp Cell Res* 2012;318:973–978.
448. Hudson BG, Reeders SI, Tryggvason K. Type IV collagen: Structure, gene organization and role in human diseases. *J Biol Chem* 1993;268:26033–26036.
449. Hudson BG. The molecular basis of Goodpasture and Alport syndromes: Beacons for the discovery of the collagen IV family. *J Am Soc Nephrol* 2004;15:2514–2527.
450. Hudson BG, Tryggvason K, Sundaramoorthy M, et al. Alport's syndrome, Goodpasture's syndrome, and type IV collagen. *N Eng J Med* 2003;348:2543–2556.
451. St. John PL, Abrahamson DR. Glomerular endothelial cells and podocytes jointly synthesize laminin-1 and -11 chains. *Kidney Int* 2001;60:1037–1046.
452. Zenker M, Aigner T, Wendler O, et al. Human laminin beta2 deficiency causes congenital nephrosis with mesangial sclerosis and distinct eye abnormalities. *Hum Mol Genet* 2004;13:2625–2632.
453. Katz A, Fish AJ, Kleppel MM, et al. Renal entactin (nidogen): Isolation, characterization and tissue distribution. *Kidney Int* 1991;40:643–652.
454. Murshed M, Smyth N, Miosge N, et al. The absence of nidogen 1 does not affect murine basement membrane formation. *Mol Cell Biol* 2000;20:7007–7012.
455. Iozzo RV. Basement membrane proteoglycans: From cellar to ceiling. *Nature Rev Mol Cell Biol* 2005;6:646–656.
456. Fraquhar MG. The glomerular basement membrane. A selective macromolecular filter. In: Hay ED, ed. *Cell Biology of Extracellular Matrix*. 2nd ed. New York: Plenum; 1991:365–418.
457. Mahan JD, Sisson-Ross SS, Vernier RC. Anionic sites in the human kidney: Ex vivo perfusion studies. *Mod Pathol* 1989;2:117–124.
458. Groffen A, Ruegg MA, Dijkman H, et al. Agrin is a major heparan sulfate proteoglycan in the human glomerular basement membrane. *J Histochem Cytochem* 1998;46:19–27.
459. Groffen AJ, Hop FW, Tryggvason K, et al. Evidence for the existence of multiple heparan sulfate proteoglycans in the human glomerular basement membrane and mesangial matrix. *Eur J Biochem* 1997;247:175–182.
460. McCarthy KJ, Wassenhove-McCarthy DJ. The glomerular basement membrane as a model system to study the bioactivity of heparan sulfate glycosaminoglycans. *Microsc Microanal* 2012;18:3–21.
461. Suleiman H, Zhang L, Roth R, et al. Nanoscale protein architecture of the kidney glomerular basement membrane. *eLife* 2013;2:e01149.
462. Arakawa M. A scanning electron microscopy of the human glomerulus. *Am J Pathol* 1971;64:457–466.
463. Ichimura K, Miyazaki N, Sadayama S, et al. Three-dimensional architecture of podocytes revealed by block-face scanning electron microscopy. *Sci Rep* 2015;5:8993.
464. Burghardt T, Hochapfel F, Salecker B, et al. Advanced electron microscopic techniques provide a deeper insight into the peculiar features of podocytes. *Am J Physiol Renal Physiol* 2015;309:F1082–F1089.

465. Neal CR, Crook H, Bell E, et al. Three-dimensional reconstruction of glomeruli by electron microscopy reveals a distinct restrictive urinary subpodocyte space. *J Am Soc Nephrol* 2005;16:1223–1235.
466. Gautier A, Bernhard W, Oberling C. [The existence of a pericapillary lacunar apparatus in the malpighian glomeruli revealed by electronic microscopy]. *C R Seances Soc Biol Fil* 1950;144:1605–1607.
467. Salmon AHJ, Toma I, Sipos A, et al. Evidence for restriction of fluid and solute movement across the glomerular capillary wall by the subpodocyte space. *Am J Physiol Renal Physiol* 2007;293:F1777–F1786.
468. Neal CR, Muston PR, Njegovan D, et al. Glomerular filtration into the subpodocyte space is highly restricted under physiological perfusion conditions. *Am J Physiol Renal Physiol* 2007;293:F1787–F1798.
469. Arkill KP, Qvortrup K, Starborg T, et al. Resolution of the three dimensional structure of components of the glomerular filtration barrier. *BMC Nephrology* 2014;15:24.
470. Schell C, Huber TB. The evolving complexity of the podocyte cytoskeleton. *J Am Soc Nephrol* 2017;28:3166–3174.
471. Andrews PM, Bates SB. Filamentous actin bundles in the kidney. *Anat Rec* 1984;210:1–9.
472. Drenckhahn D, Franke R. Ultrastructural organization of contractile and cytoskeletal proteins in glomerular podocytes of chicken, rat and man. *Lab Invest* 1988;59:673–682.
473. Holthofer H, Miettinen A, Lehto V, et al. Expression of vimentin and cytokeratin types of intermediate filament proteins in developing and adult human kidneys. *Lab Invest* 1984;50:552–559.
474. Pavenstadt H, Kriz W, Kretzler M. Cell biology of the glomerular podocytes. *Physiol Rev* 2003;83:253–307.
475. Ichimura K, Kurihara H, Sakai T. Actin filament organization of foot processes in vertebrate glomerular podocytes. *Cell Tissue Res* 2007;329:541–557.
476. Pellegrin S, Mellor H. Actin stress fibers. *J Cell Sci* 2007;120:3491–3499.
477. Suleiman HY, Roth R, Jain S, et al. Injury-induced actin cytoskeleton reorganization in podocytes revealed by super-resolution microscopy. *JCI Insight* 2017;2:e94137.
478. Falkenberg CV, Azeloglu EU, Stothers M, et al. Fargility of foot process morphology in kidney podocytes arises from chaotic spatial propagation of cytoskeletal instability. *PLoS Comput Biol* 2017;13:e1005433.
479. Perico L, Conti S, Benigni A, et al. Podocyte-actin dynamics in health and disease. *Nat Rev Nephrol* 2016;12:692–710.
480. Sever S, Schiffer M. Actin dynamics at focal adhesions: A common endpoint and putative therapeutic target for proteinuria diseases. *Kidney Int* 2018;93:1298–1307.
481. Has C, Sparta G, Kiritsi D, et al. Integrin α3 mutations with kidney, lung and skin disease. *New Eng J Med* 2012;366:1508–1514.
482. Mouawad F, Tsui H, Takano T. Role of Rho-GTPases and their regulatory proteins in glomerular podocyte function. *Can J Physiol Pharmacol* 2013;91:773–782.
483. Gu C, Lee HW, Garborcauskas G, et al. Dynamin autonomously regulates podocyte focal adhesion maturation. *Am J Soc Nephrol* 2017;28:446–451.
484. Grahammer F, Schell C, Huber TB. The podocyte slit diaphragm - from a thin grey line to a complex signaling hub. *Nat Rev Nephrol* 2013;9:587–598.
485. Rodewald R, Karnovsky MJ. Porous substructure of the glomerular slit diaphragm in the rat and mouse. *J Cell Biol* 1974;60:423–433.
486. Karnovsky MJ, Ryan GB. Substructure of the glomerular slit diaphragm in freeze-fractured normal rat kidney. *J Cell Biol* 1975;65:233–236.
487. Schneeberger EE, Levey RH, McCluskey RI, et al. The isoporous substructure of the human glomerular slit diaphragm. *Kidney Int* 1975;8:48–52.
488. Wartiovaara J, Ofverstedt LG, Khoshnoodi J, et al. Nephrin strands contribute to a porous slit diaphragm scaffold as revealed by electron tomography. *J Clin Invest* 2004;114:1475–1483.
489. Hora K, Ohno S, Oguchi H, et al. Three-dimensional study of glomerular slit diaphragm by the quick-freezing and deep-etching replica method. *Eur J Cell Biol* 1990;53:402–406.
490. Gagliardini E, Conti S, Benigni A, et al. Imaging the porous ultrastructure of the glomerular epithelial filtration slit. *J Am Soc Nephrol* 2010;21:2081–2089.
491. Rice WL, van Hoek AN, Paunescu TG, et al. High resolution helium ion scanning microscopy of the rat kidney. *PLoS One* 2013;8:e57051.
492. Tsuji K, Paunescu TG, Suleiman H, et al. Re-characterization of the glomerulopathy in CD2AP deficient mice by high-resolution helium ion scanning microscopy. *Sci Rep* 2017;7:8321.
493. Grahammer F, Wigge C, Schell C, et al. A flexible, multilayered protein scaffold maintains the slit in between glomerular podocytes. *JCI Insight* 2017;1:e86177.
494. Schnabel E, Anderson JM, Farquhar MG. The tight junction protein ZO-1 is concentrated along slit diaphragms of the glomerular epithelium. *J Cell Biol* 1990;111:1255–1263.
495. Reiser J, Kriz W, Kretzler M, et al. The glomerular slit diaphragm is a modified adherens junction. *J Am Soc Nephrol* 2000;11:1–8.
496. Kerjaschki D. Caught flat-footed: Podocyte damage and the molecular bases of focal glomerulosclerosis. *J Clin Invest* 2001;108:1583–1587.
497. Ruotsalainen V, Ljungberg P, Wartiovaara J, et al. Nephrin is specifically located at the slit diaphragm of glomerular podocytes. *Proc Natl Acad Sci USA* 1999;96:7962–7967.
498. Putaala H, Soininen R, Kilelainen P, et al. The murine nephrin gene is specifically expressed in kidney, brain and pancreas:inactivation of the gene leads to massive proteinuria and neonatal death. *Hum Mol Genet* 2001;10:1–8.
499. Huber TB, Benzing T. The slit diaphragm: A signaling platform to regulate podocyte function. *Curr Opin Nephrol Hypertens* 2005;14:211–216.
500. Lehtonen S, Ryan JJ, Kudlicka K, et al. Cell junction-associated proteins IQGAP1, MAG1-2, CASK, spectrins, and α-actinin are components of the nephrin multiprotein complex. *Proc Natl Acad Sci USA* 2005;102:9814–9819.
501. Hirabayashi S, Mori H, Kansaku A, et al. MAGI-1 is a component of the glomerular slit diaphragm that is tightly associated with nephrin. *Lab Invest* 2005;85:1528–1543.
502. Donoviel DB, Freed DD, Vogel H, et al. Proteinuria and perinatal lethality in mice lacking NEPH1, a novel protein with homology to NEPHRIN. *Mol Cell Biol* 2001;21:4829–4836.
503. Ciana L, Patel A, Allen ND, et al. Mice lacking the giant protocadherin mFAT1 exhibit renal slit junction abnormalities and a partially penetrant cyclopia and anophthalmia phenotype. *Mol Cell Biol* 2003;23:3575–3582.

504. Roselli S, Heidet L, Sich M, et al. Early glomerular filtration defect and severe renal disease in podocin-deficient mice. *Mol Cell Biol* 2004;24:550–560.
505. Shih NY, Li J, Karpitskii V, et al. Congenital nephrotic syndrome in mice lacking CD2-associated protein. *Science* 1999;286:312–315.
506. Kaplan JM, Kim SH, North KN, et al. Mutations in ACTN4, encoding α-actinin-4, cause familial focal segmental glomerulosclerosis. *Nat Genet* 2000;24:251–256.
507. Kos CH, Le TC, Sinha S, et al. Mice deficient in α-actinin-4 have severe glomerular disease. *J Clin Invest* 2003;111:1683–1690.
508. Winn MP, Conlon PJ, Lynn KL, et al. A mutation in the TRPC6 cation channel causes familial focal segmental glomerulosclerosis. *Science* 2005;308:1801–1804.
509. Reiser J, Polu KR, Moller CC, et al. TRPC6 is a glomerular slit diaphragm-associated channel required for normal renal function. *Nat Genet* 2005;37:739–744.
510. Hinkes B, Wiggins RC, Gbadegesin R, et al. Positional cloning uncovers mutations in PLCE1 responsible for a nephritic syndrome variant that may be reversible. *Nat Genet* 2006;38:1397–1405.
511. Brown EJ, Schondorff JS, Becker DJ, et al. Mutations in the forming gene INF2 cause focal segmental glomerulosclerosis. *Nat Genet* 2010;42:72–77.
512. Mele C, Iatropoulos P, Donadelli R, et al. MYO1E mutations and childhood familial focal segmental glomerulosclerosis. *New Eng J Med* 2011;365:295–306.
513. New LA, Martin CE, Jones N. Advances in slit diaphragm signaling. *Curr Opin Nephrol Hypertens* 2014;23:420–430.
514. Asanuma K, Kim K, Oh J, et al. Synaptopodin regulates the actin-bundling activity of α-actinin in an isoform-specific manner. *J Clin Invest* 2005;115:1188–1198.
515. Jones N, Blasutig IM, Eremina V, et al. Nck adaptor proteins link nephrin to the actin cytoskeleton of kidney podocytes. *Nature* 2006;440:818–823.
516. Verma R, Kovari I, Soofi A, et al. Nephrin ectodomain engagement results in Src kinase activation, nephrin phosphorylation, Nck recruitment and actin polymerization. *J Clin Invest* 2006;116:1346–1359.
517. Okrut J, Prakash S, Wu Q, et al. Allosteric N-WASP activation by an inter-SH3 domain linker in Nck. *Proc Nat Acad Sci USA* 2015;112:E6436–E6445.
518. New LA, Martin CE, Scott RP, et al. Nephrin tyrosine phosphorylation is required to stabilize and restore podocyte foot process architecture. *J Am Soc Nephrol* 2016;27:2422–2435.
519. Jones N, New LA, Fortino MA, et al. Nck proteins maintain the adult glomerular filtration barrier. *J Am Soc Nephrol* 2009;20:1533–1543.
520. Schell C, Baumhakl L, Salou S, et al. N-WASP is required for stabilization of podocyte foot processes. *J Am Soc Nephrol* 2013;24:713–721.
521. Martin CE, Peterson KA, Aoudjit L, et al. ShcA adaptor protein promotes nephrin endocytosis and is upregulated in proteinuric nephropathies. *J Am Soc Nephrol* 2018;29:92–103.
522. Regele HM, Fillipovic E, Langer B, et al. Glomerular expression of dystroglycans is reduced in minimal change nephrosis but not in focal segmental glomerulosclerosis. *J Am Soc Nephrol* 2000;11:403–412.
523. Hannigan GE, Leung-Hagesteijn C, Fitz-Gibbon L, et al. Regulation of cell adhesion and anchorage-dependent growth by a new β1-integrin-linked protein kinase. *Nature* 1996;379:91–96.
524. Barisoni L, Mundel P. Podocyte biology and the emerging understanding of podocyte diseases. *Am J Nephrol* 2003;23:353–360.
525. Sawada H, Stukenbrok H, Kerjaschki D, et al. Epithelial polyanion (podocalyxin) is found on the sides but not the soles of the foot processes of the glomerular epithelium. *Am J Pathol* 1986;125:309–318.
526. Wiggins RC, Wiggins JE, Goyal M, et al. Molecular cloning of cDNAs encoding human GLEPP1, a membrane protein tyrosine phosphatase. *Genomics* 1995;27:174–181.
527. Takeda T, McQuistan T, Orlando RA, et al. Loss of glomerular foot processes is associated with uncoupling of podocalyxin from the actin cytoskeleton. *J Clin Invest* 2001;108:289–301.
528. Orlando RA, Takeda T, Zak B, et al. The glomerular epithelial cell anti-adhesion podocalyxin associates with the actin cytoskeleton through interactions with ezrin. *J Am Soc Nephrol* 2001;12:1589–1598.
529. Doyonnas R, Kershaw DB, Duhme C, et al. Anuria, omphalocele and perinatal lethality in mice lacking the CD34-related protein podocalyxin. *J Exp Med* 2001;194:13–27.
530. Akchurin O, Reidy KJ. Genetic causes of proteinuria and nephrotic syndrome: Impact on podocyte pathobiology. *Pediatr Nephrol* 2015;30:221–233.
531. Stamenkovic I, Skalli O, Gabliani G. Distribution of intermediate filament proteins in normal and diseased human glomeruli. *Am J Pathol* 1986;125:465–475.
532. Moll R, Hage C, Thoenes W. Expression of intermediate filament proteins in fetal and adult human kidney: Modulation of intermediate filament patterns during development and in damaged tissue. *Lab Invest* 1991;65:74–86.
533. Oosterwijk E, van Muijen GNP, Oosterwijk-Wakka JC, et al. Expression of intermediate-sized filaments in developing and adult human kidney and in renal cell carcinoma. *J Histochem Cytochem* 1990;38:385–392.
534. Yaoita E, Franke WW, Yamamoto T, et al. Identification of renal podocytes in multiple species: Higher vertebrates are vimentin positive/lower vertebrates are desmin positive. *Histochem Cell Biol* 1999;111:107–115.
535. Floege J, Alpers CE, Sage EH, et al. Markers of complement-dependent and complement-independent glomerular visceral epithelial injury in vivo. *Lab Invest* 1992;67:486–497.
536. Shankland SJ, Eitner F, Hudkins KL, et al. Differential expression of cyclin-dependent kinase inhibitors in human glomerular disease: role in podocyte proliferation and maturation. *Kidney Int* 2000;58:674–683.
537. Pritchard-Jones K, Fleming S, Davidson D, et al. The candidate Wilms tumor gene is involved in genitourinary development. *Nature* 1990;346:194–197.
538. Mundlos S, Pelletier J, Darveau A, et al. Nuclear localization of the protein encoded by the Wilms tumor gene WT1 in embryonic and adult tissues. *Development* 1993;119:1329–1341.
539. Pelletier J, Brucning W, Kashatn CE. Germline mutations in the Wilms tumor suppressor gene are associated with abnormal urogenital development in Denys-Drash syndrome. *Cell* 1991;67:437–447.
540. Schumacher VA, Schlotzer-Schrehardt U, Karumanchi SA, et al. WT1-dependent sulfatase expression maintains the normal glomerular filtration barrier. *J Am Soc Nephrol* 2011;22:1286–1296.

541. Kann M, Ettou S, Jung YL, et al. Genome-wide analysis of Wilms tumor 1-controlled gene expression in podocytes reveals key regulatory mechanisms. *J Am Soc Nephrol* 2015;26:2097–2104.
542. Warejko JK, Tan W, Dga A, et al. Whole exome sequencing of ptainets with steroid-resistant nephrotic syndrome. *Clin J Am Soc Nephrol* 2018;13:53–62.
543. Rinschen MM, Godel M, Grahammer F, et al. A multi-layered quantitative *in vivo* expression atlas of the podocyte unravels kidney disease candidate genes. *Cell Reports* 2018;23:2495–2508.
544. Deen WM. What determines glomerular capillary permeability? *J Clin Invest* 2004;114:1412–1414.
545. Haraldsson B, Nystrom J, Deen WM. Properties of the glomerular barrier and mechanisms of proteinuria. *Physiol Rev* 2008;88:451–487.
546. Kanwar YS. Continuum of historical controversies regarding structural-functional relationship of the glomerular ultrafiltration unit (GUU). *Am J Physiol Renal Physiol* 2015;308:F420–F424.
547. Edwards A, Daniels BS, Deen WM. Ultrastructural model for size selectivity in glomerular filtration. *Am J Physiol* 1999;276: F892–F902.
548. Rossi M, Morita H, Sormunen R, et al. Heparan sulfate chains of perlecan are indispensable in the lens capsule but not in the kidney. *EMBO J* 2003;22:236–245.
549. Harvey SJ, Jarad G, Cunningham J, et al. Disruption of glomerular basement membrane charge through podocyte-specific mutation of agrin does not alter glomerular permeability. *Am J Pathol* 2007;171:39–52.
550. Jarad G, Cunningham J, Shaw AS, et al. Proteinuria precedes podocyte abnormalities in Lamb2 -/- mice, implicating the glomerular basement membrane as an albumin filter. *J Clin Invest* 2006;116:2272–2279.
551. Dijkman H, Smeets B, van der Laak J, et al. The parietal epithelial cell is crucially involved in human idiopathic focal segmental glomerulosclerosis. *Kidney Int* 2005;68:1562–1572.
552. Ohtaka A, Ootaka T, Sato H, et al. Phenotypic change of glomerular podocytes in primary focal segmental glomerulosclerosis: Developmental paradigm? *Nephrol Dial Transplant* 2002;17(Suppl 9):11–15.
553. Peissel B, Geng L, Kalluri R, et al. Comparative distribution of the alpha 1(IV), alpha 5(IV), and alpha 6(IV) collagen chains in normal human adult and fetal tissues and in kidneys from X-linked Alport syndrome patients. *J Clin Invest* 1995;96:1948–1957.
554. Ohse T, Chang AM, Pippin JW, et al. A new function for parietal epithelial cells: A second glomerular barrier. *Am J Physiol Renal Physiol* 2009;297:F1566–F1574.
555. Shankland SJ, Smeets B, Pippin JW, et al. The emergence of the glomerular parietal epithelial cell. *Nat Rev Nephrol* 2014;10:158–173.
556. Alcorn D, Ryan GB. The glomerular peripolar cell. *Kidney Int Suppl* 1993;42:S35–S39.
557. Gibson IW, Downie I, Downie TT, et al. The parietal podocyte: A study of the vascular pole of the human glomerulus. *Kidney Int* 1992;41:211–214.
558. Bariety J, Mandet C, Hill GS, et al. Parietal podocytes in normal human glomeruli. *J Am Soc Nephrol* 2006;17:2770–2780.
559. Smeets B, Stucker F, Wetzels J, et al. Detection of activated parietal epithelial cells on the glomerular tuft distinguishes early focal segmental glomerulosclerosis from minimal change disease. *Am J Pathol* 2014;184:3239–3248.
560. Miesen L, Steenbergen E, Smeets B. Parietal cells-new perspectives in glomerular disease. *Cell Tissue Res* 2017;369: 237–244.
561. Shankland SJ, Freedman BS, Pippin JW. Can podocytes be regenerated in adults? *Curr Opin Nephrol Hypertens* 2017; 26:154–164.
562. Appel D, Kershaw DB, Smeets B, et al. Recruitment of podocytes from glomerular parietal epithelial cells. *J Am Soc Nephrol* 2009;20:333–343.
563. Berger K, Schulte K, Boor P, et al. The regenerative potential of parietal epithelial cells in adult mice. *J Am Soc Nephrol* 2014;25:693–705.
564. Wanner N, Hartleben B, Herbach N, et al. Unraveling the role of podocyte turnover in glomerular aging and injury. *J Am Soc Nephrol* 2014;25:707–716.
565. Lasagni L, Angelotti ML, Ronconi E, et al, Podocyte regeneration driven by renal progenitors determines glomerular disease remission and can be pharmacologically enhanced. *Stem Cell Reports* 2015;5:248–263.
566. Hackl MJ, Burford JL, Villanueva K, et al. Tracking the fate of glomerular epithelial cells in vivo using serial multiphoton imaging in new mouse models with fluorescent lineage tags. *Nat Med* 2013;19:1661–1666.
567. Schulte K, Berger K, Boor P, et al. Origin of parietal podocytes in atubular glomeruli mapped by lineage tracing. *J Am Soc Nephrol* 2014;25:129–141.
568. Kaverina NV, Eng DG, Schneider RRS, et al. Partial podocyte replenishment in experimental: FSGS derives from nonpodocyte sources. *Am J Physiol Renal Physiol* 2016;310: F1397–F1413.
569. Barajas L. Anatomy of the juxtaglomerular apparatus. *Am J Physiol* 1979;237:F333–F343.
570. Barajas L, Bloodworth JMB Jr, Hartroft PM. Endocrine pathology of the kidney. In: Bloodworth JMB Jr, ed. *Endocrine Pathology*. 2nd ed. Baltimore, MD: Williams & Wilkins; 1982:723–766.
571. Barajas L, Salido EC, Smolens P, et al. Pathology of the juxtaglomerular apparatus including Bartter's syndrome. In: Tisher CC, Brenner BM, eds. *Renal Pathology*. 2nd ed. Philadelphia, PA: JB Lippincott; 1994;948–978.
572. Cantin M, Gutkowska J, Lacasse J, et al. Ultrastructural immunocytochemical localization of renin and angiotensin II in the juxtaglomerular cells of the ischemic kidney. *Am J Pathol* 1984;115:212–224.
573. Taugner R, Mannek E, Nobiling R, et al. Coexistence of renin and angiotensin II in epithelioid cell secretory granules of rat kidney. *Histochemistry* 1984;81:39–45.
574. Barajas L, Wang P. Localization of tritiated norepinephrine in the renal arteriolar nerves. *Anat Rec* 1979;195:525–534.
575. Kopp UC, DiBona GF. Neural regulation of renin secretion. *Semin Nephrol* 1993;13:543–551.
576. Gomez RA, Sequeira-Lopez MLS. Renin cells in homeostasis, regeneration and immune defense mechanisms. *Nat Rev Nephrol* 2018;14:231–245
577. Pippin JW, Sparks MA, Glenn ST, et al. Cells of renin lineage are progenitors of podocytes and parietal epithelial cells in experimental glomerular disease. *Am J Pathol* 2013;183: 542–557.
578. Pippin JW, Kaverina NV, Eng DG, et al. Cells of renin lineage are adult pluripotent progenitors in experimental glomerular disease. *Am J Physiol Renal Physiol* 2015;309:F341–F358.

579. Lichtnekert J, Kaverina NV, Eng DG. Renin-angiotensin-aldosterone system inhibition increases podocyte derivation from cells of renin lineage. *J Am Soc Nephrol* 2016;27:3611–3627.
580. Kaverina NV, Kadoya H, Eng DG, et al. Tracking the stochastic fate of cells of the renin lineage after podocyte depletion using multicolor reporters and intravital imaging. *PLoS One* 2017;12:e0173891.
581. Eng DG, Kaverina NV, Scneider RRS, et al. Detection of renin lineage cell transdifferentiation to podocytes in the kidney glomerulus with dual lineage tracing. *Kidney Int* 2018;93:1240–1246.
582. Kurt B, Paliege A, Schwarzensteiner I, et al. Deletion of von Hippel-Lindau protein converts renin-producing cells into erythropoietin-producing cells. *J Am Soc Nephrol* 2013;24:433–444.
583. Kurt B, Gerl K, Karger C, et al. Chronic hypoxia-inducible transcription factor-2 activation stably transforms juxtaglomerular renin cells into fibroblast-like cells in vivo. *J Am Soc Nephrol* 2015;26:587–596.
584. Gerl K, Miqwerol L, Todorov VT, et al. Inducible glomerular erythropoietin production in the adult kidney. *Kidney Int* 2015;88:1345–1355.
585. Pricam C, Humbert F, Perrelet A, et al. Gap junctions in mesangial and lacis cells. *J Cell Biol* 1974;63:349–354.
586. Taugner R, Schiller A, Kaissling B, et al. Gap junctional coupling between the JGA and the glomerular tuft. *Cell Tissue Res* 1978;186:279–285.
587. Wagner C, Kurtz A. Distribution and functional relevance of connexins in renin-producing cells. *Pflugers Arch-Eur J Physiol* 2013;465:71–77.
588. Yao J, Oite T, Kitamura M. Gap junctional intercellular communication in the juxtaglomerular apparatus. *Am J Physiol Renal Physiol* 2009;296:F939–F946.
589. Kaissling B, Kriz W. Variability of intercellular spaces between macula densa cells: A transmission electron microscopic study in rabbits and rats. *Kidney Int* 1982;22(suppl):9–17.
590. Salido EC, Barajas L, Lechago J, et al. Immunocytochemical localization of epidermal growth factor in mouse kidney. *J Histochem Cytochem* 1986;34:1155–1160.
591. Sikri KL, Foster CL, MacHugh N, et al. Localization of Tamm-Horsfall glycoprotein in the human kidney using immunofluorescence and immunoelectron microscopical techniques. *J Anat* 1981;132:597–605.
592. Kirk KL, Bell PD, Barfuss DW, et al. Direct visualization of the isolated and perfused macula densa. *Am J Physiol* 1985;248:F890–F894.
593. Schnermann J. The juxtaglomerular apparatus: From anatomical peculiarity to physiological relevance. *J Am Soc Nephrol* 2003;14:1681–1694.
594. Schnermann J. Concurrent activation of multiple vasoactive signaling pathways in vasoconstriction by tubuloglomerular feedback: A quantitative assessment. *Annu Rev Physiol* 2015;77:301–322.
595. Wilcox CS, Welch WJ, Murad F, et al. Nitric oxide synthase in macula densa regulates glomerular capillary pressure. *Proc Natl Acad Sci USA* 1992;89:11993–11997.
596. Mundel P, Bachmann S, Bader M, et al. Expression of nitric oxide synthase in kidney macula densa cells. *Kidney Int* 1992;42:1017–1019.
597. Harris RC, McKanna JA, Akai Y, et al. Cyclooxygenase-2 is associated with the macula densa of rat kidney and increases with salt restriction. *J Clin Invest* 1994;94:2504–2510.
598. Welch WJ, Wilcox CS, Thomson SC. Nitric oxide and tubuloglomerular feedback. *Semin Nephrol* 1999;19:251–262.
599. Harris RC, Breyer MD. Physiological regulation of cyclooxygenase-2 in the kidney. *Am J Physiol* 2001;281:F1–F11.
600. Rouillier C. General anatomy and histology of the kidney. In: Rouillier C, Muller AF, eds. *The Kidney: Morphology, Biochemistry, Physiology.* New York: Academic Press; 1969:61–156.
601. Swann HG. The functional distention of the kidney: A review. *Tex Rep Biol Med.* 1960;18:566–596.
602. Hodson CJ. Physiological change in size of the human kidney. *Clin Radiol.* 1961;12:91–94.
603. Parker MV, Swann HG, Sinclair JG. The functional morphology of the kidney. *Tex Rep Biol Med* 1962;20:424–458.
604. Genest DR, Williams MA, Greene MF. Estimating the time of death in stillborn fetuses: I. Histologic evaluation of fetal organs; an autopsy study of 150 stillborns. *Obstet Gynecol* 1992;80:575–584.
605. Tomita Y, Nihira M, Ohno Y, et al. Ultrastructural changes during in situ early postmortem autolysis in kidney, pancreas, liver, heart and skeletal muscle of rats. *Legal Medicine* 2004;6:25–31.
606. Kocovski L, Duflou J. Can acute tubular necrosis be differentiated from autolysis at autopsy? *J Forensic Sc* 2009;54:439–442.
607. Ichimura T, Bonventre JV, Bailly V, et al. Kidney injury molecule-1 (KIM-1), a putative epithelial cell adhesion molecule containing a novel immunoglobulin domain, is upregulated in renal cells after injury. *J Biol Chem* 1998;273:4135–4142.
608. Han WK, Bailly V, Abichandani R, et al. Kidney injury molecule-1 (KIM-1): A novel biomarker for human renal proximal tubule injury. *Kidney Int* 2002;62:237–244.
609. Rodman JS, Mooseker M, Faruhar MG. Cytoskeletal proteins of the rat kidney proximal tubule brush border. *Eur J Cell Biol* 1986;42:319–327.
610. Farraggiana F, Malchiodi F, Prado A, et al. Lectin-peroxidase conjugate reactivity in normal kidney. *J Histochem Cytochem.* 1982;30:451–458.
611. Hennigar RA, Schulte BA, Spicer SS. Heterogeneous distribution of glycoconjugates in human kidney tubules. *Anat Rec* 1985;211:376–390.
612. Silva FG, Nadasdy T, Laszik Z. Immunohistochemical and lectin dissection of the human nephron in health and disease. *Arch Pathol Lab Med* 1993;117:1233–1239.
613. Skinnider BF, Folpe AL, Hennigar RA, et al. Distribution of cytokeratins and vimentin in adult renal neoplasms and normal renal tissue. *Am J Surg Pathol* 2005;29:747–754.
614. Paul R, Ewing CM, Robinson JC, et al. Cadherin-6, a cell adhesion molecule specifically expressed in the proximal renal tubule and renal cell carcinomas. *Cancer Res* 1997;57:2741–2748.
615. Letts RFR, Zhai XY, Bhikka C, et al. Nephron morphometry in mice and rats using tomographic microscopy. *Am J Physiol Renal Physiol* 2017;312:F210–F229.
616. Maunsbach AB, Christensen EI. Functional ultrastructure of the proximal tubule. In: Windhager EE, ed. *Handbook of Physiology. Section 8: Renal Physiology.* New York: Oxford University Press; 1992:41–107.
617. Zhai XY, Birn H, Jensen KB, et al. Digital three-dimensional reconstruction and ultrastructure of the mouse nephron. *J Am Soc Nephrol* 2003;14:611–619.
618. Christensen EI, Grann B, Kristoffersen IB, et al. Three-dimensional reconstruction of the rat nephron. *Am J Physiol Renal Physiol* 2014;306:F664–F671.

619. Tisher CC, Bulger RE, Trump BF. Human renal ultrastructure. I. Proximal tubule of healthy individuals. *Lab Invest* 1966;15:1357–1394.
620. Mount DB, Yu ASL. Transport of sodium, chloride, potassium. In: Brenner BM, ed. *Brenner & Rector's The Kidney*. 10th ed. Philadelphia, PA: Elsevier; 2016:144–184.
621. Welling LW, Welling DJ. Shape of epithelial cells and intercellular channels in the rabbit proximal nephron. *Kidney Int* 1976;9:385–394.
622. Welling LW, Welling DJ. Relationship between structure and function in renal proximal tubule. *J Electron Microsc Tech* 1988;9:171–185.
623. Ahn KY, Madsen KM, Tisher CC, et al. Differential expression and cellular distribution of mRNAs encoding α- and β-isoforms of Na^+-K^+-ATPase in rat kidney. *Am J Physiol* 1993;265:F792–F801.
624. Clapp WL, Bowman P, Shaw GS, et al. Segmental localization of mRNAs encoding Na^+-K^+-ATPase α- and β-subunit isoforms in rat kidney using RT-PCR. *Kidney Int* 1994;46:627–638.
625. Biemesderfer D, Pizzonia J, Abu-Alfa A, et al. NHE3: A Na^+/H^+ exchanger isoform of renal brush border. *Am J Physiol* 1993;265:F736–F742.
626. Amemiya M, Loffing J, Lotscher M, et al. Expression of NHE-3 in the apical membrane of rat proximal tubule and thick ascending limb. *Kidney Int* 1995;48:1206–1215.
627. Riquier-Brison AD, Leong PK, Pihakaski-Maunsbach K, et al. Angiotensin II stimulates trafficking of NHE3, NaPi2 and associated proteins into the proximal tubule microvilli. *Am J Physiol Renal Physiol* 2010;298:F177–F186.
628. Bergeron M, Guerette D, Forget J, et al. Three-dimensional characteristics of the mitochondrial of the rat nephron. *Kidney Int* 1980;17:175–185.
629. Agre P, King LS, Yasui M, et al. Aquaporin water channels-from atomic structure to clinical medicine. *J Physiol* 2002;542:3–16.
630. King LS, Kozono D, Agre P. From structure to disease: The evolving tale of aquaporin biology. *Nat Rev Mol Cell Biol* 2004;5:687–698.
631. Nielsen S, Smith BL, Christensen EI, et al. CHIP28 water channels are localized in constitutively water-permeable segments of the nephron. *J Cell Biol* 1993;120:371–383.
632. Maunsbach AB, Marples D, Chin E, et al. Aquaporin-1 water channel expression in human kidney. *J Am Soc Nephrol* 1997;8:1–14.
633. Christensen EI, Nielsen R, Birn H. Renal filtration, transport and metabolism of albumin and albuminuria. In: Alpern RJ, Moe OW, Caplan M, eds. *Seldin and Giebisch's The Kidney: Physiology and Pathophysiology*. 5th ed. Amsterdam; Elsevier, Inc; 2013:2457–2474.
634. Christensen EI, Rennke HG, Carone FA. Renal tubular uptake of protein: Effect of molecular charge. *Am J Physiol* 1983;244:F436–F441.
635. Park CH, Maack T. Albumin absorption and catabolism by isolated perfused proximal convoluted tubules of the rabbit. *J Clin Invest* 1984;73:767–777.
636. Park CH. Time course and vectorial nature of albumin metabolism in isolated perfused rabbit PCT. *Am J Physiol* 1988;255:F520–F528.
637. Clapp WL, Park CH, Madsen KM, et al. Axial heterogeneity in the handling of albumin by the rabbit proximal tubule. *Lab Invest* 1988;58:549–558.
638. Larsson L, Clapp WL, Park CH, et al. Ultrastructural localization of acidic compartments in cells of isolated rabbit proximal convoluted tubule. *Am J Physiol* 1987;253:F95–F103.
639. Christensen EI. Rapid membrane recycling in renal proximal tubule cells. *Eur J Cell Biol* 1982;29:43–49.
640. Christensen EI, Birn H. Megalin and cubilin: Synergistic endocytic receptors in renal proximal tubule. *Am J Physiol* 2001;280:F562–F573.
641. Birn H, Fyfe JC, Jacobsen C, et al. Cubilin is an albumin binding protein important for renal tubular albumin reabsorption. *J Clin Invest* 2000;105:1353–1361.
642. Nielsen R, Christesen EI, Birn H. Megalin and cubilin in proximal tubule protein reabsorption: From experimental models to human disease. *Kidney Int* 2016;89:58–67.
643. Russo LM, Sandoval RM, McKee M, et al. The normal kidney filters nephrotic levels of albumin retrieved by proximal tubules cells: Retrieval is disrupted in nephrotic states. *Kidney Int* 2007;71:504–513.
644. Sandoval RM, Wagner MC, Patel M, et al. Multiple factors influence glomerular albumin permeability in rats. *J Am Soc Nephrol* 2012;23:447–457.
645. Weyer K, Andersen PK, Schmidt K, et al. Abolishment of proximal tubule albumin endocytosis does not affect plasma albumin during nephrotic syndrome in mice. *Kidney Int* 2018;93:335–342.
646. Jiang M, Wei Q, Dong G, et al. Autophagy in proximal tubules protects against acute tubular injury. *Kidney Int* 2012;82:1271–1283.
647. Olsen S, Solez K. Acute tubular necrosis and toxic renal injury. In: Tisher CC, Brenner BM, eds. *Renal Pathology*. 2nd ed. Philadelphia, PA: JB Lippincott; 1994:769–809.
648. Nadasdy NT, Laszik Z, Blick KE, et al. Proliferative activity of intrinsic cell populations in the normal human kidney. *J Am Soc Nephrol* 1994;4:2032–2039.
649. Droz D, Zachar D, Charbit L, et al. Expression of the human nephron differentiation molecules in renal cell carcinomas. *Am J Pathol* 1990;137:895–905.
650. Gerdes J, Becker MHG, Key G, et al. Immunohistochemical detection of tumor growth fraction (Ki-67 antigen) in formalin fixed and routinely processed tissues. *J Pathol* 1992;168:85–87.
651. Witzgall R, Brown D, Schwarz C, et al. Localization of proliferating cell nuclear antigen, vimentin, c-fos, and clusterin in the postischemic kidney. *J Clin Invest* 1994;93:2175–2188.
652. Kliem V, Johnson RJ, Alpers CE, et al. Mechanisms involved in the pathogenesis of tubulointerstitial fibrosis in 5/6-nephrectomized rats. *Kidney Int* 1996;49:666–678.
653. Hansson J, Hultenby K, Cramnert C, et al.. Evidence for a morphologically distinct and functionally robust cell type in the proximal tubules of human kidney. *Hum Pathol* 2014;45:382–393.
654. Smeets B, Boor P, Dijkman H, et al. Proximal tubular cells contain a phenotypically distinct, scattered cell population involved in tubular regeneration. *J Pathol* 2013;229:645–659.
655. Kusaba T, Lalli M, Kramann R, et al. Differentiated kidney epithelial cells repair injured proximal tubule. *Proc Natl Acad Sci USA* 2014;111:1527–1532.
656. Berger K, Bangen J-M, Hammerich L, et al. Origin of regenerating tubular cells after acute kidney injury. *Proc Natl Acad Sci USA* 2014;111:1533–1538.
657. Gobe GC, Axelsen RA, Searle JW. Genesis of renal tubular atrophy in experimental hydronephrosis in the rat. Role of apoptosis. *Lab Invest* 1987;56:273–281.

658. Gobe GC, Axelsen RA, Searle JW. Cellular events in experimental unilateral ischemic renal atrophy and in regeneration after contralateral nephrectomy. *Lab Invest* 1990;63:770–779.
659. Schumer M, Colombel MC, Sawczuk IS, et al. Morphologic, biochemical and molecular evidence of apoptosis during the reperfusion phase after brief periods of renal ischemia. *Am J Pathol* 1992;140:831–838.
660. Schimizu A, Yamanaka N. Apoptosis and cell desquamation in repair process of ischemic tubular necrosis. *Virchows Arch B Cell Pathol Incl Mol Pathol* 1993;64:171–180.
661. Dieterich HJ, Barrett JM, Kriz W, et al. The ultrastructure of the thin limbs of the mouse kidney. *Anat Embryol (Berl)* 1975;147:1–13.
662. Bulger RE, Tisher CC, Myers CH, et al. Human renal ultrastructure. II. The thin limb of Henle's loop and the interstitium in healthy individuals. *Lab Invest* 1967;16:124–141.
663. Sands JM, Layton HE, Fenton RA. Urine concentration and dilution. In: Skorecki K, Chertow GM, Marsden PA, et al, eds. *Brenner & Rector's The Kidney*. 10th ed. Philadelphia, PA: Elsevier; 2016:258–280.
664. Nielsen S, Pallone T, Snith BL, et al. Aquaporin-1 water channels in short and long loop descending thin limbs and in descending vasa recta in rat kidney. *Am J Physiol* 1995;268:F1023–F1037.
665. Zhai XY, Fenton RA, Andeason A, et al. Aquporin-1 is not expressed in descending thin limbs of short-loop nephrons. *J Am Soc Nephrol* 2007;18:2937–2944.
666. Uchida S, Sasaki S, Nitta K, et al. Localization and functional characterization of rat kidney-specific chloride channel, ClC-K1. *J Clin Invest* 1995;95:104–113.
667. Takeuchi Y, Uchida S, Marumo F, et al. Cloning, tissue distribution, and intrarenal localization of ClC chloride channels in human kidney. *Kidney Int* 1995;48:1497–1503.
668. Ma T, Yang B, Gillespie A, et al. Severely impaired urinary concentrating ability in transgenic mice lacking aquaporin-1 water channels. *J Biol Chem* 1998;273:4296–4299.
669. King LS, Choi M, Fernandez PC, et al. Defective urinary-concentrating ability due to a complete deficiency of aquaporin-1. *New Eng J Med* 2001;345:175–179.
670. Matsumura Y, Uchida S, Kondo Y, et al. Overt nephrogenic diabetes insipidus in mice lacking the ClC-K1 chloride channel. *Nat Genet* 1999;21:95–98.
671. Kokko JP, Rector FC Jr. Countercurrent multiplication system without active transport in inner medulla. *Kidney Int* 1972;2:214–223.
672. Stephenson JL. Concentration of urine in a central core model of the renal counterflow system. *Kidney Int* 1972;2:85–94.
673. Pannbecker TL, Layton AT. Targeted delivery of solutes and oxygen in the renal medulla: Role of microvessel architecture. *Am J Physiol Renal Physiol* 2014;307:F649–F655.
674. Dantzler WH, Layton AT, Layton HE, et al. Urine-concentrating mechanism in the inner medulla: Function of the thin limbs of the loops of Henle. *Clin J Am Soc Nephrol* 2014;9:1781–1789.
675. Wei G, Rosen S, Dantzler WH, et al. Architecture of the human renal inner medulla and functional implications. *Am J Physiol Renal Physiol* 2015;309:F626–F637.
676. Kone BC, Madsen KM, Tisher CC. Ultrastructure of the thick ascending limb of Henle in the rat kidney. *Am J Anat* 1984;171:217–226.
677. Allen F, Tisher CC. Morphology of the ascending thick limb of Henle. *Kidney Int* 1976;9:8–22.
678. Shen SS, Krishna B, Chirala R, et al. Kidney-specific cadherin, a specific marker for the distal portion of the nephron and related renal neoplsams. *Mod Pathol* 2005;18:933–940.
679. Garg LC, Knepper MA, Burg MB. Mineralocorticoid effects on Na-K-ATPase in individual nephron segments. *Am J Physiol* 1981;240:F536–F544.
680. Nielsen S, Maunsbach AB, Ecelbarger CA, et al. Ultrastructural localization of Na-K-2Cl cotransporter in thick ascending limb and macula densa of rat kidney. *Am J Physiol* 1998;275:F885–F893.
681. Bachmann S, Velazquez H, Obermuller N, et al. Expression of the thiazide-sensitive Na-Cl cotransporter by rabbit distal convoluted tubule cells. *J Clin Invest* 1995;96:2510–2514.
682. Plotkin MD, Kaplan MR, Verlander JW, et al. Localization of the thiazide-sensitive Na-Cl cotransporter, rTSC1, in the rat kidney. *Kidney Int* 1996;50:174–183.
683. Woodhall PB, Tisher CC. Response of the distal tubule and cortical collecting duct to vasopressin in the rat. *J Clin Invest* 1973;52:3095–3108.
684. Gross JB, Imai M, Kokko JP. A functional comparison of the cortical collecting tubule and the distal convoluted tubule. *J Clin Invest* 1975;55:1284–1294.
685. Kaissling B. Structural aspects of adaptive changes in renal electrolyte excretion. *Am J Physiol* 1982;243:F211–F226.
686. Kaissling B, Bachmann S, Kriz W. Structural adaptation of the distal convoluted tubule to prolonged furosemide treatment. *Am J Physiol Renal Physiol* 1985;248:F374–F381.
687. Dorup J, Morsing P, Rasch R. Tubule-tubule and tubule-arteriole contacts in rat distal kidney distal nephrons. A morphologic study based on computer-assisted three-dimensional reconstructions. *Lab Invest* 1992;67:761–769.
688. Ren Y, Garvin JL, Liu R, et al. Crosstalk between the connecting tubule and the afferent arteriole regulates renal microcirculation. *Kidney Int* 2007;71:1116–1121.
689. Myers CH, Bulger RE, Tisher CC, et al. Human renal ultrastructure. IV. Collecting duct of healthy individuals. *Lab Invest* 1966;15:1921–1950.
690. Kaissling B, Kriz W. Structural analysis of the rabbit kidney. *Adv Anat Embryol Cell Biol* 1979;56:1–123.
691. Loffing J, Korbmacher C. Regulated sodium transport in the renal connecting tubule (CNT) via the epithelial sodium channel (ENaC). *Pflugers Arch* 2009;458:111–135.
692. Wade JB, Fang L, Coleman RA, et al. Differential regulation of ROMK (Kir1.1) in distal nephron segments by dietary potassium. *Am J Physiol Renal Physiol* 2011;300:F1385–F1393.
693. Boros S, Bindels RJ, Hoenderop JG. Active Ca(2+) reabsorption in the connecting tubule. *Pflugers Arch* 2009;458:99–109.
694. Coleman RA, Wu DC, Liu J, et al. Expression of aquaporins in the renal connecting tubule. *Am J Physiol Renal Physiol* 2000;279:F874–F883.
695. Kortenoeven ML, Pedersen NB, Miller RL, et al. Genetic ablation of aquaporin-2 in the mouse connecting tubules results in defective renal water handling. *J Physiol* 2013;591:2205–2219.
696. Fine LG. Eustachio's discovery of the renal tubule. *Am J Nephrol* 1986;6:47–50.
697. Welling LW, Evan AP, Welling DJ. Shape of cells and extracellular channels in rabbit cortical collecting ducts. *Kidney Int* 1981;20:211–222.

698. Duc C, Farman N, Canessa CM, et al. Cell-specific expression of epithelial sodium channel alpha, beta, and gamma subunits in aldosterone-responsive epithelia from the rat: Localization by in situ hybridization and immunocytochemistry. *J Cell Biol* 1994;127:1907–1921.
699. Hager H, Kwon TH, Vinnikova AK, et al. Immunocytochemical and immunoelectron microscopic localization of alpha-, bata-, and gamma-ENaC in rat kidney. *Am J Physiol* 2001;280: F1093–F1096.
700. Stanton BA, Biemesderfer D, Wade JB, et al. Structural and functional study of the rat nephron. Effects of potassium adaptation and depletion. *Kidney Int* 1981;19:36–48.
701. Petty KJ, Kokko JP, Marver D. Secondary effect of aldosterone on Na-K-ATPase activity in the rabbit cortical collecting tubule. *J Clin Invest* 1981;68:1514–1521.
702. Mujais SK, Chekal MA, Jones WJ, et al. Regulation of renal Na-K-ATPase in the rat: Role of the natural mineralo- and glucocorticoid hormones. *J Clin Invest* 1984;73:13–19.
703. Kaissling B, Le Hir M. Distal tubular segments of the rabbit kidney after adaptation to altered Na- and K-intake. I. Structural changes. *Cell Tissue Res* 1982;224:469–492.
704. Wade JB, O'Neil RG, Pryor JL, et al. Modulation of cell membrane area in renal collecting tubules by corticosteroid hormones. *J Cell Biol* 1979;81:439–445.
705. Kirk KL, Buku A, Eggena P. Cell specificity of vasopressin binding in renal collecting duct: Computer-enhanced imaging of a fluorescent hormone analog. *Proc Natl Acad Sci USA* 1987;84:6000–6004.
706. Nielsen S, Digiovanni SR, Christensen EI, et al. Cellular and subcellular immunolocalization of vasopressin-regulated water channel in rat kidney. *Proc Natl Acad Sci USA* 1993;90:11663–11667.
707. Nielsen C, Chou CL, Marples D, et al. Vasopressin increases water permeability of kidney collecting duct by inducing translocation of aquaporin-CD water channels to plasma membrane. *Proc Natl Acad Sci USA* 1995;92:1013–1017.
708. Ecelbarger CA, Terriis J, Frindt G, et al. Aquaporin-3 water channel localization and regulation in rat kidney. *Am J Physiol* 1995;269:F663–F672.
709. Hasegawa H, Ma T, Skach W, et al. Molecular cloning of a mercurial-insensitive water channel expressed in selected water-transporting tissues. *J Biol Chem* 1994;269:5497–5500.
710. Schuster VL, Bonsib SM, Jennings ML. Two types of collecting duct mitochondria-rich (intercalated) cells: Lectin and band 3 cytochemistry. *Am J Physiol* 1986;251:C347–C355.
711. Verlander JW, Madsen KM, Tisher CC. Effect of acute respiratory acidosis on two populations of intercalated cells in the rat cortical collecting duct. *Am J Physiol* 1987;253: F1142–F1156.
712. Teng-umnuay P, Verlander JW, Yuan W, et al. Identification of distinct subpopulations of intercalated cells in the mouse collecting duct. *J Am Soc Nephrol* 1996;7:260–274.
713. Kim J, Kim YH, Cha JH, et al. Intercalated cell subtypes in connecting tubule and cortical collecting duct of rat and mouse. *J Am Soc Nephrol* 1999;10:1–12.
714. Lonnerholm G. Histochemical demonstration of carbonic anhydrase activity in the human kidney. *Acta Physiol Scand* 1973;88:455–468.
715. McKinney TD, Burg MB. Bicarbonate absorption by rabbit cortical collecting tubules in vitro. *Am J Physiol* 1978;234: F141–F145.
716. McKinney TD, Burg MB. Bicarbonate secretion by rabbit cortical collecting tubules in vitro. *J Clin Invest* 1978;61:1421–1427.
717. Brown D, Gluck S, Hartwig J. Structure of the novel membrane-coating material in proton-secreting epithelial cells and identification as an H^+ATPase. *J Cell Biol* 1987;105: 1637–1648.
718. Brown D, Hirsh S, Gluck S. An H^+-ATPase in opposite plasma membrane domains in kidney epithelial cell subpopulations. *Nature* 1988;331:622–624.
719. Alper SL, Natale J, Gluck S, et al. Subtypes of intercalated cells in rat kidney collecting duct defined by antibodies against erythroid band 3 and renal vacuolar H^+ ATPase. *Proc Natl Acad Sci USA* 1989;86:5429–5433.
720. Drenckhahn D, Schluter K, Allen DP, et al. Colocalization of band 3 with ankyrin and spectrin at the basal membrane of intercalated cells in the rat kidney. *Science* 1985;230:1287–1289.
721. Verlander JW, Madsen KM, Low PS, et al. Immunocytochemical localization of band 3 protein in the rat collecting duct. *Am J Physiol* 1988;255:F115–F125.
722. Weiner ID, Hamm LL. Regulation of intracellular pH in the rabbit cortical collecting tubule. *J Clin Invest* 1990;85: 274–281.
723. Royaux IE, Wall SM, Karniski LP, et al. Pendrin, encoded by the Pendred syndrome gene, resides in the apical region of renal intercalated cells and mediates bicarbonate secretion. *Proc Natl Acad Sci USA* 2001;98:4221–4226.
724. Soleimani M, Greeley T, Petrovic S, et al. Pendrin:an apical $Cl^-/OH^-/HCO_3^-$ exchanger in the kidney cortex. *Am J Physiol*. 2001;280:F356–F364.
725. Frische S, Kwon TH, Frokiaer J, et al. Regulated expression of pendrin in rat kidney in response to chronic NH_4Cl or $NAHCO_3$ loading. *Am J Physiol* 2003;284:F584–F593.
726. Romero MF. Molecular pathophysiology of SLC4 bicarbonate transporters. *Curr Opin Nephrol Hypertens* 2005;14:495–501.
727. Everett LA, Glaser B, Beck JC, et al. Pendred syndrome is caused by mutations in a putative sulphate transporter gene (PDS). *Nat Genet* 1997;17:411–422.
728. Wall SM, Hassell KA, Royaux IE, et al. Localization of pendrin in mouse kidney. *Am J Physiol* 2003;284:F229–F241.
729. Wall SM. Recent advances in our understanding of intercalated cells. *Curr Opin Nephrol Hypertens* 2005;14: 480–484.
730. Verlander JW, Kim YH, Shin W, et al. Dietary Cl(-) restriction upregulates pendrin expression within the apical plasma membrane of type B intercalated cells. *Am J Physiol Renal Physiol* 2006;291:F833–F939.
731. Wall SM, Weinstein AM. Cortical distal nephron Cl transport in volume homeostasis and blood pressure regulation. *Am J Physiol Renal Physiol* 2013;305:F427–F438.
732. Nanami M, Pham TD, Kim YH, et al. The role of intercalated cell Nedd4-2 in BP regulation, ion transport and transporter expression. *J Am Soc Nephrol* 2018;29:1706–1719.
733. Chen L, Lee JW, Chou CL, et al. Transcriptomes of major renal collecting duct cell types in mouse identified by single-cell RNA-seq. *Proc Natl Acad Sci USA* 2017;114: E9989–E9998.
734. Park J, Shrestha R, Qiu C, et al. Single-cell transcriptomics of the mouse kidney reveals potential cellular targets of kidney disease. *Science* 2018;360:758–763.
735. LeFurgey A, Tisher CC. Morphology of rabbit collecting duct. *Am J Anat* 1979;115:111–124.

736. Hansen GP, Tisher CC, Robinson RR. Response of the collecting duct to disturbances of acid-base and potassium balance. *Kidney Int* 1980;17:326–337.
737. Madsen KM, Tisher CC. Cellular response to acute respiratory acidosis in rat medullary collecting ducts. *Am J Physiol* 1983;245:F670–F679.
738. Madsen KM, Tisher CC. Response of intercalated cells of rat outer medullary collecting duct to chronic metabolic acidosis. *Lab Invest* 1984;51:268–276.
739. Garg LC, Narang N. Ouabain-insensitive K^+ adenosine triphosphatase in distal nephron segments of the rabbit. *J Clin Invest* 1988;81:1204–1208.
740. Wingo CS. Active proton secretion and potassium absorption in the rabbit outer medullary collecting duct: Functional evidence of $H^+ K^+$ ATPase. *J Clin Invest* 1989;84:361–365.
741. Wingo CS, Madsen KM, Smolka A, et al. $H^+ K^+$ ATPase immunoreactivity in cortical and outer medullary collecting duct. *Kidney Int* 1990;38:985–990.
742. Ahn KY, Kone BC. Expression and cellular localization of mRNA encoding the "gastric" isoform of H^+-K^+-ATPase α-subunit in rat kidney. *Am J Physiol* 1995;268:F99–F109.
743. Campbell-Thomson ML, Verlander JW, Curran KA, et al. In situ hybridization of H-K-ATPase β-subunit mRNA in rat and rabbit kidney. *Am J Physiol* 1995;269:F345–F354.
744. Weiner ID, Verlander JW. Ammonia transport in the kidney by Rhesus glycoproteins. *Am J Physiol Renal Physiol* 2014;306:F1107–F1120.
745. Madsen KM, Clapp WL, Verlander JW. Structure and function of the inner medullary collecting duct. *Kidney Int* 1988;34:441–454.
746. Sands JM, Knepper MA. Urea permeability of mammalian inner medullary collecting duct system and papillary surface epithelium. *J Clin Invest* 1987;79:138–147.
747. Sands JM, Nonoguchi H, Knepper MA. Vasopressin effects on urea and H_2O transport in inner medullary collecting duct subsegments. *Am J Physiol* 1987;253:F823–F832.
748. Clapp WL, Madsen KM, Verlander JM, et al. Intercalated cells of the rat inner medullary collecting duct. *Kidney Int* 1987;31:1080–1087.
749. Clapp WL, Madsen KM, Verlander JW, et al. Morphologic heterogeneity along the rat inner medullary collecting duct. *Lab Invest* 1989;60:219–230.
750. Nielsen S, Terris J, Smith CP, et al. Cellular and subcellular localization of the vasopressin-regulated urea transporter in rat kidney. *Proc Natl Acad Sci USA* 1996;93:5495–5500.
751. Shayakul C, Knepper MA, Smith CP, et al. Segmental localization of urea transporter mRNAs in rat kidney. *Am J Physiol* 1997;272:F654–F660.
752. Terris JM, Knepper MA, Wade JB. UT-A3; localization and characterization of an additional urea transporter isoform in the IMCD. *Am J Physiol* 2001;280:F325–F332.
753. Wall SM, Truong AV, DuBose TD Jr. H^+-K^+-ATPase mediates net acid secretion in rat terminal inner medullary collecting duct. *Am J Physiol* 1996;271:F1037–F1044.
754. Silverblatt FJ. Ultrastructure of the renal pelvic epithelium of the rat. *Kidney Int* 1974;5:214–220.
755. Khorshid MR, Moffat DB. The epithelia lining the renal pelvis in the rat. *J Anat* 1974;118:561–569.
756. Lucien N, Bruneval P, Lasbennes F, et al. UT-B1 urea transporter is expressed along the urinary and gastrointestinal tracts of the mouse. *Am J Physiol Regul Integr Comp Physiol* 2005;288:R1046–R1056.
757. Verlander JW, Moudy RM, Cambell WG, et al. Immunohistochemical localization of H-K-ATPase a2 subunit in rabbit kidney. *Am J Physiol Renal Physiol* 2001;281:F357–F365.
758. Madsen KM, Zhang L, Shamat AR, et al. Ultrastructural localization of osteopontin in the kidney: Induction by lipopolysaccharide. *J Am Soc Nephrol* 1997;8:1043–1053.
759. Bonventre JV, Karnovsky MJ, Lechene CP. Renal papillary epithelial morphology in antidiuresis and water diuresis. *Am J Physiol Renal Fluid Electrolyr Physiol* 1978;235:F69–F76.
760. Lemley KV, Kriz W. Anatomy of the interstitium. *Kidney Int* 1991;39:370–381.
761. Bohman SO. The ultrastructure of the renal medulla and the interstitial cells. In: Cotran RS, ed. *Tubulo-Interstitial Nephropathies*. New York: Churchill Livingstone; 1983:1–34.
762. Hestbech J, Hansen HE, Amdisen A, et al. Chronic renal lesions following long-term treatment with lithium. *Kidney Int* 1977;12:205–213.
763. Bohle A, Grund KE, MacKensen S, et al. Correlations between renal interstitium and level of serum creatinine. *Virchows Arch A Pathol Anat Histol* 1977;373:15–22.
764. Pfaller W. Structure function correlation in rat kidney. Quantitative correlation of structure and function in normal and injured rat kidney. *Adv Anat Embryol Cell Biol* 1982;70:1–106.
765. Mounier F, Foidart JM, Gubler MC. Distribution of extracellular matrix glycoproteins during normal development of human kidney: An immunohistochemical study. *Lab Invest* 1986;54:394–401.
766. Zeisberg M, Kalluri R. Physiology of the interstitium. *Clin J Am Soc Nephrol* 2015;10:1831–1840.
767. Kaissling B, Hegyi I, Loffing J, et al. Morphology of interstitial cells in the healthy kidney. *Anat Embryol (Berl)* 1996;193:303–318.
768. Kaissling B, Lr Hir M. The renal interstitium: Morphological and functional aspects. *Histochem Cell Biol* 2008;130:247–262.
769. Bachmann S, LeHir M, Eckardt KU. Colocalization of erythropoietin mRNA and ecto-5-nucleotidase immunoreactivity in peritubular cells of the rat renal cortex suggests that fibroblasts produce erythropoietin. *J Histochem Cytochem* 1993;41:335–341.
770. Maxwell PH, Osmond MK, Pugh CW, et al. Identification of the renal erythropoietin-producing cells using transgenic mice. *Kidney Int* 1993;44:1149–1162.
771. Asada N, Takase M, Nakamura J, et al. Dysfunction of fibroblasts of extrarenal origin underlies renal fibrosis and renal anemia in mice. *J Clin Invest* 2011;121:3981–3990.
772. Kobayashi H, Liu Q, Binns TC, et al. Distinct subpopulations of FOXD1 stroma-derived cells regulate renal erythropoietin. *J Clin Invest* 2016;126:1926–1938.
773. Di Carlo SE, Peduto L. The perivascular origin of pathological fibroblasts. *J Clin Invest* 2018;128:54–63.
774. Humphreys BD. Mechanisms of renal fibrosis. *Annu Rev Physiol* 2018;80:309–326.
775. Sims DE. The pericyte-A review. *Tissue Cell* 1986;18:153–174.
776. Lemos DR, Marsh G, Huang A, et al. Maintenance of vascular integrity by pericytes is essential for normal kidney function. *Am J Physiol Renal Physiol* 2016;311:F1230–F1242.
777. Kriz W, Kaissling B, Le Hir M. Epithelial-mesenchymal transition (EMT) in kidney fibrosis: Fact and fantasy?. *J Clin Invest* 2011;121:468–474.

778. Humphreys BD, Lin SL, Kobayashi A, et al. Fate tracing reveals the pericyte and not epithelial origin of myofibroblast in kidney fibrosis. *Am J Pathol* 2010;176:85–97.
779. Kramann R, Schneider RK, DiRocco DP, et al. Perivascular Gli1 progenitors are key contributors to injury-induced organ fibrosis. *Cell Stem Cell* 2015;16:51–66.
780. Viehmann SF, Bohner AMC, Kurts C, et al. The multifaceted role of the renal mononuclear phagocyte system. *Cell Immunol* 2018;pii:S0008-8749(18)30180-1.
781. Brahler S, Zinselmeyer BH, Raju S, et al. Opposing roles of dendritic cell subsets in experimental glomerulonephritis. *J Am Soc Nephrol* 2018;29:138–154.
782. Muirhead EE. The medullipin system of blood pressure control. *Am J Hypertens* 1991;4:556s–568s.
783. Folkow B. Incretory renal functions-Tigerstedt, renin and its neglected antagonist medullipin. *Acta Physiol* 2007;190:99–102.
784. Kurtz A. Endocrine functions of the renal interstitium. *Pflgers Arch Eur J Physiol* 2017;469:869–876.
785. Fourman J, Moffat DB. *The Blood Vessels of the Kidney*. Oxford: Blackwell Scientific; 1971.
786. More RH, Duff GL. The renal arterial vasculature in man. *Am J Pathol* 1951;27:95–117.
787. Edwards JG. Efferent arterioles of glomeruli in the juxtamedullary zone of the human kidney. *Anat Rec* 1956;125:521–529.
788. Casellas D, Mimran A. Shunts in renal microvasculature of the rat. A scanning electron microscopic study of corrosion casts. *Anat Rec* 1981;201:237–248.
789. Ljungqvist A. Ultrastructural connection between afferent and efferent arterioles in juxtamedullary glomerular units. *Kidney Int* 1975;8:239–244.
790. Ljungqvist A. Fetal and postnatal development of the intrarenal arterial pattern in man. *Acta Paediatr* 1963;52:443–464.
791. Mukai K, Rosai J, Burgdorf WH. Localization of factor VIII related antigen in vascular endothelial cells using an immunoperoxidase technique. *Am J Surg Pathol* 1980;4:273–276.
792. Sanfilippo F, Pizzo SV, Croker BP. Immunohistochemical studies of cell differentiation in a juxtaglomerular tumor. *Arch Pathol Lab Med* 1982;106:604–607.
793. Fina L, Molgard HV, Robertson D, et al. Expression of the CD34 gene in vascular endothelial cells. *Blood* 1990;75:2417–2425.
794. Civin CL, Trischmann TM, Fackler MJ, et al. Summary of CD34 cluster workshop section. In: Knapp W, ed. *Leucocyte Typing IV*. London: Academic Press; 1989:818–825.
795. Gabbiani G, Schmid E, Winter S, et al. Vascular smooth muscle cells differ from other smooth muscle cells: Predominance of vimentin filaments and a specific α-type actin. *Proc Natl Acad Sci USA* 1981;78:298–302.
796. Rollhauser H, Kriz W, Heinke W. Das gefass–system der rattenniere. *Z Zellforsch* 1964;64:381–403.
797. Kriz W, Barrett JM, Peter S. The renal vasculature: Anatomical–functional aspects. In: Thurau K, ed. *Kidney and Urinary Tract Physiology II*. Baltimore, MD: University Park Press; 1976:1–21.
798. Beeuwkes R, Bonventre JV. Tubular organization and vascular-tubular relations in the dog kidney. *Am J Physiol* 1975;229:695–713.
799. Beeuwkes R. Vascular-tubular relationships in the human kidney. In: Leaf A, Giebisch G, Bolis L, et al, eds. *Renal Pathophysiology*. New York: Raven Press; 1980:155–163.
800. Pierce EC. Renal lymphatics. *Anat Rec* 1944;90:315–335.
801. Bell RD, Keyl MJ, Shrader FR, et al. Renal lymphatics: The internal distribution. *Nephron* 1968;3:454–463.
802. Kriz W, Dieterich HJ. Das lymphagefass system der niere bei einigen saugetieren: Licht-und elektronenmikroskipische untersuchungen. *Z Anat Entwickl Gesch* 1970;131:111–147.
803. Ishikawa Y, Akasaka Y, Kiguchi H, et al. The human renal lymphatics under normal and pathological conditions. *Histopathology* 2006;49:265–273.
804. Kriz W. A periarterial pathway for intrarenal distribution of renin. *Kidney Int* 1987;31(suppl 20):551–556.
805. Yang Y, Oliver G. Development of the mammalian lymphatic vasculature. *J Clin Invest* 2015;124:888–897.
806. Zheng W, Aspelund A, Alitalo K. Lymphangiogenic factors, mechanisms and applications. *J Clin Invest* 2015;124:878–887.
807. Kenig-Kozlovsky Y, Scott RP, Onay T, et al. Ascending vasa recta are angiopoietin/Tie2-dependent lymphatic-like vessels. *J Am Soc Nephrol* 2018;29:1097–1107.
808. Mitchell GAG. The nerve supply of the kidneys. *Acta Anat (Basel)* 1950;10:1–37.
809. Gosling JA. Observations on the distribution of intrarenal nervous tissue. *Anat Rec* 1969;163:81–88.
810. Stefansson K, Wollmann RL, Jerkovic M. S-100 protein in soft tissue tumors derived from Schwann cells and melanocytes. *Am J Pathol* 1982;106:261–268.
811. Nakajima T, Uatanabe S, Sato Y, et al. An immunoperoxidase study of S-100 protein distribution in normal and neoplastic human tissues. *Am J Surg Pathol*. 1982;6:715–727.
812. Trojanowski JQ, Lee VMY, Schlaepfer WW. An immunohistochemical study of human central and peripheral nervous system tumors, using monoclonal antibodies against neurofilaments and glial filaments. *Hum Pathol* 1984;15:248–257.
813. Lee VMY, Carden MJ, Schlaepfer WW. Structural similarities and differences between neurofilament proteins from five different species as revealed using monoclonal antibodies. *J Neurosci* 1986;6:2179–2186.
814. Barajas L. Innervation of the renal cortex. *Fed Proc* 1978;37:1192–2001.
815. Fourman J. The adrenergic innervation of the efferent arterioles and the vasa recta in the mammalian kidney. *Experientia* 1970;26:293–294.
816. Barajas L, Powers K, Wang P. Innervation of the renal cortical tubules: A quantitative study. *Am J Physiol* 1984;247:F50–F60.
817. Barajas L, Powers K. Innervation of the thick ascending limb of Henle. *Am J Physiol* 1988;255:F340–F348.
818. Barajas L, Liu L, Poers K. Anatomy of the renal innervation: Intrarenal aspects and ganglia of origin. *Can J Physiol Pharmacol* 1992;70:735–749.
819. Sakakura K, Ladich E, Cheng Q, et al. Anatomic assessment of sympathetic peri-arterial renal nerves in man. *J Am Coll Cardiol* 2014;64:635–643.

Urinary Bladder, Ureter, and Renal Pelvis

Victor E. Reuter ■ Hikmat Al-Ahmadie ■ Satish K. Tickoo

EMBRYOLOGY 949

ANATOMICAL CONSIDERATIONS 950
   Bladder 950
   Ureters 952
   Renal Pelvis 952
   Microscopic Anatomy 953

Urothelium 953
Urothelial Variants and Benign Urothelial Proliferations 954
Lamina Propria 957
Muscularis Propria 958

REFERENCES 961

The urinary bladder is an epithelial-lined muscular viscus which has the ability to distend and accommodate up to 400 to 500 mL of urine without a change in intraluminal pressure. In addition, it is able to initiate and sustain a contraction until the organ is empty. Interestingly, micturition may be initiated or inhibited voluntarily despite the involuntary nature of the organ by activating skeletal muscles of the pelvis. The ureters are epithelial-lined muscular tubes designed to transport urine from the kidneys to the urinary bladder with the aid of peristalsis. The renal pelvis represents the expanded proximal end of the ureter and will serve to collect the urine excreted from the kidney and transport it to the ureter proper.

EMBRYOLOGY

The cloaca is divided by the urorectal septum into a dorsal rectum and a ventral urogenital sinus (1,2). It is this urogenital sinus which will give rise to the majority of the urinary bladder, aided by the caudal migration of the cloacal membrane which will close the infraumbilical portion of the abdominal wall. The caudal portions of the mesonephric ducts become dilated and eventually fuse with the urogenital sinus in the midline dorsally, contributing to the formation of the bladder trigone. While these ducts contribute initially to the formation of the mucosa of the trigone, this is subsequently entirely replaced by the endodermal epithelium of the urogenital sinus. The gradual absorption of the mesonephric ducts brings about the separate opening of the ureters into the urinary bladder in the area of the trigone. During embryologic development, the allantois regresses completely forming a thick, epithelial-lined tube, the urachus, which extends from the umbilicus to the apex (dome) of the bladder (1). Before or shortly after birth, the urachus involutes further becoming simply a fibrous cord. Pathologists commonly refer to this fibrous cord which extends from the dome of the bladder to the umbilicus as the urachal remnant but it should be called the median umbilical ligament since urachal remnant refers to remnants of the epithelial lining of the urachus which occasionally persist within the median umbilical ligament (Fig. 34.1). The epithelial lining of the urachus is urothelium, similar to that of the urinary bladder and the ureter, but it frequently undergoes metaplastic change, mostly glandular.

The epithelium of the urinary bladder is endodermally derived from the cranial portion of the urogenital sinus in continuity with the allantois. The lamina propria, the muscularis propria, and the adventitia develop from the adjacent splanchnic mesenchyme. These facts are important in understanding the histogenesis and nomenclature of lesions arising from the epithelial surface, as well as the bladder wall. For example, glandular features within benign (cystitis glandularis, nephrogenic adenoma/metaplasia) and malignant (adenocarcinoma) urothelium are not due to mesodermal or müllerian rests within the trigone but come about through a process of metaplasia or neometaplasia and are a reflection of histologic plasticity (multipotentiality) of the urothelium. Since the mesonephric ducts involute totally during embryologic development, it is incorrect to refer to tumors with mixed epithelial and sarcomatoid features arising in the

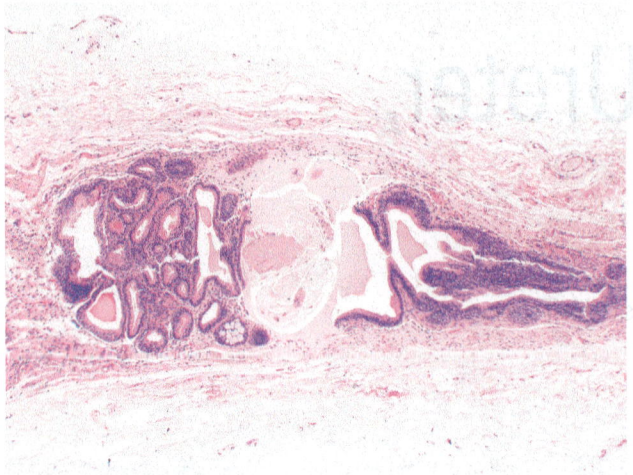

FIGURE 34.1 Urachal remnants within the median umbilical ligament.

bladder epithelium as mesodermal mixed tumors. They are, in fact, "endodermal mixed" tumors and usually called sarcomatoid carcinomas (3). Very rarely müllerian rests may be identified in the wall of the bladder and ureters or in the surrounding soft tissues in the form of endometriosis, endocervicosis, or endosalpingiosis (the so-called müllerianosis) (Fig. 34.2) (4–7). Mesonephric rests may occasionally be encountered within the bladder.

The ureters develop by branching and elongation of the ureteric bud (metanephric diverticulum), which begins as a dorsal bud from the mesonephric duct (1,2). The stalk of the ureteric bud becomes the ureter, whereas the cranial end forms the renal pelvis, as well as the calyces and the collecting tubules. The epithelium of the ureter and renal pelvis, although histologically identical to that of the bladder, is of mesodermal derivation.

ANATOMICAL CONSIDERATIONS

Bladder

In the adult, the empty urinary bladder lies within the anteroinferior portion of the pelvis minor, inferior to the peritoneum. In infants and children, it is located in part within the abdomen, even when empty (8). It begins to enter the pelvis major at about 6 years of age and will not be found entirely within the pelvis minor until after puberty. Nevertheless, in adults as the bladder fills it will distend, ascending into the abdomen at which time it may even reach the level of the umbilicus.

The bladder lies relatively free within the fibrofatty tissues of the pelvis except in the area of the bladder neck where it is firmly secured by the pubovesical ligaments in the female and the puboprostatic ligaments in the male (8,9). The relative freedom of the rest of the bladder allows for expansion superiorly as the viscus fills with urine.

The empty bladder in an adult has the shape of a four-sided inverted pyramid and is enveloped by the vesical fascia (8). The superior surface faces superiorly and is covered by the pelvic parietal peritoneum (Figs. 34.3 and 34.4). The posterior surface, also known as the base of the bladder, faces posteriorly and inferiorly. It is separated from the rectum by the uterine cervix and the proximal portions of the vagina in females and by the seminal vesicles and the ampulla of the vasa deferentia in males. These posterior anatomic relationships are very important clinically. Since the majority of bladder neoplasms arise in the posterior wall adjacent to the ureteral orifices, invasive tumor may extend into adjacent soft tissue and organs (Fig. 34.5A). The intimate relationship to the previously mentioned organs explains why hysterectomy and partial vaginectomy

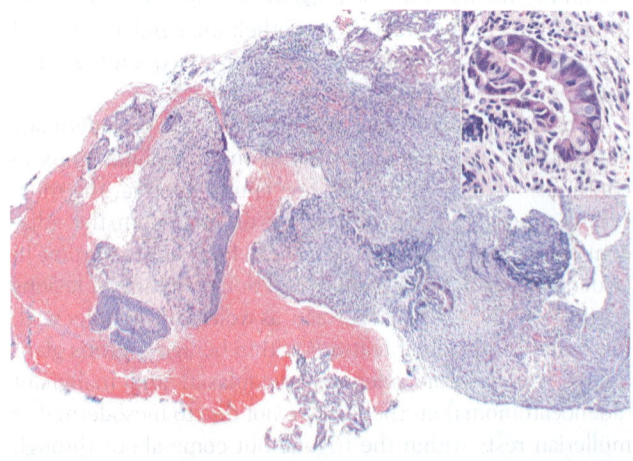

FIGURE 34.2 Endometriosis involving the ureteral wall. This female patient was presented with hematuria and was thought to have a primary ureteral neoplasm. *Inset* shows an endometriotic gland at higher magnification.

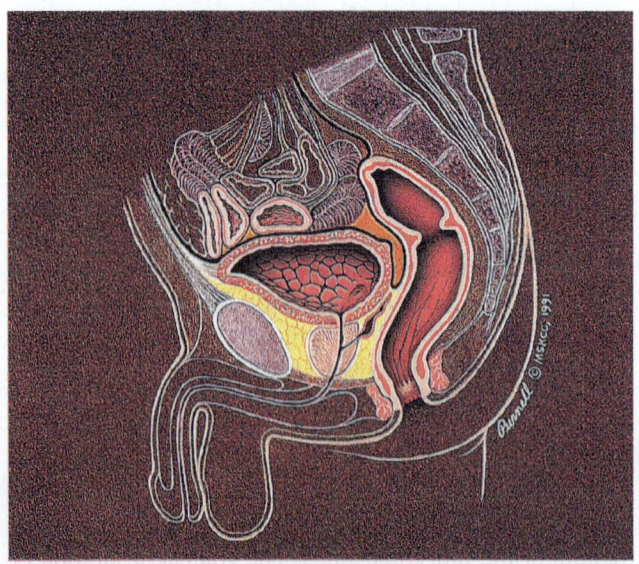

FIGURE 34.3 Anatomical relationships of the urinary bladder in males.

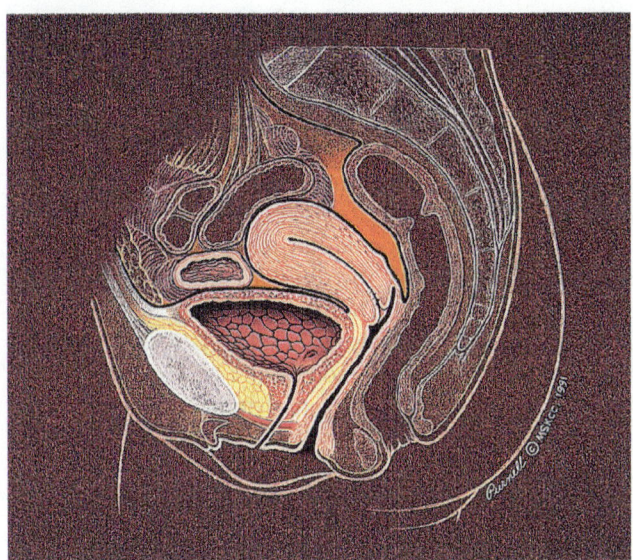

FIGURE 34.4 Anatomical relationships of the urinary bladder in females.

are commonly performed at the time of radial cystectomy in women. Similarly, we know that perivesical and seminal vesical involvement is a bad prognostic sign in bladder carcinoma in males (10–12), a reflection of high pathologic stage. It is important to note that seminal vesicles may contain carcinoma without invasion and this occurs in cases of in situ urothelial carcinoma involving prostatic, as well as ejaculatory ducts and extending into the seminal vesicle epithelium. The latter is a rare occurrence but these patients do not appear to have a similarly bad prognosis unless prostatic stromal invasion is present. The two inferolateral surfaces of the bladder face laterally, inferiorly and anteriorly and are in contact with the fascia of the levator ani muscles. The most anterosuperior point of the bladder is known as the apex and it is located at the point of contact of the superior surfaces and the two inferolateral surfaces. The apex (dome) marks the point of insertion of the median umbilical ligament and consequently is the area where urachal carcinomas are located (Figs. 34.3 and 34.4).

The trigone is a complex anatomic structure located at the base of the bladder and extending to the posterior bladder neck. In the proximal and lateral aspects of the trigone, the ureters enter into the bladder (ureteral orifices) obliquely. The muscle underlying the mucosa in this region is a combination of smooth muscle of the longitudinal layer of the intramural ureter and the detrusor muscle (13–17). The intramural ureter is surrounded by a fibromuscular sheath (Waldeyer sheath) which is fused into the ureteral muscle. This fibromuscular tissue fans out in the area of the trigone and mixes with the detrusor muscle, thus fixing the intramural ureter to the bladder. As the bladder distends, the surrounding musculature exerts pressure on the obliquely oriented intramural ureter, producing closure of the ureteral lumen and thus avoiding reflux of urine. The most distal portion of the bladder is called the bladder neck and it is the area where the posterior and inferolateral walls converge and open into the urethra. In the male, the bladder neck merges with the prostate gland. It is important to recognize the existence of occasional presence of prostatic ducts in this area since their involvement by urothelial carcinoma should not be mistaken with invasive carcinoma. The bladder neck is formed with contributions from the trigonal musculature (inner longitudinal ureteral muscle and Waldeyer sheath), the detrusor musculature, and the urethral musculature (13–18). The internal sphincter is located in this general area, with major contributions from the middle circular layer of the detrusor muscle (Fig. 34.5B).

The bladder bed (structures on which the bladder neck rests) is formed posteriorly by the rectum in males and vagina in females (Figs. 34.3 and 34.4). Anteriorly and laterally it is

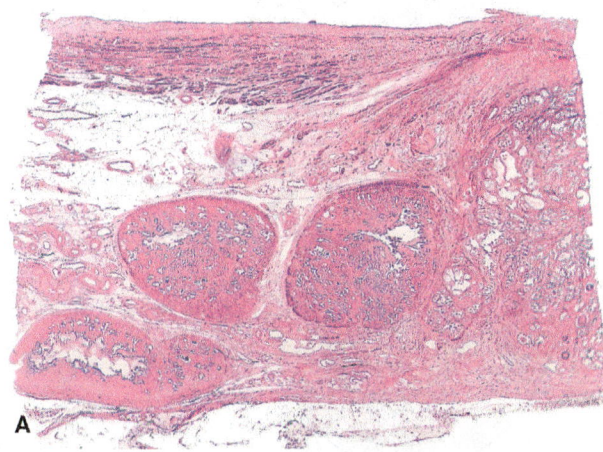
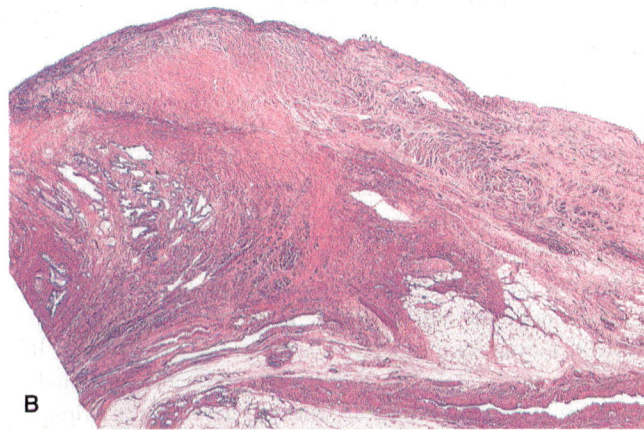

FIGURE 34.5 Bladder neck and distal trigone. **A:** The seminal vesicles are separated from the muscularis propria of the trigone by a scant amount of soft tissue. **B:** The muscularis propria merges with the prostate in the bladder neck area. The central (circular) fibers will predominate in this area and form the internal sphincter. The outer longitudinal layer contributes somewhat to the formation of the prostate musculature.

formed by the internal obturator and levator ani muscles, as well as the pubic bones. These structures may be involved in advanced tumors occupying the anterior, lateral, or bladder neck regions and render the patient inoperable.

The main arterial blood supply of the bladder comes from the inferior vesical arteries which are branches of the internal iliacs (19,20). The umbilical arteries through their branches (the superior vesical arteries) also supply the bladder as do the obturator and inferior gluteal arteries and, in females, the uterine and vaginal arteries. The veins of the urinary bladder drain into the internal iliac veins and form the vesical venous plexus. In the male, this plexus envelops the bladder base, prostate, and seminal vesicles and connects with the prostatic venous plexus. In females, it covers the bladder neck and urethra and communicates with the vaginal plexus. Lymphatic drainage is through the external and internal lymph nodes although drainage of portions of the bladder neck region may be through the sacral or common iliac nodes.

The urinary bladder is supplied by both sympathetic and parasympathetic nerves which form the vesical nerve plexus (19,20). The former are derived from T_{11}–L_2 nerves and play no role in micturition. On the other hand, the parasympathetic nerves come from S_2–S_4 and travel to the bladder via the pelvic nerve and the inferior hypogastric plexus. These nerves are important to micturition since they contract the fibers of the muscularis propria which in turn produce traction upon the bladder neck, opening the internal sphincter of the bladder. In fact, it is believed that micturition is initiated by voluntary relaxation of the perineal muscles and the striated muscle of the external sphincter located along the urethra. This action decreases urethral resistance as well as triggers contraction of the smooth muscle of the trigone and the remaining bladder, closing the ureteral orifices and increasing the hydrostatic pressure within the viscus (9,21). The bladder also contains sensory nerves which travel along the pelvic and hypogastric nerves and account for the sensation of pain as the bladder becomes too distended.

Ureters

The ureters measure approximately 30 cm in length, equally divided between the abdomen (retroperitoneum) and pelvis (22–27). The abdominal ureter takes a vertical course downward and medially on the anterior surface of the psoas muscle. It is covered by adventitia which is an extension of Gerota fascia. The pelvic ureter can be subdivided into a longer parietal and a shorter intravesical portion. The parietal portion is intimately related to the peritoneum. It descends posterolaterally and, as it approaches the bladder base, it becomes medially directed to reach the urinary bladder. The ureters enter the base of the bladder obliquely and empty into the bladder at the ureteral orifices. The distal parietal portion and the intravesical segments are enveloped in a fibromuscular sheath (Waldeyer sheath) which aids in fixing the ureter to the bladder (see description of the Trigone).

The ureteral blood supply is quite diverse (19,22). Depending on the anatomic level, it receives blood from branches of the renal, abdominal aortic, gonadal, hypogastric, vesical, and uterine arteries which form a richly intercommunicating plexus of vessels surrounding the tube. Venous drainage is variable but tends to follow a pattern similar to the arterial distribution. Lymphatic drainage is also quite complex. The upper portions drain into the lateral aortic lymph nodes, the middle portion drains into the common iliac lymph nodes, and the inferior portion drains into either the common, external, or internal iliac lymph nodes.

Renal Pelvis

As previously mentioned, the renal pelvis has its origin in the cranial portion of the ureteric bud, together with the calyces and collecting ducts. The renal pelvis lies primarily within the renal hilum, a space formed medially when one draws a vertical plane through the medial aspects of the upper and lower poles of the kidney (Fig. 34.6). Within the hilum is the renal sinus, a space within the medial and antral portions of the kidney occupied by the renal pelvis, renal vessels and nerves, renal calyces, and fat. The fibrous capsule which lines the kidney passes over the lips of the hilum and lines the renal sinus, becoming continuous with the renal calyces. Within the renal sinus, the renal pelvis divides into two and rarely three major calyces, which in turn divide into 7 to 14 minor calyces. Urine from the distal collecting ducts within the renal medulla (ducts of Bellini) flows into the minor calyces at

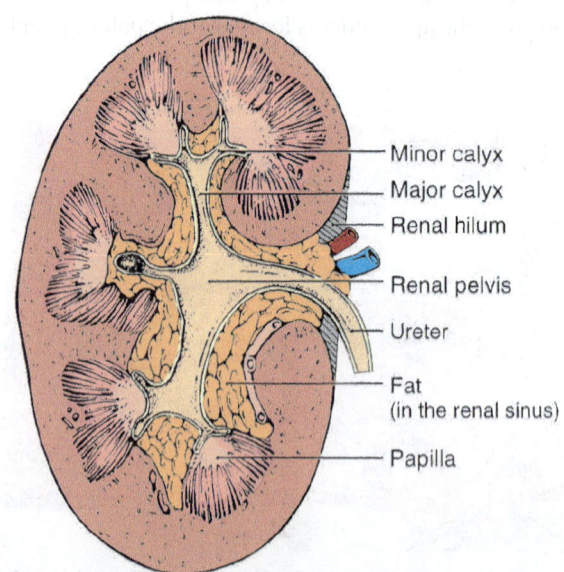

FIGURE 34.6 Anatomical relationships of the renal pelvis. Notice that the pelvis is mostly within the renal hilum (medial shaded area) and the renal sinus.

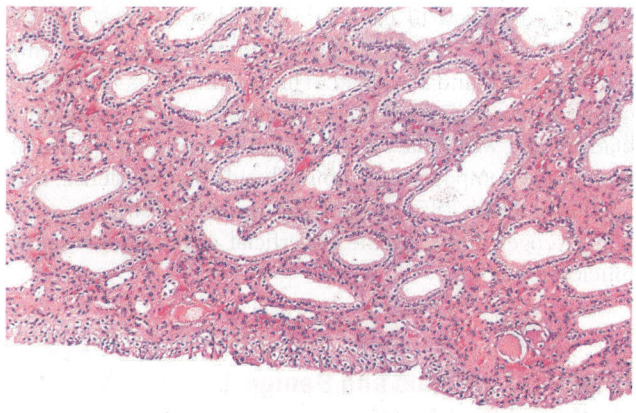

FIGURE 34.7 Renal papilla. Distal collecting ducts open into the urothelium covering the papillae.

the tips of the renal papillae (area cribrosa) (Fig. 34.7). The blood supply of the renal pelvis comes from branches of the renal arteries and the venous drainage follows a similar distribution. Its lymphatic drainage is into the renal hilar lymph nodes.

Microscopic Anatomy

The urinary bladder, ureter, and renal pelvis for the most part have a similar anatomic composition, the innermost layer being an epithelial lining and, extending outward, a lamina propria or subepithelial connective tissue, smooth muscle (muscularis propria), and adventitia. The superior surface of the bladder comes in contact with the parietal peritoneum and hence has a serosal lining. The anatomic landmarks are used clinically and pathologically to stage patients with urothelial cancer in order to choose therapy and estimate survival (Fig. 34.8). For this reason, it is important to accurately identify them microscopically.

Urothelium

The urinary bladder, ureters, and the renal pelvis are lined by the urothelium, which formerly was referred to as "transitional epithelium." The thickness of the urothelium will vary according to the degree of distention and anatomical location. It may be only two or three cell layers thick along the minor calyces. In the contracted bladder, it is usually six to seven cells thick and in the ureter three to five cells thick. One can identify three regions: the superficial cells which are in contact with the urinary space, the intermediate cells, and the basal cells which lie on a basement membrane (Fig. 34.9) (28,29). In the distended bladder, the urothelium may be only two to three cells thick and flattened with their long axis horizontal to the basement membrane. In practice, the thickness of the urothelium is dependent not only on the degree of distention but also on the plane on which the tissue is cut. If the cut is tangential to the basement membrane, it is possible to generate an artificially thick mucosa. For these and other reasons, we feel that urothelial thickness is of marginal or no utility in the assessment of urothelial neoplasms.

Superficial cells are in contact with the urinary space. They are large, elliptical cells which lie umbrella-like over the smaller intermediate cells (28–31). They may be binucleated and have abundant eosinophilic cytoplasms (Fig. 34.10). In the distended bladder, they become flattened and barely discernible. While the presence of these cells is taken as a sign of normalcy of the urothelium, one must be aware that they may become detached due to superficial erosion, during instrumentation or tissue processing in the prosecting room. Conversely, it is possible to see umbrella cells overlying frank carcinoma. Thus, the presence or absence of superficial cells cannot be used as a determining factor of normalcy or malignancy. Ultrastructural studies have shown superficial urothelial cells to be quite unique. The luminal surface is lined by a cytoplasmic membrane which is three layers thick; two electron-dense layers and a central lucent layer. The two dense layers are

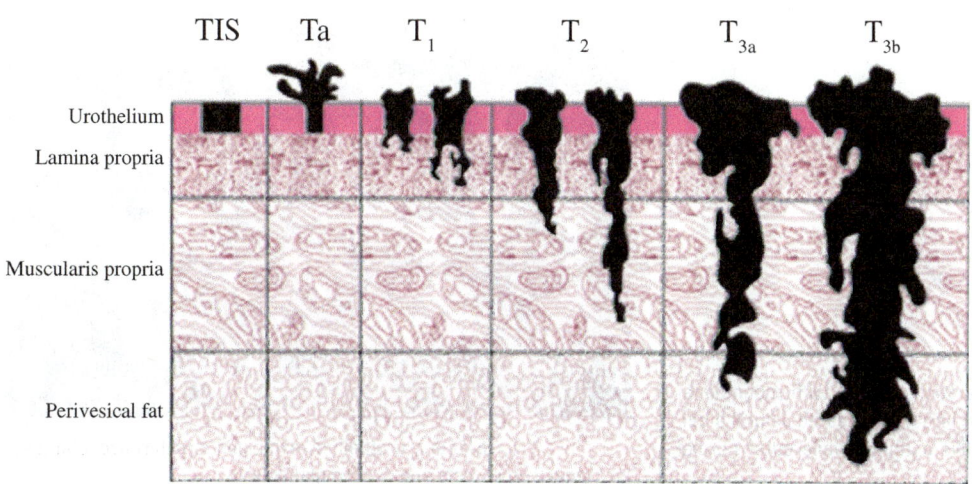

FIGURE 34.8 Pathologic staging of bladder cancer. This classification follows the recommendations of the American Joint Committee on Cancer (AJCC). Prostatic stromal invasion by direct extension is considered stage pT4.

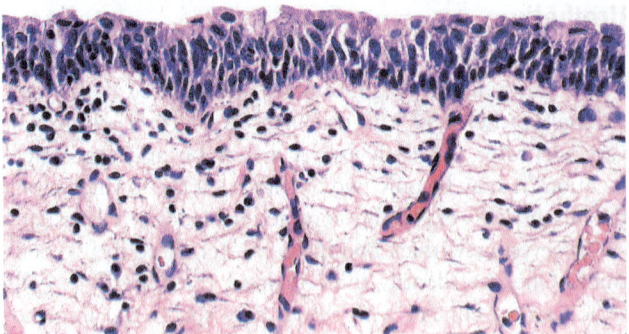

FIGURE 34.9 Normal urothelium. The mucosa may be up to seven cells thick in the bladder but thickness will vary as a consequence of distention and other factors. The superficial (umbrella) cells have ample eosinophilic cytoplasm.

said to be of unequal thickness and for this reason the membrane is known as the "asymmetric unit membrane" (AUM) (30–34). In reality, while the trilaminar arrangement of the cytoplasmic membrane can be readily observed, it is difficult to see the asymmetry of the dense layers. The membrane contains frequent invaginations giving it a scalloped appearance. The superficial (luminal) cytoplasm contains vesicles which are also lined by AUM. During the process of distention, these invaginations and vesicles are incorporated into the surface membrane, thus increasing the surface area and maintaining the structural integrity of the urothelium.

The intermediate cell layer may be up to five cells thick in the contracted bladder, where they are oriented with the long axis perpendicular to the basement membrane. The nuclei are oval and have finely stippled chromatin with absent or minute nucleoli. Longitudinal nuclear grooves are common. There is ample cytoplasm which may be vacuolated. The cytoplasmic membranes are distinct and these cells are attached to each other by desmosomes. In the distended state, this layer may be inconspicuous or only one cell thick and flattened. The basal layer is composed of cuboidal cells which are evident only in the contracted bladder and which lie on a thin but continuous basement membrane composed of a lamina lucida, lamina densa, and anchoring fibrils (35). All normal urothelial cells may contain glycogen but only the superficial cells are occasional mucicarminophilic.

Urothelial Variants and Benign Urothelial Proliferations

While the above microscopic and ultrastructural features describe normal urothelium, we know there are many benign morphologic variants. Koss et al. studied 100 grossly normal bladders obtained at postmortem (36). Of these, 93% had either Brunn nests, cystitis cystica, or squamous metaplasia.

The most common urothelial variant is the formation of Brunn nests, which are invaginations of the surface urothelium into the underlying lamina propria (Fig. 34.11). In some cases these solid nests of benign-appearing urothelium may lose continuity with the surface. They may become cystic due to accumulation of cellular debris or mucin and the term cystitis cystica has been coined to describe this phenomenon. The lining epithelium of these small cysts is composed of one or several layers of flattened "transitional" or cuboidal epithelium. In some cases the epithelial lining undergoes glandular metaplasia, giving rise to what is called cystitis glandularis (Fig. 34.11). The cells become cuboidal or columnar and mucin secreting; some are transformed into goblet cells. These processes also occur in the renal pelvis and the ureter, where they are called pyelitis or ureteritis cystica or glandularis, respectively (Fig. 34.12).

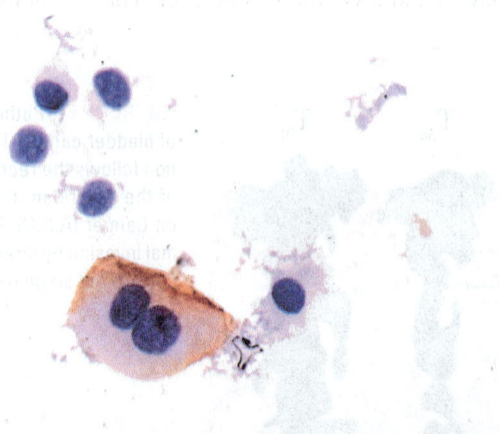

FIGURE 34.10 Urine cytology preparation stained with monoclonal antibody BG-7 (Signet Laboratories). A large, binucleated umbrella cell expresses the antigen identified by this antibody while other normal urothelial cells do not.

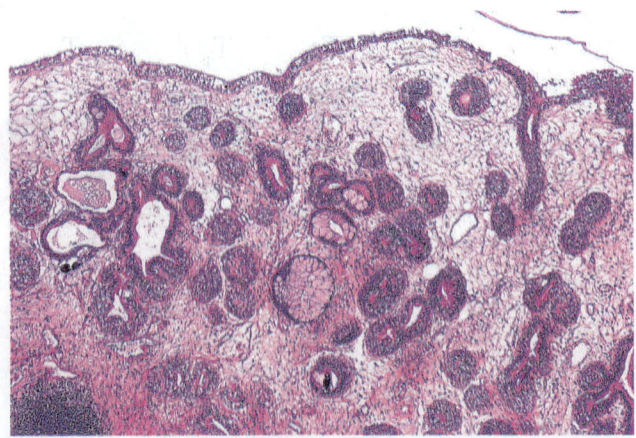

FIGURE 34.11 Bladder urothelium exhibiting proliferative changes, including Brunn nests and cystitis glandularis.

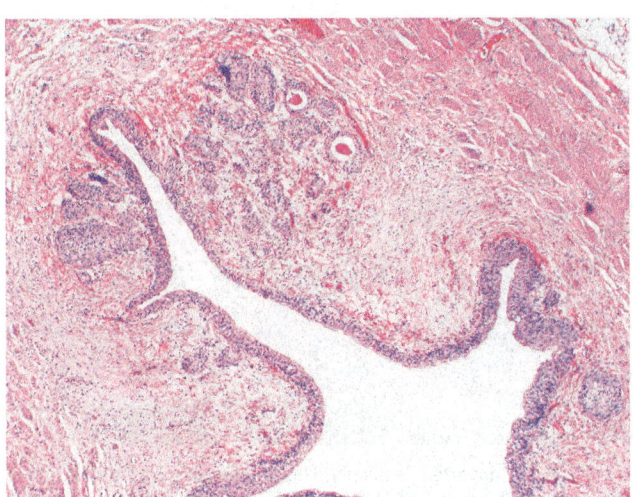

FIGURE 34.12 Brunn nests involving a ureter. Notice that the nests are more numerous and irregularly oriented compared to what is commonly seen in the bladder.

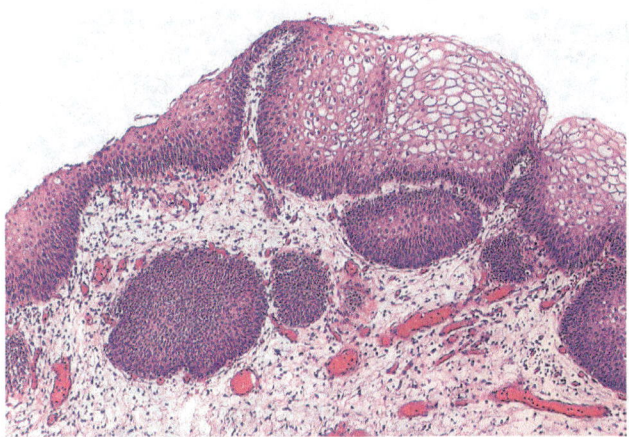

FIGURE 34.13 Squamous epithelium in the trigone of a woman. In this setting squamous epithelium is so common that it is considered to be a normal urothelial variant.

Brunn nests, cystitis cystica, and cystitis glandularis represent a continuum of proliferative or reactive changes seen along the entire urothelial tract, and it is common to see all three in the same tissue sample (Fig. 34.11). Most investigators believe that they occur as a result of local inflammatory insult (36–38). Nevertheless, these proliferative changes are seen in the urothelium of patients with no evidence of local inflammation, so that it is possible that they also represent either normal histologic variants or the residual effects of old inflammatory processes (39,40). The high incidence of these proliferative changes in normal bladder suggests that they are not likely to be premalignant changes and that there is no cause-and-effect relationship between their presence and the development of bladder cancer. It is true that one or all of these changes are commonly present in biopsy specimens containing bladder cancer, but the coexistence may be coincidental or the cancer itself may be producing the local inflammatory insult that gives rise to them. The fact that exceptional cases may occur in which carcinoma clearly arises within the epithelium of these reactive lesions does not alter this argument (41,42).

Metaplasia refers to a change in morphology of one cell type into another which is considered aberrant for that location. Urothelium frequently undergoes either squamous or glandular metaplasia, presumably as a response to chronic inflammatory stimuli such as urinary tract infection, calculi, diverticula, or frequent catheterization (37,40).

Squamous epithelium in the area of the trigone is a common finding in women. It is characterized by abundant intracytoplasmic glycogen and lack of keratinization, making it histologically similar to vaginal or cervical squamous epithelium (Fig. 34.13). In this particular setting, most of us believe that squamous epithelium should be regarded as a normal variant of urothelium rather than metaplasia. Squamous metaplasia may occur at other sites and at times may undergo keratinization and even exhibit parakeratosis and a granular layer. Squamous metaplasia is not preneoplastic per se but patients with keratinizing squamous metaplasia must be monitored closely since some may progress to squamous carcinoma (43).

The most common site of glandular metaplasia of the urothelium is the bladder, in the form of cystitis glandularis. Nevertheless, it may also occur within surface urothelium elsewhere in the urinary tract, usually as a response to chronic inflammation or irritation and also in cases of bladder exstrophy (44,45). The epithelium is composed of tall columnar cells with mucin-secreting goblet cells (Fig. 34.14), strikingly similar to colonic or small intestinal epithelium in which one might identify even Paneth cells. As with squamous metaplasia, glandular metaplasia is not of itself a precancerous lesion but may eventually undergo neoplastic transformation in exceptional cases (45). Patients should be monitored accordingly.

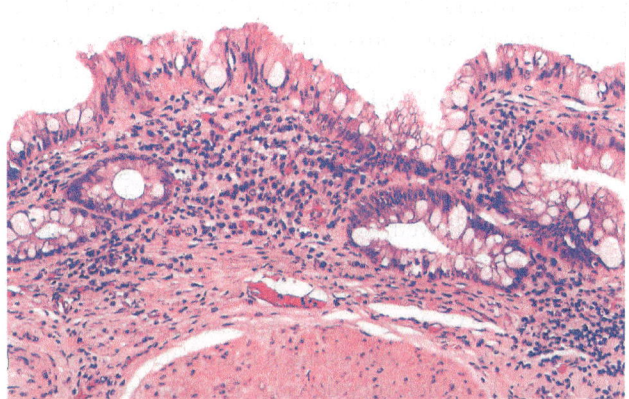

FIGURE 34.14 Intestinal metaplasia. The individual cells are morphologically identical to intestinal-type epithelium, even at the electron microscopic level.

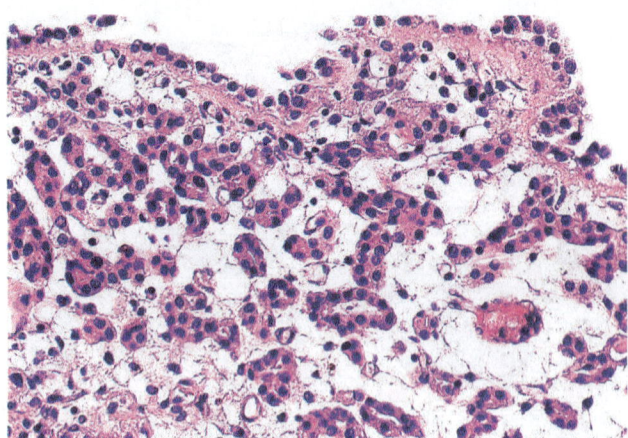

FIGURE 34.15 Nephrogenic adenoma. This proliferative urothelial lesion is characterized by aggregates of cuboidal cells with scant eosinophilic cytoplasm forming small tubules within the lamina propria. It may exhibit an exophytic, papillary growth.

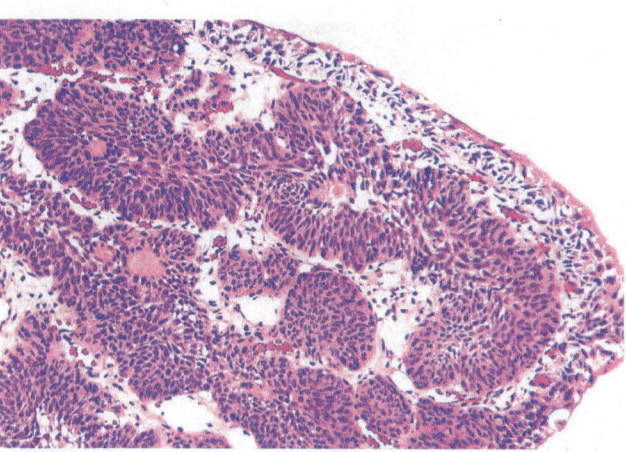

FIGURE 34.16 Inverted papilloma. This proliferative urothelial lesion is characterized by invaginated cords and nests of transitional epithelium within the lamina propria.

The so-called nephrogenic adenoma is a distinct metaplastic lesion characterized by aggregates of cuboidal or hobnail cells with clear or eosinophilic cytoplasm and small discrete nuclei without prominent nucleoli (46). These cells line thin papillary fronds on the surface or form tubular structures within the lamina propria of the bladder (Fig. 34.15). The tubules are often surrounded by a thickened and hyalinized basement membrane. Variable numbers of interspersed acute and chronic inflammatory cells are commonplace, as is associated stromal edema.

Nephrogenic adenoma/metaplasia is thought to be secondary to an inflammatory insult or local injury (46–50). It was originally described in the trigone and given its name because it was thought to arise from mesonephric rests. We now know that nephrogenic adenoma may occur anywhere along the urothelial tract, although it is most common in the bladder. It is important in that it may present as an exophytic mass mimicking carcinoma grossly and suggesting adenocarcinoma microscopically. The benign histologic appearance of the cells arranged in characteristic tubules surrounded by a prominent basement membrane should provide the correct diagnosis. A very interesting publication described nephrogenic adenomas of the bladder in patients that underwent renal transplantation (51). The authors demonstrated that the adenomatous lesions and the donor kidneys were clonal, suggesting that they developed through a process of shedding of donor renal tubule cells followed by implantation and proliferation within the bladder. Additional support for this hypothesis is postulated by other authors who have shown immunoreactivity for PAX-2, an antigen expressed in renal tubules (52,53). While this is interesting, it is unlikely to be the sole mechanism by which they develop. The true specificity of PAX-2 or PAX-8 expression in this setting remains to be determined since it may very well be due to differentiation rather than histogenesis.

Inverted papillomas are relatively rare lesions that may occur anywhere along the urothelial tract and may be confused clinically and pathologically with transitional cell carcinoma (54,55). In order of decreasing frequency, they occur in the bladder, renal pelvis, ureter, urethra, and renal pelvis (56–62). Patients usually present with hematuria. Cystoscopically, the lesions are polypoid and either sessile or pedunculated. The mucosal surface is smooth or nodular without villous or papillary fronds. Microscopically, the surface transitional epithelium is compressed but otherwise unremarkable. It is undermined by invaginated cords and nests of transitional epithelium which occupy the lamina propria (Fig. 34.16). The accumulation of these endophytic growths gives the lesion its characteristic polypoid gross appearance. The urothelial cells forming the cords are cytologically benign, exhibiting normal maturation and few if any mitoses. They are similar to the cells of bladder papillomas, differing only in that the epithelial cords are endophytic and consequently more closely packed. Frequently the cells are oval or spindle shaped. Epithelial nests may become centrally cystic, dilated, and even lined by cuboidal epithelium.

These cords of transitional epithelium in the lamina propria represent invagination, not invasion. As such, there are no fibrous reactive changes within the stroma. Although mitotic figures can be seen, they are rare, regular, and located at or near the basal layer of the epithelium. Inverted papillomas are discrete lesions and do not exhibit an infiltrative border or a fibrous stromal reaction (56,57). One must be careful not to confuse a nested type of urothelial carcinoma infiltrating lamina propria with an inverted papilloma.

The etiology of inverted papilloma is unclear. Most investigators feel that, similar to other proliferative lesions such as Brunn nests and cystitis cystica, they are a reactive, proliferative process secondary to a noxious insult. They are not premalignant per se, although in exceptional cases they

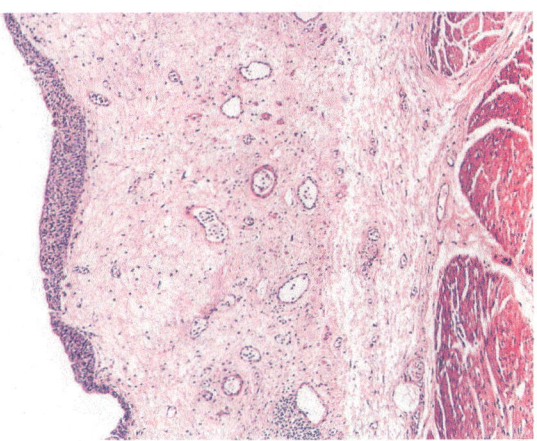

FIGURE 34.17 Lamina propria. It is composed of connective tissue, vascular structures, sensory nerves, and elastic fibers. Notice that the superficial connective tissue is denser than the deep portion.

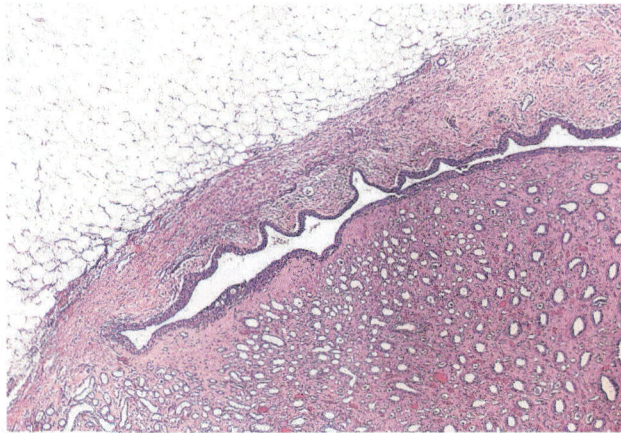

FIGURE 34.19 Junction of the renal papilla with the minor calyx. Notice the absence of the lamina propria along the papilla and a very thin lamina propria and muscularis propria along the minor calyx.

have been associated with carcinoma (58–60). Given the rarity of this association, we consider it incidental. Nevertheless their etiology remains controversial with recent studies suggesting recurring genetic abnormalities qualifying them as neoplastic although benign (63,64).

Lamina Propria

The lamina propria lies between the mucosal basement membrane and the muscularis propria. It is composed of dense connective tissue containing a rich vascular network, lymphatic channels, sensory nerve endings, and a few elastic fibers (20,28,32). In the deeper aspects of the lamina propria of the urinary bladder and the ureter, the connective tissue is loose, allowing for the formation of thick mucosal folds when the viscus is contracted (Figs. 34.17 and 34.18). Its thickness varies with the degree of distention and is generally thinner in the areas of the trigone and bladder neck. In fact, in patients with urinary outflow obstruction (i.e., prostatic hyperplasia) the bladder neck may contain muscularis propria directly beneath the mucosa with the lamina propria being virtually indiscernible (Fig. 34.5B). Lamina propria is also absent beneath the urothelium lining the renal papillae in the renal pelvis and is quite thin along the minor calyces (Fig. 34.19). In the midportion of the lamina propria of the bladder lie intermediate-sized arteries and veins. Specifically within the urinary bladder, wisps of smooth muscle are commonly found in the lamina propria, usually associated with these vessels (Figs. 34.20A,B) (65,66). These fascicles of smooth muscle are not connected to the muscularis propria and appear as isolated bundles but may form a discontinuous thin layer of muscle. The anatomic relationship of these fibers to the overlying urothelium can be severely disrupted by inflammation or prior therapeutic intervention (transurethral resection) when they may be seen juxtaposed to the basement membrane (Fig. 34.20C). Uncommonly, these muscle fibers may present as a continuous layer of muscle within the lamina propria, thus forming a true muscularis mucosae (66). In evaluating surgical and biopsy materials, every effort should be made to distinguish these superficial muscle fascicles from muscularis propria since a failure to do so will lead to errors in tumor staging and treatment. A pathologist should not sign out a biopsy as "transitional cell carcinoma invading muscle" because he/she is not giving useful information as to the depth of invasion. In fact, many urologists are unaware of the existence of a superficial muscle layer (muscularis mucosae) so that the above diagnosis will lead the urologist to treat the patient as a deeply invasive tumor (stage pT2 or greater) when in fact the patient has superficially invasive disease (stage pT1).

Recent reports have evaluated the ability of an antibody directed to smoothelin, a smooth muscle–specific contractile protein, in differentiating smooth muscle of the lamina

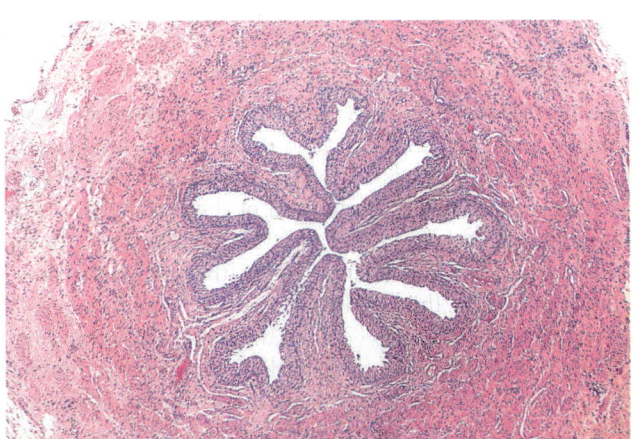

FIGURE 34.18 Cross section of mid-ureter. The elastic fibers and loose connective tissue within the lamina propria impart a festooned appearance to the urothelium. Notice that the different layers of the muscularis propria are indiscernible.

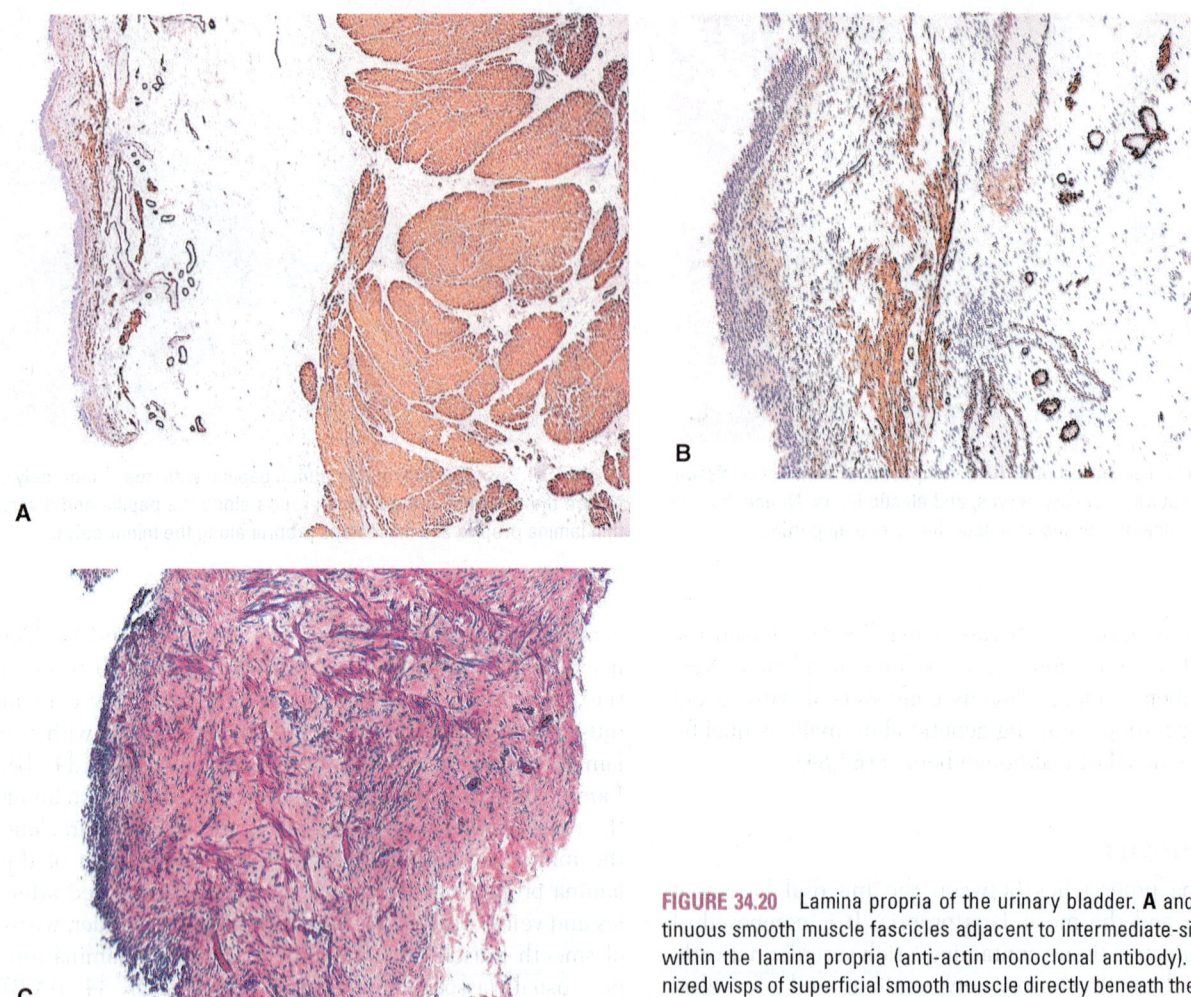

FIGURE 34.20 Lamina propria of the urinary bladder. **A** and **B:** Discontinuous smooth muscle fascicles adjacent to intermediate-sized vessels within the lamina propria (anti-actin monoclonal antibody). **C:** Disorganized wisps of superficial smooth muscle directly beneath the urothelium at the site of a prior biopsy. TURB specimen.

propria from muscularis propria (Fig. 34.21). At this point its utility remains controversial since some authors find it to be very useful while others do not (67,68). Occasionally one may encounter fat within the lamina propria and muscularis (Fig. 34.22) (69). At this time it is unclear whether this is due to the patient's body habitus but its presence should not be misinterpreted by pathologists as evidence of perivesical fat. Since muscularis mucosa is never seen along the renal pelvis and ureter the term subepithelial connective tissue is the favored term for this anatomical site, rather than lamina propria.

Pathologists are surprised to learn that, in terms of prognosis and treatment, urologists and urologic oncologists group noninvasive (Ta) and superficially invasive (T1) into a single category. It is our opinion that this is greatly due to the fact that there is significant interobserver variability among pathologists as to what constitutes lamina propria invasion. There are many cases of pT1 disease which are unequivocal but there is an equal number of cases in which invasion is, at best, questionable. Pathologist's interpretation in the latter group is inconsistent and not reproducible. While this confusion is partly due to the lack of orientation of transurethral biopsy specimens and to disruption of the normal histologic architecture by tumor or prior therapy, it is clear that applying strict parameters to diagnose lamina propria/subepithelial connective tissue invasion is a must.

Muscularis Propria

The muscularis propria is said to be composed of three smooth muscle coats, inner and outer longitudinal layers, and a central circular layer. In fact, these layers can only be identified consistently in the area of the bladder neck. In other areas, the longitudinal and circular layers mix freely and have no definite orientation. In the ureter, the muscularis propria is thicker distally and the proximal portion contains only two layers (70). In the renal pelvis the muscularis propria becomes thinner along the major and minor calyces and no orientation of the muscle fibers is evident (Fig. 34.23). No muscular fibers are evident between the urothelium and the renal medulla at the level of the renal papillae (Fig. 34.7). Within the renal sinus, the muscularis propria is surrounded by variable amounts of fat (Figs. 34.6 and 34.23). This fact is rarely mentioned by pathologists at

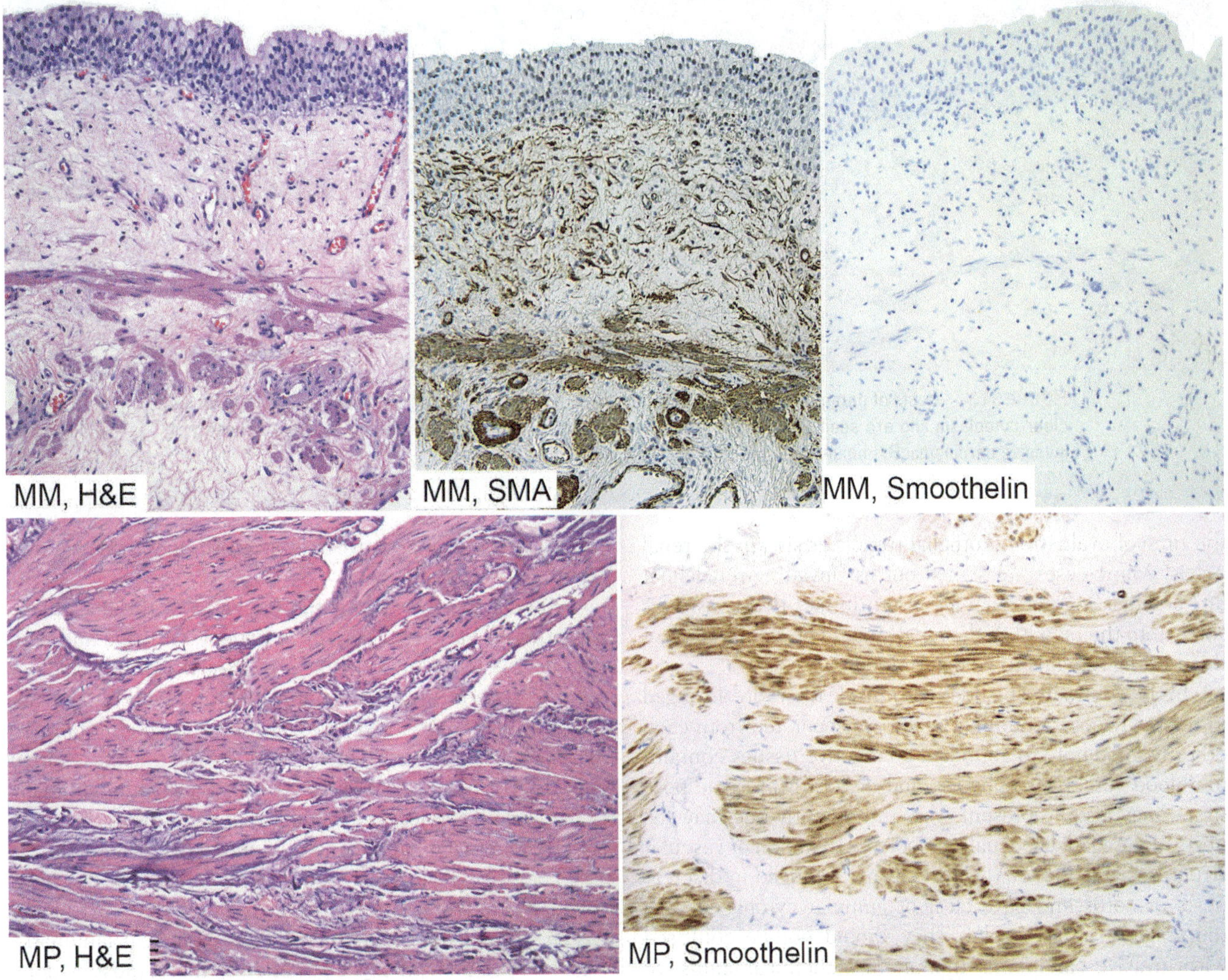

FIGURE 34.21 An example of bladder depicting staining characteristics of muscularis mucosa (MM) and muscularis propria (MP) with smooth muscle actin (SMA) and smoothelin, a marker of terminally differentiated smooth muscle cells. Both MM and MP express SMA, whereas smoothelin is expressed only in muscle fibers of MP.

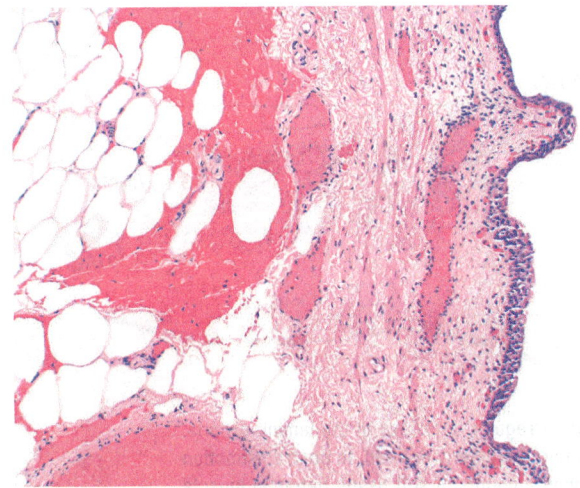

FIGURE 34.22 Mature adipose tissue within the lamina propria of the urinary bladder.

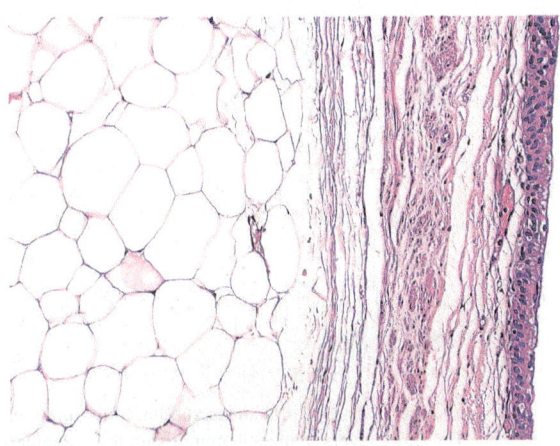

FIGURE 34.23 Urothelial wall along the minor calices. Thin layers of lamina propria and muscularis propria are surrounded with fat within the renal sinus.

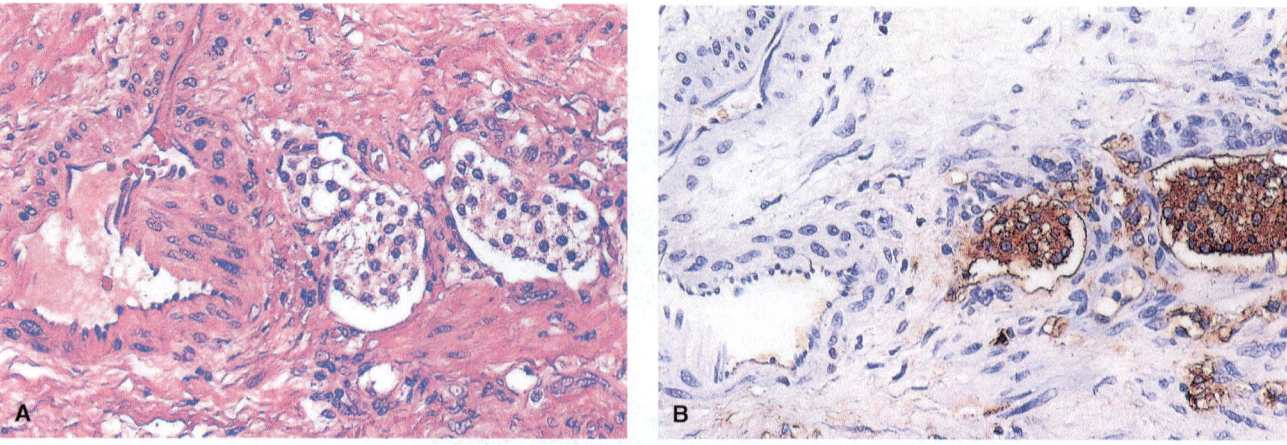

FIGURE 34.24 Nests of paraganglia within the bladder wall. **A:** The cells are small, have vesicular nuclei and clear cytoplasm and are seen adjacent to neural or vascular structures. They should not be confused with invasive carcinoma. **B:** Immunostain for chromogranin A can clarify the issue.

the time of evaluating urothelial tumors arising in the renal pelvis. Many cases are signed out as "invading renal hilar fat" or "invading perirenal fat" when in fact the invasion is solely into the fat within the renal sinus. The significance of this finding remains to be determined (71).

In the contracted bladder, the muscle fibers are arranged in relatively coarse bundles which are separated from each other by moderate to abundant connective tissues containing blood vessels, lymphatics, and nerves. Mature adipose tissue may also be present. Very infrequently one may see nests of paraganglia, usually associated to neural or vascular structures (Fig. 34.24A). The cells are arranged in discrete nests or cords and have clear or granular cytoplasm with round or vesicular nuclei. They should not be confused with invasive carcinoma. Immunohistochemical stains for cytokeratins are negative but positive for chromogranin (Fig. 34.24B).

Similar to other layers, the thickness of the muscularis propria will vary from patient to patient, with age and with the degree of distention (Figs. 34.25A, B). In fact, Jequier et al. (72) performed sonographic measurements of the bladder wall thickness in 410 urologically normal children and 10 adults. They found that the bladder wall thickness varied mostly with the state of bladder filling and only minimally with age and gender. The bladder wall had a mean thickness of 2.76 mm when empty and 1.55 mm when distended.

For staging purposes, the muscularis propria has been divided into two segments, superficial and deep (pT2a and pT2b respectively) (Fig. 34.8). No anatomical landmarks can be used to make this distinction so that it must be done

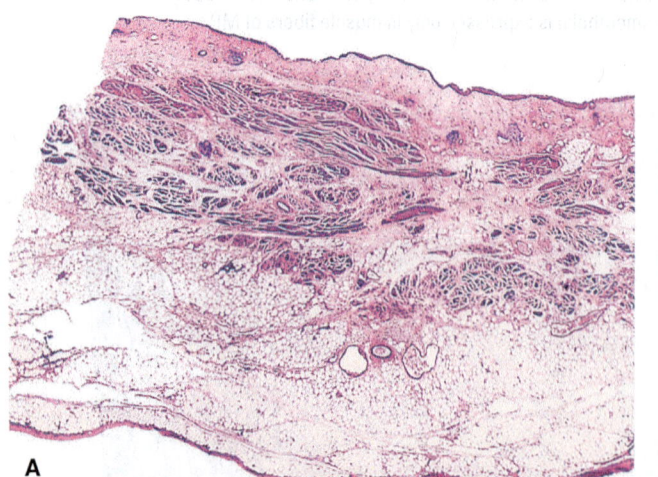
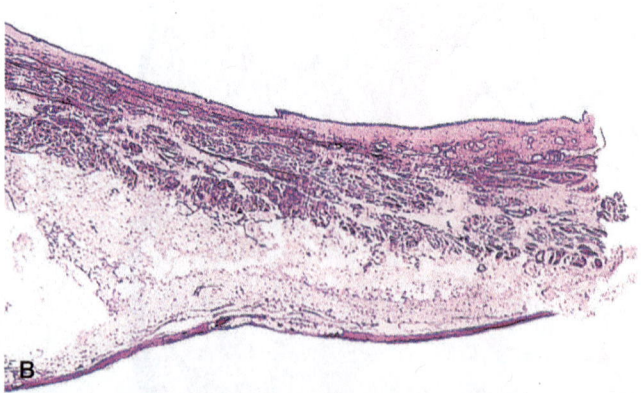

FIGURE 34.25 Full-thickness section of the bladder. **A:** Notice the irregular thickness of the lamina propria. The three layers of muscle comprising the muscularis propria cannot be clearly defined. In contradistinction to the muscularis propria of the gut in the bladder, there are ample amounts of soft tissue between muscle bundles. **B:** Cross section of distended bladder. The overall thickness of the viscus is diminished as compared to the contracted bladder. Both the lamina propria and the muscularis propria become more compact.

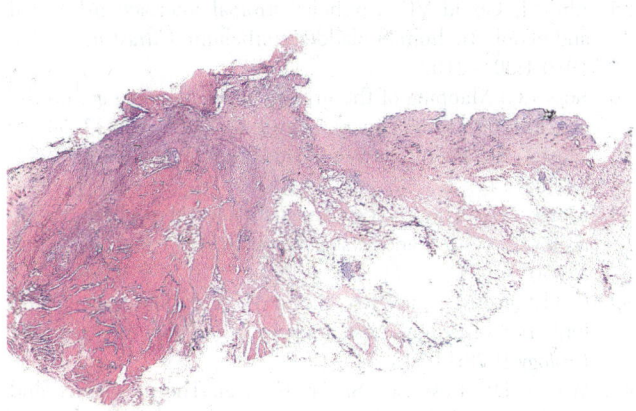

FIGURE 34.26 Bladder diverticulum. To the *left* is inflamed but anatomically normal bladder wall while in the *center* and to the *right* one sees total absence of the muscularis propria. Perivesical soft tissue comes in contact with the inflamed, fibrotic, and thickened lamina propria.

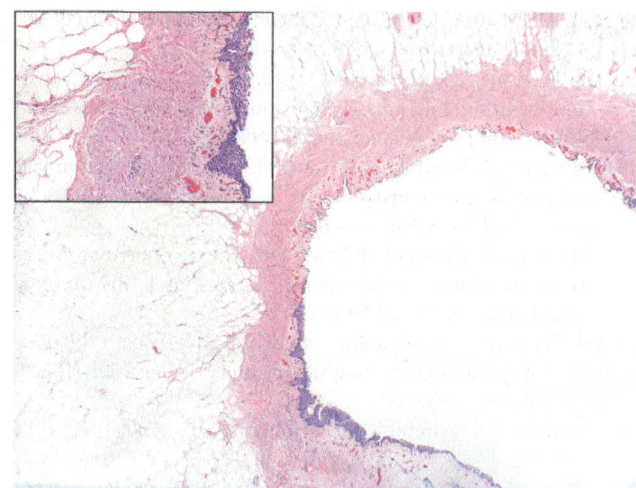

FIGURE 34.27 Wall of bladder diverticulum exhibits hyperplastic muscularis mucosa within the lamina propria but no muscularis propria. *Inset* shows higher magnification.

direct visualization on the light microscope at the time of cystectomy. Prior transurethral resection will alter the anatomy of the site and mask normal landmarks, making proper staging difficult, if not impossible.

Bladder diverticula are relatively common, yet their etiology remains controversial. Most investigators agree that they occur secondary to increased intravesical pressure as a result of obstruction distal to the diverticulum (73–75). The obstruction brings about compensatory muscle hypertrophy and eventual mucosal herniation in areas of weakness. Others feel that at least some diverticula are a consequence of congenital defects in the bladder musculature, citing as evidence cases of diverticula in young patients without evidence of obstruction (75,76). The most common sites of diverticula are: (a) adjacent to the ureteral orifices; (b) the bladder dome (probably related to a urachal remnant); and (c) the region of the internal urethral orifice. Grossly, one sees distortion of the external surface of the bladder. The diverticula may be widely patent but are usually narrow in symptomatic patients. The mucosa adjoining the diverticulum is usually hyperemic or ulcerated. There may be epithelial hyperplasia and hypertrophy of the muscularis propria of the urinary bladder at the os of the diverticulum (Fig. 34.26). Very commonly, there is inflammation involving the lamina propria and muscularis. The wall of the diverticulum itself consists of urothelium and underlying connective tissue, virtually identical to the bladder mucosa with lamina propria. At this site one commonly encounters a hyperplasia muscularis mucosae but no muscularis propria since few, if any of these muscle bundles will be identified in cases of acquired diverticula (Fig. 34.27). The true "congenital" diverticulum contains a thinned outer muscle layer. Infrequently, the epithelium lining the sac will undergo squamous or glandular metaplasia due to local irritation associated with urine stasis, infection, or stone. In these cases it is not unusual for the diverticular wall to become extensively fibrotic (Fig. 34.27).

Major complications of bladder diverticula include infection, lithiasis, and carcinoma. It is believed that 2% to 7% of patients with bladder diverticula will develop an associated neoplasm, presumed secondary to the chronic inflammatory stimuli mentioned above (77,78). Ureteral diverticula are rare, and asymptomatic if uncomplicated (79). They are not seen in the renal pelvis.

REFERENCES

1. Moore K. The urinary system. In: Moore K, ed. *The developing human*. Philadelphia, PA: WB Saunders; 1982.
2. Kissane JM. Development and structure of the urogenital system. In: Murphy WM, ed. *Urological Pathology*. Philadelphia, PA: WB Saunders; 1989.
3. Eble J, Sauter G, Epstein J, et al. *Pathology and Genetics of Tumours of the Urinary System and Male Genital Organs*. Lyon: IARC Press; 2004.
4. Clement PB, Young RH. Endocervicosis of the urinary bladder. A report of six cases of a benign mullerian lesion that may mimic adenocarcinoma. *Am J Surg Pathol* 1992;16:533–542.
5. Young RH, Clement PB. Mullerianosis of the urinary bladder. *Mod Pathol* 1996;9:731–737.
6. Comiter CV. Endometriosis of the urinary tract. *Urol Clin North Am* 2002;29:625–635.
7. Chapron C, Boucher E, Fauconnier A, et al. Anatomopathological lesions of bladder endometriosis are heterogeneous. *Fertil Steril* 2002;78:740–742.
8. Moore KL. The pelvis and perineum. In: Moore KL, ed. *Clinically Oriented Anatomy*. Baltimore, MD: Williams & Wilkins; 1985.
9. Tanagho E. Campbell's urology. In: Walsh PC, Retik AB, Stamey TA, eds. *Anatomy of the Lower Urinary Tract*. Philadelphia, PA: WB Saunders; 1992.
10. Mahadevia PS, Koss LG, Tar IJ. Prostatic involvement in bladder cancer. Prostate mapping in 20 cystoprostatectomy specimens. *Cancer* 1986;58:2096–2102.

11. Utz DC, Farrow GM, Rife CC, et al. Carcinoma in situ of the bladder. *Cancer* 1980;45:1842–1848.
12. Ro JY, Ayala AG, el-Naggar A, et al. Seminal vesicle involvement by in situ and invasive transitional cell carcinoma of the bladder. *Am J Surg Pathol* 1987;11:951–958.
13. Tanagho EA, Smith DR, Meyers FH. The trigone: Anatomical and physiological considerations. 2. In relation to the bladder neck. *J Urol* 1968;100:633–639.
14. Tanagho EA, Meyers FH, Smith DR. The trigone: Anatomical and physiological considerations. I. In relation to the ureterovesical junction. *J Urol* 1968;100:623–632.
15. Shehata R. A comparative study of the urinary bladder and the intramural portion of the ureter. *Acta Anat (Basel)* 1977;98:380–395.
16. Politano VA. Ureterovesical junction. *J Urol* 1972;107:239–242.
17. Elbadawi A. Anatomy and function of the ureteral sheath. *J Urol* 1972;107:224–229.
18. Tanagho EA, Smith DR. The anatomy and function of the bladder neck. *Br J Urol* 1966;38:54–71.
19. Moore KL, Dalley AF, Agur AMR. *Clinically Oriented Anatomy*. Baltimore, MD: Lippincott Williams & Wilkins; 2006.
20. Weiss L. *Cell and Tissue Biology: A Textbook of Histology*. Baltimore, MD: Urban & Schwarzenberg; 1988.
21. Fletcher TF, Bradley WE. Neuroanatomy of the bladder-urethra. *J Urol* 1978;119:153–160.
22. Olson CA. Anatomy of the upper urinary tract. In: Walsh PC, Gittes RE, Perlmutter AD, et al., eds. *Campbell's Urology*. Philadelphia, PA: WB Saunders; 1986.
23. Hanna MK, Jeffs RD, Sturgess JM, et al. Ureteral structure and ultrastructure. Part I. The normal human ureter. *J Urol* 1976;116:718–724.
24. Kaye KW, Goldberg ME. Applied anatomy of the kidney and ureter. *Urol Clin North Am* 1982;9:3–13.
25. Motola JA, Shahon RS, Smith AD. Anatomy of the ureter. *Urol Clin North Am* 1988;15:295–299.
26. Notley RG. Ureteral morphology: Anatomic and clinical considerations. *Urology* 1978;12:8–14.
27. Crelin ES. Normal and abnormal development of ureter. *Urology* 1978;12:2–7.
28. Koss LG. *Tumors of the Urinary Bladder. Fascicle 11*. Washington, DC: Armed Forces Institute of Pathology; 1975.
29. Fawcett DW. *Bloom and Fawcett: A Textbook of Histology*. Philadelphia, PA: WB Saunders; 1986.
30. Hicks RM. The function of the golgi complex in transitional epithelium. Synthesis of the thick cell membrane. *J Cell Biol* 1966;30:623–643.
31. Battifora H, Eisenstein R, McDonald JH. The human urinary bladder mucosa. An electron microscopic study. *Invest Urol* 1964;12:354–361.
32. Fawcett DW, Bloom W, Raviola E. *A Textbook of Histology*. New York: Chapman & Hall; 1994.
33. Koss LG. The asymmetric unit membranes of the epithelium of the urinary bladder of the rat. An electron microscopic study of a mechanism of epithelial maturation and function. *Lab Invest* 1969;21:154–168.
34. Newman J, Antonakopoulos GN. The fine structure of the human fetal urinary bladder. Development and maturation. A light, transmission and scanning electron microscopic study. *J Anat* 1989;166:135–150.
35. Alroy J, Gould VE. Epithelial-stromal interface in normal and neoplastic human bladder epithelium. *Ultrastruct Pathol* 1980;1:201–210.
36. Koss LG. Mapping of the urinary bladder: Its impact on the concepts of bladder cancer. *Hum Pathol* 1979;10:533–548.
37. Mostofi FK. Potentialities of bladder epithelium. *J Urol* 1954;71:705–714.
38. Morse HD. The etiology and pathology of pyelitis cystica, ureteritis cystica and cystitis cystica. *Am J Pathol* 1928;4:33–50.
39. Goldstein AM, Fauer RB, Chinn M, et al. New concepts on formation of Brunn's nests and cysts in urinary tract mucosa. *Urology* 1978;11:513–517.
40. Wiener DP, Koss LG, Sablay B, et al. The prevalence and significance of Brunn's nests, cystitis cystica and squamous metaplasia in normal bladders. *J Urol* 1979;122:317–321.
41. Edwards PD, Hurm RA, Jaeschke WH. Conversion of cystitis glandularis to adenocarcinoma. *J Urol* 1972;108:568–570.
42. Lin JI, Yong HS, Tseng CH, et al. Diffuse cystitis glandularis. Associated with adenocarcinomatous change. *Urology* 1980;15:411–415.
43. Tannenbaum M. Inflammatory proliferative lesion of urinary bladder: Squamous metaplasia. *Urology* 1976;7:428–429.
44. Engel RM, Wilkinson HA. Bladder exstrophy. *J Urol* 1970;104:699–704.
45. Nielsen K, Nielsen KK. Adenocarcinoma in exstrophy of the bladder—the last case in Scandinavia? A case report and review of literature. *J Urol* 1983;130:1180–1182.
46. Bhagavan BS, Tiamson EM, Wenk RE, et al. Nephrogenic adenoma of the urinary bladder and urethra. *Hum Pathol* 1981;12:907–916.
47. Navarre RJ Jr, Loening SA, Platz C, et al. Nephrogenic adenoma: A report of 9 cases and review of the literature. *J Urol* 1982;127:775–779.
48. Molland EA, Trott PA, Paris AM, et al. Nephrogenic adenoma: A form of adenomatous metaplasia of the bladder. A clinical and electron microscopical study. *Br J Urol* 1976;48:453–462.
49. Ford TF, Watson GM, Cameron KM. Adenomatous metaplasia (nephrogenic adenoma) of urothelium. An analysis of 70 cases. *Br J Urol* 1985;57:427–433.
50. Satodate R, Koike H, Sasou S, et al. Nephrogenic adenoma of the ureter. *J Urol* 1984;131:332–334.
51. Mazal PR, Schaufler R, Altenhuber-Muller R, et al. Derivation of nephrogenic adenomas from renal tubular cells in kidney-transplant recipients. *N Engl J Med* 2002;347:653–659.
52. Fromont G, Barcat L, Gaudin J, et al. Revisiting the immunophenotype of nephrogenic adenoma. *Am J Surg Pathol* 2009;33:1654–1658.
53. Tong GX, Melamed J, Mansukhani M, et al. PAX2: A reliable marker for nephrogenic adenoma. *Mod Pathol* 2006;19:356–363.
54. DeMeester LJ, Farrow GM, Utz DC. Inverted papillomas of the urinary bladder. *Cancer* 1975;36:505–513.
55. Henderson DW, Allen PW, Bourne AJ. Inverted urinary papilloma: Report of five cases and review of the literature. *Virchows Arch A Pathol Anat Histol* 1975;366:177–186.
56. Caro DJ, Tessler A. Inverted papilloma of the bladder: A distinct urological lesion. *Cancer* 1978;42:708–713.
57. Anderstrom C, Johansson S, Pettersson S. Inverted papilloma of the urinary tract. *J Urol* 1982;127:1132–1134.

58. Lazarevic B, Garret R. Inverted papilloma and papillary transitional cell carcinoma of urinary bladder: Report of four cases of inverted papilloma, one showing papillary malignant transformation and review of the literature. *Cancer* 1978;42: 1904–1911.
59. Whitesel JA. Inverted papilloma of the urinary tract: Malignant potential. *J Urol* 1982;127:539–540.
60. Stein BS, Rosen S, Kendall AR. The association of inverted papilloma and transitional cell carcinoma of the urothelium. *J Urol* 1984;131:751–752.
61. Assor D. Inverted papilloma of the renal pelvis. *J Urol* 1976; 116:654.
62. Lausten GS, Anagnostaki L, Thomsen OF. Inverted papilloma of the upper urinary tract. *Eur Urol* 1984;10:67–70.
63. Cheng L, Davidson DD, Wang M, et al. Telomerase reverse transcriptase (TERT) promoter mutation analysis of benign, malignant and reactive urothelial lesions reveals a subpopulation of inverted papilloma with immortalizing genetic change. *Histopathology* 2016;69(1):107–113.
64. Jørgensen PH, Vainer B, Hermann GG. A clinical and molecular review of inverted papilloma of the urinary tract: how to handle? *APMIS* 2015;123(11):920–929.
65. Dixon JS, Gosling JA. Histology and fine structure of the muscularis mucosae of the human urinary bladder. *J Anat* 1983;136:265–271.
66. Ro JY, Ayala AG, el-Naggar A. Muscularis mucosa of urinary bladder. Importance for staging and treatment. *Am J Surg Pathol* 1987;11:668–673.
67. Paner GP, Shen SS, Lapetino S, et al. Diagnostic utility of antibody to smoothelin in the distinction of muscularis propria from muscularis mucosae of the urinary bladder: A potential ancillary tool in the pathologic staging of invasive urothelial carcinoma. *Am J Surg Pathol* 2009;33:91–98.
68. Miyamoto H, Sharma RB, Illei PB, et al. Pitfalls in the use of smoothelin to identify muscularis propria invasion by urothelial carcinoma. *Am J Surg Pathol* 2010;34:418–422.
69. Philip AT, Amin MB, Tamboli P, et al. Intravesical adipose tissue: A quantitative study of its presence and location with implications for therapy and prognosis. *Am J Surg Pathol* 2000; 24:1286–1290.
70. Notley RG. The musculature of the human ureter. *Br J Urol* 1970;42:724–727.
71. Olgac S, Mazumdar M, Dalbagni G, et al. Urothelial carcinoma of the renal pelvis: A clinicopathologic study of 130 cases. *Am J Surg Pathol* 2004;28:1545–1552.
72. Jequier S, Rousseau O. Sonographic measurements of the normal bladder wall in children. *AJR Am J Roentgenol* 1987;149:563–566.
73. Miller A. The aetiology and treatment of diverticulum of the bladder. *Br J Urol* 1958;30:43–56.
74. Kertsschmer HL. Diverticula of the urinary bladder: A clinical study of 236 cases. *Surg Gynecol Obstet* 1940;71:491–503.
75. Fox M, Power RF, Bruce AW. Diverticulum of the bladder: Presentation and evaluation of treatment of 115 cases. *Br J Urol* 1962;34:286–298.
76. Barrett DM, Malek RS, Kelalis PP. Observations on vesical diverticulum in childhood. *J Urol* 1976;116:234–236.
77. Abeshouse BS. Primary carcinoma in a diverticulum of the bladder: A report of four cases and a review of the literature. *J Urol* 1943;49:534–547.
78. Faysal MH, Freiha FS. Primary neoplasm in vesical diverticula. A report of 12 cases. *Br J Urol* 1981;53:141–143.
79. Cochran ST, Waisman J, Barbaric ZL. Radiographic and microscopic findings in multiple ureteral diverticula. *Radiology* 1980;137:631–636.

35

Prostate

Samson W. Fine ■ Jesse K. McKenney

- EMBRYOLOGY AND DEVELOPMENT OF THE PROSTATE 964
- GENERAL TOPOGRAPHIC RELATIONSHIPS: McNEAL'S ZONAL ANATOMY 965
- SECTIONING OF RADICAL PROSTATECTOMY SPECIMENS 966
- ANATOMY OF THE PROSTATE GLAND IN SURGICAL PATHOLOGY SPECIMENS 967
    - Gross Anatomy 967
    - Histologic Variation by Anatomic Region 967
    - Nonglandular Components of Prostatic and Extraprostatic Tissues 969
- ARCHITECTURAL AND CYTOLOGIC FEATURES OF THE GLANDULAR PROSTATE 973
    - Architectural Patterns 973
    - Cytologic Features 974
- DEVIATIONS FROM NORMAL HISTOLOGY 976
- CONSIDERATIONS IN TRANSURETHRAL RESECTION AND NEEDLE BIOPSY SPECIMENS 978
- ACKNOWLEDGMENT 979
- REFERENCES 979

EMBRYOLOGY AND DEVELOPMENT OF THE PROSTATE

The prostate appears in early embryonic development as a condensation of mesenchyme along the course of the pelvic urethra. By 9 weeks of embryonic life, the mesenchymal condensation is most dense along the posterior (rectal) and distal (apical) aspects of the urethra (Fig. 35.1), where it is in contact with the urethral lining epithelium (1). Between its midpoint and the bladder neck, the proximal urethral segment shows a sharp anterior angulation. However, the highly condensed mesenchyme continues directly proximal to a dome-shaped prostatic base, leaving a gap between condensed prostatic mesenchyme and proximal urethra. The ejaculatory ducts penetrate this mesenchyme toward the future verumontanum, which is located at the urethral midpoint. The ejaculatory ducts are wolffian duct structures, but in the embryo their surrounding stroma is indistinguishable from the remaining prostatic mesenchyme, which is mainly derived from the urogenital sinus (2). The portion of mesenchyme that surrounds the ejaculatory ducts and expands proximally to occupy nearly the entire prostate base is distinguishable in the adult as the central zone, which like the seminal vesicles, is probably also derived from the wolffian duct (1). In this concept, the prostate is of dual embryonic derivation.

At about 10 weeks, epithelial buds begin to branch, mainly posteriorly and laterally from the walls of the distal (apex to mid) urethral segment into the condensed mesenchyme in a pattern that is essentially identical to that seen in the adult.

Postnatally, the prostate grows at a slow rate, reaching less than 2 cm in diameter by the time of puberty. During this period, the ducts and acini are lined by epithelium, which undergoes little change from the neonatal period. Gland spaces are lined by cells that are crowded with multilayered dark nuclei (Fig. 35.2).

The pubertal growth acceleration and maturation of the prostate gland appears not to be complete until at least 20 years of age. The average prostate by this time measures about 4.5 cm in width, 3.5 to 4.0 cm in length, and 3 cm in thickness. In most men older than 50 years of age, there is focal resumption of growth as benign prostatic hyperplasia (BPH). This process increases the thickness of the gland prominently. BPH typically represents enlargement of only a single region of the gland, identifiable in the adult as the transition zone. In fact, the normal mass of the glandular portion of the prostate after subtraction of the BPH-prone region remains at nearly constant mean volume until 70 years of age or more.

CHAPTER 35: Prostate 965

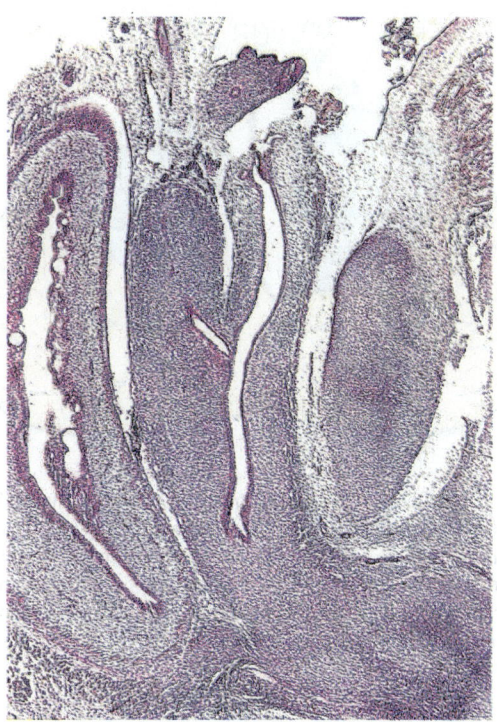

FIGURE 35.1 Embryonic prostate, age 9 weeks, in the sagittal plane of the pelvis. Urethra (narrow central lumen) is angulated to the right at the midpoint, where the ejaculatory duct approaches from above left. A vertical strip of highly condensed prostate mesenchyme contacts the posterior urethral wall only distal to the ejaculatory ducts. The prostate is flanked by the rectum (*left*) and pubis (*right*). Duct buds have not yet formed.

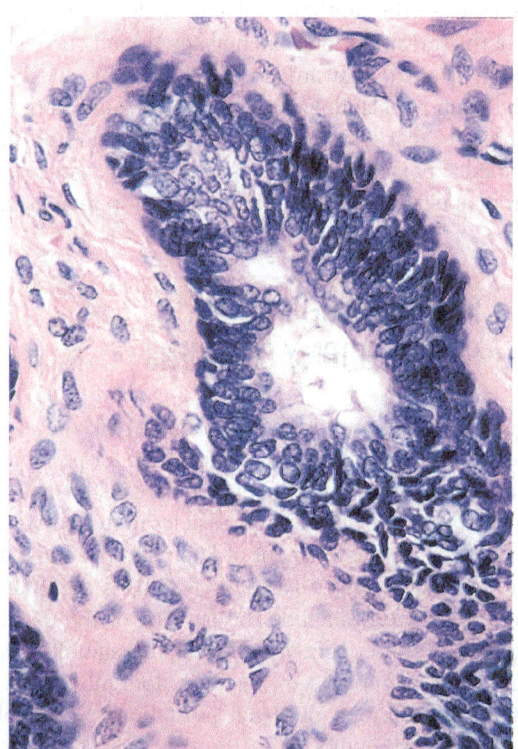

FIGURE 35.2 Prepubertal prostatic duct lined by epithelium with multiple layers of nuclei and showing no cytoplasmic differentiation.

GENERAL TOPOGRAPHIC RELATIONSHIPS: McNEAL'S ZONAL ANATOMY

The human prostate gland is a composite organ, comprised of several glandular and nonglandular components. These different "zones" are tightly fused together within a common sheath of fibromuscular tissue—the "capsule"—such that gross dissection is not possible. In a series of elegant dissections in postmortem specimens, Dr. McNeal showed that anatomic relationships are best demonstrated by examination of cut sections in the sagittal, coronal, and oblique coronal planes (3,4). From these studies, it is evident that: (a) there are three distinct glandular regions: the peripheral, central, and transition zones; and (b) the main nonglandular tissue of the prostate, termed the anterior fibromuscular stroma, is concentrated anteromedially and is responsible for much of the anterior convexity of the organ.

The urethra is a primary reference point for describing anatomic relationships. Visualized in a sagittal plane of section (Fig. 35.3), the prostatic urethra is divided into proximal and distal segments of approximately equal length by an anterior angulation at the midpoint between the prostate apex (distal) and the bladder neck (proximal) (1,5). The

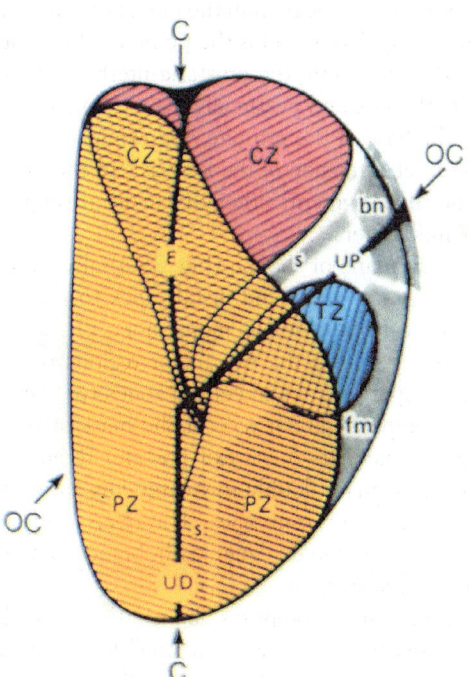

FIGURE 35.3 Sagittal diagram of distal prostatic urethral segment (*UD*), proximal urethral segment (*UP*), and ejaculatory ducts (*E*) showing their relationships to a sagittal section of the anteromedial nonglandular tissues (bladder neck [*bn*]; anterior fibromuscular stroma [*fm*]; prepostatic sphincter [*s*]; distal semicircular ["striated"] sphincter [*s*]). These structures are shown in relation to a three-dimensional representation of the glandular prostate (central zone [*CZ*]; peripheral zone [*PZ*]; transition zone [*TZ*]). Coronal plane (*C*) of Figure 35.4 and oblique coronal plane (*OC*) of Figure 35.5 are indicated by *arrows*.

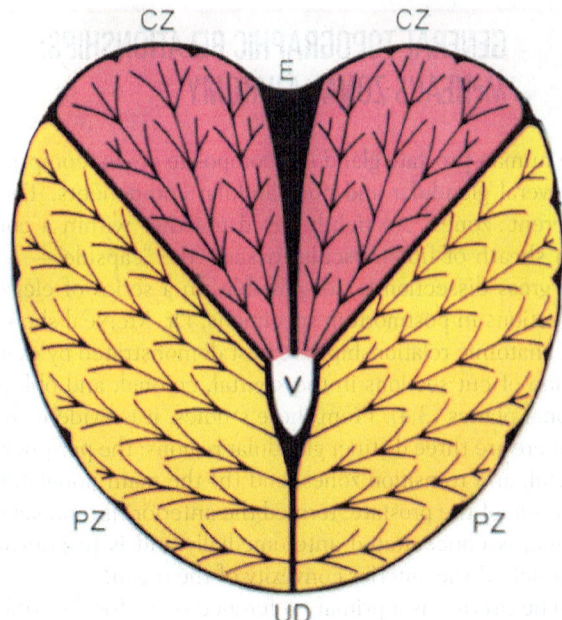

FIGURE 35.4 Coronal section diagram of prostate showing location of central zone (*CZ*) and peripheral zone (*PZ*) in relation to the distal urethral segment (*UD*), verumontanum (*V*), and ejaculatory ducts (*E*). The branching pattern of prostatic ducts is indicated; subsidiary ducts provide uniform density of acini along the entire main duct course.

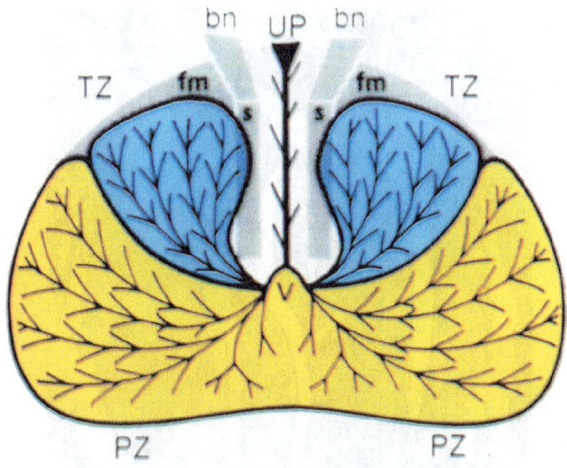

FIGURE 35.5 Oblique coronal section diagram of prostate showing location of peripheral zone (*PZ*) and transition zone (*TZ*) in relation to proximal urethral segment (*UP*), verumontanum (*V*), preprostatic sphincter (*s*), bladder neck (*bn*), anterior fibromuscular stroma (*fm*), and periurethral region with periurethral glands. Branching pattern of prostatic ducts is indicated: the medial transition zone ducts penetrate into the sphincter.

verumontanum protrudes from the posterior urethral wall at the point of angulation and is the point at which the ejaculatory ducts empty into the prostatic urethra. The ejaculatory ducts then extend proximally from the verumontanum (mid) to the base of the prostate, following a course that is nearly a direct extension of the long axis of the distal (apex to mid) urethral segment, although usually offset posteriorly by a few millimeters.

A coronal plane of section (Fig. 35.4) along the course of the ejaculatory ducts and distal (apex to mid) urethral segment provides the best demonstration of the anatomic relationships between the two major regions of glandular prostate, the peripheral and central zones (6). The peripheral zone comprises about 65% of the mass of the normal glandular prostate. Its ducts exit posterolaterally from the urethral wall along a double row extending from the verumontanum to the prostate apex. The ducts extend mainly laterally in the coronal plane, with branches that curve anteriorly and posteriorly.

The central zone comprises about 30% of the glandular prostate mass. Its ducts arise in a small focus on the verumontanum and immediately surround the ejaculatory duct orifices. The ducts branch directly toward the base of the prostate along the course of the ejaculatory ducts, fanning out to form an inverted conical structure that is flattened in the anterior–posterior plane. The base of this cone comprises almost the entire base of the prostate. The most lateral central zone ducts run parallel to the most proximal (base) peripheral zone ducts, separated only by a narrow band of stroma, which is usually imperceptible in clinical specimens.

An oblique coronal section (Fig. 35.5) along the proximal (mid to base) segment of the prostatic urethra from verumontanum to the bladder neck best defines its glandular relationships. Normally, the proximal urethral segment is intimately related to about only 5% of the prostatic glandular tissue, and almost all of this is the transition zone (7). This zone is formed by two small lobes whose ducts leave the posterolateral recesses of the urethral wall at a single point. The main ducts of the transition zone extend laterally and curve sharply anteriorly, arborizing toward the bladder neck.

The main nonglandular tissue of the prostate is the anterior fibromuscular stroma which overlies the urethra in the anteromedial prostate. Its bulk and consistency vary considerably from apex to base, as described further in this chapter.

SECTIONING OF RADICAL PROSTATECTOMY SPECIMENS

Radical prostatectomy, including removal of the seminal vesicles, is the definitive surgical procedure for patients with prostatic carcinoma. Current convention calls for inking the intact prostate gland and seminal vesicles in two colors in the fresh state to allow assessment of laterality. The most apical region of the gland (approximately 5 mm) is amputated in a transverse plane to include the opening of the distal urethra, and then subsequently sectioned parasagittally, perpendicular to the inked surface (Fig. 35.6) for embedding. This allows for visualization of apical prostatic tissue in planes that are near perpendicular to the true apical surface and hence, more accurate evaluation of cancer penetration and margin status. Handling of the bladder neck margin may be

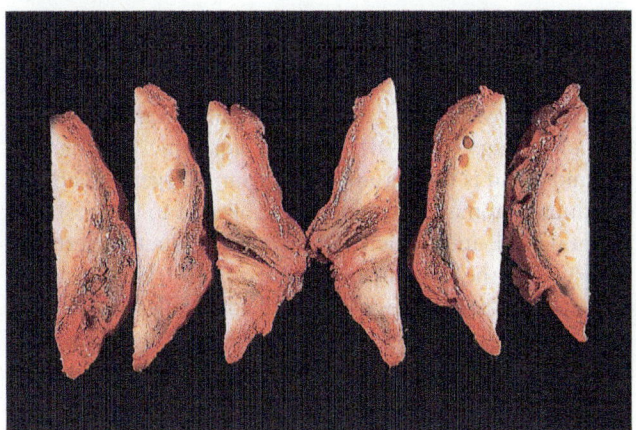

FIGURE 35.6 Apex of prostate seen grossly after 5-mm thick apical block has been subsectioned parasagittally at 3-mm intervals. Orientation of sections and localization of lesions are easily demonstrated, and cuts through the tissue are nearly perpendicular to the apical surface.

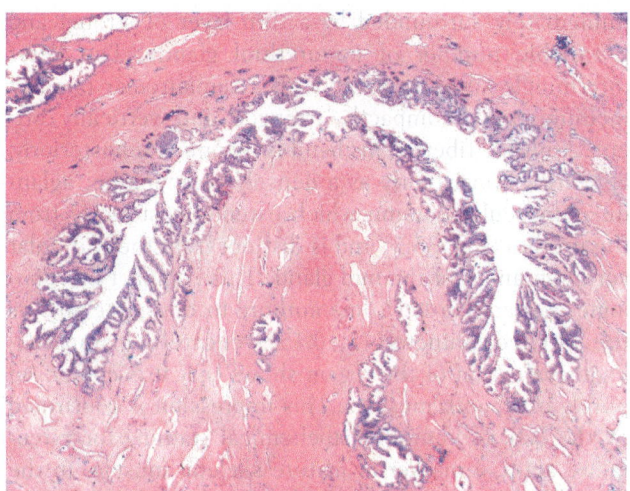

FIGURE 35.7 Distal urethra near the apex. Note the "promontory" or eversion of posterior periurethral tissue into the urethral space. The posterior portion of the semicircular sphincter (see Fig. 35.8) is present as a central muscular column.

accomplished in a similar fashion to the prostatic apex; however, some institutions shave a thin section of the most superficial muscle fragment(s) surrounding the proximal prostatic urethra and submit this tissue as an en face margin (8). While there is consensus that the junction of the seminal vesicles and the prostate should be sampled, the extent to which the remainder of the seminal vesicle should be submitted is not standardized (9). A reasonable approach may be to take two sections of each seminal vesicle, one at the prostatic junction, as well as a mid-seminal vesicle section to account for both contiguous spread of tumor from the prostatic base, as well as seminal vesicle invasion that occurs in the context of extraprostatic tumor extension. The remaining bulk of the gland is sectioned from apex to base in the anterior–posterior plane at approximately 3-mm intervals (10,11). The resulting complete transverse macrosections are submitted as either full whole mount sections or divided into half or quadrant sections using conventional tissue cassettes. Although there is debate as to the appropriate extent of sampling (8), a minimum submission of every other intervening macrosection is often recommended.

and tissue processing (12,13) is also typical, resulting in artifactual shortening of the distance from prostatic apex to verumontanum and everting the posterior periurethral tissue into the urethral space. These effects create an artificial "promontory" in the apical portions of the gland (Fig. 35.7) (14).

Histologic Variation by Anatomic Region

Apical One-Third of the Prostate (Apex)

In a surgical pathology specimen sectioned in the anterior–posterior plane, the apical (distal) urethra is located near the center of the section (Fig. 35.8). It is

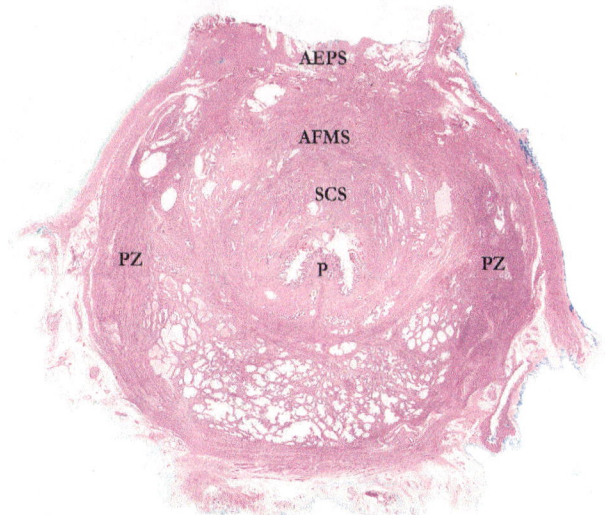

FIGURE 35.8 Whole mount section from apex of prostate. The urethra and promontory (*P*) are central and proceeding anteriorly, the semicircular sphincter (*SCS*) and anterior fibromuscular stroma (*AFMS*) are visualized. The posterior, lateral, and anterolateral portions of the apex are composed of peripheral zone (*PZ*) tissue. Most anteriorly, the anterior extraprostatic space (*AEPS*) contains vascular and adipose remnants of the dorsal vascular complex.

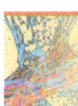

ANATOMY OF THE PROSTATE GLAND IN SURGICAL PATHOLOGY SPECIMENS

Gross Anatomy

In situ operative views of the prostate reveal a cone-shaped organ with its base surrounding the proximal urethral segment and abutting the bladder neck and its apex narrowing around the distal urethral segment as it approaches the urogenital diaphragm. Surgical manipulation and subsequent detachment of the prostate from native connective tissue leads to superior retraction of the distal (apical) urethra and yields a roughly spherical specimen at the gross dissection bench. Significant tissue shrinkage due to formalin fixation immediately surrounded by a thin layer of stroma and a variable number of periurethral glands. The latter intermingle anteromedially with a semicircular band of medium-sized, compactly arranged and vertically oriented muscle fibers. This band is incomplete posteriorly, appearing consistently as a densely eosinophilic, aglandular muscular column which extends posteriorly from the urethra (Fig. 35.7) and is distinct from the glandular verumontanum of the mid gland. This compact morphologic appearance led some authors to designate this as the "striated sphincter" (5,10,15), yet careful histopathologic evaluation of the region shows that it is composed purely of smooth muscles. This impression is confirmed by the lack of immunohistochemical staining for sarcomeric actin, a marker of mature skeletal muscle, in the muscle cells of this region (14).

Anterior to the semicircular muscle, fibers of the anterior fibromuscular stroma traverse horizontally and laterally as they extend to the anterior- and apical-most aspects of the prostate. While heightened intraprostatic pressure may cause bulging of hypertrophic transition zone acini, no normal transition zone tissue is located in the prostatic apex. The bilateral peripheral zone, which composes essentially all of the glandular tissue at the apex, occupies the posterior, lateral, and anterolateral prostates, abutting the anterior fibromuscular stroma medially and forming a nearly complete ring in histologic sections.

Middle One-Third of the Prostate (Mid Gland)

McNeal's studies revealed a 35-degree angulation of the prostatic urethra at mid gland, dividing the urethra into proximal (toward the base) and distal (toward the apex) segments (Fig. 35.9A–B). The key anatomic landmark in the mid gland is the verumontanum, an exaggerated area of glandular–stromal tissue, located subjacent to the posterior urethral wall, into which the ejaculatory ducts insert and from which the glandular zones arise (16). Histologically, the verumontanum consists of a crowded collection of prostatic glands, lined by secretory epithelium and often with abundant intraluminal corpora amylacea, directly underlying the urothelium of the prostatic urethra. When prominent, the term verumontanum gland mucosal hyperplasia is applied (Fig. 35.10) (17). At mid gland, the transition zone becomes evident as bilateral lobes in the anteromedial region of the gland. The ducts of the transition zone appear to arise from the posterior boundary of the periurethral space and course anterolaterally to serve as a boundary between transition and peripheral zones. A stromal boundary between these two zones has also been described (7), but may be difficult to identify in individual cases. In the normal mid gland, the peripheral zone still composes the posterior, lateral, and the majority of anterolateral tissues (Fig. 35.9A). In prostates with BPH, this tissue may be significantly compressed toward the lateral most portions of the gland (Fig. 35.9B). The anterior fibromuscular stroma in this region may be less evident owing to the increased

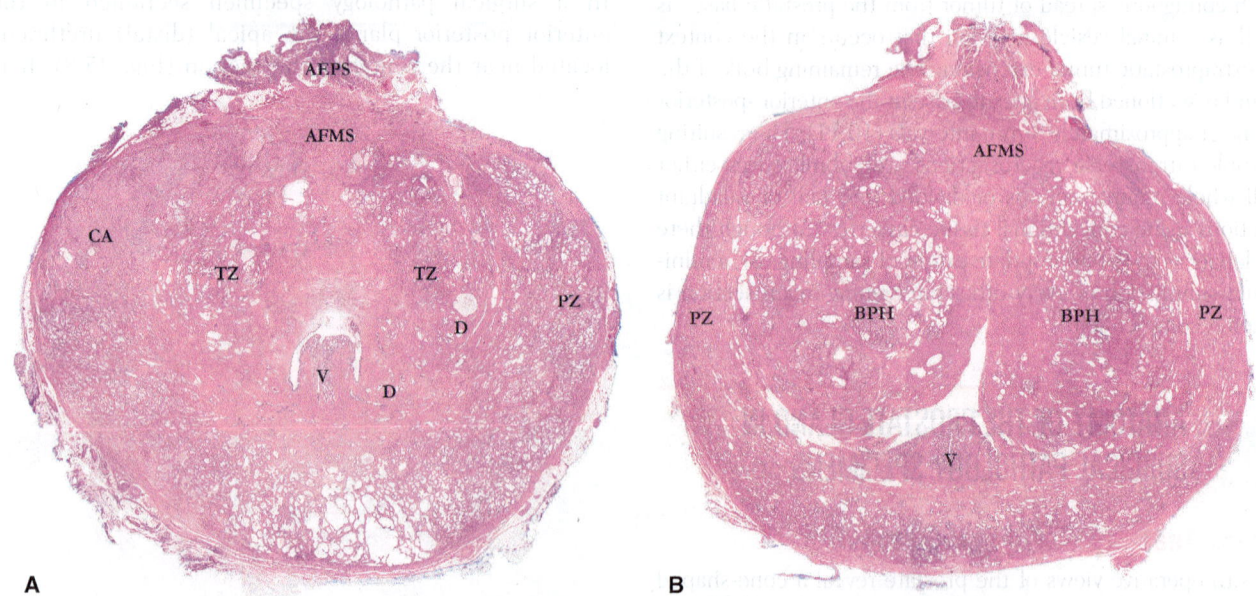

FIGURE 35.9 A: Whole mount section from mid prostate at the level of the verumontanum (*V*). Note the bilobed transition zone (*TZ*) arising from elongated ducts (*D*) which course anterolaterally. The peripheral zone (*PZ*) still occupies the posterior, lateral, and anterolateral portions of the gland, with a cancer nodule (*CA*) evident in the right anterior peripheral zone. In the mid prostate, the anterior fibromuscular stroma (*AFMS*) is much condensed and the anterior extraprostatic space (*AEPS*) largely retains its apical consistency. **B:** Whole mount section from mid prostate at the level of the verumontanum (*V*) in a gland with extensive benign prostatic hypertrophy (*BPH*). Anterolateral "horns" of the peripheral zone (*PZ*) are compressed laterally by the expanded transition zone tissue and the *AFMS* is diminished in extent.

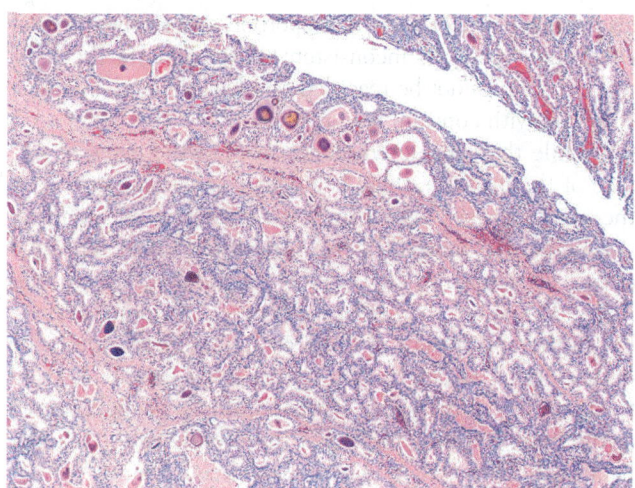

FIGURE 35.10 The verumontanum often contains densely packed prostatic glands lined by benign secretory cells, often with abundant intraluminal corpora amylacea.

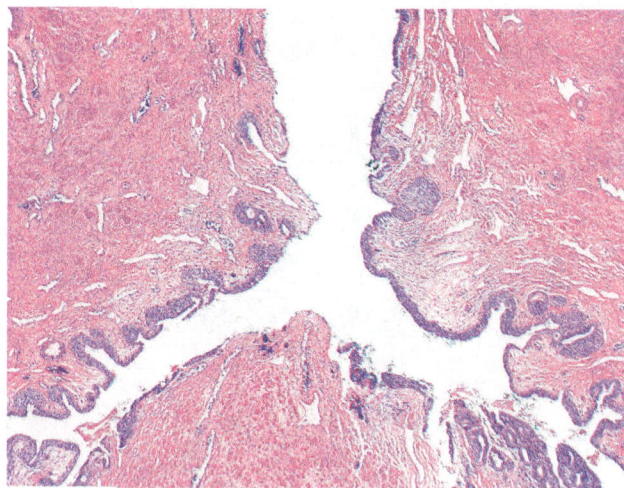

FIGURE 35.12 Preprostatic sphincter investing the proximal urethra in section from the base of prostate. The sphincter is composed of compact, short smooth muscle fibers distinct from prostatic smooth muscle and conveying a paler appearance to the periurethral zone as seen in Figure 35.11.

density of glandular tissue in the mid gland coupled with effects of organ contraction (14).

Basal One-Third of the Prostate (Base)

Progressing proximally from mid gland to base, the urethra becomes invested by a thick layer of short smooth muscle fibers, constituting the "preprostatic sphincter" (Figs. 35.11 and 35.12), which at its most lateral point may be in contact with the glands and acini of the transition zone (5,7). The preprostatic sphincter is thought to function during ejaculation to prevent retrograde flow of seminal fluid from the distal urethral segment and may have resting tone that maintains closure of the proximal urethral segment (18). At the base, the glands of the transition zone gradually recede and the few remaining peripheral zone acini once again comprise the anterior glandular tissue. In contrast with its apical appearance, however, the peripheral zone rarely extends anteromedially due to the abundant stroma in this region. This stroma appears as an expansive strip of tissue consisting of both preprostatic sphincter and anterior fibromuscular stroma, with the latter often merging with large smooth muscle bundles located in the anterior extraprostatic space. With increasing angulation, the prostatic urethra is identified further anteriorly in histologic sections, eventually breaching the anterior-most border of tissue sections at the level of the bladder neck. Posteriorly and posterolaterally, the central zone becomes evident surrounding the ejaculatory ducts which themselves are immediately encircled by a sheath of loose fibrous tissue with abundant lymphovascular spaces (Fig. 35.13). In the most basal portions of the gland, the well-formed muscular coat at the base of the seminal vesicles emerges and separates from the bulk of the prostatic tissue creating a fibroadipose tissue septum. The last vestiges of the central zone are present at the most lateral aspects of these emerging seminal vesicles (14).

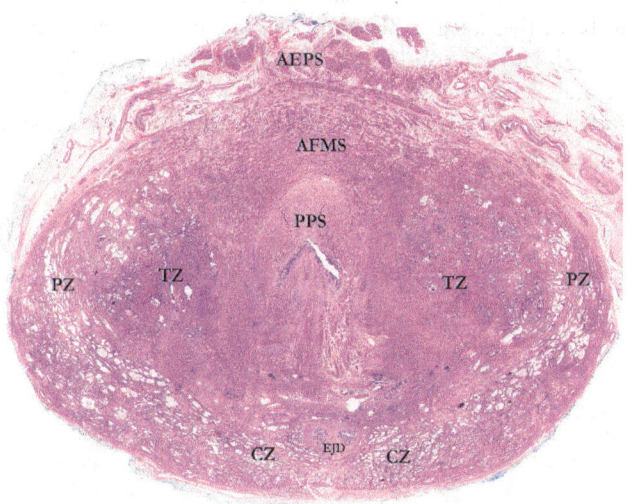

FIGURE 35.11 Whole mount section from base of prostate. The preprostatic sphincter (PPS) is evident as a pale area surrounding the proximal urethra. The transition zone (TZ) shows abortive small acini and is covered anteriorly by a vast anterior fibromuscular stroma (AFMS) which merges with smooth muscle bundles in the anterior extraprostatic space (AEPS). Posteriorly, the expansive central zone (CZ) surrounds the ejaculatory duct complex (EJD), while some peripheral zone (PZ) is still apparent posterolaterally.

Nonglandular Components of Prostatic and Extraprostatic Tissues

Prostatic Capsule and Anterior Fibromuscular Stroma

The prostatic "capsule" or condensed fibromuscular tissue (Fig. 35.14) ideally consists of an inner layer of smooth muscle fibers and an outer collagenous membrane. However, the relative and absolute amounts of fibrous and muscle

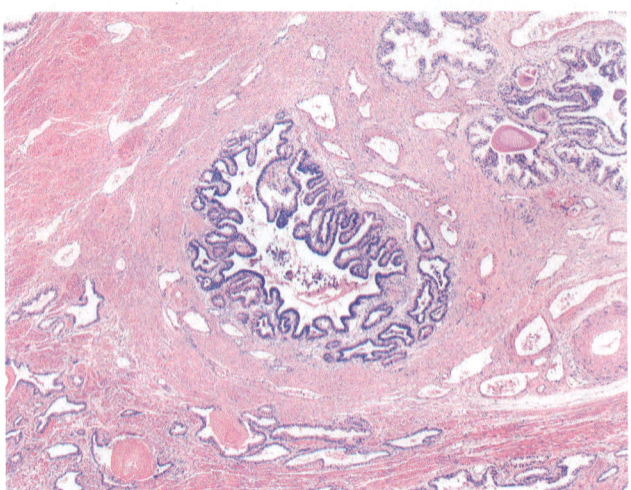

FIGURE 35.13 Ejaculatory duct encircled by a fibroconnective tissue sheath containing numerous lymphovascular spaces.

tissues and their arrangement vary considerably from region to region (19,20). At the inner capsular border, transverse smooth muscle blends with periglandular prostatic smooth muscle, and a clear separation between them cannot be identified microscopically (19). The distance from terminal acini of the peripheral and central zones to the prostate surface is

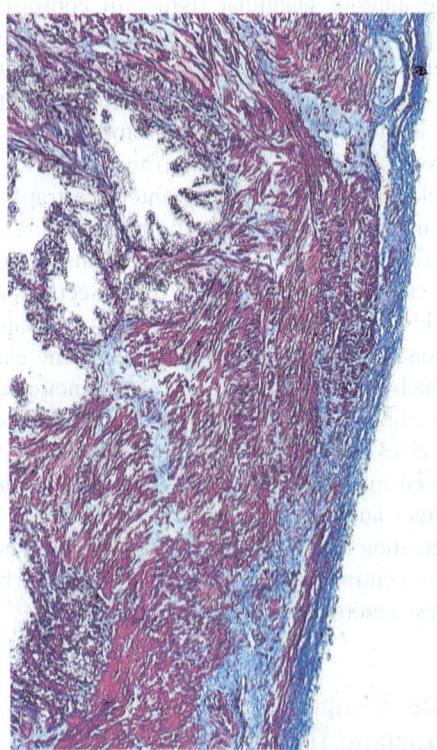

FIGURE 35.14 The prostate capsule consists of a layer of mainly transverse smooth muscle bundles (red), which is of variable thickness and blends with periacinar smooth muscle bundles at the capsule's poorly defined inner aspect (left). Collagen fibers (blue) are always present and usually concentrated in a thin compact membrane at the external capsular border (right) (trichrome stain).

also variable (7,21) and the proportion and arrangement of collagenous tissue is inconsistent. Consequently, the prostate capsule cannot be regarded as a well-defined anatomic structure with constant features.

While the capsule envelopes most of the external surface of the prostate, there is a defect of variable caliber at the prostatic apex anteriorly and anterolaterally such that the most distal (apical) fibers of the anterior fibromuscular stroma often mingle with the prostatic glandular tissue anterior and lateral to the urethra. Hence, if carcinoma is present in the apical third of the prostate anteriorly, it may be quite difficult to determine whether it has invaded beyond the boundary of the gland. Similar difficulty is encountered at the most proximal portion of the urethra in the bladder neck section, in which no clear capsule is evident.

The anterior fibromuscular stroma is an apron of tissue that extends downward from the bladder neck over the anteromedial surface of the prostate, narrowing to join the urethra at the prostate apex (Fig. 35.3) (7). Its lateral margins blend with the prostate capsule along the line where the capsule covers the most anteriorly projecting border of the peripheral zone. Its deep surface is in contact with the preprostatic sphincter and the transition zone proximally (toward the base) and with the "striated" or the semicircular sphincter distally (toward the apex). It is composed of large bundles of smooth muscle cells that may be separated by bands of dense fibrous tissue, and are more randomly oriented than those of the bladder neck and blend with the latter at its proximal (basal) extent.

Unlike the posterolateral prostate, in histopathologic sections the anterior-most region of the gland does not exhibit a distinct "capsule" (19). Rather, as one proceeds from apex to base, the anterior fibromuscular stroma is variably intertwined with skeletal muscle fibers emanating from the urogenital diaphragm (apical prostate) (Fig. 35.15) or levator ani muscles (mid prostate) and may fuse with detrusor smooth

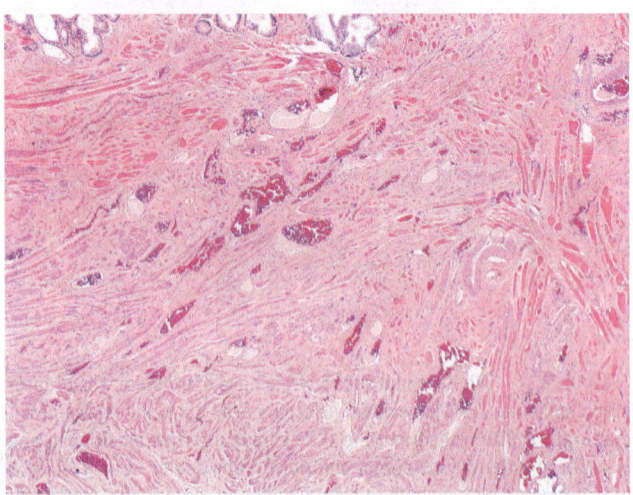

FIGURE 35.15 Anterior fibromuscular stroma showing admixture of smooth muscle bundles with skeletal muscle fibers from the urogenital diaphragm at the apex of the prostate.

muscle (mid to base). Moreover, the anterior fibromuscular stroma also contains blood vessels that supply/drain the anterior prostate throughout its extent. Due to the complex tissue composition of the anterior and anterolateral prostates and lack of a definitive border, the task of separating prostatic from extraprostatic tissue can be challenging in this region.

Extraprostatic Tissues, Prostatic Innervation, and Vascular Supply

In vivo, the tissue immediately anterior to the prostate is the dorsal venous or vascular complex, a series of veins and arteries set in fibroadipose tissue that runs over the anterior prostate and continues distally to supply/drain the penis (22). At the time of radical prostatectomy, the dorsal vascular complex is ligated and then divided, with a portion of the blood vessels and fibroadipose tissue remaining adherent to the prostate specimen. These may be identified as the anterior extraprostatic tissue from apex through mid gland. The most proximal (basal) two to three sections typically reveal medium- to large-sized smooth muscle bundles admixed with adipose tissue (Fig. 35.16). These fibers are morphologically identical to those of the detrusor muscle and possibly represent the inferior border of the bladder neck (23).

Over the medial half of the posterior (rectal) surface of the prostate, the thickness of the capsule is increased by its fusion to Denonvilliers' fascia (Figs. 35.17 and 35.18), a thin, compact collagenous membrane whose smooth

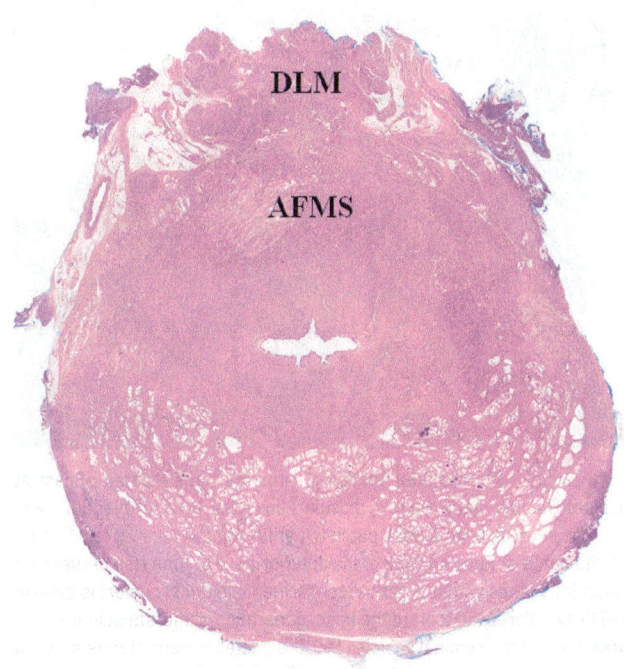

FIGURE 35.16 Prostate at mid to base of the gland—anterior extraprostatic space displays numerous medium- to large-sized discrete (detrusor-like) muscle bundles (*DLM*) admixed with adipose tissue, which merge with the anterior fibromuscular stroma (*AFMS*).

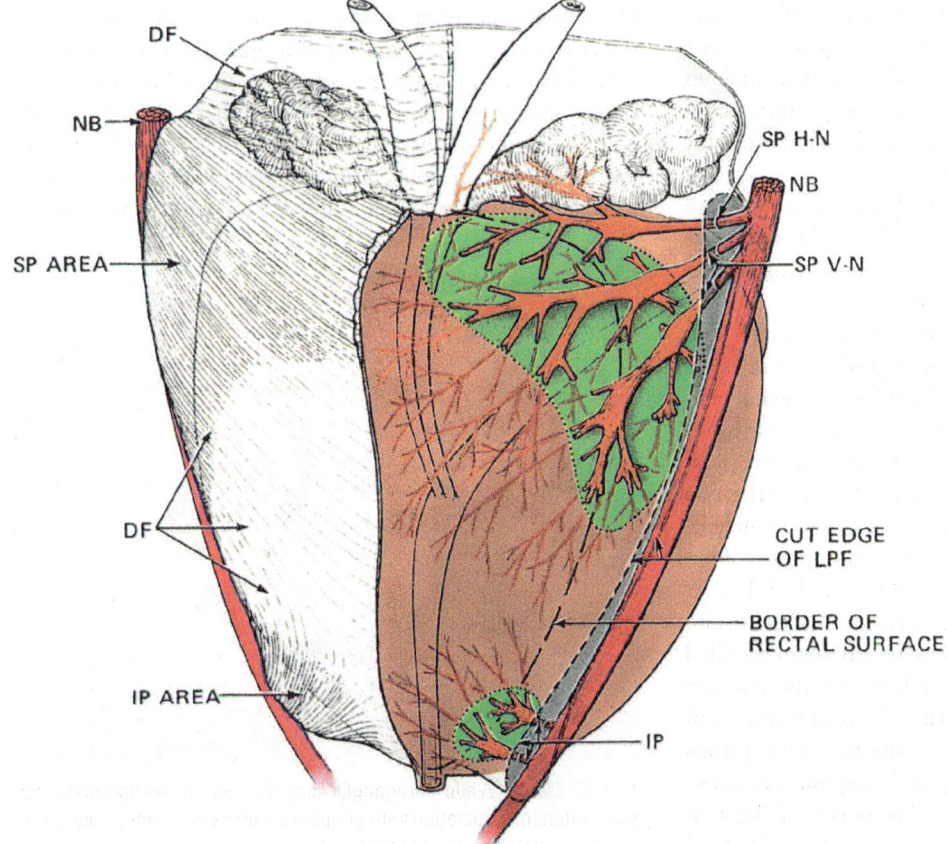

FIGURE 35.17 Distribution of nerve branches to the prostate, right posterolateral view. Nerves within the neurovascular bundle (*NB*) (*red*) branch to supply the prostate (*brown*) in a large superior pedicle (*SP*) at the prostate base and a small inferior pedicle (*IP*) at the prostate apex. Nerve branches (*orange*) leave the lateral pelvic fascia (not shown) to travel in Denonvilliers' fascia (*DF*), which has been cut away from the right half of the prostate. Nerve branches from the superior pedicle fan out over a large area. A small horizontal subdivision (*H-N*) crosses the base to midline; a large vertical subdivision (*V-N*) fans out extensively over the prostate surface as far distally as mid prostate. Branches continue their course within the prostate after penetration into the capsule within a large nerve penetration area (*green*). A small inferior pedicle has a limited ramification and nerve penetration area (*green*). *LPF*, lateral pelvic fascia.

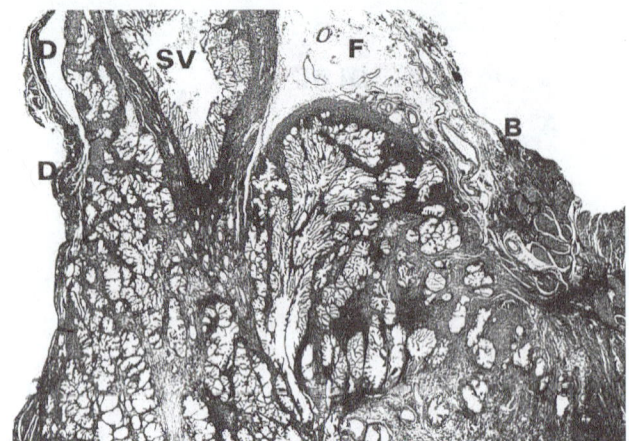

FIGURE 35.18 Parasagittal section of prostate base located almost at midline. Bladder neck smooth muscle above the level of bladder neck lumen is seen as a small dark patch (*B*) at far right. A layer of fat (*F*) covers the dome-shaped surface of the anterior central zone (*top center*). All glandular tissues within is central zone. One main duct (*center*) is seen in profile as it flares out toward the base, generating elaborate acinar structures. Behind the seminal vesicle (*SV*), the posterior central zone extends superiorly as a narrow plate. Denonvilliers' fascia (*D*) is not adherent behind the seminal vesicles but blends with the capsule below.

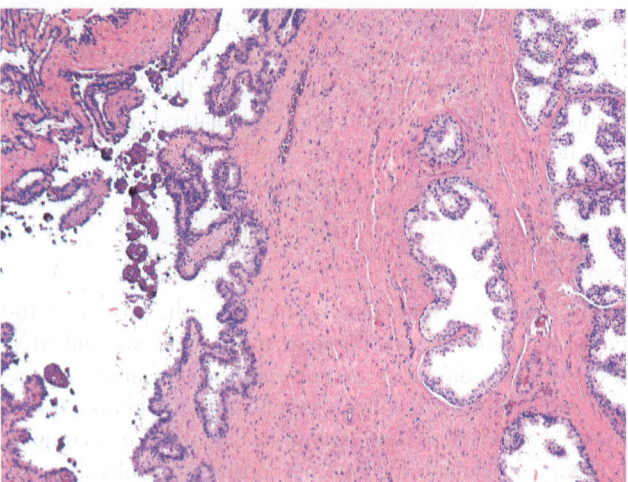

FIGURE 35.19 Minimal muscular tissue separating the prostatic central zone (*right*) from the seminal vesicles (*left*) at the base of the prostate.

posterior surface rests directly against the muscle of the rectal wall (24). The capsule is typically fused to the fascia with occasional remnants of an interposed adipose layer. In the adult, there remain only scattered microscopic islands of fat along with a variable number of smooth muscle fibers.

Superiorly (toward the base), Denonvilliers' fascia extends above the prostate to cover the posterior surface of the seminal vesicles in a loosely adherent fashion (Fig. 35.17). Laterally, the fascia leaves the posterior capsule where the prostate surface begins to deviate anteriorly, and it continues in a coronal plane to anchor against the pelvic sidewalls. Thus, the prostate and seminal vesicles are suspended along the anterior aspect of this fascial membrane in a similar fashion to the uterus being suspended from the broad ligament in the female.

As the seminal vesicles leave the prostate base, they extend laterally along its basal surface. Often there is no capsule between the two organs, at least for the medial centimeter or more of the seminal vesicle. The degree of fusion between the two muscular walls is variable between prostates, but there is frequently no boundary between the two organs medially with a minimal amount of common muscular wall separating the most basal central zone gland lumen from the seminal vesicle lumen (Figs. 35.18 and 35.19).

Where Denonvilliers' fascia separates from the prostate capsule posterolaterally, the space between them is filled with adipose tissue in a thick layer between the anterior aspect of the fascia and the posterolateral capsular surface of the prostate. The autonomic nerves, from the pelvic plexus to the seminal vesicles, prostate, and corpora cavernosa of the penis, travel in this fatty layer. The nerves, along with the blood vessels to the prostate, originate from bilateral neurovascular bundles that course vertically along the pelvic sidewalls (Fig. 35.17) (25). Most of the nerve branches to the prostate leave the neurovascular bundle just superior to the prostate base and course medially as the superior pedicle. These nerve branches fan out to penetrate the "superior pedicle insertion area" of the capsule, centered at the posterolateral aspect of the prostate base (25,26) and extend as far as mid gland. Some nerve trunks travel medially across the prostate base, sending branches into the central zone, but the majority of nerve branches fan out distally and penetrate the capsule at an oblique angle. Small microscopic paraganglia may also be seen in association with extraprostatic nerves and ganglia, reportedly identified in up to 8% of radical prostatectomies (27). They are characterized by small collections of round cells with clear or amphophilic cytoplasm, often with small cytoplasmic granules and an associated small capillary vasculature (Fig. 35.20). Some variable

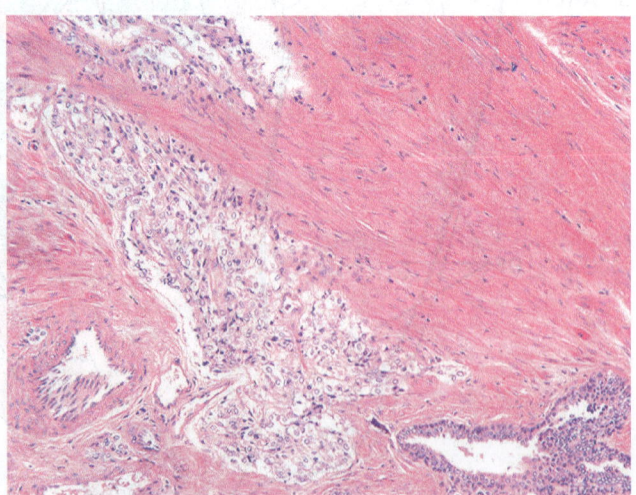

FIGURE 35.20 While paraganglia may be seen in extraprostatic tissues, often in association with peripheral nerves and ganglia, very rare examples may be intraprostatic.

cytologic atypia may be present in paraganglia, which could be confused with carcinoma, particularly in rare examples of intraprostatic paraganglia.

Before supplying the corpora cavernosa, nerve branches leave the neurovascular bundle at the prostate apex in the very small inferior pedicle and penetrate the capsule directly in a small "apical insertion area" located laterally and posterolaterally (26). Here the distance from neurovascular bundle to prostate capsule is narrowed to only a few millimeters and hence sparing the nerves involved in erectile function requires dissecting very close to the prostatic capsule in this region (28,29).

Arterial branches follow the nerve branches from the neurovascular bundle; they spread over the prostate surface and penetrate the capsule to extend directly inward toward the distal (apex to mid) urethral segment between the radiating duct systems of the central and peripheral zones (30,31). A major arterial branch enters the prostate at each side of the bladder neck and runs toward the verumontanum parallel to the course of the proximal (mid to base) urethral segment. It supplies the periurethral region and medial transition zone.

ARCHITECTURAL AND CYTOLOGIC FEATURES OF THE GLANDULAR PROSTATE

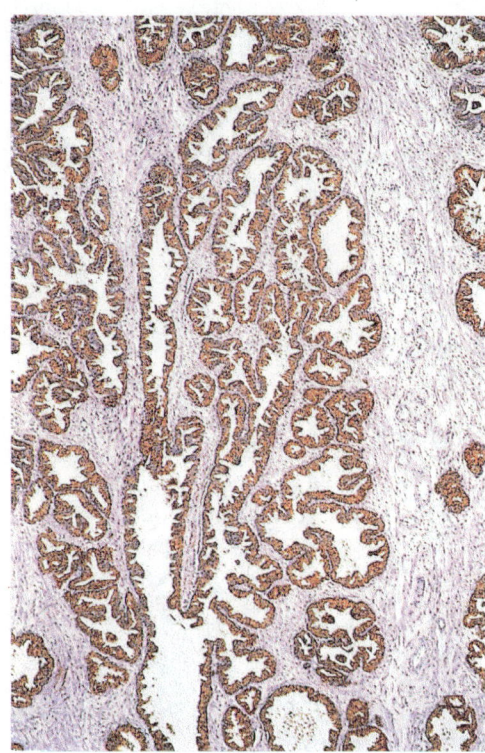

FIGURE 35.21 Ducts and acini of peripheral zone, immunohistochemically stained with anti-PSA and showing uniform distribution of protein throughout the cytoplasm of all ducts and acini.

Architectural Patterns

The biologic role of the prostate calls for the slow accumulation and occasional rapid expulsion of small volumes of fluid. These requirements are optimally met by a muscular organ having a large storage capacity and low secretory capacity. It is fitting then that the prostatic ducts are morphologically identical to the acini except for their geometry, and both appear to function as distensible secretory reservoirs. Within each prostate zone, the entire duct–acinar system, except for the main ducts near the urethra, is lined by columnar secretory cells of identical appearance between ducts and acini. Immunohistochemical staining for prostate-specific antigen (PSA) and prostatic acid phosphatase (PAP) shows uniform granular staining of all ductal and acinar cells (Fig. 35.21).

Except for the main transition zone ducts, which terminate at the anterior fibromuscular stroma, the main ducts of the prostate originate at the urethra and terminate near the capsule (3,6,7) (Figs. 35.4 and 35.5). Since ducts and acini within each zone have a similar caliber, spacing, and histologic appearance, ducts, ductules, and acini cannot reliably be distinguished microscopically. Hence, abnormalities of architectural pattern such as those seen in adenosis, prostatic intraepithelial neoplasia (PIN), and prostatic carcinoma are identified in routine sections mainly by deviations from normal size and spacing of glandular units.

The main excretory duct orifices of the peripheral zone arise every 2 mm from the distal (apex to mid) urethral segment along a double lateral line. A cluster of three or four subsidiary ducts arise about every 2 mm along each main excretory duct from urethra to capsule. These subsidiary ducts branch and extend only a short distance, rebranching and giving rise to groups of acini (Fig. 35.22). Hence, acini tend to be distributed with nearly uniform density along the course of the main duct between urethra and capsule, except that no acini are found immediately adjacent to the urethra.

In the peripheral zone and transition zone, ducts and acini have simple rounded contours that are not perfectly circular because of prominent undulations of the epithelial border (4,6). The undulations presumably allow expansion of the lumina as secretory reservoirs.

Central zone ducts and acini are distinctively larger than those of the peripheral zone and transition zone (Fig. 35.23). Both ducts and acini of the central zone become progressively larger toward the capsule at the prostate base reflecting the great expansion of central zone cross-sectional area from a small focus on the verumontanum to almost the entire prostate base. The corrugations in central zone duct/acinar walls are often exaggerated into distinctive intraluminal ridges—so-called "Roman arches."

In some specimens, there is an evident contrast in stromal morphology that delineates the boundary between peripheral zone and transition zone (21). The transition zone stroma is composed of compact interlacing smooth muscle bundles. This stromal density differs from the adjacent loose

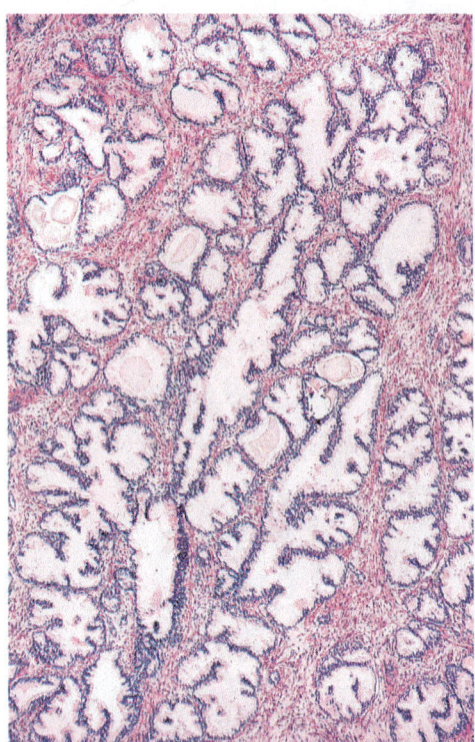

FIGURE 35.22 Subsidiary duct and branches in peripheral zone, terminating in small rounded acini with undulating borders. Ducts and acini have similar calibers and histologic appearances.

peripheral zone stroma, but blends with the stromas of the preprostatic sphincter and anterior fibromuscular stroma. Stromal distinctions are less evident in older prostates and may be obliterated by disease (32,33).

Cytologic Features

As with other glandular organs, the secretory cells throughout the prostate are separated from the basement membrane

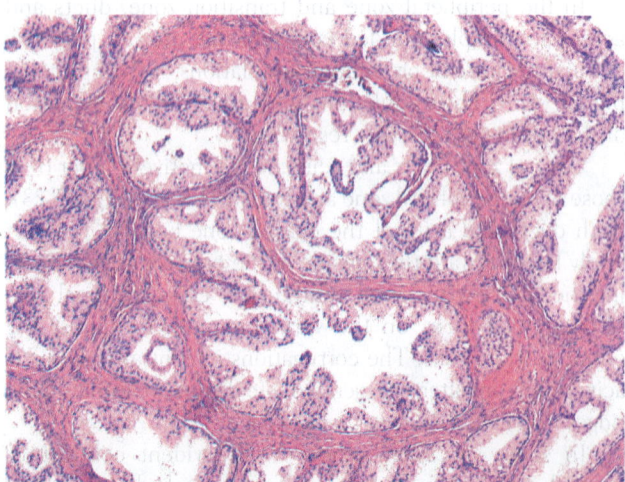

FIGURE 35.23 Low-power view of prostatic central zone architecture; large glands with complex luminal infoldings and distinct intraluminal bridges ("Roman arches").

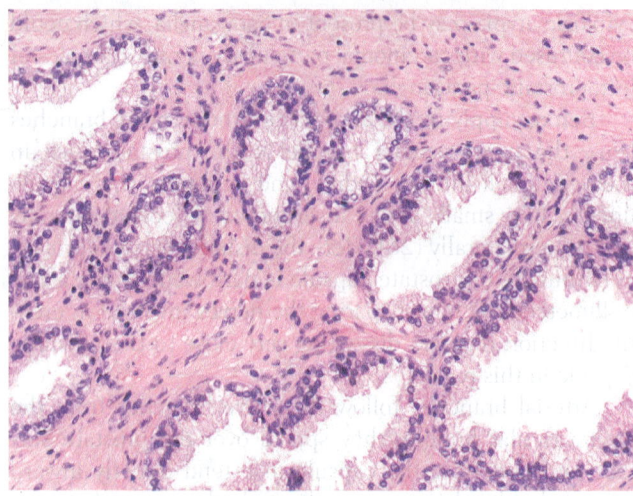

FIGURE 35.24 Prostatic acini with basal cells demonstrating little to no cytoplasm and arranged parallel to the basement membrane.

and the stroma by a layer of basal cells. The basal cells are typically elongated and flattened parallel to the basement membrane and have slender dark nuclei and usually little or no discernible cytoplasm (Fig. 35.24) (34). They are typically quite inconspicuous and, in routine preparations may appear incomplete or even absent around individual ducts or acini. Immunohistochemical labeling with high—molecular-weight cytokeratin and/or antibodies to p63 highlights the basal cell population (Fig. 35.25) (35–37). These stains are consistently negative in the cells of invasive malignant glands (36) because basal cells are absent. Basal cells are not myoepithelial cells analogous to those of the breast because, by electron microscopy, they do not contain muscle filaments (34).

In all zones of the prostate, the epithelium contains a small population of isolated, randomly scattered endocrine–paracrine cells (38) that are rich in serotonin-containing granules and contain neuron-specific enolase.

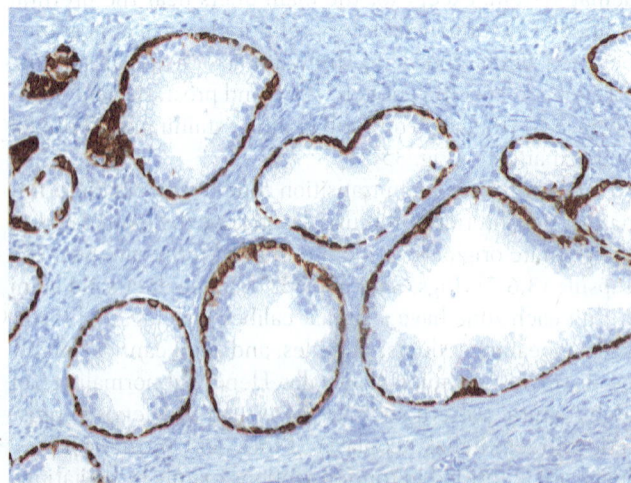

FIGURE 35.25 Same acini as in Figure 35.24 labeled with a double immunohistochemical stain for 34βE12 (cytoplasmic) and p63 (nuclear) in basal cells.

Subpopulations of these cells also contain a variety of peptide hormones, such as somatostatin, calcitonin, and bombesin. They rest on the basal cell layer between secretory cells and often have laterally spreading dendritic processes. They are not reliably identifiable microscopically except with immunohistochemical and other special stains. Their specific role in prostate biology is unknown, but they presumably have paracrine function.

The secretory cells of the prostate contribute a wide variety of products to the seminal plasma. PSA and PAP are produced by the secretory cells of the ducts and acini of all zones, while pepsinogen II (39), tissue plasminogen activator (40), and lactoferrin are normally produced only in the ducts and acini of the central zone. While PSA and PAP have historically been utilized as immunohistochemical markers of prostatic epithelium (or for prostatic origin in carcinomas), newer antibodies against the NKX3.1 protein are also frequently employed in routine clinical practice (41).

The cytoplasmic appearance of the normal secretory cell in all zones is similar and contains an abundance of small clear secretory vacuoles. Vacuoles in peripheral zone and transition zone cytoplasm are tightly packed (42), whereas in the central zone, a more abundant dense cytoplasm is associated with a somewhat wider vacuole spacing and lower vacuole density. Since the secretory vacuoles appear empty by routine microscopy, peripheral zone and transition zone cells are typically pale to clear, while central zone cells are typically somewhat darker (Figs. 35.26 and 35.27).

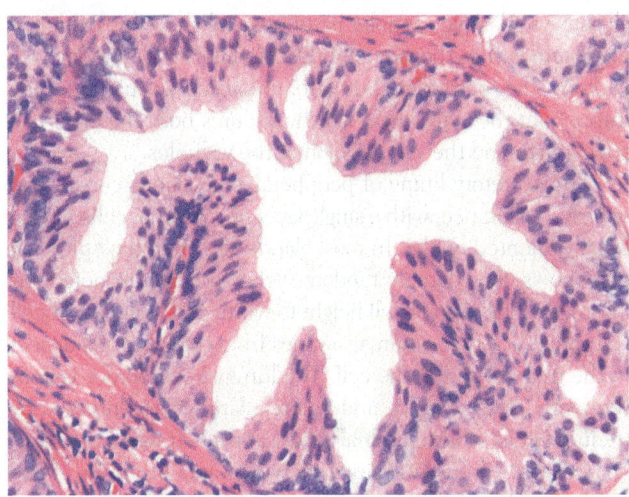

FIGURE 35.27 Central zone epithelium with eosinophilic cytoplasm and prominent basal cell layer.

The appearance of normal cell cytoplasm on tissue sections is strongly influenced by staining technique and by the type of fixative used. In the peripheral zone and the transition zone, light hematoxylin & eosin (H&E) staining after formalin fixation shows that normal cells are "clear cells" in which a faint network of pale-staining cytoplasmic partitions between vacuoles can be visualized with careful scrutiny under high magnification. Only an occasional cell shows complete outlines that define numerous intact vacuoles, but immunostaining with PSA (Fig. 35.28) or PAP on the same tissue sharply outlines

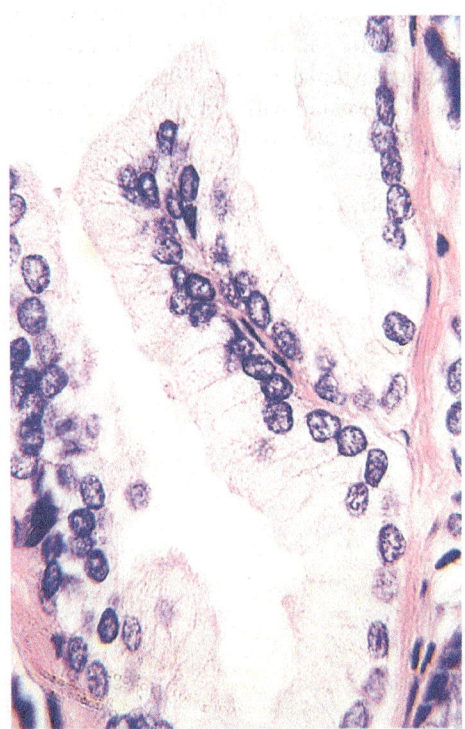

FIGURE 35.26 Peripheral zone epithelium showing clear cells in which cytoplasm is barely discernible as composed of a sheet of small empty vacuoles with delicate pale partitions.

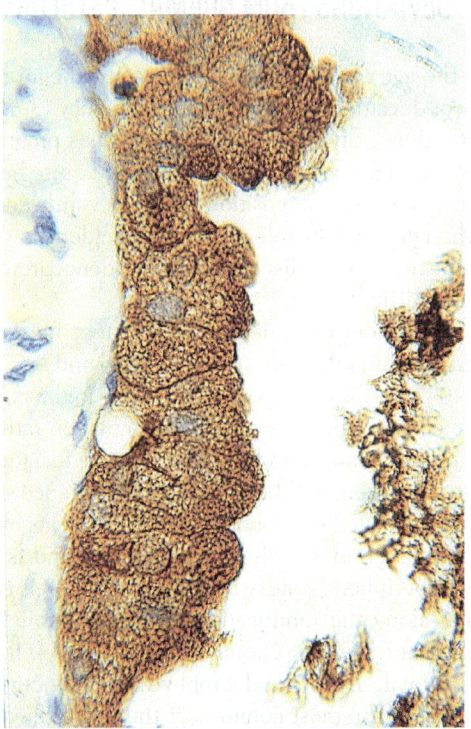

FIGURE 35.28 Peripheral zone epithelium immunostained with antibody to PSA. Protein is concentrated in a reticulated pattern that spares vacuole lumens and accentuates portions of vacuole partitions.

all the cytoplasmic vacuolar partitions and shows no evidence of protein within the vacuoles. Darker H&E staining not only darkens the partitions but also enhances diffuse staining throughout the cytoplasm, which obscures both the clear cell appearance and the visualization of the vacuoles.

The secretory lining of peripheral zone glands conveys an orderly appearance, with a single layer of columnar cells having basally oriented nuclei. In most glands, however, the epithelial row shows considerable random variation between neighboring cells in the ratio of cell height to width and in apparent cell volume. Nuclear location also varies from the basal cell aspect to the mid-portion of the cell. The luminal cell border is consequently often uneven, and its irregularity is accentuated by frequent cells whose luminal aspect appears frayed.

Central zone epithelium shows an accentuation of the mild disorder of cell arrangement of the peripheral zone/transition zone (Figs. 35.23 and 35.27). Here the epithelium is variably thickened by prominent cell crowding. Nuclei, which are usually larger than in the peripheral zone, are often displaced further from the cell base than in the peripheral zone and appear pseudostratified.

The dark cytoplasm, thickened variable epithelium, and complex architecture in the central zone may be misinterpreted as PIN on needle biopsies. However, the distinctive histologic features coupled with the absence of enlarged nuclei, nucleoli, or hyperchromasia and an often prominent basal cell layer are useful in excluding this diagnosis.

DEVIATIONS FROM NORMAL HISTOLOGY

Beyond the age of 30 years, many prostates begin to show a variety of deviations from normal morphology (3,6,32,33). Their prevalence and extent of these changes progressively increase with age so that most prostates are quite heterogeneous in histologic composition by the seventh decade of life. Although these histologic patterns seldom have clinical significance, their distinction from adenocarcinoma is sometimes difficult.

Early morphologic studies concluded that focal atrophy in the prostate was a manifestation of aging and was seen as early as 40 years of age. In fact, focal atrophy in the prostate is often the consequence of previous inflammation rather than aging (3,6). The number and extent of atrophic foci tend to be greater in older men, but their histologic appearance is identical to that of isolated foci found as early as 30 years of age.

Atrophy is an extremely common lesion and is mainly seen in the peripheral zone, where its distribution is typically segmental along the ramifications of a duct branch (3,6). Publication of a Working Group classification (43) has highlighted four patterns of focal atrophy with distinctive histologic features. The most common of these is termed *simple atrophy*, in which irregular or angulated, basophilic acini are seen at low magnification. Some degree of acinar dropout may be present. Individual acini have reduced cytoplasm,

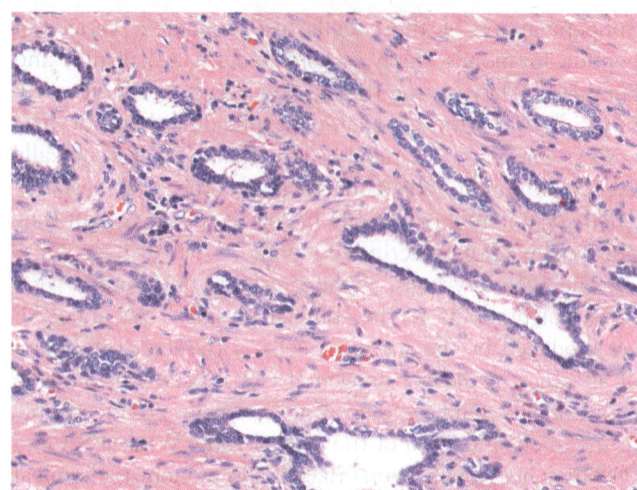

FIGURE 35.29 Simple atrophy demonstrating angulated, basophilic glands with limited to no cytoplasm and dark nuclei; scattered chronic inflammatory cells are also present.

yet nuclei often retain their usual size (Fig. 35.29). *Simple atrophy* is commonly associated with chronic inflammation that may involve the prostatic stroma or epithelium. Especially in the setting of inflammation, atrophic glands may exhibit small nucleoli. The combination of small angulated glands with variable architectural distortion and nucleoli may mimic cancer and cause diagnostic difficulty.

Simple atrophy with cyst formation is characterized by rounded acini of very large diameter which have a sieve-like gross and cyst-like microscopic appearance. Glands show back to back architecture with little intervening stroma (Fig. 35.30). Cytologically, the cyst-like acini have little to no apparent cytoplasm and unlike *simple atrophy*, are uncommonly associated with chronic inflammation.

Postatrophic hyperplasia, like *simple atrophy*, has a basophilic appearance at low magnification and is composed of small round acini in a vaguely lobular arrangement. In radical

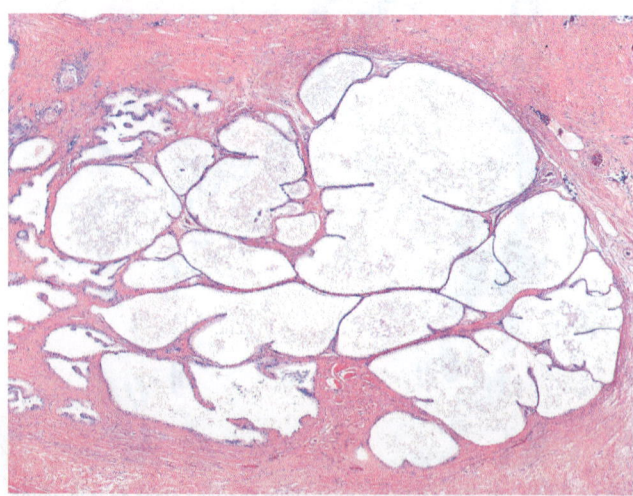

FIGURE 35.30 Back-to-back large caliber rounded acini with little to no cytoplasm characteristic of cystic atrophy.

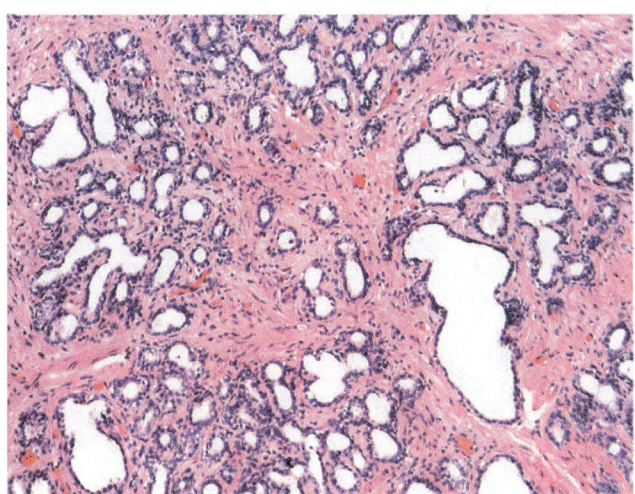

FIGURE 35.31 Postatrophic hyperplasia with atrophic acini in a lobular array surrounding a central dilated duct.

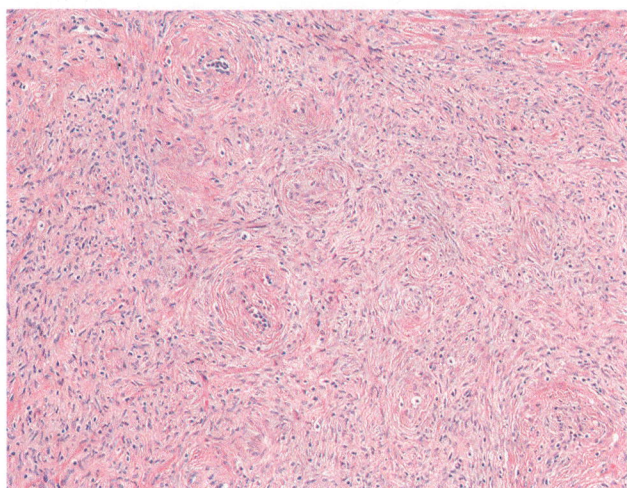

FIGURE 35.33 Prostatic stromal hyperplasia is characterized by a relatively lobular or nodular proliferation of cytologically bland spindle cells associated with prominent small round blood vessels.

prostatectomy sections, these acini often seem to surround a dilated duct (Fig. 35.31), which has led some to use the alternate term "lobular atrophy." The close packing of multiple small acini conveys a histologic impression of hyperplastic glands, yet whether this is truly a hyperplastic process or not remains unknown. The atrophic acini are often engulfed in a variable degree of fibrotic or sclerotic stroma. Cytologically, *postatrophic hyperplasia* shows low cuboidal cells with scant cytoplasm and small- to medium-sized nucleoli. Like *simple atrophy*, chronic inflammation is often present, and the differential diagnosis of adenocarcinoma is often raised, especially in needle biopsy material.

Partial atrophy is distinct from the other forms described here in that cytoplasm is attenuated, but is variably present, with a nonbasophilic appearance at low magnification. Characteristically, *partial atrophy* displays more cytoplasm lateral to the nucleus, increasing internuclear distance and imparting a pale low-power impression (Fig. 35.32). Small- to medium-sized nucleoli, as well as intraluminal dense pink sections/crystalloids may mimic carcinoma. *Partial atrophy* is frequently seen admixed with foci of *simple atrophy* suggesting that they represent a spectrum of atrophic changes.

In contrast to atrophy, the histologic hallmark of BPH is the expansile nodule, produced by the budding and branching of newly formed duct–acinar structures, by the focal proliferation of stroma (Fig. 35.33), or by a combination of both elements (Fig. 35.34) (3,4,7,44). It mainly affects the transition zone.

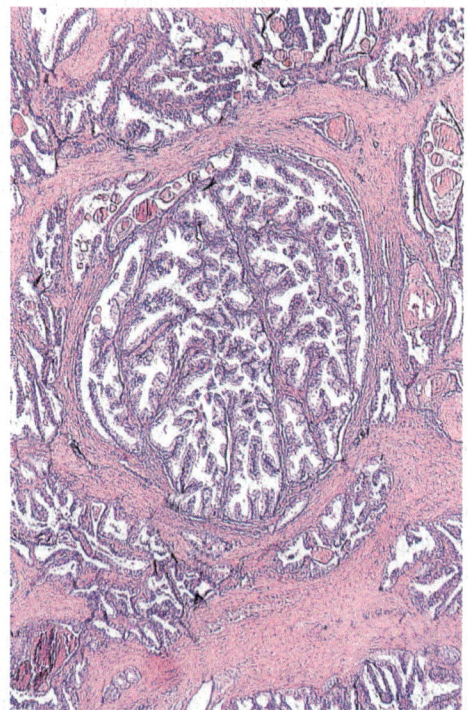

FIGURE 35.34 Nodule of glandular benign nodular hyperplasia in the prostatic transition zone.

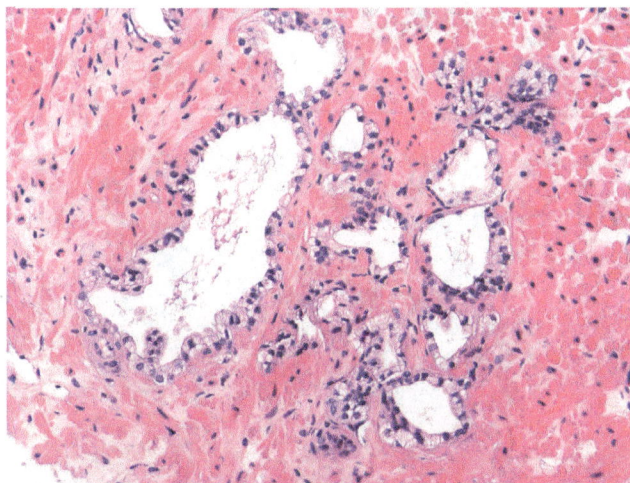

FIGURE 35.32 Focus of partial atrophy with attenuated pale cytoplasm and wispy eosinophilic intraluminal secretions. The nuclei appear relatively evenly spaced due to retention of the lateral cytoplasm.

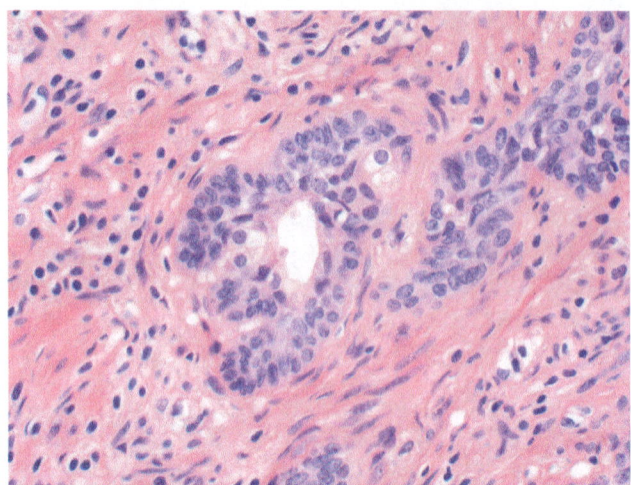

FIGURE 35.35 Focus of basal cell hyperplasia showing multiple layers of rounded basal cells with a central flattened layer of eosinophilic secretory cells. The basal cells commonly contain small prominent nucleoli.

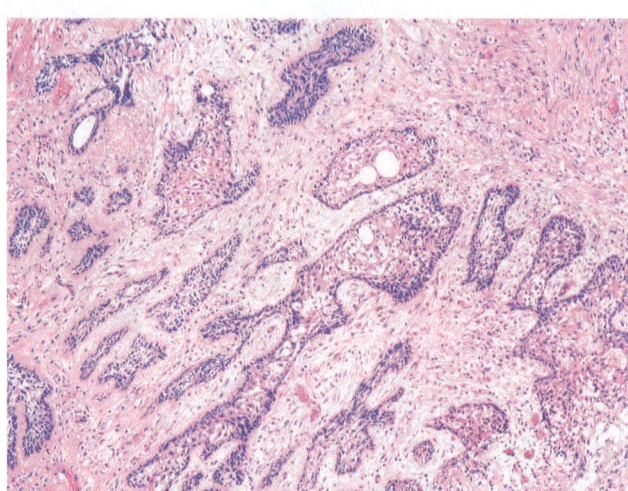

FIGURE 35.36 Prominent squamous metaplasia is often present surrounding areas of ischemia or frank infarct.

Grossly BPH is usually recognized as a globular mass replacing each transition zone and is composed of numerous individual nodules. Only the nodular component is recognizable histologically as a deviation from normal pattern; internodular tissue, even when increased in amount, is not distinguishable microscopically from normal transition zone.

The enlargement of transition zone BPH produces a characteristic progressive deformity of overall prostate contour. The expansion is chiefly anterior and toward the apex resulting in stretching and thinning of the anterior fibromuscular stroma and producing an increase in the thickness (anteroposterior dimension) of the gland. The anterolateral "horns" of the peripheral zone (Fig. 35.9B) are compressed and thinned concomitant with increase of overall prostate width.

Basal cell hyperplasia is most often seen as a secondary change in BPH nodules or inflammatory foci (45). The basal cells of ducts and acini become rounded with oval nuclei, and they form a multilayered lining (Fig. 35.35) that stains for basal cell–specific high–molecular-weight cytokeratins. There is typically a single luminal row of columnar secretory cells that stain positive for PSA. When ischemia or frank infarcts are present (often in association with BPH), squamous metaplasia may also become prominent. This benign metaplastic change may closely mimic urothelial carcinoma (Fig. 35.36) (46).

Because many men with prostate cancer are treated by radiation therapy, pathologists must be familiar with its effects on benign glands. After radiation, the normal glands typically become atrophic, but with cytoplasmic eosinophilia that imparts a "squamoid" appearance, and scattered nuclei become enlarged and hyperchromatic, albeit with degenerative-appearing, "smudgy," chromatin (Fig. 35.37). Many of the cells within these glands assume a basal cell phenotype, so the expression with basal cell markers, including GATA3, is common. Because of the cytologic atypia, the latter immunophenotypic finding may cause confusion with urothelial carcinoma (47,48).

CONSIDERATIONS IN TRANSURETHRAL RESECTION AND NEEDLE BIOPSY SPECIMENS

Tissue distortion by thermal artifact near the edges of transurethral resection (TUR) tissue fragments ("chips") can create important diagnostic problems that occasionally may be insurmountable. Basal cell hyperplasia, adenomatous hyperplasia, atrophy, and fragments of BPH nodules with small glands may be difficult to distinguish from carcinoma without utilizing adjunctive immunohistochemical stains. Loss of nuclear detail occurs more homogeneously across the tissue chips than obvious cell distortion. Hence, small foci of cancer may be more difficult to diagnose because of the artifactual absence of nucleoli.

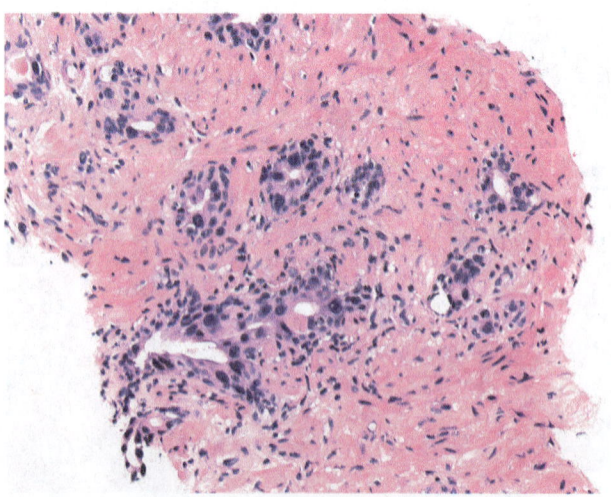

FIGURE 35.37 Radiation therapy induces atrophic changes in benign prostatic glands, often with associated cytoplasmic eosinophilia and nuclear pleomorphism.

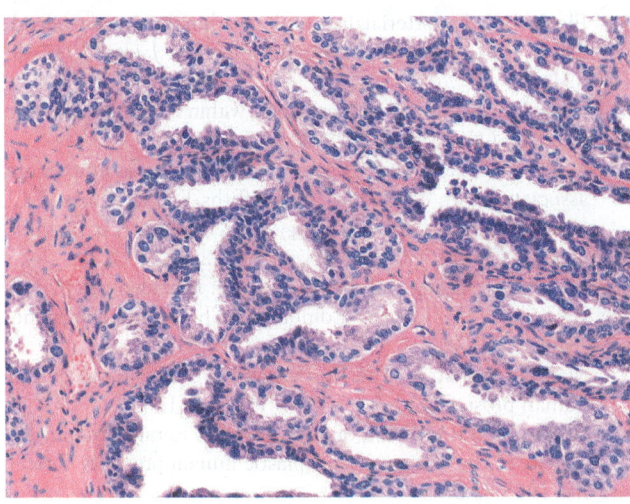

FIGURE 35.38 Benign tubular invaginations from the wall of the ejaculatory duct showing architectural (small crowded acini) and cytologic (focal prominent nucleoli) features that suggest carcinoma. Focal yellow-brown cytoplasmic pigment, as seen in the *upper right–hand portion* of the figure, is characteristic of this epithelium.

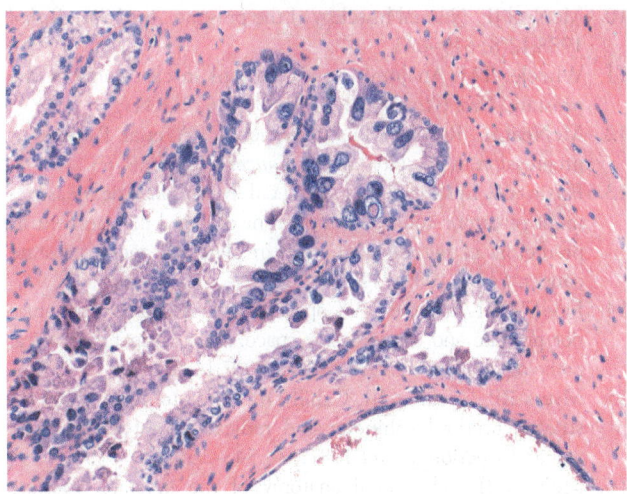

FIGURE 35.39 Benign ejaculatory duct/seminal vesicle–type epithelium demonstrating bizarre enlarged hyperchromatic nuclei.

The same problems are seen in needle biopsies, where the artifact is presumably due to compression rather than heat. The presence of artifact is usually limited to loss of nuclear detail and is more subtle because areas of severe tissue distortion are not often represented.

The regions of the prostate sampled by TUR and by needle biopsy are also quite different. Most needle biopsies represent posterior peripheral zone tissue. Unless a special effort is made, as in a transition zone–directed needle biopsy (49), the needle seldom reaches the more anterior portions of the gland.

In a majority of the cases, TUR specimens consist of transition zone tissue, urethral and periurethral tissues, bladder neck fragments, and anterior fibromuscular stroma (44) with variable amounts of peripheral zone tissue. On rare occasions, central zone fragments may be sampled and show the distinctive architectural and cytologic features described above. They may be accompanied by fragments of ejaculatory duct/seminal vesicle and the tiny tubular outgrowths from the walls of these structures may be misinterpreted as adenocarcinoma when seen in tangential sections that do not reveal the main lumen (Fig. 35.38). This impression of carcinoma may be further encouraged by the frequent presence of enlarged dark nuclei with bizarre contours in the seminal vesicle and ejaculatory duct epithelium (Fig. 35.39). The presence of golden brown cytoplasmic granules, which may be few and inconspicuous, may help to establish the benign diagnosis.

ACKNOWLEDGMENT

The content of this chapter builds upon the prodigious work of the late Dr. John E. McNeal, who in a series of manuscripts and monographs from the 1970s through the early 1990s, defined the modern approach to prostatic anatomy. Although this current iteration has been reorganized to focus on anatomic structures as they relate to the evaluation of prostate cancer in routine prostatectomy specimens today, it is based on Dr. McNeal's principles and the previous editions that he authored.

REFERENCES

1. McNeal JE. Developmental and comparative anatomy of the prostate. In: Grayhack J, Wilson J, Scherbenske M, eds. *Benign Prostatic Hyperplasia.* DHEW Publication No. (NIH) 76–1113. Washington, DC: Department of Health, Education and Welfare; 1975:1–10.
2. Cunha GR, Donjacour AA. Mesenchymal–epithelial interactions in the growth development of the prostate. In: Lepor H, Ratliff TL, eds. *Urologic Oncology.* Boston: Kluwer Academic; 1989:159–175.
3. McNeal JE, Stamey TA, Hodge KK. The prostate gland: Morphology, pathology, ultrasound anatomy. *Monogr Urol* 1988;9:36–54.
4. McNeal JE. Anatomy of the prostate and morphogenesis of BPH. *Prog Clin Biol Res* 1984;145:27–53.
5. McNeal JE. The prostate and prostatic urethra: A morphologic synthesis. *J Urol* 1972;107:1008–1016.
6. McNeal JE. Regional morphology and pathology of the prostate. *Am J Clin Pathol* 1968;49:347–357.
7. McNeal JE. Origin and evolution of benign prostatic enlargement. *Invest Urol* 1978;15:340–345.
8. Samaratunga H, Montironi R, True L, et al; ISUP Prostate Cancer Group. International Society of Urological Pathology (ISUP) Consensus Conference on Handling and Staging of Radical Prostatectomy Specimens. Working group 1: Specimen handling. *Mod Pathol* 2011;24:6–15.
9. Berney D, Wheeler TM, Grignon DJ, et al; ISUP Prostate Cancer Group. International Society of Urological Pathology (ISUP) Consensus Conference on Handling and Staging of Radical Prostatectomy Specimens. Working group 4: Seminal vesicles and lymph nodes. *Mod Pathol* 2011;24:39–47.

10. McNeal JE. Normal histology of the prostate. *Am J Surg Pathol* 1988;12(8):619–633.
11. Wheeler TM. Anatomic considerations in carcinoma of the prostate. *Urol Clin North Am* 1989;16:623–634.
12. McNeal JE, Bostwick DG, Kindrachuk RA, et al. Patterns of progression in prostate cancer. *Lancet* 1986;1:60–63.
13. Partin AW, Epstein JI, Cho KR, et al. Morphometric measurement of tumor volume and percent of gland involvement as predictors of pathological stage in clinical stage B prostate cancer. *J Urol* 1989;141:341–345.
14. Fine SW, Al-Ahmadie HA, Gopalan A, et al. Anatomy of the anterior prostate and extraprostatic space: A contemporary surgical pathology analysis. *Adv Anat Pathol* 2007;14:401–407.
15. Myers RP, Goellner JR, Cahill DR. Prostate shape, external striated urethral sphincter and radical prostatectomy: The apical dissection. *J Urol* 1987;138:543–550.
16. McNeal JE. The zonal anatomy of the prostate. *Prostate* 1981;2:35–49.
17. Gagukas RJ, Brown RW, Wheeler TM. Verumontanum mucosal gland hyperplasia. *Am J Surg Pathol* 1995;19:30–36.
18. Greene DR, Wheeler TM, Egawa S, et al. Relationship between clinical stage and histological zone of origin in early prostate cancer: Morphometric analysis. *Br J Urol* 1991;68:499–509.
19. Ayala AG, Ro JY, Babaian R, et al. The prostatic capsule: Does it exist? Its importance in the staging and treatment of prostatic carcinoma. *Am J Surg Pathol* 1989;13:21–27.
20. McNeal JE, Villers AA, Redwine EA, et al. Capsular penetration in prostate cancer: Significance for natural history and treatment. *Am J Surg Pathol* 1990;14:240–247.
21. McNeal JE, Redwine EA, Freiha FS, et al. Zonal distribution of prostatic adenocarcinoma: Correlation with histologic patterns and direction of spread. *Am J Surg Pathol* 1988;12:897–906.
22. Walsh PC. Radical retropubic prostatectomy with reduced morbidity: An anatomic approach. *NCI Monogr* 1988;7:133–137.
23. Tanagho EA, Smith DR. The anatomy and function of the bladder neck. *Br J Urol* 1966;38:54–71.
24. Villers A, McNeal JE, Freiha FS, et al. Invasion of Denonvilliers' fascia in radical prostatectomy specimens. *J Urol* 1993;149:793–798.
25. Lepor H, Gregerman M, Crosby R, et al. Precise localization of the autonomic nerves from the pelvic plexus to the corpora cavernosa: A detailed anatomical study of the adult male pelvis. *J Urol* 1985;133:207–212.
26. Villers A, McNeal JE, Redwine EA, et al. The role of perineural space invasion in the local spread of prostatic adenocarcinoma. *J Urol* 1989;142:763–768.
27. Ostrowski ML, Wheeler TM. Paraganglia of the prostate. Location, frequency, and differentiation from prostatic adenocarcinoma. *Am J Surg Pathol* 1994;18:412–420.
28. Catalona WJ, Dresner SM. Nerve-sparing radical prostatectomy: Extraprostatic tumor extension and preservation of erectile function. *J Urol* 1985;134:1149–1151.
29. Eggleston JC, Walsh PC. Radical prostatectomy with preservation of sexual function: Pathological findings in the first 100 cases. *J Urol* 1985;134:1146–1148.
30. Flocks RH. The arterial distribution within the prostate gland: its role in transurethral prostatic resection. *J Urol* 1937;37:524–525.
31. Clegg EV. The vascular arrangements within the human prostate gland. *Br J Urol* 1956;28:428–435.
32. McNeal JE. Age-related changes in the prostatic epithelium associated with carcinoma. In: Griffiths K, Pierrepoint CG, eds. *Some Aspects of the Aetiology and Biochemistry of Prostatic Cancer*. Cardiff, Wales: Tenovus; 1970:23–32.
33. McNeal JE. Aging and the prostate. In: Brocklehurst JC, ed. *Urology in the Elderly*. Edinburgh: Churchill Livingstone; 1984:193–202.
34. Mao P, Angrist A. The fine structure of the basal cell of human prostate. *Lab Invest* 1966;15:1768–1782.
35. Brawer MK, Peehl DM, Stamey TA, et al. Keratin immunoreactivity in the benign and neoplastic human prostate. *Cancer Res* 1985;45:3663–3667.
36. Hedrick L, Epstein JI. Use of keratin 903 as an adjunct in the diagnosis of prostate carcinoma. *Am J Surg Pathol* 1989;13:389–396.
37. Weinstein MH, Signoretti S, Loda M. Diagnostic utility of immunohistochemical staining for p63, a sensitive marker of prostatic basal cells. *Mod Pathol* 2002;15:1302–1308.
38. di Sant'Agnese PA. Neuroendocrine differentiation in prostatic carcinoma. *Cancer* 1995;75:1850–1859.
39. Reese JH, McNeal JE, Redwine EA, et al. Differential distribution of pepsinogen II between the zones of the human prostate and the seminal vesicle. *J Urol* 1986;136:1148–1152.
40. Reese JH, McNeal JE, Redwine EA, et al. Tissue type plasminogen activator as a marker for functional zones, within the human prostate gland. *Prostate* 1988;12:47–53.
41. Gelmann EP, Bowen C, Bubendorf L. Expression of NKX3.1 in normal and malignant tissues. *Prostate* 2003;55:111–117.
42. deVries CR, McNeal JE, Bensch K. The prostatic epithelial cell in dysplasia: An ultrastructural perspective. *Prostate* 1992;21:209–221.
43. De Marzo AM, Platz EA, Epstein JI, et al. A working group classification of focal prostate atrophy lesions. *Am J Surg Pathol* 2006;30:1281–1291.
44. Price H, McNeal JE, Stamey TA. Evolving patterns of tissue composition in benign prostatic hyperplasia as a function of specimen size. *Hum Pathol* 1990;21:578–585.
45. Cleary KR, Choi HY, Ayala AG. Basal cell hyperplasia of the prostate. *Am J Clin Pathol* 1983;80:850–854.
46. Milord RA, Kahane H, Epstein JI. Infarct of the prostate gland: Experience on needle biopsy specimens. *Am J Surg Pathol* 2000;24:1378–1384.
47. Wobker SE, Khararjian A, Epstein JI. GATA3 positivity in benign radiated prostate glands: A potential diagnostic pitfall. *Am J Surg Pathol* 2017;41:557–563.
48. Tian W, Dorn D, Wei S, et al. GATA3 expression in benign glands with radiation atypia: A diagnostic pitfall. *Histopathol* 2017;71:150–155.
49. Haarer CF, Gopalan A, Tickoo SK, et al. Prostatic transition zone directed needle biopsies uncommonly sample clinically relevant transition zone tumors. *J Urol* 2009;182:1337–1341.

Testis and Excretory Duct System

Muhammad T. Idrees ■ Thomas M. Ulbright

SUPPORTING STRUCTURES 981	RETE TESTIS 994
SEMINIFEROUS TUBULES 982	DUCTULI EFFERENTES 995
SERTOLI CELLS 983	EPIDIDYMIS 996
GERM CELLS 984	DUCTUS (VAS) DEFERENS 997
INTERSTITIUM 987	SEMINAL VESICLES 998
LEYDIG CELLS 987	EJACULATORY DUCTS 1000
VASCULAR SUPPLY 989	MESONEPHRIC AND MÜLLERIAN REMNANTS 1001
FETAL AND PREPUBERTAL TESTIS 990	GUBERNACULUM 1003
AGING TESTIS 993	REFERENCES 1003

The adult testes are paired organs that lie within the scrotum suspended by the spermatic cord (Fig. 36.1). The average weight of each is 15 to 19 g, the right usually being, on average, 10% heavier than the left (1). The left testis hangs slightly lower than the right in standing posture (2,3). The scrotal coverings are skin, dartos muscle, Colles' fascia, an external spermatic fascia, and the parietal layer of the tunica vaginalis (Fig. 36.2). The dartos muscle, of the non-striated type, is closely attached to the overlying skin and glides freely over the underlying loose fascia layer.

SUPPORTING STRUCTURES

The supporting structures of the testis consist of a tough capsule (the tunica) and a number of fibrous septa that extend from the inner surface of the tunica into the parenchyma and divide the testis into approximately 250 lobules. The posterior part of the testis is not covered by the capsule and is called the mediastinum (hilum), which contains blood and lymphatic vessels, nerves, and the extratesticular portion of the rete testis. The capsule has three distinctive layers: The outer serosa (or visceral tunica vaginalis), the thick, collagenous tunica albuginea, and the inner tunica vasculosa. The tunica vaginalis consists of a flattened layer of mesothelial cells overlying a well-developed basement membrane. It forms a sac with two components: a visceral layer, covering the testis and head of the epididymis, and a parietal layer, formed as the lining reflects posteriorly and superiorly at the mediastinum and the epididymis and then covers the internal spermatic fascia. The space between the two layers normally contains a small amount of serous fluid. Infrequently, transitional or squamous metaplasia of the surface mesothelium may be present, the former occurring as Walthard nests identical to those found more commonly on the serosa of the fallopian tubes. The tunica albuginea is composed of a layer of collagen fibers within which are embedded fibroblasts, myocytes, mast cells, and nerves. The myocytes, found mainly in the posterior region of the testis, undergo regular contractions that cause a transient increase in intratesticular pressure. The tunica vasculosa, a loose connective tissue containing blood vessels and lymphatics, sends septa into the testicular parenchyma to form the individual lobules. The tunica vasculosa is a common location to identify lymphovascular space invasion by

---

This chapter is an update of a previous version authored by Thomas D. Trainer.

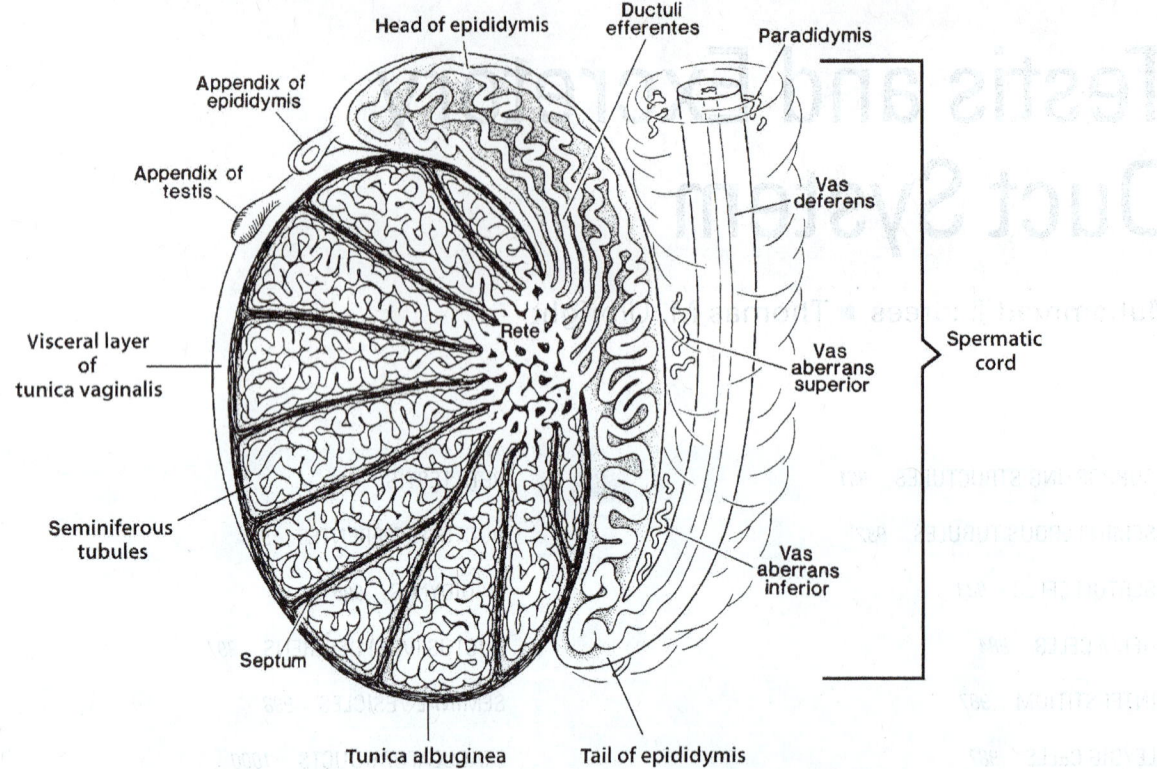

FIGURE 36.1 Diagrammatic views of testis, epididymis, and portion of ductus (vas) deferens.

germ cell tumors. The tunica overall varies greatly in thickness with age, averaging 300 µg at birth, 400 to 450 µg in young adults and 900 to 950 µg in men older than 65 years of age (4).

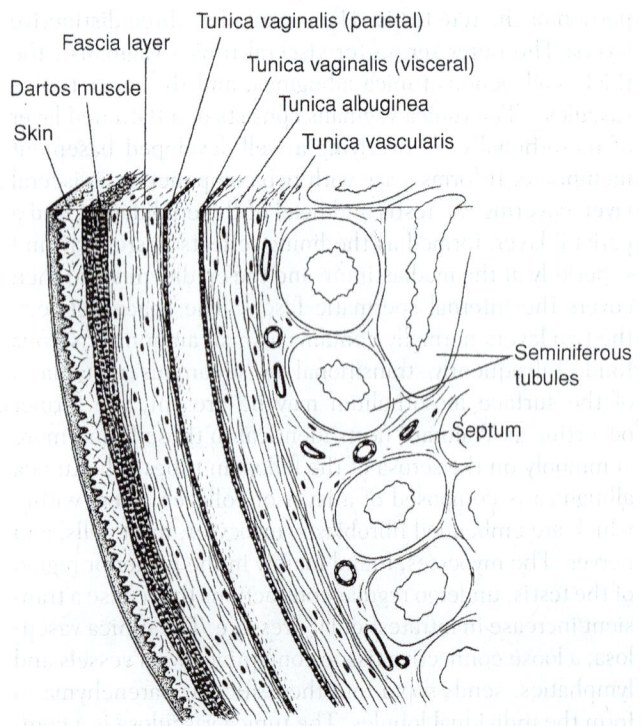

FIGURE 36.2 Scrotal covering layers and capsule of testis.

SEMINIFEROUS TUBULES

Each lobule of the testis contains one to four seminiferous tubules (Fig. 36.1). The individual tubule is a highly convoluted, closed loop structure, with numerous communications between the arms of the loop but without any blind endings or branches. The absence of branching in the tubules can help distinguish intratubular tumor from intravascular tumor, since vessels may frequently show a branched pattern. Each arm of the looped tubule empties into the septal portion of the rete testis. The collective length of the tubules in each testis has been estimated to be between 299 and 981 m, with an average of 540 m (5). The average tubule diameter in young adults is 180 µm (± 30). The usual open testicular biopsy may encompass tubules from up to five lobules along with portions of the intervening septa. It is important not to interpret the latter as foci of fibrosis. The seminiferous tubules are composed of germ cells in varying stages of differentiation and Sertoli cells. Each tubule has a distinctive basement membrane and a thin lamina propria (Fig. 36.3). At puberty, the tubule is divided into a basal compartment and an adluminal compartment via the development of a tight junction complex between adjacent Sertoli cells. The basal compartment or spermatogonial niche houses the spermatogonia and preleptotene spermatocytes and the adluminal section contains all the more developed forms. Germ cell neoplasia in situ (previously termed intratubular germ cell neoplasia unclassified) occupies the spermatogonial niche.

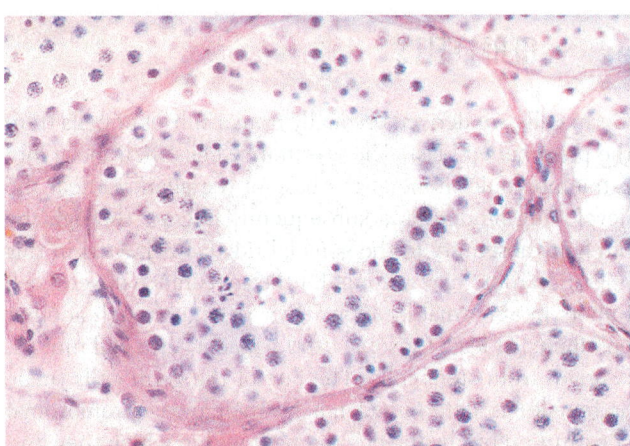

FIGURE 36.3 A cross-sectional view of seminiferous tubule and interstitium. Germ cell maturation is variable around the tubule, a normal finding.

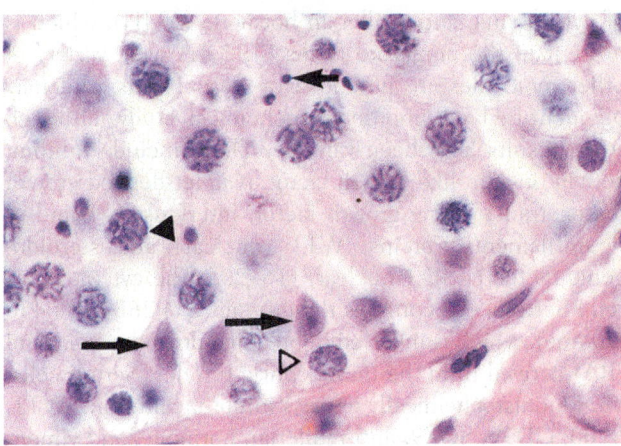

FIGURE 36.4 Seminiferous tubule with Sertoli cells (*long arrows*), spermatogonia (Δ), primary spermatocytes (▲), and spermatids (*short arrow*).

SERTOLI CELLS

Sertoli cells play important and very different roles in the fetal and adult testes, and these divergent roles are reflected in their proliferative activity, cell protein markers, and the nature of cellular intermediate filaments at these periods of the cell's life span. Adult Sertoli cells are nondividing cells. The role of Sertoli cells in spermatogenesis is indispensable. Recently it has been demonstrated that specific ablation of a single protein (Dicer, an RNAse III endonuclease) from the Sertoli cells leads to a loss of all germ cell types in the adult mouse testis (6). The number of Sertoli cells is important since they have the capacity to nurture only a finite number of germ cells. Genetic, hormonal, and environmental factors appear to play significant roles in determining the final number of Sertoli cells in the adult testis (7). These tall, irregular, columnar cells, with their bases attached to the underlying basal lamina, have an abundant but relatively inconspicuous cytoplasm and an ill-defined cytoplasmic membrane. The cells send intricate cytoplasmic extensions around the germ cell elements and continuously alter their contours to accommodate the changing size and shape of the germ cells that they cradle. Adult Sertoli cell nuclei have round to slightly irregular shapes, with a folded nuclear membrane, a homogeneous chromatin distribution, and a prominent, round nucleolus (Figs. 36.4 and 36.5). These features are in sharp contrast to those of the fetal and prepubertal Sertoli cells, which have an oval or elongated nucleus, a smoothly contoured nuclear membrane, and an inconspicuous nucleolus. The Sertoli cell nuclei represent about 10% of the nuclei in a normal adult tubule cross section. They are located toward the basal side of the tubule and lie just adluminal to the spermatogonia and preleptotene spermatocytes. The cytoplasm may contain lipid vacuoles and/or eosinophilic granular debris. Much of this material represents phagocytosed remnants of the residual bodies of the spermatids or degenerated earlier germ cell forms. Vimentin is the predominant intermediate filament in the adult Sertoli cell, whereas embryonic Sertoli cells also contain cytokeratins 8 and 18 (8,9). The transient appearance of cytokeratins is of interest in view of the report of malignant Sertoli cell tumors containing both cytokeratins and vimentin (10,11). Low–molecular-weight cytokeratins may also be identified in some of the Sertoli cells of atrophic tubules in the adult testis (12), in Sertoli cells of tubules containing germ cell neoplasia in situ (13), and in Sertoli cells of the contralateral testis of patients with germ cell neoplasms. These Sertoli cells have an immature morphologic appearance and, in the latter two instances, appear to be part of the "testicular dysgenesis syndrome" (TDS) (14). Adult Sertoli cells, unlike fetal or prepubertal Sertoli cells, express androgen receptors (AR) in their nuclei, but, at the same time, have lost their expression

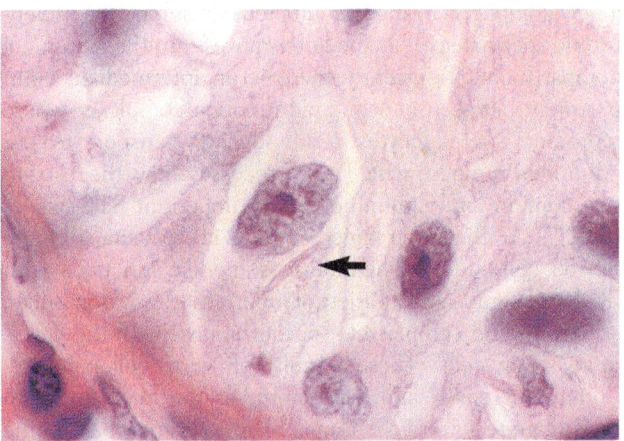

FIGURE 36.5 Sertoli cell with intracytoplasmic Charcot–Böttcher filaments (*arrow*) from a patient with germ cell aplasia. Note the prominent nucleolus and slightly wrinkled nuclear membrane.

of cytoplasmic anti-müllerian hormone (AMH), which is present in the immature forms (7,15). A wide variety of other molecules are produced by Sertoli cells, and may be identified on immunohistochemical study, although some results have been variable. These include inhibin/activin, insulin-like growth factor, platelet-derived growth factor, transforming growth factor, interleukins 1 and 6, neurofilament proteins, WT1 (nuclear) and steroidogenic factor-1 (SF-1 nuclear) (16–20). The cytoplasm of fetal Sertoli cells contains the enzyme CYP26B1 (a P450 enzyme), which is involved in breaking down retinoic acid (RA) derived from the mesonephric tubules. Sertoli cells, immunohistochemically express inhibin, calretinin, WT1, S100, CD99, SOX9, anti-müllerian hormone, and vimentin. Some studies showed variable expression of different markers (21–23). RA is a key substance in the process of directing fetal germ cells into meiosis. CYP26B1 thus acts as meiosis-inhibiting substance. Reduced levels of RA in the male may also play a role in directing the fetal male germ cell to mitotic arrest (24). The distinctive crystalloids of Charcot–Böttcher are a cytoplasmic feature of adult Sertoli cells (25). These bundles of filamentous structures, located primarily in the basal portion of the cell, are best seen on ultrastructural examination, but are occasionally large enough to be recognized by light microscopic studies (Fig. 36.5). Ultrastructurally, they appear to merge with vimentin-labeled intermediate filaments, both of which are increased in the cryptorchid testis and the Sertoli cell–only syndrome (13).

At puberty, the Sertoli cells develop a complex of intercellular junctions that divide the seminiferous tubule into two distinctive compartments: the basal compartment, containing the various stages of spermatogonia and preleptotene spermatocytes; and the adluminal compartment, which houses the primary and secondary spermatocytes and spermatids. This junction structure comprises the true blood–testis barrier (BTB). As preleptotene spermatocytes move from the basal compartment to the adluminal compartment this junction complex undergoes disassembly and a new complex is formed simultaneously behind the preleptotene spermatocyte as the latter moves into the adluminal compartment. Transiently there is an intermediate compartment between new and old junction complexes where leptotene spermatocytes reside during transport to the adluminal compartment. These processes allow the testis to maintain an intact immunologically important BTB barrier (26,27). At the same time as the BTB is being formed, Sertoli cells develop hemidesmosome-like junctions with the basal lamina and a variety of junctions (desmosome-like, adherens, and ectoplasmic specializations) with the developing germ cells. These Sertoli cell–germ cell junctions undergo assembly and disassembly as the maturing germ cells migrate toward the lumen of the seminiferous tubule (28). Still unclear is the mechanism that serves to promote the movement of germ cells from the basal compartment to the adluminal compartment.

GERM CELLS

Germ cells are derived originally from a subset of cells from the proximal epiblast. These primitive cells then move into extraembryonic tissue at the base of the allantois near the developing hindgut and subsequently migrate through the hindgut mesentery to the gonadal ridge. Deviations in this migration route may account for the appearance of germ cell tumors in abnormal locations (Fig. 36.6), although another possibility, at least for some extra-gonadal germ cell tumors, is origin from stem cells. The fate of the germ cells (male or female) is determined not by their own chromosomal constitution but by the environment within which they find themselves. If the developing gonad is destined to be a testis, the germ cell will become a spermatogonium and, if the gonad is destined to become an ovary, the germ will become an oocyte (29). The germ cell elements comprise the majority of the cells in the adult seminiferous tubule (Figs. 36.3 and 36.4). Spermatogenesis, including proliferation of committed spermatogonia, covers a period of ~74 days, with no evidence that this time requirement is altered by age or pathologic states (30). Marked morphologic transitions occur in these cells during this time period, as shown in Figure 36.7.

The undifferentiated spermatogonia lie in the basal compartment of the adult testis. Their nuclei are oval to round and, depending on the plane of section, may have one or two easily identifiable nucleoli (Fig. 36.8). Within the cytoplasm in a perinuclear location are the crystalloids of Lubarsch. These structures, best seen on electron microscopic examination, measure up to 3 µg in length. They are a mixture of parallel arrays of fibrils, 80 to100 Å in thickness, and ribosome-like granules (31). These structures are also sometimes found in primary spermatocytes and resemble Charcot–Böttcher crystalloids of Sertoli cells (32). On the basis of their nuclear chromatin staining pattern, utilizing special fixatives such as Zenker formal, spermatogonia have been divided into type A_{dark} and type A_{pale} cells. It should be pointed out that these nuclear pattern staining differences are not so evident with commonly employed fixatives such as Bouin solution, which produces coarse clumping in the nuclei of all of the spermatogonial subtypes, precluding a

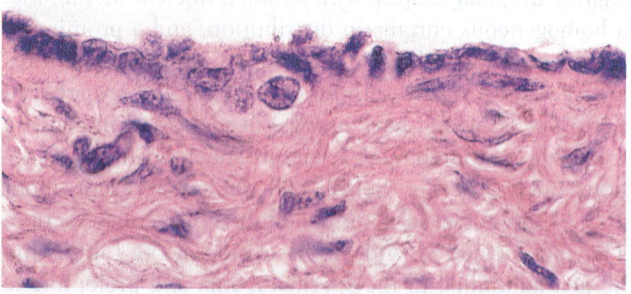

FIGURE 36.6 Germ cells located immediately beneath the mesothelial lining cells of the process vaginalis of a 16-week fetus.

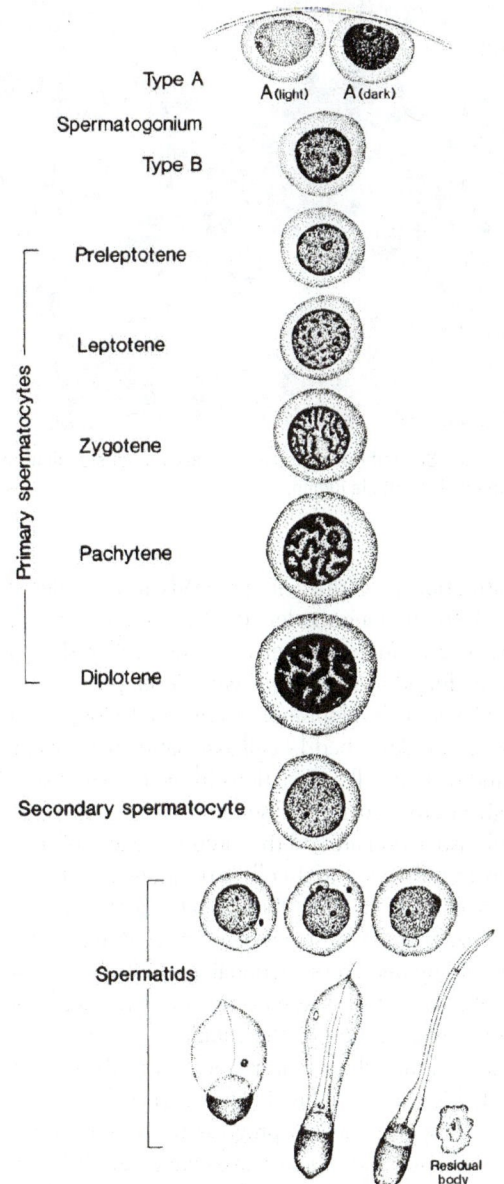

FIGURE 36.7 Steps in spermatogenesis.

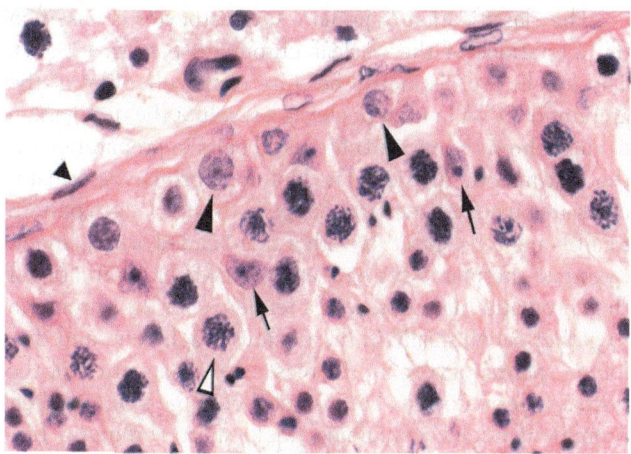

FIGURE 36.8 Portion of seminiferous tubule showing spermatogonia (*solid arrowhead*), primary spermatocytes (*open arrowhead*), Sertoli cells (*arrow*), and fibromyocyte of tunica propria (*solid triangle*). The smaller cells in the *lower right* are mainly secondary spermatocytes and early spermatids.

clear separation (33). The progenitor A_{dark} cells are considered to be the true SSCs or reserve cells, with only limited mitotic division. Undifferentiated spermatogonia in rodents have been divided into A_{single}, A_{paired}, and $A_{aligned}$ forms. Whether or not this method of identifying different stem, progenitor, and differentiating spermatogonia forms will be adapted to primates is unclear at this time.

A number of molecular markers, including OCT3/4, GFRA1, PLZF, CDH1 (E-cadherin), ID4, RET, and NEUROG3, have been found to be positive in the more undifferentiated A spermatogonia. CD117 (KIT) first appears in the later A spermatogonia forms (34–40). Several other markers including SOX3, STRA8, SOHLH1, and SOHLH2 have been shown to be expressed at different stages of differentiation (41). However, most of these studies have been performed in mice and less is known in humans. These progenitor cells are located in the so-called spermatogonial stem cell (SSC) niche. This niche is poorly defined in the testis because of the unavailability of a clear-cut marker of SSCs, but it is found in close relationship to the basement membrane of the tubule, as well as the Leydig cells and vasculature of the interstitium (42). Some of the SSCs become committed to the process of spermatogenesis. These cells undergo further division, while maintaining a narrow intercellular bridge connection among all of the offspring. This bridge allows for simultaneous maturation of these interconnected cells. Of interest is the lack of these intercellular connections in seminomas and germ cell neoplasia in situ, but their occasional presence in spermatocytic tumors (43).

The pattern of division of A_{pale} spermatogonia is still uncertain. Some of them proliferate to produce more type A_{pale} cells while others produce type B spermatogonia, which soon thereafter convert to the preleptotene form of primary spermatocytes. In humans, it appears that eight preleptotene spermatocytes are produced per each original pair of A_{pale} spermatogonia (30). The preleptotene spermatocytes then move into the adluminal compartment and start the process of the first meiotic division. How these interconnected cells move from one compartment to the other is still unclear.

In an effort to understand the process of spermatogenesis, in earlier studies the seminiferous epithelium cycle was randomly divided into six stages based on morphologic evaluation; however, it is practically impossible to assign stages by light microscopy because of difficulty in morphologic identification due to poor preservation and random distribution of germ cells in the seminiferous epithelium cycle. Moreover, more than one stage can be identified in any given section of the tubules. Recently, with high-resolution light microscopy, new germ cell characterizations within the proposed six stages have been suggested (44).

The classification of primary spermatocytes is based on the alterations of the nuclear chromatin pattern (33,44). These cells are distinctive because of the doubling of the amount of DNA in their nuclei as a result of the duplication of each chromosome into chromatid pairs in preparation for the first meiotic division. The leptotene primary spermatocytes are characterized by a change in the chromatin pattern to a filamentous structure with a fine-beaded arrangement. Zygotene spermatocytes have an even coarser granularity of the chromatin filaments, with a tendency for the chromatin to gather eccentrically in the nucleus. Pachytene and diplotene spermatocytes are the most easily recognized of the primary spermatocytes because of their large size and their prominent nuclei, containing thick, short chromatin filaments (Fig. 36.8). The primary spermatocyte phase occupies a period of 24 days (45). After this relatively long period of gametogenesis, the first meiotic division occurs, with the formation of secondary spermatocytes.

Secondary spermatocytes, have an extremely short half-life and make up only a small minority of the cells seen in a cross section of the tubule. Their nuclei, substantially smaller than those of the primary spermatocytes, have a finely granular chromatin pattern and a haploid number of chromosomes, but a diploid amount of chromatin because of the presence of the chromatid pairs. They are located near the tubule lumen, differing only slightly in appearance from the very early spermatids, with which they are closely associated (Figs. 36.4 and 36.8). They undergo the second meiotic division to produce spermatids. The spermatids have been broken down into several types based on their morphologic appearance and with particular emphasis on the nuclear and body shape and the development of the acrosome. The 6-type classification of Heller and Clermont, with designations of Sa, Sb1, Sb2, Sc, Sd1, and Sd2, is most commonly employed (46). The earlier forms have a round nucleus, similar to the secondary spermatocytes, but with a haploid number of chromosomes and half the amount of DNA that a normal cell has (Figs. 36.7 and 36.8). The late spermatid forms are characterized by a change in the nuclear shape to an oval contour and then to an elongated appearance and a marked condensation of the chromatin. At the same time, excess cytoplasm is discarded by the spermatid and is phagocytosed by the Sertoli cell. Soon thereafter, the Sertoli cell–germ cell connections are removed and the intercellular bridges that connected earlier germ cell forms are dissolved, allowing the disconnected spermatozoa to enter the tubule lumen. Abnormal sloughing of immature germ cells, often with persistent intercellular connections, may be seen in patients with varicocele or other pathologic states, suggesting a failure of Sertoli cells to regulate this maturation process. This failure of maturation may be reflected in the presence of multiheaded spermatozoa in the seminal fluid. One must take care to separate this pathological sloughing process from the artificial sloughing that frequently occurs in open biopsy specimens (Fig. 36.9).

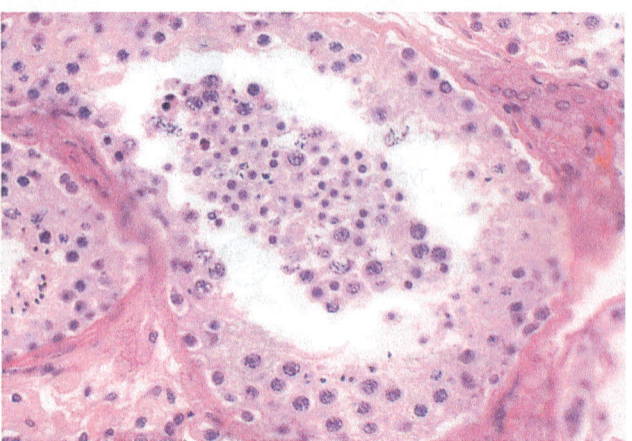

FIGURE 36.9 Seminiferous tubule, with artifactual sloughing of germ cell elements into tubule lumen.

Maturation of germ cells proceeds in an ordered, nonrandom fashion along the length of the seminiferous tubule. Groups of evolving germ cells of one level of development tend to be found in association with developing germ cells of another level of development at any point along the tubule. Clermont (33) described 14 cell association patterns in the rat testis and 6 such cell associations in the human testis. In the rat, a given cross section of seminiferous tubule shows only one cell association around the circumferences of the tubule, whereas in humans 2 to 4 cell associations may be seen in a tubule cross section (30). Of practical importance is the need to recognize that not all stages of germ cell differentiation may be seen in any one cross-sectional view of a human seminiferous tubule. Mature spermatozoa and late spermatids may be seen in one portion of the tubule cross section, and the opposite wall may show maturation only to the early spermatid level (Fig. 36.3). It has been recognized for many years that not all spermatogonia progress to become spermatozoa and that apoptotic or degenerative changes in these precursor cells can be seen regularly in the seminiferous tubules (47). This normal physiologic process should not be mistaken for maturation arrest. The broad category of germ cell elements should be recognized with relative ease and one should be able to distinguish spermatogonia, primary spermatocytes, secondary spermatocytes, and spermatids, using standard fixation/staining methods such as formalin/Bouin.

Elaborate methods have been developed for quantitative assessment of germ cell maturation and the relationship of spermatogenesis to seminal fluid sperm density (48–51). One study proposed a semiquantitative method of analysis that includes uniformity (or lack thereof) of histologic features, tubule diameter, presence or absence of a lumen, evaluation of maturity of Sertoli cells, presence or absence of germ cell elements, degree of hypospermatogenesis, and the presence of germ cell maturation arrest and stage of arrest. This study emphasized that the presence of any late spermatids, even in a small number of tubules, excludes a diagnosis of "germ cell arrest" (52).

Two relatively simple alternative methods are helpful to the surgical pathologist. The first method (53) involves establishing a germ cell to Sertoli cell ratio by counting at least 30 tubule cross sections. This ratio is approximately 13:1 in young healthy men. An average of 10 to 12 Sertoli cells per tubule cross section is considered normal and approximately half of the germ cell elements within the tubule should be in the spermatid phase. An assumption is made that the Sertoli cell population is stable throughout adult life. A reasonably good assessment of the presence or absence of hypospermatogenesis or maturation arrest can be made with this technique. A second method involves counting spermatids per tubule cross section (54). Only the more mature spermatids (those with oval or elongated nuclei and densely stained chromatin) are counted. Excellent correlations have been made with seminal fluid sperm counts. A spermatid/tubule cross-section count of 45 should correspond to a seminal fluid sperm count of 85×10^6/mL. Average spermatid/tubule cross-section counts of 40, 20, or 6 to 10 correspond to sperm counts of 45, 10, or 3×10^6/mL, respectively. A minimum of 20 tubules must be counted.

INTERSTITIUM

The interstitium of the testis accounts for 25% to 30% of the testicular mass. It can be loosely divided into interstitial and peritubular regions. Complex cellular and molecular interaction of the interstitium provides a suitable milieu to guarantee a step-wise differentiation of SSCs through the process of spermatogenesis and spermiogenesis. Cells within the tubules and outside of the tubules, including interstitial and peritubular cells, therefore, help regulate the differentiation of SSCs and are crucial for maintaining and promoting male fertility (55). Surrounding each seminiferous tubule in a sheath-like fashion is the lamina (tunica) propria, which consists of an inner basement membrane, surrounded by a thin zone of multilayered spindle cells, the peritubular myoid cells, intermingled with type 1 collagen fibrils and elastic fibers (Fig. 36.8). The outermost cells in this layer stain for vimentin, calponin, CD34, and actin, whereas the cells of the inner layer stain also for desmin, a staining pattern characteristic of fibromyocytes (56). In addition to providing structural support, their contractile function plays an important role in compressing the seminiferous tubules and moving spermatozoa into the rete testis. These cells also contain AR in their nuclei (15) which are present not only in the adult but also the fetal testis. Along with other secreted molecules, these receptors play an important role in modulating Sertoli cell functions in both the fetus and adult (57,58). There is accumulating evidence that peritubular myoid cells contribute to self-renewal of SSCs through androgen and glial cell line–derived neurotrophic factor (GDNF) signaling pathways (59,60).

The basal lamina or basement membrane is composed of type 4 collagen fibrils intermixed with laminin, fibronectin, entactin, and heparan sulfate proteoglycans. This zone plays an important role in the function of Sertoli cells, the bases of which are in juxtaposition with the basement membrane. This zone also influences Leydig cell proliferation and testosterone production (61). Within the interstitial region are Leydig cells, blood vessels, lymphatics, nerves, mast cells, and macrophages. The latter are often found in close association with the Leydig cells (62), where the two cells form complex cell–cell interactions. Cytokines (such as tumor necrosis factor alpha) and reactive oxygen species from macrophages are known to influence steroidogenesis of the Leydig cells (63) and also likely play a role in the function of the peritubular myoid cells. A direct interaction with SSCs via CSF1 and RA pathways has been proposed (64). Mast cells also are thought to have an influence on these structures (57). Elastic fibers first appear at puberty in the outermost layer of the lamina propria (65). There is a striking absence of elastic fibers in the lamina propria of the sclerotic tubules in patients with Klinefelter syndrome, in contrast to their abundance in patients with postpubertal sclerosis of multiple other causes (66).

A common finding in patients with oligospermia or azoospermia due to primary testicular failure is the accumulation of eosinophilic, acellular material in the lamina propria. This material is an admixture of increased collagen fibers, elastic fibrils, and basement membrane–like material (51). The peritubular tissue of patients with hypogonadotropic hypogonadism is underdeveloped, having only one or two layers of myoid cells mixed with a few collagen fibers. In contrast, there is a large accumulation of collagen in the lamina propria of some of the tubules of adult patients with cryptorchidism.

LEYDIG CELLS

Adult Leydig cells, the source of testicular androgens and insulin-like factor 3 (INSL3), only rarely undergo mitotic division (67,68). They are found singly and in clusters within the interstitium of the testis, some lying immediately adjacent to capillaries and others being located next to the peritubular fibromyocytes (Fig. 36.10). They may be seen in the lumen of sclerotic seminiferous tubules and in the tunica albuginea, the epididymis, the spermatic cord, and the mediastinum of the testis (69). They are often located in intimate association with nerve fibers, sometimes as a large cluster adjacent to the nerve (Fig. 36.11), but more frequently they are scattered randomly throughout the nerve fiber (66,70). They may be found at these sites in the fetus, as well as the adult. The single nucleus of the cell is round and vesicular, with one or two eccentrically located nucleoli. An occasional binucleated cell may be seen. The nuclei may exhibit a ground-glass appearance (Fig. 36.12). The cytoplasm is usually abundant and stains intensely with eosin. Lipid droplets and lipofuscin

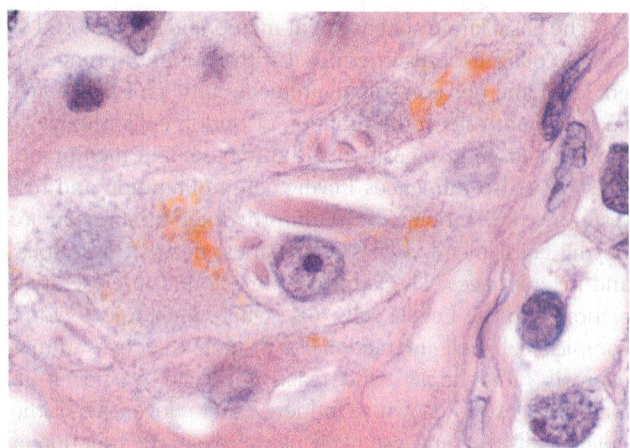

FIGURE 36.10 Leydig cells in interstitium of testis. An eosinophilic crystal of Reinke and abundant lipofuscin are prominent features in the cytoplasm of the Leydig cell in the *center* of this field. Peritubular fibromyocytes are at right.

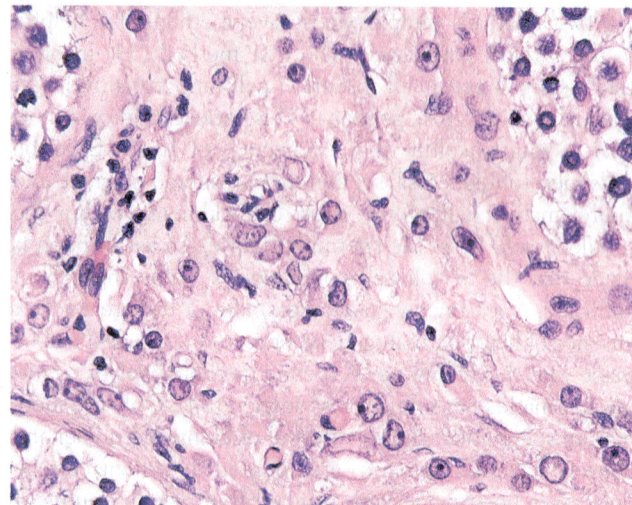

FIGURE 36.12 Leydig cells with ground-glass nuclei.

pigment are found in the cytoplasm, first appearing at the time of puberty and increasing in prominence in the aging testis. Sometimes the lipid accumulation is so intense that confusion of these cells with ectopic adrenal cortical cells may occur. Occasionally similar appearing cells occur in clusters designated as "nodular steroid cell nests" in close association with the rete testis (71). These cells make non-encapsulated aggregates with a sinusoidal and trabecular appearance. Although they are steroidogenic in type and resemble Leydig cells (but lacking Reinke crystals), they have properties similar to those of adrenal cortical cells. Nonetheless, they do not have the compact arrangement and zonation of the commonly found adrenal cortical nests, which are mostly in the spermatic cord and not the hilum (Fig. 36.13).

The characteristic Reinke crystals of the Leydig cells are present only in the postpubertal state (Fig. 36.10). Their presence is highly variable in the normal testis and they are frequently absent or difficult to find in Leydig cell tumors (present in approximately 30% of cases) (Fig. 36.14). Often these crystals are associated with globular eosinophilic intracellular material thought to be precursor of Reinke crystals (Fig. 36.15). The nature of the material is unknown but is presumed to represent a protein product of the cell (72). The crystals stain positively with PAS and trichrome stains (red), and negatively for actin, vimentin, and desmin (Fig. 36.16).

Leydig cells produce testosterone after stimulation by lutenizing hormone (LH) through interaction with luteinizing hormone receptors on the cell surface. This is accomplished by upregulating the expression of the steroidogenic enzyme 17-beta-hydroxysteroid dehydrogenase. Testosterone interacts with AR inducing local effects or exerts its effect by binding to androgen binding protein (ABP), elevating testosterone levels in seminiferous tubules and epididymis (73). AR is present in Sertoli cells, pertubular myoid cells, Leydig cells and spermatids. In the adult testis testosterone also exerts its influence by an indirect Sertoli

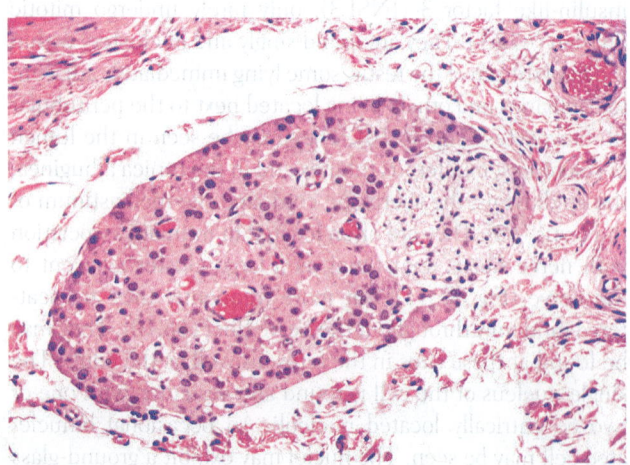

FIGURE 36.11 Leydig cells in intimate association with a nerve in the hilus of the testis.

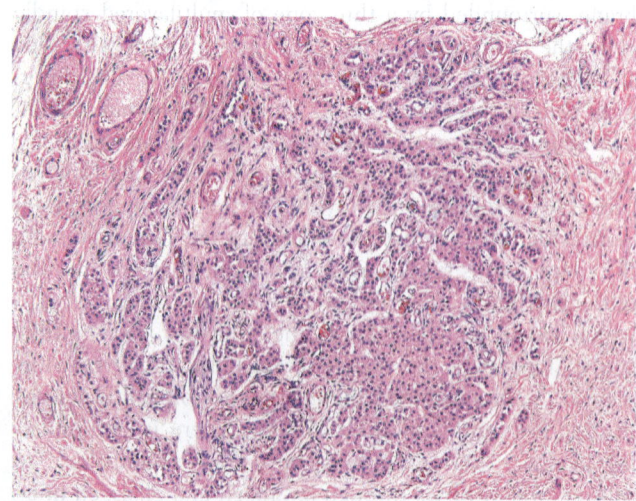

FIGURE 36.13 A nodular steroid cell nest in hilar soft tissue. These cells are different from Leydig cells and adrenal cortical cells.

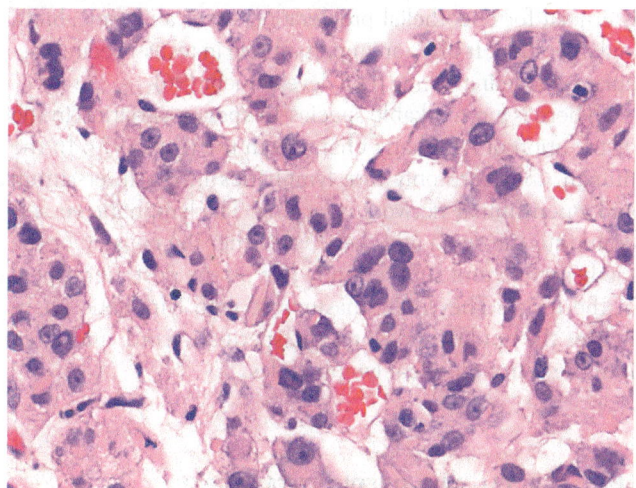

FIGURE 36.14 Leydig cell tumor with abundant Reinke crystals.

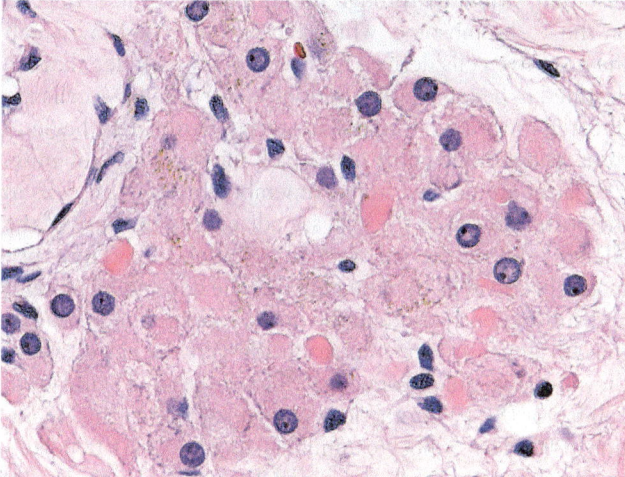

FIGURE 36.15 Leydig cells in Leydig cell tumor with Reinke crystals and globular eosinophilic intracellular material. Abundant lipofuscin is present.

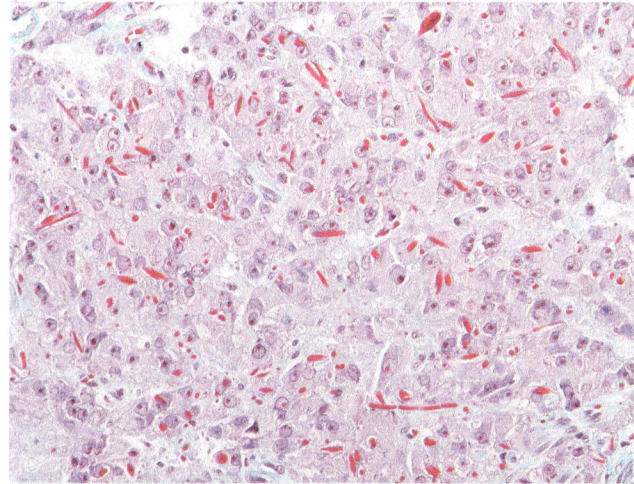

FIGURE 36.16 Trichrome stain displays intense red staining of Reinke crystals in a Leydig cell tumor.

cell regulated attachment process and through peritubular myoid cells secreted factors (74,75).

Quantitation of Leydig cells has been a difficult parameter to assess. Heller et al. (76), using a Leydig cell to Sertoli cell ratio, found a normal value of 0.39 and a range from 0.19 to 0.72. In that same study, they also determined the average number of Sertoli cells per adult tubule cross section to be 10.13 ± 0.6. They made an assumption that the Sertoli cell population in the adult testis is stable, which was later verified by others (77). As a rule, normal adult testis tissue should have four or five Leydig cells for each tubule cross section. The mean number of Leydig cells per one cross section of seminiferous tubule was defined as the "Leydig cell index." In both oligospermic and azoospermic groups, the Leydig cell index was significantly elevated as compared to normal individuals, which suggested Leydig cell hyperplasia in the infertile testis.(78) Leydig cell micronodules/hyperplasia are common in men with impaired spermatogenesis and TDS, and are associated with a decreased testosterone/LH ratio (79,80).

Vimentin is the predominant intermediate filament in Leydig cells, but actin filaments and neurofilament triplet proteins have been identified in both Leydig cells and Sertoli cells (17). Antibodies to inhibin α and calretinin stain Leydig cells intensely. Calretinin is also present in mesothelial cells and cells of the rete testis but not in Sertoli cells (81). INSL3 is a very specific marker for functioning fetal and adult types of Leydig cells (82). Leydig cells also stain positively for S100 protein, glial fibrillary acidic protein, synaptophysin, chromogranin A and B, CD99, melan A, colony stimulating factor 1 (CSF1) and neuron-specific enolase. The immunoprofile supports an important neuroendocrine function for these cells (83–85). The astrocyte-like markers in Leydig cells suggest a role similar to that of central nervous system astrocytes in inducing and maintaining a barrier feature of testicular capillaries (86). A subpopulation of cells stain intensely for nestin, an intermediate filament seen mainly in nerve and muscle progenitor cells (87). The presence of all of these substances undoubtedly indicates important paracrine functions that Leydig cells share with Sertoli cells, endothelial cells, peritubular cells, macrophages, and nerves.

VASCULAR SUPPLY

The blood supply of the testis is derived primarily from the internal spermatic (testicular) artery. A small contribution comes from the deferential artery, a branch of the inferior vesicle artery, and from the cremasteric artery, a branch of the inferior epigastric artery (88). Anastomoses between the testicular artery and these other two vessels occur regularly, prior to the entrance of the testicular artery into the testis proper (89). A few anastomoses may be seen between the parenchymal branches of the testicular artery and the deferential artery. Each testicular artery, arising from the aorta immediately distal to the renal artery, is highly coiled and extremely long relative to its diameter. The vessel has a low pulse pressure as it enters the testis (90). The artery plays an important role in thermal regulation of the testis via countercurrent heat exchange with the veins of the pampiniform plexus. The combination of this vascular heat exchange and the heat lost via the thin scrotal layer serves to maintain the testicular temperature 2° to 3°C below body temperature. The testicular artery enters the testis posteriorly, where it localizes to the tunica vasculosa. It then courses to the inferior pole, and subsequently turns back superiorly along the anterior surface, sending branches in a centripetal fashion into the septa and then to the mediastinum, where they form a dense cluster. Only a few branches of these centripetal arteries enter the lobules. From the mediastinum the small arterial segments, called "recurrent arteries," then pass in a centrifugal fashion within the parenchyma, where they branch into arterioles and then capillaries. Each recurrent artery supplies blood to only a single lobule, as defined by the septa (91). The veins run either centripetally or centrifugally to the mediastinum or capsule respectively and eventually anastomose to form the pampiniform plexus of the testicular vein. Biopsy specimens of the testis from patients with varicoceles often show a striking sclerosis of vascular walls of both arteries and veins (92). The significance of these vascular alterations with respect to seminiferous tubule function in these patients is uncertain.

At puberty, there is extensive development of the intratesticular microvasculature, the most notable feature being a marked coiling of the arteries and a great expansion of the peritubular capillary network. Unlike other capillaries of the body, the testicular capillary walls have a prominent basement membrane and an incomplete outer layer of pericytes (93).

The capillary network appears to have a very structured arrangement with respect to the Leydig cells and the seminiferous tubules. The capillaries arising from arterioles first intermingle with Leydig cells (arterial side inter-Leydig cell capillary). They then extend to the lamina propria of the seminiferous tubules (intramural capillary) and subsequently return to the interstitium, where they are again surrounded by Leydig cells (venous side inter-Leydig cell capillary). At one point in their journey through the tunica propria, the capillary basement membrane comes in close contact with the basement membrane of the seminiferous tubule. This site is the only location where the capillaries have defined fenestrations (94), thereby allowing for a significant exchange of a variety of substances between the microvasculature lumen and the seminiferous tubule. The capillaries in the testis have some similarities to those in the brain, supporting some type of biologic barriers. Both of these capillary beds have a high density of the GLUT-1 isoform of the glucose transporter and immunoreactivity for P-glycoprotein. Unlike the nervous tissue vascular bed, localized fenestrations can be found in the vessels of the testis (86). Vascular and perivascular cells play an important role in stem cell development, as well as localization in the testis (95). VEGFA secreted by Leydig and Sertoli cells is crucial for endothelial proliferation, survival, permeability, and migration. It plays an important role in testis-specific vascular remodeling during fetal development (96).

There is a remarkable species-to-species variation in the distribution of lymphatic channels in the testis (97). In the human, there are only rare lymphatics in the interstitium and a peritubular network is lacking. The lymphatic vessels drain into the septa and thence to either the capsule or the mediastinum and subsequently join on the posterior aspect of the testis. They then anastomose with lymphatic channels of the epididymis, enter the spermatic cord, and drain into the retroperitoneal lymph nodes.

FETAL AND PREPUBERTAL TESTIS

The fetal testis first becomes recognizable at 7 to 8 weeks of gestation, primarily through the influence of the *SRY* gene on the Y chromosome, which initiates a process by which the primitive cells derived from the celomic surface that are destined to become either Sertoli cells or granulosa cells are directed toward the former. Clusters of Sertoli cells begin to form recognizable cords into which the germ cells migrate. The latter are derived from extraembryonic epiblast cells in the posterior wall of the yolk sac adjacent to the base of the allantois during the 3rd week of gestation (98). These primordial germ cells then migrate into the developing hindgut and subsequently through the dorsal root mesentery during the 4th and 5th weeks to reach the gonadal ridge, where they are now called gonocytes. Signaling via KIT and stem cell factor (SCF) interactions plays a key role in this migration (99). The gonocyte numbers increase to 1,000 cells by the time they reach the gonadal ridge and up to 30,000 cells by the 9th week of gestation (100). The vast majority of these cells develop in a unipotent direction toward the production of spermatozoa, although small numbers may remain pluripotent and potentially become precursors of embryonal germ cells in culture (101).

Early in gestation, the gonocytes are mitotically active and have a round nucleus, a prominent nucleolus, and relatively little cytoplasm. They are located in basilar and suprabasilar portions of the lumenless seminiferous tubules, surrounded by the immature Sertoli cells (Figs. 36.17 and 36.18). During the latter half of fetal life and the first 6 months after birth, they undergo a maturation process in which they enter mitotic arrest, although a few Ki-67 positive cells may still be present in early postnatal life. They become larger, acquire more cytoplasm and a coarser nuclear chromatin pattern, and are now referred to as primary spermatogonia (Fig. 36.19). It should be noted that at any time after about 20 weeks of gestation, there may be a mixture of gonocytes in different stages of maturation along with primary spermatogonia. These maturing gonocytes are called "prospermatogonia" (102), "fetal spermatogonia" (103), "intermediate cells," or "prespermatogonia" (104). By the 6th postnatal month, virtually all

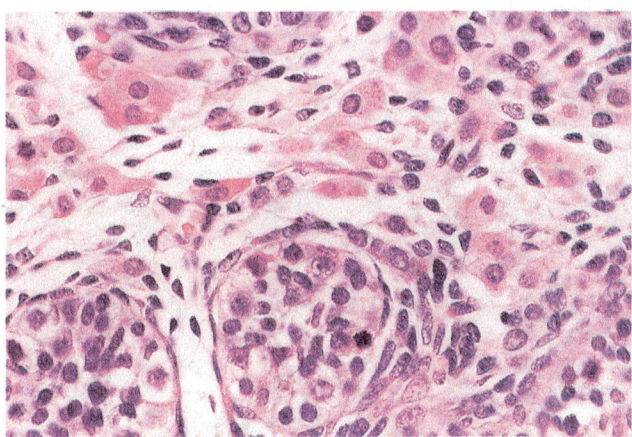

FIGURE 36.17 Fetal testis of 20 weeks' gestation, with numerous Leydig cells throughout the interstitium.

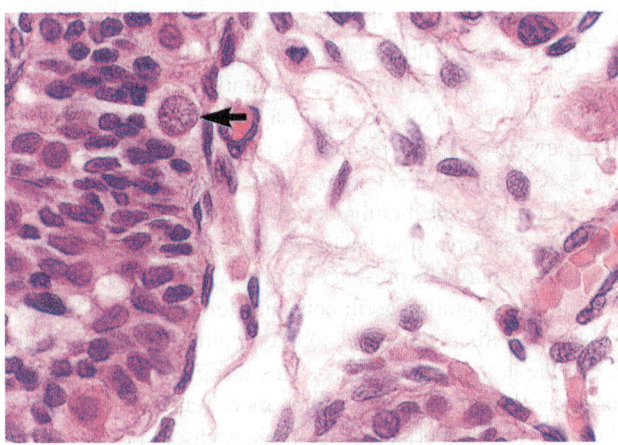

FIGURE 36.19 Testis of an 11-month-old child. A spermatogonium is presented adjacent to the basement membrane (*arrow*). The interstitium contains undifferentiated spindle cells.

of the germ cells are spermatogonia. This transition from the fetal stem cell pool to the adult stem cell pool is an important first step in the maturation process and appears to be defective in patients with the TDS and who subsequently later in life are prone to develop germ cell neoplasia (105). At birth, the germ cells average 2 to 4 per tubule cross section. From the age of 1 to 4 years, the number of germ cells averages 1 or 2 per tubule cross section and this number doubles between the ages of 5 and 8 years (106).

Early in puberty, repeated waves of incomplete spermatogenesis take place, with an orderly process of complete maturation not appearing until the end of puberty (107). Several studies have demonstrated a marked diminution in the number of germ cells in the undescended, prepubertal testis (Fig. 36.20), and a less predictable decrease of germ cells in the truly ectopic testis (31,108). Early primordial germ cells undergo striking epigenetic reprogramming during their migration, including extensive DNA demethylation, histone modifications, RNA-associated gene expression silencing, erasure of parental imprinted genes, and, in the case of the female gonocyte, reactivation of the inactivated X chromosome. Epigenetic remethylation and reestablishment of imprinted genes in a sex-specific manner occurs in an asynchronous manner in subsequent stages of gametogenesis. Although the exact timing of imprint reacquisition is still not known in humans, it generally occurs in males before meiosis begins. However, other epigenetic reprogramming events may occur in sperm cells released into the epididymis (109–111). This pattern of demethylation and loss of imprinting is also demonstrated in many of the germ cell neoplasms derived from these gonocytes (112). Epigenetic perturbations have also been demonstrated in spermatozoa of men with subfertility (113). Primordial germ cells and gonocytes acquire a number of markers that are useful in their identification and in the evaluation of germ cell neoplasms derived from these cells. These include the membranous placental alkaline phosphatase (PLAP) and CD117 (KIT) and the nuclear markers: OCT3/4, NANOG, SALL4, SOX2, SOX17,

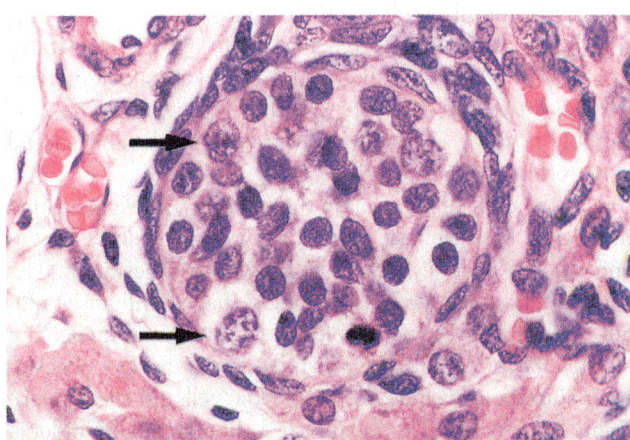

FIGURE 36.18 Same testis as shown in Figure 36.17. Note the mitotic figure, probably of a Sertoli cell. Larger cells (*arrows*) are undifferentiated germ cells. The remaining cells are immature Sertoli cells.

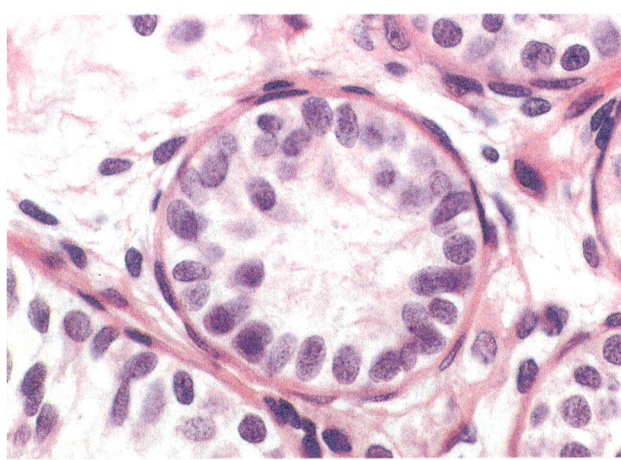

FIGURE 36.20 Thirteen-year old prepubertal boy with bilateral cryptorchidism. Mature Leydig cells are absent in the interstitium. The tubules lack a distinct lumen. The Sertoli cells are immature, and germ cells are rare.

MAGE-A4, and VASA. PLAP was one of the earliest markers employed to identify early migrating primordial germ cells. Germ cells in the first trimester of gestation are PLAP positive but by 19 weeks of gestation only a few cells remain positive. In recent years, PLAP has been largely replaced by CD117, NANOG, and OCT3/4 as markers of gonocytes. CD117, located on the cell membrane and within the cytoplasm of gonocytes, is a tyrosine kinase receptor for the ligand SCF. The latter is normally present on Sertoli cells. CD117 appears early in the migrating germ cells and tends to persist somewhat longer than the other markers; although it is usually not easily detectable in adult testes using older immunohistochemical methodologies, newer, more sensitive techniques show CD117 in spermatogonia in many cases (114).

OCT3/4 (also known as POU5F1), SALL4, and NANOG (a homeobox domain protein, regulating self-renewal) tend to parallel each other in their staining patterns. They are located in the nucleus and stain both primordial germ cells and gonocytes. At 7 weeks' postfertilization, twice as many germ cells stain positive for CD117 as there are staining for NANOG or OCT3/4. By 8 to 10 weeks, there are approximately equal numbers positive for these markers (Fig. 36.21), but by week 15, the number staining for CD117 is 16 times higher than for OCT3/4 and NANOG. At birth, only rare OCT3/4 or NANOG positive cells can be found (100). By the 4th week after birth, NANOG is no longer detected but a rare cell staining positive for OCT3/4 may still be found at 6 months after birth (115). After the 12th postnatal month, none of the germ cells should be positive for OCT3/4. There is evidence that failure of switching off expression of OCT3/4 in gonocytes leads to coexpression of testis-specific Y-encoded protein in the spermatogonial niche. This coexpression and the concomitant expression of KIT ligand (SCF) by Sertoli cells induce neoplastic conversion of immature (delayed) gonocytes to germ cell neoplasia in situ (116–120). The retained expression of OCT3/4 beyond 12 months of age is considered maturation arrest and proclivity to develop germ cell neoplasia (Fig. 36.22).

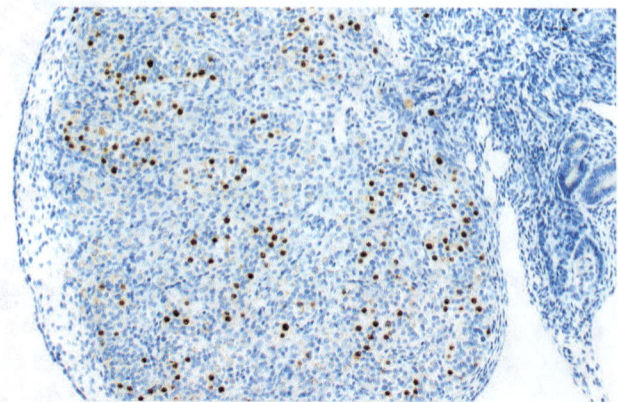

FIGURE 36.21 Fetal testis of 10 weeks' gestation. OCT 3/4 immunohistochemical stain of gonocytes. This section of testis would demonstrate an identical staining pattern of the gonocytes with CD117 (KIT).

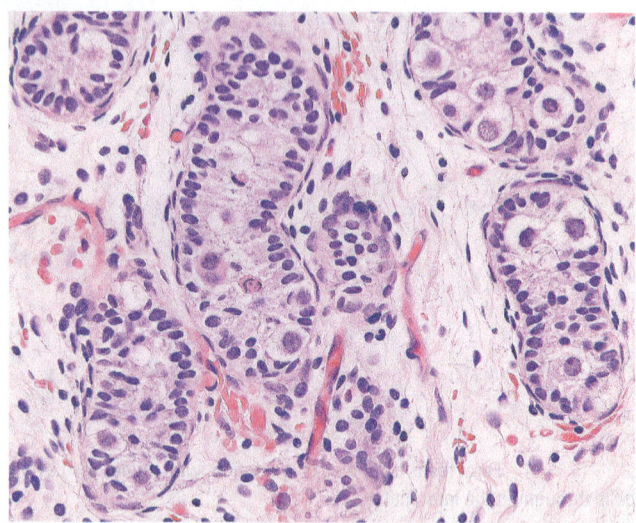

FIGURE 36.22 Delayed maturation; atypical germ cells, which immunohistochemically expressed OCT3/4, are present within the tubules.

VASA and MAGE-A4 stain more mature gonocytes, as well as primary spermatogonia. Some costaining of gonocytes with MAGE-A4 and CD117 occurs (104) and some colocalization of VASA and OCT3/4 also can be seen (121). CD30, somewhat useful in separating seminoma (−) and embryonal cell carcinoma (+), does not stain normal gonocytes (122). Corresponding to their mitotic activity and prior to their mitotic arrest soon after birth, gonocytes and spermatogonia reveal strong nuclear staining with Ki-67.

Immunohistochemical stains are critical for the diagnosis of germ cell tumors of the testis. Seminoma display expression of PLAP, c-kit (CD117), OCT3/4, and D2-40. OCT3/4 is positive in both seminoma and embryonal carcinoma; however, CD30 expression in embryonal carcinoma is helpful in sorting out this diagnosis. Several sensitive and relatively specific markers are useful for the identification of yolk sac tumor including α-fetoprotein (AFP), glypican 3, ZBTB16 and CDX2. Choriocarcinoma stains with several markers including human chorionic gonadotropin (hCG); human placental lactogen; inhibin and glypican 3 (in syncytiotrophoblasts); and GDF3, p63, and GATA3 (in cytotrophoblasts). SALL4 has emerged as a pan germ cell marker; it is sensitive but not very specific. Cytokeratins may be variably positive in different germ cell tumors and should be carefully interpreted (123–125).

Leydig cells first appear in the fetus at 7 weeks' gestation in the first of a triphasic pattern of Leydig cell development and reach a peak level at 14 to 20 weeks of gestation. The earliest fetal Leydig cells are spindle shaped and are gradually replaced by the more typical cells with round nuclei and abundant eosinophilic cytoplasm. By the 20th week of gestation, abundant, well-developed Leydig cells fill the interstitium (Fig. 36.12). The Leydig cells then gradually undergo regression with only a few recognizable cells at birth. The cell of origin of this first wave of Leydig cells is still uncertain (126), with proposals that they are derived from microvascular pericytes, epithelial components of the adjacent mesonephros, from the celomic epithelium, or even from neural crest cells. There is strong support for a common origin of all of the steroidogenic cells of the urogenital system from the adrenogenital primordium (127). Likewise, the mechanisms leading to late fetal life regression of these cells are unknown (128). The second wave of Leydig cells appears during the so-called mini-puberty at 2 to 3 months after birth, corresponding to the activation of the hypothalamus/pituitary/gonad axis (129). Equally unclear is whether this second population of Leydig cells arises from the same or from a separate mesenchymal precursor cell as the first wave of Leydig cells (130). These cells are a mix of mature-appearing Leydig cells, smaller cells with a round nucleus and a fairly prominent nucleolus but without the eosinophilic cytoplasm of mature Leydig cells, and small spindle cells. After this second phase of Leydig cell activity ends at about the 6th neonatal month, only immature spindle cells (Fig. 36.14) are recognized until just before puberty, when the third wave of adult Leydig cells begins to make its appearance.

Sertoli cells are the first cells to become recognizable in the earliest fetal testis and they play a crucial role in the differentiation of the Leydig cells, the suppression of entry into meiosis of the gonocytes, and the production of AMH (7). The conventional viewpoint is that Sertoli cells are derived from thickened celomic epithelium but, like the Leydig cell, there is also one study supporting that Sertoli cells likely arise from steroidogenic progenitor cells (127). Fetal Sertoli cells outnumber germ cells in a ratio of 7:1 (131) and undergo active mitotic division during this period. The nucleus of the earliest fetal Sertoli cell is elliptical, but later on a mixture of round and oval nuclei is present and these nuclear shapes persist until puberty. They are in sharp contrast to the irregular and highly folded nuclear membrane of the adult Sertoli cell. The nucleolus of fetal and infantile Sertoli cells is inconspicuous, in contrast to the prominent nucleolus of the adult form.

Inhibin-α and vimentin are reliable (although not specific) markers of both immature and mature Sertoli cells. AMH is present in Sertoli cells from the 7th week of gestation until puberty but is not present in mature cells. Cytokeratin 18 is present in the first 20 weeks of gestation but is completely absent thereafter. This latter marker is of interest because of its presence in some Sertoli cells in adults with TDS. In contrast, androgen receptor nuclear expression is a feature seen only in pubertal and adult Sertoli cells (7,132).

Sertoli cell nodules or tubular congeries, frequently seen in cryptorchid but also in descended testes, (Fig. 36.23) are composed of nonencapsulated immature Sertoli cell tubular nests, showing a prominent peripheral hyaline–like basement membrane, as well as central basement membrane deposits. Laminated microliths are often present and occasional spermatogonia can frequently be found in the nodules. These Sertoli cells are proliferating and stain for AMH, SOX9, only focally for cytokeratin 18, and variably for androgen receptor (132,133).

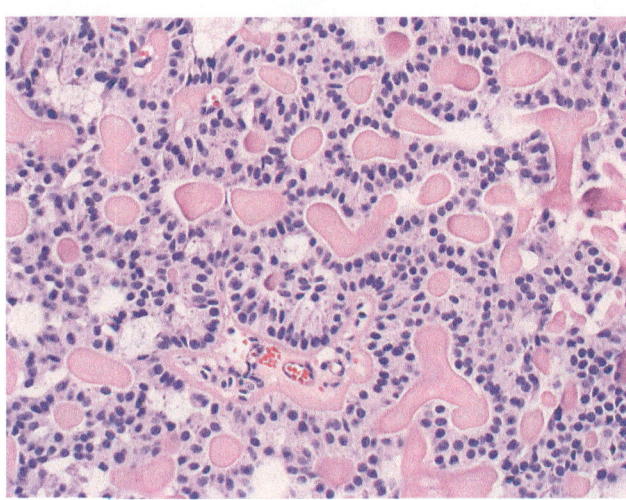

FIGURE 36.23 Sertoli cell nodule (or tubular congeries). The tubules are composed of immature Sertoli cells lack germ cells and have prominent basement membrane deposits.

Fetal Sertoli cells are mitotically active and increase in number through the first few months after birth. After the neonatal proliferative phase, the Sertoli cell population remains relatively stable until the onset of puberty when another increase in number takes place. Sertoli cells become mitotically inactive at the end of puberty and remain so throughout adult life. Stereologic studies indicate the Sertoli cell total number increases from 260 million late in fetal life to 1,500 million between 3 months and 10 years, and to 3,700 million in the adult testis (134). The testis shows a sixfold increase in size in the 1st year after birth, primarily as a result of Sertoli cell proliferation and the marked lengthening of the seminiferous tubules rather than a significant increase in tubule diameter (107). Sertoli cells per tubule cross-section average 30 in the fetal testis at 20 weeks of gestation, increase to 42 at the 4th postnatal month, then decrease to 26 at 13 years, and then to 12 to 15 in the adult (31,135). At puberty, there is fivefold increase in Sertoli cell volume and, at the same time cytoplasmic Charcot–Böttcher crystalloids first appear. The seminiferous tubules at 20 weeks of fetal life measure 45 to 50 μm in diameter, are solidly filled with Sertoli and germ cells in a ratio of 7:1, and lack a well-defined lumen (135). The postnatal tubules slowly increase in size to reach a prepubertal diameter of 64 μm (range 43 to 70 μm), at which time lumens begin to appear (131).

AGING TESTIS

There is a gradual and progressive decline in testicular volume with aging. Well et al. demonstrated a decrease in testicular volume from 16.5 cm^3 in males between 20 and 30 years to 14 cm^3 in men between 80 and 90 years (136). Histologic changes include a patchy pattern of hypospermatogenesis, peritubular fibrosis, and hyalinization of the seminiferous tubules, although an occasional sclerotic tubule may be found in an otherwise normal testis (137). A variable number of tubules will contain all elements of developing germ cells, including mature spermatozoa. Although the total number of peritubular cells is maintained in elderly men, there is a sharp decline in the proportion of cells that stain positively for desmin and actin (56).

Thickening of testicular arterial and arteriolar walls, with hyalinization, is found in over 90% of testes in which there are large zones of tubular fibrosis. The capillary bed in the aged testis becomes sparse and poorly organized (138). These vascular changes likely play a causal role in the peritubular sclerosis and tubular hyalinization.

Substantial controversy exists regarding the Leydig cell population in the aging testis (139,140). According to Neaves et al., Leydig cell numbers progressively decline from the early postpubertal state and this process continues through the life of the individual, with nearly 50% of that loss occurring in the first 30 years after puberty (141). The production of testosterone by Leydig cells is relatively maintained despite this loss, probably because of the large reserve of these cells in the adult testis. When the Leydig cell mass decreases to a certain threshold point, daily sperm production does decline. The aged Leydig cell contains large amounts of lipofuscin pigment, numerous vacuoles, and increased numbers of Reinke crystals within the cytoplasm.

Abnormal sperm maturation, sloughing of germ cells into the tubule lumen, degeneration of germ cell elements, and Sertoli cell lipid accumulation and cytoplasmic vacuolization are frequent findings in the aged testis. Earlier studies suggested that the Sertoli cell population is stable throughout adulthood (142,143). However, Johnson et al. (48) found that men of ages 20 to 48 years had significantly more Sertoli cells per tubule cross section than did men of 50 to 85 years of age, and that there was a relatively constant relationship between Sertoli cells and immature germ cells in both age groups. Sertoli cells in those tubules with hypospermatogenesis have increased amounts of vimentin and the reappearance of cytokeratins 8 and 18, suggesting that the reversion of the intermediate filament pattern to that of the fetal/prepubertal testis is related to the alteration of the spermatogenic process (144).

RETE TESTIS

The rete testis, a network of channels at the hilus of the testis, receives the luminal contents of the seminiferous tubules (Fig. 36.1). It is divided into three components; the septal portion containing the tubuli rete, the mediastinal rete, and the extratesticular portion also known as the bullae retis (145,146). The tubuli rete are short tubules, 0.5 to 1.0 mm in length, that connect the two ends of the seminiferous tubule loop to the mediastinum testis. The terminal end of the seminiferous tubule usually consists only of Sertoli cells, forming an epithelial plug–like structure as it protrudes into the rete

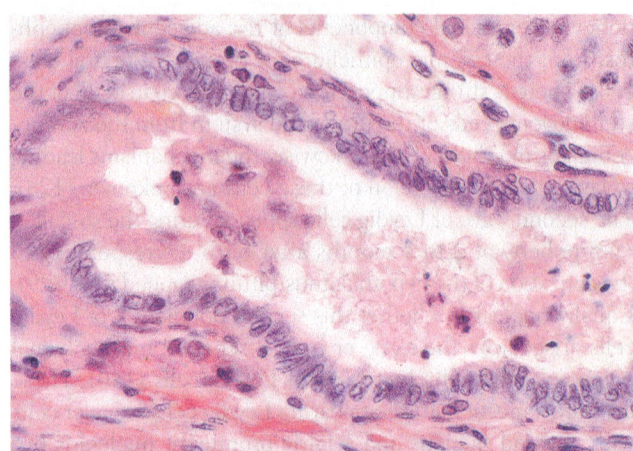

FIGURE 36.24 Junction of septal rete testis and terminal end of seminiferous tubule. Note the Sertoli cells "pouting" into the lumen of the rete. Rete epithelium is a low columnar type with frequent nuclear grooves.

lumen (Fig. 36.24). There are approximately 1,500 entrances of seminiferous tubules into the rete. A few tubules may enter the mediastinal rete directly, without intervening tubuli rete. The mediastinal rete is a cavernous network of interconnecting branching channels that exits from the testis to form several dilated, vesicular channels or antechamber-like structures called the bullae retis. These structures, measuring up to 3 mm in width, anastomose together to form the ductuli efferentia. The rete epithelium is a low columnar type with frequent nuclear grooves and with a luminal surface, which is studded with microvilli (Fig. 36.24). Each cell contains a single, central flagellum that is inconspicuous on light microscopic examination. The epithelium sits on a relatively thick basal lamina, beneath which are a few fibroblasts and myoid cells intermixed with collagen and elastic fibers. Traversing the mediastinum and the extratesticular rete are epithelium-covered columns or strands called chordae retis. These columns, often appearing as islands on a cross section of the rete testis (Fig. 36.25), vary greatly in length (15 to 100 μm)

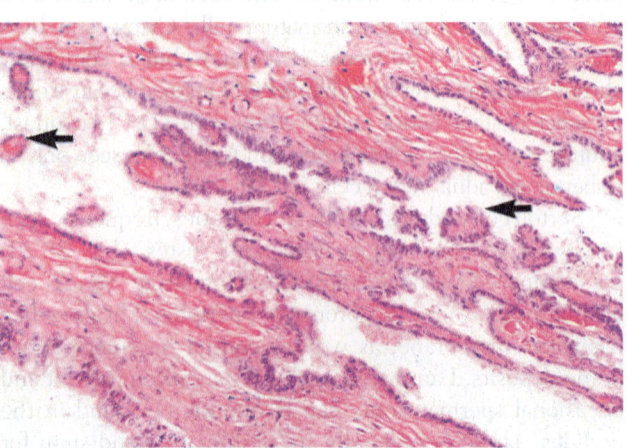

FIGURE 36.25 Rete testis, mediastinal portion, with irregular cavernous channels and cross sections of intratubular chordae (*arrows*).

and thickness (5 to 40 μm) and serve to connect opposing walls of the chambers. The cytoplasm of the rete epithelium contains keratin and vimentin intermediate filaments, the former being located primarily in the apical portion of the cell and the latter being found in the basal region. The keratins, mostly of low–molecular-weight types, can be first identified at the 10th week of fetal life and precede the appearance of vimentin by 2 to 3 weeks (147). One would expect coexpression of these two intermediate filaments in the rare carcinoma of the rete or in hyperplasia of the rete. In recent studies, the benign rete testis was shown to express androgen receptors, PAX8, WT1, CK7 and CK20, variable calretinin, and progesterone receptor (21). In our experience cytokeratin 7, AE1/AE3, EMA, CK5/6, WT1, and vimentin are often expressed in rete testis carcinomas in a patchy distribution. Calretinin, WT1, and PAX-8 have also been reported in rete testis carcinoma (21,148). A report of nine cases of hyperplasia of the rete testis showed strong cytokeratin and epithelial membrane antigen (EMA) staining but a negative reaction for vimentin (149). Hyaline, refractile, eosinophilic globules, which are periodic acid–Schiff (PAS) positive, sometimes are seen within the cells or lumen of the rete and sometimes are α1-antitrypsin positive but AFP negative (150). They are especially prominent when the rete undergoes hyperplasia, a reaction that is most frequently provoked by rete invasion by a germ cell tumor. They should not be confused with the globules produced by yolk sac tumors of the testis in the presence of germ cell tumors. The rete epithelium, as well as that of efferent ductules and the head (caput) of the epididymis, also contains receptors for estrogen, progesterone, and androgen (151). The presence of estrogen receptors perhaps accounts for the hyperplasia of the rete and efferent ductules seen in patients undergoing sex-reversal procedures (152).

The rete serves multiple functions: (a) as a mixing chamber for the contents of the seminiferous tubules; (b) as a pressure gradient between the seminiferous tubules and the epididymis; (c) as a possible source of as yet unknown components of the seminal fluid; and (d) as a reabsorptive site of proteins from the luminal contents (153).

DUCTULI EFFERENTES

The ductuli efferentes consist of 10 to 12 tubules that arise from the extratesticular rete testis (Fig. 36.1) (154). They are involved primarily in resorption of fluid and do not appear to store spermatozoa for any length of time. These tubules aggregate to form a significant portion of the head of the epididymis proper (Fig. 36.26). Unlike the body of the epididymis, the lumens of the ductuli have an undulating border. The cells are composed of ciliated and nonciliated columnar cells, basal cells, and scattered intraepithelial lymphocytes, giving the epithelium a pseudostratified appearance (Fig. 36.27). Occasional cells with a Paneth cell–like appearance are seen (Fig. 36.28), having numerous and

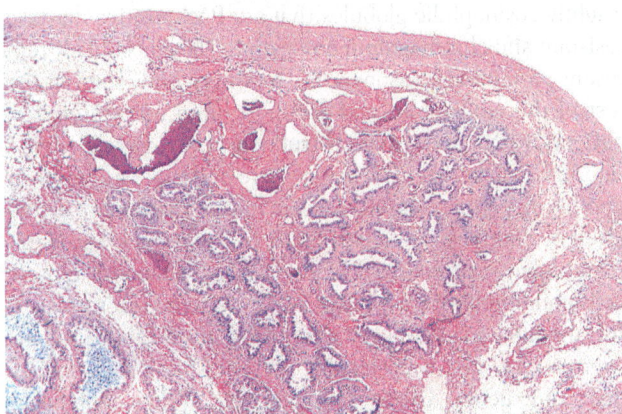

FIGURE 36.26 Head (caput) of epididymis, showing cross sections of distal portions of ductuli efferentia (*upper right*) and epididymis (*lower left*).

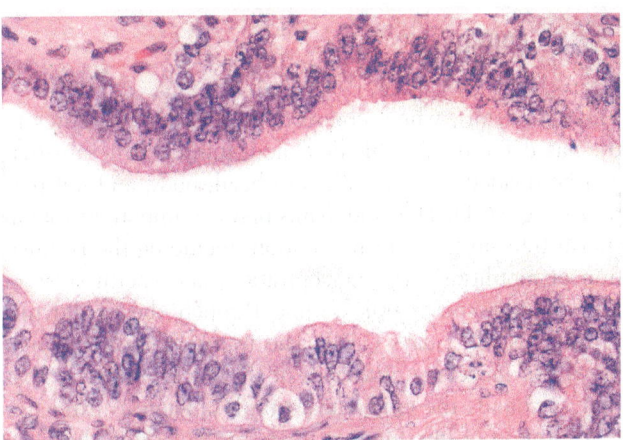

FIGURE 36.27 Epithelium of efferent ductulus. The columnar epithelial cells are mixed with basal cells and occasional intraepithelial lymphocytes, giving the epithelium a pseudostratified appearance.

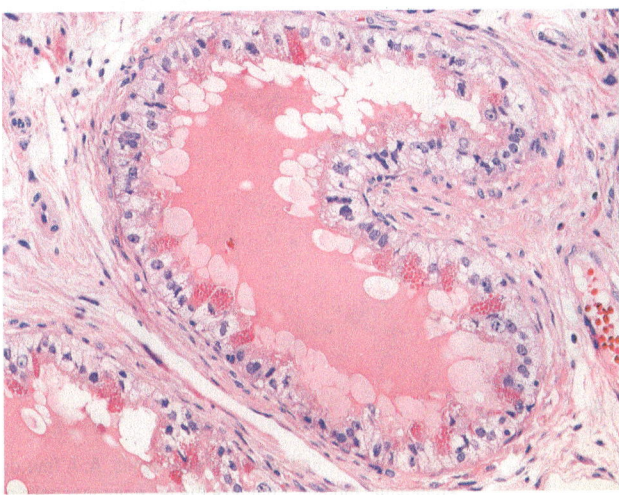

FIGURE 36.28 Epithelium of ductulus with prominent Paneth cell–like intracytoplasmic globules.

brightly eosinophilic globules that are PAS positive/diastase resistant and chromogranin A negative. They most likely represent prominent lysosomes, are less frequently seen in the rest of the epididymis, and are most often encountered in patients with epididymal obstruction (155). Rarely similar findings can be seen in benign rete testis. Golden-brown lipofuscin pigment is often seen in the cytoplasm of the efferent ductules. The epithelium sits on a thick basement membrane, surrounding which is a coat of smooth muscle cells and fibroblasts, as well as a few scattered macrophages. Intraluminal macrophages that are actively phagocytizing spermatozoa are occasionally present, particularly when duct obstruction exists. Coexpression of low–molecular-weight cytokeratins, vimentin, and EMA is evident within the epithelial cytoplasm (147). Other markers including AR, ER, PR, PAX-8, CK7, and CK20 have been reported in the epithelium (21).

EPIDIDYMIS

The epididymis, which connects the ductuli efferentes to the vas deferens, is a highly coiled, tubular structure that can be divided anatomically into head, body, and tail portions (Fig. 36.1). The epididymis plays an important role in sperm transport, sperm maturation, including the acquisition of motility, sperm concentration, and sperm storage. The average sperm transit time through the epididymis in humans is 12 days (156). The transport mechanism is by way of muscle contractions of the thick, muscular coat that surrounds the epididymal tubules. There is extensive reabsorption of intraluminal fluid, particularly in the head portion of the epididymis. Most of the sperm are stored in the tail segment until ejaculation occurs, and it is in this location in humans that final sperm maturation takes place (157). Many spermatozoa undergo senescence and degeneration in the tail via an unknown mechanism.

The epithelium of the epididymis consists of tall columnar or principal cells, basal cells, clear cells, tall slender or apical cells rich in mitochondria (apical mitochondria–rich cells), and scattered intraepithelial lymphocytes and macrophages (158). The principal cells form elaborate tight junctions that serve to regulate the intraluminal contents at different loci of the epididymis (159). Occasional large cells with atypical nuclei similar to those seen in the seminal vesicle are sometimes present. These have no clinical significance. The principal cells, comprising over 95% of the columnar cells, have straight stereocilia (Fig. 36.29), which are tall and nearly obliterate the lumen in the head but become progressively shorter as the tail is reached; these have no clinical significance. The columnar cell nuclei often show eosinophilic nuclear inclusions (Fig. 36.29). The principal cells stain strongly for vimentin, EMA, and acid phosphatase. Both basal and principal cells stain positively for low–molecular-weight cytokeratins, with more intense staining in the body and tail sections than the head region (160). In cryptorchid testes, the intensity of staining for low–molecular-weight keratins, particularly cytokeratin 18, is markedly diminished (161). The intensity of the vimentin staining progressively declines in the tail section (160). Intense CD10 apical membranous staining is evident both in the epididymis and vas deferens, a finding that has been utilized to ascertain the possible origin (positive if wolffian origin and negative if müllerian origin) of glandular structures found adjacent to the epididymis or vas deferens (162). Other immunohistochemical markers including AR, PAX8, and CK20 have recently been described (21). The apical mitochondria–rich cells, located primarily in the head, show intense staining for cytokeratins and acid phosphatase and

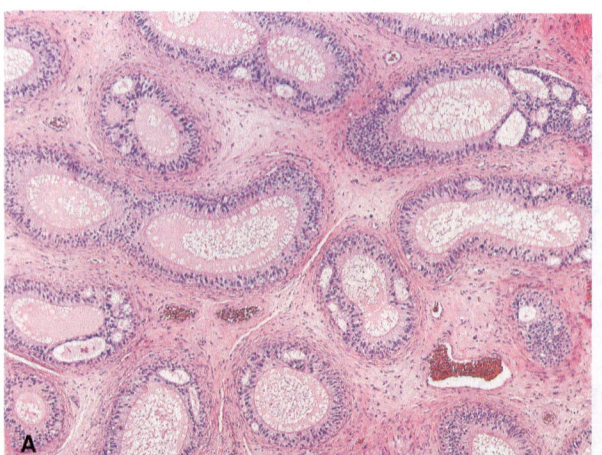
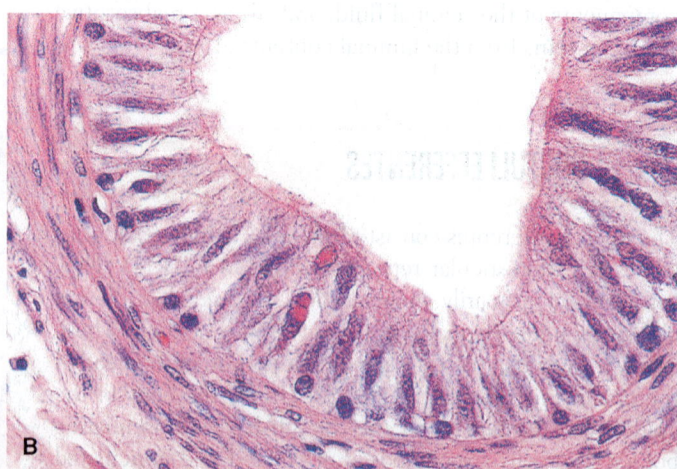

FIGURE 36.29 Epithelium of epididymis. **A:** A few ducts with cribriform architecture. **B:** High magnification of epididymal tubules. Compare the tall columnar cells of the epididymis with the pseudostratified cells of the efferent ductulus. A few intraepithelial lymphocytes are present. The stereocilia are somewhat short, indicating the tail segment. A layer of muscle cells forms the wall. Note intranuclear eosinophilic inclusions.

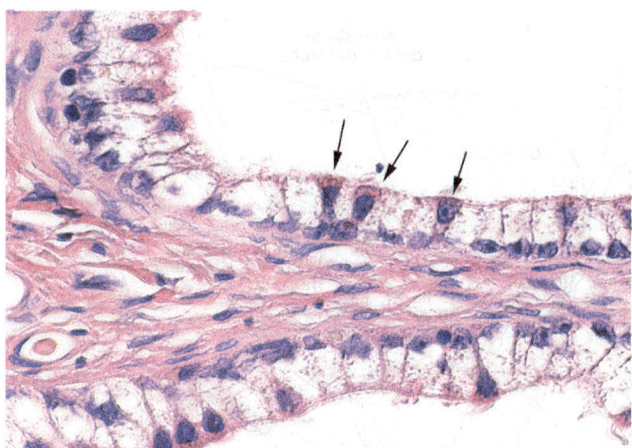

FIGURE 36.30 Epithelium of head of epididymis, demonstrating clear cells and apical mitochondria–rich cells (*arrows*).

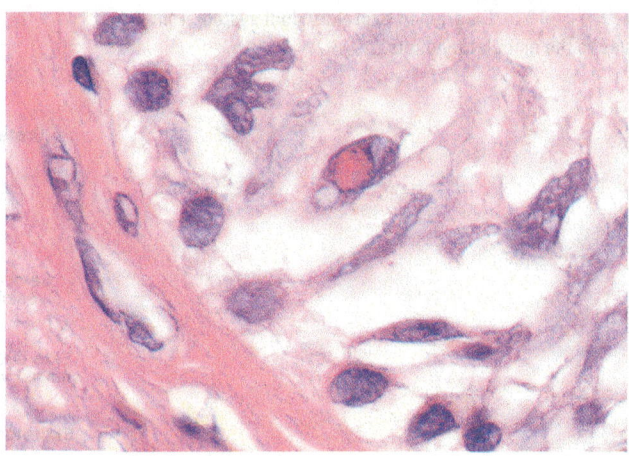

FIGURE 36.31 Intranuclear inclusions present in the epithelium of the epididymis. Similar inclusions are found in the epithelium of the ductus (vas) deferens.

less intense reactivity for EMA and vimentin. Their configuration varies from slender cells extending from the basement membrane all the way to the lumen to those that appear to be located only in the base of the duct (Fig. 36.30). Small foci of epithelium may rarely have the appearance of prostatic epithelium, including positive immunostaining for prostate-specific antigen. Whether this process represents metaplasia or ectopia is unclear (163). Epididymal cells may contain lipofuscin pigment, which tends to be more prominent in the head segment and is particularly evident when there is obstruction of the epididymis (164). The lumens are generally round and regular. In up to 50% of individuals, a focal cribriform pattern is seen (Fig. 36.29), which is considered a normal variation. Often this process is associated with cytoplasmic vacuolization and nuclear atypia (156,165). Importantly, these changes should not be mistaken for intraepididymal spread from a testicular germ cell tumor or a primary epididymal carcinoma. The focal distribution of the nuclear atypia and the absence of mitotic figures should be helpful features supporting a benign process.

Intranuclear, eosinophilic, PAS positive, and diastase-resistant inclusions (Fig. 36.31), measuring 1 to 14 μm, are found in the columnar cells of the adult epididymis, as well as throughout the vas and seminal vesicles. Electron microscopic examination shows the electron-dense globules to be enclosed by a single membrane and to lack any features suggesting viral structures (166). They are most common in the distal epididymis and adjacent vas and least common in the ampulla of the vas and seminal vesicles.

The epididymis is supported by a thick basement membrane, surrounding which is a well-defined muscular coat. The latter plays an important role in sperm movement through the epididymis. After puberty, scattered elastic fibers can be seen in both the ductuli and the epididymis. Mast cells are found throughout the connective tissue of the epididymis in a pattern similar to that seen in the tunica and interstitium of the testis (167). They are numerous in infancy, decrease in childhood, and then increase at the time of puberty. A progressive decline in numbers occurs in later adulthood. The epididymis is a rare site for carcinomas but does develop either sporadic or von Hippel–Lindau syndrome-associated papillary cystadenomas (168–170).

DUCTUS (VAS) DEFERENS

The ductus (vas) deferens, a tubular structure arising from the tail portion of the epididymis, measures about 40 cm in length. The distal 4 to 7 cm portion is enlarged to form the ampulla. The latter joins the excretory duct of the seminal vesicle to form the ejaculatory duct (Fig. 36.32). The adult vas is lined by a pseudostratified columnar epithelium composed of columnar cells and basal cells by light microscopic examination. Ultrastructural studies show four different cell types: principal cells, pencil or peg cells, mitochondria-enriched cells, and basal cells. The luminal surface of the columnar cell is lined by tall stereocilia throughout most of the vas (171). These stereocilia are substantially shorter and sparser in the ampullary region. Prominent intranuclear eosinophilic inclusions, as described above in the epididymis, may be seen (166). In addition, occasional lipid-positive vacuoles are present within the cytoplasm. The epithelium of the vas is thrown into folds, which are relatively simple in the proximal vas (Fig. 36.33) but become much more complicated in the ampullary segment (Fig. 36.34). The ampulla has highly complex infoldings and many outpocketings or diverticula that reach into the muscle coat. Beneath the epithelium of the adult vas is a loose connective tissue stroma that contains a well-defined, circumferentially oriented layer of elastic fibers (172). These fibers, lacking in infants and children, become frayed and fragmented in the aged vas. The muscle coat is an extraordinary thick

FIGURE 36.32 Diagram of excretory duct system from the vas to the ejaculatory ducts.

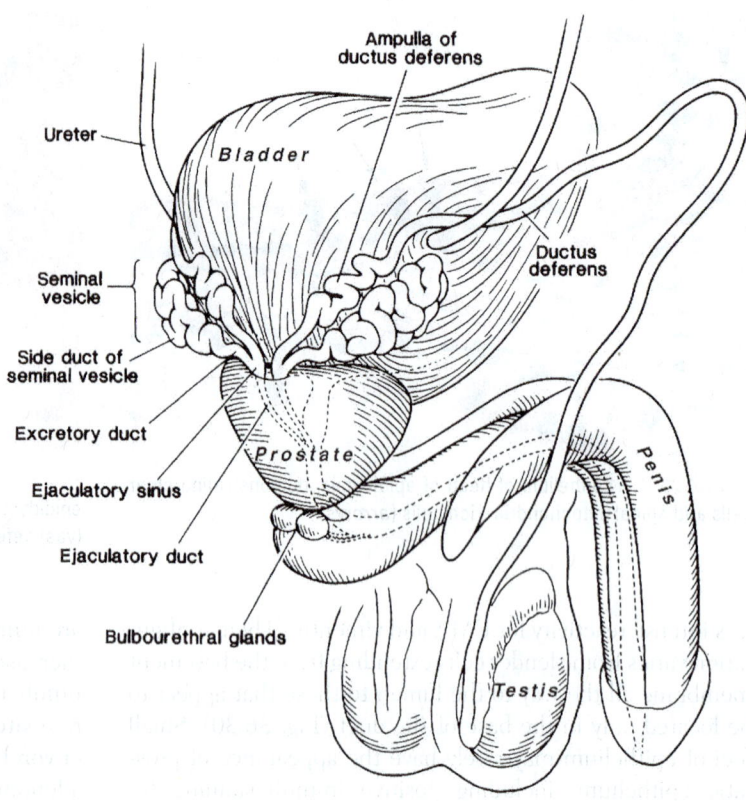

structure with inner and outer longitudinal coats and a middle oblique or circular zone. The entire muscle mass progressively decreases as the ampulla is reached, although the inner longitudinal layer becomes somewhat thicker distally (171). The epithelium in the ampulla contains significant amounts of lipofuscin pigment and rather closely resembles the epithelium seen in the seminal vesicles. Active phagocytosis of degenerated spermatozoa has been demonstrated in the ampullary region of a number of mammalian species (173). Vas deferens epithelium is immunohistochemically positive for AR, PAX8, and CK7. ER and PR may occasionally be positive (21).

SEMINAL VESICLES

The seminal vesicles are paired, highly coiled, tubular structures, lying posterolateral to the base of the bladder and in a parallel path with the ampulla of the vas deferens (Fig. 36.26).

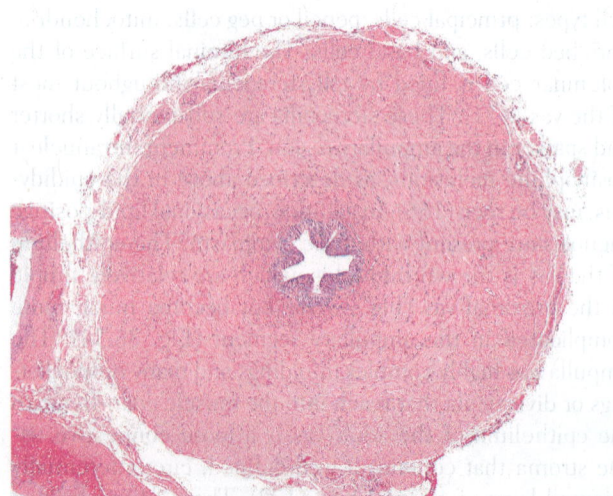

FIGURE 36.33 Proximal ductus (vas) deferens. This cross section shows a thick muscle coat, tiny lumen, and slightly folded mucosa.

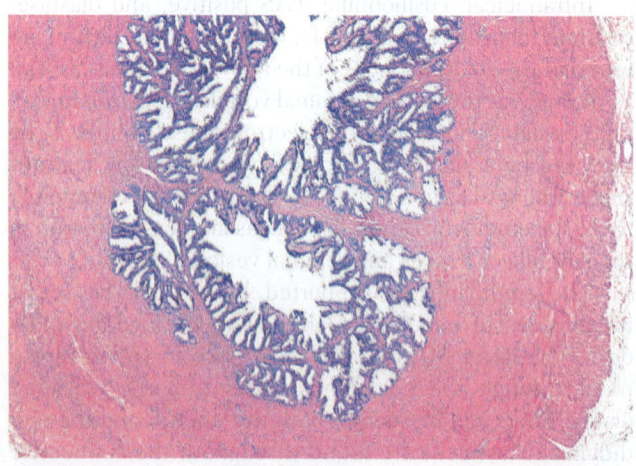

FIGURE 36.34 Ampullary region of ductus (vas) deferens. Note the complex folding and outpouching of the mucosa into the muscular coat.

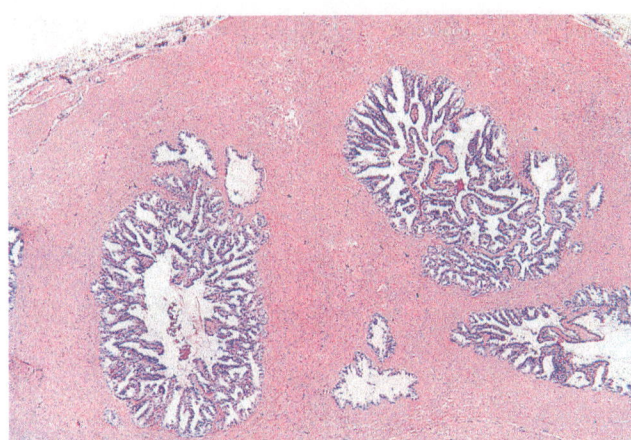

FIGURE 36.35 Seminal vesicle: alveolus-like arrangement of mucosal folds and cross sections of side ducts.

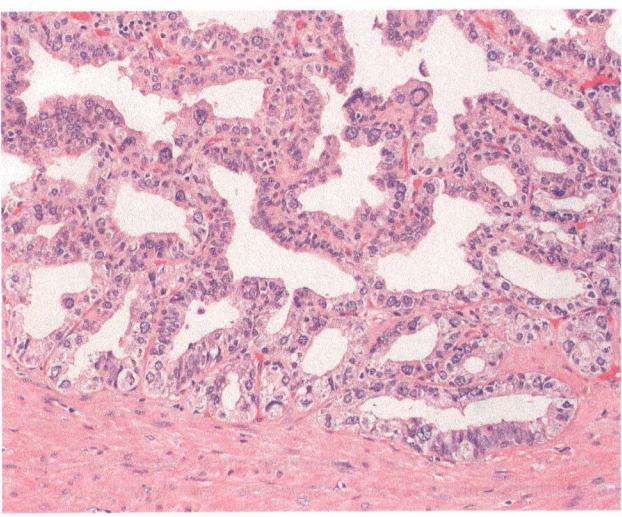

FIGURE 36.36 Seminal vesicle epithelium. Tall columnar to cuboidal cells line the lumen. Hyperchromatic "monster" cells are present. Nuclear inclusion in a large cell is present. These cells should not be mistaken for malignant cells, a distinction which is aided by the cytoplasmic lipofuscin.

Each vesicle measures 3.5 to 7.5 cm in length and 1.2 to 2.4 cm in thickness in the adult. The main duct, which is duplicated in approximately 10% of individuals, measures 10 to 15 cm in length when unraveled. Six to eight first-order side ducts extend off the main duct, and several secondary side ducts are derived from these. The upper part of the main duct is bent backward in a hook-like fashion. A short excretory duct combines with the ampulla of the vas to form the ejaculatory duct (Fig. 36.32). The wall of the seminal vesicle has a thin external longitudinal and a thicker internal circular muscle layer. The mucosal folds, relatively simple and shallow in infancy and childhood, become highly complex and alveolus-like in the reproductive years (Fig. 36.35) and are blunted in the aged vesicle. The lumen may contain a few sloughed epithelial cells and debris. Eosinophilic secretions, often with crystalloid structures, are commonly seen within the lumens. They usually have a plate-like arrangement but sometimes appear as smaller crystalloids similar to those seen in the lumens of well-differentiated prostate carcinomas. Their significance is unknown, but one should be aware of their presence in biopsies where the seminal vesicle is inadvertently sampled (174). Spermatozoa, refluxed from the ejaculatory duct, occasionally may be present, although they are not normally stored within the seminal vesicles.

The vesicle epithelium is composed of columnar and basal cells. The former have short microvilli projecting from the surface. The cytoplasm often contains a large amount of lipofuscin pigment, a feature important in recognizing these cells obtained by needle biopsy or aspiration cytology studies of the prostate. Similar lipofuscin pigment is found in the ampulla of the ductus deferens and in the epithelium of the ejaculatory ducts. The pigment has been divided into two different types, based on its appearance. Type 1 consists of coarse and highly refractile, golden-brown granules of uniform diameter (1 to 2 μg). Type 2 granules are much more variable in size (0.25 to 4 μg). Type 2 granules are further divided into type 2A and type 2B. Type 2A are poorly refractile to nonrefractile, and appear yellow-brown to gray-brown. Type 2B are nonrefractile and are dark to light purple or pink. Both type 1 and 2 granules are found in the seminal vesicle, vas, and ejaculatory ducts, whereas only the type 2 granules are found in prostatic epithelium (175).

An unusual feature of the seminal vesicle epithelium is the presence of peculiar, monstrous epithelial cells (Fig. 36.36). Similar cells may be seen in the ampulla of the vas and, less commonly, more proximally in the vas or epididymis. These cells have enlarged, hyperchromatic, and often irregularly shaped nuclei and are found in approximately three-quarters of adult seminal vesicles. They often have prominent intranuclear cytoplasmic inclusions (Fig. 36.36). They are not seen in infants or children. Their genesis is unknown but may be related to endocrine influences, similar to the Arias-Stella cells seen in gestational endometrium. Since these cells may be encountered in both needle biopsy and aspiration biopsy specimens, the surgical pathologist must be alert to avoid identifying them as malignant cells (176). Degenerative-type atypia and the presence of lipochrome pigment in the cells provide helpful clues to identify them as normal seminal vesicle epithelium, and their associated basal cells provide additional assurance that they do not represent prostate cancer.

Hyaline, pink globules (Fig. 36.37) are also encountered in the muscle portion of the seminal vesicle, thought to represent degenerating smooth muscle cells. They also may be seen occasionally in the muscular coat of the vas and within the prostate parenchyma (177). Deposits of amorphous pink material under the epithelium and variably replacing the muscle wall of the seminal vesicle is a normal phenomenon in aging individuals. This condition, usually referred to as senile amyloidosis, may also involve the vas deferens

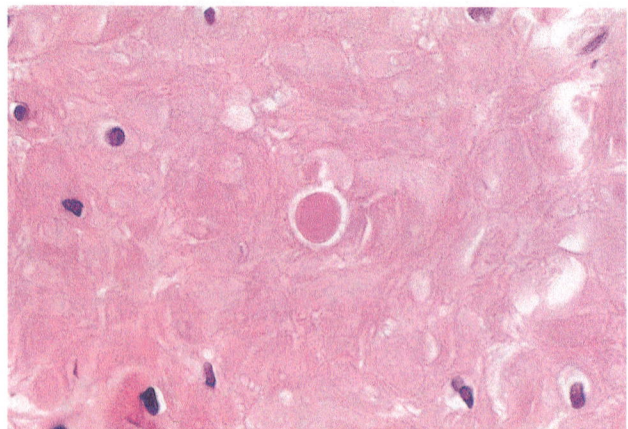

FIGURE 36.37 Muscle coat of seminal vesicle showing a hyaline globule, which probably represents a degenerated smooth muscle cell.

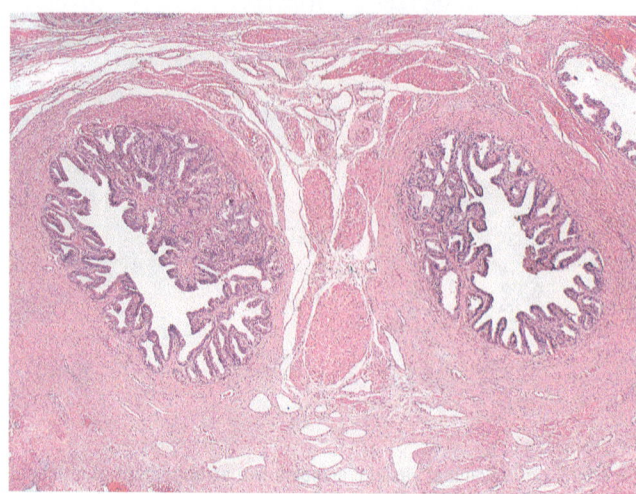

FIGURE 36.39 Paired ejaculatory ducts within the prostatic parenchyma.

and ejaculatory duct, has no association with systemic amyloidosis, and is without any clinical sequelae (Fig. 36.38). It contains semenogelin 1, a major secretory product of the seminal vesicles, and lactoferrin (178,179).

EJACULATORY DUCTS

The ejaculatory ducts are short (1.5 cm) paired ducts, arising from the confluence of the excretory duct of the seminal vesicle and the ampulla of the vas, that quickly converge and enter the prostate (Fig. 36.39). They run through the central zone of the prostate parenchyma and enter the posterior aspect of the distal prostate urethra at the verumontanum (180). The outer portions of the ejaculatory ducts have a thin muscle coat that progressively becomes more attenuated as the ducts pass through the prostate. The epithelium of the ejaculatory ducts resembles that of the seminal vesicle and ampulla of the vas (Fig. 36.40). On occasion, a needle biopsy of the prostate will sample a portion of one of these ducts, making it imperative that the surgical pathologist be aware of the characteristics of these cells. The presence and character of the lipofuscin pigment in the cytoplasm should give a clue to the cell origin. Immunoperoxidase stains for prostate-specific antigen demonstrate a sharp contrast between the positively stained prostate epithelium and the negatively stained cells of the intraprostatic ejaculatory ducts (Fig. 36.41). An opposite staining pattern is observed with PAX8 and PAX2, which are positive in the ejaculatory duct epithelium and negative in the prostatic epithelium, including prostatic carcinoma cells (181).

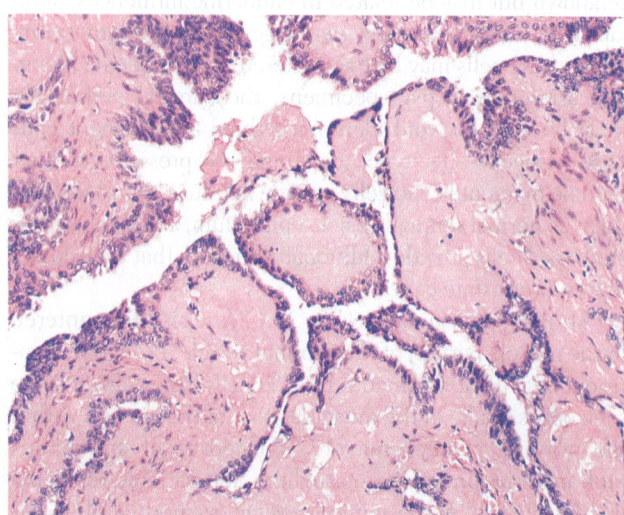

FIGURE 36.38 Senile amyloidosis in seminal vesical. Subepithelial deposits of amorphous eosinophilic amyloid.

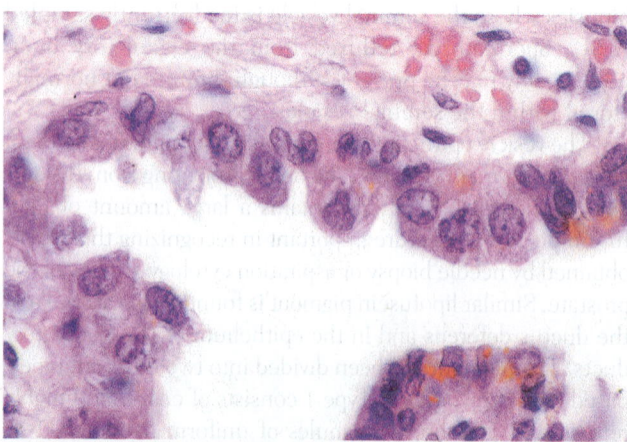

FIGURE 36.40 Epithelium of prostatic portion of ejaculatory duct. This epithelium may be encountered in a needle biopsy or aspiration biopsy of the prostate and should not be misinterpreted as malignant.

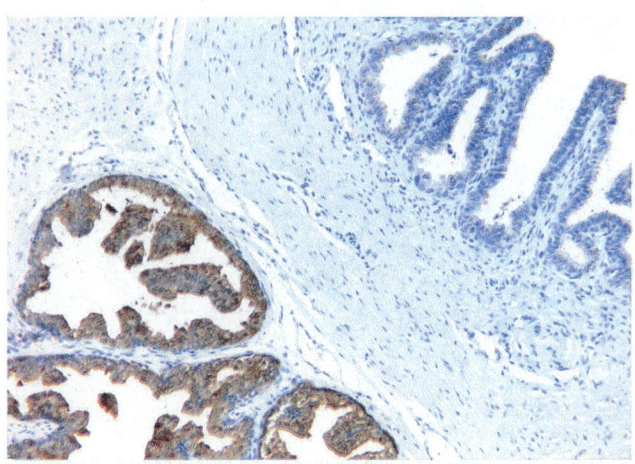

FIGURE 36.41 Intraprostatic ejaculatory duct (*right*) and adjacent prostatic tissue (*left*). Prostate-specific antigen immunoperoxidase demonstrates strongly positive cytoplasmic staining of the prostatic secretory cells and negative staining of ejaculatory duct epithelium.

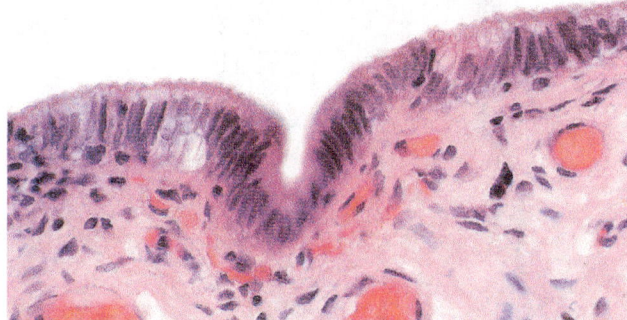

FIGURE 36.43 Appendix testis with covering of low columnar, nonciliated epithelium.

MESONEPHRIC AND MÜLLERIAN REMNANTS

Remnants of either the mesonephric (wolffian) duct or the paramesonephric (müllerian) duct are commonly encountered in tissues adjacent to the testis, epididymis, or vas deferens (146). These are the appendix testis (hydatid of Morgagni), appendix epididymis, vas aberrans (organ of Haller), and paradidymis (organ of Giraldes) (Fig. 36.1).

The appendix testis, a remnant of the cranial portion of the müllerian duct, is attached to the tunica vaginalis on the anterosuperior aspect of the testis just below the head of the epididymis. Occasionally, it is attached to both the testis and the epididymis. It is most often sessile and either oval or fan shaped (90%) and, less commonly, pedunculated (10%) and measures 0.5 to 2.5 cm in greatest dimension (Fig. 36.42). It is sometimes represented by only a slight roughening or a calcified thickening of the tunica vaginalis (182,183). Approximately 80% of individuals have an appendix testis, with bilaterality in one-third of them. The appendix testis is covered by a cuboidal or columnar epithelium, which may be ciliated (Fig. 36.43). The structure has a highly vascular fibrous core containing variable numbers of smooth muscle cells. Tubular invaginations and small gland-like structures may also be found in the stroma. Rarely, a macroscopic cyst may be present. Because of its occasionally pedunculated structure, the appendix testis can become twisted, causing hemorrhagic infarction and producing severe testicular pain (184). This event occurs most often in prepubertal or pubertal boys and may be related to the presence of androgen and estrogen receptors known to be present in the appendix epithelium and the possible growth of the appendix as a result of stimulation by androgens and estrogens at this period of time (185).

The appendix epididymis (Fig. 36.44), a remnant of the most cranial portion of the mesonephric duct, is present in ~25% of testes (183). It is almost invariably cystic, the

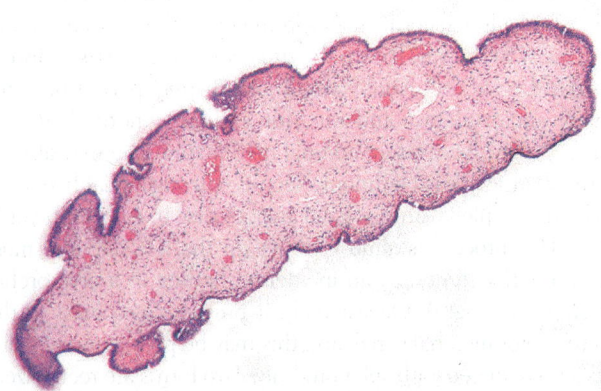

FIGURE 36.42 Appendix testis. This specimen was an incidental finding in a surgically removed testis. It was pedunculated and measures 0.9 cm in greatest length.

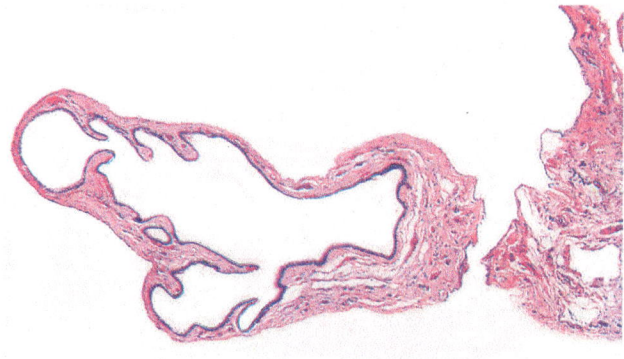

FIGURE 36.44 Appendix epididymis. A pedunculated cystic structure is attached to the head of the epididymis.

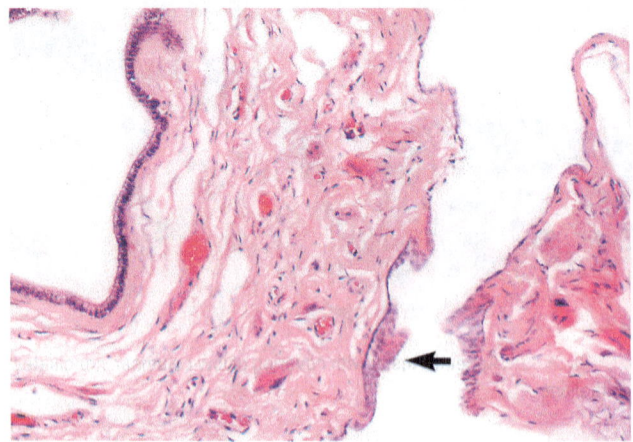

FIGURE 36.45 Appendix epididymis. Low columnar epithelium lines the cystic space. The surface is lined by focally thickened mesothelium (*arrow*).

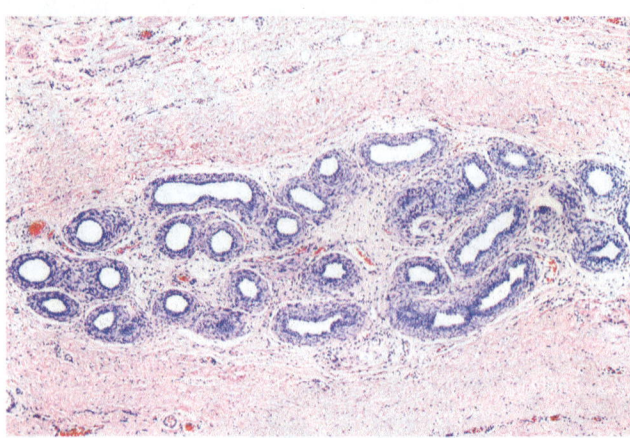

FIGURE 36.47 Epididymis-like tubules in the hernia sac of a 6 year old.

vesicle lumen being filled with amorphous protein secretions. The epithelium lining the cyst is columnar and often ciliated (Fig. 36.45). The external surface is covered by a flattened or low cuboidal layer of mesothelial cells. Since it may be pedunculated, it is also subject to torsion and infarction. Appendix testis and appendix epididymis express AR, ER, PR, PAX-8, WT1, and CK7 (21).

The other appendicular structures are derived from remnants of either the mesonephric tubules or the müllerian ducts and are variably encountered in the fat, usually as microscopic incidental findings. These are the vas aberrans inferior, the vas aberrans superior, and the paradidymis. They all have somewhat similar histologic features, with a low columnar epithelium lining a small cystic space and a thin muscular coat. Some investigators refer to these structures collectively as the paradidymis (186). The vas aberrans inferior is a tubular structure (Fig. 36.46) located near the junction of the vas and the tail portion of the epididymis and which may or may not communicate with either structure.

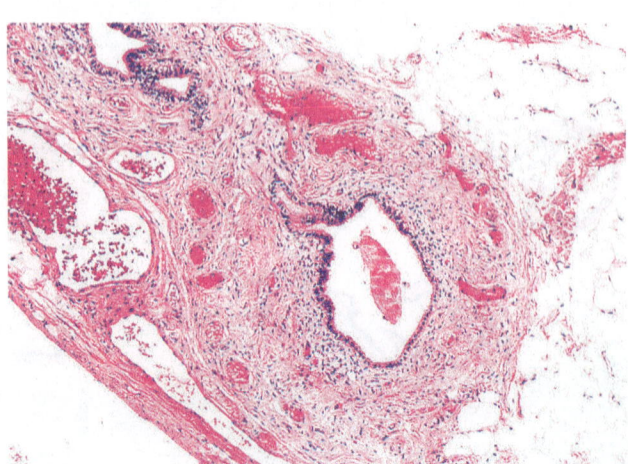

FIGURE 36.46 Vas aberrans inferior. A tubular structure is found near the tail portion of the epididymis.

The vas aberrans superior is a small collection of tubules located near the head or body of the epididymis. It may communicate with the epididymis or the rete testis. Remnants of the vas aberrans may be the origin of cord cysts, seen sporadically in isolated individuals, in patients whose mothers had been treated with diethylstilbestrol (187), or in patients with von Hippel–Lindau syndrome (188).

The paradidymis is represented by one or more tubules embedded in the spermatic cord, adjacent to the ductus (vas) deferens, and near the head of the epididymis. These tubules may be encountered in a section of the wall of an inguinal hernia sac and should not be mistaken for a portion of the ductus deferens or epididymis (189). Some of these structures mimic the epididymis (Fig. 36.47) and others resemble the vas. CD10 staining of the epithelial cells and the relatively thick muscle coat of the vas deferens may help in separating the true vas from vas-like tubules and, to a lesser degree, in separating the epididymis from epididymis-like remnants (162). Rarely, macroscopic cysts may form in the spermatic cord (190).

Although not part of the paradidymis, infrequently one may find adrenal cortical rests in the fat of the spermatic cord, adjacent to the vas, the epididymis or the rete testis. Adrenal cortical rests are usually small and display partial or complete encapsulation and zonation similar to normal adrenal (Fig. 36.48). Very rarely, adrenal medullary tissue may also be present. Even less commonly seen is splenogonadal fusion, in which the splenic and gonadal anlages fuse in early embryonic life. This process is almost always on the left side and most commonly is found as an incidental finding in a cryptorchid testis (Fig. 36.49). Occasionally, it presents as a mass in the scrotum or inguinal canal, and this may be precipitated by diseases associated with splenomegaly. Two forms are recognized: a continuous type where a fibrous cord connects the testicular splenic tissue to the eutopic spleen; and a discontinuous type, where there is no such connection. The former is associated with congenital anomalies, particularly limb defects (191).

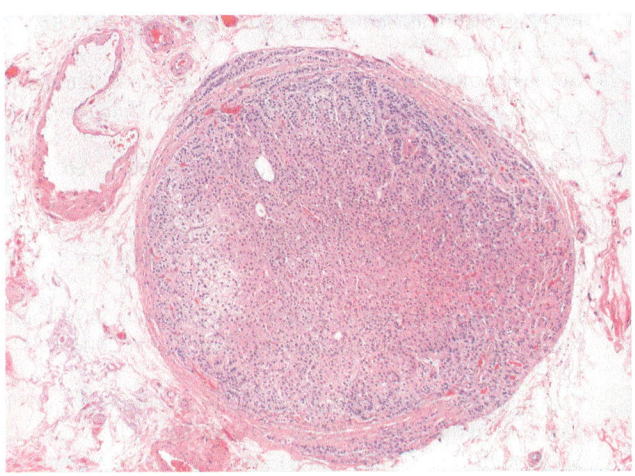

FIGURE 36.48 Adrenal cortical rest in fat adjacent to the epididymis. Note partial encapsulation and zonation similar to normal adrenal.

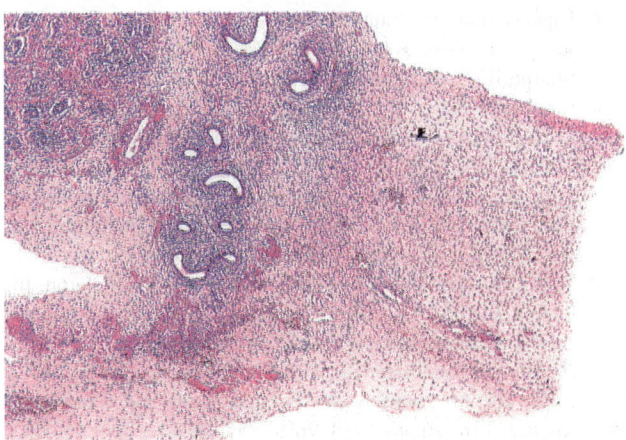

FIGURE 36.50 Gubernaculum and cranial attachment to epididymis and testis in a 26-week-old fetus.

Epididymis-like intratesticular tubular or microcystic structures are occasionally encountered, usually in elderly men (192). They are most often seen near the mediastinal rete. The epithelium is pseudostratified and stains positively for cytokeratins 8, 18, and 19, and for CD10. Vimentin staining of the basal cells and some of the columnar cells is observed. These structures most likely are derived from wolffian duct elements.

GUBERNACULUM

The gubernaculum, also known as the tail ligament of the testis, has been the center of attention with respect to the descent of the testis since it was first described by John Hunter in 1762, and its specific role is still being debated. In the fetus, this cylindrical, gelatinous structure is attached cranially to the testis and epididymis (Fig. 36.50) and caudally to the anterior abdominal wall at the site of the inguinal canal. Just before the descent of the testis through the inguinal canal, the gubernaculum increases in net weight disproportionately to the testis, supporting the theory that this structure plays a crucial role in this phase of the passage of the testis into the scrotum.

Histologically, the fetal gubernaculum is composed of a loose undifferentiated mesenchymal tissue similar to Wharton jelly. Large amounts of glycosaminoglycans fill the extracellular space and separate the individual spindle cells, most of which are fibroblasts. Fibroblasts tend to decrease with increasing gestational age. At the periphery of the distal gubernaculum, where it attaches to the inguinal wall, a few striated muscle cells, presumably derived from the cremasteric muscle, can be identified. The cranial portion of the early fetal gubernaculum is completely devoid of striated muscle. Smooth muscle cells are confined to the vessel walls. Collagen and elastic fibers increase in number later in gestation (193). After the testis descends into the scrotum, the gubernaculum undergoes degenerative changes, loses much of the intercellular matrix, and becomes infiltrated by blood vessels, collagen fibers, and striated muscle.

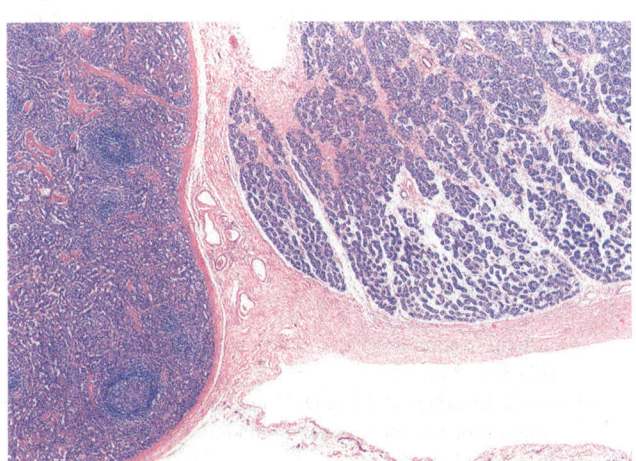

FIGURE 36.49 Splenogonadal fusion of a cryptorchid testis in a 3-year-old child. Spleen is on the *left*, and gonad, on the *right*.

REFERENCES

1. Handelsman DJ, Staraj S. Testicular size: The effects of aging, malnutrition, and illness. *J Androl* 1985;6(3):144–151.
2. Nayak BS. Why the left testis hangs at a lower level than the right? *Med Hypotheses* 2009;73(2):269–270.
3. Kumar A, Kumar CJ. Swinging high and low: Why do the testes hang at different levels? A theory on surface area and thermoregulation. *Med Hypotheses* 2008;70(3):698.
4. Sosnik H, Studies on the participation of tunica albuginea and rete testis (TA and RT) in the quantitative structure of human testis. *Gegenbaurs Morphol Jahrb* 1985;131(3):347–56.
5. Lennox B, Ahmad KN, Mack WS. A method for determining the relative total length of the tubules in the testis. *J Pathol* 1970;102(4):229–238.

6. Papaioannou MD, Pitetti JL, Ro S. Sertoli cell Dicer is essential for spermatogenesis in mice. *Dev Biol* 2009;326(1):250–259.
7. Sharpe RM, McKinnell C, Kivlin C, et al. Proliferation and functional maturation of Sertoli cells, and their relevance to disorders of testis function in adulthood. *Reproduction* 2003;125(6):769–784.
8. Franke FE, Pauls K, Rey R, et al. Differentiation markers of Sertoli cells and germ cells in fetal and early postnatal human testis. *Anat Embryol (Berl)* 2004;209(2):169–177.
9. Vogl A, Vaid K, Guttman J. The Sertoli cell cytoskeleton. In: Cheng C, ed. *Molecular Mechanisms in Spermatogenesis.* Austin: Landes Bioscience and Springer Science; 2008.
10. Nielsen K, Jacobsen GK. Malignant Sertoli cell tumour of the testis. An immunohistochemical study and a review of the literature. *Apmis* 1988. 96(8):755–60.
11. Henley JD, Young RH, Ulbright TM. Malignant Sertoli cell tumors of the testis: A study of 13 examples of a neoplasm frequently misinterpreted as seminoma. *Am J Surg Pathol* 2002;26(5):541–550.
12. Stosiek P, Kasper M, Karsten U. Expression of cytokeratins 8 and 18 in human Sertoli cells of immature and atrophic seminiferous tubules. *Differentiation* 1990;43(1):66–70.
13. Rogatsch H, Jezek D, Hittmair A, et al. Expression of vimentin, cytokeratin, and desmin in Sertoli cells of human fetal, cryptorchid, and tumour-adjacent testicular tissue. *Virchows Arch* 1996;427(5):497–502.
14. Hoei-Hansen CE, Holm M, Rajpert-De Meyts E, et al. Histological evidence of testicular dysgenesis in contralateral biopsies from 218 patients with testicular germ cell cancer. *J Pathol* 2003;200(3):370–374.
15. Suarez-Quian CA, Martínez-García F, Nistal M, et al. Androgen receptor distribution in adult human testis. *J Clin Endocrinol Metab* 1999;84(1):350–358.
16. Emerich DF, Hemendinger R, Halberstadt C R. The testicular-derived Sertoli cell: Cellular immunoscience to enable transplantation. *Cell Transplant* 2003;12(4):335–349.
17. Davidoff MS, Middendorff R, Pusch W, et al. Sertoli and Leydig cells of the human testis express neurofilament triplet proteins. *Histochem Cell Biol* 1999;111(3):173–187.
18. Comperat E, Tissier F, Boyé K, et al. Non-Leydig sex-cord tumors of the testis. The place of immunohistochemistry in diagnosis and prognosis. A study of twenty cases. *Virchows Arch* 2004;444(6):567–571.
19. Fisher JS, Macpherson S, Marchetti N. et al. Human 'testicular dysgenesis syndrome': A possible model using in-utero exposure of the rat to dibutyl phthalate. *Hum Reprod* 2003;18(7):1383–1394.
20. Sangoi AR, McKenney JK, Brooks JD, et al. Evaluation of SF-1 expression in testicular germ cell tumors: A tissue microarray study of 127 cases. *Appl Immunohistochem Mol Morphol* 2013;21(4):318–321.
21. Magers MJ, Udager AM, Chinnaiyan AM, et al. Comprehensive immunophenotypic characterization of adult and fetal testes, the excretory duct system, and testicular and epididymal appendages. *Appl Immunohistochem Mol Morphol* 2016;24(7):e50–e68.
22. Mesa H, Gilles S, Datta MW, et al. Comparative immunomorphology of testicular Sertoli and sertoliform tumors. *Hum Pathol* 2017;61:181–189.
23. Banco B, Palmieri C, Sironi G, et al. Immunohistochemical expression of SOX9 protein in immature, mature, and neoplastic canine Sertoli cells. *Theriogenology* 2016;85(8):1408–1414.e1.
24. Bowles J, Koopman P. Sex determination in mammalian germ cells: Extrinsic versus intrinsic factors. *Reproduction* 2010;139(6):943–958.
25. Schulze C. Sertoli cells and Leydig cells in man. *Adv Anat Embryol Cell Biol* 1984;88:1–104.
26. Mruk DD, Cheng CY. Tight junctions in the testis: New perspectives. *Philos Trans R Soc Lond B Biol Sci* 2010;365(1546):1621–1635.
27. Lui WY, et al. Sertoli cell tight junction dynamics: Their regulation during spermatogenesis. *Biol Reprod* 2003;68(4):1087–1097.
28. Kopera IA, Bilinska B, Yan Cheng C, et al. Sertoli-germ cell junctions in the testis: A review of recent data. *Philos Trans R Soc Lond B Biol Sci* 2010;365(1546):1593–1605.
29. Wilhelm D, Palmer S, Koopman P. Sex determination and gonadal development in mammals. *Physiol Rev* 2007;87(1):1–28.
30. Amann RP, The cycle of the seminiferous epithelium in humans: A need to revisit? *J Androl* 2008. 29(5):469–487.
31. Hadziselimovic F. Cryptorchidism. Ultrastructure of normal and cryptorchid testis development. *Adv Anat Embryol Cell Biol* 1977;53(3):3–71.
32. Nagano T. The crystalloid of Lubarsch in the human spermatogonium. *Z Zellforsch Mikrosk Anat* 1969;97(4):491–501.
33. Clermont Y. Kinetics of spermatogenesis in mammals: Seminiferous epithelium cycle and spermatogonial renewal. *Physiol Rev* 1972;52(1):198–236.
34. Hermann BP, Sukhwani M, Hansel MC, et al. Spermatogonial stem cells in higher primates: Are there differences from those in rodents? *Reproduction* 2010;139(3):479–493.
35. Tokuda M, Kadokawa Y, Kurahashi H, et al. CDH1 is a specific marker for undifferentiated spermatogonia in mouse testes. *Biol Reprod* 2007;76(1):130–141.
36. Niedenberger BA, Busada JT, Geyer CB, Marker expression reveals heterogeneity of spermatogonia in the neonatal mouse testis. *Reproduction* 2015;149(4):329–338.
37. Oatley MJ, Kaucher AV, Racicot KE, et al. Inhibitor of DNA binding 4 is expressed selectively by single spermatogonia in the male germline and regulates the self-renewal of spermatogonial stem cells in mice. *Biol Reprod* 2011;85(2):347–356.
38. Song HW, Wilkinson MF. Transcriptional control of spermatogonial maintenance and differentiation. *Semin Cell Dev Biol* 2014;30:14–26.
39. Wu X, Schmidt JA, Avarbock MR, et al. Prepubertal human spermatogonia and mouse gonocytes share conserved gene expression of germline stem cell regulatory molecules. *Proc Natl Acad Sci U S A* 2009;106(51):21672–21677.
40. Kaucher AV, Oatley MJ, Oatley JM, NEUROG3 is a critical downstream effector for STAT3-regulated differentiation of mammalian stem and progenitor spermatogonia. *Biol Reprod* 2012;86(5):164, 1–11.
41. Suzuki H, Ahn HW, Chu T, et al. SOHLH1 and SOHLH2 coordinate spermatogonial differentiation. *Dev Biol* 2012;361(2):301–312.
42. Caires K, Broady J, McLean D. Maintaining the male germline: Regulation of spermatogonial stem cells. *J Endocrinol* 2010;205(2):133–145.
43. Gondos B Ultrastructure of developing and malignant germ cells. *Eur Urol* 1993;23(1):68–74; discussion 75.

44. Nihi F, Gomes MLM, Carvalho FAR, et al. Revisiting the human seminiferous epithelium cycle. *Hum Reprod* 2017; 32(6):1170–1182.
45. Kerr JB, de Kretser D. The cytology of the human testis. In: Burger M, de Kretser D, eds. *The Testis*. New York: Raven Press; 1981.
46. Heller CH, Clermont Y. Kinetics of the germinal epithelium in man. *Recent Prog Horm Res* 1964;20:545–575.
47. Bartke A. Apoptosis of male germ cells, a generalized or a cell type-specific phenomenon? *Endocrinology* 1995;136(1):3–4.
48. Johnson L, Zane RS, Petty CS, et al. Quantification of the human Sertoli cell population: Its distribution, relation to germ cell numbers, and age-related decline. *Biol Reprod* 1984; 31(4):785–795.
49. Weissbach L, Ibach B. Quantitative parameters for light microscopic assessment of the tubuli seminiferi. *Fertil Steril* 1976;27(7):836–847.
50. Zukerman Z, Rodriguez-Rigau LJ, Weiss DB, et al. Quantitative analysis of the seminiferous epithelium in human testicular biopsies, and the relation of spermatogenesis to sperm density. *Fertil Steril* 1978;30(4):448–455.
51. de Kretser DM, Kerr JB, Paulsen CA, The peritubular tissue in the normal and pathological human testis. An ultrastructural study. *Biol Reprod* 1975. 12(3):317–24.
52. McLachlan RI, Rajpert-De Meyts E, Hoei-Hansen CE, et al. Histological evaluation of the human testis—approaches to optimizing the clinical value of the assessment: Mini review. *Hum Reprod* 2007;22(1):2–16.
53. Skakkebaek NE, Heller CG. Quantification of human seminiferous epithelium. I. Histological studies in twenty-one fertile men with normal chromosome complements. *J Reprod Fertil* 1973;32(3):379–389.
54. Silber SJ, Rodriguez-Rigau LJ. Quantitative analysis of testicle biopsy: Determination of partial obstruction and prediction of sperm count after surgery for obstruction. *Fertil Steril* 1981;36(4):480–485.
55. Potter SJ, DeFalco T. Role of the testis interstitial compartment in spermatogonial stem cell function. *Reproduction* 2017;153(4):R151–R162.
56. Arenas MI, Bethencourt FR, De Miguel MP, et al. Immunocytochemical and quantitative study of actin, desmin and vimentin in the peritubular cells of the testes from elderly men. *J Reprod Fertil* 1997. 110(1):183–193.
57. Albrecht M. Insights into the nature of human testicular peritubular cells. *Ann Anat* 2009;191(6):532–540.
58. Welsh M, Saunders PT, Atanassova N, et al. Androgen action via testicular peritubular myoid cells is essential for male fertility. *FASEB J* 2009;23(12):4218–4230.
59. Spinnler K, Köhn FM, Schwarzer U, et al. Glial cell line-derived neurotrophic factor is constitutively produced by human testicular peritubular cells and may contribute to the spermatogonial stem cell niche in man. *Hum Reprod* 2010;25(9):2181–2187.
60. Chen LY, Willis WD, Eddy EM, Targeting the Gdnf Gene in peritubular myoid cells disrupts undifferentiated spermatogonial cell development. *Proc Natl Acad Sci U S A* 2016; 113(7):1829–1834.
61. Siu MK, Cheng CY, Extracellular matrix: Recent advances on its role in junction dynamics in the seminiferous epithelium during spermatogenesis. *Biol Reprod* 2004;71(2):375–391.
62. Miller SC, Bowman BM, Rowland HG. Structure, cytochemistry, endocytic activity, and immunoglobulin (Fc) receptors of rat testicular interstitial-tissue macrophages. *Am J Anat* 1983;168(1):1–13.
63. Cheng CY, Wong EW, Yan HH, et al. Regulation of spermatogenesis in the microenvironment of the seminiferous epithelium: New insights and advances. *Mol Cell Endocrinol* 2010;315(1-2):49–56.
64. DeFalco T, Potter SJ, Williams AV, et al. Macrophages contribute to the spermatogonial niche in the adult testis. *Cell Rep* 2015. 12(7):1107–1119.
65. De Menezes AP. Elastic tissue in the limiting membrane of the human seminiferous tubule. *Am J Anat* 1977;150(2):349–373.
66. Nistal M, Paniagua R. Non-neoplastic disease of the testis. In: Bostwick D, Eble J, eds. *Urologic Surgical Pathology*. St. Louis, MO: Mosby; 1997.
67. Amat P, Paniagua R, Nistal M, et al. Mitosis in adult human Leydig cells. *Cell Tissue Res* 1986;243(1):219–221.
68. Tanaka T, Kanatsu-Shinohara M, Lei Z, et al. The luteinizing hormone-testosterone pathway regulates mouse spermatogonial stem cell self-renewal by suppressing WNT5A expression in Sertoli cells. *Stem Cell Reports* 2016;7(2):279–291.
69. Jun SY, Ro JY, Park YW, et al. Ectopic Leydig cells of testis: An immunohistochemical study on tissue microarray. *Ann Diagn Pathol* 2008;12(1):29–32.
70. Nistal M, Paniagua R. Histogenesis of human extraparenchymal Leydig cells. *Acta Anat (Basel)* 1979;105(2):188–197.
71. Paner GP, Kristiansen G, McKenney JK, et al. Rete testis-associated nodular steroid cell nests: Description of putative pluripotential testicular hilus steroid cells. *Am J Surg Pathol* 2011;35(4):505–511.
72. Nagano T, Otsuki I. Reinvestigation of the fine structure of Reinke's crystal in the human testicular interstitial cell. *J Cell Biol* 1971;51(1):148–161.
73. Smith LB, Walker WH. The regulation of spermatogenesis by androgens. *Semin Cell Dev Biol* 2014;30:2–13.
74. Schlatt S, Ehmcke J. Regulation of spermatogenesis: An evolutionary biologist's perspective. *Semin Cell Dev Biol* 2014;29:2–16.
75. Wen Q, Cheng CY, Liu YX. Development, function and fate of fetal Leydig cells. *Semin Cell Dev Biol* 2016;59:89–98.
76. Heller CG, Lalli MF, Pearson JE, et al. A method for the quantification of Leydig cells in man. *J Reprod Fertil* 1971; 25(2):177–184.
77. Weiss DB, Rodriguez-Rigau L, Smith KD, et al. Quantitation of Leydig cells in testicular biopsies of oligospermic men with varicocele. *Fertil Steril* 1978;30(3):305–312.
78. Hashimoto J, Yamamoto M, Miyake K, et al. A morphological study of the testis in patients with idiopathic male infertility—quantification and ultrastructure of Leydig cells. *Hinyokika Kiyo* 1988;34(11):1995–2011.
79. Soerensen RR, Johannsen TH, Skakkebaek NE, et al. Leydig cell clustering and Reinke crystal distribution in relation to hormonal function in adult patients with testicular dysgenesis syndrome (TDS) including cryptorchidism. *Hormones (Athens)* 2016;15(4):518–526.
80. Holm M, Rajpert-De Meyts E, Andersson AM, et al. Leydig cell micronodules are a common finding in testicular biopsies from men with impaired spermatogenesis and are associated with decreased testosterone/LH ratio. *J Pathol* 2003;199(3):378–386.

81. Cao QJ, Jones JG, Li M. Expression of calretinin in human ovary, testis, and ovarian sex cord-stromal tumors. *Int J Gynecol Pathol* 2001;20(4):346–352.
82. Anand-Ivell RJ, Relan V, Balvers M, et al. Expression of the insulin-like peptide 3 (INSL3) hormone-receptor (LGR8) system in the testis. *Biol Reprod* 2006;74(5):945–953.
83. Davidoff MS, Middendorff R, Köfüncü E, et al. Leydig cells of the human testis possess astrocyte and oligodendrocyte marker molecules. *Acta Histochem* 2002;104(1):39–49.
84. Davidoff MS, Middendorff R, Müller D, et al. The neuroendocrine Leydig cells and their stem cell progenitors, the pericytes. *Adv Anat Embryol Cell Biol* 2009;205:1–107.
85. Ulbright TM, Srigley JR, Hatzianastassiou DK, et al. Leydig cell tumors of the testis with unusual features: Adipose differentiation, calcification with ossification, and spindle-shaped tumor cells. *Am J Surg Pathol* 2002;26(11):1424–1433.
86. Holash JA, Harik SI, Perry G, et al. Barrier properties of testis microvessels. *Proc Natl Acad Sci U S A* 1993;90(23):11069–11073.
87. Lobo MV, Arenas MI, Alonso FJ, et al. Nestin, a neuroectodermal stem cell marker molecule, is expressed in Leydig cells of the human testis and in some specific cell types from human testicular tumours. *Cell Tissue Res* 2004;316(3):369–376.
88. Mostafa T, Labib I, El-Khayat Y, et al. Human testicular arterial supply: Gross anatomy, corrosion cast, and radiologic study. *Fertil Steril* 2008;90(6):2226–2230.
89. Jarow JP. Intratesticular arterial anatomy. *J Androl* 1990;11(3):255–259.
90. Kormano M, Suoranta H, Reijonen K. Blood supply to testis and excurrent ducts. In: Raspe G, ed. *Advances in Biosciences*. Vol. 10. Oxford, England: Pergamon Press; 1972.
91. Ergun S, Stingl J, Holstein AF. Segmental angioarchitecture of the testicular lobule in man. *Andrologia* 1994;26(3):143–150.
92. Andres TL, Trainer TD, Lapenas DJ. Small vessel alterations in the testes of infertile men with varicocele. *Am J Clin Pathol* 1981;76(4):378–384.
93. Fawcett DW, Leak LV, Heidger PM, Jr., Electron microscopic observations on the structural components of the blood-testis barrier. *J Reprod Fertil Suppl* 1970;10:105–122.
94. Ergun S, Davidoff M, Holstein AF. Capillaries in the lamina propria of human seminiferous tubules are partly fenestrated. *Cell Tissue Res* 1996;286(1):93–102.
95. Chan F, Oatley MJ, Kaucher AV, et al. Functional and molecular features of the Id4+ germline stem cell population in mouse testes. *Genes Dev* 2014;28(12):1351–1362.
96. Nowak DG, Woolard J, Amin EM, et al. Expression of pro- and anti-angiogenic isoforms of VEGF is differentially regulated by splicing and growth factors. *J Cell Sci* 2008;121(Pt 20):3487–3495.
97. Holstein AF, Orlandini GE, Moller R. Distribution and fine structure of the lymphatic system in the human testis. *Cell Tissue Res* 1979;200(1):15–27.
98. McLaren A. Primordial germ cells in the mouse. *Dev Biol* 2003;262(1):1–15.
99. Figueira MI, Cardoso HJ, Correia S, et al. Hormonal regulation of c-KIT receptor and its ligand: Implications for human infertility? *Prog Histochem Cytochem* 2014;49(1-3):1–19.
100. Kerr CL, Hill CM, Blumenthal PD, et al. Expression of pluripotent stem cell markers in the human fetal testis. *Stem Cells* 2008;26(2):412–421.
101. Culty M. Gonocytes, the forgotten cells of the germ cell lineage. *Birth Defects Res C Embryo Today* 2009;87(1):1–26.
102. Wartenberg H. Comparative cytomorphologic aspects of the male germ cells, especially of the "Gonia". *Andrologia* 1976;8(2):117–130.
103. Fukuda T, Hedinger C, Groscurth P. Ultrastructure of developing germ cells in the fetal human testis. *Cell Tissue Res* 1975;161(1):55–70.
104. Gaskell TL, Esnal A, Robinson LL, et al. Immunohistochemical profiling of germ cells within the human fetal testis: Identification of three subpopulations. *Biol Reprod* 2004;71(6):2012–2021.
105. Sharpe RM, Environmental/lifestyle effects on spermatogenesis. *Philos Trans R Soc Lond B Biol Sci* 2010;365(1546):1697–1712.
106. Hadziselimovic F, Thommen L, Girard J, et al. The significance of postnatal gonadotropin surge for testicular development in normal and cryptorchid testes. *J Urol* 1986;136(1 Pt 2):274–276.
107. Chemes HE. Infancy is not a quiescent period of testicular development. *Int J Androl* 2001;24(1):2–7.
108. Nistal M, Paniagua R, Queizan A. Histologic lesions in undescended ectopic obstructed testes. *Fertil Steril* 1985;43(3):455–462.
109. Weaver JR, Susiarjo M, Bartolomei MS. Imprinting and epigenetic changes in the early embryo. *Mamm Genome* 2009;20(9-10):532–543.
110. Kerjean A, Dupont JM, Vasseur C, et al. Establishment of the paternal methylation imprint of the human H19 and MEST/PEG1 genes during spermatogenesis. *Hum Mol Genet* 2000;9(14):2183–2187.
111. Laprise SL. Implications of epigenetics and genomic imprinting in assisted reproductive technologies. *Mol Reprod Dev* 2009;76(11):1006–1018.
112. Furukawa S, Haruta M, Arai Y, et al. Yolk sac tumor but not seminoma or teratoma is associated with abnormal epigenetic reprogramming pathway and shows frequent hypermethylation of various tumor suppressor genes. *Cancer Sci* 2009;100(4):698–708.
113. Boissonnas CC, Abdalaoui HE, Haelewyn V, et al. Specific epigenetic alterations of IGF2-H19 locus in spermatozoa from infertile men. *Eur J Hum Genet* 2010;18(1):73–80.
114. Aflatoonian B, Moore H. Germ cells from mouse and human embryonic stem cells. *Reproduction* 2006;132(5):699–707.
115. Mitchell RT, Cowan G, Morris KD, et al. Germ cell differentiation in the marmoset (Callithrix jacchus) during fetal and neonatal life closely parallels that in the human. *Hum Reprod* 2008;23(12):2755–2765.
116. Stoop H, Honecker F, van de Geijn GJ, et al. Stem cell factor as a novel diagnostic marker for early malignant germ cells. *J Pathol* 2008;216(1):43–54.
117. Kaprova-Pleskacova J, Stoop H, Brüggenwirth H, et al. Complete androgen insensitivity syndrome: Factors influencing gonadal histology including germ cell pathology. *Mod Pathol* 2014;27(5):721–730.
118. Oram SW, Liu XX, Lee TL, et al. TSPY potentiates cell proliferation and tumorigenesis by promoting cell cycle progression in HeLa and NIH3T3 cells. *BMC Cancer* 2006;6(1):154.
119. Oosterhuis JW, Stoop H, Dohle G, et al. A pathologist's view on the testis biopsy. *Int J Androl* 2011;34(4 Pt 2):e14–e19; discussion e20.

120. Honecker F, Stoop H, de Krijger RR, et al. Pathobiological implications of the expression of markers of testicular carcinoma in situ by fetal germ cells. *J Pathol* 2004;203(3):849–857.
121. Mitchell RT, Saunders PT, Childs AJ, et al. Xenografting of human fetal testis tissue: a new approach to study fetal testis development and germ cell differentiation. *Hum Reprod* 2010;25(10):2405–2414.
122. Berney DM, Lee A, Randle SJ, et al. The frequency of intratubular embryonal carcinoma: Implications for the pathogenesis of germ cell tumours. *Histopathology* 2004;45(2):155–161.
123. Emerson RE, Ulbright TM. Intratubular germ cell neoplasia of the testis and its associated cancers: The use of novel biomarkers. *Pathology* 2010;42(4):344–355.
124. Xiao GQ, Priemer DS, Wei C, et al. ZBTB16 is a sensitive and specific marker in detection of metastatic and extragonadal yolk sac tumour. *Histopathology* 2017;71(4):562–569.
125. Osman H, Cheng L, Ulbright TM, et al. The utility of CDX2, GATA3, and DOG1 in the diagnosis of testicular neoplasms: An immunohistochemical study of 109 cases. *Hum Pathol* 2016;48:18–24.
126. Svechnikov K, Landreh L, Weisser J, et al. Origin, development and regulation of human Leydig cells. *Horm Res Paediatr* 2010;73(2):93–101.
127. Griswold SL, Behringer RR. Fetal Leydig cell origin and development. *Sex Dev* 2009;3(1):1–15.
128. O'Shaughnessy PJ, Baker PJ, Johnston H. The foetal Leydig cell—differentiation, function and regulation. *Int J Androl* 2006;29(1):90–95; discussion 105–8.
129. Nistal M, Paniagua R, Regadera J, et al. A quantitative morphological study of human Leydig cells from birth to adulthood. *Cell Tissue Res* 1986;246(2):229–236.
130. Wu X, Wan S, Lee MM. Key factors in the regulation of fetal and postnatal Leydig cell development. *J Cell Physiol* 2007;213(2):429–433.
131. Muller J, Skakkebaek NE. Quantification of germ cells and seminiferous tubules by stereological examination of testicles from 50 boys who suffered from sudden death. *Int J Androl* 1983;6(2):143–156.
132. Brehm R, Rey R, Kliesch S, et al. Mitotic activity of Sertoli cells in adult human testis: An immunohistochemical study to characterize Sertoli cells in testicular cords from patients showing testicular dysgenesis syndrome. *Anat Embryol (Berl)* 2006;211(3):223–236.
133. Kao CS, Idrees MT, Young RH, et al. "Dissecting Gonadoblastoma" of Scully: A Morphologic Variant That Often Mimics Germinoma. *Am J Surg Pathol* 2016;40(10):1417–1423.
134. Cortes D, Muller J, Skakkebaek NE. Proliferation of Sertoli cells during development of the human testis assessed by stereological methods. *Int J Androl* 1987;10(4):589–596.
135. Waters BL, Trainer TD. Development of the human fetal testis. *Pediatr Pathol Lab Med* 1996;16(1):9–23.
136. Well D, Yang H, Houseni M, et al. Age-related structural and metabolic changes in the pelvic reproductive end organs. *Semin Nucl Med* 2007;37(3):173–184.
137. Paniagua R, Nistal M, Amat P, et al. Seminiferous tubule involution in elderly men. *Biol Reprod* 1987;36(4):939–947.
138. Suoranta H. Changes in the small blood vessels of the adult human testis in relation to age and to some pathological conditions. *Virchows Arch A Pathol Pathol Anat* 1971;352(2):165–181.
139. Kothari LK, Gupta AS. Effect of ageing on the volume, structure and total Leydig cell content of the human testis. *Int J Fertil* 1974;19(3):140–146.
140. Kaler LW, Neaves WB. Attrition of the human Leydig cell population with advancing age. *Anat Rec* 1978;192(4):513–518.
141. Neaves WB, Johnson L, Petty CS. Seminiferous tubules and daily sperm production in older adult men with varied numbers of Leydig cells. *Biol Reprod* 1987;36(2):301–308.
142. Rowley MJ, Heller CG. Quantitation of the cells of the seminiferous epithelium of the human testis employing the sertoli cell as a constant. *Z Zellforsch Mikrosk Anat* 1971;115(4):461–472.
143. Steinberger A, Steinberger E. Replication pattern of Sertoli cells in maturing rat testis in vivo and in organ culture. *Biol Reprod* 1971;4(1):84–87.
144. de Miguel MP, Bethencourt FR, Arenas MI, et al. Intermediate filaments in the Sertoli cells of the ageing human testis. *Virchows Arch* 1997;431(2):131–138.
145. Roosen-Runge EC, Holstein AF. The human rete testis. *Cell Tissue Res* 1978;189(3):409–433.
146. Srigley JR. The paratesticular region: Histoanatomic and general considerations. *Semin Diagn Pathol* 2000;17(4):258–269.
147. Dinges HP, Zatloukal K, Schmid C, et al. Co-expression of cytokeratin and vimentin filaments in rete testis and epididymis. An immunohistochemical study. *Virchows Arch A Pathol Anat Histopathol* 1991;418(2):119–127.
148. Rubegni P, Poggiali S, De Santi M, et al. Cutaneous metastases from adenocarcinoma of the rete testis. *J Cutan Pathol* 2006;33(2):181–184.
149. Hartwick RW, Ro JY, Srigley JR, et al. Adenomatous hyperplasia of the rete testis. A clinicopathologic study of nine cases. *Am J Surg Pathol* 1991;15(4):350–357.
150. Jones EC, Murray SK, Young RH, Cysts and epithelial proliferations of the testicular collecting system (including rete testis). *Semin Diagn Pathol* 2000;17(4):270–293.
151. Hittmair A, Zelger BG, Obrist P, et al. Ovarian Sertoli-Leydig cell tumor: A SRY gene-independent pathway of pseudomale gonadal differentiation. *Hum Pathol* 1997;28(10):1206–1210.
152. Sapino A, Pagani A, Godano A, et al. Effects of estrogens on the testis of transsexuals: A pathological and immunocytochemical study. *Virchows Arch A Pathol Anat Histopathol* 1987;411(5):409–414.
153. Hinton BT, Keefer DA. Evidence for protein absorption from the lumen of the seminiferous tubule and rete of the rat testis. *Cell Tissue Res* 1983;230(2):367–75.
154. Saitoh K, Terada T, Hatakeyama S. A morphological study of the efferent ducts of the human epididymis. *Int J Androl* 1990;13(5):369–376.
155. Shah VI, Ro JY, Amin MB, et al. Histologic variations in the epididymis: Findings in 167 orchiectomy specimens. *Am J Surg Pathol* 1998;22(8):990–996.
156. Rowley MJ, Teshima F, Heller CG. Duration of transit of spermatozoa through the human male ductular system. *Fertil Steril* 1970;21(5):390–396.
157. Hinrichsen MJ, Blaquier JA. Evidence supporting the existence of sperm maturation in the human epididymis. *J Reprod Fertil* 1980;60(2):291–294.
158. Regadera J, Cobo P, Paniagua R, et al. Immunohistochemical and semiquantitative study of the apical mitochondria-rich cells of the human prepubertal and adult epididymis. *J Anat* 1993;183(Pt 3):507–514.

159. Dube E, Dufresne J, Chan PT, et al. Assessing the role of claudins in maintaining the integrity of epididymal tight junctions using novel human epididymal cell lines. *Biol Reprod* 2010;82(6):1119–1128.
160. Kasper M, Stosiek P. Immunohistochemical investigation of different cytokeratins and vimentin in the human epididymis from the fetal period up to adulthood. *Cell Tissue Res* 1989;257(3):661–664.
161. De Miguel MP, Mariño JM, Gonzalez-Peramato P, et al. Epididymal growth and differentiation are altered in human cryptorchidism. *J Androl* 2001;22(2):212–225.
162. Cerilli LA, Sotelo-Avila C, Mills SE. Glandular inclusions in inguinal hernia sacs: Morphologic and immunohistochemical distinction from epididymis and vas deferens. *Am J Surg Pathol* 2003;27(4):469–476.
163. Lee LY, Tzeng J, Grosman M, et al. Prostate gland-like epithelium in the epididymis: A case report and review of the literature. *Arch Pathol Lab Med* 2004;128(4):e60–e62.
164. Rajalakshmi M, Kumar BV, Kapur MM, et al. Ultrastructural changes in the efferent duct and epididymis of men with obstructive infertility. *Anat Rec* 1993;237(2):199–207.
165. Oliva E, Young RH. Paratesticular tumor-like lesions. *Semin Diagn Pathol* 2000;17(4):340–358.
166. Madara JL, Haggitt RC, Federman M. Intranuclear inclusions of the human vas deferens. *Arch Pathol Lab Med* 1978;102(12):648–650.
167. Nistal M, Santamaria L, Paniagua R. Mast cells in the human testis and epididymis from birth to adulthood. *Acta Anat (Basel)* 1984;119(3):155–160.
168. Nozawa T, Konda R, Ohsawa T, et al. Clear cell papillary cystadenocarcinoma of the epididymis: A case report and immunohistochemistry of markers for renal cell carcinoma. *Histol Histopathol* 2013;28(3):321–326.
169. Yu CC, Huang JK, Chiang H, et al. Papillary cystadenocarcinoma of the epididymis: A case report and review of the literature. *J Urol* 1992;147(1):162–165.
170. Soria Gondek A, Julià Masip V, Jou Muñoz C, et al. Adolescent hydrocele carrying a surprise: A case of papillary cystadenoma of the epididymis. *Urology* 2017.
171. Paniagua R, Regadera J, Nistal M, et al. Histological, histochemical and ultrastructural variations along the length of the human vas deferens before and after puberty. *Acta Anat (Basel)* 1982;111(3):190–203.
172. Paniagua R, Regadera J, Nistal M, et al. Elastic fibres of the human ductus deferens. *J Anat* 1983;137(Pt 3):467–476.
173. Murakami M, Nishida T, Shiromoto M, et al. Scanning and transmission electron microscopic study of the ampullary region of the dog vas deferens, with special reference to epithelial phagocytosis of spermatozoa and latex beads. *Anat Anz* 1986;162(4):289–296.
174. Shah RB, Lee MW, Giraldo AA, et al. Histologic and histochemical characterization of seminal vesicle intraluminal secretions. *Arch Pathol Lab Med* 2001;125(1):141–145.
175. Shidham VB, Lindholm PF, Kajdacsy-Balla A, et al. Prostate-specific antigen expression and lipochrome pigment granules in the differential diagnosis of prostatic adenocarcinoma versus seminal vesicle-ejaculatory duct epithelium. *Arch Pathol Lab Med* 1999;123(11):1093–1097.
176. Kuo T, Gomez LG. Monstrous epithelial cells in human epididymis and seminal vesicles. A pseudomalignant change. *Am J Surg Pathol* 1981;5(5):483–490.
177. Kovi J, Jackson MA, Akberzie ME. Unusual smooth muscle change in the prostate. *Arch Pathol Lab Med* 1979;103(4):204–205.
178. Linke RP, Joswig R, Murphy CL, et al. Senile seminal vesicle amyloid is derived from semenogelin I. *J Lab Clin Med* 2005;145(4):187–193.
179. Rath-Wolfson L, Bubis G, Shtrasburg S, et al. Seminal tract amyloidosis: Synchronous amyloidosis of the seminal vesicles, deferent ducts and ejaculatory ducts. *Pathol Oncol Res* 2017;23(4):811–814.
180. McNeal JE. Normal histology of the prostate. *Am J Surg Pathol* 1988;12(8):619–633.
181. Tong GX, Memeo L, Colarossi C, et al. PAX8 and PAX2 immunostaining facilitates the diagnosis of primary epithelial neoplasms of the male genital tract. *Am J Surg Pathol* 2011;35(10):1473–1483.
182. Rolnick D, Kawanoue S, Szanto P, et al. Anatomical incidence of testicular appendages. *J Urol* 1968;100(6):755–756.
183. Sahni D, Jit I, Joshi K, et al. Incidence and structure of the appendices of the testis and epididymis. *J Anat* 1996;189(Pt 2):341–348.
184. Skoglund RW, McRoberts JW, Ragde H. Torsion of testicular appendages: Presentation of 43 new cases and a collective review. *J Urol* 1970;104(4):598–600.
185. Samnakay N, Cohen RJ, Orford J, et al. Androgen and oestrogen receptor status of the human appendix testis. *Pediatr Surg Int* 2003;19(7):520–524.
186. Sadler T. *Langman's medical embryology*. 7th ed. Baltimore, MD: Williams & Wilkins; 1995.
187. Whitehead ED, Leiter E. Genital abnormalities and abnormal semen analyses in male patients exposed to diethylstilbestrol in utero. *J Urol* 1981;125(1):47–50.
188. Bernstein J, Gardner K. Renal cystic disease and renal dysplasia. In: Walsh P, ed. *Campbell's Urology*. 5th ed. Vol. 2. Philadelphia, PA: WB Saunders; 1986.
189. Popek EJ. Embryonal remnants in inguinal hernia sacs. *Hum Pathol* 1990;21(3):339–349.
190. Wollin M, Marshall FF, Fink MP, et al. Aberrant epididymal tissue: A significant clinical entity. *J Urol* 1987;138(5):1247–1250.
191. McPherson F, Frias JL, Spicer D, et al. Splenogonadal fusion-limb defect "syndrome" and associated malformations. *Am J Med Genet A* 2003;120a(4):518–522.
192. Nistal M, Frias JL, Spicer D, et al. Age-related epididymis-like intratesticular structures: Benign lesions of Wolffian origin that can be misdiagnosed as testicular tumors. *J Androl* 2006;27(1):79–85.
193. Costa WS, Sampaio FJ, Favorito LA, et al. Testicular migration: Remodeling of connective tissue and muscle cells in human gubernaculum testis. *J Urol* 2002;167(5):2171–2176.

37

Penis and Distal Urethra

Elsa F. Velazquez ■ José E. Barreto ■ Sofía Cañete-Portillo ■ Antonio L. Cubilla

DISTAL PENIS 1009	VEINS 1026
Glans 1009	LYMPHATICS 1026
Coronal Sulcus 1013	NERVES 1026
Foreskin 1013	REFERENCES 1026
PROXIMAL PENIS (OR SHAFT) 1019	
DISTAL URETHRA 1022	
ARTERIES 1025	

Three cylindrical, firmly adherent, tubular erectile tissues (the corpora cavernosa [CC] and the corpus spongiosum) and the pendulous urethra are the basic constituents of the penis that can be subdivided into a distal portion that includes glans, coronal sulcus, and foreskin and a proximal portion, the corpus or shaft (Fig. 37.1) (1). Most of the penile carcinomas arise from the distal portion of the organ (Fig. 37.2).

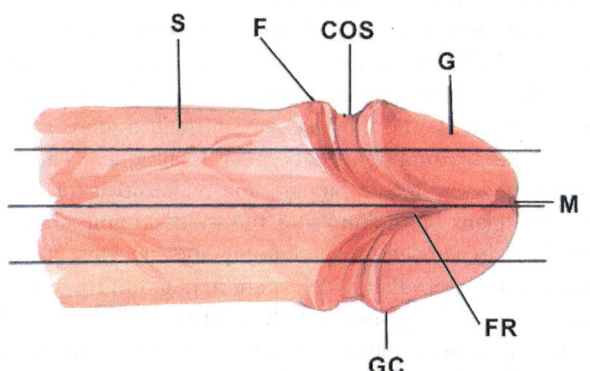

FIGURE 37.1 The penis can be subdivided in a distal portion that includes glans (*G*), coronal sulcus (*COS*), and foreskin (*F*) and a proximal portion, the corpus or shaft (*S*). *M*, urethral meatus; *GC*, glans corona; *FR*, frenulum.

This chapter is an update of a previous version authored by Elsa F. Velazquez, José E. Barreto, and Antonio L. Cubilla.

DISTAL PENIS

Glans

ANATOMIC LEVELS OF THE GLANS

Epithelium
Lamina propria
Corpus spongiosum
Tunica albuginea[a]
Corpus cavernosum[a]

[a]The distal portions of the corpora cavernosa encased by the tunica albuginea are part of the glans in 77% of the cases. The tunica albuginea is part of the corpus cavernosum.

Anatomic Features

The conically shaped glans, covered by a pink smooth mucous membrane, is the most distal portion of the organ and shows in its central and ventral region, the meatus urethralis. The expanded anterior end of the corpus spongiosum, which has the shape of an obtuse cone similar to the cap of a mushroom, is the central and main tissue of the glans. It is molded over and attached to the blunt extremity

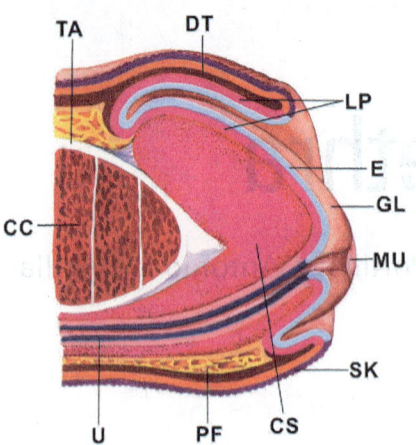

FIGURE 37.2 Diagram illustrating the distal portion of the penis, which includes glans (*GL*), coronal sulcus, and foreskin. *E*, epithelium; *LP*, lamina propria; *CS*, corpus spongiosum; *TA*, tunica albuginea; *CC*, corpus cavernosum; *DT*, dartos; *SK*, skin; *U*, urethra; *MU*, meatus urethralis; *PF*, penile, or Buck fascia.

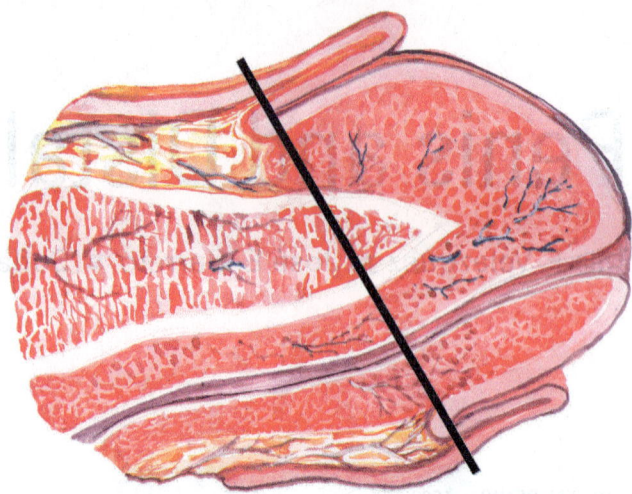

FIGURE 37.3 The distal portion of corpora cavernosa encased by the tunica albuginea is part of the glans in the majority of cases. The diagonal line passing through the coronal sulcus divides glans from shaft.

of the CC and extends farther over their dorsal than their ventral surfaces (1). The base of this conus is an elevated rim or border, the corona, occupying 80% of the circumferential head of the glans; it is interrupted in the ventral portion of the glans by the mucosal fold of the frenulum (Fig. 37.1). The diameter of the corona is wider than the shaft and the remainder of the glans. Within the corpus spongiosum, there is the distal portion of the urethra that opens at the summit of the glans as a vertical, slit-like external orifice termed the urethral meatus (Figs. 37.1 and 37.2). Anatomical structures frequently found in sexually active males and located in the proximal glans are called pearly penile papules, hirsutoid papillomas, or papillomatosis corona penis or glandis (2–5). Grossly, they appear as 1 to 3 mm skin-colored, domed papules evenly distributed circumferentially around the corona and extending proximally on each side of the frenulum. They may be mistaken for warts and be the source of much anxiety for worried adolescents (2).

Considering the glans as the tissues distal to a line passing through the coronal sulcus, the distal portions of the CC encased by the tunica albuginea extend out into the glans in approximately 77% of the cases (Fig. 37.3) (6). However, since they are the main constituents of the shaft, they are discussed in detail in that section.

It is important for the surgical pathologists to grossly recognize the cut surface anatomical levels of the glans. The epithelium is thin, soft, and white-gray. When hyperplastic, it is brightly white contrasting with the darker tissues below. Lamina propria is white-pink, and measures from 1 to 4 mm in thickness contrasting with the darker reddish color of the highly vascular corpus spongiosum. The tunica albuginea is a thick white fibrous tissue separating corpora spongiosa from cavernosa. There is a correlation of regional tumor spread and involvement of the various anatomical levels of the glans and corpus. Lymph node metastasis is very unusual in tumors involving only lamina propria and common for tumors invading CC (7,8).

Microscopic and Immunohistochemical Features

› **EPITHELIUM** Both circumcised and uncircumcised men have partially keratinized stratified squamous epithelium of five to six layers thick (Fig. 37.4). Some textbooks state that the glans squamous epithelium in circumcised men is thicker and more keratinized than the epithelium of uncircumcised individuals but well-controlled studies to support this are lacking. The normal squamous epithelium is usually positive for the cytokeratins AE1/AE3 and 34βE12. It is negative for the cytokeratins CAM5.2, CK7, and CK20. Expression of p63 is seen in basal/suprabasal cells. Langerhans cells are found scattered among keratinocytes, and they are increased in number in different inflammatory conditions. Langerhans cells express S100 protein, CD4, CD1a, and Langerin (Fig. 37.5). Rarely Merkel cells are also present, and they are very difficult to demonstrate by routine or immunohistochemical techniques. They are usually negative for chromogranin and positive for CK20 (9). The glans epithelium and the mucosal epithelium of the foreskin appear to not contain melanocytes (10,11). Rarely, mucus-producing cells can be noted in the perimeatal region of the glans epithelium (12). They may be the source of the adenosquamous carcinoma of the glans penis. Intraepithelial free nerves ending close to the surface of the epithelium are noted (13). No adnexal or glandular structures are present in the glans. Histologically, the pearly penile papules appear like fibrovascular papillary projections lined by squamous epithelium (Fig. 37.6) (2). No koilocytosis is seen in these structures.

› **LAMINA PROPRIA** The lamina propria is the prolongation of the foreskin lamina propria and separates the corpus

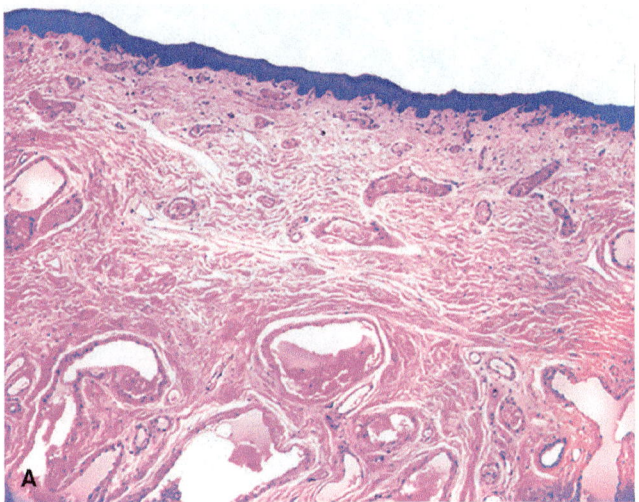
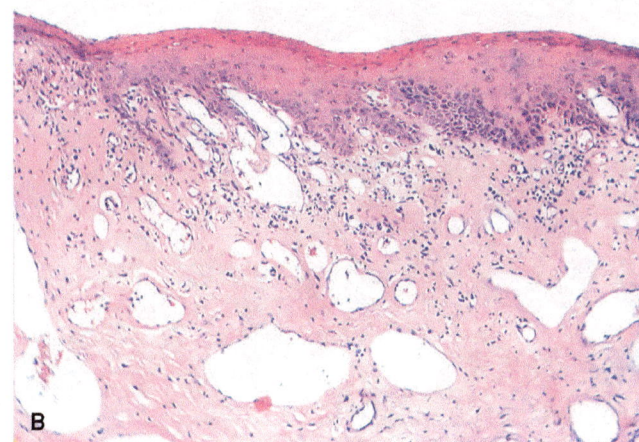

FIGURE 37.4 **A** and **B**: Low- and higher-power views of glans. The three layers of the glans are noted: partially keratinized stratified squamous epithelium, lamina propria, and corpus spongiosum.

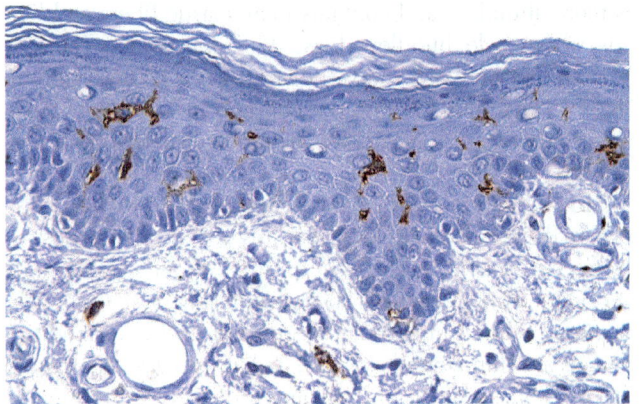

FIGURE 37.5 CD1a immunostain highlights the presence of scattered Langerhans cells in the glans epithelium.

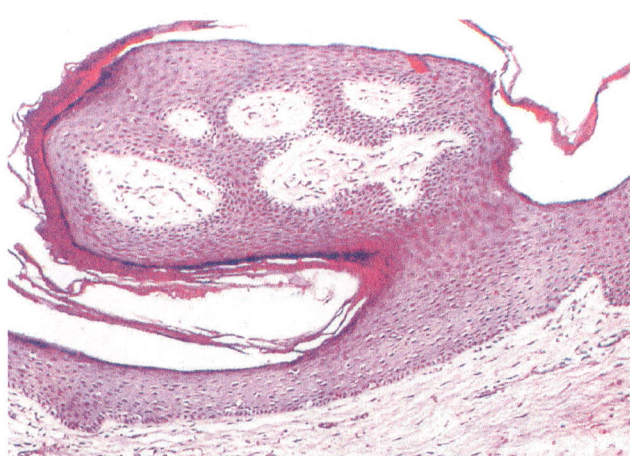

FIGURE 37.6 Pearly penile papule appears histologically as a papillary structure with a fibrovascular core lined by squamous epithelium with no evidence of koilocytosis.

spongiosum from the glans epithelium. In the glans, the loose connective tissue of the penile fascia and the fibrous tunica albuginea are lacking so that the lamina propria adheres firmly to the underlying corpus spongiosum (Fig. 37.4) (14). The connective tissue of the lamina propria is somewhat similar to that of the corpus spongiosum, although it is more compact and contains fewer peripheral nerve bundles and elastic fibers than the erectile structure. The transition between lamina propria and corpus spongiosum is sometimes difficult to determine at medium or high magnifications. However, at low power or even after a careful gross inspection or with a magnifying lens, this delimitation is evident and follows a line corresponding to the geographic limit of the extension of venous sinuses of the corpus spongiosum. The thickness of the lamina propria varies from 1 mm at the glans corona to 2.5 mm near the meatus. Scattered specialized genital corpuscles are identified in the lamina propria underneath the squamous epithelium. These genital corpuscles are found mainly in the glans corona and frenulum and may be less numerous in the glans when compared to the foreskin. Additional quantitative studies are needed to confirm or deny this belief. A predominance of free nerve endings over the genital corpuscles has been described in the glans (10,15). A few dermal Merkel cells have been identified at the end of the free nerves.

> **CORPUS SPONGIOSUM** The corpus spongiosum is the principal tissue component of the glans penis and is composed of specialized venous sinuses (Fig. 37.7). In the glans, the erectile tissue has the character of a dense, venous plexus (Fig. 37.8) (14). As compared with the CC, the interstitial fibrous connective tissue of the corpus spongiosum

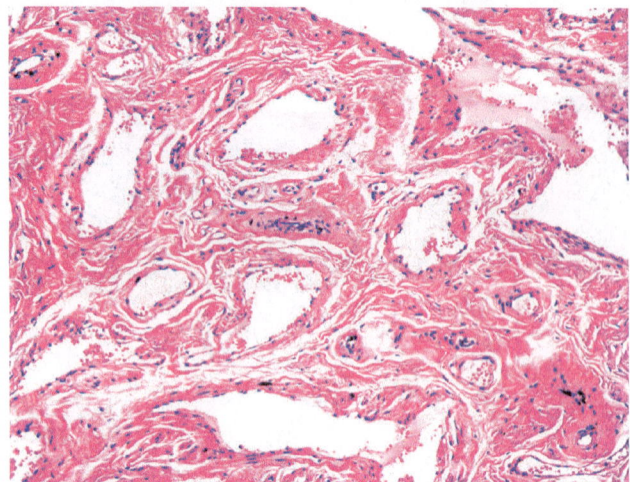

FIGURE 37.7 Glans. Higher-power view of the corpus spongiosum showing specialized venous sinuses.

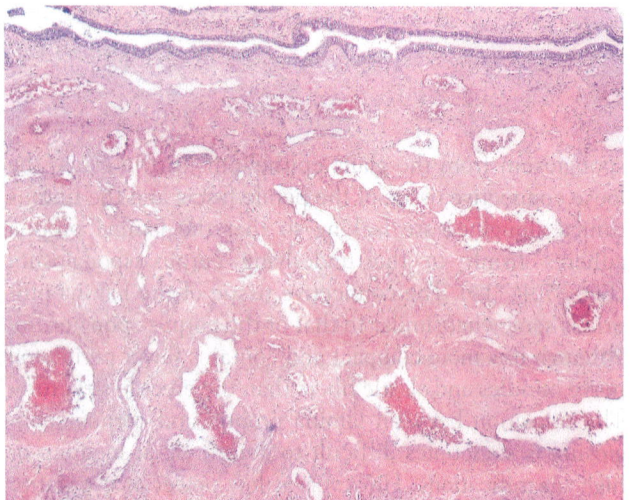

FIGURE 37.8 Corpus spongiosum. Note the dense venous plexus in corpus spongiosum periurethralis.

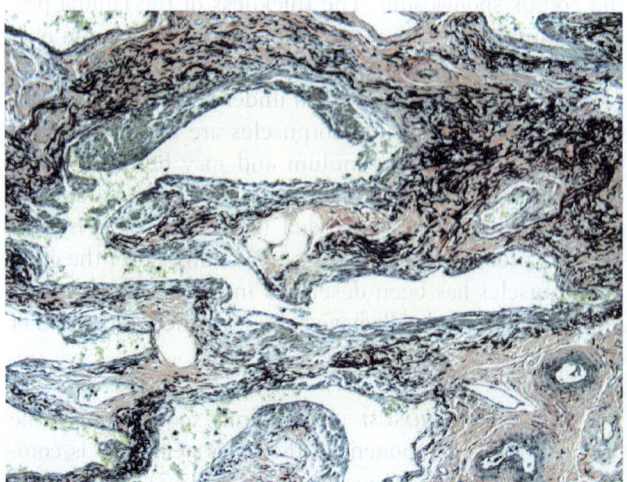

FIGURE 37.9 Corpus spongiosum. The interstitial fibrous connective tissue is more abundant and contains more elastic fibers than in the corpus cavernosum. Note the presence of nutritional veins and arteries in the interstitium of this erectile tissue (van Gieson elastic stain).

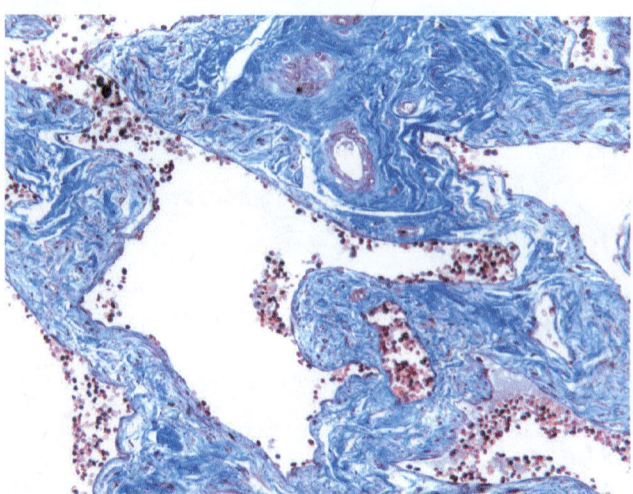

FIGURE 37.10 Corpus spongiosum. The interstitial fibrous connective tissue contains fewer smooth muscle fibers than does the corpus cavernosum (Masson trichrome).

is more abundant and contains more elastic fibers and less smooth muscle bundles (Figs. 37.9 and 37.10) (16,17). The stroma between the vascular spaces is a loose fibrous tissue containing some nerve endings and lymphatic vessels. In this erectile tissue, we also find nutritional veins and arteries (Fig. 37.9).

In poorly oriented biopsies or specimens it may be difficult to distinguish histologic features of corpus spongiosum from cavernosum. It is useful to find a wider separation of vascular lumina in corpus spongiosum (Fig. 37.8) and little or no separation in corpus cavernosum. In the former, the vessels are thinner and rounder, and in the latter the vessels are thicker, irregular, or convoluted due to the prominent smooth muscle fibers (Fig. 37.11).

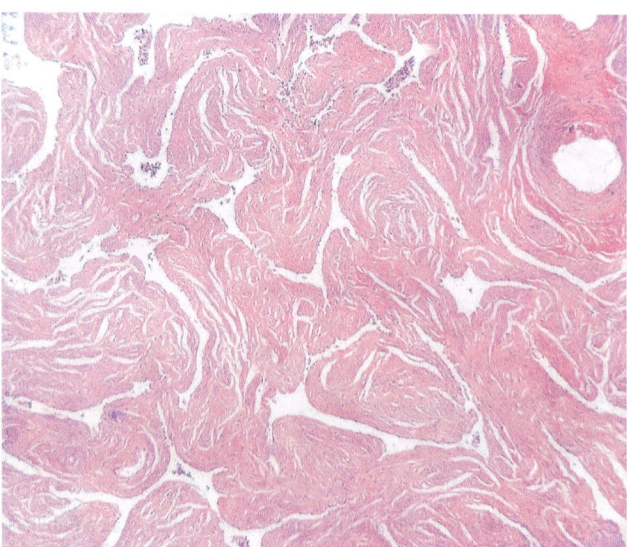

FIGURE 37.11 Corpus cavernosum: note the thick smooth muscle fibers.

Coronal Sulcus

ANATOMIC LEVELS OF THE CORONAL SULCUS
Epithelium
Lamina propria
Buck fascia

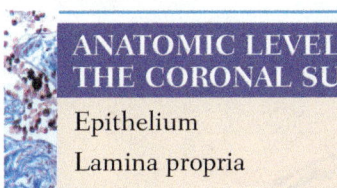

Anatomic Features

The coronal sulcus is a narrow and circumferential cul-de-sac located proximal to the glans corona (Figs. 37.1 and 37.2). It is found in both lateral and dorsal aspects of the penis, but not in the ventral region, which is occupied by the frenulum, a mucosal fold that fixes the foreskin to the inferior portion of the glans, just below the urethral meatus. The mucous membrane of the glans continues to cover this region, as well as the inner surface of the foreskin.

Microscopic and Immunohistochemical Features

Three main histologic layers are seen in the coronal sulcus: (a) The squamous epithelium, identical to the glans epithelium; (b) a thin lamina propria or chorion, which is a prolongation of the foreskin and glans lamina propria; and (c) Buck fascia and the point of insertion of some of the smooth muscle fibers coming from the penile body dartos (Fig. 37.12).

Microscopically, the **squamous epithelium** shows a stratified epithelium (5 to 12 cell layers thick) covered by a thin keratin layer with little keratinization; **lamina propria** (2- to 6-mm thick) is composed of loose connective tissue containing numerous capillary and lymphatic vessels, as well as peripheral nerves, and few Paccini bodies; and **Buck fascia** is composed of fibrous elastic connective tissue containing small- and medium-sized blood vessels and nerves. There is a fourth layer we described that can be present in more than half of specimens: **the dartos** (Fig. 37.13), which is a wide and loose layer (6- to 15-mm thick) surrounding the coronal sulcus composed of fibrous connective tissue and irregular bundles of smooth muscle. This layer is continuous with corporal and preputial dartos. There are small blood and lymphatic vessels. In primary penile carcinoma originating in the coronal sulcus, which are rare (18), the absence of the dartos could facilitate the spreading of carcinomas involving coronal sulcus by reaching more rapidly deeper level of anatomical invasion such as the loose and vascular tissue of the Buck fascia, making an easy pathway of tumor progression and consequent worse prognosis.

The coronal sulcus has been reported as the most frequent site of the so-called Tyson glands (1,3,16,17,19–22), described as modified sebaceous glands and reported as responsible for smegma production. Smegma represents epithelial debris and secretions collected in this space (23). There has been some question about the existence of Tyson glands (10,23,24). Several studies with numerous tissue sections failed to demonstrate these glands (23,25). We could not find Tyson glands in a pathologic study of 67 totally sectioned penises removed for carcinoma of the penis. Apparently the original descriptions by Tyson (26) were based on primate studies that could not be confirmed in humans. After circumcision, occasionally some sebaceous glands can be found in the mucosa adjacent to the skin. They are probably skin sebaceous glands misplaced after surgery. Sebaceous glands associated with or without hair follicles are found in the penile shaft and cutaneous aspect of the foreskin. We have observed the presence of sebaceous glands that are nonrelated to hair follicles at the mucocutaneous junction of the foreskin and adjacent mucosa, but not in the coronal sulcus. The presence of sebaceous gland hyperplasia or ectopic sebaceous glands (Fordyce condition) is more frequent on the penile shaft and foreskin, but may also occur in the glans (2).

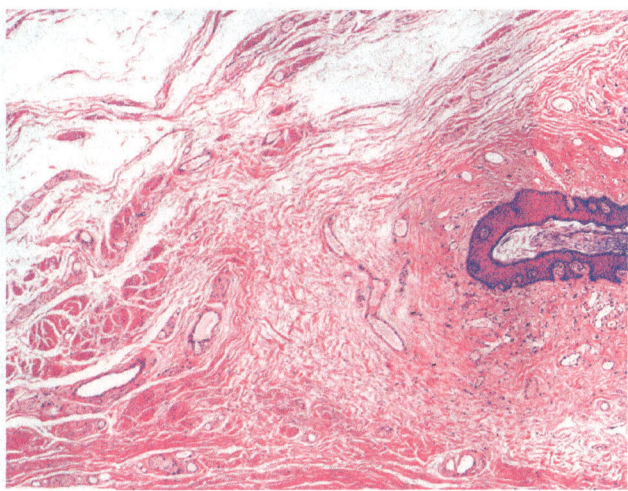

FIGURE 37.12 A section of the coronal sulcus. Histologic components of both glans and penile body are present. This specimen from an uncircumcised person (a portion of the foreskin is seen on *top*) shows the squamous epithelium (*right*), lamina propria below, then Buck fascia and dartos smooth muscle bundles (*left*).

Foreskin

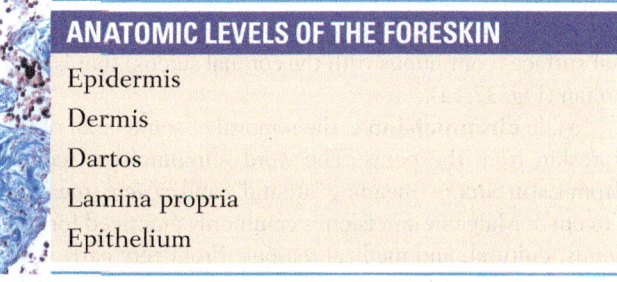

ANATOMIC LEVELS OF THE FORESKIN
Epidermis
Dermis
Dartos
Lamina propria
Epithelium

Anatomic Features and Circumcision

The foreskin or prepuce is the prolongation of the shaft's skin and normally covers most of the glans, reflecting beyond itself and transforming into a mucosal inner surface.

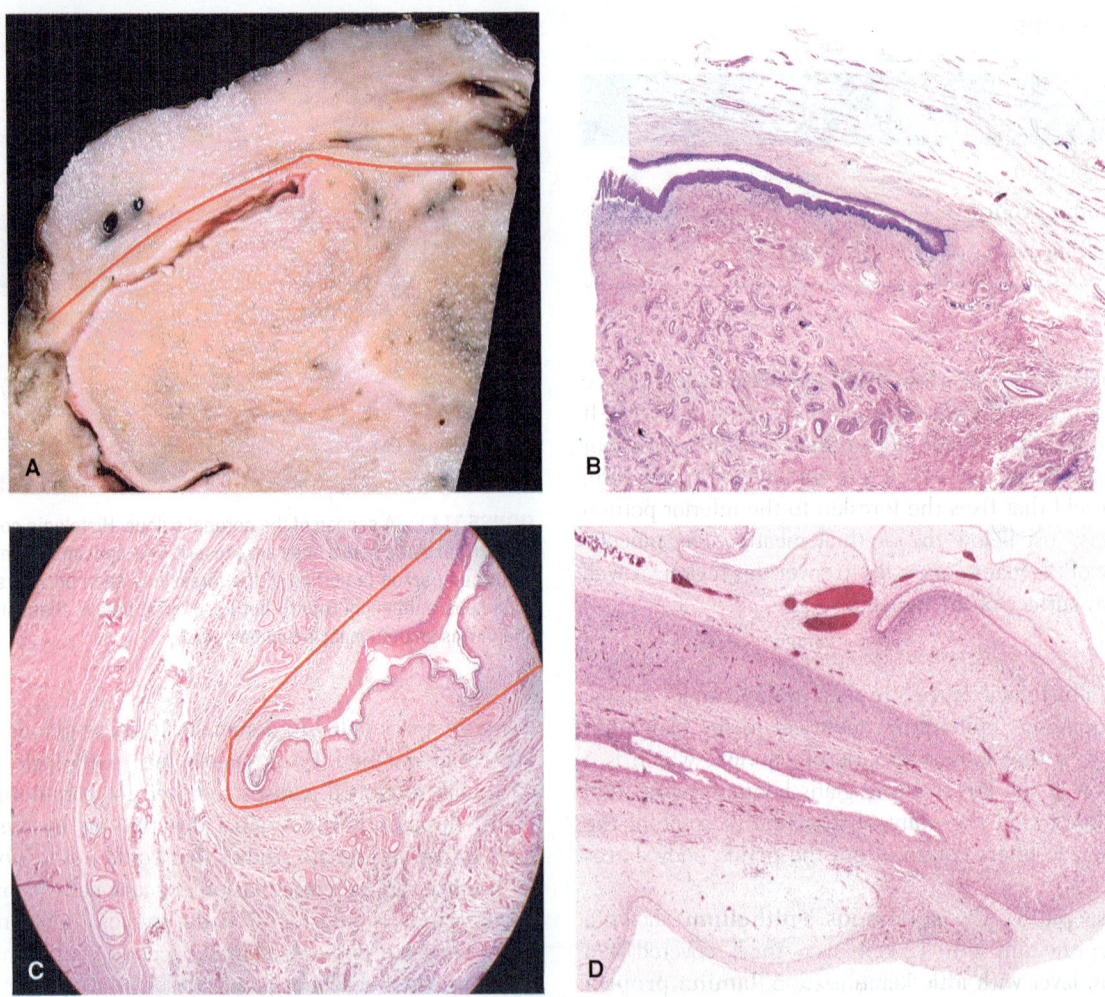

FIGURE 37.13 **A:** Cut surface of a partial penectomy specimen showing the epithelial compartments glans, foreskin, and coronal sulcus. The red line indicates the anatomical location of the dartos layer from foreskin directly to penile shaft. **B:** Low-power microscopic view of the coronal sulcus. **C:** Anatomical levels of coronal sulcus: keratinized squamous epithelium, lamina propria, and dartos. The red line indicates the mode in which the dartos encases the coronal sulcus. **D:** Fetal penis. Note the coronal sulcus formation in relation to the Buck fascia. Glans and foreskin inner surfaces are firmly adherent.

The epithelium covering the mucosal inner surface is continuous with the epithelium of the coronal sulcus, as well as the surface of the glans (Figs. 37.1 and 37.2). Grossly, the adult foreskin shows a cutaneous surface (continuous with the skin of the shaft) that is dark and wrinkled and a mucosal surface (continuous with the coronal sulcus) that is pink to tan (Fig. 37.14).

Male **circumcision** is the removal of some or all of the foreskin from the penis. The word "circumcision" comes from Latin *circum* (meaning "around") and *cædere* (meaning "to cut"). Male circumcision is commonly practiced for religious, cultural, and medical reasons. From very early years to the present, there have been controversies regarding the role of the foreskin and the importance of circumcision (27–32). Preputial functions are related to protection of the glans from external irritation or contamination, and it has been shown that the foreskin is a normal erogenous tissue (10,30,33). In addition, it has been demonstrated that the squamous mucosa of the glans, coronal sulcus, and foreskin are fused during the embryologic development of the penis (Fig. 37.15), and they can be considered as one tissue compartment. The fused mucosa of the glans and inner lining of the foreskin separate gradually over the years (10). Most newborn males show an unretracted foreskin at the time of delivery (34). When boys reach the age of 5 to 6 years, the foreskin can be completely retracted in most cases beyond the level of the glans corona. According to these observations, a tight preputial orifice due to an immature preputial plate does not represent an adhesion but a normal stage of penile development. Therefore, neonatal circumcision before the foreskin has naturally separated involves tearing the common prepuce/glans mucosa apart, with the possible complications of excoriation and injury to the glans and ablation of the frenular artery and meatal stenosis (10).

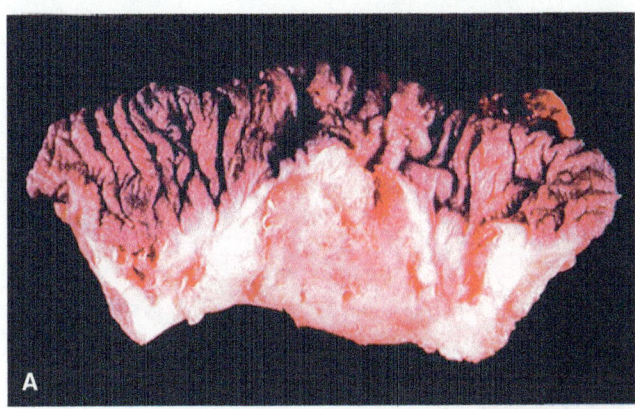 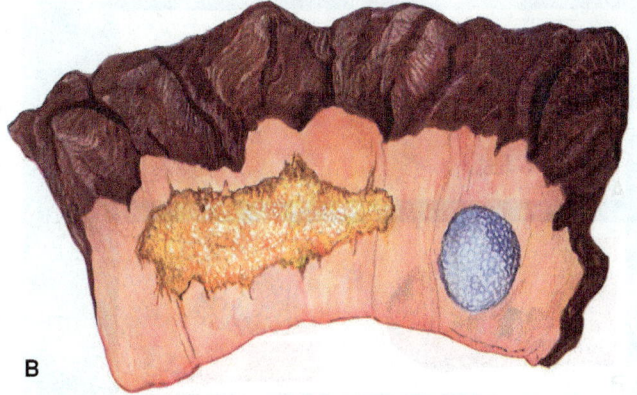

FIGURE 37.14 **A** and **B**: Gross appearance and corresponding diagram of an adult foreskin (prepuce) with multicentric carcinomas. The cutaneous surface (*top*) is darker and more wrinkled. The mucosa (*bottom*) is pale beige and slightly irregular. Two separate carcinomas (in yellow and light blue in the diagram) are present in the mucosal surface, the most common location of preputial carcinomas.

On the other hand, different studies have been published suggesting that circumcision may reduce the risk of urinary tract infection, common sexually transmitted diseases (STDs), and penile carcinoma (27,35–43). It has been proposed that the mucosal inner surface of the foreskin from newborns shows a propensity to be colonized by fimbriated bacteria, with the subsequent occurrence of serious urinary tract infection (37). Studies suggest that male circumcision is associated with a reduced risk of penile human papillomavirus (HPV) infection and, in the case of men with a history of multiple sexual partners, a reduced risk of cervical cancer in their current female partner (41–43). Furthermore, randomized controlled trials have shown that adult circumcision reduces the risk of acquiring human immunodeficiency virus (HIV) infection (44,45). However, it appears clear that the risk of sexually transmitted disease, including HPV and HIV infections, correlates with sexual behavior, and behavioral factors appear to be far more important risk factors than circumcision status. Moreover, proper hygiene and access to clean water has been shown to reduce the rate of development of squamous cell carcinoma of the penis in the uncircumcised population (43). Nevertheless, in areas where safe sexual and hygienic practices are poorly adhered to, circumcision can have a relative protective effect against the transmission of STDs (including HIV) and may lower the incidence of penile carcinoma (36). In general, complications of circumcision are minor and treatable, especially at young ages. Higher frequency of complications, and severe complications, are seen when the procedure is undertaken by inexperienced providers, in nonsterile settings or with inadequate equipment and supplies (29). Existing scientific evidence demonstrates potential medical benefits of newborn male circumcision; however, these data are not sufficient to recommend routine neonatal circumcision. Parents should be given accurate and unbiased information to determine what is in the best interest of the child in each individual case. In a policy statement, the American Academy of Pediatrics stated that "although health benefits are not great enough to recommend routine circumcision for all male newborns, the benefits of circumcision are sufficient to justify access to this procedure for families choosing it and to warrant third-party payment for circumcision of male newborns. It is important that clinicians routinely inform parents of the health benefits and risks of male newborn circumcision in an unbiased and accurate manner." But, "parents ultimately should decide whether circumcision is in the best interests of their male child. They will need to weigh medical information in the context of their own religious, ethical, and cultural beliefs and practices. The medical benefits alone, may not outweigh these other considerations for individual families" (46).

FIGURE 37.15 Fused squamous mucosa of the glans, coronal sulcus, and foreskin during the embryologic development of the penis. Note the common immature epithelial plate (*center*). The dense stromal cells of the glans will form the corpus spongiosum (*right*). The lamina propria of the glans is not yet formed. The foreskin is on the *left*.

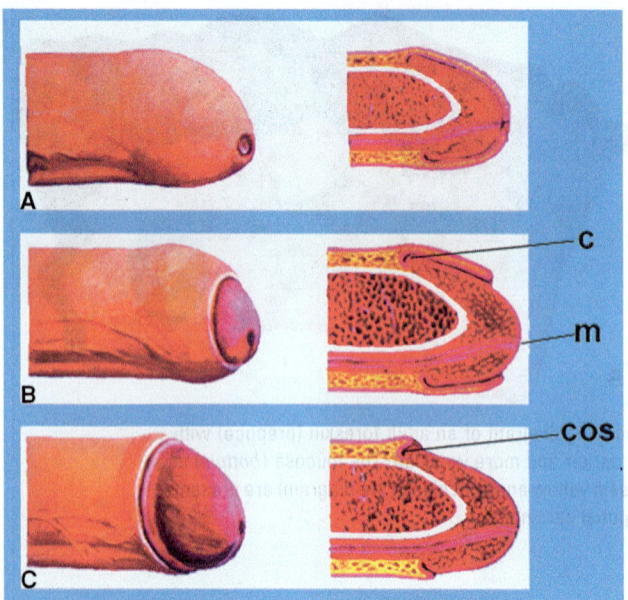

FIGURE 37.16 Foreskin length variation. **A:** most common type, long foreskin. **B:** Intermediate. **C:** Short, unusual. *c* and *cos*, coronal sulcus; *m*, meatus urethralis.

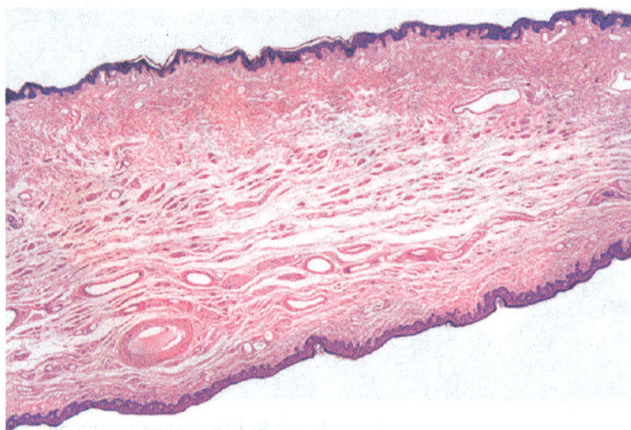

FIGURE 37.17 Full thickness of the foreskin showing all five layers: keratinized stratified squamous epithelium (*top*), dermis, dartos, submucosa, and squamous epithelium of the mucosal portion (*bottom*).

Microscopic and Immunohistochemical Features

The prepuce is formed by a midline collision of ectoderm, neuroectoderm, and mesenchyme, resulting in a pentalaminar structure (10). There are five layers in the histologic evaluation of the foreskin (Fig. 37.17):

1. The epidermis consists of a keratinized stratified squamous cell epithelium that is similar to the epidermis seen in the cutaneous tegument. Melanocytes, Langerhans cells, and Merkel cells are also present. Compared to the mucosal epithelium, the epidermis is thinner and shows better developed rete ridges and usually a pigmented basal layer (Fig. 37.18). Vellous hairs, sebaceous, and sweat glands may be seen connected to the epidermis.

2. The dermis of the foreskin consists of connective tissue with blood vessels and nerve bundles. Meissner corpuscles

In adult populations, the variable length of the foreskin has motivated some studies, especially those related to the relation of length and amount of smegma in the balanopreputial sulcus (27,47). Phimosis is found in 4% of boys 6 to 17 years of age, but with a diminishing incidence in later years (47). In nonphimotic boys, where the preputial space can be inspected, smegma is present in 5% of the cases. Production of smegma appears to increase in quantity in the 16- to 17-year-old group (47). In a recent prospective study in a high-risk population, we found a variation in foreskin length (Fig. 37.16): long phimotic foreskins were significantly more frequent in patients with penile carcinoma as compared with the general population (27). Coexistence of a long foreskin and phimosis may explain the high incidence of penile cancer in some geographic regions, and circumcision in patients with long and phimotic foreskins living in high-risk areas may be indicated (27).

The foreskin is frequently involved by carcinomas, usually as a secondary invasion from tumor originating in the glans, the most common site of penile cancer. However, there are carcinomas exclusive of the foreskin. It is important to identify these primary preputial tumors since they have a better prognosis than those of other penile sites (48). Primary foreskin squamous cell carcinomas tend to be of lower grade and multicentric (Fig. 37.14) comparing with those of the glans (49).

Like in the glans, there is a correlation of anatomical levels of invasion in the foreskin and regional cancer spread. Invasive tumors limited to lamina propria only rarely metastasized. On the contrary, transmural carcinomas with invasion of all tissue layers, lamina propria, dartos, and skin, are frequently associated with nodal metastasis (49).

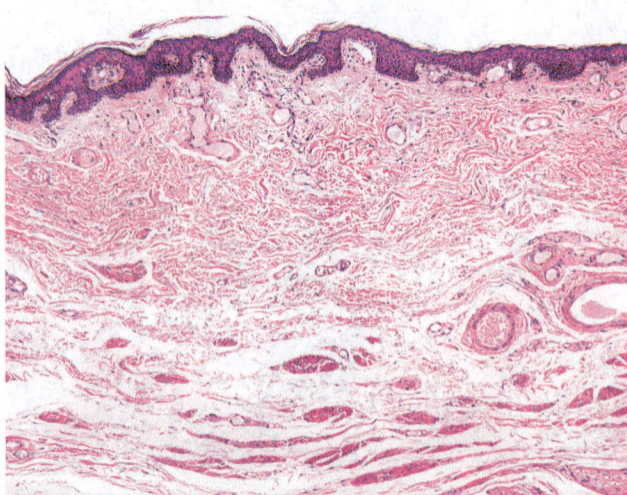

FIGURE 37.18 Cutaneous surface of the foreskin. Compared to the mucosal epithelium, the epidermis is thinner with better developed rete ridges and usually a pigmented basal layer. Underneath the dermis the smooth muscle bundles of the dartos can be appreciated.

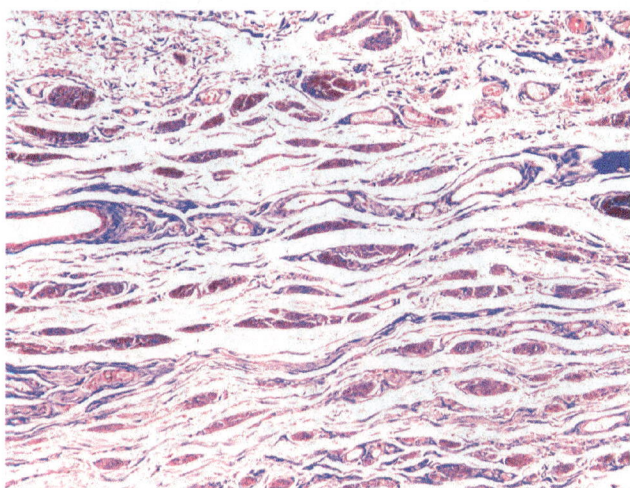

FIGURE 37.19 Smooth muscle bundles, the main component of the preputial dartos, are shown in red (Masson trichrome).

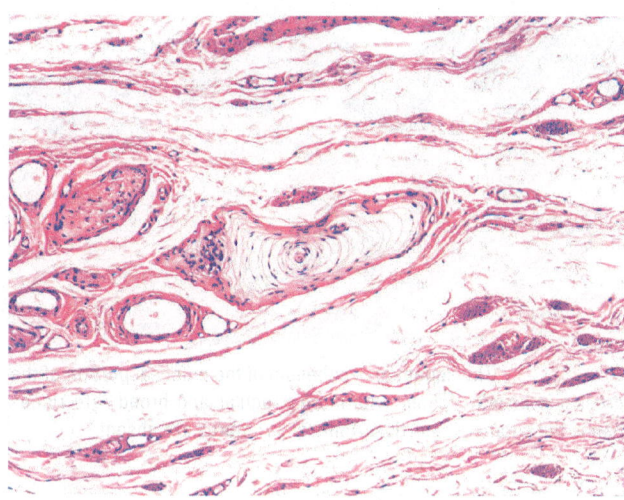

FIGURE 37.21 A Vater–Pacini corpuscle is present deep in the dartos layer of the foreskin.

are present in the dermal papillae and a few Vater–Pacini corpuscles may be found in deeper areas. Scattered vellous hairs and sebaceous and sweat glands are noted, and they are usually confined to the dermis without extension beyond the dartos. The dermis appears to have more elastic fibers than the lamina propria.

3. The dartos consists of smooth muscle fibers invested with elastic fibers, and it is the central axis of the foreskin (Fig. 37.19). From the foreskin, the delicate penile dartos surrounds the penile shaft and is continuous with the scrotal dartos. Similar to the penile body dartos, the smooth muscle fibers vary in their disposition. At the edge of the foreskin, the fibers are transversely arranged to form a sphincter to close this edge over the distal end of the glans. There are numerous nerve endings in close association with the smooth muscle fibers (Fig. 37.20).

Nerve bundle density in the foreskin was noted to be the highest in the ventral preputial tissue (mean: 17.9 bundles per nm) as opposed to lateral (8.6 per nm) or dorsal (6.2 per nm) tissues (50). A few Vater–Pacini corpuscles may be found scattered between these nerve bundles (Fig. 37.21).

4. The lamina propria, or chorion, is composed of a vascular connective tissue looser than the glans lamina propria. Scattered genital corpuscles and free nerve endings are seen in the lamina propria immediately underneath the epithelium. The genital corpuscles are usually found in clusters of three to five (Fig. 37.22). Some authors believe that the corpuscular receptors are more numerous at the mucocutaneous junction of the foreskin; however, this assertion needs further study (10,30). The mucosal lamina propria is devoid of

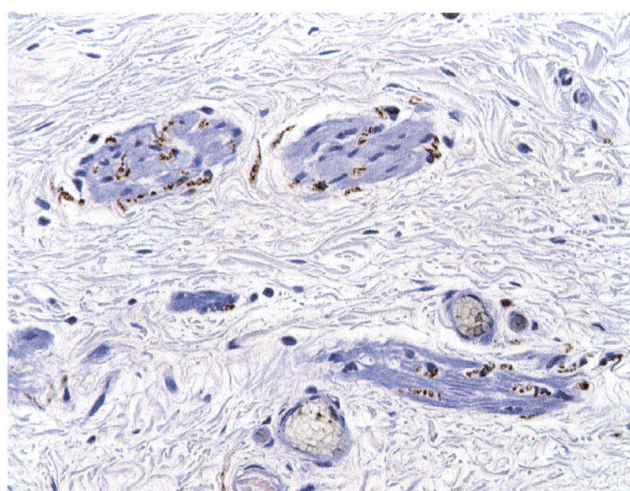

FIGURE 37.20 Neurofilament immunostain highlights numerous free nerve endings associated with smooth muscle bundles in the foreskin dartos.

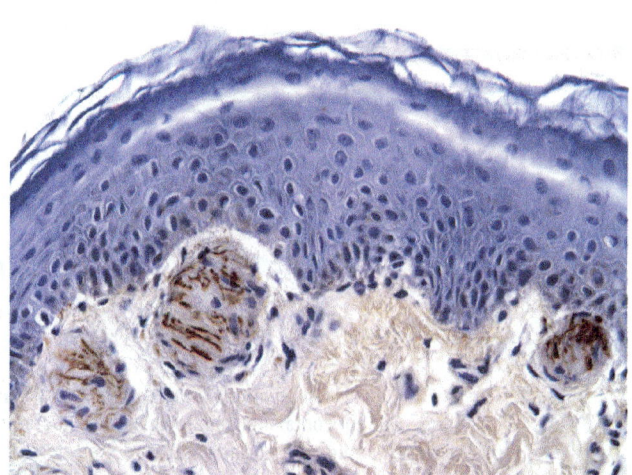

FIGURE 37.22 The genital corpuscles are usually found in clusters of three to five underneath the mucosal epithelium, in the lamina propria of the foreskin (neurofilament immunostain).

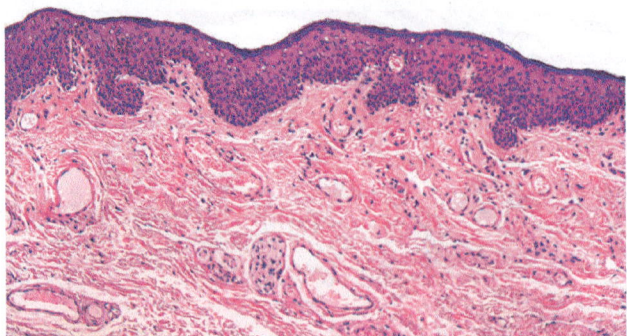

FIGURE 37.23 The squamous epithelium of the mucosal portion of the foreskin is usually thicker with more irregular and broad rete ridges than in the cutaneous portion. Adnexal structures are absent.

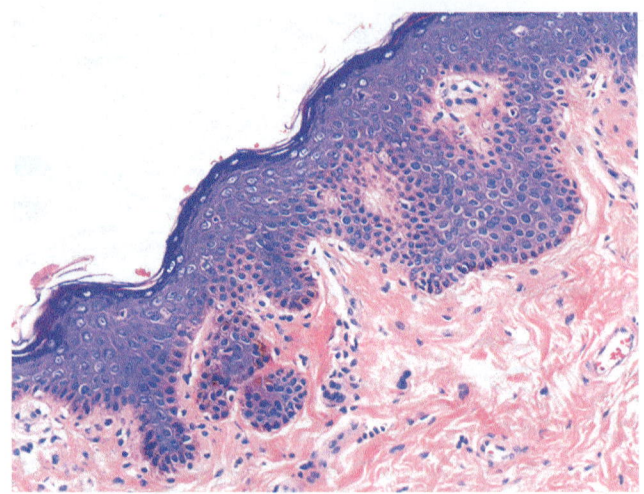

FIGURE 37.24 Foreskin showing the squamous epithelium and its pigmentation in basal layers.

hair follicles and sweat and sebaceous glands. We have observed a few specimens with rare sebaceous glands unrelated to hair structures at the mucocutaneous junction and immediately adjacent foreskin mucosa, but it is not clear if these represent ectopic glands or variation of normal anatomy.

5. The mucosal squamous epithelium (Fig. 37.23) is identical to and a prolongation of the glans and the coronal sulcus' epithelia. Toward the free edge of the foreskin and approaching the mucocutaneous junction, the basal layer shows a progressive pigmentation more similar to what is seen in the epidermis of the cutaneous portion of the foreskin (Fig. 37.24). The immunohistochemical characteristics of this epithelium are identical to the glans squamous epithelium. Langerhans and Merkel cells are present but not melanocytes. Intraepithelial nerves have been described (10,13).

Anatomical Features Related to Cancer Spread

The anatomical levels of the glans, epithelium, lamina propria, corpus spongiosum and corpus cavernosum, are important landmarks for the evaluation and prediction of cancer progression. It is the base on which the TNM system was constructed (51) and crucial for the design of the prognostic Index and nomograms, useful tools for cancer spread and outcome prediction (52–54). This correlation is illustrated in the diagrams. In a series of 51 patients with penile squamous cell carcinoma, a larger number of nodal metastasis were found in tumors infiltrating CC (Fig. 37.25A). Likewise in a series of 20 carcinomas exclusive of the foreskin the majority of the metastatic cases were tumors infiltrating deep dartos or outer dermis (Fig. 37.25B).

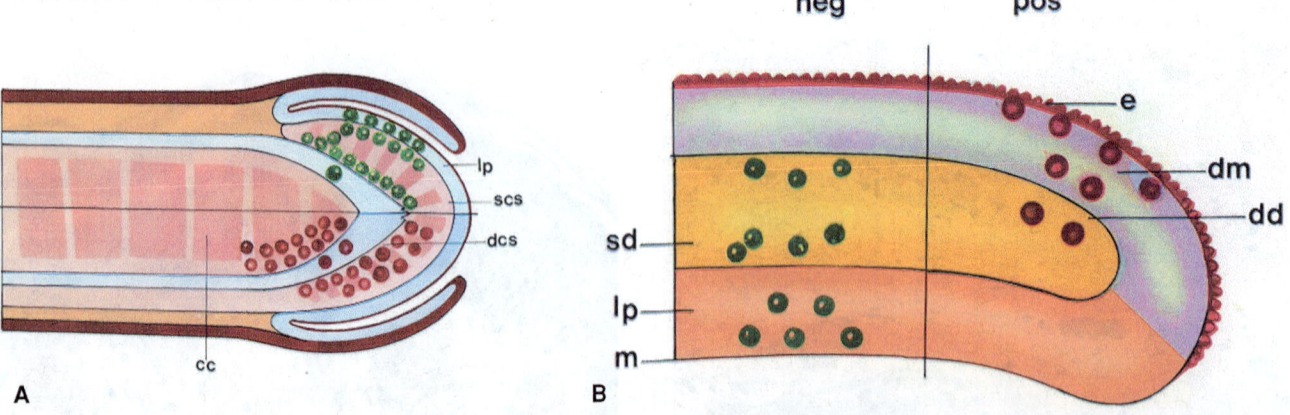

FIGURE 37.25 Anatomical features related to cancer spread. A: Diagram representing cut surface of glans. The horizontal line separates sites associated with and without nodal metastasis. Above, *green dots* represents negative nodes and below, *red dots* represent nodal metastasis. The vast majority of tumors compromising corpora cavernosa are associated with regional spread. B: This diagram represents the cut surface of the foreskin. Tumors associated with nodal metastasis were those invasive of the deep dartos or outer skin. *m*, mucosal epithelium; *lp*, lamina propria; *sd*, superficial dartos; *dd*, deep dartos; *dm*, dermis; *e*, epidermis.

PROXIMAL PENIS (OR SHAFT)

ANATOMICAL LEVELS OF THE PENILE SHAFT

Epidermis
Dermis
Dartos
Buck fascia
Tunica albuginea
Corpora cavernosa
Corpus spongiosum

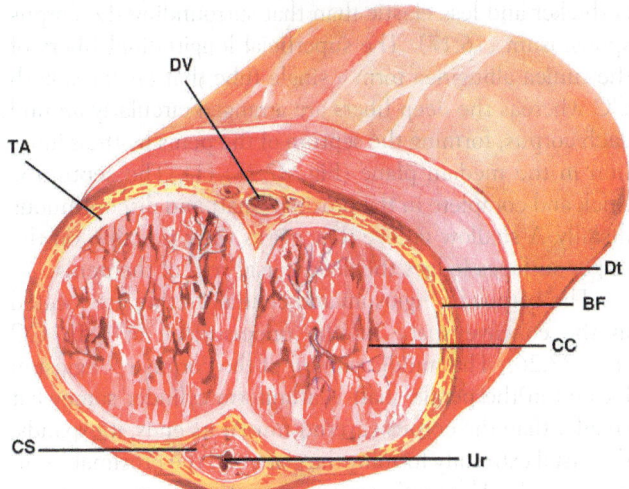

FIGURE 37.26 Cross section of the penis illustrating both corpora cavernosa (CC), each surrounded by the tunica albuginea (*TA*); they form the septum of the penis by their junction in the median plane. A shallow groove that marks their junction on the upper surfaces lodges the deep dorsal vein of the penis (DV). The dorsal arteries are located on both sides of the vein. Note the corpus spongiosum (*CS*) and central urethra (Ur) located in the concave space on the undersurface of both corpora cavernosa, buck fascia (BF) and dartos (Dt).

Anatomic Features

The penile shaft, body, or corpus, of the penis is mainly composed of three cylindrical masses of erectile tissue, the two CC and a corpus spongiosum with central urethra (Fig. 37.26). The posterior portion of the CC are two divergent and gradually tapering structures, called crura, that insert in the ischiopubic bone from where they converge to fuse at the level of the inferior portion of the pubic symphysis. The distal three-fourths of the two CC are intimately bound together and make up the greater part of the shaft of the penis. They retain a uniform diameter in the shaft and terminate anteriorly in a bluntly rounded extremity, being embedded in a cap formed by the corpus spongiosum of the glans (1). The erectile tissue of the CC is a vast, sponge-like system of irregular vascular spaces fed by the afferent arteries and drained by the efferent veins. In the flaccid condition of the organ, the cavernous spaces contain little blood and appear as collapsed irregular clefts. In erection, they become large cavities engorged with blood under pressure (16).

The CC are surrounded by a firm, thick, fibrous envelope, the tunica albuginea. In the flaccid state, the tunica albuginea measures 2 to 3 mm in thickness and becomes thinner (about 0.5 mm) during erection. On longitudinal sections of the organ, the albuginea covering the CC terminates in a ">"-shaped pattern variably ending beyond or at the level of coronal sulcus or, less frequently, behind it (Fig. 37.27) (6). The tunica albuginea enveloping the CC

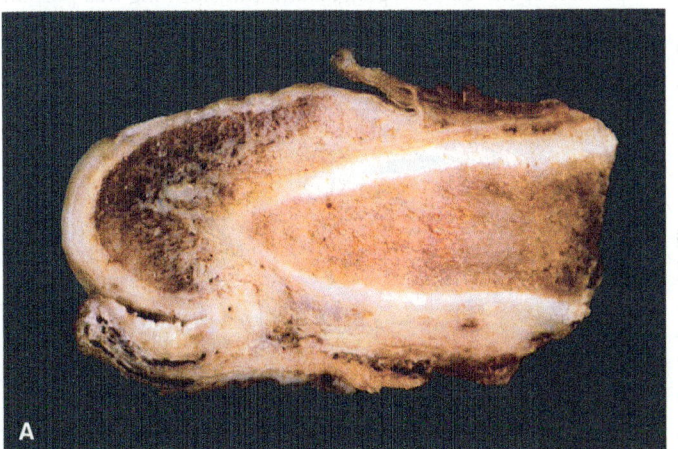
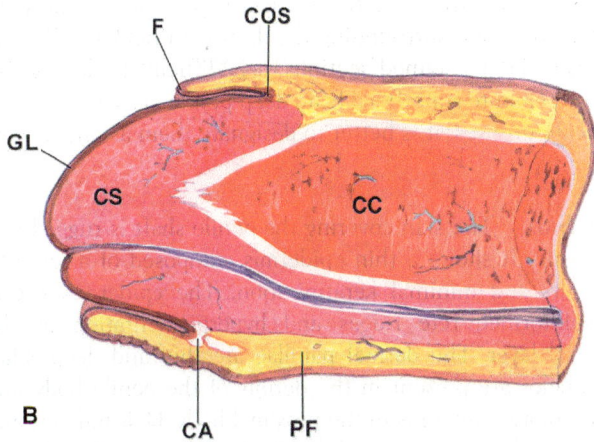

FIGURE 37.27 Gross picture (**A**) and diagram (**B**) of two longitudinal sections of a partial penectomy specimen with a small squamous cell carcinoma (*CA*) located in the coronal sulcus (*COS*). The albuginea (*in white*) surrounds the corpus cavernosum. The diagram from a parallel but more central section of the same specimen, illustrates the urethra running within the corpus spongiosum F, foreskin; GL, glans; PF, Buck fascia; CS, corpus spongiosum; CC, corpus cavernosum.

is thicker and less elastic than that surrounding the corpus spongiosum (16,17). The superficial longitudinal fibers of the tunica albuginea form a single tube that encloses both CC whereas the deep fibers are arranged circularly around each corpus, forming the septum of the penis by their junction in the median plane (Fig. 37.26) (1). The septum is thick and complete in the proximal shaft and discontinuous distally. A shallow groove that marks their junction on the upper surfaces lodges the deep dorsal vein of the penis.

The corpus spongiosum and central urethra are located in the concave space on the undersurface of both CC (Fig. 37.26). The middle portion of the corpus spongiosum located in the penile shaft is a uniform cylinder somewhat smaller than the corpus cavernosum. At its ends, it expands, the distal extremity forming the glans and the proximal forming the bulb. The urethra enters the corpus spongiosum 1 to 2 cm from the posterior extremity of the bulb by piercing the dorsal surface. The bulb is just superficial to the urogenital diaphragm, and its posterior portion projects backward toward the anus beyond the entrance of the urethra.

The three cylindrical structures forming the penile shaft are covered by a thin, delicate, and elastic skin. Beneath the dermis, there is a discontinuous smooth muscle layer called the dartos (Fig. 37.26) embedded in a thin layer of connective tissue corresponding to the superficial fascia of the classical descriptions. Between the dartos and the albuginea, there is a highly elastic yellowish tube-like sheath encasing all three CC and spongiosum; this is designated as Buck fascia (deep penile fascia of the classical descriptions) (Figs. 37.26 and 37.27). A septum of fascia extends inward between the CC and the corpus spongiosum, providing separate tubular investments for these columns of erectile tissue and dividing the penis into its dorsal (CC) and ventral (corpus spongiosum) portions as can be also seen via CT (computed tomography) or MRI (magnetic resonance imaging) (55). When using the terms *fascia* or *penile fascia* in this chapter, we are referring to Buck fascia since the superficial fascia is just part of the connective tissue surrounding the dartos. In hematoxylin and eosin (H&E)-stained sections, it is difficult to distinguish and separate superficial from deep penile fascias. For practical purposes, it is better to designate them as one fascia.

Microscopic and Immunohistochemical Features

> **Skin** The skin covering the penile shaft is rugged and elastic. It shows a thin epidermis composed of a few cell layers and minimal keratinization. The epidermis shows well-formed rete ridges and hyperpigmentation of the basal layer. The dermal papillae are thin and deep. Hair follicles are present in the dermis of the penile body and are more numerous in the proximal body. Hair follicles and other adnexa can extend out to the cutaneous foreskin in some individuals. They are scanty and contain no piloerector muscle. There are a few sebaceous glands that are not related to hair follicles. Occasionally, there are also poorly developed sweat glands.

> **Dartos** The penile dartos is composed of a discontinuous layer of smooth muscle fibers, variably arranged in transverse and longitudinal branches. Some bundles end at the balanopreputial sulcus whereas others run farther to become the preputial dartos. The dartos is embedded in a loose fibrovascular connective tissue with numerous nerve bundles that correspond to the superficial penile fascia of the classical anatomic description, and it is the penile equivalent of the skin subcutaneous tissue or hypodermis, but without adipose tissue (1). Similarly to the scrotal smooth muscle fibers, the penile dartos produces a retraction of genital structures when the exterior temperature falls.

> **Buck Fascia** Buck fascia is a well-developed and continuous fibrovascular sheath that encases the CC and the corpus spongiosum. It is composed of loose connective tissue with numerous blood vessels and peripheral nerve bundles running within and beneath it (56). Vater–Pacini corpuscles are often seen in the penile fascia. Its yellow color is due to the presence of adipose tissue and abundant elastic fibers (Fig. 37.28). The skin and dartos slide over this fascia. Buck fascia is important from the surgical pathology point of view since it is a frequent pathway of tumor invasion in penile cancer progression (57). This is most likely due to the loose quality of this tissue and the presence of numerous lymphovascular and neural structures. Some investigators point to Buck fascia as the site of origin of Peyronie disease (56).

> **Tunica Albuginea** The tunica albuginea is a thick sheath of partially hyalinized collagen fibers covering both the CC and corpus spongiosum. It is a poorly vascular structure, with only a few branches of circumflex vessels traversing through it, as demonstrated by factor VIII and CD31 immunostains. It is mainly composed of collagen fibers arranged in an outer longitudinal and an inner circular layer (16,17). The outer layer, which appears to determine the variation in the thickness and strength of the tunica, is absent in the ventral portion of the corpus spongiosum, transforming this portion

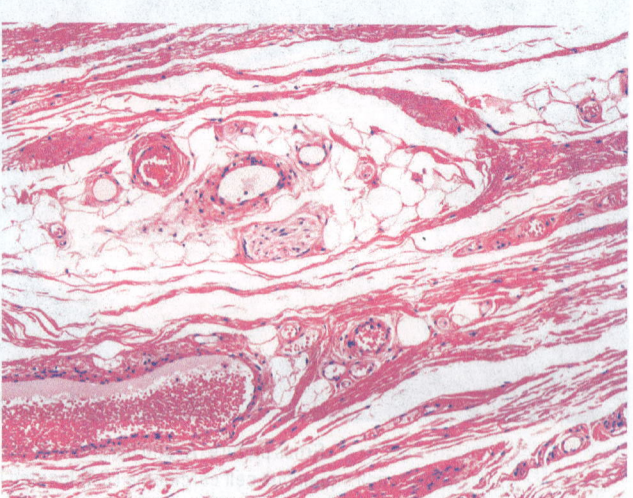

FIGURE 37.28 Buck fascia is composed of loose connective tissue with adipose cells and numerous blood vessels and peripheral nerve bundles.

of tunica into a vulnerable area to perforation. This anatomic aspect probably explains why most prostheses tend to extrude in this area (58). The tunica albuginea forms an incomplete fibrous septum separating both CC. The collagen fibers are wavy in the flaccid state and become straight during erection. The fibers are arranged in such a way so as to permit some elasticity necessary for erection. Elastic fibers are rare in the tunica albuginea of the CC. The tunica albuginea surrounding the corpus spongiosum is thinner and contains more elastic fibers than the one around the CC. In some unusual cases, an infection of the lower urinary tract can spread to the corpus spongiosum to cause Fournier gangrene (59). Eventually the tunica albuginea may be penetrated; and, with involvement of Buck fascia, the infection can rapidly spread to the dartos and directly extend to Colles' scrotal fascia and Scarpa fascia of the anterior abdominal wall. The infection can spread to the buttocks, thigh, and ischiorectal space. The tunica albuginea is probably the real barrier to the infiltration of squamous cell carcinoma, contrary to the old concept that Buck fascia was the barrier to the spread of cancer (57).

› **CORPORA CAVERNOSA** The CC are the main anatomic structures used during erection. The substance of the CC consists of a three-dimensional network of trabeculae. These are composed of connective tissue and smooth muscle and are covered by endothelium, creating a network of interanastomosing vascular spaces between them. These spaces tend to be larger in much of the central parts of each corpus cavernosum and smaller at their periphery (16,17). It seems that the smooth muscle bundles are the main component of the trabeculae in the CC (Fig. 37.29). There is a highly structured criss-crossing of interconnected fibers and spaces that are tensed as the cylinder expands during erection (60,61). This creates an internal strength and rigidity that is far greater than that possible in a hollow tube filled to equivalent pressure. This specialized network appears to be necessary for erection (61). In the flaccid state, the vascular spaces are 1-mm slits but they increase several times in diameter with erection. The interconnection between the venous sinuses is so wide that if a contrast is injected at one point, both CC can be immediately and completely visualized. The precise nature of vascular connections between the CC and corpus spongiosum remains controversial. Cavernospongious arterial anastomoses were described by different authors; however, their physiologic role in erection remains unknown (62). These arterial anastomoses could explain how drugs penetrate into the CC via the corpus spongiosum after transurethral diffusion (62,63). No arteriovenous shunts or venous connections were found between the CC and the corpus spongiosum (63).

A progressive increase of collagen fibers and decrease of smooth muscle and elastic fiber may be seen in the cavernous trabeculae over the course of time (64).

› **ADIPOSE TISSUE IN CORPORA CAVERNOSA** Adipose tissue, along with arteries, veins, and peripheral nerves are normal constituents of mesenchymal tissues present in penile fascias, which encases the CC at the level of penile shaft. We recently reported presence of adipose tissue within the CC in a study of 63 consecutive partial penectomy specimens for squamous cell carcinoma. Fat was present within the tunica albuginea in 19% and within CC in 52% of the cases (65). The fatty tissue was focal or multifocal and scant and peripherally located at the junction of the tunica albuginea with the corpora. In some cases, it was associated with small amounts of fibrous tissue, small vessels and nerves. It is possible that adipose tissue, along with small nutritional vessels and nerves perforates from the fascia, were fat is usually present, through the tunica albuginea to reach the corpora (Fig. 37.30). In previous examination of the local routes of cancer spread, we found this pathway to be one of the mechanisms of cancer invading penile corpora from penile fascia (Fig. 37.31) (66).

› **CORPUS SPONGIOSUM** In the corpus spongiosum of the shaft, there are widely interconnected, branching vascular spaces separated by trabeculae. These vascular spaces of variable caliber are lined by endothelial cells and are surrounded by a thin layer of smooth muscle fibers. These fibers coalesce in various extraluminal parts of the vessels to form the subendothelial cushions or polsters. The lacunae become continuous with a mucosal plexus of veins toward the urethra; at the periphery, they communicate with the venous network of the albuginea (14). Compared to the corpus spongiosum of the shaft, the substance of the glans corpus spongiosum is made up of convolutions of large veins rather than spaces separated by trabeculae (17).

The main differences between the corpus spongiosum and the CC from the penile shaft are that the blood spaces in the corpus spongiosum, unlike those of the CC, are the same size in peripheral and central areas and the trabeculae between them contain more elastic fibers, whereas smooth muscle bundles are relatively scarce when compared to the trabeculae of the CC (Fig. 37.32) (16,17) However, there

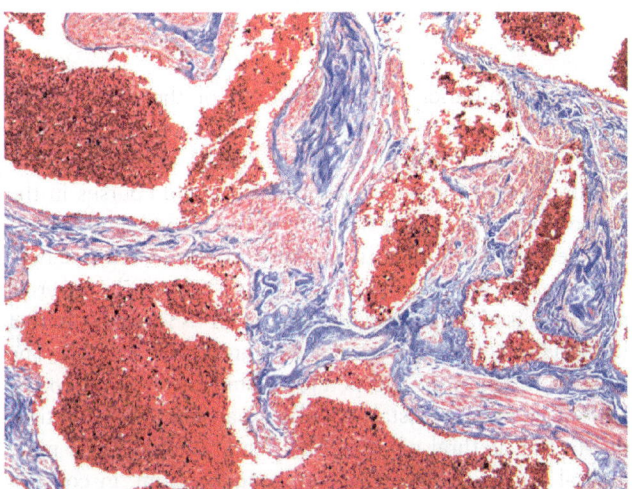

FIGURE 37.29 Corpus cavernosum. The interstitial fibrous connective tissue contains more smooth muscle fibers than in the corpus spongiosum (Masson trichrome).

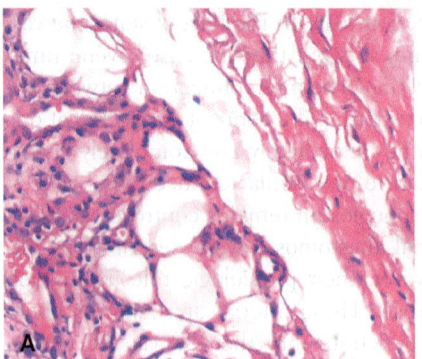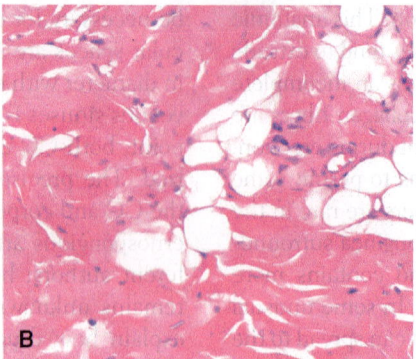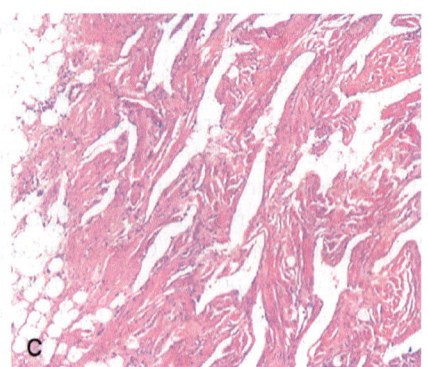

FIGURE 37.30 Adipose tissue. **A:** High-power view with adipose tissue as part of the penile fascia, which surrounds the tunica. **B:** High-power view of a cluster of adipose tissue cells within the tunica albuginea. **C:** High-power view showing adipose tissue cells within the corpus cavernosum (CC).

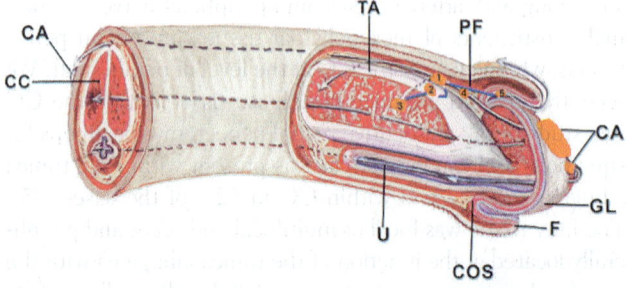

FIGURE 37.31 Diagram representing cancer spread. Cancer (*CA*) is located in the glans (*GL*). *Blue line* shows the route of invasion following penile fascia (*PF*) and the hypothetic way of invasion of corpora cavernosa (*CC*) through the tunica albuginea (*TA*). (*1*) Adipose tissue in Buck fascia. (*2*) Adipose tissue in tunica albuginea. (*3*) Adipose tissue in corpora cavernosa. *F*, foreskin; *COS*, coronal sulcus; *U*, urethra.

is variability and sometimes it can be difficult to distinguish corpus cavernosum from spongiosum by histology alone.

DISTAL URETHRA

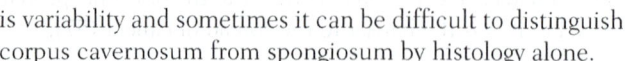

ANATOMIC LEVELS OF THE URETHRA AND PERIURETHRAL TISSUES

Urethral epithelium
Lamina propria
Corpus spongiosum
Tunica albuginea
Buck fascia

Anatomic Features

The distal (anterior) urethra consists of the bulbous and penile (pendulous) segments. The 3- to 4-cm bulbous urethra is located between the inferior margin of the urogenital diaphragm and the penoscrotal junction and courses in the root of the penis within the bulb of the corpus spongiosum. The penile urethra measures approximately 15 cm in length and extends from the penoscrotal junction to the external meatus; it is closely associated to the corpus spongiosum that forms a protective cylindrical sheath around it (1,12,22). The distal 4 to 6 mm of the penile urethra corresponds to the fossa navicularis, a distal saccular expansion that is contiguous to the urethral meatus. The penile urethra has a more central position within the corpus spongiosum, in contrast to the more dorsally positioned bulbous urethra. The mucosa of the distal urethra has numerous recesses, called Morgagni lacunae, which extend deeply into the mucin-secreting Littré

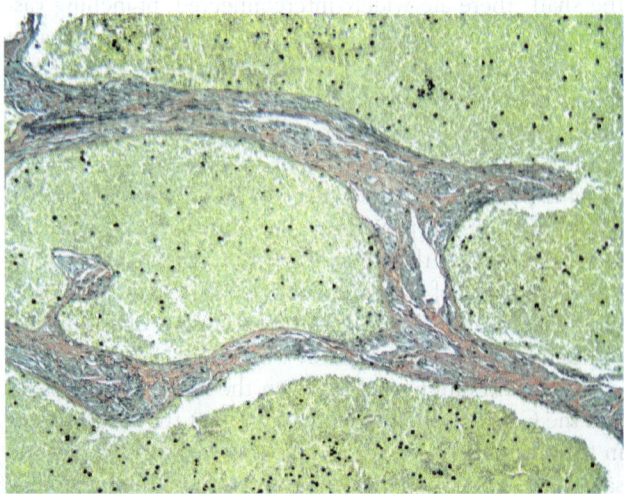

FIGURE 37.32 Corpus cavernosum. The interstitial fibrous connective tissue contains fewer elastic fibers than does the corpus spongiosum (van Gieson elastic stain).

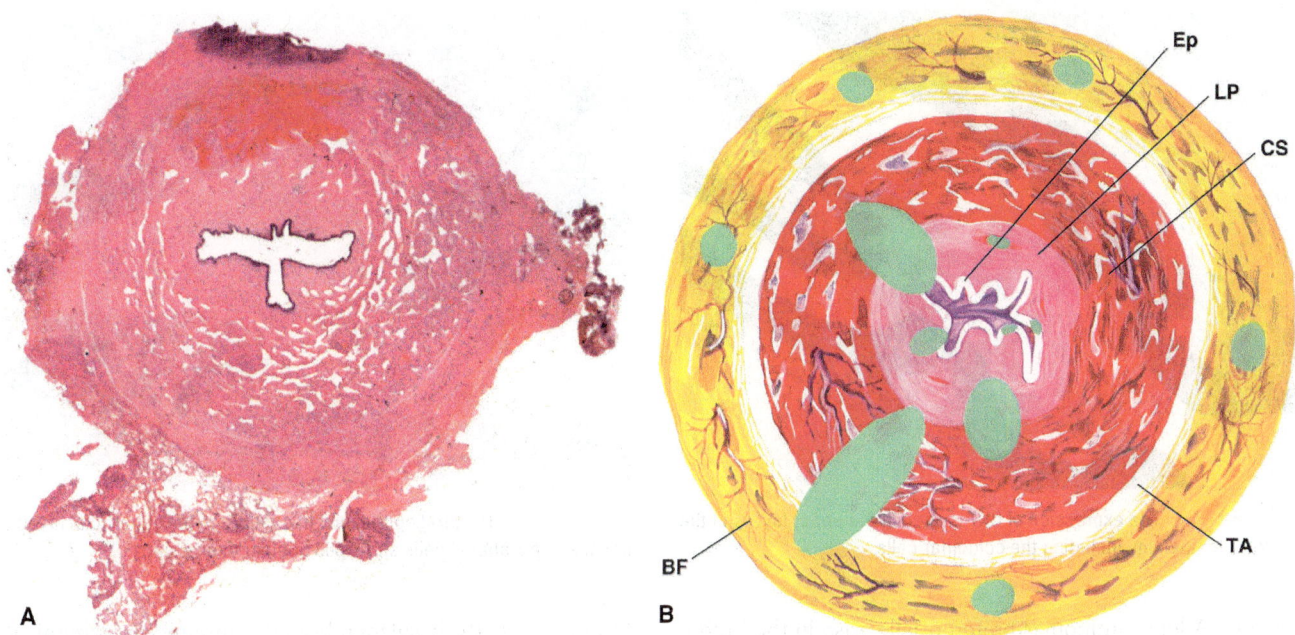

FIGURE 37.33   **A:** Cross section of the penile urethra and periurethral tissues. Note the stellate-shaped lumen at the center. **B:** Diagrammatic cross section of penile urethra and periurethral tissues. The anatomical levels at the urethral margin of resection are epithelium (*Ep*), lamina propria (*LP*), periurethral corpus spongiosum (*CS*), tunica albuginea (*TA*), and Buck fascia (*BF*).

glands that are present in the lateral walls of the bulbous and penile urethra. A stellate-shaped lumen can be noted in cross section of the penile urethra owing to these folds of epithelium and lamina propria (Fig. 37.33A). From the surgical pathology point of view, the urethra with surrounding periurethral tissues is an important resection margin and should be carefully examined in partial penectomy specimens with penile carcinoma. In a study of penectomies with carcinoma, the urethra and periurethral cylinder was found to be the most frequently involved margin of resection (57). The anatomical levels at the urethral/periurethral margin are epithelium, lamina propria, periurethral corpus spongiosum, tunica albuginea, and Buck fascia (Fig. 37.33A-B).

Microscopic and Immunohistochemical Features

▶ **URETHRAL EPITHELIUM** There are two conflicting embryologic explanations of the differentiation of the distal urethra: The ectodermal ingrowth theory (the distal urethra originates in the ectoderm, penetrating from glans to urethra) and the endodermal differentiation theory (distal urethra is formed by differentiation of endodermal tissues from urethra to glans) (67,68). Independently of the embryogenesis, there are histologic differences between the epithelium of the anterior urethra and the classical transitional urothelium of the posterior urethra and the urinary tract. The fossa navicularis is lined by nonkeratinizing squamous epithelium, and it is similar and continuous to the epithelium covering the glans penis. In the pendulous and bulbous urethra, the surface cell layer is columnar without the "umbrella" cells noted in bladder urothelium and prostatic urethra. In addition to the columnar cells, the epithelium of the anterior urethra is composed of 4 to 15 stratified layers of uniform small cells, usually categorized as stratified or pseudostratified columnar epithelium (Fig. 37.34). The distinctive epithelium appears to be related to the squamous rather than to the transitional urothelium. This would explain the high frequency of squamous metaplasias, as well as the predominance of carcinomas of squamous type in the anterior urethra compared with a much higher frequency of transitional cell carcinomas in the prostatic urethra. The tumors in the membranous portion of the posterior urethra are more similar to those of the bulbous

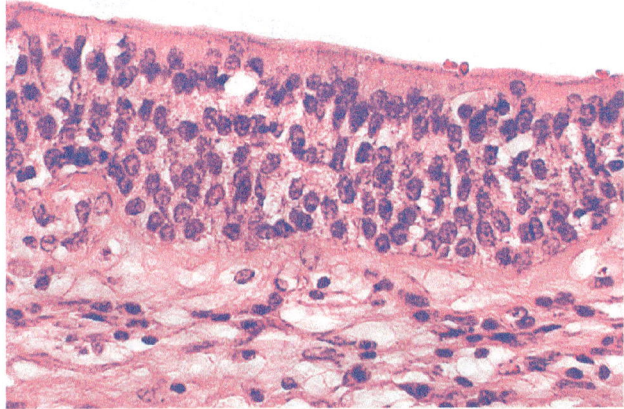

FIGURE 37.34   The epithelium of the anterior urethra is composed of columnar cells overlying 4 to 15 stratified layers of uniform small cells, usually categorized as stratified or pseudostratified columnar epithelium.

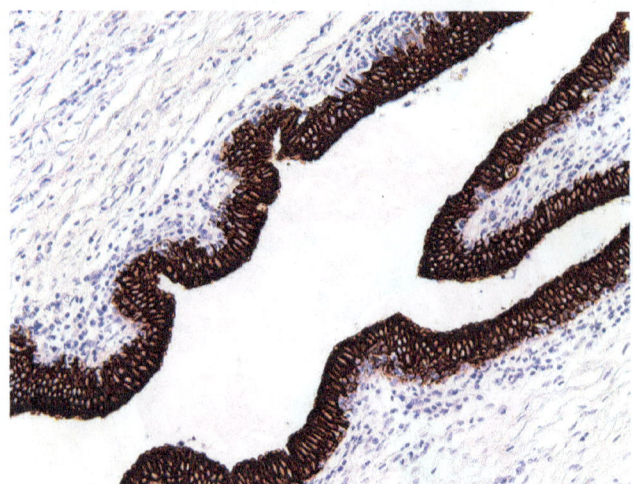

FIGURE 37.35 The expression of CK7 is seen in the upper layers of the urethral epithelium, including the columnar cells.

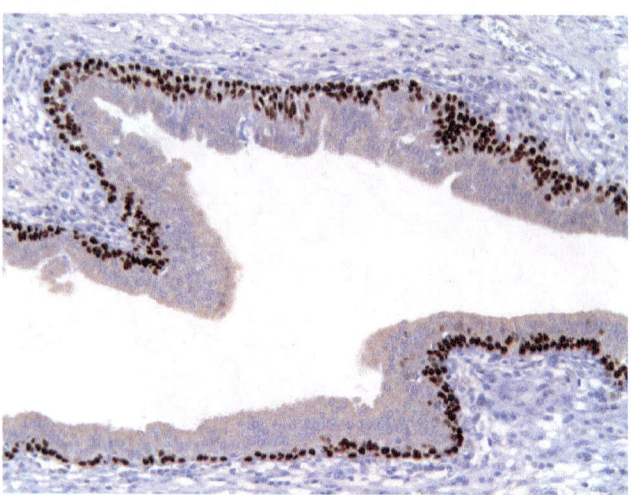

FIGURE 37.37 Urethral epithelium. In contrast to the superficial layers, basal and parabasal cells show p63 nuclear expression.

urethra. Adenocarcinomas preferentially arise in the bulbo-membranous urethra; however, squamous cell carcinomas are significantly more frequent than adenocarcinomas in these portions (12). The frequent finding of intraepithelial precancerous lesions in the penile urethras of patients with penile squamous cell carcinoma is noteworthy because it indicates that the urethra participates either as a mechanical pathway of penile cancer progression in a continuous manner or as an independent site of primary tumor growth in discontinuous lesions (68).

Immunohistochemical studies show that the penile urethral epithelium expresses CK7, 34βE12, and p63, but is negative for CK20. The CK7 immunostain is positive in the upper layers of the epithelium, including the columnar cells (Fig. 37.35), in contrast to the expression of p63 and 34βE12 that is mostly seen in basal and parabasal cells, but not in the superficial layer of columnar cells (Figs. 37.36 and 37.37). Occasional chromogranin-positive cells may be found close to the basal membrane by immunohistochemical stains.

> **URETHRAL AND PERIURETHRAL GLANDS** There are two different types of glands in the anterior urethra: The intra- or juxtaepithelial glands, with a dense eosinophilic cytoplasm and rounded basal nuclei, and the classical mucinous Littré glands, with clear mucinous cytoplasm and basally compressed nuclei resembling pyloric glands of the gastrointestinal tract (Fig. 37.38). There are histologic transitions from the intra- or juxtaepithelial glands with dense eosinophilic cytoplasm to more mucinous cells.

The recesses of the urethra (Morgagni lacunae) are lined by paraurethral mucinous Littré glands. Littré glands are tubuloacinous–mucous structures located along the full length of the corpus spongiosum, in close relation with erectile tissue (Fig. 37.39). Littré glands end in the urethra at the level of the intraepithelial lacunae. Some cysts

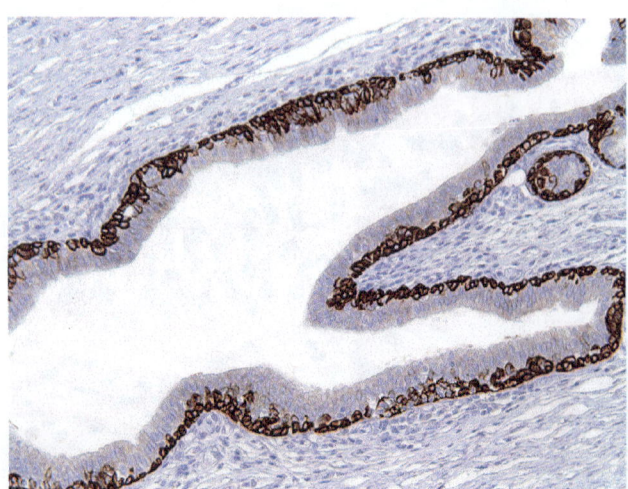

FIGURE 37.36 Urethral epithelium. Basal and parabasal cells express 34βE12. The superficial layers are negative.

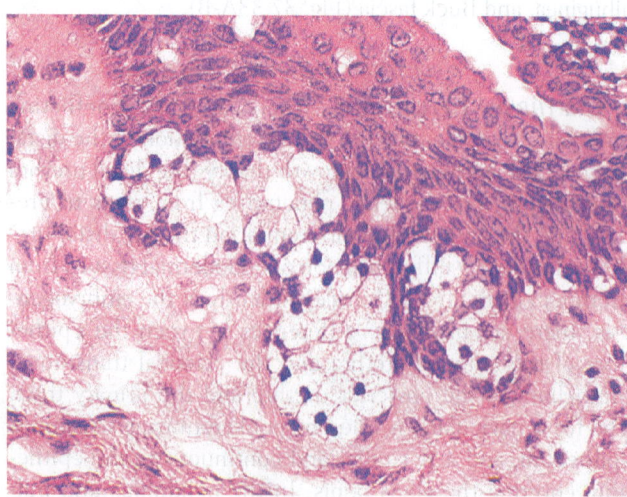

FIGURE 37.38 Penile urethra. A section illustrating intraepithelial mucinous glandular structures.

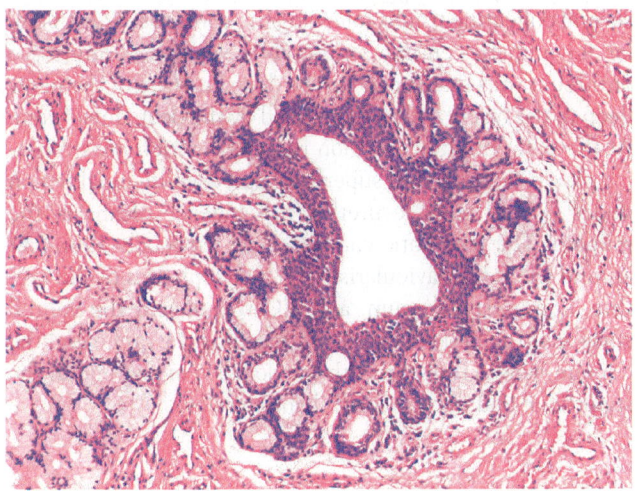

FIGURE 37.39 Penile urethra. Photomicrograph illustrating a cluster of tubular and acinar Littré mucous glands.

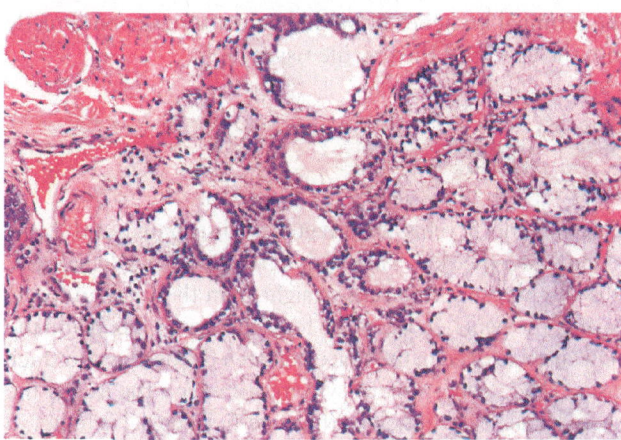

FIGURE 37.41 Bulbourethral (Cowper) gland. Specimen was taken from autopsy and shows acinous–mucous structures, which are located deeply in the membranous urethra. Courtesy of Dr. Victor Reuter, Memorial Sloan-Kettering Cancer Center.

have been described as originating in the parameatal Littré glands (69). Inflammation of Littré glands can clinically simulate a tumor (70). Cohen et al. recognized the normal presence of prostatic epithelial cells in periurethral glands along the penile urethra. These "minor prostatic glands" may be entirely composed of prostatic cells or, more commonly, mixed prostatic and mucinous epithelia (71) (Fig. 37.40). The same authors suggested that these glands may be partially responsible for the minimal, but persistently elevated levels of serum prostate-specific antigen (PSA) in some cases of successful radical prostatectomy (71).

The bulbourethral, or Cowper glands are two small structures deeply located at the level of the membranous (or bulbous) urethra where they terminate in two small ducts (72). They are mucous–acinous structures (Fig. 37.41). The clear cells of these glands can be confused with prostatic carcinoma in a core needle biopsy specimen.

> **LAMINA PROPRIA** The urethral lamina propria is a thin layer of loose fibrous and elastic tissue. Genital corpuscles are identified in the lamina propria of the most distal portion of the urethra, which is lined by squamous epithelium; however, they are not seen in other portions of the penile urethra. We have seen cases of lichen sclerosus affecting the glans and extending into the lamina propria of the anterior urethra (68).

The corpus spongiosum, tunica albuginea, and Buck fascia were discussed in a previous section.

ARTERIES

The arteries of the penis are branches of the internal pudenda, which is a branch of the iliac. There are two systems: the dorsal and the cavernous arteries. The dorsal arteries are located from the base of the penis near and on both sides of the dorsal profunda vein within Buck fascia and in the superior groove formed by the CC (Fig. 37.26). Small caliber branches, or circumflex arteries, irrigate the CC and the periurethral corpus spongiosum. They also perforate the albuginea to reach the corpora. The terminal branches irrigate the glans, and collateral branches provide the skin nutrients. Cavernous arteries penetrate the CC at the site where the corpora join, and they run longitudinally near the central septum, which divides the corpora. From the cavernous arteries originate the vasa vasorum, small arteries that irrigate the erectile tissues. The helicine branches also originate from the cavernous arteries, and they are responsible for filling the vascular spaces during the process of erection; their name derives from the fact that they are coiled and twisted along the trabeculae when the penis is flaccid (73,74). These arteries have thick muscular walls; and, in addition, many possess inner thickenings of longitudinal muscle fibers that bulge into their lumina. Many of

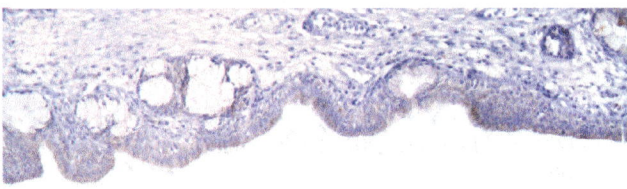

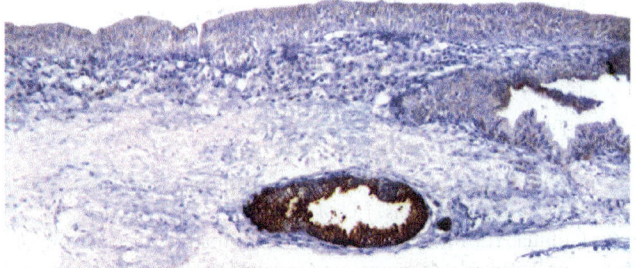

FIGURE 37.40 Some periurethral glands are positive with prostate-specific antigen (PSA) immunostain.

the terminal branches of the helicine arteries open directly into the spaces of the erectile tissue.

VEINS

The superficial veins are irregularly distributed and easily noted under the skin. They end in the superficial dorsal vein; this vascular structure runs straight from the foreskin to the base of the penis. It drains the foreskin venous blood and the skin and is located in the space between the dermis and Buck fascia. The deeper venous system, for which the axis is the deep dorsal vein, runs along the superficial dorsal vein but in a plane separated by Buck fascia (Fig. 37.26). The circumflex veins originate in the periurethral corpus spongiosum and terminate in the deep dorsal vein system. Similarly, there are veins originating in the CC that, after forming a small plexus at the base of the penis, terminate in the internal pudendal vein. The cavernous venous system, unlike the venous drainage from the glans penis, delays venous drainage and in doing so assists in maintaining erections (75).

Penile erection is a vascular phenomenon that results from trabecular smooth muscle relaxation, arterial dilation, and venous restriction. In further support of the concept of restriction of outflow is the observation that the walls of the circumflex veins are unusually muscular. In addition, these veins exhibit unique specializations of their lumina called *polsters*. These are local accumulations of fibroblasts and smooth muscle cells beneath the endothelium that form conspicuous longitudinal thickenings or ridges that can be followed throughout hundreds of serial sections. These are believed to have a role in constricting the lumen and retarding venous outflow during erection (16). There are, however, controversies regarding the real presence and significance of the polsters in the penile veins and arteries, and some authors have proposed that they represent degenerative changes (76).

The deep dorsal vein of the penis has a connection with the vertebral veins; hence it is possible for metastases to make their way to the vertebrae or even to the skull and brain without going through the heart and lungs. Pyogenic organisms may be transported by the same route (1).

LYMPHATICS

The lymphatics of the foreskin spring from a network that covers its internal and external surfaces; they arise from the lateral aspect and converge dorsally with the skin of the shaft lymphatics to form 4 to 10 vessels that run toward the pubis, where they diverge to drain into the right and left superficial inguinal lymph nodes. The lymphatics draining the glands form a rich network that, beginning in the lamina propia, course toward the frenulum, where they coalesce with two or three trunks from the distal urethra to form several collecting trunks following the coronal sulcus. A collar of lymphatics entirely surrounds the corona, forming two or three trunks that run along the dorsal surface of the penis deep to the fascia and accompanied by the deep dorsal vein. At the parasymphyseal region they form a rich anastomosing plexus draining into superficial and deep inguinal lymph nodes (77). The male urethra has a dense plexus in the mucosa. The lymphatic capillaries are especially abundant around the fossa navicularis (1). The lymphatics of the urethra, corpus spongiosum, and CC run toward the ventral surface of the body of the penis, reaching the raphe and the dorsum, where they run with the dorsal vein and end in the superficial and deep inguinal lymph nodes.

NERVES

The nerves originate in the sacral and lumbar plexuses. Peripheral nerves run along the arteries. Dorsal nerves are located external to the arteries, giving circumflex branches to the CC (78,79). The terminal branches end in the glans and the foreskin. The dorsal nerve of the penis, the principal somatosensory nerve innervating the penis, consists of two populations of axons, one to innervate the penile shaft and urethra and the other to innervate the glans. Urethral innervation by the dorsal nerve of the penis supports the view that urethral afferent impulses are a component of reflex ejaculatory activity. The pattern of glandular innervation by the dorsal nerve of the penis identifies the glans as a sensory end organ for sexual reflexes. The undulating character of the dorsal nerve of the penis is a mechanism by which the nerve can accommodate to significant changes in penile length with erection (78). The dorsal nerve of the penis supplies the glans in most men, but branches of the perineal nerve can supply the ventral penis, frenulum, and periurethral area in some men.

REFERENCES

1. Susan Standring S, ed. *Gray's Anatomy: The Anatomical Basis of Clinical Practice*. 40th ed. Churchill Livingstone, Elsevier; 2008.
2. Bunker CB. *Male Genital Skin Disease*. Philadelphia, PA: Elsevier Saunders; 2004.
3. Hyman AB, Brownstein MH. Tyson's "glands." Ectopic sebaceous glands and papillomatosis penis. *Arch Dermatol* 1969;99:31–36.
4. Tanenbaum MH, Becker SW. Papillae of the corona of the glans penis. *J Urol* 1965;93:391–395.
5. Winer JH, Winer LH. Hirsutoid papillomas of the coronal margin of glans penis. *J Urol* 1955;74:375–378.
6. Cubilla AL, Piris A, Pfannl R, et al. Anatomic levels: Important landmarks in penectomy specimens: A detailed anatomic and histologic study based on examination of 44 cases. *Am J Surg Pathol* 2001;25:1091–1094.

7. Ornellas AA, Nóbrega BL, Wei Kin Chin E, et al. Prognostic factors in invasive squamous cell carcinoma of the penis: Analysis of 196 patients treated at the Brazilian National Cancer Institute. *J Urol* 2008; 180(4):1354–1359.
8. Ficarra V, Martignoni G, Maffei N, et al. Predictive pathological factors of lymph nodes involvement in the squamous cell carcinoma of the penis. *Int Urol Nephrol* 2002;34(2): 245–250.
9. Moll I, Kuhn C, Moll R. Cytokeratin 20 is a general marker of cutaneous Merkel cells while certain neuronal proteins are absent. *J Invest Dermatol* 1995;104:910–915.
10. Cold CJ, Taylor JR. The prepuce. *BJU Int* 1999;83(Suppl 1): 34–44.
11. Tuncali D, Bingul F, Talim B, et al. Histologic characteristics of the human prepuce pertaining to its clinical behavior as a dual graft. *Ann Plast Surg* 2005;54:191–195.
12. Young RH, Srigley JR, Amin MB, et al. Tumors of the prostate gland, seminal vesicles, male urethra and penis. In: Young RH, Srigley JR, Amin MB, et al., eds. *Atlas of Tumor Pathology: Third Series, Fascicle*. Washington, DC: Armed Forces Institute of Pathology; 2000.
13. Montagna W, Kligman AM, Carlisle KS. *Atlas of Normal Human Skin*. New York: Springer-Verlag; 1992.
14. Kelly DE, Wood RL, Enders AC. *Bailey's Textbook of Microscopic Anatomy*. 18th ed. Baltimore, MD: Williams & Wilkins; 1984.
15. Halata Z, Munger BL. The neuroanatomical basis for the protopathic sensibility of the human glans penis. *Brain Res* 1986;371:205–230.
16. Fawcett DW. *Bloom and Fawcett: A Textbook of Histology*. 11th ed. Philadelphia, PA: WB Saunders; 1986.
17. Ham AW, Cormack DH. *Histology*. 8th ed. Philadelphia, PA: JB Lippincott Company; 1979.
18. Cubilla AL, Barreto J, Caballero C, et al. Pathologic features of epidermoid carcinoma of the penis. A prospective study of 66 cases. *Am J Surg Pathol* 1993;17(8):753–763.
19. Poirier P, Charpy A. *Traité d'Anatomie humaine*. Paris: Masson et Cie; 1901:183.
20. Saalfeld E. Ueber die Tyson'schen drüsen. *Arch Mikr Anat* 1899;53:212–218.
21. Tandler J, Dömeny P. Ueber Tyson'schen drüsen. *Wiener Klin Wochen* 1898;23:555–556.
22. Testut L, Latarjet A. *Tratado de Anatomía Humana*. Vol. 4. 9th ed. Barcelona: Salvat; 1959.
23. Parkash S, Jeyakumar S, Subramanyan K, et al. Human subpreputial collection: Its nature and formation. *J Urol* 1973;110:211–212.
24. Keith A, Shillitoe A. The preputial or odoriferous glands of man. *Lancet* 1904;1:146–148.
25. Sprunk H. *Ueber die vermeintlichen Tyson'schen draüsen [dissertation]*. Germany: University of Königsberg; 1897.
26. Tyson E. *The anatomy of a pygmy compared with that of a monkey, an ape and a man*. London: University of London Press; 1699.
27. Velazquez EF, Bock A, Soskin A, et al. Preputial variability and preferential association of long phimotic foreskins with penile cancer: An anatomic comparative study of types of foreskin in a general population and cancer patients. *Am J Surg Pathol* 2003;27:994–998.
28. Winberg J, Bollgren I, Gothefors L, et al. The prepuce: A mistake of nature? *Lancet* 1989;1:598–599.
29. Weiss HA, Larke N, Halperin D, et al. Complications of circumcision in male neonates, infants and children: A systematic review. *BMC Urol* 2010;10:2.
30. Taylor JR, Lockwood AP, Taylor AJ. The prepuce: Specialized mucosa of the penis and its loss to circumcision. *Br J Urol* 1996;77:291–295.
31. Lukong CS. Circumcision: Controversies and prospects. *J Surg Tech Case Rep* 2011;3(2):65–66.
32. Pinto K. Circumcision controversies. *Pediatr Clin North Am* 2012;59(4):977–986.
33. Winkelmann RK. The erogenous zones: Their nerve supply and its significance. *Mayo Clin Proc* 1959;34:39–47.
34. Ben-Ari J, Merlob P, Mimouni F, et al. Characteristics of the male genitalia in the newborn: Penis. *J Urol* 1985;134: 521–522.
35. Dillner J, von Krogh G, Horenblas S, et al. Etiology of squamous cell carcinoma of the penis. *Scand J Urol Nephrol Suppl* 2000;205:189–193.
36. Lerman SE, Liao JC. Neonatal circumcision. *Pediatr Clin North Am* 2001;48:1539–1557.
37. Fussell EN, Kaack MB, Cherry R, et al. Adherence of bacteria to human foreskins. *J Urol* 1988;140:997–1001.
38. Castellsague X, Bosch FX, Munoz N, et al. Male circumcision, penile human papillomavirus infection, and cervical cancer in female partners. *N Engl J Med* 2002;346: 1105–1112.
39. Tobian AA, Serwadda D, Quinn TC, et al. Male circumcision for the prevention of HSV-2 and HPV infections and syphilis. *N Engl J Med* 2009;360(13):1298–1309.
40. Wawer MJ, Tobian AA, Kigozi G, et al. Effect of circumcision of HIV-negative men on transmission of human papillomavirus to HIV-negative women: A randomised trial in Rakai, Uganda. *Lancet* 2011;377(9761):209–218.
41. Bailey RC, Moses S, Parker CB, et al. Male circumcision for HIV prevention in young men in Kisumu, Kenya: A randomised controlled trial. *Lancet* 2007;369:643–656.
42. Gray RH, Kigozi G, Serwadda D, et al. Male circumcision for HIV prevention in men in Rakai, Uganda: A randomised trial. *Lancet* 2007;369:657–666.
43. Frisch M, Friis S, Kjear SK, et al. Falling incidence of penis cancer in an uncircumcised population (Denmark 1943–90). *BMJ* 1995;311:1471.
44. Hines JZ, Ntsuape OC, Malaba K, et al. Scale-Up of Voluntary Medical Male Circumcision Services for HIV Prevention—12 Countries in Southern and Eastern Africa, 2013–2016. *MMWR Morb Mortal Wkly Rep* 2017;66(47):1285–1290.
45. Kalichman S, Mathews C, Kalichman M, et al. Male circumcision for HIV prevention: Awareness, risk compensation, and risk perceptions among South African women. *Glob Public Health* 2018;25:1–9.
46. American Academy of Pediatrics Task Force on Circumcision. Circumcision policy statement. *Pediatrics* 2012;130(3): 585–586.
47. Oster J. Further fate of the foreskin: Incidence of preputial adhesions, phimosis, and smegma among Danish schoolboys. *Arch Dis Child* 1968;43:200–203.
48. Oertell J, Caballero C, Iglesias M, et al. Differentiated precursor lesions and low-grade variants of squamous cell carcinomas are frequent findings in foreskins of patients from a region of high penile cancer incidence. *Histopathology* 2011;58(6): 925–933.

49. Epstein JH, Cubilla AL, Humphrey PA. Tumors of the prostate gland, seminal vesicles, male urethra, penis and scrotum. In: Epstein JH, Cubilla AL, Humphrey PA, eds. *Atlas of Tumor Pathology. 4th Series, Fascicle*. Washington, DC: Armed Forces Institute of Pathology; 2011.
50. Modwing R, Valderrama E. Immunohistochemical analysis of nerve distributions pattern within preputial tissues. *J Urol* 1989;141(Suppl 1):489A.
51. Brierly JD, Gospodarowicz MK, Wittekind C, eds. *TNM Classification of Malignant Tumours*. 8th ed. Oxford, UK; Hoboken, NJ: John Wiley & Sons, Inc.; 2017.
52. Chaux A, Caballero C, Soares F, et al. The prognostic index: a useful pathologic guide for prediction of nodal metastases and survival in penile squamous cell carcinoma. *Am J Surg Pathol* 2009;33(7):1049–1057.
53. Kattan MW, Ficarra V, Artibani W, et al. Nomogram predictive of cancer specific survival in patients undergoing partial or total amputation for squamous cell carcinoma of the penis. *J Urol* 2006;175(6):2103–2108.
54. Ficarra V, Zattoni F, Artibani W, et al. Nomogram predictive of pathological inguinal lymph node involvement in patients with squamous cell carcinoma of the penis. *J Urol* 2006;175(5):1700–1704.
55. Hricak H, Marotti M, Gilbert TJ, et al. Normal penile anatomy and abnormal penile condition: Evaluation with MR imaging. *Radiology* 1988;169:683–690.
56. Mostofi FK, Davis C Jr. Male reproductive system and prostate. In: Kissane JM, ed. *Anderson's Pathology*. Vol. 1. 8th ed. St. Louis, MO: CV Mosby; 1985.
57. Velazquez EF, Soskin A, Bock A, et al. Positive resection margins in partial penectomies: Sites of involvement and proposal of local routes of spread of penile squamous cell carcinoma. *Am J Surg Pathol* 2004;28:384–389.
58. Hsu GL, Brock G, Martínez-Pineiro L, et al. Anatomy and strength of the tunica albuginea: Its relevance to penile prosthesis extrusion. *J Urol* 1994;151:1205–1208.
59. Spirnack JP, Resnick MI, Hampel N, et al. Fournier's gangrene: Report of 20 patients. *J Urol* 1984;131:289–291.
60. Goldstein AMB, Meehan JP, Zakhary R, et al. New observations on microarchitecture of corpora cavernosa in man and possible relationship to mechanism of erection. *Urology* 1982;20:259–266.
61. Zinner NR, Sterling AM, Coleman RV, et al. The role of internal structure in human penile rigidity. *J Urol* 1989;141:221A.
62. Droupy S, Giuliano F, Jardin A, et al. Cavernospongious shunts: Anatomical study of intrapenile vascular pathways. *Eur Urol* 1999;36:123–128.
63. Vardi Y, Saenz de Tejada I. Functional and radiologic evidence of vascular communication between the spongiosal and cavernosal compartments of the penis. *Urology* 1997;49:749–752.
64. Fontana D, Rolle L, Lacivita A, et al. Modificazioni anatomo-funzionali dei corpi cavernosi nell'anziano. *Arch Ital Urol Androl* 1993;65:483–486.
65. Rodriguez IM, Cuevas M, Silvero A, et al. Novel histologic finding: Adipose tissue is prevalent within penile tunica albuginea and corpora cavernosa: An anatomic study of 63 specimens and considerations for cancer invasion. *Am J Surg Pathol* 2017;41(11):1542–1546.
66. Moch H, Humphrey PA, Ulbright TM, et al. *WHO Classification of Tumours of the Urinary System and Male Genital Organs*, 4th ed. Lyon: IARC Press; 2016.
67. Kurzrock EA, Baskin LS, Cunha GR. Ontogeny of the male urethra: Theory of endodermal differentiation. *Differentiation* 1999;64:115–122.
68. Velazquez EF, Soskin A, Bock A, et al. Epithelial abnormalities and precancerous lesions of anterior urethra in patients with penile carcinoma. A report of 89 cases. *Mod Pathol* 2005;18:917–923.
69. Shiraki IW. Parameatal cysts of the glans penis: A report of 9 cases. *J Urol* 1975;114:544–548.
70. Krawitt LN, Schechterman L. Inflammation of the periurethral glands of Littre simulating tumor. *J Urol* 1977;118:685.
71. Cohen RJ, Garrett K, Golding JL, et al. Epithelial differentiation of the lower urinary tract with recognition of the minor prostatic glands. *Hum Pathol* 2002;33:905–909.
72. Bourne CW, Kilcoyne RF, Kraenzler EJ. Prominent lateral mucosal folds in the bulbous urethra. *J Urol* 1981;126:326–330.
73. Breza J, Aboseif SR, Orvis BR, et al. Detailed anatomy of penile neurovascular structures: Surgical significance. *J Urol* 1989;141:437–443.
74. Krane RJ. Sexual function and dysfunction. In: Walsh PC, Gittes R, Perlmutter AD, Stamey TA, eds. *Campbell's Urology*. Vol. 1. 5th ed. Philadelphia, PA: WB Saunders; 1986:700–735.
75. Fitzpatrick T. The corpus cavernosum intercommunicating venous drainage system. *J Urol* 1975;113:494–496.
76. Benson GS, McConnell JA, Schmidt WA. Penile polsters: Functional structures or atherosclerotic changes? *J Urol* 1981;125:800–803.
77. Cunéo B, Marcille M. Note sur les lymphatiques du gland. *Bull Soc Anat Paris* 1901;76:671–674.
78. Yang CC, Bradley WE. Peripheral distribution of the human dorsal nerve of the penis. *J Urol* 1998;159:1912–1916.
79. Lepor H, Gregerman M, Crosby R, et al. Precise localization of the autonomic nerves from the pelvic plexus to the corpora cavernosa: A detailed anatomical study of the adult male pelvis. *J Urol* 1985;133:207–212.

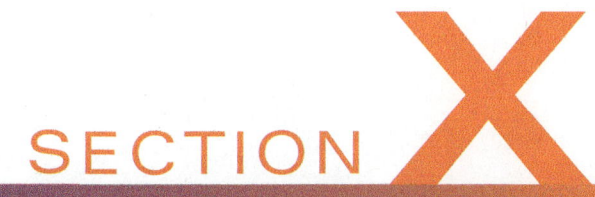

SECTION X

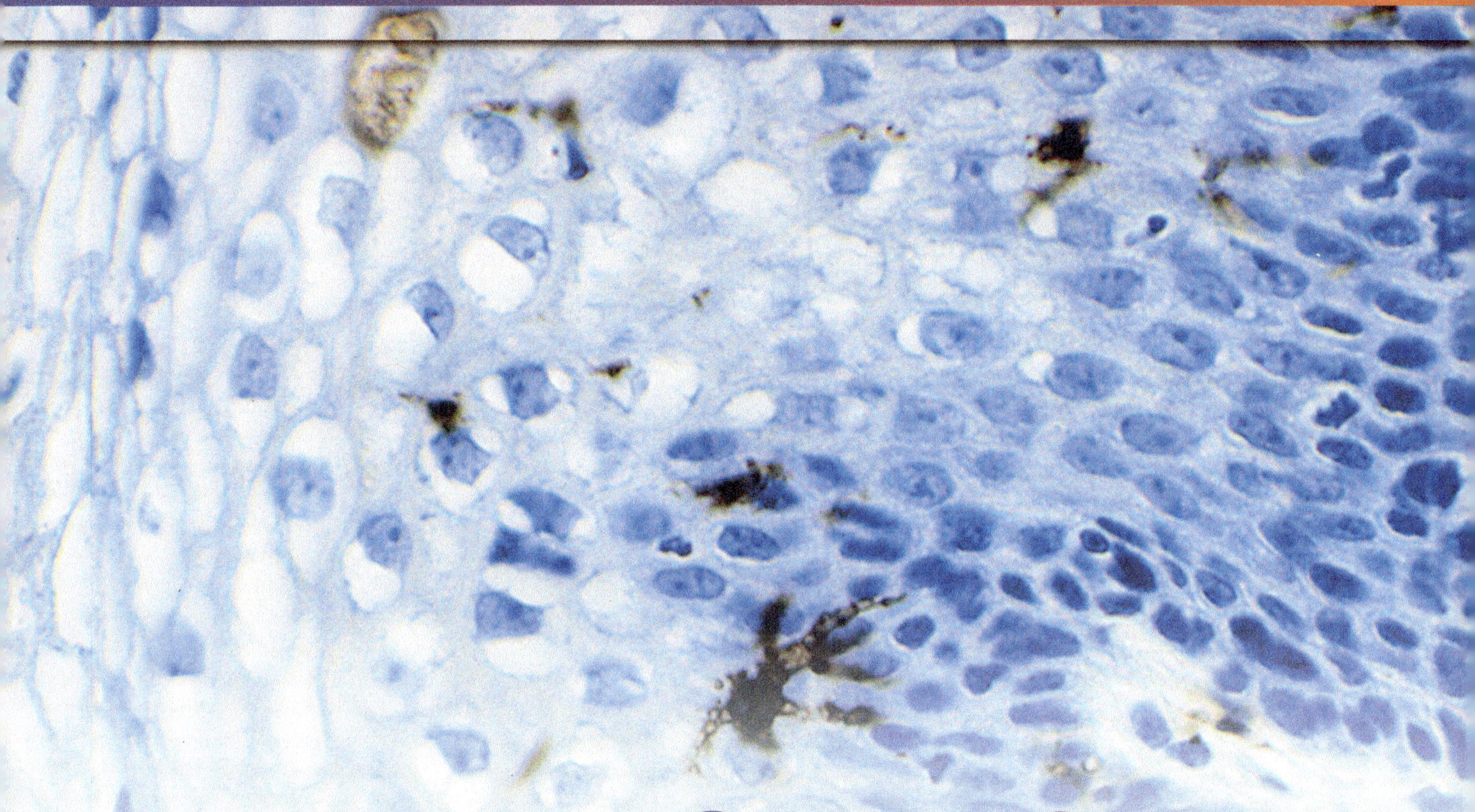

Female Genital System

Vulva

Krisztina Z. Hanley

CLINICAL PERSPECTIVE 1031	Labia Minora 1038
SPECIAL TECHNIQUES IN CLINICAL EVALUATION 1031	Labia Majora 1039
	Mons Pubis (Mons Veneris) 1043
ANATOMY 1032	Lymphatic Drainage 1043
Vulvar Biopsy 1033	Arterial Supply 1044
Vulvar Vestibule 1034	Venous Supply 1044
Urethral Orifice (Meatus Urinarius) 1036	Nerve Supply 1044
Hymen 1037	REFERENCES 1044
Clitoris 1037	

CLINICAL PERSPECTIVE

Vulvar symptoms are a common cause of clinical visits to gynecologists and family practitioners. Studies have shown that 8% to 15% of reproductive age women in the general population have symptoms related to vulvar pain (1–3). Complaints may include pruritus, burning, pain, external dyspareunia, and a visible or palpable mass (4). Vulvodynia refers to vulvar pain or burning sensation for at least 3 months, without identifiable cause (5). In postmenopausal women, vulvar pain is often attributed to atrophy of the vulvovaginal epithelium due to low levels of estrogen. Chronic vulvar pain can impact quality of life. Women often seek multiple health care providers and receive several different diagnoses and treatment modalities before experiencing any improvement of symptoms.

The majority of sexually transmitted infections, as well as granulomatous, neoplastic dermatologic diseases, may involve the vulva (6–10). Graft-versus-host disease (11) and contact dermatitis (12) may create symptoms requiring evaluation of the vulva and the vagina. The vulva (pudendum femininum) is also a crucial area for detailed examination in cases of reported rape, sexual abuse, or female circumcision (13). Ambiguous genitalia and genital anomalies challenge the clinician and demand critical examination of the patient and the external genitalia (14,15). Clitoral enlargement in the newborn resulting from adrenal genital syndrome, maternal exposure to exogenous androgens, maldevelopment of the clitoris, benign tumors, and other conditions, such as the Lawrence–Seip syndrome (8,16), may result in ambiguous-appearing external genitalia. Clitoromegaly may occur in adulthood due to benign tumors, malignancy, or endocrinopathy (14,16,17).

Surgical approaches to vulvar diseases are evolving as a result of better understanding of vulvar anatomy and sexual function, as well as tumor biology. Clitoral specimens are submitted less frequently in cases of infant genital ambiguity now that follow-up studies have indicated that permanent loss of function and sensation may result (15,18–20). In extended surgery for carcinoma of the vulva, the clitoris may be surgically spared with partial deep vulvectomy, if clinical examination does not indicate tumor involvement of that structure (15). The techniques for sentinel node evaluation used in other cancers are now applied to carcinomas of the vulva, permitting removal of less normal tissue from lymph node drainage fields (21–23).

Cytologic evaluation of the vulva may complement biopsy in special cases such as extramammary Paget disease and distinguishing disorders that may clinically resemble Paget disease (24).

SPECIAL TECHNIQUES IN CLINICAL EVALUATION

Direct examination of the vulva requires adequate illumination and is enhanced by the use of a ring light or a magnifying

---

This chapter is an update of a previous version authored by Edward J. Wilkinson and Nancy S. Hardt.

glass (25). Some practitioners routinely use colposcopy or vulvoscopy to enhance identification of areas of hypopigmentation, scarring, fissures, small condyloma acuminatum, vestibular papillae, and vulvar intraepithelial neoplasia (VIN) (25). In cases in which condyloma acuminatum or VIN is suspected, the use of 3% acetic acid (white vinegar) is of value. Gauze sponges soaked in 3% acetic acid are applied for approximately five minutes, followed by prompt examination. The principle of this technique is that abnormal epithelium, especially condyloma acuminatum and VIN, becomes white (acetowhite) immediately after exposure to acetic acid. This is related to poorly understood differences between normal epithelium and human papillomavirus–associated lesions. The color change to white after application of the dilute acetic acid is referred to as acetowhitening, and the epithelium so changed is referred to as acetowhite epithelium. This procedure has gained wide acceptance in the evaluation of the cervical transformation zone during colposcopic examination to enhance identification of cervical intraepithelial neoplasia and carcinoma. However, its use on the vulva has two serious limitations. First, when ulcers or fissures are present on the vulva, the application of 3% acetic acid may be associated with pain and thus is unacceptable to the patient. Second, the vulvar vestibular epithelium is normally somewhat acetowhite. The inexperienced clinician may misinterpret this acetowhitening as abnormal or as condyloma acuminatum. A biopsy is then performed of the vestibular epithelium and submitted as condyloma acuminatum. The vestibular epithelium in women of reproductive age is normally glycogenated (see section on Vulvar Vestibule) and can be misinterpreted by the unwary pathologist as koilocytosis suggestive of condyloma acuminatum, resulting in both improper diagnosis and improper therapy for the patient. Inflammation within the vestibule may be associated with epithelial spongiosis, which also may resemble koilocytosis.

The use of 1% toluidine blue O with a 1% acetic acid rinse also has been used to assist in the recognition of areas requiring biopsy when invasive carcinoma is suspected (7). Areas with ulceration, parakeratosis, and carcinomas without a keratinized surface retain the blue stain (6,7). This test has limited usefulness in that false-positive staining patterns occur, usually due to benign superficial ulceration or fissures. The test may be falsely negative when the carcinoma or intraepithelial neoplasm has a keratinized surface. For these reasons, the test is no longer commonly used.

Diagnostic workup of vulvodynia often includes a sensory examination, so called "cotton swab test" is performed with moist cotton swab to identify painful areas of the vestibule by applying a gentle rolling motion on the entire vestibule (26). Pelvic examination of the pelvic floor muscles, uterus, and adnexa are often performed, as causes of vulvodynia may be related to endometriosis, pelvic inflammatory disease, or increased pelvic floor muscle tone.

Clinical evaluation of the vulva to assess for trauma after reported child or adult sexual assault is important and challenging. Colposcopy and vulvovaginoscopy are of value to identify related injuries (25). Documentation of findings should occur as soon as possible after the assault, since most genital injuries heal rapidly and without grossly evident scarring. In many cases there is little or no physical evidence for prosecution of sexual offenders (27). Ecchymosis resolves in 2 to 18 days, submucosal hemorrhages resolve in 2 to 14 days, and petechiae are gone within 24 hours. Superficial lacerations heal within a few days and only deep lacerations leave a scar (28).

Commonly used outpatient laboratory techniques in the diagnosis of vulvar diseases include wet mount, potassium hydroxide preparation and assessment of vaginal pH to exclude infectious etiologies, such as candidiasis, trichomonas, or bacterial vaginosis.

In addition to direct visualization techniques, imaging studies are increasingly applied in the vulvar assessment of female sexual response and have increased our understanding of the three-dimensional anatomy of that region. These include duplex Doppler ultrasound (28) and magnetic resonance imaging (MRI) (29).

From the pathologist's perspective, the majority of vulvar specimens that are examined are either diagnostic biopsies, excisional biopsies, or partial superficial or deep, or total superficial or deep vulvectomy specimens submitted as treatment for VIN, Paget disease, carcinoma, melanoma, and other diseases (9,10). An understanding of the normal histology of the vulva enhances interpretive skills and assists in arriving at an appropriate diagnosis.

ANATOMY

The female external genitalia can be defined as that portion of the female anatomy external to the hymen, extending anteriorly to include the mons pubis, posteriorly to the anus, and laterally to the inguinal–gluteal folds. Included are the mons pubis, clitoris, labia minora, labia majora, vulvar vestibule and vestibulovaginal bulbs, urethral meatus, hymen, Bartholin and Skene glands and ducts, and vaginal introitus (Fig. 38.1). The anterior investment of the clitoris includes the prepuce, which represents the anterior fusion of the labia minora and overlays the clitoris anteriorly, and the frenulum, which passes posteriorly and ends in its attachment to the flattened posterior aspect of the clitoris. Posteriorly, the labia minora end in the fourchette, or frenulum of the labia. The labia majora lie lateral to the intralabial sulcus and medial to the inguinal–gluteal fold. Anteriorly, the hair-bearing lateral aspects of the labia majora blend with the mons pubis, and posteriorly, the labia majora end in the perineal body. The hair follicles of the labia majora are absent in its medial portion; however, the sebaceous gland elements are retained medial and posterior to the labia minora at the junction with the vulvar vestibule at Hart line (Fig. 38.2) (6,7,10,30). These sebaceous gland elements open directly to the epithelial surface in this portion of the vulva and can

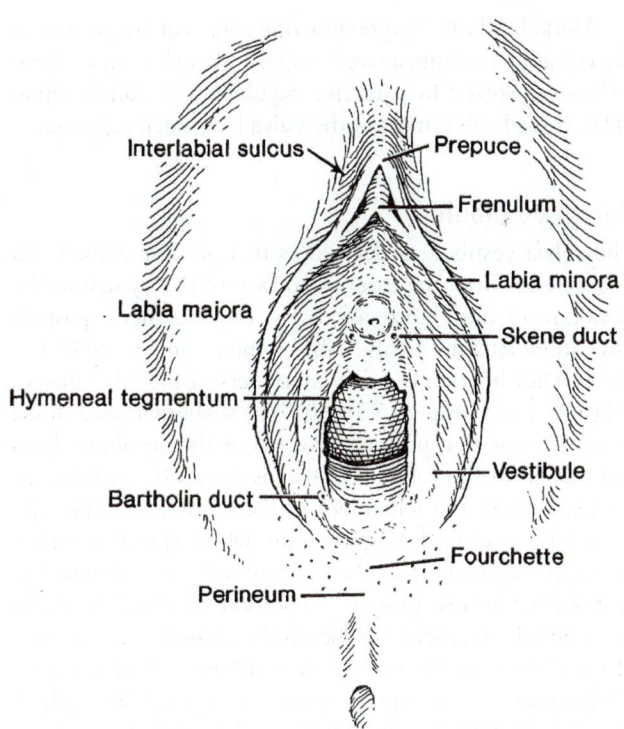

FIGURE 38.1 Topography of the vulva.

be observed as small, slightly pale to yellow elevations of the epithelium, known as Fordyce spots.

Advances in imaging techniques including MRI and digital technology have led researchers to revisit the anatomy of the vulva, and particularly the distal vagina, unifying the findings of prior research. MRI is often used in the diagnostic workup of suspected pelvic pathology, staging of vulvar malignancies, and characterization of mullerian duct anomalies (31). The vulva shows low- to intermediate-signal intensity on T1-weighted imaging and slightly higher-signal intensity on T2-weighted imaging (32).

Vulvar Biopsy

The type of lesion and its anatomic location determine which type of surgical sample is performed for histologic evaluation (33). *Punch biopsies* are excellent tools for evaluating melanocytic lesions, ulcers, tumors, or inflammatory processes. It is important that the biopsy extends below the deepest portion of tumor, since tumor depth determines stage, prognosis, and management. Special techniques may be required when sampling modified mucous membranes (e.g., labia minora) and mucous membranes (e.g., introitus) as these surfaces are difficult to grasp with instruments. Furthermore, the surface epithelium often "slips off" due to lack of skin adnexal structures (i.e., hair follicles) to hold epithelium and submucosa together. This is particularly problematic in immunobullous disorders. If immunobullous disorder is suspected, tissue sample should be obtained by a broad, long technique rather than a narrow deep biopsy to ensure tissue intactness (33).

Shave biopsy is best performed on hair-bearing, keratinized skin (e.g., labia majora). Superficial and exophytic lesions are often sampled with shave biopsies (33). Tissue sample should be placed in 10% buffered formalin, with a volume of media 10 to 20 times the amount of the specimen. Specimens requiring direct immunofluorescence (DIF) are placed in Zeus or Michel media and material for cultures placed in a sterile container. Clinical history can be extremely helpful in the diagnosis of vulvar lesions, especially in inflammatory and nonneoplastic diseases. A minimum specimen requisition should include the following: distribution, size, appearance, clinical differential diagnosis, and which part of the lesion was biopsied. Patients' electronic health records may contain digital photographs of the lesion biopsied, which can be particularly helpful. Histologic evaluation of vulvar biopsies follows a systematic approach of step by step assessment of all tissue layers, identification, localization and distribution of histopathologic changes, differential diagnosis, and clinic-pathologic correlation. Familiarity of normal histology is a key reference point.

A study on histologic evaluation of 118 normal skin and mucosal specimens from mons pubis, labia, vestibule, and perineum found site-specific differences in stratum corneum morphology and parakeratosis and the mucocutaneous junction (34). Samples from the mons pubis show basket-weave stratum corneum (open weave of keratin with clear spaces), while from the labia it can show compact (solid eosinophilic band off keratin), intermediate or basket weave. Basket-weave pattern in biopsies from the perineum is usually not seen.

Normal vulvar epithelium varies in thickness 0.27 ± 0.14 mm. Studies on normal vulvar histology show that

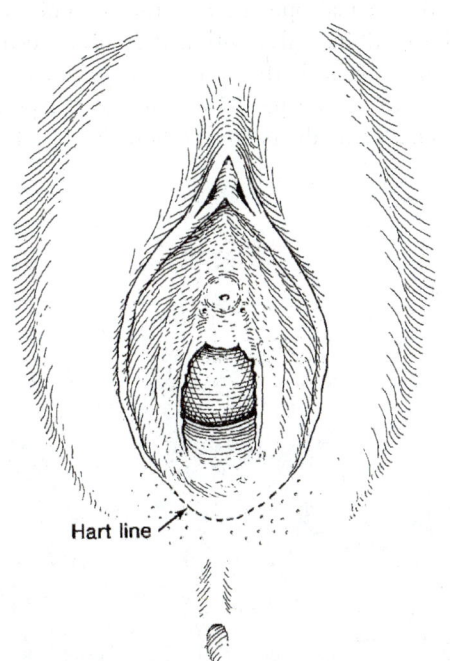

FIGURE 38.2 The vulvar vestibule and the position of Hart line. Hart line can be found on the medial aspect of the labia majora, extending in a curvilinear manner from the most inferior posterior portion of the labia minora to the vaginal fourchette.

epithelial thickness decreases from medial to lateral, coupled with changes in stratum corneum morphology (34,35). When involved by VIN, the thickness of the epithelium with VIN is reported from 0.52 ± 0.23 mm (36). The vulvar epithelium, especially that of the lateral labia minora, labia majora, and perineal body, contains melanocytes that are distributed among the basal cells of the epithelium in a ratio from 1:5 to 1:10 basal keratinocytes (37). Increased pigmentation of these areas during pregnancy relate to increased melanin production secondary to the effects of gestational hormones.

Langerhans cells are relatively abundant in the vulvar epithelium, where they are more prevalent than within the vagina or the cervix. They are present predominantly in the suprabasal layers of vulvar epithelium, with a median number of 18.7 per 100 basal squamous cells (38). They are present in keratinized and nonkeratinized epithelium, as well as within skin appendages. These dendritic cells are bone marrow derived and can express HLA-DR antigens and Fc and C3 receptors and are capable of activating T lymphocytes as an afferent component of the immune response of the vulvar epithelium (39). Langerhans cells have been thought to be associated with control of keratinocyte maturation and recent observations that Langerhans cells are present in reduced numbers in patients with vulvar squamous cell carcinoma add support to this hypothesis (40).

Lichen sclerosus (LS) is a dermatosis that is considered to be T-lymphocyte mediated. Topical corticosteroids including high potency corticosteroids have proven effective in treatment for vulvar LS and are commonly used (7,8).

Lymphocytes are also commonly found in the dermis and submucosal areas of the vulva in small numbers and are located primarily in a perivascular area within the lamina propria. These sparse lymphocytes are thought to represent normal components of skin and mucosa–associated lymphoid tissue. Intraepithelial lymphocytes are infrequently seen in normal vulvar epithelium (38).

Merkel cells are neuroendocrine cells that are present in the vulvar epithelium, as well as most other skin sites. These cells are involved in paracrine regulation of skin function (41). Merkel cell tumors of the vulva have been reported.

Vulvar Vestibule

The vulvar vestibule is defined as that portion of the vulva that extends from the exterior surface of the hymen to the frenulum of the clitoris anteriorly, the fourchette posteriorly, anterolaterally to the labia minora, and posterolaterally to Hart line, on the medial aspects of the labia majora (Figs. 38.1 and 38.2) (6,7,10,30). The vestibular fossa (fossa navicularis) is that posterior portion of the vestibule, from the hymen to the fourchette that is somewhat concave as compared with the remainder of the vestibule. Unlike the remainder of the vulvar epithelium, which is of ectodermal origin, the epithelium of the vulvar vestibule is of endodermal origin. One exception is the portion of the vulvar vestibular epithelium anterior to the urethra, which some think is of ectodermal origin. The vulvar vestibule is predominantly nonkeratinized stratified squamous epithelium, which peripherally blends with the thinly keratinized squamous epithelium of the labia minora, the medial labia majora at Hart line, the prepuce, and the fourchette. Although the vestibular epithelium has an embryonic origin similar to that of the distal urethra of the male, the epithelium is not of a typical transitional type with associated surface umbrella cells. Rather, it is a stratified squamous epithelium that is rich in glycogen in women of reproductive age, similar to the mucosa of the vagina and the ectocervix (Fig. 38.3).

Both the vaginal opening and the urethral orifice are within the vestibule. Also within the vulvar vestibule are gland openings from both the major and minor vestibular glands, as well as the paired opening of the periurethral Skene ducts. Skene ducts are the homologues of the male

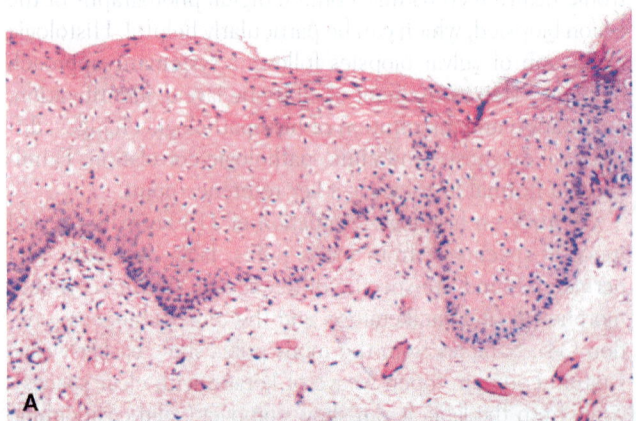
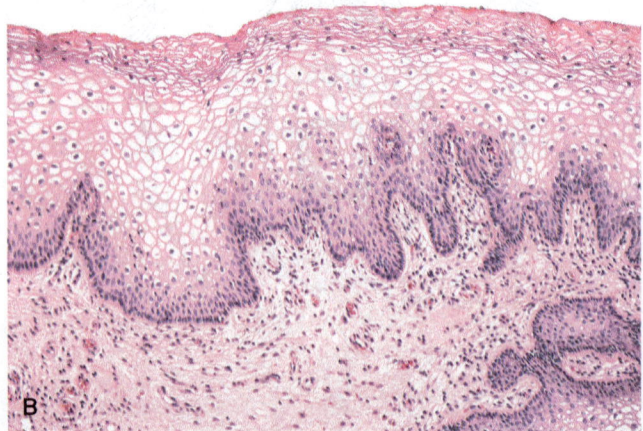

FIGURE 38.3 A: Vulvar vestibule with adjacent prominent vascular submucosa. Superficial thin-walled vessels are prominent and are found within the delicate fibrous stroma. A few lymphocytes are seen scattered in the superficial submucosa. **B:** Epithelium of the vulvar vestibule of a 27-year-old woman. Note that the epithelium is stratified squamous and that the superficial cells have cytoplasmic clearing, reflecting the glycogen-rich epithelium.

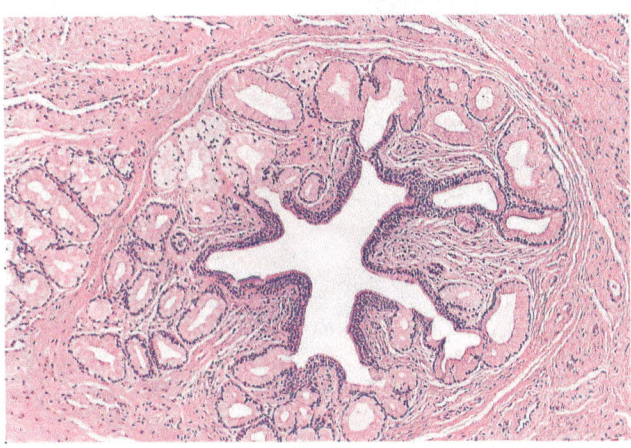

FIGURE 38.4 Bartholin gland acini are lined with a columnar epithelium. The adjacent branching Bartholin duct is present adjacent to the gland.

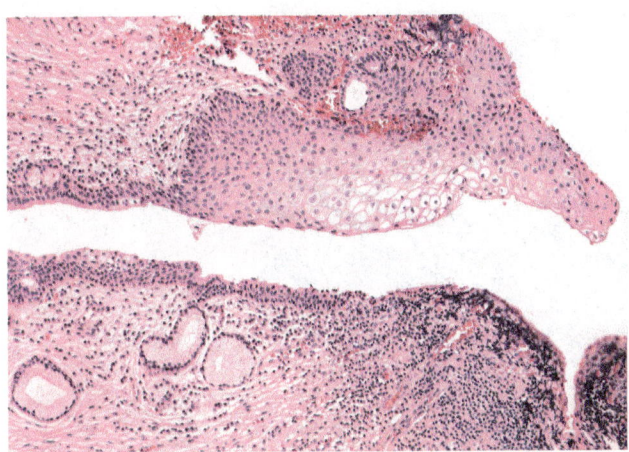

FIGURE 38.6 Bartholin duct near its exit to the vulvar vestibule. At this location the duct is lined by stratified squamous epithelium, without surface columnar cells.

prostate gland. The major vestibular glands, or Bartholin glands (glandula vestibularis major) are located symmetrically at the posterolateral region of vaginal opening beneath the hymen, labia minora, and labia majora. Its major role is mucus production for vaginal lubrication. Bartholin gland is of ectodermal origin and consists of bilateral tubuloalveolar glands that correspond to the male bulbourethral glands, or Cowper glands. The normal epithelial lining of Bartholin gland is composed of several different cell types. The acini consist of mucus-secreting columnar cells (Fig. 38.4) (6,7,10). The secretion of the acini empties into Bartholin duct, which measures approximately 2.5 cm in length and enters the vestibule immediately exterior (distal) and adjacent to the hymen in a posterolateral location. Bartholin duct is lined by transitional epithelium but sometimes may contain squamous or mucinous epithelial cells as well (Fig. 38.5). The orifice of the duct is lined by squamous epithelium to adjoin the nonkeratinized stratified squamous epithelium of the vulvar vestibule (Fig. 38.6) (6,10). Within Bartholin duct epithelium, argentaffin cells can also be identified, predominantly concentrated within the transitional ductal epithelial cell area and absent in the secretory gland area (42). Cysts that arise in the area of Bartholin gland are primarily a result of dilation of Bartholin duct, secondary to distal duct obstruction (6). Carcinoma of the Bartholin gland can arise from any of these native cell types, resulting in different type of carcinomas.

The periurethral, or Skene, glands also enter the vulvar vestibule as paired gland openings found immediately adjacent to and posterolateral to the urethra. These glands, with their adjacent ducts, are generally not more than 1.5 cm in length. These periurethral glands are analogous to the male prostate gland and are lined with a pseudostratified mucus-secreting columnar epithelium. The ducts of Skene glands are lined with transitional-type epithelium that joins with the stratified squamous epithelium of the vestibule at the gland orifices. A cyst of Skene duct may result from obstruction of the duct.

The minor vestibular glands (glandulae vestibulares minores) consist of simple tubular glands that enter directly to the mucosal surface of the vestibule (Fig. 38.7). They are analogous to the glands of Littré of the male urethra. Minor vestibular glands are small and shallow, with a maximum depth of 2.27 mm (43). These glands are lined with a mucus-secreting columnar epithelium that merges with the stratified squamous epithelium of the vestibule (43–45). We found minor vestibular glands in vulvar vestibulectomy specimens for vestibulitis in 66% of our cases (43). In women with identifiable minor vestibular glands, minor vestibular glands were identified within the vestibule in 42% of women studied in an autopsy-related series (45). When present, the number ranged from 1 to over 100, with the majority having 2 to 10 identifiable minor vestibular glands. Although these glands were found to be distributed throughout the vestibule,

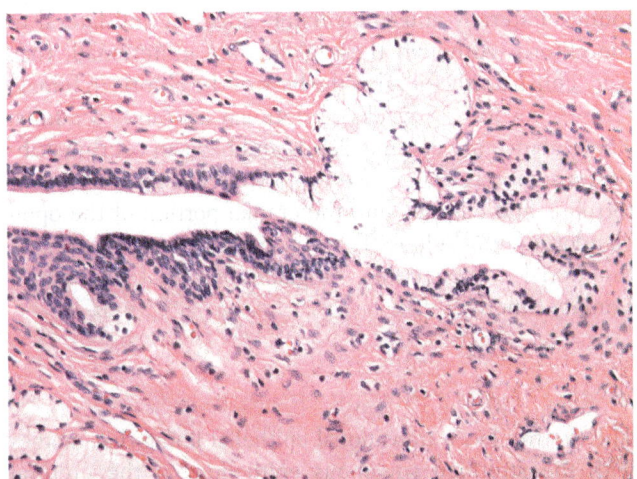

FIGURE 38.5 Bartholin duct near the gland. Bartholin duct has a transitional-like epithelial lining, with columnar cells near the surface, similar to the columnar cells lining the gland acini.

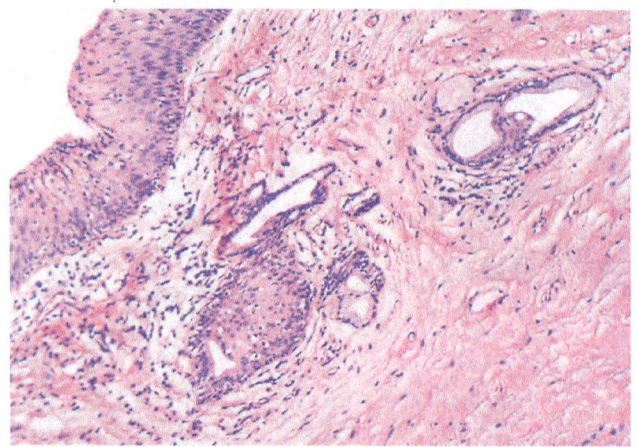

FIGURE 38.7 Minor vestibular glands of the vulvar vestibule. The vulvar vestibular glands are simple glands with a mucus-secreting columnar epithelial lining. Near their exit at the vestibular surface the glands have a stratified squamous epithelium. Vascular vestibular stroma surrounds the superficial gland elements.

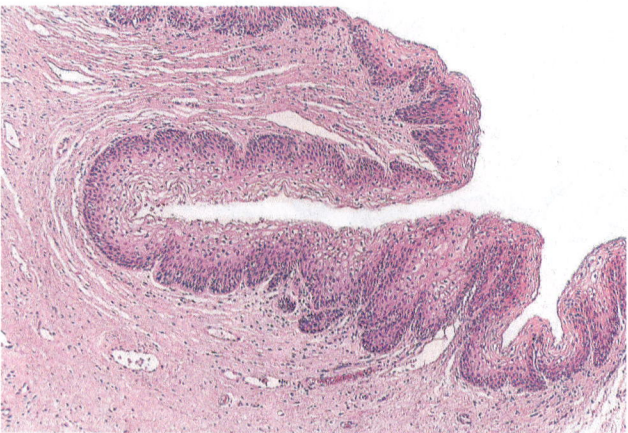

FIGURE 38.9 Vulvar vestibular cleft. The vulvar vestibular cleft has a stratified squamous epithelial lining, similar to the vulvar vestibule. These clefts appear to arise as a result of squamous metaplasia of vestibular glands.

they were found in greater numbers in the posterior vestibule, just anterior to the fourchette. Minor vestibular glands have been described as having ducts composed of transitional epithelium; this epithelium, however, is essentially the same epithelium and borders that of the adjacent vulvar vestibule, which is stratified squamous epithelium without surface umbrella cells. Several types of neuroendocrine cells are also present in these glands and those expressing serotonin and CXCR2 appear to increase in vestibulitis (46). Minor vestibular glands may undergo squamous metaplasia, similar to that seen within the endocervix, where the mucus-secreting epithelial cells lining the glandular epithelium are replaced by stratified squamous epithelium (Fig. 38.8). This metaplastic epithelium may completely replace the glandular epithelium, resulting in the formation of a vestibular cleft (Fig. 38.9) (43). Obstruction of a minor vestibular gland associated with this metaplastic process may result in accumulation of mucous secretion within the simple tubular gland, leading to the formation of a vulvar mucous cyst (43,44). Vestibular adenomas have been described arising from these minor vestibular glands (47). Severe vulvar sensitivity and tenderness, often with dyspareunia but without associated inflammation of the vestibule, is termed vulvodynia (4). It is a relatively common but poorly understood condition that is a common cause for visits to vulvar clinics (4). Histologic examination of vestibular biopsies obtained from women with vestibulitis syndrome often show proliferation of peripheral nerve bundles accompanied by neuroendocrine cell hyperplasia (48).

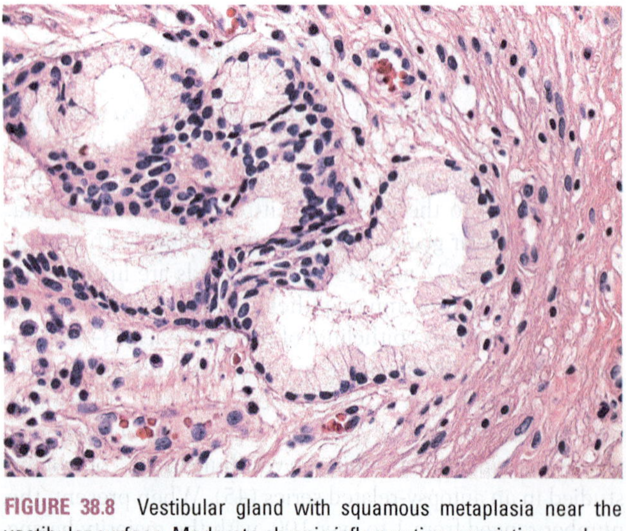

Small glandopreputial glands have been described by van der Putte within the glandopreputial sulcus that is found bilaterally and immediately adjacent and lateral to the clitoris. Although these glands are quite small, they were consistently found at the base of the clitoris in female fetuses beyond 17 weeks' gestational age and in adults. These glands are eccrine glands and have an eccrine cribriform secretory coil. The excretory duct of these glands is tortuous and empties into the cranial portion of the open glandopreputial sulcus. These glands are considered to be functional in moistening the glandopreputial sulcus as a primary function (49).

Urethral Orifice (Meatus Urinarius)

The urethra has a transitional epithelial lining that merges with the stratified squamous epithelium at the urethral orifice. The periurethral glands of Huffman enter into the urethra throughout most of its length (10,50). Obstruction or inflammation of these periurethral glands may result

FIGURE 38.8 Vestibular gland with squamous metaplasia near the vestibular surface. Moderate chronic inflammation, consisting predominantly of lymphocytes, is seen adjacent to the gland and is consistent with vulvar vestibulitis.

in a urethral diverticulum or periurethral abscess. Partial prolapse of the urethra results in a polypoid mass, often referred to as a urethral caruncle. The mucosa may become ulcerated, and the underlying stroma may become inflamed with vascular dilation and engorgement; however, it otherwise retains the normal histology of the urethra.

Hymen

The hymen marks the distal-most extent of the vagina and the most proximal boundary of the vulvar vestibule. The hymen may be imperforate, round, annular, septate, cribriform, or porous. On the vaginal surface, the hymen has a nonkeratinized stratified squamous epithelium, which is glycogenated upon estrogen exposure, as seen in women of reproductive age, newborn female infants, and postmenopausal women receiving estrogen therapy. On the vulvar surface, the vestibular epithelium appears similar to the vaginal epithelium in women of reproductive age (Figs. 38.3 and 38.10). The hymenal ring contains some Merkel tactile discs for touch and moderate numbers of free nerve endings, which are pain receptors; the hymenal ring lacks other receptors that are present in the labia majora (51).

In rare cases of imperforate hymen, the hymen lacks its normal opening. This leads to accumulation of menstrual exodus in the vagina, resulting in vaginal distension with menstrual products, a condition referred to as hematocolpos. Coitus, or the routine use of intravaginal tampons, results in tears in the hymen, which result in small soft hymenal tags referred to as carunculae hymenales or carunculae myrtiformes. On the external hymen and on the vulvar vestibule, small papillae may be identified, which are referred to as vestibular papillae. Multiple papillae are seen in the condition known as vestibular papillomatosis (6,7).

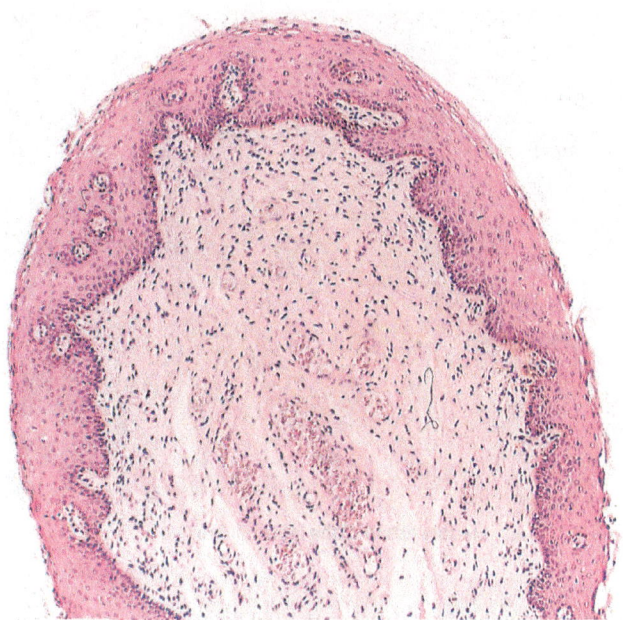

FIGURE 38.11 Vulvar vestibular papillae. The papillae have a stratified squamous epithelial surface and fibrovascular stalks.

They are usually linearly and symmetrically distributed, soft, delicate and easily separated from each other in contrast to condyloma accuminatum. Such papillae within the vestibule are generally considered a variant of normal anatomy and are not considered associated with human papillomavirus (52). Solitary or isolated asymptomatic papillae on the hymen usually represent a normal anatomic variant (Fig. 38.11) (52).

During the prepubertal period, mucosal redundancy in the lower vagina can appear near the hymen as a fold. Histologically, these mucosal redundancies have no fibrovascular cores, but may cause confusion on physical examination after sexual assault. It is thought that these redundancies disappear as the vagina enlarges with the onset of puberty (53).

Clitoris

The clitoris is the descendant of the embryonic phallus, homologous to the corpus cavernosum of the male penis. The human fetus begins differentiation into male versus female at approximately 8 weeks of gestation. The genital tubercle forms the basis for both genders, which in males develops into penis as a result of the testis determining factor protein, a product of sex determining gene of the Y chromosome. Although it is generally stated that in adults the clitoris measures approximately 2 cm in its long axis, the size of the clitoris, as well as the labia, may be highly variable in individuals.

The external components of clitoris consist of nonerectile tip and glans, while deeper structures include body, two crura and vestibular bulbs. The crura are composed of erectile tissue similar to that in the corpora cavernosa of the male (10,39). They consist of cavernous veins surrounded

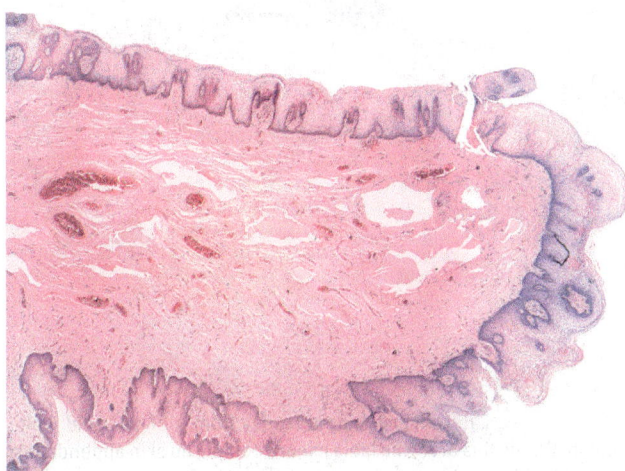

FIGURE 38.10 Cross section of the hymen of a 26-year-old woman. The epithelium of the vaginal (*upper*) and vestibular (*lower*) surfaces of the hymen is a stratified squamous epithelium, which is nonkeratinized and glycogen rich. The fibrovascular component of the hymen supports the epithelium.

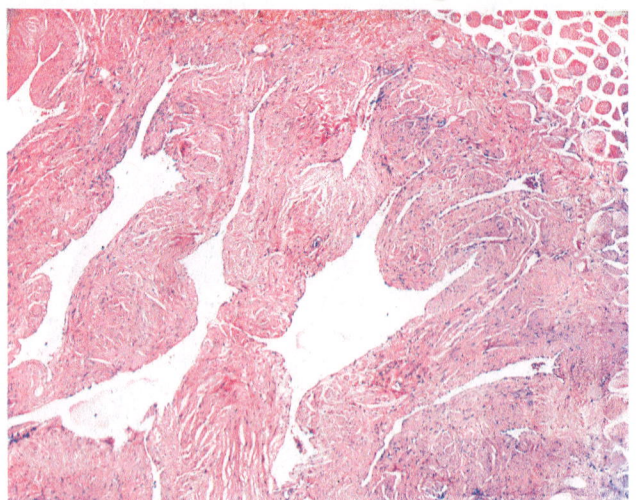

FIGURE 38.12 Erectile tissue of the labia minora.

by longitudinal smooth muscle, as well as small centrally placed muscular arteries, enveloped by the tunica albuginea. The tunica albuginea is composed of wavy collagen fibers and straight elastic fibers. Peripheral to the tunica albuginea is the loose connective tissue that supports the nerves and receptors of this area. The glans clitoridis is covered with squamous mucosa without glands, rete, or papillae (54). The cavernous tissue of the corpus spongiosum of the male does not have its counterpart in the clitoris; it is found instead in the vascular erectile tissue of the labia minora (Fig. 38.12). The clitoris contains nerve endings in lesser amount than those seen in the labia majora, although pacinian corpuscles are abundant. Peritrichous nerve endings for touch reception are absent. The other receptors are present, although their distribution is highly variable (51). Other touch receptors, namely, Meissner corpuscles and Merkel tactile disks, are present in reduced numbers in the clitoris, as compared with the labia majora or mons pubis. Pacinian corpuscles, for pressure reception, are present in large numbers (51). The free nerve endings for pain reception are found throughout the vulva and in relatively high concentrations in the clitoris, labia majora, and mons pubis (51). Ruffini and Dogiel–Krause corpuscles, which may be associated with temperature or sexual sensation, are found throughout the vulva but not in the hymenal ring (51). The rich blood supply of the clitoris is derived from the external pudendal artery, dorsal clitoral artery and perineal arteries.

Labia Minora

The bilateral labia minora derive from the embryonic medial folds (genital folds) and lie lateral to the vulvar vestibule and medial to the labia majora, bounded by the intralabial sulcus. Development of the external genitalia in both sexes is a complex process, driven by sequential expression of regulatory genes. Studies have shown that hedgehog, *Wnt* and fibroblast growth factor signaling pathways play key role in the cross-talk between epithelium and adjacent mesenchyme during the development of external genitalia (55). The labia minora have their male embryologic counterpart in the penile corpus spongiosum (39). In adult women the minora measure approximately 5 cm in length and 0.5 cm in thickness; however, their length and thickness can vary considerably between individuals, as well as in a single individual, comparing the right to the left labia (30). Labia minora enlargement or hypertrophy remains a clinical diagnosis which is poorly defined as it could be considered a variation of the normal anatomy and it is very subjective to define the "normal" vulva. Enlarged labia minora can cause functional, aesthetic, and psychosocial problems (56). The epithelium of the labia minora is of ectodermal origin, a nonkeratinizing stratified squamous type on its vestibular surface but has a thin keratin layer lateral from Hart line.

Most of the epithelium of the labia minora does not contain skin appendages; however, in some individuals, the lateral labia minora may contain sweat and/or sebaceous glands (54). The epithelium of the labia minora may be somewhat pigmented, especially in lateral and posterior areas (Fig. 38.13). Beneath the epithelium is a highly vascular, loose connective tissue that is rich in elastic fibers. Posterior and deep to the labia minora are the vestibular bulbs (bulbi vestibuli), which are composed of erectile tissue and are invested by the bulbocavernous muscles. The labia minora contain erectile tissue and thus are highly vascular, yet they lack adipose tissue. The vessels and erectile tissue are supported by a rich elastic fiber component. The nerve endings within the labia majora are similar to those found within the clitoris, yet Meissner corpuscles and Merkel tactile disks occur in larger numbers than usually identified within the clitoris (51). A recent study has

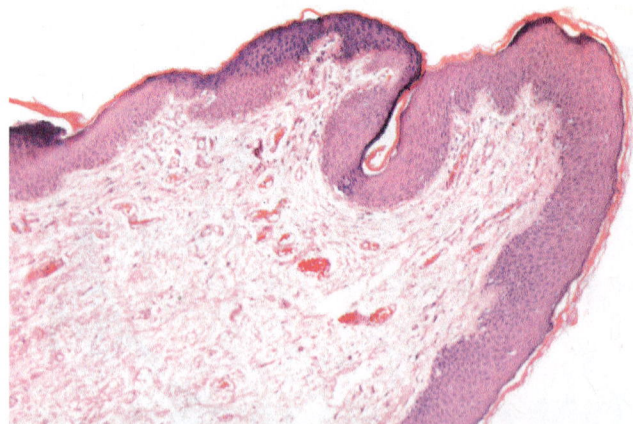

FIGURE 38.13 Lateral labia minora biopsy from a 27-year-old white woman. Within this area, the labia minora contain no skin appendages. The epithelium is pigmented, and melanocytes and pigmented basal epithelial cells are seen in the basal layer. The stratified squamous epithelium has a thinly keratinized surface. Beneath the epithelium, there is an elastic fiber–rich stroma without fat or skin appendages. Moderate numbers of small vessels can be seen. Deeper tissue is demonstrated in Figure 38.12.

shown characteristic staining patterns of free nerve endings, Meissner corpuscles, and pacinian corpuscles in the labia minora (57), where they are seen in stratum basale, spinosum, and granulosum of the epidermis.

Developmental anomalies of labia minor rare, and are often seen a clinical setting of congenital adrenal hyperplasia or rarely as part of a malformation syndrome. Genital hypoplasia has been reported in association with CHARGE syndrome and Cenani–Lenz syndrome (16).

Congenital enlargement of the labia minora may occur and may be asymmetrical. Enlargement also may be secondary to irritation, chronic edema, or minor trauma. Surgical reduction of the labia minora or local excision for therapeutic reasons does not appear to impede normal sexual function or response; however, excision of the labia minora for female circumcision is associated with introital stenosis, vulvar keratinous cysts, and sexual and urinary dysfunction (13).

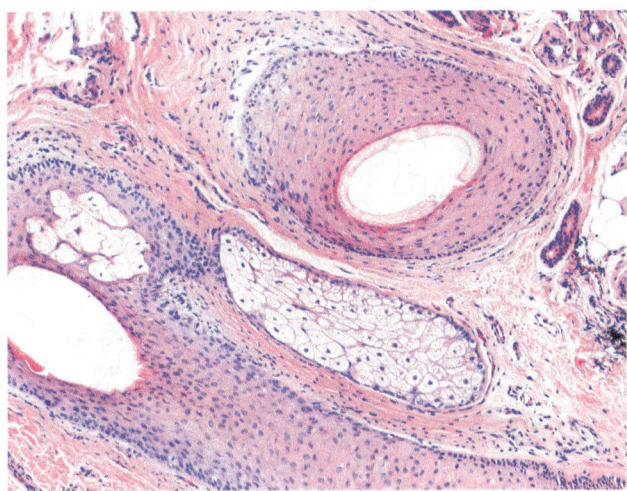

FIGURE 38.14 Pilosebaceous unit with hair follicle and adjacent sebaceous gland.

Labia Majora

The labia majora arise from the embryonic lateral folds (genital folds, labial folds), which arise lateral to the cloacal plate and do not fuse (10). The epithelium is ectodermally derived from the urogenital sinus. The endodermally derived epithelium of the vestibule joins with the ectodermally derived epithelium of the medial labial majora. This junction is apparently at Hart line, where the epithelium of the medial (inner) labia majora joins the nonkeratinized squamous epithelium of the vestibule (6,7,30). In the male, the labial (scrotal) folds fuse to form the scrotum. This fusion usually occurs by 74 days of gestation (crown–rump length approximately 71 mm) (45). In the female, the labia majora merge with the mons pubis anteriorly and with the perineal body posteriorly. The labia majora lie immediately lateral and parallel to the labia minora, separated by the interlabial sulcus. In the medial posterior positions, the labia majora are bounded by the vulvar vestibule. Laterally, they merge with the inguinal–gluteal folds, which separate the labia from the medial aspect of the thighs. The length of the labia majora can vary considerably between individuals, as well as in a single individual, comparing the right to the left labia (30). Although some asymmetry of the labia majora is normal, marked asymmetry may be early evidence of neurofibromatosis (58). Chronic inflammation, varicosities, edema, Bartholin cysts, and benign or malignant tumors also may be associated with asymmetry of the labia majora.

Aging changes related to the labia majora include an increase in size of the labia with puberty, primarily related to increased fat within the labia. In addition, there are dramatic changes in hair growth during puberty (see Mons Pubis discussion later) (59). After menopause, there is a progressive loss of hair follicles and consequent loss of labial hair (60), as well as shrinkage of the labia majora. This is primarily related to loss of fat within the labia (38).

In addition to age-related changes, changes occur in the labia majora that are related to parity. During gestation, the influence of gestational hormones, especially progesterone, results in vascular dilation and stasis within the labia (51). These gestational changes may result in the development of vulvar venous varicosities (61).

Similar to other hair follicles, each follicle of the vulva has a hair root surrounded by the dermal root sheath, which invests the root sheath of the hair follicle. The inner root sheath is composed of an external clear epithelial cell layer (Henle layer) and an inner granular epithelial cell layer (Huxley layer). The hair matrix matures to the formed hair of the hair shaft, where the hair has an outer cuticle with a cortex and medulla. The hair papilla is found at the base of the hair root, protruding into and partially surrounded by the matrix of the hair. The papilla is supported by the dermal root sheath (54). Hair follicles are a portion of the pilosebaceous unit, which includes sebaceous glands (Fig. 38.14).

In the labia majora, sebaceous glands can be found with and without associated hair follicles. The sebaceous glands are alveolar and arranged in a lobular manner, vested by collagen fibers. The cells of the sebaceous glands secrete in a holocrine manner, with the more mature cells accumulating sebaceous secretion (sebum) within their cytoplasm. The secretion is released as the cells undergo necrosis. The secretion may be released adjacent to the hair shaft in the pilosebaceous unit or directly to the surface when no hair shaft is present. There are two types of sweat gland: Apocrine and merocrine (54). Apocrine glands are tubular and have a columnar secretory epithelium characterized by a prominent eosinophilic granular cytoplasm (Figs. 38.15A and 38.15B). These glands secrete by release of cytoplasmic secretion and are associated with scent production. The scent associated with these sudoriferous glands is related to bacterial growth supported by the secretory products (54). Beneath the epithelial layer, myoepithelial cells are identified. These myoepithelial cells are arranged about the periphery of the gland, and their contraction promotes expression of the secretory

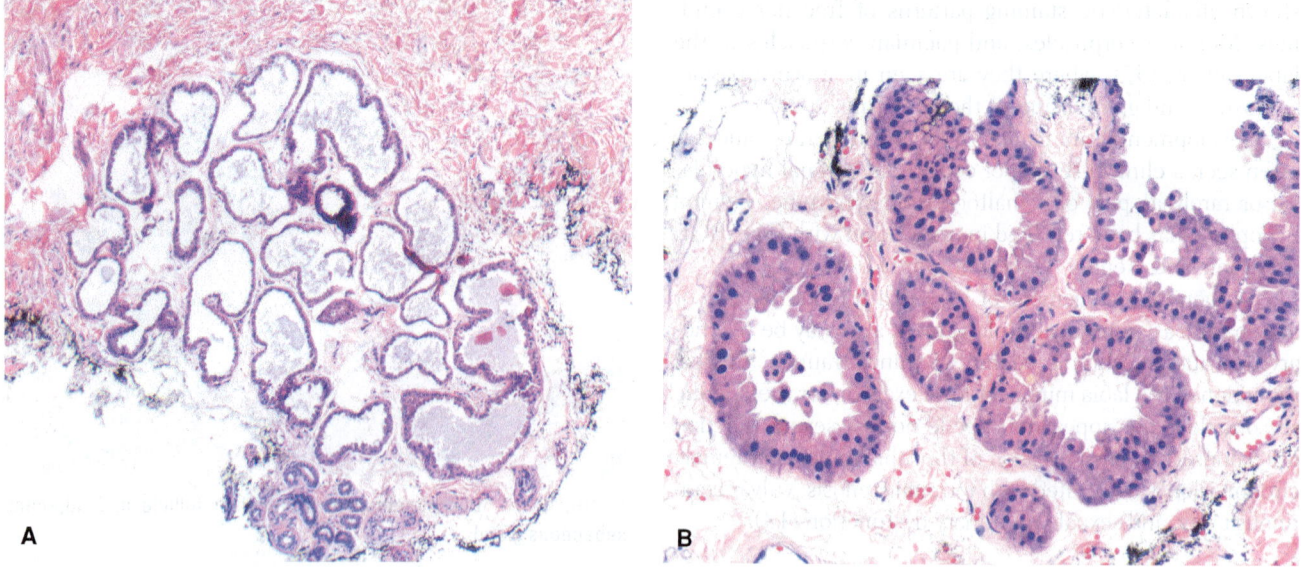

FIGURE 38.15 **A:** Apocrine tubular glands (low power). **B:** Glands are lined by columnar cells containing eosinophilic granular cytoplasm. Apical snouts are often seen (high power).

contents from the gland lumen. The ducts of the apocrine glands are similar to those of the merocrine glands but may secrete into the upper hair follicle rather than to the skin surface when present in hair-bearing skin.

The merocrine glands are eccrine glands that produce clear watery sweat. The secretory cells have a pale, slightly granular cytoplasm and an outer layer of myoepithelial cells. The glands are simple and coiled and are found deep to the reticular dermis. The sweat duct is lined by cuboidal epithelium two-cells thick, and the double epithelial cell layer is lost as it joins with the stratified epithelial surface.

Unlike sebaceous and apocrine glands, merocrine glands are not significantly stimulated by the sex hormones. (For further discussion on the histology of the skin elements, the reader is referred to Chapter 1 in this volume and to texts on histology (54).)

The epithelium of the posterolateral aspects of the labia majora, peripheral to Hart line, is thinly keratinized and pigmented (Fig. 38.16). At the posterior fourchette, the retia are relatively deeper than those in the posterior lateral area (Fig. 38.17). Pigmented cells are seen at the basal layer and rare small cells with clear cytoplasm (Toker cells) are noted at the epithelial stromal junction (Fig. 38.18). A granular layer may be present immediately beneath the keratinized surface (stratum corneum). The granular layer arises from the underlying prickle cell (spinous cell) layer of the stratified squamous epithelium, with the stratum malpighii overlying the

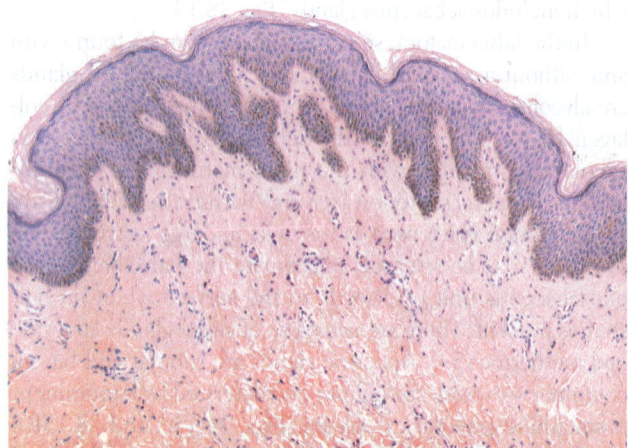

FIGURE 38.16 Posterior medial labia majora of a 27-year-old white woman peripheral to Hart line. This pigmented portion of the labia majora has a stratified squamous epithelium with a thin keratinized surface. The epithelium has deeper rete ridges than those seen in the minora. The dermis is elastic fiber rich and moderately vascular. Sebaceous gland–bearing skin was immediately adjacent to this area and has a moderately vascular dermis.

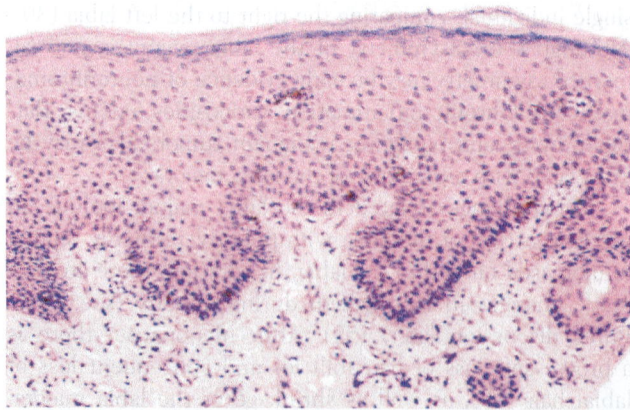

FIGURE 38.17 Posterior vulvar fourchette. The epithelium has a thinly keratinized surface, moderately deep rete, and some melanin pigmentation within the basal cells.

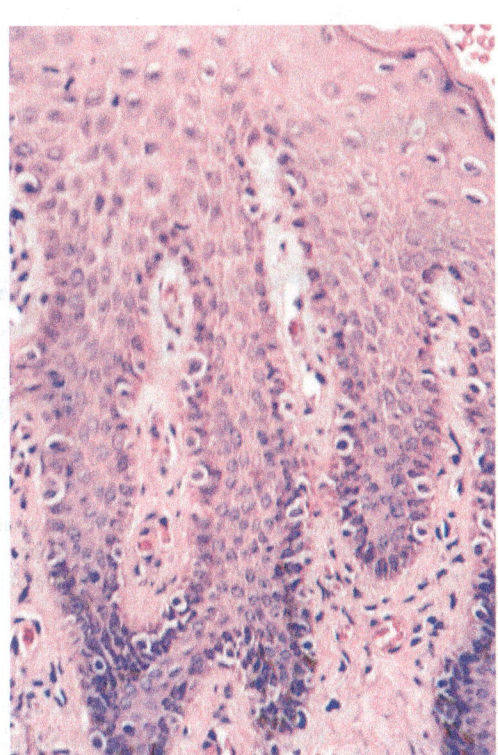

FIGURE 38.18 Posterior perineal body of a 27-year-old white woman. The skin at the perineal body is pigmented, and melanocytes and pigmented keratinocytes are present within the basal layer. The epithelium is stratified squamous epithelium, which has a thin keratin layer. The perinuclear halos present within the epithelial cells are normally seen and should not be confused with koilocytosis. Small clear cells are seen in the epithelial stromal junction within many of the retia.

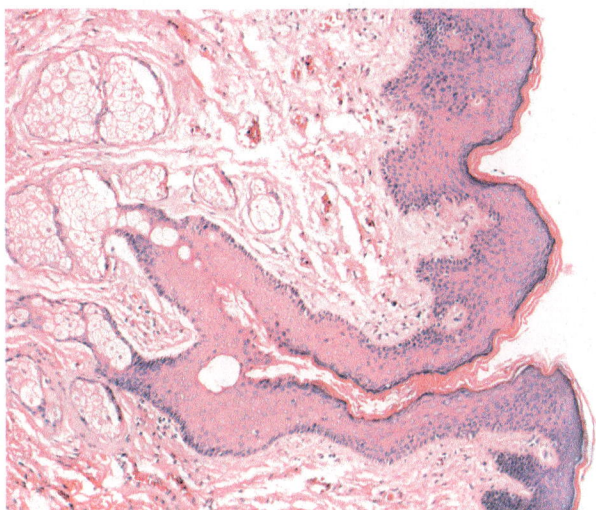

FIGURE 38.19 Labia majora, medial portion, with sebaceous gland elements exiting directly to the skin surface. The epithelium of the medial labia majora has a thin keratin and granular layer. The sebaceous glands may be seen clinically as Fordyce spots.

basal layer. The basal layer (stratum germinativum) is present immediately adjacent to the basement membrane (62). The medial hairless surfaces of the labia majora contain an abundance of sebaceous glands, which end at Hart line. These glands are not associated with hair-bearing pilosebaceous units and open directly onto the epithelial surface, with a short nonkeratinized epithelium-lined duct joining with the keratinized epithelial surface (Fig. 38.19). Sebaceous glands within the labia majora may have a depth of up to 2.03 mm (63). Keratinous (epithelial) cysts may be associated with these sebaceous gland elements (6). Sebaceous glands are not found medial to Hart line (Figure 38.2). At the midportion of the labia majora, hair follicles are associated with the sebaceous gland elements. Hair follicles within the labia majora may be as deep as 2.38 mm (Figs. 38.14 and 38.20) (63). Apocrine and eccrine sweat glands are found associated with the hair-bearing areas of the vulva but are generally absent in the vestibule and medial nonhair-bearing areas of the medial labia majora (Fig. 38.21). Deeper within the dermis of the labia majora, a delicate muscle layer (tunica dartos labialis) is present. Beneath this layer is a fascial layer that has a prominent elastic fiber component (51). The fascial layer is associated with a prominent adipose layer in women of reproductive age.

Within the deep anterior labia majora, immediately adjacent to the inguinal canal, the round ligament joins with the deep longitudinal smooth muscle layer (cremaster muscle) of the labia majora (51). The round ligament may include entrapped peritoneum (processus vaginalis), which can become cystically dilated and result in a cyst of the canal of Nuck (6). These peritoneum-lined cysts are typically encountered in the anterior portion of the labia majora, adjacent to or within the inguinal canal.

The skin of the labia majora is rich in nerve endings and contains touch receptors, including Meissner corpuscles, Merkel tactile disks, and peritrichous nerve endings (51). Pacinian corpuscles for pressure sensation are present

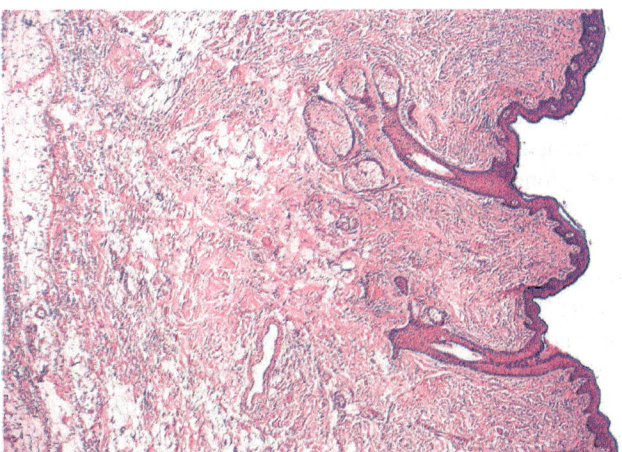

FIGURE 38.20 Labia majora, midportion, with underlying dermis and deep fatty tissue. The thickness of the dermis can be seen in this section of the labia majora. A few deep hair follicles can be seen within the elastic fiber–rich dermis. The dermal junction with the deep fatty tissue is irregular.

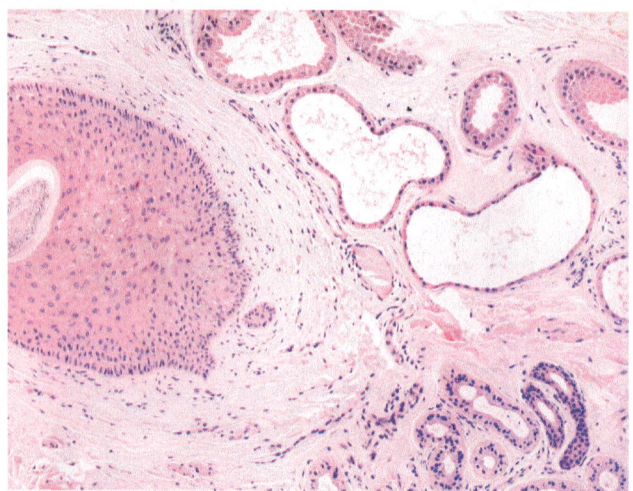

FIGURE 38.21 Labia majora with apocrine glands and sweat ducts adjacent to a hair follicle. Moderate vascularity of the collagen-rich dermis of the labia majora surrounds these sweat gland elements.

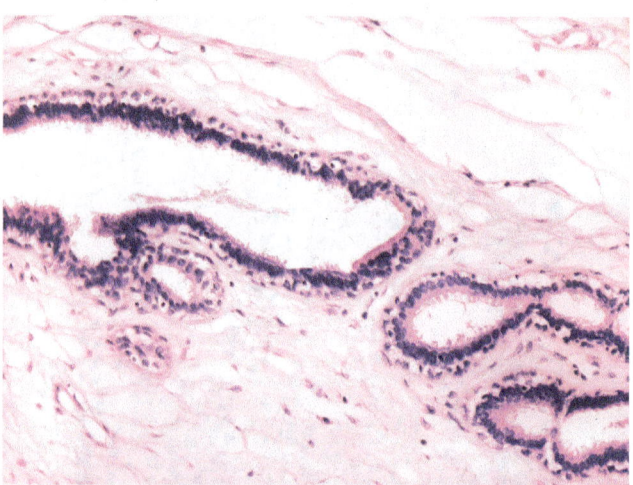

FIGURE 38.22 Mammary-like anogenital gland with duct and small acini. The epithelial lining is composed of a two-layered epithelium with an underlying myoepithelial cell layer and a low columnar epithelial luminal epithelium.

within the fatty layer of the labia majora, as well as within the labia minora, clitoris, and mons pubis. Free nerve endings for pain reception are also present within the labia majora, as well as within the associated muscle cells and blood vessels (51). Ruffini corpuscles are seen throughout the subcutaneous tissue of the labia majora, labia minora, clitoris, and mons pubis. They are absent in the hymen. Their exact function in the vulva is uncertain; however, they may be temperature receptors and/or receptors for sexual stimuli (51). Dogiel–Krause receptors have a distribution similar to that of Ruffini corpuscles; however, they are present in a relatively smaller concentration in the mons pubis and labia majora (51).

Medial to the labia majora, within the sulcus between the labia majora and the labia minora (sulcus interlabialis), anogenital mammary-like glands are present. These glands were first described by Hartung in 1872 and were thought to represent ectopic breast tissue from the caudal remnant of the milk line. Later Van der Putte proposed that these glands are normal components of the anogenital region. Current evidence also supports that the "milk line" does not extend to the vulva in the human, and that breast-like tissue in that location are histologically distinct anogenital mammary-like glands (64,65). Their histologic appearance ranges from small simple glands to complex lobular units similar to breast lobules. The stroma adjacent to lobules may be lose or fibrotic. The excretory duct system is lined by columnar epithelium containing apocrine secretion and underlying myoepithelium. As the excretory duct enters the skin surface its lining transitions into squamous epithelium and myoepithelial layer is lost. Rare Toker cells may be near the opening of the duct. The myoepithelial cells are immunoreactive for smooth muscle actin and S100 antigen, as well as low–molecular-weight keratin. The superficial luminal epithelial cells are of an apocrine type, with visible "snouts" (Fig. 38.22). These cells are immunoreactive for low–molecular-weight keratin and human milk fat globule antigen. Individual cells are also immunoreactive for carcinoembryonic antigen and S100 antigen. Estrogen and progesterone receptors have been detected in these cells. Mucus-containing or ciliated cells are not present, distinguishing the cysts of anogenital mammary-like glands from vestibular mucous cysts, müllerian-related cysts or ciliated cysts, or Bartholin gland. The lack of a stratified squamous epithelium or transitional epithelium distinguishes them from Bartholin duct cysts, keratinous cysts, or vestibular glandular cysts that have undergone squamous metaplasia (64). A recent study on comparing molecular pathways involved in pathogenesis of histologically similar lesions of the anogenital mammary-like glands and breast tissue found mutations of *PIK3CA, AKT1, MET, ABL1* and *TP53* genes. It appears that the *PI3K-AKT* cascade plays a role in the pathogenesis of tumors arising at both sites (66).

Vulvar Toker Cells

Toker cells were first described in the lower half of the epidermis of nipple, where they show predilection to the ostia of lactiferous sinuses. Similar clear cells were also identified in the epidermis of the anogenital region. They are often seen as single cells, clusters or small tubules between the epidermal keratinocytes. Toker cell precursors can be identified as early as 15 to 16.5 weeks of gestation at the interlabial sulci of the vulva (67). By 24 and 39 weeks of gestation Toker cells are readily identified as clusters of clear cells with round nuclei and scant cytoplasm with variable distribution within the lower half of the epidermis, showing the highest concentration in the deep parts of the interlabial sulci. In adults their highest number is seen in association with the ostia of mammary-type glands. Toker cells are the presumed precursors of primary extramammary

TABLE 38.1 Immunohistochemical Staining Characteristics of Various Cell Types And Paget Disease Cells in The Vulvar Epithelium (79)

Stain	Toker Cells	Melanocytes	Squamous Cells	Paget Cells
LMWCK	+	−	+/−	+
HMCK	−	−	+	−
EMA	+/−	−	+	+
S100	+/−	+	−	+/−
mCEA	−	−	−	+/−
HER2	−	−	−	+/−
Melan-A	−	+	−	−
GCDFP-15	−	−	−	+/−
Mucin	+/−	−	−	+/−

LMWCK, low–molecular-weight cytokeratin (CK7, CAM5.2); HMCK, high–molecular-weight cytokeratin (CK5/6, 34βE12, CK14, CK17); EMA, epithelial membrane antigen; S100, S100 protein; mCEA, monoclonal carcinoembryonic antigen; HER2, human epidermal growth factor receptor 2; Melan-A, melanoma antigen; GCDFP-15, gross cystic disease fluid; +, positive; −, negative; +/−, may be positive.

Paget disease (68). Immunohistochemical studies focused on the utility of various antibodies in the diagnosis of Paget disease revealed that Toker cells, similar to Paget cells and Merkel cells are also strongly positive for cytokeratin (CK) 7, but negative for CK20. Toker cells also differ from Paget cells by their expression of estrogen receptor (ER) and lack of staining for Her2-neu (Table 38.1) (69,70). When Toker cells are arranged in clusters, it can be challenging to distinguish them from extramammary Paget disease in a small biopsy specimen.

Mons Pubis (Mons Veneris)

The mons pubis has its origin in the embryonic genital medial cranial swellings. The subcutaneous tissue of mons pubis becomes more prominent with the onset of puberty, when there is a progressive increase in fat tissue beneath the mons. There is also a dramatic increase in hair growth of the mons pubis and labia majora.

Aging changes related to the mons pubis include hair growth changes that have been summarized and staged by Tanner in the following sequence (59). Stage 1 is characterized by no visible pubic hair growth. In stage 2, a small amount of pubic-type hair is seen on the midportion of the mons pubis, and some similar hair may be seen on the labia majora. In stage 3, the mons pubis hair growth is more prominent, both in the amount of hair and the coarseness of the hair. In stage 4, the hair growth over the mons pubis is similar to the adult, with the exception that the upper lateral corners of hair growth are lacking. Stage 5 characterizes the adult pubic hair pattern (59). The adult hair growth distribution is reached between the ages of 12 and 17 years (39). There can be substantial variability in the amount and character of the pubic hair (escutcheon) related to racial and genetic factors; however, pubic-type hair growth generally does not extend above a horizontal line drawn between, and 2 cm above, the uppermost limits of the genitofemoral folds (60,71). Hair follicle depth within the vulva is greatest in the mons pubis, where hair follicle depth has been measured up to 2.72 mm (63). The mons pubis is richly endowed with nerve receptor types that were previously described for the labia majora (51). Some experts believe that the function of mons pubis is to cushion the pubic bone from impact during intercourse. In addition, it is rich in oil-secreting (sebaceous) glands that release substances that are involved in sexual attraction (pheromones).

Lymphatic Drainage

The lymphatic drainage of female external genitalia is covered by a complex lymphoid network that covers the entire labia minora, fourchette, prepuce, and distal vagina below the hymen. Larger lymphoid channels run lateral to the clitoris which coalesce with lymphatics draining the mons pubis and labia majora. Radiolabeled tracer studies on lymphatic drainage of various sites of the vulva reveal that the lymphatic drainage of the perineum, clitoris, and anterior labia minora is bilateral, whereas the lymph flow from well-lateralized sites in the vulva is, predominantly, to the ipsilateral groin. From the superficial inguinal nodes, secondary lymphatic drainage is through the cribriform fascia to the deep inguinal or femoral nodes, with subsequent tertiary flow under the inguinal ligaments to the deep pelvic (external iliac and obturator) nodes. The node of Cloquet, also called Rosenmüller node, is the most cephalad of the femoral nodes, often lying in the femoral canal below Poupart (inguinal) ligament (72,73).

In some cases, lymphatic channels from a lateral site may drain to the contralateral node group, which has clinical relevance in planning therapy for malignancies of the vulva. The most common site of metastasis from vulvar malignancies are the superficial inguinal nodes. In general 8 to 10 nodes are found in this area, with superior oblique (above the ligament of Poupart) and inferior ventral (between the ligament of Poupart and the saphenous vein and fascia lata) divisions. Midline structures, such as the clitoris and the midline perineum, drain bilaterally. A second path of lymphatic drainage from the clitoris involves urethral lymphatics and lymphatics draining the dorsal vein of the clitoris. These channels lead inferior to the symphysis pubis through the anogenital diaphragm to join the lymphatic plexus of the anterior bladder surface. Ultimately, these channels terminate in the interiliac and obturator nodes or course superiorly to the femoral and internal iliac nodes. Deep pelvic nodes are not generally involved unless the superficial inguinal nodes are involved.

Sentinel lymph node mapping in the assessment of vulvar carcinoma and melanoma, employing intraoperative lymphoscintigraphy (technetium-99m–labeled nanocolloid) is gaining in application to assess inguinal lymph node status. Azulfidine blue vital dye (blue dye) has been used either alone or with the colloid, although a few clinicians have discontinued using the blue dye due to rare untoward reactions to the dye. Surgical excision with histopathologic assessment of the lymph nodes picking up the radioisotope-labeled colloid/blue dye (the sentinel nodes) is performed to plan appropriate lymph node resection related to the vulvar surgery. When these nodes are found to be free of tumor by this technique, the patient may be spared radical inguinal–femoral lymphadenectomy (21–23).

Obstruction of vulvar lymphatics related to prior surgical interruption, radiation therapy, or chronic inflammation (such as secondary to Crohn disease, hidradenitis suppurativa, etc.) may result in lymphangiectasia of the vulva. Obstruction of vulvar lymphatics may present clinically with leakage of clear fluid from the vulva and result in lymphangioma circumscriptum of the vulva where multiple small, glistening, superficial clustered vesicles on the vulvar skin, resembling frog spawn, may be found (74). Vulvar lymphatic obstruction is typically associated with some degree of epithelial and dermal edema (75). Massive vulvar edema may occur in immobilized and obese women, with bilateral labial enlargement reported up to 45 cm in diameter, related to chronic lymphatic obstruction (76).

Arterial Supply

The major arterial supply of the vulva originates from the branches of the internal pudendal artery, a division of the internal iliac (hypogastric) artery. These branches supply arterial blood to labia (labial artery) via the perineal artery, to corpora cavernosa and the vestibule via deep artery of the clitoris, and to the glands and prepuce via dorsal and deep arteries of the clitoris. Additional arterial supply originates from the superficial and deep external pudendal arteries, branches from the femoral artery, which anastomose with anterior and posterior labial branches of the perineal artery. The anterior vaginal artery supplies the vestibule and Bartholin gland areas (6,10,73).

Venous Supply

Major venous drainage of the vulva is primarily from the bilateral internal iliac veins that drain into the external iliac venous system. The internal iliac veins drain both parietal and visceral venous systems. The parietal tributaries of the internal iliac vein include the internal obturator, internal pudendal veins, superior and inferior gluteal veins, sciatic vein, and ascending lumbar veins. The visceral branches drain pelvic organs, including the uterine, ovarian, and vaginal venous systems. In a study of this drainage in 79 specimens, a single internal iliac vein was present on the side studied in 73% of the cases; in 29% of the cases, two separate iliac veins drained into the external iliac vein; and, in one case, the internal iliac vein drained directly to the inferior vena cava (10,77). Such varices correlate with insufficiency of the internal iliac venous system and also involve the tributaries of the internal iliac vein, as well as the saphenous vein (77). Varices are identified in the vulva and perivulvar area in approximately 4% of women and are more commonly identified in pregnant women. They may be related to arteriovenous malformations involving the vulva in Klippel–Trenaunary–Weber syndrome and Parkes syndrome (61). Although they are usually evident by their clinical appearance, vulvar varices may occasionally present as a "cyst" or "nodule" in the superficial dermis and be biopsied. The findings are of a dilated venous vessel with an associated organized thrombus, with an associated perivenous neutrophilic infiltrate (61).

Nerve Supply

The major nerves of the vulva are from the anterior and posterior labial nerves. The anterior nerve is a branch of the ilioinguinal nerve, and the posterior labial branch is from the pudendal nerve. The clitoral nerve supply is from the dorsal nerve of the clitoris and the cavernous nerves of the clitoris. Branches of the cavernous nerves, arising from the vaginal nerve plexus, join the clitoral dorsal nerve at the hilum of the clitoral bodies (78). The dorsal nerve of the clitoral bundle branches from the pudendal nerve. The two clitoral bodies, beneath the pubic arch, separate to form the two clitoral crura. Immunohistochemical studies have demonstrated that the dorsal nerves form two bundles that are extensively distributed along the lateral aspects of the clitoral bodies at the 11 and 1 o'clock positions and are sparse at the 12 o'clock position. These join distally to form a single clitoral body. The densest nerve groups that enter the glans clitoris are found on the dorsal aspect of the clitoris, with a concentration of nerves under the epithelium of the glans clitoris (78). The vestibule shares the clitoral nerve supply (51).

REFERENCES

1. Reed BD, Harlow SD, Sen A, et al. Prevalence and demographic characteristics of vulvodynia in a population based sample. *Am J. Obstet Gynecol* 2012;206(2):170.e1–170.e9
2. Harlow BL, Stewart EG. Population-based assessment of chronic unexplained vulvar pain: Have we underestimated the prevalence of vulvodynia? *J Am Med Womens Assoc* 2003; 58(2):82–88.
3. Arnold LD, Bachman GA, Rosen R, et al. Assessment of vulvodynia symptoms in a sample of US women: A prevalence survey with nested case control study. *Am J Obstet Gynecol* 2007;196(2): 128.e1–128.e6.
4. Haefner HK, Collins ME, Davis GD, et al. The vulvodynia guideline. *J Low Genit Tract Dis* 2005;9:40–51.

5. Vieira-Baptista P, Donders G, Margesson L, et al. Diagnosis and management of vulvodynia in postmenopausal women. *Maturitas* 2018;108:84–94.
6. Wilkinson EJ, Massoll N. Benign diseases of the vulva. In: Kurman RJ, ed. *Blaustein's Pathology of the Female Genital Tract*. 6th ed. New York: Springer-Verlag; 2011:3–46.
7. Wilkinson EJ, Stone IK. *Atlas of Vulvar Disease*. 3rd ed. Philadelphia, PA: Wolters Kluwer/Lippincott Williams & Wilkins; 2012.
8. Neill S, Lewis F. *Ridley's The Vulva*. 3rd ed. Wiley-Blackwell; 2009.
9. Wilkinson EJ. Premalignant and malignant tumors of the vulva. In: Kurman RJ, Ellenson LH, Ronnett BM, eds. *Blaustein's Pathology of the Female Genital Tract*. 6th ed. New York: Springer-Verlag; 2011:56–103.
10. Kurman RJ, Ronnett BM, Sherman ME, et al. Tumors of the cervix, vagina, and vulva. In: Rosai J, ed. *AFIP Atlas of Tumor Pathology. Series 4*. Washington, DC: American Registry of Pathology; 2010:1–22.
11. Spiryda LB, Laufer MR, Soiffer RJ, et al. Graft-versus-host disease of the vulva and/or vagina: Diagnosis and treatment. *Biol Blood Marrow Transplant* 2003;9:760–765.
12. Nardelli A, Degreef H, Goossens A. Contact allergic reactions of the vulva: A 14-year review. *Dermatitis* 2004;15:131–136.
13. Thabet SM, Thabet AS. Defective sexuality and female circumcision: The cause and the possible management. *J Obstet Gynaecol Res* 2003;29:12–19.
14. Creighton SM, Minto CL, Steele SJ. Objective cosmetic and anatomical outcomes at adolescence of feminizing surgery for ambiguous genitalia done in childhood. *Lancet* 2001;358:124–125.
15. Baskin LS. Anatomical studies of the female genitalia: Surgical reconstructive implications. *J Pediatr Endocrinol Metab* 2004;17:581–587.
16. Seely JR, Seely BL, Bley R Jr, et al. Localized chromosomal mosaicism as a cause of dysmorphic development. *Am J Hum Genet* 1984;36:899–903.
17. Hanna SJ, Kaiser L, Muneer A, et al. Squamous cell carcinoma of the bladder presenting as vulvitis and cliteromegaly. *Gynecol Oncol* 2004;95:722–723.
18. Lee PA, Witchel SF. Genital surgery among females with congenital adrenal hyperplasia: Changes over the past five decades. *J Pediatr Endocrinol Metab* 2002;15:1473–1477.
19. Crouch NS, Minto CL, Laio LM, et al. Genital sensation after feminizing genitoplasty for congenital adrenal hyperplasia: A pilot study. *BJU Int* 2004;93:135–138.
20. Minto CL, Liao LM, Woodhouse CR, et al. The effect of clitoral surgery on sexual outcome in individuals who have intersex conditions with ambiguous genitalia: A cross-sectional study. *Lancet* 2003;361:1252–1257.
21. Hakam A, Nasir A, Raghuwanshi R, et al. Value of multilevel sectioning for improved detection of micrometastases in sentinel lymph nodes in invasive squamous cell carcinoma of the vulva. *Anticancer Res* 2004;24:1281–1286.
22. Moore RG, Granai CO, Gajewski W, et al. Pathologic evaluation of inguinal sentinel lymph nodes in vulvar cancer patients: A comparison of immunohistochemical staining versus ultrastaging with hematoxylin and eosin staining. *Gynecol Oncol* 2003;91:378–382.
23. Moore RG, DePasquale SE, Steinhoff MM, et al. Sentinel node identification and the ability to detect metastatic tumor to inguinal lymph nodes in squamous cell cancer of the vulva. *Gynecol Oncol* 2003;89:475–479.
24. Brown HM, Wilkinson EJ. Cytology of secondary vulvar Paget's disease of urothelial origin: A case report. *Acta Cytol* 2005;49:71–74.
25. Mancino P, Parlavecchio E, Melluso J, et al. Introducing colposcopy and vulvovaginoscopy as routine examinations for victims of sexual assault. *Clin Exp Obstet Gynecol* 2003;30:40–42.
26. Stenson AL. Vulvodynia. Diagnosis and management. *Obstet Gynecol Clin N Am* 2017 44; 493–508.
27. Pillai M. Genital findings in prepubertal girls: What can be concluded from an examination? *J Pediatr Adolesc Gynecol* 2008;21(4):177–185.
28. McCann J, Miyamoto S, Boyle C, et al. Healing of nonhymenal genital injuries in prepubertal and adolescent girls: A descriptive study. *Pediatrics* 2007;120(5):1000–1011.
29. Bechara A, Bertolino MV, Casabe A, et al. Duplex Doppler ultrasound assessment of clitoral hemodynamics after topical administration of alprostadil in women with arousal and orgasmic disorders. *J Sex Marital Ther* 2003;29(Suppl 1):1–10.
30. Hart DB. *Selected Papers in Gynaecology and Obstetrics*. Edinburgh, Scotland: W&AK Johnston; 1893.
31. Grant LA, Sala E, Griffin N. Congenital and acquired conditions of the vulva and vagina on magnetic resonance imaging: A pictorial review. *Semin Ultrasound CT MR* 2010;31(5):347–362.
32. Griffin N, Grant LA, Sala E. Magnetic resonance imaging of vaginal and vulval pathology. *Eur Radiol* 2008;18(6):1269–1280.
33. Reuter JC. High-yield vulvar histopathology for the clinician. *Obstet Gynecol Clin North Am* 2017;44(3):329–333.
34. Day T, Holland SM, Scurry J. Normal vulvar histology: Variation by site. *J Low Genit Tract Dis* 2016;20(1):64–69.
35. Jones IS. A histological assessment of normal vulval skin. *Clin Exp Dermatol* 1983;8(5):513–521
36. Benedet JL, Wilson PS, Matisic J. Epidermal thickness and skin appendage involvement in vulvar intraepithelial neoplasia. *J Reprod Med* 1991;366:608–612.
37. Hu F. Melanocyte cytology in normal skin. In: Ackerman AB, ed. *Masson Monographs in Dermatology-1*. New York: Masson; 1981.
38. Edwards JN, Morris HB. Langerhans' cells and lymphocyte subsets in the female genital tract. *Br J Obstet Gynaecol* 1985;92:974–982.
39. McLean JM. Anatomy and physiology of the vulva. In: Ridley CM, ed. *The Vulva*. New York: Churchill Livingstone; 1988:39–65.
40. Rotsztejn H, Trznadel-Budzko E, Jesionek-Kupnicka D. Do Langerhans cells play a role in vulvar epithelium resistance to squamous cell carcinoma? *Arch Immunol Ther Exp (Warsz)* 2007;55(2):127–130.
41. Gould VE, Moll R, Moll I, et al. Biology of disease. Neuroendocrine (Merkel) cells of the skin: Hyperplasias, dysplasias, and neoplasms. *Lab Invest* 1985;52:334–352.
42. Fetissof F, Berger G, Dubois MP, et al. Endocrine cells in the female genital tract. *Histopathology* 1985;9:133–145.
43. Pyka RE, Wilkinson EJ, Friedrich EG Jr, et al. The histology of vulvar vestibulitis syndrome. *Int J Gynecol Oncol* 1988;7:249–257.
44. Friedrich EG Jr, Wilkinson EJ. Mucous cysts of the vulvar vestibule. *Obstet Gynecol* 1973;42:407–414.

45. Robboy SJ, Ross JS, Prat J, et al. Urogenital sinus origin of mucinous and ciliated cysts of the vulva. *Obstet Gynecol* 1978; 51:347–351.
46. Slone S, Reynolds L, Gall S, et al. Localization of chromogranin, synaptophysin, serotonin, and CXCR2 in neuroendocrine cells of the minor vestibular glands: An immunohistochemical study. *Int J Gynecol Pathol* 1999;18(4):360–365.
47. Axe S, Parmley T, Woodruff JD, et al. Adenomas in minor vestibular glands. *Obstet Gynecol* 1986;68:16–18.
48. Halperin R, Zehavi S, Vaknin Z, et al. The major histopathologic characteristics in the vulvar vestibulitis syndrome. *Gynecol Obstet Invest* 2005;59(2):75–79.
49. van der Putte S. Development and structure of glandopreputial sulcus of the human clitoris with a special reference to glandopreputial glands. *Anat Rec* 2011;294:156–164.
50. Huffman JW. The detailed anatomy of the paraurethral ducts in the adult human female. *Am J Obstet Gynecol* 1948;55: 86–101.
51. Krantz KE. The anatomy and physiology of the vulva and vagina and the anatomy of the urethra and bladder. In: Philipp EE, Barnes J, Newton M, eds. *Scientific Foundations of Obstetrics and Gynaecology*. Chicago: Year Book; 1977:65–78.
52. Bergeron C, Ferenczy A, Richart RM, et al. Micropapillomatosis labialis appears unrelated to human papillomavirus. *Obstet Gynecol* 1990;76:281–286.
53. Altcheck A, Wasserman B, Deligdisch L. Prepubertal distal longitudinal vaginal folds. *J Pediatr Adolesc Gynecol* 2008; 21(6):351–354.
54. Amenta PS. *Elias-Pauly's Histology and Human Microanatomy*. 5th ed. New York: John Wiley & Sons; 1987:502–503.
55. Miyagawa S, Monn A, Haraguchi R, et al. Dosage-dependent hedgehog signals integrated with Wnt/β;-catenin signaling regulate external genitalia formation as an appendicular program. *Development* 2009;136:3969–3978.
56. Clerico C, Lari A, Mojallal A, et al. Anatomy and aesthetics of the labia minora: The ideal vulva? *Aesthetic Plast Surg* 2017;41(3):714–719.
57. Schober J, Aardsma N, Mayoglou L, et al: Terminal innervation of female genital, cutaneous sensory receptors of the epithelium of the labia minora. *Clin Anat* 2015;28(3): 392–398.
58. Friedrich EG Jr, Wilkinson EJ. Vulvar surgery for neurofibromatosis. *Obstet Gynecol* 1985;65:135–138.
59. Tanner JM. *Growth at Adolescence*. 2nd ed. Oxford: Blackwell; 1962.
60. Barman JM, Astore J, Pecoraro V. The normal trichogram of people over 50 years. In: Montagna W, Dobson RL, eds. *Advances in Biology of Skin*. Vol. IX. Hair Growth. Oxford, England: Pergamon Press; 1969.
61. Bell D, Kane PB, Liang S, et al. Vulvar varicies: An uncommon entity in surgical pathology. *Int J Gynecol Pathol* 2006;26: 99–101.
62. Zelickson AS. *Electron Microscopy of Skin and Mucous Membranes*. Springfield, IL: Charles C Thomas; 1963.
63. Shatz P, Bergeron C, Wilkinson EJ, et al. Vulvar intraepithelial neoplasia and skin appendage involvement. *Obstet Gynecol* 1989;74:769–774.
64. van der Putte SC, van Gorp LH. Cysts of mammary-like glands in the vulva. *Int J Gynecol Pathol* 1995;14:184–188.
65. van der Putte SC. Mammary-like glands of the vulva and their disorders. *Int J Gynecol Pathol* 1994;13:150–160.
66. Konstantinova AM, Vanecek T, Martinek P, et al: Molecular alterations in lesions of anogenital mammary-like glands and their mammary counterparts including hidradenoma papilliferum, intraductal papilloma, fibroadenoma and phyllodes tumor. *Ann Diagn Pathol* 2017;28:12–18.
67. van der Putte SC. Clear cells of Toker in the developing anogenital region of male and female fetuses. *Am J Dermatopathol* 2011;33(8):811–818.
68. Willman JH, Golitz LE, Fitzpatrick JE. Vulvar clear cells of Toker: Precursors of extramammary Paget's disease. *Am J Dermatopathol* 2005;27:185–188.
69. Park S, Suh YL. Useful immunohistochemical markers for distinguishing Paget cells from Toker cells. *Pathology* 2009; 41(7):640–644.
70. Lundquist K, Kohler S, Rouse RV. Intraedermal cytokeratin 7 expression is not restricted to Paget cells but is also seen in Toker cells and Merkel cells. *Am J Surg Pathol* 1999;23(2): 212–219.
71. Lunde O. A study of body hair density and distribution in normal women. *Am J Phys Anthropol* 1984;64:179–184.
72. Parry-Jones E. Lymphatics of the vulva. *J Obstet Gynaecol Br Commonw* 1963;70:751–765.
73. Russel AH, Duska LR. *Cancer of Vulva in Liebel and Phillip: Textbook on Radiation Oncology*. 3rd ed. Philadelphia, PA: Elsevier Saunders; 2010, Chapter 52:1085.
74. Sims SM, McLean FW, Davis JD, et al. Vulvar lymphangioma circumscriptum: A report of 3 cases, 2 associated with squamous cell carcinoma and 1 with hidradenitis suprativa. *J Low Genit Tract Dis* 2010;14(3):234–238.
75. Handfield-Jones SE, Prendiville WJ, Norman S. Vulval lymphangiectasia. *Genitourin Med* 1989;65:335–337.
76. McCluggage WG, Nielsen GP, Young RH. Massive vulval edema secondary to obesity and immobilization: A potential mimic of aggressive angiomyxoma. *Int J Gynecol Pathol* 2008;27(3): 447–452.
77. LaPage PA, Villavicencio JL, Gomez ER, et al. The valvular anatomy of the iliac venous system and its clinical implications. *J Vasc Surg* 1991;14:678–683.
78. Yucel S, De Souza A Jr, Baskin LS. Neuroanatomy of the human female lower urogenital tract. *J Urol* 2004;172:191–195.
79. Rekthman N, Bishop JA. *Quick Reference Handbook for Surgical Pathologists*. Germany: Springer-Verlag Berlin Heidelberg; 2011:43–45.

Vagina

Stanley J. Robboy ▪ Gerald R. Cunha ▪ Takeshi Kurita ▪ Kyle C. Strickland

EMBRYOLOGIC DEVELOPMENT 1047	ULTRASTRUCTURE 1054
GROSS FEATURES 1049	DIFFERENTIAL DIAGNOSIS AND SPECIAL ANATOMY 1054
ANATOMY 1050	Wolffian Ducts 1054
Ligaments 1050	Paraurethral Glands (Skene Glands) 1054
Blood Supply 1050	G-spot (Gräfenberg Spot) 1055
Nerves 1050	Remnants of Mullerian Duct Epithelium (Adenosis) 1055
Lymphatic Drainage 1051	ACKNOWLEDGMENTS 1056
LIGHT MICROSCOPY 1051	REFERENCES 1056
Epithelium 1051	
Epithelial Responses and Functions 1052	
Vaginal Wall and Adventitia 1053	

Tissue from the vagina is infrequently examined via biopsy, owing to the fact that primary disease of the vagina is remarkably uncommon. Excluding the vaginal cuff removed for cervical disease, most biopsies and surgical operations are for infection, small intramural growths, intrauterine exposure to diethylstilbestrol (DES), or, in older women, squamous cell cancer and its precursors. More recently, the pathology associated with vaginal mesh, a prosthetic used for the treatment of stress urinary incontinence, (1) has led to an increasing number of surgical excisions being performed.

This chapter addresses the gross, microscopic, and ultrastructural anatomy of the normal vagina. The embryologic discussion focuses on developmental perturbations, which provide insights into normal gross and microscopic anatomy.

EMBRYOLOGIC DEVELOPMENT

The paired mullerian (paramesonephric) ducts appear about the 37th day postconception as funnel-shaped openings of the celomic epithelium (2). These develop into paired, undifferentiated tubes that later grow caudally, using the already formed wolffian (mesonephric) ducts as a guidewire to reach the urogenital sinus (Fig. 39.1). Absent this occurrence, the frequency of which is about 1 in 5000 newborn girls, the child is born lacking all mullerian derivatives, or at most any more than tubal remnants (Mayer–Rokitansky–Kuster–Hauser [MRKH] syndrome) (3,4). MRKH syndrome usually occurs sporadically, but it can also be hereditary, transmitted in an autosomal dominant pattern (5).

At about day 54, the paired mullerian ducts fuse caudally, becoming a straight uterovaginal canal (primordia of uterine corpus, cervix, and vagina), the lining of which is an immature simple columnar (mullerian) epithelium (Fig. 39.2) (6). The above developmental processes occur in both female and male embryos. If the fetus is a male, the indifferent gonads become anatomically distinct testes at around day 44. The testis is important for two products it makes. One, mullerian-inhibiting substance (MIS), elicits degeneration of the mullerian ducts. The other, testosterone, prevents degeneration of the wolffian ducts and stimulates their subsequent development. Shortly after the testes become distinct, Sertoli cells initiate MIS production, a protein in the transforming growth factor-β family, in amounts effective to cause the mullerian ducts to regress through a process of programmed cell death (7). If the embryo is

---

This chapter is an update of a previous version authored by Sarah M. Bean, Emanuella Veras, Rex C. Bentley, and Stanley J. Robboy.

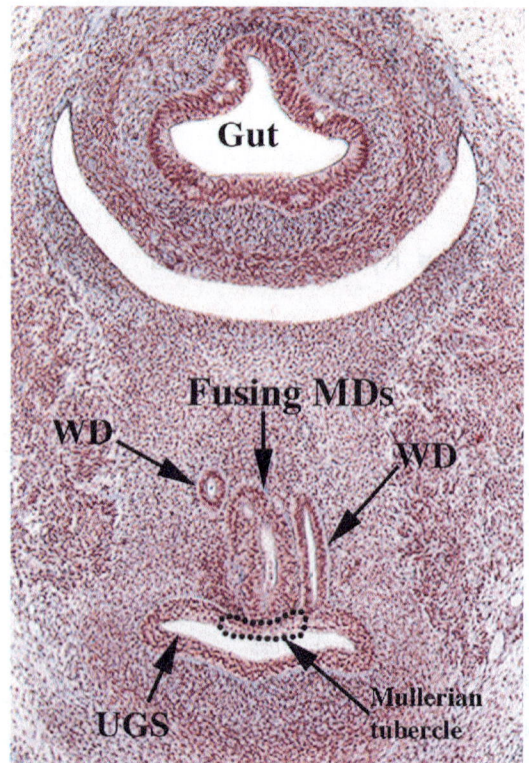

FIGURE 39.1 Pelvic section of a stage 23 Carnegie embryo (56 days) showing contact of the fusing mullerian ducts (MD) with the urogenital sinus (UGS). The point of contact of the mullerian ducts with the urogenital sinus is called the mullerian tubercle. Wolffian ducts (WD) also join the urogenital sinus just lateral to the mullerian tubercle. From the Virtual Human Embryo Project (http://virtualhumanembryo.lsuhsc.edu) with permission.

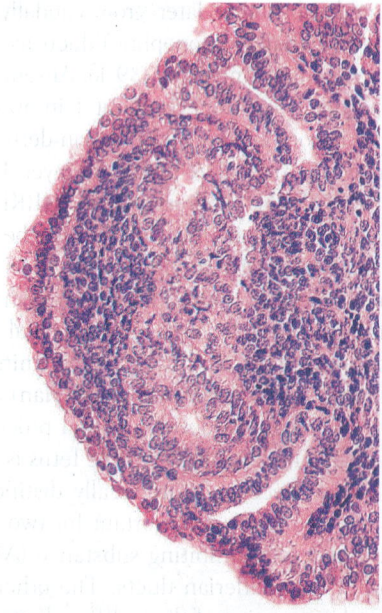

FIGURE 39.2 Region of urogenital sinus disclosing the tips of two central mullerian ducts that have grown down the (outer) paired wolffian ducts (circa day 54). The cytologic features of the cells comprising both types of ducts are indistinguishable on light microscopy at early stages of development. From Robboy SJ, Ellington KS. Pathology of the female genital tract in Kodachrome slides. Chapel Hill, NC: Robboy Associates, LLC; 1996.

female, testes do not develop. Since there is then no MIS, the mullerian ducts are not inhibited and thus grow without impedance and eventually fuse, forming the uterine tubes, the uterus, and the vagina. Failure of the mullerian ducts to fuse can cause septate vagina and uterus didelphys (i.e., double vagina and double uterus).

In contradistinction to MIS, which acts as an inhibitor, testosterone stimulates and is required to promote wolffian duct growth and development. In the male, the critical period for testosterone stimulation begins early in the 10th week and causes the embryonic wolffian ducts to differentiate into epididymis, seminal vesicle, ejaculatory ducts, and ductus (vas) deferens. If testes are absent (as in the female) and testosterone stimulation has not occurred by the close of the critical window (circa day 84), the wolffian ducts wither and become vestigial remnants, which in the adult are found deep in the vaginal wall and in the broad ligament.

At the end of week 10, the uterovaginal canal makes contact with the urogenital sinus due to caudal growth. At the point of contact with the urogenital sinus the columnar epithelium of the tubular uterovaginal canal proliferates and occludes the lumen forming the solid vaginal plate. The solid vaginal plate at 12 weeks of gestation is composed of PAX2-positive mullerian epithelium cranially and FOXA1-positive urogenital sinus epithelium caudally (Fig. 39.3). Subsequently, the FOXA1-positive urogenital sinus epithelium grows cranially to completely replace the PAX2-positive mullerian epithelium up to the level of the external cervical os (2). The transition to squamous epithelium, which reflects the urogenital sinus epithelium growing cranially to replace the original mullerian columnar epithelium, occurs at about the time when nuclear estrogen receptors appear in the vaginal stroma (9,10).

During the 13th week (91 days), cervical glands develop; they exhibit a wavy architectural appearance but cytologically are minimally differentiated. By the 14th week, the caudal vagina increases markedly in size. During the 15th week, the solid epithelial anlage of the anterior and posterior vaginal fornices appears. Starting in the 16th week, the squamous epithelium lining the vagina and the exocervix begins to mature, thus resembling the lining of the adult vagina, presumably due to elevation of endogenous estrogens. The epithelium thickens and glycogenates, features most likely related to increased maternal and hence fetal estrogen levels. As the epithelial cells mature, they lose cellular adhesiveness and desquamate, heralding the canalization of the vaginal plate and thus the onset of the final gross structure of the vagina. By the 18th to 20th week, the development of the vagina is complete.

Why columnar epithelium with an embryonic appearance should initially line the mullerian system and later be replaced by squamous epithelium remains of teleologic interest. The answer to the mechanism may lie in the vaginal wall stroma. Prior work in the mouse has shown that epithelial differentiation in the lower genital tract epithelium is dependent on the stroma on which it grows. In other

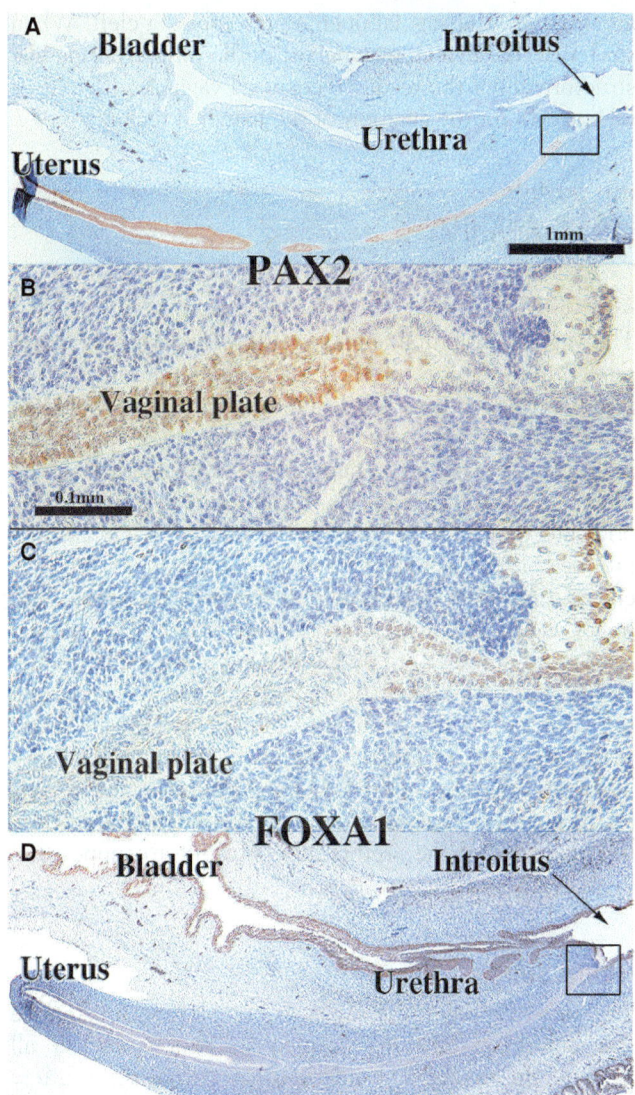

FIGURE 39.3 Sagittal sections of a 12-week human female fetal reproductive tract immunostained with PAX2 (A–B) and FOXA1 (C–D). PAX2-reactive epithelial cells extend to near the junction with the introitus/urethra (A–B). FOXA1-reactive epithelial cells extend only a short distance into the solid vaginal plate (C–D). Scale bar in A also refers to D. Scale bar in D also refers to C. From Robboy SJ, Kurita T, Baskin L, et al. New insights into human female reproductive tract development. *Differentiation* 2017;97:9–22.

most prominent in the endocervix. It is from this zone that fibroepithelial polyps seem to arise, an entity of no apparent physiologic function but which clinically should not be confused with a malignant tumor.

Should the squamous epithelium described above fail to replace the original columnar cells lining the vagina during the critical weeks of embryonic life, the epithelial columnar cells may remain in an arrested state of development until sometime around puberty, when they may further differentiate into the adult-type epithelium usually seen in biopsy material. We conjecture that the vaginal mesenchyme signals the overlying cells to develop as a tuboendometrial-type epithelium. In fact, it may be the mesenchyme throughout the entire mullerian duct programs the overlying cells to develop with cilia, manifesting the so-called serous cells in the uterine tube, endometrioid cells in the uterine corpus, and tuboendometrial cells in the vagina—epithelial cells that are quite similar histologically. In the cervix, a tuboendometrial layer of epithelium also lies deep to and as a cuff around the luminal layer of mucinous epithelium (16). The tuboendometrial layer, which is continuous with the lining of the uterine corpus, is readily observed in hysterectomy specimens but is located too deep to be detected on biopsy. In fetuses where the vaginal lining has become squamous (older than 10 weeks), the inner stromal zone is obvious in the uterine tube, endometrium, and endocervix and tapers, appearing to end at the squamocolumnar junction of the cervix and vagina. Part of this layer may correspond to the most superficial stromal layer in the adult vagina described above. The original tuboendometrial layer is the origin of glandular remnants in the vagina of adults (adenosis).

GROSS FEATURES

The vagina (from the Latin for sheath) extends from the vulvar vestibule to the uterine cervix, lying posterior (dorsal) to the urinary bladder and anterior (ventral) to the rectum. Its axis averages 30 degrees with the vertical, arching slightly posteriocranially, and more than 90 degrees with the uterus (Fig. 39.4). If the woman is standing, the lower vaginal axis is vertical and posterior, but the upper vaginal axis changes at the level of the pelvic diaphragm and becomes horizontal (17). Vaginal length was variable, ranging from 6.5 to, and depending how measured to 12.5 cm (17–19). The anterior wall is 8 cm long and the posterior wall 11 cm, with the cervix filling the 3 cm difference. Vaginal length is often slightly decreased in women with prior hysterectomy or pelvic reconstruction; in addition, every additional 10 years of age also slightly decreases total vaginal length (20). In early life, the vagina is constricted distally at the vestibule, dilated in the middle, and narrowed proximally near the exocervix. The vaginal apex surrounds the exocervix and forms vault-like fornices between its cervical attachment and the vaginal encompassing wall. In the adult, the anterior and

words, the stroma determines the fate of the overlying epithelium. For example, in the mouse, uterine epithelium, when grown in association with neonatal vaginal stroma, develops histotypic features of vagina (11) and expresses p63 (a vaginal epithelial identity marker), keratin 14, and other vaginal markers (12). In contrast, vaginal epithelium, if grown in association with neonatal uterine stroma, develops a uterine phenotype, lacks p63, and expresses uterine epithelial markers (13–15).

The developmental morphology of the vaginal mucosa and the inductive properties of the stroma supporting the vaginal mucosa are complex. For example, a band of subepithelial stroma (lamina propria) 0.5 to 5 mm thick in mature females extends from the endocervix to the vulva. It is

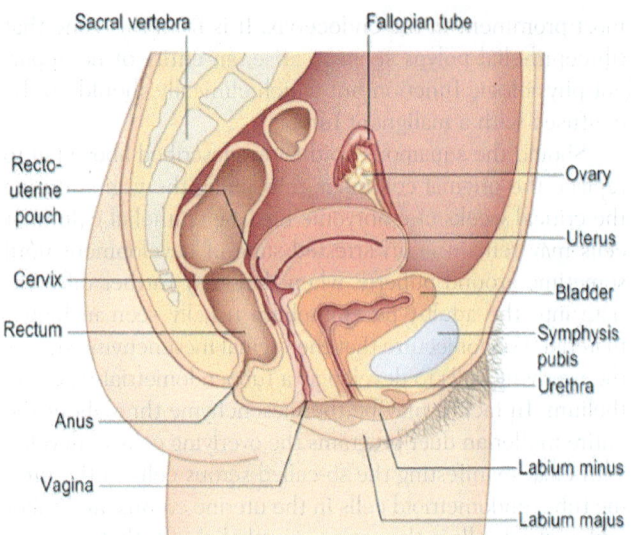

FIGURE 39.4 Structural relationships of the vagina. Its axis forms an angle of more than 90 degrees with the uterus. From Bean S, Prat J, Robboy SJ. Vagina. In: Mutter GL, Prat J, eds. Pathology of the female reproductive tract. London: Churchill Livingstone/Elsevier; 2014:132–159.

posterior vaginal walls are slack and remain in contact with each other, whereas the lateral walls remain fairly rigid and separated. This is thought to give an H-shaped appearance to the vaginal canal on cross section (21), although with three-dimensional imaging with magnetic resonance imaging (MRI), a "W" shape is now also recognized (22). During intercourse, the position of the uterus and the bladder changes relative to the vagina (23,24).

Posteriorly, the upper one-fourth of the vagina is related to the rectouterine space (i.e., the cul-de-sac or pouch of Douglas), which is covered with peritoneum. The middle half of the vagina is closely apposed to the rectum, separated only by fibrofatty adventitia and the rectovaginal septum. The lower one-fourth of the vagina is separated from the anal canal by anal and rectal sphincters, as well as the interposing perineal body, from which originates the bulbocavernosus and superficial transverse perineal muscles.

The urinary bladder and urethra lie anterior to the vagina. The urethra courses approximately one-third of its length on the vagina and then enters into the vaginal wall to become an inseparable part of it, usually terminating with its external meatus at the introitus. Typically, the urethral meatus is outwardly directed (opening just anterior to the vaginal opening), but occasionally it is directed into the outermost vagina (in the vaginal wall). The ureters course along both sides of the upper one-third of the vagina until entering the bladder wall.

The vagina opens into the vestibule formed from the urogenital sinus, and in many ways share features more in common with these areas, including blood and nerve supply, than with the rest of the vagina (26). The vagina, urethra, and ducts of Bartholin glands open into the vestibule. The size and shape of the vaginal orifice are related to the state of the hymen. When the inner edges of the hymen are apposed, the vaginal opening resembles a cleft. When stretched, the hymen may persist in the form of a ring-like structure about the readily recognized vaginal orifice. (See Chapter 38 for the anatomy of the hymenal region.)

ANATOMY

Ligaments

The vaginal structural supports (ligaments) are intimately related to the uterus, urethra, bladder, and rectum and are best described in three levels: uterosacral/cardinal ligament complex, paravaginal attachments, and perineal membrane and muscles. The lateral supports are called cardinal ligaments, the posterior supports, sacrouterine ligaments. They originate where the isthmus of the uterine cervix and the uterine corpus meet and course outward, fanlike to the lateral and posterior pelvic walls, suspending the uterus and upper vagina and maintaining vaginal length. The isthmic fibers turn upward onto the uterus and downward onto the vagina. The paravaginal attachments support the mid-anterior vagina while the perineal membrane and muscles support the urethra and distal third of the vagina (21). These ligaments, the connective tissues surrounding the vessels on the lateral vaginal walls, and the proximity of the rectum, the bladder, and the urethra all contribute to support the vagina within the pelvis.

Blood Supply

The blood supply to the vagina is complex, with extensive anastomoses maintaining an adequate blood supply to all areas of the vagina. The internal iliac (hypogastric) artery is the principal source of blood cranially as branches of the uterine arteries and caudally as branches of the middle hemorrhoidal arteries and pudendal arteries. Beginning cranially, the uterine artery gives off a descending branch, the cervicovaginal artery. Several branches supply the cervix. Lower branches supply the vagina. The vaginal arteries, which lie lateral to the vagina, send branches to both the anterior and posterior vaginal surfaces. The lower vagina receives its supply from ascending branches of the middle hemorrhoidal arteries and pudendal arteries, which also divide to send rami to the anterior and posterior vaginal walls. In toto, the extensive rami form a plexus around the vagina from which arise the median arteries, the azygos vaginal arteries on the anterior and posterior walls. A rich venous plexus also surrounds the vagina and communicates with the vesicle, pudendal, and hemorrhoidal venous plexuses, which empty into the internal iliac veins.

Nerves

The autonomic system of the pelvis originates in the superior hypogastric plexus with input from the sacral spinal cord (preganglionic parasympathetic innervation), outflow of the lower thoracic and upper lumbar spinal cord segments (preganglionic sympathetic innervation), and ventral horn of the lower spinal cord segments (somatic motor innervation from α-motor neurons) (27). It functions to coordinate sympathetic, parasympathetic, and somatic innervation activities that regulate clitoral erection, vaginal secretions, smooth muscle contractions of the vagina, and the somatic pelvic muscles that accompany orgasm. The middle hypogastric plexus, which passes into the pelvis, divides at the level of the S1 (sacral) vertebra into branches that pass to both sides of the pelvis and initiate the inferior hypogastric plexus. The inferior hypogastric plexus, a divided continuation of the middle hypogastric plexus, the superior hypogastric plexus, and the presacral nerve, descend into the pelvis in a position posterior to the common iliac artery and anterior to the sacral plexus; it curves laterally and finally enters the sacrouterine ligament. The medial segment of the sacral nerves' primary division (S2–S5), as it sends fibers into the pelvic plexus located within the sacrouterine folds, appears to contain both sympathetic (inferior hypogastric plexus) and parasympathetic (nervi erigentes) components. An extension of this plexus, located at the base of the broad ligament and supplied by the middle vesical artery, contains many ganglia. Most nerves enter the uterus near the isthmus. A lesser number descend along the lateral vagina, a pattern similar to the arteries that supply the vagina. Sensory fibers come from the pudendal nerve and pain fibers arise from the sacral nerve roots. The nerve density is relatively uniform throughout all areas of the organ (28).

Lymphatic Drainage

The vaginal lymphatic system is highly variable. The lymphatics begin as a delicate plexus of small channels involving the entire mucosa and lamina propria and then drain into a deep muscular network. They terminate in a perivaginal plexus from which arise collecting trunks, which themselves coalesce into several larger channels. Virtually all of the lymphatic vessels lie within the superficial 5 mm of the vaginal wall (29).

The lymph drainage follows patterns that reflect functionally diverse geographic regions. The lymphatics of the upper anterior wall join those of the cervix, where they follow the cervical vessels to the uterine artery and accompany it to terminate in the medial chain of the external iliac nodes. The lymph from the posterior vagina drains into deep pelvic, rectal, and aortic nodes. The lymphatics of the lower vagina, which also include the hymenal region, follow two distinct courses. One passes to the interiliac nodes. The other traverses the paravesical space, carrying lymph to the deepest portions of the pelvis and draining into the inferior gluteal nodes near the origin of the vaginal or internal pudendal artery. The channels that anastomose with those of the vulva drain to the superficial iliac nodes. In summary, as a practical matter, lymph in the upper vagina drains as the cervix to involve obturator and both internal and external iliac nodes.

In contrast, the lower vagina drains to involve superficial iliac (inguinal) and deep pelvic nodes, much like the vulva.

LIGHT MICROSCOPY

Epithelium

The vaginal wall consists of three principal layers: Mucosa (epithelial and submucosal stroma), muscle, and adventitia. The epithelium is about 0.4 mm thick and, on gross examination, exhibits a characteristic pattern of folds or rugae separated by furrows of variable depth. There are two longitudinal (anterior and posterior) and multiple transverse furrows. The rugal pattern of the vaginal mucosa, which contributes to the organ's elasticity, produces an undulating appearance on microscopic examination in contrast to the flat surface of the cervix. The rugae, which are more prominent in nulliparous than multiparous women, reinforce the gripping effect of the levator ani and vaginal constrictor muscles during intercourse. Nonkeratinized glycogenated squamous epithelium lines the luminal surface similar to the cervical epithelium. The normal vaginal mucosa lacks glands. Its surface is lubricated both by fluids that pass directly through the mucosa and by cervical mucus.

The mature, stratified squamous epithelium can be subdivided into several layers, typical of squamous epithelia elsewhere in the body (Fig. 39.5). From the base to the surface, they are the deep (basal), intermediate, and superficial

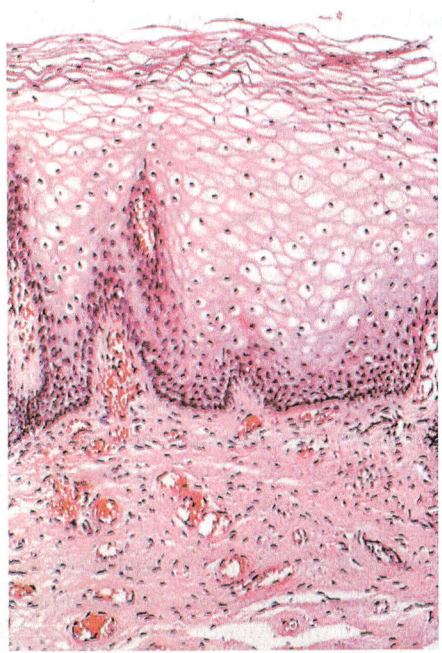

FIGURE 39.5 Mucosa of the adult vagina. Mature cells with glycogenic cytoplasm and pyknotic nuclei occupy most of the epithelial thickness. There is a single layer of dark basal cells and three to four layers of intermediate cells. From Robboy SJ, Ellington KS. Pathology of the female genital tract in Kodachrome slides. Chapel Hill, NC: Robboy Associates, LLC; 1996.

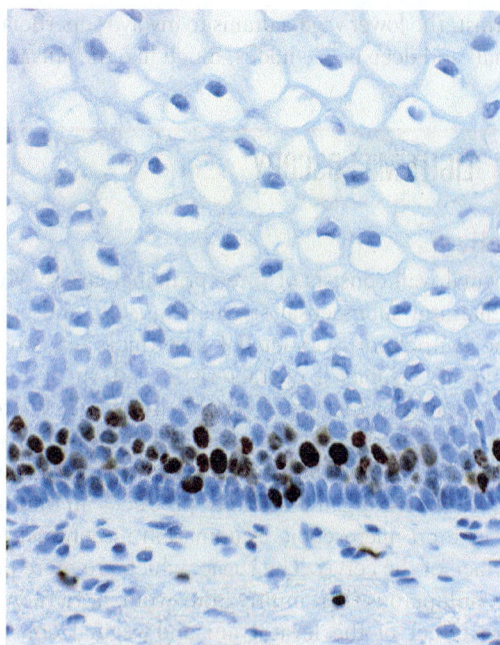

FIGURE 39.6 Ki-67 antigen, demonstrable during late G1, G2, and M phases of the cell cycle, in the basal and parabasal layers of the normal vaginal mucosa. From Robboy SJ, Ellington KS. Pathology of the female genital tract in Kodachrome slides. Chapel Hill, NC: Robboy Associates, LLC; 1996.

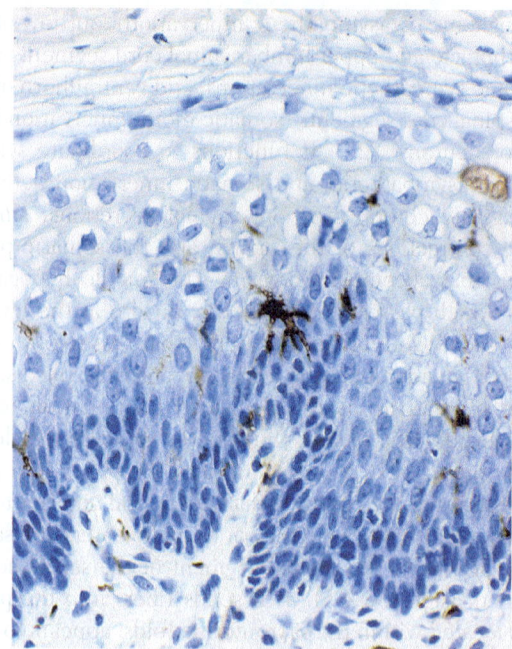

FIGURE 39.7 The dendritic processes of Langerhans cells. From Robboy SJ, Ellington KS. Pathology of the female genital tract in Kodachrome slides. Chapel Hill, NC: Robboy Associates, LLC; 1996.

zones. The deep zone contains the basal cell layer and, above this, the parabasal layer. Both are the active proliferative compartments or germinal beds, as shown by the Ki-67 antigen, which is demonstrable during late G1, G2, and M phases of the cell cycle (Fig. 39.6). The basal cell layer consists of a single layer of columnar-like cells, approximately 10 μm thick, the long axis of which is vertically arranged. The cells have a basophilic cytoplasm and relatively large oval nuclei. Mitoses may be present. Occasional melanocytes also are found.

The parabasal layer is poorly demarcated from the overlying cell layers. It usually consists of about two layers of small polygonal cells, having a total thickness of 14 μm, often with intercellular bridges. The cells have basophilic cytoplasm, a relatively large, centrally placed, round nucleus and occasional mitoses.

The intermediate cell layer is of variable thickness. The cells have prominent intercellular bridges, a naviculate configuration, and a long-cell axis paralleling the surface. The cytoplasm is basophilic, although some glycogen may be present. The nuclei are round, oval, or irregular, with finely granular chromatin. This layer of cells has about 10 rows of cells of about 100 μm thickness.

The superficial layer is also of variable thickness, commonly composed of about 10 rows of squamous cells. The cells are polygonal when viewed from above and flattened when viewed in cross-section. The cytoplasm is acidophilic and may contain keratohyalin granules. The nuclei are centrally located, small, round, and pyknotic.

Relatively little is known about the other normal components of the epithelium itself. The submucosa contains a variety of mononuclear cells demonstrable by immunocytochemical methods (30). The dendritic processes of Langerhans cells (about 4 per high-power field) are distributed throughout the mucosa (31). We have found them largely in the deeper layers, but they can extend into the superficial fields (Fig. 39.7). Both T8 and, to a lesser degree, T4 lymphocytes are also frequently found, whereas macrophages and B lymphocytes are relatively uncommon.

Epithelial Responses and Functions

The vagina may play other roles than simply serving as a conduit for intercourse and birth. As an interface between host and environment, its microbiome effectively defends against invasive microbial infections (32–35). It fosters vaginal health by maintaining a microenvironment of endogenous lactobacilli. It retains critical mediators of acquired and innate immunity (36).

Vaginal epithelial cells proliferate and mature in response to stimulation by ovarian or exogenous estrogenic hormones. But dispute exists as to whether the total number of squamous cell layers changes during the normal menstrual cycle, and also what changes occur as a woman passes through the various stages of the life cycle, that is, birth, childhood, reproduction, and the postmenopausal years. In one earlier report (37), the epithelium is thickest at ovulation (average 45 layers), building slowly during the proliferative phase. After ovulation, the number recedes to 33 on day 19 and to 23 on day 24. At the opposite end of the spectrum, the number of cell layers decrease slightly from about 28 during the proliferative phase to 26 on during the early secretory phase (31).

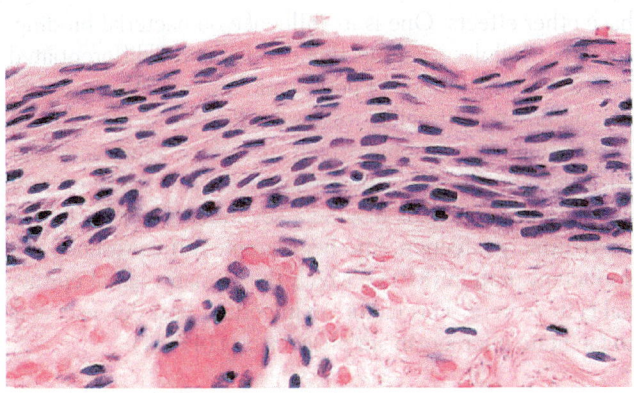

FIGURE 39.8 Atrophic vagina. From Robboy SJ, Ellington KS. Pathology of the female genital tract in Kodachrome slides. Chapel Hill, NC: Robboy Associates, LLC; 1996.

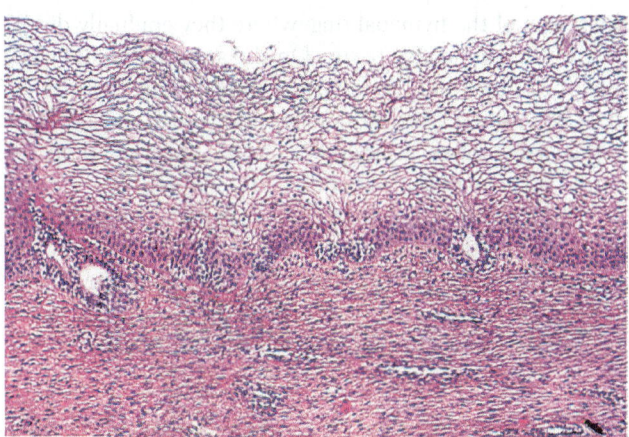

FIGURE 39.10 Vaginal mucosa of a near-term fetus. Mature cells predominate and cannot be distinguished from that of the adult (compare with Fig. 39.5). In addition, two adenotic glands of the embryonic type are present. From Robboy SJ, Ellington KS. Pathology of the female genital tract in Kodachrome slides. Chapel Hill, NC: Robboy Associates, LLC; 1996.

Without hormonal stimulation, vaginal epithelium atrophies (Fig. 39.8). Therapy with tamoxifen has a maturation effect (38). In women of reproductive age and at the peak of estrogenic activity (i.e., just before ovulation), the superficial cells with abundant intracytoplasmic glycogen predominate, both in histologic section and in vaginal smears (Fig. 39.9). Lactobacilli metabolize the glycogen normally present in the vagina to lactic acid, which maintains a vaginal acid pH (about pH 4.4 during the late proliferative and secretory phases) (39).

Progesterone inhibits maturation of the vaginal epithelium. Consequently, intermediate cells predominate when the circulating levels of progesterone are high, for example, during the postovulatory phase of the menstrual cycle or pregnancy. Estrogenic activity is low or absent before puberty and after the menopause; the vaginal epithelium fails to mature and hence remains thin. Parabasal and intermediate cells predominate in the vaginal smear. In the newborn child, the vaginal epithelium is frequently mature because of the influence of maternal estrogens (Fig. 39.10). Quantitative studies measuring the rate of change in the maturation index in the infant's vagina from birth to the atrophic state postnatally indicate that vaginal cells replace themselves in less than 2 weeks; that is, the time required for basal cells to work their way up and become desquamated superficial cells. Studies of the exocervix indicate that turnover there is also rapid (40).

The submucosa, or lamina propria, lies directly beneath the basal layer of squamous epithelium. It contains elastic fibers, which average 1.8 um in width (41), and collagen, which in disease states such as with pelvic organ prolapses, shows considerable changes from the norm (42–46). The lamina propria also contains a rich venous and lymphatic network.

Sometimes the superficial lamina propria discloses a band-like zone of loose connective tissue that contains atypical polygonal to stellate stromal cells with scant cytoplasm. Many cells are multinucleated or have multilobulated hyperchromatic nuclei. Few are mononucleate. Mitoses are not observed. These atypical stromal cells are thought to give rise to fibroepithelial polyps, which appear occasionally within the cervix, the vagina, and the vulva. They have been shown to be fibroblastic in origin.

Vaginal Wall and Adventitia

The vaginal smooth muscle musculature is continuous with that of the uterus. The outer muscular layers of both the uterus and vagina run longitudinally to pass onto the lateral pelvic wall to form the superior and inferior surfaces, respectively, of the cardinal ligaments. The longitudinal muscle fibers continue to course the length of the vagina to

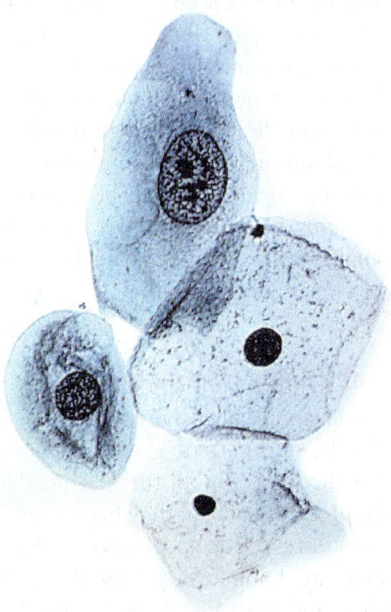

FIGURE 39.9 Vaginal smear, showing basal cell, two intermediate cells, and a superficial cell (Papanicolaou stain). From Robboy SJ, Ellington KS. Pathology of the female genital tract in Kodachrome slides. Chapel Hill, NC: Robboy Associates, LLC; 1996.

the region of the hymenal ring, where they gradually disappear in the connective tissue. On the anterior vaginal wall, the longitudinal muscle fibers are displaced by the urethra more than diminished in number. The inner muscle layer of the vagina forms a spiral-like course, appearing in microscopic sections as somewhat circular in direction.

The adventitia is a thin coat of dense connective tissue adjoining the muscularis. The connective tissue of the adventitia merges with the stroma, connecting the vagina to the adjacent structures. This layer contains many veins, lymphatics, nerve bundles, and small groups of nerve cells.

ULTRASTRUCTURE

On ultrastructural examination, the epithelial layers are not sharply demarcated from each other. Rather, they may be somewhat difficult to distinguish because each layer has ill-defined limits and displays gradual changes in structure.

On scanning electron microscopic examination, the superficial epithelial cells appear large (50 μm in greatest dimension) and polygonal (47). The intercellular edges are narrow and dense and protrude slightly. The pattern of fine webbing and anastomotic intercellular bridges typifies nonkeratinized squamous epithelium, such as that observed in buccal mucosa. The important structure on the cell surface is the microridge, or in reality myriad microridges, which are interanastomotic longitudinal elevations of the plasma membrane 0.2 nm long and 0.1 nm high. Arranged in dense convolutions, they tie one cell to another, operating in a zipper-fastener principle. They are thought to provide surface adhesion. Desmosomes are prominent in these areas.

Microridge formation in the superficial cells depends on the topographic configuration of disulfide-rich keratin or keratin precursors, which are absent in immature precursor cells (intermediate cells and young metaplastic squamous cells). From midcycle and early in the luteal phase, intercellular grooves widen. Pore-like widening (porosites) of the intercellular crevices takes place where several cells interconnect. This porosity is thought to enhance continuity of the intercellular space system of the vaginal epithelium and the vaginal surface, thus permitting free passage of vaginal lubricating fluid.

Information about changes at the biochemical and immunologic levels is sparse, but clearly the epithelial cells at various levels show dramatic differences. Part may reflect degrees of cellular maturity. Part may reflect subcellular specialization. Like other epithelia, both squamous and glandular alike, the pattern of cytokeratin expression reflects the state and nature of the epithelial cells' differentiation. The vaginal mucosa reflects that of other nonkeratinized squamous epithelium. Cytokeratin 14 (CK14) is present in the basal layer and CK13 in the parabasal layer, the latter supporting a subpopulation of cells that express CK10. In ways uncertain, the differentiating cells show changes that may

have other effects. One is its influence on bacterial binding, such that cellular receptors that develop in the differentiated cells enhance adhesion of pathogenic bacteria. As one example, differentiated vaginal mucosal cells express receptors to *Escherichia coli* type 1 pili, which are surface-adhesive organelles (48). Such colonization where fecal *E. coli* are present in the vaginal introitus may be a key initial event leading to acute urinary infection. Another example is the presence of a surfactant protein (SP-A), which the human vaginal epithelial cells secrete. This factor, an important host defense, acts to facilitate microorganism phagocytosis (49–51).

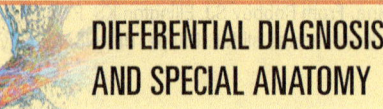

DIFFERENTIAL DIAGNOSIS AND SPECIAL ANATOMY

Wolffian Ducts

The wolffian duct, known otherwise as the mesonephric duct or Gartner duct, is vestigial in the adult female (Fig. 39.11). It begins to irreversibly wither if not stimulated to develop by testosterone before the 13th week postconception. These paired bilateral ducts are most commonly situated in the lateral vaginal walls, although we have encountered it in all areas. Where found by chance in a radical vaginectomy specimen, the ducts are virtually always invisible grossly. Mitoses are absent. Usually it is a small duct or clusters of small glands about a duct. The lumen is frequently filled with a deeply eosinophilic, hyalinized secretion. The single layer of cells lining the duct is primarily composed of the cell nucleus. The cytoplasm is scant, relatively translucent, and lacks cilia. The nuclei frequently overlap. The chromatin is strikingly bland. On a clinical basis, individual ducts occasionally become cystic and macroscopically visible. In the cervix, these ducts rarely appear diffusely throughout the wall and appear as mesonephric hyperplasia or even adenoma (52). Occasionally, even true wolffian duct carcinoma (mesonephric adenocarcinoma and malignant mixed mesonephric carcinoma) develops (53). The transcription factor, GATA3, is a highly sensitive and specific marker for both benign and malignant wolffian/mesonephric duct lesions in the lower female genital tract (54).

Paraurethral Glands (Skene Glands)

The paraurethral glands, also known as Skene glands, lesser vestibular glands, periurethral glands lie on the anterior vaginal wall at the lower end of the urethra. Although they drain into the urethra or vulva, they may be encountered in vaginal biopsies or resection specimens.

The glands are homologous with the male's prostate gland in males, and both histologically and biochemically have secretions resembling prostate (55–57). Disorders include cyst formation, bacterial infection, trichomoniasis (when the glands serve as a reservoir for the organism, *Trichomonas vaginalis*), and especially misrecognition for

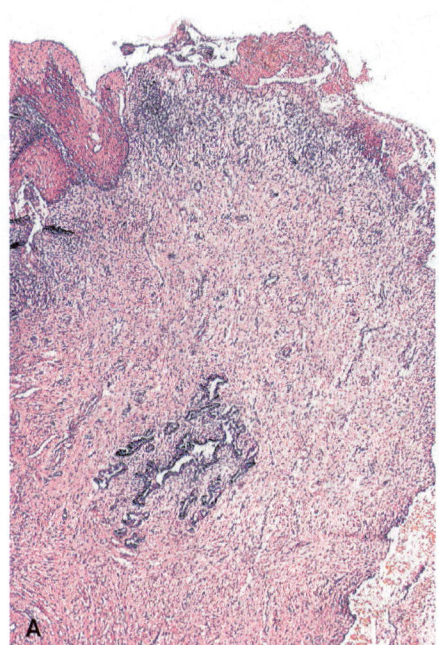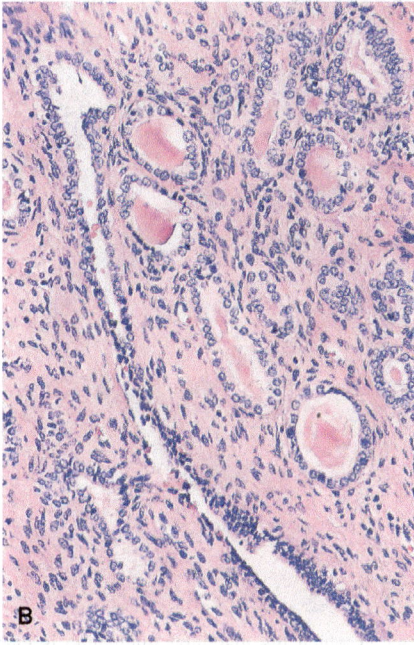

FIGURE 39.11 A: Vestigial wolffian duct remnants, deep in wall. **B:** Detail of central duct and arborized ductal terminals with eosinophilic secretions. From Robboy SJ, Ellington KS. Pathology of the female genital tract in Kodachrome slides. Chapel Hill, NC: Robboy Associates, LLC; 1996.

a normal tissue (56,58). Adenocarcinomas of Skene gland resemble prostatic adenocarcinoma histologically and immunophenotypically (59).

G-spot (Gräfenberg Spot)

The G-spot, also known as the Gräfenberg spot, is of debatable existence (60,61). Described as an erogenous area located in the anterior vaginal wall that, when stimulated, may lead to powerful orgasms and female ejaculation, a distinct morphologic entity has never been found. Some believe it may represent vascular-erectile tissue (62,63), and some paraurethral glands, that is, the female homolog of the male prostate gland.

Remnants of Mullerian Duct Epithelium (Adenosis)

The DES story began in 1938 when the nonsteroidal estrogen, DES, was synthesized and then gained popularity for the treatment of high-risk pregnancy. By 1971, up to two million women had taken the drug, at which time it was linked to the extremely rare development of clear cell adenocarcinoma of the vagina and cervix in young female offspring. Long-term follow-up studies strongly confirm the link to the genital cancer, but have some suggestion of a very tenuous connection to breast cancer (64,65).

Subsequently, about one-third of the exposed young women were found to have adenosis (presence of glandular tissue in the vagina). Both retrospective and prospective studies have shown that adenosis can be found in nonexposed women also, albeit rarely. In both exposed and nonexposed women, adenosis is related to embryonic mullerian tissue that has remained entrapped and not been replaced by squamous epithelium during fetal life. In DES-exposed mice, p63 expression is inhibited in DES-induced adenosis, at least transiently, and is related to a lack of squamous differentiation; DES-exposed mice fail to express p63 and had persistent adulthood adenosis (12,66–68).

Adenosis appears in three forms. One type, the embryonic form, is exceedingly rare. The other two are the tuboendometrial and mucinous forms. In the type of adenosis found during fetal life and in stillborns but only rarely in adults, the glands appear embryonic in character (Figs. 39.10 and 39.12). They are small, usually at the epithelial–stromal interface, and disclose individual cells with small basal nuclei and copious bland cytoplasm that does not stain with either periodic acid–Schiff or mucicarmine.

Adenosis likely takes on its adult forms in women some time during puberty (16,69). Mucinous columnar cells, which by light and electron microscopy resemble those of the normal endocervical mucosa, comprise the glandular epithelium most frequently encountered as adenosis (62% of biopsy specimens with vaginal adenosis). This epithelium, because it often lines the vaginal surface, is the type most commonly observed by colposcopy, where it presents as red granular areas distinct from the normal vaginal mucosa. Commonly, the mucinous columnar cells also line glands embedded in the lamina propria. This form of epithelium gives rise to the progestin-stimulated lesion, microglandular hyperplasia of the vagina.

Dark cells and light cells, often ciliated and resembling the lining cells of the uterine tube and endometrium, are found in 21% of specimens in the upper vagina with adenosis. This form of adenosis is called tuboendometrial, although serous might be equally appropriate. The cells are

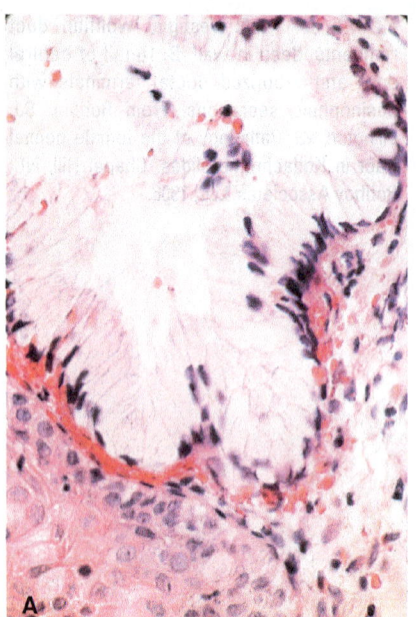 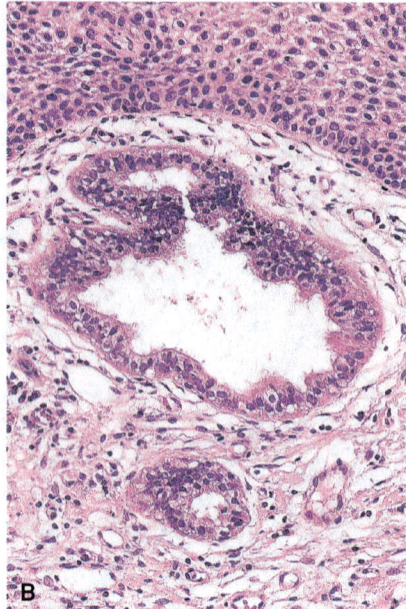 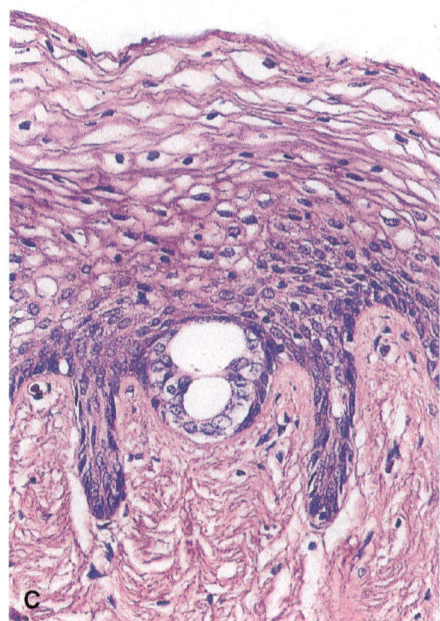

FIGURE 39.12 Vaginal adenosis in which the glandular epithelium is mucinous (**A**), tuboendometrial (**B**), or of the immature embryonic type (**C**). From Robboy SJ, Ellington KS. Pathology of the female genital tract in Kodachrome slides. Chapel Hill, NC: Robboy Associates, LLC; 1996.

usually found in glands in the lamina propria and not on the vaginal surface. Although adenosis in the lower vagina is rare in absolute number, the percentage of biopsy specimens with adenosis that exhibits tuboendometrial rather than mucinous cells increases markedly in frequency in comparison with the more cranial aspects of the vagina. The tuboendometrial cell, which is benign, is the cell that we believe is related to clear cell adenocarcinoma, possibly through atypical adenosis, a transitional form (70,71). Mucinous glands and mucinous pools or droplets are frequently encountered in the same biopsy specimen; mucinous and tuboendometrial cells are found together only occasionally in biopsy material. The tuboendometrial form of adenosis is the principal type of glandular cell in the uterine tube, uterus, or vagina. The mucinous cell, in contrast, is generally specific to the endocervix or, after DES exposure, to the deformed region of the cervix, which becomes ill defined and includes what appears to be the upper vagina.

ACKNOWLEDGMENTS

This study was supported by NIH grant DK058105 to Dr. Baskin and R01 CA154358 to Dr. Kurita.

REFERENCES

1. Li L, Wang X, Park JY, et al. Pathological findings in explanted vaginal mesh. *Hum Pathol* 2017;69:46–54.
2. Robboy SJ, Kurita T, Baskin L, et al. New insights into human female reproductive tract development. *Differentiation* 2017;97:9–22.
3. Watanabe K, Kobayashi Y, Banno K, et al. Recent advances in the molecular mechanisms of Mayer-Rokitansky-Kuster-Hauser syndrome. *Biomed Rep* 2017;7(2):123–127.
4. Bombard DS 2nd, Mousa SA. Mayer-Rokitansky-Kuster-Hauser syndrome: Complications, diagnosis and possible treatment options: A review. *Gynecol Endocrinol* 2014;30(9):618–623.
5. Herlin M, Hojland AT, Petersen MB. Familial occurrence of Mayer-Rokitansky-Kuster-Hauser syndrome: A case report and review of the literature. *Am J Med Genet A* 2014;164A(9):2276–2286.
6. Lawrence WD, Shingleton HM, Gore H, et al. Ultrastructural and morphometric study of diethylstilbestrol-associated lesions diagnosed as cervical intraepithelial neoplasia III. *Cancer Res* 1980;40(5):1558–1567.
7. MacLaughlin DT, Donahoe PK. Sex determination and differentiation. *N Engl J Med* 2004;350(4):367–378.
8. Robboy SJ, Ellington KS. *Pathology of the Female Genital Tract in Kodachrome Slides.* Chapel Hill, NC: Robboy Associates, LLC; 1996.
9. Taguchi O, Cunha GR, Robboy SJ. Expression of nuclear estrogen-binding sites within developing human fetal vagina and urogenital sinus. *Am J Anat* 1986;177(4):473–480.
10. Cunha GR, Kurita T, Cao M, et al. Molecular mechanisms of development of the human fetal female reproductive tract. *Differentiation* 2017;97:54–72.
11. Kurita T, Cooke PS, Cunha GR. Epithelial-stromal tissue interaction in paramesonephric (Mullerian) epithelial differentiation. *Dev Biol* 2001;240(1):194–211.
12. Kurita T, Mills AA, Cunha GR. Roles of p63 in the diethylstilbestrol-induced cervicovaginal adenosis. *Development* 2004;131(7):1639–1649.

13. Kurita T, Cunha GR, Robboy SJ, et al. Differential expression of p63 isoforms in female reproductive organs. *Mech Dev* 2005;122(9):1043–1055.
14. Terakawa J, Rocchi A, Serna VA, et al. FGFR2IIIb-MAPK activity is required for epithelial cell fate decision in the lower mullerian duct. *Mol Endocrinol* 2016;30(7):783–795.
15. Laronda MM, Unno K, Ishi K, et al. Diethylstilbestrol induces vaginal adenosis by disrupting SMAD/RUNX1-mediated cell fate decision in the Mullerian duct epithelium. *Dev Biol* 2013;381(1):5–16.
16. Robboy SJ. A hypothetic mechanism of diethylstilbestrol (DES)-induced anomalies in exposed progeny. *Hum Pathol* 1983;14(10):831–833.
17. Barnhart KT, Izquierdo A, Pretorius ES, et al. Baseline dimensions of the human vagina. *Hum Reprod* 2006;21(6):1618–1622.
18. Lloyd J, Crouch NS, Minto CL, et al. Female genital appearance: "normality" unfolds. *BJOG* 2005;112(5):643–646.
19. Luo J, Betschart C, Ashton-Miller JA, et al. Quantitative analyses of variability in normal vaginal shape and dimension on MR images. *Int Urogynecol J* 2016;27(7):1087–1095.
20. Tan JS, Lukacz ES, Menefee SA, et al. Determinants of vaginal length. *Am J Obstet Gynecol* 2006;195(6):1846–1850.
21. Barber MD. Contemporary views on female pelvic anatomy. *Cleve Clin J Med* 2005;72(Suppl 4):S3–S11.
22. Barnhart KT, Pretorius ES, Malamud D. Lesson learned and dispelled myths: Three-dimensional imaging of the human vagina. *Fertil Steril* 2004;81(5):1383–1384.
23. Faix A, Lapray JF, Callede O, et al. Magnetic resonance imaging (MRI) of sexual intercourse: Second experience in missionary position and initial experience in posterior position. *J Sex Marital Ther* 2002;28(Suppl 1):63–76.
24. Faix A, Lapray JF, Courtieu C, et al. Magnetic resonance imaging of sexual intercourse: Initial experience. *J Sex Marital Ther* 2001;27(5):475–482.
25. Bean S, Prat J, Robboy SJ. Vagina. In: Mutter GL, Prat J, eds. *Pathology of the Female Reproductive Tract*. London: Churchill Livingstone/Elsevier; 2014:132–159.
26. O'Connell HE, Eizenberg N, Rahman M, et al. The anatomy of the distal vagina: Towards unity. *J Sex Med* 2008;5(8):1883–1891.
27. Purves D, Augustine GJ, Fitzpatrick D, et al. *Neuroscience*. 5th ed. Sunderland, MA: Sinauer Associates; 2012:472–474.
28. Pauls R, Mutema G, Segal J, et al. A prospective study examining the anatomic distribution of nerve density in the human vagina. *J Sex Med* 2006;3(6):979–987.
29. Choo JJ, Scudiere J, Bitterman P, et al. Vaginal lymphatic channel location and its implication for intracavitary brachytherapy radiation treatment. *Brachytherapy* 2005;4(3):236–240.
30. Soloff AC, Barratt-Boyes SM. Enemy at the gates: Dendritic cells and immunity to mucosal pathogens. *Cell Res* 2010;20(8):872–885.
31. Patton DL, Thwin SS, Meier A, et al. Epithelial cell layer thickness and immune cell populations in the normal human vagina at different stages of the menstrual cycle. *Am J Obstet Gynecol* 2000;183(4):967–973.
32. Smith SB, Ravel J. The vaginal microbiota, host defence and reproductive physiology. *J Physiol* 2017;595(2):451–463.
33. Shannon B, Gajer P, Yi TJ, et al. Distinct effects of the cervicovaginal microbiota and herpes simplex type 2 infection on female genital tract immunology. *J Infect Dis* 2017;215(9):1366–1375.
34. Lewis FM, Bernstein KT, Aral SO. Vaginal microbiome and its relationship to behavior, sexual health, and sexually transmitted diseases. *Obstet Gynecol* 2017;129(4):643–654.
35. Martin DH, Marrazzo JM. The vaginal microbiome: current understanding and future directions. *J Infect Dis* 2016;214(Suppl 1):S36–S41.
36. Anderson DJ, Marathe J, Pudney J. The structure of the human vaginal stratum corneum and its role in immune defense. *Am J Reprod Immunol* 2014;71(6):618–623.
37. Burgos MH, de Vargas-Linares R. Ultrastructure of the vaginal mucosa. In: Hafez ESE, Evans TN, eds. *The Human Vagina*. Amsterdam: Elsevier/North-Holland Biomedical Press; 1978:63–93.
38. Love RR, Kurtycz DF, Dumesic DA, et al. The effects of tamoxifen on the vaginal epithelium in postmenopausal women. *J Womens Health Gend Based Med* 2000;9(5):559–563.
39. Eschenbach DA, Thwin SS, Patton DL, et al. Influence of the normal menstrual cycle on vaginal tissue, discharge, and microflora. *Clin Infect Dis* 2000;30(6):901–907.
40. Linhartova A. Extent of columnar epithelium on the ectocervix between the ages of 1 and 13 years. *Obstet Gynecol* 1978;52(4):451–456.
41. Karam JA, Vazquez DV, Lin VK, et al. Elastin expression and elastic fibre width in the anterior vaginal wall of postmenopausal women with and without prolapse. *BJU Int* 2007;100(2):346–350.
42. Sridharan I, Ma Y, Kim T, et al. Structural and mechanical profiles of native collagen fibers in vaginal wall connective tissues. *Biomaterials* 2012;33(5):1520–1527.
43. Kerkhof MH, Ruiz-Zapata AM, Bril H, et al. Changes in tissue composition of the vaginal wall of premenopausal women with prolapse. *Am J Obstet Gynecol* 2014;210(2):168.e1–168.e9.
44. Ruiz-Zapata AM, Kerkhof MH, Zandieh-Doulabi B, et al. Fibroblasts from women with pelvic organ prolapse show differential mechanoresponses depending on surface substrates. *Int Urogynecol J* 2013;24(9):1567–1575.
45. Meijerink AM, van Rijssel RH, van der Linden PJ. Tissue composition of the vaginal wall in women with pelvic organ prolapse. *Gynecol Obstet Invest* 2013;75(1):21–27.
46. De Landsheere L, Munaut C, Nusgens B, et al. Histology of the vaginal wall in women with pelvic organ prolapse: A literature review. *Int Urogynecol J* 2013;24(12):2011–2020.
47. Ferenczy A, Richart RM. *Female Reproductive System: Dynamics of Scan and Transmission Electron Microscopy*. New York: John Wiley; 1974.
48. Klumpp DJ, Forrestal SG, Karr JE, et al. Epithelial differentiation promotes the adherence of type 1-piliated Escherichia coli to human vaginal cells. *J Infect Dis* 2002;186(11):1631–1638.
49. Macneill C, de Guzman G, Sousa GE, et al. Cyclic changes in the level of the innate immune molecule, surfactant protein-a, and cytokines in vaginal fluid. *Am J Reprod Immunol* 2012;68(3):244–250.
50. Wira CR, Grant-Tschudy KS, Crane-Godreau MA. Epithelial cells in the female reproductive tract: A central role as sentinels of immune protection. *Am J Reprod Immunol* 2005;53(2):65–76.

51. Wira CR, Fahey JV. The innate immune system: gatekeeper to the female reproductive tract. *Immunology* 2004;111(1):13–15.
52. Ferry JA, Scully RE. Mesonephric remnants, hyperplasia, and neoplasia in the uterine cervix. A study of 49 cases. *Am J Surg Pathol* 1990;14(12):1100–1111.
53. Ferry JA, Scully RE. Carcinoma in mesonephric remnants. *Am J Surg Pathol* 1995;19(10):1218–1219.
54. Howitt BE, Emori MM, Drapkin R, et al. GATA3 Is a sensitive and specific marker of benign and malignant mesonephric lesions in the lower female genital tract. *Am J Surg Pathol* 2015;39(10):1411–1419.
55. Kelly P, McBride HA, Kennedy K, et al. Misplaced Skene's glands: Glandular elements in the lower female genital tract that are variably immunoreactive with prostate markers and that encompass vaginal tubulosquamous polyp and cervical ectopic prostatic tissue. *Int J Gynecol Pathol* 2011;30(6):605–612.
56. Kazakov DV, Stewart CJ, Kacerovska D, et al. Prostatic-type tissue in the lower female genital tract: A morphologic spectrum, including vaginal tubulosquamous polyp, adenomyomatous hyperplasia of paraurethral Skene glands (female prostate), and ectopic lesion in the vulva. *Am J Surg Pathol* 2010;34(7):950–955.
57. McCluggage WG, Ganesan R, Hirschowitz L, et al. Ectopic prostatic tissue in the uterine cervix and vagina: Report of a series with a detailed immunohistochemical analysis. *Am J Surg Pathol* 2006;30(2):209–215.
58. Heller DS. Lesions of Skene glands and periurethral region: A review. *J Low Genit Tract Dis* 2015;19(2):170–174.
59. Pongtippan A, Malpica A, Levenback C, et al. Skene's gland adenocarcinoma resembling prostatic adenocarcinoma. *Int J Gynecol Pathol* 2004;23(1):71–74.
60. Jannini EA, Buisson O, Rubio-Casillas A. Beyond the G-spot: Clitourethrovaginal complex anatomy in female orgasm. *Nat Rev Urol* 2014;11(9):531–538.
61. Ostrzenski A, Krajewski P, Ganjei-Azar P, et al. Verification of the anatomy and newly discovered histology of the G-spot complex. *BJOG* 2014;121(11):1333–1339.
62. Ostrzenski A. G-spot anatomy: A new discovery. *J Sex Med* 2012;9(5):1355–1359.
63. Kilchevsky A, Vardi Y, Lowenstein L, et al. Is the female G-spot truly a distinct anatomic entity? *J Sex Med* 2012;9(3):719–726.
64. Troisi R, Hatch EE, Titus L, et al. Prenatal diethylstilbestrol exposure and cancer risk in women. *Environ Mol Mutagen* 2017. https://www.ncbi.nlm.nih.gov/pubmed/?term=Troisi+R%2C+Hatch+EE%2C+Titus+L%2C+et+al.+Prenatal+diethylstilbestrol+exposure+and+cancer+risk+in+women.+Environ+Mol+Mutagen+2017.
65. Hoover RN, Hyer M, Pfeiffer RM, et al. Adverse health outcomes in women exposed in utero to diethylstilbestrol. *N Engl J Med* 2011;365(14):1304–1314.
66. Kurita T. Normal and abnormal epithelial differentiation in the female reproductive tract. *Differentiation* 2011;82(3):117–126.
67. Cunha GR, Kurita T, Cao M, et al. Response of xenografts of developing human female reproductive tracts to the synthetic estrogen, diethylstilbestrol. *Differentiation*. 2017;98:35–54.
68. Laronda MM, Unno K, Butler LM, et al. The development of cervical and vaginal adenosis as a result of diethylstilbestrol exposure in utero. *Differentiation* 2012;84(3):252–260.
69. Robboy SJ, Kaufman RH, Prat J, et al. Pathologic findings in young women enrolled in the National Cooperative Diethylstilbestrol Adenosis (DESAD) project. *Obstet Gynecol* 1979;53(3):309–317.
70. Robboy SJ, Young RH, Welch WR, et al. Atypical vaginal adenosis and cervical ectropion. Association with clear cell adenocarcinoma in diethylstilbestrol-exposed offspring. *Cancer* 1984;54(5):869–875.
71. Robboy SJ, Welch WR, Young RH, et al. Topographic relation of cervical ectropion and vaginal adenosis to clear cell adenocarcinoma. *Obstet Gynecol* 1982;60(5):546–551.

Normal Histology of the Uterus and Fallopian Tubes

Kristen A. Atkins

EMBRYOLOGY 1059

THE INDIFFERENT STAGE 1059
   Female Differentiation 1060

GROSS ANATOMY 1060
   Premenarchal Uterus and Fallopian Tubes 1060
   Adult Uterus and Fallopian Tubes 1061
   Gross Anatomic Features of the Uterus 1061
   Gross Anatomic Features of the Fallopian Tubes 1063
   Uterine and Tubal Vasculature 1063
   Uterine and Tubal Lymphatics 1064

UTERINE CERVIX 1064
   Epithelium of the Exocervix 1065
   Epithelium of the Endocervix 1066
   Epithelium of the Transformation Zone 1069
   Cervical Stroma 1073
   Cervix During Pregnancy 1073

ENDOMETRIUM 1076
   Tissue Sampling and Associated Problems 1076
   Histology of the Normal Endometrium 1076
   Relevance of Endometrial Dating to Diagnostic Surgical Pathologists 1091
   Endometrial–Myometrial Junction 1092
   Apoptosis and the Endometrium 1093

MYOMETRIUM 1093
   Pregnancy-Related Changes 1093

THE FALLOPIAN TUBE 1095
   Histology of the Fallopian Tube 1095
   Fallopian Tube in Pregnancy 1099
   Paraovarian and Paratubal Structures 1099

REFERENCES 1099

EMBRYOLOGY

The fallopian tube and the uterus, together with the ovarian surface epithelium, comprise what has been termed the extended müllerian system (1,2), which gives rise to a common set of neoplasms and non-neoplastic metaplastic epithelial changes.

The uterus and fallopian tubes have a complex developmental sequence (3–11). Both male and female internal genitalia are laid down early in each embryo known as the indifferent stage of genital development. Upon completion of this indifferent stage, definitive female differentiation is accompanied by regression of the male anlage, whereas male differentiation is accompanied by regression of the female anlage. Topographically, both of these systems are intimately related to the developing urinary tract, and, not surprisingly, anomalous development of the internal genitalia is often accompanied by anomalies of the urinary tract.

Fetal sexual differentiation is completed during the first half of gestation; the last half is marked primarily by growth of the newly established genitalia. Relevant milestones have been summarized by Ramsey (Fig. 40.1) (12).

THE INDIFFERENT STAGE

By the 6th week of fetal life the urogenital sinus and the mesonephric (wolffian) ducts are well established. At this time the paired müllerian (paramesonephric) ducts begin their development. These structures are formed by an invagination of the celomic epithelium adjacent to that investing each developing ovary. The müllerian ducts are intimately related to the mesonephric ducts, and their normal formation appears to be dependent on the presence of the mesonephros.

As the müllerian ducts grow caudally, they approach the midline where the distal portions fuse. Shortly after

AGE	GLANDS	URINARY TRACT	♂ DUCTS ♀		EXTERNAL GENITALIA
3-4 weeks	PRIMORDIAL GERM CELLS	PRONEPHROS (nonfunctional) Tubules and Ducts	PRONEPHRIC		
4-9 weeks		MESONEPHROS or WOLFFIAN BODY (temporary function) Tubules and Ducts	MESONEPHRIC or WOLFFIAN		CLOACA
5th week	UROGENITAL RIDGE				
6th week	INDIFFERENT GONAD: GERMINAL AND CORE EPITHELIUM	METANEPHROS or KIDNEY (permanent) Tubules and Ducts	PARAMESONEPHRIC or MÜLLERIAN		CLOACA SUBDIVIDES GENITAL TUBERCLE
7th week	MALE TYPE CORDS				ANAL AND URETHRAL MEMBRANES RUPTURE
8th week	TESTIS AND OVARY				URETHRAL AND LABIOSCROTAL FOLDS, PHALLUS AND GLANS
9th week			MÜLLERIAN DUCTS FUSE AT TUBERCLE		
10th week			MÜLLERIAN DUCTS DEGENERATE	WOLFFIAN DUCTS DEGENERATE	
11th week			SEMINAL VESICLES, EPIDIDYMIS, VAS DEFERENS		
12th week	OVARY DESCENT COMPLETE			WALLS FORM	SEX DISTINGUISHABLE
5 months	TESTIS AT INGUINAL RING			SINUS EPITHELIUM GROWS IN VAGINAL CLEFT	
8 months / TERM	TESTIS DESCENT COMPLETE			RAPID UTERINE GROWTH	

FIGURE 40.1 Chart showing interrelations and time sequence of events in development of genitourinary system. From Ramsey E. Embryology and developmental defects of the female reproductive tract. In: Danforth D, Scott J, eds. *Obstetrics and Gynecology.* New York: JB Lippincott; 1986:106–119.

this fusion, the apposed medial duct walls disappear, bringing the two lumina into continuity to form a single cavity. Further downward growth of the fused müllerian structures (now termed the uterovaginal primordium) brings them into contact with the urogenital sinus. At this stage the fetus has both the mesonephric ducts and the müllerian ducts.

Female Differentiation

The differentiation of the indifferent internal genitalia into male or female structures depends on whether the fetus possesses ovaries or testes. In the male fetus, the Leydig cells and the Sertoli cells in the developing testes secrete testosterone and a nonsteroidal müllerian inhibiting substance, respectively (13). The net effect of this secretory activity is to ensure the persistence, differentiation, and growth of the mesonephric ducts to form the male genital system and the regression of the müllerian system. In the absence of a secreting testis (e.g., in a normal female fetus with ovaries or in a fetus with nonfunctioning gonads) the müllerian structures persist, whereas the mesonephric ducts regress. The nonfused portions of the müllerian ducts form the fallopian tubes; the fused segments develop into the uterus and probably the upper third of the vagina. Incomplete fusion of the caudal portion of the müllerian ducts results in a spectrum of uterovaginal abnormalities (14).

By the 21st week, the uterus and vagina are well formed. In contrast to the adult cervix, the cervix of the prenatal uterus is disproportionately large and makes up two-thirds of the length of the organ. The second half of gestation is marked by uterine growth; from the 28th week to birth, the fetal uterus doubles in size. However, the earlier cervicocorpus disproportion is maintained into childhood.

The events described above are driven, at least in part, by the expression of secreted ligands of the wingless (*WNT*) gene family and transcriptional regulators of the homeobox (*HOX*) gene family (13,15).

GROSS ANATOMY

Premenarchal Uterus and Fallopian Tubes

Neonatal Period

At birth the uterus averages about 4 cm in length, and its bulk and shape are dominated by its disproportionately large cervix (the cervicofundal ratio is approximately 3 to 5:1). The maternal hormonal environment results in a markedly thickened rugal vaginal mucosa and a proliferative or weakly secretory endometrium. Maternal estrogen also results in cervical squamous cell maturation with glycogen storage. These mucosal changes regress shortly after birth (16–18).

Infancy

Uterine growth continues into the second year of life, at which time it reaches a plateau that persists until the premenarchal growth spurt at about 9 years of age. Until approximately the 13th year, the cervix continues to account for greater than half of the uterine length.

Adult Uterus and Fallopian Tubes

General Relations and Attachments

The uterus is anterior to the rectum and posterior to the bladder (Fig. 40.2). It is covered anteriorly and posteriorly by a reflection of pelvic peritoneum that continues laterally to form the anterior and posterior leaves of the broad ligament. The posterior peritoneal reflection forms the uterine wall of the pouch of Douglas and covers a longer segment of the uterine isthmus than does the anterior peritoneal reflection. The tentlike broad ligaments house the major uterine vessels, the efferent lymphatic trunks, and the apical portions of the fallopian tubes. Each ovary is attached to the ipsilateral uterine cornu by the utero-ovarian ligament, which is situated posterolateral and inferior to the uterine attachment of the fallopian tubes. The round ligaments arise anterolateral and inferior to the attachment of the fallopian tubes and pass anteriorly to insert into the canal of Nuck. These anatomic relations enable proper orientation of the hysterectomy specimen. The anterior surface of the uterus is distinguished by its longer "bare" region (i.e., lacking peritoneum) and the anteriorly directed stump of the round ligament. The posterior surface is more extensively covered by peritoneum, and the utero-ovarian ligament is attached to the posterior cornual aspect of the uterus. The uterus is anchored to its surroundings by a number of connective tissue bands; notable among them are the cardinal, uterosacral, and pubocervical ligaments (11,18–20).

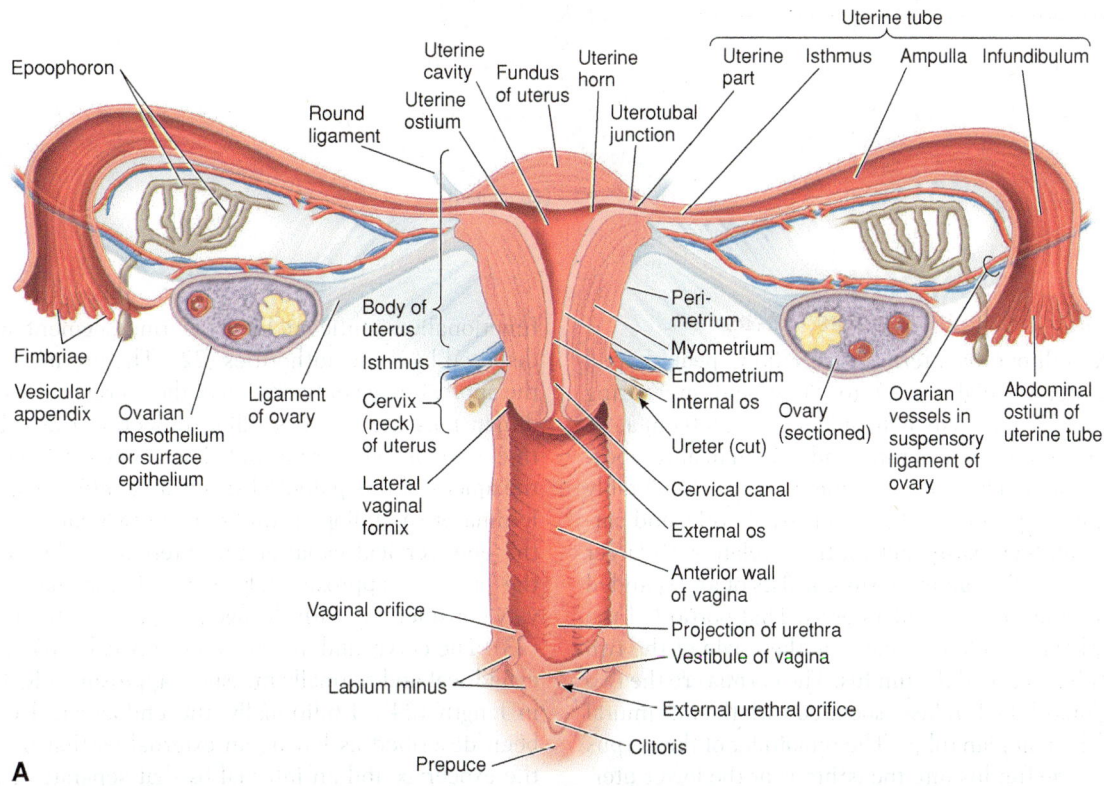

FIGURE 40.2 The normal internal female genitalia showing their relationship to other pelvic structures (**A**) and in cross section (**B**). **A**—Reprinted with permission from Dudek RW, Louis TM. *High-Yield Gross Anatomy*. Philadelphia, PA: Wolters Kluwer Health; 2015. **B**—Reprinted with permission from *Female Reproductive System Anatomical Chart*. Philadelphia, PA: Wolters Kluwer Health; 2000. (*continued*)

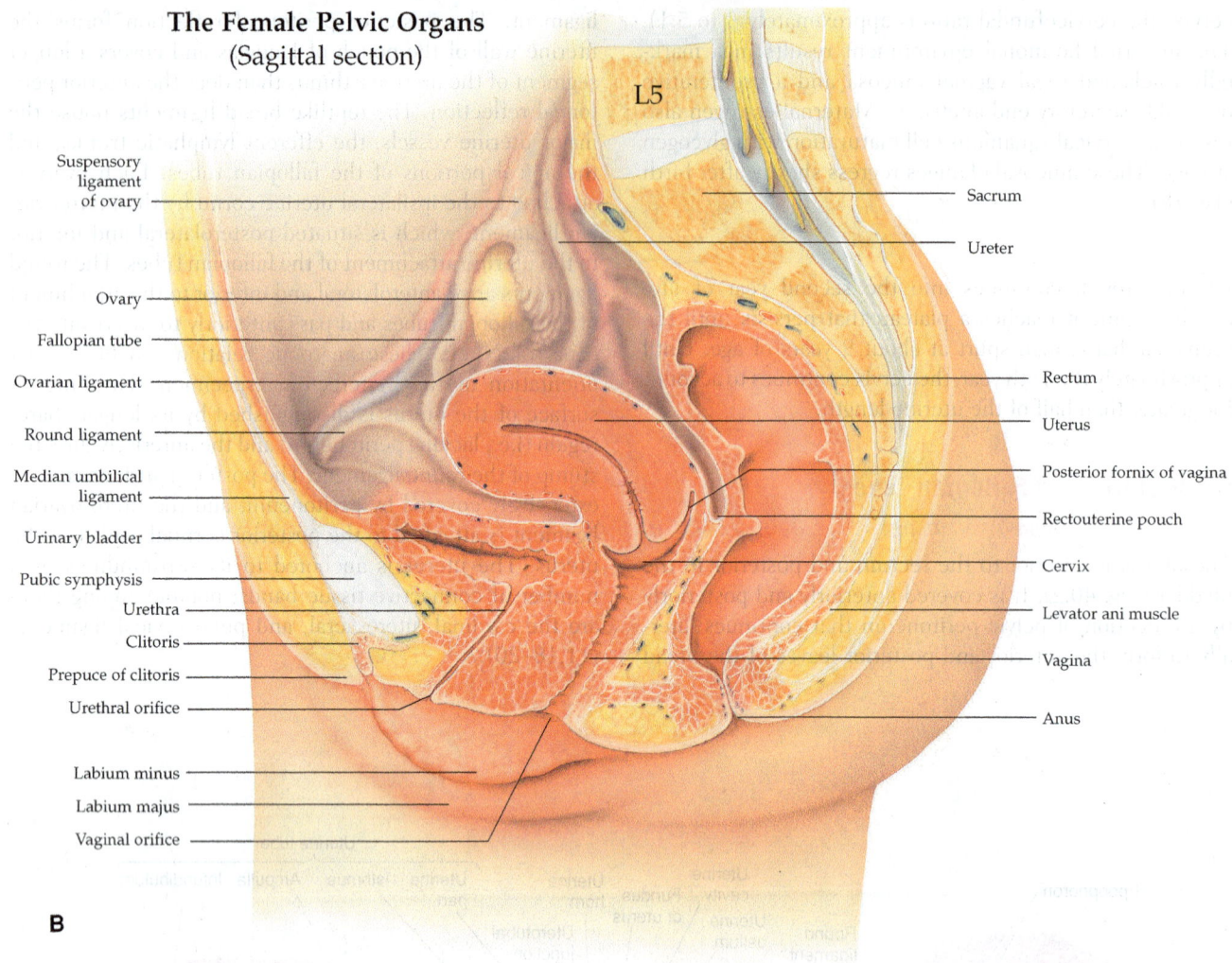

FIGURE 40.2 (Continued)

Gross Anatomic Features of the Uterus

The adult nulliparous uterus is a hollow, pear-shaped muscular organ weighing 40 to 80 g and measuring approximately 7.0 to 8 cm along its long axis, 5.0 cm at its broadest extent (cornu to cornu), and 2.5 cm in anteroposterior dimension. These measurements vary considerably as a function of age, phase of the menstrual cycle, and parity. In general, high parity and youth correlate with larger uterine size (21). The adult uterus consists of an expanded body, the corpus, and a smaller cervix. That portion of the corpus cephalad to a line connecting the origin of the two fallopian tubes is called the fundus. The cornua are the two lateral regions of the fundus associated with the intramural portion of the fallopian tubes. The remainder of the corpus tapers from the fundus into the isthmus or the lower uterine segment, which shares histologic features with both of the uterine segments that it bridges: the uterine corpus and the endocervix. The existence of an anatomically and functionally significant lower uterine segment has been disputed by some authorities (22). The uterine cavity has the approximate configuration of the uterus, but its internal dimensions are much smaller, reflecting the substantial thickness of the uterine wall. The cavity is triangular, and the apices of this potential space are continuous, with the lumina of the fallopian tubes at the two cornua and with the endocervical canal at the internal os. The length of the cavity is approximately 6 cm. These measurements vary considerably with the age and parity of the individual (23). The cervix and internal endocervical canal is roughly cylindrical and normally measures approximately 3 to 4 cm in length (24). Traditionally, the endocervical canal has been described as having an external os that opens onto the exocervix and an internal os that separates the endocervical canal from the endometrial cavity. Although the former is a reasonable anatomic landmark, the latter is not because grossly, the transition from endometrial cavity to endocervix is gradual. This is histologically mirrored by the gradual transition of the mucosa in this region from endocervical type to endometrial type. The mucosal surface of the endocervical canal is deeply clefted to form the plicae palmatae. The parametria are the lateral connective tissue attachments of the uterus, which contain vessels, nerves, lymphatics, and lymph nodes.

The normal myometrium consists of two strata: an outer longitudinal muscle layer covering the fundus and an inner circular submucosal muscle layer extending to surround the internal os and the tubal ostia. There is an interposed thick middle layer, richly populated by vessels and composed of randomly interdigitating fibers (25). The magnetic resonance imaging (MRI) correlate of these layers is the outer zone and the submucosal low intensity halo "junctional zone" (26,27). Functionally, the junctional zone appears to be more involved with menstruation while the outer zone assumes a prominent role in gestation and parturition.

Toth has described two lateral subserosally situated longitudinal bands of distinctive muscle fibers, the fasciculus cervicoangularis (28,29). On occasion, epithelium that is immunohistochemically and histologically similar to cervical mesonephric remnants is present within this bundle, suggesting that these structures represent the vestiges of the wolffian (mesonephric) duct which is more commonly encountered in the cervical stroma ("mesonephric rests") and lateral vagina (Gardner duct and derivative cysts).

Substantial deviations from the nulliparous adult uterus naturally occur throughout adult life. The uterus undergoes small-amplitude changes in size during the menstrual cycle, attaining its greatest volume during the secretory phase (27). During pregnancy, of course, the uterus enlarges much more dramatically to accommodate the growing conceptus. This growth is due largely to myocyte hypertrophy and hyperplasia, an increase in uterine vasculature and in extracellular matrix; the net weight increases 10-fold during pregnancy. After delivery, uterine size rapidly decreases, and over the ensuing weeks a striking resorption of connective tissue occurs that is associated with a decrease in the size of individual myocytes (30). However, the uterus generally does not return completely to its nulliparous size and weight. Prior pregnancy (parity) can be deduced from several gross features. The multiparous nongravid uterus tends to weigh more in consequence of its thicker and more prominently layered muscular walls; this increase in weight is proportional to the patient's parity (21). The vasculature of the multiparous uterus tends to be more prominent. The most suggestive changes of previous pregnancy, however, are seen in the cervix. The nulliparous circular small external os is transformed after pregnancy into a slit that forms prominent anterior and posterior lips. In addition, healed cervical lacerations may be pronounced, and enough endocervical tissue may reside on the exocervix to give it a red granular appearance near the os. With the waning of ovarian hormone synthesis during the menopausal years, the uterus involutes and atrophies. This is reflected by a decrease in its weight and its dimensions. On occasion the endocervical canal is almost completely obliterated. Exogenous estrogens administered during this period sometimes maintain uterine weight artificially despite the loss of ovarian hormonal support.

Gross Anatomic Features of the Fallopian Tubes

The fallopian tubes are hollow epithelium-lined muscular structures 11 to 12 cm in length that run through the apex of the broad ligament to span the uterine cornu medially and the ovary laterally. Each tube is divided into four anatomic segments. The intramural segment begins at the funnel-like uppermost recess of the uterine cornu and ends where the tube emerges from the uterine wall. The course of this 8-mm, pinpoint lumened segment varies from straight to highly convoluted (31). Beyond the uterine wall the proximal tube continues for 2 to 3 cm as the isthmus, a thick-walled, narrow-calibered segment that merges into a comparatively thin-walled expanded area, the ampulla. The distal tube ends in the trumpet-shaped infundibulum whose mouth opens into the peritoneal cavity and is fringed by approximately 25 fimbria. One of these, the ovarian fimbrium, attaches to the ovary. At the time of ovulation the infundibulum forms a cap over the ovarian surface to create the ovarian bursa. The tubal mucosa and the underlying endosalpingeal stroma are thrown up into longitudinal, branching folds (the plicae) whose branches increase in complexity from the isthmus to the infundibulum. The plicae terminate in the fimbria. At the time of ovulation the fimbria sweep over the surface of the ovary to facilitate egg capture (13,32–35).

Uterine and Tubal Vasculature

The major arterial supply of the uterus derives from the right and left uterine arteries, which arise from the corresponding hypogastric (internal iliac) arteries. The uterine artery divides into ascending and descending branches laterally at the level of the uterine isthmus. The ascending uterine artery anastomoses freely with the ovarian artery (a branch of the aorta) in the mesosalpinx, whereas the descending branch anastomoses with the vaginal arterial supply. Both the ascending and descending uterine arteries give rise to a complex network of circumferentially arranged subserosal arteries: the arcuate arteries. These in turn give rise to a series of radial arteries that penetrate the myometrium. Each of these radial vessels branches, in the inner third of the myometrium, into straight arteries (supplying the basalis) and spiral

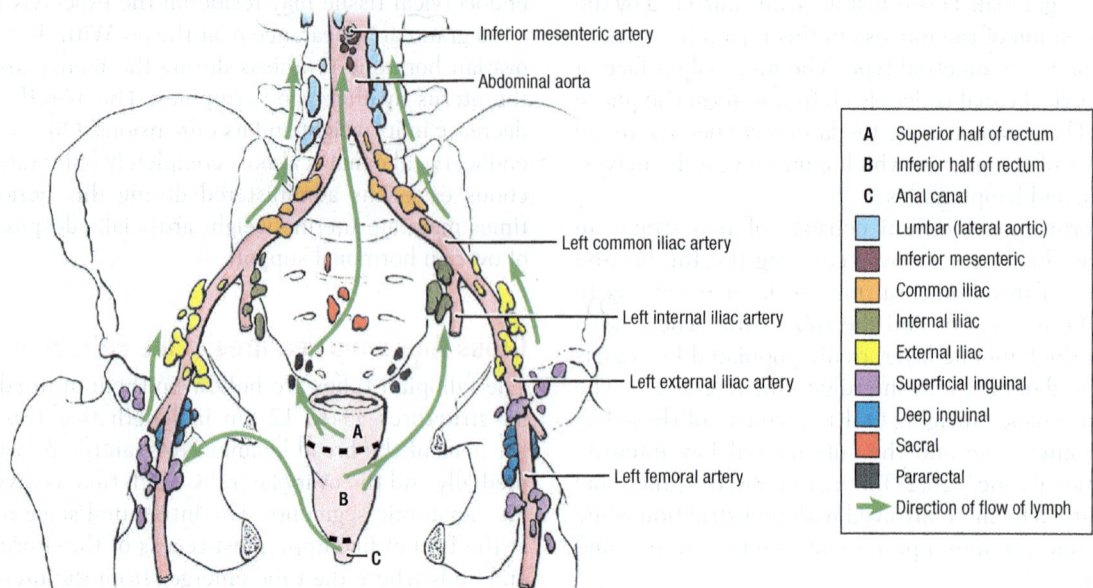

FIGURE 40.3 Lymphatic flow for the pelvis. *Green arrows* show the direction of lymphatic flow. This can be helpful in directing the pathologists to the most likely involved lymph nodes (and possible sentinel lymph nodes) by metastatic carcinoma depending on the location of the tumor. From Aqur A, Dalley A. *Grant's Atlas of Anatomy* 12th ed. Philadelphia, PA: Lippincott Williams and Wilkins; 2009:244.

arteries that become the spiral arteries of the endometrium (36–38).

A striking characteristic of the adult intramyometrial uterine arteries is their marked tortuosity. This doubtless has to do with the variation in uterine size during reproductive life. In the postmenopausal years, striking degenerative changes may be seen in the uterine arteries, including intimal proliferation, fibrosis, and medial calcification. The severity of these changes is typically out of proportion to degenerative changes in nonuterine arteries. The venous drainage of the uterus parallels its arterial supply.

Uterine and Tubal Lymphatics

Lymphatics are present in both the cervix and the corpus. In the endometrium these vessels are intimately associated with the glands of the functionalis. The myometrium and cervical stroma contain a complex labyrinth of lymphatics that course toward the subserosal plexus. The channels forming the latter ramify over the entire surface of the uterus, and the confluence of these channels forms the major efferent lymphatic trunks of the uterus. The chief interest in lymphatic drainage for the pathologist is as a guide to the dissemination of carcinoma. The major lymph node groups draining cervical and endometrial carcinoma are indicated in Figure 40.3.

In both the mucosal and muscular layers, lymphatic anastomoses exist between the cervical and corpus systems, and on occasion cervical carcinomas may take advantage of this route to spread to the corpus. Whether the converse is true is unclear. Moreover, whether or not corpus carcinoma, once having invaded the cervix, then behaves like cervical carcinoma in terms of its lymphatic metastatic distribution is also unclear, even though this is a common clinical assumption. Indeed, involvement of "cervical draining nodes" by endometrial carcinoma does not necessarily imply cervical involvement. For further detail the reader is referred to specialty works and textbooks of gynecologic oncology (39–41).

Tubal lymphatics accompany the ovarian vessels and drain into nodes near the right and left renal veins and the presacral and common iliac nodes. Lymphatic spread of tubal malignancy may reach extrapelvic sites early in its dissemination (42,43).

UTERINE CERVIX

The uterine cervix or "neck" is the elongate fibromuscular portion of the uterus that measures 2.5 to 3.0 cm. A part of this structure protrudes into the upper part of the vagina (vaginal part, portio vaginalis), whereas the remainder lies above the vaginal vault (supravaginal portion). The outer surface of the vaginal portion of the cervix is known variously as the ectocervix or exocervix. It is covered, at least in part, by stratified squamous epithelium that is continuous with, and histologically identical to, the mucosa of the vaginal fornices. That portion of the cervix in relation to the endocervical canal is known as the anatomic endocervix. The endocervical canal, lined for the most part by mucin-secreting epithelium that blends at one end with the squamous epithelium of the exocervix and with the epithelium of the lower uterine segment at its other end, brings the vagina into communication with the endometrial cavity. The anatomic opening of the endocervical canal onto the exocervix is known as the external os. In parous women, this most often takes on a slitlike configuration that serves to divide the exocervix into anterior and posterior lips (18,44). This particular geometry is thought to be important in uterine function during gestation (45). The upper limit of the endocervical canal is known as the internal os. This is not a distinct orifice; rather, there is a gradual funnel-shaped widening of the endocervical canal and a transition from endocervical epithelium into the endometrial epithelium of the lower uterine segment. The junction of the endocervical glandular mucosa with the squamous epithelium of the exocervix is known as the squamocolumnar junction. This junction does not always lie at the external os; in fact, the squamocolumnar junction typically is located on the exocervix, where it can easily be inspected with the culposcope. This is further discussed in the section devoted to the transformation zone.

The uterine cervix obviously plays an important role in the anatomic support of the internal genitalia and plays an active role in labor and delivery, but arguably its primary role is the production of cervical mucous. Cervical mucous acts as a functional gate that prevents vaginal microorganisms from gaining access to the upper genital tract and (except for a small mid-cycle window before ovulation) denies sperm access to the uterus and fallopian tubes. At mid-cycle the chemical composition of the cervical mucous changes and its viscosity decreases. This has the effect of allowing the passage of sperm into the upper genital tract. These changes are the basis of the Spinnbarkeit and fern tests. In addition, the cervical mucous plays an important role in removing seminal plasma constituents (preventing sperm phagocytosis) and in providing a suitable environment for sperm storage, capacitation, and migration (46,47).

The following discussion first focuses on the epithelium of the exocervix, the endocervix, and the transformation zone and then turns to the stroma of the cervix and the changes that occur in the cervix during pregnancy.

Epithelium of the Exocervix

The squamous epithelium covering the exocervix is normally noncornified, and it grows, matures, and accumulates glycogen in its upper layers in response to circulating estrogens, most notably estradiol (Fig. 40.4). Because low blood levels of estrogen are the rule during childhood and the postmenopausal years, the squamous cells of the cervix do not proliferate or mature, and glycogen is not stored in the upper layers of the epithelium during these periods unless estrogen is made available as a result of therapy or functioning ovarian tumors (18). In the immediate postnatal period, the squamous epithelium of the newborn cervix is fully mature due to maternal estrogen, but the epithelium quickly becomes atrophic and glycogen disappears as estrogen levels decrease.

The estrogenically stimulated cervical squamous epithelium of the sexually mature woman can be divided into three layers: the basal/parabasal cell layer, the midzone layer (or stratum spongiosum), and the superficial layer (Fig. 40.4). The basal cell layer is composed of cells with scant cytoplasm and oval to cuboidal nuclei with dense chromatin. These cells are usually mitotically inactive and do not mark immunohistochemically with proliferation markers (e.g., Ki-67 and PCNA [proliferating cell nuclear antigen]) (48). The cells immediately above the basal layer comprise the lower portion of the midzone layer and are known as parabasal cells, a term often used in cytopathology. The parabasal cells are somewhat larger than the basal cells due to their increased cytoplasm, and the nuclei have slightly less dense chromatin. In contrast to the basal layer, mitotic figures are usually present but are not abnormal or particularly numerous in the normal epithelium. This layer also displays proliferation markers (48). The midzone layer is composed of cells with even more abundant cytoplasm and somewhat smaller vesicular nuclei. These are known as intermediate cells. Glycogen accumulates in most intermediate cells, and this imparts a finely granular or clear appearance to the cytoplasm. The superficial cells contain small, rounded, regular pyknotic nuclei, and their cytoplasm is abundant and clear as a result of even greater glycogen accumulation.

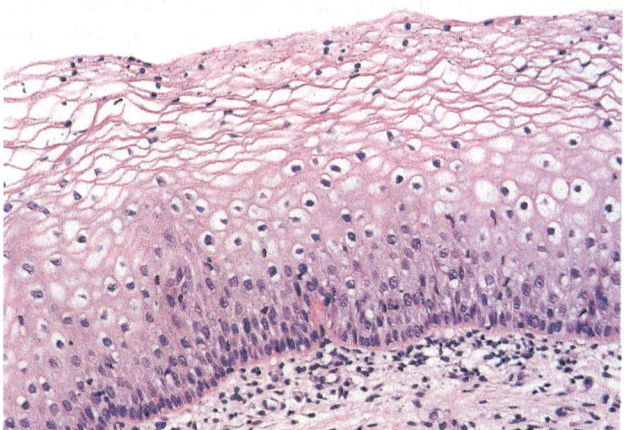

FIGURE 40.4 Mature squamous epithelium of the exocervix demonstrating a normal maturation sequence from basal cells to superficial cells. The cleared cytoplasm indicating glycogen storage should not be confused with koilocytosis.

Keratinization occurs in both the superficial and intermediate cells and renders them flat and platelike when they are spread on a slide. The cytoplasmic clearing characteristic of normal intermediate and superficial cells is often perinuclear. Because perinuclear clearing is also a feature of cells (koilocytes) infected by human papillomavirus (HPV), there is a potential for misinterpreting normal epithelial cells containing glycogen as abnormal. Nuclear abnormalities such as nuclear enlargement and membrane irregularity must be seen in order to qualify as a koilocyte (sometimes referred to as raisinoid). In contrast to the homogenous chromatin appearance in normal squamous cells the chromatin of koilocytes has a ropy texture. The cervical squamous mucosa undergoes cyclic changes during the menstrual cycle similar to the estrogen–progesterone-induced changes in the vaginal mucosa, although the cells composing the latter are a more reliable index of hormonal status. During the luteal phase and pregnancy, when progesterone levels are high, there is a predominance of intermediate cells.

The exocervical epithelium in postmenopausal women (not receiving a supplement of estrogen therapy) is composed mainly of basal and parabasal cells that feature scant cytoplasm and little or no cytoplasmic glycogen (Fig 40.5). The cells may have the same degree of nucleus-to-cytoplasm ratio shift toward the nucleus as do the cells composing cervical squamous intraepithelial lesions (SIL). Consequently, atrophic epithelium is a part of the differential diagnosis of a high-grade squamous intraepithelial lesion (HSIL), and care should be taken when a diagnosis of HSIL is contemplated in a postmenopausal woman. However, the basal and parabasal cells in atrophic epithelia do not demonstrate the nuclear abnormalities and high mitotic index usually seen in the cells constituting the neoplastic epithelium in HSIL. Immunohistochemistry for p16 can be helpful in problematic cases as HSIL will typically be positive for p16 and atrophy will be negative (49). In addition, in situ hybridization for high-risk HPV can be used for direct visualization of HPV, which will be present in HSIL and absent in atrophy (50).

Endocrine cells have been identified in the squamous epithelium of the exocervix by immunohistochemical techniques; their function is unknown, but they are thought to give rise to the rare cervical carcinoid tumors (49–56). Langerhans cells also are present in the ectocervical epithelium, as well as in the transformation zone (57–60). They are involved in antigen presentation to T lymphocytes. Melanin-containing cells have been reported in the cervical epithelium and provide a plausible cell of origin for the uncommon cervical melanoma and blue nevus (61).

Epithelium of the Endocervix

The anatomic endocervix extends from the external os to the internal os, but endocervical glandular epithelium is not exclusively limited to this anatomic area, particularly during the reproductive years. Rather, endocervical epithelium occupies significant regions of the anatomic exocervix during childhood and after the menarche. The shift of the endocervical epithelium out of the canal onto the exocervix is discussed in more detail below in the section devoted to the transformation zone.

The endocervix is lined by a single layer of mucin-secreting epithelium composed of cells with small, often basilar, nuclei above which is mucin-filled cytoplasm which imparts a "picket fence" appearance (Fig. 40.6). Goblet cells are sometimes encountered (Fig. 40.7). The nuclei are generally small and elongate with dense chromatin. When the endocervical epithelium has been damaged and is regenerating, the nuclei may become larger and more rounded, but mitotic figures are difficult to find in non-neoplastic endocervical cells (62). If mitotic figures are easily found in endocervical cells, consideration should be given to well-differentiated adenocarcinoma or carcinoma in situ, particularly if the nuclei are enlarged and nucleoli are prominent.

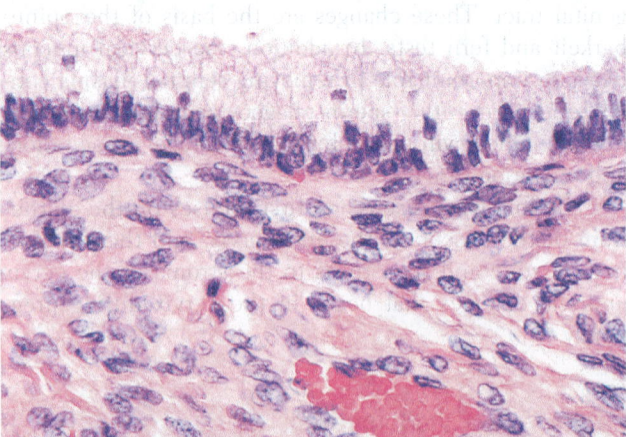

FIGURE 40.6 Normal endocervical mucosa with most nuclei in the characteristic basilar location. Enlargement of these nuclei and loss of apical mucin are features that should cause a closer inspection of the endocervical glands to ensure that neoplastic transformation is not present.

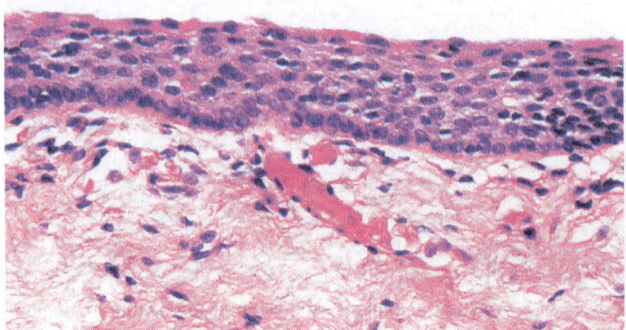

FIGURE 40.5 Postmenopausal atrophy of the cervical squamous epithelium. The immature cells can resemble the cells in high-grade SIL (CIN).

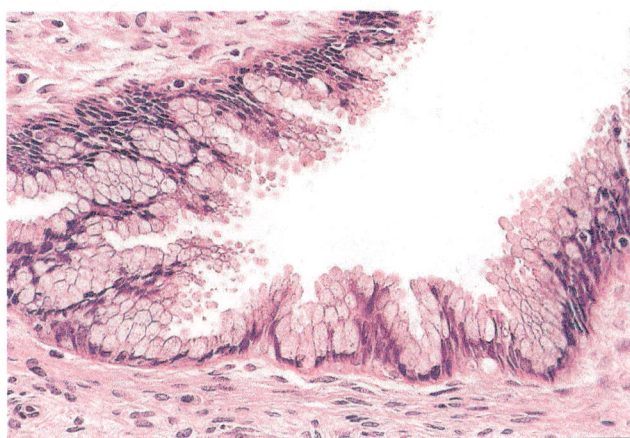

FIGURE 40.7 Goblet cells in the endocervix. Not infrequently, the nuclei of mucin-containing cells are displaced to the base of the cell and compressed by cytoplasmic mucin to produce a goblet cell. The presence of goblet cells and neuroendocrine cells in the normal endocervical mucosa tends to destabilize the conventional distinction in ovarian pathology between müllerian (i.e., cervical) mucinous and intestinal mucinous differentiation.

Nucleoli are inconspicuous in resting endocervical cells, but they may become prominent during regeneration, pregnancy, and neoplastic transformation. Mitotic figures may be found in the constituent glandular cells of cervical endometriosis.

Other types of cells may be identified in the endocervical epithelium. Ciliated cells are almost always present and can be a useful marker of a benign process when the appearance of the endocervical glandular epithelium raises concerns about well-differentiated adenocarcinoma (63). When ciliated cells are numerous, the term "ciliary (or tubal) metaplasia" is often used (Fig 40.8A to C) (62–68). Ciliated cells themselves can develop enlarged dense nuclei and thus come to resemble neoplastic cells. As a result, care should be taken to look for cilia before diagnosing in situ neoplastic transformation of the endocervix. Immunohistochemistry may be of aid in this distinction; Marques et al. found a combination of vimentin and CEA helpful: Adenocarcinoma in situ tended to be CEA positive and vimentin negative while the opposite was true for tubal metaplasia (69). In addition, since the majority of AIS is secondary to HPV infection, p16 and HPV ISH can be useful in sorting out neoplastic from ciliary metaplasia (49,50).

Subcolumnar reserve cells that have the potential to differentiate into ciliated and mucous secretory cells have been reported to populate the endocervix, even though there is evidence that the differentiated mucous cells are capable of division without the intercession of reserve cells (62,63). It is easy to confuse the lymphocytes that have populated the glandular epithelium with epithelial reserve cells (70).

Endocrine cells also are present within the endocervical epithelium. Their normal function is unclear, but it is generally held that they give rise to the endocrine neoplasms such as carcinoids and neuroendocrine carcinomas that occasionally occur in the cervix (51,56).

The endocervical epithelium not only lines the surface of the endocervical canal, it also dips, to a variable degree, into the underlying stroma to form elongate clefts (Fig. 40.9A). In histologic sections, these clefts typically are cut transversely, imparting the false impression that true endocervical glands are present within the stroma. However, true glands have different epithelia lining their ductal and secretory portions. In contrast, the endocervical mucosa has a more or less uniform appearance whether it lines the surface or the deep-lying "glands." Further evidence that these are not true glands was provided in a study conducted over 40 years ago by Fluhmann (71,72). He demonstrated by means of serial sections and three-dimensional reconstructions that what appeared to be endocervical glands within the stroma are actually complex protrusions of the endocervical lining that form clefts into the underlying stroma. When the endocervical epithelium lining the stromal clefts proliferates, side channels grow out from the clefts, giving rise to a histologic pattern that even more closely suggests acini of glands (Fig. 40.9B). Fluhmann labeled these side channels "tunnel clusters"; these are sometimes given the euphonious designation: "Fluhmann's lumens." When secretion inspissates in tunnel clusters, either because of obstruction or because of the viscosity of the secretions, it appears as bright eosinophilic material, an eye-catching pattern resembling thyroid (see Fig. 40.14). Having now discharged our obligation to anatomic accuracy, we shall continue to use the terms endocervical "gland(s)" and "cleft(s)" interchangeably.

The depth to which benign endocervical glands can extend in the cervical stroma varies from cervix to cervix. They can be found as deep as 1 cm but usually are found at a depth of less than 5 mm (73–75). This anatomic variation becomes important when considering a diagnosis of "minimal deviation adenocarcinoma" (76,77). In this form of adenocarcinoma the cytologic features differ only minimally from normal endocervical epithelium, and the diagnosis depends to a large extent on the identification of abnormally shaped glands at an inappropriate depth within the cervical stroma. The trick here is to compare the depth of the glands in question with noncontroversially benign glands in the immediate neighborhood. Additionally, useful in establishing a diagnosis of malignancy is a search for glands around nerves or vessels, an irregular "lobster claw" glandular configuration, and a granulation tissue stromal host response. Ciliated cells are extremely uncommon in malignant endocervical glandular proliferations; this finding argues strongly against a diagnosis of adenocarcinoma.

Endocervical cells show only minimal morphologic changes during the menstrual cycle, and even this amounts only to a shifting of the basally situated nuclei to a mid-cell

FIGURE 40.8 **A:** Ciliated cells in the endocervix. The normal cervical mucinous epithelium consists of an admixture of mucin-containing cells and a smaller population of ciliated cells. The population of ciliated cells undergoes cyclic variation with the menstrual cycle. **B** and **C:** Cervical tubal metaplasia. **B:** When ciliated cells are prominent they may simulate endocervical glandular dysplasia or carcinoma in situ. At low magnification the glands feature a prominence of nuclei, a feature shared with glandular dysplasia. **C:** Higher magnification shows prominent cilia, the hallmark of ciliated cell metaplasia.

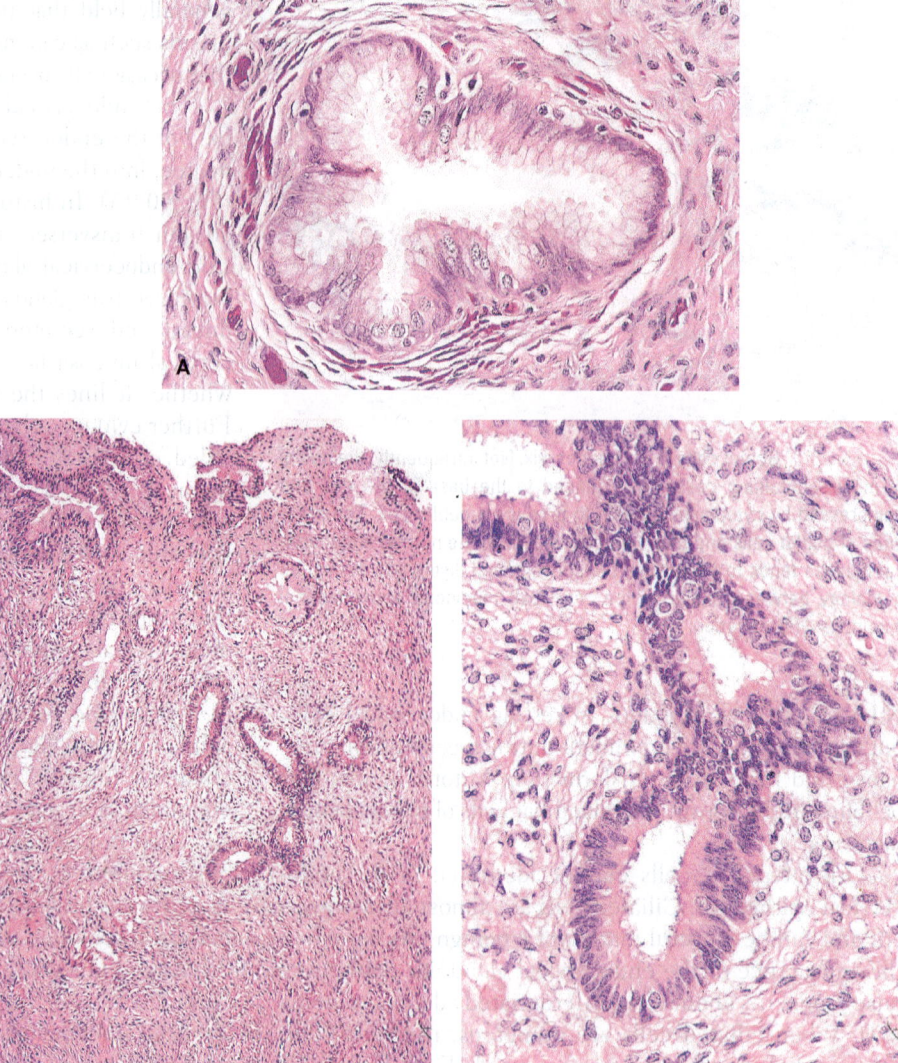

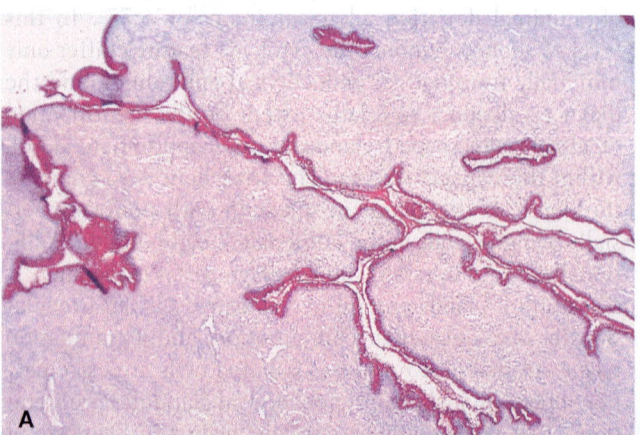
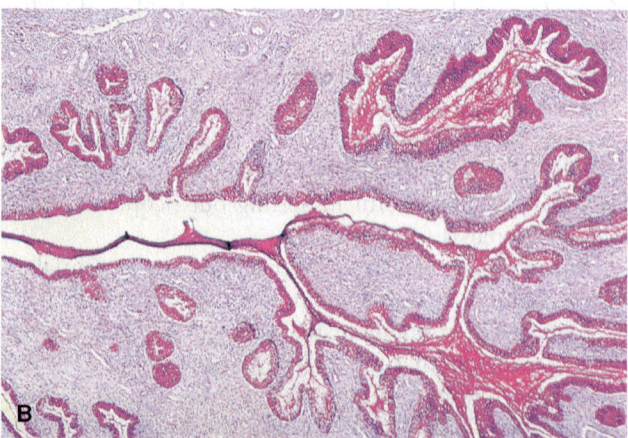

FIGURE 40.9 **A:** Tangential section of the endocervix stained with PAS to show how the gland clefts extend into the stroma and branch to form channels. **B:** When the endocervical mucosa undergoes hyperplasia and increases its surface area, as in pregnancy, the branches of the clefts proliferate and form even more collaterals ("tunnel clusters").

position at the height of the proliferative phase. These minor cytologic changes are in contrast to the dramatic biochemical changes that occur within the endometrial cells during the menstrual cycle (46). Throughout the proliferative phase of the cycle, the endocervical cells secrete mucus of lower viscosity than at other times of the cycle. This is thought to aid penetration of the cervical canal by spermatozoa (46). When progesterone levels attain their zenith during the luteal phase, the endocervical glandular secretion becomes thick and scant. It is at this stage that the secretion may become inspissated and more visible in histologic sections. During pregnancy the number of tunnel clusters increases, and when this phenomenon is extreme, the term "cervical glandular hyperplasia" is often used (78). Pregnancy also causes the secretions of the endocervical cells to thicken and form a mucous plug that blocks the endocervical canal (47,79).

Epithelium of the Transformation Zone

The endocervical mucosa shifts over the various divisions of the anatomic cervix throughout life (18,44,80). At birth the endocervical mucosa resides on the exocervix in two-thirds of infants, but it quickly moves back into the anatomic endocervical canal where in most girls it remains until near the menarche. After the onset of puberty, the endocervical mucosa again moves out onto the exocervix, usually more prominently on the anterior portion than on the posterior part (Fig. 40.10). The mechanism whereby endocervical mucosa changes location is apparently a mechanical one caused by swelling of the stroma of the cervical tissue in response to hormonal stimulation. As the lips of the cervix swell, they roll anteriorly and posteriorly, pulling the endocervical mucosa out of the canal onto the exocervix. The exposed endocervical tissue is often referred to as ectropion. Because the exposed endocervical mucosa appears red and ulcerated to the naked eye, it also has been interpreted as an erosion. There is, in fact, no erosion of the mucosa, rather the process is one of physiologic ectopy. After menarchial ectropion occurs the endocervical tissue is gradually replaced by squamous epithelium throughout the reproductive years. The area where the glandular tissue is being replaced by squamous epithelium is known as the transformation zone. The junction between the two types of epithelium is labeled the squamocolumnar junction (44,81). Two squamocolumnar junctions are usually recognized (Fig. 40.10B). The original squamocolumnar junction is the point where the native (original) exocervical squamous epithelium joins the endocervical glandular epithelium and is out on the exocervix during the reproductive years (80). This junction is usually sharply defined, and it is anatomically fixed. After squamous metaplasia has replaced endocervical tissue, the original squamocolumnar junction is the fusion point between the new squamous epithelium laid down in the transformation zone and the native squamous epithelium (Fig. 40.11). The functional squamocolumnar junction is the point of active replacement of columnar endocervical epithelium by squamous cells. This junction is often irregular and patchy, and it changes its contours and its locations during reproductive life. The functional squamocolumnar junction is usually implied when the term "squamocolumnar junction" is used without a modifier and the area between the two squamocolumnar junctions is the transformation zone. During pregnancy, particularly the first pregnancy, even more endocervical tissue moves out onto the exocervix, enlarging the area of ectopic endocervical epithelium. This phenomenon also can occur during progestogen therapy.

Because endocervical glandular epithelium is present on the exocervix, the transformation zone can be visualized with the aid of a colposcope. This is fortunate because neoplastic change begins most commonly in the transformation zone, and neoplastic transformation is accompanied by structural alterations that can be recognized using the colposcope. The combination of papilloma virus detection, cytologic preparations, colposcopic examination, biopsy, and local destruction of intraepithelial abnormalities in the transformation zone under colposcopic visualization is a powerful tool for the early detection and successful treatment of in situ neoplastic processes involving the cervix.

In the latter years of reproductive life the functional squamocolumnar junction reaches the area near the anatomic external os and, reversing its menarchal journey, begins to move up the anatomic endocervical canal. By the perimenopausal years, the squamocolumnar junction is usually concealed within the endocervical canal above the external os.

Two mechanisms are thought to be operative in transforming endocervical mucinous epithelium to squamous epithelium: (a) squamous epithelialization and (b) squamous metaplasia (3). The first involves the direct ingrowth of mature native squamous epithelium from the exocervix. This process is usually labeled "squamous epithelialization." During squamous epithelialization, mature squamous cells come to lie beneath the endocervical glandular cells. They push the endocervical cells off the basement membrane, and gradually the columnar cells degenerate and are sloughed. Squamous epithelialization initially spares the openings of the underlying endocervical glands, and at this stage the openings to the glands have the appearance of pores when examined with the colposcope. Eventually, the ingrowth of squamous epithelium involves the orifices of the glandular clefts, and then it can extend for varying distances down into the cleft spaces (Figs. 40.12 and 40.13). When this process involves the orifice, it may plug the opening, and if the mucinous epithelium below continues to secrete, a mucin-filled cyst (nabothian cyst) or tunnel clusters filled with eosinophilic secretion result (Fig. 40.14). If squamous epithelialization involves the cleft and its ramifying tunnels, squamous epithelium will be surrounded by endocervical stroma. Consequently, histologic sections taken in an area of squamous epithelialization may show nabothian cysts, mucification of tunnel clusters, and/or islands of benign squamous epithelium in the stroma beneath the surface epithelium.

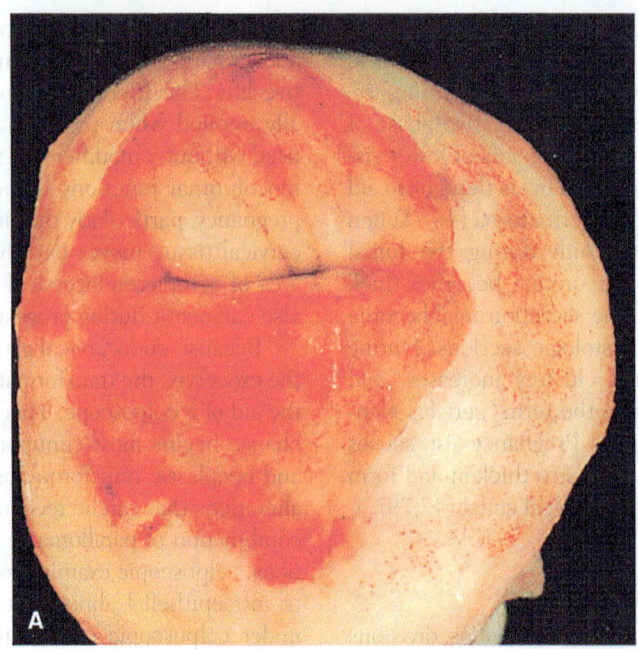
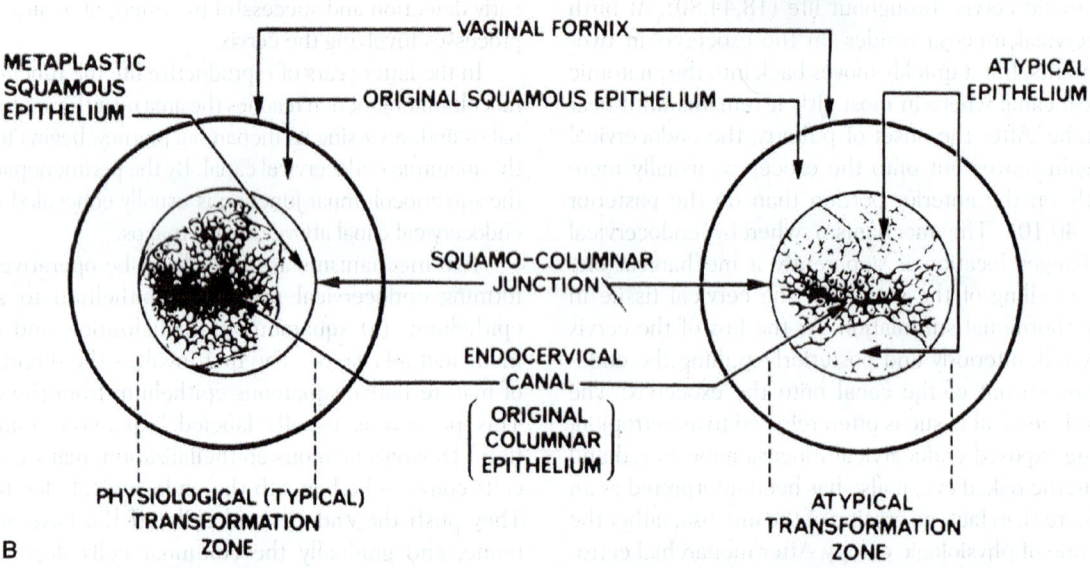

FIGURE 40.10 A: Multiparous cervix during the reproductive years. Note the slitlike configuration of the external os and the erythematous endocervical tissue out on the anatomic exocervix. This endocervical tissue undergoes conversion to squamous epithelium throughout the reproductive years. The squamocolumnar junction is visible as a sharp line between the white squamous epithelium and the erythematous glandular tissue. **B:** Diagram of the cervix demonstrating the transformation zone. On the left is a normal transformation zone in which metaplastic squamous epithelium is replacing endocervical columnar epithelium. "Squamocolumnar junction" refers to the original squamocolumnar junction. On the right the metaplastic process is composed of dysplastic squamous cells and hence the process is cervical intraepithelial neoplasia. Reprinted with permission from Fox H. *Haines and Taylor Obstetrical and Gynaecological Pathology*. 3rd ed. Philadelphia, PA: WB Saunders; 1987.

When the endocervical clefts undergo squamous epithelialization, care must be taken not to confuse the deep-lying benign squamous cells with invasive carcinoma. Although the cells in squamous epithelialization may have enlarged nuclei and prominent nucleoli, they do not demonstrate the anaplasia, the pleomorphism, the chromatin abnormalities, or the abnormal mitotic figures characteristic of invasive carcinoma. Moreover, the benign cells conform to the rounded configuration of the pre-existing cleft and do not infiltrate the stroma irregularly. Typically there is no granulation tissue host response to squamous epithelialization, although chronic inflammation may be present. If squamous epithelialization involves tunnel clusters, small groups of squamous cells come to lie deep within the cervical stroma, imparting an architectural pattern that even more resembles infiltrating squamous cell carcinoma. Squamous epithelialization

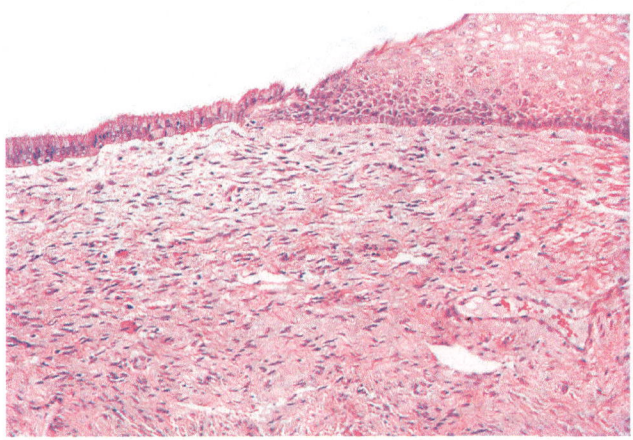

FIGURE 40.11 Squamocolumnar junction with a distinct transition from mature squamous epithelium on the right to endocervical glandular tissue on the left. Such a sharp change can be seen at the original squamocolumnar junction, as well as the junction formed by squamous epithelium with endocervical tissue in the transformation zone when squamous epithelium is mature.

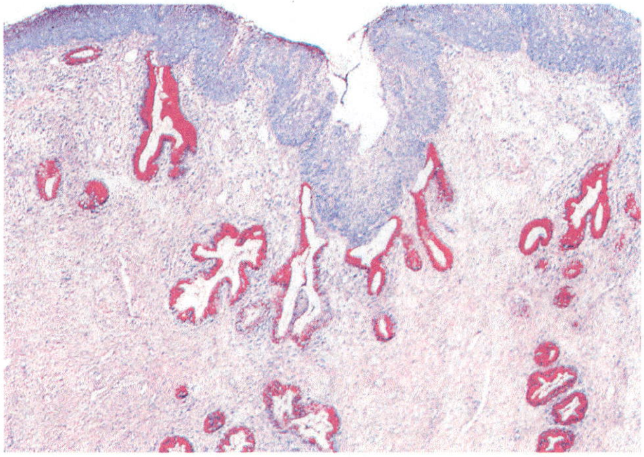

FIGURE 40.13 Conversion to squamous epithelium in the cervix may occur more rapidly on the surface than in the clefts, causing squamous epithelium to overlie endocervical gland clefts. When the newly laid down squamous epithelium blocks the orifices of the clefts, nabothian cysts, or mucification of tunnel clusters, as seen in Figure 40.14, may result.

seems to be stimulated by chronic inflammation and local trauma, including cauterization or laser surgery.

The second mechanism thought to contribute to the conversion of endocervical mucinous epithelium to squamous epithelium entails first the proliferation of endocervical "reserve cells," and then the differentiation of these cells into squamous cells rather than mucin-producing cells (82). This process, known as squamous metaplasia or prosoplasia, can be distinguished from squamous epithelialization because, unlike the cells in squamous epithelialization, the reserve cells initially do not have squamous characteristics; rather, they appear as cuboidal cells with round nuclei growing beneath the mucinous epithelium (Fig. 40.15). In fact, these cuboidal cells are identical in appearance to the basal or parabasal cells of the squamous epithelium. After the reserve cells proliferate and stratify, they differentiate into squamous cells that initially have only slightly increased amounts of cytoplasm (immature squamous metaplasia). Later the cells may fully mature to glycogen-containing squamous cells indistinguishable from the superficial cells of the exocervix (Fig. 40.11). Confusingly, "squamous metaplasia" is commonly used as a generic term for both metaplasia and squamous epithelialization.

Immature squamous metaplastic cells without fully developed squamous characteristics or glycogen accumulation can come to occupy most or all of the thickness of an epithelium (Fig. 40.16) (83,84). Because fully mature squamous cells are not present toward the surface and because the cytoplasm of the immature cells is relatively scant and their nuclei often are elongate, immature squamous metaplasia can bear a close

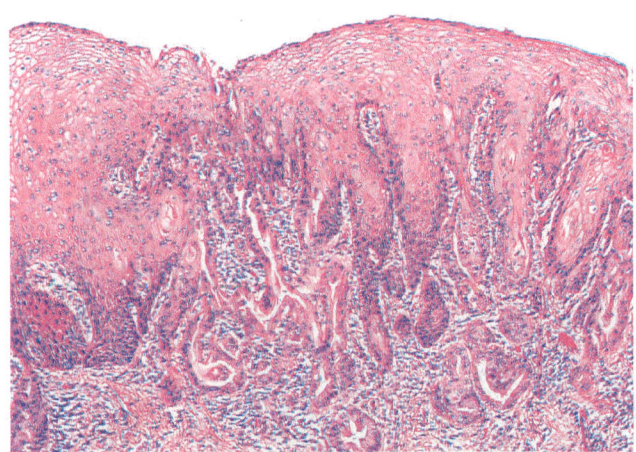

FIGURE 40.12 Squamous epithelialization of the endocervix. Note mature squamous epithelium extending into endocervical gland clefts. This process can mimic invasive carcinoma.

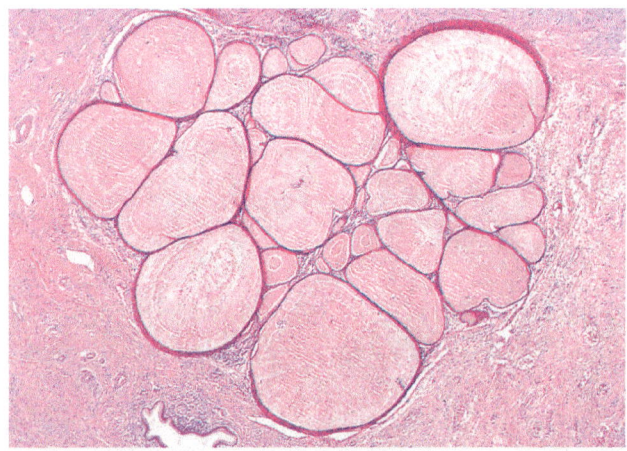

FIGURE 40.14 When the newly formed squamous epithelium in the transformation zone covers the endocervical gland cleft orifices and secretion continues, the tunnel clusters fill up with secretion that may become inspissated ("mucification").

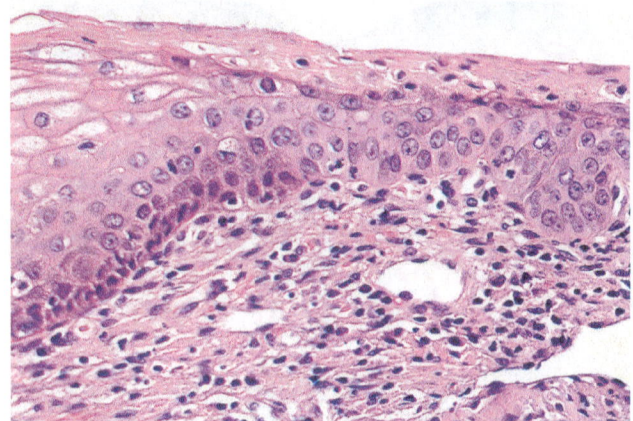

FIGURE 40.15 Functional squamocolumnar junction with metaplastic epithelium on the right. Note that in this example maturation has proceeded to the parabasal cell stage with abrupt keratinization rather than the normal maturation sequence to superficial cells as seen on the left.

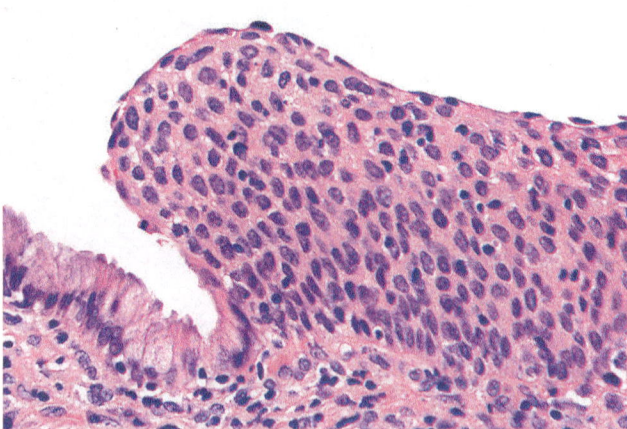

FIGURE 40.16 Immature squamous metaplasia on the right. The constituent cells do not demonstrate evidence of maturation and are similar to cells normally present in the basal layer of squamous epithelium. This type of metaplasia can be confused with high-grade squamous intraepithelial neoplasia.

resemblance to high-grade dysplasia. However, the nuclei in immature squamous metaplasia are uniform, chromatin abnormalities are minimal at most, and nuclear contours are usually smooth. Although mitotic figures may be present, in immature squamous metaplasia abnormal forms are not found and the mitoses should still be in a basilar location. The possibility of immature squamous metaplasia should be considered in each case where a diagnosis of high-grade intraepithelial lesion is contemplated.

Squamous metaplasia is usually patchy, giving rise to the characteristic irregularity of the functional squamocolumnar junction (Fig. 40.17). As squamous metaplasia proceeds, the islands of squamous cells form bridges to other centers of metaplasia, ultimately producing a solid area of squamous epithelium.

Whatever the mechanism—either squamous epithelialization or squamous metaplasia—squamous replacement of mucinous epithelium on the exocervix is a normal process that must be distinguished from in situ and invasive neoplasms. Features that are often found in neoplasia but not in metaplasia or epithelialization are moderate to marked pleomorphism, lack of maturation sequence (this may be present in immature squamous metaplasia), irregular nuclear outlines, suprabasal mitotic figures, and abnormal mitotic figures. Nucleoli are usually inconspicuous in HSIL but are often prominent in metaplasia, and epithelialization (a notable exception is immature squamous metaplasia), and reactive changes in response to cervicitis.

Recently a population of embryonic squamocolumnar junctional cells in the transformation zone has been identified. These cells are cytologically different from the endocervical and squamous cells and have a unique gene-expression profile (85). These cells are strongly cytokeratin 7 positive and able to undergo squamous metaplasia. With overlapping

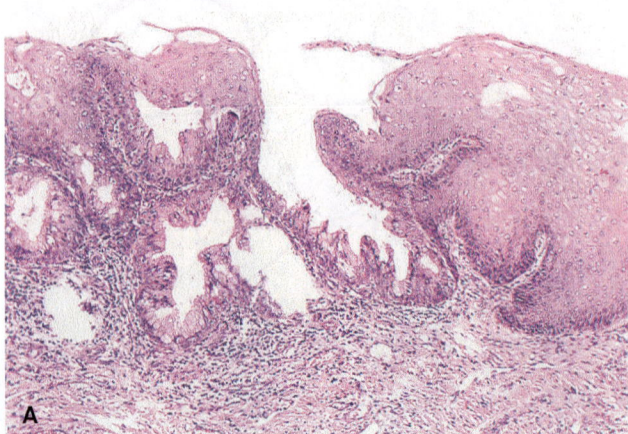
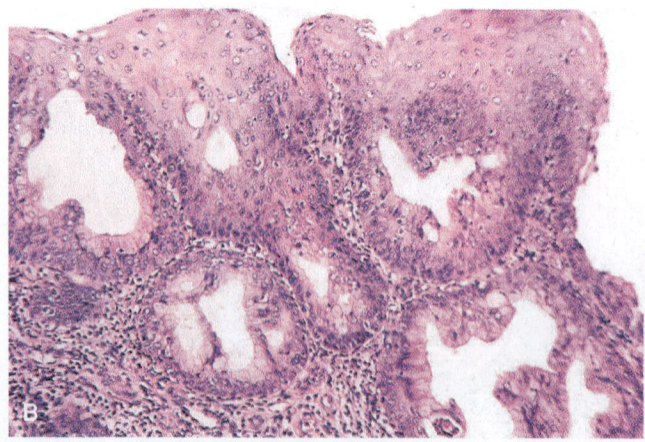

FIGURE 40.17 **A:** Islands of metaplastic squamous epithelium in the transformation zone at the functional squamocolumnar junction. These islands will eventually coalesce. **B:** Higher-power photomicrograph of the area of squamous metaplasia demonstrated in **A**.

immunophenotypic profiles to squamous and adenocarcinomas of the cervix it has been postulated that it is these squamocolumnar junctional cells that might be the nidus cell for HPV infection and HPV-related cervical neoplasia (86).

Cervical Stroma

In contrast to the wall of the uterine corpus, which is predominately muscular, the stroma of the exocervix is mainly fibrous tissue admixed with elastin through which run infrequent strands of smooth muscle (87–90). A large number of vessels course through the stroma. A rich capillary network interfaces with the epithelium at the stromal–epithelial junction. This interface is irregular and features fingers of connective tissue containing vessels overlain by a squamous cell mucosa of variable thickness. Much of the endocervical stroma is also fibroelastic tissue, but at the upper end of the endocervix the superficial fibrous stroma blends imperceptibly into the endometrial stroma of the lower uterine segment. Consequently, the superficial stroma of the upper endocervix and the stroma of the lower uterine segment have a hybrid endometrial–cervical appearance. This can cause localization problems when it is important to determine whether a neoplastic process in a curettage specimen involves the endometrium or the endocervix or both. We think the presence of unequivocal endometrial stroma, as determined by high cellularity (closely packed nuclei), should be present before interpreting tissue as originating from the endometrium on the basis of the stroma alone. Of course, if one type of normal glands is present, whether endocervical or endometrial, these glands can suggest the origin of the tissue, but both types of glands or even hybrid glands may be present in the transition area between the endocervix and lower uterine segment. The endocervix contains a greater number of smooth muscle fibers in its deeper stroma than does the exocervix, and in the lower uterine segment these blend into the myometrium.

The cervix bridges the sterile environment of the uterine cavity and the microbiologic jungle of the lower genital tract. It is not surprising that this important immunologic role (both humoral and cellular) would be marked by a conspicuous lymphoid presence (44). Thus, large numbers of T lymphocytes normally populate the endocervical stroma (91). B-lineage lymphoid cells manifest as either plasma cells or germinal centers are also commonly encountered.

In addition, dendritic cells are numerous in the cervix; a subset of these are Langerhans cells (immature dendritic cells that express MHC class II antigens and the CD4 receptor on their surface) that are involved in internalizing antigen and presenting it to T lymphocytes in the regional lymph nodes (92–95).

The relevance of these observations to the surgical pathologist is chiefly to discourage the overuse of "chronic cervicitis"; the presence of lymphoid tissue in the cervix is as normal as its presence in the small intestine.

In our opinion, a diagnosis of chronic cervicitis should be withheld unless the lymphoid infiltrate is very heavy and/or lymphoid nodules are numerous. Particularly important for the diagnosis of chronic cervicitis are large numbers of plasma cells. Scattered plasma cells are normal in the cervix. Acute cervicitis is not uncommon, but true inflammatory erosion or microabscesses are rare in the cervix.

Lymphocytes also may migrate into the endocervical epithelium, and in this location they may assume the appearance of "cleared cells." Such cells have been misconstrued as "reserve" cells in the past (70).

Remnants of the wolffian duct—commonly known as mesonephric rests—can be found in the endocervical stroma of the lateral portions of the cervix in about a third of women (96) (Fig. 40.18). Usually these are deep in the stroma, but occasionally they are found near the surface and they can even blend with the endocervical gland clefts. Mesonephric rests are tubular structures lined by a single row of cuboidal cells with a central round, cytologically bland nucleus. Typically the tubules form lumens that contain hyalin-like, eosinophilic secretions. Architecturally, there is usually a central elongate duct surrounded by smaller tubules. The combination of deep stromal location, the hyalin-like secretions, and the cuboidal cells usually serves to make identification of mesonephric rests straightforward. Even though tunnel clusters may ramify from a central cleft and contain eosinophilic secretion, they are lined by endocervical mucin-producing cells. The importance of this vestigial structure lies in its mimicry of well-differentiated adenocarcinoma. Mitotic figures are usually absent in mesonephric rests, and the chromatin of the cells is bland. Moreover, mesonephric rests do not exhibit the raggedly infiltrative growth of carcinoma even though they are located deep in the stroma. Rarely, atypical hyperplastic and neoplastic processes may involve mesonephric remnants (78,96,97). Mesonephric proliferations, benign and malignant, often express CD10 (98,99).

Multinucleated giant cells rarely are found in the normal superficial endocervical stroma. These cells have enlarged and sometimes bizarre-shaped nuclei with smudged chromatin similar to those seen in fibroepithelial stromal polyps (100). They should not be mistaken for a neoplasm (101–103).

Cervix During Pregnancy

During pregnancy the endocervical epithelium proliferates so that its mucus-secreting surface increases. This proliferation leads to both the formation of polypoid protrusions of endocervical epithelium into the endocervical canal and an increased number of tunnel clusters budding off pre-existing clefts within the cervical stroma. The overall impression is one of an increase in the amount of endocervical tissue, and consequently this normal process is often termed "endocervical glandular hyperplasia" or when numerous small glands are packed together "microglandular hyperplasia." Identical changes can be produced by artificial progestogens. The endocervical mucus during pregnancy is thick and functions as a plug to seal off the endometrial cavity from the vagina (22,104). Arias-Stella (AS) reaction may be seen in the

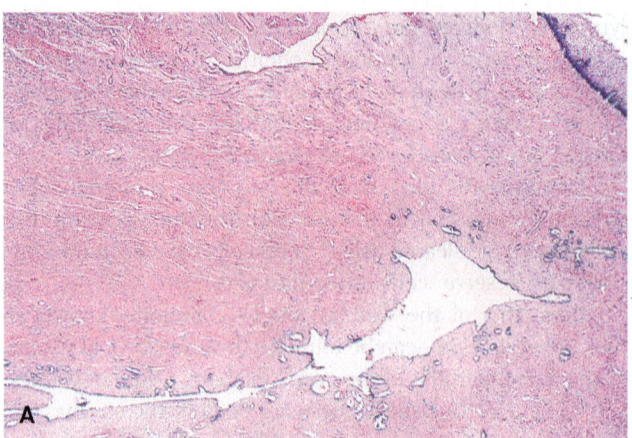
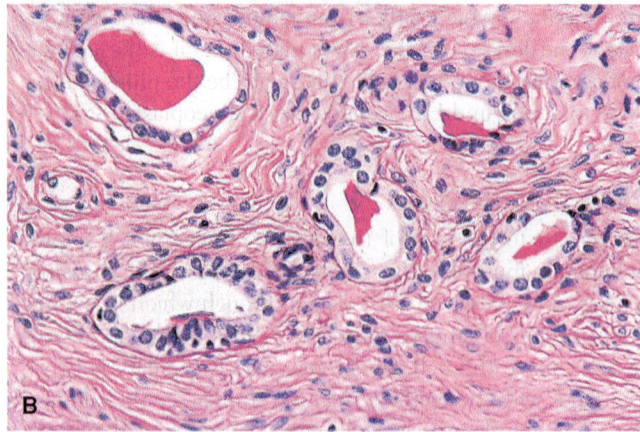

FIGURE 40.18 **A:** Mesonephric remnants in the cervix. A long cleftlike space deep in the stroma surrounded by tubules is the characteristic architectural finding. **B:** Ducts lined by bland cuboidal cells containing lumenal PAS-positive eosinophilic secretion are key features of mesonephric remnants. The blandness of the constituent cells and the organization around a central cleft are the most helpful features in distinguishing this from well-differentiated adenocarcinoma.

endocervical glandular cells (105). As in the endometrium, the large cells with prominent nucleoli characteristic of the AS reaction can raise concern about clear cell carcinoma, but the absence of mitotic figures and the gestational setting should quickly eliminate this possibility.

The stroma of the cervix undergoes a complex series of biochemical and biomechanical changes during pregnancy and parturition that taken together are known as cervical "ripening" (105). The initial change seems to be extensive destruction of collagen fibers by various collagenases accompanied by the accumulation of gel-like acid mucopolysaccharides. This process causes the cervix to soften, a process that reaches its zenith immediately before parturition. As a result, the cervix is easily effaced by the presenting part of the emerging infant. Thus, the usually cylindrical cervix is transformed into a thin saccular structure. The increased fluid in the cervical stroma during pregnancy causes the cervical lips to roll further out into the vagina, everting more of the endocervical mucosa beyond the external os. Squamous epithelialization and metaplasia rapidly ensue, and at the time of delivery there is often considerable immature squamous epithelium in the transformation zone. As noted previously, the cells in immature squamous metaplasia can closely resemble those found in intraepithelial neoplasia, so caution should be exercised when examining cervical specimens taken from pregnant women.

The cervical stromal cells, particularly those near the surface of the endocervical canal, may undergo decidual change during pregnancy (Fig. 40.19). Cervical decidual reaction is typically patchy, and at low power this focal replacement of the cervical stroma by aggregates of epithelioid cells can resemble invasive large cell nonkeratinizing carcinoma. Awareness of this physiologic process during pregnancy and close attention to the cytologic features of the suspect cells should avoid misdiagnosis (106).

Normal findings in the cervix that have relevance to histopathologic differential diagnosis are presented in Table 40.1.

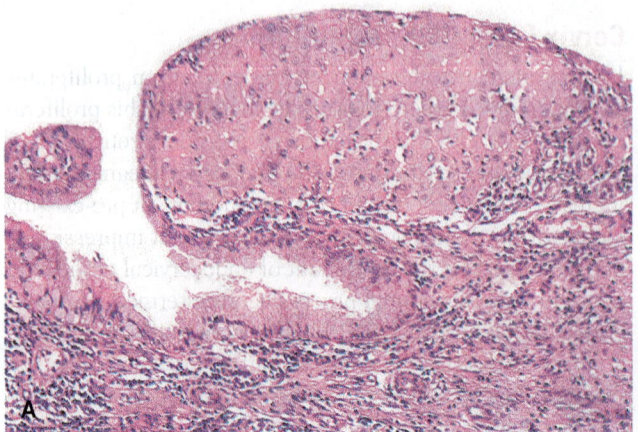
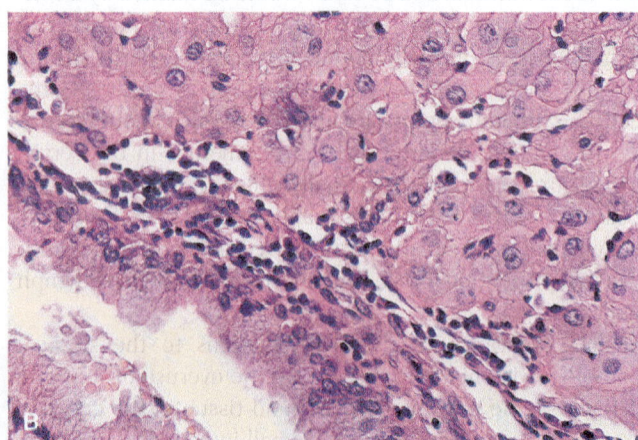

FIGURE 40.19 **A, B:** Decidual reaction in the cervix. The sheetlike arrangement of the cells can mimic squamous cell carcinoma, but the nuclei are bland.

TABLE 40.1
Normal Findings in the Cervix That Have Relevance to Histopathologic Differential Diagnosis

Finding	Diagnostic Confusion	Suggestions for Resolution	References
Deeply situated normal endocervical gland clefts or Nabothian cysts	Minimal deviation adenocarcinoma (MDC):	Lobster claw configuration in MDC Ciliated cells in benign proliferations and almost always absent in malignant cervical glandular proliferations	(69,76,77)
Easily found mitotic figures in endocervical epithelium In normal endocervical epithelium mitotic figures are rare. In squamous metaplasia and regenerating cervical epithelium mitotic figures may be numerous but abnormal forms are not present	Adenocarcinoma, invasive or in situ	Compare problematic epithelium with normal epithelium elsewhere p16 immunohistochemistry and/or high-risk HPV in situ hybridization	(49,50)
Mesonephric remnants	Minimal deviation adenocarcinoma (MDC) Mesonephric carcinoma	MDC often has an associated superficial component of ACIS The glands of mesonephric remnants are rounded and smooth contoured; those of carcinoma are usually jagged and infiltrative; the glands of Mesonephric remnants branch of a central, elongate, ductal structure, those of invasive adenocarcinoma are haphazard and lack a central originating duct.	(96)
Decidual reaction	Large cell nonkeratinizing squamous cell carcinoma	Mitotic figures, cytologic atypia in carcinoma Pankeratin negative in decidual cells and positive in squamous cell carcinoma	(107)
Arias-Stella reaction	Clear cell carcinoma of the cervix/vagina	Arias-Stella reaction usually does not feature mitotic figures that are easily found in clear cell carcinoma.	(108,109)
Lower uterine segment vs. endocervical fragments: Can make a difference when carcinoma (endocervical vs. endometrial) is found in curettings		Differential curretage; imaging studies. Immunohistochemistry for CEA, p16 and vimentin is sometimes be useful but interpret with caution.	(107)
Squamous metaplasia and epithelialization involving cervical gland clefts	Invasive carcinoma	Assess nuclear features and evaluation for the presence or absence of infiltration	
Endometriosis: Benign endometrial glands and stroma	Adenocarcinoma: When stroma inconspicuous Adenosarcoma: Look for stromal mitotic figures	Think of the possibility of endometriosis. Look for the missing component in additional levels Cytologic atypia is usually minimal in endometriosis but mitotic figures may be present	(100)
Microglandular adenosis and endocervical glandular hyperplasia	Adenocarcinoma	Prominent nucleoli and abnormal division figures are features of carcinoma. Easily found mitotic figures almost always are a carcinoma feature.	(110,69,75)
Immature squamous metaplasia	High-grade SIL; may mimic because nuclei of the cells are large and cytoplasm is relatively scant.	Look for nucleoli—often present in metaplasia, but often inconspicuous in CIN—and abnormal mitotic figures and abnormal chromatin patterns. Nucleoli may not be prominent in immature squamous metaplasia p16 immunohistochemistry or high-risk HPV in situ hybridization	(49,50)

(continued)

TABLE 40.1 Normal Findings in the Cervix That Have Relevance to Histopathologic Differential Diagnosis (Continued)			
Finding	Diagnostic Confusion	Suggestions for Resolution	References
Glycogen storage in superficial squamous cells	Koilocytosis (HPV infection)	Koilocytic nuclei: (1) enlarged, (2) irregular nuclear membranes, (3) dense ropy chromatin. High- and low-risk HPV in situ hybridization.	(49,50)
Tubal metaplasia: Endocervical epithelium lined by prominent and numerous ciliated cells may suggest adenocarcinoma in situ or endometrioid carcinoma	Cervical adenocarcinoma in situ	Numerous mitotic figures and abnormal mitotic figures are features for adeno CIS not tubal metaplasia. Look for ciliated cells; if numerous the process is almost surely benign. p16 immunohistochemistry or HPV in situ hybridization	(66,–69,73,110)
Multinucleated stromal giant cells: These may be a normal finding; probably myofibroblastic cells	Neoplasm, particularly sarcoma. Granulomatous inflammation	Look for abnormal mitotic figures, high cellularity, and granulomas	

See text for additional differential diagnostic clues (67).

ENDOMETRIUM

Tissue Sampling and Associated Problems

A variety of endometrial tissue sampling techniques are available to the clinician. These techniques differ with respect to their indications, their limitations, and their associated complications (104–106, 108, 111–119). Endometrial curettage (cervical dilation and endometrial curettage—D&C) entails the removal of most of the uterine mucosa by scraping with a sharp curette. Under ideal circumstances, the excision is complete or nearly complete. Endometrial biopsy (EMB) involves the removal of a more limited sample of tissue than does the complete curettage and is performed with a smaller curette. Single strips of endometrium are usually taken from both the anterior and the posterior fundal surfaces. Even though the sample is limited, the accuracy of diagnosis approximates that of the D&C. The chief advantage of this technique is that it does not require cervical dilation (and hence does not require anesthesia). EMB thus combines convenience and low cost, with little sacrifice in diagnostic accuracy. The major limitation of EMB lies in its inherent potential to miss focal lesions, such as polyps and localized carcinomas. Accordingly, when carcinoma is suspected clinically, a complete dilatation and curettage must follow a negative biopsy, because only this technique ensures the absence of carcinoma. Hysteroscopy in combination with endometrial sampling is thought by some to increase the detection rate of uterine abnormalities (120); others disagree (121). If EMB is performed as part of an infertility workup (but see Relevance of Endometrial Dating to Diagnostic Surgical Pathologists), tissue should be obtained well into the presumed secretory phase, that is, 2 to 3 days before the time of the next menstrual period as estimated by clinical and laboratory findings. Although in principle biopsy in the late luteal phase might destroy an early gestation, in practice this seems not to be the case (122).

Three artifacts of sectioning and tissue preparation should be mentioned at this point. A frequent finding in endometrial curettings is the "telescoped" gland, which is characterized by an "inside-out" gland within the lumen of a gland with a normal configuration. This artifact is seen when an intussuscepted or telescoped gland (produced by the traumatic removal of the tissue) is cross-sectioned, and it occurs most frequently in straight glands. Another artifact is the result of sectioning and involves the tangential cutting of a gland to produce a "pseudo-gland-within-gland" pattern. Confusion with adenocarcinoma can be avoided by attention to cytologic detail, comparison with surrounding glands, knowledge that the gland-within-gland pattern in carcinoma is usually extensive, and awareness of this topologic problem. A third artifact involves tangential sectioning of the endometrial surface to produce pseudocystic and pseudobudded glands. Poor fixation can sometimes result in the retraction of endometrial glands from their surrounding stromal envelope. Moreover, cytoplasmic vacuolization may be a result of autolysis and can simulate early secretory vacuolated epithelium.

Histology of the Normal Endometrium

The normal endometrium has a multiplicity of constantly changing normal patterns that depend on the nature and intensity of ovarian hormonal stimulation. The purpose of this section is to analyze the morphology of the normal nongravid endometrium in some detail from three points of view. First, we discuss regional variations, then the individual

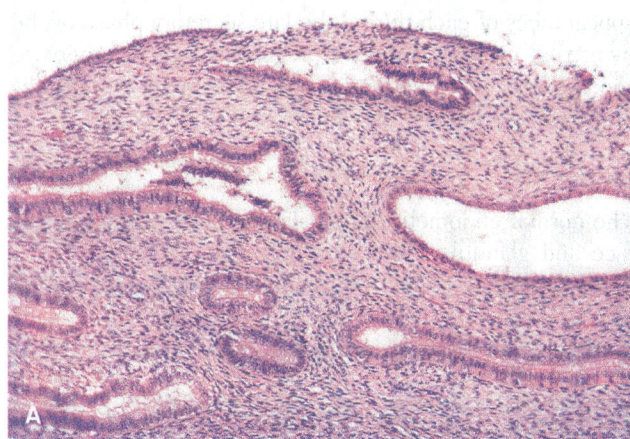
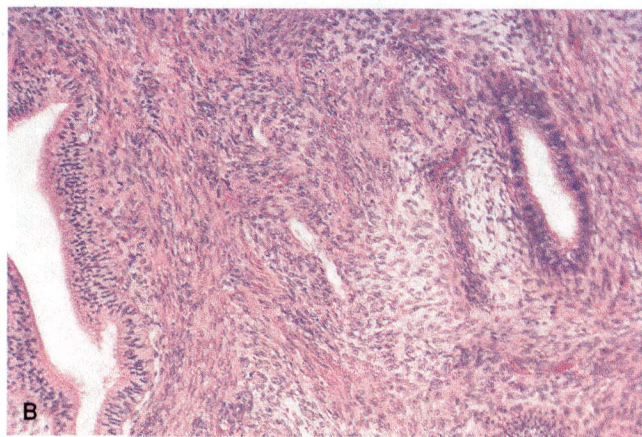

FIGURE 40.20 The lower uterine segment contains stroma and glands that are either hybrid between those seen in the endocervix and those in the fundus or a mixture of endometrial and endocervical glands and stroma. **A:** The stroma is fibrous appearing but more cellular than that typically found in the endocervix. **B:** An endometrial gland and an endocervical gland are found next to each other in this area of the lower uterine cervix.

components of the endometrium; finally, using this background, we describe the temporal variations in the histology of the endometrium that occur throughout life.

Regional Variations

The uterine lining can be divided into two regions on the basis of its morphology: the mucosa of the lower uterine segment and the mucosa of the corpus proper. The mucosa of the lower uterine segment (isthmus) is in general thinner than the fundal mucosa. The glands and stroma tend to be only sluggishly responsive to hormonal stimulation, and in consequence this portion of the endometrium most often lags behind the rest of the endometrium in its development.

The morphologic transition from endocervical mucosa to lower uterine segment mucosa is gradual, and in fact the hybrid endocervical–endometrial appearance of both the glands and the stroma of the lower uterine segment serves to identify this zone in endometrial curettings (Fig. 40.20).

The major portion of the uterine lining, the corpus mucosa proper, is normally fully responsive to hormonal stimulation. Two layers can be readily identified within the endometrium throughout this region: the lowermost is labeled the basalis and the overlying one the functionalis. The basalis is that zone of weakly proliferative glands and associated dense-spindled stroma immediately adjacent to the myometrium (Fig. 40.21). Characteristically, the

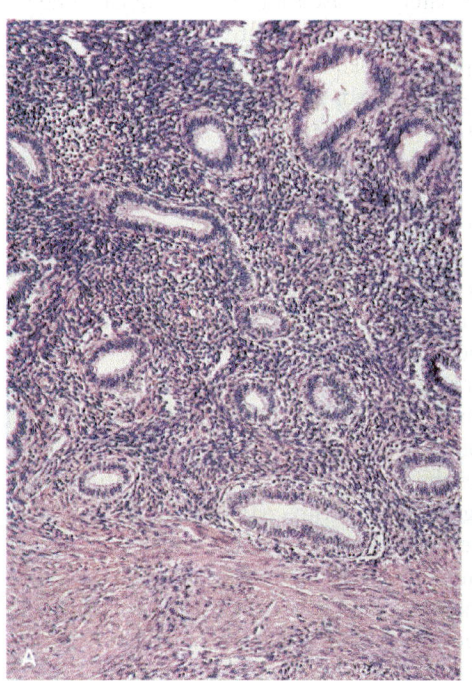
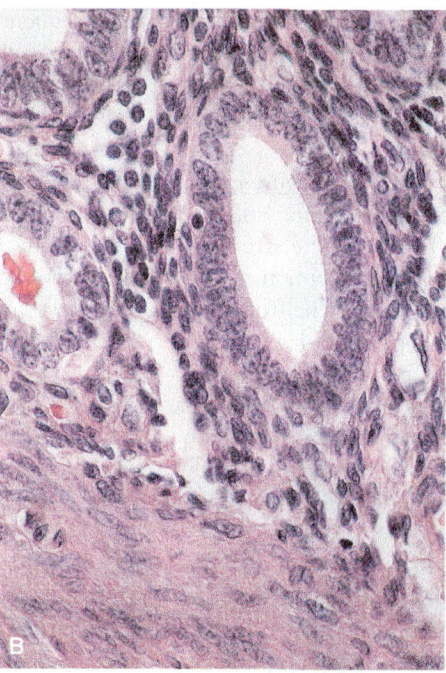

FIGURE 40.21 **A, B:** The basalis of the endometrium is demonstrated. Throughout the menstrual cycle the basalis maintains a weakly proliferative appearance. As a result, dating of endometrium should be performed on fragments containing surface epithelium.

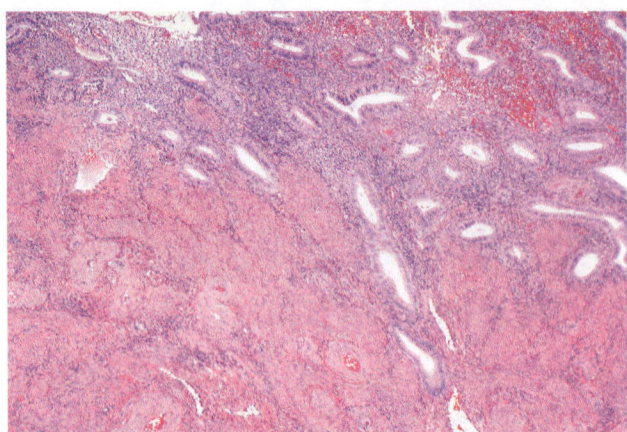

FIGURE 40.22 This is an example of an irregular endometrial–myometrial junction. This phenomenon is important to think about when determining whether or not adenocarcinoma is superficially invading the myometrium.

junction of the basalis and myometrium is irregular, and smooth muscle and endometrial stroma interdigitate and blend together at this point (Fig. 40.22). When florid, this irregularity may give the false impression that endometrial tissue is pathologically isolated within the myometrium. This deception is particularly important when evaluating the presence or absence of superficial myometrial invasion in patients with endometrial adenocarcinoma. Of less importance is the confusion it creates in the diagnosis of adenomyosis. The basalis, despite its inactive and undifferentiated appearance, plays a crucial role in the endometrial economy because it constitutes the "reserve cell layer" of the endometrium. After the bulk of the overlying functionalis is shed during menstruation, or after the functionalis is removed by curettage, the basalis and the residual deep functionalis are responsible for regenerating the endometrium. The remaining surface epithelium of the lower uterine segment also participates in this regeneration (123).

The appearance of the basalis is relatively constant throughout the menstrual cycle. Specifically, the glands usually appear weakly proliferative; that is, they possess pseudostratified elongate nuclei, rare mitotic figures, and dense intensely basophilic chromatin. Most importantly, they lack secretory change (Fig. 40.21), and the stroma is spindled and nondecidualized. A notable exception to this generalization is the basalis during the latter half of pregnancy, which usually exhibits secretory glandular changes and stromal decidualization. The importance of recognizing the basalis of the endometrium lies in not mistaking it for the functionalis in a curettage specimen. This confusion would result in an erroneous impression that this weakly proliferative appearance represented the fully developed state of the functionalis.

It is the functionalis that exhibits the protean changes so characteristic of the normal endometrium. This layer has been traditionally divided into two strata—the compactum and the spongiosum—on the basis of the morphologic appearances of each during the late secretory phase of the menstrual cycle and during pregnancy. Unless otherwise specified, the term "endometrium" refers to the functionalis in the subsequent discussion.

Individual Components of the Endometrium

The normal endometrium consists of both epithelial (surface and glandular) and mesenchymal (stromal and vascular) elements, which during reproductive years first synchronously proliferate, then differentiate, and finally disintegrate at roughly monthly intervals.

> **EPITHELIAL ELEMENTS** The endometrial glandular and surface epithelia are both composed of four morphologically distinct cells, two of which are functional variants of the same cell.

> **PROLIFERATIVE AND BASALIS-TYPE CELLS.** The basalis-type cells and the proliferative cells of the functionalis are morphologically similar. These cells both have high nucleus-to-cytoplasm ratios and elongate sausage-shaped nuclei with dense chromatin and inconspicuous nucleoli. The cytoplasm is scant and generally basophilic to amphophilic (see Figs. 40.21 and 40.33). Mitotic figures are common in the cells that compose the glands of the functionalis during the proliferative phase. When proliferative cells are the predominant cell type composing the epithelium (as in the proliferative endometrium), the nuclei appear pseudostratified.

> **SECRETORY CELLS.** The characteristic cytoplasmic differentiation of the endometrial epithelial cell is nonmucinous secretion. Shortly after ovulation, secretory products accumulate in a subnuclear location in the proliferative cells; these products gradually shift to a supranuclear position and are ultimately released into the glandular lumens. This sequence of changes results in two easily recognizable secretory cell types: Vacuolated and nonvacuolated secretory cells (see Figs 40.33B and 40.34C). Although vacuolated cells may have a nucleus similar to those seen in proliferative phase cells, the nonvacuolated secretory cells possess nuclei that are distinct from those seen in the undifferentiated proliferative phase cells. In contrast to the dense intensely basophilic elongate nuclei of the proliferative cells, the nuclei of the nonvacuolated secretory cells are rounded and vesicular, they have uniformly dispersed chromatin, and occasionally nucleoli become prominent. The nonvacuolated secretory cells have uniform, moderately dense eosinophilic cytoplasm and often a frayed luminal border (see Fig. 40.34C).

Another type of secretory cell is encountered, one that closely resembles the secretory cell of the fallopian tube. This cell has an elongate nucleus with coarse chromatin, a moderate amount of densely eosinophilic cytoplasm, and a rounded luminal bleb similar to those found in apocrine glands. These cells are common in the surface epithelium and occasionally may line an entire endometrial gland. Some of these cells may in fact represent "exhausted" ciliated cells.

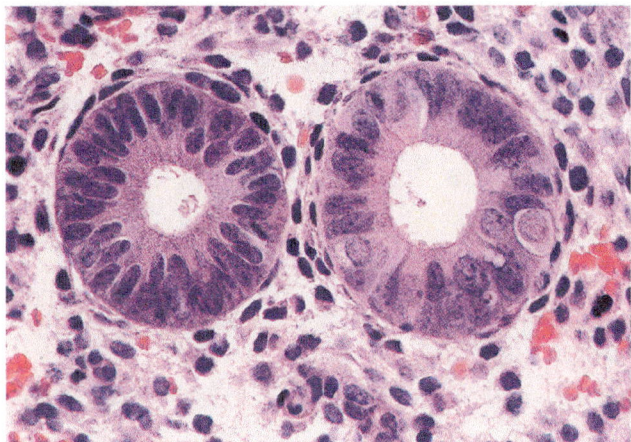

FIGURE 40.23 Proliferative phase glands with ciliated cells in the gland at the right. The round cell with clear cytoplasm at the 3:00 o'clock position has the characteristic appearance of ciliated cells before they have extruded their cilia into the glandular lumen. The other ciliated cells have a pyramidal shape.

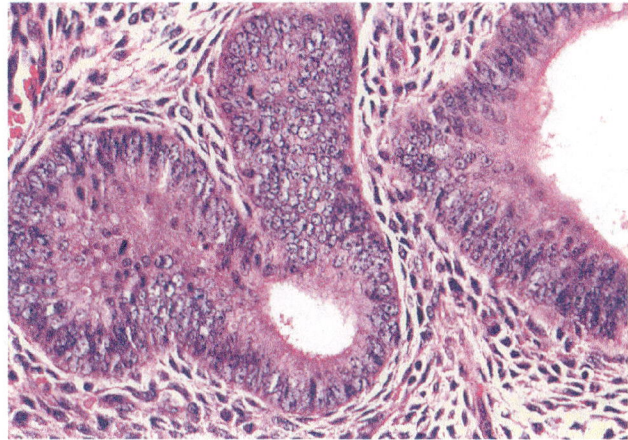

FIGURE 40.24 Proliferative phase glands and stroma. Note the elongate rather than rounded shape of the stromal cell nuclei. However, it is not uncommon for stromal cell nuclei to be elongate.

> **CILIATED CELLS.** The ciliated cells of the endometrium are consistently present in endometrial specimens and presumably represent one line of differentiation open to the basalis-type cell. These cells are more prominent near the uterine isthmus and during the proliferative phase (124,125).

Ciliated cells have distinctive round, smoothly contoured vesicular nuclei containing finely stippled chromatin (Fig. 40.23). Although the nuclear features remain relatively unchanged throughout cell development, the configuration and location of ciliated cells vary as a function of the stage of ciliogenesis. The earliest identifiable ciliated cells are situated adjacent to the basal lamina of the gland and are roughly pyramidal in shape. They possess distinctively clear cytoplasm with central round nuclei. A rounded cytoplasmic zone containing eosinophilic fibrillary material can be identified with routine stains. This zone corresponds to the intracytoplasmic cilia seen with the electron microscope. When the growing ciliated cells reach the luminal surface, the cilia are exposed to the glandular lumen. Initially the luminal surface of the ciliated cell is concave, but as the cell continues its development, this surface becomes convex, and ultimately the cilia may pinch off as a merocrine secretion. During this stage the cell has a characteristic fusiform-to-pear shape. Ciliated cells can come to predominate the cellular population of glands, and when they do the terms "ciliary metaplasia" and "ciliary change" have been used.

> **THE GLAND AS A WHOLE.** The normal endometrial gland is lined by the aforementioned cells arranged in a non-stratified cuboidal-to-columnar epithelium, which during the proliferative phase deceptively appears to be stratified (i.e., it is pseudostratified). During the early proliferative phase, the glands are straight and have narrow lumens (Fig. 40.24). Beginning in the midproliferative period and lasting throughout the rest of the cycle, the glands exhibit increasing degrees of coiling, but not branching. This culminates in the serrated saw-toothed appearance of the glands in the late secretory and menstrual endometrium. The surface epithelium is composed predominantly of apocrine-like secretory cells and ciliated cells, and has a relatively constant appearance throughout the cycle.

> **MESENCHYMAL ELEMENTS**

> **CELLULAR ELEMENTS**

> **ENDOMETRIAL STROMA.** The endometrial stromal cell is the predominant cellular component of the stroma, and its appearance varies greatly with the stage of the menstrual cycle. During the early proliferative phase these cells are small (about the size of a neutrophil) due to the scant, indistinct cytoplasm and dense oval-to-fusiform nuclei (Fig. 40.25). As the menstrual cycle proceeds, the stromal cells become

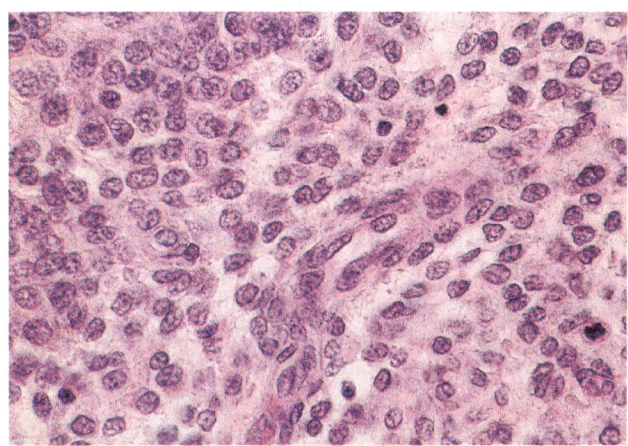

FIGURE 40.25 The proliferative phase endometrial stromal cells have scant, hard-to-discern cytoplasm and usually round nuclei (compare to Fig. 40.26). Thin walled tubular blood vessels populate the endometrial stroma.

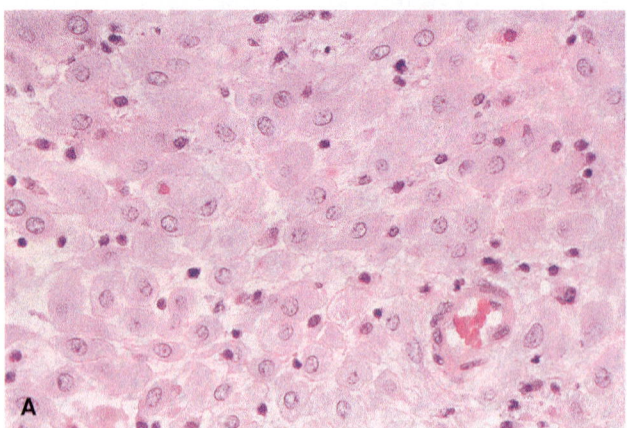
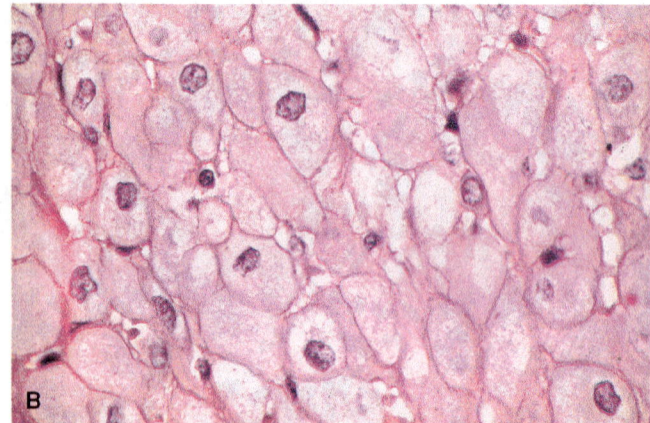

FIGURE 40.26 A, B: The decidual reaction during pregnancy is typified by cells with abundant pink cytoplasm and sharp cell margins.

more elongate and acquire more cytoplasm. During the late proliferative phase and well into the secretory phase, electron microscopy shows increasing amounts of rough endoplasmic reticulum and both intra- and extracytoplasmic collagen. Toward the end of the secretory phase, the perivascular stromal cells become rounded, acquire more cytoplasm, and develop vesicular nuclei with occasionally prominent nucleoli. Cytoplasmic borders become more fully developed and gradually the entire endometrial stroma is transformed into sheets of cells polygonal cells with sharp and distinct cytoplasmic borders, abundant cytoplasm, and centrally placed vesicular nuclei (Fig. 40.26).

This unique müllerian stromal transformation is called decidualization when fully developed (e.g., during pregnancy) and predecidualization when partially developed (e.g., during the late secretory phase of the menstrual cycle) (126). Ultrastructurally, the abundant cytoplasm of the decidual cell is populated by dilated rough endoplasmic reticulum, Golgi apparatus, and distinctly small mitochondria. Decidual cells form basal lamina and have complex intercellular interdigitations and tight junctions. The prominent intercellular borders are due to the accumulation of pericellular matrix (127).

Thus, the decidua is the specialized endometrium of pregnancy and plays an active role in implantation and in mediating the relationship between the fetoplacental unit and the mother. The decidua secretes a host of products (prolactin, relaxin, renin, insulin-like growth factors [IGFs] and insulin-like growth factor binding proteins) involved in the paracrine and autocrine regulation of the feto–maternal interface (13,128). In short, the endometrium of pregnancy functions as an endocrine organ. In addition, decidual cells appear to be capable of phagocytosis and are thought to play a role dismantling the collagen scaffolding at the implantation site (112).

> **HEMATOLYMPHOID CELLS.** A second prominent cellular constituent, particularly in the late secretory phase and during pregnancy, is what historically has been referred to as the "stromal granulocyte" but is now known to be a uterine natural killer (uNK) cell (129). These are rounded cells with bilobed nuclei, and have pale cytoplasm that contains eosinophilic granules. Their immunoprofile differs from that of blood NK cells. Their number appears to be positively correlated with the degree of predecidualization or decidualization in the surrounding endometrium; indeed, the number of such cells was used by Noyes as a dating criterion. This close association has suggested to some workers that uNKs play a role in the control of trophoblast invasion and spiral artery remodeling in human pregnancy and suggest that uNK cells in the late secretory phase and in early decidua may be important in initiating and maintaining decidualization. Alternatively, the death of uNK cells might be an early event in the onset of endometrial breakdown at menstruation (130–133).

In addition to this unique uNK cell, the endometrium contains other leukocyte subsets whose precise composition is menstrual cycle-dependent. These subsets include neutrophils and eosinophils (both rare until the premenstrual phase); macrophages; mast cells and T lymphocyte populations (present throughout the cycle but increasing perimenstrually) (13,133,134). Lymphoid follicles are commonly seen in the basalis of normal endometria (Fig. 40.27).

Plasma cells are routinely seen in postpartum endometrial samplings and as an associated feature in a variety of pathologic settings (endometrial polyps, endometrial carcinoma, etc.). It has traditionally been held that, outside these settings, plasma cells are normally not present in the endometrium and when identified suggest (usually subclinical) endometritis. Certainly this is plausible when large numbers are present, although some studies have raised questions about the clinical relevance of scattered plasma cells (135,136). In fact, small numbers of B lymphocytes and plasma cells can be detected in endometrial samples using flow cytometry (133).

Occasionally, cells with bean-shaped nuclei and abundant vacuolated lipid-containing cytoplasm are present in

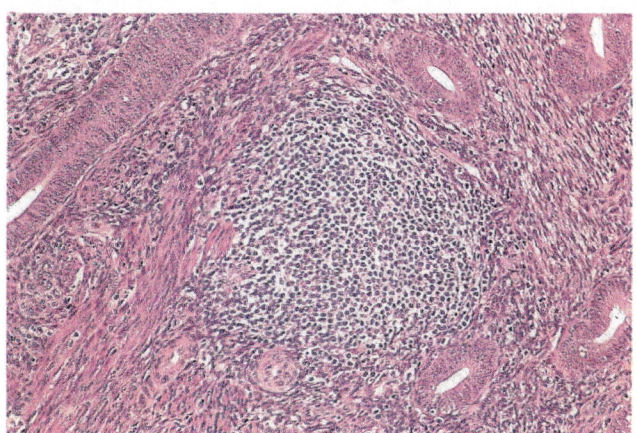

FIGURE 40.27 Lymphoid follicle. Scattered lymphoid follicles may be encountered in clinically normal women with otherwise unremarkable endometrium. When present in large numbers and when associated with plasma cells, this finding is pathologic.

the stroma of endometria stimulated by estrogen. These are termed stromal foam cells and probably represent modifications of endometrial stromal cells (Fig. 40.28). Similar appearing foam cells are seen as a component of an inflammatory infiltrate, particularly one produced by foreign material (e.g., keratin).

> **RETICULIN FRAMEWORK.** The endometrial stromal cells elaborate a reticulin framework that becomes progressively denser as the endometrium develops during the menstrual cycle, so that by the late secretory phase each stromal cell is enmeshed in reticulin. This framework undergoes dissolution during menstruation. The stromal intercellular space is also rich in high–molecular-weight mucopolysaccharides during the midproliferative and late secretory phase.

> **VASCULAR ELEMENTS.** The radial arteries of the endometrium derive from the myometrial arcuate system.

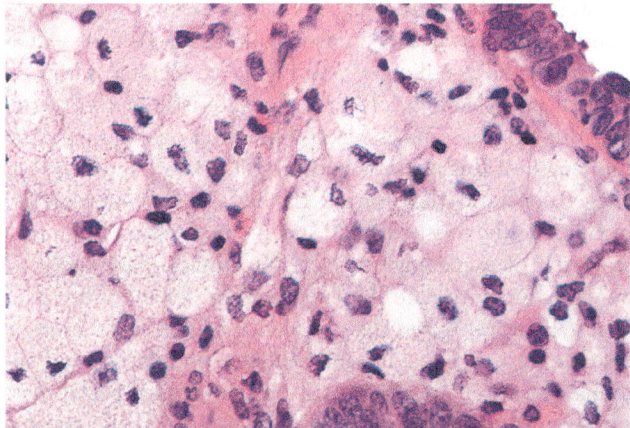

FIGURE 40.28 Stromal foam cells. Most likely these are modified endometrial stromal cells. In an inflammatory setting, stromal foam cells are probably macrophages.

As the radial arteries course toward the uterine cavity they give off basal branches and then continue as endometrial spiral arteries. The basal arteries are unresponsive to steroid hormones, whereas the spiral arteries respond to varying hormone levels both by proliferation and, during the luteal phase of the menstrual cycle, by intermittent contraction (137,138).

Angiogenesis, the formation of new vessels, is central to the menstrual cycle and to implantation and subsequent gestation. As concerns the menstrual cycle: There must be repair of the vessels ruptured during the menstrual phase, then rapid growth of vessels during the proliferative phase, further development of spiral arteries during the secretory phase and, to come full circle, the dismantling of the vasculature that leads into the menstrual phase (13). All these stages are closely monitored by activators and inhibitors (139–142).

During implantation and gestation angiogenesis is again pivotal in negotiating the hook-up of the feto-placental unit to the maternal circulation. This entails an extensive remodeling of the placental bed spiral arteries to form the utero-placental vessels (142–144).

> **ULTRASTRUCTURAL FEATURES AND IMMUNOHISTOCHEMISTRY** Both transmission and scanning electron microscopic study of the endometrium has produced an immense body of literature (115,145,146). Mention should be made of two distinctive ultrastructural features found in the early secretory glandular cell: the giant mitochondrion complex (142) and the nucleolar channel system (147). These two features seem to be the earliest postovulatory morphologic change in the endometrial glandular cell.

Normal endometrial and endocervical epithelium have some differences in their immunohistochemical profile. Endometrial glands are positive for low- and high–molecular-weight cytokeratins, vimentin, and occasionally CEA, while endocervical epithelium expresses CEA but is negative for vimentin and low–molecular-weight cytokeratin (99). The endometrial stroma and mesonephric remnants are typically strongly positive for CD10 while the endometrial and endocervical glands are not. Occasionally normal smooth muscle cells express CD10 and about 40% of leiomyomas contain CD10 positive cells usually focally. Both the endometrial stroma and smooth muscle express vimentin, muscle specific actin, smooth muscle actin, and Bcl-2. Smooth muscle cells typically express desmin and caldesmon whereas endometrial stromal cells do not. The combination of desmin (or caldesmon) and CD10 can be helpful in distinguishing smooth muscle tumors from endometrial stromal sarcoma.

The endometrium produces many secreted proteins that serve local cell signaling functions important for the developing endometrium and embryo. There is a large and growing body of literature concerning these products of endometrium, a topic beyond the scope of this chapter. However, there have been a number of excellent recent reviews of this subject (13,113,148–151).

Temporal Variations

Unlike morphologically unchanging epithelia, such as vagina or gastrointestinal mucosa, that have an essentially constant appearance throughout the cell's lifetime, the endometrium undergoes dramatic temporal morphologic changes. The changes are cyclic and particularly striking during the reproductive years. These changes can be conveniently considered under six headings: Newborn, premenarchal, perimenarchal, reproductive, perimenopausal, and postmenopausal years (113,152,153).

> **NEWBORN** The genitalia of the newborn girl respond to the high levels of circulating maternal and placental steroids by a transient burst of precocious development. The endometrium may be well developed and have either a proliferative or, less commonly, a secretory appearance. Within 2 weeks these changes have regressed, and the long hormonal quiescence of the premenarchal years begins. This quiescent period is characterized by a thin endometrium populated by inactive glands set within a spindled inactive stroma. Rarely, estrogen-secreting lesions of the ovary (follicular cysts, sex cord gonadal stromal tumors) may cause abnormal endometrial growth, with resulting abnormal bleeding as part of the syndrome of precocious pseudopuberty. The endometrium under these circumstances is proliferative or hyperplastic. This phenomenon shows that the inactive appearance of the endometrium during this period is secondary to a lack of hormonal stimulation (10).

> **MENARCHE** The onset of uterine bleeding (menarche) is one of the many changes that signal the maturation of the reproductive system. In the United States this usually occurs between 12 and 15 years of age. Characteristically, the perimenarchal period is marked by greater variability in the length of individual cycles than is seen in the reproductive years and by the occurrence of anovulatory cycles (153). Disordered proliferative endometria are commonly encountered in this setting (see section Disordered Proliferative Endometrium).

> **REPRODUCTIVE YEARS** The reproductive years are characterized by regularly occurring, roughly monthly, cycles, the end of which is signaled by menstrual bleeding (154,155). The dominant ovarian steroid secreted during the first half of the menstrual cycle is estradiol (E2), which induces endometrial proliferation. The second half of the cycle (beginning after ovulation) is hormonally dominated by both progesterone and estradiol, and this combination of hormones induces endometrial glandular secretion and stromal predecidualization. With the withdrawal of corpus luteum steroidal support, the endometrium is shed, setting the stage for the next cycle. These regularly recurring cycles may be interrupted by pregnancies, but after the termination of pregnancy, cycling is soon restored.

The biochemistry of the steroid molecules and their receptors responsible for the remarkable morphologic changes of the menstrual cycle have been the subject of intense study (156–158). Steroid molecules are hydrophobic and easily diffuse through cell membranes and freely enter all cells. The endometrium, vaginal mucosa, and other steroid-sensitive tissues are target organs by virtue of the presence of high-affinity, high-specificity, low-capacity saturable receptors for E2 and progesterone. These nucleus-based receptors are absent in nonresponsive cells. In addition to being highly responsive to circulating hormones, the endometrium also synthesizes substances such as glycoproteins that affect the hypothalamic–pituitary–ovary axis and the endometrium itself. A detailed description of hormone regulation is beyond the scope of this chapter, but several excellent reviews on the topic have been published and can be found in the general references listed at the end of the chapter. In broad terms, the steroid molecule combines with the appropriate receptor, and the steroid–receptor complex becomes associated with a nonhistone nucleoprotein. The net effect of this linkage is to alter both qualitatively and quantitatively DNA-dependent RNA transcription. The consequence is an altered profile of protein biosynthesis. Furthermore, the unique response of a particular target cell type depends on what specific growth and differentiation program is initiated by the steroidal signal. The endometrium is a major target organ for this continual barrage of steroidal information. It responds by undergoing the dramatic morphologic alterations that constitute the normal menstrual cycle, as well as producing proteins important for hypothalamic feedback, modulation of placental hormone secretion, regulation of macrophages, and regeneration after menses.

Morphology of the Normal Menstrual Cycle Endometrium

The first day of the menstrual cycle has conventionally been identified as the first day of menstrual flow. Menses usually lasts for fewer than 5 days and is followed by the endometrial proliferative phase, the length of which exhibits great variation (9 to 20 days), but on average lasts for 10 days. After ovulation, the coordinated and highly predictable series of stromal and glandular changes characteristic of the secretory (luteal) phase takes place. The traditional view is that the length of this phase is constant (14 days), and it is this alleged constancy that provides the basis for endometrial dating. Due to the sensitivity and specificity of serum hormonal studies, it is exceedingly rare for the surgical pathologist to be called upon to date the endometrium for infertility purposes. However, given the prevalence of polycystic ovarian disease, dysfunctional uterine bleeding, and iatrogenic hormonal use it remains important for the surgical pathologist to recognize when ovulation has occurred and the normal responses of the endometrium to various hormonal stimuli. The following discussion is a concise description of the normal menstrual cycle with more detailed information in the

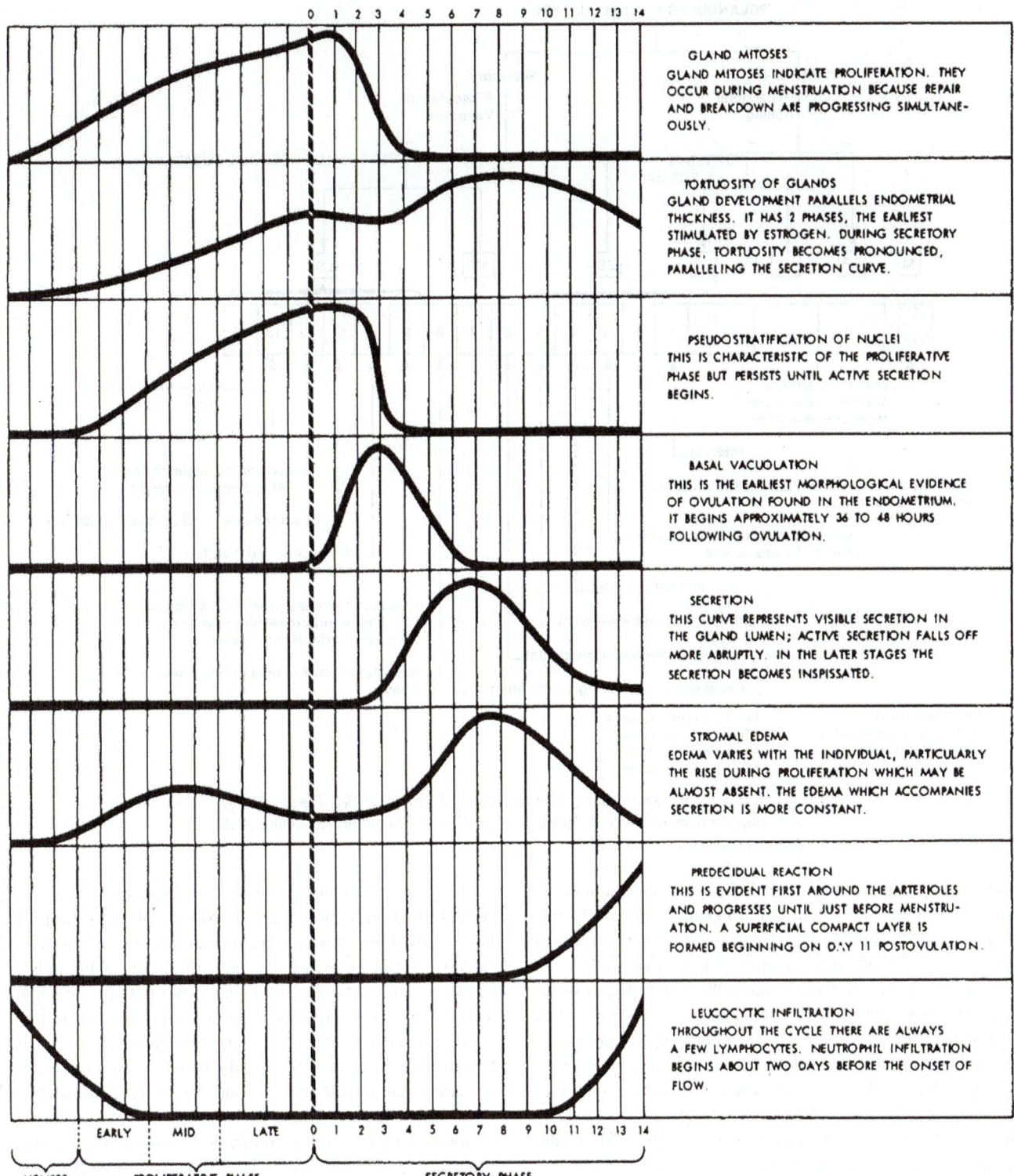

FIGURE 40.29 Approximate qualitative changes in eight morphologic criteria found to be most useful in dating human endometrium. From Marshall J. The physiology of the myometrium. In: Hertig A, Norris H, Abell M, eds. *The uterus.* Baltimore, MD: Williams & Wilkins; 1973:89–109.

accompanying figures (Figs. 40.29 and 40.30, Table 40.2) (112,113,123,159–161).

> **PROLIFERATIVE ENDOMETRIAL PHASE (OVARIAN FOLLICULAR PHASE)** The proliferative phase spans the time from the previous menstrual period to ovulation. The endometrium responds to rising estrogen levels by synchronous proliferation of glands, stroma, and vessels. During the first third of the proliferative phase (early proliferative), the rate of growth of all three of these elements is coordinated,

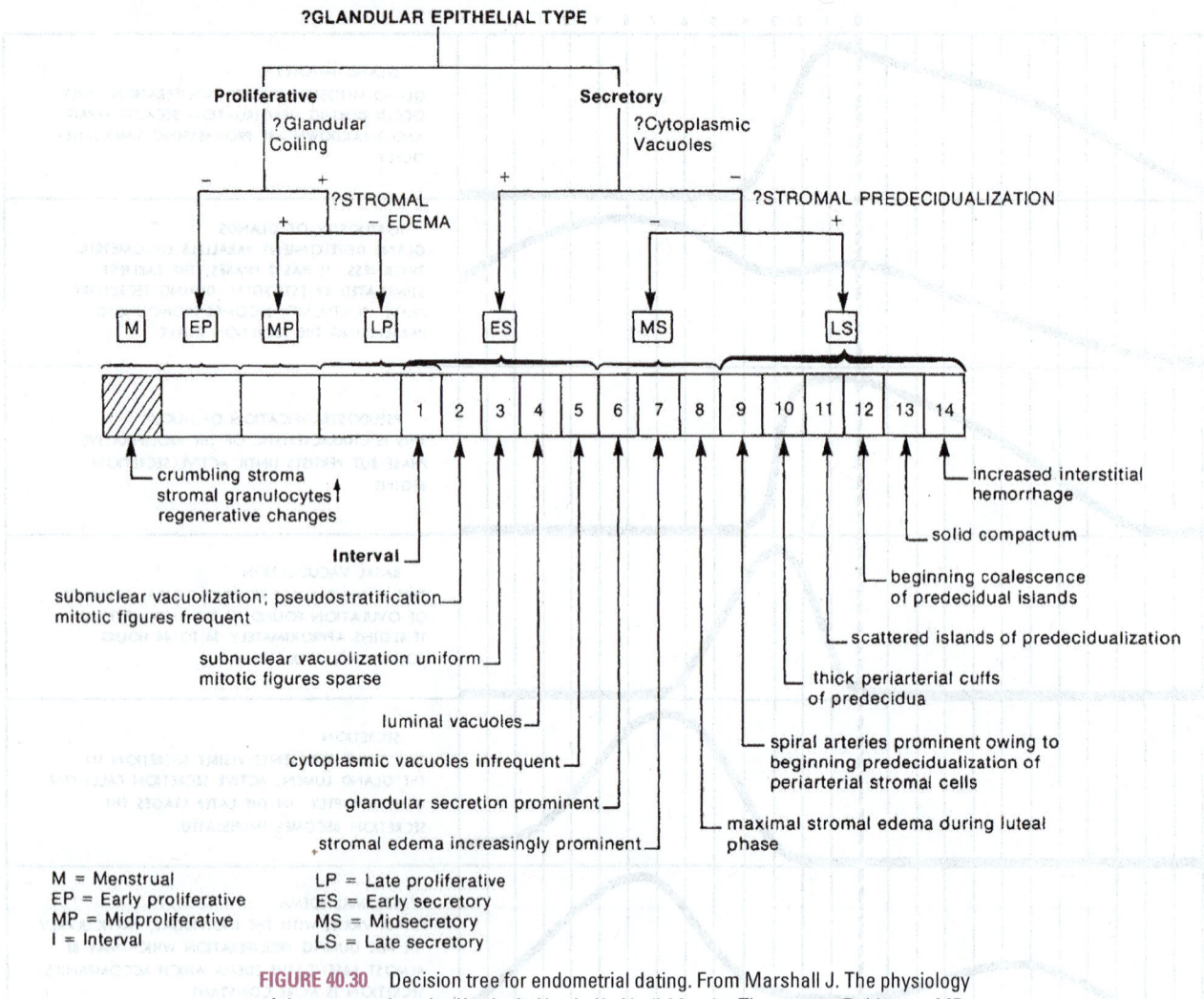

FIGURE 40.30 Decision tree for endometrial dating. From Marshall J. The physiology of the myometrium. In: Hertig A, Norris H, Abell M, eds. The uterus. Baltimore, MD: Williams & Wilkins; 1973:89–109.

and as a consequence both vessels and glands are noncoiled. After a few days the growth of both glands and vessels outstrips that of the stroma; as a result, these tubular structures become coiled (mid- and late proliferative) (Fig. 40.31).

The glands are lined by mitotically active pseudostratified columnar cells with high nuclear to cytoplasmic ratios and dense chromatin (Fig. 40.32). Mitotic figures are almost always easy to find. These cells are present throughout the proliferative phase and even into early secretion. After about 10 to 11 days, irregular subnuclear vacuoles begin to appear. During the last 2 days mitotic activity decreases, glandular coiling becomes more prominent, and vacuoles are easily found.

The interval period is the 48 hours between ovulation and the presence of uniformly vacuolated cells indicative of postovulatory day (POD) 2. Mitotic figures are present during this period, and the cells retain their proliferative nuclear features.

> ENDOMETRIAL SECRETORY PHASE (OVARIAN LUTEAL PHASE) Ovulation is mediated by the luteinizing hormone (LH) surge, a synchronous burst of LH and follicle-stimulating hormone secretion that peaks on the 14th day of a 28-day cycle. Ovulation occurs roughly 10 to 12 hours after this peak. The length of time from the last menstrual period to the day of ovulation for an individual woman is the length of her follicular phase. This surge of pituitary hormones initiates a complex series of events that results in the release of the oocyte from the developed tertiary follicle and the transformation of the follicle into a corpus luteum, which now secretes estradiol and large quantities of progesterone. The biosynthetic lifetime of the corpus luteum defines the ovarian luteal phase that corresponds to endometrial secretory development. Both ovarian and endometrial luteal phases last 14 days on the average, but this can be highly variable (see section Relevance of endometrial Dating to Diagnostic Surgical Pathologists below).

The endometrium, which has proliferated and has been primed by estrogen, responds to the simultaneous stimulation of estrogen and progesterone by differentiating in a distinctive fashion. The morphologic changes can be divided into four periods: interval, early secretory, midsecretory, and late secretory (Fig. 40.30). The first 24 to 36 hours of the secretory phase are morphologically silent because the

TABLE 40.2
Decision Tree for Endometrial Dating

What type of gland is present?
A. Proliferative gland (early proliferative, midproliferative, late proliferative, interval)
   Is the gland straight or coiled?
      Straight: Early proliferative
      Coiled: Midproliferative, late proliferative, interval
   Is there stromal edema?
      Yes: Midproliferative
      No: Late proliferative, interval
   Are there scattered subnuclear vacuoles present, but with less than 50% of the glands exhibiting uniform subnuclear vacuolization?
      No: Late proliferative
      Yes: Interval—consistent with but not diagnostic of POD 1
B. Secretory gland-vacuolated (early secretory)
   POD 2: Subnuclear vacuolization uniformly present, leading to exaggerated nuclear pseudostratification: (greater than 50% of the glands exhibit uniform subnuclear vacuolization); mitotic figures frequent
   POD 3: Subnuclear vacuoles and nuclei uniformly aligned; scattered mitotic figures
   POD 4: Vacuoles assume luminal position; mitotic figures rare
   POD 5: Vacuoles infrequent; secretion in lumen of gland, cells have a nonvacuolated secretory appearance
C. Secretory gland-nonvacuolated (midsecretory, late secretory, menstrual)
   Is there stromal predecidualization?
      No: Midsecretory
         POD 6: Secretion prominent
         POD 7: Beginning stromal edema
         POD 8: Maximal stromal edema
      Yes: Late secretory, menstrual
   Is there crumbling of the stroma?
      No: Late secretory
         POD 9: Spiral arteries first prominent
         POD 10: Thick periarterial cuffs of predecidual
         POD 11: Islands of predecidual in superficial compactum
         POD 12: Beginning coalescence of islands of predecidual
         POD 13: Confluence of surface islands; stromal granulocytes prominent
         POD 14: Extravasation of red cells in stroma; prominence of stromal granulocytes
      Yes: Menstrual
         Crumbling stroma, hemorrhage
         Intravascular fibrin thrombi
         Stromal granulocytes prominent
         Polymorphs present
         Late menstrual: Regenerative changes prominent

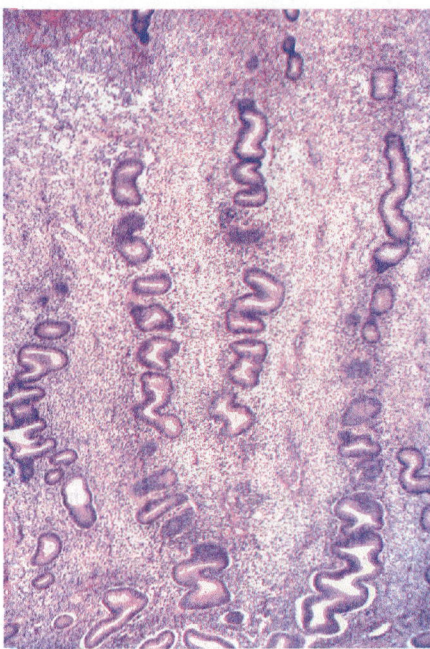

FIGURE 40.31 Midproliferative endometrium. Note the early coiling and synchronously developed glands.

The midsecretory phase lasts from PODs 5 to 9 and is characterized by nonvacuolated, prominently coiled secretory glands set within a spindled edematous stroma. Luminal secretion is most prominent during this period, and the overall appearance is one of glandular crowding (162). This glands to stroma ratio should not be mistaken for simple

endometrium for the most part retains its late proliferative appearance, although scattered nonuniform subnuclear vacuoles may appear. This morphologically indeterminate endometrium is termed "interval." The first unequivocal light microscopic indication that ovulation has occurred is the presence of uniform subnuclear vacuoles involving more than 50% of the endometrial glands. Recognizing this feature can aid the pathologist in excluding anovulatory cycling in an EMB. Over the next few days these vacuoles shift from a subnuclear to a supranuclear location. By the fifth POD, most of the secretion has been discharged into the gland lumen. The morphologic hallmark then of the early secretory phase (PODs 2 to 5) is the vacuolated gland (Fig. 40.33).

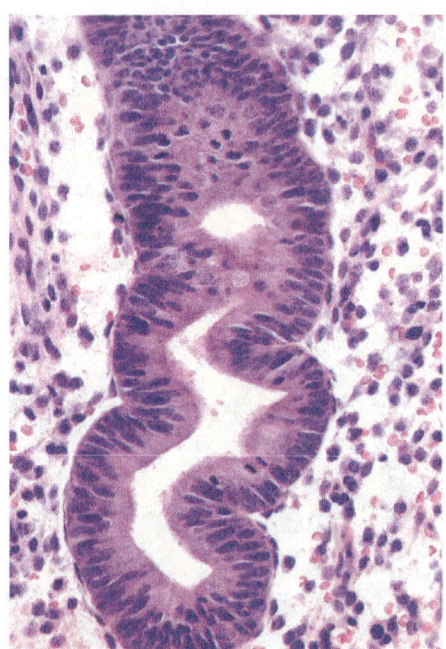

FIGURE 40.32 High-power view of a proliferative phase gland. The constituent cells are pseudostratified, and the characteristically elongate glandular nuclei have dense chromatin.

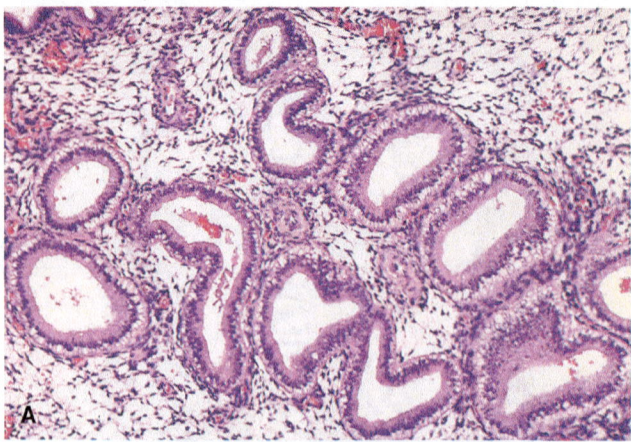
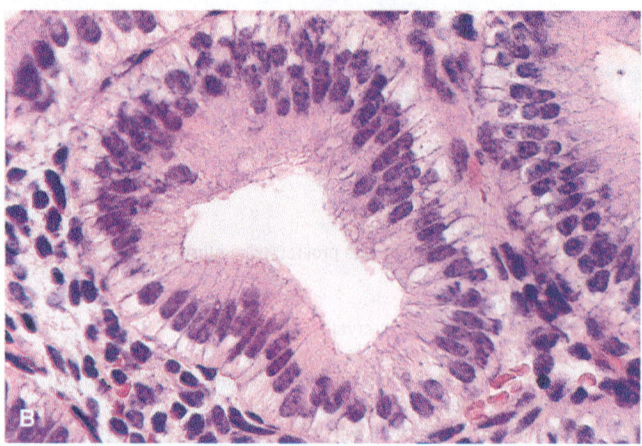

FIGURE 40.33 **A, B:** Early secretory endometrium with subnuclear vacuoles. The nuclei retain the dense chromatin of the proliferative phase. Uniformly present cytoplasmic vacuoles are the most useful marker of the first third of the secretory phase.

hyperplasia. The secretory cells usually have round somewhat vesicular nuclei. This serves to separate them from the nuclei found in early secretory phase cells (Fig. 40.34). The distinctive feature of the late secretory endometrium (PODs 10 to 14) is stromal predecidualization. This diagnostic stromal change is heralded by an increased prominence of the spiral arteries. By the tenth POD cuffs of predecidual cells are present around these arteries, initially involving the part of the vessel adjacent to the surface of the endometrium (Fig. 40.35). Subsequently, islands of predecidual cells appear in the superficial compactum. By POD 13 these islands become confluent. The extent of predecidualization is roughly paralleled by the degree of stromal infiltration by stromal granulocytes, although some investigators have

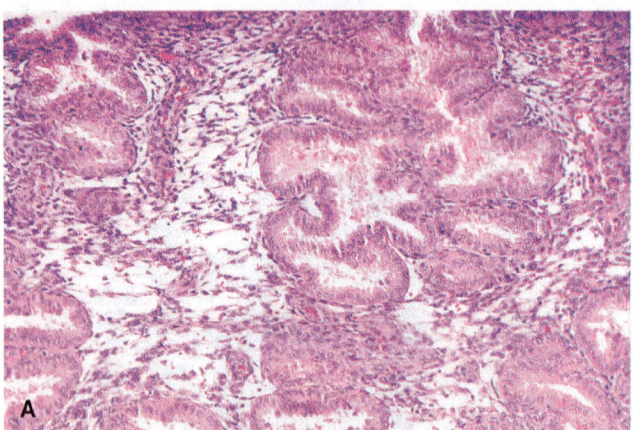
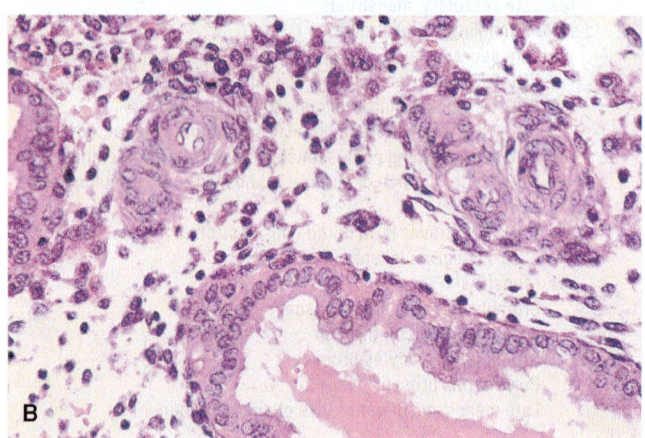
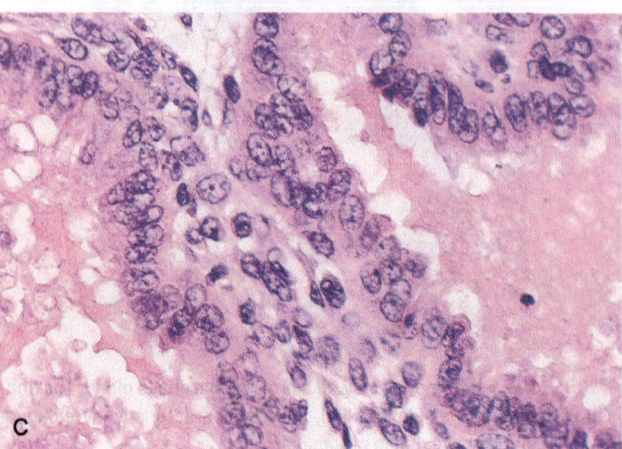

FIGURE 40.34 Midsecretory endometrium. The hallmarks of this period can be seen in these three photomicrographs. At low magnification (**A**) extreme glandular coiling and stromal edema are apparent. At a somewhat higher magnification (**B**) the coiled spiral arteries are seen within an edematous stroma. Perivascular predecidual reaction has not occurred. At yet higher magnification (**C**) the characteristically round vesicular nuclei of the midsecretory endometrium are apparent (contrast with proliferative phase nuclei in Fig. 40.23).

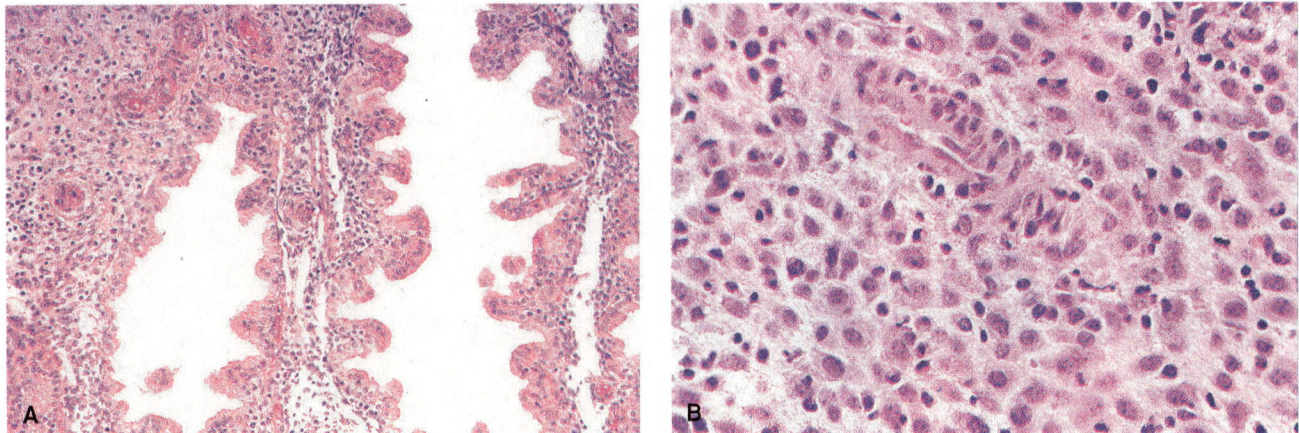

FIGURE 40.35 Late secretory endometrium. At low magnification (**A**) the serrated appearance of the gland reflects their coiled state. The stroma cells have undergone predecidual reaction. **B:** Predecidual reaction begins around the spiral arteries, and this reaction serves to distinguish midsecretory endometria from late secretory endometria.

suggested that the intensity of this infiltration is more closely correlated with the time of onset of menses (163). The appearance of the glands during the late secretory phase is not significantly different from their appearance during the midsecretory phase. They are lined by nonvacuolated secretory cells with round vesicular nuclei. During the later days of this period the glands typically have the saw-toothed appearance sometimes referred to as secretory exhaustion. As the late secretory phase progresses, the cells become apoptotic and apoptotic bodies accumulate within stromal macrophages.

> MENSTRUATION

> MENSTRUAL PHASE (CYCLE DAYS 1 TO 4). The abrupt withdrawal of both estrogen and progesterone accompanying the demise of the corpus luteum initiates menstrual bleeding. The molecular events initiating and guiding the controlled bleeding of menstruation are complex in contrast to the relatively straightforward light microscopic picture (164). The endometrium on the first day of menstrual bleeding (cycle day 1) is thin and compact. It is composed of the basalis and—relative to the fully developed secretory endometrium—a substantially shrunken, dense functionalis. The basalis maintains the relatively constant histologic appearance it has throughout the endometrial cycle. The functionalis thins mainly due to the withdrawal of interstitial fluid. The constituent glands and stroma of the functionalis fragment and crumble, often referred to as stromal breakdown. Fibrin thrombi appear in vessels and within the stroma. As the stroma disintegrates, the endometrial glands may artificially crowd together, giving the appearance of hyperplasia. In addition, the degenerative atypia of these glands and the necrotic background may suggest a diagnosis of malignancy (Fig. 40.36). The general strategy of not making a diagnosis of malignancy when well-preserved glands and stroma are absent should prevent such a mistake (Fig. 40.37).

By the second or third day the endometrium begins to repair and is completed by the fourth or fifth day. This early repair phase is thought by some to be estrogen independent as is the initial regrowth of the vasculature (165,166). Almost 50% of menstrual blood loss occurs on the first day in the majority of women (108,161,162).

> ENDOMETRIAL MORPHOLOGY DURING THE LUTEAL PHASE OF THE CYCLE OF CONCEPTION If implantation of a blastocyst occurs, it will be during the midsecretory phase (PODs 6 to 8), and this event is associated with a

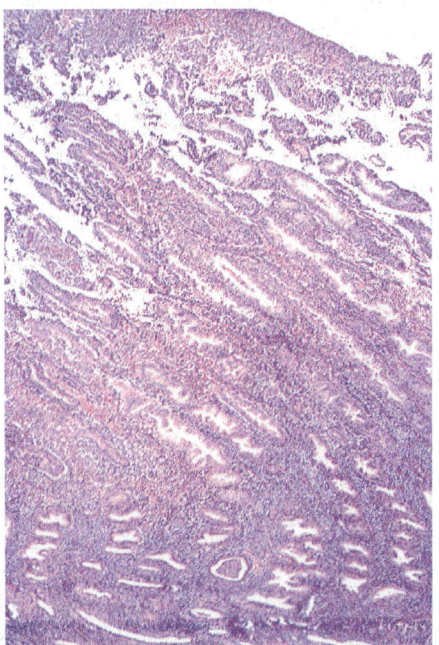

FIGURE 40.36 A low-power view of a menstrual endometrium showing the unresponsive basalis in the lower part of the photomicrograph and the functionalis disintegrating near the surface.

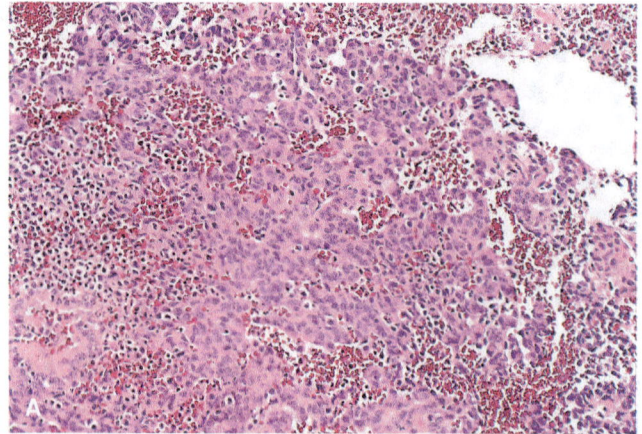
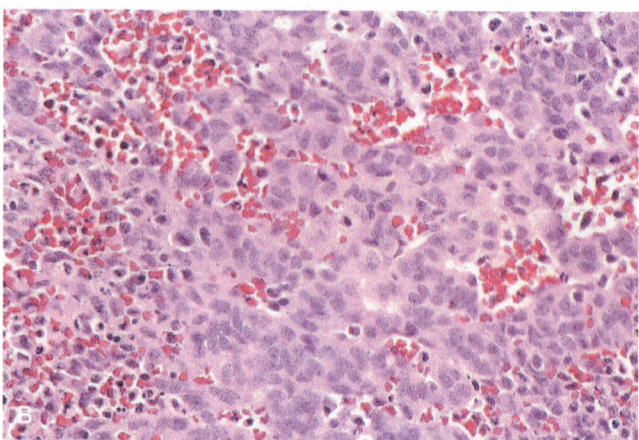
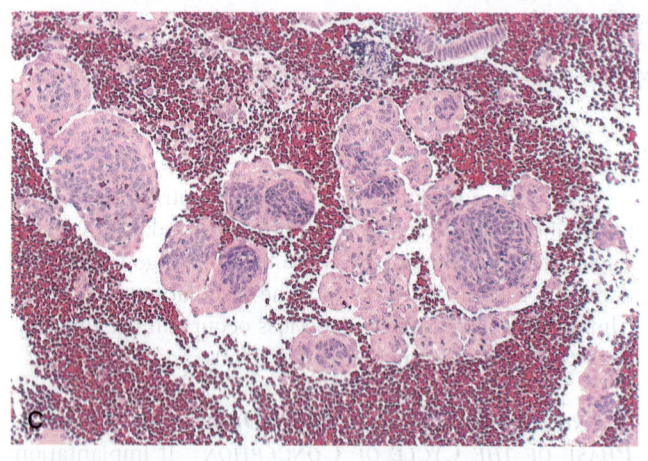

FIGURE 40.37 Stromal breakdown. Disintegrating endometrium may simulate endometrial malignancy. **A:** Sheets of disintegrating stromal cells may simulate an endometrial stromal neoplasm. **B:** Higher magnification shows individual cell necrosis and inflammation, findings that should raise the possibility of disintegrating non-neoplastic endometrium. **C:** Confirmation of this possibility is made by finding inflamed epithelium associated with degenerating stromal cells. In this case, characteristic epithelium-covered spherules are produced.

resurgence of glandular secretion and a persistence of stromal edema. After this time, biopsy findings will feature prominent glandular secretion (which in a nongravid cycle would have subsided), stromal edema, and stromal predecidualization (167,168).

The developing predecidua is gradually converted to decidua after POD 14 of the luteal phase of conception. This transformation is complete by the end of the first month of gestation. The fully developed decidual reaction is distinctive. Almost all of the endometrial stroma is converted into pavement-like sheets of epithelioid cells with prominent cytoplasmic margins and central vesicular nuclei (Fig. 40.26). In the superficial portion of the functionalis, the glands are compressed and their lining becomes flattened and endothelium-like. This compact sheetlike zone, the zona compactum, overlies saw-toothed scalloped glands, the zona spongiosum, which continue to exhibit secretory features. Many of the glands in the spongiosum are lined by cells with enlarged nuclei that often have atypical nuclear features approaching those of the AS reaction (Fig. 40.38). Scattered "stromal granulocytes" (uterine NK cells) are present. Decidual cells may exhibit substantial nuclear pleomorphism and cytologic atypia. This is particularly prominent in the region of the implantation site. In addition, this region is also infiltrated by intermediate trophoblastic cells, which normally have a bizarre cytologic appearance. These cells are positive for both keratin and human placental lactogen (hPL). The infiltration of decidua and the underlying myometrium by trophoblasts in the past has been termed "syncytial metritis," not a particularly felicitous label because the process has little to do with inflammation (Fig. 40.39). This "implantation site reaction" is diagnostic of intrauterine pregnancy (169). Both placental site reaction and decidual atypia may incorrectly suggest

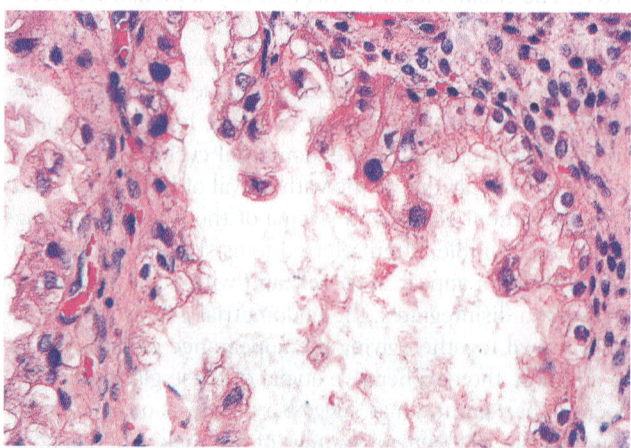

FIGURE 40.38 Gestational endometrium. This gland is lined by cells with enlarged dense nuclei characteristic of the Arias-Stella reaction.

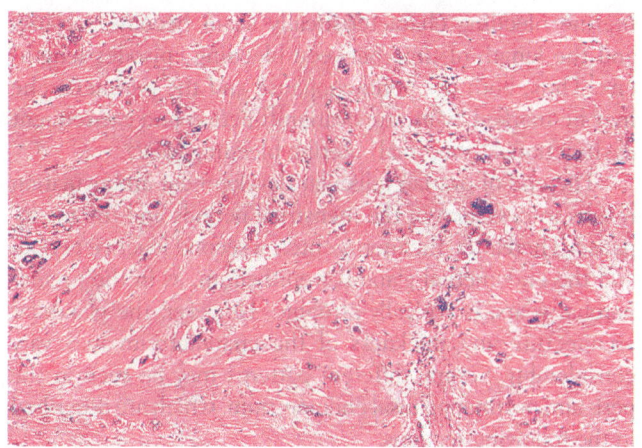

FIGURE 40.39 Myometrium beneath an implantation site containing infiltrating trophoblasts. This must not be misinterpreted as evidence of gestational trophoblastic disease.

malignancy, but confusion with adenocarcinoma is avoided by noting the secretory setting of these findings, as well as the clinical history.

This decidual reaction occurs in the setting of high progesterone stimulation and can also be seen in extrauterine (ectopic) pregnancy, iatrogenic use of progestational agents, or with persistence of the corpus luteum unassociated with pregnancy (e.g., corpus luteum cyst). For this reason, intrauterine implantation should only be diagnosed in the presence of chorionic villi or the presence of intermediate trophoblasts associated with enlarged vessels replaced by hyaline, or with fragments of fibrinoid matrix (169).

Distressingly, on rare occasions, the finding of trophoblastic tissue in a curetting does not exclude an ectopic gestation and suggests that when clinical suspicion is high the presence of either chorionic villi or an implantation site should not preclude further workup of a possible ectopic pregnancy (170).

Previous intrauterine pregnancy is strongly suggested in the postpartum endometrium by the presence of cuffs of hyalinized decidua around sclerotic ectatic spiral arteries. The decidual cells composing this cuff often have hyperchromatic smudged and degenerate nuclei, and the vessels are often thrombosed. These findings have been referred to as subinvolution of the placental site and can be responsible for postpartum hemorrhage (171). This presumably occurs because these severely altered vessels are incapable of contraction. With time the foci of hyalinization shrink and the nuclei may disappear, leaving a small pink scar resembling an ovarian corpus atreticum. These distinctive foci have been referred to as pregnancy plaques, and they may persist in the basalis for many years. Similar lesions featuring intermediate trophoblasts have been termed placental site nodule (PSN) and placental site plaque (171). Occasionally, a PSN or exaggerated placental site can be confused for a gestational trophoblastic tumor (GTT) such as placental site trophoblastic tumor (PSTT) or epithelioid trophoblastic tumor (ETT). While conventional H&E morphology is still very useful in distinguishing PSNs and plaques, immunohistochemical profiles can also be helpful. Studies over the last two decades have shown that there are a variety of intermediate trophoblasts involved in implantation and establishing vascular connections to the maternal blood flow. These trophoblasts seem to have distinct immunohistochemical properties, some of which are shared with the cells of GTTs. An exaggerated placental site is characterized by infiltration of individual cells with preservation of normal structures and mitoses are essentially absent. Placental site trophoblastic tumors are characterized by mitotically active confluent masses of cells that disrupt normal architectures. All trophoblasts express pancytokeratins, so while this may be helpful in highlighting the trophoblasts it does little to predict the aggressive potential of the proliferation. Kurman et al. have established algorithms for evaluating PSNs and trophoblastic tumors, using a combination of hPL, p63, and Ki67. Briefly, the intermediate trophoblasts of an exaggerated placental site is hPL positive, p63 negative, and has a Ki67 activity of less than 1%. A PTT will have the same immunohistochemical profile except the Ki67 is much greater. The intermediate trophoblasts in a PSN are hPL negative, p63 positive, and have a Ki67 activity of less than 10%. Epithelioid trophoblastic tumor can sometimes be confused with a PSN but has a Ki67 activity of greater than 10%. Occasionally, the diagnostic dilemma is between PSN and squamous cell carcinoma; in this scenario inhibin and cytokeratin 18 can be useful as PSN is positive for both of these antibodies while squamous cell carcinomas are negative (172–174).

Hyperprogestational states (particularly pregnancy) are sometimes associated with the distinctive glandular change to which AS first drew attention in 1954 and that now bears his name (175,176). Most commonly this change is encountered in endometrial glands, but on occasion it may be present in foci of endometriosis or adenomyosis, in endocervical glands, in fallopian tube epithelium, or in the glands within polyps. The AS phenomenon characteristically involves a focus of tightly packed glands whose extreme coiling and collapse throw the lining epithelium into prominent papillary folds. This epithelium is composed of cells exhibiting marked nuclear pleomorphism and hyperchromatism. The nuclei typically have a smudged appearance. The cell cytoplasm may be strikingly hypervacuolated and cleared (clear cells) or densely eosinophilic (dark cells) (Fig. 40.38). One or the other cell type may predominate from area to area. Occasionally, the eosinophilic cells may line the glands in a hobnail fashion. Mitotic figures are only rarely present. Elsewhere the endometrium usually exhibits the other changes one would anticipate with progestational stimulation, such as secretory glands and a stromal decidual reaction.

An endometrial AS change may be present in a variety of clinical settings, including normal intrauterine pregnancy, extrauterine pregnancy, gestational trophoblastic disease, and persistent corpus luteum. In a retrospective review of patients coded as having AS reaction, 16% had an extrauterine gestation. It also may be produced by the administration of ovulation-inducing drugs or progestational agents (175).

Because of the marked nuclear atypia of the epithelium lining the closely packed glands, the AS phenomenon can be confused with adenocarcinoma, particularly with the architectural and cytologic features of clear cell carcinoma. This difficulty largely can be avoided by remembering that the AS phenomenon occurs in a secretory setting; that is, more conventional secretory glands and decidualized or predecidualized stroma are usually found elsewhere in the specimen and the patient is premenopausal. Moreover, glandular mitotic figures tend not to be a prominent feature, although they may occasionally be encountered (177). Clear cell carcinoma (like any carcinoma) is fundamentally a proliferative process, and the constituent cells not only possess malignant features but also exhibit mitotic activity. Most importantly, clear cell carcinoma of the endometrium develops almost exclusively in postmenopausal women. Immunochemistry has been useful in separating the two; p53 and Ki-67 staining are absent in AS and present in clear cell carcinoma (178).

Occasionally in a gestational setting glandular nuclei may exhibit marked nuclear clearing reminiscent of herpetic infections (Fig. 40.40) (179).

> **ENDOMETRIAL VASCULATURE** The transition from the endometrium of early gestation to that of fully developed pregnancy is marked by the accelerated development of the endometrial vasculature, resulting in increased thickness of the spiral arteries, as reflected in their mean cross-sectional diameter (180,181).

> **PERIMENOPAUSAL AND POSTMENOPAUSAL YEARS** With the waning of hormonal function in the fifth decade of life, a woman enters the perimenopause, during which time uterine bleeding characteristically again becomes erratic, and the length of time between bleeding episodes lengthens. Thus, both the perimenopause and the perimenarche may be marked by erratic ovarian function and consequent dysfunctional (abnormal) uterine bleeding (182).

The end of ovarian follicular development and ovulation results in cessation of the menstrual periods and the menopause. Thereafter, the uterus enters a second inactive period, and the endometrial glandular epithelium, as in the premenarchal years, is typically atrophic. However, the glandular architecture and thickness of the endometrium may vary considerably. Several different patterns may be seen in the peri- and postmenopausal endometrium, which are described in the following sections.

> **ATROPHIC ENDOMETRIUM** Atrophic epithelium is nonstratified and composed of a single layer of flattened to cuboidal cells. Mitotic figures are not present, the nucleus-to-cytoplasm ratio is high, and there is usually no specific cytoplasmic differentiation, although cilia may be present. The defining and only constant feature of atrophic endometria is the atrophic epithelial lining of its constituent glands, which may have any configuration, including cystic dilatation and glandular crowding. The stroma is spindled and is neither predecidualized nor decidualized. The nuclei may be densely pyknotic (as in postmenopausal endometria or endometrial polyps) or plump (as in endometria associated with oral contraceptives). Stromal disintegration may be present (Fig. 40.41) (183–185).

Atrophic endometria can occur in a variety of clinical settings. It is the normal state during the premenarchal and later postmenopausal years. During the reproductive years, atrophic patterns may be seen in association with premature ovarian failure or, more commonly, in patients taking hormonal contraceptives.

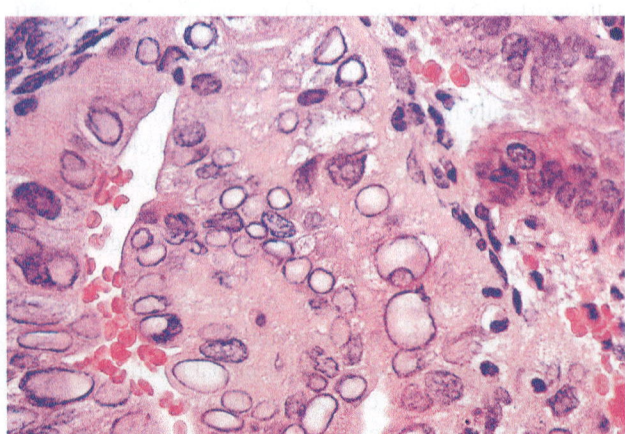

FIGURE 40.40 Nuclear clearing of the glandular cells in the endometrium may be seen in a gestational setting. This change should not be misconstrued as evidence of herpes virus infection.

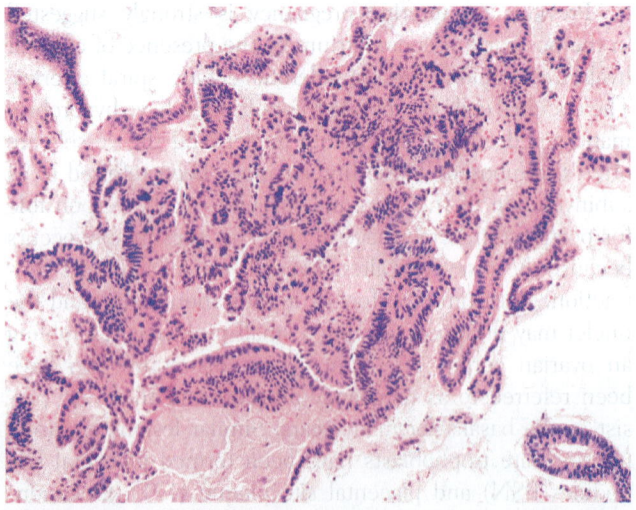

FIGURE 40.41 Endometrial atrophy as seen in an endometrial sampling. On occasion, atrophic surface epithelium may be removed in coiled masses and simulate hyperplasia because the glands are closely approximated.

❯ **WEAKLY PROLIFERATIVE ENDOMETRIUM** Weakly proliferative epithelium is nonstratified, although some degree of nuclear pseudostratification may be present, and its constituent cells are thin. In contrast to normal proliferative endometrium, atrophic endometrial cells have a paucity of mitotic figures, denser nuclear chromatin, and more disorganized glands. The glands may be of any configuration, but the glands-to-stroma ratio is almost always near unity or there can be a slight stromal predominance. The stroma is spindled; stromal cell nuclei may be densely pyknotic or plump.

The morphologic variability of the weakly proliferative endometrium parallels that of the atrophic endometrium. The difference between them is solely based on the appearance of the epithelial cells: Weakly proliferative rather than flattened or cuboidal. The clinical settings in which these two endometria occur overlap considerably and the weakly proliferative patterns are a histologic transition between normal proliferation and atrophy. Weakly proliferative endometria are most often encountered in patients in the peri- or postmenopausal years whose endometria appear to be weakly supported by low levels of endogenous or exogenous estrogen. This pattern is normal in the hormonally hyporesponsive lower uterine segment of the normally cycling premenopausal women.

During the perimenopausal period some women are prone to chronic stromal breakdown due to the inconsistent hormonal mileu and anovulatory cycles. This can result in surface metaplasias such as eosinophilic or papillary metaplasia. The former is characterized by enlarged cells with abundant pink cytoplasm with conspicuous necleoli. The later often form small papillary aggregates which layer the surface epithelium but can be detached and free floating in an endometrial sampling. When atypia is present in these cells, this benign process can be mistaken for serous papillary carcinoma or its precursor endometrial intraepithelial neoplasia. In this setting Ki67 and p53 can be useful adjuvant tests as eosinophilic metaplasia has a low Ki67 index and is usually only weakly or focally positive for p53 while EIC is often strongly and diffusely positive for both. While this panel will not give a definitive answer, it can prove helpful in confirming the histologic impression (186).

❯ **DISORDERED PROLIFERATIVE ENDOMETRIUM** Disordered proliferation is the morphologic bridge spanning normally proliferating endometrium and endometrial hyperplasia. It is the endometrial pattern encountered in women experiencing sporadic anovulatory cycles and thus is most commonly encountered in the perimenopausal and perimenarchal years. It is also commonly seen in women receiving estrogen therapy. Disordered proliferation differs from normal proliferation by virtue of a loss of synchrony of glandular development so that some glands are tubular, whereas others are cystically dilated or have complex shapes. Budding may be present so that there may be a shift in the glands-to-stroma ratio in favor of the glands, but this shift is usually focal and never more than 2:1. It is common in disordered proliferative pattern to have focal glandular crowding but when the

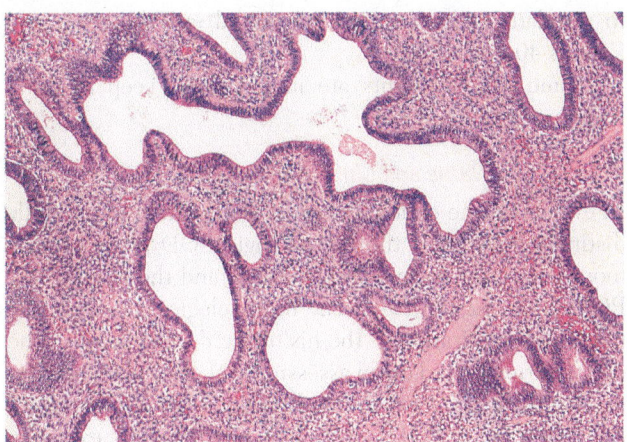

FIGURE 40.42 Disordered proliferation is the result of anovulatory cycles and is normal during the perimenopausal years. It is often found in the endometrium of women receiving estrogen therapy. Disordered proliferation is characterized by nonsynchronous growth of the glands including budding, but the glands-to-stroma ratio is unity or with a slight glandular predominance. This pattern of endometrial growth serves as a bridge between normal proliferation and hyperplasia.

glandular predominance is so marked that diffusely there is a shift in the glands to stroma ratio of 3:1 in favor of the glands, a diagnosis of hyperplasia is warranted (Fig. 40.42).

Histologically, the variously shaped glands are lined by normal proliferative cells with elongate dense nuclei that are most often pseudostratified. Mitotic figures are usually present and may be numerous. Stromal cells are spindled with plump nuclei. There is no evidence that this pattern is a marker for an increased risk for the subsequent development of endometrial carcinoma.

Relevance of Endometrial Dating to Diagnostic Surgical Pathologists

Due to the very sophisticated ability to measure serum steroid and gonadotropin levels, the EMB no longer plays the significant role it used to in the evaluation of the infertility patient. Setting aside organic causes of infertility, the EMB, functioning as a bioassay, is unreliable in separating fertile from infertile women. This is due largely to the substantial morphologic heterogeneity of the normally functioning endometrium (187–192).

On the very rare occasion an EMB is obtained for fertility evaluation, its chief function is to determine whether ovulation has occurred and documenting anovulatory cycles (which would point toward an ovarian factor in the patient's infertility). Organic reproductive tract disease may be detected on the EMB such as endometrial polyps, leiomyomas, endometritis, hyperplasia, or carcinoma (192–194).

What follows is an abbreviated version of endometrial dating for a reference and for those rare occasions a pathologist is asked to provide a fine-tuned morphologic date (i.e., more than proliferative, early, mid, or late secretory). The precise details of the morphologic patterns corresponding to standard cycle dates are presented in Table 40.2 and Figures 40.29 and 40.30.

Some general points are important to keep in mind when using these aids.

Morphologic Dates and Chronologic Dates

In evaluating the endometrium, it is important to carefully distinguish between the morphologic POD assigned to a morphologically normal endometrium and the chronologic POD (112,152,195,196). The morphologic date is a summary characterization of the histologic development of the endometrium based on an assessment of glandular and stromal features. The morphologic findings may be summarized either in terms of PODs, cycle days, or phases. For example, the morphologic pattern associated with a particular "standard" POD is assigned the number of that day; for example, POD 12 refers to the pattern seen on POD 12 of the "standard" cycle. Equivalently, this morphologic information can be conveyed using cycle day or phase (e.g., late secretory).

Endometrial Dating should be Reported as a Range of 2 Days

It is now known that both the follicular and luteal phases vary among women and not all women have a standard 28-day cycle (197). Adding to this biologic heterogeneity is the poor interobserver reproducibility of the conventional Noyes' dating.

Noyes and Haman and subsequently others reported poor agreement on single day morphologic date designation of an endometrium and significantly better agreement for a 2-day designation (154,198–201). As a consequence, the results of endometrial dating should be reported as a range of 2 days to reflect this variability.

Determining Whether the Patient has Ovulated?

During the late luteal phase the presence of a late secretory endometrium means ovulation. Deciding whether ovulation has occurred in the early luteal phase is more problematic. The characteristic light microscopic postovulatory secretory changes in the endometrium lag behind actual ovulation by at least 1 day. A biopsy on POD 2 usually reveals subnuclear vacuoles in the vast majority of glandular cells in the superficial functionalis but these may be spotty (interval pattern). Such vacuolization may be seen in late proliferative endometria, as well as in other types of nonsecretory endometria and is, for this reason, not diagnostic of ovulation. Because of the ambiguous morphologic picture in the early postovulatory period, EMBs are usually obtained well into the presumed luteal phase of the cycle, preferably on PODs 11 to 13. We require uniform subnuclear vacuolization in 50% of the glands before diagnosing the earliest morphologic evidence of ovulation, which is usually present by POD 3.

Some Practical Details

Accurate endometrial dating requires attention to a number of details (195). Dating features should be sought only in fragments of endometrial functionalis, which are lined by surface epithelium; fragments of basalis and lower uterine segment should be ignored. The assigned date should be of the most developed area and should be based on features near the surface epithelium (195).

The preconditions for assigning a morphologic date to an endometrium are described as follows. Assigning a date to an EMB is obviously not possible in the absence of an adequate specimen, in a noncycling endometrium (e.g., nonsecretory pattern other than proliferative), in a patient being treated with medication that alters the morphology of the endometrium, or in an endometrium that is inflamed or that houses an intrauterine device. Thus, a precondition for applying the dating criteria is that one is dealing with a roughly normal endometrial pattern. Scanning power examination should establish the presence of pattern uniformity (apart from the expected variation due to sectioning randomly oriented fragments and normal out of phase curettage inhabitants such as fragments of the lower uterine segment, cervical epithelium, and stratum basalis), the absence of significant budding and branching of glands, and the absence of necrosis and inflammation. Examination at higher power should exclude the presence of significant epithelial nuclear atypia and the absence of significant numbers of stromal plasma cells.

A checklist for the contents of the pathology report of EMBs is provided in Table 40.3.

Endometrial–Myometrial Junction

The endometrial–myometrial junction is normally irregular, a phenomenon that must be kept in mind when assessing the presence or absence of myoinvasion by endometrial adenocarcinoma and in diagnosing superficial adenomyosis (Fig. 40.22).

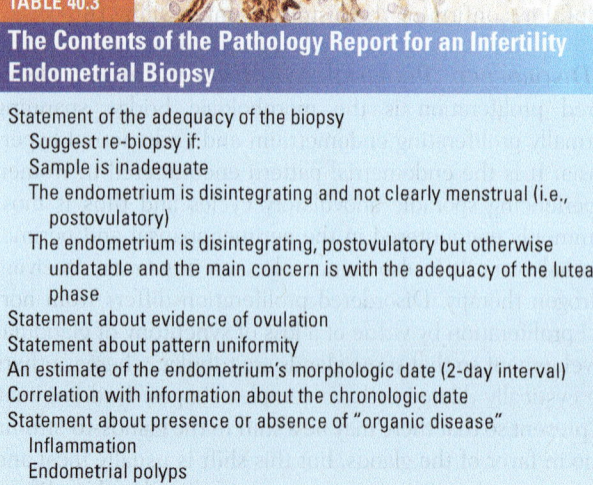

TABLE 40.3

The Contents of the Pathology Report for an Infertility Endometrial Biopsy

Statement of the adequacy of the biopsy
   Suggest re-biopsy if:
   Sample is inadequate
   The endometrium is disintegrating and not clearly menstrual (i.e., postovulatory)
   The endometrium is disintegrating, postovulatory but otherwise undatable and the main concern is with the adequacy of the luteal phase
Statement about evidence of ovulation
Statement about pattern uniformity
An estimate of the endometrium's morphologic date (2-day interval)
Correlation with information about the chronologic date
Statement about presence or absence of "organic disease"
   Inflammation
   Endometrial polyps
   Submucous leiomyomas

Apoptosis and the Endometrium

The role of programmed cell death or apoptosis in the remodeling of the endometrium was mentioned earlier in this chapter. Apoptosis and its hormonal control in both human and animal endometrium is an area of active investigation by a number of groups (202–205).

Withdrawal of progesterone in the rabbit endometrium correlates with the development of apoptosis (206–209).

Bcl-2 is a proto-oncogene initially described in the (14,18) translocation in follicular lymphoma. It has been shown to prolong cell survival by preventing apoptosis. Gompel et al. studied Bcl-2 expression immunohistochemically in the normal endometrium (210). They found that Bcl-2 predominated in glandular cells and reached a maximum at the end of the follicular phase but disappeared at the onset of secretory activity. Maia et al. found a precipitous drop in Bcl-2 after ovulation, further supporting an increase in Bcl-2 in response to estrogen and a decrease in response to progesterone (211). In addition, this group found an elevated p53 expression in the proliferative phase but a drop in the late luteal phase. These results strongly suggest hormone-dependent regulation of Bcl-2 expression and cell cycling.

The role of tumor necrosis factor alpha (TNF-α) in the induction of apoptosis was explored by Tabibzadeh et al. (212). They found that the TNF receptor, as well as Fas protein were expressed in endometrial epithelium throughout the entire menstrual cycle and were most prominent in the basalis. They concluded that endometrial epithelium, by expressing receptors for TNF-α and Fas protein can respond to ligands that regulate apoptosis.

Normal findings in the endometrium that have relevance to histopathologic differential diagnosis are shown in Table 40.4.

MYOMETRIUM

The bulk of the myometrium comprises smooth muscle cells, but an important contribution is made by extracellular components such as collagen and elastin. The smooth muscle within the corpus is more concentrated relative to collagen and elastin than the muscle in either the cervix or the lower uterine segment. This distribution of muscle is consistent with the passive role of the cervix during parturition; the uterine contents propelled by fundal contractions are thought to passively dilate a cervix previously softened by the action of collagenase. The uterine smooth muscle cells are spindled, with blunt-ended fusiform nuclei. Their cytoplasmic volume depends on the cycle and whether the patient is pregnant (214–217). Scattered normal mitotic figures may be encountered, particularly during the secretory phase of the endometrial cycle (217,218). Characteristic ultrastructural features of smooth muscle include (a) numerous dense, 60- to 80-A myofilaments without cross striations, which almost fill the cytoplasm; (b) small round dense bodies along the trajectory of the filaments; (c) dense plaques arranged along the inner aspect of the plasma membrane; and (d) plasma membrane–related vesicles that may play a role in ionized calcium movement across the plasma membrane during contraction. In addition, there is the usual complement of cytoplasmic organelles, including smooth and rough endoplasmic reticulum, mitochondria, and a Golgi apparatus. Typically these organelles arrange themselves around the nucleus, which often has an irregular shape. These ultrastructural features reflect the dual function of the uterine myocyte: Muscular contraction and collagen and elastin synthesis. The ultrastructural appearance varies with the levels of circulating steroidal hormones. In particular, estrogen appears to sharply increase myocyte protein synthesis. This correlates morphologically in an increased volume of rough endoplasmic reticulum and increased numbers of cytoplasmic contractile elements. The biochemistry and electrophysiology of the myometrium have been extensively reviewed (217,219,220). The histologic and ultrastructural appearance of smooth muscle cells differ substantially from those of the endometrial stromal cell. These differences are set out in Table 40.5. However, it should be noted that cells with a hybrid smooth muscle–stromal phenotype occur normally at the endometrial–myometrial junction and that this phenotypic ambiguity is sometimes expressed by spindle cell neoplasms of the uterine corpus (221). Some uterine smooth muscle cells have been shown to express some classes of keratins (222–225). The immunohistochemical profile of myometrial cells is presented in Table 40.5.

Pregnancy-Related Changes

To accommodate the growing fetus and to prepare for its role in fetal expulsion, the uterus undergoes a 10-fold increase in size and weight during pregnancy both by hypertrophy and to a much lesser extent by hyperplasia. Normal mitotic figures are often increased and may be present in large numbers. Uterine growth during pregnancy appears to be largely promoted by estradiol, whereas progesterone probably functions to inhibit uterine contractions during gestation. The light microscopic appearance of the hypertrophied uterine smooth muscle cells of pregnancy is distinctive. They are enlarged and have abundant, rather glassy cytoplasm and vesicular elongate nuclei with occasionally prominent nucleoli. Changes occur in the ultrastructural appearance of the smooth muscle cells as well. In addition to an increase in size and the number of myofilaments, there is a striking increase in the number of gap junctions (109,226). These establish the contact between cells required for the coordinated uterine contractions that expel the term infant (227). These myometrial changes are closely coordinated with the dramatic structural changes of the cervix required for cervical effacement (see section Uterine Cervix). In the postpartum period, the uterus undergoes an extraordinary

TABLE 40.4
Normal Findings in the Endometrium That Have Relevance to Histopathologic Differential Diagnosis

Findings	Diagnostic Confusion	Suggestions for Resolution	References
"Glands within glands" this can occur from trauma of D&C (telescoping) and tangential cutting	**Endometrial hyperplasia:** Rolled up carpet effect may simulate the architectural complexity of hyperplasia or carcinoma	This artifact is usually only focal and often at the periphery or otherwise normal fragments of functionalis. Check that epithelium is identical to architecturally normal glands in the sample.	
Strips of normal surface epithelium Commonly seen with atrophic endometrium	**Endometrial Hyperplasia/Carcinoma:** Rolled up carpet effect may simulate the architectural complexity of hyperplasia or carcinoma	In contrast to hyperplasia and carcinoma, the rolled up atrophic endometrium is cytologically bland and mitotically inactive.	(165,185)
Lower uterine segment	**Dating problem:** The glands respond weakly at best to hormones and the stroma is often fibrous	Look for mucinous epithelial component. Unless the sample is inadequate for dating the endometrium, there will be other fragments around with an appearance more typical of functionalis.	(189)
Normal basalis	**Dating problem:** The glands respond weakly at best to hormones and the stroma is inactive	When assigning a morphologic date to an endometrial fragment, use only glands in close approximation to surface epithelium	
Ciliated cells	**Adenocarcinoma:** Intraepithelial ciliated cells have rounded pear-shaped contours and open rounded nuclei with nucleoli	Look for cilia. Endometria containing ciliated cells have a polymorphous appearance; the cytologic features are uniform within each subpopulation of cells.	
Foam cells	**Endometritis:** Foam cells are commonly encountered in hypoestrogenic settings and are thought to be one differentiated form of endometrial stromal cell	Look for plasma cells to establish the diagnosis of chronic endometritis. Macrophages (xanthoma cells) with foamy cytoplasm may occur in the endometrium as a component of a chronic inflammatory process. Commonly seen as a reaction to a foreign body or to keratin (e.g., in setting of proliferations shedding keratin).	(135,213)
Arias-Stella reaction	**Adenocarcinoma:** Particularly clear cell carcinoma	Clear cell carcinoma is most frequent encountered in postmenopausal women. Arias-Stella reaction usually does not feature mitotic figures, which are almost always easily found in clear cell carcinoma. A more difficult problem is distinguishing clear cell carcinoma from Arias-Stella reaction in a postmenopausal woman who is taking progestational medication.	(174,176,177)
Implantation site	**Gestational trophoblastic disease:** Early gestations may mimic choriocarcinoma. The often bizarre shapes of trophoblastic cells may raise the possibility of choriocarcinoma a molar gestation, or PSTT	Clinical history to establish time course of gestation. Insistence on a bilaminar pattern of cytotrophoblast alternating with syncytiotrophoblast for choriocarcinoma, villi are not present in choriocarcinoma. PSTT features.	
	Clinically relevant endometritis: A mixed plasmacytic–lymphocytic infiltrate is a normal finding at the implantation site	Clinically relevant gestational endomyometritis can occur but is only rarely is diagnosed initially on endometrial samplings. The vast majority of cases of "chronic endometritis" seen in practice represent a clinically insignificant "physiologic" finding.	(135,136,213)
Irregular endometrial–myometrial junction	**Adenomyosis:** Glands and stroma surrounded by smooth muscle	Associated smooth muscle hypertrophy is a common feature of adenomyosis and not irregular junctions. Superficial myometrial location of suspected foci favors irregular junctions.	
	Myoinvasive adenocarcinoma: The irregular junction, when expanded by hyperplasia or carcinoma, often simulates myoinvasive carcinoma. Tangential sectioning often reinforces this impression	Absence of stromal host response that is usual in myoinvasive carcinoma. Presence of endometrial stroma or normal glands means irregular junction (or adenomyosis).	

TABLE 40.4			
Normal Findings in the Endometrium That Have Relevance to Histopathologic Differential Diagnosis (*Continued*)			
Findings	Diagnostic Confusion	Suggestions for Resolution	References
Menstrual endometrium	**Adenocarcinoma:** "Cytologic atypia" produced by degenerating, poorly preserved glandular elements **Endometrial stromal neoplasm:** Degenerating stroma may produce a pattern resembling endometrial stromal sarcoma with or without sex cord elements	Obtain history; menstrual fragments have degenerating not neoplastic nuclei.	
Lymphoid nodules	**Endometritis**	The presence of scattered lymphoid nodules does not correlate with significant clinical disease. Large numbers of lymphoid nodules and germinal centers are usually associated with the conventional sine qua non of "chronic endometritis," the plasma cell.	
Stromal "granulocytes"	**Acute or chronic endometritis**	"Stromal granulocytes" or uterine NK cells are a normal feature of the late secretory endometrium and serve as one of the original Noyes dating criteria (see text). Clinically significant inflammation features easily found plasma cells and is usually accompanied by acute inflammation and necrosis of the surface epithelium. Endometrial stromal cells or normal lymphoid constituents may have somewhat eccentric nuclei and amphophilic cytoplasm that mimics that of a plasma cell. This is usually a problem with one or two scattered cells in a fragment. Plasma cells have to be easily found.	(135)
Nuclear ground-glass appearance of nuclei of epithelial cells in gestational setting and with progestogen therapy	Herpes endometritis	Herpes endometritis is rare; obtain history. Immunohistochemistry may be helpful.	(179)

See text for additional differential diagnostic clues.

85% reduction in weight within 3 weeks of delivery (25). This weight loss is primarily due to a reduction in individual cell volume rather than a reduction in cell number. In addition, a large amount of collagen is degraded over this brief period. Complete return of the uterus to the nulliparous weight does not occur if gestation has proceeded beyond the second trimester.

THE FALLOPIAN TUBE

Histology of the Fallopian Tube

The fallopian tube is lined by a nonstratified epithelium that is separated from the endosalpingeal stroma by a basement membrane. Each of the tubal segments is lined by a mixture of three basic cell types: Ciliated cells, secretory cells, and intercalated (peg) cells (Figs. 40.43 and 40.44). In recent years it has become apparent that the peg cell is, in reality, a stage in the cyclic variation during the menstrual cycle of the secretory cell (228). The relative number of these cells differs in each of the anatomic regions of the tube and the variable numbers of each cell type accounts for the varied histology. In addition, many investigators believe that the numbers of the three types of cells within each of these anatomic regions undergo regular variations throughout the menstrual cycle (109,225–234). Ciliated cells are most prominent at the ovarian (distal) end of the tube—particularly in the fimbrial mucosa—and predominate during mid-cycle; their numbers diminish progressively to achieve a nadir at the time of menstruation (Fig. 40.44). In a gestational cycle the number of cilia continues to decrease. Ciliary movement rather than muscular contractions is chiefly responsible for the movement of the egg toward the site of fertilization: the ampulloisthmic junction.

Secretory cells are most prominent toward the uterine end of the tube and undergo cyclic changes in cell height and appearance, reflecting their elaboration, accumulation, and discharge of oviduct secretions as the menstrual cycle proceeds. Most often they have ovoid somewhat dense nuclei, and they may contain an apical vacuole (Fig. 40.45). The oviduct fluid secreted by these cells serves many important functions and has been the subject of a review (235).

TABLE 40.5
Comparison of Differentiated Features for Endometrial Stromal Cells and Smooth Muscle Cells

Technique	Endometrial Stromal Cell	Usual Smooth Muscle Cell	Epithelioid Smooth Muscle Cells	Endometrial Stroma with Epithelioid and/or Glandular Areas
Light microscopy Architectural features	Haphazardly arranged cells resembling normal proliferative phase endometrial stromal cells	Cells arranged in looping intersecting fascicles	Rounded or polygonal cells with moderate amount of cytoplasm	Biphasic pattern Stromal component (featuring cellular endometrial stroma or fibroblastic stroma) + Epithelioid component • Trabecular epithelial pattern or • nests or • insular pattern or • Sertoli-like tubular pattern or • glands
	Complex plexiform vascular pattern	Vascular component not complex	Foci of neoplasm often exhibit standard smooth muscle features	When the entire neoplasm has this biphasic appearance the term "uterine tumor resembling ovarian sex cord tumors" has been used When the change is focal within what is otherwise an endometrial stromal neoplasm (either stromal nodule or endometrial stromal sarcoma) the endometrial stromal diagnosis is supplemented with "epithelioid or glandular areas"
	Hyaline sometimes abundant with a tendency to be glassy			
Nuclear cytologic features	Blunt, round-to-fusiform, uniform, bland	Elongate, cigar-shaped	Round, crumpled	Small, round and regular nuclei • Minimal nuclear pleomorphism • Only rare mitotic figures
Cytoplasm	Scanty (on H&E and trichrome)	Moderate amount (on H&E and trichrome), typically fibrillar	Cytoplasm may be clear around the nucleus, clear at the periphery of the cell, or entirely clear	Scanty cytoplasm Or May have abundant eosinophilic or foamy (lipid-rich) cytoplasm
Immunohistochemistry	Normal endometrial stromal cells express CD10 and may express desmin; they are negative for cytokeratin and EMA	Uterine smooth muscle cells express desmin and caldesmon. They also express CD10 (approximately 40%), CD34 (about a third), keratin (about 20%), and EMA (roughly half)	AE1 is positive in 40% of cases, desmin is positive in 80%, and CD34 in 10%	Epithelioid areas Muscle specific actin (HHF-35) positive Vimentin positive Cytokeratin positive
Immunohistochemistry References:	(221,223)	(222,225)	(223,225)	(219)

Intercalated cells have been thought to represent either effete secretory cells or some type of reserve cells. They have a thin dense nucleus and little cytoplasm. Endocrine cells have been noted in the fallopian tube; their function is as mysterious here as it is in the uterus (236). The "basal cells" reported in the early literature have been shown to be lymphocytes, which may represent a tubal component of a mucosa-associated lymphoid system (237–241). Scattered lymphocytes and occasional lymphoid follicles should be considered to be within normal limits and constitute part of the mucosa-associated lymphoid system (242).

Ciliogenesis is promoted by estradiol and deciliation by progesterone. Prolonged exposure to progestogens (whether endogenously as in pregnancy or exogenously) or withdrawal of estrogen (as in the postmenopausal years) leads to epithelial atrophy. Postmenopausal estrogen administration leads to regrowth of cilia.

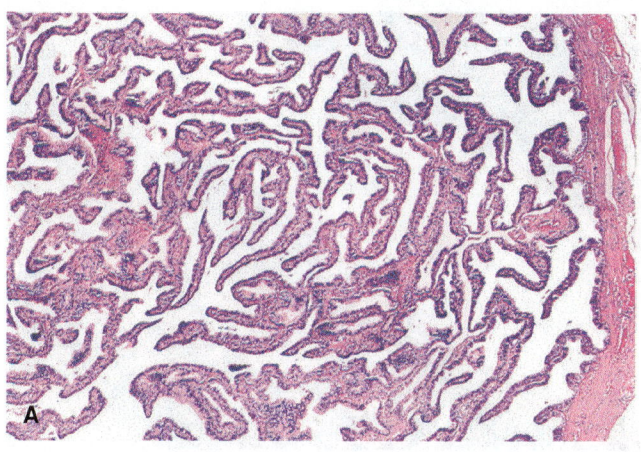
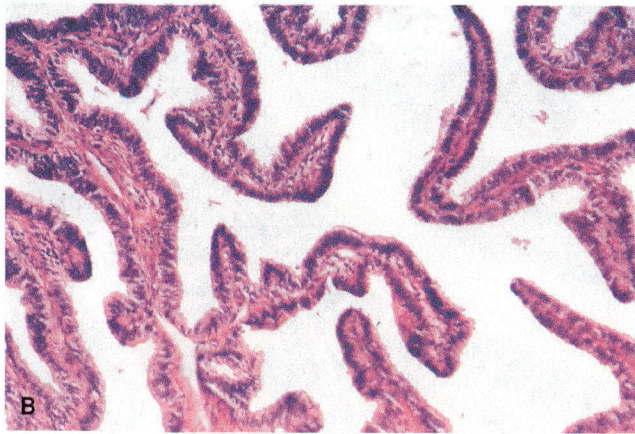

FIGURE 40.43 **A, B:** Ampulla of the fallopian tube. Note the long slender plicae or folds resting on the muscularis.

Mitotic figures are rarely seen in the fallopian tube epithelium, so no cyclic regeneration occurs as in the endometrium. Both the transmission and scanning electron microscopic appearance of the normal tubal mucosa have been extensively documented over the past three decades. The plica become blunted in the postmenopausal state secondary to contraction of the lining and decrease in epithelial cells.

Many metaplasias including mucinous, endometrioid, and transitional cell (Walthard rests) variants can arise in the fallopian tube and are benign findings.

Of interest to the diagnostic pathologist are the abnormalities of ciliogenesis found in patients with Kartagener syndrome (243,244).

With the advent of genetic testing for BRCA 1 and 2 gene mutations and an increased understanding of the fallopian tube as a nidus for serous papillary carcinoma of the ovary and peritoneum, prophylactic salpingo-oophorectomies are being performed. Although there are no inherent morphologic changes in the epithelium of a fallopian tube from a woman who harbors a BRCA-1 or 2 gene mutation, she is at an increased risk of having an in situ or invasive carcinoma. Sectioning and extensively examining the fimbriated end or the SE-FIM protocol is recommended for any patient with a family history of ovarian cancer or known genetic predisposition such as BRCA-1 or BRCA-2 mutation. The fallopian tube is entirely submitted in multiple cross sections at 3-mm intervals except for the distal 2 cm of the fimbriated end, which is cut radially/longitudinally (245) Serous tubal intraepithelial carcinoma (STIC) and its presumed precursor lesion, p53 signature and serous tubal epithelial proliferations (or lesions) of uncertain significance, will arise in otherwise normal fallopian tube and have some overlapping features with reactive atypia; recognizing this process is critical to proper patient management. For detailed evidence and categorization the reader is directed to several good review articles (Fig. 40.46) (246,247). In addition, foci of atypical hyperplasia may be seen that fall short of tubal intraepithelial carcinoma. These foci are characterized by nucleomegaly and a focal increase in p53 but also have benign features such as maintenance of the pseudostratification and polarity of cells and interdigitation by clearly benign cells. Care must be taken in not over interpreting reactive atypia as serous tubal in situ carcinoma, particularly in the setting of acute or chronic salpingitis. Identifying cilia and the maintenance of normal cell polarity support a reactive process (242).

Myosalpinx

The myosalpinx is composed of an inner circular layer and an outer longitudinal layer. The isthmus near the uterotubal junction also possesses an inner longitudinal layer. The presence of the muscular layer can be particularly helpful to the pathologist when trying to distinguish a tubo-ovarian complex from an ovarian serous neoplasm.

FIGURE 40.44 This high-power photomicrograph of tubal epithelium shows numerous ciliated cells with a compressed secretory cell nucleus above the level of the ciliated cells. The cell with clear cytoplasm is probably a lymphocyte.

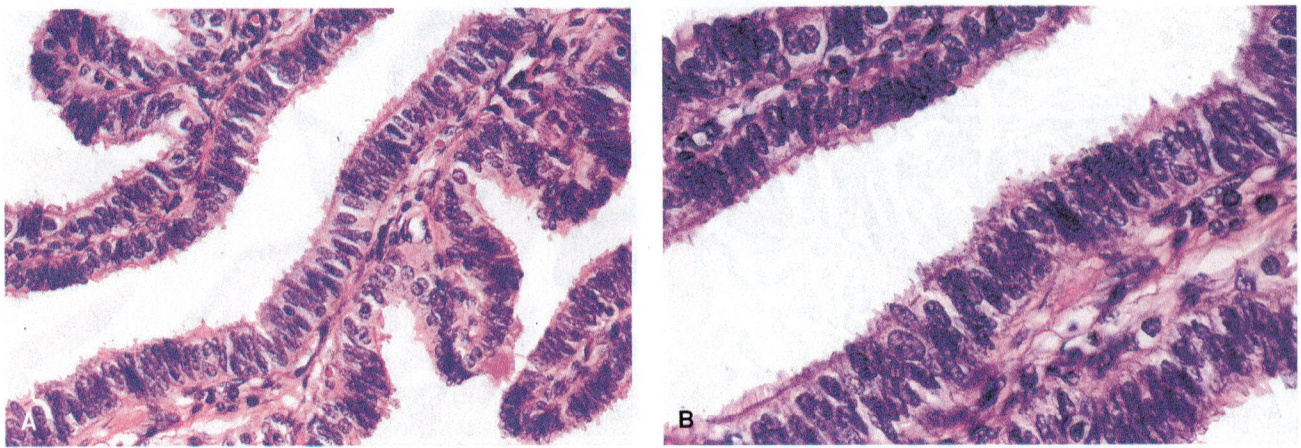

FIGURE 40.45 **A, B:** In this area the tubal epithelial cells are crowded, a pattern that is common in the fallopian tube when ciliated cells are not numerous.

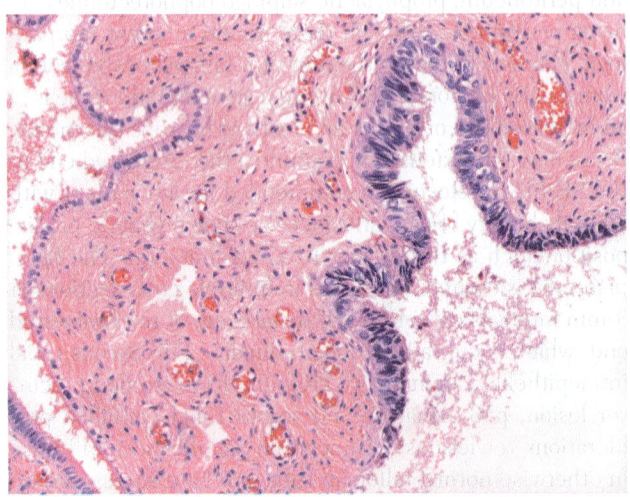

FIGURE 40.46 Fallopian tube with an area of atypical hyperplasia. p16 showed only rare positive cells and Ki67 was mildly increased. The significance of these foci is currently uncertain.

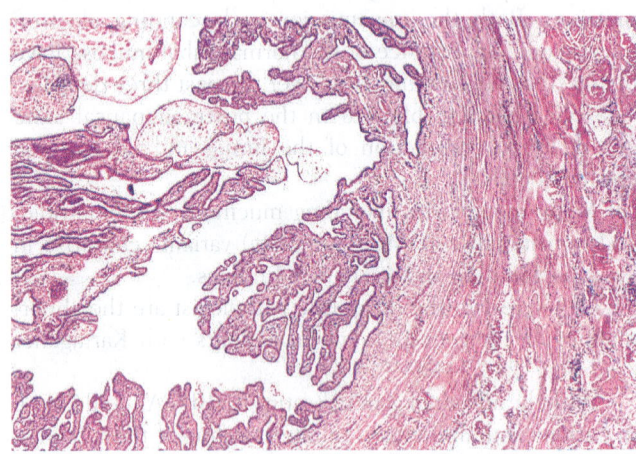

FIGURE 40.47 Fallopian tube containing decidual cells. The stromal cells of the plicae frequently undergo decidual change during pregnancy.

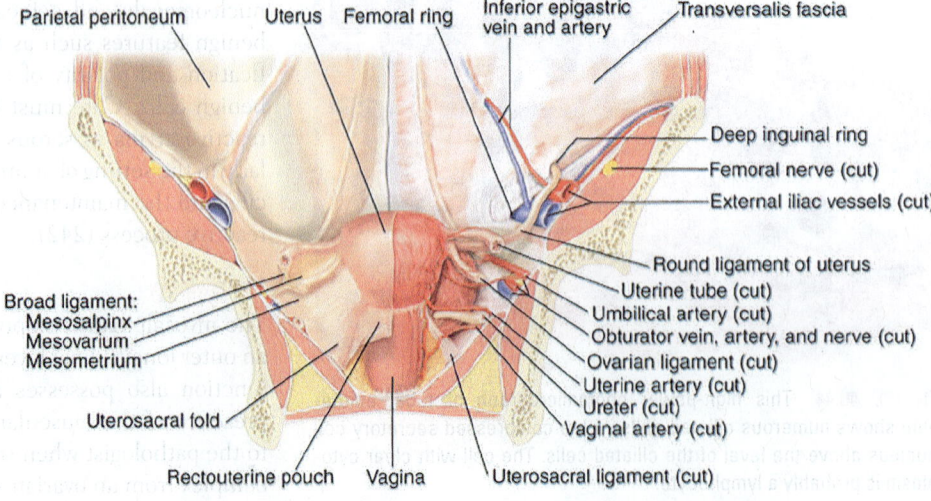

FIGURE 40.48 Topography of the supporting network for the uterus, fallopian tubes, and ovaries. Reprinted with permission from Aqur A, Dalley A. *Grant's Atlas of Anatomy* 12th ed. Philadelphia, PA: Lippincott Williams and Wilkins; 2009:244.

TABLE 40.6

Normal Findings in the Fallopian Tube and Uterine Serosa That Have Relevance to Histopathologic Differential Diagnosis

Finding	Diagnostic Confusion	Suggestions for Resolution	References when Relevant
Decidual reaction (usually encountered in postpartum tubal ligation specimens but may also be seen in the tubes of patients on progestational agents)	Do not misinterpret as carcinoma	Nuclei are bland in decidua.	(252,251)
Endosalpingiosis	Distinguish from endometriosis and ovarian serous tumor of low malignant potential (borderline tumors)	Look for endometrial stroma to confirm diagnosis of endometriosis; look for complex papillae with micropapillae to confirm diagnosis of serous LMP.	
Crowded cells and dense nuclei	Carcinoma in situ	Carcinoma in situ features prominent nucleoli and abnormal mitotic figures. Nuclear atypia and glandular complexity can be significant in chronic salpingitis.	
Mucinous and eosinophilic metaplasia (may be associated with Peutz–Jeghers syndrome)	Carcinoma	Metaplasia lacks the architectural complexity, the nuclear atypia and the mitotic activity of carcinoma.	
Squamous metaplasia Walthard cell rests	Carcinoma	Metaplasia lacks the architectural complexity, the nuclear atypia and the mitotic activity of carcinoma; immunohistochemistry for p16 and Ki67 can help	

See text for additional differential diagnostic clues.

Fallopian Tube in Pregnancy

The fallopian tube has already played its part when the fertilized ovum implants in the endometrium. It is now inactive throughout the gestational period. A muted version of endometrial decidual change often occurs in the endosalpingeal stroma during the latter part of pregnancy, while the epithelium of the fallopian tube undergoes atrophy (Fig. 40.47) (243). Occasionally AS reaction can occur. The fallopian tube is the most common site of ectopic gestation. A review of physiologic factors in its development has been presented (248). Morphologic changes in the fallopian tube can be produced by birth control pills and of course tubal ligation (249–251).

Normal findings in the fallopian tubes that have relevance to histopathologic diagnosis can be found in Table 40.6.

Paraovarian and Paratubal Structures

The broad ligament, round ligament, and mesosalpinx form a network of support to the pelvic organs (Fig. 40.48). These environs are populated by a variety of tubular and cystic structures with the propensity to form clinically or surgically noticeable cysts (38,253). Many are lined by müllerian-type epithelium. Walthard rests are universal findings over the serosal surface of the fallopian tubes. They are lined by transitional-type epithelium. A more or less constant finding in sections that include the peritubal soft tissue is the tortuous remnants of the mesonephric ducts. These are lined by cuboidal epithelium and possess a fibromyovascular cuff.

REFERENCES

1. Lauchlan SC. Metaplasias and neoplasias of Müllerian epithelium. *Histopathology* 1984;8:543–557.
2. Lauchlan SC. The secondary müllerian system revisited. *Int J Gynecol Pathol* 1994;13:73–79.
3. Moore K. *The Developing Human. Clinically Oriented Embryology*. Philadelphia, PA: W.B. Saunders Company; 2003:207–221.
4. Acién P. Embryological observations on the female genital tract. *Hum Reprod* 1992;7:437–445.
5. O'Rahilly R. *Prenatal Human Development*. New York: Plenum Medical Book Company; 1989:35–56.
6. Jost A, Vigier B, Prépin J, et al. Studies on sex differentiation in mammals. *Recent Prog Horm Res* 1973;29:1–41.
7. Gondos B. Development of the reproductive organs. *Ann Clin Lab Sci* 1985:15:363–373.
8. Szamborski J, Laskowska H. Some observations on the developmental histology of the human foetal uterus. *Biol Neonat* 1968;13:298–314.
9. Gray CA, Bartol FF, Tarleton BJ, et al. Developmental biology of uterine glands. *Biol Reprod* 2001;65:1311–1323.
10. Ramsey E. Development of the human uterus and relevance to the adult condition. In: Chard T, Grudzinskas J, eds. *The Uterus*. New York: Cambridge; 1994:41–53.

11. McLean J. Embryology and anatomy of the female genital tract. In: Fox H, Wells M, eds. *Haines and Taylor Obstetrical and Gynaecological Pathology*. Edinburgh, UK: Churchill Livingstone; 2002:1–40.
12. Ramsey E. Embryology and developmental defects of the female reproductive tract. In: Danforth D, Scott J, eds. *Obstetrics and Gynecology*. New York: JB Lippincott; 1986:106–119.
13. Strauss JF III, Barbieri RL. The structure, function, and evaluation of the female reproductive tract. In: Strauss JF III, Barbieri RL, eds. *Yen and Jaffe's Reproductive Endocrinology. Physiology, Pathophysiology, and Clinical Management*. Philadelphia, PA: Elsevier Saunders; 2004:255–306.
14. Patton G, Kistner R. *Atlas of Infertility Surgery*. Boston, MA: Little, Brown and Company; 1984.
15. Tulac S, Nayak NR, Kao LC, et al. Identification, characterization, and regulation of the canonical Wnt signaling pathway in human endometrium. *J Clin Endocrinol Metab* 2003;88:3860–3866.
16. Haber HP, Mayer EI. Ultrasound evaluation of uterine and ovarian size from birth to puberty. *Pediatr Radiol* 1994;24:11–13.
17. Nussbaum A, Sanders R, Jones M. Neonatal uterine morphology as seen on real-time US. *Radiology* 1986;160:641–643.
18. Singer A, Chow C. Anatomy of the cervix and physiological changes in cervical epithelium. In: Fox H, Wells M, eds. *Haines and Taylor Obstetrical and Gynaecological Pathology*. Edinburgh, UK: Churchill Livingstone; 2002:247–272.
19. Eddy CA, Pauerstein CJ. Anatomy and physiology of the fallopian tube. *Clin Obstet Gynecol* 1980;23:1177–1193.
20. Gray H, Williams PL, Warwick R, et al. *Grays Anatomy*. Churchill Livingstone; 1989.
21. Langlois P. The size of the normal uterus. *J Reprod Med* 1970;4:220–228.
22. Calder A. The cervix during pregnancy. In: Chard T, Grudzinskas J, eds. *The Uterus*. New York: Cambridge; 1994:288–307.
23. Kurz K, Tadesse E, Haspels A. In vivo measurements of uterine cavities in 795 women of fertile age. *Contraception* 1984;29:495–510.
24. Zemlyn S. The length of the uterine cervix and its significance. *Clin Ultrasound* 1981;9:267–269.
25. Finn C, Porter D. *The Uterus*. Acton, MA: Publishing Sciences Group; 1975.
26. Togashi K, Nakai A, Sugimura K. Anatomy and physiology of the female pelvis. MR imaging revisited. *J Magn Reson Imaging* 2001;13:842–849.
27. Hoad CL, Raine-Fenning NJ, Fulford J, et al. Uterine tissue development in healthy women during the normal menstrual cycle and investigations with magnetic resonance imaging. *Am J Obstet Gynecol* 2005;192:648–654.
28. Toth A. Studies on the muscular structure of the human uterus. II. Fasciculi cervicoangulares: Vestigial or functional remnant of the mesonephric duct? *Obstet Gynecol* 1977;49:190–196.
29. Toth S, Toth A. Undescribed muscle bundle of the human uterus: Fasciculus cervicoangularis. *Am J Obstet Gynecol* 1974;118:979–984.
30. Huszar G, Naftolin F. The myometrium and uterine cervix in normal and preterm labor. *N Engl J Med* 1984;311:571–581.
31. Merchant RN, Prabhu SR, Chougale A. Uterotubal junction–morphology and clinical aspects. *Int J Fertil* 1983;28:199–205.
32. Vizza E, Correr S, Muglia U, et al. The three-dimensional organization of the smooth musculature in the ampulla of the human fallopian tube: A new morpho-functional model. *Hum Reprod* 1995;10:2400–2405.
33. Croxatto HB. Physiology of gamete and embryo transport through the fallopian tube. *Reprod Biomed Online* 2002;4:160–169.
34. Talbot P, Geiske C, Knoll M. Oocyte pickup by the mammalian oviduct. *Mol Biol Cell* 1999;10:5–8.
35. Gordts S, Campo R, Rombauts L, et al. Endoscopic visualization of the process of fimbrial ovum retrieval in the human. *Hum Reprod* 1998;13:1425–1428.
36. Greiss FJ, Rose J. Vascular physiology of the nonpregnant uterus. In: Wynn R, Jollie W, eds. *Biology of the Uterus*. New York: Plenum; 1989:69–88.
37. Ramsey E. Vascular anatomy. In: Wynn R, Jollie W, eds. *Biology of the Uterus*. New York: Plenum; 1989:58–68.
38. Aqur A, Dalley A. *Grant's Atlas of Anatomy* 12th ed. Philadelphia, PA: Lippincott Williams and Wilkins; 2009:244.
39. DiSaia PJ, Creasman WT. *Clinical Gynecologic Oncology*. St. Louis, MO: Mosby; 1997:viii, 657.
40. Major FJ, Blessing JA, Silverberg SG, et al. Prognostic factors in early-stage uterine sarcoma. A Gynecologic Oncology Group study. *Cancer* 1992;71(4 suppl):1702–1709.
41. Plentl A, Friedman E. *Lymphatic System of the Female Genitalia. The Morphologic Basis of Oncologic Diagnosis and Therapy*. Philadelphia, PA: WB Saunders; 1971.
42. Klein M, Rosen A, Lahousen M, et al. Lymphogenous metastasis in the primary carcinoma of the fallopian tube. *Gynecol Oncol* 1994;55:336–338.
43. Klein M, Rosen AC, Lahousen M, et al. Lymphadenectomy in primary carcinoma of the Fallopian tube. *Cancer Lett* 1999;147:63–66.
44. Wright TC, Ferenczy A. Anatomy and histology of the uterine cervix. In: Kurman RJ, ed. *Blaustein's Pathology of the Female Genital Tract*. New York: Springer-Verlag; 2002:207–224.
45. Aspden RM. The importance of a slit-like lumen cross-section for the mechanical function of the cervix. *Br J Obstet Gynaecol* 1987;94:915–916.
46. Gorodeski G. The cervical cycle. In: Adashi E, Rock J, Rosenwaks Z, eds. *Reproductive Endocrinology, Surgery, and Technology*. Philadelphia, PA: Lippincott-Raven; 1996:302–324.
47. Gipson IK. Mucins of the human endocervix. *Front Biosci* 2001;6:D1245–D1255.
48. Konishi I, Fujii S, Nonogaki H, et al. Immunohistochemical analysis of estrogen receptors, progesterone receptors, Ki-67 antigen, and human papillomavirus DNA in normal and neoplastic epithelium of the uterine cervix. *Cancer* 1991;68:1340–1350.
49. Darragh TM, Colgan TJ, Cox TJ, et al. The Lower Anogenital squamous terminology standardization project for HPV-associated lesions: background and consensus recommendations from the College of American Pathologists and the American Society for Colposcopy and Cervical Pathology. *Int J Gynecol Pathol* 2013;32(1):76–115.
50. Mills AM, Dirks DC, Poulter MD, et al. HR-HPV E6/E7 mRNA In Situ Hybridization: Validation against PCR, DNA

in situ hybridization and p16 immunohistochemistry in 102 samples of cervical vulvar, anal, and head and neck neoplasia. *AM J Surg Pathol* 2017;41(5):607–615.
51. Albores-Saavedra J, Gersell D, Gilks CB, et al. Terminology of endocrine tumors of the uterine cervix: Results of a workshop sponsored by the College of American Pathologists and the National Cancer Institute. *Arch Pathol Lab Med* 1997; 121:34–39.
52. Fetissof F, Arbeille B, Boivin F, et al. Endocrine cells in ectocervical epithelium. An immunohistochemical and ultrastructural analysis. *Virchows Arch A Pathol Anat Histopathol* 1987;411:293–298.
53. Fetissof F, Berger G, Dubois MP, et al. Endocrine cells in the female genital tract. *Histopathology* 1985;9:133–145.
54. Fetissof F, Dubois MP, Heitz PU, et al. Endocrine cells in the female genital tract. *Int J Gynecol Pathol* 1986;5:75–87.
55. Fetissof F, Heitzman A, Machet MC, et al. Unusual endocervical lesions with endocrine cells. *Pathol Res Pract* 1993;189: 928–939.
56. Fetissof F, Serres G, Arbeille B, et al. Argyrophilic cells and ectocervical epithelium. *Int J Gynecol Pathol* 1991;10: 177–190.
57. Scully R, Aguirre P, DeLellis R. Argyrophilia, serotonin, and peptide hormones in the female genital tract and its tumors. *Int J Gynecol Pathol* 1984;3:51–70.
58. Chan JK, Tsui WM, Tung SY, et al. Endocrine cell hyperplasia of the uterine cervix. A precursor of neuroendocrine carcinoma of the cervix? *Am J Clin Pathol* 1989;92:825–830.
59. Hussain LA, Kelly CG, Fellowes R, et al. Expression and gene transcript of Fc receptors for IgG, HLA class II antigens and Langerhans cells in human cervico-vaginal epithelium. *Clin Exp Immunol* 1992;90:530–538.
60. Morelli AE, di Paola G, Fainboim L. Density and distribution of Langerhans cells in the human uterine cervix. *Arch Gynecol Obstet* 1992;252:65–71.
61. Osamura RY, Watanabe K, Oh M. Melanin-containing cells in the uterine cervix: Histochemical and electron-microscopic studies of two cases. *Am J Clin Pathol* 1980;74:239–242.
62. Hiersche HD, Nagl W. Regeneration of secretory epithelium in the human endocervix. *Arch Gynecol* 1980;229:83–90.
63. Gould PR, Barter RA, Papadimitriou JM. An ultrastructural, cytochemical, and autoradiographic study of the mucous membrane of the human cervical canal with reference to subcolumnar basal cells. *Am J Pathol* 1979;95:1–16.
64. Ismail SM. Cone biopsy causes cervical endometriosis and tuboendometrioid metaplasia. *Histopathology* 1991;18:107–114.
65. Jonasson JG, Wang HH, Antonioli DA, et al. Tubal metaplasia of the uterine cervix: A prevalence study in patients with gynecologic pathologic findings. *Int J Gynecol Pathol* 1992;11: 89–95.
66. Novotny DB, Maygarden SJ, Johnson DE, et al. Tubal metaplasia. A frequent potential pitfall in the cytologic diagnosis of endocervical glandular dysplasia on cervical smears. *Acta Cytol* 1992;36:1–10.
67. Pacey F, Ayer B, Greenberg M. The cytologic diagnosis of adenocarcinoma in situ of the cervix uteri and related lesions. III. Pitfalls in diagnosis. *Acta Cytol* 1988;32:325–330.
68. Suh KS, Silverberg SG. Tubal metaplasia of the uterine cervix. *Int J Gynecol Pathol* 1990, 9:122–128.
69. Marques T, Andrade LA, Vassallo J. Endocervical tubal metaplasia and adenocarcinoma in situ: Role of immunohistochemistry for carcinoembryonic antigen and vimentin in differential diagnosis. *Histopathology* 1996;28:549–550.
70. Peters WM. Nature of "basal" and "reserve" cells in oviductal and cervical epithelium in man. *J Clin Pathol* 1986;39: 306–312.
71. Fluhmann C. *The Cervix Uteri and Its Diseases*. Philadelphia, PA: WB Saunders; 1961.
72. Fluhmann CF. The nature and development of the so-called glands of the cervix uteri. *Am J Obstet Gynecol* 1957;74: 753–766; discussion 766–768.
73. Young RH, Clement PB. Pseudoneoplastic glandular lesions of the uterine cervix. *Semin Diagn Pathol* 1991;8:234–249.
74. Clement PB, Young RH. Deep nabothian cysts of the uterine cervix. A possible source of confusion with minimal-deviation adenocarcinoma (adenoma malignum). *Int J Gynecol Pathol* 1989;8:340–348.
75. Teshima S, Shimosato Y, Kishi K, et al. Early stage adenocarcinoma of the uterine cervix. Histopathologic analysis with consideration of histogenesis. *Cancer* 1985;56:167–172.
76. Bertrand M, Lickrish GM, Colgan TJ. The anatomic distribution of cervical adenocarcinoma in situ: implications for treatment. *Am J Obstet Gynecol* 1987;157:21–25.
77. Gilks CB, Reid PE, Clement PB, et al. Histochemical changes in cervical mucus-secreting epithelium during the normal menstrual cycle. *Fertil Steril* 1989;51:286–291.
78. Nucci MR. Symposium part III: tumor-like glandular lesions of the uterine cervix. *Int J Gynecol Pathol* 2002;21:347–359.
79. Lagow E, DeSouza MM, Carson DD. Mammalian reproductive tract mucins. *Hum Reprod Update* 1999;5:280–292.
80. McDonnell JM, Emens JM, Jordan JA. The congenital cervicovaginal transformation zone in sexually active young women. *Br J Obstet Gynaecol* 1984;91:580–584.
81. Burch DJ, Spowart KJ, Jesinger DK, et al. A dose-ranging study of the use of cyclical dydrogesterone with continuous 17 beta oestradiol. *Br J Obstet Gynaecol* 1995;102:243–248.
82. Forsberg J. Cervicovaginal epithelium: Its origin and development. *Am J Obstet Gynecol* 1973;115:1025–1043.
83. Crum CP, Egawa K, Fu YS, et al. Atypical immature metaplasia (AIM). A subset of human papilloma virus infection of the cervix. *Cancer* 1983;51:2214–2219.
84. Duggan MA. Cytologic and histologic diagnosis and significance of controversial squamous lesions of the uterine cervix. *Mod Pathol* 2000;13:252–260.
85. Herfs M, Yamamoto Y, Laury Y, et al. A discrete population of squamocolumnar junction cells implicated in the pathogenesis of cervical cancer. *Proc Natl Acad Sci USA* 2012; 109(26):10516–10521.
86. Yang E, Quick M, Hanamornroongruang S, et al. Microanatomy of the cervical and anorectal squamocolumnar junctions; a proposed model for anatomical differences in HPV-related cancer risk. *Mod Pathol* 2015;28(7):994–1000.
87. Aspden RM. Collagen organisation in the cervix and its relation to mechanical function. *Coll Relat Res* 1988;8:103–112.
88. Kiwi R, Neuman MR, Merkatz IR, et al. Determination of the elastic properties of the cervix. *Obstet Gynecol* 1988;71: 568–574.
89. Leppert PC, Cerreta JM, Mandl I. Orientation of elastic fibers in the human cervix. *Am J Obstet Gynecol* 1986;155:219–224.
90. Leppert PC, Yu SY. Three-dimensional structures of uterine elastic fibers: Scanning electron microscopic studies. *Connect Tissue Res* 1991;27:15–31.

91. Johansson EL, Rudin A, Wassen L, et al. Distribution of lymphocytes and adhesion molecules in human cervix and vagina. *Immunology* 1999;96:272–277.
92. Miller CJ, McChesney M, Moore PF. Langerhans cells, macrophages and lymphocyte subsets in the cervix and vagina of rhesus macaques. *Lab Invest* 1992;67:628–634.
93. Edwards JN, Morris HB. Langerhans' cells and lymphocyte subsets in the female genital tract. *Br J Obstet Gynaecol* 1985; 92:974–982.
94. Hughes RG, Norval M, Howie SE. Expression of major histocompatibility class II antigens by Langerhans' cells in cervical intraepithelial neoplasia. *J Clin Pathol* 1988;41: 253–259.
95. Roncalli M, Sideri M, Gie P, et al. Immunophenotypic analysis of the transformation zone of human cervix. *Lab Invest* 1988;58:141–149.
96. Ferry JA, Scully RE. Mesonephric remnants, hyperplasia, and neoplasia in the uterine cervix. A study of 49 cases. *Am J Surg Pathol* 1990;14:1100–1111.
97. Seidman JD, Tavassoli FA. Mesonephric hyperplasia of the uterine cervix: A clinicopathologic study of 51 cases. *Int J Gynecol Pathol* 1995;14:293–299.
98. Oliva E. CD10 expression in the female genital tract: does it have useful diagnostic applications? *Adv Anat Pathol* 2004;11: 310–315.
99. McCluggage WG, Oliva E, Herrington CS, et al. CD10 and calretinin staining of endocervical glandular lesions, endocervical stroma and endometrioid adenocarcinomas of the uterine corpus: CD10 positivity is characteristic of, but not specific for, mesonephric lesions and is not specific for endometrial stroma. *Histopathology* 2003;43:144–150.
100. Nucci MR, Young RH, Fletcher CD. Cellular pseudosarcomatous fibroepithelial stromal polyps of the lower female genital tract: an underrecognized lesion often misdiagnosed as sarcoma. *Am J Surg Pathol* 2000;24:231–240.
101. Abdul-Karim FW, Cohen RE. Atypical stromal cells of lower female genital tract. *Histopathology* 1990;17:249–253.
102. Clement PB. Multinucleated stromal giant cells of the uterine cervix. *Arch Pathol Lab Med* 1985;109:200–202.
103. Metze K, Andrade LA. Atypical stromal giant cells of cervix uteri–evidence of Schwann cell origin. *Pathol Res Pract* 1991; 187:1031–1035; discussion 1036–1038.
104. Ledger WL, Anderson AB. The influence of steroid hormones on the uterine cervix during pregnancy. *J Steroid Biochem* 1987;27:1029–1034.
105. Leppert PC. Anatomy and physiology of cervical ripening. *Clin Obstet Gynecol* 1995;38:267–279.
106. Pisharodi LR, Jovanoska S. Spectrum of cytologic changes in pregnancy. A review of 100 abnormal cervicovaginal smears, with emphasis on diagnostic pitfalls. *Acta Cytol* 1995;39: 905–908.
107. Kaspar HG, Crum CP. The utility of immunohistochemistry in the differential diagnosis of gynecologic disorders. *Arch Pathol Lab Med* 2015;139: 39–54.
108. Nucci MR, Young RH. Arias-Stella reaction of the endocervix: a report of 18 cases with emphasis on its varied histology and differential diagnosis. *Am J Surg Pathol* 2004;28: 608–612.
109. Clement PB, Young RH, Scully RE. Nontrophoblastic pathology of the female genital tract and peritoneum associated with pregnancy. *Semin Diagn Pathol* 1989;6:372–406.
110. Oliva E, Clement PB, Young RH. Tubal and tubo-endometrioid metaplasia of the uterine cervix. Unemphasized features that may cause problems in differential diagnosis: A report of 25 cases. *Am J Clin Pathol* 1995;103:618–623.
111. Manganiello PD, Burrows LJ, Dain BJ, et al. Vabra aspirator and pipelle endometrial suction curette. A comparison. *J Reprod Med* 1998;43:889–892.
112. Mutter GL, Ferenczy A. Anatomy and histology of the uterine corpus. In: Kurman RJ, ed. *Blaustein's Pathology of the Female Genital Tract*. New York: Springer-Verlag; 2002:383–420.
113. Giudice LC, Ferenczy A. The endometrial cycle. In: Adashi EY, Rock JA, Rosenwaks Z, eds. *Reproductive Endocrinology, Surgery, and Technology*. Philadelphia, PA: Lippincott-Raven; 1996:272–300.
114. Buckley CH. Normal endometrium and non-proliferative conditions of the endometrium. In: Fox H, Wells M, eds. *Haines and Taylor Obstetrical and Gynaecological Pathology*. Edinburgh, UK: Churchill Livingstone; 2002:391–442.
115. Warren M, Li T, Klentzeris L. Cell biology of the endometrium: Histology, cell types and menstrual changes. In: Chard T, Grudzinskas J, eds. *The Uterus*. New York: Cambridge; 1994: 94–124.
116. Cooper JM, Erickson ML. Endometrial sampling techniques in the diagnosis of abnormal uterine bleeding. *Obstet Gynecol Clin North Am* 2000;27:235–244.
117. Chambers JT, Chambers SK. Endometrial sampling: When? Where? Why? With what? *Clin Obstet Gynecol* 1992;35: 28–39.
118. Mihm LM, Quick VA, Brumfield JA, et al. The accuracy of endometrial biopsy and saline sonohysterography in the determination of the cause of abnormal uterine bleeding. *Am J Obstet Gynecol* 2002;186:858–860.
119. Revel A, Shushan A. Investigation of the infertile couple: Hysteroscopy with endometrial biopsy is the gold standard investigation for abnormal uterine bleeding. *Hum Reprod* 2002;17:1947–1949.
120. Tahir MM, Bigrigg MA, Browning JJ, et al. A randomised controlled trial comparing transvaginal ultrasound, outpatient hysteroscopy and endometrial biopsy with inpatient hysteroscopy and curettage. *Br J Obstet Gynaecol* 1999;106: 1259–1264.
121. Ben-Yehuda OM, Kim YB, Leuchter RS. Does hysteroscopy improve upon the sensitivity of dilatation and curettage in the diagnosis of endometrial hyperplasia or carcinoma? *Gynecol Oncol* 1998;68:4–7.
122. Hill GA, Herbert CM III, Parker RA, et al. Comparison of late luteal phase endometrial biopsies using the Novak curette or PIPELLE endometrial suction curette. *Obstet Gynecol* 1989;73:443–445.
123. Ferenczy A, Bergeron C. Histology of the human endometrium: From birth to senescence. *Ann N Y Acad Sci* 1991;622: 6–27.
124. Denholm R, More I. Atypical cilia of the human endometrial epithelium. *J Anat* 1980;131:309–315.
125. Comer MT, Andrew AC, Leese HJ, et al. Application of a marker of ciliated epithelial cells to gynaecological pathology. *J Clin Pathol* 1999;52:355–357.
126. Kearns M, Lala P. Life history of decidual cells: A review. *Am J Reprod Immunol* 1983;3:78–82.
127. Iwahashi M, Muragaki Y, Ooshima A, et al. Alterations in distribution and composition of the extracellular matrix during

decidualization of the human endometrium. *J Reprod Fertil* 1996;108:147–155.
128. Speroff L, Fritz MA. The uterus. In: Speroff L, Fritz MA, eds. *Clinical Gynecologic Endocrinology and Infertility*. Philadelphia, PA: Lippincott Williams & Wilkins; 2004:113–144.
129. Whitelaw PF, Croy BA. Granulated lymphocytes of pregnancy. *Placenta* 1996;17:533–543.
130. Bulmer JN, Lash GE. Human uterine natural killer cells: A reappraisal. *Mol Immunol* 2005;42:511–521.
131. King A. Uterine leukocytes and decidualization. *Hum Reprod Update* 2000;6:28–36.
132. Kayisli UA, Guzeloglu-Kayisli O, Arici A. Endocrine-immune interactions in human endometrium. *Ann N Y Acad Sci* 2004; 1034:50–63.
133. Gaynor LM, Colucci F. Uterine natural killer cells: Functional distinctions and influence on pregnancy in humans and mice. *Front Immunol* 2017;8:467.
134. Givan AL, White HD, Stern JE, et al. Flow cytometric analysis of leukocytes in the human female reproductive tract: Comparison of fallopian tube, uterus, cervix, and vagina. *Am J Reprod Immunol* 1997;38:350–359.
135. Tabibzadeh S. Proliferative activity of lymphoid cells in human endometrium throughout the menstrual cycle. *J Clin Endocrinol Metab* 1990;70:437–443.
136. Kiviat N, WolnerHanssen P, Eschenbach D, et al. Endometrial histopathology in patients with culture-proved upper genital tract infection and laparoscopically diagnosed acute salpingitis. *Am J Surg Pathol* 1990;14:167–175.
137. Ramsey E. *Vascular Anatomy*. New York: Plenum Press; 1977: 59–76.
138. Ramsey E. Anatomy of the uterus. In: Chard T, Grudzinskas J, eds. *The Uterus*. New York: Cambridge University Press; 1994:18–40.
139. Gargett CE, Rogers PA. Human endometrial angiogenesis. *Reproduction* 2001;121:181–186.
140. Taylor RN, Lebovic DI, Hornung D, et al. Endocrine and paracrine regulation of endometrial angiogenesis. *Ann N Y Acad Sci* 2001;943:109–121.
141. Rees MC, Bicknell R. Angiogenesis in the endometrium. *Angiogenesis* 1998;2:29–35.
142. Albrecht ED, Pepe GJ. Steroid hormone regulation of angiogenesis in the primate endometrium. *Front Biosci* 2003;8:416–429.
143. Anin SA, Vince G, Quenby S. Trophoblast invasion. *Hum Fertil Camb* 2004;7:169–174.
144. Lyall F. Priming and remodelling of human placental bed spiral arteries during pregnancy–a review. *Placenta* 2005; 26(suppl A):S31–S36.
145. Spornitz UM. The functional morphology of the human endometrium and decidua. *Adv Anat Embryol Cell Biol* 1992; 124:1–99.
146. Cornillie FJ, Lauweryns JM, Brosens IA. Normal human endometrium. An ultrastructural survey. *Gynecol Obstet Invest* 1985;20:113–129.
147. Dockery P, Pritchard K, Warren MA, et al. Changes in nuclear morphology in the human endometrial glandular epithelium in women with unexplained infertility. *Hum Reprod* 1996;11:2251–2256.
148. Paria BC, Reese J, Das SK, et al. Deciphering the cross-talk of implantation: Advances and challenges. *Science* 2002;296: 2185–2188.
149. Tazuke SI, Giudice LC. Growth factors and cytokines in endometrium, embryonic development, and maternal: Embryonic interactions. *Semin Reprod Endocrinol* 1996;14:231–245.
150. Mylonas I, Jeschke U, Wiest I, et al. Inhibin/activin subunits alpha, beta-A and beta-B are differentially expressed in normal human endometrium throughout the menstrual cycle. *Histochem Cell Biol* 2004;122:461–471.
151. Stavreus-Evers A, Koraen L, Scott JE, et al. Distribution of cyclooxygenase-1, cyclooxygenase-2, and cytosolic phospholipase A2 in the luteal phase human endometrium and ovary. *Fertil Steril* 2005;83:156–162.
152. Speroff L, Fritz MA. *Clinical Gynecologic Endocrinology and Infertility*. Philadelphia, PA: Lippincott Williams & Wilkins; 2004.
153. Treloar A, Boynton R, Behn B, et al. Variation of the human menstrual cycle through reproductive life. *Int J Fertil* 1970;12: 77–126.
154. Hall J. Neuroendocrine control of the menstrual cycle. Yen and Jaffe's Reproductive Endocrinology. In: Strauss J, Barbieri R, eds. *Physiology, Pathophysiology, and Clinical Management*. Philadelphia, PA: Elsevier Saunders; 2004:195–212.
155. Hodgen G. Neuroendocrinology of the normal menstrual cycle. *J Reprod Med* 1989;34:68–75.
156. Koehler KF, Helguero LA, Haldosen LA, et al. Reflections on the discovery and significance of estrogen receptor beta. *Endocr Rev* 2005;26:465–478.
157. Alberts B, Johnson A, Lewis J, et al. Cell communication. In: Alberts B, Johnson A, Lewis J, et al., eds. *Molecular Biology of the Cell*. New York: Garland Science; 2002:831–906.
158. Rhen T, Cidlowski JA. Steroid hormone action. In: Strauss J, Barbieri R, eds. *Yen and Jaffe's Reproductive Endocrinology. Physiology, Pathophysiology, and Clinical Management*. Philadelphia, PA: Elsevier Saunders; 2004:155–174.
159. Li T, Dockery P, Rogers A, et al. How precise is histologic dating of endometrium using the standard dating criteria? *Fertil Steril* 1989a;51:759–763.
160. Strauss JI, Gurpide E. The endometrium: Regulation and dysfunction (Chapter 9). In: Yen S, Jaffe R, eds. *Reproductive Endocrinology: Physiology, Pathophysiology and Clinical Management*. Philadelphia, PA, London, Toronto: WB Saunders Company; 1991:309–356.
161. Wynn RM. The human endometrium: Cyclic and gestational changes. In: Wynn R, Jollie W, eds. *Biology of the Uterus*. New York: Plenum Medical Book Company; 1989:289–332.
162. Milwidsky A, Palti Z, Gutman A. Glycogen metabolism of the human endometrium. *J Clin Endocrinol Metab* 1980;51: 765–770.
163. Daly D, Tohan N, Doney T, et al. The significance of lymphocytic-leukocytic infiltrates in interpreting late luteal phase endometrial biopsies. *Fertil Steril* 1982;37:786–791.
164. Critchley HO, Kelly RW, Brenner RM, et al. The endocrinology of menstruation–a role for the immune system. *Clin Endocrinol Oxf* 2001;55:701–710.
165. Rogers PA, Lederman F, Taylor N. Endometrial microvascular growth in normal and dysfunctional states. *Hum Reprod Update* 1998;4:503–508.
166. Salamonsen LA. Tissue injury and repair in the female human reproductive tract. *Reproduction* 2003;125:301–311.
167. Hertig A. Gestational hyperplasia of endometrium: A morphologic correlation of ova, endometrium, and corpora lutea during early pregnancy. *Lab Invest* 1964;13:1153–1191.

168. Parr M, Parr E. *The Implantation Reaction*. New York: Plenum Medical Book Company; 1989:233–288.
169. O'Connor D, Kurman R. Intermediate trophoblast in uterine curettings in the diagnosis of ectopic pregnancy. *Obstet Gynecol* 1988;72:665–670.
170. Gruber K, Gelven PL, Austin RM. Chorionic villi or trophoblastic tissue in uterine samples of four women with ectopic pregnancies. *Int J Gynecol Pathol* 1997;16:28–32.
171. Young RH, Kurman RJ, Scully RE. Placental site nodules and plaques. A clinicopathologic analysis of 20 cases. *Am J Surg Pathol* 1990;14:1001–1009.
172. Shih IM, Seidman JD, Kurman RJ. Placental site nodule and characterization of distinctive types of intermediate trophoblast. *Hum Pathol* 1999;30:687–694.
173. Shih IM, Kurman RJ. Ki-67 labeling index in the differential diagnosis of exaggerated placental site, placental site trophoblastic tumor, and choriocarcinoma: A double immunohistochemical staining technique using Ki-67 and Mel-CAM antibodies. *Hum Pathol* 1998;29:27–33.
174. Shih IM, Kurman RJ. p63 expression is useful in the distinction of epithelioid trophoblastic and placental site trophoblastic tumors by profiling trophoblastic subpopulations. *Am J Surg Pathol* 2004;28:1177–1183.
175. Arias-Stella J. The Arias-Stella reaction: facts and fancies four decades after. *Adv Anat Pathol* 2002;9:12–23.
176. Huettner PC, Gersell DJ. Arias-Stella reaction in nonpregnant women: A clinicopathologic study of nine cases. *Int J Gynecol Pathol* 1994;13:241–247.
177. Arias-Stella J Jr. Arias-Velasquez A, Arias-Stella J. Normal and abnormal mitoses in the atypical endometrial change associated with chorionic tissue effect [corrected]. *Am J Surg Pathol* 1994;18:694–701.
178. Vang R, Barner R, Wheeler DT, et al. Immunohistochemical staining for Ki-67 and p53 helps distinguish endometrial Arias-Stella reaction from high-grade carcinoma, including clear cell carcinoma. *Int J Gynecol Pathol* 2004;23:223–233.
179. Mazur M, Hendrickson M, Kempson R. Optically clear nuclei. An alteration of endometrial epithelium in the presence of trophoblast. *Am J Surg Pathol* 1983;7:415–423.
180. Lichtig C, Deutch M, Brandes J. Vascular changes of endometrium in early pregnancy. *Am J Clin Pathol* 1984;81:702–707.
181. Hustin J, Wells M. Pathology of the pregnant uterus. In: Fox H, Wells M, eds. *Haines and Taylor Obstetrical and Gynaecological Pathology*. Edinburgh, UK: Churchill Livingstone; 2002:1327–1357.
182. Taffe JR, Dennerstein L. Menstrual patterns leading to the final menstrual period. *Menopause* 2002;9:32–40.
183. Archer D, Mcintyreseltman K, Wilborn W, et al. Endometrial morphology in asymptomatic postmenopausal women. *Am J Obstet Gynecol* 1991;165.
184. Choo YC, Mak KC, Hsu C, et al. Postmenopausal uterine bleeding of nonorganic cause. *Obstet Gynecol* 1985;66:225–228.
185. Moodley M, Roberts C. Clinical pathway for the evaluation of postmenopausal bleeding with an emphasis on endometrial cancer detection. *J Obstet Gynaecol* 2004;24:736–741.
186. Quddus MR, Sung CJ, Zheng W, et al. p53 immunoreactivity in endometrial metaplasia with dysfunctional uterine bleeding. *Histopathology* 1999;35:44–49.
187. Haney AF. Endometrial biopsy: a test whose time has come and gone. *Fertil Steril* 2004;82:1295–1296; discussion 301–302.
188. Coutifaris C, Myers ER, Guzick DS, et al. Histological dating of timed endometrial biopsy tissue is not related to fertility status. *Fertil Steril* 2004;82:1264–1272.
189. Murray MJ, Meyer WR, Zaino RJ, et al. A critical analysis of the accuracy, reproducibility, and clinical utility of histologic endometrial dating in fertile women. *Fertil Steril* 2004;81:1333–1343.
190. Myers ER, Silva S, Barnhart K, et al. Interobserver and intraobserver variability in the histological dating of the endometrium in fertile and infertile women. *Fertil Steril* 2004;82:1278–1282.
191. Glatstein IZ, Harlow BL, Hornstein MD. Practice patterns among reproductive endocrinologists: the infertility evaluation. *Fertil Steril* 1997;67:443–451.
192. Balasch J. Investigation of the infertile couple: investigation of the infertile couple in the era of assisted reproductive technology: a time for reappraisal. *Hum Reprod* 2000;15:2251–2257.
193. Balasch J, Fabregues F, Creus M, et al. The usefulness of endometrial biopsy for luteal phase evaluation in infertility. *Hum Reprod* 1992;7:973–977.
194. Peters AJ, Lloyd RP, Coulam CB. Prevalence of out-of-phase endometrial biopsy specimens. *Am J Obstet Gynecol* 1992;166:1738–1745; discussion 1745–1746.
195. Noyes R. Normal phases of the endometrium. In: Hertig A, Norris H, Abell M, eds. *The Uterus*. Baltimore, MD: Williams & Wilkins; 1973:110–135.
196. Noyes R, Hertig A, Rock J. Dating the endometrial biopsy. *Fertil Steril* 1950;1:3–25.
197. McNeely MJ, Soules MR. The diagnosis of luteal phase deficiency: A critical review [see comments]. *Fertil Steril* 1988;50:1–15.
198. Noyes R, Haman J. Accuracy of endometrial dating. *Fertil Steril* 1953;4:504–517.
199. Li TC, Rogers AW, Lenton EA, et al. A comparison between two methods of chronological dating of human endometrial biopsies during the luteal phase, and their correlation with histologic dating. *Fertil Steril* 1987;48:928–932.
200. Gibson M, Badger GJ, Byrn F, et al. Error in histologic dating of secretory endometrium: Variance component analysis. *Fertil Steril* 1991;56:242–247.
201. Scott RT, Snyder RR, Strickland DM, et al. The effect of interobserver variation in dating endometrial histology on the diagnosis of luteal phase defects. *Fertil Steril* 1988;50:888–892.
202. Otsuki Y. Apoptosis in human endometrium: Apoptotic detection methods and signaling. *Med Electron Microsc* 2001;34:166–173.
203. Kokawa K, Shikone T, Nakano R. Apoptosis in the human uterine endometrium during the menstrual cycle. *J Clin Endocrinol Metab* 1996;81:4144–4147.
204. Konno R, Igarashi T, Okamoto S, et al. Apoptosis of human endometrium mediated by perforin and granzyme B of NK cells and cytotoxic T lymphocytes. *Tohoku J Exp Med* 1999;187:149–155.
205. Sivridis E, Giatromanolaki A. New insights into the normal menstrual cycle-regulatory molecules. *Histol Histopathol* 2004;19:511–516.

206. Rotello RJ, Lieberman RC, Purchio AF, et al. Coordinated regulation of apoptosis and cell proliferation by transforming growth factor beta 1 in cultured uterine epithelial cells. *Proc Natl Acad Sci U S A* 1991;88:3412–3415.
207. Gerschenson LE, Rotello RJ. Apoptosis: a different type of cell death. *Faseb J* 1992;6:2450–2455.
208. Rotello RJ, Hocker MB, Gerschenson LE. Biochemical evidence for programmed cell death in rabbit uterine epithelium. *Am J Pathol* 1989;134:491–495.
209. Rotello RJ, Lieberman RC, Lepoff RB, et al. Characterization of uterine epithelium apoptotic cell death kinetics and regulation by progesterone and RU 486. *Am J Pathol* 1992;140:449–456.
210. Gompel A, Sabourin JC, Martin A, et al. Bcl-2 expression in normal endometrium during the menstrual cycle. *Am J Pathol* 1994;144:1195–1202.
211. Maia H Jr, Maltez A, Studart E, et al. Ki-67, Bcl-2 and p53 expression in endometrial polyps and in the normal endometrium during the menstrual cycle. *Bjog* 2004;111:1242–1247.
212. Tabizadeh S, Zupi E, Babaknia A, et al. Site and menstrual cycle-dependent expression of proteins of the tumour necrosis factor (TNF) receptor family, and BCL-2 oncoprotein and phase-specific production of TNF alpha in human endometrium. *Hum Reprod* 1995;10:277–286.
213. Achilles SL, Amortegui AJ, Wiesenfeld HC. Endometrial plasma cells: Do they indicate subclinical pelvic inflammatory disease? *Sex Transm Dis* 2005;32:185–188.
214. Cole W, Garfield R. Ultrastructure of the myometrium. In: Wynn R, Jollie W, eds. *Biology of the Uterus*. New York: Plenum; 1989:455–504.
215. Garfield R, Yallampalli C. Structure and function of uterine muscle. In: Chard T, Grudzinskas J, eds. *The Uterus*. New York: Cambridge; 1994:54–93.
216. Huszar G, Walsh M. Biochemistry of the myometrium and cervix. In: Wynn R, Jollie W, eds. *Biology of the Uterus*. New York: Plenum; 1989:355–402.
217. Kao C. Electrophysiological properties of uterine smooth muscle. In: Wynn R, Jollie W, eds. *Biology of the Uterus*. New York: Plenum; 1989:403–454.
218. Kawaguchi K, Fujii S, Konishi I, et al. Mitotic activity in uterine leiomyomas during the menstrual cycle. *Am J Obstet Gynecol* 1989;160:637–641.
219. Pradhan N, Mohatny SK. Uterine tumors resembling ovarian sex cord tumors. *Arch Pathol Lab Med* 2013:137(12);1832–1836.
220. Marshall J. The physiology of the myometrium. In: Hertig A, Norris H, Abell M, eds. *The uterus*. Baltimore, MD: Williams & Wilkins; 1973:89–109.
221. Oliva E, Clement PB, Young RH, et al. Mixed endometrial stromal and smooth muscle tumors of the uterus: a clinicopathologic study of 15 cases. *Am J Surg Pathol* 1998;22:997–1005.
222. Azumi N, Ben-Ezra J, Battifora H. Immunophenotypic diagnosis of leiomyosarcomas and rhabdomyosarcomas with monoclonal antibodies to muscle-specific actin and desmin in formalin-fixed tissue. *Mod Pathol* 1988;1:469–474.
223. Brown D, Theaker J, Banks P, et al. Cytokeratin expression in smooth muscle and smooth muscle tumours. *Histopathology* 1987;11:477–486.
224. Gown A, Boyd H, Chang Y, et al. Smooth muscle cells can express cytokeratins of "simple" epithelium. *Am J Pathol* 1988;132(2):223–232.
225. Norton AJ, Thomas JA, Isaacson PG. Cytokeratin-specific monoclonal antibodies are reactive with tumours of smooth muscle derivation. An immunocytochemical and biochemical study using antibodies to intermediate filament cytoskeletal proteins. *Histopathology* 1987;11:487–499.
226. Silverberg S, Kurman R. *Tumors of the Uterine Corpus and Gestational Trophoblastic Disease*. Washington, DC: AFIP; 1992.
227. Garfield RE, Hayashi RH. Appearance of gap junctions in the myometrium of women during labor. *Am J Obstet Gynecol* 1981;140:254–260.
228. Brenner R, Slayden O. The fallopian tube cycle. In: Adashi E, Rock J, Rosenwaks Z, eds. *Reproductive Endocrinology, Surgery, and Technology*. Philadelphia, PA: Lippincott-Raven; 1996:326–339.
229. Bonilla-Musoles F, Ferrer-Barriendos J, Pellicer A. Cyclical changes in the epithelium of the fallopian tube. Studies with scanner electron microscopy (SEM). *Clin Exp Obstet Gynecol* 1983;10:79–86.
230. Donnez J, Casanas-Roux F, Caprasse J, et al. Cyclic changes in ciliation, cell height, and mitotic activity in human tubal epithelium during reproductive life. *Fertil Steril* 1985;43:554–559.
231. Jansen RP. Endocrine response in the fallopian tube. *Endocr Rev* 1984;5:525–551.
232. Lindenbaum ES, Peretz BA, Beach D. Menstrual-cycle-dependent and -independent features of the human Fallopian tube fimbrial epithelium: An ultrastructural and cytochemical study. *Gynecol Obstet Invest* 1983;16:76–85.
233. Verhage HG, Bareither ML, Jaffe RC, et al. Cyclic changes in ciliation, secretion and cell height of the oviductal epithelium in women. *Am J Anat* 1979;156:505–521.
234. Menezo Y, Guerin P. The mammalian oviduct: Biochemistry and physiology. *Eur J Obstet Gynecol Reprod Biol* 1997;73:99–104.
235. Leese HJ. The formation and function of oviduct fluid. *J Reprod Fertil* 1988;82:843–856.
236. Sivridis E, Buckley C, Fox H. Argyrophil cells in normal, hyperplastic, and neoplastic endometrium. *J Clin Pathol* 1984;37:378–381.
237. Constant O, Cooke J, Parsons CA. Reformatted computed tomography of the female pelvis: normal anatomy. *Br J Obstet Gynaecol* 1989;96:1047–1053.
238. de Castro A, Yebra C, Aznar F, et al. Measurement of the endometrial cavity length using Wing Sound I. *Adv Contracept* 1987;3:133–137.
239. Hricak H. MRI of the female pelvis: a review. *AJR Am J Roentgenol* 1986;146:1115–1122.
240. Morris H, Emms M, Visser T, et al. Lymphoid tissue of the normal fallopian tube–a form of mucosal-associated lymphoid tissue (MALT)? *Int J Gynecol Pathol* 1986;5:11–22.
241. Boehme M, Donat H. Identification of lymphocyte subsets in the human fallopian tube. *Am J Reprod Immunol* 1992;28:81–84.
242. Kutteh WH, Blackwell RE, Gore H, et al. Secretory immune system of the female reproductive tract. II. Local immune system in normal and infected fallopian tube. *Fertil Steril* 1990;54:51–55.

243. Lurie M, Tur-Kaspa I, Weill S, et al. Ciliary ultrastructure of respiratory and fallopian tube epithelium in a sterile woman with Kartagener's syndrome. A quantitative estimation. *Chest* 1989;95:578–581.
244. Halbert SA, Patton DL, Zarutskie PW, et al. Function and structure of cilia in the fallopian tube of an infertile woman with Kartagener's syndrome. *Hum Reprod* 1997;12:55–58.
245. Gwin K, Wilcox R, Montag A. Insights into selected genetic diseases affecting female reproductive tract and their implication for pathologic evaluation of gynecologic specimens. *Arch Pathol Lab Med* 2009; 133(7):1041–1052.
246. Meserve E, Brouwer J, Crum CP. Serous tubal intraepithelial neoplasia: the concept and its application. *Mod Pathol* 2017;30(5):710–721.
247. Mehrad M, Ning G, Chen E, et al: A pathologist's road map to benign, precancerous, and malignant intraepithelial proliferations of the fallopian tube. *Adv Anatom Pathol* 2010;17(5):293–302.
248. Pulkkinen MO, Talo A. Tubal physiologic consideration in ectopic pregnancy. *Clin Obstet Gynecol* 1987;30:164–172.
249. Donnez J, Casanas-Roux F, Ferin J. Macroscopic and microscopic studies of fallopian tube after laparoscopic sterilization. *Contraception* 1979;20:497–509.
250. Donnez J, Casanas-Roux F, Ferin J, et al. Tubal polyps, epithelial inclusions, and endometriosis after tubal sterilization. *Fertil Steril* 1984;41:564–568.
251. Mills SE, Fechner RE. Stromal and epithelial changes in the fallopian tube following hormonal therapy. *Hum Pathol* 1980;11:583–585.
252. Lindblom B, Wilhelmsson L, Wikland M, et al. Prostaglandins and oviductal function. *Acta Obstet Gynecol Scand Suppl* 1983;113:43–46.
253. Moyle P, Kataoka M, Nakai A, et al. Nonovarian cystic lesions of the pelvis. *Radiographics* 2010;30(4):921–938.

Ovary

C. Blake Gilks

EMBRYOLOGY 1107	CORPUS LUTEUM OF MENSTRUATION 1122
GROSS ANATOMY 1108	Histology 1122
Prepubertal Ovaries 1108	Ultrastructure 1124
Adult Ovaries 1108	Hormonal Aspects 1124
Postmenopausal Ovaries 1108	CORPUS LUTEUM OF PREGNANCY 1124
BLOOD SUPPLY 1109	Gross Appearance 1124
LYMPHATICS 1109	Histology 1125
NERVE SUPPLY 1109	Ultrastructure 1126
SURFACE EPITHELIUM 1110	Hormonal Aspects 1126
Histology 1110	CORPUS ALBICANS 1126
Ultrastructure 1111	ATRETIC FOLLICLES 1126
STROMA 1111	Histology 1126
Histology 1111	Hormonal Aspects 1129
Ultrastructure 1117	HILUS CELLS 1129
Hormonal Aspects 1117	Histology 1129
PRIMORDIAL FOLLICLES 1117	Ultrastructure 1130
Histology 1117	Hormonal Aspects 1130
Ultrastructure 1118	RETE OVARII 1131
MATURING FOLLICLES 1118	REFERENCES 1131
Histology and Ultrastructure 1118	
Hormonal Aspects 1121	

EMBRYOLOGY

Approximately 5 weeks after fertilization, a thickening of the coelomic epithelium (mesothelium) along the medial and ventral borders of the mesonephros leads to the formation of the genital ridge. The gonadal anlage forms as a result of continued proliferation of this epithelium and the subjacent mesenchyme (1). Simultaneously, primordial germ cells migrate to the gonad from the yolk sac endoderm, reaching the genital ridge during the fifth and sixth weeks of embryonic life (2). These cells (oogonia) undergo mitotic activity and become most numerous at mid-gestation; two-thirds of them will undergo atresia by term (1,3). At 12 to 15 weeks' gestation, the oogonia begin meiosis and arrest in meiotic prophase, and are now referred to as primary oocytes (3–5).

At 2 months, the primitive gonad is recognizable as an ovary because, in contrast to the testis, it has remained basically unaltered. At 7 to 9 weeks' gestation, the outer zone of the ovary has enlarged to form the definitive cortex, which consists of confluent sheets of primitive germ cells admixed

---

This chapter is an update of a previous version authored by Philip B. Clement.

haphazardly with a smaller number of smaller pregranulosa cells (4,6). At 12 to 15 weeks, vascular connective tissue septa begin to radiate from the medullary mesenchyme into the inner portion of the cortex, and extend into the superficial part of the cortex by 20 weeks (5,6). The cortex thereby becomes divided into cellular groups composed of oocytes and pregranulosa cells (sex cords). Simultaneously, the pregranulosa cells begin to surround individual germ cells to form primordial follicles. Folliculogenesis begins in the inner part of the cortex at 14 to 20 weeks' gestation (2,3,5,7), and gradually extends to the outer cortex by the early neonatal period (8). The occasional follicles that mature into preantral and antral follicles in late gestation become surrounded by a condensation of mesenchymal cells that become the theca interna (4,7). The rete ovarii is present in the hilus as early as 12 weeks (5).

The origin of gonadal sex cords (pregranulosa cells in the ovary and Sertoli cells in the testis) is controversial (2,4,8,9–12), but recent observations indicate that the sex cords are likely of mesonephric origin (13–16). Hummitzsch et al. have proposed that granulosa cells are derived from Gonadal-Ridge Epithelial Like (GREL) cells of the genital ridge primordium; these cells are also suggested to be the precursor of ovarian surface epithelial cells (16).

GROSS ANATOMY

The ovaries are paired pelvic organs that lie on either side of the uterus close to the lateral pelvic wall, behind the broad ligament and anterior to the rectum. Each ovary is attached along its anterior (hilar) margin to the posterior aspect of the broad ligament by a double fold of peritoneum, the mesovarium; at its medial pole to the ipsilateral uterine cornu by the ovarian (or utero-ovarian) ligament; and from the superior aspect of its lateral pole to the lateral pelvic wall by the infundibulopelvic (or suspensory) ligament. The location of the ovary posterior to the broad ligament and a similar relationship of the ovarian ligament to the ipsilateral uterine (fallopian) tube aids in the determination of the laterality of a salpingo-oophorectomy specimen.

Prepubertal Ovaries

The ovary in the newborn is a tan, elongated, and flattened structure that lies above the true pelvis. It sometimes has a lobulated appearance with irregular edges (Fig. 41.1A). It has approximate dimensions of 1.3 cm by 0.5 cm by 0.3 cm, and a weight of less than 0.3 g (17–19). Throughout infancy and childhood, the ovary enlarges, increases in weight 30-fold, and changes in shape, so that by the time of puberty it has reached the size, weight, and shape of the adult ovary, and lies within the true pelvis (18,19). Inspection of the external and cut surfaces, particularly during the first few months of life and at puberty, may reveal prominent cystic follicles (20) similar to those seen in polycystic ovary disease (Fig. 41.1B).

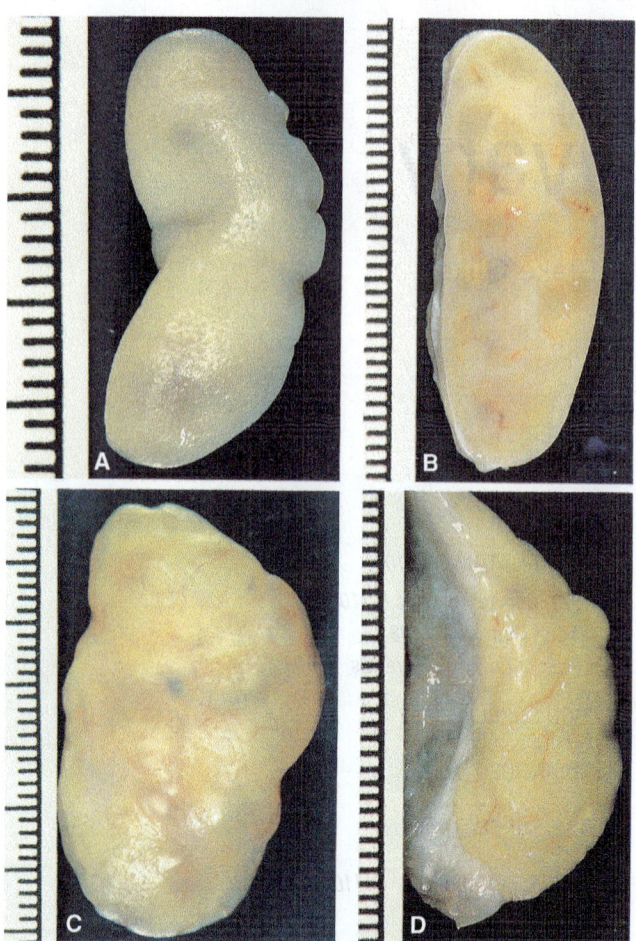

FIGURE 41.1 Gross appearance of ovary. **A:** Newborn, external aspect. **B:** Pubertal (age 15 years), sectioned surface. Note elongate shape and multiple cystic follicles. **C:** Adult (age 30 years), external aspect. **D:** Postmenopausal, external aspect. Note shrunken, gyriform appearance.

Adult Ovaries

Adult ovaries are ovoid with dimensions of approximately 3.0 to 5.0 cm by 1.5 to 3.0 cm by 0.6 to 1.5 cm, and a weight of 5 to 8 g. Their size and weight, however, vary considerably depending on their content of follicular derivatives. They have a pink-white exterior, which in early reproductive life is usually smooth (Fig. 41.1C), but thereafter becomes increasingly convoluted. Three ill-defined zones are discernible on the cut surface: an outer cortex, an inner medulla, and the hilus. Follicular structures (cystic follicles, yellow corpora lutea, white corpora albicantia) are typically visible in the cortex and medulla.

Postmenopausal Ovaries

After the menopause, the ovaries typically shrink to approximately one-half of their size in the reproductive era (21). Their size varies considerably, however, with the number of ovarian stromal cells and unresorbed corpora albicantia (22). Most postmenopausal ovaries have a shrunken, gyriform, external appearance (Fig. 41.1D), whereas some are more smooth and uniform. They have a firm consistency and a predominantly solid, pale cut surface, although occasional cysts measuring several millimeters in diameter (inclusion cysts) may be discernible within the cortex. Small white scars (corpora albicantia) are typically present within the medulla. Thick-walled blood vessels may be appreciable within the medulla and the hilus.

BLOOD SUPPLY

The ovarian artery, a branch of the aorta, courses along the infundibulopelvic ligament and the mesovarial border of the ovary where it anastomoses with the ovarian branch of the uterine artery. Approximately 10 arterial branches from this arcade penetrate the ovarian hilus, becoming markedly coiled and branched as they course through the medulla (23). These helicine arteries possess longitudinal ridges of intimal smooth muscle along their length. At the corticomedullary junction, the medullary arteries and arterioles form a plexus from which smaller, straight cortical arterioles arise and penetrate the cortex in a radial fashion, perpendicular to the ovarian surface. The cortical arterioles branch and anastomose several times, forming sets of interconnected vascular arcades (23). These arcades give rise to capillaries that form dense networks within the theca layers of the ovarian follicles. The intraovarian veins accompany the arteries, becoming large and tortuous in the medulla and forming a hilar plexus that drains into the ovarian veins; the latter traverse the mesovarium and course along the infundibulopelvic ligament (23). The ovarian veins also anastomose with tributaries of the uterine veins. The left and right ovarian veins drain into the left renal vein and the inferior vena cava, respectively.

In postmenopausal women, the medullary blood vessels may appear particularly numerous and closely packed (Fig. 41.2) and should not be mistaken for a hemangioma on microscopic examination. In addition, many of the same vessels may be calcified or have thickened walls and narrowed lumina due to medial deposition of a hyaline, amyloid-like material.

LYMPHATICS

The lymphatics of the ovary originate predominantly within the theca layers of the follicles. The granulosa layer of a maturing follicle is devoid of lymphatics in contrast to its counterpart within the corpus luteum, which possesses a rich supply of lymphatics (24). The lymphatics pass through the ovarian stroma, independent of blood vessels, to drain into larger trunks that form a plexus at the hilus. Within the hilus, the lymphatics and blood vessels converge, with the former coiled around veins in a helicoid fashion. Four to eight efferent channels pass into the mesovarium where they converge to form the subovarian plexus, which, in turn, is joined by

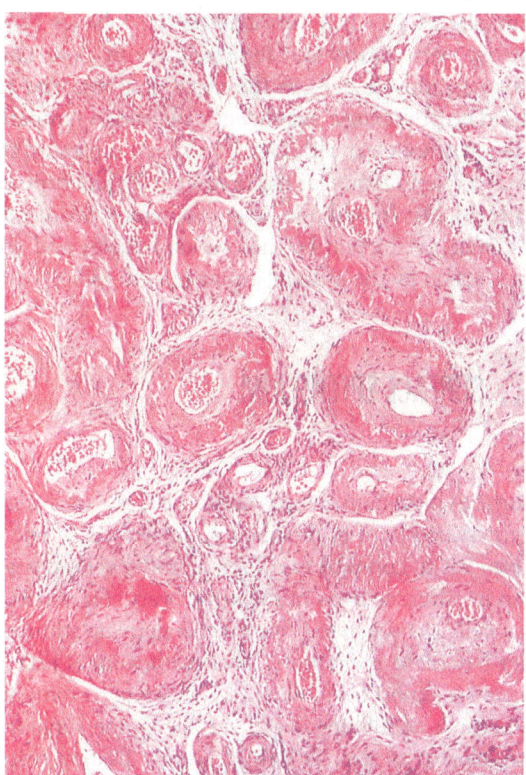

FIGURE 41.2 Numerous crowded thick-walled blood vessels within ovarian medulla of a postmenopausal woman. Some of the vessels have an eosinophilic amyloid-like material within their walls.

branches from the uterine (fallopian) tube and uterine fundus (24). Leaving the plexus, the drainage trunks diminish in number and size, passing along the free border of the infundibulopelvic ligament enmeshed with the ovarian veins. From there they accompany the ovarian vessels, juxtaposed to the psoas muscle, and drain into the upper para-aortic lymph nodes at the level of the lower pole of the kidney (24,25). The major lymphatic drainage of the ovary is therefore in a cephalad direction toward the para-aortic nodes. Accessory channels, however, may bypass the subovarian plexus, passing through the broad ligament to the internal iliac, external iliac, and interaortic lymph nodes, or in some females, via the round ligament to the iliac and inguinal lymph nodes (24,25). When the pelvic and para-aortic lymph nodes are extensively replaced by tumor, retrograde lymphatic flow may represent a rare mechanism of tumor spread to the ovaries.

NERVE SUPPLY

The nerve supply of the ovary arises from a sympathetic plexus that is enmeshed with the ovarian vessels in the infundibulopelvic ligament (26). Nerve fibers, which are predominantly nonmyelinated, accompany the ovarian artery, entering the ovary at the hilus. Delicate terminal fibers, many surrounding small arteries and arterioles, penetrate the medulla and cortex to terminate as plexuses surrounding the follicles (26,27). Adrenergic nerve fibers and terminals are in close contact with smooth muscle cells in the cortical stroma and theca externa. The physiologic significance of ovarian sympathetic innervation is not clear, although it has been suggested that it may play a role in follicular maturation, follicular rupture, or both (26,28,29). In addition, catecholamines can stimulate progesterone production by the ovarian follicles and androgen production by the ovarian stroma in vitro (30).

SURFACE EPITHELIUM

Histology

The surface epithelium of the ovary consists of a single, focally pseudostratified layer of modified peritoneal cells. The cells vary from flat to cuboidal to columnar and several types may be seen in different areas of the same ovary (Fig. 41.3). The surface cells are separated from the underlying stroma by a distinct basement membrane. This epithelium is extremely fragile and is almost always denuded in oophorectomy specimens because of rubbing of the surface by the surgeon and the pathologist, as well as lack of prompt fixation resulting in drying. Preserved epithelium is often confined to areas protected by surface adhesions or the lining of sulci.

Histochemical studies have demonstrated glycogen, as well as acid and neutral mucopolysaccharides, within surface epithelial cells (31,32). Seventeen-beta hydroxysteroid dehydrogenase activity, absent in extraovarian mesothelial cells, also has been demonstrated (31).

Epithelial inclusion glands (EIGs) are thought to arise from two sources: the surface epithelium and detached fimbrial epithelium (endosalpingiosis). The former arise from cortical invaginations of the surface epithelium that have lost their connection with the surface. They often become cystic, resulting in epithelial inclusion cysts (EICs), which may be recognized on macroscopic examination; a diameter of 1 cm has been suggested as a dividing line between an EIC and the smallest cystadenoma. Alternatively, EICs are thought to be derived from detached fimbrial epithelium. These cysts are typically multiple, scattered singly or in small clusters throughout the superficial cortex (Fig. 41.4); less commonly, extension into the deeper cortical or medullary stroma may occur. Inclusion glands and cysts (EIGCs) are typically lined by a single layer of ciliated tubal-type columnar cells; psammoma bodies within their lumina or the adjacent stroma are occasionally present. Similar glands, with or without associated psammoma bodies, encountered on the ovarian surface, within periovarian adhesions, and on the extraovarian peritoneum and omentum, are designated "endosalpingiosis" (33). EIGs have been identified on microscopic examination of ovaries from all age groups, including fetuses, infants, and adolescents (34,35). EIGCs become more numerous with age, and are common incidental findings in late reproductive and postmenopausal age groups. Less frequently, EIGCs may be lined by other müllerian epithelia (endometrioid, mucinous), or nonspecific columnar or flattened cells (36,37).

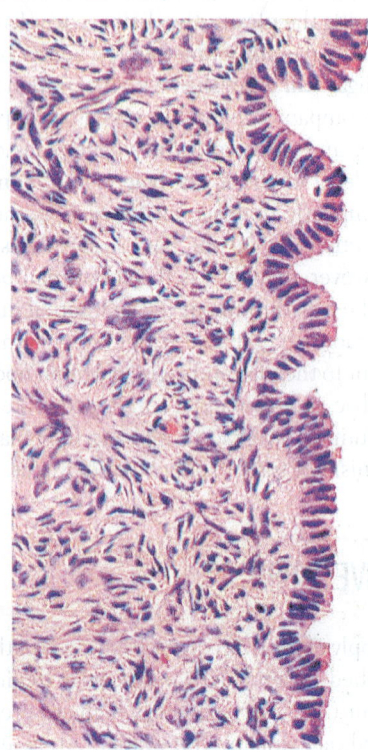

FIGURE 41.3 Ovarian surface epithelium composed of a single layer of columnar cells.

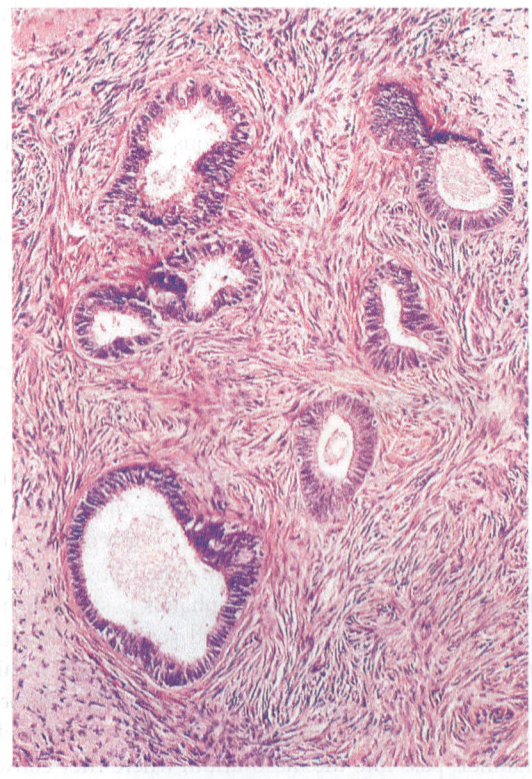

FIGURE 41.4 Epithelial inclusion glands within ovarian cortex.

It was formerly thought that EIGCs were the site of origin of most surface epithelial tumors (38), but recently there has been evidence indicating that most high-grade serous carcinomas arise from the fallopian tube, and most clear cell and endometrioid carcinomas arise from endometriosis (39–41).

The immunostaining profile of the ovarian surface epithelium (OSE) and the epithelium lining EIGCs varies depending on whether it is flattened or cuboidal and mesothelial-like, or columnar with tubal metaplasia. The former cells stain for mesothelial markers such as calretinin and mesothelin, whereas the latter columnar-ciliated cells show either focal immunoreactivity or complete absence of staining for these markers (Fig. 41.5A) (42). The cells showing columnar cell shape and tubal metaplasia, whether on the ovarian surface or lining EIGCs, stain positively for epithelial markers including oviduct-specific glycoprotein-1 and E-cadherin, whereas the flat OSE cells do not express these markers (Fig. 41.5C–F). PAX8 is expressed by all cells, flat and columnar, lining EIGCs, but not by most OSE cells on the ovarian surface (42,43).

Urothelial-like or transitional differentiation is also within the metaplastic potential of the OSE and pelvic peritoneum. Such differentiation typically takes the form of Walthard nests of transitional cells, a common microscopic finding within the serosa or the immediately subjacent stroma of the uterine (fallopian) tube, mesosalpinx, and mesovarium, or less commonly, the ovarian hilus (Fig. 41.6) (44–47). The larger nests frequently become cystic and may be lined by columnar mucinous cells. Brenner tumors are also characterized by transitional differentiation; as many as one-half of those encountered by the pathologist are of microscopic size. It has been suggested that both Brenner tumors and "ovarian" mucinous tumors (which frequently co-exist) arise from Walthard nests in most cases (48).

Hyperplastic mesothelial cells, usually a response to chronic pelvic inflammation, may involve the surface of the ovary and focally replace the OSE. Florid examples exhibiting tubulopapillary (Fig. 41.7) and pseudoinfiltrative patterns, as well as varying degrees of nuclear atypia, must be distinguished from a malignant mesothelioma or a primary ovarian or metastatic carcinoma.

Ultrastructure

The ultrastructural appearance of the OSE is similar to that of the extraovarian peritoneum (49–51). The cell surfaces by scanning and transmission electron microscopy have dome-shaped apices covered by numerous, often branching, microvilli, occasional single cilia, and pinocytotic vesicles (Fig. 41.8). The cytoplasm contains abundant polysomes, free ribosomes, abundant mitochondria, and bundles of intermediate filaments and tonofilaments. Lipid droplets are sometimes present in the basal cytoplasm. The nuclei have indented nuclear membranes and peripheral nucleoli. Straight or convoluted lateral plasma membranes (PMs) are reinforced by luminal junctional complexes, scattered desmosomes, and desmosomal–tonofilament complexes. The membranes may be widely separated in areas, creating dilated intercellular spaces (ICSs) (50). A well-developed basal lamina (BL) separates the surface epithelium from the underlying stroma.

STROMA

Histology

As the cortical and medullary stroma is continuous and similar in appearance, the boundary between these two zones is ill defined and arbitrary. The spindle-shaped stromal cells, which have scanty cytoplasm, are typically arranged in whorls or a storiform pattern (Fig. 41.9). Fine cytoplasmic lipid droplets may be appreciable with special stains, especially in the late reproductive and postmenopausal age groups (52). Immunohistochemical stains reveal cytoplasmic vimentin, actin, and desmin (53–57). Stromal cells are separated by a dense reticulin network (Fig. 41.9) and a variable amount of collagen that is most abundant in the superficial cortex. Although the latter is frequently referred to as the tunica albuginea, it lacks the densely collagenous, almost acellular appearance and sharp delineation of the tunica albuginea of the testis.

A variety of other cells may be found within the ovarian stroma, most of which are probably derived from the cells of fibroblastic type. *Luteinized stromal cells*, which lie in the stroma at a distance from the follicles, are found singly or in small nests, most often in the medulla. They are polygonal cells with abundant eosinophilic to clear cytoplasm containing variable amounts of lipid, a central round nucleus, and a prominent nucleolus (Fig. 41.10). These cells are typically immunoreactive for inhibin (58–60), calretinin (61), melan-A (62), CD10 (63), and occasionally, testosterone (64). The numbers of luteinized stromal cells increase during pregnancy and after the menopause; they are probably secondary to elevated levels of circulating gonadotropins during these periods (22,52). In one autopsy study, luteinized stromal cells were demonstrated after diligent searching in 13% of the women under the age of 55 years and in one-third of the women over that age; the frequency of their detection increased with increasing degrees of stromal proliferation (22). More exhaustive sampling might indicate that luteinized stromal cells are a normal finding in the ovary, particularly in later life. In this age group, the presence of luteinized cells is not usually associated with clinical evidence of a hormonal disturbance. In some older women, but more often in younger patients, however, more striking degrees of stromal luteinization (stromal hyperthecosis) are frequently associated with androgenic and estrogenic manifestations. Occasionally in such cases, nodules of luteinized stromal cells may be appreciable on low-power microscopic examination (nodular hyperthecosis).

Enzymatically active stromal cells are characterized by their oxidative and other enzymatic activities (52,65,66). The frequency of their detection and their numbers increase

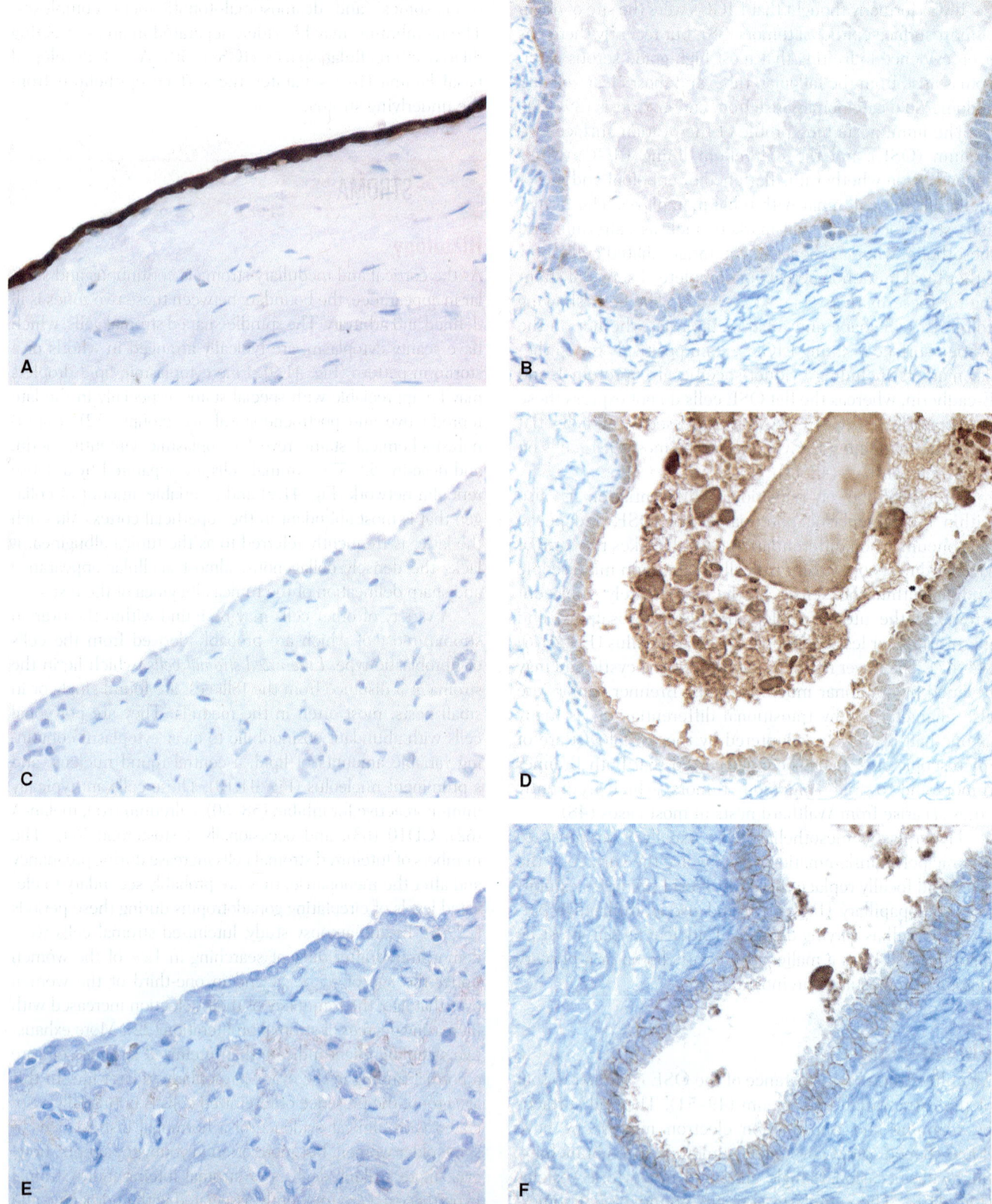

FIGURE 41.5 Immunostaining profile of normal ovarian surface epithelium and cells lining epithelial inclusion glands. The flattened and cuboidal ovarian surface epithelium cells stain positively for the mesothelial marker calretinin (**A**), and are negative for oviduct-specific glycoprotein-1 (**C**) and E-cadherin (**E**), while the columnar cells with tubal metaplasia, lining the epithelial inclusion gland, are negative for calretinin (**B**), and express both oviduct-specific glycoprotein-1 (**D**) and E-cadherin (**F**).

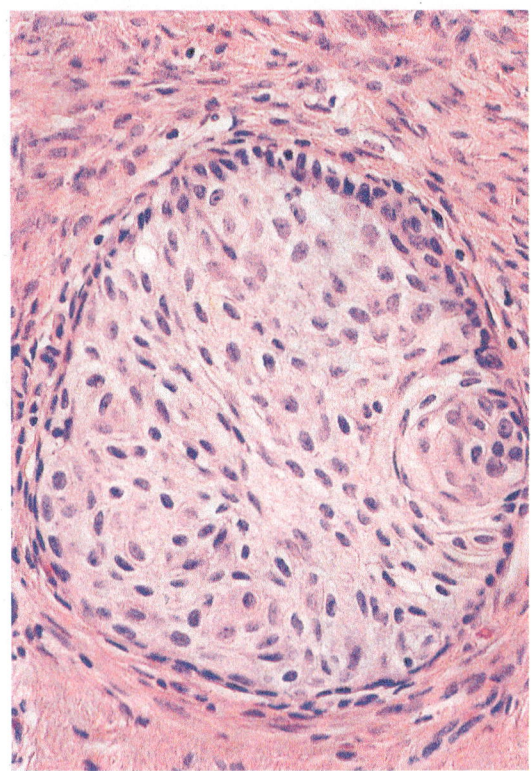

FIGURE 41.6 Walthard nest within ovarian hilus abutting medullary stroma.

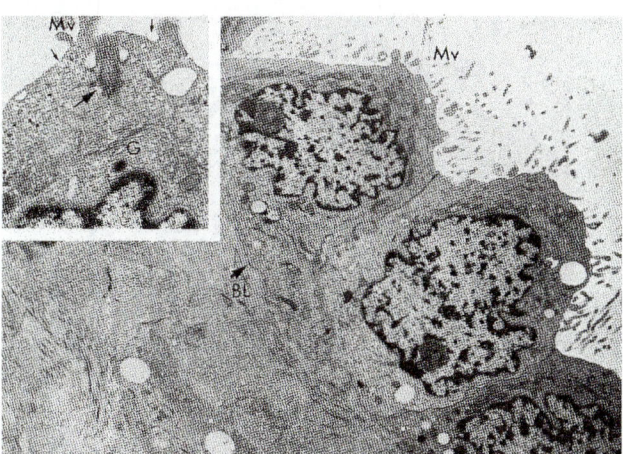

FIGURE 41.8 Electron micrograph of ovarian surface epithelium. The cells have numerous microvilli (*Mv*) and well-developed organelles in a perinuclear location. The nuclei have indented membranes and peripheral nucleoli. The lateral plasma membranes are reinforced by luminal junctional complexes and scattered desmosomes, but are occasionally widely separated producing dilated intercellular spaces. A well-defined basal lamina (*BL*) separates the cells from the underlying stroma (original magnification ×6,400). *Inset:* The surface microvilli are associated with micropinocytotic vesicles (*short arrows*) and occasional single cilia (*long arrows*). Note Golgi complex (*G*) (original magnification ×22,000). Reprinted with permission from Ferenczy A, Richart RM. *Female Reproductive System: Dynamics of Scan and Transmission Electron Microscopy.* New York: John Wiley & Sons; 1974.

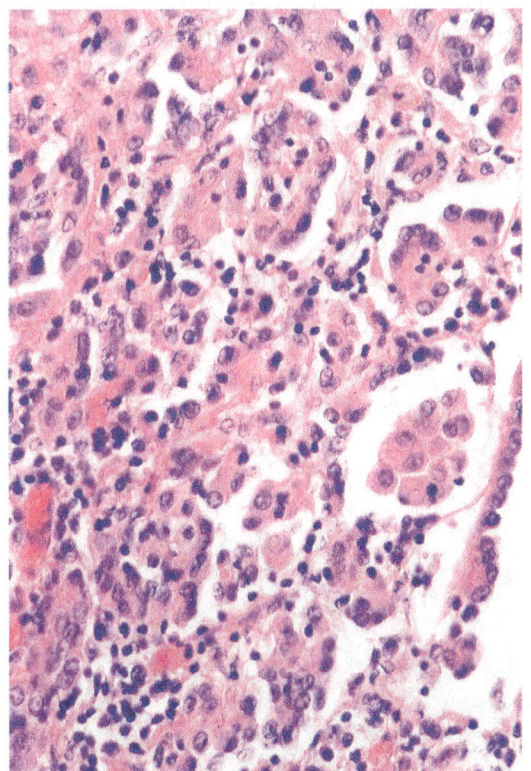

FIGURE 41.7 Hyperplastic mesothelial cells on ovarian surface. Note admixed inflammatory cells.

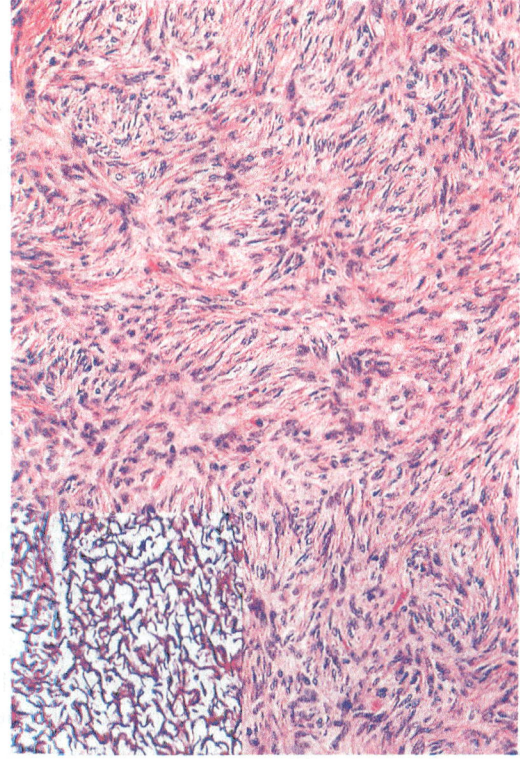

FIGURE 41.9 Ovarian stroma composed of whorls of plump spindle cells of fibroblastic type. *Inset:* Note dense reticulin network (reticulin stain).

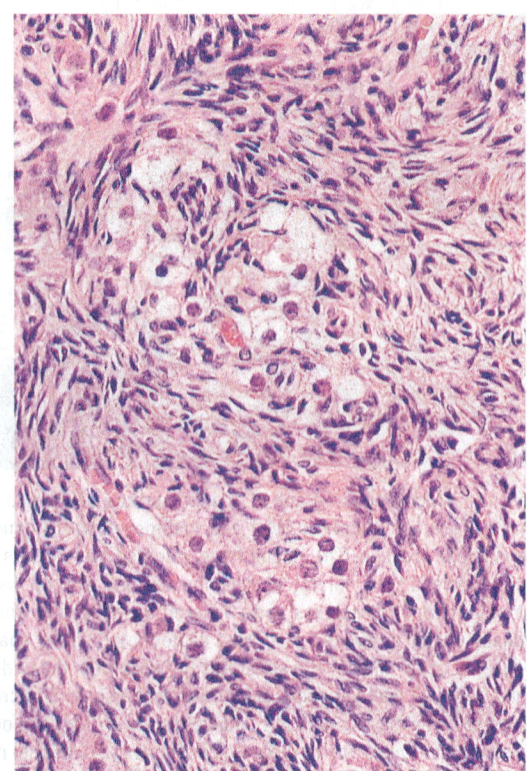

FIGURE 41.10 Luteinized stromal cells.

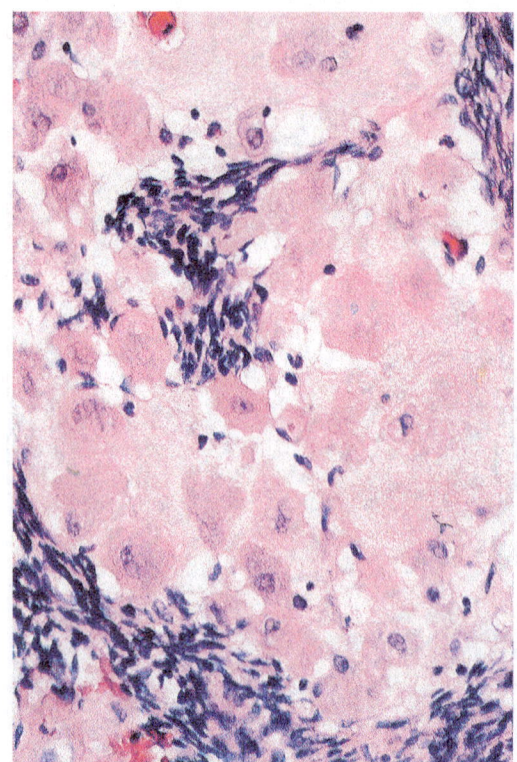

FIGURE 41.11 A nest of decidual cells within the ovarian stroma.

with age, occurring in over 80% of postmenopausal women, typically in the medulla (65,66). Some enzymatically active stromal cells correspond to luteinized stromal cells, but most cannot be distinguished from neighboring, nonreactive stromal cells in routine histologic preparations (65).

Decidual cells may occur singly, as small nodules, or as confluent sheets within the stroma of the superficial cortex or within periovarian adhesions (Fig. 41.11). The appearance of the decidual cells is usually identical to eutopic decidua, but occasional examples may exhibit cytologic atypia potentially mimicking metastatic carcinoma on histologic examination (67–72). A network of capillaries and a sprinkling of lymphocytes are typically present within the decidual foci. A decidual reaction within the ovary is almost always a response of the ovarian stromal cells to elevated circulating or local levels of progesterone; the process is seen most commonly in pregnancy, occurring as early as the ninth week of gestation and by term is present in virtually all ovaries. Less commonly it may occur in association with trophoblastic disease, in patients treated with progestins, in the vicinity of a corpus luteum, or in association with hormonally active, hyperplastic or neoplastic ovarian lesions (22,67,69). Prior pelvic irradiation may be a predisposing factor by increasing the sensitivity of the stromal cells to hormonal stimulation (69). Foci of ovarian decidua have been occasionally described in both pre- and postmenopausal women with no obvious cause (22,69).

Foci of *smooth muscle* may be seen within the ovarian stroma (Fig. 41.12), most commonly within peri or postmenopausal women (73). The smooth muscle is bilateral in about 25% of cases and usually is confined to a few microscopic fields. It is often associated with other findings in the ovary, occurring with the hyperplastic ovarian stroma

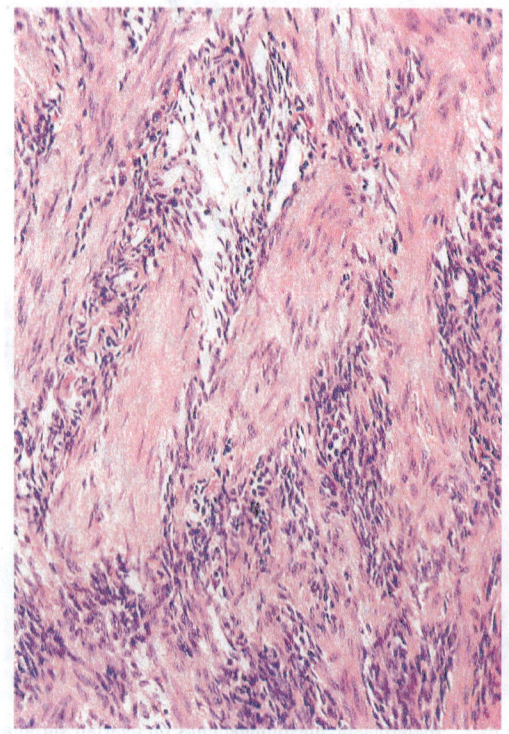

FIGURE 41.12 Smooth muscle cells within ovarian stroma.

associated with stromal hyperthecosis or sclerocystic ovaries (74), and within the stroma surrounding nonneoplastic and neoplastic cysts, including endometriotic cysts. Rare endometriotic cysts may contain prominent amounts of smooth muscle ("endomyometriosis") (75). One study (73) found that almost 90% of women with ovarian smooth muscle metaplasia had uterine leiomyomas.

Nests of cells resembling *endometrial stromal cells* ("stromal endometriosis") occur within the ovarian stroma, usually in the absence of typical endometriosis (Fig. 41.13) (76,77). Foci of mature *fat cells* may be encountered as an incidental histologic finding within the subcapsular ovarian stroma (78,79); a possible association with obesity was noted in one study (79). Reinke-crystal–containing Leydig cells, presumably representing transformed stromal cells, may occur rarely, and are typically associated with stromal hyperthecosis or within the nonneoplastic stroma in or adjacent to an ovarian neoplasm (80–82). The so-called "*neuroendocrine*" or "*APUD*" *type cells* have been demonstrated within the ovarian stroma in approximately 6% of the normal women in one study (83). The cells occur in small groups in the corticomedullary stromal junction and are argyrophilic and argentaffinic. Their clinical significance and hormonal function, if any, is unknown, but it has been suggested that they may represent the cell of origin of rare primary ovarian carcinoid tumors not associated with teratomatous or mucinous elements.

Aging Changes

Although there is typically a gradual increase in its volume from the fourth to the seventh decades (21,84), the ovarian stroma in postmenopausal women exhibits a wide spectrum of appearances (22,50,68). At one extreme, there is stromal atrophy manifested by a thin cortex and minimal amounts of medullary stroma (Fig. 41.14). At the other extreme, there is marked stromal proliferation warranting the designation "stromal hyperplasia." Most postmenopausal subjects, however, exhibit varying degrees of nodular or diffuse proliferation of the cortical and medullary stromal cells that lie between these two extremes (Fig. 41.15) (22,65), making the "normal" appearance difficult to define. Broad irregular areas of cortical fibrosis may be encountered in peri- and postmenopausal ovaries (22). When well-circumscribed, these foci resemble a small fibroma, but this designation is applied to lesions 1 cm or greater in diameter. A similar size limit could be used to distinguish between the foci of surface stromal papillarity commonly encountered in this age group (Fig. 41.16) and serous surface papillomas. Cortical "granulomas" are common incidental microscopic findings in the late reproductive and postmenopausal age groups, having been demonstrated in up to 45% of women over the age of 40 years (22,76,77,85–87). They consist of spherical circumscribed aggregates of epithelioid cells, lymphocytes, and occasionally, multinucleated giant cells and anisotropic fat crystals (Fig. 41.17). Cortical granulomas and the spherical, cloud-like, hyalin scars (Fig. 41.18)

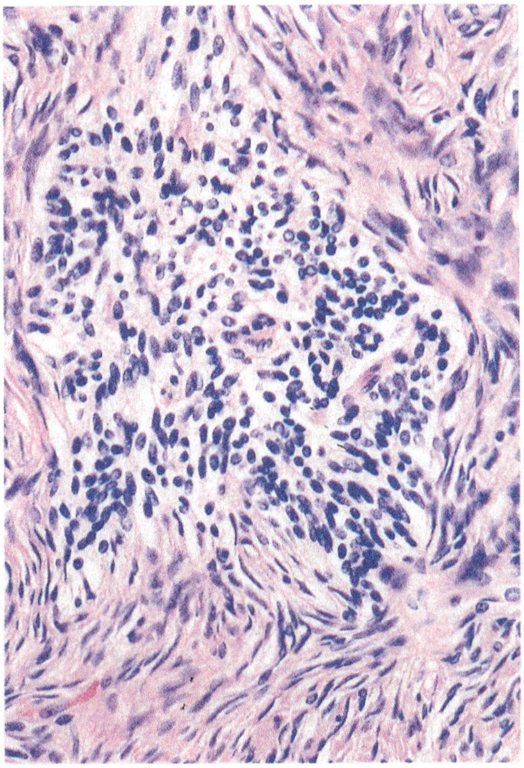

FIGURE 41.13 Focus of endometrial stromal cells ("stromal endometriosis") within ovarian cortex.

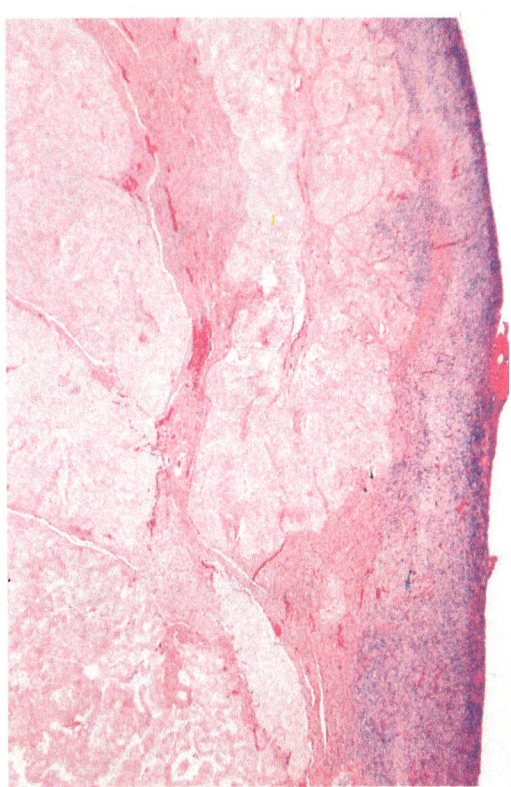

FIGURE 41.14 Atrophic postmenopausal ovary. The cortex is thin and multiple corpora albicantia are present within the medulla.

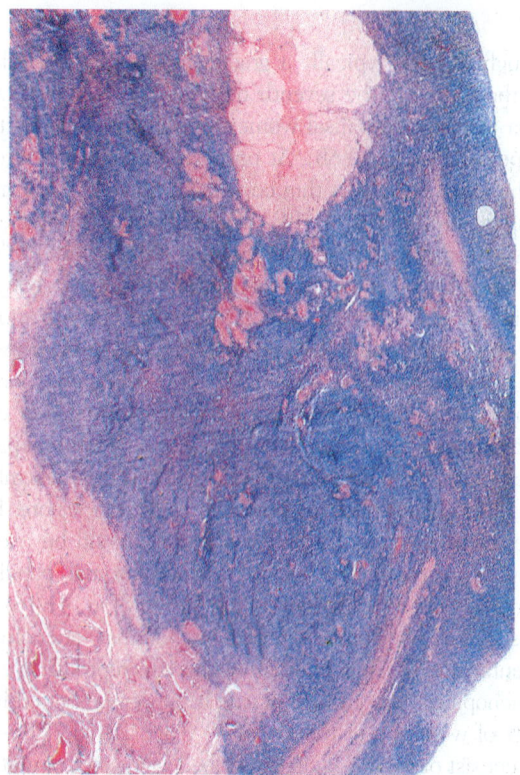

FIGURE 41.15 Postmenopausal ovary with a moderate degree of stromal proliferation.

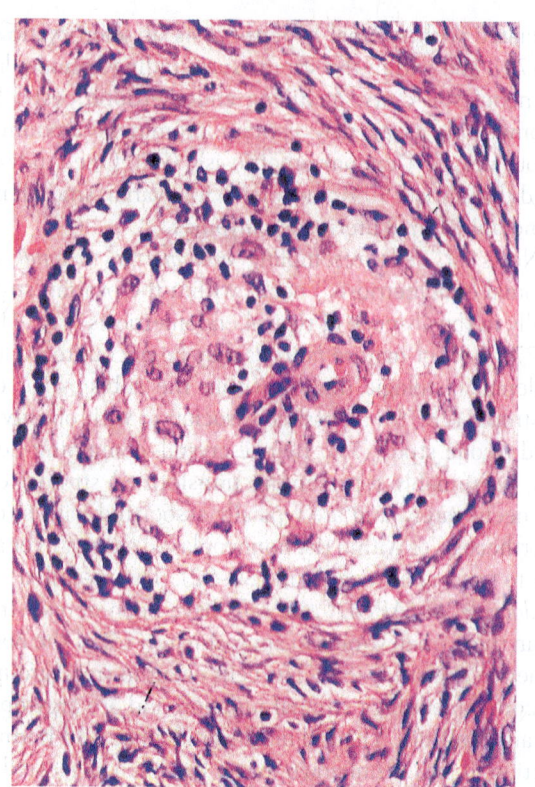

FIGURE 41.17 Cortical granuloma.

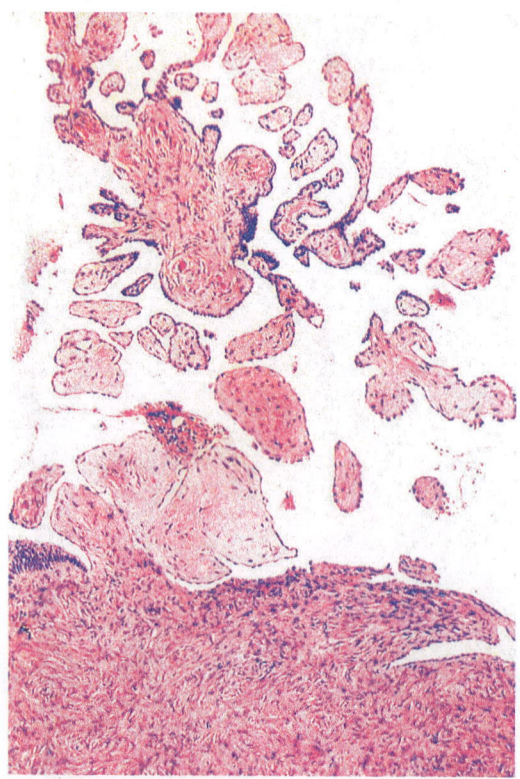

FIGURE 41.16 Papillary stromal projections from ovarian surface.

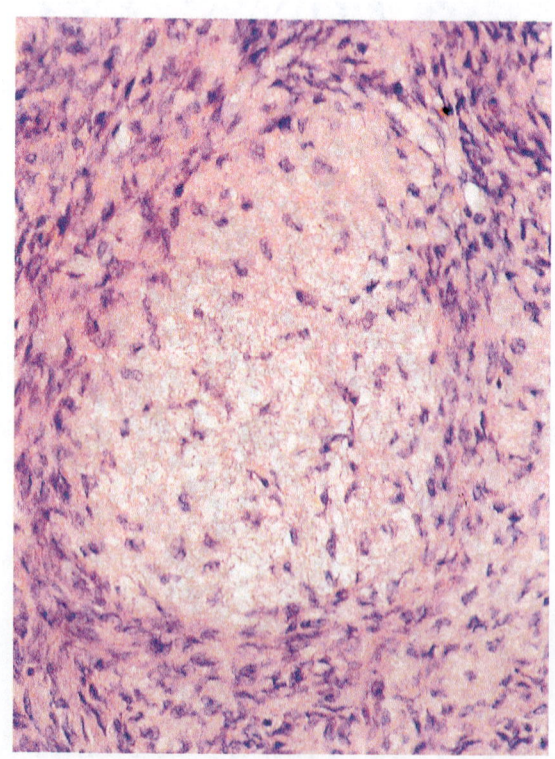

FIGURE 41.18 Hyalin scar.

present within the superficial cortical stroma of almost all postmenopausal ovaries are of uncertain histogenesis. It has been suggested that they may represent regressed foci of stromal endometriosis, ectopic decidua, or luteinized stromal cells.

Ultrastructure

Typical ovarian stromal cells have slender spindle-shaped nuclei and complex cytoplasmic processes (50,65). Their scant cytoplasm is rich in organelles required for collagen synthesis, including free ribosomes and mitochondria. Tropocollagen, concentrated at the periphery of the cytoplasm, is deposited in the extracellular space and eventually converted to collagen. Rows of micropinocytotic vesicles occur along the PM and desmosome-like attachments may be found between the cells (65). Luteinized stromal cells have abundant cytoplasm containing lipid droplets and steroidogenic organelles, including smooth endoplasmic reticulum (ER), mitochondria with tubular cristae, and Golgi (50,65,66,88).

Hormonal Aspects

Numerous studies have demonstrated the steroidogenic potential and the gonadotropin-responsiveness of the ovarian stroma in both pre- and postmenopausal women (89–101). In vitro incubation of ovarian stromal tissue indicates that its principal steroid product is androstenedione, in addition to smaller quantities of testosterone and dehydroepiandrosterone (102). In vitro production of androgens is enhanced by human chorionic gonadotropin (hCG), pituitary gonadotropins, and insulin, consistent with the presence of receptors for these hormones within the stromal cells (63,66,103). To what extent the ovarian stroma contributes to the androgen pool in normal premenopausal women is unknown, but it is likely that it is the source of small amounts of testosterone. With cessation of follicular activity at the time of the menopause, the ovarian stroma becomes, together with the adrenal glands, the major source of androgens. Testosterone and androstenedione are the major androgens secreted by the ovarian stroma in postmenopausal women (89–91,93,101), and in vitro and in vivo studies have shown that ovaries with stromal hyperplasia secrete more androstenedione, estrone, and estradiol than normal ovaries (94,96). Approximately 80% of the circulating androstenedione in postmenopausal women, however, is of adrenal origin (90). Despite a cessation of follicular synthesis of estradiol (E2) in postmenopausal subjects, small amounts of this hormone are present in the circulation (probably derived from the adrenal glands) by peripheral conversion of estrone (90,104), and from the ovarian stroma itself (89,91,105). Estrone, however, becomes the major circulating estrogen after the menopause, derived predominantly from the peripheral aromatization of androstenedione that occurs in fat, muscle, liver, kidney, brain, and adrenals (90,105,106). Increased aromatization in postmenopausal women, likely due to high endogenous LH levels in these subjects, leads to a twofold increase in the daily production rate of estrone compared to that in premenopausal women; aromatization is also higher in obese subjects. In some postmenopausal women, sufficient estrogen is elaborated by this mechanism to prevent the clinical manifestations of estrogen withdrawal and to play a role in the genesis of endometrial carcinoma (84,90). An association between the degree of stromal proliferation and postmenopausal endometrial adenocarcinoma has been noted (84), and the ovarian stroma in postmenopausal women with endometrial adenocarcinoma produces more androgens in vitro than that of control subjects without endometrial cancer (107). The variations that exist in the ovarian steroid hormone output from one postmenopausal woman to another may correspond to similar variations in the morphologic appearance of the stroma in this age group, although no correlative functional and structural studies have been performed.

PRIMORDIAL FOLLICLES

Histology

Approximately 400,000 primordial follicles present at the time of birth fill the ovarian cortex (Fig. 41.19). After this period, their numbers decrease progressively through the processes of atresia and folliculogenesis until their eventual disappearance that marks the end of the menopause.

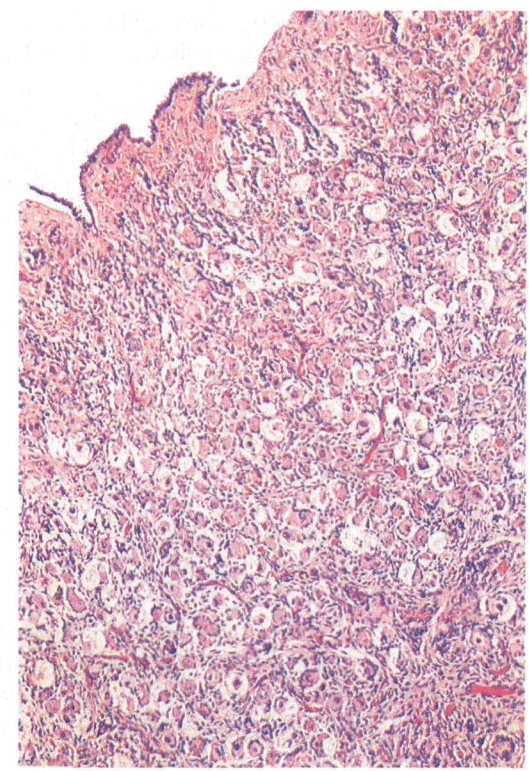

FIGURE 41.19 Newborn ovary. Multiple primordial follicles fill the ovarian cortex.

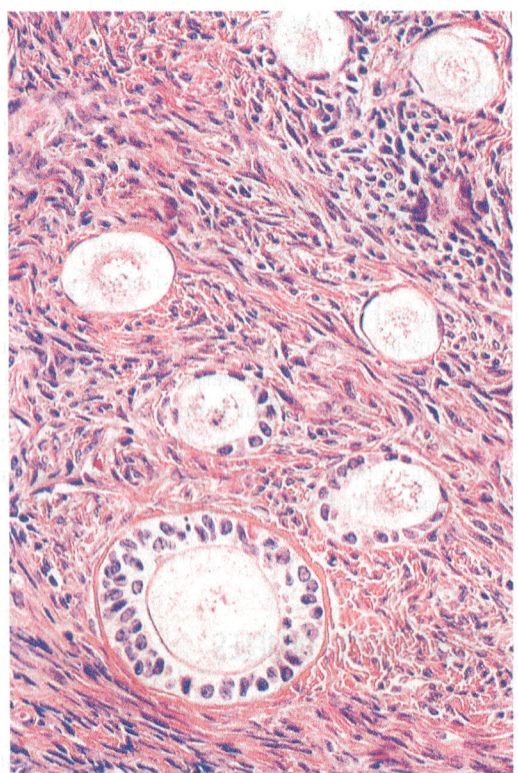

FIGURE 41.20 Primordial follicles (four at the top of the figure) and primary follicles (three at the bottom of the figure).

However, rare follicles may persist for several years after the cessation of menses, accounting for sporadic ovulation and occasional episodes of postmenopausal bleeding (108). In the reproductive era, primordial follicles are found scattered irregularly in clusters throughout a narrow band in the superficial cortex. They consist of a primary oocyte, measuring 40 to 70 μm in diameter, surrounded by a single layer of flattened, mitotically inactive, granulosa cells resting on a thin BL (Fig. 41.20). Rare primordial (and maturing) follicles may contain multiple oocytes, particularly in individuals who are less than 20 years of age (19,109–111). The oocyte is arrested at the dictyate stage of meiotic prophase at the time of birth, enters an interphase period until follicular maturation prior to ovulation, or undergoes degeneration during atresia (112). The large spherical nucleus of the oocyte has finely granular, uniformly dispersed chromatin and one or more dense, thread-like nucleoli (112); rare oocytes may have multiple nuclei (110,111). The cytoplasm of the oocyte contains a paranuclear, eosinophilic, crescent-shaped zone consisting of a complex of interrelated organelles, the so-called Balbiani vitelline body (BVB) (113,114). Within the vitelline body is a dark spot (the centrosome) surrounded by a halo, which in turn is flanked by darker, periodic acid–Schiff (PAS)-positive, granular zones rich in mitochondria (113,114). The cytoplasm of the oocyte lacks the abundant glycogen and the high alkaline phosphatase activity characteristic of the primordial germ cells and the oogonia of the embryonic gonad.

Ultrastructure

The granulosa cells of the primordial follicle have sparse organelles, occasional desmosomal attachments with each other, and microvillus projections that attach to the oocyte by tight apposition (50). Within the oocyte, the juxtanuclear centrosome (CS) of the BVB (Fig. 41.21A) consists of dense granules, closely packed vesicles, and dense fibers that form a basket-like structure at the periphery of the centrosome (Fig. 41.21B) (113,114). The centrosome is surrounded by a zone of smooth ER that represents the halo seen by light microscopy. More peripheral and constituting the rest of the BVB are a concentration of most of the oocyte's organelles, including multiple Golgi complexes, prominent compound aggregates (CAs), numerous mitochondria intimately associated with sparsely granular ER, and annulate lamellae (Fig. 41.21B) (113,114). The latter structures, which may be attached or immediately adjacent to the nucleus or free within the BVB, are constantly present in primary oocytes and other rapidly growing embryonal or neoplastic cells. They are arranged in stacks or concentric arrangements of up to 100 parallel, smooth, paired membranes that delineate greatly flattened cisternal spaces, 30 to 50 μm wide.

MATURING FOLLICLES

Histology and Ultrastructure

Folliculogenesis

Folliculogenesis refers to the continuous process occurring throughout reproductive life whereby cohorts of primordial follicles undergo maturation during each menstrual cycle. Follicular maturation begins during the luteal phase and continues throughout the follicular phase of the next cycle. Each month only one such follicle, the preovulatory (or dominant) follicle, achieves complete maturation, culminating in the release of the oocyte (ovulation). The other follicles that have begun the maturational process undergo atresia at earlier stages of their development. Folliculogenesis and atresia also occur prenatally, throughout childhood and during pregnancy, although maturing follicles rarely reach the preovulatory follicle stage during these periods (19,115–123).

The first morphologic evidence of follicular maturation is the assumption of a cuboidal to columnar shape of the granulosa cells accompanied by enlargement of the oocyte (*primary follicle*) (Fig. 41.20). Mitotic activity in the granulosa cells results in their stratification and three to five concentric layers around the oocyte (*secondary or preantral follicle*) (Fig. 41.22). At this stage an eosinophilic, PAS-positive, homogeneous, acellular layer, known as the zona pellucida, appears, encasing the oocyte. Its formation is usually attributed to the granulosa cells, but the oocyte may also play a role. At the end of its development, the zona pellucida is 20 to 25 μm thick membrane rich in acid mucopolysaccharides and glycoprotein (Figs. 41.22 to 41.25) (50). Preantral follicles measure from

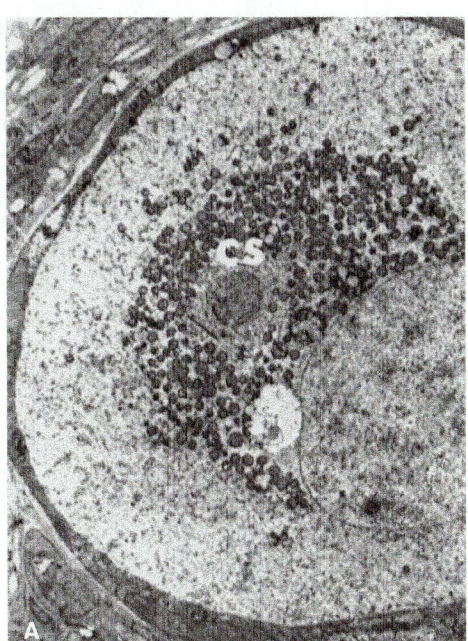
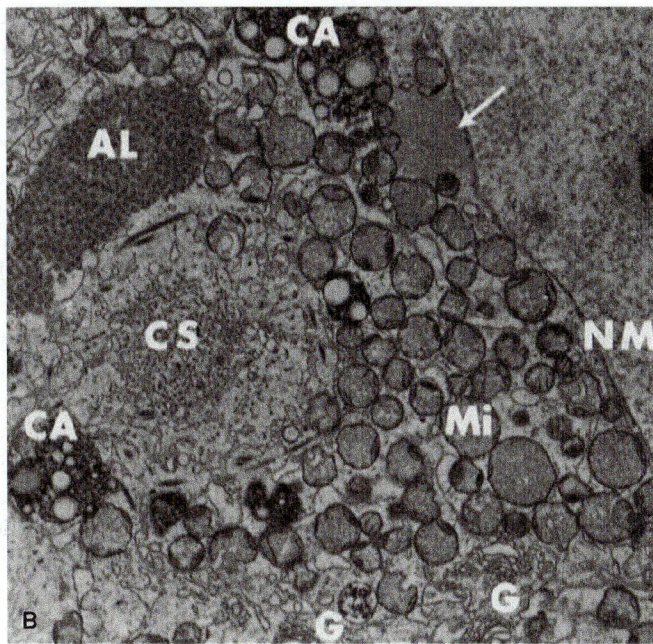

FIGURE 41.21 Electron micrograph of a primordial follicle. **A:** Balbiani vitelline body consists of a centrosome (*CS*) surrounded by a condensation of mitochondria, Golgi complexes (*G*), endoplasmic reticulum, and lysosomes (original magnification ×2,400). **B:** Detailed view of Balbiani vitelline body. A cluster of closely packed spiral fibrils (*arrow*) is attached to the nuclear envelope (*NM*). The centrosome (*CS*) is composed of dense granules, some arranged periodically on fine fibers, and small vesicles, with a peripheral zone of endoplasmic reticulum and dense fibers. Surrounding the centrosome are masses of mitochondria (*Mi*) and compound aggregates (*CAs*). A stack of annulate lamellae (*AL*) is seen tangentially. Note the prominent endoplasmic reticulum in close association with multiple Golgi complexes at the periphery of the vitelline body. Reprinted with permission from Hertig AT. The primary human oocyte: Some observations on the fine structure of Balbiani's vitelline body and the origin of the annulate lamellae. *Am J Anat* 1968;122:107–137.

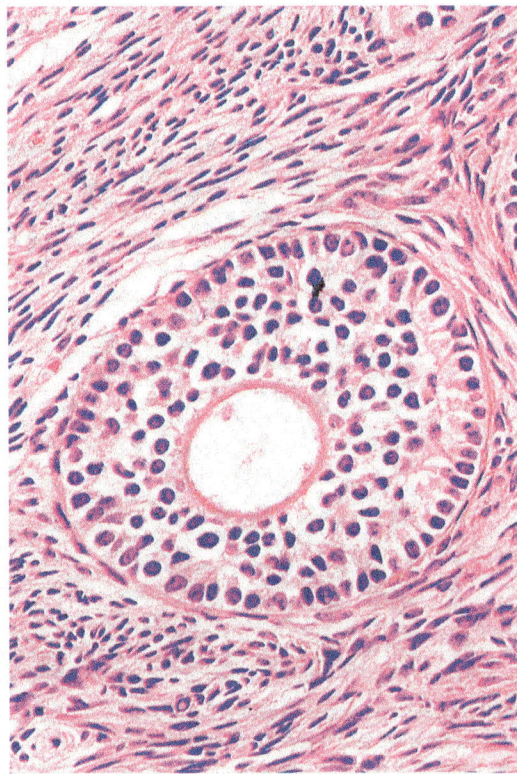

FIGURE 41.22 Preantral follicle. Several layers of granulosa cells surround the oocyte. A theca interna layer is not yet apparent.

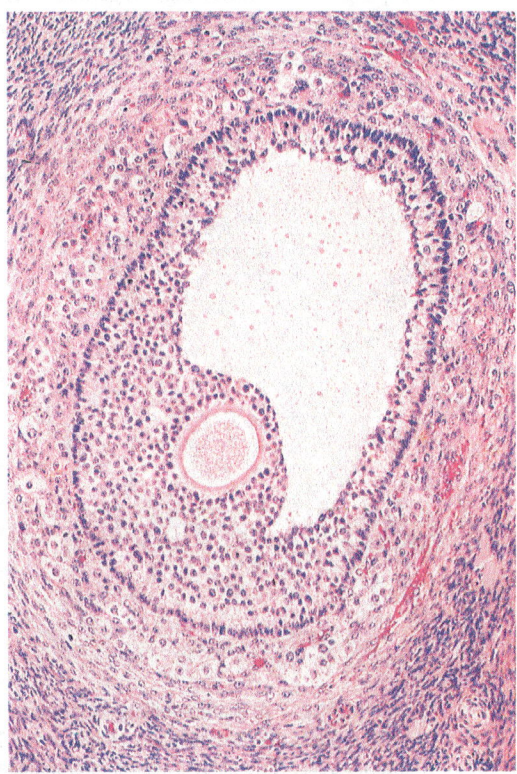

FIGURE 41.23 Mature follicle. Oocyte within cumulus oophorus projects into antrum. The theca layers are well developed.

50 to 400 μm in diameter, and as they increase in size, they migrate into the deeper cortex and medulla. Simultaneously, the surrounding ovarian stromal cells become specialized into several layers of theca interna cells and an outer, ill-defined layer of theca externa cells. Secretion of mucopolysaccharide-rich fluid by the granulosa cells results in their separation by fluid-filled clefts that eventually coalesce to form a single large cavity or antrum lined by several layers of granulosa cells (*tertiary, antral, or vesicular follicle*). The first evidence of antrum formation occurs in follicles that are from 200 to 400 μm in diameter, after which the follicles progressively enlarge due to continued fluid secretion into the antrum. Concurrently, the oocyte enlarges to its definitive size and assumes an eccentric position at one pole of the follicle. At this site, the granulosa cells proliferate to form the cumulus oophorus which, containing the oocyte in its center, protrudes into the antrum (*mature or graafian follicle*) (Fig. 41.23).

Ovulation

During each cycle, only a small number of mature follicles (<4 per ovary) reach a diameter of 4 to 5 mm by the mid- to late luteal phase; one of them will become the preovulatory follicle of the subsequent cycle (124,125). Late in follicular growth, the oocyte, its surrounding zona pellucida, and a single layer of radially disposed, columnar granulosa cells (the corona radiata) detach from the cumulus oophorus and float in the antral fluid. The preovulatory follicle, shortly before ovulation, reaches a diameter of 15 to 25 mm (28,125) and partially protrudes from the ovarian surface at the eventual rupture point, or stigma. Here the overlying surface epithelial cells exhibit progressive flattening, degeneration, and desquamation. The stroma in this area becomes attenuated and almost avascular, with degeneration of the stromal cells, fragmentation of collagen fibers, and an accumulation of intercellular fluid (28). These surface epithelial and stromal changes that immediately precede ovulation may be secondary to local ischemia and the release of proteolytic enzymes and prostaglandins into the stroma. The preovulatory follicle then ruptures with liberation of the follicular fluid and oocyte (with its surrounding granulosa cell layers, the corona radiata) into the peritoneal cavity. Following ovulation, the stigma is occluded by a mass of coagulated follicular fluid, fibrin, blood, granulosa, and connective tissue cells; it is eventually converted to scar tissue.

Shortly before ovulation, the oocyte within the ovulatory follicle enters telophase of the first meiotic division. Chromosomal reduction occurs by the migration of one-half of the oocyte chromosomes into a portion of the oocyte cytoplasm that separates from the cell as the first polar body. The first meiotic division begun in fetal life is now complete, and the oocyte is now designated the secondary oocyte. Immediately after expulsion of the first polar body, the secondary oocyte enters the second meiotic division, arresting at metaphase until fertilization occurs.

Granulosa Layer

Granulosa cells are almost entirely formed from their embryonic precursors by the time of birth (19). Those within maturing and mature follicles are polyhedral cells from 5 to 7 μm in diameter; the cells resting on the basement membrane are often columnar. The granulosa cells have pale, scanty cytoplasm, indistinct cell borders, and small, round to oval, hyperchromatic nuclei that typically lack nuclear grooves (Fig. 41.24A) (126). Mitotic figures within granulosa cells are usually numerous in maturing follicles, decreasing in numbers prior to ovulation. Until

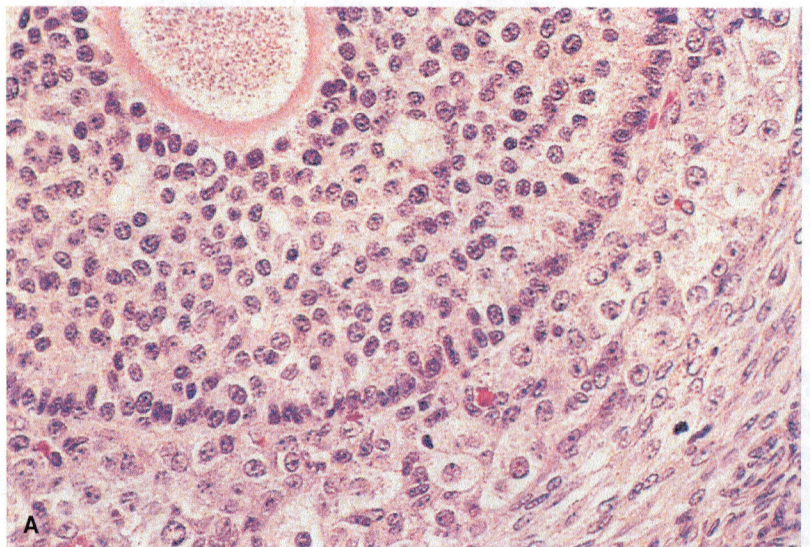 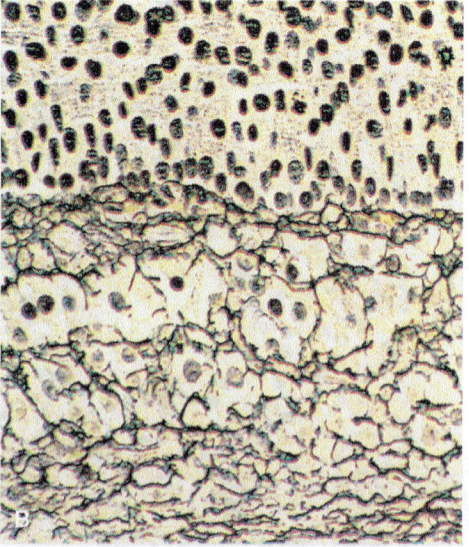

FIGURE 41.24 **A:** Mature follicle, high-power view. The granulosa layer, which contains several Call–Exner bodies, abuts the zona pellucida of the oocyte. The granulosa layer is surrounded by a layer of luteinized theca interna cells. Note mitotic figures in granulosa and theca cells. **B:** There is a reticulin network in the theca interna layer, but an absence of reticulin in the granulosa layer.

the onset of luteinization, several hours prior to ovulation, cytoplasmic lipid is absent (or sparse) as are the steroidogenic histochemical patterns (127,128). The cytoplasm of granulosa cells of primary, secondary, and mature follicles is immunoreactive for cytokeratin, vimentin, inhibin, CD99, melan-A, müllerian inhibiting substance, and desmoplakin, whereas they show nuclear immunoreactivity for WT1 and FOXL2 (53–55,58,62,129).

The granulosa cells typically surround small cavities, referred to as Call–Exner bodies (Fig. 41.24A), which have a distinctive appearance, representing one of the most specific features of granulosa cells, both normal and neoplastic. Call–Exner bodies are delimited from the granulosa cells by a BL, and typically contain a deeply eosinophilic, PAS-positive, filamentous material consisting of excess BL (50). Unlike the theca layers, the granulosa layer of the maturing and graafian follicles is avascular and devoid of a reticulin framework (Fig. 41.24B).

Mitochondria with lamelliform cristae, granular ER, free ribosomes, and Golgi gradually increase in abundance within the granulosa cells of maturing follicles. These ultrastructural features suggest active protein synthesis. Histochemical and ultrastructural features (abundant smooth ER and mitochondria with tubular cristae) indicative of steroid biosynthesis are absent until shortly before ovulation (52,65,127,128,130). The granulosa cells of follicles of varying stages contain adherens junctions, gap junctions, and desmosomes between adjacent granulosa cells (50,54,112). The slender cytoplasmic extensions of the granulosa cells of the corona radiata that traverse the zona pellucida have gap junctions and puncta adhaerentia with the PM of the oocyte (Fig. 41.25).

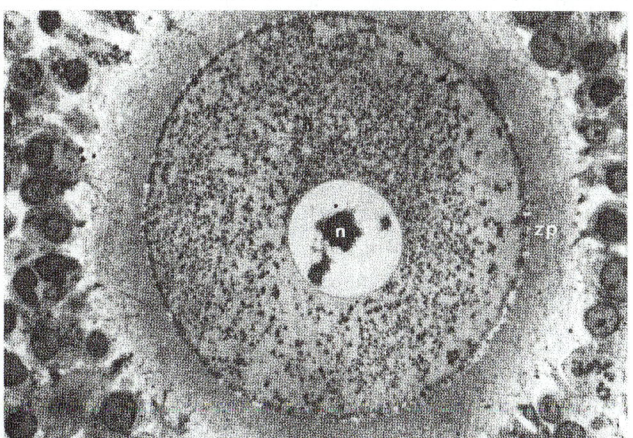

FIGURE 41.25 Maturing oocyte. Note the uniform distribution of the organelles and the row of dense granules in the cytoplasm immediately subjacent to the plasma membrane of the oocyte. A continuous zona pellucida (*zp*) surrounds the oocyte and separates it from the granulosa cells. Numerous cytoplasmic processes of the granulosa cells are visible within the zona pellucida. *n*, nucleolus. Thick section, OsO₄ fixed, Epon-embedded, toluidine blue stain. Reprinted with permission from Baca M, Zamboni L. The fine structure of the human follicular oocytes. *J Ultrastruct Res* 1967;19:354–381.

Theca Layers

In contrast to granulosa cells, theca cells differentiate continuously from the stromal cells at the periphery of developing follicles from fetal life until the end of the menopause. The thecal component of the antral follicle is characterized by a well-developed theca interna and a less well-defined theca externa. The theca interna layer is three or four cells in thickness and lies external to the granulosa layer (Fig. 41.24A) from which it is separated by a basement membrane. Unlike the granulosa cells of the developing and mature follicles, the theca interna cells typically have a luteinized or partially luteinized appearance (Fig. 41.24A) and exhibit steroidogenic histochemical patterns (52,127,128). Luteinization of the theca interna of maturing follicles is particularly prominent during pregnancy. The round to polygonal cells are from 12 to 20 micra in diameter and have abundant, eosinophilic to clear, vacuolated cytoplasm containing variable amounts of lipid; a central, round, vesicular nucleus typically contains a single, prominent nucleolus (Fig. 41.24A). The cells differ from granulosa cells but resemble stromal cells in being immunoreactive for vimentin but not cytokeratin (55); theca cells are also immunoreactive for inhibin, calretinin, melan-A, and FOXL2 (62,129). Mitotic figures are typically present with the theca cells of maturing follicles. The layer contains a rich vascular plexus consisting of dilated capillaries, as well as a dense reticulin network that surrounds each cell (Fig. 41.24B). A tangential section through the theca interna may result in seemingly isolated nodules of luteinized theca cells that may occasionally be misinterpreted as foci of stromal luteinization.

The theca externa is an ill-defined layer of variable thickness that surrounds the theca interna and merges almost imperceptibly with the adjacent ovarian stroma. It is composed of circumferentially arranged collagen bundles, blood and lymphatic vessels, and plump spindle cells that lack steroidogenic histochemical features (131). The spindle cells of the theca externa are typically highly mitotic and may be misinterpreted as fibrosarcoma, particularly when only the edge of the follicle is seen microscopically (Fig. 41.26).

Ultrastructural examination of theca interna cells reveals the organelles associated with steroidogenesis, similar to those within granulosa-lutein cells. The theca externa cells, some of which exhibit smooth muscle differentiation, lack such organelles (132).

Hormonal Aspects

The initiation of folliculogenesis and early preantral follicular development is independent of gonadotropin influence, whereas the later stages of follicular maturation are under gonadotropin control. As a small antral follicle develops into a preovulatory follicle, the sequence of endocrine events within its antral fluid differs from most, if not all, other antral follicles in the same ovary (133,134). The early stages of this development are associated with an increase

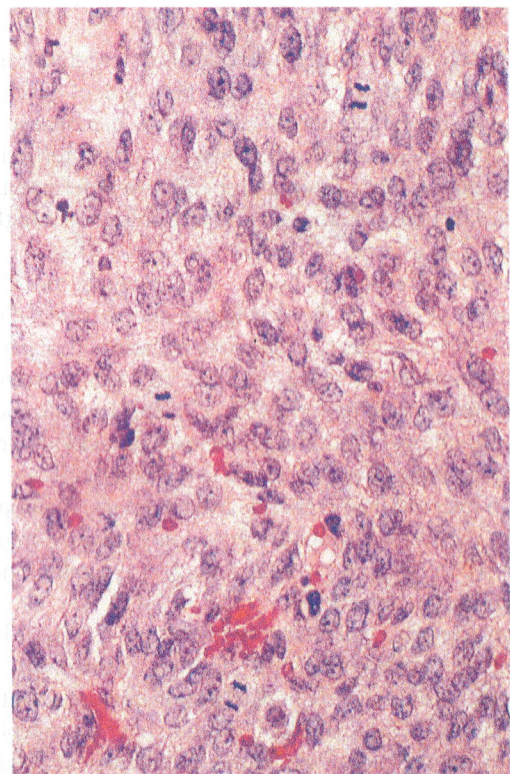

FIGURE 41.26 Theca externa of mature follicle composed of plump spindle cells. Note mitotic Figures.

in follicle-stimulating hormone (FSH) receptors and intrafollicular FSH within the preovulatory follicle (133–136). There is a concomitant increase in estradiol (E2) receptors within the granulosa cells and the E2 level within the follicular fluid. The latter reaches peak concentration (10,000 times the circulating level) during the mid- to late proliferative phase when plasma FSH falls to a basal level. At this stage the preovulatory follicle is self-sustaining, continuing to mature under the influence of intrafollicular FSH and E2 (98). During the late proliferative phase, plasma luteinizing hormone (LH) rises and LH receptors within the granulosa cells of the preovulatory follicle (but not other follicles) become apparent (136). In contrast, LH receptors are present within the theca cells of all follicles throughout the follicular phase.

Whereas circulating E2 is likely derived from both the granulosa cells and the LH-stimulated theca cells, intrafollicular E2 is derived almost exclusively from the granulosa cells by both de novo synthesis and by FSH-dependent aromatization of theca-derived androstenedione (98,137). Aromatase activity is highest in the preovulatory follicle, thereby maintaining a high E2:androstenedione ratio (133,134,138). In contrast, follicles that will undergo atresia are FSH- and aromatase-deficient and have high androstenedione:E2 ratios within their intrafollicular fluid. High circulating estrogen levels initiate a preovulatory surge of plasma LH (139,140) that induces luteinization of the granulosa cells, an increase in intrafollicular progesterone (P) concentration, and a small preovulatory rise in circulating P (133,134,141). The rising plasma P level and the peaking estrogen level further augment the LH surge, as well as initiating a smaller increase in FSH, triggering ovulation. The latter has been estimated to occur 36 to 38 hours after the onset of the LH surge, 24 to 36 hours after the estradiol peak, and 10 to 12 hours after the LH peak (141).

The ovarian follicles also produce nonsteroidal hormones. Inhibin, a glycoprotein synthesized by the granulosa cells, is secreted into the follicular fluid and ovarian venous effluent in amounts that correlate with steroid levels (141–143). Inhibin, which is predominantly under the control of LH (144), reduces, by negative feedback, FSH secretion from the hypothalamic–pituitary unit. High concentrations of prorenin are present within the fluid of mature follicles (145), and their granulosa cells, as well as theca and stromal cells, are immunoreactive for renin and angiotensin II (146). The renin–angiotensin system within the ovary has been linked to circulatory support during pregnancy (147).

CORPUS LUTEUM OF MENSTRUATION

Following ovulation on the 14th day of the typical 28-day menstrual cycle, and in the absence of fertilization, the collapsed ovulatory follicle becomes the corpus luteum of menstruation (CLM). When mature, the CLM is a 1.5 to 2.5 cm, round, yellow structure with festooned contours and a cystic center filled with a gray, focally hemorrhagic coagulum.

Histology

During the 14 days following ovulation, the CLM undergoes an orderly sequence of histologic changes that allow an approximate estimation of its age. Corner has described these stages in detail, using endometrial histology and menstrual data to establish the age of the CLM (148,149). A subsequent study that correlated the histologic date of the CLM (using Corner criteria) with the interval between the LH peak and the biopsy of the CLM, determined that the use of the histology of the CLM for retrospective timing of ovulation is subject to an error of variable magnitude due to unequal duration of each stage, as well as considerable individual variation (150).

In contrast to the granulosa cells of the maturing and preovulatory follicles, the luteinized granulosa cells of the mature CLM (granulosa-lutein cells) are large, 30 to 35 micra, polygonal cells with abundant, pale, eosinophilic cytoplasm that may contain numerous small lipid droplets (Figs. 41.27 and 41.28) (131). The spherical nucleus contains one or two large nucleoli. The histochemical pattern of these cells varies with the age of the CLM, but is generally typical of steroid hormone–producing cells (52,128,151). The cytoplasm of luteinized granulosa cells contains vimentin, but in contrast to granulosa cells of maturing and mature follicles, little or

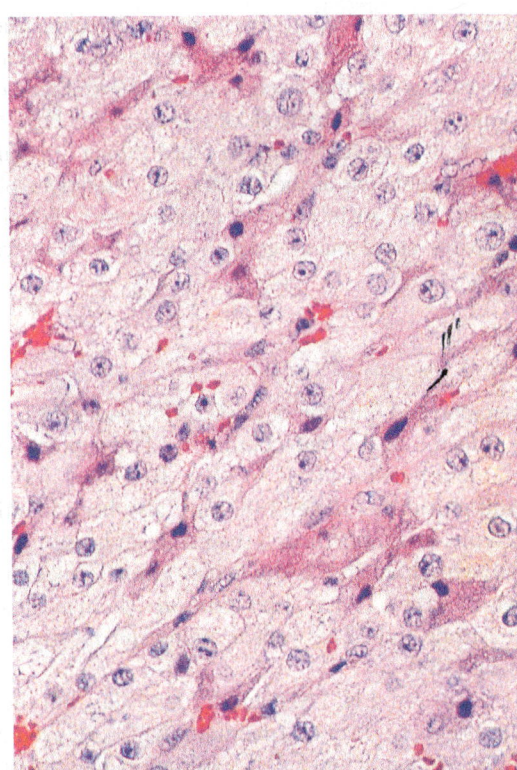

FIGURE 41.27 Mature corpus luteum of menstruation. K cells with darkly staining cytoplasm and pyknotic nuclei are interspersed between granulosa–lutein cells.

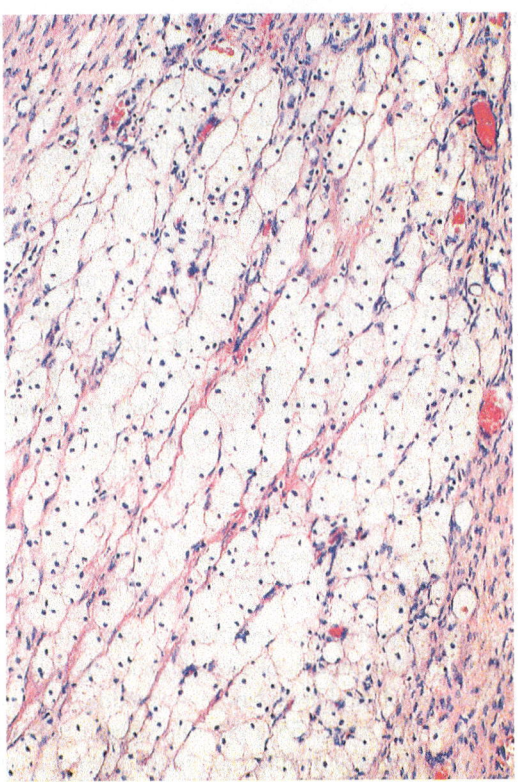

FIGURE 41.28 Degenerating corpus luteum of menstruation. Granulosa-lutein cells have pyknotic nuclei and abundant cytoplasmic lipid.

no cytokeratin (54). The luteinized granulosa cells are also immunoreactive for inhibin and calretinin (152,153).

The theca interna forms an irregular and often interrupted layer, several cells in thickness around the circumference of the CLM (Fig. 41.29), and ensheathes the vascular septa that extend into its center (131). When these septa are cut in cross section, triangular-shaped nests of theca cells appear at intervals throughout the granulosa layer. In all but the earliest stages of the CLM, the theca lutein cells are approximately half the size of granulosa-lutein cells. They contain a round to oval nucleus with a single prominent nucleolus. Their less abundant, more darkly staining cytoplasm contains lipid droplets, which are usually larger than those in granulosa-lutein cells, and exhibits steroidogenic histochemical patterns (128), and immunoreactivity for inhibin, calretinin, and melan-A (62,152,153).

A third type of cell, the so-called "K" cell, occurs in small numbers within the theca interna of the mature follicle and appears in greater numbers within the granulosa layer of the early CLM (126). K cells persist until menstruation at which time they degenerate. They are characterized by a stellate shape, a deeply eosinophilic cytoplasm, and an irregular, hyperchromatic or pyknotic nucleus (Fig. 41.27). The cytoplasm is uniformly sudanophilic due to the presence of phospholipid (126). K cells lack the histochemical patterns of steroidogenic cells and have been shown to be T lymphocytes (154).

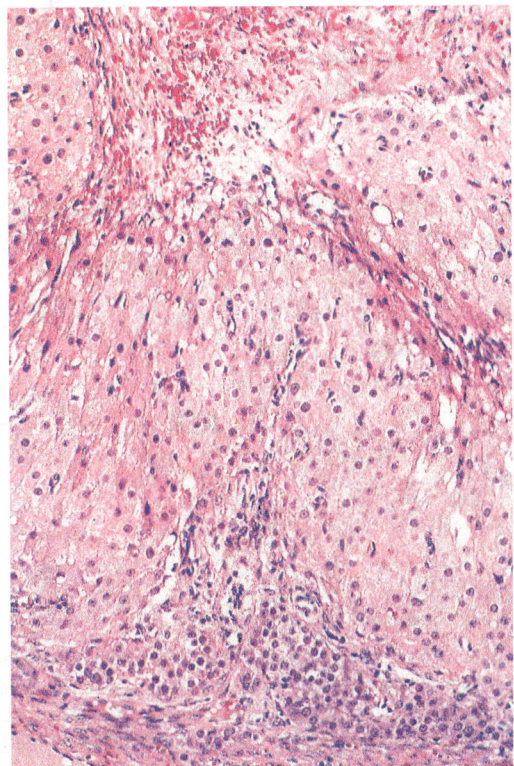

FIGURE 41.29 Mature corpus luteum of menstruation. The lining is composed of a thick layer of large granulosa-lutein cells and an outer, thinner layer of smaller theca-lutein cells. The cavity (top of the Figure) contains erythrocytes and fibrin.

During the maturation of the CLM, capillaries originating from the theca interna layer penetrate the granulosa layer and reach the central cavity. Fibroblasts that accompany the vessels form an increasingly dense reticulin network within the granulosa layer, as well as an inner fibrous layer that lines the central cavity (Fig. 41.28) (32).

Involutional changes begin on the eighth or ninth day following ovulation (148). The granulosa-lutein cells decrease in size, develop pyknotic nuclei, and accumulate abundant cytoplasmic lipid (Fig. 41.28). There is a decrease in histochemical staining of enzymes associated with steroid biosynthesis and an increase in hydrolytic enzymes (129). Eventually, the cells undergo dissolution and are phagocytosed (155). There is progressive fibrosis and shrinkage over a period of several months and eventual conversion to a corpus albicans.

Ultrastructure

At the ultrastructural level, luteinization is characterized by a gradually increasing content of steroidogenic organelles, specifically smooth ER and abundant mitochondria with tubular cristae (Fig. 41.30) (131,155–158). The smooth ER exhibits a characteristic regional modification in the form of a folded-membrane complex consisting of highly folded, radiating, tubular cisternae that communicate and interdigitate with adjacent cisternae (157). Well-developed, dispersed and perinuclear Golgi, free and bound ribosomes, lipid droplets, and lipofuscin pigment are also seen (Fig. 41.30) (131,155, 156, 157). Many irregular microvillus cytoplasmic extensions project into these pericapillary, as well as the intercellular, spaces (50,131,155,157). Theca-lutein cells are similar, ultrastructurally to granulosa-lutein cells except for the presence of localized perinuclear Golgi and the absence of folded-membrane complexes, microvilli, and a network of fine filaments (131,157). The lutein cells of the degenerating CLM exhibit disorganization and fragmentation of the smooth ER, alterations of the mitochondria, and an increase in cytolysosomes (50). Lipid droplets are increased and irregular in size and show increased osmiophilia (155).

Hormonal Aspects

The formation and function of the CLM is under the control of LH, reflected by the high content of LH receptors within the granulosa-lutein cells (136,142). Receptors for FSH (120) and growth hormone (138) have also been identified in the corpus luteum, although their roles in luteal function are unknown. Although P is the major steroid formed in vivo and in vitro by the CLM, it also synthesizes (both in vitro and in vivo) estrone and E2, as well as androgens, mostly androstenedione (159).

After ovulation, LH, FSH, and E2 levels fall, but the LH concentration is sufficient to maintain the CLM, producing a mid-luteal peak in P and E2. If fertilization does not occur, the increased levels of P and estrogen through negative feedback result in a fall of LH and FSH to basal levels, a reduction in LH and FSH receptors within the CLM, and a marked decline in P and E2 synthesis after the 22nd day of the cycle (135,136,142,160,161). These changes are reflected by the morphologic involution of the CLM and the onset of menses. Luteolysis appears to be estrogen related, possibly secondary to an estrogen-induced reduction in LH receptors or by enhancement of the luteolytic action of prostaglandins synthesized by the CLM (142,162). A nonsteroidal LH-receptor–binding inhibitor, which increases in concentration during the luteal phase, may also play a role (142).

CORPUS LUTEUM OF PREGNANCY

Gross Appearance

On gross inspection, the corpus luteum of pregnancy (CLP) may be indistinguishable from the CLM, but is usually larger and bright yellow in contrast to the orange-yellow of the late CLM (163). The larger size, which may account for up to half the ovarian volume, is due primarily to the presence of a central cystic cavity that is filled with fluid or a coagulum composed of fibrin and blood (71,121,164). The cavity size, however, can be highly variable. If the central cyst results in a corpus luteum that is over 3 cm in diameter, the CLP (or less commonly a CLM) is designated a corpus luteum cyst; if less than this size, a cystic corpus luteum. When the cavity of a CLP is large, typically in the first trimester, the wall may lose its convolutions, becoming stretched and attenuated to the extent that it may consist focally of only

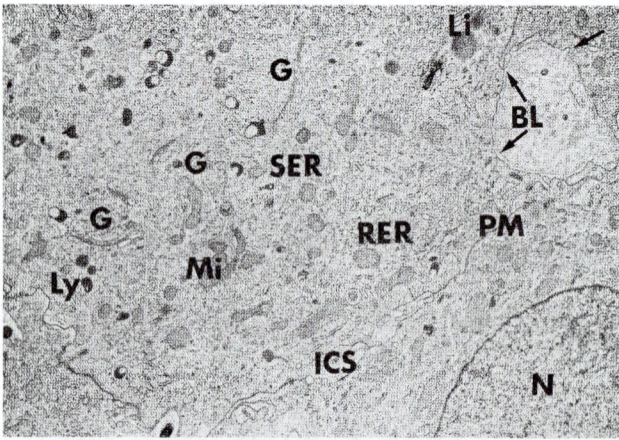

FIGURE 41.30 Electron micrograph of granulosa–lutein cell of a mature corpus luteum of menstruation. Note abundant smooth endoplasmic reticulum (*SER*), mitochondria (*Mi*), Golgi complex (*G*), rough endoplasmic reticulum (*RER*), lipid droplets (*Li*), and intercellular space (*ICS*). *BL*, basal lamina; *N*, nucleus of granulosa-lutein cell; *Ly*, lysosomes; *PM*, plasma membrane; *arrows*, micropinocytotic vesicle (original magnification ×3,600). Reprinted with permission from Ferenczy A, Richart RM. *Female Reproductive System: Dynamics of Scan and Transmission Electron Microscopy.* New York: John Wiley & Sons; 1974.

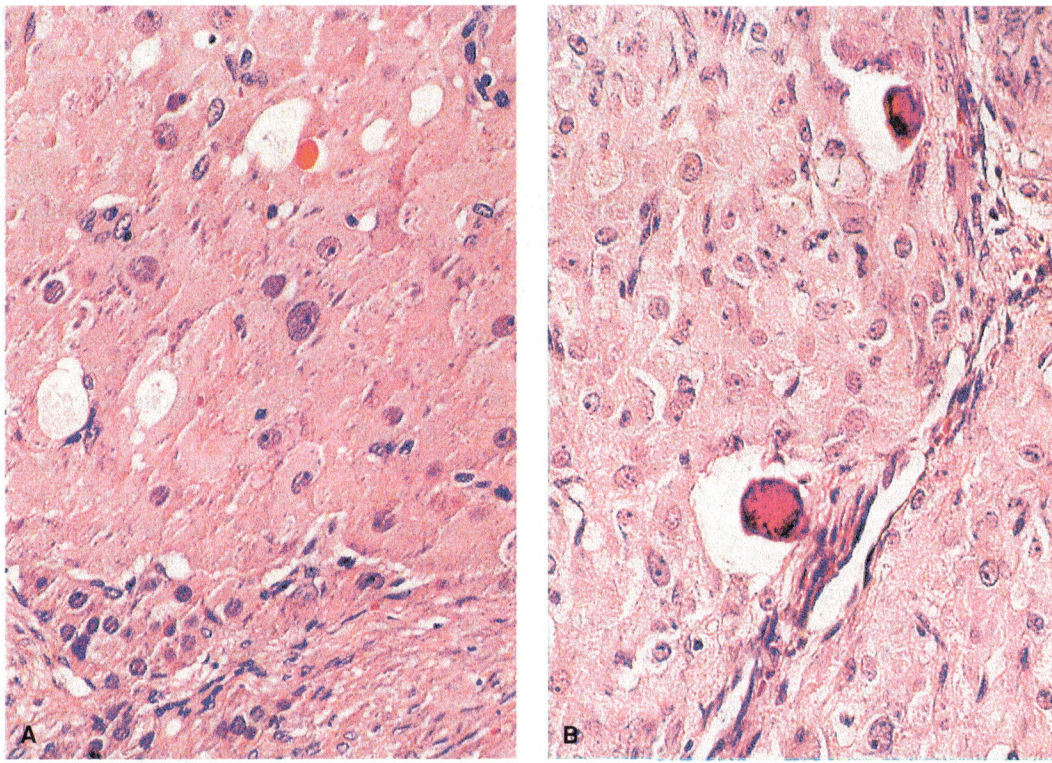

FIGURE 41.31 Corpus luteum of pregnancy. **A:** Note granulosa-lutein cells with large irregular vacuoles and densely eosinophilic hyalin body. Nests of theca cells are seen at bottom left. **B:** Focal calcification within a late CLP.

the inner fibrous layer. Obliteration of the cavity usually begins by the fifth month and is typically completed by term (122). The CLP thus gradually decreases in size, and by the last trimester, it is not a conspicuous structure. During the puerperium, the CLP undergoes involution and conversion to a corpus albicans.

Histology

The CLP, in contrast to the CLM, does not mature in an orderly sequence that allows an estimation of its age; however, early and late stages are recognizable on histologic examination.

Granulosa Layer

The first morphologic evidence within the corpus luteum that conception has occurred is the absence of the regressive changes that normally appear in the CLM on the eighth or ninth days. Instead, the granulosa lutein cells enlarge, reaching their maximum size of 50 to 60 µm by 8 to 9 weeks' gestation. They assume a round or polyhedral shape with abundant eosinophilic cytoplasm, round to oval, vesicular nuclei, and one or two prominent nucleoli (122) (Fig. 41.31A). The granulosa cells of the early CLP are characterized by cytoplasmic vacuoles that are initially tiny but eventually enlarge to occupy almost the entire cell, often with displacement and flattening of the nucleus (Fig. 41.31A). The vacuoles tend to diminish in number and size as gestation progresses, and usually disappear after the fourth month. Fine, diffusely scattered, cytoplasmic lipid droplets are also commonly seen within the cells, particularly in early CLP. With increasing age of the corpus luteum, the droplets become fewer and larger (122).

Eosinophilic colloid or hyalin droplets within the granulosa cells of a CLP, which can be identified as early as 15 days after ovulation, are almost diagnostic of pregnancy; they may occur very rarely, however, within a CLM (122). These inclusions initially appear as small, round or irregular, often multiple, droplets that enlarge, possibly by fusion of smaller droplets into one or several large bodies that may fill the entire cell (Fig. 41.31A). They become more numerous as gestation progresses (164), although by term their numbers decrease as they undergo calcification, which continues into the puerperium (Fig. 41.31B). It is likely that these calcified bodies eventually are resorbed, as they are not a feature of corpora albicantia.

K cells identical to those within CLM are typically found in the granulosa layer of the early CLP. They are most numerous in the second, third, and fourth months of gestation after which time they are rarely encountered (121,122,164).

Theca Layer

The theca interna is thickest in the early CLP at which time it resembles its counterpart in the CLM, surrounding the granulosa-lutein layer and forming triangular-shaped, vascular septa that extend into the latter. In the CLP, the theca cells are polyhedral or round and approximately one-fourth the size of the granulosa-lutein cells (Fig. 41.31A). Their cytoplasm is more darkly staining and granular than in the latter, and is typically not vacuolated. Their nuclei are central, round, and more hyperchromatic than those of the granulosa cells; one or two prominent nucleoli are usually present. The characteristic colloid inclusions seen within the granulosa cells are absent or very rare within the theca cells. Occasional K cells may be seen in early pregnancy, but in smaller numbers than in the granulosa layer (126,164). After the fourth month, the theca interna and its trabeculae become much thinner as the theca cells become smaller and fewer in number, with darker, more irregular, oblong to spindle-shaped nuclei, so that they resemble fibroblasts (164). By term, the theca interna layer has almost completely disappeared.

Connective Tissue

As in the mature CLM, the central cystic cavity is typically lined by a layer of fibrous tissue, composed of variable numbers of fibroblasts, collagen and reticulin fibers, and blood vessels (106). Its thickness is highly variable, not only within the same CLP, but also from one CLP to another and from one phase of pregnancy to another (164). As noted, in some CLP with large cystic cavities, the granulosa layer is focally absent, and its wall is formed entirely by this fibrous layer. As gestation advances, the central cyst or coagulum is eventually obliterated by connective tissue that may exhibit focal hyalinization and calcification (121).

Reticulin staining reveals a pattern similar to that of the mature CLM; that is, a dense pattern within the theca interna and inner fibrous layer, and a sparser framework within the granulosa layer (122). In the early CLP, many, often large, vessels are present in the theca externa and interna, from which emanate smaller vessels that penetrate the granulosa and inner fibrous layers. In the late CLP, the vessels develop sclerotic walls with luminal narrowing or obliteration (122,164). The amount of connective tissue around the vessels increases in proportion to the decreasing vascularization and regression of the theca interna layer.

Ultrastructure

The ultrastructural appearance of the CLP is similar to that of the CLM, and remains intact throughout pregnancy despite a reduction in its metabolic activity (165–167). The colloid or hyalin inclusions consist of homogeneous, electron-opaque material that may surround occasional needle-shaped crystals. They typically have no relationship to any organelle, although occasional smaller hyalin bodies are surrounded by rough ER.

Hormonal Aspects

Following fertilization, placental hCG stimulates P production by the granulosa-lutein cells. P concentration within the postovulatory corpus luteum increases sixfold, whereas the E2 level drops to 10% of that within the preovulatory follicle (133,134). hCG alone cannot maintain P secretion from the CLP for more than a few days, and the regulation of P secretion beyond that time is unknown. P production by the CLP begins to decline by the end of the second month of gestation with a concomitant increase of placental P production. However, in vivo and in vitro studies indicate that the CLP continues to produce P throughout the remainder of gestation, albeit in reduced amounts, consistent with the maintenance of its structural integrity until term (120,165,166,168,169). There is a rapid decline in function during the puerperium, reflecting falling hCG levels during this period.

Relaxin, a polypeptide hormone, is also produced during gestation and the puerperium by the CLP, probably under the control of hCG (170–173). The concentration of relaxin in ovarian vein plasma during pregnancy correlates with P levels. The placenta and uterus have also been suggested as additional, but less important, sources for this hormone. Its reported actions include cervical dilatation and softening, inhibition of uterine contractions, and relaxation of the pubic symphysis and other pelvic joints (170–173). Immunoreactivity for renin and angiotensin II, similar to that noted within the preovulatory follicle (see above), has been demonstrated within the CLP (147), consistent with the observation that prorenin, likely of ovarian origin, increases 10-fold in pregnant women soon after conception (146).

CORPUS ALBICANS

The regressing CLM is invaded by connective tissue that gradually converts it to a scar, the corpus albicans. The degenerating corpus luteum and the young corpus albicans may contain macrophages laden with ceroid and hemosiderin pigment (174,175). The mature corpus albicans is a well-circumscribed structure with convoluted borders composed almost entirely of densely packed collagen fibers with occasional admixed fibroblasts (Figs. 41.14 and 41.32). Focal calcification and ossification may be occasionally encountered. Most corpora albicantia are eventually resorbed and replaced by ovarian stroma. Persistent corpora albicantia are typically found in the medulla of postmenopausal women (Fig. 41.14) suggesting that this resorption process decelerates or terminates prior to the menopause.

ATRETIC FOLLICLES

Histology

Of the original 400,000 primordial follicles present at birth, approximately 400 mature to ovulation. The remaining 99.9% undergo atresia, a process that begins before birth

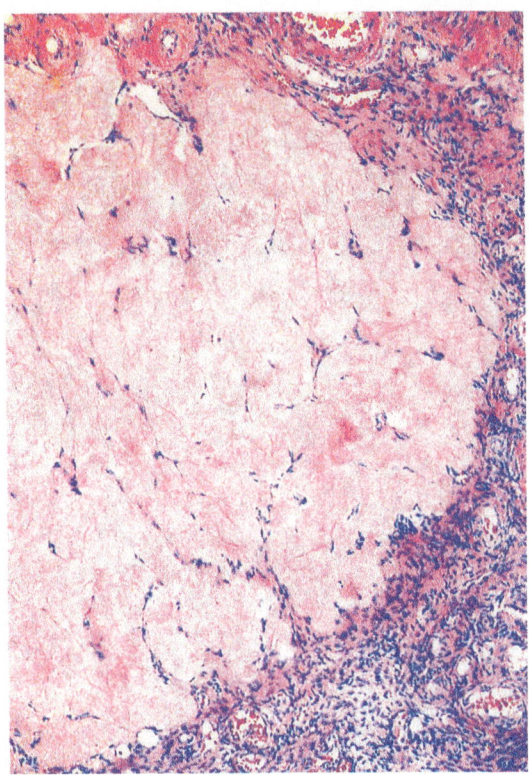

FIGURE 41.32 Corpus albicans.

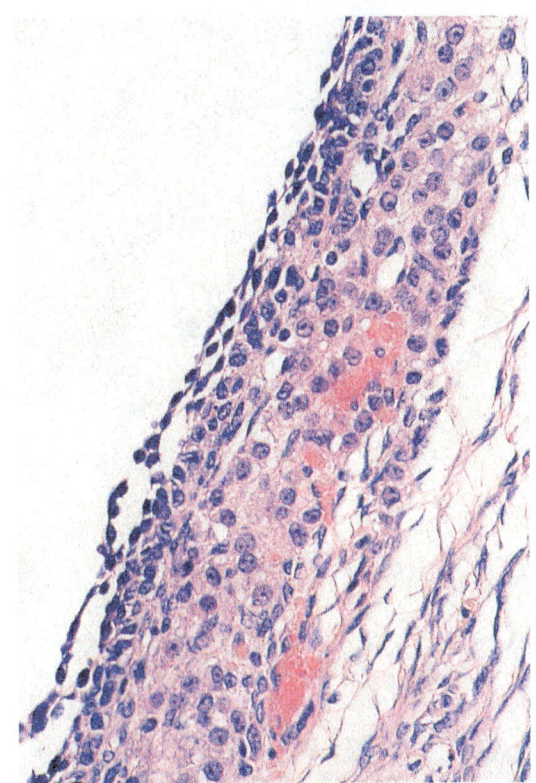

FIGURE 41.33 Lining of atretic cystic follicle composed of a thin inner layer of small, exfoliating granulosa cells and an outer, luteinized theca interna layer.

and continues throughout the reproductive life, but is most intense immediately after birth and during puberty and pregnancy (115–119,121,123). Factors that initiate atresia and determine which follicles will ultimately undergo atresia are unknown. The atretic process varies with the stage of follicular maturation that has been reached. Atresia of early follicles (primordial and preantral) begins with degeneration of the oocyte manifested by nuclear changes (chromatin condensation, pyknosis, and fragmentation) and cytoplasmic vacuolation. Degeneration of the granulosa cells soon follows and the follicle disappears without a trace. In contrast, atresia of follicles that have reached the antral stage of development is more complex and variable, but ultimately leads to obliterative atresia and the formation of a scar, the corpus fibrosum. The earliest evidence of this process is the mitotic inactivity of the granulosa cells and a decrease in their numbers, manifested by thinning and focal exfoliation of the granulosa layer. Some follicles may persist for an indefinite period of time at this stage as atretic cystic follicles (Fig. 41.33); those that exceed 3 cm are designated follicular cysts. Atretic cystic follicles and follicular cysts may persist for a number of years after the menopause (176,177). Atretic follicles are ultimately invaded by vascular connective tissue that eventually fills the central cavity (Fig. 41.34). The oocyte may persist for an indefinite period of time but eventually degenerates. Concurrent with these changes, the basement membrane between the granulosa and theca interna layers becomes transformed into a thick, wavy, eosinophilic, hyalinized band, the so-called "glassy membrane" (Figs. 41.34 and 41.35). The theca interna layer typically persists, often with prominent luteinization (Figs. 41.34 and 41.35), until the late stages of atresia at which time cords and nests of theca cells become surrounded by proliferating connective tissue (Fig. 41.35). Luteinization of both theca and granulosa layers is particularly striking in atretic follicles during infancy and childhood (178) and pregnancy (Fig. 41.36) (122).

Microscopic proliferations of persistent granulosa cells within the centers of atretic follicles of pregnant, and less commonly nonpregnant women, may mimic small granulosa cell tumors (Fig. 41.36), or rarely, Sertoli cell tumors (179). Similarly, structures resembling microscopic gonadoblastomas and sex cord tumors with annular tubules have been identified within atretic follicles in up to 35% of normal fetuses and infants (111,180,181). There is no evidence to suggest that any of these tumor-like proliferations represent early stages of neoplasia.

Continued shrinkage and hyalinization of an atretic follicle produces a serpiginous strand of hyalin tissue, the corpus fibrosum or atreticum (Fig. 41.37). Like corpora albicantia, most corpora fibrosa are probably resorbed by the ovarian stroma.

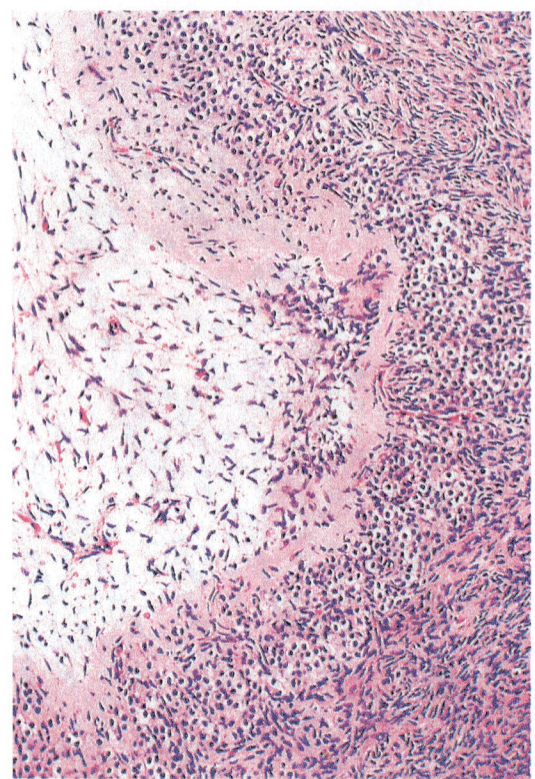

FIGURE 41.34 Atretic cystic follicle undergoing obliterative atresia. Loose connective tissue is replacing the central cavity. The wavy basement membrane ("glassy membrane") is thickened and hyalinized. A prominent layer of luteinized theca interna is evident.

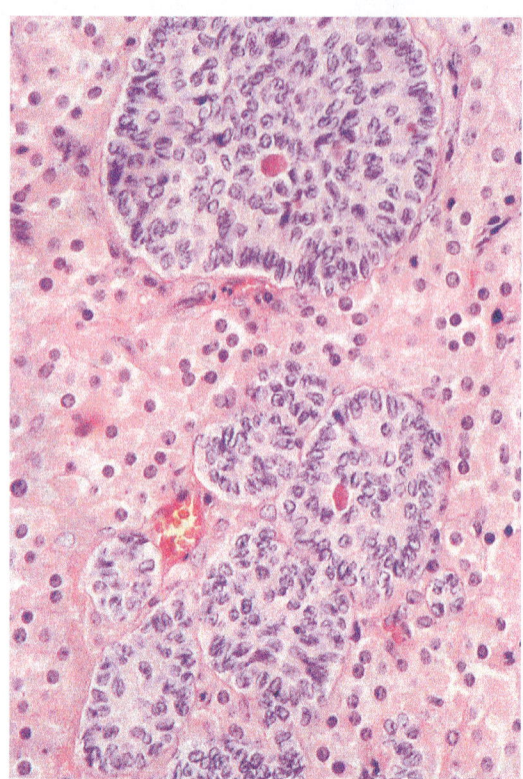

FIGURE 41.36 Atretic follicle in pregnancy. Within the center of the follicle is a proliferation of persistent granulosa cells surrounded by luteinized theca interna cells.

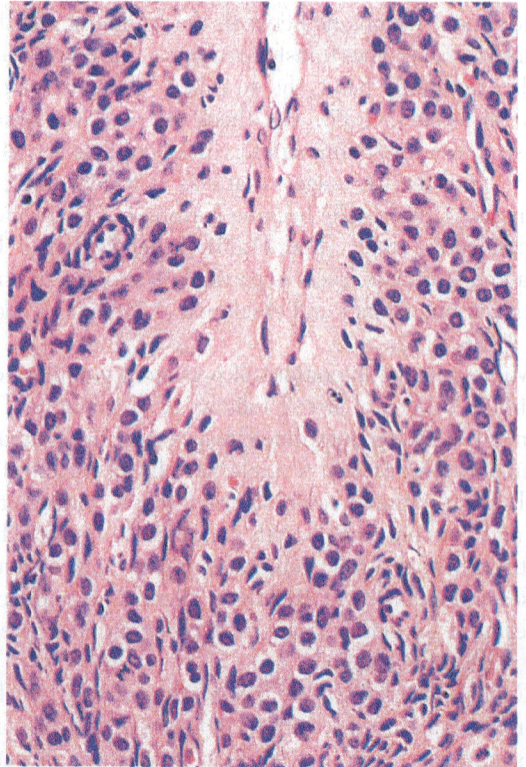

FIGURE 41.35 Edge of follicle in late stage of obliterative atresia. Hyalinized fibrous tissue occupies the central cavity and extends into the persistent luteinized theca interna layer.

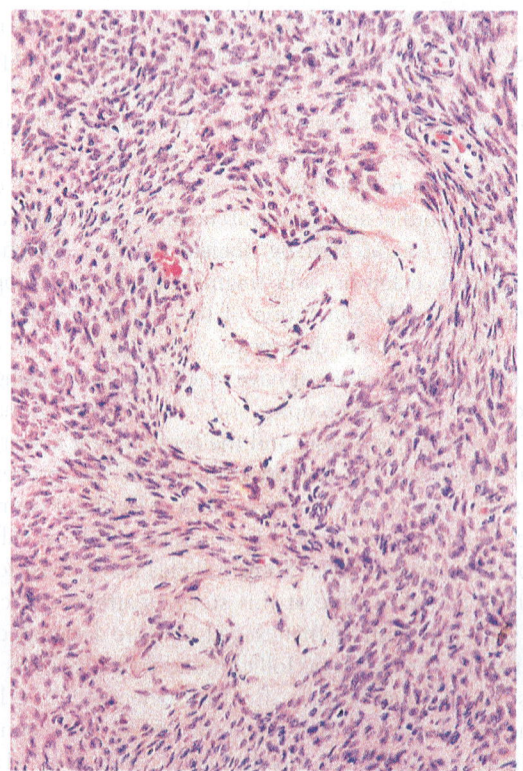

FIGURE 41.37 Two corpora fibrosa.

Hormonal Aspects

In contrast to preovulatory follicles, the microenvironment of follicles undergoing atresia is predominantly androgenic, with high concentrations of intrafollicular androstenedione and low concentrations of FSH and E2 (17,99,133,134,182). As noted, these follicles are deficient in granulosa cells, and the residual granulosa cells do not respond to FSH in vitro (125); both FSH and LH receptors are lower than in nonatretic follicles (136). Oocytes from atretic follicles are unable to complete the first meiotic division (125). It is likely that an androgenic intrafollicular milieu is the major factor that halts follicular growth and initiates atresia of that follicle.

HILUS CELLS

Histology

Ovarian hilus cells, morphologically identical to testicular Leydig cells (with the exception of a female chromatin pattern), are present during fetal life but not during childhood. They reappear at the time of puberty and are demonstrable in most postmenopausal women (183–185). Their number and location can be highly variable, and their numbers increase during pregnancy, with increasing age after the menopause, and with increasing degrees of ovarian stromal proliferation and stromal luteinization (22). Mild hilus cell hyperplasia is a relatively common incidental histologic finding in postmenopausal women (66).

Hilus cell aggregates of variable size and shape are typically found in the ovarian hilus and adjacent mesovarium (Figs. 41.38 and 41.39). They are more numerous in the lateral and medial poles of the hilus and near the junction of the ovarian ligament with the ovary, typically lying close to the junction of the hilus with the medullary stroma (Fig. 41.39) (183). The aggregates are closely associated with large hilar veins and lymphatic sinusoids, and may form nodular protrusions into their lumina. Hilus cells characteristically ensheathe, or less commonly lie within, nonmedullated nerves (Fig. 41.40), and occasionally surround the rete ovarii (183). Nests may also be present within the medullary stroma near the hilus, probably representing extensions of the hilus into the medulla. Also, as previously noted, cells of hilus type may also occur rarely within the ovarian stroma at a distance from the hilus (stromal Leydig cells). Hilus cells also may be encountered rarely in the perisalpinx and fimbrial endosalpinx (186).

Nests of Hilus cells are unencapsulated, typically lying within loose connective tissue, or rarely ovarian-type stroma, within the hilus (81). The cells are 15 to 25 micra in diameter, round to oval, less commonly elongate, with abundant eosinophilic cytoplasm and a spherical vesicular nucleus with one or two prominent nucleoli (Fig. 41.41). The nuclei, particularly in postmenopausal women, may have hyperchromatic, bizarre nuclei. Hilus cells are typically strongly immunoreactive for inhibin, calretinin, and melan-A (62,153).

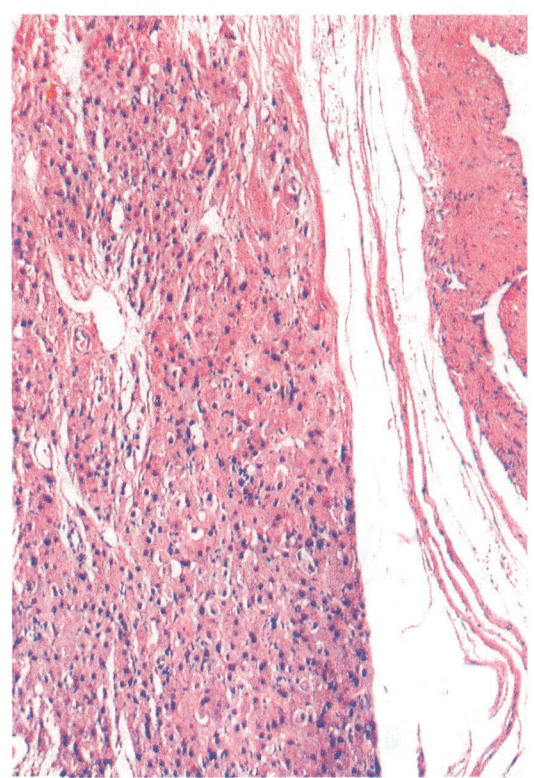

FIGURE 41.38 Nest of hilus cells adjacent to large vessel within the ovarian hilus.

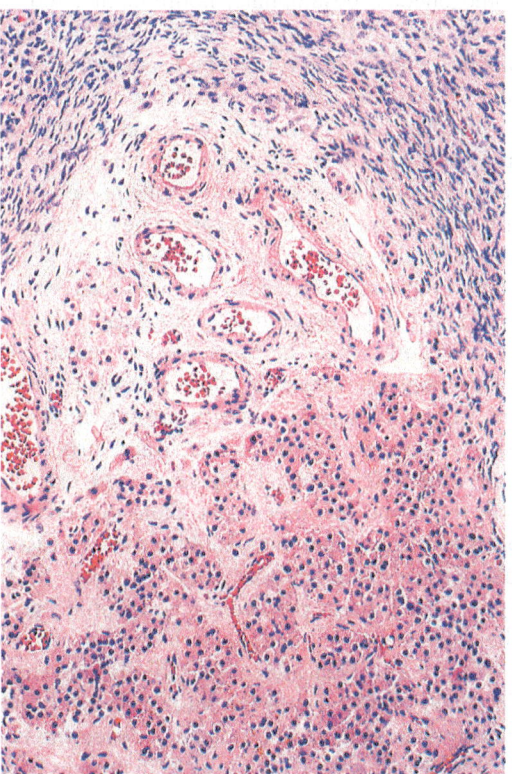

FIGURE 41.39 Nest of hilus cells with admixed small blood vessels abutting medullary stroma (top of the Figure).

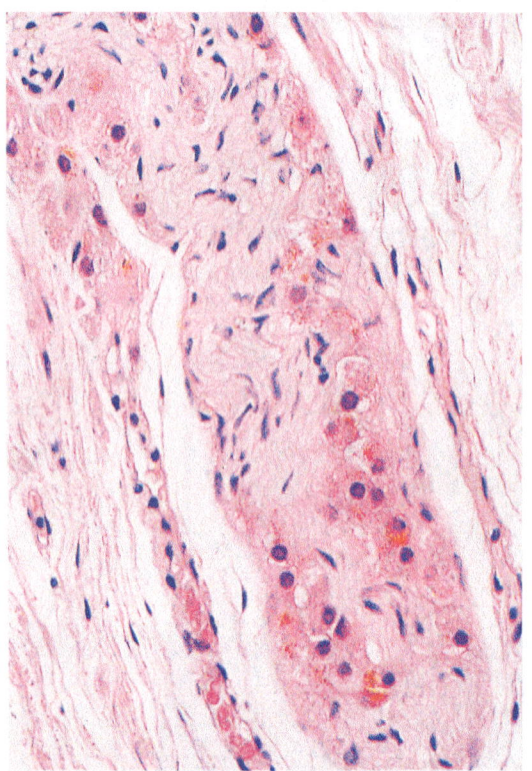

FIGURE 41.40 Perineural and intraneural hilus cells. Note fine brown lipochrome pigment within hilus cells.

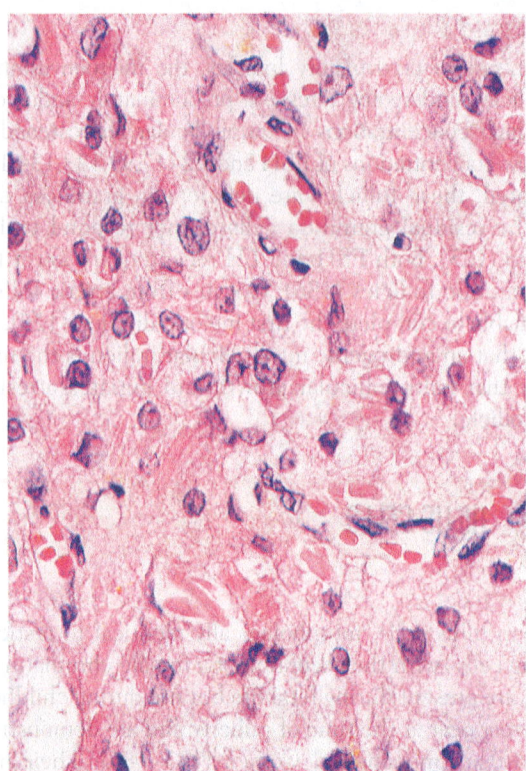

FIGURE 41.41 Hilus cells with Reinke crystals.

Hilus cells contain specific crystals of Reinke, which are homogeneous, eosinophilic, nonrefractile, rod-shaped structures, 10 to 35 μm in length, with blunt, but occasionally tapered, ends (Fig. 41.41). The crystals typically lie in a parallel or stacked arrangement within a cell, and often are surrounded by a clear halo; occasionally they appear to extend through or overlie cell membranes. The crystals are unevenly distributed and are typically present in only a minority of cells; frequently they cannot be identified (187). Their visualization may be facilitated by the use of Masson trichrome and iron hematoxylin methods that stain them magenta and black, respectively. Additionally, the crystals fluoresce yellow when hematoxylin and eosin (H&E)-stained sections are viewed by ultraviolet light (188). Also present within hilus cells, often in greater numbers than crystals, are spherical or ellipsoidal hyalin structures that have an otherwise identical appearance to crystals and probably represent their precursors. Elongated erythrocytes compressed within capillaries should not be confused with crystals and crystal precursors. The cytoplasm of Leydig cells may also contain perinuclear eosinophilic granules, peripheral lipid vacuoles, and golden-brown lipochrome pigment (Fig. 41.40). Delicate collagen fibrils surround each cell. Typically admixed with the hilus cells are fibroblasts and cells intermediate in appearance between the two cell types (189). The hilus cells and intermediate cells have intimate attachments to nerves, including true synaptic connections, suggesting that hilus cells may originate from hilar fibroblasts, possibly under the inductive influence of hilar nerves (183,189).

Hilus cells should be distinguished from adrenal cortical rests. The latter are extremely rare in the ovary (190), but are found in the mesovarium, and occasionally within the ovarian hilus, in approximately one-quarter of women (191). Their histologic appearance mimics that of the normal adrenal cortex, with most of the cells containing numerous lipid vacuoles.

Ultrastructure

Hilus cells have a steroidogenic ultrastructure consisting of prominent smooth ER and mitochondria with tubular cristae, as well as well-developed Golgi, large lysosomes, and osmiophilic lipid inclusions (189). Reinke crystals have a true crystalline appearance composed of dense parallel hexagonal microtubules with a mean thickness of 12 nm, separated by clear spaces 15 nm wide producing a "woven fabric" appearance (Fig. 41.42) (189).

Hormonal Aspects

The light and electron microscopic morphology and enzyme content of hilus cells are those of steroid hormone–producing cells, although to what extent hilus cells contribute to the steroid hormone pool in normal females is unknown (32,183). In vitro incubation studies indicate that the major

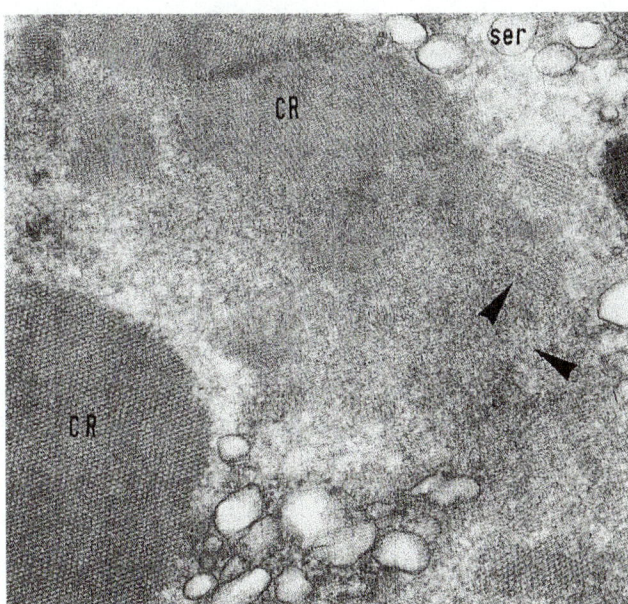

FIGURE 41.42 Reinke crystals with hexagonal internal pattern (*CR*) formed by association of precrystalline units (*arrowheads*); *ser*, smooth endoplasmic reticulum (original magnification ×25,000). Reprinted with permission from Laffargue P, Benkoel L, Laffargue F, et al. Ultrastructural and enzyme histochemical study of ovarian hilar cells in women and their relationships with sympathetic nerves. *Hum Pathol* 1978;9:649–659.

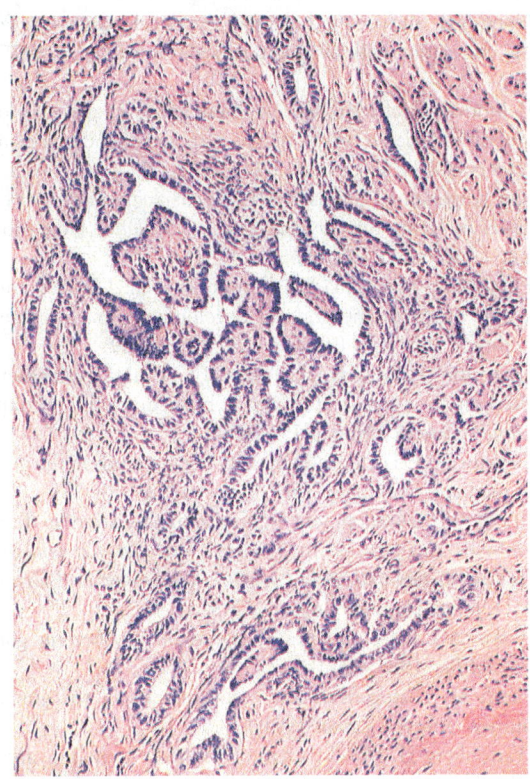

FIGURE 41.43 Rete ovarii.

steroid produced by ovarian hilus cells is androstenedione and that it is produced in amounts higher than that produced from ovarian stroma (192). Lesser amounts of E2 and P are also produced in vitro. Hilus cells are responsive in vivo to both exogenous and endogenous hCG stimulation, manifested by an increase in their numbers, cell size, and mitotic activity (193).

RETE OVARII

The rete ovarii, the ovarian analog of the rete testis, is present in the hilus of all ovaries. It consists of a network of irregular clefts, tubules, cysts, and intraluminal papillae, lined by an epithelium that varies from flat to cuboidal to columnar (Fig. 41.43) (193,194). Solid cords of similar cells may also be seen. Characteristically, the rete is surrounded by a cuff of spindle-cell stroma similar to, but discontinuous from, the ovarian stroma (Fig. 41.43).

The cytoplasm of the cells of the rete is immunoreactive for cytokeratin, EMA, vimentin, and desmoplakin (54,55,195). Ultrastructural examination has revealed two types of cells, one ciliated and the other nonciliated with apical microvilli (54). The cytoplasm contains many mitochondria, a moderate amount of rough ER, many free polyribosomes, and some glycogen. Numerous desmosomes with associated tonofilament bundles connect adjacent cells. The BL is well defined.

The rete juxtaposes and may communicate with mesonephric tubules within the mesovarium (193). Rare hilar cysts originate from the rete, and small tumor-like proliferations of the rete have been referred to as "rete adenomas" (193,196). The transitional cell metaplasia that has been encountered in the rete epithelium may account for the occasional small hilar Brenner tumors that have been contiguous with and possibly derived from the rete (194).

REFERENCES

1. Baker TG, Sum W. Development of the ovary and oogenesis. *Clin Obstet Gynecol* 1976;3:3–26.
2. Hoang-Ngoc Minh, Smadja A, Herve de Sigalony JP, et al. Etude histologique de la gonade à différenciation ovarienne au cours de l'organogenèse. *Arch Anat Cytol Pathol* 1989;37: 201–207.
3. Gondos B, Bhiraleus P, Hobel CJ. Ultrastructural observations on germ cells in human fetal ovaries. *Am J Obstet Gynecol* 1971; 110:644–652.
4. Gondos B. Cellular interrelationships in the human fetal ovary and testis. In: Federoff S, ed. *Prog Clin Biol Res. Volume 59B. Eleventh International Congress of Anatomy: Advances in the Morphology of Cells and Tissues.* New York: Alan R. Liss Inc; 1981:373–381.
5. Konishi I, Fujii S, Okamura H, et al. Development of interstitial cells and ovigerous cords in the human fetal ovary: An ultrastructural study. *J Anat* 1986;148:121–135.

6. Gondos B. Surface epithelium of the developing ovary. Possible correlation with ovarian neoplasia. *Am J Pathol* 1975;81:303–321.
7. Rabinovici J, Jaffe RB. Development and regulation of growth and differentiated function in human and subhuman primate fetal gonads. *Endocr Rev* 1990;11:532–557.
8. Van Wagenen G, Simpson ME. *Embryology of the Ovary and Testis in Homo Sapiens and Macaca Mulatta*. New Haven: Yale University Press; 1965.
9. Fukuda O, Miyayama Y, Fujimoto T, et al. Electron microscopic study of the gonadal development in early human embryos. *Prog Clin Biol Res* 1989;296:23–29.
10. Pinkerton JH, McKay DG, Adams EC, et al. Development of the human ovary—a study using histochemical techniques. *Obstet Gynecol* 1961;18:152–181.
11. Gruenwald P. The development of the sex cords in the gonads of man and mammals. *Am J Anat* 1942;70:359–389.
12. Jirasek JE. Development of the genital system in human embryos and fetuses. In: Jirasek J, ed. *Development of the Genital System and Male Pseudohermaphroditism*. Baltimore, MD: Johns Hopkins Press; 1971:3–41.
13. Byskov AG. Differentiation of mammalian embryonic gonad. *Physiol Rev* 1986;66:71–117.
14. Satoh M. Histogenesis and organogenesis of the gonad in human embryos. *J Anat* 1991;177:85–107.
15. Wartenberg H. Development of the early human ovary and role of the mesonephros in the differentiation of the cortex. *Anat Embryol (Berl)* 1982;165:253–280.
16. Hummitzsch K, Irving-Rodgers HF, Hatzirodos N, et al. A new model of development of the mammalian ovary and follicles. *PLoS One* 2013;8:e55578.
17. Nicosia SV. Morphological changes in the human ovary throughout life. In: Serra GB, ed. *The Ovary*. New York: Raven Press; 1983:57–81.
18. Pryse-Davies J. The development, structure and function of the female pelvic organs in childhood. *Clin Obstet Gynecol* 1974;1:483–508.
19. Valdes-Dapena MA. The normal ovary of childhood. *Ann N Y Acad Sci* 1967;142:597–613.
20. Merrill JA. The morphology of the prepubertal ovary: Relationship to the polycystic ovary syndrome. *South Med J* 1963;56:225–231.
21. Pavlik EJ, DePriest PD, Gallion HH, et al. Ovarian volume related to age. *Gynecol Oncol* 2000;77:410–412.
22. Boss JH, Scully RE, Wegner KH, et al. Structural variations in the adult ovary. Clinical significance. *Obstet Gynecol* 1965;25:747–764.
23. Reeves G. Specific stroma in the cortex and medulla of the ovary. Cell types and vascular supply in relation to follicular apparatus and ovulation. *Obstet Gynecol* 1971;37:832–844.
24. Plentl AA, Friedman EA. *Lymphatic System of the Female Genitalia*. Philadelphia, PA: WB Saunders; 1971.
25. Eichner E, Bove ER. In vivo studies on the lymphatic drainage of the human ovary. *Obstet Gynecol* 1954;3:287–297.
26. Jacobowitz D, Wallach EE. Histochemical and chemical studies of the autonomic innervation of the ovary. *Endocrinology* 1967;81:1132–1139.
27. Owman C, Rosenbren E, Sjoberg N. Adrenergic innervation of the human female reproductive organs: A histochemical and chemical investigation. *Obstet Gynecol* 1967;30:763–773.
28. Balboni GC. Structural changes: Ovulation and luteal phase. In: Serra GB, ed. *The Ovary*. New York: Raven Press; 1983:123–141.
29. Mohsin S. The sympathetic innervation of the mammalian ovary. A review of pharmacological and histochemical studies. *Clin Exp Pharmacol Physiol* 1979;6:335–354.
30. Dyer CA, Erickson GF. Norepinephrine amplifies human chorionic gonadotropin-stimulated androgen biosynthesis by ovarian theca-interstitial cells. *Endocrinology* 1985;116:1645–1652.
31. Blaustein A, Lee H. Surface cells of the ovary and pelvic peritoneum: A histochemical and ultrastructural comparison. *Gynecol Oncol* 1979;8:34–43.
32. McKay DG, Pinkerton JH, Hertig AT, et al. The adult human ovary: A histochemical study. *Obstet Gynecol* 1961;18:13–39.
33. Zinsser KR, Wheeler JE. Endosalpingiosis in the omentum: A study of autopsy and surgical material. *Am J Surg Pathol* 1982;6:109–117.
34. Blaustein A. Surface cells and inclusion cysts in fetal ovaries. *Gynecol Oncol* 1981;12(pt 1):222–233.
35. Blaustein A, Kantius M, Kaganowicz A, et al. Inclusions in ovaries of females aged day 1–30 years. *Int J Gynecol Pathol* 1982;1:145–153.
36. Mulligan RM. A survey of epithelial inclusions in the ovarian cortex of 470 patients. *J Surg Oncol* 1976;8:61–66.
37. Von Numers C. Observations on metaplastic changes in the germinal epithelium of the ovary and on the aetiology of ovarian endometriosis. *Acta Obstet Gynecol Scand* 1965;44:107–116.
38. Scully RE. Ovary. In: Henson DE, Albores-Saavedra J, eds. *The Pathology of Incipient Neoplasia. Major Problems in Pathology Series*. Vol 28. 2nd ed. Philadelphia, PA: WB Saunders; 1993:279–300.
39. Piek JM, Kenemans P, Zweemer RP, et al. Ovarian carcinogenesis: An alternative theory. *Gynecol Oncol* 2007;107:355.
40. Crum CP, Drapkin R, Miron A, et al. The distal fallopian tube: A new model for pelvic serous carcinogenesis. *Curr Opin Obstet Gynecol* 2007;19:3–9.
41. Singh N, Gilks CB, Wilkinson N, et al. The secondary Mullerian system, field effect, BRCA, and tubal fimbria: our evolving understanding of the origin of tubo-ovarian high-grade serous carcinoma and why assignment of primary site matters. *Pathology* 2015;47:423–431.
42. Auersperg N. The origin of ovarian carcinomas: A unifying hypothesis. *Int J Gynecol Pathol* 2011;30:12–21.
43. Bowen NJ, Logani S, Dickerson EB, et al. Emerging roles for Pax8 in ovarian cancer and endosalpingeal development. *Gynecol Oncol* 2007;104:331–337.
44. Bransilver BR, Ferenczy A, Richart RM. Brenner tumors and Walthard cell nests. *Arch Pathol* 1974;98:76–86.
45. Danforth DN. Cytologic relationship of Walthard cell rest to Brenner tumor of ovary and the pseudomucinous cystadenoma. *Am J Obstet Gynecol* 1942;43:984–996.
46. Roth LM. The Brenner tumor and the Walthard cell nest. An electron microscopic study. *Lab Invest* 1974;31:15–23.
47. Teoh TB. The structure and development of Walthard nests. *J Pathol Bacteriol* 1953;66:433–439.
48. Seidman JD, Khedmati F. Exploring the histogenesis of ovarian mucinous and transitional cell (Brenner) neoplasms, and their relationship with Walthard cell nests: A study of 120 tumors. *Arch Pathol Lab Med* 2008;132:1753–1760.

49. Papadaki L, Beilby JO. The fine structure of the surface epithelium of the human ovary. *J Cell Sci* 1971;8:445–465.
50. Ferenczy A, Richart RM. *Female Reproductive System: Dynamics of Scan and Transmission Electron Microscopy.* New York: John Wiley & Sons; 1974.
51. Blaustein A. Peritoneal mesothelium and ovarian surface cells–shared characteristics. *Int J Gynecol Pathol* 1984;3:361–375.
52. Fienberg R, Cohen RB. A comparative histochemical study of the ovarian stromal lipid band, stromal theca cell, and normal ovarian follicular apparatus. *Am J Obstet Gynecol* 1965;92:958–969.
53. Miettinen M, Lehto V, Virtanen I. Expression of intermediate filaments in normal ovaries and ovarian epithelial, sex cord-stromal, and germinal tumors. *Int J Gynecol Pathol* 1983;2:64–71.
54. Czernobilsky B, Moll R, Levy R, et al. Co-expression of cytokeratin and vimentin filaments in mesothelial, granulosa and rete ovarii cells of the human ovary. *Eur J Cell Biol* 1985;37:175–190.
55. Benjamin E, Law S, Bobrow LG. Intermediate filaments cytokeratin and vimentin in ovarian sex cord-stromal tumours with correlative studies in adult and fetal ovaries. *J Pathol* 1987;152:253–263.
56. Czernobilsky B, Shezen E, Lifschitz-Mercer B, et al. Alpha smooth muscle actin (alpha-SM actin) in normal human ovaries, in ovarian stromal hyperplasia and in ovarian neoplasms. *Virchows Arch B Cell Pathol Incl Mol Pathol* 1989;57:55–61.
57. Lastarria D, Sachdev RK, Babury RA, et al. Immunohistochemical analysis for desmin in normal and neoplastic ovarian stromal tissue. *Arch Pathol Lab Med* 1990;114:502–505.
58. Matias-Guiu X, Pons C, Prat J. Mullerian inhibiting substance, alpha-inhibin, and CD99 expression in sex cord-stromal tumors and endometrioid ovarian carcinomas resembling sex cord-stromal tumors. *Hum Pathol* 1998;29:840–845.
59. Rishi M, Howard LN, Bratthauer GL, et al. Use of monoclonal antibody against human inhibin as a marker for sex cord-stromal tumors of the ovary. *Am J Surg Pathol* 1997;21:583–589.
60. Hildebrandt RH, Rouse RV, Longacre TA. Value of inhibin in the identification of granulosa cell tumors of the ovary. *Hum Pathol* 1997;28:1387–1395.
61. McCluggage WG, Maxwell P. Immunohistochemical staining for calretinin is useful in the diagnosis of ovarian sex cord-stromal tumours. *Histopathology* 2001;38:403–408.
62. Jungbluth AA, Busam KJ, Gerald WL, et al. A103: An antimelan-a monoclonal antibody for the detection of malignant melanoma in paraffin-embedded tissues. *Am J Surg Pathol* 1998;22:595–602.
63. Oliva E, Vu Q, Young RH. CD10 expression in sex cord-stromal tumors (SCTs) and steroid cell tumors (StCTs) of the ovary. *Mod Pathol* 2002;15:204A.
64. Nagamani M, Hannigan EV, Dinh TV, et al. Hyperinsulinemia and stromal luteinization of the ovaries in postmenopausal women with endometrial cancer. *J Clin Endocrinol Metab* 1988;67:144–148.
65. Scully RE, Cohen RB. Oxidative-enzyme activity in normal and pathologic human ovaries. *Obstet Gynecol* 1964;24:667–681.
66. Loubet R, Loubet A, Leboutet MJ. The ovarian stroma after the menopause: Activity and ageing. In: de Brux J, Gautray JP, eds. *Clinical Pathology of the Ovary.* Boston, MA: MTP Press Ltd; 1984:119–141.
67. Bassis ML. Pseudodeciduosis. *Am J Obstet Gynecol* 1956;72:1029–1037.
68. Israel SL, Rubenstone A, Meranze DR. The ovary at term. I. Decidua-like reaction and surface cell proliferation. *Obstet Gynecol* 1954;3:399–407.
69. Ober WB, Grady HG, Schoenbucher AK. Ectopic ovarian decidua without pregnancy. *Am J Pathol* 1957;33:199–217.
70. Bersch W, Alexy E, Heuser HP, et al. Ectopic decidua formation in the ovary (so-called deciduoma). *Virchows Arch A Pathol Pathol Anat* 1973;360:173–177.
71. Starup J, Visfeldt J. Ovarian morphology in early and late human pregnancy. *Acta Obstet Gynecol Scand* 1974;53:211–218.
72. Herr JC, Heidger PM Jr, Scott JR, et al. Decidual cells in the human ovary at term. I. Incidence, gross anatomy and ultrastructural features of merocrine secretion. *Am J Anat* 1978;152:7–27.
73. Doss BJ, Wanek SM, Jacques SM, et al. Ovarian smooth muscle metaplasia: An uncommon and possibly underrecognized entity. *Int J Gynecol Pathol* 1999;18:58–62.
74. Hughesdon PE. Morphology and morphogenesis of the Stein–Leventhal ovary and of so-called "hyperthecosis." *Obstet Gynecol Surv* 1982;37:59–77.
75. Scully RE. Smooth-muscle differentiation in genital tract disorders. *Arch Pathol Lab Med* 1981;105:505–507.
76. Hughesdon PE. The origin and development of benign stromatosis of the ovary. *J Obstet Gynaecol Br Commonw* 1972;79:348–359.
77. Hughesdon PE. The endometrial identity of benign stromatosis of the ovary and its relation to other forms of endometriosis. *J Pathol* 1976;119:201–209.
78. Hart WR, Abell MR. Adipose prosoplasia of ovary. *Am J Obstet Gynecol* 1970;106:929–931.
79. Honoré LH, O'Hara KE. Subcapsular adipocytic infiltration of the human ovary: A clinicopathological study of eight cases. *Eur J Obstet Gynecol Reprod Biol* 1980;10:13–20.
80. Sternberg WH, Roth LM. Ovarian stromal tumors containing Leydig cells. I. Stromal–Leydig cell tumor and non-neoplastic transformation of ovarian stroma to Leydig cells. *Cancer* 1973;32:940–951.
81. Zhang J, Young RH, Arseneau J, et al. Ovarian stromal tumors containing lutein or Leydig cells (luteinized thecomas and stromal Leydig cell tumors)–a clinicopathological analysis of fifty cases. *Int J Gynecol Pathol* 1982;1:270–285.
82. Rutgers JL, Scully RE. Functioning ovarian tumors with peripheral steroid cell proliferation: A report of twenty-four cases. *Int J Gynecol Pathol* 1986;5:319–337.
83. Hidvegi D, Cibils LA, Sorensen K, et al. Ultrastructural and histochemical observations of neuroendocrine granules in nonneoplastic ovaries. *Am J Obstet Gynecol* 1982;143:590–594.
84. Snowden JA, Harkin PJ, Thornton JG, et al. Morphometric assessment of ovarian stromal proliferation–a clinicopathological study. *Histopathology* 1989;14:369–379.
85. Bigelow B. Comparison of ovarian and endometrial morphology spanning the menopause. *Obstet Gynecol* 1958;11:487–513.
86. Roddick JW Jr, Greene RR. Relation of ovarian stromal hyperplasia to endometrial carcinoma. *Am J Obstet Gynecol* 1957;73:843–852.

87. Woll E, Hertig AT, Smith GVS, et al. The ovary in endometrial carcinoma: With notes on the morphological history of the aging ovary. *Am J Obstet Gynecol* 1948;56:617–633.
88. Laffargue P, Adechy-Benkoel L, Valette C. Ultrastructure of the ovarian stroma. (Functional significance). *Ann Anat Pathol (Paris)* 1968;13:381–402.
89. Aiman J, Forney JP, Parker CR Jr. Secretion of androgens and estrogens by normal and neoplastic ovaries in postmenopausal women. *Obstet Gynecol* 1986;68:1–5.
90. Chang RJ, Judd HL. The ovary after menopause. *Clin Obstet Gynacol* 1981;24:181–191.
91. Dennefors BL, Janson PO, Knutson F, et al. Steroid production and responsiveness to gonadotropin in isolated stromal tissue of human postmenopausal ovaries. *Am J Obstet Gynecol* 1980;136:997–1002.
92. Greenblatt RB, Colle ML, Mahesh VB. Ovarian and adrenal steroid production in the postmenopausal woman. *Obstet Gynecol* 1976;47:383–387.
93. Judd HL, Judd GE, Lucas WE, et al. Endocrine function of the postmenopausal ovary: Concentration of androgens and estrogens in ovarian and peripheral vein blood. *J Clin Endocrinol Metab* 1974;39:1020–1024.
94. Judd HL, Lucas WE, Yen SSC. Effect of oophorectomy on circulating testosterone and androstenedione levels in patients with endometrial cancer. *Am J Obstet Gynecol* 1974;118:793–798.
95. Longcope C, Hunter R, Franz C. Steroid secretion by the postmenopausal ovary. *Am J Obstet Gynecol* 1980;138:564–568.
96. Lucisano A, Russo N, Acampora MG, et al. Ovarian and peripheral androgen and oestrogen levels in post-menopausal women: Correlations with ovarian histology. *Maturitas* 1986;8:57–65.
97. Mattingly RF, Huang WY. Steroidogenesis of the menopausal and postmenopausal ovary. *Am J Obstet Gynecol* 1969;103:679–693.
98. McNatty KP, Makris A, DeGrazia C, et al. The production of progesterone, androgens, and estrogens by granulosa cells, thecal tissue, and stromal tissue from human ovaries in vitro. *J Clin Endocrinol Metab* 1979;49:687–699.
99. McNatty KP, Smith DM, Makris A, et al. The intraovarian sites of androgen and estrogen formation in women with normal and hyperandrogenic ovaries as judged by in vitro experiments. *J Clin Endocrinol Metab* 1980;50:755–763.
100. Plotz EJ, Wiener M, Stein AA, et al. Enzymatic activities related to steroidogenesis in postmenopausal ovaries of patients with and without endometrial carcinoma. *Am J Obstet Gynecol* 1967;99:182–197.
101. Vermeulen A. The hormonal activity of the postmenopausal ovary. *J Clin Endocrinol Metab* 1976;42:247–253.
102. Rice BF, Savard K. Steroid hormone formation in the human ovary. IV. Ovarian stromal compartment; formation of radioactive steroids from acetate-1-14C and action of gonadotropins. *J Clin Endocrinol Metab* 1966;26:593–609.
103. Barbieri RL, Makris A, Randall RW, et al. Insulin stimulates androgen accumulation in incubations of ovarian stroma obtained from women with hyperandrogenism. *J Clin Endocrinol Metab* 1986;62:904–910.
104. Reed MJ, Beranek PA, Ghilchik MW, et al. Conversion of estrone to estradiol and estradiol to estrone in postmenopausal women. *Obstet Gynecol* 1985;66:361–365.
105. Longcope C. Metabolic clearance and blood production rates of estrogens in postmenopausal women. *Am J Obstet Gynecol* 1971;111:778–781.
106. Grodin JM, Siiteri PK, MacDonald PC. Source of estrogen production in postmenopausal women. *J Clin Endocrinol Metab* 1973;36:207–214.
107. Nagamani M, Stuart CA, Doherty MG. Increased steroid production by the ovarian stromal tissue of postmenopausal women with endometrial cancer. *J Clin Endocrinol Metab* 1992;74:172–176.
108. Dawood MY, Strongin M, Kramer EE, et al. Recent ovulation in a postmenopausal woman. *Int J Gynaecol Obstet* 1980;18:192–194.
109. Sherrer C, Gerson B, Woodruff JD. The incidence and significance of polynuclear follicles. *Am J Obstet Gynecol* 1977;128:6–12.
110. Gougeon A. Frequent occurrence of multiovular follicles and multinuclear oocytes in the adult human ovary. *Fertil Steril* 1981;35:417–422.
111. Manivel JC, Dehner LP, Burke B. Ovarian tumorlike structures, biovular follicles, and binucleated oocytes in children: Their frequency and possible pathologic significance. *Pediatr Pathol* 1988;8:283–292.
112. Baca M, Zamboni L. The fine structure of the human follicular oocytes. *J Ultrastruct Res* 1967;19:354–381.
113. Hertig AT. The primary human oocyte: Some observations on the fine structure of Balbiani's vitelline body and the origin of the annulate lamellae. *Am J Anat* 1968;122:107–137.
114. Hertig AT, Adams EC. Studies on the human oocyte and its follicle. I. Ultrastructural and histochemical observations on the primordial follicle stage. *J Cell Biol* 1967;34:647–675.
115. Curtis EM. Normal ovarian histology in infancy and childhood. *Obstet Gynecol* 1962;19:444–454.
116. Dekel N, David MP, Yedwab GA, et al. Follicular development during late pregnancy. *Int J Fertil* 1977;22:24–29.
117. Govan AD. Ovarian follicular activity in late pregnancy. *J Endocrinol* 1970;48:235–241.
118. Himelstein-Braw R, Byskov AG, Peters H, et al. Follicular atresia in the infant human ovary. *J Reprod Fertil* 1976;46:55–59.
119. Maqueo M, Goldzieher JW. Hormone-induced alterations of ovarian morphology. *Fertil Steril* 1966;17:676–683.
120. Mikhail G, Allen WM. Ovarian function in human pregnancy. *Am J Obstet Gynecol* 1967;99:308–312.
121. Nelson WW, Greene RR. The human ovary in pregnancy. *Int Abstr Surg* 1953;97:1–22.
122. Nelson WW, Greene RR. Some observations on the histology of the human ovary during pregnancy. *Am J Obstet Gynecol* 1958;76:66–90.
123. Peters H, Himelstein-Braw R, Faber M. The normal development of the ovary in childhood. *Acta Endocrinol (Copenh)* 1976;82:617–630.
124. McNatty KP, Hillier SG, van den Boogaard AM, et al. Follicular development during the luteal phase of the human menstrual cycle. *J Clin Endocrinol Metab* 1983;56:1022–1031.
125. McNatty KP, Smith DM, Makris A, et al. The microenvironment of the human antral follicle: Interrelationships among the steroid levels in antral fluid, the population of granulosa cells, and the status of the oocyte in vivo and in vitro. *J Clin Endocrinol Metab* 1979;49:851–860.

126. White RF, Hertig AT, Rock J, et al. Histological and histochemical observations on the corpus luteum of human pregnancy with special reference to corpora lutea associated with early normal and abnormal ova. *Contrib Embryol* 1951;34:55–74.
127. Jones GE, Goldberg B, Woodruff JD. Histochemistry as a guide for interpretation of cell function. *Am J Obstet Gynecol* 1968;100:76–83.
128. Sasano H, Mori T, Sasano N, et al. Immunolocalization of 3 beta-hydroxysteroid dehydrogenase in human ovary. *J Reprod Fertil* 1990;89:743–751.
129. Shah SP, Kobel M, Senz J, et al. Mutation of FOXL2 in granulose-cell tumors of the ovary. *N Engl J Med* 2009;360:2719–2729.
130. Mestwerdt W, Muller O, Brandau H. Structural analysis of granulosa cells from human ovaries in correlation with function. In: Channing CP, Marsh JM, Sadler WA, eds. *Ovarian Follicular and Corpus Luteum Function: Advances in Experimental Medicine and Biology. Vol 112.* New York: Plenum Press; 1978.
131. Gillim SW, Christensen AK, McLennan CE. Fine structure of the human menstrual corpus luteum at its stage of maximum secretory activity. *Am J Anat* 1969;126:409–427.
132. Okamura H, Virutamasen P, Wright KH, et al. Ovarian smooth muscle in the human being, rabbit, and cat. Histochemical and electron microscopic study. *Am J Obstet Gynecol* 1972;112:183–191.
133. McNatty KP. Follicular determinants of corpus luteum function in the human ovary. In: Channing CP, Marsh JM, Sadler WA, eds. *Ovarian Follicular and Corpus Luteum Function: Advances in Experimental Medicine and Biology. Vol 112.* New York: Plenum Press; 1978:465–477.
134. McNatty KP. Cyclic changes in antral fluid hormone concentrations in humans. *Clin Endocrinol Metab* 1978;7:577–600.
135. Erickson GF. Normal ovarian function. *Clin Obstet Gynecol* 1978;21:31–52.
136. Shima K, Kitayama S, Nakano R. Gonadotropin binding sites in human ovarian follicles and corpora lutea during the menstrual cycle. *Obstet Gynecol* 1987;69:800–806.
137. McNatty KP, Makris A, De Grazia C, et al. The production of progesterone, androgens and oestrogens by human granulosa cells in vitro and in vivo. *J Steroid Biochem* 1979;11:775–779.
138. Hillier SG. Intrafollicular paracrine function of ovarian androgen. *J Steroid Biochem* 1987;27:351–357.
139. Pauerstein CJ, Eddy CA, Croxatto HD, et al. Temporal relationships of estrogen, progesterone, and luteinizing hormone levels to ovulation in women and infrahuman primates. *Am J Obstet Gynecol* 1978;130:876–886.
140. Yussman MA, Taymor ML. Serum levels of follicle stimulating hormone and luteinizing hormone and of plasma progesterone related to ovulation by corpus luteum biopsy. *J Clin Endocrinol Metab* 1970;30:396–399.
141. Futterweit W. *Polycystic Ovarian Disease: Clinical Perspectives in Obstetrics and Gynecology.* New York: Springer-Verlag; 1985.
142. Tanabe K, Gagliano P, Channing CP, et al. Levels of inhibin-F activity and steroids in human follicular fluid from normal women and women with polycystic ovarian disease. *J Clin Endocrinol Metab* 1983;57:24–31.
143. Tsonis CG, Messinis IE, Templeton AA, et al. Gonadotropic stimulation of inhibin secretion by the human ovary during the follicular and early luteal phase of the cycle. *J Clin Endocrinol Metab* 1988;66:915–921.
144. McLachlan RI, Cohen NL, Vale WW, et al. The importance of luteinizing hormone in the control of inhibin and progesterone secretion by the human corpus luteum. *J Clin Endocrinol Metab* 1989;68:1078–1085.
145. Sealey JE, Glorioso N, Itskovitz J, et al. Prorenin as a reproductive hormone. New form of the renin system. *Am J Med* 1986;81:1041–1046.
146. Palumbo A, Jones C, Lightman A, et al. Immunohistochemical localization of renin and angiotensin II in human ovaries. *Am J Obstet Gynecol* 1989;160:8–14.
147. Lumbers ER, Pringle KG. Roles of the circulating renin-angiotensin-aldosterone system in human pregnancy. *Am J Physiol Regul Integr Comp Physiol* 2014;306:R91–R101.
148. Corner GW Jr. The histological dating of the human corpus luteum of menstruation. *Am J Anat* 1956;98:377–401.
149. Visfeldt J, Starup J. Dating of the human corpus luteum of menstruation using histological parameters. *Acta Pathol Microbiol Scand A* 1974;82:137–144.
150. Croxatto HD, Ortiz ME, Croxatto HB. Correlation between histologic dating of human corpus luteum and the luteinizing hormone peak—biopsy interval. *Am J Obstet Gynecol* 1980;136:667–670.
151. Wiley CA, Esterly JR. Observations on the human corpus luteum: Histochemical changes during development and involution. *Am J Obstet Gynecol* 1976;125:514–519.
152. Cao QJ, Jones JG, Li M. Expression of calretinin in human ovary, testis, and ovarian sex cord-stromal tumors. *Int J Gynecol Pathol* 2001;20:346–352.
153. Pelkey TJ, Frierson HF Jr, Mills SE, et al. The diagnostic utility of inhibin staining in ovarian neoplasms. *Int J Gynecol Pathol* 1998;17:97–105.
154. Hameed A, Fox WM, Kurman RJ, et al. Perforin expression in human cell-mediated luteolysis. *Int J Gynecol Pathol* 1995;14:151–157.
155. Adams EC, Hertig AT. Studies on the human corpus luteum. I. Observations on the ultrastructure of development and regression of the luteal cells during the menstrual cycle. *J Cell Biol* 1969;41:696–715.
156. Tamura M, Sasano H, Suzuki T, et al. Immunohistochemical localization of growth hormone receptor in cyclic human ovaries. *Hum Reprod* 1994;9:2259–2262.
157. Crisp TM, Dessouky DA, Denys FR. The fine structure of the human corpus luteum of early pregnancy and during the progestational phase of the menstrual cycle. *Am J Anat* 1970;127:37–69.
158. Green JA, Maqueo M. Ultrastructure of the human ovary. I. The luteal cell during the menstrual cycle. *Am J Obstet Gynecol* 1965;92:946–957.
159. LeMaire WJ, Conly PW, Moffett A, et al. Function of the human corpus luteum during the puerperium: Its maintenance by exogenous human chorionic gonadotropin. *Am J Obstet Gynecol* 1971;110:612–618.
160. Centola GM. Structural changes: Follicular development and hormonal requirements. In: Serra GB, ed. *The Ovary.* New York: Raven Press; 1983:95–111.
161. Rao CV. Receptors for gonadotropins in human ovaries. In: Muldoon T, Mahesh V, Perez-Ballester B, eds. *Recent Advances in Fertility Research Part A: Developments in Reproductive Endocrinology.* New York: Alan R. Liss; 1982:123–135.

162. Vijayakumar R, Walters WA. Ovarian stromal and luteal tissue prostaglandins, 17 beta-estradiol and progesterone in relation to the phases of the menstrual cycle in woman. *Am J Obstet Gynecol* 1987;156:947–951.
163. Hertig AT. Gestational hyperplasia of endometrium. A morphologic correlation ova, endometrium, and corpora lutea during early pregnancy. *Lab Invest* 1964;13:1153–1191.
164. Visfeldt J, Starup J. Histology of the human corpus luteum of early and late pregnancy. *Acta Pathol Microbiol Scand A* 1975;83:669–677.
165. Adams EC, Hertig AT. Studies on the human corpus luteum. II. Observations on the ultrastructure of luteal cells during pregnancy. *J Cell Biol* 1969;41:716–735.
166. Green JA, Garcilazo JA, Maqueo M. Ultrastructure of the human ovary. II. The luteal cell at term. *Am J Obstet Gynecol* 1967;99:855–863.
167. Pedersen PH, Larsen JF. The ultrastructure of the human granulosa lutein cell of the first trimester of gestation. *Acta Endocrinol (Copenh)* 1968;58:481–496.
168. Le Maire WJ, Rice BF, Savard K. Steroid hormone formation in the human ovary: V. Synthesis of progesterone in vitro in corpora lutea during the reproductive cycle. *J Clin Endocrinol Metab* 1968;28:1249–1256.
169. Weiss G, Rifkin I. Progesterone and estrogen secretion by puerperal human ovaries. *Obstet Gynecol* 1975;46:557–559.
170. Weiss G, O'Byrne M, Hochman JA, et al. Secretion of progesterone and relaxin by the human corpus luteum at midpregnancy and at term. *Obstet Gynecol* 1977;50:679–681.
171. Weiss G, O'Byrne EM, Steinetz BG. Relaxin: A product of human corpus luteum of pregnancy. *Science* 1976;194:948–949.
172. Schmidt CL, Black VH, Sarosi P, et al. Progesterone and relaxin secretion in relation to the ultrastructure of human luteal cells in culture: Effects of human chorionic gonadotropin. *Am J Obstet Gynecol* 1986;155:1209–1219.
173. Quagliarello J, Goldsmith L, Steinetz B, et al. Induction of relaxin secretion in nonpregnant women by human chorionic gonadotropin. *J Clin Endocrinol Metab* 1980;51:74–77.
174. Joel RV, Foraker AG. Fate of the corpus albicans: A morphologic approach. *Am J Obstet Gynecol* 1960;80:314–316.
175. Reagan JW. Ceroid pigment in the human ovary. *Am J Obstet Gynecol* 1950;59:433–436.
176. Centola GM. Structural changes: Atresia. In: Serra GB, ed. *The Ovary.* New York: Raven Press; 1983:113–122.
177. Strickler RC, Kelly RW, Askin FB. Postmenopausal ovarian follicle cyst: An unusual cause of estrogen excess. *Int J Gynecol Pathol* 1984;3:318–322.
178. Kraus FT, Neubecker RD. Luteinization of the ovarian theca in infants and children. *Am J Clin Pathol* 1962;37:389–397.
179. Clement PB, Young RH, Scully RE. Ovarian granulosa cell proliferations of pregnancy: A report of nine cases. *Hum Pathol* 1988;19:657–662.
180. Kedzia H. Gonadoblastoma: Structures and background of development. *Am J Obstet Gynecol* 1983;147:81–85.
181. Safneck JR, de Sa DJ. Structures mimicking sex cord-stromal tumours and gonadoblastomas in the ovaries of normal infants and children. *Histopathology* 1986;10:909–920.
182. Bomsel-Helmreich O, Gougeon A, Thebault A, et al. Healthy and atretic human follicles in the preovulatory phase: Differences in evolution of follicular morphology and steroid content of follicular fluid. *J Clin Endocrinol Metab* 1979;48:686–694.
183. Sternberg WH. The morphology, androgenic function, hyperplasia, and tumors of the human ovarian hilus cells. *Am J Pathol* 1949;25:493–521.
184. Sternberg WH, Segaloff A, Gaskill CJ. Influence of chorionic gonadotropin on human ovarian hilus cells, Leydig-like cells. *J Clin Endocrinol Metab* 1953;13:139–153.
185. Merrill JA. Ovarian hilus cells. *Am J Obstet Gynecol* 1959;78:1258–1271.
186. Honoré LH, O'Hara KE. Ovarian hilus cell heterotopia. *Obstet Gynecol* 1979;53:461–464.
187. Janko AB, Sandberg EC. Histochemical evidence for the protein nature of the Reinke crystalloid. *Obstet Gynecol* 1970;35:493–503.
188. Schmidt WA. Eosin-induced fluorescence of Reinke crystals. *Int J Gynecol Pathol* 1986;5:88–89.
189. Laffargue P, Benkoel L, Laffargue F, et al. Ultrastructural and enzyme histochemical study of ovarian hilar cells in women and their relationships with sympathetic nerves. *Hum Pathol* 1978;9:649–659.
190. Symonds DA, Driscoll SG. An adrenal cortical rest within the fetal ovary: Report of a case. *Am J Clin Pathol* 1973;60:562–564.
191. Falls JL. Accessory adrenal cortex in the broad ligament: Incidence and functional significance. *Cancer* 1955;8:143–150.
192. Dennefors BL, Janson PO, Hamberger L, et al. Hilus cells from human postmenopausal ovaries: Gonadotrophin sensitivity, steroid and cyclic AMP production. *Acta Obstet Gynecol Scand* 1982;61:413–416.
193. Rutgers JL, Scully RE. Cysts (cystadenomas) and tumors of the rete ovarii. *Int J Gynecol Pathol* 1988;7:330–342.
194. Sauramo H. Development, occurrence, function and pathology of the rete ovarii. *Acta Obstet Gynecol Scand Suppl* 1954;33:29–46.
195. Woolnough E, Russo L, Khan MS, et al. An immunohistochemical study of the rete ovarii and epoophoron. *Pathology* 2000;32:77–83.
196. Gardner GH, Greene RR, Peckham B. Tumors of the broad ligament. *Am J Obstet Gynecol* 1957;73:536–555.

42

Placenta

Steven H. Lewis ■ Miriam D. Post ■ Kurt Benirschke

ROUTINE STORAGE, EXAMINATION, AND PROCESSING 1138	MULTIPLE GESTATION 1155
UMBILICAL CORD 1141	VILLI 1156
Embryology 1141	Embryology 1156
Gross Morphology 1141	Gross Morphology 1158
Histology 1142	Gross Morphologic Alterations 1158
Histopathology 1143	Histology 1159
RAMIFICATION OF CHORIONIC VASCULATURE 1147	Histopathology 1160
PATHOLOGIC ALTERATIONS OF THE CHORIONIC VASCULATURE 1148	DECIDUA 1163
	Histology 1163
	Histopathology 1165
MEMBRANES 1148	GESTATIONAL TROPHOBLASTIC DISEASE 1166
Embryology 1148	REFERENCES 1168
Amnion and Chorion 1149	

Until recently, the placenta has been problematic for the pathologist. Many normal histologic variations may be mistaken for pathology and conversely, important pathologic alterations may be difficult to discern. Three decades of multispecialty education have mollified this issue (1,2).

Unique in pathology, the placental specimen provides data about two patients and has three anatomic sources. It is fetal, yet mostly extraembryonic in its differentiation and it also has maternal attachments. Principally, the placenta is important in maternal and neonatal care and can in many instances discern the etiology of medical issues affecting neonates and mothers (1–11). Noteworthy, the placenta has been deemed pivotal as "material evidence" in adjudicating the etiology of adverse pregnancy outcomes especially in cases of neonates and children who do poorly following management of labor and delivery and may result in litigation (1,3,10,12–13). Interestingly, material obtained from intrauterine curettings can also be utilized in diagnosing pathologic alterations of the placenta following fetal demise (14).

Unquestionably an objective, thorough, well-documented analysis of the placenta can provide data important for patient care which otherwise may be obscure without gross and/or histopathologic analysis. Acknowledging the placenta's many histologic and pathologic variants, its complicated derivation, its importance in patient care, and its role in legal cases, the pathologist should become accustomed to obtaining information from both pediatric and obstetrical providers to better contextualize the relevance of variants and alterations. It has been advocated that Pathologists accompany Neonatologists on "rounds" in NICUs (1).

Historically, centuries transpired from describing "suction cup" like components of placental attachment to the uterus described by Fabricius in the 1500s to now, a current modern understanding (15). The first anatomically correct drawings of various placentations (including human) and suggestions of function were brilliantly depicted by the German Physician, and Mathematician Nicholas von Hoboken and published in Utrecht, Netherlands in 1669 (16) (Fig. 42.20).

Although a variety of difficulties contributed to "placental neglect" (and the absence of submission to pathology laboratories), in recent decades massive education of Pathologists and related specialties has mitigated that difficulty. With the advent of new terms, more erudite pathology reports may cause confusion with clinicians. As a "diary of gestation" (a phrase attributed to Shirly Driscoll) education must continue. (Dr. Driscoll's recent passing is mourned by many. She illuminated countless pathologists and clinicians. The German Text, written with Benirschke and Strauss, "Handbuch Der Speziellen Anatomie und Histologie" in 1967 is a commonly cited early accurate reference defining placentology as a necessity in patient management) (17).

Concentrating on histology, the reader is directed to references describing placental pathology and pathologic alterations in extensive detail, not at all limited to those briefly listed here. (As representative texts, here referenced, the first is an encyclopedic discussion of the placenta and the second is intended as a primer) (1,3,4). Numerous other examples including consensus and scientific papers have been published recently (2,5,6,10,11,18–24).

The American College of Obstetrics and Gynecology (ACOG) "Committee Opinion" about Placental evaluation no longer exists (22). It should be noted that numerous "ACOG Clinical Opinions" covering clinical conditions such as still birth, abruption, acreta, and other pregnancy related conditions include information regarding placental assessment as a component of clinical care and follow-up (19). Also, a recent "Expert Review," compiled by Ray Redline is now a part of ACOG's educational materials (5). A new "Amsterdam" consensus panel text with terminologic addenda is in press (18) and follows its preliminary description (25). Continued education of clinicians is necessary. It is not unusual for changes in Pathologic terms to result in confusion with clinicians. Dramatic advances in the science of pathology necessitate newer terminology. Such advances at times leave clinicians with difficulty understanding how best to manage patients. In a recent study of 1500 anatomic pathology reports resulted in 35% interpretation problems among 76 clinicians (26). Another recent study showed only 21% of clinicians understanding nomenclature used in placenta reports (27).

In the not uncommon furor of a delivery room along with the absence of a requirement that all placentas (a "complex large specimen") be sent to a pathology lab, guidelines for submission are necessary to prevent their unnecessary disposal (1–3,5,7,18). The process requires operating room and delivery suite staff be familiar with the requisite complications of pregnancy and delivery which would deem placenta examination necessary. Often Labor and Delivery areas will keep lists of essential disorders posted as reminders (1,5,7,18). More about caution and how to deal with placentas postpartum is described below with placental storage, examination, and processing.

Although much has been written and is now practiced regarding the importance of placental pathology in patient care, these complex considerations cannot be addressed without a thorough understanding of the placenta's normal structure, and it is to this end that this chapter is devoted. Pathologic entities are discussed to better demonstrate normal anatomy and histology (and, especially because many gross and microscopic rarities are simply normal variants. Conversely, subtle pathologic alterations need to be excluded from what may appear as a variant of normal).

This chapter is organized as follows: embryology, gross normal morphology, histology, and its needed discussion of approximating pathologic alterations. (As the nature of this chapter is to describe histology please note: newer terminology related to the discerned-and at times difficult to distinguish pathological alterations exists (as with all advances in medicine controversy exists and older terms apply) (28). Essentially the changes add types of "malperfusion" and "gradations" of pathologic entities. Here it is advised that the reader further educate themselves about these changes and is directed to the references noted) (5–7,10,18,19,25,28–31).

Normal histology, and its histopathology are presented for each compartment of the placenta. Dividing said "compartments" into: cord, membranes, parenchyma, and decidua, avail a directed approach to the placenta's evaluation and makes the complex organ more easily understood embryologically, anatomically, and functionally. Common considerations such as storage and reporting are also described. "Compartmentalizing" the functional units of the placenta, further makes for more concise reporting.

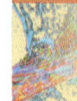

ROUTINE STORAGE, EXAMINATION, AND PROCESSING

After obstetric delivery, importantly, a decision about placental evaluation must be made (1,6,18). In most hospitals, not all placentas are sent to pathology. Because problems may often arise in neonates within the first few days of life, it is highly important to store placentas for a week following delivery. It is common for academic institutions to only perform histologic examination on approximately 10% to 20% of all delivered placentas (1). For many reasons including cost concerns, this is but a fraction of those which should be sent (2). Placentas not submitted for pathologic examination are typically "discarded." Unfortunately, this precludes gathering of useful information when problems are associated with pregnancy, labor and delivery, and the neonatal period.

Placentas may be stored fresh at 4°C in a refrigerator before examination, however the storage time should not exceed 1 week. Placentas should not be frozen before evaluation as freezing renders the gross examination difficult and histologic features are obscured. It has been advocated by some to immediately fix the placenta in 10% buffered formalin for later examination (1,3,5,6,32,33). It should be noted that when this method of processing is used, placental weights increase by a factor of approximately 10% (34).

Formalin fixation may provide information about parenchymal infarct age using criteria also readily available when fresh. It so happens that is far easier to examine a gross specimen in the fresh form (1).

Of note, although assessment of the placenta is considered in the pathologist's domain, it is the obstetrical provider who first visualizes the specimen. An educated clinician may aid the pathologist firstly by recording germane clinical and gross pathology findings; and further, by submitting it. It therefore behooves the pathologist to teach obstetrical providers important gross findings and indications for formal assessment. If a placenta does not go to the laboratory, a routine gross evaluation by the provider can document essential data, such as cord length (one example). Disposable paper tapes are easy to include in sterile delivery sets. A "compartmentalized," gross assessment by an educated obstetrical provider can become a part of a delivery note; which in turn may be exceptionally helpful when the specimen has *status post*-delivery been otherwise discarded.

The laboratory gross morphologic assessment of the placenta should be approached in a thorough, routine fashion. Our procedure for the gross evaluation and sectioning of placentas is outlined in Table 42.1. Alternative and meaningful methods exist—the importance is to be complete (1–3,5,18,27).

The placenta is removed from its container and its shape is described. It is usually discoid, but additional lobes may be present. Next, it is convenient to note the location of insertion of the umbilical cord, describe its length (There may be several portions following clamping, cutting, obtaining blood gases and even for cord blood storage. The length *in toto*, as described below, can be pathologic.), diameter, note irregularities in its contour and texture, surface aberrancies, describe its color, and note the number of vessels it contains. The cord is then amputated at its base (at the placental disk), and representative sections are immersed in fixative.

Attention is next directed to the membranes (amnion and chorion), which are inspected for completeness. When the placenta is delivered vaginally, the membranes are usually surrounding the maternal surface ("Shiny Schultze"). A few percent are delivered oppositely ("Dirty Duncan") with the parenchyma presenting and the membranes overlie the cord in a cephalad fashion. The membranes are then manually reflected to their normal anatomic position (recapitulating the anatomic amniotic "sac") and the smallest distance from the point of rupture to the placental disk (the narrowest width of membranes) is measured. When this measurement equals zero (after vaginal delivery), a low-lying or marginal placenta previa is implicated (1). The membranes are assessed for their color, transparency, sheen, and surface irregularities, as well as for the presence of membranous vessels or accessory lobes. A "membrane roll" should be taken by grasping the point of rupture with a toothed forceps (3,35) (Fig 42.1) and rolling the membrane in a concentric fashion to include the very periphery of the placental disk. With the membranes rolled in such a fashion, the point of rupture can be identified histologically. The presence of inflammatory cells confined to this region suggests early mild chorioamnionitis. Representative sections are immersed in fixative (when so taken, following fixation makes for easier sectioning of the roll for cassette placement and following processing, provides an enormous surface area to be seen in but a portion of a cassette). The remaining membranes are then removed from the placental disk margin.

The fetal surface of the placenta is next examined. Chorionic vascular thrombi, if present, and nodules or irregularities of the amnion and chorion are noted. Thrombi are enormously important when considering sources of "malperfusion" (1,5,6,7). They are very fragile and easily made unrecognizable; and, hence, care should be taken to examine this surface gently. The maternal surface of the placenta is inspected, and any blood clot that has settled in the storage container with the dependent portions of the organ is removed. Areas of blood clot that are adherent or discolored brown (indicating chronicity) and that are depressing the maternal surface are considered indicative of retroplacental hemorrhage (are clinically designated as abruption and another source of "malperfusion"). Should this be noted, the dimensions or percentage of the maternal surface involvement is recorded. The organ is next weighed free of its cord and associated membranes. The average weight of the term placenta is approximately 400 to 600 g. Placental weight varies with neonatal weight and normal weights have been reviewed for all gestational ages (1). The average dimensions of the term placenta are approximately $18 \times 16 \times 2.3$ cm.

The villous parenchyma is inspected by sectioning the placenta at 1 to 2 cm intervals looking for irregularities that indicate infarction, thrombi, or other pathologic entities. There are normally 16 to 20 cotyledonous units that do not have distinct functional correlates. An absent cotyledon may indicate a portion of retained placenta in utero. Representative sections of abnormal areas are blocked out, and areas of normal-appearing parenchyma (usually three) are placed into fixative along with the already sectioned membrane roll and umbilical cord.

The fixation of the materials for study is routine. Most laboratories use formalin. In *the past*, many placenta experts fixed tissues selected from specimens in Bouin's solution for a period of 8 to 24 hours before trimming and submission for final processing. In the past its preference was derived from excellent tissue penetration and hardening for ease of sectioning and enhanced cytologic detail. It is now rarely used as there can be interference with immunohistochemistry (contact for more than 8 hours) and if in final preparations lithium carbonate is omitted, increased extraneous pigment formation occurs (1,36).

Pathologists are accustomed to using 10% buffered formalin solution for the processing of most tissues, and this is not contraindicated in the processing of placentas (33).

TABLE 42.1 Recording Format[a]

	Unit No:
	Name:
	Date of Birth: Sex:
	Location: ED/DR/OR
	Path. No:
CLINICAL INFORMATION:	Date of Delivery:
	Date Received:
	Physician:
	Baby's Unit No:

Previous Specimens:

SPECIMEN: Placenta

CLINICAL INFORMATION: (Circle and fill in pertinent information)

NSVD	C-section	GA: _____ wk	DM class _____
Chorioamnionitis		Preeclampsia	Fetal distress
Newborn wt. _____ g		5 min Apgar <7	Other: _____

GROSS DESCRIPTION:
(Digital Image as Indicated)

Cord: _____ × _____ cm   Insertion:
            # pieces: _____   Vessel #: _____

Membranes: Complete/incomplete   Narrowest width: _____ cm
             Clear/opaque   Meconium: Old/recent/none
             Vascular Thrombi: Present/none   Other-describe below

Parenchyma: Red/pale/friable   Abruptio: _____ %
             Infarct: _____ %   Weight: _____ g
             Old/New
             Dimensions: _____ × _____ × _____ cm

Other:

MICROSCOPIC DESCRIPTION: (_____) slides evaluated.

CLINICAL DIAGNOSIS(ES):
(Photomicroscopy as Indicated)

Umbilical cord:

Membranes:

Villi:

Decidua:

Diagnosis:

Reviewed by:

Date Dictated:

Date Typed:

Print Date:

---

[a]This format is easily converted to a computerized final report that includes final microscopic diagnoses.

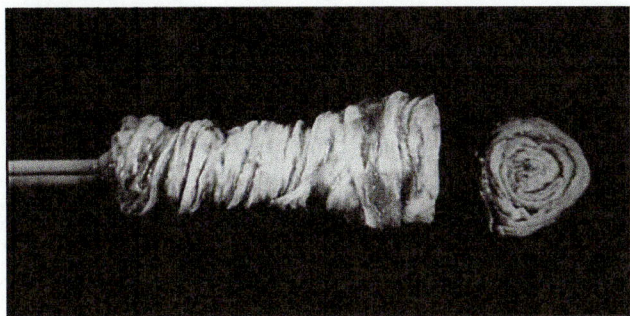

FIGURE 42.1 Proper sampling of the fetal membranes, a technique that provides the most surface area for microscopic evaluation.

It is our procedure to stain tissue sections with hematoxylin and eosin (H&E) or hematoxylin, phloxine, and saffron (HPS). Other standard special stains may be used for the detection of specific infectious agents, secretory activity, or structural composition (silver stains, periodic acid–Schiff [PAS], Masson trichrome, etc.). Furthermore, a host of immunohistochemical stains have been used to elucidate functions of specific placental cell types, possible malignancies, and malperfusion (28–30,37).

UMBILICAL CORD

Embryology

Specific embryologic considerations are germane to the understanding of the normal umbilical cord structure, including its frequent possession of embryologic remnants. The open region on the ventral surface of the developing embryo diminishes in size and then forms the early umbilicus. Through this structure extend both the yolk stalk and the body stalk, as well as the allantois. This cylindrical structure elongates, and its surface becomes covered by the expanding amnion. This is a single-layered epithelium on a layer of connective tissue. Therefore, the developing umbilical cord contains the yolk stalk, a pair of vitelline blood vessels, the allantois, and the allantoic blood vessels (two arteries and one vein) and is covered by amnionic epithelium. These anatomic relationships explain the presence of the omphalomesenteric duct (the connection between developing endoderm and the yolk sac) and the allantoic duct (which has its communication in early gestation with the urachus) within sections of proximal (fetal) umbilical cord (1,3).

Gross Morphology

The gross anatomic features of the umbilical cord that are of importance are the location of its insertion in the placental disk, its length, and the number of vessels. The presence of true knots (Fig. 42.2) may be considered normal when there is no adverse outcome, yet this occurrence may lead

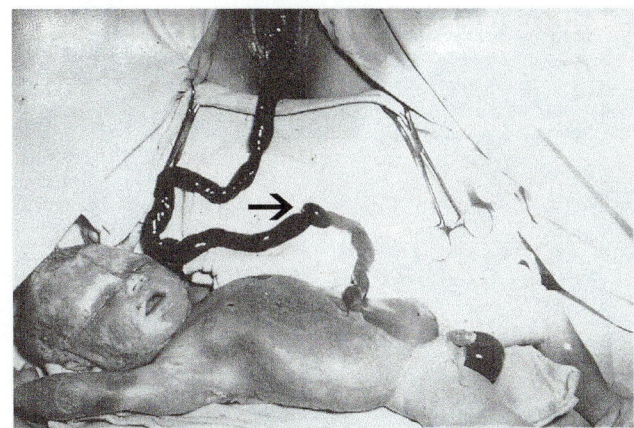

FIGURE 42.2 True knot (*arrow*), in this case, resulted in intrauterine fetal death. (Reprinted with permission from Benirschke K, Kaufmann P. *Pathology of the Human Placenta*. 3rd ed. New York: Springer-Verlag; 1995.)

to fetal demise when the knot is tight (1). The presence of vascular tortuosities (false knots) is common and rarely of clinical significance (Fig. 42.3). The finding of meconium staining and the presence of surface plaques are definitely abnormal and are described below.

The normal umbilical cord is pearly white and somewhat translucent. The length of the umbilical cord has great significance, principally when it is excessively long or excessively short. Cord length has been shown to vary with gestational age, and measurements indicate that the cord elongates as gestation proceeds. At approximately 20 weeks' gestational age, the average cord length is 32 cm (1). The normal length of the umbilical cord at term has been determined to be, on average, between 55 and 65 cm (1,7) (Fig. 42.4). Cord diameter is dependent on gestational age (35). The literature contains many articles that relate the significance of abnormal cord lengths with both in utero fetal activity and neonatal outcome. The reader is referred to an extensive review of the subject (1,38–40).

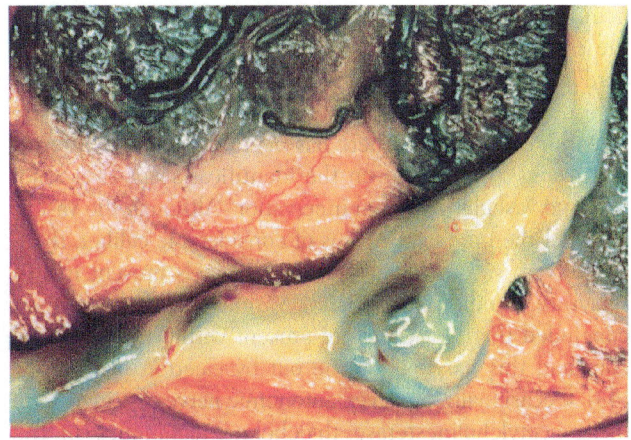

FIGURE 42.3 False knot, visible as an asymmetric dilatation of the umbilical cord and representing vascular tortuosity.

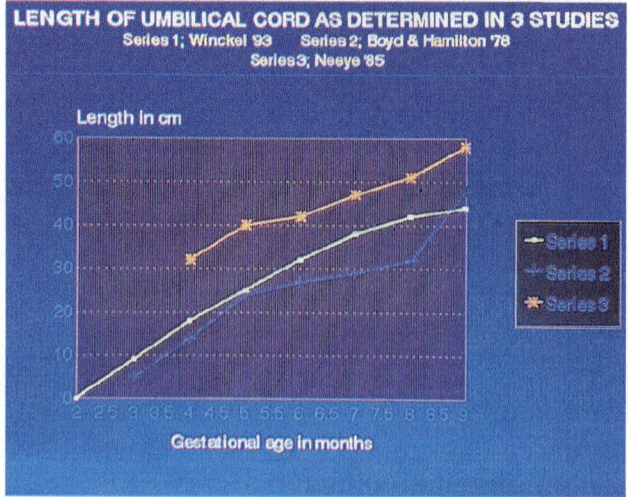

FIGURE 42.4 Normal cord length dimensions associated with changes in gestational age. (Reprinted with permission from Benirschke K, Kaufmann P. *Pathology of the Human Placenta*. 3rd ed. New York: Springer-Verlag; 1995.)

Histology

Histologic examination of the umbilical cord shows several distinct layers. On the surface is a well-defined single layer of amnionic epithelium. The epithelium is squamoid and, in the region of fetal cord insertion, often becomes multilayered and closely resembles its epidermal contiguity. Electron microscopy studies performed on cord amnionic cells have suggested that the epithelium is responsible for fluid equilibrium activities (1,2). True squamous metaplasia of the umbilical cord is considered a normal variant, and ultrastructural studies of this epithelium have shown morphologic similarities between this epithelium and the fetal epidermis (41).

Deep to the amnionic epithelium that comprises the surface of the cord is the substance of Wharton jelly. This material largely is composed of mucopolysaccharides (hyaluronic acid and chondroitin sulfate). Ultrastructural examination of this material shows the presence of delicate interlacing microfibrils and sparse collagen. Mast cells may be prominent and their frequency is increased near the periphery of the cord vasculature (42). In this same region, and in the cord in general, macrophages are rarely identified.

Embedded within the substance of Wharton jelly are the umbilical vessels. There has been considerable interest and discussion focused on the identification of vasa vasorum and vascular neuronal innervation. Although the vasculature of the umbilical cord is of considerable caliber, there are no vasa vasorum or lymphatic channels present in this structure. Studies investigating vascular innervation have concluded that no nerves are present within the umbilical cord and this has been borne out by electron microscopy (43). Occasionally, however, autonomic nerves are identified using acetylcholinesterase thiocholine techniques in the proximal (fetal) end of the cord (43–45). Such findings are compatible with the persistence of peripheral vagal neuronal elements associated with the ductus venosus, which are entrapped in the proximal portion of the umbilical cord and neuronal vestiges found within the umbilical cord are best considered as remnants; to date there has been no demonstration of their functional significance (1,45).

Since the yolk sac connects to the primitive midgut through the body stalk in early development, vestiges of this epithelium-lined duct are common in the umbilical cord. The persistence of the omphalomesenteric duct is characterized by a tubular structure present within Wharton jelly and lined by a single layer of low cuboidal to columnar, mucin-secreting epithelium (Fig. 42.5A–D). Remnants of the duct may form cystic structures that contain a variety of endodermally derived epithelia, including pancreatic, intestinal (small and large), and gastric components. Such findings are rarely of any clinical significance, although secretory products of gastric origin resulted in umbilical vascular ulceration, hemorrhage, and fetal death in a case report described by Blanc and Allan (46).

The allantois differentiates as a protuberance from the yolk sac into the body stalk and is essential for the development of the umbilical vessels. This structure is incorporated into the anterior aspect of the hindgut, where it communicates with the urachus. Remnants of the allantoic duct are often found in sections of proximal umbilical cords. Its intimate relationship with the formation of umbilical vessels explains its presence between the two umbilical arteries, when it is identified. These remnants rarely have clinical significance. The lining of this tract is often devoid of a lumen and consists of aggregates of epithelial cells with a squamoid to transitional appearance (Fig. 42.6).

The vasculature of the umbilical cord is composed of two arteries and one vein. The arteries possess no internal elastic lamina and have a double-layered muscular wall. Each of these muscular layers is composed of a network of interlacing smooth muscle bundles. The vein does have an inner elastic lamina. The umbilical vein, which generally has a larger diameter, possesses a thinner muscular coat consisting of a single layer of circular smooth muscle (Fig. 42.7A,B). As noted, no vasa vasorum are present. Remnants of the vitelline vasculature in the proximal portion of the cord sometimes may be observed in sections taken from this region. Intra-amnionic hemorrhage and fetal death have been reported (46).

Of further interest, distinguishing umbilical vasculature from other systemic vessels, is that no true vascular adventitia is found. Near the placental insertion, it is common to identify anastomotic channels between the two umbilical arteries, artifactually creating the appearance of supernumerary vessels or a single umbilical artery (47,48) (Fig. 42.8).

Transverse serial sections confirm that two umbilical arteries spiral in parallel around the umbilical vein. Often, multiple twists in the cord occur. The proposed origin of this spiraling has been extensively discussed; however, its true functional significance and origin remain to be definitively elucidated (1). As discussed and demonstrated below, when

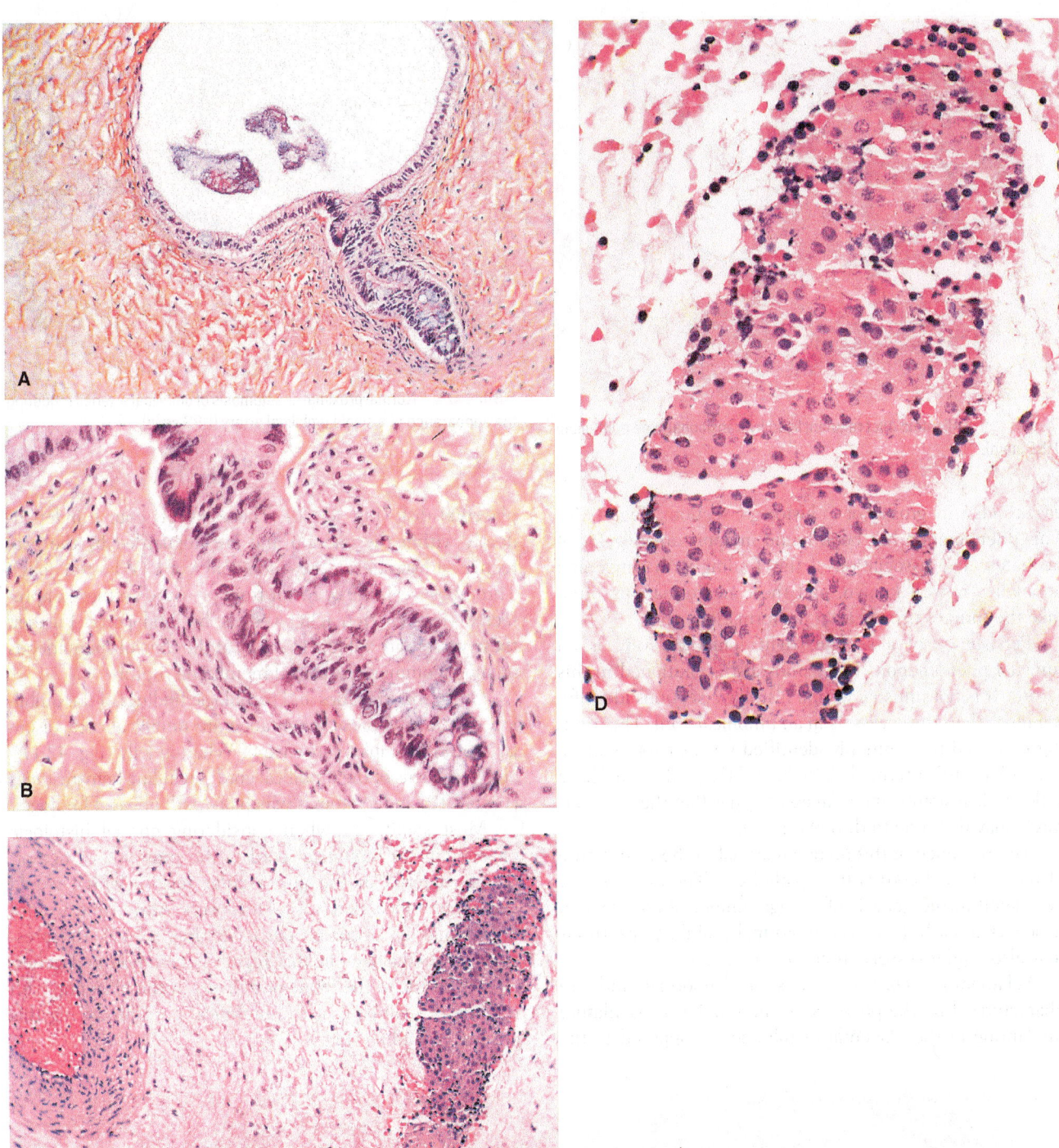

FIGURE 42.5 Omphalomesenteric duct remnant (**A**) with enteric epithelia (**B**). Omphalomesenteric duct adjacent to umbilical vein (**C**) with unusual finding of hepatic tissue (**D**).

coiling is excessive, adverse perinatal outcomes have been observed (49).

Histopathology

Distinguishing normal anatomy from pathologic entities is the essence of proper understanding of the normal anatomy and histology of the umbilical cord. Most pathology of the cord may be seen in the gross sense. Histology is confirmatory. A tight knot with notching indicating stricture associated with proximal vascular dilatation may result in fetal death. Interestingly, although true knots occur frequently and are associated with long cords, adverse outcomes are rare events; therefore, in most instances a true knot can be considered a normal variant. The absence of an umbilical artery is a well-established observation and

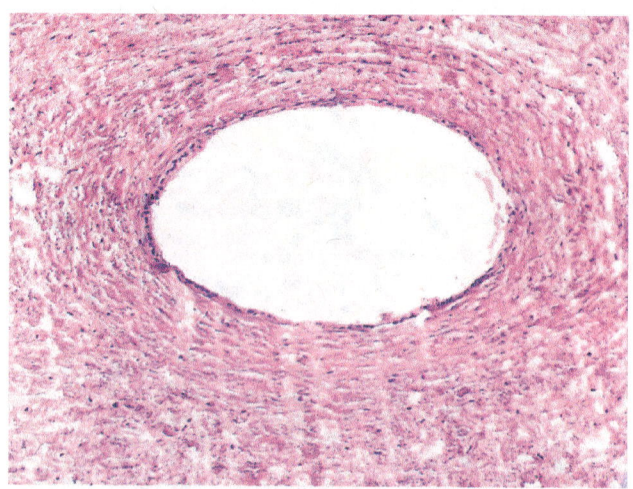

FIGURE 42.6 Allantoic duct remnant lined by transitional-type epithelium (H&E stain).

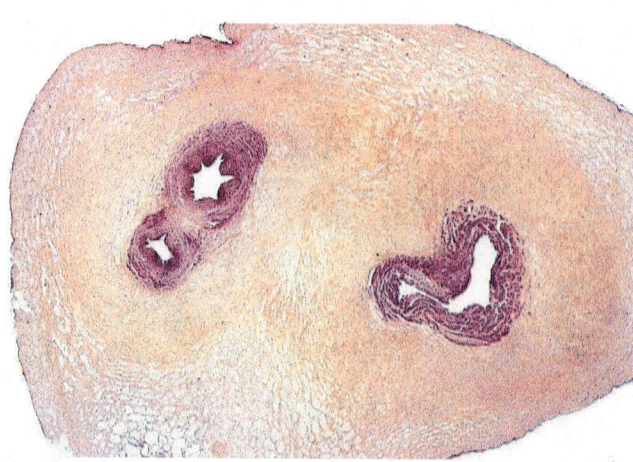

FIGURE 42.8 Normal proximal anastomosis of umbilical arteries rendering the appearance of a single umbilical artery (HPS stain).

easy to identify grossly or in histologic sections (Fig. 42.9). This phenomenon has been found in approximately 1% of neonates. The association of this finding with congenital anomalies is well known, and these malformations often take the form of urinary tract malformations (1).

Persistence of a second (right) umbilical vein is an unusual phenomenon. The pathologist is cautioned in this regard. It is not unusual to find histologic sections identifying more than three vessels in an umbilical cord. This finding is related to commonly identified vascular tortuosities, which have been termed "false knots" (Fig. 42.3) and have little clinical significance. An exception is that these vessels rarely may be prone to thrombosis (1).

The presence of thrombotic material in the vasculature of the umbilical cord is truly pathologic. The process may be related to the genesis of a single umbilical artery when it occurs in early gestation. Abnormal umbilical insertions may also render vessels prone to thrombosis.

Velamentous cord insertions are abnormal and are characterized by the presence of the umbilical vasculature implanting in the placental membranes as opposed to the placental disk (Fig. 42.10). These vessels course independently within the chorion and are unguarded by the protective substance of the umbilical cord (Wharton jelly). Thrombosis can thusly result from pressure on these unprotected (by Wharton jelly) vessels by fetal parts. Further, these vessels are subject to injury at the time of spontaneous or, more commonly, artificial membrane rupture.

Other abnormalities and pathologic findings of the umbilical cord with clinical importance are umbilical cord vascular rupture, complete absence of Wharton jelly (Fig. 42.11), and neoplasms of the umbilical cord (including hemangiomas [Fig. 42.12] and teratomas which are both unusual findings).

Most significant when considering normal histologic changes in the umbilical cord is the presence of hemorrhagic material in the perivascular region, which would suggest umbilical cord vascular rupture. Although true cord hematomas do occur on occasion (Fig. 42.13), the presence of hemorrhage in this region is common and generally attributed to the mode of delivery of the placenta, with traction or clamping of the umbilical cord producing this artifactual finding (Fig. 42.14).

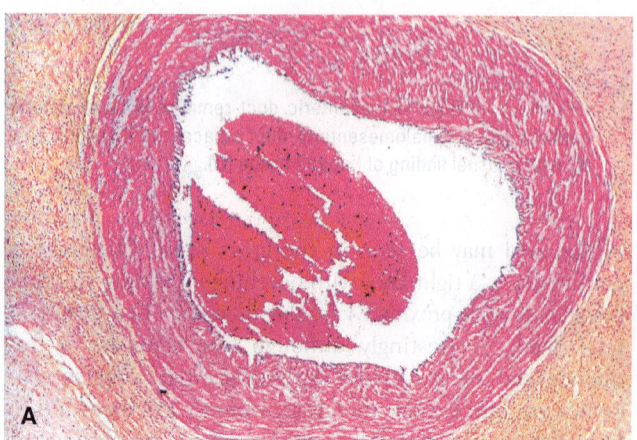
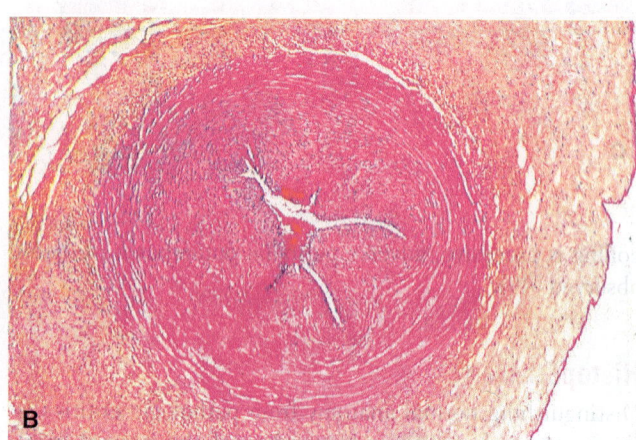

FIGURE 42.7 Umbilical vein (**A**) and artery (**B**) (HPS stain).

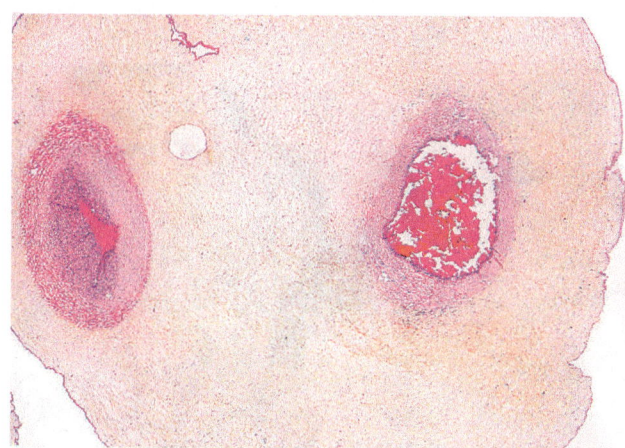

FIGURE 42.9 Single umbilical artery, frequently seen in the context of urinary tract anomalies in the neonate (HPS stain).

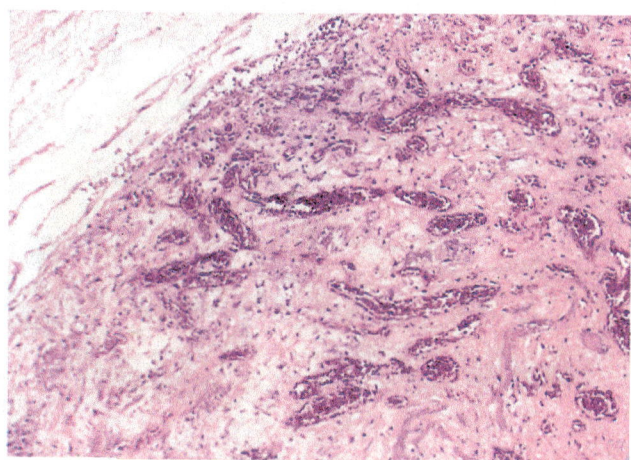

FIGURE 42.12 Dilated vascular lumina of umbilical cord hemangioma (HPS stain).

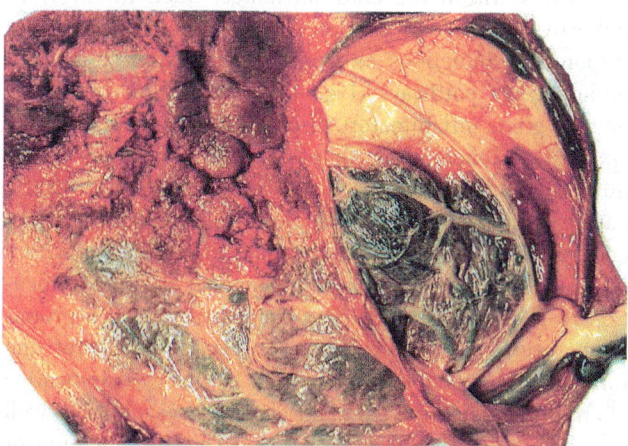

FIGURE 42.10 Velamentous insertion of umbilical cord. Umbilical vessels insert in membranes adjacent to the chorionic plate. In this case, the fetus exsanguinated after amniotomy and rupture of membranous vessels.

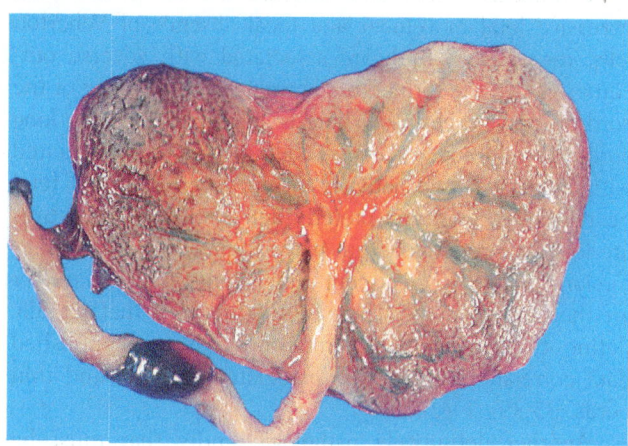

FIGURE 42.13 Hematoma of umbilical cord. This placenta was delivered by cesarean section and there was no traction or clamping of this segment of cord.

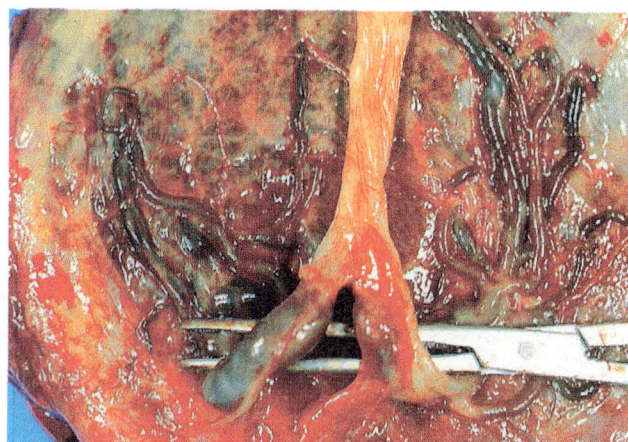

FIGURE 42.11 Furcate insertion of umbilical cord. Umbilical cord vessels insert into placental substance individually (UA, *left;* UA and UV, *right*) not surrounded by Wharton jelly.

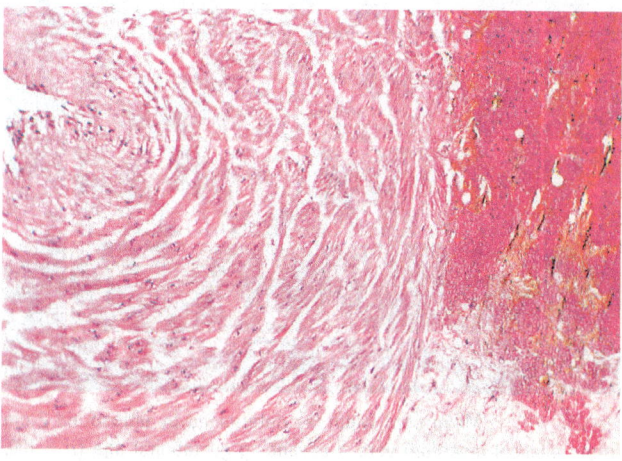

FIGURE 42.14 Perivascular hemorrhage located adjacent to umbilical artery found in the region of a cord clamp (HPS stain).

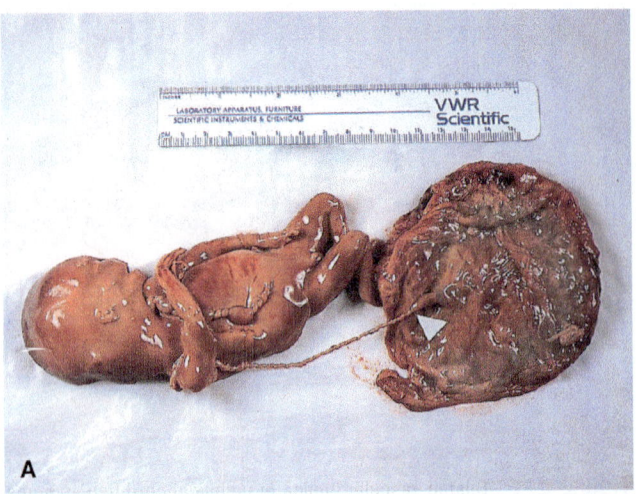
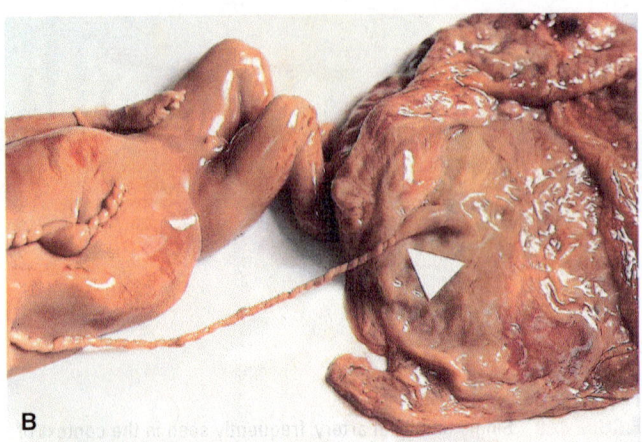

FIGURE 42.15 Excessive cord spiraling (**A**) leading to torsion (**B**) and stricture resulting in fetal death.

Umbilical torsion and stricture are associated with excessive fetal movement and focal absence of Wharton jelly, respectively. Both are associated with adverse outcomes (1). In the former, the normal twist or coiling of the cord becomes excessive. There is an association with long cords. In addition, excessive coiling has been associated with increased fetal activity, cocaine use, abnormal fetal heart rate tracings, and preterm deliveries (49). Strictures are less well understood but may at times be a function of torsion (Fig. 42.15). Nascent dimensions of cord diameter are therefore germane. There is little literature that actually defines the dimensions of normal cords, although published data correlate abnormalities associated with fat and thin cords (35,39) (Fig. 42.16).

Another definitively pathologic entity that must be distinguished from normal histology is the presence of leukocytes within the cord substance. Such findings are indicative of funisitis and are the result of inflammatory response to infectious antigens and recruitment through inflammatory pathways (Fig. 42.17). A recent trend has been to grade inflammatory disorders affecting membranes and the umbilical cord. In past studies gradation of the number of inflammatory cell may have more to do with the nature of the infectious agent (e.g., Group B Streptococcus may be associated with a paucicellular inflammatory infiltrate, yet recently a consensus panel adds quantification to description) (1,3,18). When the process is prominent (severe) and with calcifications, the term "necrotizing funisitis" is applicable. Such severe pathology is indicative of chronic inflammation and may be seen in syphilis, as well as other infections (1) (Fig. 42.18). The identification of fungal elements about the umbilical cord is often difficult to discern from an overgrowth storage phenomenon. In this regard, the difficulty lies in the usual absence of associated inflammatory infiltrate. The cord, when involved, has white surface plaques and wedge-shaped aggregates of

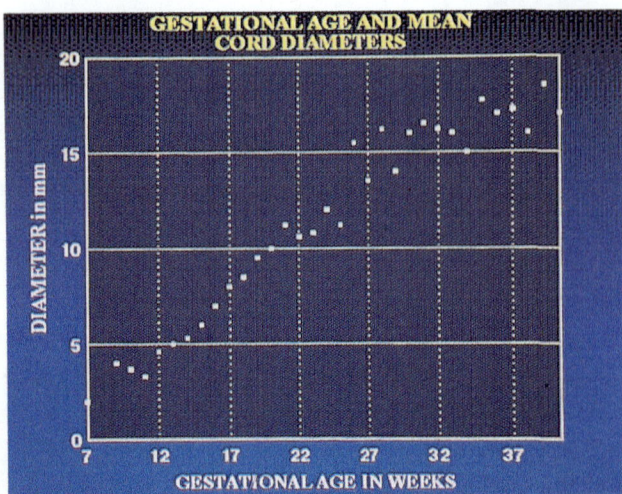

FIGURE 42.16 Mean cord width (as determined by ultrasound 2 cm from umbilical insertion) versus advancing gestational age ($n = 100$, $p < 0.05$). (Reprinted with permission from Lewis SH, Gilbert E, (Starr C.). Cord width in utero. In: Barness LA, ed. Advances in Pediatrics Vol. 45. St. Louis, MO: Mosby; 1998.)

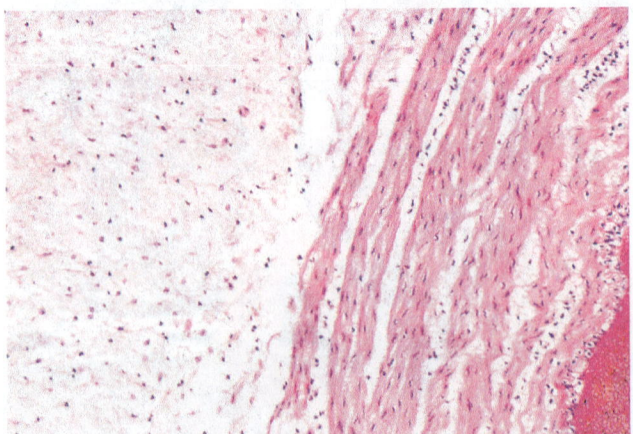

FIGURE 42.17 Acute funisitis. Polymorphonuclear leukocytes are present within the umbilical vein muscularis and adjacent Wharton jelly (H&E stain).

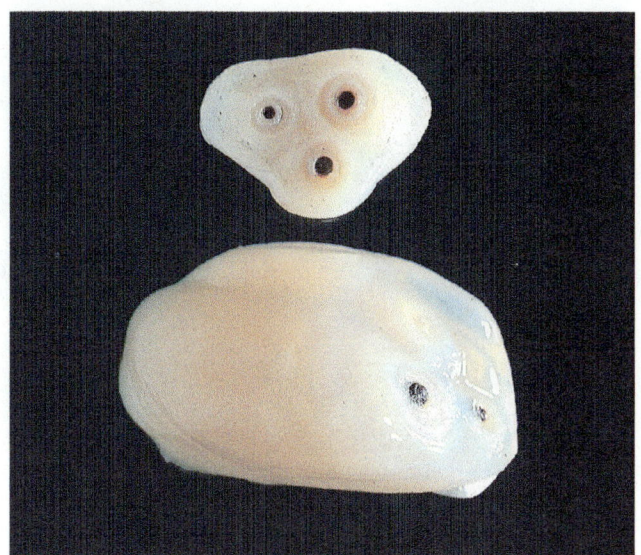

FIGURE 42.18 Necrotizing funisitis with intense concentric bands of perivascular inflammation associated with calcification (peripheral white circular bands) may be seen grossly.

acute inflammatory cells on the surface surrounding fungal elements. These (i.e., *Candida albicans*) may be identified merely with H&E stains, although special stains for fungi can be helpful when such pathology is suspected (1).

Lastly, a finding in the cord that is notably pathologic is meconium-induced medial destruction of vessels (Fig. 42.19A,B), which results from direct meconium toxicity and necrobiosis of vascular media (50). Associated vascular spasm and medial degeneration may adversely affect hemodynamics in the cord and chorionic vasculature. This finding occurs as pyknotic, hypereosinophilic cells at the periphery of the affected vessel wall, typically in that aspect closest to the umbilical cord surface and in close approximation to meconium-laden macrophages.

RAMIFICATION OF CHORIONIC VASCULATURE

At this point it is convenient to discuss the ramification of the umbilical vessels in the chorionic plate. The umbilical cord normally inserts in a central or eccentric fashion. Although abnormal insertion at the margin (Battledore) and in the membranes (velamentous) comprises a small portion of cord insertions, both should be considered pathologic and not normal variants insofar as they have been attributed to adverse outcomes when extensively analyzed (1,3,48).

The pattern of vascular ramification within the chorion is described as either magistral (characterized by large-diameter vessels, radially diminishing in caliber to the periphery of the placenta) or disperse (characterized by multiple small vessels emanating directly from the cord insertion site). It is of interest that in the chorionic vasculature, no distinction can be made between branches of the umbilical vein and umbilical arteries using histologic criteria (in counter distinction to the aforementioned description of differentiation between vein and artery in the umbilical cord). The only means of identifying which vessels are branches of

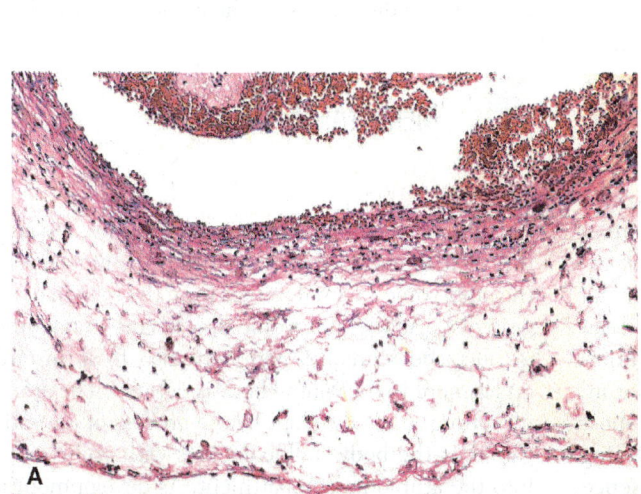
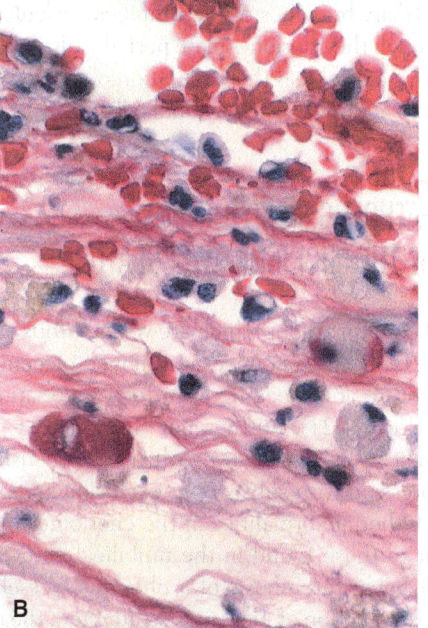

FIGURE 42.19 Globular degenerated necrobiotic medial cells secondary to meconium exposure. The process is focal and contrasts with adjacent normal myocytes (Luna Ishak stain) (**A**). Higher magnification demonstrating pigmented macrophages (**B**). (Reprinted with permission from Rana J, Ebert GA, Kappy KA. Adverse perinatal outcome with an abnormal umbilical coiling index. *Obstet Gynecol* 1995;85:573–578.)

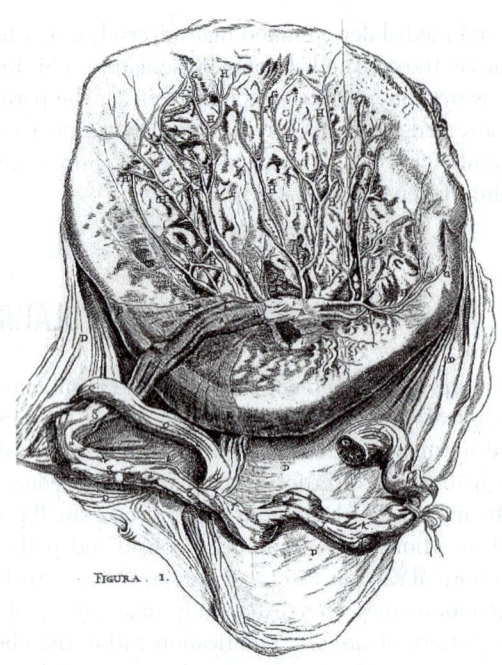

FIGURE 42.20 As early as the 1600s, Nicholas Hoboken recognized that chorionic arteries overlie veins, and this was beautifully depicted in his painstaking drawings. These are the earliest accurate drawings of the human placenta known to exist.

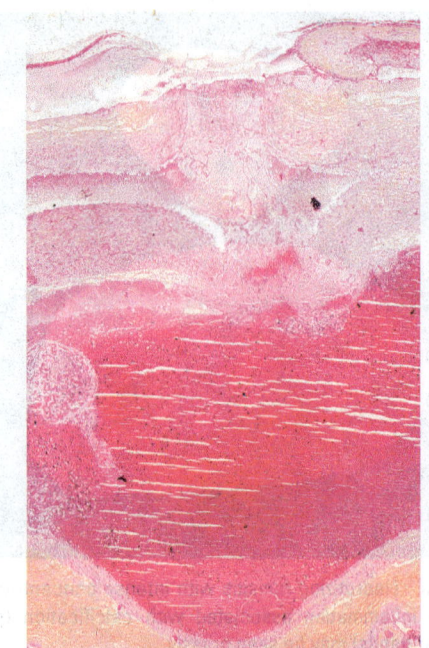

FIGURE 42.21 Iatrogenic chorionic vasculature rupture following amniocentesis for fetal lung maturation studies. The not unusual accessory lobe was several centimeters from the main body of the placenta, obscuring its presence and vasculature. Emergent cesarean section followed a "bloody tap" and fetal heart rate abnormalities.

arteries and which are veins is by noting their gross anatomic distribution. Arteries always cross over veins when observed from the fetal surface (Fig. 42.20). The notation of such vascular relationships is of extreme significance when considering vascular anastomoses, as may be seen in some twin pregnancies (1,2).

The primary branches of the umbilical vasculature that course through the chorionic plate periodically dive beneath this stratum to establish the circulation of primary vascular ramifications ending in the terminal villi.

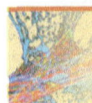
PATHOLOGIC ALTERATIONS OF THE CHORIONIC VASCULATURE

Abnormal cord insertions which are velamentous and membranous vessels which connect multilobed placentas are at risk for rupture and bleeding from fetal excoriation or iatrogenesis (Fig. 42.21). Further, not cushioned by placental parenchyma, such vessels are with increased risk of fetal part compression with subsequent occlusion and/or thrombosis (1). Other abnormalities in the chorionic vasculature are similar to those found in the umbilical cord, the most significant being thrombosis of a chorionic vessel. During the gross examination of placentas so affected, the presence of thrombotic material may readily be identified by noting dilated vessels containing firm thrombotic substance. On the other hand, vascular thrombi may be subtler and their appearance characterized only by the presence of faintly

highlighted linear white streaks that parallel the peripheral margin of vessels involved (Fig. 42.22A). These findings can be confirmed histologically (Fig. 42.22B) (1).

The presence of polymorphonuclear leukocytes migrating from the chorionic vasculature and from the umbilical vasculature is pathognomonic of chorionitis and umbilical cord vasculitis, respectively. Findings of chorionitis are histologically similar to those aforementioned in acute funisitis (Fig. 42.17) (1,3,5,32). The newer aforementioned considerations of quantification are mentioned, with consideration for both the quantity and distribution of the inflammatory cells (5–7).

MEMBRANES

Embryology

The placental membranes consist of the amnion and the chorion. The amnion, which constitutes the innermost aspect of the embryonic cavity, develops from the margin of the embryonic disk. As the embryonic disk begins to take the form of a tube, the amnionic periphery also folds inward and its attachment to the ventral body is defined. The amnionic cavity subsequently develops by the process of cavitation. Elongation of the body stalk coincides with embryonic prolapse into the amnionic compartment. As development proceeds, the resultant cavity expands, and by 12 weeks from the last menstrual period the amniotic cavity completely occupies the chorionic sac. At this point, fusion occurs with the chorionic wall. This event is commonly identified by clinicians via

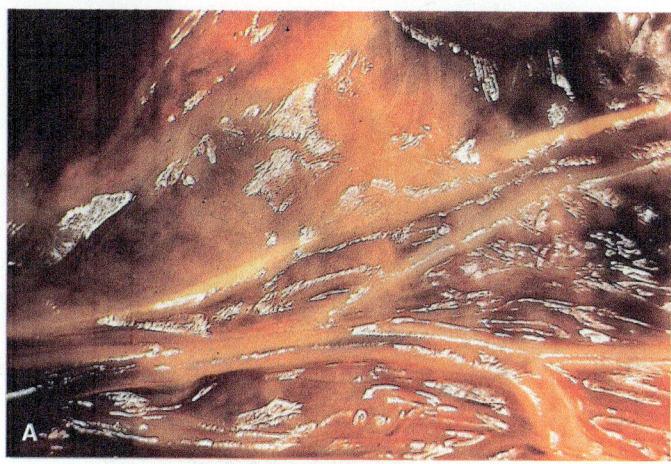
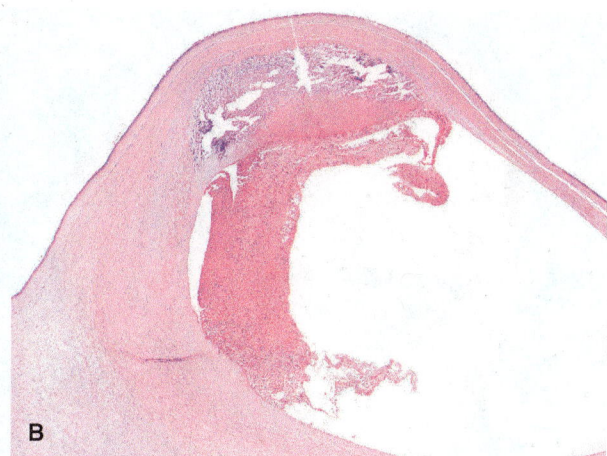

FIGURE 42.22 **A:** Chorionic vascular thrombosis characterized by a linear streak paralleling the vascular course (in this case a chorionic vein). **B:** Collection of fibrin and blood adherent to the chorionic plate vessel wall. These thrombi can be occlusive or (as in this case) nonocclusive and older lesions may calcify (H&E stain). (Reprinted with permission from Benirschke K, Kaufmann P. *Pathology of the Human Placenta*. 3rd ed. New York: Springer-Verlag; 1995.)

routine ultrasonographic analysis of advancing gestations. At this gestational age, the potential space between the chorion and the amnion is visibly obliterated. The amnionic cavity remains filled with amnionic fluid, which by the end of gestation amounts to approximately 1 L (1).

The chorion forms the base for the peripherally radiating villi and serves to encapsulate the embryo and the developing amnion. As the early implantation embryo develops, the embryonic tissues (the trophoblast and its mesodermal investments) continue to expand in a spherical fashion. The inner aspect of the condensation of mesoderm, which forms the inner capsular structure deep to the peripheral trophoblast, is also termed chorion. In the region that becomes the placental disk proper, chorionic villi continue to develop beneath these structures, and the placenta proper or the chorion frondosum is defined. The region of the chorion that covers the expanded amnionic cavity forms what has been termed chorionic laeve. This constitutes the reflected membranes and is discerned from the membranous covering of the chorionic plate. Chorionic villi in the region of the laeve (which delimits the sac containing amnionic fluid) atrophy by pressure, although remnants of villous tissue may be found in association with this structure. In the region of the chorion frondosum, the fetal blood vessels invest the chorionic plate. Such vessels only occur in the chorion; the amnion is an avascular structure.

Amnion and Chorion

Gross Morphology

The fetal membranes have a particular and characteristic appearance in normal deliveries. The sac, when viewed from the fetal surface, is clear and often has a bluish hue, and the amnion is devoid of vasculature. Remnants of atrophied vasculature may be seen in the overlying chorion and appear as filamentous streaks. The chorionic plate also has a characteristic blue sheen and, as described previously, the distribution of chorionic vessels has a characteristic appearance. The membranes of the chorionic plate are distinguished from the laeve as described above. It is not infrequent to find a peripheral nodule on the surface of the disk membranes. This normal nodule is the remnant of the fetal yolk sac (Fig. 42.23).

Gross Morphologic Alterations

Although chorionic vessels are normal in the chorion of the chorionic plate overlying the disk, the persistence of functional vasculature in the chorion laeve is aberrant and equates to membranous vessels. These vessels may connect lobes of placenta or relate to the membranous insertion of the umbilical cord (velamentous insertion as described above).

On occasion, the chorionic plate may possess a ring of fibrin that forms a concentric ridge between the insertion of the cord and the margin of the placental disk. This fibrin ring, which lies deep to the amnion, is indicative of an extrachorial placentation. Such a placentation is characterized by two

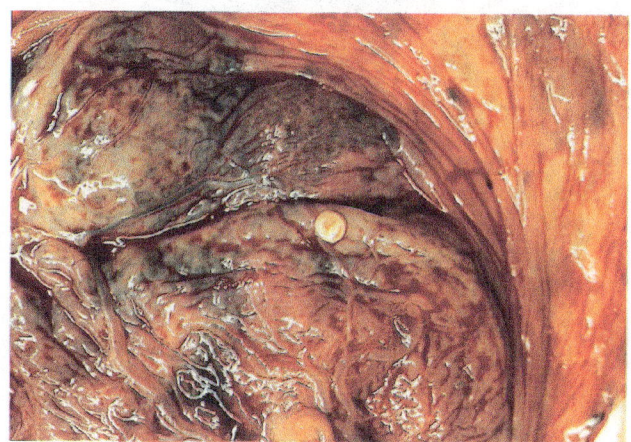

FIGURE 42.23 White nodule is the residua of the fetal yolk sac.

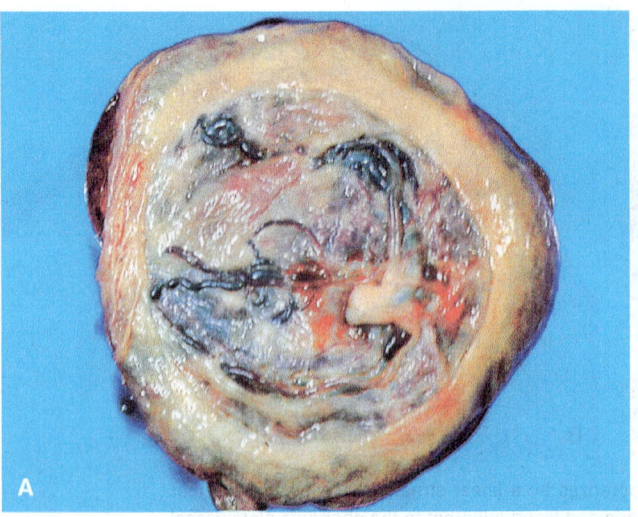
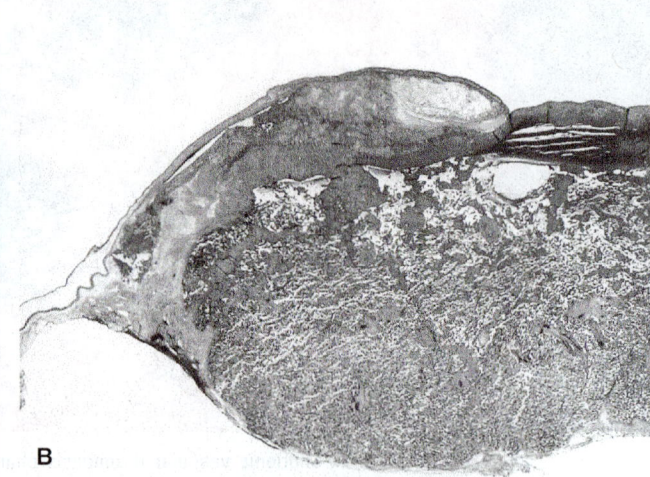

FIGURE 42.24 **A:** Circumvallate placenta. **B:** Note loose association of amnion peripheral to marginal subamnionic fibrin deposition. (Reprinted with permission from Benirschke K, Kaufmann P. *Pathology of the Human Placenta*. 3rd ed. New York: Springer-Verlag; 1995.)

forms: the circumvallate placentation and the circummarginate placentation. In the former, the membranes are reflected upon themselves at the ridge of the fibrin deposition. They then cover the remaining margin of the placental disk in a loose fashion (Fig. 42.24A,B). In the circummarginate placenta, the ring of fibrin is present over the chorion, and the overlying amnion is not reflected upon itself at this fibrinous ring (Fig. 42.25). The amnion thus extends to the margin of the placental disk, and its departure to form the amnionic sac occurs at this margin. It is currently felt that this fibrinous ring represents placental migration in conjunction with an enlarging uterus during the second trimester (the so-called "trophotropism") (1).

The common occurrence of gross squamous metaplasia is important to recognize and is a normal finding unless its presence is extensive. It is important to distinguish normal squamous metaplasia from grossly pathologic amnion nodosum. Immersion of the placental membranes in water generally defines squamous metaplasia by its failure to become moist as opposed to the normal surrounding amnion. In pathologic conditions, metaplasia in these regions may be pronounced, and large plaques and nodules may form (Fig. 42.26). These nodules are distinguished from the truly pathologic condition of amnion nodosum by their failure to be easily denuded from the surface of the amnion by slight mechanical pressure. The presence of amnion nodosum is characterized in the gross sense by the presence of multiple small papules on the amnionic surface (Fig. 42.27). The clinical history is suggestive, and oligohydramnios characterizes these gestations. The small papules are easily removed from the amnionic surface by excoriation, and their substances are confirmed histologically by the presence of debris and degenerated squames. The origin of these cells is fetal epidermis, and their presence on the amnionic surface is related to apposition of this membrane and fetal skin in conditions where there is diminished amnionic fluid. Microscopy is

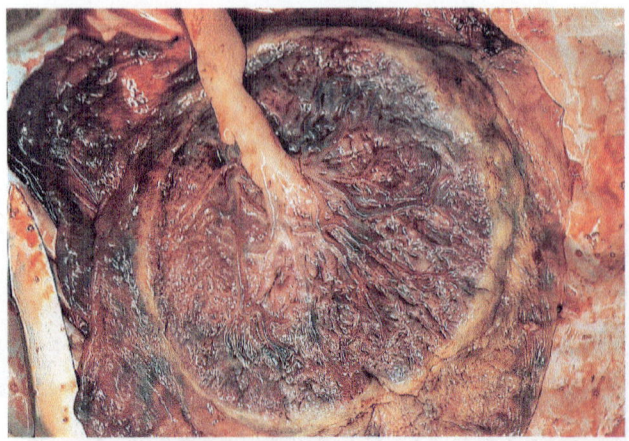

FIGURE 42.25 Circummarginate placenta. Note the close association of amnion to the disk peripheral to the fibrin ring.

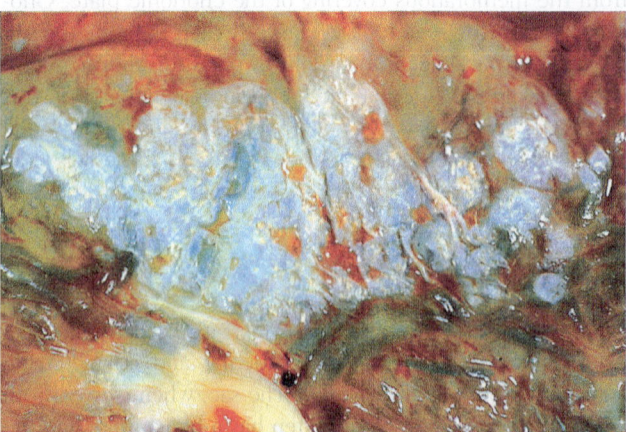

FIGURE 42.26 Extensive squamous metaplasia on the amnionic surface from a fetus with an encephalocele. It is believed that irritation from the encephalocele in this region produced the extensive metaplasia.

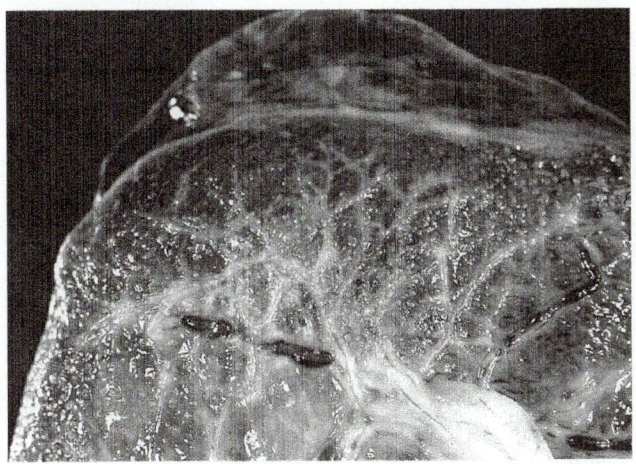

FIGURE 42.27 Multiple papules of amnion nodosum stipple the amnionic surface of this placenta from a gestation characterized by oligohydramnios.

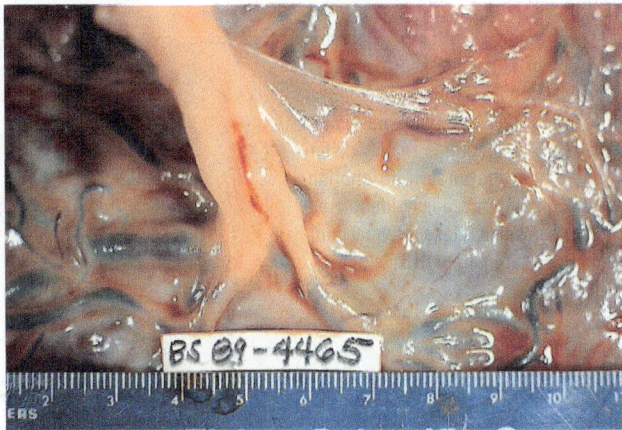

FIGURE 42.28 Amniotic web partially immobilizes the cord by limiting its movement at the cord base.

most helpful in further distinguishing squamous metaplasia from the amnion nodosum (see later).

Amnionic bands are rare. The condition is responsible for in utero fetal part amputation and trauma and is a phenomenon that occurs in approximately one in 10,000 births. The occurrence is important because it demonstrates potential difficulties from abnormal amnionic membrane development (51,52). The precise mechanism is not known in most cases, but rupture of the amnion (most probably in the first trimester) allows the fetus to enter the chorionic sac. The remnants of amnion form the substance of the resulting amnionic bands. At term these placentas have highly opaque chorionic surfaces that reflect hyperplasia of this uncovered layer. The remaining amnionic epithelium is densely coapted with the base of the umbilical cord from which it cannot be stripped. Only small amounts of amnion are present, which distinguishes this condition from artifactual disruption of the amnion from the chorionic plate during the delivery process (1,3,41,53,54). Occasionally, an abnormal "web" will be present at the base of the cord insertion, and this may limit normal cord movement (1,50) (Fig. 42.28).

Amnion Histology

The amnion, the innermost layer of the amnionic cavity, is lined by a single layer of epithelial cells that resides on a basement membrane. The basement membrane is attached to an underlying thin layer of connective tissue (55–59) (Fig. 42.29). The amnion, although adjacent to the chorion, is not truly fused to it and may be separated with minimum effort. This juxtaposition of the two membranous layers occurs at 12 weeks' gestational age (59) (Fig. 42.30). Before this time, as the amnion develops, it is separated from the chorion by the so-called magma reticulare, which is a viscous and thixotropic gelatinous fluid (1,60). Stellate mesenchymal cells may be found within this substance. These cells also have epithelial characteristics and have been stained immunohistochemically and found to be cytokeratin and vimentin positive (53).

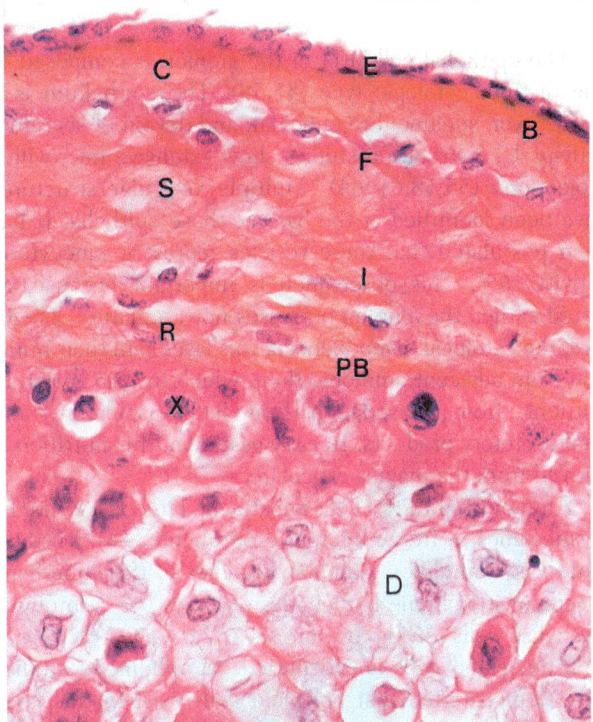

FIGURE 42.29 Flattened to cuboidal amnionic epithelial cells (*E*) adhere to their basement membrane (*B*). Beneath this is the compact layer of the amnion (*C*), which is acellular and may form a barrier to PMNs. The compact layer is rarely affected by edema and is probably the strongest amnionic layer. A fibroblastic layer (*F*) lies beneath the compact layer, and macrophages may be found. A spongy layer (*S*), relatively devoid of fibroblasts, separates the amnion from the chorion, although the two may merge imperceptibly. Often, an artifactual separation may be present near the plane of true fusion. The amnion usually measures from 0.2 to 0.5 mm in thickness (*I*). The most superficial layer of chorion is usually an incomplete cellular zone (*I*) that overlies a thick reticular layer (*R*). This layer is composed of fibroblasts and macrophages. Beneath the reticular layer is a pseudo-basement membrane (*PB*) overlying extravillous trophoblast (*X*) and then maternal decidua (*D*) (HPS stain).

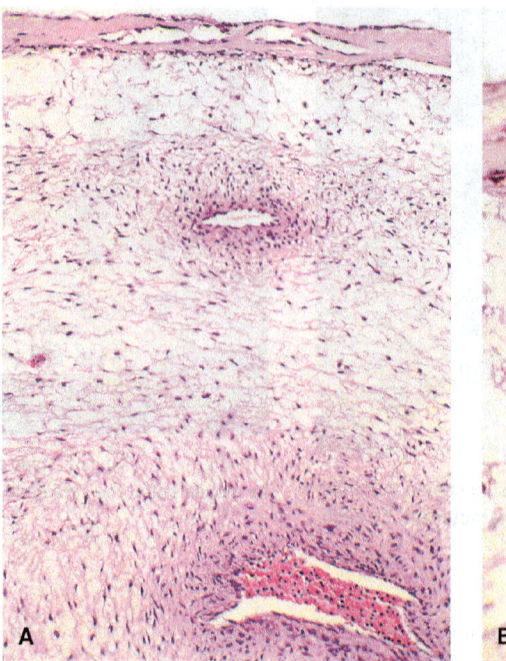
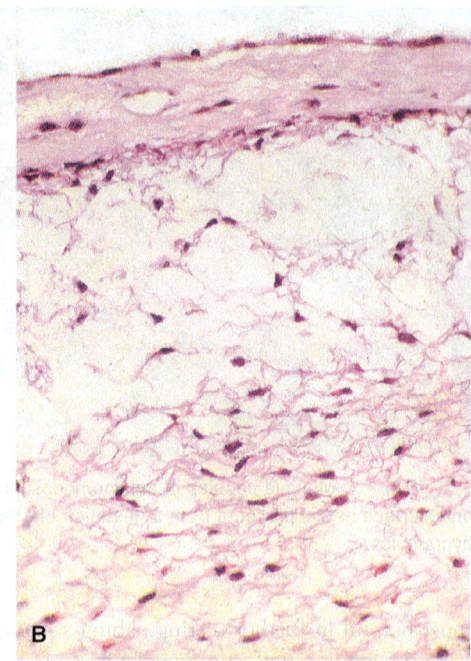

FIGURE 42.30 **A:** The separation between amnion and chorion is more apparent in early gestations as seen in this section from the chorionic plate of a 10- to 12-week placenta (*upper right*). **B:** The amnion is readily distinguished from the underlying chorion, which contains the easily identifiable chorionic vessels. Mesenchymal components are prominent (H&E stain).

The epithelial cell layer of the amnion is composed of one distinct cytologic type (57,58). The epithelium is a single layer, squamoid to cuboidal, and devoid of secretory activity. Ultrastructural studies show extensive microvillus projections (55,58,61–64). Multiple vesicular structures have been identified at the base of these epithelia. It has been postulated that these vesicles represent pinocytotic activity (65). This observation is important because, as stated earlier, the amnion possesses no vasculature. Therefore, the cytologic components of this layer gain their nutrition from adjacent amnionic fluid, which in turn is rich in nutrients from transudation (from fetal vasculature) and fetal excretory products. In early gestation, this nutrition is derived from the magma reticulare.

Amnionic epithelial cells are attached to one another by desmosomes in freeze-fracture experiments (66). Furthermore, the amnionic epithelium attaches to the underlying basement membrane by hemidesmosomes (67). Amnionic epithelial cells divide by mitosis (57,68). On occasion, multinucleated cells are identified. Morphometry studies have demonstrated that polyploid cells exist in this layer (62) and other karyotypic anomalies can occur, leading to potential false-positive results for chromosomal defects when amnionic cells contaminate amniocentesis preparations (68–71). Although the epithelium of the amnion does not actively secrete, lipid droplets have been noted within these cells, an observation that correlates with increasing gestational age (62). Glycogen also has been found within amnionic cells (72).

Squamous metaplasia is a common occurrence in the amnionic epithelium, especially near the insertion of the umbilical cord (Fig. 42.31). This epithelium may become keratinized, and keratohyalin granules can be identified. Although this appears to result from irritation of the amnionic epithelial surface, these changes can be found in more than half of all term placentas (1,67).

Beneath the basement membrane of the amnionic epithelium, an additional component of the amnion is identified. This layer principally is divided into a compact and a fibroblastic region. The connective tissue within this region may harbor macrophages, which have been identified within the first trimester of pregnancy (73).

Amnion Histopathology

Histologic abnormalities of the amnion are heralded by an abnormal gross appearance. For example, membranes that are stained green or brown may reflect deposition of meconium. Amnionic membranes that are white may be indicative of polymorphonuclear leukocyte infiltration and acute chorioamnionitis (74) and may be quantified (Fig. 42.32A,B) (18).

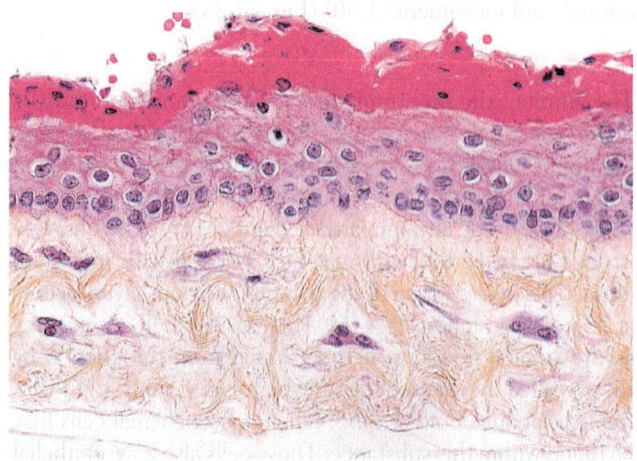

FIGURE 42.31 Squamous metaplasia of the amnion with hyperkeratosis (HPS stain).

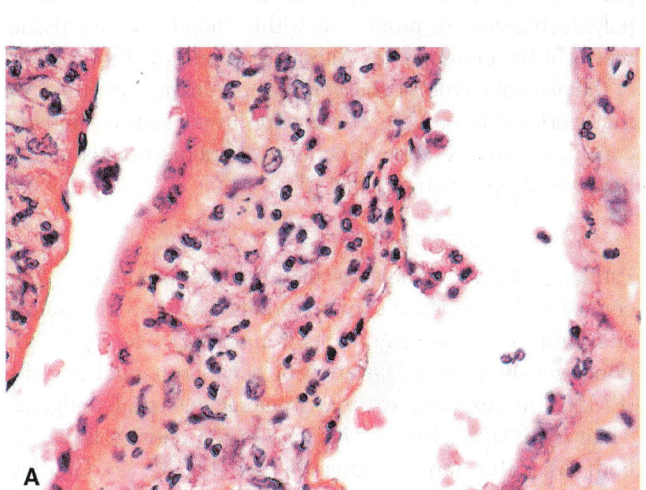
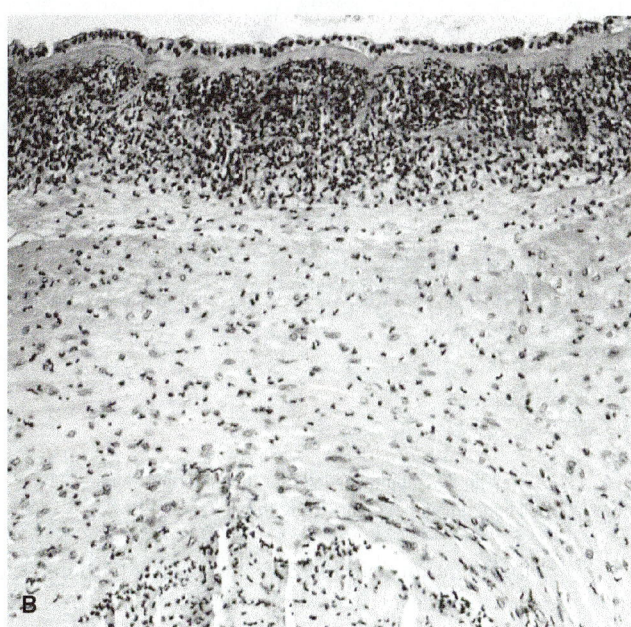

FIGURE 42.32 Acute chorioamnionitis in membrane roll (**A**) (HPS stain) and in chorionic plate (**B**) (H&E stain).

Abnormalities of amnionic epithelial cells, although suggested by gross examination, can only be confirmed by histologic assessment. Abnormalities that reflect degenerative changes are characterized by the presence of vacuolated cytoplasm and elongation to columnar forms. A rather rare and unusual finding associated with gastroschisis carries a pathognomonic histologic aberrancy of the amnion whereby amnionic epithelial cells contain innumerable vacuoles (1) (Fig. 42.33).

Amnionic epithelial degeneration (Fig. 42.34) is characteristic when meconium is present. Such findings may be confirmed when macrophages, present within the amnionic layer, contain meconium (a coarse brown pigment), which does not stain for iron (Fig. 42.35). On the other hand, hemosiderin deposition may be found within the amnionic layer in macrophages, and this can be confirmed by the use of iron stains (i.e., Prussian blue).

Although there are no true tumors of the amnion, occasional cysts representing edema may be identified. Although they may be striking in their gross appearance, it must be recognized that no clinical significance can be identified. Occasional cysts of ectodermal and mesodermal tissue have been identified deep to the amnionic layer, but such findings are not considered true neoplasms. Teratomas have been described (75). These lesions probably represent degenerative acardiac twins (1), but the lack of directed differentiation from pluripotential stem cells could account for the former.

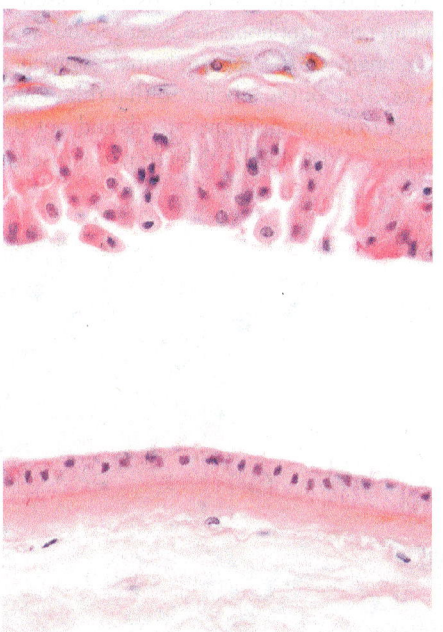

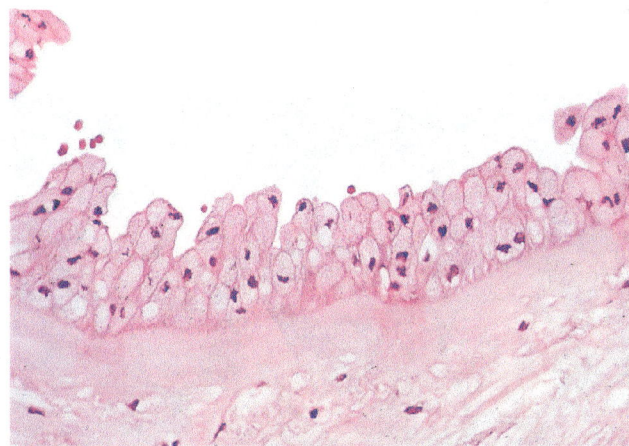

FIGURE 42.33 Unusual vacuolated elongated amnionic epithelial cells pathognomonic of gastroschisis. The pathophysiology is uncertain (H&E stain).

FIGURE 42.34 A twisted membrane roll with amnionic epithelial degeneration (*above*) and normal amnionic epithelium (*below*) (HPS stain).

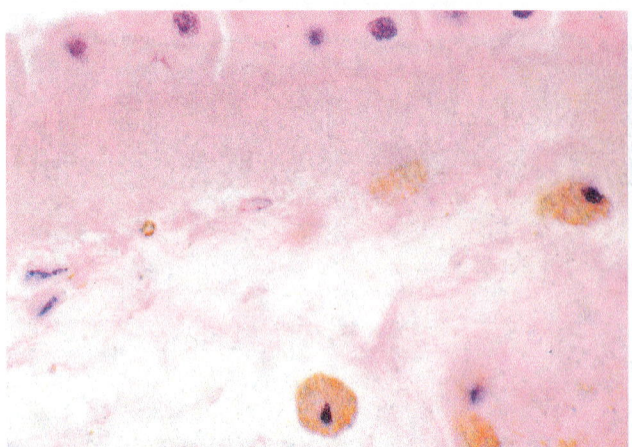

FIGURE 42.35 Amnionic epithelial degeneration overlies pigment-laden macrophages containing meconium (HPS stain).

The papules of amnion nodosum are clearly pathologic and reflect, in most cases, decreased amnionic fluid. In such instances, vernix (desquamated epithelia from the fetus) forms minute nodules on the amnionic surface in this characteristic fashion (Fig. 42.36). The lesions are composed of acellular debris and remnants of cells (76). The material within these papules is PAS and Alcian blue positive.

Chorion Histology

The chorion is composed of a connective tissue membrane that carries the fetal vasculature. Its inner aspect is bounded by the outer layer of the amnion, and the outer aspect is directly associated with the trophoblastic villi that sprout from its surface. There are two distinct aspects of the chorion: the chorion frondosum and the chorion laeve. The chorion of the reflected membranes (chorion laeve) is composed of an inner cellular layer, a "reticular" layer, a "pseudo-basement membrane," and an outer trophoblastic layer (58,60) (Fig. 42.29). The precise origin of the mesenchymal component of the chorion is not clear, but it is believed that this connective tissue is derived from the primitive streak and not the trophoblast (61,71,77) (Fig. 42.30). Electron microscopy studies have shown the connective tissue cells adjacent to the amnion to be rich in endoplasmic reticulum (60). Macrophages and degenerative endothelial cells also have been described as part of the cytologic makeup of this layer (60,78). Acid mucopolysaccharides are prominent within the connective tissue matrix of the chorion (72). Although present in other regions of the placenta, type VI collagen is a prominent constituent of the chorionic layer (79). The chorion frondosum is similarly constituted but contains functional chorionic vessels and is bordered deeply by functional villi.

Chorion Histopathology

Pathology of the chorionic vasculature (described above in the context of its umbilical cord continuity) includes chorionitis and thromboses (see comments from above). The fetal chorionic vessels allow permeation of polymorphonuclear cells (PMNs) in response to intra-amnionic bacterial antigens. Maternal PMNs also may be seen in the chorion laeve. In both cases, the amnion is later affected (Fig. 42.32). Grading and staging of inflammation is now recommended (18).

Historically (and consistent with clinical findings), chorionic cysts have been considered normal variant gross and histologic findings, even when pronounced. Such profound appearances can be described when they are extensive (18) (Fig. 42.37) and clarify their normal yet often curious appearance for the clinician. Chorionic cysts are lined with "X cells," (extravillous trophoblast) and are associated with "major basic protein (MBP)" production, a substance also found in eosinophilic granulocytes. Causation of tissue damage there from in normal implantations has not been established. Herein, such cysts are also commonly found, not just in the chorionic plate, but also within placental septa, a topic further discussed below. When considering placental site giant cells and placental site trophoblastic tumor (PSTT), the associated giant cells are vastly different from normal invasive extravillous trophoblast and better characterized with immunohistochemical stains for human placental lactogen (HPL). The associated biochemistry therein is largely beyond the scope of placental histology as described in this chapter (1).

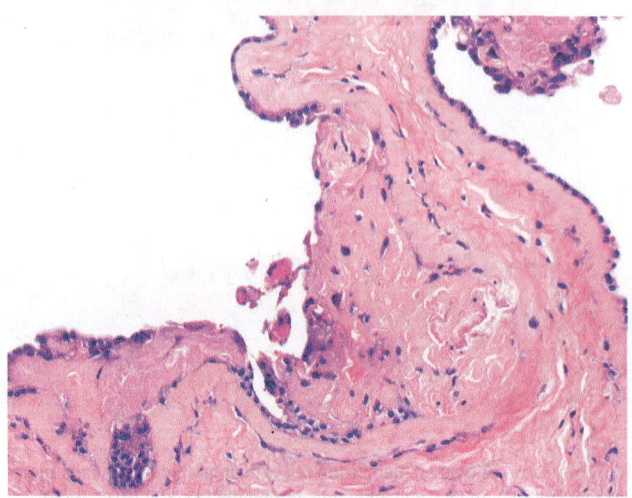

FIGURE 42.36 Amnion nodosum (H&E stain).

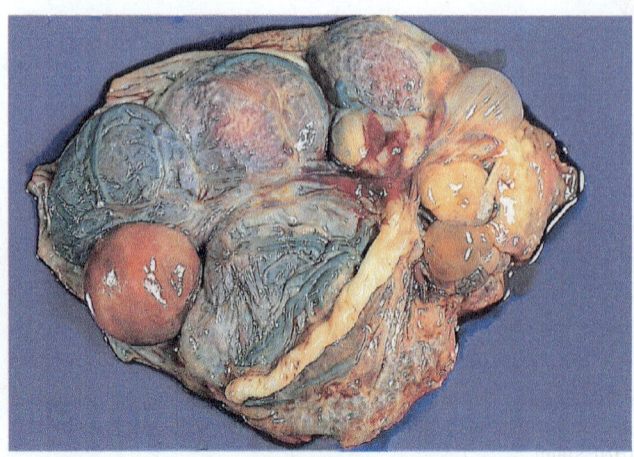

FIGURE 42.37 Multiple chorionic cysts.

MULTIPLE GESTATION

The normal relationships of the placental membranes are germane to the understanding of twin or multiple-gestations. These relationships are described briefly, but for a more complete discussion of twinning and associated pathologic conditions, readers are referred to an extensive and detailed review of the topic (1).

The majority of twin placentas (incidences show a dependence on geographic location and ethnic background) are dizygotic. The dizygotic twin placenta can present as separate or fused placental disks. In the latter, the intervening membrane should be studied to distinguish dichorionic from monochorionic twin placentas. The intervening membrane of about 70% of monozygotic twin placentas is devoid of chorion, and the term "diamnionic–monochorionic" (DiMo) is applicable (Fig. 42.38). Nearly all DiMo placentas are monozygotic. In these gestations (DiMo), the shared chorion invests only the chorionic plate and is not

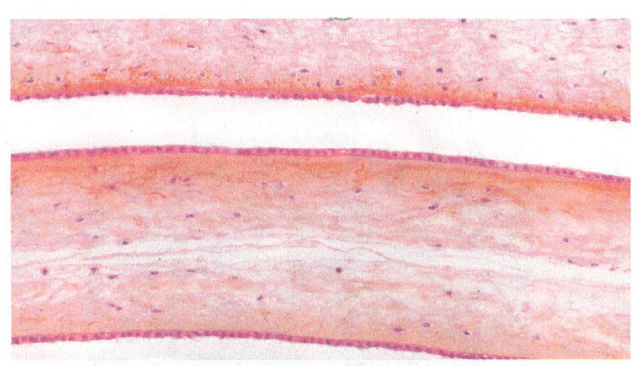

FIGURE 42.38 Intervening membrane from DiMo twin placenta. Note the absence of an intervening chorionic layer (HPS stain).

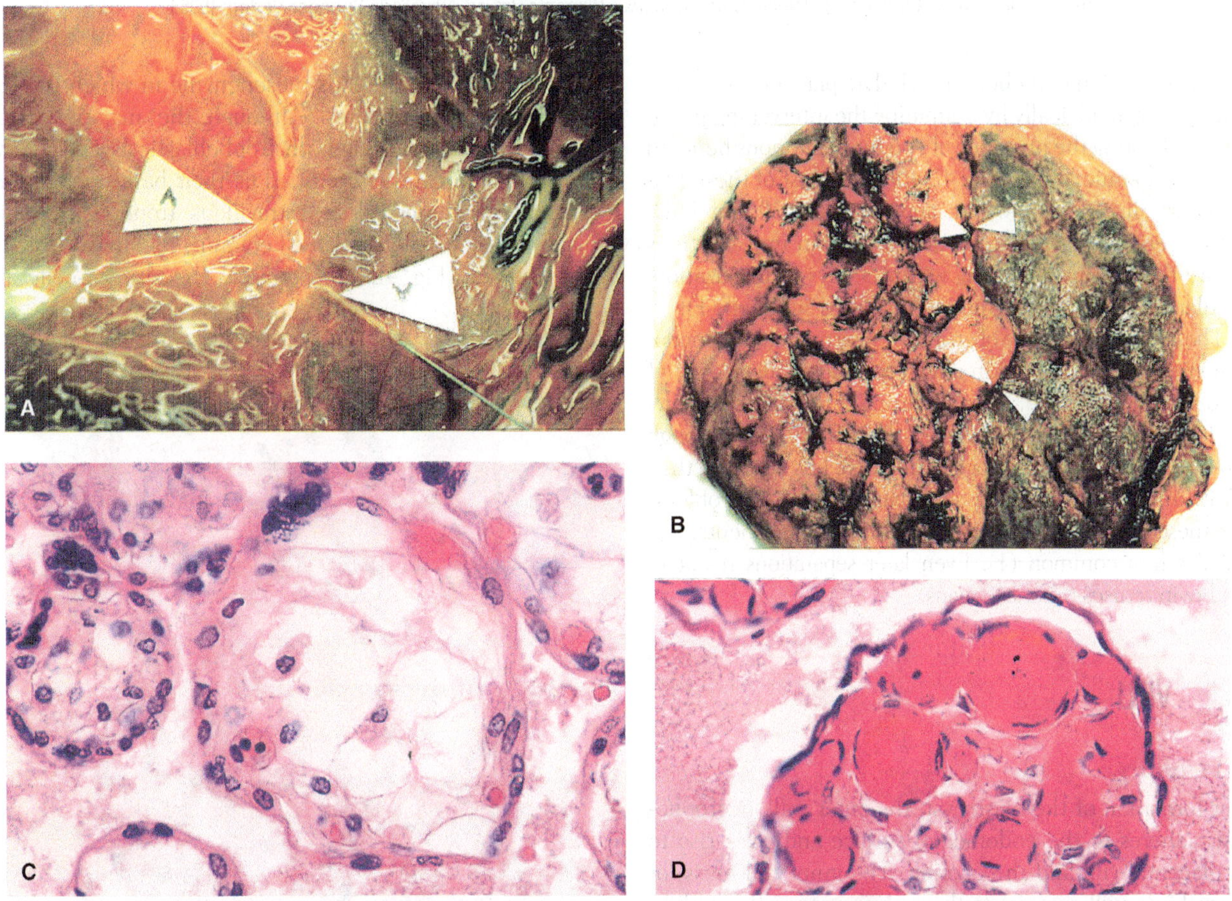

present in the intervening membrane. In DiMo placentas, shared vascular districts between placentas are possible and vein-to-vein and artery-to-artery anastomoses are the most common. Artery-to-vein anastomoses are relatively infrequent and are the etiology of the twin–twin transfusion syndrome (Fig. 42.39A–D).

FIGURE 42.39 A: Twin–twin anastomosis characterized by artery-to-vein transfusion. **B:** Note pale anemic and edematous parenchyma of donor (*left*) and dark congested parenchyma of recipient (*right*). The *arrowheads* mark the vascular equator along the maternal surface. **C:** Villi from the anemic twin are edematous with abundant macrophages, and vascular spaces contain nucleated hematologic precursors denoting high-output failure and increased red cell production, respectively. **D:** Villi from plethoric twin are markedly congested (HPS stain). Characteristic "classic" twin–twin transfusion outcomes may not always occur. Although one twin may be smaller, hemoglobin may be increased in a paradoxical fashion suggesting shifts in flow before analysis.

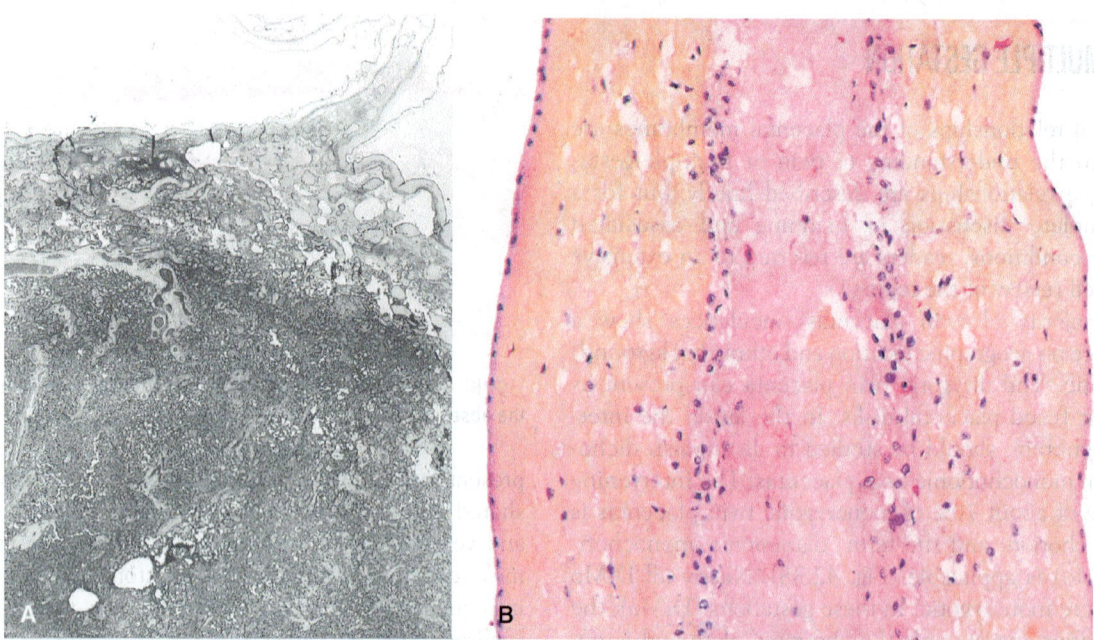

FIGURE 42.40 **A:** DiDi intervening membrane, site of fusion at chorionic plate ("T zone") (H&E stain). **B:** Note the more cellular intervening chorion separating the two layers of amnion (HPS stain). (Reprinted with permission from: Benirschke K, Kaufmann P. *Pathology of the Human Placenta*. 3rd ed. New York: Springer-Verlag; 1995.)

The diamnionic–dichorionic (DiDi) placenta is distinguished morphologically by examining the intervening membrane and noting the presence of two fused chorions beneath the two amnionic layers (Fig. 42.40A,B). Most of these placentas are dizygotic; however, approximately 30% of DiDi twin placentas result from monozygotic twin implantations and are the result of splitting within 3 days of fertilization. Vascular anastomoses are reportable in this situation (1).

The complete absence of an intervening membrane (monoamnionic–monochorionic) in a twin gestation is diagnostic of monozygotic twins (1,3). There, splitting of the embryo occurs later in gestation (at approximately 7 days of age), and although twin–twin transfusions can occur, these are less common than in DiMo placentations. The significant pathologic problems from these placentations result from cord entanglements, and fetal death is common (1). Even later separations result in fused twin fetuses (Siamese twins).

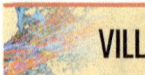
VILLI

Embryology

After formation of the blastocyst, the outer wall, or trophoblast, adheres to the endometrial surface and gives rise to the placental villi and the chorion. The inner cell mass, or embryoblast, will give rise to the embryo proper, the umbilical cord, and the amnion. The functional unit of the placenta, the villous, is initially formed by invasion of cytotrophoblast into syncytiotrophoblastic trabeculae. Throughout the first trimester, trophoblastic villi are composed of an outer syncytiotrophoblastic layer fand an inner cytotrophoblastic layer encompassing villous mesenchyme in which the fetal vasculature differentiates. Although the majority of the villous is surrounded by both trophoblastic layers, a polarity to the villi can be identified as their basal implantation regions are composed of extravillous trophoblast, which make up the trophoblastic cell columns and invade into the myometrium (Fig. 42.41). Formerly, the term "X-cells" was

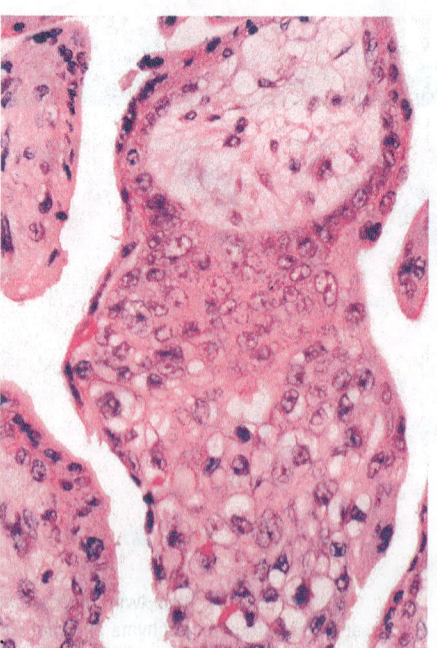

FIGURE 42.41 Polar trophoblastic proliferation comprising trophoblastic cell column. Many vacuolated extravillous trophoblasts are identified extending toward the decidual implantation site (H&E stain).

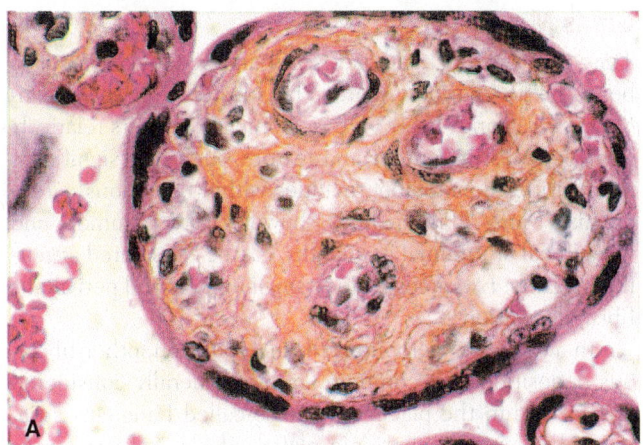 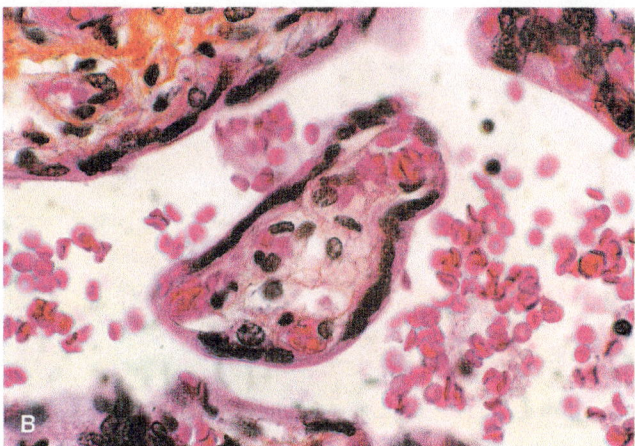

FIGURE 42.42 Third-trimester villi. Secondary villous (**A**) and tertiary villous (**B**). Note that capillary lumina are more peripherally located in the tertiary villous. Furthermore, there is less prominent villous mesenchymal substance (HPS stain).

used to describe a population of extravillous trophoblast as their origin was uncertain and more recently the term "intermediate trophoblast" has been applied to this same collection of cells. While historically notable, neither adequately captures the biologic development and the term extravillous trophoblast is currently favored by placentologists, although many pathologists use the term intermediate trophoblast interchangeably (1,18,80).

As gestation progresses, the characteristic elements of the trophoblastic villous differentiate and develop to form a more functionally efficient unit. This occurs with gradual diminution in the size of peripheral branching villi. The tertiary villi, which stem from secondary villi, which in turn are derived from major stem villi, have a characteristic appearance (Fig. 42.42A,B). The previously noted two-cell layer is less apparent, and the cytotrophoblast becomes much more difficult to identify. The overlying syncytiotrophoblast of the villous thins so that a vasculo-syncytial membrane forms the villous interface with the maternal intervillous blood. The constituents of this "membrane" separating fetal blood from maternal blood include the trophoblast surrounding the villi, the basement membrane upon which they rest, villous mesenchyme, and the fetal vessel composed of endothelial cells and surrounding basement membrane. The thickness of this membrane is critical to development, as transport of essential nutrients and waste products must occur across it.

The course of development also has an impact on the mesenchyme. Early in development, when villi have a pronounced double trophoblastic cell layer, the mesenchyme is prominent and prior to 6 weeks from the last menstrual period, capillary lumina are not readily identified (Fig. 42.43). After this point, the development of vascularization within villous tissue becomes more pronounced. The vasculature is derived from branches of the stem vessels that connect with the vasculature of the chorionic plate. By about 8 weeks' gestational age (from the last menstrual period), only nucleated hematologic precursors are evident within these villous capillary spaces (Fig. 42.44).

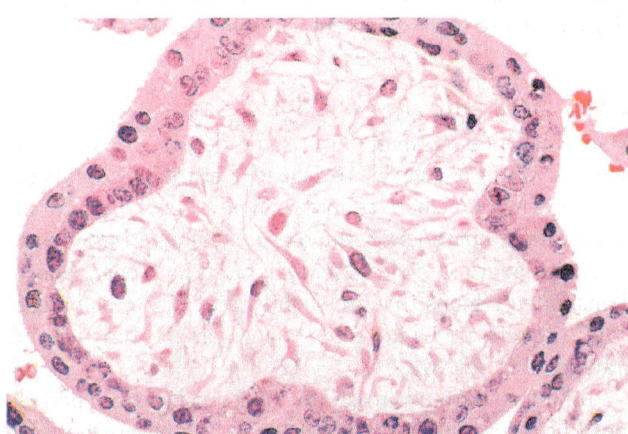 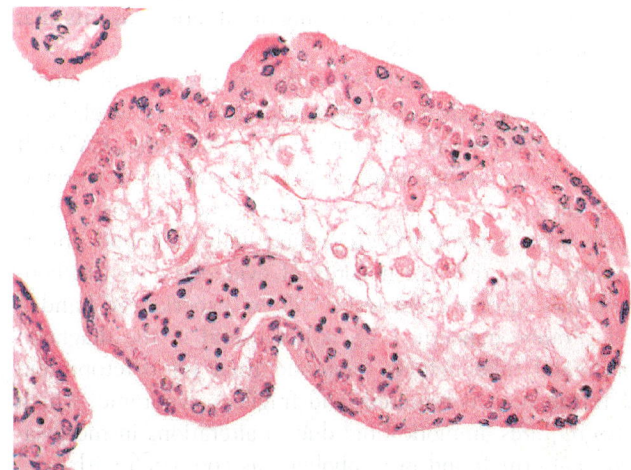

FIGURE 42.43 Villous from gestation of less than 6 weeks. No capillary lumina are present and no embryonic erythropoiesis is identified (H&E stain).

FIGURE 42.44 Villous at 8 weeks' gestation. Note the nucleated hematologic precursors present within villous capillary spaces (H&E stain).

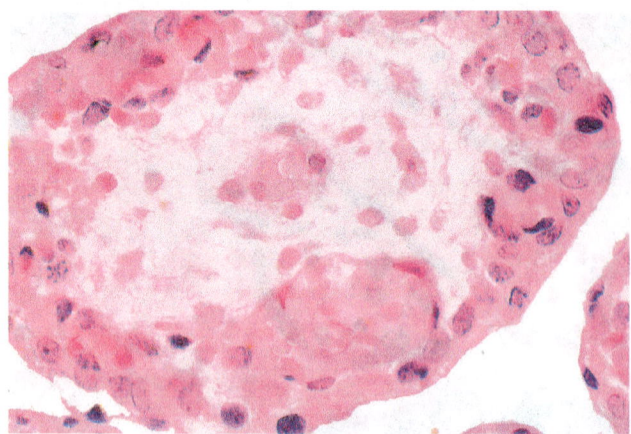

FIGURE 42.45 Near absence of nucleated hematologic precursors within villous capillaries after 12 to 20 weeks' gestation (H&E stain).

Many of these primitive blood cell precursors have their origin within the yolk sac. As gestational age progresses, there is a decrease in the number of nucleated hematologic precursors, such that between 10 and 12 weeks' gestational age (from the last menstrual period) only approximately 10% of these blood cells are nucleated and by approximately 20 weeks' gestational age, they should be virtually absent (Fig. 42.45). Other than vasculature, the remainder of the villous mesenchyme consists of primitive fibroblastic cells (about 50%), as well as members of the macrophage family. These cells bear antigens that characterize them as such (CD4, LeuM3, and a variety of macrophage markers can be identified) (1,73).

The villous macrophages or the so-called Hofbauer cells lose their prominence as gestation proceeds. The maturing tertiary villous, although it possesses this cell type, has fewer of them at term. The function of Hofbauer cells, although not completely understood, is important in water regulation activities, the transport of various nutrients and waste, and villous homeostasis via paracrine interactions with the stromal fibroblasts. This cell type also may be important to immune regulatory functions as an intermediate in the processing of infectious agents that are blood borne (1,73,81).

Chorionic villi may be useful in prenatal diagnosis. Karyotype analysis may be assessed at 10 to 12 weeks' gestational age through chorionic villous sampling (CVS). It should be noted that although early diagnosis is often preferable (to later amniocentesis), several concerns exist. There have been controversies regarding limb reduction abnormalities, but the vast majority of evidence does not confirm this adverse event, especially in "experienced hands." Of genuine concern, CVS is not useful in the diagnosis of neural tube defects (amniotic fluid for α-fetoprotein determination is required) and fragile X syndrome, which also requires amniotic fluid due to alterations in methylation patterns found in trophoblast as compared with fetal squames (82). Advances in isolation of fetal cells from maternal circulation have enhanced detection.

Gross Morphology

The villous parenchyma is discoid and occupies the space beneath the chorionic plate. The substance of the parenchyma is red and "beefy." On sectioning, it appears relatively homogeneous in contour and texture, such that significant irregularities denote abnormalities within the villous parenchyma. Many abnormalities, however, are common and when focal or minimal in quantity, can be considered as normal variants. Examples include small infarcts and perivillous fibrin deposition.

In addition to perivillous fibrin deposition, other fibrinous depositions are common and are generally considered normal within the placenta. The so-called Langhans stria, located below the chorionic plate and also referred to as subchorionic fibrin, is probably related to alterations of maternal intervillous blood flow. By virtue of its distance from the decidual vasculature, it tends to be more static in this location. Nitabuch fibrin is present between the floor of the placenta and the maternal decidua. This layer was once believed to prevent allograft rejection, but now the precise nature and functional significance of this fibrin deposition are not clear.

On occasion, the placental parenchyma has spherical defects (usually 1 to 2 cm in greatest dimension), which represent the so-called jet lesions. These cleared areas within the villous parenchyma represent pressure heads from maternal decidual vascular flow. It is not uncommon to histologically identify a small zone of acute infarction peripheral to these lesions.

Calcification is a common phenomenon in the mature placenta. Calcification has been used to diagnose placental maturity by ultrasonographic evaluation during pregnancy. Third-trimester gestations have an increase in the amount of calcium present in the placenta, and when calcifications are prominent, placentas are considered grade 3. A placenta considered mature on the basis of sonographic appearance does not necessarily denote fetal maturity. Grossly, calcium deposition is seen as fine, pinhead-sized deposits of yellow-white, gritty material. Calcification of the placenta is a normal physiologic response to development and aging (83,84).

Gross Morphologic Alterations

Many placentas normally have some degree of infarction, however when it exceeds 10% to 15% of the placental volume, or when it is more central than peripheral, this should be considered pathologic. Infarcts are characterized grossly as either acute or "old." Acute infarcts are pale, poorly demarcated regions that are slightly granular on palpation. "Old" infarcts are white, often triangular, and they too are granular (Fig. 42.46).

Infarcts evaluated grossly are distinguished from perivillous fibrin deposition. Upon palpation, infarcts are granular and firm. Perivillous fibrin, on the other hand, tends to be nodular and smooth. Further distinctions are made histologically, and these are described in detail below.

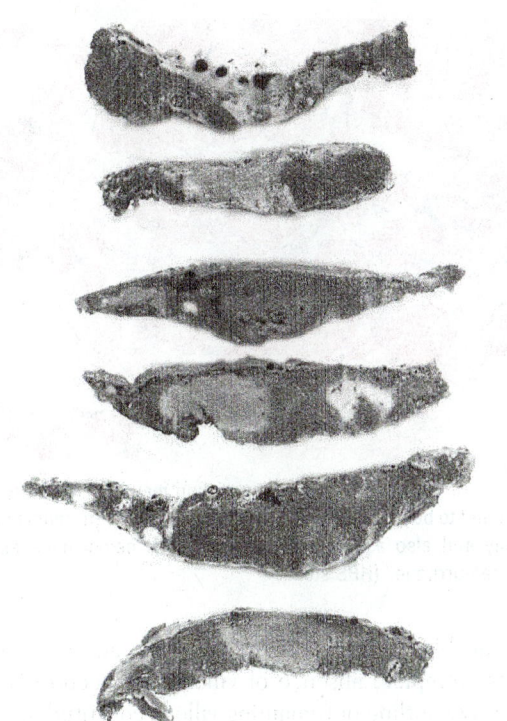

FIGURE 42.46 Multiple old infarcts from a hypertensive pregnancy.

Intervillous thrombi may be identified during the gross examination of the placenta. These triangular- or diamond-shaped lesions within the parenchyma consist of soft gelatinous red to white (depending on age of lesion) aggregates of collected blood. The lamellations of fibrin within this thrombotic material may be observed grossly and distinguish these lesions from infarcts and perivillous fibrin deposition. These lesions are associated with fetal villous capillary leakage and may result in the mixing of maternal and fetal blood, at times causing isoimmunization (1,3).

Histology

The histologic variations in placental architecture are largely dependent on the developmental state at which observations are made. The histology of the individual cell types involved directly in villous implantation is now described.

Extravillous trophoblasts are major constituents of the cell columns that form the deepest structural components of the implantation site. They are round to polygonal cells present singly or in groups and are usually associated with a fibrinous extracellular matrix. They tend to have pleomorphic and hyperchromatic nuclei with amphophilic to eosinophilic cytoplasm. Although predominantly mononuclear, they may also have multiple nuclei. They are epithelial derivatives and thus express cytokeratin, in contrast to the surrounding decidual cells. They produce human placental lactogen and major basic protein and are electron microscopically distinct insofar as they contain large numbers of mitochondria with tubular cristae (78,85–87).

Difficulty in distinguishing them from decidua has resulted in some problems with the diagnosis of intrauterine pregnancy when these are the only trophoblastic cells present in curettage specimens. In the absence of villi, most pathologists confirm their diagnosis of intrauterine pregnancy (and hence exclude the possibility of a tubal pregnancy) based on the presence of multinucleated trophoblastic derivatives, which are more readily distinguished from the surrounding decidua. Should difficulty arise with morphologic assessment of the uninuclear cells in question, immunohistochemical expression of human placental lactogen or HLA-G is helpful (78,86). Extravillous trophoblast is of important immunologic interest because factors produced by trophoblast have been shown to regulate maternal immune cells within the decidua (8). Further, an excess of immature intermediate trophoblasts has been associated with preeclampsia and eclampsia (87).

An interesting normal finding within the placenta is the so-called chorionic cyst. These cysts occur in placental septae and are composed largely of decidua and extravillous trophoblast, which line the cysts. As noted above, such cysts also may be seen in the chorionic plate (Fig. 42.37). On sectioning, gelatinous fluid may be present, and the major constituent of this fluid is one of the substances produced by extravillous trophoblast: major basic protein. The function of these cysts is not known. They should not be considered pathologic when present (1).

The syncytiotrophoblast, the outer cell layer surrounding villi, possesses a brush border. Microvilli that constitute this border are felt to be involved in pinocytotic activity. Vacuoles within the cytoplasm of these cells are indicative of the absorptive and secretory activities of the syncytiotrophoblast. Syncytiotrophoblasts are composed of pyknotic (often multiple) nuclei that are hyperchromatic. In addition to the multiple vesicles present within this cell type, ultrastructural examinations show a cytoplasm that is rich in endoplasmic reticulum, mitochondria, lipid droplets, and Golgi bodies (88).

The cytotrophoblastic nuclei are more round and open. Tritiated thymidine incorporation experiments have shown that uptake and incorporation are confined to the cytotrophoblastic layer and not the syncytiotrophoblastic layer (89). On occasion, cytotrophoblasts may possess mitotic figures (Fig. 42.47). Ultrastructurally, the cytotrophoblast has fewer organelles than does the syncytiotrophoblast. Most prominent are large mitochondria, which may be numerous.

Different antigen expression patterns help distinguish the different cell types from one another, which can be particularly useful when confronted with a trophoblastic tumor or an apparently atypical implantation site. Human placental lactogen may be localized within extravillous trophoblast and syncytiotrophoblast. Human chorionic gonadotropin can be identified within syncytiotrophoblast, but not within cytotrophoblast cells (85,90). Beta-catenin is expressed in a nuclear pattern in early cytotrophoblast and in a membranous pattern in extravillous trophoblast, while Mel-CAM is expressed exclusively in extravillous trophoblast (91).

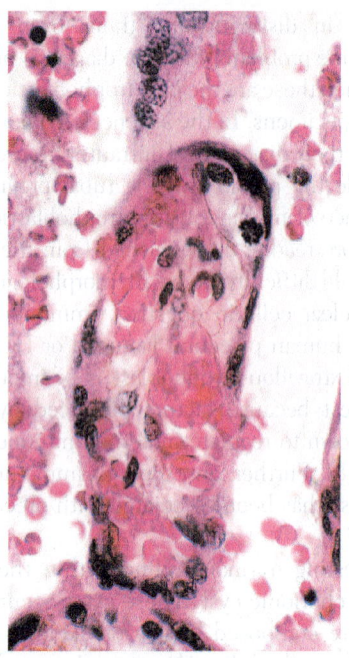

FIGURE 42.47 Sparse cytotrophoblast with rare mitotic figure in terminal villous from a third-trimester placenta (HPS stain).

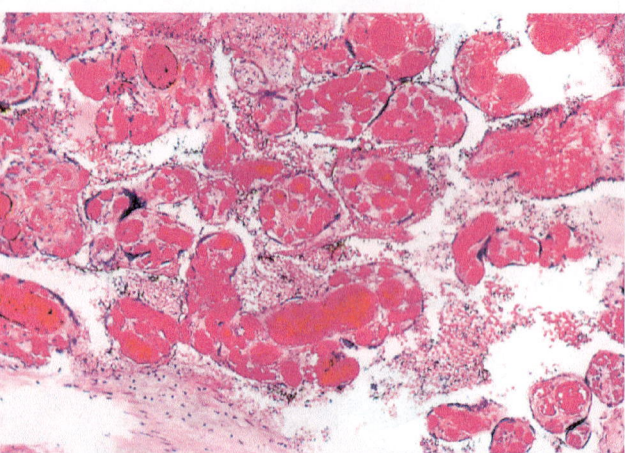

FIGURE 42.49 Villous vascular congestion may indicate early infarction or need to be more closely examined to exclude chorangiosis. Also, currently and also ascribed to retroplacental hemorrhage as "Intra villous hemorrhage" (HPS stain).

Histopathology

Various pathologic entities histologically identified within the villous parenchyma serve to better illustrate the normal histology of the placenta.

Infarcts, which are common in the placental substance, have a characteristic gross appearance. Acute infarcts are characterized histologically by the presence of faint staining villi, which are aggregated, compressed, or agglutinated to one another and have interspersed polymorphonuclear leukocytes within the intervillous space (Fig. 42.48). (As described later, it is crucial to distinguish this inflammation from that which occurs in an intravillous fashion.) Earlier forms of infarction may be characterized by the presence of villous agglutination and congestion, with lysis of intervillous maternal blood (Fig. 42.49). In very advanced ("old") infarcts, complete absence of villous architecture is noted and a fuzzy outline of remaining villous constituents can be identified (Fig. 42.50). No viable staining cells are identified, and an acute inflammatory infiltrate may persist. The placenta rarely undergoes "organization" or fibrosis. When acute infarcts resolve and become "old," fibroblasts are generally lacking. It is for this reason that organization is not a term applied to the placenta. Classic organization as might apply to other organ systems undergoing ischemic change does not occur. The variance probably relates to the two distinct vascular supplies (maternal and fetal). Disturbance in maternal flow results in placental infarction.

Infarcts are distinguished from perivillous fibrin deposition histologically in that regions of the latter contain cytotrophoblastic nuclear remnants that are often prominent (Fig. 42.51). Intervillous thrombi are identified histologically by the presence of lamellated thrombotic material displacing neighboring villi (Fig. 42.52).

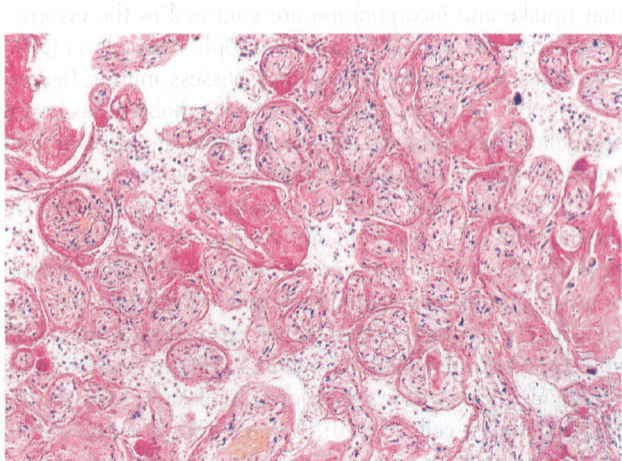

FIGURE 42.48 Acute infarct (Constituting "Malperfusion when extensive") (HPS stain).

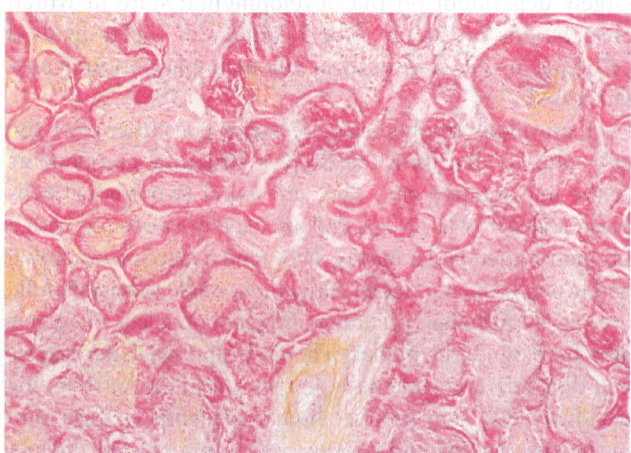

FIGURE 42.50 "Old" infarct (Constituting "Malperfusion when extensive") (HPS stain).

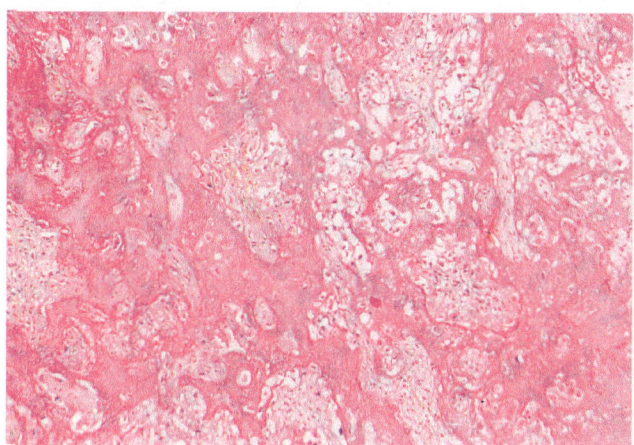

FIGURE 42.51 Increased perivillous fibrin. Note trophoblastic nuclear remnants encased in fibrin (Constituting "Malperfusion when extensive") (HPS stain).

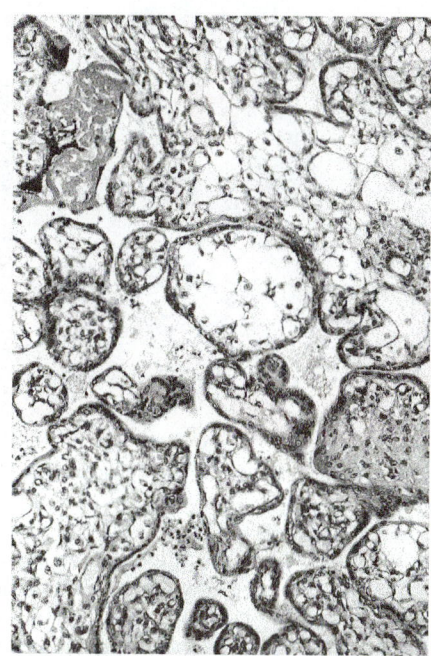

FIGURE 42.53 Focal edema (H&E stain).

Other abnormalities of the villous parenchyma include villous edema, where edema fluid displaces intravillous cytologic architecture; it is considered pathologic, especially in premature gestations (Fig. 42.53) and has been reported as a cause of fetal ischemia or malperfusion (18). Tenney-Parker change is characteristic of placentas from preeclamptic gestations (32). This change is characterized by increased syncytial knotting on villi (Fig. 42.54). Investigation has provided detailed molecular information related to placental apoptosis as pertains to hypertension, as well as the placentas normal lifespan. Considerations of the immunologically distinct organ from its maternal host and its invasive nature are areas of investigation in tumor biology (92–94).

These syncytial knots are best considered failed adaptive responses to low oxygen tension within the intervillous space. Syncytial knots are transported to the maternal lung where they undergo apoptosis and the nuclear DNA becomes the extracellular (cfDNA) of the maternal blood. It disappears in two days after delivery. As noted above, increased intermediate trophoblasts also may be seen (87). Infarcts are not uncommon (1), and in preeclamptic/eclamptic gestations, decidual vasculopathy is also encountered and is discussed below.

Unusual appearances of villous vasculature take three unrelated forms. First, villous vasculature may be congested (Fig. 42.50), and this may have no pathologic significance or may be indicative of early infarction and or malperfusion.

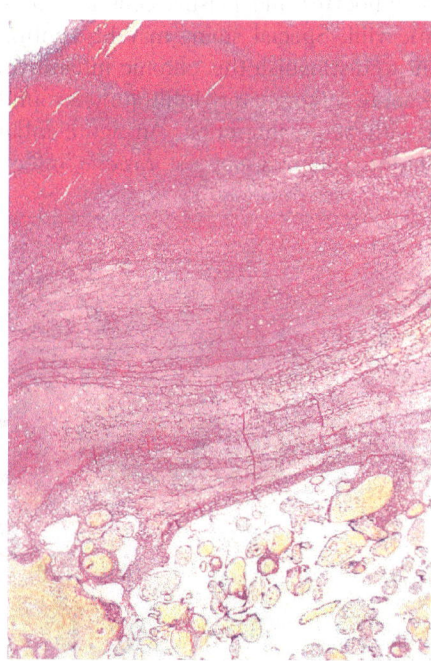

FIGURE 42.52 Intervillous thrombus. Note lamellated lines of Zahn (HPS stain).

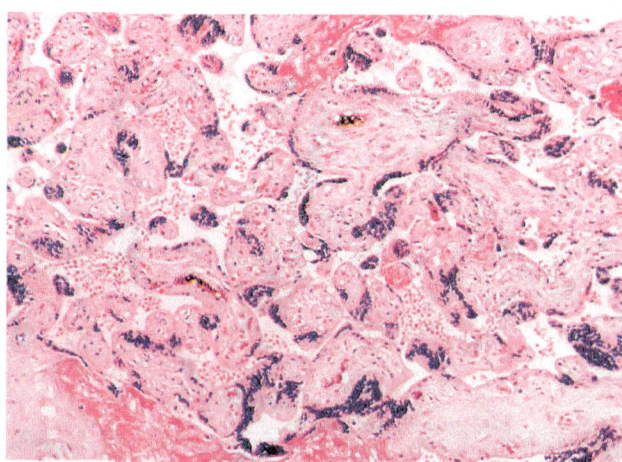

FIGURE 42.54 Increased syncytial knots in a hypertensive pregnancy (Constituting "Malperfusion when extensive") and considered a manifestation of apoptosis (98) (HPS stain).

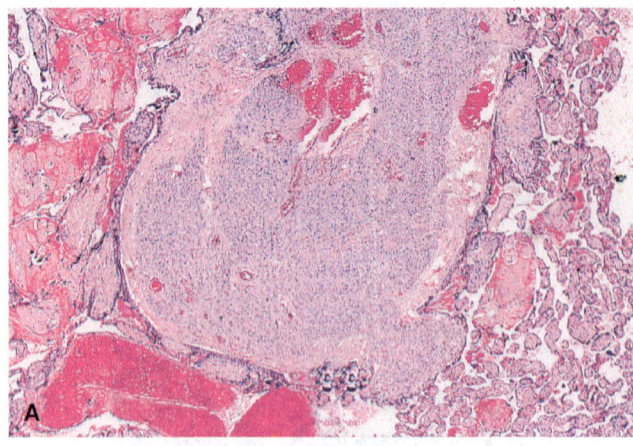
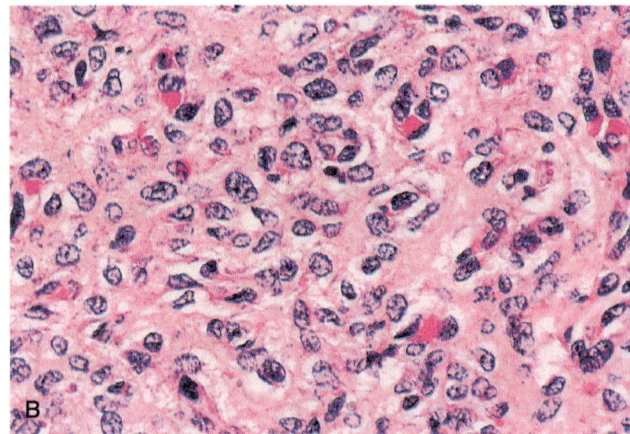

FIGURE 42.55 Chorioangioma (**A**) characterized by hemangiomatous proliferation (**B**) (HPS stain).

Second, increased numbers of villous capillaries, the so-called chorangiosis, has been considered to be indicative of chronic hypoxic changes. The definition is precise, and in histologic terms three criteria (10 vessels/10 villi/10 fields at 10×) need to be met (1) (74). Third, abnormal proliferations of villous vessels that form histologically hemangiomatous nodules are termed chorioangiomas when present in the placenta (Fig. 42.55A,B). These lesions have pathologic significance when prominent and may result in high-output cardiac failure in the fetus or microangiopathic hemolytic phenomena.

Dysmaturity of villi is also considered pathologic. Villi that show the characteristic two-cell layer of the first-trimester implantation, when present in third-trimester placentas, are indicative of abnormal developmental events. This change has been noted to occur in mothers who are diabetic.

Nucleated red blood cells in the fetal circulation are common in very early gestations, but as gestation proceeds, and especially in the third trimester, nucleated red blood cells should not be present. When present, fetal anemia with increased erythroid production should be suspected. In addition, recent investigations have addressed the presence of nucleated red blood cells (in advanced-gestation placentas), correlating such findings with erythropoietin secretion by the fetus and concomitant fetal hypoxia or malperfusion (1,18) (Fig. 42.56).

In the setting of maternal sickle cell disease or trait, it is not unusual to find sickling of maternal erythrocytes within the intervillous spaces. This is promoted by diminished oxygen tension in the setting of abnormal maternal hemoglobin S. It is wise to correlate histopathologic findings with clinical status in that it has been reported that hypoxia during and after placental separation causes sickling (95) (Fig. 42.57).

Inflammatory changes within villi are probably one of the most interesting aspects of placental pathology. These inflammatory changes herald the presence of infectious disease agents in many cases. The presence of syphilis and cytomegalovirus (CMV) should be considered when infiltrates of lymphocytes and plasma cells are found within trophoblastic villi. Special stains may be confirmatory. It is important to distinguish this chronic inflammation from that of the acute inflammatory infiltrate (surrounding villi) associated with acute infarction. An acute inflammatory infiltrate within villi may suggest *Listeria* infection with

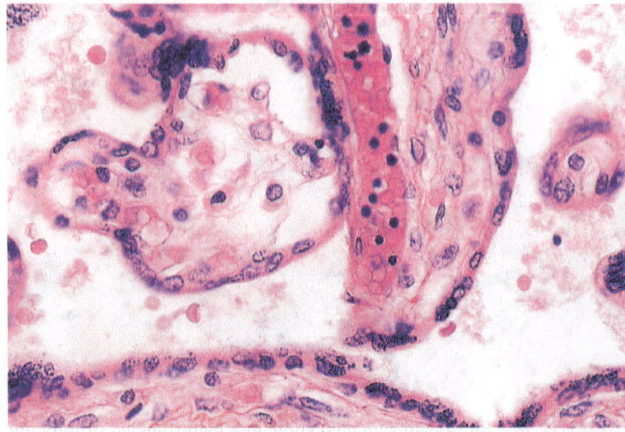

FIGURE 42.56 Fetal nucleated red blood cells are abnormal at term. There is associated focal villous edema (H&E stain).

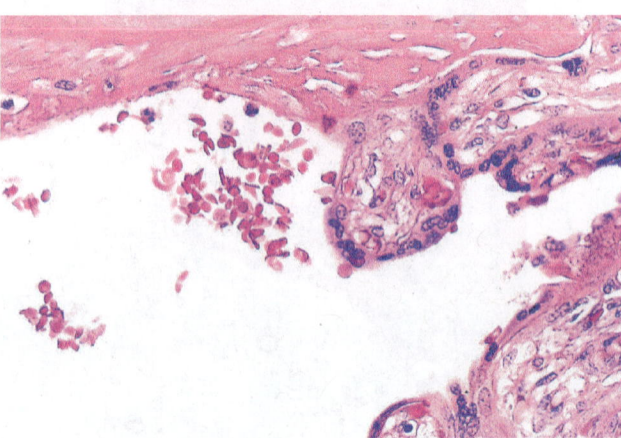

FIGURE 42.57 Intervillous maternal red cell sickling in patient with sickle cell disease (H&E stain).

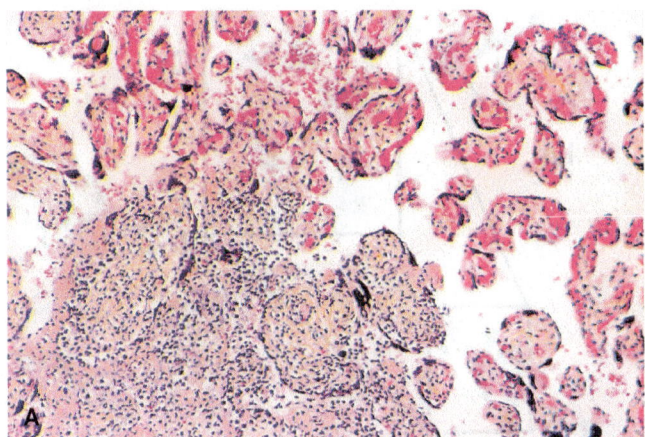
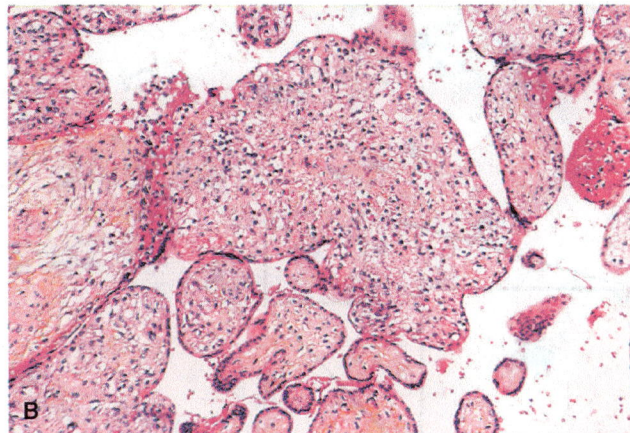

FIGURE 42.58 VUE in which a chronic inflammatory infiltrate devoid of plasma cells is present (**A**) and chronic villitis due to known syphilis infection characterized by the presence of a mononuclear infiltrate containing plasma cells (**B**) (HPS stain).

extensive microabscess formation throughout the placenta. This often can be seen grossly as innumerable white dots. The odor has been characterized as "sweet" (1). In many instances, inflammatory changes within the villi are limited to an increase in the villous cellularity (increased Hofbauer cells), and no specific infectious disease agent can be identified. Increased numbers of inflammatory cells (without plasma cells) also signify chronic villitis; however, in most instances when this occurs, no infectious disease organism can be identified. These inflammatory changes within the placenta have been termed "villitis of unknown etiology (VUE)" (32,96,97) (Fig. 42.58A,B). The infiltrate has been identified as maternal in origin (97).

The absence of inflammation does not always coincide with the absence of infection. For example, in parvovirus B19 infection, hydropic villi and the presence of villous vascular nucleated red blood cells (occasionally with "smudged" amphophilic intranuclear inclusion bodies) may herald the presence of severe congenital infection even in the absence of maternal symptoms (1) (Fig. 42.59). The virus can be detected by immunohistochemical staining or PCR for parvovirus DNA (98). Other infections have been described as evaluated through PCR examination by amniocentesis of amniotic fluid during gestation (11).

Confounding the topic of placental and neonatal infection is the entirely normal placenta, by routine examination. For instance, placentas infected with HIV-1 may have no specific pathologic findings and only special molecular studies will detect infectious materials) (Fig. 42.60A,B) (99). Increasingly, molecular techniques should be considered as an adjunct to histopathologic placental and fetal examination in cases of otherwise unexplained intrauterine or neonatal demise (31).

DECIDUA

Histology

The hypersecretory glandular epithelium of the endometrium, which is progestationally induced, affords the proper environment for implantation. At times, these hypersecretory glands may exhibit the Arias-Stella reaction in which cytologic atypia is noted (Fig. 42.61). In this condition, nuclei are often polyploid. However, nuclear cytoplasmic ratios remain low, distinguishing this normal finding from neoplasia. In this continued progestational influence, endometrial glands undergo secretory exhaustion. The endometrial stroma has undergone its characteristic "decidualization," and decidual cells of the endometrium are characterized as epithelioid and polygonal. Their small rounded nuclei are generally situated centrally in abundant pale eosinophilic, often vacuolated, cytoplasm (Fig. 42.62). The cytoplasm is rich in glycogen and glycoproteins. In regions of decidual tissue, where trophoblastic derivatives are not present, nuclear content is diploid (100). Ultrastructural examination of the decidua shows that tight junctions separate these cells (101).

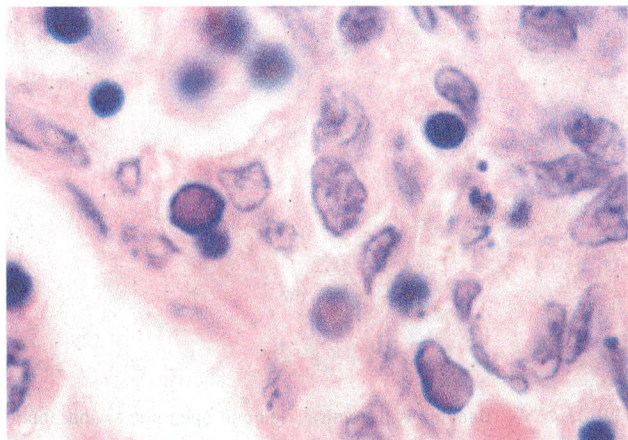

FIGURE 42.59 Parvovirus B19 infection associated with villous edema and nucleated fetal red cells with characteristic inclusions (H&E).

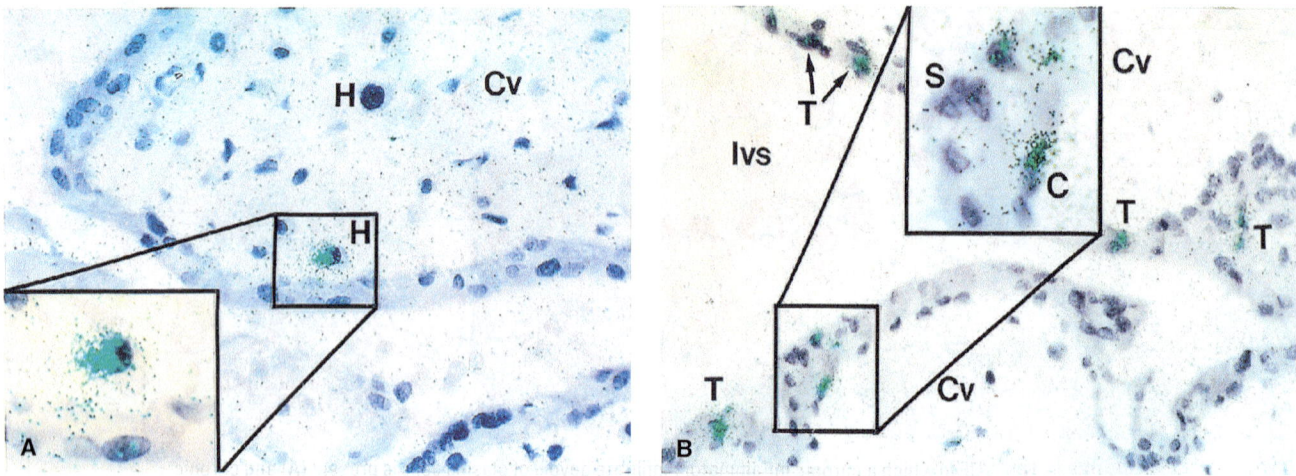

FIGURE 42.60 In situ hybridization with S^{35} probe detects HIV-1 nucleic acids in Hofbauer (*H*) cells (*A*) and trophoblast (*C, T*) of immature villi (*Cv*) (**B**). (From Lewis SH, Reynolds-Kohler C, Fox HE, et al. HIV-1 in trophoblastic and villous Hofbauer cells, and hematologic precursors in eight-week fetuses. *Lancet* 1990;355: 565–568. Reproduced with permission of THE/LANCET PUBLISHING GROUP in the format Journal via Copyright Clearance Center.)

In addition to the decidual cells, an admixture of fibroblasts and lymphocytes is also identified. An additional cell type, the "granular cell," has been shown to produce relaxin (102). The intercellular matrix contains abundant type IV collagen and laminin. Fibronectin and heparin sulfate proteins also have been identified (103). Other collagens are also present throughout the decidual matrix, and these include types I, III, and V (1).

Although prior reports suggested that the secretory activity of the decidua included the production of prolactin and human placental lactogen, it is known that this hormone is produced not by decidual cells but by invading extravillous trophoblast (85). Much of the difficulty in studying decidual tissues and their hormonal production has resulted from the inability of many investigators to distinguish decidual components from invading trophoblastic contaminants (1).

The vascularization of the decidual component of the implantation site is critical to the developing gestation. The major branches of the uterine arteries extend deeply into the myometrial substance, resulting in arcuate arteries that then branch to form radial arteries. These become the spiral arterioles, the terminal components of the endometrial vasculature. These spiral vessels have been shown by injection studies to be responsible for the intervillous blood flow within cotyledonary units (104). The precise number of spiral arterioles that serve to perfuse the placenta is a debated topic. Estimates range from 25 to 300 vascular openings (9,105).

That trophoblastic cells invade the underlying decidual vasculature is a well-known phenomenon. This finding has been documented within the decidual bed, as well as in

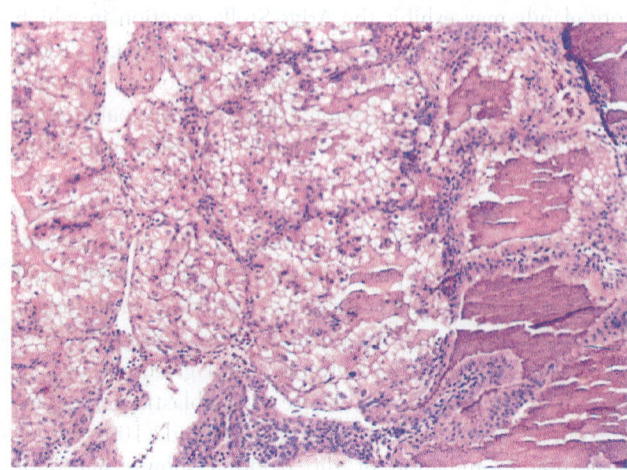

FIGURE 42.61 Arias-Stella reaction (H&E stain).

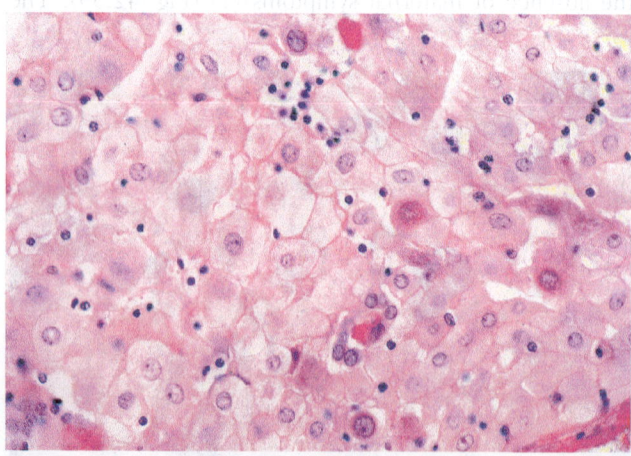

FIGURE 42.62 Decidua with centrally placed open nuclei and abundant pale cytoplasm with prominent cell borders. Note sparse normal lymphocytic infiltrate and occasional extravillous trophoblast with cytoplasm darker than decidual cytoplasm (HPS stain).

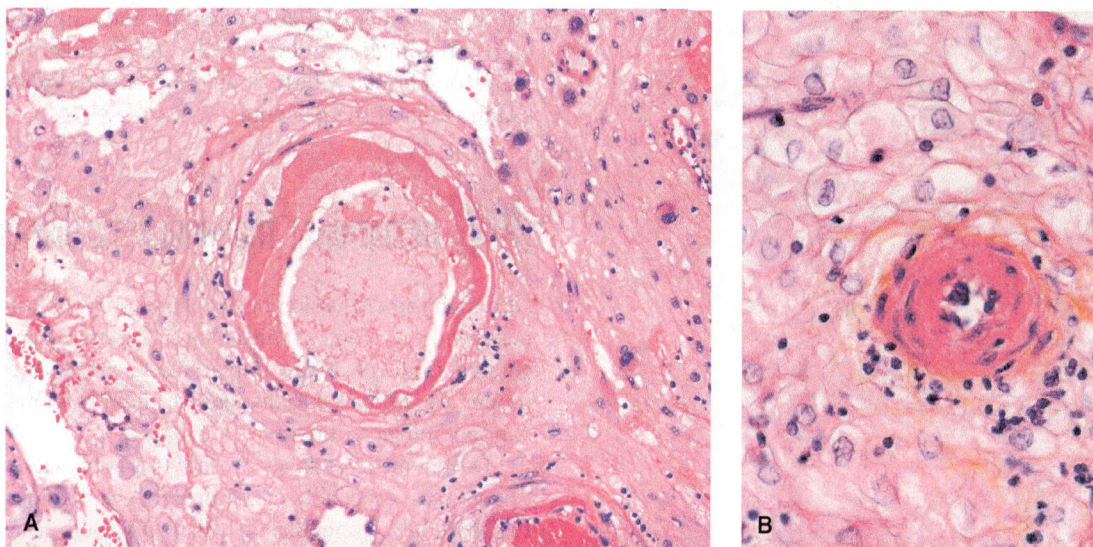

FIGURE 42.63 Decidual vascular atherosis and in recent terminology described as "Global/partial fetal vascular malperfusion" (**A**) and concentric medial hypertrophy (**B**) from a hypertensive gestation (A—H&E stain, B—HPS stain).

systemic maternal vascular compartments, most notably the lung (106). It is important to distinguish these decidual vascular changes from those abnormalities of the decidual vasculature that indicate pathologic conditions.

Gross inspection of the decidua is generally unrevealing, and important attributes and diagnoses are identified histologically. In full-thickness sections of the placenta disk, which includes the chorionic plate and the villous parenchyma, the underlying decidua is often denuded from the placental implantation site during the delivery process. Therefore, it is not uncommon to find sections of parenchyma devoid of decidual tissue. Decidual biopsy is mostly of historic note and a highly rare submission. One region in which decidua is often prominent is on the chorion laeve. Sections of "membrane rolls," which include amnion and chorion, often include sections of adherent decidua, which represent fusion of the decidua capsularis and the decidua vera during development, and decidual abnormalities may be identified in these sections. Aberrant vascular relationships of the more proximal vascular tree (radial and basal arteries) can be seen. The more proximal vessels are characterized by thicker vascular walls, and their arteries often have internal elastic laminae as evidenced by silver stains. The more distal arteries (the spiral arterioles) are thin walled and do not possess any internal elastic lamina.

Histopathology

Principal among decidual pathology is the so-called atherosis of the decidual vascular bed, which is known to accompany preeclampsia and hypertensive conditions of gestation (96). These lesions are characterized by fibrinoid necrosis and hyalinization of the vascular wall along with the deposition of foamy macrophages and should be readily distinguishable from normal trophoblastic vascular invasion. Another abnormality that may characterize hypertensive pregnancies is concentric arteriolar mural hypertrophy (Fig. 42.63A,B). These findings are both part of a constellation of placental abnormalities which indicate maternal vascular malperfusion (25).

Bleeding (retroplacental) is responsible for premature placental separation or abruptio placenta. This has been related to two maternal conditions: increased maternal blood pressure and decidual vascular necrosis (due to vasculopathies or inflammatory-bacterial decidual infections), both of which may indicate malperfusion (Fig. 42.64) (18).

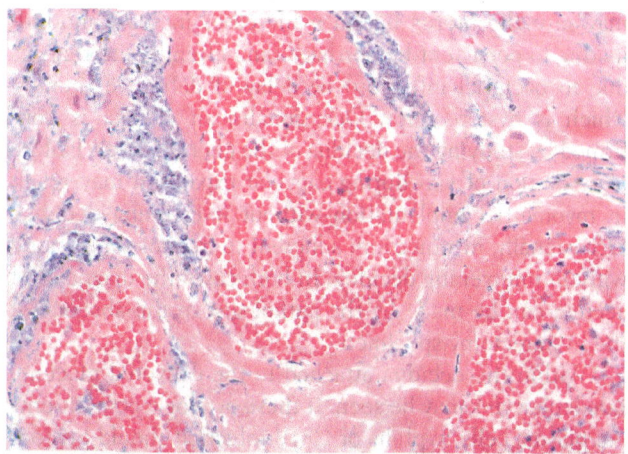

FIGURE 42.64 Decidual vascular necrosis, in this case due to a severe acute deciduitis. Note vascular wall hyalinization and necrosis, which resulted in adjacent abruptio and hence an index of "malperfusion" (H&E stain).

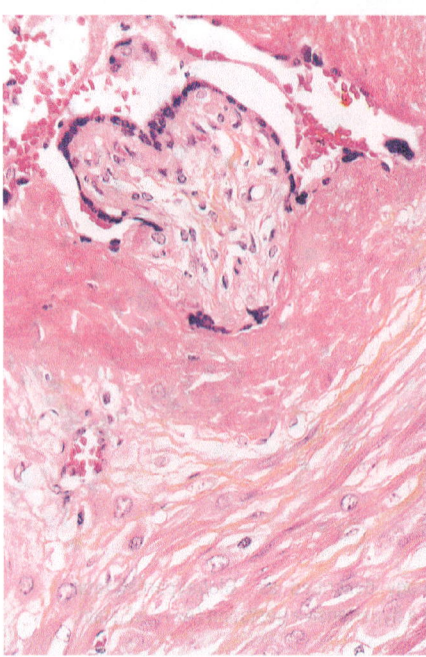

FIGURE 42.65 Placenta accreta. No decidua is present between the implanting trophoblastic villi and the uterine myometrium. The presence of small amounts of fibrin does not alter the diagnosis (HPS stain).

When trophoblastic villi implant directly on myometrial tissue and intervening decidua is absent, the pathologic condition of placenta accreta is present (Fig. 42.65). This finding is more common in low implantations of the placenta (placenta previa), especially when prior cesarean sections have been performed. Variations in which trophoblastic villi implanted within the myometrium (placenta increta) and when implantation results in the presence of villous tissue protruding through the uterine serosal surface (placenta percreta) are more severe forms of this condition. In general, all placental tissue cannot be removed from the uterus at delivery and severe hemorrhage ensues. Heroic obstetrical surgical and pharmacologic measures may save the uterus but in many cases increase morbidity due to persistent hemorrhage (and often in latter stages due to bacterial infection) by delay of definitive therapy, which is hysterectomy. Occasionally, an accreta is confirmed by studying the decidua of the chorion laeve. Failure of resolution of villi during capsular expansion may result in myometrial implantation without intervening decidua. Occasionally, myometrium adherent to frondosum is found without intervening decidua. In both cases the diagnosis of accreta can be made by the pathologist in the absence of the hysterectomy specimen.

Within the decidua attached to the delivered placenta rare leukocytes may be seen. If these cytologic constituents are plasma cells, syphilis or CMV infection should be considered. In the absence of pathologic alterations (placental, maternal, or neonatal) these rare lymphocytes within the decidua are likely physiologic or nonspecific. More distinctive inflammatory processes involving principally PMNs and plasma cells, denote deciduitis and can be associated with inflammation elsewhere. Acute chorioamnionitis and acute or chronic villitis should be sought in the further examination of the placenta.

GESTATIONAL TROPHOBLASTIC DISEASE

Although the discussion of neoplastic trophoblastic disease is beyond the scope of this chapter, several normal or exaggerated findings of the implantation site or the placenta proper are discussed to distinguish them from more significant pathologic entities.

Degenerative changes of early trophoblastic villi are not uncommon, especially in the presence of incomplete abortus material. Trophoblastic villi from such gestations are often seen in histologic sections to be swollen (hydropic). These findings are distinguished from the gestational trophoblastic neoplasm (complete hydatidiform mole) in several aspects. Principal among these distinguishing characteristics is that no trophoblastic atypia or proliferation is present along the surface of the villi (Fig. 42.66A–C). When degenerative changes have taken place and fetal components are blighted, the chorionic vasculature may be absent within the villi. However, if remnants of these vessels persist, the presence of complete hydatidiform mole is essentially excluded. The ease of identifying nucleated hematologic precursors facilitates this observation. Furthermore, should any fetal parts be identified, this too excludes the presence of complete hydatidiform mole. On the other hand, hydropic villi in the presence of fetal parts may herald genotypically abnormal gestations. This form of partial mole, which is rarely neoplastic, is characterized by scalloped trophoblastic borders and occasional trophoblastic island inclusions (representing tangential cuts of scalloped borders within the villous stroma) (Fig. 42.67A,B).

Benign abundant trophoblastic derivates, prominent within the nidus of the implantation site, need to be distinguished from choriocarcinoma and other trophoblastic neoplasms (derived from intermediate trophoblasts). The so-called syncytial endometritis—a poor term because it is not an inflammatory or infectious condition—is more appropriately diagnosed as an exaggerated placental site (EPS), and is benign. EPS is characterized by placental site–type intermediate trophoblasts which focally and superficially infiltrate the myometrium. Distinction from choriocarcinoma is based on the lack of marked cytologic atypia and hemorrhage. Further, choriocarcinoma has a characteristic mix of syncytiotrophoblasts and cytotrophoblasts (Fig. 42.68A,B). Distinction from a placental site trophoblastic tumor (PSTT) is more difficult and based on EPS's focal superficial infiltrating pattern, nonconfluent, and non–mass-forming nature. EPS is without mitotic figures, has villi present and a Ki-67 labeling index of zero. In PSTT mitoses may be present, villi are absent and the immunohistochemical labeling index for

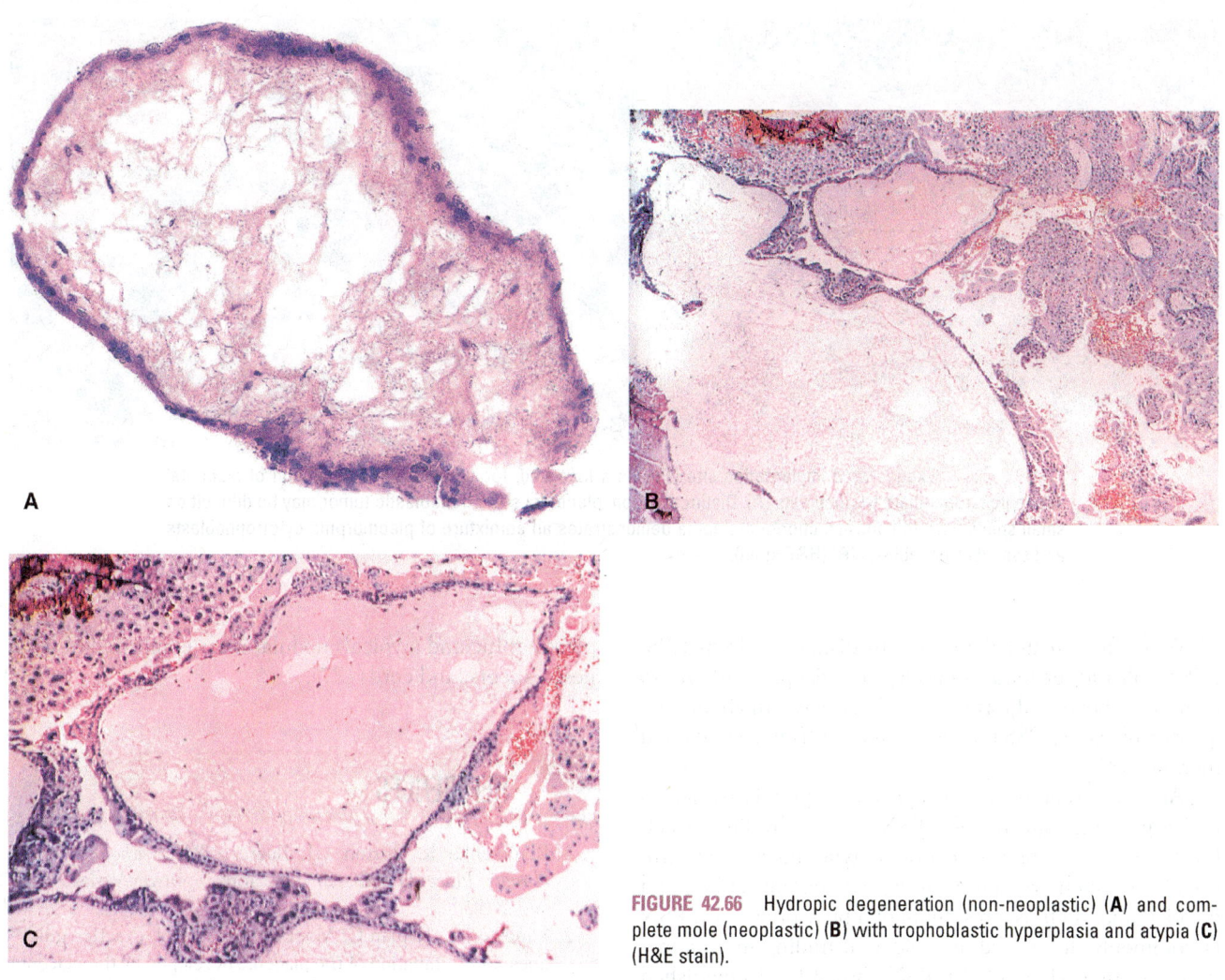

FIGURE 42.66 Hydropic degeneration (non-neoplastic) (**A**) and complete mole (neoplastic) (**B**) with trophoblastic hyperplasia and atypia (**C**) (H&E stain).

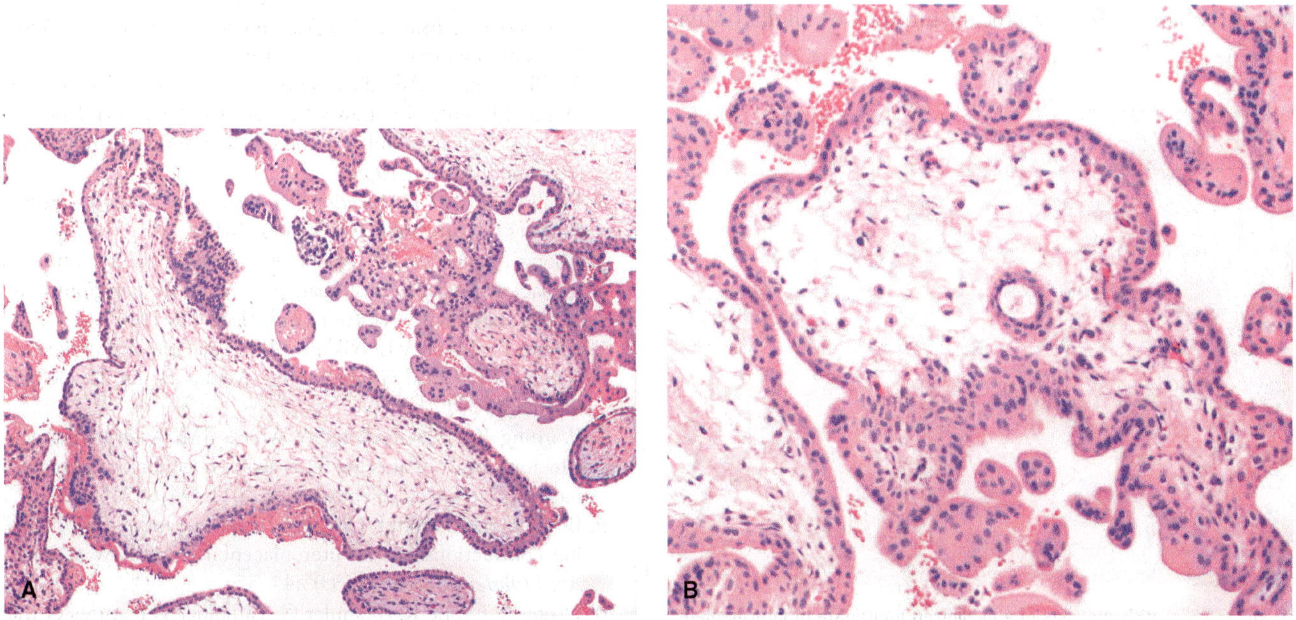

FIGURE 42.67 Triploid partial mole with scalloped trophoblastic borders (**A**) and trophoblastic inclusions (**B**), which are actually tangential cuts of scalloped borders (H&E stain).

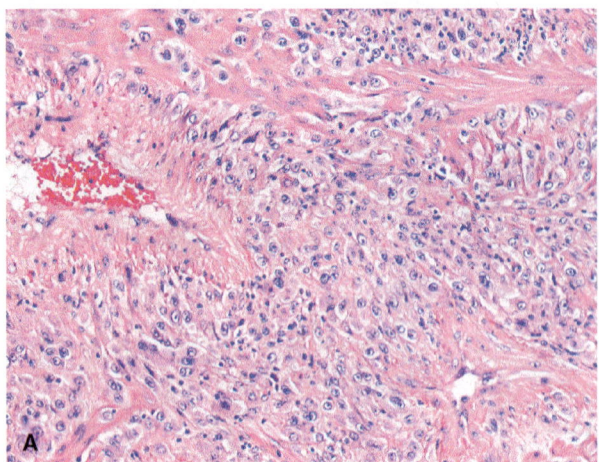 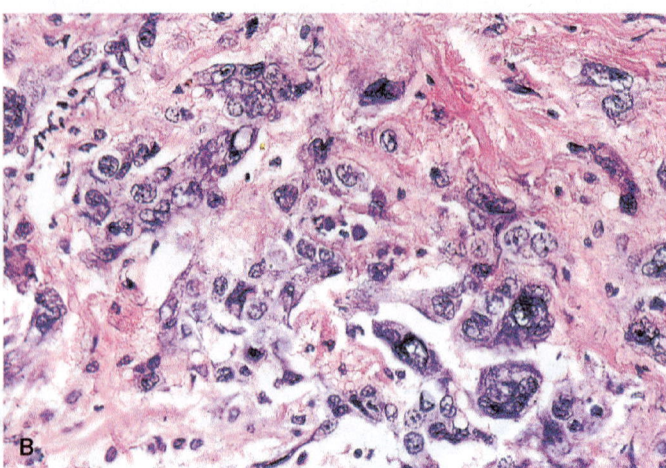

FIGURE 42.68 Exaggerated implantation site (*EIS*) is a localized, focally infiltrative collection of placental site–type intermediate trophoblasts (**A**). Distinction from placental site trophoblastic tumor may be difficult on small specimens. In contrast, choriocarcinoma demonstrates an admixture of pleomorphic cytotrophoblasts and syncytiotrophoblasts (**B**) (H&E stain).

Ki-67 is often greater than 10%. In distinction from EPS, PSST will further tend to invade more deeply, infiltrate in confluent sheets and forms a nodule or mass. In about one-quarter of cases, PSST is associated with metastases and mortality (37).

. Another common non-neoplastic trophoblastic lesion is the placental site nodule (PSN). These hyalinized cellular aggregates represent chorionic-type intermediate trophoblasts which are non-necrotic, well circumscribed and paucicellular. Left as a residuum of a prior pregnancy, PSN is commonly discovered as incidental finding in endometrial curettings (Fig. 42.69). PSN should be distinguished from epithelioid trophoblastic tumor (ETT) which may be metastatic causing death in 10% of cases. ETT differs in that it is characterized by a focally infiltrative cellular (often pleomorphic and atypical) nodular mass comprised of large nests, sheets, and cords (37).

REFERENCES

1. Benirschke K, Burton GJ, Baergen RN. *Pathology of the Human Placenta*. 6th ed. New York: Springer-Verlag; 2011 and 2012.
2. Langston C, Kaplan C, MacPherson T, et al. Practice guidelines for examination of the placenta developed by the placenta practice guidelines task force of the College of American Pathologists. *Arch Pathol Lab Med*. 1997;112:449–476.
3. Lewis SH, Perrin VDK. *Pathology of the Placenta. Vol. 23, Contemporary Issues in Surgical Pathology*. 2nd ed. New York: Churchill Livingstone; Elsevier; 1999.
4. McPherson, T. (Adjudicating the text). Review of Pathology of the Placenta. In: Lewis SH, ed. *Contemporary Issues of Surgical Pathology*. Vol. 23, 2nd ed. New York: Churchill Livingstone; Elsevier; 1999.
5. Redline RW. *Classification for Placental Lesions, Expert Reviews Classification*. ACOG.org; 2015.
6. Khong TY, Mooney EE, Ariel I, et al. Sampling and definitions of placental lesions: Amsterdam placental workshop group consensus statement. *Arch Pathol Lab Med* 2016;140(7):698–713.
7. Khong TY, Mooney E, Nikkels PJK, et al. *Pathology of the Placenta – A Practical Guide* Springer-Verlag, Berlin, Heidelber, Germany; 2017.
8. Warning JC, McCracken SA, Morris JM. A balancing act: Mechanisms by which the fetus avoids rejection by the maternal immune system. *Reproduction* 2011;141(6):715–724.
9. Borell U, Fernstrom I, Ohlson L, et al. The influence of uterine contractions on the uteroplacental blood flow at term. *Am J Obstet Gynecol* 1965;93:44–57.
10. Ornoy A, Crone K, Altshuler G. Pathological features of the placenta in fetal death. *Arch Pathol Lab Med* 1976;100(7):367–371.

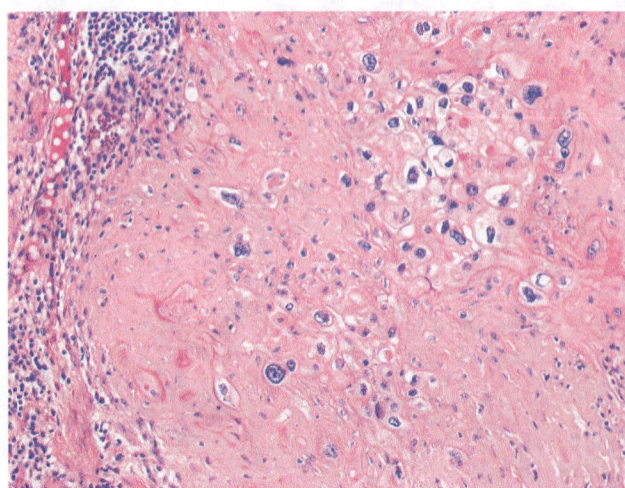

FIGURE 42.69 PSN consists of a hyalinized aggregate of intermediate trophoblastic cells, some multinucleated, representing a residua of prior pregnancy (H&E stain).

11. Stanek J. Hypoxic Patterns of Placental Injury: A review. 2013;137(5):706–720.
12. Naeye RL. *Disorders of the Placenta, Fetus and Neonate: Diagnosis and Clinical Significance*. St. Louis, MO: Mosby Year Book; 1992.
13. Werth B. *Damages*. Simon and Schuster; New York: 1998.
14. Gawron LM, Hammond C, Ernst LM. Perinatal pathologic examination of nonintact, second-trimester fetal demise specimens: The value of standardization. *Arch Pathol Lab Med* 2013;137(8):1083–1087.
15. Hieronymus Fabricus. *The Embryological Treatises of Hieronymus Fabricus of Aquapendente*. New York: Cornell University Press; 1942.
16. Nicholas von Hoboken. Anatomia secundince humance, quindecim figuris ad vivum propria authoris manu delineatis illustrata. Utrecht 1669.
17. Strauss F, Benirschke K, Driscoll SG. *Handbuch Der Speziellen Pathologischen Anatomie und Histologie*. New York: Springer-Verlag. Berlin-Heidelberg;1967.
18. Khong TY, Mooney EE, Ariel I , et al. Sampling and Definitions of Placental Lesions: Amsterdam Placental Workshop Group Consensus Statement. *Arch Pathol Lab Med* 2016;140(7): 698–713.
19. *Pathology of the Placenta. A List of Current Texts*. © Amazon.com; 2018.
20. American College of Obstetricians and Gynecologists. Practice bulletin no 151: Cytomegalovirus, parvovirus B19, varicella zoster, and toxoplasmosis in pregnancy. *Obstet Gynecol* 2015; 125(6):1510–1525.
21. ACOG Committee Opinions. *The American College of Obstetrics and Gynecology*. Washington, DC; 1998–2018.
22. Placental pathology. ACOG committee opinion: Committee on obstetrics: Maternal and fetal medicine. Number 125-July 1993 (No longer in print as an opinion reproduced in: International. *J Obstet Gynecol*. 1993; 42(3): 318–319.
23. Klebanoff MA. The collaborative perinatal project: a 50 year retrospective. *Paediatr Perinat Epidemiol* 2009;23(1):2–8.
24. Gershell DJ, Kraus FT. Diseases of the Placenta In: *Blaustein's Pathology of the Female Genital Tract*. Boston, MA: Springer; 2011:999–1073.
25. Khong TY, Mooney EE, Ariel I, et al. Sampling and definitions of placental lesions: Amsterdam Placental Workshop Group Consensus Statement. *Arch Pathol Lab Med* 2016; 140(7):698–713.
26. Lindley SW, Gillies EM, Hassell LA, et al. Pathology – research and practice communicating diagnostic uncertainty in surgical pathology reports: Disparities between sender and receiver. *Pathology Res Practice* 2014;:210: 628–633.
27. Odibo I, Gehlot A, Ounpraseuth T, et al. Pathology Examination of the Placenta and it clinical utility: A survey of Obstetrics and Gynecology Providers. *J Matern Fetal Neonatal Med* 2016;29(2):197–201.
28. Stanek J. Fetal vascular malperfusion (Letter to the Editor). *Arch Pathol Lab Med* 2018;142(6):679–680.
29. Heider A. Fetal vascular malperfusion. *Arch Pathol Lab Med* 2017;141(11):1484–1489.
30. Johnson SL, Stanek J. E-Calherin/CD34 dual immunohistochemical stain in search for placental focal fetal vascular malperfusion. *Lab Invest* 2017;97:291A–292A.
31. Stanek J. Placental examination in non-macerated stillbirth versus neonatal mortality [published online ahead of print September 15, 2017]. *J Perinat Med*. 2018;25;46(3):323–331.
32. Bartholomew RA, Colvin ED, Grimes WH Jr, et al. Criteria by which toxemia of pregnancy may be diagnosed from unlabeled formalin-fixed placentas. *Am J Obstet Gynecol* 1961;82: 277–290.
33. Schremmer BN. Gewichtsveränderungen verschiedener gewebe nach formalinfixierung. *Frank Z Pathol* 1967;77: 299–305.
34. Moghimi A, Prakash S, Dow C, et al. The effect of immersion formaldehyde fixation on placental weight. *Pathology* 2014;46:S75.
35. Lewis SH, Gilbert E. In: Barness LA, ed. *Advances in Pediatrics Vol. 45*. St. Louis, MO: Mosby; 1998.
36. Nuovo G, Richart RM. Buffered in situ hybridization analysis. *AM J Pathol* 1989;34:83723.
37. Shih IM, Kurman RJ. The pathology of intermediate trophoblastic tumors and tumor-like lesions. *Int J Gyn Pathol* 2001;20:31–47.
38. Kowalski PJ. *Long Umbilical cords*. PathologyOutlines.com, Inc; 2017,
39. Naeye RL. Umbilical cord length: Clinical significance. *J Pediatr* 1985;107:278–281.
40. Gardiner JP. The umbilical cord: Normal length; length in cord complications; etiology and frequency of coiling. *Surg Gynecol Obstet* 1922;34:252–256.
41. Hoyes AD. Ultrastructure of the epithelium of the human umbilical cord. *J Anat* 1969;105(pt 1):145–162.
42. Moore RD. Mast cells of the human umbilical cord. *Am J Pathol* 1956;32:1179–1183.
43. Nadkarni BB. Innervation of the human umbilical artery: an electron microscope study. *Am J Obstet Gynecol* 1970;107: 303–312.
44. Ellison JP. The nerves of the umbilical cord in man and the rat. *Am J Anat* 1971;132:53–60.
45. Lauweryns JM, De Bruyn M, Peuskens J, et al. Absence of intrinsic innervation of the human placenta. *Experientia* 1969;25:432.
46. Blanc WA, Allan GW. Intrafunicular ulceration of the persistent omphalomesenteric duct with intra-amniotic hemorrhage and fetal death. *Am J Obstet Gynecol* 1961;82:1392–1396.
47. Priman J. A note on the anastomosis of the umbilical arteries. *Anat Rec* 1959;134:1–5.
48. Arts NF. Investigations on the vascular system of the placenta. I. General introduction and the fetal vascular system. *Am J Obstet Gynecol* 1961;82:147–158.
49. Rana J, Ebert GA, Kappy KA. Adverse perinatal outcome with an abnormal umbilical coiling index. *Obstet Gynecol* 1995;85:573–578.
50. Altshuler G, Hyde S. Meconium-induced vasocontraction: A potential cause of cerebral and other hypoperfusion and of poor pregnancy outcome. *J Child Neurol* 1989;4:137–142.
51. Garza A, Cordero JF, Mulinare J. Epidemiology of the early amnion rupture spectrum of defects. *Am J Dis Child* 1988; 142:541–544.
52. Torpin R. *Fetal Malformations Caused by Amnion Rupture During Gestation*. Springfield, IL: Charles C Thomas; 1968.
53. Michael H, Ulbright TM, Brodhecker C. Magma reticulare-like differentiation in yolk sac tumor and its pluripotential nature [Abstract]. *Mod Pathol* 1988;1:63.

54. Wynn RM, French GL. Comparative ultrastructure of the mammalian amnion. *Obstet Gynecol* 1968;31:759–774.
55. Danforth D, Hull RW. The microscopic anatomy of the fetal membranes with particular reference to the detailed structure of amnion. *Am J Obstet Gynecol* 1958;75:536–550.
56. Boyd JD, Hamilton WJ. *The Human Placenta*. Cambridge, MA: Heffer & Sons; 1970.
57. King BF. Developmental changes in the fine structure of rhesus monkey amnion. *Am J Anat* 1980;157:285–307.
58. Bourne GL. *The Human Amnion and Chorion*. London: Lloyd-Luke; 1962.
59. Hoyes AD. Ultrastructure of the mesenchymal layers of the human amnion in early pregnancy. *Am J Obstet Gynecol* 1970;106:557–566.
60. Hoyes AD. Ultrastructure of the mesenchymal layers of the human chorion laeve. *J Anat* 1971;109(pt 1):17–30.
61. Mukaida T, Yoshida K, Kikyokawa T, et al. Surface structure of the placental membranes. *J Clin Electron Microsc* 1977; 10:447–448.
62. Bautzmann H, Hertenstein C. Zur Histogenese und Histologie des menschlichen fetalen und Neugeborenen-Amnions. *Z Zellforsch Mikrosk Anat* 1957;45:589–611.
63. Schmidt W. Struktur und Funktion des Amnionepithels von Mensch und Huhn. *Z Zellforsch Mikrosk Anat* 1963;61: 642–660.
64. Schwarzacher HG. Beitrag zur histogenese des menschilichen amnion. *Acta Anat (Basel)* 1960;43:303–311.
65. Wynn RM. Cytotrophoblastic specializations: an ultrastructural study of the human placenta. *Am J Obstet Gynecol* 1972; 114:339–355.
66. Bartels H, Wang T. Intercellular junctions in the human fetal membranes. A freeze-fracture study. *Anat Embryol (Berl)* 1983;166:103–120.
67. Robinson HN, Anhalt GJ, Patel HP, et al. Pemphigus and pemphigoid antigens are expressed in human amnion epithelium. *J Invest Dermatol* 1984;83:234–237.
68. Schwarzacher HG, Klinger HP. Die Entstehung mehrkerniger zellen durch amitose im amnionepithel des menschens und die aufteilung des chromosomalen materials auf deren einzelne zellkerne. *Z Zellforsch Mikrosk Anat* 1963;60:741–754.
69. Schindler PD. Nuclear deoxyribonucleic acid (DNA) content, nuclear size and cell size in the human amnion epithelium. *Acta Anat (Basel)* 1961;44:273–285.
70. Kalousek DK, Fill FJ. Chromosomal mosaicism confined to the placenta in human conceptions. *Science* 1983;221: 665–667.
71. Rossant J, Croy BA. Genetic identification of tissue of origin of cellular populations within the mouse placenta. *J Embryol Exp Morphol* 1985;86:177–189.
72. Sala MA, Matheus M. Histochemical study of the fetal membranes in the human term pregnancy. *Gegenbaurs Morphol Jahrb* 1984;130:699–705.
73. Goldstein J, Braverman M, Salafia C, et al. The phenotype of human placental macrophages and its variation with gestational age. *Am J Pathol* 1988;133:648–659.
74. Altshuler G. Placental infection and inflammation. In: Lewis, ed. *Pathology of the Placenta*. New York: Churchill Livingstone; 1999.
75. Nickell KA, Stocker JT. Placental teratoma: A case report. *Pediatr Pathol* 1987;7:645–650.
76. Salazar H, Kanbour AI. Amnion nodosum: Ultrastructure and histopathogenesis. *Arch Pathol* 1974;98:39–46.
77. Luckett WP. The origin of extraembryonic mesoderm in the early human and rhesus monkey embryos [abstract]. *Anat Rec* 1971;169:369–370.
78. O'Connor DM, Kurman RJ. Intermediate trophoblast in uterine curettings in the diagnosis of ectopic pregnancy. *Obstet Gynecol* 1988;72(4):665–670.
79. Hessle H, Engvall E. Type VI collagen. Studies on its localization, structure, and biosynthetic form with monoclonal antibodies. *J Biol Chem* 1984;259:3955–3961.
80. Wasmoen TL, Benirschke K, Gleich GJ. Demonstration of immunoreactive eosinophil granule major basic protein in the plasma and placentae of non-human primates. *Placenta* 1987;8:283–292.
81. Ingman K, Cookson VJ, Jones CJ, et al. Characterisation of Hofbauer cells in first and second trimester placenta: incidence, phenotype, survival in vitro and motility. *Placenta* 2010;31:535–544.
82. American College of Obstetricians and Gynecologists. *ACOG Committee Opinion (Committee on Genetics) no. 160: Chorionic Villus Sampling*; 1995.
83. Pitkin RM, Reynolds WA, Williams GA, et al. Calcium metabolism in normal pregnancy: A longitudinal study. *Am J Obstet Gynecol* 1979;133:781–790.
84. Tsang RC, Donovan EF, Steichen JJ. Calcium physiology and pathology in the neonate. *Pediatr Clin North Am* 1976;23:611–626.
85. Kurman RJ, Main CS, Chen HC. Intermediate trophoblast: A distinctive form of trophoblast with specific morphological, biochemical and functional features. *Placenta* 1984;5: 349–370.
86. Lunghi L, Ferretti ME, Medici S, et al. Control of human trophoblast function. *Reprod Biol Endocrinol* 2007;5:6.
87. Redline RW, Patterson P. Pre-eclampsia is associated with an excess of proliferative immature intermediate trophoblast. *Hum Pathol* 1995;26:594–600.
88. Wislocki GB, Dempsey EW. Electron microscopy of the human placenta. *Anat Rec* 1955;123:133–167.
89. Richart R. Studies of placental morphogenesis. I. Radioautographic studies of human placenta utilizing tritiated thymidine. *Proc Soc Exp Biol Med* 1961;106:829–831.
90. Pierce GB Jr, Midgley AR Jr. The origin and function of human syncytiotrophoblastic giant cells. *Am J Pathol* 1963; 43:153–173.
91. Mao TL, Kurman RJ, Huang CC, et al. Immunohistochemistry of choriocarcinoma: An aid in differential diagnosis and in elucidating pathogenesis. *Am J Surg Pathol* 2007; 31(11):1726–1732.
92. Allaire AD, Ballenger KA, Wells SR, et.al. Placental apoptosis in preeclampsia. *Obstet Gynecol* 2000;96:(2);271–276.
93. Louwen F, Muschol-Steinmetz C, Reinhard J, et al. A lesson for cancer research: Placental microarray gene analysis in preeclampsia. *Oncotarget* 2012;3(8):759–773.
94. Sharp AN, Alexander EP. Heazell AE, et al. Placental apoptosis in health and disease. *Am J Reprod Immunol* 2010; 64(3):159–169.
95. Fujikura T, Froehlich L. Diagnosis of sickling by placental examination. Geographic differences in incidence. *Am J Obstet Gynecol* 1968;100:1122–1124.

96. Knox WF, Fox H. Villitis of unknown aetiology: Its incidence and significance in placentae from a British population. *Placenta* 1984;5:395–402.
97. Redline RW, Patterson P. Villitis of unknown etiology is associated with major infiltration of fetal tissue by maternal inflammatory cells. *Am J Pathol* 1993;143:473–479.
98. Al-Adnani M, Sebire NJ. The role of perinatal pathological examination in subclinical infection in obstetrics. *Best Pract Res Clin Obstet Gynaecol* 2007;21(3):505–521.
99. Lewis SH, Reynolds-Kohler C, Fox HE, et al. HIV-1 in trophoblastic and villous Hofbauer cells, and hematologic precursors in eight-week fetuses. *Lancet* 1990;355:565–568.
100. Sachs H. *Quantitativ histochemische Untersuchung des Endometrium in der Schwangerschaft und der Placenta (Cytophotometrische Messungen).* Arch Gynecol Obstet 1968;205:93–104.
101. Lawn AM, Wilson EW, Finn CA. The ultrastructure of human decidual and predecidual cells. *J Reprod Fertil* 1971;26:85–90.
102. Dallenbach FD, Dallenbach-Hellweg G. Immunohistologische Untersuchungen zur Lokalisation des Relaxins in menschlicher Placenta und Decidua. *Virchows Arch Pathol Anat Physiol Klin Med* 1964;337:301–316.
103. Wewer UM, Faber M, Liotta LA, et al. Immunochemical and ultrastructural assessment of the nature of pericellular basement membrane of human decidual cells. *Lab Invest* 1985;53:624–633.
104. Freese UE. The uteroplacental vascular relationship in the human. *Am J Obstet Gynecol* 1968;101:8–16.
105. Haller U. Beitrag zur Morphologie der Utero-placentargefaesse. *Arch Gynaekol* 1968;205:185–202.
106. Attwood HD, Park WW. Embolism to the lungs by trophoblast. *J Obstet Gynaecol Br Commonw* 1961;68:611–617.

SECTION XL

Endocrine

Thyroid

Maria Luisa Carcangiu

EMBRYOLOGY 1175

GROSS ANATOMY 1177

MICROSCOPIC ANATOMY 1178

FOLLICULAR CELLS 1179
    Immunohistochemistry 1180
    Physiology 1181
    Microscopic Variations 1182

C CELLS 1184
    Histochemistry and Immunohistochemistry 1186
    Physiology 1186

STROMA 1186
    Lymphocytes 1186
    Fibrous Tissue 1187
    Adipose Tissue and Skeletal Muscle 1187
    Calcifications 1188

BRANCHIAL POUCH–DERIVED AND OTHER RELATED ECTOPIC TISSUES 1188
    Parathyroid Tissue 1191
    Thymic Tissue 1191
    Salivary Gland–type Tissue 1192
    Ectopic Cartilage 1192

BENIGN THYROID TISSUE IN ABNORMAL LOCATIONS 1192
    Midline Structures 1192
    Pericapsular Soft Tissues and Skeletal Muscle 1193
    Lateral Neck 1193
    Thyroid Inclusions in Cervical Lymph Nodes 1193
    Other Sites 1193

REFERENCES 1194

EMBRYOLOGY

The human thyroid first appears as a median anlage (the main anlage), and two lateral anlagens. The median anlage develops in the floor of the primitive pharynx at the foramen cecum (a dimple-like depression at the base of the tongue) from a median duct–like invagination that grows caudally, the *thyroglossal duct*. This formation contains at its base the developing thyroid gland, which is at first spherical but later, after the involution of the thyroglossal duct when approaching its definitive position in the neck in front of the trachea at about 7 weeks of gestation, becomes bilobed (1).

During this downward migration, the thyroglossal duct undergoes atrophy, leaving as a vestige the pyramidal lobe in about 40% of individuals. Faulty downward migration of the thyroid medial anlage or persistence of parts of the thyroglossal duct can give rise ectopic thyroid tissue in the neck, thyroglossal duct cysts, and cervical fistulae. Microscopically, the initially solid thyroid *anlage* begins to form cords and plates of follicular cells during the ninth week of gestation. Small follicles appear by the tenth week. Inside these primitive follicles, a finely granular material begins to collect, which by the 20th week acquires the morphologic features of colloid. By week 14, there are well-developed follicles with a central lumen containing colloid (Fig. 43.1A). Secondary follicles arise by budding from the primary follicles; they increase in number until the embryo reaches a length of about 160 mm. After this time the follicles increase in size, but the number remains the same. Under intense stimulation, the adult thyroid can form new follicles. Both the cytoplasm of the follicular cells and the intraluminal colloid are thyroglobulin (TGB) positive (Fig. 43.1B). Labeled amino acid studies have shown that TGB synthesis actually begins at a much

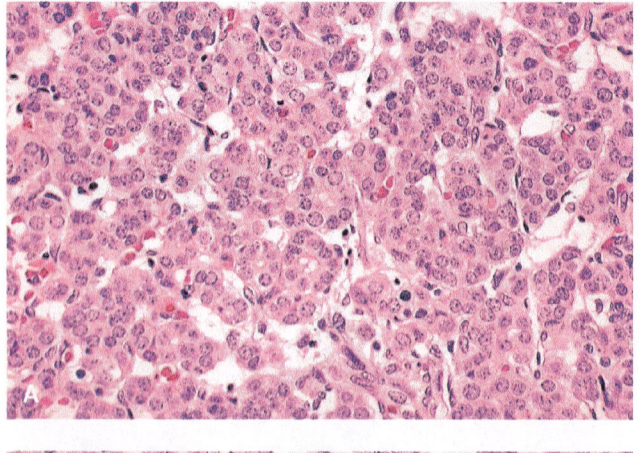
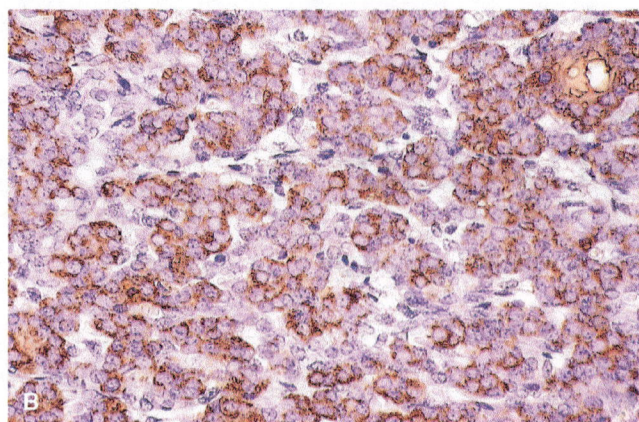
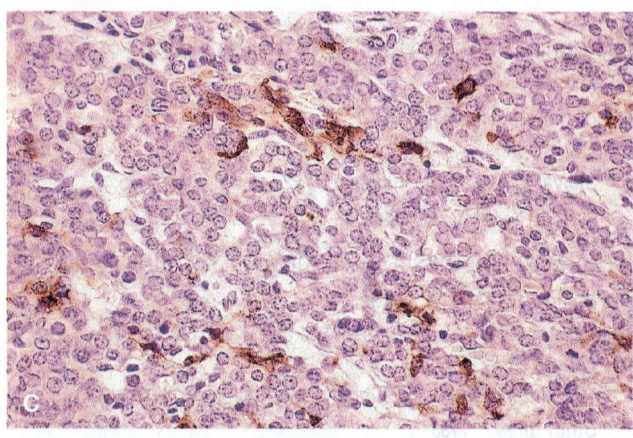

FIGURE 43.1 Developing thyroid gland in a 14-week fetus. **A:** Rare primitive follicles are seen within a mostly solid proliferation. **B:** The cytoplasm of the follicular cells and the material contained in the lumen of the primitive follicles are immunoreactive for TGB. **C:** C cells, as seen in a calcitonin immunostain preparation, are scattered within follicles.

earlier stage, when the thyroid is still a solid mass at the base of the tongue and long before follicle formation and colloid secretion can be identified morphologically (2–5). The fetal thyroid gland develops rapidly until the fourth month of intrauterine growth (crown–rump length 18 mm). After birth, the thyroid growth rate parallels that of the body, reaching the normal adult weight at around 15 years of age.

A series of intrinsic or cell-autonomous transcription factors have been shown to contribute to thyroid gland morphogenesis and follicular cells differentiation (6,7), while thyroid-stimulating hormone (TSH) influences thyroid differentiation only after the anatomic outline of the thyroid gland is well established.

The most important of these transcription factors are Hhex, TTF-1 (Nkx2-1), Pax8, and TTF-2 (Foxe1) which may be considered, collectively, as a thyroid signature within the anterior foregut endoderm (8).

Although these factors are also expressed and influence differentiation in other developing tissues, all four are co-expressed and involved in a transcriptional network of interactions of mutual dependence only in the thyroid anlage (9). Given that they regulate the expression of thyroid-specific genes, such as those responsible for the production of thyroid peroxidase and TGB, they are important not only for organogenesis but also for the functional differentiation of the thyroid gland in later stages of prenatal development, as well as postnatally (4,10–12).

Pax8 has been demonstrated in the human median thyroid anlage, in the thyroglossal duct, and in the ultimobranchial bodies (UBBs) (13). Thyroid transcription factor 1 (TTF-1), also is expressed in the median thyroid anlage (14). Immunohistochemically, *ghrelin*, a growth hormone–releasing hormone, has been shown in the follicular cells of fetal thyroid (from 8 to 38 weeks of gestational age) (15). Fetal thyroid stromal tissue is immunoreactive for galectin 1 but not for galectin 3 (16).

The two lateral anlagens of the thyroid derive from the UBBs which in turn originate from the IVth to the Vth branchial pouch complex before the incorporation of the latter in the thyroid. The UBBs, while still connected to the pharynx, start their migration downward on each side of the neck together with the parathyroid IV anlage (branchial pouch stage, 3 to 12 mm, 5 to 7 weeks); at 7 to 8 weeks, they separate from the pharynx and the parathyroid (separation stage, 13 to 17 mm, 7 to 8 weeks); their lumens become obliterated by proliferating cells, so that at 8 to 9 weeks they appear as solid masses that fuse with the dorsolateral aspects of the median thyroid anlage and become incorporated into the developing lateral lobes (incorporation stage, 18 to 27 mm, 8 to 9 weeks). After its fusion with the medial thyroid (at 9 weeks to term) the UBB enters in the dissolution phase and divides into a central thick-walled stratified epithelial cyst and a peripheral component composed of cell groups dispersed among the follicles, the C cells, dissolution stage (28 to 520 mm, 9 weeks to term) (Fig. 43.1C). The central portion is represented by a stratified epithelial-lined cyst, whereas the peripheral portion is dispersed into a few cell groups that eventually become cystic. In postnatal life, the central epithelial cyst largely disappears, its occasional remnants corresponding to the so-called solid cell nests (SCNs) (17,18).

Although plentiful embryologic, histochemical and immunohistochemical studies have led to the conclusion that mammalian and avian C cells are derived from the neural crest and that they migrate to the UBBs before their incorporation into the thyroid (19–23) the very concept of a neural crest origin of thyroid C cells is currently undergoing a major reconsideration. Thus, recent lineage tracing data from genetic studies in mice postulate that the true progenitors to C cells arise in the endodermal germ layer, pointing to a unifying origin of all cells of the UBBs. According to this hypothesis, the UBBs may turn out to be the embryonic source of C-cell precursors and not only their carriers, not differently from other organs such as lung, gall bladder, and pancreas, all of which contain neuroendocrine cells of endodermal origin. Several transcription factors and signaling molecules involved in the development of C cells have been identified, and genes expressed in the pharyngeal pouch endoderm, neural crest-derived mesenchyme in the pharyngeal arches, and UBB have been demonstrated to play critical roles for the development of C cells. Immunohistochemically, E-cadherin, an epithelial cell marker which is expressed in thyroid C cells, has been demonstrated to be colocalized with calcitonin in C cells and to be present in C-cell precursors, like the fourth pharyngeal pouch and the UBB (24–28).

It has been pointed out that a unifying origin of thyroid follicular cells and C cells, even though from different endoderm domains, might contribute to clarify the histogenesis of mixed thyroid tumors (28). Furthermore, the discovery that thyroid C cells developed from endoderm may open up new directions in the search for potential targets to treat C cell–derived tumors (29).

GROSS ANATOMY

The normal adult thyroid gland is located in the midportion of the neck, immediately in front of the larynx and trachea, where it is attached to the anterior trachea by loose connective tissue.

The two lateral lobes surround the ventral and lateral aspects of the larynx and trachea, reaching the lower halves of the thyroid cartilage and covering the second, third, and fourth tracheal rings.

The parathyroid glands are usually located adjacent to the posterior surface of the thyroid lobes. The recurrent laryngeal nerves run in the cleft between the trachea and esophagus just medial to the thyroid lobes.

The normal thyroid has a shape reminiscent of a butterfly, with two bulky lateral lobes connected by a thin isthmus. Each lateral lobe is 2 to 2.5 cm wide, 5 to 6 cm long, and 2 cm deep. Their upper and lower extremities (one having a pointed shape and the other featuring blunt contours) are referred to as upper and lower thyroid poles, respectively. One lobe may be larger than the other (mostly the right) and the isthmus may be exceptionally wide. The pyramidal lobe, a vestige of the thyroglossal duct, is found in about 40% of thyroids; it appears as a narrow projection of thyroid tissue that extends upward from the isthmus to lie on the surface of the thyroid cartilage. A gross enlargement of the pyramidal lobe may result from a diffuse pathologic process such as hyperplasia or Hashimoto thyroiditis.

The normal weight of the adult thyroid is 15 to 25 g in nongoitrous areas. However, there are significant individual variations, most of them related to gender, age, corporal weight, hormonal status, functional status of the gland, and iodine intake (30). For instance, the thyroid gland is larger and heavier in women than in men, and it becomes even larger during pregnancy and in the secretory phase of the menstrual cycle (31).

A thin fibrous capsule invests the thyroid. Connected to this capsule are numerous fibrous septa that penetrate the thyroid parenchyma and divide it into lobules (the so-called thyromeres). The microscopic integrity of the thyroid capsule was assessed in a study on 138 specimens from autopsies of adults (ages 20 to 40 years) by Komorowski and Hanson (32). Although grossly all of these capsules seemed complete, microscopically they were focally incomplete in 62% of the cases. Furthermore, thyroid follicles were found within the thyroid capsule in 14% of cases and in the pericapsular connective tissue in 88%. In the latter location, they were mostly seen as nodular aggregates.

The color of the normal thyroid is red-brown. A phenomenon exceptionally seen in otherwise normal thyroid glands of elderly individuals is the accumulation in the follicular cells of a melanin-like pigment that imparts to the gland a characteristic coal black stain, easily apparent on gross examination. The terms *melanosis thyroidi* and *black thyroid* are used to refer to this phenomenon. These changes are qualitatively identical to those seen in more florid form in thyroids of patients on chronic minocycline therapy (33). Ultrastructurally some of the granules contain lipofuscin type pigment, but in most of them is also present colloid, thus becoming ambilysosomes (34). An association between black thyroid and thyroid carcinoma has been reported. Kandil found thyroid carcinoma, predominantly of papillary type, in 65% of patients with black thyroid (35,36). Typically in papillary carcinomas arising within black thyroids there is a decreased pigmentation of the malignant cells compared to the surrounding thyroid tissue. An abnormal thyroid peroxidase of the tumor cells has been suggested as a possible cause of this phenomenon (37).

Nodularity of thyroid parenchyma is identified grossly in about 10% of the glands of endocrinologically normal individuals and its prevalence is increased in older patients (38).

The blood supply of the thyroid gland derives primarily from the inferior thyroid artery (which originates from the thyrocervical trunk of the subclavian artery) and the superior thyroid artery (which arises from the external carotid). A thyroid middle artery also may be present, which varies widely in size from an inconspicuous vessel to one the size of the inferior thyroid artery. The superior and medial thyroid veins and the inferior vein drain (via a venous plexus in the thyroid capsule) into the internal jugular and the brachiocephalic vein, respectively (39,40).

An intricate lymphatic network permeates the thyroid gland, encircling the follicles and connecting the two lateral lobes through the isthmus. In neonates and children, these lymph vessels may appear as empty, elongated, tortuous spaces that simulate a retraction artifact but which are lined by lymphatic endothelial cells positive for D2-40 (41). This network empties into subcapsular channels, which in turn give rise to collecting trunks within the thyroid capsule in close proximity to the veins to empty into the regional lymph nodes, which are the following:

- The *pericapsular* nodes. Whole organ sections of the thyroid have shown that the intraglandular lymph vessels penetrate the capsule and merge with the pericapsular lymph nodes, forming a plexus around the gland (42).
- The *internal jugular chain* nodes (including the *subdigastric* nodes) collecting lymph vessels draining the superior portion of the thyroid lobes and isthmus.
- The *pretracheal*, *paratracheal*, and *prelaryngeal* nodes collecting lymph vessels draining the inferior portion of the gland. The pretracheal node located near the thyroid isthmus is sometimes referred to as the *Delphian node* (43).
- The *recurrent laryngeal nerve chain* nodes.
- The *retropharyngeal* and *retroesophageal* nodes.

The *anterosuperior mediastinal* nodes are secondary to the recurrent laryngeal nerve chain and pretracheal groups; however, studies have shown that dye injected into the thyroid isthmus can also drain directly into them (44).

Some correlations exist between the site of a thyroid tumor within a given lobe and the location of the initial lymph node metastasis. However, the degree of anastomosing between these various nodal groups is such that any of them can be found to be the site of disease regardless of the precise location of the primary tumor. Thus in papillary thyroid carcinoma, the most common thyroid malignancy, the most frequent pattern of lymph node spread is initially to the central lymph node compartment (Level VI) followed by the lateral neck. In a retrospective study of patients who presented with clinically positive neck lymph nodes, 95% of patients had Level VI lymph node involvement, while between 54% and 68% of the patients had Levels II–IV involvement (45).

Vasomotor nonmedullated postganglionic neural fibers originating from the superior and midline cervical sympathetic ganglia influence indirectly the secretory activity of the thyroid gland through their action on the blood vessels. In addition, adrenergic receptors in follicular cells and a network of adrenergic fibers ending near the follicular basement membrane have been demonstrated (46). It has been hypothesized, therefore, that the thyroid secretion is regulated both by direct neural signals and by indirect vascular nerve signals (47–49). A role for direct neural influences in the secretion of calcitonin and other C cell–derived hormones is supported by the demonstration in chickens of a rich cholinergic network encircling the C cells (50).

Small *paraganglia* are normally present close to the thyroid and are occasionally found beneath the thyroid capsule (51). Their presence explains the rare occurrence of peri- and intrathyroidal paragangliomas (52,53).

MICROSCOPIC ANATOMY

The fundamental unit of the thyroid is the follicle, a round to slightly oval structure lined by a single layer of epithelial cells resting on a basement membrane. The lumen of the follicle contains colloid, a viscous material that is mostly composed by proteins secreted by the follicular cells, including TGB. The follicles, which are separated from each other by a loose fibroconnective tissue, have an average diameter of 200 µm. Their size may vary even within the same gland depending on the functional status of the thyroid and the age of the individual. Variations in the shape of follicles exist, but elongated follicles are a feature of hyperplastic or neoplastic conditions or are the result of compression adjacent to an expansile mass. A characteristic structure present in the normal thyroid but more often seen in hyperplastic conditions is the *Sanderson polster* (see page 1182).

The colloid, which is pale eosinophilic in the actively secreting gland, acquires a deeply eosinophilic staining quality in resting follicles. Often, numerous clumps with

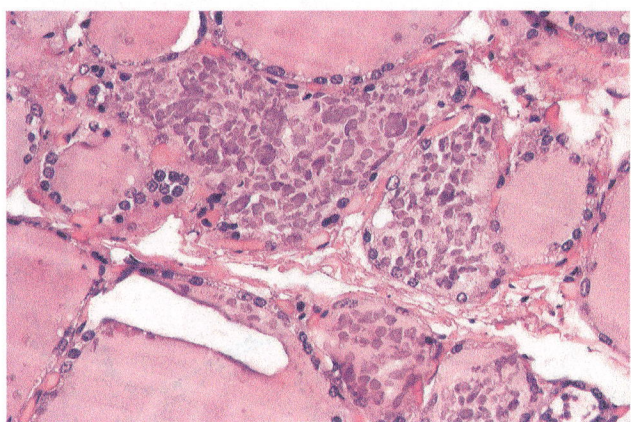

FIGURE 43.2 Clumps of condensed colloid within follicular lumina.

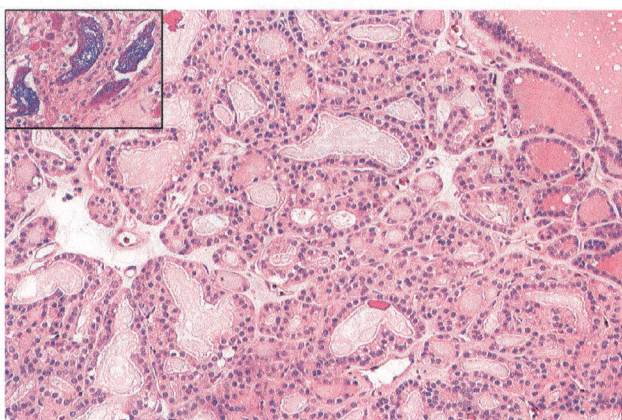

FIGURE 43.4 The basophilic colloid present in most of these follicles contrasts with the more typical red colloid present in the follicles on the right upper corner. *Inset:* The Alcian blue–PAS stain highlights the mucinous character of the basophilic colloid.

various shapes appear within the colloid of resting follicles, suggesting an artifactual coagulation-type phenomenon (Fig. 43.2). In some follicles, the colloid may have an amphophilic or basophilic staining quality, probably the result of an increase in the amount of acidic groups in the TGB molecule (Fig. 43.3). In the most advanced expression of this phenomenon, the intraluminal material acquires a distinct mucin–like appearance (Fig. 43.4). The glycoprotein material present within the follicles stains for periodic acid–Schiff (PAS) and Alcian blue and is immunoreactive for TGB. A row of small vacuoles is seen at the interface between the follicular epithelium and the colloid in actively functioning glands; these are referred to as reabsorbing vacuoles. In addition, it is not unusual to find a large round or oval clear space within the colloid; this often appears empty but it may contain *birefringent calcium oxalate crystals* (see page 1184).

Another morphologic variation of the colloid is represented by collections of round basophilic acellular corpuscles clustering at one pole of the follicle.

The epithelial glandular cells lining the follicle are known as follicular cells or thyrocytes; among them, there is a second cellular component known as C cells.

FOLLICULAR CELLS

The cells lining the follicles—follicular cells or thyrocytes—show variations in their shape and size according to the functional status of the gland. Three major types, expressions of a morphologic continuum, are described: flattened (endothelioid), cuboidal, and columnar (cylindrical) (Fig. 43.5A). Flattened cells are relatively inactive. Cuboidal cells (their height equaling their width) are the most numerous and their major function is to secrete colloid. The rarer columnar cells reabsorb the TGB-containing colloid, liberate the active hormones, and excrete these hormones into blood vessels; they may feature an apical cuticle, apical lipid droplets, and one or more basilar vacuoles (vacuoles of Bensley).

Functional polarity is apparent at the level of the follicle and the follicular cell. A single follicle may have flattened cells on one side and cuboidal or low columnar cells on the other (Fig. 43.5B), the best expression of this phenomenon being the already mentioned *Sanderson polster*. At the cellular level, all follicular cells manifest a definite polarity, resting with their bases on the basement membrane and having the apexes directed toward the lumen of the follicle. Size and position of the nucleus and some components of the cytoplasm may vary considerably. In the resting thyroid, the nucleus is round or oval, is located toward the center of the cell, and usually contains one nucleolus that is eccentrically located. Its chromatin may be finely granular or clumped. In actively secreting cells, the nucleus is enlarged; because of the mostly apical enlargement of the cytoplasm, it acquires a basal position. The cytoplasm is usually weakly eosinophilic; only exceptionally in an otherwise normal thyroid does it appear granular and intensely eosinophilic, that is, oncocytic (*the so-called*

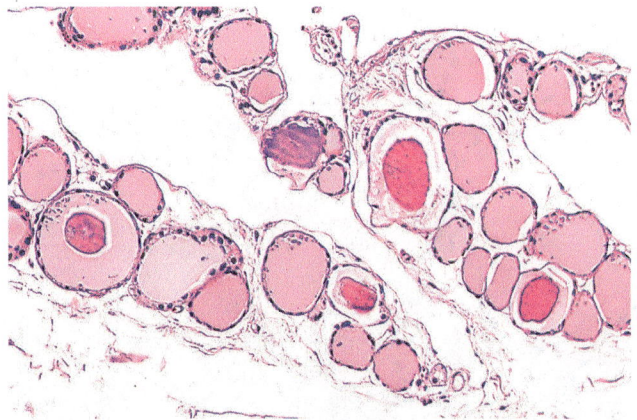

FIGURE 43.3 The colloid accumulated in these follicles exhibits different densities and tinctorial qualities, the latter ranging from acidophilic to basophilic.

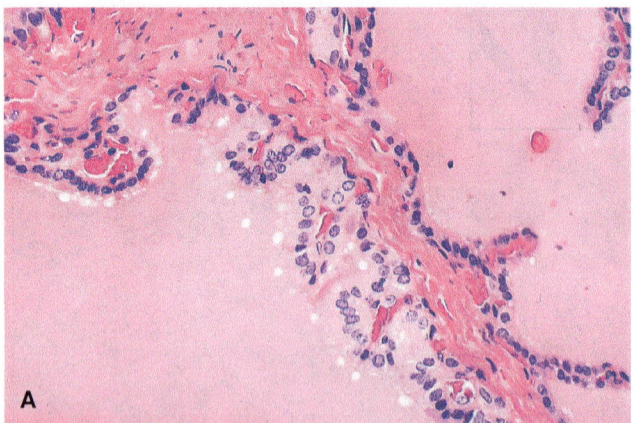 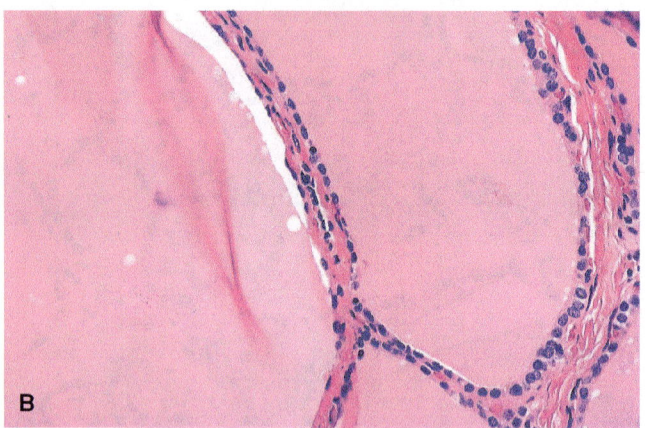

FIGURE 43.5 **A:** The epithelium of one follicle is low cuboidal and relatively inactive. The adjacent follicle shows a taller epithelium and reabsorption vacuoles. **B:** The epithelium of the same follicle is flattened on one side and cuboidal on the other, as an expression of functional polarization.

Hurthle cells). In contrast to parathyroid cells, little or no intracytoplasmic glycogen is present in them. Occasionally, the follicular cell cytoplasm contains a golden brown pigment of lipofuscin type (Fig. 43.6A), which should be distinguished from the melanin-like pigment (Fig. 43.6B).

Ultrastructurally, the follicular cells are arranged in a single layer around the colloid and rest on a basement membrane, approximately 35 to 40 nm in thickness, that separate them from the microvilli which emanate from the surface of the cells, their number being increased and their length greater in actively functioning cells. Cell membranes of adjacent cells interdigitate in a complex fashion and are joined by junctional complexes toward the apex (54,55). The cytoplasm contains variable amounts of endoplasmic reticulum, mitochondria of usually small size, and lysosomes. When the number of mitochondria is highly increased, the cell acquires at the light microscopic level an intensely eosinophilic granular cytoplasmic appearance (corresponding to the above-mentioned Hurthle cells).

Immunohistochemistry

A wide variety of markers with various degrees of specificity and diagnostic significance are expressed by the normal adult follicular cells.

Thyroglobulin (TGB)

This is probably the most specific immunohistochemical marker for normal follicular cells and the tumors composed of them. It can be demonstrated with either monoclonal or polyclonal antibodies and the reactivity is both in the cytoplasm and in the colloid (56,57). Oncocytes show a much lesser degree of positivity. Despite its high specificity, thyroxin-binding globulin (TBG) can give rise to a common pitfall. Because of its tendency to leak out from the cytoplasm of the follicular cells and to diffuse into the adjacent tissues, it can be incorporated into the cytoplasm of other types of cells (e.g., metastatic carcinoma) and cause a false positivity (58).

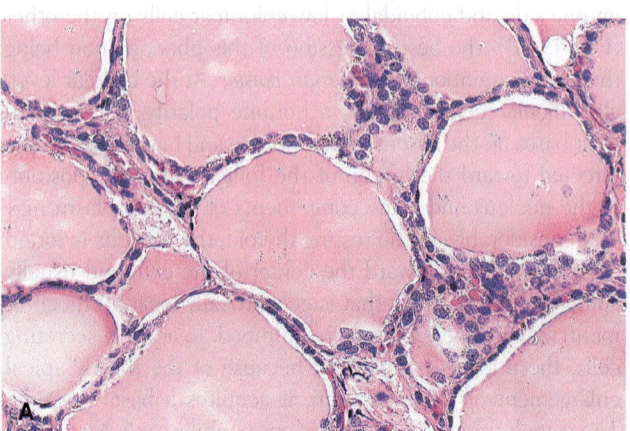 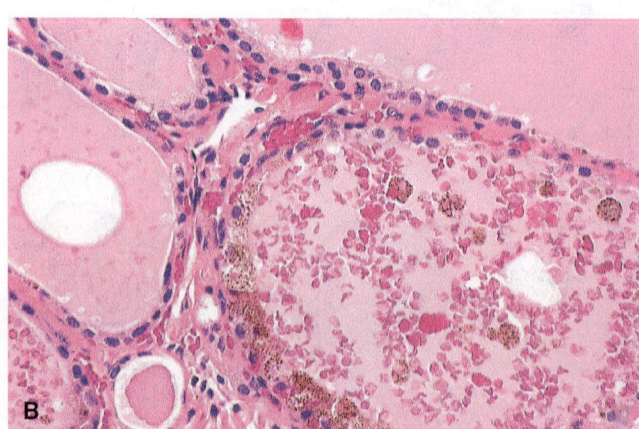

FIGURE 43.6 **A:** Lipofuscin in the cytoplasm of the follicular cells. **B:** Granular black pigment in the follicular epithelium and colloid of the thyroid of a 73-year-old patient who was not on minocycline therapy.

Thyroid Transcription Factor 1 (TTF-1)

This is another very useful marker for thyroid follicular cells and tumors composed of them. This nuclear transcription factor, first identified in thyroid follicular cells and later in lung epithelium (pneumocytes), together with TTF-2 and Pax8, is necessary for thyroid organogenesis and differentiation (6–8). In the normal adult thyroid, its distribution is related to that of TGB and thyroperoxidase (6–8,59). It is consistently expressed in all types of primary and metastatic thyroid carcinomas (including medullary carcinoma), except for the anaplastic type (59).

Keratins

The normal thyroid gland strongly expresses simple epithelial-type CKs 7 and 18 and, to a lesser degree, CKs 8 and 19, but not stratified epithelial-type CKs (60). Papillary and follicular carcinomas share the expression of simple epithelial-type CKs 7, 8, 18, and 19. CK19 is expressed particularly strongly by papillary carcinoma. The latter also usually express stratified-type CKs 5/6 and 13. This reactivity pattern of papillary carcinoma is useful to identify small tumor foci not easily identified by conventional histologic examination and is maintained in the metastatic foci. Unfortunately, this rather distinct pattern of CK distribution in papillary carcinoma is often shared, at least focally, by the thyroid follicles of Hashimoto thyroiditis (61).

Vimentin

Some normal follicular cells occasionally express this intermediate filament in conjunction with keratin, although less commonly than in neoplastic conditions (62,63).

Epithelial Membrane Antigen (EMA)

Follicular cells are variably positive, with accentuation of the cell membranes.

Galectin

The galectins constitute a family of lactose-binding soluble lectins sharing affinity for β-galactoside residues and a significant sequence similarity in their carbohydrate-binding site. They have been implicated in cell growth and differentiation, intercellular recognition, and adhesion. The most extensively studied galectins are galectin-1 and galectin-3. The latter has been studied in great detail in the thyroid gland, where it stains carcinomas (especially those of papillary type) in a stronger and more consistent fashion than adenomas (64). It is also often focally expressed in the follicles of lymphocytic/Hashimoto thyroiditis, nodular hyperplasia, and follicular adenoma (65).

Triiodothyronine (T3) and Thyroxine (T4)

These hormones can be detected immunohistochemically both in the cytoplasm of the follicular cells and in the intraluminal colloid, but they are rarely used for diagnostic purposes, having been replaced for this purpose with TGB.

Estrogen and Progesterone Receptors

Estrogen and progesterone receptors positivity, restricted to the follicular cell nuclei, shows some correlation with the age and sex of the individual (66,67).

S100 Protein

This marker, which is mainly detected in inflammatory/hyperplastic and neoplastic thyroid conditions, is only focally and weakly expressed by normal follicular cells (68).

Claudins

Claudins and occludin are integral constituents of tight junctions and are deregulated in a variety of malignancies. They are present in the normal thyroid and in most thyroid neoplasms with different levels of expression (69).

Epidermal Growth Factor Receptor (EGFR)

In normal follicular cells, and because of their functional polarization, the location of this receptor is mainly basal or basolateral (70).

Thyroid Peroxidase

This enzyme is responsible for the oxidation of iodide to iodine. Immunohistochemically, it shows a pattern of staining correlated with the age of the individual. A cytoplasmic pattern of staining with apical membrane accentuation is seen in children and young adults, and a perinuclear ring distribution is seen in older individuals (71).

Sodium Iodide Symporter

At the immunohistochemical level, this molecule, responsible for the active iodide intake into the follicular epithelium, is localized mainly to the lateral basal portion of the cells (72,73).

Physiology

The main function of the thyroid gland is the production of thyroid hormones, the most important being thyroxin (T4) and triiodothyronine (T3). These hormones regulate metabolism, increase protein synthesis in every tissue of the body, and increase O_2 consumption. Thyroid hormones are particularly important for body development and for the normal maturation of the central and peripheral nervous systems.

Steps in thyroid hormone biosynthesis include ingestion of iodine ions from water and food, their absorption and transport as iodide into the extracellular fluid, and their concentration within the thyroid, where their intracellular levels are 30 times higher than in peripheral blood. The active iodide uptake across the basement membrane is mediated by human sodium iodide symporter (hNIS) in a process coupled with the flow of sodium (72). The intrathyroidal iodide is then oxidized to iodine. This last step is dependent on the action of iodide peroxidase, which oxidates the iodine ion to a highly reactive form of iodine, which in turn binds to tyrosine. The results are monoiodotyrosine (MIT) when one iodine molecule is attached, and diiodotyrosine (DIT) when two iodine molecules are attached. The iodotyrosine residues are condensed to form the biologically active thyroid hormones *thyroxin (T4)* and *triiodothyronine (T3)*. Thyroxin results from the coupling of two molecules of DIT, and triiodothyronine from the coupling of one molecule of MIT with a molecule of DIT (73). Thyroid hormones with numerous iodinated tyrosine residues, including biologically active T4 and T3 are stored in *thyroglobulin* (TGB) which plays an essential role as a carrier protein of these hormones.

TGB, a large protein with a 19 S sedimentation coefficient and a molecular weight of 670,000, is formed by two identical subunits with a 12 S sedimentation coefficient to which many oligosaccharides are linked. Variations in the sugar chains of the TGB molecule have been evaluated by the analysis of reactivity to various lectins and found to differ between the normal gland and various pathologic states, including neoplasms (74).

TGB is encoded by a gene spreading over more than 200 kilobases in the bovine genome (75). The molecular mechanisms involved in the tissue-specific and hormone-dependent expression of the TGB gene have been studied in follicular cells in primary cultures and cell lines (76,77). TGB is collected at the center of the thyroid follicles and is the main constituent of colloid.

Ultrastructural studies have correlated the morphologic changes that accompany thyroid hormone production and secretion. The synthesis of TGB begins in the endoplasmic reticulum and continues in the Golgi apparatus, where the end sugars of the carbohydrate site are incorporated; it is then packaged in small apical microvesicles, the contents of which are discharged into the follicular lumen after fusion of the vesicle membranes with the luminal side of the plasma membrane.

Resorption of TGB takes place through cytoplasmic pseudopodia (streamers) which engulf minute portions of colloid, which are then drawn into the cell in the form of membrane-bound colloid droplets. These subsequently fuse with lysosomes, and their content is digested by the lysosomal enzymes. The breakdown products, including T3 and T4, diffuse through the cell membrane and the basement membrane into the adjacent capillaries and most of the molecules become bound to a specific carrier protein known as TBG (77–79). TBG normally transports more than 70% of thyroid hormones (78–80). Approximately 20% of circulating thyroid hormones are carried by transthyretin (prealbumin) and albumin (81).

Only a small portion of circulating thyroid hormones (approximately 0.05% of T3 and 0.015% of T4) is unbound and, therefore, biologically active. Free, circulating, biologically active T3 and T4 are in equilibrium with the hormones bound to the carrier proteins. The amount of circulating T4 is much larger than that of T3; however, T3 is about four times more active biologically; as a result, the final contribution of T3 to the biologic activity of thyroid hormones equals that of T4 (80).

Thyroid hormones acts by binding to specific thyroid hormone receptors present in nearly all tissues. Thyroid hormones stimulate metabolism, increase oxygen consumption, and cause a rise in heat production, cardiac output, and heart rate. They are essential for normal development, growth, and maturation. The acceleration of growth may result from a direct action on the cells to increase their rate of division, by acting permissively for other hormones, or by inducing the synthesis of a variety of growth-promoting hormones (78,80,82–87).

Thyroid biosynthetic and secretory activities are controlled by the blood level of TSH, a glycoprotein synthesized and secreted by the anterior pituitary gland (88). TSH binds to thyrotropin receptors located on the basolateral surface of the follicular cell membrane, and by activating the adenylate–cyclase pathway regulates the complex mechanism responsible for T3 and T4 synthesis (81,89,90).

Stimulation of the thyroid gland by thyrotropin increases its secretory activity and vascularity and results in both hypertrophy and hyperplasia of follicular cells, accompanied by reduction of colloid storage. At the functional level, this is reflected by an increase in iodide concentration and organic binding, hormone synthesis, and hormone secretion (80,91,92).

TSH release is in turn regulated by a tripeptide secreted by the hypothalamus, thyrotropin-releasing hormone (TRH which is produced by the neurons of the medial-basal hypothalamus and carried into the pituitary gland via the hypophyseal portal vessels.). TSH and TRH releases are regulated by the circulating levels of free T3 and T4, via a negative feedback on the pituitary and hypothalamus (low levels of free T3 and T4 stimulate the release of TSH and TRH). In contrast, TSH and TRH releases are inhibited by high levels of circulating free T3 and T4 (88,91,92).

Microscopic Variations

Sanderson Polster

A characteristic structure, present in the normal thyroid and accentuated in hyperplastic conditions, is the so-called *Sanderson polster* (Fig. 43.7). This refers to an aggregate of small follicles lined by flattened epithelium and covered by an undulating layer of columnar epithelium that is seen bulging into the lumina of larger follicles. This perfectly benign and to some extent physiologic change, most likely the morphologic expression of the functional polarization of the thyroid follicle, needs to be distinguished from intracystic papillary microcarcinoma.

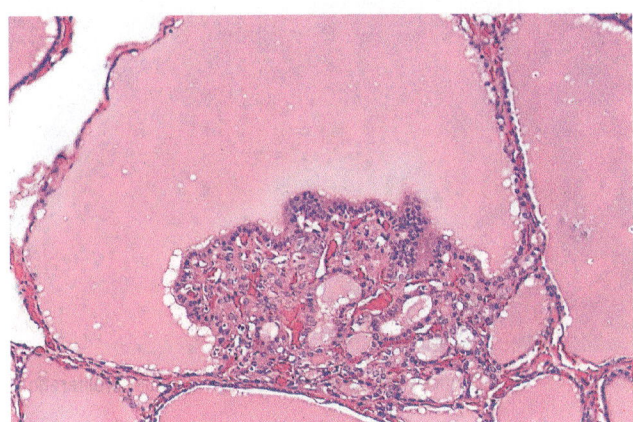

FIGURE 43.7 Sanderson polster protruding into the lumen of a follicle.

Granulomas

Granulomas are a relatively common finding in otherwise normal surgically resected thyroids and in autoptic specimens. Both foreign material and colloid may elicit this process. Suture material is the most frequent cause of formation of granulomas in completion thyroidectomy specimens. Larger foreign-body granulomas sometimes clinically simulating a thyroid nodule have been reported in thyroids of patients who underwent the laryngeal injection of Polytef (polytetrafluoroethylene) (93,94). This material may migrate through the lymphatics into adjacent tissues, where it may start an inflammatory process.

Rarely, interstitial granulomas are seen as a reaction to oxalate crystals that have been released by broken follicles (95).

Granulomatous lesions originated by the rupture of follicles and their invasion by macrophages and leukocytes as a reaction to the extruded colloid are a common incidental finding in surgically resected thyroids. Carney et al. (96) referred to this process as *multifocal granulomatous folliculitis* or *palpation thyroiditis*, and attributed it to the minor trauma resulting from physical examination of the gland. Support for this interpretation comes from the observation that the number and size of the granulomas is related to the intensity of the palpation and the fact that similar changes have been described in individuals engaged in martial arts (the picturesque called *martial-arts thyroiditis*) (96,97).

Grossly, a gland affected by palpation thyroiditis appears normal or shows tiny foci of hemorrhage. Histologically, multiple small granulomas centered in disrupted follicles and composed of histiocytes, lymphocytes, and plasma cells are seen scattered in the thyroid gland (Fig. 43.8A). Some of the histiocytes are foamy, while others have the appearance of multinucleated giant cells. The appearance depends on the stage of the process, a common picture being a cluster of foamy macrophages hanging from the follicular epithelium into the lumen (Fig. 43.8B). Necrosis, hemosiderin, and iron deposition are seen only rarely. Sometimes up to four or five follicles are involved in a single granuloma.

Immunohistochemically, most of the lymphocytes are T cells; among the plasma cells, K-positive cells predominate (98).

Palpation thyroiditis seems to represent a variation in the theme of *colloidophagy*, a process described many years ago and characterized by a granulomatous reaction to colloid in follicles allegedly undergoing spontaneous rupture in thyroids affected by goiter or thyroiditis (99).

Palpation thyroiditis needs to be distinguished from *interstitial giant cell thyroiditis* in which the granulomas are centered in the interstitium rather than in the follicles, *necrotizing granulomas* following surgical procedures (similar

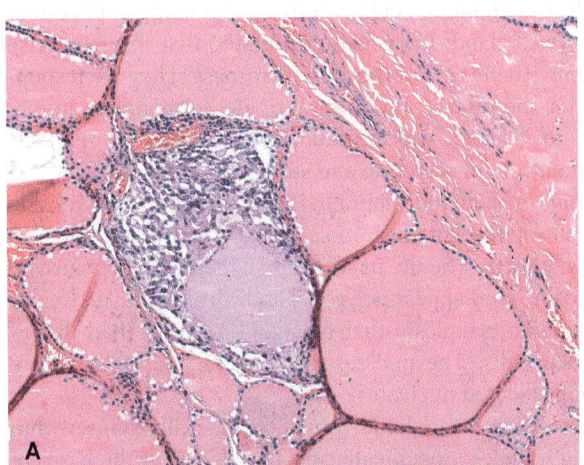
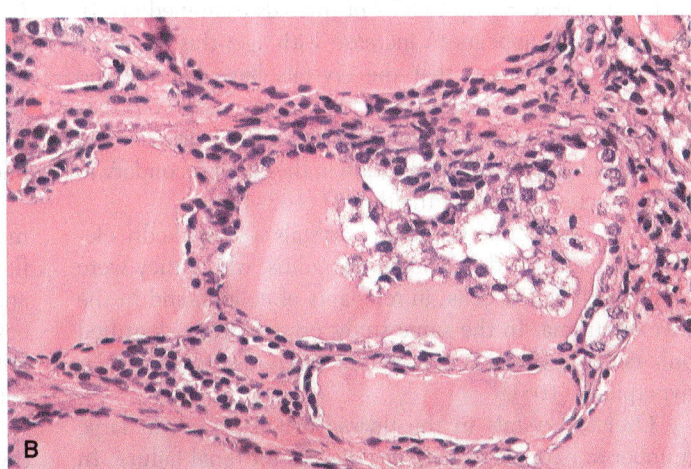

FIGURE 43.8 Palpation thyroiditis. **A:** The thyroid follicle in the center is packed with histiocytes and other inflammatory cells, with a clump of residual colloid in the center. The follicular epithelium is barely discernible. **B:** In this case, the follicle is only partially involved. Inflammatory cells and desquamated follicular cells protrude into the lumen.

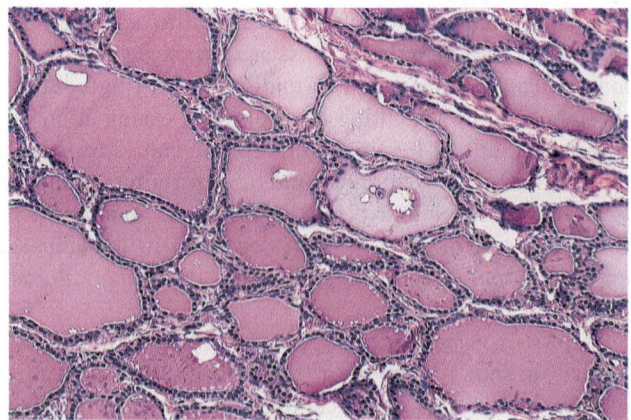

FIGURE 43.9 Multiple birefringent calcium oxalate crystals are seen in the lumina of normal thyroid follicles (polarized light).

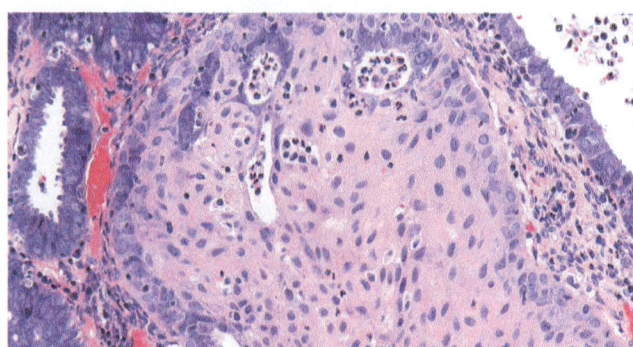

FIGURE 43.10 Squamous metaplasia in a benign follicular proliferation.

to those more commonly seen in the bladder and the prostate and characterized by a central area of necrosis surrounded by a palisading of epithelioid cells), and aggregates of C cells (which are immunoreactive for calcitonin) (100,101).

Crystals

Anisotropic crystals of calcium oxalate may be present within the colloid in normal adult thyroid glands, particularly in older and/or less active glands. They may be seen in ordinary light, but are more easily identified under polarized light (Fig. 43.9). Their shape varies from rhomboid to irregular plaques and their size shows wide variations (102).

In an autopsy study, Katoh et al. found intraluminal crystals in 88% of nodular goiters, 60% of follicular adenomas, 33% of follicular carcinomas, and only 5% of papillary carcinomas (103). The overall prevalence was 69.4% in benign nodules and 7.6% in malignant nodules. A heavy deposit of these crystals was seen almost exclusively in benign conditions. In same study, they have been found with a frequency of up to 85% of thyroids examined (103). Their number appears to increase with age; this, together with the observation that the crystals have been found more frequently in colloid with low positivity for TGB, has prompted the suggestion that they result from variations in colloid and calcium concentration in the gland secondary to a low functional state of the thyroid (102–104).

In one study, the number of crystals was markedly elevated in glands with subacute thyroiditis, where they were found in the giant cells, in remnants of colloid, and in the thyroid stroma. In the same study, crystals were identified only rarely in thyroids with chronic thyroiditis or glandular hyperplasia (105).

Oxalate crystals in the thyroid are also seen in large number in patients undergoing dialysis for renal failure. In this setting, the thyroid is just another site of oxalate deposition, together with the kidney, myocardium, and other sites (106). Rarely, crystals released by follicular breakdown may elicit a granulomatous reaction in the nearby thyroid stroma

(95). At the time of frozen section, their identification within a follicular structure can be useful in distinguishing thyroid from parathyroid gland tissue (107,108).

Squamous Metaplasia

Benign squamous cells occur as an expression of squamous metaplasia of follicular cells in various benign and malignant thyroid lesions and, under exceptional circumstances, in an otherwise normal thyroid (Fig. 43.10) (109–111). They need to be distinguished from transversally cut follicles and from the SCNs of UBB derivation. It also should be mentioned that squamous epithelium is regularly observed as a component of the epithelium of thyroglossal duct cysts. In ultrasound-guided fine-needle aspiration biopsies squamous metaplasia may represent a diagnostic pitfall in the differential diagnosis of thyroid nodules, particularly those with potentially benign cystic changes (112).

C CELLS

C cells (parafollicular cells) represent a minor component of the thyroid gland. It has been estimated that they comprise not more than 0.1% of the glandular mass. They are responsible for the production of the peptide hormone calcitonin. The term "C cells" was introduced by Pearse (113) to underline their role in secreting and storing this hormone.

Immunostain for calcitonin is at present the most reliable method for the demonstration of C cells which are identified only with difficulty in sections stained with hematoxylin and eosin. They appear polygonal and with a granular, weakly eosinophilic cytoplasm that is larger and paler than that of follicular cells. The nucleus is round to oval, pale, with a centrally located nucleolus.

C cells are located, individually or in small groups, within thyroid follicles. Specifically, most are found at the bases of the follicular cells (hence the qualifier parafollicular) without contact with the follicular lumen. Electron microscopy has shown that C cells occupy an intrafollicular (rather than interfollicular) position, and that they are separated from the thyroid interstitium by the follicular basal lamina. The presence of C cells in the interfollicular stroma has never been convincingly demonstrated ultrastructurally (114).

Occasional C cells have prominent cytoplasmic processes that extend beyond the adjacent follicular cells. In normal adults and neonates, C cells are restricted to the mid-upper and upper thirds of the lateral lobes of the thyroid, in the area where UBBs (from which they are thought to derive) fuse with the thyroid median anlage. The number of C cells varies with the development of the gland, being more numerous in early age. In one study, up to 100 C cells per low-power field were demonstrated in neonates and children, whereas in adults only a maximum of 10 cells per low-power field were counted (115). In another study, no difference in the number of C cells was found between young and middle-aged groups, but in the elderly the number of such cells was variable, with groups of up to 20 or more cells sometimes being observed (116). However, no statistically significant differences among the various age groups in adults were demonstrated. Other studies have since confirmed that normal adult thyroid glands may contain numerous C cells, sometimes in the form of large nodules (Fig. 43.11) (117). Gibson et al. suggested that such nodules of C cells, more common in men, particularly in patients over 50 years, in the absence of disturbances in calcium metabolism and of a family history of medullary carcinoma, do not constitute a precursor of medullary carcinoma but may be instead the expression of either a partial failure of embryonic C-cell migration and dispersion within the gland or of age-related hyperplasia (117). As already mentioned, C cells tend to aggregate in the vicinity of SCNs.

C-cell hyperplasia occurs in patients with MEN2A and MEN2B syndromes (*primary or "neoplastic" C-cell hyperplasia*) and in association with a variety of other disorders (*secondary or "physiologic" C-cell hyperplasia*).

Primary (neoplastic) C-cell hyperplasia is caused by a germline mutation associated with specific mutations in *RET* proto-oncogene (exon 10,11,16) and is seen in the setting of familial diseases, such as MEN2.

Secondary (physiologic) C-cell hyperplasia has been observed in the immediate periphery of nonmedullary thyroid neoplasms (papillary and follicular carcinoma; lymphoma), in association with sporadic medullary carcinoma, Hashimoto thyroiditis, in secondary hyperparathyroidism, in other hypercalcemic states with hypergastrinemia, goitrous hypothyroidism, PTEN-associated tumor syndromes with the assumption of some drugs, such as cimetidine and estrogens, and after partial removal of the thyroid (118–123). Patients with secondary (physiologic) C-cell hyperplasia, including cases of microdissected C-cell hyperplasia adjacent to sporadic medullary carcinoma, lack evidence of *RET* point mutations, despite the presence of codon 918 mutations in the tumors (124). Physiologic C-cell hyperplasia is characterized by the presence of ≥50 C cells cytologically normal, identified only on the basis of immunostains for calcitonin, per low-power (100× magnification) microscopic field (125,126).

Patients with *primary (neoplastic) C-cell hyperplasia* have elevated serum levels of calcitonin and CEA. The typical location of the C-cell hyperplasia is in the upper two-thirds of the lateral lobes although may be found in other areas of the gland. According to the most recent criteria, *primary (neoplastic) C-cell hyperplasia* is defined by the presence of >6 to 8 C cells per cluster in several foci with >50 C cells per low-power field (126). The hyperplasia may be diffuse or nodular. The C cells appear as groups of large cells, with round to ovoid centrally located nuclei, clear cytoplasm. With further progression, the follicles are filled with expansile foci of proliferating C cells (*nodular C-cell hyperplasia*). Ultrastructurally basal lamina defects are also seen more commonly in nodular hyperplasia.

The term "neoplastic" hyperplasia has been proposed by Perry on the basis of the atypia of the proliferating C cells (125). Other authors have interpreted C-cell hyperplasia associated with MEN2 as an authentic preinvasive carcinoma which represents a carcinoma in situ of the thyroid gland parafollicular cells (127). Molecular studies of microdissected foci of thyroid glands from patients with MEN2A have given further evidence in favor of the neoplastic nature of C-cell hyperplasia in the setting of MEN2A, by demonstrating that foci of C-cell hyperplasia are monoclonal, with inactivation of the same allele in both thyroid lobes and that they have different secondary alterations involving the tumor suppressor genes p53, RB1, WT1, and NF1 (128).

The distinction of this preneoplastic disorder from a small medullary carcinoma (*microcarcinoma*) is based on the nesting expansile pattern, the destruction of the follicular basement membrane, seen with PAS stain or collagen IV immunostain, the areas of early fibrosis between the infiltrating C cells into the thyroid interstitium and the diminished intensity of calcitonin immunostaining.

Foci of nodular C-cell hyperplasia occasionally may be difficult to distinguish from a variety of other changes, including squamous metaplasia, SCNs, intrathyroidal thymic or parathyroid rests, palpation thyroiditis, tangential cuts of follicles, and foci of metastatic carcinoma.

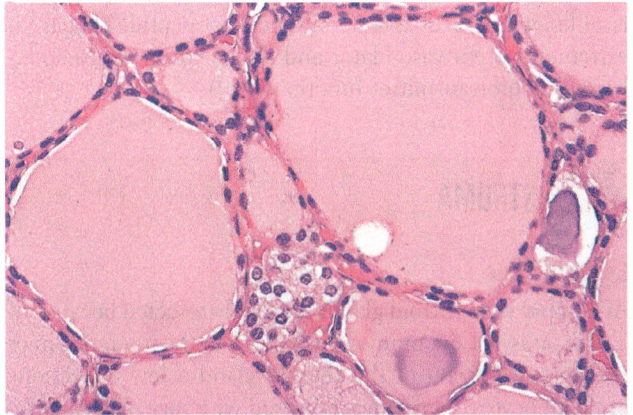

FIGURE 43.11 Clusters of C cells in the thyroid of an elderly individual with no known clinical or laboratory evidence of calcium disturbance.

The main ultrastructural characteristic of C cells is the presence of neuroendocrine-type secretory granules, which range in diameter from 60 to 550 nm (129). Two main types of granules have been identified. Type I granules have an average diameter of 280 nm and a moderately electron-dense, finely granular content which is closely applied to the limiting membranes of the granules. Type II granules are smaller (average diameter of 130 nm) with a more electron-dense content, which are separated from the limiting membranes by a small but distinct electron-lucent space. Most normal C cells are filled with type I secretory granules, with no or few type II granules. Immunocytochemical studies performed at the ultrastructural level have shown that both type I and II secretory granules contain immunoreactive calcitonin (129).

Histochemistry and Immunohistochemistry

Histochemically, normal C cells are characterized by *Argyrophilia* (130); *Lead hematoxylin* (131); *Toluidine blue, coriophosphine O* (131), and *Lectin Ulex Europaeus Agglutinin* (132). These methods, widely used in the past for the identification of C cells, have been largely replaced by the use of immunohistochemical techniques.

Immunohistochemically, C cells have been found to be reactive to:

Calcitonin (Fig. 43.12) (130,131,133,134); *calcitonin gene–related peptide* (CGRP) (135); *katacalcin* (136); *somatostatin* (137–139), *substance P* (140); *helodermin* (141); *gastrin-releasing peptide* (142,143); *thyrotropin-releasing hormone* (144); *serotonin* and other biologically active amines (145); low–molecular-weight *keratin* (146); *chromogranin A* and *synaptophysin* (146); *carcinoembryonic antigen* (CEA) (130); *vimentin* (146); *TTF-1*: normal, hyperplastic and neoplastic C cells are variably positive for this marker, in contrast to follicular cells which are more uniformly positive (147,148); *galectin-3*: hyperplastic C cells are negative, whereas MEN2A and 2B medullary carcinomas are usually positive for this marker (149).

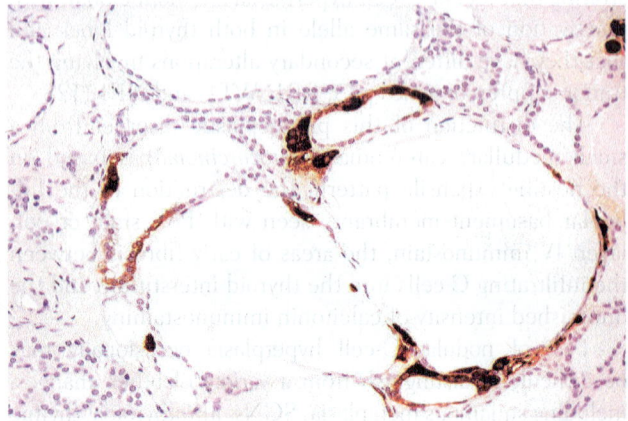

FIGURE 43.12 Immunostain for calcitonin demonstrates C cells within follicles, arranged either individually or in small groups.

It is possible that neuroendocrine cells other than C cells exist in the thyroid and that they represent the cells of origin of the rare thyroid "neuroendocrine carcinomas" having histologic and immunohistochemical features different from those of medullary carcinoma.

Physiology

Calcitonin is a 32–amino acid peptide whose main function is the regulation of the level of calcium in the plasma by a feedback mechanism. This is brought about by the inhibition of osteoclastic activity. When calcium plasma levels are increased, calcitonin is released from the thyroid. Calcitonin also acts in the kidney to enhance the production of vitamin D.

The major physiologic role of calcitonin is most likely the protection of the skeleton during periods of calcium stress such as growth, pregnancy, and lactation (150). However, the absence of calcitonin is not associated with hypercalcemia, nor does a marked excess of the hormone (as seen in patients with medullary thyroid carcinoma) produce hypocalcemia. In addition to calcium, both gastrin and cholecystokinin induce the secretion of calcitonin, as does the chronic administration of estrogenic hormones.

The calcitonin gene is located on the short arm of chromosome 11 and consists of six axons that encode katacalcin (C-terminal flanking peptide) and CGRP (136,150,151). The primary transcript of the calcitonin gene gives rise to two different mRNAs by tissue-specific alternative splicing events, leading to the production of calcitonin and CGRP mRNAs. The calcitonin–CGRP gene is expressed both in thyroid and nervous tissues, but calcitonin is produced in large quantities only in the thyroid.

In normal male adults, basal calcitonin levels range from 3 to 36 pg/mL (0.9 to 10.5 pmol/L). Plasma levels in females range from 3 to 17 pg/mL (0.9 to 5.0 pmol/L). Normal values after pentagastrin stimulation are less than 106 pg/mL (30.9 pmol/L) for males and less than 29 pg/mL (8.5 pmol/L) for females.

Katacalcin, the C-terminal flanking peptide of calcitonin, is a 21–amino acid peptide that is cosecreted with calcitonin in equimolar amounts (136). Its function, however, is unknown. CGRP is a 37–amino acid peptide that is an extremely potent vasodilator and also serves a neuromodulator or neurotransmitter function (150).

STROMA

Lymphocytes

At autopsy or in thyroid glands surgically resected because of a mass, it is not uncommon to observe in the interstitium of the normal portion of the thyroid gland a few collections of lymphocytes, sometimes admixed with rare plasma cells. *Simple chronic thyroiditis* and *focal lymphocytic thyroiditis* are the names given to this process, which is more common

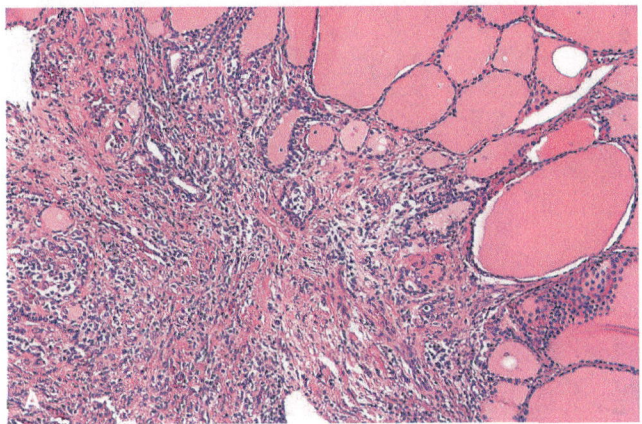
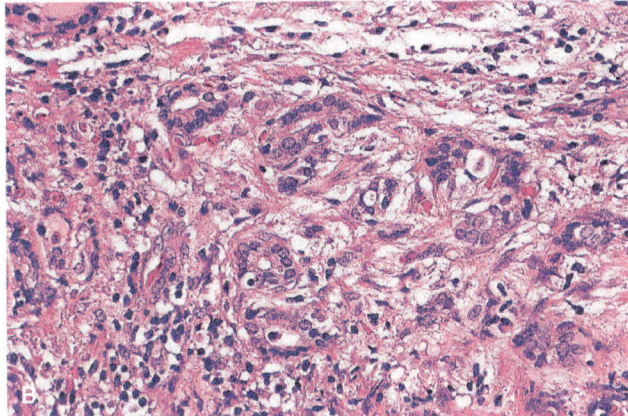

FIGURE 43.13 **A:** Multifocal sclerosing thyroiditis. On low power, the appearance resembles that of a papillary microcarcinoma. **B:** At higher power, the follicles entrapped in the fibrosis are irregularly shaped but do not show any of the cytologic features of papillary carcinoma.

in females and which most likely represents the epiphenomenon of several etiologically different conditions rather than a nosologic entity. Similar changes may in fact be seen in the proximity of neoplasms, in thyroids of patients taking lithium, or in individuals who have received low-dose external radiotherapy (152).

Fibrous Tissue

The usually thin fibrous septa that separate the thyroid lobules may exhibit microscopic variations. In a study on normal thyroids collected at autopsy from young adults, Komorowski and Hanson (32) found that 8% of the thyroid glands showed extensive fibrosis. According to their description, dense and largely acellular collagen fibers divided the thyroid into small nodules, giving it an appearance akin to micronodular cirrhosis of liver.

Another change that may occur in the thyroid interstitium, albeit rarely, is the so-called *multifocal fibrosing (sclerosing) thyroiditis* (153). It is characterized histologically by numerous microscopic of stellate-shaped foci composed of cellular fibroblastic tissue frequently entrapping few thyroid follicles in the center. Even if at low power the individual lesions appear similar to those of papillary microcarcinoma, the epithelial component of such lesions lack the cytoarchitectural features of a papillary neoplasm (Fig. 43.13A,B) (153). Furthermore, the number of lesions in multifocal sclerosing thyroiditis greatly exceeds that seen in the usual case of papillary microcarcinoma. The etiology and pathogenesis of this process are not known. Because of the occasional presence of a papillary microcarcinoma at the edge of one of these lesions has been suggested that multifocal fibrosing thyroiditis may be a precursor of papillary thyroid carcinoma development. However, in a series of PTC associated with multifocal fibrosing thyroiditis, BRAF analysis in the areas of multifocal fibrosing thyroiditis showed that all of the multifocal thyroiditis lesions and normal thyroid tissue were negative for BRAF mutations. The authors concluded that multifocal fibrosing thyroiditis is likely an incidental bystander in the process and a reflection of the background thyroiditis (154).

Adipose Tissue and Skeletal Muscle

Thyroid stroma may undergo adipose metaplasia, resulting in the presence of islands of mature adipose tissue between follicles (Fig. 43.14). Mature fat also occasionally may be seen in proximity to the thyroid gland capsule, its presence in this location most likely resulting from the close relationship of fat and thyroid tissue during fetal life (155). Only exceptionally this will result in a clinically noticeable mass ("localized adiposity"), to be distinguished from lipoadenoma (156).

Other tissues that grow in close proximity to the thyroid gland during their development and that can be found within the capsule of adults are cartilage and striated muscle. In one study, striated muscle was found within the thyroid parenchyma of 19 glands, usually in the region of the isthmus or in the pyramidal lobe of the gland. Conversely, in 10 specimens, thyroid follicles were found within fascicles of strap muscle from the same areas (Fig. 43.15) (32).

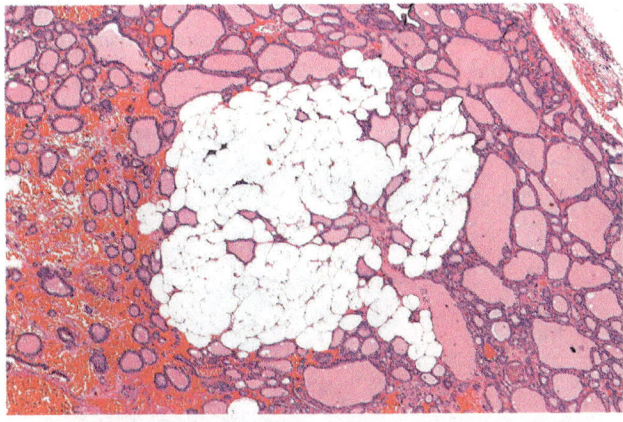

FIGURE 43.14 Adipose metaplasia of thyroid stroma. Mature adipocytes are seen between follicles.

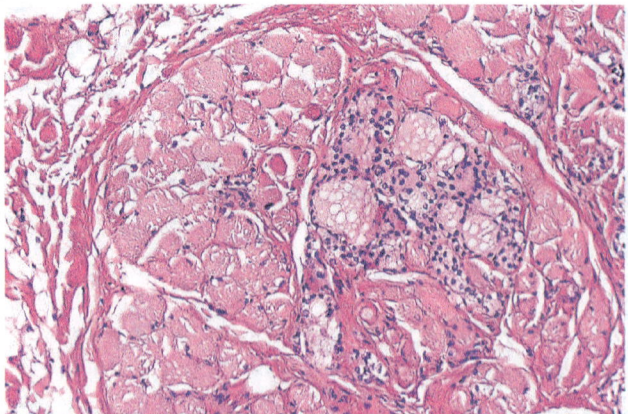

FIGURE 43.15 Clusters of thyroid tissue intimately admixed with bundles of skeletal muscle adjacent to the thyroid gland.

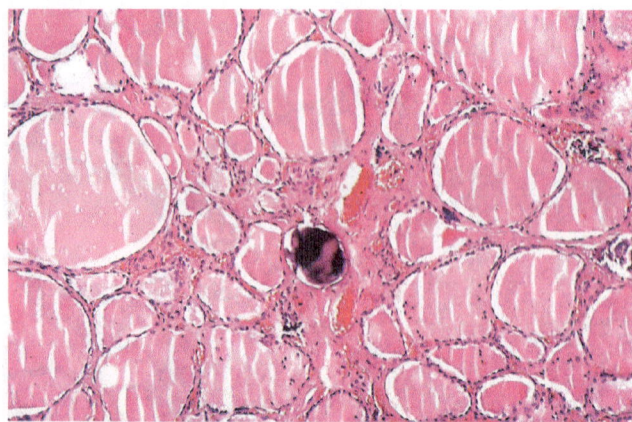

FIGURE 43.17 Psammoma body in nonneoplastic thyroid tissue adjacent to a papillary carcinoma (not shown in the picture).

Pancreatic tissue, a representative of foregut remnants, has been described in the wall of a perithyroidal epithelial cyst by Langlois et al. (157).

Calcifications

Dystrophic calcifications may be seen in normal thyroid of old age, particularly in relation to vessels. They can easily be distinguished from psammoma bodies because of the lack of laminations and the irregularity of their contours (Fig. 43.16).

Psammoma bodies have been described only exceptionally in benign thyroid lesions but even more rarely in normal thyroids (158–160). Therefore finding psammoma bodies in an otherwise normal thyroid or in a cervical lymph node should always prompt a careful search for an occult thyroid papillary carcinoma (Fig. 43.17).

BRANCHIAL POUCH–DERIVED AND OTHER RELATED ECTOPIC TISSUES

Branchial pouch–related structures are found within the thyroid in various forms: *Solid cell nests (rests)* (a remnant of the UBB or branchial pouch complex IV–V), *epithelium-lined cysts, parathyroid glands, thymic tissue, salivary gland–type tissue,* and *heterotopic cartilage.*

The so-called *solid cell nests (rests)* usually considered as the embryonic remnants of the UBB, are clusters of epithelial cells composed of a biphasic cell population that are referred to as "main cells" and "C cells," interspersed among the follicles.

A UBB origin, for what in retrospect are clearly the same formations, had already been suggested by Erdheim in 1904 and Getzowa in 1907, following their demonstration of clusters of epithelial cells with solid or rarely cystic appearance in individuals with thyroid aplasia (161,162). Additional evidence along these lines was provided by the demonstration of marked similarities of human SCNs with the normal UBB of the rat and the hyperplastic or neoplastic UBB remnants in bulls (163–165). SCNs are relatively common in the normal thyroid and can be detected in almost 90% of neonatal thyroid glands; the probability of finding them increasing with the number of sections examined. In one study, SCNs were found in only 3% of routinely examined thyroids but in as many as 61% of specimens when the gland was blocked serially at 2- to 3-mm intervals (166). For unknown reasons SCNs are more common in males than in females. Most SCNs measure an average 0.1 mm in diameter, but occasionally they can reach a large size (Fig. 43.18) (167). They may be single or multiple. They are usually surrounded by stroma and more or less demarcated by the adjacent thyroid follicles. Adipose tissue, cartilage or rarely salivary gland tissue, may be present in their vicinity (Fig. 43.19A–C).

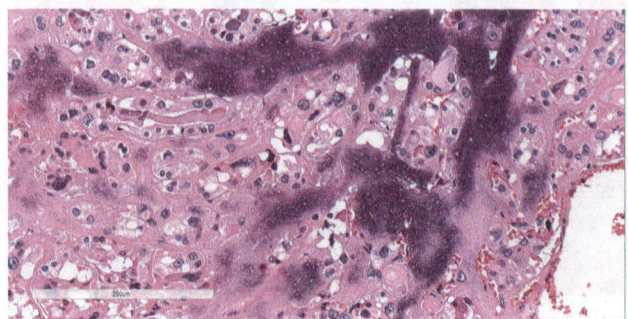

FIGURE 43.16 Dystrophic calcification.

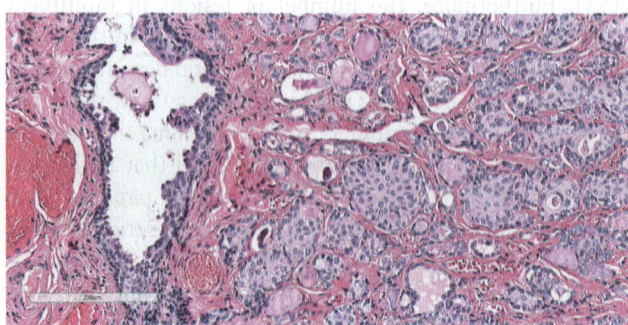

FIGURE 43.18 Hyperplastic solid cell nests adjacent to a cystic structure.

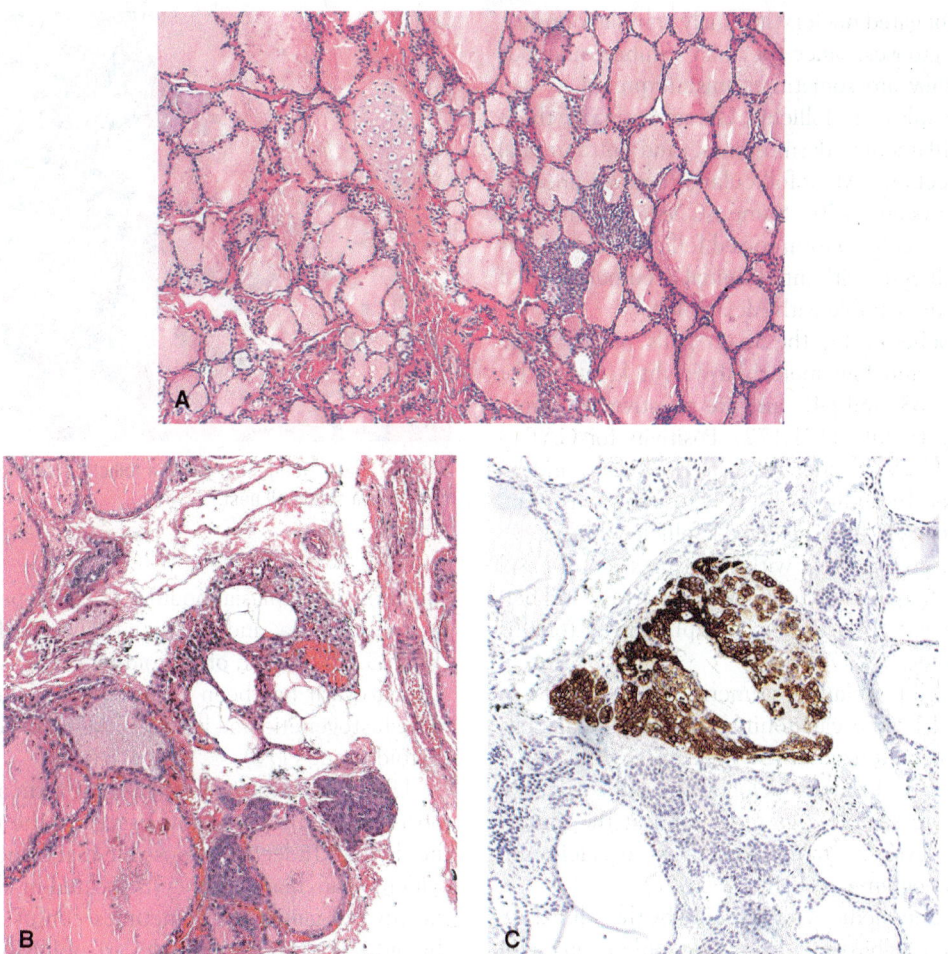

FIGURE 43.19 **A:** Cartilage island is seen in the proximity of solid cell nests. **B:** Solid cell nests with adjacent parathyroid gland. **C:** Strong PTH staining of the parathyroid gland.

Most SCNs are found along the central axis of the middle and upper third of the lateral lobes (i.e., in the same area where C cells usually occur); this constitutes additional proof for their close topographic relationship with the UBB, as it does the fact that the number of C cells is increased in the vicinity of SCNs (168,169). SCNs are often grouped in clusters featuring a multilobed shape on low-power examination within the interstitium of the thyroid gland (Fig. 43.20A). The main component is made up of epithelial cells of polygonal-to-oval shape, with acidophilic

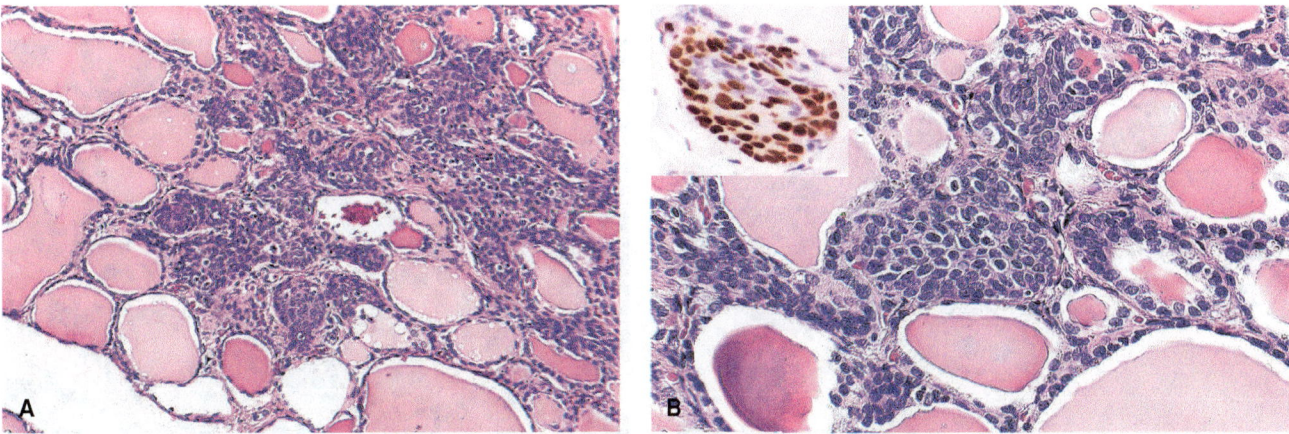

FIGURE 43.20 **A:** Low-power view shows the multilobed shape often exhibited by groups of solid cell nests. **B:** Solid cell nest in normal thyroid. Note the uniform appearance of the epithelial cells. *Inset:* Strong nuclear immunoreactivity for p63.

cytoplasm and elongated nuclei with finely granular chromatin and frequent grooves. Since they may exhibit squamous differentiation, they are sometimes misinterpreted as foci of squamous metaplasia in follicles. Ultrastructurally, these cells have tonofilaments, desmosomes, and intraluminal cytoplasmic projections. Microfollicular structures lined by ciliated cells also occur (170). Some SCNs are connected to thyroid follicular cells to form mixed follicles. The SCNs may contain small cysts with intraluminal accumulations of acidic mucins demonstrable with Alcian blue.

Immunohistochemically, the main cells of SCN are positive for high- and low–molecular-weight keratins, for TTF-1 (SPT24), p63, and p40, and are negative for monoclonal Pax8 (Fig. 43.20B) (171,172). Positivity for GATA3 and monoclonal CEA was identified in 41 (73.2%) and 36 (64.3%) of SCNs. In addition, TTF-1 positivity has been described in rare cells forming mixed follicles (171,173). The positivity for p63 together with the expression of basal cell–type keratins (such as 34betaE12), telomerase and bcl-2, is compatible with a basal/stem cell phenotype for this cellular component (174,175).

The second cell population, numerically less conspicuous, is composed by the calcitonin containing clear cells (22). They are characterized at the light microscopic level by clear cytoplasm and round nuclei, at the ultrastructural level by dense-core secretory granules, and at the immunohistochemical level by immunoreactivity to calcitonin, CGRF, and chromogranin (168,170,173,176).

A variation in the theme is represented by the admixture of SCNs (pure or combined with a cystic component) with groups of small follicles lined by low cuboidal TGB-immunoreactive epithelium, forming the so-called *mixed follicles* (Fig. 43.21). The fact that a similar admixture is seen in mixed medullary–follicular carcinomas has led some investigators to suggest that these rare tumors may arise from uncommitted stem cells of the UBBs that have the potential to differentiate into C cells, follicular cells, or both (177). SCNs need to be distinguished from follicles with

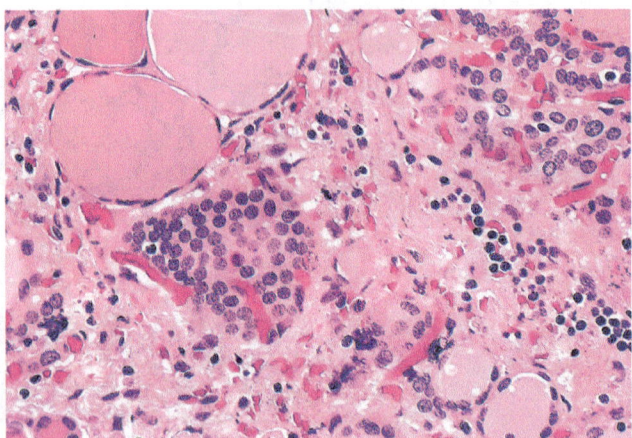

FIGURE 43.22 Tangential cut of a follicle. This should not be misinterpreted as a solid cell nest.

squamous metaplasia, nodular C-cell hyperplasia, papillary microcarcinoma, and tangential sections of normal follicles (Fig. 43.22). A case of thyroid-type SCNs associated with struma ovarii has been reported supporting the idea of a close histogenetic link between the main cells of SCNs and thyroid tissue (178).

UBB remnants may also take the form of cysts occurring most commonly in the soft tissues of the neck adjacent to the thyroid. Indeed, it is possible that some of the clinically evident branchial pouch cysts located in close proximity to the thyroid gland and sometimes confused clinically with thyroid lesions or lymph nodes are of UBB origin. They may also develop within the thyroid itself (171). In the latter instance, they may occur by themselves, may be adjacent to SCNs, or may be intimately admixed with them (Fig. 43.23). These cysts are lined most frequently by a flattened multilayered epithelium of squamous type, and less commonly by a ciliated columnar epithelium and often contain clumps of eosinophilic material in their lumen (Fig. 43.24 A,B). They are especially common in neonates. Cystic UBB remnants

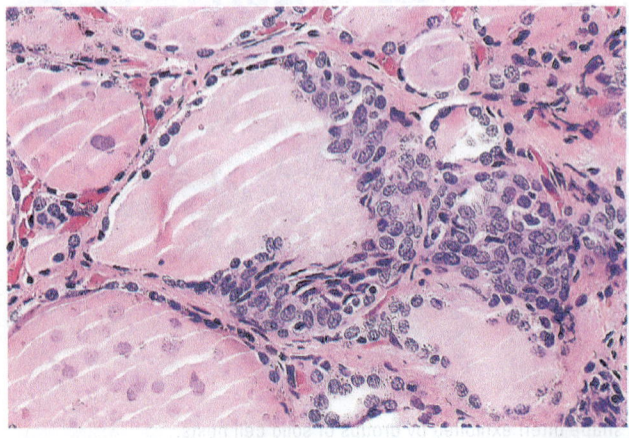

FIGURE 43.21 The so-called mixed follicle. A solid cell nest merges with a follicle lined by a flattened epithelium with colloid in the lumen.

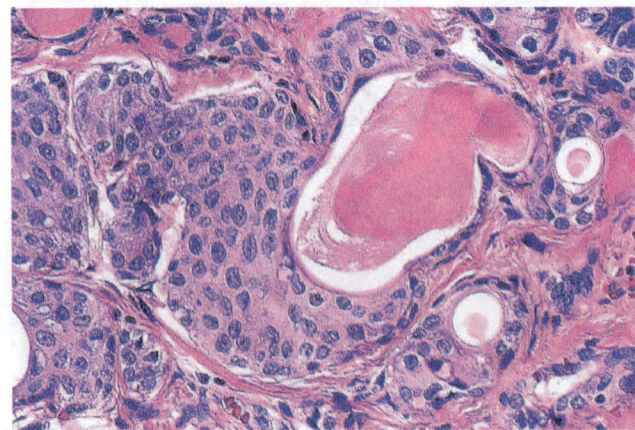

FIGURE 43.23 Solid cell nest with associated cystic formation. A dense eosinophilic material fills the lumen of the cyst.

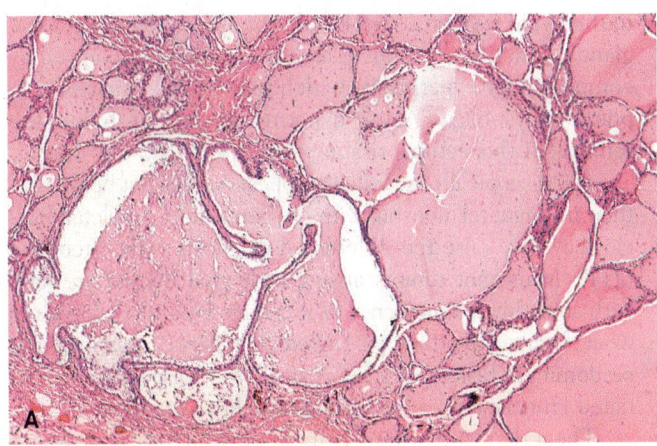
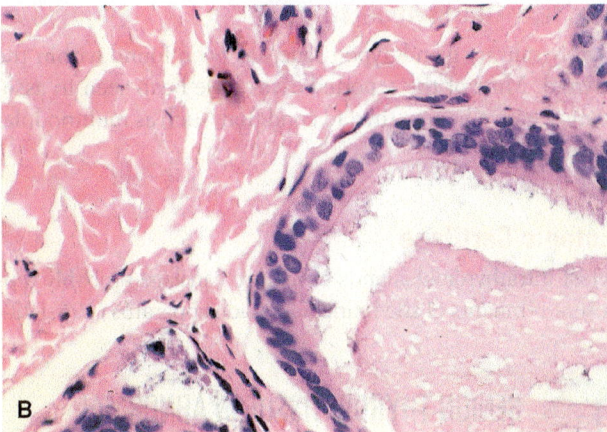

FIGURE 43.24 **A:** Intrathyroidal cyst of probable branchial pouch derivation. **B:** Higher-power view showing ciliated epithelium.

may have an associated lymphoid component (lymphoepithelial cysts) and are more commonly seen in glands with Hashimoto thyroiditis (179–182).

An intrathyroidal branchial cleft-like cyst associated with unusual heterotopic tissues including salivary gland type tissue, fat, and cartilage has been described in a 7-year-old girl. Histologically, the cyst lined by squamous or respiratory-type epithelium was intimately associated with SCN and heterotopic tissues, including seromucinous salivary glands (183).

Parathyroid Tissue

The development of the parathyroid glands and the thymus from the branchial pouches in close proximity to the thyroid gland explains why these organs occasionally may be found adjacent to the thyroid capsule or even within the thyroid itself.

True intrathyroidal parathyroid glands in adults are rare. However, in a study where 58 human fetal thyroid glands obtained at autopsy were systematically studied for the presence of intrathyroidal parathyroid tissue, the latter was found in 13 thyroid lobes from 12 fetuses (22.4%). It was located subcapsularly in 9 of 58 cases (15.5%), and it was lying deep in thyroid tissue in four (68%) (184). These intra- and perithyroidal parathyroid structures can be affected by adenoma, primary or secondary chief cell hyperplasia or carcinoma, and represent an often overlooked cause of surgical failure in primary hyperparathyroidism (185,186).

Thymic Tissue

Most of the thymus derives embryologically from the third branchial pouch, together with the lower pair of parathyroid glands. There is also a small and inconstant portion that derives from the fourth branchial pouch together with the upper pair of parathyroid glands and the UBB, which form the lateral thyroid anlage. It is from the latter source that the islands of thymic tissue occasionally found in or around the thyroid are thought to derive (Fig. 43.25) (187). The fact that ectopic thymic tissue is observed more frequently in neonates and infants supports this hypothesis. Harach and Vujanic searched systematically for the presence of intrathymic tissue in 58 thyroid glands obtained at autopsy from fetuses with proven retrosternal thymus (188). Subcapsular thymic tissue was found in two cases (3.4%) and intrathyroid thymic tissue in one (1.7%). An entire thymic gland within the thyroid of an infant has been described by Neill (189). Damiani et al. found thymic rests in 1.4% of 2,575 adult thyroid glands that they examined (190).

Mizukami et al. reported thymic tissue in the interlobular septum of the thyroid of a patient with Graves disease (191). Ectopic intrathyroidal thymic tissue, with coinciding intrathymic parathyroid tissue, was found incidentally during surgery in 23-year-old female who presented with Graves disease refractory to medical treatment (192).

Ectopic thymic tissue may show cystic changes and present clinically as a cystic neck mass. It may also be the source of peri- and intrathyroidal thymomas (193,194).

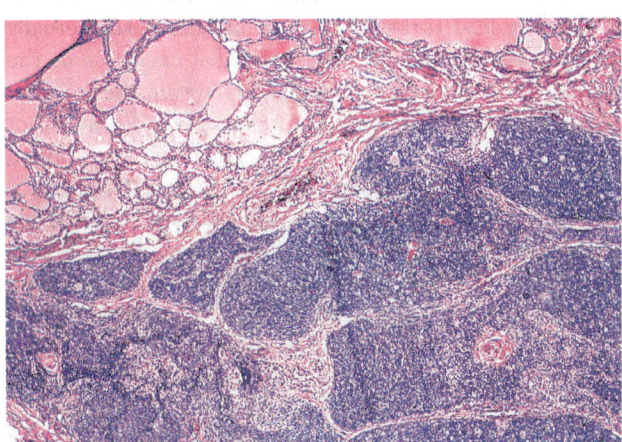

FIGURE 43.25 Intrathyroidal thymic tissue.

Salivary Gland–type Tissue

Rarely salivary gland–type tissue has been found within the thyroid. Most of the reported cases have been seen in association with a benign thyroid condition, such as multinodular goiter (195).

Ectopic Cartilage

Most intrathyroidal islands of mature cartilage probably represent remnants of the branchial pouch apparatus (196,198).

BENIGN THYROID TISSUE IN ABNORMAL LOCATIONS

The presence of nonneoplastic thyroid tissue outside the normal anatomical confines of the gland, and anatomically separate from the thyroid gland may be caused by a variety of mechanisms, ranging from congenital abnormalities to acquired processes. Their main practical interest resides in the fact that lack of knowledge of their occurrence may lead to a mistaken diagnosis of metastatic thyroid carcinoma.

Midline Structures

Most cases of *ectopic thyroid* are derived from abnormalities in migration patterns of the medial anlage and are, therefore, more commonly found in the neck in a midline position, at any point in the normal pathway of descent of the thyroglossal duct from the foramen cecum at the base of the tongue and the normal site of the gland (197–199). The reported estimated frequency of ectopic thyroid is 0.17 per 1,000 patients, with lingual thyroid accounting for 90% of cases (200,201). In most cases the ectopy is partial, clinically insignificant, and discovered accidentally. The most common sites are (1) at the base of the tongue (lingual thyroid), (2) beneath the tongue (sublingual thyroid), and (3) in or around the hyoid bone (as a component of thyroglossal duct cyst).

The opposite phenomenon is represented by exaggerated descent of the median anlage into the mediastinum, which may lead to location of thyroid tissue substernally in the preaortic area, in the pericardial cavity, or in the substance of the heart (202–204). However, the majority of mediastinal goiters represent a dislocation downward of originally orthotopic (cervical) glands that have been pulled down by the hyperplastic changes that occurred in them.

Lingual thyroid is unusual as a clinical issue but relatively common as an incidental microscopic finding. In one series, almost 10% of tongues examined at autopsy had remnants of thyroid tissue in them (205). When of large size they may cause dysphagia, bleeding, and dyspnea (199,206). In most instances, the diagnosis is made during adolescence, and a preponderance in women has been noted (205,207). In over 75% of the cases, the migration failure is complete and thyroid tissue, absent in the normal location may be found in the hyoid region (208–210). In this condition the ectopic glands, functionally inadequate, are frequently followed by compensatory hyperplasia, which may be the cause of dyspnea or dysphagia. Acute hypothyroidism may follow the removal of this ectopic tissue.

Microscopically the follicles appear normal but because of their intimate relationship with the surrounding skeletal muscle they may raise the differential diagnosis with carcinoma (211). Malignant tumors arising in lingual thyroid are rare, with an estimated incidence of less than 1% and analogous to what observed in orthotopic thyroid. Papillary carcinoma is the predominant histotype (212). A single case of poorly differentiated Hurthle cell carcinoma has also been reported (213).

The other site where ectopic thyroid tissue is found commonly is the wall of *thyroglossal duct cysts*. It appears in the form of small group of follicles and is present in 25% to 65% of cysts examined histologically, its frequency being related to the number of sections submitted for histologic examination (214). The medial location and the presence of thyroid tissue in the wall distinguish thyroglossal duct cysts from the rarer bronchial pouch cysts.

Thyroglossal cyst is the most common congenital anomaly in the neck region. Most patients present with painless mass in the midline of the neck, only rarely accompanied by dysphagia or dyspnea. Being the thyroglossal duct cyst practically always connected with the hyoid bone upward movement of the mass on swallowing is characteristic of this condition (215). Most cysts measure from 1 to 2 cm in diameter. The original lining epithelium of the duct, cuboidal ("transitional") or columnar and often ciliated tends to become squamous or to disappear as a result of secondary inflammatory changes (216). Immunoreactivity for TTF-1 (but not TGB) has been described in the lining epithelium (217). Ectopic thyroid tissue is found commonly is the wall of *thyroglossal duct cysts*. It appears in the form of irregular small groups of follicles and is present in 25% to 65% of cysts examined histologically, its frequency being related to the number of sections submitted for histologic examination (214).

This tissue may have a normal appearance, or it may exhibit inflammatory and hyperplastic nodular changes. It may also be the site of a malignancy. Nearly all of the reported cases have been PTC but there are also scattered reports of other tumor types, including follicular carcinoma and undifferentiated/squamous carcinoma (214,218–221).

The medial location and the presence of thyroid tissue in the wall distinguish thyroglossal duct cysts from the rarer branchial pouch cysts. Ectopic thyroid derived from abnormalities in migration of the medial anlage typically does not contain C cells. In one study of median anlage anomalies including 23 cases of thyroglossal cysts with adjacent thyroid tissue and one case of lingual thyroid, not a single C cell was found in either the thyroid tissue or the epithelium lining the cysts (222).

The treatment of thyroglossal duct cyst includes the removal of the middle third of the hyoid bone and the suprahyoid tract up to the foramen cecum (223).

It should be emphasized here that all instances of ectopic thyroid related to the thyroglossal duct appear as midline lesions, in keeping with the path of descent of this embryologic structure (see above). Thyroid tissue located laterally in the neck may still be of benign nature (parasitic nodules) but cannot be ascribed to the developmental abnormality discussed here.

Pericapsular Soft Tissues and Skeletal Muscle

The presence of thyroid tissue in these locations is not a rare event. It most likely results from the intimate relationship of the thyroid gland with the mesodermal structures of the neck during development.

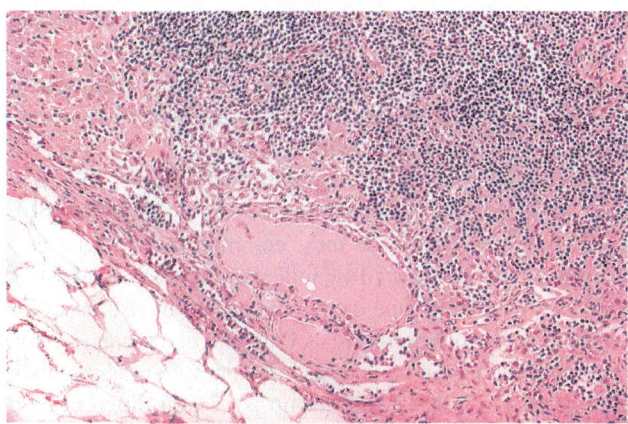

FIGURE 43.26 A group of benign-appearing thyroid follicles is seen close to the marginal sinus of a cervical lymph node. The patient did not have a carcinoma in the thyroid gland.

Lateral Neck

This phenomenon, frequently referred in the past as *lateral aberrant thyroid*, has different pathogeneses. It has been suggested that surgery and trauma may cause implantation of thyroid tissue in the lateral neck. Typically when this is the case, a few nodules of normal-appearing thyroid tissue, always of microscopic size and frequently surrounded by a fibrous capsule, are seen in the lateral neck close to the cervical lymph nodes (224–226). History of previous trauma or surgery on the neck, the presence of suture material (in cases of previous surgery), and the benign appearance of the dislocated thyroid tissue are useful in distinguishing them from metastatic carcinoma. It should be kept in mind that the latter may appear deceptively benign on microscopic examination. Spontaneous separation of thyroid tissue with subsequent implant in the lateral neck may occur in nodular goiter or Hashimoto thyroiditis (227,228). In both of these conditions, nodules of thyroid tissue extrude and separate from the surface of the gland and deposit in the extrathyroidal soft tissue, where they may acquire an autonomous blood supply (the so-called *parasitic nodules*). The differential diagnosis with metastatic lymph nodes may be very problematic, especially in the presence of Hashimoto thyroiditis.

Thyroid Inclusions in Cervical Lymph Nodes

Normal-appearing thyroid tissue in medially located cervical lymph nodes is rarely the result of a developmental anomaly (229). When this is the case, a few small follicles located immediately beneath the nodal capsule are seen (Fig. 43.26). The follicular cells that compose them should lack all the cytologic features typical of papillary carcinoma (230). Psammoma bodies and papillae should also be absent. Numerous sections are sometimes needed to rule out a metastasis from a papillary microcarcinoma, which is by far the most frequent cause of thyroid tissue in cervical nodes and may actually presents in a cervical node in the absence of an obvious thyroid nodule. Furthermore the microscopic appearance of metastasis may closely resemble nonneoplastic thyroid tissue. The criteria for diagnosing benign thyroid inclusions need to be very rigorous, to wit: cases in which the involvement includes the nodal parenchyma (as opposed to the capsular/subcapsular region); cases in which the thyroid tissue has replaced one third or more of the node; cases in which several nodes are affected, the diagnosis of metastasis should be preferred. This is also true whenever the intranodal thyroid tissue shows any of the cytoarchitectural features of papillary carcinoma (e.g., abortive papillae or ground-glass nuclei) or psammoma bodies are present. In doubtful cases, molecular analysis—especially for BRAF—can be of help. Immunostains for CK19, HBME-1, and galectin-3 could support a diagnosis of papillary carcinoma if positive.

Well-documented examples of ectopic benign tissue in lymph nodes include salivary gland, müllerian epithelium ("endosalpingiosis"), breast, nevus cells, and mesothelial cells.

Other Sites

Rarely, one can find thyroid tissue in other locations outside its place of embryonic development and occasionally quite distantly from it.

These locations include larynx (231), trachea (232), submandibular region (233), aortic arch (234), heart and pericardium (235), lung (236,237), mediastinal esophagus (238), stomach, duodenum (239,240), diaphragm, region of gallbladder/common bile duct/porta hepatis (241–243), pancreas (244,245), liver (246), spleen (247), adrenal gland (248), retroperitoneum (249), vagina (250), uterus (251), and sella turcica (252).

In the ovary, thyroid tissue represents a relatively common component of a teratoma, whereas it is very rare to find thyroid tissue in testicular or extragonadal teratomas. Sometimes the thyroid tissue is the predominant component or is the only teratoma component, the latter interpreted as a monodermal form of teratoma and designated as *struma ovarii* (253). The thyroid tissue may be normal or show diffuse or nodular hyperplastic changes which rarely can cause hyperthyroidism. The tumor cells should show immunohistochemical expression of TGB and TTF-1.

Malignant neoplasms composed of thyroid follicular cells developing in struma ovarii are rare (252,254–256). Papillary carcinoma is the most common thyroid type carcinoma to occur followed by follicular carcinoma. Most of the cases of thyroid type carcinoma arising in struma ovarii reported in the old literature as follicular carcinomas, using current criteria would qualify as follicular variant of papillary carcinoma (257,258). The diagnosis of well-differentiated thyroid-type follicular carcinoma because of the absence of a capsule in the follicular ovarian lesions is difficult to make. Identification of invasion into the surrounding ovarian tissue, vascular invasion, or metastasis is employed as evidence of malignancy. The less-differentiated forms show significant architectural abnormalities, nuclear atypia, and mitotic activity. The outcome of histologically and biologically malignant thyroid-type tumors in struma ovarii is overall favorable with only a small number of patients dying of disease (256,257,259–261). An unresolved issue concerns cases of struma ovarii associated with peritoneal implants, histologically resembling nonneoplastic thyroid tissue, which can be very extensive. This entity, considered benign strumosis in the past has been designated "highly differentiated follicular carcinomas" (262,263). In carcinomas arising in struma ovarii have been described the same molecular alterations, *BRAF* mutations and *RET/PTC* rearrangements, typical of orthotopic thyroid tumors (264,265).

REFERENCES

1. Hoyes AD, Kershaw DR. Anatomy and development of the thyroid gland. *Ear Nose Throat J* 1985;64:318–333.
2. Shepard TH. Onset of function in the human fetal thyroid: Biochemical and radioautographic studies from organ culture. *J Clin Endocrinol Metab* 1967;27:945–958.
3. Gitlin D, Biasucci A. Ontogenesis of immunoreactive thyroglobulin in the human conceptus. *J Clin Endocrinol Metab* 1969;29:849–853.
4. Fagman H, Nilsson M. Morphogenesis of the thyroid gland. *Mol Cell Endocrinol* 2010;323:35–54.
5. Nilsson M, Fagman H. Mechanisms of thyroid development and dysgenesis: An analysis based on developmental stages and concurrent embryonic anatomy. *Curr Top Dev Biol* 2013;106:123–170.
6. Trueba SS, Auge J, Mattei G, et al. PAX8, TITF1, and FOXE1 gene expression patterns during human development: New insights into human thyroid development and thyroid dysgenesis-associated malformations. *J Clin Endocrinol Metab* 2005;90:455–462.
7. Fernandez LP, Lopez-Marquez A, Santisteban P. Thyroid transcription factors in development, differentiation and disease. *Nat Rev Endocrinol* 2015;11:29–42.
8. Fernandez LP, Lopez-Marquez A, Gomez-Lopez G, et al. New insights into FoxE1 functions: Identification of direct FoxE1 targets in thyroid cells. *PLoS ONE* 2013;8:e62849.
9. Parlato R, Rosica A, Rodriguez-Mallon A, et al. An integrated regulatory network controlling survival and migration in thyroid organogenesis. *Dev Biol* 2004;276:464–475.
10. Meeus L, Gilbert B, Rydlewski C, et al. Characterization of a novel loss of function mutation of PAX8 in a familial case of congenital hypothyroidism with in-place, normal-sized thyroid. *J Clin Endocrinol Metab* 2004;89:4285–4291.
11. De Felice M, Di Lauro R. Thyroid development and its disorders: Genetics and molecular mechanisms. *Endocr Rev* 2004;25:722–746.
12. Nilsson M, Fagman H. Development of the thyroid gland. *Development* 2017;144:2123–2140.
13. Pasca di Magliano M, Di Lauro R, Zannini M. Pax8 has a key role in thyroid cell differentiation. *Proc Natl Acad Sci U S A* 2000;97:13144–13149.
14. Lau SK, Luthringer DJ, Eisen RN. Thyroid transcription factor-1: A review. *Appl Immunohistochem Mol Morphol* 2002;10:97–102.
15. Volante M, Allia E, Fulcheri E, et al. Ghrelin in fetal thyroid and follicular tumors and cell lines: Expression and effects on tumor growth. *Am J Pathol* 2003;162:645–654.
16. Savin SB, Cvejic DS, Jankovic MM. Expression of galectin-1 and galectin-3 in human fetal thyroid gland. *J Histochem Cytochem* 2003;51:479–483.
17. Norris EH. The parathyroid glands and the lateral thyroid in man: Their morphogenesis, histogenesis, topographic anatomy and prenatal growth. *Contrib Embryol Carnegie Inst* 1937;159:249–294.
18. Sugiyama S. The embryology of the human thyroid gland including ultimobranchial body and others related. *Ergeb Anat Entwicklungsgesch* 1971;44:3–111.
19. Pearse AG, Polak JM. Cytochemical evidence for the neural crest origin of mammalian ultimobranchial C cells. *Histochemie*. 1971;27:96–102.
20. Le Douarin NM, Teillet MA. The migration of neural crest cells to the wall of the digestive tract in avian embryo. *J Embryol Exp Morphol* 1973;30:31–48.
21. Le Douarin N, Fontaine J, Le Lievre C. New studies on the neural crest origin of the avian ultimobranchial glandular cells—interspecific combinations and cytochemical characterization of C cells based on the uptake of biogenic amine precursors. *Histochemistry* 1974;38:297–305.
22. Nadig J, Weber E, Hedinger C. C-cell in vestiges of the ultimobranchial body in human thyroid glands. *Virchows Arch B Cell Pathol* 1978;27:189–191.
23. Ito M, Kameda Y, Tagawa T. An ultrastructural study of the cysts in chicken ultimobranchial glands, with special reference to C-cells. *Cell Tissue Res* 1986;246:39–44.
24. Kameda Y, Nishimaki T, Chisaka O, et al. Expression of the epithelial marker E-cadherin by thyroid C cells and their precursors during murine development. *J Histochem Cytochem* 2007;55:1075–1088.
25. Johansson E, Andersson L, Örnros J et al. Revising the embryonic origin of thyroid C cells in mice and humans. *Development* 2015;142:3519–3528.
26. Schmid KW. Histopathology of C Cells and medullary thyroid carcinoma. *Recent Results Cancer Res* 2015;204:41–60.

27. Kameda Y. Cellular and molecular events on the development of mammalian thyroid C cells. *Dev Dyn* 2016;245:323–341.
28. Nilsson M, Williams D. On the origin of cells and derivation of thyroid cancer: C cell story revisited. *Eur Thyroid J* 2016;5:79–93.
29. Andersson L, Westerlund J, Liang S, et al. Role of EphA4 receptor signaling in thyroid development: Regulation of folliculogenesis and propagation of the C-cell lineage. *Endocrinology* 2011;152:1154–1164.
30. Hegedus L, Perrild H, Poulsen LR, et al. The determination of thyroid volume by ultrasound and its relationship to body weight, age, and sex in normal subjects. *J Clin Endocrinol Metab* 1983;56:260–263.
31. Hegedus L, Karstrup S, Rasmussen N. Evidence of cyclic alterations of thyroid size during the menstrual cycle in healthy women. *Am J Obstet Gynecol* 1986;155:142–145.
32. Komorowski RA, Hanson GA. Occult thyroid pathology in the young adult: An autopsy study of 138 patients without clinical thyroid disease. *Hum Pathol* 1988;19:689–696.
33. Bell CD, Kovacs K, Horvath E, et al. Histologic, immunohistochemical, and ultrastructural findings in a case of minocycline-associated "black thyroid." *Endocr Pathol* 2001;12:443–451.
34. Veinot JP, Ghadially FN. Melanosis thyroidi. *Ultrastruct Pathol* 1998;22:401–406.
35. Kandil E, Khalek MA, Ibrahim WG, et al. Papillary thyroid carcinoma in black thyroids. *Head Neck* 2011;33:1735–1738.
36. Bann DV, Goyal N, Crist H, et al. Black thyroid. *Ear Nose Throat J* 2014;93:E54–E55.
37. Thompson AD, Pasieka JL, Kneafsey P, et al. Hypopigmentation of a papillary carcinoma arising in a black thyroid. *Mod Pathol* 1999;12:1181–1185.
38. Brown RA, Al-Moussa M, Beck J. Histometry of normal thyroid in man. *J Clin Pathol* 1986;39:475–482.
39. Imada M, Kurosumi M, Fujita H. Three-dimensional imaging of blood vessels in thyroids from normal and levothyroxine sodium-treated rats. *Arch Histol Jpn* 1986;49:359–367.
40. Imada M, Kurosumi M, Fujita H. Three-dimensional aspects of blood vessels in thyroids from normal, low iodine diet-treated, TSH-treated and PTU-treated rats. *Cell Tissue Res* 1986;245:291–296.
41. Drut R, Altamirano E, Ollano AM. Lymphatic vessels in the thyroid gland of children. *Rev Esp Patol* 2009;42:159–160.
42. Russell WO, Ibanez ML, Clark RL, et al. Thyroid carcinoma. Classification, intraglandular dissemination, and clinicopathological study based upon whole organ sections of 80 glands. *Cancer* 1963;16:1425–1460.
43. Feind C. The head and neck. In: Haagensen CD, Feind C, Herter FP, et al., eds. *The Lymphatics in Cancer*. Philadelphia, PA: WB Saunders; 1972:59–222.
44. Crile G Jr. The fallacy of the conventional radical neck dissection for papillary carcinoma of the thyroid. *Ann Surg* 1957;145:317–320.
45. Yanir Y, Doweck I. Regional metastases in well-differentiated thyroid carcinoma: Pattern of spread. *Laryngoscope* 2008;118:433–436.
46. Uchiyama Y, Murakami G, Ohno Y. The fine structure of nerve endings on rat thyroid follicular cells. *Cell Tissue Res* 1985;242:457–460.
47. Melander A, Ericson LD, Sundler F, et al. Sympathetic innervation of the mouse thyroid and its significance in thyroid hormone secretion. *Endocrinology* 1974;94:959–966.
48. Tice LW, Creveling CR. Electron microscopic identification of adrenergic nerve endings on thyroid epithelial cells. *Endocrinology* 1975;97:1123–1129.
49. Ingbar SH. The thyroid gland. In: Wilson JD, Foster DW, eds. *Williams Textbook of Endocrinology*. 7th ed. Philadelphia, PA: WB Saunders; 1985:682–815.
50. Kameda Y, Okamoto K, Ito M, et al. Innervation of the C cells of chicken ultimobranchial glands studied by immunohistochemistry, fluorescence microscopy, and electron microscopy. *Am J Anat* 1988;182:353–368.
51. Zak FG, Lawson W. Glomic (paraganglionic) tissue in the larynx and capsule of the thyroid gland. *Mt Sinai J Med* 1972;39:82–90.
52. LaGuette J, Matias-Guiu X, Rosai J. Thyroid paraganglioma: A clinicopathologic and immunohistochemical study of three cases. *Am J Surg Pathol* 1997;21:748–753.
53. Lee SM, Policarpio-Nicolas ML. Thyroid Paraganglioma. *Arch Pathol Lab Med* 2015;139:1062–1067.
54. Heimann P. Ultrastructure of human thyroid. A study of normal thyroid, untreated and treated diffuse goiter. *Acta Endocrinol (Copenh)* 1966;53(suppl 110):1–102.
55. Klinck GH, Oertel JE, Winship T. Ultrastructure of normal human thyroid. *Lab Invest* 1970;22:2–22.
56. Kurata A, Ohta K, Mine M, et al. Monoclonal antihuman thyroglobulin antibodies. *J Clin Endocrinol Metab* 1984;59:573–579.
57. Stanta G, Carcangiu ML, Rosai J. The biochemical and immunohistochemical profile of thyroid neoplasia. *Pathol Annu* 1988;23(Pt 1):129–157.
58. Rosai J, Carcangiu ML. Pitfalls in the diagnosis of thyroid neoplasms. *Pathol Res Pract* 1987;182:169–179.
59. Katoh R, Kawaoi A, Miyagi E, et al. Thyroid transcription factor-1 in normal, hyperplastic, and neoplastic follicular thyroid cells examined by immunohistochemistry and nonradioactive in situ hybridization. *Mod Pathol* 2000;13:570–576.
60. Henzen-Logmans SC, Mullink H, Ramaekers FC, et al. Expression of cytokeratins and vimentin in epithelial cells of normal and pathologic thyroid tissue. *Virchows Arch A Pathol Anat Histopathol* 1987;410:347–354.
61. Fonseca E, Nesland JM, Hoie J, et al. Pattern of expression of intermediate cytokeratin filaments in the thyroid gland: An immunohistochemical study of simple and stratified epithelial-type cytokeratins. *Virchows Arch* 1997;430:239–245.
62. Coclet J, Lamy F, Rickaert F, et al. Intermediate filaments in normal thyrocytes: Modulation of vimentin expression in primary cultures. *Mol Cell Endocrinol* 1991;76:135–148.
63. Viale G, Dell'Orto P, Coggi G, et al. Coexpression of cytokeratins and vimentin in normal and diseased thyroid glands. Lack of diagnostic utility of vimentin immunostaining. *Am J Surg Pathol* 1989;13:1034–1040.
64. Xu XC, El-Naggar AK, Lotan R. Differential expression of galectin-1 and galectin-3 in thyroid tumors. Potential diagnostic implications. *Am J Pathol* 1995;147:815–822.
65. Herrmann ME, LiVolsi VA, Pasha TL, et al. Immunohistochemical expression of galectin-3 in benign and malignant thyroid lesions. *Arch Pathol Lab Med* 2002;126:710–713.

66. Bur M, Shiraki W, Masood S. Estrogen and progesterone receptor detection in neoplastic and non-neoplastic thyroid tissues. *Mod Pathol* 1993;6:469–472.
67. Kawabata W, Suzuki T, Moriya T, et al. Estrogen receptors (alpha and beta) and 17beta-hydroxysteroid dehydrogenase type 1 and 2 in thyroid disorders: Possible in situ estrogen synthesis and actions. *Mod Pathol* 2003;16:437–444.
68. Nishimura R, Yokose T, Mukai K. S-100 protein is a differentiation marker in thyroid carcinoma of follicular cell origin: An immunohistochemical study. *Pathol Int* 1997;47:673–679.
69. Tzelepi VN, Tsamandas AC, Vlotinou HD, et al. Tight junctions in thyroid carcinogenesis: Diverse expression of claudin-1, claudin-4, claudin-7 and occludin in thyroid neoplasms. *Mod Pathol* 2008;21:22–30.
70. Westermark K, Lundqvist M, Wallin G. EGF-receptors in human normal and pathological thyroid tissue. *Histopathology* 1996;28:221–227.
71. Lima MA, Gontijo VA, Schmitt FC. Thyroid peroxidase and thyroglobulin expression in normal human thyroid glands. *Endocr Pathol* 1998;9:333–338.
72. Lin JD, Hsueh C, Chao TC, et al. Expression of sodium iodide symporter in benign and malignant human thyroid tissues. *Endocr Pathol* 2001;12:15–21.
73. Ringel MD, Anderson J, Souza SL, et al. Expression of the sodium iodide symporter and thyroglobulin genes are reduced in papillary thyroid cancer. *Mod Pathol* 2001;14:289–296.
74. Maruyama M, Kato R, Kobayashi S, et al. A method to differentiate between thyroglobulin derived from normal thyroid tissue and from thyroid carcinoma based on analysis of reactivity to lectins. *Arch Pathol Lab Med* 1998;122:715–720.
75. de Martynoff G, Pohl V, Mercken L, et al. Structural organization of the bovine thyroglobulin gene and of its 5′-flanking region. *Eur J Biochem* 1987;164:591–599.
76. Christophe D, Gerard C, Juvenal G, et al. Identification of a cAMP-responsive region in thyroglobulin gene promoter. *Mol Cell Endocrinol* 1989;64:5–18.
77. Lee NT, Nayfeh SN, Chae CB. Induction of nuclear protein factors specific for hormone-responsive region during activation of thyroglobulin gene by thyrotropin in rat thyroid FRTL-5 cells. *J Biol Chem* 1989;264:7523–7530.
78. Deiss WP, Peake RL. The mechanism of thyroid hormone secretion. *Ann Intern Med* 1968;69:881–90.
79. Brent GA. Mechanisms of thyroid hormone action. *J Clin Invest* 2012;122:3035–3043.
80. Liddle GW, Liddle RA. Endocrinology. In: Smith LH, Thier SO, eds. *Pathophysiology: The Biological Principles of Disease*. Philadelphia, PA: WB Saunders; 1981.
81. Sterling K. Thyroid hormone action at the cell level (first of two parts). *N Engl J Med* 1979;300:117–123.
82. Bernal J, Liewendahl K, Lamberg BA. Thyroid hormone receptors in fetal and hormone resistant tissues. *Scand J Clin lab Invest* 1985;45:577–583.
83. Müller MJ, Seitz HJ. Thyroid hormone action on intermediary metabolism. Part I. Respiration, thermogenesis and carbohydrate metabolism. *Klin Wochenschr* 1984;62:11–18.
84. Müller MJ, Seitz HJ. Thyroid hormone action on intermediary metabolism. II. Lipid metabolism in hyper- and hypothyroidism. *Klin Wochenschr* 1984;62:49–55.
85. Müller MJ, Seitz HJ. Thyroid hormone action on intermediary metabolism. Part III. Protein metabolism in hyper- and hypothyroidism. *Klin Wochenschr* 1984;62:97–102.
86. Oppenheimer JH. Thyroid hormone action at the nuclear level. *Ann Intern Med* 1985;102:374–384.
87. Oppenheimer JH, Samuels HH, eds. *Molecular Basis of Thyroid Hormone Action*. New York: Academic Press; 1983.
88. Larsen PR. Thyroid–pituitary interaction: Feedback regulation of thyrotropin secretion by thyroid hormones. *N Engl J Med* 1982;306:23–32.
89. Davies T, Marians R, Latif R. The TSH receptor reveals itself. *J Clin Invest* 2002;110:161–164.
90. Atassi MZ, Manshouri T, Sakata S. Localization and synthesis of the hormone-binding regions of the human thyrotropin receptor. *Proc Natl Acad Sci USA* 1991;88:3613–3617.
91. Pittman JA Jr. Thyrotropin-releasing hormone. *Adv Intern Med* 1974;19:303–325.
92. Wilber JF. Thyrotropin releasing hormone: Secretion and actions. *Annu Rev Med* 1973;24:353–364.
93. Walsh FM, Castelli JB. Polytef granuloma clinically simulating carcinoma of the thyroid. *Arch Otolaryngol* 1975;101:262–263.
94. Sanfilippo F, Shelburne J, Ingram P. Analysis of a polytef granuloma mimicking a cold thyroid nodule 17 months after laryngeal injection. *Ultrastruct Pathol* 1980;1:471–475.
95. Chaplin AJ. Histopathological occurrence and characterization of calcium oxalate: A review. *J Clin Pathol* 1977;30:800–811.
96. Carney JA, Moore SB, Northcutt RC, et al. Palpation thyroiditis (multifocal granulomatous folliculitis). *Am J Clin Pathol* 1975;64:639–647.
97. Blum M, Schloss MF. Martial-arts thyroiditis. *N Engl J Med* 1984;311:199–200.
98. Harach R, Jasani B. Thyroid multifocal granulomatous folliculitis (palpation thyroiditis): An immunocytochemical study. *Endocr Pathol* 1993;4:105–109.
99. Hellwig CA. Colloidophagy in the human thyroid gland. *Science* 1951;113:725–726.
100. Manson C, Cross P, De Sousa B. Post-operative necrotizing granulomas of the thyroid. *Histopathology* 1992;21:392–393.
101. Harach HR. Palpation thyroiditis resembling C cell hyperplasia. Usefulness of immunohistochemistry in their differential diagnosis. *Pathol Res Pract* 1993;189:488–490.
102. Richter MN, McCarty KS. Anisotropic crystals in the human thyroid gland. *Am J Pathol* 1954;30:545–553.
103. Katoh R, Suzuki K, Hemmi A, et al. Nature and significance of calcium oxalate crystals in normal human thyroid gland. A clinicopathological and immunohistochemical study. *Virchows Arch A Pathol Anat Histopathol* 1993;422:301–306.
104. Reid JD, Choi CH, Oldroyd NO. Calcium oxalate crystals in the thyroid. Their identification, prevalence, origin, and possible significance. *Am J Clin Pathol* 1987;87:443–454.
105. Gross S. Granulomatous thyroiditis with anisotropic crystalline material. *Arch Pathol* 1955;59:412–418.
106. Fayemi AO, Ali M, Braun EV. Oxalosis in hemodialysis patients: A pathologic study of 80 cases. *Arch Pathol Lab Med* 1979;103:58–62.
107. Isotalo PA, Lloyd RV. Presence of birefringent crystals is useful in distinguishing thyroid from parathyroid gland tissues. *Am J Surg Pathol* 2002;26:813–814.
108. Wong KS, Lewis JS Jr, Gottipati S, Chernock RD. Utility of birefringent crystal identification by polarized light microscopy in distinguishing thyroid from parathyroid tissue on intraoperative frozen sections. *Am J Surg Pathol*. 2014;38:1212–1219.

109. Klinck G, Menk K. Squamous cells in the human thyroid. *Mil Surgeon* 1951;109:406–414.
110. Harcourt-Webster JN. Squamous epithelium in the human thyroid gland. *J Clin Pathol* 1966;19:384–388.
111. LiVolsi VA, Merino MJ. Squamous cells in the human thyroid gland. *Am J Surg Pathol* 1978;2:133–140.
112. Pellicer DL, Sadow PM, Stephen A, Faquin WC. Atypical squamous metaplasia in a benign cystic thyroid nodule mimicking high-grade carcinoma. *Diagn Cytopathol*. 2013;4:706–709.
113. Pearse AG. The cytochemistry of the thyroid C cells and their relationship to calcitonin. *Proc R Soc Lond B Biol Sci* 1966;164:478–487.
114. Teitlebaum SL, Moore KE, Shieber W. Parafollicular cells in the normal human thyroid. *Nature* 1971;230:334–335.
115. Wolfe HJ, DeLellis RA, Voelkel EF, et al. Distribution of calcitonin-containing cells in the normal neonatal human thyroid gland: A correlation of morphology with peptide content. *J Clin Endocrinol Metab* 1975;41:1076–1081.
116. O'Toole K, Fenoglio-Preiser C, Pushparaj N. Endocrine changes associated with the human aging process. III. Effect of age on the number of calcitonin immunoreactive cells in the thyroid gland. *Hum Pathol* 1985;16:991–1000.
117. Gibson WCH, Peng TC, Croker BP. Age-associated C-cell hyperplasia in the human thyroid. *Am J Pathol* 1982;106:388–393.
118. Guyétant S, Wion-Barbot N, Rousselet M-C, et al. C-cell hyperplasia associated with chronic lymphocytic thyroiditis: A retrospective quantitative study of 112 cases. *Hum Pathol* 1994;25:514–521.
119. Scopsi L, Di Palma S, Ferrari C, et al. C-cell hyperplasia accompanying thyroid diseases other than medullary carcinoma: An immunocytochemical study by means of antibodies to calcitonin and somatostatin. *Mod Pathol* 1991;4:297–304.
120. Libbey NP, Nowakowski KJ, Tucci JR. C-cell hyperplasia of the thyroid in a patient with goitrous hypothyroidism and Hashimoto's thyroiditis. *Am J Surg Pathol* 1989;13:71–77.
121. Biddinger PW, Brennan MF, Rosen PP. Symptomatic C-cell hyperplasia associated with chronic lymphocytic thyroiditis. *Am J Surg Pathol* 1991;15:599–604.
122. Tomita T, Millard DM. C-cell hyperplasia in secondary hyperparathyroidism. *Histopathology* 1992;21:469–474.
123. Zambrano E, Holm F, Glickman J et al. Abnormal distribution and hyperplasia of thyroid C-cells in PTEN associated tumor syndromes. *Endocr Pathol* 2004;15:55–64.
124. Saggiorato E, Rapa I, Garino F et al. Absence of RET gene point mutations in sporadic thyroid C-cell hyperplasia. *J Mol Diagn* 2007;9:214–219.
125. Perry A, Molberg K, Albores-Saavedra J. Physiologic versus neoplastic C cell hyperplasia of the thyroid. Separation of distinct histologic and biologic entities. *Cancer* 1996;77:750–756.
126. Lloyd RV, Osamura RY, Kloppel G, et al. *WHO classification of Tumours of Endocrine Organs. International Agency for Research on Cancer*. Lyon: 2017.
127. Carney JA, Sizemore GW, Hayles AB. Multiple endocrine neoplasia, type 2b. *Pathobiol Annu* 1978;8:105–153.
128. Diaz-Cano SJ, de Miguel M, Blanes A, Tashjian R, Wolfe HJ. Germline RET 634 mutation positive MEN 2A-related C-cell hyperplasias have genetic features consistent with intraepithelial neoplasia. *J Clin Endocrinol Metab* 2001;86:3948–3957.
129. DeLellis RA, Nunnemacher G, Wolfe HJ. C-cell hyperplasia. An ultrastructural analysis. *Lab Invest* 1977;36:237–248.
130. DeLellis RA, Wolfe HJ. The pathobiology of the human calcitonin (C)-cell: A review. *Pathol Annu* 1981;16(pt 2):25–52.
131. Pearse AG. Common cytochemical and ultrastructural characteristics of cells producing polypeptide hormones (the APUD series) and their relevance to thyroid and ultimobranchial C cells and calcitonin. *Proc R Soc Lond B Biol Sci* 1968;170:71–80.
132. Gonzalez-Cámpora R, Sanchez Gallego F, Martin Lacave I, et al. Lectin histochemistry of the thyroid gland. *Cancer* 1988;62:2354–2362.
133. Bussolati G, Pearse AG. Immunofluorescent localization of calcitonin in the 'C' cells of pig and dog thyroid. *J Endocrinol* 1967;37:205–209.
134. McMillan PJ, Hooker WM, Deptos LJ. Distribution of calcitonin-containing cells in the human thyroid. *Am J Anat* 1974;140:73–79.
135. Schmid KW, Kirchmair R, Ladurner D, et al. Immunohistochemical comparison of chromogranins A and B and secretogranin II with calcitonin and calcitonin gene-related peptide expression in normal, hyperplastic and neoplastic C-cells of the human thyroid. *Histopathology* 1992;21:225–232.
136. Ali-Rachedi A, Varndell IM, Facer P, et al. Immunocytochemical localization of katacalcin, a calcium-lowering hormone cleaved from the human calcitonin precursor. *J Clin Endocrinol Metab* 1983;57:680–682.
137. Van Noorden S, Polak JM, Pearse AG. Single cellular origin of somatostatin and calcitonin in the rat thyroid gland. *Histochemistry* 1977;53:243–247.
138. Yamada Y, Ito S, Matsubara Y, et al. Immunohistochemical demonstration of somatostatin-containing cells in the human, dog and rat thyroids. *Tohoku J Exp Med* 1977;122:87–92.
139. Kusumoto Y. Calcitonin and somatostatin are localized in different cells in the canine thyroid gland. *Biomed Res* 1980;1:237–241.
140. Kakudo K, Vacca LL. Immunohistochemical study of substance P-like immunoreactivity in human thyroid and medullary carcinoma of the thyroid. *J Submicrosc Cytol* 1983;15:563–568.
141. Sundler F, Christophe J, Robberecht P, et al. Is helodermin produced by medullary thyroid carcinoma cells and normal C-cells? Immunocytochemical evidence. *Regul Pept* 1988;20:83–89.
142. Kameya T, Bessho T, Tsumuraya M, et al. Production of gastrin releasing peptide by medullary carcinoma of the thyroid. An immunohistochemical study. *Virchows Arch A Pathol Anat Histopathol* 1983;401:99–107.
143. Sunday ME, Wolfe HJ, Roos BA, et al. Gastrin-releasing peptide gene expression in developing hyperplastic, and neoplastic human thyroid C-cells. *Endocrinology* 1988;122:1551–1558.
144. Gkonos PJ, Tavianini MA, et al. Thyrotropin-releasing hormone gene expression in normal thyroid parafollicular cells. *Mol Endocrinol* 1989;3:2101–2109.
145. Nunez EA, Gershon MD. Thyrotropin-induced thyroidal release of 5-hydroxytryptamine and accompanying ultrastructural changes in parafollicular cells. *Endocrinology* 1983;113:309–317.

146. DeLellis RA, Shin SJ, Treaba D. Immunohistochemistry of endocrine tumors (Chapter 10). In: Dabbs DJ, ed. *Diagnostic Immunohistochemistry. Theranostic and Genomic Applications.* Philadelphia, PA: Saunders; 2010:291–330.
147. Katoh R, Miyagi E, Nakamura N, et al. Expression of thyroid transcription factor-1 in human C-cells and medullary thyroid carcinoma. *Hum Pathol* 2000;31:386–393.
148. Bejarano PA, Nikiforov YE, Swenson ES, et al. Thyroid transcription factor-1, thyroglobulin, cytokeratin 7 and cytokeratin 20 in thyroid neoplasms. *Appl Immunohistochem Mol Morphol* 2000;8:189–194.
149. Faggiano A, Talbot M, Lacroix L. et al. Differential expression of galectin-3 in medullary thyroid carcinoma and C-cell hyperplasia. *Clin Endocrinol (Oxf)* 2002;57:813–819.
150. MacIntyre I. Calcitonin: Physiology, biosynthesis, secretion, metabolism and mode of action. In: DeGroot LJ, ed. *Endocrinology.* 2nd ed. Vol 2. Philadelphia, PA: WB Saunders; 1989: 892–901.
151. Amara SG, Jonas V, Rosenfeld MG, et al. Alternative RNA processing in calcitonin gene expression generates mRNAs encoding different polypeptide products. *Nature* 1982;298:240–244.
152. Kontozoglou T, Mambo N. The histopathologic features of lithium-associated thyroiditis. *Hum Pathol* 1983;14:737–739.
153. Fellegara G, Rosai J. Multifocal fibrosing thyroiditis: report of 55 cases of a poorly recognized entity. *Am J Surg Pathol.* 2015;39:416–424.
154. Frank R, Baloch ZW, Gentile C, et al. Multifocal fibrosing thyroiditis and its association with papillary thyroid carcinoma using BRAF pyrosequencing. *Endocr Pathol* 2014;25: 236–240.
155. Carpenter GR, Emery JL. Inclusions in the human thyroid. *J Anat* 1976;122(pt 1):77–89.
156. Morizumi H, Sano T, Tsuyuguchi M, et al. Localized adiposity of the thyroid, clinically mimicking an adenoma. *Endocr Pathol* 1991;2:226–229.
157. Langlois NE, Krukowski ZH, Miller ID. Pancreatic tissue in a lateral cervical cyst attached to the thyroid gland–a presumed foregut remnant. *Histopathology* 1997;31:378–380.
158. Klinck GH, Winship T. Psammoma bodies and thyroid cancer. *Cancer* 1959;12:656–662.
159. Batsakis JG, Nishiyama RH, Rich CR. Microlithiasis (calcospherites) and carcinoma of the thyroid gland. *Arch Pathol* 1960;69:493–498.
160. Dugan JM, Atkinson BF, Avitabile A, et al. Psammoma bodies in fine needle aspirate of the thyroid in lymphocytic thyroiditis. *Acta Cytol* 1987;31:330–334.
161. Erdheim J. I. Uber Schilddrusenaplasie. II. Geschwulste des Ductus Thyreoglossus. III. Uber einige menschliche Kiemenderivate. *Beitr Pathol Anat* 1904;35:366–433.
162. Getzowa S. Zur Kenntnis des postbranchialen Korpers und der branchialen Kanalchen des Menschen. *Virchows Arch* 1907;88:181–235.
163. Calvert R, Isler H. Fine structure of a third epithelial component of the thyroid gland of the rat. *Anat Rec* 1970;168:23–41.
164. Black HE, Capen CC, Young DM. Ultimobranchial thyroid neoplasms in bulls. A syndrome resembling medullary thyroid carcinoma in man. *Cancer* 1973;32:865–878.
165. Ljungberg O, Nilsson PO. Hyperplastic and neoplastic changes in ultimobranchial remnants and in parafollicular (C) cells in bulls: A histologic and immunohistochemical study. *Vet Pathol* 1985;22:95–103.
166. Harach HR. Solid cell nests of the human thyroid in early stages of postnatal life. Systematic autopsy study. *Acta Anat (Basel)* 1986;127:262–264.
167. Fellegara G, Dorji T, Bajimeta MR, et al. "Giant" solid cell nest of the thyroid: A hyperplastic change? *Int J Surg Pathol* 2009;17:268–269.
168. Janzer RC, Weber E, Hedinger C. The relation between solid cell nests and C cells of the thyroid gland: An immunohistochemical and morphometric investigation. *Cell Tissue Res* 1979;197:295–312.
169. Chan JK, Tse CC. Solid cell nest–associated C-cells: Another possible explanation for "C-cell hyperplasia" adjacent to follicular cell tumors. *Hum Pathol* 1989;20:498–499.
170. Martin V, Martin L, Viennet G, et al. Ultrastructural features of "solid cell nest" of the human thyroid gland: A study of 8 cases. *Ultrastruct Pathol* 2000;24:1–8.
171. Ríos Moreno MJ, Galera-Ruiz H, De Miguel M, et al. Inmunohistochemical profile of solid cell nest of thyroid gland. *Endocr Pathol* 2011;22:35–39.
172. Gucer H, Mete O. Positivity for GATA3 and TTF-1 (SPT24), and negativity for monoclonal PAX8 expand the biomarker profile of the solid cell nests of the thyroid gland. *Endocr Pathol* 2018;29:49–58.
173. Cameselle-Teijeiro J, Varela-Durán J, Sambade C, et al. Solid cell nests of the thyroid: Light microscopy and immunohistochemical profile. *Hum Pathol* 1994;25:684–693.
174. Preto A, Cameselle-Teijeiro J, Moldes-Boullosa J, et al. Telomerase expression and proliferative activity suggest a stem cell role for thyroid solid cell nests. *Mod Pathol* 2004;17: 819–826.
175. Reis-Filho JS, Preto A, Soares P, et al. p63 expression in solid cell nests of the thyroid: Further evidence for a stem cell origin. *Mod Pathol* 2003;16:43–48.
176. Yamaoka Y. Solid cell nest (SCN) of the human thyroid gland. *Acta Pathol Jpn* 1973;23:493–506.
177. Ljungberg O, Nilsson PO. Intermediate thyroid carcinoma in humans and ultimobranchial tumors in bulls: A comparative morphological and immunohistochemical study. *Endocr Pathol* 1991;2:24–39.
178. Cameselle-Teijeiro J, Caramés N, Romero-Rojas A, et al. Thyroid-type solid cell nests in struma ovarii. *Int J Surg Pathol* 2011;19:627–631.
179. Louis DN, Vickery AL Jr, Rosai J, et al. Multiple branchial cleft–like cysts in Hashimoto's thyroiditis. *Am J Surg Pathol* 1989;13:45–49.
180. Apel RL, Asa SL, Chalvardjian A, et al. Intrathyroidal lymphoepithelial cysts of probable branchial origin. *Hum Pathol* 1994;25:1238–1242.
181. Streutker CJ, Murray D, Kovacs K, et al. Epithelial cyst of thyroid. *Endocr Pathol* 1997;8:75–80.
182. Manzoni M, Roversi G, Di Bella C, et al. Solid cell nests of the thyroid gland: Morphological, immunohistochemical and genetic features. *Histopathology;* 2016;68:866–874.
183. Park JY, Kim GY, Suh YL. Intrathyroidal branchial cleft-like cyst with heterotopic salivary gland-type tissue. *Pediatr Dev Pathol* 2004;7:262–267.
184. Harach HR, Vujanic GM. Intrathyroidal parathyroid. *Pediatr Pathol* 1993;13:71–74.

185. Spiegel AM, Marx SJ, Doppman JL, et al. Intrathyroidal parathyroid adenoma or hyperplasia. An occasionally overlooked cause of surgical failure in primary hyperparathyroidism. *JAMA* 1975;234:1029–1033.
186. Chen CL, Lin SH, Yu JC, et al. Persistent renal hyperparathyroidism caused by intrathyroidal parathyroid glands. *J Chin Med Assoc* 2014;77:492–495.
187. LiVolsi V. Branchial and thymic remnants in the thyroid and cervical region: An explanation for unusual tumors and microscopic curiosities. *Endocr Pathol* 1993;4:115–119.
188. Harach HR, Vujanic GM. Intrathyroidal thymic tissue: An autopsy study in fetuses with some emphasis on pathological implications. *Pediatr Pathol* 1993;13:431–434.
189. Neill J. Intrathyroid thymoma. *Am J Surg Pathol* 1986;10: 660–661.
190. Damiani S, Filotico M, Eusebi V. Carcinoma of the thyroid showing thymoma-like features. *Virchows Arch A Pathol Anat Histopathol* 1991;418:463–466.
191. Mizukami Y, Nonomura A, Michigishi T, et al. Ectopic thymic tissue in the thyroid gland. *Endocr Pathol* 1993;4:162–164.
192. O'Connor K, Alzahrani H, Murad F, et al. An ectopic intrathyroidal thymic tissue and intrathymic parathyroid tissue in a patient with Graves disease. *Gland Surg* 2017;6:726–728.
193. Miyauchi A, Kuma K, Matsuzuka F, et al. Intrathyroidal epithelial thymoma: An entity distinct from squamous cell carcinoma of the thyroid. *World J Surg* 1985;9:128–135.
194. Weissferdt A, Moran CA. Ectopic primary intrathyroidal thymoma: A clinicopathological and immunohistochemical analysis of 3 cases. *Hum Pathol* 2016;49:71–76.
195. Cameselle-Teijeiro J, Varela-Duran J. Intrathyroid salivary gland-type tissue in multinodular goiter. *Virchows Arch* 1994; 425:331–334.
196. Finkle HI, Goldman RL. Heterotopic cartilage in the thyroid. *Arch Pathol* 1973;95:48–49.
197. Guimaraes SB, Uceda JE, Lynn HB. Thyroglossal duct remnants in infants and children. *Mayo Clin Proc* 1972;47: 117–120.
198. Ellis PD, Van Nostrand AW. The applied anatomy of thyroglossal tract remnants. *Laryngoscope* 1977;87(5 Pt 1): 765–770.
199. Larochelle D, Arcand P, Belzile M, et al. Ectopic thyroid tissue– a review of the literature. *J Otolaryngol* 1979;8:523–530.
200. Williams ED, Toyn CE, Harach HR. The ultimobranchial gland and congenital thyroid abnormalities in man. *J Pathol* 1989;159:135–141.
201. Ibrahim NA, Fadeyibi IO. Ectopic thyroid: Etiology, pathology and management. *Hormones (Athens)* 2011;10:261–269.
202. De Andrade MA. A review of 128 cases of posterior mediastinal goiter. *World J Surg* 1977;1:789–797.
203. de Souza FM, Smith PE. Retrosternal goiter. *J Otolaryngol* 1983;12:393–396.
204. Kantelip B, Lusson JR, De Riberolles C, et al. Intracardiac ectopic thyroid. *Hum Pathol* 1986;17:1293–1296.
205. Baughman RA. Lingual thyroid and lingual thyroglossal tract remnants. A clinical and histopathologic study with review of the literature. *Oral Surg Oral Med Oral Pathol* 1972;34: 781–799.
206. Reaume CE, Sofie VL. Lingual thyroid. Review of the literature and report of a case. *Oral Surg Oral Med Oral Pathol* 1978;45:841–845.
207. Kansal P, Sakati N, Rifai A, et al. Lingual thyroid. Diagnosis and treatment. *Arch Intern Med* 1987;147:2046–2048.
208. Nienas FW, Gorman CA, Devine KD, et al. Lingual thyroid. Clinical characteristics of 15 cases. *Ann Intern Med* 1973;79:205–210.
209. Strickland AL, Macfie JA, Van Wyk JJ, French FS. Ectopic thyroid glands simulating thyroglossal duct cysts. *JAMA* 1969;208:307–310.
210. Talib H. Lingual thyroid. *Br J Clin Pract* 1966;20:322–323.
211. Wapshaw H. Lingual thyroid. A report of a case with unusual histology. *Br J Surg* 1974;30:160–165.
212. Sturniolo G, Violi MA, Galletti B, et al. Differentiated thyroid carcinoma in lingual thyroid. *Endocrine* 2016;5: 189–198.
213. Seoane JM, Cameselle-Teijeiro J, Romero MA. Poorly differentiated oxyphilic (Hürthle cell) carcinoma arising in lingual thyroid: A case report and review of the literature. *Endocr Pathol* 2002;13:353–360.
214. LiVolsi VA, Perzin KH, Savetsy L. Carcinoma arising in median ectopic thyroid (including thyroglossal duct tissue). *Cancer* 1974;34:1303–1315.
215. Allard RH. The thyroglossal cyst. *Head Neck Surg* 1982;5: 134–146.
216. Soucy P, Penning J. The clinical relevance of certain observations on the histology of the thyroglossal tract. *J Pediatr Surg* 1984;19:506–509.
217. Kreft A, Hansen T, Kirkpatrick CJ. Thyroid transcription factor 1 expression in cystic lesions of the neck: An immunohistochemical investigation of thyroglossal duct cysts, branchial cleft cysts and metastatic papillary thyroid cancer. *Virchows Arch* 2005;447:9–11.
218. Jaques DA, Chambers RG, Oertel JE. Thyroglossal tract carcinoma. A review of the literature and addition of eighteen cases. *Am J Surg* 1970;120:439–446.
219. Joseph TJ, Komorowski RA. Thyroglossal duct carcinoma. *Hum Pathol* 1975;6:717–729.
220. Mobini J, Krouse TB, Klinghoffer JF. Squamous cell carcinoma arising in a thyroglossal duct cyst. *Am Surg* 1974;40: 290–294.
221. Nussbaum M, Buchwald RP, Ribner A, et al. Anaplastic carcinoma arising from median ectopic thyroid (thyroglossal duct remnant). *Cancer* 1981;48:2724–2728.
222. Ljungberg O. *Biopsy Pathology of the Thyroid and Parathyroid*. London: Chapman & Hall; 1992.
223. Solomon JR, Rangecroft L. Thyroglossal-duct lesions in childhood. *J Pediatr Surg* 1984;19:555–561.
224. Block MA, Wylie JH, Patton RB, et al. Does benign thyroid tissue occur in the lateral part of the neck? *Am J Surg* 1966; 112:476–481.
225. Klopp CT, Kirson SM. Therapeutic problems with ectopic non-cancerous follicular thyroid tissue in the neck: 18 case reports according to etiological factors. *Ann Surg* 1966;163: 653–664.
226. Moses DC, Thompson NW, Nishiyama RH, et al. Ectopic thyroid tissue in the neck. Benign or malignant? *Cancer* 1976;38:361–365.
227. Hathaway BM. Innocuous accessory thyroid nodules. *Arch Surg* 1965;90:222–227.
228. Sisson JC, Schmidt RW, Beierwaltes WH. Sequestered nodular goiter. *N Engl J Med* 1964;270:927–932.

229. Meyer JS, Steinberg LS. Microscopically benign thyroid follicles in cervical lymph nodes. Serial section study of lymph node inclusions and entire thyroid gland in 5 cases. *Cancer* 1969;24:302–211.
230. Frantz VK, Forsythe R, Hanford JM, et al. Lateral aberrant thyroids. *Ann Surg* 1942;115:161–183.
231. Bone RC, Biller HF, Irwin TM. Intralaryngotracheal thyroid. *Ann Otol Rhinol Laryngol* 1972;81:424–428.
232. Donegan JO, Wood MD. Intratracheal thyroid—familial occurrence. *Laryngoscope* 1985;95:6–8.
233. Babazade F, Mortazavi H, Jalalian H, et al. Thyroid tissue as a submandibular mass: A case report. *J Oral Sci* 2009;51:655–657.
234. Williams RJ, Lindop G, Butler J. Ectopic thyroid tissue on the ascending aorta: An operative finding. *Ann Thorac Surg* 2002;73:1642–1643.
235. Pollice L, Caruso G. Struma cordis. Ectopic thyroid goiter in the right ventricle. *Arch Pathol Lab Med* 1986;110:452–453.
236. Simon M, Baczako K. Thyroid inclusion in the lung. Metastasis of an occult papillary carcinoma or ectopia? *Pathol Res Pract* 1989;184:263–267; discussion 268–270.
237. Di Mari N, Barbagli L, Mourmouras V, et al. Ectopic thyroid of the lung. An additional case. *Pathologica* 2010;102:102–103.
238. Postlethwait RW, Detmer DE. Ectopic thyroid nodule in the esophagus. *Ann Thorac Surg* 1975;19:98–100.
239. Takahashi T, Ishikura H, Kato H, et al. Ectopic thyroid follicles in the submucosa of the duodenum. *Virchows Arch A Pathol Anat Histopathol* 1991;418:547–550.
240. Hammers YA, Kelly DR, Muensterer OJ, et al. Giant polypoid gastric heterotopia with ectopic thyroid tissue: Unusual cause of jejuno-jejunal intussusception. *J Pediatr Gastroenterol Nutr* 2007;45:484–487.
241. Cassol CA, Noria D, Asa SL. Ectopic thyroid tissue within the gall bladder: Case report and brief review of the literature. *Endocr Pathol* 2010;21:263–265.
242. Sekine S, Nagata M, Hamada H, et al. Heterotopic thyroid tissue at the porta hepatis in a fetus with trisomy 18. *Virchows Arch* 2000;436:498–501.
243. Fushimi H, Kotoh K, Nakamura H, Tachibana T, Yutani C. Ectopic thyroid tissue adjacent to the gallbladder, *Histopathology* 1998;32:90–91.
244. Eyuboglu E, Kapan M, Ipek T, et al. Ectopic thyroid in the abdomen: Report of a case. *Surg Today* 1999;29:472–474.
245. Seelig MH, Schonleben K. Intra-abdominal ectopic thyroid presenting as a pancreatic tumour. *Eur J Surg* 1997;163:549–551.
246. Salam M, Mohideen A, Stravitz RT. Ectopic thyroid presenting as a liver mass. *Clin Gastroenterol Hepatol* 2012;10.
247. Cicek Y, Tasci H, Gokdogan C, et al. Intra-abdominal ectopic thyroid. *Br J Surg* 1993;80:316.
248. Shiraishi T, Imai H, Fukutome K, et al. Ectopic thyroid in the adrenal gland. *Hum Pathol* 1999;30:105–108.
249. Tamaki S, Miyakura Y, Someya S, et al. Laparoscopic resection of retroperitoneal ectopic thyroid tissue. *Asian J Endosc Surg* 2017;10:331–333.
250. Kurman RJ, Prabha AC. Thyroid and parathyroid glands in the vaginal wall. *Am J Clin Pathol* 1973;59:503–507.
251. Yilmaz F, Uzunlar AK, Sogutcu N. Ectopic thyroid tissue in the uterus. *Acta Obstet Gynecol Scand* 2005;84:201–202.
252. Ruchti C, Balli-Antunes H, Gerber HA. Follicular tumor in the sellar region without primary cancer of the thyroid. Heterotopic carcinoma? *Am J Clin Pathol* 1987;87:776–780.
253. Woodruff JD, Rauh JT, Markley RL. Ovarian struma. *Obstet Gynecol* 1966;27:194–192.
254. Rosenblum NG, LiVolsi VA, Edmonds PR, et al. Malignant struma ovarii. *Gynecol Oncol* 1989;32:224–227.
255. Willemse PH, Oosterhuis JW, Aalders JG, et al. Malignant struma ovarii treated by ovariectomy, thyroidectomy, and 131I administration. *Cancer* 1987;60:178–182.
256. Brunskill PJ, Rollason TP, Nicholson HO. Malignant follicular variant of papillary struma ovarii. *Histopathology* 1990;17:574–476.
257. Garg K, Soslow RA, Rivera M, et al. Histologically bland "extremely well differentiated" thyroid carcinomas arising in struma ovarii can recur and metastasize. *Int J Gynecol Pathol* 2009;28:222–230.
258. Zhang X, Axiotis C. Thyroid-type carcinoma of struma ovarii. *Arch Pathol Lab Med* 2010;134:786–791.
259. Robboy SJ, Shaco-Levy R, Peng RY, et al. Malignant struma ovarii: An analysis of 88 cases, including 27 with extraovarian spread. *Int J Gynecol Pathol* 2009;28:405–422.
260. Roth LM, Miller AW 3rd, Talerman A. Typical thyroid-type carcinoma arising in struma ovarii: A report of 4 cases and review of the literature. *Int J Gynecol Pathol* 2008;27:496–506.
261. Shaco-Levy R, Bean SM, Bentley RC, et al. Natural history of biologically malignant struma ovarii: Analysis of 27 cases with extraovarian spread. *Int J Gynecol Pathol* 2010;29:212–227.
262. Karseladze AI, Kulinitch SI). Peritoneal strumosis. *Pathol Res Pract* 1994;190:1082–1085; discussion 1086–1088.
263. Roth LM, Karseladze AI. Highly differentiated follicular carcinoma arising from struma ovarii: A report of 3 cases, a review of the literature, and a reassessment of so-called peritoneal strumosis. *Int J Gynecol Pathol* 2008;27:213–222.
264. Flavin R, Smyth P, Crotty P, et al. BRAF T1799A mutation occurring in a case of malignant struma ovarii. *Int J Surg Pathol* 2007;15:116–120.
265. Boutross-Tadross O, Saleh R, Asa SL. Follicular variant papillary thyroid carcinoma arising in struma ovarii. *Endocr Pathol* 2007 Fall;18:182–186.

Parathyroids

Sylvia L. Asa ■ Ozgur Mete

HISTORY AND NOMENCLATURE 1201	VARIATIONS WITH GENDER AND AGE 1212
DISTRIBUTION OF PARATHYROID GLANDS 1201	PHYSIOLOGY AND PATHOPHYSIOLOGY 1212
EMBRYOLOGY 1202	SPECIAL PROCEDURES 1213
ANATOMY—GROSS FEATURES 1204	ACKNOWLEDGMENTS 1221
HISTOLOGY AND ULTRASTRUCTURE 1206	REFERENCES 1221

The parathyroid glands are endocrine organs composed of small clusters of neuroendocrine cells that are present in the neck adjacent to the thyroid, embedded within the thyroid pseudocapsule or in the upper mediastinum. They are the principal regulators of calcium homeostasis through the synthesis and secretion of parathyroid hormone (PTH).

These small glands are the source of common pathology, since asymptomatic hyperparathyroidism is now recognized as a frequent event with the advent of routine serum calcium testing (1). In addition, parathyroids are routinely removed during thyroid surgery, making them a common finding in surgical pathology.

The interpretation of parathyroid structure is highly dependent on understanding the normal anatomy, histology, and development of parathyroid glands. As in all endocrine tissues, the pathologist must also understand the function of these glands to appreciate the context of structure–function correlations.

In this chapter, we will review the embryology, anatomy, and microscopic morphology of parathyroid glands to provide a clear understanding of the variability and factors that influence structure of these glands in normal and abnormal circumstances.

HISTORY AND NOMENCLATURE

The first description of a parathyroid gland was in 1850 by Professor Richard Owen who reported to the Royal College in London the presence of "a small, compact yellow glandular body attached to the thyroid at the point where the veins emerge" in the Indian rhinoceros. The paper was only published 12 years later (2) and in the interim, Remak described similar glands in the cat (3). In 1855, Virchow identified the human counterparts (4). The name "glandulae parathyroidae" was coined by Ivar Sandström in 1880; as a medical student, he studied the parathyroid glands of several species (5). These studies attributed a relationship of the parathyroid glands to the thyroid, both structurally and embryologically, and it was only when Kohn identified an independent origin of parathyroids and proposed the name "Epithelkörperchen" (6,7) that they were recognized to be distinct and separate from their larger neighbor.

The function of the parathyroid glands was described in careful studies by Gley and Erdheim who showed an association between lack of these glands and death by tetany (8–10). The mechanism of action through regulation of calcium by PTH was debated for many years until proven by the work of Hanson (11) and Collip (12) and ultimately by the discovery of PTH itself by Aurbach in 1959 (13).

DISTRIBUTION OF PARATHYROID GLANDS

The normal adult has four parathyroid glands, but up to 13% of people have at least one supernumerary gland (14,15). These data are derived from autopsy studies but also from clinical studies of patients with hyperparathyroidism (1). Reports of fewer than four glands in normal adults are attributable to failure to identify these very small structures that can be confused with lymph nodes

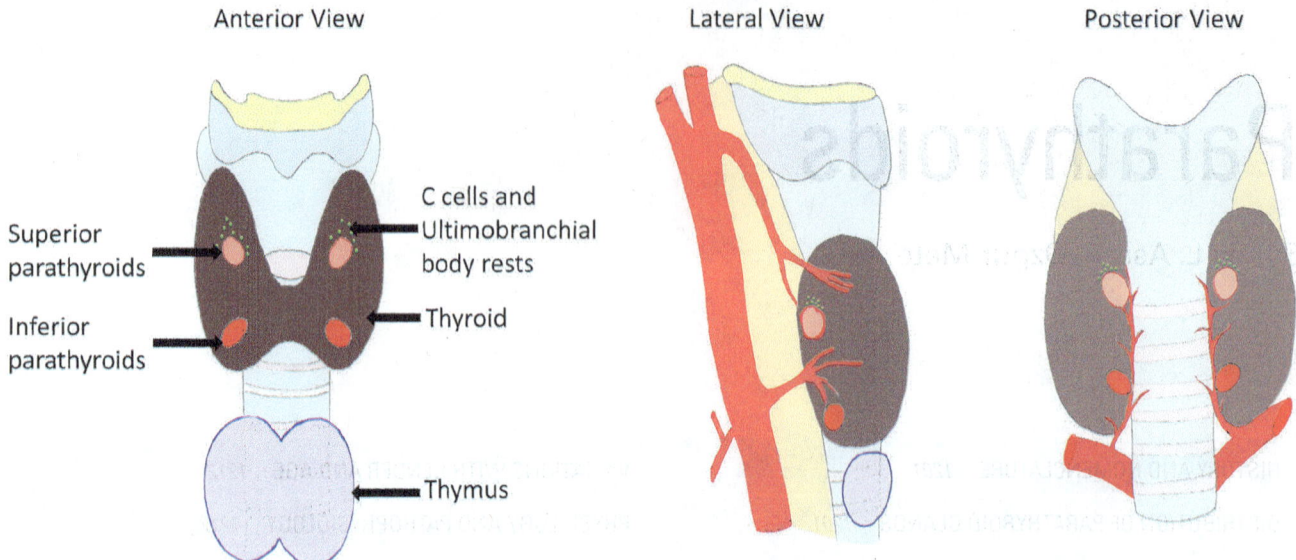

FIGURE 44.1 Location of parathyroid glands. There are four parathyroid glands, two on each side of the neck, behind the thyroid gland. The superior glands are at the junction of the upper and middle third of each lateral lobe; the inferior glands are usually near the inferior pole of the thyroid as illustrated, but are often lower, associated with the thymus, and may be found anywhere between the hyoid bone and the mediastinum. (Drawings courtesy of Paolo Batoni, PhD and Zoya Volynskaya, PhD.)

and ganglia in the neck and can be hidden within the thyroid gland itself.

The superior glands are usually located near the cricothyroid junction (Fig. 44.1), deep to the recurrent laryngeal nerve and superior to its junction with the inferior thyroid artery (Fig. 44.2) (16). They are usually intimately associated with the posterior thyroid at the junction of the upper and middle third of each lateral lobe; they may even be in the perithyroidal fascia or completely intrathyroidal (Fig. 44.3), and therefore easily missed until the thyroid is dissected. Less frequently, they may be retropharyngeal or retroesophageal.

The inferior glands are more anterior and ventral to the recurrent laryngeal nerve (16) and may be associated with the thymus. There is significant variation in their anatomical position, and they may be near the inferior pole of the thyroid, within the thyrothymic ligament, higher in the neck, as high as the hyoid bone, at the carotid bulb, or associated with thymus (Fig. 44.4) and within the mediastinum; they have been reported anywhere from the jaw to the pericardium. The distribution tends to be symmetrical in any given patient.

Ectopic parathyroid glands have been reported in up to 22% of patients undergoing parathyroid surgery but these reports include glands that are found within the thymus, in the retroesophageal space and mediastinum, as well as intrathyroidal glands that are not truly "ectopic" (17). This term should be restricted to undescended glands in a high cervical position and those trapped within the carotid sheath.

The importance of supernumerary glands is evident when surgery is performed for hyperparathyroidism and indeed the most common reason for failed parathyroidectomy is the inability to find a supernumerary or ectopic parathyroid gland (1).

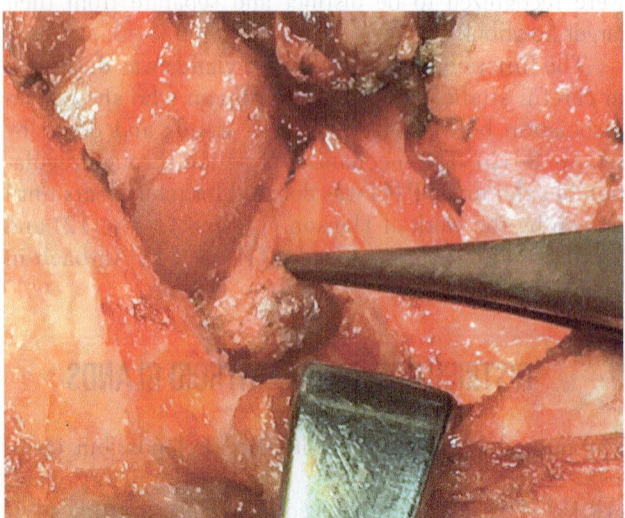

FIGURE 44.2 Localization of a parathyroid gland. A normal right superior parathyroid gland is embedded in perithyroidal fat posterior to the thyroid that has been removed in this intraoperative image taken post hemithyroidectomy. (Photo provided by Dr. Lorne Rotstein.)

EMBRYOLOGY

The parathyroid glands arise from the third and fourth pharyngeal pouches (also known as branchial pouches) of the endoderm between the fifth and twelfth week of gestation (Fig. 44.5) (18–20). The embryology can be confusing

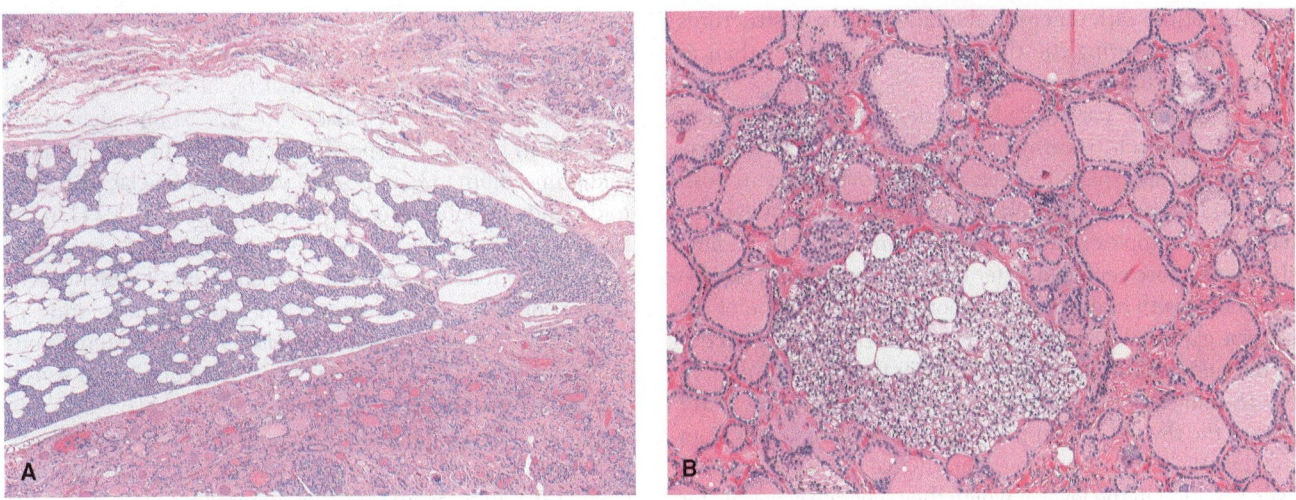

FIGURE 44.3 Intrathyroidal parathyroid glands. Parathyroids can be found within the thyroid parenchyma as in these examples (**A** and **B**) where parathyroids are completely embedded within the thyroid and surrounded by thyroid parenchyma.

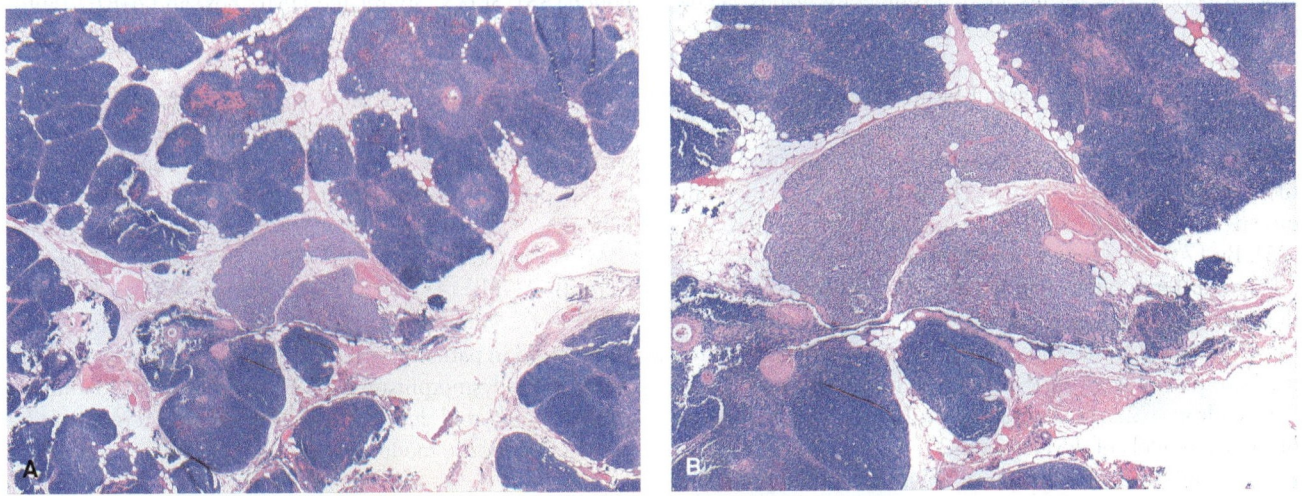

FIGURE 44.4 Intrathymic parathyroid glands. The lower or inferior parathyroid glands can sometimes be found within the thymus (**A** and **B**).

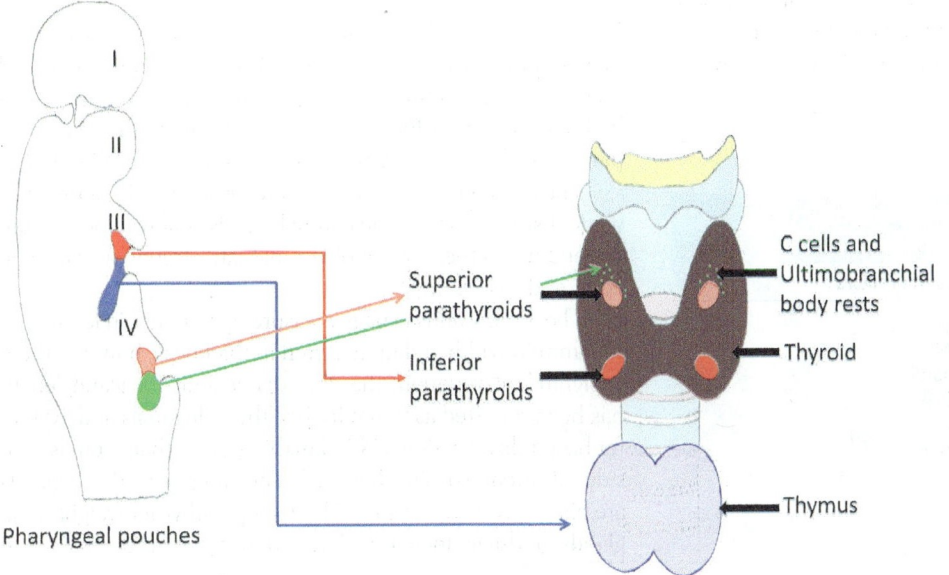

FIGURE 44.5 Embryology of parathyroid glands. The parathyroid glands derived from the third and fourth pharyngeal pouches. The superior glands originate from the fourth pouch and migrate almost directly to the junction of the upper third and lower two thirds of the thyroid lobes along with the ultimobranchial body that gives rise to calcitonin-producing C cells of the thyroid. The lower parathyroids originate higher with the thymus in the third pouch and migrate further caudally, explaining their more variable location and frequent association with the thymus. (Drawings courtesy of Paolo Batoni, PhD and Zoya Volynskaya, PhD.)

because of the differences in migration of these structures that ultimately bring the third pouch to lie lower than or caudal to the fourth pouch.

The superior parathyroids are derived from the fourth pharyngeal pouch (parathyroid IV) that has a short embryonic migration, explaining their relative consistency in position. In contrast, the third pharyngeal pouch (parathyroid III) has a more complex pattern of descent and since the midline structures move cephalad faster than the lateral ones, the differential growth rates result in a more variable location of the inferior glands. They migrate with the thymus that attaches to the pericardium and comes to lie in the mediastinum; in the 18-mm embryo, parathyroid III is at the level of the lower pole of the thyroid, and at this stage it usually separates from the thymus, forming the lower parathyroid glands (21). However, variation in the level at which they separate accounts for the anatomic variations in the position of the inferior glands.

During migration of parathyroid III, small fragments of parathyroid tissue may become separated from the main pharyngeal pouch; this results in supernumerary glands. They occur most commonly in the thymus but have also been described in several locations including but not limited to the carotid sheath (22), carotid bifurcation (23), paraaortic region (23), esophagus, hypopharynx, and vagus nerve (24).

PTH production has been demonstrated by immunohistochemistry as early as $8^{3}/_{7}$ weeks gestational age (3.1 cm crown–rump length) (21) and is readily identified at 10 weeks (25). By 17 to 20 weeks, immunoreactivity is abundant.

The differentiation and growth of parathyroid glands is dependent on a number of genes (Table 44.1) that have been identified from studies of patients with hypoparathyroidism, particularly the DiGeorge syndrome/velocardiofacial syndrome (22q11.2 deletion syndrome), and by studies of mouse models of development.

A number of transcription factors are required for parathyroid differentiation. *Hoxa3*, a member of the *Hox* (homeotic genes) family, is required for development of the organs arising from the third and fourth pharyngeal pouches (26,27). *Pax9* (paired box 9) deficiency also results in lack of thymus, parathyroid glands, and ultimobranchial bodies (28), while *Pax1* deficiency is associated with reduced parathyroid development (29). *Tbx1* (T-box gene 1) knockout mice exhibit hypoplasia of the thymus and parathyroid glands, cardiac outflow tract abnormalities, abnormal facial structures, abnormal vertebrae and cleft palate (30–32). Mammalian *gcm2* (*GCMB* in humans) is specifically restricted to the parathyroid primordium (33) and *Gcm2* deficient mice lack parathyroid glands (34); however they have expression of PTH in the thymus driven by *Gcm1*, another homolog of the Drosophila *gcm* family that functions in placental development (34). Expression of *gcm* is absent in *Hoxa3* mutant mice, indicating that it acts downstream of *Hoxa3* (29). Heterozygous mutations of *GATA3* cause hypoparathyroidism with sensorineural deafness and renal dysplasia (35); *GATA3*-deficient mice fail to develop parathyroids and lack *Gcm2* expression, indicating that this transcription factor is also upstream of *Gcm2* (36). *Eyes absent (Eya)1* is required for the initiation of thymus and parathyroid gland formation downstream of the *Hoxa3* and *Pax* genes (37) and *Six1/4* (sine oculis homeobox homolog) also regulate patterning of the third pharyngeal pouch (38). *SOX3* (Sry-related HMG box) and *AIRE1* (autoimmune regulator) have also been implicated in parathyroid development in humans (35).

Growth factors and their signaling pathways modulate migration of the pharyngeal pouch endoderm, its interaction with the mesenchyme, and the balance between proliferation and apoptosis. The critical factors include expression of *fibroblast growth factor (Fgf8)* (39,40), *bone morphogenetic proteins (BMPs)* (41), *Chordin (Chrd)* (42), and *transforming growth factor β (TGFβ)* (43), as well as silencing of *Sonic hedgehog (Shh)* (44). Mutations in tubulin chaperone E (*Tbce*) have been found in patients with the human hypoparathyroidism–retardation–dysmorphism (HRD) syndrome (45,46) but its role in parathyroid development and function remains to be proven in a mouse model.

ANATOMY—GROSS FEATURES

Parathyroid glands are smooth, soft, flattened ovoid or bean-shaped structures (Fig. 44.6) that vary in shape based on their relationship with surrounding structures; they can be bilobed or multilobulated in some individuals. The lower parathyroid glands may be larger than the upper glands.

The capsule is smooth, shiny and gray and with a fine network of small vessels. The parenchyma is yellow to orange-tan depending on the amount of stromal fat, percent of oncocytic cells, and vascularity (5).

The adult glands usually measure up to 6 mm in length, up to 4 mm in width and up to 2 mm in thickness, however there is significant variation; the 95% upper limit for gland length has been reported as 9 mm for healthy individuals and 10 mm for hospitalized patients (47); anything larger than 1 cm is considered unequivocally abnormal. The weights of these glands are also extremely variable. The total parathyroid weight of all glands gradually increases during development, reaching 5 to

TABLE 44.1
Transcription and Growth Factors Involved in the Development of Parathyroid Glands

Transcription Factors	Growth Factors
Hoxa3	Fgf8
Pax9	BMPs
Pax1	Chordin
Tbx1	TGFβ
Gcm2	Shh
Eya1	Tbce
GATA3	
SOX3	
AIRE1	

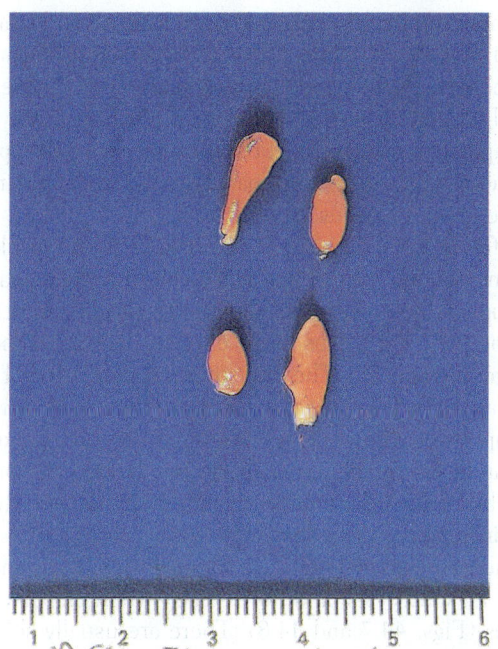

FIGURE 44.6 Gross appearance of parathyroid glands. Four normal parathyroid glands removed at autopsy from a 53-year-old man. The glands are variable in size, shape, and weight. At the tip of the right lower gland is a small area of yellow thymus. (Courtesy of Dr. S. I. Roth)

Because these glands have a significant amount of interspersed fat, the parenchymal content of the glands is extremely variable and difficult to evaluate. It has been reported that the parenchyma averages 74% of the weight of the gland in adults (53,54). Parenchymal content is a better indicator of gland function than gland weight alone but requires careful morphometric and densitometric analysis (55). The average parenchymal weight per gland has been calculated as 21.6 mg for men and 18.2 mg for women and mean total parenchymal weight for all four glands has been estimated at 82.0 ± 2.6 mg for men and 88.9 ± 3.9 mg for women (51).

Importantly, the amount of stromal fat is known to be dependent on body composition and constitutional fat. In young patients, parathyroid glands have scant fat and parenchymal weight is almost the same as gland weight (49). In adulthood, parenchymal weight stays relatively constant but stromal adipose tissue increases. There may be variation in stromal fat content of different glands in any given individual (49,56).

A number of studies of patients with hyperparathyroidism have examined the nontumorous glands to determine normal parameters (57). These studies are not entirely relevant for normal size, weight, and histology since some glands may be enlarged due to germline abnormalities and others may be reduced in size due to feedback inhibition. Parathyroid weight is likely to be inversely related to serum calcium concentration and directly related to serum phosphorus and renal function.

9 mg at 3 months of age (48) and a mean of 120 ± 3.5 mg in men and 142 ± 5.2 mg in women in adults (48,49). Mean weight per gland has been reported to be approximately 32 mg (49–51), has been reported to be lower in Caucasians than in blacks (51), and is higher in hospitalized patients (mean weight of 46.2 g) than in those who died suddenly (47). Pathologists should consider 60 mg to be the upper limit of normal weight for a parathyroid gland (49,52).

The arterial supply to the parathyroid glands is derived from the superior and inferior thyroid arteries, sometimes with anastomosing branches from both arteries. Venous drainage of the upper glands flows to the superior and/or lateral thyroid vein and that of the lower glands to the lateral and/or inferior thyroid vein. Lymphatic drainage is to the superior and inferior deep cervical, pretracheal, paratracheal, and retropharyngeal lymph nodes (49). The site of entry/exit of the main vascular supply forms a hilum of the gland (Fig. 44.7);

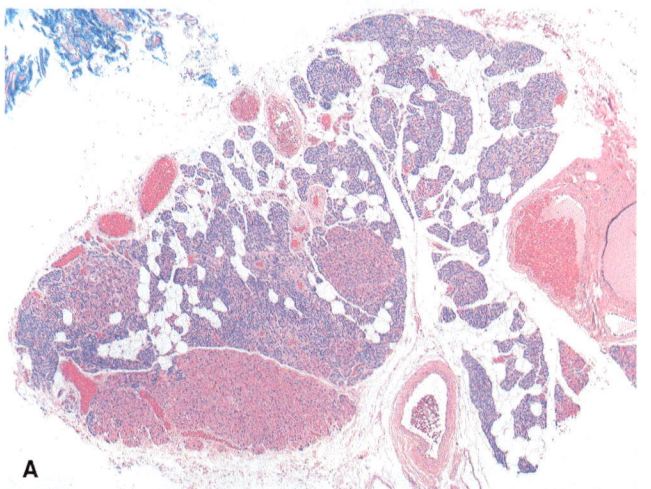
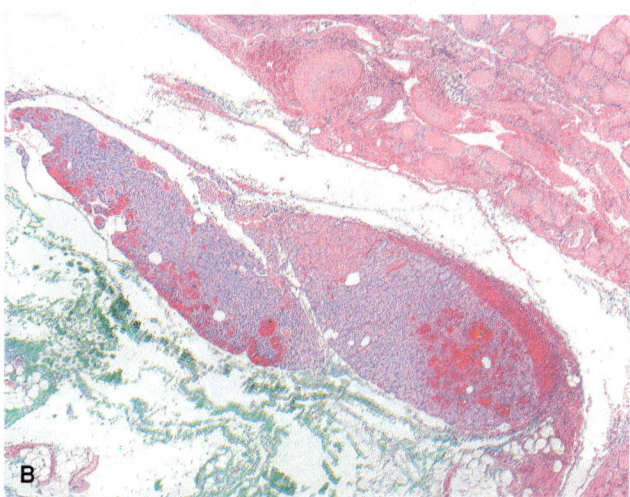

FIGURE 44.7 Vascular hilum of parathyroid glands. Parathyroid glands are well delineated but lack a true capsule; there is an incomplete thin fibrous pseudocapsule that carries the vasculature around the periphery of lobules. Histology allows clear identification of the vascular hilum of parathyroid glands (**A**). This is the region most likely to harbor nontumorous parathyroid tissue in glands with neoplasms (**B**).

this is important to identify when examining abnormal glands, since it is usually the site where nontumorous parenchyma (usually present as an atrophic rim around the lesion) can be identified in the case of neoplasia and allows the distinction of parathyroid neoplasia from hyperplasia.

HISTOLOGY AND ULTRASTRUCTURE

The embryonic parathyroid gland is a highly vascular sheet of pure chief cells with clear amphophilic cytoplasm and peripheral nuclear palisading. No oxyphil cells are present. The stroma is composed of prominent vessels but lacks fibrous tissue and adipose cells.

The normal mature parathyroid gland has a thin but incomplete, fibrous pseudocapsule (Fig. 44.7). The vascular pole, or hilum, contains an artery and a vein surrounded by fibrous tissue (Fig. 44.7). The arteries branch into a complex network of smaller arteries and veins that mainly follow the capsule; these capsular arteries and veins are connected by arterioles, capillaries, and venules located in the fibrous septa between the parenchymal cells; as in all endocrine tissues, the capillary endothelium is fenestrated (21,49) and the endothelial cells have dense bodies, pinocytotic vesicles, and Weibel–Palade bodies, as well as tight junctions. Due to the rich capillary network, the cut surface bleeds readily, providing an easy way to distinguish parathyroids from lymph nodes, adipose tissue, thymus, and thyroid, which do not bleed as profusely from their cut surfaces (21). The capsule also contains two interconnecting plexuses of lymphatic capillaries: loops of the inner plexus dip into the gland parenchyma, whereas the outer plexus forms efferent drainage associated with the thyroid (58). The interstitium is composed of collagen, elastic fibers and the basement membranes of chief cells and capillaries with pericytes, scattered fibroblasts and mast cells, and a few lymphocytes. Nerve bundles in close proximity to chief cells suggest autonomic innervation that is thought to originate in the vagus nerve (59–61).

The parenchymal cells are found in lobules composed of sheets, solid nests, and trabeculae with interspersed adipocytes (Figs. 44.7 and 44.8). There are usually scattered cysts (Figs. 44.8 and 44.9) and small gland-like follicles that are filled with pink eosinophilic homogeneous material

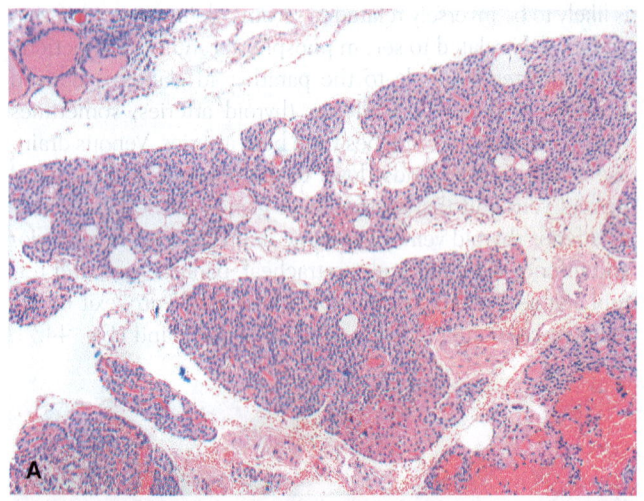
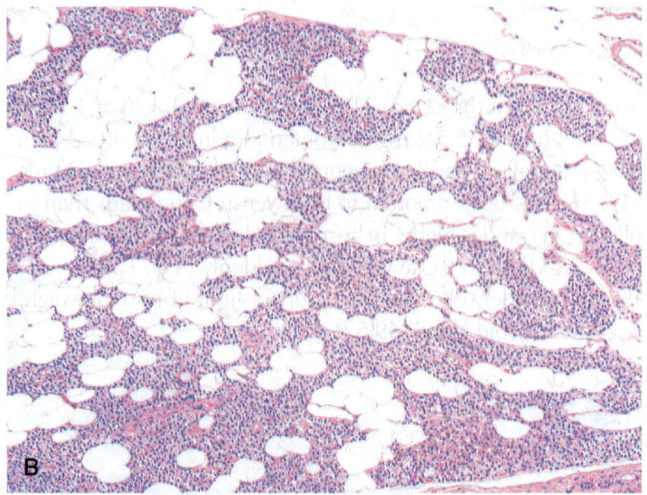
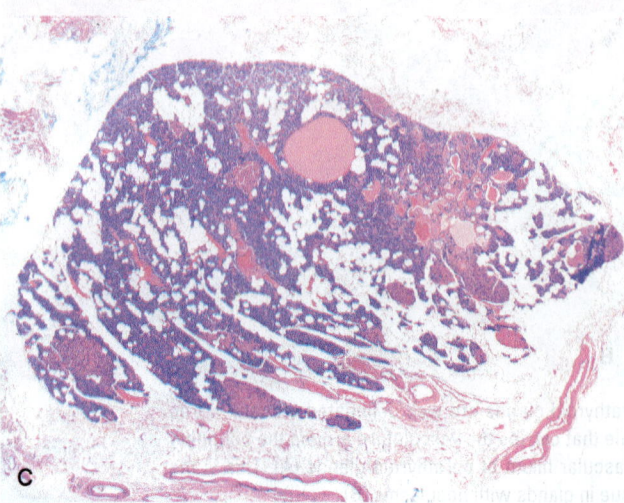

FIGURE 44.8 Variation in normal parathyroid glands. Parathyroid glands are composed of lobules of parenchymal cells with interspersed fat. **(A)** They may have scant stromal fat, **(B)** there may be an approximately equal amount of fat and cellular parenchyma or **(C)** stromal fat may be abundant.

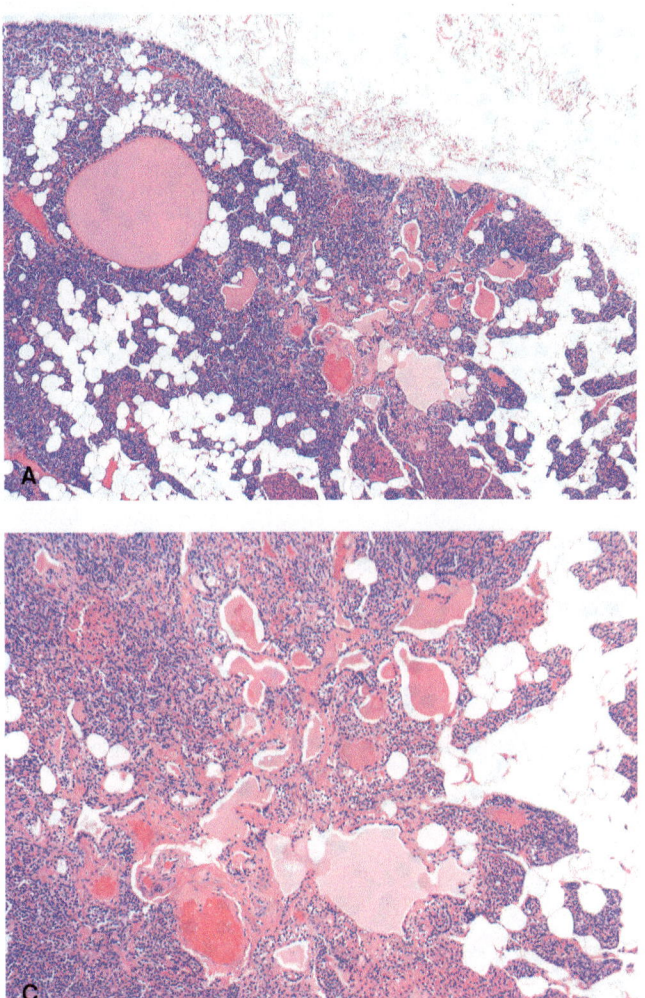
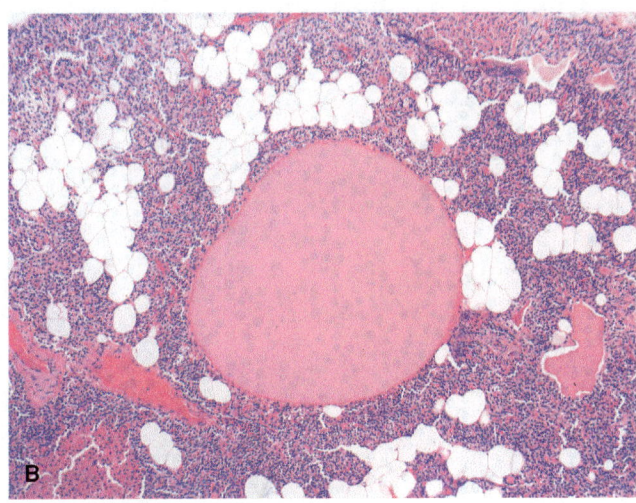

FIGURE 44.9 Colloid-like material in normal parathyroid glands. Parathyroid glands may have cysts (**A**, **B**) and follicles (**A**, **C**) filled with proteinaceous material that resembles colloid of the thyroid gland; proliferations with this colloid-like material can resemble thyroid neoplasms and may require special techniques to verify as of parathyroid origin. Note: Figures 44.9A, B and C are all higher magnifications of areas in the gland shown in 44.8C.

resembling the colloid of thyroid follicles; this material contains glycoproteins, and therefore stains with periodic acid–Schiff (PAS) (62), and is positive for PTH by immunohistochemistry. Thyroid follicles often contain birefringent calcium oxalate crystals; these are not seen in the colloid of parathyroid glands, and this feature is helpful to distinguish thyroid from parathyroid at the time of intraoperative consultation. Amyloid-like features of this colloid have been reported (63). The parenchyma has been described to have three cell types: chief cells, oxyphils, and transitional cells (49). These are all variants of the chief cells that have differing degrees of oncocytic change. Another cell variant, found usually only in pathologic states, is the clear cell or "water clear cell" (49). Fundamentally, there is a single cell type that is responsible for synthesis and secretion of PTH; this cell can exhibit variability in morphology due to functional alterations and can undergo oncocytic change.

Normal chief cells are round to polygonal cells that measure 8 to 12 μm in diameter. The nuclei are round, centrally located within the cell, and have a well-defined nuclear membrane with evenly distributed chromatin and small nucleoli. The cells have well-defined cell borders and their cytoplasm varies from clear to amphophilic or faintly eosinophilic (Fig. 44.10). The clear vacuolated appearance of significant parts of the chief cell cytoplasm is due to accumulation of glycogen that stains with PAS and lipid that can be identified with fat stains such as oil red O. The intracellular content of fat is thought to be inversely correlated with their endocrine activity; increased cytoplasmic lipid is a feature of inactive or suppressed chief cells whereas fat is minimal in hormonally active cells.

The ultrastructural features of parathyroid chief cells (Fig. 44.11) are similar to those of other neuroendocrine cells and vary with their functional activity (64,65). The organelles for hormone synthesis include rough endoplasmic reticulum where peptide hormone is translated from mRNA, the Golgi apparatus where packaging occurs, and the membrane-bound secretory granules that store hormone and carry it to the cell surface for secretion. Resting cells have poorly developed synthetic organelles, accumulation of glycogen and lysosomes, as well as large lipid bodies that correspond to the lipid seen by light microscopy; variable numbers of small dense-core secretory granules accumulate at the cell periphery. The cell membranes are relatively

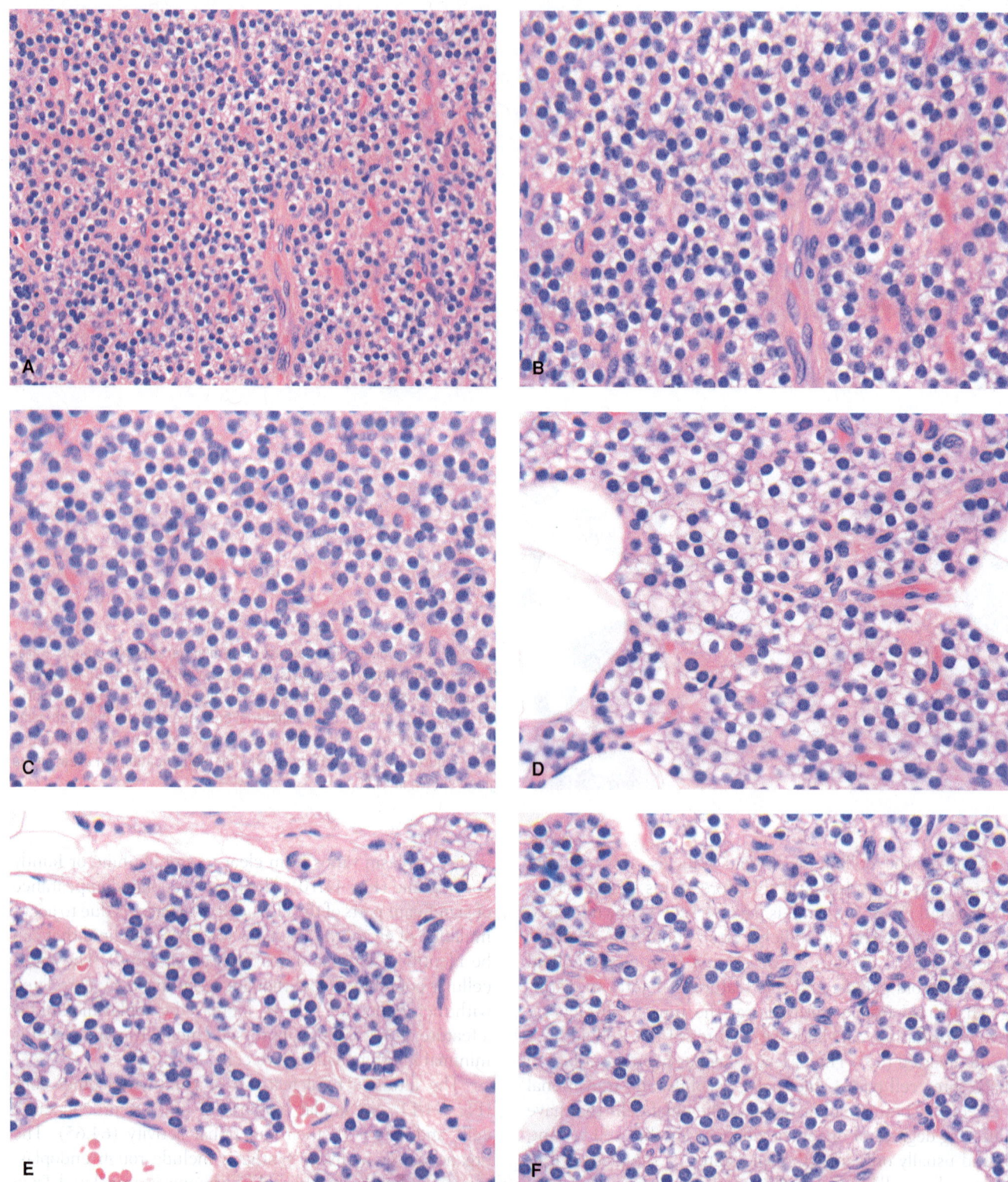

FIGURE 44.10 Histology of chief cells. Chief cells (illustrated in figures **A** through **F**) are round to polygonal with centrally located nuclei that have evenly distributed chromatin and small nucleoli and well defined cell borders. The cytoplasm varies from clear to amphophilic or faintly eosinophilic. The clear vacuolated appearance is due to accumulation of glycogen and/or lipid. Note: Figure B is a higher magnification of a portion of Figure A.

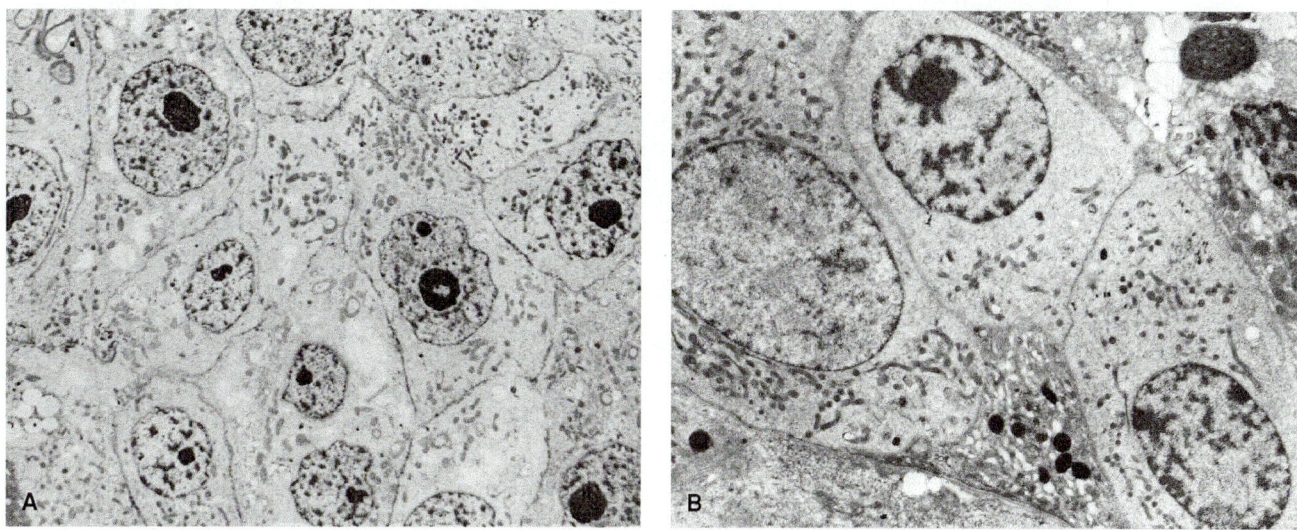

FIGURE 44.11 Ultrastructure of chief cells. By electron microscopy, parathyroid chief cells have short profiles of rough endoplasmic reticulum, scattered small secretory granules, mitochondria (**A, B**), variably developed Golgi complexes (**A**), and vacuoles that may represent lysosomes with lipid content (**B**).

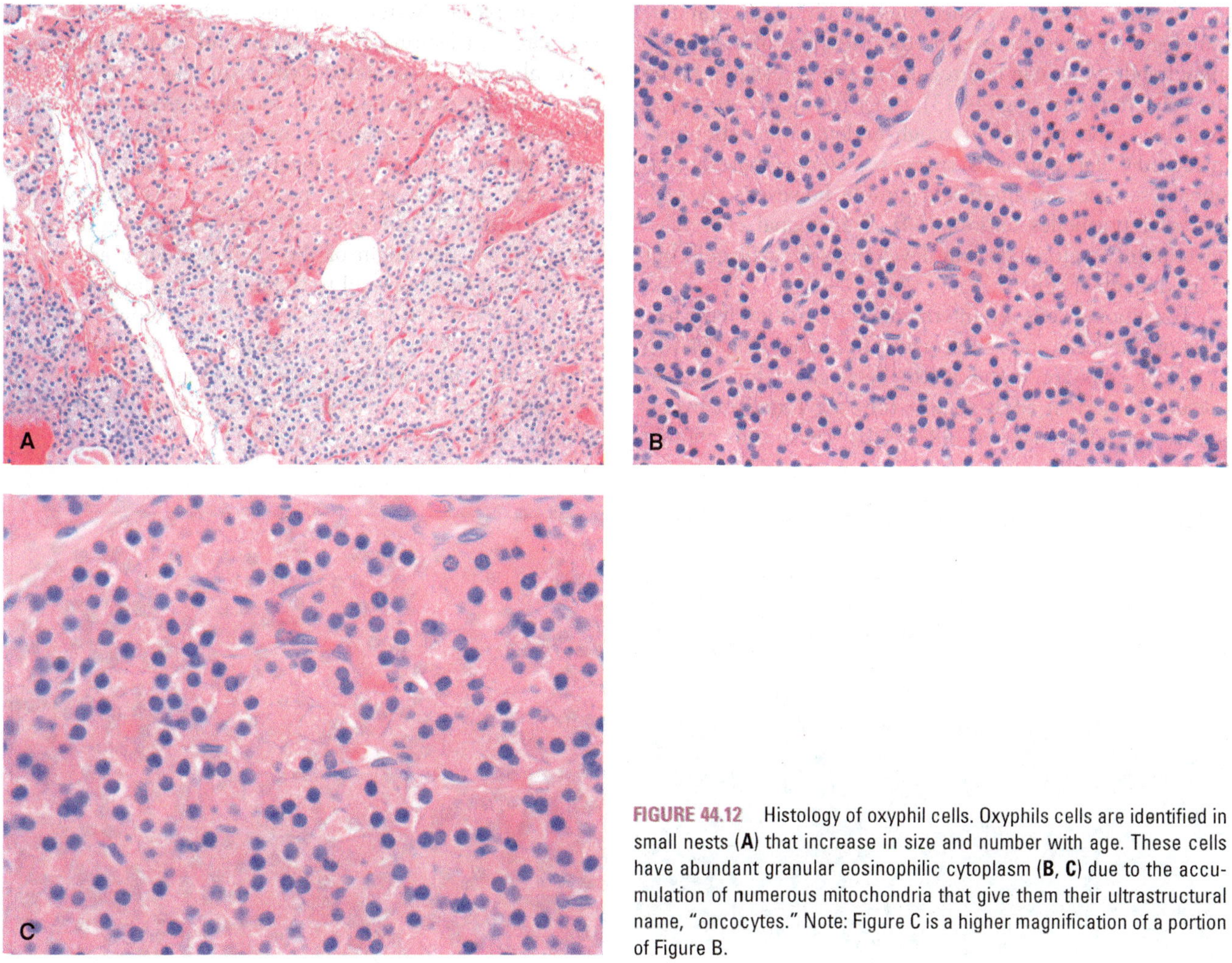

FIGURE 44.12 Histology of oxyphil cells. Oxyphils cells are identified in small nests (**A**) that increase in size and number with age. These cells have abundant granular eosinophilic cytoplasm (**B, C**) due to the accumulation of numerous mitochondria that give them their ultrastructural name, "oncocytes." Note: Figure C is a higher magnification of a portion of Figure B.

straight with few interdigitations and desmosomes connecting adjacent cells. In contrast, actively synthesizing and secreting cells have well-developed parallel arrays of rough endoplasmic reticulum, usually in a perinuclear location, prominent Golgi complexes with immature forming secretory granules of different electron densities with electron-lucent halos, and larger dense-core secretory granules throughout the cytoplasm that is depleted of glycogen and lipid bodies. The cell borders are more complex with interdigitations and occasionally one can see fusion of the secretory granule membrane with the plasma membrane and emptying of secretory product into the extracellular space.

The oxyphil cell is a chief cell that has undergone oncocytic change, accumulation of mitochondria that can be increased in both number and size. The stimulus for oncocytic change is not known but these cells increase gradually with age in the parathyroid as they do in other organs including pituitary and thyroid (66). Oxyphils are found singly, in small clusters or as large nodules and sheets (Fig. 44.12). These cells are larger than chief cells, measuring 12 to 20 μm in diameter, due to the abundant eosinophilic granular cytoplasm that is filled with mitochondria.

Oxyphils, known as oncocytes in ultrastructural terminology, are characterized by the presence of numerous mitochondria that can be irregular in size and shape, filling the cell cytoplasm (Fig. 44.13); other organelles are scant, including short profiles of rough endoplasmic reticulum, involuted Golgi complexes, sparse secretory granules, occasional lysosomes and lipofuscin granule, however some lack synthetic organelles entirely (64). Transitional cells have fewer mitochondria than fully developed oncocytic cells but more than chief cells.

Transitional cells are intermediate forms that have features of chief cells and partial oncocytic change (Fig. 44.14).

Clear cells are found in the fetal gland but are not present in normal adult glands; they are found in hyperplasias and adenomas (Fig. 44.15A,B). These cells contain

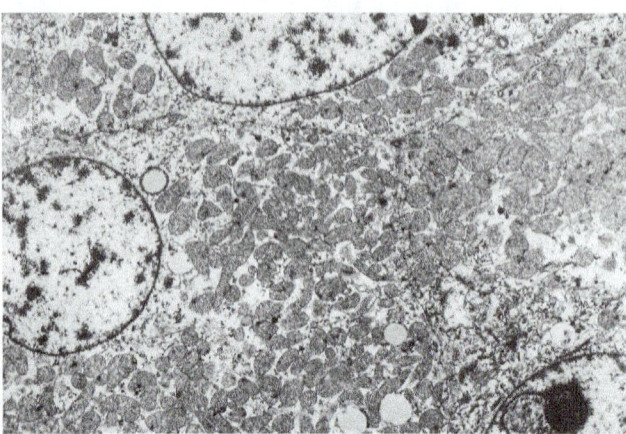

FIGURE 44.13 Ultrastructure of oxyphil cells. By electron microscopy, the cytoplasm of parathyroid oncocytic cells is almost completely replaced by the numerous mitochondria that can be enlarged and dilated; the residual rough endoplasmic reticulum, small Golgi complexes, few secretory granules and lipid vacuoles are trapped within the accumulation of mitochondria or pushed to the perinuclear or peripheral areas.

abundant cytoplasmic glycogen. A distinct variant of clear cells, known as "water clear cells" (wasserhelle cells), are very large, measuring 15 to 20 μm and up to 40 μm, and have abundant vacuolated cytoplasm that is filled with glycogen that surrounds large membrane-bound vacuoles (Fig. 44.15C). The granular component of the cytoplasm of the water clear cells is typically positive for PAS but not after diastase pretreatment, proving that this diastase-sensitive material is glycogen (67). Several hypotheses were proposed for the origin of the vacuoles. They are generally thought to be related to the Golgi complex given their resemblance to the Golgi vesicles (68,69); however, some proposed a link to dilated cisternae of the granular endoplasmic reticulum given the identification of ribosomes on the surfaces of the vacuoles (70) and others questioned a possible link to secretory granules (71).

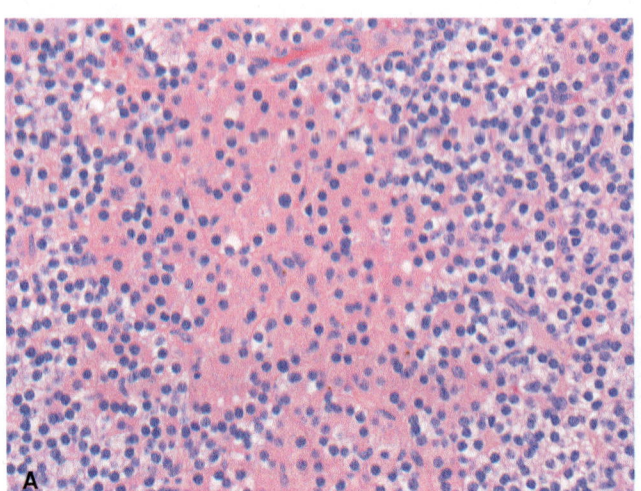
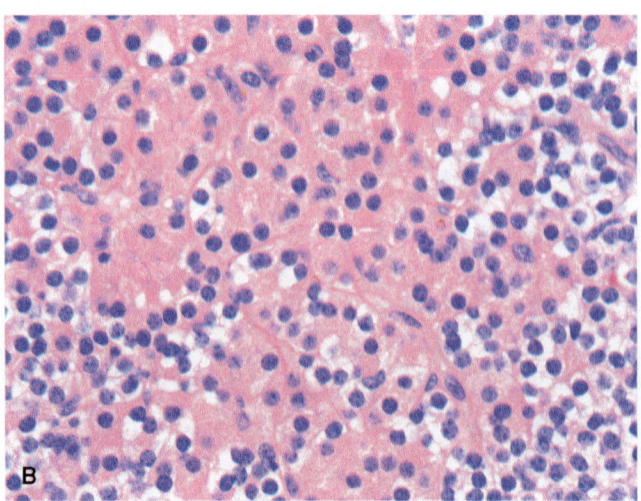

FIGURE 44.14 Histology of transitional cells. Transitional cells are chief cells with partial oncocytic change (**A, B**). Note: Figure B is a higher power image of a portion of Figure A.

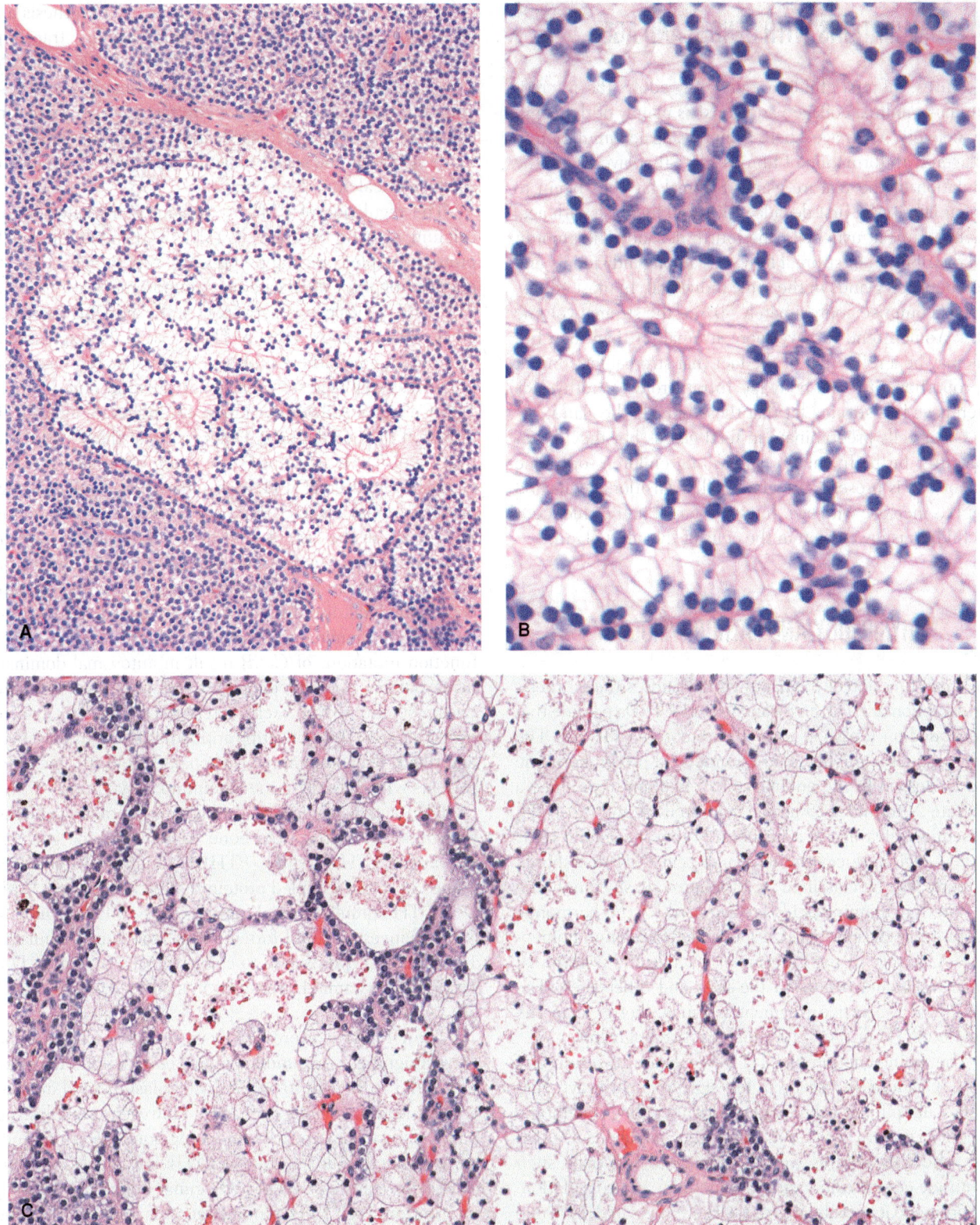

FIGURE 44.15 The spectrum of clear cell change in parathyroids. Clear cells are not usually found in normal parathyroids but are present in hyperplasias (**A** and **B**) and adenomas. A distinct form of clear cell change due to massive accumulation of glycogen and lipid gives rise to "water clear cell" morphology (**C**). Note: Figure B is a high power image from a portion of Figure A.

VARIATIONS WITH GENDER AND AGE

In fetuses, infants, children and young adults the interstitium has minimal collagen and consists mainly of the capillary network. With age, there is increasing accumulation of collagen with formation of fibrous septa that give rise to the lobulation of the mature gland. Stromal fat cells begin to appear late in the first decade of life and increase with age, reaching a peak usually in the fourth decade. The amount and distribution of stromal fat varies among individuals and even between glands in the same individual. In most adults, at cells comprise approximately 50% of the stromal volume (48). Women tend to have more stromal fat than men but this may be a reflection of the fact that stromal fat content is proportional to total body fat. Intrathyroidal parathyroids often have less stromal fat that those outside the gland.

Clear cells predominate in fetal glands but they disappear after birth. In infants and young children, only one type of cell is present, the chief cell. Transitional cells and oxyphils increase with age. Intracellular fat in the chief cells of children is lower than in the cells of the adult gland.

PHYSIOLOGY AND PATHOPHYSIOLOGY

The main function of the parathyroid glands is the synthesis and secretion of PTH, an 84 amino acid 9.4 kDa peptide that is encoded on the short arm of chromosome 11 (72). The gene product is initially a 115 amino acid pre-prohormone that is cleaved in the endoplasmic reticulum to produce a separate N-terminal 25 amino acid product and pro-PTH; subsequent cleavage of a further 6 N-terminal amino acids in the Golgi produces the 84 amino acid PTH that should correctly also be classified as a prohormone since only the 34 N-terminal amino acids are required for the hormone–receptor interaction that is responsible for calcium homeostasis. Cleavage of the C-terminal inactive and N-terminal active fragments occurs in the liver and other sites. The half-life of the active fragment is much shorter than the complete PTH or the C-terminal inactive fragment.

The main function of PTH is regulation of serum calcium. Calcium is essential for signaling pathways that control ubiquitous cellular functions including membrane integrity, protein secretion, glycogen metabolism, division, and adhesion, as well as specialized functions such as muscle contraction, neuron excitability, and coagulation. Accordingly, its levels are also closely regulated by three main hormones: PTH, calcitriol (1,25[OH]2D3) and calcitonin. Approximately 99% of calcium in the human is in bones as hydroxyapatite and only 1% is present in extracellular fluids and soft tissues. In extracellular fluid, including serum, almost half, 48%, of total calcium is ionized calcium, 46% is bound to protein and the remainder is associated with diffusible ion complexes (49). The level of ionized calcium $[Ca^{2+}]$ is the main regulator of PTH synthesis and secretion; increased ionized calcium inhibits transcription, translation, and secretion of PTH by chief cells and decreased ionized calcium results in enhanced synthesis and secretion. This is in direct contrast to other endocrine cells that respond to increased calcium with increased hormone synthesis and secretion and have reduced signaling in the face of calcium depletion.

The regulation of PTH by calcium is mediated by the calcium sensing receptor (CaSR), a member of the G protein–coupled receptor (GPCR) superfamily (73–75) encoded by the *CaSR* gene on chromosome 3 at 3q13.3 to 21 (75). Hypocalcemia activates CaSR, inducing increased PTH synthesis and secretion. The CaSR is also expressed in the renal tubules where it plays a role in calcium resorption (74,75), as well as in stomach, small intestine, and skin (76). 1,25-Calcitriol (dihydroxyvitamin D) indirectly alters PTH secretion by modulating the expression of the CaSR. Inactivation of CaSR signaling is the cause of familial hypocalciuric hypercalcemia (FHH, also known as familial benign hypercalcemia) characterized by inappropriately normal PTH levels in the face of mild hypercalcemia and hypocalciuria due to heterozygous inactivating mutation, and neonatal severe primary hyperparathyroidism, a more severe and potentially fatal disorder due to homozygous inactivation or heterozygous dominant negative mutations (76,77). Gain-of-function mutations of *CaSR* result in autosomal dominant hypocalcemia, sporadic idiopathic hypoparathyroidism, and Bartter syndrome type V, characterized by hypocalcemia and hypercalcuria (76). Activating antibodies to CaSR have been described in autoimmune hypoparathyroidism including patients with polyendocrine autoimmune syndromes (76).

PTH acts by directly and indirectly promoting calcium resorption into blood from bone, kidney, and the gut. Acting on the PTH receptor (PTHR1), another 7 transmembrane G protein–coupled protein that increases cyclic AMP (78), PTH stimulates renal tubular reabsorption of calcium, and enhances calcitriol formation in kidney by stimulating 1α-vitamin D hydroxylase to convert 25(OH) vitamin D to 1α25(OH)2 vitamin D, resulting in increased gut absorption of calcium.

The PTHR1 is expressed by osteoblasts, a feature that caused significant misunderstanding of its action. Activation of PTHR1 is thought to prolong osteoblast life and increase activity, leading to bone formation. However, osteoblast signaling activates osteoclasts, inducing bone resorption indirectly, since they do not express PTHR1. PTH also activates osteocytes, causing lysis of perilacunar bone. Paradoxically, intermittent high PTH administration is anabolic for bone, while continuous elevation is catabolic. It is postulated that the transient stimulation can stimulate the osteoblast anabolic activity without triggering the catabolic response through osteoclasts. For this reason, PTH is paradoxically used in the treatment of osteoporosis (72).

Mobilization of calcium from bone results in increased phosphate as well. Phosphate has no direct role in PTH regulation but PTH promotes excretion of phosphate by blocking its resorption in the kidney. Fibroblast growth factor 23 (FGF23) is a critical regulator of serum phosphorus; it depresses 1α-hydroxylase in the renal tubules. FGF23 produced by osteocytes and osteoblasts downregulates the type II sodium–phosphate co-transporters (NPTi2a and NPTi2c) causing phosphate wasting. FGF23 also down-regulates the activity of the renal 25(OH)2 vitamin D 1α hydroxylase decreasing the serum level of 1α,25(OH)2D.

The PTHR1 signals through the Gsα encoded by *GNAS*. Inactivating mutations of *GNAS* result in pseudohypoparathyroidism (PHP) types IA, IB, IC, and pseudopseudohypoparathyroidism (PPHP). The complex *GNAS* locus on chromosome 20q13.3 undergoes parent-specific methylation at several sites (79). Heterozygous inactivating mutations of maternal *GNAS* cause PHP type 1A with PTH-resistant hypocalcemia and hyperphosphatemia; reduced paternal *GNAS* expression in proximal renal tubules result in little or no Gsα protein, leading to PTH-resistant hypocalcemia and hyperphosphatemia. The same or similar *GNAS* mutations in the paternal allele are the cause of PPHP (79). Autosomal dominant PHP type IB is caused by heterozygous maternal deletions within *GNAS* or *STX16*, associated with loss-of-methylation (LOM) reducing Gsα expression. Epigenetic changes are also observed in sporadic PHP 1B, and rare cases have been reported to have paternal uniparental isodisomy or heterodisomy of chromosome 20q (79).

SPECIAL PROCEDURES

A number of special procedures can be used in the evaluation of parathyroid glands. These include histologic stains and immunohistochemistry, as well as molecular testing.

Histologic special stains include the Grimelius silver technique that identified the parathyroid chief cells as neuroendocrine. This stain is of historical interest and has been largely supplanted by immunohistochemistry.

The PAS stain is widely available in most laboratories and can serve to assess the amount of glycogen in chief cells, a feature that is helpful in assessing function, as well as the significance of cytoplasmic clearing. Glycogen stains strongly with the PAS stain (Fig. 44.16) but is not diastase-resistant, therefore is not identified in tissue stained with PAS-D (PAS after diastase digestion). The colloid material in cysts and follicles of the parathyroid is not composed of glycogen (Fig. 44.16).

The same is true for fat stains that have been applied to evaluate the intracytoplasmic lipid content of chief cells that is higher in resting cells and lower in active cells. This has been applied to distinguish hyperplastic and adenomatous cells from normal cells (Fig. 44.17). A significant limitation of this tool is the need for fresh and/or frozen tissue; since lipid is lost in formalin-fixed, paraffin-embedded tissues, the oil red O stain cannot be used on permanent sections. Its main application was at the time of intraoperative consultation when frozen sections or imprints could be studied with this tool. However, the use of intraoperative PTH assays to guide the extent of surgery has revolutionized the operative approach to patients with hyperparathyroidism (1) and the need for classification of a gland as abnormal is less critical than simply the identification of tissue as parathyroid rather than lymph node or other neck structures.

In contrast to the declining role of histochemistry, immunohistochemistry has emerged as a valuable method of improving diagnosis and pathologist input into clinical care. The applications fall into three main categories: confirmation of parathyroid differentiation, distinction of benign from malignant proliferations, and determination of genetic predisposition to parathyroid disease.

Parathyroid lesions may be obvious and within parathyroid glands, but given the common intrathyroidal and mediastinal location of parathyroids and their tendency to form follicles, they can be easily misdiagnosed. Immunostains including synaptophysin and chromogranin, as well as vesicle-associated membrane protein (VAMP), synaptosomal-associated protein 23 (SNAP-23) that is part of a soluble N-ethylmaleimide–sensitive fusion attachment protein receptor (SNARE), are all characteristic of neuroendocrine lineage. GATA-3 (80), GCM2 (81) and PTH define parathyroid cells and can distinguish them from other neuroendocrine cells that give rise to tumors in this regions, including C cells that develop into medullary thyroid carcinomas, thymic neuroendocrine tumors, and paragangliomas, or in the case of clear cells, renal carcinoma, and other large clear cell tumors (Table 44.2, Fig. 44.18). Paragangliomas are also negative for keratins whereas the other neuroendocrine tumors including parathyroid tumors express various cytokeratins including those identified by the AE1/AE3 cocktail and cytokeratins 8/18 identified by Cam 5.2. Chief cells are also positive for cytokeratin 19, and are negative for TTF-1, PGP 9.5 and neurofilaments. The use of multiple biomarkers is encouraged, since some parathyroid lesions may have reduced staining for GCM2 (81) and PTH expression can be reduced in some lesions.

The distinction of parathyroid hyperplasia from normal parathyroid can be difficult since the degree of stromal and even cytoplasmic fat is variable in normal glands. This was a major problem in the era of parathyroid dissections to identify all glands. However, the use of limited parathyroidectomy based on imaging and intraoperative PTH assays has reduced the need for this distinction. Clonality studies have shown that most adenomas and carcinomas are monoclonal, whereas secondary hyperplasia is not (82–84). The concept of clonality in multiple endocrine neoplasia (MEN) is more complex and it appears that nodules in the "hyperplastic" glands of patents with MEN1 syndrome are indeed clonal proliferations (85), consistent with the concept that each cell at risk of loss of the intact tumor suppressor gives rise to a neoplastic proliferation. Therefore, affected parathyroid glands are considered to display multiple multiglandular parathyroid

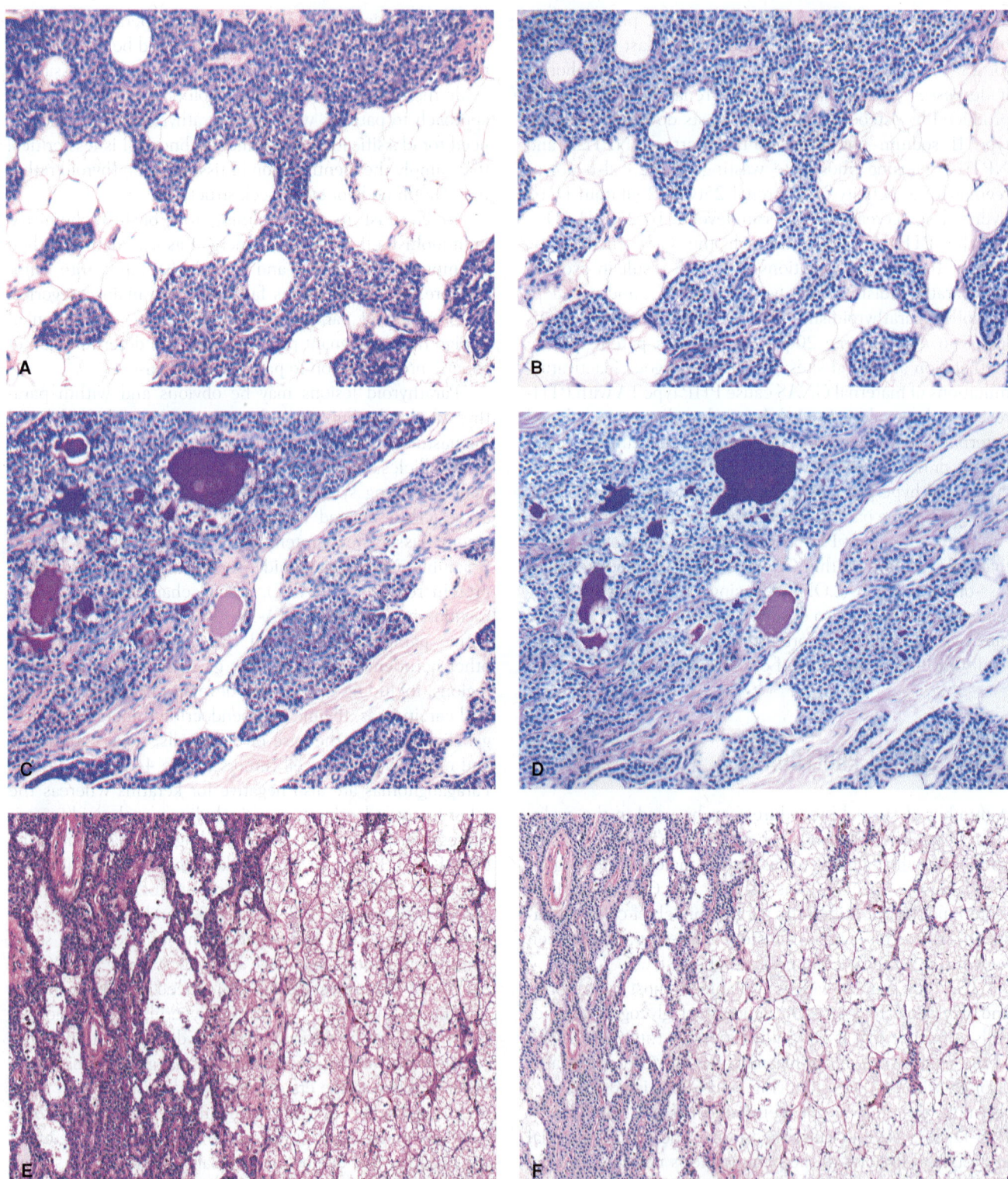

FIGURE 44.16 Histochemistry of parathyroid: PAS and PAS-D. Normal parathyroid chief cells contain abundant glycogen that stains with PAS (**A**) and is not diastase resistant (**B**). The colloid-like material in cysts and follicles stains intensely with PAS (**C**) and is diastase resistant, showing strong positivity in the PAS-D stain (**D**). Water clear cells have clear vacuoles that are not filled with glycogen but there is abundant PAS-positive glycogen in the cytoplasm surrounding them (**E**) that is lost after diastase treatment (**F**).

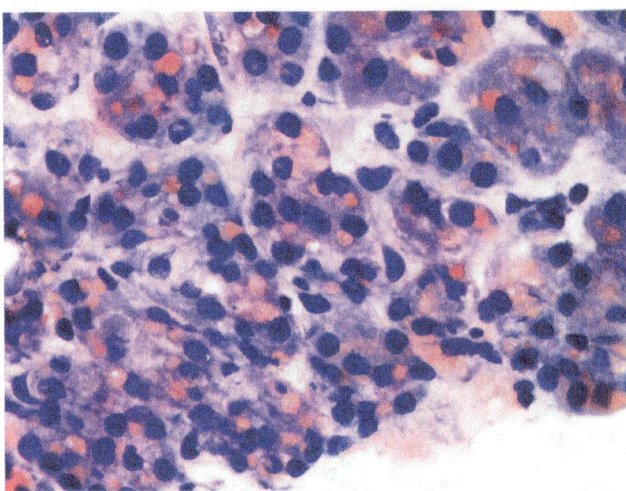

FIGURE 44.17 Histochemistry of parathyroid: Oil red O. Normal chief cells with intracytoplasmic lipid droplets in approximately 90% of the cells (frozen section Oil-Red-O stain with hematoxylin counterstain). (Courtesy of Dr. S. I. Roth)

TABLE 44.2

Immunohistochemical Biomarkers Used to Confirm Parathyroid Differentiation

Biomarkers	Reactivity Pattern
Chromogranin-A	Cytoplasmic[b]
Synaptophysin	Cytoplasmic[b]
PTH[a]	Cytoplasmic
GATA-3	Nuclear
GCM-2	Nuclear
Polyclonal PAX8	Nuclear
Monoclonal PAX8	Negative
TTF-1	Negative
Keratins (AE1/AE3, 7, 8/18, 19)	Cytoplasmic[b]

[a]Parathyroid cysts can be negative for PTH.
[b]May be negative in some tumors.

adenomas. Tertiary hyperparathyroidism is often attributed to emergence of a clonal neoplasm from the background of hyperplastic tissue in secondary hyperparathyroidism.

The distinction of benign from malignant parathyroid neoplasms can be straightforward when a lesion is either completely bland and surrounded by normal tissue, clearly an adenoma, or highly infiltrative and angioinvasive (Fig. 44.19) with perineural invasion as an obvious carcinoma. However, it is not uncommon that a patient has a fine needle biopsy of a neck mass and in that scenario, benign tumors can develop fibrosis, become infiltrative, even infiltrate into surrounding tissues, and look worrisome

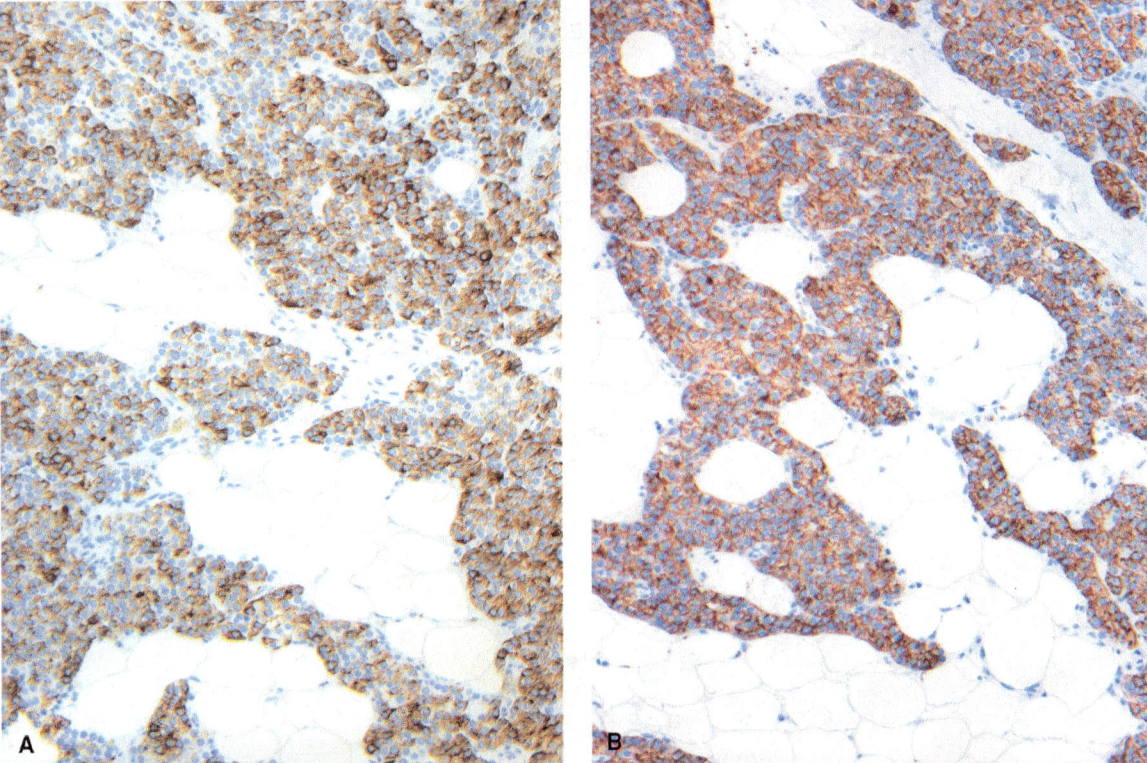

FIGURE 44.18 Immunohistochemistry: Markers of parathyroid differentiation. Normal parathyroid chief cells stain for chromogranin A (**A**) and parathyroid hormone (**B**) (*continued*)

FIGURE 44.18 (*Continued*), as well as GATA-3 (**C**). Clear cell tumors can be confirmed to be of parathyroid differentiation when they stain for GATA-3 (**D**) and parathyroid hormone (**E**). Water clear cells also express nuclear GATA-3 (**F**).

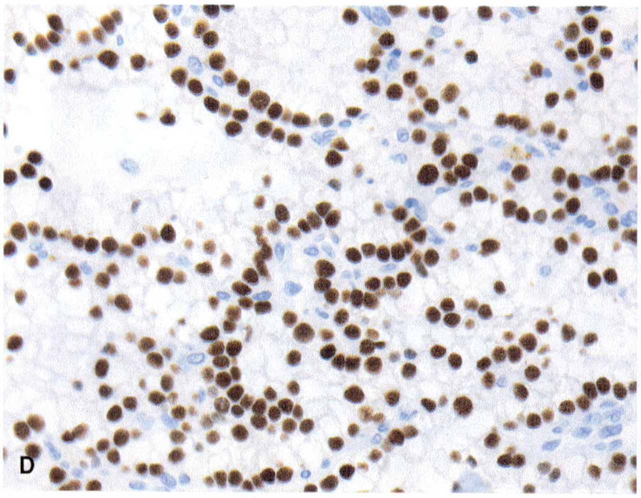

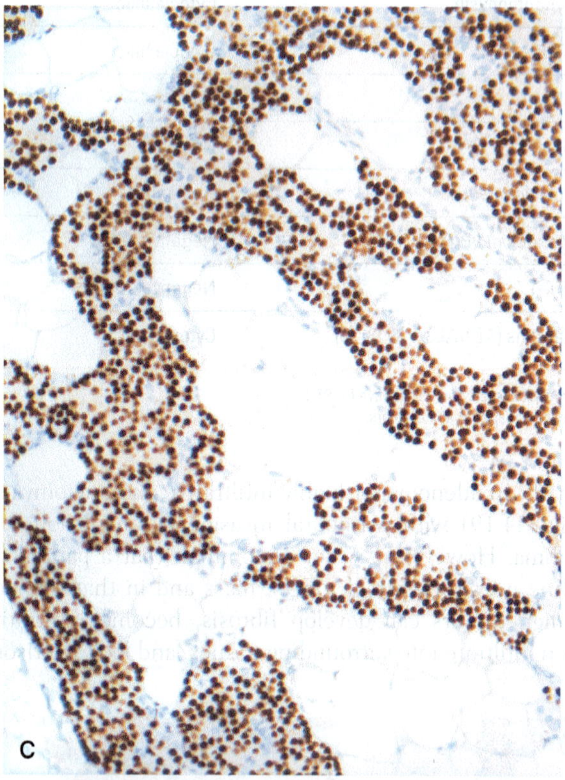

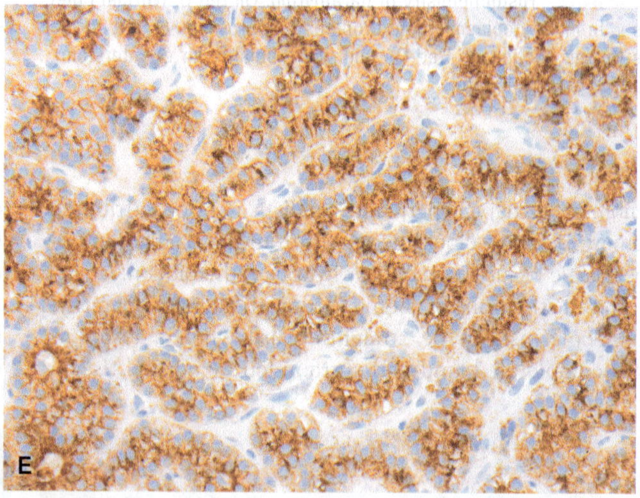

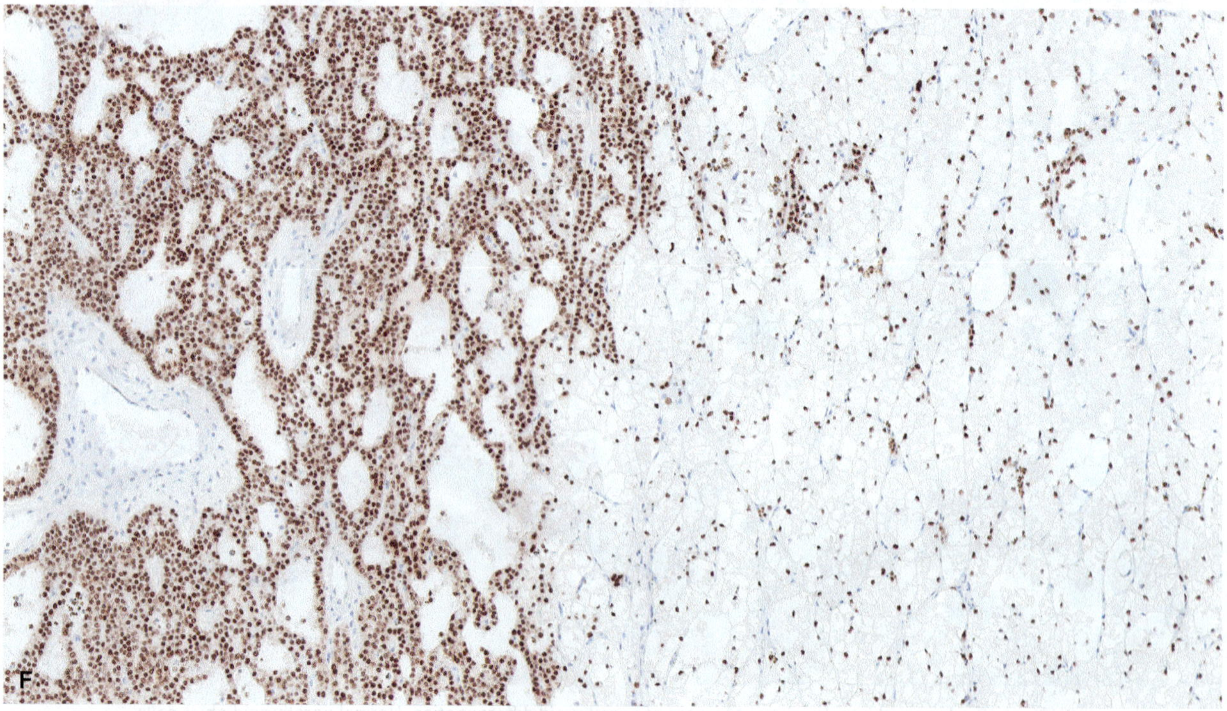

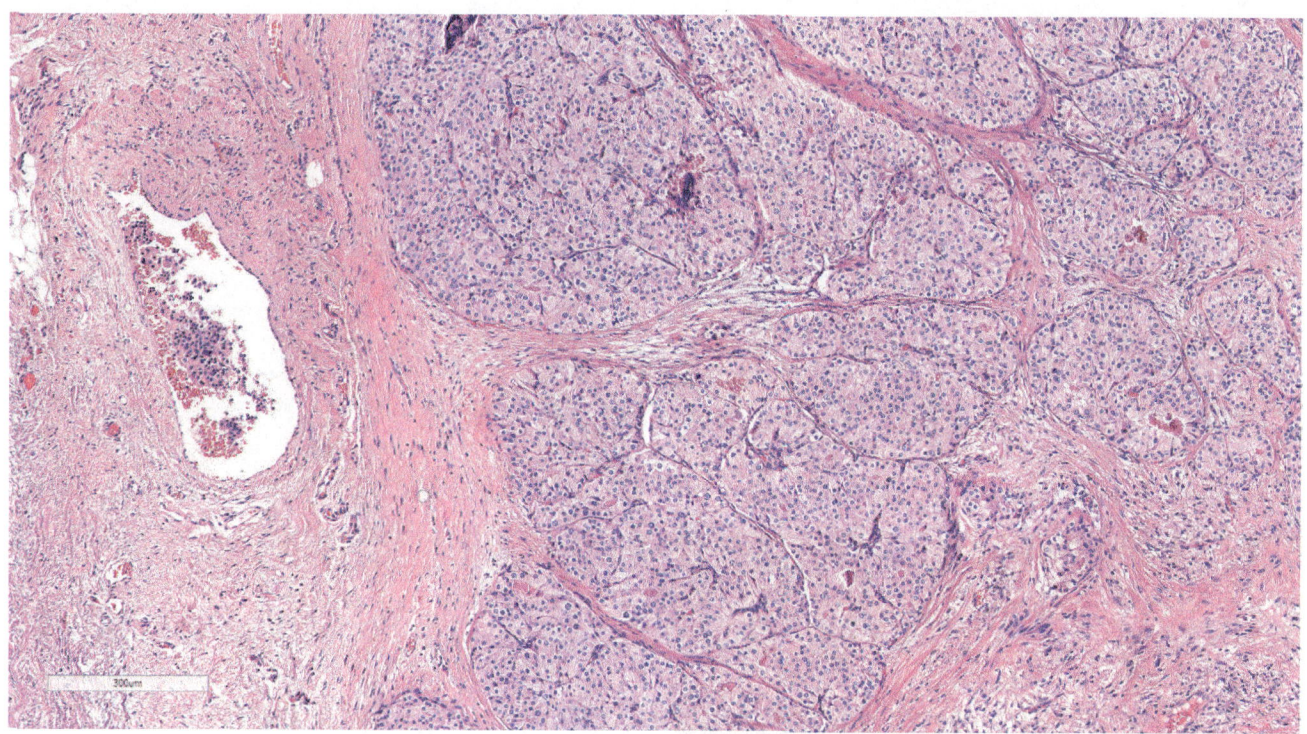

FIGURE 44.19 Vascular invasion in parathyroid carcinoma. Parathyroid carcinoma can be diagnosed on histology by the identification of unequivocal angioinvasion defined as tumor cells in a vascular lumen with associated thrombus.

as a reactive change (86,87). In this setting, it is helpful to have biomarkers of normal and benign neoplastic cells and biomarkers of malignancy (Table 44.3).

The gene initially called *Hyperparathyroidism 2* (*HRPT2*), now known as *CDC73*, encodes a protein called parafibromin, a tumor suppressor that was initially associated with the hyperparathyroidism–jaw tumor syndrome (88). Mutations inactivate this gene in that disorder and in sporadic parathyroid carcinomas. Parafibromin is immunolocalized to the nuclei and nucleoli of normal parathyroid glands (Fig. 44.20A). Decreased nuclear and/or nucleolar parafibromin staining provide evidence of the malignant potential of parathyroid proliferations (Fig. 44.20B) (89,90). Some studies have also shown the reverse pattern of staining for PGP 9.5 that is not expressed in normal parathyroid and is upregulated in parathyroid carcinoma (Fig. 44.20C).

Alterations in other tumor suppressor genes, including *p27*, *Rb*, and *Tp53*, have been reported in parathyroid carcinomas (91–95); loss of these tumor suppressors is seen in some carcinomas but not in hyperplasia or adenoma (Fig. 44.21). In contrast, activation of cyclic AMP by *GNAS* mutation (96) or overexpression of *cyclin D1*, the latter through the *CCND1/PRAD1* rearrangement involving 1p15.3 to 15.1 where the PTH gene promoter upregulates cyclin D1 (84,97), are features of adenomas (Fig 44.22). Other biomarkers of malignancy include Bcl-2 loss (Fig. 44.23) and galectin-3 overexpression (Fig. 44.23) (98), as well as loss of expression for mdm2 (99) and APC (89,100). While some authors reported that parathyroid adenomas are typically associated with a Ki67 labeling index less than 5% (100), the diagnostic role of Ki67 as a biomarker of parathyroid tumor classification remains unclear (101) (Fig. 44.24). Another ancillary tool that is helpful in

TABLE 44.3
Immunohistochemical Biomarkers Used in the Distinction of Parathyroid Adenoma and Carcinoma

Biomarker	Adenoma	Carcinoma
Parafibromin	Positive	Negative[a]
APC	Positive	Negative[b]
Bcl-2	Positive	Negative[b]
Mdm2	Positive	Negative
Rb	Positive	Negative[b]
p53 overexpression	Absent	Rare
CyclinD1	Positive	Negative
Ki67 (MIB1)	Often <5%	Often >5%
Galectin-3	Negative	Positive
PGP 9.5	Negative	Positive

[a]Nuclear expression may be retained in some parathyroid carcinomas.
[b]Can be reduced in some carcinomas.

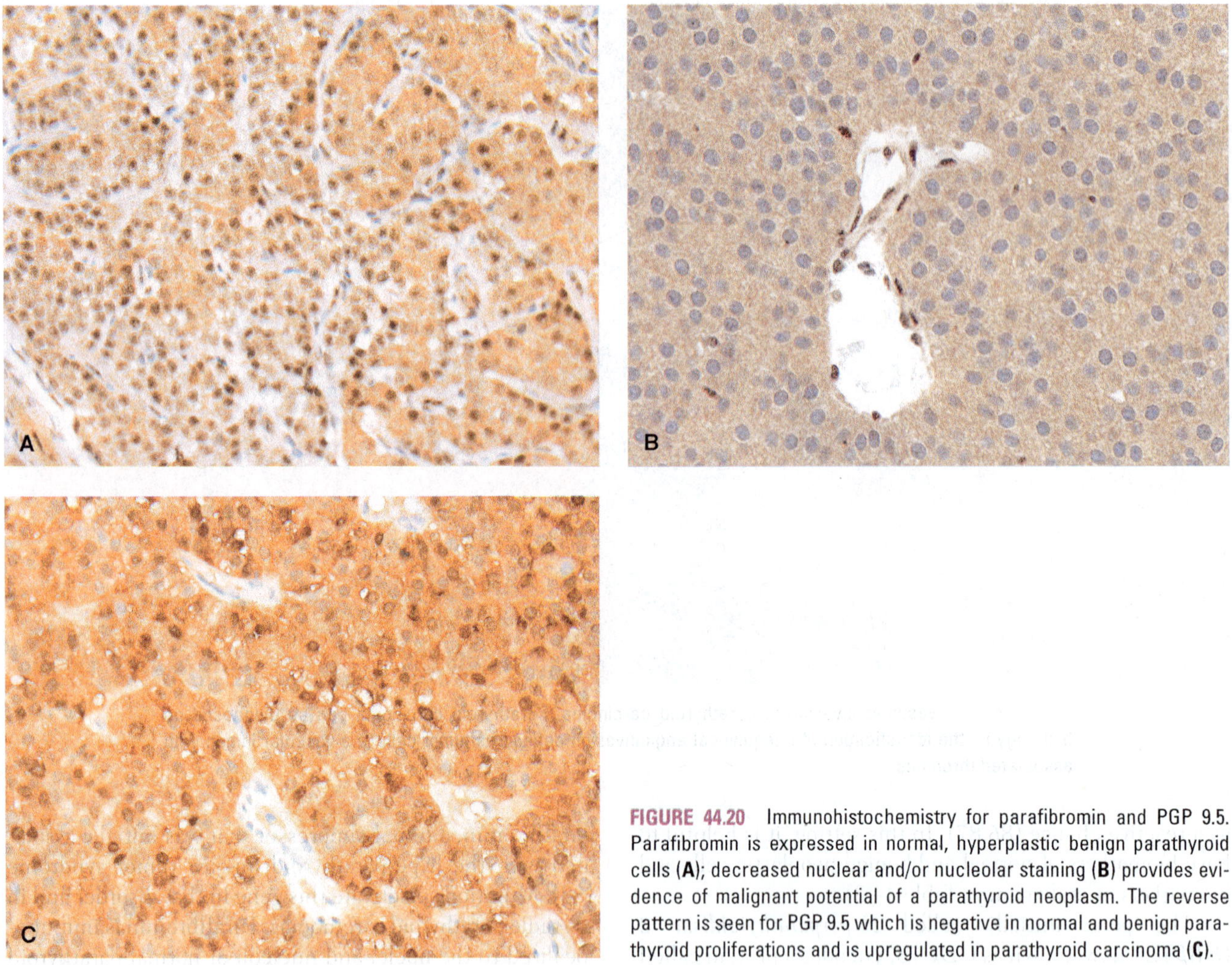

FIGURE 44.20 Immunohistochemistry for parafibromin and PGP 9.5. Parafibromin is expressed in normal, hyperplastic benign parathyroid cells (**A**); decreased nuclear and/or nucleolar staining (**B**) provides evidence of malignant potential of a parathyroid neoplasm. The reverse pattern is seen for PGP 9.5 which is negative in normal and benign parathyroid proliferations and is upregulated in parathyroid carcinoma (**C**).

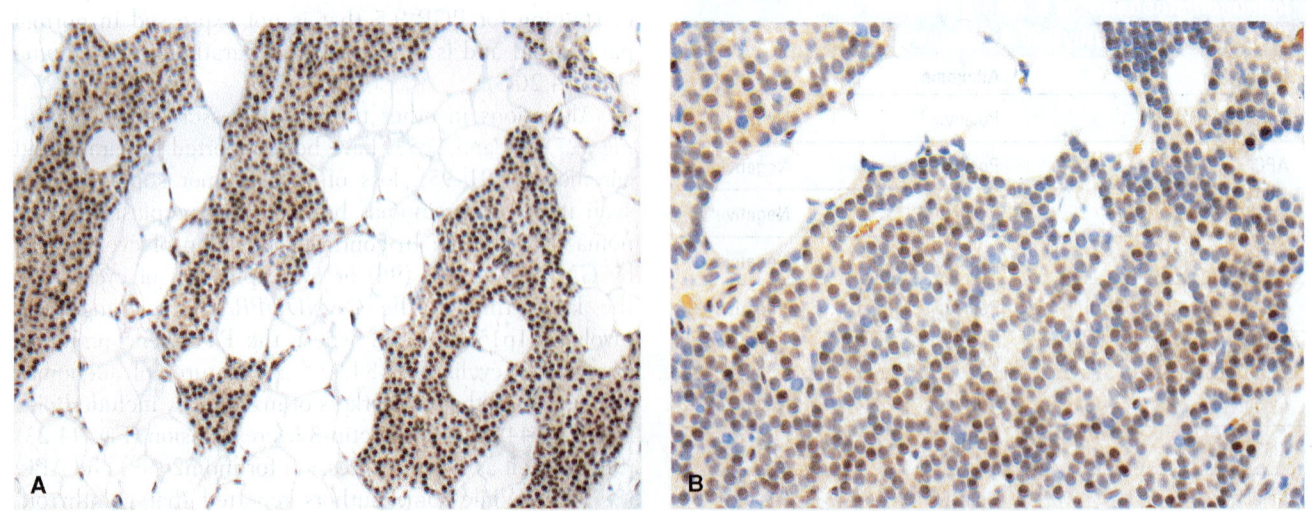

FIGURE 44.21 Dysregulation of p27, Rb, and p53 in parathyroid proliferations. Normal parathyroid stains strongly for p27 (**A**) and while there may be reduction, staining is preserved in hyperplasia (**B**) and adenomas. (*continued*)

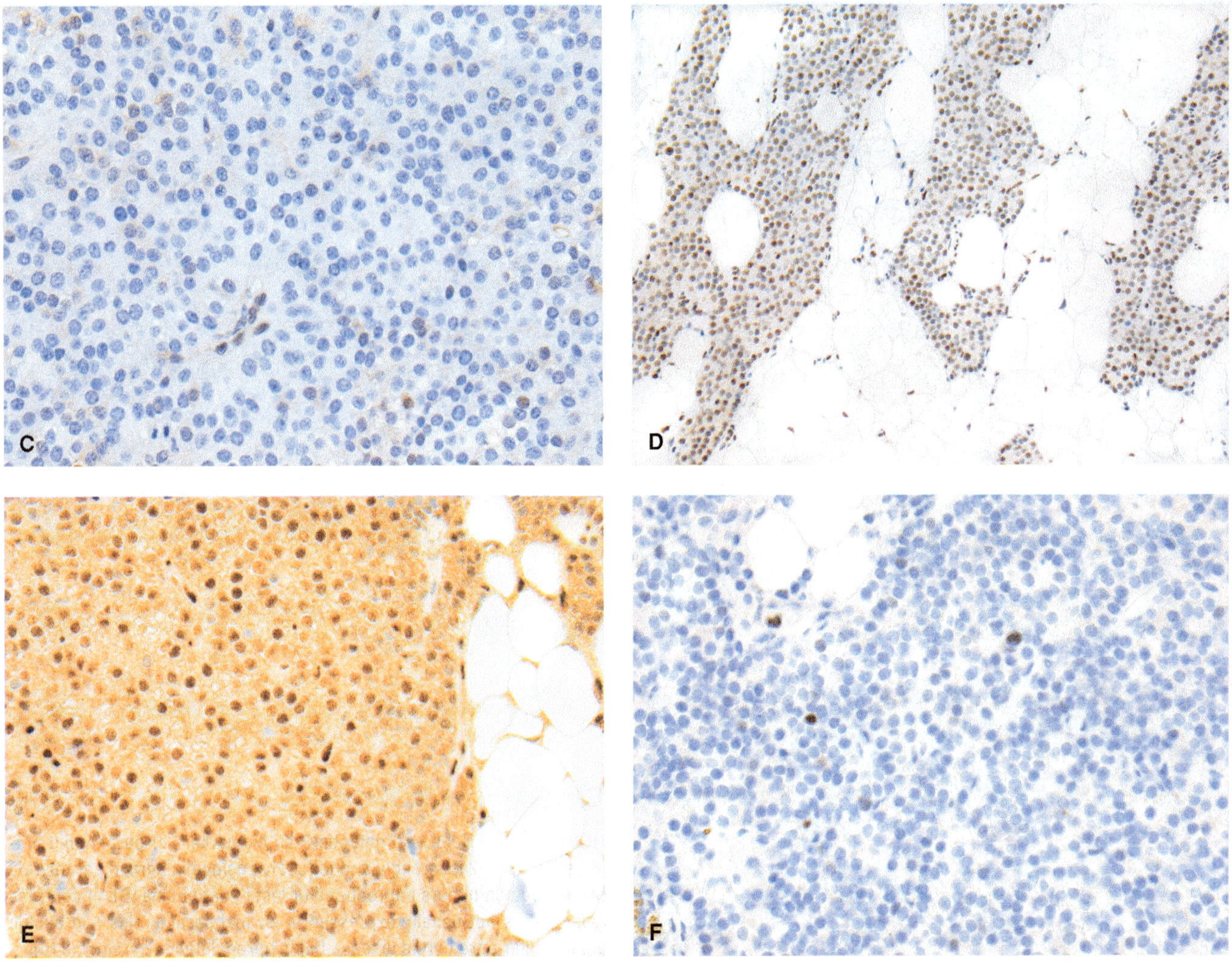

FIGURE 44.21 (*Continued*) There can be global loss in carcinoma (**C**) but this may also be a feature of benign lesions in patients with MEN4. Rb is also expressed in normal parathyroid (**D**) and hyperplasia (**E**); p53 can be focally positive in hyperplasia (**F**) and adenoma.

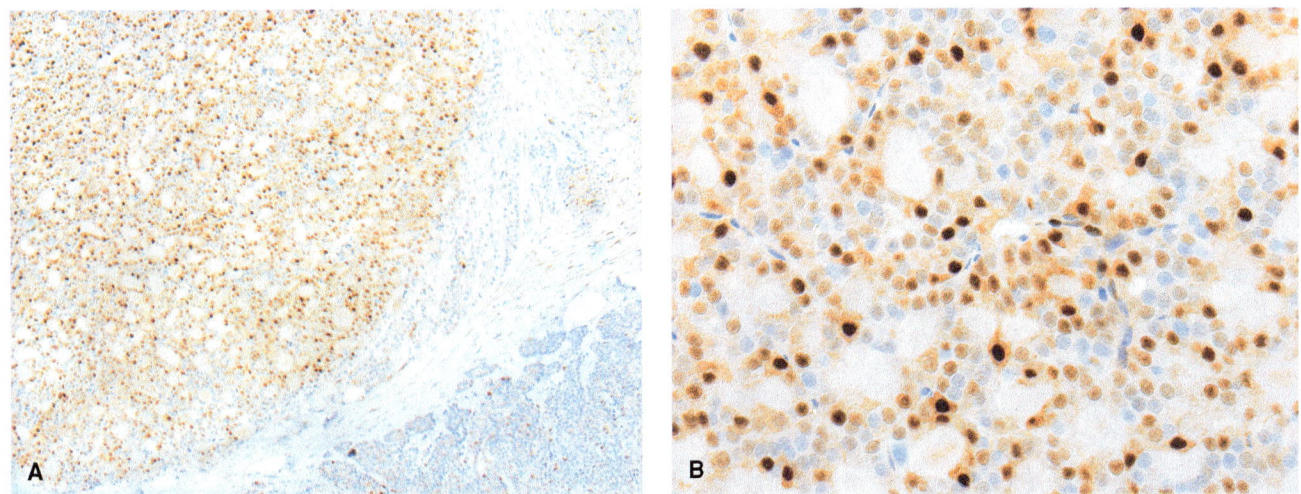

FIGURE 44.22 Cyclin D1 upregulation in parathyroid adenoma. Cyclin D1 upregulation is a feature of adenomas with PRAD1 rearrangements. It is diffusely positive in the tumor but not in the adjacent nontumorous parenchyma (**A**) and is seen in the majority of tumor nuclei with variable intensity (**B**).

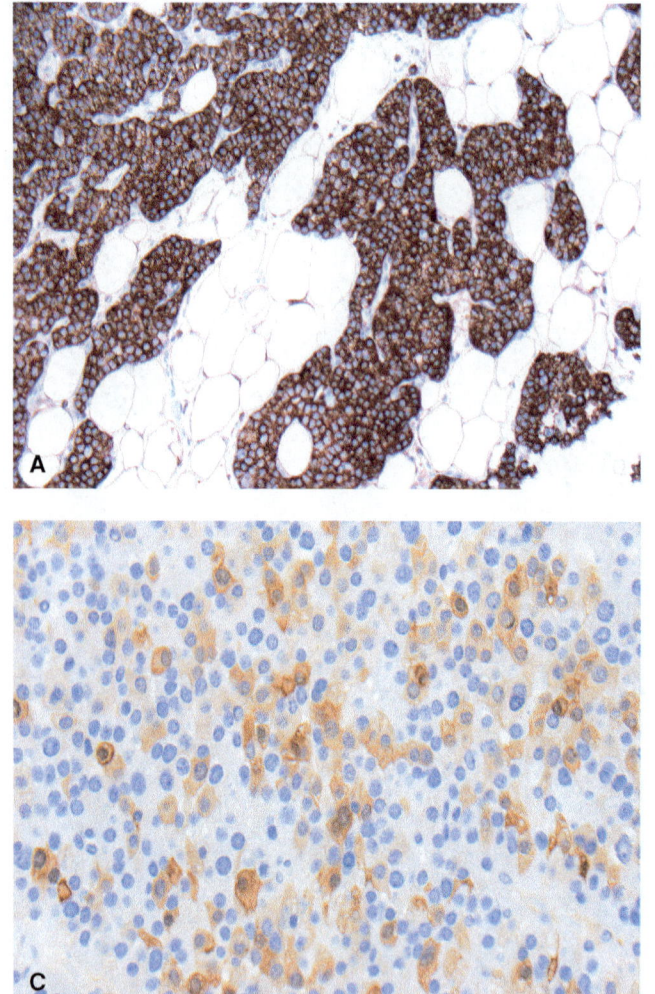
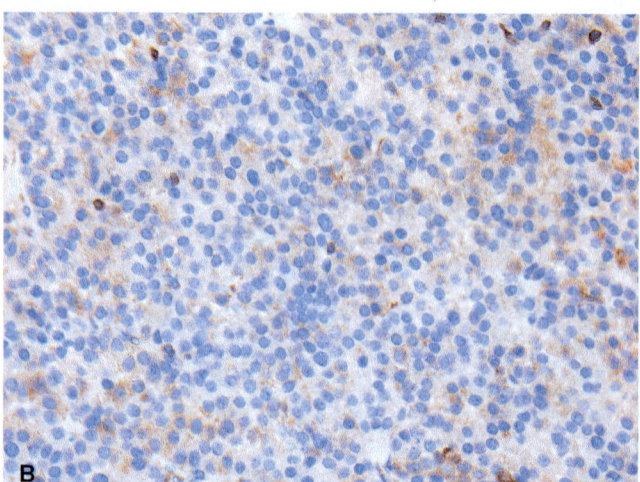

FIGURE 44.23 Bcl-2 and galectin-3 as biomarkers of parathyroid proliferations. Bcl-2 is strongly and diffusely positive in normal parathyroid (**A**) and benign tumors but reduced or lost in carcinoma (**B**). In contrast, galectin-3 is not usually expressed in normal parathyroids and benign uniglandular parathyroid disease but is upregulated in carcinoma (**C**).

identifying and counting mitoses is phosphoHistone-H3 immunohistochemistry (Fig. 44.25).

Genetic predisposition of parathyroid proliferative lesions is largely associated with MEN type 1, type 2, and type 4. MEN1 can be proposed as a likely etiologic agent when there is loss of expression of the gene product of the *MEN1* gene, menin, identified by immunohistochemistry (Fig. 44.26) and MEN4 should be considered when

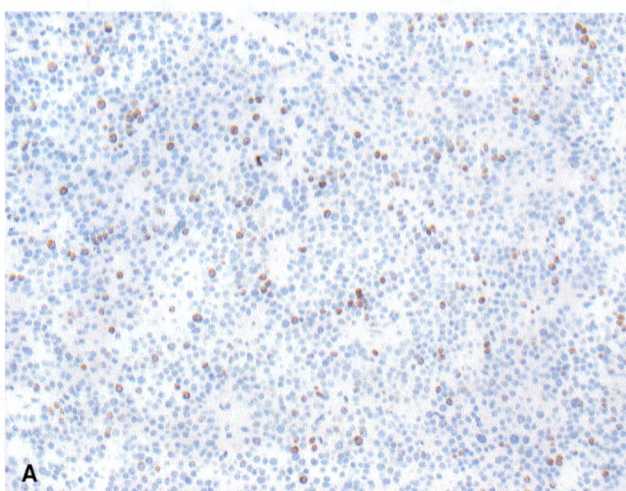
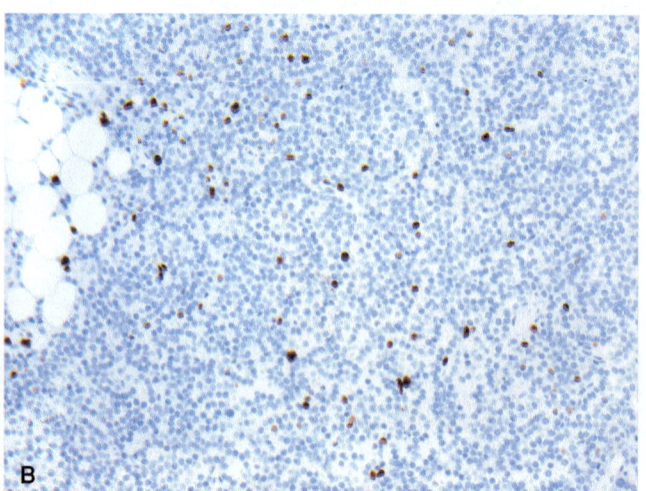

FIGURE 44.24 Ki67 labeling in hyperplasia and carcinoma. A high Ki67 labeling index is characteristic of carcinoma (**A**) but can also be seen in hyperplasia (**B**) and is therefore not specific.

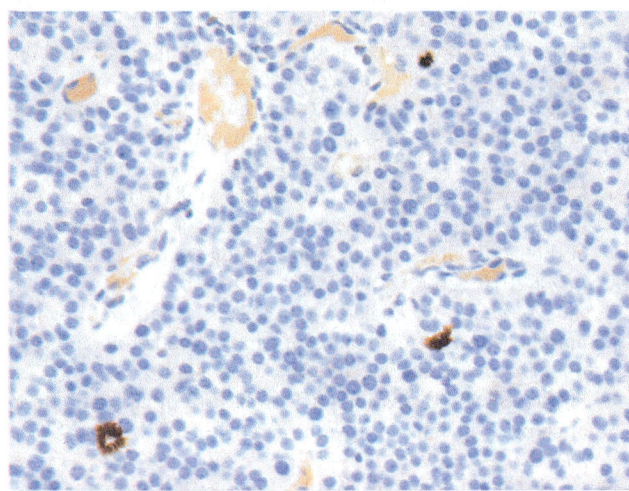

FIGURE 44.25 PhosphoHistone-H3 (pHH3)-assisted mitotic counts. The use of immunohistochemistry for pHH3 facilitates identification and quantification of mitoses.

there is global loss of the cyclin-dependent kinase inhibitor $p27^{kip1}$ (102,103). As discussed above, parafibromin loss may indicate germline predisposition, especially when found in a young patient. A recent series expanded genotype–phenotype correlations of parafibromin-deficient parathyroid neoplasms (104) that are more frequent in younger individuals with larger tumors and may display certain morphologic characteristics including microcystic change, thick capsule, arborizing vasculature, extensive sheet-like growth pattern, eosinophilic cytoplasm, nuclei with coarse chromatin, and perinuclear clearing (104).

The classification of parathyroid neoplasms as members of the larger family of neuroendocrine neoplasms is important when considering therapeutic options for the rare malignancies that can be lethal (49,105,106). These tumors are candidates for the targeted use of peptide receptor radiotherapy (PRRT) that is dependent of expression of somatostatin receptors, a ubiquitous feature of neuroendocrine cells (107,108).

ACKNOWLEDGMENTS

The authors gratefully acknowledge Paolo Batoni, PhD and Zoya Volynskaya, PhD, for contribution of the artwork in Figures 44.1 and 44.5, Lorne Rotstein, MD for contribution of Figure 44.2, and Dr. S. I. Roth who prepared Figures 44.6 and 44.17 for the previous edition of this book.

REFERENCES

1. Wilhelm SM, Wang TS, Ruan DT, et al. The American Association of Endocrine Surgeons guidelines for definitive management of primary hyperparathyroidism. *JAMA Surg* 2016;151(10):959–968.
2. Owen R. On the anatomy of the Indian rhinoceros (Rh. unicornus, L.). *Trans Zool Soc (London)* 1852;4(2):31–58.
3. Remak R. *Untersuchungen über die Entwickelung der Wirbelthiere*. Berline: G. Reimer; 1855.
4. Virchow R. *Die krankhaften Geschewülste*. Berlin: Hirschwald; 1863.
5. Sanderström I. Om en ny Körtel hos menniskan och ätskilliga däggdjur. *Upsala Läkareförenings Förhandlingar* 1880;15:441–471.
6. Kohn A. Studien über die Schilddrüse. *Arch Mikr Anat* 1895;44:366–422.
7. Kohn A. Die Epithelkörperchen. *Ergeb Anat Entwicklungsgeshch* 1899;9:194–252.
8. Gley E. Sur la toxicité des urines des chiens thyroidectomisés: contribution à l'étude des fonctions du corps thyroide. *Comptes Rendus de la Société de Biologie* 1891;3:366–368.
9. Erdheim J. Ueber tetania parathyreopriva. *Weiner Klinishe Wachenschrift* 1906;19:716–717.
10. Erdheim J. Beiträge zur pathologischen anatomie der menschlichen epithel-körperchen. *Zeitschrift für Heilkunst* 1904;25:1–15.
11. Hanson AM. The hydrochloric X sicca: a parathyroid preparation for intramuscular injection. *Military Surgery* 1924;259:218–219.
12. Collip JB. The extraction of a parathyroid hormone which will prevent or control parathyroid tetany and which regulates the level of blood calcium. *J Biol Chem* 1925;63:395–438.
13. Aurbach GD. Isolation of parathyroid hormone after extraction with phenol. *J Biol Chem* 1959;234:3179–3181.

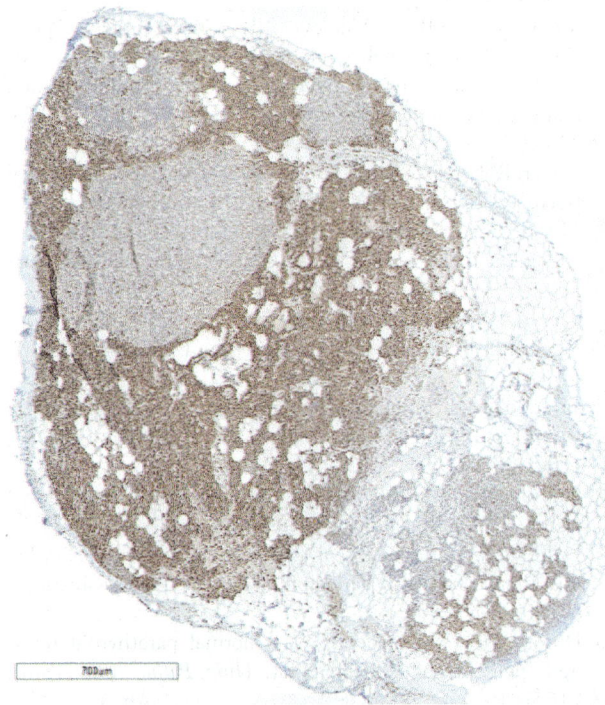

FIGURE 44.26 Menin loss in parathyroid adenoma of MEN1 patient. The loss of menin nuclear reactivity identifies multiple small neoplasms in the parathyroid of a patient with MEN1.

14. Wang C. The anatomic basis of parathyroid surgery. *Ann Surg* 1976;183(3):271–275.
15. Akerstrom G, Malmaeus J, Bergstrom R. Surgical anatomy of human parathyroid glands. *Surgery* 1984;95(1):14–21.
16. Rodgers SE, Hunter GJ, Hamberg LM et al. Improved preoperative planning for directed parathyroidectomy with 4-dimensional computed tomography. *Surgery* 2006;140(6):932–940, discussion 940–941.
17. Roy M, Mazeh H, Chen H, et al. Incidence and localization of ectopic parathyroid adenomas in previously unexplored patients. *World J Surg* 2013;37(1):102–106.
18. Weller GLJ. Development of the thyroid, parathyroid and thymus glands in man. *Contrib Embryol* 1933;24:95–138.
19. Gilmour JR. The embryology of the parathyroid glands, the thymus and certain associated rudiments. *J Pathol Bacteriol* 1937;45:507–522.
20. Norris EH. The parathyroid glands and the lateral thyroid in man: their morphogenesis, histogenesis, topographhic anatomy and prenatal growth. *Contrib Embryol* 1938;26:247.
21. Roth SI, Sadow PM, Johnson NB, et al. Parathyroid. In: Mills SE, ed. *Histology for Pathologists*. Philadelphia, PA: Wolters Kluwer Lippincott Williams & Williams; 2012.
22. Sanders CD, Kirkland JD, Wolin EA. Ectopic parathyroid adenoma in the carotid sheath. *J Nucl Med Technol* 2016;44(3):201–202.
23. Okuda I, Nakajima Y, Miura D, et al. Diagnostic localization of ectopic parathyroid lesions: developmental consideration. *Jpn J Radiol* 2010;28(10):707–713.
24. Lack EE, Delay S, Linnoila RI. Ectopic parathyroid tissue within the vagus nerve. Incidence and possible clinical significance. *Arch Pathol Lab Med* 1988;112(3):304–306.
25. Leroyer-Alizon E, David L, Anast CS, et al. Immunocytological evidence for parathyroid hormone in human fetal parathyroid glands. *J Clin Endocrinol Metab* 1981;52(3):513–516.
26. Manley NR, Capecchi MR. Hox group 3 paralogs regulate the development and migration of the thymus, thyroid, and parathyroid glands. *Dev Biol* 1998;195(1):1–15.
27. Kameda Y, Arai Y, Nishimaki T, et al. The role of Hoxa3 gene in parathyroid gland organogenesis of the mouse. *J Histochem Cytochem* 2004;52(5):641–651.
28. Peters H, Neubuser A, Kratochwil K, et al. Pax9-deficient mice lack pharyngeal pouch derivatives and teeth and exhibit craniofacial and limb abnormalities. *Genes Dev* 1998;12(17):2735–2747.
29. Su D, Ellis S, Napier A, et al. Hoxa3 and pax1 regulate epithelial cell death and proliferation during thymus and parathyroid organogenesis. *Dev Biol* 2001;236(2):316–329.
30. Jerome LA, Papaioannou VE. DiGeorge syndrome phenotype in mice mutant for the T-box gene, Tbx1. *Nat Genet* 2001;27(3):286–291.
31. Lindsay EA, Vitelli F, Su H, et al. Tbx1 haploinsufficieny in the DiGeorge syndrome region causes aortic arch defects in mice. *Nature* 2001;410(6824):97–101.
32. Merscher S, Funke B, Epstein JA, et al. TBX1 is responsible for cardiovascular defects in velo-cardio-facial/DiGeorge syndrome. *Cell* 2001;104(4):619–629.
33. Gordon J, Bennett AR, Blackburn CC, et al. Gcm2 and Foxn1 mark early parathyroid- and thymus-specific domains in the developing third pharyngeal pouch. *Mech Dev* 2001;103(1–2):141–143.
34. Gunther T, Chen ZF, Kim J, et al. Genetic ablation of parathyroid glands reveals another source of parathyroid hormone. *Nature* 2000;406(6792):199–203.
35. Grigorieva IV, Thakker RV. Transcription factors in parathyroid development: lessons from hypoparathyroid disorders. *Ann N Y Acad Sci* 2011;1237:24–38.
36. Grigorieva IV, Mirczuk S, Gaynor KU, et al. Gata3-deficient mice develop parathyroid abnormalities due to dysregulation of the parathyroid-specific transcription factor Gcm2. *J Clin Invest* 2010;120(6):2144–2155.
37. Xu PX, Zheng W, Laclef C, et al. Eya1 is required for the morphogenesis of mammalian thymus, parathyroid and thyroid. *Development* 2002;129(13):3033–3044.
38. Zou D, Silvius D, Davenport J, et al. Patterning of the third pharyngeal pouch into thymus/parathyroid by Six and Eya1. *Dev Biol* 2006;293(2):499–512.
39. Frank DU, Fotheringham LK, Brewer JA, et al. An Fgf8 mouse mutant phenocopies human 22q11 deletion syndrome. *Development* 2002;129(19):4591–4603.
40. Gardiner JR, Jackson AL, Gordon J, et al. Localised inhibition of FGF signalling in the third pharyngeal pouch is required for normal thymus and parathyroid organogenesis. *Development* 2012;139(18):3456–3466.
41. Gordon J, Patel SR, Mishina Y, et al. Evidence for an early role for BMP4 signaling in thymus and parathyroid morphogenesis. *Dev Biol* 2010;339(1):141–154.
42. Bachiller D, Klingensmith J, Shneyder N, et al. The role of chordin/Bmp signals in mammalian pharyngeal development and DiGeorge syndrome. *Development* 2003;130(15):3567–3578.
43. Wurdak H, Ittner LM, Lang KS, et al. Inactivation of TGFbeta signaling in neural crest stem cells leads to multiple defects reminiscent of DiGeorge syndrome. *Genes Dev* 2005;19(5):530–535.
44. Moore-Scott BA, Manley NR. Differential expression of Sonic hedgehog along the anterior-posterior axis regulates patterning of pharyngeal pouch endoderm and pharyngeal endoderm-derived organs. *Dev Biol* 2005;278(2):323–335.
45. Parvari R, Hershkovitz E, Grossman N et al; HRD/Autosomal Recessive Kenny-Caffey Syndrome Consortium. Mutation of TBCE causes hypoparathyroidism-retardation-dysmorphism and autosomal recessive Kenny-Caffey syndrome. *Nat Genet* 2002;32(3):448–452.
46. Parvari R, Diaz GA, Hershkovitz E. Parathyroid development and the role of tubulin chaperone E. *Horm Res* 2007;67(1):12–21.
47. Ghandur-Mnaymneh L, Cassady J, Hajianpour MA, et al. The parathyroid gland in health and disease. *Am J Pathol* 1986;125(2):292–299.
48. Gilmour JR, Martin WJ. The weight of the parathyroid glands. *J Pathol Bacteriol* 1937;44:431–462.
49. DeLellis RA. *Atlas of Tumor Pathology-Tumors of the Parathyroid Gland*. 3rd ed. Washington, DC: Armed Forces Institute of Pathology; 1993.
50. Dufour DR, Wilkerson SY. The normal parathyroid revisited: percentage of stromal fat. *Hum Pathol* 1982;13(8):717–721.
51. Dufour DR, Wilkerson SY. Factors related to parathyroid weight in normal persons. *Arch Pathol Lab Med* 1983;107(4):167–172.

52. Grimelius L, Akerström G, Bondeson L et al. The role of the pathologist in diagnosis and surgical decision making in hyperparathyroidism. *World J Surg* 1991;15(6):698–705.
53. Grimelius L, Akerstrom G, Johansson H, et al. Estimation of parenchymal cell content of human parathyroid glands using the image analyzing computer technique. *Am J Pathol* 1978;93(3):793–800.
54. Akerstrom G, Grimelius L, Johansson H, et al. The parenchymal cell mass in normal human parathyroid glands. *Acta Pathol Microbiol Scand A* 1981;89(5):367–375.
55. Akerstrom G, Grimelius L, Johansson H, et al. Estimation of the parathyroid parenchymal cell mass by density gradients. *Am J Pathol* 1980;99(3):685–694.
56. Akerström G, Malmaeus J, Grimelius L, et al. Histological changes in parathyroid glands in subclinical and clinical renal disease. An autopsy investigation. *Scand J Urol Nephrol* 1984;18(1):75–84.
57. Yao K, Singer FR, Roth SI, et al. Weight of normal parathyroid glands in patients with parathyroid adenomas. *J Clin Endocrinol Metab* 2004;89(7):3208–3213.
58. Balashev VN, Ignashkina MS. Lymphatic system of parathyroid glands in man. *Fed Proc Transl Suppl* 1965;24(4):603–604.
59. Altenahr E. Electron microscopical evidence for innervation of chief cells in human parathyroid gland. *Experientia* 1971;27(9):1077.
60. Yeghiayan E, Rojo-Ortega JM, Genest J. Parathyroid vessel innervation: an ultrastructural study. *J Anat* 1972;112(Pt 1):137–142.
61. Isono H, Shoumura S. Effects of vagotomy on the ultrastructure of the parathyroid gland of the rabbit. *Acta Anat (Basel)* 1980;108(3):273–280.
62. Cinti S, Balercia G, Zingaretti MC, et al. The normal human parathyroid gland. A histochemical and ultrastructural study with particular reference to follicular structures. *J Submicrosc Cytol* 1983;15(3):661–679.
63. Lieberman A, DeLellis RA. Intrafollicular amyloid in normal parathyroid glands. *Arch Pathol* 1973;95(6):422–423.
64. Roth SI, Capen CC. Ultrastructural and functional correlations of the parathyroid gland. *Int Rev Exp Pathol* 1974;13(0):161–221.
65. Roth SI, Au WY, Kunin AS, et al. Effect of dietary deficiency in vitamin D, calcium, and phosphorus on the ultrastructure of the rat parathyroid gland. *Am J Pathol* 1968;53(4):631–650.
66. Hamperl H. Über das Vorkommen von Onkocyten in verschiedenen Organen und ihren Geschwülsten (Mundspeicheldrüsen, Bauschpeicheldrüse, Epithelkörperchen, Hypophyse, Schilddrüse, Eileiter). *Virchows Arch* 1936;25:327–375.
67. Bai S, LiVolsi VA, Fraker DL, Bing Z. Water-clear parathyroid adenoma: report of two cases and literature review. *Endocr Pathol* 2012;23(3):196–200.
68. Grenko RT, Anderson KM, Kauffman G, et al. Water-clear cell adenoma of the parathyroid. A case report with immunohistochemistry and electron microscopy. *Arch Pathol Lab Med* 1995;119(11):1072–1074.
69. Roth SI. The ultrastructure of primary water-clear cell hyperplasia of the parathyroid glands. *Am J Pathol* 1970;61(2):233–248.
70. Emura S, Shoumura S, Utsumi M et al. Origin of the water-clear cell in the parathyroid gland of the golden hamster. *Acta Anat (Basel)* 1991;140(4):357–361.
71. Cinti S, Sbarbati A. Ultrastructure of human parathyroid cells in health and disease. *Microsc Res Tech* 1995;32(2):164–179.
72. Potts JT. Parathyroid hormone: Past and present. *J Endocrinol* 2005;187(3):311–325.
73. Brown EM, Gamba G, Riccardi D et al. Cloning and characterization of an extracellular Ca(2+)-sensing receptor from bovine parathyroid. *Nature* 1993;366(6455):575–580.
74. Riccardi D, Park J, Lee WS, et al. Cloning and functional expression of a rat kidney extracellular calcium/polyvalent cation-sensing receptor. *Proc Natl Acad Sci U S A* 1995;92(1):131–135.
75. Aida K, Koishi S, Tawata M, et al. Molecular cloning of a putative Ca(2+)-sensing receptor cDNA from human kidney. *Biochem Biophys Res Commun* 1995;214(2):524–529.
76. Alfadda TI, Saleh AM, Houillier P, et al. Calcium-sensing receptor 20 years later. *Am J Physiol Cell Physiol* 2014;307(3):C221–C231.
77. Chou YH, Pollak MR, Brandi ML et al. Mutations in the human Ca(2+)-sensing-receptor gene that cause familial hypocalciuric hypercalcemia. *Am J Hum Genet* 1995;56(5):1075–1079.
78. Juppner H, Abou-Samra AB, Freeman M et al. A G protein-linked receptor for parathyroid hormone and parathyroid hormone-related peptide. *Science* 1991;254(5034):1024–1026.
79. Tafaj O, Juppner H. Pseudohypoparathyroidism: one gene, several syndromes. *J Endocrinol Invest* 2017;40(4):347–356.
80. Ordonez NG. Value of GATA3 immunostaining in the diagnosis of parathyroid tumors. *Appl Immunohistochem Mol Morphol* 2014;22(10):756–761.
81. Nonaka D. Study of parathyroid transcription factor Gcm2 expression in parathyroid lesions. *Am J Surg Pathol* 2011;35(1):145–151.
82. Arnold A, Brown MF, Urena P, et al. Monoclonality of parathyroid tumors in chronic renal failure and in primary parathyroid hyperplasia. *J Clin Invest* 1995;95(5):2047–2053.
83. Arnold A, Kim HG. Clonal loss of one chromosome 11 in a parathyroid adenoma. *J Clin Endocrinol Metab* 1989;69(3):496–499.
84. Arnold A, Staunton CE, Kim HG, et al. Monoclonality and abnormal parathyroid hormone genes in parathyroid adenomas. *N Engl J Med* 1988;218:658–652.
85. Friedman E, Sakaguchi K, Bale AE, et al. Clonality of parathyroid tumors in familial multiple endocrine neoplasia type I. *N Engl J Med* 1989;321(4):213–218.
86. Alwaheeb S, Rambaldini G, Boerner S, et al. Worrisome histologic alterations following fine-needle aspiration of the parathyroid. *J Clin Pathol* 2006;59(10):1094–1096.
87. Kim J, Horowitz G, Hong M, et al. The dangers of parathyroid biopsy. *J Otolaryngol Head Neck Surg* 2017;46(1):4.
88. Carpten JD, Robbins CM, Villablanca A, et al. HRPT2, encoding parafibromin, is mutated in hyperparathyroidism-jaw tumor syndrome. *Nat Genet* 2002;32(4):676–680.
89. Juhlin CC, Nilsson IL, Johansson K et al. Parafibromin and APC as screening markers for malignant potential in atypical parathyroid adenomas. *Endocr Pathol* 2010;21(3):166–177.
90. Gill AJ, Clarkson A, Gimm O, et al. Loss of nuclear expression of parafibromin distinguishes parathyroid carcinomas and hyperparathyroidism-jaw tumor (HPT-JT) syndrome-related adenomas from sporadic parathyroid adenomas and hyperplasias. *Am J Surg Pathol* 2006;30(9):1140–1149.

91. Erickson LA, Jin L, Wollan P, et al. Parathyroid hyperplasia, adenomas, and carcinomas: differential expression of p27Kip1 protein. *Am J Surg Pathol* 1999;23(3):288–295.
92. Arnold A. Molecular mechanisms of parathyroid neoplasia. *Endocrinol Metab Clin North Am* 1994;23(1):93–107.
93. Cryns VL, Rubio MP, Thor AD, et al. p53 abnormalities in human parathyroid carcinoma. *J Clin Endocrinol Metab* 1994;78(6):1320–1324.
94. Cryns VL, Thor A, Xu HJ. Loss of the retinoblastoma tumor-suppressor gene in a parathyroid carcinoma. *N Engl J Med* 1994;330(11):757–761.
95. Arnold A. Genetic basis of endocrine disease 5. Molecular genetics of parathyroid gland neoplasia. *J Clin Endocrinol Metab* 1993;77(5):1108–1112.
96. Arnold A, Staunton CE, Kim GH, et al. Monoclonality and abnormal parathyroid hormone genes in parathyroid adenomas. *N Engl J Med* 1988;318:658–662.
97. Arnold A, Kim HG, Gaz RD, et al. Molecular cloning and chromosomal mapping of DNA rearranged with the parathyroid hormone gene in a parathyroid adenoma. *J Clin Invest* 1989;83(6):2034–2040.
98. Erovic BM, Harris L, Jamali M, et al. Biomarkers of parathyroid carcinoma. *Endocr Pathol* 2012;23(4):221–231.
99. Stojadinovic A, Hoos A, Nissan A, et al. Parathyroid neoplasms: clinical, histopathological, and tissue microarray-based molecular analysis. *Hum Pathol* 2003;34(1):54–64.
100. Hosny Mohammed K, Siddiqui MT, Willis BC, et al. Parafibromin, APC, and MIB-1 Are Useful Markers for Distinguishing Parathyroid Carcinomas From Adenomas. *Appl Immunohistochem Mol Morphol* 2017;25(10):731–735.
101. Abbona GC, Papotti M, Gasparri G, et al. Proliferative activity in parathyroid tumors as detected by Ki-67 immunostaining. *Hum Pathol* 1995;26(2):135–138.
102. Georgitsi M. MEN-4 and other multiple endocrine neoplasias due to cyclin-dependent kinase inhibitors (p27(Kip1) and p18(INK4C)) mutations. *Best Pract Res Clin Endocrinol Metab* 2010;24(3):425–437.
103. Georgitsi M, Raitila A, Karhu A et al. Germline CDKN1B/p27Kip1 mutation in multiple endocrine neoplasia. *J Clin Endocrinol Metab* 2007;92(8):3321–3325.
104. Gill AJ, Lim G, Cheung VKY, et al. Parafibromin-deficient (HPT-JT Type, CDC73 Mutated) Parathyroid Tumors Demonstrate Distinctive Morphologic Features. *Am J Surg Pathol* 2018.
105. Duan K, Mete O. Parathyroid Carcinoma: Diagnosis and Clinical Implications. *Turk Patoloji Derg* 2015;31 Suppl 1:80–97.
106. Erovic BM, Goldstein DP, Kim D, et al. Parathyroid cancer: Outcome analysis of 16 patients treated at the princess margaret hospital. *Head Neck* 2013;35(1):35–39.
107. Gulenchyn KY, Yao X, Asa SL, et al. Radionuclide therapy in neuroendocrine tumours: A systematic review. *Clin Oncol (R Coll Radiol)* 2012;24(4):294–308.
108. Opalinska M, Hubalewska-Dydejczyk A, Sowa-Staszczak A. Radiolabeled peptides: current and new perspectives. *Q J Nucl Med Mol Imaging* 2017;61(2):153–167.

Adrenal

J. Aidan Carney

- ANATOMY 1225
- EVOLUTION 1225
- DEVELOPMENT 1226
  - Cortex 1226
  - Medulla 1228
- GLAND WEIGHT AND CORTICAL THICKNESS 1229
- ADRENAL GLANDS FOR HISTOLOGIC STUDY 1229
  - Ideal Adrenal Glands 1229
  - Adrenal Glands Studied 1229
- HISTOLOGY 1230
  - Capsule 1230
  - Cortex 1232
  - Zona Glomerulosa 1233
  - Zona Fasciculata 1234
  - Zona Reticularis 1234
  - Medulla 1235
- IMMUNOHISTOCHEMISTRY 1239
  - Cortex 1239
  - Medulla 1239
- ULTRASTRUCTURE 1240
  - Cortex 1240
  - Medulla 1241
- OTHER ANATOMICAL STRUCTURES 1242
  - Blood Vessels 1242
  - Arteries 1242
  - Intraglandular Vasculature 1243
  - Veins 1243
  - Nerves and Ganglia 1244
  - Lymphatics 1245
  - Accessory (Heterotopic) Adrenal Cortex 1245
  - Adrenocortical Nodules 1247
- REFERENCES 1248

The paired adrenal glands are a composite of two endocrine organs—one steroid producing and the other catecholamine producing—that are located in the retroperitoneum, superomedial to the kidneys. The two organs have a different embryonic origin, histology, and function.

ANATOMY

The main portions of the adrenal gland are easily recognized on the fresh or formalin-fixed cut surface (Fig. 45.1). Externally, a relatively thick yellow layer is applied to a narrow dark brown band that abuts on a solid, pearly gray interior. The former two zones correspond histologically to the zona fasciculata and zona reticularis of the cortex, and the latter to the medulla of the organ.

The anatomic location of the human adrenal glands, which sandwiches them between several organs, is responsible for their particular shape: pyramidal on the right and crescentic on the left. The depression and ridge (crest) on the posterior surfaces (Fig. 45.2) result from their close relationship to the kidneys. When a kidney is congenitally absent, the corresponding adrenal is round and the characteristic longitudinal ridge on the posterior surface is missing.

EVOLUTION

The anatomic relationship of the adrenal cortex to the medulla that exists in mammals is not found in lower animals. In the shark, for example, the cortex and medulla are topographically completely separate; in amphibians,

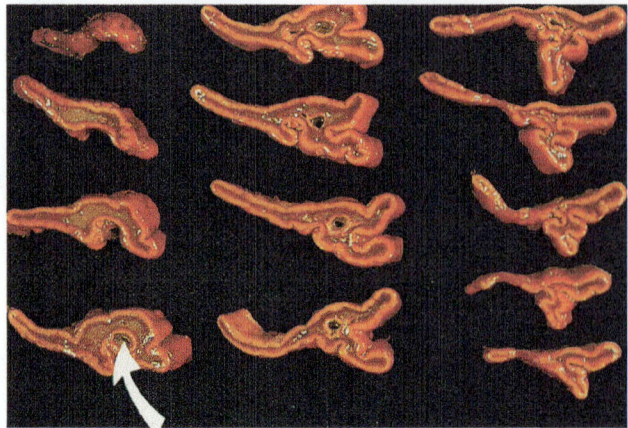

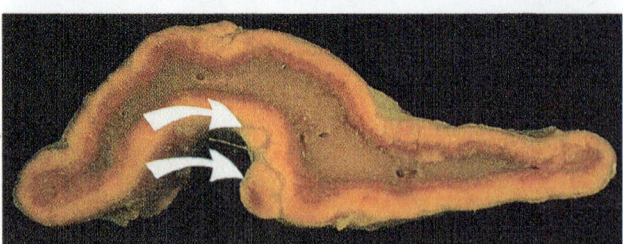

FIGURE 45.1 Normal adrenal gland. **Top:** Fresh gland sliced from head (*upper left*) through body (*center*) to tail (*lower right*). The *yellow* cortex and *pearly gray* medulla are visible in the head (*left*). *Yellow* zona fasciculata surrounds *dark brown* zona reticularis in the tail (*right*), where medulla is absent. The gland can be identified as the left adrenal because on this side the adrenal vein runs in a well-developed groove on the surface of the gland at the junction of the head and body (*arrow*). Invaginated cortex surrounds the central vein in the interior of the body. **Bottom:** Slice of formalin-fixed adrenal gland showing, from exterior inward, cortical zona fasciculata (*yellow*), zona reticularis (*brown*), and medulla (*gray*). The cortex is about 1 mm in thickness. Dilated tributaries of the central vein are seen in the medulla. The adrenal vein has been removed from its groove. Nodules of accessory cortex are present (*arrows*).

FIGURE 45.2 Topographic anatomy. There is a difference in the surface anatomy of right and left adrenal glands. IVC, inferior vena cava. (Reprinted with permission from Kawamura D, Nolan T. *Abdomen and Superficial Structures.* Philadelphia, PA: Wolters Kluwer Health; 2017.)

the two structures are in close contact; in birds, they are intermingled. Only in mammals does the intimate proximity seen among the human adrenal cortex and medulla occur. In a prototypic mammal (e.g., the rat), the medulla forms a central core that is uniformly surrounded by the cortex. The distribution of the two zones in the human adrenal is different. In the human adrenal (Fig. 45.3), most of the medulla is in the head of the gland (medial), some occurs in the body, and there is usually none in the tail (lateral) (1). Two bands of cortex applied one to the other form the alae of glands.

DEVELOPMENT

Cortex

The adrenal cortex is of mesodermal origin. Its primordia appear at the 9-mm embryo stage (sixth week of gestation) as bilateral cellular aggregations (Fig. 45.4) at the mesenteric root, medial to the developing gonad and anterior to the kidney (mesonephros) (2,3). These primordia are composed of two groups of mesenchymal cells: one destined to be the precursor of the transitory provisional or fetal cortex, the other to become the adrenal capsule and its supporting connective tissue framework (3). By the seventh week of gestation, the primordia have become more defined, have separated from the coelomic lining, and include polyhedral cells with eosinophilic, lipid-poor cytoplasm.

These cells increase in size and proliferate rapidly, forming a series of parallel columns and cords of cells that ultimately compose the bulk of the fetal cortex. The inner eosinophilic core of the gland is composed of moderately

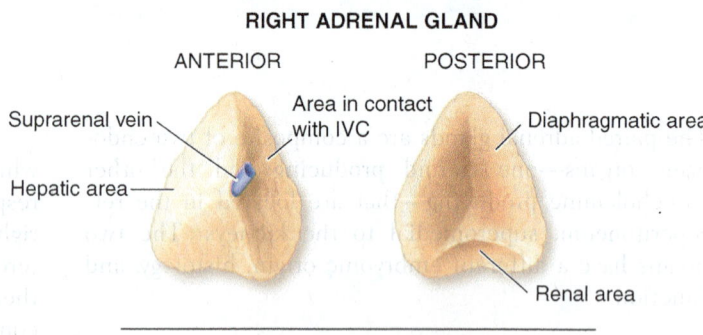

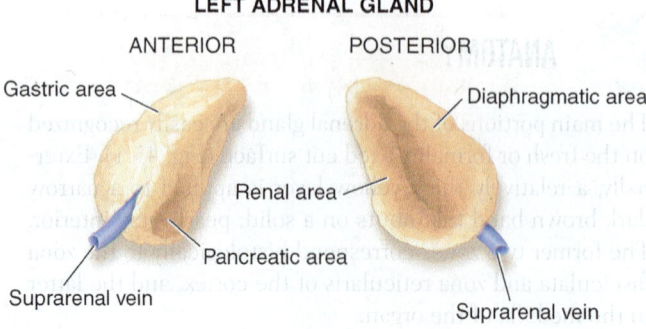

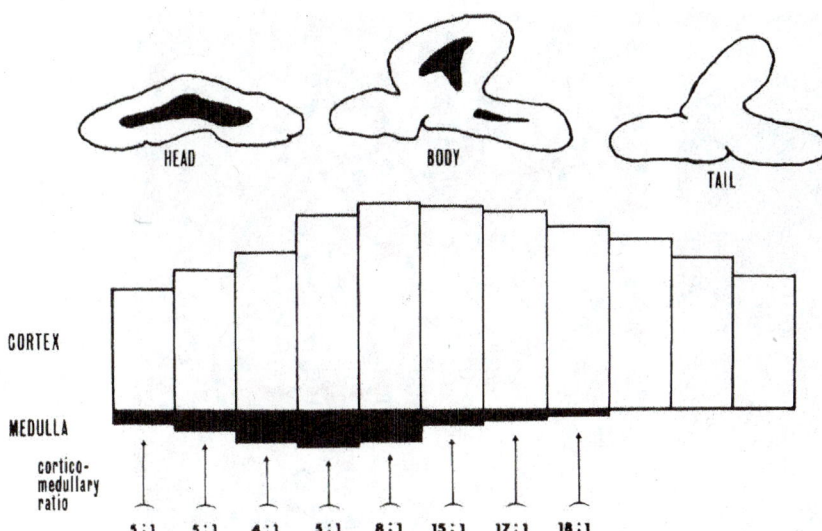

FIGURE 45.3 Diagrammatic illustration of the distribution of medulla (black) in the head, body, and tail of the adrenal gland (*above*) and corresponding corticomedullary ratios (*below*). Reprinted with permission from: Symington T. *Functional Pathology of the Human Adrenal Gland.* Baltimore, MD: Williams & Wilkins; 1969.

large cells, arranged in tightly packed cords toward the outer aspect of the zone but more widely spaced in its innermost regions where there is increased prominence of the vascular sinusoidal spaces. External to this dominant mass, a thin subcapsular rim of smaller cells (the precursor of the adult or permanent cortex) appears (Fig. 45.5). These cells are arranged in nests and arches that cap the columns of deeper cells. They have hyperchromatic, closely packed, overlapping nuclei. The nuclei are larger, more vesicular, and less hyperchromatic in the cords. Continuous, spottily distributed degeneration of the cells is found in the cords, and dead (apoptotic) cells are continuously replaced by the proliferation of cells in the narrow subcapsular band. Growth of the developing cortex is therefore centripedal (from outside inward).

The adrenals enlarge during the second trimester in direct proportion to the total increase in body weight. By the sixth month of gestation, each gland weighs about 1.5 g, the weight increase being largely due to the expansion of the inner fetal zone. At birth, each gland weighs just over 4 g. There is no sex difference in adrenal size, shape, or weight during development. At the end of gestation, the provisional cortex accounts for the bulk of the glands (Fig. 45.6).

In the newborn, the cut surface of the adrenal glands shows a relatively narrow yellow rim of permanent cortex over a deep brownish-red, hyperemic, provisional zone. Within hours of birth, the latter becomes acutely congested and starts to degenerate. At the end of 7 to 10 days, the provisional cortex is largely disorganized and necrotic. The narrow peripheral band of cell clusters survives and becomes the source of the permanent cortex. Involution of the provisional cortex is substantial at 2 weeks and well established by the end of the first month when about 50% of the gland weight has been lost. This loss of weight converts the plump-distended gland of the neonate into a relatively shrunken, leaf-like organ, which weighs on average only about 1 g at the end of the first year of life. The gland grows slowly thereafter to reach 2 g by the tenth year, but doubles in weight during puberty and adolescence to reach the mean adult weight of just over 4 g by 15 to 18 years. No sex differences have been noted in this process. The key events in the prepubertal cortex development are, first, the involution of the fetal zone, second, the establishment of zonation in the outer cortex and, finally, the emergence of a recognizable zona reticularis.

The zona glomerulosa remains diffuse during childhood and adolescence. At some time during early adult life it assumes the focal distribution characteristic of adult glands, presumably being displaced by the outward extension of lipid-rich zona fasciculata columns. The final stage in the development of the adult cortex involves evolution of the zona reticularis. A zona reticularis is seldom seen in

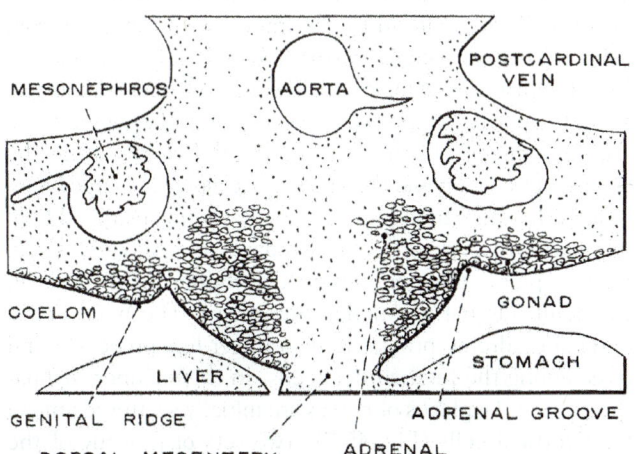

FIGURE 45.4 Diagrammatic representation of a human embryo at 6 weeks' gestation showing the anatomic relationship of developing adrenal gland to coelomic cavity, gonad, and kidney (mesonephros). Reprinted with permission from: Dahl EV, Bahn RC. Aberrant adrenal cortical tissue near the testis in human infants. *Am J Pathol* 1962;40:587–598.

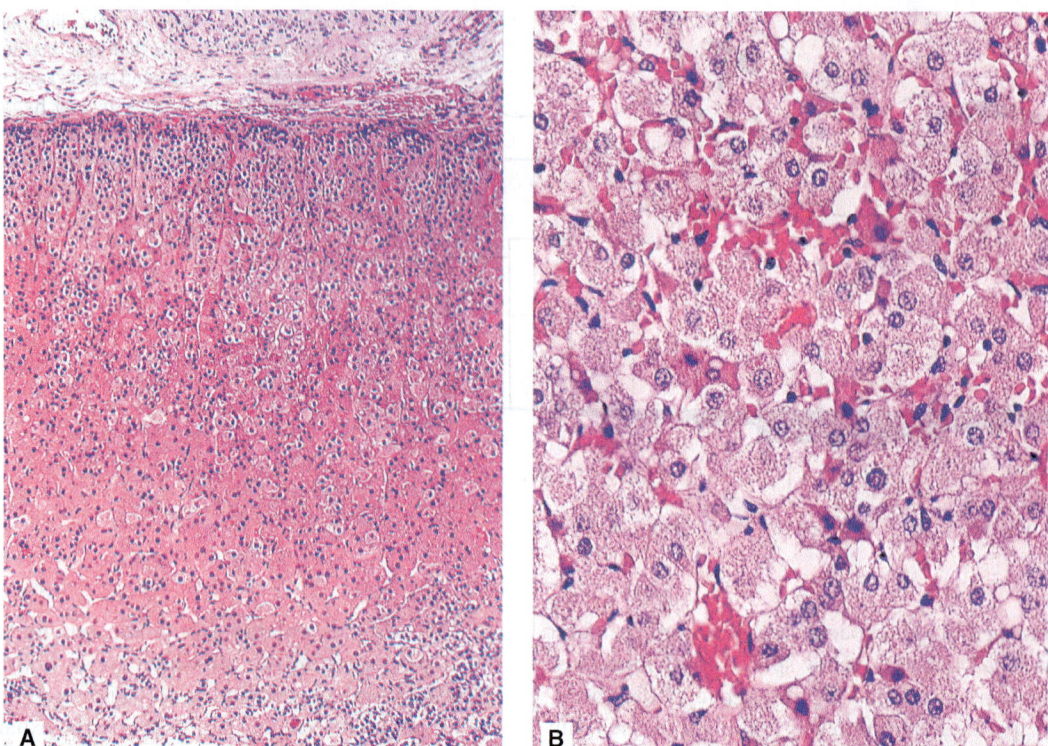

FIGURE 45.5 **A:** Provisional (fetal) cortex (29 weeks' gestation, stillborn infant). Cortex is dominated by large cells with eosinophilic cytoplasm in vague columns and solid sheet with prominent capillaries. Just beneath the tenuous capsule, there is a rim of smaller cells, the source of the permanent cortex. A sympathetic ganglion and a small nerve are present in the periadrenal connective tissue (*top*). **B:** The cortex contains large cells with voluminous granular cytoplasm. Nuclei are vesicular with a single nucleolus. Vascularity is prominent.

adrenals up to the age of 3 years. By the age of 5 years, focal accumulations of compact cells on the innermost aspect of the cortex are present in most of the glands. In a further year or 2, some glands already show a continuous zona reticularis. By the age of 14 years, virtually all glands possess a continuous, concentric zona reticularis. Lipofuscin pigment increases with age.

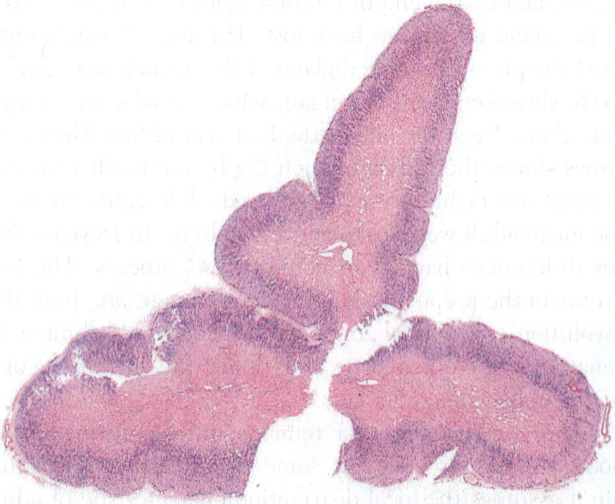

Medulla

The adrenal medulla is of neuroectodermal origin (3). Precursor cells originate in the neural crest and migrate from primitive spinal ganglia (sixth thoracic to first lumbar) to form the primitive sympathetic nervous system situated dorsal to the aorta. Sympathogonia cells (from the sympathetic anlagen) migrate further into nerves that sprout from the sympathetic chain and then they move alongside large blood vessels that penetrate into the (as yet) unencapsulated fetal adrenal cortex, primarily at its caudal pole (head). (This very likely explains the nonuniform distribution of medulla in the adult adrenal mentioned previously.) The neural cells enter the adrenal primordium as finger-like processes and pass among the fetal cortical cells. In this manner, sympathogonia and a plexus of nerves are initially scattered among fetal cortical cells (Fig. 45.7). Two sets of progeny of the sympathogonia, the precursors of the medulla, emerge. At birth, the medulla comprises a central, very thin core of these cells with offshoots stretching a short distance into the peripheral degenerating provisional cortex. The medullary cells are arranged in irregularly sized clumps containing both cell types, the larger cells now predominating. The

FIGURE 45.6 Adrenal cortex at birth (35 weeks' gestation; infant died at 2 days). The central, degenerating, eosinophilic provisional cortex is surrounded by the developing, darkly staining outer rim of permanent cortex.

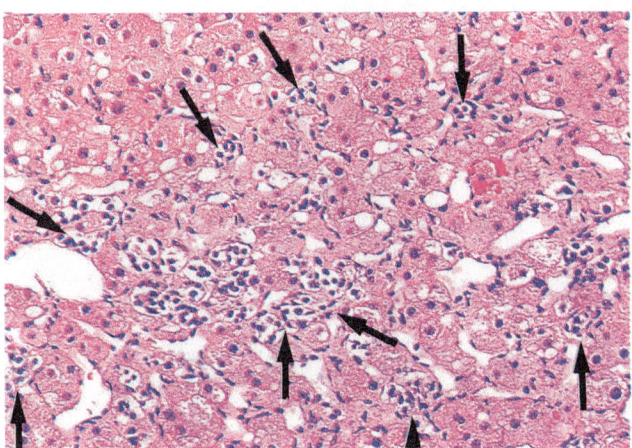

FIGURE 45.7 Developing adrenal medulla (29 weeks' gestation, stillborn infant). Clusters of small medullary cells with deeply staining nuclei (*arrows*) irregularly distributed in very vascular provisional cortex. When the latter degenerates, the clusters of medullary cells survive and, lacking the support of the cortical cells, aggregate together.

postnatal collapse of the provisional cortex and its stroma removes the framework that supported the medullary offshoots and their associated nerve plexus in the cortex. With this loss of scaffolding, these structures coalesce around the central veins.

GLAND WEIGHT AND CORTICAL THICKNESS

Although not a structural feature of the adrenal, the weight of the glands is important because assessment of the adrenal normalcy takes this feature into account. Information on truly normal adrenal weight is difficult to obtain because the organ (specifically the cortex) responds rapidly to stress by an increase in mass. Therefore, accurate normal adrenal weight can be determined only from selected autopsy material (e.g., healthy individuals who die suddenly). The combined adrenal weight in these circumstances is about 8 to 9 g (1). Exceptionally, a gland weighs as little as 2 g or as much as 6 g. Sex differences are not apparent. Formalin fixation has little effect on the gland weight.

Relative to the body weight, the adrenals are actually largest at the fourth month of gestation (4). In cases of sudden death in adults without prior illness, the mean weight of the individual glands is 4.0 to 4.2 g. The cortex accounts for 90% of the total weight of the gland. There is no correlation between absolute body weight and adrenal weight and no significant differences in the mean weight of the normal left and right glands. Neither pregnancy nor the menopause appears to result in significant adrenal weight changes. If death is preceded by a prolonged illness, there is a significant increase in mean adrenal weight. Series in this category give individual mean gland weights ranging from 5.8 to 6.2 g.

The thickness of the normal adult adrenal cortex is approximately 1 mm and ranges from about 0.7 to 1.3 mm. For accuracy, the thickness should be determined microscopically with an ocular micrometer; it is impractical to detect small alterations in the thickness using a metric scale.

ADRENAL GLANDS FOR HISTOLOGIC STUDY

Ideal Adrenal Glands

Ideally, for the reasons already mentioned, adrenal glands used for the study of normal histology of the organ should be obtained from healthy patients. Results obtained from the study of glands of patients with primary adrenal disease or disorders that might affect the adrenal histology secondarily should be used with caution. Nevertheless, since the two portions of the adrenal gland, cortex and medulla, are separate functional units that apparently do not affect each other, it is not unreasonable (until shown to be otherwise) to study, for example, the histology of the adrenal medulla (thinking of it as being normal) in a gland surgically removed for a clinically and biochemically nonfunctioning small adrenocortical adenoma. Similar considerations apply to the cortex.

For the study of cytologic details, material should be fresh and not autolysed and therefore obtained at surgery or shortly after death. The zona reticularis of the cortex quickly begins to show the effects of anoxia (degeneration). However, glands that are less than optimally preserved for the study of cell details are satisfactory for the determination of general microanatomy of the organ. In practice, fresh (and to a variable extent "normal") adrenal is most often available at the time of radical nephrectomy, in the course of which an adrenal gland is removed with the kidney. However, many such glands are torn during the surgical procedure, limiting to some extent their use for the study of normal histology. Their usefulness is also limited in that they are representative only of the gland appearance in a particular age range (middle-aged or older patients). In practice, it is difficult to get the complete range of normal adrenal specimens (fetal to aged) that would be ideal for the study of normal histology.

Adrenal Glands Studied

The actual tissue used for the histologic description that follows included adrenals from all the foregoing categories. Autopsy material was obtained from individuals (mostly male) who died suddenly (homicide, suicide, or traumatic injury) and from premature and neonatal infants. For some cases there was minimal or no medical history available, and the autopsy protocol and other autopsy slides could not be reviewed. Thus, the state of health of these patients and the condition of other organs could not be determined. A number of normal glands were available from patients undergoing nephrectomy. Also, opportunity was taken to study apparently normal extratumoral medulla and cortex in cases of adrenalectomy for certain primary adrenal neoplasms that were small or relatively small (adrenocortical adenomas producing aldosterone, nonfunctioning adrenocortical adenomas, and pheochromocytoma).

HISTOLOGY

Capsule

The capsule of the adrenal gland is composed of hypocellular fibrous tissue in the form of coarse, hyalinized collagen bundles and elastic fibers (Fig. 45.8). Usually, the capsule is thin, but it varies considerably in thickness from gland to gland and even within the same gland (Fig. 45.9). It is tough and hard to cut but tears easily and does not support the unfixed gland, which is limp and readily bends. The soft consistency of the fresh glands makes them difficult to section; cooling them for 15 minutes in a refrigerator facilitates this operation.

Because of the propinquity of development of adrenals and kidneys and the liver (on the right side), there is occasional fusion or sharing of a common capsule among the adrenal and kidney and the adrenal and liver (Fig. 45.10). The common capsule may be deficient focally, and then

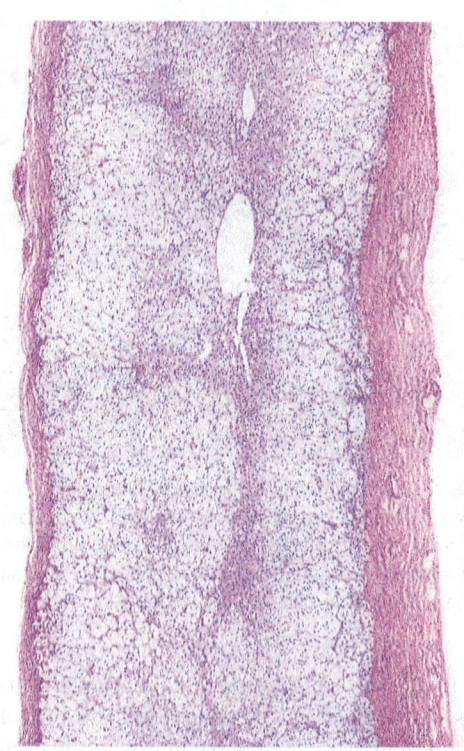

FIGURE 45.9 Adrenal capsule. Fourfold variation in the thickness of the capsule, which at its maximum thickness measures 0.3 mm.

parenchymal cells of two organs come into direct contact. The adrenal capsule is surrounded by adult-type fat (brown fat in the fetus and newborn) that features small arteries, veins, nerves, accessory cortex, excrescences of cortex, sympathetic ganglia, and an occasional paraganglion (Fig. 45.11).

The capsule is penetrated by blood vessels supplying and draining the glands, the nerves to the medulla, and lymphatic channels. In random sections of the glands, only the site of exit of the adrenal vein is regularly encountered (because of its relatively large size); occasionally, the site of penetration of a large nerve is seen; the entry sites of the small arteries into the glands are also sometimes seen. Commonly found are narrow (occasionally wide) defects in the capsule through which the cortex protrudes into the periadrenal fat to form small nodules of cells that are sometimes delimited by a distended and attenuated adrenal capsule and sometimes not (Fig. 45.12). These excrescences are composed predominantly of epithelial cells with normal zonation pattern of the cells. The protrusions may contain a connective tissue component, and sometimes there is an equal mixture of cords of epithelial cells and fibrous tissues. Single rows and groups of cortical cells, small and oval or large and round, are commonly found here and there in capsular "pockets" (Fig. 45.13). Larger oval aggregates cause a slight depression in, and thinning of, the underlying cortex, so that the total width of the two portions of cortex—that in the capsular pocket and that normally situated—is about normal (Fig. 45.13).

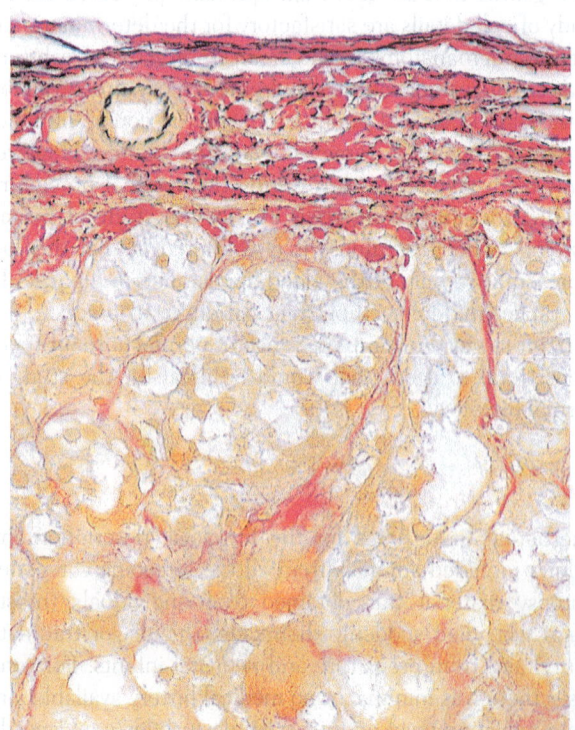

FIGURE 45.8 Adrenal capsule. Elastic-van Gieson stain shows collagen bundles (*red*) and intermingled elastic fibers (*black*). A small artery is present in the capsule.

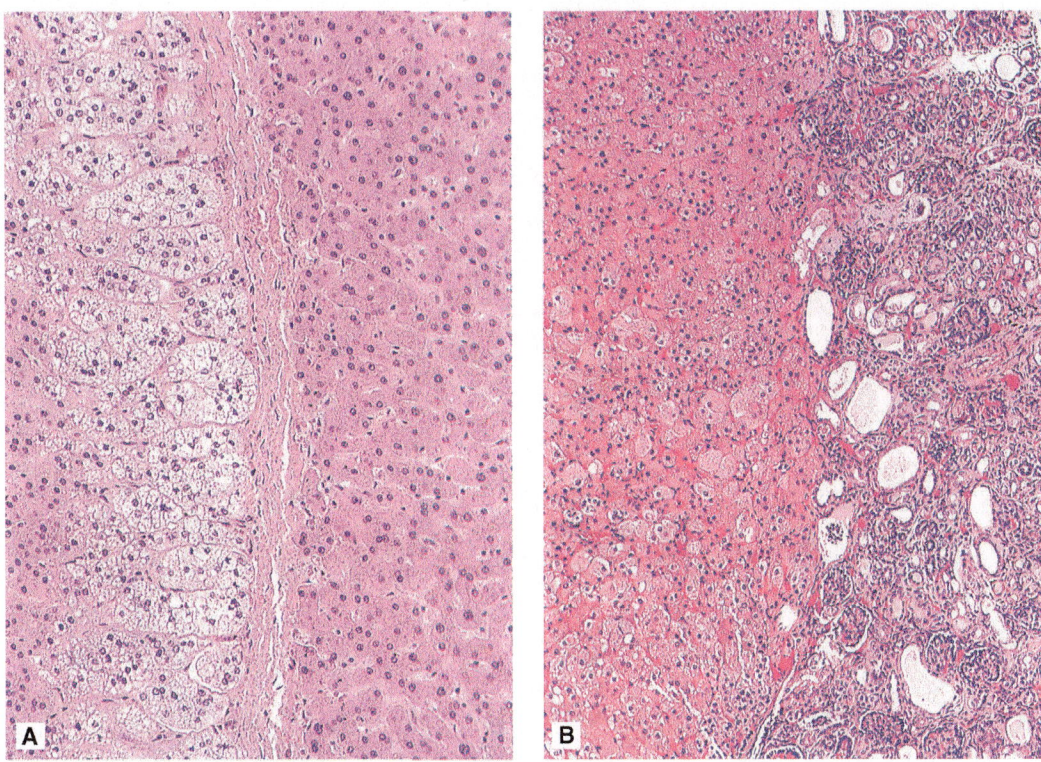

FIGURE 45.10 Adrenal capsule. **A:** Common capsule of adrenal (*left*) and liver (*right*). Note that a zona glomerulosa is not evident in the adrenal cortex. **B:** Absence of an adrenal and kidney capsule results in direct contact of adrenal cortex (provisional) and renal parenchyma.

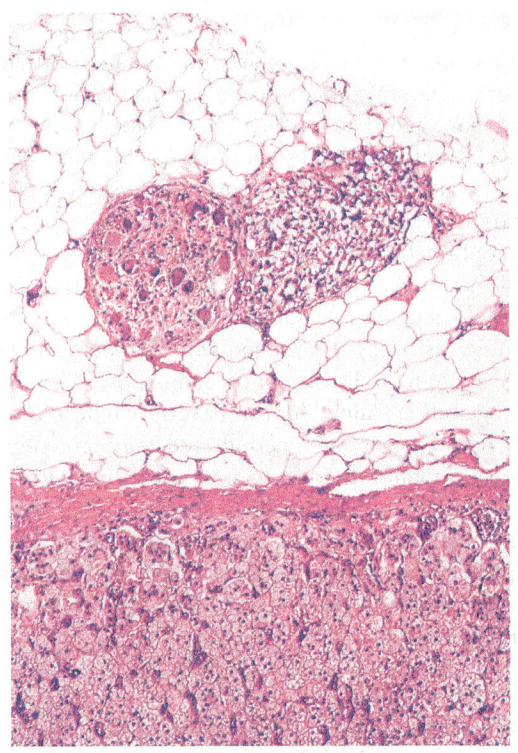

FIGURE 45.11 Normal adrenal gland. Juxtaposed sympathetic ganglion (*above left*) and paraganglion (*above right*) in periadrenal adipose tissue. The adrenal cortex features cells with clear cytoplasm (zona fasciculata). Zona glomerulosa is not evident.

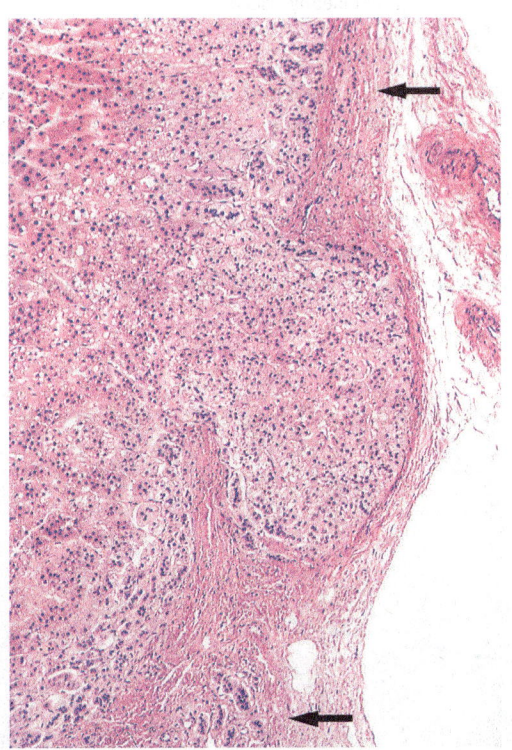

FIGURE 45.12 Normal adrenal gland. Protrusion of cortical cells surrounded by attenuated capsule through a "wide" defect in the adrenal capsule. A few cortical cells in rows and small aggregates are present in the capsule (*arrows*). A suggestive zona glomerulosa is present deep to the adrenal capsule (*top*).

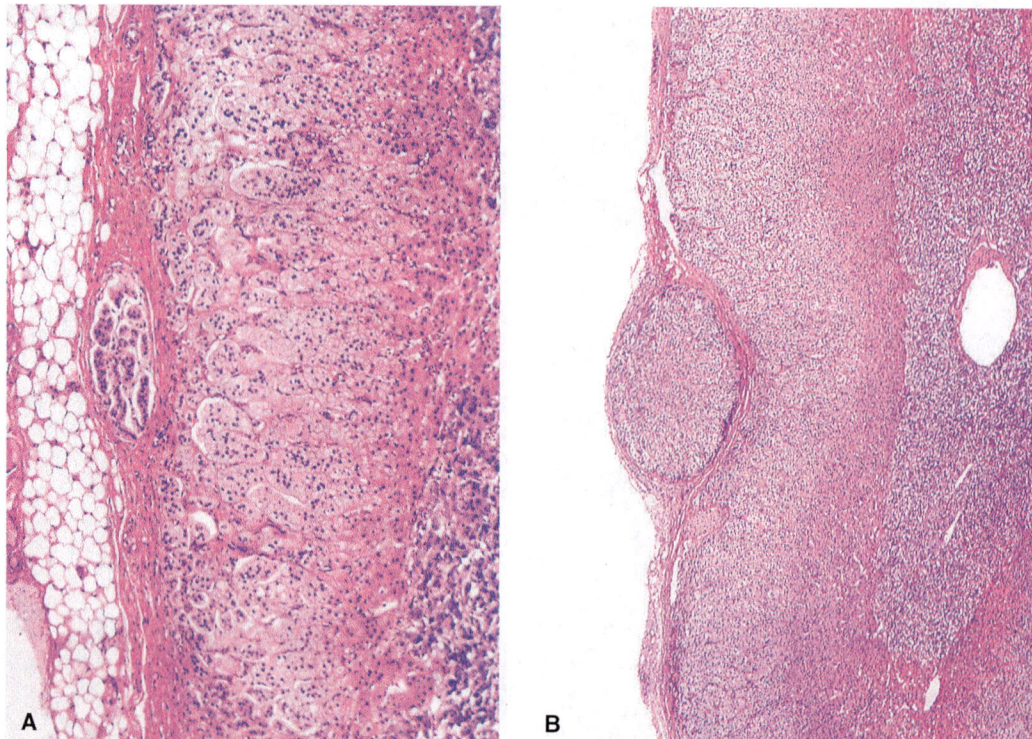

FIGURE 45.13 Normal adrenal gland. **A:** Aggregate of cells with features of zona glomerulosa type is present in a "pocket" in the capsule. **B:** Cortex featuring zona fasciculata (clear cells) and zona reticularis (compact cells) abuts medulla. A larger aggregate of cortical cells with clear (peripheral) and compact cytoplasm (central) is present in a pocket in the capsule. The cortex deep to the pocket is slightly attenuated. A zona glomerulosa is not clearly visible.

Sometimes, seen attached to the capsule are wedge-shaped foci of small, plump spindle cells with hyperchromatic nuclei. These protrude into the cortex to varying depths and may be present bilaterally (Fig. 45.14). The cells are arranged in interlacing bundles and whorls. Largely because of their light microscopic resemblance to ovarian cortical stroma, these aggregates have been termed "ovarian thecal metaplasia"; an alternative interpretation is that they represent areas of adrenocortical blastema that for unknown reasons have failed to mature (5–7). These foci undergo fibrosis, hyalinization, and sometimes calcification. Nests of cortical cells are occasionally found in the spindle cell proliferation, presumably entrapped.

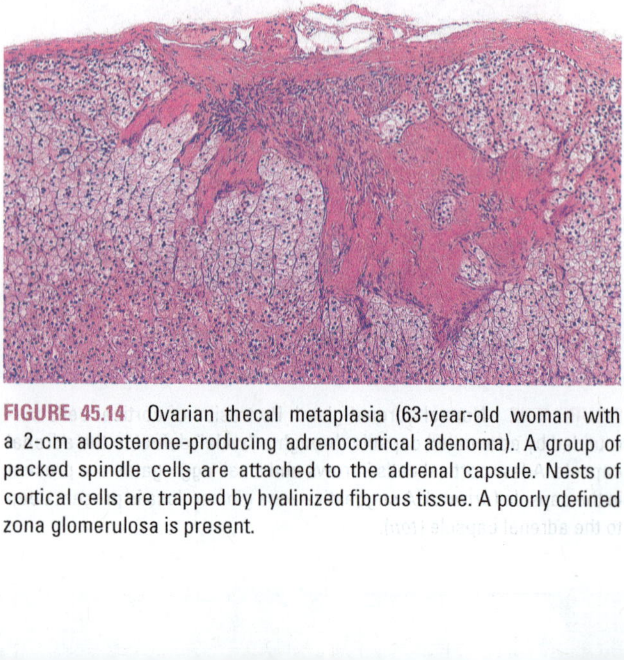

Exceptionally, the proliferations penetrate into the medulla as increasingly narrow tongues of tissue. Ovarian thecal metaplasia is said to occur in postmenopausal women, occasionally in premenopausal women, and exceptionally in old men. It was not present in any of the normal adrenal glands examined for this description despite a good search. However, it was encountered fairly commonly in the extratumoral cortex associated with a range of functioning adrenocortical adenomas and in adrenals removed for other pathology, cortical and medullary, always in perimenopausal or postmenopausal females. The "lesions" are generally incidental microscopic findings that were not recognized grossly.

FIGURE 45.14 Ovarian thecal metaplasia (63-year-old woman with a 2-cm aldosterone-producing adrenocortical adenoma). A group of packed spindle cells are attached to the adrenal capsule. Nests of cortical cells are trapped by hyalinized fibrous tissue. A poorly defined zona glomerulosa is present.

Cortex

The permanent or adult adrenal cortex consists of three readily recognizable parenchymal cell types, arranged in concentric zones or layers—the outer zona glomerulosa (glomus = ball), the inner zona reticularis (rete = net), and between them,

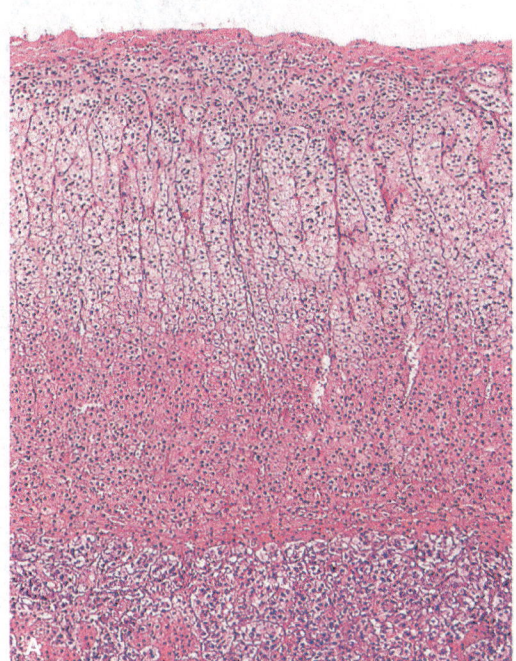 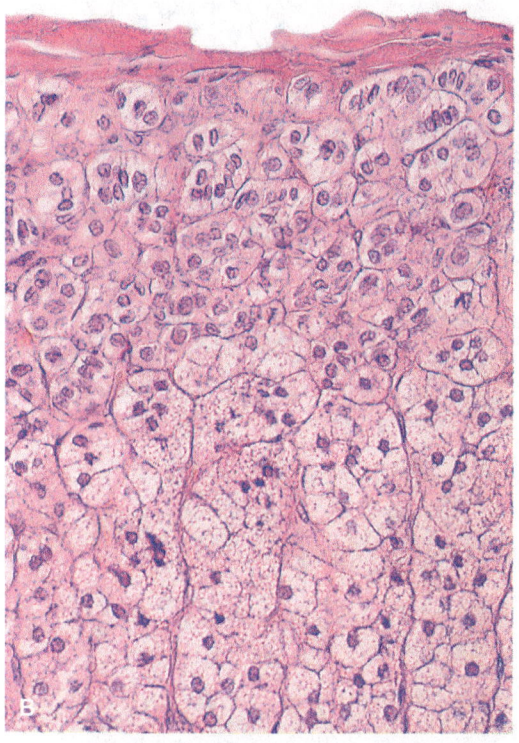

FIGURE 45.15 Normal adrenal gland. **A:** The normal pattern of zonation of the cortex is seen (clusters of cells with stainable cytoplasm in the zona glomerulosa, columns of cells with clear cytoplasm in the zona fasciculata, and cells with acidophilic cytoplasm in the zona reticularis). There is a sharp interface between the cortex (zona reticularis) and medulla (clusters of cells with basophilic cytoplasm). **B:** Zona glomerulosa composed of packed clusters and short trabeculae of cells beneath the adrenal capsule and superficial to the columns of vacuolated cells of the zona fasciculata. The zona glomerulosa nuclei tend to be oval; those of the zona fasciculata are round.

the zona fasciculata (fascis = bundle) (Figs. 45.15 and 45.16). The appearance of the different zones is dictated by their respective cellular arrangements, differential lipid distribution, and pigment accumulation. The normal zona glomerulosa seldom occupies more than 5%, the fasciculata about 70%, and the reticularis 25% of the cortex.

Zonation becomes increasingly irregular with advancing years, although the zona reticularis is always preserved as a well-developed zone, irrespective of age. Irregularity of cortical zonation is, in part, associated with the increased frequency with which cortical nodules are observed in older patients.

The functional significance of this morphologic separation is questionable, but the zona glomerulosa is the site of aldosterone production and is responsive to angiotensin and potassium, and the zona fasciculata and zona reticularis synthesize glucocorticoids and sex hormones. Cells of all zones respond to adrenocorticotropic hormone (ACTH). Division figures are rare in the normal adult cortex; in fact, the zone(s) of normal proliferation for replacement of effete cells is not known, although it is believed to be near the periphery of the cortex. (Under the influence of increased circulating levels of ACTH [Cushing disease], mitotic figures may be seen in the zona fasciculata and zona reticularis, indicating that cells in the deeper areas of the cortex are also capable of proliferating.)

A number of modern techniques for studying cell proliferation and programmed cell death (apoptosis), specifically, KI-67 immunostaining and 3-OH nick end-labeling method, respectively, have been applied to the study of the human adrenal cortex (8). Cell proliferation as indicated by KI-67 immunoreactivity occurred principally in the zona fasciculata. Cortical cells positive for nick-end labeling (apoptotic) were uniformly present in the zona reticularis and in the zona glomerulosa in one-third of cases. The findings suggest that cortical cells may disperse in two directions, centripetally and centrifugally, from the zona fasciculata to the zona reticularis and from the zona fasciculata to the zona glomerulosa, in some cases. Biochemically, apoptosis features chromatin cleavage. Morphologically, there is shrinkage of cytoplasm, condensation, and fragmentation of nuclei and membrane blebbing. Adrenocortical cells undergoing apoptosis are believed to be phagocytosed by histiocytes and cells lining the sinusoids.

Zona Glomerulosa

The zona glomerulosa is the narrow, inconstant band of cortex situated immediately beneath the capsule and superficial to the zona fasciculata (Fig. 45.15). As has been mentioned, the zona glomerulosa remains diffuse during childhood and adolescence. But in the adult it is discontinuous. Sometimes

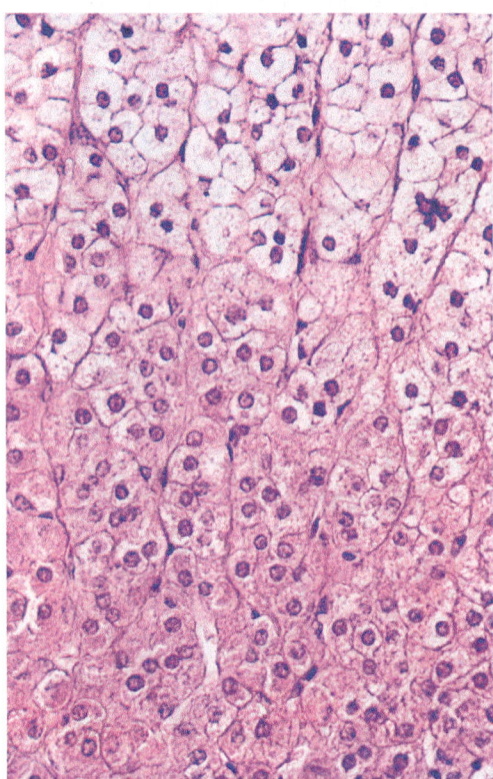

FIGURE 45.16 Normal adrenal cortex. Zona fasciculata (*upper*) features two-cell wide columns of cells with clear cytoplasm, and zona reticularis (*lower*) consists of cells having acidophilic granular cytoplasm that do not form a distinct pattern. Nuclei are vesicular, and nucleoli are small.

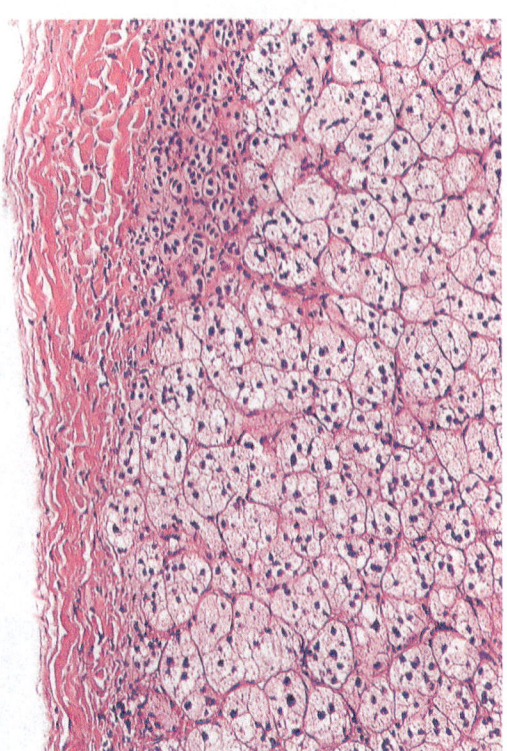

FIGURE 45.17 Normal adrenal cortex with discontinuity of zona glomerulosa. Zona glomerulosa (*upper half*) composed of clusters of cells with amphophilic cytoplasm forms a distinct band beneath the capsule and is sharply demarcated from the deeper zona fasciculata with its clustered cells having clear cytoplasm. Where the zona glomerulosa is absent (*lower half*), the zona fasciculata extends to the capsule.

it can be identified throughout a section or over a large portion of one as a distinct rim beneath the capsule; more often it cannot. Where it is deficient, the zona fasciculata extends to the capsule (Fig. 45.17). The zone is often easier to identify in autopsy material. In routine hematoxylin and eosin preparations, the band may merge with and be separated with difficulty from the outer cells of the zona fasciculata.

The zona glomerulosa cells are well outlined and aggregated into small clusters that are supported by a minimal amount of fibrovascular stroma (Fig. 45.15). The clusters occasionally merge into short trabeculae, straight, bent, or hairpin shape. The cells that tend to be columnar also occur in short cords or one-cell rows set parallel to the capsule. The cytoplasm is faintly acidophilic or amphophilic and minimally to distinctly vacuolated. The round nuclei sometimes are indistinguishable from those of the other zones of the cortex, but often they appear slightly smaller and more deeply staining. Commonly, they are ellipsoidal and elongated and display a longitudinal groove, a nuclear configuration not seen in the deeper areas of the cortex. The nuclear to cytoplasmic ratio is high.

Zona Fasciculata

The zona fasciculata is a broad band, more than half the thickness of the cortex, that lies between the zona glomerulosa (superficial) and the zona reticularis (deep) (Figs. 45.15 to 45.17). The transition between the zones is not sharp. The zona fasciculata cells are large, have distinct cell membranes, are arranged in two-cell wide cords (with the cord axes perpendicular to capsule) and are bounded laterally by parallel-running capillaries. The nuclei are more vesicular and less chromatic than those of the zona glomerulosa, feature a single small nucleolus, and are central in the cells. The nuclear to cytoplasmic ratio is low. Especially in the outer two-thirds of the zone, the cells are filled with lipid (cholesterol, fatty acids, and neutral fat), much of which is birefringent (Fig. 45.18). Since this lipid is dissolved with the usual technical procedures, the fasciculata cells have a spongy, vacuolated, clear appearance, and are often referred to as clear cells. When frozen, and sections are stained with a vital dye or stained for fat, the large amount of intracellular lipid can be appreciated (Fig. 45.18). The yellow color of the zone seen grossly is due to this high lipid content.

Zona Reticularis

The zona reticularis lies deep to the zona fasciculata, and in the head and body of the gland abuts on the medulla (Fig. 45.15). In the tail of the gland, where there is no medulla, the zona reticularis is in contact with zona reticularis

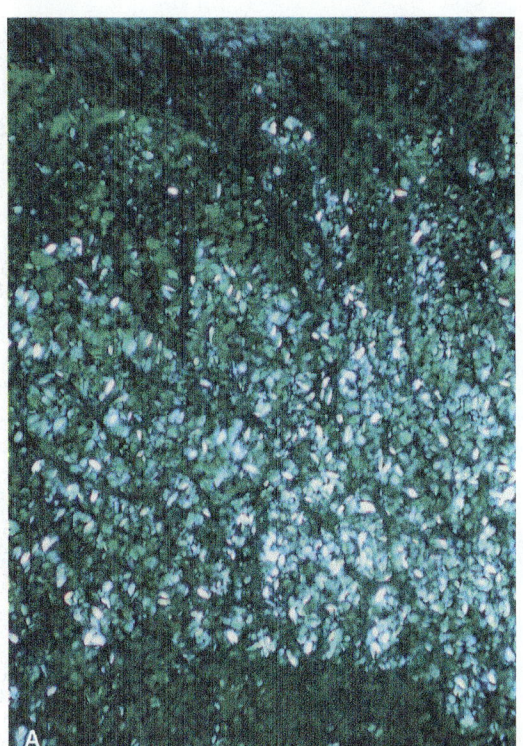 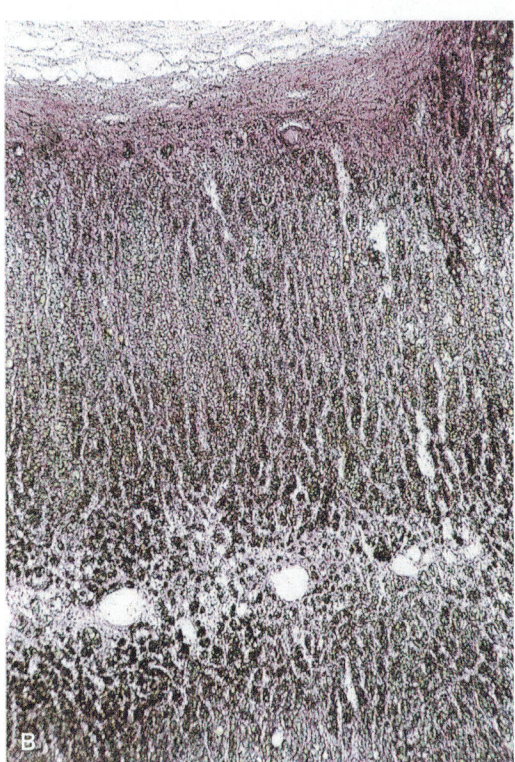

FIGURE 45.18 Normal adrenal cortex. **A:** Partial polarization shows high lipid content of zona fasciculata and low content of zona glomerulosa (*above*) and zona reticularis (*below*). **B:** Fresh-frozen section of adrenal cortex stains with polychrome methylene blue. One complete band of cortex (*above*) and portion of another (*below*) is seen; the junction point between the two is located by the dilated sinusoidal tributaries of the central adrenal vein. Zona fasciculata cells are packed with lipid globules. There are fewer globules in the zona glomerulosa (beneath the adrenal capsule) and in the zona reticularis (on either side of the sinusoidal vessels).

forming a lateral raphe. It constitutes approximately one-quarter of the thickness of the cortex. Zona reticularis cells are arranged in a sponge-like meshwork of gently buckled anastomosing one-cell wide rows of cells that are separated by dilated capillaries. The well-outlined cells are smaller than those of the zona fasciculata and have cytoplasm that is granular, acidophilic, and relatively lipid sparse. The cytoplasm is sometimes referred to as "compact" and the reticularis cells as "compact cells." The deepest cells adjacent to the medulla usually contain yellow lipochrome pigment (lipofuscin), diffusely distributed as coarse granules in the cytoplasm or localized in a single body (Fig. 45.19). The yellow pigmentation of the cytoplasm extends outward into the reticularis for a variable distance. The solid granular eosinophilic cytoplasm and the lipochrome pigment combine to produce the dark brown coloration of the zone seen on cut surface of a fresh or formalin-fixed gland.

Medulla

The medulla is situated in the interior of the organ in the head and body of the gland, deep to the zona reticularis (Figs. 45.15, 45.19 to 45.23). Its area and weight are one-tenth those of the cortex (1,9). The medulla rarely measures more than 2 mm in thickness. Because of the different staining of cells of the two tissues—acidophilia in zona reticularis and basophilia in the medulla—the interface between cortex and medulla is readily visible on low-power microscopic examination. The junction is sharp, with no or minimal intervening connective tissue, leaving cortical and medullary cells in direct contact (Figs. 45.15 and 45.19).

The medulla extends to a variable degree into the crest of the gland (the ridge on the posterior surface) and into one or both of the alae (Fig. 45.24). Areas of the medulla in the alae are not necessarily in direct continuity with the main mass of the medulla around the central veins. The medulla sometimes extends into the tail of the gland. The finding of medulla in this location therefore does not automatically equate with pathologic abnormality—specifically, medullary hyperplasia. Rarely, a narrow tongue of medulla accompanied by a vessel or nerve or unaccompanied extends through the cortex to contact the capsule of the gland.

The medulla, for practical purposes, is composed of a single cell population, the pheochromocytes (medullary or chromaffin cells) (Fig. 45.20). Among the dominant population are scattered small groups of cortical cells and clusters and individual ganglion cells (Fig. 45.21). Not uncommonly, the ganglion cells feature cytoplasmic, round, lightly acidophilic, hyalin bodies, with concentrically arranged fibrillar appearance, up to 30 μm in diameter

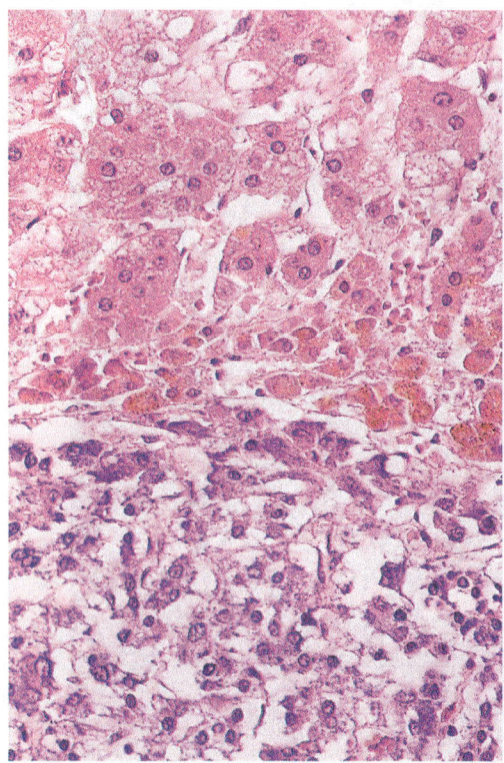

FIGURE 45.19 Corticomedullary junction. The zona reticularis of the cortex (*upper*) is sharply demarcated from the medulla (*lower*). The deepest cells of the zona reticularis contain granular *yellowish* pigment (lipofuscin).

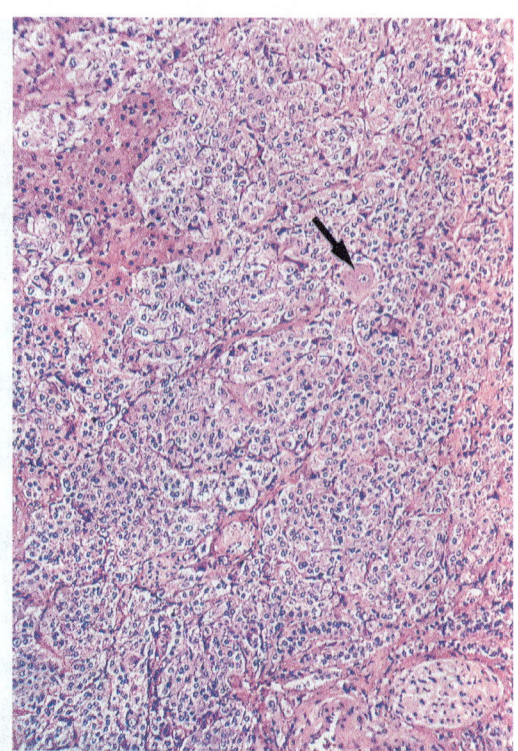

FIGURE 45.21 Normal adrenal medulla. Pheochromocytes are arranged in poorly delineated clusters. An irregularly shaped group of cortical cells (*upper left*) and an isolated ganglion cell (*arrow*) are present.

(Fig. 45.25). Sometimes these bodies appear to be external to the ganglion cells and to indent them; in immunostain preparations (vimentin and S100) they are separated from the cells by a small amount of intercellular substance. It is unusual to observe these bodies in ganglion cells outside the adrenal medulla. Their nature has not been investigated. The pheochromocytes are arranged in tight clusters and short trabeculae, supported by delicate fibrovascular stroma (Figs. 45.20 and 45.22). Sustentacular cells at the periphery of the clusters and trabeculae are not seen in routine histologic preparations, but are readily demonstrated by immunostaining for S100 protein.

The pheochromocytes are moderately large cells, polygonal to columnar, and slightly to considerably larger than cortical cells. Poorly outlined, their complete cell borders are visible only occasionally. Although the cytoplasm of most medullary cells is basophilic, finely granular, and occasionally vacuolated, sometimes it is amphophilic or slightly acidophilic. Rarely, it is partly basophilic and partly acidophilic. The resulting variability and unevenness of medullary cytoplasmic staining and cytoplasmic vacuolization often impart an overall mottled light and dark appearance at intermediate magnification. A rare normal cell has one or more periodic acid–Schiff positive cytoplasmic colloid droplets (Fig. 45.26). Most of the medullary cells are roughly similar in size, but occasionally standard-sized cells merge with groups of cells that are much smaller or much larger (Fig. 45.22).

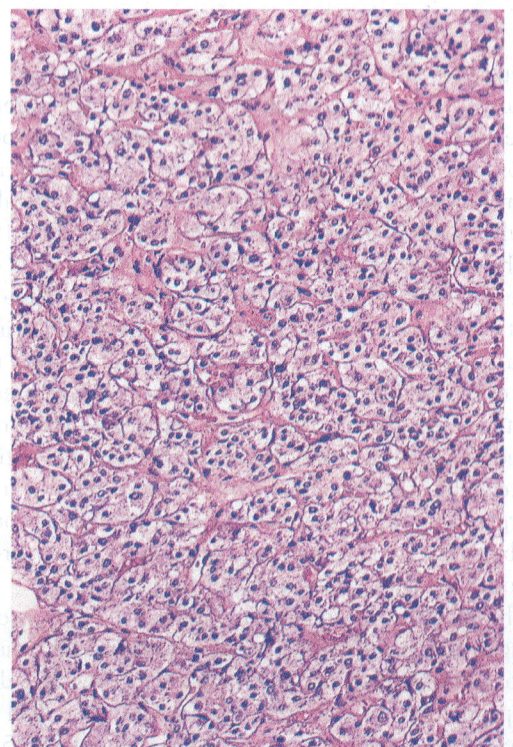

FIGURE 45.20 Normal adrenal medulla. Clusters of poorly outlined cells with basophilic cytoplasm are separated by a vascularized supporting stroma. There is some variation in nuclear size and shape.

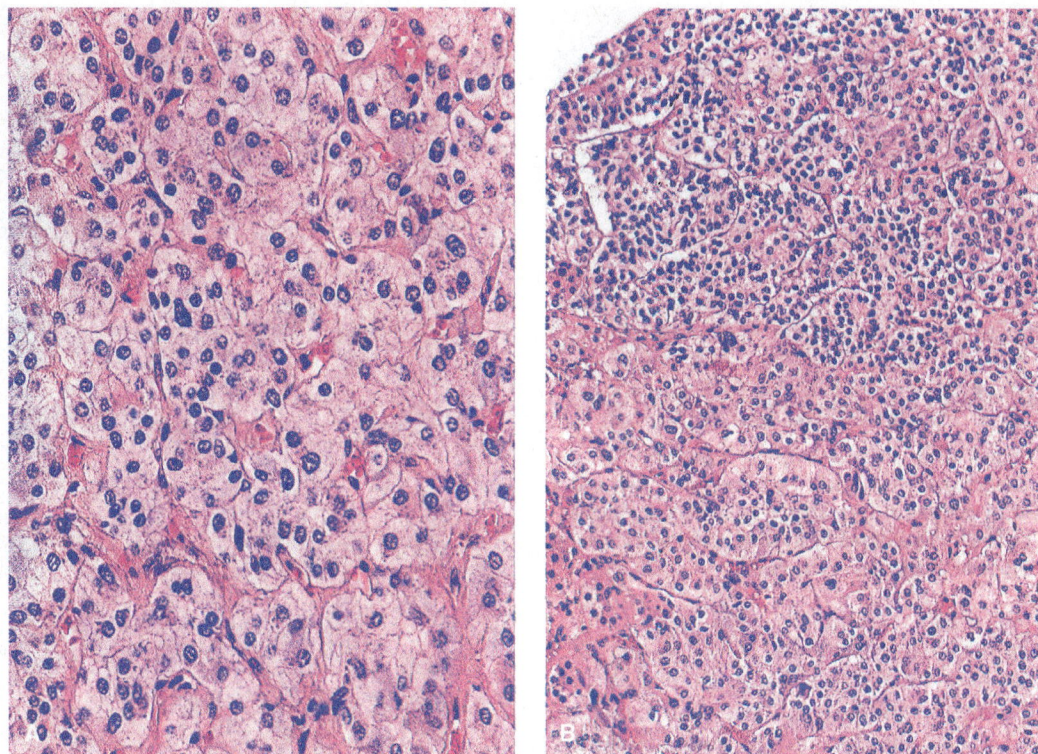

FIGURE 45.22 Normal adrenal medulla. **A:** Pheochromocytes arranged in vague clusters. Cell outlines are visible here and there. Nuclear variation in size and shape is typical. The nuclear chromatin is coarsely clumped and often marginated at the nuclear membrane. **B:** Variation in cell size, nuclear size, and cell pattern.

The nuclei of medullary cells characteristically have slight but definite variability of size, shape, and location in the cell. Most pheochromocyte nuclei are slightly larger than those of cortical cells, but nuclei that are larger and smaller than the usual ones are common. The usual nucleus has a finely or coarsely clumped chromatin pattern with a relatively clear nuclear background (Fig. 45.22). The chromatin tends to be peripherally disposed and separated into irregular clumps. Larger nuclei often have a prominent eosinophilic nucleolus and smaller nuclei are deeply staining. A rare cell has two or more nuclei.

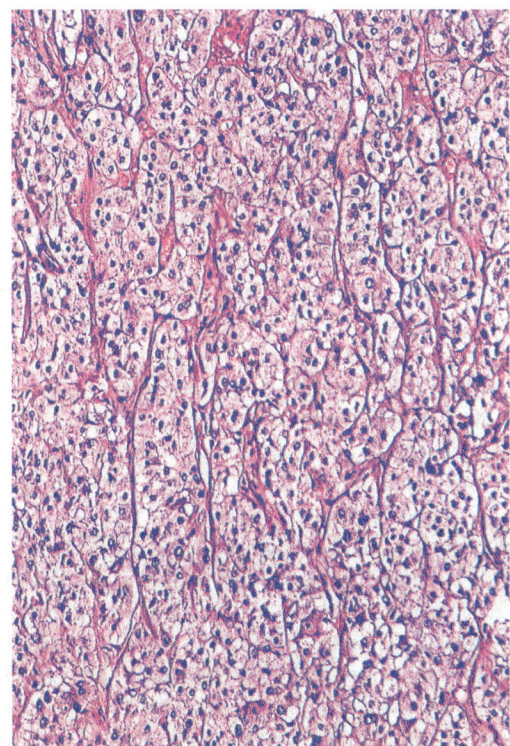

FIGURE 45.23 Normal adrenal medulla. Pheochromocytes arranged in trabecular pattern outlined by a delicate vascular supporting stroma.

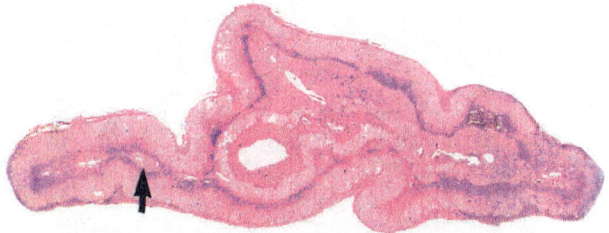

FIGURE 45.24 Normal adrenal gland. A thick capsule surrounds the adrenal cortex (outer clear zona fasciculata and inner eosinophilic zona reticularis) that encloses the basophilic adrenal medulla. An area of medulla in the ala (*arrow*) is not in continuity with the main mass of medulla. The adrenal vein is surrounded by a cuff of invaginated cortex.

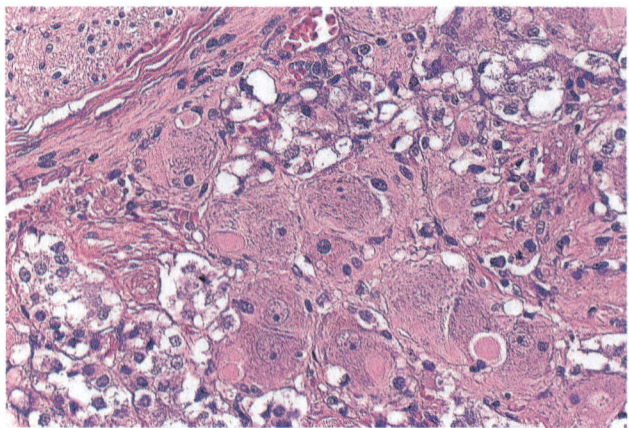

FIGURE 45.25 Normal adrenal medulla. A group of ganglion cells are demarcated by pheochromocytes (*upper right and lower left*) and a nerve (*upper left*). A number of the ganglion cells feature cytoplasmic acidophilic bodies, some outlined by a rim of retracted cytoplasm (*arrows*). There are two such bodies in one cell.

Most of the nuclei are spheroidal, but many are ellipsoidal, and some have other shapes. Large, intensely hyperchromatic and sometimes pleomorphic nuclei are common, usually single and located close to the corticomedullary junction (Fig. 45.27). The positions of the nuclei in the cells are not fixed; most are central, but some tend to be eccentric, located away from the vascular pole (Fig. 45.28).

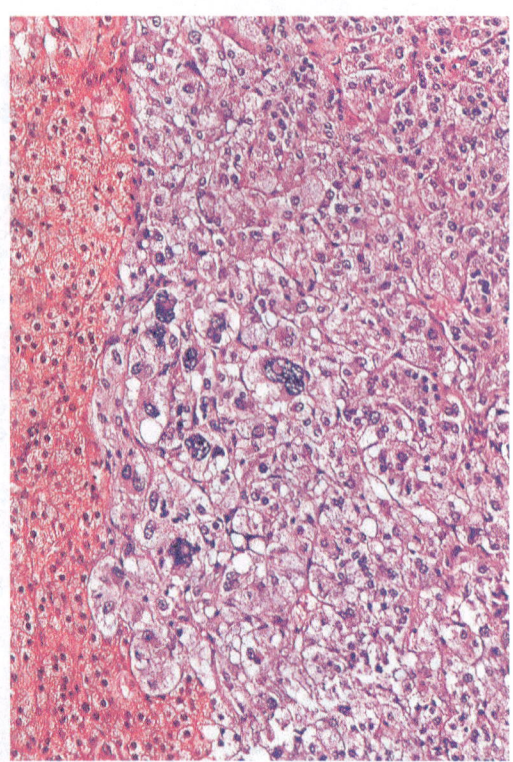

FIGURE 45.27 Normal adrenal medulla. Variability of pheochromocyte nuclei at the corticomedullary junction. The number of atypical pheochromocyte nuclei crowded together here is unusual; ordinarily, such nuclei are seen one to a medium-power field. The pheochromocytes have basophilic granular cytoplasm. The zona reticularis (*left*) features cells with granular eosinophilic cytoplasm and lipofuscin.

The medullary cells have several distinctive histochemical reactions related to their content of secretory granules. The granules contain catecholamines, dihydroxy derivatives of tyrosine, that are converted to colored polymers by oxidizing agents such as potassium dichromate, ferric chloride, ammoniacal silver nitrate, and osmium tetroxide. The oxidized and polymerized derivatives are termed adrenochromes. This staining has been called the chromaffin reaction.

Ganglion cells are scattered randomly among the pheochromocytes or in groups (Fig. 45.21), often associated with a nerve. Their number varies greatly from medulla to medulla; accordingly, they are found easily or not. Cortical cells also are a regular component of the medulla, found in irregularly shaped groups, sometimes in continuity with the zona reticularis, but more often not (Fig. 45.21).

Single or multiple small-to-large accumulations of round cells, plasma cells, and lymphocytes (positive for leukocyte common antigen), often paravascularly located, are common in the normal medulla (Fig. 45.29). They have no known significance. The delicate vascular stroma of the medulla is not conspicuous. Sometimes it is augmented focally by prolongations of the musculature of the central veins that separate groups of medullary cells (Fig. 45.30).

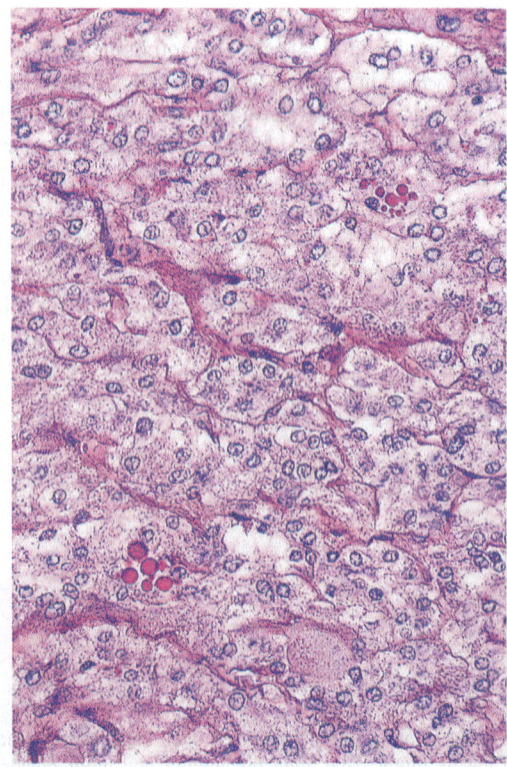

FIGURE 45.26 Normal adrenal medulla. Cytoplasmic globules, a rare finding in normal pheochromocytes, stains with periodic acid–Schiff. Condensation of the nuclear chromatin at the nuclear membrane is well demonstrated.

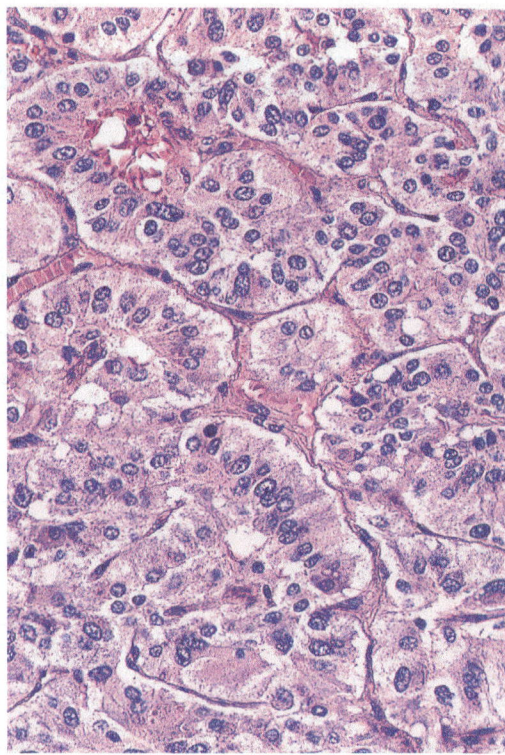

FIGURE 45.28 Normal adrenal medulla. Uncommon pattern in which pheochromocytes are columnar in shape with nuclei that are located away from the vascular pole. The variations in size and shape of the nuclei are typical. Cytoplasmic staining is uneven and ranges from almost clear to basophilic and granular.

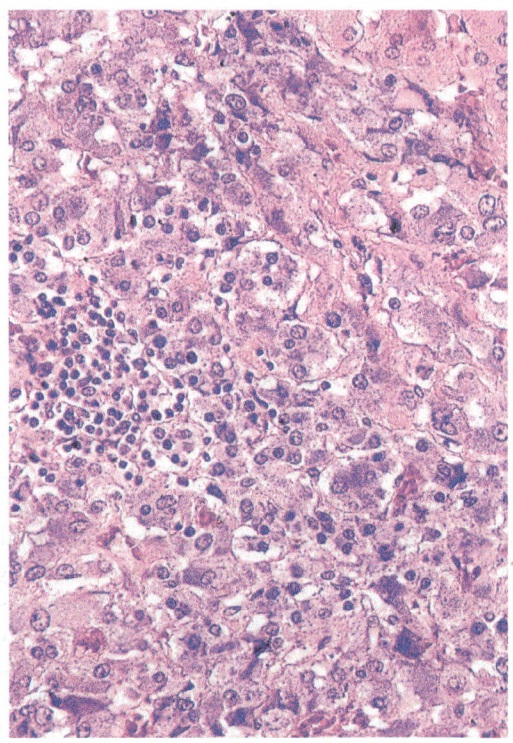

FIGURE 45.29 Normal adrenal medulla. Aggregates of lymphocytes and plasma cells are often encountered.

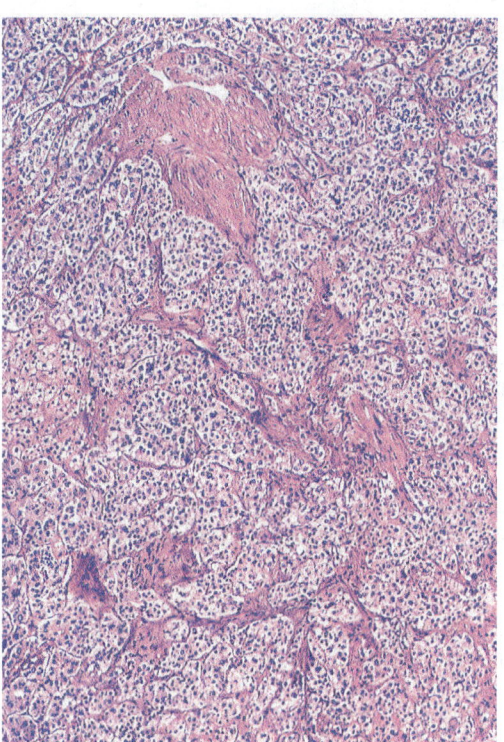

FIGURE 45.30 Normal adrenal medulla. Bundles and strands of smooth muscles are derived from the smooth muscles of central vein.

IMMUNOHISTOCHEMISTRY

Cortex

The results of immunostaining of the prenatal and postnatal adrenal cortex and postnatal medulla are presented in Table 45.1 and illustrated in Figures 45.31 and 45.32. Staining with the antibodies varied in its intensity and character (type of granularity, cell membrane involvement, and paranuclear [Golgi] pattern). With some antibodies the cortex stained diffusely, with others the outer portion was stained and the inner portion was unstained; with others, the reverse was the case. Some antibodies stained the cortex or medulla diffusely; with others the cortical staining was patchy, especially in older individuals.

Cells of the normal adrenal cortex are reported to be immunoreactive against a cytokeratin cocktail and AE1 (10). In this study, there was no staining with AE1/AE3 and minimal focal staining with OSCAR. Cells of the outer zona fasciculata and the zona reticularis were positive for melan-A and inhibin, respectively (Fig. 45.32). Cells of the three zones were variably synaptophysin positive. Cortical cells did not stain chromogranin or S100 antibodies.

Medulla

Pheochromocytes label with antibodies to chromogranin, synaptophysin, and CD56 (Figs. 45.32 and 45.33). Some

SECTION XI: Endocrine

TABLE 45.1 Immunostaining of Prenatal and Postnatal Adrenal Cortex and Medulla

Immunostain	Cortex - Prenatal Fetal (provisional)	Cortex - Prenatal Adult (permanent)	Cortex - Postnatal Neonatal	Cortex - Postnatal Teenage	Cortex - Postnatal Adult	Medulla Prenatal	Medulla Postnatal
Vimentin	Negative (neuro-blasts positive)	Negative	Negative	Strongly positive, outer one-third	Patchy positivity, strongest outer one-third	Positive[a]	Sustentacular cells positive
Synaptophysin	Positive, paranuclear globular	Positive, finely granular	Weakly positive, paranuclear globular, and cytoplasmic finely granular	Rare positivity, subcapsular, paranuclear globular, and finely granular	Negative	Positive[a]	Strongly positive
Inhibin	Strongly positive, coarsely granular	Weakly positive, finely granular	Positive, inner one-half, finely granular	Strongly positive, inner one-third, finely granular	Strongly positive, inner one-third, finely granular	Negative	Negative
Melan-A	Strongly positive, very coarsely granular	Strongly positive, coarsely granular	Weakly positive, outer half, finely granular	Positive, outer one-third, coarsely granular	Positive, outer rim, coarsely granular	Negative	Negative
CD56	Intracapsular cells positive	Negative	Strongly positive outer one-half, cell membrane	Strongly positive, outer one-third cell membrane	Discontinuous positivity outer rim, cell membrane	Weakly positive[a]	Strongly positive, membranous
MIB1	Many subcapsular nuclei stained	Scattered nuclei stained	Scattered nuclei stained, subcapsular	Scattered nuclei stained, outer one-third	Scattered nuclei stained, outer one-half	Negative[a]	Negative
Chromogranin	Negative	Negative	Negative	Negative	Negative	Negative	Strongly positive
S100	Negative	Negative	Negative	Negative	Negative	Positive[a]	Sustentacular cells positive
Keratin AE1/AE3	Negative	Negative	Negative	Negative	Negative	Negative[a]	Negative

[a]Neuroblasts.

pheochromocytes react with antibodies to S100 protein. The sustentacular cells that mantle the clusters and trabeculae of pheochromocytes are S100 protein positive (Fig. 45.33), as are nerves in the medulla.

ULTRASTRUCTURE

Cortex

There are ultrastructural features shared by the three layers of the cortex relating to their common function—synthesis of steroid hormones. The cells feature voluminous endoplasmic reticulum, stacks of rough endoplasmic reticulum, a well-developed Golgi apparatus, lysosomes, and many mitochondria. The distribution and internal structure of some of the organelles (eg, the mitochondria) vary from zone to zone. Using the electron microscope, the usually distinct transition seen between the zones is not apparent; rather, a gradual alteration from one organelle distribution and type to another being observed. Mitochondria in the zona glomerulosa are round, oval, or elongate, with lamellar infolded cristae, resulting in a ladder-like internal structure similar to that found in many other tissues (Fig. 45.34). In the zona fasciculata, these organelles are large, spherical, and feature tubular cristae (Fig. 45.34). Lipid droplets are large and numerous. The mitochondria in the zona reticularis (Fig. 45.34) tend to be more elongated and exhibit tubular and vesicular cristae that are a feature of steroid-producing cells. Lipofuscin granules, membrane-bound organelles with a moderately dense

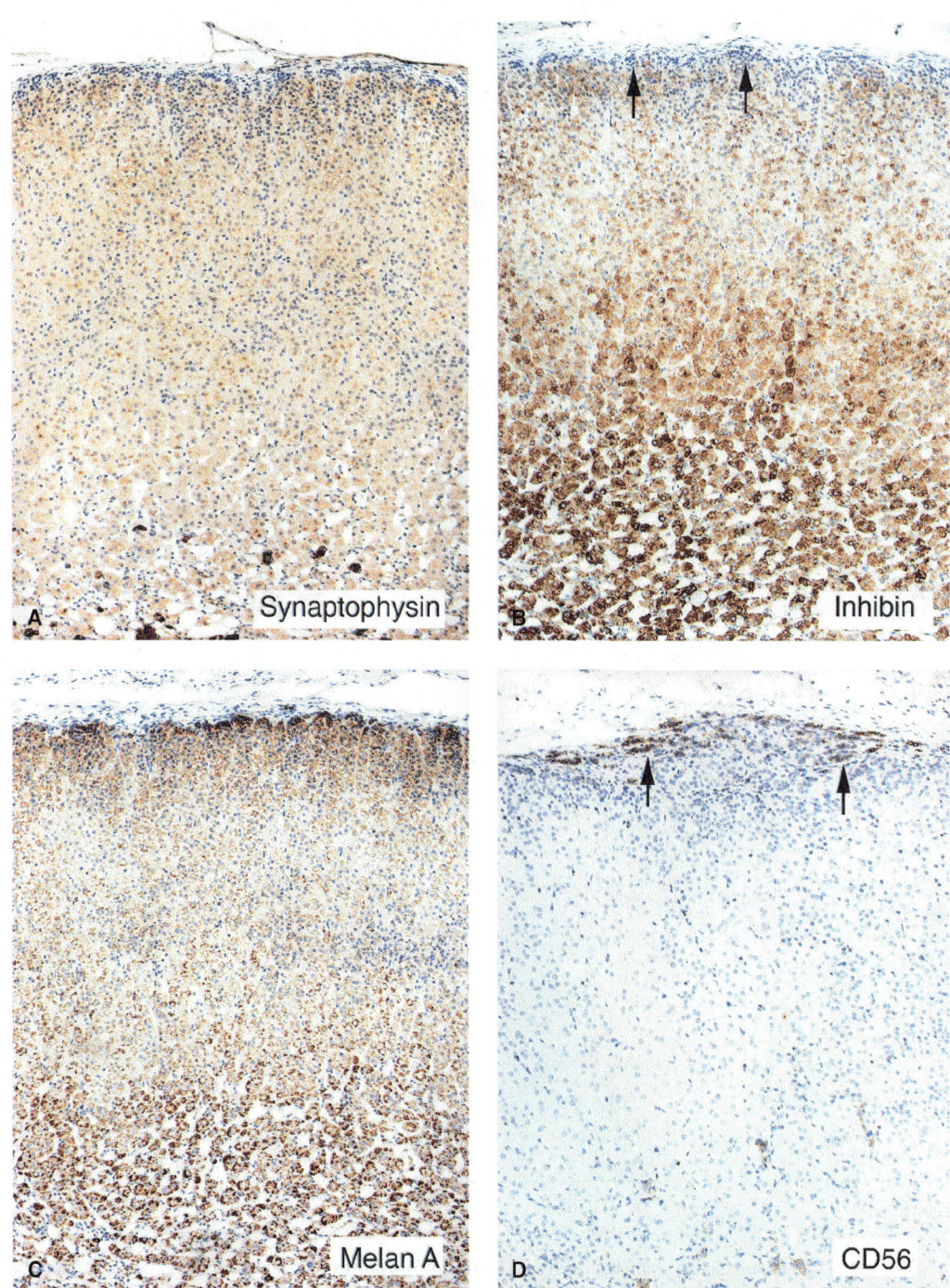

FIGURE 45.31 Immunostaining of the prenatal adrenal cortex. **A:** Synaptophysin stains almost the entire cortex leaving a narrow band of subcapsular cells unstained. **B:** Inhibin stains most of the cortex to a variable degree but do not stain a narrow subcapsular band (*arrows*). **C:** Melan A stains the entire cortex to a variable degree. **D:** CD56 labeled a peripheral band of elongated cells, some in the capsule (*arrows*).

matrix that contains dense granules and clear lipid globules, are prominent. Glycogen is present.

Medulla

Catecholamine-secreting cells dominate the medulla. Two cell types, epinephrine and norepinephrine, distinguished by granule type are present. In tissue fixed in glutaraldehyde, cells that contain epinephrine feature granules (Fig. 45.35) measuring about 190 μm in diameter, with a moderately dense but not opaque finely granular texture fills the enclosing membrane. Norepinephrine-secreting cells have granules (Fig. 45.35) that are electron opaque, often located eccentrically within a dilated sac, and measure about 250 μm in diameter.

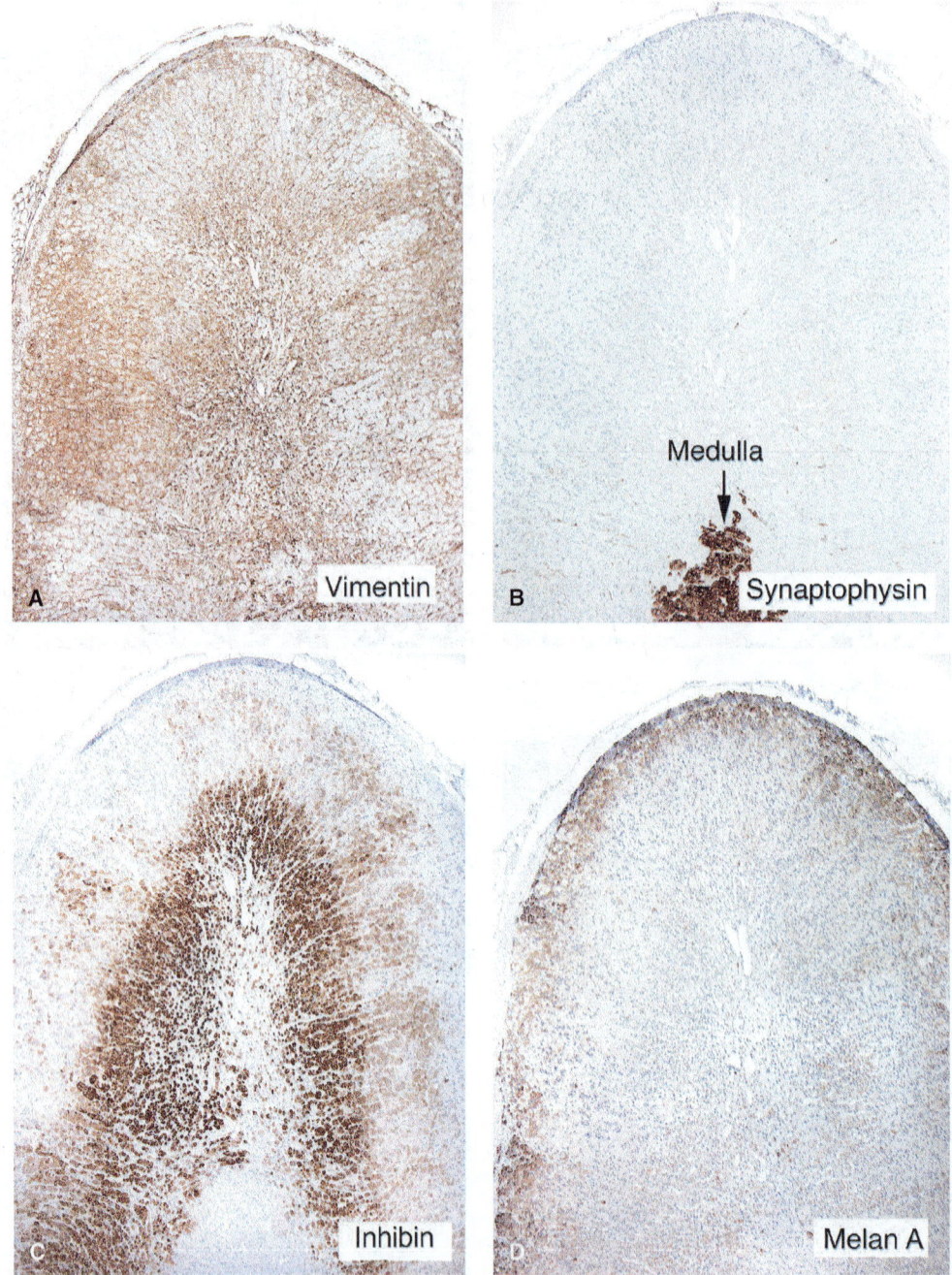

FIGURE 45.32 Immunostaining of the adult adrenal cortex. **A:** The cortex diffusely and unevenly stains with vimentin. **B:** There is no staining of the cortex with synaptophysin. The medulla stains heavily. **C:** Inhibin stains the inner cortex heavily and the outer half less heavily. **D:** Melan A stains a subcapsular band of cortical cells. (*continued*)

OTHER ANATOMICAL STRUCTURES

Blood Vessels

The blood supply of the adrenal glands has been studied mostly from the anatomic point of view, often by observing the distribution of injected material in the vasculature. The tone of the subcapsular vascular plexus controls circulation through the organ. The histologic appearance of the vessels distal to the plexus suggests that the intravascular pressure in the organ is low.

Arteries

Three separate groups of arteries—superior, middle, and inferior—arising from the inferior phrenic artery, the aorta, and the renal artery, supply each adrenal gland

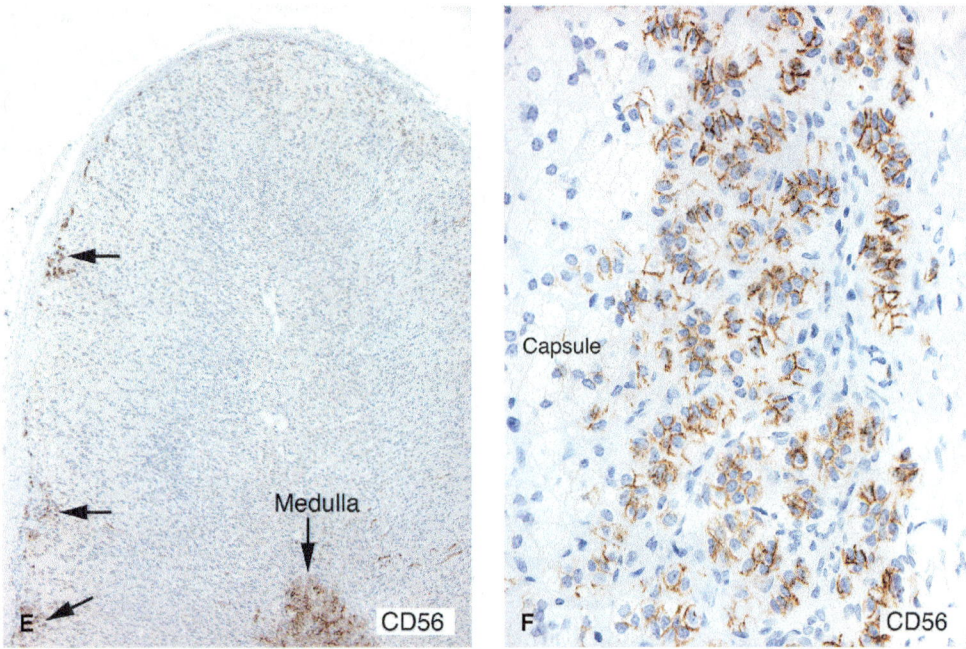

FIGURE 45.32 (Continued) **E:** CD56 scatter aggregates of subcapsular cells. The medulla stains. **F:** A subcapsular aggregate showed a membranous pattern of staining.

(Fig. 45.36). The main vessels divide into 50 to 60 small feeder vessels that penetrate the anterior and posterior surfaces of the glands and form a plexus beneath the capsule of the glands. The former are commonly encountered close to the capsule of the glands; in older patients, they frequently exhibit atherosclerotic changes. The subcapsular plexus, important in regulation of the circulation in the gland, is not conspicuous in routine histologic preparations.

Intraglandular Vasculature

Capillary loops from the subcapsular plexus surround the cells of the zona glomerulosa, then extend toward the interior of the organ between the columns of cells of the zona fasciculata, and ultimately open into wide interconnecting channels in the zona reticularis to form a second vascular plexus. This ends abruptly in a vascular dam at the corticomedullary junction that finally drains into the sinusoids of the medulla by relatively fewer channels. The marked vascular congestion commonly seen at the corticomedullary junction of adrenal glands obtained at autopsy may be a reflection of this vascular barrier. Although the medulla receives some arterial blood supply, most of its vascular supply has already nourished the cortex.

The venous drainage from the organs occurs via a single vein that emerges from the anterior surface of each gland (Fig. 45.2). Inside the organs, the central adrenal vein (which ultimately becomes the adrenal vein as it leaves the organ) and its tributaries have a unique muscle coat, two to six longitudinally running muscle bundles, varying in size and eccentrically situated around the vein lumen (Fig. 45.37). The bundles are heavily laden with elastic fibers that extend into tributaries of the larger central veins and in some instances outline clusters and trabeculae of medullary cells.

The eccentricity of the muscle bundles results in a vein wall that varies greatly in thickness and focally is devoid of muscles. In the zones, where the muscle bundles are deficient (and these may be extensive), medullary cells (and sometimes cortical cells) are separated from the bloodstream by intima and a minimal amount of subintimal connective tissue only. This peculiar anatomic structure permits medullary cells or cortical cells to occasionally form polypoid endothelium–covered projections into the lumen of the central vein (Fig. 45.38). (This ready access of pheochromocytes to the venous lumen explains the occasional finding of an intravenous tumor plug of pheochromocytoma.) A thick cuff of invaginated cortical cells surrounds the intramedullary central vein and its larger tributaries (Figs. 45.24 and 45.37). (Development of a neoplasm in this "displaced" cortex probably explains the occasional cortical neoplasm that appears to have developed in the medulla of the organ. There is another possible source for a cortical neoplasm in this location—from cortical cells that occur among cells of the medulla.)

Veins

The left adrenal vein, 2 to 4 cm in length, initially lies in a groove on the anterior surface of the gland and terminates in the left renal vein (Figs. 45.2 and 45.36). The right adrenal vein is short (1 to 5 mm) and drains into the inferior vena cava (Figs. 45.2 and 45.36). Histologically, the extra-adrenal and immediately intra-adrenal portions of the veins have a muscular coat composed of large, similarly sized, evenly

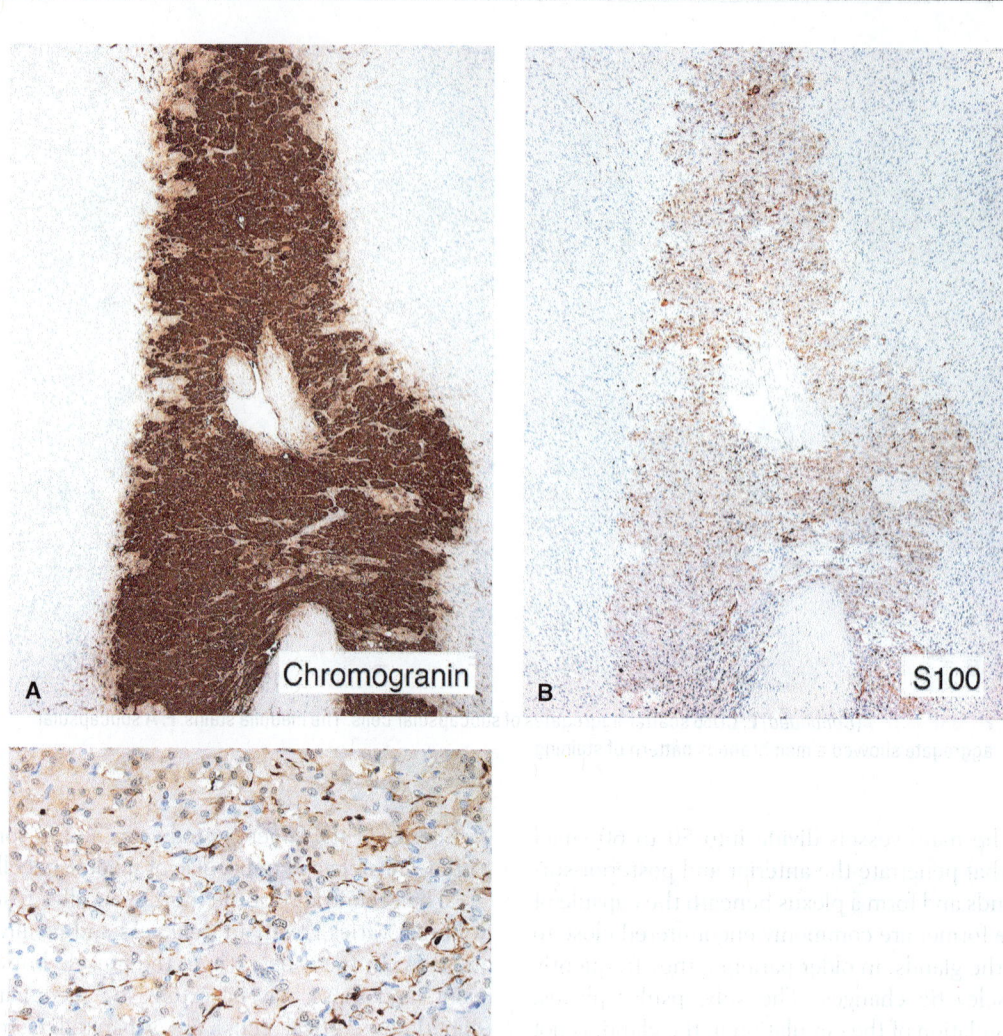

FIGURE 45.33 Immunostaining of the adrenal medulla. **A:** The medulla is heavily labeled by antibodies to chromogranin, the cortex is not labeled. **B:** Antibodies to S100 protein label the medulla and do not label the cortex. **C:** Sustentacular cells mantling groups of pheochromocytes show a linear discontinuous pattern.

disposed smooth muscle bundles, arranged side by side—a structure found in other veins of this size.

Nerves and Ganglia

The innervation of the adrenal gland, specifically of the medulla, emanates from the lower thoracic segments of the spinal cord and passes through the greater splanchnic nerve and the upper lumbar sympathetic ganglia via the celiac plexus. This nerve supply forms a plexus of medullated and nonmedullated nerves on the capsule of the gland, primarily on its posterior aspect. Thus, the largely preganglionic nerve fibers pass into the medulla following either the course of emerging or penetrating vessels or connective tissue trabeculae. Occasionally, a large nerve penetrates directly into the medulla. The number of nerves visible in the medulla varies greatly from case to case; some feature a perineurium, whereas others do not (Fig. 45.39); frequently, they have associated ganglion cells. Ganglion cells are also commonly seen singly or in clusters among the pheochromocytes (Figs. 45.21 and 45.25). The cells of the cortex do not have a nerve supply.

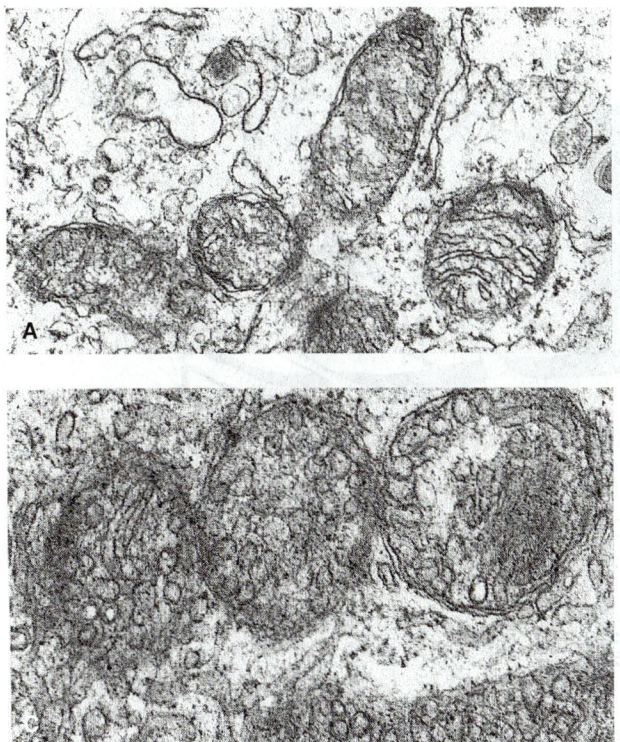
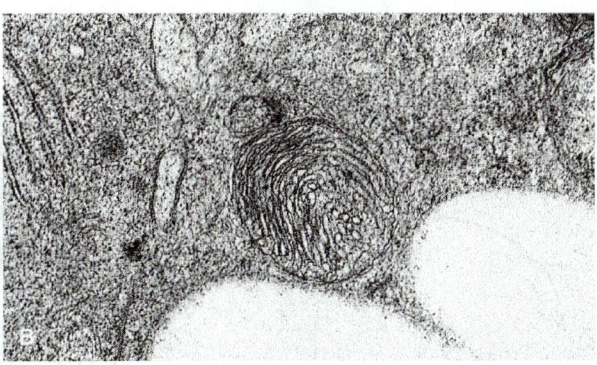

FIGURE 45.34 Normal adrenal cortex. **A:** Mitochondria in the zona glomerulosa have a lamellar pattern. **B:** Mitochondria in the zona fasciculata have a tubular and vesicular pattern. **C:** Mitochondria in the zona reticularis are elongated and have a vesicular appearance.

Lymphatics

Injection studies have demonstrated that there is a rich plexus of lymphatic channels in the capsule of the glands. Lymphatics are distributed to the adventitia of the central vein and its main tributaries. There is no lymphatic supply to the cortex. The lymphatics drain into aortic lymph nodes.

Accessory (Heterotopic) Adrenal Cortex

The adrenocortical primordium initially is unencapsulated and develops, as has been mentioned, close to the emerging gonad. Therefore, it is not surprising that (a) some cells of the unencapsulated adrenocortical primordium may become associated with and migrate alongside the gonad (testis or

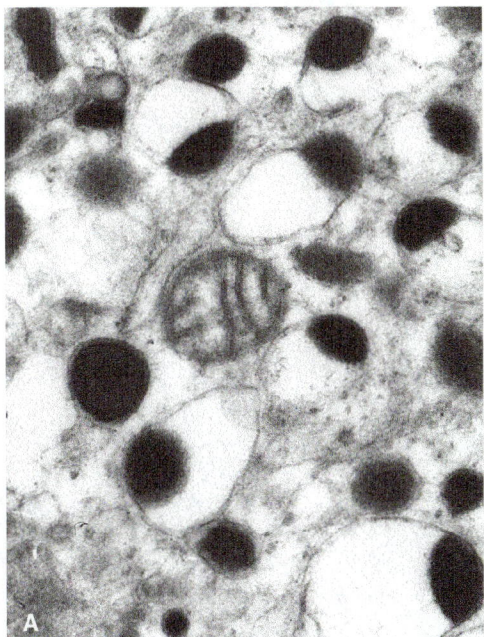
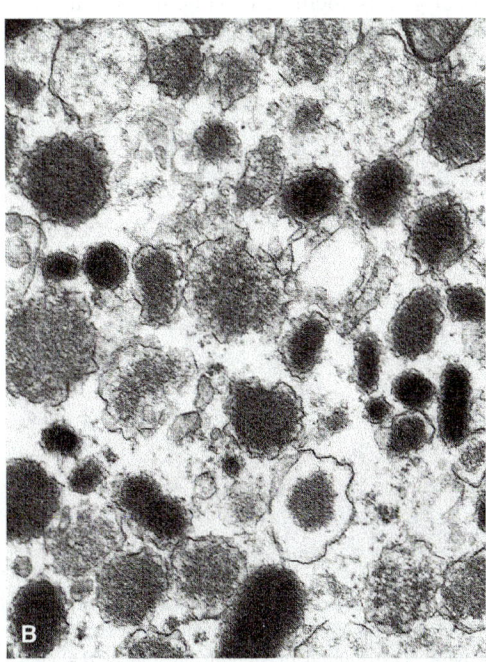

FIGURE 45.35 Normal adrenal medulla. Electron micrographs of medullary secretory granules. **A:** Content of norepinephrine granules is electron dense and often eccentrically located. **B:** Epinephrine granules with a variable electron-dense content that fill most of the sacs.

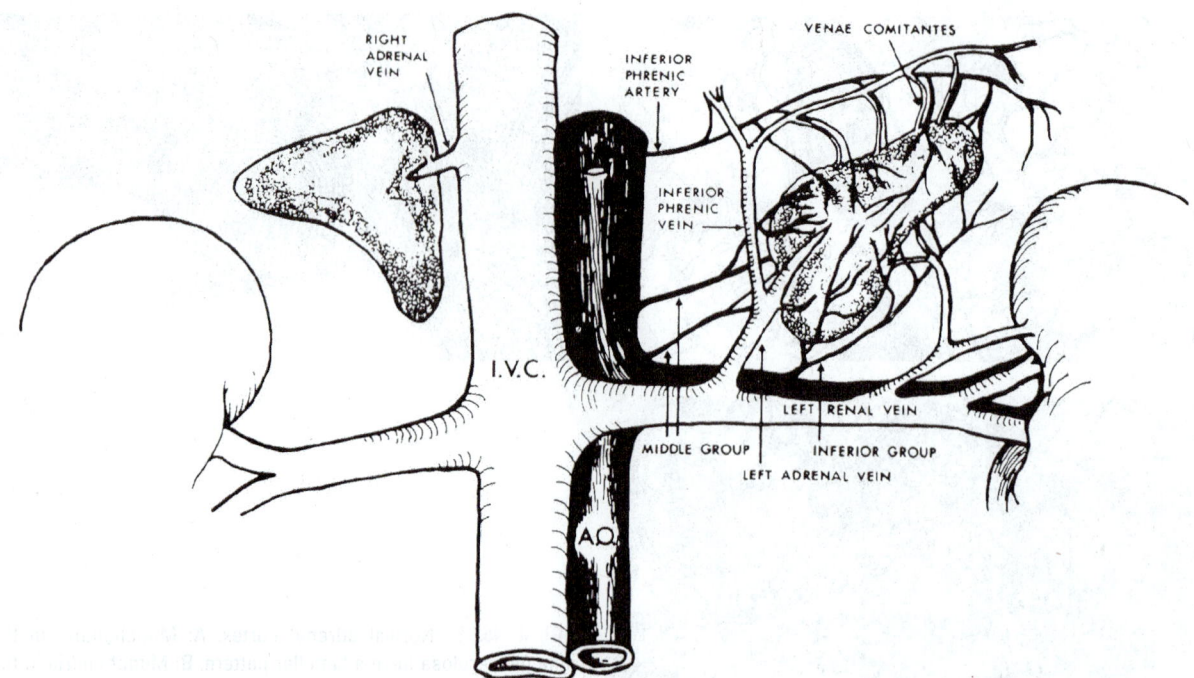

FIGURE 45.36 Diagrammatic representation of the arterial supply (*black*) and venous drainage (*light and hatched*) of the left adrenal gland. Reprinted with permission from Symington T. *Functional Pathology of the Human Adrenal Gland*. Baltimore, MD: Williams & Wilkins; 1969.

ovary) to be found postnatally distant from the adrenal in the path of gonad descent, and (b) cortical cells not sequestered by adrenal capsule formation are subsequently found in the retroperitoneal fat close to the adrenal glands. In practice, accessory adrenocortical tissue is most often encountered around the adrenal glands themselves (Fig. 45.40); it also occurs in the inguinal region and around the ovary, fallopian

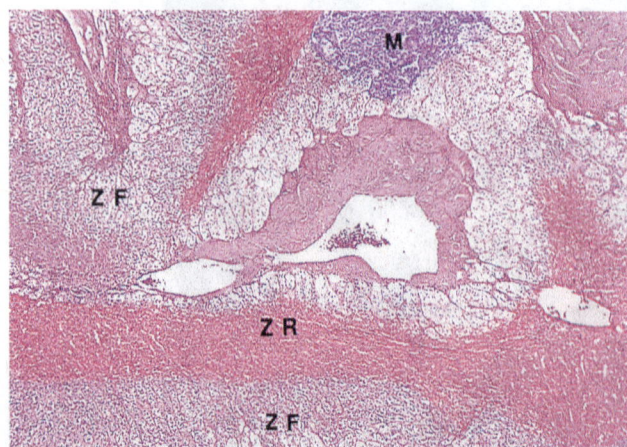

FIGURE 45.37 Central adrenal vein. Low-power view of the vein surrounded by an invaginated cuff of cortical cells with clear cytoplasm (zona fasciculata type). Distribution of smooth muscle in the vein wall is uneven. The zona fasciculata (*ZF*) and zona reticularis (*ZR*) of the cortex are evident, and there is a small amount of basophilic medulla (*M*).

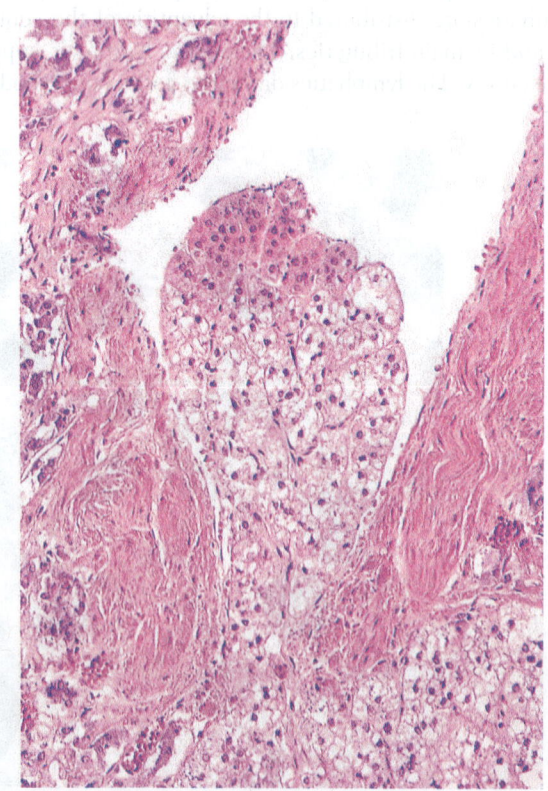

FIGURE 45.38 Central adrenal vein. Intraluminal protrusion of endothelium-covered adrenocortical cells between the discontinuous muscle bundles of a tributary of the central adrenal vein.

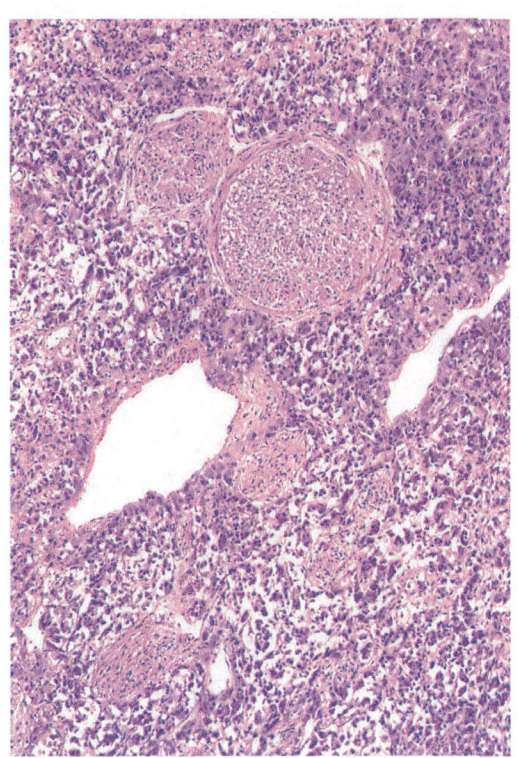

FIGURE 45.39 Adrenal medulla. Unusual concentration of nerves, some with perineurium and others without.

tube, epididymis, and rete testis. Microscopically, accessory cortex shows normal zonation and responds to ACTH. Rarely, medulla is also present (Fig. 45.40).

Adrenocortical Nodules

Adrenocortical nodules, roughly spherical, uncapsulated areas of hypertropic and hyperplastic cortical cells, are not regarded as true neoplasms. They range in size from microscopic to grossly obvious lesions (11). Before the fourth decade of life, they are rare; thereafter, they are encountered with increasing frequency. Although regarded by some as an aging phenomenon, they are not invariably found in older individuals. Usually, multiple nodules commonly consist of large, lipid-laden clear cells; some nodules are composed of clear and compact cells; a minority feature reticularis-type cells only (Fig. 45.41). The smallest nodules may be found at any level of the cortex, but usually they occur in the zona fasciculata. Initially, they appear to be the result of hypertrophy of contiguous cells in three or more adjacent cords. The smallest ill-defined nodules thus have the cord structure of the parent tissue. As they enlarge further due to cell proliferation, this organized appearance is lost, and larger nodules are patternless. Large nodules cause compression and distortion of the surrounding cortex.

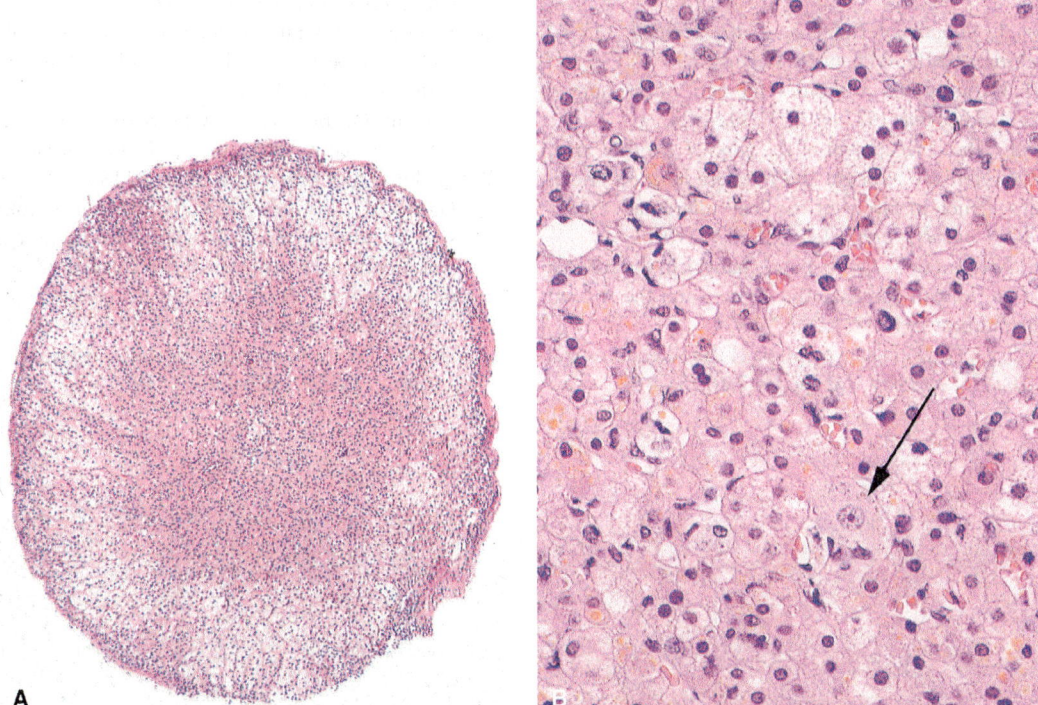

FIGURE 45.40 Accessory adrenal cortex in retroperitoneal fat. **A:** Normal zonation is suggested by the narrow rim of cells with clear cytoplasm that surrounds the main mass of cells with light eosinophilic cytoplasm. **B:** Ganglion cell (*arrow*) indicating the presence of medulla among cortical "clear" and "compact" cells. The latter contain lipofuscin.

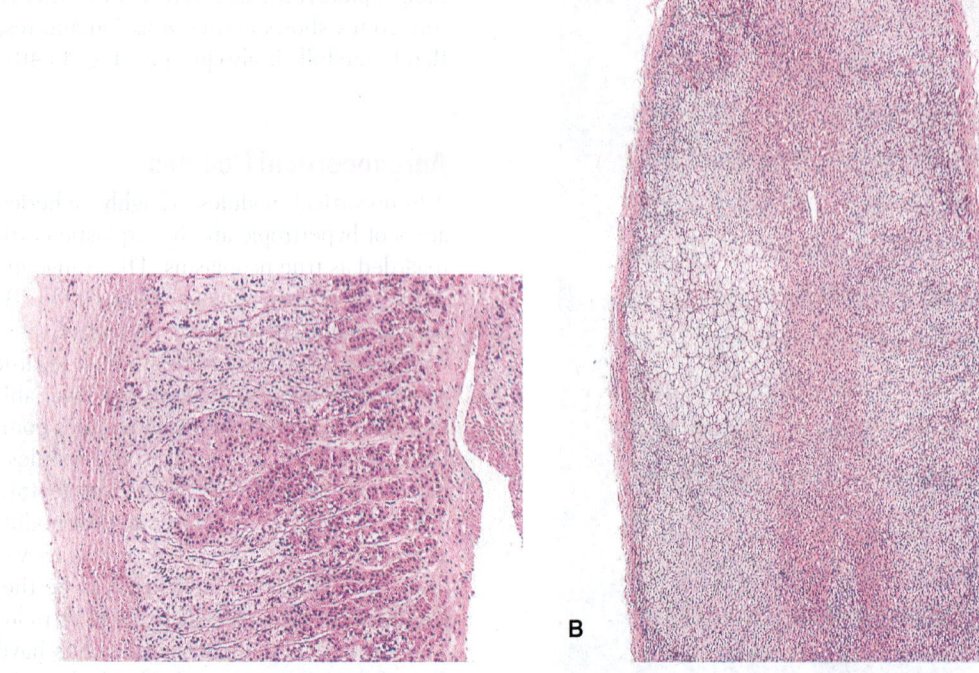

FIGURE 45.41 Cortical nodules (36-year-old man). **A:** Suggestive nodule in the mid-cortex. **B:** Distinct nodule composed of clear cells in outer cortex.

REFERENCES

1. Symington T. *Functional Pathology of the Human Adrenal Gland*. Baltimore, MD: Williams & Wilkins; 1969.
2. Keene MF. Observations on the development of the human suprarenal gland. *J Anat* 1927;61(Pt 3):302–324.
3. Crowder RE. The development of the adrenal gland in man, with special reference to origin and ultimate location of cell types and evidence in favour of the "cell migration" theory. *Carnegie Inst Contrib Embryol* 1957;26:193–210.
4. Ekholm E, Niemineva K. On prenatal changes in the relative weights of the human adrenals, the thymus and the thyroid gland. *Acta Paediatr* 1950;39(1–2):67–86.
5. Reed RJ, Patrick JT. Nodular hyperplasia of the adrenal cortical blastema. *Bull Tulane Univ Med Fac* 1967;26:151–157.
6. Wong TW, Warner NE. Ovarian thecal metaplasia in the adrenal gland. *Arch Pathol* 1971;92(5):319–328.
7. Fidler WJ. Ovarian thecal metaplasia in adrenal glands. *Am J Clin Pathol* 1977;67(4):318–323.
8. Sasano H, Imatani A, Shizawa S, et al. Cell proliferation and apoptosis in normal and pathologic human adrenal. *Mod Pathol* 1995;8(1):11–17.
9. Quinan C, Berger AA. Observations on human adrenals with especial reference to the relative weight of the normal medulla. *Ann Intern Med* 1933;6:1180–1192.
10. Gaffey MJ, Traweek ST, Mills SE, et al. Cytokeratin expression in adrenocortical neoplasia: An immunohistochemical and biochemical study with implications for the differential diagnosis of adrenocortical, hepatocellular, and renal cell carcinoma. *Hum Pathol* 1992;23(2):144–153.
11. Dobbie JW. Adrenocortical nodular hyperplasia: The ageing adrenal. *J Pathol* 1969;99(1):1–18.

Neuroendocrine

Ronald A. DeLellis ■ Shamlal Mangray

HISTORICAL PERSPECTIVES AND NOMENCLATURE 1249	DISTRIBUTION OF NEUROENDOCRINE CELLS 1261
EMBRYOLOGY 1251	Bronchopulmonary and Upper Respiratory System 1261
MOLECULAR ASPECTS OF NEUROENDOCRINE CELL DEVELOPMENT 1252	Thyroid and Thymus 1262
	Skin 1263
LIGHT MICROSCOPY AND HISTOCHEMISTRY 1252	Breast 1264
ULTRASTRUCTURE 1255	Gastrointestinal System 1264
APOPTOSIS 1255	Urogenital System 1265
FUNCTION OF NEUROENDOCRINE CELLS 1256	AGING CHANGES 1266
MARKERS OF NEUROENDOCRINE CELLS 1257	SPECIAL PROCEDURES 1266
Cytosolic Constituents 1257	ARTIFACTS 1267
Secretory Granule Constituents 1258	DIFFERENTIAL DIAGNOSIS 1267
Synaptic Vesicle and Vesicle Fusion/Release Constituents 1259	SPECIMEN HANDLING 1267
Transcription Factors 1260	REFERENCES 1267
Somatostatin Receptors 1261	

Numerous studies have established that there are many striking similarities between neurons and peptide hormone-producing neuroendocrine cells. Both cell types have polarized membrane orientations, separately regulated secretory pathways, secretory granules and vesicles that serve as storage sites for various peptides and amines, neurotransmitter-synthesizing enzymes, neural cell adhesion molecules and, in many cases, the necessary molecular machinery for the uptake and release of neurotransmitters and neuropeptide hormones (1). Detailed biochemical and molecular studies have demonstrated a commonality of biosynthetic products that may act as classical hormones, neurotransmitters, and paracrine or autocrine factors. Accordingly, concepts of the endocrine system have been expanded to include not only the traditional endocrine glands but also the peptidergic neurons and the system of neuroendocrine cells that is dispersed throughout many tissues of the body. Although neuroendocrine cells are discussed in the context of different tissues and organs in other chapters of this volume, this chapter will provide a more focused overview of these fascinating cell types.

HISTORICAL PERSPECTIVES AND NOMENCLATURE

Current concepts of the neuroendocrine system evolved from a series of observations that were initiated more than a century ago. Heidenhain in 1870 demonstrated a population of chromate positive cells in the gastric mucosa of rabbits and dogs and suggested that they might have an endocrine function (2,3). Subsequently, Kulchitsky (4) identified similar

---

This chapter is an update of a previous version authored by Ronald A. DeLellis and Yogeshwar Dayal.

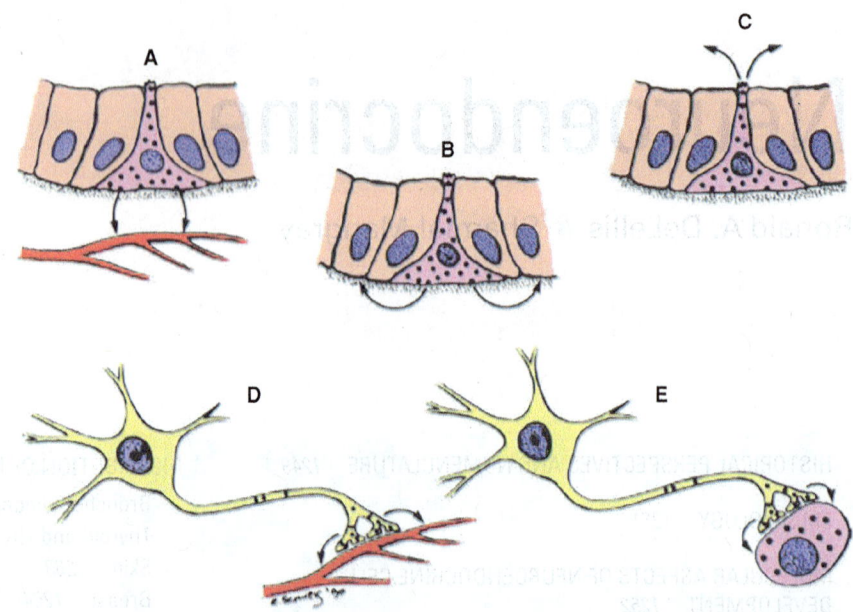

FIGURE 46.1 Secretory activities of neuroendocrine cells and neurons. **A:** Neuroendocrine cells may secrete their products through the basement membranes into adjacent capillaries for interactions with target tissues at distant sites (endocrine function). **B:** Neuroendocrine cells may secrete their products locally to influence the activities of adjacent epithelial cells (paracrine function). **C:** Neuroendocrine cells may secrete their products within a glandular lumen (luminal secretion). **D:** Neurons may secrete their products into the circulation for interactions with target tissues at distant sites (neuroendocrine function). **E:** Neurons also may secrete products that serve as neurotransmitters or neuromodulators. Adapted from Ito T, Udaka N, Yazawa T, et al. Basic helix-loop-helix transcription factors regulate the neuroendocrine differentiation in fetal mouse pulmonary epithelium. *Development* 2000;127(18):3913–3921 and Fujita T, Kobayashi S. The cells and hormones of the GEP endocrine system. In: Fujita T, ed. *Gastroenteropancreatic Cell System*. Tokyo: Igaku-Shoin; 1973:1–16.

cells in the crypts of Lieberkukn of the small intestine and noted their presence at the basal aspects of the epithelial cells, adjacent to small blood vessels. Based on the latter observation, Kulchitsky also suggested a possible endocrine role for these cells, and Ciaccio proposed that the term "enterochromaffin" be adopted to describe these cells (5). Gosset and Masson (6) demonstrated that the intestinal chromaffin cells were also argentaffin positive, and subsequent studies by Hamperl using argyrophilic-staining techniques led to the identification of a second and more extensive population of putative endocrine cells within the intestine and a variety of extraintestinal sites (7). Feyrter suggested that the clear cells (helle Zelle) of the gastrointestinal tract corresponded, in part, to the chromaffin and argentaffin/argyrophil positive cells and that they formed a diffuse epithelial endocrine system ("diffuse epitheliale endokrine Organe") (8,9). He also hypothesized that some of these cells might have a paracrine or local hormonal action (8,9). Similar groups of clear cells were illustrated by Frolich within the bronchial tree, and Feyrter also considered them to be a part of the diffuse epithelial endocrine system (9,10). Ultimately, the argentaffin, argyrophil, and clear cells were recognized as components of a diffusely distributed system of endocrine cells. These observations formed the basis of the concept of a diffuse regulatory network as opposed to the then current doctrine of maintenance of homeostasis by discrete endocrine glands.

The modern view of the neuroendocrine cell and neurosecretory neuron was based on observations that oxytocin and antidiuretic hormone were synthesized by hypothalamic neurons and were stored within neuronal processes in the posterior pituitary, prior to their release into the circulation (11). Additionally, the discovery that hormone-releasing and -inhibiting factors were synthesized by hypothalamic neurons, transported via axonal transport to the median eminence, and secreted into the pituitary portal system for interactions with specific adenohypophyseal cell types established without doubt that neurons could function as endocrine cells (Fig. 46.1) (11). These cells essentially could serve as neuroendocrine transducers by converting electrical input directly into chemical or hormonal signals (12).

The discovery that the argyrophil/argentaffin cells and the cells of Feyrter's diffuse epithelial endocrine system did, indeed, have an endocrine function originated from studies conducted in the early to mid-1960s on the source of the hormone calcitonin (13,14). The thyroid glands of many species were known to contain parafollicular cells, which occasionally appeared clear in hematoxylin and eosin (H&E)–stained sections and which also had varying degrees of argyrophilia or argentaffinity (15,16). The parafollicular cells were ultimately shown to be the source of calcitonin, for which they were subsequently renamed C cells (17,18). These studies also led to the discovery that certain endocrine cells shared a series of remarkable functional and morphologic similarities with neurons (17).

In addition to the presence of calcitonin, C cells had the ability to synthesize and store catecholamines or indolylethylamines after uptake and decarboxylation of precursors of these substances (17). The latter property led to the introduction of the descriptive acronym APUD (Amine Precursor Uptake and Decarboxylation) (15). The APUD mechanism was subsequently identified in certain cells of the anterior pituitary and pancreatic islets. Cholinesterase, nonspecific esterases, α-glycerophosphate dehydrogenase, and certain endogenous amines were also present variably

TABLE 46.1
Markers[a] of Neuroendocrine Cells

1. Fluorogenic amine content
2. Amine precursor (5-hydroxytryptophan and DOPA) uptake
3. Aromatic amino acid decarboxylase
4. Nonspecific esterase or cholinesterase
5. Alpha glycerophosphate dehydrogenase
6. Peptide hormone content
7. Cytosolic enzymes
   Neuron-specific enolase, protein gene product 9.5 (PGP 9.5), histaminase, some enzymes involved in amine synthesis
8. Secretory granule/membrane proteins
   Chromogranins/secretogranins, prohormone convertases, peptidylglycine alpha-amidating monooxygenase, and related enzymes
9. Synaptic vesicle membrane and vesicle fusion/docking/release proteins
   (Soluble N-ethylamide sensitive fusion [NSF] protein; [SNAPS]; soluble NSF receptors [SNARES]); synaptophysin; synaptic vesicle protein 2 (SV2); vesicular monoamine transporters (VMAT-1, VMAT-2); synaptosomal protein-25 (SNAP-25); vesicle-associated membrane protein/synaptobrevin (VAMP 1–3); synaptotagmin; syntaxin; Rab3a; Sec1-Munc18-1 family; Munc13s; Sec17/SNAP synaptosomal protein-25 (SNAP-25)
10. CD56 and CD57
    Transcription factors (mammalian homolog of achaete–scute complex [mASH], human homolog of achaete–scute complex [hASH], thyroid transcription factor 1 [TTF-1], forkhead box protein A1 [FoxA1], insulinoma associated 1 [INSM1], Islet 1, caudal type homeobox 2 [CDX2], pituitary transcription factor-1 [pit-1], T-box transcription factor [T-pit], steroidogenic factor 1 [SF-1])
11. Somatostatin receptors

[a]The first six markers in this listing were described by Pearse in the original formulation of the APUD concept; however, endogenous amine content and the capacity for amine precursor uptake and decarboxylation are present in only some members of the dispersed neuroendocrine cell system.

across diverse animal species and among different neuroendocrine cell types (16) (Table 46.1).

In comparing the APUD cells of the thyroid, pancreas, and pituitary to cells of known neural ancestry, Pearse concluded that "the amine storing mechanism and presence of cholinesterase together pointed towards a common ancestral cell of neural origin, perhaps coming from the neural crest" (17). The list of APUD cells was then expanded to include almost all the peptide- and amine-producing cells throughout the body, including the adrenal medulla, extra-adrenal paraganglia, and parathyroid glands.

As the numbers of candidate APUD cells increased (19), it was recognized that the synthesis of regulatory peptides was a more consistent functional parameter than was synthesis of amines, and amine synthesis was ultimately eliminated from the definition of these cells. In view of the many similarities between APUD cells and neurons, the essentially synonymous term, "paraneuron" was introduced by Fujita and Kobayashi (20). Paraneurons, according to Fujita, were endocrine and sensory cells that shared structural, functional, and metabolic features with neurons and that produced substances identical with or related to neurohormones and neurotransmitters (21). The paraneurons also possessed neurosecretory-like granules and synapse-like vesicles, and they recognized stimuli on specific receptors and released their products via the secretory portion of the cell. Many investigators also began to apply the term "neuroendocrine" to these cells (19).

EMBRYOLOGY

Embryologic data using the chick-quail chimera system have refuted the neural crest or epiblastic origin of the majority of the dispersed neuroendocrine cells, including those of the lung, pancreas, gastrointestinal tract, and a variety of other sites (22,23). Studies of normal, chimeric, and transgenic mice have established that all gut epithelial cells, including endocrine cells, originate from multipotential stem cells present within the base of the intestinal crypts (24), whereas pancreatic endocrine cells originate from the ductal epithelium. It is now recognized that genotypic switches are present in cells previously thought to be irrevocably differentiated as a result of cellular plasticity (25). Examples of this phenomenon include production of neuropeptides by immune cells and cardiomyocytes. For example, the biosynthesis of chromogranins, enkephalins, or proconvertases can be upregulated during an immune challenge.

Studies based on the chick-quail chimera system led to the concept that C cells represented one of few remaining examples of neural crest–derived dispersed neuroendocrine cells, and this conclusion was incorrectly extrapolated to mammalian species. However, more recent investigations have challenged the neural crest origin of C cells in mammals (26,27). These studies have demonstrated that Wnt+ neural crest cells contribute to the thyroid connective tissue but are not the source of C cells in embryonic mouse thyroid (26). Further lineage tracing experiments have demonstrated that mouse thyroid C cells are derived from SOX17+ progenitors originating in anterior (pharyngeal pouch) endoderm. The development of C cells in mammals is a multistep process that involves: (1) patterning of the 4th pharyngeal pouch; (2) budding of the ultimobranchial analage from the 4th pharyngeal pouch; (3) migration of the ultimobranchial body; (4) fusion of the ultimobranchial body within the thyroid primordium; and (5) C-cell differentiation and proliferation within the thyroid (28). Given these observations, the only neuroendocrine cells of proven neural crest origin in mammals are those of the adrenal medulla, extra-adrenal paraganglia, ganglion cells of the submucosal and myenteric plexus, and sympathetic ganglia (22,23).

In contrast, the ultimobranchial anlage of nonmammalian vertebrates and monotremes does not merge with the thyroid gland and remains as a separate organ throughout adulthood. Moreover, avian ultimobranchial C cells may have dual origins from neural progenitors and endodermal epithelium (29).

In its current context, therefore, the term "neuroendocrine" does not imply an embryologic origin from the neuroectoderm but rather implies a shared phenotype characterized by the concurrent expression of multiple genes encoding a wide variety of neuronal and endocrine traits.

MOLECULAR ASPECTS OF NEUROENDOCRINE CELL DEVELOPMENT
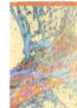

The mechanisms for the acquisition of the neuroendocrine phenotype are not fully understood; however, recent studies suggest important roles for both positively and negatively acting transcription factors. An important class of regulatory proteins includes those with common DNA binding and dimerization domains, the basic helix-loop-helix (b-HLH) region. The genes encoding these proteins are analogous to the achaete–scute complex like1 (ASCL1) which has been identified during neuronal differentiation in *Drosophila* (30). The homologous mammalian genes have been referred to as mammalian achaete–scute homologues (mASH) while the homologous human genes have been termed hASH. In Drosophila, one group of b-HLH factors encoded by genes such as ASCL1 activates neural/neuroendocrine differentiation, while another group of b-HLH factors encoded by Hes-1 (hairy enhancer of split) represses neuronal differentiation (31–33).

The Notch pathway, which plays a crucial role in the development of neuroendocrine cells, is mediated by ASCL1. Notch receptors are transmembrane proteins that regulate cell survival, proliferation and differentiation after binding to the appropriate ligand(s). Hes-1 is one of the downstream targets of Notch activation and it controls the expression of a variety of target genes, including ASCL1. Achaete–acute homolog like 1 is highly expressed in developing C cells and other neuroendocrine cell types, but it is lost when these cells reach maturity (28,34).

Notch signaling in the embryo is important in the determination of neuroendocrine differentiation pathways of precursor cells. Notch expression directs developing cells to a non-neuroendocrine pathway while the absence of such signaling and subsequent increased expression of ASCL1 directs precursor cells to the neuroendocrine phenotype. In addition to the Notch pathways, other pathways such as sonic hedgehog also play important roles in the differentiation of neuroendocrine cells (33,34).

Similar to many gastrointestinal tract endodermal derivatives, embryonic C cells co-express pioneer factors forkhead box (Fox) a1 and Foxa2 before neuroendocrine differentiation takes place. The Hes-1/mASH-1 signaling pathway plays a key role in the differentiation of C cells (28,35). In addition, a variety of other transcription factors and signaling molecules, including: Pax8 (paired box 8), Tbx1 (paired box transcription factor 1), Pbx1 (pre B-cell leukemia factor 1), nrx2.1 (neurexin-1)/TTF-1 (thyroid transcription factor 1),

Shh (sonic hedgehog), FRS2α (fibroblast growth factor receptor), Ripply3 (Ripply transcription receptors) and Hox3 (homeobox3 paralogs), Eya1 (eyes absent homolog), and EphA (ephrin receptor gene family) are involved with the formation of the 4th pharyngeal pouch and the migration, differentiation, survival, and dispersion of C cells (28,29).

Knockout ASCL1−/− mice have markedly reduced numbers of C cells as determined by staining for calcitonin. Similar observations have been made with other neuroendocrine and neural cell types, consistent with the hypothesis that the development of this phenotype is dependent on ASCL1. Knockout of ASCL1 also results in reduction of the numbers of pulmonary neuroendocrine cells, while knockout of Hes-1 results in a 10-fold increase in neuroendocrine cells with a concomitant decrease in Clara cells (33). Increased numbers of gastrointestinal neuroendocrine cells have also been observed in Hes-1 −/− mice.

The STAT-Ser/Hes-3 signaling axis was first described as a major regulator of neural stem cells and later, as a regulator of cancer stem cells. This signaling axis also regulates several cell types with stem cell properties in the adrenal gland and pancreatic islets, consistent with a potentially important role in the endocrine and neuroendocrine cell systems (36).

LIGHT MICROSCOPY AND HISTOCHEMISTRY

Neuroendocrine cells may form grossly visible structures (e.g., adenohypophysis, parathyroid glands, adrenal medulla, extra-adrenal paraganglia) or distinct microscopic structures, such as the islets of Langerhans and pulmonary neuroepithelial bodies. The so-called dispersed neuroendocrine cells are often difficult to recognize in routinely prepared H&E-stained sections, where they may appear as oval, pyramidal, or flask-shaped, with variably clear cytoplasm (Figs. 46.2 and 46.3). In some instances, the cytoplasm may contain fine eosinophilic granules (Fig. 46.2B) that are often difficult to resolve with usual microscopic preparations. Some neuroendocrine cell types, such as those of the intra- and extra-adrenal paraganglia and gastrointestinal tract (enterochromaffin cells) develop a characteristic brown to yellow coloration after primary fixation in potassium dichromate or chromic acid. This pigment results from oxidation of cellular stores of catecholamines, serotonin, or histamine.

Some neuroendocrine cells exhibit a characteristic yellow–green fluorescence after fixation in formaldehyde and other aldehyde fixatives (Fig. 46.4) (37). In some instances, the cells may become fluorescent only after administration of L-dihydroxyphenylalanine (DOPA) or 5-hydroxytryptophan. Formaldehyde forms highly fluorescent tetrahydroisoquinoline condensation products with catecholamines and β-carboline derivatives with tryptamines such as serotonin. In some instances, freeze-dried tissues or fresh-frozen sections must be used for the demonstration of cellular stores of amines (37).

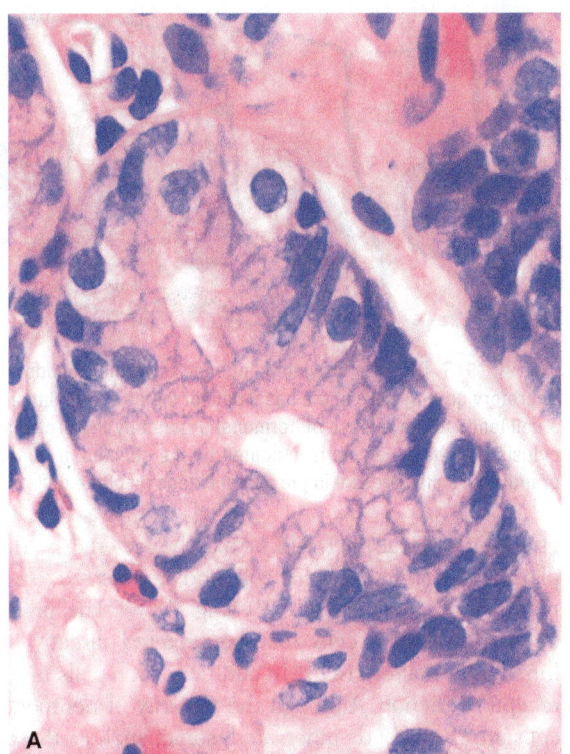
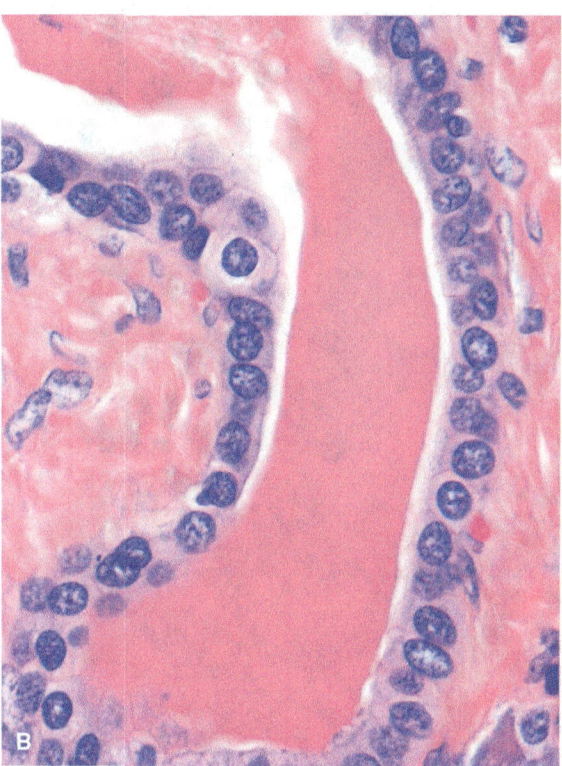

FIGURE 46.2 **A:** Neuroendocrine clear cells (helle Zelle) of gastric gland (*arrows*). **B:** Eosinophilic neuroendocrine cells of colon (*arrows*) that resemble Paneth cells but are triangular rather than columnar and the granules are smaller than those seen in Paneth cells.

Subsets of neuroendocrine cells, including those of the gastrointestinal tract, have the ability to directly reduce ammoniacal silver to the metallic state and have been referred to as "argentaffin cells" (Fig. 46.5) (6,7). In many other neuroendocrine cells, silver positivity is evident only after the addition of an exogenous reducing agent to the staining solution, and such cells are said to be argyrophilic. The chromaffin and argentaffin reactions of neuroendocrine cells in the gastrointestinal tract are due primarily to the presence of serotonin. While argentaffin cells are also

FIGURE 46.3 C cells of the thyroid (*arrows*) that are pale and are considered as clear cells and are easily identified in association with the solid cell nests (*upper left*).

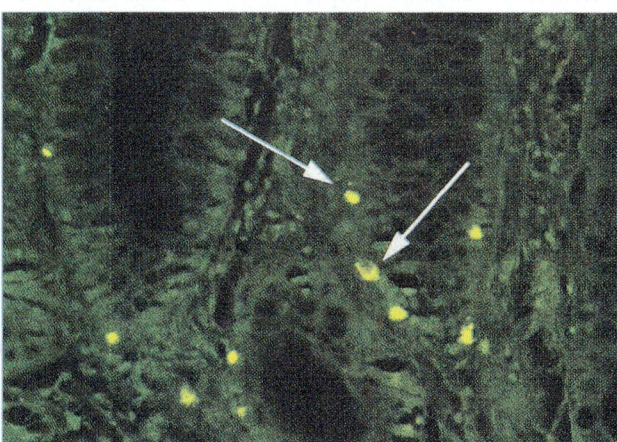

FIGURE 46.4 Formalin-fixed rectal mucosa photographed in ultraviolet light. The strongly fluorescent cells (*arrows*) correspond to the serotonin-containing enterochromaffin-type cells.

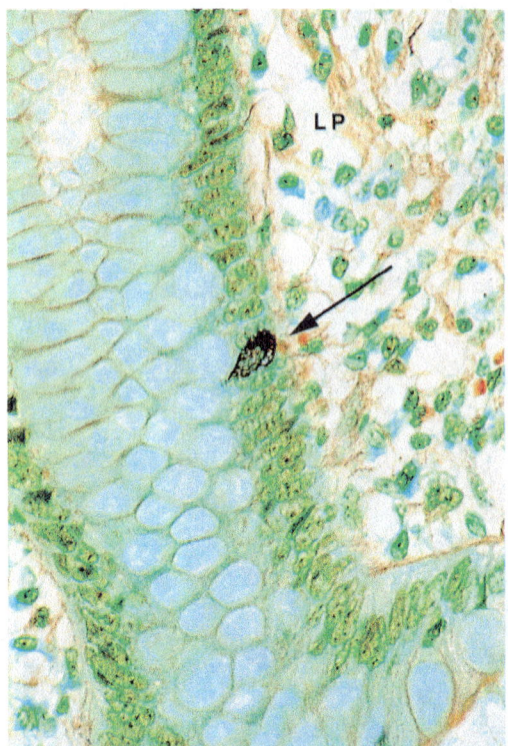

FIGURE 46.5 Colonic mucosa stained for argentaffin cells with the Masson-Fontana technique and methyl green counterstain. The argentaffin cell (*arrow*) illustrated in this field is characterized by the presence of black cytoplasmic granules. LP, lamina propria.

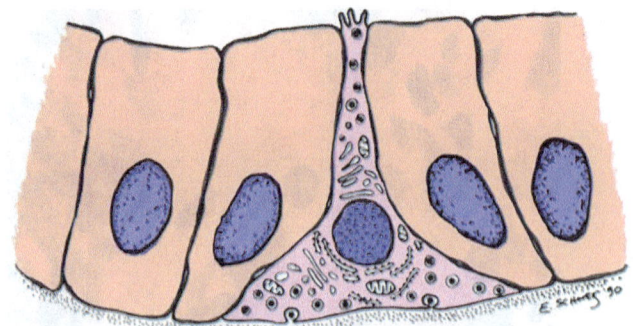

FIGURE 46.6 Diagram of typical "opened"-type neuroendocrine cell. Secretory granules are at the basal pole of the cell. Stimulation of such a cell leads to the release of hormonal product by the process of exocytosis. The basal lamina is indicated by the stippled area. Secretory granules are also present in the apical extension of the cell.

often with apical microvilli or may be covered by the cytoplasm of adjacent epithelial cells and are referred to as closed neuroendocrine cells (45–47) (Fig. 46.7). The products of opened endocrine cells may be secreted directly into the lumen of a hollow viscus. In addition, such cells may have a receptor function. Although the majority of neuroendocrine cells are not directly innervated, some, such as those of the skin and bronchial tree, may be innervated (Fig. 46.7B).

In the gastrointestinal tract, scattered neuroendocrine cells are also found within the lamina propria (48,49) without attachment to the overlying epithelium. Such cells are

argyrophilic, only a subset of argyrophil cells is argentaffin positive (38). The chemical basis of the argyrophil reaction is unknown, but it is apparent that reduced silver salts have an affinity for a nonamine constituent of neuroendocrine secretory granules, most likely chromogranin proteins (39).

It should be recognized that argyrophil stains are nonspecific. Cellular products such as lipofuscin, glycogen, and certain proteins including α-lactalbumin may be argyrophilic (40). Some neuroendocrine cells are argyrophilic only with certain silver-staining sequences. Most neuroendocrine cells stain metachromatically with toluidine blue and coriophosphine O after acid hydrolysis of tissue sections (41). Lead hematoxylin also has been used for the demonstration of neuroendocrine cells (42). However, none of the histochemical stains discussed in this section is used currently in practice, having been replaced by immunohistochemical methods.

Neuroendocrine cells are dispersed among other cell types as single cells or as aggregates of three to four cells. The basal aspects of the cells are separated from the adjacent capillaries by the subjacent epithelial basement membrane (Fig. 46.6). Processes often extend from the cytoplasm to surround adjacent epithelial cells, and such neuroendocrine cells are referred to as "paracrine cells" (43,44). The products of paracrine cells are thought to be released locally where they modulate the activities of adjacent endocrine and nonendocrine cells (43). The apex of the neuroendocrine cell may extend directly to the glandular lumen (opened-type cell),

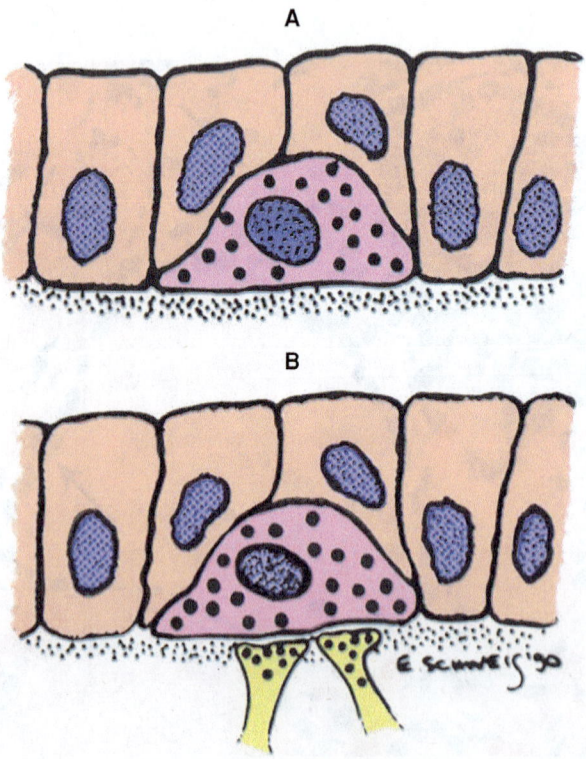

FIGURE 46.7 Closed cells are also widely distributed. **A:** The thyroid C cells are typically of the closed type. **B:** The Merkel cells of the skin are innervated closed-type neuroendocrine cells.

typically surrounded by Schwann cells and unmyelinated nerve fibers to form an enterochromaffin cell (EC)–nerve fiber complex. The EC–nerve complexes are especially prominent in appendices with chronic inflammation and neural hyperplasia (49). Stromal endocrine cells also have been identified in the prostate gland (50).

Phylogenetic and ontogenetic studies have suggested that neurons are the earliest component of the neuroendocrine system, since they are present in the most primitive organisms (coelenterates) (51). The next most likely evolutionary step is the appearance of opened-type neuroendocrine cells in the gut, which are present in the most highly developed invertebrates. Such cells become extensively diversified in vertebrates. The presence of microscopic gastroenteropancreatic neuroendocrine cell aggregates, such as the pancreatic islets, on the other hand, is a feature that is restricted to true vertebrates (51).

ULTRASTRUCTURE

The most characteristic ultrastructural feature of neuroendocrine cells is the presence of membrane-bound secretory granules, which may vary from 50 to 500 nm in diameter (Fig. 46.8). In addition, the cells are well endowed with granular endoplasmic reticulum and prominent Golgi regions, which are characteristic of secretory cells. Because of their relatively large size, the secretory granules have also been referred to large dense core vesicles or granules (1). Immunoelectron microscopic studies have shown that the granules represent storage sites of peptide and amine hormones. Granules storing different types of hormones are characterized in some instances by differences in size, density of contents, and substructure (52). Although most neuroendocrine secretory granules are round, others, such as those of the gastrointestinal EC and EC-like cells, are pleomorphic with elongated, reniform, round, oval, or pear-shaped forms.

Secretory granules tend to be concentrated at the basal aspects of the cells in relatively close proximity to the basement membrane (Fig. 46.6). They are also prominent in cytoplasmic processes and in the apical extensions of the "opened" cells (Fig. 46.6). In addition to secretory granules, many neuroendocrine cells contain synaptic-type vesicles (SSVs) which have been referred to as small synaptic vesicle analogs (1). The SSVs are responsible for the release of amino acid neurotransmitters (gamma amino butyric acid, glutamate, glycine) and various biogenic amines in a regulated fashion in response to a variety of different stimuli (1).

APOPTOSIS

Apoptosis plays a critical role in the physiology of many endocrine tissues. For example, deprivation of growth factors, including thyrotropin, epidermal growth factor, and

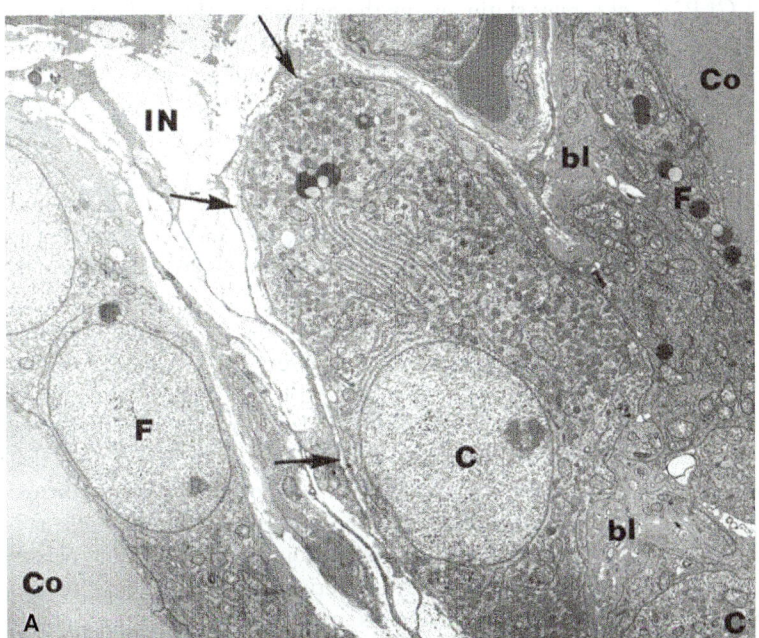
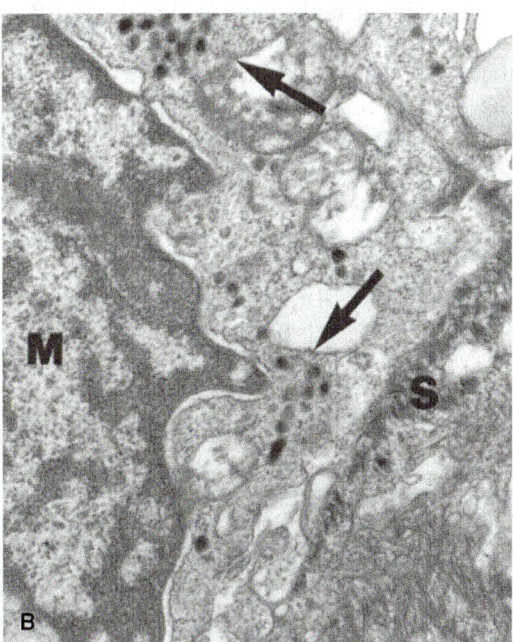

FIGURE 46.8 Ultrastructure of neuroendocrine cells. **A:** Electron micrograph of a C-cell from a patient with mild C-cell hyperplasia associated with the type 2A MEN syndrome. The C-cell is present at the base of the follicle, where it is in direct contact with the basal cytoplasm of the overlying follicular cell. The basal lamina (*bl*) is focally thickened at the junction of the C-cell and overlying follicular cells. The C-cell is separated from the interstitium by the follicular basal lamina (*arrows*). C, C-cell; Co, colloid; F, follicular cell; IN, interstitium (original magnification ×14,000). **B:** Electron micrograph of Merkel cell. Clusters of secretory granules (*arrows*) are present within the Merkel (*M*) cells. S, squamous cell (original magnification ×27,000).

serum from cultures of thyrocytes, leads to DNA fragmentation and morphologic changes of apoptosis (53). Studies of estrogen-induced prolactin cell hyperplasia in the rat have shown that withdrawal of estrogen results in increased numbers of apoptotic cells (54). This effect is enhanced by the administration of bromocriptine after estrogen withdrawal.

Although there are few published studies of apoptosis in neuroendocrine cells of the gut and other sites, this process is initiated in neurons when the concentrations of target-derived neurotrophic factors are reduced. Garcia and coworkers have demonstrated that overexpression of the *bcl-2* proto-oncogene in cultured sympathetic neurons prevents apoptosis, which is normally induced by deprivation of nerve growth factor (55). It is likely that changes in neuroendocrine cell populations influenced by variations in trophic signals in the gastrointestinal system, pancreas, and other sites may be mediated by apoptosis. However, other mechanisms also may be operative. For example, Kaneto et al. have demonstrated that both exogenous nitrous oxide and nitric oxide generated endogenously by interleukin (IL)-1 leads to apoptosis of isolated rat pancreatic islet cells (56). The action of streptozotocin appears to be mediated by a similar mechanism (56). These findings suggest that nitric oxide–induced inter-nucleosomal DNA cleavage is an important initial step in the destruction and dysfunction of pancreatic β cells induced by inflammatory stimuli or by the action of streptozotocin. The Notch signaling pathway has also been implicated in apoptosis throughout the development of neural/neuroendocrine cells (57).

The glucagon-like peptides 1 and 2 (GLP-1 and GLP-2), are released by subsets of gut endocrine cells in response to food intake and other stimuli and regulate energy absorption and disposal, as well as cell proliferation and survival. GLP-1 enhances glucose dependent insulin secretion and suppresses glucagon release. Both GLP-1 and -2 exhibit antiapoptotic actions in vivo and result in preservation of β-cell mass and gut epithelium, respectively (58). Additionally, GLP-1 and -2 promote direct resistance to apoptosis in cells expressing GLP-1 and -2 receptors (58).

FUNCTION OF NEUROENDOCRINE CELLS

The function of neuroendocrine cells has been established by the use of immunohistochemical and in situ hybridization techniques for the localization of specific hormones and their corresponding messenger RNAs. In many instances, the use of region-specific antisera also permits the localization of hormone precursors, as well as mature hormones (59). Previous studies suggested that single neuroendocrine cells were responsible for the production of a unique hormonal product (one-cell, one-hormone hypothesis); however, more recent studies indicate that these cells are multimessenger units (60). Peptide hormones are synthesized within the granular endoplasmic reticulum and are packaged into secretory granules by way of the Golgi region. Multiple different peptide products may be synthesized via this route in single neuroendocrine cells. Other nonpeptide hormone constituents such as biologically active amines are synthesized within the cytosol and are then taken up into secretory granules and small synaptic vesicles (61). Any individual neuroendocrine cell can, therefore, vary the biosynthesis and secretion of its products in response to different signals in normal and pathologic states.

Immunohistochemical and molecular biologic studies have led to many interesting insights into the functional interrelationships of the various components of the neuroendocrine system. For example, peptide hormones first isolated from the gastroenteropancreatic axis have been found subsequently in neurons of the central and peripheral nervous systems, where they may function as neurotransmitters or neuromodulators (12). Other peptides initially isolated from the brain have been localized to the neuroendocrine cells of the gut, pancreas, and lung, where they may have a paracrine or autocrine function (62). Furthermore, such studies have shown that the microarchitecture of endocrine organs, which may appear homogeneous in H&E-stained sections, is often organized in a manner that permits paracrine interactions. For example, somatostatin cells of the pancreatic islets are located between the insulin and glucagon cells and typically extend short branching processes, which are in apposition to both cell types. Regulation of the secretion of insulin and glucagon may, therefore, be mediated by the local paracrine effects of somatostatin and by the endocrine effects of somatostatin reaching the islets by the circulation (63,64). In the stomach, branching processes extending from somatostatin cells interdigitate with the adjacent gastrin cells, thereby regulating the secretion of gastrin in response to food intake and other stimuli (65).

Neuroendocrine cells in different tissues may produce identical peptides. Somatostatin, for example, is present in certain hypothalamic neurons (Fig. 46.9A), pancreatic D cells, gastrointestinal D cells (Fig. 46.9B), bronchopulmonary endocrine cells, thymic endocrine cells, and a subset of thyroid C cells, where it is colocalized with calcitonin (63–66). Calcitonin is present in thyroid C cells, bronchopulmonary and thymic endocrine cells, and certain urogenital endocrine cells. Gastrin-releasing peptide, a 27–amino acid peptide that is the mammalian homolog of bombesin, is present in thyroid C cells, small intensely fluorescent cells of sympathetic ganglia, neuronal cells of the gastrointestinal myenteric plexus, and bronchopulmonary endocrine cells (67,68).

Neuroendocrine cells may produce multiple distinct peptides from a common precursor molecule. For example, adrenocorticotropin (ACTH) is synthesized from the large precursor molecule pro-opiomelanocortin (POMC) (69). In the adenohypophysis, POMC is processed to yield ACTH, β-lipotropin, and a 16KD N-terminal fragment. In the intermediate lobe, ACTH and β-lipotropin are processed to yield α-MSH and β-endorphin–related peptides, respectively.

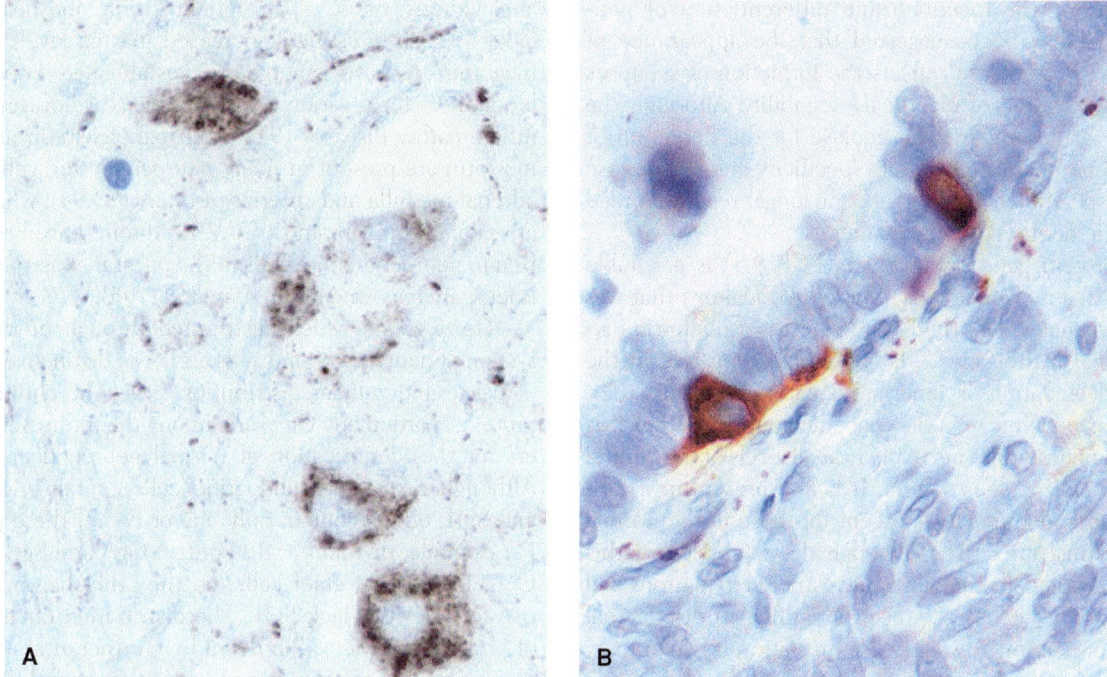

FIGURE 46.9 Somatostatin staining of hypothalamus and small intestine. **A:** Median eminence of the hypothalamus immunostained for somatostatin demonstrating positive staining of the neurons and their processes. **B:** The process of a closed neuroendocrine cell beneath the epithelium.

Hormonal diversity in neuroendocrine cells also may result from alternative splicing pathways that produce different messenger RNAs from a single gene. Both calcitonin and the calcitonin gene–related peptide (CGRP) are produced from a primary RNA transcript that is spliced to produce two different forms of mature messenger RNA (70). More than one gene may also encode closely related peptides (71).

Molecular studies have led to the identification of multiple related or associated novel peptide hormones encoded by DNA sequences of known or novel hormones (72). The individual hormone gene frequently has multiple phenotypes, as a result of alternative splicing, tandem organization, or differentiated maturation of the prohormone (73). As a result of these mechanisms, more than 100 different hormonally active peptides are released from the gut. For instance, the identification of several high–molecular-weight proteins that also contained the glucagon sequence was established by the molecular identification of glicentin, oxyntomodulin, GLP-1, and GLP-2 in addition to two intervening peptides, all of which were generated by post-translational processing in the L cell (72,73).

MARKERS OF NEUROENDOCRINE CELLS

Neuroendocrine cells can be classified into those of neural (neurons, paraganglioma cells) and epithelial types. The former contain neurofilaments as their major intermediate filament type while the latter contain cytokeratins with or without neurofilaments. Both cells groups can be identified on the basis of their contents of specific hormones and neurotransmitter substances (74–76), as discussed in other chapters in this volume and by the presence of a variety nonhormonal products. The nonhormonal constituents of neuroendocrine cells include a wide array of cytosolic, secretory granule and vesicle membrane, and plasma membrane constituents. These products can be identified effectively via immunohistochemistry with polyclonal antisera or monoclonal antibodies. This approach is of particular importance when evaluating tissues for the presence of neuroendocrine cells when the specific hormonal product is unknown.

Cytosolic Constituents

A variety of different enzymes can be demonstrated by immunohistochemistry in neuroendocrine cells. Although some of the enzymes are present in most neuroendocrine cells, others have a more restricted distribution. In the past, neuron specific enolase was used widely as a generic neuroendocrine marker for neurons and neuroendocrine cells (77). The enolases are products of three independent gene loci which have been designated α, β, and γ (78–80). Non-neuronal enolase ($\alpha\alpha$) is present in fetal tissues, glial cells, and many nonendocrine tissues. Beta ($\beta\beta$)-enolase is present in muscle tissue, whereas hybrid enolases ($\alpha\gamma$, $\alpha\beta$) have been identified in megakaryocytes and a variety of other cell types. Neuron-specific enolase ($\gamma\gamma$) replaces non-neuronal enolase during the migration and differentiation of neurons, and it has been suggested that the appearance of neuron-specific enolase reflects the formation of synapses and the acquisition of electrical excitability. Although the sensitivity of neuron-specific enolase for the detection of neuroendocrine cells is high, its specificity is low. Because of its low specificity, this marker is no longer recommended as a generic neuroendocrine marker.

The protein gene product 9.5 (PGP 9.5) is a soluble protein with a molecular weight of 27,000 Daltons that was isolated originally from the brain (81). It is a ubiquitin carboxyterminal hydrolase (UCH-L1) that plays a role in the catalytic degradation of abnormal denatured proteins (82). Immunohistochemical studies have demonstrated that it is present in neurons and nerve fibers at all levels of the central and peripheral nervous system. It is also present in a variety of neuroendocrine cells, except for those in the normal gastrointestinal tract (81). Although the expression of this marker was originally thought to be restricted to neurons and neuroendocrine, it has also been identified in distal renal tubular epithelium, Leydig cells, prostatic and mammary epithelium, and other cell types (83). Additional enzymes that have a predominant cytosolic distribution include those involved in catecholamine biosynthesis (76).

Secretory Granule Constituents

The chromogranins/secretogranins (Cg/Sg) represent a widely distributed family of soluble proteins that represent the major constituent by weight of neurosecretory granules or large dense core vesicles (LDCVs) (Table 46.1) (84–87). Three major granins have been identified and have been designated chromogranin A, chromogranin B, and to a lesser extent, secretogranin II (chromogranin C). Additional members of the granin family (numbers in parentheses refer to antibodies used for their detection) include secretogranins III (1B1075), IV (HISL-19) and V (7B2), VI (NESP55), and VII (VGF) (88). The chromogranins are calcium-binding proteins that play important roles in the packaging and processing of regulatory peptides. These proteins contain multiple dibasic residues that are potential sites for proteolytic cleavage and processing producing a wide range of smaller peptides (89,90). For example, bovine Cg A is a 439–amino acid protein that contains highly hydrophilic and acidic amino acids sequences and multiple paired basic residues that form cleavage sites that generate biologically active peptides. Chromogranin A is processed by the action of proteases, in addition to post-translational modifications, to vasostatins, chromacin, chromofungin, prochromacin, pancreastatin, catestatin, chromostatin, parastatin, serpinin, and the vasoconstrictive inhibitory factor (91). There are numerous functional roles for the granins and their smaller derivative peptides, including; stabilization of the intragranular core complex, regulatory effects on the secretion of hormones and metabolites, effects on innate immunity, antimicrobial effects, vascular homeostasis,

angiogenesis, tissue repair, inflammation, and heart physiology (91). Interestingly, increased plasma levels of chromogranin A have emerged as established or potential biomarkers for a variety of neoplastic, cardiovascular, and inflammatory diseases (92). Both pancreastatin and chromostatin are present in many neuroendocrine cells, in the adrenal medulla and anterior pituitary (93,94), while derivatives of chromogranin B (GAWK protein) have been localized to neuroendocrine cells in the pituitary, gastrointestinal tract, pancreas, and adrenal medulla (95).

The Cgs are widely distributed throughout the entire system of neuroendocrine cells and have distinctive patterns of tissue and cellular distribution (96). The chromogranin proteins, particularly CgA, are among the most useful markers for the identification of normal neuroendocrine cells. Although many neuroendocrine cells contain CgA, CgB, and SgII, others contain only one or two of these proteins. For example, thyroid C cells contain CgA and SgII but lack CgB. Parathyroid chief cells, on the other hand, are positive for CgA but lack SgII. The distribution of this family of proteins is reviewed in detail by Huttner et al. (96). The chromogranins are cosecreted with other granule contents, but their replenishment is regulated differentially.

Prohormone Convertases and Peptidylglycine Alpha-Amidating Monooxygenase

A variety of endopeptidases and carboxypeptidases are required for the formation of biologically active peptides from precursor molecules and are present in the trans-Golgi region and secretory granules of neuroendocrine cells. They include the prohormone convertases, PC1/PC3 and PC2, and carboxypeptidases H&E (97,98). The proconvertases are widely distributed in neuroendocrine cells, while other types of endocrine cells (thyroid follicular cells, parathyroid chief cells, adrenal cortical cells, and testis) are negative. Neuroendocrine cells with a neural phenotype (adrenal medullary cells) contain a predominance of PC2 while epithelial neuroendocrine cells contain a predominance of PC1/PC3. With the exception of parathyroid cells, the presence of PC2 and PC3 correlates with the presence of chromogranin and secretogranins. PC2 and PC1/PC3 are present in normal pituitaries and adenomas, with ACTH-producing adenomas containing a predominance of PC1/PC3 and other adenomas expressing a predominance of PC2.

Peptidylglycine alpha-amidating monooxygenase (PAM), peptidyl-glycine alpha-hydroxylating monooxygenase (PHM), and peptidylamidaglycolate lyase (PAL) are present in neuroendocrine secretory granules (99,100). These enzymes are responsible for the alpha amidation of the C-terminal regions of peptide hormones, a function which is critical for the biologic function of peptides. These enzymes are not restricted in their distribution to neuroendocrine cells. For example, they have also been found in the lung in cells of the airway epithelium and submucosal glands, vascular endothelium, some chondrocytes of bronchial cartilage, alveolar macrophages, and smooth muscle cells.

Synaptic Vesicle and Vesicle Fusion/Release Constituents

Synaptophysin (Mol. wt 38,000) was one of the earliest markers developed to visualize small synaptic vesicle analogs in neurons and neuroendocrine cells (101–103). Together with the chromogranin proteins, synaptophysin has emerged as an important marker for the identification of neuroendocrine cells. This protein is widely distributed in nerve terminals in the central and peripheral nervous system and is also present in neuroendocrine cells that are specialized for the regulated secretion of peptide hormones. Synaptophysin is the most abundant integral membrane protein of neuronal vesicles. It is localized in a punctate pattern in synaptic regions of neurons and has a diffuse cytoplasmic distribution in neuroendocrine cells. Ultrastructurally, synaptophysin is present predominantly in smooth-surface synaptic-type vesicles. Although synaptophysin was originally thought to be specific for neuroendocrine cells, it is also expressed in other cell types, including the adrenal cortex (104,105).

Synaptic vesicle protein 2 (SV2), an integral membrane protein that mediates calcium-stimulated neurotransmitter release, is present in the central and peripheral nervous system and in a wide variety of neuroendocrine cell types (106). This glycoprotein regulates the expression and trafficking of the calcium sensor protein, synaptotagmin, in addition to other functions related to neurotransmitter release and homeostasis (107,108). Immunoreactivity for SV2 is present in neuroendocrine cells in the gastrointestinal tract, pancreas, anterior pituitary, thyroid (C cells), parathyroid, and adrenal medulla. Chief cells of the gastric oxyntic mucosa are also positive for SV2. Interestingly, gastrointestinal stromal tumors have been reported to be positive for SV2 (109). Comparison of SV2, synaptophysin, and chromogranin A immunoreactivities has shown variations in these constituents in different neuroendocrine cell types.

The vesicular monoamine transporters (VMAT1 and VMAT2) are integral membrane proteins that mediate the transport of amines into vesicles of neurons and neuroendocrine cells (110,111). These two isoforms show broad selectivity for different amines and are distributed differently in various cell types. They play critical roles in the sorting, storing, and release of neurotransmitters and in regulating the neuronal and endocrine informational output (112). VMAT2 facilitates the uptake of dopamine, norepinephrine, epinephrine, histamine, and serotonin into neurons and neuroendocrine cells of the ECL type. VMAT1 does not recognize histamine as a substrate, it is absent from neurons, and its major functional activity is in endocrine cells, particularly EC cells (113). In the pancreas, VMAT1 is present in endocrine cells of the ductal epithelium, while VMAT2 is present primarily in the β cells of the islets (114). VMAT2, on the other hand, is present in histamine producing ECL cells and in central and peripheral neurons. VMAT1 and VMAT2 are both expressed by adrenal medullary cells to varying extents. In some studies, the VMATs have been used as surrogate markers for other types of neuroendocrine cells, such as those in the breast (115).

The process of regulated secretion in neurons and neuroendocrine cells is highly complex and involves a large number of molecules (1,11,116–119). Factors that govern neurotransmitter release include N-ethylmaleimide sensitive factor (NSF), soluble NSF adaptor proteins (SNAPs), the SNAP receptors (SNAREs), Munc18-1, Munc13s, and Rab3s. According to the SNARE (SNAP-receptor) hypothesis, the selective docking of a transport vesicle with the appropriate target membrane occurs via the formation of a complex between a vesicle membrane protein (v-SNARE) and the corresponding target membrane protein (t-SNARE) (116). The resulting SNARE complex ultimately leads to membrane fusion. Three families of SNARE proteins are currently recognized. They include the VAMP (vesicle associated membrane protein)/synaptobrevin family of v-SNAREs and two families of t-SNAREs, the syntaxin family and the SNAP-25 family. In the initial phases of exocytosis, NSF and soluble NSF attachment protein (α-SNAP) act on synaptobrevin, syntaxin, and SNAP-25. This leads to dissociation of the SNARE complexes, activation of the SNARE proteins and removal of the negative regulators of exocytosis. Subsequently, the vesicle protein Rab3 promotes reversible vesicle attachment (tethering) to the presynaptic membrane. Tethering permits the formation of the SNARE complex which consists of synaptobrevin, syntaxin, and SNAP-25. This series of events brings the vesicle into a docked position, immediately adjacent to the plasma membrane and calcium channels. Docking is an irreversible step in which there is some degree of membrane fusion. At some time during docking, synaptotagmin is recruited to the SNARE complex (118). The SNAREs play a key role in membrane fusion and other proteins are considered to be SNARE regulators. However, some of the regulator proteins may have direct roles in membrane fusion and neurotransmitter release. Additional proteins involved in this process include Sec1-Munc18 family and the Sec17/SNAP proteins (119).

Some of the proteins involved in the process of regulated secretion can be visualized in immunohistochemical formats and have been utilized as neuroendocrine cell markers. While some of these proteins are localized within the plasma membranes (SNAP-25 [synaptosomal protein of 25kDa] and syntaxin), others (synaptobrevin, synaptophysin, Rab3a, and synaptotagmin) are present in the synaptic vesicle membranes. The soluble proteins involved in this process include NSF and SNAPs.

The vesicle-associated membrane proteins (VAMPs) play important roles in docking and/or fusion of secretory vesicles with their target membranes. VAMP, which is also known as synaptobrevin, occurs in three isoforms which are designated VAMP-1, VAMP-2, and VAMP-3 (cellubrevin). VAMP-2 and VAMP-3 are expressed in pancreatic islets (120) and are involved in calcium-mediated insulin secretion. VAMP-1 is present primarily in pancreatic acinar cells (121).

The synaptotagmins (p65) include a large family of calcium-binding proteins that are constituents of the membranes of synaptic vesicles in neurons and neuroendocrine cells (122). In the normal pancreatic islets, synaptotagmins are colocalized with insulin in β cells and are involved with calcium-induced insulin secretion (123).

Rab proteins, are low–molecular-weight members of the Ras superfamily of monomeric G-proteins. The Rab3 isoforms are involved in the exocytosis of synaptic vesicles and secretory granules in the CNS and anterior pituitary. In normal human pituitary, Rab3 isoforms are present primarily within the cytoplasm of growth hormone–producing cells with rare expression in other cell types. Among pituitary adenomas, Rab 3 is most commonly expressed in growth hormone–producing adenomas but also occurs in adenomas of other types (124,125).

SNAP-25 has been studied most extensively in the pituitary gland. This protein is localized predominantly to the plasma membranes of both normal and neoplastic adenohypophyseal cells (126–128). Similar patterns of localization have been documented in the adrenal and pancreatic islets (129,130). Additionally, SNAP-25 is present in ECL cells, together with syntaxin and synaptobrevin (131).

CD56 and CD57

CD57 recognizes epitopes in natural killer lymphocytes, myelin-associated glycoprotein (MAG), neuronal cell adhesion molecules, and a granule matrix constituent of chromaffin cells (132–134). The largest of the MAGs (MAG-72) is related to the immunoglobulin supergene family proteins, as well as neural adhesion molecules. CD57 also reacts with a subset of neuroendocrine cells in the anterior pituitary, lung, adrenal gland, pancreatic islets, and gastrointestinal tract (134). In addition, CD57 immunoreactivity has been identified in a variety of non-neuroendocrine cells and is expressed, together with S100 protein, in Schwann cells and other supporting elements (sustentacular cells) in the anterior pituitary, adrenal medulla, and paraganglia (135).

The neural cell adhesion molecules (NCAMs) represent a family of glycoproteins that play key roles in cell-binding, migration, differentiation, and proliferation (136,137). The NCAM family includes several major peptides that are generated by alternative splicing of RNA from a gene that is a member of the immunoglobulin super gene family. The peptide sequences that are external to the plasma membrane contain five regions that are similar to those present in immunoglobulins. The molecules are modified posttranslationally by phosphorylation, sulfation, and glycosylation. The homophilic-binding properties of NCAMs are modulated by differential expression of homopolymers of α2, 8-linked N-acetylneuraminic acid (polysialic acid).

CD56 recognizes a 140kDa isoform of NCAM which is expressed on resting and activated NK cells and a subset of CD3+ cells. Although initial studies had suggested that NCAM was restricted in its distribution to the brain, subsequent studies indicate that it is also present in a variety of neuroendocrine cells, including the pancreatic islets of adenohypophysis, and adrenal medulla, as well as in a variety of non-neuroendocrine cells. Studies using a monoclonal antibody reactive with a long chain from of α2, 8-linked polysialic acid present on NCAMs demonstrated positive staining in cases of familial medullary thyroid carcinoma, both in the neoplastic cells and in hyperplastic C cells adjacent to the tumor foci (138). Cases of primary C-cell hyperplasia unassociated with medullary thyroid carcinoma were also positively stained, whereas most normal C cells and C cells in secondary hyperplasia were nonreactive.

Transcription Factors

Transcription factors are proteins that bind to regulatory elements in the promotor and enhancer regions of DNA, thereby regulating gene expression and protein synthesis. They may be cell specific or may be present in a variety of different cell types. Both the mammalian (M) and human (H) homologs of the achaete–scute complex (mASH and hASH), respectively, are expressed in a subset of thymic epithelial cells, thyroidal C cells, and fetal pulmonary neuroendocrine cells (139,140). FoxA1, which regulates the development of a variety of different tissues, is expressed in adult C cells and solid cell nests in the adult thyroid gland (141) INSM1 (insulinoma-associated 1) is involved in the terminal steps of neuroendocrine differentiation (142). In fetal tissues, INSM1 is present in gastrointestinal epithelium and the enteric nervous system, pancreas, thyroid, respiratory epithelium, thymus, and cerebellum. In adult tissues, INSM1 immunoreactivity is present in adrenal medulla, pancreatic islets, and GI EC cells; additionally, positive staining is present in scattered cells in bronchial epithelium and non-neoplastic prostate (142). An additional transcription factor that is present in GI and pancreatic neuroendocrine cells is Histone HIx (143). Islet-1 is a homeobox gene that is involved in the embryogenesis of the pancreatic islets. Although studies have demonstrated that it is a sensitive marker of pancreatic endocrine cell development, it is also expressed in endocrine neoplasms of the duodenum and colon/rectum (144). CDX2 is a transcription factor that has been used extensively as a marker of intestinal adenocarcinoma (145). In addition to its presence in normal enterocytes, CDX2 is present in all serotonin-producing EC cells, 10% of gastrin-producing G cells, 30% of gastric inhibitory peptide cells, and in a small proportion of motilin-producing cells, while other gastrointestinal endocrine cells are negative (145). Thyroid transcription factor 1 (TTF-1) is present both in thyroid (follicular cells and C cells) and in the lung (type II epithelial cells, subsets of respiratory nonciliated bronchiolar epithelial cells and pulmonary neuroendocrine cells at various stages of development) (146–148).

Studies of transcription factors have demonstrated three major pathways of cell differentiation and hormone production in the adenohypophysis (149–151). The pituitary transcription factor 1 (Pit-1) is expressed by the growth hormone precursors from which somatotrophs, lactotrophs, mammo-somatotrophs, and thyrotrophs are also derived. The expression of estrogen receptor-α correlates with the expression of prolactin or gonadotropins. Promelanocortin expression in corticotrophs is dependent on the T-box transcription factor (T-pit), while steroidogenic factor 1 (SF-1) regulates expression of cytochromes in steroidogenic tissues and is expressed by gonadotrophs (151). These discoveries have led to the reclassification of hormone negative adenomas, based on patterns of transcription factor expression (151). SF-1 protein and its corresponding mRNA are also expressed in adrenocortical, Leydig, and granulosa cells (152).

Somatostatin Receptors

Somatostatin receptors (sst1–sst5) have attracted considerable attention because of clinical applications related to their overexpression in certain tumors, including those of the neuroendocrine system (153). Because of the metabolic instability of natural somatostatin, a number of synthetic analogs/agonists (e.g., octreotide, lanreotide, pasireotide) have been developed (154). Radionuclide conjugates of these analogs have been used successfully for imaging and, in some cases, treatment of tumors. More recently, somatostatin receptor antagonists have also been developed and used both for imaging and therapy (154). The ability of tumors to express somatostatin receptors can be assessed with antibodies to the specific receptors. Positive staining of normal gastrin producing cells for sst-2A has been documented in gastric antrum, duodenum, jejunum, and ileum (155). In addition, occasional sst-2A positive cells have been recognized in the basal cell component of bronchi. A comprehensive study of the distribution of somatostatin receptor subtypes has revealed their presence in a wide variety of neuroendocrine and non-neuroendocrine cell types, including, adrenal cortex, myocardium, skeletal muscle, ovary, and testis (156). Different neuroendocrine cells have different expression patterns of somatostatin receptors. For example, C cells are positive for sst5, while the pancreatic islets are positive for sst1–3 and sst5, albeit in different distributions (156).

DISTRIBUTION OF NEUROENDOCRINE CELLS

Bronchopulmonary and Upper Respiratory System

The neuroendocrine components of the lung occur singly as solitary cells (Fig. 46.10) or Kulchitsky (K) cells and as small aggregates composed of 4 to 10 cells that have been

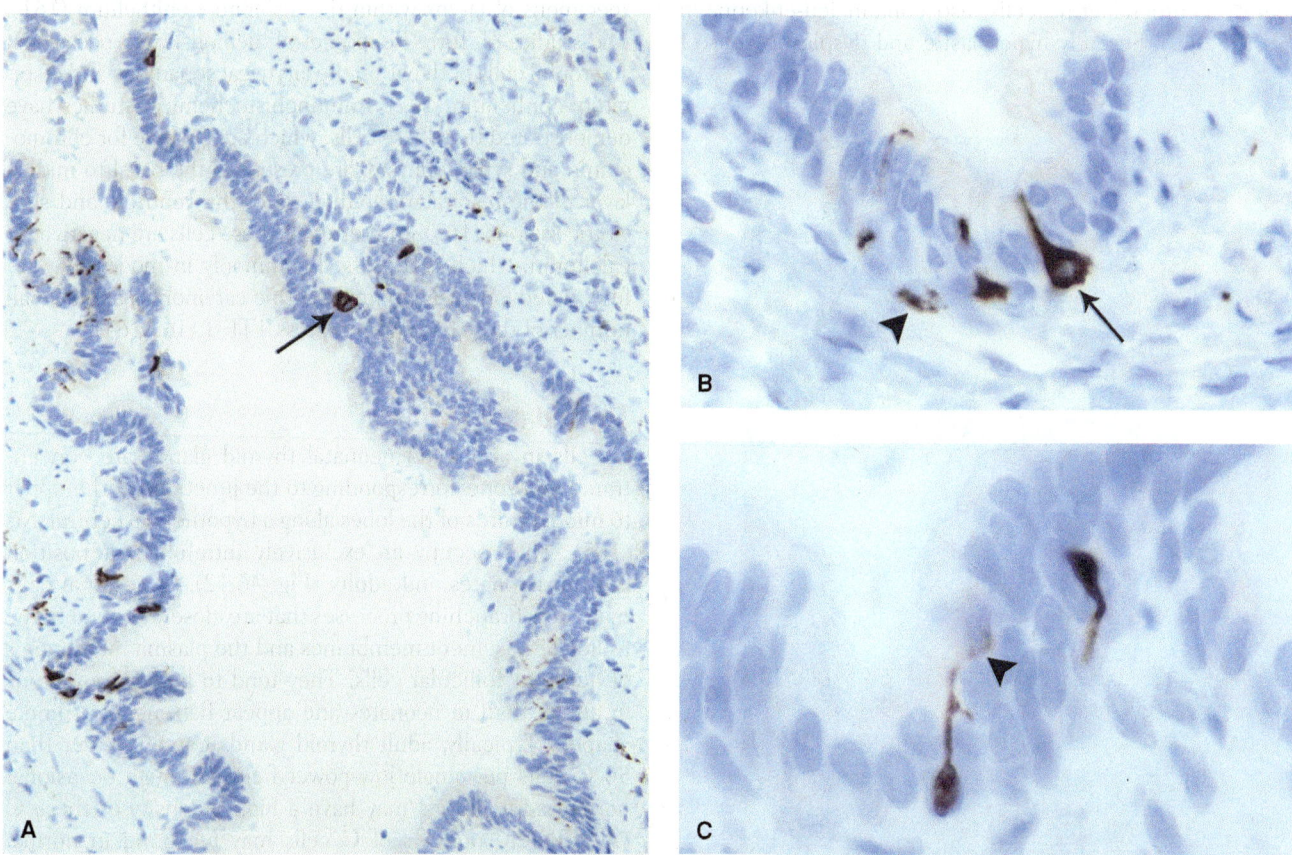

FIGURE 46.10 Neuroendocrine cells of the lung immunostained for synaptophysin. **A:** Individual neuroendocrine cells and part of a neuroepithelial body (*arrow*) are present. **B:** Open (*arrow*) and closed (*arrowhead*) neuroendocrine cells are present. **C:** The processes of the neuroendocrine cells (*arrowhead*) are interdigitating between the epithelial cells and are partially encircling a luminal cell.

designated neuroepithelial bodies (NEBs) (Fig. 46.10A) (33,157). Solitary neuroendocrine cells, which are present predominantly in bronchi, may be of the opened or closed type (Fig. 46.10B). NEBs are extensively innervated and are composed of clear to faintly eosinophilic cells that are present adjacent to the bronchial basement membranes. The NEBs tend to occur adjacent to sites of airway bifurcation. Although the functions of the two neuroendocrine components are not known with certainty, NEBs most likely act as modulators of lung growth and development during early phases of lung organogenesis and as intrapulmonary tactile- and/or chemo-receptors later in fetal growth and in the postnatal period (33).

The secretory granules of pulmonary neuroendocrine cells vary in size and density (157–159). On the basis of granule size, they have been divided into three types. The P1 cells have granules that measure 40 to 50 nm in diameter, and similar cells have been noted in fetal lung. The P2 cells have granules that measure 120 to 130 nm in diameter, whereas the P3 granules measure 180 to 200 nm. The granules of Pa cells, which are found in the adult lung, measure 100 to 120 nm in diameter. Both NEBs and solitary neuroendocrine cells are positive for chromogranin, synaptophysin, and SV2 and also contain serotonin, gastrin-releasing peptide (GRP) (Fig. 46.11), and calcitonin, while the solitary neuroendocrine cells also contain leu-enkephalin (68,158,160). Severely hyperplastic and dysplastic cells of the NEBs may also produce adrenocorticotropin, vasoactive intestinal peptide, and somatostatin (52). The NEBs are particularly conspicuous in fetal lung tissue but are sparse in the adult (33,160). The neuroendocrine components of the lung are also prominent in adults with hypoxic states, including chronic pulmonary diseases such as chronic obstructive pulmonary disease (33,158,160).

The human counterpart of achaete–scute complex, mASH 1 is essential for the development of the pulmonary neuroendocrine cell system (160). In early phases of development neuroendocrine markers are co-expressed with epithelial markers, consistent with a common cellular origin (33). Both in situ hybridization and immunohistochemical studies have shown GRP and its corresponding messenger RNA (mRNA) as early as 8 weeks of gestation in solitary neuroendocrine cells and NEBs. The numbers of cells reach a peak by 16 to 30 weeks of gestation and decline at about 6 months of age. These findings suggest that GRP may be involved in the growth and development of normal lung. Increased numbers of GRP-containing cells have been found in infants with bronchopulmonary dysplasia and in children with cystic fibrosis or prolonged assisted ventilation (160).

Neuroendocrine cells, as defined initially by their argentaffinity or argyrophilia, are rare in the larynx. Pesce et al. were able to identify scattered argyrophil cells in only 2 of 43 specimens of larynx within the respiratory epithelium (161). The studies of Torre-Rendon et al. demonstrated occasional argyrophil cells both within the laryngeal squamous and respiratory epithelium (162). Immunohistochemical studies have demonstrated that these cells, which are positive for chromogranin and synaptophysin, are present in the basal to middle layer of the respiratory epithelium of the ventricle and subglottic regions (163). Interestingly, these cells are negative for calcitonin, which is expressed commonly in moderately differentiated laryngeal neuroendocrine carcinomas and a small number of these cases also express TTF-1 (163,164).

Thyroid and Thymus

C cells in adult and neonatal thyroid glands are concentrated in a zone corresponding to the junctions of the upper to middle thirds of the lobes along a hypothetical central axis (165). They occupy an exclusively intrafollicular position both in neonates and adults (Fig. 46.12). Occasional cells may show branching processes that are closely applied to the follicular basement membranes and the plasma membranes of adjacent follicular cells. They tend to be less numerous in adults than in neonates and appear flattened or spindle shaped. Typically, adult thyroid glands contain fewer than 50 C cells per single low-power field, although occasional normal adult glands may have a higher density of these C cells. Rarely, nodules of C cells may be found in normal adult glands, as discussed in the section on aging.

Two types of calcitonin containing secretory granules ranging from 130 to 280 nm are present in normal, as well as hyperplastic C cells (165–167). Some of the C cells in normal

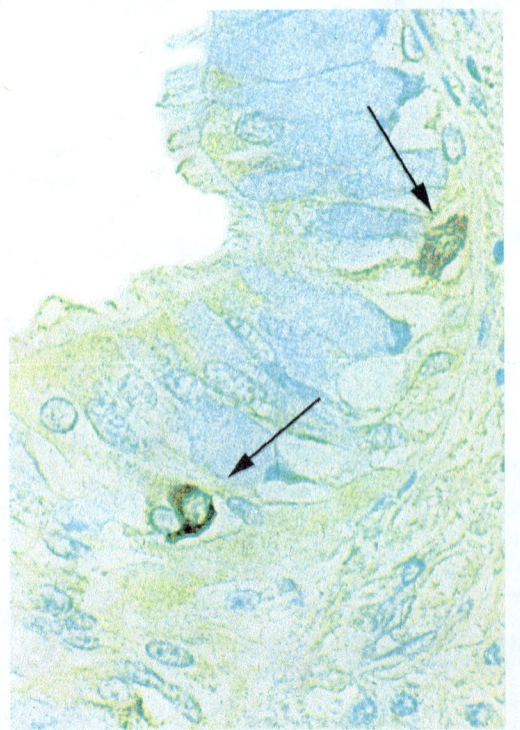

FIGURE 46.11 Adult lung immunostain for gastrin-releasing peptide (GRP) bombesin with methyl green counterstain. Two GRP-positive cells (arrows) are present within the bronchial epithelium. (Courtesy of Dr. Y. Tsutsumi, Tokai University School of Medicine, Japan.)

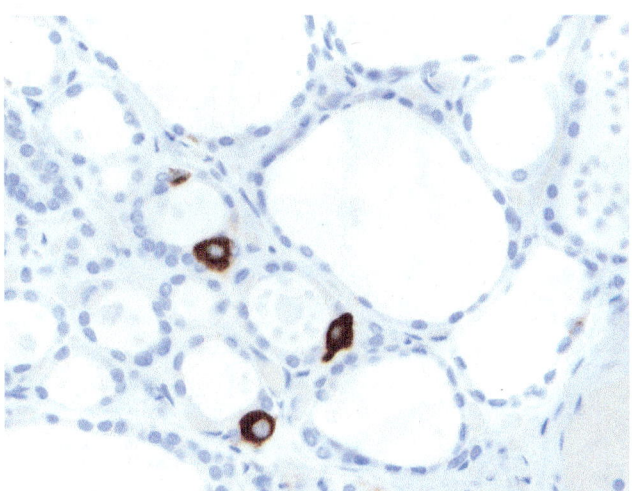

FIGURE 46.12 Adult thyroid immunostained for chromogranin with hematoxylin as the counterstain. C cells are present within the follicle as closed-type endocrine cells.

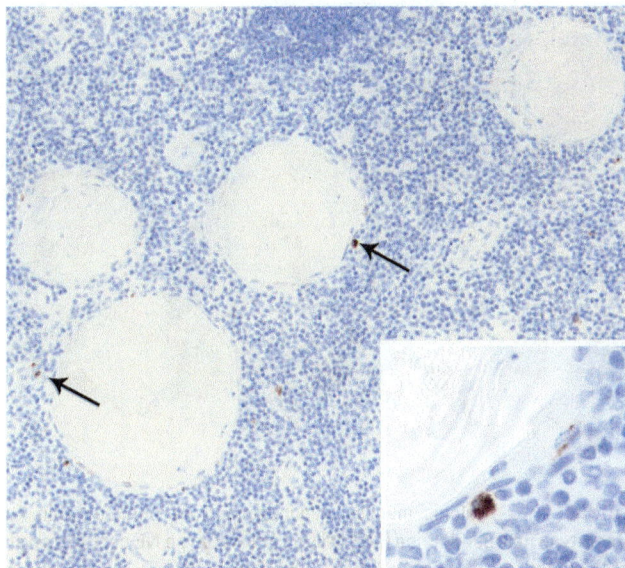

FIGURE 46.13 Thymus immunostained for chromogranin demonstrates neuroendocrine cells (*arrows*) associated with Hassall corpuscle. An NE cell is demonstrated at high power (*Inset*).

adult and neonatal glands also contain somatostatin or GRP (68,165). Approximately 70% of fetal and neonatal C cells contain GRP peptide and mRNA, whereas less than 20% of adult C cells are positive for this peptide. These observations suggest that GRP may play a role as a thyroid growth factor analogous to its presumed role in the developing lung (33).

Although neuroendocrine cells are found commonly in the thymus glands of many animal species, they are sparse in human thymic tissue. In human glands, the neuroendocrine cells may be found within the perivascular connective tissue and in association with Hassall corpuscles (168) (Fig. 46.13). Thymic neuroendocrine cells may regulate early T-cell differentiation by the transcription of neuroendocrine genes in the stromal network and expression of cognitive receptors by immature T cells (169).

Skin

Merkel cells represent the neuroendocrine components of the skin (Fig. 46.7 and 46.14). These cells occur singly and in small clusters throughout the epidermis, particularly in

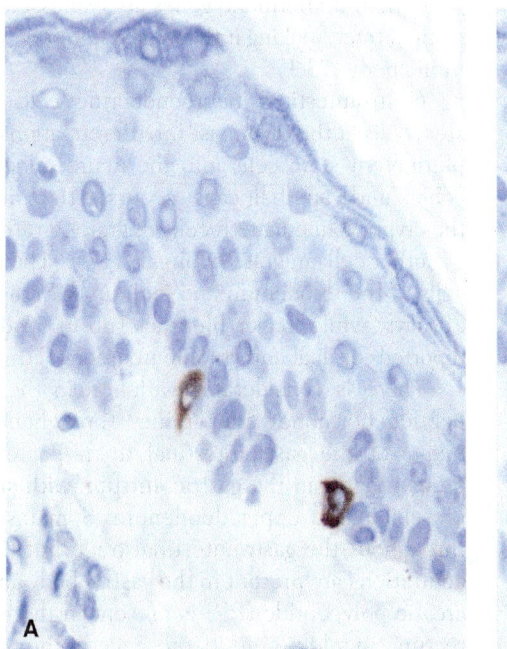
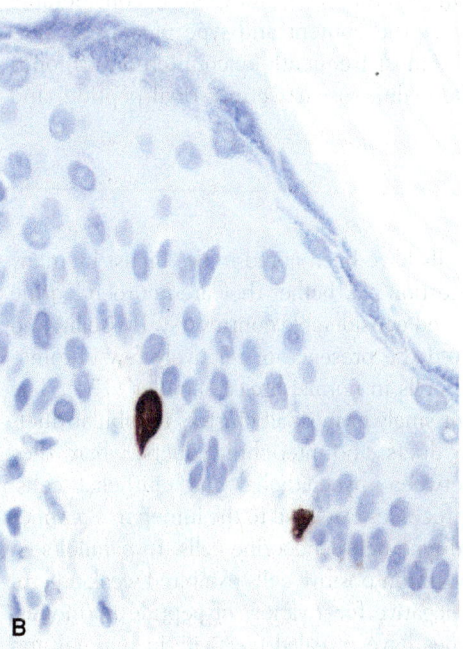

FIGURE 46.14 Merkel cells of skin immunostained for synaptophysin (**A**) and cytokeratin 20 (**B**). Note the oval and triangular appearance of the Merkel cells.

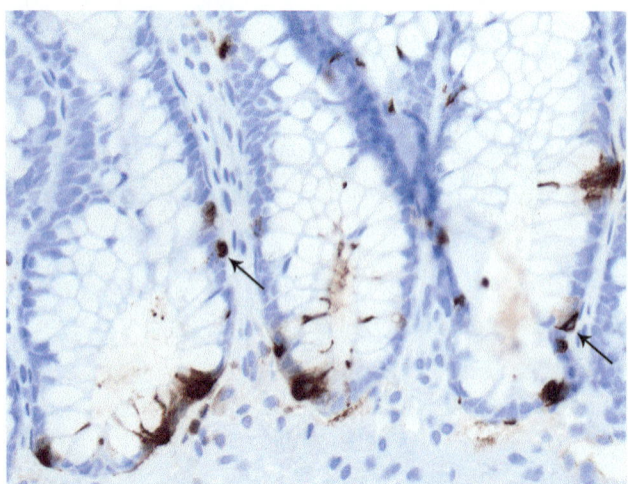

FIGURE 46.15 Colonic mucosa immunostained for chromogranin A. Open-type neuroendocrine (*NE*) cells and closed-type NE cells (*arrows*) are present.

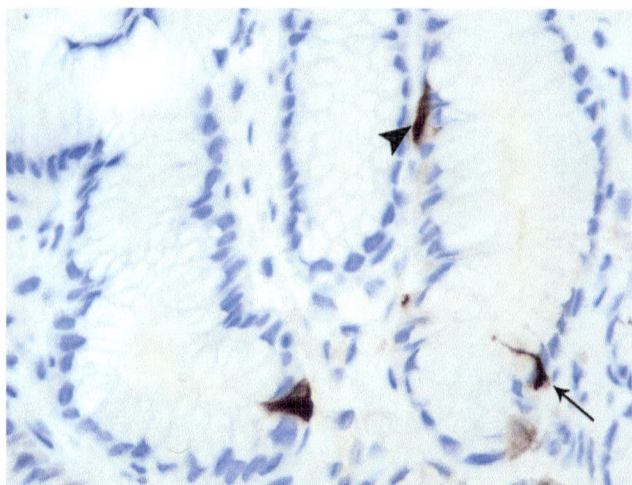

FIGURE 46.16 Gastric antrum immunostained for gastrin. The G-cells are primarily in the lower third of the gastric glands. Both open-type (*arrow*) and closed-type (*arrowhead*) G cells are present.

the basal layer. The clusters are prominent in foci of specialized epithelial differentiation, such as the touch domes (170,171). Individual cells have elongate processes that surround neighboring keratinocytes. The Merkel cells are innervated by long type I myelinated fibers. Secretory granules are abundant and range from 80 to 130 nm in diameter and are particularly prominent in cytoplasmic processes. Aggregates of intermediate filament proteins are predominantly of the cytokeratin 20 (Fig. 46.14B) and 8/18 types, but neurofilament proteins, predominantly of low-to-intermediate molecular weights, may also be present. There is variation in the distribution of epithelial and neural markers in Merkel cells in different sites and there is considerable species variation in the content and type of peptide hormones (172). The most frequently encountered hormones include met-enkephalin, vasoactive intestinal peptide, and GRP (173).

Breast

Although clear cells have been noted in the breast by many observers, the question of whether they are neuroendocrine cells has engendered considerable controversy. Bussolati and coworkers reported the presence of relatively few chromogranin A-positive cells in normal breast samples (174). The cells were present singly or in small clusters in lobular ductules, intralobular ducts, and interlobular ducts, where they were located between myoepithelial and epithelial cells. Occasional cell processes extended to the lumen in a manner typical of opened-type neuroendocrine cells. In parallel sections, the chromogranin-positive cells exhibited weak argyrophilia but were negative for a variety of peptide hormones. Subsequent studies have revealed positivity in luminal and lobular epithelium for the vesicular monoamine transporter 2 (VMAT2), chromogranin B, and several regulatory peptides, including obestatin, ghrelin, adrenomedullin, and apelin; however, stains for chromogranin A and synaptophysin were negative (115).

Gastrointestinal System

The gastrointestinal tract, from the stomach to the anal canal, is richly populated by a heterogeneous collection of peptide hormone and amine-producing neuroendocrine cells that are also referred to as enteroendocrine cells (46–48). The gut neuroendocrine cells are responsible for the production of a wide array of different hormones (Figs. 46.15 to 46.17). More than 30 hormone genes are expressed in the gastrointestinal tract, making it the largest hormone producing organ in the body (73,175).

Gastrointestinal neuroendocrine cells originate from stem cells at the crypt bases. Differentiation of the migrating pluripotent stem cells into the neuroendocrine, absorptive goblet, and Paneth lineages occurs in the transitional zone of the crypt. While Paneth cells migrate toward the crypt base, the other cells migrate luminally (175). The neuroendocrine cells of the duodenum and jejunum have a lifespan of 3 to 20 days, while longer lifetimes (up to 60 days) have been reported for ileal and colonic neuroendocrine cells (65).

There is considerable variation in the distribution of peptide hormones and amines throughout different segments of the gastrointestinal tract. For example, gastrin predominates in the gastric antrum, with smaller amounts present in the upper duodenum. Somatostatin is present throughout the gastrointestinal tract, but the highest concentrations are present in the gastric body and antrum. Pancreatic polypeptide (PP) is present in the distal colon and rectum, in addition to its presence in the pancreatic islets. Serotonin is present throughout the GI tract in different subsets of EC cells (enterochromaffin) and similar cells are

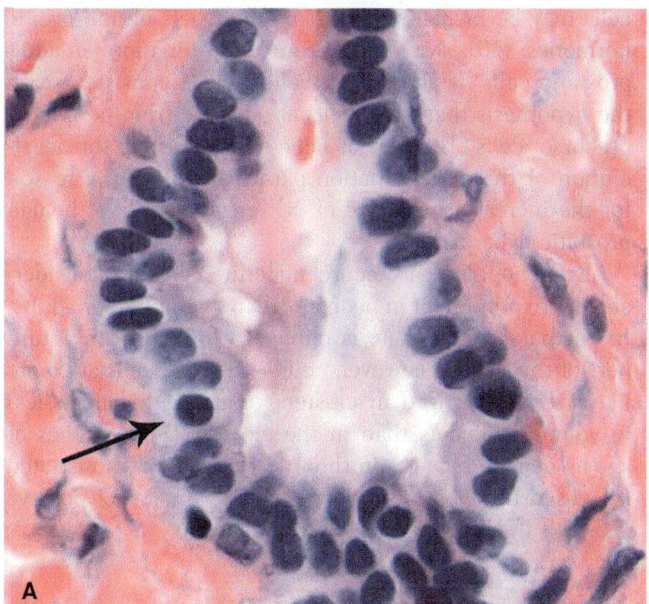 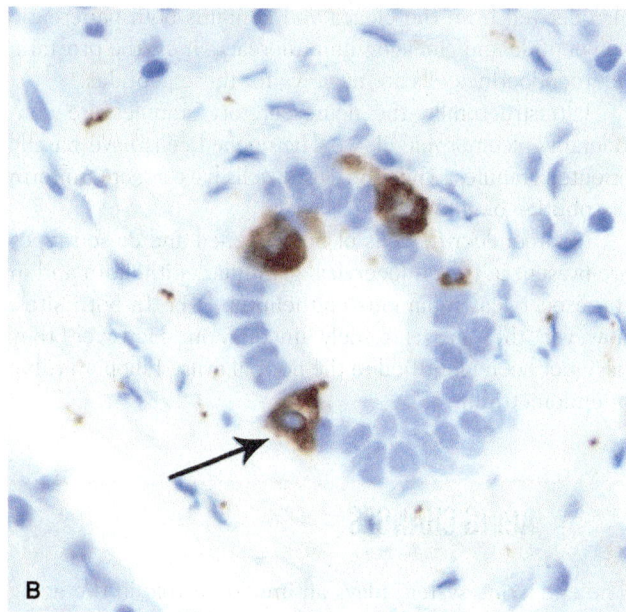

FIGURE 46.17 Neuroendocrine cell of pancreatic duct **A:** H&E section of pancreatic duct with neuroendocrine clear cell (*arrow*). **B:** Immunostain for synaptophysin demonstrates open type (*arrow*) and closed-type neuroendocrine cells the epithelium.

also present within the intra- and extrahepatic bile ducts and the pancreatic ductal system.

Individual neuroendocrine cells are generally classified according to their major secretory product(s) and by letter designations. In the stomach, the EC cells produce 5-HT/serotonin, while the ECL cells produce histamine. In addition, there are somatostatin (D), gastrin (G), and ghrelin (P/D1) cells. In the duodenum, large numbers of cells produce glucose-dependent insulinotropic polypeptide/ or gastric inhibitory polypeptide (GIP) ((K cells), cholecystokinin (I cells), and secretin (S cells). In addition, varying numbers of P/D1, D, and M (motilin) cells are present. More distally, there are increasing numbers of neurotensin (N) cells and L cells that produce glucagon-like peptide 1 and 2 (GLP-1, GLP-2), and peptide YY (PYY). Some gut hormone genes are expressed in extraintestinal neuroendocrine cells and in neurons and may also be expressed in other cell types. It has been suggested that extraintintestinal neuroendocrine cells may synthesize fragments of the same prohormone as a result of cell specific processing pathways (73).

Peptide hormones are also present within neuroendocrine cells of submucosal glands. Brunner's glands, for example, contain neuroendocrine cells positive for somatostatin, gastrin-cholecystokinin, and peptide YY. Peptidergic nerve structures containing vasoactive intestinal peptide, peptide histidine methionine, substance P, neuropeptide Y, and gastrin-releasing peptide also have been identified around Brunner glands. All of these peptides, with the exception of gastrin-releasing peptide, have been found in nerve cell bodies of the submucosal ganglia adjacent to the acini of Brunner glands (48). These findings reflect the fact that multiple peptides are involved in the control of secretion from these glands.

Urogenital System

Although argyrophil cells are not present in the adult renal parenchyma, rare argyrophilic cells have been reported in the renal pelvis. These cells may be particularly prominent in areas of glandular metaplasia. Neuroendocrine cells, as defined by their argentaffinity or argyrophilia, were first described in the urinary bladder by Feyrter (5,6). Later studies by Fetissof et al. (176) established that the endocrine cells in the urothelium were predominantly of the closed type. Immunohistochemical analyses showed that the cells were positive for serotonin but did not contain peptide hormones such as ACTH, gastrin, glucagon, or somatostatin.

The neuroendocrine cells of the prostate are present in all zones and include both opened and closed types with a predominance of the latter forms (177–179). However, detailed quantitative studies have demonstrated that these cells predominate in the transition zone, as compared to the central and peripheral zones (180). Many of the cells have prominent dendritic processes extending between adjacent epithelial cells and occasionally abutting other neuroendocrine cells. The neuroendocrine cells tend to be more prominent in normal or atrophic prostate than in hyperplastic foci. Most of the cells contain serotonin, and some also contain somatostatin. Both calcitonin and GRP also have been observed in the normal prostate, but these hormones are present in considerably less than 5% of the neuroendocrine cells. In contrast to the anorectal canal, which is also derived from the cloaca and contains both pancreatic polypeptide and glucagon immunoreactivities, the prostatic neuroendocrine cells are negative for these peptides.

Ultrastructurally, the neurosecretory granules are considerably pleomorphic (177). The opened cells have basally oriented granules, while the closed cells have a more uniform distribution of granules.

Neuroendocrine cells of both opened and closed types are present in the endocervical glandular epithelium and in the exocervical squamous epithelium (181). In both sites, however, they are extremely uncommon. However, they have not been identified in the normal ovary, fallopian tube, or endometrium.

AGING CHANGES

The endocrine system plays an important role in the aging process; however, there have been relatively few systematic studies of the effects of aging in neuroendocrine cell populations in humans. In the pituitary, Sun et al. have demonstrated a significant age-related decline in the number and size of growth hormone–producing cells that was most marked in the transition from youth to middle age (182). Prolactin cells, on the other hand, did not show age-related changes. Hypertrophy and relative hyperplasia of thyrotroph cells have been demonstrated in pituitaries from older individuals (183).

O'Toole et al. have studied the effects of the aging process on C-cell populations in the thyroid gland (184). Although C cells appeared to be more numerous in thyroid glands of elderly individuals, as compared with young and middle-aged individuals, the results were not statistically significant because of the large standard deviations. One study has demonstrated gender-related differences in the numbers of C cells, with male subjects having significantly more C cells than females (185). This difference is reflected in the higher concentrations of plasma calcitonin levels in males, as compared to females. However, the latter study failed to find any correlations between C-cell density and age. In one study, there was a positive correlation between age and C-cell density in males; however, this study is biased by the inclusion of a significant number of males under the age of 10 years (186). The same group reported that C cells more often tended to form clusters or nodules in thyroids from older individuals (187).

Age-related changes in neuroendocrine populations have been characterized in a few other sites. Although the numbers of prostatic neuroendocrine cells of the periurethral glands and ducts remain relatively constant throughout life, those in the peripheral acini are present in highest numbers in the neonatal and postpubertal periods (50). With advancing age, there is a fall in their total numbers and the number per square millimeter (188). Cohen et al. have suggested that variations in prostatic neuroendocrine cells may be mediated in part by the levels of androgenic hormones (50). Neuroendocrine differentiation of adult prostatic cells has been observed in vitro, consistent with the hypothesis that these cells are derived from peripheral precursor cells (189). It has been suggested that the acceleration of this differentiation pathway may be the reason for the increased presence of NE cells in areas of benign prostatic hyperplasia.

Bronchopulmonary neuroendocrine cells are considerably more prominent in neonates than in children or adults. In postnatal lungs, there is minimal variation in the numbers of these cells; however, neuroendocrine cells are more likely to be arranged in clusters (neuroepithelial bodies) in younger subjects than in the elderly (190). Studies of age-associated changes in the intestine have demonstrated increased numbers of chromogranin A and Ki-67 positive NE cells in elderly individuals (191,192).

SPECIAL PROCEDURES

In addition to the histochemical and immunohistochemical approaches that have been discussed throughout this chapter, molecular methodologies including in situ hybridization provide important approaches for analyzing the distribution and function of neuroendocrine cells (193,194). In contrast to immunohistochemistry, which is dependent on the peptide content of neuroendocrine cells, in situ hybridization techniques permit the identification of cells on the basis of their contents of specific mRNAs. For example, neuroendocrine cells that are acutely stimulated or are secreting their products constitutively often produce a negative immunohistochemical signal for the particular peptide. However, studies using nucleic acid probes for the corresponding mRNAs often provide an intensely positive signal in the same cells (193). Extensive posttranslational processing and intracellular degradation of peptide products also may lead to positive hybridization signals with negative immunohistochemical reactions for the corresponding peptides. Additionally, in situ hybridization methods are of particular value for demonstrating hormone receptor mRNAs in target cells and for distinguishing de novo synthesis from uptake of hormonal peptides (193–195). The combination of in situ hybridization and immunohistochemistry has the potential for providing the maximal amount of information on the highly dynamic processes of gene transcription and translation.

The in situ hybridization method also has been combined with polymerase chain reaction (PCR) methods for demonstration of low copy number DNAs and RNAs (196,197). Detection of intracellular PCR products may be achieved indirectly by in situ hybridization using PCR product-specific probes (indirect in situ PCR) or without in situ hybridization through direct incorporation of labeled nucleotides into the PCR amplificants (direct in situ PCR). Although most protocols are designed for the demonstration of DNA, low copy RNA sequences have been demonstrated by the addition of a reverse transcriptase (RT) step to generate cDNA from RNA templates before in situ PCR. This technique, which has been called in situ RT-PCR, may be of particular value when there are fewer than 20 copies of mRNA per cell. This technique is of great potential value for the identification of cells with low levels of mRNA-encoding hormones, hormone receptors, cytokines, growth factors, and growth factor receptors. The technical details and potential pitfalls of these methods are discussed in detail in several publications (196,198–200).

ARTIFACTS

Since neuroendocrine cells often have a clear appearance, they must be distinguished from a variety of other cell types that also may appear clear in H&E-stained, formalin-fixed, paraffin-embedded sections. Cytoplasmic clearing may result from intracellular accumulations of lipids or glycogen; alternatively, this change may represent a shrinkage artifact analogous to that seen in the lacunar cells of nodular sclerosing Hodgkin lymphoma. Clear cells in the intestinal epithelium may represent lymphocytes or epithelial cells with retraction of the cytoplasm from the nucleus. In general, shrinkage artifact is less pronounced in tissues that have been fixed in nonaqueous fixatives. Neuroendocrine cells can be distinguished conclusively from other clear cells by the presence of neuroendocrine markers, including chromogranins or synaptophysin.

Significant artifacts may be associated with the use of immunohistochemical procedures for the demonstration of peptide hormones and nonhormonal markers. Appropriate positive and negative controls must, therefore, be used in conjunction with these procedures, as discussed in standard textbooks of immunohistochemistry (200). Nonspecific binding of immunoglobulins to neuroendocrine secretory granules also may result from ionic interactions that may be suppressed to some extent by the use of buffers containing high concentrations of salt (201). Endogenous biotin-like activity may also contribute to nonspecific staining in neuroendocrine cells and other cell types, particularly following microwave-induced antigen retrieval (202–203). This problem can be circumvented by the use of biotin-blocking steps or by the use of biotin-free polymer-based detection systems. Diffusion of antigens from neuroendocrine cells to adjacent cells may also occur (Fig. 46.18), particularly in specimens that have not been fixed promptly.

Artifacts also may occur in in situ hybridization procedures. For example, Pagani et al. have demonstrated that oligonucleotides used for in situ hybridization procedures bind to neuroendocrine cells as a result of the presence of endogenous NH_2 groups (204). This type of nonspecific interaction can be blocked effectively by treating the sections with acetic anhydride. Controls for standard in situ hybridization and PCR-based in situ hybridization are discussed in detail in several reviews (196–199).

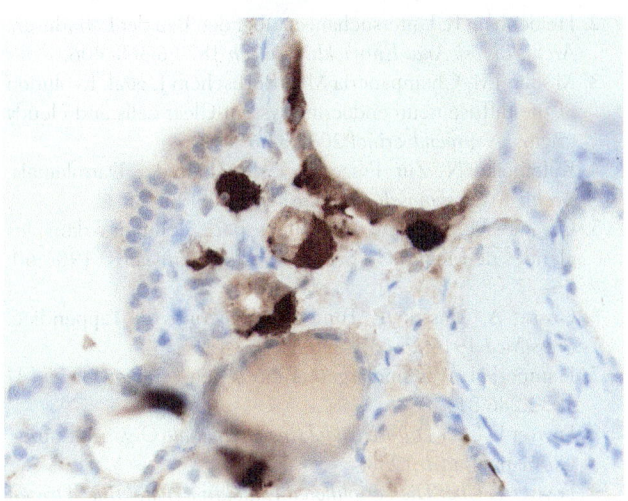

FIGURE 46.18 Immunostain for calcitonin highlighting C cells. There is artifactual diffusion of the antibody into the follicular cells and colloid which can give rise to problems with interpretation.

DIFFERENTIAL DIAGNOSIS

The differential diagnosis of various neuroendocrine cell populations is discussed in the chapters dealing with the specific organ systems in this volume.

SPECIMEN HANDLING

Most histochemical and immunohistochemical procedures for the demonstration of hormones and nonhormonal constituents of neuroendocrine cells can be performed in formalin-fixed and paraffin-embedded tissues. Other fixatives, including carbodiimide, acrolein, and diethyl pyrocarbonate, also have been used in place of formalin, and these fixatives have been reported to achieve optimal fixation of low concentrations of regulatory peptides such as those occurring in peptidergic nerve fibers (205–208).

The tissue preparative techniques for in situ hybridization studies are discussed in several review articles (193,199). In general, these methods may be performed on frozen samples that are postfixed in paraformaldehyde or in formalin-fixed samples that have been embedded in paraffin.

REFERENCES

1. Wiedenmann B, John M, Ahnert-Hilger G, et al. Molecular and cell biological aspects of neuroendocrine tumors of the gastroenteropancreatic system. *J Mol Med (Berl)* 1998;76(9): 637–647.

2. Heidenhain R. Untersuchangen über den Bau der Labüdusen. *Arch Mikrosk Anat Entwicklungsmech* 1870;6:368–406.
3. Modlin IM, Champaneria MC, Bornschein J, et al. Evolution of the diffuse neuroendocrine system-Clear cells and cloudy origins. *Neuroendocrinol* 2006;84:69–82.
4. Kulchitsky N. Zur Frage über den Bau der Darmkanals. *Archiv Microskopisch-anatomishe*. 1897;49:7–35.
5. Ciaccio M. Sur une nouvelle espece cellulaire dans les glandes de Lieber. *CR Seances Soc Biol Fil (Paris)* 1906;60:76–77.
6. Gosset A, Masson P. Tumeurs endocrines de l'appendice. *Press Med* 1914;25:237–240.
7. Hamperl H. Was sind argentaffine Zellen? *Virchows Arch [A]* 1932;286:811–833.
8. Feyrter F. *Uber Diffuse Endokrine Epithaliale Organe*. Leipzig, Germany: Barth; 1938.
9. Feyrter F. *Uber Die Periphheren Endokrine (Parakrine) Drusen Des Menshen*. Vienna: Maudrich; 1954.
10. Frolich F Die. "Helle Zelle" der bronchialschleinhaut und ihre beziehungen zum problem der chemoreceptoren. *Frankfurter Z Pathol* 1949;60:517–558.
11. Scharrer B. The neurosecretory neuron in neuroendocrine regulatory mechanisms. *Am Zool* 1967;7(1):161–169.
12. Snyder SH. Brain peptides as neurotransmitters. *Science* 1980;209(4460):976–983.
13. Copp DH, Cameron EC, Cheney BA, et al. Evidence for calcitonin–a new hormone from the parathyroid that lowers blood calcium. *Endocrinology* 1962;70:638–649.
14. Pearse AG. The cytochemistry of the thyroid C-cells and their relationship to calcitonin. *Proc R Soc Lond Biol Sci* 1966;164(996):478–487.
15. Pearse AG. The cytochemistry and ultrastructure of polypeptide hormone producing cells (the APUD series) and the embryologic, physiologic and pathologic implications of the concept. *J Histochem Cytochem* 1969;17(5):303–313.
16. Pearse AG. 5-Hydroxytryptophan uptake by the dog thyroid C-cells and its possible significance in polypeptide hormone production. *Nature* 1966;211(5049):598–600.
17. Pearse AG. Common cytochemical properties of cells producing polypeptide hormones with particular reference to calcitonin and the thyroid C-cells. *Vet Rec* 1966;79(21):587–590.
18. Bussolati G, Pearse AG. Immunofluorescent localization of calcitonin in the C-cells of the pig and dog thyroid. *J Endocrinol* 1967;37(2):205–209.
19. Pearse AG. The diffuse neuroendocrine system and the APUD concept: Related endocrine peptides in brain, intestine, pituitary, placenta and anuran cutaneous glands. *Med Biol* 1977;55(3):115–125.
20. Fujita T, Kobayashi S. Current reviews on the paraneuron concept. *Trends Neurosci* 1979;2:27–30.
21. Fujita T. Present status of the paraneuron concept. *Arch Histol Cytol* 1989;52(suppl):1–8.
22. LeDouarin N, Teillet MA. The migration of neural crest cells to the wall of the digestive tract in the avian embryo. *J Embryol Exp Morphol* 1973;30(1):31–48.
23. LeDouarin N. *The Neural Crest*. Cambridge, England: Cambridge University Press; 1982.
24. Thompson EM, Fleming KA, Evans DJ, et al. Gastric endocrine cells share a clonal origin with other gut cell lineage. *Development* 1990;110(2):477–481.
25. Day R, Salzet M. The neuroendocrine phenotype, cellular plasticity, and the search for genetic switches; redefining the diffuse neuroendocrine system. *Neuorendocrinol Lett* 2002;23(5–6):447–451.
26. Johansson E, Andersson L, Ornros J, et al. Revising the embryonic origin of thyroid C-cells in mice and humans. *Development* 2015;142(20):3519–3528.
27. Nilsson M, Williams D. On the origin of cells and derivation of thyroid cancer. C-cell story revisited. *Eur Thyroid J* 2016;5(2):79–93.
28. Kameda Y. Cellular and molecular events on the development of mammalian thyroid C-cells. *Dev Dyn* 2016;245(3):323–341.
29. Kameda Y. Morphological and molecular evolution of the ultimobranchial gland of nonmammalian vertebrates, with special reference to the chicken C-cells. *Dev Dyn* 2017;246(10):719–739.
30. Johnson JE, Birren SJ, Anderson DJ. Two rat homologues of Drosophila achaete–scute specifically expressed in neuronal precursors. *Nature* 1990;346(6287):858–861.
31. Ball DW. Achaete-scute homolog-1 and Notch in lung neuroendocrine development and cancer. *Cancer Lett* 2004;204(2):159–169.
32. Ito T, Udaka N, Yazawa T, et al. Basic helix-loop-helix transcription factors regulate the neuroendocrine differentiation in fetal mouse pulmonary epithelium. *Development* 2000;127(18):3913–3921.
33. Linniola RI. Functional facets of the pulmonary neuroendocrine system. *Lab Invest* 2006;86(5):425–444.
34. Cook M, Yu XM, Chen H. Notch in the development of thyroid C-cells and the treatment of medullary thyroid carcinoma. *Am J Transl Res* 2010;2(1):119–125.
35. Lanigan TM, DeRaad SK, Russo AF. Requirement of the MASH-1 transcription factor for neuroendocrine differentiation of thyroid C-cells. *J Neurobiol* 1998;34(2):126–134.
36. Nikolakopoulou P, Poser SW, Masjkur J, et al. STAST3-Ser/Hes 3 signaling: A New molecular component of the neuroendocrine system? *Horm Metab Res* 2016;48(2):77–82.
37. Falck B, Owman CA. A detailed methodological description of the fluorescence method for the cellular distribution of biogenic monoamines. *Acta Univ Lund* 1965;7:5–23.
38. Grimelius L. A silver nitrate stain for A2 cells of human pancreatic islets. *Acta Soc Med Upsal* 1968;73(5–6):243–270.
39. Grimelius L, Wilander E. Silver stains in the study of endocrine cells of the gut and pancreas. *Invest Cell Pathol* 1980;3(1):3–12.
40. Aguirre P, Scully RE, Wolfe HJ, et al. Endometrial carcinomas with argyrophil cells. A histochemical and immunohistochemical study. *Hum Pathol* 1984;15(3):210–217.
41. Cecilia M, Rost M, Rost FW. An improved method for staining cells of the endocrine polypeptide (APUD) series by masked metachromasia: Application of the principle of 'fixation by excluded volume'. *Histochem J* 1976;8(1):93–98.
42. Rode J, Dhillon AP, Papadaki L. Serotonin immunoreactive cells in the lamina propria plexus of the appendix. *Hum Pathol* 1983;14:464–469.
43. Larsson LI, Goltermann N, De Magistris L, et al. Somatostatin cell processes as pathways for paracrine secretion. *Science* 1979;205(4413):1393–1395.
44. Dockray GJ. Evolutionary relationships of the gut hormones. *Fed Proc* 1979;38(9):2295–2301.

45. Fujita T, Kobayashi S. The cells and hormones of the GEP endocrine system. In: Fujita T, ed. *Gastroenteropancreatic Cell System*. Tokyo: Igaku-Shoin; 1973: 1–16.
46. Dayal Y. Endocrine cells of the gut and their neoplasms. In: Norris HT, ed. *Pathology of the Colon, Small Intestine and Anus*. New York: Churchill Livingstone; 1983: 267–300.
47. Lechago J. The endocrine cells of the digestive and respiratory systems and their pathology. In: Bloodworth JMB Jr, ed. *Endocrine Pathology General and Surgical*. 2nd ed. Baltimore, MD: Williams & Wilkins; 1982: 513–555.
48. Bosshard A, Chery-Croze S, Cuber JC, et al. Immunohistochemical study of peptidergic structures in Brunner's glands. *Gastroenterology* 1989;97(6):1382–1388.
49. Aubock L, Ratzenhofer M. "Extraepithelial enterochromaffin cell complexes" in the normal human appendix and neurogenic appendicopathy. *J Pathol* 1982;136(3):217–226.
50. Cohen RJ, Glezerson G, Taylor LF, et al. The neuroendocrine cell population of the human prostate gland. *J Urol* 1993; 150(2 Pt 1):365–368.
51. Falkmer S. Phylogeny and ontogeny of the neuroendocrine cells of the gastrointestinal tract. *Endocrinol Metab Clin North Am* 1993;22(4):731–752.
52. Gould VE, DeLellis RA. The neuroendocrine cell system: Its tumors, hyperplasias and dysplasias. In: Silverberg S, ed. *Principles and Practice of Surgical Pathology*. New York: Wiley; 1983.
53. Dremier S, Golstein J, Mosselmans R, et al. Apoptosis in dog thyroid cells. *Biochem Biophys Res Commun* 1994;200(1): 52–58.
54. Drewett N, Jacobi JM, Willgoss DA, et al. Apoptosis in the anterior pituitary gland of the rat: Studies with estrogen and bromocriptine. *Neuroendocrinology* 1993;57(1):89–95.
55. Garcia I, Martinou I, Tsujimoto Y, et al. Prevention of programmed cell death of sympathetic neurons by the *bcl-2* proto-oncogene. *Science* 1992;258(5080):302–304.
56. Kaneto H, Fujii J, Seo HG, et al. Apoptotic cell death triggered by nitric oxide in pancreatic beta-cells. *Diabetes* 1995; 44(7):733–738.
57. Schwanbeck R, Martini S, Bernoth K, et al. The Notch signaling pathway; Molecular basis of cell context dependency. *Eur J Cell Biol* 2011;90(6–7):572–581.
58. Drucker DJ. Glucagon-like peptides: Regulators of cell proliferation, differentiation, and apoptosis. *Mol Endocrinol* 2003; 17(2):161–171.
59. Roth J, Kasper M, Stamm B, et al. Localization of proinsulin and insulin in human insulinoma: Preliminary immunohistochemical results. *Virchows Arch B Cell Pathol Incl Mol Pathol* 1989;56(5):287–292.
60. Hakanson R, Sundler F. The design of the neuroendocrine system: A unifying concept and its consequences. *Trends Pharmacol Sci* 1983;4:41–44.
61. Tischler AS. The dispersed neuroendocrine cells: The structure, function, regulation and effects of xenobiotics on this system. *Toxicol Pathol* 1989;17(2):307–316.
62. Pearse AG, Polak JM, Bloom SR. The newer gut hormones. Cellular sources, physiology, pathology and clinical aspects. *Gastroenterology* 1977;72(4 Pt 1): 746–761.
63. Reichlin S. Somatostatin (part 1). *N Engl J Med* 1983;309(24): 1495–1501.
64. Reichlin S. Somatostatin (part 2). *N Engl J Med* 1983;309(25): 1556–1563.
65. Gribble FM, Reimann F. Enteroendocrine cells: Chemosensors in the intestinal epithelium. *Ann Rev Physio* 2016;78: 277–299.
66. Kameda Y, Oyama H, Endoh M, et al. Somatostatin immunoreactive C-cells in thyroid glands from various mammalian species. *Anat Rec* 1982;204(2):161–170.
67. Tsutsumi Y, Osamura RY, Watanabe K, et al. Immunohistochemical localization of gastrin releasing peptide and adrenocorticotropin releasing cells in the human lung. *Lab Invest* 1983;48(5):623–632.
68. Sunday ME, Kaplan LM, Motoyama E, et al. Gastrin releasing peptide (mammalian bombesin) gene expression in health and disease. *Lab Invest* 1988;59(1):5–24.
69. Kruger DT. Pituitary ACTH hyperfunction: Pathophysiology and clinical aspects. In: Commani F, Mueller EE, eds. *Pituitary Hyperfunction: Pathophysiology and Clinical Aspects*. New York: Raven Press; 1984: 221–234.
70. Rosenfeld MG, Mermod JJ, Amara SG, et al. Production of a novel neuropeptide encoded by the calcitonin gene via tissue specific RNA processing. *Nature* 1983;304(5922):129–135.
71. Warren TG, Shields D. Cell free biosynthesis of somatostatin precursors: Evidence for multiple forms of preprosomatostatin. *Proc Natl Acad Sci U S A* 1982;79(12):3729–3733.
72. Bouillon R, Drucker DJ, Ferrennini E, et al. The past 10 years-new hormones, new functions, new endocrine organs. *Nat Rev Endocrinol* 2015;11(11):681–686.
73. Rehfeld JF. Gastrointestinal hormones and their targets. *Adv Exp Med Biol* 2014;817:157–175.
74. Polak JM, Bloom SR. Immunocytochemistry of regulatory peptides. In: Polak JM, Vaan Noordern S, eds. *Immunocytochemistry. Practical Applications in Pathology and Biology*. Wright PSG; 1983:184–211.
75. Verhofstad AAJ, Steinbusch HWM, Joosten HWJ, et al. Immunocytochemical localization of noradrenaline, adrenaline and serotonin. In: Polak JM, Van Noorden S, eds. *Immunocytochemistry. Practical Applications in Pathology and Medicine*. Bristol, England: Wright PSG; 1983: 143–168.
76. Lloyd RV. Immunohistochemical localization of catecholamines, catecholamine synthesizing enzymes and chromogranins in neuroendocrine cells and tumors. In: DeLellis RA, ed. *Advances in Immunohistochemistry*. New York: Raven Press; 1988: 317–340.
77. Schmechel D, Marangos PJ, Brightman M. Neuron specific enolase is a molecular marker for peripheral and central neuroendocrine cells. *Nature* 1978;276(5690):834–836.
78. Lloyd RV, Warner TF. Immunohistochemistry of neuron specific enolase. In: DeLellis RA, ed. *Advances of Immunohistochemistry*. New York: Masson; 1984: 127–140.
79. Haimoto H, Takahashi T, Koshikawa T, et al. Immunohistochemical localization of gamma enolase in normal human tissues other than nervous and neuroendocrine tissue. *Lab Invest* 1985;52(3):257–263.
80. Schmechel D. Gamma subunit of the glycolytic enzyme enolase: Nonspecific or neuron specific. *Lab Invest* 1985;52:2.
81. Thompson RJ, Doran JF, Jackson P, et al. PGP 9.5—a new marker for vertebrate neurons and neuroendocrine cells. *Brain Res* 1983;278(1–2):224–228.
82. Li GL, Farooque M, Holtz A. et al. Expression of the ubiquitin carboxyl-terminal hydrolase PGP 9.5 in axons following spinal cord compression trauma. *APMIS* 1997;105(5): 384–390.

83. Campbell LK, Thomas JR, Lamps LW et al. Protein gene product 9.5 (PGP 9.5) is not a specific marker of neural and nerve sheath tumors: An immunohistochemical study of 95 mesenchymal neoplasms. *Mod Pathol* 2003;16(10):963–969.
84. Blaschko H, Comline RS, Schneider FH, et al. Secretion of a chromaffin protein, chromogranin, from the adrenal medulla after splanchnic nerve stimulation. *Nature*. 1967; 215(5096):58–59.
85. Schober M, Fischer-Colbrie R, Schmidt KW, et al. Comparison of chromogranins A, B and secretogranin II in human adrenal medulla and pheochromocytoma. *Lab Invest* 1987;57(4):385–391.
86. Troger J, Theurl M, Kirchmair R, et al. Granin-derived peptides. *Prog Neurobiol* 2017;154:37–61.
87. Lloyd RV, Jin L, Kulig E, et al. Molecular approaches for the analysis of chromogranins and secretogranins. *Diagn Mol Pathol* 1992;1(1):2–15.
88. Borges R, Diaz-Vera J, Dominguez N et al. Chromogranins as regulators of exocytosis. *J Neurochem* 2010;114(2):335–343.
89. Portela-Gomes GM, Stridsberg M. Selective processing of chromogranin A in the different islet cells in human pancreas. *J Histochem Cytochem.* 2001;49(4):483–490.
90. Portela-Gomes GM, Hacker GW, Weitgassser R. Neuroendocrine cell makers for pancreatic islets and tumors. *Appl Immunohistochem Mol Morphol* 2004;12(3):183–192.
91. Helle KB, Metz-Boutigue MH, Cerra MC, et al. Chromogranins: From discovery to current times. *Pflugers Arch* 2018; 470(1):143–154
92. Corti A, Marcucci F, Bachetti T. Circulating chromogranin A and its fragments as diagnostic and prognostic disease markers. *Pflugers Arch* 2018;470(1):199–210.
93. Kimura N, Funakoshi A, Aunis D, et al. Immunohistochemical localization of chromostatin and pancreastatin, chromogranin A derived bioactive peptides, in normal and neoplastic neuroendocrine tissues. *Endocr Pathol* 1995;6(1):35–44.
94. Schmidt WE, Siegel EG, Lamberts R, et al. Pancreastatin: Molecular and immunocytochemical characterization of a novel peptide in porcine and human tissues. *Endocrinology* 1988;123(3):1395–1404.
95. Bishop AE, Sekiya K, Salahuddin MJ, et al. The distribution of GAWK-like immunoreactivity in neuroendocrine cells of the human gut, pancreas, adrenal and pituitary glands and its colocalization with chromogranin B. *Histochemistry* 1989;90(6):475–483.
96. Huttner WB, Gerdes HH, Rosa P. Chromogranins/secretogranins—widespread constituents of the secretory granule matrix in endocrine cells and neurons. In: Gratzl M, Langley K, eds. *Markers for Neural and Endocrine Cells. Molecular and Cell Biology, Diagnostic Applications.* Weinheim, Germany: VCH; 1991: 93–131.
97. Lloyd RV, Jin L, Qian X et al. Analysis of the chromogranin A post-translational cleavage product pancreastatin and the prohormone convertases PC2 and PC3 in normal and neoplastic human pituitaries. *Am J Pathol* 1995;146(5): 1188–1198.
98. Scopsi L, Gullo M, Rilke F et al. Proprotein convertases (PC1/PC3 and PC2) in normal and neoplastic tissues: Their use as markers of neuroendocrine differentiation. *J Clin Endocrinol Metab* 1995;80(1):294–301.
99. Scopsi L, Lee R, Gullo M, et al. Peptidylglycine alpha amidating monooxygenase in neuroendocrine tumors: Its identification, characterization, quantification and relation to the grade of morphological differentiation, amidated peptide content and granin immunocytochemistry. *Appl Immunohistochem* 1998;6:120–132.
100. Saldise L, Martinez A, Montuenga LM, et al. Distribution of peptidyl-glycine alpha-amidating monooxygenase (PAM) enzymes in normal human lung and in lung epithelial tumors. *J Histochem Cytochem* 1996;44(1):3–12.
101. Weidenmann B, Franke WW, Kuhn C, et al. Synaptophysin: A marker protein for neuroendocrine cells and neoplasms. *Proc Natl Acad Sci U S A* 1986;83(10):3500–3504.
102. Gould VE, Lee I, Wiedenmann B, et al. Synaptophysin: A novel marker for neurons, certain neuroendocrine cells and their neoplasms. *Hum Pathol* 1986;17(10):979–983.
103. Jahn R, DeCamilli P. Membrane proteins of synaptic vesicles: Markers for neurons and endocrine cells: Tools for the study of neurosecretion. In: Gratzl M, Langley K, eds. *Markers for Neurons and Endocrine Cells. Molecular, Cell Biology and Diagnostic Applications.* Weinheim, Germany: VCH; 1991: 25–91.
104. DeLellis RA. The neuroendocrine system and its tumors. An overview. *Am J Clin Pathol* 2001;115(Suppl):S5–S16.
105. Lloyd RV. Practical markers used in the diagnosis of neuroendocrine tumors. *Endocrin Pathol* 2003;14(4):293–301.
106. Portela-Gomes GM, Lukinius A, Grimelius L. Synaptic vesicle protein 2, a new neuroendocrine marker. *Am J Pathol* 2000;157(4):1299–1309.
107. Nowack A, Yao J, Custer KL, et al. SV2 regulates neurotransmitter release via multiple mechanisms. *Am J Physiol Cell Physiol* 2010;299(5);C960–C967.
108. Dunn AR, Stout KA, Ozawa M et al. Synaptic vesicle glycoprotein 2C (SV2C) modulates dopamine release abd is disrupted in Parkinson disease. *Proc Natl Acad Sci USA* 2017; 114(11):E2253–E2262.
109. Nilsson O, Jakobsen AM, Kolby L, et al. Importance of vesicle proteins in the diagnosis and treatment of neuroendocrine tumors. *Ann NY Acad Sci* 2004;1014:280–283.
110. Jakobsen AM, Andersson P, Saglik G, et al. Differential expression of vesicular monoamine transporter (VMAT) 1 and 2 in gastrointestinal endocrine tumors. *J Pathol* 2001;195(4): 463–471.
111. Rindi G, Paolotti D, Fiocca R, et al. Vesicular monoamine transporter 2 as a marker of gastric enterochromaffin-like cell tumors. *Virchows Arch* 2000;436(3):217–223.
112. Wimalasena K. Vesicular monoamine transporters: Stucture-function, pharmacology, and medicinal chemistry. *Med Res Rev* 2011;31(4):483–519.
113. Schafer MK, Weihe E, Eiden LE. Localization and expression of VMAT2 across mammalian species: A translational guide for its visualization and targeting in health and disease. *Adv Pharmacol* 2013;68:319–334.
114. Anlauf M, Eissele R, Schafer MK et al. Expression of the two isoforms of the vesicular monoamine transportere (VMAT1 and VMAT2) in the endocrine pancreas and pancreatic endocrine tumors. *J Histochem Cytochem* 2003;51(8): 1027–1040.
115. Gronberg M, Amini RM, Stridsberg M, et al. Neuroendocrine markers are expressed in human mammary glands. *Regul Pept* 2010;160(1–3): 68–74.
116. Sollner T, Bennett MK, Whiteheart SW, et al. A protein assembly–disassembly pathway in vitro that may correspond

117. to sequential steps of synaptic vesicle docking, activation and fusion. *Cell* 1993;75(3):409–418.
117. Elferink LA, Scheller RH. Synaptic vesicle proteins and regulated exocytosis. *J Cell Sci Suppl* 1993;17:75–79.
118. Rizo J, Xu J. The synaptic vesicle release machinery. *Ann Rev Biophys* 2015;44:339–367.
119. Wickner W, Rizo J. A cascade of multiple proteins and lipids catalyzes membrane fusion. *Mol Biol of Cell* 2017;28(6):707–711.
120. Regazzi R, Wolheim CB, Lang J, et al. VAMP2 and cellubrevin are expressed in pancreatic beta cells and are essential for Ca(2+) but not for GTP gamma S-induced insulin secretion. *EMBO J* 1995;14(12):2723–2730.
121. Braun JE, Fritz BA, Wong SM, et al. Identification of a vesicle associated membrane protein (VAMP)-like membrane protein in zymogen granules of the rat exocrine pancreas. *J Biol Chem* 1994;269(7):5328–5335.
122. Moghadam PK, Jackson MB. The functional significance of synaptotagmin diversity in neuroendocrine secretion. *Front Endocrinol (Laussane)* 2013;18:124.
123. Brown H, Meister B, Deeney J, et al. Synaptotagmin III isoform is compartmentalized in pancreatic beta cells and has a functional role in exocytosis. *Diabetes* 2000;49(3):383–391.
124. Tahara S, Sanno N, Teramoto A, et al. Expression of Rab3, a Ras-related GTP-binding protein in human non tumorous pituitaries and pituitary adenomas. *Mod Pathol* 1999;12(6):627–634.
125. Rotondo F, Scheithauer BW, Kovacs K, et al. Rab3B immunoexpression in human pituitary adenomas. *Appl Immunohistochem Mol Morphol* 2009;17(3):185–188.
126. Matsuno A, Mizutani A, Okinaga H, et al. Functional molecular morphology of anterior pituitary cells, from hormone production to intracellular transport and secretion. *Med Mol Morphol* 2011;44(2):63–70.
127. Majo G, Ferrer I, Marsal J, et al. Immunocytochemical analysis of the synaptic proteins SNAP-25 and Rab3A in human pituitary adenomas. Overexpression of SNAP-25 in the mammosomatotroph lineages. *J Pathol* 1997;183(4):440–446.
128. Nishioka H, Haraoka J. Significance of immunohistochemical expression of Rab3B and SNAP-25 in growth hormone producing pituitary adenomas. *Acta Neuropathol* 2005;109(6):598–602.
129. Roth D, Burgoyne D. SNAP-25 is present in a SNARE complex in adrenal chromaffin cells. *FEBS Lett* 1994;351(2):207–210.
130. Sadoul K, Lang J, Montecucco C, et al. SNAP-25 is expressed in islets of Langerhans and is involved in insulin release. *J Cell Biol* 1995;128(6):1019–1028.
131. Hocker M, John M, Anagnostopoulos J, et al Molecular dissection of regulated secretory pathways in human enterochromaffin-like cells; an immunohistochemical analysis. *Histochem Cell Biol* 1999;112(3):205–214.
132. Seeger RC, Danon YL, Rayner SA, et al. Definition of thy-1 on human neuroblastoma, glioma, sarcoma and teratoma cells with a monoclonal antibody. *J Immunol* 1982;128(2):983–989.
133. Lipinski M, Braham K, Cailland JM, et al. HNK-1 antibody detects an antigen expressed on neuroectodermal cells. *J Exp Med* 1983;158(5):1775–1780.
134. Tischler AS, Mobtaker H, Mann K, et al. Anti-lymphocyte antibody leu-7 (HNK-1) recognizes a constituent of neuroendocrine granule matrix. *J Histochem Cytochem* 1986;34(9):1213–1216.
135. Lloyd RV, Blaivas M, Wilson BS. Distribution of chromogranin and S100 protein in normal and abnormal adrenal medullary tissue. *Arch Pathol Lab Med* 1985;109(7):633–635.
136. Heitz PU, Roth J, Zuber C, et al. Markers for neural and endocrine cells in pathology. In: Gratzl M, Langley K, eds. *Markers for Neural and Endocrine Cells. Molecular and Cell Biology, Diagnostic Applications*. Weinheim, Germany: VCH; 1991: 203–215.
137. Jin L, Hemperly JJ, Lloyd RV. Expression of neural cell adhesion molecule in normal and neoplastic human neuroendocrine tissues. *Am J Pathol* 1991;138(4):961–969.
138. Komminoth P, Roth J, Saremaslani P, et al. Polysialic acid of the neural cell adhesion molecule in the human thyroid: A marker for medullary thyroid carcinoma and primary C cell hyperplasia: An immunohistochemical study on 79 thyroid lesions. *Am J Surg Pathol* 1994;18(4):399–411.
139. Jiang SX, Kameya T, Asamura H, et al. hASH1 expression is closely correlated with endocrine phenotype and differentiation extent in pulmonary neuroendocrine tumors. *Mod Pathol* 2004;17(2):222–229.
140. Altree-Tacha D, Tyrrell J, Li F. mASH1 is highly specific for neuroendocrine carcinomas: An immunohistochemical evaluation on normal and various neoplastic tissues. *Arch Pathol Lab Med* 2017;141(2):288–292.
141. Nonaka D. A study of FoxA1 expression in thyroid tumors. *Hum Pathol* 2017;65:217–224.
142. Rosenbaum JN, Guo Z, Baus RM, et al. INSM1 A novel immunohistochemical and molecular marker for neuroendocrine and neuroepithelial neoplasms. *Am J Clin Pathol* 2015;144(4):579–591.
143. Warneboldt J, Haller F, Horstmann O, et al. Histone H1x is expressed in human neuroendocrine cells and tumours. *BMC Cancer* 2008;8:388–407.
144. Graham RP, Shrestha B, Caron BL, et al. Islet-1 is a sensitive but not entirely specific marker for pancreatic neuroendocrine neoplasms and their metastases. *Am J Surg Pathol* 2013;37(3):399–405.
145. LaRosa S, Rigoli E, Uccella S, et al. CDX2 as a marker of intestinal EC-cells and related well differentiated endocrine tumors. *Virchows Arch* 2004;445(3):248–254.
146. Hosgor M, Ijzendoorn Y, Mooi WJ, et al. Thyroid transcription factor-1 expression during normal human lung development and in patients with congenital diaphragmatic hernia. *J Pediatr Surg* 2002;37(9):1258–1262.
147. LaRosa S, Chiaravalli AM, Placidi C, et al. TTF1 expression in normal lung neuroendocrine cells and related tumors: Immunohistochemical study comparing two different monoclonal antibodies. *Virchows Arch* 2010;457(4):497–507.
148. Miskovic J, Brekalo Z, Vukojevic K, et al. Co-expression of TTF-1 and neuroendocrine markers in the human fetal lung and pulmonary neuroendocrine tumors. *Act Hisochem* 2015;117(4–5):451–459.
149. Lloyd RV, Osamura RY. Transcription factors in normal and neoplastic pituitary tissues. *Microsc Res Tech* 1997;39(2):168–181.
150. Asa SL. *Tumors of the Pituitary Gland. AFIP Atlas of Tumor Pathology, Fourth Series Fascicle 15.* American Registry of Pathology in collaboration with the Armed Forces Institute of Pathology. Washington, DC: 2011.
151. Asa SL, Mete O. What's new in pituitary pathology? *Histopathol* 2018;72(1):133–141.

152. Ikeda Y, Lala DS, Luo X, et al. Chartacterization of the mouse FTZ-F1 gene, which encodes a key regulator of steroid hydroxylase gene expression. *Mol Endocrinol* 1993; 7(7):852–860.
153. Reubi JC. Somatostatin and other peptide receptors as tools for tumor diagnosis and treatment. *Neuroendocrinology* 2004;80(Suppl 1):51–56.
154. Fani M, Nicolas GP, Wild D. Somatostatin receptor antagonists for imaging and therapy. *J Nucl Med* 2017;58 (Suppl 2): 61S–66S.
155. Gugger M, Wasser B, Kappeler A, et al. Immunohistochemical localization of somatostatin receptor sst2A in human gut and lung tissue. Possible implications for physiology and carcinogenesis. *Ann NY Acad Sci* 2004;1014:132–136.
156. Unger N, Ueberberg B, Schulz S, et al. Differential expression of somatostatin receptor subtype 1–5 proteins in numerous human normal tissues. *Exp Clin Endocrinol Diabetes* 2012;120(8):482–489.
157. Bensch KG, Gordon GB, Miller LR. Studies on the bronchial counterpart of the Kultschitzky (argentaffin) cells and innervation of the bronchial glands. *J Ultrastruct Res* 1965; 12(5):668–686.
158. Cutz E. Neuroendocrine cells of the lung. An overview of morphologic characteristics and development. *Exp Lung Res* 1982;3(3–4):185–208.
159. Lauweryns JM, Peuskens JC. Neuroepithelial bodies (neuroreceptor or secretion organs?) in human infant bronchial and bronchiolar epithelium. *Anat Rec* 1972;172(3):471–481.
160. Cutz E. Hyperplasia of pulmonary neuroendocrine cells in infancy and childhood. *Sem Diagn Pathol* 2015;32(6): 420–437.
161. Pesce C, Tobia-Gallelli F, Toncini C. APUD cells of the larynx. *Acta Otolaryngol* 1984;98(1–2):158–162.
162. Torre-Rendon FE, Cisneros-Bernal E, Ochoa-Salas JA. Carcinoma indifferenciadio de cellular pequenas de la laringe. *Patologica* 1979;17:47–57.
163. Chung JH, Lee SS, Shim YS, et al. A study of moderately differentiated neuroendocrine carcinomas of the larynx and an examination of non-neoplastic larynx tissue for neuroendocrine cells. *Laryngoscope* 2004;114(7):1264–1270.
164. Hirsch M, Faqquin WC, Krane JF. Thryoid transcription factor-1, but not p53, is helpful in distinguishing moderately differentiated neuroendocrine carcinoma of the larynx from medullary carcinoma of the thyroid. *Mod Pathol* 2004; 17(6):631–636.
165. DeLellis RA, Wolfe HJ. The pathobiology of the human calcitonin (C)-cell. A review. *Pathol Annu* 1981;16(Pt 2):25–52.
166. DeLellis RA, Nunnemacher G, Wolfe HJ. C-cell hyperplasia: An ultrastructural analysis. *Lab Invest* 1977;36(3):237–248.
167. DeLellis RA, May L, Tashjian AH Jr, et al. C-cell granule heterogeneity in man. An ultrastructural immunocytochemical study. *Lab Invest* 1978;38(3):263–269.
168. Bearman RM, Levine GD, Bensch KG. The ultrastructure of the normal human thymus. A study of 36 cases. *Anat Rec* 1978;190(3):755–781.
169. Varga I, Mikusova R, Pospislova V, et al. Morphologic heterogeneity of human thymic non-lymphocytic cells. *Neuro Endocrine Lett* 2009;30(3):275–283.
170. Gould VE, Moll R, Moll I, et al. Neuroendocrine (Merkel) cells of the skin: Hyperplasias, dysplasias and neoplasms. *Lab Invest* 1985;52(4):334–353.
171. Munde PB, Khandekar S, Dive AM, et al. Pathophysiology of the Merkel cell. *J Oral Maxillofac Pathol* 2013;17(3): 408–412,.172.
172. Eispert AC, Fuchs F, Brandner JM, et al. Evidence for distinct populations of Merkel cells. *Histochem Cell Biol* 2009; 132(1):83–93.
173. Tachibana T, Nawa T. Immunohistochemical reactions of receptors to met-enkephalin, VIP, substance P, and CGRP located on Merkel cells in the rat sinus hair follicle. *Arch Histol Cytol* 2005;68(5):383–391.
174. Bussolati G, Gugliotta P, Sapino A, et al. Chromogranin reactive endocrine cells in argyrophilic carcinomas (carcinoids) and normal tissue of the breast. *Am J Pathol* 1985;120(2): 186–192.
175. Gunawardene AR, Corfe BM, Staton CA. Classification and functions of enteroendocrine cells of the lower gaqstrointestinal tract. *Int J Exp Path* 2011;92(4):219–231.
176. Fetissof F, Dubois MP, Arbeille-Brassart B, et al. Endocrine cells in the prostate gland, urothelium and Brenner tumors. Immunohistological and ultrastructural studies. *Virchows Arch B Cell Pathol Incl Mol Pathol* 1985;42(1):53–64.
177. di Sant'Agnese PA, De Mesy, Jensen KL. Endocrine paracrine cells of the prostate and prostatic urethra. An ultrastructural study. *Hum Pathol* 1984;15(11):1034–1041.
178. di Sant'Agnese PA, de Mesy, Jensen KL. Somatostatin and/or somatostatin-like immunoreactive endocrine–paracrine cells in the human prostate gland. *Arch Pathol Lab Med* 1984; 108(9):693–696.
179. di Sant'Agnese PA. Calcitonin-like immunoreactive and bombesin-like immunoreactive endocrine paracrine cells of the human prostate. *Arch Pathol Lab Med* 1986;110(5): 412–415.
180. Santamaria L, Martin R, Martgin JJ, et al. Stereologic estimation of the number of neuroendocrine cells in normal human prostate detected by immunohistochemistry. *Appl Immunohistochem Mol Morphol* 2001;10(3):275–281.
181. Scully RE, Aguirre P, DeLellis RA. Argyrophilia, serotonin and peptide hormones in the female genital tract and its tumors. *Int Rev Gynecol Pathol* 1984;3(1):51–70.
182. Sun YK, Xi YP, Fenoglio CM, et al. The effect of age on the number of pituitary cells immunoreactive to growth hormone and prolactin. *Hum Pathol* 1984;15(2):169–180.
183. Zegarelli-Schmidt E, Yu XR, Fenoglio-Preiser C, et al. Endocrine changes associated with the human aging process: II. Effect of age on the number and size of thyrotropin immunoreactive cells in the human pituitary. *Hum Pathol* 1985;16(3): 277–286.
184. O'Toole K, Fenoglio-Preiser C, Pushparaj N. Endocrine changes associated with the human aging process: III. Effect of age on the number of calcitonin immunoreactive cells in the thyroid gland. *Hum Pathol* 1985;16(10):991–1000.
185. Guyetant S, Rousselet MC, Durigon M, et al. Sex-related C-cell hyperplasia in the normal human thyroid: A quantitative autopsy study. *J Clin Endocrinol Metab* 1997;82(1): 42–47.
186. Gibson WG, Peng TC, Croker BP. Age associated C-cell hyperplasia in the human thyroid. *Am J Pathol* 1982:106(3): 388–393.
187. Gibson WC, Peng TC, Croker BP. C-cell nodules in adult human thyroid. A common autopsy finding. *Am J Clin Pathol* 1981;75(3):347–350.

188. Algaba F, Trias I, Lopez L, et al. Neuroendocrine cells in peripheral prostatic zone: Age, prostatic intraepithelial neoplasia and latent cancer related changes. *Euro Urol* 1995; 27(4):329–333.
189. Rumpold H, Heinrich E, Untergasser G, et al. Neuroendocrine differentiation of human prostatic primary epithelial cells in vitro. *Prostate* 2002;53(2):101–108.
190. Gosney JR. Neuroendocrine cell populations in postnatal human lungs: Minimal variation from childhood to old age. *Anat Rec* 1993;236(1):177–180.
191. Kvetnoy I, Popuichiev V, Mikhina L, et al. Gut neuroendocrine cells: Relationships to the proliferative activity and apoptosis of mucous epitheliocytes in aging. *Neuro Endocrinol Lett* 2001; 22(5):337–341.
192. Trofimov AV, Sevostianova NN, Linkova NS, et al. *Bull Exp Biol Med* 2011;150(6):735–738.
193. DeLellis RA, Wolfe HJ. Analysis of gene expression in endocrine cells. In: Fenoglio-Preiser CM, Wilman CL, eds. *Molecular Diagnostic in Pathology*. Baltimore, MD: Williams & Wilkins; 1991: 299–322.
194. Lloyd RV. Introduction to molecular endocrine pathology. *Endocr Pathol* 1993;4:64–78.
195. Speel EJ, Ramaekers FC, Hopman AH. Cytochemical detection systems for in situ hybridization and the combination with immunohistochemistry. "Who is still afraid of red, green and blue?" *Histochem J* 1995;27(11):833–858.
196. Komminoth P, Long AA. In situ polymerase chain reaction. An overview of methods, applications and limitations of a new molecular technique. *Virchows Arch B Cell Pathol Incl Mol Pathol* 1993;64:67–73.
197. Komminoth P, Long AA. In situ polymerase chain reaction and its application to the study of endocrine diseases. *Endocr Pathol* 1995;6:167–171.
198. Sällström JF, Alemi M, Spets H, et al. Nonspecific amplification in in situ PCR by direct incorporation of reporter molecules. *Cell Vision* 1994;1:243–251.
199. Nuovo G. *PCR In Situ Hybridization*. New York: Raven Press; 1992.
200. Taylor CR, Cote RJ. *Immunomicroscopy: A Diagnostic Tool for the Surgical Pathologist*. 2nd ed. Philadelphia, PA: WB Saunders; 1994: 23–28.
201. Grube D. Immunoreactivities of gastric (G-) cells. II. Nonspecific binding of immunoglobulins to G cells by ionic interactions. *Histochemistry* 1980;66(2):149–167.
202. Bussolati G, Gugliotta P, Volante M, et al. Retrieved endogenous biotin: a novel marker and potential pitfall in diagnostic immunohistochemistry. *Histopathology* 1997;31(5):400–407.
203. Srivastava A, Tischler AS, DeLellis RA. Endogenous biotin staining as an artifact of antigen retrieval with automated immunostaining. *Endocr Pathol* 2004;15(2):175–177.
204. Pagani A, Cerrato M, Bussolati G. Nonspecific in situ hybridization reaction in neuroendocrine cells and tumors of the gastrointestinal tract using oligonucleotide probes. *Diagn Mol Pathol* 1993;2(2):125–130.
205. Kendall PA, Polak JM, Pearse AG. Carbodiimide fixation for immunohistochemistry. Observations on the fixation of polypeptide hormones. *Experimentia* 1971;27(9):1104–1106.
206. King JC, Lechan RM, Kugel G, et al. Acrolein: A fixative for immunohistochemical localization of peptides in the central nervous system. *J Histochem Cytochem* 1983;31(1):62–68.
207. Pearse AG, Polak JM, Adams C, et al. Diethyl pyrocarbonate, a vapor phase fixative for immunofluorescence studies on polypeptide hormones. *Histochem J* 1974;6(3):347–352.
208. Pearse AG, Polak JM. Bifunctional reagent as vapor and liquid phase fixatives for immunohistochemistry. *Histochem J* 1975;7(2):179–186.

47

Paraganglia

Arthur S. Tischler ■ Sylvia L. Asa

HISTORY AND NOMENCLATURE 1274	ULTRASTRUCTURE 1283
SYMPATHETIC VERSUS PARASYMPATHETIC PARAGANGLIA: A CLINICOPATHOLOGIC PERSPECTIVE 1275	FUNCTION 1284
	Physiologic Roles 1284
	Secretory Products 1286
DISTRIBUTION OF PARAGANGLIA 1276	GENDER DIFFERENCES 1286
EMBRYOLOGY 1278	AGING CHANGES 1286
POSTNATAL AND DEVELOPMENTAL CHANGES 1280	SPECIAL PROCEDURES 1286
PHENOTYPIC PLASTICITY 1280	Immunohistochemistry 1286
GROSS FEATURES AND ORGAN WEIGHTS 1281	Immunohistochemical Artifacts 1290
	Other Special Procedures 1291
ANATOMY 1281	DIFFERENTIAL DIAGNOSIS 1291
LIGHT MICROSCOPY 1281	ACKNOWLEDGMENTS 1291
Cell Types 1281	REFERENCES 1291
Lobular Architecture of the Carotid Body 1282	

Paraganglia are anatomically dispersed neuroendocrine organs associated with the autonomic nervous system and characterized by morphologically and cytochemically similar neurosecretory cells derived from neural crest precursors. For many physiologic and pathophysiologic purposes, they may be considered to comprise two groups, associated with either sympathetic or parasympathetic nerves. Sympathetic paraganglia are distributed along the prevertebral and paravertebral sympathetic chains and along sympathetic nerve branches that innervate the organs of the pelvis and retroperitoneum. The adrenal medulla is the most extensively studied and best understood example of sympathetic paraganglia. Parasympathetic paraganglia are predominantly distributed along cervical and thoracic branches of the glossopharyngeal and vagus nerves. The prototypical parasympathetic paraganglion is the carotid body.

This chapter is an update of a previous version authored by Arthur S. Tischler.

HISTORY AND NOMENCLATURE

The interesting and controversial history of the paraganglia is addressed in detail in several excellent reviews (1–4). The concept of a unitary paraganglionic system was first proposed by Alfred Kohn at the beginning of the 20th century (5). Several earlier investigators had developed histochemical reactions demonstrating that the adrenal medulla contained substances chemically different from those in the adrenal cortex. The reaction that proved most significant from a historical perspective, development of brown coloration in the presence of chromate salts, was apparently first discovered by Bertholdus Werner in 1857 (3). Kohn coined the terms "chromaffin reaction" for the color change and "chromaffin cells" for the reactive cells, which he described in several extra-adrenal locations in the retroperitoneum. He further noted that some cells in the carotid body exhibited a chromaffin reaction, confirming an earlier report by

Stilling (3). Kohn believed that the reactive carotid body cells were derived from precursors of sympathetic ganglia and were innervated by sympathetic axons, and he suggested that they were, therefore, embryologically, histochemically, and functionally comparable to retroperitoneal chromaffin cells. He proposed a new term to encompass all the tissues composed of cells that were analogous to neurons, but not neuronal: "Since the chromaffin tissue complexes form ganglion-like bodies, since their elements are derived from ganglion anlagen, since they are connected to the sympathetic nervous system and still are not genuine ganglia, I have called them paraganglia" (5) (translated from German by Dr. Miguel Stadecker).

Obstacles to acceptance of Kohn's concept soon arose from DeCastro's finding that the innervation of the carotid body is primarily derived from the glossopharyngeal nerve (4) and from observations by many investigators that carotid body cells are usually nonchromaffin. Consequently, Watzka (4) divided the paraganglion system into chromaffin and nonchromaffin paraganglia, associated respectively with the sympathetic or parasympathetic nervous systems, and paraganglia of mixed type. Discovery of the chemoreceptor function of the carotid bodies created further difficulties because it implied that the nonchromaffin paraganglia served physiologically in a sensory role, in contrast to the endocrine function of the adrenal medulla. The suggestion was, therefore, made by Kjaergaard that the parasympathetic paraganglia be referred to by the term "chemodecton" (from the Greek *dechesthai*, to receive) (6). This name was never widely accepted, despite the earlier application by Mulligan of its counterpart, "chemodectoma," to paraganglionic tumors (4).

An additional synonym for the parasympathetic paraganglia is "glomus" (from the Latin *glomus*, ball). This term is a vestige of a 19th-century hypothesis that the carotid body is of vascular origin (4). Although it aptly describes the microscopic *Zellballen* characteristic of paraganglia, it has caused confusion because it is also applied to thermoregulatory structures in the skin and other locations (e.g., glomera cutanea and glomus coccygeum) and to their corresponding tumors (glomus tumors or glomangiomas). Those structures are modified arteriovenous anastomoses unrelated to paraganglia developmentally or functionally (7).

It is now possible to return to a unitary concept of paraganglia with a synthesis of new and old information. Paraganglia are composed of a very similar basic type of neuroendocrine cell that may be used differently in different anatomic locations (8). All of these cells are probably derived from neural crest precursors (9), although the origin of those precursors now seems not as straightforward as previously believed (10). All produce catecholamines detectable by more sensitive methods than the chromaffin reaction, and all express multiple additional neuroendocrine markers, including both generic markers and regulatory peptides (11). Further, chemosensory properties previously considered specific to parasympathetic paraganglia have also been documented in cells derived from sympathetic paraganglia (12). The term "paraganglion" connotes a constellation of generic characteristics of this type of cell without being dependent on a single histochemical reaction. Because it was intended by Kohn to imply analogy, rather than merely proximity, to autonomic ganglia, it continues in this context to be both conceptually helpful and literally correct.

While the chromaffin reaction is now obsolete as a basis for classification of paraganglia, reference to the reaction persists for historical reasons. "Chromaffin cell" is the name generally accepted for the neuroendocrine cells of the normal adrenal medulla and sometimes still applied to their extra-adrenal counterparts associated with the sympathetic nervous system. Similarly, "pheochromocytoma" (from the Greek *phaios*, dusky + *chroma*, color), refers to the color change imparted by the chromaffin reaction. The current World Health Organization classification of endocrine tumors reserves the term pheochromocytoma for intra-adrenal sympathetic paragangliomas. By arbitrary convention, even functionally similar extra-adrenal tumors are classified as paragangliomas (13,14).

SYMPATHETIC VERSUS PARASYMPATHETIC PARAGANGLIA: A CLINICOPATHOLOGIC PERSPECTIVE

Sympathetic and parasympathetic paraganglia differ from a clinicopathologic standpoint despite their similarities at the cellular level. This contrast might result from pre-programming or differences in the type, timing, or intensity of signals to which the two classes of paraganglia are exposed during development or in adult life.

The only pathologic changes known to be clinically important in paraganglia are hyperplasia and neoplasia. Several generalizations concerning these proliferative lesions underscore the differences between sympathetic and parasympathetic paraganglia. Although normal paraganglia of both types can produce catecholamines, proliferative lesions that produce sufficient quantities of catecholamines to cause clinical signs and symptoms usually arise in sympathetic paraganglia, and lesions that produce significant amounts of epinephrine are almost invariably in the adrenal medulla. Dopamine excess is present in a considerable percentage of patients with clinically silent parasympathetic paragangliomas in the head and neck (15). In addition, sympathetic paraganglia give rise to both neuronal tumors (neuroblastomas, ganglioneuroblastomas, and ganglioneuromas) and paragangliomas, while parasympathetic paraganglia give rise only to paragangliomas. Lesions that occur in patients with prolonged hypoxemia or hypercapnia almost invariably arise in parasympathetic paraganglia. The precise developmental basis for these differences is unclear.

Despite the differences in the contexts in which they arise, sympathetic and parasympathetic paragangliomas strongly resemble each other microscopically and are often indistinguishable. They also exhibit a widely overlapping range of secretory products and other neuroendocrine markers, reflecting the similarities of the neuroendocrine cells that are their normal counterparts. A morphologic foundation for the study of paraganglionic pathology, therefore, requires familiarity with both systemic differences and cellular similarities.

A need for deeper understanding of the differences between normal paraganglia in different locations has become apparent as a result of advances in the study of hereditary pheochromocytomas and extra-adrenal paragangliomas. Germline mutations of at least 19 genes are now known to lead to the development of these tumors (16,17) and more than 40% of pheochromocytomas and paragangliomas (PCC/PGLs) are associated with inherited cancer susceptibility syndromes, the highest among all tumor types (17). The major hereditary disorders are multiple endocrine neoplasia 2A and 2B (MEN2A, MEN2B), von Hippel–Lindau (VHL) disease, neurofibromatosis type 1 (NF1), and familial paraganglioma syndromes caused by mutations of genes encoding subunits of succinate dehydrogenase (*SDHA, SDHB, SDHD, SDHC*). Rarer syndromes are caused by mutations in transmembrane protein 127 (*TMEM127*), fumarate hydratase (*FH*), the tumor suppressor MYC-associated factor X (*MAX*) gene, hypoxia-inducible factor 2 alpha (*HIF2A* or *EPAS1*), prolyl hydroxylase (*PHD1*), and *EGLN1* (formerly known as *PHD2*), and the Succinate Dehydrogenase Assembly Factors (*SDHAF1, SDHAF2*) (18). Tumors that arise in each of the familial syndromes show distinctive distribution, function, and metastatic potential (18). For example, VHL tumors are usually noradrenergic even when intra-adrenal, while MEN2 and NF1 tumors in the adrenal typically produce both epinephrine and norepinephrine (19). Pheochromocytomas in patients with MEN2 often arise in a background of adrenal medullary hyperplasia, but hyperplasia usually does not occur in the other syndromes. Pheochromocytomas and paragangliomas metastasize infrequently except for those with *SDHB* mutations, where the metastasis rate is 30% to 50%. Corresponding to these phenotype differences, transcriptional and proteomic analyses show different clusters of markers in tumors with specific genetic backgrounds (20,21). A "transcription signature" associated with *VHL* or *SDH* mutations shows increased activity of hypoxia-driven signaling pathways, while the signatures of tumors with *RET* or *NF1* mutations suggest increased activity of the RAS-mediated MAPK pathway (21).

Some genotype–phenotype correlations may be accounted for by characteristics of the predominant anatomic sites of tumor origin, for example, the fact that epinephrine production is normally confined to the adrenal medulla where there is an environment rich in adrenal cortical steroids (22). However, the basis for different gene expression clusters in tumors at any given location is for the most part poorly understood. An attractive but speculative theory to account for genotype–phenotype correlations proposes that mutations of different susceptibility genes act at different times in embryogenesis to cause defective "developmental culling" of paraganglionic progenitors that would normally undergo programmed death, and that those surviving cells later give rise to tumors (23). The theory is consistent with the fact that the adrenal medulla matures much later than extra-adrenal paraganglia, potentially providing different developmental windows (23) in which tumorigenic events can occur. Other hypotheses include differential sensitivities to hypoxia (24) and tissue-specific effects of specific mutated genes (25).

DISTRIBUTION OF PARAGANGLIA

Sympathetic paraganglia are found predominantly in the para-axial regions of the trunk along the prevertebral and paravertebral sympathetic chains and in connective tissue in or near the walls of the pelvic organs. In adult humans, they are especially numerous along the fibers of the inferior hypogastric plexuses leading to and entering the urogenital organs, in the wall of the urinary bladder, and among the nerve fibers of the sacral plexus (Fig. 47.1) (26–29). They are not generally known by individual names, and their precise locations are variable. Exceptions are the adrenal medulla and the organ of Zuckerkandl, located at the origin of the inferior mesenteric artery (Figs. 47.1 and 47.2) (30). The distinctive characteristic of the organ of Zuckerkandl is that it is the only extra-adrenal sympathetic paraganglion that is macroscopic. Historically, it is said to have initially been shown to Alfred Kohn as an unusual lymph node by his pupil, Emil Zuckerkandl (4,31). In its most frequent anatomic configuration, it is divided into a set of paired organs (Fig. 47.2), and it is, therefore, often referred to by the plural, "organs of Zuckerkandl" (1). Since its fragmentation and its proximity to numerous smaller paraganglia may make it difficult to identify precisely, some investigators have used the plural to encompass all preaortic paraganglia between the inferior mesenteric artery and the aortic bifurcation (32). This chapter maintains the traditional, more specific, macroscopic usage.

Neuroendocrine cells are present both within and adjacent to the ganglia of human sympathetic chains. The former have been referred to in neurobiology literature as small intensely fluorescent (SIF) cells (33), intraganglionic chromaffin cells (34), or small granule-containing (SGC) cells (35), depending on the particular technique used to detect them. In pathology literature, SIF cells are often regarded as intraganglionic paraganglia (36). In anatomy literature, on the other hand, some investigators reserve the term "paraganglia" for extraganglionic sites (33).

In contrast to sympathetic paraganglia, their parasympathetic counterparts are distributed almost exclusively along

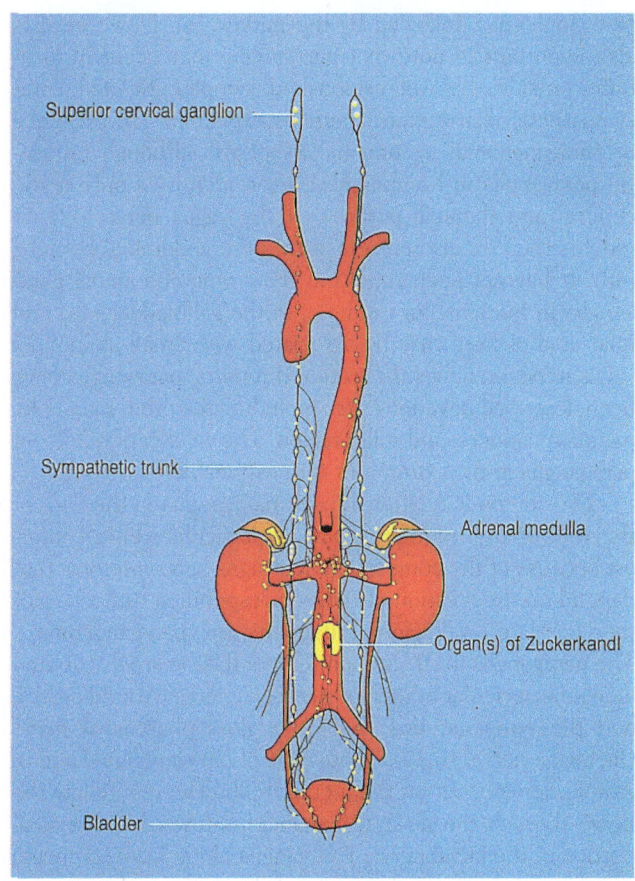

FIGURE 47.1 The distribution of sympathetic paraganglia in the human fetus. Adapted from Coupland RE. *The Natural History of the Chromaffin Cell*. London: Longmans Green; 1965; Glenner GG, Grimley PM. *Tumors of the Extra-adrenal Paraganglion System (Including Chemoreceptors)*. Washington, DC: Armed Forces Institute of Pathology; 1974.

the cranial and thoracic branches of the glossopharyngeal and vagus nerves (Fig. 47.3). With the exception of the carotid bodies, which are located between the carotid arteries just above the carotid bifurcation (Fig. 47.4), parasympathetic paraganglia are highly variable in both number and location (4). Their names refer to general locations, rather than to specific structures. The middle ear, for example, contains 0 to 12 jugular and tympanic paraganglia, with an average of 2.8 (37). The principal paraganglia of the glossopharyngeal nerve are the tympanic paraganglia in the wall of the middle ear and the carotid bodies (4,37). Those of the vagus nerve include the jugular paraganglia in the floor of the middle ear (4,37), the superior and inferior laryngeal paraganglia (4,38), and the subclavian and aorticopulmonary or cardioaortic paraganglia near the bases of the great vessels of the heart. They sometimes also may be found in the interatrial septum (39). In addition, "intravagal" paraganglia are located within or adjacent to the vagal trunk in or near the nodose and jugular ganglia (4). These two vagal ganglia are the only sensory ganglia known to contain neuroendocrine cells comparable to the SIF cells of sympathetic ganglia. These cells are described as SIF cells in some publications (40).

Knowledge of the distribution of normal paraganglionic tissue is important because of its value in predicting the sites of origin of paragangliomas. These tumors have been reported at virtually all locations where normal paraganglia are found during fetal or adult life and tend to be most frequent in areas where paraganglionic tissue is most abundant. For example, in early childhood, paraganglionic tissue is largely extra-adrenal (see "Embryology" and "Postnatal and Developmental Changes"). Approximately 30% to 60% of

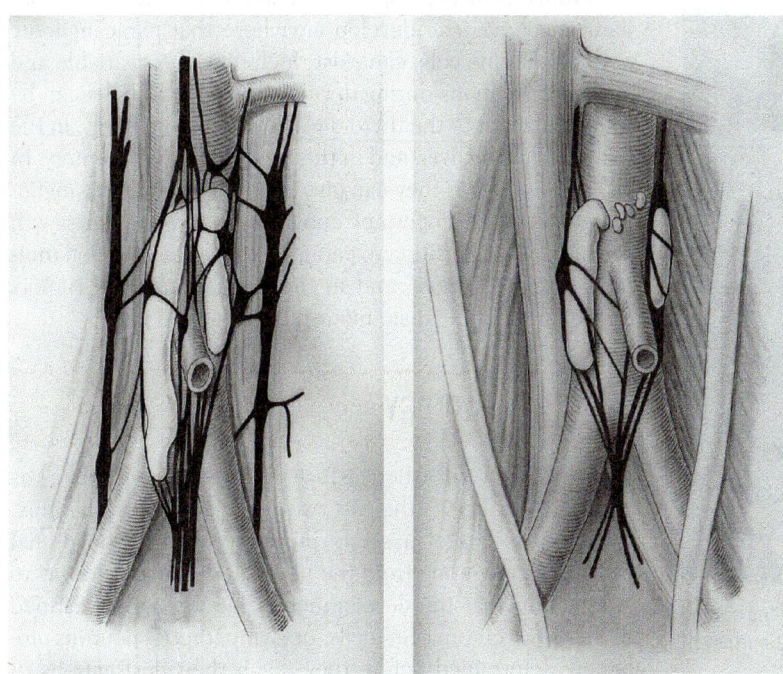

FIGURE 47.2 Modified renditions of original illustrations by Zuckerkandl representing the anatomic structure that bears his name. The bilobed configuration with a fragmented isthmus (*right*) is the most frequent variation. (Courtesy of Dr. E. E. Lack.)

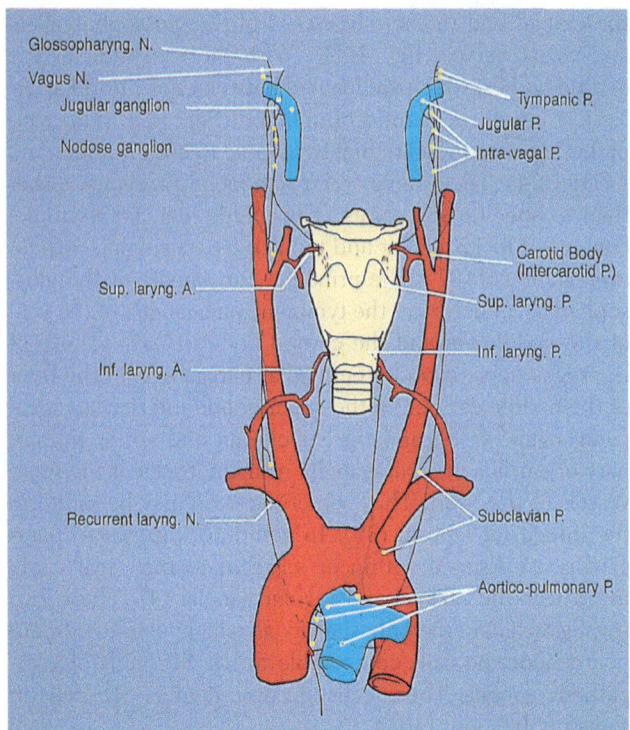

FIGURE 47.3 The distribution of the principal parasympathetic paraganglia. *P*, paraganglion; *A*, artery; *N*, nerve. Adapted from Glenner GG, Grimley PM. *Tumors of the Extra-adrenal Paraganglion System (Including Chemoreceptors)*. Washington, DC: Armed Forces Institute of Pathology; 1974.

paragangliomas in children are also extra-adrenal (41), most frequently arising in the vicinity of the organ of Zuckerkandl, while closer to 10% are extra-adrenal in adults. Similarly, the carotid body is the most frequent site of parasympathetic

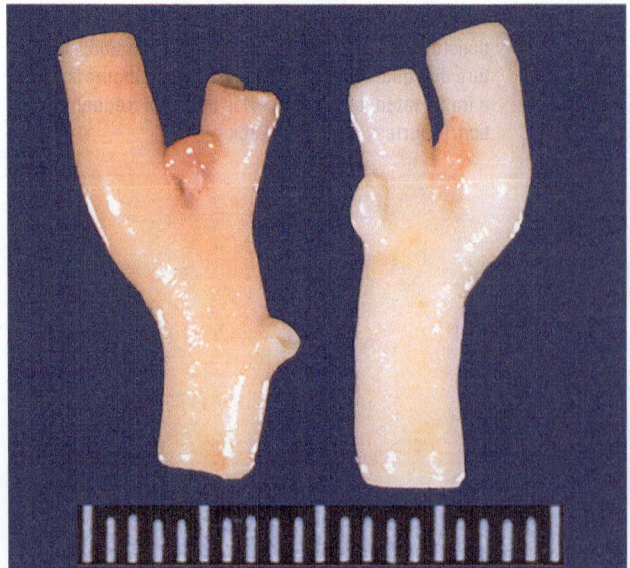

FIGURE 47.4 Gross specimens from a 5-year-old girl, illustrating normal carotid bodies and their relationship to the carotid arteries. (Courtesy of Dr. E. E. Lack.)

paragangliomas, followed by the middle ear. However, it is also important to note that paraganglia may occur in locations outside the well-established sympathetic and parasympathetic distributions, perhaps explaining the existence of paragangliomas in unusual locations. Although intravagal paraganglia in humans have been identified only in the cervical and thoracic portions of the vagus nerve (42), in rodents they are also present within the abdominal portions (43). It has not been ruled out that some abdominal paraganglia in humans, for example, in the gallbladder (44) and hilar area of liver, may be associated with small abdominal vagus nerve branches. In scattered reports, paraganglia have been described in various sites including the orbit, mandible, paranasal sinuses, and sellar region. The validity of reports of paraganglia in the extremities is questionable.

The anatomic relationships of paraganglia in the floor or the wall of the middle ear are of particular clinical interest because of the complex clinical signs and symptoms that depend on the location of their corresponding tumors ("glomus jugulare" and "glomus tympanicum" paragangliomas). The paraganglia in the human temporal bone are distributed along the auricular branch of the vagus nerve (Arnold nerve), and the tympanic branch of the glossopharyngeal nerve (Jacobson nerve) (6,37). About 70% of paraganglia related to Arnold nerve occur on the jugular bulb. The rest follow the nerve through the mastoid canaliculus toward the vertical portion of the facial nerve. Paraganglia along Jacobson nerve occur anywhere from the origin of the nerve at the petrosal ganglion (10%) to the jugular bulb (28%), tympanic canaliculus (40%), promontory of the middle ear (20%), and beyond (2%). Glomus jugulare tumors may, therefore, be associated with either Arnold or Jacobson nerve, although the former is more likely. Glomus tympanicum tumors are almost always associated with Jacobson nerve (4).

From a clinical perspective, a take-home message is that paragangliomas can develop anywhere that paraganglionic neuroendocrine cells can exist, including their variable and transient locations during development. Paraganglia can be found adjacent to the thyroid gland, within the lungs, in the hilar area of the liver, and in the pancreas and mesentery. In all these locations they can give rise to primary paragangliomas. This is an important consideration, as patients with germline predisposition to paragangliomas can develop multiple primary tumors, and in these locations such tumors may be misclassified as "metastatic."

EMBRYOLOGY

Understanding of the histogenesis of paraganglia has changed greatly over the past two decades and is still in flux. The 1970's idea of a single pluripotent sympathoadrenal progenitor migrating from the neural crest first gave way to recognition that the developmental fates of cells destined to become chromaffin cells or sympathetic neurons are largely determined before they reach their destinations in the adrenal gland or ganglia. This concept has now further evolved with the recognition of two largely separate routes of migration.

While sympathetic ganglia are directly derived from neural crest cells that reach their destinations without axonal guidance, new findings suggest that the adrenal medulla originates from a different wave of cells that migrate first to the dorsal root ganglia (DRG). Derivatives of those cells termed "Schwann cell precursors (SCPs)" subsequently migrate along the DRG axons to preganglionic sympathetic axons that have emerged from the spinal cord, and migrate along those axons to the adrenal. In essence, this model posits that adrenal chromaffin cells originate from peripheral glial stem cells, and that peripheral nerves may serve as a stem cell niche (10). It remains to be determined how this will relate to extra-adrenal sympathetic paraganglia, parasympathetic paraganglia, the nature of sustentacular cells (45), and empirical observations including phenotype plasticity and composite tumors that contain both chromaffin cells and neurons.

The new model is consistent with classic anatomic studies showing that some primitive medullary cells appear to penetrate the adrenal cortex along preganglionic nerve fibers (1,46), but may also need to be reconciled with other classic studies reporting that the medulla can form in adrenal primordia from 4- or 5-day chick embryos explanted to chorioallantoic membranes before the onset of innervation (47). It is of interest that early anatomic studies also describe primitive cells apparently migrating to developing parasympathetic paraganglia along branches of the glossopharyngeal and vagus nerves (6). In addition, later histochemical studies suggest an origin of carotid body neuroendocrine cells from the sympathetic progenitors of the superior cervical ganglion (48). These observations, including the "neuronal émigré" hypothesis, are now at least partly supported by modern lineage-tracing techniques showing multiple contributions to carotid body chief cells (49).

During embryogenesis, the paraganglia are first populated by small, primitive cells that include precursors of neuroendocrine, neural, and glial cell lineages in adult paraganglia (49,50,51) (see "Light Microscopy"). They appear to be able to produce some catecholamines at the earliest stages of paraganglionic development (48,51) (see "Function"), and express biomarkers of immature neurons or glia (51) (see "Special Procedures"). They are readily recognized in the paraganglia at about 7 weeks' gestation, although they first arrive somewhat earlier (1), and they are progressively superseded by larger, differentiated, cells. Extra-adrenal sympathetic (1) and parasympathetic (6,48) paraganglia mature cytologically earlier in development than the adrenal medulla. Primitive cells usually disappear from these locations by week 25 but may persist in small numbers in the adrenal medulla until after birth (1) (compare Figs. 47.5 and 47.6).

Classic, descriptive, embryologic studies (46,52) show primitive sympathetic cells in large numbers around the spinal nerves and branches of the developing sympathetic trunks before the formation of the paraganglia, and along the renal and spermatic arteries (46). The adrenal medulla is apparently colonized by invasion of medullary progenitor cells into the cortex through the medial aspect of the capsule (Fig. 47.7). The invading cells initially form nodular aggregates in the cortex (Fig. 47.5) and gradually coalesce around the central vein. They may form rosettes or pseudorosettes early in gestation. Chromaffin cells are identifiable among these aggregates from about week 8 on (1) and

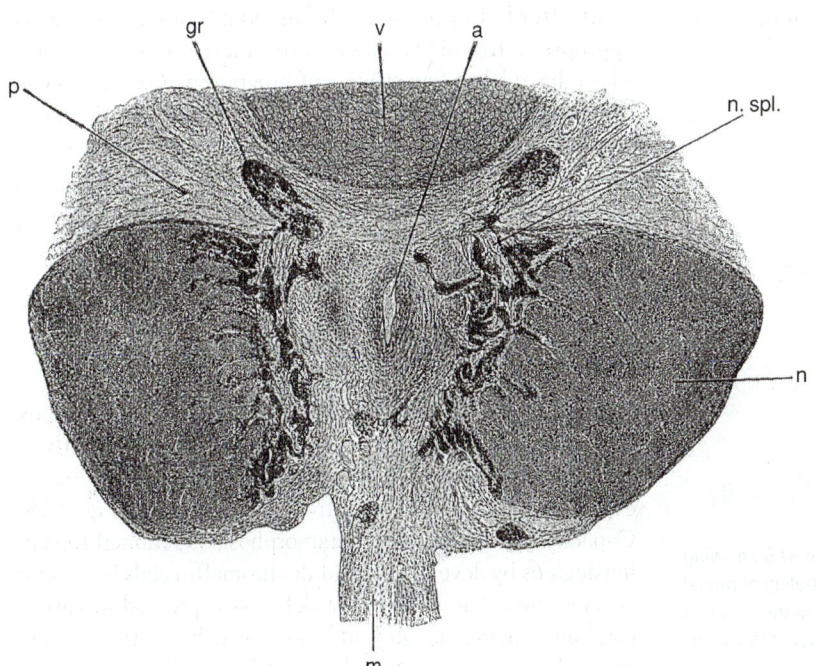

FIGURE 47.5 Original illustration by Zuckerkandl of a transverse section of a human embryo (17 mm crown–heel length) showing presumed migration of primitive sympathetic cells into the adrenal glands. The darkly stippled masses traversed by nerves are the primitive sympathetic cells. *a*, aorta; *gr*, developing sympathetic ganglia; *n. Spl.*, splanchnic nerve; *v*, vertebra; *p*, peritoneal cushion; *m*, mesentery; *n*, adrenals. Reprinted with permission from Zuckerkandl E. The development of the chromaffin organs and of the supra-renal glands. In: Keibel F, Mall FP, eds. *Manual of Human Embryology*. Philadelphia, PA: J B Lippincott; 1912.

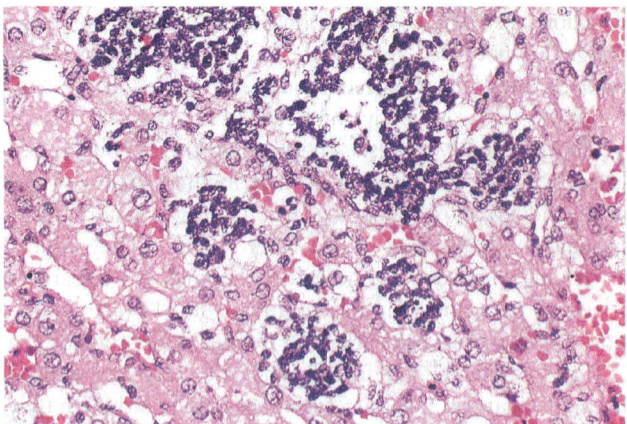

FIGURE 47.6 Section of adrenal gland from a 16-week human fetus showing typical aggregates of primitive sympathetic cells that are precursors of the medulla. Pyknotic nuclei and nuclei with changes consistent with apoptosis are present within the aggregates. Many of the small cells express immunoreactive TH, the rate-limiting enzyme in catecholamine synthesis, but do not stain for CgA or synaptophysin, which are characteristic of larger, mature or maturing chromaffin cells (39). Scattered S100-positive cells consistent with the sustentacular cell lineage are observed at about week 20 (38). From Dahlqvist A, Carlsoo B, Hellstrom S. Paraganglia of the human recurrent laryngeal nerve. *Am J Otolaryngol* 1986;7(5):366–369

gradually increase in number. The centripetal pattern of migration may result in subcapsular and intracortical chromaffin cell rests.

Nodular aggregates of primitive medullary cells, up to 400 μm in greatest dimension, can be demonstrated in the adrenal glands of all human fetuses between the ages of 10 and 30 weeks if the glands are thoroughly sectioned (52). Aggregates with a diameter of over 1 mm may occasionally be observed (52). Nerve fibers may connect intra- and extra-adrenal aggregates (53). The nodules peak in size and number between the ages of 17 and 20 weeks and then decline. Intranodular cystic degeneration is common from the age of 20 weeks onward (53). Occasional postnatal persistence of the nodules, apparently first described by Wiesel in 1902, may account for some erroneous diagnoses of "in situ neuroblastoma" half a century later (53–55) (see "Differential Diagnosis").

POSTNATAL AND DEVELOPMENTAL CHANGES

The amount or distribution of paraganglionic tissue is known to change during development and aging. Sympathetic paraganglionic tissue in fetuses and neonates is primarily extra-adrenal, with the greatest volume in the organ of Zuckerkandl. The organ of Zuckerkandl develops maximally in humans by the age of about 3 years, when its greatest dimension may be more than 20 mm. Thereafter, the organ involutes (1,29,56) while the adrenal medulla enlarges until maturity. Similarly, SIF cells are present in all human sympathetic ganglia at birth but are rare in adults (1). Parasympathetic paraganglionic tissue also appears to decrease in some locations and to increase in others. Subclavian and intrapulmonary paraganglia, for example, have been identified as prominent in human fetuses but not in adults (4), while the number of jugular and tympanic paraganglia apparently increases after birth (37). The carotid bodies, which are the only parasympathetic paraganglia that are macroscopic, increase in size between infancy and adult life, when they are normally about 3 mm in greatest dimension (4) (Fig. 47.4).

The mechanisms involved in developmental remodeling of the paraganglionic system may hold a number of clues to the pathobiology of paraganglionic tumors. It is generally accepted that apoptosis plays a critical role in the development of both the central and peripheral nervous systems, where excess neural progenitor cells undergo apoptotic death after failing to establish functional contacts or receive appropriate trophic substances from target tissues (57,58). There have been few studies of programmed death specifically focused on the paraganglia. However, apoptotic bodies can be identified within the aggregates of primitive sympathetic cells in the adrenal medulla (Figs. 47.6 and 47.7). Autophagy may be involved is the involution of the Organ of Zuckerkandl (56).

PHENOTYPIC PLASTICITY

Adult human adrenal chromaffin cells are able to "transdifferentiate" into cells closely resembling sympathetic neurons when removed from their in vivo environment and exposed to appropriate neurotrophic signals (59) (Fig. 47.8). Capacity to undergo this metamorphosis is retained to varying degrees by developing or adult chromaffin cells from other species (60). The extent to which it is expressed in various extra-adrenal paraganglia, and its relationship to the development of composite tumors, have not been fully explored.

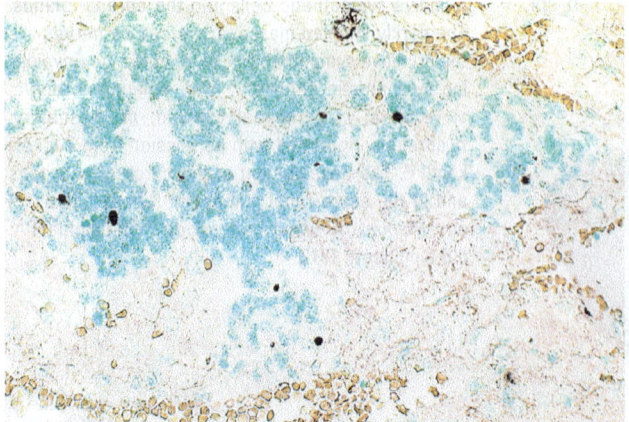

FIGURE 47.7 Section of the same adrenal as in Figure 47.6 showing terminal deoxynucleotidyl transferase–mediated end-labeling of nuclei within a neuroblastic aggregate (black nuclei). This method, which detects fragmented DNA, can be helpful in locating apoptotic cells. (Courtesy of Dr. Salvador Diaz-Cano.)

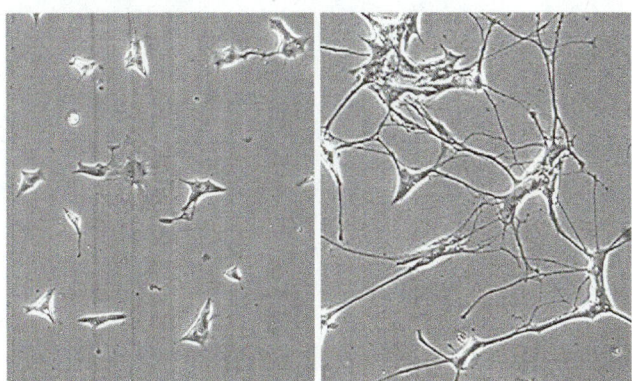

FIGURE 47.8 Phenotypic plasticity of normal adult human adrenal chromaffin cells demonstrated by acquisition of neuron-like morphology in cell culture. Cells at left were maintained in control medium for 2 weeks and those at right were in medium supplemented with nerve growth factor (50). (Courtesy of Dr. James F. Powers.) Capacity to undergo this "trans-differentiation" is exhibited to varying degrees by chromaffin cells from other species and from other normal or neoplastic paraganglia (51).

A somewhat different type of plasticity has been ascribed to sustentacular cells, which are reported to be the progenitors of newly derived chief cells in hypoxia-induced carotid body hyperplasia (45).

GROSS FEATURES AND ORGAN WEIGHTS

The paraganglionic tissue of the grossly identifiable paraganglia is gray or gray-pink. Recognition of this feature is particularly important in the adrenal gland because the medulla is normally confined to the head and body of the gland but extends into the tail and alae in adrenal medullary hyperplasia (61,62). An accurate gross examination requires that the brown tissue of the cortical zona reticularis not be misidentified as medulla.

Because of the anatomic variability of the microscopic paraganglia and the organ of Zuckerkandl, meaningful weights can be ascribed only to the adrenal medulla and carotid bodies. Extensive morphometric studies (61,63) have shown that the neonatal adrenal medulla accounts for approximately 0.4% of the total volume of the gland and weighs approximately 0.012 g. These values increase to 4.2% and 0.08 g at 2 years of age, 7.0% and 0.28 g between the ages of 10 and 13 years, and 9.9% and 0.46 g in adults up to the age of 40 years. After the age of 40 years, there is a small decline in medullary weight and volume (63). The weight of the carotid bodies appears to correlate more closely with body weight than with age. Lack (64) proposed an equation to estimate carotid body weight from body weight for any age group: Combined weight of carotid bodies (mg) = 0.29 × body weight (kg) + 3.0. Standard deviations for any age group are large (60), but in normal adults the combined weight is usually less than 30 mg (65).

ANATOMY

All paraganglia are highly vascular, a characteristic that permits them to be localized by leakage of systemically injected dye in animal studies (66). However, the details of their blood supply are highly varied according to their location and function. For example, the adrenal medulla receives arterial blood from three arteries—the inferior phrenic artery, aorta, and renal arteries—and drains via a single adrenal vein that empties into the renal vein on the left and the aorta on the right. In contrast, the carotid body receives arterial blood from one or occasionally two small arteries arising from the vicinity of the carotid bifurcation and drains via several small veins into the pharyngeal, superior laryngeal, and lingual veins (4).

The innervation of paraganglia is comparably site specific. In general, sympathetic paraganglia receive preganglionic cholinergic sympathetic innervation and variable amounts of noradrenergic and/or peptidergic innervation from intrinsic neurons, nearby sympathetic ganglia, and other sources. Most of the neuroendocrine cells in the adrenal medulla and abdominal paraganglia are innervated (67,68), although it has been suggested that the ability of paraganglia to attract or maintain innervation might determine the extent to which they persist or involute at different sites (69). Parasympathetic paraganglia generally receive their innervation from branches of either the vagus or glossopharyngeal nerves but also may receive some functional and/or vasomotor input from the nearby superior cervical ganglion and a small number of intrinsic neurons (70). Multiple neurotransmitters have been identified in both afferent and efferent nerve endings in the carotid body, and dynamic alterations of innervation occur in response to hypoxic stress (71). Multiple neurotransmitters are also present in adrenal medullary nerve endings and play a variety of roles in regulating both the development and function of adrenal chromaffin cells (71).

LIGHT MICROSCOPY

Cell Types

Paraganglia contain two characteristic cell types: Neuroendocrine cells and "sustentacular" cells (from Latin *sustinere*, to hold up, to support). The neuroendocrine cells in sympathetic paraganglia are often referred to as "chromaffin cells" or "chromaffin-like cells." Additional terms for the subset of chromaffin like cells within sympathetic ganglia are "small granule-containing cells" and "small intensely fluorescent (SIF) cells." In humans, there is only one type of SIF cell, resembling chromaffin cells in the adrenal (2). A second type, present in rodents but not in humans, has features intermediate between neuroendocrine cells and neurons and is possibly a type of

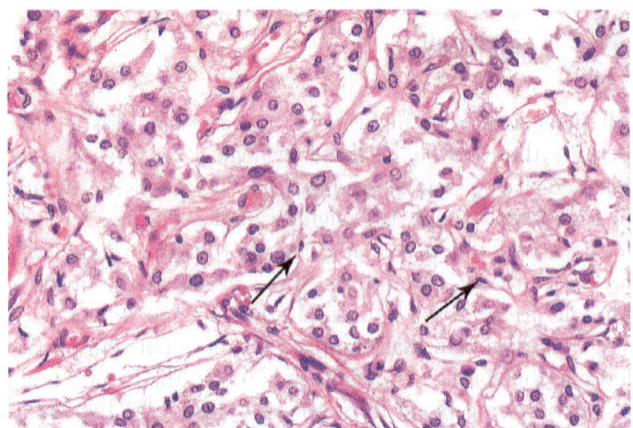

FIGURE 47.9 Section of organ of Zuckerkandl from a mid-trimester human fetus, demonstrating typical cords and nests of chief cells with rounded or oval nuclei and amphophilic cytoplasm, and occasional interspersed sustentacular cells with flattened nuclei and inconspicuous cytoplasm (*arrows*). Note that the organ of Zuckerkandl is cytologically mature while the adrenal medulla in the same developmental period is still at an early formative stage (see Fig. 47.5).

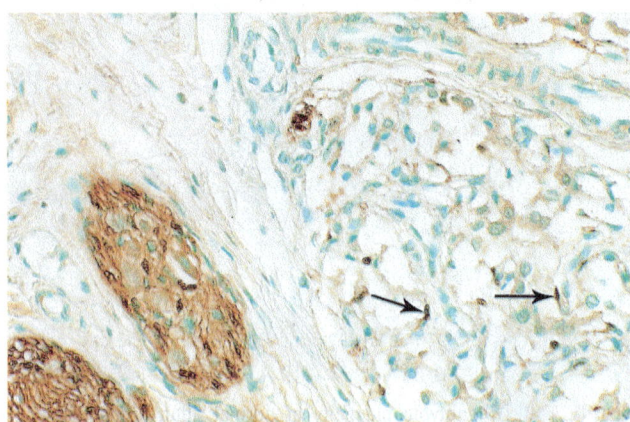

FIGURE 47.10 Organ of Zuckerkandl and adjacent sympathetic ganglion (same specimen as in Figs. 47.21 to 47.24), stained for S100 protein. Immunoreactivity for this antigen is typically localized in both nuclei and cytoplasm. Scattered sustentacular cells are stained in the organ of Zuckerkandl (*right, arrows*), where they tend to be located at the periphery of cell nests. Schwann cells are stained in the ganglion (*left*).

interneuron (2). Additional terms often applied to the principal cell types especially in parasympathetic paraganglia are "glomus cells," "type I cells" or "chief cells," and "type II cells." In addition to the two major cell types, there are variable numbers of connective tissue cells, vascular cells, Schwann cells, myelinated or unmyelinated nerve fibers, and intrinsic neurons. An additional commonly encountered cell type is the mast cell, which may be abundant in both ganglia and paraganglia (4,72).

In hematoxylin and eosin (H&E)–stained sections, paraganglionic neuroendocrine cells are polygonal cells with amphophilic or basophilic cytoplasm and small, spherical or ovoid, pale-staining nuclei (Fig. 47.9). Immunocytochemical stains for neuroendocrine markers can easily confirm their identity (see "Special Procedures"). Electron microscopy or argyrophil-type silver stains to demonstrate secretory granules or fluorescence methods to demonstrate catecholamines are employed in older publications. The neuroendocrine cells in paraganglia tend to form clusters and cords, described as *Zellballen* and *Zellsträngen* by Alfred Kohn (5), and may be partially or completely surrounded by sustentacular cells. The latter are glial cells, possibly related to non–myelin-forming Schwann cells elsewhere in the peripheral nervous system. They are usually flattened, with less conspicuous cytoplasm than chromaffin cells and more deeply basophilic nuclei with coarsely clumped chromatin. Immunohistochemically they can be identified by staining for S100 protein (73) (see "Special Procedures") (Fig. 47.10). A subset will also stain for glial fibrillary acidic protein (74). Sustentacular cells are present in both parasympathetic (75) and sympathetic (73) paraganglia but are more numerous in the former, where they may cause the *Zellballen* to appear more pronounced. The concept that they are stem cells that can give rise to chief cells has been proposed (10,45). They might also play a direct role in chemoreception (71).

Lobular Architecture of the Carotid Body

The carotid body is architecturally distinctive in that it consists of lobules separated by connective tissue septa (Figs. 47.11 to 47.13). Each lobule is individually reminiscent of the microscopic paraganglia that occur in other sites and is composed of nests of chief cells surrounded by other cell types. The amount of connective tissue between lobules tends to increase with age. This lobular arrangement is important to pathologists because carotid body hyperplasia is generally defined as an increase in mean lobule diameter (64,76).

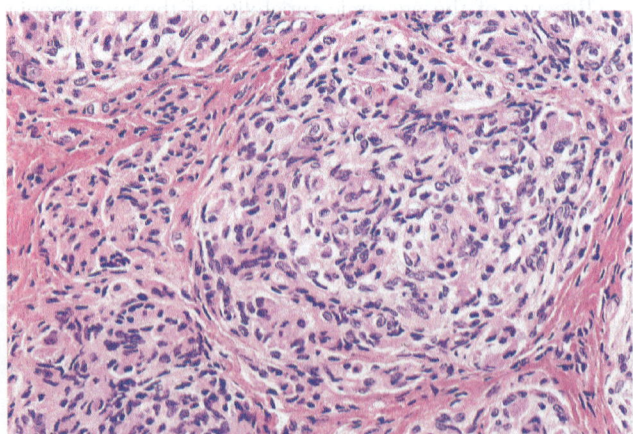

FIGURE 47.11 Section of carotid body from a 6-day-old infant demonstrating a characteristically more heterogeneous cell population than in Figure 47.6. Small nests of chief cells are highlighted by surrounding sustentacular cells and other cell types.

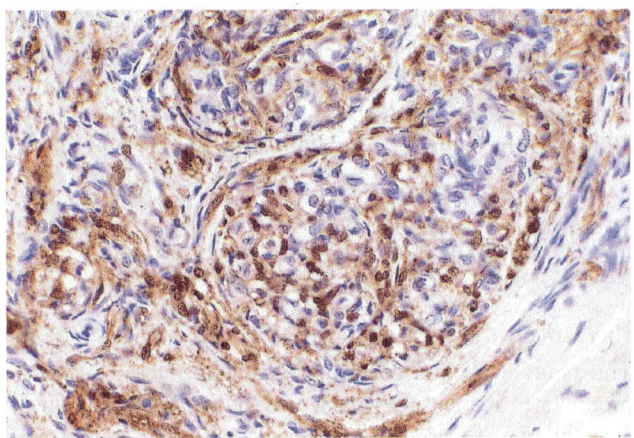

FIGURE 47.12 Lobule of a carotid body from a 16-day-old infant stained for S100 protein. In contrast to the relatively sparse S100-positive cells in the organ of Zuckerkandl (see Fig. 47.10), there are numerous stained sustentacular cells within the lobule, accentuating the *Zellballen*, and numerous stained Schwann cells both within and adjacent to the lobule, as diagrammed in Figure 47.16.

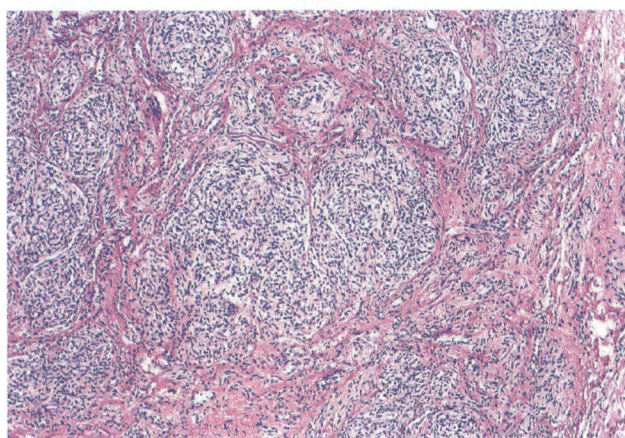

FIGURE 47.13 Carotid body from a 10-day-old infant, illustrating lobules separated by connective tissue septa.

The carotid body increases in size and weight in individuals living at high altitudes (77) and in patients with hypoxemia due to various ailments (78). Some conditions are reported to result in proliferation of sustentacular cells rather than chief cells, suggesting different mechanisms (78). While chief cell hyperplasia is associated with high altitude (77), some studies have reported that sustentacular cell proliferation is the pathognomonic feature of lobular hyperplasia in elderly patients with emphysema or hypertension (78) (Fig. 47.14). Still others studying specimens predominantly from patients with congenital heart disease have reported proportional proliferation of sustentacular cells and chief cells (64). Schwann cell proliferation and axonal sprouting also may occur at the periphery of lobules (79). Lobular architecture similar to that of the carotid body is occasionally observed in other parasympathetic paraganglia, particularly if they are enlarged (64).

ULTRASTRUCTURE

At the ultrastructural level, paraganglionic neuroendocrine cells are characterized by numerous membrane-bound granules or "dense-core vesicles" approximately 60 to 400 nm in greatest dimension. They sometimes also contain small synaptic-like vesicles that may accumulate in clusters near the plasma membrane (80). Neuroendocrine secretory granules may vary in size, shape, and electron density, reflecting differences in the secretory products stored, the functional state of individual cells, and fixation conditions. In the rodent adrenal medulla, where epinephrine and norepinephrine are mostly stored in separate cells, fixation in glutaraldehyde and postfixation in osmium tetroxide cause

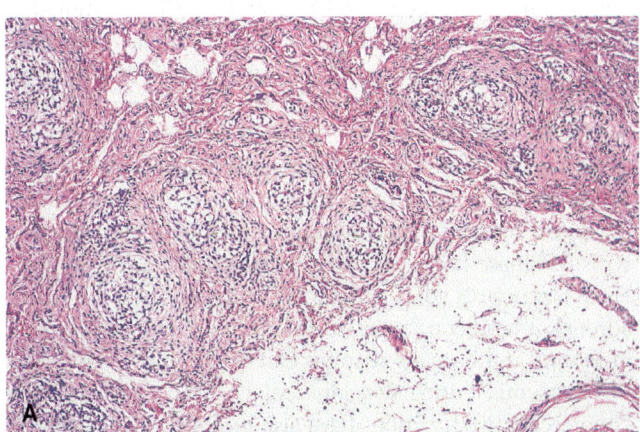
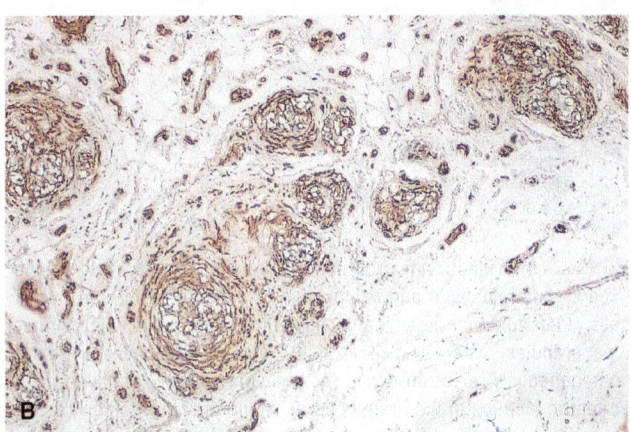

FIGURE 47.14 A: Carotid body from a 55-year-old woman with hypertension and emphysema. Lobules are separated by greater amounts of connective tissue than in Figure 47.13. In addition, there is a circumlobular proliferation of Schwann cells, demonstrable by staining for S100 protein (**B**). The latter change has been reported by some investigators to be characteristic of lobular hyperplasia in patients with hypertension (59).

granules in norepinephrine cells to appear homogeneously electron dense, whereas those in epinephrine cells are lighter and finely particulate. The mechanism for these differences involves formation of an insoluble reaction product between glutaraldehyde and norepinephrine, which is subsequently darkened by osmium (81). Because epinephrine does not similarly react with glutaraldehyde, it diffuses out of the granules, leaving behind other granule constituents that are less osmiophilic. To be successful, this method requires adequate fixation of fresh tissue. Although some human adrenal medullary cells exhibit homogeneous populations of epinephrine- or norepinephrine-type granules (1) (Fig. 47.15) most have mixed granule populations (82) and synthesize both epinephrine and norepinephrine (83). The electron density of most granules in extra-adrenal paraganglia is comparable to that of norepinephrine-type granules in the adrenal.

The ultrastructural organization of paraganglia and the proportions of their constituent cell types vary in different sites, apparently to suit different physiologic needs. Both sympathetic and parasympathetic paraganglia contain numerous small capillaries. In the former, portions of the surfaces of neuroendocrine cells closest to these vessels are usually separated from the capillary endothelium only by basal laminae and occasional collagen fibrils, suggesting that sympathetic paraganglia in most instances function as endocrine glands (67). In some locations, their secretory products also appear to be provided for local use (8). In contrast, the neuroendocrine cells in parasympathetic paraganglia tend to be separated from the capillary lumina by sustentacular cells, pericytes, or both (Figs. 47.16 to 47.18), consistent with a major role of their secretory products being to act directly on sensory parasympathetic nerve endings rather than to enter circulating blood (84,85).

FUNCTION

Physiologic Roles

The neuroendocrine cells in paraganglia release secretory products in response to neural or chemical stimuli. These products may be used for endocrine, paracrine, neurotransmitter, or neuromodulatory functions, depending on their anatomic context. Although their secretory products are similar, sympathetic and parasympathetic paraganglia generally appear to differ in the major types of stimuli to which they respond. Responses to different types of stimuli also may delineate subsets of paraganglia within the sympathetic and parasympathetic groups.

Based mostly on studies of the adrenal medulla and carotid body, the sympathetic paraganglia are considered to be essentially motor organs that respond principally to signals from spinal cord neurons via trans-synaptic stimulation, while parasympathetic paraganglia are sensory organs that respond to low pO_2, low pH, and high pCO_2 as portions of reflex loops involving the central nervous system that stimulate breathing. However, there is evidence for functional overlap, including oxygen sensing by chromaffin cells (12). Several recent reviews detail current understanding of the physiology of these two organs (71,86).

In the adult adrenal medulla, stress-induced discharges of splanchnic nerve endings that synapse on chromaffin cells, cause release of secretory granules by Ca^{2+}-mediated exocytosis. This secretory response is accompanied by ancillary effects including activation of proto-oncogenes (87), activation and induction of enzymes involved in replenishing granule constituents (88,89), and possibly stimulation of chromaffin cell proliferation (90). Cellular responses to neural-derived signals may be modulated by chemical signals, including corticosteroids and other hormones (88), growth factors (91), and secreted chromogranin fragments (89). Studies of the rat adrenal medulla suggest that neural-derived signals can increase the expression of receptors that regulate chromaffin cell function, including the receptor tyrosine kinase RET (92), which is expressed at very low levels in the normal adult adrenal (92). In contrast to the adult adrenal, it has been suggested that the organ of Zuckerkandl in rabbits and humans secretes catecholamines in response to hypoxemia during development (93). In other species, chemoreceptive functions have also been postulated for certain SIF cells (94), and for the immature adrenal medulla before the establishment of functional innervation (12).

Chemoreception was first established as a function of parasympathetic paraganglia. It was shown in the 1930s

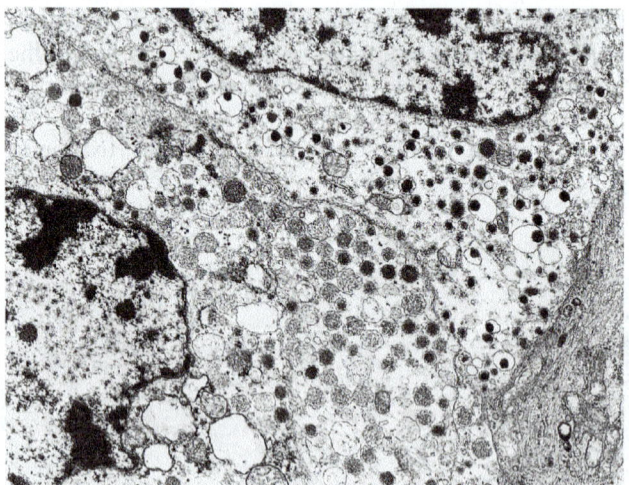

FIGURE 47.15 Electron micrograph of normal human adrenal medulla fixed in glutaraldehyde and postfixed in osmium tetroxide. Portions of cells at left contain predominantly light, finely particulate epinephrine-type granules, whereas cell at right contains predominantly dark, homogeneously electron dense norepinephrine-type granules. The eccentric location of the granule cores within their surrounding membranes is a fixation artifact most commonly observed with granules of the latter type (original magnification ×9,677). Reprinted with permission from Tischler AS. The adrenal medulla and extra-adrenal paraganglia. In Kovacs K, Asa SL, eds. *Functional Endocrine Pathology*. Cambridge, MA: Blackwell; 1990 and Springer Science+Business Media.

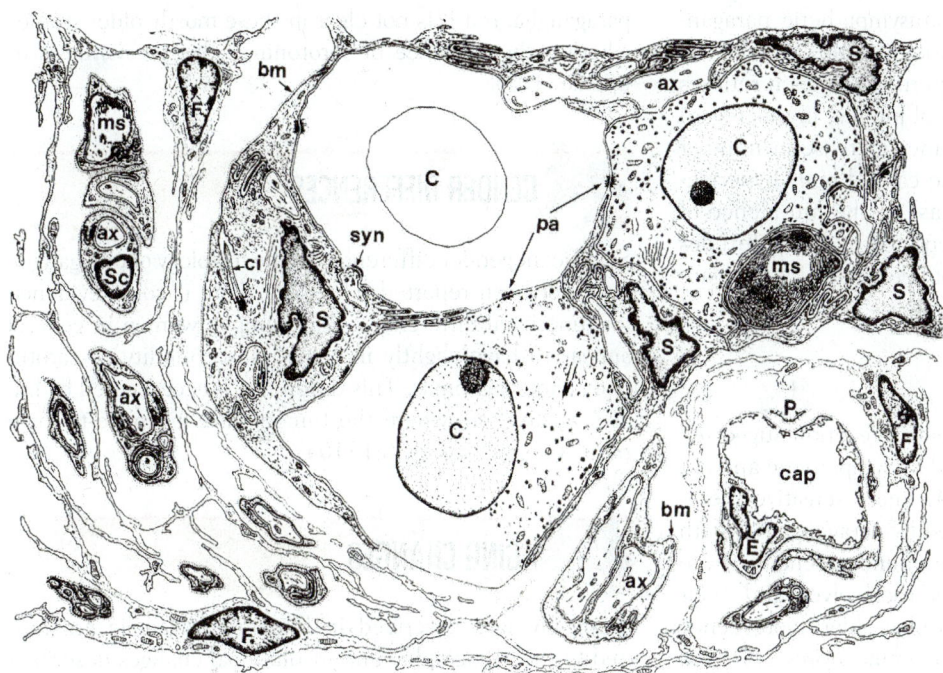

FIGURE 47.16 Diagram of the architecture of the human carotid body at the periphery of a lobule. Chief cells (*C*) in a small nest are insulated from the lumen of a nearby capillary (*cap*) by sustentacular cells (*S*), fibroblasts (*F*), and pericytes (*P*) and form synapses (*syn*) with parasympathetic axons (*ax*). They are also joined to each other by simple "puncta adherentia" type junctions (*pa*). Axons surrounded by Schwann cells (*Sc*) are present at the periphery of the lobule. Other illustrated structures are basement membrane (*bm*), endothelial cells (*E*), cilia (*ci*), and mitochondrion-rich axonal dilations termed "mitochondrial sacs" (*ms*). Reprinted with permission from Böck P, Stockinger L, Vyslonzil E. The fine structure of the human carotid body. *Z Zellforsch Mikrosk Anat* 1970;105:543–568 and Springer Science+Business Media.

that the carotid bodies and aortic paraganglia function as portions of reflex loops involving the central nervous system, whereby low pO_2, low pH, and high pCO_2 stimulate breathing (4). However, it was long debated whether the neuroendocrine cells in the carotid body are the primary receptor elements or whether their function is to modulate chemoreceptor properties intrinsic to the sensory nerve endings. Electrophysiologic studies of the mechanism of chemoreception subsequently demonstrated that the three major chemosensory stimuli depolarize dissociated carotid body chief cells. As in chromaffin cells, this leads to influx of calcium through voltage-gated calcium channels and to calcium-dependent release of secretory products to stimulate sensory nerve endings. However, the subsequent events in transduction of chemosensory information are complex and still incompletely understood. Recent evidence implicates participation of secretory products from sustentacular cells in a "tripartite synapse" (71). Chemoreceptor reflexes

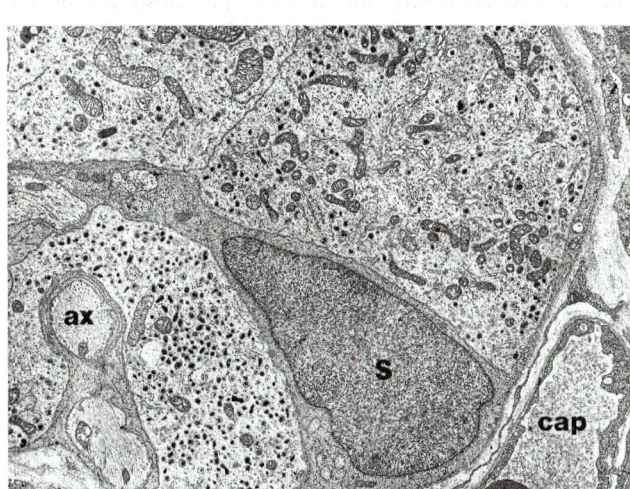

FIGURE 47.17 Electron micrograph of human carotid body from an area similar to that illustrated in Figure 47.16. S, sustentacular cell; cap, capillary; ax, axon (original magnification ×8,000). Adapted with permission from Böck P, Stockinger L, Vyslonzil E. The fine structure of the human carotid body. *Z Zellforsch Mikrosk Anat* 1970;105:543–568 and Springer Science+Business Media.

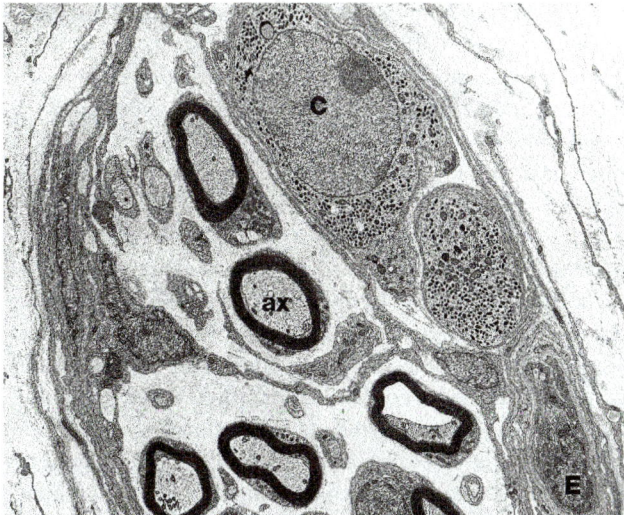

FIGURE 47.18 Electron micrograph of two chief cells enclosed within the perineurium of a small myelinated nerve in the vicinity of a human carotid body. This configuration has been described for intravagal paraganglia (56). As in the carotid body (see Figs. 47.16 and 47.17), the chief cells are separated from the lumen of a nearby capillary (original magnification ×5,400). *C*, chief cells; *E*, endothelial cell; *ax*, axons. (Courtesy of Professor P. Böck.)

have been postulated for other parasympathetic paraganglia on the basis of their similarities to the carotid body (35,95,99), but the nature and importance of such reflexes in vivo have not been defined. It is of interest in this regard that vagal paraganglia only sometimes increase in number or size under conditions that cause carotid body hyperplasia (64). Although a 10-fold increase in the prevalence of carotid body paragangliomas is reported at high altitudes (96), this strong association has not been made for paragangliomas at other sites.

Secretory Products

Although studies using the chromaffin reaction suggested that catecholamines were produced by sympathetic and not by parasympathetic paraganglia (4), more sensitive methods indicate that they are produced by paraganglia of both classes. Those methods include immunocytochemistry to demonstrate both catecholamines themselves and their biosynthetic enzymes (97,98), as well as older fluorescence techniques to demonstrate catecholamine stores (99) (see "Special Procedures"). Most of the body's epinephrine production is in the adrenal medulla, where the epinephrine-to-norepinephrine ratio is approximately 4:1. In contrast, over 90% of the catecholamine content of extra-adrenal sympathetic paraganglia is norepinephrine. Parasympathetic paraganglia produce almost no epinephrine but may produce significant quantities of dopamine. These differences in catecholamine profiles are reflected in paragangliomas that arise at different sites (100), with an important exception. Although most pheochromocytomas produce either epinephrine alone or epinephrine plus norepinephrine, approximately 1/3 produce almost exclusively norepinephrine. The noradrenergic phenotype, which is often associated with VHL disease, might arise from the small population of noradrenergic-type cells that can be found in the human adrenal either by electron microscopy (1) or immunohistochemistry (83). However, tumor genotype might also influence biochemical phenotype independently of cell of origin (25).

In addition to producing catecholamines, both sympathetic and parasympathetic paraganglia synthesize regulatory peptides (11), the most prevalent of which are enkephalins (83,101). Regulatory peptides and amines usually coexist in the same cells and in the same secretory granules, which also contain granin proteins, adenine nucleotides, peptide-cleaving and -amidating enzymes, dopamine beta-hydroxylase (DBH), and numerous other constituents of both known and unknown functions. Peptide growth factors that might exert autocrine, paracrine, and neurotrophic effects also may be present (100). Together these granule constituents comprise a "secretory cocktail," the composition of which can be varied in different physiologic and pathologic states (102).

Serotonin has been reported in addition to catecholamines in some sympathetic and parasympathetic human paraganglia, but it is not clear in these mostly older studies whether the presence of serotonin is due to synthesis or uptake (103).

GENDER DIFFERENCES

Significant gender differences in the histology of paraganglia have not been reported. However, there is some evidence for functional differences. For example, women in general appear to have slightly increased susceptibility to carotid body paragangliomas. This difference is accentuated by life at high altitude, where the tumors have a female-to-male ratio of approximately 8:1 (104).

AGING CHANGES

Aging changes described in human paraganglia are limited to the topographic and involutional changes described in the sections on "Distribution of Paraganglia," "Gross Features and Organ Weights," and "Lobular Architecture of the Carotid Body." More dramatic changes in the form of hyperplasia and neoplasia occur in the adrenal medulla of aging laboratory rats (105). In the near future rats may provide new pre-clinical models for understanding the development of human disease.

SPECIAL PROCEDURES

Immunohistochemistry

Immunohistochemistry now replaces previously useful but more cumbersome or less specific techniques such as electron microscopy, catecholamine fluorescence, or silver stains for most studies of normal and abnormal paraganglia. In normal paraganglia, immunohistochemistry can reveal subtleties such as differential expression of hormones or other markers (Figs. 47.19 to 47.31) (83) that contribute to understanding pathologic conditions. For pathologists, the major application of immunohistochemistry to the paraganglionic system has until recently been diagnosis and functional characterization of pheochromocytomas and paragangliomas. The identification of predisposition genes underlying familial paraganglioma syndromes has paved the way for immunohistochemical identification of genetic alterations (18). Loss of immunoreactivity for SDHB is a feature of any SDH-related (SDHx) tumor, and additional staining for SDHA can identify tumors related to SDHA mutations (106). Similarly, staining for MAX (107) and FH (108) has been shown to identify tumors with mutations of the respective genes. Potential future applications include identification of markers that may be applicable to targeted therapy, such as specific somatostatin receptor subtypes (109).

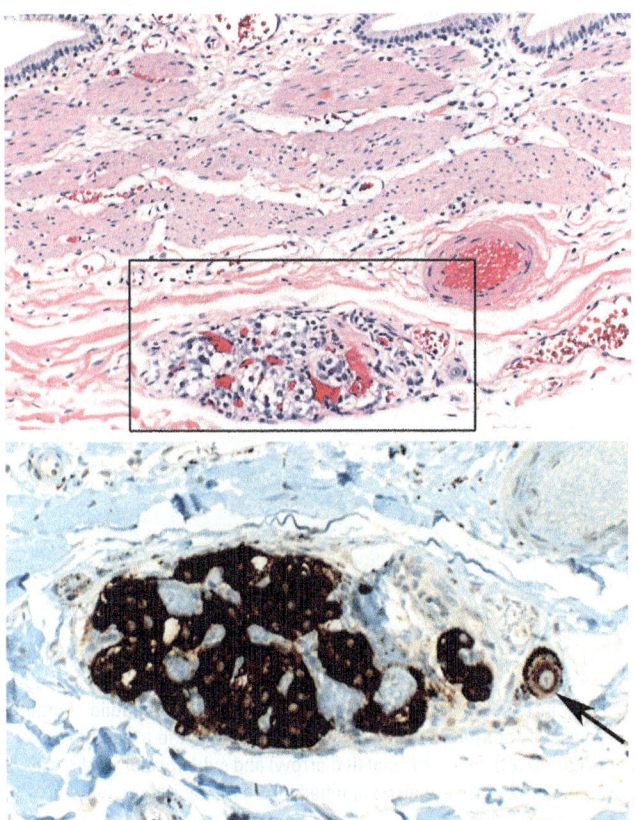

FIGURE 47.19 A microscopic paraganglion (box in top panel) discovered as an incidental finding in the gallbladder of a 53-year-old woman. The paraganglion is characterized by somewhat clear cells and prominent capillaries, and contains a single neuron at right. For bottom panel, shown at higher magnification, the slide was decolorized, stained immunohistochemically for synaptophysin and re-photographed. The neuroendocrine cells show intense immunoreactivity while the neuron (*arrow*) stains more weakly because it contains sparser secretory vesicles.

Paraganglia express a plethora of markers shared to varying degrees with other neural and endocrine tissues. A partial categorization includes amines, regulatory peptides, granins, and other constituents of the secretory granule matrix, secretory granule membrane and cell membrane components, and cytoskeletal proteins. Proteins known as "SNAPs" and "SNAREs" (SNAP receptors) that are involved in docking of secretory granules at the cell membrane in preparation for exocytosis also comprise an important class of markers. Those proteins include synaptobrevin, synaptotagmin, syntaxin, and SNAP-25 (110). Developmental biologists using revolutionary new techniques for tracing cell lineage have many new markers to offer (10).

For diagnostic purposes, care must be taken to select from the large number of available markers those that are the most specific. For example, immunoreactivity for synaptophysin, a secretory vesicle membrane protein, is characteristically present in paraganglia and can be very helpful in confirming a neuroendocrine phenotype in appropriate contexts. However, it is also present in adrenal cortex and can, therefore, not be relied on to discriminate adrenal

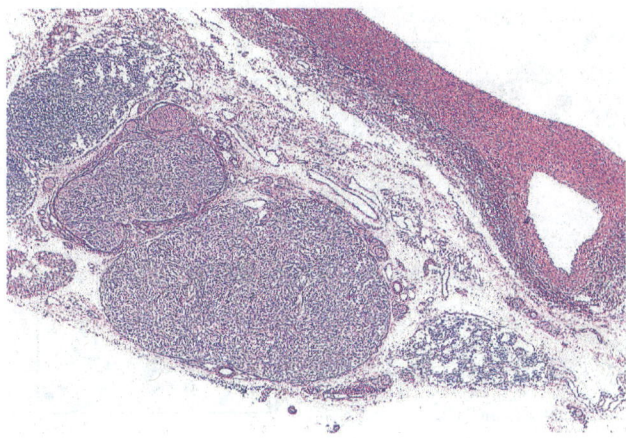

FIGURE 47.20 Transverse section through the aorta of a mid-trimester human fetus at the level of the inferior mesenteric artery, demonstrating organ of Zuckerkandl and adjacent sympathetic ganglion, related as diagrammed in Figure 47.2.

cortical carcinoma from pheochromocytoma (111). Similarly, certain SNAP and SNARE proteins are present in normal lymphoid cells. Markers that have been particularly valuable in histopathology of paraganglia are chromogranin A (CgA), catecholamine biosynthetic enzymes, S100 protein and GATA-3 (112). However, each of these has its own diagnostic caveats when extrapolating from normal to pathologic tissue and the expression of these biomarkers in other cell and tumor types must be considered.

CgA is an acidic protein that constitutes more than half the weight of many types of neuroendocrine secretory granules. It appears to be present in most neuroendocrine cells and is, therefore, a useful generic marker that can, in most instances, serve to establish the neuroendocrine nature of particular cells or tissues in the paraganglionic system (Figs. 47.20 to 47.22 and 47.24 to 47.27) (113–115). Since it is concentrated mostly in secretory granules, it may fail to

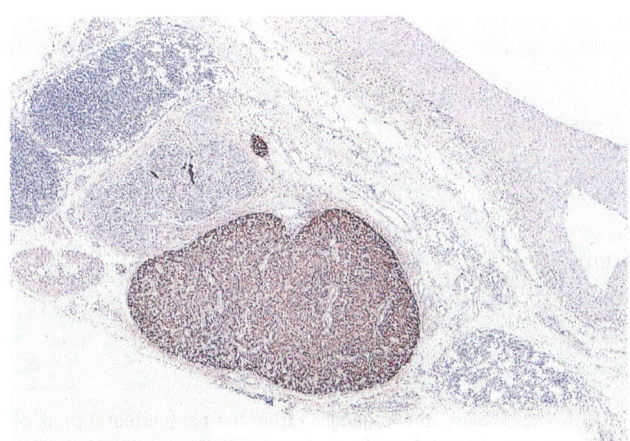

FIGURE 47.21 Section adjacent to that shown in Figure 47.20, stained for CgA. Staining is intense in the organ of Zuckerkandl and in small nests of neuroendocrine cells within and adjacent to the ganglion, but not in neurons.

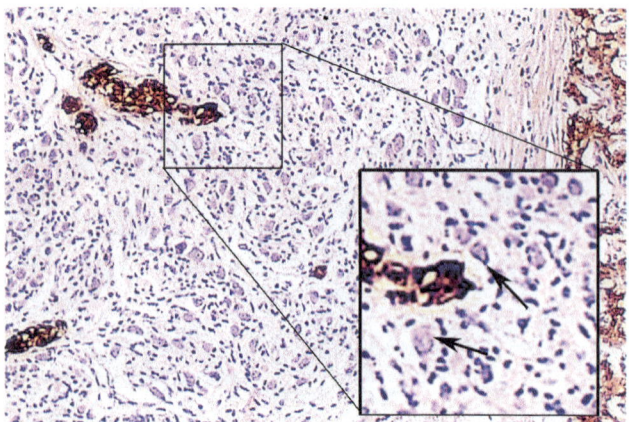

FIGURE 47.22 Higher magnifications of central area of the section shown in Figure 47.21. Organ of Zuckerkandl is on right, ganglion on left. *Arrows* in inset indicate neurons with little or no immunoreactive CgA.

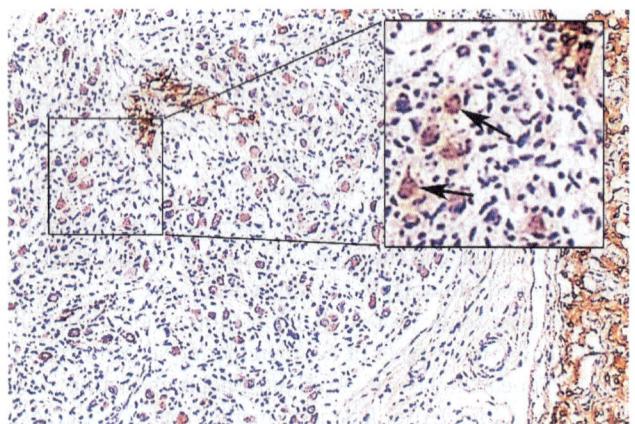

FIGURE 47.23 Section adjacent to that shown in Figure 47.22, stained for TH. Intense TH immunoreactivity is present in both sympathetic neurons (*arrows* in inset) and paraganglionic neuroendocrine cells.

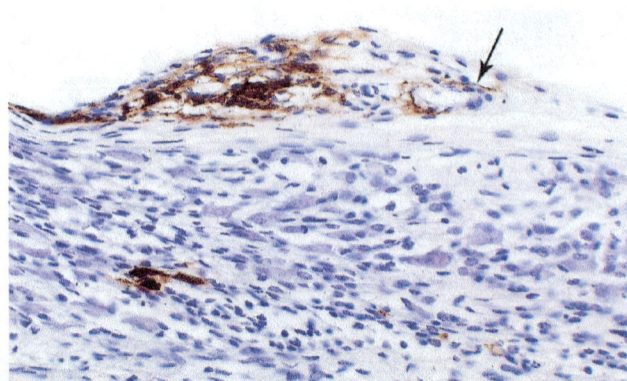

FIGURE 47.24 Sympathetic ganglion from the paravertebral trunk of a mid-trimester human fetus (same fetus as in Figures 47.21 to 47.24), stained for CgA. Neuroendocrine cells are identified both within and adjacent to the ganglion. CgA-positive processes, which might be derived from either neurons or neuroendocrine cells, surround a small blood vessel (*arrow*).

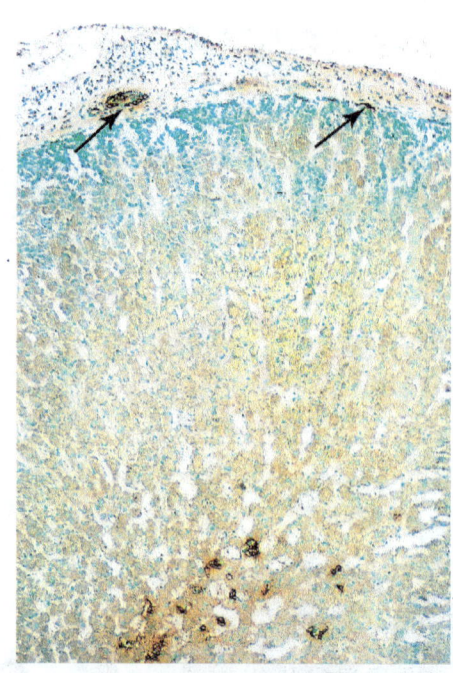

FIGURE 47.25 Adrenal gland from a mid-trimester human fetus (same fetus as in Figs. 47.21 to 47.24), stained for CgA. The medulla (*bottom*) contains only scattered positive cells, in contrast to the organ of Zuckerkandl (Fig. 47.21). Extra-adrenal (*left arrow*) and subcapsular (*right arrow*) paraganglionic cells are also identified by their immunoreactivity.

stain cells that are degranulated due to low rates of synthesis, high rates of secretion, or low storage capacity. In sympathetic ganglia, it can be used to conveniently discriminate SIF cells from principal sympathetic neurons, which produce CgA but have few perikaryal secretory granules (116). CgA was the first described member of the granin family of proteins, which now includes seven members (CgA and B, secretogranin II and III, 7B2, NESP55, and VGF) (117). The roles of granins include sorting of proteins to the

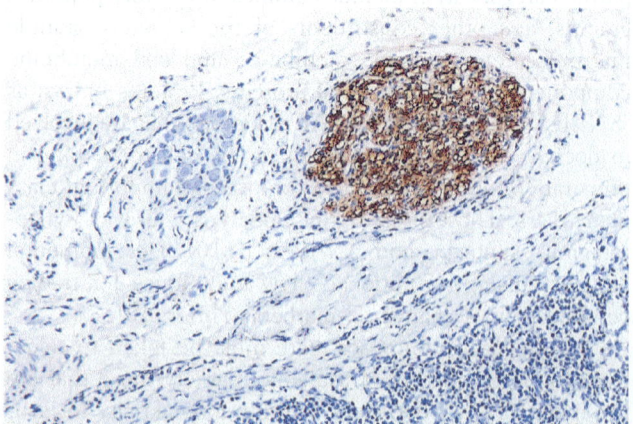

FIGURE 47.26 A small retroperitoneal paraganglion similar to that in Figure 47.20, incidentally removed along with adjacent ganglion and lymph node from a 5-month-old infant during resection of Wilms' tumor. Soaking the coverslip off a routine H&E-stained histologic section and re-staining for CgA confirmed the identity of the paraganglion.

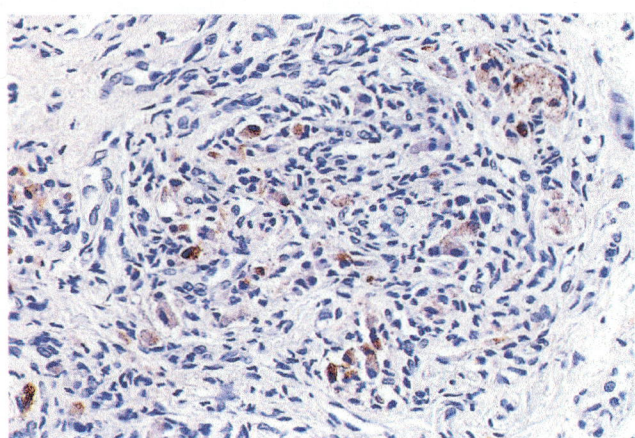

FIGURE 47.27 Lobule of a carotid body stained for CgA, demonstrating nests of immunoreactive chief cells surrounded by unstained cells of other types.

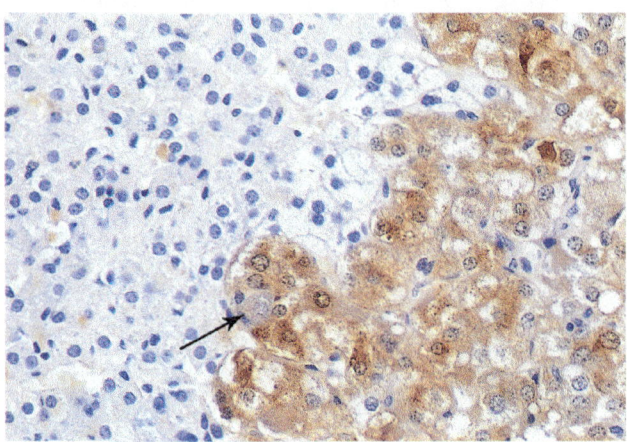

FIGURE 47.29 Adult adrenal gland stained for PNMT. The ability of almost all neuroendocrine cells in the adrenal medulla to synthesize epinephrine is inferred from their positive staining. Occasional cells are unstained (*arrow*) as previously reported (80) and as suggested by the electron micrograph in Figure 47.15.

regulated secretory pathway and directing secretory granule biogenesis. In addition, they serve as multifunctional prohormones, giving rise to cleavage fragments that exert a variety of autocrine, paracrine, and systemic effects. The various granins are differentially expressed in neuroendocrine tissues. Although most are present in the adrenal medulla, their distributions in other paraganglia are incompletely mapped (117). This is important for pathologists because some head and neck paragangliomas preferentially express CgB and are negative or only focally positive for CgA (115). Immunostaining for synaptophysin can be positive in such cases.

Antibodies against the catecholamine-synthesizing enzymes tyrosine hydroxylase (TH), DBH, and phenylethanolamine-N-transferase (PNMT) are important tools that can be used to infer from a paraffin section not only whether a tumor was producing catecholamines, but also what catecholamines were produced. TH is the rate-limiting enzyme in catecholamine synthesis and is therefore found in all catecholamine-producing cells (Figs. 47.23 and 47.28), whereas DBH is found only in cells that produce norepinephrine, and PNMT is found only in cells that can convert norepinephrine to epinephrine. This immunocytochemical approach provides a cellular correlate to biochemical data by demonstrating that only rarely do extra-adrenal paraganglionic cells stain for PNMT (97), in contrast to the adrenal medulla where the great majority of cells are stained (Figs. 47.29 and 47.30). It also has been useful in demonstrating catecholamine-synthesizing ability in pheochromocytomas and extra-adrenal paragangliomas (98). Because TH and PNMT are cytosolic enzymes (102) staining is not dependent on storage of secretory granules. Sympathetic neurons, for example, stain strongly for TH

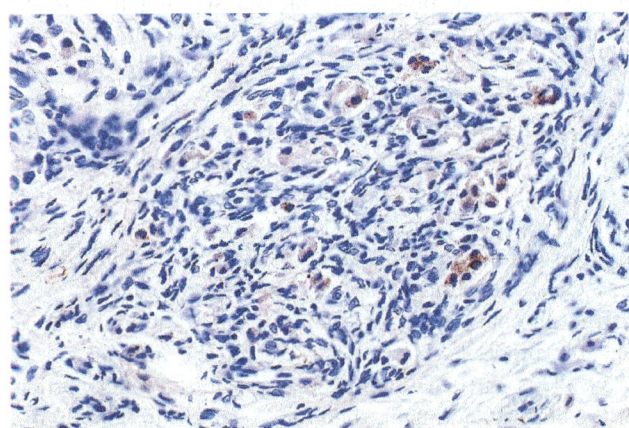

FIGURE 47.28 Lobule of a carotid body stained for TH. The catecholamine-synthesizing ability of chief cells is inferred by positive staining of chief cell nests, which are surrounded by unstained cells of other types.

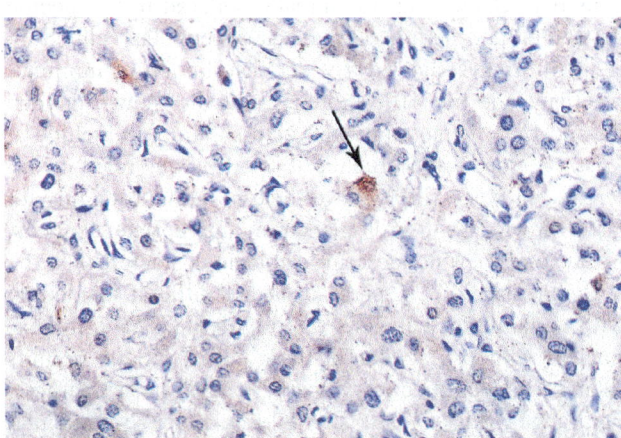

FIGURE 47.30 Organ of Zuckerkandl (same specimen as in Figs. 47.20 to 47.23) stained for PNMT. Although all the neuroendocrine cells stain for TH and can produce catecholamines (Fig. 47.23), only rare cells (*arrow*) contain immunoreactive PNMT. This finding is consistent with the limited ability of extra-adrenal paraganglia to synthesize epinephrine, the final step in the catecholamine biosynthetic pathway.

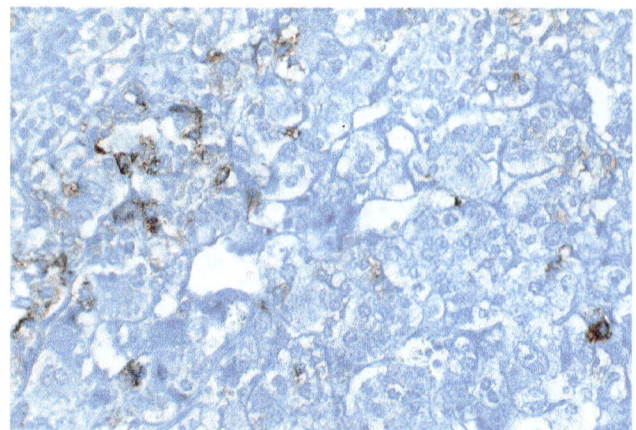

FIGURE 47.31 Adult adrenal gland stained for somatostatin, illustrating strongly immunoreactive cells scattered among cells with no detectable immunoreactivity. Immunohistochemical staining of paraganglionic neuroendocrine cells for regulatory peptides can suggest functional heterogeneity despite the fact that all of the cells produce catecholamines.

(Fig. 47.24), in contrast to their weak or absent staining for CgA. In contrast to chromogranins, which are present in many types of neuroendocrine cells, catecholamine biosynthetic enzymes in adult humans are normally present only in paraganglia and neurons (97). In addition to their biosynthetic enzymes, catecholamines themselves may be localized by immunohistochemistry. However, the presence of catecholamines without biosynthetic enzymes under some circumstances (98) suggests that synthesis cannot be distinguished from uptake by this approach. As with CgA, parasympathetic paragangliomas in the head and neck can be negative for TH (118) and, therefore, truly nonfunctional in terms of catecholamine production.

S100 protein was initially described as a calcium-binding dimer consisting of alpha–alpha, alpha–beta, or beta–beta chains and was initially believed to be specific for central and peripheral nervous system glial cells. Subsequent studies showed a wider distribution of immunoreactivity, and the S100 protein family has now expanded beyond the original alpha and beta subunits to include at least 17 members postulated to play various roles in different cell types (119). Nevertheless, immunostaining for S100 provides a useful marker in appropriate contexts. Because of their nondescript cytologic characteristics, the sustentacular cells in paraganglia are difficult to identify with certainty in sections stained with H&E. The intense nuclear immunoreactivity of these cells for S100 permits them to be identified in sympathetic and parasympathetic paraganglia (Figs. 47.10 and 47.12). Both sustentacular cells and Schwann cells contain predominantly the beta subunit of S100 (120).

Since sustentacular cells are frequently present in paragangliomas (73,121), immunohistochemical staining for S100 can sometimes be helpful in differential diagnosis. A caveat is that sustentacular cells must be distinguished from Langerhans cells and interdigitating reticulum cells of the immune system, which also express S100. Further, other types of neuroendocrine tumors can contain *bona fide* sustentacular cells (122). Genetic studies of isolated sustentacular cells from paragangliomas suggest that these cells are in fact normal (123), suggesting that their presence in paragangliomas is caused by ingrowth from nearby normal tissue rather than bidirectional differentiation.

GATA-3 is a transcription factor that plays a role in the development of multiple tissues, including breast, urothelium, lymphocytes, and parathyroid glands, as well as sympathoadrenal cells (124). It is also expressed in paraganglia and their tumors (112).

Immunohistochemical Artifacts

Important artifacts that must be borne in mind in immunohistochemical studies of paraganglia are the nonspecific interactions of some, but not all, antibodies with the secretory granules of mast cells (125,126) and of certain neuroendocrine cells (127). These artifacts may be particularly troublesome because, due to their inconstancy, negative controls consisting of irrelevant antibodies or normal sera are not adequate. The mast cell artifact has undoubtedly resulted in erroneous published reports of neuroendocrine secretory products in nonendocrine tissues, and also could produce incorrect results in studies of paraganglia because of their sometimes-high mast cell content (75). The mechanism of the mast cell artifact is not known (126), but in some cases the staining may be eliminated by dilution in the presence of normal serum proteins (125) or commercial blocking kits. Nonspecific binding of immunoglobulins to neuroendocrine secretory granules appears to result from ionic interactions and may be reduced by high concentrations of salt in the buffer (127).

Other artifacts not specific to neuroendocrine cells may also be encountered in studies of paraganglia. In immunohistochemical protocols that employ a biotin bridge, such as the "ABC" technique, artifactual staining may result from the presence of endogenous biotin. This problem may be exacerbated by heat-based antigen retrieval, which can unmask endogenous biotin in addition to specific antigens (128). Commercial biotin-blocking kits offer some remedy, but a preferable solution may be to discontinue the use of biotin-based systems and switch to newer methods that employ secondary antibodies conjugated to polymer-bound reporter enzymes. Various types of artifactual staining with less clear mechanisms are also sometimes encountered. In the adrenal gland, for example, some antibodies inexplicably produce spurious staining in the adrenal cortex (129). This particularly tends to occur in the inner portion of the cortex, and might, therefore, result from nonspecific interactions of some antibodies with lipochrome pigments. Cells that are rich in mitochondria occasionally also show weak nonspecific staining. In addition to spurious staining caused by these and other artifacts, the possibility of actual immunologic cross-reactivity of an antibody with different proteins must always be considered.

In general, immunohistochemical studies should be performed with optimally diluted antibodies and verified, when practical, with antibodies from more than one source. Ideally, adsorption controls and immunoblots should also be employed for validation, particularly in research studies or when new markers or antibodies are introduced. Controls consisting solely of primary antibody omission should not be considered adequate even for routine studies. Buffer composition, blocking proteins, and controls are now becoming standardized in automated staining procedures, but should still be optimized for each new antibody as discussed in many textbooks and reviews.

Other Special Procedures

Fluorescence methods for detection of catecholamines or other biogenic amines now have very little use in routine pathology. However, literature searches of PubMed or other databases continue to demonstrate the value of these techniques in occasional, sometimes novel (130) research applications. Catecholamines can be demonstrated in freeze dried or frozen sections or in touch preparations either by formaldehyde vapor (99) or glyoxylic acid–induced (131) fluorescence. The glyoxylic acid method is usually preferable because it produces non-diffusing fluorophores.

DIFFERENTIAL DIAGNOSIS

Paraganglia must be discriminated from normal but similar-appearing non-paraganglionic structures and from a variety of malignant tumors. The ampulloglomerular organ (132), glomus coccygeum (7), and glomera cutanea (133) are thermoregulatory structures, respectively located in the suboccipital and coccygeal regions and in the skin, resembling but unrelated to paraganglia. Lobules of fetal fat may at times appear reminiscent of paraganglia. All of these structures can be readily distinguished from paraganglia by their absence of staining for CgA, TH, or other neuroendocrine markers. Reports of paraganglia in anomalous locations are also now amenable to immunohistochemical verification.

Normal paraganglia can present diagnostic pitfalls as mimics of unrelated malignant tumors. Prostatic paraganglia can be misinterpreted as prostatic adenocarcinoma (134), bladder paraganglia can be confused with transitional cell carcinoma (135), and retroperitoneal paraganglia can be confused with metastatic clear cell carcinoma (136). Numerous mitoses, glandular or squamous differentiation, or stromal reaction are not features of paraganglia or paragangliomas. Questionable cases can be readily resolved by immunohistochemistry. For very small paraganglia that might be depleted by cutting sections, an H&E slide can be decolorized and re-stained for either CgA or synaptophysin. The stability and abundance of those antigens make them particularly suitable for such procedures.

Cases in which paraganglia or paragangliomas must be distinguished from other normal or neoplastic neuroendocrine tissues that express many of the same markers are more problematic. Knowledge of the distribution and morphology of paraganglia is therefore essential. In addition, the presence of GATA-3 and TH in paragangliomas or of distinguishing markers in other types of tumors, for example, keratins, transcription factors, and hormones in neuroendocrine tumors, may be helpful. Tumors showing glandular or squamous differentiation are almost certainly not paraganglionic.

In the adrenal gland, developmental neuroblastic nests (see "Embryology") must be distinguished from in situ neuroblastoma (54,55). Cortical invasion, mitoses, and necrosis are all characteristic of normal cells in this instance. In addition, the nuclei of normal adrenal medullary progenitors are reported to be smaller on average than those of neuroblastoma cells (53).

ACKNOWLEDGMENTS

We thank Drs. Peter Böck, Ernest Lack, and James Powers for contributing illustrative material and Dr. Harold Kozakewich for contributing tissue blocks.

REFERENCES

1. Coupland RE. *The Natural History of the Chromaffin Cell.* London: Longmans Green; 1965.
2. Coupland RE. The natural history of the chromaffin cell–twenty-five years on the beginning. *Arch Histol Cytol* 1989; 52 Suppl:331–341.
3. Carmichael SW, Rochester. The history of the adrenal medulla. *Rev Neurosci* 1989;2(2):83–100.
4. Zak FG, Lawson W. *The Paraganglionic Chemoreceptor System. Physiology, Pathology and Clinical Medicine.* New York: Springer-Verlag; 1982.
5. Kohn A. Die Paraganglien. *Arch Mikr Anat* 1903; 52:262–365.
6. Kjaergaard J. *Anatomy of the Carotid Glands and Carotid Glomus-like Bodies (Non-Chromaffin Paraganglia).* Copenhagen: F.A.D.L.'s Forlag; 1973.
7. Rahemtullah A, Szyfelbein K, Zembowicz A. Glomus coccygeum: report of a case and review of the literature. *Am J Dermatopathol* 2005;27(6):497–499.
8. Furness JB, Sobels G. The ultrastructure of paraganglia associated with the inferior mesenteric ganglia in the guinea-pig. *Cell Tissue Res* 1976;171(1):123–139.
9. Pearse AG, Polak JM, Rost FW, et al. Demonstration of the neural crest origin of type I (APUD) cells in the avian carotid body, using a cytochemical marker system. *Histochemie* 1973; 34(3):191–203.

10. Furlan A, Dyachuk V, Kastriti ME, et al. Multipotent peripheral glial cells generate neuroendocrine cells of the adrenal medulla. *Science* 2017;357(6346):eaal3753.
11. Heym C, Kummer W. Regulatory peptides in paraganglia *Prog Histochem Cytochem* 1988;18(2):1–95.
12. Nurse CA, Salman S, Scott AL. Hypoxia-regulated catecholamine secretion in chromaffin cells. *Cell Tissue Res* 2018; 372(2):433–441.
13. Lloyd R, Osamura R, Klöppel G, et al., eds. *WHO Classification of Tumours of Endocrine Organs, Fourth Edition*. IARC; 2017.
14. Turchini J, Gill AJ, Tischler AS. Pathology of pheochromocytoma and paraganglioma. In: Landsberg L, ed. *Pheochromocytomas, Paragangliomas and Disorders of the Sympathoadrenal System, Contemporary Endocrinology*. London: Springer International Publishing AG; 2018.
15. Van Der Horst-Schrivers AN, Osinga TE, Kema IP, et al. Dopamine excess in patients with head and neck paragangliomas. *Anticancer Res* 2010;30(12):5153–5158.
16. Flynn A, Dwight T, Harris J, et al. Pheo-Type: A diagnostic gene-expression assay for the classification of pheochromocytoma and paraganglioma. *J Clin Endocrinol Metab* 2016; 101(3):1034–1043.
17. Dahia PL. Pheochromocytoma and paraganglioma pathogenesis: Learning from genetic heterogeneity. *Nat rev Cancer* 2014;14(2):108–119.
18. Turchini J, Cheung VKY, Tischler AS, et al. Pathology and genetics of phaeochromocytoma and paraganglioma. *Histopathology* 2018;72(1):97–105.
19. Eisenhofer G, Lenders JW, Timmers H, et al. Measurements of plasma methoxytyramine, normetanephrine, and metanephrine as discriminators of different hereditary forms of pheochromocytoma. *Clin Chem* 2011;57(3):411–420.
20. Brouwers FM, Glasker S, Nave AF, et al. Proteomic profiling of von Hippel-Lindau syndrome and multiple endocrine neoplasia type 2 pheochromocytomas reveals different expression of chromogranin B. *Endocr Relat Cancer* 2007;14(2):463–471.
21. Fishbein L, Leshchiner I, Walter V, et al. Comprehensive molecular characterization of pheochromocytoma and paraganglioma. *Cancer Cell* 2017;31(2):181–193.
22. Cole TJ, Blendy JA, Monaghan AP, et al. Targeted disruption of the glucocorticoid receptor gene blocks adrenergic chromaffin cell development and severely retards lung maturation. *Genes Dev* 1995;9(13):1608–1621.
23. Lee S, Nakamura E, Yang H, et al. Neuronal apoptosis linked to EglN3 prolyl hydroxylase and familial pheochromocytoma genes: developmental culling and cancer. *Cancer Cell* 2005;8(2):155–167.
24. Fliedner SMJ, Brabant G, Lehnert H. Pheochromocytoma and paraganglioma: genotype versus anatomic location as determinants of tumor phenotype. *Cell Tissue Res* 2018;372(2): 347–365.
25. Fishbein L, Wilkerson MD. Chromaffin cell biology: inferences from The Cancer Genome Atlas. *Cell Tissue Res* 2018; 372(2):339–346.
26. Hervonen A, Partanen S, Vaalasti A, et al. The distribution and endocrine nature of the abdominal paraganglia of adult man. *Am J Anat* 1978;153(4):563–572.
27. Hervonen A, Vaalasti A, Partanen M, et al. Effects of ageing on the histochemically demonstrable catecholamines and acetylcholinesterase of human sympathetic ganglia. *J Neurocytol* 1978;7(1):11–23.
28. Baljet B, Boekelaar AB, Groen GJ. Retroperitoneal paraganglia and the peripheral autonomic nervous system in the human fetus. *Acta Morphol Neerl Scand* 1985;23(2):137–149.
29. Coupland RE. The development and fate of catecholamine-secreting endocrine cells. In: Parvez H, Parvez S, eds. *Biogenic Amines in Development*. Amsterdam: Elsevier/North-Holland; 1980:3–28.
30. Zuckerkandl E. Ueber nebenorgane des sympathicus im Retroperitonealraum des menschen. *Verh Anat Ges* 1901;15: 85–107.
31. Ober WB. Emil Zuckerkandl and his delightful little organ. *Pathol Annu* 1983;18 Pt 1:103–119.
32. Lack EE, Cubilla AL, Woodruff JM, et al. Extra-adrenal paragangliomas of the retroperitoneum: A clinicopathologic study of 12 tumors. *Am J Surg Pathol* 1980;4(2):109–120.
33. Helen P, Alho H, Hervonen A. Ultrastructure and histochemistry of human SIF cells and paraganglia. *Adv Biochem Psychopharmacol* 1980;25:149–152.
34. Kohn A. Die chromaffinen Zellen des sympathicus. *Anat Anz* 1898;15:399–400.
35. Matthews MR. Ultrastructural studies relevant to the possible functions of small granule-containing cells in the rat superior cervical ganglion. *Adv Biochem Psychopharmacol* 1980;25:77–86.
36. Glenner GG, Grimley PM. *Tumors of the Extra-adrenal Paraganglion System (Including Chemoreceptors)*. Washington, DC: Armed Forces Institute Of Pathology; 1974.
37. Guild SR. The glomus jugulare, a nonchromaffin paraganglion, in man. *Ann Otol Rhinol Laryngol* 1953;62(4): 1045–1071; concld.
38. Dahlqvist A, Carlsoo B, Hellstrom S. Paraganglia of the human recurrent laryngeal nerve. *Am J Otolaryngol* 1986;7(5): 366–369.
39. Gobbi H, Barbosa AJ, Teixeira VP, et al. Immunocytochemical identification of neuroendocrine markers in human cardiac paraganglion-like structures. *Histochemistry* 1991;95(4): 337–340.
40. Grillo MA, Jacobs L, Comroe JH Jr. A combined fluorescence histochemical and electron microscopic method for studying special monoamine-containing cells (SIF cells). *J Comp Neurol* 1974;153(1):1–14.
41. Sarathi V. Characteristics of pediatric pheochromocytoma/paraganglioma. *Indian J Endocrinol Metab* 2017;21(3): 470–474.
42. Plenat F, Leroux P, Floquet J, et al. Intra and juxtavagal paraganglia: a topographical, histochemical, and ultrastructural study in the human. *Anat Rec* 1988;221(3):743–753.
43. Goormagtigh N, Heymans C. On the existence of abdominal vagal paraganglia in the adult mouse. *J Anat* 1936;71:77–90.
44. Kuo T, Anderson CB, Rosai J. Normal paraganglia in the human gallbladder. *Arch Pathol* 1974;97(1):46–47.
45. Lopez-Barneo J. Oxygen sensing and stem cell activation in the hypoxic carotid body. *Cell Tissue Res* 2018;372(2): 417–425.
46. Zuckerkandl E. The development of the chromaffin organs and of the supra-renal glands. In: Keibel F, Mall FP, eds. *Manual of Human Embryology*. Philadelphia, PA: J B Lippincott; 1912.
47. Willier BH. A study of the origin and differentiation of the suprarenal gland in the chick embryo by chorio-allantoic grafting. *Phys Zool* 1930;3:201–225.

48. Korkala O, Hervonen A. Origin and development of the catecholamine-storing cells of the human fetal carotid body. *Histochemie* 1973;37(4):287–297.
49. Hockman D, Adameyko I, Kaucka M, et al. Striking parallels between carotid body glomus cell and adrenal chromaffin cell development. *Dev Biol*. 2018. pii: S0012-1606(17)30905-3. doi: 10.1016/j.ydbio.2018.05.016.
50. Cooper MJ, Hutchins GM, Israel MA. Histogenesis of the human adrenal medulla. An evaluation of the ontogeny of chromaffin and nonchromaffin lineages. *Am J Pathol* 1990; 137(3):605–615.
51. Molenaar WM, Lee VM, Trojanowski JQ. Early fetal acquisition of the chromaffin and neuronal immunophenotype by human adrenal medullary cells. An immunohistological study using monoclonal antibodies to chromogranin A, synaptophysin, tyrosine hydroxylase, and neuronal cytoskeletal proteins. *Exp Neurol* 1990;108(1):1–9.
52. Kuntz A. The development of the sympathetic nervous system in man. *J Comp Neurol* 1920;32:173–229.
53. Ikeda Y, Lister J, Bouton JM, et al. Congenital neuroblastoma, neuroblastoma in situ, and the normal fetal development of the adrenal. *J Pediatr Surg* 1981;16(4 Suppl 1):636–644.
54. Turkel SB, Itabashi HH. The natural history of neuroblastic cells in the fetal adrenal gland. *Am J Pathol* 1974;76(2): 225–244.
55. Beckwith JB, Perrin EV. In situ neuroblastomas: A contribution to the natural history of neural crest tumors. *Am J Pathol* 1963;43:1089–1104.
56. Schober A, Parlato R, Huber K, et al. Cell loss and autophagy in the extra-adrenal chromaffin organ of Zuckerkandl are regulated by glucocorticoid signalling. *J Neuroendocrinol* 2013;25(1):34–47.
57. Vogel KS. Development of trophic interactions in the vertebrate peripheral nervous system. *Mol Neurobiol* 1993;7(3–4): 363–382.
58. Garcia I, Martinou I, Tsujimoto Y, et al. Prevention of programmed cell death of sympathetic neurons by the bcl-2 proto-oncogene. *Science* 1992;258(5080):302–304.
59. Tischler AS, DeLellis RA, Biales B, et al. Nerve growth factor-induced neurite outgrowth from normal human chromaffin cells. *Lab Invest* 1980;43(5):399–409.
60. Anderson DJ. Cellular 'neoteny': a possible developmental basis for chromaffin cell plasticity. *Trends Genet* 1989;5(6): 174–178.
61. DeLellis RA, Wolfe HJ, Gagel RF, et al. Adrenal medullary hyperplasia. A morphometric analysis in patients with familial medullary thyroid carcinoma. *Am J Pathol* 1976;83(1): 177–196.
62. Carney JA, Sizemore GW, Sheps SG. Adrenal medullary disease in multiple endocrine neoplasia, type 2: pheochromocytoma and its precursors. *Am J Clin Pathol* 1976;66(2): 279–290.
63. Kreiner E. Weight and shape of the human adrenal medulla in various age groups. *Virchows Arch A Pathol Anat Histol* 1982; 397(1):7–15.
64. Lack EE. Hyperplasia of vagal and carotid body paraganglia in patients with chronic hypoxemia. *Am J Pathol* 1978; 91(3):497–516.
65. Smith P, Jago R, Heath D. Anatomical variation and quantitative histology of the normal and enlarged carotid body. *J Pathol* 1982;137(4):287–304.
66. McDonald DM, Blewett RW. Location and size of carotid body-like organs (paraganglia) revealed in rats by the permeability of blood vessels to Evans blue dye. *J Neurocytol* 1981; 10(4):607–643.
67. Parker TL, Kesse WK, Mohamed AA, et al. The innervation of the mammalian adrenal gland. *J Anat* 1993;183(Pt 2): 265–276.
68. Mascorro JA, Yates RD. Innervation of abdominal paraganglia: An ultrastructural study. *J Morphol* 1974;142(2):153–163.
69. Matthews MR. Synaptic and other relationships of small granule-containing cells. In: Coupland RE, Fujita T, eds. *Chromaffin, Enterochromaffin and Related Cells*. Amsterdam: Elsevier; 1976.
70. McDonald DM, Mitchell RA. The Innervation of glomus cells, ganglion cells and blood vessels in the rat carotid body: A quantitative ultrastructural analysis. *J Neurocytol* 1975;4(2):177–230.
71. Leonard EM, Salman S, Nurse CA. Sensory processing and integration at the carotid body tripartite synapse: Neurotransmitter functions and effects of chronic hypoxia. *Front Physiol* 2018;9:225.
72. Kraus R, Bezdicek P. The incidence of mastocytes in paraganglia. *Folia Morphologica* 1988;36(2):211–213.
73. Lloyd RV, Blaivas M, Wilson BS. Distribution of chromogranin and S100 protein in normal and abnormal adrenal medullary tissues. *Arch Pathol Lab Med* 1985;109(7): 633–635.
74. Achilles E, Padberg BC, Holl K, et al. Immunocytochemistry of paragangliomas–value of staining for S-100 protein and glial fibrillary acid protein in diagnosis and prognosis. *Histopathology* 1991;18(5):453–458.
75. Habeck JO, Kummer W. Neuronal and neuroendocrine markers in the human carotid body in health and disease. *Adv Exp Med Biol* 1993;337:31–35.
76. Lack EE, Perez-Atayde AR, Young JB. Carotid body hyperplasia in cystic fibrosis and cyanotic heart disease. A combined morphometric, ultrastructural, and biochemical study. *Am J Pathol* 1985;119(2):301–314.
77. Arias-Stella J, Valcarcel J. Chief cell hyperplasia in the human carotid body at high altitudes; physiologic and pathologic significance. *Hum Pathol* 1976;7(4):361–373.
78. Heath D, Smith P, Jago R. Hyperplasia of the carotid body. *J Pathol* 1982;138(2):115–127.
79. Fitch R, Smith P, Heath D. Nerve axons in carotid body hyperplasia. A quantitative study. *Arch Pathol Lab Med* 1985; 109(3):234–237.
80. Verna A. Ultrastructure of the carotid body in the mammals. *Int Rev Cytol* 1979;60:271–330.
81. Coupland RE, Hopwood D. The mechanism of the differential staining reaction for adrenaline-and noreadrenaline-storing granules in tissues fixed in glutaraldehyde. *J Anat* 1966;100(Pt 2):227–243.
82. Brown WJ, Barajas L, Latta H. The ultrastructure of the human adrenal medulla: with comparative studies of white rat. *Anat Rec* 1971;169(2):173–183.
83. Lundberg JM, Hamberger B, Schultzberg M, et al. Enkephalin- and somatostatin-like immunoreactivities in human adrenal medulla and pheochromocytoma. *Proc Natl Acad Sci U S A* 1979;76(8):4079–4083.
84. Bock P, Stockinger L, Vyslonzil E. [The fine structure of the human carotid body]. *Z Zellforsch Mikrosk Anat* 1970; 105(4):543–568.

85. Hervonen A, Korkala O. Fine structure of the carotid body of the midterm human fetus. *Z Anat Entwicklungsgesch* 1972;138(2):135–144.
86. Lymperopoulos A, Brill A, McCrink KA. GPCRs of adrenal chromaffin cells & catecholamines: The plot thickens. *Int J Biochem Cell Biol* 2016;77(Pt B):213–219.
87. Greenberg ME, Ziff EB, Greene LA. Stimulation of neuronal acetylcholine receptors induces rapid gene transcription. *Science* 1986;234(4772):80–83.
88. Sietzen M, Schober M, Fischer-Colbrie R, et al. Rat adrenal medulla: levels of chromogranins, enkephalins, dopamine beta-hydroxylase and of the amine transporter are changed by nervous activity and hypophysectomy. *Neuroscience* 1987;22(1):131–139.
89. Mahata SK, Mahapatra NR, Mahata M, et al. Catecholamine secretory vesicle stimulus-transcription coupling in vivo. Demonstration by a novel transgenic promoter/photoprotein reporter and inhibition of secretion and transcription by the chromogranin A fragment catestatin. *J Biol Chem* 2003;278(34):32058–32067.
90. Tischler AS, Riseberg JC, Cherington V. Multiple mitogenic signalling pathways in chromaffin cells: a model for cell cycle regulation in the nervous system. *Neurosci Lett* 1994;168(1–2):181–184.
91. Penberthy WT, Dahmer MK. Insulin-like growth factor-I-enhanced secretion is abolished in protein kinase C-deficient chromaffin cells. *J Neurochem* 1994;62(5):1707–1715.
92. Powers JF, Brachold JM, Ehsani SA, et al. Up-regulation of ret by reserpine in the adult rat adrenal medulla. *Neuroscience* 2005;132(3):605–612.
93. Hervonen A, Korkala O. The effect of hypoxia on the catecholamine content of human fetal abdominal paraganglia and adrenal medulla. *Acta Obstet Gynecol Scand* 1972;51(1):17–24.
94. Dalmaz Y, Borghini N, Pequignot JM, et al. Presence of chemosensitive SIF cells in the rat sympathetic ganglia: A biochemical, immunocytochemical and pharmacological study. *Adv Exp Med Biol* 1993;337:393–399.
95. Dahlqvist A, Neuhuber WL, Forsgren S. Innervation of laryngeal nerve paraganglia: an anterograde tracing and immunohistochemical study in the rat. *J Comp Neurol* 1994;345(3):440–446.
96. Saldana MJ, Salem LE, Travezan R. High altitude hypoxia and chemodectomas. *Hum Pathol* 1973;4(2):251–263.
97. Hervonen A, Pickel VM, Joh TH, et al. Immunocytochemical demonstration of the catecholamine-synthesizing enzymes and neuropeptides in the catecholamine-storing cells of human fetal sympathetic nervous system. *Adv Biochem Psychopharmacol* 1980;25:373–378.
98. Lloyd RV, Sisson JC, Shapiro B, et al. Immunohistochemical localization of epinephrine, norepinephrine, catecholamine-synthesizing enzymes, and chromogranin in neuroendocrine cells and tumors. *Am J Pathol* 1986;125(1):45–54.
99. Falck B, Bjorklund A, Lindvall O. Recent progress in aldehyde fluorescence histochemistry. *Brain Res Bull* 1982;9(1–6):3–10.
100. Kantorovich V, Pacak K. Pheochromocytoma and paraganglioma. *Prog Brain Res* 2010;182:343–373.
101. Varndell IM, Tapia FJ, De Mey J, et al. Electron immunocytochemical localization of enkephalin-like material in catecholamine-containing cells of the carotid body, the adrenal medulla, and in pheochromocytomas of man and other mammals. *J Histochem Cytochem* 1982;30(7):682–690.
102. Winkler H. The adrenal chromaffin granule: a model for large dense core vesicles of endocrine and nervous tissue. *J Anat* 1993;183(Pt 2):237–252.
103. Kent C, Coupland RE. On the uptake and storage of 5-hydroxytryptamine, 5-hydroxytryptophan and catecholamines by adrenal chromaffin cells and nerve endings. *Cell Tissue Res* 1984;236(1):189–195.
104. Rodriguez-Cuevas S, Lopez-Garza J, Labastida-Almendaro S. Carotid body tumors in inhabitants of altitudes higher than 2000 meters above sea level. *Head Neck* 1998;20(5):374–378.
105. Tischler AS, Powers JF, Alroy J. Animal models of pheochromocytoma. *Histol Histopathol* 2004;19(3):883–895.
106. Papathomas TG, Oudijk L, Persu A, et al. SDHB/SDHA immunohistochemistry in pheochromocytomas and paragangliomas: a multicenter interobserver variation analysis using virtual microscopy: a Multinational Study of the European Network for the Study of Adrenal Tumors (ENS@T). *Mod Pathol* 2015;28(6):807–821.
107. Roszko KL, Blouch E, Blake M, et al. Case Report of a Prolactinoma in a Patient With a Novel MAX Mutation and Bilateral Pheochromocytomas. *J Endocr Soc* 2017;1(11):1401–1407.
108. Udager AM, Magers MJ, Goerke DM, et al. The utility of SDHB and FH immunohistochemistry in patients evaluated for hereditary paraganglioma-pheochromocytoma syndromes. *Hum Pathol* 2018;71:47–54.
109. Korner M, Waser B, Schonbrunn A, et al. Somatostatin receptor subtype 2A immunohistochemistry using a new monoclonal antibody selects tumors suitable for in vivo somatostatin receptor targeting. *Am J Surg Pathol* 2012;36(2):242–252.
110. Rizo J. Mechanism of neurotransmitter release coming into focus. *Protein Sci* 2018.
111. Li H, Hes O, MacLennan GT, et al. Immunohistochemical distinction of metastases of renal cell carcinoma to the adrenal from primary adrenal nodules, including oncocytic tumor. *Virchows Arch* 2015;466(5):581–588.
112. Miettinen M, McCue PA, Sarlomo-Rikala M, et al. GATA3: a multispecific but potentially useful marker in surgical pathology: a systematic analysis of 2500 epithelial and non-epithelial tumors. *Am J Surg Pathol* 2014;38(1):13–22.
113. O'Connor DT. Chromogranin: widespread immunoreactivity in polypeptide hormone producing tissues and in serum. *Regul Pept* 1983;6(3):263–280.
114. Lloyd RV, Wilson BS. Specific endocrine tissue marker defined by a monoclonal antibody. *Science* 1983;222(4624):628–630.
115. Schmid KW, Schroder S, Dockhorn-Dworniczak B, et al. Immunohistochemical demonstration of chromogranin A, chromogranin B, and secretogranin II in extra-adrenal paragangliomas. *Mod Pathol* 1994;7(3):347–353.
116. Fischer-Colbrie R, Lassmann H, Hagn C, et al. Immunological studies on the distribution of chromogranin A and B in endocrine and nervous tissues. *Neuroscience* 1985;16(3):547–555.
117. Helle KB, Metz-Boutigue MH, Cerra MC, et al. Chromogranins: from discovery to current times. *Pflugers Arch* 2018;470(1):143–154.
118. Tischler AS. Pheochromocytoma and extra-adrenal paraganglioma: updates. *Arch Pathol Lab Med* 2008;132(8):1272–1284.
119. Schafer BW, Heizmann CW. The S100 family of EF-hand calcium-binding proteins: functions and pathology. *Trends Biochem Sci* 1996;21(4):134–140.

120. Iwanaga T, Takahashi Y, Fujita T. Immunohistochemistry of neuron-specific and glia-specific proteins. *Arch Histol Cytol* 1989;52 Suppl:13–24.
121. Schroder HD, Johannsen L. Demonstration of S-100 protein in sustentacular cells of phaeochromocytomas and paragangliomas. *Histopathology* 1986;10(10):1023–1033.
122. Gosney JR, Denley H, Resl M. Sustentacular cells in pulmonary neuroendocrine tumours. *Histopathology* 1999;34(3):211–215.
123. Douwes Dekker PB, Corver WE, Hogendoorn PC, et al. Multiparameter DNA flow-sorting demonstrates diploidy and SDHD wild-type gene retention in the sustentacular cell compartment of head and neck paragangliomas: chief cells are the only neoplastic component. *J Pathol* 2004;202(4):456–462.
124. Moriguchi T, Takako N, Hamada M, et al. Gata3 participates in a complex transcriptional feedback network to regulate sympathoadrenal differentiation. *Development* 2006;133(19):3871–3881.
125. Simson JA, Hintz DS, Munster AM, et al. Immunocytochemical evidence for antibody binding to mast cell granules. *Exp Mol Pathol* 1977;26(1):85–91.
126. Spicer SS, Spivey MA, Ito M, et al. Some ascites monoclonal antibody preparations contain contaminants that bind to selected Golgi zones or mast cells. *J Histochem Cytochem* 1994;42(2):213–221.
127. Grube D. Immunoreactivities of gastrin (G-) cells. II. Non-specific binding of immunoglobulins to G-cells by ionic interactions. *Histochemistry* 1980;66(2):149–167.
128. Srivastava A, Tischler AS, Delellis RA. Endogenous biotin staining as an artifact of antigen retrieval with automated immunostaining. *Endocr Pathol* 2004;15(2):175–178.
129. Powers JF, Brachold JM, Tischler AS. Ret protein expression in adrenal medullary hyperplasia and pheochromocytoma. *Endocr Pathol* 2003;14(4):351–361.
130. Roshchina VV. The fluorescence methods to study neurotransmitters (biomediators) in plant cells. *J Fluoresc* 2016;26(3):1029–1043.
131. de la Torre JC. Standardization of the sucrose-potassium phosphate-glyoxylic acid histofluorescence method for tissue monoamines. *Neurosci Lett* 1980;17(3):339–340.
132. Parke WW, Valsamis MP. The ampulloglomerular organ: an unusual neurovascular complex in the suboccipital region. *Anat Rec* 1967;159(2):193–198.
133. Bailey OT. The cutaneous glomus and its tumors-glomangiomas. *Am J Pathol* 1935;11(6):915–936, 917.
134. Ostrowski ML, Wheeler TM. Paraganglia of the prostate. Location, frequency, and differentiation from prostatic adenocarcinoma. *Am J Surg Pathol* 1994;18(4):412–420.
135. Rode J, Bentley A, Parkinson C. Paraganglial cells of urinary bladder and prostate: Potential diagnostic problem. *J Clin Pathol* 1990;43(1):13–16.
136. Makinen J, Nickels J. Paraganglion cells mimicking metastatic clear cell carcinoma. *Histopathology* 1979;3(6):459–465.

Index

Note: Page number followed by f and t indicates figure and table respectively.

A

Abdominal aortic aneurysms, 193–194
Abrikossoff tumor, 324
Acervuli cerebri, 249
Acetic acid zinc formalin (AZF), 814
6-Acetylmorphine, 40
Achaete–scute complex like1 (ASCL1), 1252
Achilles tendon, 122
Acidophilic and apoptotic bodies, 699f
Acinar cells, 458, 747, 748f
    cystadenoma, 764
    minor alterations in, 760–761
Acinar cystic transformation. See Acinar cell cystadenoma
Acinar ectasia, 760
Acinar enzymes, 755
Acini, 443–444, 443f, 444f, 746–749, 747f
Acinic cell carcinoma, 457
Acinus, lobule and, 475–478, 476f, 477f
Acquired immunodeficiency syndrome (AIDS), 518
Acral skeleton, 87, 88t
Acrosyringium, 14f
Actin microfilaments, 34
Acute pancreatitis, 148t
Acute respiratory distress syndrome (ARDS), 484
Adenocarcinomas, 491
    bulbomembranous urethra, 1024
    intestinal-type, 434
    of Skene gland, 1055
Adenohypophysis, 270
    age-related changes of, 294–295, 295f
    corticotrophs, 288–289, 289f
    folliculostellate cell, 292, 293f
    gonadotrophs, 289, 291, 291f
    lactotrophs, 287–288, 288f
    pars tuberalis, 291–292, 292f
    physiology and histology, 283–292
    somatotrophs, 283, 285–287
    thyrotrophs, 289, 290f, 291f
    variation in normal morphology, 292–294, 293f, 294f
Adenomatoid salivary gland hyperplasia, 455
Adenomyoma, 746, 746f
Adenosine triphosphatase (ATPase), 446
Adherens junctions, 207
Adipocytes. See also Adipose tissue
    atrophy of, 144, 145f
    brown (see Brown adipose tissue (BAT))
    capillaries and, 135
    subcutaneous tissue, 16, 18
    white (see White adipose tissue (WAT))
Adipophilin, 24
Adipose-derived stem cells, 141
Adipose tissue, 133
    beige fat, 141
    biopsy analysis of, 147
    brown, 139–141
    cytogenetics of lipomas, 155–156
    developmental stages of, 134f
    fatty infiltration, 147, 148t
    histochemistry
        enzyme, 141–142
        lipid, 142
    immunohistochemistry, 143
        obesity, 143–144
    inflammations
        calciphylaxis, 149
        fat necrosis, 147–149, 149f
        lipogranuloma, 150
        mesenteritis, 149–150
        panniculitis, 149
    lesions, 144
        atrophy, 144, 145f
        cellulite, 144–145
        degeneration, 144
        ischemia, 145–146, 146f
        metaplasia, 146, 146f
    lipodystrophy, 146
    mimics of fat cells
        lipoblasts, 157–158, 157f, 158f
        mature fat cells, 156–157
    stem cells in, 141
    syndromes associated with fatty lesions, 148t, 156
    tumors and tumor-like lesions
        adipose tissue within nonfatty lesions, 150
        ectopic adipose tissue, 151
        hamartomas containing fat cells, 151
        hibernoma, 150
        intramuscular lipoma, 152–153, 153f
        lipoblastoma, 155
        lipomas, 151–155, 152f
        massive localized lymphedema, 151
        mesenchymomas, 151
        myxoid lipoma, 152, 153f
        special lipoma types, 155, 155f
    types of, 134–141
    white, 134–139
Adnexal carcinoma, 23f, 24
Adolescent, breast, 70–71, 71f
Adrenal cortex. See also Adrenal gland
    development, 1226–1228
    evolution, 1225–1226
    histology, 1229–1238
    immunohistochemistry, 1239
    nodules, 1247
    thickness, 1229
    ultrastructure, 1240–1241
Adrenal gland. See also Adrenal cortex
    accessory adrenal cortex, 1245–1247
    adrenocortical nodules, 1247, 1248f
    anatomy, 1225, 1226f
    arteries, 1242–1243
    blood vessels, 1242
    capsule, 1230–1232, 1230f–1232f
    cortex, 1226–1228, 1227f, 1228f, 1239
    cortical thickness, 1229
    corticomedullary junction, 1236f, 1238, 1238f, 1243
    development of, 1226–1229, 1227f–1229f
    evolution, 1225–1226
    histologic study, 1229–1230
    histology, 1230–1238
    ideal, 1229
    immunohistochemistry, 1239–1240
    intraglandular vasculature, 1243
    lymphatics, 1245
    medulla, 1228–1229, 1229f, 1235–1239, 1236f–1239f
    nerves and ganglia, 1244
    prenatal and postnatal adrenal cortex and medulla, 1240t
    studied, 1229–1230
    ultrastructure, 1240–1241
    vasculature, 1243
    veins, 1243–1244
    weight, 1229
    zona fasciculata, 1233f, 1234, 1234f
    zona glomerulosa, 1231f–1233f, 1233–1234
    zona reticularis, 1233f, 1234–1235
Adrenal medulla, 1274
    development, 1228–1229
    evolution, 1225–1226
    histology, 1230
    immunohistochemistry, 1239–1240
    medullary cells, 1235
    ultrastructure, 1241
    weight, 1229
Adrenocortical nodules, 1247, 1248f
Adrenocorticotropic hormone (ACTH), adrenal cortex, 1233
Adrenocorticotropin (ACTH), 1256
Adventitia, 546
Adventitial cells, 819
Adventitial dermis, 15
Age-related changes
    anal canal, 681
    aorta, 191, 192t
    arteries, 195, 196f
    blood vessels, 190, 191t
    human conduction system, 545
    intracardiac valves, 541
    liver, 706–707
    lungs, 500, 500f
    neuroendocrine cell, 1266
    paraganglia, 1286–1287
    pulmonary vessels, 200
    skeletal muscle, 181–183
    thymic hyperplasia, 517–518, 518t
    thymic involution, 517
    vessels, 500f

Agglutinin, 443
Aggrecan, 115
Aging testis, 993–994
Airways, 470–475, 471f, 472f, 473t–474t, 474f–476f. *See also* Lungs
Albinism, 9
Alcian blue, 23, 323, 750
Alexander disease, 242
α-adrenoreceptors, 140
α-1-antitrypsin deficiency, 149
α-Bungarotoxin, 181
Alpha cell granules, 756
Alveolar–capillary membrane, 477
Alveolar microvasculature, 478
Alzheimer astrocytes, in hyperammonemia, 242, 242f
Alzheimer disease, 233
   intraneuronal inclusions in, 233
Amelogenesis, 397
Ammon horn, 225–226, 227f, 233
Amnion
   bands, 1151
   epithelial cells, 1152
   epithelium, 1151
   gross morphologic alterations, 1149–1151
   histologic abnormalities of, 1152–1154
      epithelial degeneration, 1154f
   histology, 1151–1152
Amphiarthrodial joints, 113, 115–116, 116f
Ampullae of Vater, 627, 719, 738, 741, 745, 764
Amputation neuromas, 323
Amyloidosis, fat biopsy for, 147
Amyloid precursor protein (APP), 237
Anagen phase of hair growth, 11, 12
Anal canal
   aging, 681
   anal glands, 679
   anal transitional zone, 684t
   anatomy, 679–681
   blood supply, 681
   boundaries, 677
   cell types, 684t
   colorectal carcinoma, 685t
   cytokeratins, 683f
   definitions of, 677
   diagnostic considerations, 687–689
   embryology, 677–679, 678f
   epithelial metaplasia and heterotopia, 687
   epithelial mucins, 679
   external anal sphincter, 678f
   function, 679–681
   gross and functional anatomy, 679–681, 679f
   heterotopia, 687
   histology, 687
   inflammatory conditions, 687
   innervation, 680–681
   internal anal sphincter, 678f
   keratin, 683
   lamina propria and muscularis mucosae, 682
   light microscopy, 681–687
   metaplasia, 687
   mucosa, 682–684
   muscle cells and nerves, 679
   musculature, 680
   neoplasia, 687–689
   neoplastic disease, 687
   pathologic processes, 685t
   pecten, 679f
   perianal skin, 684t
   structures of, 678f
   surgical specimen, 679f
   vasculature, 681
   zones, 679
Anal glomeruli, 202
Anastomoses, 202–203, 203f
Anatomy
   adrenal gland, 1225, 1226f
   anal canal, 679–681
   appendix, 664–665
   applied
      cardiac skeleton, 532
      interatrial septum, 535
      of intracardiac valves, 540–541
      left ventricle, 538
      pericardium, 532
      right ventricle, 538
   brain, 222f
   colon, 641–642
   external ear, 364–365
   gallbladder, 719–720
   inner ear, 374–378
   larynx, 424–432
   middle ear, 367–369
   nail, gross, 37–39
   nail plates, 39–40
   ovary, 1108–1109
   paraganglia, 1281–1282
   peripheral nerves, 302–303
   pharynx, 434–437
   pituitary and sellar region, 271–276
   skeletal muscle, 170–171, 171f
   thymus, 508–509
   thyroid gland, 1177–1179
   vulva, 1032–1033, 1033f
Angiodysplasia, 203–204
   of colon, 204, 204f
Angiofibromas, 434
Angiogenesis, 1081
Angiolipoma, 154, 154f
Angiomyolipoma, 151
Angioplasty, 205, 206f
Angle of His. *See* Incisura
Ankyrin-binding proteins, 315
Annular/ring pancreas, 745, 745f
Annulus fibrosus, 115
Anogenital mammary-like glands, 1042, 1042f
Antemortem ischemia, 226
Anterolateral commissure, 539
Anterosuperior mediastinal node, 1178
Anthracosis, 482
Anti-amyloid antibodies, 213
Antidiuretic hormone (ADH), 281
Anti-endoglin (CD105), 209
Antigens, 516
Anti-HECA 452, 210
Anti-müllerian hormone (AMH), 984
Aorta, 190–195, 191t, 192f–195f
   aging changes, 191, 192t
   aortic aneurysms, 193–194
   calcification, 191, 193f
   coarctation of, 194–195, 195f
   cystic medial degeneration, 191, 192f, 193
   degenerative changes, 191, 192f
   inflammatory aggregates in aortic wall, 194, 194f
   Marfan syndrome and aortic wall, 193, 193f
Aortic media, 208, 208f
Aortic valve from normal heart, 538f
Aortic valve sclerosis, 541
aP2 (adipocyte lipid-binding protein), 143
Apical caps, 482
Apocrine glands, 4, 15, 15f, 1039, 1040f, 1041
Apoeccrine glands, 15
Apophyses, 89
Apoptosis, 32, 168, 441, 508, 801, 801f, 1280. *See also* Thymus
   nails, 32
   in neuroendocrine cells, 1255–1256
APP. *See* Amyloid precursor protein (APP)
Appendicular skeleton, 87, 88t
Appendix
   appendiceal lumen, 672–673
   function, 665
   gross anatomy/surgical perspective, 664–665
   histology, 665–672
   mucocele of, 674
   mucosal architecture and design, 665–671, 665f–667f
   mucosal inflammation *vs.* acute appendicitis, 672
APUD (Amine Precursor Uptake and Decarboxylation), 1250–1251
Aquaporins, 40
Arabesque profiles, 146
Arachnoid cap cells, 260
Arachnoiditis ossificans, 260
Arachnoid trabeculae, 260
Areae gastricae, 602
Argentaffin cells, 1253, 1254f
Arnold nerve, 1278
Arrhythmogenic right ventricular dysplasia/cardiomyopathy (ARVD/CMP), 537, 538
Arteries, 195–197, 196f–197f
   adrenal gland, 1242–1243
   aging changes in, 195, 196f
   atheromatous, 196
   fibrinoid necrosis, 197, 197f
   healed vasculitis, 197, 198f
   intimal fibrosis, 195, 196f
   intima of, 195
   vasa vasorum, 196, 197f
   vulnerable plaque, 196–197
Arterioles, 197–198, 546
Arterioluminal vessels, 537
Arteriovenous fistula, 204
Arthritis, 122, 124
   affect of
      on articular cartilage, 124–126, 125f–127f
      on bone, 126–129, 128f, 129f
   causes of, 124f
   change in joint shape, 124
   types of, 122

Articular cartilage, 116–121
  adult, 117
  arthritis and, 124–126
  basophilic line (tidemark), 117, 120f
  calcification of cartilage matrix, 119
  cartilage turnover and articular remodeling, 120–121, 121f
  collagen fibers in, 116–117, 119f
  histomorphogenesis of, 121
  microscopic examination, 116, 117f
  mineralization with replicated tidemark, 117, 120f
  morphology, 116–120, 117f–121f
  nonviable cells in calcified zone, 116, 118f
  proteoglycans in, 117, 119f
  subchondral bone plate with irregular interface, 117, 120f
  zones, 116, 118f
Articulating cartilage, 114–115
Artifact of fixation (infant eye), 354, 354f
Artifacts, 21–22, 795
  bone, 109–110, 110f
  CNS, 264–269, 264t, 265f–268f
  freezing, 22f
  intrinsic, 795
  in lung biopsy/resection material, 484–488, 484f–487f, 484t
  neuroendocrine cell, 1267
  paraganglia, 1290–1291
  peripheral nerve, 317f
  retina, 351–352, 352f
  in salivary gland, reactive changes, 456
  skin, 21–22
  technical, 795, 795f
  thymus, 519, 519f
  tissue, and biopsy limitations, 547–549, 548f
Arytenoid cartilage, 425, 432
Asteroid bodies, 494, 495f
Asthmatics, 489
Astrocytes, 239–243
  age-related inclusions in, 241, 241f
  Creutzfeldt, 242, 242f
  normal microscopic anatomy, 239–241, 240f
  reactions to injury, 241–243, 242f, 243f
  reactive, 239f–240f
Asymmetric unit membrane (AUM), 954
Atelectasis, 486f
Atheromatous lesions, modified American Heart Association classification of, 196–197, 197t
Atherosclerosis, 190
  immunohistochemical staining in, 213, 213f
Atretic follicles, of ovary, 1126–1129
  cystic follicles, 1127
  granulosa cells of, 1127
  histology, 1126–1127, 1127f–1128f
  hormonal aspects, 1129
  shrinkage and hyalinization of, 1127, 1128f
Atrial appendage, 536
Atrial myocytes, 534
Atrioventricular (AV) nodal apparatus, 544f
Atrioventricular node (AV node), conduction system, 542, 544f, 545
Atrioventricular valves (AV valves), 539–540, 540f
Atrophy, 455, 455f, 768–772, 769f–772f

Atypical adenomatous hyperplasia (AAH), 490, 491f
Auditory epithelial migration, 365–366
Auricular appendage, 535
Autoimmune lymphoproliferative syndrome, 801
Autonomic ganglia, 545
Autonomic nerves, 303
Axial skeleton, 87, 88t
Axonal spheroids, 237, 238f
Axonal varicosities, 545
Axons, growth of, 301
Axoplasmic flow, 311
Azulfidine blue vital dye, 1044

B
Balls of thread, 275
Bannayan syndrome, 148t
Barrett esophagus, 587, 591–593, 592f, 593f
Bartholin duct, 442, 1035, 1035f
Bartholin glands, 1035
  acini, 1035, 1035f
Basal cell carcinoma (BCC)
  tissue defects in, 22f
  vs. squamous cell carcinoma, 26t
Basal cell hyperplasia, 978, 978f
Basal cells, 458, 459
  carcinoma, 22, 22f
  and cytokeratin, 6
  plasma membrane of, 7
  skin, 5
Basal ganglia, 225, 226f
Basal layers, of epidermis, 5. See also Keratinocytes
  melanocytes in, 8, 8f
  Merkel cell in, 10, 10f
Basaloid epithelium, 437
Basement membrane zone, 7, 8f
Basophil invasion, 293, 293f, 294f
BAT. See Brown adipose tissue (BAT)
BCC. See Basal cell carcinoma (BCC)
BCL10, 748
Bcl-2/caspase-9 pathway, 168
Bcl-2 immunostain, in nail matrix, 53
Bcl-2 protein, 801
Beau line, 41, 60
Beckwith hemihypertrophy, 148t
Beige fat, 141
Bell–Magendie law, 302
Benign mesenchymomas, 151
Benign prostatic hyperplasia (BPH), 964
Benign tumors, 449t
Berardinelli lipodystrophy, 148t
BerEP4, 24
Bergmann astrocytes, 238f, 239, 241
β-1 and β-2 adrenoreceptors, 140
β-catenin, in nail matrix, 51
Beta cells, 756
Betz cells, 227
Bile canaliculi, 699
Biliary intraepithelial neoplasia (BilIN), 733–734
Biopsy
  endomyocardial (see Endomyocardial biopsy)
  excisional, 21, 22f
  limitations and tissue artifacts, 547–549, 548f

  lung
    appearing normal, 500–501, 500t, 501f
    artifacts in, 484–488, 484f–487f, 484t
  of nail, 61
  skin, 20–21
  vestibular, 1036
  vulvar, 1033–1034
Biopsy trauma, 634–635
Birbeck granule, 4, 9, 10f, 16
Black spots, 553
Bladder cancer, staging of, 953f
Bladder diverticulum, 961, 961f
Blebs, 483
Blood supply, 437, 442, 509
  breast, 79–80
  kidney, 880
  nail, 58–59, 58f, 59f
  ovary, 1109
  peripheral nerve, 308
  skeletal muscle, 169
  thyroid gland, 1178
  ureters, 952
  urinary bladder, 952
  vagina, 1050
Blood vessels, 190
  adrenal gland, 1242
  aging changes in, 190, 191t
  anastomoses, 202–204, 203f
  angiodysplasias, 204
  antigen expression
    endothelium, 208–210, 209f–212f
    smooth muscle, 210, 212–213, 212f
  aorta, 190–195, 191t, 192f–195f
  arteries, 195–197, 196f–197f
  arterioles, 197–198
  capillaries, 198–199
  gross and light microscopic features, 190–206
  immunohistochemical staining of, 211f
  pulmonary arteries and veins, 199–200, 201f, 201t, 202f
  sinusoids, 199
  ultrastructural features of, 206, 207t
    adventitia and supporting cells, 208
    endothelial cells, 206–207
    inclusions of endothelial cells, 207–208
    lymphatics and veins, 208
    media, 208
  vascular malformations, 204
  vascular surgery, and pathologic changes, 204, 205t
    angioplasty, 205, 206f
    bypass grafts, 204–205, 205t
    endarterectomy, 204, 205t
    prosthetic vessels, 205–206
  veins, 199, 200f
  venules and lymphatics, 199
Blue bodies, 493, 494f
Blue spot, 235, 236f
Bodian stain, 181
Bone, 87
  basic multicellular unit of, 108–109, 109f
  cancellous, 94, 94f
  characteristics of, 87–88
  composition, 90
  cortical, 91–93, 92f–93f

Bone (continued)
  formation, growth, and remodeling, 101
    appositional and interstitial growth, 101
    endochondral ossification, 101–108, 101f
    intramembranous ossification, 108, 108f
    modeling and remodeling, 108–109, 109f
  functions of, 88
  hierarchical structure of, 87, 88f
  histologic artifacts, 109–110, 110f
    bone dust, 110, 110f
    decalcification agents, 109, 109f
    overdecalcification, 109, 110f
    underdecalcification, 109–110, 110f
  inorganic component, 96
    mineral, 100–101
  lamellar, 90–91, 90f–92f
  as organ, 89–96
    microscopic anatomy, 89–90, 89f
    size and shape, 89
  organic component, 96
    osteoblasts, 97–98, 97f, 98f
    osteoclasts, 99–100, 99f
    osteocytes, 98–99, 98f, 99f
    osteoprogenitor cells, 97
    proteins, 96–97
  pathologic conditions of, 109
  periosteum, 94, 95f
  of skeleton, 88t
    acral skeleton, 87, 88t
    appendicular (peripheral) skeleton, 87, 88t
    axial skeleton, 87, 88t
  tubular, 89
  vascular supply and innervation, 95, 95f
  woven, 90–91, 90f
Bone dust, 110, 110f
Bone marrow, 96
  fat in, 96, 96f
  functions of, 813
  gelatinous transformation of, 96, 96f
  hematopoiesis
    in embryo and fetus, 817–818
    general features of, 815–816
    regulation of, 816–817
  hematopoietic cells
    eosinophil and basophil precursors, 831–832
    lymphocytes and plasma cells, 843–847
    megakaryocytes, 840–843
    monocyte precursors, 832–835
    neutrophil precursors, 826–831
    red cell precursors, 835–840
  hematopoietic marrow, structural organization of, 818–826
  lineage antigens, 814t
  marrow cellularity, 847–848
  marrow differential count, 848, 849t
  marrow monocytes, 834
  marrow reticulocytes, 836
  marrow smears, 814
  mass of, 813
  postnatal changes, 818
  red marrow, distribution of, 818
  structural organization
    blood supply, 818–819
    extracellular matrix, 819–820
    nerve supply, 819
    stromal cells, 820–826
  techniques for studying, 813–815
  transplantation of, 815
Bone marrow embolus, 496, 496f
Bone morphogenetic proteins, 870
Bone remodeling unit of Frost, 108–109, 109f
Bony sella, 271–272, 272f, 273f
Bouin's fixative, 814
Bowel preparation effects, 654. See also Colon
Bowman capsule, 905
Brain sand, 249
Brain stem, 221–222, 222f
  base, 221
  long tracts, 221
  medulla, 223f
  midbrain, 222f
  pons, 223f
  surface anatomy of brain, 222f
  tectum, 221
  tegmentum, 221
Branching morphogenesis, 743
Bread-loafing technique, 21
Breast, 69
  adolescence, 70–71, 71f
  adult female, 71–78 (see also Female breast)
  adult male breast, 80
  biomarkers, 80–81
  blood supply, 79–80
  embryology, 69–70, 70f
  immunophenotypic features, 81
  infant, 70, 70f
  lymphatic drainage, 80
  menopause, 79, 80f
  molecular markers, 81
  neuroendocrine cells of, 1264
  pregnancy and lactation, 78–79
  steroid and peptide hormonal influences on, 70t
Breast carcinoma, microvasculature in, 209–210, 210f
Brodmann map, 227
Bronchi, 470
Bronchial cartilage, 469
Bronchial epithelium, 471f, 475f
Bronchial mucosa, 471
Bronchial submucosal glands, 476f
Bronchiolarization, 472
Bronchioles, 471, 471f
Bronchopulmonary neuroendocrine cells, 1266
Bronchpulmonary segments, 470t
Bronchus, 471f
Bronchus-associated lymphoid tissue (BALT), 479
Brown adipose tissue (BAT), 18, 139–141
  function of, 140
  histology, 141, 141f
  lesions, 150
  normal adult brown fat, 141f
  postnatal development, 140
  prenatal development, 139
  regulation, 140–141
Brown fat. See Brown adipose tissue (BAT)
Brown pigments, 714–716
Bruch membrane, 346–347, 347f
Brunner gland, 627, 634, 746
Brunner's glands, 1265
Brunn nests, 954, 955, 955f
Bubble artifact, 484, 485f
Buccopharyngeal membrane, 434
Buck fascia, 1013, 1020, 1020f
Bulbourethral glands, 1025, 1025f
Bullae, 483
Bullous emphysema, 488
Butyrate esterase, 747
Bypass grafts, 204–205, 205t

C

Calciphylaxis, 149
Calcitonin, 1186, 1256
Calcium, in nail plates, 40
Calcium oxalate crystals, 495f
Caliber-persistent artery, 204
Calretinin, 557, 557f, 989
Calyces formation, 857–858
CAM5.2 antibody, 748
CAM5.2 immunostaining, 23f
Canal of Corti, 380, 380f
Cancellous bone, 94, 94f
  macerated portion of, 94, 94f
  small trabeculae, 94
Cap, 859
Capillaries, 198–199, 546
Capsule, of adrenal gland, 1230–1232, 1230f–1232f. See also Adrenal gland
Carbonic anhydrase, 446, 752, 752f
Carbon monoxide poisoning, 225
Carboxyl ester hydrolase, 748
Carcinoembryonic antigen (CEA), 459, 621
Carcinoid tumorlets, 489
Carcinoma
  adnexal, 23f, 24
  of Bartholin gland, 1035
  basal cells, 22, 22f, 26t
  squamous cell, 24, 26t
  of vulva, 1031
Cardiac congestion, chronic, 810
Cardiac ganglia (parasympathetic), 545
Cardiac innervation, 545, 545f
Cardiac skeleton
  about, 532, 532f
  applied anatomy, 532
Cardiac valves. See also Heart
  aging changes of intracardiac valves, 541
  applied anatomy of intracardiac valves, 540–541
  atrioventricular valves (AV valves), 539–540, 540f
  chordae tendineae, 540, 541f
  papillary muscles, 541–542, 542f
  semilunar valves, 538–539, 538f
Carney complex, 324
Carney syndrome, 148t
Carotid artery, 204
Carotid body, 1274
  lobular architecture of, 1282–1283, 1283f
Carotid endarterectomy, 204
Carpal tunnel syndrome, 148t
Cartilage regeneration, 125
Caruncle, 343, 343f
Carunculae hymenales/carunculae myrtiformes, 1037
Catagen phase of hair growth, 11–12
Cataract of rubella, 354
Catecholaminergic neurons, 235

Catecholamines, 1286, 1291
Caval blood, 530
Caveolae, 207, 207f
Cavernous arteries, 1025
Cavernous nerves, 1044
Cavitational ultrasonic surgical aspirator (CUSA), 264–265
CC. See Corpora cavernosa (CC)
C cells (parafollicular cells), 1184–1186
    granules, 1186
    histochemistry and immunohistochemistry, 1186
    hyperplasia, 1185
    location of, 1184–1185
    ultrastructural characteristic of, 1186
CD1, 516
CD8, 516
CD14, 516
CD38, 516
CD56, 1260
CD57, 1260
CD99, 516
CD146, 562
CD1a, 4, 516
CD30 antigen, 3
CD34+ hematopoietic precursor cell, 4
CDX2, 1260
CEA. See Carcinoembryonic antigen (CEA)
Celiac trunk, 739
Cell junction proteins, 3–4, 314
Cell type differentiation, 873
Cellular schwannoma, 324
Cellulite, 144–145
Cement lines, lamellar bone, 91, 92f
Central chromatolysis, 235, 237, 237f
Central muscular portion of heart, 532
Central nervous system (CNS), 219
    artifacts, 264–269, 264t, 265f–268f
    brown pigment in, 263t
    cellular constituents of
        astrocytes, 239–243
        ependyma, 245–246
        gray matter and white matter, 228–229, 229f
        microglia and monocyte, 246–248
        neurons, 230–239, 230f
        oligodendroglia, 243–245
        response to injury, 248–249
    fetal brain, 263
    granular bodies in, 252t
    specialized organs of
        choroid plexus, 253–254
        circumventricular organs, 254–256
        median eminence and infundibulum, 249, 251–252
        olfactory bulbs and tracts, 252–253
        pineal gland, 249, 249f, 250f
    spinal cord and brain stem, organization of, 220–228, 220f
        basal ganglia, 225, 226f
        brain stem, 221–222, 222f
        cerebellum, 222, 224f, 225
        cerebral cortex, 227–228
        cerebrum, 225
        diencephalon, 225
        hippocampal formation, 225–226, 227f
        spinal cord, 220–221, 221f

Centriacinar (centrilobular) emphysema, 482
Centroacinar cells, 749, 749f
Cerebellopontine angle (CPA), 253
Cerebellum, 222–223, 224f, 225
    cerebellar cortex, 224f
Cerebral cortex, 227–228
Cerebrospinal fluid (CSF) rhinorrhea, 273
Cerebrum, 225
Cervical glandular hyperplasia, 1069
Cervical lymph nodes, thyroid inclusions in, 1193
Cervical stroma, 1073
Cervix, uterine
    cervical stroma, 1073
    decidual reaction in, 1074f
    differential diagnosis, 1075t–1076t
    endocervix epithelium, 1066–1069
    exocervical epithelium, 1065–1066, 1065f
    mesonephric remnants in, 1074f
    during pregnancy, 1073
    transformation zone epithelium, 1069–1073, 1071f–1072f
CFU-GEMM, 816
Charcot–Böttcher crystalloids of Sertoli cells, 984, 993
Charcot–Marie–Tooth (CMT4F), 314
Cheeks, 409
Chemoreception, 1286
Chiari network, 535, 536f
Chick-quail chimera system, 1251
Children
    epidermis of, 18
    histologic differences of skin in, 18
Cholecystokinin (CCK) receptors, 591
Cholesterol granulomas, 496, 496f, 519
Chondrocyte cloning, 125–126, 126f
Chondrocyte necrosis, 125, 126f
Chondroid lipoma, 155
Chondroid metaplasia, 122, 432, 432f
Chondrolipoma, 154, 154f
Chordae tendineae, 540, 541f
Chordomas, 158
Chorion
    chorionic cysts, 1154, 1154f
    frondosum, 1154
    histology, 1154
    histopathology, 1154
    laeve, 1154
Choroid, 346–348, 346f, 347f
Choroid plexus, 253–254, 253f, 254f
Chromaffin cell, 1275, 1282
Chromaffin reaction, 1238
Chromogranin, 26
Chromogranin A (CgA), 1258
    in histopathology of paraganglia, 1287–1289, 1287f–1289f
Chromogranins/secretogranins (Cg/Sg), 1258
Chromophobic cells, 287
Ciliary body, 345–346, 345f, 346f
Ciliated cells of endometrium, 1067, 1068f
Ciliated columnar epithelium, 429f
Ciliogenesis, 1096
Circumcision, male, 1014
Circumvallate placenta, 1150, 1150f
Circumventricular organs (CVOs), 254–256, 255f–256f
Civinini–Morton metatarsalgia, 323

CK7 immunostain, 1024
CK-5–8 immunostain, nail matrix, 47, 48f
CK-14 immunostain, nail matrix, 47, 48f
CK-KL1 immunostain, nail matrix, 47, 49f
Claudin-1 (CLDN-1), 306
    in normal nail matrix, 47, 50f
Claudins, 304, 1181
Clear cell, 449
    eccrine glands, 13, 13f
    papulosis, 6
    squamous layer of, 6
Clitoral specimens, 1031
Clitoris, 1037–1038, 1038f
Clitoromegaly, 1031
Cloaca, 949
Clonality in multiple endocrine neoplasia (MEN), 1213
Club cells, 472, 475f
CM. See Confocal microscopy (CM)
CN0. See Cranial nerve zero (CN0)
Coarctation of aorta, 194–195, 195f
Collagen, 96
Collagen fibers
    in connective tissue, 115
    in skin, 4
Collagen-IV (Col-IV) immunostains, of nail matrix, 57f
Collagen type IV, 480
Collecting duct
    cortical (CCD), 861, 917–920
    medullary (MCD), 861, 872f, 920–921, 921f
    morphogenesis of, 858
    organogenetic processes of, 858
Colloidophagy, 1183
Colon
    anatomy, 641–642
    basement membrane, 649
    bowel preparation effects, 654
    cancer, 654
    cecum and rectum, 641
    colonocytes, 642
    common artifacts and variants, 644t
    embryology, 640–641
    endoscopy, 655
    epithelium, mucosal, 618
    function, 642
    lamina propria, 642
    light microscopy, 642–654
    mucosa, 642–652
    muscularis externa, 653–654
    physiologic inflammation, 642
    regional variations, 642
    regions of, 641f
    right and left, variations in, 640
    serosa, 653–654
    staining patterns of cell types, 645t
    submucosa, 652–653
    subserosal zone, 653–654
    tissue orientation and tangential sectioning, 654
    tissue trauma, 655
Colony-forming cells (CFC), 816
Colony-forming units (CFU), 816
Communicating nerve, 433
Compact bone. See Cortical bone
Compact islets, 753

Compression-induced nuclear smearing artifact, 485
Compression of airways, 485
Concanavalin A mesothelial cell reactivity, 557
Conduction system. *See also* Heart
    aging changes in human conduction system, 545
    atrioventricular node (AV node), 542, 544f, 545
    sinoatrial node (SA node), 542, 543f
Confocal microscopy (CM), 55
    of nails, 55, 55f, 56f
Congenital asplenia, 800
Congenital cysts, 532
Congenital esophageal rings, 575–576
Congenital short pancreas, 745
Congenital tumors, 449t
Congo red stain, 500
Conjunctiva, 342–343, 342f
Connecting tubule (CNT), 858, 858t
Connecting tubule glomerular feedback (CTGF), 916
Connective tissue, 757–758
    elements, 513
    nevus, 20
    stains, 542, 547
Contractile fibers, 542
Contraction artifact, 184, 184f
Copper-associated protein, 716
Corneal epithelium, 336–337, 338f
Corneocytes, of nail plates, 40
Corneoscleral limbus, 340–342, 340f, 341f
Cornified layers, keratinocytes, 7, 7f
Cornu Ammonis (CA), 225–226, 227f
Corona, 805
Coronal sulcus, 1013, 1013f
Coronary angiography, 197
Coronary artery
    ectasia, 196
    stented, 205, 206f
Coronary CT angiography (CCTA), 530
Corpora amylacea, 241, 241f, 493
Corpora arenacea, 249
Corpora cavernosa (CC), 1019, 1019f, 1021, 1021f
    adipose tissue in, 1021, 1022f
    and corpus spongiosum, differences between, 1021–1022
Corpus albicans, 1126, 1127f
Corpus luteum
    of menstruation (CLM), 1122–1124
        degenerating, 1123f
        histology, 1122–1124
        hormonal aspects, 1124
        K cells, 1123
        lutein cells of, 1124
        mature, 1123f
        ultrastructure, 1124
    of pregnancy (CLP), 1124–1126, 1125f
Corpus spongiosum, 1011–1012, 1012f, 1021–1022
Cortex corticis, 883
Cortical bone, 91–93, 92f–93f
    cement lines, 93
    circumferential, concentric, and interstitial lamellae, 91, 92f
    endosteum, 93
    haversian systems, 91–93, 92f
    interstitial bone, 93
    Volkmann canal, 92, 93f
Cortical cells, nests of, 1232
Cortical granuloma, 1115, 1116f
Cortical map, 227
Cortical radial arteries, 924
Corticotrophs, 288–289, 289f
Cotton swab test, 1032
Cowden disease, 148t
Cowden syndrome, 578
Cowper glands. *See* Bulbourethral glands
Cracking of cartilage, 125, 125f
Cranial nerve zero (CN0), 256–257, 257f
Creutzfeldt astrocytes, 242, 242f
Cricoid, 425
Cricothyroid muscle, 432
Crooke cell, 290f
Crooke hyaline change, 288, 290f
Crush artifact, 235, 237f
Cryobiopsies, 487
Crypt epithelium, 619–621, 620f
Cryptorchid testis, 984
Crypts of Henle, 343
Crypts of Lieberkühn, 617
Crystal deposition disease, 130
CUSA. *See* Cavitational ultrasonic surgical aspirator (CUSA)
Cushing disease, 289, 1233
Cutaneous–mucosal junctions, 19
Cutaneous vasculitis, 17, 17f
Cutting cone, 91
CVOs. *See* Circumventricular organs (CVOs)
Cyclin-dependent kinase (CDK), 887
Cystic dilatation of Hassall corpuscles, 523
Cystic fibrosis transmembrane conductance regulator (CFTR), 753
Cystic medial degeneration (CMD), 191, 192f, 193
    in connective tissue disorders, 191
Cystitis glandularis, 954, 954f
Cyst of Skene duct, 1035
Cytochrome oxidase (COX)-deficient fibers, 178
Cytokeratin 5/6, 24, 502f, 557
Cytokeratin 7, 24
Cytokeratin 14 (CK14), 1054
Cytokeratin 20, 24
Cytokeratins, 458
Cytokines, 137
Cytomegalovirus (CMV), 26
Cytoplasmic bodies, 187, 187f
Cytoplasmic marker, 4

D

D2-40 antibody, 616
Dark cells, 13, 14
    with granular cytoplasm, 14, 14f
Dartos, 1013, 1014f, 1017
Decidua
    histology, 1163–1165
    histopathology, 1165–1166
Deciduoid reaction, 559
Déjerine–Sottas disease, 314
Delphian node, 1178
Delta cell granules, 757
Demarcation membrane system (DMS), 842
Demodex folliculorum mites, 11, 11f
Dendritic cells, 16
Dendritic reticulum cells. *See* Follicular dendritic cells (FDC)
Dental follicle stem cells, 397
Dental papilla, 397
Dercum disease, 148t
Dermal fibrosis and umbilicus, 19f
Dermal papillae, 683
Dermatophytosis, 20
Dermis
    adventitial, 15
    age, histologic differences of skin due to, 18
    cells of, 16
    collagen fibers, 4
    in elderly, 18
    embryology, 4
    histologic variations according to anatomic sites, 18–19
    nail, 56–58, 57f
    papillary, 4, 15, 15f
    reticular, 4, 15–16, 19, 19f
    solar elastosis in, 18, 18f
Dermoepidermal junction, 5
Descemet membrane, 338
Desert Hedgehog (Dhh), 304, 743
Desmoplastic mesothelioma, 562
Desmosomes, 5
Developmental change
    adrenal cortex, 1226–1228
    adrenal gland, 1226–1229, 1227f–1229f
    adrenal medulla, 1228–1229
    nail, 32t, 33f
    pediatric kidney, 856
Dextrose–thiamine diet, 144
Diabetic microangiopathy, 198
Diamnionic–dichorionic (DiDi) placenta, 1156, 1156f
Diamnionic–monochorionic (DiMo) placenta, 1155, 1155f
Diarthrodial joints, 113–115
    extracellular matrices mechanical properties, 114–115
    neuromuscular coordination, 115
    shape, 113–114, 114f
Diencephalon, 225
Dieulafoy lesion, 204
Diffuse idiopathic pulmonary neuroendocrine cell hyperplasia (DIPNECH), 489
Diffuse islet, 753, 754f
Diffuse mammary steatonecrosis, 148t
Diffuse microgliosis, 248
Diffuse pulmonary meningotheliomatosis, 490
DiGeorge syndrome, 508
Diiodotyrosine (DIT), 1182
D2-40 immunoreactivity, 557, 558f
Direct immunofluorescence (DIF), 1033
Distal convoluted tubule (DCT), 859, 916
Distal lung parenchyma, 477f
Distal tubule, 915
Disuse atrophy, 121
Dizygotic twin placenta, 1155
DNA hybridization, 516
Dogiel–Krause corpuscles, 1038
Dogiel–Krause receptors, 1042
Dorsal arteries, penis, 1025
Dorsal root ganglia (DRG), 303, 1279

Dorsal veins, penis, 1026
Drug eluting stents, 205
D2-40 staining, 210
Dubin–Johnson syndrome, 715
Duchenne muscular dystrophy, 185
Ductal cells, minor alterations in, 761–765
Duct ectasia, 765f, 769
Duct of Santorini, 728, 742, 743, 745
Duct of Wirsung, 728, 741, 745
Ducts, 444–446, 444f, 445f, 446f, 749–753, 749f–752f. See also Pancreas
Ductuli efferentes, 995–996, 995f
Ductus (vas) deferens, 997–998, 998f
Duodenum, 626–628, 626f
Dura mater, 257–259, 258f–259f
Dystrophic myopathies, 179, 180f

E

Ear, 363f
  acquired cholesteatoma, 387–388
  cholesteatoma, 387–388
  cochlea, 379
  cochlear duct, 375–376
  compartments of, 363
  conduction of sound, 383–384
  congenital cholesteatoma, 388
  drum, 364
  embryology of, 363
  endolymphatic duct and sac, 382
  external ear
    anatomy, 364–365
    auditory epithelial migration, 365–366
    embryology, 363–364
    histology, 365
  inner ear
    anatomy, 374–378
    embryology, 373–374
    innervation, 378–379
    perilymph and endolymph, 383
    presbycusis, 391–392
  keratoma, 387–388
  mastoid air cells, 371
  membranous labyrinth, 379
  Ménière's disease, 391–393
  middle ear
    anatomy, 367–369
    embryology, 366–367
    Eustachian tube, 370
    histology, 370–373
    joints, 372–373
    muscles and ossicles, 369–370
    otitis media, 385–387
  nerves and paraganglia, 381
  osseous labyrinth, 379
  otosclerosis, 389–390
  pathology, 384–385
  perilymph and endolymph, 383
  petrous apex, cholesteatoma of, 387
  saccule, 377
  semicircular canals, 380–381
  utricle, 377
Ecchymosis, 1032
Eccrine duct, 14, 14f
Eccrine glands, 5, 154
  clear cell, 13, 13f
  dark cells, 13, 14, 14f
  intercellular canaliculi, 13, 13f

  myoepithelial cells, 13
  secretory portion of, 13
  types of cells in, 13
Ectatic ducts, 765
Ectodermal dysplasias, 3, 37
Ectodermal ingrowth theory, 1023
Ectodysplasin, 441
Ecto-5-nucleotidase (5-NT), 923
Ectopic adipose tissue, 151
Ectopic glomeruli, 888, 888f
Ectopic sebaceous glands, 507
Ejaculatory ducts, 1000
Elastic cartilage, 119–120, 121f
Elastic tissue stains, 480
Elastic van Gieson (EVG) stain, 23, 542, 547
Elderly
  dermis in, 18
  histologic differences of skin in, 18
Electrocautery, 185
Electron microscopy, 442
Elephantiasis neuromatosa, 327
EMA. See Epithelial membrane antigen (EMA)
Embryo, hematopoiesis in, 817–818
Embryology, 949–950
  anal canal, 677–679, 678f
  anatomic landmarks, 953
  breast, 69–70, 70f
  colon, 640–641
  ear, 363
  larynx, 424
  liver, 693
  lymph nodes, 784
  mouth, 396–398
  nail, 32–34
  parathyroid gland, 1202–1204
  pharynx, 434
  pituitary and sellar region, 270–271, 271f
  prostate development, 964–965
  renal pelvis, 952–953
  skeletal muscle, 166–168, 167f
  skin, 3–5
  thymus, 506–507
  umbilical cord, 1141
  ureters, 952
  urinary bladder, 950–952
  urothelium, 953–954
  uterus and fallopian tubes, 1059
  vagina, 1047–1049
Embryonic kidney, 856
Empty sella, 273, 277f, 278f
Endarterectomy, 204, 205t
Endocardium, 532, 533f, 545
Endocervix epithelium, 1066–1069
Endochondral ossification, 101–108, 101f–108f, 120
  bone growth regulation by hormones, 107
  cartilage anlage of os calcis, 101, 101f
  cut back zone, 106
  growth of anlage, 102, 102f
  growth plate (physis), 104, 104f–105f, 105t
  primary center of ossification, 103, 103f
  ring of Ranvier, 104f, 106
  secondary centers of ossification, 104, 104f, 107f
  tidemark, 108, 108f
Endocrine cell–nonmyelinated fiber complex, 317

Endocrine cells and esophagus, 583
Endodermal differentiation theory, 1023
Endometrial gland, 1078
Endometrial–myometrial junction, 1092
Endometrial stroma, 1079–1080
  reticulin framework of cells, 1081
Endometriosis, 564–565, 564f, 565f. See also Reactive mesothelium
Endometrium
  apoptosis, 1093
  atrophic, 1090, 1090f
  changes in menarche, 1082
  ciliated cells of, 1079
  dating, 1083f–1084f, 1085t
    relevance of, 1091–1092
  differential diagnosis, 1094t–1095t
  disordered proliferative, 1091, 1091f
  early secretory phase, 1085–1086, 1086f
  endometrial vasculature, 1090
  epithelial elements, 1078
  histology of, 1076–1091
  late secretory phase, 1087, 1087f
  menstrual cycle, 1082–1083
  midsecretory phase, 1085, 1085f–1086f
  of newborn, 1082
  proliferative and basalis-type cells of, 1078
  proliferative phase, 1083–1084
  radial arteries of, 1081
  during reproductive years, 1082
  secretory cells of, 1078
  secretory phase, 1084–1087
    interval, 1084
  stroma and mesonephric remnants, 1081
  ultrastructural features, 1081
  vascular elements, 1081
  weakly proliferative, 1091
Endomyocardial biopsy
  about, 546
  biopsy limitations/tissue artifacts, 547–549, 548f
  tissue handling/processing, 547
Endomysial connective tissue, 186
Endoneurium, 307–308
Endosalpingiosis, 564–565, 564f, 565f. See also Reactive mesothelium
Endotenon, 122
Endothelial cells, 169, 206–207, 208–210
  antigens in, 209, 209f
  inclusions of, 207–208, 207f
Enkephalins, 1286
Enterochromaffin cell (EC)–nerve fiber complex, 1255
Enzyme histochemistry, 141–142
Eosinophil and basophil precursors, 831–832, 832f, 833f
Eosinophil cytoplasmic granules, 622
Eosinophilic esophagitis (EOE), 591, 595
Eosinophilic inclusions, 235, 236f
Eosinophils, 483, 622
Ependyma, 245–246
  central canal of spinal cord lined by, 246, 246f
  ependymal rosettes, 246, 246f
  granular ependymitis, 245f, 246
  plicae, 245f, 246
  response to injury, 246
  and subependymal plate, 245f

Epicardium, 532, 545
Epidermal growth factor receptor (EGFR), 1181
Epidermis, skin, 5f
  age, histologic differences of skin due to, 18
  apocrine glands, 15, 15f
  basal layers, 3, 4, 5
  basement membrane zone, 7, 8f
  cornified layers, 7, 7f
  eccrine glands, 1315
  of elderly, 18
  embryology, 3–4
  granular layers, 6–7
  hair follicles, 5, 10–12, 11f, 12f
  keratinocytes, 5–7
  Langerhans cells, 8, 8f
  melanin in, 8, 8f
  melanocytes, 7–9, 8f
  Merkel cells, 9–10, 10f
  of newborns and children, 18
  nipple, 6, 6f
  pilar unit, 10–15
  sebaceous glands, 12–13, 13f
  squamous layers, 5–6, 6f
Epididymis, 996–997, 996f–997f
Epinephrine, 1283
Epineurium, 303–304, 303f
Epiphyseal vessels (bone), 95
Epitenon, 122
Epithelial cells, thymic, 510, 514, 514t
Epithelial inclusion cysts (EICs), 1110
Epithelial inclusion glands (EIGs), 1110, 1110f
Epithelial inclusion glands and cysts (EIGCs), 1110–1111
Epithelial membrane antigen (EMA), 259, 306, 459, 1181
  in normal nail matrix, 47, 50f
Epithelial, mesenchymal, and melanocyte antibodies, 25t
Epithelial–mesenchymal transition (EMT), 923
Epithelial remnants in involuting thymus, 519f
Epithelial skin appendages, 4–5
Epithelioid trophoblastic tumor (ETT), 1168
Epithelium, glans, 1010, 1011f
Epitheloid venules, 789
Eponychium, 37
Epstein–Barr virus (EBV), 547
Erdheim–Chester disease, 150
Erosion of cartilage, 125
Erythropoietin receptor, 817
Escherichia coli type 1 pili, 1054
Esophagus
  abdominal portion of, 577
  acute necrotizing esophagitis, 595
  adenocarcinomas, 596
  arterial supply, 589–590
  Barrett's esophagus, 591–593
  cervical, 577
  cervical portion of, 577
  developmental defects of, 574
  diagnostic considerations, 591–596
  distal, 588f
  embryology, 573–576
  eosinophilic esophagitis, 595
  esophageal constrictions, 577f
  esophageal webs, 575–576
  exfoliative esophagitis, 595
  feline, 594f, 595
  fetal, 574f, 575f
  gastroesophageal junction, 581–582
  gastroesophageal reflux disease, 593–595
  gastroesophageal region, adenocarcinomas, 596
  glycogenic acanthosis, 578
  heterotopias, 578
  histology
    mucosa, 583–586
    muscularis propria, 588–589
    serosa, 589
    submucosa, 586–588
  immunostained with MIB-1, 585f
  innervation, 590–591
  lower esophageal rings, 575–576
  lower esophageal sphincter, 581
  lymphatic drainage, 590
  lymphocytic esophagitis, 595
  macroscopic/endoscopic features, 578–582
  mucosa, 583–586
  musculature, 579–580
  proximal, 578f, 579f
  regions of, 576f
  sebaceous glands, 578, 579f
  segments of, 574
  serosa, 589
  thoracic segment of, 577
  topography and relations, 576–578, 576f
  venous drainage, 590
Estrogen and progesterone receptor, 501
Estrogen receptor (ER), in normal breast tissue
  ERα, 80–81
  ERβ, 81
Eustachian valve, 535
Evolution, of adrenal gland, 1225–1226
Exaggerated placental site (EPS), 1166
Exchange vessels, 198. *See also specific type*
Exfoliative esophagitis, 595
Exocervical epithelium, 1065–1066, 1065f
External band of Baillarger, 228, 228f
External portion of heart, 532
Extrahepatic biliary system
  arterial supply and venous drainage, 726
  histology, 727–728
  lymphatic drainage, 726
  nerve supply, 727
Extrainsular neuroendocrine cells, 757, 757f
Extralymphatic heterotopias, 452
Extramedullary hematopoiesis, fetal breast, 70, 70f
Extranodal salivary heterotopias, 452f
Extrinsic muscles of larynx, 425
Eye and ocular adnexa, 335–336, 336f
  caruncle and plica semilunaris, 343, 343f
  conjunctiva, 342–343, 342f
  cornea, 336–339, 337f, 338f
  corneoscleral limbus, 340–342, 340f, 341f
  crystalline lens, 353–354, 353f, 354f
  external landmarks, 335, 336f
  extraocular muscles, 335
  eyelids, 355–357, 356f
  intraocular compartments, 355, 355f
  aqueous humor, 355, 355f
  vitreous humor, 355, 355f
  lacrimal drainage apparatus, 357–360, 359f, 360f
  optic nerve, 352–353, 352f, 353f
  orbit, 357
  retina, 348–350, 348f–350f
    artifacts of, 351–352, 352f
  sclera, 339–340, 339f, 340f
  tissue layers and chambers, 336, 337f
  uveal tract, 343
    choroid, 346–348, 346f, 347f
    ciliary body, 345–346, 345f, 346f
    iris, 343–345, 343f, 344f
Eyelid epidermis, 19

F
Factor VIII antibodies, 209
Fallopian tubes, 1059, 1098f, 1099t
  adult, 1061
  ampulla of, 1097f
  atypical hyperplasia of, 1098f
  BRCA-1 or 2 gene mutation and, 1097
  ciliated cells, 1095, 1098f
  gross anatomic features of, 1063
  histology, 1095–1097
  intercalated (peg) cells, 1096
  paraovarian and paratubal structures, 1099
  in pregnancy, 1099
  premenarchal, 1060–1061
  secretory cells, 1095
Familial multiple lipomas, 148t
Fat biopsy, for amyloidosis, 147
Fat cells, 821–822, 821f, 822f
Fat digestion and lingual lipase, 616
Fat fractures, 151
Fat necrosis
  infarction type of, 149
  ordinary type, 147, 149f
  pancreatic type, 148–149, 149f
Fatty infiltration, 147, 148t, 454
Fatty metaplasia, of cardiac valve, 146, 146f
Female breast
  clear cells in nipple epidermis, 77, 77f
  ductal-lobular system, 71–72, 72f
    basal lamina, 74–75, 75f
    epithelium lining, 73, 73f
    mammary stem cells, 74
    myoepithelial cells, 73, 73f
    normal breast luminal epithelium, 74
  intralobular and extralobular stroma, 75, 76f
  intramammary lymph nodes, 78
  lobular acini, 75
  lobule types, 75
  menstrual cycle–related changes in lobules, 76, 77t
  microanatomy of, 71, 72f
  Montgomery areolar tubercle, 78, 78f
  multinucleated stromal giant cells, 75, 76f
  nipple–areola complex, 76–78
  nipple dermis/stroma, 77, 78f
  segments in, 71–72
  sites of origin of pathologic lesions, 75, 75f
  size and location, 71–78
  stroma, 71, 72f
  terminal duct lobular unit (TDLU), 73, 75

Female external genitalia, 1032, 1033f. See also Vulva
Fenestrations, 199
Ferruginized neurons, 237, 237f
Ferruginous bodies, 494
Fetal brain, 263
Fetal gubernaculum, 1003
Fetal mammary gland, 70
Fetal sexual differentiation, 1059
  female differentiation, 1060
Fetal spermatogonia, 990
Fetal testis, 990–993, 991f
Fetus, hematopoiesis in, 817–818
Fibril-associated collagens with interrupted triple helices (FACIT) collagens, 96
Fibrillation of cartilage, 124–125, 125f
Fibrinoid necrosis of arteriolar media, 197, 197f, 198
Fibroblast growth factor, 869
Fibroblast growth factor-23 (FGF-23), 99
Fibroblastic reticulum cells (FRC), 784
Fibroblasts, 3, 16
Fibrocartilage, 119
Fibrocongestive splenomegaly, 810
Fibrolipomas, 154
Fibrosa, 539
Fibrosis, 768–772, 769f–772f
Fibrous pleurisy, 562, 562f. See also Reactive mesothelium
Fibrous synarthroses, 113
Filum terminale, 261, 261f
Fingernails, 31. See also Nail
FISH. See Fluorescent in situ hybridization (FISH)
Fishman syndrome, 148t
Fistulae, 204
Fite stain, 23
Floret tumor giant cells, 155, 155f
Fluhmann's lumens, 1067
Fluorescein isothiocyanate–conjugated (FITC), 23
Fluorescent in situ hybridization (FISH), 26–27, 136, 562, 563
Focal chronic pancreatitis, 768
Focal lymphocytic thyroiditis, 1186
Focal myocarditis, 547
Follicles, 786
  primary, 786
  secondary, 786
Follicular dendritic cells (FDC), 784, 786
Follicular hyperplasia, 793
Follicular infundibulum, 11, 11f
Follicular lymphoma, 793
Follicular (dermal) papilla, of hair follicle, 10, 11f
Folliculogenesis, 1118–1120
Folliculostellate cell, 292, 293f
Fontana–Masson silver stains, 9, 23, 498
Foramina of Luschka, 253, 253f
Fordyce spots, 1033, 1041f
Foreskin, 1013–1018
  anatomic features and circumcision, 1013–1016
  cutaneous surface of, 1016f
  microscopic and immunohistochemical features, 1016–1018
  squamous epithelium, 1018f

Fossula fenestrae vestibuli, 369
Fournier gangrene, 1021
Foveolae granulares, 259
Fox–Fordyce disease, 15
FRC conduit system, 791
Freeze–fracture electron microscopy, 171, 181
Fröhlich syndrome, 148t
Fuchs corneal dystrophy, 339
FXIIIa (AC-1A1), 24

G
Galectins, 1181
Gallbladder
  anatomy, 719–720
  blood supply, 720–721
  histology, 720
  lymphatic drainage, 720–721
  nerve supply, 721
  physiology, 720
  ultrastructure, 724–725
Ganglioneuromas, 327
Gap junctions, 207, 208
Gardner syndrome, 148t
Gartner duct, 857
Gas exchange, 476
Gastric heterotopia, 631
Gastric metaplasia, 631
Gastric oxyntic mucosa, 603f
Gastrin-releasing peptide, 1256, 1262
Gastroesophageal junction (GEJ), 601
Gastroesophageal reflux disease (GERD), 593–595
Gastrointestinal neuroendocrine cells, 1264–1265, 1265t
Gastrointestinal stromal tumors (GIST), 157, 590
GATA-3, 1290
Gdnf/Ret signaling, 867–870, 868f, 872
Gelatinous transformation, 144
Gemistocytes, 241
Genetics, nail, 34–37
Genital corpuscles, 1017, 1017f, 1025
Genitourinary Developmental Molecular Anatomy Project (GUDMAP), 861
Gerlach tonsil, 436
Germ cell neoplasia in situ, 982
Germ cells, 513
Germline deletion of BAP-1, 563
Gestational endometrium, 1088f
Gestational trophoblastic disease, 1166–1168, 1167f–1168f
Gestational trophoblastic tumor (GTT), 1089
GFAP. See Glial fibrillary acidic protein (GFAP)
Giant cell aortitis, 194
Giemsa, 23, 789
Gingiva, 412–413
Gitter cells (lattice cells), 248f
Glandopreputial glands, 1036
Glands of Krause, 343
Glands of Wolfring, 343
Glands of Zeiss and Moll, 355, 356f
Glandular metaplasia, 955
Glans, 1009–1012
  anatomic features, 1009–1010, 1010f
  microscopic and immunohistochemical features

  corpus spongiosum, 1011–1012, 1012f
  epithelium, 1010, 1011f
  lamina propria, 1010–1011
Glial fibrillary acidic protein (GFAP), 239, 239f, 292, 350, 350f, 709
Glial/Schwann junction, 302
Global glomerulosclerosis, 897
Glomera, 17
Glomerular maturation and growth, 884–887, 885f–886f
Glomerulomegaly, 884
Glomerulosclerosis in infants, 887–888, 888f
Glomerulus, 895–906
  endothelial cells, 897–898
  glomerular basement membrane, 899–901
  glomerular filtration barrier, 905
  mesangial cells, 898–899
  parietal epithelial cells, 905–906
  podocytes, 901–905
Glomus, 17, 856–857
Glomus jugulare tumors, 1278
Glomus tympanicum tumors, 1278
Glottic compartment, 426
Glucagon-like peptides 1 and 2 (GLP-1 and GLP-2), 1256
Glucose transporter protein I (Glut-1), 306, 562
  antibodies, 210
Glycocalyx proteins, 207
Glycogen, 177
Glycogenic acanthosis, 578. See also Esophagus
Glycophorin A, 213
Glycosaminoglycans, 540, 559
Glycosylated proteins, 559
Glyoxylic acid, 1291
Goblet cells, 647, 682, 727, 761
  bronchial epithelium, 472
  conjunctival epithelium, 342–343, 342f
  endocervix, 1066, 1067f
Goitrous hypothyroidism, 1185
Goldenhar–Gorlin syndrome, 148t
Golgi pattern, 287
Golgi tendon organ, 176, 176f
Gomitoli, 279f
Gomori methenamine silver (GMS), 23
Gomori reticulin stain, 810
Gomori trichrome, 173, 185
Gout, 127
Gram stains, 23
Granular cell nests, 296
Granular cell tumor (GCT), 324, 326
Granular ependymitis, 245f, 246
Granular layers, keratinocytes, 6–7
Granulovacuolar degeneration (GVD), 233–234, 234f
Gray matter and white matter, CNS, 228–229, 229f
Growth-associated protein 43 (GAP 43), 320
Growth differentiation factor 8 (GDF8), 181
Growth hormones (GH), 285–287
G-spot (Gräfenberg spot), 1055
Gubernaculum, 1003, 1003f
Guillian–Barré syndrome, 317, 321
GVD. See Granulovacuolar degeneration (GVD)
Gynecoid habitus, 136

H

Haarscheibe, 12
Hair follicle, 10–12
 follicular (dermal) papilla of, 10, 11f
 function of, 10
 hair shaft, 10, 11f
 inferior segment, 10, 11f
 infundibulum, 10
 isthmus, 10
 microanatomy of, 10
 regeneration, 4
Hair shaft, 10, 11f
Hamartomas containing fat cells, 151
Hamazaki–Wesenberg bodies, 498, 499f
Hart line, 1032, 1033f
Hartmann pouch, 720
Hashimoto thyroiditis, 1177, 1181, 1185, 1193
Hassall corpuscles, 509–510, 510f, 511f
Hassall–Henle warts, 338, 339
Haversian canals, 819
Haversian systems, 91–93, 92f
Heart
 cardiac innervation, 545, 545f
 cardiac skeleton
  about, 532, 532f
  applied anatomy, 532
 cardiac valves
  aging changes of intracardiac valves, 541
  applied anatomy of intracardiac valves, 540–541
  atrioventricular valves (AV valves), 539–540, 540f
  chordae tendineae, 540, 541f
  papillary muscles, 541–542, 542f
  semilunar valves, 538–539, 538f
 conduction system
  aging changes in human conduction system, 545
  atrioventricular node (AV node), 542, 544f, 545
  sinoatrial node (SA node), 542, 543f
 endomyocardial biopsy
  about, 546
  biopsy limitations/tissue artifacts, 547–549, 548f
  tissue handling/processing, 547
 interatrial septum
  about, 534–535, 535f
  applied anatomy, 535
 internal structure of heart wall, 532–534, 533f, 534f
 intramural coronary arteries, small, 546, 546f
 left atrium, 535–536
 left ventricle
  about, 538
  applied anatomy, 538
 lymphatics, 545–546, 546f
 pericardium
  about, 531–532, 531f, 532f
  applied anatomy, 532
 postnatal circulation, 531
 prenatal fetal circulation, 530–531
 right atrium, 535, 536f
 right ventricle
  about, 536–537, 537f
  applied anatomy, 538
 weight of, 530

Heart wall, internal structure of, 532–534, 533f, 534f
HECA 452 staining, 790f
Hedgehog signaling pathway, 743
Helicine arteries, 1025–1026
Hematocolpos, 1037
Hematologic antibodies, 26
Hematolymphoid cells, 1080–1081
Hematopoiesis, 800, 809
 in embryo and fetus, 817–818
 extramedullary, 800
 model of, 815f
 regulation of, 816–817
Hematopoietic cells
 eosinophil and basophil precursors, 831–832
 lymphocytes and plasma cells, 843–847
 megakaryocytes, 840–843
 monocyte precursors, 832–835
 neutrophil precursors, 826–831
 red cell precursors, 835–840
Hematopoietic foci, 817
Hematopoietic precursor cell, 4
Hematopoietic progenitor cells, 816
Hematoxylin and eosin (H&E), 480, 519, 547, 807
 paraganglionic neuroendocrine cells, 1282
 white fat cell, 138
Hemidesmosomes, 5, 7
Hemopoietic stem cell (HSC), 317
Hemosiderin, 715–716
Henle layer, 10
Hepatic artery, 739
Hepatic pseudolipoma, 147
Hepatoportal sclerosis, 714
Heritable demyelinating neuropathies (HDNs), 322
Herpes simplex virus, 26
Herpes virus type 8, 26
Herring bodies, 251, 251f, 280, 282f, 296
Hertwig's epithelial root sheath, 397
Hes-1/mASH-1 signaling pathway, 1252
Heterotaxy syndrome, 744
Heterotopia, 451, 452t, 578
Heterotopic pancreas tissue, 631
Heterotopic salivary tissue, significance of, 451–453, 452f, 452t
Heterotopic thyroid tissue, 532
HHF-35, 26
Hibernoma, 150
High-resolution computed tomography (HRCT), 476, 480, 481t
Hilus cells, of ovary, 1129–1131
 histology, 1129–1130
 hormonal aspects, 1130–1131
 ultrastructure, 1130
Hippocampal fissure, residual, 226
Hippocampal formation, 225–226, 227f
Hirano bodies, 233–234, 234f
Hirschsprung disease, 869
Histatins, 443
Histiocyte clusters in hilar nodes, 498f
Histochemical stains, 22–23
Histochemistry, mesothelial cells, 555, 557
Histologic artifact, in peripheral nerve, 317f
Histology
 adrenal gland, 1230–1238

 correlative normal/neoplastic, 456–458, 457f, 458t
 thymus
  about, 509–510, 509f
  epithelial cells, 510
  Hassall corpuscles, 510, 510f, 511f
  thymic lymphocytes (thymocytes), 510–513, 511f, 512f
HIV treatment–associated lipodystrophy, 137, 146
Hodgkin's disease, 3
Hollande fixative, 635
Homeobox genes, 101
Homeodomain protein PDX1, 743
Howell–Jolly (H-J) bodies, 808, 839
Howship lacunae, 99, 99f
Hoxd13, 679
Hox genes, 166
Human carcinoembryonic antigen (CEA), 51
Human leukocyte antigen (HLA), 621
Human papillomavirus (HPV), 26, 27f, 429
Hurthle cells, 1180
Huxley layer, 10
Hyaline cartilage, 113, 116, 117f, 120, 425
Hyaline fibers, 184–185
Hyaline (colloid) inclusion, 235, 235f
Hyaline plaques, of spinal leptomeninges, 260
Hyalinization, 198
Hyalin or plasmacytoid cells, 449
Hydromyelia, 246
Hymen, 1037, 1037f
 imperforate, 1037
Hypergastrinemia, 1185
Hyperparathyroidism 2 (HRPT2), 1217
Hyperplasia, 454–455
Hyperplastic pneumocytes, 476
Hypertrophic neuropathy, 322
Hypodermis. See Subcutaneous tissue
Hyponychium, 32, 35f, 45, 45f, 58
Hypopharynx, 433
Hypophysial portal system, 276
Hypothalamic hormones, 283, 283t
Hypothalamic nuclei, 280f

I

Iatrogenically introduced foreign material, 265, 267t
Ichthyosiform dermatosis, 20
Idiopathic hypertrophic subaortic stenosis (IHSS), 538
Idiopathic portal hypertension. See Hepatoportal sclerosis
Idiopathic thrombocytopenic purpura (ITP), 810
Ileum, 629–630
Immotile cilia syndrome, 800
Immune myopathies with perimysial pathology (IMPP), 178
Immunohistochemical markers of salivary glands, 458t
Immunohistochemical stains, 23–27
 for keratin (AE1/AE3), 560
Immunohistochemistry, 23, 179
 adipose tissue, 143, 143f
 lungs, 501–503, 501f–503f, 503t
 mesothelial cells, 557–558, 557f, 558f
 nail, 46–53

neurons, CNS, 231, 232f
paraganglia, 1287–1290
salivary glands, 458–459, 458f
skeletal muscle diseases, 179, 180t
thymic epithelial cells, 514, 514t
thymic lymphocytes, 515–516
Immunoperoxidase stain for BAP-1 stains, 563f
Immunostains for epithelial markers, 480
Imperforate hymen, 1037
Incidental parenchymal scar, 492f
Incisura, 577
Indian hedgehog (IHH), 743
Infantile glomerulosclerosis, 888, 888f
Infantile spinal muscular atrophy, 187
Infective arthritis, 122
Inferior laryngeal nerve, 432
Inferior vena cava (IVC), 530
Infiltrating lipomas, 152–153, 153f
Infundibulum, 249, 251–252, 251f
InGaAs photodiode array detector, 40
Inner medullary collecting duct (IMCD), 921–922, 921f
cells, 922f
role in urinary concentration, 921–922
terminal, 923f
Innervation
cardiac, 545, 545f
derivation of, 442
In situ T-cell differentiation, 517
Insulinoma-associated 1 (INSM1), 1260
Integrins, 870
in nail matrix, 52, 53t
Interatrial septum. *See also* Heart
about, 534–535, 535f
applied anatomy, 535
Intercalated duct, 445f
Intercellular canaliculi, 13, 13f
Interdigitating dendritic cells (IDC), 784, 790, 790f
Interferon (IFN)-γ, 517
Interleukin (IL), 517
Interleukin-6 (IL-6), 137
Interlobular ducts, 446f, 750, 750f, 751f
Intermediate epithelium, 435
Intermediate mesoderm (IM), 856
Internal carotid artery, 274
Internal jugular chain nodes, 1178
Internal mammary artery, 79
Internal mammary lymph node, 560f
International Classification of Diseases (ICD), 576
International Spleen Consortium, 799, 810
Interpapillary basal layer (IBL), 585
Interstitial air, 497, 498f
Interstitial cells of Cajal (ICC), 574, 758
Interstitial giant cell thyroiditis, 1183
Interstitial granulomas, 1183
Interstitium of testis, 987
Intervertebral disc, 115, 116f
Intestinal immune system, 622
Intestinal metaplasia, 955f
Intima, 546
Intra-alveolar hemorrhage, 486
Intracardiac valves, applied anatomy of, 540–541
Intraductal papillary mucinous neoplasm (IPMN), 746

Intraepidermal atypical pagetoid cells, 26t
Intraepithelial eosinophils (IEE), 593
Intraepithelial inflammatory cells (IEL), 583, 648, 648f
Intraepithelial lymphocytes (IEL), 583, 646
Intraepithelial neutrophils (IEN), 593
Intraepithelial nonkeratinocytes, 413–414
Intraganglionic chromaffin cells, 1276
Intralobular ducts, 750, 750f, 751f, 752f
Intramembranous ossification, 108, 108f
Intramural coronary arteries, structure of, 546, 546f
Intramural ureter, 951
Intramyocardial accumulations of mature adipose tissue, 547
Intraparotid lymph nodes, 459
Intrapulmonary lymph nodes, 492, 492f
Intrapulmonary peribronchial lymph nodes, 479
Intravagal paraganglia, 1277
Intravascular foreign material, 497
Intrinsic muscles of larynx, 425
Intussusception, 547
Inverted papillomas, 956, 956f
Iris, 343–345, 343f, 344f
Iron deposition on elastic tissue, 497f
Ischemia, accentuated fat lobules in, 145–146, 146f
Islet cells, 744
minor alterations in, 765–768, 766f, 767f
Islet hyperplasia, 765
Islet of Langerhans, 753–757, 753f–756f
Isolated idiopathic aortitis, 194
Ito cells of liver, 147

J
Jacobson nerve, 1278
Jawbone, 399
Jejunum, 628–629
Joints, 113
amphiarthrodial, 115–116
arthritic, 122, 124
close-packed position, 114
diarthrodial, 113–115
dysfunction, 113
function, factors affecting, 113
load on, 114, 114f
response to injury, 124
bone, 126–129, 128f, 129f
cartilage, 124–126, 125f–127f
ligaments and tendons, 129, 129f
synovial fluid, 130
synovial membrane, 129–130, 130f
tissues
articular cartilage, 116–121
ligaments and tendons, 122
synovial membrane, 121, 122f
types of, 113
Jugular paraganglia, 1277
Junctional complexes between endothelial cells, 207
Juvenile capillary angioma, 210, 211f
Juvenile pilocytic astrocytoma, 242
Juxtaglomerular apparatus, 906–908
Juxtamedullary glomeruli, early, 887
Juxtaoral Organ of Chievitz, 409–410

K
Kaposi's sarcoma, 26, 154, 210, 212f
Karyorrhexis, 235
Katacalcin, 1186
Keratin expression, in normal nail unit, 46–47, 46f
Keratinocytes, 4, 4f
basal layers, 5
cornified layers, 7, 7f
granular layers, 6–7
melanin in, 8, 8f
squamous layers, 5–6, 6f
vertical elongation of, 22f
Keratins, 34–37, 35, 748, 1181. *See also* Nail
actin microfilaments, 34
immunohistochemical labeling for, 748f
intermediate filaments, 34
microtubules, 34
role of, 34
Keratohyalin granules, 403
Kernicterus, 225
K17 gene, 37
K6hf, expression of, 37
Ki-67, 26
Kidney
adult
architecture, 893–895
gross anatomy, 889–892
nephrons, 892–893
aglomerular arterioles, 924
anatomy
blood supply, 880
configuration, 880–881
gross appearance of newborn kidney, 881f
position, 880
weight, 880–881, 881f
bone morphogenetic proteins, 870
calyces formation, 857–858
collecting system differentiation
cell types, 872–873
ureteral tip and trunk, 871–872
collecting system, formation, 858–859
connecting tubule, 916–917
cortical radial arteries, 924
development, 856
convergent extension in, 871
Gdnf/Ret signaling, 867–870, 868f, 872
gene involved in, 862t–866t
intermediate mesoderm specification, 867
molecular regulation of, 861–869
nephric duct, 867
ureteral branching, 868–869
distal convoluted tubule, 916
distal tubule, 915
efferent arterioles, 925
embryonic, 856
fetal lobations, 881–882, 881f
fibroblast growth factor, 869
glomerulus, 895–906
endothelial cells, 897–898
glomerular basement membrane, 899–901
glomerular filtration barrier, 905
mesangial cells, 898–899
parietal epithelial cells, 905–906
podocytes, 901–905
histology
of cortex corticis, 883, 883f
cortical architecture, 882–884

Kidney (*continued*)
   of developing renal cortex, 882
   of glomerular generations, 883
     medullary ray nodules, 883–884, 884f
   of preterm neonates, 882
  inner medullary collecting duct (IMCD), 921–922
  integrins, 870
  interstitium, 922–924, 924f
  juxtaglomerular apparatus, 906–908
  laminins, 870
  lymphatic networks, 927
  lymphatic networks in, 927, 927f
  maturation and growth of tubules, 889
    loops of Henle, 889
    ratio of glomerular surface area to proximal tubular volume, 889
  mesonephros, 857
  metanephric mesenchyme
    nephron progenitor population, 874–876, 875f
    specification, 873–874
  metanephros, 857–859
  nephron endowment, 884
  nephron formation, 859
  nephron number
    early juxtamedullary glomeruli, 887
    ectopic glomeruli, 888, 888f
    glomerular maturation and growth, 884–887, 885f–886f
    glomerulosclerosis in infants, 887–888, 888f
  nephron, patterning of
    glomerulogenesis, 878–879
    interstitium, 877–878
    juxtaglomerular apparatus, 880
    pretubular aggregate and renal vesicle, 876–877
    proximal and distal tubules, 877
    renal vascularization, 879–880
  nephrostomes, 856
  nerve supply to, 927–928, 927f
  outer medullary collecting duct, 920–921
  papillary surface epithelium, 922
  pediatric
    anatomy, 856
    developmental changes, 856
    histologic peculiarities of, 856
  peg-sockets, 923
  pronephros, 856–857
  proximal tubule, 908–913
  renal parenchyma, 895
  renal pelvis formation, 857–858
  renin–angiotensin system, 870
  sempahorins, 870–871
  thin limbs of Henle loop, 913–915
  ureteric branch growth, 871
  vasculature, 924–927, 925f–926f
  Wnt signaling pathways, 871
Kinocilia project, 752
Klippel–Trenaunary–Weber syndrome, 1044
Krabbe leukodystrophy, 317
KRAS oncogene, 761
Kulchitsky cells, 472
Kulchitsky (K) cells, 1261
Kupffer cells, 698, 715

L

Labial artery, 1044
Labial nerves, 1044
Labia majora, 1039–1043, 1039f–1042f
  age-related changes, 1039
  apocrine glands, 1039, 1040f, 1041
  gestational changes, 1039
  hair follicles, 1039
  length of, 1039
  mammary-like anogenital gland, 1042, 1042f
  merocrine glands, 1040
  nerve endings in skin of, 1041–1042
  posterior fourchette, 1040, 1040f
  posterior medial, 1040f
  round ligament, 1041
  sebaceous glands, 1039, 1039f, 1041
  Toker cells, 1042–1043
  tunica dartos labialis, 1041
Labia minora
  congenital enlargement of, 1039
  enlargement, 1038
  lateral, biopsy, 1038f
Lacrimal drainage apparatus, 357–360, 359f, 360f
Lactating breast tissue, 79, 79f
Lactotrophs, 287–288, 288f
Lacunar infarction, 225
Lambert canals, 472
Lambertosis, 472
Lamellar bone, 90–91, 90f
  cement lines, 91, 92f
  collagen fibers in, 90, 90f
  mineralization of, 91, 91f
  and woven bone, 90–91
Lamina densa, 7
Lamina lucida, 7
Lamina propria, 428, 585–586, 621–623, 649, 668–671, 957–958, 957f, 1010–1011, 1025
Laminins, 870, 901
Lange fold, 351–352, 352f
Langerhans cell histiocytosis, 484
Langerhans cell–like dendritic cells, 16
Langerhans cells (LCs), 4, 8, 8f, 337, 476, 512, 1010, 1034
Lanugo hair, 4
Large dense core vesicles (LDCVs), 1258
Laryngeal artery, 433
Laryngeal biopsies, 430
Larynx. *See also* Pharynx
  anatomy
    gross and functional, 424–426, 425f, 426f
    microscopic, 426–432, 427f–432f
  compartments of, 426
  definition and boundaries, 424
  embryology, 424
  neural, vascular, lymphatic components, 432–433
  seromucinous gland, 429–431, 429f, 430f, 431f
Larynx paraganglion, 431, 432
Lateral aberrant thyroid, 1192
Lateral horn, 220
Lateral nail folds, 45–46, 46f
Lateral plate mesoderm (LPM), 856
Laurence–Moon–Biedl syndrome, 148t
Lawrence–Seip syndrome, 1031

LCs. *See* Langerhans cells (LCs)
Left atrium, 535–536
Left ventricle
  about, 538
  applied anatomy, 538
Leishmania, 23
Lens (eye), 353–354, 353f, 354f
Leptin, 137, 143
Leptomeningeal melanocytes, 261–262, 262f
Leukonychia, 37
Lewy bodies of Parkinson disease, 235
Leydig cell index, 989
Leydig cells, 987–989, 988f–999f
  aged, 994
  astrocyte-like markers in, 989
  in fetus, 992–993
  micronodules/hyperplasia, 989
  production of testosterone, 988
  quantitation of, 989
  Reinke crystals of, 988
Lichen amyloidosis, 20, 21f
Lichen sclerosus (LS)
  glans, 1025
  vulvar, 1034
Ligament of Treitz, 615, 738
Ligaments, 122
Light microscopy, 443
Limiting plate, 696
Line of Gennari, 228
Lingual lipase, 616
Linguogingival sulcus, 442
Lipid
  accumulation, 142
  histochemistry, 142
  in nail plates, 40
Lipoblastoma, 155, 156f
Lipoblastomatosis, 155
Lipoblasts, 157–158, 157f
Lipochondromatosis, 154
Lipodystrophy, 146
Lipofibromatous hamartoma, 304
Lipofuscin, 144, 187, 231, 233f, 715, 1180, 1180f
  granules, 1240
Lipogranuloma, 150, 496
Lipohyperplasia, 629
Lipoid cells, 449
Lipolymph nodes, 147
Lipoma arborescens, 153
Lipomas, 151–152
  with accentuated lobulation, 152, 152f
  cytogenetics of, 155–156
  epithelial components, 154
  fat cell size in, 152, 152f
  increased cellularity of, 152, 153f
  intramuscular, 152–153, 153f
  lymphocytes in, 155
  mesenchymal component, 154, 154f
  with myxoid change, 152, 153f
Lipomatosis, 147, 772
Lipomatous hypertrophy, 535
  of interatrial septum, 147
Lipomatous pseudohypertrophy. *See* Lipomatosis
Lipopeliosis, 147
Lipoprotein lipase (LPL), 135
Lisch nodules, 327

Littré glands, 1024–1025, 1025f
Liver
   aging changes, 706–707
   apoptosis, 698
   autopsy, 710–711
   bile, 716
   bile ducts, 704–706
   biopsy, 699–700
   brown pigments, 714–716
   congestion, 708
   copper-associated protein, 716
   Dubin–Johnson syndrome, 715
   electron microscopy, 710
   embryology, 693
   extracellular matrix, 706
   and gallbladder, 693
   Glisson capsule, 694
   hemosiderin, 715–716
   hepatic alterations, 711–714
   hepatic hilum, 703
   hepatic lipocytes, 700
   hepatocytes, 695–699
   hepatoportal sclerosis, 714
   histology
      bile canaliculi, 699
      bile ducts, 704–706
      blood supply and drainage, 702–704
      hepatic artery, 703–704
      hepatocytes, 695–699
      lymphatics, 704
      nerve supply and innervation, 706
      portal tracts, 701–702
      portal vein, 702–703
      sinusoidal lining cells, 699–701
      structural organization, 694–695
   immunohistologic studies, 708–710
   lipofuscin, 715
   methodology, 707–710
   mild acute hepatitis and residual hepatitis, 712
   molecular studies, 710
   morphology, gross, 694
   nodular regenerative hyperplasia, 713
   and non-neoplastic diseases, 708–709
   nonspecific reactive hepatitis, 712
   and pancreatic carcinoma, 697
   portal tracts, 701–702
   sinusoidal dilatation, 712–713
   space-occupying lesions, 714
   specimens handling, 707
   stains, 707–708
   stellate cells, 700
   surgical biopsy, 711
   systemic macrophage, 715
Lobes, 469
Lobular atrophy, 977
Lobule, 883
Lobule and acinus, 475–478, 476f, 477f
Localized hypertrophic neuropathy, 306, 323
Longitudinal elastic tissue fibers, 500
Loose bodies, 128–129, 128f
Lower esophageal sphincter (LES), 575, 581
Loyez stain, 313
LS. See Lichen sclerosus (LS)
Lungs
   aging on, effects of, 500, 500f
   artifacts in lung biopsy/resection material, 484–488, 484f–487f, 484t
   biopsy appearing normal, 500–501, 500t, 501f
   biopsy, incidental findings in, 488–498, 488t, 489f–499f
   development
      phases of, 470t
      regulatory factors, 470t
   immunohistochemistry, 501–503, 501f–503f, 503t
   incidental findings
      in lung biopsy/resection tissue, 488–498, 488t, 489f–499f
      in transbronchial biopsies, 499–500, 499f, 500t
   neuroendocrine cells of, 1261–1262, 1261f
   normal structure and histology
      airways, 470–475, 471f, 472f, 473t–474t, 474f–476f
      general, 469, 470t
      lobule and acinus, 475–478, 476f, 477f
      lymphatics and lymphoid tissue, 478–479
      pleura, 479–480, 479f
      vasculature, 478, 478f
   pathologists, 486
   pattern recognition, 480–481, 481f, 481t
   site-specific changes, in surgical pathology material, 481–484, 481t, 482f, 483f
   stains/evaluation of lung histology, 480
Lunula, 38, 43
Luschka ducts, 724
Luxol fast blue, 313, 353
Lymphangioleiomyomatosis (LAM), 484, 492
Lymphatics. See also Heart
   adrenal gland, 1245
Lymphatic drainage of breast, 80
Lymphatic malformations, 204
Lymphatics, 199, 208, 784
   in heart, 545–546, 546f
   and lymphoid tissue, 478–479
Lymphedema, massive localized, 151
Lymph nodes
   anatomy, 784
   artifacts, 795
      intrinsic, 795
      technical, 795, 795f
   benign compartmental enlargement, 793t
   benign vs. malignant lesions, 792
   blood supply, 784
   combined patterns, 794
   compartments, 784–792
   developmental changes, 784
   embryology, 784
   features, 784
   follicular changes, 793
   immune system, part of, 783
   light microscopy, 784–792
      epithelioid venules, 789
      follicles, 786
      follicular dendritic cells, 786
      interdigitating dendritic cells, 790
      lymphoid cells, 786–787
      macrophages, 789
      medullary cords, 793–794, 793f
      paracortex, 794
      sinuses, 791–792
      tingible body macrophages, 787–788
   lymphatics, 784
   mediastinal, 783
   medullary cords
      changes in, 793–794
      lymph nodes, light microscopy of, 784–792
   medullary hyperplasia, 793t
   paracortex, changes in, 794
   parotid gland, 451f
   sinusoidal changes, 794
   specimens, handling of, 795
   techniques and procedures, 795–796
Lymphocytes
   and plasma cells, 843–847
   thymic, 515–516
   of thyroid gland, 1186–1187
   in vulvar epithelium, 1034
Lymphocytic esophagitis, 595
Lymphoepitheliomas, 434
Lymphoid aggregate, 634
Lymphoid cells, 786–787, 790
Lymphoid follicle, 512f
Lymphoid hyperplasias, 632
Lymphoid markers, 26
Lymphoid proliferations, 631–632
Lymphoid tissue, 451, 451f
Lymphoplasmacytoid cells, 810
Lysosomes, 207

M

MacCallum patch, 536
Macrophages, 16, 248f, 249, 512. See also Phagocytic reticular cells
Macula lutea, 351
Macular and lichen amyloidosis, 20, 21f
Madelung disease, 148t, 156
Magnetic resonance imaging (MRI), 38, 530
MAGs. See Myelin-associated glycoproteins (MAGs)
Major histocompatibility complex (MHC) antigens, 516
Male breast, 80
Malignant peripheral nerve sheath tumors (MPNSTs), 326, 327
Malignant tumors, 449t
Mallory–Denk hyalins, 709
Mallory hyaline, 494, 495f
Malnutrition, changes in fat lobules during, 144
Mammary ridges, 69
Mantle hair of Pinkus, 11, 12f
Marchi technique, 313, 319
Marfan syndrome, 208f
   clinical abnormalities in, 193, 193f
Marginal zone, 806
Marinesco bodies, 235, 236f
Marrow cellularity, 847–848
Martial-arts thyroiditis, 1183
Masson trichrome, 352, 352f, 542, 547, 559
Mast cells, 16, 307, 326, 825–826, 1282
Mastocytosis, 16
Matrical fibroblasts, 51
Mature-appearing salivary gland acini, 507, 507f
Maturing follicles, of ovary
   folliculogenesis, 1118–1120
   granulosa cells, 1120–1121
   hormonal aspects, 1121–1122
   morphologic evidence of follicular maturation, 1119f
   ovulation, 1120
   theca interna layer, 1121

Mayer–Rokitansky–Kuster–Hauser (MRKH) syndrome, 1047
May–Grünwald–Giemsa (MGG), 814
MC. See Merkel cells (MC)
M-cadherin, 167
McArdle disease, 173
McNeal's zonal anatomy, 965–966, 965f
Meatus urinarius. See Urethral orifice
Meckel cartilage, 367
Media, 546
Median eminence, 249, 251–252, 251f
Mediastinum (hilum), 981
Medullary cords, 789f
  changes in, 793–794, 793f
Medullary epithelial cells, 514
Medullary interstitium, 924
Megakaryocytes, 496f, 840–843
Meibomian glands, 355, 356f
Meissner corpuscles, 312
Meissner plexus, 603
Melan-A/MART-1 antigen, 9
Melanin, 8–9
Melanocytes, 7–9, 8f, 583
  with brown melanin pigment, 24f
  with MART-1, 24f
  nail, 51–52, 52f, 52t, 53t
Melanocytic hyperplasia, 9
Melanosis esophagi, 583
Melanotic schwannomas, 324
Membranocystic lesions, 146
Membranous fat necrosis, 148
Membranous lipodystrophy, 146, 148t
Menarche, 1082
Ménière's disease, 391–393
Meninges
  dura mater, 257–259, 258f–259f
  leptomeningeal melanocytes, 261–262
  optic nerve, 262
  pia-arachnoid, 259–261
Meningiomas, 259
Meningohypophysial trunk, 275
Meningothelial cells, 260
Menisci
  damage to, 114
  distribution of collagen fibers in, 117, 119f
  fibrocartilage in, 119
Menstruation
  corpus luteum of (CLM), 1122–1124, 1123f
  luteal phase, 1087–1090
  menstrual phase, 1087
  perimenopausal and postmenopausal years, 1090
Merkel cells (MC), 4, 51, 1034
  of epidermis, 9–10, 10f, 1263, 1263f, 1264
  and esophagus, 583
Merkel tactile disks, 1037
Merlin, 327
Mesenchymal condensates, 859
Mesenchymal stem cells, 97
Mesenchymomas, 151
Mesenteric panniculitis, 149
Mesonephric and müllerian remnants, 1001–1003. See also Testis and excretory duct system
Mesonephric duct, 857
Mesonephric ducts, 949

Mesonephros, 856, 857
  excretory function of, 857
Mesothelial cells, 554–555, 554f–556f. See also Serous membranes
  histochemistry, 555, 557
  immunohistochemistry, 557–558, 557f, 558f
  morphology, 554–555, 554f–556f
  ultrastructure, 558–559, 558f–560f
Mesothelial hyperplasia, 560
Messenger RNA (mRNA), 508
Metanephric mesenchyme (MM), 857
  nephron progenitor population, 874–876, 875f
  specification, 873–874
Metanephros, 856, 857–859
Metaphyseal vessels (bone), 95
Metaplasia, 955
  adipocytic, 146, 146f
  salivary ducts, 454, 454f
Metaplastic bone, 489
Metarterioles, 546
Methylene blue, 181
Michel's medium, 21, 23
Microglia and monocyte, 246–248, 247f
Microglial nodules, 248
Micronodular pneumocyte hyperplasia (MNPH), 492, 493f
Microtubule-associated proteins (MAPs), 311
Microtubules, 34
Microvilli, 618
Milk let-down reflex, 281
Milky spots, 553
Mineralization, bone
  primary mineralization, 100–101
  secondary mineralization, 101
Mineralized axons, 237, 237f
Minimal deviation adenocarcinoma, 1067
Minor prostatic glands, 1025
Minor vestibular glands, 1035–1036, 1036f
Minute pulmonary meningothelial-like nodules, 490
Mitral cells, 252
Mixed acini, 444
Mixed tumor, 449
MNPH. See Micronodular pneumocyte hyperplasia (MNPH)
Molecular biology, thymus, 516
Molecular studies, 23–27
Moll's glands, 15, 19
Monckeberg' sclerosis, 191, 193f
Monocyte precursors, 832–835
Monocytoid B cells, 792
Monoiodotyrosine (MIT), 1182
Mons pubis, 1033, 1043
Mons veneris. See Mons pubis
Morgagni lacunae, 1022–1023, 1023f, 1024
Motilin, 616
Motor nerves, 302–303
Mouth
  cheeks, 409
  embryology of, 396–398
  floor of, 405
  gingiva, 412–413
  intraepithelial nonkeratinocytes, 413–414
  juxtaoral organ of Chievitz, 409–410
  lips and vermilion border, 402
  microscopy of, 402–416

oral mucosa and submucosa, 402–404
palate, 404–405
rests of Serres and Malassez, 416
salivary glands, minor, 407–409
teeth and supporting structures, 414–416
tongue, 410–412
tonsils, 405–407
uvula, 404–405
MPIC. See Multilocular peritoneal inclusion cyst (MPIC)
Mucicarmine, 23
Mucicarmine stain, 750
Mucins, 748
Mucosa, 617–623. See also Small intestine
  architecture and design, 617–618
  components and their composition, 618–623
Mucosa-associated lymphoid tissue (MALT), 479, 512, 783
Mucosal eosinophils, 622
Mucostasis, 489
Mucous acini, 454
Mucous metaplasia, 454
Mucus secreting cells, 427
Müllerian ducts, 1059–1060
  epithelium, 1055–1056
Müllerianosis, 950
Müllerian-type epithelium, 1099
Müller muscle, 355
Multicystic mesothelioma, 566
Multidetector-row computed tomography (MDCT), 530
Multifocal fibrosing (sclerosing) thyroiditis, 1187, 1187f
Multifocal granulomatous folliculitis, 1183
Multilocular peritoneal inclusion cyst (MPIC), 565–566, 565f, 566f. See also Reactive mesothelium
Multiple endocrine adenomatosis 1 (MEA-1), 148t
Multiple endocrine neoplasia-1 (MEN-1), 768
Multiple gestation, 1155–1156
Multiple symmetrical lipomatosis (MSL) syndrome, 156
Mural hyalinization, 500
Muscle biopsy, handling of, 188–189
Muscle spindles, 175, 175f
Muscularis externa, 624–625, 624f. See also Small intestine
Muscularis mucosae, 586, 623, 671
Muscularis propria, 958–961, 959f–960f
Mycobacterium, 26
Mycobacterium avium–intracellulare, 623
Mycobacterium leprae, 316
Myelin-associated glycoproteins (MAGs), 302, 312, 313, 1260
Myelin debris, 319
Myelin, in peripheral nervous system, 312–314
Myeloblast, 826
Myoblast, 167
Myocardial fibers, 542
Myocardial nerves, 545
Myocardial sinusoids, 537
Myocardial sleeves, 200, 203f
Myocardium, 532, 534f, 537, 546
Myocyte disarray, 536

Myoepithelial cells. *See also* Salivary Glands
    characteristics of, 448, 448f
    in salivary gland tumors, role of, 449, 449t, 450f
Myofibrils, 177
Myogenesis, 167
Myogenic regulatory factors (MRFs), 167
Myoid cells, 449, 513, 514
Myometrium, 1089f, 1093–1095
    pregnancy-related changes, 1093–1095
Myosalpinx, 1097
Myosin ATPase reaction, 173
Myotubes, 167–168, 167f
Myxofibrosarcoma, 157
Myxoid liposarcoma (MLS), 136
Myxomatous degeneration, 541

N

Nail, 31–32
    anatomy
        gross, 37–39
        microscopic, 39–46
    apoptosis in, 32
    blood supply, 58–59, 59f
    and bone regrowth, 58
    confocal microscopy of, 55, 55f, 56f
    cross section, 37f
    dermis, 56–58, 57f
    developmental of, 32t, 33f
    embryology of, 32–34
    fibrillar phase, 34f
    folds, proximal, 40–41, 41f
    functions, 31
    genetics, 34–37
    granular phase, 35f
    growth, 59–61, 59t
    handling and processing of, 61
    histochemistry of, 44t
    historical aspects, 31–32
    immunohistochemistry of
        immunology and inflammatory cells, 53
        keratinocytes, 46–51
        melanocytes, 51–52, 52f, 52t, 53t
        Merkel cells, 51
        nail plate, 46
    isthmus, 37
    keratin of, 34–37
    microscopic anatomy
        hyponychium, 45, 45f
        lateral nail folds, 45–46, 46f
        matrix, 41–43, 42f
        nail bed, 43–45, 44f
        nail plate, 39–40, 39f
        proximal nail fold, 40–41, 41f
    pathologic specimens from, 31
    psoriasis, 40
    sagittal section, 37f
    schematic diagram of, 38f
    shotgun proteomic analysis of, 34
    squamous phase, 36f
    ultrastructural anatomy, 53–55, 54f, 55f
Nailfold capillaroscopy (NFC), 59
Nail growth, 59–61, 59t, 61f
    diseases affecting, 59–60, 59t
    normal, 59
Nail matrix, 41–43, 42f
    epithelial cells, 41, 42f
    Langerhans cells, 43

    lunula, 43
    melanocytes, 41–43, 43f
    Merkel cells, 43
Nail plates, 39f, 60
    anatomy of, 39–40
    biochemical composition of, 40
    calcium in, 40
    corneocytes of, 40
    dorsal, horizontal section of, 39f
    keratin analysis, 40
    lipids in, 40
    water content of, 40
Nail stem cells, 61
Nail unit, 32. *See also* Nail
Napsin-A, 501, 502f, 503
Nasolacrimal duct, 359
Nasopharyngeal cysts, 436f
Nasopharyngeal mucosa, 435
Nasopharynx, 433, 434
Near-infrared spectrometer, 40
NEBs. *See* Neuroepithelial bodies (NEBs)
Necrotizing granulomas, 1183
Necrotizing sialometaplasia, 454, 454f
Neonatal circumcision, 1014
Neoplastic diseases, 709–710
Nephrectomy, 1229
Nephric duct (ND), 857
    development of, 867
Nephrogenesis, 856
Nephrogenic adenoma, 956, 956f
Nephrogenic zone, 859, 860f
Nephron development, 858f, 859
    developing podocytes, 885
    Huber's schematic drawings of, 859f
    intrauterine growth retardation and, 884
    rate of nephron induction, 884
    sclerotic glomeruli, 888
    stages
        induction, 859
        morphogenetic, 859
Nephron number
    early juxtamedullary glomeruli, 887
    ectopic glomeruli, 888, 888f
    glomerular maturation and growth, 884–887, 885f–886f
    glomerulosclerosis in infants, 887–888, 888f
Nephron, patterning of
    glomerulogenesis, 878–879
    interstitium, 877–878
    juxtaglomerular apparatus, 880
    pretubular aggregate and renal vesicle, 876–877
    proximal and distal tubules, 877
    renal vascularization, 879–880
Nephron progenitor population, 874–876, 875f
Nephrostomes, 856
Nerve growth factor (NGF), 301
Nerve loop of Axenfeld, 339
Nerves
    urinary bladder, 952
    vagina, 1050–1051
Nerve twigs, demonstration of, 181
Nesidioblastosis, 765
Neu–Laxova syndrome, 144
Neural cell adhesion molecule (NCAM), 709
Neural cell adhesion molecules (NCAMs), 1260

Neural crest, 300
Neurilemma, 307
Neuritic plaques, 233, 234f
Neuroendocrine cells, 26, 472, 512, 1249, 1276, 1282. *See also* Paraganglia
    aging changes, 1266
    apoptosis in, 1255–1256
    artifacts, 1267
    closed, 1254, 1254f
    development, molecular aspects, 1252
    differential diagnosis, 1267
    distribution of
        breast, 1264
        bronchopulmonary and upper respiratory system, 1261–1262, 1261f, 1262f
        gastrointestinal tract, 1264–1265, 1265f
        skin, 1263–1264
        thyroid and thymus, 1262–1263, 1263f
        urogenital system, 1265–1266
    EC–nerve complexes, 1255
    embryology, 1251–1252
    function of, 1256–1257
    historical perspectives and nomenclature, 1249–1251, 1250f, 1251t
    light microscopy and histochemistry, 1252–1255, 1253f, 1254f
    markers of, 1251t, 1257
        cytosolic constituents, 1257–1258
        secretory granule constituents, 1258
        somatostatin receptors, 1261
        synaptic vesicle and vesicle fusion/release constituents, 1259–1260
        transcription factors, 1260–1261
    opened-type cell, 1254, 1254f
    secretory activities of, 1250f
    special procedures, 1266–1267
    specimen handling, 1267
    ultrastructure, 1255, 1255f
Neuroepithelial bodies (NEBs), 472, 1262
Neurofibrillary tangles, 233, 234f
Neurofibromas, 326
Neurofibromatosis, 327
    type I, 300, 327
    type II, 327
Neurofilament proteins (NFPs), 231, 232f
Neurofilaments, 310–311
Neurohypophysis, 270, 295–296, 295f
Neuromuscular junctions (NMJs), 312
Neuronal contraction, as tissue-handling artifact, 235, 237f
Neuronal nuclei (NeuN), 231, 232f
Neurons, CNS, 230–239, 230f
    age-related neuronal inclusions, 231, 233–235, 233f–236f
    autolysis and basic neuronal reactions to injury, 235–239
    immunohistochemistry, 231, 232f
    neurofilament proteins, 231, 232f
    neuronal nuclei, 231, 232f
    normal microscopic anatomy, 230–231, 230f
    synaptophysin, 231, 232f
    unipolar neurons, 230–231, 231f
Neuron-specific enolase (NSE), 231
Neuropathic abnormalities, 182–183, 182f
Neuropathic (Charcot) joints, loose bodies in, 129

Neuropil, 229, 229f
Neurotrophins, 302
Neurotropic viruses, 311
Neurotubules, 311
Neurovascular foramina, in sellar region, 272, 273f
Neutrophil bands, 828
Neutrophil precursors, 826–831
Neutrophil promyelocytes, 826
Nevus lipomatosis superficialis, 151
Newborns
   epidermis of, 18
   histologic differences of skin in, 18
   subcutaneous tissue in, 18
Nezelof syndrome, 508
NFPs. See Neurofilament proteins (NFPs)
Nidogen, 901
Nipple epidermis, 6, 6f
Node of Cloquet, 1043
Nodes of Ranvier, 303, 314–315
Nodular lymphoid hyperplasia, 632
Nodular regenerative hyperplasia, 713
Nodules of C cells, 1262
Nonmyelinating (Remak) Schwann cells, 316, 317
Nonnecrotizing epithelioid granuloma, 496
Nonrespiratory bronchioles, 471
Nonshivering thermogenesis, 140
Norepinephrine, 140, 1283
Nose
   embryology of, 396–398
   external, 399, 416
   microscopy, 416–420
   nosebleeds, 418
   olfactory mucosa, 419, 419f
Notch of Rivinus, 365
Notch pathway, 1252
Notch signaling pathway, 743
Nuclear internalization, 186, 186f
Nuclear vacuolization, 185, 185f
Nucleus pulposus, 115
Nutrient arteries (bone), 95

O

Obersteiner-Redlich zone (ORZ), 256f, 302
Obesity, 143–144
Occludin, 1181
Odontogenesis, 397
Oil red O, 142, 173
   positive carcinomas, 143t
Olfactory bulb, 252, 252f
Olfactory ensheathing cell (OEC), 312
Olfactory tracts, 252–253, 252f
Oligodendroglia, 243–245, 243f
   immunopositivity for S100 protein, 244, 245f
   perinuclear halos, 244, 245f
   satellite, 243, 245
Omentum, 551
Oncocytes, 449, 453–454, 453f
Oncocytic metaplasia, 430
Oncocytosis, 453
Onion-bulb whorls, 322
Onodi air cell, 400
Onychodermal band, 38, 38f, 40, 45
Onychodermis, 51, 57
Onychomycosis, 39, 40
Optical microscopy, usage of, 32

Optic nerve, 262, 352–353, 352f, 353f
Orbit, 357
Organ of Zuckerkandl, 1276, 1280–1281
Organogenesis, 856
Oropharynx, 433, 434
Orphan G-protein coupled receptor (oGPCR), 50
Ossification, 492f, 500
Osteoarthritis (OA), 122, 127, 128f, 129
Osteoblast differentiation and function, regulators of, 97t
Osteoblastic and myoepithelial cells, 449
Osteoblasts, 91, 97–98, 97f, 98f, 818, 820–821, 820f
Osteocalcin, 97
Osteoclasts, 99–100, 99f, 820–821, 820f
Osteocytes, 98–99, 98f, 99f
Osteocytic osteolysis, 99
Osteons. See Haversian systems
Osteoprogenitor cells, 97
Osteoprotegerin (OPG), 99, 100
Otosclerosis, 389–390
Outer medullary collecting duct, 920–921, 921f
Ovarian surface epithelium (OSE), 1111
Ovarian thecal metaplasia, 1232
Ovary
   adult, 1108
   atretic follicles, 1126–1129
   atrophic postmenopausal, 1115f
   blood supply, 1109
   corpus albicans, 1126, 1127f
   corpus luteum of menstruation (CLM), 1122–1124
   corpus luteum of pregnancy (CLP), 1124–1126, 1125f
   embryology, 1107–1108
   gross anatomy, 1108–1109
   hilus cells, 1129–1131
   lymphatics of, 1109
   maturing follicles, 1118–1122
   nerve supply of, 1109–1110
   newborn, 1117f
   postmenopausal, 1108–1109, 1116f
   prepubertal, 1108
   primordial follicles, 1117–1118, 1118f
   rete ovarii, 1131, 1131f
   stroma, 1111–1117
      aging changes, 1115–1117
      decidual cells, 1114
      endometrial stromal cells, 1115, 1115f
      enzymatically active stromal cells, 1111–1114
      hormonal aspects, 1117
      luteinized stromal cells, 1111
      Reinke-crystal–containing Leydig cells, 1115
      smooth muscle, 1114–1115, 1114f
      ultrastructure, 1117
   surface epithelium, 1110–1111
Ovulation, 1084
Oxyphil cells, 1209f, 1210
Oxytocin, 279, 281
Oxytocin-induced contraction, 448

P

Pacchionian foveolae, 259
Pachymenix. See Dura mater

Pacinian corpuscles, 176, 176f, 1041–1042
Paget disease, extramammary, 6, 6f, 1031
Palatine tonsils, 401, 434
Palisaded encapsulated neuroma (PEN), 323
Palisades of Vogt, 343
Palpation thyroiditis, 1183
Palpebral conjunctiva, 343
Pancreas, 738
   acinar cells, minor alterations in, 760–761
   acini, microscopic features of, 746–749
   anatomic factors, 738, 739f
   annular, 745, 745f
   appearance of, 741f
   atrophy, 768–772
   and biliary ducts, 742f
   cancers, 771
   chronic pancreatitis, 768–772, 769f–772f
   congenital short, 745
   connective tissue, 757–758
   cytogenesis, 743–744
   cytologic features, 758–759, 759f
   developmental anomalies, 744–746
   development of, 742–746, 743f
   ductal cells, minor alterations in, 761–765
   ducts, 749–753, 749f–752f
   duodenum, 749–753
   enzymes, 748
   extrainsular neuroendocrine cells, 757, 757f
   fetal, 753f
   fibrosis, 768–772
   heterotopia, 744–746
   heterotopic pancreatic tissue, 745
   islet cells, minor alterations in, 765–768
   islet of Langerhans, 753–757
   lipomatosis, 772
   location and relationship, 738–741, 739f
   luminal necrosis, 762
   microscopic features, 746–759
   minor alterations, 759–768
   neuroendocrine tumor, 746
   organogenesis, 742–743
   pancreaticoduodenal veins, 740
   pancreatic polypeptide, 744
   pancreatic tissue, 745
   pancreatitis, 768–772
   regions of, 741
   ventral, 745
Pancreas divisum, 745
   classical, 745
   dominant dorsal drainage, 745
Pancreatica magna, 740
Pancreatic artery
   great, 740
   inferior, 740
   superior, 740
Pancreatic cystic neoplasms, 746, 746f
Pancreatic fat necrosis, 148–149, 149f
Pancreatic heterotopia, 745
Pancreatic hypoplasia, 745
Pancreatic intraepithelial neoplasia (PanIN), 746, 761, 761f, 762f
Pancreatic lipomatosis, 147
Pancreatic metaplasia, 578
Pancreaticoduodenal veins, 740
Pancreatic polypeptide (PP), 1264
Pancreatitis, chronic, 768–772, 769f–772f
Pancreatoduodenal artery, 739, 740

Pancreatoduodenal sulcus, 739
Pancreatoduodenectomy, 739
Pancytokeratin (CAM5.2), 501f
Pancytokeratin antibodies, 47
Paneth cell, 618, 621, 647–648
Pan-keratin AE-1/AE-3, in normal nail matrix, 47, 47f
Panniculitis, 149
Papanicolaou stain, 759
Papillary basal layer (PBL), 585
Papillary dermis, 4, 15, 15f
Papillary microcarcinoma, 1187
Papillary muscles, 541–542, 542f
Papillary surface epithelium, 922
Papulosis clear cell, 6
Paracortex, 789, 790f
  immunohistochemistry of, 791f
Paracrine cells, 1254
Paraffin-section immunohistochemistry, 547
Parafibromin, 1217
Paraganglia, 758, 1178, 1274
  aging changes, 1286
  anatomy, 1281
  cell types
    neuroendocrine cells, 1282
    sustentacular cells, 1282
  developmental changes, 1280–1281
  differential diagnosis, 1291
  distribution of, 1276–1278, 1277f
  embryology, 1278–1280, 1279f, 1280f
  function
    physiologic roles, 1284–1286
    secretory products, 1284–1286
  gender differences, 1286
  genotype–phenotype correlations, 1276
  gross features and organ weights, 1281
  history and nomenclature, 1274–1275
    Kohn's concept, 1275
  immunohistochemistry, 1286–1290
    artifacts, 1290–1291
  innervation of, 1282
  light microscopy, 1281–1283, 1282f
  lobular architecture of carotid body, 1282–1283
  parasympathetic, 1274
  phenotypic plasticity, 1280–1281
  postnatal changes, 1280–1281
  sympathetic, 1274
    vs. parasympathetic, 1275–1276
  ultrastructural organization, 1283–1284, 1285f
  unitary concept of, 1275
Paragangliomas, 1275, 1278
Parakeratosis, 38
Paranasal sinuses, 399–400, 416–420
Paraneurial component, 304
Paraneurons, 1251
Parasitic nodules, 1193
Parasympathetic paraganglia, 1274. See also Paraganglia
Paratenon, 122
Parathyroid gland, 1177
  adenoma and carcinoma, 1213, 1213f–1221f, 1215, 1217t
  age-related changes, 1212
  chief cells, 1207, 1208f–1209f
  clear cells, 1211f

distribution of, 1201–1202
embryology, 1202–1204
function of, 1201, 1212
gross appearance, size, and shape, 1204–1206
histochemistry of, 1214f–1215f
histology, 1206–1210, 1211f
historical review, 1201
hyperplasia, 1213
mature, 1206
oxyphil cells, 1209f, 1210
parenchymal cells, 1206
physiology and pathophysiology, 1212–1213
regulation of PTH, 1201, 1212
transcription and growth factors, 1204, 1204t
transitional cells, 1210, 1210f
ultrastructural features of, 1207
variations in, 1206f
Parathyroid hormone (PTH), 97
Parathyroid hyperplasia, 147
Paratracheal node, 1178
Paraurethral glands (Skene glands), 1054–1055
Paraventricular nuclei (PVN), 270
Parietal pericardium, 531
Parietal pleura, 553
Parkes syndrome, 1044
Parotid gland, 440–442, 441f, 459
Parotid intralobular ducts, 444f
Pars intermedia, 284
Pars tuberalis, 291–292, 292f
p53-associated—high-grade carcinomas, 81
Patellar ligament, rupture of, 129f
Patent foramen ovale, 534
Pattern recognition, lungs, 480–481, 481f, 481t
PDE10A gene, 802
PDX1, 755
Peanut agglutinin receptor antigen (PNA-r), 514
Pectinate muscles, 535
Pediatric kidney
  anatomy, 856
  developmental changes, 856
  histologic peculiarities of, 856
Pedunculated lipofibroma, 151
Pelitis, 954
Pelvic examination, 1032
Pencil cells, 725
Penile dartos, 1020
Penile erection, 1026
Penis and distal urethra, 1009, 1009f
  arteries, 1025–1026
  distal penis
    anatomical features related to cancer spread, 1018, 1018f
    coronal sulcus, 1013, 1013f
    foreskin, 1013–1018
    glans, 1009–1012
  lymphatics, 1026
  nerves, 1026
  penile shaft, anatomical levels of, 1019–1022
    anatomic features, 1019–1020, 1019f
    Buck fascia, 1020
    corpora cavernosa, 1021, 1021f
    dartos, 1020
    skin, 1020
    tunica albuginea, 1020–1021

urethra and periurethral tissues, anatomic levels of, 1022–1025
veins, 1026
Peptide growth factors, 1286
Peptidylamidaglycolate lyase (PAL), 1258
Peptidylglycine alpha-amidating monooxygenase (PAM), 1258
Peptidyl-glycine alpha-hydroxylating monooxygenase (PHM), 1258
Percutaneous coronary angioplasty (PTCA) with stent emplacement, 205
Periarteriolar lymphoid sheath (PALS), 802
Periaxin, 313–314
Periaxonal space of Klebs, 310, 310f, 311–312
Peribronchial lymph nodes, 498
Peribronchiolar metaplasia, 472
Pericapsular node, 1178
Pericardiectomy, 530
Pericardium. See also Heart
  about, 531–532, 531f, 532f
  applied anatomy, 532
Pericytes, 198
Periderm, 3
Perifascicular atrophy, 187
Perifollicular zone (PFZ), 802, 807
Perineurial cells, 304
Perineuriomas, 324
Perineurium, 304–306
Perineuronal satellitosis, 243, 244f
Periodic acid-Schiff (PAS) stain, 472, 555, 583, 618, 618f, 747, 810, 814
  positive zymogen granules, 443, 444
  white fat cell, 138, 138f
Periosteal dura, 272
Periosteal lipoma, 154
Periosteal vessels (bone), 95
Periosteum, 94, 95f
Periparotid lymph nodes, 459
Peripheral glomus tumors, 203
Peripheral nerves, 300. See also Peripheral nervous system
  anatomy of, 302–303
  blood supply of, 308
  damaged, 303
  histologic artifact in, 317f
  histologic techniques for, 309t
  immunocytochemistry of, 305f–306f
  nerve fibers, 308–309
    myelinated, 310–311, 310f
  pathologic reactions of, 318
  sheaths and compartments, 303, 303f, 304f
  traumatic lesions of, 323–324
Peripheral nervous system, 300
  axonal growth, 301
  development of, 300–301
  GFAP immunoreactivity in, 312
  intradural elements of, 256–257
  nerve sheath components, 303, 303f
    axoplasmic flow, 311
    blood supply of nerves, 308
    endoneurium, 307–308
    epineurium, 303–304, 303f
    myelin, 312–314
    myelinated nerve fibers, 310–311, 310f
    nerve fibers, 308–309
    node of Ranvier, 314–315
    periaxonal space of Klebs, 311–312

Peripheral nervous system (*continued*)
    perineurium, 304–306
        Schmidt–Lanterman incisure, 314, 314f
        Schwann cells, 312
        unmyelinated axons, 315–317, 316f
    normal histology with pathology, correlation of
        axonal degeneration and regeneration, 318–321, 318f, 319f
        general pathologic reactions, 318
        hypertrophic neuropathy, 322
        peripheral nerve biopsy and autopsy specimens, 317–318, 317f
        peripheral neuropathies, 318
        segmental demyelination and remyelination, 321–322, 322f
        traumatic lesions of nerve, 323–324
        tumors, 324–328, 325f
    peripheral nerves, anatomy of, 302–303
    Schwann cells and myelination, 301–302
Peripheral neuropathies, 300, 318. *See also* Peripheral nervous system
Peripheral skeleton, 87, 88t
Peritoneum, 551
Peritubular cells, 817
Periurethral glands, 1035
Perivascular clearing, 243, 243f
Perivascular fibrosis, 295, 295f
Periventricular nucleus, 282f
Perls' acid ferrocyanide method, 837
Persistent neonatal hyperinsulinemic hypoglycemia (PNHH), 766
Pertinax bodies, 39
Petubular aggregate (PTA), 859
Peyer patches, 622, 629
Peyronie disease, 1020
PGs. *See* Proteoglycans (PGs)
Phagocytic macrophages, 4
Phagocytic reticular cells, 822–824
Phagocytosis, 800
Phakomatoses, 327
Phalanx, 32, 33
Pharyngeal bursa, 436
Pharyngeal tonsil, 401
Pharyngobasilar fascia, 434
Pharynx. *See also* Larynx
    anatomy
        gross, 434, 434f
        microscopic, 435–437, 435f–437f
    definition and boundaries, 433, 433f
    embryology, 434
    neural, vascular, lymphatic components, 437–438, 437f
Phenylethanolamine-N-transferase (PNMT), 1289
Pheochromocytes, 1239
Pheochromocytoma, 1275, 1276
Pheromones, 1043
Phimosis, 1016
Pia-arachnoid (Leptomeninges), 259–261, 260f, 261
Piecrust artifact, 185, 186f
Pierson syndrome, 905
Pigment donation, 8
Pilar unit
    apocrine glands, 15, 15f
    eccrine glands, 13–15, 13f, 14f
    hair follicle, 10–12, 11f, 12f
    sebaceous glands, 12–13, 13f
Pilocytic astrocyte, 239
Pilosebaceous units, 19
    skin of face with, 19f
Pineal gland, 249, 249f, 250f
    histology, 250f
    immunohistochemistry, 250f
Pineocytes, 249
Pinna, 363
Pinocytotic vesicles, 725
Piriform sinuses, 433f
Pituicytes, 296
Pituitary and sellar region
    anatomy
        arterial supply, 275–276
        bony sella, 271–272, 272f, 273f
        cavernous sinuses, 273–275, 275f, 276f
        hypophysial portal system, 276
        meninges, 272–273
    differential diagnosis, 296–298
    embryology, 270–271, 271f
        adenohypophysis, 270
        neurohypophysis, 270
    physiology and histology
        adenohypophysis, 283–292
        age-related changes, 294–295
        hypothalamus, 277–283
        neurohypophysis, 295–296, 295f, 296f
        normal histologic variations, 292–294
    transsphenoidal approach to, 277f
    ultrastructural features, 286t
Pituitary organogenesis, 271
Pituitary stalk, granular cell tumorlets, 297f
Pituitary transcription factor 1 (Pit-1), 1260
Pityrosporum yeast, 11, 11f
Placenta
    amnion and chorion, 1149–1154
    chorionic vasculature pathology, 1148
    chorionic vasculature, ramification of, 1147–1148
    decidua, 1163–1166
    gestational trophoblastic disease, 1166–1168
    membranes, 1148–1154
    multiple gestation, 1155–1156
    storage, examination, and processing, 1138–1141
    umbilical cord, 1141–1147
    villi, 1156–1163
Placenta accreta, 1166, 1166f
Placental site nodule (PSN), 1168
Placental site trophoblastic tumor (PSTT), 1089, 1154
Placenta percreta, 1166
Plasmacytoid cells, 449
Plasmacytoid dendritic cells, 650
Plasmacytoid myoepithelial cells, 449
Plasmalemmal vesicles, 207, 207f
Plasma membrane, of basal cells, 7
Plasminogen activator inhibitor 1 (PAI-1), 137
Plasminogen activator inhibitor type 2 (PAI-2), 51
Plastic sponges, 487
Platelet peroxidase (PPO), 843
Pleura, 479–480, 479f, 551. *See also* Lungs
Pleural elastic tissue (elastic stains), 479f
Pleuroparenchymal fibroelastosis (PPFE), 482
Plexiform schwannoma, 324
Plicae, 245f, 246
PLS regression, 40
Pneumocystis carinii, 23
Pneumocytes, 490
Pneumothorax, 483f
PNF. *See* Proximal nail fold (PNF)
Polsters, 1026
Polyclonal anticarcinoembryonic antigen (pCEA), 699
Polymerase chain reaction (PCR), 26, 429, 1266
Polymorphous low-grade adenocarcinoma (PLGA), 449
Ponephros, 856–857
Postatic hyperplasia, 957
Postatrophic hyperplasia, 976–977, 977f
Postmenopausal breast, 79, 80f
Postnatal circulation, 531
Posttransplant lymphoproliferative disorders (PTLD), 547
Poximal tubule, 908–913
PP cell granules, 757
p40 protein, 24
p53 protein, 26
p63 protein, 24
Preadipocyte, 135–136
Prearterioles, 197
Precapillary sphincters, 546
Pregnancy
    atretic follicle in, 1128f
    breast development in, 78–79
    corpus luteum of pregnancy (CLP), 1124–1126, 1125f
        connective tissue, 1126
        granulosa layer, 1125
        gross appearance, 1124–1125
        histology, 1125–1126
        theca layer, 1125–1126
        ultrastructure, 1126
    related changes
        myometrium, 1093–1095
        uterine cervix, 1073
Pregnancy cells, 287, 294, 295f
Preleptotene spermatocytes, 985–986
Prenatal fetal circulation, 530–531
Prepancreatic arcade, 740
Prepubertal testis, 990–993
Prepuce. *See* Foreskin
Presumptive sensory nerve terminals, 545
Pretarsal fat pad, 357
Primary (neoplastic) C-cell hyperplasia, 1185
Primary empty sella syndrome, 277f
Primary myotubes, 167
Primary thymic neoplasms, 523
Primary visual cortex, 228, 228f
Primordial follicles, of ovary, 1117–1118, 1118f
    granulosa cells of, 1118
    histology, 1117–1118
    ultrastructure, 1118
Primordial lungs, 469
Procedural atelectasis, 485
Progressive multifocal leukoencephalopathy (PML), 243
Prohormone convertases, 1258
Prolapsed orbital fat, 155
Proline-rich proteins, 443

Prospermatogonia, 990
Prostate gland, 964–965, 965f
 anatomy, 967f
 anterior fibromuscular stroma, 969–971
 apical one-third of the prostate, 967–968, 967f
 atrophy in, 976–978, 976f–977f
 basal one-third of the prostate, 969, 969f
 ejaculatory ducts, 964, 965f–966f, 966
 extraprostatic tissues, prostatic innervation and vascular supply, 971–973
 glandular prostate
  architectural patterns, 973–976, 973f
  cytologic features, 974–976, 974f–975f
 McNeal's zonal anatomy, 965–966, 965f
 middle one-third of the prostate, 968–969, 968f
 prostatic capsule, 969–971
 pubertal growth acceleration and maturation, 964
 transurethral resections, 978–979, 979f
Prostate neuroendocrine cells, 1265–1266
Prostate-specific antigen (PSA), 1025
Prostatic paraganglia, 1291
Prostatic stromal hyperplasia, 977f
Prosthetic vessels, 205–206
Protease inhibitors, 450
Protein gene product 9.5 (PGP 9.5), 1258
Proteins (bone), 96–97
Proteoglycans (PGs), 115, 540
 in articular cartilage, 117, 119f
Proximal nail fold (PNF), 32, 38, 40–41, 41f
 dorsal portion, 41f
 ventral portion, 41f
Proximal nail groove, 32
Proximal nail matrix (PNM), 37
Prussian blue stain, 814
Psammoma bodies, 254, 254f, 353, 353f, 562, 562f, 1188, 1188f
Pseudointima, 206
Pseudolipoma, 147
Pseudolipomatosis cutis, 156
Pseudomelanosis duodeni, 628
Pseudounipolar cells, 303
Psoralen-UV-A (PUVA), 40
Psoriasis, 20
 nail, 40
PTEN-associated tumor syndromes, 1185
Pterygium inversum unguis, 38
Puberty, breast development occurs, 70
Pulmonary corpora amylacea, 494f
Pulmonary edema, 501f
Pulmonary hypertension, 199–200
Pulmonary lobules, 476, 476f
Pulmonary macrophages, 476
Pulmonary neuroendocrine cells (PNC), 489
Pulmonary vasculature, 478f
Pulmonary vessels, 199–200
 aging changes in, 200
 elastic pulmonary artery, 201f
 histologic features of, 201t
 myocardial sleeves in pulmonary vein, 200, 203f
 normal pulmonary veins, 202f
 pulmonary hypertensive changes, 199–200, 202f
Punch biopsies, 1033

R
Rab proteins, 1260
Radical parotidectomy, 459f
Radical prostatectomy, 966–967, 967f
Ragged blue fiber, 188, 188f
Ragged red fibers, 187–188, 188f
Rathke cleft cysts, 270
Rathke cleft remnants, 284
Rdiation therapy, 978, 978f
Reactive alveolar cell hyperplasia, 477f
Reactive mesothelium. See also Serous membranes
 about, 561–562, 561f
 endosalpingiosis/endometriosis, 564–565, 564f, 565f
 fibrous pleurisy, 562, 562f
 multilocular peritoneal inclusion cyst, 565–566, 565f, 566f
 reactive mesothelium vs. carcinoma, 563–564, 564t
 reactive mesothelium vs. mesothelioma, 562–563, 562t, 563t
 vs. carcinoma, 563–564, 564t
 vs. mesothelioma, 562–563, 562t, 563t
Receptor activator for nuclear factor κβ (RANK), 97, 99, 100
Receptor activator for nuclear factor κβ ligand (RANKL), 97, 100
Red cell precursors, 835–840
Red neuron, 235, 236f
Red pulp, 804–805, 804f. See also Pancreas
Reed–Sternberg cells, 794
Regeneration, capacity of salivary glands, 455, 456f
Regulatory peptides, 1286
Reinke crystals, 1130, 1130f–1131f
Reinke space, 428
Remodeling, 108–109, 109f
Renal interstitium, 922–924, 924f
 extracellular matrix of, 923
 fibroblasts of, 923
 immune cells of, 923–924
 pericytes of, 923
Renal microvasculature, 926f
Renal pelvis
 anatomical relationships of, 951f
 formation, 857–858
 lamina propria, 957–958, 957f
 microscopic anatomy, 953
 muscularis propria, 958–961, 959f–960f
 renal papillae, 953, 953f
 urothelium variants and benign proliferations, 954–957
Renal vascularization, 879–880
Renaut bodies, 308, 308f
Renin–angiotensin system, 870
Renomedullary interstitial cells, 924
Respiratory bronchioles, 471
Respiratory bronchiolitis, 487
Respiratory tract epithelia, 474f
Restenosis, 205
Rete ovarii, 1131, 1131f
Rete testis, 994–995, 994f
Reticular dermis, 4, 15–16
Reticulocyte, 836
Reticuloepithelial cells, 510
Retina, 348–350, 348f–350f
 artifacts of, 351–352, 352f
 cellular components, 348, 348f
 external limiting membrane, 349
 immunopositivity to synaptophysin and NeuN, 349, 350f
 layers, 348, 348f
 microvasculature of, 31f, 351
 neuronal cells of, 349, 350f
 neurosensory, 348
 ora serrata, 348, 349f
 photoreceptors, 349
 retinal pigment epithelium, 348–349
Reticularis cells, 1235
Retractile mesenteritis, 148t, 149
Retroesophageal node, 1178
Retrograde transport, 311
Retroperitoneal xanthogranulomatosis, 150
Retropharyngeal node, 1178
Rheumatoid arthritis, 122, 127
Ribonucleoproteins, 747
Right atrium, 535, 536f
Right ventricle. See also Heart
 about, 536–537, 537f
 applied anatomy, 538
Ring fibers, 186, 186f, 804
Ring of Nemiloff, 315
Rivinus' ducts, 442
Rokitansky–Aschoff sinuses, 724
Romanowsky method, 815
Romanowsky stain, 759
Romanowsky-stained marrow smears, 824
Rosenmüller fossa, 434
Rosenmüller node, 1043
Rosenthal fibers, 239, 240f, 242
Rough endoplasmic reticulum (RER), 747, 819
Rubbery plaques, 144
Ruffini corpuscles, 1038, 1042
Russell bodies, 789

S
Saccules, 426
Sacculi of Beale, 727
Salivary gland rests, 294, 295f
Salivary glands
 aging changes
  fatty infiltration, 454
  oncocytes, 453–454, 453f
 embryologic/postnatal developmental changes
  parotid gland, 440–442, 441f
  sublingual gland, 442
  submandibular gland, 442
 heterotopic salivary tissue, significance of, 451–453, 452f, 452t
 histology, correlative normal/neoplastic, 456–458, 457f, 458t
 hyperplasia, 454–455
 immunohistochemistry, 458–459, 458f
 light microscopy, 443
 lymphoid tissue, 451, 451f
 myoepithelial cells, 448, 448f
 myoepithelial cells in salivary gland tumors, role of, 449, 449t, 450f
 reactive changes
  artifacts, 456
  atrophy, 455, 455f

Salivary glands (continued)
   metaplasia, 454, 454f
   regeneration, 455, 456f
  sebaceous glands, 446–448, 447f
  secretory units
   acini, 443–444, 443f, 444f
   ducts, 444–446, 444f, 445f, 446f
  specimen handling, 459–460, 459f
Sampling error, 547
Sanderson polster, 1179, 1182–1183, 1183f
S-100 and Melan-A immunostains, in nail matrix, 52f
Saphenous vein, 199, 200f
  grafts, 204, 205
Sarcomatoid carcinomas, 950
Sarcoplasmic reticulum (SR), 177
Satellite cells, 177, 303
Satellitosis, 243, 244f
Schatzki ring, 575, 576, 581
Schaumann bodies, 494, 495f
Schlemm canal, 341, 341f
Schmidt–Lanterman incisure (S–L I), 313, 314, 314f
Schneiderian papillomas, 434
Schwalbe ring, 340, 341f
Schwann cell precursors (SCPs), 1279
Schwann cells, 4, 17, 256, 301, 312, 545, 624
  and myelination, 301–302
Schwannomas, 300, 324, 325f–326f
Schwannomatosis, 327
Sclera, 339–340, 339f, 340f
Sclerema adiposum neonatorum, 144
Scrotum, 552
Sea nomads, 802
Sebaceous glands, 4, 12–13, 446–448, 447f, 578
  with peripheral germinative cells, 13f
Secondary (physiologic) C-cell hyperplasia, 1185
Secondary lobule, 476
Secretomotor nerves, 442
Secretory cocktail, 1286
Secretory ducts, 444
Secretory units, salivary glands
  acini, 443–444, 443f, 444f
  ducts, 444–446, 444f, 445f, 446f
Segmental demyelination and remyelination, 321–322, 322f
Segmentectomy, 71
Semilunar fold, 343, 343f
Semilunar valves, 538–539, 538f
Sempahorins, 870–871
Senile amyloidosis, 1000f
Senile scleral plaques, 340
Sentinel lymph node mapping, 1044
Septa. See Trabeculae
Septicemia, 810
Seromucinous gland, of larynx, 429–431, 429f, 430f, 431f
Seronegative arthritis, 122
Serotonin, 1286
Serous atrophy, 144
  of bone marrow, 95, 95f
Serous membranes
  anatomy, 551–552
   functional anatomy, 552–554, 552f, 553f
  mesothelial cells

   histochemistry, 555, 557
   immunohistochemistry, 557–558, 557f, 558f
   morphology, 554–555, 554f–556f
   ultrastructure, 558–559, 558f–560f
  reactive mesothelium
   about, 561–562, 561f
   endosalpingiosis/endometriosis, 564–565, 564f, 565f
   fibrous pleurisy, 562, 562f
   multilocular peritoneal inclusion cyst, 565–566, 565f, 566f
   reactive mesothelium vs. carcinoma, 563–564, 564t
   reactive mesothelium vs. mesothelioma, 562–563, 562t, 563t
  submesothelial layer
   histochemistry, 559
   immunohistochemistry, 561
   mesothelial and submesothelial cells, interactions of, 561, 561f
Sertoli cell–germ cell junctions, 984
Sertoli cell–only syndrome, 984
Sertoli cells, 983–984, 993f
  in fetus, 993
Sexually transmitted diseases (STDs), 1015
Sézary syndrome, 794
Sharpey fibers, 94, 115
Shave biopsy, 1033
Shotgun proteomic analysis, of human nail plate, 34
Shwachman syndrome, 147, 148t
Sialomucin, 14, 14f
Sick lobe hypothesis of breast cancer, 71
Sideroblasts, 837
SIF cells. See Small intensely fluorescent (SIF) cells
Signaling pathways
  bone morphogenetic proteins, 870
  fibroblast growth factor, 869
  integrins, 870
  laminins, 870
  Notch signaling, 873, 876
  renin–angiotensin system, 870
  sempahorins, 870–871
Simple chronic thyroiditis, 1186
Sinoatrial (SA node) node, conduction system, 542, 543f
Sinuses, 791–792, 791f
Sinus histiocyte, immature, 792
Sinus-lining cell, 792
Sinusoidal changes, 794
Sinusoidal lining cells, 699–701
Sinusoids, 199
Site-specific changes in lung tissue, 481–484, 481t, 482f, 483f
Sjögren syndrome, 451
Skeletalized graft, 205
Skeletal muscle, 166
  aging, effect of, 181–183
  anatomy, 170–171, 171f
  artifacts, 183–185, 184f
  blood supply to, 169
  differential diagnosis, 185–188
  embryology, 166–168, 167f
  exercise and training on, effect of, 181
  fiber type determination, 173, 174f

  gender and, 181
  light microscopy, 171–176
  nerve supply to, 169–170
  postnatal and developmental changes, 168–170
  specialized techniques for, 178–181
  specimen handling, 188–189
  ultrastructural examination, 177–178, 177f
Skeletal system, 87. See also Bone
Skene ducts, 1034–1035
Skin
  age, histologic differences with, 18
  anatomic sites, histologic variations with, 18–19, 19f
  artifacts, 21–22
  biopsies, pathologic changes in, 20–21
  blood vessels, lymphatics, nerves, and muscle, 16–18
  composition, 3
  degenerative diseases of, 20
  embryology, 3–5
  excisional biopsies, 21, 22f
  functions of, 3
  histologic variations, 18–19
  histomorphology, 5–18
  lymphatics of, 17
  neuroendocrine cells, 26, 1263–1264
  pathology interpreted as normal, 20–21
  punch and shave biopsies, 21
  smooth muscle in, 18
  specimen handling, 21
  staining methods, 22–27
  striated muscle in, 18
  subcutaneous tissue, 16, 17f
Small granule-containing (SGC) cells, 1276
Small intensely fluorescent (SIF) cells, 1276–1277, 1282
Small intestine
  age-related changes, 631
  diet, 631
  duodenum, 626–628, 626f
  environmental factors, 631
  functions of, 616
  gross anatomy and surgical perspective, 615–616
  histology
   mucosa, 617–623
   muscularis externa, 624–625
   serosa and subserosal region, 625
   submucosa, 623–624
  ileum, 629–630
  jejunum, 628–629
  lymphoid proliferations, 631–632
  malabsorptive states, 633
  metaplastic and heterotopic tissue, 631
  morphologic changes, 632–633
  physiology, 616
  specimen interpretation and common artifacts, 633–635
  specimen procurement and processing, 633
  surgical perspective, 615–616
Smegma, 1013
Smoking-related interstitial fibrosis (SRIF), 488
Smooth muscle actin (SMA-1)
  immunostaining, 26, 210, 212–213, 212f
Smooth muscle cells, 208

SNARE proteins, 1259
Sodium iodide symporter, 1181
Solar elastosis, in dermis, 18, 18f
Solitary circumscribed neuroma, 323
Somatostatin, 1256
Somatostatin receptors, 1260
Sommer's sector, 226
Sonic hedgehog (SHH), 679, 743
Sophora japonica agglutinin receptor antigen (SJA-r), 514
Southern blot, 136
Spermatogenesis, 984, 985, 985f
Spermatogonial stem cells (SSC), 985
Sphincter muscle, 344
Sphincter of Oddi, 730, 742
Spinal cord, anatomy of, 220–221, 221f
Spinal epidural lipomatosis, 148t
Spinal nerve roots, anatomy of, 301. *See also* Peripheral nervous system
Spindle cell lipoma, 155
Spindle morphology, 558
Spindle-shaped or myoid cells, 449
Spirochete, 26
Splanchnic nerves, 741
Spleen
 aging differences, 809
 anatomy, 802
 apoptosis, 801, 801f
 blood supply, 802
 compartments, 800t
 differential diagnosis, 809–810
 flow cytometry, 807
 functions, 807–809
 gross features and weight, 802
 hematopoiesis, 809
 histologic technique, 810
 histology, function, and compartments, 800t
 immunologic function, 808–809
 light microscopy, 802–807
 lymphatics, 802
 nerves, 802
 perifollicular zone, 807
 prenatal and developmental changes, 800–801
 red pulp, 804–805, 804f
 red pulp function, 804–805
 reservoir function, 809
 special procedures, 810–811
 specimen handling, 810
 splenectomy, 807
 splenitis, 810
 splenogonadal fusion, 801f
 surface and intracellular markers expression, 808t
 traumatically ruptured, 803f
 ultrastructure, 807
 vascular tree, 802–804
 white pulp, 805–806, 806f, 807f
 white pulp function, 805–806
Splenic myeloid metaplasia, 809
Spleniculi, 800
Splenogonadal fusion, 800–801, 801f
Sponge artifact, 487
Spongiosa, 539, 540
Spongiotic pericytoma, 147
Spongy bone. *See* Cancellous bone
S100 protein, 9, 143, 143f, 1181, 1260, 1290

Squamocolumnar junction, 1069
Squamous cell carcinoma, 24
 penile, 1023–1024
 vs. basal cell carcinoma, 26t
Squamous cell nests, 293
Squamous cells, 449
Squamous epithelialization, 1069–1071, 1071f
Squamous epithelium, 426, 428, 428f, 436, 955
 coronal sulcus, 1013
Squamous layers, keratinocytes, 5–6, 6f, 19
Squamous metaplasia, 454, 722, 955, 978, 1069, 1150, 1152, 1152f
 of follicular cells, 1184, 1184f
Squiggle cell, 583
Staging laparotomy, 810
Stains and evaluation of lung histology, 480
Stalk effect, 288
Staphylococcus epidermis, 11, 11f
Starvation, changes in fat lobules during, 144, 145f
STAT-Ser/Hes-3 signaling axis, 1252
Steatosis, 142
Steiner stain, 23
Stellate cells, 758
Stellate-dendritic cells, 4
Stellate or myxoid cells, 449
Stensen duct, 442
Stents, 205
Sternal aspirates, 813
Sternocleidomastoid muscle, 442
Stomach
 age-related changes, 609
 anatomical zones of, 602f
 artifacts, 609
 blood supply, 602
 cardiac and pyloric mucosa, 604–605
 differential diagnosis, 609–613
 embryology and postnatal development, 601
 endocrine cells, 606–607
 gastric function, 608–609
 gross morphologic features, 601–603
 histologic features, 603–608
 inferolateral margin, 601
 lamina propria, 607
 lymphatics, 603
 metaplasia, 612–613
 mucosal zones of, 602f
 muscular components, 607–608
 nerve supply, 602–603
 oxyntic gland mucosa, 605–606
 pancreatic acinar metaplasia, 613
 regions of, 601
 special procedures and techniques, 609
 specimen handling, 613
 submucosa, 607
 superomedial margin, 601
 surface epithelium, 604
 ultrastructure, 608
Stomodeal prominence, 396
Stomodeum, 434
Stratum lucidum, 7, 19
Striated ducts, 445f
Striated muscle, 18
Stroma, 738, 1111–1117
 aging changes, 1115–1117
 decidual cells, 1114

endometrial stromal cells, 1096t, 1115, 1115f
enzymatically active stromal cells, 1111–1114
hormonal aspects, 1117
luteinized stromal cells, 1111
Reinke-crystal–containing Leydig cells, 1115
smooth muscle, 1114–1115, 1114f
of thyroid gland
 adipose metaplasia of, 1187f
 adipose tissue, 1187–1188
 calcifications, 1188
 fibrous tissue, 1187
 lymphocytes, 1186–1187
 skeletal muscle, 1187–1188
ultrastructure, 1117
Stromal cells, 820–826
Subarachnoid space, 260f
Subarticular cysts, 127
Subcapsular cortical epithelial cells, 514
Subconjunctival herniated orbital fat, 155
Subcutaneous fat, 17, 17f, 18–19, 19f
Subcutaneous tissue, 16, 17f
Subcutis. *See* Subcutaneous tissue
Subepithelial myofibroblast (SEM) syncytia, 651
Subfascial muscle, 175, 175f
Subglottic compartment, 426
Subglottic lymphatics, 433
Sublamina densa zone, 7
Sublingual gland, 442
Submandibular (submaxillary) gland, 442
Submandibular gland tumors, 460
Submesothelial layer. *See also* Serous membranes
 histochemistry, 559
 immunohistochemistry, 561
 mesothelial and submesothelial cells, interactions of, 561, 561f
Submesothelial mesenchymal cell, 560
Submucosal lymphoid, 435f
Subpleural emphysematous change in smoking, 482, 483f
Succinate dehydrogenase (SDH), 178, 446
Sucquet–Hoyer canals, 17
Sudan black, 142, 313
Sulcus limitans, 220, 220f
Sulfur matrix protein, 40
Superficial parotidectomy, 459, 459f
Superior vena cava (SVC), 530
Supraglottic compartment, 426
Supraoptic nuclei (SON), 270
Sural nerve, 317
Surface epithelium, of ovary, 1110–1111
 histology, 1110–1111
 ultrastructure, 1111
Suspensory ligaments of Cooper, 69
Swiss cheese brain, 268f, 269
Sympathetic paraganglia, 1274. *See also* Paraganglia
Sympathogonia cells, 1228
Synaptic-type vesicles (SSVs), 1255
Synaptic vesicle protein 2 (SV2), 1259
Synaptophysin, 26, 231, 232f, 1259, 1287
Synaptotagmins, 1259
Syncytium, 651

Synovial fluid, 114
  in arthritis, 130
  normal, 130
Synovial inflammation, 130
Synovial membrane, 121, 122f
  hypertrophic and hyperplastic, 129, 130f
  inflammatory response, 130, 130f
  pannus in OA, 130, 130f
  response to injury, 129–130, 130f
  synovial fibroblasts and immune cells, interactions between, 130

T

Tamm–Horsfall glycoprotein (THGP), 338
Tamoxifen, 1053
Tanycytes, 246
Targetoid fibers, 183
T-cell receptor (TCR)/CD3 complex, 508
Telangiectasia macularis eruptive perstans, 20
Telescoping of vessels, 485f
Telogen phase of hair growth, 11, 12
Tendons, 122, 123f
Tenon capsule, 339
Teratoma, 1154
Terminal bronchioles, 471
Terminal crest, 535
Terminal duct lobular unit (TDLU), 73, 75, 79
Terminal Schwann cells, 312
Tertiary granules, 830
Tertiary hyperparathyroidism, 1215
Testis and excretory duct system
  aging testis, 993–994
  appendix epididymis, 1001–1002, 1001f
  appendix testis, 1001, 1001f
  capillary network, 990
  ductuli efferentes, 995–996, 995f
  ductus (vas) deferens, 997–998
  ejaculatory ducts, 1000
  epididymis, 996–997, 996f–997f
  fetal testis, 990–993, 991f
  germ cells, 984–987, 984f
  gubernaculum, 1003
  interstitium, 987
  Leydig cells, 987–989, 988f–999f
  mesonephric and müllerian remnants, 1001–1003
  molecular markers, 985
  prepubertal testis, 990–993
  rete testis, 994–995, 994f
  seminal vesicles, 998–1000, 999f
  seminiferous tubules, 982, 983f
  Sertoli cells, 983–984, 983f
  spermatocytes, 986
  supporting structures, 981–982
  vascular supply, 989–990
TGB. See Thyroglobulin (TGB)
Thermogenin, 140
Thick ascending limbs (TAL), 915
Thin limbs of Henle loop, 913–915
Thromboemboli in acute lung injury, 497f
Thymic cortex, 511f
Thymic dysplasia, 508
Thymic epithelial cells, 514–515, 514t
Thymic lymphocytes, 510–513, 511f, 512f, 515–516
Thymocytes, 510–513, 511f, 512f
Thymolipoma, 154

Thymosin α1, 517
Thymus
  abnormalities, developmental, 507, 507f
  age-related/trophic changes
    thymic hyperplasia, 517–518, 518t
    thymic involution, 517
  anatomy, 508–509
  apoptosis, 508
  artifacts, 519, 519f
  embryology, 506–507
  function, 516–517
  histology
    about, 509–510, 509f
    epithelial cells, 510
    Hassall corpuscles, 510, 510f, 511f
    thymic lymphocytes (thymocytes), 510–513, 511f, 512f
  immunohistochemistry
    thymic epithelial cells, 514, 514t
    thymic lymphocytes, 515–516
  molecular biology, 516
  neuroendocrine cells in, 1262–1263, 1263f
  ultrastructure, 513–514, 513f, 514f
Thyroarytenoid muscle, 425
Thyroglobulin (TGB), 1180
  microscopic variants, 1182–1184
  resorption of, 1182
  synthesis of, 1182
Thyroid gland
  anterosuperior mediastinal nodes, 1178
  blood supply of, 1178
  branchial pouch–related structures, 1188–1194
  C cells (parafollicular cells), 1184–1186
  color, 1177
  Delphian node, 1178
  embryology, 1175–1177
  epithelium of follicle, 1180f
  estrogen and progesterone receptors, 1181
  follicular carcinoma, 1184, 1185, 1190, 1192, 1194
  follicular cells, 1179–1182
    malignant neoplasms of, 1194
    squamous metaplasia of, 1184, 1184f
  granulomas of, 1183–1184
  gross anatomy, 1177–1178
  immunohistochemistry, 1180
  internal jugular chain nodes, 1178
  lymphatic network, 1178
  microscopic anatomy, 1178–1179
  neuroendocrine cells in, 1262–1263, 1263f
  nodularity of thyroid parenchyma, 1178
  oxalate crystals in, 1184, 1184f
  paratracheal node, 1178
  pericapsular node, 1178
  physiology, 1181–1182
  retroesophageal node, 1178
  retropharyngeal node, 1178
  shape, 1177
  size, 1177
  stroma, 1186–1188
    adipose tissue, 1187–1188
    calcifications, 1188
    fibrous tissue, 1187
    lymphocytes, 1186–1187
    skeletal muscle, 1187–1188

  thyrocytes, 1179
  thyroglobulin (TGB), 1180
  thyroid peroxidase, 1181
  thyroid transcription factor-1 (TTF-1), 1181
  thyroxine (T4), 1181
  triiodothyronine (T3), 1181
  ultimobranchial bodies (UBBs), 1176–1177
Thyroid neuroendocrine carcinomas, 1186
Thyroid tissue in abnormal locations
  in cervical lymph nodes, 1193
  in lateral neck, 1193
  in midline structures, 1192–1193
  in other locations, 1193–1194
  in pericapsular soft tissues, 1193
Thyroid transcription factor 1 (TTF-1), 251, 1260
Thyroid-type follicular carcinoma, 1194
Thyromeres, 1177
Thyrotrophs, 289, 290f, 291f
Tight junctions, 207, 558
Tingible body macrophages (TBM), 786, 787–788
Tissue artifacts, biopsy limitations and, 547–549, 548f
Tissue handling/processing, 547
Tissue-specific nuclear transcription protein TTF-1, 564
Tissue trauma, 655
T-lymphocyte recirculation, 199
Toker cells, 6, 77, 1042–1043
Tonsilloliths, 401
Tonsils, 401–402
Toothpaste artifact, 268f, 269, 353
Torpedoes, 239
Total parotidectomy, 459
Trabeculae, 802
Trabecular arteries, 802
Trabecular bone. See Cancellous bone
TRAIL death ligand signaling pathway, 168
Transbronchial biopsy, 487
  incidental findings in, 499–500, 499f, 500t
Transcription factors, 1260–1261
Transformation zone epithelium, 1069–1073, 1071f–1072f
Transglutaminases, 35
Transitional cells, 1210, 1210f
Transitional epithelium, 435, 953, 956
Transonychial water loss (TOWL), 40
Transvenous endomyocardial biopsy, 546
Transverse (T) tubules, 177
Traumatic hemorrhage, 486f
Treg cells, 622
Trephine biopsies, 814
Treponema pallidum, 26
Trichilemmal keratinization, 11
Trichohyalin granules, 11
Trichotillomania, 20
Trichrome staining, 480
Tricuspid valve, 540
Trite syndrome, 148t
Tropocollagen, 1117
True splenitis, 810
True thymic hyperplasia, 517–518
Trypsin, 748, 748f
TTF-1/Napsin-A, 501, 502f
Tuberoinfundibular tract, 281
Tuberous sclerosis, 148t

Tubular acini, 747
Tubular maturation and growth, 889
Tumorlet, 489f
Tumor necrosis factor alpha (TNF-α), 137
Tunica albuginea, 981, 1010, 1020–1021
Tunica vaginalis, 981
Tunica vasculosa, 981–982
Tympanic paraganglia, 1277
Type 5 glycogen storage disease, 173
Type I collagen, 15, 115
Type II collagen, 115
Type III collagen, 15
Tyrosine hydroxylase (TH), 1289
Tyson glands, 1013

U

Ultimobranchial bodies (UBBs), 1176–1177
Umbilical cord
    allantoic duct remnant, 1144f
    embryology, 1141
    epithelium of, 1142
    gross anatomic features, 1141, 1141f
    hematoma of, 1145f
    histology, 1142–1143
    histopathology, 1143–1147
    length of, 1141, 1142f
    omphalomesenteric duct remnant, 1143f
    umbilical torsion and stricture, 1146
    vascular neuronal innervation of, 1142
    vasculature of, 1142
Umbilicus with dermal fibrosis, 19f
Ureteral branching, 868–869
Ureteric branch growth, 871
Ureteric bud (UB), 857, 858f
    formation, 867–868
Ureters, 952
    blood supply, 952
    development of, 950
    epithelium of, 950
    intramural, 951
    longer parietal and shorter intravesical portion, 951
    lymphatic drainage, 952
    venous drainage, 952
Urethra, 965, 1050
    partial prolapse of, 1037
Urethra and periurethral tissues, penile, 1022–1025, 1023f–1025f
Urethral caruncle, 1037
Urethral orifice, 1036–1037
Urinary bladder, 950–952, 1050
    anatomical relationships of, 951f
    bladder bed, 951–952
    bladder neck, 951
    blood supply, 952
    empty bladder in adult, 950
    epithelium of, 949
    lymphatic drainage of, 952
    neoplasms, 950
    sympathetic and parasympathetic nerves of, 952
Urogenital system, 856
Urothelium, 953–954, 954f
Urticaria, 20, 21f
Urticaria pigmentosa, 16
Uterine cervix
    cervical stroma, 1073
    differential diagnosis, 1075t–1076t
    endocervix epithelium, 1066–1069
    exocervical epithelium, 1065–1066, 1065f
    during pregnancy, 1073
    transformation zone epithelium, 1069–1073, 1071f–1072f
Uterus, 1098f
    adult uterus and fallopian tubes, 1061
    embryology, 1059
    gross anatomic features of, 1062–1063
    growth, infancy stage, 1061
    indifferent stage, 1059–1060
    premenarchal uterus and fallopian tubes, 1060–1061
    uterine and tubal lymphatics, 1064–1065
    uterine and tubal vasculature, 1063–1064
Uveal tract, 336
    choroid, 346–348, 346f, 347f
    ciliary body, 345–346, 345f, 346f
    iris, 343–345, 343f, 344f

V

Vacuolar artifact, 184, 184f
Vagal ganglia, 1277
Vagina
    adenosis, 1056f
        embryonic form, 1055
        mucinous form, 1055
        during puberty, 1055
        tuboendometrial form, 1055–1056
    anatomy, 1050–1051
    blood supply to, 1050
    dendritic processes of Langerhans cells, 1052, 1052f
    embryology, 1047–1049
    epithelial responses and functions, 1052–1053
    epithelium, 1051–1052
    epithelium atrophies, 1053, 1053f
    gross features, 1049–1050
    G-spot (Gräfenberg spot), 1055
    ligaments, 1050
    lymphatic drainage, 1051
    mucosa of, 1049, 1051f
    müllerian duct epithelium, remnants of, 1055–1056
    nerves, 1050–1051
    paraurethral glands (Skene glands), 1054–1055
    ultrastructure, 1054
    vaginal wall and adventitia, 1053–1054
    wolffian ducts, 1054
Vagus nerve, 741
Valves of Santorini, 742
Varicella-zoster virus, 26
Varices, in vulva, 1044
Vas aberrans, 1002, 1002f
Vasa nervorum, 304, 308
Vasa vasorum, 196, 197f
Vascular calcification, 191
Vascular cell adhesion molecule (VCAM)-1, 820
Vascular endothelial growth factor (VEGF), 898
Vascular endothelial growth factor A (VEGFA), 898
Vascular endothelium, site-specific staining of, 210, 211f
Vascular malformations, 204
Vascular surgery, 204, 205t
    angioplasty, 205, 206f
    bypass grafts, 204–205, 205t
    endarterectomy, 204, 205t
    prosthetic vessels, 205–206
Vascular tissues, ultrastructural features of, 206, 207t
    adventitia and supporting cells, 208
    endothelial cells, 206–207
    inclusions of endothelial cells, 207–208, 207f
    lymphatics and veins, 208
    media, 208
Vascular tree, 802–804
Vasculature, 478, 478f. *See also* Lungs
    kidney, 924–927, 925f–926f
    pituitary gland, 278f
    umbilical cord, 1142
Vasculitis, 17, 17f
Vasitis nodosa, 306
Vasoactive intestinal peptide (VIP), 591
Vasopressin, 279, 281
Vater–Pacini corpuscles, 17, 17f, 18, 1017, 1017f, 1020
Vein bypass grafting, 204–205, 205t
Veins, 199, 200f, 208
Vellus hair, 18, 19
Ventilator-associated injury, 484f
Ventricular assist device (VAD), 530
Ventricularis, 539, 540
Ventricular perforation, 547
Vermiform appendix, 664
Verocay bodies, 324
Vesicle-associated membrane proteins (VAMPs), 1259
Vesicular monoamine transporters, 1259
Vestibular adenomas, 1036
Vestibular fossa, 1034
Vestibular gland with squamous metaplasia, 1036, 1036f
Vestibular papillae, 1037
Vestibular papillomatosis, 1037
Victorian waistband effect, 547
Video-assisted thoracoscopic surgery (VATS) biopsy, 482, 487
Villi, 617
    embryology, 1156–1158
    gross morphologic alterations, 1158–1159
    gross morphology, 1158
    histology, 1159
    histopathology, 1160–1163
Villous edema, 156–157
Vimentin, 292, 306, 989, 1181
Virchow–Robin space, 256, 783
Visceral fasciae, 559
Visceral pleura, 552f
    in transbronchial biopsies, 499f
Vitiligo, 20, 20f, 21f
Vitreous humor, 355, 355f
Vocal cords, 426, 429f
Volkmann canal, 92, 93f
Von Hippel–Lindau syndrome, 1002
von Kossa, 23
Von Willebrand factor, 26
Vortex veins, 339

Vulva, 1031
   anatomy, 1032–1033, 1033f
      arterial supply, 1044
      clitoris, 1037–1038, 1038f
      hymen, 1037, 1037f
      labia majora, 1039–1043, 1039f–1042f
      labia minora, 1038–1039, 1038f
      lymphatic drainage, 1043–1044
      mons pubis, 1043
      nerve supply, 1044
      urethral orifice, 1036–1037
      venous supply, 1044
      vulvar vestibule, 1034–1036, 1034f–1036f
   biopsy, 1033–1034
   clinical evaluation, 1031–1032
   clinical perspective, 1031
Vulvar edema, 1044
Vulvar intraepithelial neoplasia (VIN), 1032
Vulvar lymphatics, obstruction of, 1044
Vulvar vestibule, 1034–1036, 1034f–1036f
Vulvodynia, 1031, 1032

W

Wallerian degeneration, 302
Walthard nests, 981, 1111, 1113f
Warthin–Starry stain, 23
Warthin tumor, 453
Weber–Christian disease, 148t, 149
Wedge biopsies, 500
Weibel–Palade bodies, 207, 207f, 1206
Weight of heart, 530
Wernicke encephalopathy, 225
Wharton duct, 442
Wharton jelly, 1142
White adipocytes. *See* White adipose tissue (WAT)
White adipose tissue (WAT), 134–139
   functions, 136–137
   gender differences, 136
   gross aspects, 138
   histology, 138, 138f–140f
   lesions, 150–155
   molecular biology, 136
   postnatal development, 136
   prenatal development, 134–136, 134f, 135f
   regulation, 137–138
   ultrastructure, 138–139
White pulp, 805–806, 806f, 807f. *See also* Pancreas
Wilson's disease, 40
Wohlfart type B fibers, 168
Wolffian ducts, 857, 1054
Wolff law, 87, 90, 98, 120
Woven bone, 90–91, 90f
WT-1 immunoreactivity, 558f

X

XIIIa+ dermal dendrocytes, 16
X-linked hypohydrotic ectodermal dysplasia, 441
X-linked inhibitor of apoptosis protein (XIAP), 562
X-ray microdiffraction, 39

Y

Yolk sac erythropoiesis, 817

Z

Z band (skeletal muscle), 177, 177f
Zebrafish pronephric kidney, 856
Zellballen, 1282
Zenker's solution, 814
Zeus medium, 547, 1033
Ziehl–Neelsen stain, 23
Zimmerman sign, 351
Zona fasciculata, 1233f, 1234, 1234f. *See also* Adrenal gland
Zona glomerulosa, 1231f–1232f, 1233–1234. *See also* Adrenal gland
Zona reticularis, 1227, 1233f, 1234–1235. *See also* Adrenal gland
Zonulae occludentes, 304
Zonules, 345, 345f
Zymogen granules, 747, 747f, 749